D1569315

CLINICAL HEMATOLOGY

CLINICAL HEMATOLOGY

NEAL S. YOUNG, MD
Chief, Hematology Branch
National Heart, Lung, and Blood Institute
National Institutes of Health
Bethesda, Maryland

STANTON L. GERSON, MD
Shiverick Professor of Hematological Oncology
Director, Case Comprehensive Cancer Center and
Ireland Cancer Center
Case Western Reserve University
Cleveland, Ohio

KATHERINE A. HIGH, MD
William H. Bennett Professor of Pediatrics
Investigator, Howard Hughes Medical Institute
The Children's Hospital of Philadelphia
Philadelphia, Pennsylvania

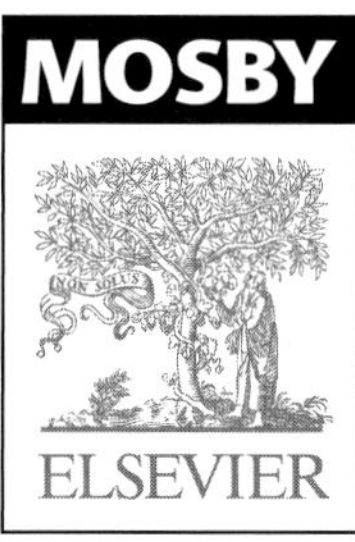

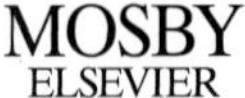

MOSBY
ELSEVIER

Four Penn Center, Suite 1800
1600 John F. Kennedy Boulevard
Philadelphia, Pennsylvania 19103

CLINICAL HEMATOLOGY
ISBN 13: 978-0-323-01908-8
ISBN 10: 0-323-01908-0

NOTICE

Knowledge and best practice in this field are constantly changing. As new research and experience broaden our knowledge, changes in practice, treatment and drug therapy may become necessary or appropriate. Readers are advised to check the most current information provided (i) on procedures featured or (ii) by the manufacturer of each product to be administered, to verify the recommended dose or formula, the method and duration of administration, and contraindications. It is the responsibility of the practitioner, relying on their own experience and knowledge of the patient, to make diagnoses, to determine dosages and the best treatment for each individual patient, and to take all appropriate safety precautions. To the fullest extent of the law, neither the Publisher nor the Editors assumes any liability for any injury and/or damage to persons or property arising out or related to any use of the material contained in this book.

The Publisher

Library of Congress Cataloging-in-Publication Data

Clinical hematology / [edited by] Neal S. Young, Stanton L. Gerson, Katherine A. High.
p. cm.
ISBN 0-323-01908-0
1. Blood – Diseases. 2. Hematology. I. Young, Neal S. II. Gerson, Stanton L. III. High, Katherine A.
RC636.C548 2006
616.1′5-dc22 2005054386

Printed in Canada

Last digit is the print number: 9 8 7 6 5 4 3 2 1

DEDICATION

To my wife, Genoveffa--bella e valente donna
NSY

Thank you Deb for many understanding hours of support and advice
during this and a life of deadline-ridden projects
and to Ruth, James and David
who always want to listen and learn
SLG

To my husband George
Nobilitas sola est atque unica virtus
KAH

CONTRIBUTORS

Janis L. Abkowitz, MD
Professor of Medicine, Division of Hematology, and Chief, Hematology Section, University of Washington Medical Center, University of Washington School of Medicine, Seattle, Washington
Pure Red Cell Aplasia and Diamond-Blackfan Anemia

Charles S. Abrams, MD
Associate Professor of Medicine, University of Pennsylvania School of Medicine; Staff Physician, Division of Hematology-Oncology, University of Pennsylvania Hospital, Philadelphia, Pennsylvania
Megakaryocyte Development and Disorders of Thrombopoiesis

Lauren E. Abrey, MD
Assistant Professor of Neurology, Department of Neurology and Neuroscience, Cornell University Medical College; Assistant Attending Neurologist, Training Program Director, and Director of Clinical Research, Memorial Sloan-Kettering Cancer Center, New York, New York
Primary and Secondary Central Nervous System Lymphomas in Immunocompetent and Human Immunodeficiency Virus–Positive Patients

Richard S. Ajioka, PhD
Division of Hematology, University of Utah School of Medicine, Salt Lake City, Utah
Hemoglobin and Heme Biosynthesis

Doru T. Alexandrescu, MD
Hematology/Oncology Fellow, and Clinical Instructor, New York Medical College, Valhalla, and Our Lady of Mercy Medical Center, Bronx, New York
Chemotherapy Toxicities and Complications

Harvey J. Alter, MD
Clinical Professor of Medicine, Georgetown University Medical School, Washington, D.C.; Chief, Infectious Diseases Section, and Associate Director for Research, Department of Transfusion Medicine, National Institutes of Health, Bethesda, Maryland
Hepatitis C Virus

Firoozeh Alvandi, MD
Fellow, Department of Transfusion Medicine, Warren G. Magnuson Clinical Center, National Institutes of Health, Bethesda, Maryland
Practice of Blood Component Transfusion

David J. Araten, MD
Assistant Professor, NYU School of Medicine, New York, New York
Paroxysmal Nocturnal Hemoglobinuria

Robert J. Arceci, MD, PhD
King Fahd Professor of Pediatric Oncology, Visiting Professor of Oncology, and Visiting Professor of Pediatrics, Johns Hopkins University; Director of Pediatric Oncology, The Sidney Kimmel Comprehensive Cancer Center at Johns Hopkins, Baltimore, Maryland
Histiocytosis

Elina Armstrong, MD, PhD
Instructor in Medicine, University of Pennsylvania School of Medicine, Philadelphia, Pennsylvania
Von Willebrand Disease

Barbara J. Bain, MBBS, FRACP, FRCPath
Professor of Diagnostic Haematology, Imperial College; Consultant Haematologist, St. Mary's Hospital, London, United Kingdom
Eosinophilic Leukemia

John Barrett, MD, FRCP, FRCPath
Chief, Allogeneic Stem Cell Transplantation Section, Hematology Branch, National Heart, Lung, and Blood Institute, National Institutes of Health, Bethesda, Maryland
Myelodysplastic Syndrome; Allogeneic Bone Marrow Transplantation

Karolin Behringer, MD
Assistant Doctor, Internal Medicine, and Study Physician of the German Hodgkin Study Group, Department I of Internal Medicine/Hematology and Oncology, University Hospital Cologne, Cologne, Germany
Hodgkin's Lymphoma

Joel S. Bennett, MD
Professor of Medicine and Pharmacology, University of Pennsylvania School of Medicine; Attending Physician, Hospital of the University of Pennsylvania, Philadelphia, Pennsylvania
Inherited and Acquired Disorders of Platelet Function

Nathan A. Berger, MD
Hanna-Payne Professor of Experimental Medicine, Professor of Medicine, Oncology and Biochemistry, and Director, Center for Science, Health and Society, Case Western Reserve University, School of Medicine; University Hospitals of Cleveland, Cleveland, Ohio
Geriatric Hematology

Nancy Berliner, MD
Professor, Internal Medicine and Genetics, Yale University School of Medicine; Attending Physician, Yale-New Haven Hospital, New Haven, Connecticut
Granulocytopoiesis

Ernest Beutler, MD
Professor and Chairman, Department of Molecular and Experimental Medicine, The Scripps Research Institute, La Jolla, California
Red Blood Cell Enzymopathies

Clara D. Bloomfield, MD
William G. Pace III Professor of Cancer Research, Cancer Scholar and Senior Advisor, Comprehensive Cancer Center, and James Cancer Hospital and Solove Research Institute, The Ohio State University, Columbus, Ohio
Leukemias: Diagnosis and Classifications

Paula H. B. Bolton-Maggs, FRCP, FRCPCH, FRCPath
Honorary Clinical Lecturer, University of Manchester; Doctor and Consultant Haematologist, Central Manchester and Manchester Children's University Hospitals, Manchester, United Kingdom
Hereditary Spherocytosis, Hereditary Elliptocytosis, and Related Disorders

Franklin A. Bontempo, MD
Associate Professor of Medicine, Division of Hematology and Oncology, University of Pittsburgh, School of Medicine; Medical Director, Coagulation Laboratory, The Institute for Transfusion Medicine, and Medical Staff, University of Pittsburgh Medical Center—PUH/SSH/Hillman Cancer Pavilion, Pittsburgh, Pennsylvania
Hematologic Abnormalities in Liver Disease

Henning Bredenfeld, MD
Consultant of Internal Medicine, and Study Physician of the German Hodgkin Study Group, Department I of Internal Medicine/Hematology and Oncology, University Hospital Cologne, Cologne, Germany
Hodgkin's Lymphoma

Gary M. Brittenham, MD
Professor of Pediatrics and Medicine, Department of Pediatrics, Columbia University College of Physicians and Surgeons; Staff Physician, Department of Pediatrics, Babies and Children's Hospital of New York-Presbyterian, New York, New York
Iron Overload

Kevin E. Brown, MD
Senior Investigator, Hematology Branch, National Heart, Lung, and Blood Institute, National Institutes of Health, Bethesda, Maryland
Parvovirus B19

Margaret Brown, BS, ASCP
Immunology Service, DLM, Clinical Center, National Institutes of Health, DHHS, Bethesda, Maryland
Flow Cytometry

Eric J. Burks, MD
Resident Physician, Department of Pathology, Penn State University, School of Medicine, The Milton S. Hershey Medical Center, Hershey, Pennsylvania
Large Granular Lymphocyte Leukemia

James B. Bussel, MD
Professor of Pediatrics, Professor of Pediatrics in Obstetrics and Gynecology, Professor of Pediatrics in Medicine, Weill Medical College of Cornell University; Attending, and Director, Platelet Research and Treatment Program, Division of Pediatric Hematology and Oncology, New York Presbyterian Hospital, New York, New York
Immune, Posttransfusional, and Neonatal Thrombocytopenia

John C. Byrd, MD
Associate Professor, The Ohio State University, Columbus, Ohio
Chronic Lymphocytic Leukemia

Michael A. Caligiuri, MD
Director of Division of Hematology and Oncology, and Professor of Medicine and Director, Comprehensive Cancer Center, The Ohio State University, Columbus, Ohio
Lymphocyte Biology

Katrin M. Carlson, PhD
Assistant Professor of Pathology, Northwestern University, Feinberg School of Medicine; Scientific Director, Cytogenetics Laboratory, Department of Pathology and Laboratory Medicine, Children's Memorial Hospital, Chicago, Illinois
Cytogenetics/Fluorescent In Situ Hybridization

Melody C. Carter, MD
Staff Clinician, Laboratory of Allergic Diseases, National Institute of Allergy and Infectious Diseases, National Institutes of Health, Bethesda, Maryland
Mastocytosis

J. C. Cawley, MBChB, MD, PhD, FRCP, FRCPath, F Med Sci
Professor and Head of University Department of Haematology, University of Liverpool; Honorary Consultant Haematologist, Royal Liverpool & Broadgreen University Hospitals NHS Trust, Liverpool, United Kingdom
Hairy Cell Leukemia

Mario Cazzola, MD
Professor of Hematology, University of Pavia Medical School; Attending Physician, Division of Hematology, IRCCS Policlinico San Matteo, Pavia, Italy
Sideroblastic Anemias

John K. Choi, MD, PhD
Assistant Professor, Department of Pathology and Laboratory Medicine, University of Pennsylvania; Director of Pediatric Hematopathology, Department of Pathology and Laboratory Medicine, The Children's Hospital of Philadelphia, Philadelphia, Pennsylvania
Blood and Bone Marrow Morphology

Douglas B. Cines, MD
Professor, and Vice-Chair, Academics, Department of Pathology and Laboratory Medicine, University of Pennsylvania; Director, Coagulation Laboratory, Hospital of the University of Pennsylvania, Philadelphia, Pennsylvania
Heparin-Induced Thrombocytopenia

Jeffrey I. Cohen, MD
Head, Medical Virology Section, Laboratory of Clinical Infectious Diseases, National Institute of Allergy and Infectious Diseases, National Institutes of Health, Bethesda, Maryland
Epstein-Barr Virus

Raymond L. Comenzo, MD
Director, Cytotherapy Laboratory, Memorial Sloan-Kettering Cancer Center, New York, New York
Amyloidosis

James R. Cook, MD, PhD
Assistant Professor of Pathology, Cleveland Clinic Lerner College of Medicine; Staff Pathologist, Department of Clinical Pathology, Cleveland Clinic Foundation, Cleveland, Ohio
Diseases of the Spleen

Megan A. Cooper, MD, PhD
Resident Physician, Washington University School of Medicine; St. Louis Children's Hospital, St. Louis, Missouri
Lymphocyte Biology

Mark A. Crowther, MD, MSc, FRCPC
Associate Professor and Hematology Residency Program Director, McMaster University; Head of Service, Hematology, St. Joseph's Hospital, Hamilton, Ontario, Canada
Anticoagulant and Thrombolytic Therapy

Melody J. Cunningham, MD
Instructor in Pediatrics, Harvard Medical School; Director, Thalassemia Program, Children's Hospital Boston, Boston, Massachusetts
Thalassemia

David C. Dale, MD
Professor of Medicine, University of Washington School of Medicine; Attending Physician, General Internal Medicine, University of Washington Medical Center, Seattle, Washington
Congenital Neutropenia

Sandeep S. Dave, MD, MS
Senior Fellow, National Cancer Institute, National Institutes of Health, Bethesda, Maryland
Gene Expression Methods

Laurence de Leval, MD, PhD
Research Associate, National Fund for Scientific Research (F.N.R.S.), University of Liège; Associate Pathologist, C.H.U. Sart-Tilman, Liège, Belgium
Biology of Lymphoid Malignancy

Volker Diehl, MD
Chairman of the German Hodgkin Study Group, Consultant of Internal Medicine/Hematology and Oncology, and Former Director of Department I of Internal Medicine, German Hodgkin Study Group, University Hospital Cologne, Cologne, Germany
Hodgkin's Lymphoma

Hartmut Döhner, MD
Professor of Medicine, Department of Internal Medicine III, University Hospital of Ulm, Ulm, Germany
Leukemias: Diagnosis and Classifications

Konstanze Döhner, MD
Department of Internal Medicine III, University Hospital of Ulm, Ulm, Germany
Leukemias: Diagnosis and Classifications

Inderjeet Dokal, MD, FRCPCH, FRCP, FRCPath
Professor of Haematology, Imperial College London; Department of Haematology, Hammersmith Hospital, London, United Kingdom
Constitutional Aplastic Anemias

Cynthia E. Dunbar, MD
Chief, Molecular Hematopoiesis Section, Hematology Branch, National Heart, Lung, and Blood Institute, National Institutes of Health, Bethesda, Maryland
Hematopoiesis

Janice P. Dutcher, MD
Professor of Medicine, New York Medical College, Valhalla; Associate Director, Clinical Affairs, Our Lady of Mercy Cancer Center, Bronx, New York
Chemotherapy Toxicities and Complications

Richard Edelson, MD

Department of Dermatology, Yale University School of Medicine, New Haven, Connecticut

Cutaneous Lymphoma

Khaled El-Shami, MD, PhD

Hematology/Oncology Fellow, Johns Hopkins Hospital, and The Sidney Kimmel Comprehensive Cancer Center at Johns Hopkins, Baltimore, Maryland

Hematologic Complications of Pregnancy

Timothy P. Endy, MD, MPH

Assistant Professor, Department of Medicine, Uniformed Services University School of Medicine, Bethesda, Maryland; Director, Communicable Diseases and Immunology, Walter Reed Army Institute of Research, Silver Spring, Maryland; Infectious Disease Staff, Walter Reed Army Medical Center, Washington, D.C.

Dengue and Hemorrhagic Fever Viruses

Juan I. Esteban, MD

Professor of Medicine, Universitari Vall d'Hebron; Attending Physician, Liver Unit, Hospital General Universiti Vall d'Hebron, Barcelona, Spain

Hepatitis C Virus

Elihu H. Estey, MD

Hubert and Olive Stringer Professorship in Medical Oncology, and Internist, University of Texas M.D. Anderson Cancer Center, Houston, Texas

Acute Myelogenous Leukemia

Anna Falanga, MD

Division of Hematology, Azienda Ospedaliera Ospedali Riuniti di Bergamo, Bergamo, Italy

Hematologic Abnormalities in Chronic Kidney Disease

Carolyn A. Felix, MD

Associate Professor of Pediatrics, Department of Pediatrics, University of Pennsylvania School of Medicine; Attending Physician, Division of Oncology, The Children's Hospital of Philadelphia, Philadelphia, Pennsylvania

Secondary Myelodysplasia/Acute Myeloid Leukemia

James L. M. Ferrara, MD

Professor, Department of Pediatrics, University of Michigan, Ann Arbor, Michigan

Graft-Versus-Host Disease

Andrés J. M. Ferreri, MD

Registrar, Medical Oncology Unit, San Raffaele H. Scientific Institute, Milan, Italy

Primary and Secondary Central Nervous System Lymphomas in Immunocompetent and Human Immunodeficiency Virus–Positive Patients

Clodoveo Ferri, MD

Professor of Rheumatology (Chair), Department of Internal Medicine, University of Modena and Reggio Emilia School of Medicine, Modena, Italy

Cryoglobulinemia

Thomas A. Fleisher, MD

Chief, Department of Laboratory Medicine, Clinical Center, National Institutes of Health, DHHS; Adjunct Professor, Department of Pediatrics, Uniformed Services University of the Health Sciences, Bethesda, Maryland

Flow Cytometry

Lindy P. Fox, MD

Department of Dermatology, Yale University School of Medicine, New Haven, Connecticut

Cutaneous Lymphoma

Charles W. Francis, MD

Professor of Medicine and of Pathology and Laboratory Medicine, University of Rochester School of Medicine and Dentistry, Rochester, New York

Venous and Arterial Thrombosis

Peter Gaines, PhD

Associate Research Scientist, Internal Medicine, Yale University School of Medicine, New Haven, Connecticut

Granulocytopoiesis

Patrick G. Gallagher, MD

Associate Professor, Department of Pediatrics, Yale University School of Medicine; Attending Physician, Yale New Haven Hospital, New Haven, Connecticut

Hematology of the Newborn

Arnold Ganser, MD

Professor of Medicine, Chief, Department of Hematology, Hemostasis and Oncology, and Head, Tumor Center, Hannover Medical School, Hannover, Germany

Cytokine Therapy and Its Complications

James N. George, MD

Professor of Medicine, University of Oklahoma Health Sciences Center, Oklahoma City, Oklahoma

Drug-Induced Thrombocytopenia

Alan M. Gewirtz, MD

Professor, Departments of Medicine and Pathology, University of Pennsylvania School of Medicine, University of Pennsylvania; Attending Physician, Hospital of the University of Pennsylvania, Philadelphia, Pennsylvania

Megakaryocyte Development and Disorders of Thrombopoiesis

Amy S. Gewirtz, MD

Medical Director, Clinical Laboratories, and Interim Director, Hematopathology, The Ohio State University Medical Center, Columbus, Ohio

Chronic Lymphocytic Leukemia

John M. Goldman, DM, FRCP, FRCPath
Fogarty Scholar, Hematology Branch, National Heart, Lung, and Blood Institute, National Institutes of Health, Bethesda, Maryland
Chronic Myeloid Leukemia

Xylina T. Gregg, MD
Clinical Instructor, Baylor College of Medicine; Chief of Hematology/Oncology, Kelsey-Seybold Clinic, Houston, Texas
Polycythemia Vera and Essential Thrombocythemia

Michael R. Grever, MD
Chairman and Charles A. Doan Professor of Medicine, and Professor of Pharmacology, The Ohio State University College of Medicine, and The Ohio State University, Columbus, Ohio
Chronic Lymphocytic Leukemia

Katherine A. Hajjar, MD
Professor and Chairman, Department of Cell and Developmental Biology, and Professor of Pediatrics, Weill Medical College of Cornell University; Attending Pediatrician, New York Presbyterian Hospital, New York, New York
Vascular Biology

William J. Harrington, Jr., MD
Professor of Medicine, University of Miami, Miami, Florida
Human Immunodeficiency Virus Type 1– and Human T-Lymphotropic Virus Type 1–Associated Lymphomas

Nancy Lee Harris, MD
Austin L. Vickery Professor of Pathology, Harvard Medical School; Director of Hematopathology, Massachusetts General Hospital, Boston, Massachusetts
Biology of Lymphoid Malignancy

John A. Heit, MD
Professor of Medicine, and Director of Coagulation Laboratories, Mayo Clinic, Rochester, Minnesota
Thrombotic Complications in Patients with Malignancy

Jay L. Hess, MD, PhD
Carl V. Weller Professor and Chair, University of Michigan Medical School, Ann Arbor, Michigan
Blood and Bone Marrow Morphology

Michael Heuser, MD
Department of Hematology, Hemostasis and Oncology, Hannover Medical School, Hannover, Germany
Cytokine Therapy and Its Complications

McDonald K. Horne, III, MD
Senior Clinical Investigator, Hematology Service, Department of Laboratory Medicine, W.G. Magnuson Clinical Center, National Institutes of Health, Bethesda, Maryland
Mechanical Hemolytic Anemia

Richard B. Hostetter, MD
Clinical Assistant Professor, Department of Surgery, Indiana University School of Medicine, Indianapolis; Associate Medical Director, and Director of Surgical Oncology, Center for Cancer Care, Goshen Health Systems, Goshen, Indiana
Surgery in Specific Hematologic Conditions

Lewis L. Hsu, MD, PhD
Associate Professor, Pediatric Hematology, Marian Anderson Comprehensive Sickle Cell Center, St. Christopher's Hospital for Children, Drexel University College of Medicine, Philadelphia, Pennsylvania; Guest Researcher/Contractor, National Institute of Diabetes and Digestive and Kidney Diseases/National Heart, Lung, and Blood Institute/Clinical Center, Bethesda, Maryland
Sickle Cell Disease

Rosangela Invernizzi, MD
Associate Professor of Internal Medicine, University of Pavia Medical School; Attending Physician, Department of Internal Medicine, IRCCS Policlinico San Matteo, Pavia, Italy
Sideroblastic Anemias

David K. Jin, MD, PhD
Chief Clinical Fellow, Division of Hematology-Medical Oncology, Department of Medicine, New York-Presbyterian Hospital, Weill Medical College of Cornell University, New York, New York
Immune, Posttransfusional, and Neonatal Thrombocytopenia

Carol L. Johnson, BS, MT(ASCP)SBB
Manager, Education Programs, New York Blood Center, New York, New York
Red Cell Antigens and Antibodies

Robin M. Joyce, MD
Instructor in Medicine, Harvard Medical School; Attending Physician, Hematologic Malignancy/Bone Marrow Transplant Program, Beth Israel Deaconess Medical Center, Boston, Massachusetts
Waldenström's Macroglobulinemia

Siripen Kalayanarooj, MD
Medical Officer, Level 10, Queen Sirikit National Institute of Child Health, Department of Medical Services, Ministry of Public Health, Bangkok, Thailand
Dengue and Hemorrhagic Fever Viruses

Karen L. Kaplan, MD, PhD
Professor of Medicine, and Director, Apheresis Program, University of Rochester School of Medicine and Dentistry, Rochester, New York
Venous and Arterial Thrombosis

James W. Kazura, MD

Professor of International Health, Medicine, and Pathology, Center for Global Health and Disease, Case School of Medicine, Case Western Reserve University; Physician, University Hospitals of Cleveland, Cleveland, Ohio

Malaria

Siobán Keel, MD

University of Washington School of Medicine; Hematology Fellow, University of Washington, Seattle, Washington

Pure Red Cell Aplasia and Diamond-Blackfan Anemia

Karen E. King, MD

Assistant Professor, Pathology and Oncology, Johns Hopkins University School of Medicine; Director, Hemapheresis and Transfusion Support Service, and Associate Director, Transfusion Medicine, Johns Hopkins Hospital, Baltimore, Maryland

The Autoimmune Hemolytic Anemias

May-Jean King, BSc, PhD

Senior Research Biochemist, Clinical Scientist, International Blood Group Reference Laboratory, Bristol, United Kingdom

Hereditary Spherocytosis, Hereditary Elliptocytosis, and Related Disorders

Harvey G. Klein, MD

Adjunct Professor of Pathology, Johns Hopkins School of Medicine, Baltimore; Chief, Department of Transfusion Medicine, National Institutes of Health, Bethesda, Maryland

Practice of Blood Component Transfusion

Beate Klimm, MD

Assistant Doctor of Internal Medicine (2nd year), and Study Physician of the German Hodgkin Study Group, Department I of Internal Medicine/Hematology and Oncology, University Hospital Cologne, Cologne, Germany

Hodgkin's Lymphoma

Catie E. Kobbervig, MD

Instructor, Hematology, University of Wisconsin Medical School; Staff, Meriter Hospital, Madison, Wisconsin

Thrombotic Complications in Patients with Malignancy

Omer N. Koç, MD

Associate Professor of Medicine, Case Western Reserve University; Staff, University Hospitals of Cleveland, Cleveland, Ohio

Non-Hodgkin's Lymphoma

Barbara A. Konkle, MD

Associate Professor of Medicine, and Director, Penn Comprehensive Hemophilia and Thrombosis Program, University of Pennsylvania School of Medicine, Philadelphia, Pennsylvania

Von Willebrand Disease

Margot S. Kruskall, MD*

Professor of Pathology, and Associate Professor of Medicine, Harvard Medical School, Boston, Massachusetts

Complications of Transfusion: Transfusion Reactions and Transfusion-Transmitted Diseases

James P. Kushner, MD

M.M. Wintrobe Distinguished Professor of Medicine, Division of Hematology, Department of Medicine, University of Utah School of Medicine; Chief, Division of Hematology, and Program Director—General Clinical Research Center, Division of Hematology, Department of Medicine, University Hospital, Salt Lake City, Utah

Hemoglobin and Heme Biosynthesis

Hillard M. Lazarus, MD, FACP

Professor of Medicine, and Professor of General Medical Sciences (Oncology), Case Western Reserve University, Comprehensive Cancer Center; Director, Blood and Marrow Transplant Program, and Director, Clinical Trials Core Unit, Ireland Cancer Center, University Hospitals of Cleveland, Cleveland, Ohio

Supportive Care for the Hematopoietic Stem Cell Transplant Patient

Michelle M. Le Beau, PhD

Professor, Department of Medicine, Section of Hematology/Oncology, University of Chicago, Chicago, Illinois

Cytogenetics/Fluorescent In Situ Hybridization

Agnes Y. Y. Lee, MD, BSc

Associate Professor, Medicine, McMaster University; Full Time Staff, Hamilton Health Sciences Henderson Hospital, Hamilton, Ontario, Canada

Thrombotic Complications in Patients with Malignancy

Marcel Levi, MD, PhD

Professor of Medicine, University of Amsterdam; Chairman, Department of Medicine, Academic Medical Center, Amsterdam, The Netherlands

Inherited Thrombophilia

Alan Lichtin, MD

Associate Professor of Internal Medicine, Cleveland Clinic Lerner College of Medicine; Staff Hematologist/Medical Oncologist, Cleveland Clinic Foundation, Cleveland, Ohio

Diseases of the Spleen

Richard F. Little, MD, MPH

HIV and AIDS Malignancy Branch, Center for Cancer Research, National Cancer Institute, Bethesda, Maryland

Epstein-Barr Virus–Related and Kaposi's Sarcoma–Associated Herpesvirus–Related Neoplasms

*Deceased

Johnson M. Liu, MD, FACP
Albert Einstein College of Medicine, Bronx; Head, Les Nelkin Memorial Laboratory for Pediatric Oncology, Schneider Children's Hospital, New Hyde Park, New York
Constitutional Aplastic Anemias

Alison W. Loren, MD, MS
Instructor of Medicine, University of Pennsylvania School of Medicine, Philadelphia, Pennsylvania
Megakaryocyte Development and Disorders of Thrombopoiesis

Karen L. LoRusso, MD
Medical Oncologist, The Cancer Institute of New Mexico, Santa Fe, New Mexico
Chronic Bruising and Bleeding Diathesis

Thomas P. Loughran, Jr., MD
Director, Penn State Cancer Institute, and Professor of Medicine, Penn State University, School of Medicine, The Milton S. Hershey Medical Center, Hershey, Pennsylvania
Large Granular Lymphocyte Leukemia

Mario Luppi, MD, PhD
Associate Professor of Hematology, Department of Oncology and Hematology, University of Modena and Reggio Emilia Azienda Policlinico, Modena, Italy
Human Cytomegalovirus, Human Herpesvirus 8, and Other Herpesviruses

Lucio Luzzatto, MD
Professor of Hematology, University of Genova, Genova; Scientific Director, Istituto Toscano Tumori, Firenze, Italy
Paroxysmal Nocturnal Hemoglobinuria

Alice D. Ma, MD
Assistant Professor of Medicine, Division of Hematology/Oncology, University of North Carolina School of Medicine; Attending Physician, UNC Hospitals, Chapel Hill, North Carolina
Antiphospholipid Antibody Syndrome

Jaroslaw P. Maciejewski, MD, PhD
Associate Professor of Medicine, Cleveland Clinic Lerner College of Medicine of Case Western Reserve University; Head, Experimental Hematology and Hematopoiesis Section, Taussig Cancer Center, Cleveland Clinic Foundation, Cleveland, Ohio
Human Cytomegalovirus, Human Herpesvirus 8, and Other Herpesviruses

B. Gail Macik, MD
Associate Professor of Medicine and Pathology, University of Virginia Health System, Charlottesville, Virginia
Chronic Bruising and Bleeding Diathesis

Harry L. Malech, MD
Laboratory Chief, Laboratory of Host Defenses, National Institute of Allergy and Infectious Diseases, National Institutes of Health, Bethesda, Maryland
Chronic Granulomatous Disease

Peter Mattei, MD
Assistant Professor, Department of Surgery, University of Pennsylvania; Attending Physician, General, Thoracic, and Fetal Surgery, The Children's Hospital of Philadelphia, Philadelphia, Pennsylvania
Surgery in Specific Hematologic Conditions

Edward E. Max, MD, PhD
Associate Director for Research, Office of Biotechnology Products, Center for Drug Evaluation and Research, Bethesda, Maryland
Lymphocyte Biology

John H. McVey, BSc (Hons), PhD
Haemostasis and Thrombosis, MRC Clinical Sciences Centre, Imperial College London, Hammersmith Hospital Campus, London, United Kingdom
Coagulation Factors

Robert T. Means, Jr., MD
Professor of Medicine, Division of Hematology, Oncology, and Blood and Marrow Transplantation, and Associate Chair for Research, Department of Internal Medicine, University of Kentucky College of Medicine; Chief, Medical Service, Veterans Affairs Medical Center, Lexington, Kentucky
Anemia of Chronic Disease

Dean D. Metcalfe, MD
Chief, Laboratory of Allergic Diseases, National Institute of Allergy and Infectious Diseases, National Institutes of Health, Bethesda, Maryland
Mastocytosis

Saskia Middeldorp, MD, PhD
Assistant Professor of Medicine, University of Amsterdam; Clinical and Research Affiliate, Department of Vascular Medicine, Academic Medical Center, Amsterdam, The Netherlands
Inherited Thrombophilia

Joseph Mikhael, MD, MEd, FRCPC
Assistant Professor, University of Toronto, Division of Hematology-Oncology, Princess Margaret Hospital, Toronto, Ontario, Canada
Multiple Myeloma and Related Diseases

Narla Mohandas, DSc
Vice President for Research, New York Blood Center, New York, New York
Erythrocyte Structure; Red Cell Antigens and Antibodies

Krzysztof Mrózek, MD, PhD
Research Scientist, Comprehensive Cancer Center, and James Cancer Hospital and Solove Research Institute, The Ohio State University, Columbus, Ohio
Leukemias: Diagnosis and Classifications

Khin Saw Aye Myint, MD
Head, Emerging Pathogens, Department of Virology, United States Army Medical Component, Armed Forces Research Institute of Medical Sciences, Bangkok, Thailand
Dengue and Hemorrhagic Fever Viruses

Paul M. Ness, MD
Professor, Pathology, Medicine, and Oncology, Johns Hopkins University School of Medicine; Director, Transfusion Medicine, Johns Hopkins Hospital, Baltimore, Maryland
The Autoimmune Hemolytic Anemias

Ellis J. Neufeld, MD, PhD
Associate Professor of Pediatrics, Harvard Medical School; Associate Chief, Division of Hematology/Oncology, Children's Hospital, Boston, Boston, Massachusetts
Thalassemia

João B. Oliveira, MD
Visiting Fellow, Immunology Service, DLM, Clinical Center, National Institutes of Health, DHHS, Bethesda, Maryland
Flow Cytometry

Roger G. Owen, MB BCh, MD, MRCP, MRCPath
Consultant Haematologist/Haematopathologist, Leeds Teaching Hospitals NHS Trust, Leeds, United Kingdom
Monoclonal Gammopathy of Undetermined Significance

Jan E. W. Palmblad, MD, PhD
Professor of Medicine, Karolinska Institutet; Karolinska University Hospital, Huddinge, Stockholm, Sweden
Acquired Neutropenia and Agranulocytosis

Simrit Parmar, MD
Fellow, Division of Hematology-Oncology, Northwestern University, Feinberg School of Medicine, Chicago, Illinois
Acute Promyelocytic Leukemia

Kimberly Perez, MD
Internal Medicine Resident (2nd year), Brown University, Providence, Rhode Island
Hematologic Complications of Pregnancy

Effie W. Petersdorf, MD
Professor of Medicine, University of Washington School of Medicine; Member, Fred Hutchinson Cancer Research Center; Attending Physician, Seattle Cancer Care Alliance, Seattle, Washington
Human Leukocyte Antigen and Transplantation

LoAnn C. Peterson, MD
Professor of Pathology, Feinberg Medical School of Northwestern University; Director of Hematopathology, Northwestern Memorial Hospital, Chicago, Illinois
Acute Promyelocytic Leukemia

Stefano A. Pileri, MD
Full-Professor of Pathology, and Director of the Research Doctorate in Clinical and Experimental Haematology and Haematopathology, Bologna University School of Medicine; Head of the Haematopathology Unit, St. Orsola Hospital, Bologna, Italy
Cryoglobulinemia

Mortimer Poncz, MD
Professor of Pediatrics, University of Pennsylvania School of Medicine, and The Children's Hospital of Philadelphia, Philadelphia, Pennsylvania
Heparin-Induced Thrombocytopenia

Jonathan Powell, MD, PhD
Department of Oncology, The Sidney Kimmel Comprehensive Cancer Center at Johns Hopkins, Baltimore, Maryland
Lymphocyte Biology

Josef T. Prchal, MD
Professor, Department of Hematology-Oncology, Baylor College of Medicine, Houston, Texas
Polycythemia Vera and Essential Thrombocythemia

Ching-Hon Pui, MD
American Cancer Society F.M. Kirby Clinical Research Professor, and Professor of Pediatrics, University of Tennessee Health Science Center; Director, Leukemia/Lymphoma Division, St. Jude Children's Research Hospital, Memphis, Tennessee
Acute Lymphoblastic Leukemia

Margaret V. Ragni, MD, MPH
Professor of Medicine, Division of Hematology/Oncology, Department of Medicine, University of Pittsburgh School of Medicine; Director, Hemophilia Center of Western Pennsylvania, Pittsburgh, Pennsylvania
The Hemophilias: Factor VIII and Factor IX Deficiencies

V. Koneti Rao, MD
Staff Physician, Laboratory of Clinical Infectious Diseases, National Institute of Allergy and Infectious Diseases, National Institutes of Health, Bethesda, Maryland
Autoimmune Lymphoproliferative Syndrome

Marion E. Reid, PhD
Director of Immunohematology, New York Blood Center, New York, New York
Erythrocyte Structure; Red Cell Antigens and Antibodies

Scot C. Remick, MD
Professor of Medicine, Oncology, and Global Health and Diseases, Division of Hematology/Oncology, and Associate Director for Clinical Research, Case Comprehensive Cancer Center, Case School of Medicine, Cleveland, Ohio
Human Immunodeficiency Virus Type 1– and Human T-Lymphotropic Virus Type 1–Associated Lymphomas

Giuseppe Remuzzi, MD
Director, Division of Nephrology, Azienda Ospedaliera Ospedali Riuniti di Bergamo, and Mario Negri Institute for Pharmacological Research, Bergamo, Italy
Hematologic Abnormalities in Chronic Kidney Disease

Raul C. Ribeiro, MD
Professor of Pediatrics, University of Tennessee; Member (Professor), Hematology/Oncology Department, St. Jude Children's Research Hospital, Memphis, Tennessee
Acute Lymphoblastic Leukemia

Margaret E. Rick, MD
Assistant Chief, Hematology Service, Department of Laboratory Medicine, National Institutes of Health; Clinical Professor of Medicine, Uniformed Services University of the Health Sciences, Bethesda, Maryland
Coagulation Testing

Griffin P. Rodgers, MD, MACP
Chief, Molecular and Clinical Hematology Branch, and Deputy Director, National Institute of Diabetes, Digestive and Kidney Diseases, National Institutes of Health, Bethesda, Maryland
Sickle Cell Disease

Daniel Rosenblum, MD, FACP
Clinical Reviewer, Office of Cellular, Tissue, and Gene Therapies, Center for Biological Evaluation and Research, U.S. Food and Drug Administration, Rockville, Maryland
Geriatric Hematology

Tracey Rouault, MD
Chief, Section on Human Iron Metabolism, National Institute of Child Health and Human Development, Bethesda, Maryland
Iron Deficiency

Robert A. S. Roubey, MD
Associate Professor of Medicine, Division of Rheumatology, University of North Carolina School of Medicine; Attending Physician, UNC Hospitals, Chapel Hill, North Carolina
Antiphospholipid Antibody Syndrome

Robin Russell-Jones, MA, FRCP, FRCPath
Skin Tumour Unit, St. John's Institute of Dermatology, St. Thomas' Hospital, London, United Kingdom
Cutaneous Lymphoma

J. Evan Sadler, MD, PhD
Professor of Medicine, Biochemistry and Biophysics, Washington University School of Medicine; Investigator, Howard Hughes Medical Institute, St. Louis, Missouri
Thrombotic Thrombocytopenic Purpura and Hemolytic-Uremic Syndrome

Jean-Marie Saint-Remy, MD, PhD
Center for Molecular and Vascular Biology, University of Leuven, Leuven, Belgium
Acquired Inhibitors to Clotting Factors

Sabah Sallah, MD
Medical Director, Novo Nordisk Pharmaceuticals, Athens, Greece
Acquired Inhibitors to Clotting Factors

Shigeru Sassa, MD, PhD
Associate Professor Emeritus, The Rockefeller University, New York, New York
Porphyrias

Geraldine P. Schechter, MD
Professor of Medicine, George Washington University; Chief, Hematology Section, Washington Veterans Affairs Medical Center, Washington, D.C.
Differential Diagnosis of Anemia

Alan N. Schecter, MD
Chief, Laboratory of Chemical Biology, National Institutes of Health; Senior Medical Staff, National Institutes of Health Clinical Centers, Bethesda, Maryland
Hemoglobin and Heme Biosynthesis

Arrigo Schieppati, MD
Division of Nephrology, Azienda Ospedaliera Ospedali Riuniti di Bergamo, Bergamo, Italy
Hematologic Abnormalities in Chronic Kidney Disease

Lowell Schnipper, MD
Berenson Professor of Medicine, Harvard Medical School; Chief, Division of Hematology/Oncology, Beth Israel Deaconess Medical Center, Boston, Massachusetts
Waldenström's Macroglobulinemia

Douglas J. Schwartzentruber, MD
Clinical Associate Professor of Surgery, Indiana University School of Medicine, Indiana University, Indianapolis; Medical Director, Center for Cancer Care at Goshen Health System, Goshen, Indiana
Surgery in Specific Hematologic Conditions

J. Paul Scott, MD
Professor of Pediatrics, Medical College of Wisconsin; Attending Physician, Department of Hematology and Oncology, Children's Hospital of Wisconsin, Milwaukee, Wisconsin
Pediatric Hematology

Paul A. Seligman, MD
Professor of Medicine, Division of Hematology, University of Colorado Health Sciences Center, Denver, Colorado
Iron Deficiency

Robert S. Siegel, MD
Professor of Medicine, and Director, Division of Hematology/Oncology, George Washington University Cancer Center; Director, Division of Hematology/Oncology, George Washington University Medical Center Medical Faculty Associates, Washington, D.C.
Hematologic Complications of Pregnancy

Elaine M. Sloand, MD
National Heart, Lung, and Blood Institute, National Institutes of Health, Bethesda, Maryland
Myelodysplastic Syndrome; Human Immunodeficiency Virus: Hematologic Complications

Jerry L. Spivak, MD
Professor of Medicine and Oncology, Johns Hopkins University School of Medicine; Attending Physician, Johns Hopkins Hospital, Baltimore, Maryland
Erythrocytosis

Sally P. Stabler, MD
Co-Division Chief of Hematology, and Professor of Medicine, University of Colorado Health Sciences Center, Denver, Colorado
Megaloblastic Anemias: Pernicious Anemia and Folate Deficiency

Edward A. Stadtmauer, MD
Associate Professor of Medicine, University of Pennsylvania School of Medicine; Director, Bone Marrow Transplant Program, Abramson Cancer Center, University of Pennsylvania, Philadelphia, Pennsylvania
Autologous Transplantation of Hematopoietic Stem Cells

Louis M. Staudt, MD, PhD
Chief, Lymphoid Malignancies Section, Metabolism Branch, National Cancer Institute, Bethesda, Maryland
Gene Expression Methods

Maryalice Stetler-Stevenson, MD, PhD
Medical Officer, Lab of Pathology, National Cancer Institute, National Institutes of Health, Bethesda, Maryland
Flow Cytometry

A. Keith Stewart, MBChB, FRCPC, MRCP
Professor, Faculty of Medicine, University of Toronto; Medical Oncologist, Princess Margaret Hospital, Toronto, Ontario, Canada
Multiple Myeloma and Related Diseases

Stephen E. Straus, MD
Senior Investigator, Laboratory of Clinical Infectious Diseases, National Institute of Allergy and Infectious Diseases, National Institutes of Health, Bethesda, Maryland
Autoimmune Lymphoproliferative Syndrome

Martin S. Tallman, MD
Professor of Medicine, Division of Hematology-Oncology, Northwestern University, Feinberg School of Medicine; Attending Physician, Northwestern Memorial Hospital, Chicago, Illinois
Acute Promyelocytic Leukemia

Ayalew Tefferi, MD
Professor of Medicine, Mayo Clinic, Rochester, Minnesota
Myelofibrosis with Myeloid Metaplasia

Arthur R. Thompson, MD, PhD
Professor of Medicine, Hematology, University of Washington; Director of Hemophilia Care and Coagulation Laboratories, Puget Sound Blood Center, Seattle, Washington
Congenital Bleeding Disorders from Other Coagulation Protein Deficiencies

John F. Tisdale, MD
Senior Investigator, Molecular and Clinical Hematology Branch, National Institute of Diabetes and Digestive and Kidney Diseases, National Institutes of Health, Bethesda, Maryland
Hematopoiesis

Cheng Hock Toh, MD, FRCP (London), FRCPath (UK)
Reader in Hematology, University of Liverpool; Consultant in Hematology, Royal Liverpool University Hospital, Liverpool, United Kingdom
Disseminated Intravascular Coagulation

Giuseppe Torelli, MD
Full Professor of Hematology, and Chief, Division of Hematology, Department of Oncology and Hematology, University of Modena and Reggio Emilia Azienda Policlinico, Modena, Italy
Human Cytomegalovirus, Human Herpesvirus 8, and Other Herpesviruses

Giovanna Tosato, MD
Center for Cancer Research, National Cancer Institute, National Institutes of Health, Bethesda, Maryland
Epstein-Barr Virus–Related and Kaposi's Sarcoma–Associated Herpesvirus–Related Neoplasms

Dimitrios Tzachanis, MD, PhD
Hematology and Oncology Fellow, Harvard Medical School, and Beth Israel Deaconess Medical Center, Boston, Massachusetts
Waldenström's Macroglobulinemia

Lynne Uhl, MD
Assistant Professor of Pathology, Harvard Medical School; Interim Director, Division of Laboratory and Transfusion Medicine, Beth Israel Deaconess Medical Center, Boston, Massachusetts
Complications of Transfusion: Transfusion Reactions and Transfusion-Transmitted Diseases

Riccardo Valdez, MD
Assistant Professor, Department of Pathology, University of Michigan, Ann Arbor, Michigan
Graft-Versus-Host Disease

Theodore E. Warkentin, MD
Professor, Department of Pathology and Molecular Medicine, and Department of Medicine, McMaster University; Associate Head, Transfusion Medicine, Hamilton Regional Laboratory Medicine Program; Hematologist, Service of Clinical Hematology, Hamilton Health Sciences, Hamilton, Ontario, Canada
Heparin-Induced Thrombocytopenia; Anticoagulant and Thrombolytic Therapy

Jill M. Watanabe, MD, MPH
Associate Professor, University of Washington, School of Medicine; Attending Physician, Harborview Medical Center, Seattle, Washington
Congenital Neutropenia

Herbert H. Watzke, MD
Faculty Member and Professor of Medicine, University of Medicine Vienna, Vienna, Austria
Evaluation of the Acutely Bleeding Patient

Alan S. Wayne, MD
Part Time Visiting Associate Professor of Pediatrics, Johns Hopkins University School of Medicine, Baltimore; Clinical Director and Clinical Tenure Track Investigator, National Institutes of Health, Pediatric Oncology Branch, Center for Cancer Research, National Cancer Institute, Bethesda, Maryland
Pediatric Leukemias

Mitchell J. Weiss, MD, PhD
Assistant Professor of Pediatrics, University of Pennsylvania School of Medicine, and The Children's Hospital of Philadelphia, Philadelphia, Pennsylvania
Thalassemia

Sean Whittaker, MD, FRCP
Skin Tumour Unit, St. John's Institute of Dermatology, St. Thomas' Hospital, London, United Kingdom
Cutaneous Lymphoma

Peter H. Wiernik, MD
Professor of Medicine and Radiation Oncology, New York Medical College, Valhalla; Director, Our Lady of Mercy Cancer Center, Bronx, New York
Chemotherapy Toxicities and Complications

Wyndham H. Wilson, MD, PhD
Senior Investigator, National Cancer Institute, Bethesda, Maryland
Non-Hodgkin's Lymphoma

Daniel G. Wright, MD
Professor of Medicine and Pathology, Boston University School of Medicine, Boston, Massachusetts
Acquired Neutropenia and Agranulocytosis

Gregory Yanik, MD
Associate Professor, Department of Pediatrics, University of Michigan, Ann Arbor, Michigan
Graft-Versus-Host Disease

Robert Yarchoan, MD
Chief, HIV and AIDS Malignancy Branch, Center for Cancer Research, National Cancer Institute, National Institutes of Health, Bethesda, Maryland
Epstein-Barr Virus–Related and Kaposi's Sarcoma–Associated Herpesvirus–Related Neoplasms

Neal S. Young, MD
Chief, Hematology Branch, National Heart, Lung, and Blood Institute, National Institutes of Health, Bethesda, Maryland
Acquired Aplastic Anemia; Myelodysplastic Syndrome; Parvovirus B19

X. Long Zheng, MD, PhD
Assistant Professor of Pathology and Laboratory Medicine, University of Pennsylvania; Medical Director of Coagulation Laboratory, The Children's Hospital of Philadelphia, Philadelphia, Pennsylvania
Thrombotic Thrombocytopenic Purpura and Hemolytic-Uremic Syndrome

Barbara Zieger, MD
Professor, Department of Pediatrics and Adolescent Medicine, University Hospital Freiburg, Freiburg, Germany
Pediatric Hematology

Anna Linda Zignego, MD
Professor of Medicine, Department of Internal Medicine, University of Florence, School of Medicine, Florence, Italy
Cryoglobulinemia

PREFACE

Production of a new textbook in hematology, daunting at inception and often frustrating in execution, nevertheless provides opportunities to its editors and authors.

First, in organizing *Clinical Hematology,* we have redrawn some of the indistinct borders of the field of hematology. Recent editions of established hematology texts suffer weight problems, often running to many thousands of pages and to multiple volumes. They offer primers in biochemistry, cell biology, and molecular biology, and massive chapters with hundreds of appended references—testimonials to the basic science foundation of hematology and to the scholarship of its academic leaders. But is the role of a subspecialty text to instruct on the performance of a Southern blot or to provide primer on the basics of cell biology? Conversely, in many important respects the compass of hematology has remained fixed for decades, with definitions and nosology still grounded in 19th and early 20th century pathology. An astute modern reader of the classical textbook will note many gaps, such as the absence of discussions dedicated to parvovirus B19 or of agranulocytosis, and a hematologist in Asia or Africa might miss the hematological manifestations of common, serious infections, such as malaria, hemorrhagic fevers, or hepatitis C. These omissions result from unchanged tradition, based on antique definitions of blood diseases that are slow to adopt pathophysiologic insights, do not address some of the real problems facing the consulting or treating hematologist in private or academic practice, and fail to recognize the enormity of hematologic complications of global (and expanding) diseases of the modern world. They cannot be justified today.

Second, *Clinical Hematology* has been created with a mind to "the reader over the shoulder" of the authors. Textbooks frequently suffer, in the editors' opinion, from their role as compendia not just of knowledge but of much esoteric data—culminating as showcases for the display of the authorial erudition rather than as efficient conduits for the transfer of processed, essential, and proven information. In a digital era when abstracts of the most recent scientific papers and medical reviews, many of highly variable quality and uncertain origin and validity, are available by desktop computer or handheld device, the role of textbooks as encyclopedias seems less required. Instead, textbooks must serve as accurate summaries of collective professional experience, critical distillations of a vast published literature, and thoughtful discussions of the scientific and clinical evidence that shape our knowledge of diseases, their diagnosis and treatment.

Third, the publisher has encouraged us to include unlimited color illustrations "on the page" drawn by excellent graphic artists. *Clinical Hematology* may be the first medical textbook to be based on Edward Tufte's provocative principles for the effective visual presentation of quantitative information—our graphics are intended to clarify and even replace text, not merely to decorate it. We encourage the reader to utilize the accompanying compact disk, which provides the book's table and figures not only for purposes of review and, teaching but for office education of an increasingly sophisticated patient population. The CD also includes a searchable, linked full bibliography for every chapter. Space constraints and aesthetic considerations also have led us to strive, even in a multi-authored book, for a style of writing that is concise and precise, yet lively and direct.

The end result of our plans for *Clinical Hematology* is, we hope, a textbook of moderate length that can be read–even enjoyed–and yet will meet completely the needs of the hematologist in training, for Board preparation, and the hematologist, oncologist, internist, and pediatrician in practice. We hope it will serve as both resource and inspiration.

THE EDITORS

Acknowledgments

Our publisher, Elsevier, has provided generous support and extraordinary resources for developing *Clinical Hematology*. The idea for *Clinical Hematology* arose from conversations between the senior editor and Marc Strauss when he was at W.B. Saunders, over many lunches; he deserves credit for the book's origin. All the editors are especially grateful to Dolores Meloni, acquisitions editor, and Catherine Carroll, our managing editor, for their enthusiasm, skill, and perseverance. Craig Durant and Dragonfly Media provided exceptional graphic design. Berta Steiner has been a very capable and *very* patient production director. Finally, our many colleagues in hematology and oncology departments throughout the world have provided constructive criticism, counseling, and, eventually, all their chapters—this work obviously would have been impossible without their active participation.

CONTENTS

Section 5
Diseases of Altered Coagulation 767

Part III
CONSULTATIVE HEMATOLOGY 901

Section 1
Hematology of Growth, Development, and Aging 902

Section 2
Infections of Marrow and Blood 956

Section 3
Hematologic Problems of Medical Practice 1037

PART I

Basic Science of Hematology

CHAPTER 1

HEMATOPOIESIS

John F. Tisdale, MD, and Cynthia E. Dunbar, MD

KEY POINTS

Hematopoiesis

- There is an ordered progression of hematopoietic development during ontogeny: blood elements are first produced by precursor cells in the yolk sac, then in the fetal liver, and finally in the bone marrow.
- A wide variety of informative experimental assays exist for hematopoietic stem and progenitor cells. Each assay has limitations. The only true assay for long-term repopulating stem cells is reconstitution of hematopoiesis in vivo.
- Hematopoietic stem cells can be defined by the expression pattern of specific cell surface proteins, cell cycle quiescence, and telomerase activity.
- Hematopoiesis occurs in a specialized bone marrow microenvironment, composed of cellular and noncellular elements critical to localization and control of blood cell production.
- The processes of stem cell mobilization and homing are governed by modulation of interactions between primitive hematopoietic cells and their microenvironment.
- Populations of nonhematopoietic stem cells in the bone marrow, including mesenchymal stem cells, are capable of generating bone, cartilage, and other tissues, along with more undifferentiated cell populations that potentially contribute to a wide variety of adult tissues.

INTRODUCTION

Hematopoiesis is defined as the process by which pluripotent hematopoietic stem cells both self-renew and differentiate into all of the specialized circulating blood cells, including white blood cells, red blood cells, and platelets. It was not until the mid-19th century that the marrow was proposed as the source of blood production. The primary cellular components of the blood were delineated consequent to Ehrlich's development of techniques for drying, fixing, and staining blood and marrow specimens, ultimately culminating in their full morphologic characterization. The recognition that marrow cells shared features of mature cells of the blood allowed segregation of precursor cells into various differentiation lineages and led to the concept of an ancestral hierarchy of blood cell production, emanating from a mononuclear cell type that shared none of the features of mature blood cells or their intermediates.

In the mid-20th century, experiments examining the effects of radiation on various tissues led to the observation that lethally irradiated mice could recover blood counts and survive if they were grafted with bone marrow from a normal mouse.[1,2] A humoral factor was originally favored as containing a critical stimulatory factor.[3] Unequal reciprocal translocations between two chromosomes present in some mice allowed tracking of the origin of cells by cytogenetics,[4] and, with these animals serving as donors, the majority of dividing cells within the marrow of lethally irradiated recipients were marked, establishing finally that the donor cellular component of the graft was responsible for the radiation protection.[5] The creation of a "chimera," a concept that dates to antiquity, was thus established as feasible and a potential therapeutic modality for the treatment of hematologic diseases.

A BRIEF ONTOGENY OF HEMATOPOIESIS

Historic morphologic studies of blood cell formation also helped to shape our current view of hematopoietic ontogeny. Red blood cells of lower vertebrates share some features of erythrocytes in developing mammalian embryos, especially the presence of nuclei in mature red cells; this observation led to the distinction of "primitive" (as in lower animals) erythropoiesis from "definitive" erythropoiesis. Red blood cells are the first lineage produced during embryogenesis, initially detected in yolk sac blood islands at gestational day 8–8.5 in murine embryos and approximately days 18–24 in humans.[6] These early red cells express embryonic hemoglobins with higher oxygen-binding affinity than found in adult hemoglobins, and thus are able to confront the major challenge of transfer of oxygen to the embryo from the maternal circulation despite low oxygen tension. By gestational day 10, murine hematopoiesis shifts to the fetal liver. Erythrocytes produced within the liver lack nuclei and synthesize adult-type hemoglobin in mice and an intermediate fetal hemoglobin in humans, constituting "definitive hematopoiesis" (see Chapter 2). Finally, during the last third of gestation, the site of hematopoiesis gradually moves from the fetal liver to the bone marrow. Hematopoietic progenitor cells can be found within the yolk sac of murine embryos as early as gestational day 8, suggesting that the yolk sac is the source not only of primitive erythropoiesis but also of hematopoietic stem cells.[7–9] Primitive cells were hypothesized to migrate to the liver to initiate definitive hematopoiesis, but this issue remains controversial because the aorto-gonad-mesonephros region of the embryo itself, not the yolk sac, may contain the cells responsible for initiating definitive hematopoiesis.[10,11]

HIERARCHICAL AND LINEAGE RELATIONSHIPS

Postnatally, the blood cell production process occurs in the three-dimensional space of the bone marrow, which includes not only hematopoietic stem cells and their progeny but vascular structures lined with specialized endothelial cells, supporting stromal cells, and extracellular matrix molecules. Within this environment, hematopoietic stem cells undergo the process of lineage commitment and differentiation through a series of maturational steps that result in the production of the mature blood elements.

The hierarchy of differentiated progenitors downstream of HSCs has been the subject of extensive investigation. Terminal maturation events of distal unilineage progenitors such as erythroid precursors are described in other chapters in this volume. Conceptually, each successive developmental stage loses the potential to contribute to other lineages or classes of cells,[12] a process at once linear and irreversible, meaning that, once a progenitor cell undergoes this commitment process, it cannot revert to an earlier stage or begin producing cells along an alternative pathway. Order hierarchies have relied primarily on clonal in vitro assays (described later), particularly within the myeloid lineages. Cell surface phenotypic characteristics define each progenitor category, with in vitro or in vivo functional assays employed to demonstrate loss or gain of function by depletion or enrichment of cells with a specific cell surface phenotype.

Using these approaches, Weissman and colleagues published a series of pioneering studies identifying the earliest lymphoid-restricted (common lymphoid progenitor [CLP]) and earliest myeloid-restricted (common myeloid progenitor [CMP]) cells in murine bone marrow (Fig. 1–1).[13–15] Cells with the phenotype of a CLP generate both T and B lymphocytes in vivo, and those with the phenotype of a CMP give rise to either megakaryocyte/erythrocyte or granulocyte/macrophage progenitors in vivo. The commitment of these progenitors is believed to be a mutually exclusive process. However, in fetal liver, cells with a CMP phenotype can also generate B cells, and cells with a CLP phenotype can produce macrophages.[16,17] The fact that children with severe combined immunodeficiency (SCID) who are transplanted with parental marrow frequently engraft only in the T-cell lineage suggests that, at least in vivo, either hematopoietic stem cells (HSCs) can generate daughter cells restricted to one lineage pathway or that CLP or a T-restricted progenitor can survive over the long term under certain conditions.[18] Purified CLP or CMP cells have been shown to have therapeutic potential in murine disease models.[19,20]

Clonal human hematologic disorders also offer insights into lineage relationships. Many blood diseases only appear to involve myeloid lineages, or myeloid and B-lymphoid lineages, while rarely affecting T-lymphoid or natural killer cells. Possibly this discordance reflects disruption of normal lineage development by specific mutations in HSCs or progenitors, but the finding of the same pattern in so many diverse conditions, including myelodysplasia, chronic myelogenous leukemia, juvenile myelomonocytic leukemia, and paroxysmal nocturnal hemoglobinuria, suggest that, in human adults, the B lineage may be more closely related to myeloid developmental programs than to T-lymphoid pathways.[21–24] Analysis of mitochondrial DNA sequence patterns in individual T, B, and myeloid cells has directly confirmed the common lineage of at least some of these cells in humans.[25]

TISSUE CULTURE ASSAYS OF HEMATOPOIETIC STEM CELLS

Protection from lethal irradiation through the establishment of multilineage hematopoiesis remains the standard for defining and quantifying HSCs. In vitro assays that would allow more rapid and practical assessment of hematopoietic function have long been sought for human HSCs because of the obvious barriers to experimental repopulation studies in humans. Over time, most of the available tests have been found to measure progenitor cells that are already committed to a particular lineage, as opposed to true HSCs; nevertheless, in many situations these assays are valuable surrogates for global hematopoietic function, have contributed immeasurably to the study of lineage-specific pathways of hematopoietic differentiation, and allowed purification and identification of hematopoietic cytokines (Fig. 1–2).

Initial attempts to culture marrow in vitro were hampered by lack of knowledge of the factors required to maintain or stimulate primitive hematopoietic cells, and the rarity of cells with proliferative potential and multipotency within an enormous number of differentiating or fully mature cells. Rapid progress was made when functional assays for primitive cells via culture in semisolid media were developed by Bradley and Metcalf as well as Pluznik and Sachs in the mid-1960s.[26–28] Individual primitive cells with proliferative potential (colony-forming units [CFU]) are defined by their ability to produce a clonal colony of 50 to several thousand mature or maturing hematopoietic cells in agar or methylcellulose after 7–14 days in culture (see Fig. 1–2). Progenitors furthest along the differentiation pathway form colonies

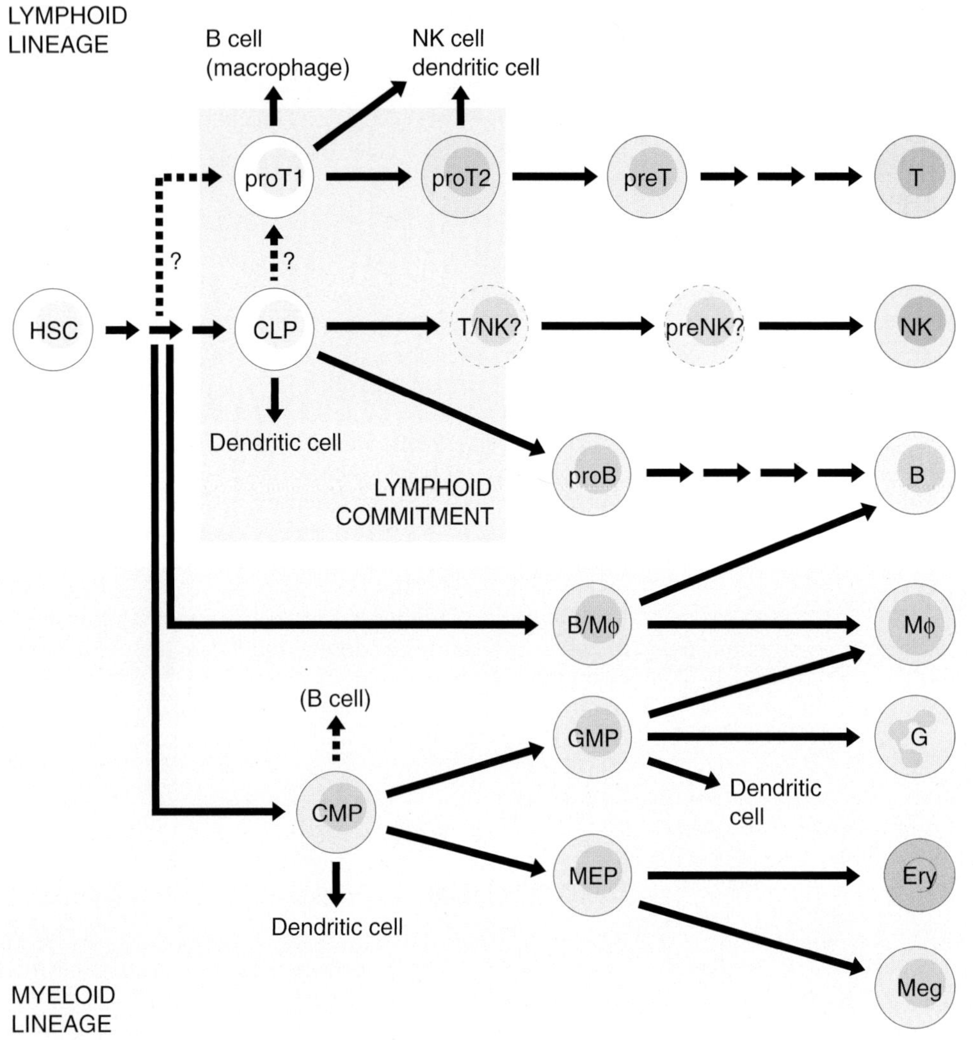

Figure 1–1. Hematopoietic lineage hierarchies. Schematic showing current concepts regarding the pathways of hematopoiesis in adult mice. Differentiation from the most primitive hematopoietic stem cell (HSC) through the common lymphoid progenitor (CLP) and common myeloid progenitor (CMP) to more lineage-restricted progeny cells and end-stage blood elements is shown. Abbreviations: B, B cell; Ery, erythroid; G, granulocyte; GMP, granulocyte-macrophage progenitor; Mϕ, macrophage; Meg, megakaryocytic; MEP, megakaryocytic-erythroid progenitor; NK, natural killer cell; PreNK, pre-natural killer cell; proB, pro-B cell; T, T cell. (Based on concepts from Kondo M, Wager AJ, Manz MZ, et al: Biology of hematopoietic stem cells and progenitors: implications for clinical application. Annu Rev Immunol 21:759–806, 2003.)

most rapidly (colony-forming units–erythroid [CFU-E]), whereas less mature progenitors form colonies more slowly, but these colonies are usually much larger and more complex in their cellular constitution (burst-forming units–erythroid [BFU-E] or multipotent colony-forming units such as CFU-mix). The inclusion in the culture media of hematopoietic cytokines able to support the survival and proliferation of progenitors of different lineages results in an array of uni- and multilineage colonies: BFU-E and CFU-E with erythropoietin, granulocyte and macrophage progenitors (CFU-GM, CFU-G, and CFU-M) with granulocyte-macrophage colony-stimulating factor (GM-CSF) or interleukin-3, and multilineage colonies (CFU-GEMM) with interleukin-3[29,30] (Fig. 1–3). Mapping of the cellular components and cytokine responsiveness of different colony types delineates hematopoietic differentiation pathways and contributes to our current understanding of lineage hierarchies.

Despite extraordinary insights into hematopoiesis from in vitro progenitor assays, it became clear by the 1980s that all types of CFU, even those containing multiple lineages, were already irreversibly differentiated and many steps removed from true repopulating HSCs. Most CFU are not self-renewing, and cells of lymphoid lineages, particularly T cells, are not detected in these colonies. Cell separation based on size, density, and surface characteristics or genetic marking studies placed CFU into different fractions than cells with in vivo repopulating activity.[31–33]

Thus attempts to re-create the marrow microenvironment in a culture dish were pursued, based upon the hypothesis that cellular and matrix components could help support the viability, proliferation, and multilineage differentiation of HSCs. As first described by Dexter, stromal elements (including macrophages, fibroblasts, and adipocytes) were allowed to develop as an adherent layer, with mononuclear cells adhering and producing maturing hematopoietic cells and CFU for 5 or more weeks[34,35] (see Fig. 1–2). Cells able to rescue irradiated mice were retained in these cultures, consistent with the presence of true HSCs. By shifting culture media and splitting the contents of wells after initial culture, Whitlock and Witte discovered a precursor able to produce both myeloid and lymphoid B cells in vitro, but none of various long-term cultures generated T cells.[36]

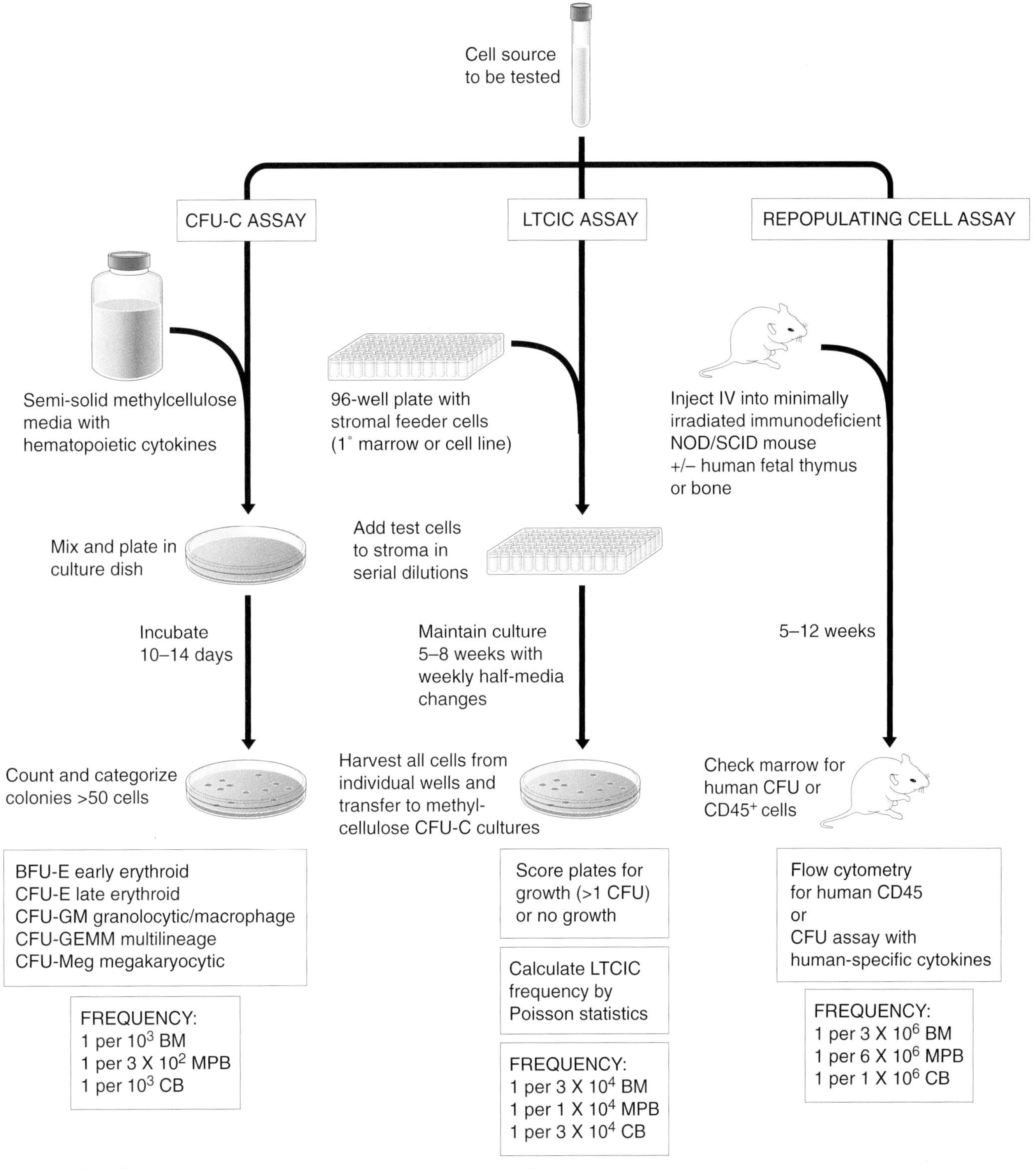

Figure 1–2. Assay systems for hematopoietic stem and progenitor cells.

Enumeration of the number of primitive cells able to support multilineage hematopoiesis became possible by limiting dilution plating of a test population of cells on preformed stroma in multiwell plates, followed by transfer of contents of each well to methylcellulose culture after at least 5 weeks to assess for cells able to produce CFU after prolonged culture (see Fig. 1–2). Application of Poisson statistics allows estimation of the frequency of "long-term culture initiating cells" (LTCIC) in the original plated cell population, even if the output of CFU per LTCIC is not homogeneous.[37] LTCIC assays are laborious and technically demanding, but because these cells are multipotent and able to self-renew, for a decade they were the standard assay for putative human HSCs. However, the LTCIC was eventually discredited as a true 1:1 representative of an HSC as phenotypic and func-

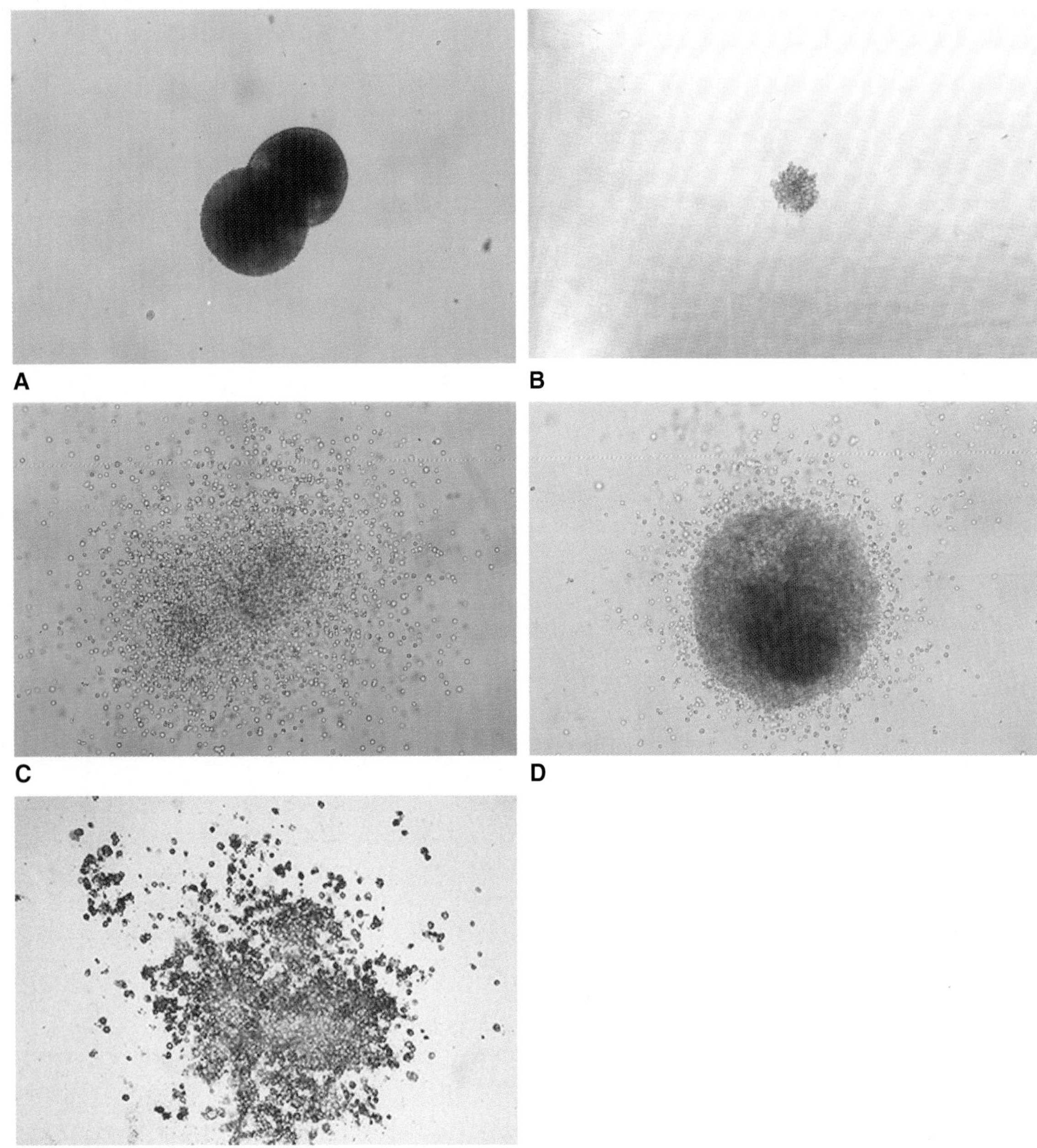

■ **Figure 1–3.** Hematopoietic-progenitor derived colony-formation. Depicted in five panels are the clonogenic output of murine hematopoietic cells plated in semisolid media. Each colony represents the result of proliferation of a single cell 7–14 days following plating in semisolid methylcellulose media plus hematopoietic cytokines. ***A,*** BFU-E (burst-forming unit–erythroid), an early erythroid progenitor. ***B,*** CFU-E (colony-forming unit–erythroid), a later erythroid progenitor. ***C,*** CFU-GM (colony-forming unit–granulocyte/macrophage), a myeloid progenitor. ***D,*** CFU-GEMM (colony-forming unit–granulocyte, erythroid, monocyte, macrophage), a multilineage progenitor. ***E,*** CFU-Meg (colony-forming unit–megakaryocyte), a megakaryocyte progenitor. (Courtesy of StemCell Technologies, Vancouver, BC, Canada.)

tional assays demonstrated that LTCIC and HSC were contained in different physically separate fractions.[38,39]

STEM CELL ASSAYS: THE REPOPULATING CELL

In parallel with the development of more sophisticated tissue culture assays for primitive cells, transplantation of human hematopoietic cells into immunodeficient mice was also employed as a potential surrogate human hematopoietic stem cell assay[40] (see Fig. 1–2). Initially, engraftment in these animal systems was inefficient and transient, but injection of mice with human cytokines and the use of progressively more immunodeficient strains ultimately allowed measurable levels of human hematopoietic engraftment.[41–43] Quantitation of human SCID-repopulating cell (SRC) activity in these assays is possible by calculation of the percentage of human cell engraftment in the marrow, by Southern blotting for human repetitive DNA sequences, or by flow cytometry for cells expressing human CD45, a pan-hematopoietic antigen. Actual assessment of the frequency of engrafting cells requires limiting dilution analysis in cohorts of animals transplanted with varying human cell doses.[44] Human cells with SRC capabilities can be separated from those forming CFU or LTCIC by cell surface phenotype and dye exclusion characteristics, as well as by genetic marking strategies using retroviral vectors.[45] The frequencies of SRCs in cord blood, bone marrow, and mobilized peripheral blood are within the range of HSC frequency estimated using other approaches, such as phenotypic analysis or genetic marking.

However, there are qualifications to the simple equation of SRCs to human long-term repopulating HSCs. Most immunodeficient mouse strains have a limited lifespan due to development of lymphoma, and therefore repopulating activity can be assessed for only 5–8 weeks after transplantation. Genetic marking studies indicate distinct populations of early versus late repopulating cells, and the SRC activity usually assayed likely represents only a short-term repopulating cell.[46] As an alternative, transplantation of human cells into other xenogeneic models has been employed to enumerate human HSCs. In experiments with preimmune second-trimester fetal sheep, lambs had low levels of human hematopoietic cells detectable in the marrow and blood over the long term.[47,48] The nonhuman primate model represents an ideal system to study hematopoietic stem cell behavior because stem cell characteristics and frequency are very similar between monkeys and humans.[49,50] Tracking the behavior of hematopoietic cells in these large animal models requires genetic marking, for instance with retroviral vectors, because allogeneic transplantation is difficult as a result of incomplete knowledge of the major histocompatibility complex in monkeys and lack of inbred strains.[51]

CELL SURFACE AND PHYSICAL CHARACTERISTICS OF PRIMITIVE HEMATOPOIETIC CELLS

The physical properties and the cell surface characteristics of HSCs and their progeny have been intensely studied in both murine and human systems, allowing purification of HSCs to near homogeneity in the mouse as dramatically demonstrated by single-cell reconstitution of hematopoiesis.[52,53] In humans, purification strategies utilize monoclonal antibodies for positive selection of stem and progenitor cells, and/or depletion of maturing cells, resulting in "designer" grafts for allogeneic or autologous transplantation, retaining hematopoietic function but with removal of elements such as mature T cells or tumor cells.

Morphologically, primitive hematopoietic cells are similar to small but immature-appearing lymphocytes. Density-gradient centrifugation, generally the first step in purification, removes mature granulocytes and red blood cells. Counterflow elutriation can further separate the smaller and more dense primitive cells from maturing lineage-committed elements.[54] Purified murine HSCs have been defined by studies based on (1) depletion of cells expressing lineage-specific cell surface markers found on T, B, monocytic, granulocytic, and erythroid lineage cells ("lin-"); and (2) positive selection by multiparameter flow-cytometric sorting for antigens found on the surface of HSCs but not their more mature progeny, including c-Kit (the stem cell factor [SCF] receptor), Sca-1, and Thy-1.[55,56]

Similar approaches have been pursued for human cells, but their antigenic profiles are not identical to those of the mouse HSC. The first cell surface marker found to be highly enriched in human progenitor cell populations was CD34. Antibodies against CD34 were initially produced using primitive human leukemic blasts as immunogens, and the 1–3% of marrow cells positive for this antigen contained all CFU and repopulating cells (tested in baboons).[57,58] Because $CD34^+$ cells include CFU and LTCIC along with repopulating HSCs, $CD34^+$ cells were further separated into more primitive subgroups using negative selection of cells expressing HLA-DR or CD38. $CD34^+/CD38^-$ cells represent less than 0.01% of marrow mononuclear cells but contain all NOD/SCID repopulating activity—but even this population is not homogeneous[39] (Fig. 1–4*A*).

In mice, a significant fraction of adult HSCs do not express CD34, but HSCs from young mice, or HSCs present following mobilization into the peripheral blood or recovery from stress such as chemotherapy, acquire CD34 positivity.[59–62] In nonhuman primates and humans, there is no evidence that significant numbers of HSCs lack CD34 expression, particularly in mobilized peripheral blood stem cell (PBSC) grafts.[58,63] Further refinement of the characterization of human lineage relationships has been challenging because of lack of robust assays for lymphoid development. All bipotent lymphoid and myeloid progenitors are $CD34^+/CD38^-$.[64,65] To date, the best candidate for human CLP cells from human bone marrow are $lin^-/CD34^+/CD38^+/CD10^+$ cells. This fraction generates no myeloid progeny but can clonally produce B, natural killer, and dendritic cells, and can reconstitute fetal thymus with human T cells.[66]

Functional Characteristics of Hematopoietic Stem and Progenitor Cells

HSCs, in contrast to committed progenitor cells, have the property of effluxing chemotherapeutic agents and vital dyes such as rhodamine via the *MDR1* gene product P-glycoprotein or other ATP-binding cassette (ABC) proteins,[67,68] and this activity may serve an important protective role for HSCs.[69] The exclusion of Hoechst 33342 dye by a very small fraction of cells termed *side population* or "SP" cells has been used to further purify murine and now human HSCs (Fig. 1–4*B*).[70,71] SP cells engraft at very high efficiency, with the majority of lethally irradiated mice rescued by a single infused SP cell.[72] SP cells characterized by Hoechst exclusion are also found in other tissues, and they may serve as a defining characteristic of cells with extensive self-renewal potential.[73]

The quiescence of the primitive hematopoietic cells has been exploited for purification, using cytokine stim-

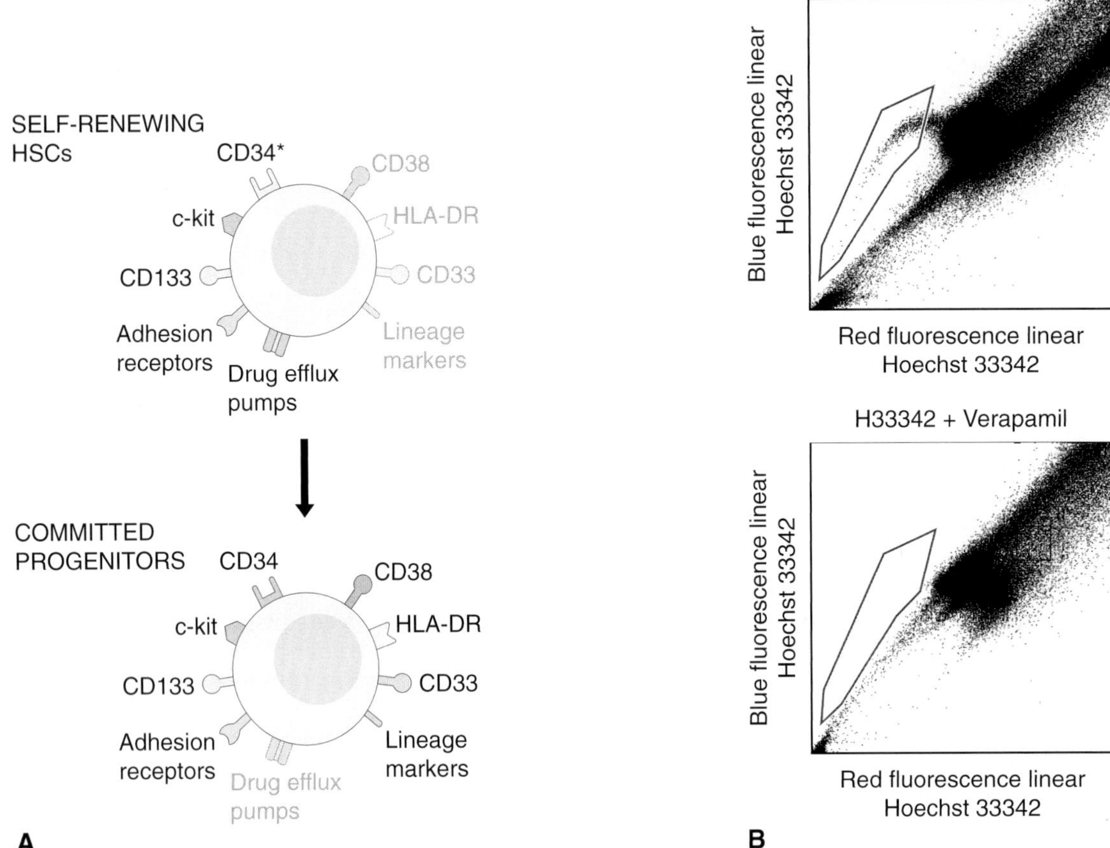

Figure 1–4. Phenotype of hematopoietic stem and progenitor cells. ***A***, Summary of the cell surface antigen profiles used to delineate human committed progenitor cells from more primitive long-term repopulating cells. ***B***, Example of staining for "side population" (SP) cells. After staining with the dye Hoechst 33342, a distinct "tail" of dull-staining cells is seen via flow-cytometric excitation with two different wavelengths of light. The cells that most efficiently efflux the dye via a membrane pump appear as a tail (gated population) in the *left panel*, with the tip of the tail representing the most primitive fraction. Efflux can be blocked by verapamil *(right panel)*, with disappearance of the population via blocking the drug efflux pump. SP cells are highly enriched for long-term repopulating ability when sorted from the bone marrow.

ulation followed by in vitro killing of responding cells, and resulting in a highly enriched HSC population.[74] The membrane intercalating dye CSFE can be used to stain marrow cells enriched for HSCs, and HSCs able to reconstitute a second mouse can be isolated from a primary transplanted mouse based on homing to the marrow and lack of cell division, as defined by retention of CFSE staining.[75,76] However, in vivo there is evidence that HSCs will eventually all cycle: after feeding mice the DNA intercalating agent BrdU, virtually all phenotypically defined HSCs were labeled within about 30 days, with 8% of HSCs cycling each day.[77] Primitive baboon cells cycle less frequently.[78]

The ends of chromosomes are capped by telomeres, consisting of hundreds to thousands of repeats of a guanine-rich sequence. Because of the incomplete replication of the lagging strand during DNA replication, telomeres shorten with each cell division, and in somatic tissues the length of human telomeres can be shown to decrease over time.[79–81] A complex of ribonucleoproteins termed *telomerase* is active in germline cells and is able to maintain telomere length despite cell division. Low-level telomerase activity can be detected in purified HSCs, as well as in some differentiated cells with high proliferative potential such as lymphocytes.[82,83] The constitutional bone marrow failure syndrome, dyskeratosis congenita is caused by mutations in genes that are part of the telomerase complex,[84–86] and patients with late-onset, apparently acquired aplastic anemia have recently been found also to have mutations in telomerase component genes.[86,87] Telomerase activity must be important for HSC self-renewal and lifelong effective hematopoiesis. Telomeres in both peripheral blood granulocytes and lymphocytes shorten with aging, most rapidly during early childhood, followed by slower loss throughout adulthood until more rapid loss in old age.[88] Allogeneic transplant recipients' donor hematopoietic cells have shorter telomeres than do the same hematopoietic cells in the original donors, suggesting that rapid expansion from a limited starting HSC dose to reconstitute hematopoiesis results in accelerated telomere loss despite some level of telomerase activity in primitive cells.[89,90]

Measurements of telomere loss have been used to estimate the replicative history of primitive hematopoietic cells.[91] Telomere shortening may eventually limit HSC self-renewal and contribute to loss of serial transplantation ability in murine models.[92]

FREQUENCY, BEHAVIOR, AND LIFESPAN OF HSCs

The "semi"-random and stable integration of replication-incompetent retroviral vectors into chromosomes of HSCs allows direct tracking of the activity of individual stem cells by identification of proviral integration sites.[93] Early retroviral tagging studies in the mouse demonstrated that a single hematopoietic stem cell could, remarkably, repopulate all hematopoietic lineages over the long term and even contribute to hematopoiesis in secondary and tertiary transplants, directly proving both self-renewal and differentiation of individual primitive cells.[93–96] Marking studies also allowed estimation of HSC frequency in murine bone marrow, by combination with limiting dilution analysis of congenic cells in transplantation models. The frequency of murine stem cells is 1 to 8 HSCs per 10^5 nucleated marrow cells.[97,98] With a marrow cellularity per mouse of approximately 10^8 nucleated marrow cells, the total number of HSCs per mouse is 10,000–20,000.[99]

Quantification and characterization of HSCs in larger animals and humans have been more challenging. Using random inactivation of polymorphic X chromosome genes during early embryonic development as a tool, HSC numbers in cats heterozygous for glucose-6-phosphate dehydrogenase protein variants could be tracked as the output of cells expressing each allele following transplantation of limiting cell numbers; computer modeling suggested that HSCs were 100-fold less frequent in cats than in rodents, with only 6 HSCs per 10^7 marrow cells, despite the animals' much greater hematopoietic demand.[100,101] Additionally, a model of polyclonal hematopoiesis in which clones contribute randomly fit the experimental data, supporting a stochastic model of hematopoiesis. These results agreed with observations in humans heterozygous for X-chromosome alleles, and in transplant recipients engrafted with marrow from heterozygous donors.[102,103] Genetic marking studies in rhesus macaques allowed more direct quantification and characterization of individual stem or progenitor cells. Many marked clones contributed to the various lineages at each time point assayed, and extrapolation to the number of cells transplanted resulted in an estimate of 5 long-term repopulating cells per 10^7 mobilized peripheral blood mononuclear cells.[104–106] These frequency estimates are considerably lower than those derived from LTCIC or even SCID-repopulating assays, further evidence that these latter methods may not accurately assay true HSC activity.

Initial genetic marking and polymorphism studies in mice and cats produced a model of sequential stem cell activation and exhaustion, with support of hematopoiesis over time by activity from waves of previously quiescent HSCs.[100,107] However, longer term analysis and the use of more modern marking techniques instead suggested that, following the initial several months of engraftment derived from short-term repopulating cells, long-term repopulation is stably derived from continuously but slowly cycling HSCs.[100,108] Even prolonged cytokine stimulation in rhesus macaques did not "exhaust" individual clonal contributions.[109]

HEMATOPOIETIC CYTOKINES

Hematopoietic cytokines comprise an increasing number of glycoprotein hormones that exist in soluble and/or membrane bound forms and act individually or in concert to exert their influence on survival, proliferation, and differentiation of hematopoietic stem and progenitor cells. The advent of molecular cloning techniques has allowed the continual discovery of such cytokines, along with their large-scale production and the elucidation of their effects in vitro and in vivo. Additional insights have been gained by the development of mice with targeted disruptions of the various cytokine genes and observations from clinical studies of recombinant human cytokines. Hematopoietic cytokines possess some degree of lineage specificity, yet they often have overlapping biologic activity, and can act synergistically with other cytokines. Hematopoietic cytokines also share structural features and signaling mechanisms. A partial list of the well-characterized hematopoietic cytokines as well as their known effects is given in Table 1–1. The receptors for hematopoietic growth factors belong to a group of cytokine receptor superfamilies divided into six types based upon unique features of each group (Fig. 1–5). The class I receptors constitute the receptor superfamily responsible for the majority of the hematopoietic growth factors, including most of the interleukins, granulocyte colony-stimulating factor (G-CSF), GM-CSF, erythropoietin, and thrombopoietin.

Many cytokines are produced at relatively low levels by marrow microenvironmental cells (see later) or by developing hematopoietic cells themselves, and they thus can exert their effects in a paracrine or autocrine fashion, respectively. One such example is SCF, which is produced by bone marrow stromal cells and which, acting through its receptor c-Kit, is important for survival of hematopoietic stem and progenitor cells. SCF, which exists in both a soluble and membrane-bound form, and its receptor were identified in part through elegant studies in natural mutant anemic strains, Steel and W/W^v mice, deficient in function of the ligand SCF and the receptor c-Kit, respectively.[110–112] Additionally, neutralizing antibodies to c-Kit produce rapid and severe depletion of bone marrow progenitors.[113] Other cytokines are produced by distant organs and act in an endocrine fashion, such as erythropoietin,[114] which in response to hypoxia is produced within the kidney to drive increased production of red blood cells in the circulation. Thrombopoietin,[115,116] which is synthesized predominantly by the liver and is regulated by megakaryocyte mass,[117] drives the production of platelets. Despite its importance in platelet production, thrombopoietin, like many other cytokines, is not essential for survival, because mice deficient in thrombopoietin or its receptor

TABLE 1–1. Hematopoietic Cytokines

Cytokine	Site(s) of Production	Predominant Action(s)	Deficiency State
Erythropoietin	Kidney	Erythropoiesis	Anemia
Thrombopoietin	Liver	Megakaryocytopoiesis	Thrombocytopenia
Interleukin (IL)-11	Stromal cells	Megakaryocytopoiesis and erythropoiesis; acts in synergy with multiple other cytokines	None known
Granulocyte colony-stimulating factor (G-CSF)	Endothelial cells, monocytes, macrophages	Myelopoiesis; granulocyte differentiation	Neutropenia
Granulocyte-macrophage colony-stimulating factor (GM-CSF)	Endothelial cells, T cells, mast cells	Myelopoiesis; eosinophil differentiation	Infection diathesis with intracellular organisms
Stem cell factor (SCF)	Stromal cells, endothelial cells, fibroblasts	Proliferation and differentiation of primitive hematopoietic stem cells (HSCs); mast cell differentiation	Anemia and reduced stem cell content
Fetal liver tissue (FLT)-3 ligand	Stromal cells, spleen, and widely	Early hematopoiesis; synergizes with other cytokines	Decreased pre- and pro-B cells
IL-1 (two forms, α and β)	Most tissues	Pyrogenic factor; inflammatory response mediator through induction of multiple other cytokines	IL-1β demonstrates impaired febrile responses
Tumor necrosis factor (TNF)-α	B cells, natural killer (NK) cells, macrophages	Inflammatory response mediator through induction of multiple other cytokines	Lack of splenic primary B-cell follicles, follicular dendritic cell (FDC) networks, germinal centers
IL-6	Endothelial cell, T cells, macrophages	Early hematopoiesis; synergizes with other cytokines; dampens inflammation; autocrine and paracrine factor in multiple myeloma	Impaired immune and acute-phase reactions
IL-3	T cells, mast cells	Proliferation and differentiation of primitive HSCs	None known
IL-7	Stromal cells, spleen, thymus	Lymphopoiesis	Lymphopenia
IL-2	T cells	T-cell proliferation and function	Immunoproliferative syndrome
IL-15	Monocytes, macrophages, stromal cells	T-cell proliferation and function, overlap with IL-2	Absent $V\gamma 3^{+}$ fetal thymic and dendritic epidermal T cells
IL-4	T cells	B-cell proliferation	Impaired mucosal immunity
IL-10	T cells, activated B cells	Inhibition of T_H1 cytokines with resulting immune suppression	Lethal immune responses to infection, autoimmune bowel disease
IL-12	Mononuclear phagocytes	Differentiation of naive helper T cells to T_H1 cells; stimulation of proliferation and activity of NK cells	Defective type 1 cytokine responses

still produce platelets, albeit at markedly reduced levels.[118,119]

G-CSF stimulates the proliferation of neutrophil precursors, activates neutrophils, and, with prolonged supraphysiologic dosing, mobilizes hematopoietic stem and progenitor cells into the circulation. G-CSF exemplifies the clinical utility of recombinant hematopoietic growth factors, with widespread application in congenital marrow failure syndromes,[120,121] chemotherapy-induced neutropenia,[122] and HSC mobilization,[123] and, in combination with other cytokines, in the treatment of myelodysplastic syndrome.[124]

The interleukins represent an expanding list of hematopoietic cytokines that are principally active in lymphopoiesis.[125] The overlapping and synergistic effects of hematopoietic cytokines are exemplified by dependence upon both SCF and interleukin (IL)-7 for T-cell development, thymic stromal lymphopoietin and IL-7 for B-cell development, and IL-15 and fetal-liver kinase 2 ligand for natural killer cell development, among others. Many of the interleukins, however, also exert effects outside of the lymphoid lineage. IL-3, encoded in close proximity to the GM-CSF gene on chromosome 5q (where a number of such factors are clustered),[126] is produced predominantly by lymphocytes and acts on cells such as hematopoietic progenitors, mature neutrophils, and megakaryocytes. Hematopoietic cytokines can also influence cell fate conversion, with redirection of a lymphoid progenitor to the myeloid lineage through the actions of exogenous IL-2 and GM-CSF.[127] Recently, hematopoietic cytokines have been discovered to have effects outside of the hematopoietic compartment, an example being the actions of erythropoietin on both skeletal and cardiac muscle.[128–130]

REGULATION OF HEMATOPOIESIS

The choice between self-renewal, in which one or both daughter cells retains the properties of the parent HSC,

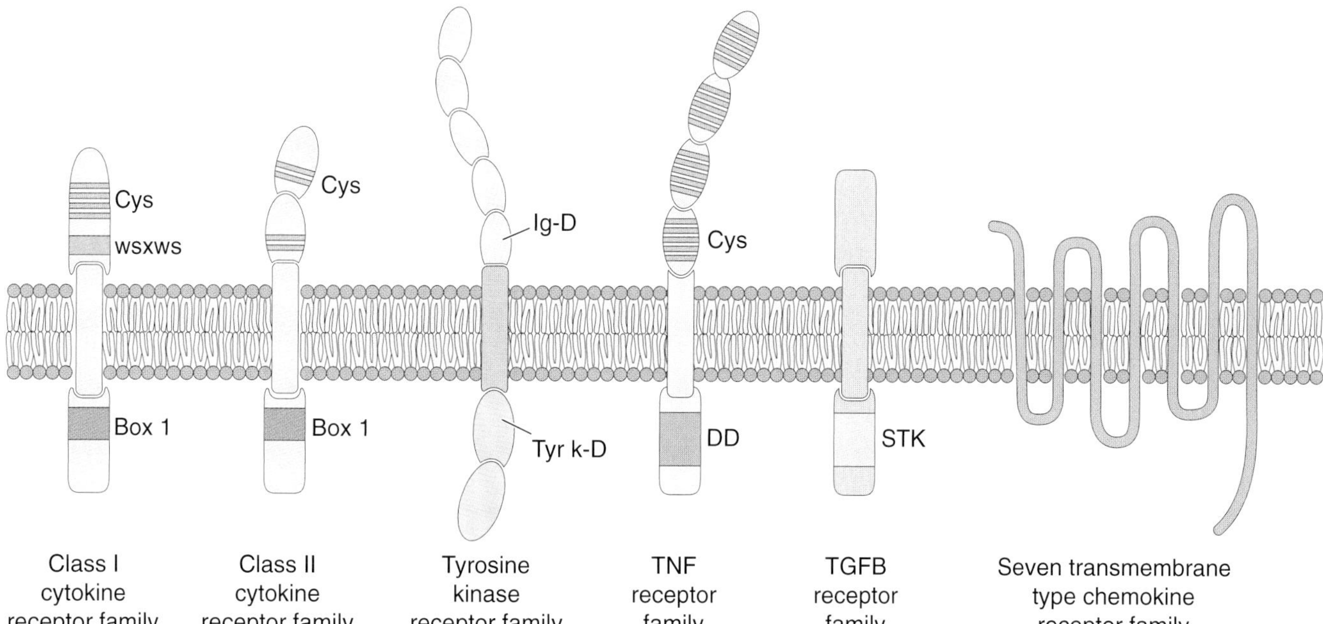

Figure 1–5. The six families of cytokine receptors. The majority of hematopoietic growth factors utilize *class I cytokine receptors.* These receptors are characterized by four cysteine (Cys) residues in the extracellular domain, a WSXWS sequence in the ligand- binding domain, and the presence of an extracellular fibronectin-type domain. A conserved motif known as Box1 is present in the cytoplasmic domain. Class I cytokine receptors constitute the receptors for the majority of interleukins and colony-stimulating factors. *Class II cytokine receptors* share many features of the class 1 cytokine receptors, including the Cys residues and the Box1 motif. The *tyrosine kinase receptor family* of receptors possesses large extracellular domains with immunoglobulin-like domains (Ig-D), but possess neither Cys residues nor WSXWS motifs. The cytoplasmic domain possesses at least one tyrosine kinase domain (TyrK-D). This class includes receptors for SCF, Flt-3 ligand, and platelet-derived growth factor (PDGF). The *tumor necrosis factor (TNF) receptor family* is rich with Cys residues in the extracellular domain along with a cytoplasmic portion containing a death domain (DD). These receptors transduce signals that can induce programmed cell death. The *transforming growth factor-β (TGF-β) receptor family* is characterized by the presence of a serine-threonine kinase cytoplasmic domain. The *chemokine receptors* are G protein–linked receptors that are seven-transmembrane-spanning–type receptors predominantly involved in chemotaxis.

versus differentiation, in which the daughter cell or cells lose capacity to self-renew and become irreversibly committed down a differentiation pathway, controls hematopoietic homeostasis. Understanding how fate decisions are controlled is central to manipulation of normal hematopoietic cells for clinical applications such as expansion of HSCs ex vivo for transplantation or genetic manipulation. Abnormal fate decisions likely underlie leukemogenesis and other abnormalities of hematopoiesis.[131,132] The two major models have been characterized as "instructive" and "stochastic"[133]: the central question is whether self-renewal versus commitment is controlled intrinsically by a property of the HSC itself (stochastic), or whether external cues such as hematopoietic cytokine signaling can directly influence HSC cell fate decisions (instructive). In the stochastic model, HSCs are proposed to randomly commit to differentiate or self-renew, with cytokines present in the microenvironment functioning only to allow survival and proliferation of lineage-committed cells, a "permissive" role. In the strict instructive model, cytokines actually influence cell fate decisions.

Early HSC events appear to be primarily stochastic, with coexpression of a number of transcription factors in individual cells that eventually influence lineage decisions; the ratio of the levels of these transcription factors to each other eventually results in direction of the daughter cells into a lineage pathway.[134,135] "Basal" HSC self-renewal and initial differentiation would then permit rapid expansion of any particular lineage with exposure of these cells moving down one pathway to lineage-specific cytokines, without loss of the potential to produce cells of other lineages. Pathways central to these early events include HOXB4, Wnt, Notch, and Sonic hedgehog.[136–139]

THE HEMATOPOIETIC ENVIRONMENT

Both the enormous productive capacity of the hematopoietic compartment and the precise regulation of blood cell production are dependent on complex three-dimensional relationships among (1) hematopoietic stem and progenitor cells and their progeny, (2) the non-hematopoietic cellular components of the environment, and (3) the noncellular matrix molecules and their complex supportive structures. Normal hematopoietic activity beyond the neonatal stage in humans occurs exclusively in the highly vascular central marrow cavities of bones, or "red pulp." The cavity is surrounded by dense compact bone and partitioned by fine bony trabeculae into millions of chambers.[140] Bony surfaces are covered by a cellular layer known as the endosteum, composed of osteoblasts and osteoclasts able to form new bone or reabsorb existing bone, respectively.

The marrow cavity receives oxygenated blood from nutrient arteries, which penetrate the midshaft and epiphyses of long bones and bifurcate repeatedly. The vascular network terminates in an array of thin-walled vascular sinuses with diameters of 50–75 μm. These simple tubes consisting of endothelial cells have the unique characteristic of lacking a basement membrane, and they are instead structurally supported by contact with surrounding but discontinuous stromal cells. Thus the "marrow-blood" barrier consists only of the monolayer of specialized endothelial cells that allows passage of newly matured blood cells through transient fenestrations in their cytoplasm into the circulation.[141] Despite accounting for a significant percentage of cardiac output, the marrow hematopoietic space is a relatively hypoxic environment, and primitive hematopoietic cells are damaged by higher oxygen tension.[142–144]

Specialized microenvironments within the marrow have critical roles in the control of hematopoiesis. Cells of nonhematopoietic origin, including adipocytes, mesenchymal stromal or smooth muscle cells, endothelial cells, and osteoblasts, all intimately contact hematopoietic precursor cells, secrete cytokines with hematopoietic activities, and express cell surface molecules that can bind receptors on HSCs and progenitors. Osteoclasts, macrophages, and T lymphocytes are present at high numbers in the marrow space, and they affect hematopoiesis locally through cytokine production and by phagocytosis of apoptotic cells. Matrix components such as fibronectin, elastin, collagen, and laminin support the three-dimensional structure of the compartment, bind and concentrate cytokines for localized presentation to target cells, and directly attach to signaling receptors on hematopoietic cells.[145–147] The cell surface presentation of certain cytokines, such as SCF, provides required signals distinct from those stimulated by soluble forms of the same cytokines, as demonstrated by the phenotype of Steel-Dickie mutant mice, which are severely anemic[148]: a mutation in the *SCF* gene results in normal production of the secreted form of SCF but no cell surface expression of SCF by marrow stromal cells.

Figure 1–6 diagrams the interactions between primitive hematopoietic cells and the cellular and matrix components central to the localization and retention of primitive cells in the marrow. Within the marrow compartment, the most primitive cells are localized along the endosteal surface, with a gradient of differentiation moving toward the central axis of the marrow cavity.[149,150] Recent elegant experiments prove that osteoblasts are central to the control of HSCs self-renewal, via the production of the protein Jagged 1, which binds to and activates the receptor Notch present on HSCs.[130]

STEM CELL MOBILIZATION AND HOMING

The ability of cells to exit one hematopoietic tissue and to relocate in another, acquired early in embryonic development, is retained by HSCs in neonatal and adult life, and has been harnessed clinically for applications in transplantation. The initial clue that HSCs reside at least transiently in the circulation was reported in 1945, when bovine fraternal twins sharing a common placenta and thus blood supply were found to have chimeric bone marrow and circulating lymphohematopoietic cells after birth.[151] Migration of HSCs from the spleen to the marrow was proven by the survival of mice following ablative total-body irradiation if the spleen was shielded.[152] The creation of parabionts by linking the circulations of two animals most conclusively demonstrated HSCs in adult peripheral blood; lethal irradiation of one animal resulted in reconstitution of the marrow of that animal from its parabiont partner, facilitating survival even after severing of the vascular link.[153]

The concentration of HSCs in steady-state blood is very low, only 10–30 in the total blood volume of an adult mouse, as compared to 2600 HSC in the bone marrow; therefore, the peripheral blood contains only 0.01% of total murine HSCs.[154] The role of circulating HSCs in hematopoietic homeostasis, if any, is unclear. The surprisingly high rate of cell division of HSCs, coupled with results from parabiosis experiments show only very slow and incomplete mixing of marrow HSC populations, has suggested that egress from the marrow into blood may normally constitute a death pathway for unneeded HSCs.[155,156]

The first observation regarding circulation of primitive hematopoietic cells in humans was in 1971, when low concentrations of committed progenitors (CFU) were measured in the peripheral blood.[157] Patients with chronic myelogenous leukemia were found to have a greatly increased concentration of circulating CFU, and cryopreserved blood buffy coat cells from patients in chronic-phase chronic myelogenous leukemia could even rescue hematopoiesis following ablative chemoradiotherapy.[158] As autologous marrow transplantation was developed to allow dose intensification in the treatment of malignancies, difficulties in harvesting an adequate bone marrow graft in patients with marrow fibrosis led to investigations of blood as an actual source for autologous stem cells. Infusion of large numbers of apheresis collections supported hematopoietic recovery of lymphoma and leukemia patients following high-dose chemotherapy.[159–161] An early concern was that the circulation did not contain sufficient numbers of HSCs or true HSCs able to sustain long-term engraftment, because some patients transplanted only with blood cells had poor trilineage recovery or late pancytopenias; however, most poor-mobilizing patients had been heavily pretreated with chemotherapy and likely had sustained permanent marrow and HSC damage.[160] Proof of long-term engraftment from infused PBSCs was established first by retroviral genetic marking studies using autologous PBSCs and then by successful allogeneic transplants.[162,163]

The concentration of CFU in the blood increases markedly during recovery from myelosuppressive chemotherapy, peaking during the early hematopoietic recovery phase.[164] Collection of PBSCs following cytotoxic drug administration, in particular after moderate-

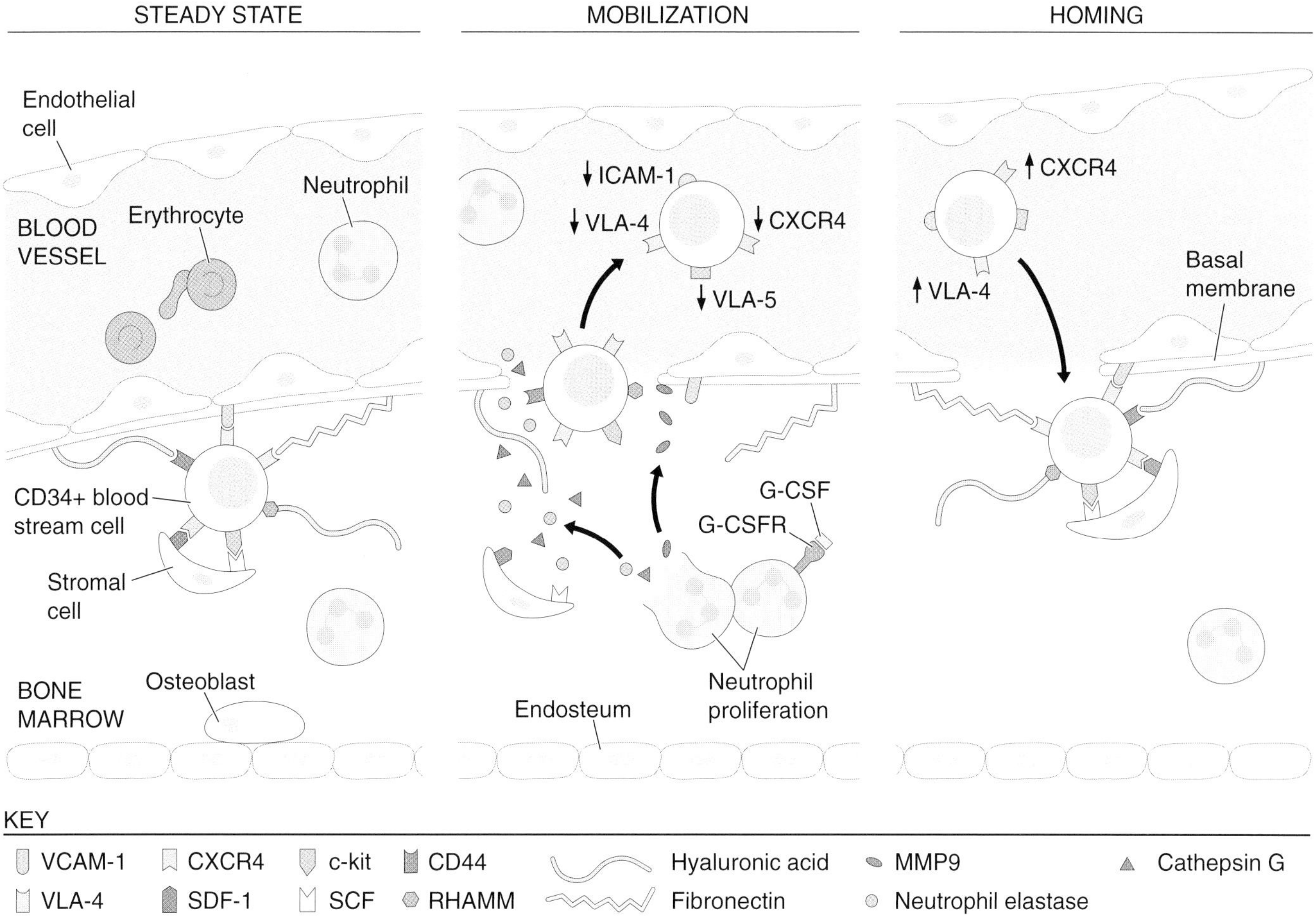

Figure 1–6. Hematopoietic stem cell (HSC) and progenitor cell (HPC) mobilization and homing. *Left,* The proposed steady-state interactions between key cell surface molecules present on HPCs/HSCs and both cellular and noncellular components of the bone marrow microenvironment. *Center,* Mobilization via release of HPCs/HSCs from the marrow microenvironment into the peripheral blood following G-CSF, with signaling via the G-CSF receptor on neutrophils resulting in release of proteases, which cleave the interactions between HPCs/HSCs and tethering molecules in the microenvironment. *Right,* The mirror image process of homing, with reengagement of cell surface molecules on HPCs/HSCs.

dose cyclophosphamide, was found to support hematopoietic recovery with many fewer apheresis collections than required for steady-state PBSCs. The administration of cytokines such as G-CSF or GM-CSF immediately following chemotherapy further increased the concentration of primitive cells in the blood.[164] Finally, when G-CSF clone was shown to induce the circulation of large numbers of progenitor cells, cytokine mobilization was introduced for the collection of PBSCs from normal volunteers and is the current preferential utilization of PBSCs as a stem cell source for almost all transplantation applications.[165–167]

Calculations from the murine model estimated that the entire marrow HSC pool could be transiently mobilized into the blood by cyclophosphamide treatment.[168] Proliferation of marrow HSCs precedes mobilization with cyclophosphamide or with G-CSF, but the primary pathway is not "overflow" of excess HSCs from the marrow but a shift of the cells out of the marrow into the peripheral blood, with a transient decrease in functional HSC marrow content.[169–171] Cells mobilized with G-CSF are more quiescent than are marrow progenitor and stem cells, with a higher fraction in the G_0 phase of the cell cycle, compared to steady-state bone marrow.[169,172]

Mobilization and homing are complementary processes: specific interactions between HSCs and the marrow environment must be disconnected for release into the blood, and these interactions must be reestablished in order to retain cells within marrow niches following transplantation. Many specific interactions between receptors on hematopoietic stem and progenitor cells and ligands within the niche microenvironment have now been identified (see Fig. 1–6); the relative importance of each component in this complex network of overlapping and redundant interactions remains unclear.

Very late antigen-4 (VLA-4), an integrin expressed on hematopoietic stem and progenitor cells, is central to the interaction of these cells with the marrow environment.[173] VLA-4 binds both cellular ligands, such as vascular cell adhesion molecule-1 (VCAM-1) on stromal and endothelial cells, and extracellular matrix components, most importantly fibronectin.[174,175] Administration of antibodies against either VLA-4 or VCAM-1 results in rapid mobilization of hematopoietic progenitors into the blood, consistent with a central role for VLA-4 in the marrow retention of primitive cells.[176,177] Blocking VLA-4 on the surface of hematopoietic cells prevents homing, and mice lacking VLA-4 and VLA-5 have abnormal migration of hematopoiesis during fetal development.[178,179] A second class of receptor-ligand interactions involves binding of CD44 and RHAMM, two receptors on primitive hematopoietic cells, to matrix glycosaminoglycans such as hyaluronic acid or to E-selectin, a cell surface protein found on marrow endothelial cells.[180,181] In a third important interaction, the receptor c-Kit binds to the transmembrane form of its ligand SCF presented by marrow stromal cells. There are complex relationships between the c-Kit/SCF receptor-ligand pair and other receptor-ligand interactions important in the processes of mobilization and homing.[177]

The most important interaction in mobilization and homing appears to be the binding of the chemokine receptor CXCR4 (the coreceptor for human immunodeficiency virus-1) on hematopoietic cells to its ligand, stromal-derived factor-1 (SDF-1).[182] SDF-1 is a potent chemoattractant for purified HSCs.[183–185] Blocking CXCR4 prevents homing, and local injection of SDF-1 attracts primitive hematopoietic cells to any tissue.[186,187] The small molecule AMD3100, a CXCR4 antagonist, can rapidly mobilize HSCs into the peripheral blood.[188,189]

The movement of primitive cells from the marrow into the blood has been studied in mice lacking the G-CSF receptor. Mobilization was impaired not only following G-CSF but also after infusion of cyclophosphamide and other agents.[190] Mice transplanted with a mixture of normal and G-CSF receptor-deficient HSCs mobilized both cell types with G-CSF, suggesting that the action of G-CSF was indirect.[191] Further experiments implicated the release of proteases from neutrophil granules, including elastase, cathepsin G, and matrix metalloproteases, with cleavage of ligands and/or receptors, such as VCAM-1, CXCR4, SDF-1, and SCF, with resultant release of HSCs from their tethers in the marrow niches.[192–195]

ADULT STEM CELLS AND TISSUE REGENERATION

As in the hematopoietic compartment, putative stem cells within a variety of adult tissues have now been identified by phenotype and function, opening new areas of investigation that may ultimately support the development of novel therapeutic strategies for disorders affecting these organs. Conventional dogma dictates that such stem cells are tissue-restricted, but the demonstration that the nucleus from a committed end-stage adult cell could direct embryogenesis in nuclear transfer models refuted the notion of irreversible commitment. Observations from other models also have challenged this paradigm.[196] Adult HSCs appeared to contribute differentiated daughter cells to a number of seemingly unrelated tissues and organs, including cardiac muscle,[197] skeletal muscle,[198] liver,[199,200] and the central nervous system,[201,202] particularly in the context of tissue injury and regeneration. The initial observations resulted in intense investigation and perhaps premature initiation of clinical testing in humans, particularly in acute and chronic myocardial ischemia.[203,204]

Focus on the potential of adult HSCs has resulted primarily in controversy. Many of the initial studies lacked sufficient rigor to substantiate a true change in stem cell fate, because of the transplantation of heterogenous cell populations rather than single cells, and generally very low levels of putative HSC-derived cells contributing to regeneration of other tissues, often at the limit of detection for the assay employed. In a landmark study, cultured muscle-derived cells (MDCs) contributed unambiguously to circulating blood cells, successfully competing with bone marrow cells.[73] Speculation that myogenic satellite cells were responsible for the hematopoietic reconstitution followed. Experiments in large animals failed to demonstrate a high-level contribution by MDCs toward hematopoiesis.[205] Subsequent observations in mice suggested that the hematopoietic potential of MDCs derives from hematopoietic stem cells residing within muscle.[206,207] Fusion between hematopoietic stem and progenitor cells and target organs also complicates interpretation of data: fusion proved to be the principal mechanism by which highly purified HSCs rescued $Fah^{-/-}$ mice, a model of hereditary tyrosinemia in which correction by HSC transplantation had previously represented the most rigorous demonstration of stem cell plasticity.[208,209] Some investigators have used sophisticated molecular techniques to exclude fusion as the source of apparent conversion events between hematopoietic cells and regenerating tissues such as pancreatic β cells and epithelial cells in the lung, liver, and skin.[210,211] Nevertheless, cell fusion accounts for at least some of the accounts of stem cell plasticity. Also possible is that completely uncommitted stem cells persisting in many tissues in the adult are responsible for regeneration under certain conditions; alternatively, tissue-committed stem cells may be distributed throughout all organs postnatally but available for organ-specific homing only in response to injury or cell death. Single-cell transplantation experiments resulting in regeneration of two diverse tissues from the same cell argue against this explanation, but retroviral insertion site analysis is the only unequivocal proof of clonal derivation of diverse cell populations.[212–215]

Marrow-Derived Mesenchymal Stem Cells or Multipotent Adult Stem Cells

A population of adherent stromal cells grown from the bone marrow is capable of extensive population doublings in vitro and differentiation toward all somatic mesenchymal lineages; these cells are known as "mesenchymal stem cells" (MSCs).[216] A much rarer adherent marrow population, "multipotent adult progenitor cells" (MAPCs), described in murine and human marrow, can differentiate into cells with endodermal, mesodermal, and ectodermal characteristics in vitro.[217] Furthermore, injection of murine MAPCs into blastocysts results in a contribution of MAPCs to virtually all tissues.[218] Both MSCs and MAPCs are being investigated as an alternative to the more controversial embryonic stem cells (see later) for regenerative medicine; however, the in vivo clinical potential of these cell types remains to be established.

HEMATOPOIETIC POTENTIAL OF EMBRYONIC STEM CELLS AND THERAPEUTIC CLONING

Fetal stem cells that retain the potential to differentiate into all cell types have been pursued as potential clinical tools for regenerative medicine. Embryonal carcinoma cells, highly proliferative cells within teratocarcinomas, are capable of differentiation into all three germ layers, but their utility is restricted because they regenerate teratomas or teratocarcinomas in vivo.[219] Embryonic stem cells (ES cells) derived from preimplantation embryos were isolated over two decades ago from mice, and they can be propagated in vitro indefinitely while maintaining their pluripotency.[220,221] Following injection into blastocysts, murine ES cells contribute normal cells to all tissues, and genetic manipulation of murine ES cells in vitro has been a very useful approach for understanding the function of individual gene products; methods based on homologous recombination produce "knockout" of individual genes in ES cells prior to blastocyst injection and then generation of adult mice with germline interruption of the gene of interest.[222]

The derivation of ES cells able to be propagated long-term in culture, first from nonhuman primates and then from gestational day 6 human blastocysts, has generated enthusiasm and also public controversy.[223–225] The use of human ES cell lines for developmental biology research and drug testing is active and scientifically valuable, but even aside from less contentious applications for tissue regeneration and more divisive practices such as reproductive cloning, ethical and political debates continue to heavily influence their availability to scientists.

Although the hematopoietic potential of cultured murine ES cells was documented early, at least in vitro, efficient in vivo recapitulation of hematopoiesis in an adult recipient has generally required genetic manipulation of these cells through overexpression of *HOXB4*, a homeobox gene implicated in HSC self-renewal.[226,227] Thus genetic modification of ES cells, followed by somatic cell nuclear transfer, might create autologous ES cells useful for treatment of hematologic diseases. In one example of therapeutic cloning by nuclear transplantation, immunedeficient $Rag2^{-/-}$ mice were used as donors for nuclear transfer, creating $Rag2^{-/-}$ ES cells.[228] These ES cells were then corrected by homologous recombination and manipulated to overexpress *HoxB4*; hematopoietic precursors generated from the corrected ES cells were then infused into immune-deficient $Rag2^{-/-}$ mice, with hematopoietic engraftment and restoration of immunity. The hematopoietic potential of human ES cells is less well characterized, so far only demonstrated at low efficiency in vitro.[229,230]

CURRENT CONTROVERSIES & FUTURE DIRECTIONS

Hematopoiesis

- Can HSCs be expanded safely and feasibly, given constraints resulting from telomere length, irreversibility of differentiation program, and potential risk of selection for cells with mutations in pathways that normally maintain homeostasis?
- Can microenvironmental niches be manipulated to enhance engraftment?
- If hematopoietic lineage cells can contribute to other tissues, is there any physiologic or therapeutic relevance to these events?
- Will human embryonic stem cells be able to efficiently differentiate into HSCs and reconstitute hematopoiesis?

Selected Readings*

Broccoli D, Young JW, de Lange T: Telomerase activity in normal and malignant hematopoietic cells. Proc Natl Acad Sci U S A 92:9082–9086, 1995.

Enver T, Heyworth CM, Dexter TM: Do stem cells play dice? Blood 92:348–351, 1998.

Kamel-Reid S, Dick JE: Engraftment of immune-deficient mice with human hematopoietic stem cells. Science 242:1706–1709, 1988.

Lemischka IR, Raulet DH, Mulligan RC: Developmental potential and dynamic behavior of hematopoietic stem cells. Cell 45:917–927, 1986.

Orkin SH: Diversification of haematopoietic stem cells to specific lineages. Nat Rev Genet 1:57–64, 2000.

Peled A, Petit I, Kollet O, et al: Dependence of human stem cell engraftment and repopulation of NOD/SCID mice on CXCR4. Science 283:845–848, 1999.

Spangrude GJ, Heimfeld S, Weissman IL: Purification and characterization of mouse hematopoietic stem cells. Science 241:58–62, 1988.

Tisdale JF, Dunbar CE: Plasticity and hematopoiesis: Circe's transforming potion? Curr Opin Hematol 9:268–273, 2002.

Weissman IL, Anderson DJ, Gage F: Stem and progenitor cells: origins, phenotypes, lineage commitments, and transdifferentiations. Annu Rev Cell Dev Biol 17:387–403, 2001.

Full references for this chapter can be found on accompanying CD-ROM.

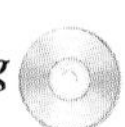

CHAPTER 2

Hemoglobin and Heme Biosynthesis

Alan N. Schecter, MD, Richard S. Ajioka, PhD, and James P. Kushner, MD

INTRODUCTION

The hemoglobin protein and its nonprotein iron-containing porphyrin cofactor, heme, are so central to the evolution of our understanding of blood diseases that the field of hematology takes its name from these molecules. This chapter provides an overview of both the globin proteins and the heme prosthetic groups; abnormalities of either constitute the basis for much of "red cell hematology," especially the inherited and acquired anemias.

We first address the function, structure, genetics, and developmental expression of the globin proteins. In the second part, the focus is on studies of the heme biosynthetic enzymes and our current view of the heme biosynthetic pathway. Both these molecular processes occur throughout evolution, and much useful information about the human molecules has come from comparative studies. Furthermore, neither the globin proteins nor the heme groups are restricted to the erythrocyte but are used in many other mammalian cells. Understanding of the hemoglobin molecule underlies the pathophysiology of many of the red cell diseases that are covered in later chapters in this book (see Chapters 20 and 21).

PART I: HEMOGLOBIN FUNCTION, STRUCTURE, GENETICS, AND DEVELOPMENT

KEY POINTS

Hemoglobin

- Hemoglobin has multiple functions in addition to oxygen transport, including transport of carbon dioxide and other gases and control of vascular dynamics.
- Oxygen affinity is finely regulated by intramolecular interactions as well as interactions with other molecules, including 2,3-bisphosphoglycerate and protons.
- Cooperative oxygenation is triggered by structural changes of the heme iron upon binding oxygen, which lead to tertiary conformational alterations within that globin subunit and changes in the orientation of the α/β dimers with respect to each other.
- Nitric oxide produced in the vasculature oxidizes oxyhemoglobin to methemoglobin; intraerythrocytic hemoglobin can destroy or preserve nitric oxide bioactivity, thus contributing to the regulation of vascular tone and oxygen delivery.
- The three human α-like globin genes are clustered on chromosome 16 in a relatively open chromatin domain; the five β-like globin genes are in a more closed chromatin domain on chromosome 11, which is activated by signals not yet understood.
- Developmental control of globin gene expression occurs via transcriptional and posttranscriptional mechanisms; transcriptional control depends on the action of distant enhancers, especially the locus control region, and silencers as well as several DNA sequences in the immediate promoter of each gene, which interact with transcription factors.

TABLE 2–1. Some Major Advances in Understanding Hemoglobin

Approximate Date	Scientist	Discovery
1862	Felix Hoppe-Seyler	Chemical identification of hemoglobin
1904	Christian Bohr	Oxygen dissociation curve
1935	Linus Pauling	Chemical nature of oxygen binding
1949	Linus Pauling	Molecular basis of sickle cell anemia
1956	Vernon Ingram	Amino acid change in sickle cell anemia
1960	Max Perutz	X-ray structure of hemoglobin
1967	Ruth & Reinhold Benesch	Effect of 2,3-bisphosphoglycerate on oxygenation
1970	M. Perutz & Herman Lehmann	Molecular pathology of hemoglobin
1978	Yuet Wai Kan	DNA-based diagnosis of sickle cell anemia

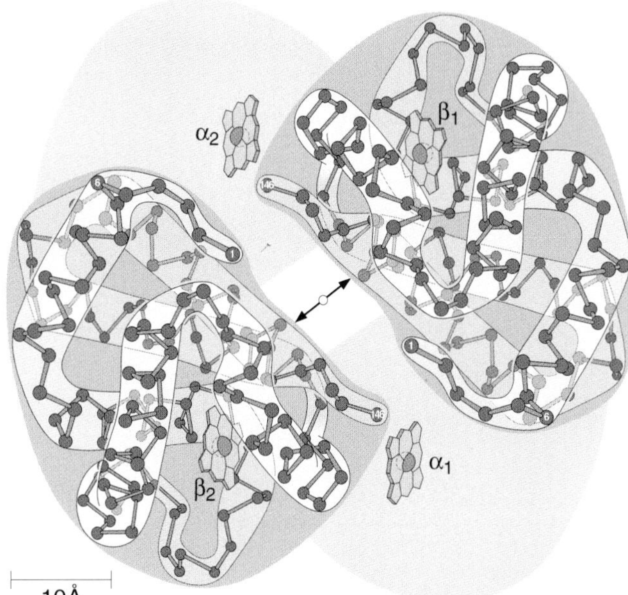

Figure 2–1. Molecular structure of oxyhemoglobin. A view of the structure of the oxyhemoglobin tetramer, based on high-resolution x-ray crystallographic analyses, drawn looking down the dyad symmetry axis with the β chains on top. Hemoglobin polypeptide chains are shown as *orange solids* with the α-carbon backbone of the β chains superimposed on the top two structures. The dimers forming the tetramer are designated $\alpha_1\beta_1$ and $\alpha_2\beta_2$. The orientations of the four heme groups are shown, as is the location of the β_6 residues where the sickle mutation occurs. Upon deoxygenation, the dimers rotate and translate with respect to each other, allowing 2,3-bisphosphoglycerate to bind in the space between the β chains (shown by *arrows*) but decreasing access to the iron atoms. (The diagram was based on the structure of horse hemoglobin but the human structure is almost identical; courtesy of the Estate of Irving Geis.)

Function

Despite its restriction to one cell type, hemoglobin is the single most abundant intracellular protein. The human erythrocyte contains about 280 million molecules of hemoglobin tetramer. Each tetramer is composed of two pairs of globin polypeptide chains, each bound to a heme moiety (Fig. 2–1). The ability of hemoglobin molecules to bind oxygen reversibly on the iron atoms of the heme groups allows erythrocytes to transport oxygen from the lungs to tissues, where it is crucial for most metabolic reactions. Erythrocytes also participate actively in other essential processes: removal of carbon dioxide, acid-base buffering, and control of vascular dynamics by regulation of nitric oxide bioavailability. The molecular understanding of the quintessential function of intraerythrocytic hemoglobin—delivering oxygen to tissues in a precisely regulated manner—has been the subject of major scientific advances for more than a century (Table 2–1).

Oxygen Transport

The oxygen binding curve for normal, adult hemoglobin (hemoglobin A) under physiologic conditions is sigmoidal (Fig. 2–2); this characteristic shape confers great physiologic benefit, including the ability to finely adjust oxygen delivery depending on need.[1,2] In the range from normal values of arterial partial pressure of oxygen (PO_2) (about 100 mm Hg) to organ tissue PO_2 values (about 40 mm Hg), about 23%, or a quarter of a billion molecules, of hemoglobin-transported oxygen will be delivered by each erythrocyte. However, actual PO_2 varies greatly in different tissues and may be markedly lowered by physiologic and pathologic stresses to values of 10 mm Hg or less. The steep midsection of the oxygen binding curve results in additional delivery of a very large volume of oxygen in response to pronounced tissue hypoxia.

The sigmoidal or cooperative shape of the oxygen binding curve and the fact that its midpoint—the P_{50}, about 28 mm Hg—is close to normal tissue PO_2 values are the result of the interactions of the four polypeptide chains with each other (homotropic interactions) and with other molecules in the cell (heterotropic interactions). Without these interactions, oxygen affinity would be expected to be much higher (with the binding curve shifted markedly to the left), as exists for other related heme proteins, such as the single globin chain of myoglobin, and could not be easily adjusted to varying physiologic conditions. The degree of cooperativity is measured through analysis of the slopes of oxygen binding curves and is designated the Hill coefficient; normally its value is about 2.8.

Acidity long has been recognized to decrease oxygen affinity, shifting the binding curve to the right. The pH range from 7.6 to about 7.0 is the most relevant physiologically because red cell contents (primarily hemoglobin) effectively buffer any more extreme plasma pH values, and the increased binding of protons as pH is lowered decreases oxygen affinity at the P_{50} by almost 20 mm Hg. However, carbon dioxide itself, the usual cause of acidosis, has a small effect in decreasing oxygen

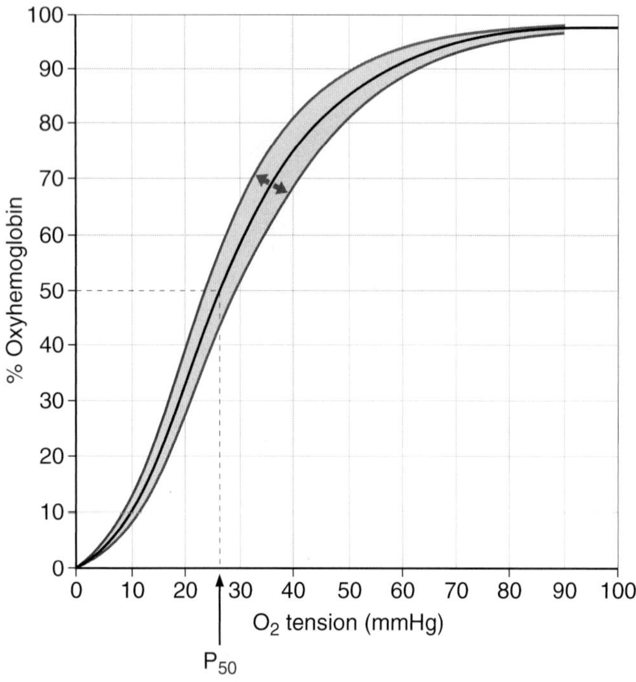

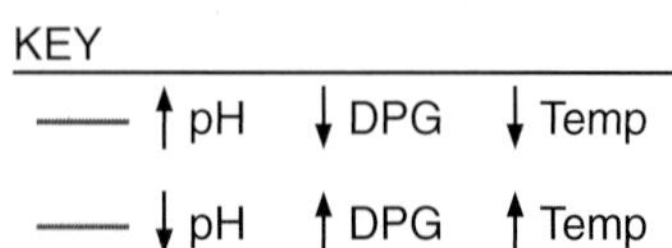

Figure 2–2. Oxygen binding curves for human hemoglobin under physiologic conditions. The normal binding curve (identical for adult red cells and hemoglobin A solutions adjusted to physiologic solution conditions) is shown with the *dark line*. The sigmoidal shape is indicative of cooperative oxygen binding. At a Po_2 of 100 mm Hg, the oxygen saturation is about 98%; at a Po_2 of 40 mm Hg, it is about 75%. The effects of changes in 2,3-BPG levels, pH, and temperature are also shown. (From Bunn HF, Forget BG: Hemoglobin: Molecular, Genetic and Clinical Aspects, Philadelphia: WB Saunders Co, 1986.)

affinity independent of proton binding, sometimes called the CO_2 Bohr effect to distinguish it from the pH Bohr effect.[1] Increasing temperature in the physiologic range also decreases the oxygen affinity of hemoglobin, to an extent intermediate between these two Bohr effects.

The other main modulator of the oxygen affinity of hemoglobin is 2,3-bisphosphoglycerate (2,3-BPG; also called 2,3-diphosphoglycerate), a molecule almost unique to the red cell and present in the cell at approximately equimolar concentrations with hemoglobin, to which it binds with a stoichiometry of one molecule of 2,3-BPG per hemoglobin tetramer. Other anions, such as phosphate and chloride ions, have similar but weaker effects. As with the binding of protons, the binding of 2,3-BPG decreases the oxygen binding of hemoglobin and thus also right-shifts the oxygen binding curve. Variations of red cell 2,3-BPG levels, in response to acute or chronic stress such as at high altitudes, are a major mechanism for adjusting the affinity parameter of oxygen transport: as the oxygen concentration falls, 2,3-BPG levels rise and oxygen affinity falls. The shape of the binding curve produces little change of arterial saturation but significantly increased tissue delivery of oxygen. The slightly higher oxygen affinity of fetal hemoglobin (see later) as compared to hemoglobin A is due primarily to decreased 2,3-BPG binding; this difference in oxygen affinity aids the fetus in transferring oxygen from the maternal circulation to itself.

Transport of other Gases

In addition to oxygen, several other gases interact physiologically with hemoglobin. Carbon dioxide, which, with water, is a common product of oxidative metabolism, binds to hemoglobin as a carbamino complex, especially on the amino-terminal residues of the polypeptide chains. However, this weak binding probably only accounts for the transport of a small fraction (20%) of the carbon dioxide that is produced in the body; most carbon dioxide is transported as bicarbonate ions and dissolved in the blood.

Carbon monoxide is also produced physiologically in the body as a result of the degradation of heme groups, especially those of hemoglobin itself, in addition to being inhaled as a frequent air pollutant.[3] Carbon monoxide binds to the heme iron atoms more tightly than does oxygen and causes severe toxicity if its levels rise significantly above the usual occupation of about 0.5% of all the oxygen-binding sites of hemoglobin. Toxicity appears to be largely due to the effects of carbon monoxide on increasing the overall oxygen affinity of the hemoglobin tetramers, which have carbon monoxide bound to a fraction of the heme-binding sites.

More recently, it has been realized that nitric oxide, which is produced in many tissues but especially endothelial cells and is a potent vasodilator and ubiquitous signaling molecule, also interacts in complex ways with hemoglobin.[4] Nitric oxide oxidizes oxyhemoglobin to methemoglobin, in which the heme iron is ferric (Fe^{III}) rather than the normal ferrous (Fe^{II}), and itself is oxidized to nitrate (NO_3^-). Nitric oxide also reacts reversibly with the iron atoms of deoxyhemoglobin to form nitrosylhemoglobin, in which nitric oxide is bound to ferrous iron, a compound with a stability between that of oxygen and of carbon monoxide. These and other nitric oxide reactions allow erythrocytes to regulate vascular tone and blood flow and thus oxygen delivery throughout the body.

Structure

Heme Chemistry

Oxygen Binding

Elucidation of the molecular structure of hemoglobin by x-ray diffraction methods in the 1960s and 1970s (see Fig. 2–1) complemented information which had been performed by spectroscopic analysis of hemoglobin solutions, to clarify the mechanisms by which the heme iron atoms of hemoglobin bind oxygen reversibly.[5-7] These spectroscopic analyses explain at the level of electronic

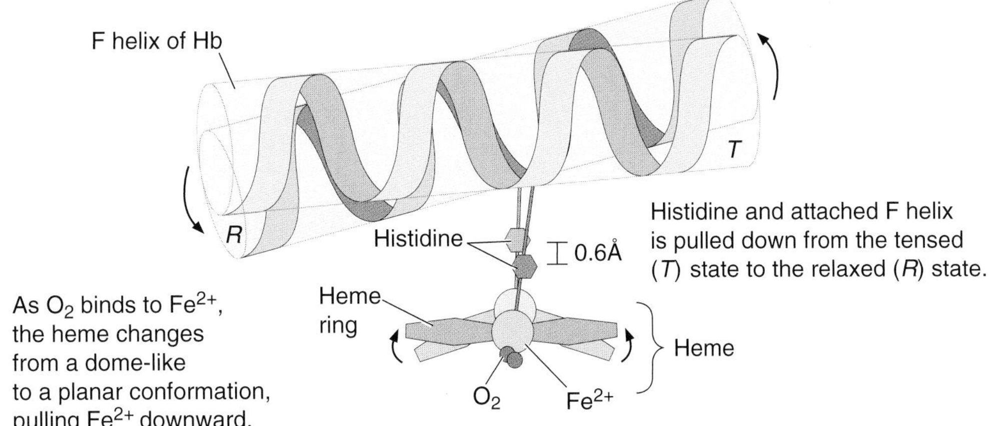

Figure 2–3. Structural changes at the heme site upon oxygen binding. A schematic diagram of the electrostatic bond between the F8 proximal histidine, on the F helix of each of the globin polypeptides, and the iron linked to the four pyrrole rings of the heme moiety. In the deoxy structure, the iron is domed above the plane of the heme; upon oxygen binding, it is pulled into the plane, changing the orientation of the histidine and of the F helix itself. These small changes are transmitted through the structure of the protein, altering in particular the contacts between the two α/β dimers and thus the overall quaternary structure (see Fig. 2–1). Note that the oxygen molecule is bent with respect to the histidine (nitrogen)–iron bond. The remainder of the heme pocket (not shown) has the distal histidine and several hydrophobic amino acid side chains (valine and phenylalanine), which tend to exclude water molecules, thus allowing oxygenation without oxidation. (From Boron WF, Boulpaep EL: Medical Physiology. Philadelphia: Elsevier Saunders, 2005.)

structure the red color of oxygenated hemoglobin and the blue-red color of deoxyhemoglobin.

Each of the four heme groups is bound to one of the four globin polypeptides through multiple weak forces between the protoporphyrin's four linked pyrrole rings and the peptide backbone and side chains of the amino acid residues in the globin heme-binding pockets. In addition, a histidine amino acid side chain at position 8 of one of the long α-helices (called the F helix) of the globin polypeptides (residue 87 on the α chains and residue 92 on the β chains) makes a strong bond to the iron atom (Fig. 2–3). The iron atom is also ligated to four nitrogen atoms of the pyrroles and, more weakly, to one other histidine side chain on the E helix. The F8 histidine residue is referred to as the proximal histidine and the other is called the distal histidine.

The energetics of this arrangement of atoms causes the iron atoms to be pulled slightly (0.6 Å) out of the plane of the porphyrin toward the proximal histidine. When the iron is in the ferrous (Fe^{II}) valence state, its resistance to oxidation is enhanced by the relative absence of water from the heme pocket, and oxygen is reversibly bound, allowing its transport. The oxygen molecule (O = O) binds in a "bent" configuration relative to the porphyrin plane, neither parallel or at right angles to that plane; the creation of space for a weak hydrogen bond with the distal histidine also contributes to the adjustment of oxygen affinity.

Other gases can also bind to the iron and be similarly transported by intracellular hemoglobin, but because they bind much more tightly than does oxygen (due to a much slower dissociation rate), they accumulate on hemoglobin and impair its oxygen delivery function. However, this problem would be much worse if not for the "selective" affinity for oxygen resulting from the detailed atomic arrangement described previously. Mutations that affect the architecture of the heme pockets of the globin proteins will perturb these sensitive atomic interactions and change hemoglobin's oxygen affinity; alterations that are large enough produce clinical manifestations of high or low oxygen affinity or other disease states.[8–10]

Methemoglobin

Under physiologic conditions, especially resulting from normal endothelial production of nitric oxide, and under pathologic states, such as exposure to oxidizing agents, the ferrous iron atoms are oxidized to the ferric form, resulting in the formation of methemoglobin.[11] This brownish form of hemoglobin does not bind oxygen. The enzyme methemoglobin reductase reduces methemoglobin, using reduced nicotinamide adenine dinucleotide (NADPH), back to the ferrous form so that normally methemoglobin levels are less than 1%. Water molecules can enter the heme pocket and bind to the ferric iron atoms, in contrast to the tightly closed ferrous hemoglobin, causing instability of the heme-protein linkage, leading to denaturation of the protein and resulting hemolytic anemia. Structural mutations in the hemoglobin molecule, especially in the heme pocket, or mutations of methemoglobin reductase can lead to hereditary forms of methemoglobinemia. The enzyme mutations are generally recessive, in contrast to structural mutations, which are apparent even in the heterozygous condition.

Nitric Oxide

There has been recent interest in the mechanism of interaction of nitric oxide with hemoglobin. In addition to oxidizing oxyhemoglobin and binding directly to the ferrous iron in deoxyhemoglobin, as described earlier, nitric oxide can react with amino acids in the globin protein, such as tyrosine and cysteine residues, to form nitrosation products. Of these nitric oxide reactions with hemoglobin, the most widely investigated is nitrosation of the cysteine residues at position 93 of each of the β chains; the biochemical function of this residue, apparently important because it is strongly conserved in evolution, has never been fully understood. Nitrosation of these cysteine residues has been proposed to be reversible, dependent on the state of oxygen binding, thus allowing hemoglobin to deliver nitric oxide to hypoxic tissues,[12,13] but this model of "S-nitrosohemoglobin" function is controversial.[14] In an alternative hypothesis, nitric oxide delivery to tissues is based on reduction of nitrite ions to nitric oxide by deoxyhemoglobin.[15,16] Whatever molecular mechanism(s) ultimately prove valid, it seems likely that intracellular hemoglobin evolution optimized its role in the transport and regulation of nitric oxide in the tissues, thus again adjusting oxygen delivery by strongly modulating blood flow.

Conversely, cell-free hemoglobin—as occurs with hemolysis—avidly binds nitric oxide, converting almost all of it to inactive nitrate ions. The resultant deficiency of bioavailable nitric oxide likely is a major reason for the toxicity of most hemoglobin-based blood substitutes.[17]

Globin Proteins

In the normal adult, hemoglobin A constitutes about 97% of the total hemoglobin, hemoglobin A_2 constitutes about 2%, and hemoglobin F (fetal) about 1%. The polypeptides of each of these hemoglobin species are composed of dimers, each of an α/β-like globin pair. These dimers themselves associate weakly to form the various hemoglobin tetramers (Fig. 2–4). In normal adult humans, the composition of these dimers is α/β for hemoglobin A, α/δ for hemoglobin A_2, and α/γ for hemoglobin F (the γ chains have two forms, differing in one amino acid but of identical function). An additional α-like globin, the ζ chain, and an additional β-like globin, the ε chain, are both present in the early embryo and combine in various combinations to produce the several embryonic hemoglobins (see Fig. 2–4). Two potential globin-coding genes, designated θ and μ, recently have been detected in the globin gene clusters (see later) but do not appear to be translated into protein.

Other globin proteins in humans and vertebrates, such as myoglobin, and also invertebrate, plant, and microorganism globins, are homologous to the α- and β-like globin polypeptides and exist in the characteristic globin-fold architecture; their evolutionary relationships have been elucidated in detail (Fig. 2–5).[18] These proteins have functions like that of hemoglobin[19] generally in the metabolism of gases, but many ancillary roles have evolved for this family of genes, including recently discovered truncated hemoglobins which have a strongly conserved three-dimensional folding pattern.[20–23] Single-chain globins expressed in tissues other than erythrocytes, analogous to myoglobin-neuroglobin in neurons and cytoglobin in many tissues, are currently the focus of much study.[24,25]

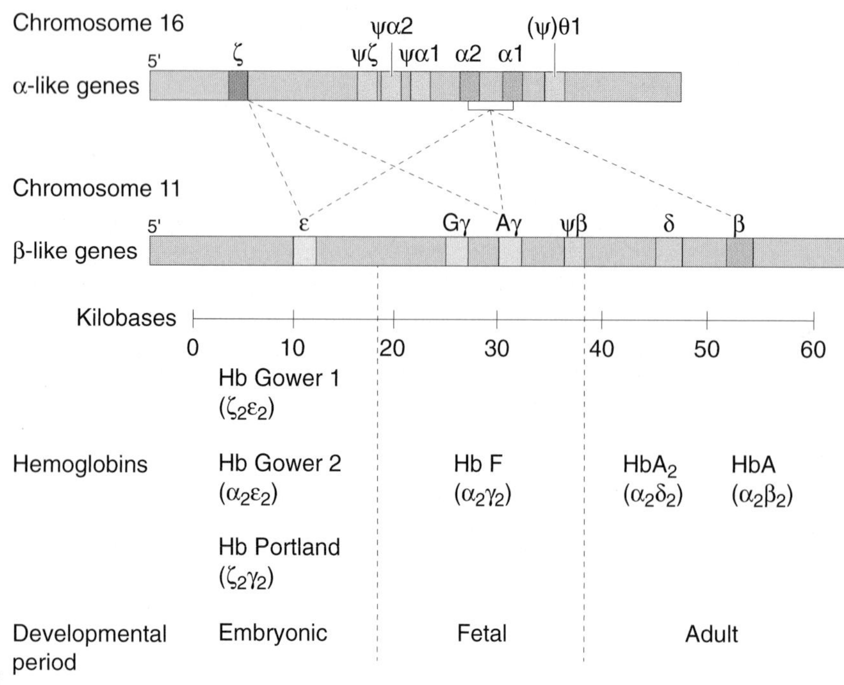

Figure 2–4. Schema of the human globin genes and proteins. The three genes coding for α-like globin proteins are shown in their arrangement on chromosome 16; the five genes coding for β-like globin proteins are shown on chromosome 11. A number of pseudo genes (genes not producing protein and generally not even transcribed) are also indicated. (Recently another dormant gene, μ, has been found near the α genes.) The seven globin polypeptides (including the two very similar forms of γ-globin) assort in any cell in which they are expressed into the six electrophoretically identifiable types of hemoglobin denoted in the bottom half of the figure. Their expression roughly correlates to the developmental periods shown.

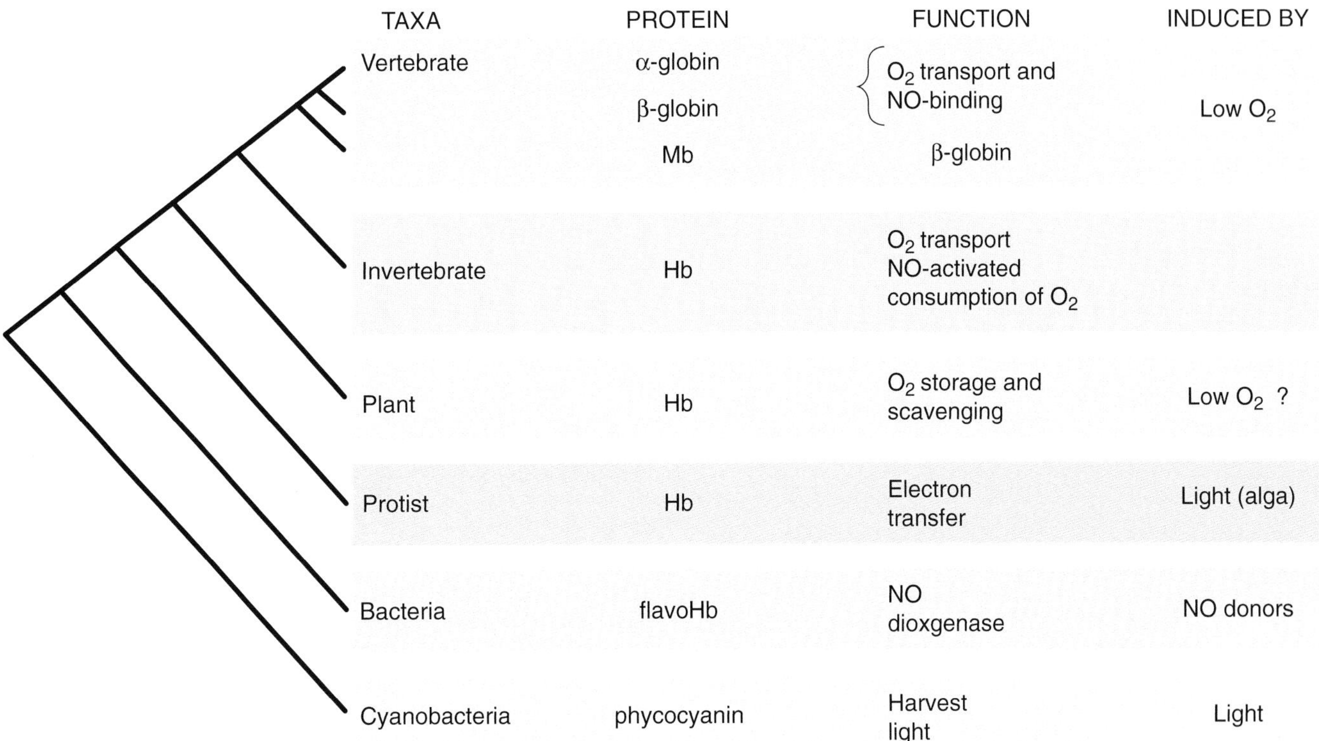

Figure 2–5. Proposed evolution of the globin proteins. This phylogenetic tree shows the apparent relations among the globin coding genes throughout approximately 2 billion years of evolution of living organisms. In vertebrates, myoglobin, and probably other proteins such as neuroglobin, evolved before the split into the α-like and β-like globins. Heme binding and conservation of the globin fold and, usually, involvement with gas metabolism characterize this family. Distance along the horizontal is roughly proportional to evolutionary time. (From Hardison R: *In* Steinberg MH, Forget BG, Higgs DR, Nagel RL [eds]: Disorders of Hemoglobin: Genetics, Pathophysiology, and Clinical Management. Cambridge: Cambridge University Press, 2001.)

Molecular Architecture

Each of the hemoglobin tetramers is arranged in a tightly packed globular structure with one true symmetry axis relating the two dimers (see Fig. 2–1),[5–7] resulting in the formation of a central cavity in the hemoglobin molecule that contains water and electrolytes. At one end of this cavity, near the amino-terminal ends of the β chains, a single 2,3-BPG molecule can bind to the deoxy form of the tetramer, particularly to histidine 2, lysine 82, and histidine 146 of each of the β chains. In addition, protons and anions bind to hemoglobin, which contributes to its strong buffering effect in the erythrocyte. The binding of these molecules and of water itself all modulate oxygen affinity, as described earlier, and are considered heterotropic effectors. In contrast to these noncovalent interactions, hemoglobin can undergo a variety of covalent modifications. Most important is glycosylation to form hemoglobin A_{1C}; the amount of this species is proportional to total exposure to blood glucose (and thus is a very good measure of control of diabetes mellitus).

Each of the individual globin chains assumes the characteristic tightly packed globin fold of dimensions about 44 × 44 × 25 Å. The α-like chains, of 141 amino acids, and the β-like chains, of 146 amino acids, are assembled into a structure made largely of α-helix regular twists of the polypeptide chain, designated A to H (with the α chains lacking helix D), separated by short stretches of amino acids without a conventionally recognized folding motif. All of these folds are extensively stabilized by noncovalent bonds, such as hydrogen bonds among the amino acid backbones and side chains, so that the individual globin folds and the globin dimers are extremely stable. The individual α and β polypeptides interact with each other to form an extremely stable α/β (or α/β-like) dimer; in contrast, much weaker interactions hold the dimers together into $\alpha_2\beta_2$ or other tetramers (subscripts in this notation referring to the numbers of each chain in the tetramer). In solution within the red cell, dissociation of tetramers into dimers allows intermolecular exchanges of dimers to occur; if two types of hemoglobin occur in a cell, the actual distribution of dimers will follow a binomial distribution (a mixture of hemoglobin A and F will result in $\alpha_2\beta_2$, $\alpha_2\gamma_2$, and $\alpha_2\beta\gamma$ species in the erythrocyte). This phenomenon is important in understanding the properties of cells containing sickle (S) hemoglobin ($\alpha_2\beta_2^S$) and other non-S hemoglobins, such as hemoglobin F.[26]

Mechanism of Cooperative Oxygen Binding

The sigmoidal oxygen binding curve is indicative of the cooperative nature of oxygen binding: after the first oxygen molecule binds to a tetramer, it is easier for a second oxygen to bind, and so on. This behavior, observed almost a century ago, indicates that there must be chemical interactions among the four heme oxygen-binding groups, despite their relatively great separation (>25 Å) in the tetramer structure. It is now recognized that these interactions are forces transmitted from the heme pocket of one subunit to the other subunits. The accepted mechanism to explain cooperativity is based on the change in the position of the ferrous iron atom in relation to the porphyrin plane upon binding oxygen; the iron moves into the plane in oxyhemoglobin.[6,7,27] These atomic movements transmit energy throughout that globin subunit, tilting the F8 histidine and moving the F helix 1 Å, which has little effect on the structure of the α/β dimer itself but which affects strongly the relative positions of the two α/β dimers with respect to each other. In this way, the effect of oxygen binding to one subunit is transmitted throughout the molecule.

The allosteric theory (from *allo* [= other] and *steric* [= arrangement of atoms in space]) provides an explanation of cooperative oxygen binding and the effects of other molecules on oxygen binding. Hemoglobin is postulated to exist in two types of molecular conformations (Fig. 2–6).[27,28] The deoxygenated form has a particular arrangement of the heme groups with respect to each of their subunits (the tertiary structure; see Fig. 2–3) and of the subunit dimers with respect to each other (the quaternary structure). This relatively "tensed" or T structure is stabilized by binding 2,3-BPG, protons, and carbon dioxide and by increasing temperature, explaining the effects of these compounds and of temperature on lowering oxygen affinity. In contrast, upon binding of one or more oxygen molecules (or binding of other gas ligands), the structure shifts to a more "relaxed" or R form. The small changes in the tertiary structure of the subunit binding the oxygen cause a major rotation and translation of the two dimers with respect to each other, opening up the structure and facilitating oxygen binding. The molecules that bind and stabilize the T form bind the R form much more weakly; these relative affinities account for the energetics of the T-to-R transition. With oxygenation of each hemoglobin tetramer, the changes and energies involved in the T-to-R transition occur in a few discrete steps rather than gradually. The only relevant oxygen affinities are those of the T and R structures themselves, not those of the intermediate forms. This allosteric model, which is in part based on symmetrical movements in the tetramer, differs strongly from an alternative "sequential" model (and other variants of these two models). Clinically, the allosteric model accounts for much of the cooperative nature of the oxygen equilibrium curves, as well as the effects of the heterotropic modulators of oxygen binding. Mutations that affect intermolecular contacts between dimers can markedly alter oxygen affinity and be clinically important.

The allosteric model was first formulated in the 1970s; more recently, the model has been recognized to be an oversimplification with respect to the number of major quaternary states, as well as to the mechanism of transition from one state to the other.[7,29] The T and R states are each composed of ensembles of several closely related (in terms of structure and energy) conformational states. A second R state (called R2) was identified by x-ray crystallography, and there is spectroscopic evidence

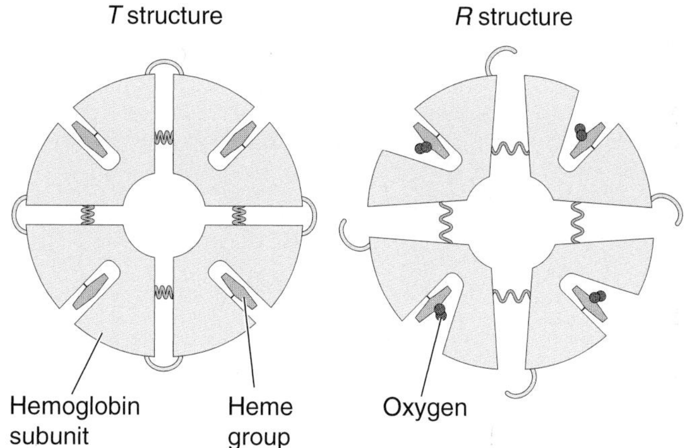

Figure 2–6. Schematic representation of the allosteric model of hemoglobin oxygenation. *Left,* In the tensed (T) structure, subunit interactions, especially between the α/β dimers, are "clamped" by many strong bonds, including with 2,3-BPG in the cavity formed between the β chains. Access to the heme pocket is restricted in this "deoxy" state and thus its affinity for oxygen is low. *Right,* In the relaxed (R) state, with a high oxygen affinity, the clamps are loosened and the molecule springs open, facilitating oxygen binding. In this model, oxygen affinity is thus dependent on the quaternary structure and not on the actual number of oxygen atoms bound to any tetramer, which can range between 0 and 4. As noted in the text, recent work has resulted in more complex forms of this model, but it still serves in its original form to explain most structure-function relations in hemoglobin. (From Perutz MF: Sci Am 259:92, 1978.)

for other R, and even other T, states. The exact atomic mechanisms by which heterotropic effectors, such as protons, act are still not fully resolved, especially with respect to whether effectors act by binding to one or a few sites or more extensively throughout the molecule. For example, the Bohr effect was originally thought to be primarily due to protonation of the histidine 146 residue of the β chains, but other sites of proton binding have been identified.[7] However, from a medical point of view, the allosteric theory in its simplest form—with two major conformations of hemoglobin and a few structural "triggers" for this interconversion—has successfully explained virtually all the physiologic and pathologic properties encountered with normal and mutant hemoglobins.

Genetics

Globin Molecular Genetics

α- and β-Globin Gene Clusters

The chromosomal arrangement of the globin genes is shown in Figure 2–7.[30,31] The human α-like genes are grouped or clustered on chromosome 16p13.3 and the β-like genes are clustered on chromosome 11p15.5. The α-cluster is near the telomere and located in a region with a number of so-called housekeeping genes that are expressed ubiquitously; the β-cluster is proximate to some olfactory genes but otherwise well delineated from the remainder of the chromosome by regions that are very specific enhancers and insulators of its function. This difference in genomic geography probably accounts in general terms for why the α-globin genes are "on" during most of development while the β-globin genes have a more stringent developmental sequence.

The genes for the α-globin proteins are in two functional copies that code for identical polypeptides; the gene for the embryonic ζ-globin gene is 5′ to these two genes, separated by several pseudoglobin genes that are no longer functional with respect to being transcribed. On the 3′ end of the β-cluster are single alleles for the β-globin gene and, to its 5′, the δ-globin gene, which is expressed at levels of only a small fraction of the β-globin gene; functionally, the δ gene has evolved as a "thalassemic" globin gene. 5′ to these genes are the pair of γ-globin genes, which are identical except for a coding change for glycine to alanine at position 136. Further 5′, close to a cluster of regulatory sites, is the lone ε-globin gene, which is expressed primarily in the embryonic period. As shown in Figure 2–7, these genes are expressed in general in a 5′-to-3′ sequence during development (see later). The globin clusters of gene have been sequenced in many species of vertebrates; there has been surprising divergence in these families despite the conservation of the primary function of globin for oxygen transport.[18] These genetic differences presumably relate to developmental constraints or other factors not fully understood.

Globin Gene Structure and Transcription

The coding regions for the amino acids of each of the globin genes (see Fig. 2–7) are interrupted by intervening sequences of DNA that are spliced out of the premessenger RNA (mRNA) after its transcription. This process, along with posttranscriptional modification of other aspects of the pre-mRNA and the effects of *cis*-acting transcription factors (discussed later), are all subject to genetic mutations. These mutations generally affect the levels of the globin proteins, secondary to transcriptional and immediate posttranscriptional effects, and are manifested clinically as thalassemia syndromes,[32] resulting from differential levels of the α-like and β-like globin proteins. A deficiency of one type of globin generally results in instability and precipitation of the globin that is in excess, leading to ineffective erythropoiesis and hemolysis. In contrast, mutations in the DNA encoding the globin proteins themselves are manifested as structural and functional changes in the hemoglobin molecule, leading to that class of diseases known as hemoglobinopathies.[9,10] The hemoglobinopathies include the prevalent sickle cell anemia ($\alpha_2\beta_2^S$)[26] and the less common methemoglobinemia, as well as oxygen affinity and stability mutants. Problems related to translation of globin mRNAs are less common but have been observed in response to heme or iron deficiencies.

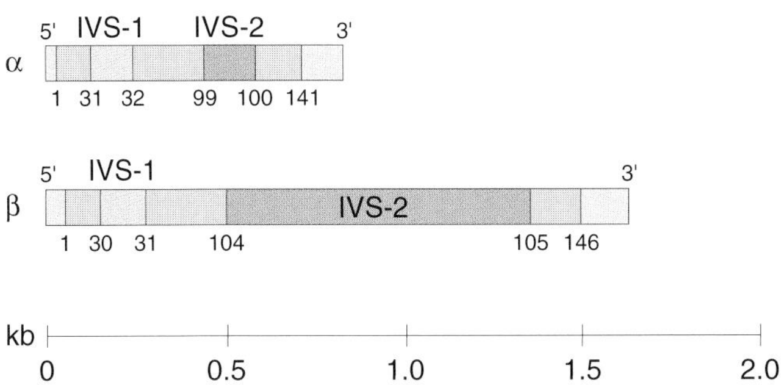

Figure 2–7. Structure of the human α- and β-globin genes. The *black blocks* are the DNA sequences coding for globin proteins; the *open blocks* correspond to the intervening sequences (IVS-1 and -2) that are spliced from the pre-mRNA; the 5′ and 3′ untranslated sequences are *hatched*. Corresponding amino acid numbers are shown for each gene. (From Bunn HF, Forget BG: Hemoglobin: Molecular, Genetic and Clinical Aspects. Philadelphia: WB Saunders, 1985.)

Regulatory Mechanisms

Globin Enhancers

Specific DNA sequences enhance the expression of the α-like and β-like globin genes. Initially, a DNA sequence 3′ to the β-globin gene was postulated as a major regulator of transcription; subsequently, it was observed that a group (originally four and now thought to be as many as seven) of DNAse I hypersensitive sites 5′ to the whole β-cluster are strong enhancers of all the genes in that cluster. These sites, now termed the *locus control region,* have been studied intensely for 2 decades, but their function is still controversial.[33] Confusion has centered on whether the locus control region has a role in the developmental control of the β-globin gene cluster, perhaps by opening a chromatin "domain,"[34] or functions primarily as a set of strong enhancers without much specificity. Among the elements in this group, one hypersensitive site appears to act as an insulator to shield the globin genes from transcription factors distal to the site.[35]

A DNA region 5′ to the α-globin gene cluster has been identified as a strong enhancer of the genes in the α-cluster, but its function differs in many ways from the locus control region; this region is called HS 40.[36]

Promoters

More closely flanking each of the globin genes are DNA sequences that act as proximal promoters and more distal effectors of gene expression.[37,38] All of them, in addition to the sequences that control processing of the pre-mRNA, are subject to mutations that control the levels of the mRNA and thus of the globin protein. These DNA sequences include the mRNA cap site, initiator codon, dinucleotide splicing sites, termination codons, and polyadenylation signals. Immediately 5′ of the gene are ATA, CCAAT, and CACCC nucleotide sequences that are very important for initiation of transcription quite generally. Further 5′ and 3′ are GATA sequences [(A/T)GATA(A/G)], which have erythroid specificity; binding sites for the EKLF transcription factor, which has specificity for the β-globin gene; and a large number of other sequences that appear to be binding sites for regions that enhance or silence gene transcription.

Regulation of Globin Gene Expression

In the adult, levels of globin gene expression are tightly regulated to ensure a precise balance between the α-like and β-like chains and to maintain the concentration of hemoglobin within a cell constant at about 34 gm/dL. The mechanism of the latter effect is not understood. Transcription, posttranscriptional processing, and degradation of mRNA and translation can all be adjusted to maintain chain balance.[39,40] Heme itself modulates translation and balances iron and protein levels; presumably the sharing of ubiquitous and erythroid-specific transcription factors (GATA motifs, in particular) facilitates coordination of transcription between the polypeptides.

Except for erythropoietin effects, signaling mechanisms affecting globin gene expression have not been elucidated. Erythropoietin is a polypeptide hormone, largely produced in the kidney in response to hypoxia, that can markedly stimulate the production of hemoglobin.[41,42] However, its major effect, through phosphorylation of a tyrosine kinase receptor, is to stimulate the production of erythroblasts that then produce hemoglobin as they mature into erythrocytes; erythropoietin does not directly affect globin gene expression.

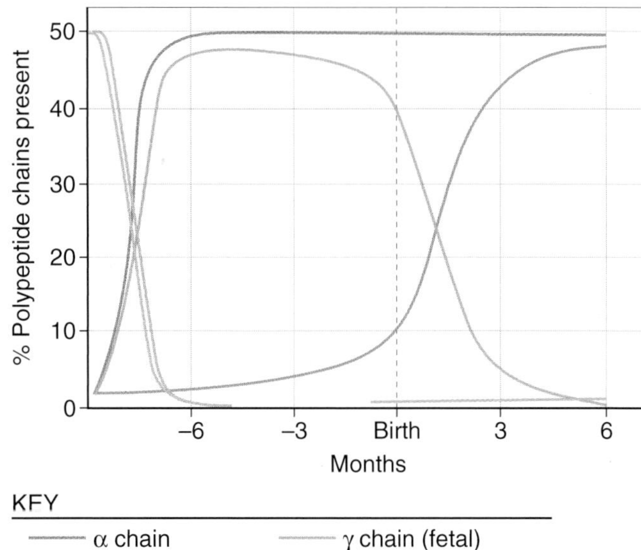

Figure 2–8. Developmental control of human globin chain expression. A diagram of the relative abundance of various human globin chains during development. The data upon which the diagram is based are incomplete because of the difficulty of obtaining fetal material. (From Bunn HF, Forget BG: Hemoglobin: Molecular, Genetic, and Clinical Aspects. Philadelphia: WB Saunders, 1985.)

Development

Developmental Biology of Globin

Figure 2–8 is a diagram of the sequence of expression of the human globin genes during ontogeny. The relatively precise sequence of control of these seven genes has been of interest as a fundamental question of developmental biology and as a basis of possible therapy of the genetic hemoglobin diseases because altering this pattern—by stopping the changes that occur at birth or reversing these processes to reactivate embryonic or fetal globin genes in the adult. The developmental pattern, which is partially controlled by changes in globin gene transcription (in contrast to posttranscriptional mechanisms), is referred to as "hemoglobin switching." Clinically, the major relevant switch is the marked decrease in γ-globin gene expression, relative to that of the β-globin gene, that occurs at the time of birth, followed by a slow decrease in fetal hemoglobin as fetal red cells reach the end of their life. This switch is likely related to the change in oxygen levels with birth, but the detailed mechanism has not been clarified.

Primitive and Definitive Erythropoiesis

Early information on the developmental modulations of the hemoglobins derived from examination of human fetuses and newborns; modern data have come from studies of erythroid cells in culture or of various animal models, especially mice. Unfortunately, differences of these experimental systems from human ontogeny have markedly limited the progress of this field. From investigations in mice and, to some extent, in humans, erythropoiesis can be divided into a "primitive" stage in the yolk sac and early in the embryo and then a "definitive" stage that takes place sequentially in the liver, spleen, and then bone marrow of the developing fetus. In the normal adult, most erythropoiesis occurs in the marrow spaces. Hematopoietic factors affecting primitive erythropoiesis and potential signaling pathways in the cellular maturation events leading to primitive erythropoiesis have been identified.

The mechanisms of sequential control of the globin genes during definitive erythropoiesis are much less clear. Specificity of expression is not related to the organ site (liver or bone marrow) of production of the erythroid cells, to clonal replacement of cell types, to identified growth factors or signaling molecules, or even to specific cascades or patterns of transcription factor expression. Although at various times and in different experimental models a temporal role in transcription has been ascribed to the locus control region, to the GATA and EKLF families of transcription factors, or to proteins that bind various enhancers or silencers, none of these processes clearly explains the observed developmental control.[31,44–48] Despite the absence of a firm conceptual basis, many therapeutic advances aimed at altering the developmental pattern—in particular hydroxyurea and, more experimentally, butyric acid—have been successful in inducing fetal hemoglobin production in order to treat sickle cell disease.[49,50]

PART II: HEME

KEY POINTS

Heme Biosynthesis

- Genes encoding enzymes of the heme biosynthetic pathway are highly conserved. The pathway includes eight enzymatic steps and can be considered as four general processes:
  - Formation of the pyrrole
  - Assembly of the tetrapyrrole macrocycle
  - Modification of the tetrapyrrole side chains
  - Oxidation of protoporphyrinogen IX to protoporphyrin IX and insertion of iron
- Four of the enzymatic steps occur in the mitochondrion and four occur in the cytoplasm. Mitochondrial enzymes require mitochondrial targeting domains in a leader peptide.
- Six of the eight enzymes of the heme biosynthetic pathway are active as homomultimeric proteins.
- The pathway in erythrocytes is regulated by the generation and export of iron-sulfur clusters by mitochondria. In other cells, regulation occurs through feedback inhibition by heme.
- Mutations in each of the eight heme biosynthetic enzymes result in a distinct disease. Reduced activity in any of the last seven enzymes result in the accumulation of porphyrin intermediates or porphyrin precursors and cause the porphyrias (see Chapter 54).

Heme is an essential molecule for both prokaryotes and eukaryotes. In addition to its central role as the oxygen-binding moiety of hemoglobin, heme serves as the prosthetic group for a number of enzymes, in particular, the cytochromes. The unique properties of an iron molecule coordinated within a tetrapyrrole enable heme to function in an array of reactions as an electron carrier and as a catalyst for redox reactions. Heme is formed in the mitochondrial matrix by the insertion of ferrous iron into the tetrapyrrole macrocycle of protoporphyrin IX. Protoporphyrin IX is generated by a highly conserved metabolic pathway that requires pyridoxine (vitamin B_6) and zinc for the initial steps leading to formation of the pyrrole ring. The enzymatic assembly of the tetrapyrrole macrocycle yields compounds designated as porphyrins. The word *porphyrin,* derived from the Greek *porphuros,* meaning purple, aptly describes the intensely colored compound first isolated from iron-free hemoglobin. Porphyrins display a characteristic absorption at approximately 400 nm, the region of the spectrum known as the Soret band. All porphyrins fluoresce, but this property is generally lost when metals are bound; exceptions are the Mg- and Zn-porphyrins, which fluoresce despite their metal content. Although the first and the last three enzymes in the pathway are located in the mitochondria, all the genes in the heme biosynthetic pathway are encoded and translated in the nucleus.

Most heme is produced in the bone marrow and the liver, but the regulatory mechanisms controlling synthesis differ between the two organs. Heme biosynthetic enzymes in the liver are characterized by rapid turnover and synthesis, which ensure the ability to respond to metabolic requirements. Approximately 15% of the daily production of heme in humans is hepatic and destined for heme-containing enzymes. In contrast, the pathway in erythroid progenitor cells permits a high steady-state level of heme synthesis. Regulation of the erythroid and "housekeeping" nonerythroid heme biosynthetic pathways differs because of the unique demand for heme synthesis in the developing red cell. For example, the first four genes in the biosynthetic pathway have dual promoters allowing both erythroid-specific and nonerythroid regulation.[51–54]

The heme biosynthetic pathway is complex, consisting of eight enzymatic steps; it is helpful to consider it as four basic synthetic processes:

1. Formation of the pyrrole
2. Assembly of the tetrapyrrole macrocycle
3. Modification of the tetrapyrrole side chains
4. Oxidation of protoporphyrinogen IX to protoporphyrin IX and insertion of iron

Formation of the Pyrrole by Aminolevulinate Synthase

The first and rate-limiting enzyme in the pathway, δ-aminolevulinate synthase (ALAS), is encoded by two separate genes that catalyze the same reaction, condensation of glycine and succinate to form δ-aminolevulinic acid (ALA) (Fig. 2–9). The nonerythroid or "housekeeping" form (*ALAS1*) maps to human chromosome 3p21.1,[55] is expressed in hepatocytes and other cells, and is regulated by cellular heme content. The erythroid-specific form (*ALAS2*) is encoded on chromosome Xp11.21.[56] Both the erythroid-specific and housekeeping forms of ALAS require pyridoxal 5′-phosphate as a cofactor (see Fig. 2–9). Mutations of *ALAS2* that affect binding of pyridoxal 5′-phosphate are responsible for most cases of X-linked sideroblastic anemia (see Chapter 55).

Both ALAS-1 and ALAS-2 are synthesized in the cytoplasm and contain an amino-terminal mitochondrial targeting sequence that is cleaved upon mitochondrial import. The targeting sequence also contains a heme-binding motif. Binding of heme to the targeting sequence inhibits import of the protein to the mitochondrial matrix.[57] The ability of heme to block mitochondrial import of ALAS represents a point of feedback inhibition for the heme synthetic pathway in the liver. Erythroid cells are probably unaffected by this mechanism because virtually all heme generated in red cells either is immediately bound to globin or is exported via a heme-specific exporter expressed by erythroblasts.[58] Alternatively, the heme regulatory motifs in ALAS-2 may not be functional, because transfected rat ALAS-2 was not inhibited by hemin in cultured fibroblasts.[59] Under identical conditions, transfected rat ALAS-1 exhibited hemin-dependent inhibition.

Both ALAS-1 and ALAS-2 also are regulated at the level of transcription.[60–62] Transcription of ALAS-1 is

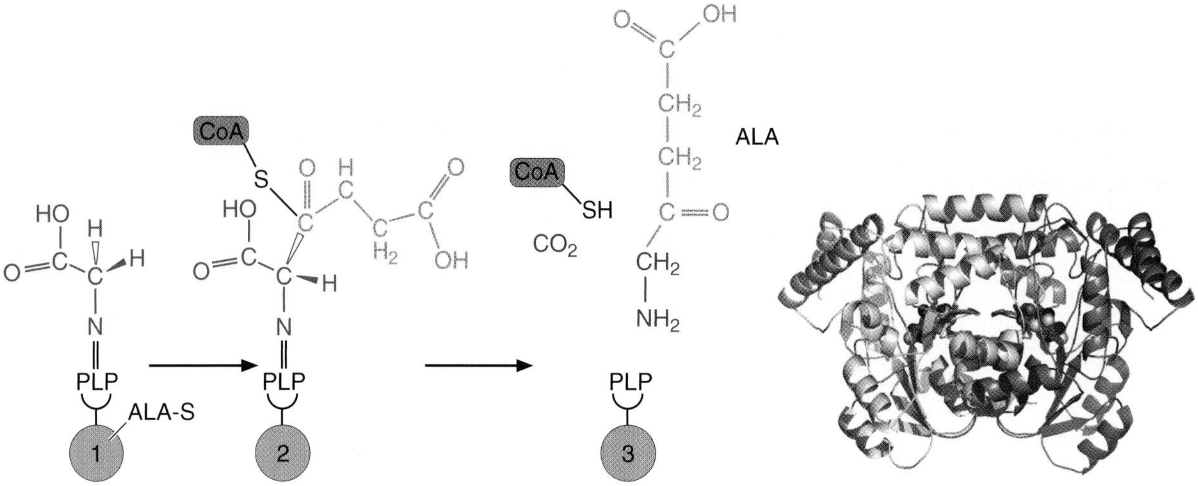

■ **Figure 2–9.** *Left,* Synthesis of δ-aminolevulinic acid (ALA). The *green sphere* represents the mitochondrial δ-aminolevulinate synthase (ALAS) enzyme and PLP represents the pyridoxal 5′ phosphate cofactor.
1. Formation of the PLP-glycine Schiff base complex (glycine is shown in *blue*).
2. Succinyl-CoA *(red box—orange)* reacts with the complex.
3. Decarboxylation of the glycine carboxyl group, stereospecific addition of a proton, and release of ALA *(orange-blue)*, CoASH *(red box)*, and carbon dioxide *(blue)*.

Right, The crystal structure of the *R. capsulatus* ALAS homodimer is shown. The bacterial protein is highly homologous with the human. Monomers in the crystal structure are shown in *gray* and *blue.*

downregulated by heme, but this effect does not occur for ALAS-2. Transcriptional regulation of ALAS-2 in erythroid cells is mediated by erythroid-specific factors, including GATA-1, that interact with sequences in the promoter region of the gene—sequences contained in many genes expressed in red cells. There is little evidence to suggest translational regulation of ALAS-1 but the ALAS-2 transcript contains a 5′ iron regulatory element (IRE) that binds a protein designated IRE-binding protein (IRP-1). The IRE–IRP-1 complex prevents translation of the ALAS2 mRNA. Addition of an iron-sulfur cluster to IRP-1 abolishes the protein's ability to bind to the iron regulatory element and permits translation to occur. Iron-sulfur clusters are generated and exported by mitochondria. These mitochondrial functions regulate the heme biosynthetic pathway in erythroid precursors.[63]

ALAS-2 from *Rhodobacter capsulatus* has been crystallized (D. Jahn, personal communication) and is highly homologous with murine and human ALAS-2, which is expressed as a homodimer.[64,65] The human *ALAS2* gene spans 22 kb and encodes 11 exons. The mRNA encodes a polypeptide of 587 amino acids. Exon 2 encodes the amino-terminal signal sequence for mitochondrial import, and exons 5–11 encode the highly conserved carboxy-terminal portion of the protein. Two mRNA isoforms are found as a result of alternative splicing of exon 4 (resulting in a 37–amino acid deletion), but the exon 4 deleted form produces functional enzyme.[66] In addition to motifs that bind erythroid-specific transcription factors, the ALAS-2 promoter region also contains elements that respond to hypoxia.[67] Hypoxia additionally upregulates the genes encoding erythropoietin, transferrin, and the transferrin receptor. Collectively, these effects of hypoxia lead to increased erythropoiesis.

Aminolevulinic Acid Dehydratase

The mechanism by which ALA exits mitochondria is not known but, once in the cytosol, two molecules of ALA are condensed to form the monopyrrole porphobilinogen (Fig. 2–10). This condensation reaction is catalyzed by δ-aminolevulinate dehydratase (ALAD). The human enzyme has been crystallized and is a homo-octamer formed from eight identical 36-kDa subunits.[68] The holoenzyme contains four catalytic sites and can be viewed as a tetramer of dimers with one active site per dimer. Each of the four active sites binds two molecules of ALA at two distinct positions. One molecule of ALA contributes the acetate and the amino-methyl group of porphobilinogen; the other contributes the propionate side chain and the pyrrole nitrogen (see Fig. 2–10). Each active site of the octamer contains two lysine residues. One (Lys252 in human ALAD) forms a Schiff base with the ALA molecule, contributing the propionate chain to porphobilinogen. Human ALAD binds eight zinc atoms, one per subunit, and the enzyme is inactivated by reversible replacement of zinc with lead. The clinical symptoms of lead poisoning are similar to those of hereditary ALAD deficiency (see Chapter 54), and it is likely that inhibition of ALAD is responsible for most of the clinical effects of lead poisoning. Four of the zincs are essential for catalysis. The other four are "structural" zincs that serve to stabilize the tertiary structure of the enzyme.[69–71] In both the red cell and the liver, ALAD activity greatly exceeds the activity of ALAS.

In humans, there is a single *ALAD* gene located on chromosome 9q34.[72] The human *ALAD* gene consists of 2 alternatively spliced noncoding exons (see Fig. 2–9) and 11 coding exons (2–12) (Fig. 2–11*A*). There are two promoter regions, a nonerythroid "housekeeping" pro-

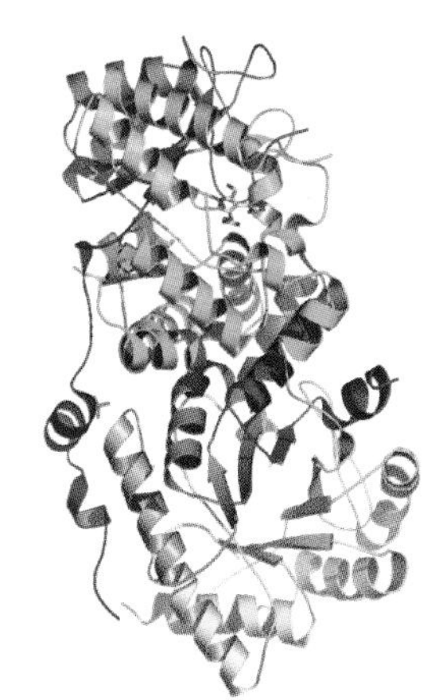

Figure 2–10. *Left,* Synthesis of porphobilinogen (PBG). Two molecules of ALA are condensed to form PBG, a monopyrrole, by the cytosolic enzyme δ-aminolevulinate dehydratase (ALAD). *Right,* The crystal structure of a monomer of human ALAD (Protein Data Bank entry 1PV8) (*http://www.rcsb.org/pdb/*). The protein in solution is an octamer of four homodimers. The amino terminus is shown in *blue* and the carboxyl terminus in *red.*

A

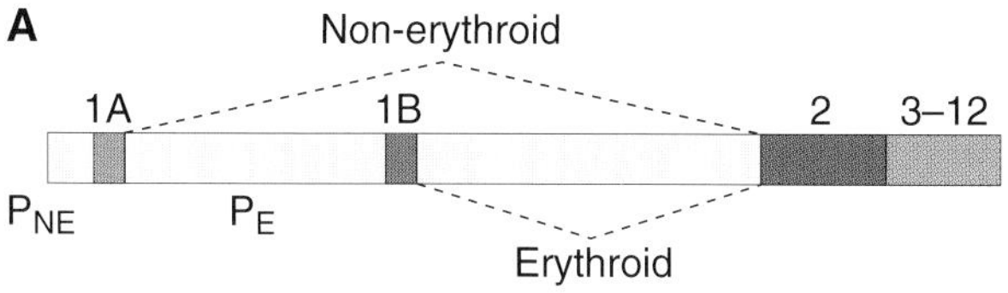

B

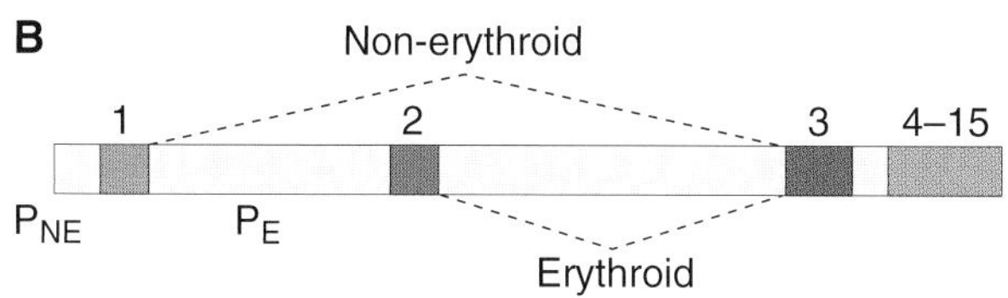

C

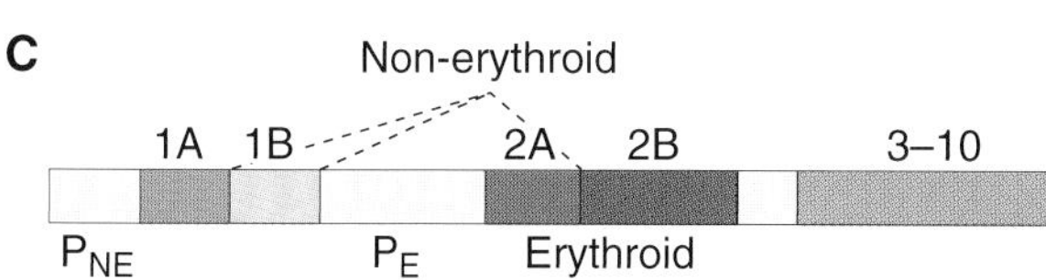

Figure 2–11. *A,* Alternate splicing of ALAD. Exon 1A *(green)* is spliced to exon 2 *(red)* in the nonerythroid transcript. Exon 1B *(blue)* is spliced to exon 2 *(red)* in the erythroid transcript. Exons 3–12 are shown in *purple.* P_E, erythroid promoter; P_{NE}, nonerythroid promoter. *B,* Alternate splicing of PBGD. Exon 1 *(green)* is spliced to exon 3 *(red)* in the nonerythroid transcript. Exon 2 *(blue)* is spliced to exon 3 *(red)* in the erythroid transcript. Exons 4–15 are shown in *purple.* P_E, erythroid promoter; P_{NE}, nonerythroid promoter. *C,* Alternate splicing of UROS. Either exon 1A *(green)* or the entire exon 1 *(green and light green)* are spliced to exon 2B *(red)* in the nonerythroid transcript. Exon 2A *(blue)* remains adjacent to exon 2B *(red)* in the erythroid transcript. Exons 3–10 are shown in *purple.* P_E, erythroid promoter; P_{NE}, nonerythroid promoter.

moter upstream of exon 1A and an erythroid-specific promoter region in the intervening sequence between exons 1A and 1B. The erythroid-specific promoter contains a GATA-1–binding site and binding sites for other erythroid-specific transcription factors found in β-globin gene promoters.[53] The organization of the murine *ALAD* gene is essentially the same as the human.[73] Mutations of the human *ALAD* gene are responsible for a rare, autosomal recessive porphyric disorder designated ALAD-deficiency porphyria (see Chapter 54).

Assembly of the Tetrapyrrole Macrocycle

Formation of the tetrapyrrole macrocycle begins with the generation of a polymer of four molecules of porphobilinogen by the enzyme porphobilinogen deaminase (PBGD). The polymer is an unstable "linear" tetrapyrrole designated hydroxymethylbilane (Fig. 2–12). PBGD is a cytosolic enzyme and functions as a monomer with an approximate molecular mass of 37 kDa.[74] The crystal structure of human PBGD has been solved[75] (see Fig. 2–12). Purification of PBGD from both mammalian and bacterial sources yields an enzyme with a dipyrromethane cofactor in the catalytic site. This dipyrrole is derived by the binding of hydroxymethylbilane to an apoenzyme (apo-PBGD). The resultant holoenzyme then deaminates and polymerizes two additional molecules of porphobilinogen to form a hexapyrrole. The final step of the reaction is cleavage of the distal tetrapyrrole from the dipyrromethane and the release of hydroxymethylbilane. The dipyrromethane remains covalently bound to the enzyme.[76]

The single human *PBGD* gene has been cloned and mapped to chromosome 11q23–11qter.[77] The *PBGD* gene contains coding regions for 15 exons. Two separate promoters control transcription (Fig. 2–11*B*). The housekeeping promoter lies upstream of the region encoding exon 1, an erythroid promoter is upstream of the region encoding exon 2. The presence of dual promoters results in two different transcripts. When transcription is initiated by the housekeeping promoter, the resulting transcript contains all 15 exons. Exon 2 is lost by splicing of exon 1 to exon 3. When transcription is initiated by the erythroid promoter, the resulting transcript contains exons 2–15. The erythroid promoter shares structural characteristics with other erythroid-specific promoters, including a CACCC motif, two GATA-1 sites, and an NF-E2–binding site.[78] Exon 2 lacks an AUG sequence, and translation of the erythroid mRNA is initiated at an AUG located in exon 3.[79] The AUG in exon 1 of the housekeeping transcript is spliced in-frame with the AUG in exon 3 and produces a protein 17 amino acids longer at the amino terminus compared to the erythroid protein.[51] Mutations of the human *PBGD* gene are responsible for acute intermittent porphyria (see Chapter 54).

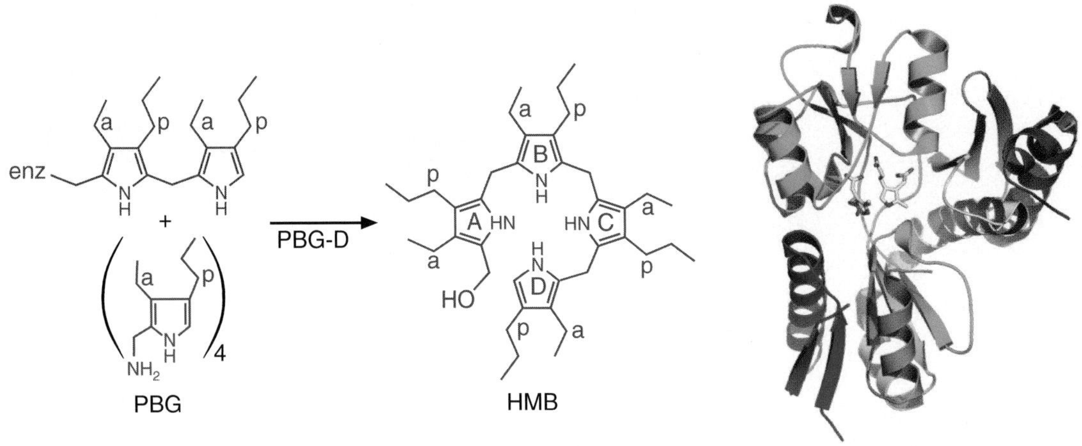

■ **Figure 2–12.** *Left,* Synthesis of hydroxymethylbilane (HMB). The reaction is catalyzed by the cytosolic enzyme porphobilinogen deaminase (PBGD). A dipyrromethane cofactor *(red)* is covalently bound to the enzyme in the catalytic site. Four additional molecules of PBG *(blue)* are deaminated and polymerized to form a hexapyrrole. The distal tetrapyrrole is then cleaved and released as HMB *(blue). Right,* The crystal structure of the human PBGD monomer (Protein Data Bank entry 1GTK). Blue to red color shading as in Figure 2–9. Abbreviations: a, acetate; p, propionate.

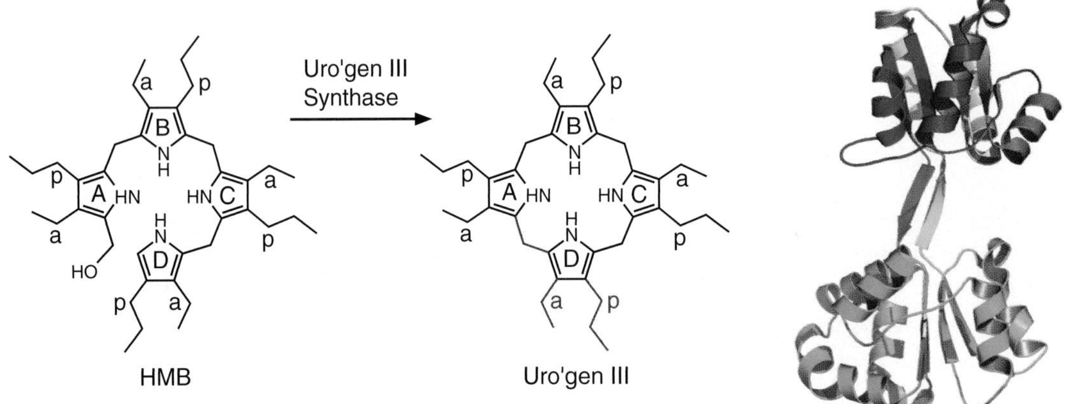

■ **Figure 2–13.** *Left,* Synthesis of uroporphyrinogen III. The reaction is catalyzed by the cytosolic enzyme uroporphyrinogen III synthase (UROS). The enzyme catalyzes ring closure of hydroxymethylbilane (HMB) with concurrent "flipping" of the D ring to generate uroporphyrinogen III. *Right,* The crystal structure of the human UROS monomer (Protein Data Bank entry 1JR2). Abbreviations: a, acetate; p, propionate.

Closure of the Tetrapyrrole Ring

Uroporphyrinogen III synthase (UROS) catalyzes the conversion of hydroxymethylbilane to uroporphyrinogen III by inversion of the D ring of hydroxymethylbilane followed by closure of the tetrapyrrole macrocycle (Fig. 2–13). Only the asymmetrical III isomer is subsequently metabolized to heme. In the absence of UROS activity, hydroxymethylbilane spontaneously cyclizes to form the symmetrical I isomer of uroporphyrinogen. Although uroporphyrinogen I can serve as a substrate for uroporphyrinogen decarboxylase (UROD), the next enzyme in the pathway, it cannot ultimately be converted to heme. Crystallized human UROS is a monomeric protein with an apparent molecular mass of 29.5 kDa.[80] Purified UROS has the highest specific activity of any enzyme in the heme biosynthetic pathway (over 3×10^5 nmol/hr/mg).[81] Mutations of UROS are responsible for congenital erythropoietic porphyria (see Chapter 54), which is transmitted as an autosomal recessive trait. Because of the high specific activity of the wild-type protein, mutations yielding enzymes with less than 5% activity are compatible with life.

Humans have a single *UROS* gene localized to chromosome 10q25.2–26.3.[82] The human *UROS* gene encodes 10 exons.[54] Exon 2 is divided into two parts, the 5′ exon 2A and 3′ exon 2B (Fig. 2–11*C*). The ATG translational start site is located within exon 2B. As with the previous two enzymes, both nonerythroid and erythroid-specific mRNAs exist. The nonerythroid transcript is ubiquitous and results from a splicing event that joins either the entire exon 1 or exon 1A to exon 2B (see Fig. 2–11*C*). The nonerythroid promoter upstream of the exon 1 coding region lacks a TATA box and contains binding sites for Sp-1, NF-1, AP-1, Oct-1, and NRF-2. The functional basis of the two nonerythroid transcripts is not known. The erythroid-specific mRNA contains the entire second exon. The TATA-less erythroid promoter lies upstream of the exon 2A coding region and contains 8 GATA-1–binding sites and is active only in erythrocytes. Thus the nonerythroid and erythroid-specific transcripts are expressed from alternative promoters of the single human *UROS* gene but produce the identical protein.

The four genes reviewed to this point share a common theme, the existence of housekeeping and erythroid-specific transcripts. In the case of *ALAS,* a red cell–specific variant exists. *ALAD, PBGD* and *UROS* are single genes that generate tissue-specific transcripts and alternate splicing.

Modification of the Peripheral Side Chains

Uroporphyrinogen III is a branch point for the pathways leading to heme, chlorophyll (Mg protoporphyrin), and corrins (cobalamins). In mammalian cells, uroporphyrinogen III is converted to coproporphyrinogen III by the sequential removal of the four carboxylic groups of the acetic acid side chains to yield coproporphyrinogen[83] (Fig. 2–14). This reaction is catalyzed by the cytosolic enzyme UROD. UROD is an unusual decarboxylase because it does not require a cofactor for enzymatic activity. Both uroporphyrinogen III and uroporphyrinogen I may serve as substrates, but uroporphyrinogen III is preferred.[84] The order of decarboxylation of the acetate groups of uroporphyrinogen III begins at the D ring and proceeds in a clockwise manner.[83,85] UROD has been purified from a number of sources and the crystal structure has been solved.[86,87] The enzyme functions as a homodimer with an apparent molecular mass of 82 kDa. Each monomer contains an active site cleft. Only porphyrinogens serve as substrates for UROD; the oxidized porphyrins do not. Structural studies of the active site revealed that only the "flexible" porphyrinogen macrocycle can be accommodated.

Mutations in *UROD* are responsible for the familial form of porphyria cutanea tarda, which is inherited as an autosomal dominant trait (see Chapter 54). In rare instances, homozygous or compound heterozygous mutations result in a disease termed *hepatoerythropoietic porphyria* (see Chapter 54). Complete loss of UROD activity is incompatible with life, because knockout mutations in mice are lethal.[88] Mutations in the *UROD* gene have not been identified in the sporadic form of porphyria cutanea tarda[89] (see Chapter 54).

Human *UROD* gene has been cloned and mapped to chromosome 1p34.[90,91] The *UROD* gene is 3 kb in length and contains 10 exons. There are two transcriptional start sites, one major and one minor, that are separated by 6 bp and do not appear to be differentially utilized in different tissues. The upstream untranslated region contains a pseudo TATA box and a unique Sp-1–binding site.[92] In contrast to the erythroid-specific and nonerythroid regulation found in the first four enzymes in the pathway, the *UROD* gene contains a single promoter. The level of *UROD* mRNA is markedly increased in tissues or cell lines of erythroid origin, but the molecular basis of erythroid-specific upregulation is not characterized.[93]

Biosynthesis of Protoporphyrinogen IX

The second side chain modification of the tetrapyrrole macrocycle is the oxidative decarboxylation of the propionate groups of pyrrole rings A and B of coproporphyrinogen to form two vinyl groups and the release of two molecules of carbon dioxide[94] (Fig. 2–15). This reaction is catalyzed by coproporphyrinogen oxidase (CPO), which in mammals is located in the mitochondrial intermembrane space. The mechanism by which coproporphyrinogen III is transported across the outer mitochondrial membrane may be mediated by peripheral-type benzodiazepine receptors.[95] Like UROD, CPO does not require a cofactor. CPO activity, however, is stimulated by phospholipids.[96] The reaction proceeds in a clockwise manner beginning with the A ring propionate.[97]

The human *CPO* gene maps to chromosome 3q12, consists of seven exons, and spans approximately 14 kb.[98,99] The human *CPO* transcript has an open reading frame of 1062 bp and encodes a protein of 354 amino acids. The mature protein of 323 amino acids has a puta-

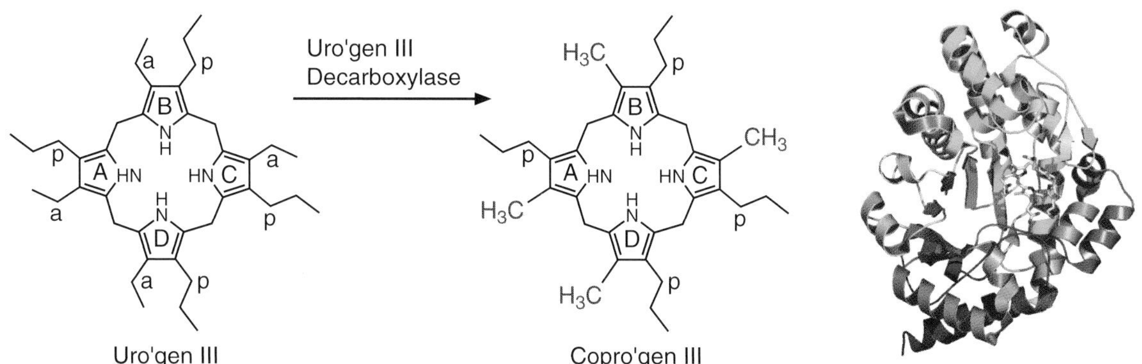

Figure 2–14. *Left,* Synthesis of coproporphyrinogen III. The reaction is catalyzed by the cytosolic enzyme uroporphyrinogen decarboxylase (UROD). The enzyme sequentially decarboxylates the four acetate side chains (a) of uroporphyrinogen III, starting at the asymmetrical D ring, to generate the tetracarboxylic, tetramethyl coproporphyrinogen III. *Right,* The crystal structure of a monomer of human UROD (Protein Data Bank entry 1URO). The enzyme is a homodimer in solution.

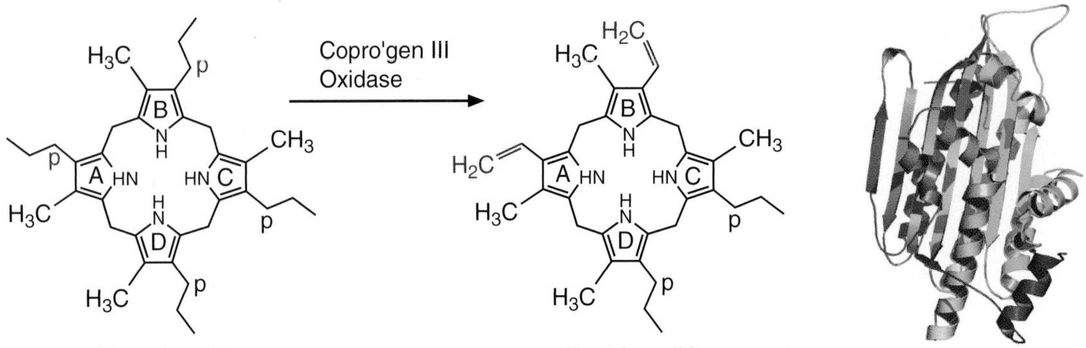

Figure 2–15. *Left,* Synthesis of protoporphyrinogen IX. This reaction is catalyzed by the enzyme coproporphyrinogen oxidase (CPO), which resides in the mitochondrial intermembrane space. The enzyme oxidizes the propionate groups *(red p)* of the A and B rings of coproporphyrinogen to form two vinyl groups (shown in *red*) with the release of two molecules of carbon dioxide. *Right,* The crystal structure of a monomer of yeast CPO (Protein Data Bank entry 1TKL). The yeast enzyme is highly homologous to the human. The enzyme is a homodimer in solution. Blue to red shading as in Figure 2–9.

tive 31–amino acid leader peptide, but the complete 120-residue amino-terminal region appears necessary for proper targeting.[94,100,101] Purified human CPO exists as a homodimer with a subunit molecular mass of 39kDa.[102] *Saccharomyces cerevisiae* CPO, which is highly homologous to the human enzyme, has been crystallized, and mapping of human mutations associated with hereditary coproporphyria (see Chapter 54) indicate that most changes result in destabilization of the protein structure or distortion of the active site.[103] There is differential regulation of CPO between erythroid and nonerythroid cells, but there is only a single promoter. The promoter region encodes an Sp-1–like element, a GATA site, and a novel regulatory element that interact in a synergistic manner in erythroid cells.[104] In nonerythroid cells, the GATA site is not necessary, but the CPO promoter regulatory element is required. This is consistent with tissue-specific expression of CPO with erythroid upregulation mediated by the GATA site.[105]

Oxidation of Protoporphyrinogen IX and Insertion of Iron

The oxidation of protoporphyrinogen IX to protoporphyrin IX is catalyzed by the enzyme protoporphyrinogen oxidase (PPO), with oxygen required as the electron acceptor (Fig. 2–16). The human enzyme has been crystallized and is active as a homodimer with a subunit molecular mass of 51kDa.[106] PPO is synthesized in the cytosol but is transported to the outer surface of the inner mitochondrial membrane. It lacks an identifiable mitochondrial targeting leader peptide, but GFP fusion proteins containing the amino-terminal 178, 59, 34, and 17 amino acids successfully targeted GFP to the mitochondria.[101] The enzyme contains one noncovalently bound FAD per dimer. PPO cannot use coproporphyrinogen III as a substrate and is inhibited by bilirubin and micromolar concentrations of the herbicide acifluorfen, which act as competitive inhibitors.[107,108] Mutations in the *PPO* gene produce the autosomal dominant disease variegate porphyria (see Chapter 54).

The human *PPO* gene, which maps to chromosome 1q22-q23,[109,110] is approximately 5.5kb in length with 1 noncoding and 12 coding exons,[111] the coding sequence is 1431bp in length and codes for a 477–amino acid polypeptide. Northern blot analysis indicates a single transcript of approximately 1.8kb in all tissues.[108] The protein contains a major mitochondrial targeting sequence between 151 and 175 residues from the amino-terminus, along with a minor sequence within the first 150 amino acids.[112] Tobacco *PPO* has been crystallized, and the active site architecture is consistent with a substrate-binding mode compatible with the unusual six-electron oxidation.[106] Mutations of *PPO* are responsible for variegate porphyria (see Chapter 54).

Insertion of Iron into Protoporphyrin IX

The final step in the heme biosynthetic pathway, the insertion of iron into protoporphyrin IX, is catalyzed by the enzyme ferrochelatase (Fig. 2–17). Ferrochelatase is synthesized in the cytosol and imported to the mitochondrion, a mitochondrial targeting sequence is cleaved during mitochondrial localization of the protein precursor.[101,113] Human ferrochelatase has been crystallized and is active as a homodimer with a molecular mass of approximately 86kDa.[114] The enzyme is associated with the inner surface of the inner mitochondrial membrane, and each subunit contains a nitric oxide–sensitive 2Fe-2S cluster.[115] Comparison of PPO and ferrochelatase structures are compatible with a model wherein the two molecules can be docked together on opposite sides of the inner mitochondrial membrane, permitting protoporphyrin IX to be directly transferred to ferrochelatase.[106]

The human ferrochelatase gene has been cloned and mapped to chromosome 18q21.3.[116] The gene contains 11 exons and spans approximately 45kb.[117] A major transcriptional start site was identified 89 bases upstream from the translational initiation ATG. The promoter

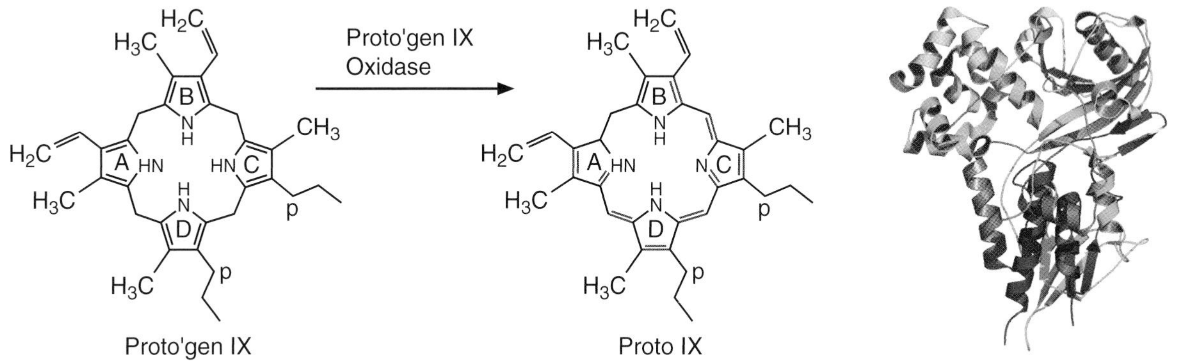

Figure 2–16. *Left,* Synthesis of protoporphyrin IX. The reaction is catalyzed by protoporphyrinogen oxidase (PPO), which is located on the outer surface of the inner mitochondrial membrane. The six-electron oxidation to the planar macrocycle protoporphyrin IX requires oxygen as the terminal electron acceptor. *Right,* The crystal structure of a monomer of tobacco PPO (Protein Data Bank entry 1SEZ). The enzyme, which is highly homologous to the human, is a homodimer in solution. Shading from blue to red as in Figure 2–9.

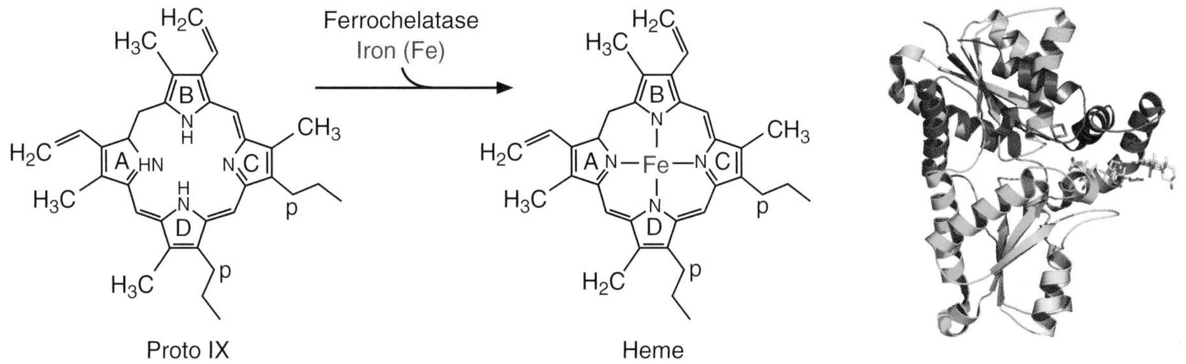

Figure 2–17. *Left,* Synthesis of heme. The final step in heme synthesis is catalyzed by the mitochondrial enzyme ferrochelatase. The enzyme catalyzes the insertion of one atom of ferrous iron into the protoporphyrin IX macrocycle. *Right,* The crystal structure of a monomer of human ferrochelatase monomer (Protein Data Bank entry 1HRK). The enzyme is a homodimer in solution. Blue to red shading as in Figure 2–9.

region contains potential binding sites for Sp-1, NF-E2, and the erythroid-specific transcription factor GATA-1 and lacks a typical TATAA or CCAAT sequence. The same transcriptional start site was found in the hepatoma cell line HepG2 and the erythroleukemia cell line K 562, consistent with a single transcript being made in both nonerythroid and erythroid cells.[117] Expression of ferrochelatase is regulated by intracellular iron levels. Activity was lost in Cos7 cells treated with the iron chelator desferrioxamine and increased in cells treated with Fe(III)NTA. When *E. coli* ferrochelatase (which lacks an iron-sulfur cluster) was expressed in Cos7 cells, neither desferrioxamine nor Fe(III)NTA affected its activity.[118] Ferrochelatase is regulated by hypoxia, two hypoxia-inducible factor-1 (HIF-1)–binding motifs are located in the ferrochelatase promoter sequence, and exposure of both nonerythroid and erythroid-derived cell lines to hypoxia result in increased ferrochelatase mRNA. A dominant negative HIF-1α blocked ferrochelatase promoter activity, consistent with regulation of the ferrochelatase gene by HIF-1 during hypoxia.[119] Mutations of the ferrochelatase gene result in the disease erythropoietic protoporphyria (see Chapter 54).

Summary

The heme biosynthetic pathway has unique, tissue-specific regulatory features. The pathway in nonerythroid cells undergoes feedback inhibition by heme, but in erythroid cells the pathway is regulated by the availability of iron (as iron-sulfur clusters). The first four enzymes in the pathway are regulated differently in erythroid and nonerythroid cells, primarily based on *cis*-acting elements that bind tissue-specific transcription factors. Six of the eight enzymes are active as homomultimers.

The heme biosynthetic pathway is highly conserved between prokaryotes and eukaryotes. In eukaryotic cells, the pathway is divided between mitochondrial and cytosolic compartments (Fig. 2–18). Despite the similarity of substrates for the final four enzymatic steps (tetrapyrrole macrocycles), the structures of the enzymes that catalyze these steps are remarkable for their diversity. It is unlikely that these enzymes evolved as a result of gene duplication. Even though the steps involved in heme synthesis are well characterized, much remains unknown about the physical distribution of substrates and enzymes in the pathway.

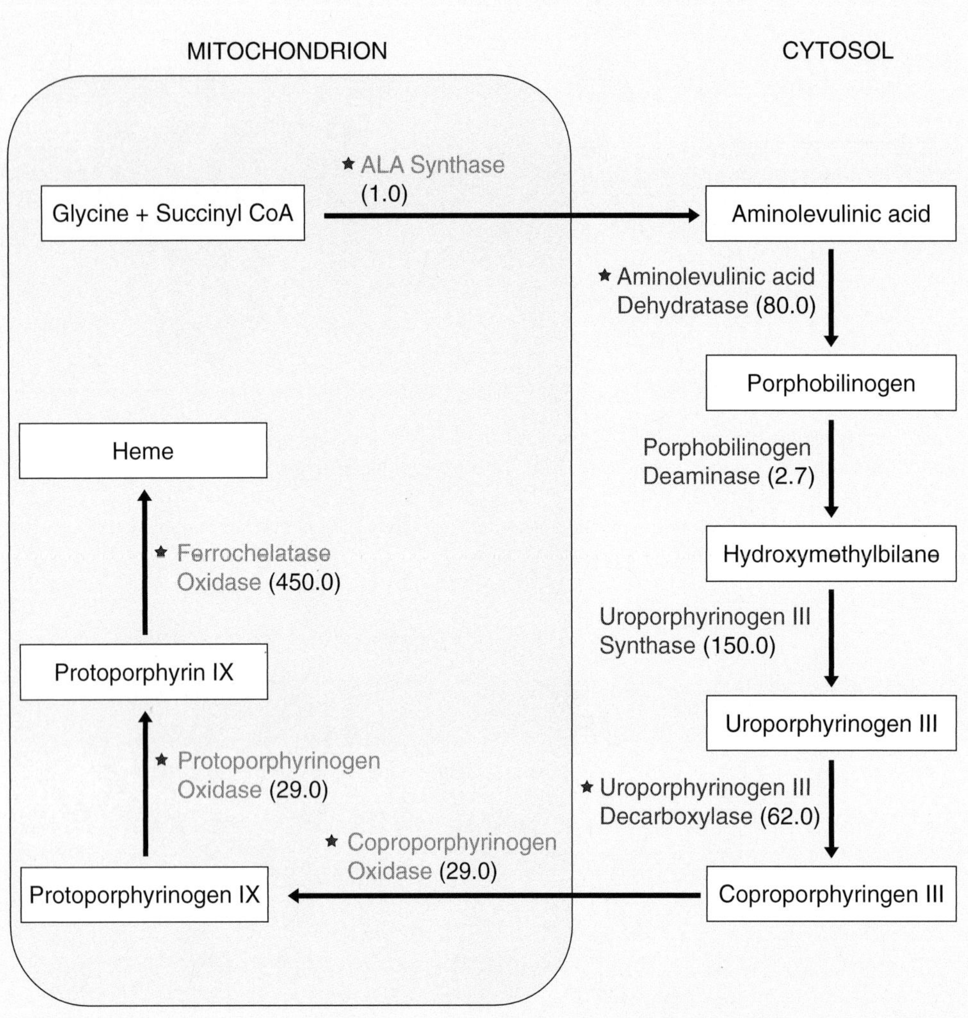

Figure 2–18. The heme biosynthetic pathway. Mitochondrial enzymes are depicted in *green* and cytosolic enzymes in *red. Stars* indicate enzymes that occur as homomultimers. Numbers in parentheses represent the relative activity of the enzyme (one unit of activity is defined as the amount of enzyme required to form 1 nmol of product per hour).

Current Controversies & Future Considerations

Hemoglobin and Heme

- What is the role of the erythrocyte in modulating nitric oxide control of blood flow? Is nitric oxide storage as S-nitrosohemoglobin or nitrite bioactivation key pathways?
- Are the known toxicities of cell-free, hemoglobin-based blood substitutes due primarily to nitric oxide destruction or increased oxygen delivery to arterioles?
- What are the important functions of myoglobin, neuroglobin, and cytoglobin?
- Will further refinement of the allosteric theory of hemoglobin's cooperative oxygen binding significantly improve our understanding of hemoglobin function?
- How is intraerythrocytic globin chain balance maintained, and how are total levels of hemoglobin controlled so closely?
- What are the molecular genetic mechanisms controlling the ontogeny or genetic "switches" of globin expression? What is the mechanism of downregulating fetal hemoglobin at birth?
- Can we use our knowledge of hemoglobin to design new therapies for its many severe and prevalent diseases?
- Are reactions taking place in the cytosolic compartment of the heme biosynthetic pathway localized to facilitate transfer of product of one enzyme to the next enzyme in the pathway?
- Models for the spatial relationship of enzymes involved in the mitochondrial reactions have not been firmly established.
- What transporter is responsible for importing iron into mitochondria in the ferrochelatase reaction?

Acknowledgment

The authors thank John D. Phillips, PhD, for his thoughtful comments, helpful criticisms, and crystallographic expertise, which contributed immensely to this chapter.

Suggested Readings*

Hemoglobin

Boron WF, Boulpaep EL: Medical Physiology, Updated Edition. Philadelphia: Elsevier Saunders, 2005, Ch 28.

Bunn HF, Forget BJ: Hemoglobin: Molecular, Genetic and Clinical Aspects. Philadelphia: WB Saunders, 1986.

Dickerson RE, Geiss I: Hemoglobin: Structure, Function, Evolution and Pathology. Menlo Park, CA: Benjamin/Cummings, 1983.

Eaton WA, Henry ER, Hofrichter J, Mozzarelli A: Is cooperative oxygen binding by hemoglobin really understood? Nat Struct Biol 6:351–358, 1999.

Embury SH, Hebbel RP, Mohandas N, Steinberg MH (eds): Sickle Cell Disease: Basic Principles and Clinical Practice. New York: Raven Press, 1994.

Lukin JA, Ho C: The structure-function relationship of hemoglobin in solution at atomic resolution. Chem Rev 104:1219–1230, 2004.

Perutz M: Science Is Not a Quiet Life: Unraveling the Atomic Mechanism of Haemoglobin. Singapore: World Scientific Publishing Company, 1997.

Perutz MF, Wilkinson AJ, Paoli M, Dodson GG: The stereochemical mechanism of the cooperative effects in hemoglobin revisited. Annu Rev Biophys Biomol Struct 27:1–34, 1998.

Stamatoyannopoloulos G, Majerus PW, Perlmutter RM, Varmus H (eds): The Molecular Bases of Blood Disease. Philadelphia: WB Saunders, 2001, Chs 5–7.

Steinberg MH, Forget BG, Higgs DR, Nagel RL (eds): Disorders of Hemoglobin: Genetics, Pathophysiology, and Clinical Management. Cambridge: Cambridge University Press, 2001.

Weatherall DJ, Clegg JB: The Thalassemia Syndromes (ed 4). Oxford: Blackwell Publishing, Ltd., 2001.

Heme Synthesis

Anderson KE, Sassa S, Bishop DF, Desnick RJ: Disorders of heme biosynthesis: X-linked sideroblastic anemia and the porphyrias. *In* Scriver CR, Beaudet AL, Sly WS, Valle D (eds): The Metabolic & Molecular Bases of Inherited Disease, Vol II (ed 8). New York: McGraw-Hill, 2001.

Dailey HA: Biosynthesis of Heme and Chlorophylls. New York: McGraw-Hill, 1990.

Phillips JD, Whitby FG, Kushner JP, Hill CP: Structural basis for tetrapyrrole coordination by uroporphyrinogen decarboxylase. EMBO J 22:6225–6233, 2003.

Ponka P: Cell Biology of heme. Am J Med Sci 318:241–256, 1999.

Wingert RA, Barout B, Foott H, et al: Glutaredoxin 5 deficiency reveals Fe/S clusters are required for vertebrate heme synthesis. Nature 2005 (in press).

Full references for this chapter can be found on accompanying CD-ROM.

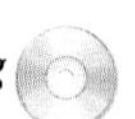

CHAPTER 3

Erythrocyte Structure

Narla Mohandas, DSc, and Marion E. Reid, PhD

KEY POINTS

Erythrocyte Structure

- Maintenance of normal cellular deformability and membrane mechanical stability of the discoid human red cell is critical for optimal oxygen delivery to tissues. Cell shape or geometry, cytoplasmic viscosity, and membrane deformability and mechanical stability are key regulators of cellular deformability.
- Decreased cell surface area or increased cell volume leads to stomatocytosis and/or spherocytosis. Loss of membrane surface area caused by inherited defects in membrane proteins or partial phagocytosis of antibody-coated red cells results in spherocytosis. In contrast, increased cell volume caused by membrane cation permeability defects leads to stomatocytosis. Reduction in lifespan of red cells is related to the extent of the decrease in the ratio of cell surface area to cell volume.
- Increased cytoplasmic viscosity resulting from cell dehydration hinders the ability of the red cell to enter capillaries in the microcirculation. Cell dehydration is a feature of red cells with membrane permeability defects and of red cells with abnormal hemoglobins (Hb), such as Hb S and Hb C.
- Decreased membrane deformability hinders the ability of red cells to undergo the rapid shape change required to enter the capillaries. Decreased membrane deformability is a feature of red cells in hereditary ovalocytosis and irreversibly sickled cells.
- Decreased mechanical stability leads to red cell fragmentation in the circulation as a result of the inability of red cells to withstand the fluid forces encountered in the circulation. Red cells in hereditary elliptocytosis exhibit diminished membrane mechanical stability.
- The basic structural organization of the red cell membrane is a spectrin-based membrane skeleton tethered to the lipid bilayer through interactions with cytoplasmic domains of transmembrane proteins. Defects in tethering of the membrane skeleton to the lipid bilayer (vertical interactions) lead to membrane loss and generation of spherocytic red cells. Defects in lateral interactions among skeletal proteins lead to decreased mechanical stability, cell fragmentation, and generation of elliptocytes.

INTRODUCTION

To optimally deliver oxygen to tissues, the human red cell during its 120-day lifespan undergoes extensive deformation as it navigates through the microcirculation but maintains its structural integrity. Loss of cellular deformability, a feature of red cells in a number of inherited and acquired red cell disorders, compromises the ability of red cells to perform their function and can also lead to their premature removal from the circulation.[1–3]

The ability of red cells to undergo marked deformation during passage through capillaries was first reported by van Leeuwenhoek in 1675: "when he was greatly disordered, the globules of his blood appeared hard and rigid, but grew softer and more pliable as his health returned: whence he infers, that in healthy body it is requisite they should be soft and flexible, that they may be capable of passing through the capillary veins and arteries, by changing their round figures into ovals, and also reassuming their former roundness when they come into vessels where they find larger room." These prescient observations were confirmed in the 20th century by elegant studies of Krögh,[4] Branemark and Bagge,[5] Chen and Weiss,[6] and others who studied red cell deformations in the capillaries using improved microscopic and imaging technologies.

Three key factors regulate red cell deformability:

1. Cell shape or cell geometry, which determines the ratio of cell surface area to cell volume; higher ratios facilitate deformation.
2. Cytoplasmic viscosity, which is primarily regulated by cell hemoglobin concentration and is therefore influenced by alterations in cell volume. The higher the cell hemoglobin concentration, the slower the ability of the red cell to enter capillaries in the microcirculation.
3. Membrane deformability and mechanical stability, which are regulated by structural organization of the various membrane proteins. Decreased membrane deformability hinders the ability of red cells to undergo the rapid shape change required to enter the capillaries, and decreased mechanical stability leads to red cell fragmentation in the circulation as a result of

the decreased ability of red cells to withstand the fluid forces encountered during circulation.

Either directly or indirectly, membrane components and their organization play an important role in regulating each of the factors that influence cellular deformability.

This chapter reviews the key factors that regulate normal red cell deformability and how alterations in various factors account for reduced deformability of cells in various red cell pathologies and thus compromise red cell function. The structural organization of red cell membrane components, their role in regulating normal membrane function, and alterations leading to loss of membrane function in red cell pathologies are summarized.

DETERMINANTS OF RED CELL FUNCTION

During its 120-day lifespan, a human red cell that is 8 microns in diameter must undergo extensive shape changes to pass through 3 micron diameter capillaries and 1 to 2 micron slits in the reticuloendothelial sinusoids while resisting cell fragmentation (Fig. 3–1*A*). The ability to undergo the necessary deformations is influenced by three distinct cellular determinants:

- Cell shape or cell geometry, which determines the ratio of cell surface area to cell volume.
- Cytoplasmic viscosity, which is primarily regulated by the cell hemoglobin concentration and is therefore influenced by alterations in cell volume.
- Membrane deformability and mechanical stability, which are regulated by structural organization of the various membrane proteins.

Cell Shape

The biconcave disc shape of the normal red cell creates an advantageous surface area/cell volume ratio, allowing the red cell to undergo marked deformation while maintaining a constant surface area (Fig. 3–2*A*). The normal human adult red cell has a volume of 90 fL and a surface area of 140 μ^2. If the red cell were a sphere of identical volume, it would have a surface area of only 98 μ^2. Thus, the discoid shape provides approximately 40 μ^2 of excess surface area, or an extra 43%, that allows the red cell to undergo extensive shape changes while maintaining constant surface area. Most deformations occurring in vivo and in vitro involve no increase in surface area: the normal red cell can undergo large linear extensions of up to 230%, but an increase of even 3–4% in surface area results in cell lysis.[2,3]

The acquisition and maintenance of a favorable surface area/volume ratio is crucial to red cell function.[7] The immediate precursor of the mature discocytic red cell is the non-nucleated reticulocyte, which is produced when the normoblast extrudes its nucleus (Fig. 3–3). In contrast to red cells, immature reticulocytes are multilobular and motile, contain mitochondria and ribosomes, and synthesize proteins (see Fig. 3–3). Compared to mature red cells, immature reticulocytes are less deformable and have decreased membrane mechanical stability.[7] Both deformability and mechanical stability of reticulocytes improve during maturation. In 2–3 days, motile reticulocytes evolve first to become deep cup-shaped nonmotile cells that still contain ribosomes, and finally to mature, fully hemoglobinized discocytic red blood cells lacking organelles (see Fig. 3–3). Major structural changes accompany acquisition of the discoid shape and enhanced deformability: loss of membrane lipids and of integral proteins, such as transferrin receptors, insulin receptors, and various adhesion proteins; a reorganization of the skeletal protein network; and a decrease in cell volume and membrane surface area.[8–11]

Having acquired the discoid shape, the mature red cell must maintain this favorable surface area/volume ratio during its circulating lifespan. Either membrane loss, leading to a reduction in surface area, or an increase in cell water content, leading to an increase in cell volume, will create a more spherical shape with less redundant surface area. As the discoid red cell loses its advantageous surface area/volume ratio, it progressively becomes more stomatocytic and finally acquires spherocytic morphology (see Fig. 3–2*A*). Therefore, varying degrees of stomatocytosis and spherocytosis are features of red cells with reduced redundant surface area. Loss of surface area redundancy results in reduced cellular deformability (see Fig. 3–2*A*) and diminished lifespan. Increased osmotic fragility is a characteristic feature of all red cell populations with less than normal surface redundancy.

During its 120-day lifespan in the circulation, the human red cell progressively loses cell surface area, and there is a concomitant reduction in cell water content leading to cell dehydration.[12,13] Removal of senescent red cells from the circulation involves recognition of cell surface modifications including clustering of band 3 molecules and increased binding of immunoglobulin G and complement.[12,14–17]

Loss of the favorable surface area/volume ratio is a feature of red cells in hereditary spherocytosis, which results from membrane loss caused by inherited defects in a number of membrane proteins.[18–33] Partial phagocytosis of the red cell by macrophages also leads to reduced surface area and the generation of spherocytes in immune hemolytic anemias.[9,34] In some forms of hereditary stomatocytosis, undefined molecular defects cause an increase in cell volume as a result of impaired volume regulation.[35–37] The extent of decrease in surface area/volume ratio is a major determinant in the reduced lifespan of spherocytes, which are removed by the spleen. Thus splenectomy increases the survival of red cells in the circulation in hereditary spherocytosis.[38–42]

In other disorders, the surface area/volume ratio is increased above normal. In patients with liver disease, increased membrane cholesterol content raises the cell surface area, which, in the context of normal cell volume, increases the degree of surface area redundancy.[43,44] This excess surface area is manifested morphologically by target or spur cells and functionally by increased osmotic resistance (decreased osmotic fragility). In certain hemoglobinopathies (thalassemia, hemoglobin CC, and hemoglobin EE) (see Chapter 21), red cells exhibit more favorable surface area/volume ratio as a result of a

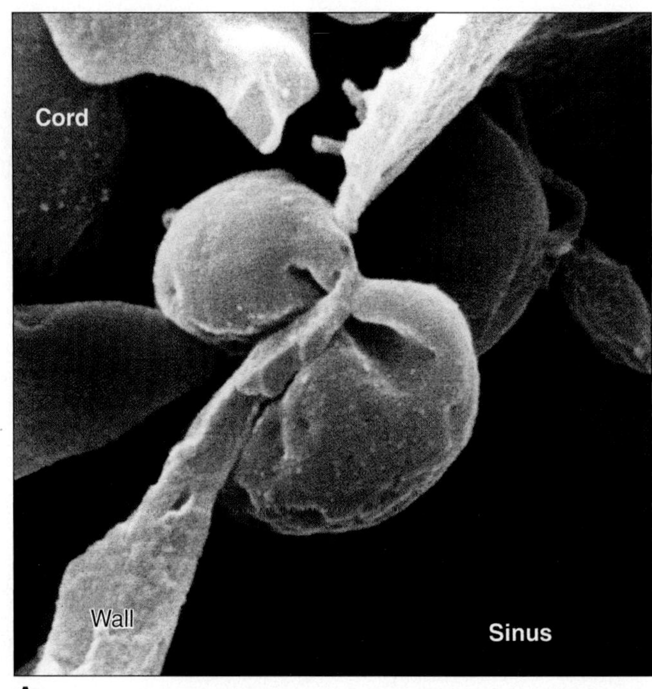

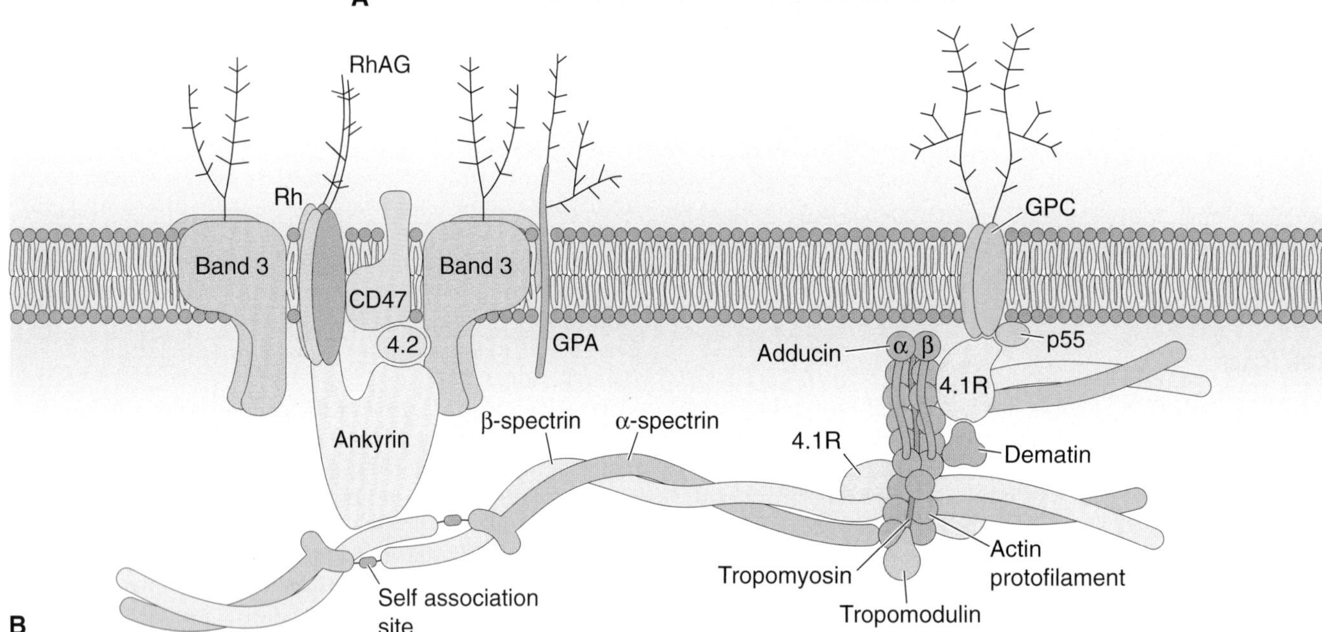

Figure 3–1. ***A,*** Scanning electron microphotograph of a red blood cell passing from a splenic cord into the splenic sinusoid through the sinusoidal barrier. Note the marked deformation that the cell undergoes to traverse the narrow fenestration in the sinusoidal wall. ***B,*** Schematic model of the structural organization of the red cell membrane (the protein and lipids are not drawn to scale). In the two-dimensional, spectrin-based membrane skeleton, dimers of α- and β-spectrin self-associate to form spectrin tetramers. The β-spectrin also assembles a multiprotein complex with actin, protein 4.1R, adducin, tropomyosin, and tropomodulin. The spectrin-based membrane skeleton is linked to the lipid bilayer through β-spectrin–ankyrin–band 3 interactions and through β-spectrin–protein 4.1R–glycophorin C interactions.

decrease in cell volume without a concomitant decrease in membrane surface area.[34,45–47]

Cytoplasmic Viscosity

Cytoplasmic viscosity, another determinant of red cell deformability, is largely determined by the cell hemoglobin concentration, which is determined in part by cell water content. As the hemoglobin concentration rises, so also does the viscosity of the hemoglobin solution (Fig. 3–4*B*). As the hemoglobin concentration increases from 27 to 35 gm/dL (the range for hemoglobin concentration of red cell populations in normal blood), the viscosity of hemoglobin solution increases from 5 to 15 centipoise (cP), which is 5–15 times greater than that of water.[48] At

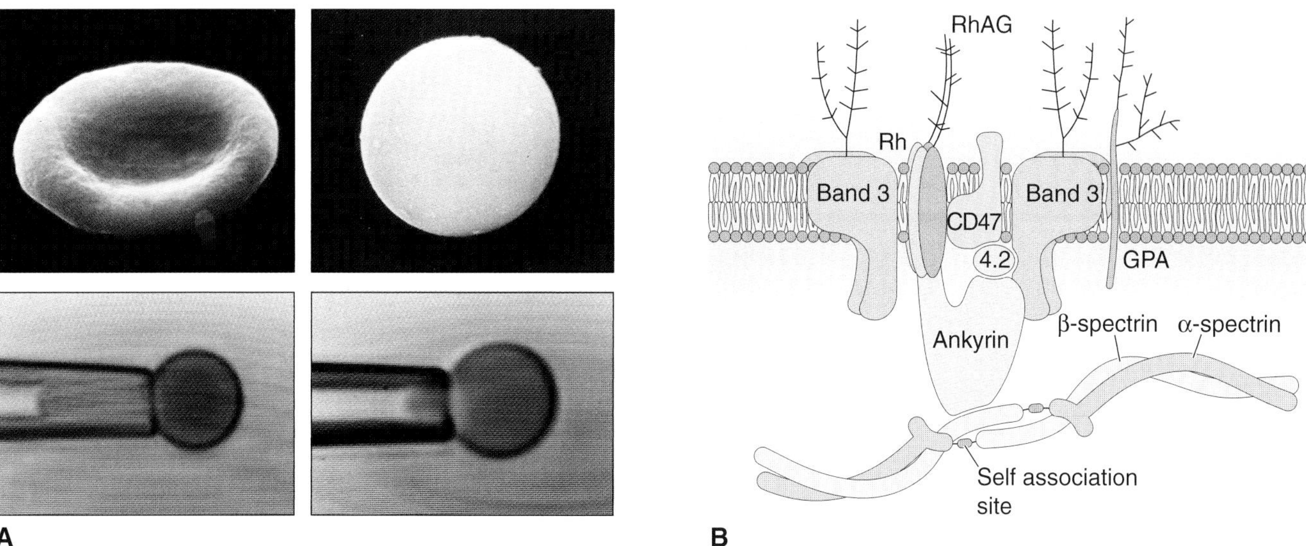

Figure 3–2. ***A,*** Scanning electron microphotographs of a discoid *(top left panel)* and a spherocytic *(top right panel)* human red cell. The discoid red cell is easily deformed when aspirated into a micropipet *(bottom left panel)*, whereas the spherocytic cell undergoes much less deformation when aspirated into the same micropipet at an equivalent aspiration pressure *(bottom right panel)*. ***B,*** Schematic representation of the macromolecular complex of band 3, RhAg, Rh, CD47, and glycophorin A linked to the spectrin-based membrane skeleton by ankyrin and protein 4.2. Loss of this vertical linkage as a result of deficiency of either band 3, ankyrin, protein 4.2, or RhAg leads to membrane surface area loss and generation of spherocytic red cells.

these levels, the contribution of cytoplasmic viscosity to cellular deformability is negligible. However, viscosity correlates exponentially to hemoglobin concentrations greater than 37 gm/dL, reaching 45 cP at 40 gm/dL, 170 cP at 45 gm/dL, and 650 cP at 50 gm/dL. At these levels, cytoplasmic viscosity becomes the primary determinant of cellular deformability. Cellular dehydration, usually caused by the failure of normal volume homeostasis mechanisms, can severely impair the rapidity with which the cell can undergo the required deformations to enter the capillaries in the microcirculation.[49]

Mutations in proteins involved in transport processes, acquired alterations in these proteins resulting from membrane oxidation, or other changes induced by mutant hemoglobin interacting with the membrane can lead to marked cellular dehydration. As examples, cellular dehydration reduces red cell deformability in hereditary xerocytosis, sickle cell anemia, hemoglobin SC, hemoglobin CC, and β-thalassemia[49–54] (see Chapters 20 and 21).

In addition to determining cytoplasmic viscosity, cell hemoglobin concentration has a profound effect on the kinetics of sickle hemoglobin polymerization (see Fig. 3–4*A*). Red cell dehydration decreases the functional ability of red cells with nonsickling hemoglobins, but it has a significant additional effect on the deformability of sickle red cells upon deoxygenation.[55–57] Increased hydration of sickle cells and the consequent reduction in cell hemoglobin concentration prolongs red cell lifespan in sickle cell disease.[58,59] Recent studies have suggested that hemoglobin can also bind and transport nitric oxide and thus play an important role in regulating vascular tone.[60] Although the precise physiologic role of nitric oxide transport by hemoglobin remains to be fully defined, there may be implications for hypertension associated with red cell disorders such as sickle cell disease.[61]

Membrane Deformability and Mechanical Stability

The two important membrane properties related to the passage of red cells through the circulation are deformability and mechanical stability. Deformability determines the extent of membrane deformation that can be induced by a defined level of applied force. The more deformable the membrane, the less is the force that needs to be applied to the cell to enable its passage through the capillaries and other narrow openings, such as fenestrations in the splenic cords (see Fig. 3–1*A*). Membrane mechanical stability is defined as the maximum extent of deformation that a membrane can undergo beyond which it cannot completely recover its initial shape at which point membrane failure occurs. Normal membrane mechanical stability allows red cells to circulate for months without fragmenting, but decreased mechanical stability leads to cell fragmentation under normal circulating stresses and premature destruction of fragmented red cells.

For both biochemically perturbed normal membranes and membranes from various red cell pathologies, deformability and stability change independently of each other, indicating that these two properties are differentially regulated by various membrane protein interactions.[62] Decreased membrane deformability can result from an increase in intermolecular or intramolecular associations of the skeletal proteins or by augmented association of integral membrane proteins such as band 3 with the skeletal network.[62,63] Decreased membrane deforma-

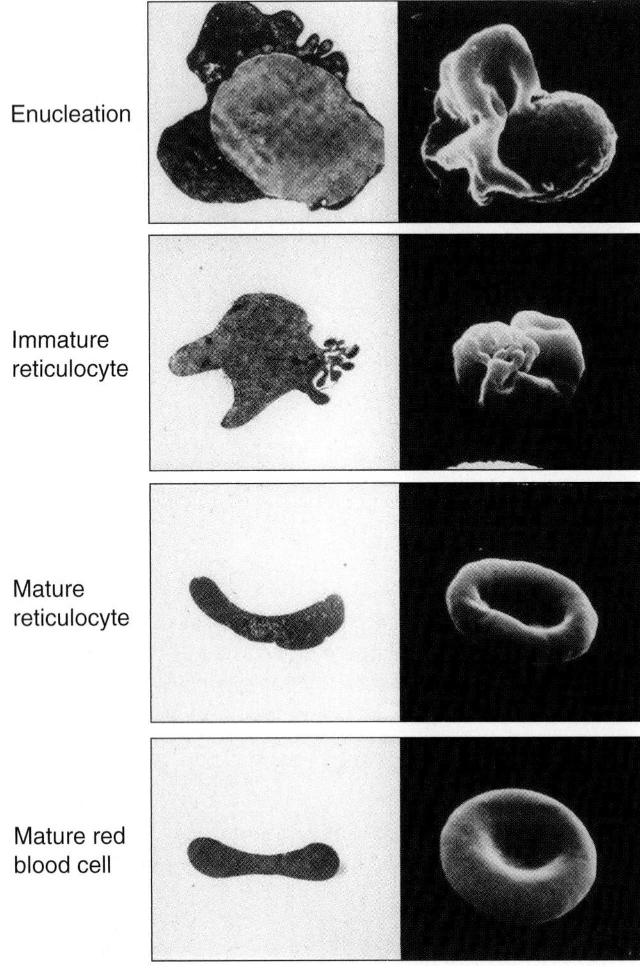

Figure 3–3. Transmission *(left row)* and scanning *(right row)* electron micrographs showing the various stages during the evolution of the mature discocytic red cell. The non-nucleated immature reticulocyte is produced when the normoblast extrudes its nucleus. The immature reticulocyte is multilobular and motile and contains mitochondria and ribosomes. These motile reticulocytes evolve first to deep cup-shaped nonmotile mature reticulocytes that contain ribosomes, and finally to mature, fully hemoglobinized discocytic red blood cells lacking organelles.

bility of irreversibly sickled cells is the result of altered skeletal protein interactions, whereas that of hereditary ovalocytosis is the result of increased association of band 3 with the skeletal network.[63,64]

Normal red cells completely recover their shape following repeated cycles of deformation in the circulation. Pathologic red cells with mutations in skeletal proteins that weaken the lateral protein-protein associations in the spectrin-based membrane skeleton exhibit membrane fragmentation (Fig. 3–5). Decreased membrane mechanical stability caused by weakening of either the spectrin-spectrin junction or the spectrin-actin–protein 4.1 junction, is a feature of red cells in hereditary elliptocytosis.[2,3] Irreversibly sickled cells in sickle cell anemia are the result of inelastic or plastic deformation of the membrane resulting from skeletal protein reorganization during repeated cycles of sickling and unsickling in the circulation.

STRUCTURAL ORGANIZATION OF THE RED CELL MEMBRANE

The basic structure of the red cell membrane is a spectrin-based membrane skeleton tethered to the lipid bilayer through interactions with cytoplasmic domains of transmembrane proteins (see Fig. 3–1*B*). This composite enables the red cell to maintain its cell shape and is critical for regulating the membrane properties of deformability and mechanical stability.[2,3] The schematic diagram in Figure 3–1 does not represent all the red cell membrane proteins, only those whose interactions with other membrane proteins have been well documented to play an important structural role. This section focuses on the membrane components that are relevant to regulation of structural integrity, function, and lifespan of the red cell.

Lipid Bilayer

The lipid bilayer provides physical continuity to the membrane, which is responsible for solute impermeability. The lipid bilayer also serves as the matrix in which the transmembrane proteins reside. Approximately 40% of the membrane mass is lipid, 52% is protein, and 8% is carbohydrate. The major lipid components of the red blood cell membrane are unesterified cholesterol and phospholipids, which are present in nearly equimolar quantities, and small amounts of free fatty acids and glycolipids.[65] The membrane phospholipid primarily consists of phosphatidylcholine (30%), sphingomyelin (25%), phosphatidylethanolamine (28%), and phosphatidylserine (14%). These phospholipids are asymmetrically distributed in the membrane: more than 75% of the choline-containing uncharged phospholipids (phosphatidylcholine and sphingomyelin) are in the outer monolayer of the lipid bilayer, whereas 80% of phosphatidylethanolamine and all of the phosphatidylserine, the charged phospholipids, are in the inner monolayer.[66] Recent studies have suggested the existence of cholesterol and sphingomyelin–enriched microdomains, or lipid "rafts," in various biologic membranes, including the human red cell.[67,68] Although there is still significant debate about the nature and size of these domains, protein complexes associated with these microdomains may play a role in cell signaling events.

The maintenance of asymmetrical phospholipid distribution in the normal red cell membrane requires active transport of the aminophospholipids (phosphatidylserine and phosphatidylethanolamine) by an ATP-dependent aminophospholipid translocase, or "flipase," from the outer to the inner monolayer.[69] Partial loss of organization occurs in sickle and β-thalassemic red cells. In both disorders, in a fraction of circulating red cells the phospholipid bilayer is scrambled so that some phosphatidylserine moves to the outer leaflet.[70,71] Phosphatidylserine on the outer leaflet is recognized by macrophages as a signal for attachment and phagocytosis, thereby contributing to reduced survival of thalassemic and sickle red cells.[72,73]

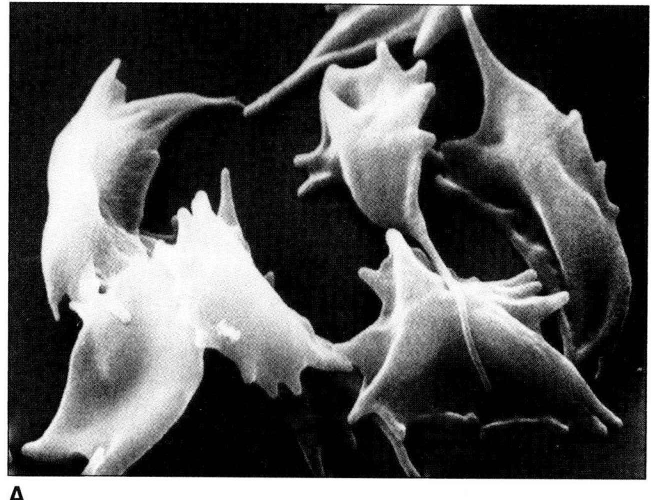

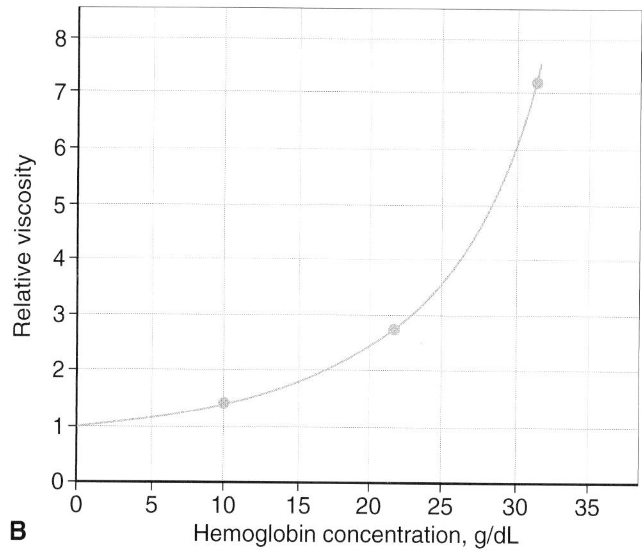

Figure 3–4. ***A,*** Scanning electron microphotograph of deoxygenated sickle red cells. Polymerization of sickle hemoglobin upon deoxygenation leads to marked changes in red cell shape. ***B,*** Relationship between viscosity and hemoglobin concentration: experimentally determined relative viscosities of hemoglobin solutions at various concentrations are shown. Note the marked increase in relative viscosities at concentrations greater than 35 gm/dL.

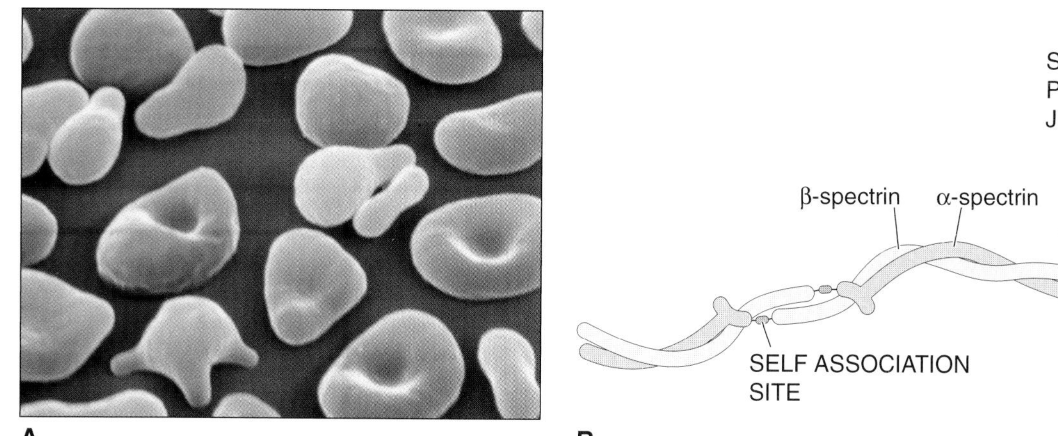

Figure 3–5. ***A,*** Scanning electron microphotograph of elliptocytic and fragmented red cells in hereditary elliptocytosis. ***B,*** Schematic representation of the two lateral junctional complexes in the spectrin-based membrane skeleton. The first complex results from self-association of dimers of α- and β-spectrin to form spectrin tetramers, and the second from interaction of spectrin dimer with actin, protein 4.1R, adducin, tropomyosin, and tropomodulin. Weakening of either of these two lateral interactions leads to decreased membrane mechanical stability and generation of elliptocytic and fragmented red cells.

Membrane Proteins

Three classes of membrane proteins are relevant to the regulation of structural integrity and function of the red cell membranes:

1. *Integral proteins* embedded in the membrane through hydrophobic interactions with lipids and whose cytoplasmic domains link the bilayer to the membrane skeleton (band 3, Rh-associated glycoprotein [RhAg], CD47, and glycophorin C).
2. *Linking proteins* that link the cytoplasmic domains of membrane proteins with membrane skeleton (ankyrin, protein 4.1R, and protein 4.2).
3. *Skeletal proteins* that constitute the two-dimensional membrane skeleton (spectrin, actin, protein 4.1R, p55, adducin, dematin, tropomyosin, and tropomodulin).

Integral Proteins

Three integral proteins—band 3, RhAg, and glycophorin C—link the lipid bilayer to the spectrin-based membrane skeleton (see Fig. 3–1*B*); deficiency of these proteins leads to abnormal cell shape and functional membrane alterations.[74–77] Other integral proteins, such as CD47 and Lu, also are linked to the membrane skeleton,[78,79] but the importance of their interactions have not been established. Integral proteins involved in regulating cation permeability of the red cell membrane are yet to be fully defined. Characterization of these integral proteins is required for detailed understanding of red cell volume regulation and for defining the molecular basis for hereditary xerocytosis (cell dehydration and increased cell hemoglobin concentration) and hereditary hydrocytosis (cell hydration and decreased hemoglobin concentration).[80]

Band 3, the anion exchange 1 protein, is the major integral protein, constituting about 25% of total membrane protein. Band 3 is composed of three dissimilar and functionally distinct domains.[81] The hydrophilic amino-terminal cytoplasmic domain interacts with peripheral membrane and cytoplasmic proteins, including ankyrin, protein 4.1R, protein 4.2, hemoglobin, and a number of glycolytic enzymes.[82–87] The hydrophobic transmembrane region contains multiple membrane-spanning domains and forms the anion transporter.[81,88] The acidic carboxy-terminal cytoplasmic domain binds carbonic anhydrase.[89] There are two clearly established functions of band 3 in the red cell membrane: (1) anion transport, resulting in one-for-one exchange of bicarbonate for chloride across the membrane; and (2) physical linkage of the lipid bilayer to the underlying membrane skeleton, primarily through interaction with ankyrin and protein 4.2 and secondarily through binding to protein 4.1R. The main structural function of band 3 is prevention of membrane surface loss. Quantitative deficiencies of band 3 caused by genetic mutations are responsible for 15–25% of cases of hereditary spherocytosis,[18,90] a disorder that is associated with progressive membrane loss (see Fig. 3–2*B*) (see Chapter 22). A qualitative defect that causes deletion of 9 amino acids at the interface of the amino-terminal cytoplasmic domain and the first transmembrane domain results in increased association of mutant band 3 with the membrane skeleton, leading to the decreased membrane deformability of hereditary ovalocytosis.[63,91]

The Rh protein complex consists of two nonglycosylated but palmitoylated membrane proteins, RhD and RhCE polypeptides, and RhAg,[92,93] which is not palmitoylated. Although the Rh protein complex is associated with the membrane skeleton, recent evidence suggests that this association may be mediated by interaction of the cytoplasmic domain of RhAg with ankyrin.[94] Red cells deficient in Rh protein complex, like band 3–deficient red cells, are stomatocytic and spherocytic because of membrane loss as a result of reduced linkages between the bilayer and the membrane skeleton (see Fig. 3–2*B*).[77]

Glycophorin C interacts with p55 and protein 4.1R and, through this association, it regulates the membrane content of both these proteins.[95,96] Red cell membranes that are completely deficient in glycophorin C have reduced protein 4.1 (approximately 70% of normal) and are completely deficient in p55.[76,97] As a consequence of protein 4.1R deficiency, red cells exhibit elliptocytic morphology and decreased membrane mechanical stability.[98]

Linking Proteins

Ankyrin, protein 4.2, and protein 4.1R link the cytoplasmic domains of membrane proteins with the membrane skeleton (see Fig. 3–1*B*). Deficiency of any of these proteins leads to abnormal cell shape and functional alterations in membrane properties.

The coupling of the membrane skeleton to the lipid bilayer is accomplished by ankyrin, which simultaneously interacts with spectrin in the membrane skeleton and band 3 in the bilayer.[99–101] This linkage is strengthened by protein 4.2, which binds both to band 3 and to ankyrin.[102–104] Deficiency of either ankyrin or protein 4.2 leads to membrane loss and spherocytosis (see Fig. 3–2*A*). Quantitative deficiency of ankyrin caused by various mutations is responsible for as many as 50% of cases of hereditary spherocytosis, and quantitative deficiency of protein 4.2 accounts for approximately 5% of cases of hereditary spherocytosis[18,19,105] (see Chapter 22).

Protein 4.1R has dual roles in the red cell membrane: it links the membrane skeleton to the lipid bilayer through its interaction with the cytoplasmic domain of glycophorin C, and it reinforces the interaction of spectrin with actin.[106–108] Deficiency of protein 4.1R decreases the membrane content of glycophorin C by 80%.[76] The elliptocytic morphology and decreased membrane stability of both glycophorin C– and protein 4.1R–deficient red cells is the direct consequence of decreased membrane content of protein 4.1R, and not of glycophorin C.

The integral proteins band 3 and RhAg, as well as proteins involved in linking them to the membrane skeleton (ankyrin and protein 4.2), are critical for maintaining membrane cohesion. Defective tethering of the membrane skeleton to the lipid bilayer (vertical interactions) caused by deficiencies of these proteins results in membrane loss and generates spherocytic red cells (see Fig. 3–2*B*).

Skeletal Proteins

The red cell membrane skeleton can be modeled as an irregular network in which the basic unit is a hexagonal lattice of six spectrin molecules. High- resolution electron micrographs show a highly repeated and remarkably regular organization of spectrin-actin–protein 4.1R complexes in which each complex is linked to adjacent complexes by multiple spectrin tetramers.[109,110] Although spectrin, actin, and protein 4.1R are the major constituents of this junctional complex in membrane skeleton, adducin, dematin, tropomyosin, and tropomodulin also have been identified as constituents of the multiprotein junctional complex (see Fig. 3–1*B*).[111–114] Functionally, lateral interactions among skeletal proteins, spectrin dimer-dimer interaction, and spectrin-actin–protein 4.1R interactions in the membrane skeleton (see

Fig. 3–5) regulate cell shape and membrane mechanical stability.[2,3] Defective lateral interactions among the skeletal proteins leads to decreased membrane mechanical stability and hereditary elliptocytosis (see Chapter 22).

Spectrin, a flexible, rodlike molecule, is composed of two nonidentical subunits (α-spectrin and β-spectrin), intertwined side to side. Spectrin heterodimers associate head to head to form tetramers through the interaction of the amino terminus of α-spectrin with the carboxyl terminus of β-spectrin.[115–119] Over 90% of spectrin exists in the tetrameric form in the normal red cell membrane. In addition to its interaction with α-spectrin, β-spectrin has several binding sites for interaction with other membrane proteins. Near the tail end (amino terminus) of β-spectrin is an attachment site for protein 4.1R and for actin.[120–122] Near the carboxyl terminus of β-spectrin is an attachment site for ankyrin, which through its binding to the cytoplasmic domain of band 3 links the membrane skeleton to the lipid bilayer.[123]

Qualitative defects that diminish the ability of spectrin dimers to self-associate to form tetramers result in decreased membrane mechanical stability, elliptocytosis, and cell fragmentation (see Fig. 3–5).[124–130] The extent of cell fragmentation and hence the clinical severity of the anemia is related to the extent of defective spectrin tetramerization.[131,132] The lower the membrane spectrin tetramer content, the greater the cell fragmentation. The vast majority of mutations resulting in defective spectrin tetramerization in hereditary elliptocytosis are in the α-spectrin gene.[130] In contrast to the elliptocytic phenotype, quantitative deficiency of spectrin resulting from reduced synthesis of either α- or β-spectrin leads to spherocytes, likely the result of decreased anchoring of the lipid bilayer to the membrane skeleton. Approximately 20–25% of cases of hereditary spherocytosis are the result of decreased spectrin synthesis[18] (see Chapter 22).

Actin in the red cell is unusual in being organized into short, highly uniform filaments of approximately 35 nm in length that align parallel to the lipid bilayer.[133] The length of actin filaments is tightly regulated by tropomyosin and tropomodulin and adducin function as actin-capping proteins in red cells.[112] Red cells with deficiencies in actin or any of the three actin-regulating proteins have not been identified.

Protein 4.1R has a dual function in the red cell membrane: it links the membrane skeleton to the lipid bilayer through its interaction with the cytoplasmic domain of glycophorin C, as discussed earlier, and stabilizes the weak binary interaction between β-spectrin and actin.[107,108] Stabilization occurs through direct interaction of protein 4.1R with both spectrin and actin.[134,135] Qualitative defects and quantitative deficiencies of protein 4.1R resulting in weakening of the spectrin-actin–protein 4.1R interaction lead to loss of mechanical stability, elliptocytosis, and cell fragmentation (see Fig. 3–5).[130,136–138]

In general, defects in either α-spectrin, β-spectrin, or protein 4.1R that weaken either spectrin-spectrin or spectrin-actin–protein 4.1R interactions (lateral interactions) induce decreased mechanical stability, cell fragmentation, and generation of elliptocytes and fragmented red cells.

RELATED DISEASES

Inability to maintain normal cellular deformability and membrane mechanical stability, key requirements for performance of the erythrocyte's function of oxygen delivery, is a feature of a number of hereditary and acquired disorders. The three factors that regulate red cell deformability—cell shape or cell geometry, cytoplasmic viscosity, and membrane deformability and mechanical stability—provide a rational basis for classification in terms of the dominant cell changes responsible for the pathobiology of abnormal red cells (Table 3–1).

TABLE 3–1. Molecular Basis and Mechanisms for Loss of Cell Deformability in Hereditary and Acquired Red Cell Disorders

	Mechanism	Molecular Defect
Cell Geometry: Stomatocytic/Spherocytic Red Cells		
Hereditary spherocytosis	Loss of cell surface area as a result of loss of vertical interactions between integral proteins and spectrin-based membrane skeleton	Deficiency of ankyrin, band 3, spectrin, protein 4.2, or RhAg
Hereditary stomatocytosis	Increased cell volume as a result of altered membrane cation permeability	Yet-to-be-defined defect in red cell membrane transport protein(s)
Immune spherocytosis	Loss of cell surface area as a result of partial phagocytosis of red cells by macrophages	Immunoglobulin G and complement binding to red cell surface proteins
Cell Dehydration: Red Cells with Increased Cell Hemoglobin Concentration		
Hereditary xerocytosis	Loss of cell water as a result of altered membrane cation permeability	Yet-to-be-defined defect in red cell membrane transport protein(s)
Sickle cell disease	Loss of cell water as a result of sickling-induced membrane permeability changes	Activation of KCl cotransporter and Gardo's channel
Altered Membrane Deformability and Decreased Membrane Mechanical Stability		
Hereditary ovalocytosis	Increased membrane rigidity	Deletion of 9 amino acids in the cytoplasmic domain of band 3
Hereditary elliptocytosis	Decrease membrane mechanical stability as a result of decreased affinity of lateral junctional complexes in spectrin-based membrane skeleton	Mutations in α- and β-spectrin and in protein 4.1R

CURRENT CONTROVERSIES & FUTURE CONSIDERATIONS

Erythrocyte Structure

- Reduced surface area/volume is dominant in determining red cell lifespan in the circulation, but the contribution of cell dehydration and increased membrane rigidity to red cell lifespan remains controversial.
- The relevance of mechanisms described for recognition and removal of senescent human red cells from the circulation needs to be resolved.
- The mechanism of nitric oxide transport by red cells remains controversial.
- Various red cell membrane protein interactions are dynamically regulated, potential mechanisms include phosphorylation, phosphatidylinositol 4,5-bisphosphate, variations in intracellular magnesium and 2,3-diphosphoglycerate during the oxygenation/deoxygenation cycle, and calmodulin effects caused by elevated intracellular calcium.
- The function of a large number of integral membrane proteins, including adhesion molecules and putative transport proteins has yet to be defined.
- Cell signaling is a feature of mature red cells, but the functional significance of such events is not known.
- The molecular basis for red cell disorders involving loss of cation homeostasis—hereditary xerocytosis and hereditary hydrocytosis—needs to be defined.

Suggested Readings*

Ballas SK, Mohandas N: Sickle red cell microrheology and sickle blood rheology. Microcirculation 11:209–225, 2004.

Bennett V, Baines AJ: Spectrin and ankyrin-based pathways: metazoan inventions for integrating cells into tissues. Physiol Rev 81:1353–1392, 2001.

Discher DE: New insights into erythrocyte membrane organization and microelasticity. Curr Opin Hematol 7:117–122, 2000.

Eber S, Lux SE: Hereditary spherocytosis—defects in proteins that connect the membrane skeleton to the lipid bilayer. Semin Hematol 41:118–141, 2004.

Gallagher PG: Hereditary elliptocytosis: spectrin and protein 4.1R. Semin Hematol 41:142–164, 2004.

Mohandas N, Chasis JA: Red cell deformability, membrane material properties and shape: regulation by transmembrane, skeletal and cytosolic proteins and lipids. Semin Hematol 30:171–192, 1993.

Mohandas N, Phillips WB, Bessis M: Red cell deformability and hemolytic anemias. Semin Hematol 16:95–114, 1979.

Mohandas N, Evans E: Mechanical properties of the red cell membrane in relation to molecular structure and genetic defects. Annu Rev Biophys Biomol Struct 23:787–818, 1994.

Full references for this chapter can be found on accompanying CD-ROM.

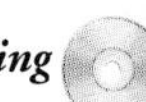

CHAPTER 4
RED CELL ANTIGENS AND ANTIBODIES

Marion E. Reid, PhD, Carol L. Johnson, BS, MT(ASCP)SBB, and Narla Mohandas, DSc

KEY POINTS

Red Cell Antigens and Antibodies

- Blood group antigens are carbohydrate or protein determinants that are carried on various red blood cell (RBC) membrane components. Antigens shown to be alternative forms inherited from one gene locus are organized into a single blood group system.
- Null phenotype cells lack a specific membrane structure and consequently all its antigens. Discovery of these natural "knockouts" has been key to our understanding of the function of many cell membrane components.
- Functions of RBC structures carrying blood group antigens include structural integrity, transport, receptor for extracellular ligands, cell adhesion, extracellular enzymes, complement regulation, and maintenance of surface charge in the glycocalyx.
- Because of blood group polymorphisms, antibodies to non-self RBC antigens may be produced by transfusion recipients or by women who have been exposed to RBCs during pregnancy. These antibodies have led to the serologic discovery of most known antigens.
- Blood group antibodies have clinical relevance because they may cause hemolysis of transfused antigen-positive RBCs, and during pregnancy they may result in hemolytic disease of the newborn. Testing to detect antibody in a patient's serum is required before selection of donor blood for transfusion; it is also performed during pregnancy as a part of standard prenatal care.
- The usual method for antigen typing and antibody detection is hemagglutination. All transfusion candidates are matched with ABO- and Rh-compatible donor blood. Detected antibodies in a patient's serum must be investigated to determine their specificity and potential to cause hemolysis. Antigen-negative blood is provided in the presence of a clinically significant antibody, especially for transfusion-dependent patients, who are likely to produce an increasing number of antibodies and thus require transfusion with more precisely matched RBC products.
- Immunoglobulin G blood group antibodies are clinically significant because they bind to their antigens at body temperature. Antibody-sensitized cells are then destroyed by extravascular hemolysis. Antibodies to ABO antigens, although largely immunoglobulin M, are by far the most significant. They react with their antigens over a broad thermal range, and their pentameric structure allows activation of vast quantities of complement, leading to acute intravascular hemolysis.
- Aside from ABO, the most commonly detected antibodies are directed toward antigens in the Rh, MNSs, Kell, Kidd, and Duffy blood group systems. In most cases, they are clinically significant, except for anti-M and anti-N, which react at room temperature or colder.
- Awareness of the racial mix of a donor population is helpful in screening for certain blood group phenotypes.

INTRODUCTION

Blood group antigens are of relevance in transfusion medicine when a patient who requires a transfusion, or is pregnant , is found to have unexpected blood group antibodies (see Chapter 98). Over 50 years of transfusion medicine practice, detection of alloantibodies has led to the identification of many blood group antigens, and to the so-called null phenotypes (natural "knockouts") and eventually to determination of the structure and function of the red blood cell (RBC) component carrying the antigen.

Our ability to detect and identify blood group antigens and antibodies has contributed enormously to the safe, supportive blood transfusion practices used today. Blood groups are clinically important in the immune destruction of RBCs in allogeneic blood transfusions, maternal-fetal blood group incompatibility, autoimmune hemolytic anemia, and organ transplantation. The polymorphisms of blood groups have been exploited as a tool to monitor in vivo survival of transfused RBCs. By virtue of their ease of detection by hemagglutination and simple mode of inheritance, blood group antigens have been used in genetic, forensic, and anthropologic investigations. Blood group profiles can predict inheritance of diseases encoded by genes in close proximity to the locus encoding the antigens. In the postgenomic era, knowledge of the molecular basis of blood group antigens and phenotypes is applied to microarray technology, which may revolutionize the practice of transfusion medicine. This chapter reviews the structural aspects of the molecules that express RBC blood group antigens, the function of these molecules, and the potential biologic significance of blood group polymorphisms and antibodies to clinical practice.

TERMINOLOGY FOR BLOOD GROUPS

The notation used to describe a blood group antigen has evolved over time, and antigens have been named by various terminologies: examples are a single letter (A, D, K), a symbol with a superscript (Fy^a, Jk^b, Kp^a), a symbol with a number (Rh17, Fy3, K12), and three or four letters (DAK, MAR, FPPT, TSEN). Sometimes all four types of notation are used within the same blood group system.[1] In order to reduce confusion, the Committee for Terminology of RBC Surface Antigens of the International Society for Blood Transfusion (ISBT) introduced a system of upper case letters and numbers to represent blood group systems and antigens in a format that allows both infinite expansion and computer-based storage.[2] The blood group antigens were placed into four categories:

- *Blood Group Systems:* genetically discrete clusters of antigens encoded by alternative forms at one gene locus (001 to 029 Series). Many components carrying blood group systems have been assigned CD (cluster of differentiation) numbers (see Table 4–1).[2]
- *Blood Group Collections:* serologically, biochemically, or genetically related antigens (200 Series)
- *Series of Low-Incidence Antigens:* antigens that occur in less than 1% of most populations studied and are not known to belong to a blood group system (700 Series)
- *Series of High-Incidence Antigens:* antigens that occur in more than 90% of most populations studied and are not known to belong to a blood group system (901 Series)

Nevertheless, confusing terminology persists; for example, the P1 antigen is the sole antigen in the P blood group system, and the P antigen is the only antigen in the GLOB system. There is also a GLOB Collection, with P^k and LKE antigens. In clinical practice, the traditional terminology is still extensively employed, and this nomenclature is used throughout this chapter.

Collectively, there are over 260 antigens recognized by the ISBT and only a handful that are not. We describe here the more commonly encountered antibodies and antigens.

TABLE 4–1. Blood Group Systems, in ISBT Order, and Associated Antigens

ISBT Name (Number)	Gene Name: ISGN (ISBT)	Gene Product Name (CD Number)	Null Phenotype	Function	Disease Association
ABO (001)	*ABO* (*ABO*)	*N*-Acetylgalactosaminyltransferase; galactosyltransferase	Group O Bombay (O^h)		Altered expression in some hematologic disorders—leukemia Absent in LAD II
MNS (002)	*GYPA* *GYPB* (*MNS*)	GPA (CD235a) GPB (CD235b)	En(a–) U – M^kM^k	Carrier of sialic acid; Complement regulation; receptor for microbes	Decreased *P. falciparum* invasion, may be receptor for *E. coli*
P (003)	*P1* (*P1*)	Galactosyltransferase			
Rh (004)	*RHD* *RHCE* (*RH*)	RhD (CD240D) RhCE (CD240CE)	Rh_{null}	Possible NH_4^+/H^+ counter-transport	Hemolytic anemia, hereditary stomatocytosis, reduced expression and mosaicism—hematologic malignancies, Rh_{null} syndrome
Lutheran (005)	*LU* (*LU*)	Lutheran glycoprotein B-CAM (CD239)	Recessive type Lu(a–b–)	Binds laminin	Increased expression possibly involved in vaso-occlusion in sickle cell disease
Kell (006)	*KEL* (*KEL*)	Kell glycoprotein (CD258)	K_0 or $Kell_{null}$	Cleaves big endothelin-3 to ET-3 (a potent vasoconstrictor)	
Lewis (007)	*FUT3* (*LE*)	Carbohydrate adsorbed from plasma	Le(a–b–)		Increased expression in fucosisdosis Absent in LAD II

TABLE 4–1. Blood Group Systems, in ISBT Order, and Associated Antigens—cont'd

Duffy (008)	*DARC (FY)*	Fy glycoprotein (CD234)	Fy(a–b–)	Chemokine/ *Plasmodium vivax* receptor	Resistance to *P. vivax*
Kidd (009)	*SLC14A1 (JK)*	Kidd glycoprotein	Jk(a–b–)	Urea transport	Impaired urea transport, urine concentrating defect
Diego (010)	*SLC4A1 (DI)*	Band 3, AE1 (CD233)	1 case: transfusion dependent	Anion transport	Southeast Asian ovalocytosis, hereditary spherocytosis, renal tubular acidosis
Yt (011)	*ACHE (YT)*	Acetylcholinesterase		Enzymatic	Absent from PNH III RBCs
Xg (012)	*XG (XG) MIC2*	Xg^a glycoprotein (CD99)		Adhesion	
Scianna (013)	*ERMAP (SC)*	ERMAP	Sc: −1, −2, −3	Adhesion	
Dombrock (014)	*DO (DO)*	Do glycoprotein; ART 4 (CD297)	Gy(a–)	Enzymatic	Absent from PNH III RBCs
Colton (015)	*AQP1 (CO)*	Channel-forming integral protein	Co(a–b–)	Water transport	Monosomy 7, congenital dyserythropoietic anemia
Landsteiner-Wiener (016)	*ICAM (LW)*	LW glycoprotein (ICAM-4) (CD242)	LW(a–b–) Also Rh_{null}	Ligand for integrin	Depressed in pregnancy and in some malignant diseases
Chido/ Rodgers (017)	*C4A, C4B (CH/RG)*	C4A; C4B adsorbed from the plasma		Part of the complement cascade	Certain phenotypes have increased susceptibility to autoimmune conditions and infections. C4-deficient RBCs predisposes for SLE
Hh (018)	*FUT1 (H)*	Fucosyltransferase (CD173)	Bombay (O^h)		Altered expression in some hematologic disorders—leukemia Absent in LAD II
Kx (019)	*XK (XK)*	Xk glycoprotein	McLeod phenotype	Transport; possible neurotransmitter	Acanthocytosis, muscular dystrophy, hemolytic anemia, McLeod syndrome
Gerbich (020)	*GYPC (GE)*	GPC (CD236) GPD	Leach phenotype	Interacts with protein 4.1 and p55. *P. falciparum* receptor	Hereditary elliptocytosis with mild hemolytic anemia Decreased protein 4.1 and p55
Cromer (021)	*DAF (CROM)*	DAF (CD55)	Inab	Complement regulation; binds C3b; disassembles C3/C5 convertase	Absent from PNH III RBCs Dr^a is the receptor for uropathogenic *E. coli*
Knops (022)	*CR1 (KN)*	CR1 (CD35)	Helgeson phenotype	Complement regulation; binds C3B and C4b; mediates phagocytosis	Antigens depressed in certain autoimmune and malignant conditions
Indian (023)	*CD44 (IN)*	Hermes antigen (CD44)	1 case: congenital dyserythropoietic anemia	Binds hyaluronic acid, mediates adhesion of leukocytes	
Ok (024)	*BSG (OK)*	Neurothelin, basoglin (CD147)	Ok(a–)	Adhesion	
Raph (025)	*MER2 (MER2)*	Tetraspanin (CD151)	Raph–	Adhesion	
JMH (026)	*SEMA-L (JMH)*	H-Sema-L (CD108)		Adhesion molecule; function in RBCs not known	Absent from PNH III RBCs
I (027)	*IGNT (IGNT)*	*N*-Acetylglucosaminyltransferase	I– (i adult)		Cataracts in Asians
Globoside (028)	*B3GALT3 (βGalNAcT1)*	Gb_4, globoside *N*-acetylgalactosaminyltransferase	P^k, p		Receptor: *E. coli* and parvovirus B19
GIL (029)	*AQP3 (GIL)*	AQP-3	GIL–	Glycerol/water/urea transport	

Note: Color associations with each structure in this table are the same as those in Figure 4–1.

Abbreviations: ISBT, International Society for Blood Transfusion; ISGN, International Society for Gene Nomenclature; LAD II, leukocyte adhesion deficiency II; PNH, paroxysmal nocturnal hemoglobinuria.

COMPONENTS OF THE RBC MEMBRANE

Specific protein components of the RBC membrane skeleton, which is associated with the inner leaflet of the lipid bilayer, interact with the cytoplasmic domains of some antigen-carrying transmembrane proteins.[3–5] Two major and well-defined interactions are (1) ankyrin, which binds to spectrin in the membrane skeleton and the cytoplasmic domain of the multipass transmembrane protein band 3 (anion exchanger, AE1)[6–14]; and (2) protein 4.1, which provides a link between spectrin, actin, and P55 in the membrane skeleton and the single-pass transmembrane proteins glycophorin (GP) C and GPD.[15–22] Some integral transmembrane proteins interact with other transmembrane proteins, forming either small or large macromolecular complexes: (1) GPA with GPB; (2) band 3 with GPA[23–27]; (3) Kell with Kx[28,29]; and (4) RhD, RhCE, RhAG, LW (intercellular adhesion molecule-4 [ICAM-4]), CD47, and GPB.[4,30]

Carbohydrates are restricted to the extracellular surface of the RBC membrane, where they collectively form a negatively charged environment, the glycocalyx. The glycocalyx, which is 10–15 nm deep, prevents spontaneous aggregation of circulating RBCs and their adhesion to endothelium, and also protects against microbial invasion. The majority of carbohydrates are attached to lipids on a ceramide backbone and to proteins by linkage either to asparagine (N-linked) or to serine or threonine (O-linked) residues.[31–34]

RBC BLOOD GROUP ANTIGENS

Blood group antigens are polymorphic, inherited carbohydrate or protein structures located on the extracellular surface of the RBC membrane. Recognition of a blood group antigen begins with discovery of an antibody. When an individual whose RBCs lack an antigen is exposed to RBCs that possess the antigen (usually through pregnancy or transfusion), an immune response may occur, producing antibodies that react with the antigen in an observable manner.

Carbohydrates attached to proteins or lipids in specific linkages define antigens in six blood group systems (*http://www.bioc.aecom.yu.edu/bgmut/index.htm*). Antigens of two systems (LE and CH/RG) are absorbed by the RBC membrane from the plasma. Antigens of the remaining 24 blood group systems are located on integral RBC membrane proteins or on glycosylphosphatidylinositol-linked (GPI) proteins (Fig. 4–1). Genes encoding 28 of the blood group systems have been cloned and sequenced[35] (Fig. 4–2) and the molecular bases of many antigens and phenotypes have been delineated.[36,37] Only the genes encoding for the P system remain to be fully characterized.

Years of meticulous hemagglutination studies not only have provided a vast knowledge base regarding the nature of the various blood group antigens but also identified blood samples with unusual characteristics for detailed genetic analyses. Genes encoding blood group

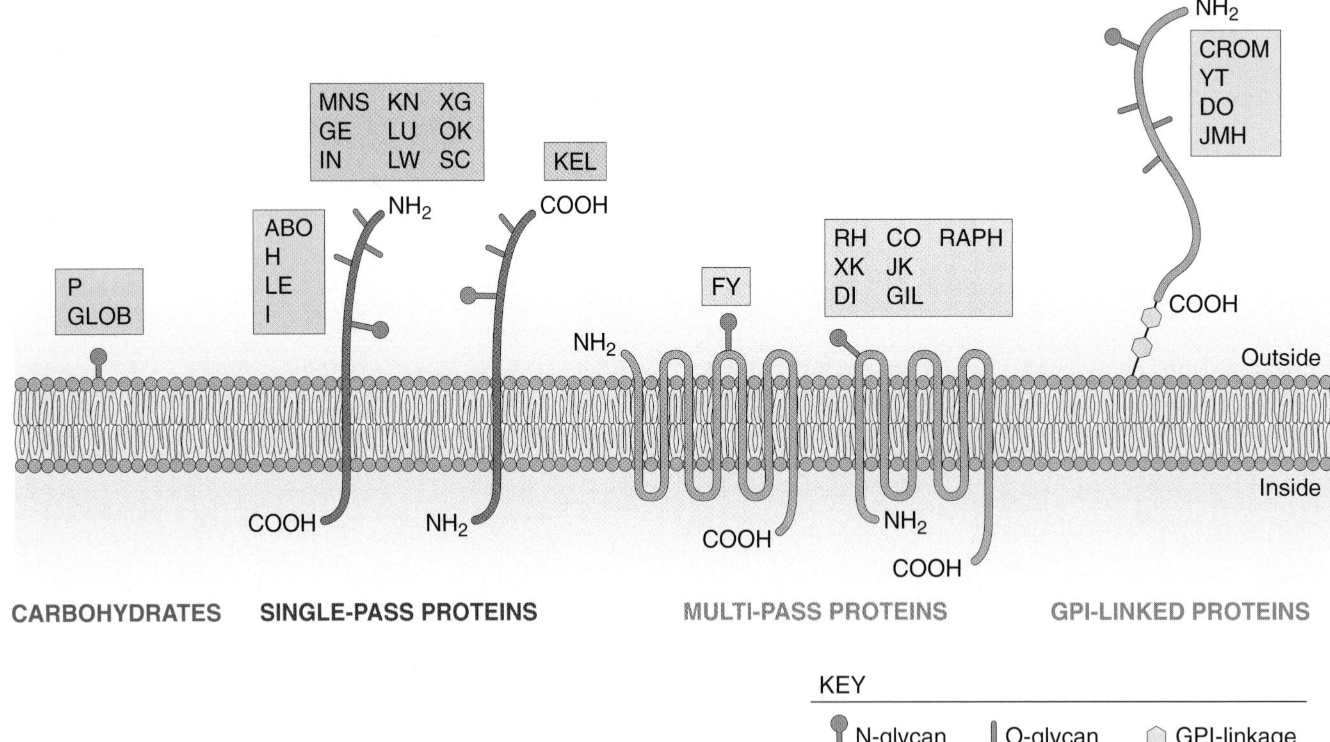

Figure 4–1. Model of RBC membrane components that carry blood group antigens. Carbohydrate antigens *(blue)* are attached to lipids (P, GLOB), or to lipids and proteins (ABO, H, LE, I). Of the blood group antigens present on single-pass proteins *(red),* most are on type I while Kell is on type II. Of the blood group antigens carried on multipass proteins *(orange),* most have both termini oriented toward the inside of the lipid bilayer, while the protein carrying Duffy antigens has its amino terminus oriented to the outside of the membrane. Antigens in the remaining systems are carried on proteins *(green),* which are attached to the lipid bilayer by carbohydrate moieties (glycosylphosphatidylinositol [GPI]-linked). CH/RG antigens are carried on C4d, which is absorbed onto the RBC membrane (not shown).

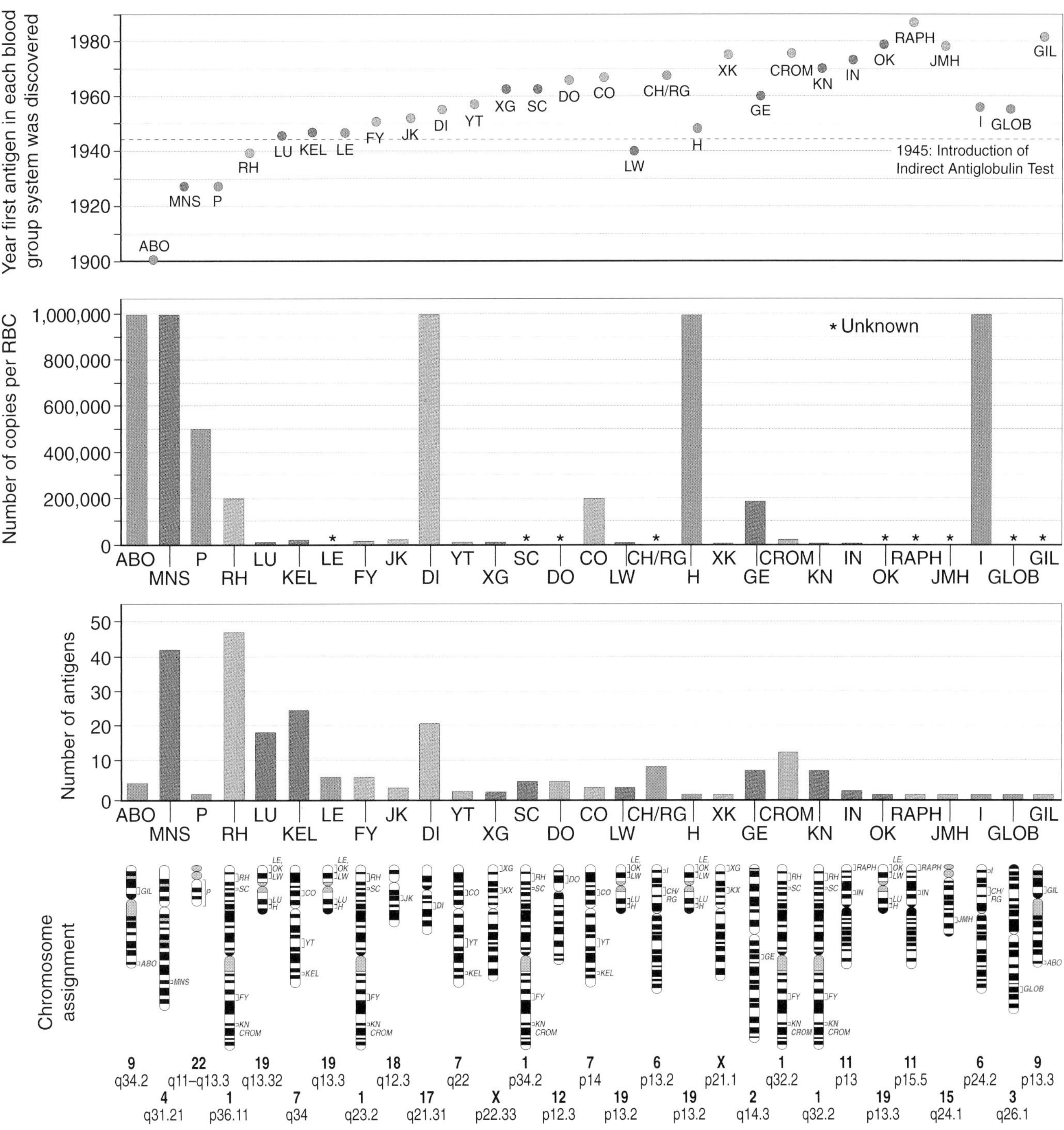

Figure 4–2. Blood group systems. *Bottom,* The first panel depicts the chromosome location of the gene encoding each blood group system. The second panel indicates the number of known antigens within each system. More than a third of the antigens are contained in only two systems (MNS and RH), and nearly a third (9) of the systems contain only one antigen each. *Middle,* The number of copies of each blood group per RBC. Clearly shown is the high copy number of carbohydrate antigens (ABO, P, H, and I), which contributes to the ability of their immunoglobulin M antibodies to effect direct agglutination. Also, there are high numbers of glycophorin A (which carries MN) and of band 3 (which carries the Diego blood groups). *Top,* The year that the first antigen of each system was discovered. Antigens M, N, and P_1 were described early, but using the serum of immunized animals, not with human antibody. Nearly 40 years elapsed between the discovery of ABO and the finding of a maternal antibody that detected the first antigen reported in the Rh system. The antihuman globulin method described in 1945 allowed discovery of the vast majority of protein-based blood group antigens. Some antigens (LW and H) were discovered years before they were assigned to a blood group system by the ISBT. *Note:* Color associations with each structure in this figure are the same as in Figure 4–1.

TABLE 4–2. Structure and Function of RBC Membrane Components Carrying Blood Group Antigens

	Structure of Component				
Function	**Carbohydrate**	**Single-Pass**	**Multipass**	**GPI-Linked**	**Adsorbed**
Glycocalyx	ABO GLOB H I P	MNS			LE
Structural		GE	DI RH XK		
Transport			CO DI GIL JK RH XK		
Adhesion/Receptor		IN LU LW MNS OK SC XG	FY RAPH	JMH	
Enzyme		KEL		DO YT	
Complement Regulator		KN MNS		CR	CH/RG

Note: Color associations with each structure in this table are the same as those in Figure 4–1.
Abbreviation: GPI, glycosylphosphatidylinositol.

antigens have been identified and the amino acid sequences predicted from the nucleotide sequence, provide insights into the topology and functions of proteins carrying the blood group antigens. In general, polymorphisms, which are recognized as blood group antigens and are significant in transfusion practice, do not alter the function of the specific component. Mechanisms of action predicted from sequence homology with proteins in other tissues may not apply to mature RBCs, altered forms may function as recognition signals in senescent RBCs, or important roles may be played during early stages of erythroid development.[38] Blood group antigens can be divided into broad physiologic categories: membrane structural integrity, transport, receptor for extracellular ligands, adhesion, extracellular enzyme, complement regulation, and maintenance of surface charge in the glycocalyx[4,39–43] (Tables 4–1 and 4–2).

Natural Knockouts and Related Diseases

The detection of an alloantibody to a high-incidence antigen during compatibility or prenatal testing has led to the discovery of RBCs with null phenotypes. Null phenotype RBCs lack the specific carbohydrate or carrier protein, and therefore all the blood group antigens within one system. These RBCs serve as natural "knockout" models and provide insights into the function of membrane proteins.

Rh Blood Group System and Hemolytic Anemia

The proteins RhD and RhCE express Rh blood group antigens. With an associated protein, RhAG, they form a core complex in the erythrocyte membrane that is stabilized by amino-terminal and carboxy-terminal domain associations. This Rh complex also contains LW glycoprotein (ICAM-4), integrin-associated protein (CD47), GPB, and possibly Duffy blood group glycoprotein.[44]

Although the function of the Rh protein complex in the normal RBC has yet to be completely defined, a structural role is suggested by evidence of an attachment site to the cytoskeleton,[45] and a transport function is indicated by the potential involvement of RhAG in the movement of ammonium.[46,47] The importance of the Rh protein complex in regulating red cell membrane structure was first revealed by the rare Rh_{null} phenotype; patients exhibit stomatocytic and spherocytic morphology with loss of membrane surface area, cell dehydration, cation permeability abnormalities, and shortened red cell survival, leading to a compensated hemolytic anemia.[48]

Lutheran and LW Blood Group Systems and Erythropoiesis

The Lutheran blood group glycoprotein is the receptor on erythrocytes for the extracellular matrix protein laminin.[49–51] Lutheran glycoprotein mediates adhesion of sickle RBCs to laminin.[52] Lutheran glycoprotein is expressed late in erythroid differentiation and may mediate erythroblast–extracellular matrix interactions in the bone marrow, regulating egress of reticulocytes into the circulation.[38]

The LW glycoprotein (also known as ICAM-4)[53] interacts with lymphocyte function–associated antigen-1 (CD11/CD18) and $\alpha_4\beta_1$ and α_V integrins.[54,55] LW glycoprotein also is expressed early in erythropoiesis and may function in erythroblast-macrophage interactions (in erythroblastic islands) that are critical for erythropoiesis.[56] Rare individuals with LW_{null} phenotype are apparently normal. Transient loss of LW antigen from the RBCs has been reported in pregnancy and in lymphoma, leukemia, sarcoma, and other malignancies.

Kell Blood Group System and Endopeptidases

The Kell glycoprotein, which has sequence homology with a family of neutral endopeptidases, is an endothelin-3–converting enzyme. Kell glycoprotein cleaves the precursor of endothelin-3, and less effectively the precursors of endothelin-1 and endothelin-2.[57] Endothelins are potent vasoactive peptides involved both in the regulation of vascular tone and in the differentiation of neural crest–derived cells during development. Kell glycoprotein is expressed in brain, testes, lymphoid tissue, and heart, but no phenotypic changes have been reported in these tissues or in erythroid cells from a lack of Kell glycoprotein.

Duffy Blood Group System and Malaria

The Duffy glycoprotein is a chemokine receptor in RBCs[58] and is expressed in many cells, including endothelium and epithelium.[59] Duffy glycoprotein binds a variety of pro-inflammatory cytokines of both the CXC class (acute inflammation) and the CC class (chronic inflammation), including interleukin-8, melanoma growth-stimulatory activity, monocyte chemotactic protein-1, and RANTES (regulated on activation, normal T cell expressed and secreted).[60–62]

The function of Duffy glycoprotein in normal RBC physiology is undefined. Duffy-null phenotype individuals have no obvious hematologic or immunologic abnormalities. The Duffy glycoprotein may have a role in enhancing leukocyte recruitment to sites of inflammation by facilitating movement of chemokines across the endothelium.[63] Duffy glycoprotein is the receptor for the malarial parasite, *Plasmodium vivax*.[64] Because Duffy-null RBCs are refractory to invasion by *P. vivax* merozoites, this phenotype, at least in Africa, likely is under selective pressure to circumvent the infection.

Kidd Blood Group System and Urinary Concentrating Defects

The Kidd glycoprotein is the major urea transporter in the RBC membrane.[65,66] It rapidly transports urea into and out of RBCs and prevents red cell dehydration as erythrocytes transit the renal medulla, which has a high concentration of urea. Urea transport across Kidd-null red cell membranes is approximately 1000 times slower than across normal membranes, but no phenotypic changes in either red cell shape or survival have been observed in the absence of Kidd glycoprotein.[67] Two Kidd-null individuals exhibited an impaired ability to maximally concentrate urine.[68]

Diego Blood Group System and Hereditary Spherocytosis

Band 3 (anion transporter), which carries antigens of the Diego blood group system, is a major integral transmembrane protein, comprising 25–30% of the RBC membrane protein content.[6] The 43-kDa amino-terminal cytoplasmic domain functions as an anchor point for the membrane skeleton through interactions with the peripheral membrane proteins ankyrin, protein 4.1R, and protein 4.2. In addition, this region serves as a binding site for the glycolytic enzymes glyceraldehyde-3-phosphate dehydrogenase, phosphofructokinase, and aldose, as well as for hemoglobin and hemichromes.[69] The transmembrane domain forms a channel that exchanges HCO_3^- and Cl^-, which enables the red cell to perform the critical function of uptake of CO_2 in the lungs. The carboxyl terminus is on the cytoplasmic side of the membrane and binds carbonic anhydrase II.[8]

Band 3 deficiency results in membrane surface area loss because of the disruption of membrane cohesion and the resultant generation of spherocytic RBCs (see Chapter 22). Approximately one fifth of human cases of hereditary spherocytosis result from a deficiency of band 3.[12,70,71] A qualitative defect resulting in deletion of amino acids 401 to 408 causes Southeast Asian ovalocytosis, which is characterized by unusually rigid ovalocytes with mild or absent hemolysis.[72–74] These ovalocytes resist invasion by malarial parasites. Ovalocytosis is predominant in Melanesia and Malaya, with an incidence as high as 25% in some populations.

Band 3 may play a role in physiologic RBC senescence. Hemichromes, a partially denatured form of hemogloblin, bind to band 3 more avidly than does hemoglobin, resulting in the formation of hemichrome-band 3 aggregates.[75] This clustering of band 3 generates a cell surface epitope identified by autologous immunoglobulin G (IgG) antibodies; this complex may act as a signal for the removal of aged or defective RBCs from the circulation by phagocytosis.[76–79]

Band 3 is also expressed in kidney. Mutations in transmembrane domains 6 and 7 and an 11–amino acid deletion in the carboxy-terminal domain of band 3 have been independently associated with the autosomal dominant form of distal renal tubular acidosis, a syndrome characterized by impaired distal nephron secretion of hydrogen ions.[80–83] The phenotype results from faulty targeting of band 3 to the apical rather than the basolateral membrane of collecting tubule type A intercalated cells, rather than from a defect in anion transport. A different mutation located in the intracellular loop between transmembrane domains 8 and 9 occurs in the autosomal recessive form of distal renal tubular acidosis, a phenotype also driven by faulty band 3 trafficking.[27]

Colton Blood Group System and Renal and Pulmonary Defects

The Colton blood group system is expressed on the protein aquaporin-1 (AQP-1), a major RBC water channel,[84,85] that functions to rehydrate red cells after their shrinkage in the hypertonic renal medulla. Human RBCs lacking AQP-1 (and consequently all Colton antigens) exhibit markedly reduced osmotic water permeability but no obvious phenotypic abnormality; patients are apparently healthy.[85]

AQP-1 is also expressed in kidney, lung, vascular endothelium, brain, and eye. Both defective urinary concentrating ability and decreased pulmonary vascular permeability occur in otherwise healthy individuals with complete deficiency of AQP-1.[86,87]

Kx Blood Group System and McLeod Syndrome

The McLeod syndrome is caused by mutations in the X-linked gene and thus is carried by females but only affects males. When the mutations include deletions encompassing other X-linked genes, diseases such as chronic granulomatous disease can be present.[88] In the red cell membrane, the Xk protein is covalently linked to the Kell glycoprotein by a disulfide bond, forming a stable complex.[28] The Xk protein is structurally analogous to a family of proteins involved in transport of neurotransmitters, but its transport substrate(s) have not yet been defined. Male hemizygotes who lack Xk on their red cells (McLeod syndrome) have weak expression of Kell antigens, variable acanthocytosis (8–85%), and mild, compensated hemolytic anemia (3–7% reticulocytes).[89,90] Female heterozygotes have occasional acanthocytes (as expected with X-chromosome inactivation) and very mild hemolysis.[89,90] Xk protein is also expressed in adult skeletal muscle, heart, and brain. Patients with McLeod syndrome may show elevated serum creatinine kinase and late-onset muscular (fourth decade), cardiac (fifth decade), and neurologic (sixth decade) defects that include skeletal muscle atrophy, diminished deep tendon reflex, choreiform movements, and cardiomyopathy[29,57,91–94] (*www.nefo.med.uni-muechen.de/~adenek/McLeod.html*).

Gerbich Blood Group System and Elliptocytosis

Red cells deficient in GPC (Leach phenotype, the Gerbich null) are elliptocytic and exhibit decreased membrane mechanical stability.[17,95] GPC is also expressed in renal endothelium, brain, cerebellum, and ilium, although at lower levels than in erythrocytes. No specific pathology resulting from GPC deficiency has been identified.

Knops Blood Group System and Complement

The membrane glycoprotein CR1 is a member of the complement control protein family and carries antigens of the Knops blood group system.[96] CR1 helps to protect RBCs from hemolysis by inhibiting the classic and alternative complement pathways through cleavage of C4b and C3b.[97] CR1 binds immune complexes, which are removed by the reticuloendothelial system in the liver and spleen without damaging red cell integrity. Acquired deficiencies of CR1 have been described in systemic lupus erythromatosus and other malignant, rheumatologic, and inflammatory disorders. Lowered levels of CR1 on RBCs may cause deposition of immune complexes on blood vessel walls, with subsequent vascular damage.

RAPH Blood Group System and Renal Failure

An absence of tetraspanin protein CD151, which carries the RAPH blood group system, does not result in observable RBC changes. CD151 is widely expressed in many cells and tissues. It forms stable laminin-binding complexes with integrins $\alpha_3\beta_1$ and $\alpha_6\beta_1$ in kidney and $\alpha_3\beta_1$ and $\alpha_6\beta_4$ in skin. Three MER-2–negative (MER-2 is the only antigen in the RAPH system) patients without CD151 had end-stage kidney disease; they also suffered sensorineural deafness and pretibial epidermolysis bullosa.[98] CD151 may be important for the proper assembly of the glomerular and tubular basement membrane in the kidney and may have as yet undefined functional roles in the skin and inner ear.

GIL Blood Group System and Transport of Glycerol, Water, and Urea

Aquaporin-3 (AQP-3), which carries the GIL blood group system, transports not only water but also glycerol and, to a lesser extent, urea.[85] AQP-3 is expressed in kidney, skin, lung, eye, and colon. The absence of significant changes in glycerol permeability in AQP-3–deficient RBCs suggests that an additional protein may also transport glycerol across the membrane, consistent also with lack of functional defects in GIL_{null} (AQP-3–deficient) RBCs.

ABO, I, and H Carbohydrate Blood Group Antigens

The blood group systems previously discussed are protein-based, and each is expressed on a unique component of the RBC membrane. In contrast, ABO, I, and H are carbohydrate blood group systems, and, although they are inherited independently, their specific carbohydrates are in single sequential chains attached to proteins and/or lipids in the RBC membrane.[36,39,41,99] Determinants of the I blood group provide a substrate for formation of H antigens, which in turn act as a precursor for ABO. The I antigen is expressed only weakly at birth but, as the carbohydrate chains branch, it reaches full expression by 2 years of age. The null phenotype in the H system, known as Bombay, expresses no H and therefore does not allow formation of ABO antigens. As a result, these rare individuals phenotype as group O, even though they may genetically be any ABO type.

BLOOD GROUP ANTIBODIES

Immune Response

Alloimmunization to RBC antigens occurs in about 1% of individuals who receive a blood product and in as many as a third of multiply transfused patients[100–102] (Fig. 4–3). A serologically identifiable primary response is transient and therefore usually observed only in patients who are chronically transfused and repeatedly tested. If a primary antibody response is no longer detectable during pretransfusion testing, then antigen-positive donor blood will appear compatible in laboratory tests and, if trans-

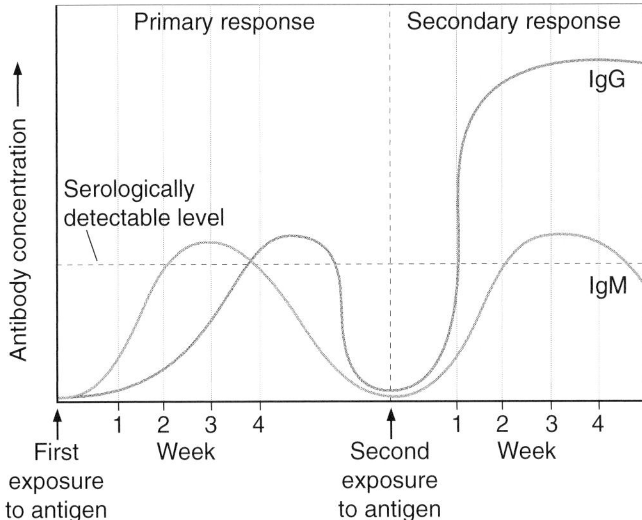

Figure 4–3. Immune response to non-self blood group antigens. The primary response slowly develops over a period of weeks, whereas the secondary response appears within days (and sometimes hours) of exposure. The secondary response is primarily immunoglobulin G and rapidly reaches a sustainable titer.

fused, will provoke a rapid secondary antibody response that may mediate hemolysis of the transfused cells. These delayed hemolytic transfusion reactions are usually not severe and may be unnoticed, except that the increment in hematocrit achieved by transfusion is short-lived.

Secondary immunization in women during pregnancy can potentially cause hemolytic disease of the newborn. Routine use of Rh immune globulin prophylaxis in Rh-negative women has greatly reduced the incidence of anti-D; however, there is no available prophylaxis to prevent production of other antibody specificities, which also are capable of causing severe hemolytic disease of the newborn. Maternal antibody to K, the major antigen of the Kell system, suppresses erythropoiesis and may cause severe anemia in a K-positive infant.[103–105]

Antibodies to some RBC antigens may appear without any exposure to red cells; these antigens are expressed on plants or bacteria and are first encountered at birth in the digestive tract.[106] These "naturally occurring" antigens are generally carbohydrates and produce immunoglobulin M (IgM) antibodies. Most common are anti-A and anti-B antibodies, which are found normally in all individuals who lack the corresponding antigens.

Clinical Relevance

Specific criteria define the characteristics of a clinically significant blood group antibody:

- Temperature range of reactivity (thermal amplitude)
- Concentration (titer)
- Immunoglobulin class or subclass
- Ability to bind complement
- Accessibility to antigen

In general, blood group antibodies of clinical importance are IgG, which bind optimally with their antigens at body temperature. Once sensitized with antibody, RBCs are marked for extravascular hemolysis. In high concentration, IgG antibodies are more likely to bind to adjacent antigen sites, thereby activating complement. Hemolysis is then amplified as reticuloendothelial cells in the liver and spleen recognize and destroy the complement-coated RBC.[107–110]

Most IgM antibodies react best with their antigens at ambient or colder temperatures and therefore are not likely to be clinically significant. They are also of no concern during pregnancy because IgM does not cross the placenta. Occasional IgM antibodies react at higher temperatures, and if their thermal range reaches 30° C or more, they may bind to antigen-positive RBCs in vivo. Once bound to RBCs, the pentameric structure of IgM allows activation of vast amounts of complement, resulting in intravascular hemolysis in acute episodes that may be fatal, as can occur with major antibodies within the ABO system. The high number of antigen sites also contributes to the severe transfusion reactions with ABO-incompatible transfusions (see Fig. 4–2). All individuals have these antibodies in their serum, except the 3–4% who are group AB, and therefore nearly all transfusion recipients are at potential risk.

ABO incompatibility is a primary cause of preventable transfusion-related fatalities.[111–113] The overwhelming majority of these adverse events are due to patient misidentification or other clerical mistakes, and not to technical errors (see Chapter 99). Approximately half occur when blood is transfused into the wrong patient; sample collection error, obtaining blood from the wrong patient, or mislabeling the sample are also responsible.[114]

Antibody Specificities

The antibodies most commonly encountered in a transfusion service are to major antigens in five blood group systems (Rh, Kell, Duffy, Kidd, and MNS), a consequence of their polymorphisms.[99,101,102] The antibodies produced are nearly always IgG and clinically significant, with the exception of anti-M and anti-N, which are rarely of medical importance because they are cold-reactive IgG. Other specificities are less common because the antigens occur with either very high or very low prevalence[107,108] (Tables 4–3 and 4–4) (*www.nybloodcenter.org*).

Hemagglutination Testing

The standard serologic method for immunohematology is hemagglutination in test tubes.[99] Automated assays based on agglutination and manual or automated solid-phase adherence assays are used in some laboratories today, but they have not replaced the use of test tubes in most settings. Direct agglutination was first described over 100 years ago and indirect agglutination 50 years later.[115] The method does not require sophisticated equipment and is simple, inexpensive, sensitive, specific, and reproducible (Figs. 4–4 and 4–5). Hemagglutination is influenced by the:

Characteristics of the antibody
Copy number and topology of the RBC membrane component carrying the antigen

TABLE 4–3. Characteristics of Some Blood Group Alloantibodies (Listed in Approximate Order of Clinical Significance)

Alloantibody within Blood Group System	IgM	IgG	Clinical Significance	
			Transfusion Reaction	**Hemolytic Disease of the Newborn**
ABO	Most	Some	Immediate; mild to severe	Common; mild to moderate
H in Bombay	Most	Some	Immediate; mild to severe	Mild to severe
Rh	Some	Most	Immediate/delayed; mild to severe	Common; mild to severe
Kell	Some	Most	Immediate/delayed; mild to severe	Sometimes mild to severe
Kidd	Few	Most	Immediate/delayed; mild to severe	Rare; mild
Duffy	Rare	Most	Immediate/delayed; mild to severe	Rare; mild
M	Some	Most	Delayed (rare)	Rare; mild
N	Most	Rare	None	None
S	Some	Most	Delayed/mild	Rare; mild to severe
s	Rare	Most	Delayed/mild	Rare; mild to severe
U	Rare	Most	Immediate/delayed; mild to severe	Rare; severe
$PP1P^k$	Most*	Most*	Mild to severe	Mild to severe†
Lutheran	Some	Most	Delayed	Rare; mild
Diego	Some	Most	Delayed; none to severe	Mild to severe
Dombrock	Rare	Most	Immediate/delayed; mild to severe	Rare; mild
Yt^a	Rare	Most	Delayed (rare); none to mild	None
Ch/Rg	Rare	Most	Anaphylactic (3 cases)	None
JMH	Rare	Most	Delayed (rare in genetic variants); none to mild	None
P1	Most	Rare	None (rare)	None
Le^a	Most	Few	Immediate (rare)	None
Le^b	Most	Few	None	None
Knops	Rare	Most	None	None

*Most examples of these antibodies have both IgM and IgG.
†Seldom hemolysis of fetal cells but high incidence of recurrent spontaneous abortions.

TABLE 4–4. Clinical Significance of Some Alloantibodies to Blood Group Antigens

Usually Clinically Significant	Sometimes Clinically Significant	Clinically Insignificant If Not Reactive at 37°C	Usually Clinically Insignificant
A and B	At^a	A1	Chido/Rodgers
Diego	Colton	AnWj	Cost
Duffy	Cromer	H	JMH
H in O^h	Dombrock	Lewis	HLA/Bg
Kell	Gerbich	Lutheran	Knops
Kidd	Indian	M, N	Le^b
P, $PP1P^k$	Jr^a	P1	Xg^a
Rh	Lan	Sd^a	
S, s, U	Landsteiner-Wiener		
Vel	Scianna		
	Yt		

Figure 4–4. Hemagglutination testing. At the top of the figure, the generic method for all agglutination testing is shown. Direct agglutination is compared with indirect agglutination (antihuman globulin test). Indirect agglutination includes the indirect antiglobulin test (IAT), which detects in vitro sensitization, and the direct antiglobulin test (DAT), which detects in vivo sensitization. In both the DAT and IAT procedures, thorough washing before adding antihuman globulin reagent is essential to remove free globulins that might inhibit the antiglobulin reagent, leading to a false-negative result. The procedure can be used to test unknown RBCs with reagent antibodies, and for unknown plasma/serum with reagent RBCs. During incubation, IgM antibodies will bind to their antigen and, because of their size, cross-link RBCs and induce agglutination (direct agglutination). When the test involves IgG antibodies (a much smaller molecule), antigen-positive RBCs are sensitized, but cross-linkage rarely occurs. A second antibody, antihuman globulin (AHG; anti-IgG), is required to cross-link the antibody-sensitized RBCs, and allow visualization of agglutination (indirect agglutination).

SET UP:

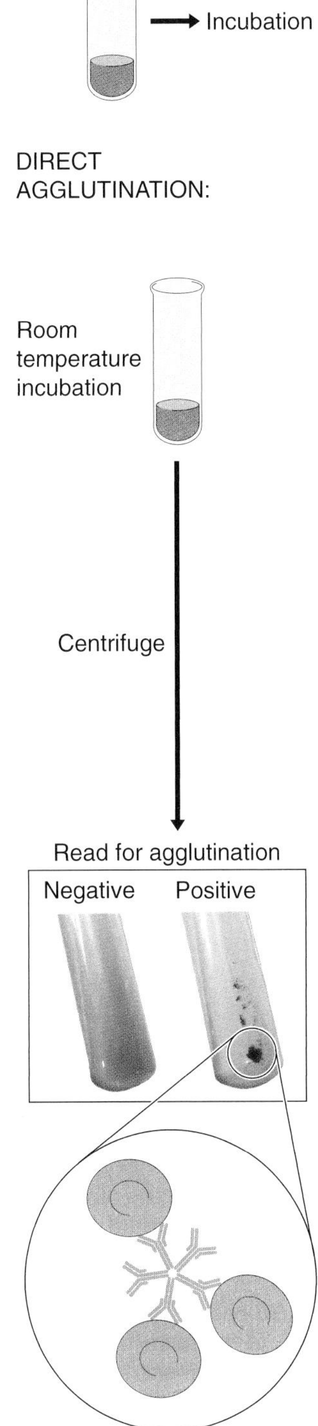

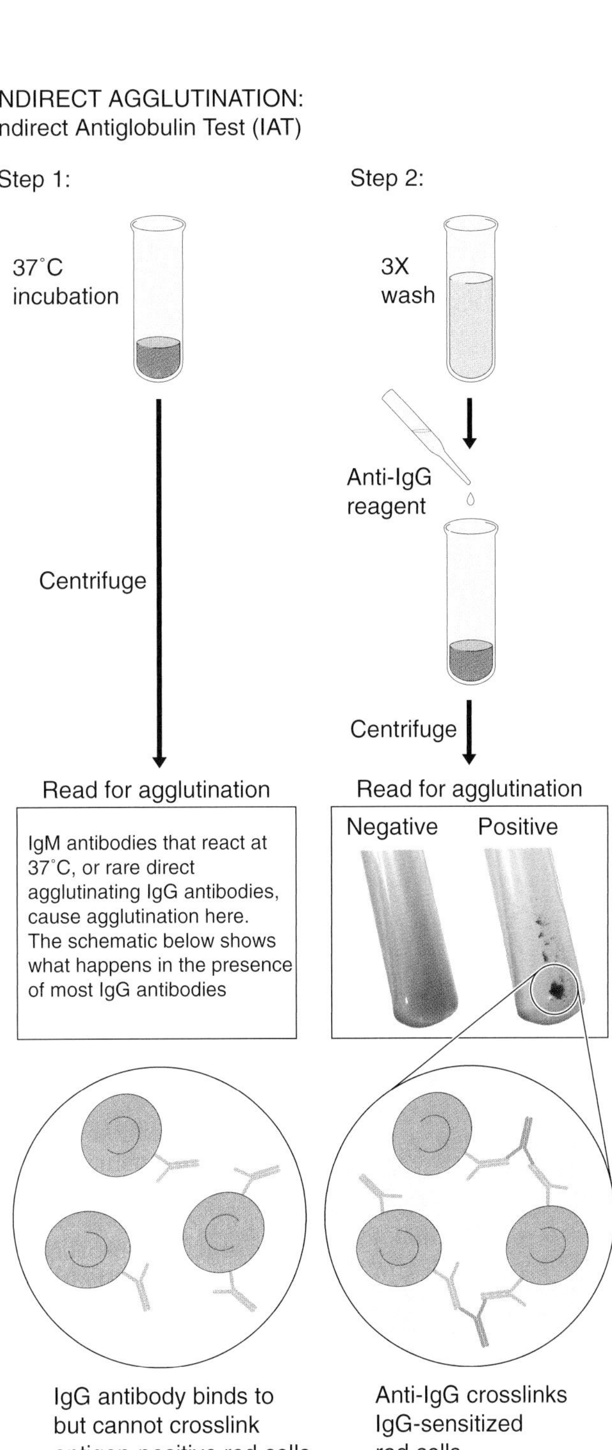

INDIRECT AGGLUTINATION:
Direct Antiglobulin Test (DAT)

3X wash

Anti-IgG reagent

Centrifuge

Read for agglutination

Negative Positive

Anti-IgG crosslinks red cells sensitized *in vivo* with IgG (C3 sensitized red cells detected with anti-C3)

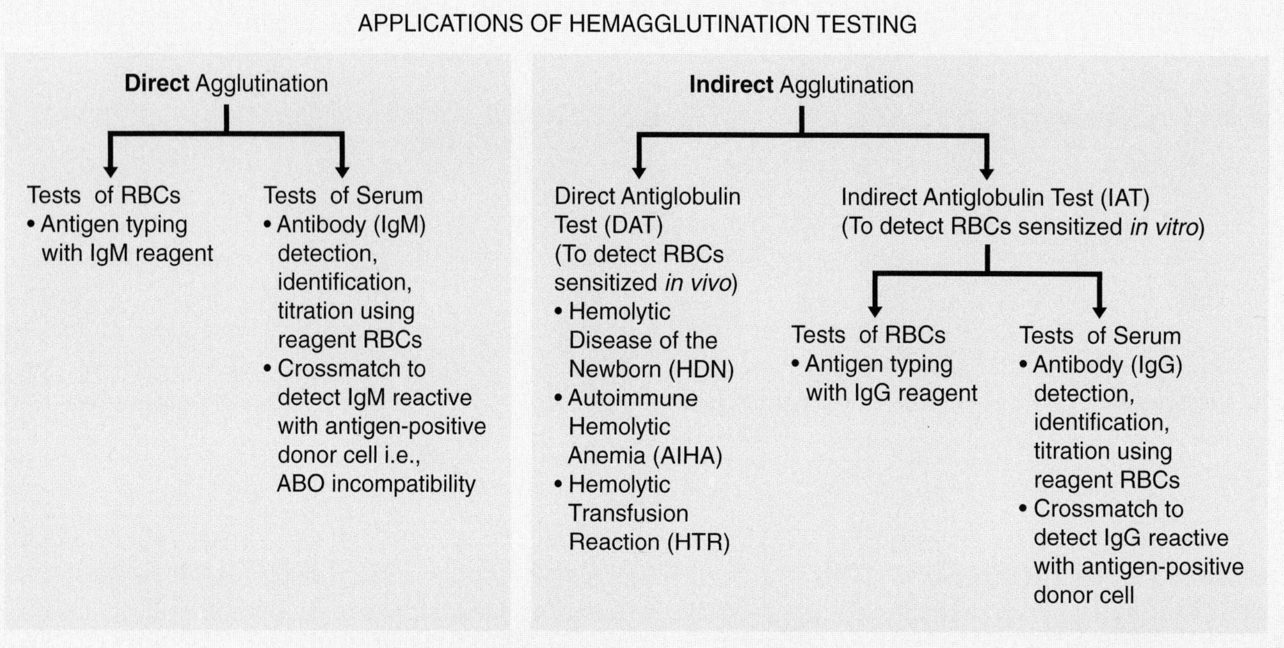

Figure 4–5. Applications of direct and indirect hemagglutination. These include detection of serum antibody using reagent RBCs, identification of an antibody specificity using a panel of reagent RBCs, and crossmatch testing of patient serum with donor cells. Both direct and indirect agglutination tests are also employed for antigen typing of RBCs using known antibodies.

The direct antiglobulin test (DAT) is a diagnostic assay that determines if a patient's RBCs have been sensitized with antibody or complement. Sensitization occurs in vivo, so the DAT consists of only one step. A positive reaction with anti-IgG would be expected in patients with warm-reactive autoimmune hemolytic anemia, in neonates with hemolytic disease of the newborn, and in recent transfusion recipients whose serum contains an alloantibody for an antigen on the donor RBCs and who may be experiencing a hemolytic transfusion reaction. RBCs from a patient whose serum contains cold autoantibodies may also have a positive DAT as a result of C3 bound by the IgM antibody and detected by anti-C3.

TABLE 4–5. ABO and Rh Typing

"Front" or "Forward" Typing: Tests of RBCs with			"Back" or "Reverse" Typing: Tests of Serum with		Interpretation		Prevalence in U.S. Donor Population
Anti-A	**Anti-B**	**Anti-D**	**A_1 Cells**	**B Cells**	**ABO Type**	**Rh Type**	
O	O	+	+	+	O	Positive	38%
+	O	+	O	+	A	Positive	36%
O	+	+	+	O	B	Positive	8%
+	+	+	O	O	AB	Positive	2%
O	O	O	+	+	O	Negative	7%
+	O	O	O	+	A	Negative	6%
O	+	O	+	O	B	Negative	2%
+	+	O	O	O	AB	Negative	<1%

Distance of the antigen from the lipid bilayer
Physical interactions

Pretransfusion Testing of Recipient

The protocol for pretransfusion testing of the recipient includes determining the ABO and Rh type and performing an antibody detection test (Fig. 4–6), followed by a crossmatch. Expected results for ABO and Rh typing are listed in Table 4–5. A flow chart summarizing appropriate action to be taken depending on results of the antibody detection test is shown in Figure 4–7.

Resolving ABO and Rh Typing Discrepancies

Any discrepancy between ABO red cell typing (forward typing) and serum typing (back typing) must be resolved.

ABO AND RH TYPING

Anti-A reagent
Anti-B reagent
Anti-D reagent
Patient serum
Patient serum
A
B
D
A_1
B
5% patient cells
5% patient cells
5% patient cells
A_1 cells reagent
B cells reagent
A
B
D
A_1
B
Centrifuge and read for agglutination

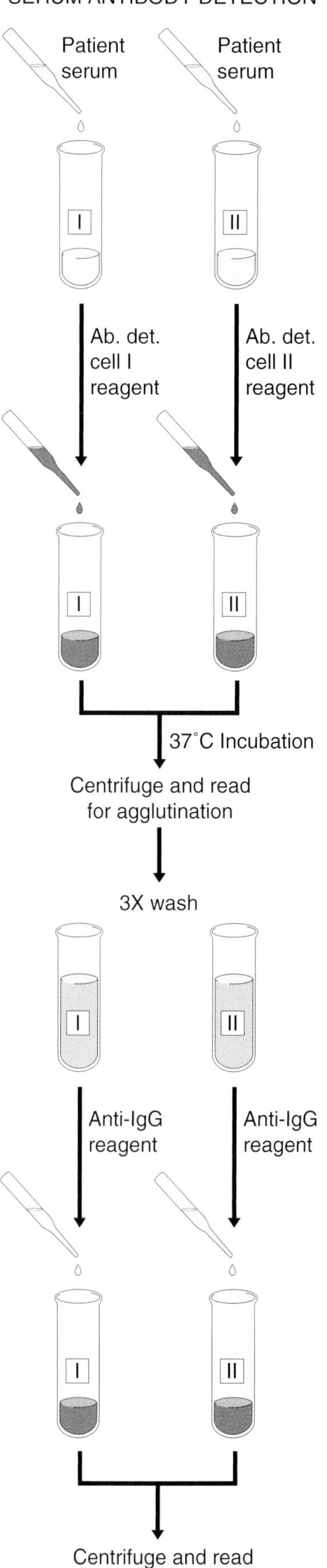

Figure 4–6. Pretransfusion testing of recipient. The protocol includes typing the recipient's RBCs for ABO and Rh, and testing of the recipient's serum (or plasma) for clinically significant blood group antibodies (antibody screen). Because the antibodies involved in ABO and Rh typing are IgM, the method used is direct agglutination. Because clinically significant antibodies are usually IgG, an indirect antiglobulin method is used. The final step is a match between patient and donor either by computer, or by physically testing the patient's serum against the selected donor's RBCs. Abbreviation: Ab. Det., antibody detection.

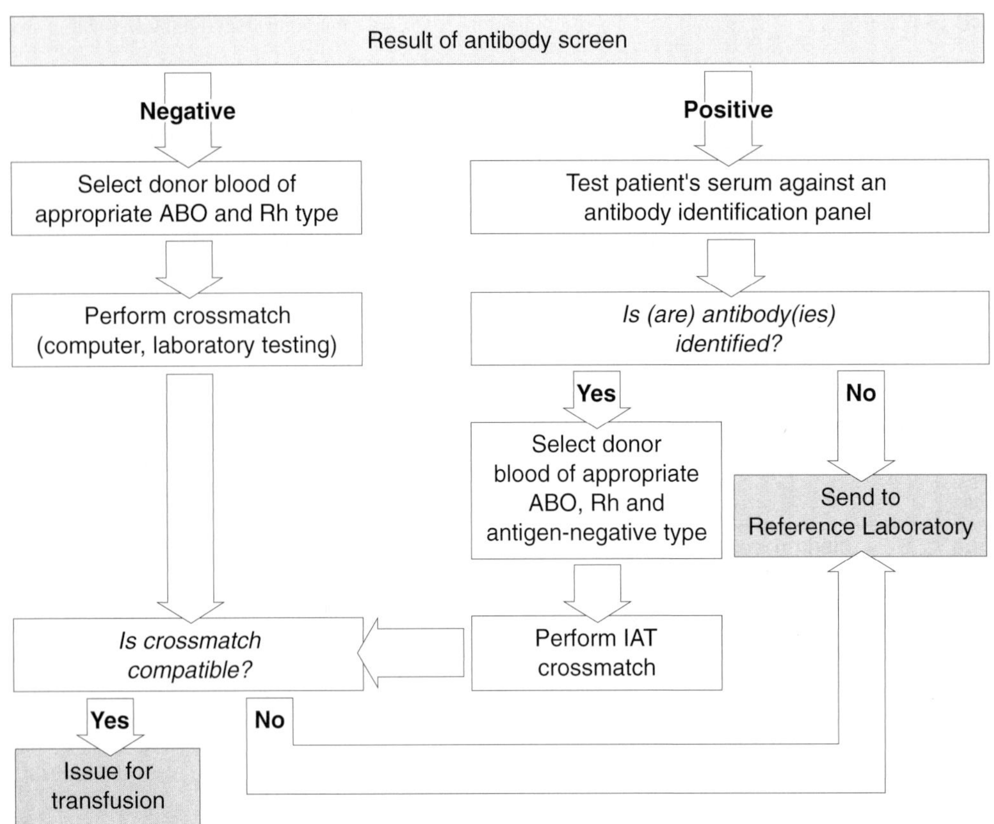

Figure 4–7. Flow chart for interpretation of the results of antibody detection test. When no antibody is detected and there is no record of the patient having an antibody, donor blood may be selected electronically ("computer crossmatch"). Alternatively, a direct agglutination test of the patient's serum with the donor's cells ("immediate spin crossmatch") may be performed to ensure ABO compatibility. If the patient has a clinically significant serum antibody in the current sample or identified in the past, antigen-negative donor blood is selected and an indirect antiglobulin test (IAT) crossmatch must be performed.

If transfusion is necessary before resolution, group O blood can be safely used (except in the rare Bombay patient, in which case the antibody detection test will be positive), because it carries neither A nor B antigens, which would be incompatible with anti-A and anti-B in the patient's serum. Some causes of ABO discrepancies are:

- Mixed cell population resulting from transfusion or transplant
- Weak antigen expression
  genetic variant
  altered by disease
- Lack of expected back-typing reaction(s)
  age of individual (neonate or elderly)
  low gamma globulin levels as a result of disease
- Unexpected back-typing reaction(s) caused by serum antibody to other RBC antigens

Atypical Rh typing results may also occur, often as a result of the complexity of the Rh blood group system.

Resolving Positive Antibody Tests

Antibodies detected by screening test are identified using an identification panel (Fig. 4–8). Complex cases in which a serum contains multiple antibodies may require tests with more RBCs of selected phenotypes in a reference laboratory (see Fig. 4–7). Special serologic techniques are available to analyze complicated patient samples. Considerations such as strength of antigen expression on reagent cells and the likelihood of certain specificities to react in a particular phase of testing figure in the analysis.[99]

In hemolytic anemia caused by warm-reactive autoantibodies, compatibility may be difficult to establish. It is more important to be sure that there are no clinically significant alloantibodies underlying the warm-reactive autoantibodies[100,116–119] (see Chapter 24).

Selection of Appropriate Donor Blood

Donor blood is typed for ABO and Rh by the blood collection facility. The plasma is also tested for the presence of clinically significant antibodies in order to eliminate the need to test the patient's RBCs with the donor plasma, and to prevent passive transfer of antibody to the recipient.

Donor RBCs selected for a recipient must be ABO identical or compatible with the patient's existing anti-A and/or anti-B antibodies (Table 4–6). Because of the immunogenicity and prevalence of the major Rh antigen (D), D-negative (Rh-negative) patients are given Rh-negative RBC products. In emergencies, when a large transfusion requirement cannot be met by the available O Rh-negative inventory, Rh-positive blood can be transfused if the patient has not made anti-D. Some volume of ABD-incompatible plasma can be, and often is, transfused until the level of passively transfused antibody becomes significant and may hemolyze patient RBCs.

When a patient's serum contains a potentially clinically significant antibody, blood for transfusion is further selected to lack antigens that correspond to the antibodies[99,120] (Table 4–7). Depending on the antigen-negative combination needed, it may be efficient to screen donors from certain ethnic populations (Fig. 4–9).

	Rh-hr					Kell		Kidd		Duffy		Lewis		MNSs				Test results	
cells	D	C	E	c	e	K	k	Jk^a	Jk^b	Fy^a	Fy^b	Le^a	Le^b	M	N	S	s	37°C	IAT
I	+	+	O	O	+	+	+	+	O	+	O	O	+	+	+	+	O	O	2+
II	+	O	+	+	O	O	+	+	+	O	+	+	O	O	+	+	+	O	O

A Antibody detection test

	Rh-hr					Kell		Kidd		Duffy		Lewis		MNSs				P	Test results		
cells	D	C	E	c	e	K	k	Jk^a	Jk^b	Fy^a	Fy^b	Le^a	Le^b	M	N	S	s	P_1	RT	37°C	IAT
1	+	+	O	O	+	+	+	+	O	O	+	O	+	O	+	O	+	+	O	O	2+
2	+	+	O	O	+	O	+	O	+	+	O	+	O	+	O	+	+	+	O	O	2+
3	+	O	+	+	O	O	+	+	O	O	+	O	+	O	+	O	+	O	O	O	O
4	+	O	+	+	O	O	+	+	O	O	+	O	O	+	O	+	O	+	O	O	O
5	O	+	O	+	+	O	+	+	O	O	+	O	+	+	+	+	+	+	O	O	O
6	O	O	+	+	+	O	+	+	+	+	+	O	+	+	+	+	+	+	O	O	2+
7	O	O	O	+	+	+	+	+	O	O	+	O	+	+	+	O	+	+	O	O	2+
8	O	O	O	+	+	O	+	O	+	+	O	O	+	O	+	O	+	+	O	O	2+
9	O	O	O	+	+	O	+	O	+	O	+	+	O	+	O	O	+	O	O	O	O
10	O	O	O	+	+	O	+	+	+	+	O	O	O	+	O	+	+	+	O	O	2+

B Antibody identification panel

Figure 4–8. Detection and identification of antibodies. *A,* Antibody detection test. Reagent RBCs used for antibody detection (antibody screening test) are selected so that at least one of the RBCs will be agglutinated if a patient's serum contains antibody to a major blood group antigen. In the antibody screening test, two reagent RBCs, numbered I and II in the first column of the sample, are used. The extended blood group phenotype of each RBC sample is indicated in the rows. Cell I, for example, is positive for antigens D, C, e, K, k, and Jk^a among others; and is negative for antigens E, c, Jk^b, and others. The two right-hand columns indicate the test results of the patient's serum with each reagent red cell sample after incubation at 37°C and after the indirect antiglobulin test. In this case, the positive reaction with RBC I indicates that the patient's serum contains an antibody. Detected antibodies are identified by using an antibody identification panel.

B, Antibody identification panel. When the antibody detection (screening) test is positive, testing of a panel of RBCs of varying phenotypes is necessary to reveal the specificity of the antibody. Panels may be incubated at ambient (room) room temperature (RT), and then centrifuged and read for agglutination to detect IgM antibodies. Lewis, P1, and sometimes MNS antibodies are IgM, and although they are not of clinical significance, their serologic activity may carry into other test phases and obscure analysis of those results. Tests are then incubated at 37°C and, after results are read for that phase of testing, moved into the antiglobulin phase. Positive reactivity in the antiglobulin phase indicates that IgG is present.

In the initial analysis, considerable information is provided by negative reactions. In this panel, four RBC samples are nonreactive, so antibody specific for any antigen expressed on those cells can be excluded. Cell #3 allows elimination of antibodies to antigens D, E, c, k, Jk^a, Fy^b, Le^b, N, and s. Additional rule-outs are made based on antigens expressed on the other nonreactive cells. The only remaining antibody possibilities are anti-K and anti-Fy^a. Each of the cells that react with the patient's serum are positive for one of these antigens, and the cells that are nonreactive with the patient's serum are negative for both of these antigens, confirming that both antibodies are present. In general, at least three RBC samples expressing the antigen must react and at least three RBC samples that are antigen-negative should not react, in order to identify an antibody. Antibody identification must also include a test of the patient's own cells and serum, called an autocontrol, to ensure that the antibody present is an alloantibody (especially with a mixture of alloantibodies or an antibody to a high-prevalence antigen) and not an autoantibody. Extended phenotyping of the patient's RBCs is often helpful in analysis of test results because, in general, alloantibody can be produced only against those antigens that the patient does not express.

Selection of blood for transfusion to patients with blood group alloantibodies is the joint responsibility of hospital staff and donor blood center. The transfusion service is needed for communication between the patient's physician or consultant hematologist and the donor center staff in order to determine predicted immediate and continuing transfusion needs and to ensure that appropriate antigen-negative blood is available. Clinical information that can be helpful for immunohematology problem solving includes

- Patient demographics: diagnosis, age, sex, ethnicity
- Medical history: previous transfusions, pregnancies, drugs, intravenous fluids used (Ringer's lactate, intravenous IgG, antilymphocyte globulin, antithrombocyte globulin), infections, malignancies, hemoglo-

TABLE 4–6. Selection of ABO-Compatible Donor Blood*

Recipient's Type	Donor RBC Type				Donor Plasma Type			
O	—	—	—	O	O	A	B	AB
A	—	A	—	O	—	A	—	AB
B	—	—	B	O	—	—	B	AB
AB	AB	A	B	O	—	—	—	AB

*Group O RBC donors are called "universal donors."

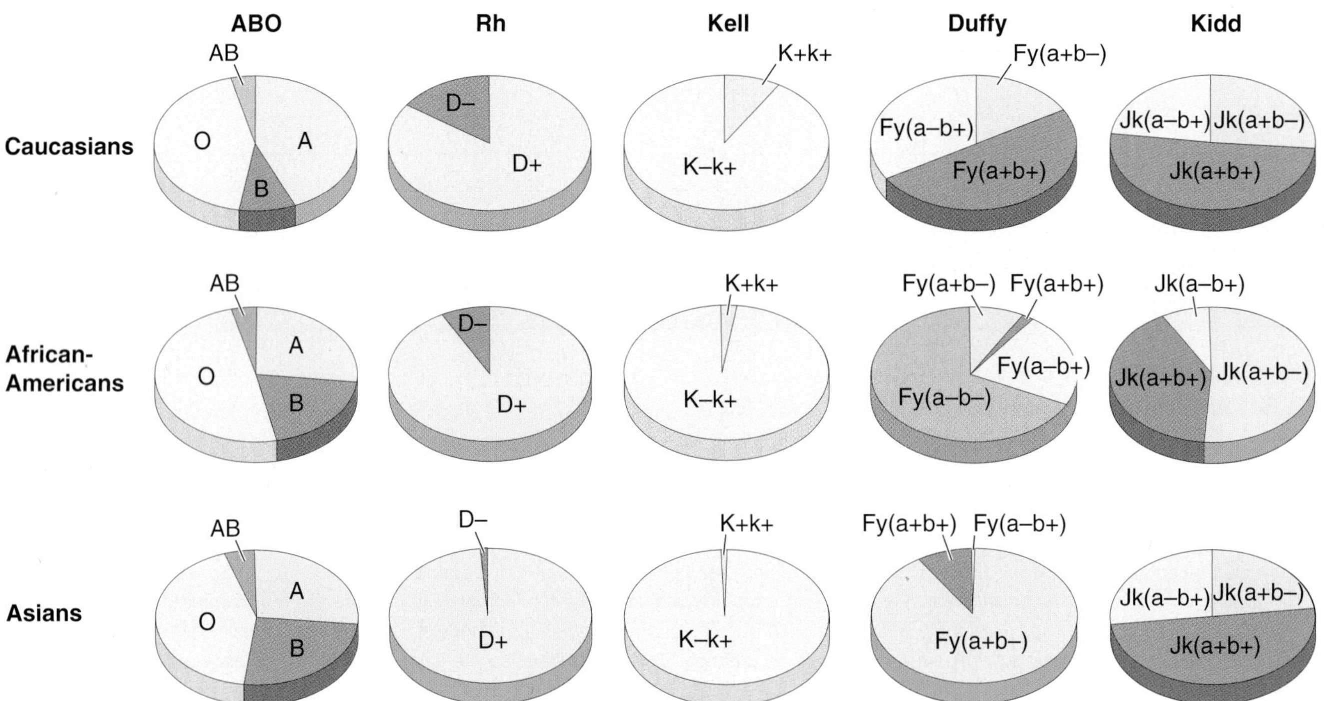

Figure 4–9. The distribution of selected phenotypes of the major blood groups in three populations. D– is rare in Asians; Fy(a–b–) (the null phenotype) is present in approximately two thirds of African Americans but effectively nonexistent in Caucasians and Asians; Fy(a+b–) is most common in Asians; and Jk(a+b–) is most common in African Americans. Thus, if a patient requires transfusion with K–, Fy(a–), Jk(b–) RBCs, the best population in which to search is African Americans, because this extended phenotype is found in 44% of African Americans but in only 8% of Caucasians and less than 1% of Asians.

binopathies, stem cell transplantation, records of previous hospitalizations

- Laboratory values: hemoglobin, bilirubin, lactate dehydrogenase, reticulocyte count, haptoglobin, hemoglobinuria, albumin/globulin ratio, RBC morphology

Antigen-negative blood can be obtained from several sources: screened hospital inventory, screened donor center inventory, available donors of known phenotype, autologous donation (with or without erythropoietin therapy), family members (particularly siblings), an extensively typed frozen blood inventory, and national and international rare donor registries. Blood-salvage procedures and methods to reduce blood use ("bloodless surgery") may be helpful for the surgical patient. In urgent situations, the use of antigen-positive RBCs may be an option after consideration of the risks involved.

Chronically Transfused Patients

Provision of antigen-matched blood to prevent antibody formation in patients who require chronic transfusion therapy, in particular for sickle cell disease (SCD), has been the subject of controversy,[121–125] and there is no consensus as to the best and most practical approach. The goal is to not only provide blood that will survive maximally but also to avoid immunization to blood group antigens. Three strategies are currently in practice[126–130]:

- Antigen-negative blood after the patient has made the alloantibody (traditional approach)
- Extended phenotype-matched blood after the patient makes the first antibody
- Blood matched for D, C, E, and K antigens only, as in the Stroke Prevention Trial (STOP) program

TABLE 4–7. Antigen-Negative Prevalence for Common Polymorphic Antigens

		Prevalence*	
System	**Antigen**	**Caucasian**	**Black**
Rh	C	0.32	0.73
	E	0.71	0.78
	c	0.20	0.04
	e	0.02	0.02
MNS	S	0.48	0.69
	s	0.11	0.06
Kell	K	0.91	0.98
	k	0.002	<0.001
Duffy	Fy^a	0.34	0.90
	Fy^b	0.17	0.77
Kidd	Jk^a	0.23	0.08
	Jk^b	0.26	0.51

*To calculate the prevalence of compatible donors, multiply the prevalence of antigen-negative donors for each antibody; for example, the prevalence of K−, S−, Jk(a−) donors in the general donor pool is 0.91 × 0.48 × 0.23 = 0.10 in 100, or 1 in 10.

TABLE 4–8. Serologic Tests as an Aid to the Diagnosis of Disease

Disease	**Diagnostic Test**
Rh_{null} syndrome	D−, C−, E−, c−, e−
McLeod syndrome	Kx−
LAD II (CDG II)	Le(a−b−), Bombay
HDN	DAT+
AIHA (WAIHA & CHAD)	DAT+ plus serum antibody
PNH (PNH III RBCs)	Cr(a−), Yt(a−), Do(a−b−)
PCH	Donath-Landsteiner test
Sepsis	Polyagglutination
Several hematologic malignancies	Altered expression of certain blood groups

Abbreviations: AIHA, autoimmune hemolytic anemia; CDG II, congenital disorder of glycosylation; CHAD, cold hemagglutinin disease; DAT, direct antiglobulin test; HDN, hemolytic disease of the newborn; LAD II, leukocyte adhesion deficiency II; PCH, paroxysmal cold hemoglobinuria; PNH, paroxysmal nocturnal hemoglobinuria; WAIHA, warm autoimmune hemolytic anemia.

Although it may be desirable to transfuse only phenotypically matched blood, it is not usually possible for the community to meet this request; indeed, in some regions it is a challenge to provide antigen-negative blood even to patients who are already alloimmunized.

Because the incidence of antigens differs in various ethnic groups, appropriate antigen-negative blood for patients with SCD is most likely to be found among African American donors[121–124,131] (see Fig. 4–9). However, RBCs from African American donors are also more likely to express immunogenic antigens that are not routinely tested: V/VS, Js^a, Go^a, and DAK. These antigens may provoke antibodies that would not ordinarily be detected because the antigens are not present on screening cells. We recommend in this group of patients that blood always be crossmatched using the indirect antiglobulin test in order to detect incompatible donor cells and to prevent a potential transfusion reaction in an alloimmunized patient.

Chronic transfusion in thalassemia, aplastic anemia, and steroid-resistant Diamond-Blackfan anemia does not elicit as many antibodies as in patients with SCD. Chronic inflammation associated with SCD appears to act as an immunologic stimulant.

RELATED DISEASES

Hemagglutination can directly diagnose syndromes that are caused by the absence of a component carrying blood group antigens (null phenotypes) (see Table 4–1). For example, an absence of the Rh proteins causes stomatocytosis and compensated hemolytic anemia (Rh syndrome)[30,132,133] and absence of Xk protein causes the McLeod syndrome.[28,91,93,134] Individuals with these conditions can be identified with a simple test of their RBCs with antibody to common Rh antigens and to Kx antigen, respectively. RBCs and white blood cells (WBCs) from patients with leukocyte adhesion deficiency II (also known as congenital disorder of glycosylation) lack antigens that are dependent on fucose; thus, their RBCs have the Bombay, Le(a−b−) phenotype and their WBCs lack $sialyLe^x$, which explains the high WBC count and infections.[135,136] Hemagglutination is also a valuable aid in the diagnoses (Table 4–8).[36,39,41]

Box 4–1. Potential Uses of DNA-Based Assays

- To type patients who have been recently transfused
- To identify a fetus at risk for hemolytic disease of the newborn
- To type patients whose RBCs are coated with immunoglobulin (positive direct antiglobulin test)
- To type patients with autoimmune hemolytic anemia in order to select antigen-negative RBCs for absorption of autoantibodies when searching for underlying alloantibodies
- To type donors, including mass screening for antigen-negative donors, when appropriate antisera are not readily available
- To type donors for use on antibody identification panels when antisera are not available
- To type patients who have an antigen that is expressed weakly on RBCs
- To resolve blood group A, B, and D discrepancies

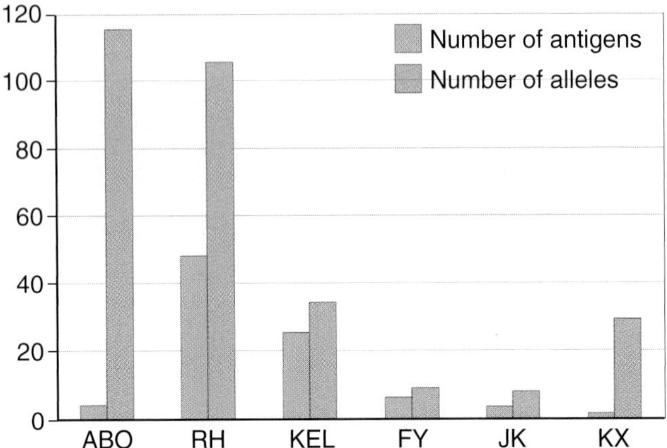

Figure 4–10. Alleles versus antigens. The number of known alleles relative to the number of antigens in the selected systems shows the high degree of diversity in ABO, RH and XK. Each antigen in each system must have at least one associated allele, and the extra alleles encode a multitude of variant phenotypes and null phenotypes within the system.

PERSPECTIVES ON DNA-BASED ASSAYS

Selection and provision of antigen-negative blood depends upon having sufficient reagents, which are often expensive or in short supply, and personnel to perform the labor-intensive testing and data entry. DNA-based assays provide knowledge of the molecular bases associated with blood group polymorphisms, making it possible to infer an antigen type.[137] DNA testing on microarrays has the potential to revolutionize transfusion practice (Box 4–1).[138] There is little difference in the cost and labor involved in testing a few or many polymorphisms, and data entry can be automated. This technology has not yet been approved by the Food and Drug Administration. Microarrays could serve as an invaluable screen for donor blood of particular phenotypes, followed by verification by classic hemagglutination. Some patients with extremely unusual phenotypes (especially in Rh) can make antibodies that are difficult to identify. The challenge of location of compatible blood for such patients may be met by mass screening using microarray technology, thereby allowing extensive phenotype matching of the donor and patient.

Although DNA-based assays have tremendous potential, they are unlikely to replace hemagglutination but will be a valuable adjunct. Genotype is not phenotype.[137] As examples, the ABO system consists of four basic phenotypes (A, B, AB, and O) but over 115 alleles that encode numerous variations; the many assays required to correctly identify a given ABO phenotype for the purpose of transfusion practice are unnecessary. Because the McLeod syndrome is associated with at least 29 alleles, DNA-based assays are more complex than is a single test with one antibody (anti-Kx) (Fig. 4–10).

CURRENT CONTROVERSIES & FUTURE CONSIDERATIONS

Red Cell Antigens and Antibodies

- Will hemagglutination ever be replaced as the standard testing method in transfusion medicine? Can any other practical technique be as specific and sensitive?
- Is providing antigen-negative RBC products before production of alloantibody(ies) feasible in the management of chronically transfused patients?
- Will molecular testing allow mass screening of donor populations and the provision of more precisely matched blood, even if genotype is not phenotype?
- What processes can eliminate clerical errors that result in serious transfusion reactions?
- What role do blood groups play in early erythroid development and removal of senescent RBC?
- Knowledge acquired about blood groups for over half a century has provided insights into human biology and disease. Modern technology ensures that this will continue.

Suggested Readings*

Blaney KD, Howard KD: Basic and Applied Concepts of Immunohematology. St. Louis: Mosby, 2000.

Brecher ME, Combs MR, Drew MJ, et al (eds): Technical Manual (ed 14). Bethesda, MD: American Association of Blood Banks, 2002.

Daniels GL, Fletcher A, Garratty G, et al: Blood group terminology 2004. Vox Sang 87:316, 2004.

Issitt PD, Anstee DJ: Applied Blood Group Serology (ed 4). Durham, NC: Montgomery Scientific Publications, 1998.

Lögdberg L, Reid ME, Lamont RE, Zelinski T: Human blood group genes 2004: chromosomal locations and cloning strategies. Transfus Med Rev 19:45–57, 2005.

Mollison PL, Engelfriet CP, Contreras M: Blood Transfusion in Clinical Medicine (ed 10). Oxford, UK: Blackwell Science, 1997.

Reid ME, Øyen R, Marsh WL: Summary of the clinical significance of blood group alloantibodies. Semin Hematol 37:197–216, 2000.

Woodfield DG, Anstee DJ, Flegel WA, et al: Rare blood: an updated report from the International Society of Blood Transfusion Working Party on Rare Blood Donors. Vox Sang (in press).

Web Sites

New York Blood Center: Immunohematology reference laboratory. Available at: *http://www.nybloodcenter.org/.* (description of clinical and technical aspects of blood group antibodies)

Albert Einstein College of Medicine for the Human Genome Variation Society: Blood group antigen gene mutation database. Available at: *http://www.bioc.aecom.yu.edu/bgmut/index.htm,* 2005. (comprehensive information about blood group genes and alleles)

***Full references for this chapter can be found on accompanying CD-ROM.**

CHAPTER 5

GRANULOCYTOPOIESIS

Peter Gaines, PhD, and Nancy Berliner, MD

KEY POINTS

Granulocytopoiesis

- Neutrophils circulate in the peripheral blood for only 3–6 hours, requiring a constitutive high level of neutrophil production by the bone marrow.
- Neutrophils arise from pluripotent stem cells under the influence of cytokines, notably granulocyte and granulocyte-macrophage colony-stimulating factors, which induce an intricate transcriptional program that drives morphologic maturation and neutrophil-specific gene expression.
- Neutrophils have a critical role in the innate immune response. They respond to bacterial and fungal infection through the processes of chemotaxis, endothelial adhesion, phagocytosis, and release of microbicidal enzymes, proteases, and reactive oxygen species.
- Disruption of neutrophil homeostasis can result in serious disease reflecting abnormalities of neutrophil number, maturation, or function.
- Neutropenia may be congenital or acquired. Evidence linking neutrophil elastase to congenital neutropenic syndromes has both provided new insights and raised new controversies regarding control of neutrophil production.
- Disruption of transcriptional control of myeloid differentiation is an important contributor to myelodysplasia and leukemia.
- Abnormalities in neutrophil function may arise either from defects in functionally important proteins (as seen in chronic granulomatous disease and leukocyte adhesion deficiency), or as a reflection of abnormal neutrophil differentiation (as in specific granule deficiency or myelodysplasia).

NEUTROPHILS

Neutrophils are highly specialized cells mediating both antimicrobial and inflammatory responses. They are produced in the bone marrow under the influence of an array of cytokines that induce a complex transcriptionally regulated program of differentiation. Mature neutrophils circulate in the peripheral blood for only 3–6 hours, placing a demand on the marrow for an impressive capacity for constitutive neutrophil production that can be rapidly upregulated in response to acute bacterial, fungal, or inflammatory stresses. The regulation of neutrophil number and the integrity of the neutrophil maturation program are both critical to normal homeostasis, and disruption of either can lead to serious disease. Deficits in neutrophil number and functional defects of mature neutrophils both predispose to life-threatening infection, and disruption of the maturation sequence underlies the pathophysiology of myelodysplasia and leukemia.

Neutrophil Ontogeny

Neutrophils arise from committed progenitors in the bone marrow through a series of maturational stages marked by morphologic changes, sequential acquisition of surface markers, and stage-specific production of phagocytic and secretory granules. This process takes 7–10 days, during which undifferentiated myeloblasts mature into fully functional neutrophils.[1,2]

Morphologic Changes

The earliest morphologically identifiable neutrophil precursor is the myeloblast, with a high nuclear/cytoplasmic ratio, prominent nucleolus, and minimal granules (Fig. 5–1). This is followed by the promyelocyte stage, which is characterized by the acquisition of primary granules. As discussed in detail later, these granules, common to both monocytes and granulocytes, fuse with phagocytic

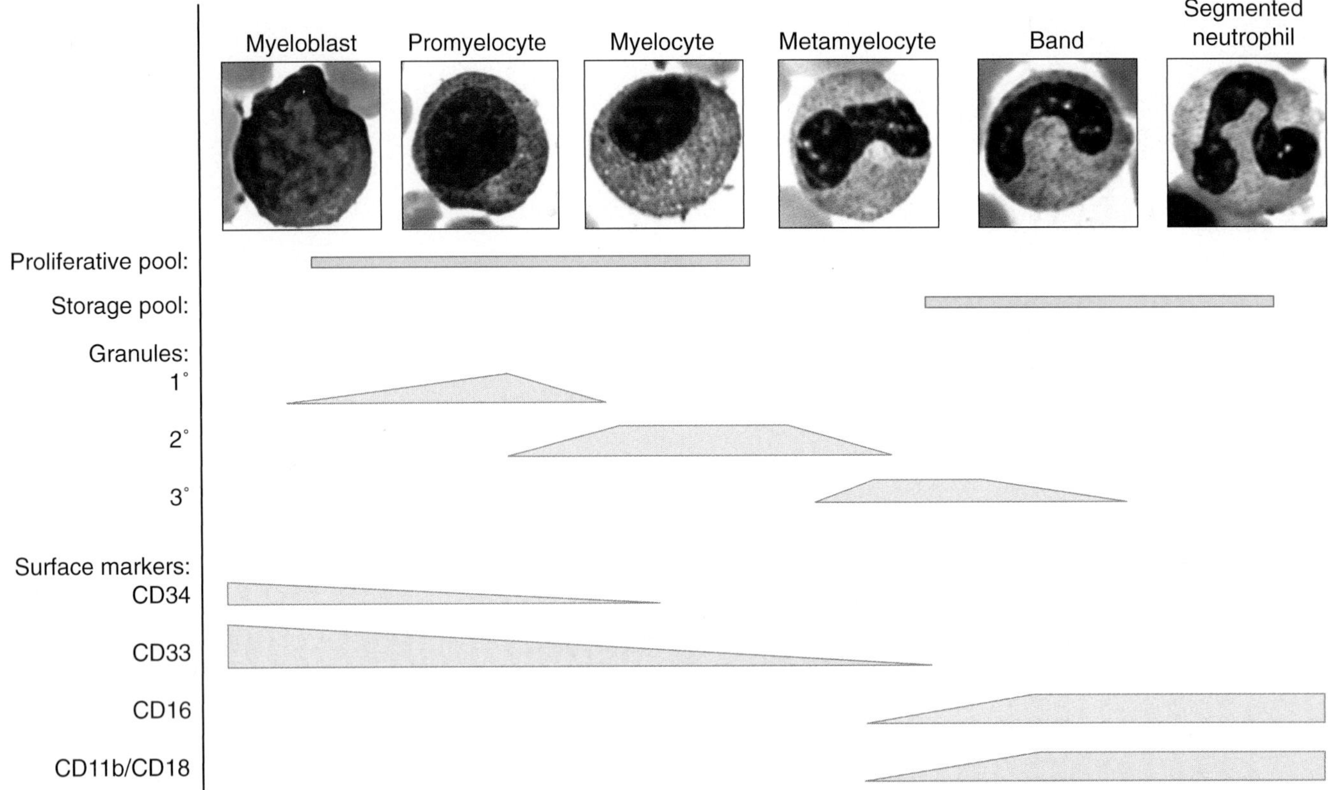

Figure 5–1. Differentiation schema of the neutrophil. The morphologic stages of neutrophil maturation are correlated with marrow pool distribution, stage-specific granule production, and characteristic surface marker expression.

vacuoles and contain many of the proteins that mediate intracellular microbial killing. The myelocyte stage is the last proliferative stage of differentiation, after which neutrophils mature as nondividing cells. Upon transition to the myelocyte stage, the neutrophils acquire the secondary granules that give them their characteristic appearance and serve to distinguish them morphologically from basophils and eosinophils.

Surface Marker Changes

Hematopoietic precursors are distinguished by characteristic antigenic proteins that are expressed on the cell surface (see Fig. 5–1). Many of these surface markers are important for normal cellular differentiation and function. They also allow the more precise identification of cell populations within the differentiating hematopoietic compartment. Early hematopoietic stem cells are $CD34^+/CD33^-$, and lack lineage-specific markers. This is the subpopulation of cells from which bone marrow engraftment is presumed to occur. The expression of CD33 is the marker that characterizes the common myeloid progenitor (colony-forming unit–granulocyte, erythrocyte, megakaryocyte, macrophage [CFU-GEMM]) and is expressed on early granulocytic and monocytic progenitors.[3] Unlike many of the surface markers expressed later in maturation, the functions of CD34 and CD33 remain unclear. Commitment to the neutrophil lineage and morphologic differentiation toward the myeloblast is associated with high-level expression of CD45RA,[4–6] myeloperoxidase, and CD38.[7] Further differentiation is associated with the expression of adhesion molecules (CD16, CD11a/CD18, CD11b/CD18),[5,8] which are expressed at high levels on mature neutrophils and are critically important to neutrophil trafficking and adhesion at sites of infection or inflammation. Defects in adhesion molecules cause predisposition to infection, as discussed later in this chapter.

Granule Protein Production

Granule protein production occurs in a sequential fashion throughout neutrophil maturation (see Fig. 5–1).[9,10] Primary granules arise at the transition from the myeloblast to the promyelocyte stage, and contain a wide array of antibacterial proteins.[10–12] These include myeloperoxidase, defensins, cathepsins, and elastase.[13,14] As discussed later, mutations in elastase have been implicated in the pathogenesis of cyclic and congenital neutropenia. At the transition to the myelocyte stage, neutrophils acquire secondary granules, and are considered a marker of commitment to terminal neutrophil differentiation. Secondary granules give neutrophils their characteristic staining properties, as do the corresponding eosinophilic and basophilic specific granules in other granulocytes. Neutrophil secondary granules contain lactoferrin, the cobalamin (vitamin B_{12})–binding protein transcobalamin I, neutrophil collagenase, neutrophil gelatinase, and gelatinase-associated lipocalin. Tertiary granules arise late in neutrophil maturation, and contain primarily gelatinase.[15,16] Secretory granules are formed in maturing neutrophils by endocytosis and contain plasma proteins.[17,18] It is hypothesized that the content of the primary, secondary, and tertiary granules is determined by the timing of synthesis of the various content proteins rather than by any more specific sorting mechanism.[19,20]

Neutrophil Kinetics

Over 95% of the neutrophil mass is sequestered within the bone marrow, where maturing and mature neutrophil precursors comprise approximately half of the marrow populating cells.[21] Over half of these are a mobilizable pool of bands and mature neutrophils, and the rest are precursors at various stages of granulocyte differentiation. The remaining 5% represent the circulating pool of neutrophils, of which 40% circulate freely in the intravascular space and the rest are adherent to vessel walls and sequestered within the spleen. These marginated cells are the most rapidly mobilizable population of mature neutrophils, and are released by a variety of stresses. The marginated pool provides the source of mature cells that allow the neutrophil count to double immediately in response to steroids, infection, and acute stress. Although the circulating pool represents only a small percentage of the neutrophil mass, its short lifespan demands that it be continuously replenished, and even a brief cessation in neutrophil cell production can cause a rapid fall in the peripheral white blood cell count.

Neutrophil Function

The mature neutrophil plays a critical role in the innate immune response, roaming the body in search of invading microorganisms. Exposure of the mature neutrophil to bacteria-derived products or inflammatory mediators, such as chemoattractants released from sites of infection, induces a complex series of functional responses culminating in microbial destruction. These neutrophil functional responses include chemotaxis toward the site of infection, adhesion to vascular endothelium, transmigration across endothelial cells, phagocytosis of microbial pathogens, and finally the release of potent microbicidal enzymes, proteases, and reactive oxygen species. Some of the key molecular mechanisms that mediate these functional responses are briefly discussed.

Engagement of Neutrophils with Endothelium and Transmigration

Recruitment of neutrophils to sites of infection begins with the activation of capillary endothelium. This activation is typically initiated by tissue injury and/or microbial invasion. Following injury, inflammatory mediators released by injured tissue, such as interleukin (IL)-1, tumor necrosis factor-α, and interferon-γ, activate the expression of endothelial selectins, type 1 membrane glycoproteins that interact with corresponding neutrophil surface proteins (Fig. 5–2). The earliest selectin to be expressed by activated endothelial cells is P-selectin, released from Weibel-Palade bodies, which engages P-selectin glycoprotein ligand-1, expressed on the surface of neutrophils.[22] This interaction initiates the early phase of rolling, a loose attachment of neutrophils onto capillary endothelium. Shortly thereafter, chemokines stimulate endothelial expression of E-selectins, which attach with low affinity to L-selectins also expressed on the surface of circulating neutrophils. Activated endothelial cells also release neutrophil-stimulating factors, including platelet-activating factor and chemokines such as IL-8, both of which lead to neutrophil activation.[23,24] Once activated, neutrophils shed L-selectin and mobilize secretory vesicles, leading to a rapid increase in cell surface β_2 integrin expression. These β_2 integrins, specifically CD11a/CD18 (lymphocyte function–associated antigen-1) and CD11b/CD18 (membrane attack complex-1), provide firm attachment to the endothelial cell by binding to their ligands, intercellular adhesion molecule-1 and -2 (reviewed by Wang and Doerschuk[25]). Following a concentration gradient of chemoattractants emanating from the underlying extravascular tissue, the neutrophil then transmigrates across endothelial cell junctions, mediated primarily by interactions between lymphocyte function–associated antigen-1 and intercellular adhesion molecules (see Fig. 5–2).[26] The importance of the β-integrins in neutrophil adhesion and transmigration is evidenced by the neutrophil functional defects seen in patients with leukocyte adhesion deficiency. This deficiency is caused by a lack of CD18 expression that renders neutrophils deficient in their adhesive and migratory capacity (reviewed by Roos and colleagues[27] and discussed later). Adhesion proteins expressed by endothelial cells and/or neutrophils also support transmigration. These include the platelet–endothelial cell adhesion molecule-1 (PECAM-1), the integrin-associate protein, and junctional adhesion molecule family members, such as JAM-C, expressed at the interendothelial junctions in association with tight junctions.[28–31] During the final stages of extravasation, neutrophils release granule proteases that lead to subendothelial basement membrane degradation and passage into the infected tissue. Two factors important to this process are gelatinase B, a metalloproteinase that degrades type IV collagen, and the gelatinase B activator neutrophil elastase.[32,33]

Chemotaxis of Neutrophils to Inflammatory Foci

Injured or infected endothelial cells release potent chemoattractants into the bloodstream, creating a concentration gradient that emanates from the site of infection. This concentration gradient of chemoattractants provokes a chemotactic response, a directed migration of neutrophils toward the site of chemoattractant release. Chemoattractants are composed of host-derived products, including chemoattraction-inducing cytokines (chemokines), the cleavage product of the fifth component of complement (C5a), or bacteria-derived products, such as the *N*-formylated tripeptide formyl-methyl-leucyl-phenylalanine (fMLP). Chemokines are small proteins characterized by four conserved cysteine residues that form key disulfide bonds; chemokines specific to neutrophil activation are the CXC chemokines, in which the first two cysteines are separated by one amino acid, and include IL-8, neutrophil activating peptide-2, growth-

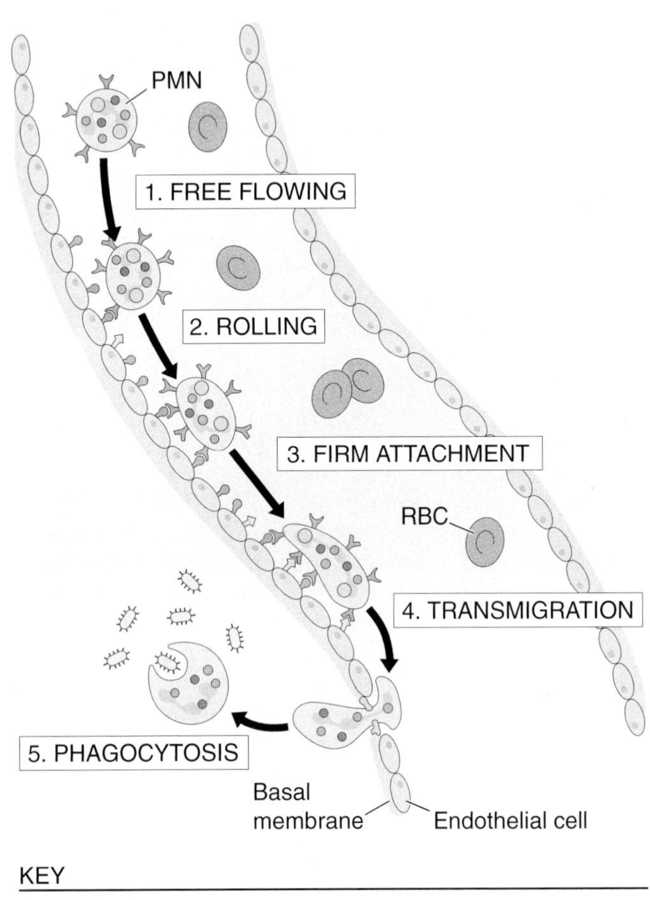

Figure 5–2. Sequence of neutrophil activation, showing process of rolling, engagement with the vessel wall, attachment, diapedesis, and phagocytosis. Abbreviations: PMN, polymorphonuclear cell; RBC, red blood cell.

related oncogene α, and epithelial cell–derived neutrophil activating protein-78.[34,35] These small molecules, referred to as "intermediary" chemoattractants, are released into capillaries at the site of inflammation and initiate the early stage of neutrophil chemotaxis. Once neutrophils have migrated into the vicinity of the infection, they bind to additional chemokines released by endothelial cells, promoting firm adherence and extravasation of neutrophils into the underlying tissue.

Each chemoattractant induces a chemotactic response by binding with high affinity to a specific seven-transmembrane-domain receptor, which in turn activates an intracellular signaling cascade via heterotrimeric G proteins that result in directional F-actin polymerization.[36,37] Interestingly, each type of chemoattractant receptor may utilize different intracellular signaling pathways to elicit the chemotactic response. For example, fMLP has been shown to induce primarily the activation of the p38 mitogen-activated protein kinase cascade,[38] whereas chemokines predominantly activate the phosphatidylinositol-3-kinase signaling pathway.[39–41] Furthermore, stimulation of neutrophils with fMLP can inhibit IL-8–induced phosphatidylinositol-3-kinase activation.[41] These differences in signaling pathways between chemoattractants have been suggested to create a hierarchy of migratory signals that help guide the neutrophil toward its final target. In this model, intermediary chemoattractants provide positional cues that guide neutrophils to the general vicinity of the infection, but thereafter, end-product chemoattractants dominate the chemotactic response, ensuring migration toward the pathogen.[42] This notion, however, is complicated by reports demonstrating that inhibition of phosphatidylinositol-3-kinase signaling disrupts fMLP-induced neutrophil migration, suggesting significant overlap between intracellular signaling pathways activated by each chemoattractant (see Niggli[43] and references therein).

Phagocytosis of the Pathogen

Phagocytosis by neutrophils is activated by direct binding of opsonized bacteria to specialized receptors expressed on the neutrophil cell surface (Fig. 5–3). The opsonins that coat bacteria are host-derived products found in serum, comprising immunoglobulins, typically immunoglobulin G, and complement fragments C3b and iC3b. Shortly after bacterial invasion, these particles coat the bacterial cell wall, labeling the pathogen for neutrophil digestion. Each immunoglobulin G molecule is bound to the bacteria via the F(ab′)2 domains, leaving the Fc domain exposed for direct interaction with Fcγ receptors expressed on the neutrophil. Complement factors also facilitate binding via CD11b/CD18, the β integrins that are rapidly transported to the neutrophil membrane during activation by fusion of secretory vesicles and specific granules. During the initial step of phagocytosis, the bound receptors cluster together, which initiates the activation of intracellular protein tyrosine kinases, including Src-family kinases and Syk/ZAP-70 kinases.[44–46] A progression of receptors are then recruited by the opsonins covering the pathogen, creating a zippering of the neutrophil membrane around the particle, coincident with increased particle binding and additional neutrophil activation (see Kwiatkowska and Sobota[45] and references therein). Once opposing membranes meet, engulfment is completed with the formation of the phagosome (see Fig. 5–3). This entire process is driven by actin polymerization and the formation of actin microfilaments, and can be directly inhibited by cytochalasin B, a well-known actin assembly inhibitor.[47–49]

Activation of Respiratory Burst in the Neutrophil

Shortly after formation of the phagosome, actin filaments disassemble, allowing fusion of the phagosome with primary and secondary granules, each armed with an arsenal of potent microbicidal proteases. The fusion

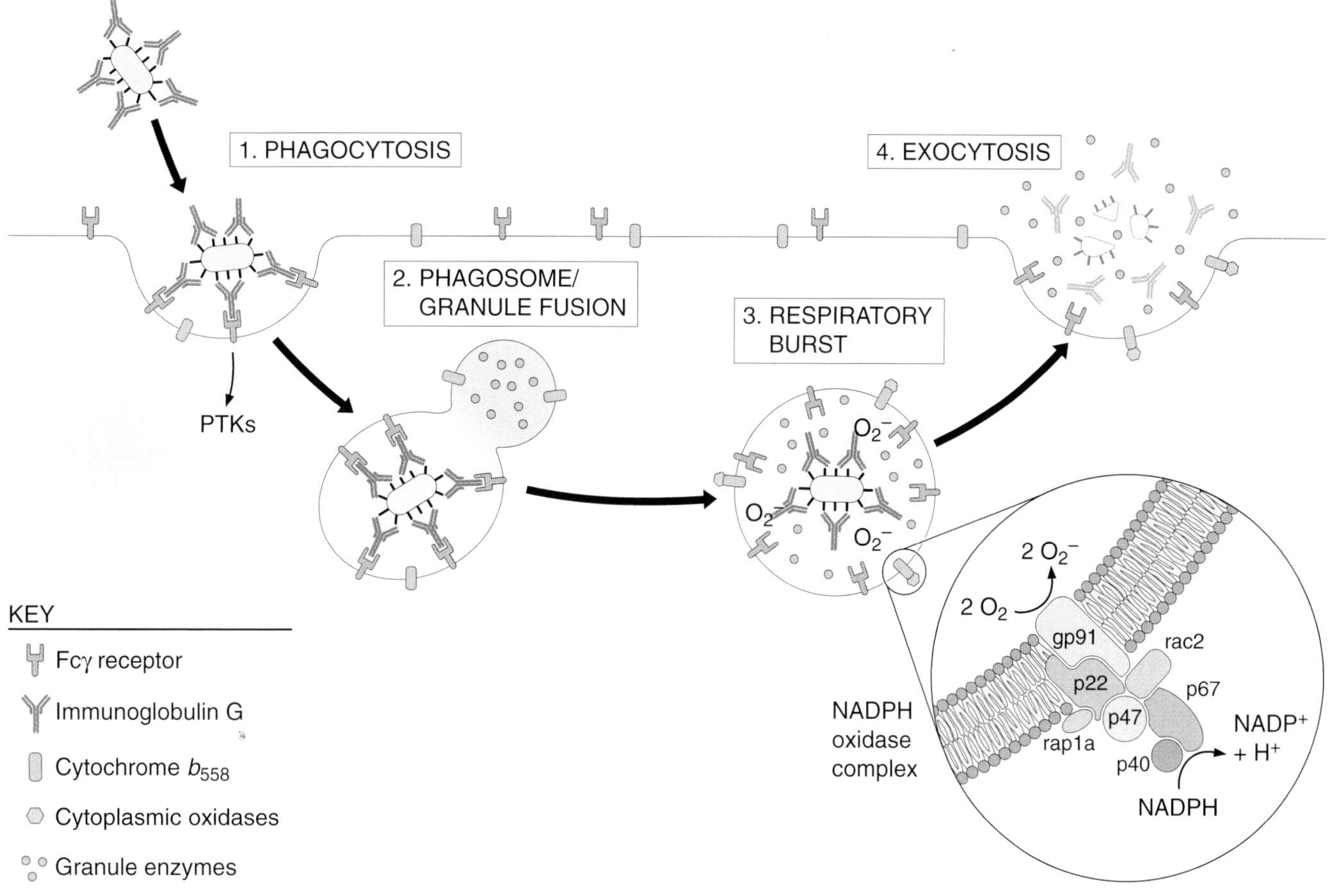

Figure 5–3. Events of functional intracellular killing of opsonized organisms by neutrophils, illustrating formation of the phagolysosome, fusion with granules, activation of the respiratory burst, and extrusion of debris. Abbreviation: PTKs, protein tyrosine kinases.

process also facilitates the assembly of NADPH oxidase, a complex that generates O_2^- within the phagocytic vacuole. NADPH oxidase is composed of a membrane-bound subunit, cytochrome b_{558}, and cytoplasmic subunits. Assembly of NADPH oxidase begins when cytochrome b_{558}, a heterodimer of $gp91^{phox}$ and $p22^{phox}$, becomes incorporated into the membrane of the phagocytic vacuole during the fusion process (see Fig. 5–3). Throughout this process, two intracellular components, $p47^{phox}$ and $p67^{phox}$, become phosphorylated by the actions of protein kinase C and the extracellular signal-regulated kinase 1/2 pathway.[50–53] Once phosphorylated, these components, together with $p40^{phox}$ and two GTP-binding proteins, Rap1A and Rac2, translocate to cytochrome b_{558} located within the phagocytic vacuole membrane, and to a lesser extent the plasma membrane, to complete the assembly of the NADPH oxidase complex.

Once fully assembled, NADPH oxidase functions to transfer electrons from cytosolic NADPH to molecular oxygen within the phagolysosome. This reaction generates superoxide anion (O_2^-) that is converted to hydrogen peroxide (H_2O_2) via the actions of superoxide dismutase. In a process catalyzed by myeloperoxidase, hydrogen peroxide reacts with additional superoxide anion to form the potent microbicidal product hydroxyl radical (·OH), which in turn can react with chloride ion (Cl^-) to form hypochlorous acid, also a potent antibacterial agent.[27,54] Together these reactive oxygen species kill the engulfed particles but are also released into the surrounding tissue, causing substantial tissue destruction and inflammation. This process is therefore tightly associated with neutrophil activation. Each member of the oxidase complex is essential to reactive oxygen species production, and reactive oxygen species production is critical to normal neutrophil function, as illustrated by the clinical syndrome of chronic granulomatous disease, a disease caused by disrupted expression of any one of the components of NADPH oxidase (reviewed by Goebel and Dinauer[55]).

Control of Neutrophil Production

Cytokine Regulation of Myelopoiesis

Neutrophil production is under the control of cytokines that induce a complex program of gene expression that specifies neutrophil-specific development (Fig. 5–4). The major cytokines implicated in neutrophil differentiation are granulocyte colony-stimulating factor (G-CSF) and granulocyte-macrophage colony-stimulating factor (GM-CSF).[56] The G-CSF receptor is expressed on myeloid progenitors at all stages of differentiation, contributing to the

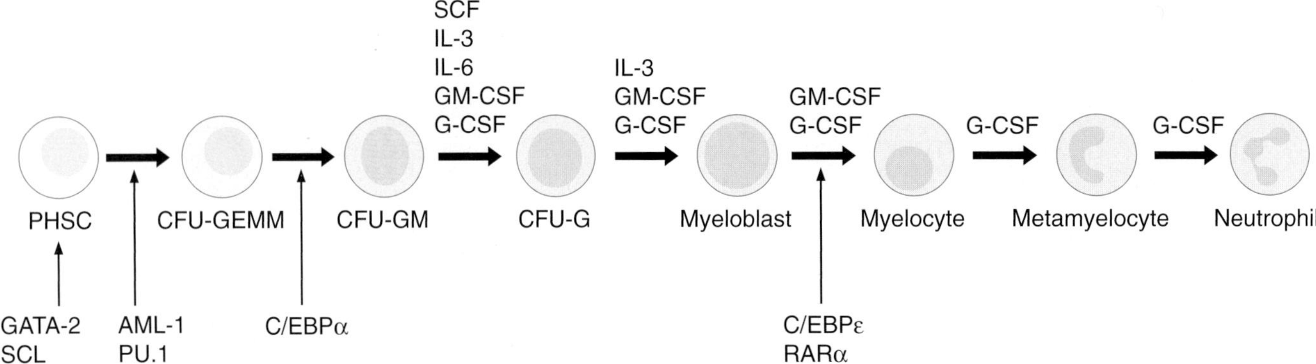

Figure 5–4. Neutrophil maturation. Cytokine mediators of maturation are noted above, and most important stage-specific transcription factors below. Abbreviation: PHSC, pluripotent hematopoietic stem cell.

survival, maturation, and functional activity of the granulocyte lineage. G-CSF receptors are also expressed very early in hematopoietic cell differentiation on a wide range of lineages, including platelets, monocytes, and lymphocytes, as well as on nonhematopoietic cells including endothelial cells.[57–60] This wide expression on multiple cell types is thought to explain the success of G-CSF in mobilizing early progenitors for stem cell collection and in speeding platelet recovery as well as neutrophil recovery following chemotherapy or transplantation.[61] The importance of G-CSF in neutrophil production is underscored by studies in G-CSF and G-CSF receptor knockout mice, which have decreased myeloid progenitors, are neutropenic, and have increased neutrophil apoptosis.[62,63] Nevertheless, such mice do maintain the ability to produce about 20% of the normal number of neutrophils, suggesting that other cytokine pathways can support neutrophil production.[63]

GM-CSF also influences myeloid differentiation through the induction of proliferation and differentiation of myeloid precursors. The cytokine binds to the GM-CSF receptor, a heterodimeric receptor with a unique α subunit and a β subunit that is shared by GM-CSF, IL-3, IL-5, and IL-6 receptors. The α subunit binds GM-CSF and the β subunit mediates high-affinity binding to the heterodimer. GM-CSF binding to its receptor induces signaling through Jak 2, and activates the Ras–mitogen-activated protein pathway (reviewed in[64]). GM-CSF has been shown to induce proliferation and differentiation of myeloid cells in vitro and has been used clinically to speed neutrophil recovery following chemotherapy or stem cell transplantation. Consequently, it is surprising that the GM-CSF–null mouse has no hematopoietic defects,[65] and that adult mice with combined null mutations in G-CSF and GM-CSF have no more neutropenia than mice lacking G-CSF alone.[66]

Transcriptional Regulation of Myelopoiesis

Myeloid maturation is a complex process that depends on the proliferation and survival of pluripotent hematopoietic stem cells, the differentiation to lineage-committed progenitors, and the granulocyte-specific maturation of myeloid precursors to mature neutrophils. Transcription factors are hypothesized to play the major role in determining the changes in gene expression that govern all aspects of this hematopoietic differentiation program.[67,68] The proliferation, survival, and lineage choice of pluripotent stem cells is influenced by a small number of broadly acting transcription factors, including SCL, GATA-2, and AML-1.[67] The process of commitment and maturation to the granulocyte lineage is driven by the expression of myeloid-specific genes, whose tissue- and stage-specific expression is regulated by a small number of lineage-specifying transcription factors, including PU.1, C/EBPα, and C/EBPε.[67] These factors influence gene expression that modulates both the phenotypic maturation and the acquisition of mature functional properties of the developing neutrophil. Studies in knockout mice and the dissection of gene defects underlying diseases affecting neutrophils have demonstrated that the transcriptional pathways governing phenotypic maturation overlap significantly with those that influence neutrophil function, such that diseases affecting neutrophil production and maturation also have an impact on the functional capabilities of the mature phagocyte. The main transcription factors governing myeloid maturation are outlined in Figure 5–4.

Transcription Factors Regulating Myeloid Differentiation and Myeloid-Specific Gene Expression

The specific transcription factors required for hematopoiesis have largely been defined by demonstrating loss of the granulocytic lineage upon targeted disruption of the genes in knockout mice. Many of these null mutations result in embryonic lethality, usually secondary to hematopoietic failure. Although an extensive discussion of myeloid-specific transcription factors is beyond the scope of this chapter, a few of the most important transcriptional regulators are mentioned briefly.

AML-1

AML-1 forms the α subunit of the core binding factor transcription complex, and has broad importance in hematopoietic differentiation.[69] AML-1–null mutations result in embryonic lethality because of a failure of establishment of definitive hematopoiesis in the liver in the developing fetus.[70] In addition, in vitro studies have demonstrated that AML-1 influences the expression of many myeloid-specific genes, including those encoding for the receptors for GM-CSF and macrophage colony-stimulating factor and for the early primary granule proteins myeloperoxidase and neutrophil elastase.[70–73] As discussed below, translocation of *AML1* is a common finding in human myeloid and lymphoid leukemia.[74]

C/EBPα

CCAAT/enhancer binding protein-α (C/EBPα) is a member of the C/EBP family of transcriptional activators that recognize a common consensus DNA binding sequence and bind as homo- or heterodimers to target genes in a wide range of tissues. C/EBPα has been proposed to be the "master regulator" of granulocyte development. C/EBPα-null mice die at birth from metabolic derangements induced by failure to express the gene in the liver; however, they also have a failure of development of both the monocyte-macrophage and the granulocyte lineages.[75] C/EBPα has been shown to bind to and regulate the expression of a wide range of neutrophil-specific genes expressed at all stages of neutrophil maturation, including the G-CSF receptor.[76–78] Genetic alterations that inhibit the expression C/EBPα have also been implicated in the development of acute myeloid leukemia (AML).[79,80]

C/EBPε

CCAAT/enhancer binding protein-ε (C/EBPε) is unique among the C/EBP family members in that its expression appears to be restricted to the granulocyte lineage. C/EBPε is expressed in the later stages of neutrophil differentiation, where it regulates the expression of late neutrophil-specific genes.[81] C/EBPε-null mice produce morphologically abnormal granulocytes that lack secondary granules and display multiple defects in neutrophil function.[82] These mice go on to develop myelodysplasia and have a shortened life expectancy, dying of low-pathogenicity bacterial infections.[82] Truncation mutations in the human C/EBPε gene have been shown to be the cause of disease in a subset of patients with specific granule deficiency, a rare neutrophil disorder associated with a propensity to bacterial infection and the absence of specific granules and their content proteins.[83,84]

PU.1

PU.1 is a member of the Ets family of transcription factors.[85] It is widely expressed in multiple hematopoietic lineages, and the relative level of PU.1 expression appears to influence lineage choice in hematopoietic cells. Knockout of PU.1 expression results in perinatal lethality with absence of the monocyte-macrophage lineage and delayed development and reduction in the granulocytic lineage.[86] Granulocyte precursors from PU.1$^{-/-}$ mice show defective late maturation. Like C/EBPα, PU.1 binds to the promoters of nearly all myeloid-specific promoters, including those for macrophage colony-stimulating factor, GM-CSF, and G-CSF.[87] Studies suggest that PU.1 expression is modulated by C/EBPα, and that the relative level of expression of the two transcription factors plays a role in modulating monocyte-macrophage versus neutrophil differentiation.[88]

RARα

The retinoic acid receptor α is a member of the nuclear receptor superfamily that specifically binds all-*trans* retinoic acid (ATRA), a lipophilic molecule derived from vitamin A (retinol). RARα regulates the transcription of retinoic acid target genes as a heterodimer with the retinoid X receptor (RXR). In the absence of ligand, the RARα/RXR heterodimer recruits corepressor complexes that include N-CoR, Sin3a, and histone deacetylases to RARα binding sites. Upon binding retinoic acid, conformational changes in the RARα/RXR complex causes dissociation of the repressor complex and recruitment of coactivators, resulting in transcriptional activation of retinoic acid target genes.[89] The importance of RARα in mediating neutrophil differentiation beyond the promyelocyte stage is suggested by the observations of patients with chromosomal translocations involving the *RARA* locus in acute promyelocytic leukemia. The most common of these, the t(15;17), results in fusion of the promyelocytic leukemia (*PML*) gene with *RARA*. In the case of PML/RARα, pharmacologic doses of ATRA can overcome the block in myeloid differentiation. Interestingly, all of the translocations involving *RARA* that have been identified in acute promyelocytic leukemia patients cause fusion of the identical region of the RARα protein, which includes the DNA-binding domain (reviewed by Zelent and coworkers[90] and Pandolfi[91]). The important functional targets of RARα remain to be determined, although both C/EBPα and C/EBPε are upregulated by ATRA-induced differentiation of leukemic HL-60 and NB4 cells.[92–95] Despite the inhibition to neutrophil maturation induced by *RARA*-containing translocations, mice bearing a null mutation for RARα are viable and exhibit normal hematopoiesis. This may be due to redundant functions of RAR isoforms, such as RARβ and γ.[96,97]

Disruption of Neutrophil Production, Differentiation, and Function in Disease

The complex process of neutrophil differentiation leads to a cell that is capable of diverse functions, including adherence to the vascular wall, transmigration, oxidative killing, and granule release. Disruption of any of the complex processes involved in the acquisition of this mature granulocytic phenotype can disrupt the critical role of the neutrophil in the innate immune response. The study of naturally occurring mutations in the genes mediating these processes and human disease has contributed to our understanding of the role these genes play in normal neutrophil maturation and function. The major disease manifestations of neutrophil-specific gene dysfunction are abnormalities in neutrophil number, failure of neutrophil differentiation, or a propensity to infection reflecting a failure of neutrophil functional competence. As described later, the link between disease phenotype and neutrophil-specific genotype often reflects the

TABLE 5–1. Selected Disorders Induced by Neutrophil-Specific Gene Expression Abnormalities

Disease	Gene(s) Implicated	Disease Manifestations	Pathophysiology
Abnormalities of Neutrophil Number			
Severe congenital neutropenia (SCN)	*NE*	Neutropenia May progress to MDS/AML in up to 10% of patients	Unknown. Elastase is subject to aberrant intracellular trafficking, but relationship to neutrophil number is unclear.
Cyclic neutropenia	*NE*	Cyclic neutropenia No MDS/AML	As above.
Chédiak-Higashi syndrome	*LYST*	Neutropenia Platelet dysfunction Oculocutaneous albinism Lymphoid infiltration	Abnormality of membrane and granule trafficking; relationship to neutrophil number is unclear.
Hermansky-Pudlak syndrome	*AP3B1*	Neutropenia Platelet dysfunction Oculocutaneous albinism	Abnormality of Golgi-ER transport, resulting in abnormal trafficking of granule proteins. Relationship to neutrophil number is unclear.
Abnormalities of Neutrophil Maturation			
Acute myelogenous leukemia	*AML1*, *CBFB* (core binding factor β), *CEBPA* (C/EBPα), etc.	Acute leukemia with accumulation of undifferentiated blasts	Heterogeneous mechanisms for disruption of transcriptional regulatory pathways governing neutrophil maturation.
Abnormalities of Neutrophil Function			
Leukocyte adhesion deficiency	Common β chain, integrin receptors	Increased infections Leukocytosis Early mortality	Loss of expression of LFA-1, MAC-1, and gp150;95, all of which include the common β chain. Results in inability to ingest and kill opsonized organisms.
Chronic granulomatous disease	Components of the NADPH oxidase complex	Increased infections	Loss of oxidative burst, with failure to kill encapsulated organisms, fungi.
Secondary granule deficiency	*CEBPE* (C/EBPε)	Increased infections	Failure of development of secondary granules and their contents.

Abbreviations: ER, endoplasmic reticulum; LFA-1, lymphocyte function–associated antigen-1; MAC-1, membrane attack complex-1; MDS/AML, myelodysplastic syndrome/acute myeloid leukemia.

known role of the target gene in the neutrophil maturation and functional program; however, in other cases, the connection between mutation and disease remains a puzzle. Although each of these syndromes will be discussed in detail elsewhere in this text, they are mentioned here to place them in the context of the neutrophil maturation program (Table 5–1).

Abnormalities in Neutrophil Number

The genes implicated in the pathogenesis of the inherited neutropenic syndromes have been recently identified. However, the link between the known function of those genes and the diseases induced by mutations in them has proved elusive. The primary granule protein neutrophil elastase has been linked to two diseases. Mutations in *NE* have been found in essentially 100% of patients with cyclic neutropenia, and in approximately half of patients with severe congenital neutropenia.[98,99] These heterozygous mutations have pleomorphic effects on the NE protein, suggesting that the phenotype is not related to altered enzymatic function of the cognate protein.[100] There is increasing evidence that part of the phenotype may be related to abnormalities of trafficking of the granule protein within neutrophil progenitors.[101] This is supported by the observation that two other neutropenic syndromes, Chédiak-Higashi syndrome[102] and Hermansky-Pudlak syndrome,[103,104] have also been linked to genes involved in protein trafficking within the cell.[105] However, how these abnormalities become linked to changes in neutrophil mass, and what determines the phenotypic differences between severe congenital neutropenia and patients with cyclic neutropenia remains a mystery.

Abnormalities in Neutrophil Maturation

The disruption of transcriptional regulatory pathways is an important mechanism of leukemogenesis, and acquired mutations in transcription factors implicated in neutrophil differentiation have been linked to the development of acute leukemia. Nearly half of patients with AML have translocations that fuse neutrophil-specific transcription factors with tissue-specific genes, creating fusion proteins that interfere with the normal process of neutrophil differentiation.[67,68] The most common translocations involve the t(8;21) in *AML1* in M2 AML,[106] the inv(16) in *CBFB* in M4 AML,[107] and the t(15;17) in *RARA* in M3 acute promyelocytic leukemia.[68] The role of the translocations in leukemogenesis is still under intensive investigation; studies in animal models strongly suggest that the fusion proteins play a necessary but insufficient role in the pathogenesis of AML.[108,109] Other mutations affect the expression of transcription factors such as C/EBPα.[68] The role of these genetic alterations in the pathogenesis of leukemia is discussed in further detail in Chapter 27.

Abnormalities in Neutrophil Function

Abnormalities in neutrophil function may arise either from defects in functionally important proteins or by changes that disrupt granulocytic maturation. It is self-evident that mutations disrupting the formation of integrin receptors on the neutrophil surface should cause leukocyte adhesion deficiency,[110] or that abnormalities of components of the respiratory burst should lead to the defects in bacterial killing seen in chronic granulomatous disease.[111] More surprising was the observation that the rare disorder known as specific granule deficiency is caused in some cases by a defect in the transcription factor C/EBPε.[84,112] As previously noted, most of the transcription factors regulating neutrophil differentiation are important in inducing neutrophil-specific gene expression at many stages throughout the maturation program. Therefore, in addition to directing the differentiation of the cells, they contribute to the functional competence of the mature neutrophil as well. Consequently, separation of the processes of neutrophil maturation and the acquisition of functional properties is somewhat artificial. Defects in transcription factors that do not completely abrogate differentiation can induce functional abnormalities in the mature cells, and mutations in functional proteins can lead to unexplained consequences in the regulation of neutrophil proliferation. Hence, increasing understanding of how defects in C/EBPε can cause specific granule deficiency and defects in the granule protein neutrophil elastase can induce severe neutropenia will continue to highlight the close relationship between the neutrophil maturation sequence and the acquisition of functional competence of the innate immune system.

EOSINOPHILS AND BASOPHILS

Eosinophils and basophils are minor granulocyte populations with characteristic staining properties inferred by the contents of their unique secondary granules. The characteristic staining properties of eosinophils results from their secondary granules, which contain major basic protein, eosinophil cationic protein, eosinophil peroxidase, and eosinophil-derived neurotoxin. Eosinophils are produced in response to IL-3, IL-5, and GM-CSF, and are characteristically increased in the setting of allergic reactions (Fig. 5–5).[113] It is hypothesized that eosinophil proliferation and release is stimulated by cytokines elaborated by T cells in that setting.

Although platelet-derived growth factor is not thought to be critical to normal eosinophil production, recent studies of the idiopathic hypereosinophilic syndrome have demonstrated activating mutations in the platelet-derived growth factor receptor that induce constitutive tyrosine kinase activity and eosinophilia. This appears to mediate the pathogenesis of the disease, because imatinib induces remission in these patients by direct platelet-derived growth factor receptor inhibition.[114]

PU.1, C/EBPα, and C/EBPβ, all of which have also been implicated in neutrophil differentiation, mediate transcriptional regulation of eosinophil maturation. The factors that serve to "sort" these signals to direct eosinophil rather than neutrophil production are unknown, although it has been proposed that levels of GATA-1 may influence this lineage choice.

Basophils and mast cells mediate immunoglobulin E–induced immune responses.[115,116] The secondary granule proteins of basophils are rich in glycosaminoglycans, predominantly heparin. Basophils have a cytokine profile similar to that of eosinophils, with maturation and proliferation in response to IL-3, IL-5, and GM-CSF (see Fig. 5–5).[117] They differentiate in the marrow, and circulate briefly in tissues in a manner

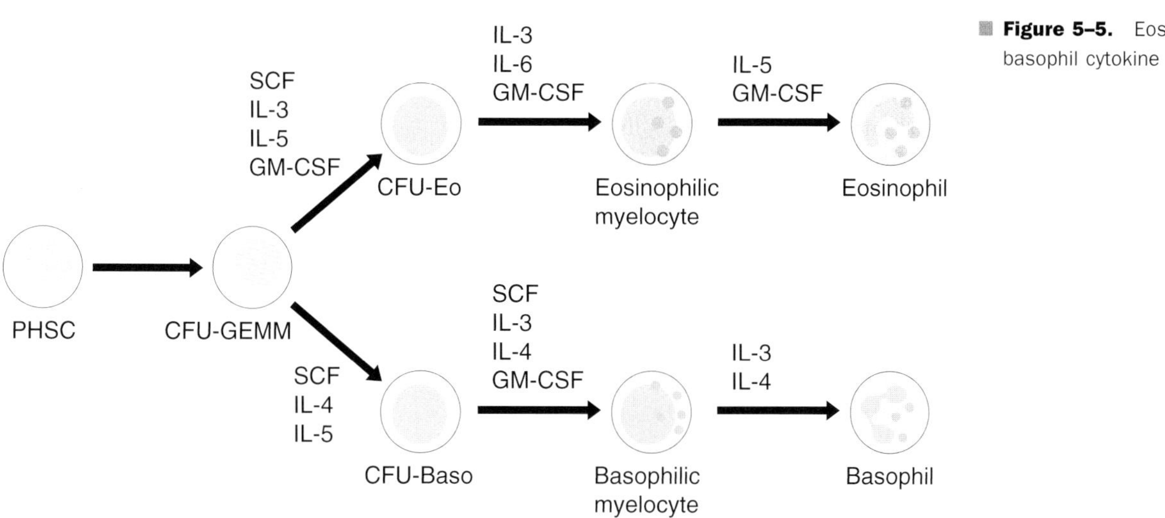

Figure 5–5. Eosinophil and basophil cytokine profile.

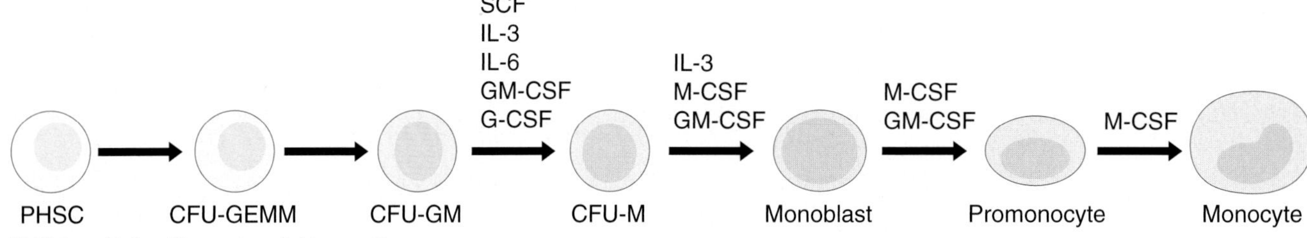

Figure 5–6. Monocyte cytokine profile.

similar to that of neutrophils. Mast cells, however, are released as immature cells, completing their maturation in the peripheral tissues after release from the marrow.[116] Stem cell factor is a particularly potent inducer of mast cell proliferation, and activating mutations in c-Kit, the stem cell factor receptor, have been demonstrated to induce mast cell proliferation in the majority of cases of systemic mastocytosis.[118]

MONOCYTES

Monocytes are bone marrow–derived granulocytes that are the precursors of tissue macrophages. They differentiate in the bone marrow, with a brief maturation period of 2–3 days, following which they circulate briefly in the peripheral blood and then enter the tissues, where they mature to macrophages that may survive 2–3 months.[21,119,120] Monocytes are also the precursors to dendritic cells, professional antigen-presenting cells that can arise from either myeloid or lymphoid precursors.[121]

Monocytes contain both primary and secondary granules. The primary granules are very similar to those in neutrophils, and contain myeloperoxidase.[122] Monocyte secondary granules fuse with the membrane when the monocyte is stimulated, increasing the expression of adhesion molecules.[123]

Monocyte precursors respond to macrophage colony-stimulating factor, receptors for which are expressed on the surface of the promonocyte (Fig. 5–6).[124,125] It has been difficult to identify monocyte-specific surface markers because many of the same proteins are expressed on both neutrophils and monocytes. CD14, the receptor for lipopolysaccharide, is a functionally important surface protein that may be expressed uniquely on the monocyte-macrophage lineage.[126] Monocytes also express lysozyme and the Fcγ receptor (II, III),[127] both of which are also expressed by neutrophils.

CURRENT CONTROVERSIES & FUTURE CONSIDERATIONS

Granulocytopoiesis

- What is the role of elastase in neutrophil production, and how do mutations in this granule protein have a profound impact on neutrophil number?
- Since the GM-CSF–null mouse has no hematopoietic phenotype, what is the importance of GM-CSF in regulating neutrophil homeostasis?
- What are the defects in transcriptional regulation that contribute to the development of the myelodysplastic syndrome?

Suggested Readings*

Berliner N, Horwitz M, Loughran TP Jr: Congenital and acquired neutropenia. Hematology (Am Soc Hematol Educ Program) 63–79, 2004.

Borregaard N, Cowland JB: Granules of the human neutrophilic polymorphonuclear leukocyte. Blood 89:3503–3521, 1997.

Dinauer MC, Lekstrom-Himes JA, Dale DC: Inherited neutrophil disorders: molecular basis and new therapies. Hematology (Am Soc Hematol Educ Program) 303–318, 2000.

Khanna-Gupta A, Berliner N: Granulocytopoiesis and monocytopoiesis. *In* Benz EJ, Cohen HJ, Furie B, et al (eds): Hematology, Basic Principles and Practice (ed 4). 2005, pp 289–301.

Tenen DG, Hromas R, Licht JD, Zhang DE: Transcription factors, normal myeloid development, and leukemia. Blood 90:489–519, 1997.

Full references for this chapter can be found on accompanying CD-ROM.

CHAPTER 6

Lymphocyte Biology

Megan A. Cooper, MD, PhD, Michael A. Caligiuri, MD, Edward E. Max, MD, PhD, and Jonathan Powell, MD, PhD

KEY POINTS

Lymphocyte Biology

- Immunity can be divided into innate and adaptive immune responses.
- Major effector cells of the innate immune response include natural killer (NK) cells, NK/T cells, dendritic cells (DCs), macrophages, and granulocytes.
- NK cells develop within the bone marrow, and mature NK cells produce immunoregulatory cytokines and lyse target cells.
- DCs are important antigen-presenting cells (APCs) of the immune system and exhibit a great deal of heterogeneity.
- Immunoglobulins are "Y"-shaped proteins that are produced by B lymphocytes and that convey immune protection by binding to foreign molecules called antigens.
- The amino-terminal domains of immunoglobulin proteins are highly variable as a result of mutations arising though assembly of separate V, D, and J elements and somatic hypermutation.
- Soluble immunoglobulins protect against infections through virus (or toxin) neutralization, complement activation, and enhancement of phagocytosis.
- T cells recognize antigen in the form of peptides presented by MHC molecules. T-cell activation requires T-cell receptor (TCR) recognition of antigen and the engagement of costimulatory molecules.
- $CD4^+$ T cells can be categorized into T_H1 and T_H2 cells.
- $CD8^+$ T cells kill infected target cells.
- T-cell tolerance to self antigens is maintained centrally in the thymus as well as in the periphery.

INTRODUCTION

The immune response to infection can broadly be divided into two arms, the innate (or nonadaptive) and the adaptive immune systems. The adaptive immune system exhibits immunologic memory, antigen specificity, and a delayed response, whereas the innate immune system lacks memory and is less specific, but rapidly responds to infection. The property of immunologic memory implies that the adaptive immune system becomes more efficient upon repeated exposure to the same pathogen. By contrast, cellular components of the innate immune system have a set repertoire of recognition receptors, and repeated exposures to antigens produce equivalent responses.[1] Interactions between these two arms of the immune system are critical for an efficient immune response, and deficiencies in either will lead to significant defects in host immunity.[2–4] Innate immunity has often been considered to be more primitive and nonspecific as compared to adaptive immunity.[4]

INNATE IMMUNITY

Upon initial infection, the innate immune response—consisting of soluble mediators such as complement (see later discussion under "Functions of Immunoglobulin") and antimicrobial peptides in addition to cellular effectors—is quickly mounted. Cellular components of the innate immune response, including natural killer (NK) cells, NK/T cells, macrophages, dendritic cells (DCs), and granulocytes (see Chapter 5) work through lysis or phagocytosis of pathogens and infected cells as well as production of immunoregulatory cytokines to rapidly control infections (Fig. 6–1). In addition, these cells alert the adaptive immune B and T lymphocytes to the presence of infection through antigen presentation, upregulation of costimulatory molecules, and production of immunostimulatory cytokines.[3] As is discussed later in this chapter, B and T lymphocytes undergo receptor rearrangement, producing millions of distinct receptors to specifically recognize antigens from nearly any pathogen. Following processing and presentation of anti-

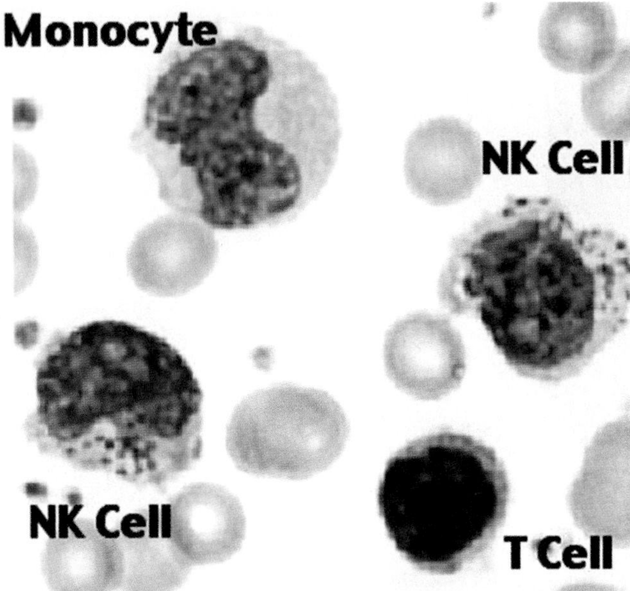

Figure 6–1. Innate immune cells found in the peripheral blood. Shown are a monocyte, two natural killer (NK) cells, and a T lymphocyte.

gens from pathogens by antigen-presenting cells (APCs) of the innate immune system, adaptive immune cells expressing the correct receptors with high affinity for a particular antigen are selected and expanded.[5] Once adaptive immune cells are present in sufficient numbers, various types of specific B- and T-cell immune responses can occur.

Macrophages and DCs of the innate immune system express pattern recognition receptors for the identification of pathogen-specific molecules.[6–8] These receptors, called Toll-like receptors based on their homology to the *Drosophila toll* gene, can recognize specific components of infectious organisms such as viral RNA, bacterial CpG DNA motifs, fungal wall components, and bacterial cell wall products.[7–9] Furthermore, NK cells, lymphocytes of the innate immune system, express activating receptors for ligands that are induced by viral infection, cellular stress, and perhaps malignant transformation, thereby allowing specific recognition of target cells and activation of lysis.[10–13]

Cellular Mediators of the Innate Immune System

Natural Killer Cells

NK cells are lymphocytes that were first identified functionally by their ability to lyse target cells without prior sensitization or activation.[14] NK cells express an array of receptors (NK receptors [NKRs]) for recognition of infected, cancerous, and otherwise transformed cells, resulting in production of a variety of cytokines.[15–17] In addition to their cytotoxic effects, rapid production of a variety of cytokines by NK cells is crucial for host defense against a variety of pathogens including viruses, parasites, and bacteria.[15–17]

NK cells comprise 10–15% of all peripheral blood lymphocytes and are also found in marrow, spleen, tonsils, and lymph nodes. Human NK cells are defined phenotypically by the presence of CD56 and the lack of the CD3 antigen.[14] Two subsets of human NK cells, $CD56^{dim}$ and $CD56^{bright}$ NK cells, with distinct functional and phenotypic properties have been described.[18] The majority (~90%) of peripheral blood NK cells have low-density expression of CD56 ($CD56^{dim}$) and express high levels of the Fcγ receptor III (FcγRIII, or CD16), whereas approximately 10% of circulating NK cells are $CD56^{bright}CD16^{dim/neg}$. This minor $CD56^{bright}$ NK cell population produces high levels of immunoregulatory cytokines, and in particular interferon-γ (IFN-γ), but has a limited NKR repertoire and relatively low cytotoxic activity. By contrast, the major population of circulating $CD56^{dim}$ NK cells produces lower levels of cytokines but has broader expression of NKRs and is highly cytotoxic. Whereas the $CD56^{dim}$ population predominates in the periphery, within lymphoid organs (including tonsils and lymph nodes) a $CD56^{bright}$ NK cell population predominates.[19,20] These NK cell populations may represent either mature subsets or different stages of a common human NK differentiation pathway.[18,21]

NK Cell Development and Homeostasis

Both NK cell differentiation and survival are dependent upon the cytokine interleukin (IL)-15. NK cells develop within the bone marrow from a common lymphoid progenitor under the influence of several cytokines and growth factors.[21–23] IL-15 is a widely expressed cytokine and a product of normal bone marrow stromal cells as well as APCs and epithelial cells.[21] IL-15 shares signaling receptor subunits with IL-2—the shared IL-2/IL-15 receptor β chain (IL-2/15Rβ) and common γ chain (also shared by IL-4, -7, -9, and -21)—and also utilizes its own unique receptor, IL-15Rα, which binds this cytokine with high affinity and is utilized for presentation of IL-15 by cells producing the cytokine.[21,24] Mice and humans with defects in genes affecting IL-15, but not IL-2, production or signaling have severe defects in NK cells.[25–32] However, IL-2 can also drive NK cell differentiation in vitro and expands NK cells when administered in vivo (Fig. 6–2).

The receptor tyrosine kinases c-Kit and Flt-3 present on progenitors drive the development of IL-15R–positive NK cell precursors from hematopoietic stem cells and potentiate NK cell expansion when administered in vivo.[23] The current paradigm for NK cell development suggests two phases of NK cell differentiation: (1) an early phase, during which the hematopoietic stem cell generates a common lymphoid progenitor that then, under the influence of factors such as c-Kit and Flt-3 ligands, is committed to becoming an NK cell precursor that expresses IL-15R, and (2) a maturation phase, during which stromal cell interactions, IL-15, and perhaps other cofactors such as IL-12 and IL-21 induce the development of functionally mature NK cells with NKRs, cytolytic activity, and the ability to produce cytokines[22,23,33] (Fig. 6–3). Once in the periphery, various cytokines and growth factors contribute to NK cell activation and function;

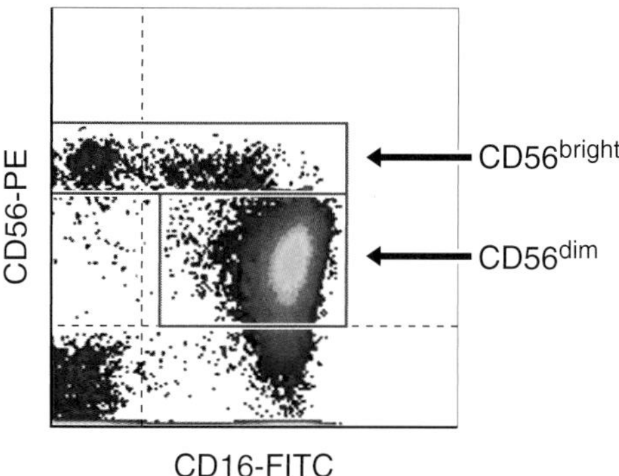

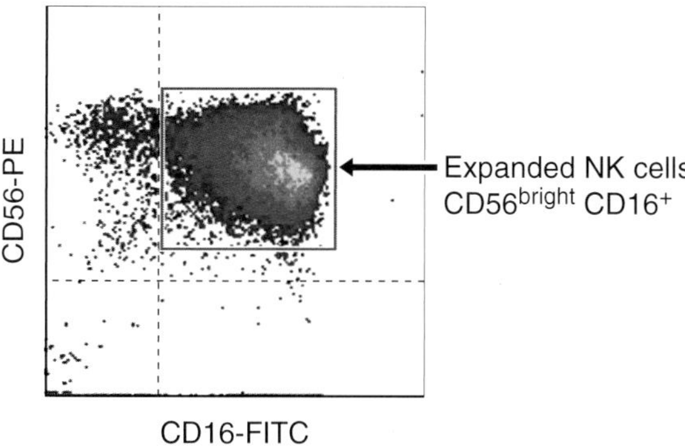

Figure 6–2. IL-2 expansion of natural killer (NK) cells. Human NK cells can be divided into two subsets based on cell surface density expression of CD56. ***A,*** Flow cytometric analysis of normal donor-enriched NK cells (CD56 vs. CD16) shows typical ratios of approximately 10% CD56^{bright} and 90% CD56^{dim}. ***B,*** Flow cytometric analysis of NK cells from a patient receiving low-dose IL-2 therapy shows a large expansion of CD56^{bright}CD16^{pos} cells. Quadrants are drawn based upon background staining of appropriate isotype control antibodies. (Adapted from Fehninger TA, Caligiuri MA: Ontogeny and expansion of human natural killer cells: clinical implications. Int Rev Immunol 20:503–534, 2001.)

however IL-15 is requisite for the continued survival of these cells.[33]

NK Cell Cytotoxicity and Receptors

NK cells mediate two main types of cytotoxicity, natural cytotoxicity and antibody-dependent cellular cytotoxicity (ADCC). Natural cytotoxicity is regulated by NKRs and the presence of target cell major histocompatibility complex (MHC) class I molecules and stimulatory ligands. In certain circumstances preactivation of NK cells in vitro with cytokines such as IL-2 is necessary for lysis of target cells, known as lymphokine-activated killing activity. ADCC refers to the ability of NK cells to recognize immunoglobulin (Ig)G antibody–coated target cells. Both mechanisms of NK cell activation lead to a common end pathway resulting in perforin- and granzyme-mediated lysis of target cells.[34]

Natural cytotoxicity relies on the ability of an NK cell to recognize self versus non-self cells (i.e., transformed cells), and NKRs for MHC class I molecules are critical for this recognition. Three major superfamilies of NKRs have been described in humans: the killer-cell immunoglobulin-like receptor (KIR) superfamily, which primarily recognizes human lymphocyte antigen (HLA)-A, -B, and -C; the C-type lectin superfamily, which includes CD94 and NKG2 receptors recognizing HLA-E; and natural cytotoxicity receptors with unknown ligands.[35,36] Activation of natural cytotoxicity is mediated by a balance of inhibitory and activating NKRs, as well as various adhesion and costimulatory molecules[37,38] (Fig. 6–4).

ADCC is mediated by the CD16 molecule (FcγRIII), a low-affinity Fc receptor on the surface of NK cells that binds to antibody-coated (opsonized) targets and signals through associated subunits containing an immunoreceptor tyrosine-based activation motif (ITAM) to direct killing.[38] Most CD56^{bright} NK cells (~50–70%) lack CD16, and the remaining cells have low-density expression of this activating Fc receptor. By contrast, nearly all CD56^{dim} NK cells have high expression of CD16 and are efficient mediators of ADCC.[39]

NK Cell Cytokine Production

In contrast to resting T lymphocytes, NK cells constitutively express receptors for numerous cytokines, and rapidly produce IFN-γ and other NK-derived cytokines and chemokines in response to cytokine stimulation.[40–42] These early pro-inflammatory cytokines and chemokines can promote activation of other innate immune cells such as macrophages and DCs, recruit immune cells to sites of infection, and set the stage for the induction of an adaptive immune response based on the cytokine milieu produced. Activated CD56^{bright} NK cells appear to have an intrinsic capacity for high cytokine production when compared to CD56^{dim} NK cells. In addition, the CD56^{bright} NK cell subset, present in lymph nodes, constitutively expresses the high-affinity IL-2 receptor and can produce IFN-γ in response to IL-2 produced by antigen-activated T cells, promoting the adaptive immune response.[19]

NK/T Cells

NK/T cells comprise a small, heterogeneous population of lymphocytes that express both NK-cell and T-cell markers, including restricted T-cell receptors (TCRs) that recognize lipid antigens associated with the non–classical antigen-presenting molecule CD1d,[43,44] T-cell markers CD4 or CD8, and NK cell markers CD161 and NKRs[43] (Table 6–1). In vivo models have shown that NK/T cells modulate the immune response through rapid production of cytokines, in particular IL-4 and IFN-γ, and may prevent autoimmunity and tumor immunity.[44–46]

Macrophages

Macrophages are critical components of the innate immune response for the elimination of intracellular pathogens. Macrophages are one of the first cell types to recognize infection because they are resident in lymphoid and nonlymphoid organs, including thymus,

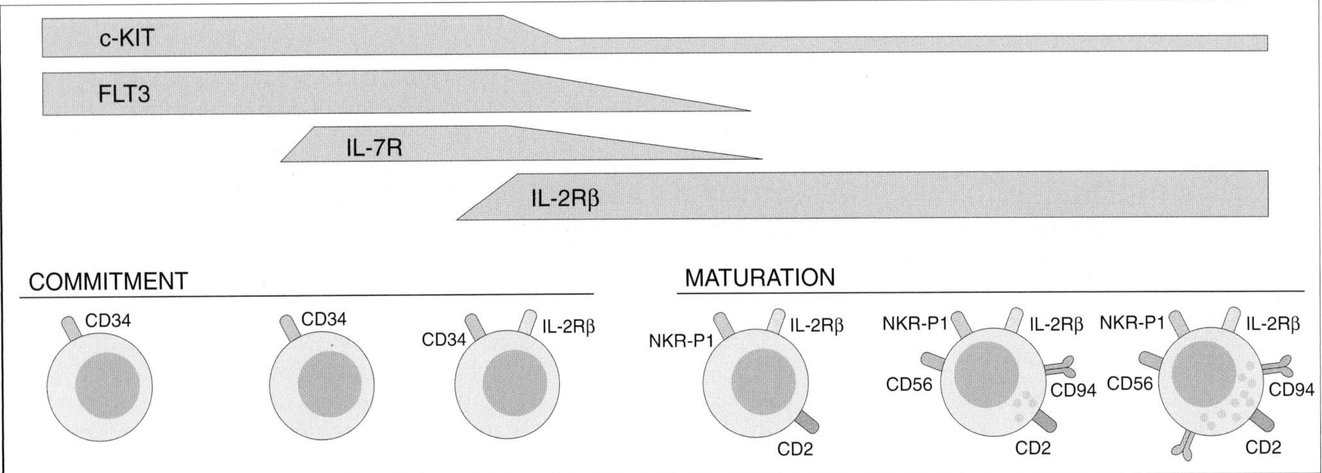

A Human NK cell differentiation

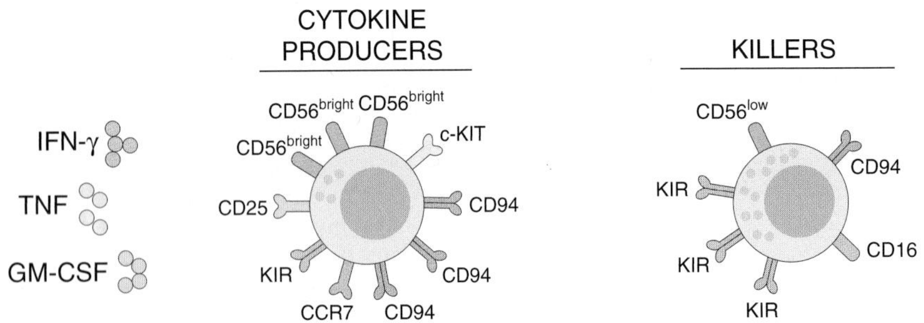

B Human NK cell subsets

Figure 6–3. Human natural killer (NK) cell differentiation in vitro. ***A,*** NK cells develop from hematopoietic ($CD34^+$) progenitor cells within the bone marrow. Commitment to NK cell development depends on maturation signals from cytokines and growth factors, including c-Kit and Flt-3, and is marked by the upregulation of the shared IL-15/IL-2 receptor β chain (IL-2/15Rβ). Maturation of NK cells from IL-$2R\beta^{pos}$ precursors is dependent on signals from IL-15, and perhaps other cofactors such as IL-12 and IL-21. ***B,*** Mature peripheral blood human NK cells can be divided into two subsets based on cell surface density of CD56, each with differential phenotype and function. $CD56^{bright}$ NK cells have a high capacity for cytokine production and a lower innate cytotoxic capacity. By contrast, the more abundant $CD56^{dim}$ NK cell population are potent cytotoxic cells with a lower capacity for cytokine production. (Adapted from Colucci F, Caligiuri MA, Di Santo JP: What does it take to make a natural killer? Nat Rev Immunol 3:413–425, 2004.)

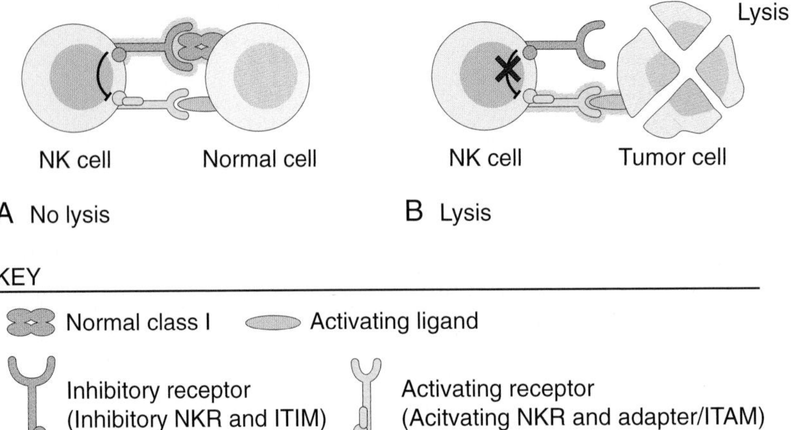

Figure 6–4. Natural killer (NK) cell receptor-mediated target lysis. NK cells recognize cells through a variety of inhibitory and activating NK receptors (NKRs) for major histocompatability complex (MHC) class I and class I–like molecules that are critical for recognition of normal versus transformed and/or foreign cells. ***A,*** Class I molecules expressed on the surface of normal host cells are engaged by surveying the inhibitory receptors of NK cells, and normally a strong inhibitory signal prevents NK cell activation and any consequent tissue destruction. ***B,*** When inhibitory NKRs fail to recognize class I molecules on a foreign, malignant, or infected cell, the inhibitory signal is interrupted. Activating NKRs, when engaged by their ligands, can then initiate the cytolytic pathways that allow NK cell lysis of target cells.

TABLE 6–1. Innate Immune Antigens*

Antigen	NK	NKT	DC	Mφ
CD2	+	+	+/–	–
CD3	–	+	–	–
CD4	–	+/–	+/–	+
CD8	+/–	+/–	+/–	–
CD11b	+	na	+/–	+
CD11c	+	na	+/–	+
CD13	–	–	+/–	+
CD14	–	–	–	+
CD16 (FcγRIII)	+/–	+/–	+/–	+
CD19	–	–	+/–	–
CD20	–	–	–	–
CD32 (FcγRII)	+/–	–	+/–	+
CD33	–	–	+/–	+
CD40	–	–	+	+
CD45	+	+	+	+
CD56	+	+	–	–
CD64 (FcγRI)	–	–	+/–	+
CD83	–	–	+	–
CD161	+/–	+	–	–
NKRs	+	+/–	–	–
MHC Class II	–	–	+/–	+/–

Major antigens expressed by innate immune cells and used for the identification of human natural killer (NK) cells, NK/T cells, dendritic cells (DCs), and monocytes/macrophages (Mφ):
+, expressed by most cells
+/–, expressed by a subset of cells, including activated cells
–, not typically expressed
na, unknown
Abbreviations: MHC, major histocompatibility complex; NKRs, natural killer receptors (see text for further details).

lymph nodes, lung, spleen, liver, and skin. The main roles of these cells are recognition of infection; initiation and regulation of the innate and adaptive immune responses through production of immunoregulatory cytokines and chemokines and small molecules such as nitric oxide; and phagocytosis and lysis of pathogens and abnormal (i.e., infected and/or necrotic) cells.[47] Following phagocytosis of pathogens, macrophages can present antigen for the initiation of an adaptive immune response, although to a lesser extent than monocyte-derived DCs. Macrophage activation is mediated by a variety of receptors, including complement, scavenger, Toll-like, and Fc receptors, allowing these cells to recognize a wide variety of pathogens and injured cells.[47–49]

Dendritic Cells

DCs are the major APCs of the immune system and are key to the success of both the early innate immune response and later adaptive immune responses.[50] Human DCs are heterogeneous in phenotype (see Table 6–1).[50,51] Similar to macrophages, DCs express Toll-like receptors and other pattern recognition receptors that allow them to recognize a variety of pathogens. Following uptake of antigens, immature DCs begin a process of maturation and activation with eventual migration to lymphoid organs. Once in the lymph nodes, DCs stimulate adaptive immune lymphocytes through presentation of antigens to T lymphocytes, upregulation of costimulatory molecules, and production of immunoregulatory cytokines to guide the initiation of B- and T-cell adaptive immune responses.[52] Additional DC interactions with NK and NK/T cells through direct contact and/or soluble mediators (i.e., cytokines) activate these cells to promote an innate immune response.[53,54] In addition to their role in immune defense, DCs are important for immunologic tolerance to self antigens and prevention of autoimmunity.

Dendritic Cell Differentiation and Maturation

Precursor DCs are found in the peripheral blood and arise from myeloid and lymphoid progenitors.[51] Human DCs can be derived in vitro from bone marrow hematopoietic cells and peripheral blood monocytes under the influence of growth factors including granulocyte-macrophage colony-stimulating factor, Flt-3 ligand, IL-4, and tumor necrosis factor (TNF)-α. Whereas DCs can be effectively expanded ex vivo for use in cancer immunotherapy, the pathways and growth factors required for human DC differentiation in vivo are not entirely clear. Studies suggest that precursor DCs migrate to tissues where they become resident immature epidermal and dermal DCs, lying in wait for activation by pathogens and other signals of danger. Additional immature DCs can be quickly recruited to sites of inflammation via production of local immune mediators, including chemokines. Immature DCs, but not mature DCs, are efficient at capturing antigen through several processes, including macropinocytosis, endocytosis, and phagocytosis.[55] Uptake of antigen, signals such as inflammatory cytokines and molecules, and interactions with local immune cells such as NK cells initiates the process of DC maturation. DC structure and function evolve as these cells mature, resulting in an efficient APC. A variety of homing receptors, including the chemokine receptor CCR7, are upregulated, triggering the migration of maturing DCs from tissues to endolymphatics for travel to lymph nodes[55] (Fig. 6–5).

Mature DCs acquire the ability to effectively process and present antigen and upregulate costimulatory molecules necessary for interactions with antigen-specific T cells. DCs present antigen in the context of MHC class I, MHC class II, and CD1 molecules and can activate both $CD8^+$ and $CD4^+$ T cells in addition to CD1-restricted T and NK/T cells. Additionally, mature DC interactions with B cells induce differentiation and isotype switching in these adaptive immune cells.

Dendritic Cell Cytokine Production

Different subsets of DCs have differential capacities for cytokine production. Indeed, a specialized subset of DCs—plasmacytoid DCs, also known as interferon-producing cells—produce high levels of type I interferons (IFN-α and -β) in response to viruses. Plasmacytoid DCs appear to have a lesser role in antigen presentation and may be more important in activating immune cells, including T, DC, and NK cells, via production of type I IFNs and IL-12.[50,56] Production of pro-inflammatory cytokines and chemokines in the periphery by immature DCs activates and recruits additional immune cells, including NK cells

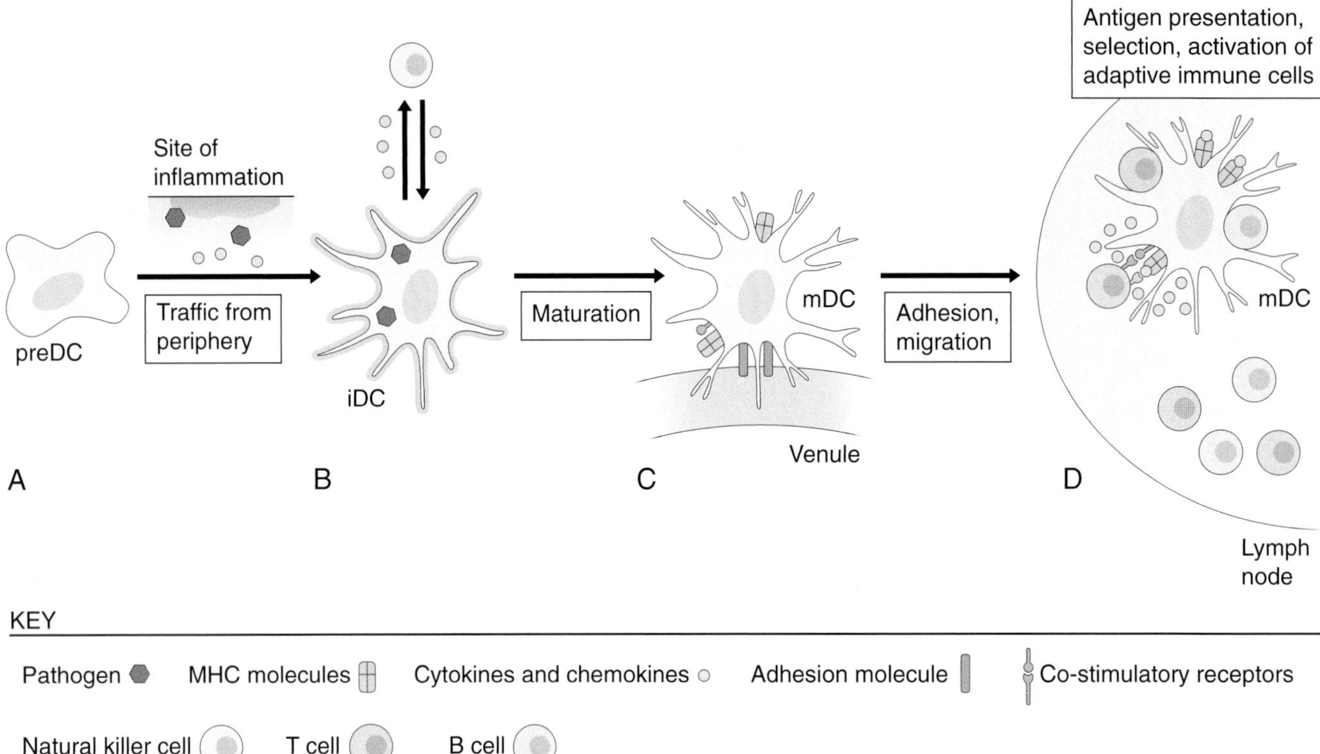

■ **Figure 6–5.** Dendritic cell (DC) activation and maturation. ***A,*** Peripheral blood precursor DCs (pre-DCs) traffic to sites of inflammation in response to inflammatory signals. ***B,*** Activation signals from pathogens, cytokines, and other cells, including natural killer (NK) cells, induce DC activation and uptake of antigens by immature DCs (iDCs). ***C,*** Maturing DCs express adhesion and homing receptors that allow them to travel to lymph nodes. ***D,*** Once in the lymph nodes, mature DCs present antigen to T cells and activate T and B cells through cytokines and cell surface molecules.

and macrophages. Mature DCs within lymph nodes produce cytokines, such as IL-12 or IL-10, during the process of T-cell activation that help to guide the initiation of type 1 and 2 helper T cell (T_H1 and T_H2) adaptive immune responses (discussed later in this chapter).

Innate Immune Cells in Immunotherapy

In the setting of HLA-haplomismatched bone marrow transplantation for relapsed acute myelogenous leukemia, NK cell "mismatch" (i.e., donor-derived NK cells that lack inhibitory receptors for recipient MHC class I molecules) can result in a beneficial NK-versus-leukemia effect.[57,58] Patients with acute myelogenous leukemia who received NK cell–mismatched transplants have a significantly lower rate of rejection and graft-versus-host disease and increased disease-free survival when compared with those patients without an NK cell mismatch.[58] DCs have shown considerable potential as therapeutic agents for cancer vaccines and are being used in Phase I/II clinical trials to induce immunity to patients' tumors.[59] Critical to the success of any immunotherapeutic strategy is an improved understanding of the biology of immune cells and the ways in which they interact. For instance, elucidation of growth factors involved in immune cell differentiation led to the use of low doses of IL-2 to expand functional NK cells in cancer patients and human immunodeficiency virus–infected patients.[60,61]

ADAPTIVE IMMUNITY: B CELLS

Whereas the innate immune system evolved to immediately recognize a set of molecular determinants commonly associated with pathogens, the adaptive immune system develops specific recognition proteins targeted to virtually any molecule but takes 4–7 days to mount an effective response. However, unlike innate immunity, the adaptive immune system retains a "memory," so that a second exposure to the same determinant triggers an almost immediate protective response.

The cells of the adaptive immune system are B (or *b*one marrow-derived) and T (or *t*hymus-derived) lymphocytes, and their recognition molecules are TCRs and B-cell receptors (BCRs). BCRs also exist in a secreted form known as antibodies or immunoglobulins. Both T and B lymphocytes use "clonal selection" to generate a response targeted against a specific pathogen (or experimentally administered antigen). Before antigen exposure, T and B lymphocytes circulate in the body in an inactive "resting" state. Each lymphocyte expresses a single type of surface BCR or TCR, with a particular antigen-binding specificity. As a result of the recombinational mechanism described later in this chapter, the repertoire of distinct receptors in the population of resting lymphocytes is astoundingly diverse, so that virtually any pathogen will encounter (in a healthy individual) some lymphocytes bearing surface receptors that can bind to the pathogen. Binding of the BCR or TCR to an antigen under appropriate conditions awakens a lymphocyte from its resting state, triggering clonal proliferation and various maturational changes that occur over several days, amplifying the immune response. Some of the activated T lymphocytes become effector cells capable of secreting cytokines and killing either infectious microbes or host cells bearing intracellular pathogens; some effector B lymphocytes mature into plasma cells secreting large amounts of antibody with the same recognition specificity of the originally triggered B lymphocyte. Other members of the clone of activated lymphocytes serve as memory cells that persist after the infection resolves, ready to proliferate rapidly on reexposure to the same antigen.

To protect against autoimmunity, B or T lymphocytes capable of recognizing self antigens are subject to several mechanisms, collectively known as tolerance, that eliminate autoreactive cells or render them ineffectual. Failures of tolerance account for autoimmune diseases such as type 1 diabetes mellitus and systemic lupus erythematosus.[62]

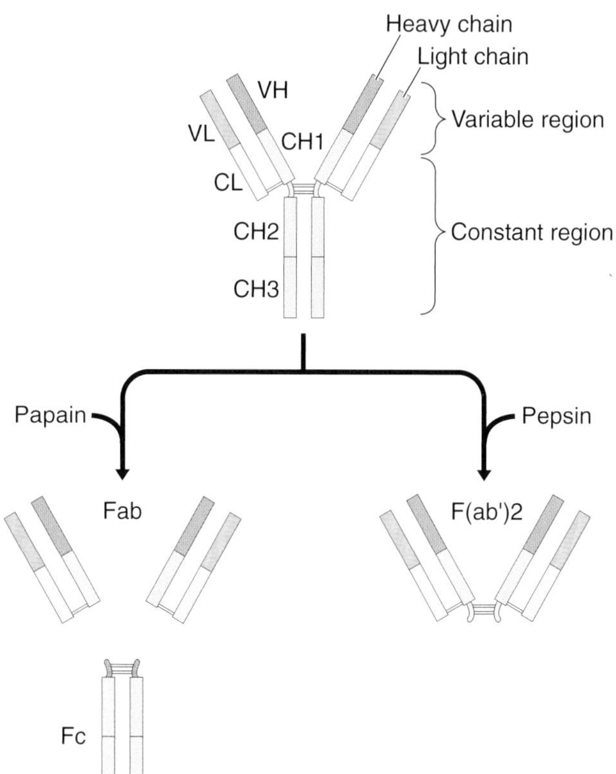

Figure 6–6. Immunoglobulin structure diagram. An IgG molecule is shown in the center. Its two identical heavy (H) chains are composed of four immunoglobulin domains (shown as *grey rectangles*): V_H, C_H1, C_H2, and C_H3. C_H1 and C_H2 are joined by a flexible hinge, which contains two disulfide bonds that hold the heavy chains together. The two identical light (L) chains each have two immunoglobulin domains *(white rectangles)*—V_L and C_L—and the C_L domain is linked near its carboxyl terminus to the heavy chain C_H1 domain by disulfide bonds. The amino-terminal domains of heavy and light chains are highly variable in amino acid sequence (V_H and V_L domains), whereas the remaining domains are constant (C_L or C_H) for proteins of the same isotype. The figure also shows the cleavage site of the protease papain, and its products (at left in diagram), Fab and Fc. The cleavage site of pepsin and its product, F(ab')2 (at right in diagram), are also shown.

Structure of Immunoglobulin

The prototype immunoglobulin molecule is a "Y"-shaped protein. The two tips of the "Y" contain identical antigen recognition domains. The stem of the "Y" anchors it to the membrane of the lymphocyte or, in the case of secreted immunoglobulin, accounts for the several effector functions of these proteins. As shown in Figure 6–6, four separate chains form the antibody molecule: two identical heavy (H) chains and two identical light (L) chains, a structure designated H_2L_2. There are nine different classes or "isotypes" of human heavy chains, which determine the nine human immunoglobulin isotypes: IgM, IgD, IgG1, IgG2, IgG3, IgG4, IgA1, IgA2, and IgE. Each isotype has a characteristic structure and particular functional roles in immunity[63] (Table 6–2). Heavy chains are linked by disulfide bonds to either of the two light

TABLE 6–2. Isotypes of Human Heavy Chains

	Isotype								
	M	**D**	**G1**	**G2**	**G3**	**G4**	**A1**	**A2**	**E**
Serum concentration (mg/mL)	0.25–3	0.03	5–12	2–6	0.5–1	0.2–1	1.5–4	0.2–0.5	<0.0005
Half-life (days)	5		23	23	7	23	6	6	2
Transplacental transfer	–	–	++	+	++	++	–	–	–
Complement activation	++++	–	+++	+	++++	–	–	–	–
Mucosal expression	–	–	–	–	–	–	+	+++	–
Mast cell degranulation	–	–	–	–	–	–	–	–	++++
Biologic role	Primary antibody response	Uncertain					Mucosal defense	Mucosal defense	Allergy, antihelminth response

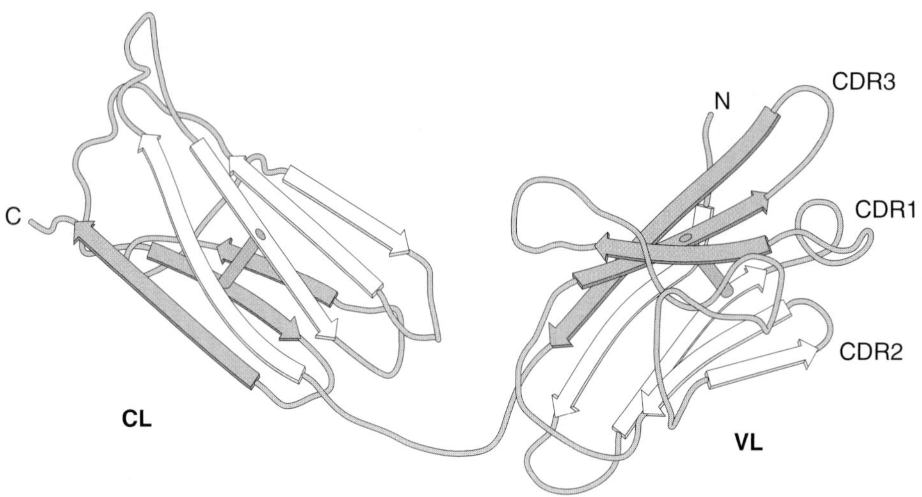

■ **Figure 6–7.** Light chain immunoglobulin domains. A ribbon diagram of a human λ light chain is shown, illustrating the β-pleated sheet structure (*white and green arrows,* representing two parallel β-pleated sheets) and internal disulfide bond (*blue bars*) characteristic of an immunoglobulin domain. The three complementarity-determining residue (CDR) loops from the V_L domain that would contact antigen are shown at right. (Modified from Schiffer A, Girling RL, Ely KR, Edmundson AB: Structure of a lambda-type Bence-Jones protein at 3.5-A resolution. Biochemistry 12:4620–4631, 1973.)

chain classes—κ or λ—but these classes do not have distinct effects on immunoglobulin function.

Immunoglobulin chains are composed of several domains, each composed of roughly 100 amino acids containing an internal disulfide bond and having a characteristic three-dimensional folding. TCRs are composed of similar domains, as are a large number of other proteins that form the immunoglobulin superfamily. The amino-terminal domains of immunoglobulin light and heavy chains have highly variable (V) amino acid sequences. Included within the V regions are three segments that are "hypervariable." These regions—three from the light chain and three from the heavy chain—form amino acid loops that contact the diverse antigens bound by antibodies[64] (Fig. 6–7); they are therefore sometimes called complementarity-determining residues (CDRs).[65] In contrast to the V domains, the sequences of other domains of light and heavy chains are constant (C) within a given class of chain. The number of C region domains varies with isotype; IgM and IgE have four, the other heavy chain isotypes have three, and the κ and λ light chains have only one. Each heavy chain isotype has characteristic covalently linked oligosaccharides. The membrane immunoglobulin expressed on the surface of B lymphocytes differs from the secreted form at its carboxyl terminus, where an extended segment containing hydrophobic residues anchors the molecule into membrane lipids. This difference is a result of alternative splicing of immunoglobulin heavy chain messenger RNA to include one or more additional exons omitted from the version encoding secreted heavy chain.[66] Table 6–3 compares some features of immunoglobulins and T cell receptors.

The binding of an antibody to its antigen results from several molecular binding forces, including attraction between positive and negative charges, hydrophobic interactions, hydrogen bonds, and van der Waals forces. X-ray crystallography of several antigen-antibody pairs has revealed contact surfaces with complementary three-dimensional structures and charged residues. The number and quality of these contact interactions determine the binding affinity. The multivalency of IgM—

TABLE 6–3. Immunoglobulins versus T-Cell Receptors

	Immunoglobulin (B-Cell Receptor)	T-Cell Receptor
Location	Surface or secreted	Surface only
Valency	2 (IgG, IgE), 4 (IgA), or 10 (IgM)	1
Chains	Heavy (VDJ) and light (VJ)	α (VDJ) and β (VJ)
Recognition target	Proteins, carbohydrates, or small molecules (haptens)	Peptide-MHC
Somatic mutation	Active in generating affinity maturation	None

which is typically pentameric, with 10 binding sites—is functionally important because early in an infection IgM is the dominant isotype, and its monomeric binding affinity is often low; however, its multivalency can induce effective binding to repeated epitopes on a pathogen. IgA exists primarily as a dimer, with four binding sites. Since the spacing between repeated epitopes on a pathogen may vary, it is important that antibody molecules are flexible to allow variable spacing between the two antigen binding tips; this is achieved by a flexible "hinge" region between the first and second constant domains of each isotype.

As shown in Figure 6–6, papain cleaves IgG into two identical fragments with antigen-binding function, known as Fab (fragment, antigen-binding), which can be used to study monomeric binding. A third fragment representing the C_H2 and C_H3 domains without the diversity of the V regions can sometimes be crystallized from polyclonal antibody preparations and is therefore known as Fc (fragment, crystallizable). The Fc regions of immunoglobulins bind isotype-specific immunoglobulin Fc receptors on macrophages, neutrophils, and other white blood cells. The protease pepsin cleaves immunoglobulin into two disulfide-linked Fab fragments, known as $F(ab')_2$. This can be used to study dimeric antibody binding in the absence of effector functions conferred by the Fc fragment.

Genetic engineering of immunoglobulin variants has led to the development of single-chain molecules carrying the structure of the V domains of both heavy and light chains covalently linked by a spacer of about 15 amino acids.[67] These "Fv" molecules may penetrate tissues better than the much larger intact antibody molecules. Immunoglobulin Fv proteins have been engineered with links to other functional domains, such as toxins, to target tumor antigens as a potential cancer therapy.

Functions of Immunoglobulin

Immunoglobulin performs several different functions, depending on whether it resides on the lymphocyte surface as a BCR or is secreted as soluble antibody.

As a BCR, immunoglobulin serves as an antigen-specific trigger for B-cell activation or, in the case of self antigen, tolerance. The cytoplasmic residues at the carboxyl terminus of the heavy chain are quite short and apparently do not contribute significantly to signaling. Each H_2L_2 molecule of membrane immunoglobulin is associated with a disulfide-linked heterodimer of signaling proteins known as Igα and Igβ.[68] Each of these proteins contains a single extracellular immunoglobulin domain and a cytoplasmic ITAM. Similar ITAMs mediate signal transduction in TCR complexes and in various other receptors of the immune system including Fc receptors on NK cells, as discussed earlier. In BCRs, crosslinking by multivalent antigen epitopes brings Igα-Igβ proteins in close proximity to kinases that phosphorylate the ITAMs and trigger a cascade of downstream phosphorylation events similar in many respects to that seen in T cells as a result of TCR ligation.[69] Certain BCR signaling events trigger several maturation steps early in B-cell development, so individuals genetically deficient in a signaling protein can suffer from profound B lymphocytopenia and agammaglobulinemia (e.g., patients with Bruton's agammaglobulinemia, caused by a mutation in the kinase Btk).[70] B cells act as efficient APCs for their cognate antigen (i.e., the protein recognized by their surface immunoglobulin)[71] or, at high concentrations, for other soluble antigens they happen to internalize.

The three major functions of secreted immunoglobulin in immune defense are neutralization of toxins and viruses, complement activation, and opsonization. Toxins and viruses typically attach to a host cell receptor before they can trigger their damaging consequences. If antibodies bind to the same surface regions of the toxin or virus that contact their respective receptors, this binding can block attachment and thereby prevent toxin function or viral entry into host cells. This protective function relies exclusively on the antigen-binding properties of antibodies, but antigen clearance is enhanced by the Fc portion (see later).

Complement is a system of serum proteins that can lyse bacteria and trigger various local inflammatory changes to promote immune defense. These proteins circulate in an inactive state but can be activated by proteolytic cleavage, in many cases by other specific complement components. The complement cascade can be triggered by certain pathogens through pathways that are part of the innate immune system, but complement can also be activated by antibodies of certain isotypes binding on the surface of a bacterium. The ability to fix complement in this way is dependent on amino acid residues in the Fc portion of certain immunoglobulin isotypes (see Table 6–2).[72] Several complement proteins deposited on a bacterium form an "attack complex" that lyses the cell. Certain other complement components enhance B-cell activation through a membrane complement receptor protein, CD21. Because of the potency of complement to induce cell lysis and inflammation, the system is tightly controlled by complement regulatory proteins. Defects in complement or complement regulatory proteins can cause symptoms of inflammation (e.g., hereditary angioedema), recurrent infections (from various complement factor deficiencies), or cell lysis (paroxysmal nocturnal hemoglobulinuria; see Chapter 25).

The third function of antibody in immune defense is to promote phagocytosis and killing of bacteria by NK cells, macrophages, and granulocytes. This ADCC function results from antibodies that bind to antigens on the surface of bacteria; these bound antibodies are said to "opsonize" the bacteria by tagging them for destruction by phagocytes. ADCC depends on the Fc portion of the antibody, which binds to isotype-specific Fc receptors on the surface of phagocytes, thus activating these cells.[73] Binding of antibody Fc regions to Fc receptors also facilitates phagocytosis of soluble protein antigens, toxins, and viruses that are bound to antibody.

V Region Gene Assembly during B-Lymphocyte Development in Bone Marrow

Lymphocytes develop in the bone marrow from a common lymphoid progenitor, which gives rise to NK cells and T and B lymphocytes. The common origin of B and T lymphocytes correlates with their common mechanism for generating V region diversity of antigen receptors. The genes for these receptors are unique in that they exist in the germline in several segments that must be assembled during the development of individual lymphocytes in order to be expressed. For heavy chains, a V region is formed from one germline variable (V_H) segment; one diversity (D) segment, and one joining (J_H) segment, and light chain V regions are formed from a V_κ (or V_λ) segment plus a J_κ (or J_λ) segment. The assembly of a complete immunoglobulin gene region occurs through the process of VDJ recombination, which proceeds in ordered steps during the maturation of the B-cell lineage in the bone marrow.[74] Each recombination is initiated by DNA cleavage catalyzed by the two recombinase-activating genes, *RAG1* and *RAG2*. These enzymes recognize cleavage sites just outside the V, D, and J segments via a conserved heptamer (CACAGTG) and nonamer (ACAAAAACC) present on one or the other of the DNA strands. The RAG proteins are expressed almost exclusively in the lymphoid lineage, at specific stages of early B- and T-cell development; however, most subsequent steps of DNA processing and rejoining are accomplished by ubiquitous enzymes of the nonhomologous end joining pathway.

The germline diversity of the three human immunoglobulin gene loci (heavy chain, κ and λ) can be approximated by counting V segments available in the germline DNA before VDJ recombination. However, in all three loci an exact enumeration of germline V segments is complicated by variations in different haplotypes, by the presence of multiple pseudogenes and V segments that have never been shown to be expressed, and by some V segments that do not increase effective sequence diversity because they are nearly identical to other V segments. With these caveats, the heavy chain locus on chromosome 14q32 contains about 40 different functional V_H segments, 27 D segments, and 6 J_H segments. The κ locus at chromosome 2p12 contains about 29 different V_κ regions and 5 J_κ segments, and the λ locus at chromosome 22q11 contains about 30 V_λ segments and 4 J_λ segments. This germline diversity could theoretically yield 1.7 million VDJ_H/VJ_L combinations. Additional diversity is provided because, after RAG-mediated cleavage, the DNA ends of the V, D, or J segments may be shortened to a variable extent by exonuclease trimming before being joined.[75] Conversely, variable numbers of nucleotides may be added to the DNA ends by the enzyme terminal deoxynucleotide transferase; these added nucleotides are known as N (nucleotide) regions.[76] The trimming and nucleotide addition create extra diversity at the boundaries of the V, D and J segments, although at the cost of creating some useless out-of-frame sequences. However, human D regions can be utilized in all three reading frames, so an assembled VDJ region can be functional as long as the reading frames of V and J match. The residues at the V-J and V-D-J junctions correspond to CDR3 of the light and heavy chains, respectively, so the junctional diversity contributes significantly to the diversity of antigen-binding specificities.

The steps of VDJ recombination are tightly regulated during B-cell development in such a way that each B cell expresses only one species of immunoglobulin; of the two chromosomal copies of each locus the silent one is said to be allelically excluded. When the RAG proteins are expressed beginning in pro-B cells, the initial recombination occurs in the heavy chain locus, joining one D and one J_H and deleting all the intervening DNA. Usually DJ_H recombinations occur on both chromosomal copies. Then recombination joins a V_H to the DJ_H on one chromosome. If the recombination is nonproductive, yielding an out-of-frame VDJ sequence, then recombination continues on the other chromosome. However, if the first VDJ sequence is in frame and can produce a functional μ heavy chain, then this protein is expressed on the surface (of what is now a pre-B cell) along with a surrogate light chain to form a pre-BCR. This surface molecule shuts off RAG expression, preventing further heavy chain recombination that might lead to expression of the second chromosomal heavy chain locus.[77] (The surrogate light chain comprises a V-like and a C_λ-like protein, which together supply a light chain–like function necessary to allow the heavy chain to reach the surface of the

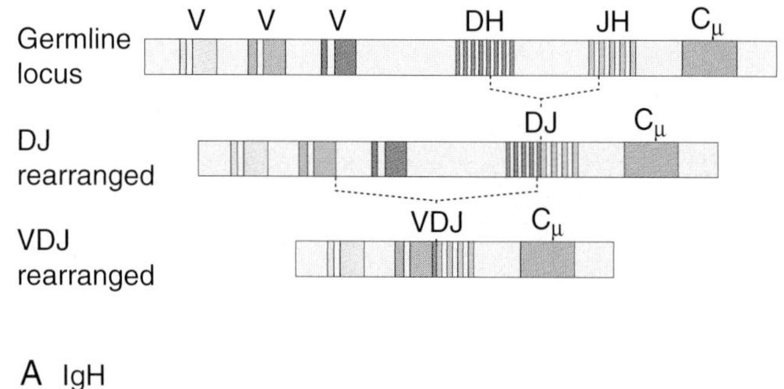

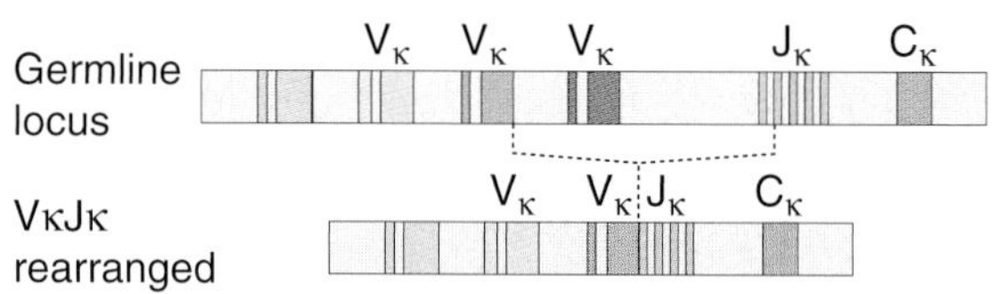

Figure 6–8. V(D)J recombination. ***A,*** The heavy chain locus, IgH, comprises V regions, D_H regions, J_H regions, and multiple heavy chain constant (C) regions, of which C_μ is the one first expressed. An initial recombination event joins one D_H and one J_H to create a DJ segment, which subsequently joins to one of the V_H regions to complete V region assembly. ***B,*** Light chain gene rearrangement joins one V and one J segment to assemble a contiguous variable region gene.

pre-B cell.[78]) After further maturation of the pre-B cell, RAG expression is reactivated and light chain gene recombination begins, usually at the κ locus. When a productive κ recombination occurs, surface expression of the completed H_2L_2 IgM protein generates similar negative feedback of further light chain recombination to insure light chain allelic exclusion. The appearance of surface IgM defines the cell as an immature B cell. After further maturation, the cell expresses surface IgD along with IgM. The RNA transcript for IgD is produced by alternative splicing of a transcript that reads through the C_μ gene, past its downstream termination site, and continues through the C_δ gene. With IgD expression, the cell becomes a mature B cell (Fig. 6–8).

More than 50% of newly created B cells express an antibody that binds to a self antigen.[79] Such autoreactive cells risk causing autoimmune disease, but are restrained by several mechanisms. These cells can be deleted by triggering apoptosis[80]; they can be silenced ("anergized") so that, though alive, they are unable to secrete antibody; or they can revise their antibody by light chain "editing."[81] Mature B cells must pass a screening "checkpoint" that tests autoreactivity before they are released from the bone marrow, and at least one other checkpoint in the periphery before they become functional in antibody secretion.[82] The nature of these checkpoints is cur-

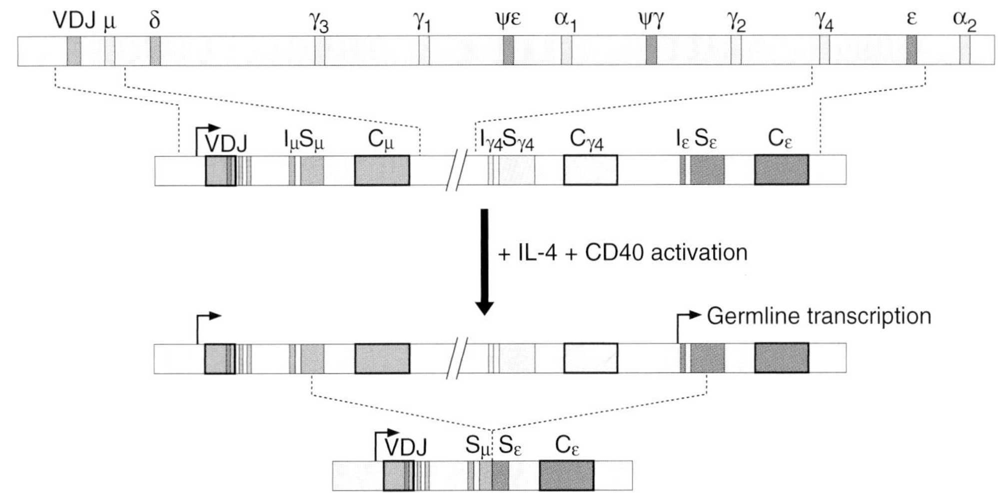

Figure 6–9. Heavy chain isotype switching. The *top line* depicts the human heavy chain locus as it exists in a B cell expressing IgM; a rearranged VDJ segment lies upstream of the C_μ gene, which in turn lies upstream of C_δ, $C_\gamma 3$, $C_\gamma 1$, a pseudo-C_ε, $C_\alpha 1$, pseudo-C_γ, $C_\gamma 2$, $C_\gamma 4$, C_ε, and $C_\alpha 2$. As shown in the expanded segments in the *second line* of the figure, upstream of the C regions lies a switch (S) region and an untranslated exon known as an I region. (In this and subsequent lines, the rectangles outlined in bold represent coding regions, and rectangles with thin outlines represent noncoding segments.) When the B cell is activated by stimuli suitable for inducing isotype switching, new transcription is driven by a promoter upstream of the targeted I region *(third line),* which leads to recombination between the associated S region and S_μ. The product of the switch recombination is a composite S region, which leaves a new C region downstream of VDJ in the position formerly occupied by C_μ *(fourth line).*

rently unknown, but defects in the checkpoints presumably underlie autoimmune disease. For example, defects in apoptosis of autoreactive cells triggered by the membrane protein Fas are found in the autoimmune lymphoproliferative syndrome (see Chapter 58).

B-Cell Development in the Periphery

Mature resting B cells circulate in the periphery and can be activated when the BCR is cross-linked by the binding of multivalent antigen. In addition to stimulation by antigen, most B-cell responses require T-cell "help" consisting of stimulation by cytokines and contact between surface molecules on the B and T cells. This interaction is efficient in germinal centers of the spleen, lymph nodes, and tonsils, and under appropriate conditions (typically including antigen presentation by follicular dendritic cells) leads to mutual activation of B and T cells. The germinal center environment also promotes two further alterations in immunoglobulin gene structure: isotype switching and somatic mutation.

In isotype switching, a recombination mechanistically distinct from VDJ recombination leads to deletion of the C_μ gene and its replacement downstream of the expressed VDJ segments by a different C region gene, which is then expressed[83] (Fig. 6–9). The breakpoints for this class switch recombination (CSR), fall within highly repetitive "switch regions" located upstream of Cμ and of each constant region gene (except Cδ). A key participant is the protein referred to as "activation-induced deaminase,"[84] which is specifically expressed in activated B cells in germinal centers and which is required for somatic mutation as well as CSR. This protein is homologous to enzymes that deaminate cytosine, and it has in vitro cytosine deaminase activity. Activation-induced deaminase expression is believed to lead to DNA cleavage in switch regions; the resulting DNA ends might then be joined by some ubiquitous DNA repair factors. Patients (and mice) with null mutants of activation-induced deaminase, CD40, or CD40 ligand are defective in CSR and often show increased IgM levels ("hyper-IgM") and immunodeficiencies related to inadequate secretion of IgG and other isotypes.[85] Mutations in several other genes (e.g., *H2AX,* exonuclease-1, *53BP1,* uracil deglycosylase, DNA-PK) also impair CSR, although their exact roles in the mechanism of CSR remain unknown.

The other major modification of immunoglobulin genes in the germinal center is somatic hypermutation.[86] This process specifically targets V_H and V_L genes for DNA mutations that occur at a frequency about a million times higher than the background mutation frequency. Most of these mutations are inconsequential, but a few increase binding affinity to antigen. These favorable mutations are efficiently selected in the germinal center by a process that induces apoptosis in B cells except those triggered most efficiently by the interaction of their surface BCR with antigen.[87] Multiple rounds of mutation and selection can yield antibodies with 100-fold increases in binding affinity compared with unmutated antibodies.

These high-affinity B cells proliferate over several days and mature into plasma cells, which secrete very high levels of antibody. Plasma cells are terminally differentiated, with an eccentric nucleus owing to proliferation of endoplasmic reticulum supporting high level protein synthesis; and most have a life span of about 3 days. But a small population of plasma cells live longer, providing a sustained antibody level for several weeks after challenge. A population of memory cells derived from the high-affinity mutated B cells circulates for months or years, able to respond to a subsequent antigen challenge with almost immediate high-affinity antibody production.[88]

Immunoglobulin Genes in Lymphomas and Leukemias

Chromosomal translocations are known to play a role in many malignancies. Immunoglobulin (and TCR) genes are uniquely prone to translocations through errors in the normal recombination mechanisms that are required for their function. A classic example of a malignancy triggered by a faulty immunoglobulin gene rearrangement is Burkitt's lymphoma. A translocation most commonly found in this cancer brings the c-*myc* gene from chromosome 8 into the proximity of the heavy chain immunoglobulin gene regulatory regions on chromosome 14, leading to dysregulation of c-*myc* expression (see Chapter 43).[89] Similarly, translocation of the *bcl2* gene on chromosome 18 into the IgH locus causes upregulation of this antiapoptotic gene, leading to follicular lymphoma (see Chapter 43). The polymerase chain reaction can be used to amplify the specific translocation in a given lymphoma or leukemia, so presence of the translocation can serve as a marker for detection of residual disease during remission. Similarly, specific VDJ or VJ recombined segments can be used as markers because they should be unique to the malignant clone.[90] In addition, characteristic features of various stages in B-cell (or T-cell) development can be used in the diagnosis or characterization of malignancies derived from those stages. For example, V genes are typically unmutated in acute lymphocytic leukemia (corresponding to lymphoid progenitor cells), but often actively mutating in follicular and Burkitt's lymphomas (corresponding to germinal center cells), and mutated without clonal variation in Waldenström's macroglobulinemia and multiple myeloma (corresponding, respectively, to post–germinal center IgM-secreting B cells and plasma cells).

Apart from the status of their immunoglobulin genes, leukemias and lymphomas share many cell surface markers with normal cells of the corresponding lymphoid maturation state, allowing tumor typing by staining with antibodies against such markers. Recently, attempts to link specific lymphoid malignancies to corresponding stages of normal development have been enhanced by the availability of microarray technology to quantitate and compare expression of thousands of genes simultaneously between malignant cells and subsets of normal cells (see Chapter 104).

ADAPTIVE IMMUNITY: T CELLS

The T-Cell Receptor

T cells recognize antigen via their antigen-specific TCRs. The TCR is composed of a heterodimer consisting of either α/β or γ/δ gene products.[91] As shown in Figure 6–10, each chain consists of a C region that is proximal to the T-cell membrane and a distal V region. γ/δ T cells are less clonally diverse and appear to play an important role in the innate immune response. α/β TCRs, in contrast, demonstrate greater diversity, and this accounts for the ability of T cells to recognize the vast array of potential pathogens. Most T cells express a single TCR that is generated by recombination of germline DNA V, D, and J elements similar to those described for BCR expression.[92] Diversity is enhanced by random insertion/deletion of residues,[93] and by the combination of the rearranged α and β chains.

T Cells Recognize Peptides Complexed to MHC Molecules

The TCR recognizes antigens in the form of peptides presented by MHC molecules, expressed on the cell surface.[94] Class I MHC molecules are expressed on almost all cells in the body and interact primarily with T cells that express the CD8 coreceptor molecule. Class II MHC molecules interact with $CD4^+$ T cells and in general are only expressed on APCs such as DCs, macrophages, and B cells. For both classes of MHC molecules, processed antigens are presented as peptides bound to a groove in the MHC molecules and displayed on the surface of cells (see Fig. 6–10). MHC molecules are highly polymorphic, especially in the peptide-binding region. At any one time, a cell may express between 10^4 and 10^6 MHC molecules on its surface, and each MHC allele may present between 1000 and 2000 different self peptides.[95] During an infection, between 100 and 10,000 pathogen-derived peptides may be displayed per cell.[96]

MHC Restriction

The V region of the TCR binds both to the MHC molecule and to exposed residues of the peptide residing in the groove of the MHC molecule.[97] The interaction between TCR and peptide-MHC is facilitated by the binding of the coreceptor CD8 to the nonpolymorphic region of class I molecules or CD4 to class II. Because the TCR recognizes the composite structure of a peptide-MHC molecule, a TCR specific for one peptide-MHC combination will generally not bind to the same peptide in the context of a different MHC protein. This fact, along with the differential peptide-binding affinities of allelic MHC proteins, explains why T cells from one individual will not recognize peptide presented by infected cells from an MHC-discrepant individual, a property known as MHC restriction.

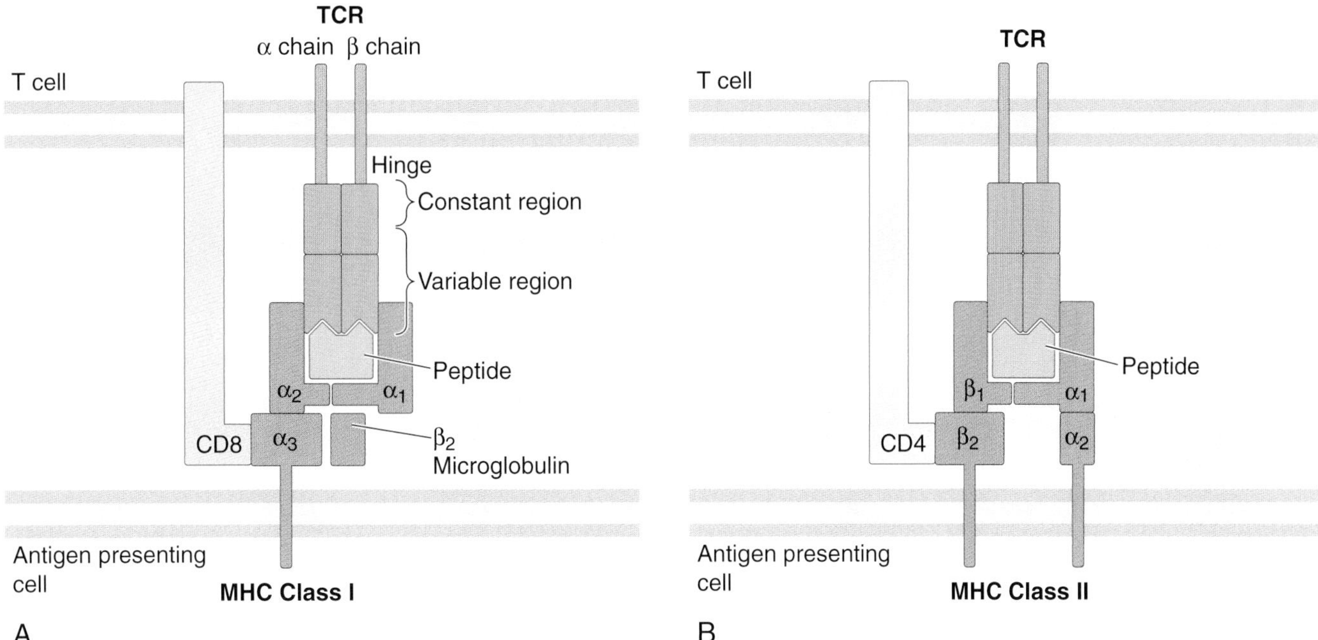

Figure 6–10. T-cell receptor–major histocompatability complex (TCR-MHC) interaction. The TCR consists of an α chain and a β chain. Each chain has a constant region proximal to the T-cell membrane and a variable region that interacts with both MHC and peptide. ***A,*** $CD8^+$ cells recognize peptide presented by MHC class I molecules that consist of a single chain that is associated with β_2-microglobulin. The peptide-binding groove of class I is composed of both the α1 and α2 domains, while CD8 binds to a site on the α3 domain. ***B,*** $CD4^+$ T cells recognize peptide presented by MHC class II molecules that consist of an α and β chain. The peptide-binding groove is formed by the α1 and β1 domains, while the CD4 binding site lies at the base of the β2 domain.

T-Cell Development

Anatomy of Thymic Development

Precursors of T cells migrate from the bone marrow to the thymus, where T-cell development occurs. These precursors enter the thymus at the corticomedullary junction as $CD4^-CD8^-$ double-negative (DN) cells.[98] On the cell surface, these cells are $CD44^+CD25^-$ and are known as DN1 stage cells. Next, the cells migrate toward the subcapsular epithelium, where they upregulate CD25 (DN2 stage) and then downregulate CD44 (DN3 stage). Thymocytes at the DN3 stage have evidence of rearrangement of the β locus of the TCR. In addition, at this stage there is evidence of γδ locus rearrangement. In order for a thymocyte to successfully advance to the next stage (DN4), $V_\beta DJ_\beta$ rearrangement must be in frame so that β chain protein can pair with an invariant form of the α chain known as pre-TCRα. Signaling through the V_β/pre-TCRα heterodimer results in the downregulation of CD25, proliferation and maturation marked by rearrangement of the V_α chain, and the simultaneous expression of CD4 and CD8, known as double-positives (DPs).

Positive Selection

Because the generation of the TCR is a stochastic process, it is crucial that each receptor be tested for its ability to interact with host MHC molecules. Most TCRs cannot make proper contact with host MHC molecules and die of "neglect" in the thymus. As the DP thymocytes migrate from the cortex to the medulla, they encounter MHC molecules on the surface of the thymic cortical epithelial cells.[99] The TCRs on the DP T cells interact with the MHC molecules presenting self peptides.[100] Because the thymocyte is both $CD4^+$ and $CD8^+$, this interaction can occur with either class I or class II MHC molecules. When a TCR and its coreceptor adequately engage an MHC molecule downregulates its unused coreceptor, a process known as positive selection. If a DP cell interacts with a class I molecule on the surface of a thymic epithelial cell, then this cell is positively selected to become a $CD8^+$ single-positive (SP) T cell. Likewise, if the DP thymocyte should encounter a fit with a class II molecule via its TCR and CD4 coreceptor, then the cell will downregulate its CD8 coreceptor and become a $CD4^+$ SP T cell (Fig. 6–11). Upon being positively selected to become a SP cell, the thymocyte continues to migrate toward the medulla of the thymus.[101]

Negative Selection

It is potentially dangerous to the host if the TCR has high affinity for and becomes activated as a result of interacting with self peptides.[102] If a TCR engages a self peptide-MHC complex with high affinity the T cell is deleted. This process is known as negative selection and serves to greatly reduce the odds of self reactive T cells from emerging from the thymus. This process can occur in the cortex,

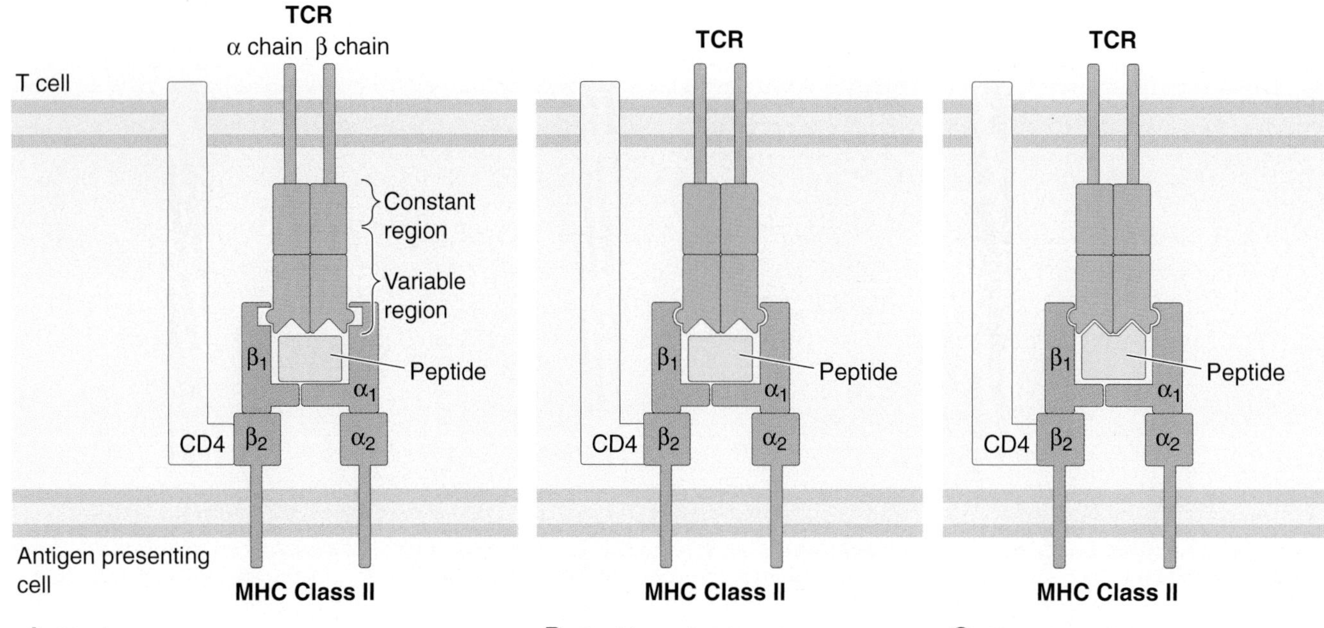

Figure 6–11. Positive and negative selection *A,* The majority of developing thymocytes do not receive adequate survival signals through the TCR. As depicted in the figure, the shape of this TCR does not permit it to adequately interact with the MHC molecules. This in turn prevents the T cell from receiving the (low-affinity) interaction necessary to promote its survival. As a result, T cells bearing "useless" TCRs die. *B,* In positive selection, the TCR interacts with the MHC-peptide complex in a low-affinity interaction. This interaction is adequate to deliver survival signals via the TCR. As depicted in the figure, this TCR is able to contact the MHC molecule but does not have a strong interaction with the peptide. *C,* In negative selection, the affinity for the MHC-peptide complex is great and the TCR-mediated signaling leads to apoptosis.

but in general it is thought that negative selection takes place in the medulla, where bone marrow–derived APCs efficiently present self peptides to SP thymocytes.[103]

T-Cell Signaling

The Immunologic Synapse

The interaction between the TCR and the MHC molecule results in a defined cytoskeletal reorganization in which cell surface receptors, actin filaments, and lipids become polarized at the T cell–APC interface at a structure known as the immune synapse. Microscopic sections of the T cell–APC interface have revealed supramolecular activation complexes (SMACs) composed of the TCR, adhesion molecules and signaling machinery.[104] At the center (cSMAC) of this "bull's eye–like" structure is the TCR along with key signaling elements such as protein kinase C (PKC)-θ. The region peripheral to the cSMAC (termed the pSMAC) is enriched with adhesion molecules such as lymphocyte function antigen-1. Finally, most distal from the center (the dSMAC) are large molecules such as CD43, CD44, and CD45, which actually enter the cSMAC during the course of activation.

Lipid Rafts

The recognition of antigen by the TCR and the formation of the immunologic synapse with accessory molecules promote signal transduction. Signaling in T cells is greatly facilitated by the recruitment of detergent-resistant microdomains termed *lipid rafts* that are rich in cholesterol, sphingolipids, and GPI-anchored proteins.[105] These lipid rafts are enriched for Src family kinases (Lck) and the adapter protein referred to as "linker for activated T cells" (LAT), which play a critical role in initiating and amplifying TCR-induced signaling.[106] In naive T cells, raft components are predominately found scattered throughout the cell, whereas in previously activated/memory cells, these signaling molecule–laden microdomains can be found preexisiting the plasma membrane. This observation may account for the fact that memory cells are more rapidly activated than naive cells.

The TCR-associated protein CD3 mediates TCR-induced signaling through phosphorylation of its ITAM motifs by protein tyrosine kinases such as Lck. These in turn act as docking sites for proximal signaling molecules, leading to the attraction of rafts bearing Lck and LAT.[107] The mobilization of the rafts to the synapse is dependent upon actin reorganization involving Vav-1, Rac, Cdc42, and Wiskott-Aldrich syndrome protein.[108,109] Upon phosphorylation by ZAP-70, LAT acts as a docking site for phospholipase C-γ (PLC-γ), phosphatidylinositol-3-kinase, and other adapter proteins. Finally, ITK, SLP-76, Grb2, and PKC-θ, all of which play critical roles in TCR-induced signaling, are also found in the rafts (Fig. 6–12).

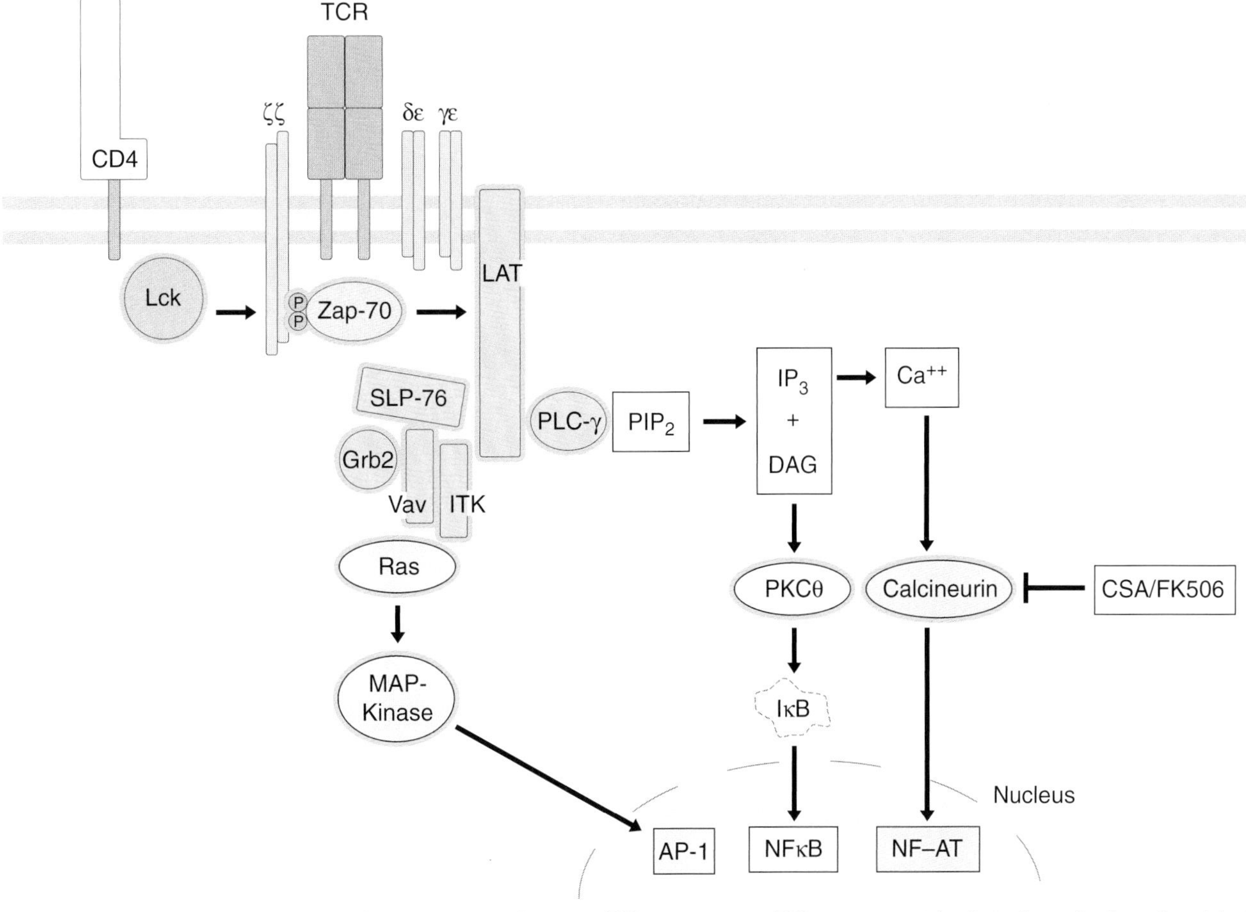

Figure 6–12. Outline of the flow of signal transduction upon TCR engagement. TCR engagement leads to the activation of protein tyrosine kinases such as Lck. This in turn leads to the phosphorylation of immunoreceptor tyrosine-based activation motifs (ITAMs) on the chains of CD3 and the phosphorylation and activation of ZAP-70 *(yellow)*. Next, depicted in *green,* the adapters LAT and SLP-76 become activated, and this facilitates the activation of PLC-γ, ITK, and Vav Grb2. PLC-γ facilitates the generation of IP_3 and DAG. DAG + Ca^{2+} promote PKC activation, while Ca^{2+} promotes calcineurin activation *(pink)*. At this point *(blue)*, signaling begins to diverge into three general pathways. The activation of the calcineurin pathway leads to the dephosphorylation and translocation of NF-AT to the nucleus. The activation of PKC ultimately leads to the degradation of the inhibitor of κB (IκB) and the translocation of NF-kB to the nucleus. The activation of Ras in turn leads to the activation of mitogen-activated protein kinases (MAP kinases) and ultimately the production and activation of Jun and Fos, which together make up activator protein-1.

TCR-Induced Signaling Pathways

The phosphorylation of LAT and SLP-76 provides the scaffolding for the molecules that will promote the downstream events responsible for TCR-induced signaling (see Fig. 6–12).[107] In particular, PLC-γ recruitment causes the hydrolysis of phosphatidylinositol-4,5-bisphosphate into 1,4,5-triphosphate (IP_3) and diacylglycerol (DAG). DAG serves to activate PKC and IP_3 leads to the release of intracellular Ca^{2+}.[110] The Ca^{2+}-dependent activation of the phosphatase calcineurin leads to the dephosphorylation of nuclear factor of activated T cells (NF-AT) and its translocation to the nucleus. Notably, calcineurin is inhibited by the potent immunosuppressive agents cyclosporin A and FK506.[111] PKC-θ leads to degradation of inhibitor of κB and the activation of the transcription factors that make up the nuclear factor-κB (NF-κB) family.[112] Activation of the Ras/mitogen-activated protein kinase pathway leads to the generation of active forms of the transcription factors Jun and Fos, which make up activator protein-1.[113] The transcription factors NF-AT, NF-κB, and activator protein-1 are involved in the upregulation of many T-cell–produced cytokines, in particular IL-2.

Costimulatory Molecules

TCR engagement is referred to as signal 1, whereas costimulatory signals are referred to as signal 2.[114] A major component of signal 2 is the engagement of CD28 on the surface of the T cell by B7.1 or B7.2 on the surface of the APC. Resting "professional" APCs do not display significant levels of B7 on their surface, and thus, when antigen is presented by a resting APC, the outcome is the induction of T-cell tolerance.[115] When APCs become activated by infectious products such as lipopolysaccharide, CpG, or viral RNA or by other cells via CD40 stimulation, they upregulate B7.1 and B7.2 and become potent T-cell stimulators.

CD28 engagement enhances T-cell activation, whereas engagement of the related protein cytotoxic T-lymphocyte antigen-4 (CTLA-4) inhibits T-cell activation.[116] CTLA-4 has a 10-fold higher affinity for B7.1 and B7.2 compared with CD28 and is upregulated upon T-cell activation at the transcriptional level as well as through the rapid cell surface migration of CTLA-4–laden vesicles. The B7–CTLA-4 interaction increases the threshold of TCR-induced activation and attenuates T-cell responses. The importance of this negative regulation is demonstrated by the death of CTLA-4 knockout mice from a lymphoproliferative disorder. In addition, the blockade of CTLA-4–B7 interactions in vivo in mice promotes tumor immunity.[117]

Additional costimulatory molecules have been identified by searching for molecules that share sequence similarity with B7.[118] These include B7-H1, B7-DC, B7-H3, and B7-H4. B7-H1 appears to mediate negative regulation by binding to a specific receptor (PD-1) on T cells. In addition to B7 family members, member of the TNF receptor family have also been shown to play a role in providing costimulation[119] (Fig. 6–13).

T-Cell Effector Functions

Anatomy of a T-Cell Response

Naive T cells emerge from the thymus and traffic through the blood and in and out of lymph nodes (see Fig. 6–5). The naive T cells enter the lymph via specialized portals consisting of high endothelial venules.[120] They are attracted to the secondary lymphoid organs by chemokines (e.g., CCL21, the ligand for CCR7).[121] Once in the lymph node, T cells localize in a region known as the T zone that is rich in DCs expressing a high density of peptide-MHC complexes. When an antigen-specific naive T cell encounters its cognate antigen, it clonally expands and differentiates into an effector memory cell. Such cells then leave the lymph node via the efferent lymph and migrate to the site of infection. In addition, these newly activated cells interact with antigen-specific B cells and provide the "help" necessary for humoral responses. A key aspect of this response is the activation of B cells by CD40 ligand interacting with CD40 on the surface of the B cell.

A subset of T cells emerging from the primary immune response will persist as memory cells. Such cells

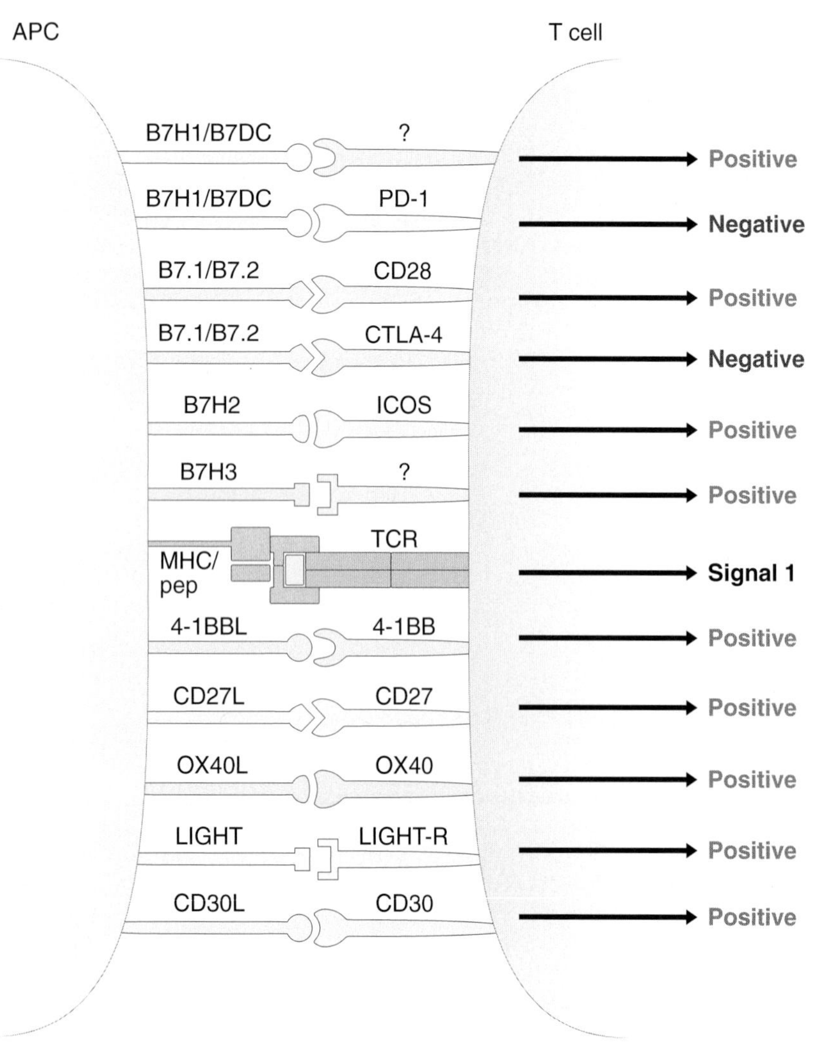

Figure 6–13. Costimulatory molecules. Signal 1 refers to TCR engagement of the MHC-peptide complex. Signal 2 can be derived from a number of ligand-receptor interactions that can either enhance or inhibit T-cell activation. B7 family members are shown in *pink* and TNF receptor family members are shown in *blue*. (Adapted from Pardoll DM: Spinning molecular immunology into successful immunotherapy. Nat Rev Immunol 2:227–238, 2002.)

respond rapidly upon stimulation in terms of the secretion of cytokines such as IL-4 and IFN-γ and, in the case of CD8$^+$ T cells, possess cytotoxic granules.[121] A second subset, CCR7$^+$ memory cells, are termed *central memory T cells*. Central memory T cells circulate throughout secondary lymphoid tissues and may represent a pool of memory T cells from which effector memory T cells are derived.

CD4$^+$ Helper T Cells as T_H1 Cells and T_H2 Cells

CD4$^+$ T cells mediate their effector function through the release of cytokines. When a naive T cell is stimulated by an APC, it produces IL-2. Upon antigen recognition, the T cell upregulates its IL-2 receptor and responds to autocrine IL-2 by proliferating. IL-2 can also promote proliferation and differentiation of NK cells as well as enhance their cytolytic function. Alternatively, IL-2 can also negatively regulate immune responses by promoting activation-induced cell death.[121a]

The resulting stimulated CD4$^+$ T cells became either T_H1 or T_H2 cells.[122] T_H1 cells secrete IL-2, IFN-γ, and TNF, and T_H2 cells secrete IL-4, IL-5, IL-9, IL-13, and IL-15. T_H1 T cells help in combating intracellular bacteria and parasites as well as viral infections.[123] The IFN-γ released from these cells activates macrophages, promotes the production of IgG from B cells, activates NK cells, and, along with IL-2, promotes the differentiation of CD8$^+$ cytotoxic T lymphocytes (CTLs). TNF promotes the activation of neutrophils. Cumulatively, these functions promote the eradication of intracellular pathogens.

The T_H2 response is essential for antibody production and combating extracellular organisms such as helminthes.[124] IL-4 promotes antibody production by B cells (IgG4 and eventually IgE) and, along with IL-10 (which is often grouped with T_H2 cytokines), suppresses macrophage function. IL-5 activates eosinophils. Taken together T_H2 cells enhance the production of neutralizing antibodies and mast cell and eosinophil function. In addition, T_H2 responses are associated with allergies, atopy, and asthma (Table 6–4).

The fate of a CD4$^+$ T cell (whether it is destined to become a T_H1 or T_H2 cell) is dictated by the context in which the cell is stimulated.[124] Intracellular bacteria (e.g., *Listeria*), parasites such as *Leishmania*, or viruses promote T_H1 responses due to the release of IL-12 by macrophages. Virally stimulated NK cells can skew T-cell polarization to a T_H1 response by releasing IFN-γ, which in turn acts on macrophages to release IL-12. In addition, CD8α$^+$ DCs produce IL-12 and preferentially skew T cells toward T_H1 responses, whereas CD8α$^-$ DCs promote T_H2 responses.[125]

CD8$^+$ T-Cell Effector Function

When a cell is infected by a pathogen, peptides derived from the pathogen will be displayed by MHC class I molecules on the surface of the cell. CD8$^+$ T cells (CTLs) specific for the pathogen-derived peptides can then recognize the infected cell and destroy it. Thus, the CD8$^+$ CTLs play an important role in the immunity to viruses, intracellular pathogens such as *Listeria monocytogenes*, mycobacteria, and parasites such as *Toxoplasma gondii*.[126]

When CD8+ T cells emerge from the thymus they are not capable of lysing targets. They are preCTLs that circulate between the blood and the lymph. In order to be activated and differentiated into CTLs, they must first be activated by antigen in the presence of costimulation. This can occur in a number of ways. First, the CD8$^+$ T cell can recognize antigen presented by an infected, activated, professional APC. Since the APC is activated, it will express high levels of costimulatory molecules such as B7, and the CD8$^+$ T cell will thus be stimulated via its TCR (signal 1) and by CD28 engagement (signal 2).[127] This "full activation" will result in the differentiation of the CD8+ T cell such that now it begins to express molecules associated with the ability to lyse targets.[127] In some cases, the APC itself does not necessarily have to be infected but simply activated (for example, by TLR engagement). In this process, known as cross presentation, pathogen-derived peptides are picked up by bone marrow–derived APCs and presented by class I molecules.

In some instances, full activation and differentiation of pre-CTLs into activated killers can be facilitated by CD4$^+$ T cells. For example, if a CD4$^+$ T cell recognizes a pathogen-derived peptide presented in the context of a class II molecule and a CD8$^+$ pre-CTL is engaged with a class I molecule on the same APC, then cytokines such

TABLE 6–4. T_H1 versus T_H2 Helper T Cells

	T_H1	T_H2
Promoted by	IL-12, IFN-γ	IL-4
Inhibited by	IL-4	IFN-γ
Cytokines	IL-2, IFN-γ, TNF; also IL-3, GM-CSF	IL-4, IL-5, IL-9, IL-13, IL-15; also IL-3, GM-CSF, IL-10.
Effect on antibody production	Promotes IgG1, IgG3 (humans)	Promotes naive B cells to differentiate and produce IgM. Promotes production of Ig (other than IgG1 & IgG3).
Effect on immune cells	Activates macrophages, neutrophils, NK cells, CTLs	Inhibits macrophage function, promotes growth of mast cells and growth and differentiation of eosinophils.
Promotes immunity	Viruses, intracellular pathogens	Extracellular organisms such as parasites

Abbreviations: CTLs, cytotoxic T lymphocytes; GM-CSF, granulocyte-macrophage colony-stimulating factor; IFN, interferon; Ig, immunoglobulin; IL, interleukin; NK, natural killer; TNF, tumor necrosis factor.

as IL-2 and IFN-γ from the $CD4^+$ T cell can serve to promote the $CD8^+$ differentiation process. Finally, $CD4^+$ T cells can facilitate $CD8^+$ T-cell activation by activating APCs. In this scenario, an activated CD4+ T cell, expressing CD40L can engage CD40 on the surface of an APC thus activating the APC. Later, that same activated APC can present antigen in the context of costimulation to a CD8 T cell and thus promote its full activation.

When the preCTLs are fully stimulated in the lymph node they proliferate and differentiate. In particular, the cells assemble membrane bound cytoplasmic granules that contain preforin and granzymes (see below). In addition, the differentiated CTLs now have the ability to produce IFN-γ and TNF that activate macrophages and enhance inflammation. They next migrate to the site of the infection. Here they will recognize antigen presented by Class I of the infected cell and initiate target cell lysis. The process of CTL killing does not require costimulation.

There are two general mechanisms by which CTLs kill their targets.[128] First, recognition of the target cell leads to the fusing of cytoplasmic granules within the CTL with the plasma membrane and subsequent exocytosis. Perforin is released and polymerizes to form pores in the plasma membrane of the target cell. Perforin facilitates the transfer of granzymes, which are serine proteases that activate caspases and thus promote apoptosis of the target cell. Additionally, CTLs can kill their targets when FasL on the CTL interacts with Fas on the target cell.

Mechanisms of T-Cell Tolerance

Horror autotoxicus is the term coined by Ehrlich and Morgenroth to describe the consequences of the immune system unleashing its effector function on one's own body.[129] Several mechanisms of peripheral tolerance protect against self-reactive T cells that escape negative selection:

- **Ignorance:** In this mechanism of peripheral tolerance, the autoreactive T cells can be found in the periphery. However, since the level of autoantigen expression is so low or is hidden from the immune system (by the blood brain barrier for example) the T cells do not respond and thus do not cause autoimmunity.[130]
- **Clonal deletion:** Autoreactive T cells can be deleted in the periphery,[131] especially if the autoantigen is present at high levels.
- **Anergy:** T cells that receive signal 1 in the absence of signal 2 not only fail to produce IL-2 and proliferate but do not respond to subsequent full rechallenge; they are said to be anergic.[132]
- **T regulatory cells:** A subset of $CD4^+CD25^+$ T cells have the ability to inhibit activation of other T cells.[133,134]
- **Immunoregulation:** Mechanisms by which the immune system negatively regulates antipathogen immune responses might also play a role in preventing horror autotoxicus, and in this sense may be considered mechanisms of peripheral tolerance. For example, IL-10, originally described as cytokine synthesis inhibitory factor, negatively regulates active immune responses, but can also play a role in inhibiting autoimmune responses and thus promote tolerance.[135–137]

Suggested Readings*

Colucci F, Caligiuri MA, Di Santo JP: What does it take to make a natural killer? Nat Rev Immunol 3:413–425, 2004.

Cooper MA, Fehniger TA, Caligiuri MA: The biology of human natural killer-cell subsets. Trends Immunol 22:633–640, 2001.

Germain RN, Stefanova I: The dynamics of T cell receptor signaling: complex orchestration and the key roles of tempo and cooperation. Annu Rev Immunol 17:467, 1999.

Jenkins MK: Peripheral T-lymphocyte responses and function. *In* Paul WE (ed): Fundamental Immunology (ed 5). Philadelphia: Lippincott Williams & Wilkins, 2003, pp 303–319.

Meffre E, Casellas R, Nussenzweig MC: Antibody regulation of B cell development. Nat Immunol 1:379–385, 2000.

Melchers F, ten Boekel E, Seidl T, et al: Repertoire selection by pre-B-cell receptors and B-cell receptors, and genetic control of B-cell development from immature to mature B cells. Immunol Rev 175:33–46, 2000.

Moser M: Dendritic cells. *In* Paul WE (ed): Fundamental Immunology (ed 5). Philadelphia: Lippincott Williams & Wilkins, 2003, pp 455–480.

Rajewsky K: Clonal selection and learning in the antibody system. Nature 381:751–758, 1996.

Starr TK, Jameson SC, Hogquist KA: Positive and negative selection of T cells. Annu Rev Immunol 21:139, 2003.

Full references for this chapter can be found on accompanying CD-ROM.

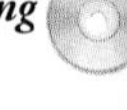

CHAPTER 7

Megakaryocyte Development and Disorders of Thrombopoiesis

Alison W. Loren, MD, MS, Charles S. Abrams, MD, and Alan M. Gewirtz, MD

KEY POINTS

Megakaryocyte Development and Disorders of Thrombopoiesis

- Peripheral blood smear and bone marrow examination are crucial components of the evaluation of the patient with thrombocytopenia.
- Autosomal dominant causes of mild thrombocytopenia should be considered in adults who are incidentally diagnosed with low platelet levels, because these patients require no medical therapy but should receive genetic counseling.
- The genetic bases for inherited thrombocytopenias provide further insight into megakaryocytopoiesis and thrombopoiesis, and highlight opportunities for future interventions with genetic or other targeted therapies.

INTRODUCTION: OVERVIEW OF MEGAKARYOCYTOPOIESIS AND THROMBOPOIESIS

Megakaryocyte Developmental Biology

Formed elements in peripheral blood are generated within the bone marrow by primitive, undifferentiated hematopoietic cells that exist in a developmental continuum.[1,2] Stem cells are the most primitive of these marrow elements.[3–5] By definition, they are noncycling and lineage indifferent, and have the capacity to self-renew. Through a series of still incompletely described molecular and biochemical events, stem cells give rise to more differentiated progenitor cells, which are characterized by decreased self-renewal capacity, commitment to development within a given hematopoietic lineage, and increased proliferative activity. Progenitor cell proliferation and acquisition of lineage-specific phenotypic markers initially accompany one another, but proliferative activity eventually subsides as cytoplasmic maturation proceeds. With continued cytoplasmic development, cells become morphologically identifiable as belonging to a given lineage and are then classified as precursor cells. Precursor cells may undergo one or two divisions as they complete their maturation into the fully functional elements that circulate in the peripheral blood.

Where megakaryocytes are concerned, lineage commitment begins when a marrow stem cell gives rise to a bipotent erythro-megakaryocytic progenitor cell (Fig. 7–1). This cell, as the name implies, can then further commit to development of either erythrocytes or megakaryocytes. How this fate decision is made is as yet uncertain, though transcriptional regulation of megakaryocyte development is an area of active investigation.

The primary purpose of the progenitor cell compartment is to exponentially amplify the number of cells that are available to enter the precursor compartment. Three types of megakaryocyte progenitor cells have been defined on the basis of their physical properties, the types of colonies they give rise to in vitro, and how long they take to develop in culture. The burst-forming unit–megakaryocyte (BFU-MK) is the least mature of the megakaryocyte progenitor cells, as demonstrated by the fact that it takes the longest to develop in culture and has the greatest proliferative capacity of all the megakaryocyte progenitor cells.[6–9] BFU-MK colonies are "buckshot" in appearance and are composed of hundreds of cells. The BFU-MK is likely the direct antecedent of the colony-forming unit–megakaryocyte (CFU-MK).[10–13] CFU-MK give rise in 10 to 12 days to single cluster colonies containing minimally 3 cells with an average of 10 cells. The most mature progenitor is the light-density CFU-MK.

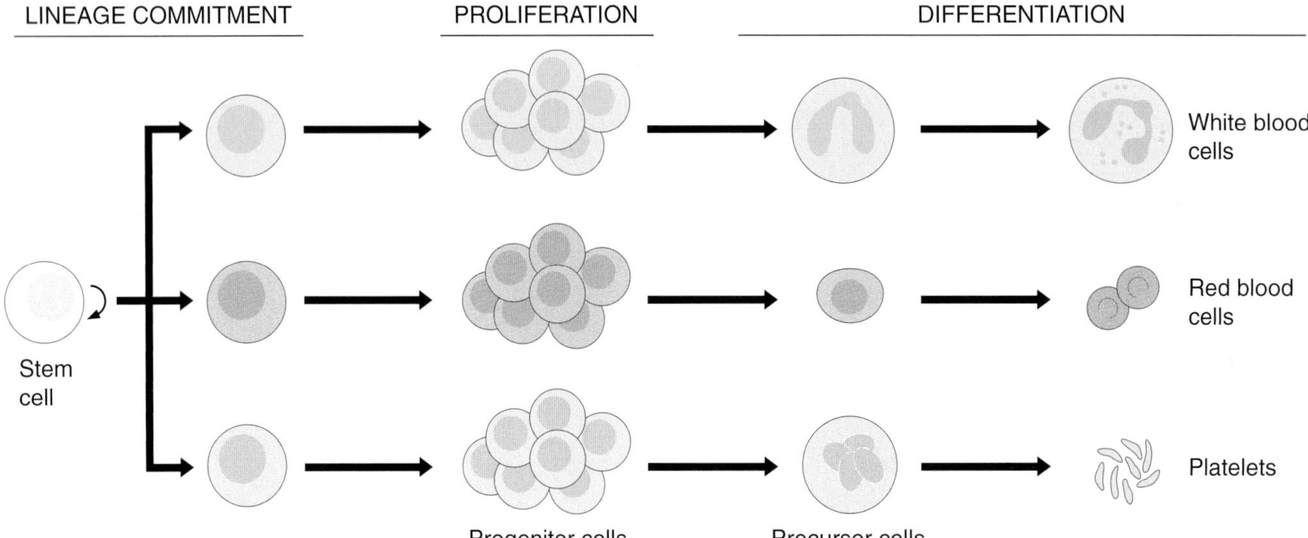

Figure 7–1. Hematopoiesis.

Light-density CFU-MK have very little proliferative capacity and therefore give rise to small colonies. The progeny of the light-density CFU-MK tend to have higher ploidy than the cells derived from the earlier progenitor cells.

Mature megakaryocytes are visible by light microscopy. Terminal development is accomplished by increasing cell ploidy and completing cytoplasmic maturation.[14,15] The microanatomic description of these stages has been well characterized in other sources.[16,17] During the initial stages of terminal maturation, DNA replication continues to occur. However, in marked contrast to the proliferative stage of cell development, DNA replication is no longer accompanied by cell division. In fact, neither karyokinesis nor cytokinesis occurs. This type of DNA replication, called endoreduplication, is unique to megakaryocytes. The result of endoreduplication is a large, lobed, convoluted nucleus. On cessation of the endoreduplicative process, megakaryocyte cytoplasm undergoes terminal maturation, in which formation of the demarcation membrane system (DMS) is a critical event. The DMS likely plays a vitally important role in thrombopoiesis by providing the redundant membrane needed for pseudopod formation. Pseudopods are the structures from which platelets are ultimately formed and shed.

Regulation of Megakaryocyte Development

Thrombopoietin (TPO) is the major regulator of megakaryocyte development. It is synthesized at site(s) remote from the bone marrow, and circulates in plasma. The term *thrombopoietin* was initially used in 1958 by Kelemen and colleagues[18] to describe a factor found in the plasma of thrombocytopenic animals that was able to increase the number of circulating platelets by increasing megakaryocyte production in the bone marrow.

Human TPO is a 70-kDa molecule consisting of 332 amino acids and two distinct domains: an amino-terminal domain of 153 amino acids with 23% homology to erythropoietin and a glycosylated 181–amino acid carboxy-terminal domain whose function is unclear. The human gene maps to the long arm of chromosome 3 (3q 26–27), which is perhaps not surprising because this locus has been implicated in diseases associated with abnormal thrombopoiesis.[19–21] Patients with inversions, insertions, and translocations involving the long arm of chromosome 3 have an associated megakaryocyte hyperplasia and thrombocytosis.[22–24] The primary source of TPO is the liver,[25] though the kidney makes some contribution to serum levels.[26]

With the advent of molecularly cloned growth factors and serum-free culture systems, more definitive studies on the role of specific cytokines in regulating megakaryocytopoiesis became possible. Although TPO appears to be the major factor in regulating megakaryocyte and platelet production, several recombinant cytokines and growth factors also appear to affect megakaryocyte cell development, probably in concert with TPO. Detailed effects of recombinant cytokines on human megakaryocytopoiesis have been published.[27–33]

Transcription Factors in Megakaryocyte Development

The transcriptional regulation of megakaryocyte and platelet development has become much better understood in recent years (Fig. 7–2). Members of the GATA family of transcription factors, in particular GATA-1, along with its obligate cofactor FOG-1 (friend of GATA-1), are of particular importance.[34] GATA-1 was initially identified as a 413–amino acid nuclear protein with two highly conserved zinc finger regions needed for DNA binding.[35] GATA-1 is expressed in erythroid, megakaryocyte, and mast cell lines.[36] In the absence of GATA-1 and FOG-1, megakaryocytopoiesis fails at the level of the bipotent progenitor cell.[37]

Mice that are deficient in GATA-1, or that express GATA-1 mutant genes, are severely thrombocytopenic and have marrow megakaryocytes with abnormally high nuclear/cytoplasmic ratios and poorly developed demar-

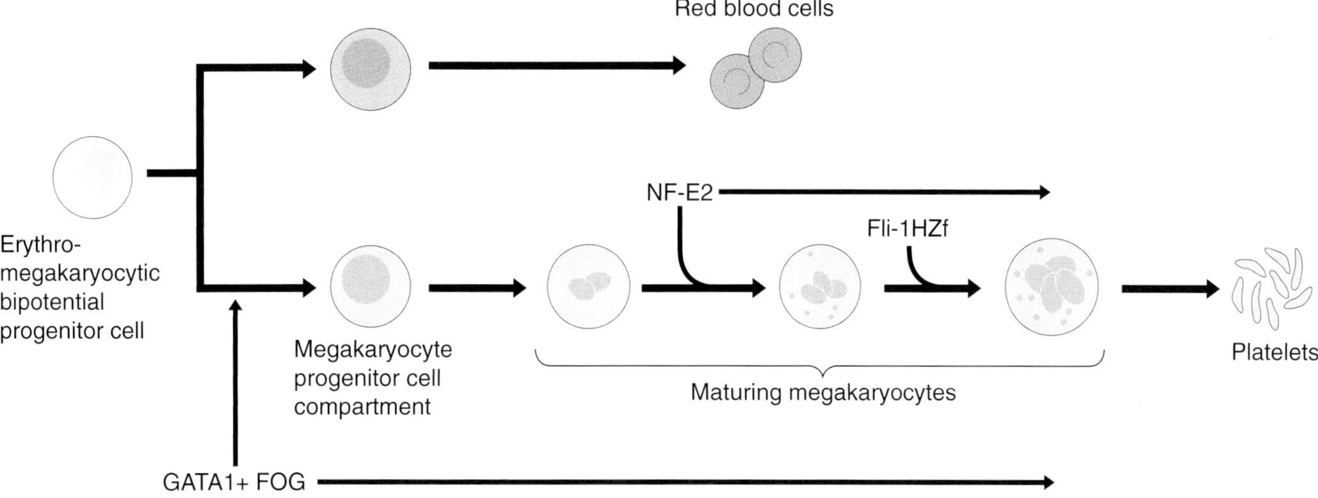

Figure 7–2. Transcriptional regulation of megakaryocytopoiesis.

cation membrane systems and granules. These observations suggest an important role for GATA-1 in terminal megakaryocyte differentiation in addition to its role in early megakaryocyte development.[38] In support of such a role, it is known that several megakaryocyte/platelet-specific genes (those for platelet factor 4, glycoprotein [GP] IIb and GPIX, thrombomodulin) contain GATA sequences in their promoter regions.[39–41]

The importance of two additional transcription factors has been unexpectedly revealed by other murine knockout studies. Megakaryocytes that develop in animals deficient in Fli-1, a member of the Ets family, have poorly developed membrane systems and few granules in their cytoplasm.[42,43] A "gray platelet"–like syndrome characterized by diminished α-granule content is seen in animals deficient in Hzf, a zinc finger protein transcription factor.[44]

Regulation of Nuclear Endoreduplication and Polyploidization

The initial phases of megakaryocytopoiesis are characterized by progenitor cell proliferation and mitotic division. When cells are ready to begin terminal maturation, mitotic division ceases. As previously noted, megakaryocytes are unique because DNA synthesis continues in these cells in the absence of nuclear division, a process called endomitosis. Endomitosis leads to cells that are polyploid, that is, cells that have more than the diploid complement of DNA. In fact, megakaryocytes can acquire a DNA content of 2 to 64 times the normal 2N complement of somatic cells.[45–49] The mechanism by which polyploidization occurs is still under study, but recent studies suggest that it involves more than simply skipping mitosis; in fact, mitotic spindles can be seen during TPO-induced polyploidization of megakaryocytes[50] (Fig. 7–3). Gain in cellular DNA takes place primarily at the level of the promegakaryoblast. The biologic imperative that drives megakaryocytes to become polyploid is mysterious. It is appealing to assume that some evolutionary advantage derives from the ability to make platelet-producing cells in this manner. It is likely that higher ploidy cells produce more platelets because they have more cytoplasm, but whether actual platelet production and release is more efficient from a single large cell than from several smaller ones is unknown.

Thrombopoiesis

A detailed discussion of this fascinating topic is beyond the scope of this chapter. The interested reader is referred to a recent detailed review by Italiano and Shivdasani.[51] There are two general hypotheses explaining thrombopoiesis (platelet formation) and platelet delivery into the peripheral blood.[52,53] The major distinction between them relates to the origin of the megakaryocyte demarcation membrane system (DMS) and its role in platelet formation. The DMS is known to arise early during megakaryocyte development, probably by invagination of megakaryocyte plasma membrane.[54]

It has been suggested that platelets are formed from "proplatelets."[53] According to this theory, the DMS is organized in the megakaryocyte cytoplasm into discrete platelet domains, probably by partial fusion of parallel channels of DMS. This model is now less popular than the so-called flow model, which suggests that the DMS represents a storage form of highly redundant, invaginated megakaryocyte plasma membrane. According to this theory, the DMS does not delineate platelet territories but is still crucial for platelet formation and release. It is postulated that, during the process of platelet release, the redundant membrane is extruded from the megakaryocyte in the form of a pseudopod. Shear forces induced by flow in the capillary sinus cause constrictions to develop in these pseudopods, which eventually attenuate enough to break, thereby releasing platelets into the circulation. A fully mature megakaryocyte produces approximately 1–1.5 × 10^3 platelets, which have a half-life of 7 to 10 days in the circulation.

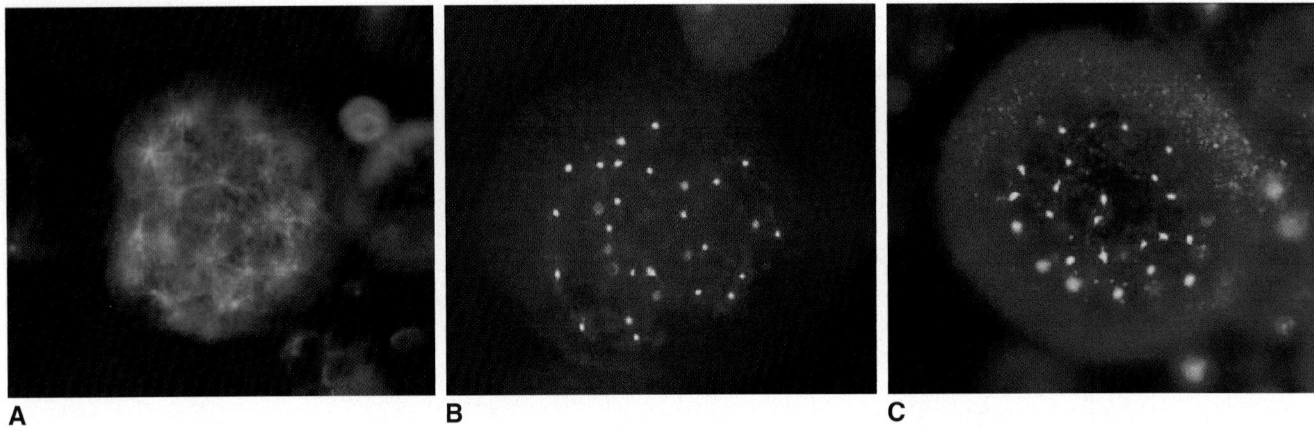

Figure 7–3. Multiple mitotic spindle pole formation during TPO-induced polyploidization of primary megakaryocytes. Mitotic spindle poles were detected by immunofluorescent light microscopy in TPO-induced primary mouse megakaryocytes. Megakaryocytes cultured with TPO were fixed in methanol for probing with anti–α-tubulin antibody ***(A)***, anti–γ-tubulin antibody ***(B)***, and anticentriole antibody ***(C)***, followed by incubation with a fluorescein isothiocyanate–labeled F(ab′)2 fragment ***(A)*** or a Cy3-conjugated F(ab′)2 fragment (***B*** and ***C***). (From Nagata Y, Muro Y, Todokoro K: Thrombopoietin-induced polyploidization of bone marrow megakaryocytes is due to a unique regulatory mechanism in late mitosis. J Cell Biol 139:449–457, 1997, with permission.)

STRUCTURE AND FUNCTION: PLATELET MORPHOLOGY AND SHAPE CHANGE

The resting platelet is an oval-shaped cell that contains mitochondria, glycogen, peroxisomes, and three types of granules: lysosomes, α-granules, and dense (or δ) granules (Fig. 7–4). Lysosome contents include enzymes that may facilitate the physiologic breakdown of thrombi; the contents of the latter two types of granules are described in Table 7–1. The shape of the quiescent platelet is maintained by three major structures: a cytoplasmic actin network,[55] a marginal band consisting of a microtubule coil,[56] and a rim of membrane-associated cytoskeleton. Upon exposure to collagen fibrils in the subendothelial matrix, or upon activation by thrombin or ADP[57] (see later), the platelet becomes spherical, rather than discoid, and develops cytoplasm-filled filopodial projections (Fig. 7–5). These long spines increase the surface area of the platelet, which facilitates the interaction of the activated platelet with nearby cells.[58]

The cytoplasmic actin network is composed of actin filaments and associated proteins. Actin is a 42-kDa protein that accounts for as much as 20% of total platelet protein.[59] In resting platelets, 40–50% of the actin is present as filamentous F-actin, and the remainder is present as globular monomeric G-actin. The shift to increase the proportion of F-actin to 70–80% during platelet activation involves a coordinated sequence of events in which the actin filaments present in resting platelets are severed and the resultant smaller fragments used as the nidus for new, longer actin filaments. This process is thought to be regulated in part by the increase in levels of phosphatidylinositol 4,5-bisphosphate and calcium that accompanies platelet activation.[60] At the same time, myosin is phosphorylated by myosin light chain kinase and becomes associated with F-actin, forming filaments that are anchored to the platelet plasma membrane by attachment (via actin-binding protein) to the GPIb-IX complex.

TABLE 7–1. Platelet Granule Contents

	Content	Function
α-Granule	Fibrinogen	Adhesion, aggregation, coagulation
	Fibronectin	Adhesion
	Vitronectin	Adhesion
	von Willebrand factor	Adhesion
	Thrombospondin	Adhesion, aggregation, cell proliferation
	Platelet-derived growth factor	Growth of smooth muscle
	Transforming growth factor-β	Control of cellular proliferation
	Platelet factor 4	Growth
	Factor V	Coagulation
	High-molecular-weight kininogen	Coagulation
	Factor XI	Coagulation
	Protein S	Anticoagulation
	Plasminogen-activator inhibitor-1	Coagulation
Dense (δ) granule	Adenosine diphosphate	Platelet activation and recruitment
	Adenosine triphosphate	Leukocyte activation
	Serotonin	Vascular tone
	Calcium	Activation and coagulation

The cytoskeletal rim is composed of actin, filamin, P235 (talin), vinculin, spectrin, α-actinin, and several membrane glycoproteins. Filamin is an elongated 280-kDa protein that is present in platelets and functions as an actin-binding protein. In resting platelets, filamin is part of a semirigid array that helps to maintain the platelet's discoid shape and limits the lateral movement of GPIb. This role is analogous to that performed by spectrin in erythrocytes. When platelets are activated, actin filaments form and attach to actin-binding protein. Later, the rising cytoplasmic Ca^{2+} concentration

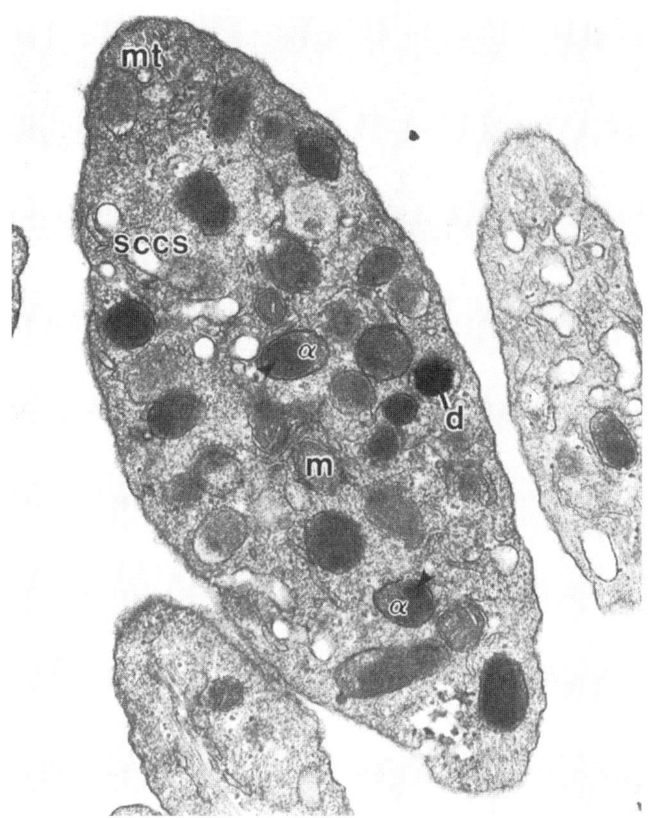

■ **Figure 7–4.** Circulating platelet. Platelets are discoid structures that contain numerous α-granules (α) with nucleoids *(arrowheads)*, dense bodies (d), and mitochondria (m). The surface-connected canalicular system (sccs) is in continuity with the extracellular milieu. Each platelet contains a circumferential microtubular coil (mt), cut in cross section (×37,500). (From Isenberg WM, Bainton DF: Megakaryocyte and platelet structure. *In* Hoffman R, Benz EJ, Shattil SJ, et al [eds]: Hematology: Basic Principles and Practice [2nd ed]. New York: Churchill Livingstone, 1995, pp 1516–1524, with permission.)

activates calpain that cleaves actin-binding protein, severing the link to GPIb. The third major structural element in platelets is the marginal band.[61] This microtubule coil is a single tightly wound polymer of tubulin that encircles the platelet perimeter and helps to maintain its discoid shape. During platelet activation, the microtubule coil contracts. Initially it was thought that contraction of the marginal band was required for stable adhesion of platelets under arterial shear pressures; however, recent evidence has challenged this theory.[61]

RELATED DISEASES: DISORDERS OF PLATELET PRODUCTION

Disorders of platelet production are addressed here because they highlight important features of megakaryocyte and platelet developmental biology. Diseases related to disruptions in platelet function are addressed in Chapter 59.

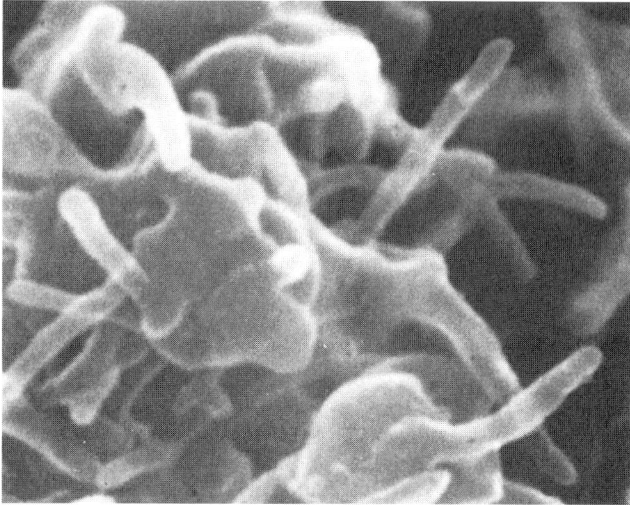

■ **Figure 7–5.** Platelet activated with ADP develops long, slender filopodial projections (scanning electron micrograph, ×21,000). (From Isenberg WM, Bainton DF: Megakaryocyte and platelet structure. *In* Hoffman R, Benz EJ, Shattil SJ, et al [eds]: Hematology: Basic Principles and Practice [2nd ed]. New York: Churchill Livingstone, 1995, pp 1516–1524, with permission.)

An examination of the peripheral blood smear is always indicated in the initial assessment of the patient with thrombocytopenia. Platelet clumps, indicative of pseudothrombocytopenia, or abnormally large or small platelets can be very useful in generating a differential diagnosis, as can the presence of inclusion bodies in neutrophils (Fig. 7–6), as discussed later. A bone marrow biopsy and aspirate, however, is required for the diagnosis of thrombocytopenia resulting from ineffective platelet production, because this provides a direct visualization of the quantity and the "quality" of the megakaryocyte population. It is convenient to group disorders of platelet production according to whether they are congenital (typically hereditary) or acquired (Tables 7–2 and 7–3).

Failures of either megakaryocytopoiesis or thrombopoiesis will result in peripheral blood thrombocytopenia. Under either circumstance, platelet production is characterized as "ineffective," either because there is an absolute decrease in available megakaryocyte cytoplasm (failure of megakaryocytopoiesis), or because conversion of cytoplasm to platelets is impaired (failure of thrombopoiesis). Selective impairment of megakaryocytopoiesis may result from damage to the progenitor cell compartment (the BFU-MK and/or CFU-MK) or, rarely, from a compromised ability to synthesize TPO, the chief cytokine regulator of this compartment.[62,63] Inherent or acquired defects in megakaryocyte precursor cells may lead to ineffective thrombopoiesis.[64]

Congenital Disorders of Megakaryocytopoiesis or Thrombopoiesis Resulting in Thrombocytopenia

Recognition of congenital or hereditary thrombocytopenias is growing, as is our understanding of their molecu-

TABLE 7–2. Thrombocytopenia Caused by Decreased Platelet Production: Congenital Causes

	Genetic Locus	Bleeding?	Platelet Size	Other Features
Autosomal Dominant				
MYH9 gene mutations	22q12-13	No	Large	
May-Hegglin anomaly				Döhle-like bodies
Sebastian syndrome				Abnormal Döhle-like bodies (EM)
Epstein's syndrome				Döhle-like bodies absent
Fechtner syndrome				Nephritis, sensorineural hearing loss, cataracts
Mediterranean macrothrombocytopenia	17	No	Large	
Velocardiofacial/DiGeorge syndrome	22q11	No	Large	Cardiac, thymic, facial abnormalities
Familial platelet disorder with associated myeloid malignancy	21q22	Yes	Normal	AML
Paris-Trousseau/Jacobsen syndrome	11q23	No	Large	Psychomotor retardation, facial and cardiac abnormalities
Gray platelet syndrome	Unknown	No	Large, gray	No α-granules
Autosomal Recessive				
Congenital amegakaryocytic thrombocytopenia	1p34	Yes	Normal	Absent megakaryocytes
Thrombocytopenia with absent radii syndrome	Unknown (possible role for *HOX* genes)	Yes	Normal	Absent radii with intact thumbs
Bernard-Soulier syndrome	Unknown	Variable	Large	Abnormal GPIb/IX
X-Linked				
Wiskott-Aldrich syndrome	Xp11	Yes	Small	T-cell immunodeficiency, eczema
Wiskott-Aldrich–like syndrome	Unknown	Yes	Small	Girls affected
GATA1 mutation		Yes	Normal–large	No immunodeficiency; dyshematopoiesis

Abbreviations: AML, acute myelogenous leukemia; EM, electron microscopy.

lar and genetic bases. Not surprisingly, the most severe forms of congenital thrombocytopenia are generally diagnosed in newborns and infants, whereas syndromes with minimal clinical significance are diagnosed, often incidentally, in adults. The congenital thrombocytopenia syndromes have recently been reviewed in detail.[65,66] Congenital thrombocytopenia is classified here by mode of inheritance and genetic mutation, when known, primarily for ease of reference,[66] because a more physiologic classification still eludes the field.

Autosomal Dominant Thrombocytopenias

Autosomal dominant thrombocytopenia may be encountered with or without other congenital abnormalities.[67–72] Patients with isolated thrombocytopenias usually have only a modest decrement in platelet counts, normal platelet morphology, and normal number of megakaryocytes. They are generally asymptomatic, although exceptions have been reported.[73]

Autosomal dominant causes of thrombocytopenia may be more common than previously believed. The most important reason for recognizing these disorders is that patients may be misdiagnosed as having immune thrombocytopenic purpura (ITP) and treated for that disorder.[66,67] A detailed family history may be useful. One study identified 54 patients with autosomal dominant thrombocytopenia, characterized by large platelets, normal megakaryocytes, and normal platelet survival, from a group of patients referred with a diagnosis of refractory ITP.[69]

Thrombocytopenia Syndromes Associated with *MYH9* Gene Mutations

May-Hegglin anomaly (Online Mendelian Inheritance in Man [OMIM] 155100), first described almost 100 years ago, is associated with mutations of the nonmuscle myosin heavy chain IIA gene, *MYH9,* on chromosome 22q12–13.[74,75] *MYH9* encodes nonmuscle myosin heavy chain that is expressed in platelets and is upregulated during granulocyte differentiation.[73,76–78] These disorders share a characteristic triad of thrombocytopenia, macrothrombocytes, and neutrophil inclusions called "Döhle-like" bodies.

The thrombocytopenia associated with May-Hegglin anomaly, also called familial thrombocytopenia with leukocyte inclusions, is usually mild to moderate, with giant platelets whose volume may exceed that of red blood cells.[65,79] Marrow megakaryocytes appear normal and platelet survival is slightly decreased or normal,[80,81] leaving ineffective production as the probable etiology of thrombocytopenia. The mechanism by which the giant platelets are formed is unknown; most likely, there is a defect in fragmentation of megakaryocyte pseudopods.[80]

The other characteristic of the May-Hegglin anomaly is the presence of cytoplasmic inclusions in the patient's granulocytes. Morphologically, the inclusions resemble the classical Döhle bodies found in neutrophils from

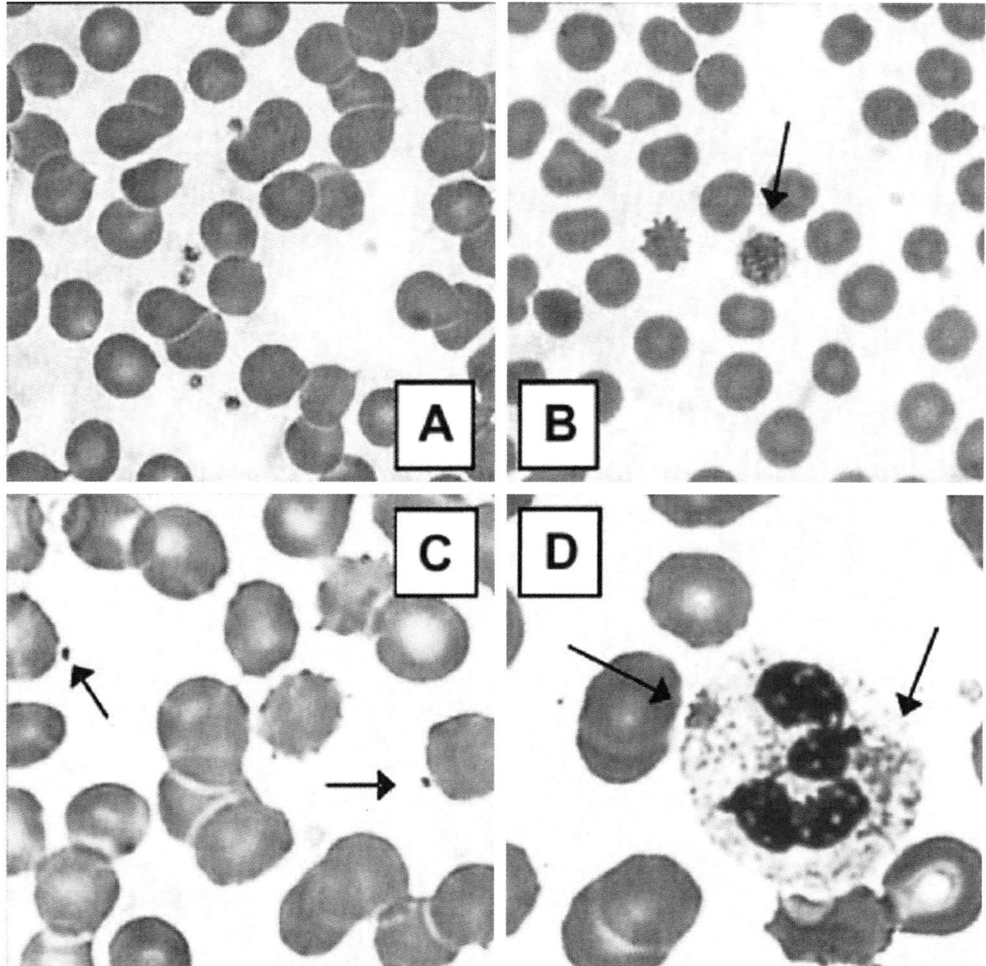

■ **Figure 7–6.** Peripheral blood platelets. ***A,*** Normal blood smear. ***B,*** Macrothrombocyte. The platelet depicted *(arrow)* is larger than the average erythrocyte. ***C,*** Microthrombocytes *(arrows)* are typical of those seen in Wiskott-Aldrich syndrome or X-linked thrombocytopenia. ***D,*** Döhle-like bodies in the cytoplasm of neutrophils *(arrows)* are seen in the May-Hegglin anomaly. (All photomicrographs ×100; Wright-Giemsa stain.) (From Drachman JG: Inherited thrombocytopenia: when a low platelet count does not mean ITP. Blood 103:390–398, 2004 with permission.)

TABLE 7–3. Thrombocytopenia Caused by Decreased Production: Acquired Causes

Selective megakaryocytic aplasia
Infection
Chemotherapy/irradiation
Nutritional deficiency
Iron deficiency
Bone marrow infiltration
Ethanol
Drugs
Paroxysmal nocturnal hemoglobinuria
Myelodysplastic syndromes
Cyclic thrombocytopenia

patients with acute inflammatory conditions, but unlike Döhle inclusions, they are present chronically (see Fig. 7–6). The inclusions are bright blue after Wright-Giemsa staining, and are composed largely of mutated nonmuscle myosin heavy chain IIA, which appears to be an important cytoskeletal contractile protein in hematopoietic cells.[77]

Three May-Hegglin–like syndromes have been described—Fechtner (OMIM 153640), Sebastian (OMIM 605249), and Epstein's (OMIM 153650) syndromes—that likely represent variants of a single entity with a spectrum of clinical manifestations.[74] All have mild macrothrombocytopenia, but are otherwise distinguished by variations in the quantity or ultrastructural quality of Döhle-like inclusion bodies (inclusion bodies are absent in Epstein's syndrome, and possess fewer ribosomes and dispersed microfilaments in Sebastian syndrome), or the presence of an Alport's syndrome–like triad of nephritis, sensorineural hearing loss, and cataracts (Fechtner syndrome).[82–84]

Macrothrombocytopenia is frequently discovered during routine testing of an asymptomatic individual. Individuals with mutations of *MYH9* and associated syndromes do not have life-threatening bleeding events. Because the thrombocytopenia is modest and bleeding times are variable, treatment is usually not required,[85] although platelet transfusions have been given if patients are bleeding.[86,87] Platelet inhibitors should be avoided.[66] Genetic counseling should be offered to affected kindreds.

Mediterranean Macrothrombocytopenia

Mediterranean macrothrombocytopenia (OMIM 153670),[88,89] a cause of macrothrombocytopenia in individuals of southern European descent, has been assigned through linkage analysis to an unidentified gene mutation on the short arm of chromosome 17.[90] The degree of thrombocytopenia is generally mild to moderate, with platelet counts ranging from 70,000 to 150,000/μL, and patients do not have a bleeding diathesis. Flow cytometric analysis of platelets has shown decreased expression of the GPIb-IX-V complex in a high percentage of affected individuals, and sequencing of the *GPIbα* gene has revealed an Ala156Val mutation in the GPIb protein in almost all families.[90] The clinical phenotype and the molecular genetics of the condition are essentially identical to those of carriers of the Bernard-Soulier syndrome (see later; also discussed in Chapter 59). As in May-Hegglin anomaly, identification of patients with this disorder is important to prevent potentially harmful therapies for ITP, and to provide genetic counseling because these patients are at risk for having a child with a bleeding risk similar to those with Bernard-Soulier syndrome.

Macrothrombocytopenia Associated with Velocardiofacial Syndrome and DiGeorge Syndrome

Patients with velocardiofacial syndrome (OMIM 192430) and DiGeorge syndrome (OMIM 188400) have a host of congenital abnormalities affecting their skeletal, cardiac, endocrine, neurologic, and immune systems.[91–95] Collectively, these disorders are known by the acronym "CATCH22" (*c*ardiac *a*bnormality, *T*-cell deficit, *c*left palate, and *h*ypocalcemia caused by Chr*22* deletion).[96–99] Mild thrombocytopenia, unassociated with a bleeding disorder, is frequently observed. Similar to Mediterranean macrothrombocytopenia, the platelet abnormality found in these conditions appears to be due to a deletion in one of the four genes that comprise the von Willebrand factor receptor locus (*GPIbα, GPIbβ, GPV,* and *GPIX*) on chromosome 22q11[100,101]; in these cases, *GPIbβ* is deleted.[101] Again, although therapy is unnecessary, genetic counseling is recommended.

Familial Platelet Disorder with Associated Myeloid Malignancy

This autosomal dominant thrombocytopenia (OMIM 601399) was first described in 1985,[68] but its genetic basis has only recently been understood.[102–104] Patients with this disorder have mild to moderate thrombocytopenia with normal platelets, but bleeding times are prolonged and an aspirin-like defect in aggregation studies has been found. The abnormal gene is *AML1,* now known as *CBFA2,*[103] located on chromosome 21q22.1–22.2. CBFA2 is a hematopoietic transcription factor that plays an important role in regulating cell development, and nonsense mutations or an intragenic deletion of one *CBFA2* allele are responsible for the condition. CFU-MK are diminished, but not the progenitors of other lineages.[103] These defects predispose patients to developing acute myeloid leukemia.[104] Although bleeding in these patients may be treated with platelet transfusions, the high likelihood of leukemic transformation has led some to suggest that these patients should undergo bone marrow transplantation.[66] However, based on its inheritance pattern, siblings have a 75% chance of also having the condition, and there is at least one reported case of a sibling transplant in which both the donor and recipient subsequently developed donor-derived leukemia.[105]

Paris-Trousseau and Jacobsen Syndrome

Paris-Trousseau syndrome (OMIM 188025) and Jacobsen syndrome (OMIM 147791) are autosomal dominant macrothrombocytopenias that are associated with deletions of the distal portion of chromosome 11 (11q23–24).[43,106–108] Children with Jacobsen syndrome have psychomotor retardation and facial and cardiac abnormalities,[109] but only a mild bleeding diathesis. These platelets have giant granules that stain red with Giemsa. There is an increased number of dysplastic micromegakaryocytes with small hypolobulated nuclei in the marrow[43,108]; the paucity of larger, more mature cells is thought to be due to spontaneous lysis of normal megakaryocytes. Mutations of *FLI1,* a member of the Ets family of transcription factors located on 11q, have been implicated in the etiology of Paris-Trousseau thrombocytopenia because of similarities to the megakaryocytes of mouse embryos in which *fli1* has been deleted.[43]

Gray Platelet Syndrome

The gray platelet syndrome (OMIM 139090) is a rare congenital bleeding disorder in which thrombocytopenia is associated with increased platelet size and decreased α-granule contents,[110–112] causing the platelets to appear "gray" after histochemical staining. The decrease in granule contents results from a failure to transport and incorporate proteins into the granules,[113–115] a defect that may occur in neutrophils as well.[116] The responsible genes have not been identified. The bleeding tendency in this syndrome is mild to moderate, and generally no treatment is needed.[112,117]

Autosomal Recessive Thrombocytopenias

Because profound thrombocytopenia is a common problem in sick newborns, it is important to note that, in this population, thrombocytopenia is typically due to sepsis, viral infections, perinatal asphyxia, or immunologic causes.[118] It has been estimated that fewer than 5% of cases are due to inherited or congenital disorders of platelet production.[119]

Maternal ITP may result in transient neonatal thrombocytopenia, because antiplatelet antibodies may be transferred either in utero or during delivery. Alternatively, neonatal alloimmune thrombocytopenia may occur. This neonatal thrombocytopenia results from incompatibility between maternal and fetal platelet antigens, resulting in the formation of maternal antiplatelet alloantibodies that cross the placenta (see Chapters 60 and 70). These disorders are self-limited and resolve as the maternal antibodies degrade.

Congenital Amegakaryocytic Thrombocytopenic Purpura

Profound thrombocytopenia in an otherwise well newborn (<10,000 platelets/μL) raises the possibility of congenital amegakaryocytic thrombocytopenic purpura (OMIM 604498).[120–122] A bone marrow examination reveals markedly diminished or absent megakaryocytes. Congenital amegakaryocytic thrombocytopenic purpura is a progressive disorder that results in worsening thrombocytopenia, as well as leukopenia and anemia, toward the end of the first decade of life. If the initial presentation is at this stage, other marrow failure syndromes such as Fanconi's anemia, aplastic anemia, or dyskeratosis congenita could be confused with this disorder.

The differential diagnosis for severe congenital thrombocytopenia includes thrombocytopenia with absent radii syndrome[123] and Wiskott-Aldrich syndrome (see later). These can often be distinguished from congenital amegakaryocytic thrombocytopenic purpura on the basis of associated skeletal hypoplasia of the arms in the case of thrombocytopenia with absent radii, and microthrombocytes in the case of Wiskott-Aldrich syndrome. Immune thrombocytopenias should be considered as well (see Chapter 60).[124]

Composite mutations affecting both alleles of the TPO receptor gene, *c-mpl* (chromosome 1p34), are responsible for congenital amegakaryocytic thrombocytopenic purpura.[71,125–127] The identification of one of these mutations is diagnostic of the disorder. Nonsense or frameshift mutations completely abrogate receptor function, whereas single amino acid substitutions may allow some function to remain. The severity of the disease correlates directly with the degree of receptor impairment. Because TPO is also required for maintenance of the stem cell compartment,[124,128] it is not surprising that congenital amegakaryocytic thrombocytopenic purpura—even mild forms—progresses to marrow failure.[124]

Treatment options for children with congenital amegakaryocytic thrombocytopenic purpura are limited. Platelet transfusions are used to treat acute bleeding episodes, but allogeneic stem cell transplantation is the only curative therapy.[129] Because the genetic defect is well described, patients with this thrombocytopenia are good candidates for gene therapy to replace or correct defective Mpl.

Thrombocytopenia with Absent Radii

Thrombocytopenia with absent radii syndrome (OMIM 274000) is usually transmitted in an autosomal recessive manner, although dominant transmission from an affected parent to offspring has been described.[130,131] There is a pathognomonic absence of radii with intact thumbs[132] (Fig. 7–7). Other skeletal malformations, including absence or malformation of the ulnar bones and abnormalities of the humerus, shoulder, and lower extremities, are also frequent. Cardiac malformations, especially tetralogy of Fallot and atrial septal defects, occur in one third of patients. Symptomatic milk allergy has been observed frequently and may cause severe bloody diarrhea.[132,133] Thrombocytopenia in these patients is most severe in the perinatal period, with platelet counts ranging from 15,000 to 30,000/μL. The low platelet count may be exacerbated by any significant stress, including infection, surgery, or even the gastrointestinal disturbances that accompany milk allergies. Such episodes are often accompanied by a leukemoid reaction. Eosinophilia is noted in approximately 50% of patients and is particularly common in patients with milk allergy. Anemia related to bleeding or hemolysis is typical in the first year of life. The thrombocytopenia improves with age: children who survive the first year or two of life have a normal lifespan.[131,134]

A bone marrow aspirate will show decreased or absent megakaryocytes. When present, megakaryocytes are small, basophilic, and vacuolated. Recent studies on the megakaryocyte progenitor cell compartment and *c-mpl* expression in six patients have found markedly reduced numbers of CFU-MK and increased numbers of very primitive progenitor cells, suggesting an inability of primitive cells to differentiate into the megakaryocyte lineage.[135] There were no abnormalities in *c-mpl* or its promoter. Although some studies identify decreased levels of Mpl RNA and protein in the platelets of these patients, others have found normal Mpl receptor level expression and structure, suggesting abnormalities in TPO signaling.[136]

The diagnosis of thrombocytopenia with absent radii is suspected when the typical skeletal malformations are encountered. Prenatal diagnosis is possible using ultrasonography, skeletal radiography, and fetal blood sampling.[137,138] Thrombocytopenia with absent radii is distinguished from Fanconi's anemia by the presence of thumbs and by the lack of chromosomal abnormalities. There is no specific treatment for this syndrome; steroids, splenectomy, and intravenous immunoglobulin G treatments are usually ineffective.[132,139] Thrombocytopenia may rarely first manifest in adulthood. Splenectomy has been reported to be useful under such circumstances.[140] In the unusual case in which thrombocytopenia does not remit, stem cell transplantation may be considered for children who suffer from recurrent significant bleeding episodes.[141,142]

Bernard-Soulier Syndrome

Bernard-Soulier syndrome (OMIM 231200) is characterized by mild to moderate macrothrombocytopenia (see Chapter 59). Patients with Bernard-Soulier syndrome generally have a mild bleeding diathesis that requires no treatment,[143] although some may have significant bleeding, often out of proportion to the thrombocytopenia alone, because of the functional defects displayed by the platelets in this syndrome.[144] Bernard-Soulier syndrome

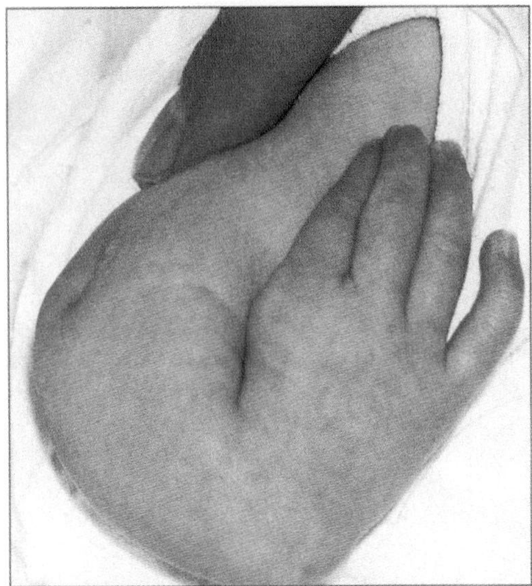
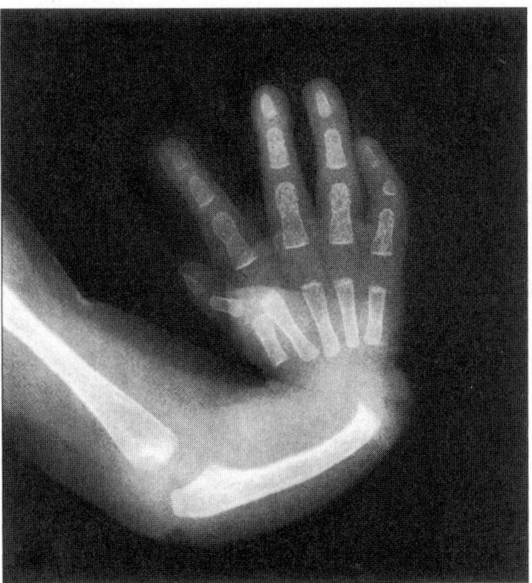

Figure 7–7. Thrombocytopenia with absent radius syndrome. *Left,* A typical upper extremity deformity. *Right,* Radiograph showing complete absence of the radius. (Adapted from Hoffbrand AV, Pettit JE: Color Atlas of Hematology. London: Mosby, 2000.)

platelets have decreased or absent expression of the von Willebrand factor receptor.[145] Large platelets in decreased number are often seen in ITP. Thus, Bernard-Soulier syndrome should be considered in patients who are presumed to have ITP, but bleed out of proportion to their thrombocytopenia, or those who do not respond to the usual ITP treatments. Platelet function studies will provide the correct diagnosis.

It remains unclear why a defect in the von Willebrand factor receptor leads to macrothrombocytopenia. One speculation is that the lack of this receptor prevents proper anchoring of the cytoskeleton to the plasma membrane.[146] Alternatively, a production deficit is possible, because platelet survival studies are often normal, though shortened survival has also been reported.[147,148] However, the numbers of bone marrow megakaryocytes may be increased or decreased; thus, ineffective thrombopoiesis may also play a role.[148,149] Megakaryocytes fail to express the GPIb-IX complex,[150] and deficiencies or mutations of this complex may be important in the formation of platelet territories.[151,152] There is abnormal development of the internal membrane system, which may be one cause of large platelets. However, qualitative (i.e., functional), rather than quantitative, defects are likely more important in the pathogenesis of bleeding in this disorder (see Chapter 59). Significant bleeding is usually managed by platelet transfusions, but recently success with the use of recombinant factor VIIa has been reported.[153] For particularly difficult cases with severe recurrent bleeding, hematopoietic stem cell transplantation has also been performed.[154]

X-Linked Disorders

Wiskott-Aldrich Syndrome and X-Linked Thrombocytopenia

The Wiskott-Aldrich syndrome (OMIM 301000) is a rare X-linked disorder characterized by immunodeficiency, eczema, and microthrombocytopenia.[155,156] Platelet counts are in the 5000–50,000/μL range, with a volume approximately 50% that of normal platelets. These reductions yield an effective platelet mass equal to approximately 1% of that found in normal individuals. Biochemical abnormalities are also present that variably compromise platelet function.[79,157–161] An abnormality of GPIb, for example, has been observed in some patients.[162,163] The protease calpain is reduced in Wiskott-Aldrich syndrome platelets, but is normal in affected lymphocytes.[164] Decreased platelet calpain may lead to inappropriate platelet stimulation and subsequent increased clearance from the circulation.[165] Platelet counts in patients with Wiskott-Aldrich syndrome rise after splenectomy. Nevertheless, although platelet survival time is approximately half that of normal platelets,[166] this does not explain the degree of thrombocytopenia. Platelet turnover is about 25% of normal and the mass of megakaryocyte cytoplasm is normal.[167] Therefore, ineffective platelet production must also contribute to the thrombocytopenia observed in these patients.[168] Immunodeficiency results from dysfunctional T lymphocytes, which manifest decreased responsiveness to mitogenic stimuli. Ultrastructural and biochemical defects have also been reported.[169,170]

The gene involved in the pathogenesis of the syndrome has been localized to the short arm of the X chromosome (Xp11.22).[171] The gene, *WAS,* is composed of 12 exons and encodes a protein (WASP) of 502 amino acids.[172] WASP contains a number of functional domains that are thought to provide a critical link between the cell's cytoskeleton and signal transduction pathways.[173]

How *WASP* mutations lead to the development of microthrombocytes is still not understood. Interestingly, megakaryocytes from patients with Wiskott-Aldrich syndrome are capable of forming proplatelet processes and platelets of normal size in vitro.[174] Analysis of the X-chromosome inactivation pattern in female heterozygotes (who have no abnormalities) has revealed nonrandom inactivation of WASP in multiple hematopoietic lineages, including $CD34^+$ progenitors, suggesting that WASP plays a crucial function in hematopoietic cell development.[175] There are a variety of mutations involving the *WAS* gene that lead to either absent or mutated WASP protein.[171,172,176–178] To a large extent, the phenotypic variation of Wiskott-Aldrich syndrome can be explained by the location and nature of the genetic mutations.[179] Frameshifts, nonsense mutations, and large deletions generally cause classical Wiskott-Aldrich syndrome, whereas single amino acid substitutions, especially in exons 1 to 3, cause the milder X-linked thrombocytopenia (OMIM 313900).

The diagnosis of Wiskott-Aldrich syndrome should be considered in any male child with thrombocytopenia and immunodeficiency.[156] Classical Wiskott-Aldrich syndrome is usually recognized within the first year of life because of easy bruising, epistaxis, bloody diarrhea, and even intracranial hemorrhage. Infections, usually bacterial in origin, are also typical. The classical triad of thrombocytopenia, infections, and eczema is only seen in about 25% of patients at diagnosis, because the latter is usually not problematic until after the first 6–12 months of life.[156,180] One third of cases have no family history. In such instances, the *WAS* gene may be sequenced to ascertain the diagnosis.[66]

Children with Wiskott-Aldrich syndrome also have a significant risk of malignancy, most often lymphoid, with patients who have autoimmune manifestations at highest risk.[181] Acute myelogenous leukemia, as well as nonhematologic malignancies, may occur.[182] Life expectancy is usually less than 10 years.

As with many disorders affecting stem cells, hematopoietic stem cell transplantation, including cells from cord blood, is the most effective treatment for Wiskott-Aldrich syndrome.[183–188] Corticosteroids are not indicated because they do not ameliorate the thrombocytopenia and only contribute to the propensity for infection. Patients who exhibit significant bleeding may benefit from splenectomy.[185,189–191] Median survival in 39 untransplanted, splenectomized patients has been reported to be 25 years, but many patients are now living into their third and fourth decades, thanks primarily to advances in supportive care, particularly antibiotics and intravenous immunoglobulin.[185,191]

Wiskott-Aldrich Syndrome Variants and Other X-Linked Recessive Thrombocytopenias

Girls have occasionally been noted to have microthrombocytes, with or without other components of Wiskott-Aldrich syndrome.[192,193] In one such patient, a spontaneous mutation in one *WAS* allele, coupled with skewed X inactivation among hematopoietic cells, was demonstrated.[193] However, in other families more than one female has been affected, and no *WAS* gene mutations were detected.[194] A mutation in a gene that encodes a WASP-interacting protein might conceivably cause a similar disease phenotype.

A number of families with an isolated X-linked thrombocytopenia, or with a Wiskott-Aldrich–like syndrome consisting of variable immune deficiencies and eczema, have been described.[195,196] Family studies of patients with Wiskott-Aldrich–like disorders have suggested both autosomal recessive and autosomal dominant modes of inheritance.[192,194] The thrombocytopenia usually is mild in these families, and most cases have been discovered incidentally. Marrow megakaryocytes are normal or increased.[174,197,198] Because it is now thought that Wiskott-Aldrich syndrome, and in fact most X-linked isolated thrombocytopenias, are caused by *WAS* mutations, sequencing of the gene should prove a reliable molecular diagnostic tool. The Wiskott-Aldrich variants, like classical Wiskott-Aldrich syndrome, manifest diminished lymphocyte mitogenic response to periodate[199]; this test could also prove useful for distinguishing variant Wiskott-Aldrich syndrome from other congenital thrombocytopenias.

GATA1 Mutation: A Newly Recognized X-Linked Thrombocytopenia

Five families with an X-linked pattern of thrombocytopenia, and an accompanying mild to moderate dyserythropoiesis, were recently reported.[200–204] This *GATA1* mutation disorder (OMIM 305371) differs from Wiskott-Aldrich syndrome in that the platelets were normal to large in size, and there is no associated eczema, immunodeficiency, or malignancy. The degree of thrombocytopenia was moderate to severe (10,000–40,000/μL) and platelet function defects were identified.[201] Not surprisingly, the associated bleeding diathesis is often severe. The bone marrow of these individuals was hypercellular, with dysplastic erythroid progenitors as well as dysmegakaryopoiesis.[203]

Mutations in the *GATA1* gene, which encodes a transcription factor required for normal megakaryocyte and erythroid development, have been found in each of the five families. The mutations are clustered in the highly conserved N-zinc finger domain, introducing single amino acid substitutions at four positions (Val205Met, Gly208Ser, Arg216Gly, Asp218Gly, and Asp218Tyr). Four of these mutations result in amino acid substitutions that interfere with the ability of GATA-1 to associate with a known cofactor, FOG-1.[205,206] Interestingly, the severity of the thrombocytopenia correlates with the degree to which the GATA-1/FOG-1 interaction is impaired.[202,203,207] In contrast, Arg216Gly results in impaired binding of GATA-1 to palindromic DNA-binding sites.[204] This mutation also causes a moderate globin chain imbalance (thalassemia).[208] *FOG1* gene mutations, which would be expected to yield a similar clinical phenotype, have yet to be described. More disruptive *GATA1* mutations are unlikely to be compatible with survival of the embryo because the gene is required for normal hematopoietic cell development.

GATA1 mutations must be suspected in male children with severe thrombocytopenia, normal to large platelets, and absence of immunodeficiency and eczema. *GATA1* gene sequencing is required to make this diagnosis and would therefore require specialized laboratory studies. Bleeding episodes in these patients can be treated with platelet transfusions. If the thrombocytopenia, or less likely the anemia, become life-threatening, hematopoietic stem cell transplantation can be curative.[209] Repair of the responsible *GATA1* mutation or insertion of a normal *GATA1* gene to autologous stem cells would be an ideal therapeutic option.

Acquired Defects in Thrombopoiesis Resulting in Thrombocytopenia

Acquired thrombocytopenia may also be caused by a failure of either megakaryocytopoiesis or thrombopoiesis. Ineffective thrombopoiesis is more likely, because thrombocytopenia caused by pure megakaryocyte aplasia or hypoplasia is quite rare, and often is a prodrome of aplastic anemia or myelodysplasia. Clues to these conditions may be found in the marrow, where often subtle abnormalities of other lineages, such as macrocytosis or dyserythropoiesis, may be seen.[210]

Selective Megakaryocyte Aplasia

Acquired selective amegakaryocytic thrombocytopenia is very rare. It is almost always due to an autoimmune process. Autoantibodies[211] and T cells[212] directed against megakaryocytes or their progenitor cells have been described, as have antibodies against cytokines that regulate megakaryocyte development, such as thrombopoietin.

The pathognomonic finding is an isolated decrease or absence of megakaryocytes in an otherwise normal-appearing marrow. Platelet survival is normal. These patients may respond to treatment with cyclosporine and antithymocyte globulin, achieving durable remissions.[213] Cytotoxic antibodies directed toward the CFU-MK may be treated with corticosteroids, plasmapheresis, intravenous immunoglobulin G, danazol, cyclosporine, or cyclophosphamide.[214] A review of 30 patients found that sustained remissions were achieved in 8 patients with immunosuppressive agents,[215] but most patients do not respond to treatment. Intensive immunosuppressive therapy may not prevent progression to aplastic anemia.[216]

Infection

Infection is likely the most important noniatrogenic cause of ineffective platelet production.[217] Infectious agents associated with decreased platelet counts include many viruses as well as *Mycoplasma,* mycobacteria,[218] *Ehrlichia,*[219] and malaria.[220] In these disorders, the etiology of the thrombocytopenia is thought to be diminished platelet production,[221] but immune-mediated thrombocytopenia has also been described.[218]

Viruses are by far the most common infectious agents associated with thrombocytopenia resulting from ineffective megakaryocyte or platelet production. Thrombocytopenia has been reported in mumps, rubella, measles, varicella, cytomegalovirus, infectious mononucleosis, varicella, dengue and other hemorrhagic fevers, hepatitis, parvovirus infections, and infusion of adenoviral vectors.[222–225] Live measles virus vaccination can also induce thrombocytopenia resulting from decreased production.[226] The mechanism responsible for viral suppression of platelet counts is not clear. Viruses are capable of infecting megakaryocytes, which may appear dysplastic with inclusion bodies, vacuoles, or degenerating nuclei. Naked megakaryocyte nuclei may be seen in particular after human immunodeficiency virus (HIV) infection.[221]

Perhaps the best studied viral-induced thrombocytopenia is that associated with HIV infection.[227] Mild to moderate decreases in platelet count are quite common: in a large study (738 patients) of HIV-positive patients with hemophilia, 27% of children and 43% of adults were thrombocytopenic 10 years after seroconversion.[228] Platelet counts rarely drop below 50,000/μL and thus bleeding is rare, except for patients who acquire HIV in the setting of hemophilia. Thrombocytopenia may precede frank immunodeficiency but it does correlate with viral load and depletion of the $CD4^+$ T-cell population.[229,230]

The principal cause of thrombocytopenia appears to vary with the stage of disease. A retrospective study of 85 patients with HIV and thrombocytopenia suggested that platelet destruction is predominant in early stages of infection, whereas in patients with acquired immunodeficiency syndrome, thrombocytopenia is more often due to a production deficit.[231,232] Production thrombocytopenia may be related directly to HIV infection, adverse effects of drug therapy, or secondary malignancy or myelodysplasia. Platelet kinetics studies have shown that patients infected with HIV have a moderate reduction in platelet survival, but all have decreased platelet production regardless of the degree of thrombocytopenia.[232,233] HIV can infect megakaryocytes directly, as evidenced by finding HIV messenger RNA and p24 antigen in megakaryocyte cytoplasm.[234–236]

Bone marrow aspiration can establish the presence of a granulomatous infection or lymphoma, which may contribute to, or cause, thrombocytopenia. Assuming no other obvious cause for thrombocytopenia, and the presence of typical megakaryocyte changes, antiretroviral therapy is the principal treatment. For patients with severe and/or symptomatic thrombocytopenia, ITP regimens may well be effective, including splenectomy if medical therapies are ineffective or contraindicated.[237]

Chemotherapy and Irradiation

Chemotherapy and irradiation commonly damage bone marrow in a dose-dependent fashion. Megakaryocytes and their progenitors seem to be particularly sensitive to the effects of these agents. As a result, thrombocytopenia is one of the most frequent adverse effects of total-body irradiation[238] and chemotherapy. Hematopoietic stem cell transplantation is often complicated by prolonged thrombocytopenia, which may persist long after restoration of neutrophil and red blood cell counts. Attempts have been made to expand megakaryocyte progenitor cells, either with a recombinant form of TPO[239] or with other cytokines.[240] Although not yet successful,[241] the future of these therapies remains promising.[242]

Alkylating agents in general produce more prolonged thrombocytopenia than do antimetabolites. Agents such as busulfan, the nitrosoureas, or platinum may cause cumulative damage in the more primitive progenitors. Mechanisms for the relative sparing of platelets by chemotherapeutic drugs such as vinca alkaloids have recently been investigated.[243]

For patients who suffer from severe or prolonged thrombocytopenia, reducing the intensity of the chemotherapy is the most appropriate approach to management. It had been hoped that use of recombinant TPO might significantly ameliorate this problem, but unfortunately this has not yet been demonstrated.[244] The formation of antibodies to a TPO derivative, with resulting profound thrombocytopenia in patients in whom such antibodies developed, has significantly slowed clinical investigations of this material.[245] A number of other cytokines have also been reported to raise platelet counts in this setting, including interleukin (IL)-1, IL-3, IL-6, and IL-11, but most are no longer available and their clinical utility was not clearly demonstrated.[246–252]

Supportive therapy with platelet transfusions, and drugs such as ε-aminocaproic acid for patients who become refractory to platelet transfusion, remain the mainstays of therapy. Amifostine, a phosphorylated aminothiol agent, has been reported to have a cytoprotective effect, but in a recent study, there was no significant reduction in thrombocytopenia or neutropenia.[253]

Nutritional Deficiencies

Ineffective platelet production of varying degrees may be observed with either folate or vitamin B_{12} deficiency.[254–259] Megakaryocyte numbers are normal or increased in the marrow, and platelet survival is normal or slightly shortened.[260] Vitamin B_{12} deficiency was reported to be causal in a case of amegakaryocytic thrombocytopenia.[261] Folate deficiency is frequently associated with ethanol abuse, and the etiology of the thrombocytopenia in patients who abuse ethanol is often complex (see later).

Examination of a peripheral blood smear will typically show macrocytosis and hypersegmented neutrophils, with megaloblastic changes in the erythroid and myeloid lineages on bone marrow biopsy. Megakaryocytes are normal in number and in appearance, although they may appear large, with multiple disconnected nuclear lobulations. Rapid recovery of the platelet count can be achieved with administration of the appropriate vitamin.

Iron Deficiency

Patients with iron deficiency typically exhibit thrombocytosis, but rare patients may become thrombocytopenic.[262] The number of megakaryocytes in the marrow may be decreased[263] or increased.[264] Curiously, thrombocytopenia has been caused by iron therapy in a patient with severe iron deficiency. It was suggested, but not addressed experimentally, that initiation of iron therapy resulted in preferential development of erythroid cells with concomitant decrease in megakaryocytes because they share a common progenitor.[265]

Marrow Infiltration

Marrow infiltrative diseases of any type, including metastatic cancer, lymphoma, or leukemia, may cause ineffective hematopoiesis. Physical replacement of marrow is the etiology of the thrombocytopenia in many cases, but it is also possible that inhibitory factors produced by infiltrating cells are toxic to the cells of the megakaryocytic lineage or interfere with normal regulatory mechanisms. The diagnosis of infiltrative disease is made by marrow examination, although diagnostic clues are usually provided by history, physical examination, and a leukoerythroblastic blood smear. The marrow shows decreased megakaryocytes, which may be larger than normal because of a compensatory physiologic response to the thrombocytopenia. The treatment approach is specific to the infiltrative process.

Ethanol

Ethanol abuse is commonly associated with thrombocytopenia that may be multifactorial.[254,266–272] Mechanisms include increased splenic pooling from portal hypertension, ineffective production related to folate deficiency, and direct marrow toxicity from ethanol itself.[270,273,274] In vitro studies have shown that alcohol concentrations achievable in vivo inhibit megakaryocyte maturation but do not inhibit CFU-MK.[270,273] Megakaryocytes are usually normal in number, but decreased numbers have been observed.[270] Rarely, marrow panhypoplasia has been observed in association with alcohol ingestion.[274] Anemia and macrocytosis accompanied by megaloblastic changes and ringed sideroblasts in the erythroid marrow are typically observed in the marrow of patients who abuse ethanol. However, the severity of the anemia is not correlated with the thrombocytopenia.[268] Treatment consists of withdrawal of ethanol and administration of a normal diet. Recovery of the platelet count, often with a rebound thrombocytosis, usually occurs within 2 weeks.

Other Drug-Related Disorders

A variety of drugs and toxins have been implicated in isolated platelet production defects. Estrogen, for example, has been reported to decrease platelet counts through an unknown mechanism.[275] Thrombocytopenia caused by thiazide diuretics has been reported frequently.[276] Although the etiology of the thrombocytopenia in most cases is probably increased clearance, decreased megakaryocytes have been noted.[277] Interferons and IL-2 may induce thrombocytopenia,[278,279] most likely via inhibition of CFU-MK. Anagrelide, a very useful drug for lowering platelet counts in patients with myeloproliferative disorders, appears to work by reducing megakaryocyte size and ploidy, and by disrupting maturation.[280]

Paroxysmal Nocturnal Hemoglobinuria

Paroxysmal nocturnal hemoglobinuria is a clonal disorder resulting from mutations in the X-linked gene *PIGA* that encodes an enzyme required in the initial step of biosynthesis of glycosylphosphatidylinositol anchors[281] (see Chapter 26). Approximately 25% of patients with paroxysmal nocturnal hemoglobinuria have significant marrow aplasia.[282] Thrombocytopenia at diagnosis is a poor prognostic indicator. Because platelet survival is usually normal in paroxysmal nocturnal hemoglobinuria,[283] the mechanism of the thrombocytopenia is decreased or ineffective production. Megakaryocyte progenitors show decreased proliferative activity and exhibit increased sensitivity to complement.[284,285] Treatment with antithymocyte globulin or granulocyte colony-stimulating factor and cyclosporine has ameliorated the thrombocytopenia in some patients,[286,287] whereas marrow transplantation has resulted in long-term remissions in patients with aplasia associated with paroxysmal nocturnal hemoglobinuria.[288]

Refractory Thrombocytopenia Caused by Myelodysplasia

Myelodysplastic syndromes may present with isolated thrombocytopenia in a very small number of cases.[289] The diagnosis of refractory thrombocytopenia can be considered when there are clonal chromosomal abnormalities. Typically, they involve chromosomes 3, 5, 7, 8, or 20, but partial deletions of other chromosomes have also been reported.[290] The usual laboratory findings include macrocytosis of platelets and red cells. Mononuclear megakaryocytes, sometimes present in increased numbers, are most typical[289,291,292]; dysplastic erythroblasts or myeloid cells may also be seen.

The clinical course is progressive, with additional cytopenias invariably developing.[289] Some patients with a full-blown myelodysplastic syndrome associated with marked thrombocytopenia and less than 10% blasts have shown an increase in platelet count after androgen therapy.[293] It has been reported that some of these cases have been misdiagnosed as having ITP, and treated for this disease. Because such therapy is not useful or helpful, it is important to recognize this entity.

Cyclic Thrombocytopenia

Cyclic oscillations in the platelet count have been reported sometimes associated with a woman's menstrual cycle.[294–301] The fluctuations can be extreme, with thrombocytopenic bleeding.[302] Various etiologies have been reported, including cyclic variations in platelet production[303] and autoantibodies to megakaryocytes.[304] Fluctuating cytokine levels may contribute to the pathogenesis, although it is difficult to discern cause from effect.[213,305,306] Cyclic thrombocytopenia may rarely be a presenting manifestation of myelodysplasia.[307] Treatment has included low-dose contraceptives and intravenous gamma globulin.[296,308]

Suggested Readings*

Drachman JG: Inherited thrombocytopenia: when a low platelet count does not mean ITP. Blood 103:390–398, 2004.

Hoffman R, Mazur E, Bruno E, Floyd V: Assay of an activity in the serum of patients with disorders of thrombopoiesis that stimulates formation of megakaryocytic colonies. N Engl J Med 305:533–538, 1981.

Kaushansky K, Drachman JG: The molecular and cellular biology of thrombopoietin: the primary regulator of platelet production. Oncogene 21:3359–3367, 2002.

Shivdasani RA: Molecular and transcriptional regulation of megakaryocyte differentiation. Stem Cells 19:397–407, 2001.

Song WJ, Sullivan MG, Legare RD, et al: Haploinsufficiency of *CBFA2* causes familial thrombocytopenia with propensity to develop acute myelogenous leukaemia. Nat Genet 23:166–175, 1999.

Full references for this chapter can be found on accompanying CD-ROM.

CHAPTER 8

Coagulation Factors

John H. McVey, BSc (Hons), PhD

KEY POINTS

Coagulation Factors

- Blood coagulation is a delicately balanced process whose central feature is the conversion of fibrinogen to fibrin by the serine protease thrombin.
- The plasma factors VII, IX, X, and XI, protein C, and prothrombin are zymogens of serine proteases that act in a coordinated fashion to control this process.
- The coagulation network of zymogen activations that leads to clot formation is initiated by exposure of blood to cells expressing the integral membrane glycoprotein tissue factor.
- To be effective, factors IXa and Xa require assembly into complexes with nonenzymatic cofactors, factors Va and VIIIa, that are also activated by limited proteolysis.
- Factors V and VIII are activated by trace amounts of thrombin formed in the "initiation" stage of coagulation.
- The back-activation of these cofactors leads to the explosive generation of thrombin that occurs in the propagation phase of coagulation.

INTRODUCTION

Blood coagulation is normally initiated in response to injury in order to preserve the integrity of the vascular system. The ability to stem the loss of body fluids from a site of injury is a basic defense mechanism that is essential for the survival of any multicellular organism. In some organisms tissue contraction is the principal method of wound closure, in others this is accompanied by mucus secretion or supplemented by cellular aggregation that forms plugs at sites of injury, and in some species there is a coagulation system that ultimately leads to deposition of specialized "clottable" proteins. Vertebrates and invertebrates have both evolved analogous responses to injury but, although they share some organizational features, it is unlikely that invertebrate coagulation systems are evolutionarily related to those found in vertebrates.[1] Rather, they appear to have arisen independently and are an example of convergent evolution. Vertebrates have evolved a complex system to prevent blood loss that involves coordinate muscle contraction, cellular aggregation, and deposition of an insoluble polymer (fibrin) that results in the formation of a stable clot at the site of injury (Fig. 8–1). Recent analysis of the coagulation network in bony fish suggests that the coagulation network leading to fibrin deposition is present in all vertebrates and must have evolved over 430 million years ago prior to the divergence of the bony fish from tetrapods.[2–4]

The critical need to rapidly form a stable localized clot in response to injury must be balanced with the need to maintain blood flow within the vessel. Furthermore, the process of blood coagulation must be intimately linked with cellular processes that ultimately lead to controlled clot removal and wound/tissue repair. The coagulation network has therefore evolved a complex, highly integrated series of interacting activation or inhibitory feedback or feed-forward pathways that integrate these processes.

This chapter reviews current understanding of the regulation of hemostasis. The chapter is divided into two parts; the first explains the series of molecular interactions that maintain the fluid state of blood, or, in response to injury, result in formation of the fibrin clot, and the second discusses structure and function of the coagulation factors in detail. For details on specific factors, the reader should consult the second part of the chapter. A fuller grasp of coagulation can be obtained by reading the whole chapter through once and re-reading the first part again after becoming acquainted with the information presented in the second part.

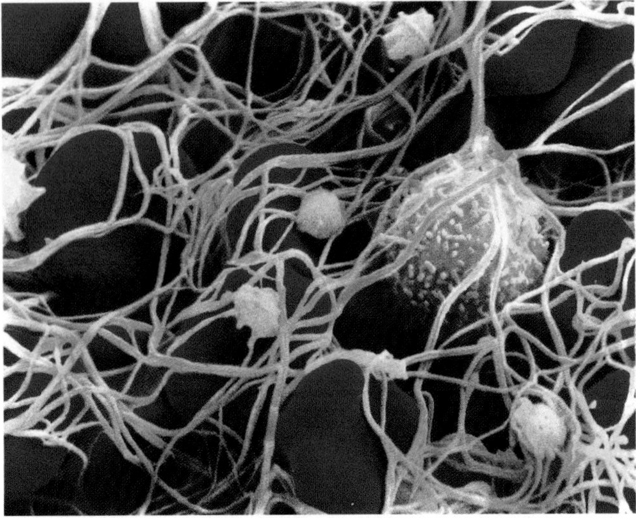

■ **Figure 8–1.** A colored scanning electron micrograph of a blood clot or thrombus. Red blood cells (erythrocytes) are seen trapped in a web of insoluble fibrin polymer *(white)*. Platelets *(green)* and a white blood cell *(yellow)* have become enmeshed in the clot. (Courtesy of the Science Photo Gallery.)

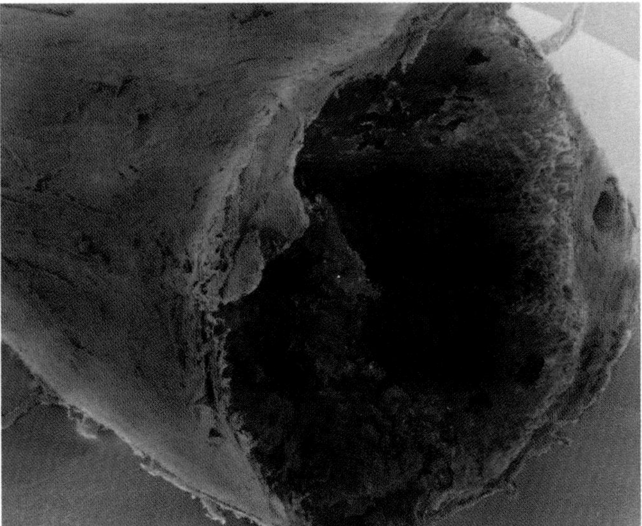

■ **Figure 8–2.** A colored scanning electron micrograph of a blood clot or thrombus inside a coronary artery of the human heart. The artery has been cross-sectioned, showing its wall *(brown)* and inner lumen *(blue)*. A blood clot *(red)* is seen, blocking about 30% of the diameter of the artery. A clot in either of the two coronary arteries that supply blood to the heart limits blood flow to the heart, leading to a heart attack. Thrombus formation occurs following disruption of an atherosclerotic plaque, exposing tissue factor on monocytes to flowing blood, which leads to initiation of blood coagulation. (Courtesy of the Science Photo Gallery.)

THE COAGULATION NETWORK

The "Resting" State

Blood coagulation occurs when the enzyme thrombin is generated and proteolyses soluble plasma fibrinogen, forming the insoluble fibrin polymer, or clot (see Fig. 8–1). In order to minimize blood loss, particularly from the high-pressure arterial circulation, an almost instantaneous response is required. In the absence of vascular damage, the coagulation network therefore exists in a "primed" state; however, checks and balances have also evolved that ensure that inappropriate coagulation does not normally occur (Fig. 8–2). The pathophysiologic consequences of inappropriate intravascular coagulation include thrombotic events following atherosclerotic plaque rupture[5] (see Chapter 86) and disseminated intravascular coagulation, seen in sepsis[6] (see Chapter 89).

Blood coagulation is initiated by the exposure of factor (F) VII to cells that express the integral membrane protein tissue factor (TF). The primary control of hemostasis is therefore the anatomic segregation of cells that express functional tissue factor from other components of the coagulation network present in blood (Fig. 8–3). Tissue factor is constitutively expressed at biologic boundaries such as skin, organ surfaces, vascular adventitia, and epithelial-mesenchymal surfaces.[7] The tissue factor expression pattern has been described as forming a "hemostatic envelope," which ensures that, following disruption of vascular integrity, FVII/FVIIa in blood is exposed to cells that express tissue factor, leading to the initiation of blood coagulation. Conversely, it also ensures that inappropriate initiation of intravascular coagulation does not occur.

The endothelial cells that line the blood vessels of the vasculature tree in the "resting state" present an anticoagulant surface (see Fig. 8–3), firstly through expression of thrombomodulin (TM) and endothelial cell protein C receptor (EPCR), which play a pivotal role in the activation of the anticoagulant pathway; secondly through expression of glycosaminoglycans on their surface that promote the action of inhibitors of coagulation factors; and finally by the expression of the protease inhibitor tissue factor pathway inhibitor (TFPI) and of protein S (PS), a cofactor in the anticoagulant pathway. The endothelium should not, however, be regarded as a simple homogeneous cell type.[8] Endothelial cell phenotypes are differentially regulated; at any given point in time, at any given location, the endothelial phenotypes may change from one moment to the next. Endothelial heterogeneity occurs between different organs, within the vascular loop of a given organ, and even between neighboring endothelial cells of a single vessel. For example, in contrast to thrombomodulin, which is abundant both in large vessels and most capillaries, in most organs EPCR expression is restricted primarily to veins and arteries, with most capillary endothelial cells expressing little if any EPCR.[9,10]

The serine proteases of the coagulation system (factors VII, IX, X, and XI, protein C [PC], and prothrombin) are all synthesized in the liver and circulate in plasma as inactive zymogens that require proteolytic cleavage for activation. Cleavage generates a neo–amino terminus that then folds into a cleft in the protease domain, creating a conformation essential for substrate binding and catalytic function. The cofactors factor V and factor VIII are also synthesized primarily in the liver and also circulate as

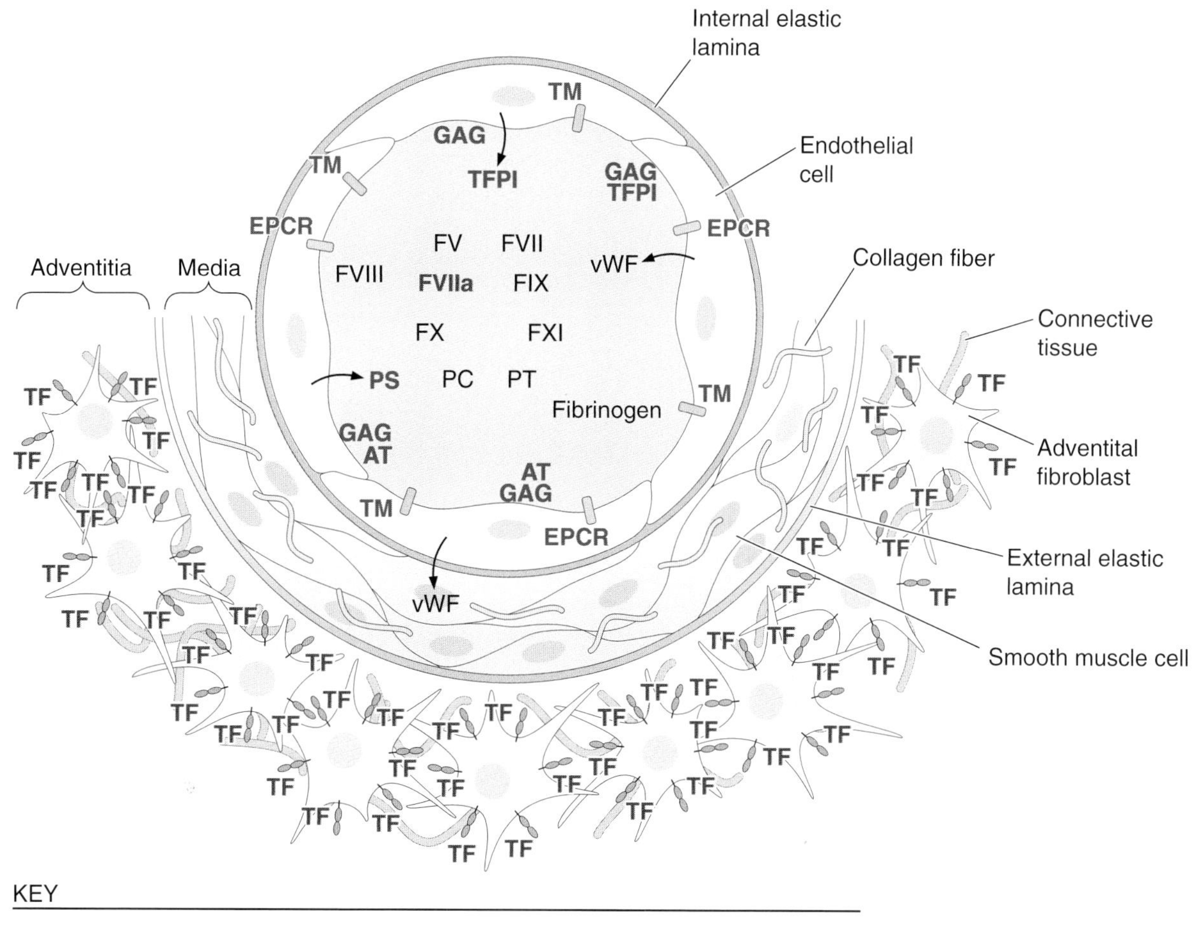

■ **Figure 8–3.** The anatomy of a generic vessel in the resting state; the layer thicknesses vary widely between arterial and venous circulation and between large and small vessels. The three main layers (adventitia, media, and intima) are shown. In the absence of vessel damage, cells expressing tissue factor are anatomically separated from components of the blood coagulation network, preventing initiation of coagulation. The endothelium (intima) may also present an anticoagulant surface through expression of glycosaminoglycans, TFPI, protein S, thrombomodulin, and EPCR.

inactive forms that require limited proteolytic cleavage for activation. Small amounts of activated (a) factors (IXa, Xa, XIa) and thrombin are continuously generated in asymptomatic individuals, but these are rapidly inactivated by the protease inhibitor antithrombin (AT), a serpin (serine protease inhibitor), found at high concentrations in blood. The rate of inhibition by antithrombin is substantially increased by binding glycosaminoglycans expressed on the surface of endothelial cells.

Factor VIIa is not inhibited by antithrombin, and circulating levels of factor VIIa average 4% of total factor VII in blood. The levels of circulating factor VIIa are influenced by both genetic and environmental factors. Triglyceride levels are a major determinant of factor VIIa levels in blood, and levels increase acutely in the postprandial phase after a high-fat meal. This increase is due to activation of zymogen rather than an increase in total factor VII concentration and appears to be dependent on factor IX, because this rise is not observed in patients with factor IX deficiency (hemophilia B).[11] Factor VIIa has little activity in the absence of its cofactor, tissue factor, but this pool of factor VIIa most likely serves to prime the system to respond upon exposure of tissue factor.

The protease inhibitor TFPI, a Kunitz-type inhibitor, found primarily on the surface of endothelial cells, plays a key role in inhibiting the TF-FVIIa complex by forming a quaternary complex with TF-FVIIa-FXa (Fig. 8–4). It should be noted, however, that TFPI first forms a complex with factor Xa, which then interacts with the TF-FVIIa complex to form the quaternary complex in which both proteases are inhibited. Therefore, TFPI can only function as an inhibitor of the initiation complex (TF-FVIIa) once some factor Xa has been generated. TFPI acts to downregulate the initiation complex (TF-FVIIa) of the coagulation network once it is activated rather than as an inhibitor of blood coagulation per se.

Endothelial cells constitutively express thrombomodulin, which binds thrombin and, by an allosteric mechanism, alters its substrate specificity. The procoagulant substrates of thrombin, including factor V, factor VIII, and fibrinogen, are no longer efficiently proteolyzed. The preferred substrate of the thrombin-thrombomodulin

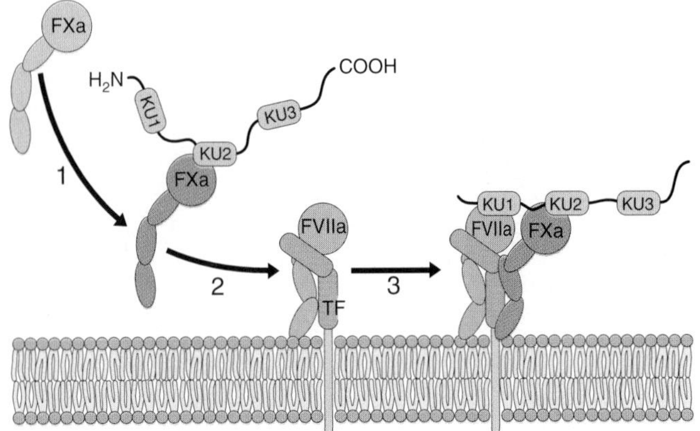

Figure 8–4. Inhibition by tissue factor pathway inhibitor (TFPI). Free factor Xa initially forms a complex with TFPI (step 1) by binding the second Kunitz domain (KU2) of TFPI. This binary complex then forms a quaternary complex with the TF-FVIIa complex (steps 2 and 3), with the first Kunitz (KU1) domain of TFPI binding to factor VIIa. The role of the third Kunitz domain (KU3) is not known. The positively charged carboxy-terminal tail is believed to interact with glycosaminoglycans (GAGs) on the endothelial cell surface.

complex is protein C. Thrombin converts protein C to activated protein C by a single proteolytic cleavage, which is enhanced by protein C binding to EPCR, its receptor present on endothelial cells. Activated protein C in complex with its cofactor, protein S, rapidly inactivates the procoagulant cofactors factor Va and factor VIIIa by specific proteolytic cleavages in a negative feedback loop. Homozygous protein C and homozygous protein S deficiencies are rare but are associated with severe, often fatal thrombosis, and heterozygous individuals have a high risk of venous thrombosis (see Chapter 67). These observations indicate the crucial role for the protein C anticoagulant pathway in maintaining balanced hemostasis.[12]

Platelets actively participate in regulating thrombin production following injury to vessels. Thrombin is the most potent physiologic activator of platelets, and thrombin-activated platelets release and/or recruit coagulation factors necessary both for accelerating thrombin generation and inhibiting prothrombin activation. Platelets store a number of procoagulant proteins within their α-granules, including fibrinogen, factors V, IX, and XI, and von Willebrand factor, that are rapidly released upon activation. Activated platelets also release TFPI and the protease nexin II, an inhibitor of factor XIa.

Thus, in the absence of injury, the balance of hemostasis is toward the maintenance of vascular blood flow by preventing or inhibiting blood coagulation through the secretion or expression of anticoagulant molecules. However, all the factors necessary for a procoagulant response have been presynthesized and circulate in blood in inactive forms or are stored in secretory granules within endothelial cells or platelets ready for a rapid response following vascular damage.

The Procoagulant Response

Following disruption of vasculature integrity, blood is immediately exposed to cells expressing tissue factor, leading to the initiation of blood coagulation (Fig. 8–5). The formation of the TF-FVII complex promotes the activation of factor VII. Activation is catalyzed by many proteases in vitro, but the most efficient catalyst in vivo is most probably autoactivation by the TF-FVIIa complex formed from the pool of factor VIIa within the circulation. The formation of the TF-FVIIa complex results in the activation of factors IX and X. In the absence of its cofactor, factor Va, factor Xa generates only trace amounts of thrombin. Although insufficient to initiate significant fibrin polymerization, trace amounts of thrombin formed in this "initiation" stage of coagulation are able to activate factors V and VIII by limited proteolysis in a positive feedback loop (Fig. 8–6). In the "propagation" phase of coagulation, factor VIIIa forms a complex with factor IXa (the tenase complex) and activates sufficient factor Xa, which in complex with factor Va (the prothrombinase complex) leads to the explosive generation of thrombin that ultimately leads to the formation of a fibrin clot. Thrombin also activates factor XI to factor XIa in a further positive feedback loop, resulting in further generation of factor IXa independent of the TF-FVIIa complex.

Hereditary factor VII deficiency is a rare autosomal recessive bleeding disorder that in severe cases is often associated with life-threatening gastrointestinal and central nervous system bleeds, reflecting the pivotal role of factor VII in the initiation of coagulation (see Chapter 66). Deficiency of factor VIII (hemophilia A) and factor IX (hemophilia B) share an indistinguishable clinical phenotype, being characterized by bleeding into muscles, joints, and other organs with consequent damage that, untreated, leads to progressive arthropathy, musculoskeletal deformity, and early death (see Chapter 63). The severity of the bleeding in hemophilia A and B supports a key role for the tenase complex (FIXa–FVIIIa) in the propagation phase of blood coagulation. In contrast, the relatively mild bleeding associated with factor XI deficiency (see Chapter 66) suggests that the back activation of factor XI by thrombin may only be required in severe trauma.

A key feature of these processes is the assembly of multiprotein complexes on a negatively charged phospholipid surface. Each of these complexes consists of a cofactor (tissue factor, factors Va and VIIIa), an enzyme (factors VIIa, IXa, and Xa), and a substrate that is a zymogen (factors IX and X and prothrombin) of a serine protease. The product of one reaction becomes the enzyme in the next complex.

Platelets activated at sites of vascular injury play key roles in normal hemostasis. By adhering to the exposed subendothelium and aggregating, they create a physical barrier that limits blood loss. In addition, platelets accelerate thrombin generation by providing a surface that promotes the activation of factor X and prothrombin. Furthermore, they release procoagulant factors that contribute to the local coagulation response.

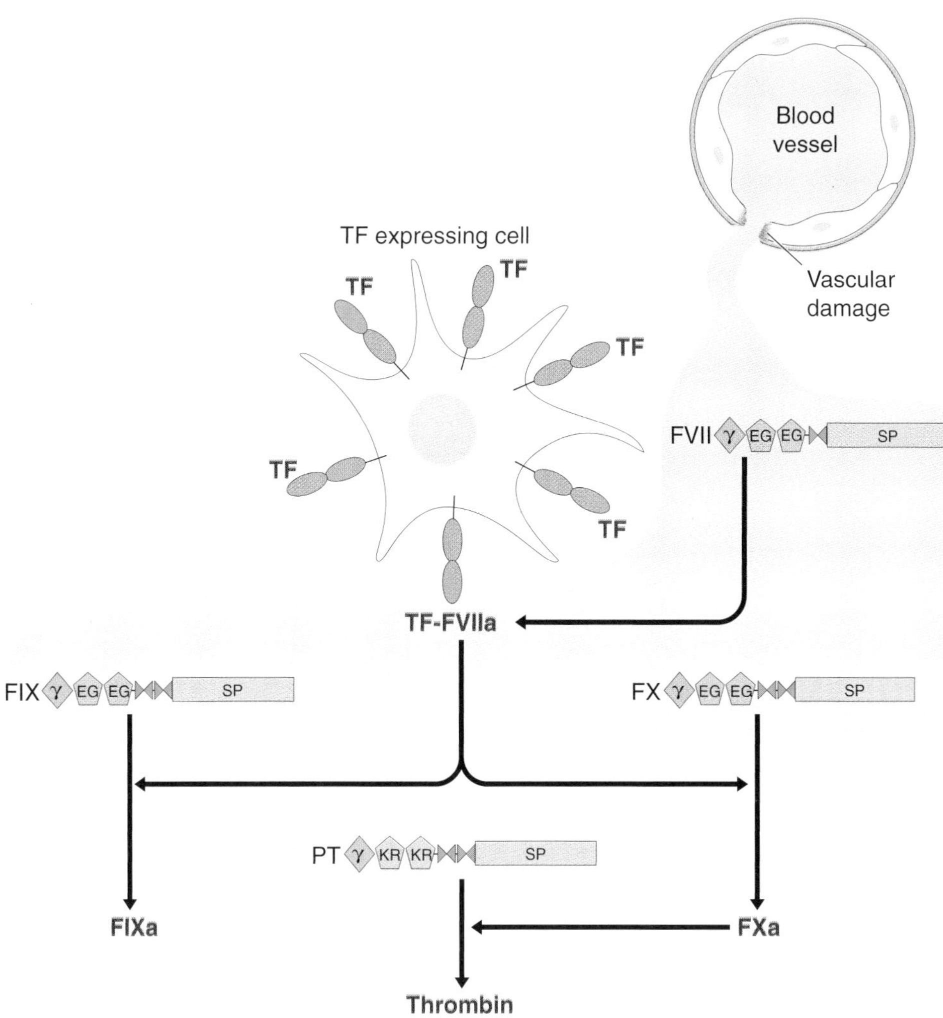

Figure 8–5. The initiation phase of coagulation. Following vascular damage, blood is exposed to cells expressing tissue factor on their surfaces. Formation of the TF-FVII/FVIIa complex initiates coagulation by activating factors IX and X. In the absence of its activated cofactor, factor Va, factor Xa generates only trace amounts of thrombin in this initiation phase of blood coagulation. Module organization of proteins is indicated (see "Structure and Function" and Fig. 8–9) and all abbreviations are given in the text. Protein names are colored: functionally active proteins are *red*; inactive proteins, *black*.

The importance of providing a negatively charged phospholipid surface for the assembly of the procoagulant response is seen in Scott syndrome, an extremely rare bleeding disorder that is characterized by a failure to expose phosphatidylserine on the outer leaflet of the plasma membrane and is associated with a moderate bleeding tendency.[13]

The Anticoagulant Response

Following the initiation of coagulation, various inhibitory mechanisms prevent extension of the coagulation process beyond the site of vascular injury, which might otherwise result in unnecessary occlusion of the blood vessel (see Figs. 8–2 and 8–7). TFPI associated with the endothelial cell surface rapidly inactivates the initiation complex by forming a quaternary inhibited complex (TF-FVIIa-FXa-TFPI) (see Fig. 8–4). Thrombin stimulates both endothelial cells and platelets to release further TFPI. Thrombin generated at the endothelial surface binds thrombomodulin and activates protein C. The activation of protein C is promoted by EPCR, which provides a direct binding site for protein C on endothelial cells and increases the affinity of the thrombin-thrombomodulin complex for protein C. Activated protein C in complex with its cofactor, protein S, rapidly inactivates the procoagulant cofactors factor Va and factor VIIIa by specific proteolysis, forming a negative feedback loop. The activated coagulation proteases factor IXa, factor Xa, factor XIa, and thrombin are all inhibited by antithrombin. The rate of inhibition by antithrombin is substantially increased by binding glycosaminoglycans on the surface of endothelial cells.

The relevance of protein C activation by thrombin-TM/PC-EPCR complexes is evident from the severe hypercoagulable condition associated with deficiencies of protein C or protein S, and the strong risk of venous thrombosis in individuals with the factor V Leiden polymorphism (FV R506Q), which renders factor Va resistant to inactivation by APC[14] (see Chapter 67).

The Fibrinolytic Response

Formation of fibrin triggers activation of the fibrinolytic system and generation of the active fibrinolytic enzyme plasmin that degrades fibrin into soluble fragments,

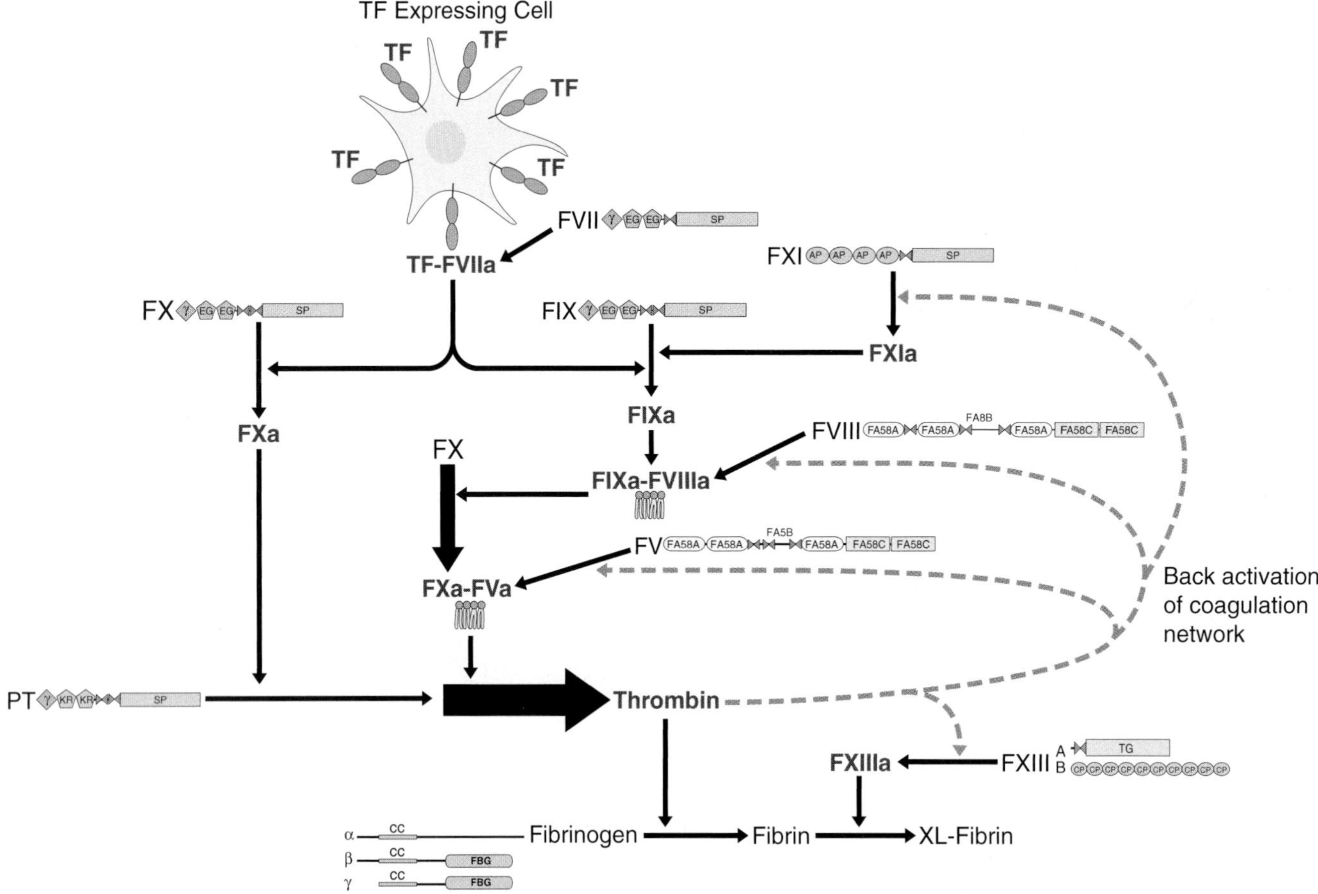

■ **Figure 8–6.** The propagation phase of coagulation. The trace amounts of thrombin generated in the initiation phase of coagulation are insufficient to initiate significant fibrin polymerization. However, the trace amounts of thrombin generated in this initiation phase are able to activate factors V and VIII by limited proteolysis in a positive feedback loop *(dashed red arrows)*. In the propagation phase of coagulation, factor VIIIa forms a complex with factor IXa and activates sufficient factor Xa, which in complex with its cofactor, factor Va, leads to the explosive generation of thrombin that ultimately leads to the generation of a fibrin clot. Thrombin also activates factor XI in a further positive feedback loop *(dashed red arrow)*. Factor XIa is then able to activate further factor IX independent of the TF-FVIIa complex. The FIXa-FVIIIa (tenase) and the FXa-FVa (prothrombinase) complexes assemble on phospholipid surfaces.

disintegrating the clot[15] (Fig. 8–8). Plasmin is formed from plasminogen by limited proteolysis by the action of tissue plasminogen activator (tPA) or urokinase (urinary-type plasminogen activator). tPA is the most important activator in the circulation. Plasminogen activator inhibitor (PAI)-1 and PAI-2 inhibit the activities of these activators, whereas plasmin is primarily inhibited by plasmin inhibitor (α_2-antiplasmin) and to a lesser extent by α_2-macroglobulin.

tPA is a serine protease synthesized, stored, and secreted by endothelial cells. In the absence of fibrin, tPA displays a low activity toward plasminogen; however, in the presence of fibrin this activity is increased by up to three orders of magnitude. The rate-enhancing effect of fibrin on plasminogen activation may be divided into two phases. In the first, slow phase, single-chain tPA activates plasminogen on the intact fibrin surface. Plasmin generated in this phase cleaves fibrin at many different positions, but always after a lysine or arginine residue. The carboxy-terminal lysine and arginine residues provide additional binding sites for plasmin and possibly tPA and thus propagate fibrinolysis in the second phase. Fibrinogen does not display any of these properties, and therefore the formation of plasmin and the generation of fibrinolytic activity are restricted to the location of a fibrin blood clot.

More recently, a new inhibitor, thrombin-activatable fibrinolysis inhibitor (TAFI), was described that down-regulates fibrinolysis by removing the carboxy-terminal lysine residues from fibrin generated in the first phase of fibrinolysis, and therefore limits plasmin formation. TAFI is a carboxypeptidase synthesized in the liver that circulates in blood as a zymogen and is activated by a single proteolytic cleavage mediated by thrombin in complex with thrombomodulin.[16]

The plasmin-generating potential of plasma is sufficient to degrade completely all of the fibrinogen in the body in a very short time. It is prevented from doing so by primarily PAI-1 and α_2-antiplasmin, which both belong to the serpin family. PAI-1 is secreted by endothelial cells and is also found in α-granules of platelets. The PAI-1 concentration can increase 10-fold at sites of injury following

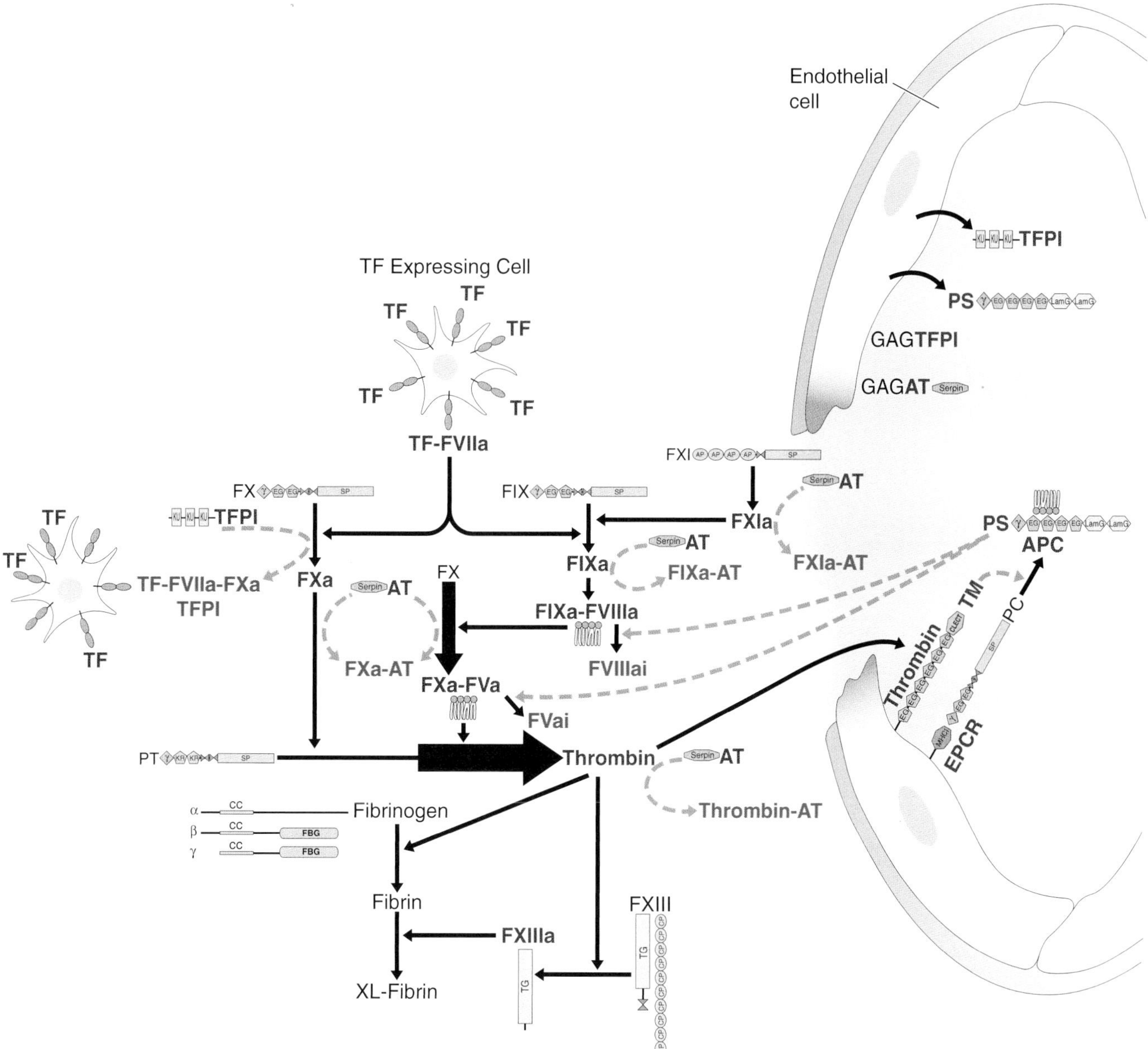

Figure 8–7. The inhibition of coagulation. The initiation of blood coagulation via generation of factors IXa (FIXa) and Xa (FXa) by the tissue factor (TF)–factor VIIa (FVIIa) complex is shut down by the action of TFPI, which forms a quaternary complex with the TF-FVIIa-FXa complex. Functional TFPI is principally associated with the endothelial cell surface or is released from activated platelets. The serine proteases FIXa, FXa, factor XIa (FXIa), and thrombin are all inhibited by antithrombin. Thrombin bound to thrombomodulin (TM) on endothelial cell surfaces activates protein C (PC) bound to its receptor, EPCR. APC in complex with its cofactor, protein S (PS), inactivates factor Va (FVa) and factor VIIIa (FVIIIa) by further proteolytic cleavages. *Dashed blue arrows* indicate negative feedback loops. Module organization of proteins is indicated (see "Structure and Function" and Fig. 8–9) and all abbreviations are given in the text. Protein names are colored: functionally active proteins are *red*; inactive proteins *black*; inactivated or inhibited proteins, *blue*.

platelet activation. Deficiency of PAI-1 results in a hyperfibrinolytic state associated with abnormal bleeding only after trauma or surgery. α_2-Antiplasmin inhibitor is the most potent and rapidly acting of the plasmin inhibitors, forming a 1:1 complex with plasmin in which the protease is completely inactivated. Deficiency of α_2-antiplasmin (also known as Miyasato disease) is associated with a significant bleeding tendency, supporting its importance in preventing uncontrolled fibrinolytic activity.

STRUCTURE AND FUNCTION

Coagulation Factor Modules

The coagulation factors are assembled from a small number of modules or domains. A module always adopts the same three-dimensional structure or fold despite differences in the primary amino acid sequences. The different component modules are illustrated in Figure 8–9.

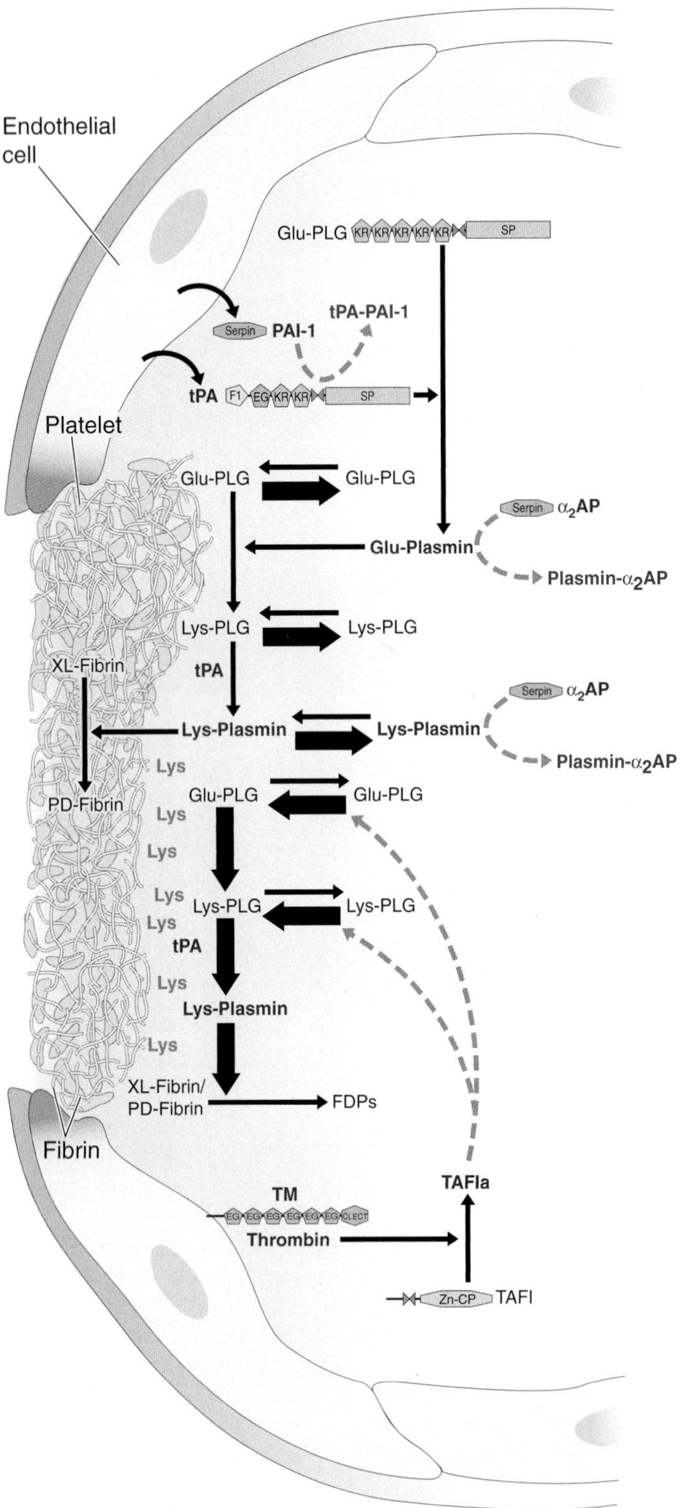

Figure 8–8. Fibrinolysis. TPA is secreted by endothelial cells but has a short half-life in blood as a result of inhibition by PAI-1. tPA and Glu-plasminogen (PLG) (the native circulating form) both interact with fibrin in a lysine-dependent manner; interaction with fibrin results in efficient generation of plasmin. Plasmin in blood is inhibited by α_2-antiplasmin (α_2AP). Lys-PLG is formed when plasmin cleaves Glu-PLG. tPA more readily activates Lys-PLG. Degradation of extra-large fibrin (XL-Fibrin) to partially degraded fibrin (PD-Fibrin) exposes additional carboxy-terminal lysine residues (Lys) that present new binding sites for tPA and plasminogen, increasing the amount of plasmin generated and the degradation of fibrin to fibrin degradation products (FDPs). Thrombin in complex with thrombomodulin (TM) activates TAFI, which inhibits plasminogen association with fibrin by cleaving carboxy-terminal lysine residues. Module organization of proteins is indicated (see "Structure and Function" and Fig. 8–9) and all abbreviations are given in the text. Protein names are colored: functionally active proteins are *red*; inactive proteins *black*; inactivated or inhibited proteins, *blue*. *Dashed blue arrows* indicate negative feedback loops.

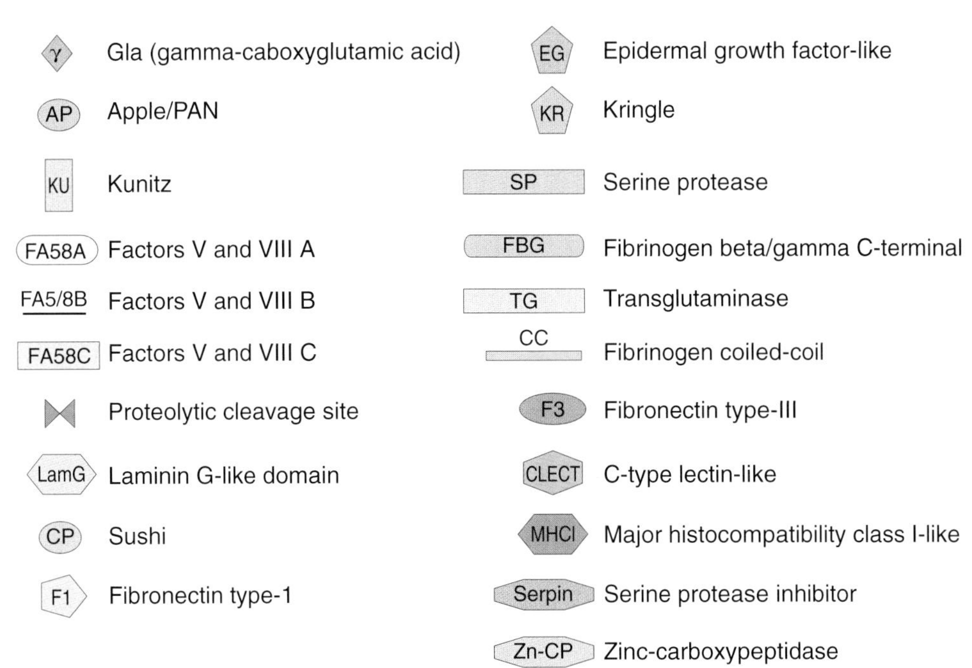

Figure 8–9. Blood coagulation factor modules. The coagulation factors have a modular organization. The different modules or domains that are present in these factors and the cartoon representations of the modules used throughout this chapter are listed.

Tissue Factor: The Initiator of Blood Coagulation

Tissue factor is structurally organized in three domains: an extracellular domain extends from the mature amino terminus to residue 219, a 23-residue hydrophobic sequence that follows represents the transmembrane-spanning segment, and a cytoplasmic domain of 21 residues contains a cysteine that may be acylated to palmitate or stearate on the inner leaflet of the membrane. The extracellular domain consists of two fibronectin type III modules oriented at an angle of 125 degrees to each other.[17] The extracellular domain of tissue factor is necessary and sufficient for procoagulant activity, because recombinant variants lacking either the intracellular domain or both the intracellular and transmembrane domains retain full procoagulant activities.[18] Tissue factor functions as a cellular receptor and cofactor for FVII/FVIIa, enhancing the proteolytic activity of the bound protease several thousandfold. It achieves this in several different ways: binding of factor VII to tissue factor makes it exquisitely sensitive to proteolytic activation; through an allosteric effect on the active site, it enhances the proteolytic activity of the enzyme; and it localizes factor VIIa on the cell surface at an appropriate distance from the membrane, enabling its macromolecular substrates, factor IX and factor X, to dock with the TF-FVIIa complex, thereby allowing efficient cleavage.[19]

Tissue factor has been implicated in a number of coagulation-independent functions, including inflammation, angiogenesis, and tumor metastasis, and it has been proposed to have a role in cell signaling.[20–22] Tissue factor is structurally related to the cytokine receptor family. Cell signaling via these receptors usually involves participation of the cytoplasmic domain; however, although the 21–amino acid cytoplasmic domain of tissue factor contains serine residues that are phosphorylated when cells are stimulated with phorbol esters, evidence for a role in signal transmission is limited. The cytoplasmic domain has however, been shown to interact with the cell cytoskeleton through binding to nonmuscle filamin (actin-binding protein 280). It is still unclear how formation of the TF/FVIIa complex influences various biologic processes; however, emerging evidence suggests that TF/FVIIa participates in cell signaling through its proteolytic activity, either directly activating receptors or indirectly by generating factor Xa and/or thrombin that then activates cellular receptors. The receptors responsible for transducing the extracellular proteolytic activity are the protease-activated receptors (PARs), which belong to the family of seven-transmembrane-domain, G protein–coupled receptors.[23,24] The PARs, of which there are four known members (PAR-1, -2, -3, and -4), are activated by proteolytic cleavage, leading to the exposure of a neo–amino terminus that folds back and activates the receptor.

Mutations in the gene encoding tissue factor have been predicted to lead to either a bleeding (loss of function) or a prothrombotic (gain of function) phenotype; however, no congenital abnormalities have been described to date. Targeted disruption of the mouse tissue factor gene (*f3*) results in embryonic lethality of $f3^{-/-}$ embryos at embryonic days 9.5–10.5, most probably as a result of a failure of vasculogenesis.[25–27] Hence loss in early pregnancy most probably accounts for the lack of *TF*-null individuals seen in clinical practice.

Factors VII, IX, and X, Protein Z, and Protein C

Factors VII, IX, and X, protein Z, and protein C share a common protein structure: they are all zymogens of vitamin K–dependent serine proteases composed of a Gla–EGF-1–EGF-2–SP (γ-carboxylated glutamic acid, epidermal growth factor-1 and -2–like, and serine protease) domain structure. Although they have distinct functional properties within the coagulation network, analysis of the gene organizations, protein structures and sequence identities suggest they have resulted from gene duplication events. Indeed, factor VII, factor X, and protein Z are tandemly linked on chromosome 13 (q34), suggesting they have arisen through tandem gene duplication. Protein Z lacks the critical histidine and serine residues of the catalytic triad of the protease domain and therefore is not a zymogen of a serine protease. It has been shown to negatively regulate blood coagulation through the formation of a complex with factor Xa and protein Z–dependent protease inhibitor, a member of the serpin superfamily, thereby inhibiting the catalytic activity of factor Xa.

The Gla domain consists of a number (9–12) of glutamic acid residues that are posttranslationally modified by the addition of a carboxyl group to the γ-carbon by a vitamin K–dependent carboxylase. Blocking this posttranslational modification with coumarin derivatives such as warfarin represents the current therapy of choice for the long-term treatment and prevention of thromboembolic events (see Chapters 86 and 88). The module forms a Ca^{2+}-dependent fold that confers affinity to negatively charged phospholipid membranes, promoting the assembly of functional complexes on these surfaces.

The EGF modules are widely dispersed in nature and are often involved in protein-protein interaction. The typical structure is a β-pleated sheet maintained by a characteristic 1–3, 2–4, 5–6 arrangement of three disulfide bonds.

The serine protease domain is homologous to that of chymotrypsin and contains the archetypal catalytic triad: a serine, histidine, and aspartate that are critical for catalytic activity of these enzymes. Although the structural elements responsible for the trypsin fold are highly conserved, amino acid substitutions to surface loops that border the active site and the substrate recognition pocket confer the diverse functional properties to these proteases.

Factor VII

Factor VII is synthesized in the liver and circulates in blood as a single-chain molecule that is activated by a single proteolytic cleavage (▶◀) between residues Arg152 and Ile153, yielding a two-chain disulfide-linked molecule. Factor VIIa has little activity in the absence of its cellular receptor and its cofactor, tissue factor. Factor VIIa is not inhibited by antithrombin; however, TF-FVIIa is inhibited by TFPI in a quaternary complex with factor

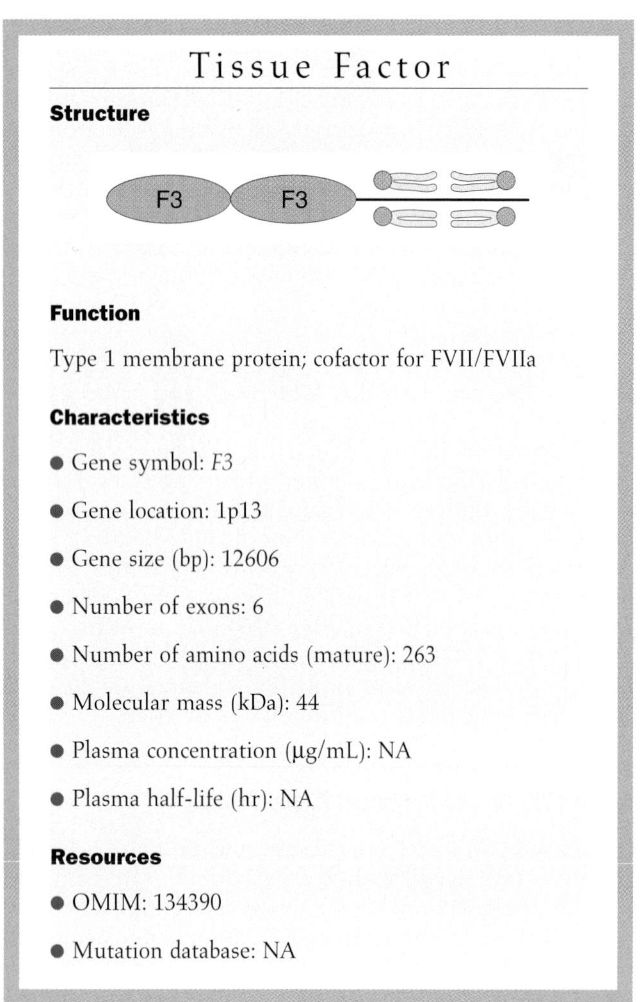
Tissue Factor

Structure

Function

Type 1 membrane protein; cofactor for FVII/FVIIa

Characteristics

- Gene symbol: *F3*
- Gene location: 1p13
- Gene size (bp): 12606
- Number of exons: 6
- Number of amino acids (mature): 263
- Molecular mass (kDa): 44
- Plasma concentration (μg/mL): NA
- Plasma half-life (hr): NA

Resources

- OMIM: 134390
- Mutation database: NA

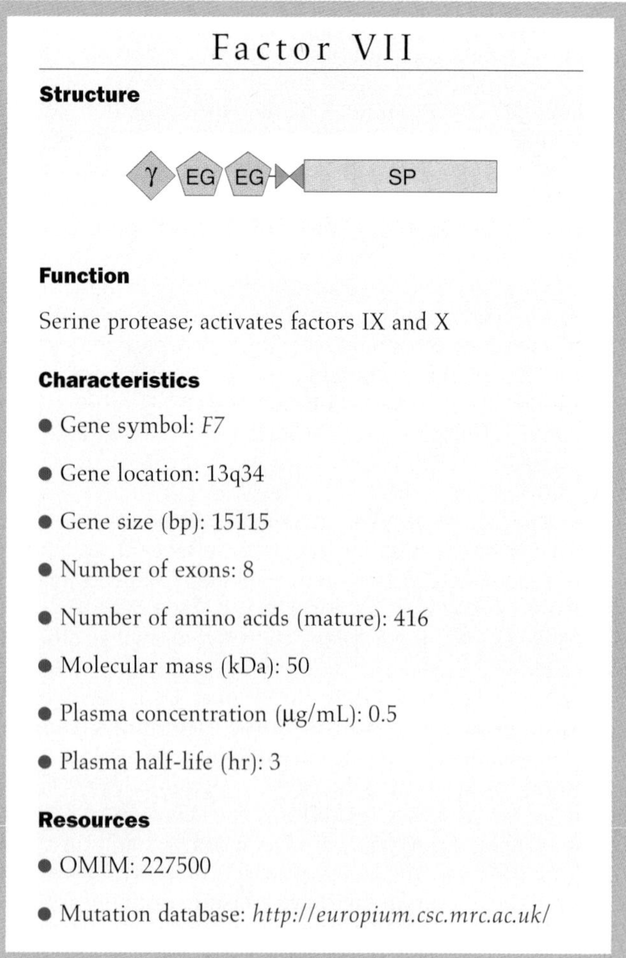
Factor VII

Structure

Function

Serine protease; activates factors IX and X

Characteristics

- Gene symbol: *F7*
- Gene location: 13q34
- Gene size (bp): 15115
- Number of exons: 8
- Number of amino acids (mature): 416
- Molecular mass (kDa): 50
- Plasma concentration (μg/mL): 0.5
- Plasma half-life (hr): 3

Resources

- OMIM: 227500
- Mutation database: *http://europium.csc.mrc.ac.uk/*

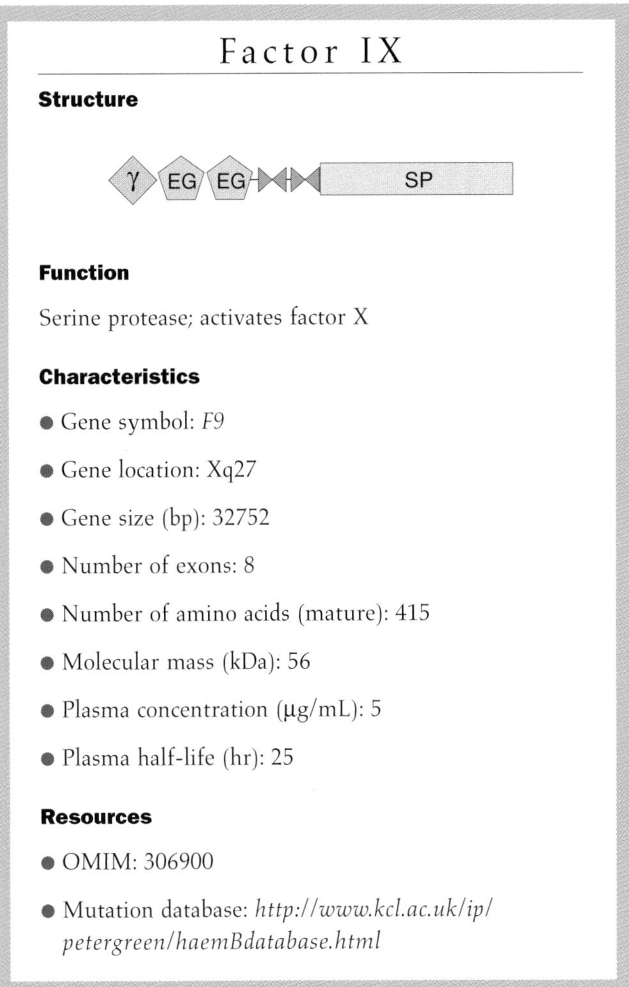

Factor IX

Structure

Function

Serine protease; activates factor X

Characteristics

- Gene symbol: *F9*
- Gene location: Xq27
- Gene size (bp): 32752
- Number of exons: 8
- Number of amino acids (mature): 415
- Molecular mass (kDa): 56
- Plasma concentration (μg/mL): 5
- Plasma half-life (hr): 25

Resources

- OMIM: 306900
- Mutation database: *http://www.kcl.ac.uk/ip/petergreen/haemBdatabase.html*

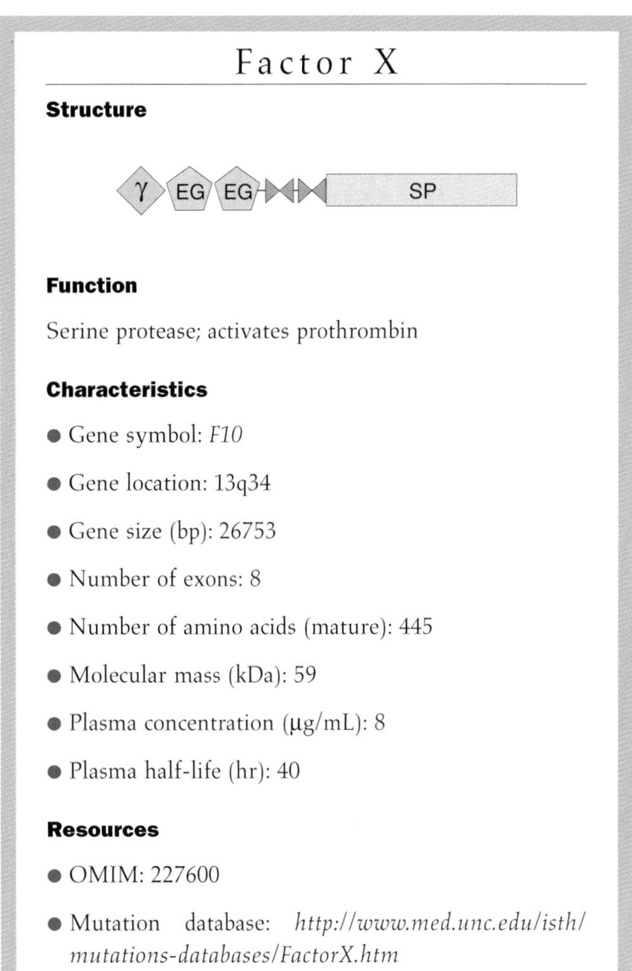

Factor X

Structure

Function

Serine protease; activates prothrombin

Characteristics

- Gene symbol: *F10*
- Gene location: 13q34
- Gene size (bp): 26753
- Number of exons: 8
- Number of amino acids (mature): 445
- Molecular mass (kDa): 59
- Plasma concentration (μg/mL): 8
- Plasma half-life (hr): 40

Resources

- OMIM: 227600
- Mutation database: *http://www.med.unc.edu/isth/mutations-databases/FactorX.htm*

Xa (see Fig. 8–4). Deficiency of factor VII is an autosomal recessive bleeding disorder with a highly variable phenotype (see Chapter 66). Neonatal central nervous system bleeds that are often fatal are characteristic of severely affected individuals.

Factor IX

Factor IX is synthesized in the liver and circulates in blood as a single-chain molecule that is activated by proteolytic cleavages between residues Arg145-Ala146 and Arg180-Val181, releasing an activation peptide. Factor IX is activated by the TF-FVIIa complex or factor XIa. Factor IXa is inhibited by antithrombin. Deficiency of factor IX, also known as hemophilia B, is a sex-linked recessive bleeding disorder affecting primarily males (see Chapter 63).

Factor X

Factor X is synthesized in the liver and circulates in blood as a two-chain disulfide-linked molecule. During biosynthesis, the primary translation product is proteolytically processed at residues 139–141, releasing the tripeptide Arg-Lys-Arg. Factor X is activated by either the TF-FVIIa complex or the FIXa-FVIIIa complex (tenase complex) by a single proteolytic cleavage between residues Arg194 and Ile195, releasing a 52-residue activation peptide. It is inhibited by antithrombin and TFPI. Factor X deficiency is a rare autosomal recessive bleeding disorder (see Chapter 66).

Protein C

Protein C is synthesized in the liver and circulates in blood as a two-chain disulfide-linked molecule. During biosynthesis, the primary translation product is proteolytically processed at residues 156–157, releasing the dipeptide Lys-Arg. Protein C is activated by the thrombomodulin-thrombin complex by a single proteolytic cleavage at Arg169-Leu170, releasing a 12–amino acid activation peptide; this process is markedly accelerated by binding to the receptor EPCR. Activated protein C is inhibited by antithrombin. Deficiency of protein C is an autosomal recessive prothrombotic disorder; homozygous protein C deficiency is associated with lethal purpura fulminans, and heterozygous individuals have a high risk of venous thrombosis (see Chapter 67).

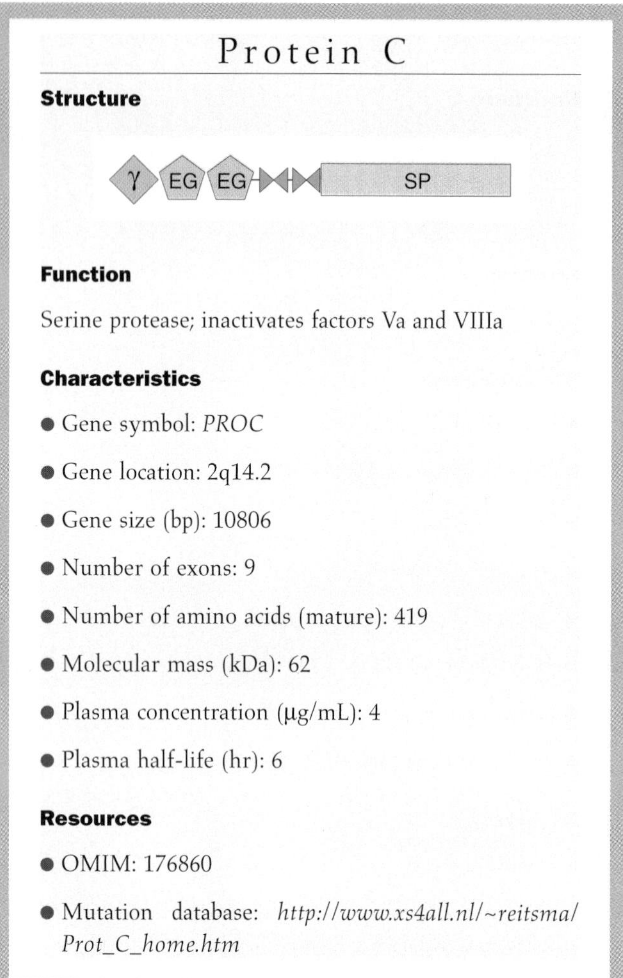

Protein C

Structure

Function

Serine protease; inactivates factors Va and VIIIa

Characteristics

- Gene symbol: *PROC*
- Gene location: 2q14.2
- Gene size (bp): 10806
- Number of exons: 9
- Number of amino acids (mature): 419
- Molecular mass (kDa): 62
- Plasma concentration (μg/mL): 4
- Plasma half-life (hr): 6

Resources

- OMIM: 176860
- Mutation database: *http://www.xs4all.nl/~reitsma/Prot_C_home.htm*

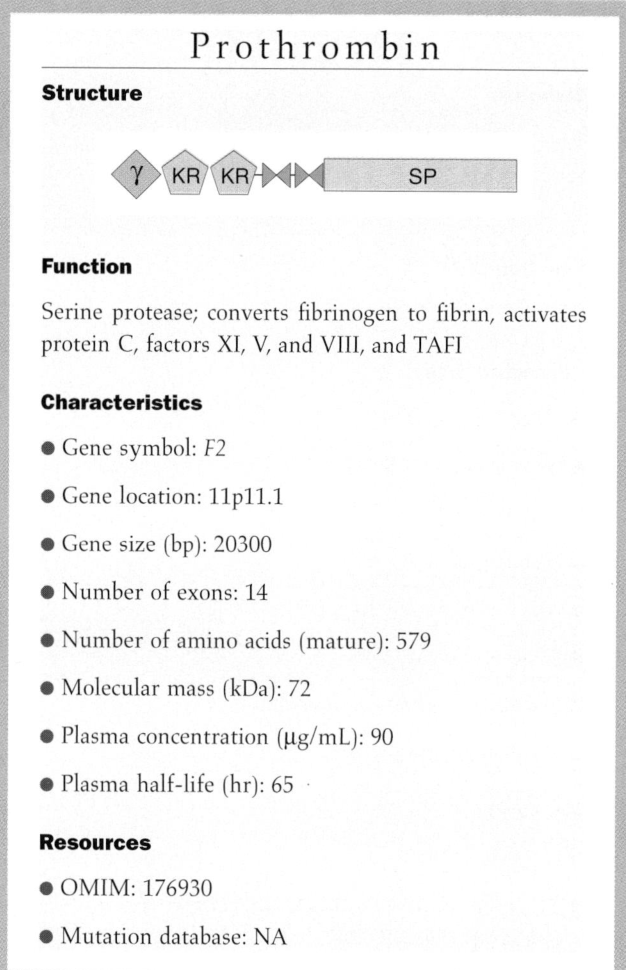

Prothrombin

Structure

Function

Serine protease; converts fibrinogen to fibrin, activates protein C, factors XI, V, and VIII, and TAFI

Characteristics

- Gene symbol: *F2*
- Gene location: 11p11.1
- Gene size (bp): 20300
- Number of exons: 14
- Number of amino acids (mature): 579
- Molecular mass (kDa): 72
- Plasma concentration (μg/mL): 90
- Plasma half-life (hr): 65

Resources

- OMIM: 176930
- Mutation database: NA

Prothrombin

Prothrombin is also a zymogen of a vitamin K–dependent serine protease but has two "kringle" (KR) domains in place of the EGF domains in factors VII, IX, and X and protein C. It has been hypothesized that a primitive prothrombin may have had EGF domains but that these were replaced during gene duplication and exon shuffling.[28] The serine protease domain is homologous to that of the other clotting factors; however, analysis of amino acid residues and codon usage at highly conserved residues linked to active site function in the serine protease distinguishes prothrombin from factors VII, IX, and X and protein C, and suggests thrombin was the ancestral blood coagulation enzyme.[29]

Prothrombin is synthesized in the liver and circulates in blood as a single-chain molecule. The "prothrombinase" complex (factor Xa complexed with factor Va on a phospholipid surface) activates it by sequential cleavage of two peptide bonds at Arg271-Thr272 and Arg320-Ile321. The first cleavage releases the protease domain from the Gla-Kr-Kr modules; the second generates the active catalytic site of thrombin. The soluble, fully cleaved thrombin is termed α-thrombin and is active against many procoagulant substrates, including fibrinogen and factors V, VIII, and IX. In complex with thrombomodulin, it is active against protein C (anticoagulant) and TAFI (antifibrinolytic). Thrombin is also active against PARs, eliciting various cellular responses, including platelet activation.[23]

Prothrombin deficiency is always partial, presumably because total deficiency is embryonic lethal. It is exceedingly rare, with only about 50 case reports. Those few cases that have been studied have hypoprothrombinemia or dysprothrombinemia and present with a mild or moderate bleeding tendency (see Chapter 66).

FV and FVIII

Factors V and VIII share a common protein domain structure, A1-A2-B-A3-C1-C2. They also share sequence similarity with the copper-binding plasma protein ceruloplasmin and the enterocyte transmembrane protein hephastin, which share the domain structure A1-A2-A3. They are involved in protein-protein interactions that permit the assembly of the tenase and prothrombinase complexes. The C domains share sequence similarity with milk fat globule binding protein and have been implicated in phospholipid binding. The B domains of factors V and VIII do not share any apparent sequence

Factor V

Structure

FA5B

FA58A FA58A FA58A FA58C FA58C

Function

Membrane-bound cofactor for factor Xa

Characteristics

- Gene symbol: *F5*
- Gene location: 1q23
- Gene size (bp): 72409
- Number of exons: 25
- Number of amino acids (mature): 2196
- Molecular mass (kDa): 330
- Plasma concentration (μg/mL): 10
- Plasma half-life (hr): 15

Resources

- OMIM: 227400
- Mutation database: *http://www.med.unc.edu/isth/mutations-databases/Factor_V.htm*

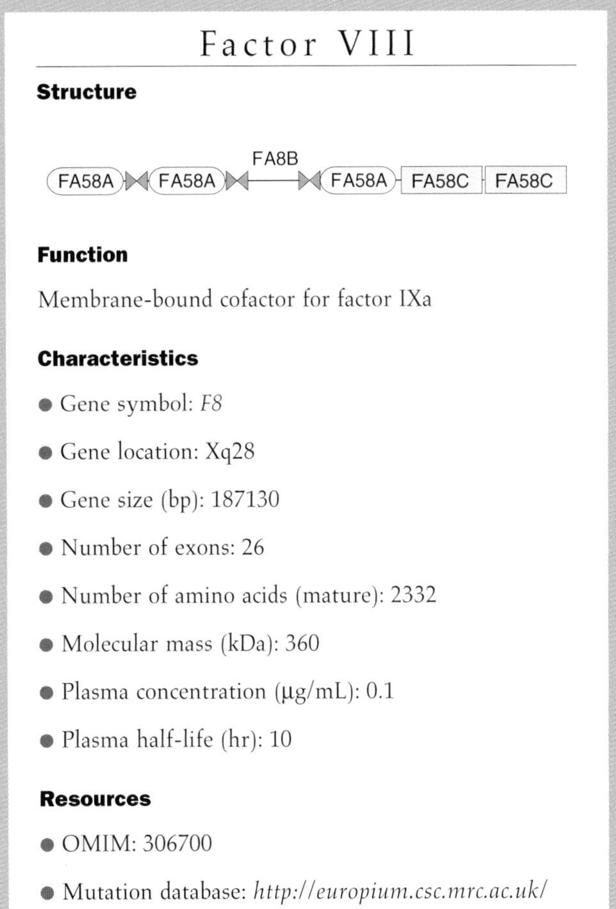

Factor VIII

Structure

FA8B

FA58A FA58A FA58A FA58C FA58C

Function

Membrane-bound cofactor for factor IXa

Characteristics

- Gene symbol: *F8*
- Gene location: Xq28
- Gene size (bp): 187130
- Number of exons: 26
- Number of amino acids (mature): 2332
- Molecular mass (kDa): 360
- Plasma concentration (μg/mL): 0.1
- Plasma half-life (hr): 10

Resources

- OMIM: 306700
- Mutation database: *http://europium.csc.mrc.ac.uk/*

similarity; however, both contain high numbers of potential amino-linked glycosylation sites. The B domain is dispensable for procoagulant activity, because recombinant B-domainless versions of these factors retain full activity and have pharmacokinetic profiles similar to full-length proteins.[30]

Factor V

Factor V is synthesized in the liver and circulates in blood as a single-chain molecule. An additional pool comprising 18–25% of total factor V in blood is sequestered in the α-granules of platelets.[31] Factor V is activated by limited proteolytic cleavage by thrombin at Arg709-Ser710, Arg1018-Thr1019, and Arg1545-Ser1546, resulting in the noncovalently associated heterodimer composed of A1-A2 and A3-C1-C2. The B domain is released upon activation. Factor Va is inactivated by activated protein C through proteolytic cleavage at Arg506-Ser507 and Arg1765-Leu1766. The cleavage at Arg506 is rate limiting, and the mutation FV Arg506Gln (factor V Leiden) that is resistant to cleavage by APC is associated with venous thrombosis. Factor V deficiency is a very rare autosomal recessive condition that affects about 1 in 1 million of the population (see Chapter 66).

Factor VIII

Factor VIII is synthesized in the liver and circulates in blood as a two-chain disulfide-linked molecule. Factor VIII is activated by limited proteolytic cleavage by thrombin at Arg372-Ser373 and Arg1689-Ser1690, resulting in the noncovalently associated heterotrimer composed of A1, A2, and A3-C1-C2. The B domain is released upon activation. Factor VIIIa is inactivated by activated protein C through proteolytic cleavage at Arg336-Ser337 and Arg562-Ser563; however, functional activity of factor VIIIa also decays rapidly through dissociation of the A2 subunit. Factor VIII deficiency (hemophilia A) is a sex-linked recessive disorder affecting about 1 in 5000 males worldwide (see Chapter 63).

Fibrinogen

Fibrinogen is synthesized by the liver and circulates in blood as a symmetrical dimer of a disulfide-linked α-β-γ trimer (Fig. 8–10). The molecule has distal globular domains connected by three-stranded coiled coils to the central domain, which contains the carboxyl termini of all six chains tethered together by disulfide bonds. Polymerization of fibrinogen occurs through the thrombin-catalyzed removal of fibrinopeptides A and B from the

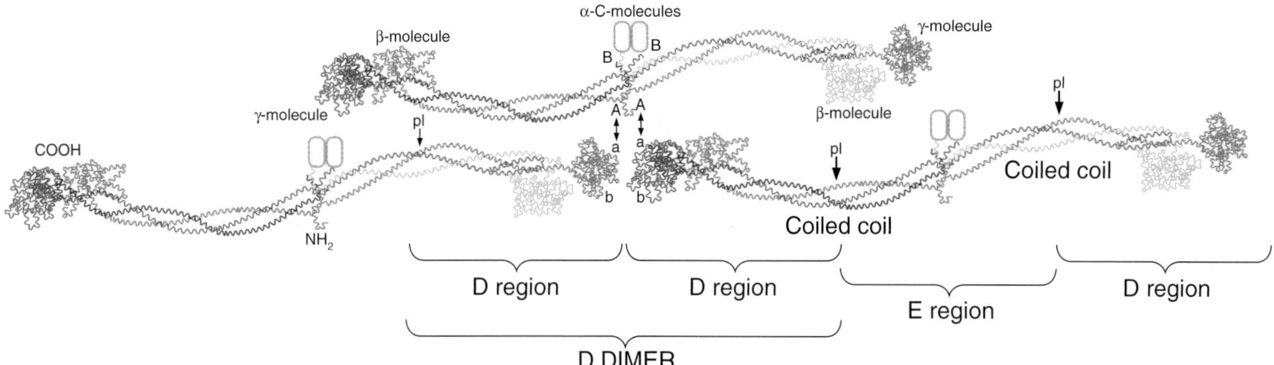

Figure 8–10. Fibrinogen structure and fibrin assembly. Fibrinogen circulates in blood as a symmetrical dimer of a disulfide-linked α-β-γ trimer. A ribbon model of chicken fibrinogen based on its crystal structure illustrates the structure of fibrinogen. Fibrinogen can be divided into structural regions: the central E region, two identical D regions, and the αC domain. The amino-terminal portions of the α and β chains and the αC domains were not resolved in this structure, and the αC domains are shown schematically. Thrombin converts fibrinogen to fibrin by cleavage of short amino-terminal peptides from the α and β chains to yield fibrinopeptides A and B. This cleavage exposes polymerization sites or "knobs." The interaction of the knobs with corresponding "holes" in the D regions of adjacent molecules promotes fibrin polymerization. Each D region, consisting of the β and γ modules, is connected by a triple-helical coiled-coil that is cleaved by plasmin (pl) to yield D and E fragments.

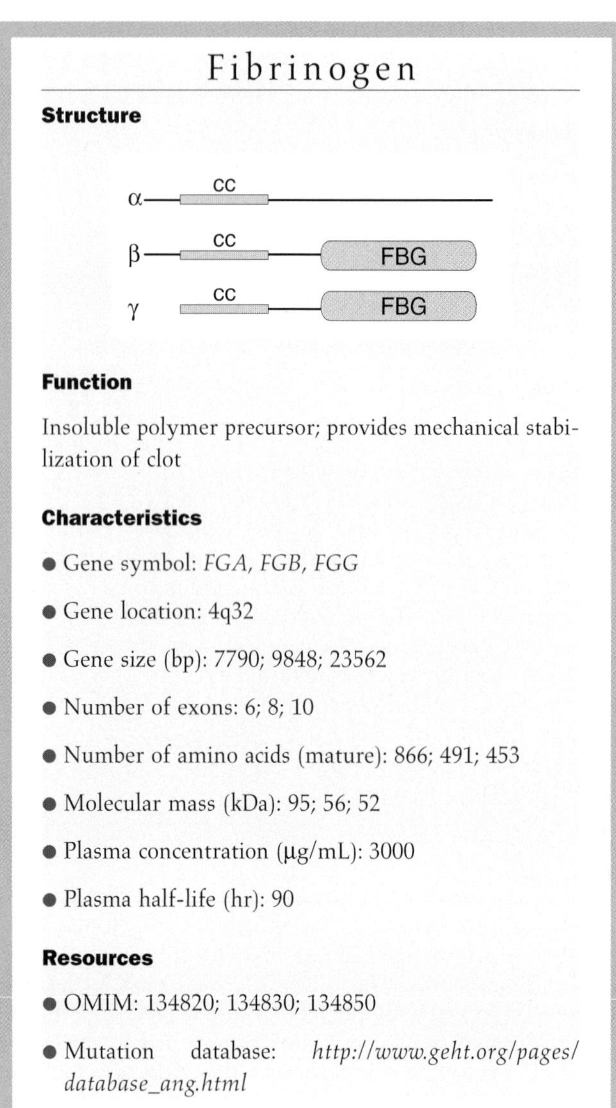

Fibrinogen

Structure

Function

Insoluble polymer precursor; provides mechanical stabilization of clot

Characteristics

- Gene symbol: *FGA, FGB, FGG*
- Gene location: 4q32
- Gene size (bp): 7790; 9848; 23562
- Number of exons: 6; 8; 10
- Number of amino acids (mature): 866; 491; 453
- Molecular mass (kDa): 95; 56; 52
- Plasma concentration (μg/mL): 3000
- Plasma half-life (hr): 90

Resources

- OMIM: 134820; 134830; 134850
- Mutation database: *http://www.geht.org/pages/database_ang.html*

amino termini of the α and β chains, respectively. The release of the fibrinopeptides exposes new amino-terminal sequences, the A and B "knobs," that fit into their appropriate "holes," leading to spontaneous polymerization that can elongate indefinitely in either direction.[32]

Perhaps surprisingly, total fibrinogen deficiency is compatible with normal in utero development.[33] The disorder is rare but responds well to treatment with infusions of plasma-derived fibrinogen. Some types of dysfibrinogenemia are associated with thrombotic tendency rather than bleeding.

Factor XI

Factor XI is a zymogen of a serine protease. It is synthesized in the liver and circulates in blood as a disulfide-linked homodimer. Factor XI is homologous to prekallikrein, sharing a common protein structure composed of four "apple" (AP) domains or PAN domains, which are important for protein-protein interactions, and a serine protease domain. Homodimerization occurs through the A4 domain. Factor XI is activated by thrombin by a single proteolytic cleavage at Arg369-Ile370, yielding a four-chain disulfide-linked heterodimer. Factor XI deficiency is an autosomal recessive bleeding dis-order that is generally mild even in homozygous cases with very low residual factor XI (see Chapter 66).

Thrombomodulin

Thrombomodulin is an integral membrane receptor expressed constitutively on endothelial cells in virtually all tissues with the exception of the brain vasculature and in hepatic sinusoids and lymph node venules. Throm-

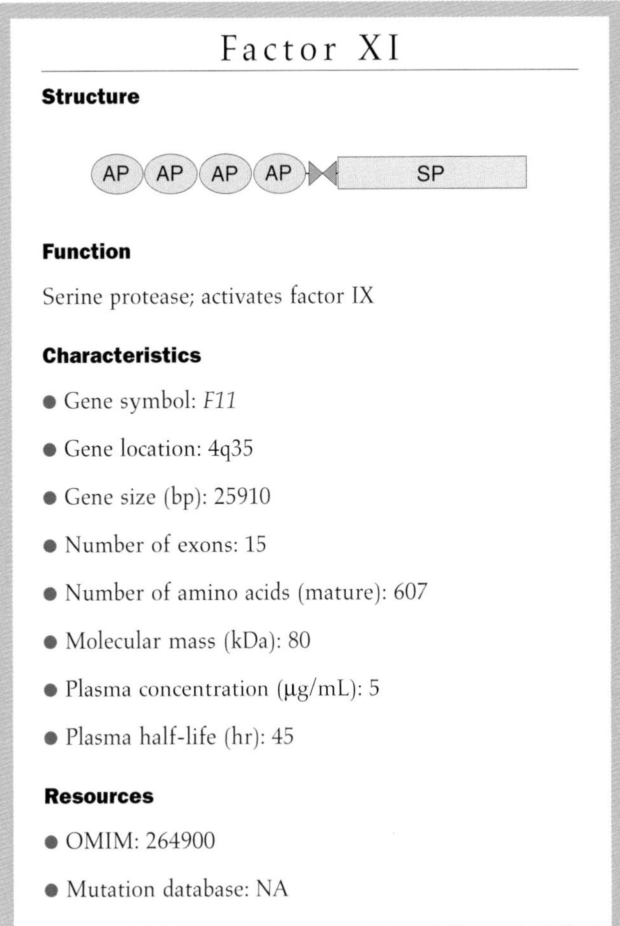

Factor XI

Structure

Function

Serine protease; activates factor IX

Characteristics

- Gene symbol: *F11*
- Gene location: 4q35
- Gene size (bp): 25910
- Number of exons: 15
- Number of amino acids (mature): 607
- Molecular mass (kDa): 80
- Plasma concentration (μg/mL): 5
- Plasma half-life (hr): 45

Resources

- OMIM: 264900
- Mutation database: NA

bomodulin is structurally organized in three domains: the extracellular portion of the molecule consists of an amino-terminal lectin-like (CLECT) domain and six EGF modules, a transmembrane sequence of 23 amino acids, and a cytoplasmic domain of 38 amino acid residues. Thrombomodulin functions as a cellular receptor for thrombin, forming a complex via EGF modules 4–6 and the protease's anion-binding exosite 1, thus preventing the protease from binding to its various procoagulant substrates (factors V, VIII, and XIII and fibrinogen). Formation of the thrombomodulin-thrombin complex also increases the rate of activation of protein C.

Endothelial Cell Protein C Receptor

EPCR is an integral membrane protein that is constitutively expressed on endothelial cells. The extracellular domain of EPCR is homologous to that of the major histocompatibility complex class I/CD1 family of proteins. EPCR is thought to interact with the Gla domain of protein C and, by localizing the protein C molecule to the endothelial cell surface, increases the activation rate of protein C by the thrombomodulin-thrombin complex. Recent data implicate the EPCR-APC complex in cell signaling through activation of PAR-1, leading to

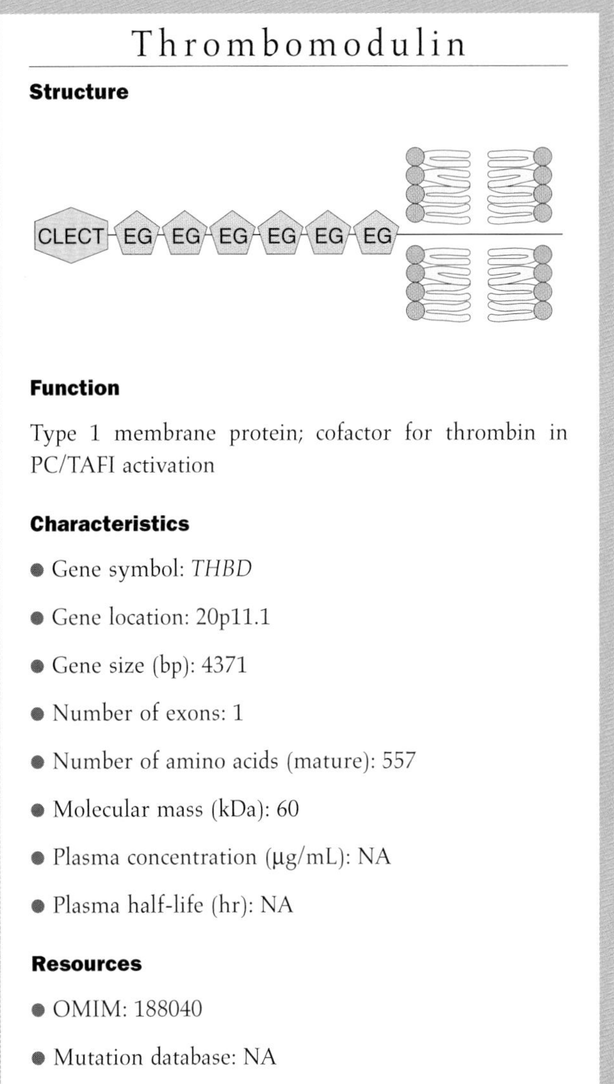

Thrombomodulin

Structure

Function

Type 1 membrane protein; cofactor for thrombin in PC/TAFI activation

Characteristics

- Gene symbol: *THBD*
- Gene location: 20p11.1
- Gene size (bp): 4371
- Number of exons: 1
- Number of amino acids (mature): 557
- Molecular mass (kDa): 60
- Plasma concentration (μg/mL): NA
- Plasma half-life (hr): NA

Resources

- OMIM: 188040
- Mutation database: NA

induction of antiapoptotic and endothelial protective genes.[34]

Tissue Factor Pathway Inhibitor

TFPI is synthesized by endothelial cells and megakaryocytes. Circulating concentrations are approximately 2.5 nM, but this pool of TFPI is largely truncated at the carboxyl terminus and has poor anticoagulant activity. The largest pool of TFPI is associated with the endothelial cell surface. Heparin therapy induces a large increase in the plasma concentration of TFPI, suggesting that TFPI binding to endothelial cells is mediated by surface glycosaminoglycans; however, recent evidence indicates that a significant portion of TFPI associates with the cell surface through interaction with a glycosylphosphatidylinositol-anchored protein.[35] TFPI is also found in platelets and is released in response to stimulation by thrombin. TFPI has an acidic amino-terminal sequence followed by three tandem domains with homology to the

Endothelial Cell Protein C Receptor

Structure

MHCI

Function

Type 1 membrane protein; cofactor for protein C activation by thrombomodulin-thrombin

Characteristics

- Gene symbol: *PROCR*
- Gene location: 20p11.1
- Gene size (bp): 16693
- Number of exons: 7
- Number of amino acids (mature): 220
- Molecular mass (kDa): 27
- Plasma concentration (μg/mL): NA
- Plasma half-life (hr): NA

Resources

- OMIM: 600646
- Mutation database: NA

Tissue Factor Pathway Inhibitor

Structure

–KU–KU–KU–

Function

Kunitz-type inhibitor; inhibits TF-FVIIa-FXa complex

Characteristics

- Gene symbol: *TFPI*
- Gene location: 2q33
- Gene size (bp): 90289
- Number of exons: 12
- Number of amino acids (mature): 304
- Molecular mass (kDa): 35
- Plasma concentration (μg/mL): 0.08
- Plasma half-life (hr): NA

Resources

- OMIM: 152310
- Mutation database: NA

Kunitz-type protease inhibitors (Ku) and a basic carboxy-terminal region. KU1 and KU2 are required for binding to TF-FVIIa and factor Xa, respectively, whereas KU3 has no protease substrate but is necessary for full anticoagulant activity. The basic carboxyl terminus is required for rapid inhibition of factor Xa by KU2 and interaction with the cell surface.

Antithrombin

Antithrombin is a serpin synthesized by the liver. It forms a stable 1:1 complex with several serine protease coagulation factors, most importantly factor Xa and thrombin. The importance of antithrombin is demonstrated by the high association of deficiency with venous thrombosis (see Chapter 67) and by the success of heparin anticoagulant therapy. The anticoagulant effect of heparin is mediated principally through the activation of antithrombin.

Protein S

Protein S is a single-chain vitamin K–dependent glycoprotein that is synthesized by the liver and endothelial cells. Four EGF domains and two carboxy-terminal LamG domains follow the amino-terminal Gla domain. About 40% of protein S in blood is in the free form, which can form a Ca^{2+}-dependent complex with activated protein C, enhancing its anticoagulant activity toward factors Va and VIIIa. The remaining 60% of protein S is in a 1:1 complex with C4b-binding protein, which does not enhance the activity of activated protein C. C4b-binding protein may therefore serve to modulate the activated protein C pathway. Protein S deficiency is associated with thrombophilia (see Chapter 67).

Plasminogen

Plasminogen is synthesized primarily in the liver and circulates in blood as a single-chain glycoprotein. It is a zymogen of a serine protease, plasmin. It is structurally organized into five kringle (KR) domains and a serine protease domain. The KR domains contain lysine-binding sites that are critical for its interaction with its substrates, its activators and inhibitors. Plasminogen is activated

Antithrombin

Structure

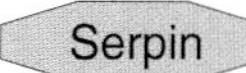

Function

Serpin; inhibits thrombin, factors IXa, Xa, and XIa

Characteristics

- Gene symbol: *SERPINC1*
- Gene location: 1q23
- Gene size (bp): 21005
- Number of exons: 9
- Number of amino acids (mature): 464
- Molecular mass (kDa): 58
- Plasma concentration (μg/mL): 140
- Plasma half-life (hr): 5

Resources

- OMIM: 107300
- Mutation database: *http://www.med.ic.ac.uk/divisions/7/antithrombin/*

Protein S

Structure

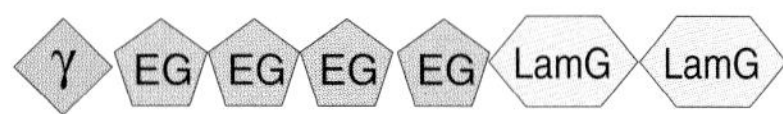

Function

Membrane-bound cofactor for activated protein C

Characteristics

- Gene symbol: *PROS1*
- Gene location: 3q11.2
- Gene size (bp): 101884
- Number of exons: 15
- Number of amino acids (mature): 676
- Molecular mass (kDa): 75
- Plasma concentration (μg/mL): 10 (free)
- Plasma half-life (hr): ?

Resources

- OMIM: 176880
- Mutation database: *http://www.med.unc.edu/isth/SSC/communications/plasma_coagulation/proteins.htm*

Plasminogen

Structure

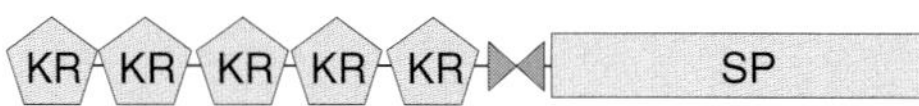

Function

Serine protease; acts in dissolution of clot

Characteristics

- Gene symbol: *PLG*
- Gene location: 6q27
- Gene size (bp): 51056
- Number of exons: 14
- Number of amino acids (mature): 791
- Molecular mass (kDa): 90
- Plasma concentration (μg/mL): 200
- Plasma half-life (hr): 50

Resources

- OMIM: 173350
- Mutation database: NA

by a single proteolytic cleavage at Arg561-Val562 to generate a disulfide-linked two-chain molecule. Subsequent autolysis results in cleavage at the carboxyl side of Lys62, Arg68, and Lys77 to generate new amino termini resulting in forms that are collectively termed Lys-plasmin(ogen) to differentiate them from native plasmin(ogen), which is referred to as Glu-plasmin(ogen). Lys-plasminogen exhibits a more open conformation than Glu-plasminogen and as a result is more readily activated by plasminogen activators.[36]

Tissue Plasminogen Activator

tPA is a serine protease synthesized, stored, and secreted by endothelial cells. The native molecule is a single chain structurally composed of a fibronectin type I (F1) domain, an EGF domain, two KR domains, and a serine protease domain. The single-chain molecule is converted into a two-chain disulfide-linked molecule by plasmin by cleavage at Arg275-Ile276. Both the single-chain and the two-chain form possess very little serine protease activity until they bind fibrin. tPA binds fibrin, and the subsequent binding of plasminogen to fibrin leads to ternary complex formation and activation of plasminogen. Fibrin thus fulfills a dual function, both as a cofactor of plasminogen activation and as a substrate of generated plasmin. The half-life of tPA in blood is extremely short because of its rapid uptake by the liver and rapid inhibition by PAI-1.

Plasminogen Activator Inhibitor-1

PAI-1 is a serpin and is the primary inhibitor of tPA. It is synthesized and secreted by endothelial cells; however, the major pool is contained within platelets, where it is stored and released from α-granules upon stimulation. PAI-1 plays a regulatory role in fibrinolysis by limiting production of plasmin. Deficiency of PAI-1 results in a hyperfibrinolytic state.

α_2-Antiplasmin

α_2-Antiplasmin is the primary inhibitor of plasmin. It is a single-chain serpin synthesized and secreted by the liver. It forms a 1:1 complex with plasmin, in which the protease is completely inactivated. Fibrin-bound plasmin is protected from rapid inactivation by α_2-antiplasmin.

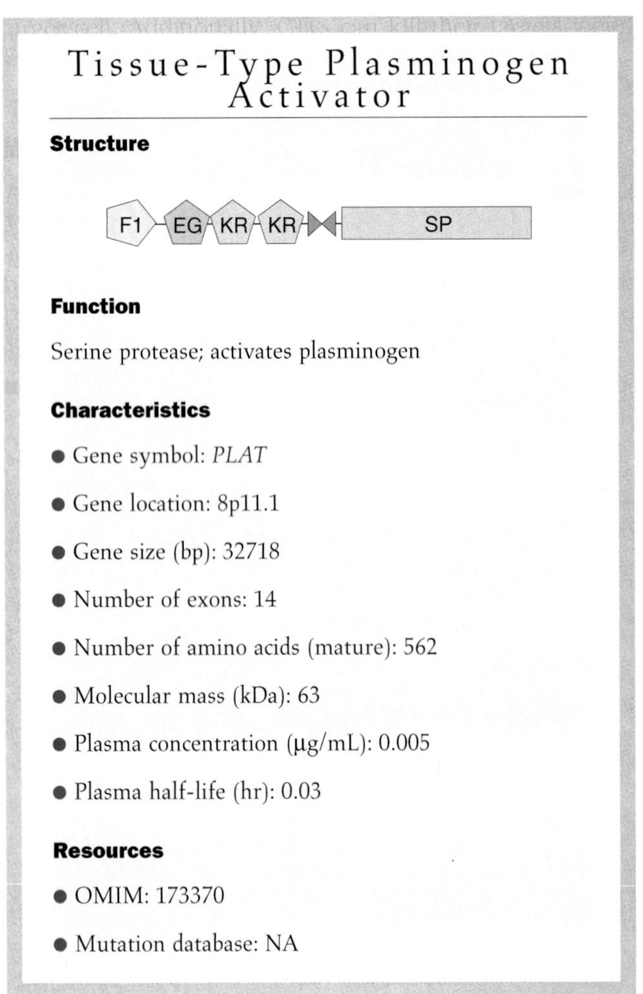

Tissue-Type Plasminogen Activator

Structure

Function

Serine protease; activates plasminogen

Characteristics

- Gene symbol: *PLAT*
- Gene location: 8p11.1
- Gene size (bp): 32718
- Number of exons: 14
- Number of amino acids (mature): 562
- Molecular mass (kDa): 63
- Plasma concentration (μg/mL): 0.005
- Plasma half-life (hr): 0.03

Resources

- OMIM: 173370
- Mutation database: NA

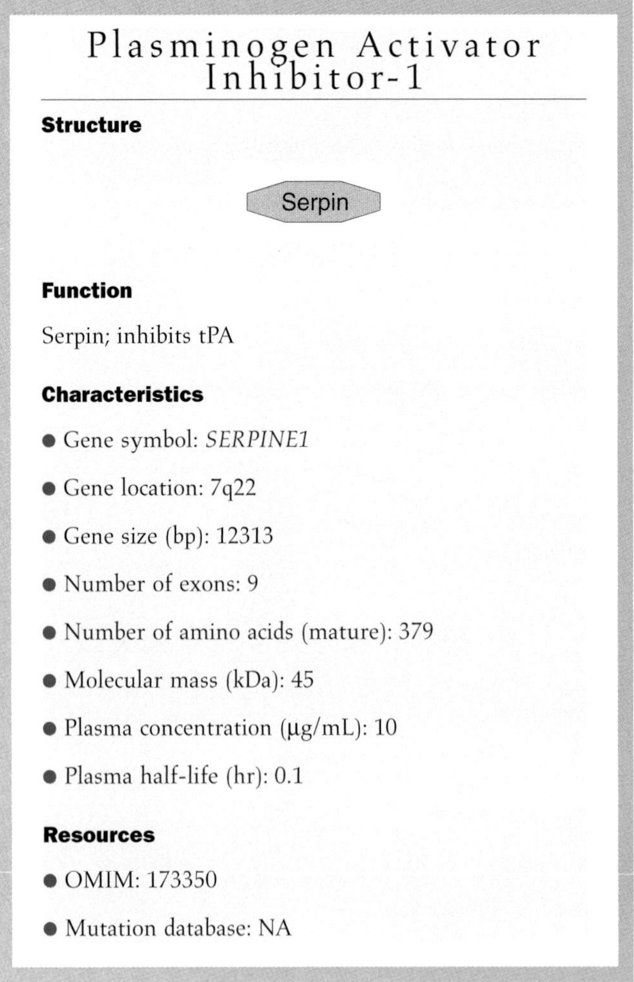

Plasminogen Activator Inhibitor-1

Structure

Function

Serpin; inhibits tPA

Characteristics

- Gene symbol: *SERPINE1*
- Gene location: 7q22
- Gene size (bp): 12313
- Number of exons: 9
- Number of amino acids (mature): 379
- Molecular mass (kDa): 45
- Plasma concentration (μg/mL): 10
- Plasma half-life (hr): 0.1

Resources

- OMIM: 173350
- Mutation database: NA

α_2-Antiplasmin

Structure

Serpin

Function

Serpin; inhibits plasmin

Characteristics

- Gene symbol: *SERPINF2*
- Gene location: 17p13
- Gene size (bp): 13322
- Number of exons: 9
- Number of amino acids (mature): 452
- Molecular mass (kDa): 55
- Plasma concentration (μg/mL): 70
- Plasma half-life (hr): 72

Resources

- OMIM: 262850
- Mutation database: NA

Thrombin-Activatable Fibrinolysis Inhibitor

Structure

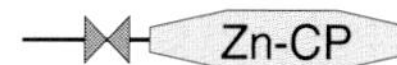

Function

Carboxypeptidase (CP); inhibits fibrinolysis

Characteristics

- Gene symbol: *CPB2*
- Gene location: 13q14
- Gene size (bp): 52423
- Number of exons: 11
- Number of amino acids (mature): 401
- Molecular mass (kDa): 60
- Plasma concentration (μg/mL): 5
- Plasma half-life (hr): 0.2

Resources

- OMIM: 603101
- Mutation database: NA

Factor XIII

Structure

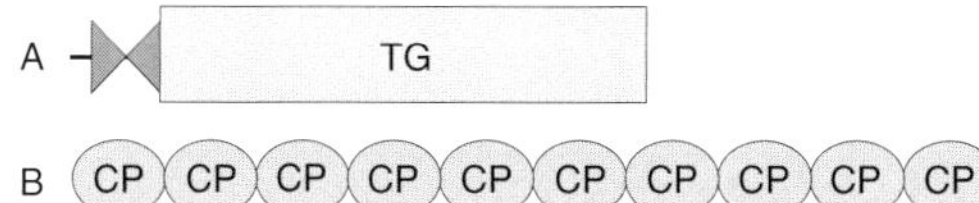

Function

Transglutaminase (TG); cross-links fibrin

Characteristics

- Gene symbol: *F13A1; F13B*
- Gene location: 1q31
- Gene size (bp): 177817; 28045
- Number of exons: 15; 12
- Number of amino acids (mature): 731; 641
- Molecular mass (kDa): 83; 75
- Plasma concentration (μg/mL): 10
- Plasma half-life (hr): 200

Resources

- OMIM: 134570; 134580
- Mutation database: NA

RECURRENT THEMES IN THE BLOOD COAGULATION NETWORK

- The proteases (factors VIIa, IXa, Xa, and XIa, APC, thrombin, tPA, and plasmin) that function in the coagulation network are serine proteases that are members of the chymotrypsin superfamily.
- Factors VIIa, IXa, Xa, and XIa, APC, thrombin, and plasmin circulate in plasma as zymogens that are activated by limited proteolysis.
- Insertion of the neo–amino terminus, generated by proteolytic activation, into a cleft in the protease domain generates a conformation essential for substrate binding and catalytic activity.
- For maximal activity, factors VIIa, IXa, and Xa and APC require cofactors (tissue factor, factor VIIIa, factor Va, and protein S, respectively).
- The complexes assemble on surfaces of either phospholipids or fibrin clots.

Thrombin-Activatable Fibrinolysis Inhibitor

TAFI is a procarboxypeptidase synthesized and secreted by the liver. Activation occurs by a single proteolytic cleavage at Arg92 by the thrombomodulin-thrombin complex, releasing an activation peptide. TAFIa inhibits fibrinolysis by removing carboxy-terminal lysine residues in fibrin that provide binding sites for plasminogen and tPA. Thus the fibrin cofactor function in plasminogen activation is reduced, downregulating fibrinolysis.

Factor XIII

Factor XIII is a protransglutaminase that circulates in blood as a noncovalently bound tetramer (A_2B_2). The B subunit is synthesized and secreted by hepatocytes and serves as a carrier for the hydrophobic A subunit. In contrast, the A subunit is found in monocytes/macrophages and megakaryocytes/platelets, with only trace amounts in hepatocytes. The A subunit contains the active site of the transglutaminase that catalyzes the formation of amide bonds between γ-carbonyls of glutamine residues and ε-amino groups of lysine residues, cross-linking the γ chains and also the α chains of fibrin to form a mesh of covalently linked fibrin. It is activated by thrombin by proteolytic cleavage of a 37–amino acid activation peptide from the A subunit. Consequently, the B subunits dissociate to completely unmask the active site. Activation of factor XIII is tightly controlled by the presence of its substrate, fibrin(ogen).

Suggested Readings*

Davidson CJ, Tuddenham EGD, McVey JH: 450 million years of haemostasis. J Thromb Haemost 1:1487–1494, 2003.

Esmon CT: Inflammation and thrombosis. J Thromb Haemost 1:1343–1348, 2003.

Mackman N: Role of tissue factor in hemostasis, thrombosis and vascular development. Arterioscler Thromb Vasc Biol 24:1015–1022, 2004.

Ruf W, Dorfleutner A, Riewald M: Specificity of coagulation factor signalling. J Thromb Haemost 1:1495–1503, 2003.

Van de Wouwer M, Collen D, Conway EM: Thrombomodulin-protein C-EPCR system. Arterioscler Thromb Vasc Biol 24:1–10, 2004.

Full references for this chapter can be found on accompanying CD-ROM.

CHAPTER 9

Vascular Biology

Katherine A. Hajjar, MD

KEY POINTS

Vascular Biology

- During embryologic development, endothelial cells give rise to the entire cardiovascular system, which reaches functional maturity before any other organ system.
- In the adult, endothelial cells are heterogeneous in terms of their structure, protein synthesis profiles, and responses to environmental stimuli.
- Endothelial cells possess several surface-oriented systems that impart thromboresistance to the blood vessel wall. They also secrete thromboregulatory molecules.
- Inflammatory mediators perturb endothelial thromboresistance mechanisms.
- Both primary and secondary endotheliopathies are expressed as disorders of vascular occlusion.

INTRODUCTION

In the adult, the endothelium is a 1-kg organ containing over 1 trillion cells and covering a surface area of up to 7 m^2.[1,2] Endothelial cells provide a conduit for flowing blood, as well as a barrier that separates the tissues from blood-borne toxins, drugs, and infectious agents (Fig. 9–1). The intimate association of the endothelium with the circulation allows it to regulate blood pressure and vascular tone; participate in immune responses; transport nutrients, macromolecules, and gases; modulate hemostasis; and initiate angiogenesis. In these processes, endothelial cells respond to an unremitting barrage of stimuli induced by fluid dynamic forces, soluble mediators, infectious agents, and physical contact with other cells.

STRUCTURE AND FUNCTION OF THE ENDOTHELIUM

Embryonic Origin of Endothelial Cells

During development, the heart and blood vessels reach functional maturity before any other organ system.[3] Endothelial cell precursors arise within the mesoderm of the yolk sac and the embryo immediately following gastrulation (Fig. 9–2). In the mammalian yolk sac, hemangioblasts develop within "blood islands" and give rise to both hematopoietic precursors and early endothelial cells. In the embryo itself, angioblasts appear to differentiate without associated hematopoietic cells and aggregate to form a primitive tubular network in a process called vasculogenesis.[4,5]

As the embryo develops, new blood vessels undergo extensive remodeling.[6] Neovessels can emerge either as branches of preexisting vascular elements (sprouting angiogenesis) or by subdivision of preexisting vessels (intussusceptive angiogenesis). Regression of blood vessels through activation of apoptotic pathways is also an important component of vascular maturation. In fact, it is likely that only a fraction of blood vessels formed during embryonic development persists to adulthood. Thus, the primitive capillary plexus, consisting of vessels of relatively uniform size and shape, differentiates into an arborized vascular system of graduated diameters, variable wall thickness, and diverse functional properties.

Vascular endothelial growth factor-A (VEGF-A) promotes the development, maintenance, and remodeling of the vascular tree. Multiple alternatively spliced forms of VEGF-A signal via tyrosine kinase receptors known as VEGFR-1/Flt-1 (Fms-like tyrosine kinase) and VEGFR-2/Flk-1 (fetal liver kinase-1)/Kdr (kinase-inserted domain receptor) found on endothelial cells and their precursors.[7] VEGF-A stimulates endothelial cell replication and migration upon receptor dimerization and autophosphorylation. Haploinsufficiency for VEGF-A is incompatible with embryonic life, and heterozygous embryos die from abnormal vascular development.[8,9] Active endothelial

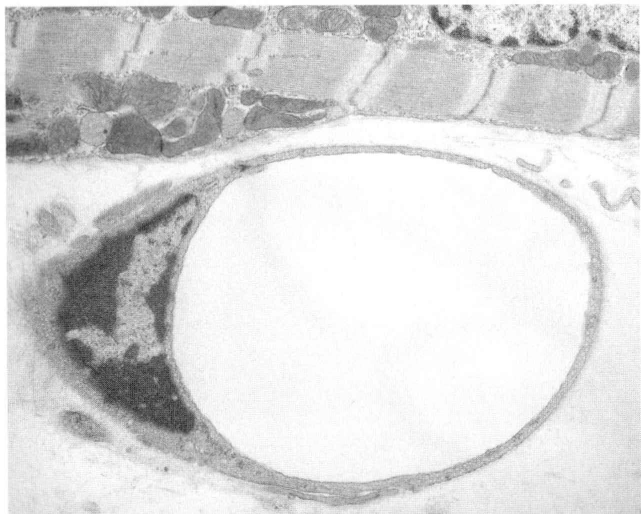

■ **Figure 9–1.** Endothelial cell ultrastructure. Electron micrograph showing a capillary endothelial cell in mouse left ventricular myocardium. Note the eccentric endothelial cell nucleus, the thin capillary wall devoid of investing cells, and the large surface area available to circulating blood. (Courtesy of Patrick Nahirney, PhD.)

cell proliferation, which is ubiquitous in the embryo, occurs only under special circumstances in the adult organism.

Subsequent recruitment of pericytes and smooth muscle cells, which invest and stabilize nascent blood vessels, requires additional tyrosine kinase receptors and their ligands. Tie-1 and Tie-2 (tyrosine kinase with immunoglobulin [Ig] and epidermal growth factor homology domains) are receptors for the angiopoietins.[10] Both angiopoietin-1 and -2 interact with Tie-2, the former being stimulatory and the latter, inhibitory.[11,12] The ligand for Tie-1 remains unidentified.

There is increasing evidence that circulating endothelial precursor cells may participate in neovessel formation beyond embryonic life[13,14] (Fig. 9–3). These precursor cells may be identifiable by their coexpression of specific markers such as Flk-1 and AC133.[15] Although small numbers of circulating endothelial precursor cells appear to circulate in the peripheral blood of normal adults,[16] increased numbers are evident in the blood following trauma,[17] in response to tissue ischemia,[18] and in umbilical cord blood.[19]

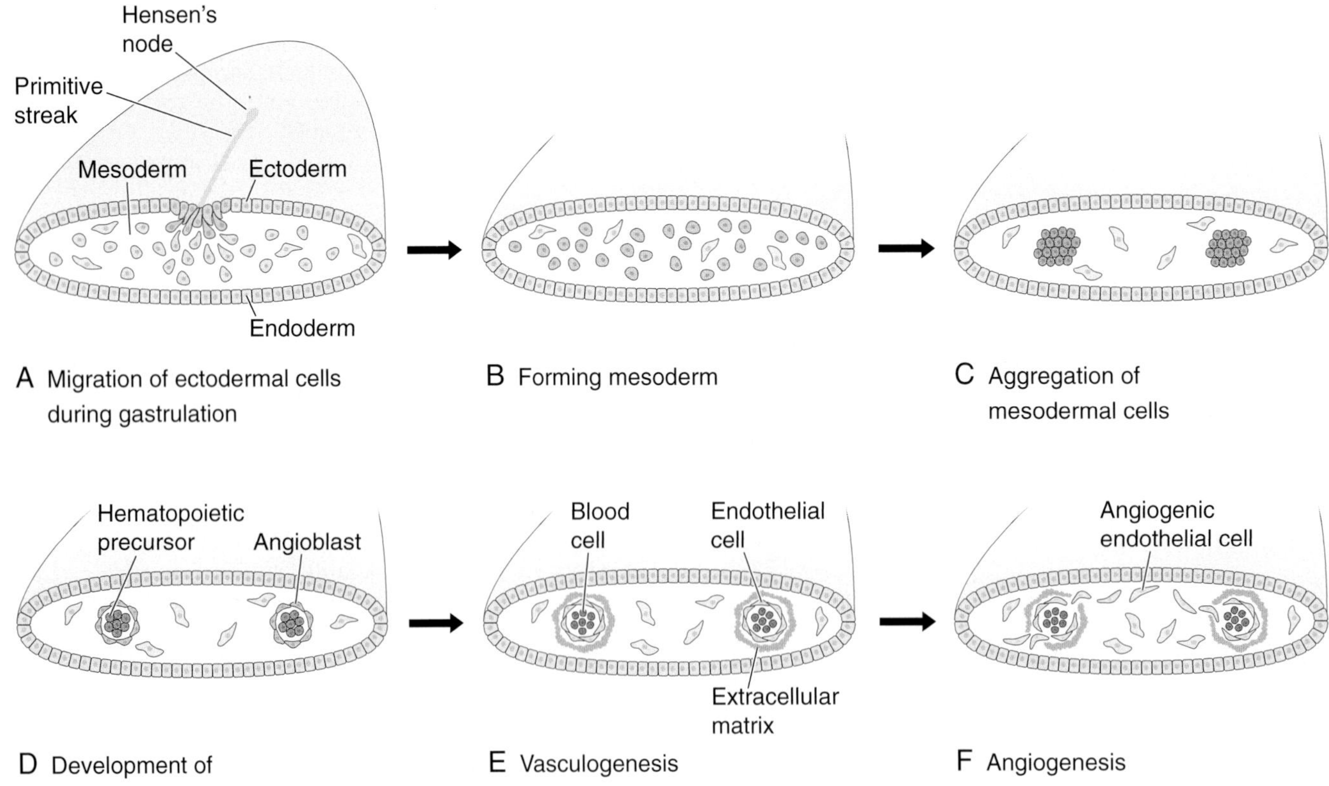

■ **Figure 9–2.** Origin of endothelial cells and blood vessels. During gastrulation, ectodermal cells migrate through the primitive streak *(A)* and occupy the space between ectoderm and endoderm, creating a third layer called mesoderm *(B)*. In a process known as vasculogenesis, mesodermal cells aggregate into clusters *(C)*, and differentiate into endothelial cell precursors, known as angioblasts, and hematopoietic precursor cells *(D)*. Differentiating endothelial cells produce extracellular matrix that stabilizes the developing blood vessel *(E)*. During angiogenesis, endothelial cells may break away from an existing blood vessel, and proliferate and migrate to form new vasculature *(F)*. (Adapted from Mikawa[186] and Cleaver and Krieg.[6])

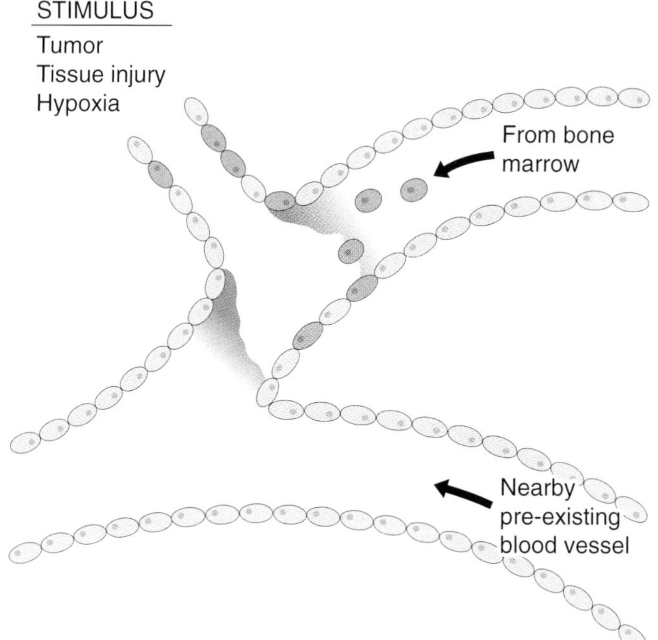

Figure 9–3. Circulating endothelial precursor cells. In response to tissue injury, tumors, or hypoxia, angiogenic growth factors are produced. New blood vessels may form by either of two mechanisms. The stimulus may induce proliferation and migration of endothelial cells originating within a nearby preexisting blood vessel. Alternatively, the stimulus may recruit circulating endothelial cell precursors from a bone marrow niche to create the new vessel. (Adapted from Rafii S: Circulating endothelial precursors: mystery, reality, and promise. J Clin Invest 105:17–19, 2000.)

Endothelial Cell Heterogeneity

As the organism differentiates, its endothelial cells acquire highly diverse phenotypes that correlate with their arterial and venous nature.[20–27] Expression of the growth factor ephrin B2 is seen in arterial endothelial cells, whereas expression of its tyrosine kinase receptor Eph-B4 is restricted to the venous side; this pattern suggests a role for these signaling partners in the demarcation of the venous and arterial vascular trees during development.[28–31] EDG-1, the G protein–coupled receptor for sphingosine 1-phosphate, which contributes to smooth muscle cell and pericyte recruitment during embryonic development, is expressed only on arterial endothelial cells.[32] In the adult, constitutive nitric oxide synthase, an enzyme critical for the regulation of vascular tone, is expressed predominantly on arterial, rather than venous, endothelial cells.[1]

Blood vessel size may also correlate with endothelial cell expression patterns. Thrombomodulin (TM), for example, is widely expressed by endothelial cells of both small and large vessels.[33] Endothelial cell protein C receptor (EPCR) and von Willebrand factor (vWF), in contrast, are produced mainly by macrovascular endothelial cells, and expression of tissue plasminogen activator (tPA) is largely restricted to the microvasculature.[34–38]

Microvascular endothelial cells can be subclassified further according to their ultrastructural morphology[3,22,23] (Fig. 9–4). "Continuous" endothelia serve a barrier function in the brain, lymph nodes, and skeletal muscle, and have uniform membrane structure and tight intercellular junctions. "Discontinuous" endothelia, in contrast, possess membrane pores that allow liver, bone marrow, and spleen to participate in hematopoiesis, particle exchange, and blood cell processing. Finally, "fenestrated" endothelia possess diaphragms that facilitate secretion, absorption, or filtration of macromolecules in endocrine organs, the gastrointestinal tract, the choroid plexus, and renal glomeruli.

ENDOTHELIAL CELLS AND THROMBORESISTANCE

As defined by Virchow's triad, the fluid state of blood results from an exquisite balance that involves the mechanical flow of blood, the reactivities of soluble circulating coagulant factors, and the modulating influence of the blood vessel wall.[39] The endothelium contributes to this homeostasis by modulating blood flow, procoagulant reactivity, and cell-cell interactions.[3]

Modulation of Platelet Reactivity (Fig. 9–5)

Prostacyclin

A potent vasodilator and inhibitor of platelet aggregation, prostacyclin (prostaglandin $[PG]I_2$) is produced by the endothelium in response to hormones, biochemical agents, or physical forces.[40–42] Increases in intracellular calcium activate phospholipases A_2 and C, which release free arachidonate from membrane phospholipids. Cyclooxygenase (COX) catalyzes the oxygenation and cyclization of free arachidonate, giving rise to the endoperoxide known as PGG_2, which is then reduced to PGH_2 via the peroxidase activity of COX. Prostacyclin (PGI_2) is formed upon isomerization of PGH_2 by PGI synthase.[43] With an exceedingly short half-life, PGI_2 is cleared within 3 minutes by chemical hydrolysis to 6-keto-$PGF_{1\alpha}$. The biochemical effects of PGI_2 are mediated mainly through G proteins and result in increased intraplatelet cyclic AMP, abolition of platelet shape change and secretion, and impaired binding of vWF and fibrinogen to the platelet surface.

Although both the constitutive COX-1 and inducible COX-2 are expressed by endothelial cells, regional specificities appear to govern PGI_2 synthesis and responsiveness within the vasculature.[43,44] Although COX-2 is induced in a general sense upon exposure to prothrombotic, inflammatory, mitogenic, or hypoxic stimuli,[45–48] its baseline activity in an animal model is two- to threefold higher in coronary arteries than in other large vessel endothelia.[49] Similarly, systemic infusion of PGI_2 results in vasorelaxation of coronary, mesenteric, and pericranial, but not cerebral, vessels.[50]

Nitric Oxide

Nitric oxide (NO) was the first gas to be characterized as an intracellular messenger. A highly reactive, slightly water-soluble, colorless substance with a half-life of

Figure 9-4. Heterogeneity of Microvascular Endothelial Cells

Morphology	Tissue or Organ	Properties	Function
Continuous 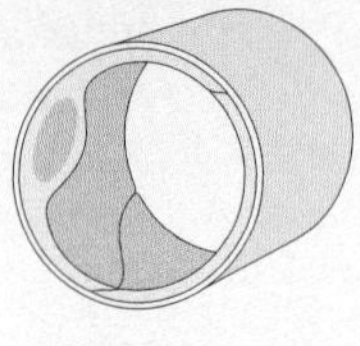	CNS	Complex tight junctions	Blood-brain barrier
	Lymph nodes	High endothelial venules	Lymphocyte homing
	Muscle	High number of vesicles	Exchange/transport
Discontinuous: Fenestrated 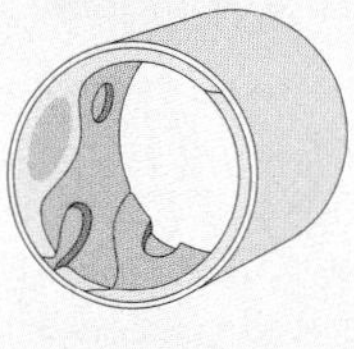	Endocrine glands	Fenestrae	Secretion
	GI tract	Fenestrae	Absorption
	Choroid plexus	Fenestrae	Secretion
	Renal glomeruli	Pores	Filtration
Discontinuous: Non-fenestrated 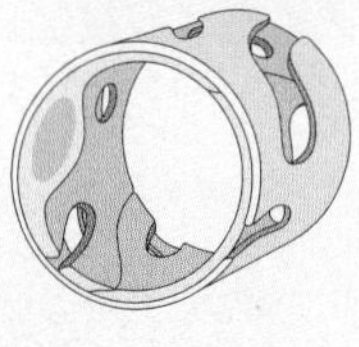	Liver	Large gaps	Exchange of particles
	Spleen	Splenic sinus of red pulp	Blood cell processing
	Bone marrow	Marrow sinus	Hematopoiesis; delivery of blood cells

Figure 9–4. Heterogeneity of microvascular endothelial cells. Within different organs and tissues, endothelial cells acquire specific structural adaptations. Continuous endothelial cells serve primarily a barrier function. Fenestrated endothelial cells promote secretion, absorption, and filtration. Nonfenestrated discontinuous endothelial cells possess gaps that allow exchange of particles and cells between blood and the extravascular space. (Adapted from Hajjar KA: The endothelium in thrombosis and hemorrhage. *In* Loscalzo J, Schaefer AI [eds]: Thrombosis and Hemorrhage. Philadelphia: Lippincott, Williams & Wilkins, 2003, pp 206–219.)

about 6 seconds,[51,52] NO is formed in vascular endothelial cells from L-arginine by the constitutively active endothelial nitric oxide synthase (eNOS).[52] NO production is accelerated by ADP, thrombin, bradykinin, and shear stress, all of which elevate intracellular calcium. In particular, shear forces induce transcriptional activation of the eNOS gene via a shear response consensus sequence (GAGACC) within its promoter.[53–55] Whereas constitutive eNOS is regulated by Ca^{2+} and calmodulin, inducible nitric oxide synthase is stimulated by agonists such as cytokines.[56]

NO binds to the heme prosthetic group of guanylyl cyclase, inhibiting platelet activation, inducing vasodilation, inhibiting leukocyte adhesion to the endothelial surface, blocking smooth muscle cell migration, and reducing smooth muscle cell proliferation. Systemic overproduction of NO may contribute to the hypotension of endotoxic shock, and low levels in the lung circulation may be pathogenetic in pulmonary hypertension.[57] Inhibition of NO synthase in the conscious rat elevates skeletal muscle vascular resistance but has little effect on cerebellar vascular tone.[24,58] Similarly, basal release of NO in the rabbit appears to be greater in mesenteric and femoral arteries than in the aorta,[59] and release in the carotid artery exceeds that in the jugular vein,[60] possibly reflecting different patterns of shear stress in specific vascular beds.[61] These findings suggest that regional differences in regulation of endothelial cell NO synthase activity may control local vasoreactivity and platelet responses.

Ecto-ADPase/CD39

Endothelial cells express CD39, a cell surface ADP/ATPase[24,62] of the E-type apyrase family (EC3.6.1.5) (Table 9–1). CD39 metabolizes ADP released from activated platelets, thereby inhibiting ADP-induced platelet recruitment, release, and aggregation. Intravenous injection of a recombinant soluble form of CD39 in mice decreases platelet aggregation in response to ADP and other agonists. In the CD39-null mouse, fibrin deposition was most prominent in the lung and heart, with accentuation in the lung upon induction of hypoxia.[63] In studies suggesting potential therapeutic value, recombi-

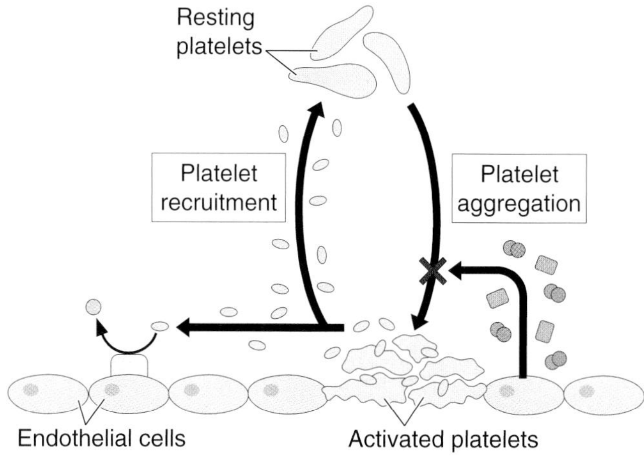

KEY

CD39/ADPase ADP Adenosine NO PGI_2

Figure 9–5. Endothelial cell control of platelet reactivity. CD39/ADPase, expressed on the surface of endothelial cells, metabolizes adenosine diphosphate (ADP), which is secreted by activated platelets for the further recruitment of platelets to an evolving thrombus. Endothelial cells also secrete prostacyclin (PGI_2), which inhibits platelet aggregation by blocking shape change and granule secretion. Finally, nitric oxide (NO) interferes with G protein–mediated signaling, thereby inhibiting platelet reactivity.

nant soluble CD39 reduced the infarct volume in mice undergoing transient occlusion of the middle cerebral artery.[64]

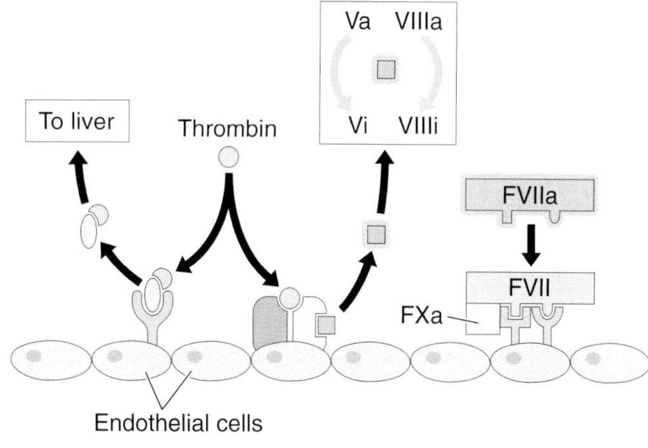

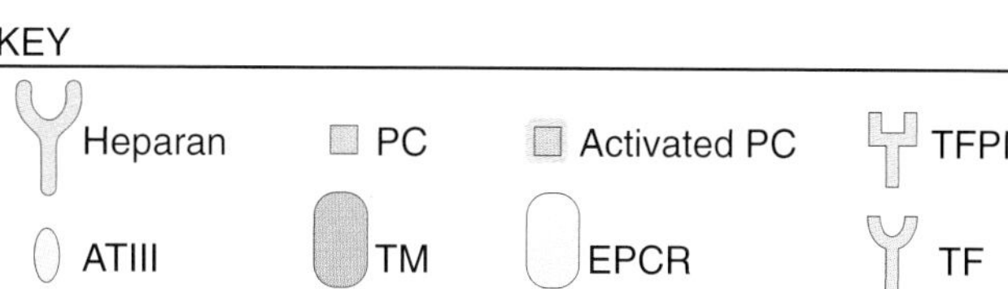

Figure 9–6. Endothelial cell anticoagulant pathways. The transmembrane protein thrombomodulin (TM) binds thrombin and alters its substrate specificity. Thrombomodulin-bound thrombin then converts protein C, bound to its own cell surface receptor (endothelial cell protein C receptor [EPCR]), to activated protein C (aPC). aPC can then convert the activated procoagulant cofactors, factors Va and VIIIa, to their respective inactive forms (Vi and VIIIi). The serpin antithrombin III (ATIII) resides on the endothelial cell surface in association with heparan or other glycosaminoglycans. In this configuration, AT III can form a covalent complex with thrombin (or factor Xa), which is then cleared in the liver. Tissue factor pathway inhibitor (TFPI) is present on the endothelial cell surface and neutralizes the tissue factor (TF)–factor VIIa (FVIIa)–factor Xa catalytic complex.

Endothelial Anticoagulant Pathways (Fig. 9–6)

Tissue Factor

Tissue factor (TF), the primary initiator of coagulation, is expressed on the adventitia of blood vessels and by cells, such as monocytes and macrophages, beyond the confines of the blood vessel (see Table 9–1).[65] Blood coagulation is initiated when vascular injury allows blood to come in contact with extravascular sources of TF; binding of factor VII to TF leads to activation of factor VII, and a nearly 1000-fold increase in its proteolytic activity.[66,67] Although endothelial cell expression of TF can be induced in vitro by exposure to bacterial products[68] or by shear stress,[69] in vivo studies involving infusion of *Escherichia coli* into baboons show that induction of TF expression is confined to the splenic microvasculature.[68,70] Thus, although monocytes, macrophages, and epithelial cells respond to inflammatory mediators with dramatic increases in TF expression, the endothelial cell response is highly restricted.[70]

von Willebrand Factor

Expression of vWF by endothelial cells varies significantly from one tissue to another, providing an important paradigm for the molecular basis of endothelial cell heterogeneity (see Table 9–1).[21] Functionally, vWF serves as a carrier for factor VIII in plasma and as a platelet adhesion molecule in endothelial cell matrix. Although vWF is synthesized by endothelial cells throughout the body,[71] expression by venous macrovessels predominates over that in arterial microvessels.[72–75] Within the heart, vWF is expressed more strongly in the endocardium than in myocardial capillaries,[37] and in the mouse embryo, vWF is generally expressed in aortic arches, intersomitic arteries, and cardinal veins, but not in angioblasts and capillaries.[76] In humans with deficiency of vWF, bleeding occurs most often in skin, mucous membranes, and joints.[77]

Tissue Factor Pathway Inhibitor

Tissue factor pathway inhibitor (TFPI) is a serine protease antagonist produced by microvascular endothelial cells. TFPI regulates activity of factor Xa and factor VIIa/TF.[78,79] Although small amounts of TFPI are associated with platelets and may also circulate in plasma, about 85% is associated with the endothelial cell surface.[80] Infusion of lipopolysaccharide reduces TFPI expression on pulmonary capillaries in vivo.[70]

TABLE 9–1. Some Endothelial Cell Surface Molecules, Their Functions, and Their Expression Patterns

Molecule	Function	Pattern of Expression	Location
Platelet Modulators			
ADPase/CD39	Platelet inhibition	Constitutive	Ubiquitous
Procoagulants			
Tissue factor	Procoagulant activity	Stimulated	Splenic microvessels
von Willebrand factor	Procoagulant activity	Constitutive	Venous > arterial; macro- > microvessels
Anticoagulants			
Thrombomodulin	Anticoagulant activity	Constitutive	Ubiquitous
EPCR	Anticoagulant activity	Constitutive	Macrovessels
AT III/heparan	Anticoagulant activity	Constitutive	Ubiquitous
Fibrinolytic Receptors			
Annexin 2	Fibrinolytic surveillance	Constitutive	Ubiquitous
uPAR	Fibrinolytic surveillance?	Stimulated	Macro- and microvessels
Adhesion Molecules			
P-selectin	Leukocyte adhesion	Stimulated	Postcapillary venule
PECAM-1	Leukocyte adhesion	Stimulated	Postcapillary venule
VCAM-1	Leukocyte adhesion	Stimulated	Postcapillary venule
ICAM-1	Leukocyte adhesion	Stimulated	Postcapillary venule
LFA-3	Leukocyte adhesion	Stimulated	Postcapillary venule
Histocompatibility Antigens			
HLA-DR	Antigen presentation	Stimulated	Ubiquitous?
HLA-DQ	Antigen presentation	Stimulated	Ubiquitous?

Thrombin activation leads to a two- to threefold increase in plasma TFPI concentration as a result of its release from the cell surface.[81] Low levels of heparin-releasable TFPI have been reported in young individuals with thrombosis.[82]

Thrombomodulin

The TM–protein C pathway is a major anticoagulant system that is oriented on the endothelial cell surface (see Table 9–1).[83] High levels of TM, an integral membrane protein, are found in human lung and placenta; moderate levels in heart, liver, spleen, kidney, and pancreas; low levels in aorta and skin; and nearly undetectable levels in brain.[84] Thrombomodulin is expressed by both macro- and microvascular endothelial cells, but it may act more effectively in the microcirculation because of the higher endothelial cell–to-blood ratio in smaller vessels.[34] Thrombomodulin converts thrombin from a procoagulant protease to an anticoagulant activator of protein C, which, in turn, inactivates coagulation cofactors Va and VIIIa. Thrombomodulin-bound thrombin–mediated activation of protein C is facilitated by its binding to EPCR.[85–91] The profoundly altered nature of TM-bound thrombin is further illustrated by its inability to clot fibrinogen, aggregate platelets, activate factors V and VIII, or interact with protease-activated receptors.[86,92,93] Thrombomodulin-bound thrombin is, nevertheless, readily inactivated by either antithrombin III (AT III) or protein C inhibitor, with a reduction in half-life to 2–3 seconds.[87]

Endothelial Cell Protein C Receptor

EPCR binds protein C to the endothelial cell or platelet surface, allowing protein C to be activated by TM-associated thrombin (see Table 9–1).[94] EPCR expression is specific to large vessel endothelium,[34–36,76] with higher density on the arterial, as opposed to venous, side of the circulation.[35] Infusion of endotoxin in the rat, or sepsis or systemic lupus erythematosus in humans, is associated with increased EPCR plasma levels as a result of the apparent release of soluble receptor by a thrombin-like, hirudin-sensitive serine protease.[35,88] Because soluble EPCR binds circulating protein C, its liberation from the cell surface may result in sequestration of protein C away from the cell surface, thereby preventing its activation and leading to a hypercoagulable state.[88] Depletion of protein C, as is seen in congenital protein C deficiency, is associated with consumption coagulopathy, with fibrin deposition in brain and liver.[95]

Antithrombin III

In association with heparin or other glycosaminoglycans in the vicinity of the endothelial cell surface, AT III constrains the enzymatic activity of thrombin, factor Xa, and factor IXa (see Table 9–1).[34] Heparin and other glycosaminoglycans serve to localize AT III on the endothelial cell surface. Once thrombin is neutralized, AT III–thrombin complexes dissociate from the endothelial cell surface and are cleared in the liver. Antithrombin III is constitutively expressed and does not seem to be

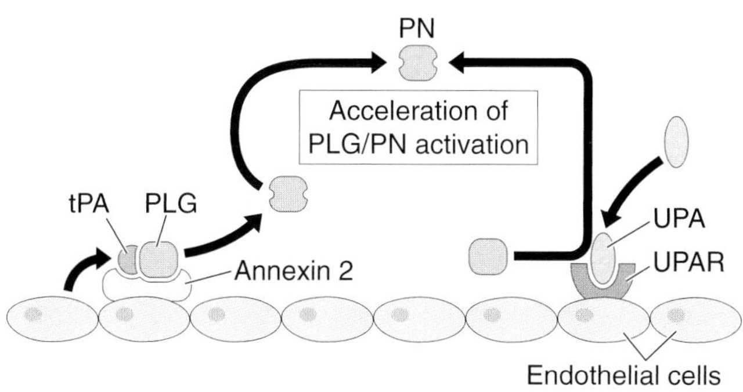

Figure 9–7. Endothelial cell fibrinolytic surveillance. Endothelial cells express a cell surface receptor, annexin 2, that binds both plasminogen (PLG), which circulates in plasma, and tissue plasminogen activator (tPA), which is secreted by the endothelial cell. Upon assembly of PLG and tPA on annexin 2, activation of PLG to the serine protease plasmin is greatly accelerated. Under conditions of cytokine stimulation, the urokinase (uPA) receptor (uPAR) may be expressed on the endothelial cell, bind uPA, and promote activation of PLG to plasmin.

subject to regulation by inflammatory mediators or endothelial cell injury.

Endothelial Cell Fibrinolytic Surveillance (Fig. 9–7)

Plasmin is the primary fibrin-degrading protease in humans. In a reaction influenced by multiple endothelial cell–related mechanisms, the two-chain serine protease plasmin is activated upon hydrolysis of a single peptide bond within the one-chain parent zymogen plasminogen.[98,99] Plasmin may act intravascularly to clear fibrin-containing thrombi, or extravascularly to activate proteases, remodel matrix proteins, or liberate matrix-associated growth factors.

Tissue Plasminogen Activator

Circulating tPA is produced primarily by microvascular endothelial cells.[96,97] tPA is a poor fluid-phase plasminogen activator, but its effectiveness is enhanced on a fibrin surface or when associated with its cellular receptor. In the mouse, levels of tPA messenger RNA (mRNA) are highest in brain; moderately high in kidney, heart, lung, testis, adrenal, aorta, and adipose tissue; and barely detectable in liver, spleen, thymus, muscle, and gut.[98] In the baboon, tPA antigen and mRNA are restricted to 7- to 30-μm diameter precapillary arterioles, postcapillary venules, and vasa vasora, but not femoral artery, femoral vein, carotid artery, or aorta.[38] In the mouse lung, bronchial artery endothelial cells express tPA antigen, especially at branch points, and pulmonary blood vessels are uniformly negative.[99–102] In addition, endotoxin, desmopressin acetate (DDAVP), bradykinin, platelet-activating factor, endothelin, and thrombin all induce a burst of fibrinolytic activity as a result of the acute release of tPA.[98,103] Tumor necrosis factor (TNF) infusion is also associated with increased plasma tPA in patients with malignancy.[104] Low-level release of tPA in response to venous occlusion has been associated with venous thrombosis,[105] atrophie blanche, and other cutaneous vasculitides.[106]

Urokinase

Under resting conditions, expression of urokinase (urinary-type plasminogen activator; uPA) appears to be highest in renal endothelial cells,[107,108] with moderate levels in thymus and adipose tissue, and barely detectable levels in liver, heart, lung, brain, spleen, testis, adrenal, aorta, muscle, and gut.[98] Production of uPA in the mouse kidney can be interrupted by intraperitoneal injection of endotoxin.[98] However, endothelial cell synthesis of uPA within ovarian follicles, corpus luteum, and maternal decidua is strongly enhanced during wound healing and during physiologic angiogenesis.[109]

Urokinase Receptor

The urokinase receptor (urinary-type plasminogen activator receptor; uPAR), a glycosylphosphatidylinositol-linked cell surface protein, may function as a profibrinolytic agent only under special circumstances (see Table 9–1). uPAR mRNA is not detected in resting mouse heart, brain, liver, or kidney endothelium, but does appear following infusion of endotoxin.[110] uPAR also appears to be induced in migrating endothelial cells stimulated with angiogenic agents.[111] Aside from a potential role in fibrinolysis, uPAR plays important roles in cellular signaling and adhesive events because it interacts specifically with vitronectin, and co-localizes with integrins at focal adhesion contacts.[99]

Plasminogen Activator Inhibitor-1

The major, rapidly acting modulator of fibrinolysis is plasminogen activator inhibitor-1 (PAI-1), which neutralizes the activity of both tPA and uPA.[112,113] Whereas quiescent endothelial cells in vivo express little or no PAI-1, endotoxin and other inflammatory cytokines induce a dramatic 10- to 100-fold increase in PAI-1 mRNA in the mouse kidney, adrenal, lung, and heart, but not brain.[98] At rest, the liver is a major source of plasma PAI-1,[114,115] and inflammatory cytokines are also powerful stimuli for induction of PAI-1 in this organ.[115] A noncirculating, stabilized form of PAI-1 in association with vitronectin is present in extracellular matrix. In both rats and humans with active malignancy, injection of TNF dramatically increases plasma PAI-1.[103,104] PAI-1 deficiency in humans, a rare hereditary disorder, is characterized by excessive bleeding associated with surgery or trauma.[116]

Annexin 2

Annexin 2 is an endothelial cell coreceptor for tPA and plasminogen that stimulates the catalytic efficiency of tPA-dependent plasmin generation by 1–2 log orders (see Table 9–1).[117–119] Through the action of calcium-regulated phospholipid-binding sites, annexin 2 binds avidly to the surface of endothelial cells as well as monocytes and macrophages.[120] In the adult mouse, rat, and human, endothelial cells of nearly all tissues show constitutive annexin 2 expression by immunohistology.[121,122] Evidence that annexin 2 may be physiologically important in fibrin homeostasis first came from studies of patients with acute promyelocytic leukemia in whom circulating blast cells overexpressed very large quantities of annexin 2 in association with excessive plasmin generation and a hemorrhagic diathesis.[123] Soluble annexin 2 can attenuate the thrombotic effect of vascular injury in an animal model.[124] Annexin 2 can be derivatized by the prothrombotic, atherogenic amino acid homocysteine, with resultant impairment of tPA binding and loss of plasmin generation.[125] In addition, plasminogen binding to annexin 2 can be specifically blocked by the atherogenic low-density lipoprotein–like particle lipoprotein(a).[126] Mice deficient in annexin 2 display widespread fibrin deposition in microvasculature and impaired lysis of acute arterial thrombi; in addition, these mice have severe defects in growth factor–induced angiogenesis in the cornea, retina, and skin.[127] To date, no humans with annexin 2 deficiency have been reported.

TABLE 9–2. Some Disorders Associated with Endothelial Cell Dysfunction

Primary Endotheliopathies
Vascular dysmorphogenesis
Hemangioma
Vascular malformation
Venous
Capillary
Arteriovenous
Lymphatic
Vascular neoplasms
Kaposi's sarcoma
Hemangioendothelioma
Angiosarcoma
Infectious endotheliitis
Rickettsiae
Hepatitis C
Parvovirus
Human immunodeficiency virus
Ebola/Marburg virus
Dengue virus
Bartonella
Immune vasculitis
Systemic lupus erythematosus
Progressive systemic sclerosis
Kawasaki disease
Wegener's granulomatosis
Rheumatoid arthritis
Behçet's disease
Nonvasculitic immune injury
Antiphospholipid syndrome
Heparin-induced thrombocytopenia
Secondary Endotheliopathies
Secondary immune injury
Sepsis
Graft rejection
Atherosclerosis-related
Oxidized lipoproteins
Homocysteine
Hyperglycemia
Shear stress
?Infectious agents
Chlamydia
Herpesviruses
Adenovirus
Trauma

DISORDERS OF THE ENDOTHELIUM (Table 9–2)

Primary Endotheliopathies

Vascular Dysmorphogenesis

Hemangioma, the most common tumor of infancy, arises as a benign, transient monoclonal proliferation of endothelial cells, which eventually resolves via involution.[128–130] Hemangioma-derived endothelial cells appear to have normal morphology, but demonstrate a two- to threefold increase in proliferative rate, enhanced directed migration, and upregulation of angiopoietin-2 and Tie-2 transcripts. In addition, hemangiomas in the proliferative phase appear to contain endothelial precursor cells that express CD133 and the endothelial cell marker Kdr (VEGFR-2, Flk-1).

Vascular malformations, which encompass venous, capillary, and arteriovenous malformations, in addition to lymphatic malformations, are a heterogeneous group of lesions that persist throughout life.[131] Vascular components frequently lack a complete smooth muscle layer, and an inherited form of venous malformation has been linked to an activating mutation in the Tie-2 receptor on endothelial cells, which is crucial to the recruitment of smooth muscle cells and pericytes during vascular development.[132] Other molecules proposed to play a role include the angiogenic growth factors fibroblast growth factor and VEGF, endoglin, transforming growth factor-β–binding proteins, activin receptor–like kinase 1, and phosphatidylinositol-3–like kinase.[131]

Primary endothelial cell neoplasms are rare disorders characterized by proliferation of transformed endothelial cells and the potential for metastasis. Kaposi's sarcoma represents the proliferation of spindle-shaped endothelial cells latently infected with the Kaposi's sarcoma herpesvirus; it is rare in the absence of human immunodeficiency virus.[133] Hemangioendothelioma is often multifocal and can exist as epithelioid, spindle-cell, and malignant endovascular papillary subtypes.[134] Angiosarcomas are rare and aggressive sinusoidal or solid tumors in which component cells retain endothelial cell marker antigens.[135]

Infectious Endotheliitis

Agents that directly infect endothelial cells can severely impair endothelial cell thromboresistance.[136,137] The endothelium, especially in brain and lungs, is specifically targeted by *Rickettsiae*, leading to increased vascular permeability, edema, and immune-mediated injury.[138] Hepatitis C virus infection is associated with endotheliitis within small portal veins,[139] and parvovirus infection of endothelial cells may be associated with mononuclear vasculitis in rheumatoid arthritis.[140] Endothelial cells within the bone marrow, liver sinusoids, or brain microvasculature are variably permissive to human immunodeficiency virus infection, and undergo activation in response to cytokines released by activated mononuclear or adventitial cells.[141,142] Ebola virus, and its close relative Marburg virus, are cytotoxic for endothelial cells in vivo, leading to increased vascular permeability and hemorrhage.[143,144] Endothelial cells are also a target for the Dengue arbovirus infection in vitro, although it is not yet clear whether they play a central pathogenetic role in vivo.[145] Finally, pathogenic *Bartonella* species can invade endothelial cells and induce them to undergo angiogenic proliferation.[146]

Immune-Mediated Vasculitis

The immune vasculitides, such as systemic lupus erythematosus, progressive systemic sclerosis, Kawasaki disease, Wegener's granulomatosis, rheumatoid arthritis, and Behçet's disease, are characterized by production of anti–endothelial cell antibodies of the IgG, IgM, or IgA classes.[20] Binding of anti–endothelial cell antibodies and/or complement components to cultured endothelial cells can result in activation leading to adherence of platelets, induction of procoagulant activity, and inhibition of fibrinolytic activity. The degree to which such antibodies play a primary pathogenic role in vivo is currently under investigation.

Nonvasculitic Immune Injury

Antiphospholipid Syndrome

In antiphospholipid syndrome, antibodies directed against a variety of proteins associated with the endothelial cell surface may be detected, sometimes in association with thrombotic complications.[147] Reported antigenic targets include β_2 glycoprotein, prothrombin, activated protein C, oxidized low-density lipoprotein, annexin V, phosphatidylethanolamine, and kininogens.[148] However, it is not yet clear whether such antibodies are causal in thrombosis, and, if so, whether thrombosis results from inhibition of cell surface anticoagulant proteins, from immune-mediated activation of the endothelial cell, or both.[149]

Heparin-Induced Thrombocytopenia

Heparin-induced thrombocytopenia occurs in 1–5% of patients exposed to heparin, and leads to a moderate drop in platelet count, about 30% risk of either venous or arterial thrombosis, and about 20% risk of death in individuals with a thrombotic event.[150] Antibodies are directed against platelet factor 4 in complex with heparin and bind to an Fc receptor subtype (FcRIIA) on the platelet surface, thereby activating the thrombocyte and causing further release of platelet factor 4. On the endothelial cell surface, platelet factor 4 may bind to endothelial cell heparan sulfate proteoglycan, leading to immune activation of the endothelial cell, TF expression, and platelet adhesion, thereby further exacerbating the thrombotic tendency.[151]

Secondary Endotheliopathies

Immune Perturbation

Inflammatory stimuli are invariably also prothrombotic.[3] In an inflammatory milieu, cytokines, growth factors, and other mediators not only stimulate the adhesion of platelets and leukocytes to the endothelial cell surface, but also induce changes that dampen its anticoagulant and fibrinolytic properties. In addition, cell-cell and cell-matrix interactions initiated by inflammatory stimuli promote the thrombotic process.

Leukocyte Adhesion

Within seconds of exposure to histamine or thrombin, endothelial cells degranulate their Weibel-Palade bodies and translocate P-selectin to the cell surface (Fig. 9–8; see Table 9–1).[3] At the cell surface, P-selectin binds its ligand, P-selectin glycoprotein ligand 1, which is expressed on neutrophils, monocytes, and T, B, and natural killer lymphocytes.[152,153] This reversible, low-affinity interaction results in the tethering and rolling of circulating leukocytes along the endothelial cell surface, as a prelude to their emigration into tissues. Leukocytes rolling along the luminal surface of the blood vessel are exposed to additional tissue-specific bioactive molecules, such as chemokines, platelet-activating factor, and additional molecules that establish tighter adhesive interactions.[154–156] Inflammatory stimuli also induce expression of mucosal addressin cell adhesion molecule-1 (MadCAM-1), which interacts with L-selectin expressed constitutively on lymphocytes; the molecular nature of MadCAM-1 has not yet been elucidated.[3]

Over minutes to hours, leukocytes undergo repeated cycles of forward adhesion and rearward disadhesion, as they migrate toward interendothelial cell junctions.[157] At this location, homotypic interactions involving platelet/endothelial cell adhesion molecule-1 (PECAM-1) on both the migrating leukocyte and the activated endothelial cell lead to increased intracellular calcium, remodeling of cell-cell junctions, and leukocyte transmigration (see Table 9–1).[158–160] Additional molecules implicated in this process include endothelial cell receptors, vascular cell adhesion molecule-1 (VCAM-1) and intercellular adhesion molecule-1 (ICAM-1), and their cognate leukocyte ligands, $\alpha_4\beta_1$ (vascular leukocyte adhesion molecule-4) and $\alpha_L\beta_2/\alpha_M\beta_2$ (lymphocyte function–associated antigen [LFA]/Mac-1), respectively.[157] Ultimately, the leukocyte traverses the interendothelial cell junction without disrupting the vascular permeability barrier, a process known as diapedesis.[161]

Within hours of exposure to cytokines such as endotoxin, interleukin-1, or TNF-α, the adhesion molecules E-selectin, ICAM-1, and VCAM-1 appear on the endothelial cell surface (see Table 9–1).[162,163] Expression of E-selectin appears to be further sustained by interferon-γ, while expression of P-selectin, initiated by thrombin or histamine in the immediate inflammatory response, can be prolonged for hours to days by interleukin-3, interleukin-4, or oncostatin M. Leukocytes bearing sialylated, fucosylated carbohydrates bind to E-selectin.

Loss of Thromboresistance

Although endothelial cell perturbation can result in a profound loss of thromboresistance, the pathophysiologic effects of this change may reflect regional diversity of endothelial cell function.[21] Plasma from patients with thrombotic thrombocytopenic purpura, for example, induces apoptosis in endothelial cells of renal and cerebral, but not pulmonary or hepatic, origin.[68] Similarly, activation of TF during gram-negative sepsis in baboons is confined to endothelial cells of the splenic vasculature.[68] Although mice deficient in CD39 demonstrate significant fibrin deposition in multiple organs, accentuation of this deposition by hypoxic stress occurs only in the lung.[63] Similarly, mice with mutations in the thrombomodulin, uPA, tPA, or plasminogen genes display fibrin accumulation in selected tissues.[164–166]

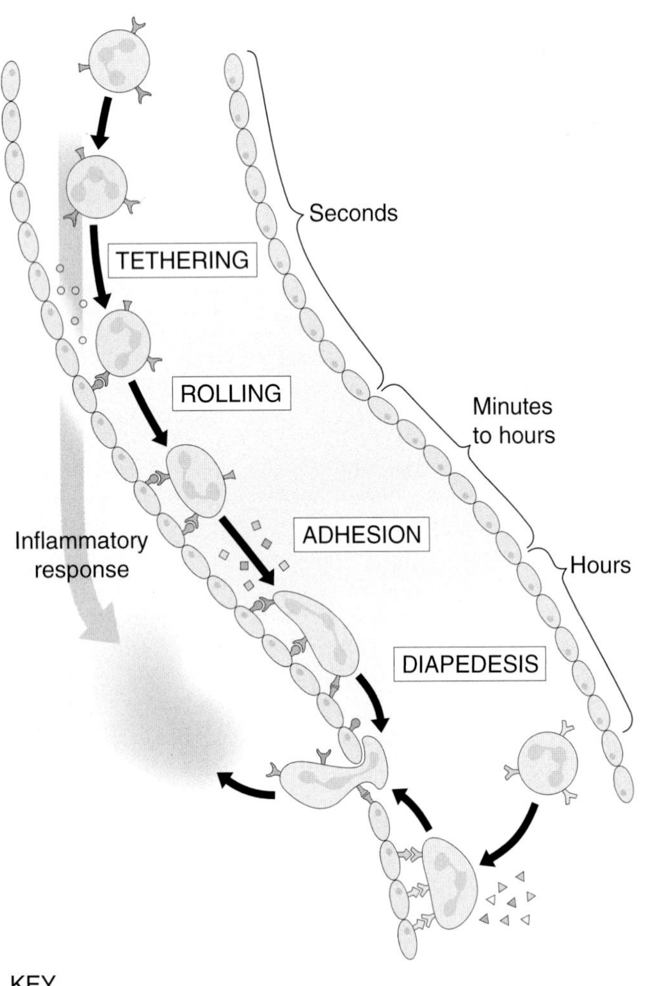

Figure 9–8. Leukocyte adhesion to endothelium during inflammation. Within seconds of their release, histamine and thrombin induce expression of P-selectin, which interacts with P-selectin glycoprotein ligand-1 (PSGL-1) on leukocytes, resulting in tethering of the leukocyte to the endothelial cell surface. Leukocyte rolling along the vessel surface is initiated thereafter by ligation of mucosal addressin cell adhesion molecule-1 (MadCAM-1) by L-selectin on the leukocyte surface. Within minutes to hours, interleukins-3 (IL-3) and -4 (IL-4), and perhaps oncostatin M (Onc M), stimulate platelet/endothelial cell adhesion molecule (PECAM) expression on the endothelial cell, and enable homotypic interactions between leukocytes and endothelial cells. This adhesion at intercellular junctions is followed by diapedesis into the subendothelial space. Over the ensuing hours, cytokines such as lipopolysaccharide (LPS), tumor necrosis factor (TNF), interleukin-1 (IL-1), and interferon-γ (IFN γ) stimulate expression of intercellular adhesion molecule (ICAM-1), vascular cell adhesion molecule (VCAM-1), and E-selectin that interact with lymphocyte function–associated antigen-1 (LFA1), vascular leukocyte adhesion molecule-4 (VLA-4), and sialyl carbohydrate moieties, respectively, on the leukocyte surface.

Antigen Presentation and Graft Rejection

Stimulation of endothelial cells over a period of days with interferon-γ leads to expression of major histocompatibility complex class II molecules (human lymphocyte antigen [HLA]-DR and HLA-DQ) on the cell surface (see Table 9–1).[167–169] When costimulatory molecules such as CD40, ICAM-1, and LFA-3 are also expressed on endothelial cells, such as during allograft placement, $CD4^+$ memory T cells can also be activated. Under these circumstances, the endothelial cell may function as an antigen-presenting cell, and initiate graft rejection.

Donor endothelial cells are a major target of the host immune system following organ transplantation.[170] Alloantibodies can develop against a variety of endothelial cell antigens, including histocompatibility molecules (MHC-1), blood group antigens, and tissue-specific alloantigens.[171] Some may cause acute endothelial cell lysis, whereas others may induce a more restricted endothelial cell injury.[172] In addition, antibodies to endothelial-specific antigens have been implicated in hyperacute graft rejection, in which platelet consumption is accompanied by the development of microvascular thrombi.

Atherosclerosis

Atherosclerosis represents a common response to endothelial cell injury caused by oxidants, shear stress, homocysteine, hyperglycemia, hyperlipidemia, or infectious agents.[173] Oxidized forms of low-density lipoprotein can signal endothelial cells to express leukocyte adhesion molecules, and diminish their thromboresistance properties.[174] Similarly, reactive oxidant species, generated at sites of inflammation or injury, can trigger leukocyte adhesion and increasing vascular permeability through activation of redox-regulated transcription factors such as activator protein-1 and nuclear factor-κB.[175]

Shear stress not only can induce cytoskeletal rearrangements and shape change, but also can modify the endothelial cell's expression of proteins such as eNOS, basic fibroblast growth factor, platelet-derived growth factor-A and -B, tPA, VCAM-1, and ICAM-1.[176–178] As an independent risk factor for occlusive cardiovascular disease, homocysteine induces endothelial cell expression of TF in vitro and inhibits expression of TM and heparan sulfate, and tPA binding to annexin 2.[179] Hyperglycemia induces endothelial cell dysfunction via nonenzymatic glycation of macromolecules, production of reactive oxygen intermediates, activation of protein kinase C, and accumulation of sorbitol and reduced myoinositol.[180] Advanced glycation end products may also interact with the endothelial cell receptor for advanced glycation end products (RAGE) and stimulate oxidant stress reactions, activation of nuclear factor-κB, expression of VCAM-1, and induction of vascular hyperpermeability.[181] In adults, infectious processes implicated in the etiology of atherogenesis include cytomegalovirus and *Chlamydia* endotheliitis,[182–184] and, in pediatric transplantation patients, adenoviral infection is a strong predictor of accelerated arteriosclerosis.[185]

Suggested Readings*

Cleaver O, Krieg PA: Molecular mechanisms of vascular development. *In* Harvey RP, Rosenthal N (eds): Heart Development. New York: Academic Press, 1999, pp 221–252.

Hajjar KA: Molecular basis of fibrinolysis. *In* Nathan DG, Orkin SH, Ginsburg D, Look AT (eds): Nathan and Oski's Hematology of Infancy and Childhood. Philadelphia: WB Saunders, 2003, pp 1497–1514.

Hajjar KA, Esmon NL, Marcus AJ, Muller WA: Vascular function in hemostasis. *In* Beutler E, Lichtman MA, Coller BS, et al (eds): Williams Hematology. New York: McGraw-Hill 2005 (in press).

Hansson GK: Inflammation, atherosclerosis, and coronary artery disease. N Engl J Med 352:1685–1695, 2005.

Pober JS: Immunobiology of human vascular endothelium. Immunol Res 19:225–232, 1999.

Full references for this chapter can be found on accompanying CD-ROM.

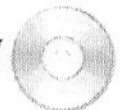

PART II

Hematologic Diseases

SECTION 1
DISEASES OF HEMATOPOIETIC CELL PRODUCTION

CHAPTER 10

ACQUIRED APLASTIC ANEMIA

Neal S. Young, MD

KEY POINTS

Aplastic Anemia

- Severe aplastic anemia is a fatal disease that demands rapid recognition and institution of both immediate treatment of low blood counts and attempts at long-term restitution of adequate hematopoiesis.
- Most aplastic anemia is the result of T-cell–mediated destruction of hematopoietic target cells of the marrow.
- Aplastic anemia must be distinguished from other, more common causes of pancytopenia.
- Bone marrow examination is required for diagnosis: low cellularity on the biopsy and residual but largely normal hematopoietic precursors on the aspirate smear are typical.
- The difficult differential diagnosis is between aplastic anemia and closely related hematologic syndromes, especially myelodysplasia and paroxysmal nocturnal hemoglobinuria.
- Definitive treatments are stem cell transplantation, preferred for all children and for younger severely neutropenic patients with a histocompatible sibling, and immunosuppression, using an antithymocyte globulin–based regimen.
- Relapse after successful immunosuppression is frequent but treatable. A minor proportion of patients develop late clonal hematologic disease: abnormal cytogenetics, myelodysplasia, and even leukemia.

INTRODUCTION

Aplastic anemia is pancytopenia and a hypocellular bone marrow (Fig. 10–1). One of the classic blood diseases, often manifesting dramatically and in its severe form, invariably fatal, aplastic anemia can now be successfully treated in most cases. The pathophysiology of bone marrow failure applies to other hematologic syndromes and to immune-mediated organ dysfunction in general.

The disease was first described in 1888 by Paul Ehrlich, in a report of an autopsy of a young woman who died after a brief, catastrophic illness marked by profound anemia, bleeding, and high fever.[1] Vaquez and Aubertin provided a name in 1904, noting "la forme aplastique" of pernicious anemia with yellow marrow[2]; the etymology of "aplastic" is the Greek verb *plắtho*, to create and give shape to. A relationship of aplastic anemia to the environment was inferred by early observers from important clinical associations: with benzene from studies of Swedish bicycle tire workers in the 1890s[3] and with medical drugs, first through dipyrone's role in agranulocytosis in the 1930s[4] and then in an apparent epidemic of aplastic anemia following the introduction of chloramphenicol as an antibiotic in the 1960s.[5] Marrow aplasia also was appreciated as a rare complication of other environmental agents, such as prior infection (especially hepatitis), and conditions (occurring during pregnancy and with other diseases such as systemic lupus). The link between confusingly diverse environmental triggers and aplastic anemia is an immune pathophysiology in which lymphocytes destroy hematopoietic stem and progenitor cell targets. This type of T-cell–mediated, organ-specific damage is similar to that in human autoimmune diseases such as multiple sclerosis, ulcerative colitis, and type 1 diabetes. Aplastic anemia in the modern view is also intimately related to other hematologic syndromes (Fig. 10–2).

Untreated aplastic anemia in its severe form is invariably fatal (Fig. 10–3). Corticosteroids and then androgens were employed early but in retrospect were of uncertain benefit (Fig. 10–4). Bone marrow replacement was obviously ideal for a disease of failed hematopoiesis, and by the 1970s transplantation was demonstrated to be curative for most matched siblings and feasible also from unrelated donors. The use of antilymphocyte sera was pioneered at about the same time, and immunosuppressive regimens that address the immune pathophysiology are now applied to the majority of patients with aplastic anemia. Aplastic anemia remains a serious disease but, if managed appropriately, in most patients marrow failure can be effectively ameliorated or cured.

EPIDEMIOLOGY AND RISK FACTORS

Aplastic anemia often affects young people (see Fig. 10–3); there is no sex preference.

Aplastic anemia is relatively rare in Western countries. In the International Aplastic Anemia and Agranulocyto-

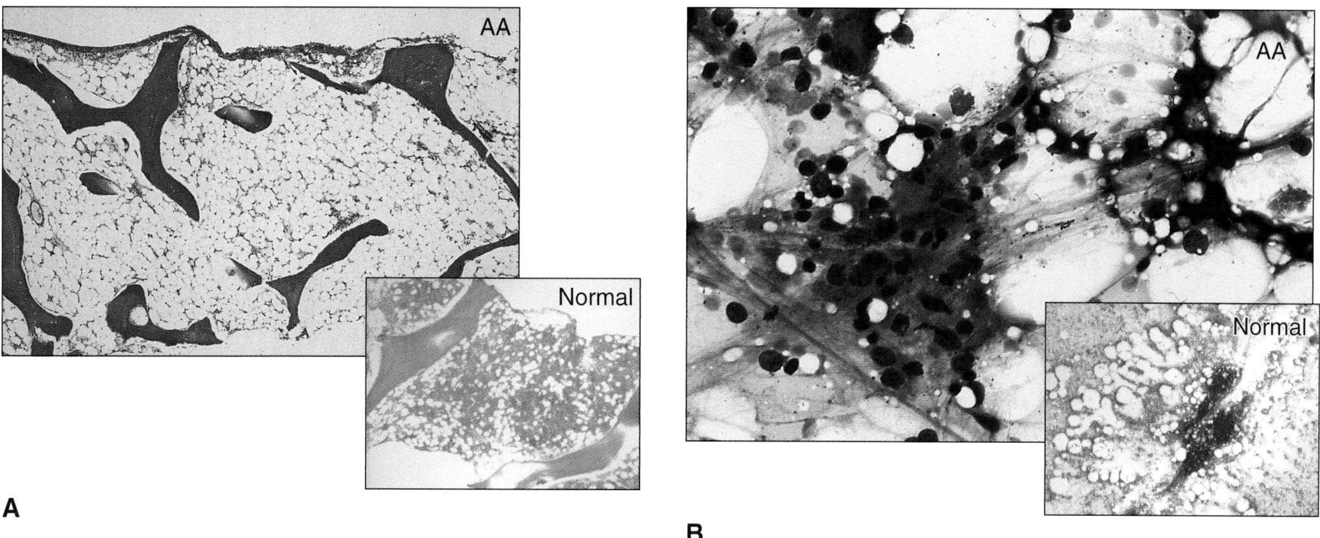

Figure 10–1. Bone marrow morphology in severe aplastic anemia. *A,* Biopsy, showing replacement of normal hematopoietic cells with fat. *B,* Aspirate smear, with an overall paucity of cells; myeloid and erythroid precursors and megakaryocytes are absent, and only lymphocytes, plasma cells, and stromal elements are seen.

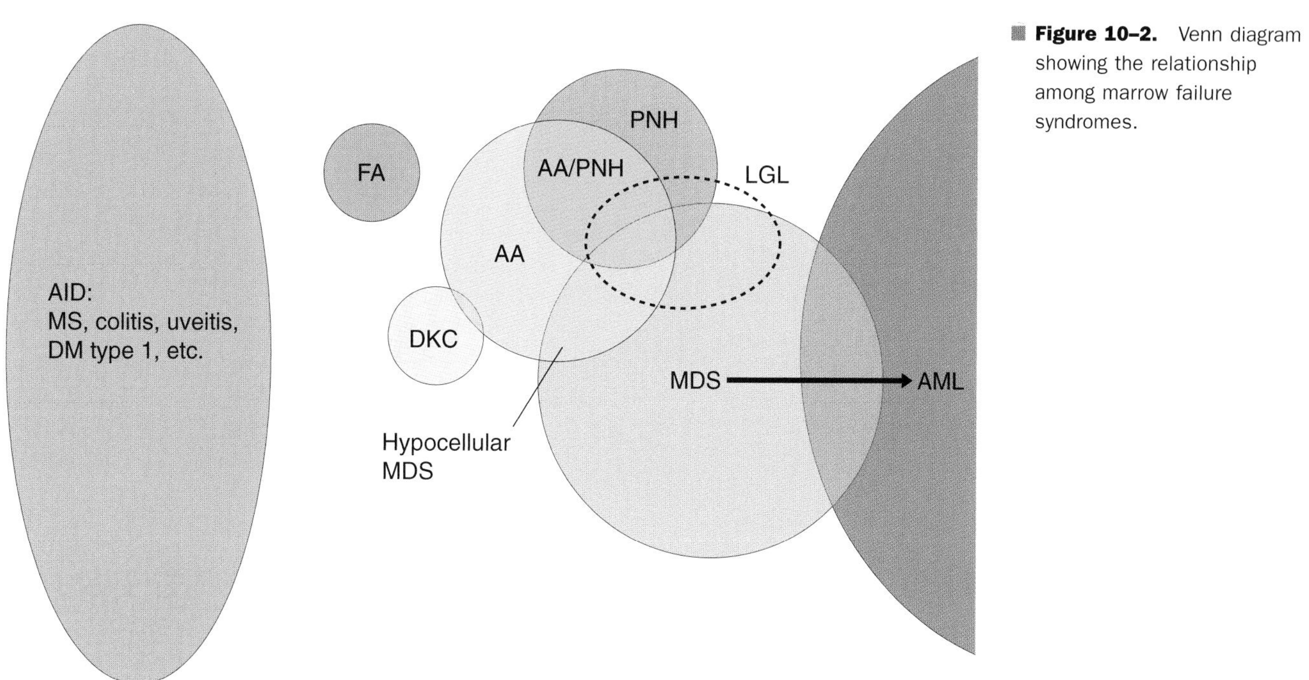

Figure 10–2. Venn diagram showing the relationship among marrow failure syndromes.

sis Study (IAAAS), the incidence was two new cases per million population each year for Europe and Israel in the years 1980–1984.[6] This figure has been confirmed for other proximate regions.[7] However, the most remarkable feature of the epidemiology of aplastic anemia is the marked geographic variation in its incidence. In striking contrast to European and American hospitals, in hematology clinics in Asia, aplastic anemia as an admitting diagnosis may rival in frequency acute myeloid leukemia. The incidence of aplastic anemia in Thailand using the same methods as in the IAAAS was higher, 4.0 per 10^6 in the capital and 5.6 per 10^6 in a rural province.[8] A large Chinese study yielded an estimated annual incidence rate of 7.4 per 10^6.[9] Aplastic anemia is almost certainly more prevalent in Malysia,[10] Vietnam, and Indonesia; in Russia, Iran, Iraq, Pakistan,[11] and India; in Mexico and other regions of Latin America[12]; and in Africa, where it is likely underdiagnosed.[13,14]

Environmental Risk Factors

Population-based studies have investigated causal associations. Drugs were implicated in about 25% of

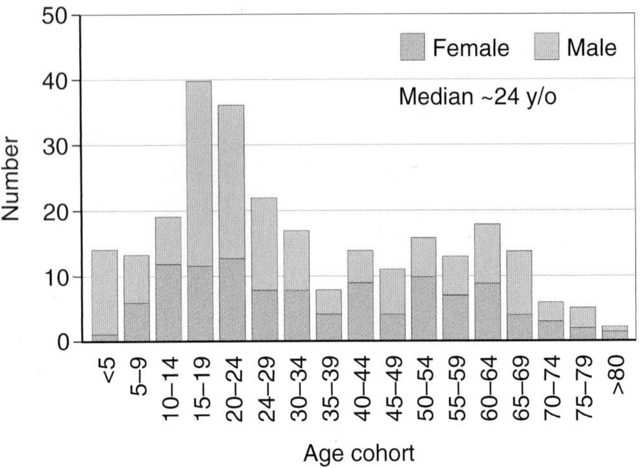

Figure 10–3. Age distribution at presentation of patients admitted to the National Institutes of Health Clinical Center.

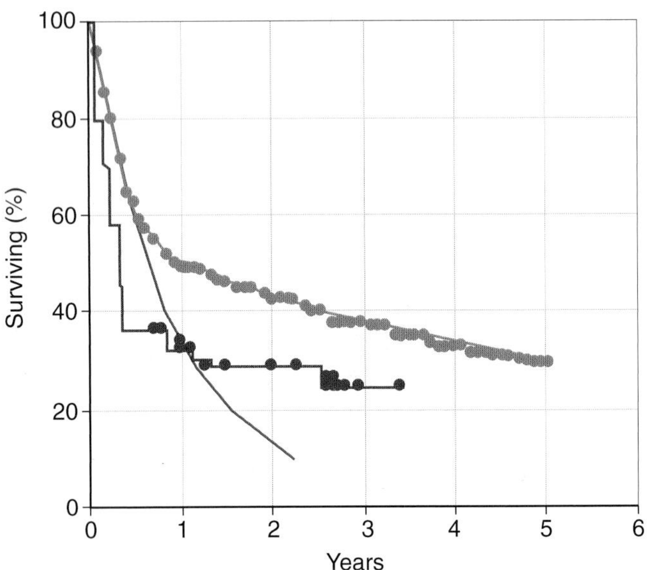

Figure 10–4. "Natural" history of aplastic anemia, in the era when treatment was transfusion, antibiotics, corticosteroids, and androgens.[116,507]

European cases in the IAAAS[6] (Table 10–1). Smaller studies have shown relationships to chemical exposures and to viruses through transfusions, hepatitis, and occupation.[15] In Thailand, medical drug use accounted for only about 15% of cases, but neither chloramphenicol nor household pesticide exposure were significantly related[16]; high relative risk ratios were established for benzene and agricultural exposure to pesticides, use of nonbottled water, and prior exposure to hepatitis A.[17,18] The explanation for the geographic variation in aplastic anemia might be environmental. Japanese in Hawaii seemed to have aplastic anemia at the American rate,[19] and American soldiers in the Pacific theater during World War II had a high incidence of aplastic anemia.[20]

TABLE 10–1. Drugs Associated with Aplastic Anemia in the International Aplastic Anemia and Agranulocytosis Study*

Drug	Stratified Risk Estimate (95% Confidence Interval)	Multivariate Relative Risk Estimate (95% Confidence Interval)
Nonsteroidal analgesics		
Butazones	3.7 (1.9–7.2)	5.1 (2.1–12)
Indomethacin	7.1 (3.4–15)	8.2 (3.3–20)
Piroxicam	9.8 (3.3–29)	7.4 (2.1–26)
Diclofenac	4.6 (2.0–11)	4.2 (1.6–11)
Antibiotics		
Sulfonamides†	2.8 (1.1–7.3)	2.2 (0.6–7.4)
Antithyroid drugs	16 (4.8–54)	11 (2.0–56)
Cardiovascular drugs		
Furosemide	3.3 (1.6–7.0)	3.1 (1.2–8.0)
Psychotropic drugs		
Phenothiazines	3.0 (1.1–8.2)	1.6 (0.4–7.4)
Corticosteroids	5.0 (2.8–8.9)	3.5 (1.6–7.7)
Penicillamine	—	
Allopurinol	7.3 (3.0–17)	5.9 (1.8–19)
Gold	29 (9.7–89)	

*The multivariate model included the following factors: age, sex, geographic area, date of interview, reliability of the patient, person interviewed, transfer from another hospital, history of blood disorder or tuberculosis, exposure to benzene and related chemicals, and suspected use of other drugs.
†Other than trimethoprim/sulfonamide combination.
Adapted from Kaufman DW, Kelly JP, Levy M, Shapiro S: The Drug Etiology of Agranulocytosis and Aplastic Anemia. New York: Oxford University Press, 1991.

Genetic Factors

As with many autoimmune diseases, aplastic anemia has been linked to specific human lymphocyte antigens (HLAs), most consistently HLA-DR2.[21,22] In Japanese patients, a class II haplotype (DRB*1501) that determines HLA-DR2 presentation was strongly associated with a hematologic response to cyclosporine.[23,24] In a recent study, Asian-ethnicity children resident in British Columbia suffered a much higher rate of disease (an incidence of about 7 per million compared to 1.7 per million in the total population), and the antigens HLA-B75, -DRB1*0901, -DRB*1301, and -DRB*1501 were greatly overrepresented in these patients.[25] Polymorphisms in cytokine gene sequences, important in regulating the immune response, also have been associated with acquired aplastic anemia: with the *TNF2* allele and the presence of an adenine at position 308 of the tumor necrosis factor (TNF)-α promoter[26,27] (correlated with increased TNF production); with homozygosity for dinucleotide repeats in the first intron of the interferon (IFN)-γ gene encoded by allele 2[28] (correlated with high in vitro production of interferon); and in the interleukin (IL)-6 gene,[27] another pro-inflammatory pathway involved in autoimmunity.

Genetic risk factors for hematopoiesis recently have also been identified, involving genes of the telomere repair complex: functionally disabling mutations for the RNA template gene (*TERC*; abnormal also in autosomal dominant dyskeratosis congenita [see Chapter 11])[29] and the gene encoding the telomerase enzyme (*TERT*).[30] Remarkably, genetically affected family members may show minimal or no hematologic manifestations despite evidence of a much diminished hematopoietic compartment.

PATHOPHYSIOLOGY

Hematopoiesis

By all measures, hematopoiesis is severely reduced in aplastic anemia: morphologically, radiographically, phenotypically, and functionally.[31] By flow cytometry, the CD34$^+$ cell population, containing most of the committed progenitor cells and stem cells, is very small.[32,33] Hematopoietic progenitor cells—CFU-GM (granulocytic-macrophagic), BFU-E and CFU-E (erythroid), and pluripotent progenitors (CFU-GEMM)—are severely reduced.[32,34] In stem cell surrogate assays, primitive progenitors also are virtually absent.[35,36] Combining progenitor number and marrow cellularity leads to an estimate that stem cells are reduced to less than 1% of normal in severe aplastic anemia.

The stroma is not usually defective in aplastic anemia.[31] In vitro, stroma from patients supported hematopoiesis by normal CD34$^+$ cells, whereas no hematopoietic colonies developed when patients' CD34$^+$ cells were cultured in the presence of normal stroma.[37,38] Stromal cells from patients' bone marrow produce normal quantities of hematopoietic growth factors, measured as protein,[39] as messenger RNA,[40] or functionally.[41] Serum levels of erythropoietin,[42] thrombopoietin,[43–45] IL-11,[46] granulocyte colony-stimulating factor (G-CSF),[47] and granulocyte-macrophage colony-stimulating factor (GM-CSF)[48] are usually much elevated. Cytokines that act at very early stages of hematopoiesis include FLT-3 (FMS-like tyrosine kinase 3) ligand, for which blood levels are highly elevated in aplastic anemia,[49] and stem cell factor, levels of which have been modestly decreased.[50]

Mechanisms of Hematopoietic Cell Destruction

Direct Toxicity

The most common form of aplastic anemia is iatrogenic—the transient marrow failure that follows on cytotoxic chemotherapy or irradiation for cancer. Chemical or physical agents can directly act to injure both proliferating and quiescent hematopoietic cells; the introduction of sufficient damage to DNA leads to the process of apoptosis. Among the drugs that are idiosyncratically associated with marrow failure may be a few that also directly cause marrow damage. However, patients with community-acquired aplastic anemia rarely have a history of exposure to consistently toxic physicochemical agents.

Immune-Mediated Marrow Failure

Mathé in the 1970s observed unexpected improvement of pancytopenia after failed marrow transplantation, and he speculated that the immunosuppressive conditioning regimen, intended to allow engraftment of the donor marrow, instead promoted the return of host marrow function.[51] The effectiveness of immunosuppressive therapies is a strong argument for an underlying immune-mediated pathophysiology (Fig. 10–5*A*).

Laboratory support for the immune hypothesis first came from co-culture experiments: mononuclear cells from patients' blood or bone marrow suppressed colony formation, and removal of T cells from the patient samples could improve recovery of hematopoietic progenitor cells in these in vitro assays.[52] Eventually, these T cells were shown to act by secretion of specific cytokines (Fig. 10–5*B*). Aplastic anemia patients' T cells[53–55] overproduced IFN-γ and also TNF.[56,57] IFN-γ messenger RNA, evidence of gene activity, was detectable in samples from most aplastic anemia patients but not in normal individuals or in other hematologic diseases.[58,59] Blood and marrow of aplastic anemia patients also contain elevated numbers of activated cytotoxic lymphocytes that could be assayed phenotypically (by expression of activation markers), functionally (by suppression of colony formation),[60] and molecularly (by measurement of T-cell receptor skewing in expanded subsets of T cells and sequencing of the antigen-binding region CDR3)[61]; the number and activity of these cells decreased appropriately with successful immunosuppressive therapy.[62,63]

In vitro, IFN-γ and TNF-α suppress proliferation of early and late hematopoietic progenitor and stem cells.[64] Cell killing is effected by induction of apoptosis: IFN-γ and TNF-α induce expression of Fas receptor on CD34$^+$ progenitor cells, and triggering by Fas ligand initiates programmed cell death.[65,66] Microarrays of CD34$^+$ cells in aplastic anemia showed activation of immune response as well as apoptosis and death receptor pathway genes.[67] Lymphokines increase nitric oxide synthase and nitric oxide production by marrow cells,[68] which would contribute to immune-mediated cytotoxicity and elimination of hematopoietic cells. In an animal model, inoculation of parental lymph node cells into F1 mice produces rapid aplasia of the marrow, pancytopenia, and death; monoclonal antibodies to murine IFN-γ and TNF-α abrogated this destructive process,[69] and these cytokines are the probable mediators of a potent "innocent bystander" effect, in which even cells genetically identical to the effector T cells become targets of the immune response.[70]

The early immune system events that precede the global destruction of hematopoietic cells are not well elucidated: specific target antigens remain largely unidentified and the reasons for breached tolerance and the subsequent process of spreading autoimmunity are unknown. Oligoclonal expansion of a limited number of T-cell subfamilies, as defined by flow cytometry, spectratyping, and sequencing of the antigen-binding region of the T-cell receptor,[61,71] is strong evidence of an antigen-driven immune response. Examination of the transcrip-

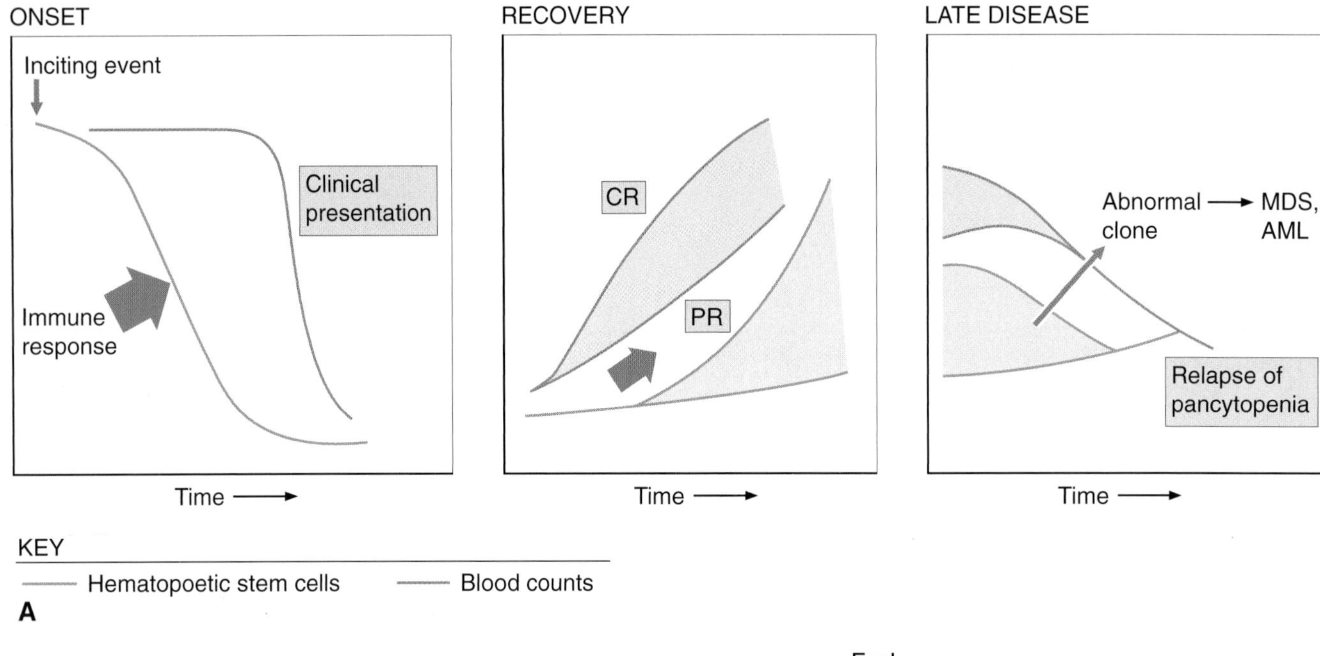

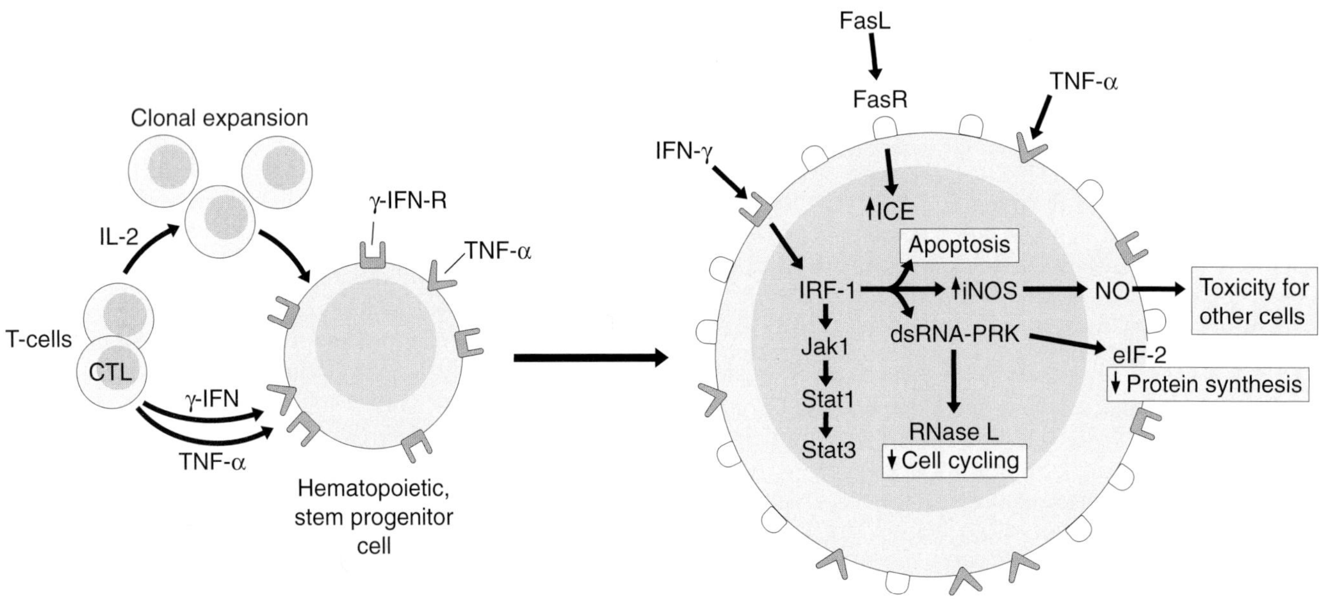

■ **Figure 10–5.** Pathophysiology of acquired aplastic anemia. ***A,*** Three phases of disease, showing the relationship of the aberrant immune response to hematopoietic cell number. Complete response (CR) and partial response (PR) refer to hematologic recovery. Abbreviations: AML, acute myelogenous leukemia; MDS, myelodysplastic syndrome. ***B,*** Proximal events; important signaling pathways in T-cell–mediated marrow failure are shown. Abbreviations: CTL, cytotoxic T lymphocyte; ICE, interleukin converting enzyme; IFN, interferon; IL-2, interleukin-2; iNOS, inducible nitric oxide synthase; IRF-1, interferon response factor-1; L, ligand; NO, nitric oxide; R, receptor; TNF, tumor necrosis factor.

tome of T cells in aplastic anemia by microarray has implicated multiple pathways of immune system activation.[72] In a few individual cases, T-cell clones have been shown to specifically proliferate in response to or to effect cytotoxicity of autologous hematopoietic targets,[73,74] but which peptides do they recognize? Autoantibodies can be measured in aplastic anemia,[75] and molecular screening of sera has uncovered antibodies to a few proteins, but their apparent antigens (kinectin,[75] diazepam-binding inhibitor–related protein[76]) are not obvious tissue-specific initiating candidate peptides analogous to myelin basic protein in multiple sclerosis, islet cell proteins for diabetes, or keratin in uveitis.

Specific Etiologic Associations

Aplastic anemia is conventionally classified by its presumed etiology, and, although in practice it is usually idiopathic, marrow failure may occur secondary to

TABLE 10–2. A Classification of Aplastic Anemia

Acquired Aplastic Anemia	Inherited Aplastic Anemia
Secondary aplastic anemia	Fanconi's anemia
Radiation	Dyskeratosis congenita
Drugs and chemicals	Shwachman-Diamond syndrome
Regular effects:	Reticular dysgenesis
cytotoxic agents (benzene)	Amegakaryocytic thrombocytopenia
Idiosyncratic reactions:	Familial aplastic anemias
chloramphenicol	Preleukemia (monosomy 7, etc.)
nonsteroidal anti-inflammatories	Nonhematologic syndromes:
antiepileptics	Down, Dubowitz, Seckel
gold	
other drugs and chemicals	
Viruses	
Epstein-Barr virus (infectious mononucleosis)	
Hepatitis C virus (non-A, non-B hepatitis)	
Parvovirus (transient aplastic crisis, some pure red cell aplasia)	
Human immunodeficiency virus (acquired immunodeficiency syndrome)	
Immune diseases	
Eosinophilic fasciitis	
Hypoimmunoglobulinemia	
Thymoma and thymic carcinoma	
Graft-versus-host disease in immunodeficiency	
Paroxysmal nocturnal hemoglobinuria	
Pregnancy	
Idiopathic aplastic anemia	

various proximate causes, including not only obvious physical and chemical toxins but also medical drugs and viruses (Table 10–2).

Autoimmune Diseases and Immune System Abnormalities

Immune cell destruction of the bone marrow is most dramatically exemplified by transfusion-associated graft-versus-host disease (and modeled in animals by "runt" disease; see earlier) in which aplastic anemia is the invariant cause of death.[77] Very small numbers of effector cells mediate disease under these conditions, which have been conveyed by residual lymphocytes contained in plasma or with solid organ transplants, and a single amino acid difference in an HLA molecules has sufficed to induce graft-versus-host disease after marrow transplant between twins. Aplastic anemia is associated with rheumatic syndromes, especially eosinophilic facsciitis[78] but also rheumatoid arthritis (in which the role of medical drugs used in treatment is confounding), and systemic lupus erythematosus (associated with a serum inhibitor of hematopoiesis).[79,80] A particularly interesting parallel exists between aplastic anemia and hemophagocytic syndrome, in which immune-mediated pancytopenia develops during convalescence from a wide variety of viral infections, especially herpesviruses such as Epstein-Barr virus but also B19 parvovirus.[81–85] Cytotoxic T-cell activation and circulating IFN-γ have been measured in these patients, who can respond to immunosuppressive therapies. Hemophagocytosis is an occasional morphologic feature of bone marrow in typical aplastic anemia.[86]

Pregnancy

Marrow failure appearing or worsening with pregnancy has been reported since the 1950s,[87–89] although the association has been questioned as coincidental rather than causal.[90] Remissions have occurred after termination by spontaneous delivery and spontaneous or therapeutic abortion, but the course is highly variable and there is no standard of management.[88,89,91,92] Pregnant women have been successfully treated by stem cell transplantation[93] and immunosuppression.[94] Pregnancy poses a risk of relapse and death for women who have recovered from aplastic anemia after immunosuppression.[95]

Radiation

Aplastic anemia is a feared outcome of radiation exposure, historically from carelessness in handling sources and immediately following the atomic bombs exploded over Japanese cities, now usually secondary to industrial accidents and manipulation of improperly discarded radiation sources. Very large doses of radiation can result in acute and massive physical and thermal injury, but aplasia figures as the major cause of mortality in those who survive such damage.[96,97]

All components of the marrow are susceptible, including stem and progenitor cells and the stroma. Mitotically active hematopoietic tissue is exquisitely sensitive, with a rough correlation to cycling status. The dose-related occurrence of pancytopenia 2–4 weeks following exposure to radiation is due to injury to the actively replicating progenitor cell pool. Mortality from hematologic toxicity is a function of the marrow's ability to tolerate both depletion of hematopoietic cells and damage to the stem cell. The capacity for recovery of hematopoietic function following even massive single radiation exposures is considerable, reflecting resistance of the quiescent stem cell and the enormous regenerative capacity of even a greatly reduced stem cell pool.

Bone marrow hypoplasia occurs with radiation doses above 1.5–2 Gy to the whole body. The median lethal dose in humans is highly dependent on the quality of medical care: improved support may double the tolerated radiation dose.[98] Autopsies of atomic bomb victims in Japan showed acellular bone marrows in the first weeks after the explosions, but there frequently was regenerating bone marrow in those who survived longer.[99] From the outcome of radiation accidents and after high-dose therapeutic irradiation, the median lethal dose has been estimated at about 4.5 Gy.[100,101] Survival of some of the Chernobyl nuclear plant workers who received doses greater than 9 Gy indicates that autologous marrow reconstitution can occur if the immediate consequences of radiation exposure are survived.[102]

The type and intensity of the source of radiation and the distance and shielding of the subject are major determinants of radiation injury. Cells are most affected by high-energy γ-rays, and secondarily by α and β particles. Because lymphocytes are particularly sensitive to radiation, their rate of fall can be used to estimate dose to a total body exposure of about 3 Gy. At higher doses, the fall in granulocytes and the severity of thrombocytopenia and reticulocytopenia can be used as gauges[103]; at Chernobyl, dicentric chromosomes provided an estimate of dose.[104,105]

Aplastic anemia is not well documented as a delayed sequela of radiation exposure. Of 156 cases of aplastic anemia in Japan in the 20 years following the atom bomb explosions, only 13 had received more than a 1-rad dose, and, of the 3 persons who had been heavily irradiated, only one had typical aplastic anemia.[106] Repeated low-dose irradiation can damage bone marrow and has been associated with aplastic anemia. Excessive numbers of deaths from aplastic anemia were reported after therapeutic irradiation of the spine for ankylosing spondylitis[107,108] and among American radiologists who worked during the early part of the century with inadequate shielding.[109,110] Despite occasional instances in which marrow failure developed years after radiation and chemotherapy,[111] aplastic anemia was not found in unexpected numbers in a large population of cancer patients who had received therapeutic irradiation,[112] among nuclear power plant or thorium processing factory workers,[113] or with higher natural background radiation.[114] With radiation, as with benzene (see later), late marrow failure referred to in the older literature as "aplastic" might in fact be classified now as myelodysplasia, and therefore represent delayed manifestation of genetic damage rather than depletion of a limited stem cell reserve.

Drugs and Chemicals

Drugs are the most familiar clinical associations with aplastic anemia.[115] Initially suggested by the accumulation of case reports, specific drug associations have been established in formal case-control, population-based epidemiologic studies. In the IAAAS, relative risks were established for individual drugs and classes of pharmaceutical agents[6] (see Table 10–1).

Drug associations between chemicals and marrow aplasia are divided into two classes. Drugs used in chemotherapy are selected for their cytotoxicity and their regular, dose-dependent induction of marrow aplasia is expected. In contrast, most aplastic anemia associated with medical drug use in the community is idiosyncratic, meaning that it occurs unexpectedly in rare individuals. Mechanisms that might lead to the very occasional development of aplastic anemia after drug exposure include direct chemical toxicity and immune-mediated destruction. These pathophysiologic pathways have been better described for agranulocytosis, which is more commonly associated with prior medical drug use than is aplastic anemia (see Chapter 14). The clinical course, including the favorable response to immunosuppressive therapy, of patients with histories of drug exposure is the same as in idiopathic disease[116,117]; serum assays are also unhelpful because antibodies to either drugs or cells have only occasionally been identified in aplastic anemia.[118]

The low probability of developing aplastic anemia with a course of a drug may be a reflection of the gene frequency for metabolic enzymes (for direct chemical effects) or immune response genes (for immune-mediated marrow failure) in the human population. Many drugs and chemicals, especially those of limited water solubility, must be enzymatically degraded before conjugation and excretion. Highly reactive intermediate metabolites of degradation pathways may be the toxins responsible for adverse effects of the primary agents. Examples of detoxifying enzyme systems directly applicable to bone marrow failure and also demonstrating genetic variability include arylhydrocarbon hydroxylase (benzene toxicity), epoxide hydrolases (phenytoin toxicity), *S*-methylation (6-mercaptopurine, 6-thioguanine, and azathioprine), and *N*-acetylation (sulfa drugs). In a patient with carbamazepine-associated aplastic anemia, generation of reactive metabolites of the incriminated agent killed patient cells while there was no toxicity for normal donors' cells, and intermediate killing of cells of the patient's mother.[119] The rarity of idiosyncratic drug reactions would be a function of genetic variation in drug metabolism systems,[120] differences in major histocompatibility antigens,[121–123] and the available repertoire of potentially self-reactive lymphocytes.

Benzene

Benzene is a ubiquitous chemical strongly linked to bone marrow failure and leukemia.[115,124–126] Benzene myelotoxicity falls between the regular effects of chemotherapeutic agents and idiosyncratic drug reactions. The concentrations of benzene to which consumers are exposed, in the ambient air or at the gas pump, are orders of magnitude lower than those historically implicated in hematologic disease, and the effect on a population of chronic exposure to low doses of benzene, as with most "threshold" phenomena, is unknown.

Water-soluble products of benzene metabolism—phenols, hydroquinones, and catechols—and not the parent compound mediate marrow toxicity. These intermediate metabolites covalently and irreversibly bind to bone marrow DNA, inhibit DNA synthesis, and introduce DNA strand breaks. Benzene acts as a "mitotic poison" and as a mutagen; both DNA damage responses and apoptosis induction can now be measured at the molecular level.[127] Administration of benzene to animals produces bone marrow depression.[128,129] Acutely, the more mature, actively cycling marrow precursor cells are preferentially damaged compared to more primitive progenitors.[130] Intermittent exposure is more damaging to stem cell number than is continuous exposure,[130,131] and the stroma also can be damaged.[132]

Hematologic disease attributable to benzene ranges from relatively frequent but modest alterations in blood counts to marrow failure or leukemia. Studies of exposed American workers earlier in this century suggested that the risk of aplastic anemia was 3–4% in men exposed to concentrations higher than 300 ppm, and 50% of individuals exposed to 100 ppm showed some blood count depression.[133–135] The prevalence of some form of marrow suppression with heavy exposure can be high: over 10% of workers showed leukopenia; with improved hygiene the figure was lowered to 0.5%, a proportion that still resulted in a prevalence of 1 in 250.[136] Leukopenia, anemia, thrombocytopenia, and lymphocytopenia are common consequences of benzene exposure; other manifestations include macrocytosis, Pelger-Huët anomaly, eosinophilia, and basophilia. The appearance of the marrow is usually normocellular but may be hypo- or hypercellular[135]; necrosis, fibrosis, edema, and hemorrhage have been described.[137] Pancytopenia not infrequently precedes acute leukemia.[138]

Aromatic Hydrocarbons

That other molecules resembling benzene or containing a benzene ring must also cause marrow suppression is not well supported by available evidence. In contrast to benzene, neither closely related alkylbenzenes nor pure toluene and xylene are established marrow toxins. In total, the number of aplastic anemia cases reported is small considering the very large populations exposed to this heterogeneous group of chemicals. Surveys found only 2%[139] to 6%[140] of cases associated with insecticide exposure, and the significance of a handful of individual reports in the context of vast use of these compounds may be questioned. Pesticides and insecticides have been associated with aplastic anemia in almost 300 case reports[141]: most frequently cited are chlordane, lindane, and dichlorodiphenyltrichloroethane (DDT). A similarly diverse list of agricultural chemicals was significantly associated with aplastic anemia in rural Thailand[142] (although not with household use[143]). For the miscellaneous aromatic hydrocarbons, case reports also greatly outnumber series of patients and the results of systematic epidemiologic surveys are mixed. That many quite different chemical structures of pesticides have been incriminated is not readily explained on the basis of direct toxicity, and insecticide exposure could be a surrogate for another risk factor, such as an insect-borne virus.

Chloramphenicol

During its period as a widely available and extremely popular antibiotic, chloramphenicol was considered the most common cause of aplastic anemia in the United States,[144,145] blamed for 20–30% of total cases and 50% of drug-associated cases.[146–148] However, the assumption that the introduction of chloramphenicol greatly increased the number of cases of aplastic anemia is only weakly supported by epidemiologic data, and the death rate from aplastic anemia remained constant during the period of the drug's introduction, extensive use, and fall from favor in the prescription market. In recent series in the United States and Europe, in a total of 394 patients, only 1 was found who had ingested the drug.[15,149] Chloramphenicol has not appeared as a risk factor in Thailand, despite its high rate of use there, nor in Hong Kong, where utilization of chloramphenicol is almost 100 times greater than in the West but drug-associated aplastic anemia is infrequent.[150,151] The early epidemiologic surveys stressed excessive dosage, high blood levels, repeated or intermittent courses, young age, and oral route of administration as particular risks for chloramphenicol marrow toxicity. However, in a later collection of 600 cases, most patients had received a dose of less than 10 gm.[152]

At ordinary doses of chloramphenicol, a stereotypical pattern of reversible alterations in erythropoiesis occurs secondary to the drug's action as a ribosomal poison.[153] However, no in vitro study, including hematopoietic colony formation, stromal function, or biochemical activities, has provided a satisfactory mechanism of action operative for idiosyncratic aplastic anemia with chloramphenicol exposure.

Nonsteroidal Anti-inflammatory Drugs

Following on recognition of an association of phenylbutazone with aplastic anemia,[154] estimates of mortality rates ranged from 1 per 100,000 to 1 per 10^6 treatment courses.[155] The IAAAS identified even higher risks of marrow failure with other nonsteroidal anti-inflammatory drugs.[156]

Neuroleptics and Psychotropic Drugs

A variety of drugs with activity for the central nervous system but extremely diverse chemical structures have been associated with aplastic anemia: the hydantoins and carbamazepine, different antidepressants, tranquilizers, and, most recently, felbamate, the marketing of which was severely affected by the occurrence of aplasia in more than 30 patients.[157] Blood level and peripheral blood count monitoring of carbamazepine regimens were recommended despite fewer than two dozen aplastic anemia cases reported by 1982,[158] doubt about the validity of many cases in the literature, multiple large series of patients without hematologic toxicity,[159,160] and an estimated marrow complication case rate of only about 1 per 200,000 treated patients.[161] "Bundling" of a monitoring system for blood counts with the marketing of clozapine, because of the occurrence of agranulocytosis, greatly increased the price of this drug.

Gold and Other Heavy Metals

Gold salts have an extraordinarily high frequency of fatal adverse reactions, estimated at 1.6 per 10,000 prescriptions. Dose-dependent leukopenia is common, but several dozen cases of aplastic anemia have been reported[162] and gold figured prominently in the IAAAS, with an estimated excess risk of 23 cases per 10^6 users in 1 week.[6] Spontaneous recovery rarely can occur,[163] and patients have been successfully treated by transplantation or immunosuppression; chelation has not been generally helpful.[164,165] High concentrations of gold salts inhibit hematopoietic colony formation in vitro,[166] and there is some evidence for a dose relationship in vivo.[167]

Arsenic poisoning can result in neutropenia, anemia, and thrombocytopenia,[168,169] with characteristic basophilic stippling. Organic arsenicals, originally used in the treatment of syphilis (arsphenamine) and now as antihelminthics (arsenamide), historically were associated with aplastic anemia.[170]

Viruses

Viral infections frequently suppress marrow function and typically cause mild neutropenia. In the Thailand epidemiologic study, aplastic anemia was associated with use of nonbottled water, exposures to certain animals,[18] and prior hepatitis A,[17] all consistent with an infectious etiology. Viruses can damage the bone marrow directly, by cytolysis of hematopoietic cells, as exemplified by B19 parvovirus infection (see Chapter 76). Viruses commonly produce pathology indirectly, by induction of secondary immune pathways; initiation of an autoimmune process in the marrow could lead to depletion of progenitor and stem cells or destruction of supporting stroma.

Aplastic anemia is a rare sequela of Epstein-Barr virus infection: pancytopenia may accompany or follow infectious mononucleosis,[171,172] or there may be evidence of new or reactivated viral infection in a patient with typical aplastic anemia[173] (see Chapter 45). There is a genetic basis for an aberrant immune response to this virus in boys with X-chromosome–linked lymphoproliferative disease syndrome, in whom aplastic anemia is often responsible for a fatal outcome.[174,175]

Aplastic anemia follows closely on acute hepatitis in 5–10% of Western cases[176,177] but more frequently in some circumstances—almost one third of Indian patients admitted to a large Mumbai hospital[164] and 25% of cases undergoing stem cell transplant in Israel[178] had preceding hepatitis. In stereotypical posthepatitis aplasia, young males suffer an episode of acute, apparently viral hepatitis; in the convalescent phase, severe pancytopenia and marrow aplasia develop, which are uniformly fatal if untreated.[179,180] The syndrome has not been linked to any know hepatitis virus.[178,180,181] There is a striking association with fulminant hepatitis of childhood, which is also seronegative, and with marrow failure manifesting after liver transplantation[182,183] or in association with about 10% of cases of acute liver failure.[184,185] Postviral aplastic anemia can respond to immunosuppressive therapy[180,186]; posthepatitis aplastic anemia shows T-cell repertoire skewing at the molecular level.[187]

CLINICAL FEATURES

Aplastic anemia may vary in its clinical presentation and course, from a fulminant illness marked by hemorrhage and infection to an indolent process manageable by transfusions alone. Granulocyte, platelet, and red blood cell levels may not be uniformly affected, especially at presentation, and less drastic degrees of marrow hypoplasia and odd combinations of bicytopenias and even monocytopenias occur. The degree of marrow hypocellularity is variable and does not correlate with blood counts: hematopoietic cells may be seen in the marrow aspirated from the sternum, even with the severest pancytopenia, and conversely, profound marrow aplasia may be accompanied by only moderate blood count depression.

Symptoms and Signs

History

Patients' complaints derive from their low blood counts. Even minor bleeding is an alarming symptom: gum oozing, nosebleeds, easy bruising, or heavy or irregular menses often precipitate the first visit to a physician. Dark urine from the presence of hemoglobin may accompany paroxysmal nocturnal hemoglobinuria (PNH), but frank blood in the urine or stool is not otherwise observed early in the course of aplastic anemia. Frequent are the nonspecific symptoms of chronic anemia: fatigue or lassitude, shortness of breath, and ringing in the ears; older patients may have chest pain or congestive heart failure. Surprisingly, serious infection is unusual at presentation. Notably absent also are systemic symptoms of weight loss, failed appetite, or fever.

In a few instances in which blood counts have been serially monitored, the time interval between exposure to a medical drug or a viral infection and the onset of pancytopenia is about 6–8 weeks.[188] The interval may be more prolonged if the low blood counts are well tolerated. A careful and directed history should be obtained to elicit possible inciting events, but their identification rarely has an impact on choice of therapy. Exceptions are the rare cases of acute exposure to high doses of radiation or cytotoxic drugs, and chronic benzene exposure. A past history of chemotherapy points toward secondary myelodysplasia, and familial hematologic diseases or blood count abnormalities to Fanconi's anemia and dyskeratosis congenita.

Physical Examination

Findings range from a well-appearing patient with minimal abnormalities to an acutely ill individual with signs of systemic toxicity. Cachexia, lymphadenopathy, and splenomegaly are not seen with aplastic anemia and suggest an alternative diagnosis. Petechiae are usually located over dependent surfaces such as the pretibial surface and dorsal aspects of the ankles and wrists, as well as within the oropharynx and on the palate. Ecchymoses of differing sizes and hues may be found on areas that ordinarily suffer minor trauma. With severe degrees of thrombocytopenia, active hemorrhage may be observed in the retina, from the nares, and as gingival oozing; the stool guaiac will be positive and blood may be present at the cervical os. Pallor of the mucous membranes and nail beds is common. Less frequently there is fever, usually without localizing signs of infection. Areas of hyper- or hypopigmentation as well as typical anomalies lead to a diagnosis of Fanconi's anemia, and peculiarly misshapen nails are pathognomonic of dyskeratosis congenita.

Laboratory Tests

Blood

At classic presentation, all the blood counts are low. The blood smear lacks platelets and granulocytes but shows normal red cell morphology. Automated cell counting indicates little variation in erythrocyte size, but macrocytosis is the rule. Platelets are not enlarged. Automated counting has sharpened the accuracy of the reticulocyte count, which is markedly decreased. Monocyte and lymphocyte numbers also are reduced. Prior transfusions temporarily alter platelet values as well as the hemoglobin. Coexistent expansion of a clone of PNH cells is revealed by flow cytometry for glycosylphosphoinositol-linked surface proteins[189] (see Chapter 25). Serum transaminases point to prior or concurrent hepatitis, but specific viral serologies are negative.[180] A fetal pattern of erythrocyte i antigen expression and low sialic acid content, like macrocytosis, reflects stressed erythropoiesis. Lymphocytes cultured in vitro can be analyzed for the characteristic susceptibility of Fanconi's anemia cells to cytogenetic damage in the presence of DNA-damaging agents. Short telomeres are suggestive of mutations in genes of the telomere repair complex.

Bone Marrow

Cellularity is estimated from a biopsy, a core sample obtained using a Jamshidi needle of sufficient length (at least 1 cm) and undistorted by crush artifact (see Fig. 10–1A). Point counting and comparison to age-matched control data are ideal, but visual estimation is the practice; generally the biopsy is so preponderantly fatty that precise quantitation is unnecessary. The aspirate smear is preferred to assess individual cells (see Fig. 10–1*B*). Hematopoietic cells are drastically reduced in number and may be totally lacking. Residual erythroid precursors may be megaloblastic or even dysplastic, but there are no myeloblasts and megakaryocytes are absent. Hemophagocytosis may be observed. Instead of hematopoietic cells, the few spicules of the fatty aspirate show fibroblastic cells of presumably stromal origin, plasma cells, and lymphocytes.

Cytogenetic analysis of marrow cells is important in the bone marrow failure syndromes. In aplastic anemia at presentation, chromosomes are almost always normal,[190–192] whereas they are frequently abnormal in myelodysplasia (see Chapter 15). At some centers, normal cytogenetic testing is required for the diagnosis of aplastic anemia, but other investigators accept certain recurrent chromosomal abnormalities, especially trisomy 6[193–195] and trisomy 8,[196] if the marrow is hypocellular without dysplasia. The low numbers of cells capable of undergoing mitosis often limit the applicability of this test in a hypocellular marrow specimen.

Differential Diagnosis

The differential diagnosis is best considered in two stages that follow from the blood count results initially and the bone marrow examination later. Pancytopenia has many etiologies, of which aplastic anemia is not the most frequent (Table 10–3). The history and physical examination can quickly lead to an obvious diagnosis: a history of recent chemotherapy for cancer or a long course of systemic lupus; the stigmata of alcoholic liver disease, especially splenomegaly; or overwhelming sepsis. Although the typical presentation of aplastic anemia offers little diagnostic confusion, aplastic anemia may closely resemble other important hematologic diseases. Leukemia can occasionally be accompanied by a hypocellular bone marrow and the absence of circulating blast cells ("aleukemic leukemic"); pancytopenia is not uncommon at presentation of acute lymphoblastoid leukemia of childhood, and in some cases the marrow also is hypoplastic.[197–199] Abnormal leukemia and lymphoma cells should always be sought close to the marrow spicule. Pancytopenia occurs in myelofibrosis or myeloid metaplasia, and the "dry tap" on marrow aspiration is sometimes mistaken for aplasia; the leukoerythroblastic appearance of the blood smear and fibrosis of the marrow biopsy specimen allow an accurate diagnosis. Most confusing is the distinction between aplastic anemia and hypocellular myelodysplasia, for which absolute distinguishing criteria have not yet been developed.

TABLE 10–3. Differential Diagnosis of Pancytopenia

Pancytopenia with Hypocellular Bone Marrow
Acquired aplastic anemia
Inherited aplastic anemia (Fanconi's anemia, dyskeratosis, and others)
Some myelodysplasia syndromes
Rare aleukemic leukemia (acute myeloid leukemia)
Some acute lymphoblastic leukemia
Some lymphomas of bone marrow
Pancytopenia with Cellular Bone Marrow
Primary Bone Marrow Diseases
Myelodysplasia syndromes
Paroxysmal nocturnal hemoglobinuria
Myelofibrosis
Some aleukemic leukemia
Myelophthisis
Bone marrow lymphoma
Hairy cell leukemia
Secondary to Systemic Diseases
Systemic lupus erythematosus, Sjögren's syndrome
Hypersplenism
Vitamin B_{12}, folate deficiency (familial defect)
Overwhelming infection
Alcohol
Brucellosis
Ehrlichiosis
Sarcoidosis
Tuberculosis and atypical mycobacteria
Hypocellular Bone Marrow + Cytopenia
Q fever
Legionnaires' disease
Toxoplasmosis
Mycobacteria
Tuberculosis
Anorexia nervosa, starvation
Hypothyroidism

TABLE 10–4. Recent Results of Allogeneic Stem Cell Transplantation in Aplastic Anemia*

Institution/Study	Years of Study	N	Age (median)	Rejection/Failure	Chronic GVHD	Actuarial Survival
Vienna[500]	1982–1996	20	17–37 (25)	0	53	95 (at 15 yr)
IBMTR[219]	1988–1992	471	1–51 (20)	16	32	66 (at 5 yr)
EGBMT[222]	1991–1998	71	4–46 (19)	3	35	86 (at 5 yr)
Seattle and three other centers[221]	1988–1999	94	2–59 (26)	4	32	88 (at 6 yr)
Korea[357]	1990–2001	64	—	18	19	
Hamburg[501]	1990–2001	21	7–43 (25)	5	5	86 (at 5 yr)

*Only studies reporting 20 patients are tabulated (for smaller studies, see also Osman et al.,[502] Meidlinger et al.,[503] and Goldenberg et al.[504]). Graft-versus-host disease (GVHD) results are generally for grades III/IV and in patients at risk.

About 20% of myelodysplasia cases present with a predominantly fatty marrow.[200–203] Morphology, chromosome testing, and radiographic studies are most helpful (see Chapter 15). Marrow morphology in aplastic anemia is usually normal or shows only erythroid changes, and cytogenetics are normal. In myelodysplasia, megakaryocytes are preserved and can be aberrantly micro- and mononuclear. Myeloid precursors are often hypogranulated, there may be an increased representation of blasts and other young forms, and nuclear morphology may be abnormal. Extreme megaloblastic changes, bizarre erythroid morphology, and ringed sideroblasts are not consistent with a diagnosis of aplastic anemia. Chromosomes 5, 7, 9, and others show characteristic abnormalities in myelodysplasia. Magnetic resonance imaging of a few vertebral bodies can distinguish a uniformly fatty marrow from a spotty mixture of hypo- and hypercellularity.[204,205]

A final difficult differential diagnosis is between acquired and constitutional hematopoietic failure, because the marrow appearance is the same. Physical anomalies, especially café au lait lesions, bony abnormalities of the hands, and unexpectedly short stature or peculiar facies, point to Fanconi's anemia, which can be confirmed by stressed cytogenetic testing of peripheral blood (see Chapter 11). Shoddy nails and leukoplakia are clues to the diagnosis of dyskeratosis congenita, which is established by telomere length measurements and genetic testing.

TREATMENT

Options for therapy differ based on the prognosis, which is almost entirely dependent on early blood counts. The popular "Camitta" criteria define severe disease as the presence of two of three diminished blood counts: neutrophils less than 500/L, platelets less than 20,000/μL, and corrected reticulocytes less than 1% (<40,000–60,000/μL).[206,207] Patients with severe aplastic anemia are treated either by stem cell transplantation or by immunosuppressive drugs. Patients with less severe blood count depression but hypocellular bone marrows are diagnosed with moderate aplastic anemia; depending on the levels of blood counts and their stability, they can be offered the choice of simple observation, modest modalities of immunosuppression, androgens, and growth factors (Fig. 10–6).

Hematopoietic Stem Cell Transplantation

Allogeneic stem cell transplantation from a fully histocompatible sibling cures the large majority of aplastic anemia patients who are able to undergo the procedure[176,208–213] (Table 10–4; Fig. 10–7) (see Chapter 102). Bone marrow and also peripheral blood from cytokine-primed donors can serve as a stem cell source; the faster rate of engraftment, and convenience to the hematologist and donor, have made the use of blood increasingly popular.[214–217] One retrospective analysis suggested that the higher lymphocyte dose present in mobilized peripheral blood, while not affecting the rate of occurrence of chronic graft-versus-host disease, might be associated with a more protracted and less responsive course of this syndrome.[218]

Early studies conclusively demonstrated the superiority of allogeneic marrow transplants compared to supportive care; in an international multicenter controlled study, patients with severe disease who were transplanted early had actuarial survival of greater than 60% compared to about 20% in patients who received androgens and blood transfusions only.[206] The results of marrow transplantation have steadily improved over time, due to a combination of factors: progressive modification of conditioning regimens and lower procedure-related early mortality; improved transfusion medicine support and antibiotic regimens; and the introduction of cyclosporine in graft-versus-host disease regimens. Five-year survival rates in the International Bone Marrow Transplant Registry data have climbed from 48% in the years 1976–1980 to 66% for 1988–1992[219] and to 77% in the most recent cohort.[212] In favorable subgroups—children and younger untransfused or minimally transfused and uninfected patients—survival of 80–90% may be routinely achieved. Some individual hospitals now report very high long-term survival, credited to the addition of antithymocyte globulin (ATG) to the cyclophosphamide regimen,[220,221] to the combination of methotrexate and cyclosporine for the prevention of graft-versus-host disease[222] (although neither modifica-

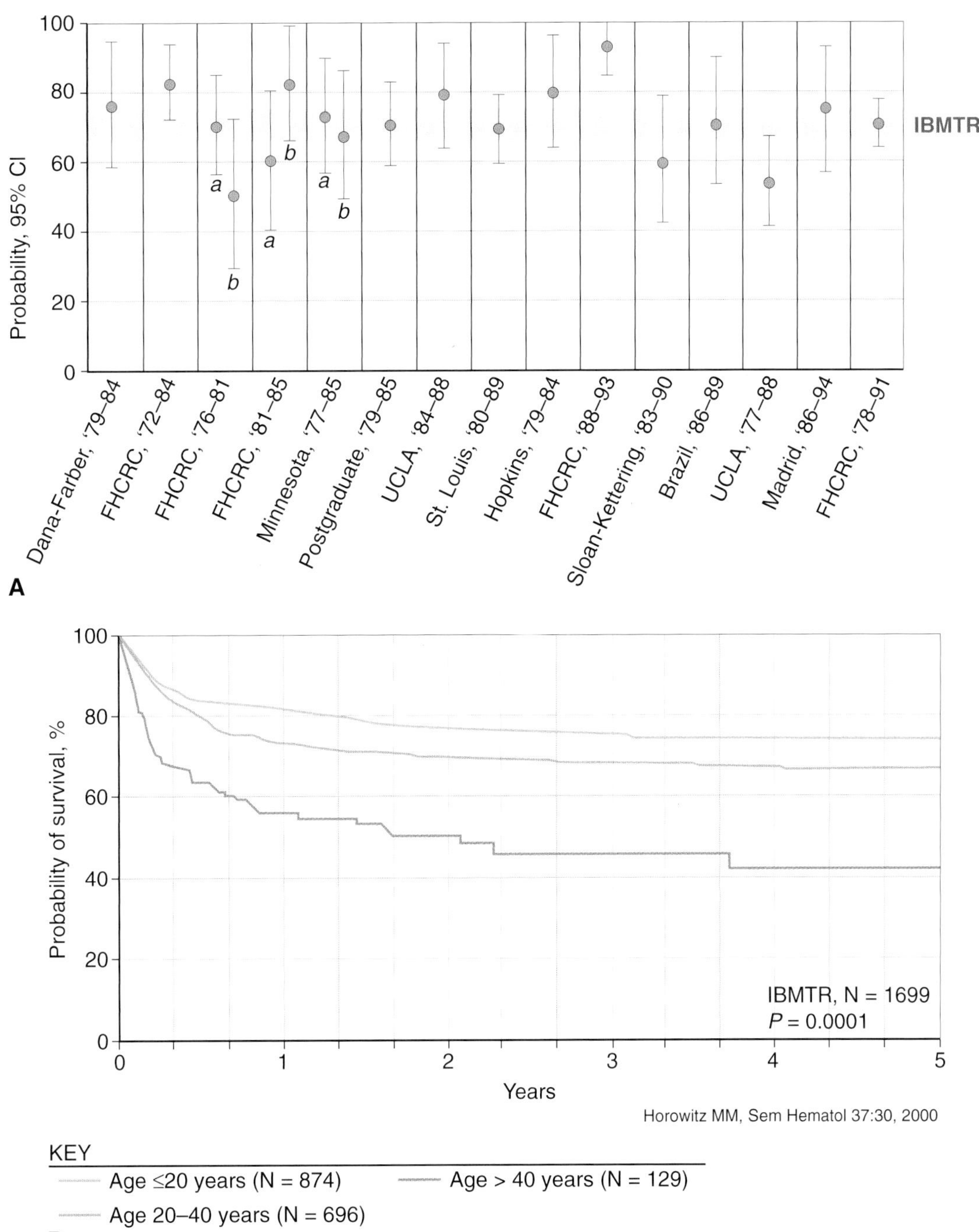

Figure 10–6. Allogeneic bone marrow transplantation for severe aplastic anemia. ***A,*** Summary of survival data from many centers, in comparison to results from the International Bone Marrow Transplant Registry (see Horowitz[508] for details and references). ***B,*** Survival by age cohort (data from Horowitz[508]).

tion is convincingly supported by randomized trials), and to omission of irradiation in conditioning.[223]

Graft rejection and graft-versus-host disease are the major complications of allogeneic transplantation in aplastic anemia. Graft rejection was a major predictor of survival for transplantations performed in the 1980s and the most common single fatal event.[224] Graft rejection rates have fallen with intensification of immunosuppressive conditioning, from 15% to 4% in Europe[224] and from 35% to 9% in Seattle.[225] Outcomes after second transplantation for primary graft failure have improved but still vary widely, from 20% to 80% survival.[225–228] That rejection might be intrinsic to the pathophysiology of aplastic anemia has been inferred from the unexpectedly high proportion of graft failure in unprepared syngeneic twin transplants,[229–232] even with adequate precondition-

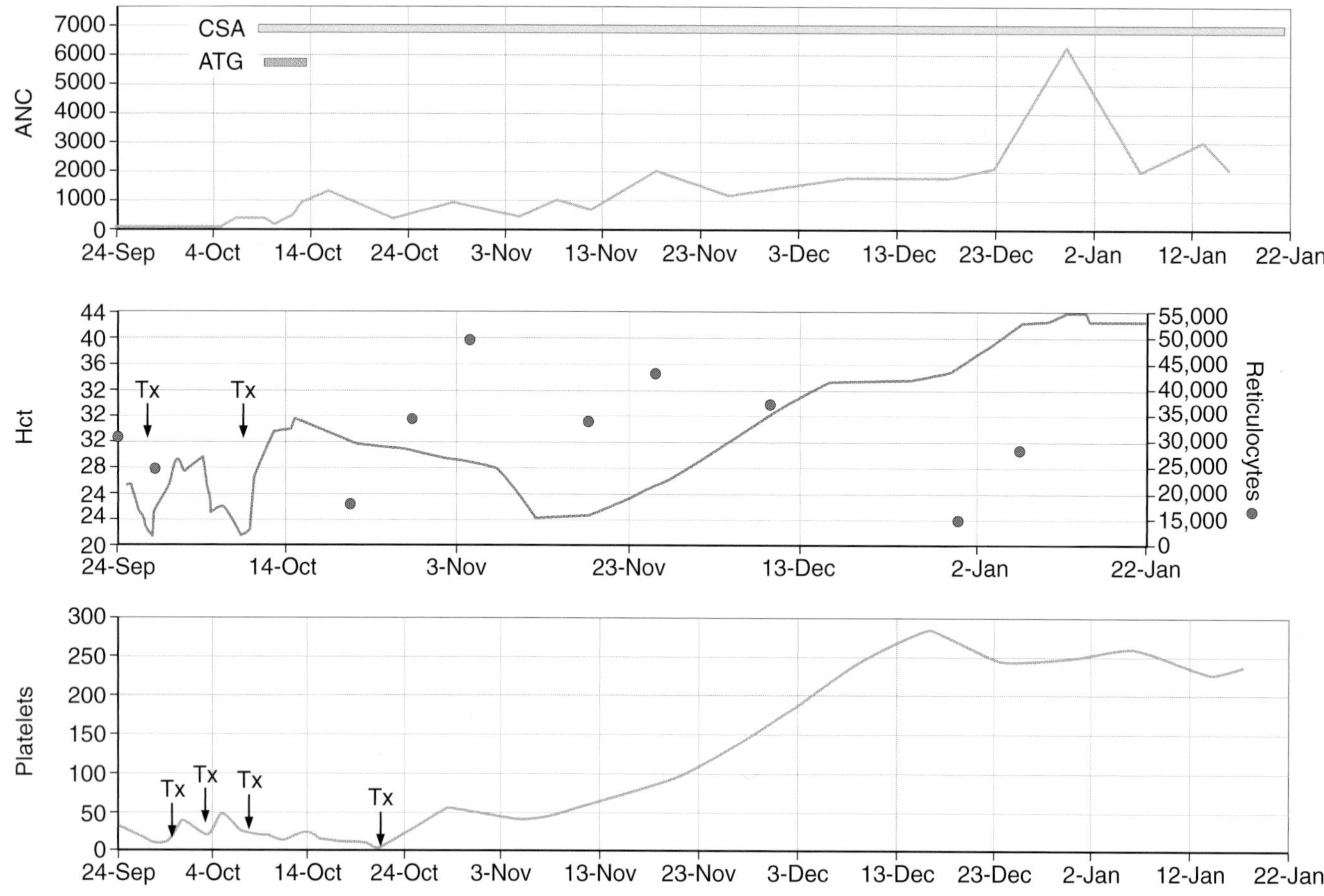

■ **Figure 10–7.** Immunosuppression for severe aplastic anemia, showing dramatic response of a 16-year-old boy with posthepatitis syndrome to ATG and cyclosporine (CSA); he remains with normal blood counts more than a decade after treatment. Abbreviations: ANC, absolute neutrophil count; Hct, hematocrit; Tx, transfusion.

ing.[233,234] In untransfused patients who received allogeneic stem cells, the incidence of graft rejection was only 10%.[235] The influence of prior transfusion on graft rejection is relative, and modest numbers of blood donations (<40 units in the International Registry experience[226] and <10 units of erythrocytes or 40 units of platelets in Seattle patients[236]) likely do not greatly increase the risk of graft rejection. Modern platelet transfusion practice has reduced the risk of allosensitization.

Rates and severity of chronic graft-versus-host disease vary, related to patient selection and treatment regimens. Age is the major risk factor, with rates of severe chronic graft-versus-host disease rising from 19% for patients 0–10 years old to 46% at 11–30 years, and 90% in patients over 31 years old in a historic Seattle series.[237] Recent data confirm a higher incidence and more serious disease in older adults: for 212 patients treated in Seattle who survived for more than 2 years after transplant, 41% had developed chronic graft-versus-host disease, with a mortality three times higher than in those patients without this complication. Age was a significant univariate risk factor for the development of chronic graft-versus-host disease in this study, with an increased relative risk of 1.04 per year.[238] In a European Group analysis, a significant difference was observed in survival for those younger than 20 years (65%) compared to patients older than 20 years (56%), but there was no difference between patients 21–30 and those 31–55 years.[239] For the International Bone Marrow Transplant Registry, rates of severe graft-versus-host disease (acute and chronic combined; acute disease is a major risk factor for the development of chronic disease) were 15–20% in children but 40–45% in adults.[212] Deaths from chronic graft-versus-host disease can occur many years after transplantation, and about a third of patients require long-term treatment.[238] Although graft-versus-host disease resolves slowly in most patients, it remains a major risk factor for many of the late complications of transplantation, including effects on growth and development and on endocrine, neurologic, and other organ systems[238] (see Chapter 94).

An increased rate of secondary malignancies has been registered after transplantation in general as well as for aplastic anemia. In a National Cancer Institute retrospective analysis of almost 20,000 transplantations, the risk of late cancer was eightfold at 10 years than anticipated in the general population, and even higher for young patients at the time of transplantation (about 40-fold).[240] For aplastic anemia, among 320 patients with aplasia transplanted in Seattle, 4 developed cancer, leading to a calculated risk 7 times greater than expected[241]; chronic graft-versus-host disease was a risk factor for late malignancy.[238] In a French survey, 4 of 147 aplastic patients developed solid tumors, an 8-year cumulative incidence rate of 22%, equivalent to a relative risk of 41.[242] Secondary solid tumors can develop in the penumbra of the thoracoabdominal irradiation field.[243] Associated risk factors have been acute graft-versus-host disease, treatment with ATG or monoclonal antibody, and total-body irradiation.[241] A significant risk of late malignancy exists in aplastic anemia patients, with relative risks equivalent for immunosuppression and transplantation.[244]

Excellent survival and low morbidity in younger patients make allogenic transplantation the treatment of choice for children and adolescents. Older patients have a higher risk of transplant-related morbidity and mortality. Young adults in the intermediate age group have a good opportunity for cure with bone marrow transplantation but also face more complications than do children. In addition to age, a prolonged interval between diagnosis and transplantation, multiple transfusions, and serious infections before transplantation adversely impact outcomes.

Hematopoietic Stem Cell Transplantation from Alternative Donors: Mismatched Family, Matched Unrelated, and Umbilical Cord Blood

Until recently, the lack of an HLA genotypically identical sibling donor precluded marrow transplantation, thus excluding this therapeutic option in about 70% of patients with aplastic anemia.[245] Alternative potential donors include either relatives who are phenotypically matched or partially matched and HLA phenotypically matched but unrelated volunteers.

Phenotypically identical family donors are available in only 1–2% of cases, but haplotype sharing between parents occasionally has allowed identification and successful transplantation between matched relatives.[246,247] Full phenotypic matches fare well (about 50% survival), but even a one-locus, and especially a two- or three-antigen, disparity yields inferior survival rates (<20% survival), because of the familiar problems of graft rejection and graft-versus-host disease.[245,247] In the large European experience, for phenotypically identical family matches actuarial survival was 45%; for patients with a single locus mismatch, 25%; and for two or three loci mismatched, 11%.[248,249] In a Seattle report, although all patients who received transplants that were fully HLA-matched survived, those with one or more loci mismatched had poorer outcomes, with survival of only 50%.[247] Satisfactory engraftment and low graft-versus-host disease incidence have been achieved in partially matched related donors with conditioning that includes total-body irradiation and multiple and high doses of cytotoxic drugs in combination with T-cell depletion.[250] A few aplastic anemia patients have received transplants from family members in which only a single haplotype was shared between donor and recipient: 3 of 10 rejected the graft, but survival in the "low-risk" group was about 50%.[245]

Many more donors histocompatible at the major HLA loci are available outside the family, but in comparison to standard HLA-matched sibling transplantation, most large studies have shown inferior long-term survival and higher rates of complications of graft rejection,[245,251] graft-versus-host disease,[252,253] and delayed immune reconstitution.[254] Age is a crucial risk factor and probably more important even than the level of match, conditioning regimen, or use of T-cell depletion.[249,255–257] Historically, survival for aplastic anemia patients after unrelated transplantation has been poor: 29% at 2 years for the National Marrow Donor Program,[258] and 34% in the European Group registry 1994 report.[259] Superior results were initially obtained at Children's Hospital in Milwaukee in a protocol of T-cell depletion of the donor graft combined with a rigorous conditioning program of cytosine arabinoside, cyclophosphamide, and total-body irradiation: for 28 transfused and previously treated children with severe aplastic anemia, survival was 54% with no chronic graft-versus-host disease.[260] In a British study intensive immunosuppression with a combination of cyclophosphamide, Campath (a monoclonal antibody to the T-cell antigen CD52), and either irradiation or fludarabine led to survival in all of eight aplastic anemia patients.[261] Recently, diverse protocols that use large inocula of highly purified peripheral blood CD34 cells, T-cell depletion, and aggressive conditioning with radiation and highly immunosuppressive drugs have led to engraftment with very little graft-versus-host disease in children with severe aplastic anemia.[262–264] Registry data reflect general improvement in outcomes,[265–267] credited to briefer intervals from diagnosis to transplant, better genotyping for HLA matching, and improved immunosuppressive regimens to overcome graft rejection.[266]

Experience with umbilical cord blood transplantation is more limited.[268] The number of stem cells available from a single cord donor is inadequate for most adults, and the engraftment period is prolonged in all recipients. Of 21 aplastic anemia patients transplanted with cord blood, only 8 of 19 who were evaluable engrafted, almost all of whom then suffered transplant-related events of death, autologous reconstitution, or need for a second transplant.[268] In addition to older recipient age and histoincompatibility, the diagnosis of marrow failure conferred a particularly poor prognosis.

Immunosuppression

Antithymocyte Globulin

Immunosuppression is an effective alternative treatment for patients who are not candidates for transplantation.[269–272] Immunoglobulin preparations made from the sera of horses or rabbits immunized against human thymocytes are the mainstays of current regimens. A horse ATG (ATGAM; Upjohn) and a rabbit ATG (Thymoglobulin; Sangstat) are licensed for use by the Food and Drug Administration.

The efficacy of ATG in marrow failure was discovered serendipitously in the late 1960s, when Mathé observed recovery of autologous hematopoiesis in patients who had received ATG as conditioning for marrow transplantation.[51] In a collection of European cases from Basel, Paris, and Leiden, treated with different serum preparations and in a variety of dosing regimens, sustained hematologic improvement occurred in 12 of 29 severe aplastic anemia patients and 1-year survival of the entire group was 55%.[273] In a combined-center study in the United States, Swiss antilymphocyte globulin was much superior to androgens, with significantly better response (70% vs. 18%) and 1-year survival (76% vs. 22%).[274] Similar results were also obtained in a small randomized study of ATG versus supportive care (52% vs. 0% response rate).[275] In a big multicenter American trial, 47% of patients improved.[276] Review of published results from Europe and America suggested that, overall, about half the patients treated with ATG would show hematologic improvement, broadly defined as an end to transfusion-dependence and neutrophil number levels adequate to protect from serious infection, although rates may vary with center from 20% to 85%.[277] Patient selection is important, because the likelihood of response to ATG has been inversely correlated to disease severity,[278,279] and, in particular, to neutrophil count.[239,280] Putative etiology does not predict response: virus-associated and drug-induced aplasia behave similarly to idiopathic disease. Nor do cytogenetic abnormalities preclude a hematologic response, because both aplastic anemia with chromosomal abnormalities[281–283] and frank myelodysplasia[284] may improve to transfusion-independence. The response rate to ATG was not increased by addition of androgens[285] or very high doses of corticosteroids.[286]

A hematologic response to ATG is usually apparent within several months; in some cases, all blood counts rise dramatically, and in others, increases in platelets or red cells may be delayed. The average time to improvement in neutrophil number is around 1–2 months,[276] to transfusion-independence about 2–3 months after initiating treatment.[287,288] Blood counts may return to normal, but usually recovery is partial, with levels of platelets and hemoglobin adequate to avoid transfusion and neutrophil numbers sufficient to avoid bacterial and fungal infections. Bone marrow cellularity[289] and functional measures of the hematopoietic stem cell compartment[290] often remain depressed despite clinical hematologic recovery. Continued improvement without further therapy is not uncommon, but it is hematologic status at 3 or 6 months that strongly correlates with long-term survival.[276,291]

ATG has three major toxicities: immediate allergic phenomena, serum sickness, and transient blood count depression (Fig. 10–8). Fever, rigors, and a urticaria occur on the first day or two of infusion, and these symptoms respond to antihistamines and meperidine. Anaphylaxis is rare but has been fatal.[292] A positive immediate wheal-and-flare reaction to the epicutaneous application of the 50-mg/mL stock solution of ATG may predict massive histamine release on systemic infusion, and desensitization with gradually increasing doses of ATG administered intradermally, subcutaneously, and then intravenously has permitted ATG use in allergic individuals.[292] Corticosteroids are usually administered in moderate doses (1 mg/kg of prednisone or methylprednisolone) during the first 2 weeks to ameliorate serum sickness.

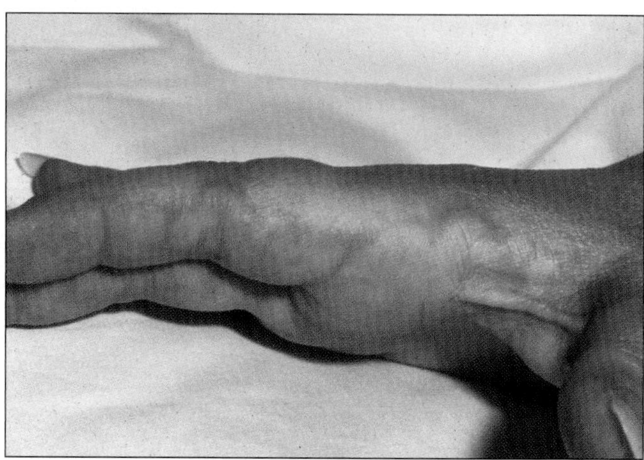

Figure 10–8. Characteristic cutaneous eruption of serum sickness, usually occurring about 10 days after initiation of ATG, the serpiginous erythema at the dorsal-volar circle may be hemorrhagic in the setting of severe thrombocytopenia.

Dosages and regimens have varied widely. It is rational to administer high doses over a short period: for horse ATG, 40 mg/kg/day for 4 days, and for rabbit ATG, 3.5 mg/kg/day for 5 days; antiserum will then have reached low levels in the circulation by the time host antibody appears.[293] A shorter course is easier to administer, associated with less serum sickness, and appears equally effective as the same dose given over more time.

Antilymphocyte globulins are immunosuppressive. ATGs contain a heterogeneous mix of antibody specificities for lymphocytes, including reactivity to antigens such as CD2, CD3, CD4, CD8, CD25 (the receptor for IL-2), and HLA-DR.[294–296] ATGs fix human complement efficiently, and all preparations are cytotoxic to T cells in vitro. Lot-to-lot differences have been difficult to demonstrate in the laboratory.[295] Commercial rabbit ATG is more potent than is horse ATG on a weight basis, and a few studies in renal transplant recipients have suggested that it might also be more effective clinically.[297,298] In vitro, antilymphocyte globulins efficiently inhibit T-cell proliferation and block IL-2 and IFN-γ production and IL-2 receptor expression[299]; ATG induced Fas-mediated apoptosis in T cells, especially after activation.[300] Monkey experiments have suggested that persisting specific antibodies are responsible for the induced chronic anergy and tolerance.[301] In patients, ATG results in rapid reduction in the number of circulating lymphocytes and lymphocytopenia persists for several days after discontinuing the last infusion. When lymphocyte numbers have returned to pretreatment values at 3 months, activated lymphocyte numbers are reduced.[62,303–305]

Reliable methods to predict a response to ATG are lacking. In some cases, lymphocyte inhibitory activity for hematopoietic progenitors disappeared after successful therapy.[305–307] Clonotyping, or the measurement of putative pathogenic clones by analysis of specific lymphocyte subpopulations bearing specific Vβ T-cell receptor subfamilies or a specific sequence of the CDR3 antigen-binding region, has also correlated with clinical response

TABLE 10–5. Large Trials of Intensive Immunosuppression in Severe Aplastic Anemia

Study, Year(s)	Regimen	*N*	Median Age in yr (range)	Median ANC/µL/% Cases <0.2/µL	Response	Survival (%)	Relapse (%)	Median Follow-up (yr)
German multicenter,[†] 1986–1992[505]	ALG + CSA	43	32 (7–80)	0.48/19%	65% at 6 mo*	58	38	>11
EGBMT, 1995[506]	ALG + CSA + G-CSF	100	16 (2–72)	0.20/50%	77% at 1 yr	87	12	~4
NIH, 1989–1998[177]	ATG + CSA	122	35 (3–79)	0.30/38%	58% at 1 yr	55	35	>7
Japan multicenter,[†,‡] 1992–1997[335]	ATG + CSA + androgen ± G-CSF	119	9 (1–18)	–/42%	68% at 1 yr	88	33	>3

*For patients with severe aplastic anemia in this study.
[†]Some values for German and Japanese studies were calculated from data presented in the publications.
[‡]Includes some moderate aplastic anemia.
Abbreviations: ALG, antilymphocyte globulin; ANC, absolute neutrophil count; ATG, antithymocyte globulin; CSA, cyclosporine; G-CSF, granulocyte colony-stimulating factor; EGBMT, European Group for Bone Marrow Transplantation; NIH, National Institutes of Health.

in a small number of cases.[308] However, other promising relationships between response and pretreatment improvement in hematopoietic colony formation after T-cell depletion,[305,309] incubation of marrow with ATG[310] or corticosteroids,[311] in co-culture assays,[312] and for lymphocyte stimulatory activities,[313] have not been generally confirmed.[291,314–318]

Cyclosporine

Cyclosporine, often combined with androgens, appeared helpful in individual patients with aplastic anemia, many of whom had failed other therapies. Subsequently, several groups reported efficacy of cyclosporine in patients refractory to ATG, with salvage rates of about 50%.[319–324] Efficacy of cyclosporine as initial therapy was promoted in a large French cooperative randomized study,[325] but in a subsequent randomized German trial, cyclosporine plus G-CSF was clearly inferior to ATG as measured by response rate and survival,[300] and in patients with moderate aplastic anemia, cyclosporine alone led to an overall response of 46% compared to 74% when it was combined with ATG[326] (and see later).

The optimal dose has not been determined. In the United States, cyclosporine has usually been employed at high doses, 12 mg/kg/day for adults and 15 mg/kg/day for children, with adjustment of doses to plasma drug concentrations, serum creatinine, or other toxicities. In Europe, lower doses (3–7 mg/kg/day) have appeared to be sufficient.[327,328] Hematologic improvement may occur in a few weeks or months. When achieved, remissions usually have been durable, but some proportion of patients relapse when cyclosporine is discontinued; although most will then respond to its reinstitution,[327–330] some may require maintenance treatment.[319,331]

Hypertension and azotemia are the most common serious side effects; hirsutism and gingival hypertrophy are also frequent. Increasing serum creatinine levels are an indication to lower the dose. Chronic nephropathy, characterized by interstitial fibrosis and tubular atrophy, can be irreversible and must be avoided; the risk of nephropathy is increased by high doses and long duration of therapy, and occurs more commonly in older than younger patients. Cyclosporine produces temporary immunodeficiency and new susceptibility to unusual infectious agents; monthly aerosolized pentamidine prophylaxis will prevent *Pneumocystis* in patients receiving cyclosporine. Convulsions, possibly related to hypomagnesemia, are also a serious complication of cyclosporine.

Combined or Intensive Immunosuppressive Therapy

The combination of an agent that lyses lymphocytes (ATG) with a drug to block T-cell function is rational, and indeed a striking increase in the response rate to immunosuppression was observed in a German randomized trial in which patients were treated initially with a combination of ATG and cyclosporine compared to ATG only: the addition of cyclosporine led to higher hematologic response rates and more complete responses than with ATG alone (65% vs. 39% and 70% vs. 46% at 3 and 6 months, respectively)[332] (Table 10–5). A single-center protocol at the National Institutes of Health[333] and a multicenter European study[334] confirmed the better response rates for the combination, which appeared to translate into better long-term survival. Responses variably defined but usually equivalent to transfusion-independence and neutrophil numbers sufficient to protect against infection, occur in two thirds to three fourths of patients. Combined immunosuppression has been especially beneficial for patients with extreme neutropenia and in children, both of which groups fared poorly with antilymphocyte globulins alone. Among 50 Japanese children with very severe aplastic anemia (<200/µL neutrophils), 73% were hematologic responders at 1 year and 83% were alive at 3 years.[335] Older patients, who have not been candidates for stem cell transplantation, also can do well: response rates of about 62% in a European Bone Marrow Transplant Registry analysis were similar for adults in cohorts from 20 to more than 60 years of age.[336] Long-term outcomes strongly correlate with blood counts at 3 months: for the approximately 50% of patients treated at the Clinical Center who achieved

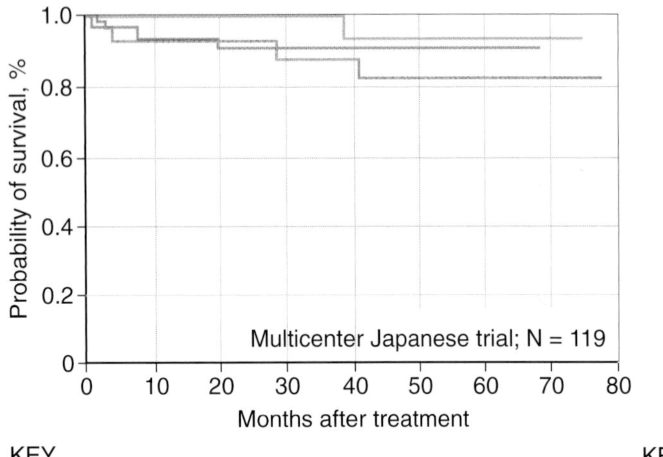

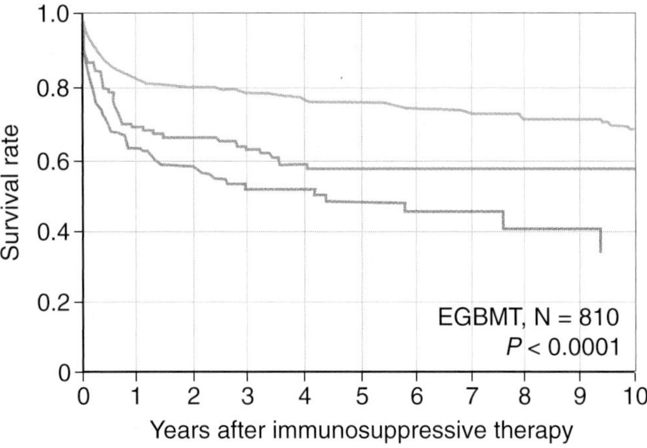

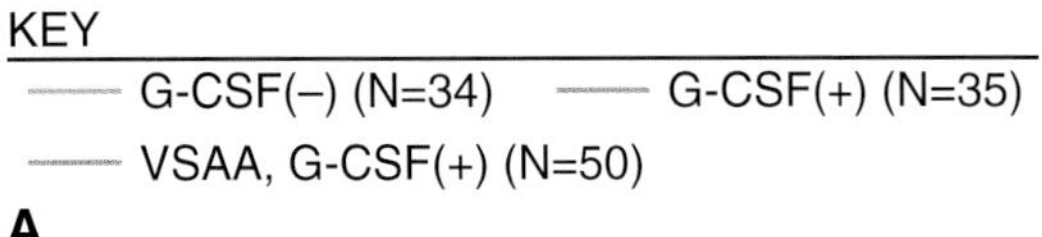

A

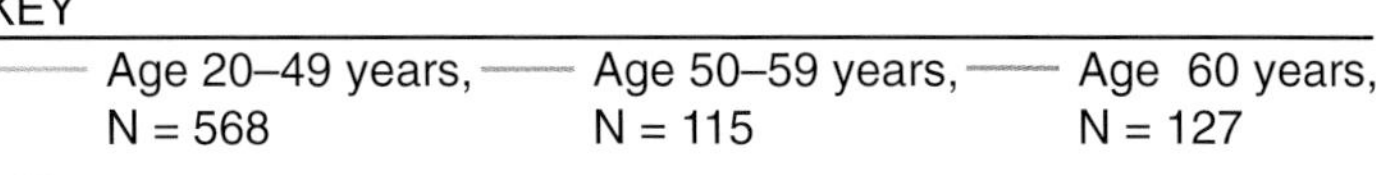

B

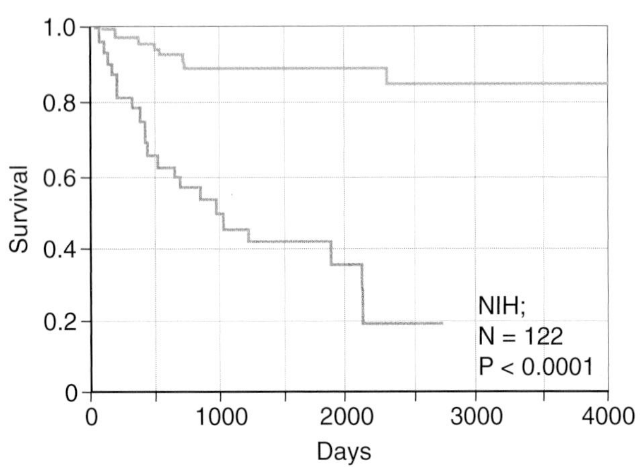

KEY

Platelets or reticulocytes ≥50 x 10^3/μL

Platelets or reticulocytes <50 x 10^3/μL

C

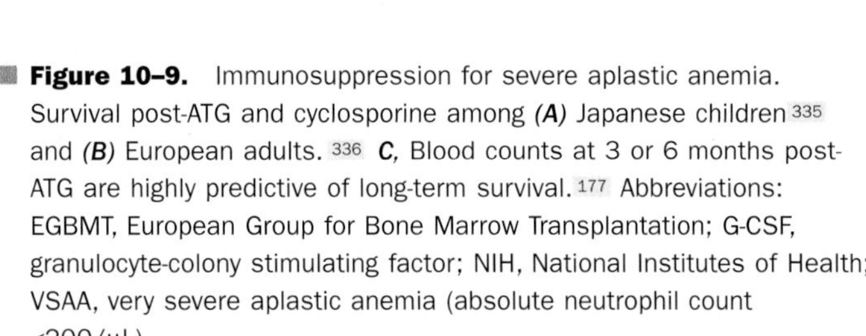

Figure 10–9. Immunosuppression for severe aplastic anemia. Survival post-ATG and cyclosporine among *(A)* Japanese children [335] and *(B)* European adults. [336] *C,* Blood counts at 3 or 6 months post-ATG are highly predictive of long-term survival. [177] Abbreviations: EGBMT, European Group for Bone Marrow Transplantation; G-CSF, granulocyte-colony stimulating factor; NIH, National Institutes of Health; VSAA, very severe aplastic anemia (absolute neutrophil count <200/μL).

counts of greater than 50,000/μL for either platelets or reticulocytes, the survival plateau was about 85% at a decade after treatment (Fig. 10–9). [177]

The use of high-dose cyclophosphamide, 45–50 mg/kg/day for 4 days without stem cell rescue, is controversial. [337] Autologous recovery after failed allogeneic transplant had been observed with cyclophosphamide conditioning as well as pretreatment with ATG. Investigators at Johns Hopkins intentionally treated 11 patients with cyclophosphamide: the overall response rate was similar to that achieved with ATG, blood counts normalized, and there were no late complications. [338] In a further 19 patients, 73% were considered responders and survival was 84% at 2 years. [339] The hematologic response to cyclophosphamide was gradual, with counts rising over many months (median of 36 months to complete remission). Applied as salvage therapy, over half of a group of 17 patients who had failed other immunosuppression regimens responded to cyclophosphamide. [340] However, in a randomized controlled trial at the National Institutes of Health, which entered 31 patients before premature termination, cyclophosphamide was associated with early deaths and invasive fungal infection, even in patients with reasonable neutrophil counts at presentation, because of the induction of prolonged neutropenia [341]; in contrast to the Baltimore experience, some cyclophosphamide-treated patients relapsed, one developed a clonal cytogsenetic abnormality, and clones of PNH cells were unaffected. [342] Cyclophosphamide is appealing because of its low cost and ease of administration, but application of this regimen to patients in China, [343] Mexico, [344,345] and elsewhere has had mixed results, with some recoveries and other deaths likely secondary to treatment. More experience is desirable, especially in the setting of another controlled trial with the addition of antifungal prophylaxis.

Corticosteroids

Methylprednisolone in modest doses is administered with ATG to ameliorate serum sickness. Very high—"industrial"—doses of corticosteroids have been administered; boluses of 6-methylprednisolone given intravenously and starting at 20 mg/kg/day may be efficacious, especially in recently diagnosed cases.[317,346,347] High-dose methylprednisolone added to ATG therapy was not helpful in a controlled trial.[286] ATGs have a better toxicity profile and are generally preferable as initial therapy. Modest doses of corticosteroids alone do not have a role in the treatment of aplastic anemia: not only is there little evidence of their effectiveness in either reversing marrow failure or improving hemostasis, but even limited courses may contribute to aseptic vascular necrosis of bones, a troubling complication in the pancytopenic patient.[348]

Relapse

Recurrence of pancytopenia is common. In 719 European patients treated with immunosuppression, the actuarial rate of relapse among 358 responders was 35% at 14 years; relapse occurred more commonly among patients who had shown initial rapid responses to treatment.[349] About half the relapsed patients could be induced to respond to a second course of immunosuppression, but survival was lower in patients who suffered a relapse compared to those who had not. In the National Institutes of Health cohort of 112 patients, relapse, defined as a need for treatment, occurred commonly but survival was unaffected by its occurrence, and most patients responded to further therapy, usually only reinstitution of cyclosporine.[350] These observations are consistent with a view of aplastic anemia as a chronic immunologic disease that is not cured by a single course of immunosuppressive therapy.

The much more serious complication of late clonal hematologic disease is discussed later.

Immunosuppression Versus Bone Marrow Transplantation

Lack of a matched sibling donor, the cost and availability of stem cell transplantation, and risk factors such as active infection, older age, or a heavy transfusion burden mean that aplastic anemia is usually treated by immunosuppression.[351] For some patients with aplastic anemia and their physicians, a choice does exist between the two different therapies. Marrow transplantation offers the opportunity of permanent cure of hematopoietic failure; its disadvantages are expense; procedure-related morbidity and mortality, especially graft-versus-host disease in older patients; and late complications such as solid organ malignancies. Immunosuppression carries less toxicity and at least initially is less costly. However, many patients do not achieve normal blood counts, they remain at high risk for relapse and the need for additional therapy, and some proportion will develop the serious complication of late clonal hematologic disease, especially myelodysplasia.

Retrospective analyses of the large number of European patients show consistently improved results with both therapies but have repeatedly failed to demonstrate a survival advantage for transplantation over immunosuppression[239,352–354]: the most recent 5-year survival figures were 75% for immunosuppression and 77% for transplantation.[355] Results of single-center studies are similar: whether immunosuppression is equivalent to transplantation or superior[289,356,357] or inferior,[353,358] the observed differences usually do not reach statistical significance. Despite similar probabilities of overall and event-free survival, the courses following immunosuppression and transplantation do differ: deaths occur earlier with transplantation and later with ATG regimens, and transplanted patients benefit from longer periods without symptoms while immunosuppressed patients often require continued close medical attention, transfusions, and drug therapy.[359] In the European group analyses, marrow transplantation yielded superior results in children age 10 years and younger with less than 400 neutrophils/μL, whereas immunosuppression was better for adults 40 years and older; for patients in the intermediate age category, a neutrophil count below 300/μL favored transplantation.[224,355] Even its enthusiasts do not recommend transplantation as first-line therapy in the elderly.[360]

In some cases, unsuccessful immunosuppression has been followed by marrow sibling donor transplant rescue.[361] The ability to predict outcome early after treatment is helpful, because long-term survival after failure to respond to a single course of ATG plus cyclosporine is sufficiently poor[177] as to make the prompt performance of unrelated transplantation attractive, especially in severely neutropenic patients. Delayed transplantation could be employed not only for aplasia refractory to standard immunosuppression but also for relapse and late clonal disease.[351]

Androgens

Testosterone and synthetic anabolic steroids seemed a major advance in the treatment of aplastic anemia in the 1960s,[362,363] but in retrospect some responses were likely due to the inclusion of patients with only moderate acquired aplastic anemia and others with unrecognized constitutional marrow failure syndromes. For severe acquired disease, modern, often controlled trials generally have failed to demonstrate efficacy, measured as survival[116] or hematologic improvement.[276] With respect to the use of androgens as adjuncts to immunosuppression, a controlled trial in the United States did not show an increase in the response rate,[285] and in a randomized study in Europe, only a modest survival advantage was observed.[364]

Certain androgen regimens have their advocates, who have argued for response rates similar to those after ATG[365] and long survivals[366] with their use. Androgens continue to be helpful in some patients as second-line therapy, and most hematologists have observed patients who appeared to respond or even to develop hormone-dependence.[367,368] Androgens are popular in the Orient[369–372] and Mexico[373] because they are inexpensive and believed to be effective. Diverse androgens in various doses have given indistinguishable response rates of 35–60% at 6 months.[374] Nevertheless, transplantation and immunosuppression are the strongly preferred options in newly diagnosed severe aplastic anemia.

Popular commercial preparations include nandrolone decanoate, oxymetholone, and danazol. The hemoglobin response is usually more impressive than increases in granulocytes or platelets. An adequate trial is at least 3 months at full doses. Despite multiple toxic effects, among long-term survivors after androgen treatment, complications are infrequent and the patients' quality of life is good. Some rare complications are more serious and may limit effective therapy, especially in the elderly.[375] The cholestatic pattern of liver function test abnormalities is usually reversible. Hepatotoxicity (bile duct proliferation, peliosis, atypical hepatocyte hyperplasia, and tumors) can occur with all preparations but is less frequent with parenteral formulations.[376] Children appear to tolerate androgens without lasting effects on growth or maturation.[377]

Hematopoietic Growth Factors

Even if hematopoietic growth factor production is normal or increased in aplastic anemia, pharmacologic stimulation with very high doses of cytokines might be effective, either through a direct effect on residual stem cells, promoting marrow recovery, or by increasing progenitor cell activity and allowing patients to survive long enough to respond to other, more definitive therapy. G-CSF and GM-CSF are also immunomodulatory.

Neutropenia can lead to serious and life-threatening infections, and both G-CSF and GM-CSF can increase neutrophil counts in some patients with aplastic anemia.[378–384] However, there is no formal demonstration that growth factor administration, even when granulocyte counts respond, ultimately either decreases serious infections or improves survival. In a European controlled trial, the addition of G-CSF to a standard immunosuppressive regimen, while increasing neutrophil responses, did not diminish infective episodes or days of hospitalization or impact either overall response rates or survival at 5 years,[385] nor did 10-μg versus 5-μg daily dosing improve outcomes.[386] Similarly, in a controlled study of Japanese children, prolonged G-CSF was without apparent benefit.[335] Neutrophils can increase with GM-CSF adminstration,[378–381,387] and GM-CSF also has been combined with immunosuppression[388–390] but without proven benefit. Case reports suggested that combining a growth factor and cyclosporine might rescue refractory patients,[391–393] but as noted earlier, a randomized trial showed G-CSF plus cyclosporine to be inferior to ATG plus cyclosporine as first-line therapy for aplastic anemia.[394]

For both G-CSF and GM-CSF, granulocyte increases are often transient, dependent on continuous growth factor administration, and mainly restricted to less severe cases. Nevertheless, some very neutropenic patients can respond[383] and occasional bi- and trilineage responses have been observed.[384,395,396]

G-CSF and GM-CSF have immediate toxicities, including bone pain and "cytokine flu." GM-CSF increases eosinophil and monocyte counts, and G-CSF can reduce platelet numbers. Of greatest concern has been the possibility that prolonged administration of G-CSF causes late clonal disease, especially monosomy 7: in retrospective analyses of Japanese children[397–400] and adults[401,402] with severe aplastic anemia, this serious syndrome appeared to occur only among patients who had received growth factor. However, this experience has not been confirmed in Europe or the United States or in prospective studies, and the utilization of G-CSF, especially in the most neutropenic patients, confounds the interpretation of results collected retrospectively.[403]

IL-3,[404–407] IL-1,[408,409] IL-6,[410] IL-11,[411] and a chimeric IL-3/GM-CSF protein[412] have been piloted in refractory aplastic anemia, without marked benefit and often with toxicity. There are case reports of improvements in anemia[50,413] and pancytopenia[414,415] with erythropoietin, with GM-CSF and erythropoietin,[282,416–418] and with IL-3 and G-CSF.[419] Stem cell factor and G-CSF raised blood counts, including trilineage recovery, in some refractory patients,[420] but stem cell factor is unlikely to be approved for use in the United States because of its allergic complications. Megakaryocyte growth factor also may be effective in some aplastic anemia patients,[421] but commercial development has been aborted by the serious toxicity of autoantibody formation. In a large randomized protocol, the combination of G-CSF and high doses of erythropoietin improved hemoglobin values, but mainly in patients with moderate disease.[422] IL-3 combined with GM-CSF[423] or IL-3 and GM-CSF administered sequentially[424] have produced responses ranging from better neutrophil counts to trilineage recovery. Hematopoietic growth factors can be offered to patients with refractory cytopenias, but G-CSF, GM-CSF, and erythropoietin are commonly and inappropriately employed as first-line therapy in aplastic anemia, where they are of unproven and unlikely utility; a "therapeutic trial" under this circumstance can delay the institution of definitive and effective treatments.[425–427]

Moderate Aplastic Anemia

A more chronic illness, and sometimes difficult to define, moderate aplastic anemia has been less well studied than severe disease. Probably around half of patients first diagnosed as moderate progress within a few weeks or months and should be treated as having severe aplastic anemia at that time.[428] The role of anticipatory intervention has never been tested, and patient with mild blood count abnormalities may only require observation. Introduction of a therapy is usually prompted by a requirement for some transfusions, by one or more blood counts approximating severe levels, or if counts are declining. As described earlier, moderate aplastic anemia may be more likely than severe disease to respond to androgens; in a European multicenter controlled trial, addition of male hormones to an ATG regimen led to a higher hematologic response rate and better survival in more neutropenic women.[364] When directly compared in a large American multicenter trial, ATG alone was clearly superior to androgens alone.[276] Cyclosporine alone led to hematologic remissions in 11 of 13 Russian children with moderate aplastic anemia.[429] In contrast, ATG plus cyclosporine produced responses in 74% of moderate disease patients compared to 46% for cyclosporine only, but no difference in the greater than 90% survival seen in both groups.[326] At the National Institutes of Health, daclizumab, a monoclonal antibody to the IL-2 receptor and specific to activated T cells, led to clinical improvement, usually transfusion-independence, in more than one third of moderate patients; toxicity was minimal for this outpatient regimen.[430]

SUPPORTIVE CARE AND LONG-TERM MANAGEMENT

The ultimate benefits of transplantation or immunosuppression will be unrealized if the patient succumbs to an early clinical catastrophe or suffers unnecessary bleeding or infectious complications. A haphazard transfusion policy increases the risk of graft rejection after a marrow transplantation, and too frugal an approach to providing blood products can jeopardize the patient's life and increase morbidity. Supportive management therefore requires both meticulous attention to the daily problems presented by pancytopenia and appreciation of their impact on the ultimate possibilities for cure or amelioration of the disease.

Bleeding

Effective use of platelet transfusions has been credited with a substantial improvement in survival in this disease (see Chapter 98). Measurable correction of the platelet count by transfusion almost always alleviates the minor mucocutaneous bleeding common in thrombocytopenic patients. The treatment of serious hemorrhage should include correction of severe anemia because red cell transfusions may lessen bleeding symptoms.[431] Other than cost and convenience, the major problem related to platelet transfusions is the development of the refractory state in the recipient, as evidenced by lack of platelet increments on transfusion.[432] The lifespan of the transfused platelet in the circulation is dramatically shortened by host antibodies, almost always directed to HLA class I antigens. Alloimmunization is suggested by poor recovery at the 1-hour posttransfusion platelet count and confirmed by finding specific HLA antibodies in serum.[433,434] Refractoriness often can be overcome by selection of HLA-matched donors; nevertheless, 6–39% of perfectly HLA-matched transfusions fail.[434] Alloimmunization can be prevented by the use of single-donor rather than pooled platelets[435] and by physical leukocyte depletion by filtration or ultraviolet treatment[436,437]; such methods have been successfully piloted in aplastic anemia patients.[438] Avoidance of platelet transfusions except when there is active bleeding is another alternative to prevent alloimmunization, but the dose relationship between exposure to different donors' platelets and the probability of developing refractoriness is not established[434] and only at greater than 40 units was the risk of alloimmunization clearly higher.[439]

Prophylactic platelet transfusions have not been shown to alter survival,[440–446] but effects on minor bleeding complications and improvement in the quality of life have been considered sufficient justification.[442] Current practice has allowed lowering of the maintenance threshold to 10,000/μL, based on hospital testing of a refined transfusion policy[447] and a randomized trial in acute myeloid leukemia.[448]

Bone marrow sampling can be performed without prior platelet transfusions. Major surgery can be accomplished in the setting of thrombocytopenia: in one study, blood loss and morbidity were low even at levels of platelets less than 30,000/μL.[449]

Anemia

Complete replacement of erythrocytes requires transfusion of about 2 units of packed red blood cells every 2 weeks. There is little rationale for allowing a patient to suffer symptoms of anemia; once equilibrium is achieved, a constant amount of blood will be required to maintain any hemoglobin concentration. With acclimation, fit individuals are usually not symptomatic at hemoglobin concentrations greater than 7 gm/dL, and patients with underlying cardiovascular disease should be maintained at a higher level, >9 gm/dL. Aplastic anemia patients show a relatively low frequency (about 11%) of alloimmunization resulting from packed red cell transfusions.[450] Iron chelation should be used in patients with unresponsive chronic anemia who have a reasonable expectation of survival, iron accumulation, and therefore benefit from chelation (see Chapter 56). Blood products from a potential marrow donor, or from another family member such as a parent, who will share histocompatibility antigens should be avoided.

Infection

Guidelines have been based on studies of chemotherapy-induced neutropenia because there are very few investigations of infections specific to aplastic anemia.[451–453] From classic observations in leukemic children, neutropenia was shown to increase susceptibility to bacterial infections, and infectious episodes correlated with the degree and duration of neutropenia, the majority occurring at neutrophil levels less than 500/μL.[454] Susceptibility to serious infection is so extremely high at an absolute neutrophil count below 200/μL that this value has been used to define a category of "super severe" aplastic anemia. Duration is the major difference between the neutropenia of marrow failure and that induced by cytotoxic chemotherapy: with longer periods of neutropenia, the probability of serious bacterial or fungal infection increases.[455]

Similar recommendations for initiation of empirical antibiotic therapy apply to aplastic anemia patients as to other patients with neutropenia: at absolute neutrophil counts less than 500/μL and with infection suspected, broad-spectrum, parenteral antibacterial therapy should be immediately undertaken. Because bacteremia is present during only a minority of febrile neutropenic episodes, and in only about 40% of cases can a microbiologic cause or localizing physical findings be identified, early discontinuation of antibiotics because cultures are unrevealing is dangerous. Sometimes patients remain febrile despite antibacterial antibiotics; fever may also recrudesce after a few days or weeks. In the absence of additional microbiologic data or clinical clues from the patient's complaints or physical examination, antifungal therapy should be instituted in patients who remain febrile despite adequate antibacterial therapy for more than 3 days. Fungemia during an initial febrile episode is rare,[456] but fungal infection becomes more likely with repeated courses of antibiotics and ultimately represent the major cause of death in aplastic anemia.[457] *Candida* and *Aspergillosis* species account for almost all fungal disease in aplastic anemia.[457] Early aggressive treatment can reverse fungal disease,[458–460] and G-CSF–mobilized granulocyte transfusions may be of clinical benefit.[461–464]

Infections can be prevented, often by simple but neglected measures such as handwashing.[465] A ward's physical surroundings should be well maintained to reduce nosocomial infection. Dental hygiene should be sustained and sources of infection removed. Nystatin oral rinses prevent thrush.[466] "Routine" rectal examinations are more likely to be harmful than helpful. Blood should not be taken from fingertips and ear lobes. Early attention to the signs of infection, especially after discharge from the hospital, can avert many of the catastrophic complications of initially minor infectious episodes. Total protective environments and selective gut decontamination are not obviously superior to simpler methods of isolation,[467] and reverse isolation accomplishes little more than compulsive handwashing.[468] Sterile diets, avoidance of fresh fruit and vegetables, and no flowers in the room are popular proscriptions of similarly unproven value.

PROGNOSIS

Collections of published cases of aplastic anemia from the era when diagnosis was made at autopsy described a disease with a fatal outcome in days to months, and entirely untreated severe disease must be almost invariably fatal. The rate of spontaneous recovery is difficult to estimate but likely low. In the IAAAS epidemiologic survey, about 5% of cases with hypoplastic marrows were excluded because their pancytopenia resolved, most within a few weeks.[289] In an older series of pediatric patients treated mainly with transfusions, only 3% of 334 were judged to be eventually cured,[145] and among more recently reported African patients treated with transfusions, corticosteroids, and androgens, mortality at 18 months was 72%,[14] similar to American case series[469] and controls in early transplantation protocols[116] collected in the 1970s. None of 21 controls randomized to supportive care only rather than ATG improved during 3 months of observation.[275]

Prognosis is correlated with presentation blood counts, and extremely severe neutropenia (<200/μL) characterizes a very high-risk group. Most patients with severe aplastic anemia treated by stem cell transplantation are cured of their marrow failure; their survival is a function of age at transplantation as the major determinant of graft-versus-host disease risk. For immunosuppression, very severe neutropenia is a negative because early fatal infection precludes the possibility of a hematologic response. In general, children and less neutropenic patients have the best outcomes. Hematologic recovery and especially robust hematologic improvement post-ATG and cyclosporine are highly prognostic of long-term survival.[177] Pretreatment special testing has not been sufficiently reproducible or reliable either to guide the choice of transplantation versus ATG or to permit prediction of recovery with immunosuppressive drugs; monitoring of putatively pathogenic T cells molecularly[308] or immunophenotypically[470] may ultimately help to predict and monitor responses and relapses.

"Late" Clonal Hematologic Disease

Both in its clinical implications and at a basic biologic level, the evolution of clonal hematologic diseases from immune-mediated bone marrow failure is one of aplastic anemia's most striking and least understood characteristics.

Paroxysmal Nocturnal Hemoglobinuria

When PNH was solely diagnosed by testing red cells in the Ham or sucrose lysis test, it appeared to be a late manifestation of aplastic anemia—now understood to be an artifact caused by the early replacement of patient cells by transfused blood. By flow cytometry of not only erythrocytes but also granulocytes and monocytes, a large proportion of patients with aplastic anemia have evidence of PNH clonal expansion at the time of first clinical presentation, with small numbers of abnormal cells detected in 50%,[471,472] 67%,[473,474] or 90% of patients,[475] depending on the method; only a few patients actually acquire a PNH clone late, and others lose their clone over time.[476] In flow cytometric assays, a proportion of circulating blood cells lack glycosylphosphoinositol-anchored proteins on their cell surface, as a result of an acquired mutation in the *PIG-A* gene in a single (or a few) hematopoietic stem cells. Stem cells with *PIG-A* lesions exist in most normal adults, but the expansion of the clone occurs only with underlying marrow failure, subtle evidence for which can be inferred from hematopoietic progenitor assays even in hemolytic PNH with a cellular marrow and relatively normal blood counts (see Chapter 25). Association of PNH clonal expansion with HLA-DR2 and its prognostic link to recovery with immunosuppressive therapy[475,477–479] imply a relationship with the immune pathophysiology of marrow failure, and PNH progenitor cells, in comparison to the phenotypically normal cells in the same marrow, appear to be spared by cytotoxic T cells,[476,480,481] but the precise mechanism of clonal selection has not been elucidated. Early in aplastic anemia the PNH clone is small, and further increase in clone size occurs slowly if at all,[476] so that most patients with the aplastic anemia/PNH syndrome do not have typical PNH manifestations of hemolysis and thrombosis. However, brisk intravascular hemolysis may become clinically dominant years after successful restoration of blood counts by immunosuppressive therapy.

Cytogenetic Abnormalities and Myelodysplasia

Dameshek first postulated a classification of aplastic anemia with malignant myeloproliferative disorders,[482] a provocative nosology much revisited.[483–485] Leukemia was described as an unusual complication of aplastic anemia in case reports before the era of immunosuppressive treatment[486–488]; among 156 patients treated with androgens, there were 5 cases of late-onset myelodysplasia and 1 of lymphoma.[366] With the success of ATG and consequent prolonged survival, clonal evolution became recognized as an important feature of aplastic anemia.[489,490] Incomplete follow-up, sporadic marrow examination, and diagnostic uncertainties make early quantitation of risk unreliable.[491] More accurate figures derive from retrospective analyses of registry data: of 223 long-term survivors after immunosuppression, 11 had myelodysplasia and 5 of them later manifested acute myeloid leukemia (combined risk of 15% at 7 years).[489] Similarly, among National Institutes of Health patients who had been treated with ATG and cyclosporine and assessed with annual marrow examination, including cytogenetics, 13 of 122 evolved to a new hematologic diagnosis, for an actuarial risk of about 16% at 7 years; myelodysplasia occurred late and usually in patients who had failed treatment and remained pancytopenic.[177] Monosomy 7 is the most frequent cytogenetic abnormality and associated with a poor outcome because of refractory pancytopenia and development of acute myeloid leukemia; trisomy 8 has a more benign course and blood counts often are stable with continued cyclosporine therapy.[177,492] Chromosomal abnormalities, even those of chromosome 7, may be transient.[191,192,493–495]

The mechanisms of clonal evolution are becoming clearer. As discussed earlier, chronic administration of G-CSF has been blamed for evolution to monosomy 7 and acute leukemia; high endogenous or exogenously administered G-CSF appears to select for cells bearing truncated G-CSF receptors, which signal for proliferation over differentiation.[495] In contrast, in trisomy 8, cytotoxic T cells specifically recognize cytogenetically aberrant hematopoietic targets, but these cells do not undergo apoptosis.[496–498]

CURRENT CONTROVERSIES & FUTURE CONSIDERATIONS

Aplastic Anemia

- The exact nature of the inciting antigens, the determinants of an aberrant, presumably autoimmune response, and the forces that drive development of the somatic genetic alterations leading to late clonal hematologic diseases remain outstanding questions of clinical and biologic importance.
- Is there an infectious agent responsible for posthepatitis aplastic anemia, fulminant hepatitis of childhood, and acute seronegative hepatitis?
- Can results with immunosuppression be improved with a longer cyclosporine course (years rather than months), addition of new immunosuppressive drugs (mycophenolate mofetil, rapamycin), or replacement of ATG with more potent agents (fludarabine, Campath)?
- Should young patients who fail ATG and cyclosporine immediately undergo stem cell transplantation from an unrelated donor?
- The role of peripheral blood as a source of hematopoietic stem cells needs formal comparison with traditional bone marrow transplantation.

Suggested Readings*

Barrett J, Sauntharajah Y, Molldrem J: Myelodysplastic syndrome and aplastic anemia: distinct entities or diseases linked by a common pathophysiology? Semin Hematol 37:15–29, 2000.

Georges GE, Storb R: Stem cell transplantation for aplastic anemia. Int J Hematol 75:141–146, 2002.

Kondo Y, Molldrem JJ: Immune-induced cytopenia: bone marrow failure syndrome. Curr Hematol Rep 3:178–183, 2004.

Kurre P, Johnson FL, Deeg HJ: Diagnosis and treatment of children with aplastic anemia. Pediatr Blood Cancer 2005 (in press).

Marsh JC: Management of acquired aplastic anaemia. Blood Rev 19:143–151, 2005.

Yamaguchi H, Calado RT, Ly H: Mutations in TERT, the gene for telomerase reverse transcriptase, in aplastic anemia. N Engl J Med 352:1413–1424, 2005.

Young NS: Hematopoietic cell destruction by immune mechanisms in acquired aplastic anemia. Semin Hematol 37:3–14, 2000.

Young NS: Immunosuppressive treatment of acquired aplastic anemia and immune-mediated bone marrow failure syndromes. Int J Hematol 75:129–140, 2002.

Full references for this chapter can be found on accompanying CD-ROM.

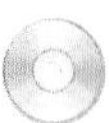

CHAPTER 11

Constitutional Aplastic Anemias

Johnson M. Liu, MD, FACP, and Inderjeet Dokal, MD, FRCPCH, FRCP, FRCPath

KEY POINTS

Constitutional Aplastic Anemias

- Historically, Fanconi's anemia (FA) and dyskeratosis congenita (DC) were viewed as marrow failure syndromes of infants and young children, associated with classic somatic stigmata. However, the heterogeneity of physical findings, family history, and age of onset make diagnosis based on clinical features alone difficult and often unreliable.
- DC and FA can both present as aplastic anemia alone, and appropriate laboratory studies should be undertaken to exclude them in older patients with bone marrow failure.
- The genes mutated in constitutional aplastic anemias serve crucial "housekeeping functions" in the cell. FA genes have a key role in preserving genomic stability, DC genes in the maintenance of telomeres.
- For the DC genes involved in telomere repair, phenotypic variability is apparent from the variable manifestations within a single family. DC gene mutations have been described also in the Hoyeraal-Hreidarsson syndrome, which produces severe multiorgan failure in infants and children, and in adult patients with apparently "acquired" aplastic anemia.
- Androgens such as oxymetholone can produce durable hematologic responses in most FA and DC patients, but their use requires careful monitoring for specific toxicities.
- Severe aplastic anemia is definitively treated by stem cell transplantation. In both FA and DC, low-intensity transplant protocols can produce prompt hematopoietic engraftment and reduce procedure-related toxicity, and they may lower the risk of late secondary malignancies.

INTRODUCTION

A number of inherited (constitutional/genetic) disorders are characterized by aplastic anemia, classically in association with one or more somatic abnormalities.[1] Fanconi's anemia (FA) and dyskeratosis congenita (DC) are the most important of these disorders. In both FA and DC, bone marrow failure may be present at birth or appear during childhood or even in adulthood in some cases. Remarkable recent advances in the understanding of the genetic basis of FA and DC have helped unravel their complex pathophysiology and provided important insights into normal hematopoiesis.

FANCONI'S ANEMIA

FA, the best defined inherited bone marrow failure disorder, was first described by the Swiss pediatrician Fanconi in three brothers with a syndrome of aplastic anemia and congenital physical anomalies.[1] In addition to the chief criteria of pancytopenia, hyperpigmentation, malformation of the skeleton, small stature, and hypogonadism noted by Fanconi, diverse malformations of the eye, ear, genitourinary and gastrointestinal tracts, and cardiopulmonary and central nervous systems can occur (Fig. 11–1). FA is notoriously heterogeneous in the degree and number of clinical manifestations,[2] and patients presenting solely with either congenital malformations or hematologic abnormalities may either be misdiagnosed or go unrecognized entirely.

The modern diagnosis of FA no longer rests upon the constellation of abnormalities described by Fanconi but is based on finding chromosomal breakage after incubation of the patient's cells with chromosome-damaging (clastogenic) agents such as diepoxybutane (DEB) or mitomycin C (MMC)[3,4] (see Fig. 11–1). This strict laboratory diagnosis has enabled the identification of affected indi-

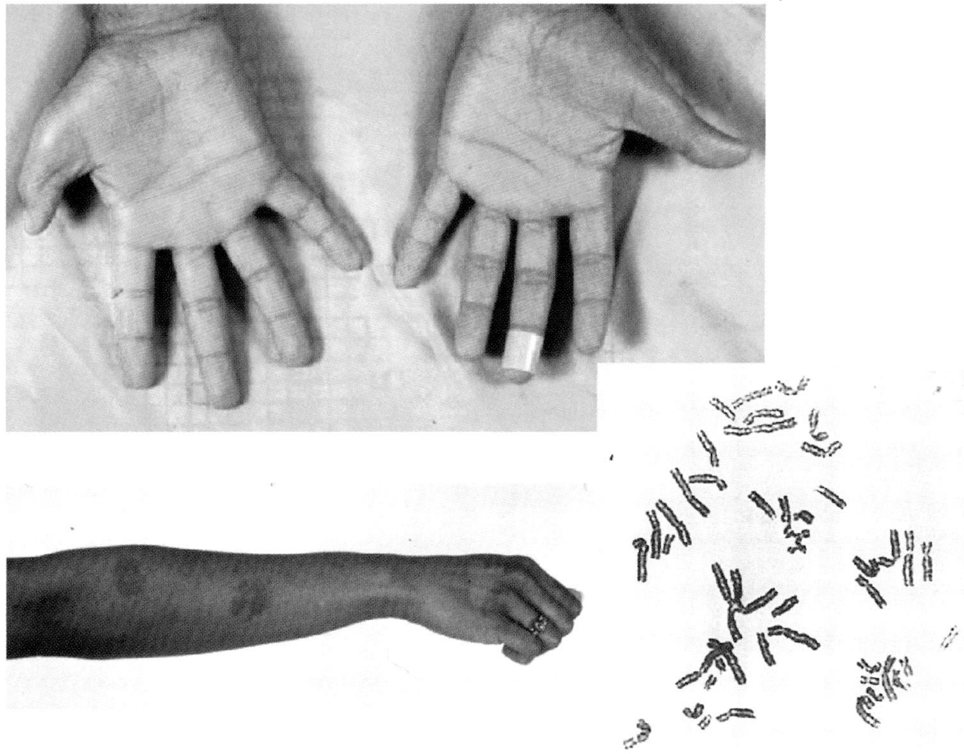

Figure 11–1. Photographs of chromosomal breakage and congenital anomalies seen in FA patients. Shown are: thumb abnormality in an adult patient who had undergone surgery in childhood and characteristic skin pigmentation changes in an African-American patient. Right inset shows characteristic chromosomal breaks and radial figures in FA cells treated with mitomycin C.

viduals, some of whom were unsuspected because of advanced age at presentation or the absence of physical anomalies. Specific testing has led to appreciation of the heterogeneity of the disease. FA usually presents with aplastic anemia, indistinguishable from the acquired type. Data from the International Fanconi Anemia Registry (IFAR) indicate that almost all FA patients will eventually develop hematologic abnormalities (thrombocytopenia or pancytopenia).[5] Thus FA is nosologically linked with acquired aplastic anemia (see Chapter 10), although the hematologic manifestations are only a part of the FA syndrome. In addition, FA patients are susceptible to both hematologic and solid organ malignancy.[6]

Diagnosis by Chromosome Breakage Analysis

Sensitivity of FA cells to DNA-alkylating (cross-linking) agents was first recognized nearly 40 years after the original clinical description.[7] At present, chromosome breakage analysis remains the basis for the diagnosis of FA. Testing is typically performed by scoring chromosome preparations for breakage after exposure to DEB or MMC[3,4] (see Fig. 11–1). At a biochemical level, monoadducts and diadducts (interstrand cross-links) are induced in DNA by bifunctional cross-linking agents such as DEB, MMC, nitrogen mustard, cyclophosphamide, cisplatin, or activated psoralens. Interstrand cross-links are thought to block DNA replication and RNA transcription, with potent effects on cell survival and function. For FA, specific cellular defects following exposure to these agents include the induction of chromosomal aberrations (breaks and rearrangements),[8] delayed transit and arrest in the G_2 phase of the cell cycle[9] with a consequent decrease in the numbers of cells synthesizing DNA,[10] and cell death.[11]

A confounding factor in the diagnosis of FA by chromosome breakage analysis is "reverse mosaicism."[12–14] In the course of testing patients' lymphocytes for sensitivity to MMC, it was noted that approximately 25% of FA patients had evidence of spontaneously occurring mosaicism, as manifested by the presence of two subpopulations of lymphocytes, one hypersensitive to MMC (as expected for FA) and a second behaving normally in response to MMC. In the initial report of eight FA patients with evidence of mosaicism, three were compound heterozygotes for a pathogenic FA gene, and the molecular mechanism of the mosaicism was attributed to recombination or gene conversion events.[13] Even FA patients initially diagnosed as a result of MMC breakage analysis could develop near-complete reversion in blood cells, raising the possibility that chromosome breakage tests could be interpreted as negative. In such circumstances, breakage analysis performed in nonhematopoietic tissues (presumably not subject to selective pressure for reversion), such as skin fibroblasts, allows the correct diagnosis to be made.[14] The prognostic significance of mosaicism is unclear at present.[15]

Epidemiology and Genetics

FA was proven to be an autosomal recessive disorder in the 1970s.[16] FA is rare, occurring in approximately 5 per 1 million births. All races and ethnic groups are affected. As the FA genes have been identified, specific mutations have been associated with particular ethnic groups as a result of a "founder effect." Because of these strong associations, the carrier frequency for certain mutations can be remarkably high in selected populations (see later), and for the general population has been estimated at approximately 1:300 in the United States, Europe, and Japan. The three most common FA genes in the Western hemisphere are *FANCA, FANCC,* and *FANCG.*

The variable clinical appearance of FA has long suggested genetic heterogeneity, because mutations in different genes could lead to alternative phenotypes. Complementation (correction of the increased sensitivity of FA cells to the cytotoxic action of DNA cross-linking agents) has been used to define this genetic heterogeneity. Many studies have been based on hybrid lymphoblast cell lines from patients: selectable markers were introduced into FA cells and used to isolate hybrids after fusion. Complementation of the FA phenotype was assessed by analysis of spontaneous and MMC-induced chromosomal breakage and of growth inhibition by MMC. Currently, there is evidence for at least 12 FA genes (*FANCA, FANCB, FANCC, FANCD1, FANCD2, FANCE, FANCF, FANCG, FANCI, FANCJ, FANCL,* and *FANCM*),[17–21] with more complementation groups being identified as the number of cell lines examined increases (Table 11–1).

Most of the FA genes were cloned by exploiting the increased sensitivity of FA cells to DNA cross-linking agents. As first successfully applied to FA-C, complementary DNA (cDNA) libraries in episomal vectors were used to isolate a series of cDNAs that complemented the cellular defects of FA-C cells.[22] These FA-C cDNAs did not correct the defects in FA-A, FA-B, or FA-D cells, and a mutation in this gene was found in the cell line used for the cloning. The cDNAs encode a novel protein known as FANCC. A splice mutation in intron 4 (IVS4 + 4 A→T) is the predominant mutation in all FA patients of Ashkenazi Jewish origin,[23] and the carrier frequency of this mutant allele in a selected Jewish population has been determined to be 1.1%.[24] FA-C patients can be divided into three subgroups based on genotype-phenotype analysis: patients with the intron 4 mutation; those with at least one exon 14 mutation (R548X or L554P); and those with at least one exon 1 mutation (322delG or Q13X) and no known exon 14 mutation.[25] In Kaplan-Meier analysis, patients with either an intron 4 or an exon 14 mutation suffered from a significantly earlier onset of hematologic abnormalities and poorer survival as compared to exon 1 patients and to the non–FA-C IFAR population.

TABLE 11–1. Fanconi's Anemia Gene Products, Mutations, Chromosomal Location, Exons, and Protein Structure

Gene	Mutations	Location	Exons	Protein (AA)
FANCA	~100	16q24.3	43	1455
FANCB	4	Xp22.31	10	859
FANCC	10	9q22.3	14	558
FANCD1	= *BRCA2?*	13q12-13	26	3418
FANCD2	5	3p25.3	44	1451
FANCE	3	6p21.3	10	536
FANCF	6	11p15	1	374
FANCG	18	9p13	14	622
FANCI				
*FANCJ**				
FANCL	= *PHF9?*	2p16	14	375
*FANCM**				

Abbreviation: AA, amino acids.
**FANCJ* (also called BRIP1/BACH1) and *FANCM* were identified in 2005. Both proteins have DNA-unwinding (Helicase) motifs. *FANCM* is a member of the FA core complex, whereas *FANCJ* acts independently of the complex (as do *FANCD1* and *FANCD2*).

Approximately 65% of FA patients from Europe and North America belong to complementation group A,[26–28] and this major FA mutant gene, *FANCA,* has been identified.[29–31] In contrast to *FANCC,* for which a few mutations account for nearly all cases, mutations in *FANCA* are widely dispersed through the gene and more likely to be unique for each patient.[32]

Pathophysiology

The FA Complex and Its Link with the BRCA Pathway

A seminal series of observations led to a model of FA function that emphasizes a role in DNA damage processing through close links with the breast cancer susceptibility gene products BRCA1 and BRCA2. The first five FA genes (*FANCA, FANCC, FANCE, FANCF,* and *FANCG*) were identified by expression cloning and have no homology either to each other or to other proteins of known function.[22,30,31,33–36] However, based on the similar clinical and cellular phenotypes among the FA complementation groups, the FA proteins were proposed to cooperate in a common cellular pathway.[37] FANCC was first found to interact with FANCA,[38] and all five FA proteins appear to cooperate to form a nuclear complex,[39–44] the so-called core complex. The formation of the FA nuclear complex was disrupted in all mutant cell lines except for FA-D cells.[45] This complementation group was also genetically heterogeneous, consisting of at least two genes, *FANCD1* and *FANCD2.*[46] Thus, FANCD1 and FANCD2 function downstream or independently of the FA protein complex.

With the positional cloning of *FANCD2* came recognition that its gene product was normally modified by posttranslational monoubiquitination in normal cells (but not in FA-A, FA-C, FA-F, or FA-G cells).[46,47] FA protein complex formation either serves as or recruits a ubiquitin ligase, whose key substrate is FANCD2. The importance of this modification was illustrated by its induction by DNA damage or cell cycle progression and its abrogation in most FA cell lines. Monoubiquitinated FANCD2 was found to target discrete, ionizing radiation–induced nuclear foci, co-localizing with the breast cancer susceptibility protein BRCA1 (Fig. 11–2). Finally, the discovery[48] of biallelic inactivation of *BRCA2* in cell lines from FA-B and FA-D1 patients suggests that *BRCA2* is either a FA gene (*FANCD1*) or a FA-like gene[49] and that BRCA2 and

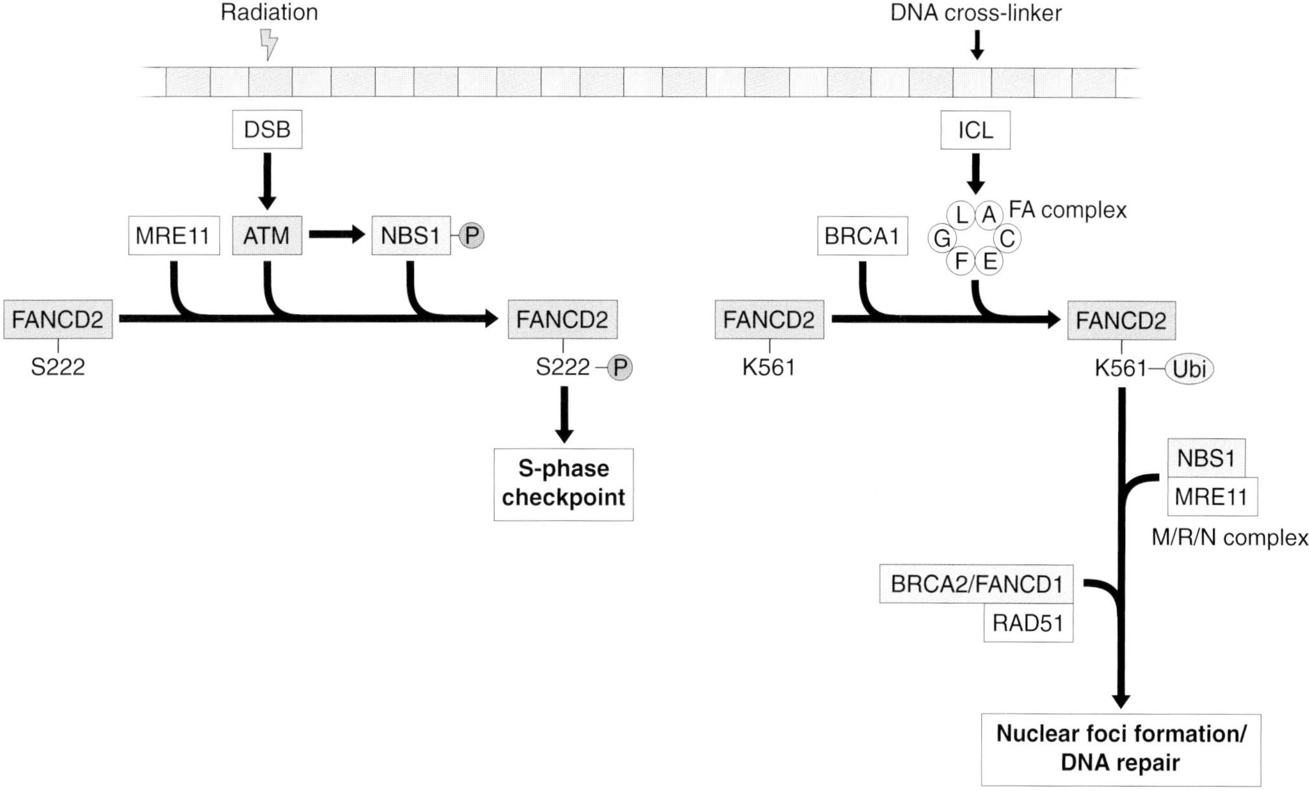

Figure 11–2. Interaction between FANCD2, ATM, and NBS1. FANCD2 undergoes phosphorylation and monoubiquitination and interacts with ATM, NBS1, and BRCA1 to respond to DNA double-stranded breaks (DSBs) and interstrand cross-links (ICLs). Other members of the DSB repair pathway include RAD51, MRE11, and the MRE11/RAD50/NBS1 (or M/R/N) complex. ATM phosphorylates FANCD2 at serine 222 (S222), and BRCA1 somehow facilitates FANCD2 monoubiquitination at lysine 561 (K561). The newly discovered PHF9, or FANCL, is a component of the FA core complex that possesses E3 ubiquitin ligase activity and appears to be essential for monoubiquitination of FANCD2.

other FA proteins cooperate in a common DNA damage-response pathway. Recently, PHF9, or FANCL,[50] was discovered as a new component of the FA core complex that possesses E3 ubiquitin ligase activity in vitro and appears to be essential for monoubiquitination of FANCD2. Another newly identified member of the FA core complex is FANCB, whose gene was unexpectedly localized to the X chromosome.[51]

To maintain genomic integrity in the face of DNA damage, cells must undergo a regulated process of DNA replication and repair, genetic recombination, cell cycle transit, chromosome segregation, and programmed cell death. Chromosomal instability occurs when these homeostatic processes fail, resulting in genetic syndromes such as ataxia-telangiectasia, Nijmegen breakage syndrome (NBS), Bloom syndrome, and FA.[52] Inactivating mutations in these syndromes all cause defects in DNA damage signaling. Double-stranded breaks (DSBs)[53] are a particular form of DNA damage that is dangerous to cells because of the difficulty in their repair.[52] DNA damage activates "checkpoints" that delay progression through the cell cycle, thus providing time for damage repair prior to the critical events of DNA replication at S phase or chromosome segregation at mitosis. Ataxia-telangiectasia cells are characteristically defective in induction of all these checkpoints in response to DSBs,[54] and the ataxia-telangiectasia protein, ATM, encodes an ionizing radiation–activated protein kinase. ATM responds to DNA damage by phosphorylation of key components of the cell cycle checkpoints, including p53 and BRCA1.[55]

The FA pathway has a remarkable interconnection with the tumor suppressors BRCA1 and BRCA2, genetic defects in which predispose individuals to familial breast and ovarian cancer.[56,57] Germline mutations in the *BRCA1* and *BRCA2* tumor suppressor genes account for approximately 5–10% of all breast cancer cases[56–58] (collectively, 70–95% of hereditary and a small percentage of sporadic breast and ovarian cancers[59–61]). *BRCA1* and *BRCA2* genes encode large proteins[56,57] bearing little sequence homology to previously identified proteins. However, several repeated motifs have been found.[62] BRCA1 contains a ring-finger domain and two BRCA1 carboxy-terminal domains, both involved in protein-protein interactions[63–69] that may explain many of its functions.[70] (The recently identified *FANCJ* or BRIP1 helicase binds to a cleft between the carboxy-terminal domains.) BRCA1 has been proposed to form a multi-subunit protein complex, referred to as the BRCA1-associated genome surveillance complex,[71] which includes DNA repair proteins as well as gene products first identified as mutated in various chromosomal breakage syndromes.[52] This suggests the existence of a dynamic and interrelated protein complex that cooperates to maintain genomic integrity in the face of various types of DNA damage. ATM was found to phosphorylate FANCD2.[72] This phosphorylation event is required for activation of an S-phase cell cycle checkpoint. Other members of the BRCA1-associated genome surveillance complex, including NBS1[73] and Bloom syndrome (BLM) protein,[74] to interact with FANCD2 and the core FA complex, respectively. These associations have led to a model of involvement of the FA pathway in processing or repair of DSBs and interstrand cross-links (see Fig. 11–2).

Activated FANCD2 and BRCA1 have been associated with chromatin.[47] FANCA, FANCC, and FANCG also localized to the nuclear matrix and chromatin, particularly following DNA damage.[75] FANCA interacts with BRG1, one of the two catalytic subunits of the SWI/SNF ATP-dependent chromatin remodeling complex.[76] In biochemical fractionation studies the FA core complex exists in different configurations in cytoplasmic, nuclear, and chromatin-associated compartments.[77]

FA Proteins, Reactive Oxygen Species, and Apoptosis

The first FA gene product to be cloned, FANCC, was initially localized predominantly to the cytoplasm.[78,79] To identify a cytoplasmic function for FANCC, investigators sought proteins that interacted with FANCC and then related their function to the FA phenotype.[80] FA proteins were hypothesized to have a role in detoxification of reactive oxygen species (ROS). Mutant FA cells appear to be hypersensitive to oxygen,[81] and ROS-scavenging enzymes[82–84] can protect FA cells from chromosomal damage and cell death. Many of the pathophysiologic features of FA might be attributed to a state of oxidative stress.[82,85] Studies of FANCC and elements of the redox metabolic pathway, such as NADPH cytochrome P-450 reductase[86] and glutathione-S-transferase P-1 (GSTP1),[87] suggest that FA proteins counter ROS-induced damage and apoptotic signaling.[88] For example, overexpression of FANCC and GSTP1,[87] a phase II detoxification enzyme that catalyzes the conjugation of glutathione with various xenobiotics, in a myeloid progenitor cell line prevented apoptosis following growth factor deprivation.[87,89] FANCC also increased GSTP1 activity after the induction of apoptosis. FA hematopoietic progenitors are hypersensitive to growth inhibition by cytokines such as interferon-γ,[90] tumor necrosis factor-α,[91,92] and macrophage inflammatory protein-1α.[92] Overexpression of FANCC protects hematopoietic progenitors from death induced by Fas (CD95)-mediated apoptosis,[93] whereas tumor necrosis factor-α and CD95 ligation suppress erythropoiesis in Fancc$^{-/-}$ mice.[91]

Cell Death Mechanisms: FANCC and FANCD2

One important function of the FA proteins is modulation of apoptosis. FANCC suppressed a DNA cross-linker–inducible apoptosis pathway in *FANCC*-mutant lymphoblastoid cell lines[94]; overexpression of wild-type FANCC protein protected hematopoietic cells from apoptosis.[89] FANCC was inferred to act downstream in the pathway regulating programmed cell death; when FANCC is absent or defective, mutant cells may be unusually susceptible to various forms of apoptotic stimuli. Bone marrow failure may be secondary to continuing and cumulative apoptosis of hematopoietic stem cells. Recent experiments on the zebrafish homologue of FANCD2 have suggested that physical anomalies in FA may also be due to inappropriate cell apoptosis in developing tissues.[95]

Clinical Features and Diagnosis

Heterogeneity of Presentation

The diagnosis of FA is usually suspected by a pediatrician when a child has classic features[96]: hyper- or hypopigmented skin lesions; short stature (poor growth); anomalies of the upper limb or thumb; male hypogonadism; microcephaly; characteristic facial features, including a broadened nasal base, epicanthal folds, and micrognathia; and structural renal abnormalities. When this constellation of physical anomalies is accompanied by bone marrow failure, confirmation of the diagnosis can be made by DEB or MMC chromosome breakage tests. The mean age at diagnosis is 8 or 9 years. With the advent of the chromosome breakage test, however, has come increasing recognition of the heterogeneity of FA in terms of clinical presentation. Based solely on definition by the DEB test, nearly 40% of the first 200 patients analyzed in the IFAR were reported to be free of major physical anomalies.[3] Such normal-appearing patients had previously been identified by noting their familial presentation with hypoplastic or aplastic anemia.[97,98] FA homozygotes with normal appearances may not be recognized unless there is a high index of suspicion for familial disease.[99] Another challenge is the diagnosis of FA in older patients. Although the mean age of diagnosis is in the first decade of life, presentation of FA has been described in a 56-year-old woman.[100]

Symptoms, Signs, and Hematologic Indices

The symptoms and signs of FA typically relate to the cytopenias. Often thrombocytopenia or leukopenia occurs first before pancytopenia, which worsens with time. Almost all FA patients will develop hematologic abnormalities in their lifetime.[5] Erythropoiesis is usually macrocytic, recognized by Fanconi as "perniziosiforme," or "pernicious-like."[1] Classically, the bone marrow is hypocellular and fatty, indistinguishable from that of acquired aplastic anemia. Microscopic examination of the marrow may show dyserythropoiesis and dysplasia. Some patients develop or present with a morphologically defined myelodysplastic syndrome (MDS) or frank acute myeloid leukemia (AML).[101]

Cancer

The risk of developing MDS and AML[102] is high: progression to AML occurs in at least 10–15% of cases, with increasing risk with age. Less commonly recognized is the probability of developing MDS (~5%), which appears also to correlate with a poor prognosis for FA patients. Clonal karyotypic abnormalities, identical to those seen in non-FA MDS and secondary AML, are frequent in FA whether or not marrow morphologic criteria for defined MDS are met. The prognostic significance of these clonal chromosomal abnormalities in FA patients is not clear, because cytogenetic changes can fluctuate over time.[103] Clonal hematopoiesis in this setting may simply reflect a reduced stem cell pool. However, gain of chromosomal segment 3q is strongly associated with a poor prognosis and is an adverse risk factor.[104]

With better supportive care and longer survival, solid organ malignancies, especially vulvar, esophageal, and head and neck cancers,[6,105] have become major causes of morbidity and mortality. In a statistical analysis of North American FA patients,[105] the cumulative incidence of a solid tumor rose to 29% by age 48. In addition, a subset of long-term survivors of stem cell transplantation will develop secondary malignancies, particularly head and neck cancer (see later). These clinical data likely reflect an intrinsic propensity of mutant FA cells to undergo malignant transformation.[106] Whether FA squamous cell carcinomas are associated with human papillomavirus is not yet established.[107]

As discussed above, BRCA2 is identical to FANCD1. Germline mutations in *BRCA2* were found in five kindreds with FA, early-onset acute leukemia, and breast cancer.[108]

Treatment

Allogeneic hematopoietic stem cell transplantation (HSCT) from a human lymphocyte antigen (HLA)-matched sibling donor is the only curative therapy for the hematologic manifestations of FA (aplasia or myelodysplasia). Decreased doses of cyclophosphamide and irradiation must be used in order to avoid severe toxicity resulting from the chemo- and radiosensitivity of FA. When FA patients early underwent standard HSCT, they suffered a uniformly poor outcome as a result of preparative-regimen toxicity, severe graft-versus-host disease, and infection.[109] Based on biologic and clinical observations, investigators from Paris championed the use of a conditioning regimen of low-dose (20 mg/kg) cyclophosphamide and 5 Gy thoracoabdominal irradiation[110] (Fig. 11–3*A*). Collected data from multiple institutions (with over 150 FA patients) yielded an overall 2-year survival rate of 66% (range, 58–73%), with lower dose cyclophosphamide and limited-field irradiation correlated with improved survival.[111] Older age at transplantation and low platelet count prior to HSCT were also associated with a lower rate of survival, mostly as a result of increased graft failure and chronic graft-versus-host disease. Umbilical cord blood transplantation from related donors also has been successfully applied to a small number of FA patients.[112,113] A few FA patients have undergone successful stem cell transplantation from cord blood of unrelated donors.[114]

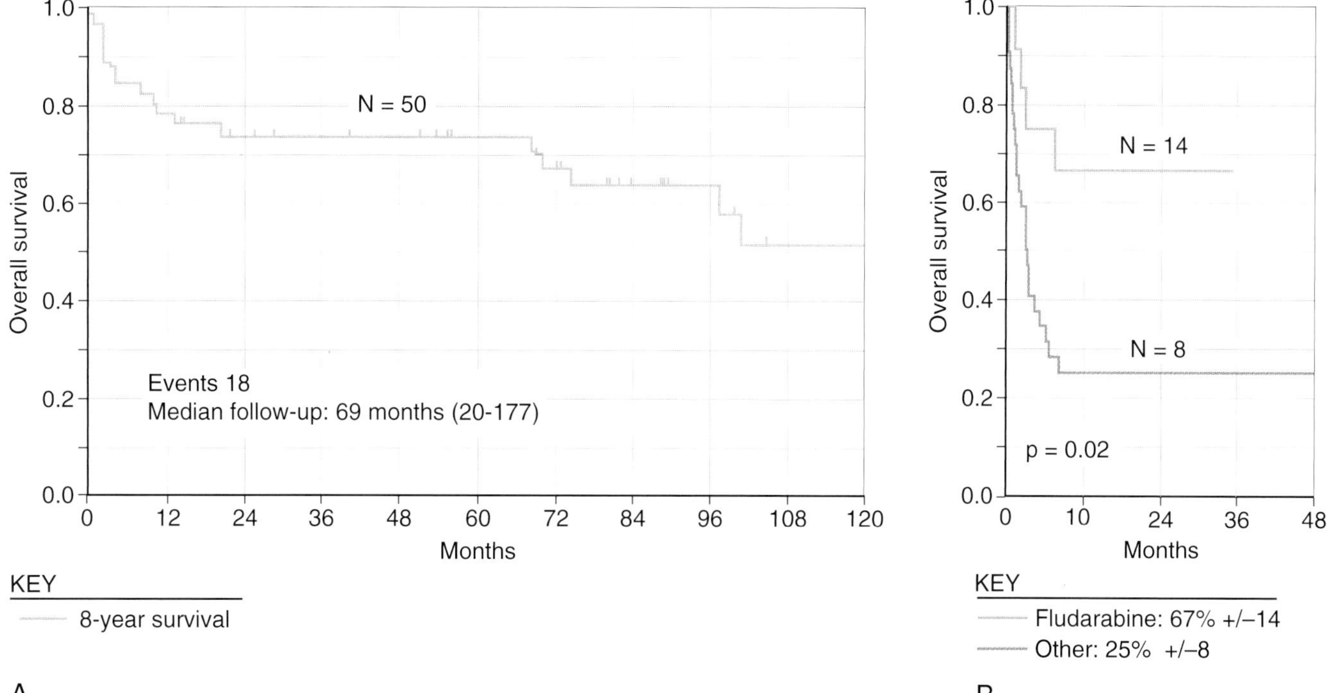

Figure 11–3. *A,* Survival of 50 FA patients who received HLA-matched sibling bone marrow transplantation according to the Paris conditioning regimen. *B,* Survival of 44 FA patients who received cord blood cell transplantation from an unrelated donor, divided into two groups according to the inclusion of fludarabine in the conditioning regimen. (Data courtesy of Prof. Eliane Gluckman, Hospital Saint Louis, Paris.)

Despite success in treating the aplasia of FA by HSCT, some survivors will suffer later secondary malignancies, particularly of the head and neck.[115–117] On long-term follow-up, 7 of a cohort of 50 patients transplanted according to the Paris conditioning regimen developed cancer (8-year projected incidence, 24%) reflective of the continued genetic susceptibility of host nonhematopoietic tissues to carcinogenesis. The role of irradiation as a cofactor for malignancy cannot be excluded, but patients transplanted at Seattle who did not receive irradiation also developed late cancers.[118] Acute graft-versus-host disease also may represent a major risk factor.[119]

Clearly, young patients with an HLA-compatible sibling should be treated by HSCT at the earliest stages of marrow failure, in preference to other therapies. However, most patients do not have an HLA-identical donor and are dependent upon finding a suitably matched nonsibling relative or unrelated donor. A small number of FA patients have undergone HSCT from alternative sources (matched unrelated and haploidentical family donors): initial analysis of 48 patients showed a 29% 2-year survival rate.[111] In a large single-institution study,[120,121] 29 patients conditioned with cyclophosphamide (40 mg/kg) and total-body irradiation (4.0–6.0 Gy) had a probability of survival of 34% at 1 year. With the advent of fludarabine-based conditioning regimens, transplantation protocols without total-body irradiation have been reported for both HLA-compatible sibling and unrelated donors; early results are promising[122] (Fig. 11–3*B*).

Supportive Care and Long-Term Management

Patients lacking a suitable HLA-compatible donor (sibling or matched unrelated) often benefit from chronic administration of androgens or hematopoietic growth factors. First used to treat FA in 1959,[123] androgens induce hematologic responses in 50–75% of patients, although their effectiveness in raising blood counts may be neither durable nor complete in all lineages.[124] Typically, androgen therapy is initiated when the platelet count is consistently below 30,000/μL and/or the hemoglobin less than 7 gm/dL. Orally administered oxymetholone, at a dose of 2–5 mg/kg/day, is usually combined with prednisone, 5–10 mg every other day, in order to counterbalance the anabolic properties of oxymetholone with the catabolic actions of corticosteroids.[125] Androgens are associated with multiple liver toxicities, including transaminase enzyme elevation, cholestasis, peliosis hepatis, and hepatic tumors (the latter only rarely seen in patients not treated with androgens). Injectable androgens have a decreased risk of hepatotoxicity, but pediatricians have sometimes objected to them over concerns of pain and local bleeding: one standard formulation is nandrolone decanoate, administered by intramuscular injection at a dose of 1–2 mg/kg/wk.

Levels of most growth factors, including the stem/progenitor cell—active Flt-3 ligand,[126] are markedly increased in FA as they are in acquired aplastic anemia, as a compensatory physiologic response. Nevertheless, chronic administration of granulocyte colony-stimulating factor may have transient beneficial effects on multiple hematopoietic lineages. In a study of 12 FA patients with neutropenia,[127] granulocyte colony-stimulating factor at 5 μg/kg/day led to an increase in neutrophils in all patients, in platelets in 4 patients, and in hemoglobin in 4 patients at week 8. Worrisome aspects of chronic growth factor administration are the theoretical risks of stimulating a leukemic clone or speeding the process of stem cell exhaustion.

Gene Therapy

Experimental trials of hematopoietic cell transduction with FA genes are rational, but because of unknown long-term consequences they should be considered only in carefully selected patients. Recombinant viral vectors have been engineered to express wild-type *FANCC* in cells from patients with *FANCC* mutations.[128–130] Phenotypic correction followed viral transduction, as shown by resistance to MMC-induced cell death and insusceptibility to induced chromosomal aberrations. CD34-enriched hematopoietic progenitors isolated from FA patients, which exhibit the same hypersensitivity to MMC as do cultured FA cells, showed improved colony formation in clonogenic assays in the absence as well as in the presence of low concentrations of MMC after gene transduction with a viral vector containing the wild-type *FANCC* cDNA.[128,129] Similarly, transduction with the *FANCA* vector also improved the viability of hematopoietic progenitor colonies from patients with *FANCA* mutations.[131] These experiments indicate that both FANCC and FANCA proteins are involved in the maintenance of hematopoietic progenitor cell viability, perhaps by countering programmed cell death. In an experimental trial of gene therapy in group-C FA patients,[132] function of the normal *FANCC* transgene was suggested by a marked increase in hematopoietic colonies following successive transduction cycles in all patients. However, despite the in vitro selective advantage resulting from *FANCC* gene transfer, long-term hematopoietic reconstitution with gene-corrected clones failed to occur. Further advances in understanding gene transfer and stem cell growth and manipulation will be needed before gene therapy becomes clinically useful in FA.

Prognosis

Because of the heterogeneous presentations and variable outcomes in FA, it is difficult to establish a prognosis for an individual. Bone marrow failure is the most likely adverse outcome in childhood, whereas a solid tumor becomes more probable in adults, and the risk of developing AML peaks during teenage years.[105] For young patients undergoing matched sibling HSCT for bone marrow failure, hematologic manifestations may be cured. However, these patients, like untransplanted patients surviving past age 20, are at risk for secondary malignancies that may not be responsive to cytotoxic therapies.

CURRENT CONTROVERSIES & FUTURE CONSIDERATIONS

Fanconi's Anemia

- Do defects in the FA pathway underlie some cases of idiopathic aplastic anemia or cancer?
- Do the FA proteins function in pathways other than DNA damage response?
- What is the basis of cancer predisposition in FA?
- What genes are mutated in the remaining complementation groups?
- What is the relationship between the FA and BRCA pathways?
- Are there functional differences between the different complementation groups?

DYSKERATOSIS CONGENITA

Epidemiology and Risk Factors

The precise incidence of DC is unknown; the prevalence is approximately 1 per 1 million persons. DC has been observed in many racial subtypes. The Dyskeratosis Congenita Registry at the Hammersmith Hospital, with information on 340 patients, distinguishes DC[133–140] into X-linked recessive (MIM 305000), autosomal dominant (MIM 127550), and autosomal recessive (MIM 224230) subtypes. Clinical heterogeneity is observed, in part related to the different mutations in DC-causing genes, but there can also be considerable variability in affected individuals in the same family, implicating other genetic and environmental factors in producing the disease phenotype.

Pathophysiology

Bone marrow cellularity is reduced in many DC patients, and the marrow morphology is similar to that in patients with idiopathic aplastic anemia; there also are reduced numbers of all hematopoietic progenitors.[141–145] Abnormalities of growth and chromosomal rearrangements in fibroblasts suggest that bone marrow failure is likely to be a consequence of dysfunction of both hematopoietic stem cells[142,145] and stromal cells.

X-chromosome inactivation patterns (XCIPs) have been examined in blood of women from X-linked DC families, using a methylation-sensitive restriction enzyme site in the polymorphic human androgen receptor locus. All carriers of X-linked DC showed complete skewing in their inactivation patterns,[146,147] suggesting that cells expressing the defective gene have a growth or survival disadvantage compared to cells expressing the normal allele. X-chromosome inactivation patterns provide information about carrier status for use in genetic counseling and also allow distinction of an inherited mutation from a new event in a sporadic male DC case, as well as of autosomal from X-linked forms of the disease.

Molecular Genetics and Link to Telomere Repair

Linkage analysis in one large family first mapped the gene for the X-linked form of the disease to Xq28.[148,149] Available genetic markers and additional X-linked families facilitated positional cloning of the gene (*DKC1*) that was mutated in X-linked DC.[150–153] Cloning of *DKC1* provided a genetic test for diagnosis in suspected cases, identification of carriers, and antenatal diagnosis in X-linked families. Extended genetic studies also led to the demonstration that the Hoyeraal-Hreidarsson syndrome[154–159] was due to mutations in *DKC1*.[160] Hoyeraal-Hreidarsson syndrome is a severe multisystem disorder in boys, characterized by profound growth failure, abnormalities of brain development, aplastic anemia, and immunodeficiency.

The *DKC1* gene and its encoded protein, dyskerin (a nucleolar protein),[161,162] are highly conserved with many homologues, including in yeast, rat, and *Drosophila*.[163–165] Like its homologues, dyskerin is associated with the H/ACA class of small nucleolar RNAs, and one of its functions is pseudouridylation of specific ribosomal RNA,[166] an essential step in ribosome biogenesis. However, subsequent studies showed that dyskerin is also associated with the human telomerase RNA component (hTERC), which also contains a H/ACA consensus sequence.[167,168] Telomerase is an enzyme complex that is important in maintaining the telomeres of chromosomes. The complete composition of the telomerase complex is unknown, but two essential components, the RNA template (hTERC) and the catalytic human telomerase reverse transcriptase (hTERT), have been well characterized.[169] Telomerase copies a short template sequence within the RNA component (hTERC) onto chromosome ends (telomeres) to counter the telomere shortening that occurs during DNA replication. Cell lines from patients with X-linked DC show reduced level of hTERC and much shorter than normal telomere lengths (but no defects in ribosomal RNA processing or pseudouridylation).[168]

Telomeres are also abnormally short in cells from patients with autosomal forms of DC.[170] Subsequent linkage analysis in one large DC family localized the gene for autosomal dominant DC to chromosome 3q, in the same area where *hTERC* had been mapped. *hTERC* mutation analysis in several families demonstrated that autosomal dominant DC is due to mutations in *hTERC*.[171] These mutations appear to give rise to the disease through haploinsufficiency, through either the absence of a 3′ end, impaired RNA accumulation, or a catalytic defect.[172]

Because *DKC1*'s encoded protein dyskerin and hTERC are both components of the telomerase complex (Fig. 11–4), DC arises principally from an abnormality in telomerase activity.[173] Affected tissues are those requiring constant renewal, consistent with a basic deficiency in stem cell activity as a result of defective telomerase activity. The effect of mutation of one allele of human telomerase RNA in families with autosomal dominant DC can be compared with the behavior of knockout laboratory mice lacking both alleles of the gene for telomerase RNA (*mTR*): significant abnormalities only arise in later generations, which show progressive telomere shortening and defects including reduced proliferative capacity of hematopoietic cells.[174–176]

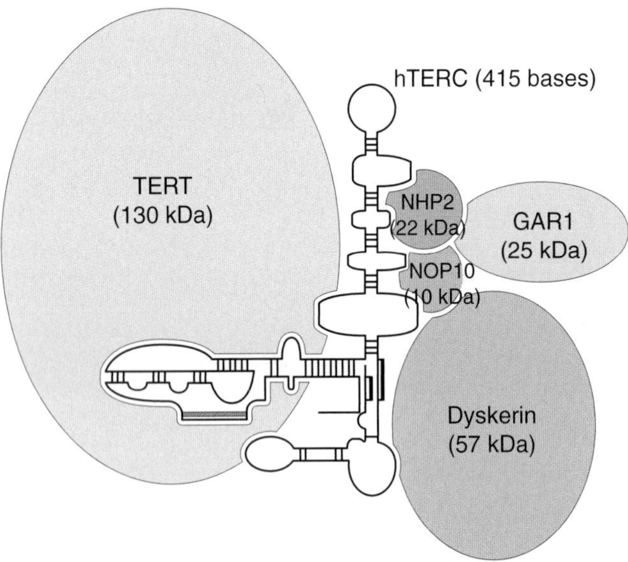

Figure 11–4. Putative associations between dyskerin and hTERC (human telomerase RNA component) in the telomerase complex and hTERT (human telomerase reverse transcriptase). GAR1, NHP2, and NOP10 are part of the ribonucleoprotein complex and are known also to associate with dyskerin and the H/ACA class of small nucleolar RNAs (snoRNAs).

In addition, DC gene mutations may underlie some cases of apparently "acquired" aplastic anemia.[177] As in DC, telomeres may be short in patients who present "sporadically" as adults. In some cases, *TERC* mutations have been found in individuals who lacked the physical anomalies diagnostic of DC; family members with the same mutation have been hematologically normal or showed only slight degrees of macrocytosis or cytopenias, although their marrows were very hypocellular and had markedly diminished hematopoietic cell function[178,179] (see Chapter 10).

Clinical Features and Diagnosis

Classic DC is an inherited bone marrow failure syndrome characterized by the mucocutaneous triad of abnormal skin pigmentation, nail dystrophy, and mucosal leucoplakia[180–182] (Fig. 11–5). Dental, gastrointestinal, genitourinary, immunologic, neurologic, ophthalmic, pulmonary, and skeletal system abnormalities, as well as hair graying or loss, also have been reported.[183–186] Marrow failure is the principal cause of early mortality, but there is an additional predisposition to malignancy and fatal pulmonary complications.[184]

Clinical manifestations in DC often occur during childhood but over a wide age range. The skin pigmentation and nail changes typically appear first, usually by the age of 10 years. Bone marrow failure usually develops before age 20 years, and 80–90% of patients will have developed hematologic abnormalities by age 30 years.[184,185] In some cases, marrow abnormalities may precede the mucocutaneous manifestations and lead to an initial diagnosis of "idiopathic" aplastic anemia.[185–189] There is considerable clinical variability among patients, even within the same family. In general, the X-linked recessive form

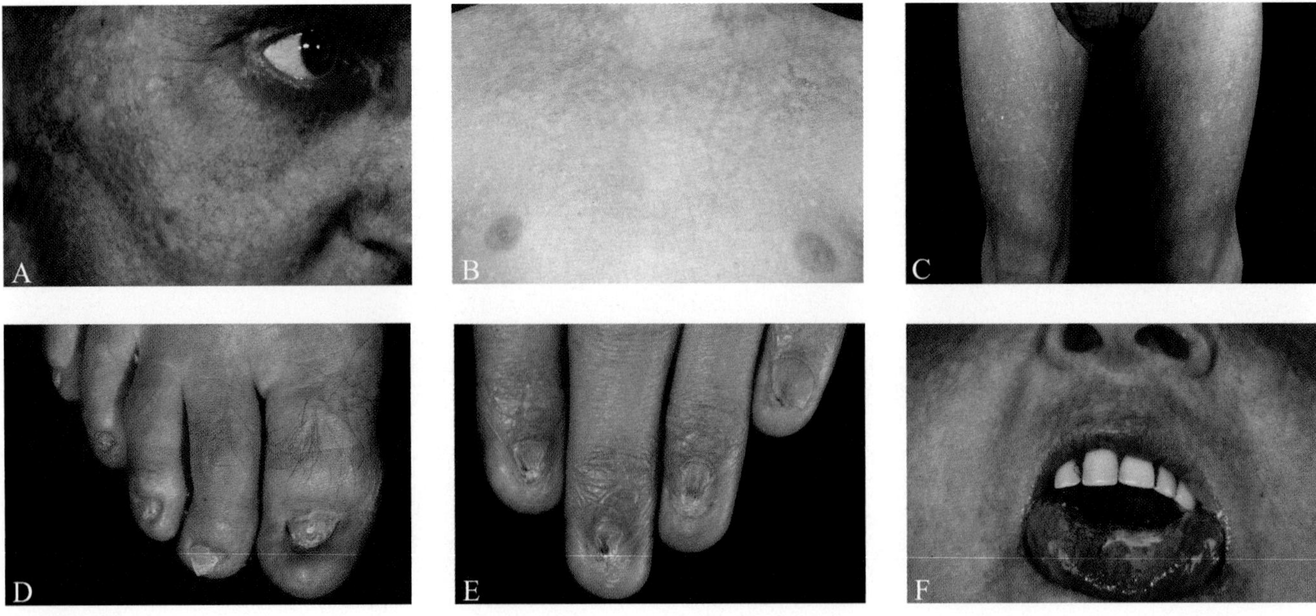

Figure 11–5. Photographs of dyskeratosis congenita patients showing abnormal skin pigmentation, nail dystrophy, and leukoplakia of the tongue.

has a worse phenotype (more abnormalities and a younger age of onset) than does autosomal dominant DC. The skin and mucosal findings in autosomal dominant DC can be mild or subtle. Autosomal recessive families show considerable heterogeneity, with some patients having severe bone marrow failure by the age of 10 years and others no hematologic abnormalities in middle age. The main causes of death in DC are bone marrow failure or immunodeficiency (~60–70%), pulmonary complications (~10–15%), and malignancy (~5–10%).[184,185]

The diagnosis of DC is easy when all the classic features are present; difficulties occur when these features are absent or the initial presentation is with aplastic anemia. With knowledge of the genes mutated in X-linked recessive (*DKC1*) and autosomal dominant (*TERC*) DC, the diagnosis can be substantiated in a significant proportion of patients. Molecular screening for *DKC1* mutations may be appropriate in males who have two of the following: abnormal skin pigmentation, nail dystrophy, leukoplakia, and bone marrow failure. For *TERC*, analysis might be undertaken in all patients with aplastic anemias; as a subgroup, these individuals clearly are known to have mutations in this gene, and screening is relatively simple.

Differential Diagnosis

Patients with DC have clinical features that overlap with FA and acquired aplastic anemia. Chromosome breakage is normal in DC, and DC should be differentiated from FA by standard clastogenic assays.[190] If the chromosomal breakage study is normal, *TERC* analysis can be undertaken. If *TERC* is normal, and depending on gender and somatic features, the *DKC1* gene may be sequenced (Fig. 11–6).

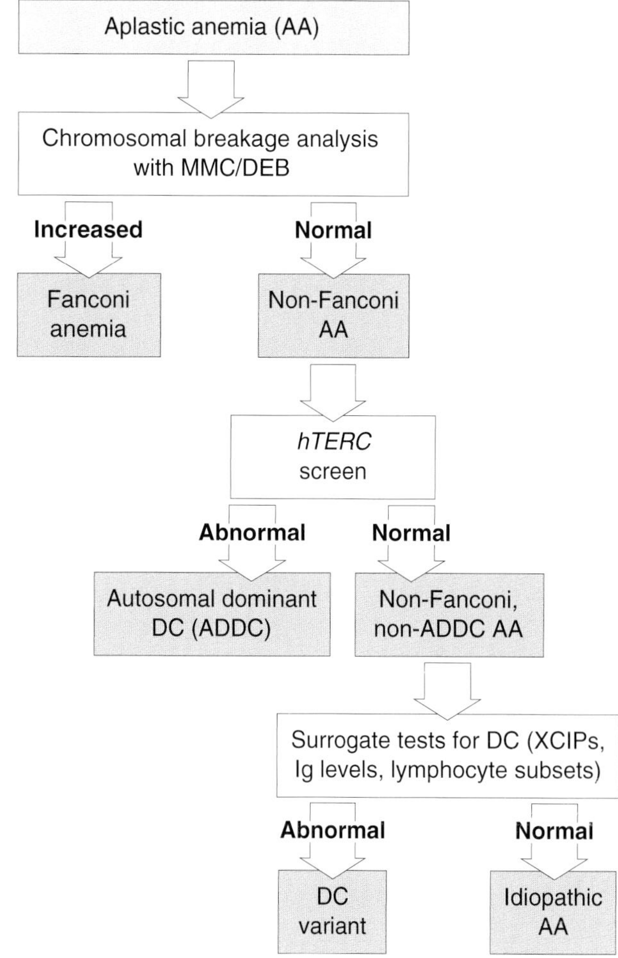

Figure 11–6. Algorithm for differential diagnosis of congenital aplastic anemias. Abbreviations: Ig, immunoglobulin; XCIPs, X-chromosome inactivation patterns.

Treatment

DC is a multisystem disorder, and optimal care may require cooperation among many subspecialists. DC patients should avoid exposure to sunlight, for example, by use of barrier creams. Smoking and alcohol should be discouraged because the livers and lungs of these individuals are more susceptible to injury. Moisturizing creams to prevent skin damage and good oral hygiene are simple prophylactic measures. Although hematologic monitoring ultimately guides therapy, the pulmonary system in particular may require periodic reassessment, and screening for malignancies, an important cause of mortality, is recommended.

Bone marrow failure is the main cause of early death in DC. The anabolic steroid oxymetholone can produce an improvement in hematopoietic function in more than half of patients for variable periods of time. Successful but usually transient responses to granulocyte-macrophage colony-stimulating factor, granulocyte colony-stimulating factor, and erythropoietin also have been reported.[191,192] The main treatment for severe bone marrow failure is allogeneic HSCT, but there is limited experience using both sibling and alternative stem cell donors in DC.[193–198] Pulmonary and vascular complications have led to early and late complications in stem cell transplantation. Preexisting lung disease in DC explains some of these toxicities and the now-recognized need to avoid agents associated with pulmonary toxicity, especially busulfan and radiotherapy. The best transplantation candidates are patients without pulmonary disease with sibling donors. Fludarabine-based, low-intensity protocols appear to produce better results than do fully ablative procedures.[199–202]

Prognosis

DC is a very heterogeneous disease, with some patients dying in infancy (Hoyeraal-Hreidarsson syndrome) and others only diagnosed in adulthood. Except for the generally more severe course of X-linked DC, accurate predictions cannot yet be inferred from genotype-phenotype correlations. Improved supportive care and low-intensity transplantation protocols likely will improve prognosis.

CURRENT CONTROVERSIES & FUTURE CONSIDERATIONS

Dyskeratosis Congenita

- What are the functions of dyskerin? Does defective ribosome generation in addition to telomere maintenance play a role in DC manifestations?
- What is the molecular basis of autosomal recessive DC?
- How much of the incidence of acquired aplastic anemia is due to defects in DC genes?
- What is the best conditioning regimen for DC patients undergoing stem cell transplantation?
- Can treatment strategies be directed to the underlying telomerase defect?

Suggested Readings*

Fanconi's Anemia

Garcia-Higuera I, Taniguchi T, Ganesan S, et al: Interaction of the Fanconi anemia proteins and BRCA1 in a common pathway. Mol Cell 7:249–262, 2001.

Howlett NG, Taniguchi T, Olson S, et al: Biallelic inactivation of BRCA2 in Fanconi anemia. Science 297:606–609, 2002.

Joenje H, Patel KJ: The emerging genetic and molecular basis of Fanconi anaemia. Nat Rev Genet 2:446–457, 2001.

Liu TX, Howlett NG, Deng M, et al: Knockdown of zebrafish Fancd2 causes developmental abnormalities via p53-dependent apoptosis. Dev Cell 5:903–914, 2003.

Liu JM, Kim S, Read EJ, et al: Engraftment of hematopoietic progenitor cells transduced with the Fanconi anemia group C gene (FANCC). Hum Gene Ther 10:2337–2346, 1999.

Dyskeratosis Congenita

Dokal I: Dyskeratosis congenita in all its forms. Br J Haematol 110:768–779, 2000.

Fu D, Collins K: Distinct biogenesis pathways for human telomerase RNA and H/ACA small nuclear RNAs. Mol Cell 11: 1361–1372, 2003.

Heiss NS, Knight SW, Vulliamy TJ, et al: X-linked dyskeratosis congenita is caused by mutations in a highly conserved gene with putative nucleolar functions. Nat Genet 19:32–38, 1998.

Vulliamy T, Marrone A, Goldman F, et al: The RNA component of telomerase is mutated in autosomal dominant dyskeratosis congenita. Nature 413:432–435, 2001.

Vulliamy T, Marrone A, Dokal I, et al: Association between aplastic anaemia and mutations in telomerase RNA. Lancet 359:2168–2170, 2002.

Full references for this chapter can be found on accompanying CD-ROM.

CHAPTER 12

Pure Red Cell Aplasia and Diamond-Blackfan Anemia

Siobán Keel, MD, and Janis L. Abkowitz, MD

KEY POINTS

Acquired Pure Red Cell Aplasia

- Pure red cell aplasia is a morphologic diagnosis, established by bone marrow findings.
- It is important to distinguish cases of myelodysplasia from other pure red cell aplasia pathophysiologies because myelodysplastic syndromes carry a significantly worse prognosis and respond poorly to immunosuppressive therapies. Clonal cytogenetics and the lack of in vitro erythroid progenitor growth assist in diagnosing myelodysplasia.
- Most patients with pure red cell aplasia will ultimately respond to an immunosuppressive drug. Cyclosporine may be the best first-line agent.
- Persistent infection with parvovirus B19 is etiologic in about 10% of cases of pure red cell aplasia. Establishing the viral diagnosis is important because immunoglobulin injections are highly effective.

Diamond-Blackfan Anemia

- Diamond-Blackfan anemia likely results from an intrinsic progenitor cell defect.
- Mutations in the *RPS19* gene, which encodes ribosomal protein S19, account for some cases of Diamond-Blackfan anemia. The precise pathophysiologic role of these mutations is unknown. Apparently normal individuals from Diamond-Blackfan families carry the gene mutations.
- Corticosteroids, blood transfusions, and iron chelation are the mainstays of therapy.

INTRODUCTION

Pure red cell aplasia is characterized by severe normochromic, normocytic or normochromic, macrocytic anemia, reticulocytopenia, and the absence of hemoglobin-containing cells in an otherwise normal marrow aspirate or with maturation arrest at the level of pronormoblasts[1] (Fig. 12–1). Pure red cell aplasia occurs as either an acquired or a congenital disorder (Diamond-Blackfan anemia). Kaznelson first described acquired pure red cell aplasia in 1922.[2] It presents as two physiologies, either an acute self-limiting illness, usually in children in the setting of a nonspecific viral infection and termed *transient erythroblastopenia of childhood,* or as a chronic, relapsing disease more frequent in adults. Acquired pure red cell aplasia is further classified as primary or secondary, depending on the absence or presence of an associated disease, infection, or drug[3] (Tables 12–1 and 12–2). The congenital counterpart of acquired pure red cell aplasia, Diamond-Blackfan anemia, first appeared in the literature in 1936 as "red cell aplasia in infancy,"[4] and Diamond and Blackfan reported four additional cases shortly thereafter.[5] Acquired pure red cell aplasia and Diamond-Blackfan anemia share common bone marrow morphologies but their pathophysiologies differ.

ACQUIRED PURE RED CELL APLASIA

Epidemiology and Risk Factors

Although pure red cell aplasia may be acquired at any age, the age of presentation in cases of secondary pure red cell aplasia follows that of the underlying disease. Of

TABLE 12–1. Classification of Pure Red Cell Aplasia

Congenital Pure Red Cell Aplasia (Diamond-Blackfan Anemia)
Intrinsic progenitor cell defect

Acquired Pure Red Cell Aplasia (PRCA)
Primary PRCA (likely immune-mediated mechanism)
- Transient erythroblastopenia of childhood
- Idiopathic

Secondary PRCA (humoral or cellular immune consequence of an underlying disorder)
- Thymoma
- Hematologic malignancies
  - Chronic lymphocytic leukemia
    - B-cell type
    - T-cell type
  - Large granular lymphocytic leukemia
  - Hodgkin's disease
  - Non-Hodgkin's lymphomas
  - Multiple myeloma
  - Waldenström's macroglobulinemia
  - Myeloproliferative diseases
    - Chronic myelocytic leukemia
    - Myelofibrosis
    - Essential thrombocythemia
  - Acute lymphoblastic leukemia
- Solid Tumors
  - Stomach carcinoma
  - Breast carcinoma
  - Lung carcinoma
  - Renal cell carcinoma
  - Skin epidermoid carcinoma
  - Kaposi's sarcoma
  - Carcinoma of unknown primary
- Infections
  - Human immunodeficiency virus
  - T-cell leukemia-lymphoma virus
  - Infectious mononucleosis
  - Viral hepatitis
  - Mumps
  - Cytomegalovirus
  - Meningococcemia
  - Staphylococcemia
  - Leishmaniasis
  - Atypical pneumonias
- Collagen vascular diseases
  - Systemic lupus erythematosus
  - Rheumatoid arthritis
  - Sjögren's syndrome
  - Mixed connective tissue disease
- Drugs and chemical
- Pregnancy
- Miscellaneous
  - Post–ABO-incompatable bone marrow transplantation
  - Autoimmune chronic hepatitis
  - Autoimmune hypothyroidism
  - Angioimmunoblastic lymphadenopathy

Parvovirus B19 (virus is directly cytotoxic to red blood cell precursors)
Myelodysplastic syndrome (hematopoietic stem cell that is unable to differentiate along the erythroid lineage)

Adapted from Dessypris EN, Lipton JM: Red cell aplasia. *In* Greer JP, Rodgers GM, Foerster J, et al (eds): Wintrobe's Clinical Hematology (ed 11). Philadelphia: Lippincott Williams & Wilkins, 2004, pp 1423–1437.

TABLE 12–2. Drugs and Chemicals Associated with Pure Red Cell Aplasia

Anesthetics	Benzene hexachloride
Halothane	Calomel
Antiarrhythmic	HIV medications
Procainamide	Lamivudine
Antibacterials	Zidovudine
Cephalothin	Hormones
Cotrimoxazole	Chlormadinone
Dapsone	Estrogens
Isoniazid	Hypoglycemics
Linezolid	Chlorpropamide
Penicillin	Tolbutamide
Rifampin	Immunosuppressant and antineoplastic agents
Thiamphenicol	Azathioprine
Anticonvulsants	Cladribine
Carbamazepine	Chloramphenicol
Diphenylhydantoin	Fludarabine
Phenobarbital	Interferon alfa
Sodium dipropylacetate	Leuprolide
Sodium valproate	Mepacrine
Antiglaucoma agent	Mycophenolate mofetil
Methazolamide	Tacrolimus
Antihyperuricemic	Miscellaneous
Allopurinol	Arsphenamine
Antirheumatics	α-Methydopa
D-Penicillamine	Erythropoietin
Gold	Pyrimethamine
Pentachlorophenol	Santonin
Salicylazosulfapyradine	NSAIDs
Sulfasalazine	Fenobufen
Chemicals	Fenoprofen
Aminopyrine	Phenylbutazone
Anagyrine	Sulindac

Abbreviations: HIV, human immunodeficiency virus; NSAIDs, nonsteroidal anti-inflammatory drugs.
Adapted from Dessypris EN, Lipton JM: Red cell aplasia. *In* Greer JP, Rodgers GM, Foerster J, et al (eds): Wintrobe's Clinical Hematology (ed 11). Philadelphia: Lippincott Williams & Wilkins, 2004, pp 1423–1437.

special note is the association between pure red cell aplasia and thymoma: pure red cell aplasia develops in approximately 5% of patients with thymoma,[6] and, conversely, thymoma occurs in approximately 8% of patients presenting with pure red cell aplasia.[7–9] Thymoma is also associated with pure white blood cell aplasia.[10] Some medications have been incriminated in pure red cell aplasia, with the anemia usually developing 3–4 months after the onset of drug exposure.

Pathophysiology

A second way to classify pure red cell aplasia is by the pathophysiology of the anemia. There are three distinct mechanisms by which erythropoiesis can fail (Fig. 12–2). In most cases of pure red cell aplasia, an aberrant immune response leads to suppression of red cell development: erythroid progenitor cells are intrinsically normal but their differentiation is inhibited. In about 10% of patients, pure red cell aplasia results from chronic parvovirus infection (the virus infects and lyses erythroid

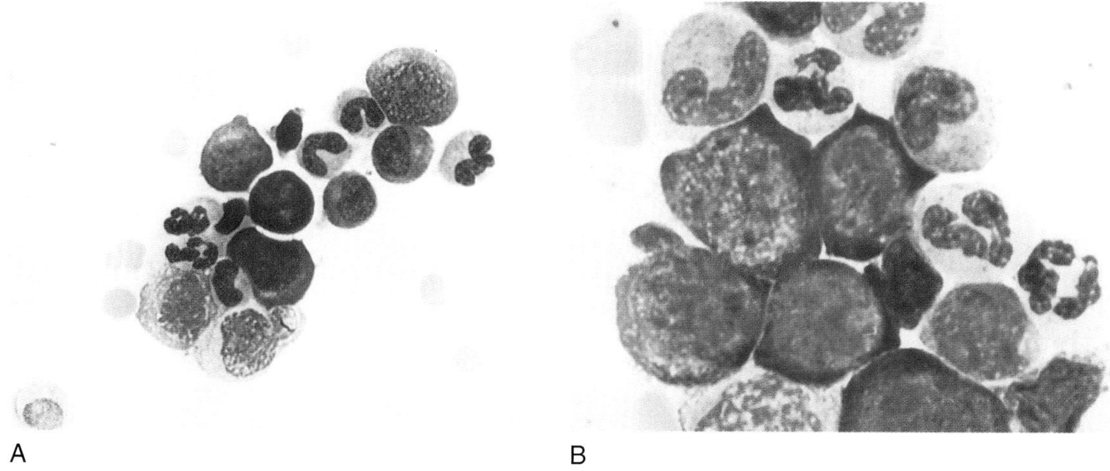

Figure 12–1. **A** and **B**, Bone marrow aspirate of pure red cell aplasia patient shows maturation arrest at the level of pronormoblasts.

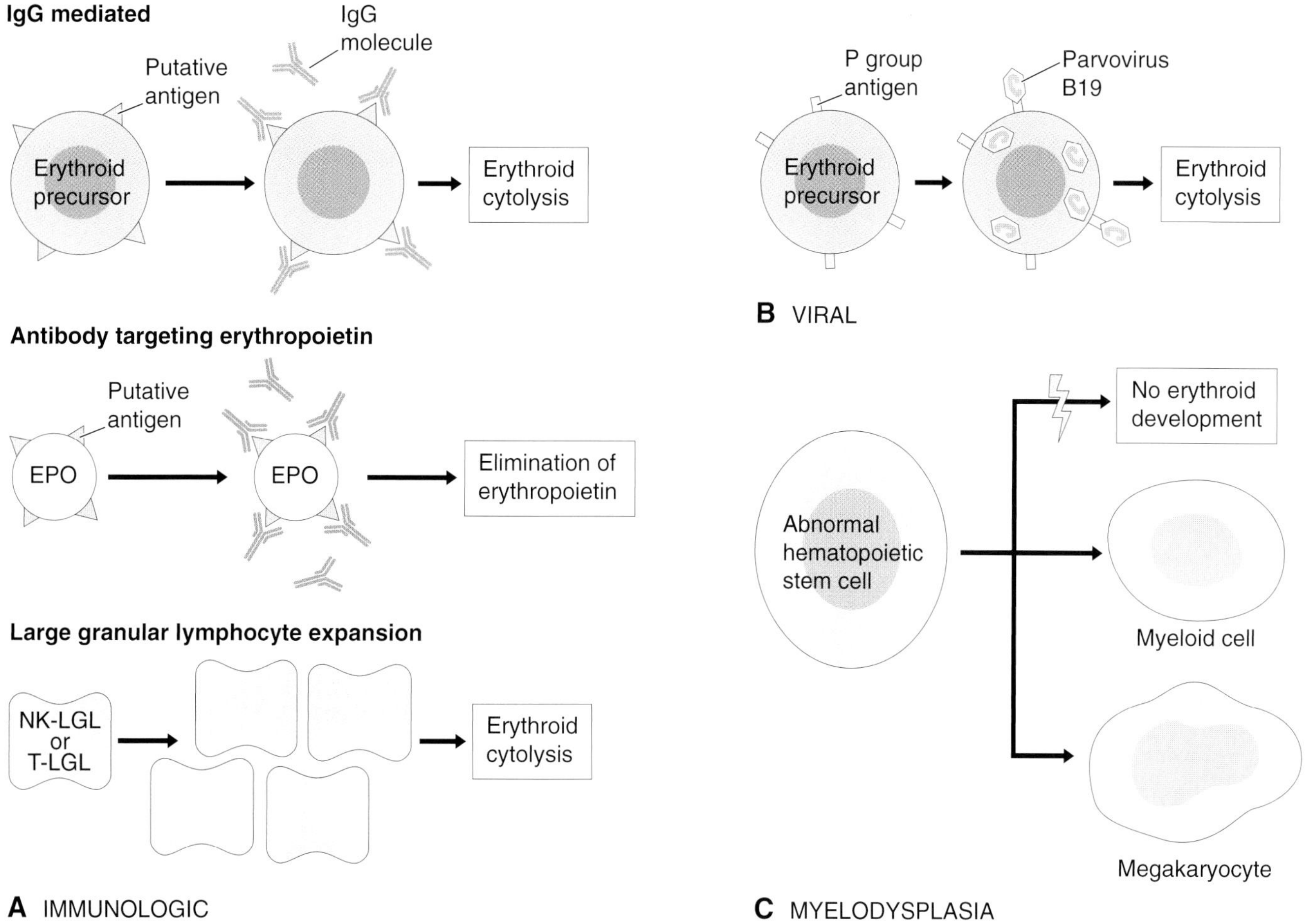

IgG mediated

Putative antigen

IgG molecule

Erythroid precursor

Erythroid cytolysis

Antibody targeting erythropoietin

Putative antigen

EPO

EPO

Elimination of erythropoietin

Large granular lymphocyte expansion

NK-LGL or T-LGL

Erythroid cytolysis

A IMMUNOLOGIC

P group antigen

Parvovirus B19

Erythroid precursor

Erythroid cytolysis

B VIRAL

No erythroid development

Abnormal hematopoietic stem cell

Myeloid cell

Megakaryocyte

C MYELODYSPLASIA

Figure 12–2. Three mechanisms of pure red cell aplasia. ***A,*** Immunologic: IgG molecule targets an antigen on an erythroid cell or erythropoietin, which leads to complement- or non-complement-mediated cytolysis. Clonal or polyclonal expansion of large granular lymphocytes (natural killer cells or T cells) causes red cell destruction through various immune pathways (further described in Fig. 12–3). ***B,*** Viral: Parvovirus binds to the blood group P antigen on erythroid cells and enters the cell, where it undergoes DNA replication and viral assembly, and ultimately causes cell lysis as the viruses are released. ***C***, Myelodysplasia: an abnormal hematopoietic stem cell is unable to differentiate into erythroid cells.

precursor cells), and it is the initial clinical manifestation of myelodysplasia in fewer than 10% of patients.[8]

Immunologic: Humoral and Lymphocyte-Mediated Suppression of Erythropoiesis

When marrow cells from cases of pure red cell aplasia are assayed in semisolid media, 60% have a normal number of erythroid progenitors.[3] This ability to proliferate in vitro, and not in vivo, suggests an inhibitor of erythropoiesis. This inhibitor can be either humoral (antibody) or cellular (T cell or natural killer cell). Erythroid progenitors have distinct growth characteristics and express different antigenic determinants at successive stages of differentiation; this variability provides multiple targets for both humoral and cell-mediated suppression.

Many cases of primary acquired pure red cell aplasia and transient erythroblastopenia of childhood are blamed on humoral suppression of erythropoiesis.[11] Early laboratory studies described a plasma inhibitor of heme synthesis[12,13] that localized to the immunoglobulin (Ig)G fraction and disappeared after successful treatment of the disease with immunosuppressive thereapies.[14–16] Although the inhibitor selectively suppressed erythroid differentiation, the antigenic targets remain unknown. In addition, antibodies have been described in patients' sera that are cytotoxic to marrow erythroid cells or are directed against erythropoietin.[5,17,18] Humoral pure red cell aplasia can also develop in the recipients of ABO-incompatible allogeneic bone marrow transplants as a result of the persistence of antibody against donor A or B determinants.[19]

In those cases of pure red cell aplasia in which an IgG inhibitor cannot be demonstrated, lymphocyte-mediated inhibition of erythropoiesis may be implicated, and an aberrant cellular immune response may be the most common pathophysiology for pure red cell aplasia.[8] Pure red cell aplasia is frequently associated with T-cell and B-cell chronic lymphocytic leukemia (CLL).[1,20,21] One early study presented a patient with T-cell CLL whose peripheral blood and bone marrow T cells suppressed erythroid colony formation by normal bone marrow cells; suppression was reversed by pretreatment of the T cells with antithymocyte globulin and complement.[21] Later investigators identified lymphocytes responsible for suppression of erythroid progenitor growth as expanded populations of large granular lymphocytes (LGLs); remission correlates with the disappearance of these cells.[7,22–28] LGL proliferations may be of T-cell type ($CD3^+$ and T-cell receptor positive) or of natural killer-cell type ($CD3^-$ and T-cell receptor negative). As in the cases associated with B-cell CLL, the expanded population of LGLs may be reactive and not "malignant." The mechanism by which lymphocytes mediate erythroid suppression in pure red cell aplasia, like humoral inhibition, is varied. A recent case of pure red cell aplasia mediated by the clonal expansion of T-cell–type LGLs is particularly instructive (Fig. 12–3). In this patient, T lymphocytes that expressed killer cell inhibitory receptors for class I human lymphocyte antigen (HLA) lysed erythroblasts, but not earlier cells, because the surface expression of class I HLA antigens decreases as erythropoiesis proceeds.[27] In some patients, erythroid progenitor suppression is not complete and the bone marrow histology reveals reduced erythropoiesis but not true pure red cell aplasia. A pathophysiology of incomplete inhibition of red cell development may account for the hypoplastic anemia seen in B-cell CLL[23] and other lymphoproliferative processes.

Parvovirus

Human parvovirus B19 infection causes a transient "aplastic" crisis when red cell survival is short and can cause pure red cell aplasia in immunosuppressed patients.[29] The virus infects erythroid cells by binding to the blood group P antigen expressed on erythroid colony-forming units (CFU-E), on all proerythroblasts, and on subsequent erythroid cells,[30] and viral infection is cytotoxic.[29] In an immunologically normal host, parvovirus persists at high titer in the blood and marrow for 2–3 weeks, but because the lifespan of a red blood cell is 120 days, infection does not result in a significant decrease in hemoglobin levels. Immunocompromised patients, including individuals with human immunodeficiency virus type 1 infection, who are unable to clear the parvovirus, develop erythroid marrow failure indistinguishable from other forms of pure red cell aplasia (see Chapter 76).

Myelodysplasia

Myelodysplasia is a clonal disorder originating in the hematopoietic stem cell or early progenitor cells[31] (see Chapter 15). Generally, all three lineages (red cells, white cells, and platelets) are affected and the marrow is hyperproliferative and dysmorphic. A variant of myelodysplasia exists in which the neoplastic stem cell has limited erythroid differentiation, resulting in the morphology of pure red cell aplasia.[7,8] In marrow culture studies, erythroid burst-forming units (BFU-E) are absent.[8,32] Clonal karyotypic abnormalities help to establish this diagnosis and may portend both a poor prognosis and a low likelihood of response to immunosuppressive therapies.[7,33] Subtle dysmorphic features of granulocytes characteristic of myelodysplasia are variably present.[8]

Clinical Features and Diagnosis

Acquired pure red cell aplasia, like its congenital counterpart, presents with symptoms related to the severity of the anemia. Apart from pallor, physical examination in acquired primary pure red cell aplasia is typically normal. In secondary pure red cell aplasia, signs related to the underlying disease such as hepatomegaly, splenomegaly, or lymphadenopathy may be present.[3]

Diagnosis of acquired pure red cell aplasia is first suggested by finding a normochromic, normocytic anemia and reticulocytopenia in the peripheral blood. The white blood cell count and differential are normal unless the condition is secondary to CLL. Bone marrow aspirate and biopsy, which establish the diagnosis, show a normocellular marrow with an almost complete absence of ery-

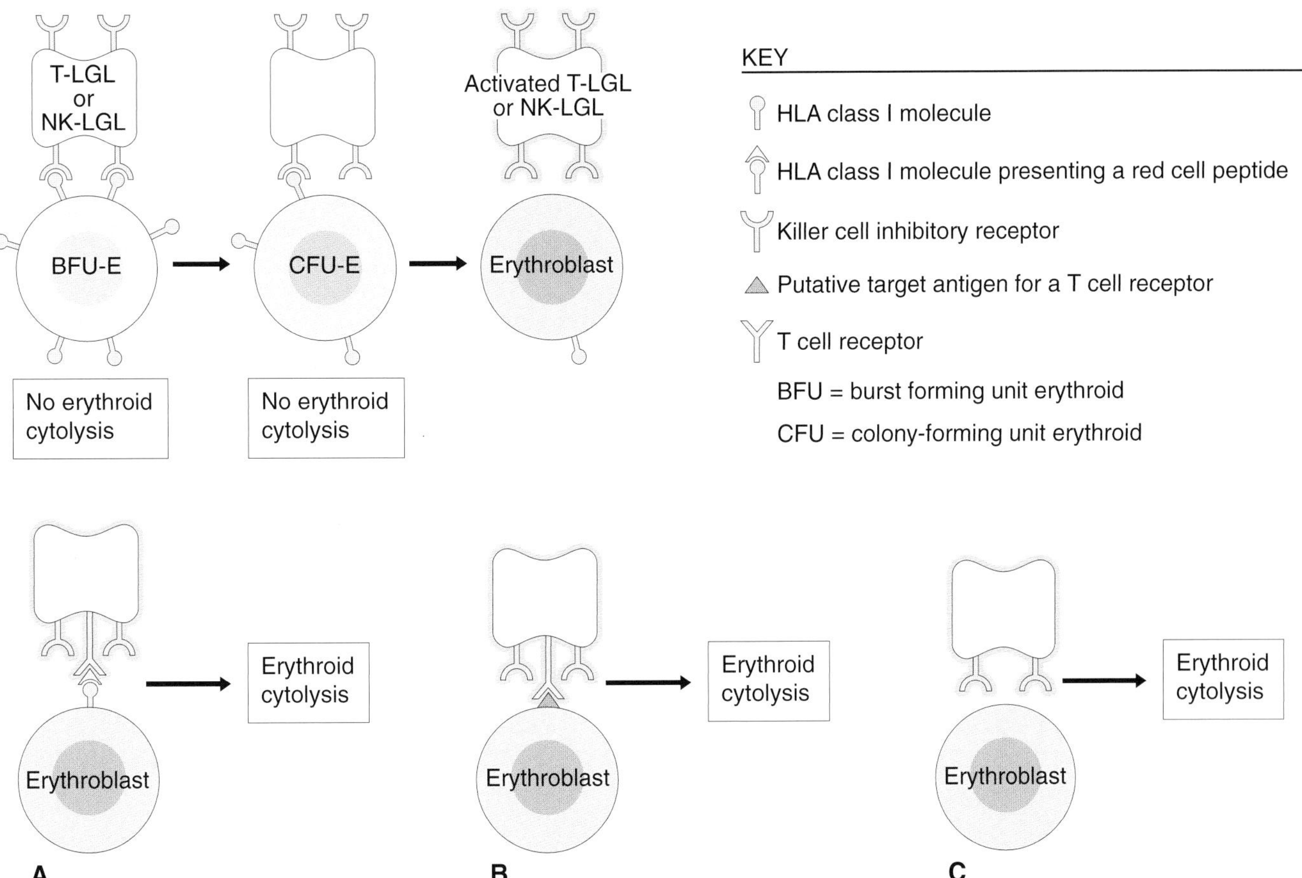

Figure 12–3. Pure red cell aplasia mediated by T-cell or natural killer–cell large granular lymphocytes (T-LGLs, NK-LGLs). When a killer cell immunoglobulin-like receptor binds to a HLA class I molecule on the surface of an erythroid precursor, the ability of the T-LGL or NK-LGL to lyse the erythroid cell is inhibited. Normal blast-forming units–erythroid express class I determinants, but this expression is downregulated as erythroid precursors mature. HLA class I antigens are expressed on all myeloid cells regardless of their maturation. ***A–C,*** Possible mechanisms for pure red cell aplasia directly mediated by T-LGLs or NK-LGLs. ***A,*** The T-cell receptor may directly recognize a red cell peptide presented by an HLA class I molecule. ***B,*** The T-cell receptor may recognize a ligand expressed on red cell precursors. ***C,*** NK-LGLs (or T-LGLs) may be positively triggered by circulating antibody against red cell antigens, activating NK receptors and adhesions molecules (not shown), and then the T-cell receptor would not be directly involved in the recognition of red cell antigens. Other possible mechanisms can be theorized including inhibited lymphokine production by LGLs that leads to erythroid cytolysis. (Adapted from Fisch P, Handgretinger R, Schaefer HE: Pure red cell aplasia. Br J Haematol 111:1010–1022, 2000.)

throid cells yet preservation of the granulocytic and megakaryocytic lineages. There may be increased numbers of proerythroblasts and "maturation arrest" at the proerythroblast stage.[34] In parvovirus B19 infection, the marrow aspirate may show giant pronormoblasts with eosinophilic nuclear inclusion bodies,[30] but this morphologic feature can also be seen in patients with human immunodeficiency virus type 1 in the absence of parvovirus B19 infection[35] and thus is not entirely pathognomonic. Additional diagnostic testing and a careful history and physical examination define whether the acquired pure red cell aplasia is primary or secondary. A computed tomography scan of the chest is performed to exclude thymoma. Parvovirus B19 should be sought by DNA assays. Serum erythropoietin, except in the rare cases of acquired pure red cell aplasia associated with antibodies to erythropoietin,[36] is elevated. A negative parvovirus B19 polymerase chain reaction assay excludes B19 as the etiology of pure red cell aplasia, whereas a positive test requires confirmation by DNA hybridization (a less sensitive assay) because only high-level viremia ($>10^6$ copies/mL) is associated with pure red cell aplasia (in normal individuals, B19 DNA can be detectable by gene amplification techniques for 6–9 months following an acute infection)[37] (see Chapter 76).

Differential Diagnosis

The differential diagnosis can be considered from findings in the peripheral blood and in the bone marrow (Fig. 12–4). In the blood, the differential diagnosis includes all causes for a normochromic, normocytic anemia with reticulocytopenia, such as endocrinopathies or marrow infiltration by cancer, granulomatous diseases, or fibrosis. In endocrinopathies, the anemia is generally not severe, and when marrow is replaced by cancer, granuloma, or fibrosis, white cell and/or platelet numbers are

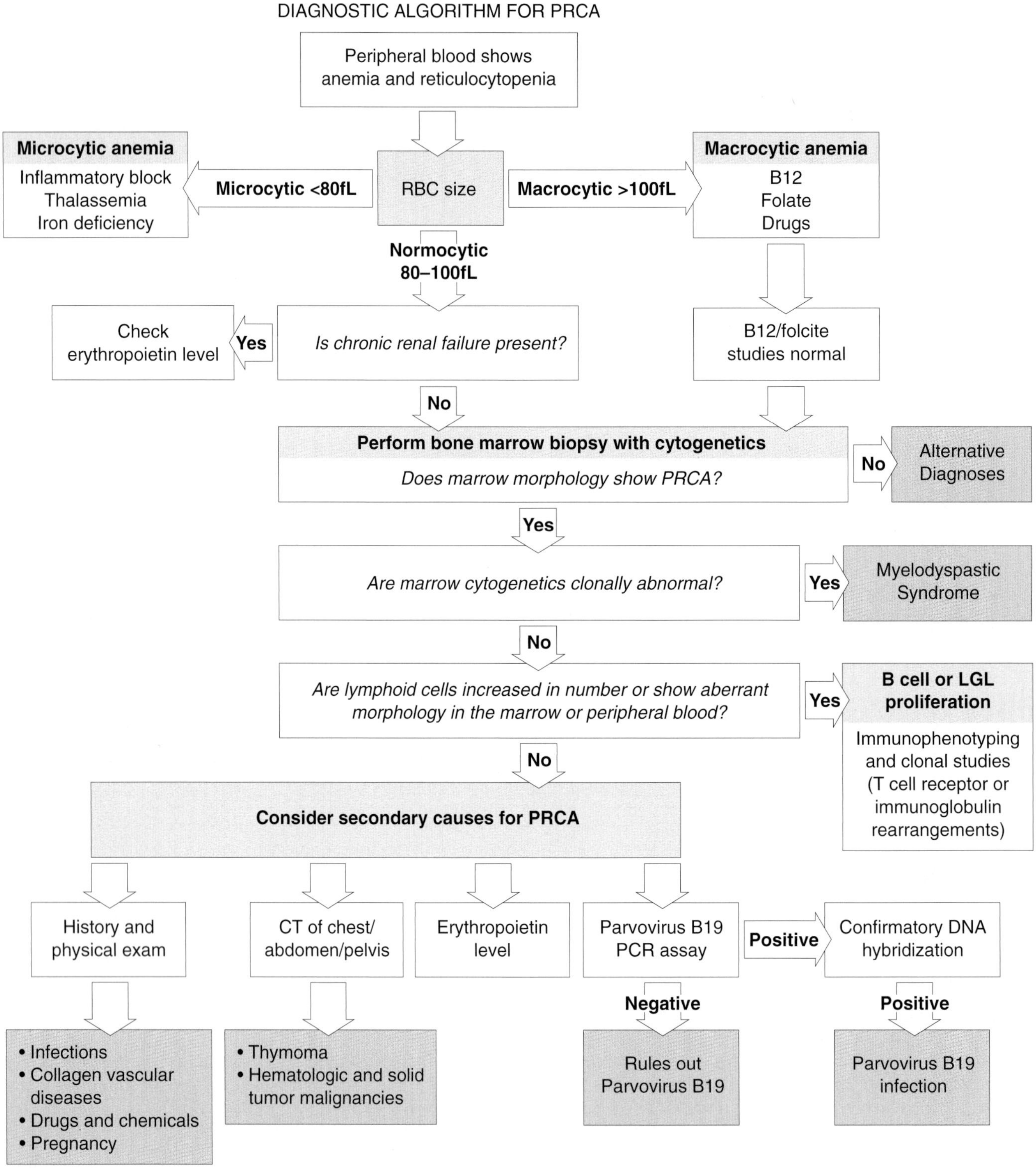

DIAGNOSTIC ALGORITHM FOR PRCA

Peripheral blood shows anemia and reticulocytopenia

RBC size

Microcytic <80fL → **Microcytic anemia**: Inflammatory block, Thalassemia, Iron deficiency

Macrocytic >100fL → **Macrocytic anemia**: B12, Folate, Drugs → B12/folcite studies normal → Perform bone marrow biopsy with cytogenetics

Normocytic 80–100fL → *Is chronic renal failure present?*

- **Yes** → Check erythropoietin level
- **No** → **Perform bone marrow biopsy with cytogenetics**

Does marrow morphology show PRCA?

- **No** → Alternative Diagnoses
- **Yes** → *Are marrow cytogenetics clonally abnormal?*

Are marrow cytogenetics clonally abnormal?

- **Yes** → Myelodyspastic Syndrome
- **No** → *Are lymphoid cells increased in number or show aberrant morphology in the marrow or peripheral blood?*

Are lymphoid cells increased in number or show aberrant morphology in the marrow or peripheral blood?

- **Yes** → **B cell or LGL proliferation**: Immunophenotyping and clonal studies (T cell receptor or immunoglobulin rearrangements)
- **No** → **Consider secondary causes for PRCA**

Consider secondary causes for PRCA

- History and physical exam →
  - Infections
  - Collagen vascular diseases
  - Drugs and chemicals
  - Pregnancy
- CT of chest/abdomen/pelvis →
  - Thymoma
  - Hematologic and solid tumor malignancies
- Erythropoietin level
- Parvovirus B19 PCR assay
  - **Negative** → Rules out Parvovirus B19
  - **Positive** → Confirmatory DNA hybridization → **Positive** → Parvovirus B19 infection

Figure 12–4. Differential diagnosis algorithm for pure red cell aplasia.

also usually decreased. Pure red cell aplasia is a morphologic diagnosis based on bone marrow examination; once the diagnosis is established, the primary process must be determined.

Treatment

Pure red cell aplasia caused by parvovirus B19 infection is treated with normal pooled serum IgG (such as 800 mg/kg/day for 3 days), which provides specific antibodies to clear the infection. (Parvovirus is a common epidemic and endemic infection, and more than 75% of adults over 50 years old have neutralizing antibodies in their serum.[38,39]) Cases of pure red cell aplasia which are associated with thymoma can respond to thymectomy, which is the primary treatment of nonmetastatic thymoma because of the tumor's tendency to be locally aggressive, within 4–8 weeks in 30–40% of cases; there is no benefit for thymectomy in the absence of a thymoma.[6] Pure red cell aplasia can develop many years after thymectomy[40]; these cases are treated with immunosuppressive therapies.

Clinical response is measured by comparing the interval between transfusions and monitoring hemoglobin levels and reticulocyte counts. Prednisone or cyclosporine is recommended for first-line treatment. Patients who fail corticosteroids or cyclosporine are treated with sequential trials of immunosuppressive therapies. No clear data favor one agent over another; the choice is influenced by coexisting diseases and by considerations of toxicity and cost. For example, cyclophosphamide is used with underlying systemic lupus erythematosus or rheumatologic disorders, and weekly methotrexate is given for pure red cell aplasia associated with LGL leukemia, a therapy first established to treat LGL-associated autoimmune neutropenia.

Corticosteroids

Prednisone is administered orally at a dose of 1 mg/kg body weight for a 10- to 12-week trial; reported response rates are 30–40%.[7–9] When the hematocrit reaches 33–35%, the dose is slowly tapered over 3–4 months. Some patients remain corticosteroid-dependent, and only 11% with steroid-induced remission continue in remission at 5 years.[9] Randomized prospective data comparing corticosteroids to other immunosuppressives as initial therapy have not been published; however, at least one study suggests that, in secondary acquired pure red cell aplasia, corticosteroids may not be as effective as other therapies.[9] The numerous complications of corticosteroids include myopathy, infection, hyperglycemia, and osteoporosis.[9]

Cyclosporine

Cyclosporine may be the most effective treatment for acquired pure red cell aplasia and may ultimately replace corticosteroids as the first drug to employ.[41–44] As reviewed earlier, T lymphocytes may be responsible for pure red cell aplasia by a direct cytotoxic effect on erythroid progenitors, by secreting lymphokines themselves, or by facilitating B-cell production of inhibitory cytokines. Cyclosporine acts by decreasing T-cell and natural killer–cell activity. Response rates in several series of cases ranged from 65% to 100%.[7,8,42,43] The optimal dose, duration of therapy, and trough blood level are not known. Dosages used for aplastic anemia of 12 mg/kg/day in adults and 15 mg/kg/day in children in two equally divided doses, adjusted to maintain a level between 200 and 400 ng/mL by radioimmunoassay, are adequate to treat pure red cell aplasia.[45] Often the drug is given with 20–30 mg of daily prednisone when used as initial therapy in pure red cell aplasia. Remission maintenance in many cases is cyclosporine-dependent.[43] Nephrotoxicity is the main complication of cyclosporine, and careful monitoring, of renal function and potassium and magnesium balance, is required.

Cytotoxic Immunosuppressants

Cyclophosphamide, 6-mercaptopurine, azathioprine, and methotrexate each can result in resolution of anemia in pure red cell aplasia.[7–9,46] Remissions may be dependent on concomitant prednisone therapy.[9] Response, as with all immunosuppressive therapies, occurs approximately 10–12 weeks after initiation of therapy; thus a therapeutic trial should continue for at least this duration of time. Fifty percent to 60% of pure red cell aplasia patients achieve remission with cytotoxic therapies.[7,9] Typical dosing for either cyclophosphamide or azathioprine is 50–100 mg by mouth daily, with adjustment should thrombocytopenia or neutropenia occur. Major concerns that limit the use of these agents are uncertainty as to the adequate dose and time-dependent leukemogenic and carcinogenic potentials.

Other Therapies

Antithymocyte globulin is an alternative for nonresponders; the response rate is about 50%.[8,9,47] The humanized monoclonal antibodies anti-CD20 (rituximab) and anti-CD52 (alemtuzumab) have also been used to treat pure red cell aplasia; experience with these agents is limited but encouraging.[48–51] Plasmapheresis and splenectomy can be considered for completely refractory patients.[52]

Prognosis

Sequential immunosuppressive therapies lead to remission in 60–70% of patients with acquired pure red cell aplasia,[7-9] and the median survival is 12–14 years.[7,9] Spontaneous remissions can occur within 5 months to 14 years after diagnosis in about 10% of cases.[1] In general, primary acquired pure red cell aplasia confers better survival than is seen with secondary disease.[9] The majority of recurrences are responsive to further therapy[7,9]; data on the durability of remission are discordant. As many as 80% of patients have been estimated to relapse within 24 months of remission[1,9]; conversely, others have reported that the great majority of patients who respond to therapy remain in remission without maintenance at a median follow-up of 5 years.[8] The prognosis for improvement of anemia in nonresponders is poor.[1] Rarely, pure red cell aplasia transforms into leukemia.[32]

Cytogenetics and erythroid progenitor growth are two valuable prognostic indicators. Clonal cytogenetic abnormalities are evidence of pure red cell aplasia arising from myelodysplasia, and they predict a low likelihood of response to immunosuppressive therapy and a poor prognosis.[7,8] In vitro erythroid hematopoietic colony formation also correlates with clinical response to therapy: in vitro BFU-E maturation has a sensitivity of 96%, a specificity of 78%, and a positive predictive value of 93%.[8,32] In patients refractory to a 10- to 12-week trial of two or three immunosuppressive agents, culture studies are particularly useful because the absence of erythroid progenitor growth helps to identify patients with myelodysplasia.

DIAMOND-BLACKFAN ANEMIA

Epidemiology and Risk Factors

More than 500 cases of Diamond-Blackfan anemia have been accrued into patient registries in Europe and North America. The prevalence of the disease among different ethnic populations is similar to its distribution in the overall population.[53] Diamond-Blackfan anemia is diagnosed in 4–7 newborns per 1 million live births, with an equal sex ratio.[53,54] Few maternal risk factors are identified, and data suggesting a seasonal variation in the incidence of Diamond-Blackfan anemia are not consistent.[53,54] There does appear to be a higher incidence of miscarriages in families with affected children.[53,55] Twenty percent of Diamond-Blackfan patients were born prematurely.[53]

Genetics

Although a congenital disorder, Diamond-Blackfan anemia has significant genetic heterogeneity. In the 10–20% of familial cases, both dominant and recessive inheritance are reported.[54,56–58] A wide variety of mutations in the *RPS19* gene on chromosome 19q13.2, which encodes a ribosomal protein, have been identified in 25% of patients with Diamond-Blackfan anemia[59–61]; pathophysiologic implications of *RPS19* are discussed later. A second locus linked to Diamond-Blackfan anemia was identified on chromosome 8 (8p23.2–23.1)[62]; its gene product is still unknown. Neither of these mutations is involved in large numbers of other familial cases, implying that other loci responsible for Diamond-Blackfan anemia are yet to be defined.

Pathophysiology

Multiple etiologies for Diamond-Blackfan anemia—a marrow microenvironment defect,[63] accessory cell dysfunction,[64] or immune cell–mediated pathogenesis[65]—have been suggested and refuted.[66,67] The currently accepted theory is that Diamond-Blackfan anemia results from an intrinsic progenitor cell defect. Bone marrow BFU-E and CFU-E are decreased in Diamond-Blackfan anemia[68–70]; progenitors also appear unable to respond normally to inducers of erythroid differentiation and proliferation. In vitro studies demonstrate insensitivity of Diamond-Blackfan progenitors to crude recombinant erythropoietin,[69,71] interleukin-3, interleukin-6, and granulocyte-macrophage colony-stimulating factor, alone or in combination.[72] In one clinical trial, hematopoiesis improved in some Diamond-Blackfan patients who were treated with interleukin-3.[73] Although this is suggestive of a possible receptor-ligand abnormality involving various growth-promoting cytokines, none has been identified, including for erythropoietin and stem cell factor.[74,75] Recent experiments using a two-phase culture system have confirmed that the commitment and early differentiation of erythroid progenitor cells in Diamond-Blackfan anemia are normal but that maturation at or following the CFU-E stage (the phase of differentiation that is erythropoietin dependent) fails.[76] A defect in completing terminal erythroid differentiation is consistent with the macrocytic anemia and increased hemoglobin F expression observed in Diamond-Blackfan anemia.

Although constitutional pure red cell aplasia likely results from an intrinsic erythroid progenitor cell defect, the variable clinical manifestations (even among affected family members) suggest that other genetic and epigenetic events, including the effects of microenvironmental cells, modulate the phenotype.

RPS19 Gene Mutations

A major advance in understanding the molecular basis for Diamond-Blackfan anemia is the recent identification in one affected girl of a balanced chromosomal translocation, 46,XX, t(X;19)(p21;q13).[77] Linkage analysis performed on families with more than one affected member identified the candidate gene at 19q13.2; both dominant and recessive patterns of inheritance were observed.[60] Positional cloning studies identified the gene as *RPS19*, which encodes ribosomal protein S19[59]; a wide variety of mutations in this gene accounts for approximately 25% of cases of DBA. *RPS19* gene mutations also were found in some apparently unaffected individuals in Diamond-Blackfan families, who had only isolated elevated erythrocyte adenosine deaminase levels.[59,78] All *RPS19* mutations identified are on a single allele (heterozygous), which suggests that homozygosity is lethal.[79] Phenotype-genotype analysis showed no correlation between the presence or nature of *RPS19* gene mutations and differences in clinical expression patterns or therapeutic responses.[59,61]

Diamond-Blackfan anemia is the first known human disease in which a defect in a ribosomal protein is involved in the pathogenesis. *RPS19* is expressed in many human tissues, including bone marrow, peripheral blood, spleen, liver, and skeletal muscle.[59] The nucleotide sequence, particularly between codons 52 and 62, is highly conserved among many species, from *Archaebacteria* to mammals.[78] *RPS19* expression normally decreases during terminal erythroid differentiation,[80] and the protein localizes to the nucleolus.[81]

TABLE 12–3. Prevalence of Malformations in Diamond-Blackfan Anemia

	Alter	Ball et al.	Janov et al.	Willig et al.
Evaluable cases (*n*)	29	65	76	229
Overall prevalence of physical anomalies	62%	58%	45%	40.6%
Head	52%	35%	8%	20.5%
Eyes	38%		9%	11.8%
Neck	17%		7%	3.5%
Thumb	17%	18%	13%	9.2%
Genitourinary	10%		9%	6.5%
Heart	3%		4%	6.9%
Bone and joint	10%		3%	8.7%
Miscellaneous	21%		18%	7.4%

From Da Costa L, Thiebaut-Noel W, Fixler J, et al: Diamond-Blackfan anemia. Curr Opin Pediatr 13:10–15, 2001, with permission.

Mutations in *RPS19* in Diamond-Blackfan anemia disrupt nucleolar localization and dramatically decrease the expression of the mutant protein.[82] Enforced expression of the *RPS19* transgene improved proliferation of CD34$^+$ cells from Diamond-Blackfan patients with mutations.[82]

The mechanism by which an abnormality of RPS19 causes Diamond-Blackfan anemia is unknown. Potentially, the RPS19 protein could have both ribosomal and extraribosomal functions, as described for other ribosomal proteins in the rat and *Drosophila melanogaster*. Alternative roles may explain the abnormalities in erythropoiesis and embryogenesis of Diamond-Blackfan anemia.[59] Although *RPS19* is ubiquitously expressed, the consequence of its mutation is generally manifest in erythropoiesis alone. That platelet and leukocyte production are unaffected may reflect the kinetics of red cell development and the dependence of early red cell precursors on efficient globin translation and hemoglobin synthesis.

Trilineage Hematopoietic Defect

Diamond-Blackfan anemia patients can present with or develop neutropenia and/or thrombocytopenia and leukemia, suggesting that, at least in some patients, the defect in this anemia affects a multilineage hematopoietic progenitor cell.[83,84] Normal stromal adherent layers, which act as the in vitro counterpart to the bone marrow microenvironment, fail to sustain Diamond-Blackfan CD34$^+$ cells in culture; furthermore, the recovery of erythroid- and granulocyte-macrophage–committed progenitors (BFU-E and granulocyte-macrophage colony-forming units) is low to absent.[70] The stem cell surrogate cell called an LTC-IC (long-term culture-initiating cell assays) in Diamond-Blackfan anemia also produces fewer BFU-E and granulocyte-macrophage colony-forming units than do primitive progenitors in normal subjects.[85]

Clinical Features

Patients present early in infancy with signs and symptoms related to the severity of the anemia. Some have congenital anomalies. The median age at diagnosis is 2–4 months, with about 75% of cases diagnosed by 3 months and 95% of cases before 2 years of age. "Failure to thrive," persistent diarrhea, and refusal to eat are characteristic. Pallor is the major finding on examination. Congenital anomalies occur in 37–47% of patients, including a myriad of malformations (Table 12–3). Short stature is present in about one third of patients.[53,55,58]

Diagnosis

Diamond-Blackfan anemia is diagnosed in early childhood based on the findings of a normochromic, usually macrocytic anemia, reticulocytopenia, and normocellular marrow with selective deficiency of red cell precursors (<5% of nucleated cells).[57] Hemoglobin values in untransfused patients range from 1.5 to 12.4 gm/dL. The anemia is macrocytic at diagnosis in 67% of patients.[53] Leukocyte and platelet counts are usually normal, but 25% of patients have neutropenia and some have thrombocytosis or thrombocytopenia.[86] Other hematologic findings may assist the diagnosis. Hemoglobin F is persistently elevated, even during remission, and red cell i antigen, which is normally absent on red cells by 1 year, is expressed at near fetal levels in older patients with Diamond-Blackfan anemia.[57,87] More important, erythrocyte adenosine deaminase activity, which reflects abnormalities in purine and pyrimidine metabolism, is increased in 80% of Diamond-Blackfan patients,[88,89] and this enzymatic determination may be a critical diagnostic study. Serum levels of erythropoietin, vitamin B_{12}, and folate are normal or increased.[57]

Differential Diagnosis

The differential diagnosis includes adult acquired pure red cell aplasia, its numerous secondary causes, and two childhood diseases: Fanconi's anemia and transient erythroblastopenia of childhood. With presentation at an older age in the absence of physical anomalies, the distinction between constitutional and acquired pure red cell aplasia may be arbitrary; a family history or the presence of *RPS19* mutations is obviously helpful. Diamond-Blackfan anemia is distinguished from transient erythroblastopenia of childhood by a number of findings (Table 12–4). Fanconi's anemia is excluded by a normal

TABLE 12–4. Criteria for Distinguishing Between Diamond-Blackfan Anemia (DBA) and Transient Erythroblastopenia of Childhood (TEC)

Criteria	DBA	TEC
Age at diagnosis	90% < 1 year	80% 1–4 years
Etiology	Constitutional	Acquired
Congenital anomalies	30–40%	No
Hemoglobin F increased at diagnosis (>250 mg/dL)	90–100%	No, except during marrow recovery
Erythrocyte adenosine deaminase activity	90% of cases increased	Normal or slightly elevated (<1.25 U/gm hemoglobin)
Treatment	Immunosuppression	Transfusion
Progression	Most frequently a chronic anemia	Spontaneous remission

TABLE 12–5. Steroid Treatment and Clinical Course in Diamond-Blackfan Anemia Cohort Studies

	Alter [87]	Ball et al. [53]	Janov et al. [55]	Willig et al. [86]
Sample size	21	69	76	222
Initial response to steroids	14/21 (66)	50/69 (72)	31/56 (55)	139/222 (62.6)
Number of patients (%) who became free of any treatment (steroids or transfusion)	1/21 (4.7)	11/69 (25.9)	24/73 (33)	46/222 (20.7) 57/222 including BMT (25.7)
Of those who initially responded to steroids, number (%) who became refractory or discontinued drug because of side effects	2/14 (14.2)	9/50 (18)	8/31 (25)	22/139 (15.8)
Number (%) who required regular transfusions	13/61 (62%)	27/69 (39)	36/72 (50)	65/222 (29.2)
Number (%) of spontaneous remissions	0	1/69 (1.4)	10/73 (13.6)	0

Abbreviation: BMT, bone marrow transplantation.

chromosome stress test. Maternal-fetal or postnatal parvovirus B19 infection may be excluded by determining maternal and child parvovirus serologies and by polymerase chain reaction analysis for the virus.

Treatment

Immunosuppression

Corticosteroids are the main therapy, producing hematologic responses in 50–70% of patients.[53–55,87] It was the misconception that Diamond-Blackfan anemia was an immune-mediated disease that initially prompted steroid treatment; there remains little understanding of the mechanism(s) of action of steroids and no predictor of corticosteroid responsiveness. Prednisone is usually initially employed at 2 mg/kg/day in divided doses. In responders, a reticulocytosis is usually apparent in 1–2 weeks. When the hemoglobin reaches 10 gm/dL, prednisone is slowly tapered to maintain a hemoglobin of 8.0–10.0 gm/dL.[57] Primary nonresponders may respond to higher doses of steroids or to the reintroduction of steroids at a later point in their disease course. Relapsed disease is variably corticosteroid-responsive. The durability or absence of response to steroids reported in the literature is summarized in Table 12–5. Toxicities of corticosteroids are numerous and include osseous complications (5.6%), growth retardation (13.3%), and, more rarely, infection-related death.[54]

Transfusions

Transfusion sustains the 20–30% of patients who fail to respond to steroids initially, become refractory, or are intolerant to corticosteroids. Transfusions are administered monthly, aiming to maintain the hemoglobin at a value compatible with normal activity (above 6–7 gm/dL). Iron overload is the major complication of regular transfusion and occurs in 69% of patients transfused long term, despite chelation therapy.[54] Secondary hemochromatosis leads to heart, liver, and endocrine dysfunction (see Chapter 56).

Other Therapies

Uncontrolled therapeutic trials have shown variable responses to other therapies in corticosteroid-refractory patients, including cyclosporine, erythropoietin, interleukin-3, and metoclopramide.[73,90–94]

Bone Marrow Transplantation

Transplantation for Diamond-Blackfan anemia was first reported in 1976, and, over the past 2 decades, multiple cases of both umbilical cord and bone marrow transplantations have been published. In contrast to HLA-matched sibling stem cell transplantation, data supporting alternative-donor transplantation are less favorable. For 10 patients in the International Bone Marrow Registry, the 2-year actuarial survival rate was 72% for the 8 HLA-matched allogeneic sibling bone marrow transplants; the 2 recipients of non-HLA-identical sibling bone marrow transplants died less than 2 weeks after transplantation.[95] In the Diamond-Blackfan Anemia Registry, including both bone marrow and umbilical cord blood transplantations, survival at greater than 5 years from transplantation in 20 patients receiving allogeneic sibling transplants was 88% ± 12% versus 14% ± 12% for alternative-donor transplantation.[96] For 13 bone marrow transplantations in the French registry, survival was 85% at 36 months, with the two reported deaths occurring in one unrelated-donor transplantation and one HLA-matched sibling transplantation.[54]

Appropriate timing for transplantation in Diamond-Blackfan anemia with a suitable donor is unclear. This decision is further confounded because 15–20% of Diamond-Blackfan patients may have a durable spontaneous remission, often in adolescence. Alternatives to transplantation, mainly chronic corticosteroids or transfusions, have inherent risks. These iatrogenic complications, coupled with a poorly defined increased risk of malignancy, may sway clinicians toward early transplantation in selected patients. For allogeneic donor selection, clinically "normal" family members of Diamond-Blackfan patients have been found to have a silent Diamond-Blackfan anemia phenotype, characterized by macrocytosis and elevated fetal hemoglobin and/or erythrocyte adenosine deaminase levels, and some potential donors have been reported who carry *RPS19* mutations.[78] Donors should be screened for these abnormalities.

Prognosis

The median survival in untreated patients is 19 years, and corticosteroid treatment improves survival to 42 years.[86] Initial steroid-responsiveness is one of the only favorable prognostic factors identified. Age at diagnosis, family history, and presence of congenital malformation have not been reproducibly verified as prognostic indicators. In the French cohort of 222 Diamond-Blackfan patients followed for a median of 112 months, 6% of the transfusion-dependent patients died: 5 from hemochromatosis, 3 from pancytopenia, 3 from infection, 2 from cancer, and 2 from bone marrow transplantation–related complications. In the steroid-dependent patients, 1 of 125 patients died of sepsis.[54]

There is a predisposition to hematologic and solid tumor malignancies in Diamond-Blackfan anemia.[55,86,97] In the Diamond-Blackfan Anemia Registry, 29 patients have developed malignancy; acute nonlymphoblastic leukemia and myelodysplastic syndrome (11 cases) and osteogenic sarcoma (5 cases) are most frequently reported. The association of leukemia and myelodysplastic syndrome with Diamond-Blackfan anemia is consistent with the hypothesis of an intrinsic hematopoietic progenitor defect. Of 28 patients followed for up to 13 years with periodic bone marrow biopsies, 75% developed moderate to severe bone marrow hypoplasia (none developed acute myeloid leukemia), which was clinically reflected in significant neutropenia and thrombocytopenia.[85]

Current Controversies & Future Considerations

Acquired Pure Red Cell Aplasia

- Should cyclosporine and not prednisone be the initial treatment of choice for patients with acquired secondary pure red cell aplasia?
- What epitopes on erythroid precursors are recognized by autoantibodies or T cells? Are these unique to individual patients or shared? Can we develop new reagents that specifically block these interactions?

Diamond-Blackfan Anemia

- What is the optimal timing for transplantation in Diamond-Blackfan anemia? Should a trial of cyclosporine precede transplantation?
- What factors influence the variable penetrance of this disease? Will insight into the pathophysiology provide a general understanding of normal erythropoiesis or promote novel therapies?
- What is the mechanism by which *RPS19* gene mutations cause Diamond-Blackfan anemia?
- Will oral iron chelators alter the long-term outcome for Diamond-Blackfan anemia, especially for transfusion-dependent patients?

Suggested Readings*

Casadevall N, Nataf J, Viron B, et al: Pure red-cell aplasia and antierythropoietin antibodies in patients treated with recombinant erythropoietin. N Engl J Med 346:469–475, 2002.

Charles RJ, Sabo KM, Kidd PG, et al: The pathophysiology of pure red cell aplasia: implications for therapy. Blood 87:4831–4838, 1996.

Draptchinskaia N, Gustavsson P, Andersson B, et al: The gene encoding ribosomal protein S19 is mutated in Diamond-Blackfan anaemia. Nat Genet 21:169–175, 1999.

Gazda H, Lipton JM, Willig T-N, et al: Evidence for linkage of familial Diamond-Blackfan anemia to chromosome 8p23.3-p22 and for non-19q non-8p disease. Blood 7:2145–2150, 2001.

Giri N, Kang E, Tisdale JF, et al: Clinical and laboratory evidence for a trilineage haematopoietic defect in patients with refractory Diamond-Blackfan anaemia. Br J Haematol 108:167–175, 2000.

Gustavsson P, Garelli E, Draptchinskaia N, et al: Identification of microdeletions spanning the Diamond-Blackfan anemia locus on 19q13 and evidence for genetic heterogeneity. Am J Hum Genet 63:1388–1395, 1998.

Hamaguchi I, Flygare J, Nishiura H, et al: Proliferation deficiency of multipotent hematopoietic progenitors in ribosomal protein S19(RPS19)-deficient Diamond-Blackfan anemia improves following *RPS19* gene transfer. Mol Ther 7:613–622, 2003.

Handgretinger R, Geiselhart A, Moris A, et al: Pure red-cell aplasia associated with clonal expansion of granular lymphocytes expressing killer-cell inhibitory receptors. N Engl J Med 340:278–284, 1999.

Kiyoshi ML, Furukawa H, Hayashi K, et al: Pure red cell aplasia associated with expansion of CD3+ CD8+ granular lymphocytes expressing cytotoxicity against HLA-E+ cells. Br J Haematol 123:147–153, 2003.

Lacy MQ, Kurtin PJ, Ayalew T: Pure red cell aplasia: associated with large granular lymphocyte leukemia and the prognostic value of cytogenetic abnormalities. Blood 87:3000–3006, 1996.

Willig T-N, Draptchinskaia N, Dianzani I, et al: Mutations in ribosomal protein S19 gene and Diamond Blackfan anemia: wide variations in phenotypic expression. Blood 94:4294–4306, 1999.

Full references for this chapter can be found on accompanying CD-ROM.

CHAPTER 13

Congenital Neutropenia

Jill M. Watanabe, MD, MPH, and David C. Dale, MD

KEY POINTS

Congenital Neutropenia

- Congenital neutropenia encompasses a heterogeneous group of inherited diseases.
- The genetic mutations causing congenital neutropenia may have an isolated effect on the bone marrow but can also affect one or more other organ systems.
- Genes implicated in the congenital neutropenia have been rapidly identified over the past decade.
- Granulocyte colony-stimulating factor has dramatically improved the prognosis for children with congenital neutropenia.

INTRODUCTION

The congenital neutropenias are inherited hematologic conditions that are usually recognized in infancy or early childhood. Congenital neutropenia is often diagnosed when a young child has a differential white blood cell count performed for symptoms and signs of a severe infection. Congenital neutropenia may also be recognized in evaluating a child with a complex congenital syndrome. The severity of the neutropenia and its clinical consequences vary considerably.

Neutropenia is defined as an absolute blood neutrophil count more than 2 standard deviations below normal. The absolute count is percent neutrophils plus bands counted on a differential multiplied by the total white blood cell count. Using this definition, the blood count to define neutropenia varies by age and race. In children 1 month to 10 years of age, neutropenia is defined by a neutrophil count less than 1500 cells/μL; beyond 10 years of age, neutropenia is defined by a neutrophil count less than 1800 cells/μL in persons of white and Asian descent.[1] In persons of African descent, neutropenia is defined by a count of 800–1000 cells/μL.[1]

The severity and duration of neutropenia are also clinically important. Mild neutropenia is usually defined by neutrophil counts of 1000–1500 cells/μL, moderate neutropenia is 500–1000 cells/μL, and severe neutropenia is less than 500 cells/μL. Acute neutropenia usually is present for only 5–10 days; neutropenia is chronic if its duration is at least several weeks. Almost all congenital neutropenias are chronic neutropenia.

The characteristics and causes of congenital neutropenia are shown in Tables 13–1 and 13–2, and an algorithm for their diagnosis is presented in Figure 13–1.

SEVERE CONGENITAL NEUTROPENIA

Patients with severe congenital neutropenia (SCN) typically present with recurrent bacterial infections and neutrophil counts persistently less than 200 cells/μL. Kostmann described SCN as an autosomal recessive disorder in 1956[2]; subsequently many sporadic cases and families with an autosomal dominant inheritance were reported. The incidence of SCN is estimated at 2 per 1 million births.[3]

Pathophysiology

The genetics of SCN are heterogeneous. Up to 80% of patients have heterozygous mutations in exons 2, 3, 4, or 5 of the gene for neutrophil elastase (NE), also known as elastase-2 (*ELA2;* locus 19p13.3)[4,5] (Fig. 13–2). *ELA2* encodes a potent protease that is synthesized at the promyelocytic stage in neutrophil development and packaged in the neutrophil's primary granules.[4] Genetic and cellular evidence is persuasive that mutations in *ELA2* cause sporadic and autosomal dominant SCN. The

TABLE 13–1. Characteristics of the Congenital Neutropenias

Disorder	Incidence	Clinical Features
Severe congenital neutropenia	2 : 1,000,000	Neutrophil counts <200 cells/μL with recurrent bacterial infections.
Cyclic neutropenia	0.5–1 : 1,000,000	Periodic oscillations of neutrophil counts, with nadirs <200 cells/μL approximately every 21 days and periodic vulnerability to infections, especially oral ulcerations.
Myelokathexis (WHIM syndrome)	~25 case reports	Neutrophil counts <500 cells/μL with lymphopenia despite hypercellular bone marrow. Neutrophils and eosinophils appear "bizarre" in bone marrow and blood. Association of warts, hypogammaglobulinemia, infections, and myelokathexis (retention in the bone marrow) defines WHIM syndrome.
Cartilage-hair hypoplasia	Finland: 1 : 23,000 Old Order Amish: 1.5 : 1,000	Short-limb dwarfism with hypoplastic hair, T-cell dysfunction. Neutropenia seen in ~24% of cases.
Shwachman-Diamond syndrome	1 : 77,000	Exocrine pancreatic dysfunction, short stature, and neutropenia (66% with absolute neutrophil count <1000 cells/μL, often with cyclic fluctuations), mild anemia.
Chédiak-Higashi syndrome	>200 case reports	Hypopigmentation of hair, eyes, and skin with neutropenia and recurrent bacterial infections. Giant peroxidase-positive lysosomal granules in granulocytes from bone marrow and blood. Vulnerability to hemophagocytic lymphohistiocytosis evolution.
Griscelli syndrome, type 2	~60 case reports (all types)	Hypopigmentation of hair and skin, neutropenia typically seen in association with pancytopenia; patients also have impaired T-cell and B-cell function. Vulnerability to hemophagocytic lymphohistiocytosis evolution.
Barth syndrome	1 : 300,000–400,000 males	Cardiomyopathy, skeletal myopathy, and neutropenia (can be cyclic).
Dyskeratosis congenita	~275 case reports	Abnormal skin pigmentation, nail dystrophy, and mucosal leukoplakia. Bone marrow failure before the first decade of life is common with pancytopenia.
Glycogen storage disease, type 1b	<1 : 100,000	Hypoglycemia, hepatomegaly, and growth retardation associated with glycogen accumulation in the liver and kidneys. Neutrophil counts typically <1000 cells/μL; neutrophil dysfunction.
Wiskott-Aldrich syndrome	4 : 1,000,000 males	Microthrombocytopenia, immunodeficiency (25% with neutropenia), and eczema; increased risk of autoimmune disease and malignancy.

TABLE 13–2. Molecular Biology of the Congenital Neutropenias

Disorder	Inheritance	Gene and Locus	Enzyme Defect
Severe congenital neutropenia	AD and S	*ELA2* at 19p13.3	Neutrophil elastase: a prominent enzyme in the primary granules
Cyclic neutropenia	AD and S	*ELA2* at 19p13.3	Neutrophil elastase: a prominent enzyme in the primary granules
Myelokathexis (WHIM syndrome)	AD and S	*CXCR4* at 2q21	CXCR4 gene product: chemokine receptor involved in leukocyte trafficking
Cartilage-hair hypoplasia	AR and S	*RMRP* at 9p13	Ribonuclease MRP: mitochondrial processing of RNA or pre-RNA
Shwachman-Diamond syndrome	AR	*SBDS* at 7q11	SBDS gene product: involved in RNA metabolism
Chédiak-Higashi syndrome	AR	*CHS1* at 1q43	LYST: a lysosomal trafficking regulatory protein
Griscelli syndrome, type 2	AR	*RAB27a* at 15q21	GTPase: expressed in melanocytes and T cells; may have a role in granule release and cytotoxicity
Barth syndrome	X-linked	*TAZ* at Xq28	Tafazzins: involved in cardiolipin synthesis; important in normal mitochondrial function
Dyskeratosis congenita	X-linked	*DKC1* at Xq28	Dyskerin: component of the telomerase complex involved in telomere synthesis
	AD	*hTERC* at 3q21–q28	hTERC gene product: RNA component of the telomerase complex involved in telomere synthesis
	AR	Not identified	
Glycogen storage disease, type 1b	AR	*G6PT* at 11q23	Glucose 6-phosphate translocase: transports glucose 6-phosphate from the cytoplasm to the lumen of the endoplasmic reticulum
Wiskott-Aldrich syndrome	X-linked	*WASP* at Xp11.22–11.23	WASP gene: cytoplasmic scaffolding protein that stabilizes actin filaments

Abbreviations: AD, autosomal dominant; AR, autosomal recessive; S, sporadic.

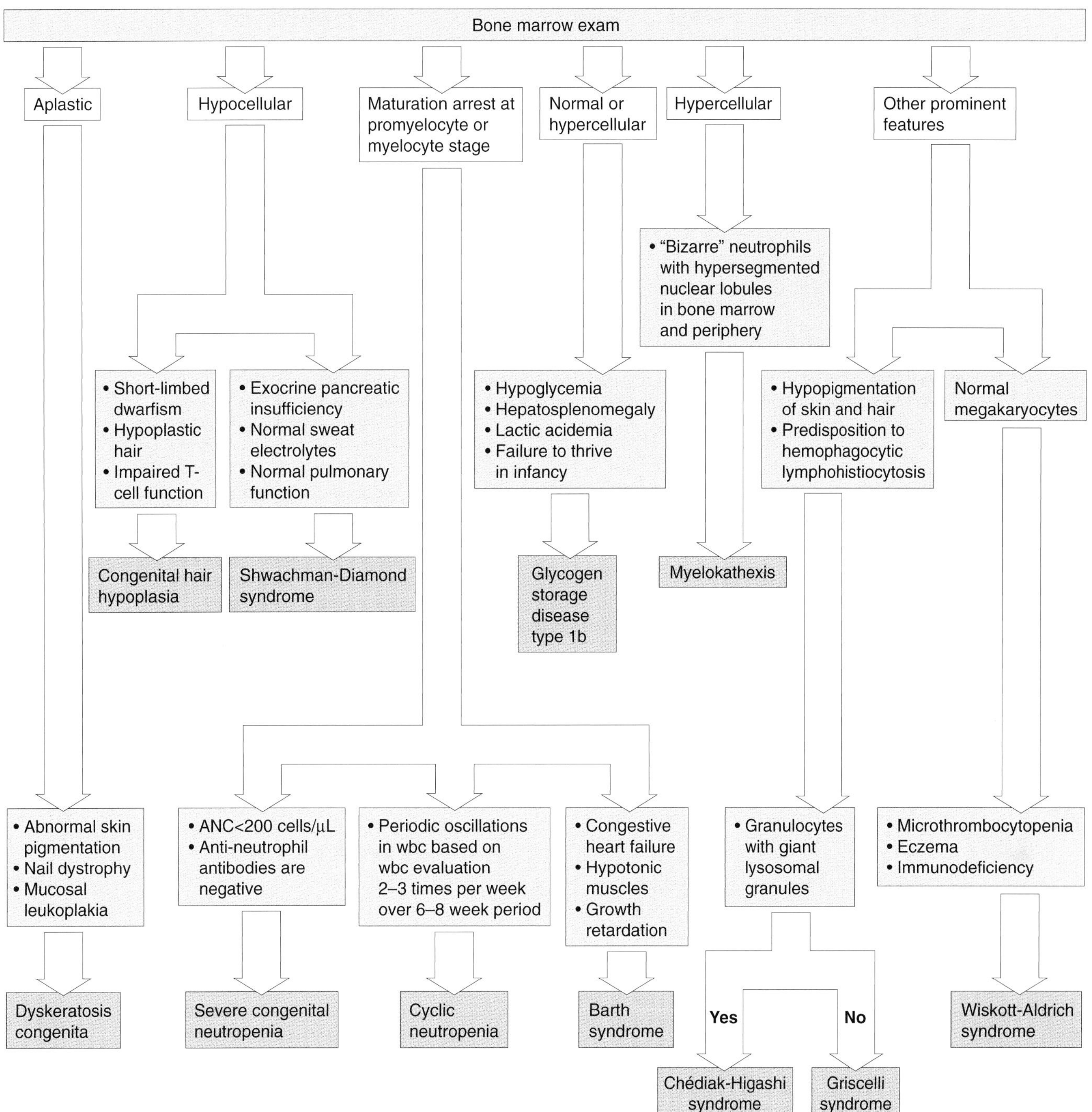

Figure 13–1. Algorithm for the diagnosis of congenital neutropenia.

cause for the autosomal recessive cases is still unknown. In autosomal dominant SCN, the same heterozygous mutation is found in all affected family members but not in normal relatives.[6] In a very informative case, the father of a patient with typical SCN showed mosaic expression of the same *ELA2* mutation; half of his somatic cells contained the mutant gene, but the mutant protease was virtually absent in circulating neutrophils. In this natural observation, neutrophils expressing the abnormal gene appeared to be destroyed in the marrow before entering the circulation.[7] Human promyelocytic leukemia cells, such as HL-60 cells, which express the neutrophil esterase mutants, exhibit accelerated apoptosis.[8] Accelerated apoptosis may be mediated through altered expression of Bcl-2 proapoptotic factors, which appear to be normalized with the administration of granulocyte colony-stimulating factor (G-CSF).[9] Several other mutations have been associated with SCN, but their causal role is uncertain. G-CSF receptor mutations, present in a few cases, were probably acquired during evolution to acute

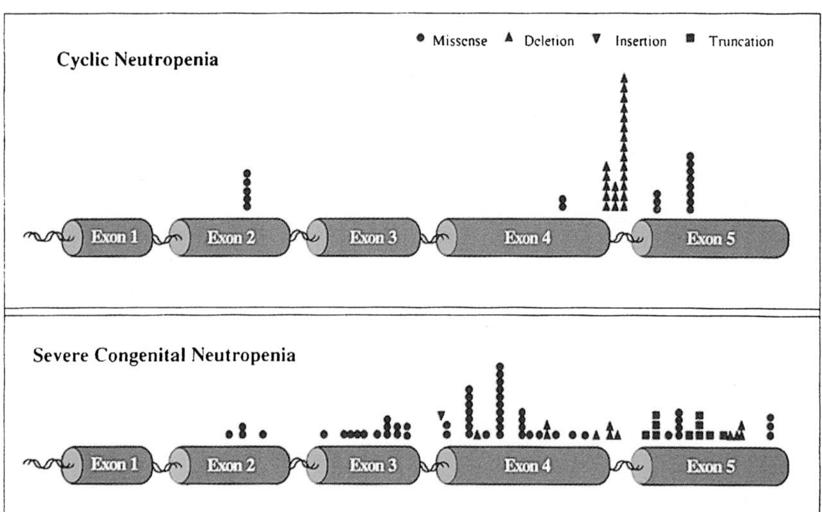

Figure 13–2. The pattern of mutations in the gene for neutrophil elastase in patients with cyclic and autosomal dominant congenital neutropenia.

myelogenous leukemia (AML).[8,10] A mutation in *GFI1* has been reported in one child.[11]

Clinical Features and Diagnosis

In addition to severe neutropenia, SCN patients usually have monocytosis, thrombocytosis, and a mild normocytic, normochromic, or hypochromic anemia. The bone marrow demonstrates "arrest" of neutrophil development at the promyelocyte and myelocyte stage, although some samples show many maturing band and segmented neutrophils, particularly in response to infections. The cellularity of the bone marrow is normal or decreased, with a reduced myeloid-to-erythroid ratio, normal megakaryocytes, and occasional eosinophilia[3] (Fig. 13–3). Anemia and thrombocytosis are probably due to chronic inflammation; monocytosis reflects growth factor stimulation of the neutrophil-monocyte lineage. At diagnosis, tests for antineutrophil antibodies and chromosomal abnormalities are absent.[3] Tests for *ELA2* mutations may be helpful but are still largely a research procedure.

Patients with SCN typically have recurrent fevers, oropharyngeal ulcers, and skin, respiratory, and perirectal infections. Deep tissue abscesses in the liver and lungs with bacteremias are not uncommon, and these infections may quickly become life-threatening. Common pathogens include *Staphylococcus aureus, Escherichia coli,* and *Pseudomonas* species. Until recently, SCN was often fatal as a result of infections in early childhood, despite prompt and aggressive antibiotic therapy. Prior to the availability of G-CSF, the mortality by the age of 2 years was estimated at 42%.

Treatment and Prognosis

The availability of G-CSF has markedly altered the outlook for SCN patients. Almost all patients respond to G-CSF with improvement in neutrophil counts and in their quality of life.[12] By contrast, corticosteroids,[13,14] lithium,[15,16] intravenous immunoglobulins,[17,18] or

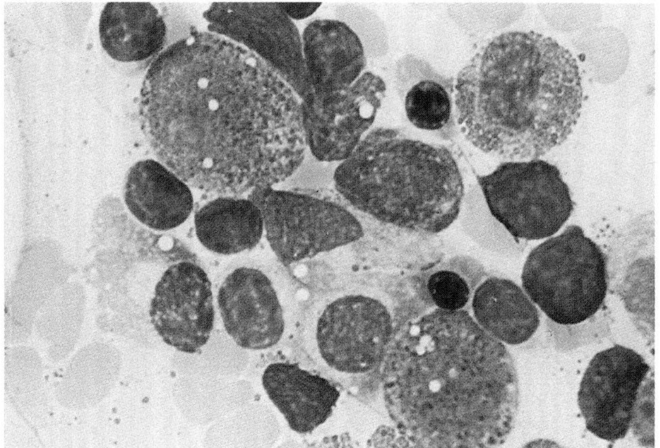

Figure 13–3. Bone marrow aspirates from a patient with severe congenital neutropenia showing neutrophil precursors; mature neutrophils are absent or greatly reduced.

granulocyte-macrophage colony stimulating factor[19] are of little benefit. The role of G-CSF in the treatment of the congenital neutropenias is summarized in Table 13–3. The effectiveness of prophylactic G-CSF was established in a randomized, controlled clinical trial[20]: the median G-CSF dose for SCN was approximately 5 μg/kg/day; starting at this dose, G-CSF was increased by 5–10 μg/kg/day every 14 days to achieve a neutrophil count greater than 1000 cells/μL. Currently, dosages higher than 50–100 μg/kg/day are not recommended because of the low likelihood of benefit and the volume of drug required.[3,21] Adverse effects are generally mild, primarily consisting of transient headache and bone pain.[20] Splenomegaly, osteoporosis, vasculitis, rashes, arthralgia, and hematuria are infrequent adverse events.[22] Allogenic hematopoietic stem cell transplantation is the only established alternative treatment for patients refractory to G-CSF.[23]

SCN patients are at risk of developing myelodysplastic syndrome (MDS) and AML, a risk recognized before the availability of G-CSF. In a population of SCN patients

TABLE 13–3. Treatment of Congenital Neutropenias with G-CSF

Disorder	General Role	Dose	Other Comments
Severe congenital neutropenia	All patients	5–50 μg/kg SQ daily	Maintain ANC > 1000 cells/μL Severe disease that requires higher doses may predict increased risk for transformation to MDS or AML
Cyclic neutropenia	Prophylactic	1–5 μg/kg SQ daily or every other day	G-CSF shortens periodicity of neutropenia Decreases the severity of neutropenia
Myelokathexis (WHIM syndrome)	Generally not necessary Use in patients with recurrent infections	1–5 μg/kg SQ daily	Normalizes ANC G-CSF corrects accelerated apoptosis of neutrophils
Shwachman-Diamond syndrome	Use in patients with severe neutropenia and recurrent infections	1–10 μg/kg SQ daily	Normalizes ANC Possible increased risk of malignant transformation
Chédiak-Higashi syndrome	Neutropenia is generally mild G-CSF may be beneficial with recurrent infections	1–10 μg/kg SQ daily	G-CSF may increase ANC
Barth syndrome	Neutropenia is generally mild G-CSF may be beneficial with recurrent infections	1–10 μg/kg SQ daily	G-CSF increases ANC
Glycogen storage disease, type 1b	90% of patients with ANC < 1000 cells/μL	1–2 μg/kg SQ daily	Maintain ANC > 1000 cells/μL Splenic enlargement is a universal complication of G-CSF use Inflammatory bowel disease improves with G-CSF therapy

Abbreviations: ANC, absolute neutrophil count; SQ, subcutaneously.

receiving G-CSF, transformation to AML or MDS occurred in about 2% per year.[24] The risk appears to be higher for patients with more severe disease, as reflected by their requirement of higher doses of G-CSF.[6] Monitoring with regular clinical evaluations, blood counts, and an annual bone marrow examination is recommended to assess histologic changes and chromosomal abnormalities, especially the acquisition of monosomy 7. Ras and G-CSF receptor mutations also have been linked to malignant transformation.[22] Survival after hematopoietic stem cell transplantation is more favorable if patients do not have MDS/AML; transplantation should be considered in patients revealing genetic transformation in their bone marrow.

CYCLIC NEUTROPENIA

Cyclic neutropenia (CN) usually presents with recurring episodes of fever, mouth ulcers, pharyngitis, and lymphadenopathy every 3 weeks, resolving spontaneously over 5–7 days. In 1910, Leale reported the first case in a 19-month-old boy.[25] CN occurs sporadically or by autosomal dominant inheritance; the estimated incidence is 0.5–1 per 1 million births.[26]

Pathophysiology

Mutations of the gene for NE (*ELA2*) were originally implicated in autosomal dominant and sporadic forms of CN prior to the discovery of the same genetic association with SCN.[4,27] *ELA2* mutations predominantly involve exon 4 at its junction with intron 4 (see Fig. 13–2).[27] In both SCN and CN, the neutrophil precursors are subjected to accelerated apoptosis, making marrow production of neutrophils ineffective. The loci of the mutations predict that they affect function of the active site of the enzyme binding to its substrates or to natural inhibitors.[4] No abnormality of the gene for the G-CSF receptor or other genes has been documented in well-characterized cases of CN.

Clinical Features and Diagnosis

In most cases, neutrophil nadirs occur every 19–21 days,[28] but some long and shorter cycles are reported, ranging from 11 to 52 days.[29] Neutrophil counts typically fall to zero at their nadir and do not increase above 200 cells/μL for 3–5 days; peaks are generally less than 2000 cells/μL. The monocyte counts also cycle, rising as the neutrophils fall; platelets, eosinophils, lymphocytes, and reticulocytes can oscillate in a pattern of "cyclic hematopoeisis"[29] (Fig. 13–4). The bone marrow histology varies cyclically. During neutropenia, there is "neutrophil maturation arrest" at the promyelocyte or myelocyte stage and the bone marrow may become "hyperplastic" during periods of neutrophil count recovery, showing large numbers of marrow neutrophils (Fig. 13–5). Tests for chromosomal abnormalities and antineutrophil antibodies are negative. Mathematical studies suggest that cyclic oscillations in cells of the marrow and blood are a natural feature of hematologic diseases with increased apoptosis of early progenitors.[30,31]

Recognition of CN is primarily based on the characteristic fluctuations of blood neutrophils in serial blood counts performed at least two to three times per week for 6–8 weeks.[28] Sequencing of *ELA2* is available and may aid in the diagnosis, but serial blood counts remain important to determine diagnosis and also prognosis.

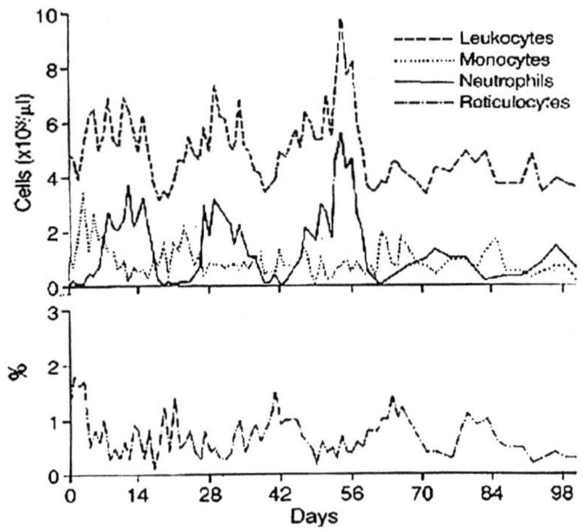

■ **Figure 13–4.** Serial blood cell counts for a patient with cyclic neutropenia. Oscillations in absolute leukocyte blood neutrophils, monocytes, and reticulocytes are shown. (From Dale DC, Hammond WP: Cyclic neutropenia: a clinical review. Blood Rev 2:178–185, 1988, with permission.)

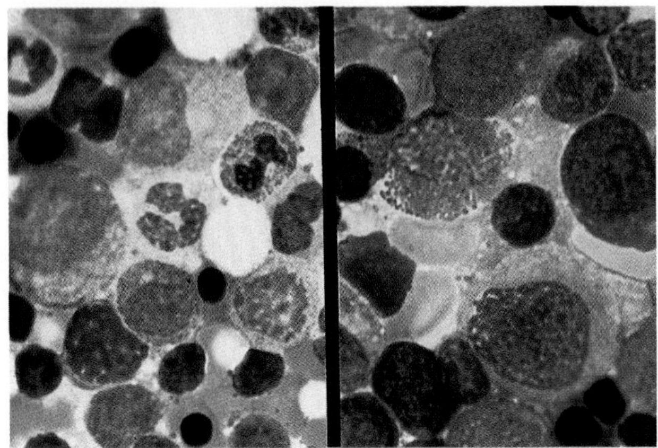

■ **Figure 13–5.** Bone marrow aspirate cells from a patient with cyclic neutropenia at the peak and the nadir of the neutrophil cycle.

Family studies and *ELA2* sequencing indicate that there are mild cases of CN with less severe neutropenia and fewer infections.

Fever, malaise, oral ulcers, and lymphadenopathy are features of almost every cycle in most cases; the mouth ulcers can be extremely deep and painful. Cellulitis, sinusitis, pneumonia, mastoiditis, and recurrent perirectal lesions are also common. Although CN is generally more benign than is SCN, about 10% of patients will die suddenly from peritonitis, necrotizing enterocolitis, and sepsis with *Clostridium perfringens* and *E. coli* bacteremias during a neutropenic period.[32]

Treatment and Prognosis

Historically, the management of CN was supportive care, intermittent antibiotics, and good oral hygiene. Now treatment with prophylactic G-CSF decreases the severity of the neutropenia, shortens the periodicity, and prevents recurrent infections.[33] A typical G-CSF dose is 1–5 µg/kg/day on a once-daily or every-other-day schedule[34] (see Table 13–3).

Neutropenia may become moderated in adulthood, when the severity and frequency of infections wane; the mechanism underlying this change is not known.[35] Patients with CN have no recognized risk of transformation to MDS or AML, with or without G-CSF treatment.[22]

MYELOKATHEXIS AND WHIM SYNDROME

Myelokathexis (a term for retention of neutrophils in the bone marrow) is a rare congenital disorder characterized by severe neutropenia and lymphocytopenia, first described by Zuezler and by Krill and colleagues in 1964.[36,37] White blood cell counts are usually less than 1000 cells/µL, and neutrophil counts less than 500 cells/µL. The neutrophils in the blood and marrow have very pyknotic nuclei, a distinctive if not entirely diagnostic feature of this disorder. Neutropenia associated with warts, hypogammaglobulinemia, infections, and myelokathexis constitute the WHIM syndrome. Both myelokathexis and WHIM syndrome have autosomal dominant inheritance,[38] although sporadic cases have also been reported. The genetic defect for WHIM syndrome has been isolated to the gene encoding a chemokine receptor (CXCR4) at chromosome 2q21.[39]

Pathophysiology and Clinical Features

Diagnosis of myelokathexis is established by examination of the blood smear and bone marrow. The marrow is hypercellular with many neutrophil precursors, despite the abnormally low peripheral count. In the blood and bone marrow, neutrophils are characterized by hypersegmentation of their nuclear lobules separated by thin filaments of chromatin; they contain cytoplasmic vacuoles and prominent granules[40] (Fig. 13–6). There is accelerated apoptosis of marrow and blood neutrophils, and their marrow precursors, attributable to depressed expression of *bcl*-x.[40] Eosinophils can also appear bizarre, but the lymphocytes, monocytes, and basophils are unaffected. Killing of bacteria by the neutrophils is normal.[41] Immune function may be primarily affected as a result of abnormal surveillance and trafficking of leukocytes, functions mediated through the CXCR4 receptor and its interactions with CXCL12 (stromal-derived factor-1α).[42]

Treatment and Prognosis

Despite severe neutropenia and lymphocytopenia, serious bacterial infections are very infrequent. Patients with WHIM syndrome have susceptibility to human papillomavirus but not to cytomegalovirus or *Toxoplasma gondii*. Treatment with G-CSF partially corrects the accelerated apoptosis of developing neutrophils[40] and normalizes blood neutrophil levels, increases immunoglobulin levels, and may reduce infections[43] (see

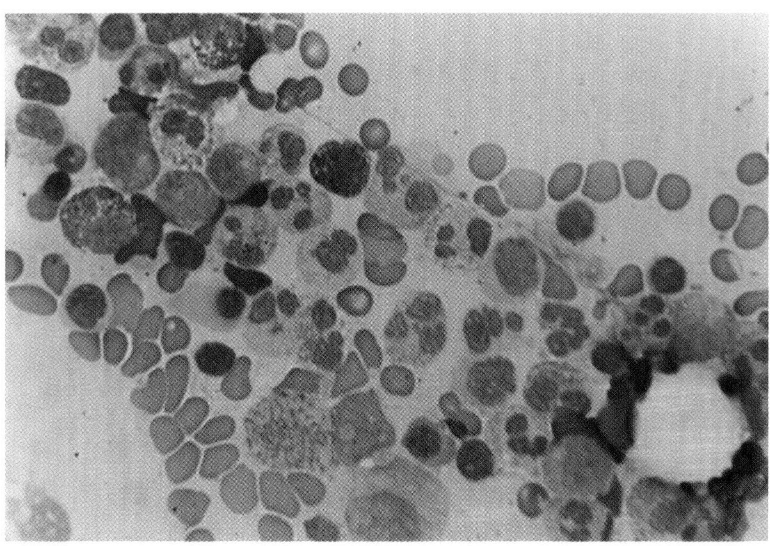

Figure 13–6. Bone marrow aspirate from a patient with myelokathexis. The marrow shows many segmented and hypersegmented neutrophils. By contrast, in the blood, there is severe neutropenia.

Table 13–3). However, for most patients, this treatment is not necessary.

CARTILAGE-HAIR HYPOPLASIA

Cartilage-hair hypoplasia (CHH) is a rare autosomal recessive disorder characterized by a short-limb dwarfism, hypoplastic hair, and impaired T-cell function with a susceptibility to viral infections, especially varicella-zoster. It was first described by McKusick and coworkers in 1965 in an isolated Old Order Amish community.[44] In Finland, the incidence of CHH is 1 : 23,000.[45] Among the Old Order Amish, an isolated religious community, the incidence has been estimated at 1.5 : 1000.[46] Sporadic cases have been described in many other ethnic populations.

Pathophysiology

The genetic defect of CHH is located at locus 9p13,[47] where mutations to the gene encoding the ribonuclease MRP have been identified.[48] Ribonuclease MRP is an endoribonuclease that cleaves RNA or pre–ribosomal RNA in mitochondrial processing. CHH is associated with increased apoptosis of T lymphocytes with altered expression of Fas and Bax, members of the Bcl-2 protein family.[49] There is remarkable variability of expression among members of affected families, suggesting that other modifying factors play a role in the expression of the CHH phenotype.

Clinical Features

In a study of 88 Finnish patients, 86% had macrocytic anemia, 62% had lymphopenia, and 24% had variable degrees of neutropenia.[50] Rare cases were associated with fatal hypoplastic anemia. Skeletal biopsies have shown cartilage hypoplasia, typically manifested as shortened limbs with increased joint laxity. The hair is characteristically fine, fragile, and sparse, and typically light-colored. Other associated features include Hirschsprung's disease (colonic aganglionosis)[51] and malignancies (lymphoma and basal cell carcinoma).[52] Between 1971 and 1995, a population register center in Finland documented that the most frequent causes of death were pneumonia and sepsis.[53]

Treatment and Prognosis

Hematopoietic stem cell transplantation corrects the immunodeficiency but not the chondrodysplasia.[54] Treatment of four patients with growth hormone was without benefit.[55]

SHWACHMAN-DIAMOND SYNDROME

Shwachman-Diamond syndrome (SDS) is a rare autosomal recessive disorder characterized by pancreatic insufficiency, neutropenia, and short stature. Shwachman and associates first described the syndrome in 1964.[56] The incidence of this disorder is 1 : 77,000,[57] with approximately 300 cases reported as of December 2000.[58]

Pathophysiology

The genetic defect is located at 7q11[59] at a site now designated the *SBDS* (Shwachman-Bodian-Diamond syndrome) gene.[60] Although the mutations in *SBDS* are not understood, indirect evidence points to abnormal RNA metabolism that could widely affect cellular function in the pancreas, bone marrow, and bone.[60] The connection between these genetic mutations and the phenotypic expression of the cellular abnormalities has not been established. Cellular manifestations include defects in neutrophil chemotaxis[61] and abnormalities of progenitor cells in the bone marrow, which have a decreased potential to form new colonies and an increased apoptosis rate.[62]

Clinical Features and Diagnosis

Neutropenia is seen in virtually all patients: approximately 66% have neutrophil counts less than 1000 cells/μL, and cyclic fluctuation is common.[58] Cellulitis, otitis media, pneumonia, and osteomyelitis are associated with the neutropenia. Mild normochromic and normocytic anemia occurs in 80% of cases.[58] Thrombocytopenia also is frequent (24–88% of cases), with recorded fatal hemorrhagic events.[58] Cell-mediated immunity can be impaired.[63] As many as one third of patients with SDS undergo malignant transformation to MDS and AML, with acquired clonal chromosomal abnormalities.[61]

SDS is a multisystem disorder with variable involvement of other organs, including the pancreas, liver, kidneys, and teeth. Malabsorption resulting from pancreatic insufficiency is often severe, particularly in young children. Growth problems occur in the first 2 years; metaphysial chondrodysplasia, metaphyseal dysostosis, rib cage abnormalities, syndactyly, kyphosis, and scoliosis are common features.

Diagnostic criteria for SDS include evidence of pancreatic insufficiency and the hematologic abnormalities.[58] Pancreatic insufficiency can be established by an elevated 72-hour fecal fat level, a decrease in serum cationic trypsinogen, and an abnormal quantitative pancreatic stimulation test. The hematologic abnormalities are manifested by neutropenia (absolute neutrophil count < 1500 cells/μL), anemia (hemoglobin more than 2 standard deviations below the age-adjusted mean), and thrombocytopenia (platelet count < 150,000 cells/mm^3).[58]

Treatment and Prognosis

Supportive therapy includes pancreatic enzyme replacement and antibiotic therapy for infections. Case studies have shown that G-CSF is effective in increasing the neutrophil count in patients with severe neutropenia[64] and decreases the rate of infections[65] (see Table 13–3). SDS patients with aplastic anemia may respond to corticosteroids[66] and cyclosporine therapy.[67] The only curative treatment following malignant transformation is a stem cell transplant.[68]

The role of annual bone marrow evaluation in long-term follow-up of patients with SDS is controversial. Frequent marrow examinations monitor for acquired chromosomal abnormalities, which may precede malignant transformation, but some abnormal clones regress without intervention.[69] If patients with SDS survive the respiratory difficulties and most serious infections of early life, both the neutropenia and the pancreatic insufficiency may improve as they age. However, aging also increases the risk for undergoing malignant transformation to MDS and AML. The projected median survival of patients is more than 35 years.[58]

CHÉDIAK-HIGASHI SYNDROME

Chédiak-Higashi syndrome (CHS) is a rare autosomal recessive disorder characterized by hypopigmentation of the hair, eyes, and skin; giant granules in several types of cells; and neutropenia with recurrent bacterial infections. CHS was first reported by Beguez-Cesar in 1943[70] and further defined by Chédiak,[71] Higashi,[72] and Sato.[73] About one half of all cases with CHS are now attributable to mutations of the *CHS1* gene at 1q43 that encodes a lysosomal trafficking regulatory protein (LYST).[74] Mutations of *CHS1* that totally abolish LYST expression cause more severe disease; milder cases are associated with missense mutations.[75]

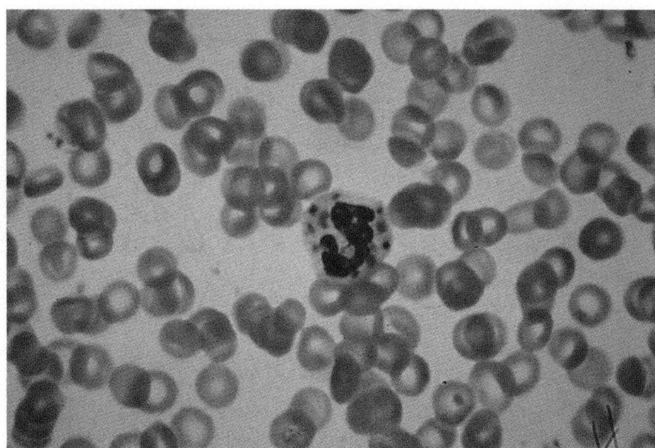

Figure 13–7. Blood smear showing typical appearance of a neutrophil of a patient with Chédiak-Higashi syndrome. The large cytoplasmic granules can be seen easily with standard Wright- or Giemsa-stained blood smears. (From the teaching collection of the American Society of Hematology.)

Clinical Features and Diagnosis

CHS is diagnosed by detection of the giant granules in neutrophils, monocytes, and lymphocytes, which are easily visible by light microscopy and are sometimes more prominent in the bone marrow than in the blood. In neutrophils, the very large granules appear to result from fusion of the primary and specific granules (Fig. 13–7).[76,77] These cells undergo intramedullary destruction resulting in neutropenia. Blood neutrophils have depressed chemotaxis[78] and diminished bactericidal potency.[79] Platelets also have abnormal granules and exhibit defective aggregation leading to easy bruising and bleeding.[80,81] Cytotoxic T-cell and natural killer cell function also are abnormal.[82,83] In the most common and severe form, young children develop recurrent, often life-threatening, bacterial infections and then progress in an "accelerated phase,"[84] characterized by diffuse lymphohistiocytic infiltration of the liver, spleen, lymph nodes, and bone marrow, and progressively worsening pancytopenia.

Treatment and Prognosis

Management is directed primarily to avoiding infections and appropriate institution of aggressive antibiotic treatment. Ascorbic acid improves neutrophil functions in vitro,[85] but its clinical benefits are uncertain.[86,87] G-CSF may increase blood neutrophil levels but is also an unproven therapy[88] (see Table 13–3). Systemic corticosteroids have been used to treat an accompanying peripheral neuropathy.[89] Treatment of the accelerated phase with vincristine and corticosteroids can induce temporary remissions, but bone marrow transplantation is the only cure.[90]

Treatment and Prognosis

The accelerated phase is lethal within months without a hematopoietic stem cell transplantation,[95,100] although immune suppression with glucocorticosteroids, antithymocyte globulin, methotrexate, etoposide, and cyclosporin have all been reported to be of benefit, at least transiently.[101–103]

GRISCELLI SYNDROME

In 1978, Griscelli and colleagues described two patients with hypopigmentation of the hair and skin, similar to CHS, but with normal-appearing neutrophils.[91] The three subtypes of this rare autosomal recessive disorder occur predominantly in persons of Turkish and Mediterranean descent.[92] In type 1, attributable to a mutation in the *MYO5a* gene at 15q21 (expressed abundantly in the brain), there is developmental delay and mental retardation without neutropenia or immune deficiency.[93] In type 2, due to mutations in *RAB27a* at 15q21, patients have neutropenia and pancytopenia and progress to an accelerated phase similar to that in CHS.[94] *RAB27a* is expressed in melanocytes and hematopoietic cells but not in brain.[95] A third form with only hypopigmentation is caused by mutations at 2q37.3 in *MLPH,* a gene encoding melanophilin that is expressed in melanosomes but not brain.[96] Melanophilin is involved in the interactions of the *MYO5a* and *RAB27a* gene products to mediate melanosome transport.[97]

Clinical Features and Diagnosis

Based on the phenotypic similarities between Griscelli syndrome and CHS, a patient with hypopigmentation and immune dysfunction should be evaluated for both conditions. The distinguishing feature of CHS is the presence of large granules in the neutrophils, melanocytes, and keratinocytes. Examination of the hair shafts in patients with CHS shows only small melanin aggregates in comparison to the large clumps seen in patients with Griscelli syndrome. Because of the defect in granule transport, melanosomes accumulate in the melanocytes but are reduced in the keratinocytes in all subtypes of Griscelli syndrome.[98] Confirmation can be provided by mutation analysis.

Patients with Griscelli syndrome have silver hair with hypopigmentation of their skin and eyes. Patients with type 2 are vulnerable to fever and recurrent infections. Hepatosplenomegaly and a combined T-cell and B-cell deficiency are common. Natural killer cell activity, delayed-type hypersensitivity, and the response to an antigenic challenge all are impaired.[99] Immunoglobulin levels may be normal or low; other features are hypofibrinogenemia, hypertriglyceridemia, and hypoproteinemia.[99] The accelerated phase with hemophagocytic lymphohistiocytosis is characterized by fever, pancytopenia, and diffuse lymphocytic infiltration of brain, spleen, liver, and lymph nodes. Neurologic deficits are associated with lymphohistiocytic infiltration in the central nervous system.[95]

BARTH SYNDROME

Barth syndrome is a rare disorder characterized by cardiomyopathy, neutropenia, and skeletal myopathy. In 1983, Barth and associates described a large family with affected males who typically died from sepsis or cardiac failure before the age of 3.[104] Mitochondria appeared normal in cardiac and skeletal muscle. A patient with a similar X-linked condition, reported by Neustein and coworkers in 1979, had abnormal mitochondria on electron microscopy.[105] Barth syndrome has an estimated incidence of 1 per 300,000–400,000 male births, based on the identification of 10 new cases annually in the United States.[106]

Pathophysiology

The locus for the Barth syndrome gene is Xq28,[107] and the disease is due to mutations to the *G4.5* gene (renamed *TAZ*).[108] The gene products of *TAZ,* the tafazzins, may share some homology with acetyltransferases involved in complex lipid metabolism,[109] and defects in cardiolipin synthesis may lead to mitochondrial dysfunction.[110] Molecular abnormalities of several phospholipids, including cardiolipin, were demonstrated in 19 of 25 children with Barth syndrome.[111]

Clinical Features and Diagnosis

Barth syndrome findings include dilated cardiomyopathy, skeletal myopathy, neutropenia, growth retardation, and elevated urinary excretion of 3-methylglutaconic acid.[112] Diagnosis is established by echocardiogram, quantitative urine organic acid analysis including quantification of 3-methylglutaconic acid (can be increased 5- to 20-fold), serial blood counts, and growth monitoring.[106] Neutropenia can be chronic, cyclic, or absent.[112] Cyclic oscillations in Barth syndrome occur at between 21 and 28 days. Peak absolute neutrophil counts are often normal, and nadirs approach zero. During infections, the neutrophil count may rise to normal or high levels.

Treatment and Prognosis

Supportive therapy is critical. Early diagnosis of Barth syndrome has been correlated with improved survival.[106] Cardiac function improves and may be normalized by treatment of congestive heart failure. Infectious complications improve with prompt recognition and aggressive treatment. G-CSF increases neutrophil levels and may be clinically beneficial[106] (see Table 13–3).

GLYCOGEN STORAGE DISEASE, TYPE 1b

Glycogen storage diseases are genetic disorders that interfere with glycogen synthesis and degradation. Glycogen storage disease (GSD) was first described by Von Gierke in 1929[113] and further defined by Cori and Cori[114] and Senior and Loridan.[115] There are several subtypes of GSD; the subtyping divides patients with primary deficiencies in glucose-6-phosphatase deficiency from those with defects in intracellular glucose transport.[116,117] Neutropenia and neutrophil dysfunction are characteristic features of GSD 1b[118] and have been documented in only a single patient with type 1a.[119] The frequency of GSD type 1 is thought to be less than 1:50,000.[120]

Pathophysiology

GSD 1b is caused by a mutation in the glucose-6-phosphatase transporter gene at 11q23. This gene encodes a protein that delivers glucose 6-phosphate from cytoplasm to the lumen of the endoplasmic reticulum, where it is catalyzed by glucose-6-phosphatase to glucose and phosphate.[121–123]

Clinical Features and Diagnosis

Patients with GSD 1b typically present with hypoglycemia, hepatomegaly, and growth retardation early in the first year of life.[124] Deficiency of the glucose 6-phosphate translocase causes hypoglycemia with irritability, seizures, and coma. Other features include hyperlipidemia, hyperuricemia, organomegaly secondary to glycogen accumulation, inflammatory bowel disease, and osteopenia.

The diagnosis of GSD 1b is established based on clinical features and the absence of an increase in serum glucose levels following the administration of glucagon or oral galactose. Mutation analysis and enzyme studies on samples obtained by open liver biopsy can confirm the diagnosis.[124]

About 90% of patients have neutrophil counts of less than 1000 cells/μL[125] at diagnosis, and usually the neutropenia gradually worsens.[125] Patients may also be anemic and experience frequent epistaxis.[124] The bone marrow may be normal or hypercellular with abundant mature neutrophils, or may show "maturation arrest."[126,127] Marrow neutrophils are predisposed to early apoptosis.[128] Neutropenia plus neutrophil dysfunction, reduced chemotaxis, and impaired respiratory burst[118,129,130] result in susceptibility to infections of the skin and perioral and perianal areas as well as pneumonia, sepsis, and meningitis. Infections are often caused by *Staphylococcus aureus*, group A streptococci, *Streptococcus pneumoniae*, *E. coli*, and *Pseudomonas* species.[127] Chronic diarrhea and inflammatory bowel disease are often severe. In these neutropenic patients, it may be difficult to determine whether new gastrointestinal symptoms represent a worsening of chronic inflammatory conditions or a new infection. Late complications of GSD 1b include predisposition to hepatic adenomas with increasing age and progressive renal disease.[124] The relationship between neutropenia and inflammatory bowel disease is unclear.[131] Neutrophil function and counts may improve following portacaval shunt anastomosis[132] and liver transplantation.[133,134]

Treatment and Prognosis

Treatment is directed toward correcting the metabolic abnormalities, as well as prevention of hypoglycemia and seizures. Liver transplantation is indicated in patients with dietary-unresponsive metabolic control and with complications of hepatic adenomas, including hemorrhage, compression, or malignant transformation.[124] G-CSF corrects the neutropenia and reduces infections (see Table 13–3); splenic enlargement is a universal complication of cytokine administration.[126,135] Low doses should be used, starting at 1–2 μg/kg/day to maintain neutrophils at 1000–2000/mm^3.[136] The inflammatory bowel disease also improves with G-CSF treatment.[135]

WISKOTT-ALDRICH SYNDROME

Wiskott-Aldrich syndrome (WAS) is characterized by microthrombocytopenia, immunodeficiency, and eczema. The first case was described by Wiskott in 1937,[137] and X-linked inheritance was reported by Aldrich and colleagues in 1954.[138] The clinical manifestations of WAS are variable, and its phenotypic expression may evolve over time. In addition to an increased susceptibility to recurrent infections, patients are at risk to develop autoimmune disorders and malignancies. In its most benign form, X-linked thrombocytopenia, patients have low platelet counts (<70,000/μL) and abnormally small platelets but no immunologic abnormalities. Rarely, isolated neutropenia can be the presenting feature of WAS.[139] WAS occurs with a frequency of 4 per 1 million males.[140]

Pathophysiology

The WAS protein (*WASP*) gene is located at Xp11.22–p11.23.[141] More than 150 unique mutations have been reported in over 340 families.[142] The wide range of genotypic manifestations likely correlates with the variability of phenotypic expression. Patients who lacked *WASP* gene expression (those with nonsense mutations, large deletions, small deletions, and small insertions) had an increased risk of infections, severe eczema, intestinal bleeding, and malignancies; these null expressions were predictive of mortality and morbidity.[143] The gene product of *WASP* is a cytoplasmic scaffolding protein that stabilizes actin filaments. The protein is believed to be important in the actin cytoskeletal rearrangement that occurs in response to immunoreceptor stimulation.[144]

Clinical Features and Diagnosis

A review of 154 patients revealed that only 27% had the classic triad of microthrombocytopenia, bloody diarrhea,

CURRENT CONTROVERSIES & FUTURE CONSIDERATIONS

Congenital Neutropenia

- The molecular pathophysiology linking the genetic defects associated with the diseases that cause congenital neutropenia to their phenotypic expression remains under investigation.
- The molecular pathophysiology must account for a wide spectrum of phenotypic expression seen with the diseases that cause congenital neutropenia.
- The risk of leukemic transformation varies substantially in various types of congenital neutropenia. Risk factors for leukemia are not yet fully defined.
- The future treatment of congenital neutropenia may be directed at correcting underlying genetic defects or may include drugs specifically designed to target abnormal molecular pathways.

and eczema; hematologic manifestations were present in 20% before the diagnosis of WAS was established. The clinical course was quite variable, even in the same kindred. Autoimmune complications were associated with the risk of future malignancy.[145] Neutropenia, probably on an autoimmune basis, occurred in up to 25% of patients.[146] Other autoimmune syndromes (arthritis, skin vasculitis, cerebral vasculitis, inflammatory bowel disease, and glomerulonephritis) were also common in early childhood.[146]

Treatment and Prognosis

General measures for management include immunizations, intravenous immunoglobulin therapy, and suppressive antibiotic therapy.[147] Immunizations against *S. pneumoniae, Haemophilus influenzae,* and *Neisseria meningitidis* and treatment with prophylactic antibiotics are recommended.[147] Splenectomy generally increases the platelet counts and reduces the risk for major hemorrhage[147–149] but increases the risk of death from sepsis. Hematopoietic stem cell transplantation is curative; best results are obtained with a sibling donor.[150,151]

Suggested Readings*

Dale DC, Person RE, Bolyard AA, et al: Mutations in the gene encoding neutrophil elastase in congenital and cyclic neutropenia. Blood 96:2317–2322, 2000.

Dale DC, Bonilla MA, Davis MW, et al: A randomized controlled Phase III trial of recombinant human granulocyte colony-stimulating factor (filgrastim) for treatment of severe chronic neutropenia. Blood 81:2496–2502, 1993.

Dale DC, Cottle TE, Fier CJ, et al: Severe chronic neutropenia: treatment and follow-up of patients in the Severe Chronic Neutropenia International Registry. Am J Hematol 72:82–93, 2003.

Full references for this chapter can be found on accompanying CD-ROM.

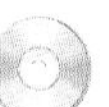

CHAPTER 14

Acquired Neutropenia and Agranulocytosis

Daniel G. Wright, MD, and Jan E. W. Palmblad, MD, PhD

KEY POINTS

Acquired Neutropenia and Agranulocytosis

- The risk of infection with acquired neutropenia depends both on the severity of the neutropenia and its clinical context.
- Risk of infection is greatest when neutropenia is severe (absolute neutrophil count < $0.5 \times 10^3/\mu L$) and when the neutropenia has developed abruptly and is associated with depletion of neutrophil marrow reserves.
- Clinical presentation is the principal determinant of management and also helps to distinguish severe neutropenias with a high risk of life-threatening sepsis from those with low risk.
- The differential diagnosis and prognosis of acquired neutropenia vary with age. Acquired neutropenia in children is often a transient condition associated with an incidental viral infection, and chronic idiopathic and immune neutropenias in children are also more likely to be self-limited than in adults.
- A drug reaction is the first diagnostic consideration to be excluded when unexplained neutropenia occurs in adults, particularly in the elderly.
- Supportive care, attentive clinical monitoring, and the appropriate use of antibiotics are the most important aspects of managing acquired neutropenia.
- Recombinant granulocyte colony-stimulating factor may be an effective drug when chronic severe neutropenia is complicated by recurrent infections.

INTRODUCTION

Neutrophils are the principal phagocytic cells responsible for host defenses against infectious bacteria and fungi (see Chapter 5). Continuous delivery of neutrophils to tissues, particularly the oropharyngeal, respiratory, and gastrointestinal mucosa and the hair follicles and glandular structures of the skin,[1–6] is critical for maintenance of health. Decreased numbers of neutrophils, or neutropenia, if sufficiently severe and prolonged, are associated with an increased risk of opportunistic infection by microorganisms that colonize these integumental sites.[7–13] This risk of infection is also influenced by the clinical context in which neutropenia occurs. Whereas leucopenia is encountered by hematologists most often as an expected complication of myelosuppressive anticancer chemotherapy (see Chapters 90 and 96), the present chapter focuses on the diagnosis and management of neutropenia that is unexpected or is a manifestation of drug toxicity or underlying systemic disease.

Definitions

Once neutrophils leave the bone marrow and enter the blood, they transit the intravascular space rapidly, with a circulation half-life of only about 7 hours,[1,3,4] unlike platelets and erythrocytes, which circulate for weeks or months, respectively. Moreover, only about 50% of intravascular neutrophils are measurable in a peripheral blood sample, because a substantial proportion of circulating neutrophils are, at any given time, reversibly adherent to the microvascular endothelium, or "*marginated.*"[14,15] Also unlike erythrocytes and platelets, neutrophils function principally in extravascular tissues. Nonetheless, clinical recognition of disturbances in neutrophil production and supply is based primarily on blood neutrophil counts.

Neutropenia is defined by an "absolute" blood neutrophil count (ANC) that is less than 2 standard deviations below the mean for a normal, healthy population. The ANC is equivalent to the total leukocyte count per microliter multiplied by the percentage of neutrophils (including both segmented and band forms) in a leukocyte differential, and is a value now reported routinely in automated blood cell counts. Population studies have shown that the lower limit of a normal ANC varies with age, particularly during the first 6 months of life, and among different ethnic groups. For individuals of European origin, the lower limit of a normal ANC is about

TABLE 14–1. Acquired Neutropenia: Severity and Clinical Context

Neutropenia Stratification	ANC ($\times 10^3/\mu L$)	Clinical Context	Risk of Infection
Mild	1.0–1.5	• General good health • Associated disease, debilitated, malnourished, newborn	Usually none Minimal to severe
Moderate	0.5–1.0	• General good health • Associated disease, debilitated, malnourished, newborn	Usually minimal Moderate to severe
Severe	<0.5	• All clinical settings	Moderate to severe

$3.5 \times 10^3/\mu L$ at birth, but decreases to $1.0 \times 10^3/\mu L$ by 6 months. It then increases to $1.5 \times 10^3/\mu L$ by 1 year and to $1.8 \times 10^3/\mu L$ after age 10, where it remains throughout the balance of childhood and adult life.[16–20] However, threshold ANC levels that define neutropenia in adults are lower (~1.0–1.2 $\times 10^3/\mu L$) in certain population groups (African Americans, African and Bedouin blacks, and Yemenite Jews[21–28]), giving rise to the term *ethnic neutropenia* to describe ANC levels of 1.0–1.5 $\times 10^3/\mu L$ in such individuals. *Leukopenia* (a low total white blood cell count) and *granulocytopenia* (reduced numbers of blood granulocytes, including eosinophils and basophils as well as neutrophils) are sometimes used as imprecise synonyms of *neutropenia*. *Agranulocytosis* implies a complete absence of neutrophils but is often used to indicate a very severe neutropenia with an ANC less than $0.2 \times 10^3/\mu L$.

Stratification and Clinical Context

Neutropenias are stratified clinically as mild (ANC = 1.0–1.5 $\times 10^3/\mu L$), moderate (ANC = 0.5–1.0 $\times 10^3/\mu L$), or severe (ANC < 0.5 $\times 10^3/\mu L$), and the significance of neutropenia is influenced by its severity as well as by its clinical context (Table 14–1). Neutrophil reserves in healthy individuals greatly exceed those required to maintain normal antimicrobial host defenses. For this reason, there is generally little or no increased risk of opportunistic infection with mild to moderate degrees of neutropenia in otherwise healthy adults, and such risks emerge only at ANC levels of less than $0.5 \times 10^3/\mu L$ (or less than ~10% of normal). In contrast, neutrophil reserves are limited in newborns and debilitated, malnourished, or alcoholic adults,[9,29–34] and in these cases even mild degrees of neutropenia may signal a potentially lethal depletion of neutrophils with sepsis.[33,35,36] Similarly, when mild or moderate neutropenia occurs in an autoimmune or lymphoproliferative disorder, with immunoglobulin or complement deficiencies, or with diabetes or renal failure, qualitative defects in neutrophil function may accentuate modest quantitative deficiencies to increase infection susceptibility.[37,38] Other host factors (polymorphisms of immunoglobulin G Fc receptors, genetic variants of mannose-binding lectins, or subtle immunoglobulin deficiencies[13,39–41]) may also influence the likelihood of infections in neutropenia.

EPIDEMIOLOGY

By definition, neutropenia may be detected by chance in approximately 2.5% of isolated blood cell counts in asymptomatic, apparently healthy individuals. Because modern blood cell counters provide automated leukocyte differentials and ANC measurements routinely, unexpected findings of neutropenia are not uncommon in general clinical practice, and an isolated finding of neutropenia should be confirmed by repeated blood cell counts. The incidence of neutropenia, like its clinical significance, is also influenced by clinical context. For example, mild to moderate neutropenia is a common feature of systemic lupus erythematosus (SLE), human immunodeficiency virus (HIV) disease, and infectious mononucleosis[42–45] and an expected feature of neoplastic, immunologic, or severe nutritional deficiency (vitamin B_{12}, folate, copper[46,47]) disorders that broadly affect hematopoiesis, as in aplastic anemia, megaloblastic anemia, and myelodysplasia. Conversely, an isolated, unexpected finding of severe neutropenia or agranulocytosis, regardless of etiology, is relatively uncommon, occurring with an estimated incidence of 5–10 per 1 million per year.[48–52]

CLINICAL PRESENTATION

The clinical presentation determines management. When severe neutropenia is discovered in an asymptomatic individual, the risk of life-threatening sepsis is usually low, and aggressive, empirical interventions are inappropriate. However, moderate to severe neutropenia with anemia and thrombocytopenia, regardless of symptoms, suggests evolving marrow failure and requires prompt evaluation for diagnosis and appropriate therapy. With mild to moderate neutropenia, signs and symptoms such as fever, malaise, pharyngitis, or arthralgia may be manifestations of an associated viral infection or autoimmune/inflammatory disorder rather than of infection, but the possibility of a potentially serious bacterial infection should nonetheless be considered and excluded. Such signs or symptoms, when associated with any degree of neutropenia in newborns or in malnourished, debilitated adults should always prompt aggressive management based on the possibility of life-threatening infection.

TABLE 14–2. Clinical Presentation of Severe Neutropenia

Subtypes of Severe Neutropenia	Characteristics of the Neutropenia	Symptoms and Signs	Risk of Life-Threatening Sepsis
Chronic (gradual onset)	Myelopoietic reserves limited but preserved Some delivery of neutrophils to tissues is maintained	Asymptomatic or mild malaise, intermittent low-grade fever, stomatitis, gingivitis, localized infections	Generally low
Acute (abrupt onset)	Depleted myelopoietic reserves Delivery of neutrophils to tissues is severely limited or absent	Fever (≥101°F), acute pharyngitis, flushing, tachycardia, inanition or prostration	High

Appropriate management also depends on whether neutropenia is acute or chronic (Table 14–2). Records of prior blood counts and clinical history are helpful in making this distinction, as are presenting signs and symptoms. Schultz in 1922 first described a syndrome of fever, pharyngitis, and prostration as the clinical presentation of acute idiopathic agranulocytosis, subsequently recognized to be caused by aminopyrine analgesics that had become widely available at that time.[53–55] In acute, symptomatic neutropenia, life-threatening sepsis must be considered likely, and hospitalization for aggressive supportive care and empirical, intravenous broad-spectrum antibiotics is required. However, this complication rarely occurs with chronic neutropenias. Studies of oral mucosal neutrophil numbers in individuals with neutropenia have shown that delivery of neutrophils to tissues is more effectively maintained when severe neutropenia develops gradually than when it occurs acutely.[56,57] Neutrophil reserves and effective delivery of neutrophils to tissues also appear to be reflected by FcγRIIIb (CD16) and granulocyte colony-stimulating factor (G-CSF) levels, because low soluble CD16 and high G-CSF levels in plasma have been associated with an increased likelihood of infection in neutropenic patients.[58,59]

TABLE 14–3. Pathophysiologic Categorization of Acquired Neutropenia

Pathophysiology	Conditions and Disorders
Impaired generation and proliferation of neutrophil precursors	Aplastic anemia,* leukemia* (hairy cell, APL) Pure white cell aplasia (thymoma) Myelotoxic chemotherapy Idiosyncratic drug reactions Nutritional deficiencies* (vitamin B_{12}, copper) Neonatal neutropenia (prematurity, preeclampsia)
Impaired myelopoiesis at multiple stages of neutrophil development	Myelodysplasia* Lymphoproliferative disorders (chronic LGL, NHL,* CLL*) Infections: Viral (HIV, EBV, HepB, CMV, parvovirus-B19) Other (mycobacteria,* *Rickettsia**) Acquired idiopathic neutropenias
Impaired maturation, survival, and distribution of neutrophils	Acute complement activation Immune neutropenias: Neonatal alloimmune neutropenia Isolated autoimmune neutropenia Neutropenia associated with systemic autoimmune disorders (e.g., SLE, RA)

*Neutropenia is a common feature of these disorders but only occasionally prompts diagnosis.
Abbreviations: APL, acute promyelocytic leukemia; CLL, chronic lymphocytic leukemia; CMV, cytomegalovirus; EBV, Epstein-Barr virus; HepB, hepatitis B virus; HIV, human immunodeficiency virus; LGL, large granular lymphocytosis; NHL, non-Hodgkin's lymphoma; RA, rheumatoid arthritis; SLE, systemic lupus erythematosus.

PATHOPHYSIOLOGY

Multiple pathophysiologic mechanisms lead to acquired neutropenia, and not all are fully understood (see later). Nonetheless, it is clinically useful to distinguish disorders in which the generation and proliferation of neutrophil progenitors and precursors is impaired from those in which the terminal maturation, survival, or distribution of neutrophils is disturbed (Table 14–3). Neutrophils and neutrophil precursors spend most of their brief lifespans in the bone marrow, and normally only a small proportion of total neutrophil reserves are in the blood[1,4–6] (Fig. 14–1). In healthy adults, nearly three times the number of neutrophils present in the intravascular space at any given time are delivered to tissues and replaced every day, and this number increases with infection. Given this rapid turnover, neutrophils are quickly depleted in the circulation and tissues if marrow reserves are abruptly compromised. Disturbances of the "proliferative" compartment of neutrophil precursors are particularly likely to deplete neutrophil reserves and cause an increased risk of serious infection. The probability that an acquired neutropenia is associated with a damaged proliferative compartment is favored when anemia, thrombocytopenia, and monocytopenia are also evident. Sequestration and destruction of cells in the splenic or peripheral circulation is less important as a cause of neutropenia than for anemia or thrombocytopenia. However, neutropenia resulting from microvascular sequestration can occur transiently with acute complement activation with endotoxemia or anaphylaxis, or from the contact of blood with extracorporeal circuits during cardiopulmonary bypass,

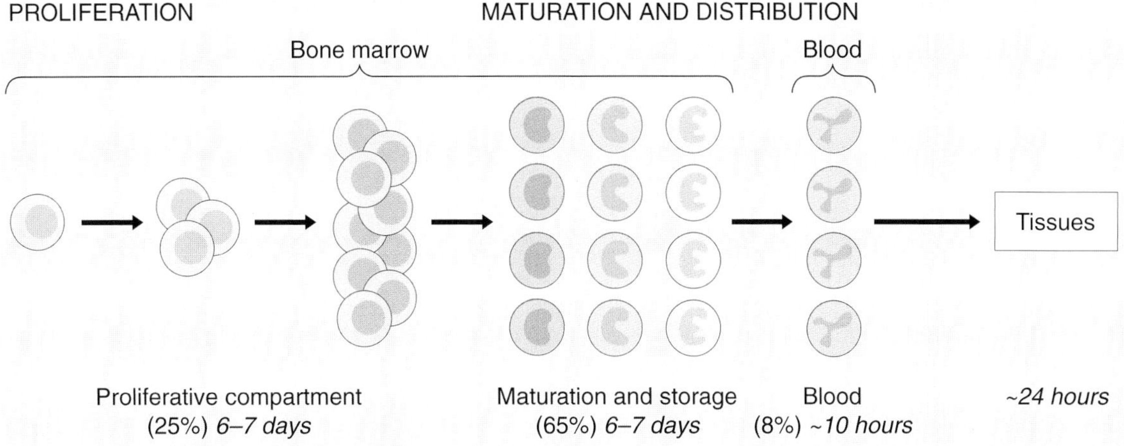

Figure 14–1. Neutrophil production and distribution. Normal proportions of total neutrophil reserves are shown in parentheses and normal transit times through successive developmental compartments are in italics.

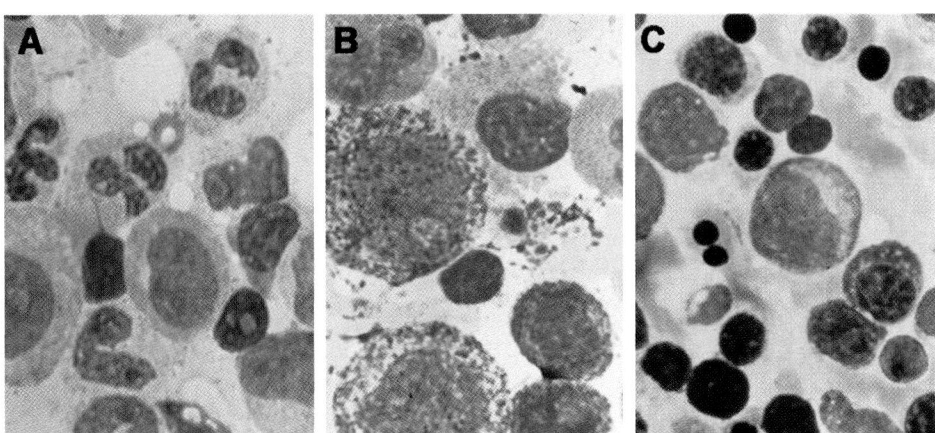

Figure 14–2. Marrow aspirates. *A*, Normal. *B*, Immune neutropenia with myeloid cells dominated by immature forms. *C*, Pure white cell aplasia with complete absence of myeloid cells.

apheresis, or hemodialysis.[60–64] Although splenomegaly and "hypersplenism" may be contributing causes of neutropenia,[65,66] suppressed neutrophil production in the marrow is required for moderate or severe neutropenia to persist, regardless of etiology.

Neutrophil precursors in the proliferative and "maturation" compartments of the marrow are not readily quantified, but they can be assessed indirectly in marrow aspirate and biopsy specimens. Marrow studies, often uninformative in cases of isolated mild or moderate neutropenia, are justified when neutropenia is severe or associated with pancytopenia, and the underlying cause of the neutropenia is not readily apparent. Normally, one half to two thirds of nucleated cells in the marrow are morphologically recognizable as neutrophils or neutrophil precursors (Fig. 14–2*A*), and they outnumber nucleated erythroid precursors by about 2:1. About two thirds of the myeloid cells in marrow are normally mature (metamyelocytes, bands, and segments) and one third are immature (myeloblasts, promyelocytes, and myelocytes). Decreased numbers of myeloid cells (Figs. 14–2*C* and 14–3), with normal or reduced marrow cellularity, indicate a depletion of neutrophil precursors in the proliferative compartment. Hypocellularity of the marrow (Figures 14–3*C* and 14–3*D*) can indicate a depleted proliferative compartment, whereas a predominance of immature myeloid cells versus mature forms (commonly referred to as "maturation arrest"; see Figs. 14–2*B* and 14–3*C*) implies that the terminal development of neutrophils is disturbed and ineffective.

CLINICAL FEATURES AND DIFFERENTIAL DIAGNOSIS

Drug-Associated Neutropenia and Agranulocytosis

With the increasingly widespread use of prescription and over-the-counter medications, idiosyncratic drug reactions and drug side effects have become frequent causes of acquired neutropenia, particularly among older adults.[49,51,52,67–72] Certain categories of drugs and individual agents within these categories are likely causes of neutropenia (Table 14–4). Although new agents have been added to the list of incriminated drugs over time, neither the basic spectrum of drugs associated with neu-

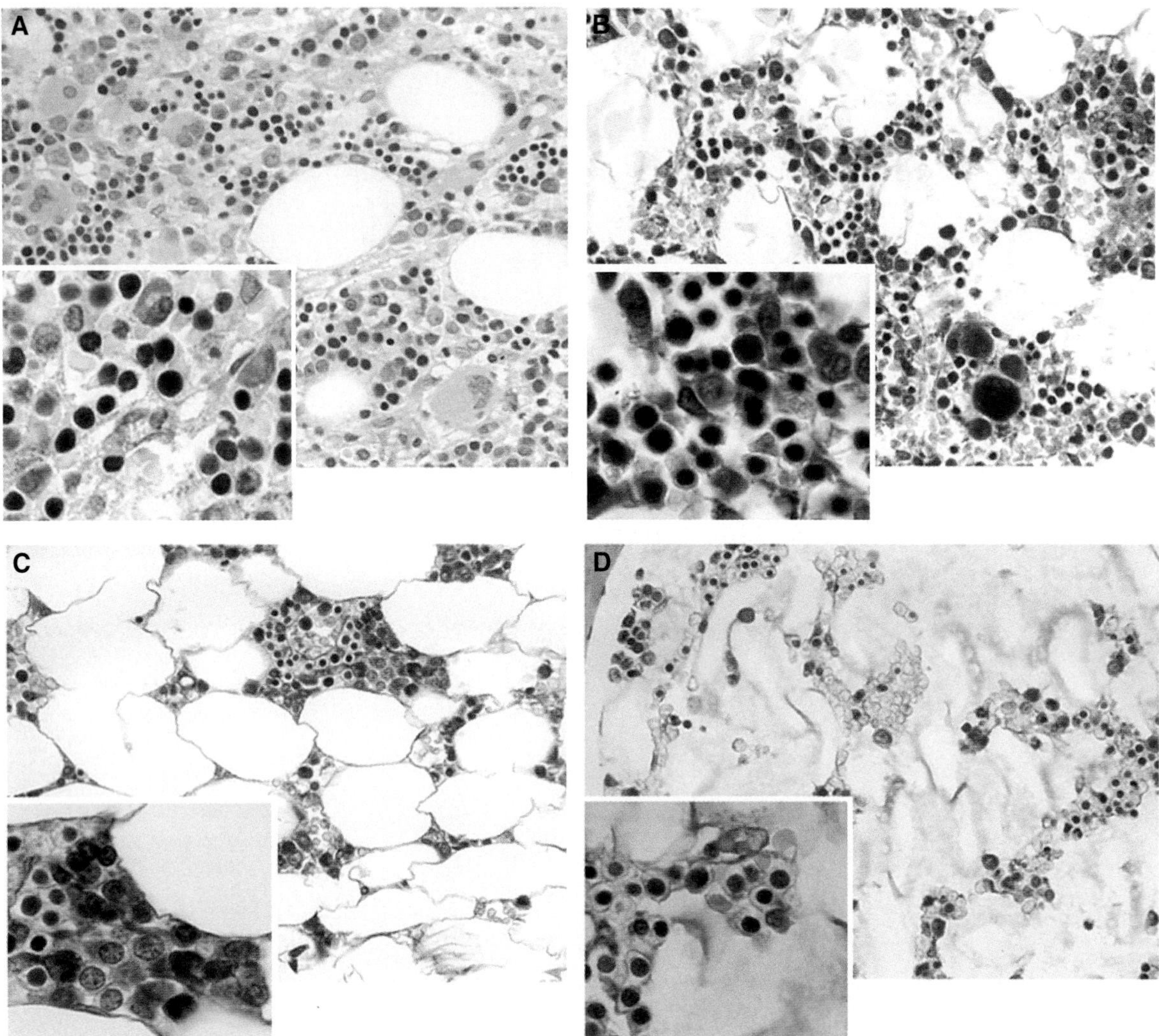

Figure 14–3. Marrow biopsies from individuals with severe neutropenia (higher power views in insets). *A,* Hypercellularity (30% fat) and decreased myeloid-to-erythroid (M:E) ratio. *B,* Normal cellularity and decreased M:E ratio. *C,* Hypocellularity (70% fat), decreased M:E ratio, and "maturation arrest." *D,* Marked hypocellularity (>90% fat) and near absence of myeloid cells.

tropenia nor the frequency of drug-induced agranulocytosis have changed substantially over the past 30 years.[49,68,72,73] Drug-induced neutropenias (other than those associated with cancer chemotherapy) are generally uncommon, except in certain specific clinical circumstances, such as with the use of trimethoprim-sulfamethoxazole or zidovudine in individuals with HIV disease, or due to clozapine or phenothiazines in psychiatric patients. Consequently, medicated individuals are generally not monitored in anticipation of neutropenia as a complication of drug treatment, and, when they do present with agranulocytosis, neutropenia may be severe with signs of infection that demand urgent management. Analgesic and anti-inflammatory pyrazolone derivatives (aminopyrine, dipyrone, phenylbutazone) remain important causes of drug-induced agranulocytosis, although they are no longer available in the United States or many Western European countries. Aminopyrine was the first widely used drug to be convincingly linked to idiosyncratic agranulocytosis, which in the 1930s was often fatal.[55,76–78] Aminopyrine is the prototype both for drugs that induce neutropenia in an unpredictable and non–dose-dependent manner and for agents (including penicillins and cephalosporins) that cause agranulocytosis by drug-dependent, hapten-mediated autoantibody reactions.[79–81] These serious, immune-mediated reactions typically occur abruptly after reexposure to the drug. The aminopyrine analogue dipyrone, a very effective oral analgesic, is still manufactured and widely available as an over-the-counter medication in many parts of the world, and individuals may acquire it as an "aspirin substitute" while traveling abroad.[82,83] Aminopyrine and phenylbutazone have also been detected as adulterants in traditional Chinese herbal medicines, especially those prepared for relief of pain or rheumatic complaints, and are likely responsible for cases of agranulocytosis reported with these medicines.[84–86]

Idiosyncratic, drug-induced neutropenia may also be caused by a dose-dependent inhibition of protein

TABLE 14–4. Drugs Associated with Idiosyncratic Neutropenia

Drug Categories	Drugs
Analgesics and anti-inflammatory agents	***Pyrazolone drugs*** *(aminopyrine,* ***dipyrone****,* phenylbutazone, oxyphenbutazone)
	Indomethacin
	***Para*-aminophenols** (acetaminophen, phenacetin)
	Gold salts
Antibiotics, antivirals, antimalarials	***Sulfonamides***
	Trimethoprim-sulfamethoxazole
	Macrolides (clindamycin, vancomycin)
	β-Lactams
	Penicillins
	Chloramphenicol
	Zidovudine, acyclovir, ganciclovir
	Dapsone, chloroquine
Anticonvulsants	**Phenytoin**
	Mesantoin
	Valproic acid
	Carbamazepine
Antidepressants, antipsychotics	***Phenothiazines***
	Clozapine
	Diazepam, chlordiazepoxide
	Meprobamate
	Haloperidol
Antithyroid drugs	***Thiouracil, propylthiouracil***
	Methimazole
	Carbimazole
Cardiovascular drugs	***Procainamide, propranolol,* quinidine**
	Captopril
	Nifedipine
	Enalapril
	Amiodarone
Other	**Antihistamines (cimetadine, ranitidine)**
	Ticlopidine
	Allopurinol, colchicine
	Diuretics (chlorothiazide, ***acetazolamide,*** spironolactone)
	Oral hypoglycemic agents (chlorpropamide, tolbutamide)

Drugs most frequently associated with neutropenia clinically are listed in bold, and those most frequently associated with agranulocytosis [51,72–75] are listed in italics.

TABLE 14–5. Infections Associated with Neutropenia

Infection Categories	Infections
Common childhood viruses	Measles, mumps
	Parvovirus B19 **(in immunocompromised individuals)**
	Roseola, rubella, respiratory syncytial virus
Other viruses	**Human immunodeficiency virus**
	Epstein-Barr virus
	Hepatitis B virus, hepatitis A and C viruses
	Cytomegalovirus
	Influenza viruses A and B
	Other viruses (varicella, herpes simplex, polio, Colorado tick fever, dengue, yellow fever, psittacosis, smallpox)
Bacteria	**Bacterial sepsis (gram-negative in particular) in neonates, alcoholics, malnourished and debilitated patients**
	Tuberculosis, brucellosis, ehrlichiosis, tularemia
	Typhoid, paratyphoid
Rickettsia	Typhus, Rocky Mountain spotted fever, rickettsial pox
Fungi	Histoplasmosis
Protozoa	Malaria, leishmaniasis

Infections that may be associated with severe, prolonged, and/or life-threatening neutropenia are listed in bold.

synthesis and cell replication, or enhanced apoptosis, as occurs with phenothiazines, chloramphenicol, clozapine, β-lactam antibiotics, and valproic acid.[87–92] The dose- and time-dependent nature of drug-induced neutropenia with these agents justifies monitoring of blood counts in patients treated for more than several weeks.[94] Drug-associated neutropenia is generally more common among women and the elderly[51,52,68,69] because of their increased exposure to multiple medications. Host factors also increase the probability of certain drug-induced neutropenias. Genetic determinants have been shown to predispose for neutropenias caused by clozapine (tumor necrosis factor gene polymorphisms and human lymphocyte antigen type) and sulfasalazine ("slow acetylator" phenotype),[94–96] and renal insufficiency increases the risk of captopril-induced agranulocytosis.[97]

Recognition of neutropenia as a potential drug reaction and discontinuation of the offending agent are most important in managing drug-induced neutropenia. Supportive care and antibiotic use are as those for severe neutropenia in general. Recovery from drug-induced agranulocytosis usually begins within 4–7 days after a causative drug is removed. However, the rate of recovery is influenced by the extent of hypocellularity evident in the marrow at the time neutropenia is discovered; with total myeloid aplasia, recovery may be delayed for weeks.

Neutropenia Associated with Infections

Viral infections are commonly associated with neutropenia, particularly in children[98,99] (Table 14–5). Neutropenia typically develops during the first several days of clinical illness, coincident with viremia, and persists for 3–7 days. Neutropenia is usually mild to moderate and generally short lived and so rarely clinically significant.[98–104] HIV, Epstein-Barr virus (EBV), and hepatitis B virus may cause severe and prolonged neutropenias associated with damage to neutrophil precursor and progenitor pools.[42–44,105–108] Occasionally, transient agranulocytosis develops during the recovery phase of infectious mononucleosis and, although self-limited, can be life-threatening.[106,109] Neutropenia with influenza infections is usually mild but can be associated with a risk of serious, secondary bacterial infections because of virus-induced neutrophil dysfunction.[38]

Neutropenia also occurs with certain bacterial, rickettsial, fungal, and protozoal infections (see Table 14–5).[110–116] Recognition and appropriate treatment of infection in these cases are keys to management. With bacterial sepsis in neonates, efforts to expand myelopoietic reserves emergently with G-CSF[117–120] or leukocyte transfusions[121–123] may be valuable adjuncts to aggressive antibiotic treatment.

Immune Neutropenias

Immune mechanisms, especially drug-dependent hapten-antibody reactions, underlie certain drug-induced neutropenias.[79–81] Both cell-mediated immune mechanisms and antineutrophil autoantibodies associated with polyclonal B-cell activation have been implicated in the etiology of neutropenia associated with HIV, EBV, cytomegalovirus, and hepatitis virus infections.[42,43,109] Alloimmune and autoimmune disorders, for which detection of antineutrophil antibodies is a key diagnostic indicator, are also important primary causes of acquired neutropenia. Premature apoptosis of neutrophils and neutrophil precursors occurs in these disorders,[124] leading to ineffective terminal maturation of neutrophils in the marrow and altered distribution and survival in the circulation. Marrow cellularity is typically normal or increased, numbers of mature myeloid forms are decreased relative to immature forms (maturation arrest), and monocyte numbers are often high, particularly in children. Infections may be recurrent but are usually not severe, as is characteristic of other types of chronic neutropenia (see Table 14–2).

A variety of methods have been developed to measure circulating antineutrophil antibodies based on the detection of either antibody-specific effects on neutrophils using functional assays or cell-surface immunoglobulin using radiolabeled or fluorescent anti-immunoglobulin.[125–132] Historically, agglutination was useful for detecting antineutrophil alloantibodies but not autoantibodies, and nonspecific binding of immunoglobulin and immune complexes via neutrophil Fc receptors has complicated the development and interpretation of tests designed to detect antineutrophil antibody reactivity by measuring cell-surface immunoglobulin binding. Recently, methods that detect antineutrophil antibodies in sera using panels of paraformaldehyde-fixed test neutrophils and flow cytometry have proven reliable and are widely available.[131,132] Moreover, substantial progress has been made in identifying specific neutrophil antigens that are targeted by antineutrophil allo- and autoantibodies associated with immune neutropenia[131,133–145] (Table 14–6). Although immune neutropenia associated with antineutrophil antibodies occurs throughout life, there are distinct syndromes in children and adults.

TABLE 14–6. Human Neutrophil Alloantigens and Autoantigens

	Nomenclature*
Alloantigens	
FcγIIIb receptor isotypes:	
Allele FCGR3B-01	HNA-1a (NA1)
Allele FCGR3B-02	HNA-1b (NA2)
Allele FCGR3B-03	HNA-1c (SH or NA3)‡
Gp 50–64 (CD177)†	HNA-2a (NB1)
Gp 70–95	HNA-3a (5b)
CD11b (integrin α_M chain)	HNA-4a (MART)
CD11a (integrin α_L chain)	HNA-5a (OND)
Autoantigens	
FcγIIIb receptors[136,147]	HNA-1a/b (NA1/NA2)
CD11b (integrin α_M chain)[138]	HNA-4a (MART)
CD18 (integrin β_2 chain)[138]	
Cell surface actin§ [137]	

*Based on Bux.[144] The previously used nomenclature is indicated in parentheses.
†Closely related to PRV-1, a member of the PAR receptor superfamily, overexpressed in polycythemia vera.[146]
‡Expression of HNA-1c is associated with triplication of the FcγRIIIb gene.[147]
§Likely bound to the surface of neutrophils via actin-binding protein scavenger receptors.

Neonatal Alloimmune Neutropenia

Antigens expressed on neutrophils and neutrophil precursors of a fetus may be genetically distinct from those expressed on maternal neutrophils, and prenatal sensitization can induce maternal immunoglobulin G antineutrophil alloantibodies that cross the placenta and cause moderate to severe neutropenia in the newborn.[133,136,140,145,147–154] Neonatal neutropenia occurs in approximately 1 in 1000 live births[153] and is analogous to Rh hemolytic disease. Studies of neonatal neutropenia prompted development of the first methods for detecting antineutrophil antibodies and led to the initial serologic classification of neutrophil antigens.[133] Characterization of these antigens, targeted by antineutrophil antibodies in both alloimmune and autoimmune neutropenias, has evolved, as has their nomenclature (see Table 14–6). The antigens most commonly involved in neonatal alloimmune neutropenia have been shown to be distinct isotypes of CD16, or the FcγIII receptor (hence, the term *isoimmune neutropenia* also used to describe this disorder),[149,151] but other less well-characterized neutrophil antigens also have been implicated.[144,150]

Passive transfer of antineutrophil autoantibodies from mother to fetus also can cause neutropenia in newborns.[126] Fever and signs of infection in a newborn shortly after birth should prompt consideration of this syndrome. Infections are usually localized to the skin, oropharynx, ears, or urinary tract and are rarely severe,[126,152] but life-threatening pneumonia and septicemia sometimes occur. Neonatal alloimmune neutropenia is self-limited and resolves within 2–3 months. It must be distinguished from the transient neutropenia occasionally seen in premature newborns or low-birth-weight infants of hypertensive mothers, and also from congenital, familial severe neutropenias (see Chapter 13).

Autoimmune Neutropenia in Children

A distinct disorder, commonly referred to as "chronic benign neutropenia of childhood," likely has an autoimmune etiology because antineutrophil autoantibodies have been reported in almost all cases.[126,154–160] In this disorder, isolated neutropenia appears in young children typically between 6 and 12 months of age and resolves spontaneously within 1–6 years. Although neutropenia is often severe, the clinical course is usually benign. There are recurrent infections of the skin, oropharynx, and respiratory tract but they are rarely serious.[32,158–160] An incidence of 1:100,000 has been reported, but recognition of the disorder in pediatric practice is more frequent with the routine reporting of automated ANC measurements in screening blood counts. Autoimmune lymphoproliferative syndrome, a distinct and uncommon childhood disorder associated with lymphadenopathy, neutropenia, and antineutrophil autoantibodies,[161,162] is discussed in Chapter 58.

Autoimmune Neutropenia in Adults

Chronic neutropenia with circulating antineutrophil autoantibodies in teenagers and adults is more likely to be associated with a systemic autoimmune disease, a viral infection (as discussed earlier), or an underlying lymphoproliferative disorder, and less likely to remit spontaneously than is chronic neutropenia in children. Neutropenia is common in SLE (>50% of cases), rheumatoid arthritis (RA), and Sjögren's syndrome (~30% of cases),[45,163–171] and also occurs in Wegener's granulomatosis and Crohn's disease.[168,171] The severity of neutropenia in SLE and Sjögren's syndrome is usually mild to moderate and seldom associated with infectious complications. In contrast, chronic neutropenia associated with RA may be severe, and recurrent localized infections are common. In RA, as in SLE, the onset of neutropenia may precede systemic inflammatory manifestations of disease.

The association of chronic neutropenia with active arthritis, splenomegaly, and elevated rheumatoid factor levels has long been referred to as "Felty's syndrome." The pathophysiology of neutropenia in this disorder is complex, and the marrow findings are variable. Abnormalities of neutrophil maturation, distribution, and survival (as in other forms of immune neutropenia), as well as impaired neutrophil precursor production and proliferation in the marrow, have been described.[172–178] Defects in neutrophil function also occur and likely contribute to the propensity for recurrent infections.[168,173] Many, if not most, patients with Felty's syndrome are now recognized as having a clonal lymphoproliferative disorder with increased numbers of circulating $CD3^+$, $CD8^+$, and $CD57^+$ large granular lymphocytes (LGLs). This is an important disorder with respect to the differential diagnosis of acquired neutropenia, particularly in older adults (age 50 and over), and has been variously called Tγ lymphocytosis and chronic LGL leukemia (see Chapter 16). Chronic severe neutropenia, usually with detectable antineutrophil autoantibodies, is a prominent manifestation of this disease.[179–182] Moreover, an acquired form of cyclic neutropenia,[181] clinically and hematologically very similar to congenital cyclic neutropenia (see Chapter 13), may occur. Common pathophysiologic mechanisms in classic RA and Tγ lymphocytosis are likely, because up to one third of patients with RA and neutropenia have been reported to have a clonal expansion of LGL, and oligoclonal $CD3^+CD8^+CD57^+$ T cells have been demonstrated in both the blood and synovial fluid of patients with active RA.[183–187]

Immune dysregulation following allogeneic bone marrow or blood stem cell transplantation, particularly in association with chronic graft-versus-host disease, is an unusual cause of acquired autoimmune neutropenia, as are reactions to repeated transfusions with blood products (particularly when not leukodepleted). Antineutrophil autoantibodies detected in chronic graft-versus-host disease are similar to those in other forms of autoimmune neutropenia; neutropenia with blood transfusions is often involve anti–human leucocyte antigen reactivities.[188,189]

Thymoma and Pure White Cell Aplasia

The unusual lymphoid neoplasm thymoma is associated with a distinct form of acquired agranulocytosis characterized by a complete and selective absence of myeloid cells in the marrow, referred to as "pure white cell aplasia" (PWCA; see Fig. 14–2*C*). Although PWCA has been reported as a rare idiosyncratic drug reaction (ibuprofen, chlorpropamide[190,191]), most cases (~70%) are associated with thymoma, and PWCA, like pure red cell aplasia, should always prompt a search for this tumor. Often, PWCA resolves after surgical removal of a thymoma, but additional treatment (cyclophosphamide or cyclosporine) may be required to induce a remission. PWCA may also appear years after the diagnosis and removal of a thymoma.[192–196] Both humoral and cell-mediated immune suppression of myeloid progenitor cells have been implicated.[192,193] Autoimmune manifestations of other lymphoid neoplasms, such as chronic lymphocytic leukemia, non-Hodgkin's lymphoma, and Hodgkin's disease, occasionally include immune neutropenia. However, neutropenia is not a frequent or prominent clinical feature of these diseases except in the context of treatment with myelosuppressive chemotherapy.[197–199]

Chronic Idiopathic Neutropenia

Chronic neutropenia is occasionally discovered in older children and adults without other hematologic abnormalities or evidence of another disease.[32,156,158,160,200–202] The neutropenia may be detected serendipitously or in the context of recurrent, localized infections. Marrow findings are typically unremarkable or show only a moderate depletion of mature myeloid forms (maturation arrest), as with immune neutropenias, but some hypoplasia may also be present. Cytogenetic studies are normal, and there is no general predisposition for eventual development of aplastic anemia or leukemia. However, chronic idiopathic neutropenia in older adults may be the first sign of myelodysplasia. Some cases are likely subclinical forms of autoimmune neutropenia[156,157,203,204]; others (in younger patients) may be mild, late-appearing phenotypes of congenital, familial neutropenias (see Chapter 13). Spontaneous remission occurs in over half of childhood cases, but is much less frequent in adults.[158,200] Recurrent fevers, periodontitis, stomatitis, and localized infections may occur. In a randomized trial, long-term treatment with low-dose G-CSF was found to be effective in ameliorating neutropenia and reducing infectious complications.[206,207]

MANAGEMENT

The characterization, diagnosis, and management of acquired neutropenia should be undertaken systematically (Fig. 14–4). Although pathogenic mechanisms underlying acquired neutropenia are diverse, a number of management principles apply generally. Because circulating neutrophil counts are subject to substantial day-to-day variability, an unexpected finding of neutropenia should always be verified with repeated blood counts and leukocyte differentials determined by direct microscopic evaluation of a blood smear. Once neutropenia is confirmed, the first rule of management is to treat the patient and not the neutropenia. Both the severity and clinical presentation of neutropenia are important. Severe neutropenia that presents with signs and symptoms of systemic infection and a clinical history suggestive of acute onset, regardless of etiology, is a medical emergency that requires hospitalization, cultures of the blood and other possible sites of infection, and preemptive treatment with intravenous broad-spectrum antibacterial antibiotics. In contrast, severe neutropenia in an asymptomatic individual or in a clinical presentation suggestive of a chronic condition (see Table 14–2), the risk of life-threatening sepsis is low; aggressive measures are inappropriate, and the use of antibiotics should be targeted to clinically evident sites of infection.

Neutropenia, regardless of severity, does not itself justify therapeutic interventions. Initial management of an unexpected finding of neutropenia is in most cases restricted to diagnostic measures aimed at defining the character and underlying cause of the neutropenia, such that subsequent management is disease-specific. The differential diagnosis of acquired neutropenia varies with age (see Fig. 14–4). Bone marrow studies are not routinely needed to establish a diagnosis and are usually uninformative in isolated mild to moderate neutropenia. Marrow examination is required when the etiology or character of the neutropenia is uncertain and the neutropenia is severe or associated with anemia, thrombocytopenia, lymphocytosis, adenopathy, and/or splenomegaly. Once an acquired neutropenia is defined, regular evaluations, supportive care, and the judicious use of antibiotics are the most important elements of management.

Granulocyte Colony-Stimulating Factor

Recombinant G-CSF is widely used to accelerate neutrophil recovery following myelosuppressive cancer chemotherapy.[205] G-CSF is also useful in the management of severe congenital and acquired neutropenias. G-CSF increases neutrophil counts rapidly in most acquired neutropenias, and in individuals with severe idiopathic neutropenia, chronic G-CSF treatment was shown to ameliorate neutropenia and prevent infectious complications in a randomized trial.[206] However, experience with G-CSF in other forms of acquired neutropenia (associated with idiosyncratic drug reactions,[208–210] HIV disease,[211] and allo- or autoimmune disorders[212–217]; see Fig. 14–4), although often dramatic, is confined to uncontrolled series and anecdotal reports. It is gratifying for both managing physicians and patients to observe increases in blood neutrophil counts induced by G-CSF, but these effects do not necessarily reflect clinical benefit for a patient with acquired neutropenia, who may have limited risks of infection. Even short-term use of G-CSF is very costly,[218] and G-CSF can induce flares of vasculitis and other inflammatory manifestations of systemic autoimmune disease.[219,220] Nonetheless, a therapeutic trial of G-CSF is justified in difficult cases that are complicated by recurrent or high-risk infections. The doses and frequency of G-CSF injections should be titrated to the minimum levels that achieve modest increases in neutrophil counts.[218] Normalization of the ANC is not required for a clinically meaningful restoration of neutrophil-dependent host defenses. G-CSF use should never preclude efforts to identify the cause of acquired neutropenia.

Other Treatments

Splenectomy, corticosteroids, and infusions of intravenous immunoglobulin have well-documented roles in autoimmune thrombocytopenia and hemolytic anemia, but they are less useful in the management of acquired immune or idiopathic neutropenias. Splenectomy can ameliorate neutropenia and decrease recurrent infections in more than 50% of RA patients with Felty's syndrome, but these effects are often transient (see Chapter 16).[178,221] Treatment regimens with methotrexate and/or cyclosporine directly affect the cytotoxic T cells involved in the pathogenesis of neutropenia in Felty's syndrome and chronic LGL lymphocytosis.[222–225] Corticosteroids, when given daily and in high doses as in immune thrombocytopenia and hemolytic anemia, have limited, unpredictable efficacy and exacerbate infection risk.[226] Corticosteroids in low doses on alternate days (prednisolone 25 mg every other day), are much less toxic and may gradually correct or ameliorate chronic immune neutropenia in some cases.[158,181,227] Intravenous immunoglobulin has been effective treating severe immune neutropenia in infants and children,[126] but this disorder is generally self-limited and G-CSF appears to be a more reliable and effective supplement to supportive care when treatment is required.[160,228]

Recent experience with leukocyte transfusions using cells harvested from G-CSF–stimulated donors has revived interest in this technique.[229–231] These transfusions may be clinically valuable in selected cases of very-high-risk acquired neutropenia, such as severe neonatal neutropenia with sepsis[121–123] (see Chapter 98).

PROGNOSIS

The prognosis of acquired neutropenia is as varied as the disorders underlying it, but most patients can be

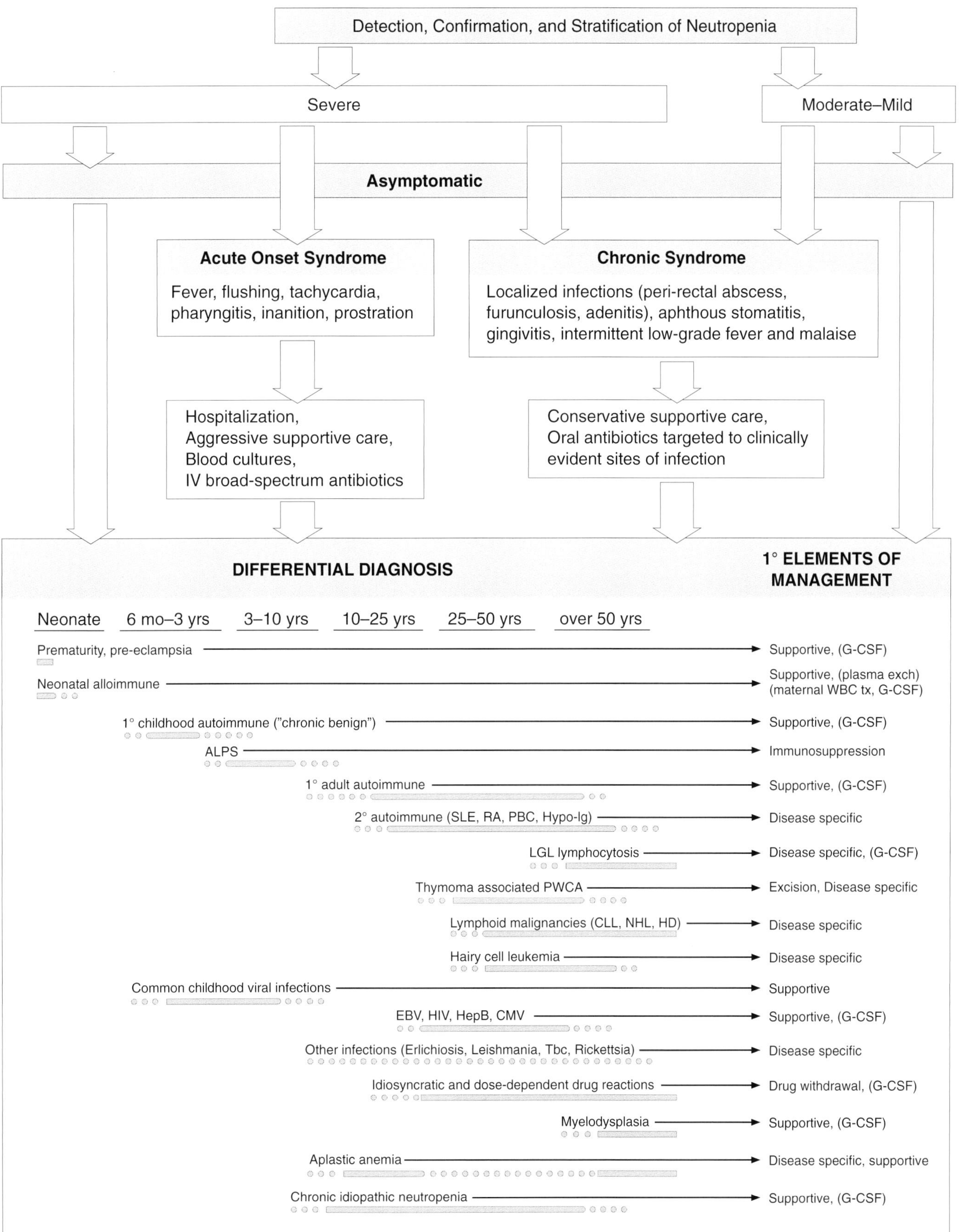

Figure 14–4. General strategy for the initial assessment, management, and differential diagnosis of acquired neutropenia and agranulocytosis.

CURRENT CONTROVERSIES & FUTURE CONSIDERATIONS

Acquired Neutropenia and Agranulocytosis

- Recombinant G-CSF is a powerful therapy that stimulates neutrophil production. However, its proper role in the management of acquired neutropenias (in particular those caused by drugs, as with the prolonged use of β-lactam antibiotics to treat osteomyelitis in diabetics) and its potential hazards have yet to be fully defined.
- Refined techniques for measuring neutrophil reserves and the effective delivery of neutrophils to tissues in acute and chronic acquired neutropenias (plasma CD16 and G-CSF levels, and mucosal neutrophil numbers) should improve our ability to predict the risks of infection associated with neutropenia more precisely.
- Techniques for detecting antineutrophil allo- and autoantibodies have improved and are useful for recognizing immune neutropenias. Further refinements based on measurements of reactivity to specific neutrophil antigens and the detection of intramedullary apoptosis induced by antineutrophil antibodies would enhance our ability to diagnose and categorize immune neutropenias.

managed effectively. Immune and idiopathic neutropenia in children is usually self-limited. In adults, most cases of acquired neutropenia and agranulocytosis are associated with idiosyncratic drug reactions that are reversible if properly diagnosed and the offending drug discontinued. Chronic autoimmune and idiopathic neutropenias rarely evolve into more serious marrow failure syndromes and may resolve spontaneously over time, particularly in younger patients. In general, acquired neutropenias that are associated with hypoplasia of the marrow and pancytopenia have the worst prognosis, in the short term because of a high risk of infection and in the long term because of overlap with evolving myelodysplastic syndromes, hematologic malignancies, and other disorders characterized by progressive hematopoietic failure.

Suggested Readings*

Boxer L, Dale DC: Neutropenia: causes and consequences. Semin Hematol 39:75–81, 2002.

Bux J, Stroncek D: Human neutrophil antigens. Transfusion 42:1523, 2002.

Koene HR, de Haas M, Kleijer M, et al: Clinical value of soluble IgG Fc receptor type III in plasma from patients with chronic idiopathic neutropenia. Blood 91:3962–3966, 1998.

Palmblad JE, von dem Borne AE: Idiopathic, immune, infectious, and idiosyncratic neutropenias. Semin Hematol 39:113–120, 2002.

Wright DG, Meierovics AI, Foxley JM: Assessing the delivery of neutrophils to tissues in neutropenia. Blood 67:1023–1030, 1986.

Young NS: Agranulocytosis. *In* Bone Marrow Failure Syndromes. Philadelphia: WB Saunders, 2000, pp 156–182.

***Full references for this chapter can be found on accompanying CD-ROM.**

CHAPTER 15

Myelodysplastic Syndrome

Neal S. Young, MD, Elaine M. Sloand, MD, and John Barrett, MD, FRCP, FRCPath

KEY POINTS

Myelodysplastic Syndrome

- The myelodysplastic syndromes (MDS) are a heterogeneous group of marrow disorders, producing low blood counts and often progressing to acute myeloid leukemia. MDS is a relatively frequent hematologic diagnosis in older persons.
- Classification of MDS into subtypes relies on a combination of marrow morphology and cytogenetic findings.
- The origin of MDS is complex, involving a combination of abnormal stem cell clones; a failed marrow environment, related in part to aging and also secondary to immune inhibition; and evolution by selection of genetically and cytogenetically altered cells of increasingly malignant phenotype.
- Clinical presentation and course are highly variable: some patients may remain asymptomatic with mild blood count abnormalities for years, whereas others progress rapidly to leukemia. Complications of pancytopenia cause most deaths from MDS. Marrow blast percentage and specific cytogenetic abnormalities are highly predictive of malignant transformation and death.
- Allogeneic stem cell transplant is curative in MDS but of limited applicability, mainly because of patient age and the risk of transplant-related complications. Immunosuppression is helpful in a subset of patients in achieving transfusion-independence. Decitabine and lenalidomide, a thalidomide analogue, also can improve blood counts in MDS.

INTRODUCTION

Difficult to define simply, myelodysplastic syndrome (MDS) is always described as heterogeneous. MDS is characterized by ineffective hematopoiesis resulting in low blood cell counts and dysplastic features of marrow morphology, but it is also a clonal stem cell disorder, in which the abnormal population of hematopoietic progenitors has a high likelihood of evolution to frank leukemia.[1] Confusion not only in defining but also in categorizing MDS has a historical origin: the propounding of MDS as a disease was an effort to simplify a variety of confusing diagnoses, usually named for an aspect of the marrow's appearance or the patient's clinical behavior, and often based on case series collected by a single investigator or institution. In one category were "refractory megaloblastic anemias" or "DiGuglielmo's syndrome," peculiar entities in which the bone marrow was normal or hypercellular rather than empty (as in aplastic anemia), and that failed to respond to vitamin replacement. Also included were "smoldering leukemia" or "preleukemia," frightening diagnoses in which blood counts were low, the marrow showed increased numbers of monocytes and myeloblasts, and slow progression to frank leukemia often occurred. A more recently observed type of MDS is iatrogenic, the result of exposure to specific cytotoxic chemotherapeutic agents; secondary MDS is discussed in Chapter 29.

A first attempt to unite a myriad of seemingly unrelated disease labels was the publication in 1982 of the French-American-British (FAB) classification (Table 15–1).[2] The FAB scheme succeeded in bringing order and focus to the diagnosis of MDS by providing specific criteria, and as hematologists became familiar with its subtypes, recognition of MDS soared. The FAB scheme relied solely on morphologic criteria to classify MDS and grouped together disorders of different hematopoietic lineages and cytogenetic abnormalities; nevertheless, there was clear prognostic value to the reorganization (see later). However, the FAB nosology created its own confusion, by suggesting stages of progression through some of its subtypes—refractory anemia (RA), RA with excess blasts (RAEB), and RAEB in transformation (RAEB-t)—and by including syndromes (chronic myelomonocytic leukemia [CMML], RA with ringed sideroblasts [RARS]) that were likely to have very different etiologies but that shared the single feature of marrow dysplasia. Marrow cellularity and fibrosis, neither unusual in MDS, were not distinguished. The FAB classification was superseded in 2001 by an attempt at rationalization on the part of World Health Organization (WHO) experts[3] (Table 15–2), refining the FAB criteria using clinical observations and data accumulated over the intervening 20-year period. Major changes effected by the WHO classification include (1) removal from MDS of diagnoses in which

TABLE 15–1. FAB Classification of MDS

Subtype	Blood	Marrow	% of Cases
Refractory anemia (RA)	Blasts <1%	Blasts <5%	27
RA w/ ringed sideroblasts	Blasts <1%	Blasts <5%	20
RA w/ excess blasts (RAEB)	Blasts ≤5%	Blasts 5–20%	26
RAEB in transformation	Blasts >5%	Blasts 20–30% (or Auer rods)	13
Chronic myelomonocytic leukemia	≥1 × 10^9/L monocytes	Any number	14

FAB Subtypes and Prognosis

Subtype	***Median Survival***	***Leukemic Evolution % of Cases***
RA	50 months	16
RARS	65	15
RAEB	15	48
RAEB (t)	9	62
CMML	23	29

TABLE 15–2. WHO Classification of MDS and Prognosis

Disease	Blood	Marrow	Frequency (%)	Course	Leukemia
RA	Anemia, no blasts	Erythroid dysplasia	5–10	Protracted	~6%
RARS	Anemia, no blasts	≥15% sideroblasts; erythroid dysplasia	10–12	Protracted	~1–2%
Refractory cytopenia with multilineage dysplasia (RCMD)	Cytopenias (2–3)	Dysplasia in ≥2 lineages	24	Variable	~11%
RCMD with ringed sideroblasts		Dysplasia in ≥2 lineages; ≥15% sideroblasts	15		
RA with excess blasts (RAEB)-1	Cytopenias; <5% blasts	Uni- or multilineage dysplasia; 5–9% blasts	40	Progressive BM failure	~25%
RAEB-2	5–19% blasts	Dysplasia; 10–19% blasts		Progressive BM failure	~33%
MDS, unclassified	Cytopenias, no blasts	Dysplasia in myeloid or platelet lineage	Unknown	Unknown	Unknown
MDS, 5q–	Anemia, <5% blasts	Normal or ↑ hypolobated megakaryocytes, 5q–	Unknown	Long survival	Unknown

leukemic proliferation is obvious (CMML and RAEB-t), essentially lowering the threshold for the diagnosis of acute myeloid leukemia (AML) to 20% marrow myeloblasts; (2) defining some subtypes based on distinctive clinical and cytogenetic features (5q– syndrome; see later); and (3) subdivision of low-grade categories of refractory anemia (RA and RARS) into separate entities depending on the number of cell lines that manifest dysplasia. Advocates argue the merits of the FAB versus WHO systems, and MDS categorization is likely to evolve as better cytogenetic and molecular methods reveal pathophysiologic mechanisms that allow more reliable discrimination than subjective microscopic examinations. Both the FAB and WHO classifications are helpful in predicting survival in MDS (Fig. 15–1).

EPIDEMIOLOGY AND RISK FACTORS

MDS is a relatively common hematologic diagnosis, especially in older patients.[4,5] In the bone marrow registry of the University of Dusseldorf, 3.2% of all cases were diagnosed as MDS (compared to 2.8% for AML).[6] For this well-defined geographic area, age-specific incidence figures were calculated for the years 1986–1990: for patients 50–70 years old, the incidence was 4.9 per 100,000 (more than twice the rate for AML), and for patients older than 70 years of age, the incidence was 22.8 per 100,000 (more than thrice that of AML; Fig. 15–2). Similar figures have been reported from Sweden (15 per 100,000 for individuals over 70 years old,[7] France (31.4 per 100,000 for those older than 80 years),[8] and England (49.0 per 100,000 for 70- to 79-year-olds),[9] but MDS may be less prevalent in Japan.[10] In general, MDS is about 100-fold less frequent in patients under the age of 50 years compared to those over 50, and it is very rare in children (see later). In almost all series, men are more often affected than are women. Over the last several decades, the prevalence of MDS has risen for three reasons: (1) awareness on the part of physicians of a new diagnostic category, (2) increasing survival of patients exposed to mutagenic drugs in the course of cancer chemotherapy, and (3) the aging of populations in developed countries.[4]

The most important environmental risk factors for MDS are exposure to specific anticancer drugs, alkylat-

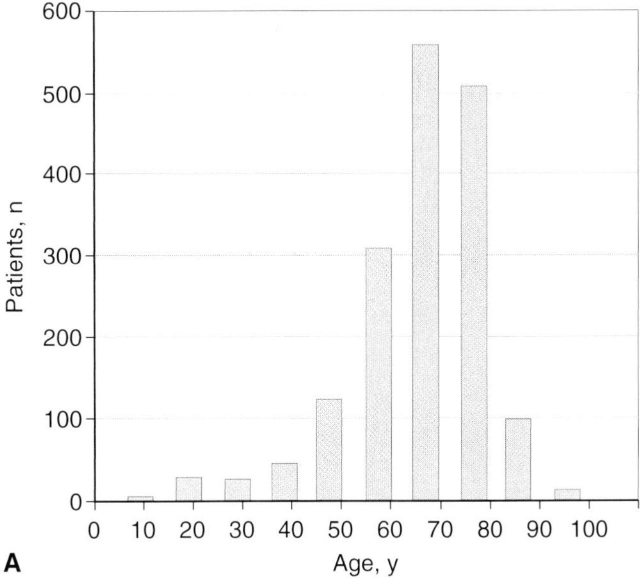

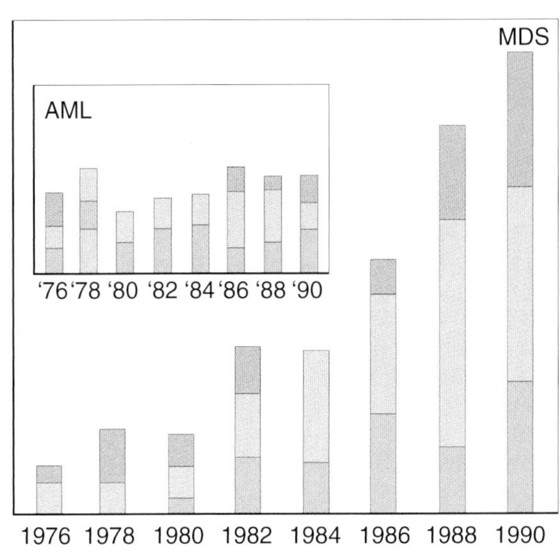

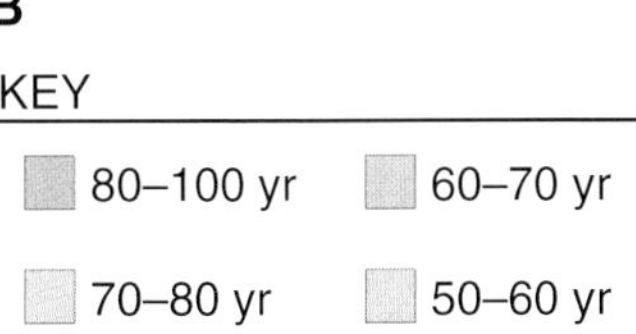

Figure 15–1. Demographics and epidemiology of MDS. ***A***, Age distribution of 1759 patients with MDS (primary and secondary) diagnosed at the University of Dusseldorf over a 20-year period.[105] ***B***, Age-specific incidence of MDS (and acute myeloid leukemia [AML], *inset*) in the same patient population; data for those greater than 70 years old are *shaded*.[6]

ing agents and etoposides[11] (see Chapter 29). Other factors have been less consistently and convincingly associated. Benzene, etiologic in both aplastic anemia and AML, was also implicated in a massive National Cancer Institute study of exposed workers in China.[12] A variety of chemical exposures and occupations involving radiation, organic solvents, and pesticides (and also metal, stone, and cereal dusts) have been related to MDS in some case-control studies.[13–17] Common exposures, such as to gasoline, hair dyes, and tobacco smoke, do not appear to play a major role in the development of MDS.

Familial MDS occurs but is rare.[18–20] Because MDS patients usually present late as older adults, testing for Fanconi's anemia is not performed, and some families may represent unusual manifestations of this constitutional marrow failure syndrome or of dyskeratosis congenita–like defects in telomere repair complex genes.[21,22] The null phenotype of genes encoding for glutathione-*S*-transferases, enzymes involved in carcinogen metabolism, has been increased in some populations of MDS patients.[23,24]

PATHOPHYSIOLOGY

The origins of MDS are understood in pieces, not as a whole. Studies of cell proliferation and death, as well as immune abnormalities and molecular defects, have provided important clues but not a broad hypothesis to account for the simultaneous or sequential development of a marrow that both has failed as an organ of hematopoiesis and is also highly susceptible to leukemic transformation.

Hematopoietic Cell Proliferation

Overall cell proliferation rates usually are high, consistent with the cellular appearance of most patients' marrows. Hematopoietic progenitors in committed lineages are often deficient; erythroid (BFU-E and CFU-E) and megakaryocytic (CFU-Meg) colony formation is decreased, whereas myeloid colony (CFU-GM) growth is more normal.[25–27] Primitive hematopoietic cells, characterized as multipotential progenitors (CFU-GEMM), blast colonies, or long-term colony initiating cells, also are numerically or functionally reduced in most MDS, although they may be normal.[28–30] Correlation of responsiveness of colony formation to hematopoietic growth factors such as erythropoietin, granulocyte colony-stimulating factor (G-CSF), and granulocyte-macrophage colony-stimulating factor have been imperfect.[28,31–33] Normal progenitor function, as occurs in 5q− syndrome, in MDS with normal cytogenetics, and in sideroblastic anemia, has been associated with a more favorable prognosis.[34–37] In many studies, clonal progenitors form small clusters of cells rather than full colonies.[38,39] The number of stem cell clones, inferred from X chromosome inactivation patterns, is more reduced in MDS with marked dysplasia or increased marrow blasts than in RA[40]; nonclonal, presumably normal hematopoiesis, can be detected in a subset of patients.[40–42] The stromal microenvironment also shows evidence of functional abnormalities in vitro.[42,43]

Apoptosis

Pancytopenia occurs in MDS despite a usually cellular bone marrow—a paradox that could be explained if

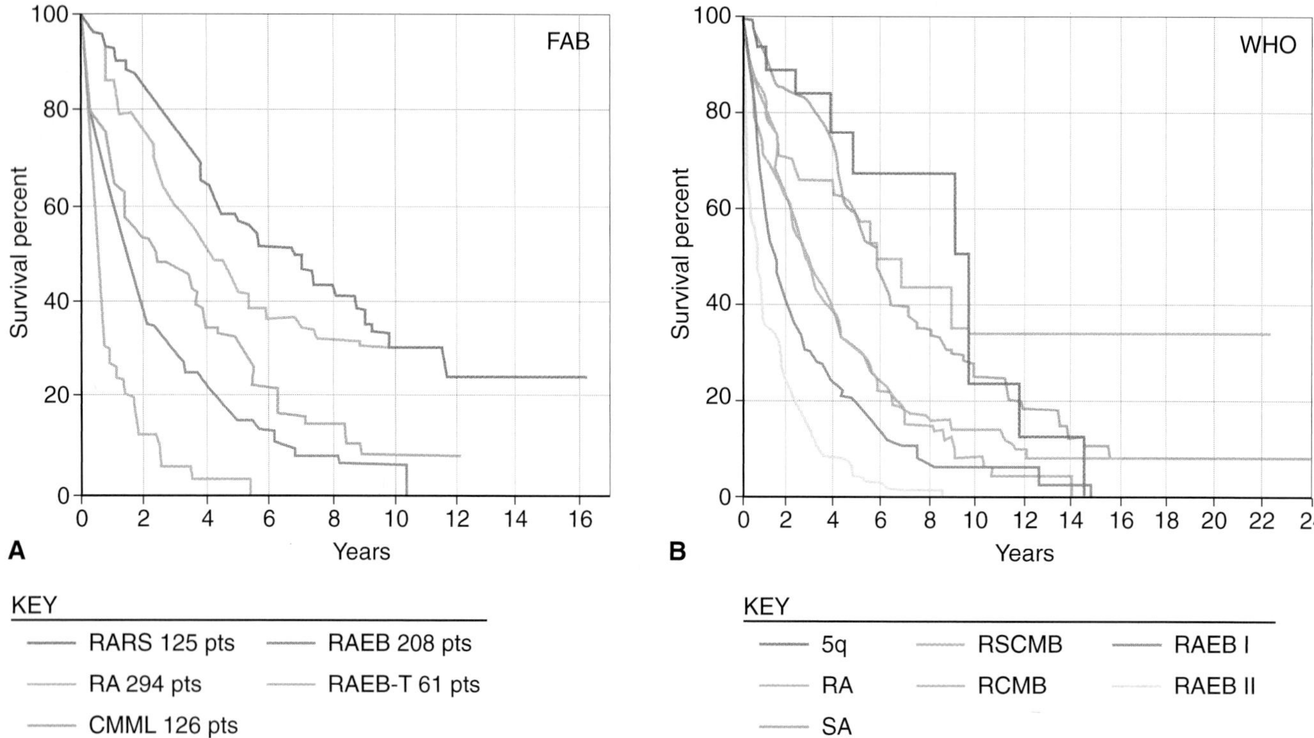

Figure 15–2. Classification and prognosis in MDS. *A*, French-American-British (FAB) subtype and survival in a group of MDS patients with FAB classification subtypes as follows: 15% RARS, 36% RA, 26% RAEB, 8% RAEB-t, and 15% CMML. The median age of all patients was 69 years, and the male : female ratio was 1.5. The median follow-up time for these patients was 1.9 years (range, 0.1–17 years). Median survival and rate of leukemic transformation are for RA, 50 months and 16%; for RARS, 65 months and 15%; for RAEB, 15 months and 48%; for RAEB-t, 9 months and 62%; and for CMML, 23 months and 29%.[199] *B*, World Health Organization (WHO) classification of diagnosis and survival.[105] Patients were stratified into four distinctive risk groups with respect to both survival and AML evolution, with risk scores as follows: low risk, 0; intermediate (INT)-1 risk, 0.5–1.0; INT-2 risk, 1.5–2.0; and high risk 2.0 or greater (see Table 15–3). The Kaplan-Meier curves depict survival without development of acute myelogenous leukemia are shown for patients in the various prognostic subgroups.

hematopoietic cell death dominated cell proliferation. This aspect of MDS pathophysiology has attracted much attention.[44–46] Programmed cell death is increased as measured in a variety of assays of apoptosis in MDS marrow: morphologic and ultrastructural changes,[47,48] molecular assessment of DNA strand breaks[49] and specific apoptotic proteins such as Bcl-2,[50] and immunohistochemistry for exposed membrane phosphatidylserine.[39] In contrast, DNA fragmentation has been harder to demonstrate, and seemingly apoptotic cells may unexpectedly proliferate in tissue culture,[51] suggesting that cell death may be incomplete and perhaps explaining the morphology of dysplasia and functional ineffective hematopoiesis. Although results of apoptosis assays are variable, as would be expected with the heterogeneity inherent in MDS, some investigators have observed cell death to be more marked in the subtypes associated with refractory pancytopenia and less marked in MDS with increased blasts,[52–54] and clinical improvements in blood counts with growth factor therapy or anti-inflammatory drugs[55] have been correlated with evidence of decreased programmed cell death in the marrow. The extent of apoptosis (modest or massive[56]) and which specific cell types are subject to destruction remain controversial.[57,58]

Altered Immunity in MDS

The immune system has been implicated as an effector of cell death in the myelodysplastic bone marrow,[59–61] in part because of clinical data, the association of MDS with autoimmune diseases and the response of patients to immunosuppressive therapies. Laboratory data also suggest a relationship. Tumor necrosis factor (TNF)-α, a suppressor of hematopoiesis through Fas induction, has been the major focus of experiments. TNF has been shown to be overexpressed in patients' cells in culture,[62] elevated in marrow biopsies,[63] and present in plasma.[64] Also elevated in some MDS hematopoietic tissues are TNF-related apoptosis-inducing ligand (TRAIL),[65] interferon-γ, and transforming growth factor-β. TNF production has not been well correlated with disease subtype.[66] Some investigators have suggested that the source of TNF, and perhaps other negative regulators, may be macrophages or other cells located within stroma.[42,43,67,68]

TNF has been linked to hematopoietic cell destruction by its receptor and downstream proapoptotic signaling pathways. Constitutive and abnormal expression of various TNF and TRAIL receptors is high,[65,69] and marrow cells of patients may be correspondingly sensitive to TNF and TRAIL inhibition of growth and cytotoxicity.[65] An alternative pathway to programmed cell death is through induction of Fas and its signaling pathway. Both Fas and Fas ligand, measured by flow cytometry, gene amplification of complementary DNA generated from messenger RNA, and immunohistochemistry, have been elevated in MDS.[52,70–73] The functional role of the Fas pathway has been more elusive to experimental confirmation, but in one recent experiment a role for the Fas-associated death domain in MDS CD34 cells was directly demonstrated in vitro.[73]

A proportion of MDS patients respond hematologically to antithymocyte globulin therapy (see later), a clinical observation that implicates T cells in marrow suppression, analogous to the pathophysiology of aplastic anemia (see Chapter 10). In many patients with MDS, there is comparable evidence of T-cell activation, as, for example, by the presence of functionally inhibitory T cells in colony assays[74] and in skewing of the T-cell repertoire, detected by spectratyping of the length of the Vβ chain of the T-cell receptor,[74–76] which correct with successful immunosuppression. Clonal expansions of T cells may be large enough to suggest a coincident diagnosis of large granular lymphocytic leukemia.[77] MDS is associated with a human lymphocyte antigen (HLA) class II antigen.[78]

The most complete description of a role of immune effectors in MDS has come from studies of MDS associated with trisomy 8; these cytogenetics predict responsiveness to immunologic therapy and prolonged survival.[79] In the trisomy 8 syndrome, the cytogenetically abnormal clones, in comparison to the normal progenitor cells, overexpress Fas on their surface, appear apoptotic in vivo, and are more susceptible to Fas-mediated apoptosis in vitro.[80] In trisomy 8 MDS, T-cell receptor skewing is consistently present, highly suggestive of an antigen-driven process, and these T cells appear to specifically recognize the cytogenetically abnormal hematopoietic progenitors.[81] Cytokines such as TRAIL also seem to target cells with aberrant chromosomes.[65] In trisomy 8, as in other MDS,[51] apoptosis may not be completed, perhaps as a result of compensatory mutations that block the apoptotic signaling pathways. One antigen putatively identified as the target of T-cell attack in trisomy 8 MDS is WT1.[81] The Wilms' tumor antigen is overexpressed in leukemia, and thus the T-cell attack in trisomy 8 MDS may be viewed as a successful control of myeloblast expansion, at the expense of "innocent bystander"[82] injury to normal hematopoiesis, but selecting also within the trisomy 8 clone for cells able to survive immune aggression.

Chromosomal and Genetic Abnormalities

Cytogenetic abnormalities are very common in MDS, present in more than half of patients at the time of clinical presentation, and they occur in stereotypical patterns that have in practice a strong relationship with clinical course, especially the probability of leukemic transformation and survival (see later). Cytogenetic abnormalities also may provide clues to molecular pathogenesis—in the specific chromosomes (5, 7, 8, 9, and 20 especially), the pattern of aberrancy (aneuploidy and large interstitial deletions), and the individual genes involved. In secondary MDS, chromosomes 5 and 7 are usually involved after exposure to alkylating agents, and the 11q23 locus following treatment with etoposides (see Chapter 29). One stereotypical karyotype in idiopathic MDS is deletion of a portion of the short arm of the fifth chromosome, or 5q− syndrome,[83] particularly revealing because of the presence of genes for multiple hematopoietic growth factors and their receptors in the affected region; in the commonly deleted region of about 1.5 megabases at 5q32 are a large proportion of genes expressed in CD34 cells, including a tumor suppressor gene (*MEGF1*), a gene that encodes a Ras-GTPase activating protein (*G3BP*), and a gene that encodes a platelet-derived growth factor receptor (PDGFR-β).[84] Larger but less consistent deletions of 5q− remove other genes encoding for hematopoietic growth factors and their receptors. The length and location of 5q deletions has been correlated with clinical behavior and survival.[85] Microarray patterns of messenger RNA expression have revealed a subset of genes that discriminate 5q− from other types of MDS.[86] Trisomy of chromosome 8 confers a good prognosis, with cytopenias often responsive to immunosuppressive therapies and a low rate of leukemic transformation (see above).[87] In trisomy 8 MDS, the cytogenetically aberrant cells appear to be targeted because of their overexpression of WT1, but apoptosis is abortive because of overexpression of CDK2.[88,89] Absence or partial deletions of chromosome 7, in contrast, confer a poor prognosis, with usually refractory cytopenias and transformation to acute leukemia. Monosomy 7 is a characteristic lesion in survivors of the bone marrow failure states of acquired aplastic anemia[79] and congenital neutropenia. Cells lacking a chromosome 7 show high expression of a short isoform of the G-CSF receptor, which preferentially signals proliferation over differentiation,[90] accounting for their clonal expansion under conditions of neutropenia or exogenous cytokine administration. Multiple loci on chromosome 7 are probably involved in producing the monosomy 7 phenotype, but a single tumor suppressor gene has not been implicated.[91,92] Monosomy 7 has been associated with *ras* mutations in vivo[93] and in vitro.[94] Microarray analysis clearly distinguishes the transcriptomes of trisomy 8 and monosomy 7 CD34 cells: marrow progenitors from trisomy 8 are more similar to normal CD34 cells and show increased expression of apoptosis and immune regulation genes, whereas the pattern of gene expression in monosomy 7 CD34 cells resembles that of leukemic blasts.[82]

Oncogenic mutations among *ras* family members occur in 5–15% of MDS patients; as in AML, N-*ras* mutations at codons 12 or 61 are most common. Some MDS patients also have mutations in the tyrosine kinase *FLT3*, resulting in constitutive activation of the receptor. FLT-3 and Ras may be therapeutic targets for FLT-3 and farnesyltransferase inhibitors, respectively. Mutations are rare in p53, except in association with 17p−; loss of one allele as a result of mutation and of the second allele from

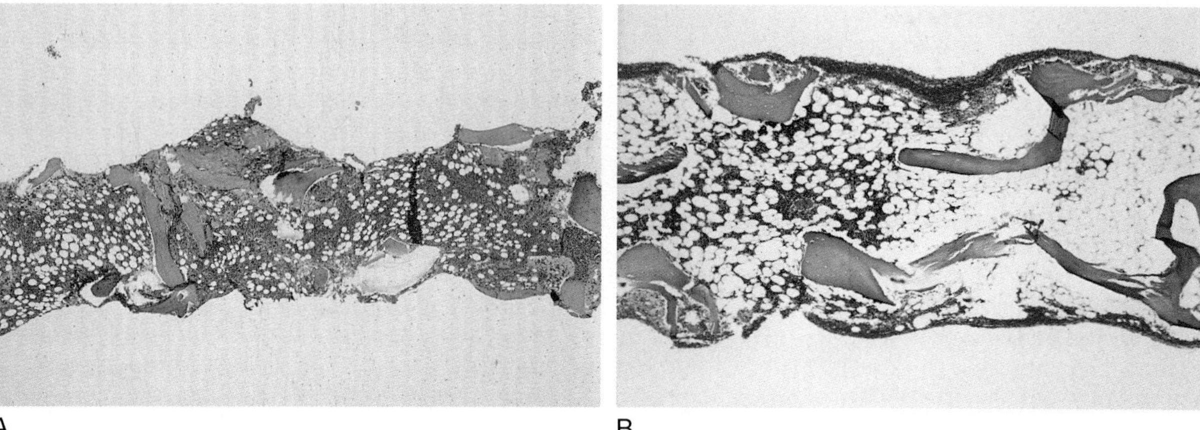

■ **Figure 15–3.** Bone marrow biopsies in MDS; low-power views. ***A***, Typical hypercellular appearance in a patient with MDS classified as RAEB. ***B***, Partially hypocellular specimen of a patient with 5q− syndrome.

a large chromosomal deletion are pathogenic in these cases.

CLINICAL FEATURES AND DIAGNOSIS

MDS is a disease of the elderly; older men and women are about equally affected. Anemia dominates the early course in most symptomatic patients, who typically complain of the gradual onset of fatigue and weakness, dyspnea, and pallor. Half the cases are asymptomatic and the myelodysplasia is discovered only incidentally, as, for example, when anemia or another cytopenia is found on a routine blood examination. A family history may indicate a hereditary form of sideroblastic anemia, or suggest a constitutional marrow failure syndrome. Previous chemotherapy or radiation exposure is an important historical fact for secondary MDS. A significant proportion of MDS patients, 12% in a large Japanese series[95] and more than half in a smaller group seen in Minnesota,[96] also suffer from autoimmune diseases: rheumatoid arthritis but also hemolytic or pernicious anemia, pure red cell aplasia, immune thrombocytopenia, eosinophilic fasciitis (also seen with aplastic anemia), hypothyroidism, erythema nodosum, pyoderma gangrenosum, Behçet's disease, and vasculitis.[5,59] Fever and weight loss point to a myeloproliferative rather than myelodysplastic process.

The physical examination is remarkable for signs of anemia. Severe thrombocytopenia may be accompanied by petechiae, ecchymoses, and frank mucosal bleeding. Splenomegaly is found in about 20% of cases. Some unusual skin lesions, such as Sweet's syndrome (febrile neutrophilic dermatosis), have been associated with MDS.[97]

Laboratory Studies

Peripheral Blood

Anemia is present in the majority of cases, either alone or as part of bi- or pancytopenia, and isolated neutropenia or thrombocytopenia is unusual. Macrocytosis is expected in the absence of transfusion, and the smear may be dimorphic with a distinctive population of large cells. Platelets are often large and agranular. Neutrophils also may be hypogranulated, show the Pelger-Huët anomaly or ringed or abnormally segmented nuclei, and contain Döhle bodies. Circulating myeloblasts usually correlate with marrow blast numbers; their quantitation is important for classification and prognosis. The total white blood cell count is usually normal or low.

Bone Marrow

The bone marrow is most often normo- or hypercellular, but in 20% of myelodysplasia cases it is sufficiently hypocellular to be confused with aplasia; fibrosis may occasionally be present. There is no single characteristic of marrow morphology to distinguish MDS, and some features of dyserythropoiesis and dysmyelopoiesis are present in a significant proportion of marrows obtained from healthy older donors.[98] In MDS, common findings include megaloblastoid and dyserythropoietic changes in red blood cell precursors; hypogranulated myeloid precursors with a preponderance of primitive cells and increased myeloblasts; and distinctly abnormal megakaryocytes that show reduced numbers of disorganized nuclei (Figs. 15–3 and 15–4). The erythroid series changes are least specific because they are seen also in aplastic anemia and paroxysmal nocturnal hemoglobinuria. Ringed sideroblasts and myeloblasts are the most striking and objective evidence of MDS in the marrow. The diagnosis of RARS requires the presence of sufficient numbers of ringed sideroblasts (see Chapter 55). The percentage of blasts must be accurately quantitated in order to discriminate MDS from acute leukemia and because of the importance of this number in determining prognosis.

Cytogenetics

Analysis of chromosomes from cultured bone marrow cells should always be performed. Cytogenetics are now

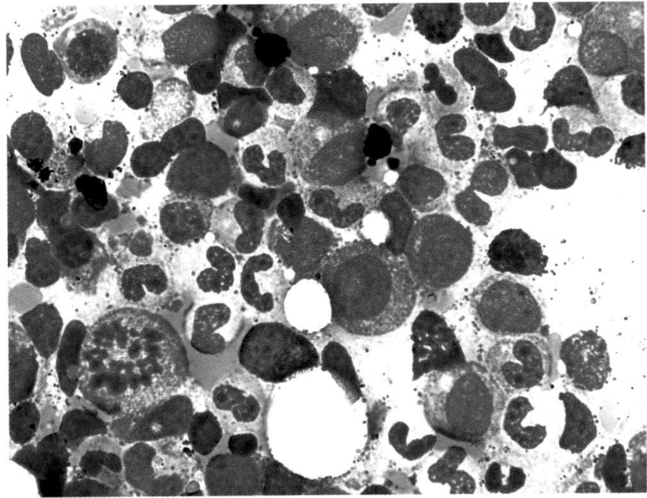

A

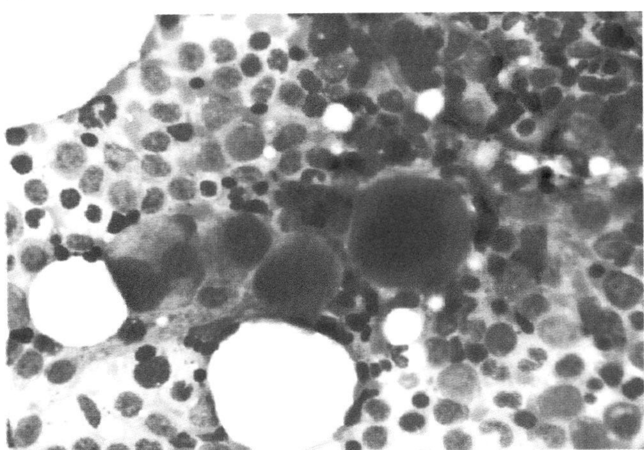

B

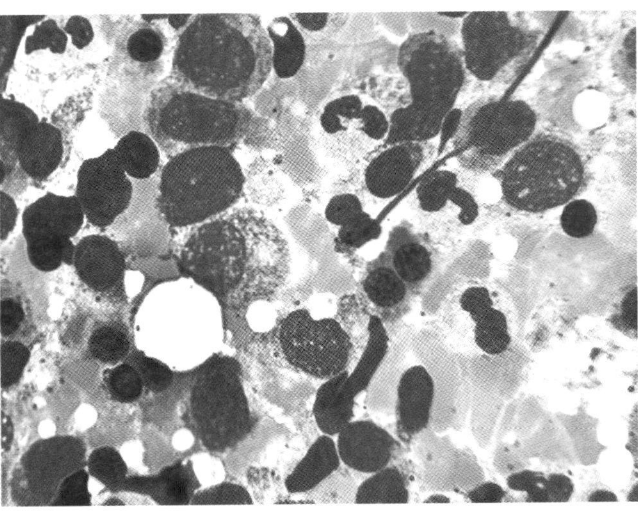

C

■ **Figure 15–4.** Dysplasia in MDS; high-power views of aspirate smears. *A*, Dysmyelopoiesis with "left shift," hypogranulation, and increased myeloblasts. *B*, Mononuclear megakaryocytes, including micromegakaryocytes. *C*, Megaloblastoid dyserythropoiesis.

often routinely supplemented by more sensitive methods such as fluorescent in situ hybridization and spectral karyotyping (see Chapter 103), which, by using chromosome-specific molecular probes and assaying nondividing cells, greatly increase detection and quantitation of abnormal cells. Cytogenetic abnormalities are detected in 40–70% of patients with MDS, depending on the series (and in virtually all treatment-related MDS). Stereotypical abnormal chromosome patterns have been detected in the absence of morphologic dysplasia during evaluation of an elderly patient with a cytopenia or other blood abnormality without necessarily heralding frank MDS.[99]

Chromosomes 5 (del 5q), 7 (del 7q or del 7), 8 (trisomy 8), 20 (del 20q), and Y (−Y) account for the majority of abnormalities. Large deletions and aneuploidy are most common, and translocations (common in AML) are infrequent in MDS. In an international study of more than 800 untreated MDS patients[100] with available cytogenetic data, a normal karyotype and deletions of 5q and 20q conferred a relatively good prognosis, and del 7 or 7q− predicted the poorest outcomes; trisomy 8 or double chromosomal abnormalities were intermediate. Current treatments that improve cytopenias or slow progression to leukemia may alter the relationship between cytogenetics and survival. For example, in MDS treated with immunosuppression, trisomy 8 as the sole cytogenetic abnormality predicted a good response to immunotherapy and prolonged survival.

Other Laboratory Studies

An expanded clonal population of glycosylphosphinositol-anchored protein-deficient cells, as seen in paroxysmal nocturnal hemoglobinuria (see Chapter 25), is most easily detected by flow cytometry; the presence of a paroxysmal nocturnal hemoglobinuria clone is a favorable factor for response to immunosuppressive treatment.[101,102] Clonal T-cell expansion, also measured by flow cytometry, can be so pronounced as to suggest large granular lymphocytic leukemia.[77,103] MDS frequently coexists with benign plasma cell expansions, also age-related, and immunoglobulin testing may show increased monoclonal gammopathy. Because of the frequent concurrence of autoimmune disease, serologic and collagen vascular panels may be abnormal. Ferritin should be monitored as patients acquire a transfusion burden. Magnetic resonance imaging measures marrow cellularity but is not generally employed to distinguish MDS from aplastic anemia.[104]

Prognosis Predicted from Laboratory Studies

The International Prognostic Staging System (IPSS)[105,106] was developed from the retrospective analysis of several thousand well-documented cases of MDS. It provides clinical evidence–based probabilities for leukemic transformation and survival, giving numerical weight to three highly predictive criteria: marrow blast percentage, cytogenetic abnormalities, and cytopenias (Table 15–3). The IPSS accurately predicts disease behavior in individual patients and permits comparisons of treatments (Fig. 15–5).

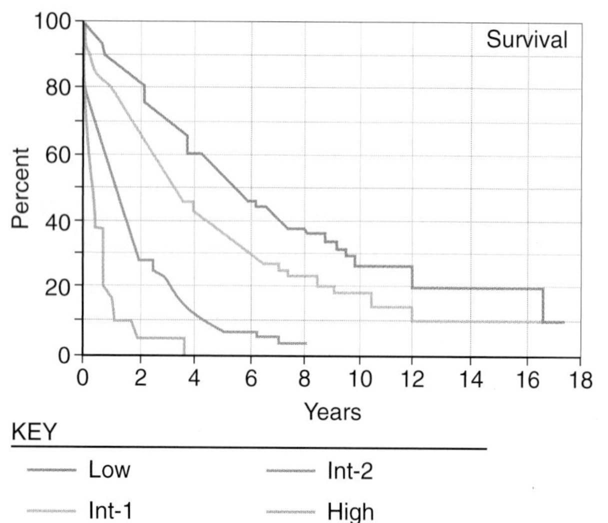

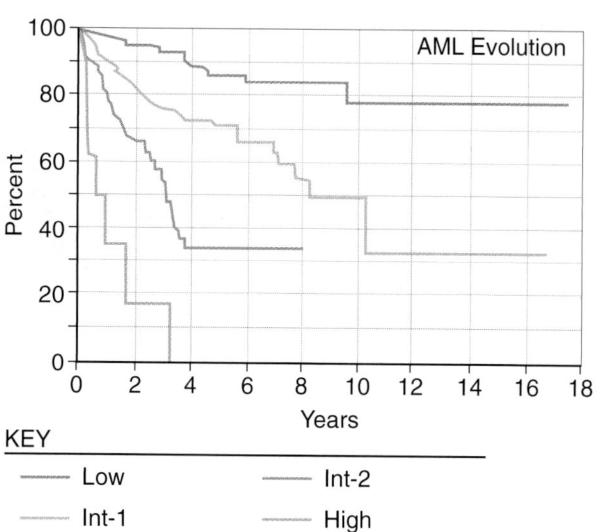

A International IPSS

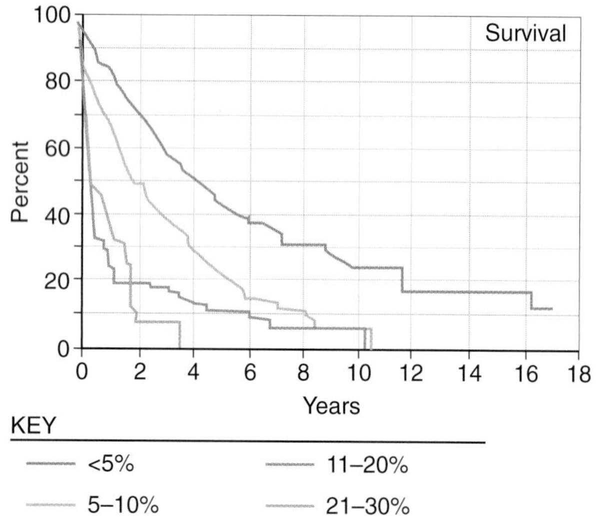

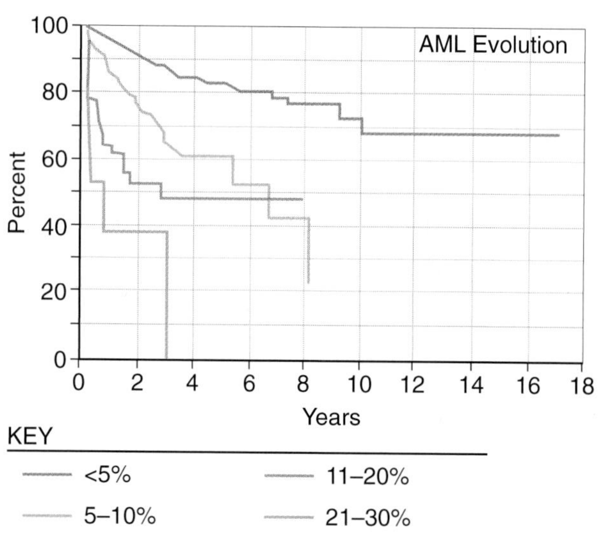

B Marrow blasts

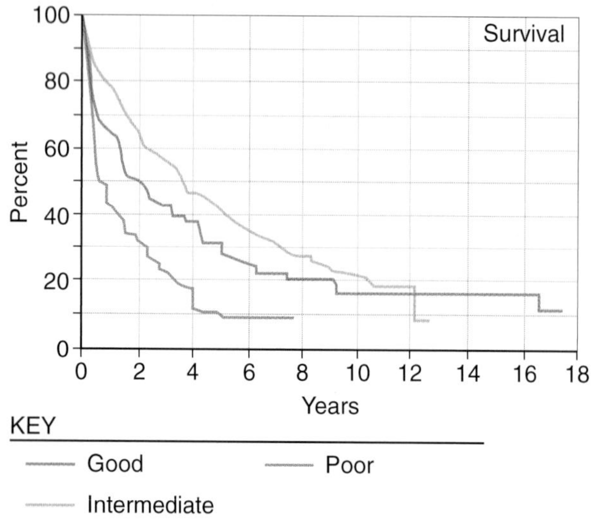

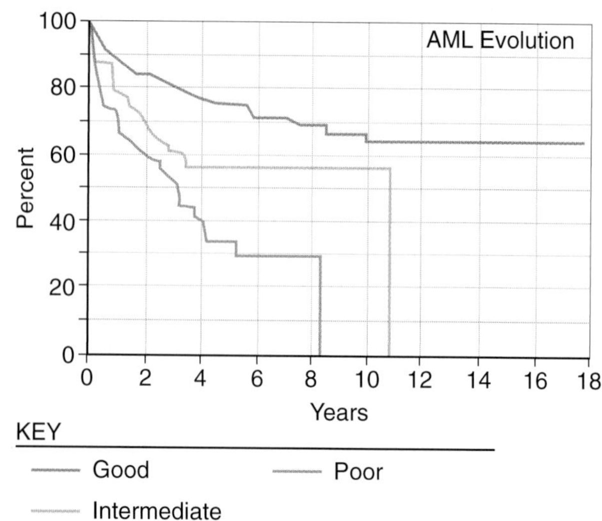

C Cytogenetics

Figure 15–5. Prognosis determined by IPSS. Survival (above) and evolution to leukemia by IPSS classification *(A)*, marrow blast percentage *(B)*, and cytogenetics *(C)*.[105]

TABLE 15–3. International Prognostic Scoring System for Myelodysplasia*

Parameter	Criteria	Score
Marrow blasts	<5%	0
	5–10%	0.5
	11–20%	1.5
	21–30%	2
Karyotype	Good (normal 46,XY; −Y; 5q−; 20q−)	0
	Intermediate (other)	0.5
	Poor (at least 3 abnormalities or chromosome 7 anomalies)	1
Cytopenias		
Hemoglobin <10 gm/dL	None or one	0
Platelet count <100,000/µL	Two or three	0.5
Neutrophil count <15,000/µL		

*Total score: 0 = low-risk group; 0.5–1.0 = intermediate-1–risk group; 1.5–2.0 = intermediate-2–risk group; >2.0 = high-risk group.

Differential Diagnosis

Inherited marrow failure in young patients can manifest as MDS. Characteristic physical anomalies should be sought by careful examination but may be absent. If suspected, Fanconi's anemia can be excluded by appropriate chromosome or genetic testing; dyskeratosis congenita requires telomere length or genetic analyses now only available in research laboratories (see Chapter 11). In older adults, the most difficult distinctions are between MDS and AML or aplastic anemia. The presence of circulating blast cells and an accurate blast count in the marrow establish the diagnosis of leukemia. In aplastic anemia, erythroid megaloblastoid changes are common but megakaryocytes are almost always absent and never mononuclear, and residual myeloid cells generally appear normal. As described earlier, MDS can occur in combination with paroxysmal nocturnal hemoglobinuria and/or large granular lymphocytic leukemia.[103] Occasional patients show features of both MDS and myeloproliferative disease. Finally, because the reading of dysplasia on microscopy is subjective, an important caution is to avoid overinterpretation of a marrow specimen in an elderly person who may have only minimal hematologic abnormalities.

Specific Myelodysplastic Syndromes

5q−

An interstitial deletion on the long arm of chromosome 5 is the sole chromosomal abnormality (see earlier)[107]; the extent of deletion is variable, although the distal breakpoint is 5q33 in 70% of cases and the proximal breakpoint is q13 in 50% of cases.[85,108] The clinical syndrome is typified by macrocytic anemia, leukopenia, and normal or even elevated platelet counts (in about one third of patients, but conspicuously absent in therapy-related MDS with 5q−). Small dysplastic, monolobulated megakaryocytes are characteristic. Patients with de novo 5q− do well, with prolonged survival and relatively infrequent transformation to acute leukemia: in one large study, the rate of leukemic transformation in 5q− was 25% over an observation period of 15 years compared to 40% in MDS with a normal karyotype.[105] The presence of additional cytogenetic abnormalities cancels the favorable prognosis.

Trisomy 8

Trisomy 8 occurs in 10–15% of MDS.[109] It is considered an intermediate prognostic marker in the IPSS,[105] and the median survival of these MDS patient ranges from 25 to 57 months.[110] MDS patients with RA and trisomy 8 respond to immunosuppressive therapy[111]: 77% of trisomy 8 patients treated at the National Institutes of Health had favorable responses to antithymocyte globulin and have predicted median survival in years. Patients often remain dependent on cyclosporine administration, and the proportion of trisomy 8 cells usually rises with hematologic remission.[112,113] As with 5q−, trisomy 8's benign character is negated by additional cytogenetic abnormalities.

Monosomy 7

Aneuploidy for chromosome 7 is frequent in MDS secondary to exposure to alkylating drugs and in pediatric MDS. Monosomy 7 is also a late evolutionary event in acquired aplastic anemia that is poorly responsive to immunosuppression[114] and in congenital neutropenia treated with G-CSF (see Chapters 10 and 13). Japanese studies linked monosomy 7 to therapeutic administration of G-CSF.[115] A molecular explanation for these relationships may be abnormalities in G-CSF receptor signaling in monosomy 7 cells (see earlier). In general, patients with monosomy 7, 7q−, or other abnormalities of this chromosome have poor overall survival, with death usually occurring secondary to leukemic progression or from refractory cytopenias. Survival statistics vary depending on whether the chromosomal abnormality is acquired from chemotherapy or radiation (<3 months), occurs following aplastic anemia (median survival 125 months[79]), or is found in new MDS (median survival 3–6 months[116]). Children with bone marrow failure may show transient expression of monosomy 7, and this cytogenetic abnormality does not adversely affect prognosis in pediatric MDS.[117] Adult patients may revert to normal cytogenetics when they respond to immunotherapy,[118] consistent with the altered sensitivity of the monosomy 7 clone to the effects of high endogenous G-CSF in bone marrow failure.[118]

MDS with Myelofibrosis

Myelofibrosis, usually slight to moderate when quantitated, is observed in about 17% of primary MDS cases, most frequently in CMML. With the presence of fibrosis, dysplastic changes may be more marked in the megakaryocyte lineage. Marrow fibrosis is associated with a poor prognosis and a rapidly progressive course.

Chronic Myelomonocytic Leukemia

Because dysplasia is frequently concurrent in the marrow specimens of CMML, this disease was included as MDS in the FAB classification,[119] but the similarity of CMML to chronic myeloid leukemia led to its exclusion in the WHO system and its transfer to the myeloproliferative diseases (see Chapter 31).

Pediatric MDS

MDS in childhood is extremely rare (see Fig. 15–2), with an estimated annual incidence of about 3 per 1 million in dedicated epidemiologic studies in Europe and North America (half that of pediatric AML, and constituting only 6% of all childhood leukemias).[120,121] MDS in children is often accompanied by an inherited or associated disorder.[122] There are major differences between MDS as it occurs in children compared to adults.[123] RAEB and RAEB-t are more frequent and monosomy 7 is the most common cytogenetic abnormality in pediatric MDS[124,125] (and also among younger adults, under 50 years of age, with MDS).[126,127] As with MDS in general, cytogenetics are predictive of outcome.[128] Leukemic transformation is expected, occurring in 32% of patients within 2 years of diagnosis in one series.[129] Monosomy 7 does not appear to alter the outcome in pediatric MDS, in contrast to pediatric AML with monosomy 7 and to adult MDS.[130,131] Pediatric MDS is a severe hematologic disease, with short overall survivals (5.5–9.9 months) and a high rate of leukemic transformation.

Because of these differences, the WHO classification for adult MDS does not apply to pediatric MDS. Separate criteria for the diagnosis of MDS in childhood have been proposed, to include (1) juvenile myelomonocytic leukemia, (2) myeloid leukemia of Down syndrome, and (3) MDS occurring de novo and as a complication of previous therapy (see Chapters 29 and 33 for details). The subgroup of MDS RAEB-t would be retained because of uncertainty as to a meaningful threshold blast percentage in this population.[131] Factors negatively impacting survival in children with MDS include hemoglobin F levels greater than 10%, platelet counts less than 40,000/μL, and complex karyotypic changes.[124]

TREATMENT

Allogeneic hematopoietic stem cell transplant can cure MDS, but this treatment has until recently only been available to younger patients with histocompatible sibling donors. Thus, most MDS patients have been treated supportively or with ameliorative medical regimens. Nevertheless, even small changes in transfusion requirements or modest increases in granulocyte number can markedly improve quality of life, particularly in an elderly population who often suffer other medical problems. Unfortunately, despite the frequency of MDS, there is a surprising paucity of adequate clinical trials of either standard or experimental regimens. Given the heterogeneity of the syndrome and the difficulties of classification, studies may be difficult to compare. Because success has often been claimed based on evidence of minimal hematologic improvement, attempts have been made to develop acceptable standardized criteria for response.[106]

5-Azacytidine and Decitabine

The nucleoside analogue 5-azacytidine recently has been licensed for use in MDS by the Food and Drug Administration based on results of a controlled, randomized clinical trial.[132] When 5-azacytidine was compared to supportive care, treated patients showed reduced transfusion requirements and a delayed time to leukemic transformation. Treated patients had improved quality-of-life measures as well.[133] However, no survival benefit was demonstrated, possibly because of the crossover design of the pivotal study. 5-Azacytidine is generally administered subcutaneously for a 7-day period, once monthly. Toxicities include nausea and vomiting as well as significant myelosuppression, and they must be balanced against the potential benefits of the drug. Thrombocytopenic patients should receive 5-azacytidine parenterally because continued subcutaneous injections result in bruising with repeated cycles.

Decitabine is similar in structure and function to 5-azacytidine and also has been studied in patients with MDS.[134] A randomized Phase III trial, similar in design to the 5-azacytidine study but without crossover, has recently been completed but not yet formally published; 10% complete response rates have not appeared to translate to improved survival. The current formulation of decitabine is for intravenous use.

The mechanism of action of 5-azacytidine and decitabine remains uncertain. Their activity has been presumed to relate to DNA demethylation, reversing the gene silencing associated with promoter hypermethylation and inactivation of tumor suppressor genes, but both drugs also are cytotoxic at higher doses.

Thalidomide and Lenalidomide

Thalidomide has been much used in MDS.[135] Thalidomide has multiple activities, including antiangiogenesis, and also inhibits production of TNF-α, a cytokine that has been implicated in pathogenesis of MDS. Despite its popularity, response rates to thalidomide have been modest. The North Central Cancer Treatment Group[136] reported responses in only 1 of 43 MDS patients with favorable IPSS scores, and in 6 of 30 high-risk patients. In another study, hematologic improvement was reported for 19 of 34 study patients but only 4 achieved a major remission with transfusion-independence.[137] Toxicities frequently lead to termination of treatment in experimental trials; fatigue, reversible neurotoxicity, rash, and constipation are most frequent. Thrombosis is a particularly worrisome complication.[138]

CC5013, or lenalidomide, is an oral analogue of thalidomide with a better toxicity profile, especially fewer neurologic side effects, and possibly additional immunomodulatory activities. In a group of 36 evaluable patients,[139] 24 responded, 20 with major responses defined as a substantial improvement in hemoglobin or a reduction/elimination of transfusion requirements. There was striking benefit in the group of patients with the 5q– cytogenetic abnormality, among whom 10 of 11 responded and 1 relapsed with a mean follow-up period of 81 weeks.

Arsenic

Arsenic trioxide targets the sulfhydryl groups present in many proteins involved in oncogenesis. Arsenic has been evaluated in small studies, in which hematologic responses were noted in 7 of 28 patients when it was combined with thalidomide[140] and in 13 of 50 patients when it was employed as a single agent.[141] Responses have been largely erythroid and usually do not produce independence from the need for transfusion. Significant myelosuppression, as well as QT interval prolongation and complete atrioventricular block, hypoxia, and back pain, have been major toxicities.

Immunosuppression

Multiple studies have demonstrated improved outcomes in patients treated with immunosuppressive drugs.[142–145] When cyclosporine was administered to 17 cytopenic Czech patients with RA and variable bone marrow cellularity, "substantial" and sustained hematologic response was observed in 14 (82%): anemia improved and transfusion-dependence resolved, and complete trilineage recovery occurred in 4 patients.[146] More than half of a small series of cases showed similar improvement in a Japanese study.[147] At the National Institutes of Health, 133 MDS patients, most with RA and in the intermediate-1 category of IPSS, have been treated, usually with antithymocyte globulin alone. Younger patients with a low transfusion burden and those with HLA-DR15 were more likely to respond; responding patients became transfusion-independent and had improved survival compared to nonresponders.[148] Marrow cellularity did not predict recovery; trisomy 8 was highly associated with response to immunosuppression, but patients with other cytogenetic abnormalities also recovered. In a confirmatory British study,[142] 20 "low-risk" MDS patients were treated with antithymocyte globulin: half responded with transfusion-independence, with median duration of response of almost 16 months.

More limited immunosuppression aimed at abnormal TNF-α production in MDS has not been successful, including administration of anti-TNF monoclonal antibodies,[149–151] the soluble form of the TNF receptor,[152] and chemical inhibitors of TNF.[137,139,153]

Farnesyltransferase Inhibitors

Farnesyltransferase inhibitors[154–157] are a novel class of potent, oral inhibitors of Ras, although their activity may be related to their modulation of other signaling pathways implicated in the pathophysiology of CMML and MDS. In Phase I/II trials of tipifarnib in MDS (and acute leukemia), 23% of patients showed partial or complete response, but without a relationship of response to *ras* mutation status. Interim results of a multicenter Phase II trial[157] in RAEB MDS patients (and elderly leukemic patients) showed 44% hematologic responses with duration of about 5.5 months; treatment-related mortality was 7%. Toxicities include significant myelosuppression, fatigue, and mental confusion.

Cytotoxic Chemotherapy

Older patients with MDS do not tolerate intensive chemotherapy; remission rates are low, relapse is common, and morbidity and mortality are high. In younger patients, the remission rate for high-risk MDS patients is comparable to that achieved in AML[158]; although the duration of remission is only about 12 months, intensive treatment might allow an alternative donor to be located for an attempt at curative stem cell transplantation. Disappointingly, consolidation with intensive treatment by autologous stem cell transplantation does not prolong relapse-free survival.[158] Some long-term remissions are associated with restoration of polyclonal hematopoiesis.[159]

The well-known toxicities of intensive chemotherapy should be balanced against the potential benefit of only modest prolongation of life. Low-dose cytosine arabinoside, utilized as a "differentiating agent" but certainly cytotoxic, can produce responses in a substantial proportion of MDS patients (37% overall in a meta-analysis), but improvement is usually short-lived and toxicity, including fatal events, relatively frequent.[160] However, the drug has its advocates.[161]

Allogeneic Hematopoietic Stem Cell Transplantation

The curative potential of hematopoietic stem cell transplantation derives from the combined effect of the cytoreductive treatment used to prepare the patient for transplantation and the immunotherapeutic properties of transplanted allogeneic donor lymphocytes—the graft-versus-leukemia effect.[162–164] Success of transplantation for MDS is limited by the advanced age of the typical patient and the tendency for MDS to relapse, especially when the procedure is undertaken late in the disease course. Results of allogeneic transplantation for MDS from large single centers and from multicenter analyses are summarized in Table 15–4: overall, long-term disease-free survival has been achieved in 30–50% of patients, using marrow from HLA-identical sibling donors. There is a high rate of non–relapse-related mortality.[165–167] Transplantation outcome is largely determined by the age of the recipient and disease status. For

TABLE 15–4. Stem Cell Transplant for MDS*

Study	N	Median Age (yr)	Transplant-Related Mortality (%)	Relapse (%)	Survival (%)	Disease- or Event-Free Survival (%)
HLA-Matched Sibling Donors						
Seattle†[194] 1981–1990	93	30	40	29	41 (at 6yr)	40 (at 5yr)
Paris[167] 1982–1991	71	37	39	48	32 (at 6yr)	32 (at 7yr)
EBMT[170] 1983–1994	131	33	44	39	46 (at 2yr)	34 (at 5yr)
Vancouver[166] 1986–1996	60	40	50	42	33 (at 6yr)	29 (at 7yr)
EBMT[195] 1983–1998	885	37	43	36	45 (at 3yr)	36 (at 3yr)
IBMTR[171] 1989–1997	452	38	37	23	42 (at 4yr)	40 (at 3yr)
Seattle[176] 1993–2000	41	46	28	16	—	56 (at 3yr)
Alternative Donors						
Seattle[196] 1987–1993	30	29	48	28	—	38 (at 2yr)
EBMT[197] 1986–1996	96	24	58‡	35‡	28% (at 2yr)‡	29 (at 2yr)‡
EBMT[195] 1983–1998	198	—	58	41	26 (at 3yr)	25 (at 3yr)
Seattle[176] 1993–2000	64	46	30	11	—	59 (at 3yr)
NMDP[198] 1988–1998	510	38	54	14	30 (at 2yr)	29 (at 2yr)

*Single-center studies are identified by city. Whenever possible, survival reports actual number of patients alive; disease- or event-free survival is actuarial.
†Includes three syngeneic transplants.
‡Includes some secondary MDS patients.
Abbreviations: EBMT, European Group for Bone Marrow Transplantation; IBMTR, International Bone Marrow Transplantation Registry; NMDP, National Marrow Donor Program.

example, up to 80% disease-free survival is possible after stem cell transplantation from matched siblings in patients less than 40 years of age with RA, whereas less than 20% survival is more usual in older patients transplanted in more advanced phases of MDS.[168] The risk factors for relapse are largely dictated by the subtype and status of the MDS at time of transplantation. Transplants for RA or RARS patients carry the lowest risk of relapse, and transplanted patients with an excess of blasts or those who have transformed to AML have the worst outcomes. Particularly unfavorable for relapse are transplants performed for CMML and in patients with high-risk karyotypic abnormalities, including therapy-related MDS.[166,169–171] Outcomes in children are similarly dependent on the MDS subcategory: among 94 pediatric MDS cases transplanted in Seattle, overall disease-free survival at 3 years was 41%, but overall survival ranged from 74% for RA and RARS to 33% in more myeloproliferative MDS diagnoses.[172] Because of the slow progression of the less severe forms of MDS, delay of transplantation for patients in good prognostic categories appears to improve outcome in Markov models, whereas immediate transplantation for higher risk disease is a better strategy.[173]

As with transplantation for other hematologic malignancies, results continue to improve because of improved supportive care and possibly also the increased use of mobilized peripheral blood rather than bone marrow allografts. Use of peripheral blood confers faster hematopoietic engraftment and may exert a more potent graft-versus-leukemia effect, although accompanied by an increase in chronic graft-versus-host disease. In a recent study, recipients of peripheral blood grafts had a 2-year relapse-free survival of 50% compared with 39% for bone marrow transplants, as a result of both less transplant-related mortality and a lower relapse risk.[174]

A major challenge for hematopoietic stem cell transplantation in MDS has been the development of effective regimens suitable for the majority of the affected population over the age of 60 years. Such regimens, which usually combine fludarabine with busulfan, melphalan, low-dose total-body irradiation, or cyclophosphamide, minimize toxicity and harness a potential graft-versus-leukemia effect by sufficient immunosuppression of the recipient to allow full engraftment of donor immune cells. Although reduced-intensity transplantation strategies have curative potential, they carry a higher risk of relapse, suggesting that conditioning regimen dose intensity may be important in disease control. Some myeloablative regimens have achieved better results in older MDS patients: combinations of fludarabine and melphalan (140–180 mg/m^2) or fludarabine and intravenous busulfan (6.5 mg/m^2) have produced relapse-free survivals of 60%.[175] Improved results in MDS are likely to come from these newer, less toxic but still myeloablative conditioning regimens.

Most patients with hematologic diseases will lack a suitable HLA-matched sibling donor. Unrelated-donor marrow transplantation can succeed in MDS, but such high-risk transplants are undertaken with some trepidation because of the enormous risks of transplant-related mortality, which is fatal in most older patients (see Table 15–4). Nevertheless, recent results with carefully selected patients and targeting of the busulfan dose have produced much improved results, with the majority of patients surviving disease-free, an outcome apparently independent of patient age.[176]

SUPPORTIVE CARE AND LONG-TERM MANAGEMENT

Supportive care is of great importance in the management of MDS. Most patients are not eligible for transplantation, and many will not be benefited by current drug therapies; furthermore, the frequently indolent course of MDS is compatible with a good quality of life for months to years in many cases. Because most MDS patients are older, attention is required to other coexisting illnesses of aging, such as cardiac insufficiency, cerebrovascular disease, and diabetes. These nonhematologic conditions can limit intensive treatment and shape the nature and relevance of the MDS management.

The elements of supportive care are (1) transfusion of red cells and platelets to control anemia and thrombocytopenia, with appropriate iron chelation; (2) prevention and treatment of bacterial and fungal infections; (3) use of growth factors and vitamins to improve marrow function; and (4) outpatient control of MDS transformed into leukemia.

Transfusions

Red Cells

The same precautions and procedures apply to MDS patients as for any individual requiring long-term transfusion support: provision of suitably matched blood, use of leukocyte-depleted products in order to minimize alloimmunization, monitoring for red cell antibody formation, and minor red cell antigen matching when necessary. Patients with MDS frequently are undertransfused; the objective should be to avoid symptoms, not to adapt to them, and generally two units of packed erythrocytes infused every 2 weeks can compensate for complete failure of red blood cell production. Elderly patients, especially those with cardiac and pulmonary compromise, may require transfusion at higher nadir hemoglobin values; 9 gm/dL is a reasonable threshold value. Iron chelation with desferrioxamine is indicated in patients when their prognosis is measured in years, usually beginning about the time of the 50th erythrocyte transfusion.[177]

Platelets

For MDS patients, who may be thrombocytopenic for months to years, platelet transfusions may be administered at the onset of fresh petechiae or in response to other spontaneous, bothersome bleeding. Prophylactic use of platelets—transfusion at a threshold of 10,000/μL—may be reserved for patients who consistently develop hemorrhagic symptoms at low levels; there are no data to show that a policy of frequent preemptive platelet transfusions improves survival, and it is both inconvenient and expensive. Conversely, platelet transfusions may be indicated at higher values, as, for example, with rapid platelet consumption during bacterial infection and when the dysplastic platelets are also dysfunctional, allowing bleeding at platelet counts higher than 10,000/μL.[53] Amicar (ε-aminocaproic acid), to a dose of 1 gm twice daily, occasionally helps reduce mucosal bleeding in thrombocytopenic MDS. Leukocyte-depleted blood products and single-donor platelet transfusions decrease the risk of alloimmunization, but a minority of patients eventually require HLA-matched platelets in order to achieve adequate increments.

Infection

MDS patients are at increased risk from bacterial and fungal infection not only because of chronic neutropenia but due to defective function of their dysplastic (usually hypogranular) neutrophils; in addition, implanted venous access devices now in routine use to facilitate transfusions offer a dangerous portal of entry to microorganisms. Frank and also suspected infection—symptoms of fever, malaise, and change in mental status—require the prompt use of parenteral antibiotics (see Chapter 10). Initial treatment with a single agent such as intravenous ceftazidime is appropriate, with vancomycin added when a staphylococcal infection is suspected (as in the presence of an intravenous catheter). The availability of oral antibiotics such as the quinolones and of effective antifungal agents such as voriconazole has improved the outpatient management of chronically neutropenic MDS patients.

Hematopoietic Growth Factors

Erythropoietin and G-CSF are often employed in MDS patients[120,178–182] (see also Chapter 91). Only a minority (<20%) of MDS patients show a meaningful erythropoietic response to erythropoietin alone, and improvement is less likely in patients who are transfusion-dependent compared to the mildly anemic. Erythropoietin plus G-CSF appeared more effective than either given alone in a randomized trial[183]; the combination produces red cell responses in about 40% of MDS patients and neutrophil improvement in almost all, but hemoglobin levels are more likely to increase in untransfused patients.[178,184,185] Trilineage improvement can occur,[186] and responses have been correlated with increased proportions of cytogenetically normal hematopoietic progenitors.[187] Growth factor treatment is generally well tolerated, and now more conveniently administered as pegylated long-acting formulations[188]; serious toxicities such as splenic rupture have been rarely reported.[189] An algorithm based on hormone levels less than 100 μ/mL and fewer than 2 units of erythrocytes transfused per month predicts benefit from a regimen of combined growth factors.[182,190] MDS patients' white cell counts can respond to G-CSF,[191] but its use is not indicated solely to increase a low neutrophil count, and in a randomized study, G-CSF treatment did not result in a survival advantage.[192] Recombinant megakaryocyte growth factor raised platelet (and hemoglobin) levels in MDS patients in a Japanese pilot study,[193] but the development of antibodies and immune thrombocytopenia in some recipients have halted clinical studies elsewhere.

Control of Transforming MDS

Aggressive chemotherapy rarely induces sustained hematologic remissions in advanced MDS and more usually

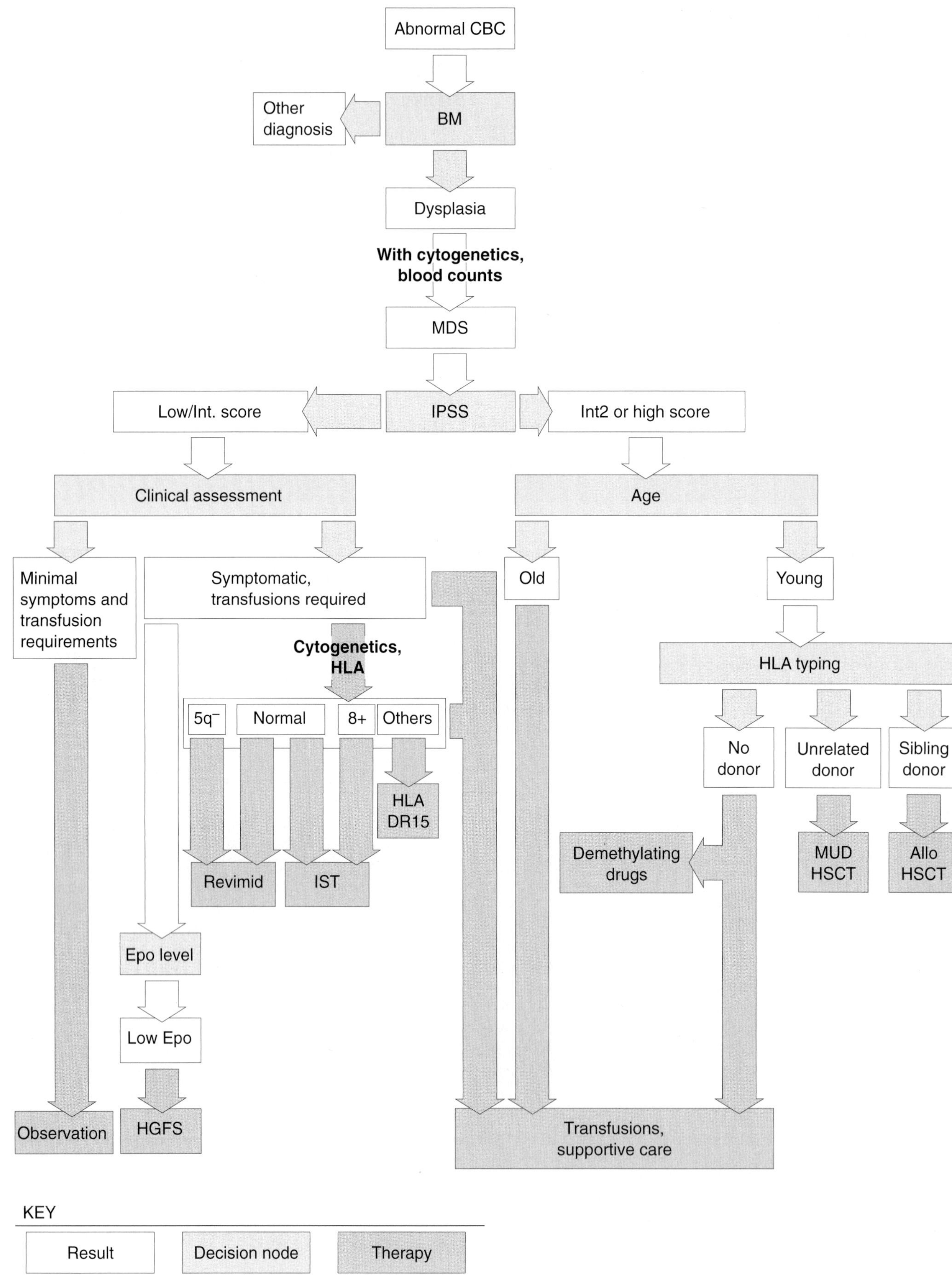
Abnormal CBC
Other diagnosis
BM
Dysplasia
With cytogenetics, blood counts
MDS
Low/Int. score
IPSS
Int2 or high score
Clinical assessment
Age
Minimal symptoms and transfusion requirements
Symptomatic, transfusions required
Old
Young
Cytogenetics, HLA
HLA typing
5q⁻
Normal
8+
Others
No donor
Unrelated donor
Sibling donor
HLA DR15
Demethylating drugs
MUD HSCT
Allo HSCT
Revimid
IST
Epo level
Low Epo
Observation
HGFS
Transfusions, supportive care
KEY
Result
Decision node
Therapy

Figure 15–6. Treatment algorithm for MDS. The pathways are complex and still cannot incorporate all possible diagnostic and treatment permutations; major directions in arriving at an appropriate choice of therapies are emphasized. Only stem cell transplantation is curative, but treatment-related morbidity and mortality are considerable. Immunosuppressive therapy provides a survival benefit in responding patients, and likely responders can be predicted based on age, IPSS, HLA type, and length of transfusion requirement. Lenolidomide (Revimid) is likely to be approved for use in MDS; it can dramatically improve anemia in some patients. The demethylating agents azacitidine (approved for use in MDS) and its active metabolite decitabine can increase blood counts, especially in high-risk patients, but these drugs are also myelosuppressive. Neither lenolidomide, azacitidine, nor decitabine has yet been shown to prolong survival in responding patients. Abbreviations: Epo, erythropoietin; HGF, hematopoietic growth factor; HSCT, hematopoietic stem cell transplant; IPSS, International Prognostic Scoring System; IST, immunosuppressive treatment; MUD, matched unrelated transplant.

compounds the cytopenias, often fatally in the elderly patient. Therefore, standard acute leukemia induction chemotherapy usually is reserved for younger patients. Alternatively, judicious use of hydroxyurea (0.5–1.5 gm/day) or oral etoposide (VP16; 100 mg × 3 days repeated every 7–10 days) can sometimes suppress blast cell proliferation and maintain residual marrow function. Advantages of such low-intensity cytotoxic chemotherapy are the ease of outpatient administration and the minimal associated toxicities. Some MDS patients develop chloromas, which usually respond to low-dose (100–600 rads) local irradiation.

PROGNOSIS AND TREATMENT DECISIONS

The care of MDS patients is complex, for many reasons: the advanced age of the patient, who often has comorbid diseases and may particularly suffer the consequences of low blood counts; a complex classification; an extremely variable prognosis overall; and the availability of multiple medical treatment options, which range from careful observation to high-risk transplant strategies (Fig. 15–6). Cure when feasible should be the intent, but harm also must be avoided. Transplantation should be discussed as a treatment option with younger MDS patients, those less than 60 years old as of this writing. Hematopoietic stem cell transplantation is the best option in most pediatric MDS cases. Marrow blast number and the chromosome pattern remain the best guide to prognosis; patients with high blast percentage and poor cytogenetics most need transplantation but also the worst outcome. The decision for transplantation depends also upon the availability of an HLA-identical related donor or a well-matched unrelated donor. The choice is ultimately the patient's, after an unbiased presentation of the probable outcomes for stem cell transplantation versus alternative treatments.

Other medical therapies can ameliorate MDS and improve the patient's hematologic and general clinical status. Many do not require hospitalization or have modest toxicities, making them suitable even for older persons. The choice among approved and experimental therapies to some extent can now be guided by convincing clinical studies (see Fig. 15–6); as the pathophysiology of MDS is better understood, therapies and their application to specific patients will also improve.

CURRENT CONTROVERSIES & FUTURE CONSIDERATIONS

Myelodysplastic Syndrome

- The value of the WHO classification will need further confirmation in retrospective analyses of large patient databases.
- Specific genetic and cytogenetic abnormalities may provide better clues to MDS pathophysiology and also clinical course and appropriate treatment. MDS provides an opportunity to clarify the earliest events in leukemic transformation.
- Promising therapeutic approaches include new thalidomide derivatives and immunosuppressive drugs that do not require hospitalization.
- Transplantation is increasingly utilized in older patients and using alternative donors; short-term success must be followed by reports of long-term survival and quality of life.

Suggested Readings*

Bennett JM, Greenberg PL: The Myelodysplastic Syndromes: Pathobiology and Clinical Management. New York: Marcel Dekker, 2005.

Deeg HJ, Appelbaum FR: Hematopoietic stem cell transplantation in patients with myelodysplastic syndrome. Leuk Res 24:653–663, 2000.

Estey EH: Current challenges in therapy of myelodysplastic syndromes. Curr Opin Hematol 10:60–67, 2003.

Hofmann W-K, Koeffler HP: Myelodysplastic syndrome. Annu Rev Med 56:1–16, 2005.

List A, Kurtin S, Roe DJ, et al: Efficacy of lenalidomide in myelodysplastic syndromes. N Engl J Med 352:549–557, 2005.

Molldrem J, Rivera M, Bahceci E, et al: Treatment of bone marrow failure of myelodysplastic syndrome with antithymocyte globulin. Ann Intern Med 137:156–163, 2002.

Silverman LR, Demakos EP, Peterson BL, et al: Randomized controlled trial of azacitidine in patients with the myelodysplastic syndrome: A study of the cancer and leukemia group B. Br J Clin Oncol 20:2429–2440, 2002.

**Full references for this chapter can be found on accompanying CD-ROM.*

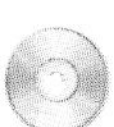

CHAPTER 16

LARGE GRANULAR LYMPHOCYTE LEUKEMIA

Eric J. Burks, MD, and Thomas P. Loughran, Jr., MD

KEY POINTS

Large Granular Lymphocyte Leukemia

- T-cell large granular lymphocyte (T-LGL) leukemia is a clonal disorder of cytotoxic T cells resulting in bone marrow failure, manifesting most commonly as severe neutropenia.
- T-LGL expansions are currently hypothesized to be an antigen-driven T-cell response in the setting of disordered programmed cell death.
- T-LGL leukemia is often associated with a second process such as autoimmune disease (especially rheumatoid arthritis), hematologic malignancies, and solid tumors.
- The diagnosis of T-LGL leukemia usually requires a multiparametric approach, including peripheral blood examination, flow cytometric immunophenotyping, bone marrow aspirate and core biopsy with immunohistochemistry, and molecular analysis for TCR gene rearrangements.
- Absolute lymphocytosis or elevations in peripheral blood large granular lymphocytes are not required to diagnose T-LGL leukemia.
- The characteristic immunophenotype is $CD3^+$, $CD8^+$, $CD16^+$, and $CD57^+$, but variants may be difficult to distinguish from a reactive lymphocytosis.
- TCR-γ gene analysis by polymerase chain reaction is the most sensitive technique for detecting T-cell clonality; TCR-β gene analysis by Southern blot remains the standard for excluding a T-cell clone.
- Although clonality is a requisite for diagnosing T-LGL leukemia, patients with benign diseases and those with non–T-cell malignancies may exhibit clonal rearrangement of their TCR in the peripheral blood, making correlation with other diagnostic features of T-LGL essential.
- The diagnostic value of bone marrow biopsy is greatly enhanced with immunohistochemical staining for T-cell– and NK cell–associated antigens.
- T-LGL leukemia must be distinguished from other mature NK/T-cell neoplasms, especially hepatosplenic T-cell lymphoma and aggressive NK cell leukemia.
- T-LGL leukemia is an indolent disorder that responds well to immunosuppressive therapies such as methotrexate and cyclosporine.

INTRODUCTION

Definition

T-cell large granular lymphocyte (T-LGL) leukemia is an antigen-driven, clonal expansion of cytotoxic T cells; its principle manifestation is bone marrow failure.[1,2] The leukemic cells are characteristically large with azurophilic granules and are immunophenotyped as $CD3^+$, $CD8^+$, $CD16^+$, and $CD57^+$. Tissue infiltration occurs primarily within the bone marrow, spleen, and liver, accounting for the clinical features of cytopenias and organomegaly.[3] Bone marrow failure typically manifests as severe chronic neutropenia with or without anemia.[4] T-LGL is frequently associated with other chronic medical conditions that involve a cytotoxic T-cell immunologic response, such as autoimmune diseases and various malignancies.[5]

Classification

Large granular lymphocyte (LGL) leukemia was defined in 1985 based on the identification of nonrecurring cytogenetic abnormalities and the demonstration of LGL infiltration of the marrow, spleen, and liver.[6] In 1993, two phenotypically and clinically distinct subtypes of LGL leukemia were recognized.[1] The most common type was designated T-LGL leukemia because it was $CD3^+$ and associated with an indolent course complicated by neutropenic infections. The less frequent form was designated natural killer cell LGL (NK-LGL) leukemia because it was $CD3^-$ and generally characterized by an aggressive clinical course. This nomenclature was subsequently adopted by the REAL classification (1994) of hematopoietic neoplasms.[7] The current (2001) World Health Organization ordering of hematopoietic neoplasms includes T-LGL leukemia as a subtype of mature T-cell neoplasms, whereas NK-LGL leukemia is now classified as aggressive natural killer (NK) cell leukemia, believed to represent the leukemic counterpart to extranodal NK/T-cell lymphomas of the nasopharynx.[8] Alternatively, chronic NK-lymphoproliferative disorder (NK-LPD) has an indolent course with less pronounced cytopenias than in T-LGL; NK-LPD is not associated with rheumatoid arthritis (RA).[9,10] Clonality is occasionally demonstrated by X-chromosome inactivation in female patients, but many cases are polyclonal. Although it shares many clinical and pathophysiologic similarities with T-LGL, it is unclear whether NK-LPD is reactive or malignant.[11–13] The designation NK-LGL leukemia is to be avoided to prevent clinical confusion with aggressive NK cell leukemia.

EPIDEMIOLOGY AND RISK FACTORS

Incidence

The incidence of T-LGL is unknown. Based on the original series description in 1977, T-LGL represented 4% of chronic lymphoproliferative disorders.[14] More recently, a community hospital-based study to establish the relative frequencies of lymphoid neoplasms under the REAL classification found T-LGL to be the most common T-cell malignancy.[15] For comparison, T-LGL was about three times as frequent as mycosis fungoides/Sézary syndrome, twice as common as anaplastic large-cell lymphoma, hairy cell leukemia, or lymphoplasmacytic lymphoma.

Age and Geographic Distribution

T-LGL presents at a median age of 60 years (range, 4–88 years). Less than 10% of cases occur before the age of 40 years, and pediatric cases are rare.[16] There is no sex predominance. All races may be affected, but the disease appears to be increased among Asians, with relative frequencies of 9–15% of chronic lymphoproliferative disorders among Chinese[17,18] and common occurrence among Japanese.[19] Bone marrow failure manifesting as T-LGL varies geographically as well: severe chronic neutropenia associated with RA represents the dominant manifestation in the West, whereas pure red cell aplasia (PRCA) without RA is more common in China and Japan.[18–20]

Risk Factors

There are no known risk factors for T-LGL. Genetic predisposition may be inferred from the different frequencies between Western and Asian populations, which are suspected also for NK/T-cell malignancies that are more common among Asians.[21] The frequency of the human leucocyte antigen (HLA)-DR4 allele is increased for T-LGL with RA (90%), but this increased allele frequency is not maintained in T-LGL without RA, suggesting association to RA rather than to T-LGL.[22–25] Infectious exposures may be a risk factor for T-LGL, because sera in many patients show reactivity to the Gag p24 and Env p21e proteins of human T-lymphotropic virus type 1 (HTLV-1). These data suggest infection with a retrovirus with homology to HTLV-1, but most patients do not have a prototypical HTLV infection (see below).[26]

PATHOPHYSIOLOGY

Antigen-Driven Clonal Expansions

Much evidence suggests that T-LGL cells are cytotoxic T lymphocytes that have undergone antigen activation in vivo. First, the cells display an immunophenotype consistent with antigen activation, which is $CD3^+$, $CD8^+$, $CD57^+$, $CD45R0^+$, and HLA-$DR27^+$,[27] and they constitutively express perforin, usually only observed after activation.[28,29] Second, functional evidence of non–major histocompatibility complex (MHC)-restricted cytotoxicity after anti-CD3 monoclonal antibody exposure supports in vivo activation.[27] Molecular evidence of common V_α usage suggests antigenic pressure in the clonal expansions.[30] Finally, DNA microarray analysis shows upregulation of cytotoxic proteases and downregulation of protease inhibitors, a transcriptome consistent with an activated phenotype.[31]

Chronic Antigenic Stimulation

Many patients with T-LGL have secondary diseases that result in chronic antigenic stimulation, such as RA and malignancies, and this may explain the in vivo activation of cytotoxic T cells. Alternatively, serologic data suggest possible infection with a retrovirus with homology to HTLV.[26]

T-Cell Homeostasis

A relatively constant number of T cells is maintained throughout life, with increases occurring during infectious stimuli but resolving after viral clearance.[32] Two mechanisms may explain an elevated T-cell number: increased cell proliferation or decreased cell death. In the case of T-LGL, the leukemic cells are in the G_0/G_1 phase of the cell cycle, therefore excluding proliferation as the mechanism of expansion.[33] Alternatively, T-LGL cells constitutively express high levels of Fas receptor and Fas ligand (FasL) but are resistant to Fas-mediated apoptosis.[34] These findings suggest a defect within the Fas-mediated apoptotic pathway to explain T-cell expansions in T-LGL leukemia (Fig. 16–1).[35]

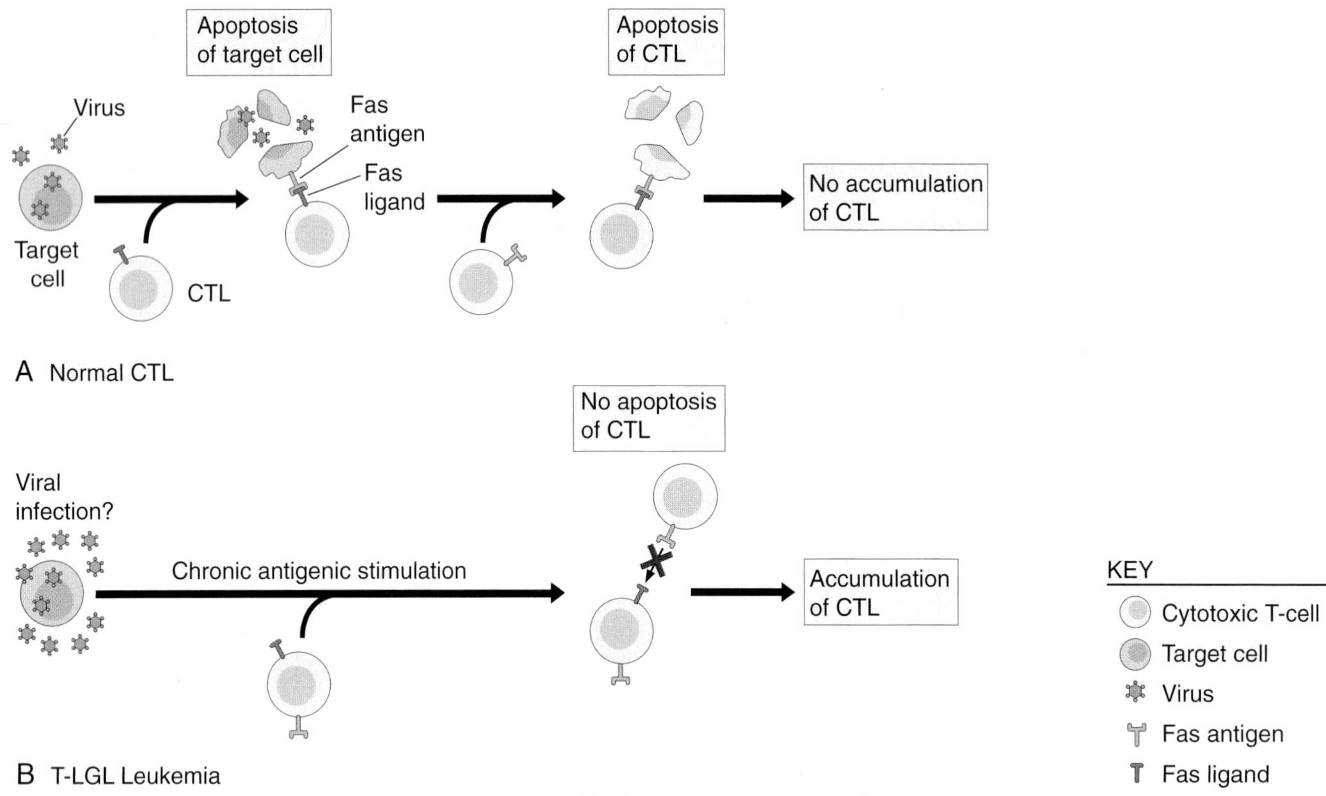

Figure 16–1. Mechanism of LGL expansion. *A,* In normal T cells, target cell destruction is mediated by Fas/Fas ligand on the target cell and T cell, respectively. After the infectious stimulus is cleared, T-cell apoptosis occurs through a similar mechanism. *B,* In T-LGL, chronic antigenic stimulation, possibly caused by a viral infection with homology to HTLV, results in expansion of cytotoxic T cells; however, defects within the Fas-mediated apoptotic pathway prevent cell clearance. (From Greer JP, Kinney MC, Loughran TP Jr: T cell and NK cell lymphoproliferative disorders. Hematology [Am Soc Hematol Educ Program] 259–281, 2001, with permission.)

Dysregulated Apoptosis

Both extrinsic and intrinsic pathways mediate apoptotic cell death.[36,37] Fas (CD95) is a surface receptor of the tumor necrosis factor family, which may initiate the extrinsic pathway of apoptosis.[38] Stimulation of Fas results in the formation of Fas receptor microaggregates followed by recruitment of intracellular proteins required to assimilate the death-inducing signaling complex (DISC).[39] The intracellular portion of Fas contains a death domain that interacts with FADD (MORT-1)[40,41] and FLICE, the inactive zymogen form of caspase 8.[42–44] Caspase 8 activation then results in the release of active subunits p20 and p10.[45] The intrinsic pathway of apoptosis serves to amplify the extrinsic signals in some cell types.[46] Cleavage and activation of Bid, a proapoptotic BH3 domain–only protein, is the link between the intrinsic and extrinsic pathways.[47]

There are several known defects in the Fas signaling pathway in T-LGL. Unlike in autoimmune lymphoproliferative syndrome (see Chapter 58), mutations within the death domain of Fas have not been identified in T-LGL.[48,49] Soluble Fas decoy receptors represent one mechanism by which LGLs escape apoptosis. Soluble Fas results after proteolytic cleavage of the Fas membrane receptors or alternative splicing of messenger RNA, with resultant truncated Fas receptors that efficiently bind FasL. Studies of messenger RNA in patients with T-LGL revealed three novel splice variants encoding soluble Fas molecules.[50] Elevated soluble Fas levels occur in autoimmune disorders associated with chronically activated T cells[51] as well as in patients with T-LGL and NK-LGL.[52] Elevated levels of soluble Fas may provide a mechanism for circumventing immunosurveillance in T-LGL, and other autoimmune diseases.[53] Another mechanism of defective apoptosis in T-LGL involves the JAK/STAT pathway. Signal transducers and activators of transcription (STAT) regulate antiapoptotic survival in some tumors.[54–57] Recently, STAT3 regulation of Mcl-1 has been shown to be important in T-LGL survival[48,49]; apoptosis was induced in T-LGL cells with inhibitors of both STAT activation (AG490) and Mcl-1 expression (antisense complementary DNA to Mcl-1).

Mechanism of Cytopenias

Chronic neutropenia in patients with T-LGL is also mediated by FasL. The leukemic cells of T-LGL constitutively express FasL gene transcripts.[58] Because membrane-bound FasL can be solubilized by a matrix metalloproteinase–like enzyme, high levels of circulating FasL are detected in most patients with T-LGL.[59] The sera of these patients triggers apoptosis of normal neutrophils in vitro. Resolution of neutropenia concurrent with methotrexate administration was temporally related to diminution of soluble FasL levels.[59] Pro-inflammatory cytokines such as FasL and interferon-γ also may inhibit myeloid progenitors in patients with idiopathic chronic neutropenia.[60] FasL thus may have multiple inhibitory effects on neutrophil development, leading to chronic neutropenia. In contrast, the pathogenesis underlying adult-onset cyclic neutropenia associated with T-LGL remains elusive. PRCA in T-LGL involves direct killing of erythroid progenitors by the leukemic LGL.[61] Two mechanisms have been proposed, involving MHC-restricted or non–MHC-restricted pathways.[62,63] In both cases, erythroid precursors are preferentially killed compared to myeloid precursors, because maturing erythroid cells downregulate HLA class I molecules and killer-cell immunoglobulin-like receptor (KIR) molecules on the LGLs bind HLA class I molecules of target cells (normally resulting in inactivation). With diminished HLA class I expression on erythroid precursors, cell lysis occurs.[64]

CLINICAL FEATURES AND DIAGNOSIS

Signs and Symptoms

Patients with T-LGL often (20–40% of cases) present with recurrent infections and fever.[1,28,65–68] Because the infections are related to neutropenia, typical sites include the skin, oropharynx, and perirectal region; pneumonia and sepsis are less frequent. Opportunistic infections are uncommon. B symptoms, including fever, night sweats, and weight loss, occur in 20–30% of patients. Fatigue, related to anemia, may be the first symptom of PRCA. Lung involvement,[69] mainly pulmonary hypertension, and neuropathy[65] have been reported but are rare. About one third of patients are asymptomatic at presentation. On physical examination, organomegaly is the most consistent finding,[4] and mild to moderate splenomegaly is present in 20–50% of patients. Hepatomegaly is less frequent (found in 10–20% of cases) and is mild to moderate in degree. Lymphadenopathy is not a prominent feature of T-LGL. Skin involvement or other sites of extramedullary/extranodal disease are rare.

Secondary Disease

T-LGL leukemia is frequently associated with an autoimmune disease (Table 16–1). The nature of this association most likely relates to chronic antigenic stimulation of cytotoxic T cells, ultimately resulting in clonal expansion (see "Pathophysiology" earlier). RA is observed in 25% of cases of T-LGL leukemia.[70] Felty's syndrome is a closely related disorder characterized by RA, neutropenia, and variable splenomegaly. The distinction between Felty's syndrome and T-LGL with RA is based on the presence of T-cell clonality, and these disorders likely represent a disease continuum rather than distinct entities. Supportive is the fact that the frequency of the HLA-DR4 allele within Felty's syndrome is 86%, compared with a frequency of 90% for T-LGL with RA and 33% in patients with T-LGL without RA.[22–25] Further understanding of

TABLE 16–1. Diseases Associated with T-LGL Leukemia

Autoimmune Disease
Systemic
Rheumatoid arthritis
Systemic sclerosis
Systemic lupus erythematosus
Endocrinopathy
Sjögren's syndrome
Ulcerative colitis
Autoimmune hepatitis
Hematologic
Hemophagocytic syndrome
Immune-mediated thrombocytopenic purpura
Autoimmune hemolytic anemia
Transplant
Bone Marrow Transplant
Allogeneic donor
Solid Organ Transplant
Liver
Kidney
Malignancies
B-Cell Malignancies
Chronic lymphocytic leukemia
Multiple myeloma
Hairy cell leukemia
Splenic lymphoma with villous lymphocytes
Non-Hodgkin's lymphoma
Myeloid Malignancies
Acquired aplastic anemia
Paroxysmal nocturnal hemoglobinuria
Myelodysplastic syndrome
Acute myeloid leukemia
Solid Tumors

how chronic antigenic stimulation in autoimmune disease relates to clonal lymphocyte expansion is illustrated in systemic sclerosis. Although systemic sclerosis with T-LGL has only occasionally been reported,[71] monoclonal rearrangements of the T-cell receptor (TCR)-γ gene may be detected by polymerase chain reaction (PCR) in the peripheral blood of almost half of systemic sclerosis patients not diagnosed with T-LGL.[72]

The association of T-LGL leukemia with other bone marrow failure syndromes, including acquired aplastic anemia, paroxysmal nocturnal hemoglobinuria (PNH), myelodysplastic syndrome (MDS), and acquired PRCA, is more than coincidental (Fig. 16–2). The key feature uniting these disorders is the combination of cytopenias with antigen-driven T-cell expansions. T-cell "microclones" have been demonstrated by sensitive PCR methods in patients with cyclosporine-dependent aplastic anemia,[73] patients with PNH,[74] and MDS patients responsive to ATG.[75] Immunosuppression in subsets of these disorders has induced loss of T-cell microclones[75] as well as diminished T-cell–mediated myelosuppression concurrent with response to therapy.[76] Concurrent T-LGL leukemia has been reported in 9 patients with aplastic

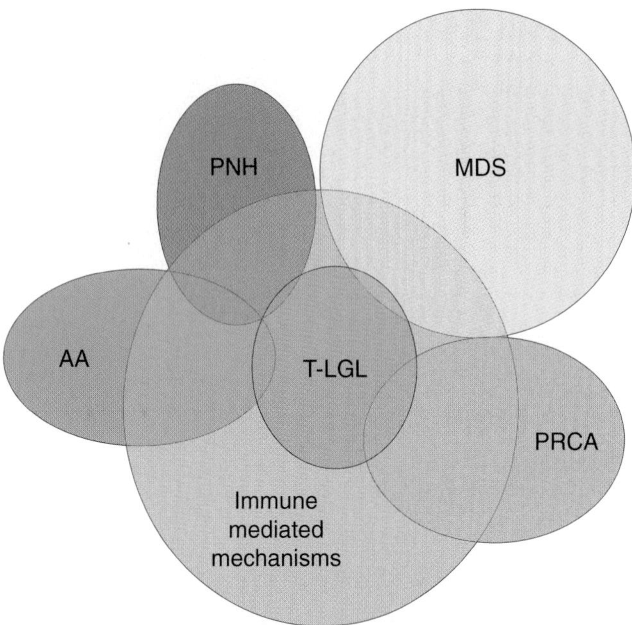

■ **Figure 16–2.** Venn diagram of the relationship of T-LGL with other bone marrow failure syndromes. Immune-mediated mechanisms are important in a percentage of each disorder, and, in some cases, clonal T-cell aberrations overlap with T-LGL. Abbreviations: AA, aplastic anemia; MDS, myelodysplastic syndrome; PNH, paroxysmal nocturnal hemoglobinuria; PRCA, pure red cell aplasia.

anemia,[77] 1 patient with PNH,[78] 14 patients with MDS,[65,79] and 19% of patients with PRCA.[80,81]

Similar associations have been observed for T-LGL and malignancies (see Table 16–1). B-cell neoplastic disorders and clonal T-cell aberrations are not uncommon.[82,83] About one third of patients with multiple myeloma had monoclonal TCR-β rearrangements by Southern blot of the peripheral blood,[84] and expanded T-cell populations in myeloma share an immunophenotype similar to T-LGL leukemia ($CD3^+CD8^+CD57^+$).[85] Likewise, monoclonal and oligoclonal TCR-γ rearrangements by PCR are detected in the peripheral blood of patients with chronic lymphocytic leukemia (CLL) in 20% and 50% of cases, respectively.[86] As expected, there are examples of T-LGL concurrent with multiple myeloma[87] and CLL.[88]

Transplantation represents another pathologic state in which chronic antigenic stimulation may result in T-cell clonal expansions. In T-LGL leukemia after allogeneic bone marrow transplantation,[89–91] the expanded T-cell populations are $CD3^+CD8^+CD57^+$ and share functional properties with those of T-LGL leukemia.[92] T-LGL leukemia has been seen after solid organ transplantation, including kidney[93,94] and liver[95] transplantation.

Diagnosis

Serologies

A variety of serologic abnormalities occur in T-LGL.[1,65,69] Increased titers of antinuclear antibodies (40%) and rheumatoid factor (60%) are common. Hypergammaglobulinemia is seen in about half of patients, but monoclonal hypergammaglobulinemia is unusual. Circulating immune complexes occur in about two thirds of cases. Antineutrophil antibodies present in approximately half of patients are of uncertain significance in the mechanism of neutropenia given the frequency of circulating immune complexes. A direct Coombs test is positive in 12% of patients, but concurrent hemolytic anemia is rare.[96,97] Antiplatelet antibodies are variably seen (25–60%). Elevated β_2-microglobulin is present in 72% of patients.[96,98] Soluble FasL can be measured in most cases.[59,99]

Blood

T-LGL presents with lymphocytosis, neutropenia, and/or anemia, lymphocytosis (absolute lymphocyte count >5.0 × 10^9/L) is present in half of patients. LGLs are usually large (15–18 μm) with round to oval nuclei composed of condensed chromatin and abundant pale blue cytoplasm containing azurophilic granules (Fig. 16–3*A*). Normal peripheral blood LGL counts range from 100 to 300 cells/μL by morphology and from 120 to 320 cells/μL by flow cytometry, gating on $CD3^+$ and $CD57^+$ lymphocytes. The original diagnostic criteria required an absolute LGL count in excess of 2000 cells/μL persisting for greater than 6 months.[68,100] The introduction of molecular analysis and multicolor flow cytometry now allows diagnosis with low numbers of circulating LGLs.[2] Historical studies reported absolute LGL counts of greater than 4000 cells/μL in most patients, and only 8% having LGL counts less than 1000 cells/μL. In contrast, more recent studies reported absolute LGL counts of less than 500 cells/μL in 25–30% of cases.[101,102] Sustained neutropenia (absolute neutrophil count <1500 cells/μL) is present in 80% and is severe (absolute neutrophil count <500 cells/μL) in 45% of patients. Most adult-onset cyclic neutropenia is associated with T-LGL.[103,104] Mild to moderate anemia (hemoglobin <11 gm/dL) is seen in about half of LGL patients, and 20% are transfusion dependent.[1,65,66] Mild thrombocytopenia (platelet count <150 × 10^9/L) occurs in about 20%, and platelet counts of less than 50 × 10^9/L are uncommon (5%).[1,2,65] Rarely, immune-mediated thrombocytopenic purpura is concurrent with T-LGL.[65]

Bone Marrow

Bone marrow biopsy and aspirate aid in the diagnosis of T-LGL leukemia (Fig. 16–3*B–D*).[3,101,102] Hypercellularity is the most consistent finding, occurring in 56–78% of patients. Left-shifted myeloid maturation is observed in 20–45% of patients and may be associated with a relative erythroid hyperplasia in 22–33%. In PRCA, complete absence of erythroid precursors or arrest at the pronormoblast stage should be observed; a large granular lymphocytosis is seen in about one third of patients. Because LGLs are difficult to recognize on aspirate preparations, a more consistent observation is simple marrow lymphocytosis. Lymphocytosis may be difficult to discern on biopsy sections, where it is typically diffuse and

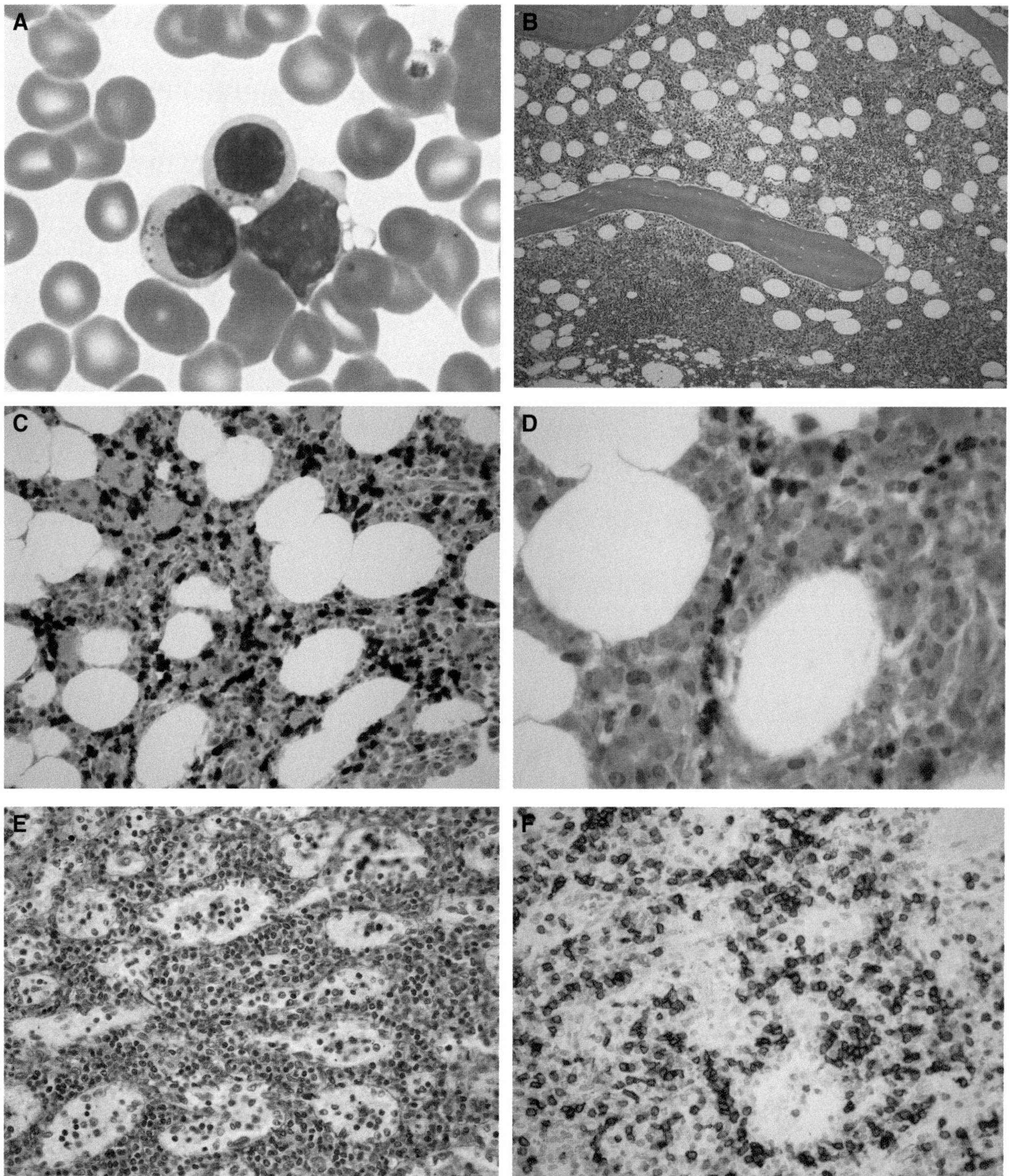

Figure 16–3. Peripheral blood, bone marrow, and splenic findings in T-LGL. *A,* Large granular lymphocytes are demonstrated near a reactive lymphocyte. *B,* A low-power view of the bone marrow biopsy reveals mild hypercellularity and lymphoid aggregates. *C,* Immunoperoxidase stain with CD8 reveals increased interstitial T cells, forming clusters of more than eight cells focally. *D,* Immunoperoxidase stain with TIA-1 reveals intrasinusoidal arrays of leukemic T-LGL. *E,* Periodic acid–Schiff stain showing spleen with distended red pulp cords containing mature lymphocytes. *F,* Immunoperoxidase stain with CD3 revealing the majority of infiltrating lymphocytes to be T cells.

interstitial, but reactive lymphoid aggregates are detectable in 14–44% of cases. Immunohistochemistry using T-cell antibodies has shown increased T cells in biopsy sections as compared to normal, reactive, and pathologic marrows,[102] staining for CD8, TIA-1, and granzyme B in interstitial clusters and intrasinusoidal linear arrays. Granzyme B appears to have the greatest diagnostic specificity, with clusters of eight cells or more occurring in 50% of cases of T-LGL but not in reactive conditions.[101]

Spleen

Splenectomy is rarely performed in current practice for T-LGL leukemia, but may be undertaken in cases posing diagnostic difficulty or for indications of traumatic rupture, immune-mediated thrombocytopenic purpura, or autoimmune hemolytic anemia. In T-LGL, spleen size varies from 450 to 1650 gm, with a mean weight of 600 gm.[3] Red pulp expansion is the usual gross pathologic finding. Histologic examination reveals an increase in LGLs within sinuses and cords, frequently accompanied by plasmacytosis (Fig. 16–3*E, F*). White pulp hyperplasia also is common. Hemosiderin deposition may be observed.

Flow Cytometry

The typical immunophenotype of T-LGL is $CD3^+$, $CD8^+$, $CD16^+$, and $CD57^+$, but variations are common, as are reactive lymphoid populations that may obscure the clonal proliferation. Almost all patients demonstrate an inverted CD4:CD8 ratio in favor of cytotoxic cells (Fig. 16–4*A*).[102] Although the vast majority of T-LGL is $CD3^+$ and $CD8^+$, rare cases may be $CD4^+$. CD16 is highly variable depending on the monoclonal antibody used (many studies of $CD16^-$ cases employed clone Leu 11, whereas clones VD2 or 8.23 are frequently positive for its detection; recently, CD16 was reported positive in 81% of cases using clone Leu 11c).[105] CD57 has been reported in almost all cases, but most exhibit only partial CD57 expression, which may be identical to the pattern seen in normal T cells (Fig. 16–4*C*).[105] Expression of NK-associated antigens CD56, CD94, and CD161 occurs in 19%, 42%, and 56% of cases, respectively.

Aberrant expression of T-cell–associated antigens (CD2, CD3, CD5, CD7) is seen in nearly all cases of T-LGL leukemia (Fig. 16–4*B*).[105] CD5 and CD7 are most consistently abnormal, in 90% and 81% of cases, respectively. Although decreased intensity of staining is most common, in about one third there is either complete or partial loss of these antigens. CD2 is abnormally

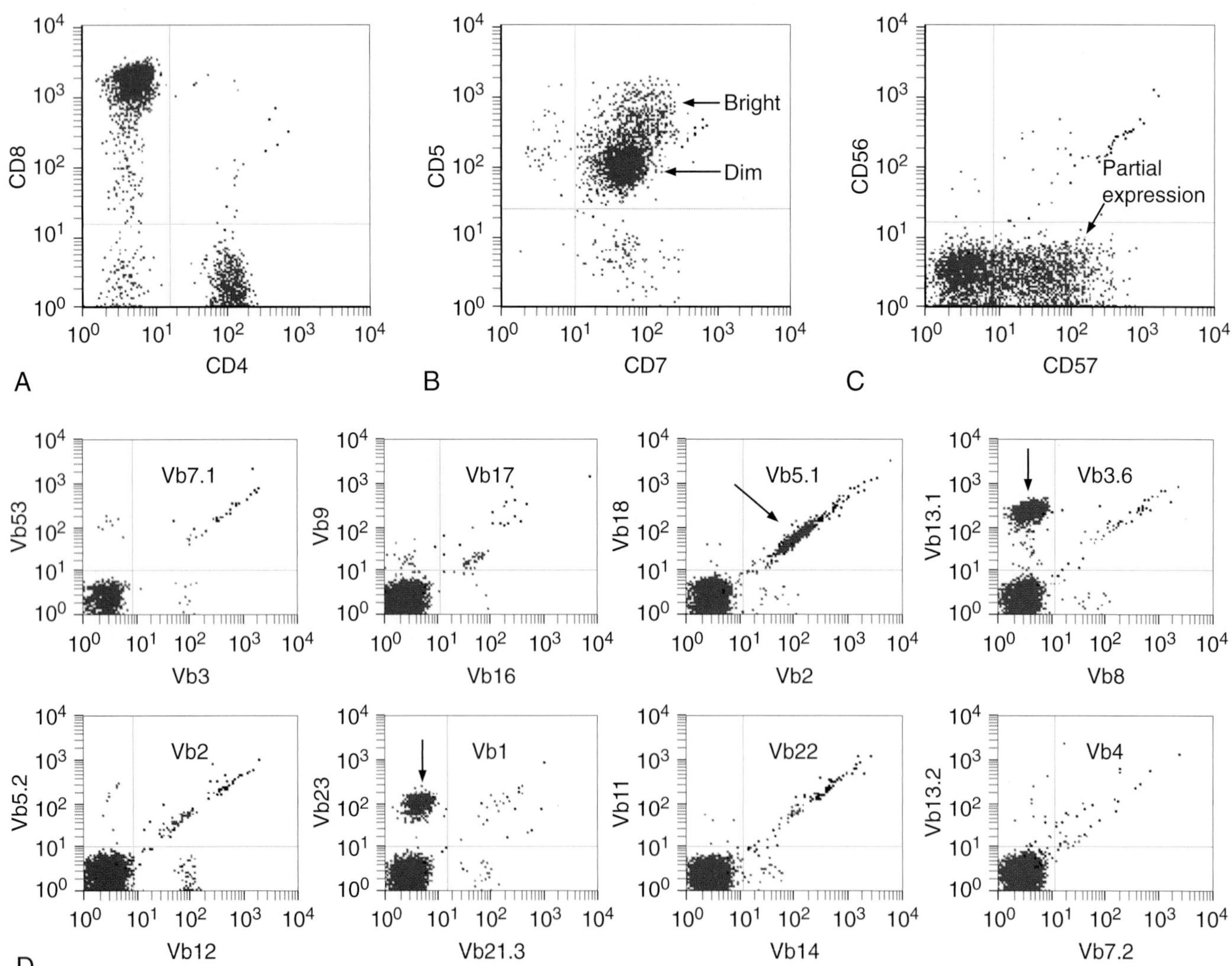

Figure 16–4. Flow cytometry in T-LGL. ***A***, A reversed CD4:CD8 ratio is typical. ***B***, Dim expression of CD5 and CD7 is a common finding in T-LGL. ***C***, CD57 is expressed in most cases of T-LGL, although usually partial. ***D***, V_β analysis reveals three clonal populations in this patient with only monoclonal rearrangement on TCR-γ by PCR analysis.

expressed in 38% of cases, usually only as diminished staining intensity, CD3 similarly may show diminished intensity with complete or partial loss uncommon.

Inferring clonality of T cells by flow cytometry is more difficult than for B cells, which exhibit light-chain restriction. TCR analysis is more problematic for immunophenotyping. Two methods have been employed for this purpose: a limited antibody panel for KIRs and an extensive antibody panel for TCR V_β analysis. KIRs are proteins of the immunoglobulin superfamily found on subsets of cytotoxic T cells and NK cells, where they function to mediate non–major histocompatibility complex (MHC)-restricted cytotoxicity.[106] In a study of 21 T-LGL patients, a monotypic pattern of KIR expression was observed in 48% using monoclonal antibodies to CD158b (7 cases), CD158a (3 cases), and CD158e (1 case), whereas the remaining 52% showed absent KIR expression. Immunophenotypic analysis of the variable region of the β chain of the TCR is a more sensitive approach to clonality but requires multiple antibodies.[107,108] Current V_β kits are available to analyze 67% of V_β rearrangements, using 24 antibodies in eight tubes for analysis in three or more color flow cytometers. Relative frequencies of V_β usage in normal controls are established for comparison.[109] For one commercial kit, a sensitivity of 89% and specificity of 88% was defined, as compared to molecular evidence of clonality utilizing TCR-γ by PCR.[110] For unclear reasons, some cases deemed monoclonal by PCR exhibited more than one V_β clone expanded by flow cytometry (Fig. 16–*4D*).

Molecular Analysis of TCR

Monoclonal TCR rearrangement is a defining feature in T-LGL leukemia.[2] The exact type of TCR analysis varies among laboratories, most common is TCR-γ sequence amplification by PCR followed by visualization of the TCR-β on Southern blot. T cells belong to the α/β (95%) or γ/δ (5%) phenotypes. During T-cell development, TCR genes are rearranged in the order γ, β, α, and δ such that all mature T cells will have a γ chain rearrangement. However, most of these rearrangements will be nonproductive, resulting in phenotypically α/β T cells. TCR analysis of the δ chain is limited because the gene coding the δ region is located within the α chain and is therefore deleted in most α chain rearrangements. TCR analysis of the α chain is of little value because of inconsistent allele inactivation, often resulting in complex bands on DNA sizing gels.

TCR-γ analysis is the most sensitive method to detect clonality in T cells, whether of the α/β or γ/δ phenotype. Use of PCR for this assay has advantages over DNA hybridization tests. First, PCR is more sensitive at detecting small or dilute populations of clonal T cells within a reactive cellular background than is Southern blotting because of selective amplification of the desired gene fragments. Second, because rearranged TCR-γ genes are smaller than rearranged TCR-β genes, partially degraded specimens, such as formalin-fixed paraffin-embedded tissue, can still be assayed with only a moderate loss of sensitivity.[111] Finally, because of the ease and routine nature of PCR, turnaround time is about 2–3 days. In standard practice, primers are only designed to cover a fraction of the variable regions within the γ gene, resulting in sensitivities of approximately 75–85% with two to three primer pairs. False-negatives may result when rearrangement involves variable regions not encompassed by the assay, or when mutations within the rearranged variable regions prevent primer binding.

TCR-β analysis by DNA hybridization is used to exclude clonal T-cell rearrangement. Unlike the PCR technique for TCR-γ analysis, TCR-β analysis is performed by restriction endonuclease enzyme digestion of nonamplified DNA. The method eliminates the possibility of missing a clonal rearrangement because of incomplete primer sets, inherent in PCR analysis of the TCR-γ gene. Southern blotting requires a relatively high-concentration (nondilute) sample of clonal T cells for detection. In addition, because the analysis assesses high-molecular-weight DNA, only fresh tissue can be studied. Finally, the technique is cumbersome, frequently requiring repeated analyses, and therefore turnaround times range from 7 to 14 days. TCR-β rearrangements are present in all α/β T cells (virtually all T-LGL cases are of the α/β phenotype) but will be negative in γ/δ T cells.

Although monoclonal TCR rearrangements define T-LGL leukemia, monoclonal rearrangements also may occur in the peripheral blood of patients with benign disorders and in malignant B-cell diseases.[112] In a study comparing the utility of TCR-γ rearrangements by PCR in the peripheral blood of 363 patients with cutaneous lymphoid infiltrates, a dominant T-cell clone was detected in 30% with cutaneous T-cell lymphoma, in 41% with non– cutaneous T-cell lymphoma malignant infiltrates, and in 34% with benign infiltrates.[113] Moreover, TCR rearrangement can be found in the peripheral blood of a large proportion of patients with autoimmune disorders such as systemic sclerosis,[72] and in lymphoid malignancies (see earlier discussion).[84,86] The term *T-cell clonality of undetermined significance* has been coined to reflect similarities with the B-cell disease known as monoclonal gammopathy of undetermined significance.[114]

DIFFERENTIAL DIAGNOSIS

Because patients with T-LGL leukemia generally have neutropenia, lymphocytosis without lymphadenopathy, or anemia, the key differential diagnostic considerations relate to these three common manifestations.

Neutropenia

Most patients in the Western world with T-LGL leukemia have early symptoms related to neutropenia. The most common etiology of neutropenia is infection (Table 16–2).[115] Viral, bacterial, and parasitic agents all can cause acute transient neutropenia, but viral infections are most likely to be accompanied by lymphocytosis and therefore to simulate LGL leukemia. In hepatitis C, for example, isolated severe neutropenia unrelated to inter-

TABLE 16–2. Disorders Causing Neutropenia in Adults That Simulates T-LGL

Disorders	Comments
Infections	
Viral	Viral infections, such as hepatitis C, most closely mimic T-LGL.
Bacterial	
Parasitic	
Idiosyncratic Drug Reactions	Distinguish by clinical history
Autoimmune Neutropenia (AIN)	
Primary	Rare in adults
Secondary	
Systemic lupus erythematosus (SLE)	SLE and Felty's syndrome are the most common causes of secondary AIN.
Felty's syndrome	
Mixed connective tissue syndrome	Sjögren's syndrome is the most likely syndrome to be overlooked when evaluating for neutropenia.
Polymyalgia rheumatica	
Sjögren's syndrome	
Immune-mediated thrombocytopenic purpura	Neutropenia in these disorders, unlike in T-LGL, is mediated by humoral mechanisms
Evans's syndrome	
Autoimmune hemolytic anemia	
Leukemia	
Lymphoma	
Miscellaneous Conditions	
Hypersplenism	Pancytopenia is more typical than isolated neutropenia.
Myelophthisic processes	
Aplastic anemia	Copper deficiency, although rare, may cause isolated neutropenia.
Nutritional deficiencies	

may resemble T-LGL leukemia with neutropenia, hepatosplenomegaly, and reactive-appearing lymphocytes.[116] Viral infections may be excluded by careful attention to the clinical history and appropriately directed serologic tests. Idiosyncratic drug reactions are the second most frequent explanation of neutropenia. The drugs causing neutropenia and their mechanisms of action are diverse (see Chapter 14).[115] A drug reaction should be considered when neutropenia is temporally related to initiating a new medication. Autoimmune neutropenia, which is very uncommon, is another consideration in the differential diagnosis.[117] Autoimmune neutropenia is difficult to assess with routine laboratory tests; it has been defined as chronic neutropenia with autoantibodies against neutrophil autoantigens detected by leukoagglutination, neutrophil immunofluorescence, or monoclonal antibody immobilization of neutrophil antigens.[118] Primary autoimmune neutropenia is rare in adults; secondary autoimmune neutropenia is related to a variety of disorders (see Table 16–2), including collagen vascular disorders, hematologic autoimmune disorders, and hematologic malignancies, and there is considerable overlap between these disorders and those associated with T-LGL. Other conditions causing neutropenia frequently present with a pancytopenic blood picture, including hypersplenism, regardless of etiology,[119] myelophthisic processes, aplastic anemia, myelodysplastic syndrome, and nutritional deficiencies.[120] Rarely, copper deficiency may cause isolated neutropenia.[121,122]

Anemia/Pure Red Cell Aplasia

Patients with T-LGL may have symptomatic or transfusion dependent anemia. T-LGL leukemia may present with PRCA (see Chapter 12), especially in Asian populations; approximately 7% of Western patients with T-LGL have PRCA.[80] In a recent study of 48 patients, T-LGL was the most commonly identified cause of PRCA in adults (19%).[81] Other considerations in PRCA include CLL, thymoma, MDS, non-Hodgkin's lymphoma, and idiopathic causes, which usually can be distinguished with adequate material for morphologic, immunophenotypic, and molecular analysis.

Lymphocytosis without Lymphadenopathy

B-cell lymphoproliferative disorders that are morphologically and clinically similar to T-LGL leukemia are easily distinguished by standard immunophenotyping using flow cytometry (Table 16–3).[123] Hairy cell leukemia (see Chapter 35) presents with splenomegaly, without lymphadenopathy, and causes cytopenias. Unlike in T-LGL, monocytopenia is pronounced in hairy cell leukemia and the cells are agranular, characteristically with cytoplasmic projections. Splenic marginal zone lymphoma may present with splenomegaly and cytopenias without lymphadenopathy. Unlike in T-LGL leukemia, neutropenia is usually not prominent and the lymphocytes are agranular, often with nucleoli, and may have bipolar cytoplasmic projections. CLL is rarely a diagnostic problem because the cells are small with scant cytoplasm and neutropenia is typical only late in the course.

Reactive lymphocytosis, as in viral infections, may result in large granular lymphocytosis, but these proliferations are transient rather than chronic. Alternatively, in chronic NK cell lymphocytosis or NK-LPD there is a history of large granular lymphocytosis exceeding 6 months, which phenotypes as NK cells ($CD3^-CD16^+$) with germline TCR rearrangements.[9,10] The course is similar to T-LGL except the cytopenias are less profound and not associated with RA. Some cases are clonal when examined by X-inactivation studies, but the significance of this finding is unclear and the diagnostic utility of this test is limited.[11–13] NK cells in NK cell lymphocytosis can have a restricted KIR phenotype, with loss of inhibitory KIR and an increase in activating KIR[124,125]—a property potentially useful to distinguish reactive NK cell proliferations from NK-LPD.

Aggressive NK/T-cell disorders pose a significant diagnostic challenge because their phenotypic, morphologic, and clinical features overlap with T-LGL, and the rarity of these disorders make confidence in their distinction low.[126] Hepatosplenic T-cell lymphoma may present with splenomegaly in the absence of lymphadenopathy.[127–129] The peripheral blood morphology consists of atypical lymphoid cells that may resemble LGLs (and some cases of T-LGL are agranular). The immunophenotype is vari-

TABLE 16–3. Differential Considerations in Lymphocytosis Mimicking T-LGL Leukemia

Disorder	Cytopenia*	LAD	SM	HM	CD19	CD3	CD8	CD57	CD56	Morphology
T-LGL	N	−	+	+/−	−	+	+	++/−	−/+	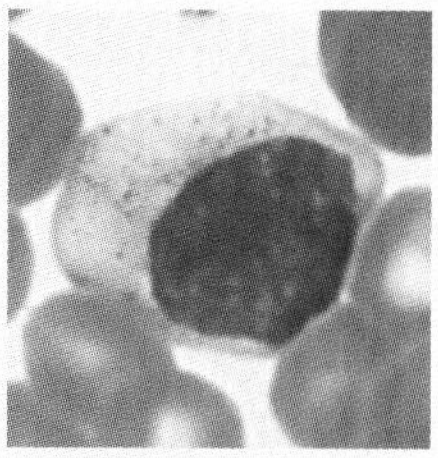
HCL	M/P	−	+	−	+	−	−	−	−	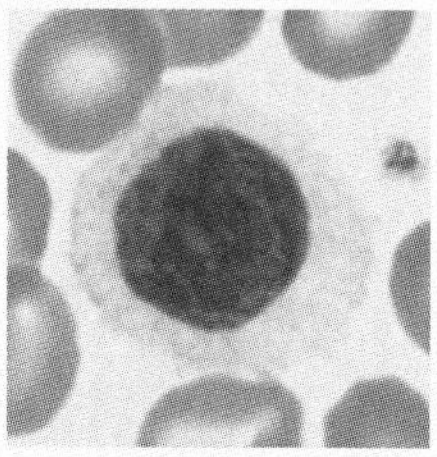
SMZL	P	−	+	−	+	−	−	−	−	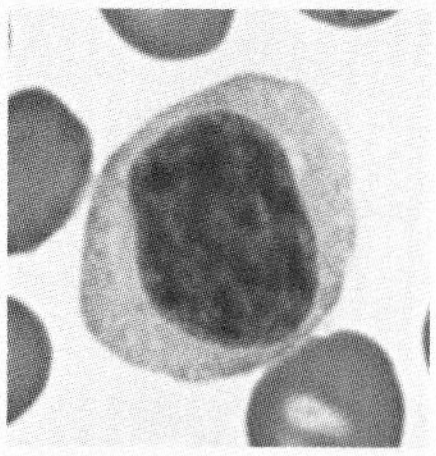
CLL	A/T	+	+	−	+	−	−	−	−	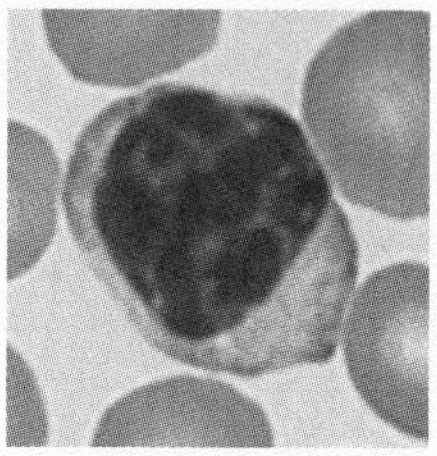
NK-LPD	V	V	V	V	−	−	+/−	−	+	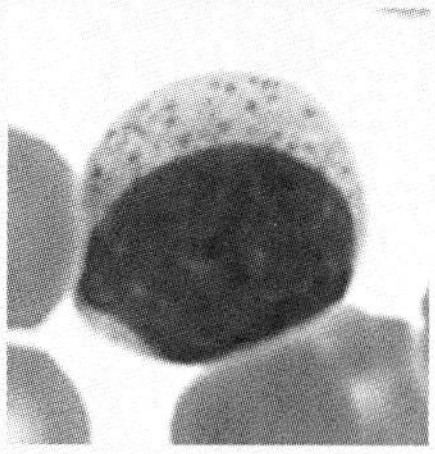
HSTCL	T/A	−	+	+	−	+	+/−	−	+	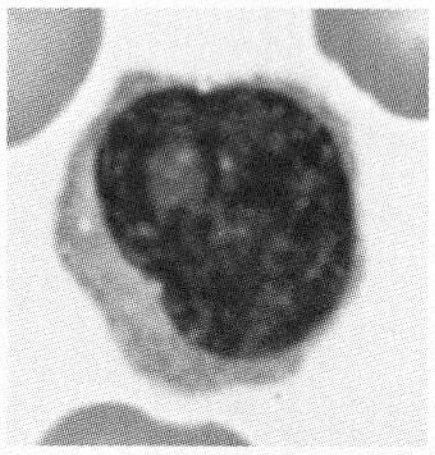
ANKL	P	−	+	+	−	−	+/−	−	+	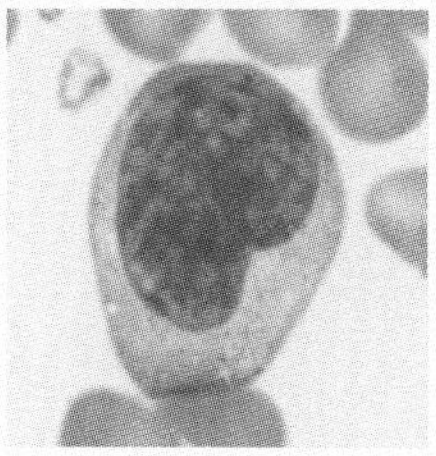

*A, anemia; M, monocytopenia; N, neutropenia; P, pancytopenia; T, thrombocytopenia; V, variable.

Abbreviations: ANKL, aggressive NK cell leukemia; CLL, chronic lymphocytic leukemia; HCL, hairy cell leukemia; HM, hepatomegaly; HSTCL, hepatosplenic T-cell lymphoma; LAD, lymphadenopathy; NK-LPD, NK cell lymphoproliferative disorder; SM, splenomegaly; SMZL, splenic marginal zone lymphoma.

able but is typically $CD3^+$, $CD5^-$, $CD7^{+/-}$, $CD8^-$, $CD56^+$, $CD57^-$, and γ/δ^+, although 10–50% of cases may be $CD8^+$, and α/β^+ hepatosplenic T-cell lymphoma has been described.[130] Hepatosplenic T-cell lymphoma is a diagnostic consideration in cases of T-LGL with an immunophenotype of $CD3^+$, $CD5^-$, $CD7^{+/-}$, $CD8^+$, $CD56^+$, $CD57^-$ and α/β^+.[131] Hepatosplenic T-cell lymphoma can be distinguished from T-LGL by its pronounced intrasinusoidal bone marrow infiltrate, the dominant cytopenias being thrombocytopenia and anemia rather than neutropenia, hepatomegaly with elevated transaminases, and the cytogenetic finding of isochromosome 7q. NK cell leukemia morphologically may simulate T-LGL leukemia, but the immunophenotype is surface $CD3^-$ and $CD56^+$ by flow cytometry and the clinical course is very aggressive.[132,133] NK cell leukemia is almost invariably associated with Epstein-Barr virus transcripts within the malignant cells.

TREATMENT

Indications for therapy of T-LGL include recurrent infections resulting from severe neutropenia and transfusion-dependent anemia. Almost three fourths of patients will require therapy over the course of their disease,[65,134] although spontaneous remissions occur rarely.[135] Uncomplicated or asymptomatic cytopenias may be simply observed over time (Fig. 16–5).

Immunosuppressive Therapies

Methotrexate, 10 mg/m^2/wk orally, induces complete remission in 50% of patients.[136] Indefinite treatment is required to prevent relapse.[16] Sometimes several months of therapy are required before counts improve. Toxicities include perturbations of liver function tests and drug-related pneumonitis.[137]

Cyclosporine occasionally ameliorates LGL cytopenias. In a study of 25 patients, 50% had response to therapy and 24% had a complete hematologic remission.[138] Improvement was independent of the quantity of T cells infiltrating the bone marrow, peripheral LGL counts, or concurrent myelodysplasia. Therapeutic response to cyclosporine is related to the HLA-DR4 haplotype.[139] LGL clones may persist despite correction of the neutrophil count, and cyclosporine has its own significant toxicities.[140]

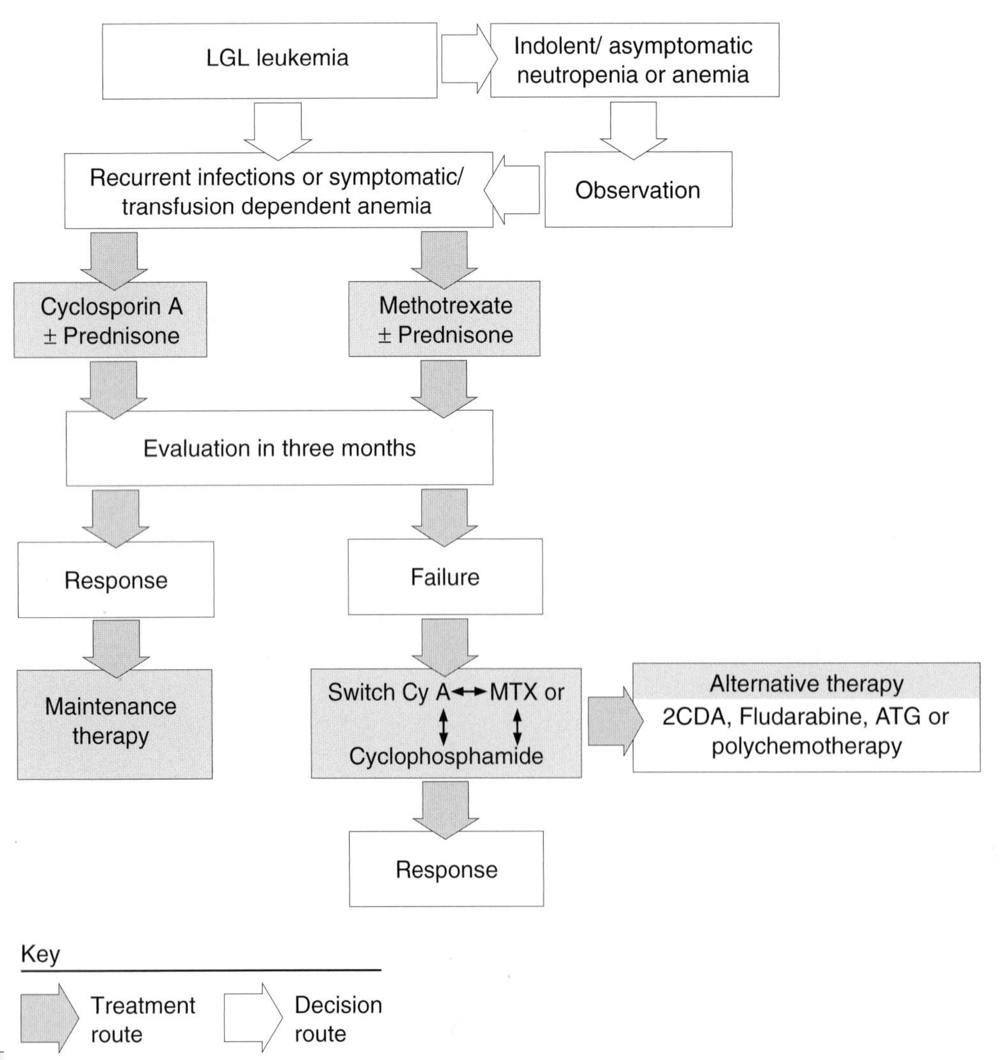

Figure 16–5. Algorithm for the management of T-LGL. (From Lamy T, Loughran TP Jr: Clinical features of large granular lymphocyte leukemia. Semin Hematol 40:185–195, 2003, with permission.)

Cyclophosphamide as an oral agent has been used with good response. Prednisone combined with cyclophosphamide increased the duration of response compared to prednisone alone; overall response to therapy was 66%, with a median duration of 32 months. The response to cyclophosphamide in patients with PRCA is 88–100%.[141]

Alternative Therapies

Complete remissions have followed second-line therapy with purine analogues such as chlorodeoxyadenosine, fludarabine, and deoxycoformycin.[65] Purine analogues may increase susceptibility to the development of opportunistic infections, and RA has been reported after deoxycoformycin treatment.[142] Campath I, a monoclonal antibody to the CD52 antigen present on T cells, or antithymocyte globulin may be considered in methotrexate- or cyclosporine-resistant patients. Bone marrow transplantation in T-LGL has only been reported anecdotally.

Surgical Therapies

Splenectomy is not effective in correcting the neutrophil count and may increase circulating LGLs. Splenectomy has no role in the management of T-LGL leukemia except for traumatic splenic rupture and concurrent immune-mediated thrombocytopenic purpura or autoimmune hemolytic anemia.

Aggressive Disease

Patients with aggressive T-LGL leukemia have received chemotherapy, including CHOP-like (cyclophosphamide, doxorubicin, vincristine, and prednisone) and etoposide/cytarabine-containing regimens. Despite such efforts, most die within 1 year of chemotherapy initiation. Aggressive T-LGL leukemia behaves similarly to aggressive NK cell leukemias. The poor response is likely related to expression of high levels of P-glycoprotein, the gene product of multidrug resistance gene 1 (*MDR1*).[143]

Clinical Trials

Two important prospective therapeutic trials are current. The Eastern Cooperative Oncology Group is evaluating the efficacy of oral methotrexate, 10 mg/m^2/wk, with crossover to cyclophosphamide in nonresponders. The Cancer and Leukemia Group B is testing cyclosporine, orally 2 mg/kg every 12 hours, as front-line therapy. Indications for both protocols are neutropenia or symptomatic or transfusion-dependent anemia.

SUPPORTIVE CARE AND LONG-TERM MANAGEMENT

Infection

Patients with severe neutropenia are at risk of serious infections. Although treatment with immunosuppressive medications can induce remission, these drugs act slowly and neutropenia may persist for months. In this setting, hematopoietic growth factors such as granulocyte-macrophage colony-stimulating factor or granulocyte colony-stimulating factor can produce partial and transient responses. Bacterial infections should be treated aggressively with parenteral, broad-spectrum antimicrobial regimens.

Anemia

Transfusions may be required for symptomatic anemia until remission can be induced with immunosuppressive regimens.

PROGNOSIS

T-LGL leukemia is an indolent chronic lymphoproliferative disorder with good long-term survival, if its cytopenias are corrected and symptoms appropriately managed. Survival rates vary, likely reflecting differences in diagnostic criteria.[2] An early study of 151 patients found 26 deaths during a median follow-up period of 23 months.[67] More recently, a median survival of greater than 10 years was reported for 68 patients.[65] Multivariant analysis has revealed that fever at diagnosis, a low percentage of CD57$^+$ cells, and low peripheral blood LGL counts predict a poor prognosis.[67]

CURRENT CONTROVERSIES & FUTURE CONSIDERATIONS

Large Granular Lymphocyte Leukemia

- Growing evidence suggests T-LGL leukemia is related to other bone marrow failure disorders, including acquired aplastic anemia, PNH, MDS, and PRCA.
- Although Felty's syndrome is distinguished from T-LGL by clonality, the clinical and immunogenetic features suggest that these diseases likely represent the ends of the spectrum of one disease.
- It is uncertain if NK-LPD is a reactive or malignant disorder, but it should be distinguished from aggressive NK cell leukemia, previously called NK-LGL leukemia, because the clinical course and treatment are markedly different.
- T-cell clonality may be detected in reactive conditions, leading some to propose the term *T-cell clonopathy of undetermined significance* and to question the malignant nature of T-LGL.

Suggested Readings*

Dhodapkar MV, Li CY, Lust JA, et al: Clinical spectrum of clonal proliferations of T-large granular lymphocytes: a T-cell clonopathy of undetermined significance? Blood 84:1620–1627, 1994.

Epling-Burnette PK, Loughran TP Jr: Survival signals in leukemic large granular lymphocytes. Semin Hematol 40:213–220, 2003.

Lamy T, Liu JH, Landowski TH, et al: Dysregulation of CD95/CD95 ligand-apoptotic pathway in $CD3^+$ large granular lymphocyte leukemia. Blood 92:4771–4777, 1998.

Lamy T, Loughran TP Jr: Clinical features of large granular lymphocyte leukemia. Semin Hematol 40:185–195, 2003.

Loughran TP Jr: Clonal diseases of large granular lymphocytes. Blood 82:1–14, 1993.

***Full references for this chapter can be found on accompanying CD-ROM.**

CHAPTER 17

Iron Deficiency

Paul A. Seligman, MD, and Tracey Rouault, MD

KEY POINTS

Iron Deficiency

- Iron deficiency is the most common cause of anemia.
- In order to ensure that serum transferrin delivers sufficient iron to the appropriate tissues without causing toxicity, specialized proteins regulate iron absorption, iron transport, and iron compartmentalization.
- New diagnostic tests for iron deficiency are not only important to identify uncomplicated iron deficiency, but they also recognize iron deficits in patients with erythropoietin-responsive anemia.
- Early iron deficiency causes cognitive and other functional defects that adversely affect quality of life before development of anemia.
- Newer intravenous iron preparations are particularly useful in patients receiving recombinant erythropoietin.

INTRODUCTION

A challenge for all organisms is to acquire and appropriately distribute iron to the numerous proteins that require the element for their function. Iron is a transition metal that can readily accept or donate single electrons. This chemical flexibility makes iron indispensable and an important constituent of a variety of proteins and prosthetic groups that participate in reactions that utilize oxygen.[1] Most of the iron in the body is incorporated into hemoglobin, a tetrameric molecule synthesized within red cells that transports oxygen from the lungs to other tissues (see Chapter 2).[1] In hemoglobin, each globin monomer binds a heme prosthetic group, which consists of a planar porphyrin ring in which a single ferrous iron atom is bound at the center. The heme-iron is oriented to allow one unpaired electron free to ligate oxygen at high oxygen concentrations. As erythrocytes move through the circulation, the lower tissue concentrations of oxygen release the oxygen bound to heme-iron.[1,2]

EPIDEMIOLOGY AND RISK FACTORS

Iron deficiency is the most prevalent nutritional disease and the most common cause of anemia worldwide.[2,3] A recent World Health Organization publication cited iron deficiency as the third greatest global health risk (after obesity and unsafe sex).[3] Anemia resulting from iron deficiency affects approximately 2 billion people worldwide (34% of the world population), most of whom live in developing countries, where the incidence is about 40%.[4,5] In developing countries, an iron-deficient diet is commonly associated with iron deficiency anemia. However, the most common cause for anemia resulting from iron deficiency is blood loss, often exacerbated by an iron-deficient diet or poor absorption of iron from the gastrointestinal tract.[6] Other causes of increased iron loss are pregnancy, when significant amounts of iron are transferred to the placenta and the growing fetus, and periods of rapid growth in young children and during adolescence.[2,4,7,8]

The incidence of iron deficiency anemia in more developed countries, including the United States, is about 10%.[5] Iron deficiency with or without anemia is particularly common in certain high-risk groups: 50% of pregnant women, 25% of menstruating females, and about 3% of adolescent males.[5] About one third to one half of these individuals have hemoglobin levels below the lower limits of the "reference range" (see later) and therefore deserve a diagnosis of anemia.

PHYSIOLOGY

Cellular Iron Homeostasis

Because excess iron is toxic (see Chapter 56), iron must be appropriately transported and compartmentalized so as to ensure its adequate delivery to tissues and to avoid the accumulation of dangerous excesses of intracellular iron species.

Mammals maintain a reservoir of bioavailable iron in the bloodstream in the form of iron-transferrin. Transferrin (Tf) is an abundant serum protein that binds two atoms of ferric iron (Fe^{3+}) with high affinity.[9–11] Normally, serum transferrin is approximately 30% saturated with iron; saturation levels decrease in iron-deficient animals and increase with iron overload.[12,13] Although the iron-transferrin pool accounts for less than 1% of total body iron, about 10 times that amount of iron flows through this pool each day. Cells remove iron from circulating mono- and deferric transferrin by expressing surface transferrin receptors (TfRs) that bind transferrin. Upon binding, cells internalize the Tf-TfR complex in an endosome.[14] Acidification of the endosome leads to release from transferrin of ferric iron, which then undergoes reduction and transport out of the endosome by a transporter known as the divalent metal transporter 1 (DMT1).[15] The apoTf-TfR complex then recycles back to the cell surface, where exposure to neutral plasma pH promotes dissociation of apoTf from transferrin receptors, allowing the intact apoTf to reenter the general circulation and engage in multiple cycles of iron uptake.[16,17]

To ensure that serum transferrin carries sufficient iron to the appropriate tissues, mammals coordinate the activities of three major tissues: the duodenal mucosa, the reticuloendothelial system, and the liver.[2,9] The duodenum regulates how much dietary iron is absorbed through the gut, whereas macrophages control the fraction of the iron acquired from heme catabolism that they return to the circulation after phagocytosis of senescent red cells. The liver regulates the iron transport activities of both the duodenal mucosa and macrophages by secreting a regulatory peptide hormone, hepcidin,[18] that acts to repress duodenal iron uptake and macrophage iron release[19] (Fig. 17–1). Transcription of the hepcidin gene increases proportionally as body iron stores increase.[20]

In iron-deficient patients, intestinal iron uptake of iron salts in the duodenum rises as a result of increased expression of iron transporters on the apical and basolateral membranes.[21,22] On the apical membrane, the transporter DMT1 transports ferrous (Fe^{2+}) iron from the intestinal lumen to the cytosol, along with a single proton.[23,24] Dietary elemental iron is mainly in the ferric oxidation state; gastric acidity and a ferric reductase known as Dcytb[25] reduces ferric iron so that ferrous iron can be transported by DMT1. Iron is then exported from intestinal mucosal cells by the iron exporter ferroportin.[26–28] Hypoxia and iron deficiency lead to transcriptional activation of DMT1, Dcytb, and ferroportin, and increased uptake of iron through the intestinal mucosa. In addition, a separate dedicated heme transporter found in the duodenum and jejunum is also transcriptionally activated; this process explains why dietary heme iron appears to be a more bioavailable nutritional source than are iron salts[5,29] (McKie, personal communication).

Identification of multiple human disease genes in which loss of function leads to iron overload have led to a description of a physiologic iron-sensing regulatory circuit in which the liver plays a central role. Genes in which loss of function leads to hereditary hemochromatosis (see Chapter 56) include those for (1) HFE,[30] a protein that influences transferrin-iron uptake by binding to transferrin receptors[31,32] and is needed for appropriate hepcidin production[33,34]; (2) TfR2, a second transferrin receptor mainly expressed in the liver[35,36]; (3) transferrin, loss of which leads to iron overload in mice and humans[37–39]; (4) hepcidin, in which mutations were recently described in juvenile-onset hemochromatosis[40]; and (5) hemojuvelin,[41] the disease gene in many families affected by severe juvenile hemochromatosis.[42] These defects suggest that a regulatory circuit exists that is highly protective of the consequences of cellular iron molecular toxicity.

The role of the broad physiologic axis defined by the hepcidin pathway is to provide sufficient iron to load circulating serum transferrin, the major source of bioavailable iron for cells throughout the body (see Fig. 17–1). Cellular iron uptake is mainly regulated by transferrin receptor expression on the cell surface.[43–45] Although these receptors are found on most cells, especially during iron-dependent proliferation, most of the total body transferrin receptors are on erythrocyte precursors. Developing erythroblasts depend almost completely on transferrin receptors to mediate iron uptake[46,47]; when serum transferrin contains little iron, developing erythroblasts cannot acquire enough iron to generate heme. Through an unknown mechanism, erythroblasts repress globin synthesis when they are unable to synthesize heme.[48] Overall hemoglobin synthesis is markedly reduced in iron-deficient erythroblasts, resulting in mature erythrocytes with low hemoglobin levels.

In many cells, including developing erythroblasts, iron regulatory proteins (IRPs) regulate iron homeostasis.[49,50] IRP1 functions both as a cytosolic aconitase, interconverting citrate and isocitrate in cytosol in iron-replete cells, or as an RNA-binding protein that posttranscriptionally regulates expression of transferrin receptor, ferritin, and other iron metabolism proteins in iron-depleted cells.[49,51] IRP2, highly homologous to IRP1, functions simply to regulate iron metabolism in iron-depleted cells; unlike IRP1, IRP2 undergoes iron-dependent degradation by the ubiquitin-proteasome system and is absent in iron-replete cells.[52–55]

IRPs regulate expression of target transcripts by binding to RNA stem-loop elements known as iron-responsive elements (IREs)[56] (Fig. 17–2). IREs are composed of a six-residue loop, a five–base pair upper stem, and a lower stem of at least four base pairs that is separated from the upper stem by an unpaired residue. IRPs bind with high affinity to IREs, but the effect of IRP binding on gene expression depends on the location of the IRE in the transcript. When IREs are near the 5′ end of transcripts, IRP binding interferes with initiation of translation, and synthesis of the protein normally encoded by the transcript is inhibited. IREs are found in the 5′ end of ferritin H and L transcripts and mitochondrial aconitase[57,58] (see Fig. 17–2). An IRE is also present at the 5′ end of a δ-aminolevulinate synthase (ALAS) transcript, expressed only in erythrocytes, known as erythroid ALAS[59,60] (see Chapter 2); ALAS catalyzes the first step of heme biosynthesis, in which succinyl coenzyme

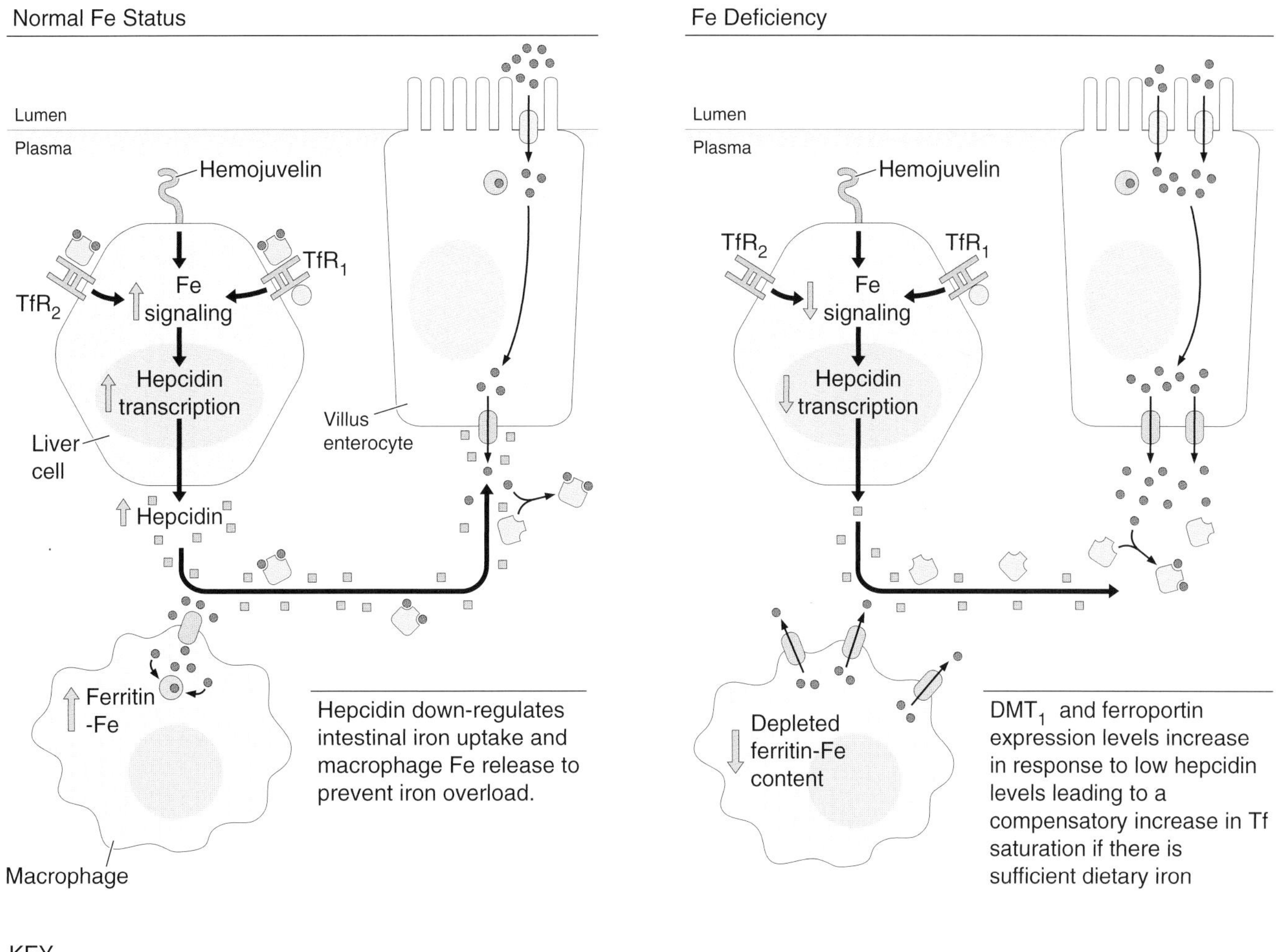

Figure 17–1. Hepatic synthesis of hepcidin to coordinate regulation of entry of iron into the systemic circulation from the duodenal mucosa and macrophages. The liver integrates information from several different iron uptake systems, including two transferrin receptors (TfRs), TfR1-HFE and TfR2, both of which bind diferric transferrin (Tf), and hemojuvelin, a membrane-linked protein with an unknown role, perhaps in a non–transferrin-dependent iron pathway. Liver cells increase hepcidin transcription in proportion to increased body iron *(left panel).* Conversely, when the body is iron deficient, hepatic hepcidin transcription decreases *(right panel).* Receptors for hepcidin likely exist in the duodenal mucosa and macrophages. As hepcidin levels decrease, iron transporter expression increases, resulting in more iron uptake through the duodenal mucosa to the circulation, and increased export of iron from macrophages that catabolize heme during red cell phagocytosis. The molecular events by which hepcidin decreases expression of iron transporters such as ferroportin in the intestinal mucosa and macrophages are not known.

A and glycine condense to form aminolevulinic acid. From evolutionary and functional perspectives, red cells have developed a mechanism for repressing the first step of heme biosynthesis in iron-deficient cells. Insertion of ferrous iron into the porphyrin ring to form heme is catalyzed by ferrochelatase in mitochondria as the final step in heme biosynthesis. Accumulation of the ferrochelatase substrate protoporphyrin IX can result in disease when ferrochelatase cannot insert iron, either because of mutations in the ferrochelatase gene[61] or because of iron deficiency. When cells are iron deficient, ferrochelatase incorporates zinc into the iron-binding site of protoporphyrin IX.[62,63] Because heme cannot be synthesized if iron is insufficient, the erythroid form of ALAS is appropriately repressed by IRP binding in iron-deficient cells,[64] enabling red cells to avoid synthesis and accumulation of potentially toxic heme precursors such as protoporphyrin IX.[65]

As red cell precursors develop, transferrin receptor expression mediates the uptake of serum transferrin-iron that is needed to supply iron for proliferation heme synthesis; TfR2 is expressed mainly in the liver and does not appear in normal differentiating erythroid cells.[66] In most iron-deficient cells, transferrin receptor expression rises

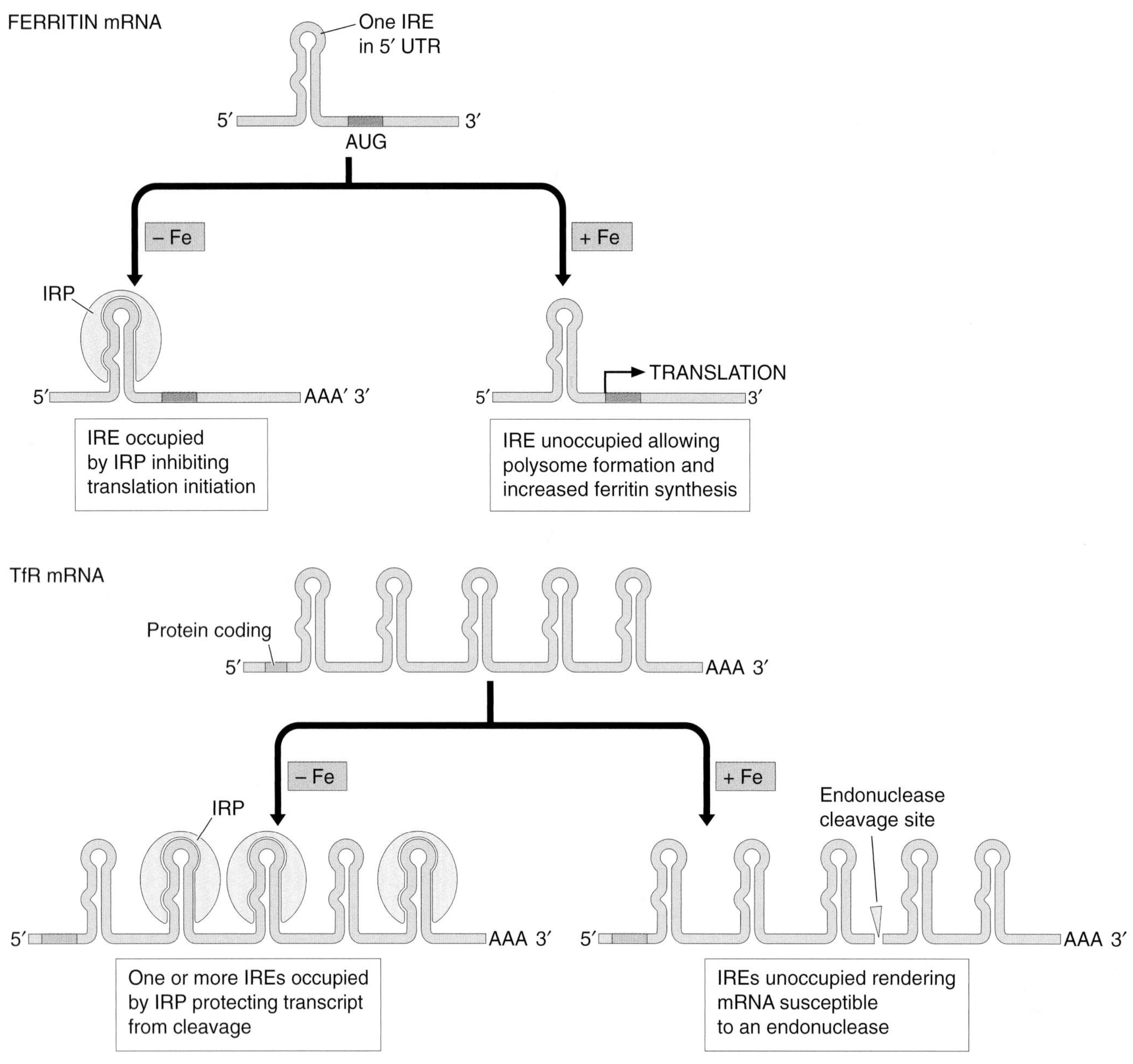

Figure 17–2. IRP regulation of ferritin and transferrin receptor (TfR) synthesis. RNA stem-loops, known as IREs, are found in the 5′ untranslated region (UTR) of ferritin transcripts and in the 3′ UTR for TfR transcripts. IRPs bind to IREs when cells are iron deficient. When they bind near the 5′ end of the transcript, they interfere with initiation of translation; when they bind to the 3′ UTR of TfR, they protect the transcript from endonucleolytic cleavage and degradation. This posttranscriptional regulation enables cells to increase iron availability by simultaneously increasing TfR-dependent iron uptake and decreasing ferritin-associated iron sequestration.

when IRPs bind to IREs in the 3′ untranslated region of the transcript; IRP binding increases the abundance of transferrin receptor transcript by protecting the transcript from cleavage and degradation[67] (see Fig. 17–1). A significant elevation in transferrin receptor transcription occurs in developing red cells,[68,69] and some of the transcriptional increase may be mediated by hypoxia inducible factor.[70,71] IRP binding facilitates high transferrin receptor expression and iron uptake at the earliest stages of red cell differentiation, before the onset of heme synthesis, an effect probably related to iron regulation of erythropoiesis rather than to heme synthesis.[72,73] Careful dissection of molecular events at each state in erythrocyte development[74,75] defines how iron metabolism evolves during red cell differentiation.

Physiology of Iron Regulation: The Iron Cycle

Iron is not a trace element; adults have an average of 2–3 gm of total body iron, most within hemoglobin in red cells. In iron-replete individuals, a significant amount of

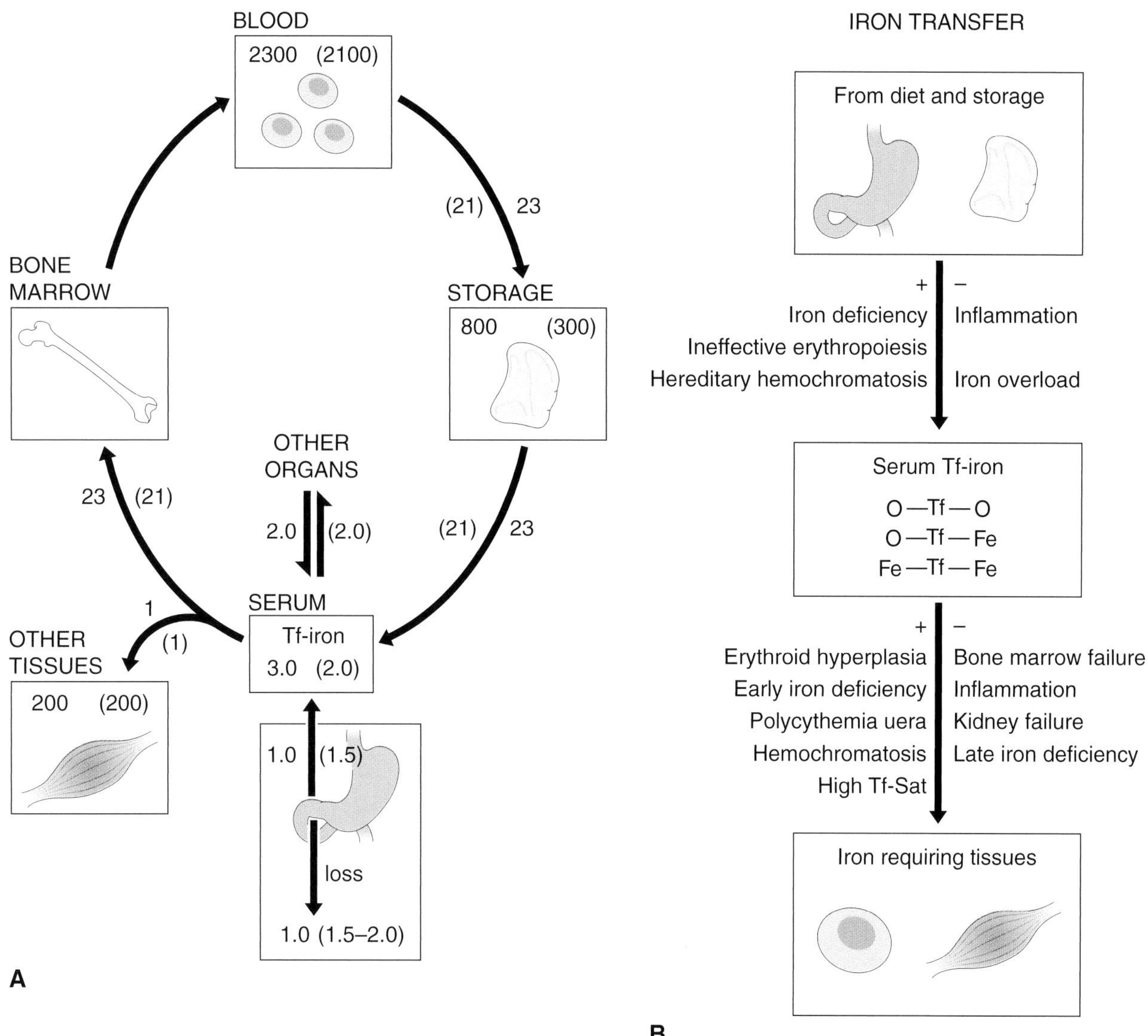

Figure 17–3. *A,* The "iron cycle." Numbers on the sides of the *arrows* indicate milligrams of iron transported between compartments over a 24-hour period; numbers in the compartments indicate the milligrams of iron they contain. For both males and nonmenstruating females, 1 mg of iron is absorbed from the gastrointestinal tracts and transferred to transferrin daily. Each day, 23 mg of iron is delivered to the bone marrow for red cell proliferation and hemoglobin production, and 1 mg goes to other tissues for iron-dependent reactions, including myoglobin production and cellular proliferation. New red cells containing 23 mg of iron are released daily from the bone marrow, and that amount of iron from senescent red cells is stored. Storage iron found in ferritin releases a similar amount of iron to transferrin in order to maintain erythropoiesis. Besides erythropoiesis, "known" iron-dependent reactions, and iron storage, a small but significant amount of iron (about 2 mg) exists in a "labile" pool, which may also allow for rapid iron-dependent reactions. The daily iron cycle is different for menstruating females (noted by numbers in parentheses), who because of blood loss have less iron in serum and less storage iron. (Adapted from Bothwell TH, Charlton RW, Cook JD, Finch CA: *In* Iron Metabolism in Man. Oxford, UK: Blackwell Scientific, 1979, p 24.) *B,* Positive and negative influences on (1) loading of iron onto transferrin and (2) transfer of transferrin-bound iron to cells. The latter process is mainly regulated by density of transferrin receptors, but low cell surface receptor concentration in the face of high transferrin iron saturation (as in hemochromatosis) will increase iron transfer to cells, and high transferrin receptor concentration, associated with low transferrin iron (as in severe iron deficiency), results in low transfer to cells.

iron is stored in ferritin.[2,8,10] The storage compartment is important to maintain daily iron balance as well as to make iron available during periods of iron loss.[2,9,10]

Regulation of iron transport at the cellular level, as detailed earlier, allows for a physiologic daily exchange of iron among the various body compartments (Fig. 17–3*A*). This movement of iron on a daily basis is the "iron cycle." In males, the daily iron cycle remains relatively constant.[2,9,10,76–78] About 1 mg of iron is absorbed from the diet daily and transferred to transferrin; transferrin-bound iron accounts for about 3 mg of iron at any one time, with most of this iron transferred to the bone marrow for red cell production, and a small but significant amount utilized for other iron-dependent reactions.

Because erythrocytes circulate for only about 120 days, iron from these cells is degraded and stored as ferritin in reticuloendothelial cells (including macrophage and Kupffer cells). About 25 mg of iron released from storage is transferred to transferrin per day. This iron makes up the vast majority of the 25–35 mg of iron that flows through the transferrin pool on a daily basis. In men, average storage iron remains stable at about 800 mg. Gastrointestinal iron absorption equals the daily loss of about 1 mg of iron from sweat and desquamated epithelial cells. With increased iron loss as with bleeding, storage iron is utilized until it becomes depleted and transferrin saturation decreases; eventually iron-deficient erythropoiesis and anemia occur (see later).

Menstruating females have a different daily iron cycle,[79] less consistent but still predictable. Menstruating women require more daily iron from their diet (1.5–2 mg) but still have lower average iron stores (300 mg) and lower levels of transferrin-bound iron in serum (2.5 mg) (see Fig. 17–3*A*).[80,81] They must therefore transport a higher percentage of serum transferrin-iron over a 24-hour period in order to maintain a hemoglobin similar to levels in men and nonmenstruating women. Because their stores are lower, they are more susceptible to iron deficiency if menstrual blood loss becomes excessive, bleeding occurs from other sites, or dietary iron is lacking. Iron loss resulting from pregnancy or from growth during adolescence also increases the likelihood of iron-deficient erythropoiesis.[5,8,82]

Iron, Erythropoietin, and Regulation of Erythropoiesis

Although most iron utilized by erythroid precursors is incorporated into hemoglobin, chronic iron deficiency is associated with decreased erythropoiesis.[72] Even before heme synthesis begins, erythropoietin induces expression of transferrin receptors on erythroid precursors as a necessary step for increased proliferation and expansion of erythropoiesis[73] (Fig. 17–3*B*). The kidney, in response to hypoxia, releases erythropoietin; increased erythropoietin gene expression is mediated by hypoxia inducible factor α.[83] In renal failure, especially for patients undergoing hemodialysis, the most common reason for resistance to pharmacologic doses of erythropoietin is inadequate iron availability; parenteral iron is usually required to optimize erythropoietin efficacy.[84–86] High erythropoietin levels associated with hemolytic anemias result in increased iron utilization; higher transferrin saturation may be necessary to maximize erythropoiesis. As in renal failure, some patients require intravenous iron even in the absence of laboratory evidence of iron deficiency.

PATHOPHYSIOLOGY

Inadequate Iron Intake and Gastrointestinal Malabsorption of Iron

Although iron is one of the most abundant elements on earth, most foods contain relatively small amounts of iron, much of which has low bioavailability.[5,87] Poor iron intake and impaired absorption of iron from the gastrointestinal tract can cause but more often contribute to iron deficiency anemia.

In general, dietary iron comes in two forms: iron salts found in plant products and heme iron bound to animal proteins, including hemoglobin and myoglobin.[5,87–89] Iron salts are difficult to absorb through the gastrointestinal tract. A "well-balanced diet" contains about 6 g of iron per 1000 calories. Diets high in grains and cereals (not supplemented) have lower iron content. When the daily intake is less than 1500 calories, an individual can become iron deficient, particularly in underdeveloped countries where even adequate caloric intake is associated with a higher proportion of nonsupplemented grains and cereals. Gastrointestinal iron absorption can be inhibited by other dietary components: tannins, phytates, and phenols found in teas, grains, and other plant products.[90]

Iron absorption is low in small bowel malabsorption syndromes. Because absorption of iron salts occurs in the duodenum, even mild celiac disease or chronic giardiasis can contribute to iron deficiency.[91] Nonheme food iron must be degraded and reduced by the acidic environment of the stomach for optimal absorption, and achlorhydria caused by conditions such as atrophic gastritis or chronic *Helicobacter pylori* infection can result in significant iron malabsorption even when blood loss is minimal or absent.[92–94] Gastric surgery that bypasses the duodenum, such as that for ulcers or for obesity, may be a significant etiology of iron deficiency, particularly in women of childbearing age.[95]

Increased Iron Loss

Inadequate intake or gastrointestinal malabsorption of iron is seldom the sole reason for iron deficiency, particularly in the United States; these problems often exacerbate iron deficiency caused by iron loss from bleeding. Therefore, any patient who presents with iron deficiency, with or without anemia, must be evaluated for blood loss. Even menstruating females should be carefully assessed to exclude another explanation for blood loss. A good menstrual history should be obtained; women often believe that their menstrual periods are normal even when bleeding is excessive.[81] A menstrual history should include the number of days of menses, the number of pads or tampons used, and, most important, whether blood clots are present, and particularly if they exceed a couple of centimeters in length. Clots provide objective evidence of excessive bleeding because the amount of hemorrhage has exceeded the lytic capacity of the urogenital tract.

Gastrointestinal bleeding is the most common cause of iron deficiency in men and in nonmenstruating females in developed countries.[96,97] Bleeding may occur anywhere from the posterior pharynx to the anus. Often the source is obvious because of a history of peptic ulcer disease, colitis, or hemorrhoids. In other cases, bleeding is not apparent and is described as "occult." Iron deficiency anemia may be the first evidence of cancers of the gastrointestinal tract, including the esophagus, stomach, small bowel, and colon. Other causes of occult bleeding are intermittent hemorrhage from small arteriovenous malformations; drugs that cause gastric irritation, such as nonsteroidal anti-inflammatory drugs; and esophagitis from reflux disease.

When a patient presents with iron deficiency without an obvious source of blood loss, gastrointestinal evaluation is indicated.[96,97] Several nomograms are available for the initial approach.[8–10] Younger individuals are usually assessed for upper gastrointestinal tract bleeding, whereas older persons should have the lower tract evaluated. Occult bleeding may not be recognized even after numerous stool samples have been collected and both esophagogastroduodenoscopy and colonoscopy have been performed. Other methodologies, such as angiography to find arteriovenous malformations, or newer techniques that utilize swallowed capsules, allowing for visualization of the entire tract, may provide a definitive diagnosis.[98] A trial of iron therapy may be necessary when iron deficiency remains undiagnosed. Failure to respond to iron in spite of adequate absorption suggests active bleeding and the need for reevaluation of the gastrointestinal tract.[99] Blood loss from intermittent gastritis, which may be difficult to detect, can result in an average of 5 mL of blood loss (about 2 mg of iron) per day and can lead to iron deficiency; withdrawal of irritant drugs, such as nonsteroidal anti-inflammatories, or treatment with acid production inhibitors may be diagnostic as well as therapeutic. A negative gastrointestinal evaluation and a complete response to iron therapy at least reassures the patient that a serious condition, such as cancer or arteriovenous malformation, has been excluded.

Other Conditions Associated with Increased Iron Loss

Iron requirements during pregnancy, the combination of iron transfer to the placenta and fetus, postpartum bleeding, and iron loss during lactation result in a net loss of more than 1000 mg of iron.[5,8,82,100] During periods of rapid growth in infants, babies, and adolescents, iron requirements double.[5,101,102]

A combination of factors can cause iron deficiency and result in suboptimal health in many individuals who otherwise appear to be normal. A 15-year-old high school girl can become iron deficient from low caloric intake, a disproportionate decrease in intake of bioavailable iron such as heme iron, menstrual blood loss, and increased iron requirements for growth and strenuous sports. There was a high incidence of iron deficiency in apparently healthy, elite female adolescent volleyball players.[103]

CLINICAL FEATURES

Most of the symptoms attributable to iron deficiency are secondary to anemia. Hemoglobin levels below 9 gm/dL also are associated with a higher risk of heart disease and death, particularly in populations at risk.[104] Studies of erythropoietin effectiveness document that many aspects of quality of life, including functional status, weakness, and overall sense of well-being, are negatively affected by hemoglobin levels below 11 gm/dL.[105]

There is controversy as to whether iron deficiency or even iron depletion causes symptoms in the absence of anemia. Anecdotal evidence suggests that vague complaints such as weakness may be more common in iron-deficient subjects even at hemoglobin levels within the reference range: a woman with a hemoglobin of 13 gm/dL but absent iron stores may have a better sense of "well-being" and feel "more energy" after iron repletion. However, even if a hemoglobin of 13 gm/dL is considered "normal," an increase to 13.8 gm/dL may provide more optimal oxygen efficiency and improvement in symptoms.

Iron depletion may produce defective thermoregulation, particularly abnormalities in thyroid hormone kinetics.[106] Rats that were transfused to normal hemoglobin levels showed improved work performance when body iron content was restored.[107] Iron repletion improves work capacity in iron-deficient females.[108] Achievement of optimal performance, as for athletes, may be an important consideration in iron-depleted individuals.[109]

Neurologic effects of iron deficiency are most pronounced in infants and children.[110] In the rat central nervous system, development of the midbrain has an important iron requirement.[111] Iron deficiency during infancy and early childhood has been associated with sensory deficits, such as auditory recognition, and cognitive deficiencies, including learning problems later in life.[112,113]

Some neuromuscular conditions may be caused or exacerbated by iron deficiency. In restless leg syndrome, involuntary nocturnal leg movements and resulting sleep disturbances[114] can respond to iron even in subjects who are only mildly iron depleted.[114] In hemodialysis patients, involuntary movements decreased after intravenous iron therapy.[115] Involuntary movements during sleep abate after iron supplementation in iron-deficient children[116] and in frequent blood donors.[117]

DIAGNOSIS

Diagnostic studies that demonstrate iron deficiency derive from the biochemical changes associated with iron utilization. For example, decreased iron uptake by cells is evidenced by increased transferrin receptor expression and decreased synthesis of intracellular ferritin.[9] This process is associated with a fall in serum ferritin, a smaller glycosylate form of ferritin that is secreted by the cell, and generally parallels cellular ferritin synthesis.[5,9,10] Levels of serum transferrin receptor, a truncated form of the cellular transferrin receptor, increase as iron deficiency develops.[118] As iron stores decline and as serum iron rises, transferrin synthesis by the liver increases.[9–11] The percentage of transferrin-binding sites saturated with iron decreases as iron deficiency develops.[5,89] When the amount of transferrin-bound iron is not sufficient to maintain red cell production commensurate with red cell loss, iron-deficient erythropoiesis occurs. Decreased erythropoiesis is manifested by reticulocytopenia and smaller cells containing less hemoglobin, described as microcytic

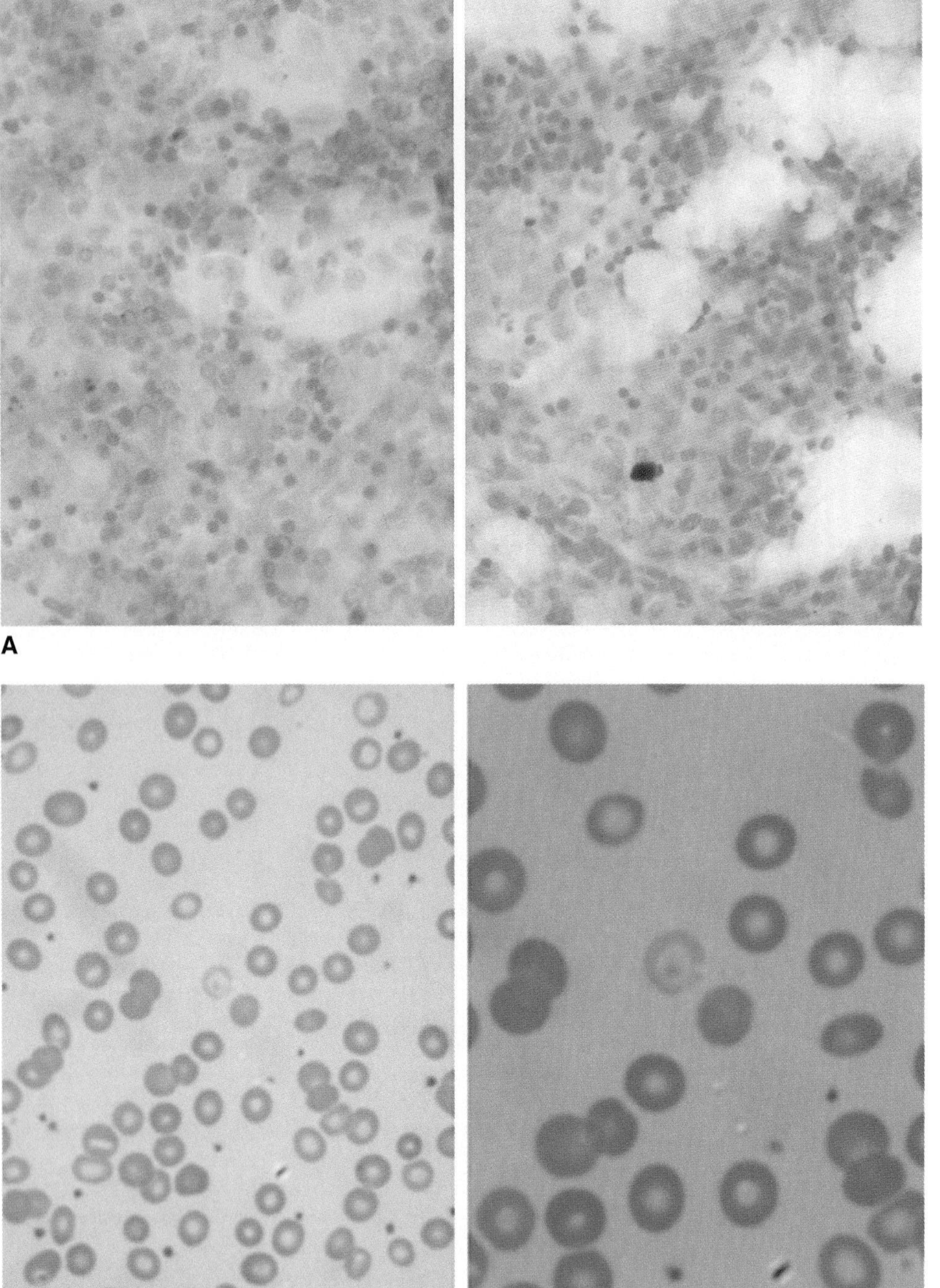

Figure 17–4. Peripheral blood smears in iron deficiency. ***A,*** Prussian blue staining for iron in the bone marrow of an iron-deficient patient is shown on the *left*; lack of stainable iron is demonstrated when compared to an iron-replete individual on the *right*. ***B,*** Low power *(left)* and high power *(right)* views. Because of variation in amount of hemoglobin relative to the degree of iron deficiency, hypochromia is variable. Cells are "floppy" or deformable, and they appear to have a large degree of size disparity when spread on a glass smear. Automated cell counters more correctly measure the most hypochromic cells as small or microcytic.

and hypochromic[119] (Fig. 17–4*A*). Because hemoglobin accounts for 90% of the protein in mature erythrocytes, loss of the osmotic pressure that it exerts in the cell results in a reduction in red cell or mean corpuscular volume[120] (see Fig. 17–4*A*). When hemoglobin levels are at 10–11 gm/dL, the mean corpuscular volume falls below 8 nL. Even earlier, the smaller cell size associated with the more deficient cells increases cell size variability, manifest as a broader red cell distribution width.[121] Newer automated assays that assess the percentage of hypochromic red cells or hypochromic reticulocytes may become useful in the diagnosis of early iron deficiency.[122]

The diagnosis of iron deficiency is based on the absence of iron stores: the standard is a bone marrow examination that shows no discernible iron present in storage cells utilizing the Prussian blue staining technique[10] (Fig. 17–4*B*). Loss of iron stores also is reflected by a serum ferritin concentration below 12 ng/mL[5,10]; because as many as 25% of women of childbearing age are iron deficient, the lower value for the serum ferritin "reference range" of this population may be below 12 ng/mL. The zinc protoporphyrin or erythrocyte protoporphyrin assay[123] can be performed rapidly, is very sensitive, and uses a small amount of whole blood, so it is often used in pediatric populations.[124]

The serum transferrin receptor assay is similar in sensitivity to the serum ferritin assay in the diagnosis of iron deficiency.[118] Serum transferrin receptor testing is especially useful when anemia is associated with a chronic inflammatory state such as infection, tumor, or collagen vascular disease[125] (see Chapter 10). Serum ferritin is an "acute-phase reactant," and, even in the face of iron-deficiency, inflammation can produce extremely high serum ferritin and low serum iron levels. The hormone hepcidin has been implicated as mediator of this low serum iron[126–128]: cytokines increase hepcidin production, which leads to less release of iron from reticuloendothelial cells and decreased intestinal iron uptake (see Fig. 17–1). Chronic inflammatory states increase cytokine production and also cause an inappropriately low erythropoietin response to anemia, and the serum transferrin receptor assay may reveal when iron deficiency coexists. In patients with Still's disease, ferritin values as high as 1000 ng/mL were observed in patients with high serum transferrin receptor levels,[129] but study patients with high transferrin receptor levels responded to parenteral iron therapy.[129] Anemia associated with chronic inflammation may require intravenous iron because the "inflammatory block" adversely affects oral iron absorption. Patients with inflammatory conditions and iron deficiency will often have only a partial hemoglobin response to intravenous therapy even when they are iron replete.[129] Multiple positive test results increase the confidence of the diagnosis of iron deficiency. In a study of geriatric patients who were admitted to the hospital with anemia, among those with serum ferritin levels between 20 and 50 ng/mL (a value that would suggest iron depletion but not deficiency), 95% had absent iron stores on bone marrow examination.[130] Combining two tests can also increase sensitivity and not change specificity: for example, an increased ratio of serum transferrin receptor to serum ferritin values can yield higher sensitivity in the diagnosis of early iron deficiency.[131]

Certain groups at risk often are screened for iron deficiency. Screening is recommended for pregnant women in the third trimester,[132–134] who require 4–6 mg/day to balance iron loss. At 28 weeks, most pregnant women are anemic, partly accounted for by the "hyperhydremia of pregnancy" resulting from increased plasma volume; however, women who are iron deficient at 20 weeks will not show increased hemoglobin level at 32 weeks, typical of iron-replete individuals.[132–134] In children, particularly in developing countries, screening studies often use the erythrocyte protoporphyrin assay because the test is rapid, the equipment relatively inexpensive, and the quantity of blood needed modest.[124] In the United States, iron studies are included during yearly physical examinations or at "health fairs." Some of the low-cost screening arrays contain a serum ferritin assay, whereas others measure only serum iron. If the serum iron is low, a repeat iron and total iron-binding capacity assay should be performed to calculate transferrin saturation. Patients receiving recombinant erythropoietin to treat anemia, particularly renal failure patients, should be regularly tested for iron bioavailability by determining transferrin saturation,[84–86] both before and shortly after the initiation of therapy; phlebotomy for laboratory testing should be obtained at least 48 hours after the last intravenous iron infusion.[84] In general, patients with transferrin saturations below 20% require iron therapy to optimize erythropoietin dosing (see later).

TREATMENT

Some foods are routinely supplemented with iron. In the United States, for example iron has been added to flour since the 1950s.[5,135] When Swedish grain manufacturers ceased iron supplementation to expand exports, the incidence of iron deficiency anemia in Swedish children and women rose sufficiently that the additive was restored for domestic consumption.[136,137] In developed countries, supplementation of other foods is controversial because the bioavailability of added iron is not standardized, raising concerns of iron overload. In developing countries where iron deficiency is much more prevalent, supplementation is appropriate, but treatment for known causes of blood loss[138] and ensuring that supplemented foodstuffs are directed toward rural areas are problems. An innovative approach is genetic engineering either to develop plants that contain more iron or to lower concentrations of inhibitors of iron absorption.[139,140]

In the United States, the Food and Drug Administration provides a recommended dietary allowance of iron: for infants and young children at 10 mg/day; for menstruating females, 15 mg/day; for pregnant females, 30 mg/day; and for all others, 8 mg/day.[5] Supplemental iron is only routinely recommended for pregnant women. The American Gynecologic Society and the Institute of Medicine recommend that pregnant women take a supplement containing 30–60 mg of iron, starting at about 12–14 weeks of pregnancy.[5,141,142] Countries in which iron supplementation is routinely recommended have a lower incidence of anemia among pregnant women.[143,144] Supplementation with lower amounts of iron (20 mg) may be equally efficacious and produce less gastrointestinal toxicities.[145] When a multivitamin-mineral compound is employed for iron supplementation, other components such as calcium carbonate or magnesium oxide may interfere with iron absorption.[146]

Iron deficiency associated with anemia or suboptimal hemoglobin levels requires treatment. Supplemental iron is available in a multitude of oral preparations. Salts that contain 30–70 mg of elemental iron are most commonly used. Most iron salts are sensitive to oxidation, and the tablets must be coated to ensure that the iron salt remains in the more bioavailable ferrous form.[5,10,147] One commonly used preparation, ferrous fumarate, does not need coating, potentially allowing for better bioavailability.[148,149]

Patients receiving supplemental iron should self-administer at least 30–60 mg of elemental iron daily in two to three divided doses.[5,10,147–149] In 1997, the Food and Drug Administration required and then later recommended that all tablets containing 30 mg or more of elemental iron be individually packaged in "blister packs" to decrease the risk of childhood iron poisoning.[150] Pharmacies do not routinely place supplements containing more than 30 mg of elemental iron "over the counter."

Iron-deficient anemic subjects receiving supplemental iron will generally respond with reticulocytosis by 7–10 days after treatment, and an increase in hemoglobin should appear within 2 weeks. The optimal time to measure the hemoglobin level varies depending on the degree of anemia at the initiation of treatment, but once the hemoglobin level has stabilized, an additional 2–3 months of oral iron therapy is recommended to replenish stores.[5,10,148,149]

Failure to respond to iron therapy or a suboptimal response may be due to lack of patient compliance, poor absorption from the gastrointestinal tract, continued blood loss, and/or another cause of anemia, such as an underlying inflammatory state.[10] Occasionally oral supplementation is inadequate because the product itself does not dissolve, as a result of a thick outer coating or overcompression of the tablets during manufacture.[146] Poor compliance is often due to the side effects of oral iron therapy, especially gastric upset and constipation.[145] "Black" stools are often described after beginning iron supplementation, but the color is actually dark green and distinguishable from the characteristic appearance following gastrointestinal hemorrhage. Ingestion of iron supplements with a meal may prevent gastric upset, but food inhibits gastrointestinal absorption. When inadequate gastrointestinal absorption is suspected, an oral iron tolerance test may help.[146,151] Typically, a fasting patient arrives in the office for a baseline (0 hour) serum iron determination, and the supplement containing 30–60 mg of elemental iron is administered under observation; about 3 hours later the patient returns, still fasting, and a posttreatment serum iron level is obtained. The amount of iron absorbed can be estimated from the following formula[146]:

$$\text{Iron absorbed (mg Fe)} = \text{change in serum iron } \mu g/dL \times 0.062 + 0.45$$

An individual receiving about 60 mg of elemental iron should absorb more than 10% of the dose or have a change in serum iron of at least 90 μg/dL or higher.[146] An iron-deficient patient whose absorption is less than 5 mg should have the iron preparation changed, and/or be evaluated for gastrointestinal malabsorption. For poor iron absorption resulting from achlorhydria, alternative therapies including intravenous administration of iron should be considered. A newer iron preparation, possibly more efficacious than iron salts, is heme iron polypeptide; this supplement does not require gastric acidity for absorption and may be better absorbed in conditions that cause a block in iron salt absorption, such as inflammatory states.[152,153]

Table 17–1 contains information related to intravenous iron products. Iron dextran is associated with high rate of both immediate and delayed allergic reactions, including a 0.5–1% incidence of life-threatening anaphylaxis.[154]

TABLE 17–1. Intravenous Iron Products

	Iron Dextran	Ferric Gluconate (Complex in Sucrose)	Iron Saccharate (Iron Sucrose)
Life-threatening reactions	0.5	<0.1	<0.1
Bio-*un*availability	30%	<10%	<10%
Elimination half-life (hr)	48	1	6
Urine elimination (%)	<2	<2	2–10 (variable)
Direct transfer to transferrin	–	–	±
Recommended single dose (mg)	100–1000	125	100

Adapted from Seligman and colleagues[156] and Silverstein and Rodgers.[162]

Newer iron preparations, such as iron saccharate and ferric gluconate, have a negligible risk of severe allergic reactions and may provide more bioavailable iron.[155,156] These newer compounds can be effective in treating iron deficiency unresponsive to oral iron therapy.[155,156]

Erythropoietin increases iron requirements. Kidney failure patients on dialysis, and even those on parenteral dialysis or who are predialysis, need iron supplementation to optimize administered erythropoietin effects. Continued blood loss, as well as poor iron absorption resulting from inflammation and/or the use of drugs that inhibit gastrointestinal absorption, often mandate parenteral iron.[84,86,155–159] Recombinant erythropoietin for cancer patients on chemotherapy and in chronic inflammatory states usually requires iron supplementation, often parenteral.[156,160,161] Despite initial adequate iron availability, a transferrin saturation less than 20% during erythropoietin administration implies a need for supplementation.[160]

CURRENT CONTROVERSIES & FUTURE CONSIDERATIONS

Iron Deficiency

- Will further recognition of the cognitive and performance effects of early iron deficiency lead to more widespread treatment of even nonanemic individuals?
- Will the increased pharmacologic and "off-label" use of erythropoietin lead to a higher prevalence of iron overload following intravenous iron therapy?
- Will iron supplementation that is more bioavailable be deemed necessary in developed countries?

Suggested Readings*

Bridle KR, Frazer DM, Wilkins SJ, et al: Disrupted hepcidin regulation in HFE-associated haemochromatosis and the liver as a regulator of body iron homoeostasis. Lancet 2361:669–673, 2003.

Brownlie T 4th, Utermohlen V, Hinton PS, et al: Tissue iron deficiency without anemia impairs adaptation in endurance capacity after aerobic training in previously untrained women. Am J Clin Nutr 79:437–443, 2004.

Ganz T: Hepcidin. Blood 103:832–838, 2003.

Hallberg L, Hulthen L: Perspectives on iron absorption. Blood Cells Mol Dis 23:562–573, 2002.

Hentze MW, Muckenthaler MU, Andrews NC: Balancing acts: molecular control of mammalian iron metabolism. Cell 30:285–297, 2004.

National Academy of Sciences: Dietary Reference Intakes for Vitamin A, Vitamin K, Arsenic, Boron, Chromium, Copper, Iodine, Iron, Manganese, Molybdenum, Nickel, Silicon, Vanadium, and Zinc. Washington, DC: National Academy of Sciences, 2000.

National Kidney Foundation: DOQI clinical guidelines for the treatment of anemia of chronic renal failure: 2000 update. Am J Kidney Dis 37:S186–S206, 2001.

Rouault TA, Klausner RD: Molecular basis of iron. *In* The Molecular Basis of Blood Diseases (ed 3). Philadelphia: WB Saunders, 2001, pp 363–387.

Full references for this chapter can be found on accompanying CD-ROM.

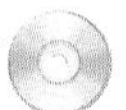

CHAPTER 18

Megaloblastic Anemias: Pernicious Anemia and Folate Deficiency

Sally P. Stabler, MD

KEY POINTS

Pernicious Anemia and Folate Deficiency

Diagnosis

- Cobalamin (vitamin B_{12}) and folate deficiency cause identical megaloblastic anemia.
- Pernicious anemia (autoimmune loss of gastric intrinsic factor) is the most common cause of megaloblastic anemia worldwide, especially in persons of African or European ancestry.
- There is a strong *inverse* correlation between the severity of anemia and neurologic disease in cobalamin deficiency.
- Serum cobalamin and folate assays have poor sensitivity and specificity.
- Elevated methylmalonic acid is the most sensitive indicator of impaired cobalamin status.
- Elevated total homocysteine is a sensitive indicator of either cobalamin or folate deficiency.
- Hyperhomocysteinemia is associated with vascular and cognitive disorders.

Treatment

- High-dose oral cobalamin therapy is as effective as are monthly injections.
- Dietary folate deficiency is rare in the United States and Canada, except in alcoholics or patients with hemolysis, skin disease, or malabsorption or those ingesting antifolate drugs.
- Breast-fed infants of cobalamin-deficient mothers risk disabling neurologic disease.

INTRODUCTION

Megaloblastic anemia refers to anemia, often pancytopenia, with macrocytic red blood cells and hypersegmented neutrophils that is thought to be due to an impairment in DNA synthesis.[1] Causes of both macrocytosis and megaloblastic anemia with macrocytosis are shown in Table 18–1. The clinical distinction between these is subtle and often irrelevant.[2–4] Cobalamin (vitamin B_{12}) deficiency and folate deficiency are the most common causes of severe megaloblastic anemia, and they are indistinguishable pathologically.

PERNICIOUS ANEMIA

Epidemiology and Risk Factors

Pernicious anemia is actually a gastric disorder: chronic atrophic gastritis type A (also known as autoimmune gastritis), which results in achlorhydria and loss of intrinsic factor (IF).[5] Although it is called pernicious *anemia*, cobalamin deficiency may manifest as severe neurologic sequelae—without anemia. A prevalence of 50–200 per 100,000 has been reported for pernicious anemia in Northern Europe and the United States,[6–12] and pernicious anemia was the main cause of severe megaloblastic anemia in reports from Africa,[13] Saudi Arabia,[14] and Hong Kong.[15] Large series from Los Angeles and New York show an even distribution of African-Americans and white Americans, and many Latino patients.[16,17] Pernicious anemia also is frequent among Native Americans.[18] The prevalence of pernicious anemia increases with age,[19] and is possibly as high as 4.3% for elderly African-American women in California.[20] There is often a delay in the diagnosis of pernicious anemia in children and young adults. Patients with pernicious anemia may have other autoimmune disorders, especially thyroid disease and type 1 diabetes mellitus.[7,11,12,21,22]

The recommended dietary allowance for cobalamin in the United States is 2.4µg/day, although omnivorous Western populations often average intakes of approximately twice that amount.[23] Cobalamin is almost exclusively found in food of animal origin, and thus vegetarianism for philosophical reasons or compelled by poverty leads to nutritional cobalamin deficiency.[6] Macrocytosis is often masked by coexisting iron deficiency, which also results from a lack of meat. Dietary cobalamin deficiency is a major problem on the Indian subcontinent and in Mexico, Central and South America, and areas of the Middle East and Africa, but is much less common in China and Southeast Asia.[6]

Pathophysiology

Cobalamin is required for the function of only two enzymes (Fig. 18–1). The block in L-methylmalonyl-CoA mutase activity leads to increased formation of methylmalonic acid (MMA), which is the most sensitive indicator of impaired cobalamin status.[24] The other cobalamin-dependent enzyme, methionine synthase, forms methionine from homocysteine by demethylating *N*-5-methyltetrahydrofolate to tetrahydrofolate. Elevated total homocysteine (tHcy) concentrations are sensitive indicators of either folate or cobalamin deficiency.[17,24,25] Megaloblastic anemia may result from a deficiency of tetrahydrofolate for DNA synthesis, because deficient methionine synthase activity will cause a "trapping" of folate as methylfolate[1,26]; indeed, folate treatment of cobalamin deficiency can correct the megaloblastic anemia.[27] Hematologic findings in florid megaloblastic anemia can be striking (Table 18–2 and Fig. 18–2). The hypercellular bone marrow with large erythroblasts may be so alarming as to lead to a false diagnosis of acute leukemia. The death of many cells in the bone marrow prior to release results in ineffective erythropoiesis[28,29]

TABLE 18–1. Causes of Macrocytosis

Megaloblastic Anemia
Cobalamin (vitamin B_{12}) or folate deficiency and related inborn errors of metabolism
Drugs affecting DNA synthesis: chemotherapy, azathioprine, zidovudine, stavudine
Nitrous oxide—impaired cobalamin metabolism
Pyridoxine- or thiamine-responsive anemia, hereditary orotic aciduria, Lesch-Nyhan syndrome
Other Causes
Reticulocytosis
Liver disease
Alcoholism
Thyroid disorders
Primary marrow disorders (megaloblastoid morphology)
Cold agglutinins
Hyperosmolarity

TABLE 18–2. Hematologic Abnormalities in Cobalamin* or Folate Deficiency

Peripheral Blood
Hypersegmented neutrophils: 1 six-lobed or 5 five-lobed per 100 cells
Oval macrocytosis with or without anemia
MCV higher than normal for the individual patient
Thrombocytopenia and/or leukopenia with immature forms
Basophilic stippling, leukoerythroblastic changes
Bone Marrow
Hypercellular
Giant bands and metamyelocytes
Nuclear-cytoplasmic dyssynchrony
Open and immature nuclear chromatin pattern
Karyorrhexis
Blood Chemistry
Increased indirect bilirubin
Increased lactate dehydrogenase

*Expect mild or no abnormalities in those with cobalamin-deficient neurologic disease.

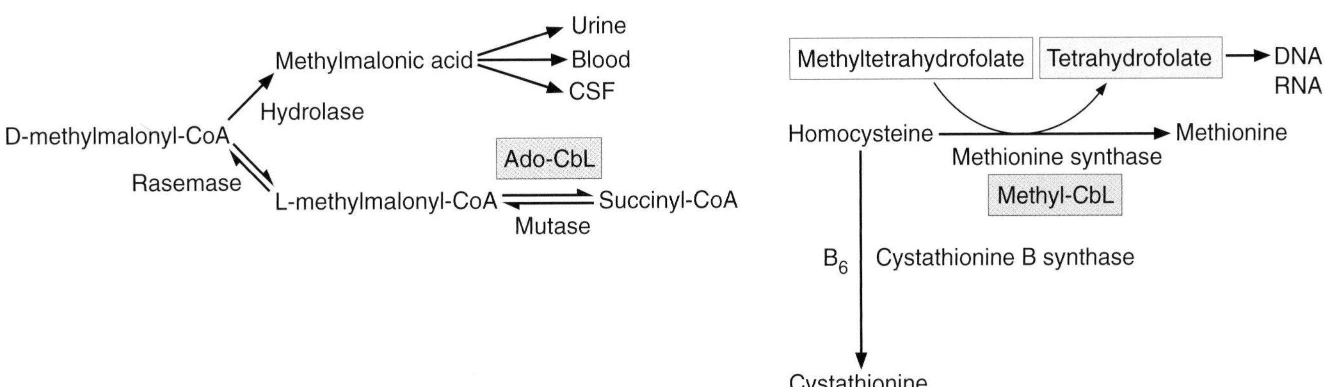

Figure 18–1. The two cobalamin-dependent enzymes, L-methylmalonyl-CoA mutase and methionine synthase are shown. Methionine synthase also requires methyltetrahydrofolate as a cofactor. Abbreviations: Ado-Cbl, adenosylcobalamin; methyl-Cbl, methylcobalamin.

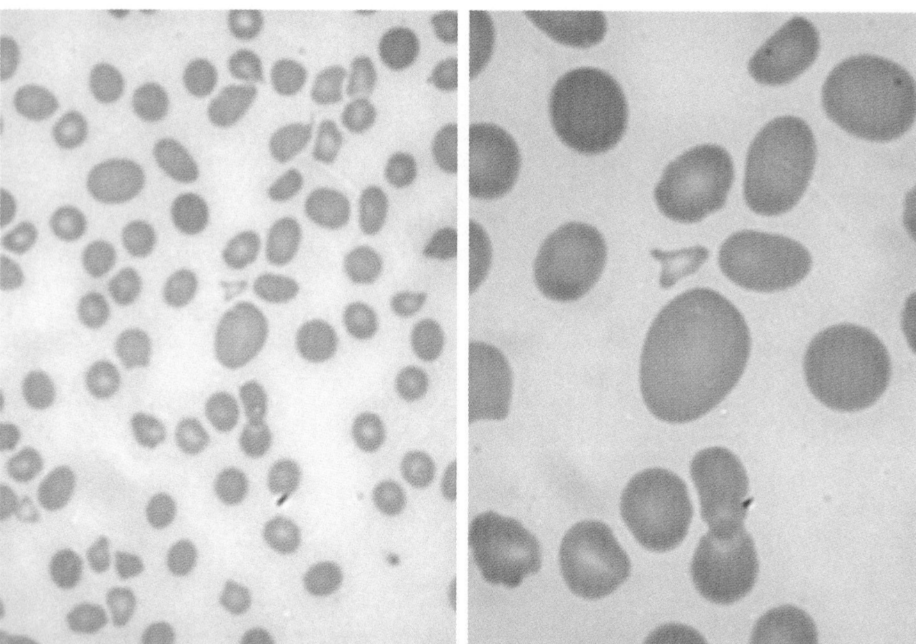

A

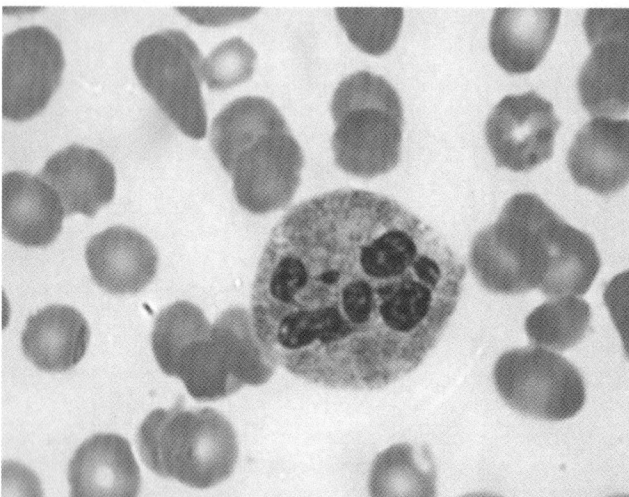

B

Figure 18–2. Characteristic hematologic abnormalities seen in megaloblastic anemia. ***A,*** Macro-ovalocytes and marked anisocytosis are seen under low and high power. ***B,*** A hypersegmented neutrophil with at least six lobes.

and laboratory findings suggestive of hemolysis.[7] Other tissues dependent on rapid proliferation also develop megaloblastic changes[7,17] (Table 18–3).

Cobalamin deficiency, but not folate deficiency, also causes a characteristic demyelinating disease of the central and peripheral nervous system with a pathologic picture of spongy degeneration of the dorsal columns of the thoracic or cervical spinal cord, progressing to the lateral columns or the brain[30–35] (Fig. 18–3). The cause of the neurologic disease is not known,[27,36–39] and patients with severe neurologic disease have elevations of MMA and tHcy similar to those who do not.[36]

TABLE 18–3. Other Clinical Manifestations of Cobalamin and Folate Deficiency

Glossitis
Secondary malabsorption caused by megaloblastic gastrointestinal changes
Weight loss or growth failure
Infertility
Thrombosis
Hyperpigmentation
Immune deficiency

Causes of Cobalamin Malabsorption

Because cobalamin is found in only trace amounts in food, there are elaborate mechanisms for its absorption[40–43] (Fig. 18–4). Requirements for absorption include gastric acid, pepsin, and IF, and the intact ileal receptor complex of cubilin and amnionless with or without megalin.[42–47] The IF-cobalamin complex is internalized in lysosomes,[48] released, and bound to

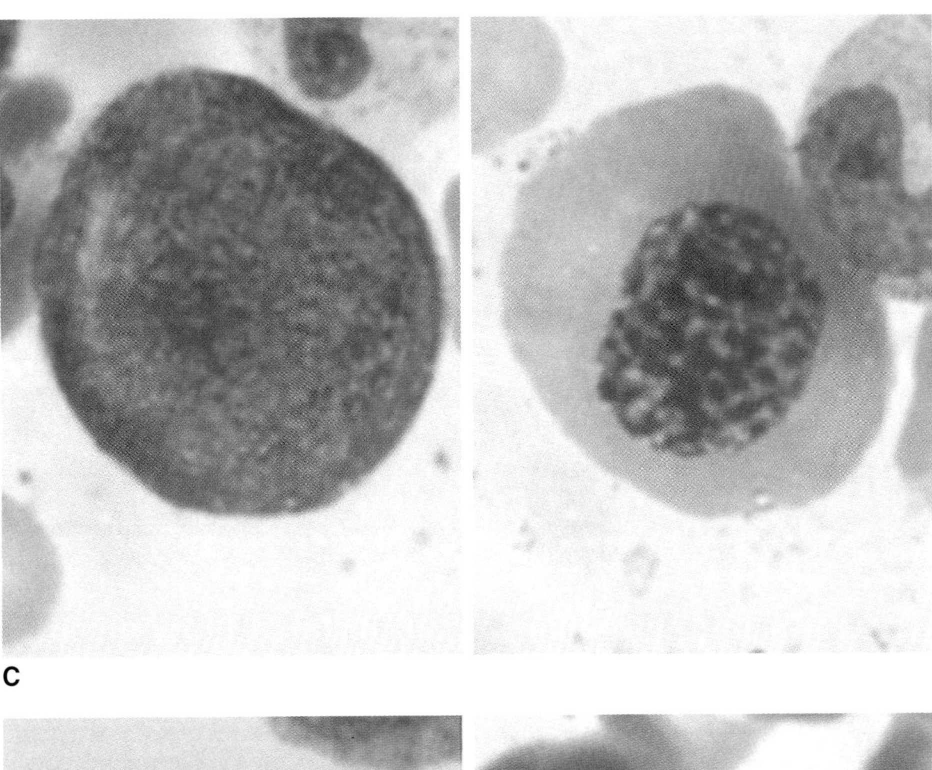

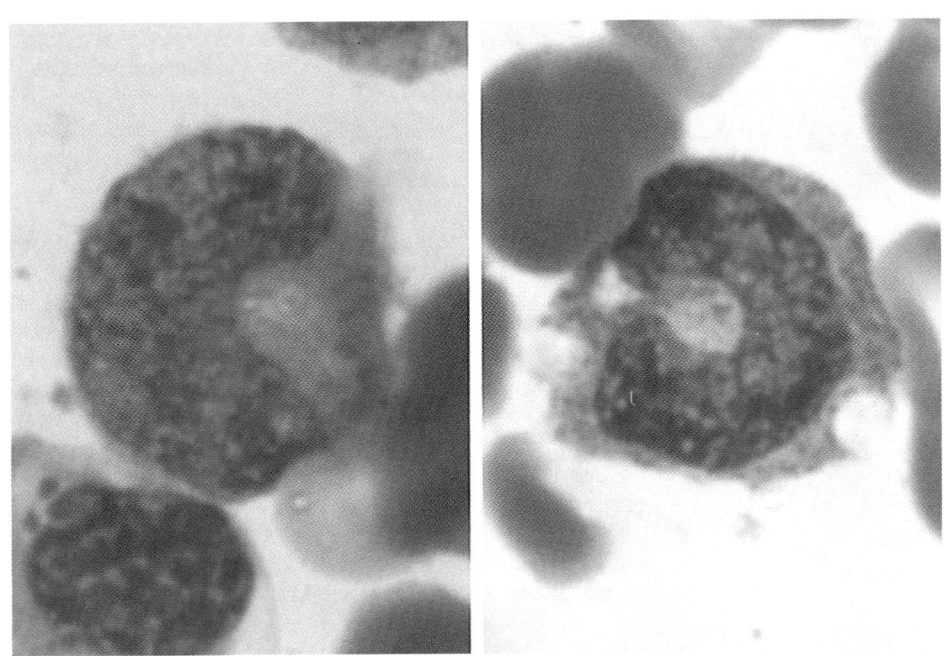

Figure 18–2, cont'd *C*, Megaloblastic pronormoblast *(left)* and megaloblastic polychromatophilic normoblast *(right)*. ***D***, Megaloblastic "giant" metamyelocyte *(left)* and band *(right)*. (Photomicrographs courtesy of John W. Ryder, MD, Department of Pathology, University of Colorado Health Sciences Center, Denver.)

transcobalamin II (TCII).[40] TCII is the physiologic delivery protein, which carries cobalamin to specific TCII receptors on all cells.[40] The enterohepatic circulation is important in conserving cobalamin, because as much as 3–9 µg of cobalamin is released into the bile daily and must be reabsorbed.[40,41] Partial or total gastrectomy,[49,50] gastric or intestinal bypass,[51–57] atrophic gastritis with or without lack of IF,[5,19,43,58–64] chronic pancreatitis, bacterial overgrowth,[43,65,66] parasites,[17,67,68] ileal resection,[69–71] sprue[17,65–67] or inflammatory bowel disease,[72,73] and defects in IF,[74–76] cubilin or amnionless,[42,44–47,77–80] or the intracellular processing of cobalamin[48,81] all will result in cobalamin deficiency. Nitrous oxide,[82–87] metformin,[88–93] and gastric acid–blocking drugs[93–97] may contribute to cobalamin deficiency syndromes.

Clinical Features and Diagnosis

With the exception of neurologic disease, the clinical features of cobalamin deficiency and folate deficiency are similar (see Tables 18–2 and 18–3 and Fig. 18–3). Hypersegmentation of neutrophils and oval macrocytosis are sensitive but not specific indicators of megaloblastic hematopoiesis.[1–4,98–100] Cobalamin or folate deficiency is more likely when the mean corpuscular volume (MCV)

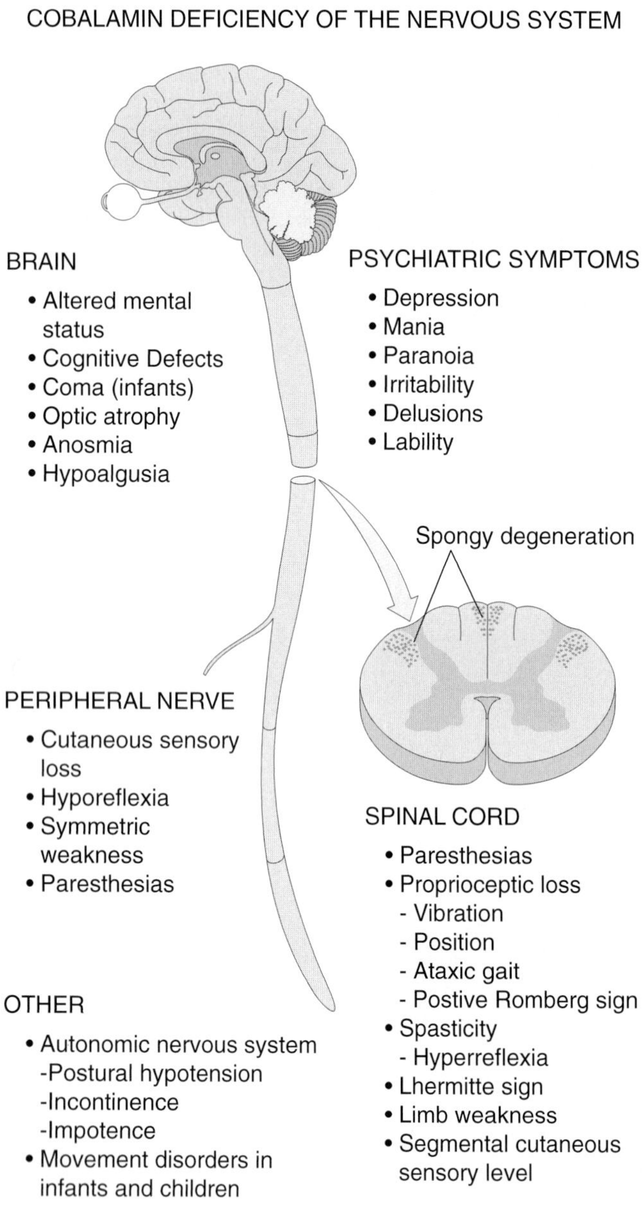

Figure 18–3. Characteristic symptoms and signs seen in cobalamin deficiency of the nervous system are shown along with a schematic demonstration of the spongy degeneration seen in the dorsal and sometimes lateral columns of the spinal cord.

is extremely elevated in the absence of medications[4]; however, no MCV value should be used to exclude megaloblastic anemia because coexisting iron deficiency is extremely common.[6,101] Even a normal MCV may fall after cobalamin or folate treatment.[99]

Unique to cobalamin deficiency is the demyelinating nervous system disease, which is completely reversible if treated early[35,99] (see Fig. 18–3). Paresthesias are the most common symptoms, and patients often have both myelopathy and neuropathy.[35] An important aspect of the neurologic syndrome of cobalamin deficiency is the strong *inverse* correlation with hematologic disease[13,31–33,35,99]: the complete blood count is helpful if abnormal but is otherwise irrelevant in screening for or diagnosing cobalamin-deficient neurologic disease. Magnetic resonance imaging scans show the spongy degeneration as a bright area on T2-weighted imaging,[102–122] which normalizes with treatment. Diffuse high-intensity signal changes can also be seen in the white matter of the brain.[103,106,116,119,121,122] These recently reported cases are notable in that they involve children,[114,116] younger adults,[102,103,105,108–110,117,118] marked delay in diagnosis,[102,103,108–110] occasional nitrous oxide exposure,[107,110,112] usually normal blood counts,[104–106,109,110,112,117,118,121,122] and serum cobalamin in the low-normal range.[105,110,117] Electrophysiology studies are often abnormal in cobalamin-deficient neurologic disease.[35,105,106,116,122–129]

For decades, the diagnosis of vitamin B_{12} deficiency has been made on the basis of a low serum cobalamin concentration. Extremely reduced values (<100 pg/mL) usually correlate with a clinical deficiency syndrome such as megaloblastic anemia or neurologic disease. However, values from 100 to 400 pg/mL overlap with measurements in normal individuals but may be associated with severe cobalamin deficiency.[24,99,100,105,117,122,129–132] False-positive low or low-normal cobalamin values also are frequent with other causes of anemia or neuropathy.[98,133,134] The many different methods for assay of serum cobalamin mean that normal ranges can vary substantially, further confusing issues of sensitivity and specificity.[135–142]

Because of these problems, most experts now recommend documentation of cobalamin deficiency with metabolite testing for serum or urine MMA and/or tHcy.[142–148] Virtually every patient with megaloblastic anemia or a neurologic syndrome that will respond to cobalamin replacement has elevated urine[149–160] or serum MMA.[13,17,24,36,82,98,99,134,161–164] tHcy also is high in the vast majority of patients with clinical cobalamin deficiency.[13,17,24,25,36,98,99,165,166] Tests must be obtained *prior* to treatment because they normalize quickly (Fig. 18–5). Serum MMA and tHcy are often very high in megaloblastic anemia[17]; MMA is usually greater than 500 nmol/L in patients with clinical abnormalities such as megaloblastic anemia. When patients with low serum cobalamin but normal MMA or tHcy values were treated intensively with cobalamin, there was no improvement, in contrast to those with elevated metabolites.[98] The serum MMA was abnormal more often than were serum cobalamin or blood counts in poorly compliant patients with pernicious anemia[24] or when intervals between cobalamin injections were lengthened.[167] tHcy and/or MMA values are elevated in vegetarians without evidence of macrocytic anemia or low serum cobalamin values[168–176]; these elevated MMA values fall and normalize after adequate cobalamin treatment.[24,25,49,82,98,99,101,117,130,134,147,149,151–153,155,157,163,167,177–179] If folate status is adequate, then tHcy also normalizes after adequate cobalamin treatment.[24,25,49,98,99,101,117,130,134,165–167,177–179] Although treatment with folic acid will improve megaloblastic anemia in cobalamin deficiency,[27] neither tHcy or MMA values will be corrected, which is helpful in differential diagnosis.[134]

The mothers of infants with cobalamin deficiency should be investigated for pernicious anemia even if they are asymptomatic and have normal blood counts.

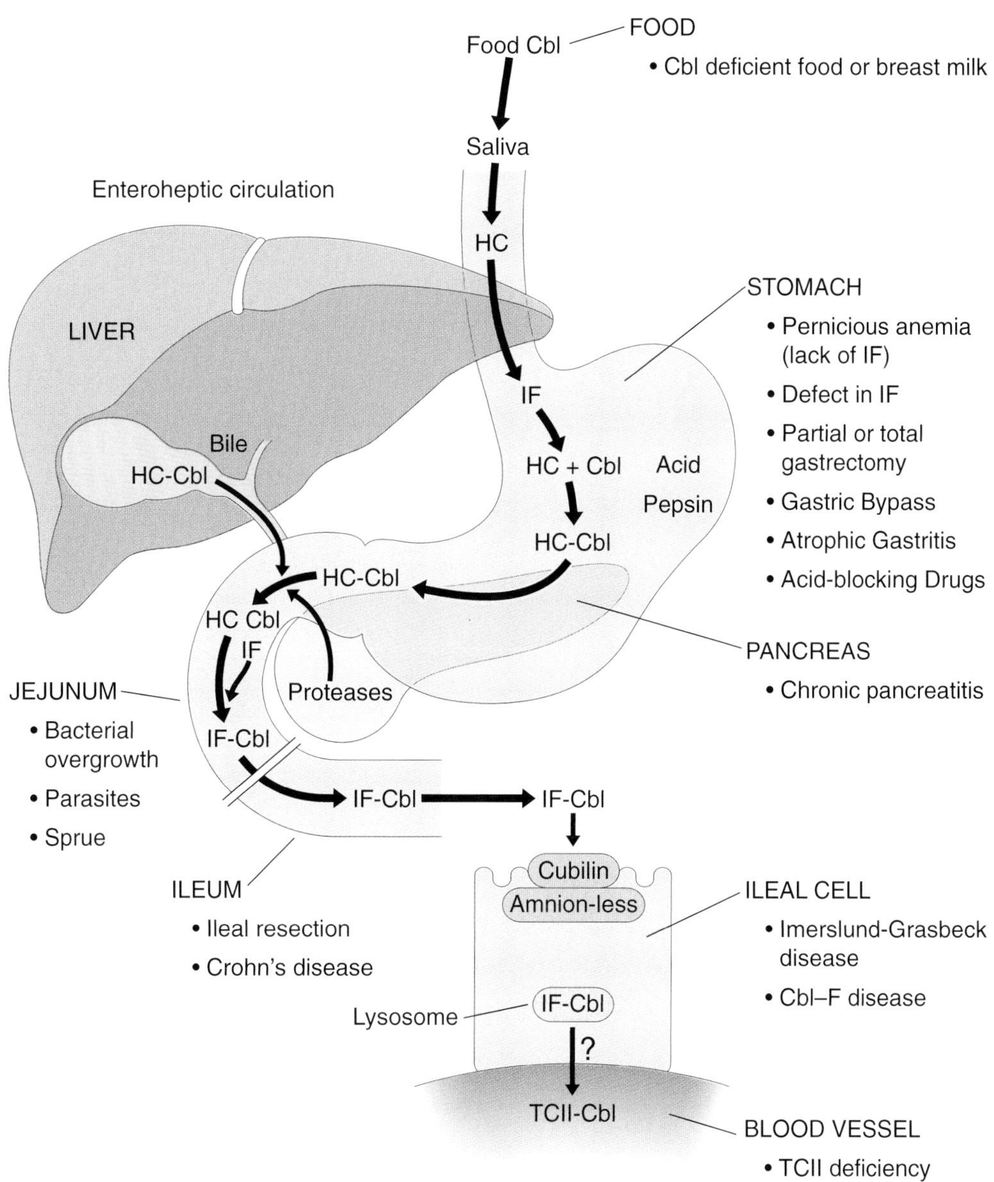

Figure 18–4. The normal processes of cobalamin absorption are shown along with the typical defects causing cobalamin deficiency.

Infants with elevated MMA and/or tHcy values must be evaluated for dietary deficiency versus an inborn error of metabolism.[48,81,116,143,180–183]

Renal insufficiency or failure causes mild elevations of serum MMA, usually less than 800 nmol/L.[184–187] Azotemia commonly coexists with cobalamin deficiency in older persons, and their MMA will decline significantly or normalize after treatment.[162] tHcy also is elevated in subjects with renal failure[188–192] and, like MMA, will decrease with cobalamin[188] and folate[192] treatment.

Recently, methods to measure holo-TCII have become commercially available, but these tests result in some false-positive and false-negative values, similar to the serum cobalamin level compared to standard MMA and/or tHcy assays.[193–195]

Specific serologic and other tests are suggestive of pernicious anemia and atrophic gastritis[5,43,60–64,135,142,144,145,148,167,182,196–199] (Table 18–4). The cobalamin absorption test (Schilling test)[200] utilizes an oral dose of radioactive cobalamin with a flushing unlabeled parenteral dose followed by collection of a 24-hour urine to quantitate the percentage of cobalamin absorbed and excreted (normal >10%).[201] If an abnormal test is corrected with exogenous IF, pernicious anemia is diagnosed. Other causes of malabsorption (including malabsorption caused by megaloblastic change of the gut) will not correct after IF. The Schilling test has become difficult to perform at many hospitals, and the assay has problems with sensitivity.[202] Because the classic Schilling test is normal with milder forms of atrophic gastritis,

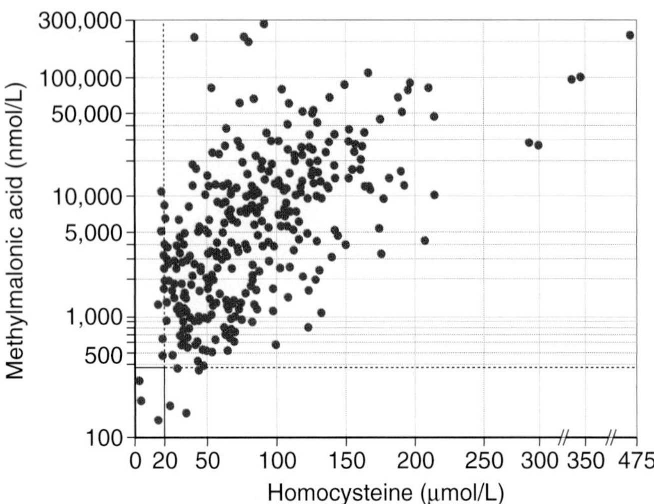

Figure 18–5. Homocysteine and methylmalonic acid values in pernicious anemia. Pretreatment serum total homocysteine is plotted against the serum methylmalonic acid in 313 episodes of megaloblastic anemia caused by cobalamin deficiency. The *dashed lines* indicate 3 standard deviations above the mean for normal controls. There were similar elevations of MMA and tHcy in 121 subjects with neurologic abnormalities who did not have either anemia or macrocytosis.[17] Note that most patients with megaloblastic anemia had serum methylmalonic acid levels greater than 500 nmol/L. (Adapted from Savage DG, Lindenbaum J, Stabler SP, et al: Sensitivity of serum methylmalonic acid and total homocysteine determinations for diagnosing cobalamin and folate deficiencies. Am J Med 96:239–246, 1994.)

TABLE 18–4. Diagnostic Tests for Pernicious Anemia

Test	Comments
Anti–parietal cell antibodies	90% sensitive but not specific
Anti–intrinsic factor antibodies	50% sensitive and very specific; obtain prior to monthly injection
Low serum pepsinogen I (<30 μg/L)	Chronic atrophic gastritis
High serum gastrin (>100 pmol/L)	Achlorhydria with antral sparing
Schilling test, stage 1 and 2	Difficult to obtain and frequent false negatives
Pentagastrin-resistant achlorhydria	Rarely utilized
Endoscopy with biopsy	Reserve for patients with gastrointestinal symptoms

as seen in the elderly,[19,50,58,59,93,127,202,203] modified food cobalamin absorption tests also have been developed[202–207] but again suffer limited sensitivity and specificity as compared to the serum metabolites. Serum antibodies to IF are highly specific for pernicious anemia but only 50–70% sensitive.[4,7,16] The diagnosis of a potential underlying cause for malabsorption does not establish cobalamin deficiency, because malabsorption must exist for many years to produce deficiency. Also, if MMA and/or tHcy are elevated or characteristic clinical abnormalities are apparent, the patient should be treated for deficiency even if an etiology cannot be demonstrated. Because few of the causes of malabsorption can be corrected, there is little enthusiasm for invasive gastrointestinal investigations.

Treatment and Long-Term Management

Any patient with megaloblastic anemia or demyelinating central nervous system disease caused by cobalamin deficiency should be assumed to have malabsorption, with a few exceptions (breast-fed infant or long-standing vegan diet). Treatment must be either parenteral or high-dose oral cobalamin therapy.[167] A regimen of either daily or weekly cyanocobalamin, 1 mg intramuscularly for 4–8 injections followed by 1 mg monthly, is commonly used in the United States. In Europe, hydroxocobalamin every 3–4 months is employed, although this regimen has not been tested with serial MMA concentrations to document adequacy. Nearly 40 years ago it was shown that approximately 1% of a radiolabeled dose of oral cobalamin is absorbed without IF.[208,209] Thus, high oral doses (about 1000 μg vitamin B_{12} daily) have long been used in Europe[210] with complete correction of pernicious anemia.[209–216] Daily oral vitamin B_{12} may be superior to monthly injections. Cobalamin was higher and MMA was lower after 4 months of therapy in a randomized trial; as the interval between the cobalamin injections lengthened, the serum cobalamin concentrations fell and MMA increased and became frankly abnormal.[167] Because cobalamin is inexpensive and nontoxic, it is better to err towards overtreatment. Patients with neurologic abnormalities may require intensive therapy on a weekly or biweekly basis for many months.[35] Whether costs, patient preference, and/or long-term compliance will be improved or worsened using high-dose oral treatment remains controversial.[167,208,216–219] Unfortunately, a major cause of the discontinuation of therapy in the patient with pernicious anemia is physician error[220]; widely available nonprescription high-dose cobalamin tablets enable informed patients to assume responsibility for their treatment.

Infants, children, and young adults should have reassay of MMA and/or tHcy after adequate replacement so that enzyme defects (Cbl-C, TCII) can be distinguished from inborn errors of absorption of cobalamin or juvenile pernicious anemia.[143] Young patients with pernicious anemia often have other severe autoimmune disorders. Gastric cancer, carcinoid tumors, and other gastrointestinal malignancies may be increased in patients with pernicious anemia,[9,221–223] but the need for screening endoscopies is controversial.[9,221,223]

Prognosis

Megaloblastic anemia caused by cobalamin deficiency should completely correct to normal hematologic parameters. Reticulocytosis occurs within days, and patients often produce more than a unit of blood per week after treatment is initiated. If there is no response to cobalamin, another diagnosis must be sought. Many elderly patients have cobalamin and folate deficiency with iron and/or erythropoietin deficiency and do not respond to vitamin B_{12} monotherapy.[101] Coexisting thyroid disorders may increase the MCV and persisting pancytopenia. If elevated MMA and/or tHcy concentrations fall after treatment, then cobalamin treatment must be continued during additional testing.

Unfortunately, the demyelinating nervous system disease is often not completely reversible with cobalamin therapy, although its progression will be halted.[3,35,99,102–105,109,116,118,122] Paresthesias usually respond first[35] and cerebral symptoms may dramatically improve.[224] The more severe and the longer the duration of the symptoms, the poorer the prognosis.[35] Neurologic symptoms recur relatively rapidly in patients with pernicious anemia who stop treatment.[220,225] Infants with nutritional cobalamin deficiency may have permanent neurologic disability.[116,143,183]

Coexisting thrombotic disease resulting from severe hyperhomocystinemia will require additional treatment and serial evaluations (see later).[106,118,226–230]

FOLATE DEFICIENCY

Folate Metabolism and Absorption

"Folate" refers to a group of related compounds that contain tetrahydropteridine linked to *para*-aminobenzoic acid and varying numbers of glutamic acid residues. These folate coenzymes are involved in the synthesis of purines, thymidine, and methionine; the metabolism of formate; and interconversions and reactions of serine, glycine, histidine, and choline.[231,232] The folate role in methionine synthesis is exploited clinically because the level of tHcy is a very sensitive indicator of folate status.[17,142,145,166,233,234] The folates are synthesized largely by plants and are present in vegetable foodstuffs, organ meats, and dairy products. Dietary folates are mostly polyglutamated and must be hydrolyzed prior to absorption in the proximal small intestine.[235–239] The monoglutamated folates are internalized by a reduced folate carrier (RFC-1).[235–237] Atrophic gastritis with hypochlorhydria leads to an increased pH in the upper small bowel and a decrease in folate absorption in the elderly.[240] Synthetic folic acid is more highly bioavailable than are natural folates in food.[241]

Epidemiology and Risk Factors

The United States, Canada, Chile, and Australia introduced grains fortified with folic acid as early as 1998.[242,243] Grain fortification, added folate in supplements and breakfast foods, and the widespread use of multivitamins in the United States and Canada have raised folate values in these populations and virtually eliminated dietary folate deficiency as a cause of megaloblastic anemia or hyperhomocysteinemia.[101,243–256] Dietary folate deficiency continues in populations worldwide whose diet is deficient in green vegetables and dairy products.[257] Megaloblastic anemia occurs only with severe, prolonged folate deficiency.[258–260] If cobalamin status is adequate, the serum tHcy is a very sensitive indicator of the folate intake of an individual or an entire population.[260–262] Mean tHcy values have fallen significantly in the United States and Canada as a result of an increase in folate intake of 200–300 μg/day.[244,246] Folate requirements are high in individuals with increased cellular turnover, as in pregnancy, hemolytic anemia, proliferative skin diseases, and cancers,[259,262] and in those taking medications that affect folate absorption or metabolism, as shown in Table 18–5.[259,261–269] Empirical folic acid to prevent hyperhomocystinemia or macrocytosis in such patients is useful.[263,266,268] Alcohol abuse is probably the most important cause of folate deficiency and the resulting megaloblastic anemia.[17,270–275] Not only is the alcoholic diet deficient, but there is decreased folate absorption and increased renal excretion and some impairment of hepatic metabolism in ethanol abusers.[271,275]

TABLE 18–5. Causes of Folate Deficiency

Diet lacking fruit and vegetables
Alcoholism
Sprue, Crohn's disease, and others
Hemodialysis
Increased cellular proliferation
Pregnancy
Skin diseases
Hemolysis
Malignancies
Drugs
Antifolates: methotrexate, pyrimethamine, sulfasalazine
Anticonvulsants: carbamazepine, phenytoin, and others

Clinical Features and Diagnosis

The megaloblastic anemia caused by pure folate deficiency is indistinguishable from pernicious anemia. However, folate deficiency is frequently accompanied by malnutrition involving other nutrients or abnormalities related to the toxicity of alcoholism.[259,270,272] tHcy is elevated in clinical folate deficiency.[17,24,25,36] The pathophysiology of folate deficiency has been discussed in an earlier section of the chapter.

Deficiency or impairment in folate metabolism is strongly implicated in the incidence of neural tube and other congenital defects.[276–279] Such defects have decreased in Canada and the United States since folate fortification of foods.[278,279] Folate deficiency may also be a risk factor for the development of epithelial and other cancers,[280–282] and neuroblastoma in children also has decreased in Canada.[283] Folate and cobalamin deficiency–induced hyperhomocysteinemia appears to contribute to vascular disease[260–262,284,285] as well as in psychiatric and cognitive disorders.[286,287] Individuals with elevated tHcy have increased mortality rates[288,289] and cardiovascular or cerebrovascular events.[289]

A variety of methods are used to measure serum and red blood cell folate, and there is often poor concordance of results.[290,291] Folate levels suffer from a lack of sensitivity and specificity in diagnosing clinical syndromes, analogous to the serum cobalamin values. For instance, approximately 25% of 123 subjects with folate-responsive megaloblastic anemia had serum folate in the low-normal range (between 2 and 4 ng/mL), yet 97.5% had elevated tHcy.[17] Since folate fortification of foods in the United States and Canada, serum folate concentrations have risen dramatically and some subjects have detectable folic acid, an unnatural form of folate in the blood.[290] The red blood cell folate assay is not recommended: the methodology is often problematic[290,291] and levels are frequently low in severe cobalamin deficiency and therefore fail to distinguish between the two disorders. The serum tHcy is more sensitive in detecting impaired folate status and is widely available from clinical laboratories[17,24,25,26,166]; tHcy is very useful in detecting drug- or alcohol-induced folate deficiency. If folate deficiency is the cause of hyperhomocysteinemia, tHcy should normalize, usually into the low-normal range,[24,164] after treatment.

A common polymorphism of methylenetetrahydrofolate reductase (677C→T), which in homozygous form (*TT*) is found in 10–30% of persons of European or Asian ancestry (rarely in Africans), increases tHcy *only* when there is deficiency of folate intake[292]; the polymorphism does not cause hyperhomocysteinemia in folate-sufficient populations. The methylenetetrahydrofolate reductase effect probably is not associated with an increased risk of vascular or thrombotic disease.[293,294] Unfortunately, testing for the polymorphism has become widespread in clinical medicine as part of the evaluation for thrombotic disease. Potential cobalamin deficiency must be investigated in every case of hyperhomocysteinemia in order to prevent tragic occurrences such as treating a cobalamin-deficient nursing mother with only folic acid.

Treatment

Folate-deficient megaloblastic anemia is treated with folic acid 1 mg/day orally, with full recovery within several months.[259] All women of childbearing age should take a supplement containing at least 400 µg of folic acid to prevent neural tube defects.[23] Patients with increased folate requirements can be treated with folic acid 1 mg per day orally. Folate-deficient patients without exposure to suspicious drugs or to alcohol should be investigated for sprue and other gastrointestinal disease because dietary folate deficiency is now so unlikely in the United States or Canada. Folate treatment can be halted when the underlying disease is corrected. Children with severe folate deficiency should be studied for congenital defects of folate absorption or metabolism.[143]

HYPERHOMOCYSTEINEMIA

Serum tHcy is frequently measured during the evaluation of hypercoagulability or cardiovascular disease.[261,295,296] If tHcy is elevated, cobalamin deficiency must be excluded by assay of serum or urine MMA (Table 18–6); if the MMA is elevated, cobalamin treatment is indicated. A normal MMA and a tHcy greater than 50 µmol/L suggest classic homocystinuria (and other inborn errors), which deserves measurement of cystathionine[189] and methionine and referral to a genetics clinic. The hyperhomocysteinemia commonly seen in older patients with vascular and cognitive disease, sometimes also associated with renal insufficiency, is best treated with both folic acid (0.4–5 mg) and high-dose oral cobalamin (at least 1000 µg), with some advocating vitamin B_6 also.[101,167,177–179,192,295–299] Whether lowering elevated homocysteine with combinations of folate, cobalamin, and vitamin B_6 therapy decreases vascular events remains unknown, although homocysteine is readily normalized in nondialysis patients. Results of homocysteine-lowering treatment protocols have been mixed, and further recommendations await results of large randomized trials.[297–299]

TABLE 18–6. Use of Metabolites in Vitamin Deficiency

Consider testing if serum cobalamin <400 pg/mL or folate <5 ng/mL
If methylmalonic acid is elevated, then cobalamin is deficient
If homocysteine is elevated, then *either* or *both* cobalamin and/or folate is/are deficient
If homocysteine >50 µmol/L *and* cystathionine is low, then cystathionine β-synthase (classic homocystinuria) should be investigated

CURRENT CONTROVERSIES & FUTURE CONSIDERATIONS

Pernicious Anemia and Folate Deficiency

- Should cobalamin deficiency be treated with high-dose oral daily versus monthly parenteral cobalamin?
- Do asymptomatic cobalamin-deficient subjects with metabolic abnormalities require treatment?
- Does lowering homocysteine prevent thrombotic and other cardiovascular events?
- Is it cost-effective to screen for gastrointestinal cancer in patients with pernicious anemia?
- Should foods be fortified with cobalamin in addition to folic acid?

Suggested Readings*

Healton EB, Savage DG, Brust JC, et al: Neurologic aspects of cobalamin deficiency. Medicine 70:229–245, 1991.

Klee GG: Cobalamin and folate evaluation: measurement of methylmalonic acid and homocysteine vs vitamin B_{12} and folate. Clin Chem 46:1277–1283, 2000.

Kuzminski AM, Del Giacco EJ, Allen RH, et al: Effective treatment of cobalamin deficiency with oral cobalamin. Blood 92:1191–1198, 1998.

Refsum H, Smith AD, Ueland PM, et al: Facts and recommendations about total homocysteine determinations: an expert opinion. Clin Chem 50:3–32, 2004.

Savage DG, Lindenbaum J, Stabler SP, Allen RH: Sensitivity of serum methylmalonic acid and total homocysteine determinations for diagnosing cobalamin and folate deficiencies. Am J Med 96:239–246, 1994.

Full references for this chapter can be found on accompanying CD-ROM.

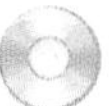

CHAPTER 19

Anemia of Chronic Disease

Robert T. Means, Jr., MD

KEY POINTS

Anemia of Chronic Disease

- Chronic disease is the most common etiology of anemia other than that resulting from blood loss with or without consequent iron deficiency.
- A significant minority of patients with anemia of chronic disease (ACD) will not suffer from chronic infectious, inflammatory, or neoplastic disease.
- ACD is a response to the cytokines involved in the host response to inflammation, infection, or malignancy.
- The first treatment should be aimed at the associated disease or clinical syndrome.
- Erythropoietin therapy is effective in ACD.
- Iron supplementation is a necessary adjunct to erythropoietin therapy in ACD.

INTRODUCTION

Anemia of chronic disease (ACD) describes a persisting anemia syndrome that is typically (although not exclusively) observed in patients with underlying infectious, inflammatory, or neoplastic disorders. Hypoferremia in the presence of adequate reticuloendothelial iron stores is characteristic of ACD. ACD does not include anemias caused by marrow replacement, blood loss, renal failure, hemolysis, hepatic disease, or endocrine deficiencies, even when these disorders are chronic. The term also may be used to describe the hypoproliferative, normocytic, hypoferremic anemia that is frequent in patients in intensive care units and during acute infections.

As ACD does not include all anemias observed in diseases that are chronic but does include some anemias that occur acutely has led to a general dissatisfaction with the syndrome's name.[1] However, use of the term remains in the absence of an adequate substitute. Alternatives have been proposed—"anemia of inflammation," "anemia of infection," and "anemia of cancer"; pathophysiologic descriptors such as "cytokine-mediated anemia" or "anemia of defective iron utilization"; and purely descriptive phrases such as "hypoferremic anemia with reticuloendothelial siderosis" or "thesauric hypoferremic anemia"[2–4]—none of which has gained general acceptance.

EPIDEMIOLOGY AND RISK FACTORS

ACD is probably the most frequent etiology of anemia other than blood loss with resultant iron deficiency.[5] When all the anemic patients without blood loss admitted to the medical service of an urban hospital at the Baylor College of Medicine in Texas were evaluated, 52% of them met laboratory diagnostic criteria for ACD: a low serum iron level and normal or elevated serum ferritin.[6]

The major risk factors for ACD are infections, inflammatory disorders, and malignancies. The precise frequency of ACD varies with clinical circumstances. In patients with infections, ACD is particularly common when the clinical course is longer than a month. Infections associated with ACD include tuberculosis, empyema and lung abscess, osteomyelitis, subacute bacterial endocarditis, cellulitis, and chronic fungal infections, as well as human immunodeficiency virus infection.[7,8] In patients with tuberculosis, anemia is apparent in 60–75% of those with active pulmonary disease[9,10] and in slightly more than half of patients with extrapulmonary or disseminated disease.[11,12] In a large single-institution series, 89 of 135 patients (65%) with infective endocarditis had hemoglobin concentrations less than 12 gm/dL; anemic individuals with infected prosthetic valves were more likely to have hemoglobin concentrations greater than 10 gm/dL than were patients with endocarditis involving native valves or in the setting of intravenous drug abuse.[13] Eighty percent of reported patients with pneumococcal vertebral osteomyelitis were also anemic.[14] In a survey of acutely infected pediatric

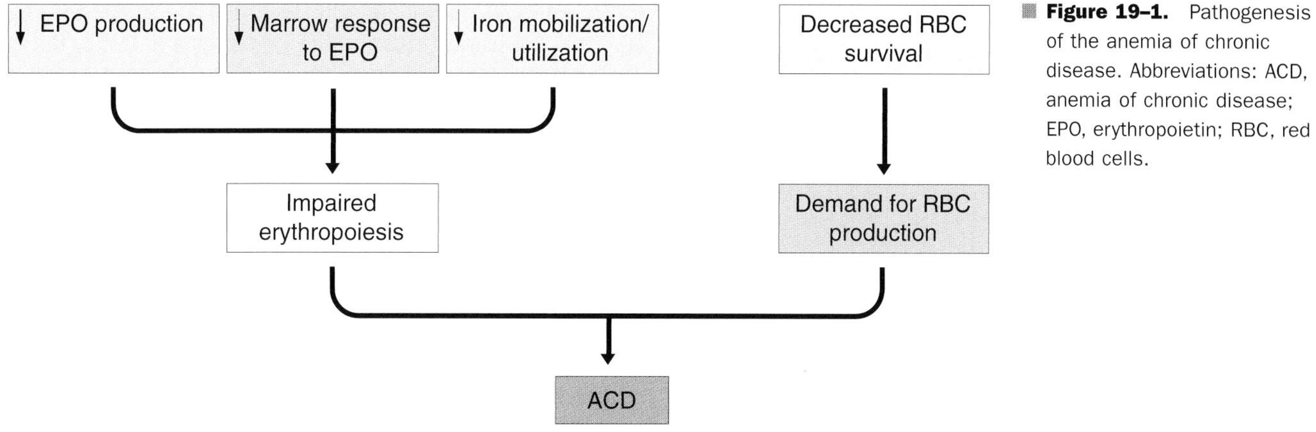

Figure 19–1. Pathogenesis of the anemia of chronic disease. Abbreviations: ACD, anemia of chronic disease; EPO, erythropoietin; RBC, red blood cells.

outpatients, 17% of children under 4 years of age and 5% of children between ages 4 and 12 were anemic.[15]

In the series from Texas, more than 80% of anemic patients with inflammatory syndromes had ACD.[6] A lower frequency is typically reported in series of patients with specific disorders. ACD was present in 27% of outpatients followed for rheumatoid arthritis,[16] and in more than 50% of newly diagnosed patients admitted to inpatient rheumatology services.[17] ACD accounted for 37% of diagnoses in anemic lupus patients.[18] In general, ACD appears more frequent among inpatients compared to outpatients.

In a series of unselected anemic hospitalized cases, 19% of ACD patients had a nonhematologic malignancy.[6] The frequency of ACD in specific malignant syndromes is difficult to define because anemia reflects underlying processes characteristic of the diseases. For example, the vast majority of anemias in colon cancer (particularly at early stages) are secondary to blood loss, with or without iron deficiency. In solid tumors without blood loss, ACD is likely to be the dominant anemia syndrome, particularly early in the course. In the Baylor series, 23% of anemic patients had a solid tumor; 44% met the study's criteria for ACD.[6] In a series of solid tumor patients referred for radiation therapy,[19] approximately half were anemic, and three fourths of the patients whose anemia was investigated further had ACD.

For hematologic malignancies, the situation is complicated by the potential effect of marrow infiltration and replacement, more prevalent than in solid tumors. About 40% of patients with Hodgkin's disease are anemic at presentation, with the majority of cases attributed to ACD.[20] For non-Hodgkin's lymphomas, anemia is initially present in 32% of patients[21] and similarly attributed to ACD. In multiple myeloma, anemia is found at diagnosis in 73% of cases,[22] but it is difficult to distinguish anemia due to marrow replacement and the proportion suffering anemia due to suppressive effects of cytokines.[23] The same pathophysiologic considerations exist for hairy cell leukemia.[24,25]

Of importance, 40% of ACD patients lack an association with a "traditional" infectious, inflammatory, or neoplastic disorder.[6]

PATHOPHYSIOLOGY

For 50 years it has been known that there are three pathophysiologic processes involved in ACD: a modest shortening of red cell survival that creates an increased demand for red cell production; an impaired erythropoietic response to this demand; and the abnormalities of iron metabolism that are the diagnostic hallmark of ACD (Fig. 19–1). The observation of a blunted erythropoietin (EPO) response to anemia in both rheumatoid arthritis and cancer provided an explanation for the poor marrow response to anemia.[26,27] However, although anemic patients with ACD do not achieve the increments in EPO production observed in similarly anemic patients with iron deficiency, they have circulating EPO concentrations higher than in healthy individuals who are not anemic.[26] ACD erythroid progenitors thus exhibit a degree of cellular "EPO resistance."

Not all of the pathophysiologic processes involved in ACD are implicated equally in all clinical situations. In children with cancer, the EPO concentration was appropriate for the degree of anemia observed[28]; the major contributor to the anemia appeared to be an impaired erythropoietic response to EPO.[28] Adult lung cancer patients also exhibit a blunted EPO response.[29] In contrast, inadequate availability of iron for erythropoiesis was dominant in the anemia of juvenile rheumatoid arthritis.[30]

A challenge to the investigation of the pathogenesis of ACD is to identify a mechanism that would link the diverse associated syndromes. The observation that the presence of ACD correlated with the activity of the associated disease[16,31] led investigators to consider mediators of the immune and inflammatory responses, such as tumor necrosis factor (TNF),[32] interleukin (IL)-1,[33] and the interferons (IFNs)[34–36] as responsible agents. Concentrations of these cytokines are increased in patients with disorders associated with ACD[36–40] and in animal models of ACD,[41] and their therapeutic administration to patients may result in anemia as well.[42,43] These mediators, other cytokines such as IL-6, and the cytokine second messengers nitric oxide and ceramide, have been implicated in all the pathophysiologic mechanisms associated with ACD.[44]

Shortened Red Cell Survival

Anemic patients with rheumatoid arthritis (a widely used model for ACD) show an inverse correlation between IL-1 levels and red cell survival.[45] Similar results were reported in mice following exposure to TNF in vivo.[46] As will be discussed later in more detail, various cytokines have been shown to decrease EPO production in response to physiologic stimuli. The recent demonstration that a reduction in EPO availability results in selective hemolysis of the youngest red cells (neocytolysis) provides another mechanism for the shortened red cell survival observed in ACD.[47] Increased generation of peroxynitrite (a byproduct of the cytokine messenger nitric oxide) in red cells may enhance membrane rigidity and shorten red cell survival.[48]

Impaired Marrow Response

As noted earlier, the inability of the marrow to compensate for the modest reduction in red cell lifespan seen in ACD results from the combination of an impaired EPO response to anemia and relative inability of the erythroid progenitors to respond to EPO.

Impaired EPO Production

Typically there is an inverse relationship between serum or plasma EPO levels and hemoglobin: as the hemoglobin decreases, the EPO level rises.[49] A similar inverse relationship between hemoglobin and EPO level was observed in anemic rheumatoid arthritis patients,[26] but for any given anemic individual with rheumatoid arthritis, the EPO level was lower than that found in equally anemic individuals with iron deficiency. Thus the EPO response to anemia was blunted in rheumatoid arthritis; similar results have been reported in anemic patients with cancer.[50] This impaired EPO response appears to be cytokine-mediated. IL-1, TNF-α, and transforming growth factor-β inhibit production of EPO in vitro by hepatoma cell lines exposed to hypoxia or by isolated perfused rat kidneys.[51,52]

Impaired Marrow Progenitor Response to EPO

Although the EPO levels of patients with ACD are not as high as those in equally anemic iron-deficient individuals, these values are still higher than in normal individuals who are not anemic. Another factor likely contributes to the impaired erythropoiesis associated with ACD. TNF, IL-1, and the IFNs all have been reported to inhibit erythroid colony formation in vivo and in vitro.[37,53–62]

Using highly purified human erythroid progenitors, the mechanisms of inhibition effects have been clarified. Recombinant human (rh) TNF was found to inhibit colony formation by erythroid colony-forming units (CFU-E) from bone marrow mononuclear cells (containing approximately 2 CFU-E/1000 cells) in a dose-dependent fashion; however, colony formation by highly purified CFU-E generated from peripheral blood cells (containing approximately 300 CFU-E/1000 cells) was not affected, indicating that rhTNF action was indirect, likely mediated by a marrow accessory cell resident in marrow stromal.[63] Inhibition was mediated by soluble factors released from stroma, including IFN-β.[64] Similarly, the inhibitory effect of rhIL-1 on CFU-E colony formation was also shown to be indirect and dependent on IFN-γ released from T lymphocytes.[65] As discussed later, treatment of ACD patients with rhEPO can result in an increased hemoglobin concentration. The in vitro inhibitory effect of rhIFN-γ, but not of IFN-β, can be reversed at high supraphysiologic concentrations of rhEPO[66,67]; explaining heterogeneity of the response to treatment with rhEPO in ACD patients.

rhIFN-γ induces apoptosis in CFU-E, a process that requires Fas activation.[68] Ceramide, a product of sphingomyelin hydrolysis, is a mediator of the apoptotic effects of TNF, IL-1, and IFN-γ and is frequently implicated in Fas-mediated events. Either endogenous ceramide, produced by exposure to bacterial sphingomyelinase, or exogenous cell-permeable ceramide significantly inhibits bone marrow CFU-E-derived colony formation. Exposure of marrow cells to rhIFN-γ led to a significant increase in ceramide content, suggesting a role for ceramide.[69] Nitric oxide, another potential second messenger in cytokine effects, directly inhibits erythroid colony formation in vitro.[70]

Cytokines may alter the expression of hematopoietic growth factor receptors during erythroid development as well. Exposure to 2500 U/mL rhIFN-γ in vitro resulted in a decrease in erythroid progenitor receptors for EPO and stem cell factor, but not insulin-like growth factor-I, probably mediated at the gene translation level.[71]

Impaired Mobilization of Reticuloendothelial Iron Stores

The impaired iron mobilization of ACD may also result from cytokine effects. A correlation between the immune activation marker neopterin and increasing ferritin levels in patients with malignancies suggests a role for immune activation in altered iron metabolism.[72] Rodents injected with recombinant TNF develop hypoferremic anemia associated with impaired reticuloendothelial iron release and incorporation into erythrocytes.[46,73] IL-1 increases translation of ferritin messenger RNA (mRNA), and additional ferritin could act as a trap for iron that might otherwise be available for erythropoiesis.[74] The acute-phase reactant protein α_1-antitrypsin inhibited erythropoiesis by impairing transferrin binding to transferrin receptor (TfR) and subsequent internalization of the TfR-transferrin complex.[75]

Hepcidin, or liver-expressed antimicrobial peptide-1 (LEAP-1), is a 25–amino acid liver-derived peptide with antimicrobial effects found in human blood and urine.[76,77] Hepcidin is a major factor in innate immunity and its structure is highly conserved among mammalian species, suggesting a key role in major biologic functions.[78] Induced iron overload leads to hepcidin mRNA overexpression in hepatocytes,[79] presumably a regulatory response defending against adverse effects of iron overload (see Chapter 56). Knockout mice lacking hepcidin exhibit severe parenchymal iron deposition.[80] In physiologic iron balance, hepcidin enhances iron uptake and retention by reticuloendothelial cells in the duodenal crypts while decreasing dietary iron absorption.[81] Hepcidin production and regulation are abnormal in hereditary hemochromatosis.[82,83] In compensated hemochromatosis urinary hepcidin excretion is normal, whereas hepcidin is elevated in patients with iron overload.[84]

In a mouse model, anemia (whether caused by acute hemolysis or iatrogenic blood loss) was associated with decreased hepatic hepcidin gene expression; hypoxia, which also increases demand for red cell production, had a similar effect.[85] A single turpentine injection, used to induce an inflammatory state,[86,87] in wild-type mice produced a sixfold increase in hepcidin mRNA, as well as a marked decrease in serum iron concentration; when hepcidin-deficient mice were injected with turpentine, however, the anticipated drop in iron concentration did not occur.[85] Low serum iron concentrations observed in inflammatory or cytokine activation states[73] was inferred to be mediated by hepcidin induction.

In humans, a cohort of patients with type 1a glycogen storage disease with large hepatic adenomas had a microcytic anemia associated with hypoferremia, refractory to iron therapy. This anemia was dependent on the presence of the adenomas, because their removal by resection or liver transplantation normalized hemoglobin concentrations.[88] Evaluation of hepcidin mRNA expression in the liver tissue from these patients showed a marked increase within the adenomas but not in adjacent normal tissue.[88] These findings support a crucial role for hepcidin in the pathogenesis of ACD. Inflammatory cytokines associated with ACD were similarly expressed in normal liver tissues as they were in the adenomas.[88] However, the clinical picture observed in these patients was not identical to ACD: the degree of anemia and hypoferremia was compatible with ACD, but the degree of microcytosis was greater and the ferritin values lower than in typical ACD.

Urinary hepcidin (normalized to creatinine) has been evaluated in patients with iron overload, compensated hemochromatosis, iron deficiency anemia (IDA), and "anemia of inflammation," defined as anemia with an elevated serum ferritin concentration in an appropriate clinical setting.[84] Urinary hepcidin excretion was strongly correlated with serum ferritin concentration, and, in a patient with epididymitis and sepsis, decreased from initially elevated level as the clinical syndrome improved. IL-6 and lipopolysaccharide induced hepcidin mRNA within 8 hours of exposure, whereas IL-1 and TNF had no similar effects.[84] This induction pattern indicates that hepcidin is a type II acute-phase protein.[84]

In measurements of hepcidin in stored sera from anemic patients undergoing diagnostic bone marrow examination and in samples submitted for ferritin determination, a very strong and similar correlation was observed between serum ferritin and hepcidin concentrations.[89] However, no correlations between serum hepcidin and any other laboratory parameters reflected iron status or degree of anemia, nor could the etiology of the anemia be related to the hepcidin concentration.[89]

In total, these studies suggest that hepcidin may be the major factor regulating iron abnormalities in ACD, but it is unclear if hepcidin measurements will be more specific than ferritin in the diagnosis of this syndrome.

CLINICAL FEATURES AND DIAGNOSIS

ACD is typically a mild or moderate anemia. In older series, hemoglobin concentrations less than 9 gm/dL were present in fewer than 5% of cases[90]; in more recent reports, approximately one quarter of patients have very low hemoglobin concentrations.[6,16] ACD is usually normocytic, but microcytosis is observed in 20–30% of cases.[6,16,19] Although the reticulocyte count expressed as a percentage of erythrocytes may be normal or only slightly decreased, the reticulocyte production index is invariably low. The erythrocyte sedimentation rate is typically elevated.[92,93] Bone marrow morphology is usually normal in ACD. The underlying inflammatory or infectious disorder may alter the relative proportions of cells in the marrow differential, causing a mildly increased myeloid-to-erythroid ratio or a reactive plasmacytosis.[7]

The diseases associated with ACD produce quantitative abnormalities in a variety of serum or plasma proteins. Transferrin (often reported as total iron-binding capacity [TIBC]) is decreased,[90] as may be serum albumin.[92] In contrast, C-reactive protein levels and polyclonal globulin concentrations are usually elevated.[92,94] In general, nonerythroid, noniron abnormalities are characteristic of the associated disease.

Although the term *anemia of inflammation* has been used to describe anemias with an infectious, inflammatory, or neoplastic syndrome and an elevated serum ferritin, without reference to iron concentration,[84] the strict diagnosis of ACD requires demonstration of a hypoproliferative anemia, in which the serum or plasma iron concentration is low despite adequate reticuloendothelial iron stores.

DIFFERENTIAL DIAGNOSIS

The major objective of diagnostic evaluation is to demonstrate the presence of iron stores in a hypoferremic patient, and the major syndrome from which ACD must be distinguished is iron deficiency anemia (Table 19–1). Patients with an ACD-associated illness also may have iron deficiency anemia as a primary diagnosis, or ACD and iron deficiency may coexist. In series evaluating iron stores in anemic patients with chronic inflammatory rheumatic diseases by bone marrow examination, the frequency of iron deficiency was 25–30%.[16,95] When iron deficiency was defined by an elevated serum soluble transferrin receptor (sTfR) concentration, its frequency was about 50%.[96,97] As discussed later, the sTfR test has limited utility when the serum ferritin is elevated.

Decreased serum iron concentration is one of several parameters that may lead to confusion between ACD and iron deficiency anemia. Serum TIBC and/or transferrin concentration is traditionally said to be elevated in IDA and normal or decreased in ACD; however, in a recent multicenter study involving complicated patients, only 1

TABLE 19–1. Laboratory Characteristics of ACD, IDA, and IDA with Inflammation

	ACD	Iron Deficiency Anemia	Iron Deficiency Anemia with Inflammation
Mean corpuscular volume	72–100 fL	<85 fL	<100 fL
Mean corpuscular hemoglobin concentration	<36 gm/dL	<32 gm/dL	<32 gm/dL
Serum iron	Decreased	Decreased	Decreased
Serum total iron-binding capacity (TIBC)	Typical below mid-normal range	Elevated	Less than upper limit of normal range
TIBC saturation	2–20%	<15% (usually <10%)	<15%
Serum ferritin	>35 μg/mL	<35 ng/mL	<200 ng/mL
Serum soluble transferring receptor concentration	Normal (may be increased if serum ferritin > 200 μg/L)	Increased	Increased
Stainable iron in bone marrow	Present	Absent	Absent

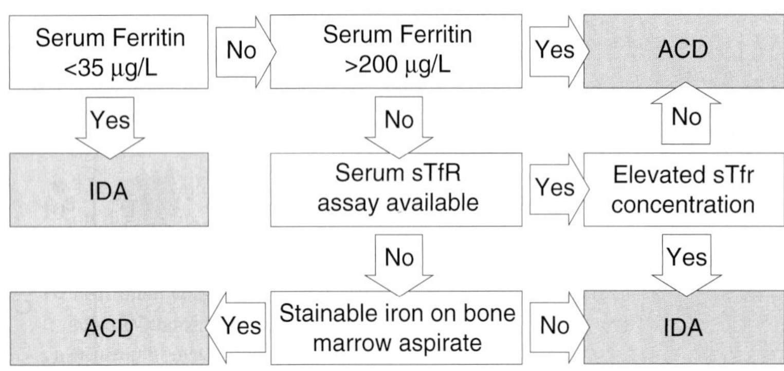

Figure 19–2. Differential diagnosis of anemia with low serum iron. Abbreviations: ACD, anemia of chronic disease; IDA, iron deficiency anemia; sTfR, soluble transferrin receptor.

of 24 patients with absent marrow iron stores had an elevated serum TIBC.[98] Although the serum ferritin concentration is the best biochemical indicator of reticuloendothelial iron status, its sensitivity is limited in patients with concurrent inflammatory disorders; the serum ferritin is frequently elevated out of proportion to iron stores. In a retrospective study correlating marrow iron stores to biochemical iron parameters, approximately 50% of patients without stainable marrow iron had serum ferritin concentrations in the normal range, and a third of these iron-deficient patients had serum ferritin concentrations greater than 100 μg/L (no patient with a serum ferritin concentration > 200 μg/L lacked stainable marrow iron).[99]

Determination of sTfR may be a partial solution to the problem of distinguishing iron deficiency anemia with inflammation from ACD when serum ferritin concentrations are in the normal range. TfRs are predominantly expressed on erythroblasts; iron deficiency anemia erythroblasts express an increased number of TfRs per cell,[100] whereas those from patients with ACD express fewer TfRs.[101] In addition, iron-deficiency may be accompanied by marrow erythroid hyperplasia, resulting in a further increment in cellular sTfR numbers. Because the serum sTfR concentration reflects the total body quantity of erythroblast cellular TfRs,[102] it should distinguish between iron deficiency anemia and ACD.[103] In one recent study, elevated sTfR concentrations were measured in individuals with serum ferritin concentrations well above normal[99]; the same result was obtained in a prospective correlation of marrow aspirate iron stores and serum sTfR concentrations in anemic patients.[98] An algorithm has been proposed in which serum ferritin concentrations below the normal range predicted a lack of stainable marrow iron, and serum ferritin concentrations outside the normal range predicted iron repletion. Thus patients with serum ferritin concentrations in the normal range should undergo serum sTfR determination; in this limited setting, an elevated sTfR concentration distinguished patients who lacked stainable marrow iron.[98] A similar discrimination is obtained by determining the ratio of the logarithm of the serum ferritin concentration to the sTfR concentration.[104]

If these noninvasive measures fail, bone marrow examination for assessment of iron stores may be necessary (Fig. 19–2). Measurement of the iron regulatory protein hepcidin, which some investigators have reported to distinguish ACD from iron deficiency,[84,89] is neither sufficiently studied nor available.

TREATMENT

The usual approach to ACD has been to direct treatment to the underlying disorder, as the degree of anemia reflects the activity of the associated disease and the anemia is generally not sufficiently severe to merit specific therapy. Implication of cytokine mediators of the immune response in the pathogenesis of ACD suggested that anticytokine therapy might be of benefit in this syndrome. In a randomized, double-blind comparison of chimeric antibody directed against TNF to placebo in rheumatoid arthritis patients, treatment reversed anemia, either as a result of a specific TNF effect on marrow erythropoiesis or overall reduction in disease activity.[105] In animals, murine IFN-γ receptor immunoadhesin (a soluble murine IFN-γ receptor attached to hinge and Fc regions of human immunoglobulin G1 heavy chains) corrected inhibition of CFU-E-derived colony formation by murine IFN-γ in vitro.[106] Because cytokines also serve biologically beneficial functions, careful assessment will be needed before anticytokine therapy is clinically applied to syndromes such as ACD.

In the mid 1980s, the demonstration that anemic patients had a blunted EPO response to anemia[16] prompted investigation of the use of rhEPO in ACD. In the initial report, two women with rheumatoid arthritis and persistent anemia for a year were treated with intravenous rhEPO, 100–150 U/kg three times weekly for several weeks, and they attained a normal hematocrit; they also received oral ferrous sulfate. Accompanying resolution of the anemia, total body red cell mass increased 250–500 mL and the marrow concentration of erythroid progenitors rose, but the arthritis was unaffected. After cessation of rhEPO therapy, both patients became anemic again, indicating that the red cell response was due to rhEPO therapy and not to iron supplementation.[107] These initial results were subsequently confirmed in a multicenter study[108] of subcutaneous rhEPO to correct ACD in anemic rheumatoid arthritis patients. Pretreatment, endogenous EPO levels did not correlate with response.[109] In a placebo-controlled study, predictors of a poor response to rhEPO were an elevated C-reactive protein concentration and failure to administer concurrent oral iron.[94] Early studies of intravenous rhEPO reported no changes in disease activity or quality of life with rhEPO therapy for rheumatoid arthritis patients with ACD.[110] Subsequently, subcutaneous rhEPO at similar or slightly lower total weekly doses produced improvements in these parameters,[111] possibly as a consequence of the combination of an increased hemoglobin and the use of the disease-modifying drugs now routine in the management of rheumatoid arthritis.

Although in published trials rhEPO in ACD is almost always administered three times weekly, weight-based dosing, most physicians in practice employ rhEPO in ACD at a fixed dose of 40,000–60,000 units subcutaneously each week (the standard dose for the anemia of

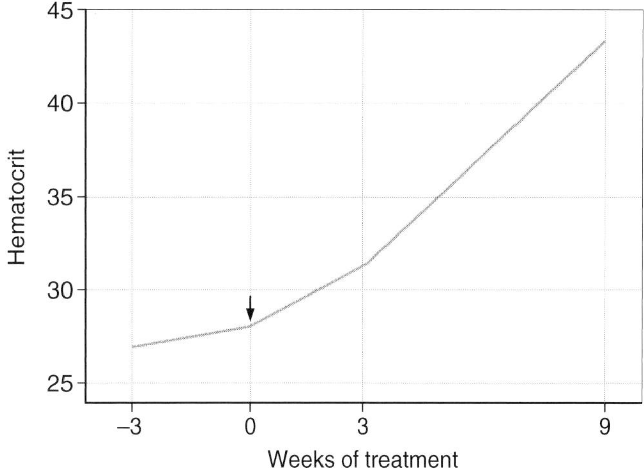

Figure 19–3. Response of an anemic rheumatoid arthritis patient to recombinant human erythropoietin, 40,000 units subcutaneously per week, and oral ferrous sulfate, 325 mg three times daily; treatment was initiated at the *arrow*.

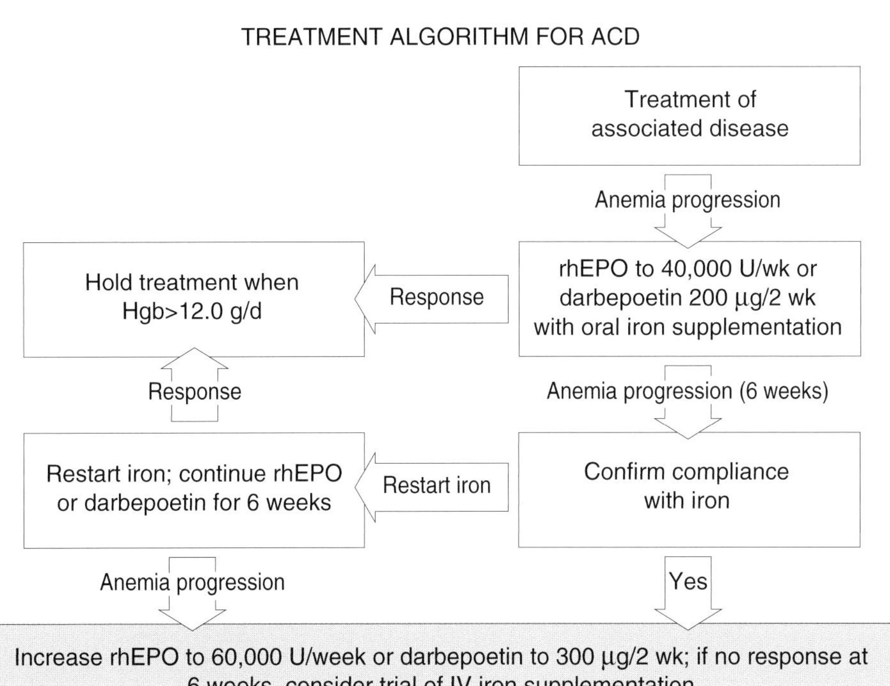

Figure 19–4. Therapeutic algorithm for the anemia of chronic disease. Abbreviations: ACD, anemia of chronic disease; rhEPO, recombinant human erythropoietin.

cancer) (Fig. 19–3). Iron supplementation is clearly important for the hemoglobin response to rhEPO and should be prescribed routinely unless contraindicated by clinical or laboratory evidence of iron overload, such as a transferrin saturation greater than 40%. In trials of rhEPO in anemic rheumatoid arthritis patients, much higher mean hemoglobin increments were achieved with more aggressive (2.5 gm/dL vs. 1.2 gm/dL) iron supplementation, dictated by the definition of serum ferritin chosen for iron deficiency.[94,111] Iron is not useful alone in ACD.

Novel erythropoiesis stimulating protein (NESP; also called darbepoetin) is an erythropoietin analogue with modified glycosylation permitting a longer half-life in the circulation; it is currently approved in the United States for the anemia of renal insufficiency and in cancer. In preclinical studies, NESP was able to reverse cytokine-mediated anemia in an animal model of ACD.[41] NESP is effective in anemic cancer patients not receiving chemotherapy,[112] and experience with other rhEPO products suggests that it will also be efficacious in patients with ACD of other etiologies. The optimal administration schedule for ACD is not yet established but is likely to be identical to that for cancer patients (a fixed dose of 200–300 μg subcutaneously every 2 weeks). Iron supplementation should be as necessary for NESP as it is for rhEPO, but whether the novel pharmacokinetics of NESP requires a different route of supplementation (intravenous vs. oral) remains to be addressed.

An algorithm for the treatment of ACD is outlined in Figure 19–4.

Current Controversies & Future Considerations

Anemia of Chronic Disease

Diagnosis

- Should ACD continue to be defined on the basis of hypoferremia with adequate iron stores, or be expanded to include normoferremic anemias with elevated ferritin in the appropriate clinical setting?
- Can hepcidin concentration (either in serum or in urine) distinguish ACD from iron deficiency anemia more effectively than does the serum ferritin?

Pathophysiology

- What are the effects of hepcidin on erythroid progenitors, the EPO response to anemia, and red cell survival?
- Are the correlations of hepcidin with various clinical and laboratory parameters mediated through ferritin or are these direct effects of hepcidin?

Treatment

- What is the optimum route of administration and dosage for iron supplementation during EPO therapy for ACD?
- Can antagonists of hepcidin correct ACD?

PROGNOSIS

Anemia is recognized as a poor prognostic sign in a variety of disease states.[113] Since ACD is an indicator of disease activity (as discussed above), it is no surprise that ACD, being reflective of a more advanced state of the underlying process, generally confers a poor prognosis; however, in and of itself, it may not be a major contributor to that prognosis.[114] In at least some reports, anemic patients with rheumatoid arthritis treated with rhEPO have shown a decrease in arthritis severity.[111] A meta-analysis of studies of anemic cancer patients treated with rhEPO noted a suggestion of improved survival in these individuals,[115] but this finding is not confirmed.[116]

Suggested Readings*

Baer AN, Dessypris EN, Krantz SB: The pathogenesis of anemia in rheumatoid arthritis: a clinical and laboratory analysis. Semin Arthritis Rheum 14:209–223, 1990.

Cash JM, Sears DA: The spectrum of diseases associated with the anemia of chronic disease: a study of 90 cases. Am J Med 87:638–644, 1990.

Ganz T: Hepcidin, a key regulator of iron metabolism and mediator of anemia of inflammation. Blood 102:783–788, 2003.

Means RT: Recent developments in the anemia of chronic disease. Curr Hematol Rep 2:116–121, 2003.

Full references for this chapter can be found on accompanying CD-ROM.

SECTION 2
DISEASES OF RED BLOOD CELL DESTRUCTION

CHAPTER 20

SICKLE CELL DISEASE

Lewis L. Hsu, MD, PhD, and Griffin P. Rodgers, MD, MACP

KEY POINTS

Sickle Cell Disease

- Sickle cell disease is due to a point mutation in the β-globin gene, leading to polymerization of deoxyhemoglobin S and instability of oxyhemoglobin S. The clinical consequences extend beyond hemolytic anemia to include vaso-occlusive pain, vasculopathy, multifocal infarcts, immune compromise, a prothrombotic state, and potential complications in nearly every system of the body.
- Sickle cell disease is now typically diagnosed by newborn screening, which permits early enrollment in preventive and comprehensive care programs.
- Recent therapeutic advances, confirmed in randomized clinical trials, include transcranial Doppler ultrasound screening, conjugated pneumococcal vaccine, incentive spirometry, and extended matching for red blood cell antigens for blood transfusion. Hydroxyurea therapy reduces the severity of sickle cell disease and prolongs survival by inducing fetal hemoglobin synthesis and through other beneficial mechanisms.
- Bone marrow or cord blood stem cell transplantation from a human lymphocyte antigen–matched sibling donor is curative. If a couple with one child with sickle cell disease have another pregnancy, banking the new baby's umbilical cord blood should be considered.
- Knowledge of the baseline hemoglobin and degree of reticulocytosis are critical for management, especially of aplastic crisis and splenic sequestration.
- Although homozygous Hb SS sickle cell disease is an example of mendelian inheritance, the disease course is significantly modified by environmental factors and by other genes (β-globin haplotypes, fetal hemoglobin, α-thalassemia), including tertiary modifiers (genes controlling bilirubin, hypertension, coagulation pathways, vascular cell adhesion molecule-1 polymorphism, morphine receptor polymorphisms).

INTRODUCTION

Sickle cell anemia is a severe hemoglobinopathy caused by a nucleotide substitution in codon 6 of the β-globin gene. This single mutation leads to the formation of the abnormal sickle hemoglobin, Hb S ($\alpha_2\beta^S_2$), which is much less soluble than normal hemoglobin A (Hb A; $\alpha_2\beta_2$) when deoxygenated.[1–3] This insolubility results in the formation of aggregates of Hb S polymer inside sickle erythrocytes as they traverse the circulation. With progressive deoxygenation, polymer become so extensive that the cells become sickled in shape, yet even at high oxygen saturation there may be sufficient quantities of Hb S polymer to alter the rheologic properties of the sickle erythrocyte in the absence of morphologic changes. Sickle erythrocytes occlude end-arterioles, leading to chronic hemolysis and microinfarction of diverse tissues and ultimately vaso-occlusive crises and irreversible organ damage.

The first clinical report of sickle cell anemia in the United States was published in 1910 by James B. Herrick. A Grenandan student attending a Chicago dental school, who presented with severe anemia and agonizing bone and joint pain, was found to have "crescent-shaped" red blood cells. Over the succeeding decades, studies of sickle cell disease have illuminated a number of broader scientific principles and stimulated seminal applications[4]: the diagnostic application of electrophoresis, x-ray crystallography of a complex protein structure, two-dimensional gel "fingerprints," prenatal diagnosis, DNA haplotype analysis, and the clinical application of the polymerase chain reaction.

EPIDEMIOLOGY

The sickle hemoglobin gene occurs in ethnic groups throughout Africa, South Asia, and the Mideast and around the Mediterranean (Fig. 20–1), and is now spread worldwide because of migration, slavery, and war. Anthropologic and genetics studies, plus animal models, indicate that the sickle trait increases survival after falciparum malaria infection of humans[5] and the murine malaria equivalent[6] (see Chapter 80). The four haplo-

A

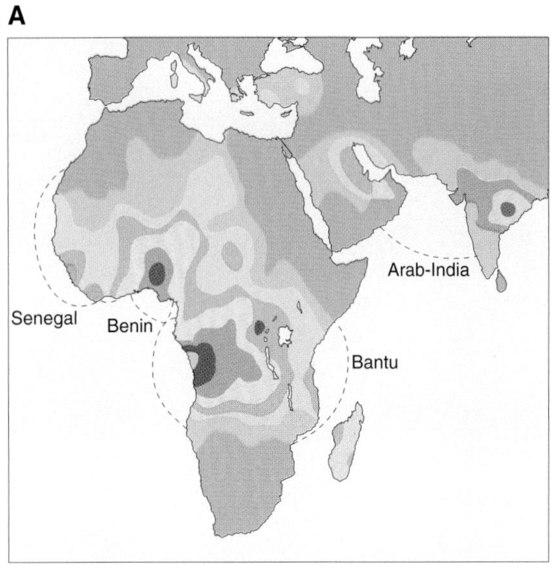

B

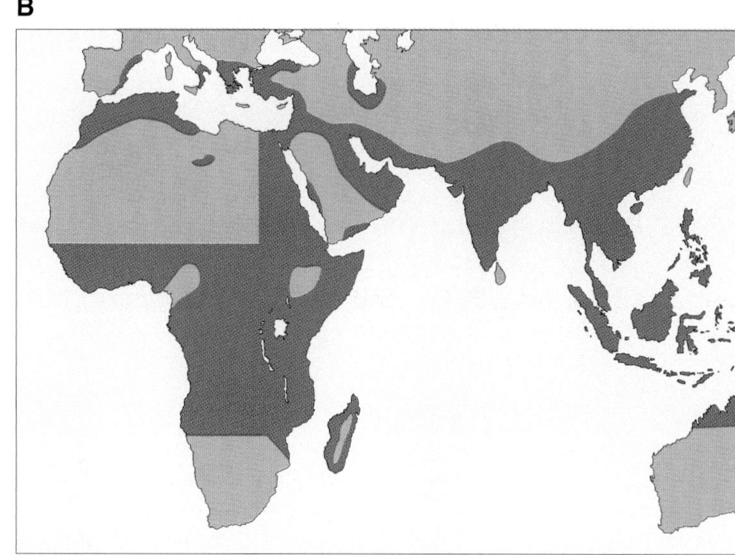

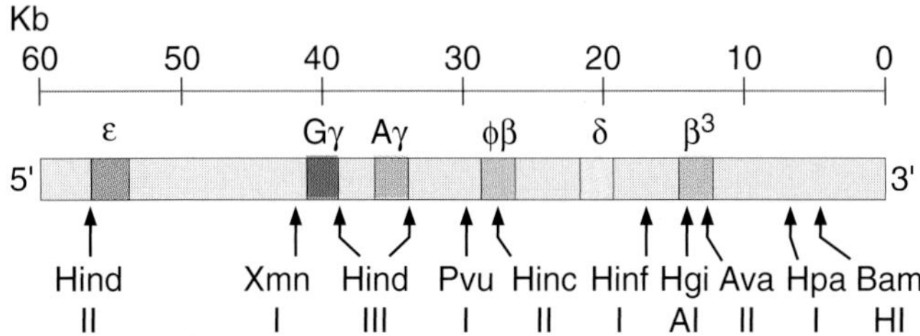

■ **Figure 20–1.** *A,* World distribution of sickle gene and its four haplotypes. Sickle hemoglobin gene frequency is high in West Africa, Central Africa, southern India, the Mediterranean, and the Middle East. Sickle β-globin haplotype analysis and anthropology indicate four separate origins for the mutation (Benin, Senegal, Central African Republic, and Indian-Arab). Haplotypes have been associated with increased risk for specific complications, with the Indian-Arab haplotype having a low frequency of pain and rare strokes, while the Senegal haplotype is associated with more frequent pain and early mortality. These associations have less utility in North American populations which have a high incidence of heterozygosity for these sickle gene haplotypes.

B, Geographic distribution of falciparum malaria. Originally the sickle gene distribution corresponded to areas susceptible to falciparum malaria, the heterozygote condition, sickle cell trait, confers a relative resistance to malaria.[9,36] Migration of people over several millennia, including through slave trading and war, have distributed the sickle gene throughout the world. The incidence of sickle cell disease in the United States is approximately 1 in 360 African Americans and 1 in 1200 Latinos in Florida. Sickle cell care and research now span the globe, including Belgium, Brazil, Cuba and the West Indies, France, Greece, Mexico, Saudi Arabia, and the United Kingdom.

types of the Hb S gene have different geographic distribution (see Fig. 20–1*A*). Coinheriting other abnormal hemoglobins with hemoglobin S creates other types of sickle cell disease. Distribution of the gene for hemoglobin C (Hb C) is high in the populations with Hb S, so that nearly one third of people followed at American sickle cell centers have Hb SC. Other compound heterozygotes are shown in Table 20–1. Globin chain variants may also be coinherited: β^0-thalassemia, β^+-thalassemia, hereditary persistence of fetal hemoglobin, and α-thalassemia (see Table 20–1; and Table 20–4 and Fig. 20–6 later).

PATHOPHYSIOLOGY AND MOLECULAR BASIS

Sickle hemoglobin (Hb S) was the first hemoglobin mutant to be characterized not biochemical and molecular levels; sickle cell anemia is most common of the hemoglobinopathies worldwide. Hemoglobin S results from a substitution of a hydrophobic valine for the normal glutamic acid at position six of the β-globin chain; a single base pair mutation (GAG→GTG) accounts for this amino acid change. The underlying pathophysiologic mechanism common to all sickle genotypes is intracellular polymerization of deoxyhemoglobin S (Fig. 20–2).

TABLE 20–1. Clinical Effects of Some Compound Heterozygotes in Modulating the Effect of Hb S*

Very Mild	Milder Than SS	Similar to SS	More Severe Than SS
Hb SS/HPFH	Hb S/β^+-thal	Hb S/β^0-thal	Hb S/Hb O Arab
Hb S/$\delta\beta$-thalassemia	Hb S/Hb C Hb S/Hb E	Hb S/Hb D Punjab Hb S/Hb C Harlem	

*These conditions also illustrate that some types of sickle cell disease can occur even if the father has no Hb S; this may be an important point during genetic counseling to forestall concerns about paternity.
Abbreviation: HPFH, hereditary persistence of fetal hemoglobin.

Release of oxygen normally produces conformational change in the hemoglobin tetramer, which for Hb S with its substituted hydrophobic valine at the β_6 position is marked by a significant decrease in intracellular solubility and a proclivity of free tetramers to aggregate or polymerize.[1–3] The extent (and rate) of intracellular polymer formation, which ultimately determines the rheologic properties of the erythrocytes as well as the familiar change in morphology, is governed principally by the intracellular hemoglobin composition (percent of S and non-S hemoglobin species), hemoglobin concentration, and percent oxygen saturation. Indeed, changes in the intracellular polymer fraction, which can be calculated from knowledge of these three variables, account for 80% of the hemolytic and overall clinical severity among large populations of patients affected with sickle cell disease and its genetic variants.[4]

The process of intracellular Hb S polymer formation is at least partially reversible as the red cells traverse the lungs and the hemoglobin oxygen tension rises. However, in the circulation, two additional erythrocyte biologic aberrations occur with repeated cycles of polymerization and depolymerization that further contribute to pathogenesis. First, polymer elongation leads to tangential forces repetitively applied to the red cell membrane that, which overcome the normal elastic properties of the membrane and progressively lead to permanent membrane-damaged cells, typified by irreversibly sickled cells.[4,7–10] Second, the abnormal hemoglobin-membrane interactions lead to the activation of a KCl cotransport pathway, a calcium-activated K^+ channel (Gardos pathway), and other deoxygenation-induced cation fluxes. The cumulative effects of these abnormally activated cation channels are profound: modest to severe cellular dehydration with potassium and water loss that increase polymerization and thus propagate a vicious cycle.

Endothelial cells also play a role in many aspects of sickle cell pathobiology.[10] Sickle cells can adhere to endothelium via surface antigens such as CD36 and CD44, integrins, and perhaps other unique features of the sickle erythrocyte membrane. Sickle cells may interact directly with endothelial cell and extracellular matrix molecules such as laminin, glycoprotein Ib, integrins, vascular cell adhesion molecule-1, and Fc receptor, or use such plasma proteins as von Willebrand factor, thrombospondin, fibrinogen, and fibronectin as intermediates to bridge attachments. This abnormal red cell–endothelium interaction induces the endothelial cell to express greater quantities of proteins including procoagulants, cytokines, and proinflammatory molecules, that then further impair bloor flow. Endothelial activation and damage may cause prostacyclin release, oxidant radical formation, inhibition of DNA synthesis, endothelin-1 expression, and disturbance of nitric oxide biology (Fig. 20–3).

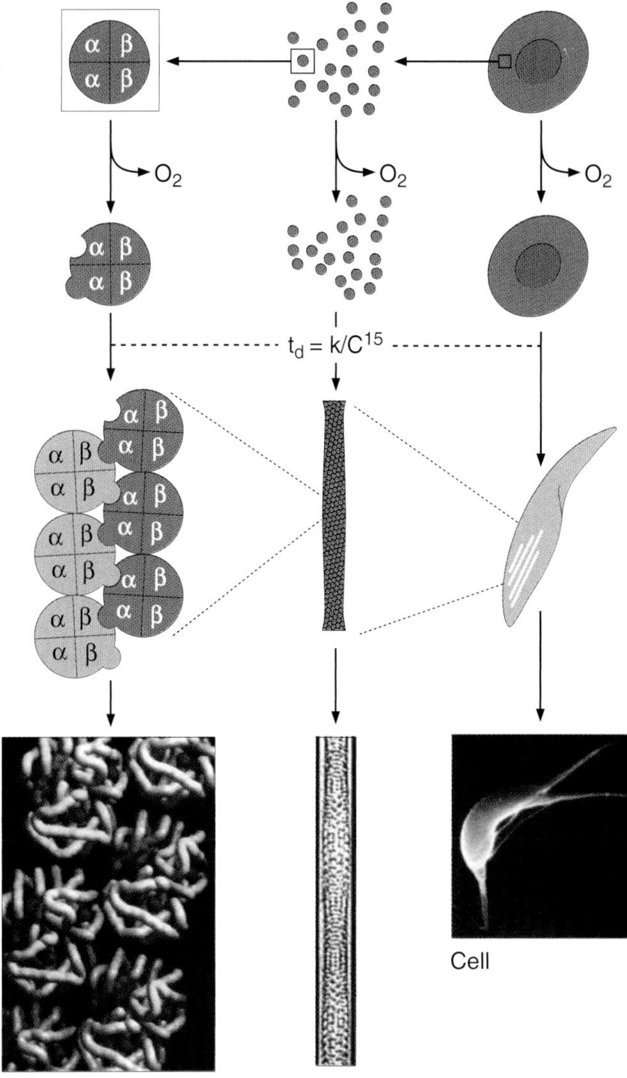

Figure 20–2. Pathophysiology of sickle cell disease.[2] The abnormal sickle hemoglobin polymerizes when deoxygenated, deforming the erythrocyte (RBC) and damaging the cell cytoskeleton. The rigid cells can obstruct or slow blood flow.

CLINICAL FEATURES AND DIAGNOSIS

Laboratory Diagnosis

In the United States, sickle cell disease now is usually diagnosed by newborn screening, universal in 46 states and targeted in the others.[11,12] Newborn blood blotted on

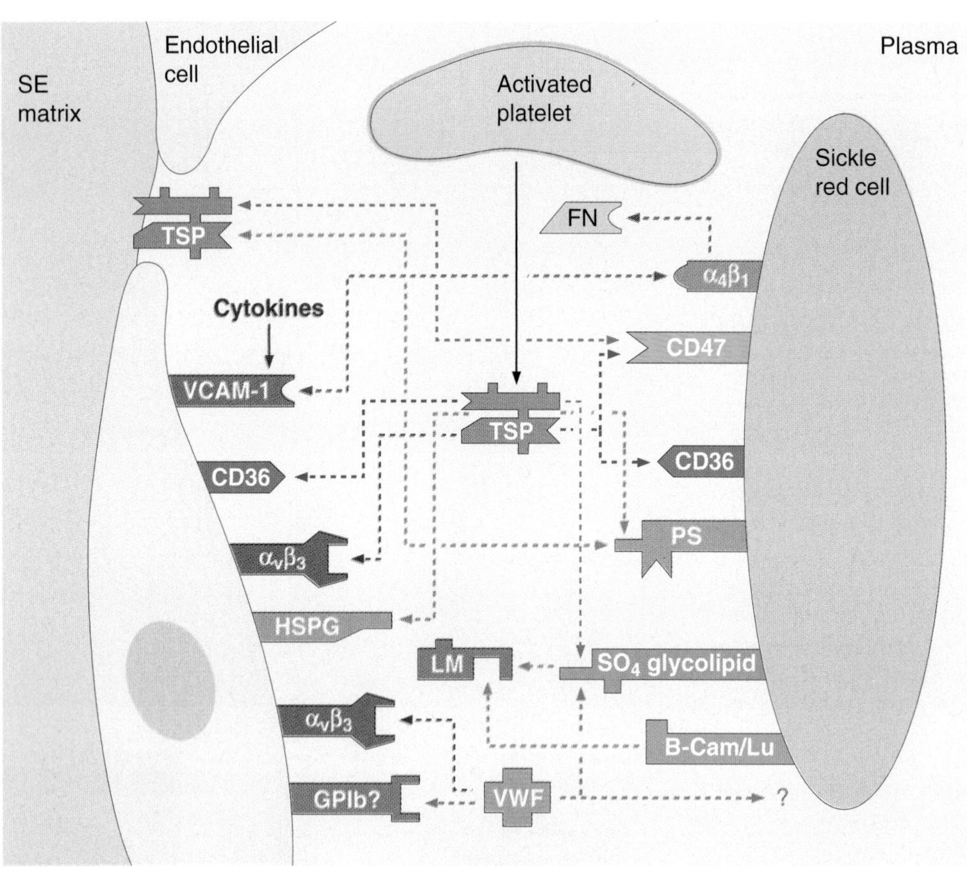

Figure 20–3. Red blood cell adhesion pathways in sickle cell disease. The abnormally increased adhesion of sickle red blood cells can be mediated by multiple molecular interactions. These can bind the red blood cell to endothelium, to subendothelial basement membrane, and to other blood cells. Some adhesive pathways appear to be related to normal adhesion mechanisms for leukocytes or platelets. Other pathways arise from abnormal sickle red blood cell surface expression of adhesion proteins and other molecules such as phosphatidylserine. (From Stuart MJ, Nagel RL: Sickle-cell disease. Lancet 364:1343–1360, 2004, with permission.)

filter paper and tested for inborn errors of metabolism is also tested for hemoglobinopathies by isoelectric focusing or high-performance liquid chromatography (Table 20–2). The public health goal is to establish a diagnosis of sickle cell disease and start the baby on prophylactic antibiotics by 4–6 weeks of age in order to prevent deaths from *Streptococcus pneumoniae* sepsis.[13–16]

Diagnosis in individuals who missed the newborn screening as new immigrants, or because of error in the testing program, depends on an alert clinician.[11,17–19] Asymptomatic anemia with reticulocytosis and anisocytosis can be detected by a routine complete blood count in toddlers or adults. Sickle deformation is readily appreciated on the blood smear and hemoglobin electrophoresis confirms the diagnosis, although exceptional cases can be confusing (see Table 20–2). Infants with sickle cell disease may present with dactylitis pain (Table 20–3) or life-threatening complications such as splenic sequestration or sepsis. Clinical presentations of sickle cell disease later in life include acute complications such as stroke and pain, described later, or chronic sequelae, as shown in Figure 20–4. Sickle cell disease of the SC type is more likely to be asymptomatic in infancy, but half of affected patients develop symptoms as preschoolers.[20]

TABLE 20–2. Special Pitfalls in Diagnosing Compound Heterozygosity with Hemoglobin S

Hb SS/Hb G-Philadelphia	α-Globin variant Hb G-Philadelphia migrates like Hb A at acidic electrophoresis, and like Hb S under alkaline conditions. Similar to Hb SS in severity.[204]
Hb S/Hb O Arab	Migrates like Hb SC on electrophoresis. Severe sickle cell disease.[205,206]
Hb S/Hb Quebec-Chori	Hb Quebec-Chori migrates like Hb A on alkaline electrophoresis and isoelectric focusing, can lead to false diagnosis of Hb AS (1 case described). Mild anemia, reticulocytosis, sickle red blood cells.[207]
Hb S/Hb San Diego	Difficult to separate from Hb A. Can arise as a new mutation in a "hot spot." High oxygen affinity causes erythrocytosis, not sickle cell disease.[208]
Hb Jamaica Plain/HbA	Mutant β sickle hemoglobin with low oxygen affinity. Heterozygote resembles Hb AS on isoelectric focusing, but still has sickle cell complications under hypoxic stress (1 case described).[209]

Sickle cell disease often involves compound β-globin heterozygosity and coinheritance of α-thalassemia. Common combinations in the United States are tabulated here. For encyclopedic discussions, see Hardison and colleagues,[210] Steinberg,[211] and (*http://globin.cse.psu.edu/*).

Hematology

The hemoglobin genotype of sickle cell disease correlates with a range of hematologic values and risks of

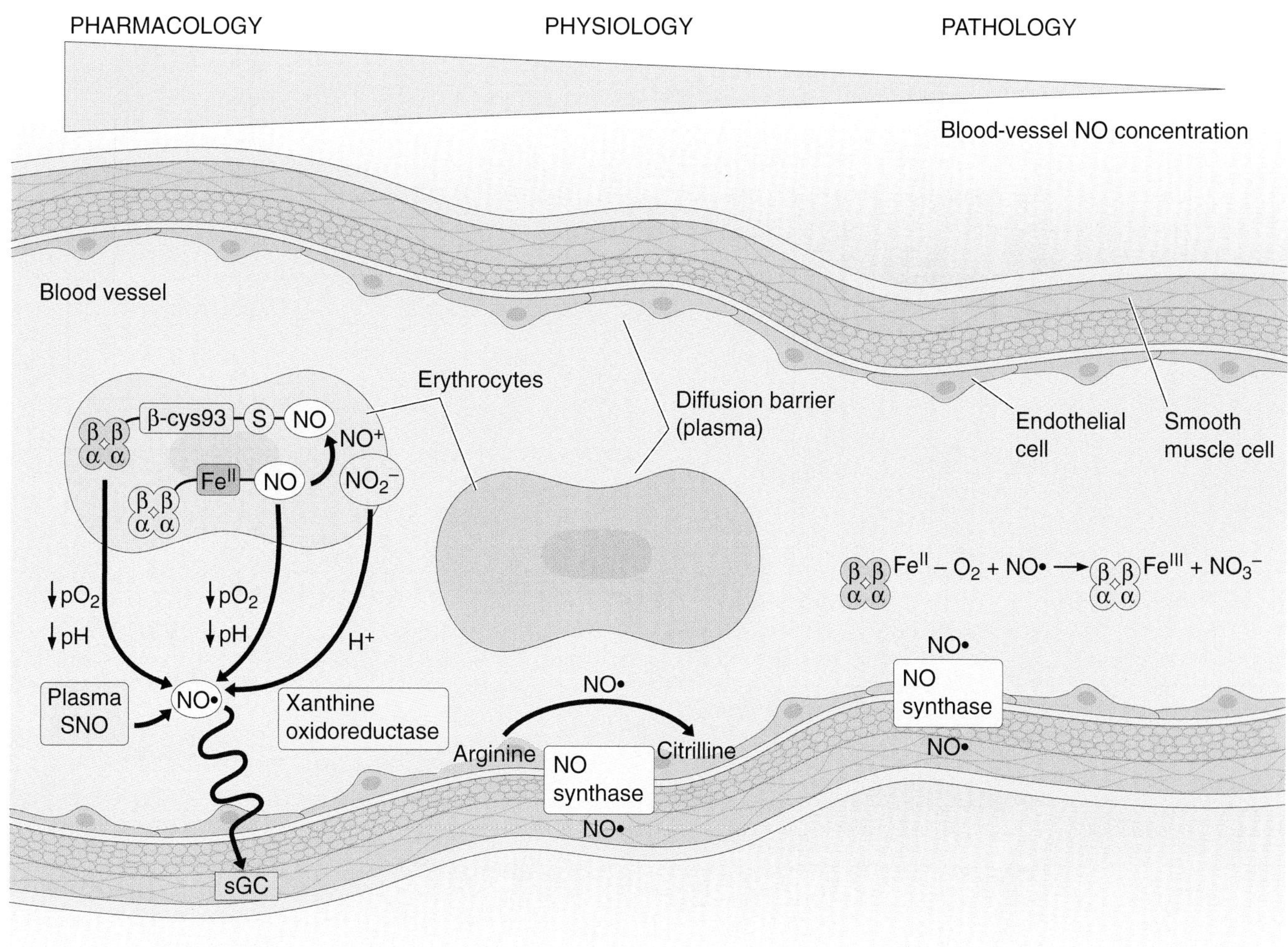

B

Figure 20–3, cont'd

complications. Hemolytic anemia is most severe for Hb SS and Hb S/β^0-thalassemia, more moderate in Hb SC and Hb S/β^+-thalassemia, and modified by inheritance of other traits such as α-thalassemia and hereditary persistence of fetal hemoglobin (Table 20–4). However, each individual appears to have a baseline level of anemia and of steady-state hemolysis. Declines below steady-state anemia should trigger a search for a new acute complication, such as parvoviral suppression of erythropoiesis (aplastic crisis), sequestration of erythrocytes in the spleen, accelerated hemolysis, or acute chest syndrome.

Leukocytosis is common in sickle cell disease, and baseline white blood cell counts may be as high as 30,000/mm^3, which can confound an evaluation for infection. Marked leukocytosis is statistically associated with worse morbidity and mortality.[21] Acute elevation of neutrophils in response to infection is similar to that in normal hosts, as is a fall in neutrophils with sepsis syndrome. Thrombocytosis also is common (and not well explained). Sudden declines in platelet count below baseline are associated with acute complications such as splenic sequestration, acute chest syndrome, and sepsis. A thrombotic diathesis in sickle cell disease[22] has been blamed on low-grade platelet activation and thrombin generation, associated with the activated surfaces of red blood cells, endothelium, and perhaps microvesicles.

Clinical Features

Sickle cell disease is characterized by unpredictability and—despite its well-described single-gene mutation—multiorgan involvement. Clinical manifestations appear to be modified by many genetic and environmental factors, plus each individual patient's course may be punctuated by a diversity of single or recurrent acute events.

Pain

Episodic severe pain is one of the most distressing features of sickle cell disease. Triggers for vaso-occlusive

SICKLE CELL DISEASE DAMAGES: NON-HEMATOLOGIC ORGAN SYSTEMS

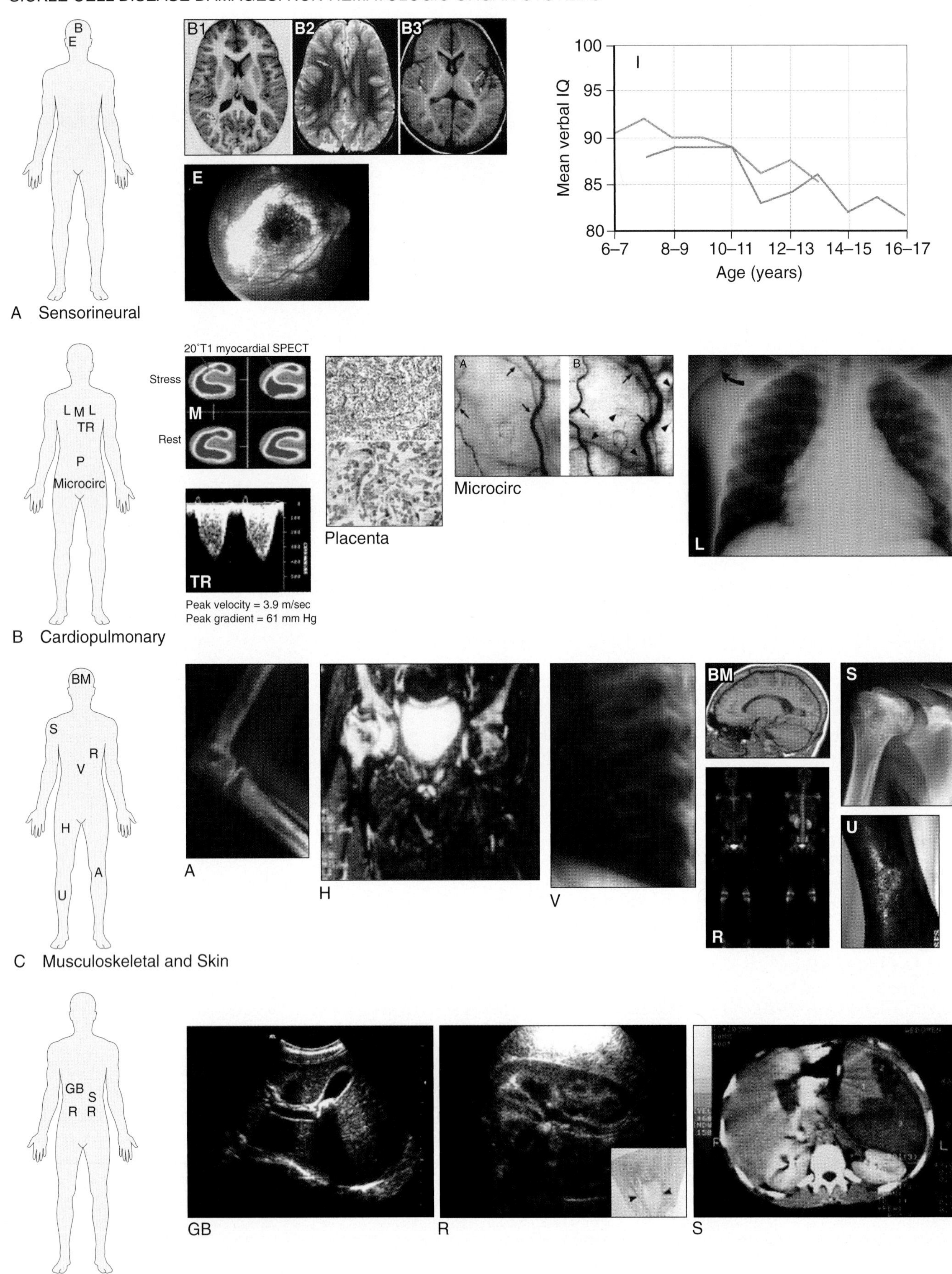

pain are often identifiable: dehydration, cold temperature or skin cooling, exhaustion and lactic acidosis, infection, emotional stress (including academic final exams), and menstruation. Changes in weather trigger pain in certain individuals[23–25]; similarly, acute inflammation from musculoskeletal trauma or mild respiratory infection acts as an inciter in a subset of patients with sickle cell disease. The pathophysiologic basis for these relationships appears to be increased Hb S polymerization, vasoconstriction, and increased endothelial activation. Why some triggers affect only some patients with sickle cell disease remains unclear, but recognizing characteristic sites and patterns of

Figure 20–4. Chronic nonhematologic complications of sickle cell disease. Classic findings on imaging are shown. Several insidious problems can be subclinical until quite severe,[197] but they can be detected by screening tests such as transcranial Doppler ultrasound[65] and echocardiogram for tricuspid regurgitant jet.[39]

A, Sensorineural complications.

B – Brain complications: B1, deep white matter infarct in brain; B2, encephalomalacia, extensive in the occipital areas; and B3, lacunar infarct. Focal ischemic damage may result from stenotic cerebral arteries and/or microcirculatory abnormalities. Tortuous arteries and collateral vessels may be demonstrated on magnetic resonance angiogram, not shown.

E – Retinopathy with infarcts and neovascularization can be caused by collateral development around areas of obstruction. Retinopathy can be subclinical until the fragile neovascular tissue bleeds to cause hyphema, or retinal detachment. Annual ophthalmology screening can detect early retinopathy.

I – Neurocognitive function may decline as shown in the trend of WISC and WISC-R scores of children serially tested during the Cooperative Study of Sickle Cell Disease.[198] This decline is partially attributable to "silent infarcts" that affect frontal lobes or memory, but also attributable to chronic anemia. However, not every individual with sickle cell disease will have decline in cognitive function.

B, Cardiopulmonary complications.

L – Chronic lung disease and cardiac hypertrophy. Chest radiograph shows chronic lung disease as a fine reticular pattern throughout both lungs, and cardiomegaly, as compensation for increased cardiac output resulting from chronic anemia.[197] Pulmonary function testing often reveals a subclinical mixed obstructive and restrictive respiratory dysfunction.

M – Myocardial strain. Dilated cardiomegaly is a typical compensation for chronic anemia. Recent studies indicate a significant incidence of myocardial ischemia, especially with exertion. This single-photon emission computed tomography scan shows abnormal strain on the myocardial wall with stress.

TR – Tricuspid valve regurgitant jet. Doppler echocardiogram detects this indirect measure of pulmonary hypertension. Pulmonary hypertension, indicated by tricuspid regurgitant jet velocity greater than 2.5 m/sec, is associated with high mortality, even though cardiologists may consider this mild pulmonary hypertension in people without chronic anemia. Mitral regurgitation can be caused by distortion of the valve ring.

Microcirc – Microvascular abnormalities. Abnormally diminished perfusion of the microcirculation, especially during crisis *(left panel)* is compared to increased flow at recovery from crisis *(right panel).* Abnormal tortuosity of the microvessels are also noted.

Placenta – Placental abnormalities in a mother with sickle cell disease. Histopathology shows sickled maternal red blood cells in the placental circulation in a primipara with Hb SC sickle cell at two levels of magnification. In contrast, fetal red blood cells in capillaries are not deformed at the same level of oxygen, in this case because the baby has sickle cell trait. A baby with sickle cell disease would be protected because of high levels of fetal hemoglobin in the newborn period.

C, Musculoskeletal complications.

BM – Bone marrow hyperplasia. Increased erythropoietic drive expands the marrow space in many patients with sickle cell disease, here shown as a thickened calvarium.

R – Rib infarcts. Rib infarcts caused by ischemia can be very painful and associated with acute chest syndrome. Infarcted ribs are highlighted white on the nuclear scan.

V – Vertebral infarction. Bony collapse of the infarcted vertebral bodies from the normal cylindrical shape with rectangular cross-section, into a bi-concave shape with a characteristic outline of the letter "H" on two-dimensional projection ("the H sign" or "fish-mouth"), seen on radiographs of the thoracolumbar spine. Similar bone infarcts in long bones such as the radius and humerus may appear as sclerotic mottling.

H – Avascular necrosis of the humeral and femoral heads. Ischemic damage can cause chronic pain, bony collapse, and dislocation of the joint. Avascular necrosis of the femur can be severely disabling.

A – Arthropathy. The knee displays osteoarthritis with a narrowed joint space, and the long bones have mottled lucencies due to infarcts.

U – Leg ulcers. Poor vascular supply of the skin near the malleoli can cause severely painful and disabling ulceration, and healing can take months to years even with appropriate treatment.

D, Gastrointestinal/genitourinary complications.

GB – Gallbladder and gallstones. Hemolysis causes increased bilirubin production, and patients with severe hemolysis are chronically jaundiced. Pigmented gallstones form in nearly three fourths of patients as a result of hemolysis, but can be asymptomatic.

S – Spleen infarct. Scattered rounded foci of low attenuation in the spleen are noted by computed tomography scan of an adult with Hb SC sickle cell disease. The spleen accumulates infarcts over time and can become a shrunken scar, or a spongy nonfunctional bag that can cause splenic sequestration. Spleen images on nuclear scan can be speckled with infarcts, or absent because of functional asplenia.

R – Hyperechoic kidney. This ultrasound finding corresponds to an abnormally heterogeneous texture of the renal cortex as a result of multiple infarcts of the medulla seen in histology (*inset* with *paired arrowheads* indicating papillary necrosis). Renal ischemic damage to tubules leads to isosthenuria early in childhood. Renal glomerulopathy includes thickened capillaries and proteinuria.

sickle cell vaso-occlusive pain (see Table 20–3) can spare the patient unnecessary medical testing.

Infection

Infection was the leading cause of death in sickle cell disease in natural history studies, but comprehensive care and acute interventions have greatly diminished mortality and morbidity.[26–28] Implicated in immunocompromise of sickle cell disease are an opsonic defect, functional asplenia, complement activation, altered lymphocyte function, impaired antibody response, impaired phagocytosis, and abnormal cytokine production.

Sepsis

Bacterial sepsis was probably responsible for the very short life expectancy of patients with sickle cell disease in the United States until the 1970s and still applies in the developing world (see Fig. 20–6*A* later). Sepsis mortality caused by *S. pneumoniae* was 100- to 400-fold greater in children with sickle cell disease than in the general childhood population in historical studies. Other encapsulated bacteria (*Haemophilus influenzae*, *Neisseria meningitidis*) also have produced high rates of sepsis in sickle cell in the past. Patients with iron overload and desferrioxamine chelation are particularly susceptible to *Yersinia* sepsis, because of the unusually high requirement for iron in this family of bacteria.

Pneumonia

Acute chest syndrome in sickle cell disease is defined as a new infiltrate on chest roentgenogram, combined with fever, cough, or chest pain.[29,30] Acute chest syndrome often results in rapid respiratory deterioration and has a mortality rate as high as 6%.[30] Multiple etiologies can trigger acute chest syndrome, but respiratory infection is common, preceding over half the episodes of acute chest syndrome in children.[30] Organisms involved include respiratory bacteria, such as *S. pneumoniae*, *H. influenzae*, *Staphylococcus aureus*, *Klebsiella*, and *Escherichia coli*; atypical bacteria, such as *Chlamydia pneumoniae*[31] and *Mycoplasma hominis*; and respiratory viruses, such as influenza, parainfluenza, respiratory syncytial virus, cytomegalovirus, and adenovirus.

Osteomyelitis and Septic Arthritis

Bacterial bone and joint infections in sickle cell disease are much more frequent than in normal hosts, attributable to the increased number of devitalized bones produced by recurrent ischemic events. Bone infections are difficult to diagnose because their symptoms and signs overlap with those following vaso-occlusion, and imaging modalities do not yet reliably distinguish infection from infarction.

The relative prevalence of *S. aureus*, *Salmonella*, and other enteric bacterial etiologies in osteomyelitis reflects the bacteria of the geographic area.[32–35] Because reptiles are usually colonized with *Salmonella*, health counselors recommend avoidance of these pets. Osteomyelitis can emerge as a complication of bone fractures, may be accompanied by sepsis syndrome, or can be slow and insidious in onset.

Other Infections

Parvovirus B19, a common respiratory virus, causes a transient erythroblastopenia that holds particular hazards for persons with sickle cell disease and other hemolytic

TABLE 20–3. Patterns of Pain*

Pain Pattern	Possible Differential Diagnosis
Dactylitis	Osteomyelitis, trauma
Rib infarct	Pulmonary embolism
Skull infarct	Skull abscess, hemorrhagic stroke
Hepatic sequestration	Hepatitis, ascending cholangitis
Priapism	
Biliary colic	Constipation
Mesenteric sickling	Acute surgical abdomen, constipation
Menstrual trigger	Unexplained recurrent pain
Avascular necrosis of femoral head	Recurrent vaso-occlusive pain, sciatica
Vaso-occlusion with joint effusion	Septic arthritis, fracture

*Sickle cell vaso-occlusive pain often involves these sites and patterns, which may be recurring. Deviations from a previous pattern can be subtle but important. For example, asymmetrical pain in the digits may be osteomyelitis rather than dactylitis, or abdominal pain that is now focal in the right lower quadrant may be acute appendicitis. Finally, some disabilities should raise concern for other complications of sickle cell disease; for example, painless limp may be due to cerebrovascular accident.

TABLE 20–4. Mixed Clinical Effects of α-Thalassemia on Hb SS

Cellular Effects	Physiologic Effects	Clinical Comparison to Hb SS Without α-Thalassemia
Reduced Hb S polymer	Decreased hemolysis	Fewer strokes
Decreased cation exchange		Fewer leg ulcers
Decreased erythrocyte density	Improved red blood cell survival, higher hematocrit, increased whole blood viscosity	Increased osteonecrosis
Increased erythrocyte deformability		Increased splenic sequestration Possible increased pain

Adapted from Steinberg MH: Compound heterozygotes and other sickle hemoglobinopathies. *In* Steinberg MH, Forget BG, Higgs DR, Nagel RL (eds): Disorders of Hemoglobin: Genetics, Pathophysiology, and Clinical Management. Cambridge: Cambridge University Press, 2001, p 801.

anemias (aplastic crisis; see "Hematology," earlier) (see Chapter 76). The sudden cessation of erythrocyte production can lead to fatal anemia, stroke, and heart failure. In parvovirus B19 aplastic crisis, reticulocyte counts are typically zero for 7–10 days. In addition, parvovirus B19 can produce thrombocytopenia, neutropenia, acute chest syndrome, and hemophagocytic syndrome.

Malaria sickle trait offers relative protection from falciparum malaria,[36] but individuals with sickle cell disease are at least as susceptible as normals.

Influenza can be complicated in sickle cell disease, including acting as a precipitant of acute chest syndrome.

Respiratory

Acute chest syndrome is a leading cause of death. The relationship between recurrent episodes of acute chest syndrome and chronic lung disease is suspected clinically, if not supported by epidemiologic studies to date. A large multicenter study demonstrated that acute chest syndrome usually involved more than one etiology,[30] with marrow fat embolism more common in adulthood and infection more frequent in children. Acute chest syndrome can be associated with neurologic complications, splenic or hepatic sequestration, and priapism. Rapid progression to severe acute chest syndrome is unpredictable and can be fatal, manifesting as acute respiratory distress syndrome and multiorgan failure syndrome.[37]

Pulmonary hypertension occurs in almost one third of adults with sickle cell disease.[38,39] Vasoconstriction of pulmonary arteries and arterioles may be reversible, but chronic remodeling can lead to hyperplasia of the medial layer of the vessel wall and plexiform vascularity.[40,41] Sequelae of pulmonary hypertension include right heart failure, arrhythmias, and sudden cardiac death. Dyspnea can limit exercise tolerance, as measured by the 6-minute walk test. Pulmonary hypertension can be diagnosed formally by cardiac catheterization or post-mortem by histopathology. One noninvasive screen is Doppler echocardiogram to detect tricuspid regurgitant jet velocity; a level greater than 2.5 m/sec is associated with 10-fold increased rate of mortality in 18 months,[39] even in patients without hemoglobinopathy. The ability of sickle cell patients to compensate for pulmonary hypertension may be impaired by chronic anemia and high cardiac output. The etiology of pulmonary hypertension has been attributed to tonic vasoconstriction resulting from abnormally low nitric oxide bioavailability.[42] Pulmonary hypertension is present in other hemolytic conditions, such as thalassemia and hereditary spherocytosis.[43–46] Tricuspid regurgitant jet velocity determination[39] by Doppler echocardiogram is recommended as a routine screening test for adults with sickle cell disease, and studies are underway to determine the prevalence of pulmonary hypertension in adolescents and pediatric patients.

Obstructive sleep apnea caused by adenoidal hypertrophy is more common in pediatric sickle cell disease than in the general population; it can be relieved surgically. Chronic hypoxia is present in as many as 40% of children followed in sickle cell centers.[47] Hyperreactive airways are present in as many as 80% of children with sickle cell disease, although pulmonary function tests can demonstrate a mixture of restrictive and obstructive dysfunction. Interpretation of abnormal pulse oximetry in sickle cell disease can be complex,[48–50] but true chronic hypoxemia is determined by arterial blood gas analysis.

Central Nervous System

Stroke

Prominent among manifestations of sickle cell disease as a vasculopathy are cerebrovascular complications, ranging from fatal hemorrhagic stroke to subtle neuropsychologic damage. Common ischemic changes in children with Hb SS and Hb S/β^0-thalassemia sickle cell disease[51] are focal segments of arterial stenosis around the circle of Willis, with the microscopic appearance of disrupted elastic lamina layer and intimal hyperplasia that can restrict the lumen of the artery.[52–54] (These stenoses are detected by magnetic resonance angiography with data acquisition adjustments to suppress artifacts of turbulent flow.) Small infarcts in the deep white matter are associated with abnormalities of smaller arteries—termed small vessel disease—and not detectable by magnetic resonance angiography. Infarcts may manifest as sensory or motor deficits or be completely silent. Infarcts of frontal cortex or deep white matter can produce diminished "executive function" responsible for organizational skills and attention to task.[55–57]

Cerebrovascular disease is one of the major phenotypic heterogeneities that provide evidence for epistatic factors that modulate the course of sickle cell disease.[58] Protective genes that reduce stroke risk include hereditary persistence of fetal hemoglobin and α-thalassemia.[59,60] Thrombophilia genes, including homocystinemia, have been much studied but few associations have emerged. Specific human lymphocyte antigen (HLA) subtypes associate with susceptibility to stroke.[58,61] Sibling studies have identified other genes,[62] but twin studies have not yet been conducted. With evidence for inflammatory triggers for stroke in other conditions,[63] there is a quest for toxins and infections as precipitants of stroke in sickle cell disease.[64]

Primary stroke prevention was demonstrated, for the first time in any disease, in the landmark STOP study.[65] This randomized controlled clinical trial used transcranial Doppler ultrasound screening to identify a high-risk group of children with sickle cell disease and then demonstrated that chronic blood transfusion protected these children from stroke, with an approximately 92% reduction in stroke in 1.5 years of study. Similar protocols now seek to identify high-risk children before stroke, using magnetic resonance imaging or neurocognitive testing for screening. Epidemiologic studies suggest that transcranial Doppler screening and transfusion intervention reduce the incidence of new strokes in children with sickle cell disease[66] (Fig. 20–5). Stroke recurrence may be more likely in children with cerebrovascular disease than in those whose stroke was due to transient anemia or a hypoxic event,[67] and some children may not require long-term transfusions.

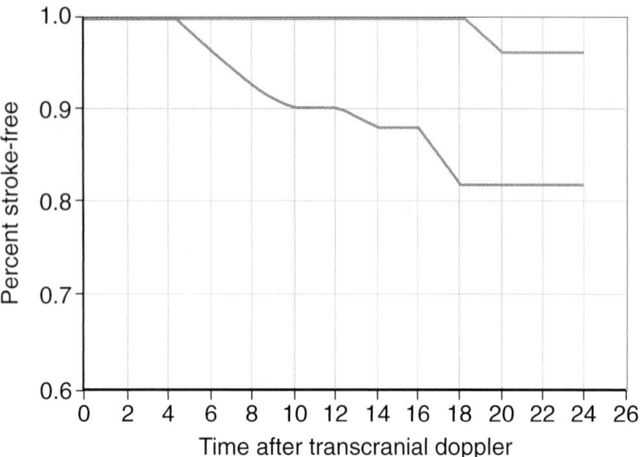

Figure 20–5. Chronic blood transfusion for primary prevention of ischemic stroke. As survival with sickle cell disease improves, morbidity is of increased interest. Kaplan-Meier plot of transcranial Doppler ultrasound and stroke demonstrates the increased risk of ischemic stroke in children with time-averaged mean velocity greater than 200 cm/sec using the STOP study methods, and decreased incidence of stroke in children randomized to chronic red blood cell transfusion to maintain Hb S less than 30%.[65] Preliminary findings of a follow-up study after transcranial Doppler ultrasound normalizes demonstrate that transfusions cannot safely be halted.

Hemorrhagic stroke is more common in adults than in children with sickle cell disease. The etiology is often an aneurysm, associated with hemodynamic stress on a weakened medial layer of the arterial medial wall.[68] Multiple aneurysms may be present, and bleeds may be prevented by a vascular clip. Bleeding may also occur from moyamoya disease collateral vessels associated with stenosis of a major vessel.

Renal

Sickle cells damage the kidneys from very early in childhood. Initial tubular damage affects the renal concentrating ability, so the urine produced all night is dilute and in a larger volume; bladder filling wakes the child or causes enuresis. Hematuria is common in sickle cell disease, as a result of papillary necrosis from red cell sickling in the renal medulla. Glomerular damage also begins early in life, with proliferative glomerulopathy on histology. Proteinuria can manifest as microalbuminuria early.[69,70] Frank albuminuria and nephrotic syndrome can occur in childhood but usually onset is in young adulthood.[71] Renal failure requiring hemodialysis develops in approximately 4% of patients with Hb SS and half as frequently in Hb SC disease.[72]

Leg Ulcers

Leg ulcers occur in 25–100% of patients with sickle cell anemia and Hb S/β-thalassemia during their lifetime, depending on geographic location, and they can cause significant physical, psychological, and social disability. In the United States, the incidence of leg ulcers is about 2–6 per 100 patient-years.[73] The skin overlying the malleoli is particularly susceptible. Venous insufficiency causes edema, then skin thinning and breakdown, a process similar to that in diabetes mellitus. Trauma, insect bites, and dry skin contribute to ulcer formation. Ulcers can be extremely painful and slow to heal, with functional disability over months to years and the potential for infectious complications such as cellulitis, lymphadenitis, or osteomyelitis. Hydroxyurea therapy either has no impact or may worsen leg ulcers.[74–76]

Bone Infarcts and Osteonecrosis of Femoral and Humeral Heads

Osteonecrosis or avascular necrosis presents as pain in the hip or shoulder, often unrelated to typical crises; pain increases with weight bearing or motion, and aching is worse at night. The head of the femur or humerus is usually involved. Avascular necrosis is more common in Hb SC and Hb S/β^+-thalassemia. Radiographs show degeneration in advanced cases, and bone scans demonstrate decreased early uptake. Magnetic resonance imaging is useful in early diagnosis.

Vertebral bone infarcts lead to a characteristic radiographic sign of the "H"-shaped vertebral body, and vertebral distortion can lead to nerve compression.

Priapism

Priapism is a prolonged, painful penile erection as a manifestation of sickle vaso-occlusion. Priapism affects over 30% of males, children as well as adults, with sickle cell disease.[77] Priapism occurs in two patterns: (1) episodic events of 2–4 hours, which are often recurrent and may precede a major episode, and (2) severe events that last more than 4 hours that can eventually result in impotence.

Other Complications

Many other organ systems are involved in sickle cell disease (see Fig. 20–4). Proliferative retinopathy can be detected in a screening ophthalmologic examination, and treatment with laser therapy can prevent complications such as hyphema or retinal detachment. Cholelithiasis with pigment stones is present in over half of adults but can remain asymptomatic for years. Impaired growth and delayed puberty are related to elevated energy expenditure and micronutrient and endocrine abnormalities.[11,78]

THERAPY

Comprehensive Care Approach

A comprehensive approach is important in maintaining continuity of care for chronic problems, individualized pain management, preventive measures, and screening, plus psychosocial support and education (Table 20–5). Patient satisfaction and financial considerations favor multidisciplinary colloboration for sickle cell disease, which can even be implemented in developing countries.[79] A comprehensive management is less expensive than episo-

TABLE 20–5. Preventing Pain and Its Complications

Immunizations	Prophylactic Medications	Environmental/Situational
Conjugated pneumococcal	Oral Penicillin VK twice daily *or* Intramuscular Pen G monthly *or* Oral Erythromycin twice daily	Maintain good hydration
23-Valent polysaccharide pneumococcal	Folate	Avoid extremes of temperature
Conjugated *Haemophilus influenzae* type b	Vitamin C	Avoid exhaustion/lactic acidosis
Influenza	Hydroxyurea	Reduce stress/epinephrine
		Avoid hypoxia (asthma, sleep apnea)

dic care.[80] Families can provide significant life-saving home assistance for infants and children with prophylactic antibiotics and spleen palpation,[26] and families also lay the foundation for home pain management and coping skills. Adolescents can develop an understanding of their disease and benefit from peer counseling. Adolescent transition to adult medical care is complex, because sickle cell complications may increase in the late teens or early adulthood, mingling with teenage psychosocial issues, change in financial status, and possibly relocation away from family and friends.[81–83] Adults continue to benefit from peer support, as well as guidance on navigating the medical and social complexities of a chronic illness. Enhanced survival in sickle cell disease (Fig. 20–6*B*) has led to an increase of geriatric patients, who require skilled medical support for the interplay of changes caused by aging and those caused by sickle cell disease.

Pain Management Principles

Pain management in sickle cell disease can be a daunting task for the clinician because the vaso-occlusion is episodic, unpredictable, and variable and may lack objective signs. However, basic principles of pain management can be applied, such as quantifying the subjective report of pain and using a "staircase" of analgesics to match the strength of combination therapy to the intensity of pain.[84,85] Gaining control of pain by rapid dose adjustments is ideal, rather than gradually titrating upward over several days. Patient-controlled analgesia pumps permit greater flexibility of pain control through the day and can be used safely by children as young as 6 years old.

Common complications of a hospitalization for sickle cell pain are acute chest syndrome, constipation, and loss of venous access. The adverse effects of cumulative parenteral opioids can be minimized by the use of agonist-antagonist agents such as nalbuphine,[86,87] or by pharmacologic management of adverse effects. Antiemetics should be employed for nausea, antihistamines for pruritus, a bowel regimen for constipation, and stimulants for sedation. A randomized clinical trial demonstrated that having hospitalized children with sickle cell chest wall pain use incentive spirometry reduced acute chest syndrome by a factor of 9,[88] leading to widespread adoption of this inexpensive interaction. Adjunct corticosteroids may provide some benefit, but a short steroid taper is needed to avoid rebound pain.[89] Individualized pain management plans can be developed, including atypical adjunct pharmacologic measures such as tricyclic antidepressants and γ-aminobutyric acid inhibitors. Nonpharmacologic pain management in the hospitalized patient can be very important: warming pads, cushioned mattress pads, recreational therapy and music for distraction, massage, hydrotherapy, hypnosis, relaxation exercise, yoga, transcutaneous electrical nerve stimulators, and biofeedback are beneficial for some patients.[90] Cuban sickle cell centers have a large experience with laser acupuncture (E. de la Torre, personal communication, 1998) (Table 20–6).

Improving Hospital Pain Management

A small subset of patients who are hospitalized frequently consume a large proportion of economic and clinical resources,[53,91–93] (Fig. 20–7) and focused individualized case management may reap more economic and clinical impact than do broad guidelines that force the majority of patients to abbreviate already short hospital stays. Psychosocial support staff are vital to such a case management approach. Some centers have established day hospitals or 18- to 24-hour urgent care centers dedicated to sickle cell pain management; 8 hours of treatment can provide sufficient pain relief to permit 80% of patients to avoid hospital admission.[87,94–96]

Improving Home Pain Management

Teaching of families to prevent sickle cell vaso-occlusive pain emphasizes avoiding the triggers for polymerization—dehydration, acidosis, hypoxia, and vasoconstriction—by lifestyle choices. Hydroxyurea reduces the frequency of sickle cell pain episodes in adults,[97] teenagers, and children[81,98–100] (Fig. 20–8). Menstruation can trigger sickle vaso-occlusive pain in some patients,[24,101,102] and some young women benefit from hormonal regulation to suspend menses.[103,104] Stereotypical pain patterns are important in individualized case management, but many pain episodes have no identifiable trigger.

Full discussion of sickle cell pain management theory and practice exceeds the scope of this chapter, and the reader may seek monographs and electronic guidelines on the topic[84,105,106] (*http://www.SCInfo.org; http://www.nhlbi.nih.gov/health/prof/blood/sickle/index.htm*) (Box 20–1).

Infection

Rapid evaluation of fever in sickle cell disease and empirical antibiotic treatments targeting *S. pneumoniae* are the current standard of care. However, the onset of sepsis

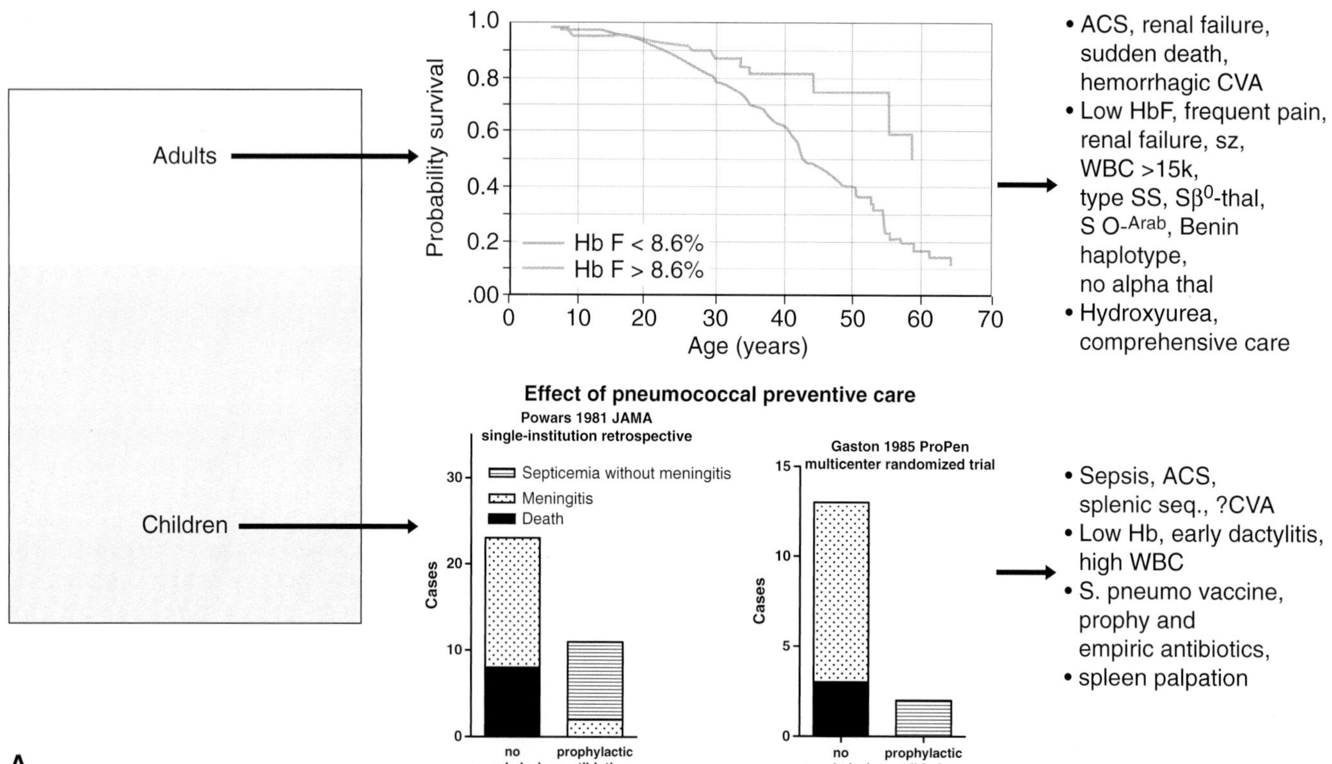

Figure 20–6. Heterogeneity of sickle cell disease mortality. Subsets of people may differ significantly in disease severity, and some of the larger subsets are contrasted in panels *A* and *B*. Pioneering work in Jamaica and the United States created a comprehensive care treatment program for sickle cell disease. Even in the absence of a randomized comparison, comprehensive care clearly reduces childhood mortality. Panels *A* and *B* show how comprehensive care for sickle cell disease changes the demographics and the clinical issues.

A, Sickle cell disease course without comprehensive care. Death in early childhood was common and only a minority of people with sickle cell disease survived to adulthood. Most caregivers focused on newborn screening and pediatric problems with prophylactic antibiotics showing a clear benefit in reducing early childhood septicemia, meningitis, and death from *Streptococcus pneumoniae*. The frequency of hospitalization for pain was recognized as a predictor of survival in the multicenter natural history study Cooperative Study of Sickle Cell Disease.[199] A small number of patients account for the majority of hospitalizations for sickle cell disease, while approximately half the patients have less than one hospitalization per year.[91]

B, Comprehensive care changes sickle cell disease. Comprehensive care programs have lowered childhood mortality due to *Streptococcus pneumoniae* sepsis and splenic sequestration, so that median survival is shifted into mid-adulthood and the majority of people with sickle cell disease are adults. Adult morbidity and mortality are reduced by hydroxyurea therapy, with gradations—depend on the details of their response to hydroxyurea therapy. Two new major risk factors for mortality have been identified in adults with sickle cell disease: pulmonary hypertension and iron overload. Pulmonary arterial hypertension was recently identified as a risk factor for death in adults with tricuspid regurgitant jet velocity greater than 2.5 m/sec by echocardiogram.[39] Based upon these findings, recommendations were made for screening adults using echocardiogram, and clinical trials are in progress to find effective intervention(s) to reduce the mortality after pulmonary hypertension is detected. Iron overload in adults (resulting from multiple red blood cell transfusions) was also identified recently as a predictor for high mortality in young adults with sickle cell disease[200] parallels the high mortality among young adults with thalassemia major who fail to adhere to iron chelation therapy. Renal compromise is a risk factor,[199,201] but renal failure may overlap significantly with pulmonary hypertension[39] and multiple transfusion.[123]

can be extremely rapid, and *S. pneumoniae* is increasingly resistant to antibiotics. Therefore, conjugated vaccines against *S. pneumoniae* and *H. influenzae* are now recommended, together with 23-valent polysaccharide vaccine against *S. pneumoniae*. The highly effective conjugated pneumococcal vaccines have not made newborn screening unnecessary because pneumococcal sepsis rates after introduction of these vaccines remain excessive.[107]

Desferrioxamine therapy should be interrupted in febrile patients, especially those with abdominal pain, diarrhea and vomiting, or fever and sore throat. Stool cultures and, if possible, serology for *Yersinia* should be obtained. If empirical antibiotics are implemented *Yersinia* susceptibility should be considered (by incorporating cotrimoxazole or aminoglycoside into the regimen).[108]

Acute Chest Syndrome

Because of the high likelihood of one or more infectious etiologies, a management recommendation for acute

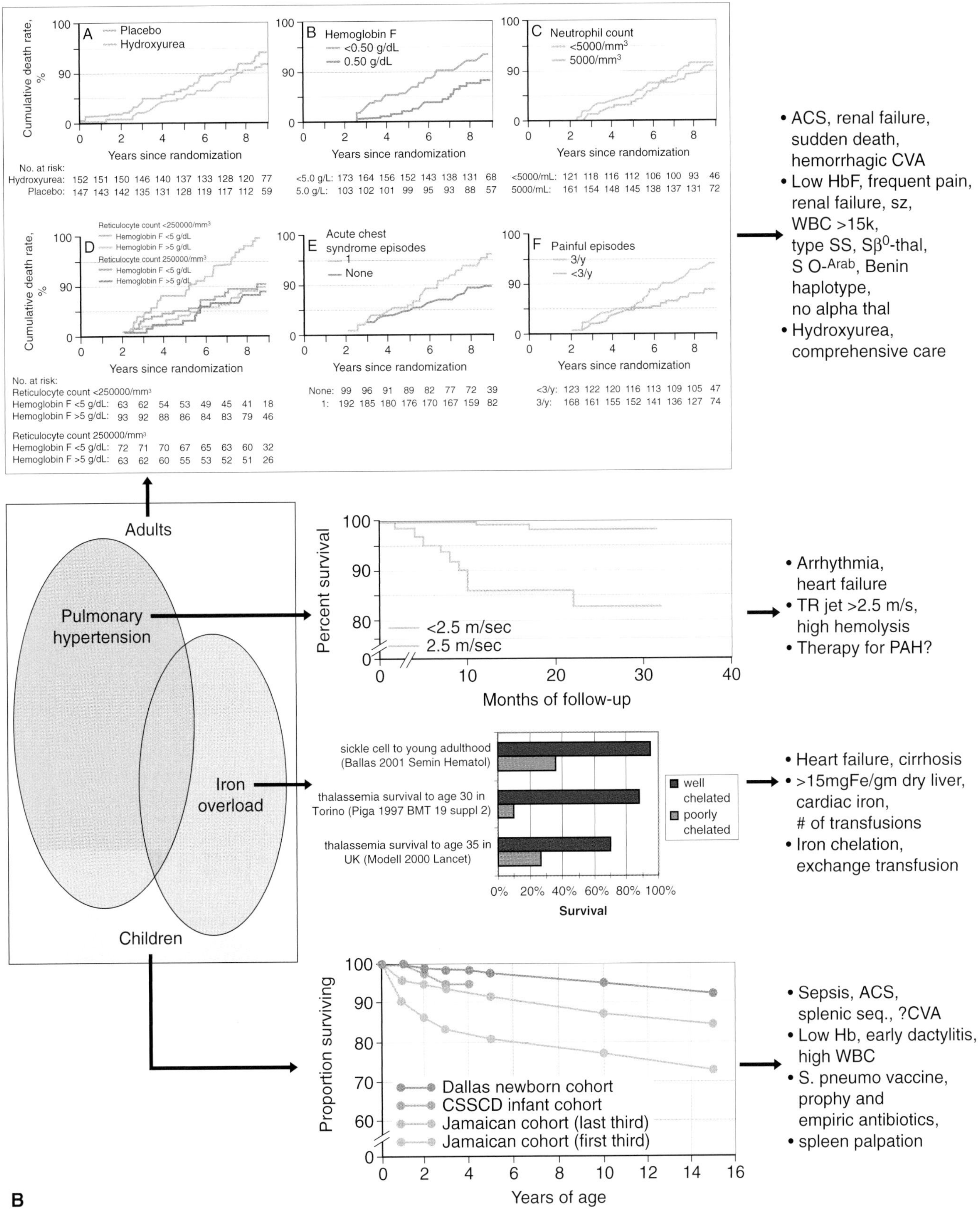

Figure 20–6, cont'd

TABLE 20–6. Complications of Sickle Cell Disease—Severity of Chronic Tissue Injury

Condition or Complication	Severity Criteria and/or Pre-symptomatic Assessment	Endstage or Overt Manifestation	Reference(s)
Hb level WBC	<8 gm/dL >20,000	Predictor for mortality	21
Early dactylitis	Onset before 12 mo		
Hb F	<20%	Predictor for morbidity & mortality	212
	>0.5 gm/dL		165
Recurrent pain	Days hospitalized >3 episodes per yr		199
Renal			
Glomerulopathy and tubular dysfunction	Microalbuminuria	Nephrotic	71
	Proteinuria	Renal failure	70,213,214
	Glomerulosclerosis		
	Concentrating defect		
Pulmonary hypertension	Tricuspid regurgitation >2.5 m/sec	Right heart failure	39
	NYHA classes I–IV	Arrhythmia	
		Sudden cardiac death	
Cerebrovascular disease	TCD Time-averaged mean velocity > 170 cm/sec	Ischemic stroke	65
		Hemorrhagic stroke	
	MRA stenosis		
	Aneurysm		
	Neurocognitive defect		
Bone infarcts	AVN Stage I–IV by MRI & radiograph	Hip prosthesis replacement	215,216
		Vertebral collapse	
Iron overload	Hepatic iron	Cirrhosis	141,142
	Portal fibrosis	Cardiomyopathy	? 217–219
Aplastic crisis	Hb drop > 1 gm/dL	Death	? 220
	Reticulocytes < X		
Splenic sequestration	Hb drop > 1 gm/dL 3 or more episodes	Splenectomy	221,222
Retinopathy	Grade	Death	
	Proliferative sickle retinopathy	Vitreous hemorrhage	? 223
Priapism	Acute, prolonged stuttering, recurrent	Impotence	
Leg ulcers	? CEAP grade		? 224
Global Severity Score	Global Severity Score to correlate with biomarkers or genotype		225–231

? For these complications, the assessment and management of similar complications in other diseases has been adopted for care of sickle cell disease.
Abbreviations: AVN, avascular necrosis; CEAP, clinical, etiologic, anatomic, and pathologic grade; MRA, magnetic resonance angiography; MRI, magnetic resonance imaging; NYHA, New York Heart Association; s.g., specific gravity; TCD, transcranial Doppler ultrasound; WBC, white blood cell count.

chest syndrome is empirical antibiotics for both respiratory bacteria and atypical bacteria (ceftriaxone or ampicillin/sulbactam, and a macrolide).

Osteomyelitis

When osteomyelitis is clinically suspected, the affected bone should be aspirated prior to the initiation of antibiotics. In patients with culture-proven bone or joint infection, surgical curettage/drainage is followed by 2–6 weeks of antibiotics treatment. Initial empirical antibiotics should be effective for *Salmonella* and *Staphylococcus*[32–35] but then adjusted specifically to the organism isolated. Most patients can be cured, but recurrences and refractory infection are observed. Sickle cell patients without culture-proven infection of bone or joint should not be overtreated with antibiotics, because bone infarction is 50 times more likely than osteomyelitis.

Parvovirus B19

Immunization for human parvovirus is entering clinical trials (see Chapter 76). Transfusion risks and benefits during a parvovirus aplastic crisis should be weighed in the context that the red blood cell production will recover within 7–10 days (unless there is an additional deficit of cell-mediated immunity). Supportive care may be sufficient in uncomplicated aplastic crisis in children without cardiopulmonary complications, especially those with milder hemolysis, and may be an option for those with red blood cell alloimmunization or religious objection to transfusion.

Therapy for Other Specific Infections

Malaria treatment should include prompt antimalarials and fluid supplements to prevent dehydration and splenic sequestration. Influenza immunization is strongly recommended in sickle cell disease.[109] Because of the theoretical risk of endocarditis, some clinicians advocate antibiotic prophylaxis for dental care.

Respiratory Complications

Therapy for acute chest syndrome needs to be expeditious and almost always requires hospital observation because of the potential for rapid deterioration. Treatment for acute chest syndrome addresses its multiple etiologies, and includes empirical antibiotics, bronchodilators, analgesics, supplemental oxygen, and measures to reduce atelectasis (incentive spirometry and

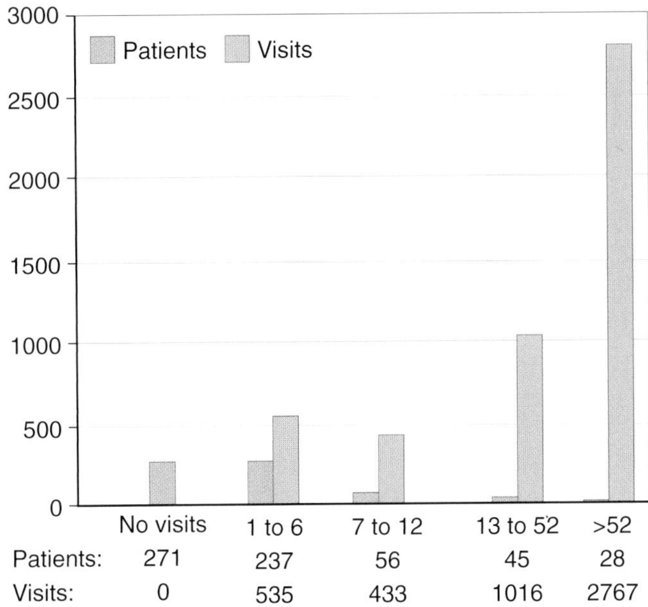

■ **Figure 20–7.** Disproportionate impact of a minority of patients. One year tally of emergency department visits in 637 adults followed at the Georgia comprehensive Sickle Cell Center illustrated that a few sickle cell disease patients accounted for a huge share of the visits. The majority of patients hardly use medical visits at all. These frequently encountered patients are candidates for hydroyxurea and other anti-sickling therapy, and for case management.

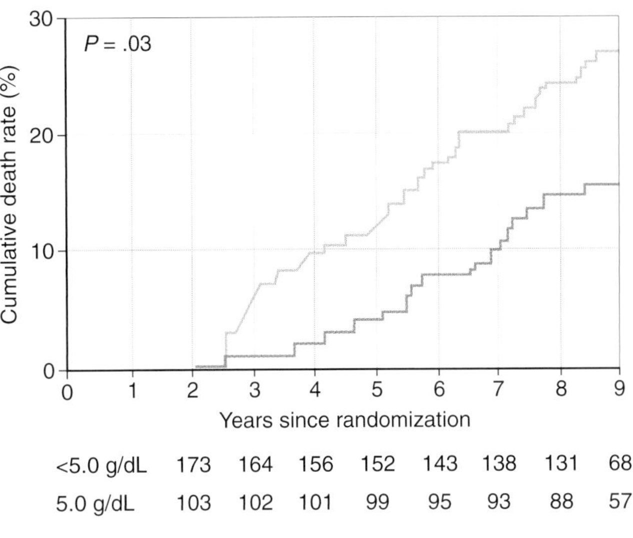

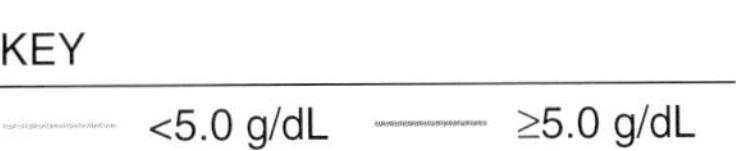

■ **Figure 20–8.** Hydroxyurea and survival in adults with sickle cell disease.[165] After the end of the multicenter double-blinded randomized MSH trial of hydroxyurea versus placebo,[97] the participants self-selected whether to continue hydroxyurea therapy. The subset whose hydroxyurea therapy resulted in an effective rise in Hb F had 40% lower mortality than those whose Hb F remained below 0.5 gm/dL (mortality 15% vs. 28%, *P* = .04) in this follow-up of 299 adults on self-selected treatment for severe sickle cell disease. A single-institution report of 226 adults on hydroxyurea showed a similar mortality rate of 17%.[166]

intermittent positive airway pressure). Red blood cell transfusion can be promptly beneficial,[30] and may be implemented when the hemoglobin declines by more than 1 gm/dL, with caution to not overtransfuse and cause hyperviscosity or volume overload. Parenteral fluid supplements should be moderate so as to avoid adding pulmonary edema to pneumonitis. A requirement for high supplemental oxygen despite red blood cell transfusion should lead to consideration of exchange transfusion in order to reduce the fraction of sickle red blood cells below 30%. Severe acute chest syndrome benefits from the same therapies as does acute respiratory distress syndrome: extracorporeal membrane oxygenation, nitric oxide, and high-frequency ventilation. Chronic management of recurrent acute chest syndrome includes pulmonology consultation or multidisciplinary evaluation with hematologists. Optimizing management of reactive airway disease can be very helpful in reducing acute chest syndrome recurrence.[110]

Pulmonary hypertension in sickle cell disease is refractory to hydroxyurea.[39] Clinical interventions under examination for this high-risk group include sildenafil, inhaled nitric oxide, and atorvastatin.

Obstructive sleep apnea can be relieved surgically by tonsillectomy and/or adenoidectomy.

Neurologic Complications

Screening of children by transcranial Doppler ultrasound to detect those at high risk for stroke and then protecting them from primary stroke by chronic blood transfusion to maintain the sickle red blood cell fraction below 30%[65] are the standard of care. Current evidence indicates that chronic transfusions need to be continued indefinitely.[111]

In acute stroke, many centers use exchange transfusion to reduce the proportion of sickle erythrocytes below 30% and limit ischemic damage. Acute anticoagulation has not been studied in this setting. Evaluation by a neurologist and vigorous rehabilitation therapy are indicated, and many neurologic deficits in children are reversible. Neurocognitive testing should be performed to help develop an individualized educational plan for a child's school. After a stroke, chronic transfusion to maintain sickle erythrocytes below 30% is widely employed in pediatric sickle cell centers, and several small studies indicate its utility in preventing recurrent stroke (secondary stroke prevention).[112] Both simple transfusion and erythrocytapheresis can achieve dilution of sickle erythrocytes; the principal benefit of chronic erythrocytapheresis is that iron accumulation is avoided and there is no need for iron chelation therapy. Disadvantages of erythrocytapheresis include increased exposure to blood donors, the need for large-bore venous access, and a requirement for a dedicated apheresis team and its resources. If an ischemic stroke has already occurred, chronic transfusion after one stroke to maintain sickle red blood cell count below 30% can be relaxed after 3 years, to maintain sickle red blood

Box 20–1 Treatment of Acute Pain Episodes

There are numerous approaches for sickle cell pain. The doses and drugs listed below are suggested; good clinical judgment and especially consideration of the characteristics of the episode in the context of the patient's particular disease manifestations and long-term course are very important in individualizing care. Management advice is based on information available on selected websites (http://scinfo.org/painepi.htm, http://scinfo.org/protpainIP.htm, http://www.nhlbi.nih.gov/health/prof/blood/sickle/sc_mngt.pdf) and the authors' experience.

- Assess the patient for the cause of pain and for complications. For the individual patient, check which treatments are usually effective, appropriate dosages and side effects, and which drugs have been recently self-administered at home for this episode.
- Rapidly assess pain intensity using a simple measurement tool.
- Begin hydration. Children often are treated with a 10-mL/kg intravenous bolus over 1 hour and then at a maintenance rate with hypotonic fluid such as 5% dextrose solution or 5% dextrose plus 0.2 normal saline. Because adults are more likely to have renal insufficiency, the bolus of fluids is usually omitted and hydration is initiated at 1.5-fold the maintenance fluid rate. The rate of infusion and the solute can be adjusted according to blood chemistries. Excessive fluids should be avoided unless the patient is dehydrated.
- Provide supplemental oxygen if pulse oximetry registers below 92% or a value lower than the patient's baseline value. A clinical explanation for a new requirement for supplemental oxygen should be investigated.
- Parenteral nonsteroidal anti-inflammatory drugs such as ketorolac are often helpful in relieving pain. For adults over 50 kg, 30 mg of ketorolac can be infused intravenously every 6 hours; in adults less than 50 kg, give 15 mg intravenously every 6 hours. For children, the dose is 1 mg/kg, to a maximum of 30 mg initially, followed by 0.5 mg/kg/dose, to a maximum of 15 mg/dose. Ketorolac should not be administered for more than 5 days in a month.
- Opioids: Many prefer parenteral morphine. Intravenous administration is the route of choice, but patients with poor venous access can receive opioids subcutaneously.
    - For loading, the typical morphine dose for adults is 5 to 10 mg and that for children, 0.1 to 0.15 mg/kg.
    - Titration of subsequent doses is based on frequent clinical assessment. Patients should be admitted to the hospital if there are other complications, pain persists for more than 8 hours despite adequate therapy, or outpatient therapy fails and the patient returns for further treatment within 48 hours. Titration strategies include the following:

        1. Reassess the patient at 30-minute intervals and, based on the results, treat with doses of 2.5 to 5 mg (0.05 to 0.1 mg/kg for children) until pain is relieved.
        2. Gradual titration may also be employed. The patient is started immediately on "by-the-clock" (BTC) doses based on prior history (e.g., morphine, 8 mg intravenously every 2 hours). "Rescue" doses are used for titration between BTC doses until relief is achieved.
        3. Titrate parenteral opioids using a patient-controlled analgesia pump. Patient-controlled injections typically are 0.018 to 0.04 mg/kg/dose with a 6-minute lockout. Continuous infusion may be given at night or around the clock, typically at 0.01 to 0.04 mg/kg/hr. Total morphine dose above 0.1 mg/kg/hr (continuous infusion plus boluses) should be used with caution but may occasionally be required.
- Adjuvant medications can reduce opioid side effects. For example, offer adults hydroxyzine 25 mg every 6 hours or promethazine 12.5 mg intramuscularly every 3 hours to prevent opioid-induced nausea and diphenhydramine, 25 to 50 mg every 6 hours, with morphine to prevent itching.
- Alternatively, a mixed agonist-antagonist opioid may be given, such as nalbuphine (0.2 mg/kg every 2 hours or 0.3 mg/kg every 3 hours; adult maximum, 20 mg/dose). Titration is limited by the analgesic "ceiling effect." Agonist-antagonists are contraindicated in patients on chronic opioids because they can precipitate withdrawal syndromes.
- Nonpharmacologic adjuncts such as heating pads and a soothing environment are also important for pain control. Atelectasis can be simply prevented by incentive spirometry (10 breaths every 2 hours when awake) or positive expiratory pressure respiratory maneuvers. Ambulation and activity should be encouraged.
- The physician or caregiver should continue to reassess pain, possible complicating medical events, and drug side effects frequently to determine the adequacy and duration of the effects of medication.

cells below 50%.[113] Bone marrow transplantation appears to halt the progressive stenosis of arteries around the circle of Willis.[114,115] Hydroxyurea has been used in patients with contraindications to chronic transfusion and appears to confer partial protection against recurrent stroke.[116] However, no randomized controlled trial has yet determined the best approach to secondary stroke prevention.[117]

Intracranial bleeding may present dramatically as sudden subarachnoid hemorrhage with severe headache, vomiting, and coma, or more subtly with hemiparesis, especially if there is intraparenchymal bleeding. A noncontrast head computed tomography scan determines whether urgent neurosurgical intervention is needed to address the site of hemorrhage, to evacuate blood, and to monitor intracranial pressure. Standard guidelines for intracranial hemorrhage should be followed,[118] with awareness of the features unique to the management of sickle cell disease. A subarachnoid hemorrhage in sickle cell disease should raise the possibility of multiple aneurysms, sometimes in unusual locations.[68] A sickle cell disease moyamoya vasculopathy can be the source of intraparenchymal or intraventricular hemorrhage.[119] If the hemoglobin is less than 10 gm/dL, a simple transfusion of packed red blood cells can improve cerebral oxygenation, but excessive transfusion to a hemoglobin level over 12 gm/dL risks hampering oxygen delivery through hyperviscosity and hypertension. Many clinicians proceed to erythrocytapheresis or manual erythrocyte exchange to reduce the Hb S percentage below 30%[120] in order to optimize blood flow and oxygenation for the ensuing weeks of critical care and recovery. Evaluation by expert neurologists and rehabilitation specialists is important. The role of long-term anticoagulation has not been evaluated. A program of chronic transfusion is recommended in a child with severe vasculopathy or unrepaired aneurysm.[106]

Renal Complications

Desmopressin and anticholinergic drugs helpful in other types of childhood enuresis produce only modest benefit in sickle cell disease, probably because of unresponsiveness of the damaged renal tubules. Behavior training can be counseled: reduced fluids for several hours before bedtime, urination just before going to bed, an alarm to have a nocturnal bathroom visit, and having the child share in washing wet sheets teach the consequences of enuresis.

Evaluation of a sickle cell disease patient with hematuria assesses for malignancy, infection, and other etiologies; sickle cell disease renal papillary necrosis is the diagnosis of exclusion. The treatment of hematuria in sickle cell disease includes bed rest, maintenance of a high urinary flow as documented by monitoring of intake and output, and, if blood loss is significant, iron replacement and/or blood transfusion.

The inability to concentrate urine in sickle cell disease leads to extreme susceptibility to dehydration. When oral replenishment is not feasible, such as before general anesthesia, intravenous fluids should be administered, and never discontinued "to promote thirst" during periods of high risk for dehydration such as the second day after tonsillectomy. Dehydration occurs easily in hot weather or dry environments, as with airline travel; sickle cell disease patients should always provide their own ample water supply. An exception to the principle of liberal hydration is acute chest syndrome; parenteral fluid supplementation should be moderate to avoid pulmonary edema (Box 20–2).

Sickle cell disease patients with renal insufficiency often need erythropoietin supplementation to increase their hemoglobin concentration; hormone therapy is preferable to chronic transfusion.[106] Angiotensin-converting enzyme inhibitors can reduce proteinuria and may have help prevent progression to end-stage renal disease.[106,121] Standard hemodialysis practice may need to be modified to allow for transfusion to a normal red blood cell count, and to address the higher risk of thrombotic complications in venous access lines. Kidney transplantation provides better survival than does chronic dialysis in sickle cell disease, and posttransplantation mortality appears to be similar to that in other types of end-stage renal disease.[122,123]

Box 20–2 Fluid Therapy

Inability to concentrate urine also leads to very high susceptibility to dehydration in people with sickle cell disease. Whenever a person with sickle cell disease cannot drink (such as prior to general anesthesia), IV fluids should be given. A prudent clinician will not shut off IV fluids "to promote thirst," in periods of high risk for dehydration as the second day after tonsillectomy. Dehydration is also easy in hot weather or dry environments such as airline travel, so that people with SCD should bring their own water along always. An exception to this principle of liberal hydration is during acute chest syndrome: parenteral fluid supplements should be moderate, to avoid adding pulmonary edema to the region of pneumonitis.

Leg Ulcers

Successful treatment of leg ulcers requires a consistent, systematic approach to maximize patient compliance over a course of weeks to months, including elevation of the legs, meticulous débridement, zinc supplements, antibiotics, and analgesics for chronic pain (see the National Heart, Lung and Blood Institute guidelines website, *http://www.SCInfo.org*). Agents that appear helpful to speed the healing include topical RGD peptide[124] and locally applied granulocyte-macrophage colony-stimulating factor.[125–128] Extrapolating from its use in diabetic ulcers,[129] hyperbaric oxygen has been applied to sickle cell leg ulcers but with mixed results and no formal clinical trial. Prevention must be stressed, especially avoiding venipuncture of the ankles and feet and occupations that involve prolonged standing for hours at a time, and awareness of the antecedent edema that can herald recurrence of a leg ulcer.

Bone Infarcts and Avascular Necrosis

Patients must be informed that the pain of bone infarct, sickle arthritis, or other joint complications may endure from days to weeks and that persistent narcotic administration may be unwise—they need to differentiate the treatment of this chronic pain from therapy of acute pain episodes. Non–weight bearing during periods of exacerbation of pain in aseptic necrosis improves acute symptoms and may slow progression. Hip replacement is generally postponed as long as possible, because of increased rates of perioperative and prosthetic complications.[130] Core decompression of the femoral head may slow joint deterioration in early aseptic necrosis in sickle cell disease[131] and is now the subject of a multicenter randomized study in progress.

Priapism

Priapism has had numerous therapeutic approaches but been subject to few randomized trials.[132,133] Recurrent priapism led to impotence in one half to one third of historical cases, but current guidelines for swift intervention[134–137] may reduce this long-term sequela as well as acute suffering. Immediate home therapy may be sufficient to relieve an episode: oral fluids, analgesics, urinating, moderate exercise, and/or bathing or showering. Priapism that fails to resolve promptly with such measures is an ischemic emergency requiring prompt aspiration of the corpora cavernosa by a urologist, who may also consider intracavernous injection of sympathomimetic drugs.[134] Intravenous hydration and analgesics are used as in other vaso-occlusive pain, and cooling is avoided because it promotes vaso-occlusion. Patients who have frequent episodes can be evaluated for priapism prophylaxis using pseudoephedrine.

Transfusion and Its Complications

Patients with sickle cell disease often receive numerous transfusions, either in a chronic transfusion program such as for stroke prevention or sporadically, for surgery or acute complications such as aplastic crisis, splenic sequestration, and acute chest syndrome.[138] Whenever possible, extended red blood cell count phenotyping and matching should be performed to avoid alloimmunization to antigens (such as C, E, Kell, and Jkb) that have low frequency among African Americans but high frequency among American blood donors. Blood banks that serve a large population of sickle cell patients often maintain packed red blood cell units that are negative for C, E, and Kell antigens for urgent use. Patients who receive fragmented medical care and transfusions at different medical institutions are at risk of red blood cell alloimmunization and hemolytic transfusion reactions unless the blood banks share information regionally. Hyperhemolysis in a transfused patient with sickle cell disease can be life-threatening and very difficult to evaluate.[139,140]

Transfusional iron overload can lead to cardiomyopathy and cirrhosis, as in β-thalassemia major, but whether sickle cell patients suffer the same endocrine complications as thalassemics is still uncertain. Compared to serum ferritin values, either liver biopsy or the cumulative number of blood transfusions appear to be better measures of tissue iron burden.[141] The threshold for portal fibrosis is probably a hepatic iron concentration of 7 mg/gm liver dry weight[142]; iron chelation therapy is usually initiated after 20 red blood cell units have been administered in chronic transfusion programs. Deferoxamine is the only chelator currently available in the United States, and the need for parenteral self-administration leads to problems with compliance, but new iron chelators for oral administration are in clinical trials (see Chapter 56). Erythrocytapheresis offers an alternative transfusion approach that may be adjusted to provide no net iron loading,[143,144] but at the cost of increased exposure to blood units, with resultant increased risks for red blood cell count alloimmunization and transfusion-transmissible infections. Venous access can become problematic for patients who are frequently transfused, but an increasing variety of indwelling subcutaneous central lines are commercially available.

Management of Pregnancy and Contraception

Pregnancy is not contraindicated in women with sickle cell disease,[145] but there are increased risks of hypertension, vaso-occlusive pain, urinary tract infections, hypercoagulability, and renal and pulmonary complications.[106,146,147] Managing the pregnancy ideally starts with preconceptual planning and genetic counseling, and gathering a multidisciplinary team with expertise in sickle cell hematology, obstetrics, nutrition, and primary care. Perinatal mortality with good medical care may still be 4.8–6 %,[148] or four to five times higher than in pregnancies without hemoglobinopathy; maternal mortality with sickle cell disease ranges from 2% to 6.7%.[145,146,149,150] Hyperemesis and dehydration in early pregnancy should be managed with preventive measures and early intervention with antiemetics. Prophylactic transfusions are reserved for women with additional high-risk features, such as twin pregnancies, a previous poor obstetric history, recurrent acute chest syndrome, or recurrent vaso-occlusion and severe anemia.[147,148,151] Postpartum care must include screening for sickle cell disease in the infant and counseling on plans for future pregnancies.[106]

Despite early theoretical concerns about oral contraceptives, there is no evidence of increased thrombotic events with low-estrogen formulations in women with sickle cell disease.[152,153] Disease-specific factors to weigh when choosing contraception include the adverse health effects of pregnancy in sickle cell disease and the potential for hormonal therapy to reduce menstrual-triggered vaso-occlusive pain.[103,104] Women and men on hydroxyurea therapy should use contraceptive methods and discontinue hydroxyurea if they plan to conceive a child,[106] because hydroxyurea is well known to be teratogenic in animal models.[154] However, if conception occurs during administration of hydroxyurea, counseling should mention that hydroxyurea has not yet been associated with birth defects in humans.[155,156]

TABLE 20–7. Antisickling Therapies

	Chronic Transfusion	Hydroxyurea	Bone Marrow/Cord Blood Stem Cell Transplantation
Indications	Ischemic CVA Recurrent ACS Splenic sequestration Severe anemia caused by renal failure	Recurrent ACS Frequent pain	Ischemic CVA Recurrent ACS Frequent pain Avascular necrosis
Contraindications	Multiple RBC alloantibodies Poor venous access	Pregnant	No matched donor
Advantages	Reduces severity of sickle cell complications Primary prevention of stroke in children	Reduces severity of sickle cell complications Improves longevity Increases Hb Gain weight	Curative Prevents further cerebrovascular disease
Disadvantages	Requires venous access RBC alloimmunization Iron overload except when using erythrocytapheresis Not curative	Requires monitoring for myelosuppression Not curative	Risk of procedure-related death: infection, organ failure, GVHD Risk of chronic GVHD

Abbreviations: ACS, acute chest syndrome; CVA, cerebrovascular accident; GVHD, graft-versus-host disease; RBC, red blood cells.

Surgery and Perioperative Care

Careful attention to the unique needs of sickle cell disease is necessary during perioperative management, and coordinating care with the anesthesia and surgery teams can significantly reduce the risk of complications. The Cooperative Study of Sickle Cell Disease reported that, in 717 nonrandomized surgical episodes, postoperative complications increased with age, with an estimated odds ratio 1.3 times increased risk of postoperative complications per ten years of age, and preoperative transfusion resulted in a lower complication rate for those undergoing low-risk surgery.[157] Regional anesthesia and abdominal surgery were associated with a greater risk of sickle cell disease–related complications.[157] Tonsillectomy for patients with sickle cell disease particularly merits carefully coordinated perioperative care, because the associated blood loss, fluid depletion, and inability to take oral hydration can easily trigger vaso-occlusive pain.[157–160] A multicenter randomized study of aggressive (exchange) versus simple transfusion in Hb SS sickle cell disease patients, with both treatments performed to achieve a hemoglobin level of 10 gm/dL, showed no difference in complication rates.[161] The perioperative protocol from that study is now generally accepted as the standard of perioperative care,[85] including preoperative hydration, close intraoperative monitoring, and postoperative oxygen, hydration, monitoring with pulse oximetry, and respiratory therapy with incentive spirometry.

Globin Modulation

Hemoglobin F is the best understood phenotypic modulator of sickle cell disease. Besides reducing the concentration of Hb S, Hb F also inhibits polymerization of Hb S. The strategy of using globin gene modulation as therapy for sickle cell disease arose from observations that Saudi Arabians with Hb SS sickle cell disease and high fetal hemoglobin suffered very few complications of sickle cell disease,[162] and infants were similarly protected until the fetal hemoglobin was developmentally down-regulated. Hydroxyurea, an S-phase cytotoxic drug that raises Hb F, moved from "bench to bedside"[97,163] and gained Food and Drug Administration approval as anti-sickling therapy for adults with severe sickle cell disease complications (Table 20–7). Results of hydroxyurea clinical trials in adolescents and children are similar to those in adults to date, and an infant study is in progress. New data indicate that hydroxyurea improves patient survival and is cost-effective.[164–166] Hydroxyurea appears to increase Hb F synthesis by premature commitment of erythroid precursors during the marrow regeneration that follows cytoreduction. Possible other mechanisms of action for hydroxyurea, and whether patients with Hb SC can benefit, are being examined. Problems of nonresponders, as well as toxicity/teratogenicity, have resulted in the search for other agents (butyrate, decitabine, 5-azacytidine), and also exploration of combining hydroxyurea with erythropoietin.

Transplantation

The only cure for sickle cell disease and other hemoglobinopathies has been transplantation of hematopoietic stem cells. After "proof of concept" with incidental cure of sickle cell disease in a child with bone marrow transplantation for leukemia,[167] Belgian and French groups pioneered the use of transplants for children with severe complications of sickle cell disease, using HLA-identical sibling donors.[168] The ethical challenge of balancing transplant-related mortality and morbidity for a disease in which severity of disease course is heterogeneous and unpredictable led to international moot court discussions.[169] The early transplant experience in the United

States included peritransplant strokes and seizures, but these complications were greatly reduced after protocol modifications for better control of hypertension, transfusion for thrombocytopenia, and the appropriate employment of anticonvulsants and electrolyte correction.[170] Current conditioning regimens used in American trials avoid total-body irradiation and include cyclophosphamide, busulfan, and T-cell depletion using either antithymocyte globulin or Campath monoclonal antibody. A combination of methotrexate and cyclosporine or cyclosporine and prednisone is used for prophylaxis against graft-versus-host disease. These modern transplant techniques have produced success rates exceeding 93%, with a graft rejection rate of 5–7%. A recent Belgian report of transplantation of asymptomatic children claimed essentially no transplant complications.[171] The graft rejection rate remains higher than in bone marrow transplantation for malignant diseases, and current speculation is that HLA sensitization or a robust host marrow may be the reasons. Transplantation of related-donor cord blood/placental blood stem cells gives results similar to those with bone marrow but the cell dose limits this type of transplant to pre-teenagers. Unintentional partial mixed chimerism was noted to provide cure due to the survival advantage of normal red blood cells compared to sickle red blood cells.[172] Attempts to achieve partial mixed chimerism through nonmyeloablative preparative transplant regimens of reduced toxicity have been unable to produce immune tolerance, and patients suffered an extremely high rate of graft rejection when immunosuppression was withdrawn. Unrelated-donor cord blood/placental blood and bone marrow transplantation have been attempted, but there is a high risk of severe chronic graft-versus-host disease and consequent significant morbidity and mortality. Transplants in adult patients have been far less successful than in children, because of organ impairment from more years of active sickle cell disease and also increased HLA sensitization. The major barrier to more cures by transplantation is the lack of HLA-identical related donors[173] (Fig. 20–9).

COMPOUND HETEROZYGOSITY WITH OTHER HEMOGLOBINS AND THALASSEMIAS

Hemoglobin C and Hemoglobin SC

Hemoglobin C is an unstable hemoglobin and also activates dehydration of the red blood cell via the KCl cotransporter. Compound heterozygotes with Hb S and Hb C (Hb SC) have sickle cell disease, with a pattern that largely overlaps with homozygous Hb S. Hemoglobin SC sickle cell disease typically produces less frequent painful crises in childhood, a lower risk of stroke, and milder anemia. However, Hb SC sickle cell disease has greater risk than does Hb SS sickle cell disease for avascular necrosis and retinopathy, and perhaps also for leg ulcers. Pilot studies of hydroxyurea in Hb SC sickle cell disease provided contradictory laboratory evidence for separate mechanisms of benefit: improved red blood cell hydration in adults[174] and increased Hb F in children.[175] Caution is necessary in dose escalation of hydroxyurea for Hb SC sickle cell disease because of the potential for hyperviscosity if the hematocrit rises.

β-Thalassemia and Hemoglobin S/β-Thalassemia

β-Thalassemia can be simply divided into β-thalassemia, in which some normal Hb A is expressed, and β^0-thalassemia, in which no β-globin is produced (see Chapter 21). Sickle cell disease compound heterozygotes with Hb S/β-thalassemia have anemia and risks of complications that are similar to those with Hb SS sickle cell disease. Distinguishing Hb S/β-thalassemia sickle cell disease from Hb SS sickle cell disease is important principally for genetic counseling; elevated Hb A_2 and microcytosis may be useful clues that prompt family studies and hemoglobin genotyping. Compound heterozygotes with Hb S/β-thalassemia have milder anemia and lower risks of complications than do patients with Hb SS, and a risk pattern similar to patients with Hb SC (more avascular necrosis and retinopathy, less pain and stroke). Compound heterozygotes are frequently misdiagnosed at newborn screening as having sickle cell trait, leading to undiagnosed sickle vaso-occlusive pain and lack of screening for complications.

Hemoglobin E

Hemoglobin E is an unstable hemoglobin of very high frequency in Southeast and South Asia. Homozygous Hb E and heterozygotes with Hb A and Hb E are generally asymptomatic. Compound heterozygotes with Hb E and Hb S have likewise been described as asymptomatic, with unusual exceptions.[175a,175b] Compound heterozygotes with Hb E and β-thalassemia (Hb E/β-thalassemia) may manifest a wide spectrum of clinical manifestations even within one family, ranging from asymptomatic microcytic anemia to transfusion dependence and resembling β-thalassemia major; impaired growth; and pulmonary hypertension.[176–178] Some of the clinical variability of Hb E/β-thalassemia can be attributed to coinherited α-thalassemia or hereditary persistence of fetal hemoglobin.[179–182] Hb E is an important hemoglobinopathy for hematologists and in newborn screening programs in Western countries with growing populations of Asian immigrants.[183]

FUTURE DIRECTIONS

New research is exploring the roles of vasoconstriction, oxidant damage, inflammation, and endothelial dysfunction in acute vaso-occlusion and chronic complications. Medications to improve erythrocyte hydration and to decrease endothelial adhesion are in clinical trials. Nutritional supplements such as L-Arginine and omega-3 fatty acids may treat the vascular abnormalities in sickle cell disease. Future therapy may combine these agents with new medications to induce higher fetal hemoglobin.

Gene therapy as practical treatment is for the future, not yet able to achieve stable high-level expression of

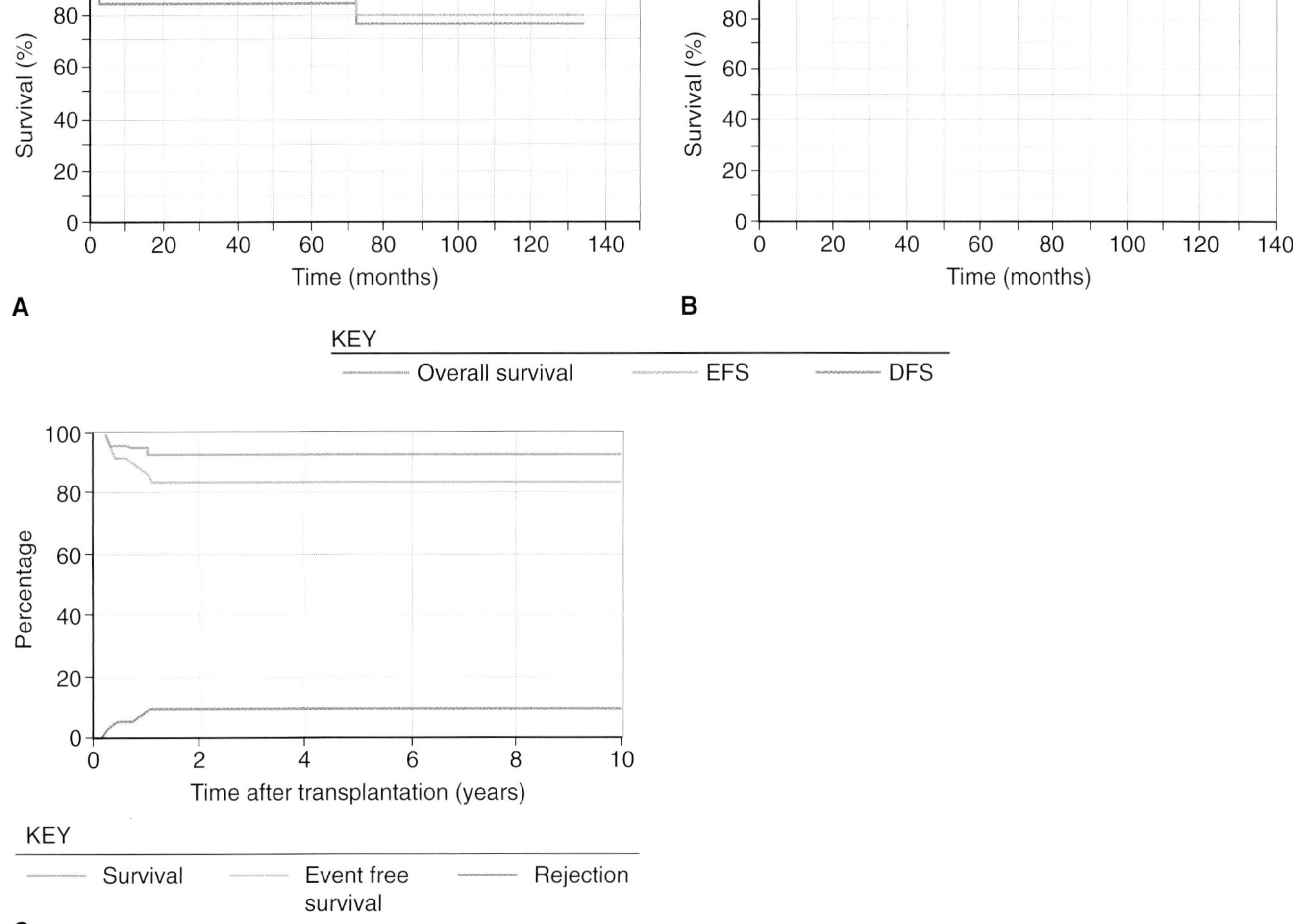

Figure 20–9. Outcomes after bone marrow transplantation for sickle cell disease. Kaplan-Meier plots of bone marrow transplantation (BMT) for children severely affected with sickle cell disease, from HLA-matched sibling donors, shows cure in more than 85% and stability over nearly 10 years of follow-up in multicenter studies by Belgian-French *(A)*[171] and North American *(C)* consortia.[170] Asymptomatic children transplanted in Belgium had over 93% disease-free survival *(B)*.[171] Graft-versus-host disease rates are low, but fatal graft-versus-host disease occurs. The BMT consortia developed a standard of supportive care specific to sickle cell disease, which markedly reduced mortality from hemorrhagic cerebrovascular accident.[170] The 8–10% rate of graft rejection in both studies, which is similar to that in other nonmalignant conditions with a history of multiple transfusions, is due to host alloimmune sensitization. A hyperactive "robust marrow" could promote rejection, and pretransplant hydroxyurea is associated with a lower rate of this complication.[203]

the modified gene without adverse consequences for the host.

In contrast, cures by transplantation of bone marrow and other hematopoietic stem cells are practical now, but only available to a small fraction of people with sickle cell disease. Ongoing clinical trials seek to determine whether curative hematopoietic stem cell transplantation can be offered to patients without a HLA-matched donor, while reducing the risks of morbidity and mortality in transplant for adult patients.

PROGNOSIS

Despite numerous attempts, no single parameter or system has become accepted as the measure of clinical severity of sickle cell disease. Four main gauges of the clinical impact of sickle cell disease have been used:

a) mortality: Kaplan-Meier analysis, odds ratios, deaths per 1000 pt-yrs)
b) functional measures: quality of life questionnaires,[187–189] medical contacts for pain,[89] absences from school[190] or work
c) clinical-pathologic scoring: for impairment of different organ systems (see Fig. 20–4 and Table 20–6)
d) cost of medical care.[78,191,192]

Part of the difficulty of this severity assessment is the heterogeneous and unpredictable nature of sickle cell disease. In addition, the complications accumulate over time, so that the full "phenotype" of an individual will not be evident in childhood. Finally, severity is probably

CURRENT CONTROVERSIES & FUTURE CONSIDERATIONS

Sickle Cell Disease

- Will new combinations of therapy have targets beyond HbS? New research is exploring the roles of vasoconstriction, oxidant damage, inflammation, and endothelial dysfunction in acute vaso-occlusion and chronic complications. Medications to improve erythrocyte hydration and to decrease endothelial adhesion are in clinical trials. Nutritional supplements such as L-Arginine and omega-3 fatty acids may treat the vascular abnormalities in sickle cell disease. Future therapy may combine these agents with new medications to induce higher fetal hemoglobin.

- Can hematopoietic stem cell transplant be offered to more patients using matched-unrelated donor transplant and reduced-intensity transplant? For patients without HLA-matched relatives as donors,[105] alternative donors such as haploidentical relatives or HLA-matched unrelated donors including cord blood have been used in pilot studies, but these transplants have had a very high rate of chronic GVHD. For patients with extensive organ damage who would fare poorly with myeloablative preparative regimens, non-myeloablative preparative regimens are being examined,[182–186] but these protocols have had enormous difficulty with graft rejection.

- Will gene therapy be feasible in practice, and should it be combined with autologous transplant? Gene therapy has advanced to testing in animal models with lentiviral and adenoviral vectors.[180,181] Some insert genes for normal Hb A or anti-sickling hemoglobins that will disrupt Hb S polymerization. Others aim for correction of the Hb S gene itself. The major challenges for gene therapy include transfection and stable expression of the modified gene in a large fraction of erythroid progenitors, without adverse consequences for the host. An amplified hematologic benefit is expected due to the survival advantage of gene-modified RBC over sickle RBC.

- Will new measures be developed based on the severity of SCD? Stratifying the SCD population by level of risks for organ failure and death is beginning to use functional tests (TCD, echocardiogram for pulmonary hypertension, proteinuria).

- Will access to healthcare be the controlling factor in determining people's longevity with SCD?

modulated by medical treatment (such as preventing pneumococcal infection, transfusions, antibiotics) and other environmental factors (bacterial osteomyelitis, leg ulcers). When a prophylactic or therapeutic strategy can be agreed upon, it will be easier to develop risk-benefit models, assess the effectiveness of therapies, and develop standards of care with quality assurance. Proper application of gene therapy and high-risk hematopoietic stem cell transplants can then be based on rational risk assessment categories, rather than the current case-by-case evaluations. In the future, polymorphisms of modifier genes will probably be identified to enhance functional stratification. The measures will permit evaluation and comparison of new therapies such as fetal hemoglobin inducers, antioxidants, nitric oxide donors/promoters, antithrombotics, anti-adhesion therapy, trace mineral supplements, educational and psychosocial therapy, traditional herbal medicines, alternative and complementary treatments. After subtypes of sickle cell disease are revealed by clinical measures and genetic profile, conceivably a customized "cocktail" of combination therapy could be mixed for one subtype.

Those with good access to comprehensive care, including preventive care, education, and combination therapy, may have few complications and nearly normal lifespan. However, most of the world's sickle cell population reside in developing nations, where access to healthcare will be very difficult and probably will suffer preventable morbidity and mortality. Americans with poor healthcare due to economics or geography will also have suboptimal care.

Suggested Readings*

Adams RJ, McKie, VC, Hsu L, et al: Prevention of a first stroke by transfusions in children with sickle cell anemia and abnormal results on transcranial Doppler ultrasonography. N Engl J Med 339:5–11, 1998.

Atkins RC, Walters MC: Haematopoietic cell transplantation in the treatment of sickle cell disease. Expert Opin Biol Ther 3: 1215–1224, 2003.

Gladwin MT, Sachdev V, Jison ML, et al: Pulmonary hypertension as a risk factor for death in patients with sickle cell disease. N Engl J Med 350:886–895, 2004.

Lee A, Thomas P, Cupidore L, Serjeant G: Improved survival in homozygous sickle cell disease: lessons from a cohort study. BMJ 311:1600–1602, 1995.

Steinberg MH, Barton F, Castro O, et al: Effect of hydroxyurea on mortality and morbidity in adult sickle cell anemia: risks and benefits up to 9 years of treatment. JAMA 289:1645–1651, 2003. [Published erratum appears in JAMA 290:756, 2003.]

Stuart MJ, Nagel RL: Sickle-cell disease. Lancet 364:1343–1360, 2004.

Vichinsky EP, Neumayr LD, Earles AN, et al: Causes and outcomes of the acute chest syndrome in sickle cell disease. National Acute Chest Syndrome Study Group. N Engl J Med 342:1855–1865, 2000. [Published erratum appears in N Engl J Med 343:824, 2000.]

Vichinsky EP, Haberkern CM, Neumayr L, et al: A comparison of conservative and aggressive transfusion regimens in the perioperative management of sickle cell disease. The Preoperative Transfusion in Sickle Cell Disease Study Group. N Engl J Med 333:206–213, 1995.

Full references for this chapter can be found on accompanying CD-ROM.

CHAPTER 21

Thalassemia

Melody J. Cunningham, MD, Mitchell J. Weiss, MD, PhD, and Ellis J. Neufeld, MD, PhD

KEY POINTS

Thalassemia

- Thalassemia syndromes are genetic disorders of globin chain synthesis that lead to unbalanced globin chain production, ineffective erythropoiesis, hemolysis, and variably severe anemia.
- Transfusion to maintain trough hemoglobin level of 9–9.5 g/dL ameliorates ineffective erythropoiesis in the majority of patients.
- Iron chelation therapy is required to prevent organ damage caused by transfusional iron overload.
- The phenotypic diversity of the thalassemia syndromes is due to the complex genotypic combinations of the α locus on chromosome 16 and the β locus on chromosome 11.
- Mortality in thalassemia patients is primarily due to heart disease and sepsis.
- Nontransfused thalassemia patients also can develop hemochromatosis as a result of exuberant iron absorption in the gut.

INTRODUCTION

Historical Perspective

The thalassemias are a phenotypically diverse group of genetic anemias caused by mutations affecting the production of α- or β-globin. The clinical syndrome of anemia, splenomegaly, and bony changes associated with β-thalassemia major was first reported by Cooley and coworkers in 1927.[1] Milder forms of the disease were described at about the same time, Weatherall and Clegg suggested that the onset of thalassemia in infancy was not noted in the Mediterranean region as a distinct disease because it was confounded by anemia and splenomegaly from malaria.[2] The history of evolving models of transfusion support for Cooley's anemia, or thalassemia major, in the 1950s and 1960s is described in comprehensive reviews.[3]

An understanding of the thalassemias and of emerging treatment strategies is important to hematologists for several reasons. First, the thalassemia syndromes are extremely common: thalassemia minor is one of the most prevalent single-gene diseases worldwide and thalassemia major is a leading cause of severe anemia in many regions of the world.[4] Second, the thalassemias were among the first diseases to be understood at the level of DNA and RNA.[5–7] Mutation analysis of α- and β-thalassemias was a paradigm for molecular approaches to other inherited diseases.[8,9] Third, the molecular analysis of thalassemias has led to individualized prenatal screening[10–12] and population-based public health strategies based on genetic screening[13] that remain important today.

Several systems for classification and nomenclature are used to describe the thalassemias, with naming based on (1) severity of clinical manifestations (thalassemia *minor* [trait], *major* [transfusion dependent], or *intermedia* [non–transfusion dependent]); (2) the hemoglobin phenotype or (3) the actual genotype. The thalassemia major syndromes lead to significant morbidity affecting nearly all organ systems, including a distinct physical appearance; untreated, they are uniformly fatal in the first few years of life.[14] However, early diagnosis, comprehensive treatment, and careful management have enabled many patients with thalassemia major to live productive, active lives well into adulthood.[15–20]

Epidemiology and Risk Factors

The evolutionary benefit that led to high prevalence of heterozygous states of both α- and β-thalassemia genotypes appears to be protection of heterozygotes against death from *Plasmodium falciparum* malaria.[21] The distribution of the thalassemia origins corresponds with areas of malarial prevalence prior to the 20th century,[22] although thalassemia trait now is found throughout the world[4] (Fig. 21–1). β-Thalassemia genes are particularly common in the Mediterranean region, parts of the Middle East, South and Southeast Asia, and southern China (Fig. 21–1*B*). α-Thalassemia arose independently in tropical Africa, the Middle East, China, India, Southeast Asia, and some regions of the South Pacific (Fig. 21–1*A*). The genotype that leads to the more severe forms of α-thalassemia (α^0-thalassemia) is found predominantly in populations of Mediterranean and Southeast Asian descent.[3] Immigration has brought thalassemia to the Western hemisphere as well.

Mode of Inheritance

Thalassemia is often described as a "recessive" disease in the sense that simple thalassemia minor never causes symptoms, and if two carrier partners with, for example, β-thalassemia minor, have children, each offspring has a 1 in 4 chance of being affected with thalassemia major. Therefore, identification of thalassemia trait in persons at risk is crucial for reproductive counseling in affected populations. However, thalassemia trait is detectable as microcytosis and trivial anemia, there are numerous modifying factors for the thalassemias,[23] and many combinations of defective α- and β-thalassemia genes are possible.[24] As with many other genetic disorders, the condition is more complex than simple mendelian recessive inheritance would predict.

PATHOPHYSIOLOGY

The molecular pathology of the thalassemia syndromes is understood in detail. More than 200 β mutations and many common α deletions have been described.[25] A paucity of one globin type (α or β) leads to a relative excess of the other.[26] The chain in excess tends to be unstable, leading to its denaturation, degradation, and ultimate precipitation within red blood cell precursors[16]; apoptosis of early erythroid cells within the bone marrow manifests functionally as ineffective erythropoiesis. In addition, many of the red blood cells that are released from the bone marrow are either damaged and removed by the spleen or hemolyzed in the circulation. These pathologic processes result in anemia and poor tissue oxygenation, signaling the kidneys to produce more erythropoietin and further stimulating ineffective marrow production.[16] Production of damaged cells and subsequent splenic trapping lead to splenomegaly, exacerbating sequestration of cells and thus the

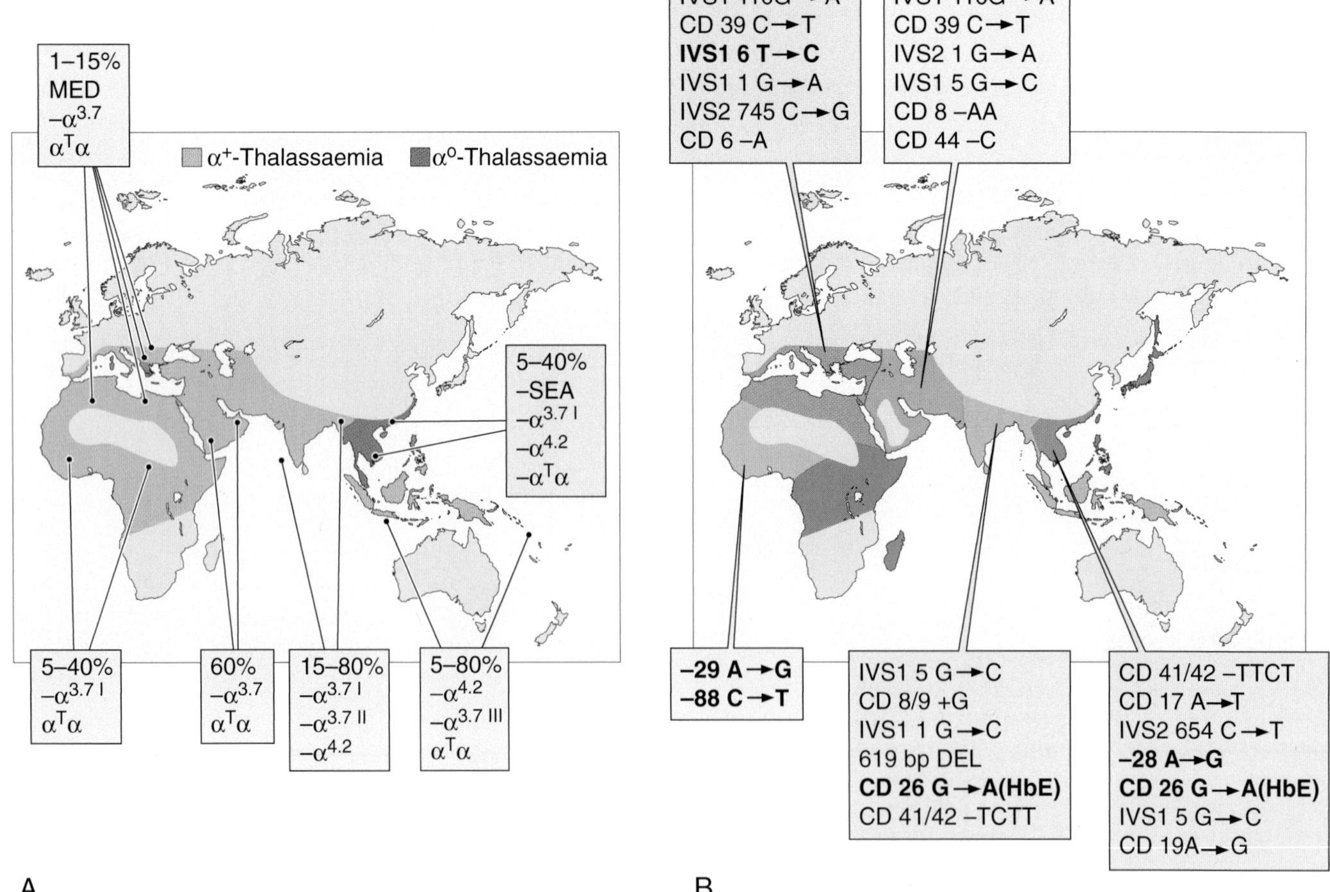

Figure 21–1. Distribution of α- and β-thalassemia mutations. The shaded areas correspond to areas of α- *(Map A)* or β- *(Map B)* thalassemia. The corresponding boxes indicate the mutations associated with the area shaded. (From Weatherall DJ: Phenotype-genotype relationships in monogenic disease: lessons from the thalassaemias. Nat Rev Genet 2:245–255, 2001.)

degree of anemia. Profound marrow expansion leads to the classic skeletal deformities in untransfused thalassemia major and "thalassemia intermedia" with severe phenotype (Fig. 21–2).

Pathophysiology of Transfusional Iron Overload

As discussed in Chapter 56, mammals have no endogenous mechanisms to rid the body of excess iron. Precisely how tissue injury results from the excess iron that inevitably accumulates with repeated erythrocyte transfusions is not perfectly understood. The damage is at least in part due to iron in excess of available transferrin (non–transferrin bound iron),[27] and the generation of free radicals and other oxidative species.[28,29] Ineffective erythropoiesis promotes increased gut absorption of iron.[30] In murine thalassemia models, and in recent studies in humans, a novel regulator of iron stores, termed *hepcidin,* has been implicated as a regulator of iron recycling and intestinal absorption.[31,32] First characterized as a small antimicrobial peptide,[33,34] hepcidin may prove to be the missing link between ineffective erythropoiesis and iron uptake in humans.

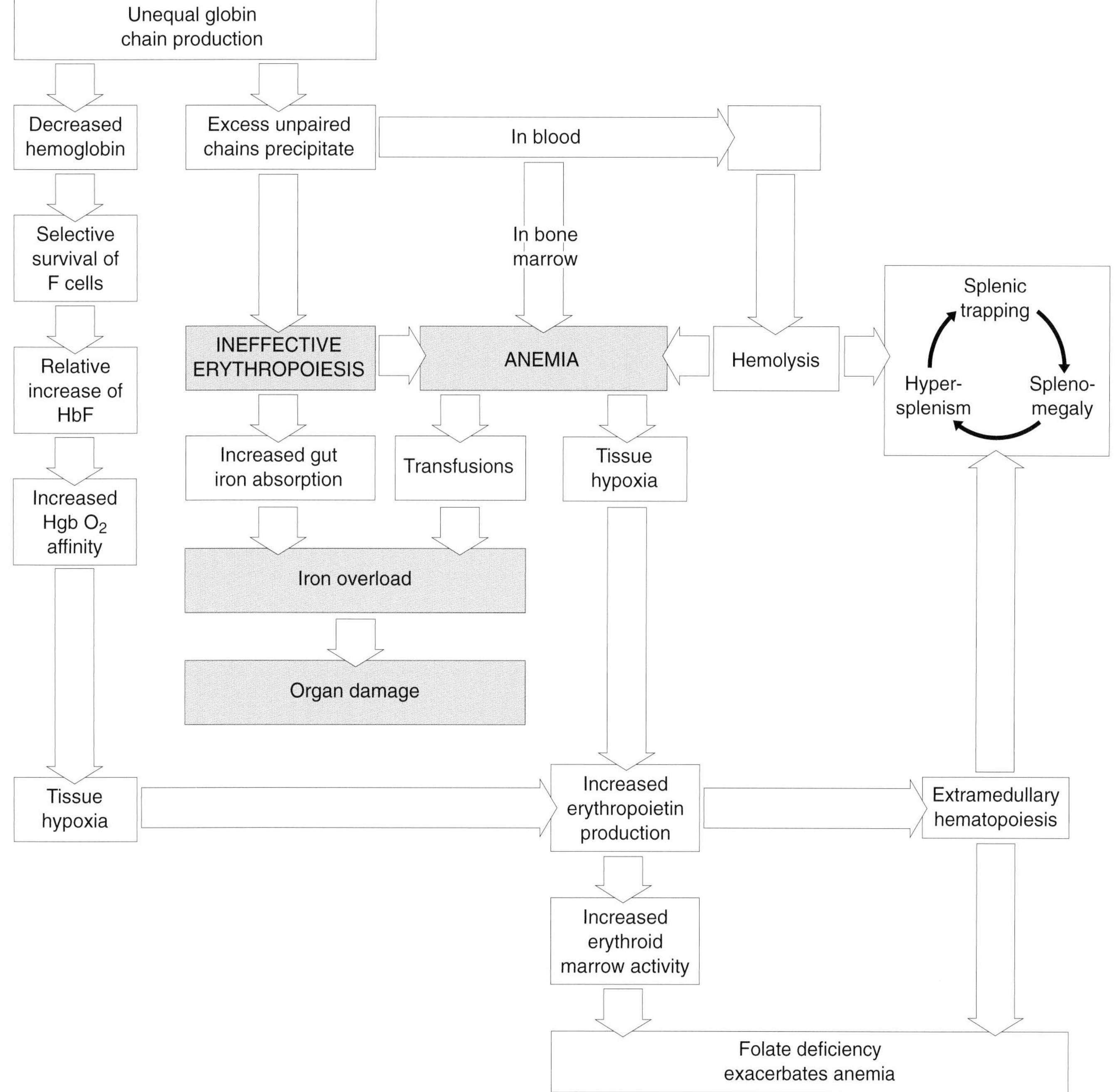

Figure 21–2. Pathophysiology of anemia and organ damage in thalassemia.

Globin Gene Organization, α-Globin Deletions, and β-Globin Mutations

Within the α-globin cluster on chromosome 16p, ζ, α2, and α1 are the functional genes[35–39] (see Chapter 2). The ζ gene is expressed during early embryonic life, and the two α genes are expressed throughout gestation and adulthood. There is no "fetal" α-like globin analogous to γ-globin in the β cluster, which is typically expressed only during late embryogenesis and within the first year after birth (Fig. 21–3*B*). Hemoglobin development progresses from hemoglobin Gower to hemoglobin A (Fig. 21–3*C*). The clinical implications of these differences are that severe α-thalassemia manifests as fetal hydrops, with prenatal or perinatal death from profound anemia, whereas severe β-thalassemia typically presents within 6–12 months after birth, when γ-globin levels decline. The two adjacent α genes are contained within highly homologous

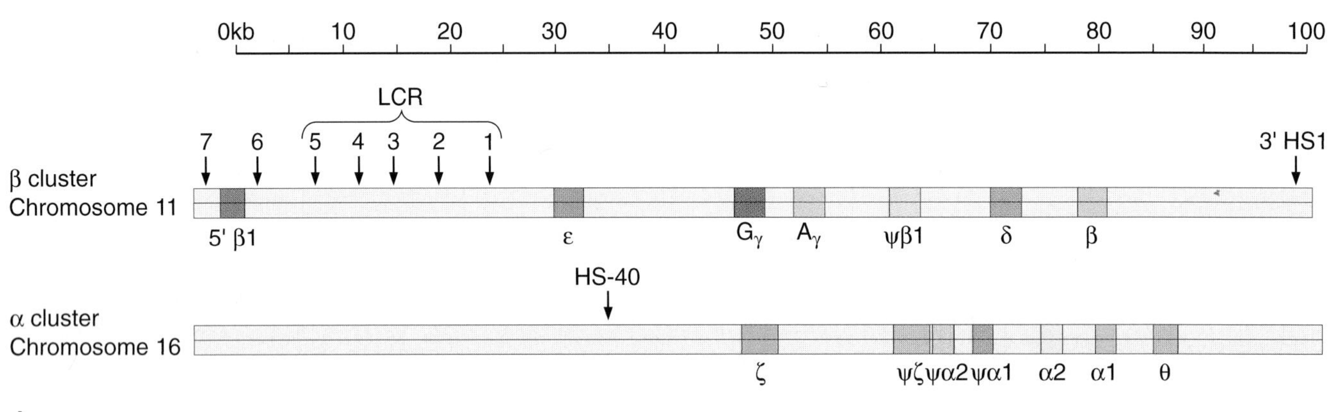

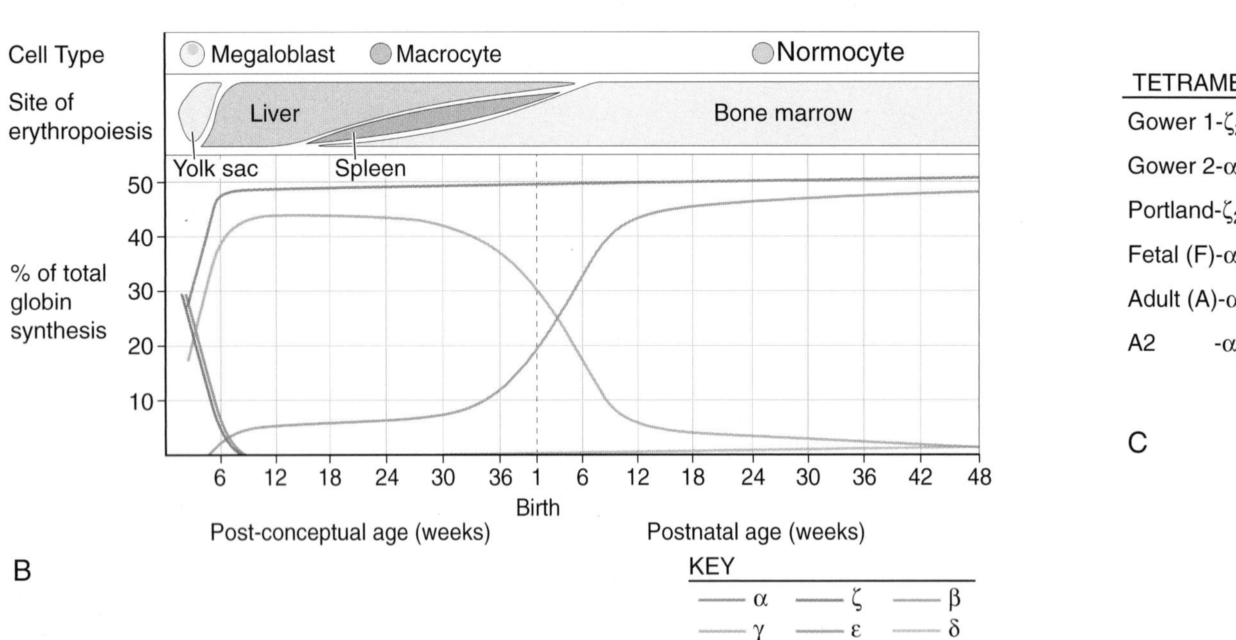

Figure 21–3. Human globin gene loci and developmental gene expression. ***A,*** Schematic of the human globin loci, with scale in kilobase pairs (kb). The β locus includes five genes with functional products, and one pseudogene (ψβ): ε (embryonic β-like gene); Aγ and Gγ (fetal β-like genes of hemoglobin [Hb] F); δ (minor β-like gene of Hb A2); and adult β of Hb A. The α locus includes three genes with functional products and three pseudogenes: ζ (embryonic α-like gene) and two α genes. Each locus has an enhancer region that directs high-level expression as described in the text (LCR for β locus, HS-40 for α locus). *Arrows* denote DNAse I–hypersensitive sites. (Adapted from Steinberg MH, Forget BG, Higgs DR, Nagel RL [eds]: Disorders of Hemoglobin: Genetics, Pathophysiology, and Clinical Management. Cambridge, MA: Cambridge University Press, 2001, p 118.) ***B,*** Developmental expression pattern of α-like and β-like genes, site of erythropoiesis, and morphologic appearance of circulating erythrocytes. For example, "primitive" erythrocytes in the early embryo are synthesized in the yolk sac and express embryonic globins ζ and ε. Specific globin genes expressed at each age are designated in the key. α-Like and β-like gene synthesis are nearly perfectly balanced, each 50% of the total. (From Wetherall DJ, Clegg JB: Historical perspectives: the many and diverse routes to our current understanding of the thalassemias. *In* The Thalassemia Syndromes. Oxford, UK: Blackwell Science, 2001, p 54.) ***C,*** Hemoglobin tetramers. At each stage of development, circulating hemoglobin is formed of pairs of two α-like and two β-like gene products.

segments of DNA, which arose by gene duplication about 60 million years ago.[40] Because these distinct closely linked regions are so similar, there is a propensity for genetic recombination to occur between them. The products of such unequal crossovers are α gene deletions and triplications. Deleted α alleles generated through this mechanism are the most common α-thalassemic mutations. In addition, triplicate α chromosomes are observed in thalassemic populations.[41,42] These mutations are significant when coinherited with β-thalassemias because they worsen clinical severity by increasing the level of unpaired cytotoxic free α chain[43,44] (discussed later).

Within the α and β clusters, the expression of each gene is regulated by its unique promoter region.[45] Naturally occurring point mutations in the β-globin gene promoter that cause mild β-thalassemia have helped to identify functionally important regions required for optimal transcription. In addition, both globin clusters contain distinct regulatory elements that are more distant from the structural globin genes and regulate the output of the locus as a whole (Fig. 21–3*A*). The β-globin locus control region (LCR) was originally identified as a cluster of erythroid-specific DNAse-hypersensitive sites situated upstream of the ε gene.[46–48] In transgenic mice and tissue culture lines, the LCR is required for sustained high-level erythroid expression of linked globin genes.[49] An analogous segment, a *cis*-acting α locus enhancer termed *HS-40,* exists within the human α-globin cluster.[50,51] Both the β LCR and the α HS-40 sequences illustrate how long-range enhancer-like elements can interact functionally with individual genes to regulate their developmental timing and level of expression. Natural mutations that delete the LCR or HS-40, but leave the structural globin genes intact, are associated with some forms of β- and α-thalassemia, respectively.[52–61]

α-Thalassemic chromosomes are designated α^0 or α^+ to indicate whether globin chain synthesis is fully or partially ablated. Because each human chromosome has two tandem α genes, a normal individual is designated αα/αα to indicate four active genes. Deletion of one α gene within a chromosome is designated –α; several common deletions are shown in Figure 21–4*A*. Nonhomologous recombination within the α-globin locus can delete both α-globin genes to produce an α^0 (–/–) chromosome (Fig. 21–4*B*). Distinct α-thalassemia syndromes result from loss of one, two, three, or four genes. The genetic configuration of α-globin deletions in individuals with α-thalassemia trait is of practical importance. In particular, two α gene deletions can exist either in *cis* (αα, –/–) or in *trans* (α/–,α/–). The α^0 (–/–) chromosome is much more common in persons of southern Chinese ancestry; two Asians with α-thalassemia trait are more likely to produce a nonviable offspring with hydrops fetalis caused by deletion of all four α-globin genes. In contrast, the α^0 chromosome is virtually never present in α-thalassemia carriers of African descent, so that a hydrops fetalis pregnancy is highly improbable.

Point mutations are a less frequent cause of α-thalassemia; they occur at multiple sites and impair various different steps in gene expression, including RNA processing, splicing, and translation. Among the most common are mutations within the α2-globin gene termination codon, with hemoglobin Constant Springs (α^{CS}) being the most well-studied example. This class of mutations produces an elongated globin that can be visualized as a distinct band in hemoglobin electrophoretic studies. In addition, the messenger RNA (mRNA) is destabilized by a unique mechanism: loss of the termination signal permits read-through of the translational machinery into the 3′ untranslated region, which

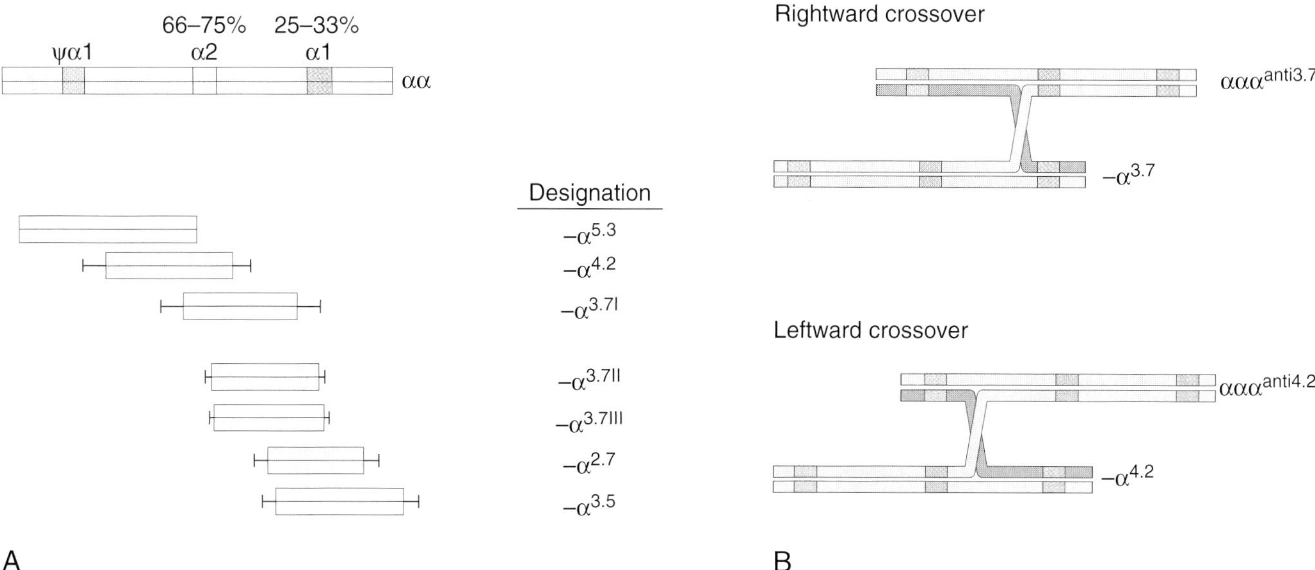

Figure 21–4. Molecular basis of α gene deletions. ***A***, Several common deletions spanning the α region have been described, denoted by shaded boxes below the genes. The numerical designations express the deletion size in kilobase pairs. ***B***, Deletions and triplications arose from non-homologous crossovers between adjacent and nearly identical α and pseudo-α (ψα) genes. (Adapted from Steinberg MH, Forget BG, Higgs DR, Nagel RL [eds]: Disorders of Hemoglobin: Genetics, Pathophysiology, and Clinical Management. Cambridge, MA: Cambridge University Press, 2001, pp 411–412.)

then disrupts the binding of a protein complex required for mRNA stability.[62,63] Compound heterozygotes for α^0 and α^{CS} (—/$\alpha\alpha^{CS}$) exhibit the phenotype of hemoglobin H disease.

β-Globin gene mutations are usually the result of point mutations, which can impair virtually every step of gene expression (Fig. 21–5): promoter function, mRNA capping, splicing, and protein translation. Splice mutations are among the most common. Some point mutations produce both qualitative and quantitative effects, termed *thalassemic hemoglobinopathies*. Most clinically important is hemoglobin E (Hb E), which is extremely common in Southeast Asia, with an allele frequency as high as 30%. The mutation results in the substitution of lysine for glutamic acid at codon 26, producing a mildly unstable hemoglobin. In addition, the mutation activates a cryptic splice site within exon 1 resulting in the production of a proportion of nonfunctional RNA. Heterozygous or homozygous hemoglobin E causes microcytosis but no clinical manifestations. However, severe thalassemia can result from Hb E/β^0-thalassemia compound heterozygous states because of the thalassemic nature of the predominant, aberrant spliced product.

Other variations of the thalassemic hemoglobinopathies are the rare, dominantly inherited β-thalassemias.[64,65] These are typically caused by β-globin exon 3 mutations that produce frameshift mutations, resulting in elongated, unstable β-globin variants; the abnormal chains precipitate, damaging erythrocytes and their precursors.

Genetic Modifiers of β-Thalassemia

Marked differences in disease severity can occur among individuals who inherit the same β-thalassemic alleles, even within families; these variations may be due to coinherited genes that modify the thalassemic phenotype. The most common genetic modifiers of β-thalassemia are other globin genes. Because free α-globin is a major determinant of disease pathophysiology (discussed later), genetic influences that minimize α/β chain imbalance lead to milder phenotypes. Mutations that prevent γ-globin from being switched off after birth alleviate β-thalassemia because γ chains can bind free α-globin to form functional fetal hemoglobin (Hb F, $\alpha_2\gamma_2$). Coinherited α-thalassemia trait ameliorates β-thalassemia severity by normalizing the α/β globin ratio; decreased overall hemoglobin synthesis is better tolerated than is globin chain imbalance.

Continued γ-globin synthesis during adulthood is caused by a group of infrequent DNA changes and termed *hereditary persistence of fetal hemoglobin*. A common mechanism for elevated Hb F in hemoglobinopathies is a C-to-T change at position 158 of the Gγ promoter, referred to as the *Xmn*I polymorphism because it creates a new *Xmn*I restriction enzyme digestion site.[66–72] Fetal hemoglobin is not affected in normal individuals with the *Xmn*I polymorphism, but when the allele is coinherited with β-thalassemia, $^G\gamma$-globin synthesis is usually elevated and the phenotype is less severe.

For many individuals and pedigrees, differences in the severity of β-thalassemia cannot be explained by these mechanisms, suggesting the existence of additional modifier genes.[73] Two candidates have been identified based on their demonstrated abilities to modulate globin structure or synthesis in erythroid cells. Heme regulated kinase (HRI) is a protein that inhibits globin mRNA translation in response to heme deficiency and a variety of stresses, including oxidant injury, which occurs in β-thalassemia. Alpha hemoglobin stabilizing protein

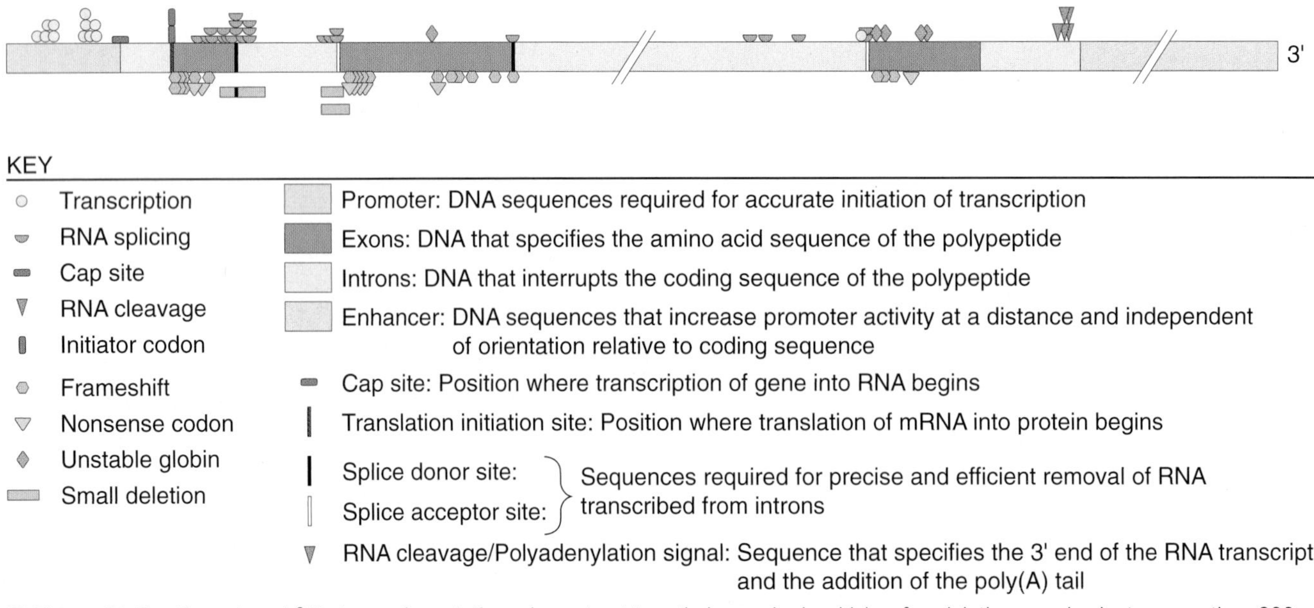

Figure 21–5. Examples of β-thalassemia mutations. In contrast to α-thalassemia, in which a few deletions predominate, more than 200 distinct β-globin mutations, mostly point mutations or small deletions, are known. These impair virtually every known step of gene expression, including transcription (promoter and enhancer mutations), RNA processing, early stop codons (nonsense), and protein mutations, as described in the key. (Adapted from Orkin SH, Nathan DG: The thalassemias. *In* Nathan DG, Orkin SH, Ginsburg D, Look AT [eds]: Nathan and Oski's Hematology of Infancy and Childhood. Philadelphia: WB Saunders, 2003, p 850.)

(AHSP) is an abundant erythroid protein that binds and stabilizes free α-globin to limit its toxicity.[74] In mice, coexisting *AHSP* or *HRI* mutations worsen the severity of β-thalassemia intermedia; whether these genes are modifiers of β-thalassemia in human populations requires further study.[75,76]

CLINICAL FEATURES AND DIAGNOSIS

Four-gene-deleted α-thalassemia presents as hydrops fetalis and is embryonic lethal without transfusions in utero.[77] *Severe β-thalassemia* syndromes (β-thalassemia major, and some patients with Hb E/β^0-thalassemia) are clinically apparent by 6–12 months of age. Pallor, lethargy, poor growth, hepatosplenomegaly, or significant anemia are presenting signs. *Thalassemia intermedia* syndromes exhibit a range of clinical presentation. At their most severe, the signs and symptoms are those of transfusion-dependent β^+-thalassemia, but with an older age of onset. *Hemoglobin H disease* (three-gene-deleted α-thalassemia, named for excess, abnormal β_4 detected in red cells) and hemoglobin H/Constant Springs may cause overt anemia in early infancy or be detected on newborn screening as elevated hemoglobin Barts[78] (excess γ_4). Some thalassemia intermedia patients are barely distinguishable from persons with thalassemia trait and may be discovered only incidentally on hemoglobin screening in infancy and childhood. Patients with borderline globin production may only be diagnosed with additional hematopoietic stress of pregnancy or intercurrent illness. Differences in severity of erythrocyte dysmorphology and number of nucleated red blood cells may help the clinician to distinguish the syndromes (Fig. 21–6).

DIFFERENTIAL DIAGNOSIS

The diagnostic approach to the thalassemias should be systematic (Fig. 21–7). Both α- and β-thalassemia trait must be distinguished especially from iron deficiency anemia and anemia of chronic disease based on laboratory findings and the response to iron therapy (Table 21–1). Iron deficiency can lower hemoglobin A2 in individuals with true β-thalassemia trait, resulting in false-negative electrophoresis studies (see Chapter 18).

TREATMENT

In thalassemia major, *chronic transfusion* is always required to prevent complications of anemia. The frequency of transfusion ranges from every 2 to every 4 weeks, based on factors including blood availability,[79] and physiologic contributors that affect the survival of the

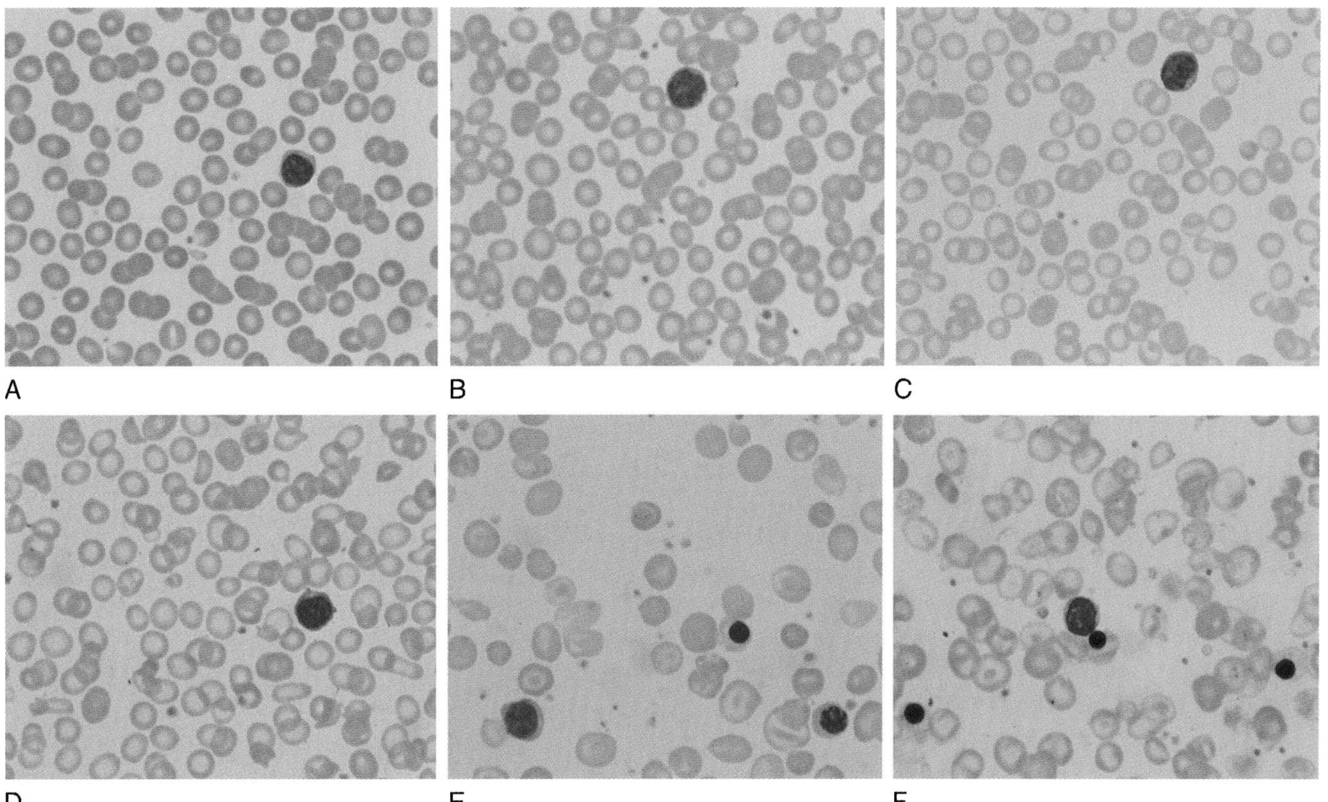

Figure 21–6. Peripheral blood in thalassemia. The blood smears of patients with thalassemia syndromes can demonstrate varying degrees of microcytosis, hypochromia, and basophilic stippling, as well as target cells and elliptocytes, but there is wide variation in RBC abnormalities, ranging from normal *(A)* to α-thalassemia single-gene deletion *(B)* and two-gene deletion *(C)*, hemoglobin H disease *(D)*, β-thalassemia intermedia *(E)*, and β-thalassemia major prior to initiation of transfusion therapy *(F)*.

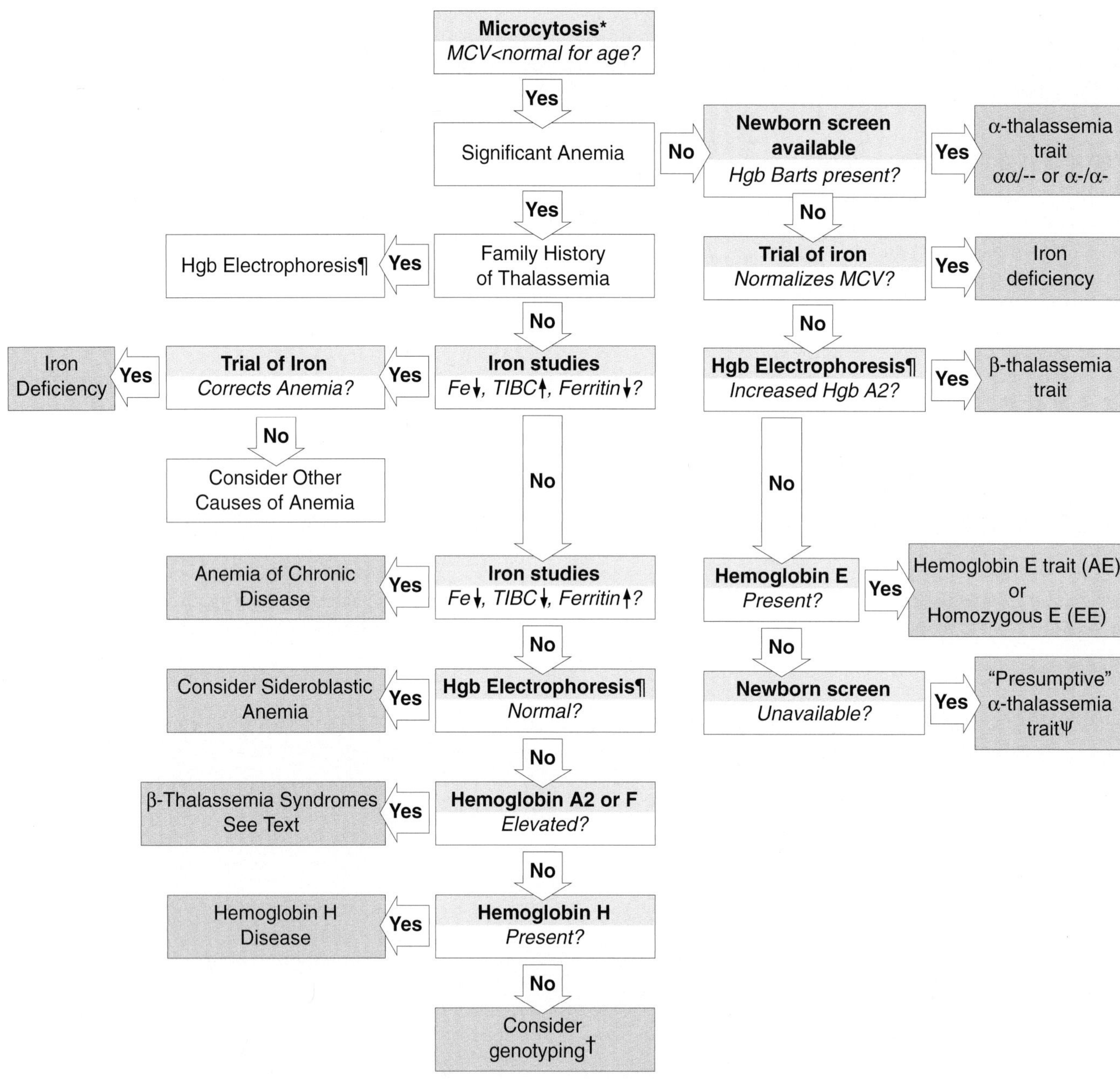

* Consider lead screening in toddlers

† To detect unstable hemoglobinopathies, β/δ thalassemia; exacerbating combinations of β-thalassemia trait/α-excess; if at risk for α and both parents microcytic

Ψ If at risk for α and both parents microcytic recommend genotyping due to risk of fetal hydrops

¶ Without family or ethnic history, trial of iron before electrophoresis is appropriate. With family or ethnic history electrophoresis with concurrent trial of iron is appropriate.

Figure 21–7. Diagnostic algorithm for thalassemia.

TABLE 21–1. Thalassemia Trait Versus Other Microcytic Anemias*

	Smear and Indices	Mentzer Index (MCV/RBC)	Hemoglobin A2	Ferritin	Response to Iron Therapy
α-Thalassemia trait	Microcytosis > hypochromia	Usually <12	Normal	Normal	None in pure thalassemia
β-Thalassemia trait	Microcytosis > hypochromia	Usually <12	Elevated	Normal	None in pure thalassemia
Iron deficiency	Microcytosis and hypochromia variable among cells	Usually >15	Normal	Low	Rapid improvement in CHR & reticulocytes; weeks for normal Hgb
Anemia of chronic disease	Some microcytosis; varies among patients		Normal	Elevated	None or modest
Iron deficiency *and* thalassemia trait	Microcytosis and hypochromia variable among cells	Indeterminate	May be normal until patient is iron replete in β-thalassemia trait; normal in α-thalassemia trait	Low	Still microcytic after repletion

*Plumbism and sideroblastic anemia are also in the differential of the microcytic anemias and are addressed in the diagnostic algorithm in Figure 21–7.
Abbreviations: CHR, corpuscular hemoglobin, reticulocyte; Hgb, hemoglobin concentration; MCV, mean corpuscular volume; RBC, red blood cell count.

transfused cells, such as hypersplenism[80] and alloimmunization.[81–84] Full antigen phenotyping of the patient's erythrocytes prior to initiation of transfusion therapy allows extended phenotypic matching for transfusions. This approach can prevent allosensitization,[84] ensure appropriate transfusions if allosensitization occurs, and eliminate the need for subsequent typing by genotypic methods.[85]

The decision to initiate transfusion in thalassemia syndromes other than homozygous β^0-thalassemia may be difficult and cannot be made based solely on an average or one-time hemoglobin measurement. The goal of transfusion is to improve the anemia, thereby diminishing the degree of ineffective erythropoiesis. Regular transfusions can prevent most of the serious clinical manifestations of thalassemia but produce also the complications of iron overload and the need for chelation therapy to prevent secondary hemochromatosis. There are presently no standards and no algorithm to guide the practitioner in initiating transfusion therapy. The decision should be based on the symptoms and signs due to anemia. Persistent tachycardia, sweating, poor feeding, or a slow rate of growth suggest the need for transfusion. Additionally, organ compromise secondary to massive ineffective erythropoiesis and subsequent massive splenomegaly or bony changes may be ameliorated by transfusions.

Iron chelation is necessary, to prevent the obligatory transfusional hemosiderosis of lifelong transfusions (see Chapter 56). Iron chelation also may be required in older thalassemia intermedia patients who have nontransfusional iron overload from inappropriate, exuberant gut uptake of iron.[86,87] Chelation with deferoxamine, a natural-product siderophore,[88] can prevent the clinical consequences of iron overlood due to transfusion therapy.[17,20] Because of the very short plasma half-life of the drug, deferoxamine must be administered intravenously or subcutaneously; intramuscular administration has some efficacy but is inferior to intravenous or subcutaneous dosing.[89,90] Initiation of chelation is recommended when the ferritin value reaches 1000 ng/mL, or at 3 years of age, or after 20 monthly transfusions in regularly transfused patients.[91] Deferoxamine therapy in children younger than 3 years of age can lead to significant growth retardation.[18] The average dose of deferoxamine recommended is 25–40 mg/kg/day in regularly transfused thalassemia major patients older than 5 years of age; for patients between the ages of 3 and 5 years, the recommended dose is 15–35 mg/kg/day on average.[91] The average dose is calculated by the total dose per day, multiplied by the number of days infused, divided by 7. Treatment for a minimum of 5 days per week is recommended.[18] The dose should be adjusted for trends in hepatic iron content over time,[18] but nomograms are not available. Adherence to lifelong deferoxamine, given subcutaneously overnight for 5 or more nights weekly, is difficult for even the most compliant patient.[18]

Two oral chelators have been developed but are not yet available in the United States. Deferiprone is approved for use in Europe for patients unable to tolerate deferoxamine.[79,92] Deferasirox, a novel tridentate iron-selective chelator,[93–95] was submitted for American regulatory approval in 2005 after a randomized Phase III trial comparing deferoxamine and deferasirox demonstrated comparable efficacy at higher doses.

Hematopoietic stem cell transplantation from human lymphocyte antigen (HLA)-identical siblings is curative for thalassemia major, if the donor cells engraft sufficiently. The source of stem cells can be bone marrow, peripheral blood, or umbilical cord blood. The procedure has been highly successful in large series from Italy. In 2003, Gaziev and Lucarelli published a review of more than 900 patients treated in Pesaro, Italy.[96] Multivariate analysis of the first 222 patients transplanted identified the presence of hepatomegaly greater than 2 cm, liver fibrosis, and irregular iron chelation as adverse risk factors.[97] Barriers to implementation of this strategy are several. Only one in four full sibs of thalassemia patients are HLA matched, and therefore a minority of patients have an unaffected sibling donor. Matched unrelated transplants may carry higher morbidity and graft failure rates. Thalassemia major patients with end-organ damage (especially cardiac or hepatic) are at high risk for morbidity and mortality from the procedure itself, although new approaches to reduce graft rejection may improve the outlook for transplantation in high-risk patients.[98] Allosensitization from innumerable transfusions may reduce engraftment. Families of young, healthy thalassemia major children may not be willing to hazard the risks of transplantation, even if these patients are potentially ideal recipients. Induction regimen–related toxicity, infertility, and acute and chronic graft-versus-host disease must be weighed against improved survival and reduced complications in younger birth cohorts.[20,99] Successful transplantation has the added advantage of allowing subsequent phlebotomy to normalize total body iron.[100,101]

SUPPORTIVE CARE AND LONG-TERM MANAGEMENT

Fastidious supportive care and long-term management must address maintenance of the ameliorative regimen of

TABLE 21–2. Recommended Studies for Regularly Transfused Thalassemia Patients

Subspecialty	Studies	Frequency	Comments
Physical examination		q 3mo	Plot on ethnically appropriate growth charts; document spleen size, because splenomegaly may increase transfusion requirement.
Laboratory	CBC	Each transfusion	Pretransfusion Hgb goal is 9–9.5gm/dL. Consider low-dose aspirin therapy w/ thrombocytosis.
	Manual differential	Each transfusion	Assess nucleated RBCs as index of erythropoiesis.
	Reticulocyte count	Each transfusion	Variably useful depending on genotype and ± spleen.
	Ferritin	q 3mo	Trends important. Underestimates iron overload in thalassemia intermedia.
	Liver enzymes, bilirubin	q 3mo	
Hematology	Total transfusion requirement	q 6mo	If greater than 200mL/kg/yr, evaluate for allo/autoimmunization; consider splenectomy.
Genetics	Hemoglobin genotype	Once	Determine α and β genotype.
	HLA typing	Once	Determine parents, patient, and full siblings.
Transfusion medicine	Full antigen phenotype	**Prior** to transfusion	Obtain before any transfusion in case of antibody development and difficulty finding matched blood. Molecular typing after transfusion may be possible in older patients.
Hepatology	SQUID or liver biopsy for hepatic iron content (HIC); R2 MRI (in development)	q 12–18mo	Biopsy if HIC **and** pathology important.
	α-fetoprotein	Annually	In patients with chronic hepatitis C.
	Hepatic ultrasound	Annually	In patients with chronic hepatitis C, and any time symptoms of biliary obstruction occur.
Cardiology	Cardiology assessment	Annually	
	Echocardiogram, ECG, Holter monitor	Biannually <12yo Annually >12yo	Initiate after 3–5yr of transfusion. Include LV function assessment, evidence for pulmonary hypertension in adults.
	T2* MRI (in development) Exercise stress test	Per cardiology	
Infectious diseases	HIV, hepatitis C Ab, and PCR	Annually	If Ab positive, PCR only yearly and only if Ab positive.
	Hepatitis A and B Ab	Once to demonstrate immunity	If hepatitis B Ab negative, check surface Ag and core Ab; if negative, immunize if not previously done. Booster no longer recommended.
Immunizations	Influenza	Annually	Safety of live nasal influenza vaccine not tested in this population.
	Pneumococcal Meningococcal	Before splenectomy	7-valent conjugated pneumococcal vaccine, as well as boost with 23-valent polysaccharide vaccine after 2yr of age.
	Hepatitis A and B	One course each	
Endocrinology	Endocrinology appointment	Annually	At 5yr of age or after 3yr of transfusion.
	Bone age	At least biannually	Until growth plate has fused.
	Growth velocity	Annually	
	Bone density (DEXA)	Annually	Initiate at 8yr of age.
Pulmonary	PFTs	Annually after splenectomy	
Dental		Regular twice-yearly prophylaxis	Assess for malocclusion from maxillary changes of marrow expansion.
Ophthalmology	Acuity, peripheral and dark-adapted vision	Annually when on DFO	Baseline at DFO initiation. New baseline if increasing DFO >10%.
	ERG	Biannually	
Audiology	Audiometry	Annually when on DFO	Baseline at DFO initiation. New baseline if increasing DFO >10%.

Abbreviations: Ab, antibody; Ag, antigen; CBC, complete blood count; DEXA, dual-energy x-ray absorptiometry; DFO, deferoxamine; ECG, electrocardiogram; ERG, electroretinogram; Hgb, hemoglobin concentration; LV, left ventricular; PCR, polymerase chain reaction; PFTs, pulmonary function tests; yo, years old.

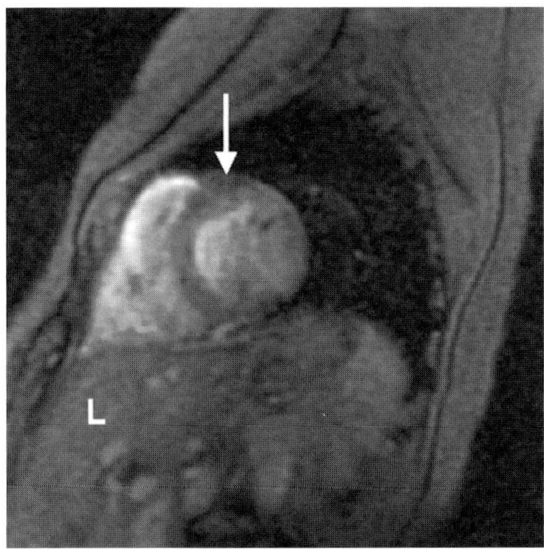

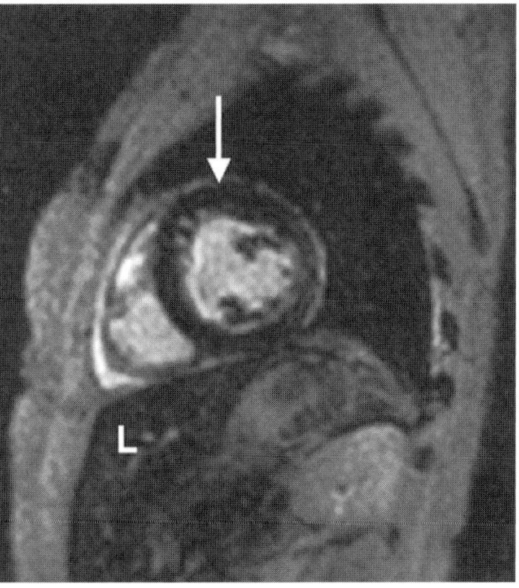

Figure 21–8. T2* MRI of the heart. The *arrows* denote the area of interest. *Left,* Normal heart. *Right,* Heart of a patient with iron overload. The darker signal is indicative of high iron and more rapid relaxation. Because iron has strong paramagnetic properties, increasing iron concentration within the liver (L) and myocardium results in a greater signal loss on T2*-weighted imaging. (Courtesy of Andrew Powell, MD, Assistant Professor of Pediatrics, Harvard Medical School.)

chronic transfusions and its myriad complications, including alloimmunization, infections and iron overload in inadequately chelated patients, and the toxicity of chelation therapy itself[20,99] (Table 21–2).

Assessment of total body iron burden is critical in both the prognosis and management of thalassemia patients.[16,18] Most nonheme iron stores are hepatic, so liver biopsy is the current standard for this measurement, but when the liver is significantly fibrotic or cirrhotic, heterogeneity in the sample may underestimate hepatic iron content. The serum ferritin is a convenient (but often unreliable) surrogate marker of hepatic iron burden,[99,102,103] and is generally assessed every 3 months.

Noninvasive measurements of organ iron content have been developed in the research setting. The superconducting quantum interference device (SQUID) is available at only four centers in the world. In the SQUID, the local magnetic field of the liver is enhanced by the iron content in the liver, allowing accurate ferrometric measures by magnetic susceptibility.[104] Magnetic resonance approaches are also being used; R2 assessment of hepatic iron measures shows great promise.[105] Cardiac T2 star (T2*) magnetic resonance imaging (MRI) has the potential to quantify cardiac iron.[106–109] Elevated iron is black on a T2* image because of the strong paramagnetic properties of iron, and increasing iron results in greater signal loss (Fig. 21–8). T2* less than 20 msec is abnormal, and may be an early marker for progressive heart disease and the need for more aggressive chelation.[110]

PROGNOSIS

Prognosis varies as a function of severity in the several thalassemia syndromes discussed in this chapter.

CURRENT CONTROVERSIES & FUTURE CONSIDERATIONS

Thalassemia

- In the absence of an HLA-matched sibling, will there be a role for unrelated HLA–matched or HLA-nonidentical stem cell transplantation in thalassemia syndromes?
- How might preimplantation genetic diagnosis (to select HLA-identical, unaffected sibling donors) be integrated with standard therapies?
- What will be the optimal strategies to enhance fetal hemoglobin production in order to ameliorate β-thalassemia major and intermedia?
- Can globin gene therapy play a role in thalassemia treatment? Can high-level, stable gene expression from globin locus constructs provide clinically relevant levels of the defective globin gene product? Are alternative gene therapies (correction of specific splice defects) feasible?
- How will new alternative oral iron chelators impact patients with transfusion-dependent thalassemia?
- Will noninvasive assessments of iron burden (by T2* MRI or SQUID) become useful for routine management in thalassemia? Can noninvasive measures elucidate variable iron loading in sensitive organs?
- Will evaluation of genetic modifier loci for thalassemia patients aid in prognosis and optimization of individualized treatment strategies?
- Could strategies to increase hepcidin levels prevent or correct nontransfusional iron overload in thalassemia intermedia syndromes?

Suggested Readings*

Angelucci E, Brittenham GM, McLaren CE, et al: Hepatic iron concentration and total body iron stores in thalassemia major. N Engl J Med 43:327–331, 2000.

Borgna-Pignatti C, Rugolotto S, De Stefano P, et al: Survival and complications in patients with thalassemia major treated with transfusion and deferoxamine. Haematologica 89:1187–1193, 2004.

Cunningham MJ, Macklin EA, Neufeld EJ, Cohen AR: Complications of β-thalassemia major in North America. Blood 104:34–39, 2004.

Olivieri NF: The beta-thalassemias. N Engl J Med ;341:99–109, 1999.

Weatherall DJ: Phenotype-genotype relationships in monogenic disease: lessons from the thalassaemias. Nat Rev Genet 2:245–255, 2001.

**Full references for this chapter can be found on accompanying CD-ROM.*

CHAPTER 22

Hereditary Spherocytosis, Hereditary Elliptocytosis, and Related Disorders

Paula H. B. Bolton-Maggs, FRCP, FRCPCH, FRCPath, and May-Jean King, BSc, PhD

KEY POINTS

Hereditary Spherocytosis, Hereditary Elliptocytosis, and Related Disorders

- Hereditary spherocytosis (HS) and hereditary elliptocytosis (HE) are common causes of inherited hemolysis.
- HS hemolysis is due to fragility of the red cell cytoskeleton.
- Laboratory investigation is usually not complicated. However, careful review of the smear and a complete clinical history are essential to diagnose the rare hereditary stomatocytic disorders, in which splenectomy is contraindicated because of an increased risk of thrombosis.
- An additional screening test for HS should be used whenever the family history is not available.
- HS is best classified by clinical severity, which predicts the need for splenectomy.
- Splenectomy is an important treatment for symptoms in severe and moderate cases of HS and HE. Splenectomy should not be undertaken without careful consideration because of the risk of postsplenectomy sepsis, which is not completely prevented by the currently available recommendations for vaccination and antibiotic prophylaxis.

INTRODUCTION

The first description of a chronically jaundiced woman with spherocytes in the peripheral blood, together with similarly affected relatives, was published in 1871.[1] This condition was indistinguishable from acquired immune hemolytic anemia until the antiglobulin test became available in 1950.[2] A shortened red cell lifespan[3] is a common feature of those inherited hemolytic anemias due to defects of the red cell cytoskeleton. The cytoskeleton is a spectrin-actin–based network attached to the membrane lipid bilayer through linker and transmembrane proteins (see Chapter 4). The tight spatial organization of the cytoskeletal and accessory proteins together with the lipid membrane not only determine the cell shape but also confer deformability and elasticity on the erythrocyte. The expression of cytoskeletal proteins during erythropoiesis is highly regulated,[4–8] and the emergence of erythroid spliceoforms for spectrin, ankyrin,[9,10] protein 4.2,[11,12] and protein 4.1[13] is developmentally controlled.

Hereditary spherocytosis (HS) (Fig. 22–1*A*) and hereditary elliptocytosis (HE) (Fig. 22–1*B* and *C*) result from defects in the vertical and horizontal modes of interaction of the red cell cytoskeleton, respectively.[14] Hereditary pyropoikilocytosis (HPP) (Fig. 22–1*D*) is a more severe form of HE. Both HS and HE/HPP are heterogeneous in clinical presentation (asymptomatic, mild, moderate, or severe types) and protein defect (single or combined deficiency). Neither is a single-gene disorder, and more than one membrane protein is affected: four proteins are known to be abnormal in HS (spectrin, ankyrin, band 3, and protein 4.2) and two in HE (protein 4.1 and spectrin). In contrast to HS and HE, red cells of Southeast Asian ovalocytosis (SAO) (Fig. 22–1*E*), also known as Melanesian elliptocytosis, are osmotically resistant. Abnormal monovalent cation permeability,[15] rather than a cytoskeletal protein defect, is the underlying defect in hereditary stomatocytosis (Fig. 22–1*F*) and its related disorders, which include hydrocytosis, xerocytosis (dehydrated), and the temperature-dependent variants pseudohyperkalaemia[16] and cryohydrocytosis. The importance of distinguishing these patients from those with HS and HE is their increased risk of thromboembolism after splenectomy.[17]

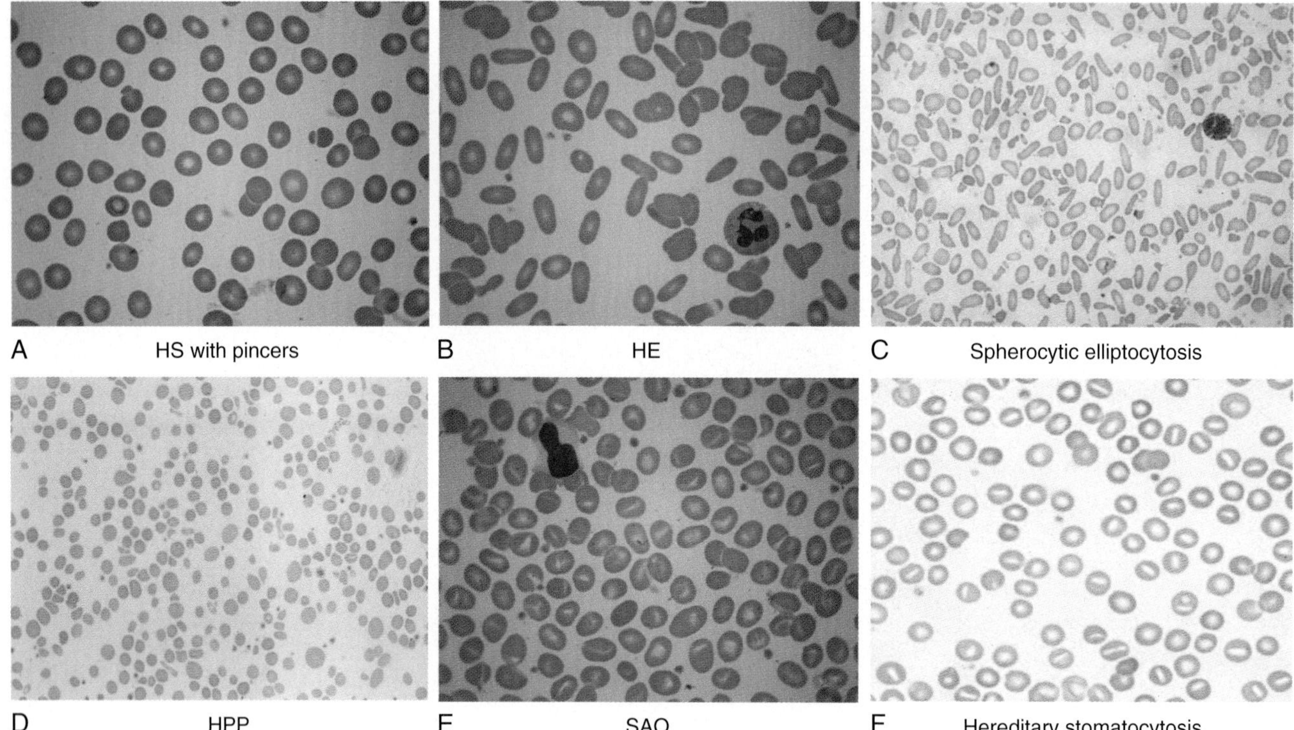

Figure 22–1. Blood smears in red cell membrane disorders. ***A,*** Hereditary spherocytosis with some pincer cells. ***B,*** Hereditary elliptocytosis. ***C,*** Spherocytic elliptocytosis. ***D,*** Hereditary pyropoikilocytosis. ***E,*** Southeast Asian ovalocytosis. ***F,*** Hereditary stomatocytosis. (***A, B,*** and ***E*** courtesy of Dr. Barbara Bain; ***C*** courtesy of Dr. Jim Murray; ***F*** from King M-J: Diagnosis of red cell membrane disorders. CME Bull Haematol 3:39–41, 2000 with permission from RILA publications.)

EPIDEMIOLOGY AND RISK FACTORS

Hereditary Spherocytosis

HS may be diagnosed from birth to old age[18,19] and can be found in all countries and races.[20–26] HS is rarely reported in blacks,[27–31] and is relatively more common in Japan.[32–41] In northern Europe and North America, the incidence is reported as 1 in 5000 births.[42] More recent studies of normal blood donors in Europe suggest that mild forms are common, with an incidence of 1 in 2000[43,44]; the laboratory finding of increased osmotic fragility alone is of uncertain clinical significance.

Hereditary Elliptocytosis

Common HE, usually a clinically mild disorder, is associated with defective spectrin (α and β) and protein 4.1 deficiencies, which segregate according to the ethnic origin of the patients. HE with α-spectrin defects is especially common in Mediterranean or African (or African-Caribbean) populations. A particular mutation of the α-spectrin gene occurs in HE in individuals of African origin worldwide, with an incidence of 1.6% in Benin, where haplotype analysis suggests a founder effect.[45] The incidence is about 10 times more frequent in West Africa and the Antilles (4–6 cases in 1000 births) than in Europe or the United States.[46] Defects in β-spectrin and protein 4.1 are found mainly among whites, who tend to have a mild anemia. One third of HE is due to partial protein 4.1 deficiency.

Southeast Asian Ovalocytosis

SAO (see Fig. 22–1*E*) is restricted to the Far East and is highly prevalent in Papua New Guinea,[47] Thailand, Malaysia, Indonesia, and the Philippines; in some tribes up to 25% of the population is affected. A selective advantage of SAO[48,49] and HE[50] in tropical countries is probably related to resistance to malaria. Outside Southeast Asia, only isolated cases have been reported.[51–53]

Hereditary Stomatocytosis

Hereditary stomatocytosis and related disorders[54] are very rare, with eight distinct families described in the United Kingdom.[55] Depending upon clinical phenotype, the frequencies vary between 1 in 10,000 and 1 in 1 million births.[56] These disorders are characterized by the appearance of stomatocytes (5–50%) on the blood film (see Fig. 22–1*F*), macrocytosis, and a low mean cell hemoglobin concentration.

MOLECULAR GENETICS

The red cell membrane disorders are usually inherited in an autosomal dominant manner.

Hereditary Spherocytosis

The molecular defect in HS is almost always due to "private" mutation(s), unique for each kindred. Inheritance is dominant[42,57] in two thirds to three quarters of HS families. Dominant HS is caused by mutations of the ankyrin (*ANK1*), band 3 (*AE1*), or β-spectrin (*SPTB*) genes.[58–60] In the remaining 25% of HS cases, inheritance is nondominant rather than classic recessive, as a result of low expression at a pathogenic HS allele from each parent. Two genetic backgrounds can give rise to nondominant HS, with a more severe clinical phenotype than in parent(s) and/or siblings who are hematologically normal. In the first, patients coinherit a low-expressed allele and a pathogenic HS allele in the α-spectrin gene (*SPTA1*). The low-expressed allele is designated as *L*ow-*E*xpressed *PRA*gue (αSp^{LEPRA}),[61] which has an estimated frequency of 3.6% in normal individuals; the α^{LEPRA} mutation reduces α-spectrin. The second type of nondominant HS results from de novo mutations leading to the loss of one haploid *SPTB*[62] or *ANK1*.[58,63]

Hereditary Elliptocytosis

Autosomal dominant HE resulting from spectrin mutations is clinically more variable than is HE with protein 4.1 deficiency. Compound heterozygosity for two different spectrin mutations or homozygosity for a single spectrin mutation can cause HPP. However, the increased severity in the biochemical, morphologic, and at times the clinical phenotype[64] is more often due to a compound heterozygous state associated with a low-expressed spectrin α^{LELY} allele (*L*ow *E*xpression allele *Ly*on)[65,66] and a HE allele carried on a separate spectrin gene (a *trans* inheritance).[67–70]

PATHOPHYSIOLOGY

Hereditary Spherocytosis

Spherocyte formation is due to loss of membrane surface area relative to intracellular volume, resulting from gradual vesiculation of circulating red cells through the microvasculature in the spleen. Hemolysis is mainly due to splenic entrapment and destruction of spherocytes by macrophages.[64] The underlying membrane protein defects are broadly classified as single or combined deficiencies in spectrin, ankyrin, band 3, and protein 4.2.

Ankyrin Deficiency

Combined deficiencies of spectrin and protein 4.2[59,71–73] and of ankyrin and spectrin indicate dominant HS with ankyrin reduction.[59,74–77] A partial B3 reduction is found when mutations occur close to or within the B3-binding domain (ankyrin Marburg and ankyrin Walsrode[58]) (Fig. 22–2). Some patients with severe HS have both ankyrin deficiency and chromosome 8 deletions.[60,78–81]

Spectrin Deficiency

Partial spectrin deficiency was the first identified biochemical abnormality in HS.[82,83] Patients with single or isolated spectrin deficiency (HS(Sp)) often have normal levels of ankyrin and band 3. The finding[61] of αSp^{Prague} inherited in *trans* to αSp^{LEPRA} uncovered the role of αSp^{LEPRA} in recessive or nondominant HS(Sp), and established that α-spectrin mutations are frequently involved in genuinely recessive HS (patients with two normal parents). The molecular basis for this type of recessive HS may be homozygosity for αSp^{LEPRA}, or a compound heterozygote coinheriting a HS allele with αSp^{LEPRA}, or a spontaneous HS resulting from de novo monoallelic expression of *SPTB*.[62,84] All mutations in *SPTB* produce dominant HS(Sp) (Fig. 22–3, bottom panel).

Band 3 Deficiency

Approximately 25% of HS patients have band 3 deficiency. Heterozygous patients with autosomal dominant inheritance exhibit mild to moderate HS, usually clinically and biochemically homogeneous within a family.

Other Band 3-Associated Red Cell Abnormalities

Two mutations are found in *AE1* of SAO: a deletion of 27 bases coding for the junction of the cytoplasmic domain and TM1 (Fig 22–4*A*), and band 3 Memphis polymorphism.[85–88] Homozygosity has never been detected, suggesting lethality. Heterozygotes are asymptomatic. Increased B3 oligomerization causes rigidity in SAO red cells[89] and may lead to defective cation transport. Distal renal tubular acidosis, an autosomal dominant disease,[90] has been detected in some individuals with SAO[91,92] or HS.[93,94] The impaired anion transport in HS[95–98] results from *AE1* mutations different from those responsible for renal tubular acidosis.[99–101]

Complete Protein 4.2 Deficiency

Patients with complete protein 4.2 deficiency were not immediately recognized as having HS because of the high incidence in ethnic Japanese, whose red cells showed predominantly ovalostomatocytes with no apparent spherocytes on blood smears,[102] a characteristic morphology attributed to the $P4.2^{Nippon}$ allele (A142T).[103] However, typical spherocytosis was observed when this allele was coinherited with either allele Fukuoka or allele Shiga (see Fig. 22–4).

Hereditary Elliptocytosis and Pyropoikilocytosis

The underlying membrane defects in common HE are spectrin variants and abnormalities of protein 4.1 (deficiency or an aberrant protein).[104–106]

Spectrin Defects

Spectrin variants of different molecular sizes are associated with distinct mutations in individuals of similar genetic backgrounds, suggesting founder effects. The

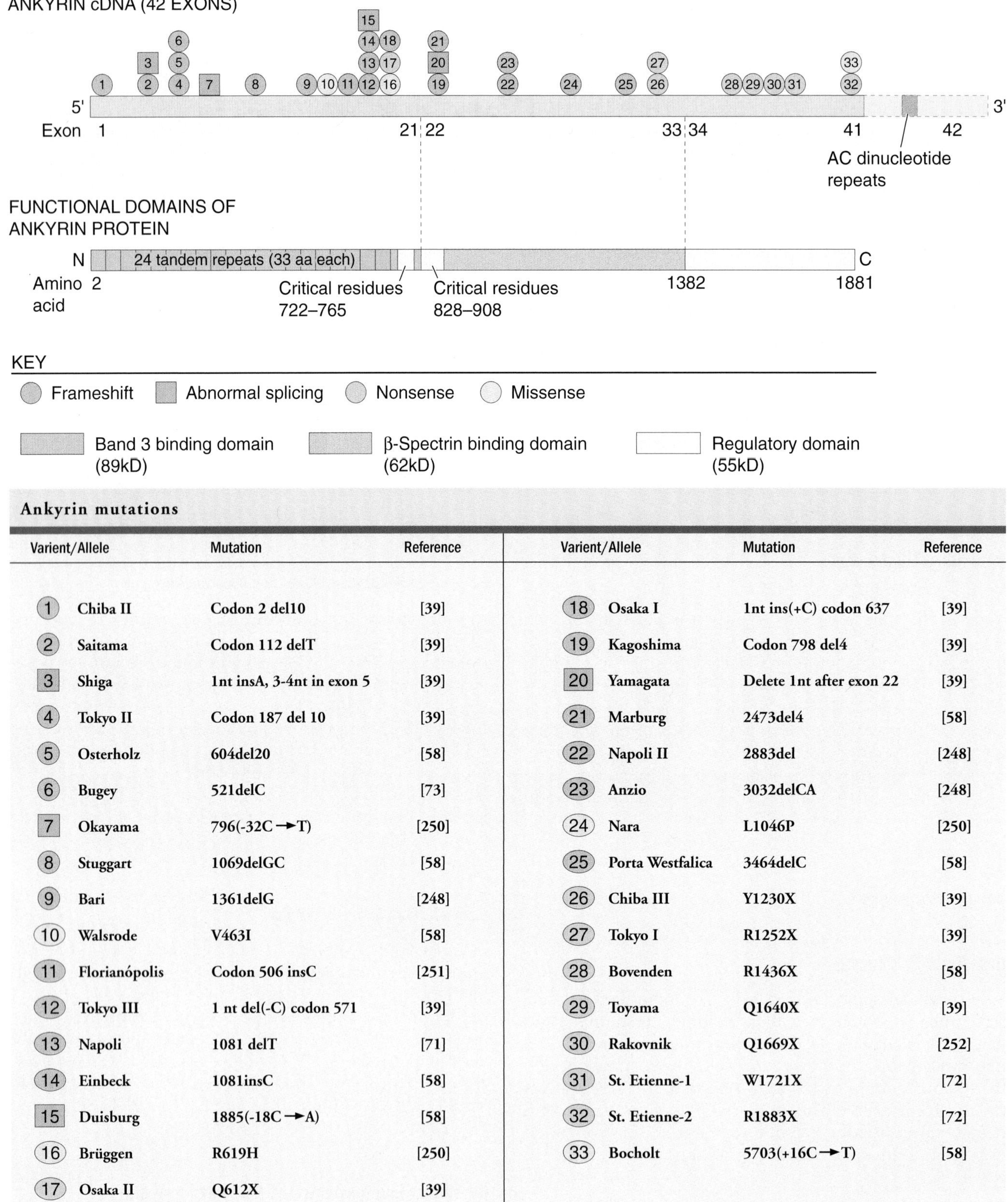

Ankyrin mutations

Varient/Allele		Mutation	Reference	Varient/Allele		Mutation	Reference
1	Chiba II	Codon 2 del10	[39]	18	Osaka I	1nt ins(+C) codon 637	[39]
2	Saitama	Codon 112 delT	[39]	19	Kagoshima	Codon 798 del4	[39]
3	Shiga	1nt insA, 3-4nt in exon 5	[39]	20	Yamagata	Delete 1nt after exon 22	[39]
4	Tokyo II	Codon 187 del 10	[39]	21	Marburg	2473del4	[58]
5	Osterholz	604del20	[58]	22	Napoli II	2883del	[248]
6	Bugey	521delC	[73]	23	Anzio	3032delCA	[248]
7	Okayama	796(-32C→T)	[250]	24	Nara	L1046P	[250]
8	Stuggart	1069delGC	[58]	25	Porta Westfalica	3464delC	[58]
9	Bari	1361delG	[248]	26	Chiba III	Y1230X	[39]
10	Walsrode	V463I	[58]	27	Tokyo I	R1252X	[39]
11	Florianópolis	Codon 506 insC	[251]	28	Bovenden	R1436X	[58]
12	Tokyo III	1 nt del(-C) codon 571	[39]	29	Toyama	Q1640X	[39]
13	Napoli	1081 delT	[71]	30	Rakovnik	Q1669X	[252]
14	Einbeck	1081insC	[58]	31	St. Etienne-1	W1721X	[72]
15	Duisburg	1885(-18C→A)	[58]	32	St. Etienne-2	R1883X	[72]
16	Brüggen	R619H	[250]	33	Bocholt	5703(+16C→T)	[58]
17	Osaka II	Q612X	[39]				

Figure 22–2. Localization of mutations in ANK-1 complementary DNA (cDNA) and the domain arrangement of the ankyrin protein. The erythroid ankyrin gene (*ANK1,* 42 exons) encodes three functional domains [9,10]: band 3 (B3)–binding [245] and spectrin-binding [246] domains, and the regulatory domain involved with erythroid stage-specific and complex alternate splicing gene arrangements. This region also modulates the affinities of both the B3- and spectrin-binding domains. Nonsense and frameshift mutations form two distinct clusters along the *ANK1* cDNA. The 3′ untranslation region (exon 42) contains the highly polymorphic AC dinucleotide repeats. Determination of the genomic distribution of the ankyrin $(AC)_n$ dinucleotide repeats has uncovered a high frequency of de novo mutations in *ANK1* gene [63,247] in probands with hematologically normal parents. [73,248,249] A mutation (108T→C; silent in heterozygotes) [58] in the *ANK1* promoter region can cause recessive HS when coinherited with an ankyrin HS allele. [26,249]

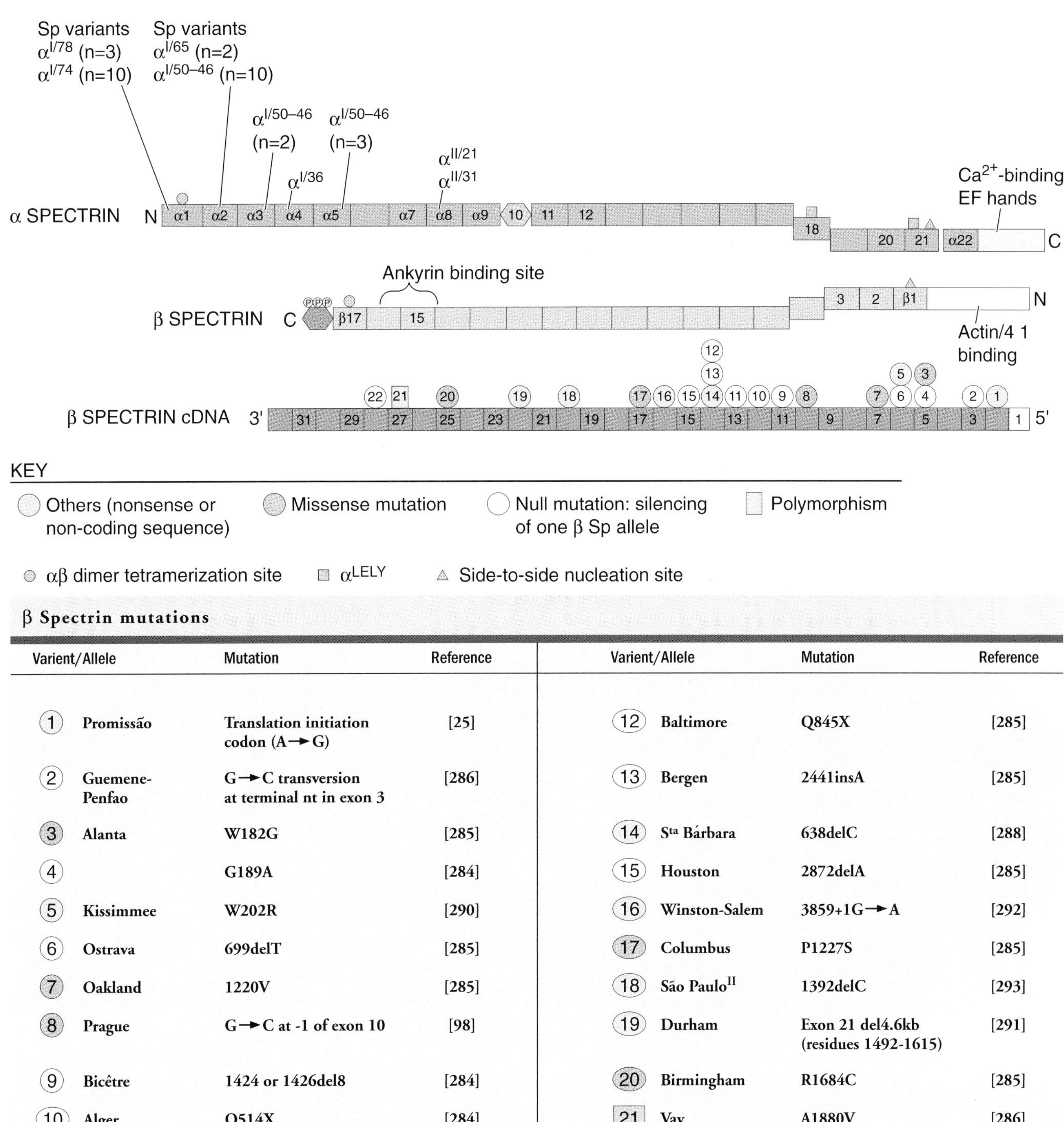

β Spectrin mutations

	Varient/Allele	Mutation	Reference		Varient/Allele	Mutation	Reference
1	Promissão	Translation initiation codon (A→G)	[25]	12	Baltimore	Q845X	[285]
2	Guemene-Penfao	G→C transversion at terminal nt in exon 3	[286]	13	Bergen	2441insA	[285]
3	Alanta	W182G	[285]	14	Sta Bárbara	638delC	[288]
4		G189A	[284]	15	Houston	2872delA	[285]
5	Kissimmee	W202R	[290]	16	Winston-Salem	3859+1G→A	[292]
6	Ostrava	699delT	[285]	17	Columbus	P1227S	[285]
7	Oakland	1220V	[285]	18	São Paulo II	1392delC	[293]
8	Prague	G→C at -1 of exon 10	[98]	19	Durham	Exon 21 del4.6kb (residues 1492-1615)	[291]
9	Bicêtre	1424 or 1426del8	[284]	20	Birmingham	R1684C	[285]
10	Alger	Q514X	[284]	21	Vay	A1880V	[286]
11	Philadelphia	1862insA	[285]	22	Tabor	Q1946X	[285]

Figure 22–3. Location of α-spectrin (α-Sp) variants for HE and mutations of β-spectrin (β-Sp) gene (*SPTB*) for HS. *Top,* α-Sp (comprising 22 units) and β-Sp (17 units) are structurally similar but nonidentical proteins. The first attachment of α-Sp to β-Sp occurs at the nucleation site. This process is affected by the mutations of α^{LELY} localized to repeating units α18 to α21. Pairing of αβ dimers proceeds in an antiparallel manner, and their self-association occurs at the tetramerization site (repeat α1 and β17). In HE, common tryptic Sp variants ($\alpha^{I/78}$, $\alpha^{I/74}$, $\alpha^{I/65}$, and $\alpha^{I/50\text{-}46}$) are derived from the αI domain of Sp, [109,253] indicating that amino acid substitutions occur either within or in the vicinity of the Sp tetramerization site. The result is probably an altered conformation in the triple helical unit, affecting Sp dimer self-association. Sp variants are detected only in selected repeat segments ($\alpha^{I/74}$ [107,253–259] and $\alpha^{I/78}$ [260–262] on repeat αI); the others are located on α2, [263–266] α3, [267] α4, [268] α5, [267,269,270] and α8. [271,272] Variant Sp$\alpha^{I/74}$ is associated with a mutational hot spot Arg28 in the repeating segment αI [107,254,255]; the same Sp variant produced by mutations in exon 30 (i.e., repeat β-17) or its exon-intron boundaries of *SPTB*. [273–283] *Bottom,* Localization of mutations on β-Sp cDNA. Frameshift, nonsense, missense, and abnormal splicing cause premature termination of translation, [284,285] aberrant messenger RNA (mRNA) splicing, [286] and unstable or no protein product. [25,287,288] The lack of expression of one β-Sp allele as a result of a null mutation (or inactivation) of the *SPTB* gene is invariably associated with dominant HS. [62,284,285] Some mutant proteins were found to have impaired Sp dimer association, [289] impaired binding to actin/protein 4.1R, [285,290] or impaired binding to ankyrin. [291]

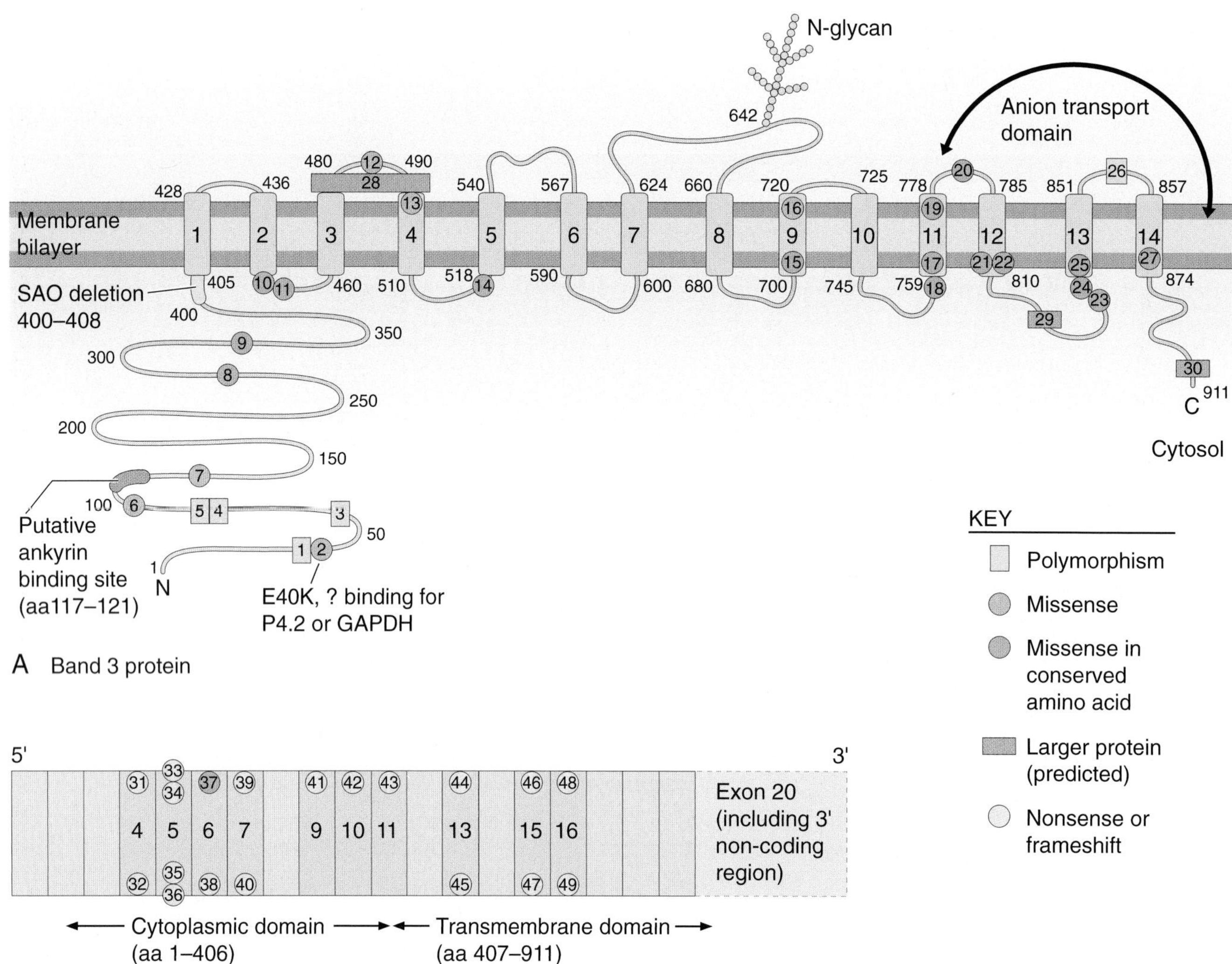

B Band 3 cDNA (20 exons)

Figure 22–4. Localization of mutations in band 3 (B3) protein and B3 complementary DNA (cDNA). ***A,*** Human red cell B3 (AE1, EPB3; 911 amino acids) has two functionally and structurally distinct regions that span 14 transmembrane domains (TM) connected by extracellular and cytoplasmic loops. The NH_2-terminal domain (43 kDa) interacts with protein 4.1, protein 4.2 (P4.2),[34,294,295] ankyrin,[296,297] glycolytic enzymes, and hemoglobin.[298] The membrane-spanning carboxy-terminal domain (52 kDa) functions as a HCO_3^-/Cl^- exchange channel, and the antigens of the Diego blood group system and senescent antigen are localized on the outer loops.[299,300] Missense mutations in the amino acids conserved throughout evolution are prevalent. The mutant B3 proteins are often not incorporated into the red cell membrane, although mutant transcripts are detected. These mutations occur mainly in the carboxy-terminal domain of B3 and are clustered around TM9 to TM14 or the region in the connecting inner or outer loop. An additive effect of two B3 alleles (a HS allele inherited in *trans* to a silent allele) can aggravate hemolysis by producing a greater reduction of B3 in the propositus.[95,301–303] A compound heterozygote of band3[Okinawa] and band 3[Fukuoka] exhibited a P4.2(–) phenotype.[37] ***B,*** Mutations in the numbered exons of B3 cDNA (total 20 exons) produce no detectable mutant messenger RNA (mRNA). The affected red cells showed reduction in normal B3 content.

A

	Varient/Allele	Mutation	Reference		Varient/Allele	Mutation	Reference
1	Damstadt	D38A	[58, 301]	16	Okinawa	G714R	[37]
2	Montefiore	E40K	[295]	17	Prague II or Kumamoto	R760Q	[98, 250]
3	Memphis I	K56E	[304]	18	Hradec Kralove or Tochigi I	R760W	[98, 250]
4	Okayama	E72D	[250]	19	Chur	G771D	[305]
5		L73M	[301]	20	Napoli II	I783N	[301]
6	Cape Town	E90K	[95]	21	Jablonec	R808C	[98]
7	Fukuoka	G130R	[34]	22	Nara	R808H	[250]
8	Boston	A285D	[296]	23	Birmingham	H834P	[296]
9	Tuscaloosa	P327R	[294]	24	Philadelphia	T837M	[250, 296, 306]
10	Prague V	G455E	[296]	25	Nagoya	T837R	[250]
11	Yamagata	G455R	[250]	26	Diego	P854L	[250, 307, 308]
12	Coimbra	V488M	[302]	27	Prague III	R870W	[98]
13	Bicêtre I	R490C	[309]	28	Milano	Duplicate 478-499	[310]
14	Dresden	R518C	[58]	29	Prague I	Duplicate 10 nts	[97]
15	Prague VIII	L707P	[296]	30	Vesuvio	Codon 894delC	[311]

B

	Varient/Allele	Mutation	Reference		Varient/Allele	Mutation	Reference
31	Foggia	162delC	[301]	41	Princeton	InsC273	[296]
32	Kagoshima	AAG→STOP	[250]	42	Noirterre	Q330X	[96]
33	Prague IV	W81X	[296]	43	Brüggen	1369delC	[58]
34	Fukuyama	I-AC or -CA112	[250]	44	Bicêtre II	1476delG	[306]
35	Bohain	355delT	[306]	45	Evry	1600delT	[306]
36	Napoli I	InsT100	[301]	46	Prague VII	delC616	[296]
37	Hradec Kralove II	117del5 [ankyrin binding]	[296]	47	Trutnov	Y628X	[296]
38	Lyon or Osnabruck I	R150X	[58, 303]	48	Hobart	delG646	[296]
39	Worcester	InsG170	[296]	49	Osnabruck II	delM633	[58]
40	Fukuyama II	InsA183	[250]				

Figure 22–4, cont'd

severity of HE correlates both with the estimated amount of spectrin variant incorporated into red cell membranes and the increase in spectrin dimers detected. Above a threshold in the amount of spectrin variant, the red cell membrane becomes unstable and the clinical manifestations very severe.[107]

When compared with HE, HPP red cells show a greater increase of spectrin dimer and marked spectrin deficiency.[14,108] Three genetic effects can alter the spectrin composition: homozygosity for a single structural mutation, compound heterozygosity for two different structural mutations or one HE mutation coinheriting with α^{LELY} allele, and the synthesis of an unstable mutant spectrin protein.[109]

Protein 4.1 Abnormalities

Red cells with a partial or complete deficiency of protein 4.1 (4.1(−) phenotype) have a uniform smooth elliptocytic morphology and a mild reduction of glycophorin (GP) C.[110] Those 4.1-deficient HE red cells should be distinguished from elliptocytic red cells of the blood group Leach phenotype, which lack both GPC and GPD[111] and have approximately 20% reduction of protein 4.1.[112] HE patients heterozygous for partial protein 4.1 deficiency do not suffer the hemolytic anemia observed in those with the null phenotype.[113] HE 4.1(+) individuals have been found to have elongated or truncated protein 4.1 variants[114,115] or a variant with altered binding to spectrin-actin complex of the cytoskeleton.[113]

Several molecular mechanisms can produce the 4.1(−) phenotype: a deletion or defect in a downstream translation codon[116–119] and gene rearrangement resulting in the synthesis of a nonerythroid form of protein 4.1.[120] An absence of erythroid protein 4.1 affects both the horizontal interaction between actin and spectrin[121] and the vertical interaction between the spectrin network and the complex of protein 4.1, protein p55, and GPC.[122]

Hereditary Stomatocytosis and Related Disorders

In contrast to the structural protein defects in HS and HE, hereditary stomatocytosis (HSt) and related disorders have a functional abnormality in membrane permeability to monovalent cations Na^+ and K^+.[56] Red cells of the overhydrated form (OHSt) have a net increase of Na^+ flux, causing an inflow of water. A lipid raft–associated protein, stomatin (band 7.2),[123] is absent from these red cells.[124] Stomatin is present in erythroid progenitors but is gradually lost on maturation. The loss of stomatin is not genetically determined because the stomatin gene in OHSt was apparently normal.[125]

Red blood cells of dehydrated stomatocytosis (DHS) have an increased K^+ efflux exceeding the Na^+ influx. These erythrocytes lack deformability, which may be the cause of their premature destruction in the microcirculation. Dehydrated stomatocytosis has been included in a broader syndrome comprising a particular form of perinatal edema (designated as PE^{DHS}) and familial pseudohyperkalemia.[126] Familial pseudohyperkalemia is characterized by an increase of the K^+ concentration in plasma when freshly drawn blood stands at temperature below 37°C. These allied disorders map to chromosome 16q23-q24.[127]

CLINICAL FEATURES AND DIAGNOSIS

Hereditary Spherocytosis

The diagnosis of HS is usually simple and most often made in childhood. However, the classic clinical features of hemolysis—pallor, jaundice, and splenomegaly—are not specific for HS. HS is usefully divided by clinical criteria into severe, moderate, mild, and asymptomatic (trait) forms (Table 22–1). Generally, more severe cases present at a younger age (Table 22–2). Anemia and jaundice are absent in mild cases (about 30%, with compensated hemolysis), but mild to moderate splenomegaly is usual. The severity of anemia, and probably also spleen size, correlate with the degree of hemolysis. Severe HS is uncommon (5%), presents early in life, and can be life-threatening. Milder HS may be diagnosed incidentally after a blood count is obtained for another reason either in childhood, later in life (even in the ninth decade!),[19] or during pregnancy.[128]

The diagnosis of HS may be difficult in the neonatal period because spherocytes are present on blood smears from normal newborns.[129] Neonates with HS often have normal hemoglobin levels at birth; they may become pro-

TABLE 22–1. Classification of Spherocytosis and Indications for Splenectomy

Classification	Trait	Mild	Moderate	Severe
Hemoglobin (gm/dL)	Normal	11–15	8–12	6–8
Reticulocyte count (%)	Normal (<3%)	3–6	>6	>10
Bilirubin (μmol/L)	<17	17–34	>34	>51
Spectrin* per erythrocyte (% of normal)	100	80–100	50–80	40–60
Splenectomy	Not required	Usually not necessary during childhood and adolescence	Necessary during school age before puberty	Necessary—delay until 6 yr if possible

*Data on spectrin content are provided for interest; it is not necessary to measure this.

Modified from Eber SW, Armbrust R, Schroter W: Variable clinical severity of hereditary spherocytosis: relation to erythrocytic spectrin concentration, osmotic fragility and autohemolysis. J Pediatr 177:409–411, 1990.

TABLE 22–2. Presentation of HS by Patient Age

Age Group	Presentation	Likely clinical severity of HS
Neonatal period	Hydrops fetalis (rare)	Severe
	Neonatal anemia (rare)	Severe
	Neonatal jaundice	Not necessarily related to severity
Early childhood	Severe hemolytic anemia	Severe
Childhood	Anemia, jaundice	Moderate
	Parvovirus infection	Mild or moderate
	Incidental finding on blood count	Mild
Adulthood	Parvovirus infection	Mild
	Incidental finding on blood count	Mild
	Extramedullary hemopoiesis [135]	Mild
	Anemia unmasked by pregnancy	Mild

gressively more anemic during the first month of life as a result of a poor erythropoietic response. Jaundice does not necessarily predict disease severity. Jaundice is usually evident within the first 48 hours and may become more severe over several days, warranting exchange transfusion[130]; the risk is increased when HS is coinherited with Gilbert syndrome.[131,132] Transfusion may be temporarily required for anemia, and treatment with erythropoietin has reduced the transfusion need in some infants[133,134] but not in all studies.[135] Hydrops fetalis was reported in an infant homozygous for a β-spectrin mutation.[136]

HS may coexist with and complicate or modify the clinical expression of other red cell disorders, such as sickle cell trait or disease[27,137,138] or thalassemia.[139–145] HS has also been linked with retinal angioid streaks,[146,147] which may require treatment.[148] Iron absorption is increased in anemic states, which potentiates iron loading in those at risk for hereditary hemochromatosis.[149–152]

Hereditary Elliptocytosis

Although HE is usually a mild and clinically insignificant disorder (often noted only incidentally, as in the original description[153]), some affected individuals may have severe hemolysis or present with hydrops fetalis (Table 22–3). Mild HE may be difficult to differentiate from other hematologic disorders, but only true HE produces more than 35% elliptocytes on a blood smear (see Table 22–3). The clinical phenotype can be quite variable even within a single kindred. Patients with hemolytic HE may display pyknocytes rather than elliptocytes early in life.

Hereditary Stomatocytosis

Patients with overhydrated stomatocytosis may present as atypical HS. Red cells in dehydrated stomatocytosis have a high mean cell hemoglobin concentration and are less deformable. Perinatal edema and ascites have been associated with dehydrated hereditary stomatocytosis; the mechanism is not understood.[126,154] A family history of splenectomy failure, postsplenectomy thrombosis, recurrent high plasma K^+ values that may indicate pseudohy-

TABLE 22–3. Classification of HE and Related Disorders

Type	Clinical and Laboratory Features
Silent carrier state	Normal morphology; asymptomatic, but in relative of affected person, detectable membrane abnormality or gene mutation.
Mild HE	Most common group. Asymptomatic, incidental finding. Impressive elliptocytosis on blood film (>30–100%).
Common HE with chronic hemolysis	A more bizarre blood film appearance with poikilocytes and budding of red cells.
Common HE with sporadic hemolysis	May develop hemolysis under conditions of marrow stress (pregnancy, vitamin B_{12} deficiency) or increased reticuloendothelial activity (e.g., viral hepatitis, bacterial infections, infectious mononucleosis).
HE with infantile poikilocytosis	Moderately severe hemolytic anemia, red cell budding, fragmentation, poikilocytosis, neonatal jaundice that may require exchange transfusion. Can cause diagnostic confusion, but examination of parents will show one with typical HE. By 4 mo to 2 yr the blood picture evolves to classic mild HE.
HE with dyserythropoiesis	A rare subgroup reported only from Italy.[210]
Homozygous common HE	Range of clinical disease—moderate to severe hemolysis with marked fragmentation and poikilocytosis. Good response to splenectomy.
Hereditary pyropoikilocytosis	An uncommon disorder presenting in early life with severe hemolysis (Hb 4–8 gm/dL) with a dramatic blood film appearance; marked poikilocytosis, fragmented cells and spherocytes. Can be confused with homozygous HE or HE with infantile poikilocytosis. Very low MCV. Improved by splenectomy. One parent or sibling typically has common HE. Characterized by severe spectrin deficiency.
Spherocytic HE	Hybrid of HE and HS. Only reported in white Europeans, and rare. Improved by splenectomy.

Abbreviations: Hb, hemoglobin; MCV, mean cell volume.
From Gallagher PG, Lux SE: Disorders of the erythrocyte membrane. *In* Nathan DG, Orkin SH, Ginsburg D, Look AT (eds): Nathan and Oski's Hematology of Infancy and Childhood. Philadelphia: WB Saunders, 2003, pp 561–684.

TABLE 22–4. Diagnostic Parameters for HS and HE/HPP

Parameters	HS	HE/HPP [211]
Clinical features	Splenomegaly almost always	Splenomegaly in HE with overt hemolysis
Blood film	Spherocytes; pincer cells in some nonsplenectomized HS cases	Elliptocytes In hemolytic HE, poikilocytes, cell fragmentation, microspherocytes (<60 fL)
Laboratory parameters	↓ Hb, ↓ MCV, ↑ MCHC, ↑ hyperdense cells ↑ RDW, ↑ reticulocyte count	Hb and reticulocytes in normal range for nonhemolytic HE ↓ Hb, ↑reticulocytes in hemolytic HE
Best indicator of disease severity	% microcytes* and % hyperdense cells† [212] or combined % hyperdense cells and RDW [213] Combined MCHC and RDW (or HDW) significantly higher in HS.[214,215] Combined MCHC and % hyperdense cells are a discriminating feature of the HS phenotype.[212]	% microcytes (dehydrated, mainly mature red cells) and % dense hyperchromic cells

*Physiologic microcytosis occurs in children.[216]
†Hyperdense cells are also present in Hb SC disease, Hb CC disease, and xerocytosis.
Dual-angle laser light–scattering hematology analyzer.[212–215]
Electronic aperture impedance hematology analyzer.[214,215]
Abbreviations: Hb, hemoglobin; HDW, hemoglobin distribution width; MCHC, mean cell hemoglobin concentration; MCV, mean cell volume; RDW, red cell distribution width.

perkalemia, or perinatal problems may suggest a diagnosis of stomatocytosis.[155] The increased risk of thrombosis after splenectomy in stomatocytosis[156] is possibly due to altered endothelial adherence of these abnormal red cells.[157]

Parvovirus Infection in Hemolytic Disorders

Parvovirus B19 infection[158] (see Chapter 76) may unmask clinically silent HS (and HE) in children and adults.[159–163] The infectious nature of the transient aplastic crisis was suggested by the occurrence of multiple cases in single families.[164,165] During acute infection in patients with HS, there is commonly an associated thrombocytopenia and neutropenia, perhaps related to the enlarged spleen. The diagnosis is made in the laboratory by demonstrating immunoglobulin M antibodies or parvovirus B19 DNA in serum.[166] Infection produces lifelong immunity. Development of a recombinant parvovirus B19 vaccine may prevent infection in susceptible groups in the future.[167]

Laboratory Diagnosis

The diagnosis of HS or HE should be uncomplicated (Table 22–4). A combination of clinical features, classic laboratory findings, and careful examination of the blood smear (see Fig. 22–1*A* and *B*) is usually sufficient to make a firm diagnosis without the need for further tests (Fig. 22–6). Blood films of neonates with microspherocytes, cell fragments, and poikilocytes can be difficult to differentiate from those of neonates with both recessive and nondominant HS and HPP. The blood smear of HPP (see Fig. 22–1D) has marked microspherocytosis (as a result of spectrin reduction), micropoikilocytosis, fragmentation, and elliptocytosis; the mean cell volume of HPP red cells can be as low as 50–60 fL. Irregularly contracted

TABLE 22–5. Classification of Red Cell Membrane Disorders by Predominant Morphology

Spherocytes
ABO incompatibility in neonate
Immune hemolytic anemia
Acute oxidant injury
Hemolytic transfusion reactions
Hereditary spherocytosis
Clostridial sepsis
Severe burns or other thermal injuries
Spider, bee, and snake venoms
Severe hypophosphatemia

Bizarre Poikilocytes
Red cell fragmentation syndromes
Acute oxidant injury
HE in neonates
Hereditary pyropoikilocytosis
Homozygous HE

Elliptocytes
HE
Iron deficiency
Thalassemias

Stomatocytes
Hereditary stomatocytosis and related disorders (including hydrated, dehydrated, pseudohyperkalemia, and cryohydrocytosis)
Rh_{null} or Rh_{mod} blood group
Adenosine deaminase hyperactivity with low red cell ATP (sometimes)

From Gallagher PG, Lux SE: Disorders of the erythrocyte membrane. *In* Nathan DG, Orkin SH, Ginsburg D, Look AT (eds): Nathan and Oski's Hematology of Infancy and Childhood. Philadelphia: WB Saunders, 2003, pp 561–684.

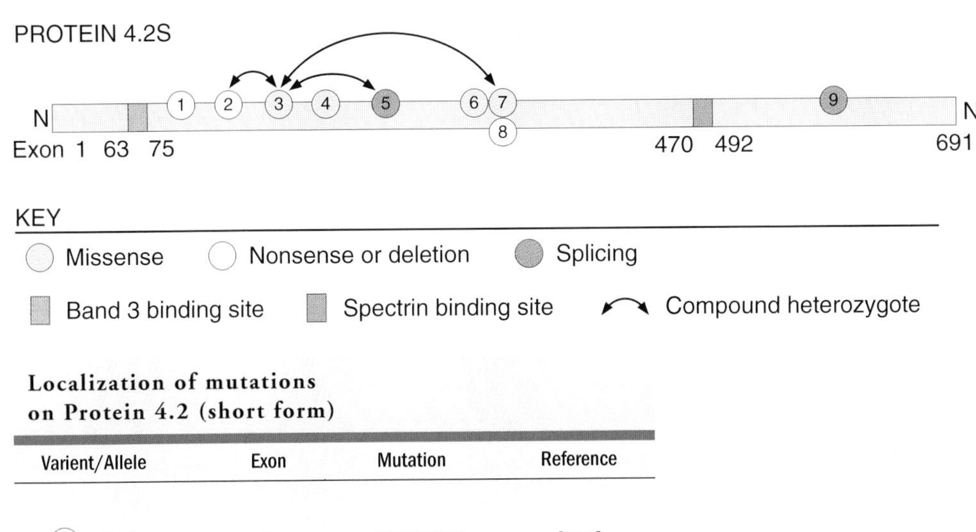

Localization of mutations on Protein 4.2 (short form)

	Varient/Allele	Exon	Mutation	Reference
1	Lisboa	2	KV88KW	[315]
2	Fukuoka	3	W119X	[316]
3	Nippon	3	A142T	[103]
4	Komatsu	4	D175Y	[317]
5	Notame	6 (spliced)	1st nt of intron 6 G→C	[38]
6	Tozeur	7	R310Q	[318]
7	Shiga	7	R317C	[36]
8	Nancy	7	949delG	[319]
9	Hammersmith	11	E583X	[320]

Figure 22–5. Localization of mutations for protein 4.2 (short form). The short form P4.2S (72 kDa, 691 amino acids) is found mainly in mature red cells, whereas the larger P4.1L (74 kDa), comprising an insert of amino acids 4–33, predominates in erythroid precursors.[102] P4.2 has distinct binding sites for band 3,[312] spectrin,[313] and ankyrin.[314] Patients with alleles Tozeur and Nancy exhibited severe hemolytic anemia, whereas those carrying alleles Shiga, Fukuoka, Notame, Lisboa, and Hammersmith had mild to moderate anemia.

cells may also be seen in microangiopathic hemolysis, alcoholic liver disease, and Wilson's disease.[168,169] Coexisting iron, folate, or vitamin B_{12} deficiency can mask some of the laboratory features of HS.[170,171]

If there is no family history, HS must be distinguished from acquired spherocytic hemolytic anemias (Table 22–5), the most important being autoimmune (see Chapter 24). Autoimmune hemolytic anemia is usually, but not always, excluded by a negative direct antiglobulin test.[172] Autoimmune hemolytic anemia is uncommon in childhood[173] and is a more important consideration in adults. If there are atypical features, and a hereditary disorder appears likely, some of the less common membrane disorders should be considered.

Additional Tests for the Diagnosis of HS

Additional testing is indicated when diagnostic criteria are not met and other causes of hemolysis have been excluded: for example, the blood film appearances are atypical, there is no clear pattern of inheritance, or the proband has a mild hemolytic process but an apparently normal blood count result. All current laboratory screening tests can detect typical HS[174] (Table 22–6). Sodium dodecyl sulfate–polyacrylamide gel electrophoresis of erythrocyte membrane proteins determines the specific membrane defect; the result allows molecular genetic analysis of the defective protein gene to establish the mode of inheritance (Fig. 22–6). The identification of spectrin or protein 4.1 deficiency may help to gauge disease severity in HE/HPP.

TREATMENT

Most cases of HS and HE do not require specific therapy because affected individuals are asymptomatic. Folate therapy historically has been prescribed in all chronic hemolysis, based on experience in sickle cell disease, but megaloblastic anemia in HS is extremely rare and there is no consensus concerning dosage.[175] Most children in developed countries consume well above the recommended daily requirement for folic acid.[175] Folate therapy can be reserved for those cases with severe or moderate hemolysis but is indicated for all pregnant women with inherited hemolytic diseases.

Baseline hemoglobin, reticulocyte count, and bilirubin levels help determine the need for splenectomy in HS. If the initial diagnosis is precipitated by parvovirus infection, the values at full recovery should be assessed to avoid a false impression of severity. Families need to be

TABLE 22–6. Screening Tests for the Diagnosis of HS

Test	Evaluation (Sensitivity, Specificity, Precaution)
Osmotic fragility (OF) test [217]	Normal result does not exclude HS,[218] detecting about 66% of the nonsplenectomized HS patients.[212] Increased OF found in immune-mediated and other hemolytic conditions. Reticulocytosis gives normal results (e.g., recovery from aplastic crisis).[219]
Acidified glycerol lysis test (AGLT)[220] The Pink test[221] is a modified AGLT.	Also detects autoimmune hemolytic anemia, hereditary persistence of fetal hemoglobin, pyruvate kinase deficiency, severe glucose-6-phosphate dehydrogenase, pregnant women (one third), chronic renal failure on dialysis (some), and myelodysplastic syndrome. Reagent preparation: special attention to the pH and osmolality.
Osmotic gradient ektacytometry[222]	Distinct deformability curves for red cells from patients with HS, HE, HPP, stomatocytosis, and sickle disease.[223]
Hypertonic cryohemolysis test[224]	Positive results for HS, some congenital dyserythropoietic anemia II (CDA II) and Melanesian elliptocytosis.
Eosin-5-maleimide (EMA) binding[225,226]	Distinct histograms for red cells of HS (sensitivity of 92.7% for HS and specificity of 99.1%) and HPP. HPP and HE can be differentiated from HS based on the graded reduction in fluorescence intensity for HPP (the lowest) < HS < HE ≤ normal controls. Reduced fluorescence with CDA II, cryohydrocytosis, SAO. Normal results for patients with a reticulocytosis and autoimmune hemolytic anemia. Reagent: A solution of EMA (light sensitive) must be stored at −20°C (max. 3 mo).

From Bolton-Maggs PH, Stevens RF, Dodd NJ, et al: Guidelines for the diagnosis and management of hereditary spherocytosis. Br J Haematol 126:455–474, 2004.

BOX 22–1. COMPLICATIONS OF HS

- Increase in hemolysis and/or exacerbation of jaundice as a result of intercurrent infection
- Aplastic crisis resulting from parvovirus B19
- Pigment gallstones (symptomatic or asymptomatic)
- Splenomegaly (rarely symptomatic)
- Transfusion-transmitted infection (very rare)
- Extramedullary hemopoiesis (adults with mild HS)
- Leg ulcers (very rare)
- Postsplenectomy complications (see text)

informed about their disorder and advised of the possibility of aplastic crisis related to parvovirus infection, of exacerbation of anemia by other infections, and the risk of gallstone development (Box 22–1). The likelihood of gallstones increases with severity of HS; they may cause symptoms in the first decade, particularly with coincidental Gilbert syndrome.[176,177] Abdominal complaints need to be reported and appropriately investigated; ultrasound examination has 96% accuracy for detection of stones.[178] Symptomatic stones are best treated by cholecystectomy together with splenectomy, but if stones are an incidental finding at splenectomy, it may be reasonable only to remove the stones, with subsequent evaluation by ultrasound, particularly in a young patient.[174]

There are no good longitudinal studies of cholelithiasis in HS, and surgical techniques (especially laparoscopy) are improving, complicating the decision for cholecystectomy versus simple removal of stones.[135,174]

The key therapeutic decision in HS concerns splenectomy. Because the spleen is the major site of red cell destruction, its removal results in improvement in erythrocyte lifespan (although not always completely to normal[179]). Spherocytes persist, but hemolysis is reduced or eliminated, as is the risk of pigment gallstones. However, splenectomy is associated with an increased risk of infection (Table 22–7)[180–194] that is lifelong, and not completely eliminated by immunization against pneumococcal species and postsplenectomy antibiotic prophylaxis.[195–197] Splenectomy therefore should generally be reserved for those individuals with severe HS (see Table 22–1), and if symptomatic gallstones develop. Splenectomy is an effective treatment for severe HE, with indications similar to those in HS (see Table 22–1). Precautions must be taken to prevent or reduce the risk of postsplenectomy sepsis (Table 22–8).

Splenectomy has traditionally been total and performed in open surgery; recently, the laparoscopic route has been successful.[198–202] There is also limited experience with partial splenectomy, which may benefit the very young child with severe, transfusion-dependent HS.[3,203–205] Partial splenectomy aims to leave enough splenic tissue to protect against overwhelming sepsis while ameliorating the hemolysis, but full splenectomy may be required later. Partial embolization has also been suggested.[206]

Postsplenectomy Thrombosis

There is little evidence of a long-term increased risk of venous thrombosis after splenectomy for HS (only isolated case reports) despite sometimes spectacular in-

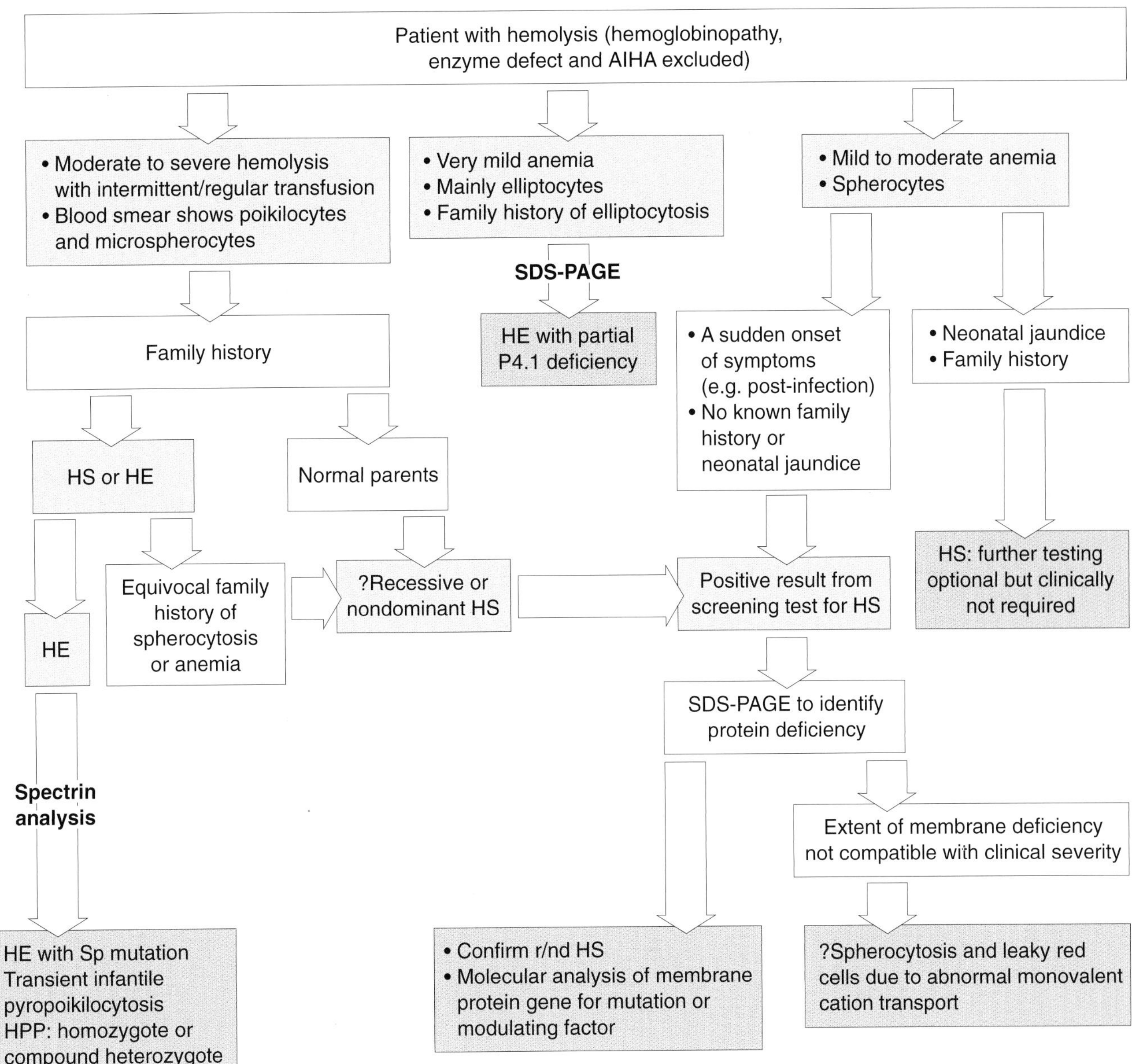

Figure 22–6. Algorithm for the diagnosis of HS and HE.

TABLE 22–7. Risks and Benefits of Splenectomy

Benefit	Refs	Risks	Refs
Improved red cell survival, often to normal.	179, 227	Overwhelming postsplenectomy sepsis, particularly caused by pneumococcal species.	181, 182, 184, 186–190, 192, 227, 229, 230
Correction of anemia (in most cases).		Risk greatest at young age and within first few years after splenectomy, but persists lifelong.	
Reduction to normal of risk of gallstone development.	228		
Resolution of leg ulcers (a very rare complication of HS).	135	Increased risk from other encapsulated organisms (*Haemophilus* and meningococcal spp.).	
		Increased risk of invasive malaria, and babesiosis.	231, 232
		Increased risk of infection from dog bites.	233, 234
		Increased risk of pulmonary hypertension and ischemic heart disease.	227, 235–240

TABLE 22–8. Guidelines for Prevention of Postsplenectomy Sepsis

Recommendation	Source	Reference
Defer splenectomy until after age 6 if possible	Scandinavia,	241
After 5–9 yr and after 3 yr of age in all children.	UK	174
	USA	135
Presplenectomy vaccination with pneumococcal, *Haemophilus*, and meningococcal vaccines.	UK Guidelines	242, 243
	Update of UK Guidelines	243
Postsplenectomy antibiotic prophylaxis (variable):		
Penicillin (or erythromycin) for life	UK Guidelines	242, 243
Penicillin for 3 yr		
Penicillin until age 16–18 yr (because of higher risk of sepsis of 4.4% under 16 yr vs. 0.9% in adults)		197
No regular antibiotic, keep a broad-spectrum antibiotic at home and start if febrile.	USA, Hungary	135, 244
Concern about pneumococcal resistance to penicillin (more than 50% in Hungary and 35% in United States).	Update of UK Guidelines	243
Give advice to obtain prompt medical attention when febrile, warn of risk of invasive malaria, and warn of risks associated with dog bites and other parasites such as *Babesia*.	UK Guidelines	242, 243
Asplenic individuals should be given written information and carry a medical information card to alert professionals to the risk of overwhelming infection.	UK Guidelines	242, 243

CURRENT CONTROVERSIES & FUTURE CONSIDERATIONS

Hereditary Spherocytosis, Hereditary Elliptocytosis, and Related Disorders

- In which individuals is folate therapy essential?
- Is splenectomy of value in all cases of mild HS?
- What is the role of partial splenectomy?
- What is the best way to manage postsplenectomy infection risk:

  Which pneumococcal vaccine should be used?

  When should boosters be given?

  Antibiotic prophylaxis—for how long and which antibiotic?

creases in platelet count. There are experimental data in mice demonstrating an association between severe HS (or HE) and thrombosis,[207,208] which is abrogated by the presence of a small number of normal stem cells,[209] approximating more closely to the majority of human patients. There is no indication to treat a high platelet count postsplenectomy. Adults should receive perioperative thromboprophylaxis according to standard guidelines. There may be a long-term increased risk of pulmonary hypertension (see Table 22–7). There is a significant risk of thrombosis after splenectomy for hereditary stomatocytosis, and the procedure should be avoided in these conditions.[56,155]

Suggested Readings*

Bolton-Maggs PH, Stevens RS, Dodd N, et al: Guidelines for the diagnosis and management of hereditary spherocytosis. Br J Haematol 126:455–474, 2004.

Cynober T, Mohandas N, Tchernia G: Red cell abnormalities in hereditary spherocytosis: relevance to diagnosis and understanding of the variable expression of clinical severity J Lab Clin Med 128:259–269, 1996.

Delaunay J: The hereditary stomatocytoses: genetic disorders of the red cell membrane permeability to monovalent cations. Semin Hematol 41:165–172, 2004.

Eber S, Lux SE: Hereditary spherocytosis—defects in proteins that connect the membrane skeleton to the lipid bilayer. Semin Hematol 41:118–141, 2004.

Gallagher PG: Hereditary elliptocytosis: spectrin and protein 4.1R. Semin Hematol 41:142–164, 2004.

Stewart GW: Hemolytic disease due to membrane ion channel disorders. Curr Opin Hematol 11:244–250, 2004.

Full references for this chapter can be found on accompanying CD-ROM.

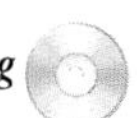

CHAPTER 23

Red Blood Cell Enzymopathies

Ernest Beutler, MD

KEY POINTS

Red Blood Cell Enzymopathies

- Glucose-6-phosphate dehydrogenase (G6PD) deficiency is the most common red cell enzymopathy; the A− variant is present on the X-chromosomes of 11% of African Americans, and other variants are very common in the Mediterranean region and in Asia.
- G6PD deficiency causes sensitivity to hemolysis when certain drugs are administered, neonatal jaundice, and hemolytic anemia as a response to infection.
- Some G6PD variants can cause chronic hemolytic anemia (hereditary nonspherocytic hemolytic anemia).
- Chronic hemolytic anemia can be the result of a deficiency of erythrocyte G6PD, pyruvate kinase, glucose-6-phosphate isomerase, pyrimidine 5′-nucleotidase, and, rarely, other enzymes.
- The diagnosis of enzyme deficiencies requires assay of red cell enzymes; red cell morphology is of little value.

INTRODUCTION

Once it leaves the marrow, the human red cell circulates for an average of 120 days. Its hemoglobin is loaded with oxygen and unloaded every few minutes, sometimes generating an active, harmful form of oxygen in the process. The erythrocyte must defend against these potentially damaging molecules, and when its hemoglobin iron is oxidized from ferrous to ferric, the iron must be reduced so that it can again bind oxygen. The red cell is a biconcave disk with a diameter larger than the capillaries that it must traverse; therefore, it must be deformable. The potassium concentration within the red cell is high, and that of sodium is low[1]; to survive, the cell must pump out the sodium that leaks in and pump in potassium to replace that which has leaked out. The calcium content of the cell is extremely low, and any calcium ions that gain entry also must be pumped out.[2,3] The membrane phospholipids are dispersed in an asymmetrical fashion, with phosphatidylserine on the inner face of the membrane and phosphatidylcholine on the outer face.[4] When a phospholipid molecule is on the wrong face in the membrane, it must be translocated by an energy-requiring enzyme. All these activities require that energy be extracted from glucose and be utilized by the required enzymes. Deficiencies of the enzymes that generate the energy for these processes are designated red cell enzymopathies, and they may result in disease, particularly hemolytic anemia.

EPIDEMIOLOGY AND RISK FACTORS

Most red cell enzymopathies are inherited; only a few instances of acquired deficiencies of red cell enzymes, particularly of pyruvate kinase, have been described.[5–7]

Glucose-6-Phosphate Dehydrogenase Deficiency

Glucose-6-phosphate dehydrogenase (G6PD) deficiency is the most common erythrocyte enzymopathy.[8–10] G6PD deficiency may be polymorphic or sporadic. The polymorphic forms occur in several different populations, each with one or more variants that are characteristic of that population. In persons of African origin, the most common is G6PD A−, which, in reality, is composed of three different pairs of mutations[11] (Table 23–1).

In southern Europe, G6PD Mediterranean is the most common variant, but G6PD A− and G6PD Seattle are encountered as well. In Asia, still other variants are found, including G6PD Canton, Viangchan, Chinese-4, and Union. G6PD Union is a rare exception to the rule that most polymorphic variants are limited to a single geographic region, as it presents both in Asia and in Europe. When they have been investigated, most of the

TABLE 23–1. Prevalence of G6PD Deficiency in Various Populations*

Population	Gene Frequency	Mutations Encountered†	References
U.S. black	0.112		12,13
Nigerian (Yoruba)	0.239	A–	14
Mexican Mestizos	0.011	A–202A/376G; A–376G/968C	15
Kurdish Jews	0.582	Mediterranean	16,17
Sardinians	0.072		18
Africans (Brazzaville, Congo)	0.225	A–	19
Hawaiian Chinese	0.037	95G; 835T; 1388A	20
Hawaiian Filipino	0.134	493G; 871A; 1003A	20
Hawaiian Laotians	0.203	487A; 871A; 1360T; 1388A	20
Singaporian Chinese	0.0162		21
Singaporian Malay	0.018		21
Singaporian Indian	0.008		21
Greek	0.045		22
Italy (Conzesa Province)	0.012	Mediterranean; A–	23
Arab (Kuwait, Syria, Egypt, Jordan, Lebanon)	0.038	Mediterranean?; A–	24
Iran	0.12		24

*A comprehensive tabulation of studies performed prior to 1978 may be found in Beutler.[25]
†When known.

polymorphic variants exist in a single haplotype,[15,26,27] implicating a single founder, but there are exceptions.[28]

The prevalence of G6PD deficiency varies greatly among different populations (see Table 23–1). High gene frequencies are due to the selective pressure that has been exerted by malaria during human evolution.[29,30] Thus, polymorphic G6PD mutations are common in Southeast Asia, southern Europe, the Middle East, Africa, and wherever people with ancestry in these regions subsequently have migrated. Sporadic mutations of G6PD may occur in any ethnic group, and predominate in populations in which no selective pressure in favor of G6PD mutations has been exerted, as in northern Europeans. Conversely, most G6PD-deficient individuals in southern Europe or in Africa carry the mutations that are characteristic of those regions.

Other Red Cell Enzyme Deficiencies

Mutations of red cell enzymes other than those of G6PD are all uncommon or very rare. Surprisingly, they also show evidence of a founder effect. For example, almost half of European patients with pyruvate kinase deficiency share the same mutation, a G→A transition at cDNA nucleotide 1529.[31] Similarly, although triose-phosphate isomerase deficiency is very unusual, about one half of the affected patients have the same mutation at complementary DNA nucleotide 315.[32,33]

Because of their infrequency, little is known about the prevalence of these mutations. However, in the case of pyruvate kinase deficiency, the least uncommon of these disorders, homozygotes have been estimated at 51 per 1 million in the white population.[34]

PATHOPHYSIOLOGY

Energy Metabolism of the Red Cell: Glucose Metabolism

The primary source of metabolic energy utilized by the erythrocyte is glucose, and most of the known enzymatic defects that result in hemolytic anemia are lesions that affect glucose metabolism. As shown in Figure 23–1, two pathways of glucose metabolism are active in the red cell, the direct glycolytic pathway (Embden-Meyerhof pathway) and the hexose monophosphate shunt.

The Direct Glycolytic Pathway

This ancient metabolic pathway, present in yeast, bacteria, and all lower plants and animals, metabolizes glucose to pyruvate and lactic acids. The breakdown of glucose yields metabolic energy by the phosphorylation of ADP to ATP and reducing equivalents by the reduction of NAD to NADH.

Glucose enters the erythrocyte through a facilitated glucose transporter, GLUT1.[35] Glucose then undergoes phosphorylation at the 6 position in the hexokinase reaction. Hexokinase deficiency is an uncommon cause of hereditary nonspherocytic hemolytic anemia.[36–41] The glucose 6-phosphate formed represents the branch point between the Embden-Meyerhof pathway and the hexose monophosphate shunt.

Red cell glucose 6-phosphate is in equilibrium with fructose 6-phosphate through the enzyme glucose-6-phosphate isomerase. A deficiency of this enzyme is associated with hemolytic anemia.[42–45]

The phosphorylation of fructose 6-phosphate to fructose 1,6-phosphate by phosphofructokinase commits glucose to the Embden-Meyerhof pathway. A deficiency of this enzyme results in mild hemolysis—with erythrocytosis as a consequence of the lowered 2,3-bisphosphoglycerate (2,3-BPG; also known as 2,3-diphosphoglycerate) levels that result from the metabolic block.[46] Another phosphofructokinase enzyme phosphorylates fructose 6-phosphate to fructose 2,6-phosphate[47,48]; this sugar phosphate presumably plays a regulatory role in glycolysis. The cleavage of fructose 1,6-phosphate into two triose molecules, glyceraldehyde phosphate and dihydroxyacetone phosphate, is accomplished by aldolase A. Aldolase A deficiency is a rare cause of hereditary hemolytic anemia.[49–51] The red cell is not able to further metabolize dihydroxyacetone phosphate without isomerizing it to glyceraldehyde phosphate, a reaction that is catalyzed by triose-phosphate isomerase. Deficiency of triose-phosphate isomerase is among the most devastating red cell enzymopathies, less due to its effect on the erythrocyte than because all tissues are affected and death almost always occurs in childhood.[32,52–55]

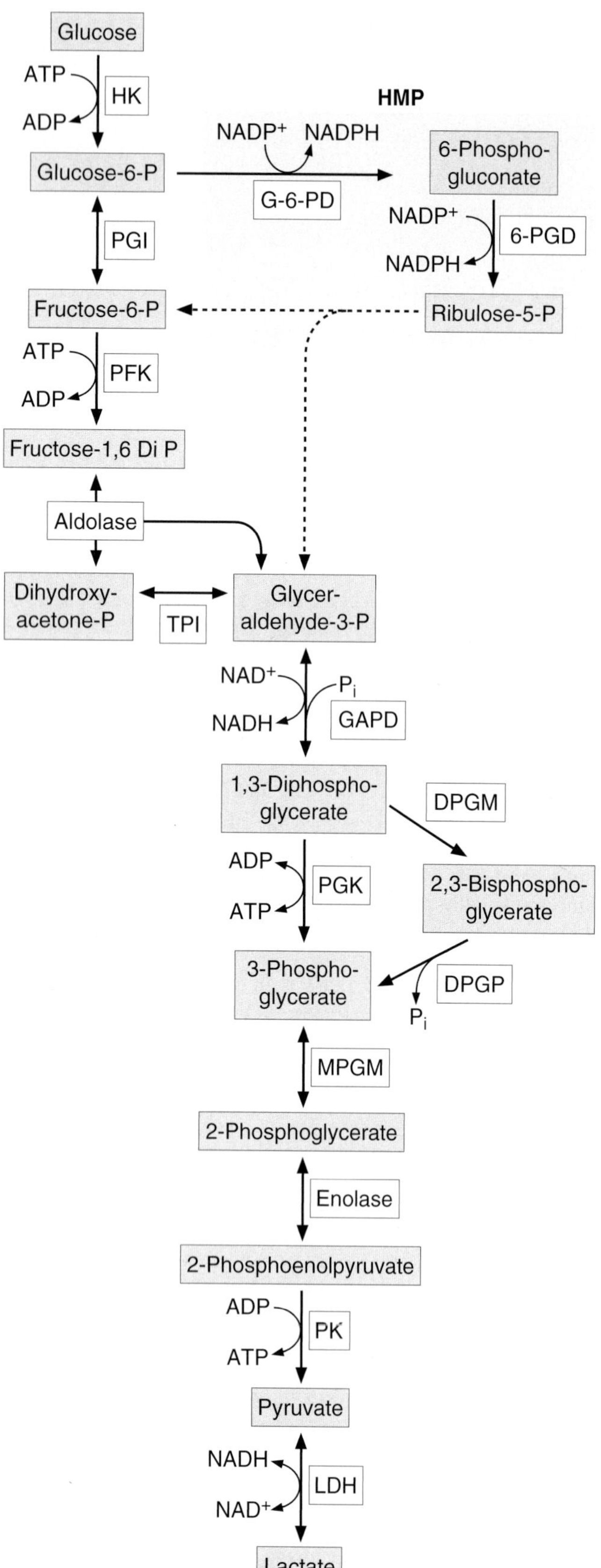

Figure 23–1. The metabolism of glucose by erythrocytes. Abbreviations: DPGM, diphosphoglycerate mutase; DPGP, diphosphoglycerate phosphatase; GAPD, glyceraldehyde phosphate dehydrogenase; G-6-PD, glucose-6-phosphate dehydrogenase; HK, hexokinase; LDH, lactate dehydrogenase; MPGM, monophosphoglycerate mutase; 6-PGD, glucose-6-phosphogluconic dehydrogenase; PGI, phosphoglycerate isomerase; PGK, phosphoglycerate kinase; PK, pyruvate kinase; TPI, triosephosphate isomerase.

Erythrocytes contain an extraordinarily high level of 2,3-BPG. This highly acidic sugar diphosphate binds to hemoglobin, stabilizing it in the low-affinity confirmation, and thus modulating the oxygen dissociation curve (see Chapter 2). Decreased levels of 2,3-BPG cause an increase of the oxygen affinity of hemoglobin, leading to erythrocytosis. As noted earlier, phosphofructokinase deficiency is one such defect. The greatest effect on 2,3-BPG levels is exerted by a deficiency of the enzyme diphosphoglycerate mutase/phosphatase, which results in its formation from 1,3-diphosphoglyceric acid. Deficiency of this mutase/phosphatase enzyme is rare but more generally leads to erythrocytosis[56,57] although in some patients hemolytic anemia results.[58,59]

After 2,3-BPG is hydrolyzed to 3-phosphoglyceric acid, it is metabolized in two steps by monophosphoglycerate mutase and enolase to 2-phospho*enol*pyruvate. Deficiencies of these enzymes have not been clearly documented, but defects in the subsequent metabolic step, catalyzed by pyruvate kinase, are the most common cause of hereditary nonspherocytic hemolytic anemia.[60–62]

The Hexose Monophosphate Pathway

The hexose monophosphate pathway oxidizes glucose 6-phosphate, in the process reducing NADP to NADPH. Because NADPH serves as an electron donor for the reduction of oxidized glutathione, this pathway plays an essential role in protecting the red cell against oxidative damage.[63] G6PD deficiency results in inability to maintain an adequate level of NADPH, leading to red cell damage when the erythrocyte is exposed to oxidative stress. The hexose monophosphate pathway also provides pentose needed for nucleotide synthesis in the salvage pathway.

Other Metabolic Processes

Many other metabolic processes exist in the erythrocyte. Defects in some cause hemolytic anemia or methemoglobinemia, but others, although not producing hematologic disease, afford the opportunity to make a diagnosis by merely obtaining a blood sample.

Pyrimidine 5′-nucleotidase catabolizes pyrimidine nucleotides in reticulocytes,[64,65] and its deficiency causes a hereditary nonspherocytic hemolytic anemia. Stippling of erythrocytes on blood films is characteristic; stippling occurs also in lead poisoning, and pyrimidine 5′-nucleotidase is remarkably sensitive to inhibition by lead

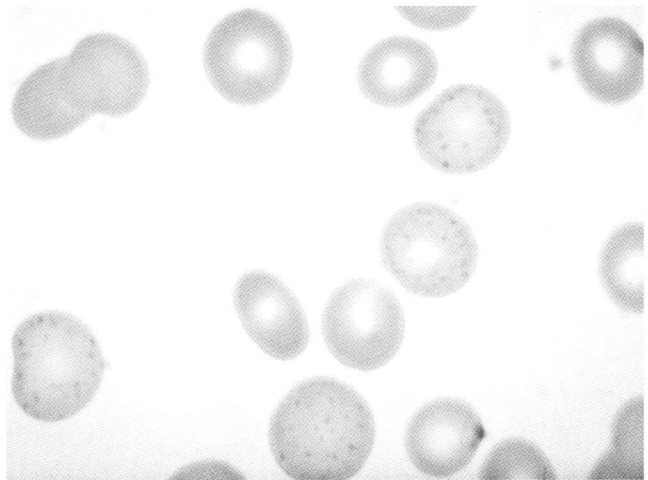

Figure 23–2. Stippled red cells from a patient with pyrimidine 5′-nucleotidase deficiency.

(Fig. 23–2). The tripeptide glutathione is synthesized in red cells in two steps. First, γ-glutamylcysteine is formed from glutamic acid and cysteine, a step catalyzed by the enzyme γ-glutamylcysteine synthetase. Next, glutathione synthetase catalyzes the formation of a peptide bond between γ-glutamylcysteine and glycine. A deficiency of either enzyme causes hemolytic anemia.[66–72] When glutathione synthetase deficiency affects not only erythrocytes but other tissues as well, overproduction of 5-oxoproline (pyroglutamic acid) results, with 5-oxoprolinuria and neurologic abnormalities.

The erythrocyte has the capacity to synthesize purine nucleotides from preformed adenine in the adenine phosphoribosyltransferase (APRT) reaction and from preformed guanine or hypoxanthine in the hypoxanthine guanine phosphoribosyltransferase (HGPRT) reaction. Deficiencies do not result in hematologic disease, but the detection of the enzyme can be useful in the diagnosis of gout caused by APRT deficiency[73,74] or of Lesch-Nyhan syndrome, a neurologic disorder caused by HGPRT deficiency.[75] A deficiency of another enzyme of purine metabolism, adenosine deaminase, causes severe combined immunodeficiency,[76] and an excess of the enzyme causes a dominantly inherited hemolytic anemia.[77–79] Deficiency of galactose-1-phosphate uridyltransferase, or galactokinase, does not produce hematologic disease but is useful in the diagnosis of galactosemias.[80–82]

The reduction of methemoglobin to hemoglobin is achieved in erythrocytes by generating NADH in the glycolytic pathway and utilizing this reduced coenzyme to reduce cytochrome b_5, which, in turn, reduces the iron of the methemoglobin nonenzymatically. A deficiency of cytochrome b_5 reductase (also known as methemoglobin reductase or NADH diaphorase) results in hereditary methemoglobinemia.[83–88]

Red Cell Enzyme Deficiencies

The mechanism by which red cell enzyme deficiencies produce their clinical consequences is not always clear. In the case of mutations involving the hexose monophosphate pathway, particularly those of G6PD, inability to maintain glutathione in the reduced state is probably the most important pathogenic mechanism. Reduced glutathione plays an important role in the detoxification of hydrogen peroxide in the erythrocyte; in its absence, the cell is vulnerable to oxidative damage. For mutations that affect enzymes of the direct glycolytic pathway, inability to generate ATP may be important. Conversely, impediments to the normal flow of metabolites result in distortion of the concentration of the various metabolic intermediates in the cell, and abnormal levels of some metabolites may interfere with red cell functions. For example, a deficiency of methemoglobin reductase impairs the ability of the cell to reduce cytochrome b_5 and therefore to maintain hemoglobin in the ferrous state.

Mutations of genes encoding enzymes of important metabolic pathways may affect tissues other than the red cell. However, in most red cell enzyme deficiencies, clinical manifestations are largely limited to the erythrocyte. This apparent sparing of other tissues is probably a function of ascertainment bias. Severe defects of glycolytic enzymes are presumably not compatible with postfetal life. As discussed later, some deficiencies do have marked phenotypic effects in other tissues, most prominently in the case of triose-phosphate isomerase deficiency, in which widespread neuromuscular involvement usually leads to early death.

CLINICAL FEATURES AND DIAGNOSIS

Hemolytic Anemia

The clinically most frequent result of red cell enzyme deficiencies is hemolytic anemia. The clinical and routine laboratory features of hemolytic anemia secondary to red cell enzyme defects do not distinguish them from other forms of hemolytic anemia. Reticulocytosis is usually present, although, in severe forms of pyruvate kinase deficiency, the red cells may be destroyed in the marrow before they ever gain entry into the circulation. The spleen may be enlarged. Onset of the disorder may be at birth, and in the case of some deficiencies, particularly that of glucose-6-phosphate isomerase, hydrops fetalis may be present.[89] Conversely, some patients with mild manifestations are not diagnosed until late in life.

In the most common forms of G6PD deficiency, hemolysis follows a triggering event: treatment with a medical drug[90–117] (Table 23–2), infection,[118–127] ingestion of fava beans,[128–138] and possibly physiologic stresses such as diabetic ketoacidosis [139–141] or cardiopulmonary bypass.[142] Genetic variants of G6PD have been divided into four classes based upon the functional severity of the enzyme deficiency. Class 4 variants cause no clinical manifestations, whereas class 1 variants comprise a subset of patients with uncommon, sporadic variants of G6PD resulting in chronic hemolytic anemia. Thus, G6PD deficiency is one of the causes of hereditary nonspherocytic hemolytic anemia. The mutations that cause chronic hemolysis usually are located at the interface of the two identical subunits, near the site where structural NADP is bound[9,143,144] (Fig. 23–3). The clinical manifestations of different variants are summarized in Table 23–3.

Other Manifestations

The most dangerous manifestation of G6PD deficiency is neonatal icterus.[145–151] Hemolysis of enzyme-deficient cells seems to play only a small role; a defect in bilirubin conjugation in the G6PD-deficient liver is mainly responsible. Only a subset of G6PD-deficient infants develops jaundice, and these babies usually have co-inherited a promoter polymorphism in the UDPglucuronosyltransferase gene. Some patients deficient in NADH diaphorase,[152] aldolase,[49] or phosphoglycerate kinase[153] have developed mental retardation or behavior problems. Erythrocytosis and myopathies are found in phosphofructokinase deficiency. Severe neuromuscular defects lead to early death in most patients with triosephosphate isomerase deficiency.

TABLE 23–2. Drugs and Chemicals That Should Be Avoided by Persons with G6PD Deficiency*

Acetanilid[90]
Dimercaptosuccinic acid[91 ‡]
Furazolidone (Furoxone)[92,93]
Glibenclamide[94 ‡]
Henna[95,96 †]
Isobutyl or amyl nitrite[97–99]
Menthol[100,101]
Metformin[102 ‡]
Methylene blue[103]
Nalidixic acid (NegGram)[104,105 ‡]
Naphthalene[106,107]
Nimesulide[108]
Niridazole (Ambilhar)[109,110 ‡]
Nitrofurantoin (Furadantin)[111]
Phenazopyridine (Pyridium)[112]
Phenylhydrazine[90]
Primaquine[90]
Propacetamol[113,114]
Sulfacetamide[90]
Sulfanilamide[90]
Sulfapyridine[90]
Thiazolesulfone[90]
Toluidine blue[115 ‡]
Trinitrotoluene (TNT)[116]
Urate oxidase[117]

*Further details may be found in Beutler.[25]
†A leaf extract containing lawsone (2-hydroxy-1,4-naphthoquinone).
‡Single report; cause-and-effect relationship is not certain.

Diagnosis

The diagnosis of red cell enzyme deficiencies is definitively established by measurement of the enzyme in a freshly prepared hemolysate. Screening tests are available for the detection of some of the more common enzyme defects, particularly of G6PD deficiency.[154–157] In some cases, the diagnosis may best be established by demonstrating the presence in the patient's DNA of a mutation known to cause an enzyme deficiency. Mutation analysis is particularly useful when the patient has been transfused, because the DNA is prepared from peripheral blood white cells. Because DNA is very stable, whereas most red cell enzymes are relatively unstable, DNA testing has the advantage that samples can be shipped long distances to a specialty laboratory. However, a normal sequence of the entire coding region does not preclude an enzyme deficiency, because mutations upstream of the coding region can affect gene expression and may not be detected. DNA analysis is easiest to perform and most useful when a specific mutation is suspected, as, for example, the A− mutation of G6PD in a black patient. DNA analysis is the preferred approach to prenatal diagnosis.

Microscopic examination of the blood film is of very little value in the diagnosis of red cell enzyme defects. The appearance of basophilic stippling in the erythrocytes of patients with pyrimidine 5′-nucleotidase deficiency is an exception (see Fig. 23–2). A commonly held misconception is that pyruvate kinase–deficient red cells

TABLE 23–3. The Clinical Manifestations of Different Classes of G6PD Mutants

	Class 4 (Nondeficient)	Class 3 (Mild Deficiency)	Class 2 (Severe Deficiency)	Class 1* (NSHA)
G6PD activity	over 60%	10–60%	0–10%	0–35%
Example	A	A−	Mediterranean Canton	Duarte Alhambra
Drug-induced hemolysis	0	+	+	+
Infection-induced	0	+	+	+
Favism	0	0	+	+
Icterus neonatorum	0	±	+	+
Red cell lifespan in the absence of stress	N	N or sl ↓	N or sl ↓	↓
Anemia in the absence of stress	0	0	0	+

*Class 1 mutants have the most severe clinical phenotype.
Abbreviations: 0, absent; ±, absent or present; +, present; N, normal; NSHA, nonspherocytic hemolytic anemia; sl ↓, slightly decreased; ↓, decreased.

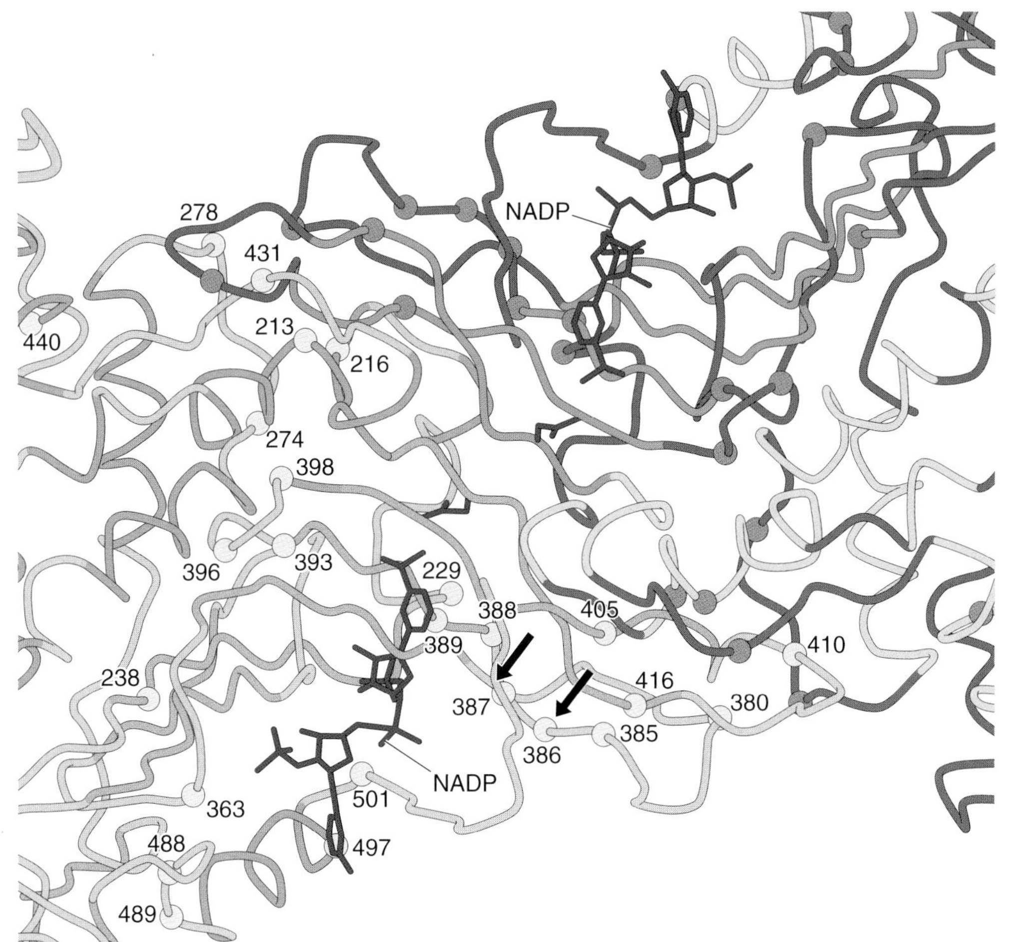

Figure 23–3. The crystal structure of human G6PD, showing the two molecules of structural NADP. These molecules are close to the dimer interface of the molecule. The *red arrows* point to the sites of two mutations that cause hereditary nonspherocytic hemolytic anemia: G6PD Iowa (Lys386Glu) and G6PD Beverly Hills (Arg387His). (Modified from Au SWN, Gover S, Lam VMS, et al: Human glucose-6-phosphate dehydrogenase: the crystal structure reveals a structural NADP$^+$ molecule and provides insights into enzyme deficiency. Struct Fold Des 8:293, 2000.)

show echinocytic changes. Similarly, the autohemolysis test is of no value in the diagnosis of hemolytic anemia caused by red cell enzyme defects.

DIFFERENTIAL DIAGNOSIS

Hemolytic anemia secondary to red cell enzyme deficiencies presents similarly to hemolytic anemia resulting from an unstable hemoglobin. Unstable hemoglobins are inherited as autosomal dominant disorders. An isopropanol stability test will detect most unstable hemoglobins. The clinical manifestations of hereditary spherocytosis may also resemble those of hereditary nonspherocytic hemolytic anemia. Hereditary spherocytosis also is usually inherited in an autosomal dominant fashion. The osmotic fragility of the red cells of patients with hereditary spherocytosis is increased; that of patients with red cell enzyme defects is normal.

Methemoglobinemia resulting from NADH diaphorase deficiency is an autosomal recessive disorder and therefore can be rather readily distinguished from the dominantly inherited hemoglobin M diseases. The optical spectrum of hemoglobin is normal in NADH diaphorase deficiency and abnormal in hemoglobin M disease.

TREATMENT

Some but not all patients with hereditary nonspherocytic hemolytic anemia respond well to splenectomy.[158–177] Splenectomy appears to be most beneficial in glucose-6-phosphate isomerase deficiency, but responses are also frequent in pyruvate kinase deficiency, and occasional improvement is seen in patients with G6PD deficiency. Splenectomy is usually undertaken to relieve a substantial transfusion requirement. Stem cell transplantation has been successful in a patient with pyruvate kinase deficiency.[178] Iron storage disease can complicate pyruvate kinase deficiency[179–183] and may require chelation therapy.

G6PD-deficiency with neonatal icterus should be managed as in infants jaundiced from other causes. The bilirubin must be prevented from reaching levels that damage the central nervous system by employing phototherapy or exchange transfusion as appropriate. The administration of *sn*-mesoporphyrin between the ages of 12 and 36 hours can prevent the development of severe jaundice in G6PD-deficient infants.[184]

Hereditary methemoglobinemia secondary to NADH diaphorase deficiency may be treated by the administration of ascorbic acid, 300–600 mg orally daily, divided into three or four doses.

SUPPORTIVE CARE AND LONG-TERM MANAGEMENT

G6PD-deficient individuals and those with glutathione deficiency should avoid drugs that are known to produce hemolysis. Many drugs have been falsely implicated as the cause of hemolysis in G6PD deficiency. Unfounded warnings not only may deprive the patient of a needed medication but may erode confidence in the physician's advice. Aspirin, for example, is sometimes listed as being hemolytic, but, because it does not produce hemolysis in normal doses, many G6PD-deficient patients will know that they can take this drug with impunity.

Apart from avoidance of some drugs by such individuals, the care given to patients with red cell enzyme deficiencies is that appropriate for any other patients with anemia. Splenectomized patients need to observe the usual precautions related to their susceptibility to certain bacterial infections.

PROGNOSIS

The prognosis in red cell enzyme deficiencies depends upon the specific abnormality. For example, the polymorphic forms of G6PD deficiency are usually very mild and have no effect on health except under rare circumstances. Hereditary methemoglobinemia is also a benign disorder. At the other extreme, triose-phosphate isomerase deficiency is usually fatal before the age of 5 years. Pyruvate kinase deficiency can be severe and life-threatening; it can also be very mild and have very little effect on quality of life. In pyruvate kinase deficiency as well as in many of the other red cell enzyme deficiencies, the correlation between the mutation present and the severity of the clinical phenotype is weak: among patients with identical pyruvate kinase mutations, some suffer very severe hemolysis and others only mild disease.[185]

CURRENT CONTROVERSIES & FUTURE CONSIDERATIONS

Red Blood Cell Enzymopathies

- Most patients with hereditary nonspherocytic hemolytic anemia do not have a demonstrable red cell enzyme deficiency. Most of the causes of this syndrome remain to be discovered.
- The clinical phenotype of patients with genetically identical red cell enzyme deficiencies can differ widely. The molecular basis for these differences are not established.

Suggested Readings*

Beutler E (ed): Hemolytic Anemia in Disorders of Red Cell Metabolism. New York: Plenum Press, 1978.

Beutler E: G6PD: population genetics and clinical manifestations. Blood Rev 10:45, 1996.

Fujii H, Miwa S: Red blood cell enzymes and their clinical application. Adv Clin Chem 33:1, 1999.

Jacobasch G, Rapoport SM: Hemolytic anemias due to erythrocyte enzyme deficiencies. Mol Aspects Med 17:143, 1996.

Full references for this chapter can be found on accompanying CD-ROM.

CHAPTER 24

The Autoimmune Hemolytic Anemias

Karen E. King, MD, and Paul M. Ness, MD

KEY POINTS

The Autoimmune Hemolytic Anemias

Diagnosis

- The major types of autoimmune hemolytic anemia include warm autoimmune hemolytic anemia, cold agglutinin syndrome, and paroxysmal cold hemoglobinuria. These diseases are distinguished based on the serology of the causative autoantibody and the clinical presentation.
- Warm autoimmune hemolytic anemia is characterized by immunoglobulin (Ig) G autoantibody directed against red cell antigens optimally reactive at 37°C.
- Cold agglutinin syndrome is due to IgM autoantibody, which is optimally reactive between 0° and 5°C.
- Paroxysmal cold hemoglobinuria is caused by a biphasic cold hemolysin, the Donath-Landsteiner antibody, an IgG that binds to red cells at lower temperatures, activating complement, and causes hemolysis at warmer temperatures.
- Other less common autoimmune hemolytic anemias include mixed-type (warm and cold autoimmune), direct antiglobulin test–negative autoimmune hemolytic anemia, and autoimmune hemolytic anemia mediated by warm IgM antibodies.
- Drugs can induce an autoimmune hemolytic anemia that is clinically indistinguishable from warm autoimmune hemolytic anemia.

Treatment

- Initial therapy for warm autoimmune hemolytic anemia is corticosteroids.
- Splenectomy should be considered if steroids fail in warm autoimmune hemolytic anemia.
- Additional immunosuppressive agents can be used, if corticosteroids and splenectomy fail to achieve a durable remission.
- Avoidance of the cold is generally effective in treating cold agglutinin syndrome.
- Paroxysmal cold hemoglobinuria is usually a self-limited disease that requires supportive care only. However, patients may present with severe anemia requiring urgent transfusion.
- Mixed-type (warm and cold) autoimmune hemolytic anemia responds to corticosteroid therapy.
- In drug-induced autoimmune hemolytic anemia, the offending agent must be discontinued immediately.

INTRODUCTION

All of the autoimmune hemolytic anemias are characterized by shortened red blood cell survival and autoantibodies directed against red blood cell antigens. Patients with any of the autoimmune hemolytic anemias will have symptoms and signs of anemia; the severity depends on the time course of the disease. Patterns of presentation can help define specific types. The autoimmune hemolytic anemias may be idiopathic or secondary to an underlying disease.

The autoimmune hemolytic anemias are classified on the basis of the in vivo and in vitro characteristics of the causative autoantibody (Table 24–1). This classification system not only reflects our understanding of the diseases and their pathogenesis, but the distinctions are clinically significant—prognosis and management of the various types of autoimmune hemolytic anemia differ significantly. Serology allows classification into the autoimmune hemolytic anemias associated with warm antibodies, reacting optimally at 37°C, and those with cold-reacting antibodies, having optimal reactivity at 0° to 5°C. The cold autoantibody syndromes can be further

TABLE 24–1. Classification and Typical Serologic Features of the Autoimmune Hemolytic Anemias

	Warm Autoimmune Hemolytic Anemia	Cold Agglutinin Syndrome	Paroxysmal Cold Hemoglobinuria
Direct antiglobulin test	IgG, IgG and C3	C3 only	C3 only
Immunoglobulin class	IgG (sometimes IgA)	IgM	IgG
Eluate	IgG	Nonreactive	Nonreactive
Serum	IgG agglutinating red cells at the anti–human globulin phase (panagglutinin)	IgM agglutinating antibody, often with titers >1000, reacting at 30° C in albumin	IgG biphasic hemolysin (Donath-Landsteiner antibody)
Specificity	Rh	I, i	P

subdivided into the more common cold agglutinin syndrome and the rare paroxysmal cold hemoglobinuria. Typically, warm autoimmune hemolytic anemia is due to immunoglobulin (Ig) G autoantibodies; cold agglutinin syndrome is most often caused by IgM autoantibodies. The pathogenic autoantibody in paroxysmal cold hemoglobinuria is an IgG autoantibody known as a biphasic cold hemolysin or the Donath-Landsteiner antibody, which is capable of binding to red cells at low temperatures, activating complement, and leading to hemolysis at 37°C.

WARM AUTOIMMUNE HEMOLYTIC ANEMIA

Epidemiology and Risk Factors

The incidence of autoimmune hemolytic anemia has been estimated to be 1 in 75,000 to 1 in 80,000 per year.[1] Warm autoimmune hemolytic anemia accounts for 60–70% of all the autoimmune hemolytic anemias.[2–4] About half of all cases of warm autoimmune hemolytic anemia are idiopathic or primary,[3–8] with the remainder secondary to underlying lymphoproliferative diseases, immunodeficiency states, solid tumors, connective tissue disorders, or infectious diseases. Warm autoimmune hemolytic anemia may occur after an allogeneic transfusion.[9] Warm autoimmune hemolytic anemia has been diagnosed in individuals of all ages, from 1 month to the elderly.[10] The incidence of disease increases with age, especially after 50 years[4]; idiopathic disease has a peak incidence between the ages of 40 and 70, with a mean of approximately 49 years.[11] Secondary cases have the age distribution of the underlying disease. Approximately 60% of patients with the idiopathic syndrome are women.[3,11,12]

Pathophysiology

Extravascular hemolysis and intravascular hemolysis are two distinct mechanisms of immune-mediated red blood cell destruction. In warm autoimmune hemolytic anemia, the hemolysis is usually extravascular. The causative antibody in warm autoimmune hemolytic anemia is typically an IgG autoantibody with optimal reactivity at 37°C. The pathogenic IgG autoantibody binds to the red cells. Antibody-coated red cells circulate through the spleen and liver, where extravascular hemolysis occurs by adherence and phagocytosis of the antibody-coated erythrocytes by macrophages of the reticuloendothelial system (Fig. 24–1). Macrophages may only remove a portion of the antibody-coated red cell, resulting in formation of microspherocytes as a result of the loss of red cell membrane. Alternatively, the entire red cell may be engulfed and removed from circulation. Extravascular hemolysis often results in hyperbilirubinemia.

In severe hemolysis, there may be evidence of intravascular hemolysis. When antibody-coated red cells are capable of activating complement, the classic pathway of complement activation destroys them through formation of the membrane attack complex, lysing the cell. Free hemoglobin is released into the blood, leading to hemoglobinemia and hemoglobinuria; hemoglobin in the blood forms complexes with haptoglobin, decreasing serum haptoglobin (Fig. 24–2).

Although the distinction between intravascular and extravascular hemolysis appears clear, many cases of warm autoimmune hemolytic anemia demonstrate both mechanisms of hemolysis, sometimes with a predominance of one type of red cell destruction but with overlapping laboratory findings (Fig. 24–3).

Clinical Features and Diagnosis

Symptoms and Signs

More severe symptoms and signs are seen in patients with rapid onset of brisk hemolysis; less severe symptoms occur with a more indolent course and lower level of hemolysis. The same degree of anemia may be better tolerated if the pace of the disease has allowed for compensation or in patients without underlying cardiopulmonary disease. Fatigue, weakness, malaise, dizziness, fever, back pain, dyspnea on exertion, and even angina can be presenting complaints if the hemolytic process has produced severe anemia. Patients may report having jaundice, pallor, or discolored urine, consistent with hemoglobinuria.

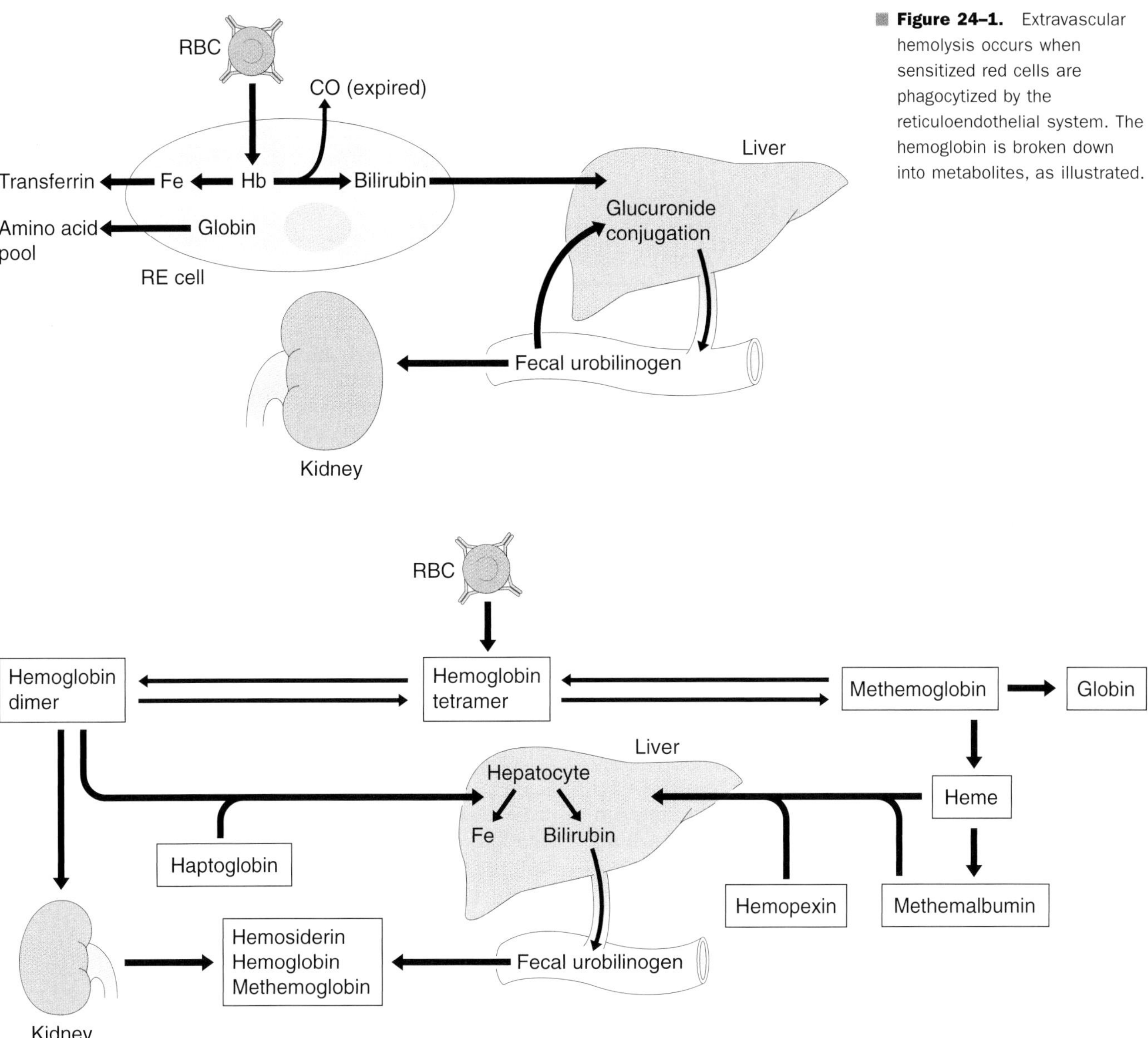

Figure 24–1. Extravascular hemolysis occurs when sensitized red cells are phagocytized by the reticuloendothelial system. The hemoglobin is broken down into metabolites, as illustrated.

Figure 24–2. When intravascular hemolysis occurs, hemoglobin is released into the circulation, where it binds to haptoglobin and then is metabolized by the liver. If the available haptoglobin is depleted, hemoglobin dimers are eliminated by the kidneys as free hemoglobin.

Physical Examination

The examination of the patient may reveal jaundice and/or pallor. Hepatosplenomegaly is the most common physical finding in autoimmune hemolytic anemia, present in greater than 50% of cases.[1,11]

Thromboembolism can be a complication of autoimmune hemolytic anemia, but published reports can be difficult to interpret. Secondary autoimmune hemolytic anemia may occur in association with diseases that have an increased risk of thromboembolism, such as systemic lupus erythematosus, with anticardiolipin antibodies and/or the lupus anticoagulant.[13]

Laboratory Findings

The diagnosis of warm autoimmune hemolytic anemia is based on laboratory findings indicative of shortened red cell survival and serologic evidence of autoantibodies directed against red cell antigens, optimally reactive at 37°C.

Routine blood counts confirm the presence of anemia with decreased hemoglobin and hematocrit, ranging from only moderate to severe anemia with hemoglobin and hematocrit as low as 5 gm/dL and 15%, respectively.[14] When thrombocytopenia accompanies warm autoimmune hemolytic anemia, Evans's syndrome is diagnosed.[15] Like the hemolytic anemia, the thrombocytopenia is autoimmune, an immune-mediated idiopathic thrombocytopenic purpura (ITP).

Evaluation of the peripheral smear is important in the diagnosis. Classically, the smear reveals evidence of immune-mediated hemolysis and bone marrow compensation. The red cell morphology shows anisocytosis with microspherocytes and polychromatophilic macro-

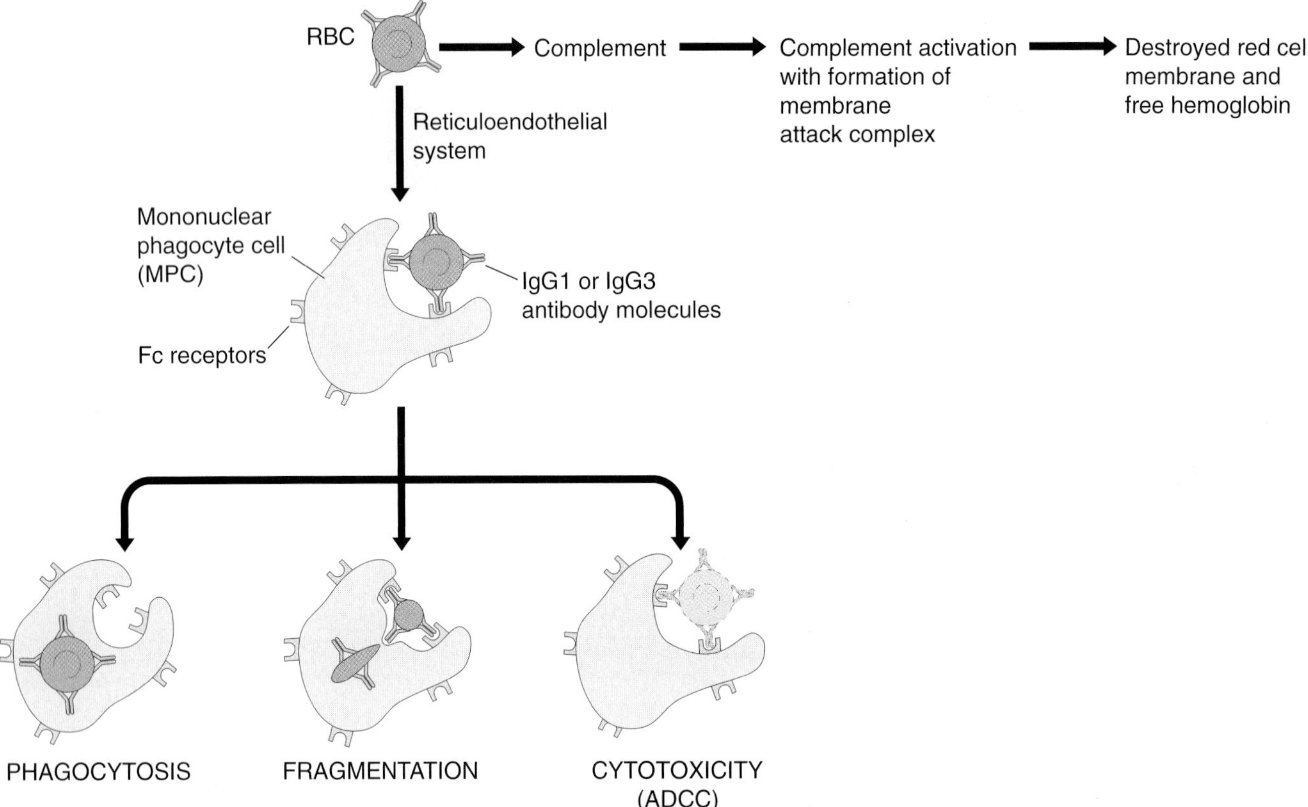

Figure 24–3. Immune red cell destruction by complement activation and cellular mechanisms.

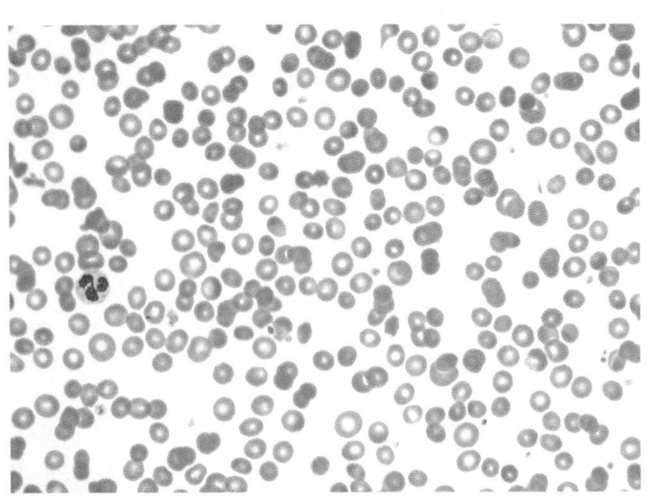

Figure 24–4. A characteristic peripheral blood smear from a patient with warm autoimmune hemolytic anemia shows microspherocytes and some polychromatophilia.

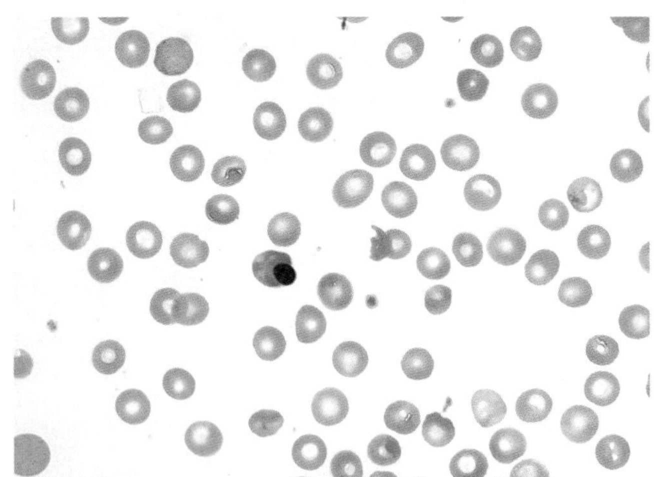

Figure 24–5. Peripheral blood smear shows both polychromatophilia and a nucleated red cell in a patient with warm autoimmune hemolytic anemia.

cytes, suggestive of reticulocytes (Fig. 24–4). Nucleated red cells appear when the rate of hemolysis is brisk (Fig. 24–5).

Reticulocytes are generally elevated, indicative of bone marrow compensation for the anemia and of the shortened red cell survival. However, not infrequently there is reticulocytopenia—a hematologic emergency because life-threatening anemia can develop.[16,17] Laboratory evidence of hemolysis includes elevated total bilirubin and serum lactate dehydrogenase, and decreased haptoglobin. Hemoglobinuria and hemoglobinemia indicate intravascular hemolysis.

Serologic evaluation determines that the hemolytic process is immune mediated. Studies should begin with routine pretransfusion testing, including determination of ABO group, Rh type, and antibody screening tests. Direct antiglobulin tests using anti-IgG and anti-C3 (C3d) identify the presence of IgG and/or complement coating red blood cells. Direct antiglobulin tests revealing IgG alone occur in 20–66% of warm autoimmune hemolytic anemia.[2,4] Both IgG and C3 coating of red cells are observed in 24–63% of cases, and C3 alone in 7–14% of patients.[2,4]

Eluate studies confirm the presence of IgG autoantibody when the direct antiglobulin test indicates IgG binding to red blood cells. The eluate typically reacts with all cells in a panel representing a diversity of antigenic phenotypes, thus demonstrating a panagglutinin, but may occasionally reveal additional information about the specificity of the autoantibody. Enhanced reactivity will be seen with enzyme-treated test cells.

Indirect antiglobulin tests, using either untreated or enzyme-treated red blood cells at 20°C and 37°C, will demonstrate IgG antibody in the serum. Again, panel studies show a panagglutinating antibody in the serum; selected cell panels may indicate a specific autoantibody. Some autoantibodies have broad specificity in the Rh system. Less frequent, the autoantibody will bind to a simple Rh antigen or a glycophorin-associated antigen.

Direct antiglobulin tests are negative in 2–4% of cases.[18,19] Several possible explanations account for direct antiglobulin test–negative warm autoimmune hemolytic anemia: very low levels of IgG bound to the erythrocyte, an IgG autoantibody of low affinity, and autoantibody that is IgA. About 14% of patients with warm autoimmune hemolytic anemia have IgA class antibodies.[20] Often, an IgG and/or IgM antibody can also be identified, and cases solely attributable to IgA autoantibody are rare (less than 1%).[21] IgA warm autoimmune hemolytic anemia should be considered when despite otherwise typical signs and symptoms, the direct antiglobulin test is negative for IgG. Patients with IgA-mediated hemolysis respond to therapy for warm autoimmune hemolytic anemia, which relieves clinical symptoms and transfusion-dependence.

Differential Diagnosis

Other causes of anemia should be considered and excluded, including blood loss and bone marrow failure. Once hemolysis is established, other processes should be eliminated, including the microangiopathic hemolytic anemias such as thrombotic thrombocytopenic purpura. The immune-mediated pathophysiology should be confirmed, and the serologic features of the causative autoantibody can be used to determine the type of autoimmune hemolytic anemia (warm autoimmune hemolytic anemia versus cold agglutinin syndrome versus paroxysmal cold hemoglobinuria). Medications recently administered should be assessed for possible drug-induced autoimmune hemolytic anemia.

Treatment

Corticosteroids

Corticosteroids are the initial therapy of choice for warm autoimmune hemolytic anemia. A standard approach is to treat adults with prednisone, 60–100 mg/day for 1–3 weeks. Clinical improvement may be seen within several days to 1 week, approximately 80% of patients have a good initial response.[1,11] After stabilization of hematologic parameters, the dosage of corticosteroids can be gradually reduced. If relapse occurs, the dose should be increased. Most clinicians consider a maintenance dose of prednisone of greater than 15 mg daily a therapeutic failure.

The explanation for clinical response to corticosteroids is likely multifactorial. Steroids have been shown to have an early effect on tissue macrophages, which become less efficient at clearing IgG- and C3-coated red blood cells within the first 8 days of therapy.[22] Steroids may also affect antibody avidity.[23] Only after several weeks of therapy is there a significant decrease in antibody production. Permanent remission of autoimmune hemolytic anemia occurs in only 20–35% of adult patients.[8,24] Consequently, additional therapy is generally planned because clinical relapse is likely.

Splenectomy

Approximately 50% of patients will have an excellent initial response to splenectomy, although low doses of prednisone (<15 mg/day) may still be needed to maintain adequate hemoglobin levels.[25] Late relapses do occur, presumably as a result of enhanced antibody synthesis and increased hepatic sequestration.[11,24]

Patients who have had a splenectomy need to be educated about the risks of overwhelming postsplenectomy sepsis syndrome. Infections with encapsulated bacteria are the special problem and represent a medical emergency because there may be rapid progression from an apparent flulike illness to bacteremic shock. The risk of overwhelming postsplenectomy sepsis syndrome has been quantitated as 3.2% with a mortality rate of 1.4%.[26] The risks of both infection and mortality can be reduced by the use of pneumococcal and meningococcal vaccines. Prophylactic antibiotic regimens are controversial, however; many advocate the use of penicillin (250 mg twice a day); amoxicillin or bactrim can be used as alternatives. Febrile illnesses in splenectomized patients must be given prompt attention and antibiotics administered expeditiously.

Immunosuppressive Therapy

Several immunosuppressive agents have been reported to be successful in the treatment of warm autoimmune hemolytic anemia, but mainly in case reports and small series. These more intensive regimens should be considered: (1) when there is lack of response to splenectomy or relapse after splenectomy, (2) when splenectomy is an unacceptable medical risk, and (3) when corticosteroid therapy cannot be tolerated.

Azathioprine has been used with success in warm autoimmune hemolytic anemia,[27] but its adverse effects can be limiting, including gastrointestinal intolerance and bone marrow suppression. Because azathioprine is cytotoxic, its prolonged administration is not advised. Some case reports describe the successful use of cyclosporine in treating warm autoimmune hemolytic anemia,[28,29] and others, its failure.[30] Monitoring for nephrotoxicity is important. Mycophenolate mofetil is used to prevent kidney allograft rejection; a few case reports suggest efficacy in the treatment of warm autoimmune hemolytic anemia.[31,32] High-dose cyclophosphamide (50 mg/kg/day for 4 days) followed by granulocyte colony-stimulating factor has reversed refractory disease: complete remission in 6 patients and partial remission in 3 patients of 9 treated.[33]

Rituximab is a genetically engineered chimeric murine/human monoclonal anti-CD20 antibody that targets B-cell precursors and mature B cells; plasma cells do not carry the CD20 antigen. Success of rituximab has not been limited to warm autoimmune hemolytic anemia secondary to B-cell neoplasms. Patients with idiopathic warm autoimmune hemolytic anemia, including those with refractory disease[34] and children with the syndrome, have responded.[35–37] The typical dosing regimen of rituximab for this indication is 375 mg/m^2, once a week for 2–4 weeks. One series of 15 patients showed continuous remission in 10 cases, relapse after remission in 3 cases, and failure to respond in 2 cases.[37]

ITP, a hematologic disease with many similarities to autoimmune hemolytic anemia but much more common in clinical practice, offers opportunities to test the increasing number of new immunosuppressive drugs and biologic agents. Many that prove useful in refractory ITP should be evaluated in autoimmune hemolytic anemia.

Additional Therapies

Danazol, an attenuated androgen, has been helpful in a few cases of warm autoimmune hemolytic anemia.[38,39] In this clinical setting, its mechanism of action is uncertain. Intravenous immunoglobulin is effective in ITP, and there are mixed case reports of success, failure, and indifferent response in warm autoimmune hemolytic anemia. Plasmapheresis has been used as a temporizing measure but is impractical for long-term management.

Supportive Care and Long-Term Management

Transfusion Therapy

Red blood cell transfusion is a significant component of the supportive care of autoimmune hemolytic anemia. Although mild to moderate anemia usually does not require transfusion, an occasional patient presents with life-threatening anemia and the need for red blood cell replacement is emergent.

Careful communication between the clinician and the transfusion service is imperative. On occasion, a transfusion may be required before the serologic evaluation is completed. Even after thorough serologic evaluation, the optimal blood for transfusion may be incompatible. The clinician must understand that, in some cases, serologically incompatible blood is safe for transfusion and should have in vivo survival comparable to the patient's own red cells. Reluctance to transfuse patients because of serologic incompatibility or an incomplete evaluation can be devastating. Patients with very severe anemia may appear to be hemodynamically stable, but they have life-threatening anemia and should be transfused immediately regardless of the serologic tests or compatibility. The onset of confusion in a patient with worsening anemia is a particularly important clinical indication for immediate transfusion.

Selection of Blood for Transfusion

Transfusion management can be complicated by serologic complexities (see Chapter 99). An ABO discrepancy requires removal of IgG autoantibody in order to perform accurate ABO typing. In urgent situations or if ABO typing results are not clear, group O donor red cells can be administered. Rh typing may also be problematic. Low-protein, monoclonal reagents for Rh typing are available for use in the setting of immunoglobulin-coated red cells.

With a history of previous pregnancy or transfusion, it is critical to detect and identify any coexistent alloantibody, which may be hidden or obscured by the autoantibody. The exclusion of underlying clinically significant alloantibodies requires time-consuming and labor-intensive adsorption techniques.[40] A critical clinical situation may not permit completion of these studies before transfusion is necessary. In the patient who has not been transfused in the last 3 months, autologous adsorption studies must be performed to identify the presence of underlying alloantibodies.[41] In the recently transfused patient, more complex differential allogeneic adsorption studies may be required.[42,43]

In patients who have not recently been transfused, determination of the red cell phenotype is invaluable. Techniques are available to dissociate autoantibody in order to allow for accurate phenotyping. The erythrocyte phenotype then can guide the exclusion of alloantibodies by indicating which antigen specificities might elicit an alloantibody. When they are available, phenotypically matched red blood cells should be safe for transfusion.[44] When autoimmune hemolytic anemia requires chronic transfusion support, determination of the patient's red cell phenotype can help to identify alloantibodies if they develop.

When compatible blood cannot be located, many clinicians request "least incompatible" blood in the hope of additional safety, but these maneuvers only delay needed blood transfusions and offer no additional protection for the patient.[45] The clinician and the transfusion medicine physician together assess and manage the transfusion needs for patients with severe autoimmune hemolysis and worsening anemia.

Prognosis

The prognosis of warm autoimmune hemolytic anemia is not well established. Mortality rates of 38% for patients treated between 1955 and 1965,[11] and of 38% for idiopathic autoimmune hemolytic anemia between 1958 and 1966,[1] indicate a historically poor outcome. Recent reports are more encouraging: in one review of 117 patients, actuarial survival at 1 year was 91%, at 5 years was 76%, and at 10 years, 73%.[46] The prognosis of disease among children is even better.[47–49]

COLD AGGLUTININ SYNDROME

Epidemiology and Risk Factors

Cold agglutinin syndrome is less frequent than is warm autoimmune hemolytic anemia, representing 15–25% of cases of autoimmune hemolytic anemia.[2,3] Cold agglutinin syndrome can be acute or chronic. The acute form is often secondary to a lymphoproliferative syndrome or *Mycoplasma pneumoniae* infection. Chronic cold agglutinin syndrome occurs in elderly patients and not children.

Pathophysiology

In cold agglutinin syndrome, the red blood cells are sensitized with IgM antibody. These sensitized red cells can activate complement and undergo intravascular hemolysis. More commonly, they may be removed from the circulation by extravascular hemolysis, following passage through the spleen and liver and interaction with the reticuloendothelial system.

Clinical Features and Diagnosis

Symptoms and Signs

Patients with cold agglutinin syndrome often present with clinical symptoms of a progressive chronic anemia.[50] Typically, the disease is indolent, with a slower hemolytic rate than in warm autoimmune hemolytic anemia. There is an association between the thermal amplitude of the pathogenic autoantibody and the severity of symptoms: with autoantibody reactive at higher temperatures, patients may have worse symptoms of hemolysis.[51] Anemia can be exacerbated in the winter, when the extremities are more likely to be exposed to colder temperatures, and acute hemolytic crises can be accompanied by frank hemoglobinuria.

Physical Examination

On examination, patients may demonstrate evidence of a chronic hemolytic anemia with pallor and jaundice. Acrocyanosis involving the tip of the nose, fingers, toes, and ears resolves with warming.[50] Hepatosplenomegaly is not a major feature.

Laboratory Findings

Often the initial laboratory finding suggesting the diagnosis of cold agglutinin syndrome is progressive agglutination of the blood sample with cooling, which is reversible by warming the sample to 37°C. Agglutination can be problematic when attempting to analyze the sample on automated equipment: the return of spurious blood counts and inconsistent indices suggests the diagnosis.

Serologic evaluation reveals the presence of a cold-reactive, IgM autoantibody. The direct antiglobulin test shows complement coating of the red cells. Because the autoantibody is IgM, it will not be detected by routine direct antiglobulin tests using anti-IgG anti–human globulin reagent; consequently, eluate studies are rarely indicated. Serum evaluation should include a cold agglutinin titer and thermal amplitude measurement; these studies are helpful in determining and confirming the clinical significance of the cold autoantibody. In general, the cold autoantibodies that cause clinical cold agglutinin syndrome have a high titer (>1000) and/or serum studies using 30% bovine albumin (a media which enhances agglutination) that show reactivity at 30°C.[52] The specificity of the antibody is most often directed against I antigen. Less frequent is specificity for i antigen, which usually appears in patients with infectious mononucleosis. Rarely, other antigen specificities have been reported.

Many healthy individuals have cold agglutinins in their sera that are typically low titer and clinically benign. During evaluation for anemia, these benign cold agglutinins should not be mistaken for clinically important pathogenic antibodies.

Blood

The ability of cold reactive antibody to agglutinate red cells as a blood sample cools is reflected by agglutination on the peripheral blood smear (Fig. 24–6). In other respects, the morphologic features of hemolysis are more subtle in cold agglutinin syndrome as compared to warm autoimmune hemolytic anemia: there is less anisocytosis and fewer microspherocytes and polychromatophilic

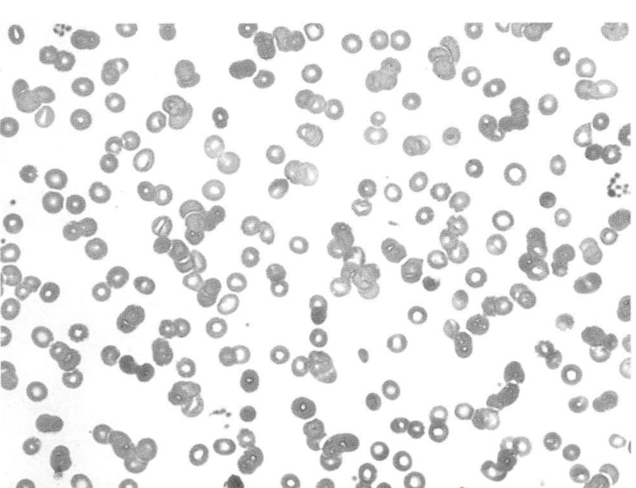

Figure 24–6. In patients with cold agglutinin syndrome, the peripheral blood smear typically reveals red cell agglutination.

macrocytes because of the decreased severity of red blood cell destruction.

Examination of the bone marrow can be useful in cold agglutinin disease. In many cases, the disorder is secondary to a lymphoproliferative disease that is clinically obvious. In others, the cold agglutinin syndrome appears to be primary or idiopathic, but a bone marrow examination will reveal that it is truly a manifestation of indolent lymphoproliferation. Sophisticated immunologic studies may be required to reveal a subtle clonal proliferation of B cells, resulting in monoclonal IgM cold agglutinins.[53]

Differential Diagnosis

Other etiologies of anemia must be considered. Once hemolysis is established, nonimmune causes, such as microangiopathic hemolytic anemias and hemolytic anemias that are due to mechanical causes, must be excluded. Once an immune-mediated process is established, the necessary distinction is between alloimmune and autoimmune hemolytic anemia. Alloimmune hemolytic anemias may be related to recent transfusion. Autoimmune hemolytic anemias can be distinguished by serologic findings. "Benign" cold agglutinins should not be overinterpreted!

Treatment

Avoidance of Cold

The mainstay of therapy for cold agglutinin syndrome is avoidance of the cold. Acute hemolytic crises can be prevented by maintaining a high temperature in the indoor environment and wearing additional clothing outdoors. By diligent avoidance of the cold, many patients are managed without transfusions. Patients with mild, compensated anemia are often not treated for prolonged periods of time and may only require episodic transfusions.

Additional Therapy

For patients with more severe, partially compensated idiopathic cold agglutinin syndrome, medical therapy is generally unsatisfactory. Corticosteroids are not efficacious in most patients with cold agglutinin syndrome. Similarly, splenectomy is not usually effective, presumably because the liver is the dominant site of sequestration of red cells heavily sensitized with C3. Chlorambucil has been used with some success, but the consequent bone marrow suppression can be limiting.[54] In patients without an underlying hematologic malignancy, the therapeutic results of rituximab treatment have been encouraging.[55] One study treated 27 patients with primary chronic cold agglutinin disease with 37 courses of rituximab and achieved complete remission in 1 course of therapy, partial remission in 19 and no remission in 17 courses of therapy.[55] As with warm autoimmune hemolytic anemia, plasmapheresis may have a role as a temporizing measure. For this procedure, special attention is required to maintain the core body temperature at 37°C, and use of an in-line blood warmer is recommended.

Supportive Care and Long-Term Management

Similar to warm autoimmune hemolytic anemia, patients with cold agglutinin syndrome may have a complex serology that complicates transfusion management. ABO discrepancies may make determination of their major blood group difficult. Warm washing of red cells to remove the IgM autoantibody may be necessary to facilitate determination of an accurate ABO group. If ABO typing remains uncertain, group O red cells can be administered. A blood warmer is generally recommended for transfusion.

Prognosis

Idiopathic cold agglutinin syndrome has a better prognosis as compared to warm autoimmune hemolytic anemia. Most patients have a long and indolent course. In the rare reported cases of severe and even fatal cold agglutinin disease,[56,57] the unusually high thermal amplitude of the causative antibody has suggested the possibility of warm autoimmune hemolytic anemia caused by IgM antibodies as the cause; this entity carries a poor prognosis.

PAROXYSMAL COLD HEMOGLOBINURIA

Epidemiology and Risk Factors

Paroxysmal cold hemoglobinuria is an uncommon autoimmune hemolytic anemia, accounting for approximately 2% of cases.[2] The disease was the first of the autoimmune hemolytic anemias to be described, in part because of its often dramatic appearance of hemoglobin in the urine. Paroxysmal cold hemoglobinuria was commonly seen in association with syphilis; as the incidence of syphilis has decreased, so has paroxysmal cold hemoglobinuria. Paroxysmal cold hemoglobinuria is now more usually seen in children than in adults. One study found no cases of paroxysmal cold hemoglobinuria in 531 adults but 22 cases in 68 children (32%) with autoimmune hemolytic anemia.[58] Paroxysmal cold hemoglobinuria often occurs in association with viral infections.

Pathophysiology

The pathogenic antibody in paroxysmal cold hemoglobinuria is a biphasic, IgG antibody known as the Donath-Landsteiner antibody. The Donath-Landsteiner antibody binds to red cells in the cold, causing irreversible binding of C3 and C4. At warmer temperatures, the antibody dissociates from the red cell and complement activation leads to hemolysis.

Clinical Features and Diagnosis

Symptoms and Signs

The typical patient with paroxysmal cold hemoglobinuria is a young child who has had a recent upper respiratory tract infection. Clinical presentation can be dramatic, with hemoglobinuria, jaundice, pallor, and fever.[59] A history of cold exposure is usually not obtained. Hepatosplenomegaly is not prominent.

Diagnosis

The anemia may be severe.[58,59] Reticulocytes may be variably present at diagnosis. The peripheral blood smear can be dramatic, showing red cell morphologic features of immune hemolysis: spherocytes, fragmented forms, polychromatophilia, anisocytosis, and poikilocytosis. Erythrophagocytosis by neutrophils may be observed.

Routine direct antiglobulin tests reveal the presence of complement (C3) coating of erythrocytes. IgG does not bind to the red cells, and eluate studies are negative. The Donath-Landsteiner antibody usually is specific for erythrocyte P antigen. A Donath-Landsteiner test demonstrates the biphasic nature of the hemolysin in vitro. On addition of normal serum as a source of fresh complement, the patient's serum and test red cells expressing P antigen are placed in the cold and then at 37°C; a positive test result is the final demonstration of hemolysis.

Differential Diagnosis

Other diseases causing severe, acute intravascular hemolysis must be considered and excluded.

Treatment

The majority of cases of paroxysmal cold hemoglobinuria are postinfectious and self-limited. Patients require only supportive care during their acute disease. Severe intravascular hemolysis can result in life-threatening anemia requiring urgent blood transfusions. Many clinicians administer corticosteroids, but their utility has never been established.

Supportive Care and Long-Term Management

Transfusions are required for severe hemolysis. The Donath-Landsteiner antibody does not react above 4°C and therefore does not interfere with routine compatibility testing. The transfusion of red cells of p phenotype has been advocated, but donors are uncommon and their blood is difficult to obtain under urgent circumstances, often being available only through rare red blood cell registries. The use of p red blood cell transfusion may be considered if routine donor blood fails to elevate the hemoglobin level, but typically it is more important to expeditiously replace blood, and the nature of the anti-P antibody should be ignored. Whether blood warmers are required is uncertain, but their use may reassure the clinician in dealing with a life-threatening anemia in a child.

Prognosis

Paroxysmal cold hemoglobinuria has an excellent prognosis. The disease typically resolves within a few days to weeks. The highest risk associated with paroxysmal cold hemoglobinuria is at initial presentation and diagnosis, when patients may have severe anemia and require prompt medical attention and urgent transfusions.

OTHER TYPES OF AUTOIMMUNE HEMOLYTIC ANEMIA

Warm and Cold, or Mixed-Type, Autoimmune Hemolytic Anemia

Epidemiology and Risk Factors

Occasional patients may not be easily classified as having either warm autoimmune hemolytic anemia or cold agglutinin syndrome, and they may appear to have a combination of both, or mixed-type autoimmune hemolytic anemia. Such unusual cases comprise approximately 7% of all cases of idiopathic autoimmune hemolytic anemia.[4]

Diagnosis

Serologic studies reveal the presence of both a warm-reactive IgG autoantibody and an IgM autoantibody, with a lower titer than is usually seen in cold agglutinin syndrome but a high thermal amplitude.

Treatment

Patients with mixed-type autoimmune hemolytic anemia frequently have a rapid response to corticosteroid therapy. The serologic diagnosis is of special importance, because a patient with mixed-type autoimmune hemolytic anemia who is mistakenly labeled as having cold agglutinin syndrome ordinarily would not receive steroids.

Autoimmune Hemolytic Anemia Caused by Warm IgM Antibodies

Epidemiology

Hemolytic anemia is rarely seen in association with warm-reactive IgM autoantibodies, which are capable of activating complement and agglutinating in vivo. Most reported cases are adults,[60,61] but this entity has been observed in a few children as well.[62,63]

Pathophysiology

In autoimmune hemolytic anemia caused by warm IgM autoantibodies, the IgM antibodies coat the red cells. The IgM antibody is capable of activating complement and causing intravascular hemolysis. Additionally, the IgM can form agglutinates of multiple red cells linked by antibody, resulting in sludging of the red cells, poor organ perfusion, and ultimately tissue necrosis. The clinical hallmark of autoimmune hemolytic anemia caused by warm IgM antibodies is concomitant intravascular hemolysis and tissue ischemia. Ischemia is life-threatening and, when widespread to involve the brain, heart, and kidneys, can culminate in multiorgan failure.

Diagnosis

The symptoms and signs of severe hemolytic anemia may be accompanied by findings of marked intravascular agglutination leading to ischemia and tissue infarction. Ischemic infarcts can be identified by various radiologic studies. Cutaneous ischemia and tissue necrosis can result in visible gangrene.

Serologic studies reveal spontaneous agglutination in vitro that cannot be dispersed despite repeated warm washes. The diagnostic finding is an IgM autoantibody with high thermal amplitude.

Treatment

Whole blood exchange, immunosuppressive drugs, and cytotoxic agents are usually unsuccessful. The goals of therapy should be the rapid reduction of antibody and temporary relief of ischemia by plasma or whole blood exchange.

Prognosis

Autoimmune hemolytic anemia caused by IgM antibodies is virtually always fatal.[60]

Drug-Induced Autoimmune Hemolytic Anemia

Epidemiology and Risk Factors

Acquired hemolytic anemia can develop in association with various medications. In investigating the possibility of a drug-induced hemolytic anemia, not only prescription drugs but also over-the-counter medications and even potential chemical exposures should be considered.

Although patterns change over time as new drugs are introduced into the market, the cephalosporins are most often implicated in drug-induced autoimmune hemolytic anemia and should always be considered a potential culprit.[64]

Pathophysiology

Three pathophysiologies traditionally have been offered to explain autoantibodies in association with drugs, without very much laboratory support for any mechanisms. Some patients have features suggesting more than one mechanism. As a result, a unifying theory has been proposed (Fig. 24–7).[64,65]

In the drug adsorption mechanism, the drug binds to the surface of the red cell, and an antibody directed against the drug is formed. The antigen-antibody reaction occurs at the surface of the red cell, leading to its destruction. The prototypic drug is penicillin. Hemolysis is typically extravascular.

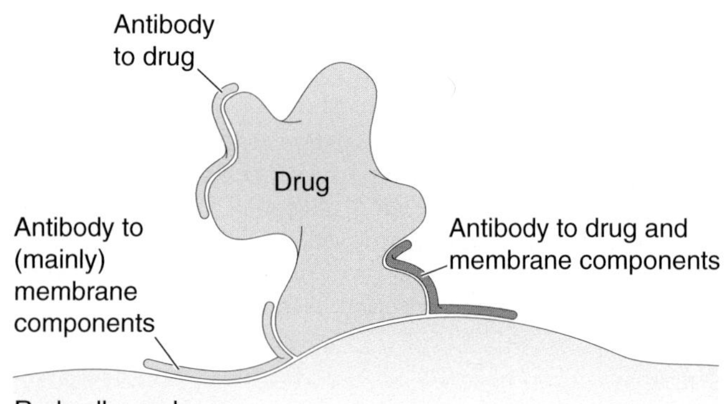

Figure 24–7. Proposed unifying theory of drug-induced antibody reactions. The thicker, darker lines represent antigen-binding sites on the F(ab) region of the drug-induced antibody. Drugs (haptens) bind loosely or firmly to cell membranes, and antibodies may be made to the drug (producing in vitro reactions typical of a drug adsorption [penicillin-type] reaction); the membrane components, or mainly membrane components (producing in vitro reactions typical of autoantibody); or part-drug, part-membrane components (producing an in vitro reaction typical of the so-called immune-complex mechanism). (From Garratty G: Review: drug-induced immune hemolytic anemia—the last decade. Immunohematology 20:142, 2004.)

In the immune complex mechanism, free drug within the circulation stimulates the production of drug-specific antibody. The antibody and drug form immune complexes that can bind to red cells, although it is unclear whether this is specific or nonspecific binding. The prototypic drug demonstrating this mechanism is quinidine. Hemolysis can be brisk and is often intravascular.

In the drug-independent mechanism, the drug induces a red blood cell destruction with serologic similarities to idiopathic warm autoimmune hemolytic anemia. The autoantibody may persist and be detected for prolonged periods of time, even after the drug has been discontinued. Here the prototypic drug is α-methyldopa.

In the unifying theory, depending on the specific interaction between the drug and red cell, antibody may be directed against any of the following: predominantly red cell membrane, predominantly drug, or a portion of the membrane and the drug. Consequently, antibodies directed against all of these may be identified, explaining patients who appear to have multiple pathophysiologies operating simultaneously.[64,65]

Clinical Features and Diagnosis

Patients may present with severe hemolysis and even life-threatening anemia. Their clinical signs and symptoms are indistinguishable from those of warm autoimmune hemolytic anemia.

The serologic findings may be suggestive of a mechanism. For drug adsorption, the antibody is generally a warm-reactive IgG antibody. The direct antiglobulin test is positive because of IgG coating of the red cells. Complement may or may not be present on red cells.

When the immune complex mechanism is implicated, the antibody may be IgG, IgM, or both. The direct antiglobulin test is usually positive, revealing complement coating of the red cells. There is often severe intravascular hemolysis.

When drug-independent autoantibodies are formed, the serology is suggestive of idiopathic warm autoimmune hemolytic anemia. The autoantibody may show relative specificity for the Rh blood group antigens, and antibodies may persist after the drug is discontinued.

Serologic testing can be performed with the addition of specific drugs or drug metabolites. If positive, these studies confirm the drug association of the autoimmune hemolytic anemia. Such testing requires expertise that is only available through an immunohematology reference laboratory.

Differential Diagnosis

The differential diagnosis is that of a hemolytic anemia. The drug exposure history should be carefully elicited and reviewed in all patients with autoimmune hemolytic anemia. Careful consideration should be given to drugs that are new to the patient's regimen. Although large lists of causative drugs are available, most reflect only single cases. A convincing case history should prompt discontinuation of the drug even in the absence of previous reports.

Treatment

The implicated drug must be discontinued immediately. Although there are no supportive data, empirical corticosteroid therapy is commonly employed.

Supportive Care and Long-Term Management

There may be massive intravascular hemolysis and hemoglobinemia, hemoglobinuria, and even renal failure; transfusion support may be necessary. This severe clinical presentation is most commonly associated with the immune complex mechanism. In cases of drug-independent autoantibody formation, a prolonged period of transfusions may be required because of the persistence of the autoantibody.

Prognosis

The prognosis of drug-induced hemolytic anemia is excellent. The patient should expect a full recovery with resolution of the hemolysis, but the implicated drug or any chemically related agent should be avoided.

CURRENT CONTROVERSIES & FUTURE CONSIDERATIONS

The Autoimmune Hemolytic Anemias

- What is the therapeutic role of the newer pharmacologic agents? Initial experience with rituximab is encouraging; will anti-CD2O monoclonal antibody or other designer antibodies become the initial therapy of choice? Can agents that have been successfully applied to ITP be proven useful in autoimmune hemolytic anemia?
- What is the potential role for blood substitutes in serologically complex patients who often require transfusions? Case reports suggest the value of substitutes to provide hematologic support in the absence of compatible blood.[66]
- Are there clinically useful measures to determine when a patient with severe and worsening anemia requires emergency transfusion?
- A formal link between hemolysis (autoimmune and other) and thrombosis has not been convincingly established. Is there a potential role for antithrombotic therapy in autoimmune hemolytic anemia?
- What is the role of intensive immunosuppressive therapy to prevent relapses of autoimmune hemolytic anemia?
- Can an assay be developed to better measure the success of therapy, since the direct antiglobulin test does not determine or predict the severity of ongoing hemolysis?

Suggested Readings*

Buetens OW, Ness PM: Red blood cell transfusion in autoimmune hemolytic anemia. Curr Opin Hematol 10:429–433, 2003.

King KE: Transfusion of the patient with autoimmune hemolysis. *In* Hillyer CA, Strauss R, Luban N (eds): Handbook of Pediatric Transfusion Medicine. San Diego: Academic Press, 2004, pp 245–251.

King KE, Ness PM: Autoimmune hemolytic anemias. *In* Rackel RE, Bope ET (eds): Conn's Current Therapy 2004. Philadelphia: WB Saunders, 2004, pp 405–409.

Petz LD: A physician's guide to transfusion in autoimmune haemolytic anaemia. Br J Haematol 124:712–716, 2004.

Petz LD, Garratty G: Immune Hemolytic Anemias (ed 2). Philadelphia: Churchill Livingstone, 2004.

***Full references for this chapter can be found on accompanying CD-ROM.**

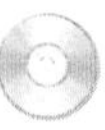

CHAPTER 25

Paroxysmal Nocturnal Hemoglobinuria

Lucio Luzzatto, MD, and David J. Araten, MD

KEY POINTS

Paroxysmal Nocturnal Hemoglobinuria

- Paroxysmal nocturnal hemoglobinuria is an acquired chronic hemolytic anemia caused by an intrinsic abnormality of the membrane of red blood cells, which makes them exquisitely sensitive to the hemolytic action of activated complement.
- The membrane abnormality of paroxysmal nocturnal hemoglobinuria is present in cells of all hematopoietic lineages: it consists in deficiency of all proteins that are anchored to the membrane via a glycosylphosphatidylinositol (GPI) anchor, including the complement regulator CD59.
- The biochemical abnormality in paroxysmal nocturnal hemoglobinuria is caused by an inactivating somatic mutation of the X-linked gene *PIG-A,* which encodes one subunit of an enzyme required for an early step of the biosynthesis of GPI.
- In order to produce clinical paroxysmal nocturnal hemoglobinuria, a hematopoietic clone with a *PIG-A* mutation must expand; thus, in the patient's blood there will be characteristically a dual cell population, with a variable proportion of residual non-PNH cells.
- A major determinant of the rate of expansion of a PNH clone is significant depression of normal hematopoiesis: an element of bone marrow failure exists in every patient with paroxysmal nocturnal hemoglobinuria.
- Bone marrow failure in paroxysmal nocturnal hemoglobinuria can be cryptic, masked by vigorous paroxysmal nocturnal hemoglobinuria–derived erythropoiesis to frank aplastic anemia.
- Venous thrombosis, especially in the abdominal veins, is a frequent, serious manifestation of paroxysmal nocturnal hemoglobinuria. Although thrombosis does not occur in all patients, a single event can have a major impact on survival and quality of life.
- Hematopoietic stem cell transplantation is currently the only form of definitive treatment for paroxysmal nocturnal hemoglobinuria. A proportion of patients may experience spontaneous recovery after more than 10 years. Patients with paroxysmal nocturnal hemoglobinuria and pancytopenia, like patients with aplastic anemia, may benefit from intensive immunosuppressive treatment.

INTRODUCTION

Paroxysmal nocturnal hemoglobinuria (PNH) is a bone marrow disorder characterized by a clonal population of blood cells with a unique phenotypic abnormality; at the same time, normal hematopoiesis is markedly reduced. The abnormality of red cells can cause severe intravascular hemolysis and the hemoglobinuria that names the disease (Fig. 25–1).

EPIDEMIOLOGY AND RISK FACTORS

Paroxysmal nocturnal hemoglobinuria is rare, and there are no accurate incidence data. Paroxysmal nocturnal hemoglobinuria is less diagnosed than aplastic anemia, the rate of which has been estimated to be 1.5 cases per million population per year in France[1] and about twice that figure in Thailand,[2] where paroxysmal nocturnal hemoglobinuria is also more common.[3] Paroxysmal nocturnal hemoglobinuria tends to follow a more protracted course than does aplastic anemia, and a crude estimate of its prevalence might be between 1 per million and 1 per 100,000 population.

PATHOPHYSIOLOGY

Two points are cardinal in understanding paroxysmal nocturnal hemoglobinuria: the mechanism of hemolysis and the pathophysiology responsible for the origin and the expansion of the mutant blood cell population.

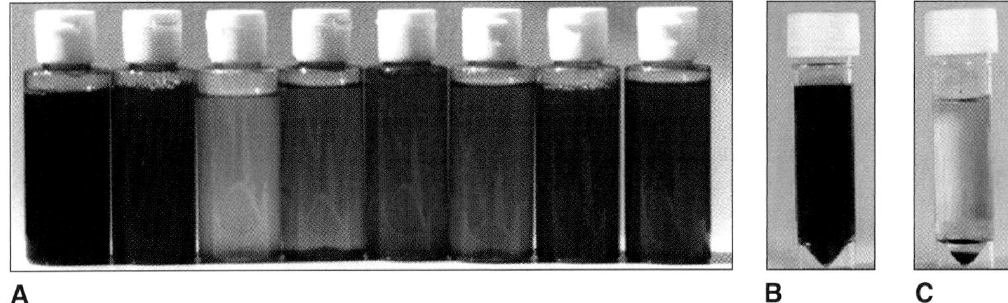

Figure 25–1. *A,* Urine samples from a patient with paroxysmal nocturnal hemoglobinuria within the short time span of 3 days. Extremely dark urine was first observed in the morning, but this cleared in the course of the day. The term *nocturnal* is a reflection of this finding. Elevated lactate dehydrogenase and a normal creatine phosphokinase in this patient were suggestive of hemolysis and excluded myoglobinuria. Depending on the degree of oxidation of the hemoglobin, the urine can appear red or black. Several weeks later, the urine looked completely normal, suggesting to the eye that the hemoglobinuria is "paroxysmal." However, biochemical evidence of hemoglobinuria persists, and hemosiderin was consistently present in the urine sediment. *B,* It is crucial to differentiate hemoglobinuria from hematuria. After centrifugation of the patient's urine, the color—caused by free hemoglobin—remains in the supernatant. *C,* In contrast, after centrifugation of a specimen darkened due to red cells, a red cell pellet appears, and the supernatant is clear. These simple maneuvers can preempt unnecessary invasive urologic work-ups.

PNH Phenotype in Red Cells

The unique hypersusceptibility to activated complement (C) of red cells in patients with paroxysmal nocturnal hemoglobinuria results from the absence on the erythrocyte surface of a complement-regulatory protein called membrane inhibitor of reactive lysis, currently identified as CD59.[4] In normal red cells, this surface protein prevents the polymerization of C9, which produces pores in the lipid bilayer of the red cell membrane (Fig. 25–2). In PNH red cells, CD59 is absent or markedly decreased: as a result, C9 polymerization is unimpeded and red cells will be destroyed when complement is activated.[5] A single patient with paroxysmal nocturnal hemoglobinuria who also had inherited deficiency of C9 never developed massive hemolysis.[6]

Clonal Origin of Paroxysmal Nocturnal Hemoglobinuria Cells

The coexistence of two distinct blood cell populations (Fig. 25–3) characteristic of paroxysmal nocturnal hemoglobinuria has suggested that the abnormal population is clonal.[7,8] This notion was first tested in female patients heterozygous for the X-linked gene encoding glucose-6-phosphate dehydrogenase (G6PD), in whom the entire abnormal PNH population was homogeneous in expressing only one of the two G6PD alleles,[9] implying that, in a cell expressing that allele, a somatic mutation had produced the PNH phenotype. The mutant clone coexists with a variable number of preexisting normal cells, and the ratio between normal and PNH cells in the bone marrow is a measure of the relative size of the PNH clone. Because PNH erythrocytes have a much shorter lifespan in the circulation than do normal cells,[10] the proportion of PNH red cells underestimates the size of the PNH clone, which correlates better with the proportion of PNH granulocytes.

Molecular Basis of the PNH Phenotype

How does a somatic mutation cause hypersusceptibility to activated complement?[2] The phenotype of PNH cells is complex; in addition to CD59, other proteins are deficient on the surface of PNH red cells (Fig. 25–4), including acetylcholinesterase[11,12] and CD55[13] (another complement regulator).[14] These and other surface proteins are deficient also in all other lineages of blood cells,[14–17] suggesting an underlying somatic mutation has taken place in a hematopoietic stem cell. All of the proteins implicated are normally anchored to the cell surface through a glycophospholipid molecule, glycosylphosphatidylinositol (GPI).[18] In normal cells, the polypeptide chains of these proteins and the GPI anchor are synthesized independently in the endoplasmic reticulum (Fig. 25–5). After synthesis, each protein is covalently linked to the anchor by a transpeptidation reaction. The GPI anchor remains embedded in the cell membrane and the protein moiety is exposed on the external side of the membrane.

The biochemical lesion responsible for the failure of PNH cells to express GPI-linked proteins on the cell surface is a metabolic block at an early step of the complex pathway of the biosynthesis of the GPI molecule, the transfer of acetylglucosamine onto phosphatidylinositol.[19–21] The somatic mutation that underlies this block is in a gene called *PIG-A*[22,23] (Fig. 25–6), which maps to the short arm of the X chromosome.[24–26] *PIG-A* encodes one of the subunits of the acetylglucosamine transfer enzyme,[27] and the PNH phenotype can be corrected by transfecting PNH lymphoblastoid cells with the *PIG-A* complementary DNA.[28] To produce the PNH phenotype, the mutation must cause loss of *PIG-A* function—completely in some cases, partially in others,[29] explaining why some PNH cells totally lack GPI-linked proteins (PNH III phenotype) and in others the deficiency is incomplete[30] (PNH II phenotype). Because *PIG-*

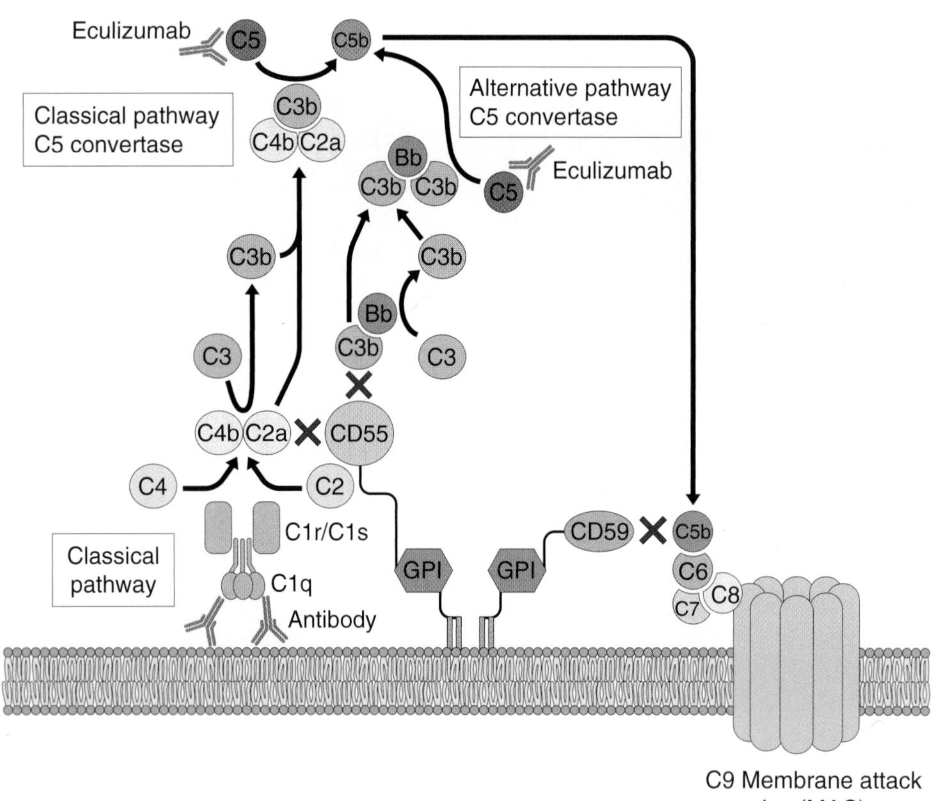

Figure 25–2. Complement activation. GPI-linked complement inhibitors CD55 (DAF) and CD59 (MIRL) inhibit the activation of early and late complement proteins, respectively. CD55 promotes the disassociation of the C3 convertases C3bBb and C4b2a as well as the C5 convertases C4b2a3b and C3bBb3b. CD59 blocks the ability of the C5b-8 complex to mediate the assembly of C9 into a membrane attack complex. PNH red cells, which do not express CD55 and CD59, are susceptible to complement-mediated lysis (a similar abnormality in platelets may result in their inappropriate activation). The monoclonal anti-C5 antibody eculizumab blocks complement-mediated hemolysis by binding to C5 and preventing its activation by C5 convertases.

A mutations are somatically acquired, almost every patient has a different mutation[31–34] (see Fig. 25–6); the majority are either small insertions or deletions causing frameshift or nonsense mutations, all of which will lead to a truncated, functionally inactive PIG-A protein, and therefore a PNH III phenotype. Numerous missense mutations may cause the PNH II phenotype.[29]

Unlike in inherited X-linked conditions, which affect males more than females, there is no significant sex difference in the prevalence of paroxysmal nocturnal hemoglobinuria. Because of X-chromosome inactivation, there is only a single functional *PIG-A* gene in each somatic cell in both males and females.[35] The PNH phenotype might arise from a metabolic block elsewhere in the GPI synthetic pathway, but this is unlikely because the other enzymes are encoded by autosomal genes (an inactivating mutation in an allele would only cause a 50% loss of activity and not significantly reduce the ultimate output of GPI).

PNH Phenotype in Nonerythroid Cells

There are several dozen GPI-linked proteins,[36,37] and they have a wide range of functions in different cells. In the mouse, *Pig-A* inactivation leads to fetal death[38,39]; tissue-specific inactivation of the *Pig-A* gene in the skin produces a form of icthiosis,[40] and in the oocyte it interferes with fertilization.[41] Nonhematopoietic cells are not affected in paroxysmal nocturnal hemoglobinuria, but the consequences of GPI deficiency are not confined to red cells. PNH neutrophils are competent for phagocytosis, but they are impaired in adhesion and migration,[42] probably as a result of deficiency in the GPI-linked protein CD157. GPI-deficient T lymphocytes in mice are functionally abnormal, including in delayed-type hypersensitivity.[43] Abnormalities in platelets may lead to the release of thromboplastin-like substances,[44,45] which might be responsible in part for the tendency to venous thrombosis.

Bone Marrow Failure and Paroxysmal Nocturnal Hemoglobinuria

Multiple lines of evidence indicate that hematopoiesis is not normal in paroxysmal nocturnal hemoglobinuria. First, in many patients non-PNH cells in the bone marrow are in a minority; erythroid and granulocyte-monocyte colony-forming cells are always markedly reduced.[46–48] Non-PNH $CD34^+$ cell have decreased growth and increased expression of Fas,[49] while granulocytes have shortened telomeres, suggesting an excessive number of rounds of cell division.[50] These data indicate that "normal" hematopoiesis is deficient in paroxysmal nocturnal hemoglobinuria. Second, paroxysmal nocturnal hemoglobinuria may develop in patients who had an original diagnosis of aplastic anemia, and conversely, some patients with paroxysmal nocturnal hemoglobinuria subsequently "convert" to aplastic anemia.[51–53] Third, experiments in mice provide evidence that knocking out the *PIG-A* gene is insufficient to cause paroxysmal nocturnal hemoglobinuria: a population of PNH blood cells

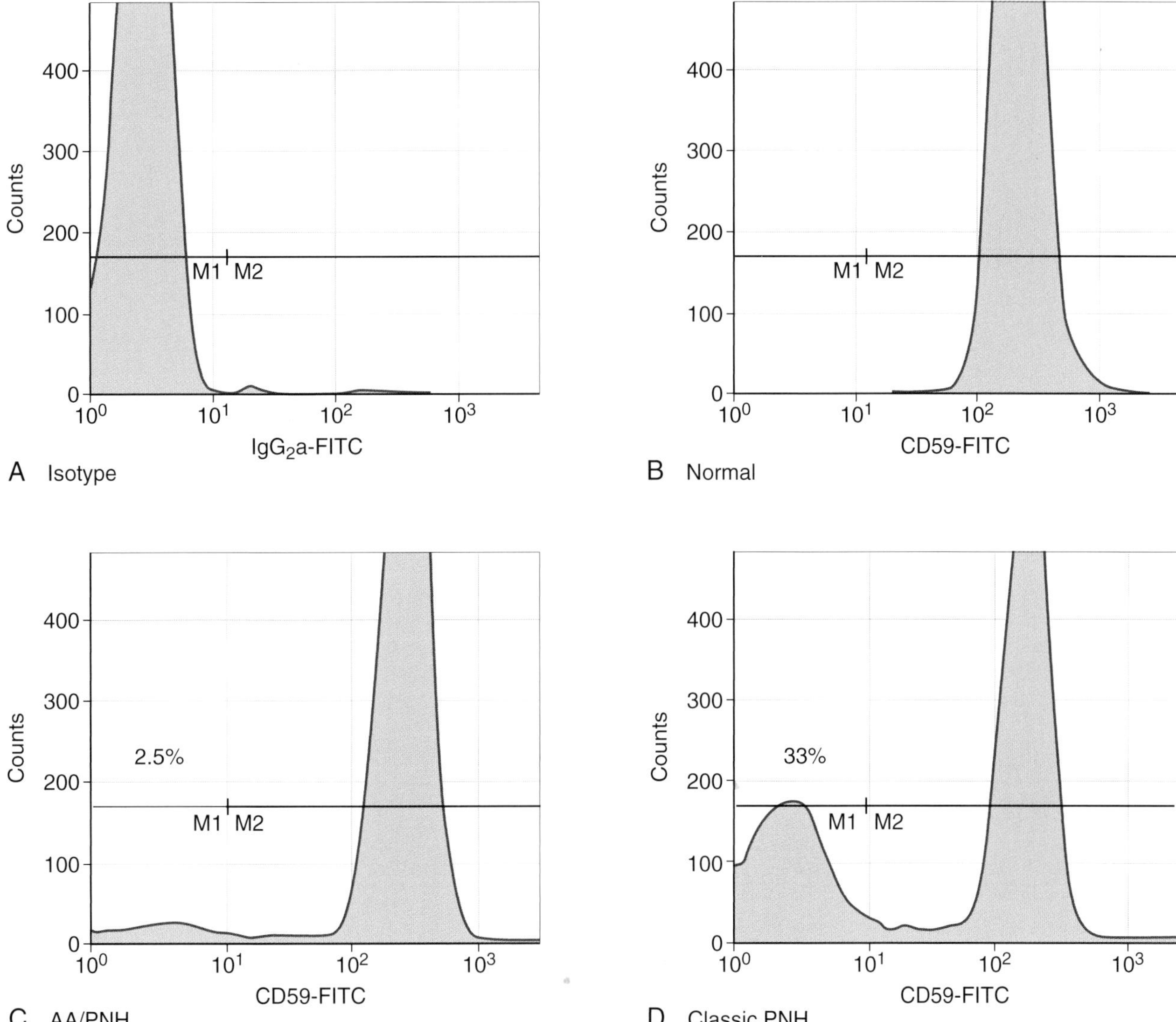

Figure 25–3. Identification of PNH cell populations by flow cytometry analysis. Cells are stained with a fluorescent antibody specific for CD59 (a GPI-linked protein). The vertical axis represents the number of cells expressing a given level of fluorescence intensity (shown on the horizontal axis on a log scale). Histograms from a normal individual demonstrate a unimodal population of red cells that strongly express CD59, about 100-fold brighter than isotype control antibody (***A*** and ***B***). The patient with aplastic anemia/paroxysmal nocturnal hemoglobinuria has a small population of red cells that do not express CD59 (2.5% of total cells; ***C***), whereas the patient with classic paroxysmal nocturnal hemoglobinuria has a large population of CD59-negative red cells (33% of cells; ***D***). Similar results can be obtained by analysis of circulating granulocytes. The proportion of PNH granulocytes (which is not affected by red cell transfusions) is usually much higher than that of PNH red cells, and it reflects more accurately the size of the hematopoiesis caused by PNH cells in the patient. Flow cytometric analysis of bone marrow cells does not yield information beyond that which is obtained with peripheral blood.

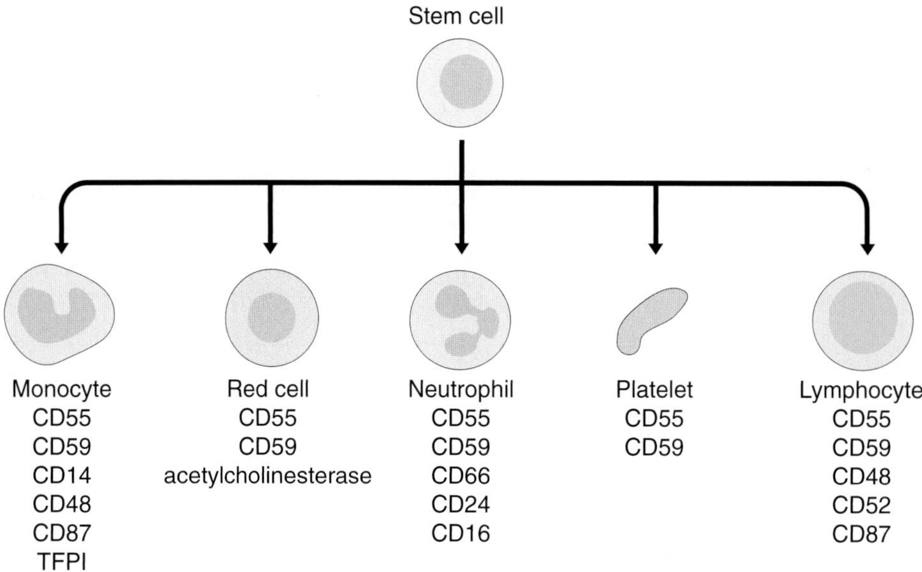

Figure 25–4. Paroxysmal nocturnal hemoglobinuria is a stem cell disorder. Cells of multiple lineages are derived from a hematopoietic stem cell with a deficiency in GPI anchor production. Their progeny lack all the GPI-linked proteins that are normally expressed on those cells. The lack of complement inhibitors CD55 and CD59 on the red cell surface results in complement-mediated red cell lysis. This defect on the platelet surface may lead to complement deposition and platelet activation; abnormalities in the urokinase receptor (CD87) and the tissue pathway factor inhibitor on monocytes may also contribute to the tendency to thrombosis characteristic of patients with paroxysmal nocturnal hemoglobinuria.

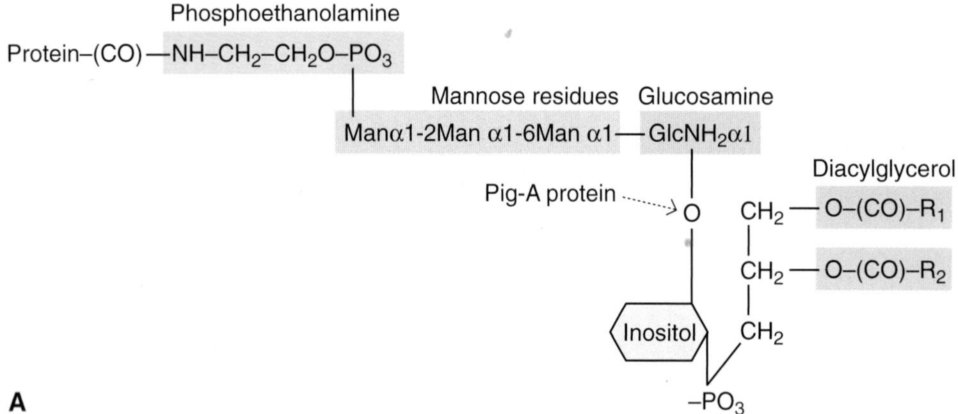

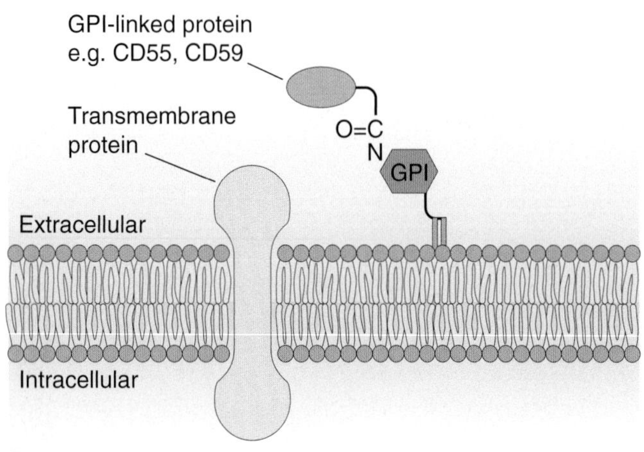

Figure 25–5. *A,* Structure of GPI. Many membrane proteins lack a transmembrane domain; instead, they are linked to the cell surface by a glycosylphosphatidylinositol anchor, the diacylglycerol moiety of which is held by the force of hydrophobic bonds in the lipid bilayer of the plasma membrane. The carboxyl terminus of the protein is covalently linked to the phosphoethanolamine moiety of GPI by a peptide bond. The PIG-A protein is one of the subunits of an enzyme (an acetylglucosamine transferase), located in the endoplasmic reticulum, that is required for an early step in the biosynthetic pathway of the GPI anchor (see *arrow*). ***B,*** Cells that cannot produce GPI do not express any of the GPI-linked proteins on their surface, although they do express proteins with transmembrane domains.

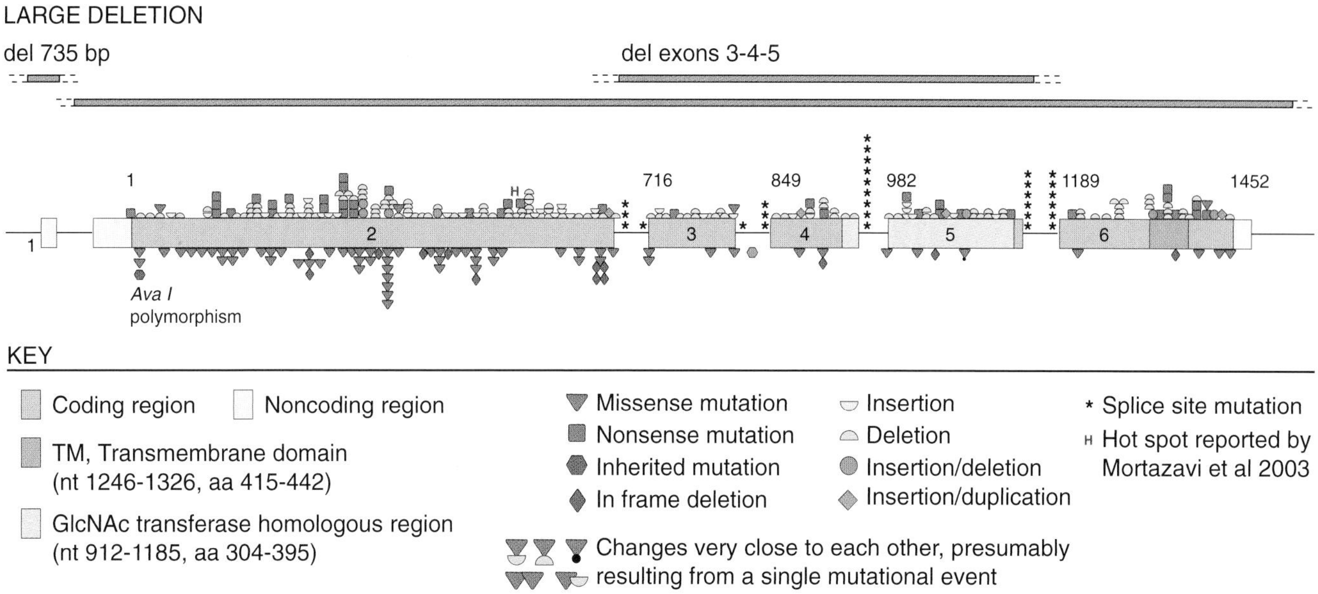

LARGE DELETION

del 735 bp

del exons 3-4-5

Ava I polymorphism

KEY

Coding region | Noncoding region

TM, Transmembrane domain (nt 1246-1326, aa 415-442)

GlcNAc transferase homologous region (nt 912-1185, aa 304-395)

Missense mutation

Nonsense mutation

Inherited mutation

In frame deletion

Insertion

Deletion

Insertion/deletion

Insertion/duplication

* Splice site mutation

H Hot spot reported by Mortazavi et al 2003

Changes very close to each other, presumably resulting from a single mutational event

Figure 25–6. Structure and mutations of the *PIG-A* gene. The coding region is represented by *boxes;* introns are depicted by *lines* (not drawn to scale). Nucleotide numbers are shown above the exons starting with the first nucleotide of the first coding exon. Null mutations (frameshift, nonsense, and splicing) are indicated above the exons. Missense mutations and in-frame deletions are indicated below the exons. All mutations are somatic, except for the two shown as hexagons. The *PIG-A* gene product has a transmembrane domain at its carboxyl terminus, by which it is inserted in the membrane of the endoplasmic reticulum, where GPI anchor biosynthesis occurs. The enzymatic domain catalyzes the transfer of *N*-acetylglucosamine to phosphatidylinositol. Mutation detection in individual patients is an important aspect of clinical investigation in paroxysmal nocturnal hemoglobinuria but is not a routine part of patient care, because the diagnosis of paroxysmal nocturnal hemoglobinuria can be made by flow cytometry alone. (Adapted from Luzzatto L, Nafa K: Genetics of PNH. *In* Young NS, Moss J [eds]: Paroxysmal Nocturnal Hemoglobinuria and the GPI-Linked Proteins. New York: Academic Press, 2000, pp 21–47; the *PIG-A* mutations database was updated in 2004.)

is present in embryonic life but disappears after birth.[54] Thus, if the bone marrow is normal, the disease does not develop, although PNH hematopoietic cells are present. There is always a component of bone marrow failure in paroxysmal nocturnal hemoglobinuria.[55–57]

PIG-A Mutation and Paroxysmal Nocturnal Hemoglobinuria

In patients with aplastic anemia, even in those who do not subsequently develop paroxysmal nocturnal hemoglobinuria, there may be a very small proportion of granulocytes of the PNH phenotype[58–60] (see Chapter 10). By high-sensitivity flow cytometric analysis, it has been possible to detect in normal subjects a minute number of PNH granulocytes (5–30 per million) and to demonstrate that they have *PIG-A* mutations, in some cases identical to those found in patients with paroxysmal nocturnal hemoglobinuria.[61] PNH-like lymphocytes also are present in normal subjects[62] and in patients with chronic lymphocytic leukemia.[63]

Mechanism of Expansion of the PNH Clone(s)

A critical factor in the pathogenesis of paroxysmal nocturnal hemoglobinuria must be the expansion of PNH clone(s) to a size sufficient to cause clinical disease. There are several theoretical possibilities:

1. The PNH clone has an intrinsic growth advantage. This is argued against by the data presented previously.
2. PNH clones that expand have an additional mutation in another gene. Cytogenetic abnormalities may be present in patients with paroxysmal nocturnal hemoglobinuria,[64] and a mutation in the *TERC* telomerase gene has been reported in 1 of 12 such patients tested,[65] but it is unclear whether these genetic events have contributed to clonal expansion.
3. PNH clones expand only under certain environmental conditions in the bone marrow.[66–68] Supporting this hypothesis are the consistent findings of depressed hematopoiesis in all patients with paroxysmal nocturnal hemoglobinuria; the presence of multiple PNH clones, either simultaneously or sequentially[69–72]; and the lack of expansion of PNH clones in mouse experiments.[73]

A crucial issue is what factor in the bone marrow is so specific as to damage normal cells while sparing PNH hematopoietic cells, thus conferring upon them a conditional growth advantage. One possible explanation is autoimmune attack (Fig. 25–7), as probably underlies acquired aplastic anemia (see Chapter 10). In both aplastic anemia and paroxysmal nocturnal hemoglobinuria, there are abnormalities in the T-cell repertoire similar to those associated with autoimmune disorders.[74] Certain HLA-DR2 alleles figure prominently in paroxysmal noc-

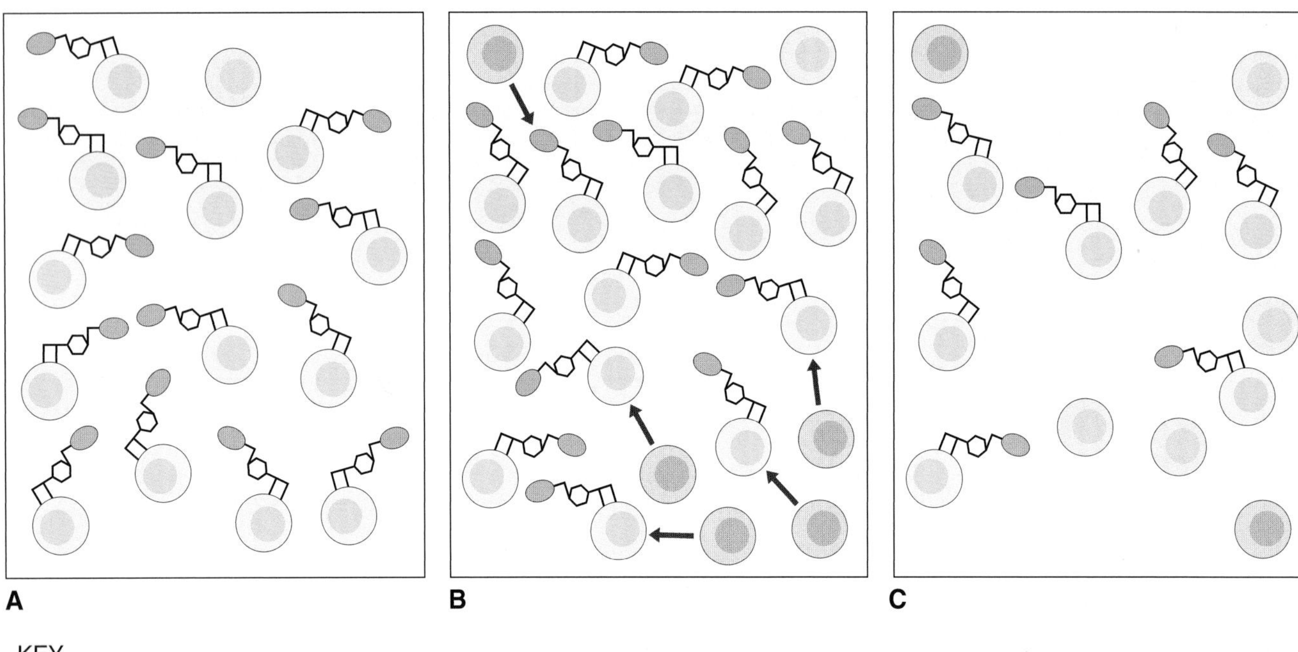

Figure 25–7. Immune escape model of paroxysmal nocturnal hemoglobinuria. Normal hematopoietic stem cells can produce GPI anchors and express GPI-linked proteins on the cell surface. Rare GPI⁻ stem cells arise as a result of spontaneous somatic mutation of the *PIG-A* gene. In the normal individual, these *PIG-A*⁻ stem cells have no selective advantage and remain rare ***(A)***. If there is an autoimmune attack on the hematopoietic stem cells mediated by T cells (or natural killer cells), stem cells will be lost, often resulting in aplastic anemia ***(B)***. If target recognition or effector mechanisms of stem cell killing are dependent on the expression of GPI-linked proteins, *PIG-A*⁻ stem cells will have a selective advantage and may be able to provide a recovery of hematopoiesis ***(C)***. Although proliferation of *PIG-A* mutant stem cells may protect the patient from severe cytopenias, this protection comes at the expense of circulating mature red cell (and platelet) progeny with the PNH phenotype, resulting in hemolysis (and thrombosis). The ability of the *PIG-A*⁻ stem cell to recover in this environment will dictate whether the patient develops aplastic anemia/paroxysmal nocturnal hemoglobinuria or classic paroxysmal nocturnal hemoglobinuria.

turnal hemoglobinuria.[75] Damage to hematopoietic stem cells caused by autoreactive T cells, perhaps of the $CD8^+CD57^+$ (natural killer–like) subset,[76,77] might spare PNH cells if a GPI-linked molecule were targeted. GPI^- cells, under certain experimental conditions, are less prone to apoptosis[49,78–81] and less sensitive to natural killer effector cells.[82] Thus, the expansion of the PNH cell population, arising through a spontaneous *PIG-A* mutation, would then result by negative selection against normal hematopoietic stem cells. In this sense, failed hematopoiesis may be rescued by a PNH clone.[83]

Additional Features of PNH Clones

Multiple *PIG-A* mutations are frequently present in the same patient, which is understandable because small *PIG-A* mutant clones exist normally, and may be co-selected independently with marrow failure. Two different *PIG-A* mutant clones have been detected in the same patient 20 years apart.[72] A *PIG-A* mutation is a valuable "natural" marker of the stem cell in which it has arisen; in this patient, a single stem cell supported hematopoiesis for at least a decade.[71]

CLINICAL FEATURES AND DIAGNOSIS

Typical paroxysmal nocturnal hemoglobinuria is a chronic hemolytic anemia in which red cell destruction is largely intravascular; the tendency to severe exacerbations results in the paroxysms of hemoglobinuria.[84,85] Venous thrombosis is a common manifestation of paroxysmal nocturnal hemoglobinuria; in several series it ultimately affected nearly one half of patients.[53,86] In addition, in about one third of cases blood counts reveal not only anemia but also decreased neutrophils or platelets, or both.[87]

Probably the first record of paroxysmal nocturnal hemoglobinuria is that written in 1678 in Gdansk by Johann Schmidt[88]: he wrote, in Latin, that the deputy mayor of his town had summoned him because one morning, when he passed urine, "he saw it coming out black; and this frightened him." This "classic" presentation is not unusual, and can still frighten a patient today. In other cases, the onset is insidious: hemoglobinuria may not have been evident and the clinical presentation is with fatigue and pallor (without jaundice), and a blood count reveals anemia. An attack of abdominal pain may be the first symptom. Rarely, persistent dysphagia is the initial complaint.

The physical examination is unremarkable except for pallor. Tachycardia is usually not present, because of the hemodynamic adjustment expected with chronic anemia, but there may be a systolic heart murmur. Even in the absence of pain, there may be tenderness on deep palpation of the abdomen, especially midline just above the umbilicus. The spleen is usually not enlarged (it is not a major site of hemolysis); splenomegaly almost invariably indicates thrombosis of the splenic or portal veins. Liver enlargement is usually the result of hepatic vein thrombosis. In the acute phase, there may be full Budd-Chiari syndrome, including ascites (often less prominent in paroxysmal nocturnal hemoglobinuria cases because of the coexistence of portal vein thrombosis).

Hematologic Findings

The anemia can be mild to very severe and is usually moderately macrocytic (unless there is superimposed iron deficiency; see later) and normochromic. The reticulocyte count is elevated and may be very high (absolute counts of 200,000–300,000/μL are not unusual). The blood smear shows anisocytosis, macrocytes, and polychromasia but not poikilocytosis (Fig. 25–8*D*); nucleated red cells are rare. White cells and platelets may be normal but there also may be neutropenia and/or thrombocytopenia. In spite of hemolysis, the bilirubin is usually only mildly elevated and may be normal; by contrast, the lactate dehydrogenase is markedly elevated (values in the thousands are common) and haptoglobin is low or even undetectable.

The bone marrow is classically cellular (Fig. 25–8*A*), with marked erythroid hyperplasia (Fig. 25–8*B*), although at certain stages of the disease it may have been or may become hypocellular (Fig. 25–8*C*). Morphologic findings of myelodysplasia (see Fig. 25–8*B*) are seen frequently in paroxysmal nocturnal hemoglobinuria,[64] and cytogenetic abnormalities similar to those of aplastic anemia and myelodysplasia can occur.[64,89] Although not required for the diagnosis of paroxysmal nocturnal hemoglobinuria, a bone marrow examination is appropriate at presentation in order to assess hematopoiesis, and aspiration and biopsy should be repeated in certain clinical circumstances during the course of the disease.

Clinical Course

The clinical manifestations of paroxysmal nocturnal hemoglobinuria are very variable among patients, and

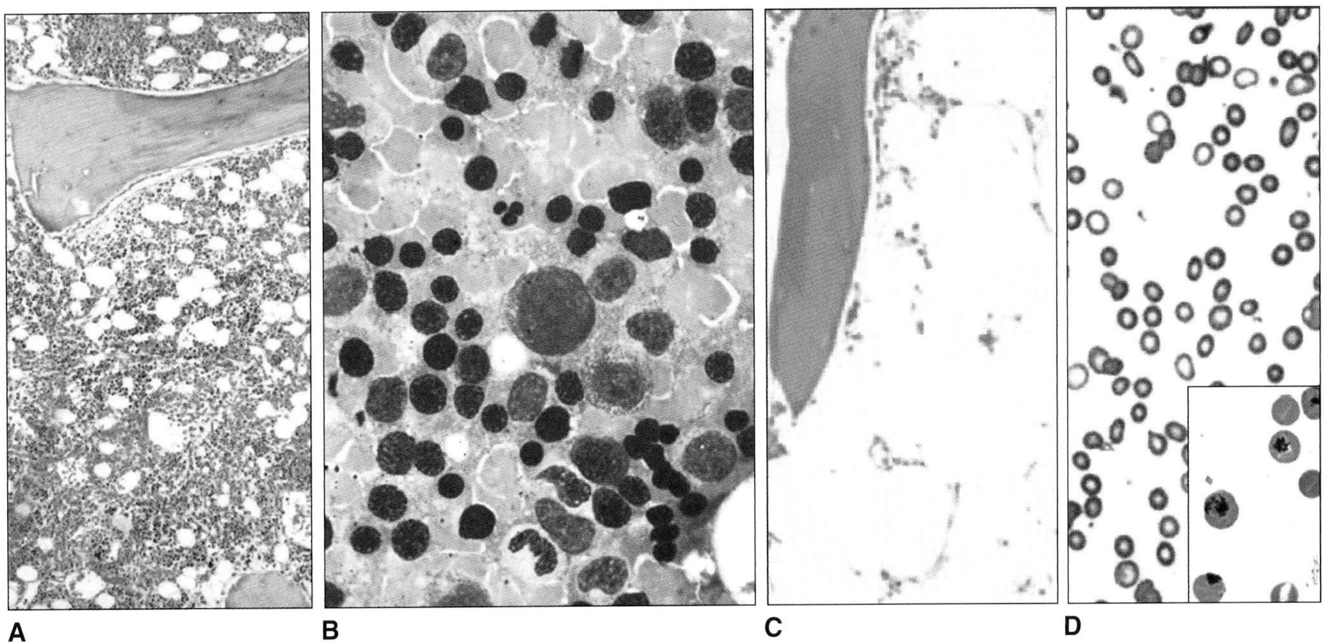

Figure 25–8. Bone marrow and peripheral blood findings in paroxysmal nocturnal hemoglobinuria. ***A,*** Histologic section demonstrating that the cellularity in classic paroxysmal nocturnal hemoglobinuria is increased. ***B,*** Smear from an aspirate from the same patient, indicating that the increased cellularity is largely accounted for by compensatory erythroid hyperplasia, as seen in chronic hemolytic anemia from any cause. Note that "dysplastic features" are commonly associated with the erythroid hyperplasia in paroxysmal nocturnal hemoglobinuria and do not mandate a concurrent diagnosis of myelodysplasia. ***C,*** Histologic section from a patient who presented with aplastic anemia and a small PNH clone. Sometimes, especially in patients with the aplastic anemia/paroxysmal nocturnal hemoglobinuria syndrome, the marrow can appear patchy in cellularity, with some areas resembling panel ***A*** and some areas resembling panel ***C*** even within the same biopsy specimen. ***D,*** Peripheral blood Wright's stain and *(inset)* reticulocyte stain in a patient with severe hemolytic paroxysmal nocturnal hemoglobinuria. Note the marked anemia (hemoglobin 5.5 gm/dL), anisocytosis, and macrocytes, in large part resulting from reticulocytosis (25% in this patient), indicating a vigorous erythropoietic response to anemia. Hypochromasia resulted from mild iron deficiency—which this patient has developed despite numerous transfusions, indicating the massive loss of iron consequent to hemoglobinuria. There is also poikilocytosis, regarded as nonspecific in paroxysmal nocturnal hemoglobinuria, but probably in this case reflecting iron deficiency. (Courtesy of Dr. Peter Maslak.)

because the course may span decades, they may also vary in an individual patient. Certain patterns in individual patients are stable for years. At one end of the spectrum is the patient who has daily macroscopic hemoglobinuria, accompanied by frequent attacks of abdominal pain and episodes of venous thrombosis; who has a hemoglobin level of 6 gm/dL; and who requires 1–2 units of red cells per month. At the other end is the patient whose urine is usually almost clear, who has a hemoglobin level of 9–11 gm/dL, and who has never required blood transfusion. The proportion of PNH red cells also tends to be constant over years in most patients.[90]

Venous Thrombosis

In any patient with paroxysmal nocturnal hemoglobinuria, venous thrombosis is always a threat—and a potentially fatal event. Although thrombosis can occur at any site, for reasons not clear, in paroxysmal nocturnal hemoglobinuria typical limb thrombosis is far less common than is thrombosis in any of the abdominal veins (Fig. 25–9). In one young woman, the hepatic veins, the splenic vein, the portal vein, the superior mesenteric, and the inferior vena cava were all affected within the space of 3 days. The most remarkable feature of venous thrombosis in paroxysmal nocturnal hemoglobinuria is its unpredictability and the possibility of an occurrence even years after diagnosis. The cranial veins can be involved, and thrombosis of the sagittal sinus is ominous.

Why about one half of the patients with paroxysmal nocturnal hemoglobinuria do not develop venous thrombosis is unknown. Inherited factors may play a role; venous thrombosis is more common in patients who

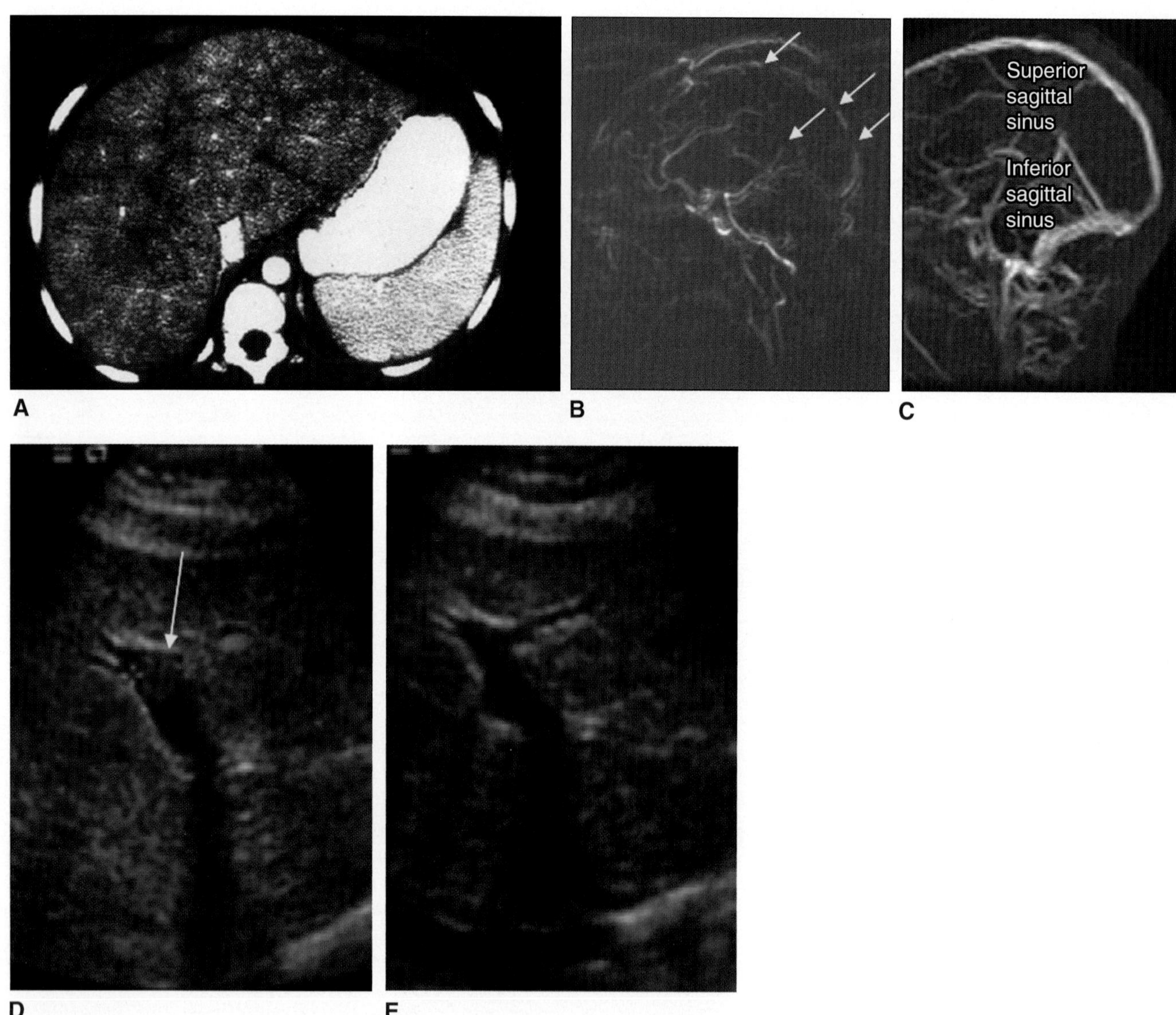

Figure 25–9. *A,* Contrast computed tomography scan of the liver in a patient with Budd-Chiari syndrome. The hepatic veins are not visualized and there is centrilobular congestion (nutmeg liver). *B,* Magnetic resonance venogram demonstrating multiple thromboses of the superior and inferior sagittal sinuses, in comparison with a normal individual *(C)*. *D,* Thrombosis in the portal vein demonstrated by sonogram, which is no longer present after infusion of tissue plasminogen activator *(E)*.

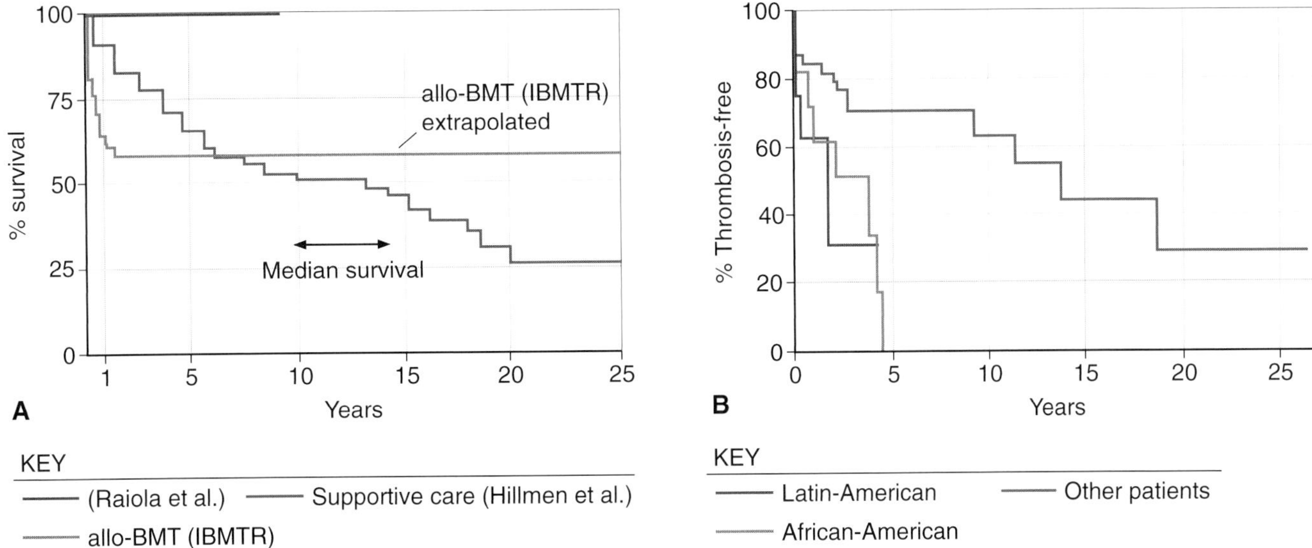

Figure 25–10. *A,* Prospects for paroxysmal nocturnal hemoglobinuria patients as a function of management. The survival curve of the natural history of paroxysmal nocturnal hemoglobinuria[53] is superimposed on the results of patients treated with bone marrow transplantation from a multicenter study[120] and a single-center study.[126] It can be seen that prospects for survival in the short term may be better with supportive care, whereas long-term survival may be better with transplantation. *B,* In the United States, the risk of thrombosis in paroxysmal nocturnal hemoglobinuria is highest among African American and Latin American patients.[93] Note that thromboses can occur even in patients who have been thrombosis free for decades.

have factor V Leiden.[91] Thrombosis in paroxysmal nocturnal hemoglobinuria is much rarer in Asian populations than in those of European ancestry[92] but more common in African Americans[93] (Fig. 25–10).

Other Manifestations

The cause for frequent episodes of abdominal pain is not clear. When extensive imaging studies are unrewarding, the presumption is of an underlying pathology described as "microthrombosis." Dysphagia is usually associated with exacerbation of hemolysis and may be caused by free hemoglobin binding nitric oxide.[94] Erectile dysfunction also is usually present with massive hemolysis.

Relation Between Paroxysmal Nocturnal Hemoglobinuria and Aplastic Anemia

The more common sequence is an initial diagnosis of aplastic anemia with gradual development of hemolysis into full paroxysmal nocturnal hemoglobinuria. In many cases, aplastic anemia has been treated with antithymocyte globulin (ATG), and therefore this evolution has been regarded as an adverse effect of ATG.[95] However, there are well-documented cases of aplastic anemia evolving to paroxysmal nocturnal hemoglobinuria without ATG treatment.

In some cases, a patient with classic paroxysmal nocturnal hemoglobinuria, with or without a previous history of aplastic anemia, may become more pancytopenic, and the bone marrow more hypocellular—referred to as "spent PNH." The transfusion requirement may increase or, if already high, remain high. Patients with hemolytic paroxysmal nocturnal hemoglobinuria do not develop iron overload because of the massive loss of iron through hemoglobinuria. When the serum ferritin increases, a deficiency in erythropoietin production rather than hemolysis should be suspected.

Whether aplastic anemia evolves to paroxysmal nocturnal hemoglobinuria or paroxysmal nocturnal hemoglobinuria to spent PNH, there are intermediate stages that may last months or years; this clinical-hematologic picture has been termed *aplastic anemia/paroxysmal nocturnal hemoglobinuria syndrome* (see Chapter 10). As already discussed, there is an element of bone marrow failure in every patient with paroxysmal nocturnal hemoglobinuria.

Very Small PNH Populations

Standard practice is to test all patients with aplastic anemia for the presence of a PNH cell population. Depending on the sensitivity of the method, as many as one half of aplastic anemia patients may register positive. Clinical manifestations of paroxysmal nocturnal hemoglobinuria do not occur when the clonal cell population of erythrocytes is less than 5% and PNH granulocytes are less than 10%.

Development of Acute Myeloid Leukemia

The evolution of acute myeloid leukemia (AML) from paroxysmal nocturnal hemoglobinuria has been reported recurrently in the literature.[96] In unselected series the frequency of leukemic transformation is less than 2%, and from a recent meta-analysis was estimated to be between 1% and 5%,[97,98] a rate sufficiently high to regard paroxysmal nocturnal hemoglobinuria as a preleukemic condition. AML M6 type is overrepresented,[97,99,100] and the AML clone can arise from within the PNH clone or from residual non-PNH cells.[101] The small risk of AML likely is related to the abnormal bone marrow that exists in paroxysmal nocturnal hemoglobinuria. AML often is preceded by myelodysplasia, and also follows aplastic anemia (see Chapter 10).

Paroxysmal Nocturnal Hemoglobinuria and Myelodysplasia

Both paroxysmal nocturnal hemoglobinuria and myelodysplasia can present with anemia or pancytopenia. Both are clonal disorders, and both have some relationship to aplastic anemia, in that a certain fraction of patients with myelodysplasia responds to immunosuppressive treatment with ATG.[102,103] In addition, when the bone marrow of a patient with paroxysmal nocturnal hemoglobinuria has trilineage morphologic abnormalities, paroxysmal nocturnal hemoglobinuria/myelodysplasia may be regarded as another “overlap” syndrome. However, paroxysmal nocturnal hemoglobinuria/myelodysplasia may not be a discrete entity, because morphologic abnormalities indistinguishable from myelodysplasia are commonly seen in classic paroxysmal nocturnal hemoglobinuria.[64]

Pregnancy in Paroxysmal Nocturnal Hemoglobinuria

Each of the main clinical features of paroxysmal nocturnal hemoglobinuria is relevant to pregnancy, and both maternal and fetal complications are above average.[104] Anemia worsens in pregnancy but can be managed by blood transfusion. Neutropenia and thrombocytopenia, if present, also entail risks. Pregnancy is a physiologic thrombophilic state, which adds to the pathologic thrombotic proclivity of paroxysmal nocturnal hemoglobinuria. Thrombosis is the major threat to the pregnant woman with paroxysmal nocturnal hemoglobinuria,[104] and pregnancy in paroxysmal nocturnal hemoglobinuria must be regarded as high risk, and often advised against; nevertheless, numerous pregnancies have been successfully completed, and sometimes the paroxysmal nocturnal hemoglobinuria was diagnosed during pregnancy. In our experience, full explanation of the risks to the patient is required to reach a considered decision, including the possibility of termination of pregnancy, should serious complications develop, and the possibility of irreversible organ damage as a result of a catastrophic thrombosis event.

Spontaneous Recovery from Paroxysmal Nocturnal Hemoglobinuria

In a series of 80 patients followed for at least 25 years, 12 had a full clinical and hematologic recovery,[53] corresponding to about one third of those surviving for 10 years or more. In another recent group of 23 patients, 2 had full recovery, again after 15 years or more.[105] That about 10% of long-term survivors can spontaneously result is cause for optimism, but which patients will recover cannot be predicted. In three patients who spontaneously remitted, flow cytometry of lymphocytes (the blood cells with the longest lifespan) showed persistence of the PNH clone,[53] consistent with the dependence of PNH clonal expansion on the marrow environment.

DIFFERENTIAL DIAGNOSIS

With the full triad of intravascular hemolysis, thrombosis, and pancytopenia, the diagnosis of paroxysmal nocturnal hemoglobinuria is simple. However, because paroxysmal nocturnal hemoglobinuria may present initially with a variety of signs and symptoms, it has been also called a great impostor. Once hemolysis is recognized, the differential diagnosis is among chronic hemolytic anemias; hemoglobinuria limits these possibilities by indicating that the hemolysis is intravascular. Other causes of hemoglobinuria include blackwater fever in *Plasmodium falciparum* malaria, fava bean or drug-induced hemolytic anemia in G6PD deficiency, paroxysmal cold hemoglobinuria, “march” hemoglobinuria, and ABO-incompatible blood transfusion (see Chapter 24).

There are two valid diagnostic tests for paroxysmal nocturnal hemoglobinuria, both based on the unique abnormalities in the surface of blood cells. For 50 years the diagnosis has been based on the acidified serum test developed by Ham[106] and Dacie and colleagues,[107] which is based on the high susceptibility to activated complement of PNH red cells. Other than paroxysmal nocturnal hemoglobinuria, only the rare inherited condition congenital dyserythropoietic anemia type II (also called HEMPAS; see Chapter 66) tests positive in these tests because of the presence in some but not all normal sera of a naturally occurring anti-HEMPAS antibody that binds complement. Although the acidified serum test is reliable, simple, and cheap, it is no longer performed in most laboratories, especially in the United States and Europe. Today the diagnosis of paroxysmal nocturnal hemoglobinuria is established by flow cytometry.[108,109] By “staining” cells with appropriate fluorescent-conjugated antibodies, a dual population of cells, normal and PNH, can be easily visualized. The main advantage of this methodology is that the dual population can be displayed not only for red cells but also for individual white cells. The proportion of PNH red blood cells correlates roughly with the severity of hemolysis, and the proportion of PNH granulocytes with the size of the PNH clone(s) (see later).

TREATMENT

Management of a chronic complex disease such as paroxysmal nocturnal hemoglobinuria requires physician expertise and a willingness to fully engage with the patient. Treatment options can range from simple supportive measures to major intervention such as allogeneic stem cell transplantation.

TABLE 25–1. Management of Paroxysmal Nocturnal Hemoglobinuria

Hemolytic Anemia	Thrombosis/Thrombophilia	Bone Marrow Failure
• Folic acid (in view of increased rate of erythropoiesis) • Iron supplementation whenever there is iron deficiency • Transfusion of red cells (via white cell filter) as clinically indicated • Erythropoietin may be helpful in selected cases • Complement blockade (anti-C5): in clinical trial	• Long-term anticoagulation is imperative for patients who have already sustained thrombosis • Testing for thrombophilic factors (factor V Leiden, antiphospholipid, etc.) • Primary anticoagulation for high-risk patients; controversial for others • Low threshold for diagnostic imaging • Avoiding potentially thrombogenic hormones • Thrombolytic therapy with tissue plasminogen activator whenever appropriate	• Platelet transfusion support as needed • When patient is neutropenic, appropriate surveillance and immediate medical care for fever

Supportive Treatment

Most supportive measures are summarized in Table 25–1.

Folic acid supplementation (at least 3 mg/day) should always be provided. Patients often are iron deficient on presentation, especially if they have abundant hemoglobinuria, and for them iron administration is also indicated. The antique claim (since Strübing's classic paper[110] of 1882) that iron was contraindicated because it exacerbated hemolysis is incorrect; iron repletion alone can produce significant hemoglobin increments, and even relieve the need for transfusions.

The decision to use blood transfusion must be based on (1) objective clinical assessment, (2) rate of decline in hemoglobin level since the previous blood count, and (3) subjective state and quality of life acceptable to the patient. In general, because of its chronicity, the anemia in paroxysmal nocturnal hemoglobinuria is well tolerated, but individual variation is considerable. Transfusion reactions can be almost always effectively prevented by the use of white cell filters, and washing of cells now is unnecessary and wasteful. In most patients with paroxysmal nocturnal hemoglobinuria, iron overload does not occur because of iron wastage in the urine.

Erythropoietin levels are very high in paroxysmal nocturnal hemoglobinuria[111,112]; nevertheless, anecdotal reports suggest occasional efficacy of high doses of erythropoietin in reducing or abolishing a blood transfusion requirement.[105,113,114]

For recurrent attacks of abdominal pain, oral hydration and mild analgesics often suffice. There should be a low threshold for a clinic visit or hospital admission, where parenteral fluids and more powerful analgesia, including opiates, can be administered.

Male patients with paroxysmal nocturnal hemoglobinuria who experience erectile dysfunction may benefit from the cautious administration of sildenafil.

Control of Hemolysis

Chronic intravascular hemolysis is the most distinctive and dramatic feature of paroxysmal nocturnal hemoglobinuria, and yet, despite a complete understanding of its mechanism,[115] therapies of proven value have not been developed until recently. Corticosteroids have been used extensively in paroxysmal nocturnal hemoglobinuria,[116] but without evidence that pharmacologic doses of prednisone reduce complement-dependent hemolysis in vitro, and no longitudinal study has been published demonstrating control of in vivo hemolysis. Serious toxicities, including adrenal suppression, cushingoid features, mood and affect alterations, aseptic necrosis of the hip, and fungal infections, all have occurred in patients with paroxysmal nocturnal hemoglobinuria who have received prednisone for months to years; therefore, long-term administration of corticosteroids is contraindicated in paroxysmal nocturnal hemoglobinuria. A short course of prednisone (0.5–1 mg/kg/day) may be helpful during an episode of severe exacerbation of hemolysis when an acute inflammatory process is suspected as a trigger.

Very recently, a humanized antibody against the C5 component of complement has been tested in a pilot study in 11 transfusion-dependent paroxysmal nocturnal hemoglobinuria patients; 7 of them became transfusion-independent.[117] Convincing evidence was provided that this antibody effectively prevented complement-mediated hemolysis of PNH red blood cells, because the proportion of defective cells increased markedly during antibody treatment. The availability of a specific antihemolytic agent is a major advance in the clinical management of paroxysmal nocturnal hemoglobinuria. An international multicenter, double-blind trial of anti-C5 in paroxysmal nocturnal hemoglobinuria is underway.

Management of Thrombosis

Paroxysmal nocturnal hemoglobinuria can produce a vicious acquired thrombophilic state. A proven thrombosis requires anticoagulant prophylaxis, to be continued as long as the patient has paroxysmal nocturnal hemoglobinuria. Normally this is accomplished with coumadin (warfarin), although subcutaneous heparin has been used in a few cases. In view of an actuarial risk of thrombosis that may reach a plateau of about 45% (see Fig. 25–10), and because the first episode of thrombosis can be devastating, the more difficult issue is the advisability of anticoagulant prophylaxis from the time of diagnosis. In a recent report, thrombosis was effectively prevented but at the cost of two episodes of serious hemorrhage.[118] A conservative approach is to undertake baseline investigations, including a full thrombophilia screen (antithrombin III, protein S, protein C, activated protein C resistance, prothrombin G20210A, methylene tetrahydrofolate reductase, and the "lupus anticoagulant"); if one of these tests is abnormal, anticoagulant prophylaxis can be recommended in the absence of a history of thrombosis.

Any abdominal vein thrombosis in paroxysmal nocturnal hemoglobinuria is an indication for prompt thrombolytic therapy[119] with tissue plasminogen activator, even if the patient is thrombocytopenic. Unlike with arterial thrombosis, tissue plasminogen activator treatment several days after the clinical onset of the thrombotic event may be highly effective and prevent irreversible damage (see Fig. 25–9).

Hematopoietic Stem Cell Transplantation

Hematopoietic stem cell transplantation (HSCT) is the only approach to medical cure of paroxysmal nocturnal hemoglobinuria.[120] HSCT has several actions: (1) elimination of the abnormal clone(s), (2) provision of normal hematopoietic stem cells, and (3) elimination of autoreactive immune cells. The first mechanism may be the least critical because, unlike in leukemia, relapse does not occur after allo-HSCT for paroxysmal nocturnal hemoglobinuria. Complete remission following engraftment is the rule even when using conditioning regimens that are inadequate for leukemia (cyclophosphamide or cyclophosphamide plus ATG). Relapses have occurred after syngeneic recipients were minimally conditioned,[72,121] suggesting that the immunosuppression provided by conditioning is critical.

A range of regimens have been used, generally without total-body irradiation; a common protocol uses busulfan and cyclophosphamide. Less myeloablative approaches, such as those used to treat patients with aplastic anemia (cyclophosphamide plus ATG) also have been successful and are indicated particularly in patients with hypocellular marrow morphology. Patients with aplastic anemia/paroxysmal nocturnal hemoglobinuria should be treated as are those with aplastic anemia; the presence of a small PNH clone does not mandate a more intensive conditioning regimen. Recently, "minitransplants" have been reported. Overall, the results of allo-HSCT generally have been inferior in paroxysmal nocturnal hemoglobinuria compared to aplastic anemia, possibly because of the longer interval between diagnosis and the procedure. As for other conditions, outcomes of transplantation for paroxysmal nocturnal hemoglobinuria have improved as a result of better supportive care.[120,122–123]

The decision for bone marrow transplantation in paroxysmal nocturnal hemoglobinuria is difficult, especially in cases in which there is no perception of an immediate threat to life. Nevertheless, a patient with florid paroxysmal nocturnal hemoglobinuria, at high risk of thrombosis, transfusion-dependent, and with a 50% risk of mortality within a decade (see Fig. 25–10) may have both quality of life and life expectancy restored to normal by HSCT. Conversely, a patient who dies of a transplant-related complication may have otherwise lived for decades. Delaying tactics (supportive treatment while the patient is well, transplantation for the development of refractory cytopenias or thromboses) might appear to be a reasonable compromise, but transplant-related mortality increases with age and as a result of the same complications prompting the transplant (although there are two case reports of successful transplantation in paroxysmal nocturnal hemoglobinuria complicated by Budd-Chiari syndrome[128,129]). HSCT should be offered to every young patient with paroxysmal nocturnal hemoglobinuria who has a human lymphocyte antigen–identical sibling donor. By contrast, bone marrow transplantation from unrelated donors must be regarded as experimental in paroxysmal nocturnal hemoglobinuria because of an extremely poor record of success.[127,128,130–132]

For the subset of patients with paroxysmal nocturnal hemoglobinuria and severe cytopenias, treatment should be promptly initiated with either intensive immunosuppression (see Chapter 25) or transplantation, as in aplastic anemia. Transplantation is more complicated in the older patient, and the probability of survival with immunosuppression is lower with severe neutropenia (as for aplastic anemia). Absent a matched sibling donor, ATG infusions followed by cyclosporine are recommended. Recently published tabular summaries of outcomes[133] provide a rational basis to choose between sibling transplantation and immunosuppression.

Intensive Immunosuppressive Treatment

Protocols used for aplastic anemia (see Chapter 10), consisting of ATG, methylprednisolone, and cyclosporine, are usually employed. The most compelling indication for ATG is severe pancytopenia.[105,134–136] ATG treatment cannot be expected to influence hemolysis directly: there may be little effect on hemoglobin levels, and response to treatment is measured by neutrophils and platelets. Acutely, ATG can exacerbate red blood cell destruction; immune complex formation and subsequent C′ activation can produce massive hemolysis in a patient with paroxysmal nocturnal hemoglobinuria. A majority of patients will respond with improved blood counts. Cyclosporine can be administered for years, aiming to maintain blood levels of 100–150 ng/mL. Although immunosuppression does not directly affect the PNH clone, it relieves the immune cytotoxicity for hematopoietic cells, and may limit if not eliminate the abnormal marrow environment in which the PNH clone thrives.

CURRENT CONTROVERSIES & FUTURE CONSIDERATIONS

Paroxysmal Nocturnal Hemoglobinuria

- There is circumstantial evidence that bone marrow failure in paroxysmal nocturnal hemoglobinuria is due to an autoimmune process damaging normal hematopoietic stem cells. The target molecule; the precise mechanism; and differences between aplastic anemia and paroxysmal nocturnal hemoglobinuria are unknown.
- Expansion of PNH clone(s) may result from negative selection against non-PNH hematopoietic stem cells; however, an alternative possibility is that there may be an additional unknown somatic mutation in PNH clones that do expand.
- The PNH phenotype can be rescued by transduction with *PIG-A* complementary DNA, tempting consideration of gene therapy for paroxysmal nocturnal hemoglobinuria; however, the corrected cells might become vulnerable to the same autoimmune attack that initially destroyed normal cells and may not be clinically useful.
- The precise mechanism that triggers venous thrombosis—especially in the abdominal veins—in patients with paroxysmal nocturnal hemoglobinuria must be identified, in order to rationalize the prophylactic use of anticoagulants.
- The clinical course of paroxysmal nocturnal hemoglobinuria in those patients suffering hemolysis may be radically modified by the use of an anticomplement (anti-C5) antibody, currently in clinical trial.
- Definitive treatment may become available for more patients with paroxysmal nocturnal hemoglobinuria as methodologies for transplant improve, especially with respect to the use of unrelated donors and conditioning regimens that are not myeloablative but strongly immunoablative/suppressive.

Suggested Readings*

Araten DJ, Nafa K, Pakdeesuwan K: Clonal populations of hematopoietic cells with paroxysmal nocturnal hemoglobinuria genotype and phenotype are present in normal individuals. Proc Natl Acad Sci U S A 96:5209–5214, 1999.

Bessler M, Mason PJ, Hillmen P, et al: Paroxysmal nocturnal haemoglobinuria (PNH) is caused by somatic mutations in the *PIG-A* gene. EMBO J 13:110–117, 1994.

Boccuni P, Del Vecchio L, Di Noto R, Rotoli B: Glycosyl phosphatidylinositol (GPI)-anchored molecules and the pathogenesis of paroxysmal nocturnal hemoglobinuria. Crit Rev Oncol Hematol 33:25–43, 2000.

Dacie JV: Paroxysmal nocturnal haemoglobinuria. *In* The Haemolytic Anaemias: Drug and Chemical Induced Haemolytic Anaemias, Paroxysmal Nocturnal Haemglobinuria, and Haemolytic Disease of the Newborn. London: Churchill Livingston, 1999, pp 139–330.

Hillmen P, Hall C, Marsh JCW, et al: Effect of eculizumab on hemolysis and transfusion requirements in patients with paroxysmal nocturnal hemoglobinuria. N Engl J Med 350:552–559, 2004.

Luzzatto L, Bessler M, Rotoli B: Somatic mutations in paroxysmal nocturnal hemoglobinuria: a blessing in disguise? Cell 88:1–4, 1997.

Rosse WF, Parker CJ: Paroxysmal nocturnal hemoglobinuria. Clin Hematol 105:125–120, 1985.

Takeda J, Miyata T, Kawagoe K, Kinoshita T: Deficiency of the GPI anchor caused by a somatic mutation of the *PIG-A* gene in paroxysmal nocturnal hemoglobinuria. Cell 73:703–711, 1993.

Young NS: The problem of clonality in aplastic anemia: Dr Dameshek's riddle, restated. Blood 79:1385–1392, 1992.

Full references for this chapter can be found on accompanying CD-ROM.

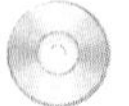

CHAPTER 26

Mechanical Hemolytic Anemia

McDonald K. Horne, III, MD

KEY POINTS

Mechanical Hemolytic Anemia

- Mechanical hemolysis results from physical forces exerted on circulating red cells. It is primarily intravascular and is characterized by elevated lactate dehydrogenase, urine hemosiderin, and red cell fragments in the peripheral blood.
- Leaks around prosthetic heart valves and microvascular pathology associated with metastatic carcinoma or renal vasculopathy lead to mechanical hemolysis.
- Mechanical hemolysis also is characteristic of thrombotic thrombocytopenic purpura/hemolytic-uremic syndrome (see Chapter 62) and disseminated intravascular coagulation (see Chapter 89).
- Curative therapy is directed at the primary disease.
- Iron deficiency may arise because of urinary iron loss; iron supplements may be beneficial.

INTRODUCTION

"Mechanical" hemolytic anemia results from physical stresses placed on circulating red blood cells, causing them to rupture and spill their contents. This phenomenon was first recognized in marching soldiers and long-distance runners, who literally crush red cells in the microvasculature of their feet.[1,2] Any pathology in small, high-shear vessels that roughens the smooth endothelial surface or creates intravascular obstruction can also strain the red blood cell membrane to its breaking point. The residue from the broken erythrocytes is cleared by a combination of renal and reticuloendothelial mechanisms, producing laboratory features of both intra- and extravascular hemolysis.

EPIDEMIOLOGY AND RISK FACTORS

Because mechanical hemolysis is always a secondary process, its incidence depends upon the associated primary diseases. Although estimates of the frequency of mechanical hemolysis in different clinical settings are not available, it would be considered uncommon in any population of patients.

PATHOPHYSIOLOGY

Red Cell Rupture

The pathologic feature common to all mechanical hemolysis is the intravascular rupture of red blood cells by physical force. In "march" hemoglobinuria, red cells are crushed by external pressure repetitively applied to microvascular beds, such as in the soles of the feet.[1,2] In the heart, red cells can be ripped apart by excessive shear forces across valvular stenoses or high-pressure leaks around prosthetic valves.[3]

Other forms of mechanical hemolysis have a more complex pathophysiology. "Microangiopathic" hemolysis occurs in microvessels that have been partially obstructed by fibrin thrombi or platelet aggregates.[4] Hence mechanical hemolysis is observed with disseminated intravascular coagulation (DIC) (see Chapter 89) and is characteristic of thrombotic thrombocytopenic purpura and the hemolytic-uremic syndrome (TTP/HUS) (see Chapter 62).

Fibrin deposits in microvessels also are common in microangiopathic hemolytic anemia associated with carcinoma, even in the absence of typical DIC.[5,6] Red cells are sheared as they traverse the vessels narrowed by thrombi or tumor emboli. An electron micrograph from one patient with metastatic cancer dramatically revealed the process: a red cell about to be cleaved on a fibrin strand in the microvasculature[7] (Fig. 26–1). These patients appear to have heightened coagulability but suppressed fibrinolytic capacity. Therefore, diffuse microthrombi develop but are only slowly removed. Thrombocytopenia occurs because of platelet consumption in the thrombi. Fibrinogen turnover is increased despite normal plasma fibrinogen concentrations.[5] Occasionally patients show a reduction in hemolysis in response to heparin, implying that thrombosis is part of the pathogenesis.[6]

Microangiopathic hemolysis can also occur in vessels narrowed or roughened by inflammation and necrosis and secondarily laced with fibrin.[4] This process has been observed in the setting of microvascular inflammation and thrombosis experimentally induced with endotoxin.[8] Fibrin deposits are found in these microvascular beds, and thrombocytopenia may develop.

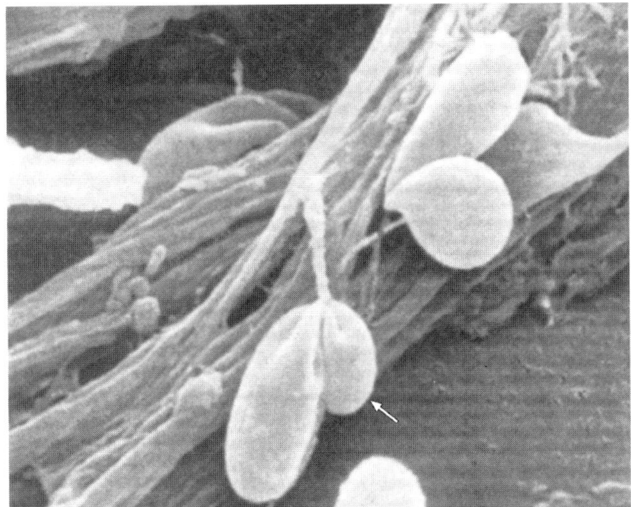

Figure 26–1. Electron micrograph of a red cell *(arrow)* snared by a fibrin strand in the microvasculature of a patient who died from metastatic adenocarcinoma of the stomach. (From Bull BS, Kuhn IN: The production of schistocytes by fibrin strands [a scanning electron microscope study]. Blood 35:104–111, 1970. Copyright American Society of Hematology, used with permission.)

The Fate of Cleaved Red Cells and Their Contents

The red cell destruction that results from mechanical force occurs both intravascularly and extravascularly. At the instant a red cell is ruptured, its contents are partially released directly into the bloodstream (intravascular hemolysis), but the fractured cell membrane reseals around its residual cytoplasm and continues to circulate. The cell fragment (Fig. 26–2), however, is rigid and is quickly removed and degraded by splenic phagocytes (extravascular hemolysis).

The catabolic pathways taken by the intravascular hemoglobin and the intraphagocytic hemoglobin are different. Macrophages degrade the heme of intraphagocytic hemoglobin to elemental iron, which becomes bound to plasma transferrin and recirculates to developing erythroid precursors in the marrow, and to unconjugated bilirubin, which is taken up by hepatocytes, conjugated, and excreted in the bile (Fig. 26–3).

The fate of intravascular hemoglobin is more complex (Fig. 26–4). In plasma, the hemoglobin tetramer disintegrates into dimers, which bind to haptoglobin.[9,10] Haptoglobin-hemoglobin complexes are also cleared by hepatocytes, but this clearance provides no stimulus for accelerated haptoglobin synthesis. Therefore, haptoglobin quickly becomes depleted.[11,12] Unbound plasma hemoglobin is oxidized to methemoglobin, which denatures to free metheme and globin chains. The metheme binds either to hemopexin, which is in limited supply and also becomes depleted, or to albumin, which is abundant and becomes the principal metheme-binding

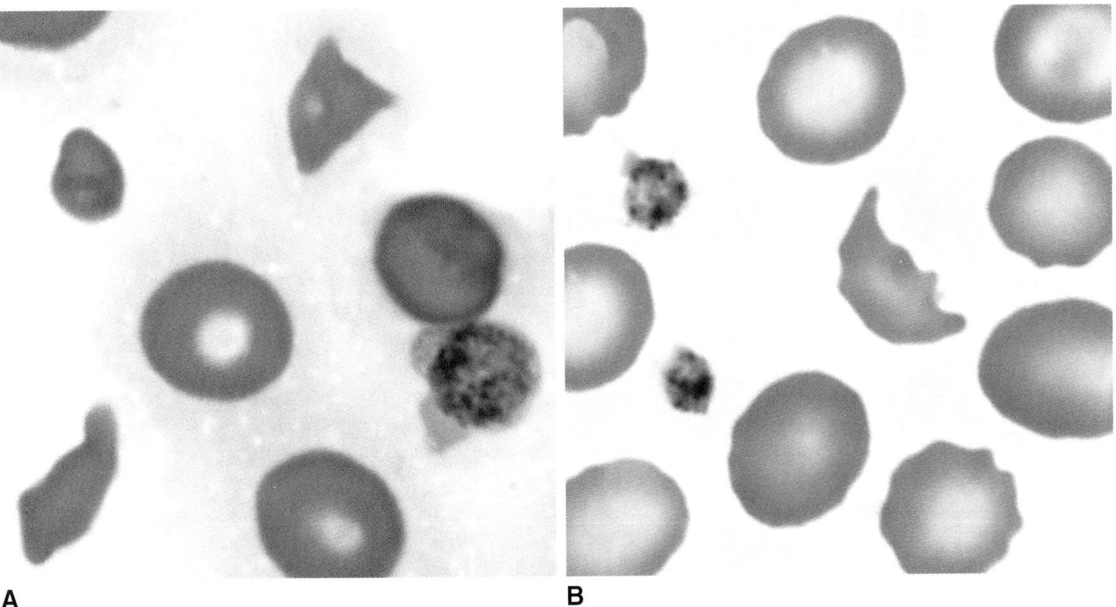

Figure 26–2. Red cell fragments. *A,* From a patient with microangiopathic hemolytic anemia, with red cell fragments and platelets approximately the same size. *B,* From a patient recovering from iron deficiency anemia.

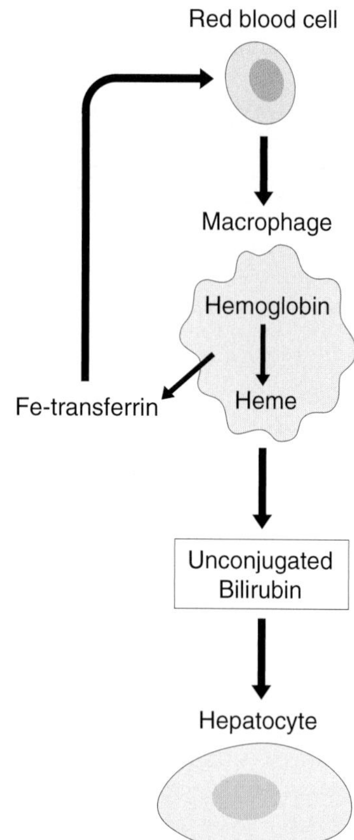

Figure 26–3. Catabolism of hemoglobin during extravascular hemolysis.

protein during mechanical hemolysis. All of these metheme complexes are eventually removed by hepatocytes and degraded to iron and bilirubin.

With brisk and sustained mechanical hemolysis, free hemoglobin dimers appear in the urine. In less severe states, free hemoglobin is taken up by renal tubular epithelium and metabolized to hemosiderin, which is retained in the epithelial cells. As these cells slough into the urine, their hemosiderin accompanies them into the urinary sediment (Fig. 26–5).

CLINICAL FEATURES & DIAGNOSIS

Clinical Settings (Table 26-1)

Cardiac Mechanical Hemolysis

Aortic stenosis can cause mechanical hemolysis if the pressure gradient is high enough.[13] The original mechanical prosthetic heart valves also commonly produced chronic hemolytic anemia, but modern valves rarely produce more than subclinical (compensated) hemolysis if they are functioning normally.[31] Bileaflet prosthetic valves (St. Jude) cause hemolysis more frequently than do pivoting disc valves (Medtronic Hall), and aortic valve protheses tend to be more hemolytic than are mitral valve protheses.[32] Porcine xenograft valves rarely cause hemolysis when they are working properly.[14,15] The most common cardiac cause of hemolytic anemia is a periprosthetic leak related to infection or surgical technique (Fig. 26–6). Chronic valve hemolysis can lead to iron deficiency that worsens the anemia.[17]

Microangiopathic Hemolytic Anemia Secondary to Metastatic Malignancy

Metastatic adenocarcinomas are by far the most common malignancies associated with mechanical hemolysis (Fig. 26–7).[6] Rarely microangiopathic hemolytic anemia is the presenting sign of an occult malignancy.[30] Thrombocytopenia and evidence of a coagulopathy (DIC) often accompany the anemia, which can be particularly severe because of inadequate marrow function due to metastases, chemotherapy, and secondary infections.

Renal Vasculopathy/Vasculitis

Mechanical hemolysis associated with renal disease should suggest the possibility of TTP or HUS (see Chapter 62), especially if thrombocytopenia is also present.[24] However, mechanical hemolysis also occurs with primary renal diseases.[4] Because renal insufficiency reduces erythropoietin production and chronic inflammation suppresses the erythron's response to erythropoietin, patients with mechanical anemia secondary to renal disease are likely to have relatively severe anemia as a result of a reduced ability to produce new red cells.

Primary Pulmonary Hypertension

Only a few cases have been reported of microangiopathic hemolytic anemia caused by primary pulmonary hypertension.[25] The lung capillaries and arterioles in this disease are laced with proliferating endothelial cells and fibrin deposits. Hemolysis is generally a preterminal event.

"March" (Exercise-Induced) Hemoglobinuria

This condition acquired its name as many of the cases first described were soldiers returning from long marches.[1] However, it is also seen in marathon runners and even after prolonged walking, and has been reported after activities involving hand pounding, such as karate exercises and conga drumming.[26–29] A limited degree of exercise-induced hemolysis can be considered physiologic.[2] The most dramatic manifestation of march hemoglobinuria is indeed hemoglobinuria, which appears as dark urine after vigorous exercise and disappears within hours. Increases in plasma hemoglobin and reductions in haptoglobin can also be detected, and urine hemosiderin may be present. The mean corpuscular volume may be somewhat increased because the turnover of the red cell mass is high and more young (larger) cells are present.[26] The hemolysis is so mild and transient, however, that it does not cause anemia. Conversely, long-distance runners often have small amounts of gastrointestinal blood loss that can lead to iron deficiency and limit compensation for hemolysis.[33]

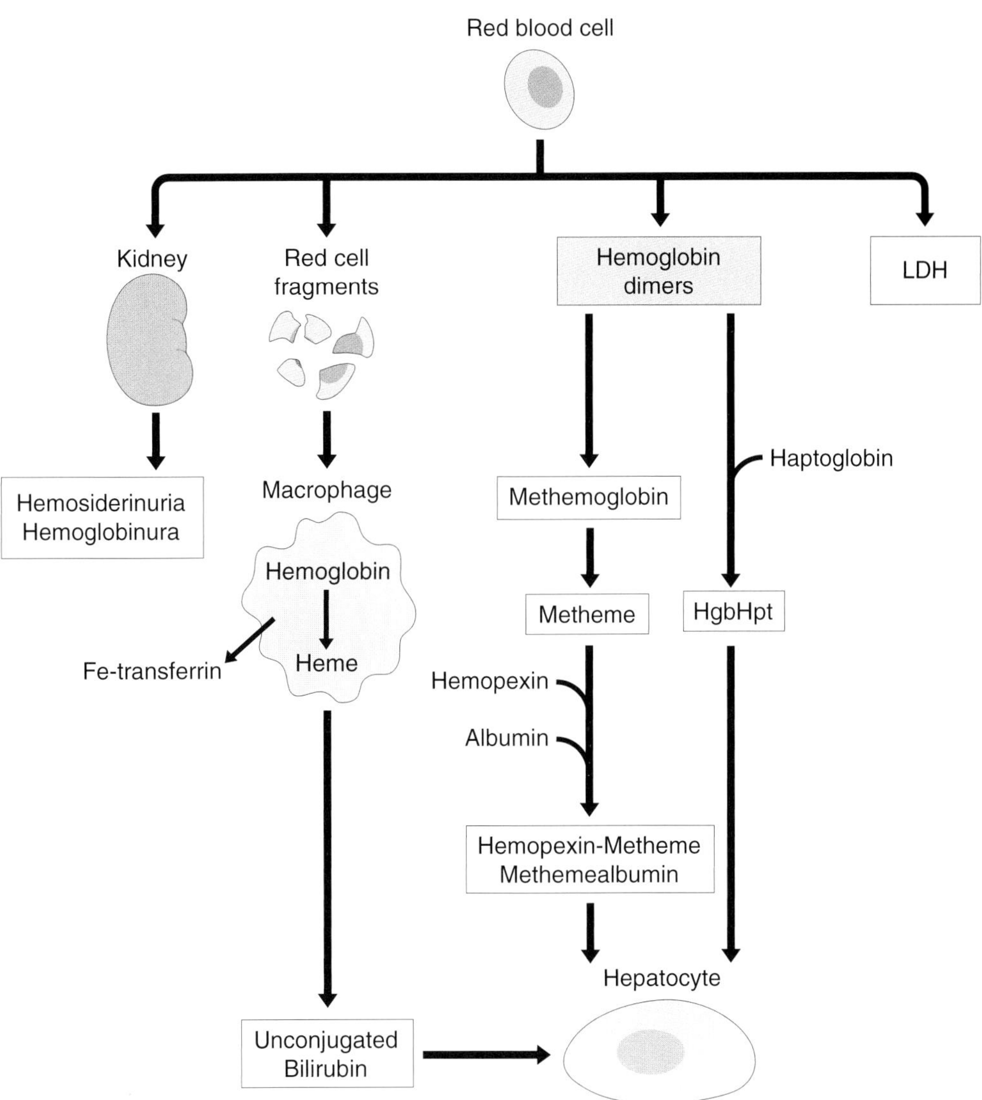

Figure 26–4. Catabolism of hemoglobin during intravascular hemolysis.

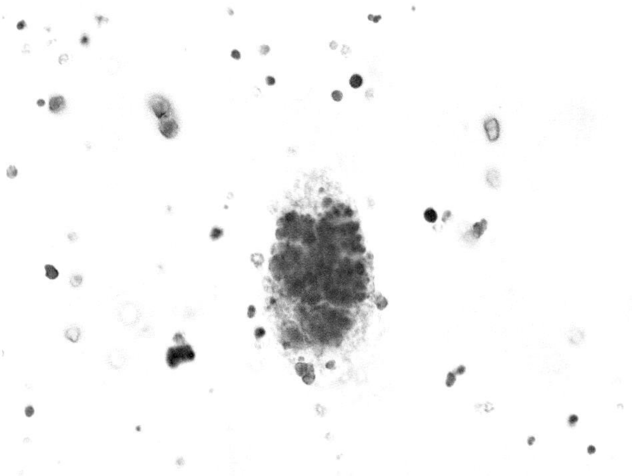

Figure 26–5. Prussian blue staining of the urinary sediment of a patient with intravascular hemolysis. Hemosiderin stains blue-green.

TABLE 26–1. Causes of Mechanical Hemolysis

Cardiac etiologies
Prosthetic heart valves
Normal function: subclinical hemolysis [13]
Malfunction: hemolytic anemia [2,14,15]
Perivalvular leak: subclinical hemolysis, hemolytic anemia [2,16]
Aortic stenosis [12]
Metastatic adenocarcinoma [4,5,6,17,18]
Renal vasculopathy/vasculitis
Renal cortical necrosis [3]
Glomerulonephritis [3]
Renal transplants [19]
Malignant hypertension [3,20]
Diabetes [21]
Scleroderma [22,23]
Primary pulmonary hypertension [24]
Traumatic exercise ("March" hemoglobinuria): subclinical hemolysis [25–29]
TTP/HUS [30]

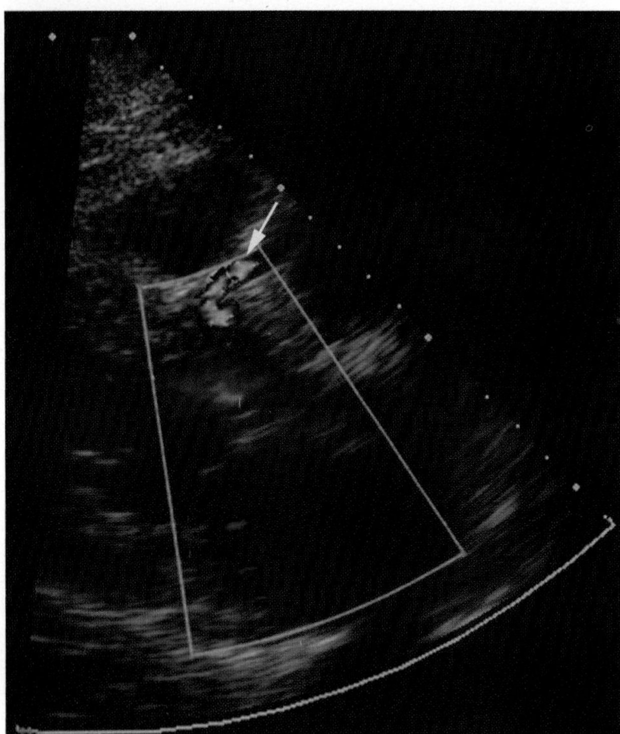

■ **Figure 26–6.** Echocardiogram of a patient with a perivalvular leak around a Starr-Edwards valve in the aortic position. The retrograde jet of blood is red *(shown by the arrow)*. (Courtesy of Inez Ernst, RN, NHLBI.)

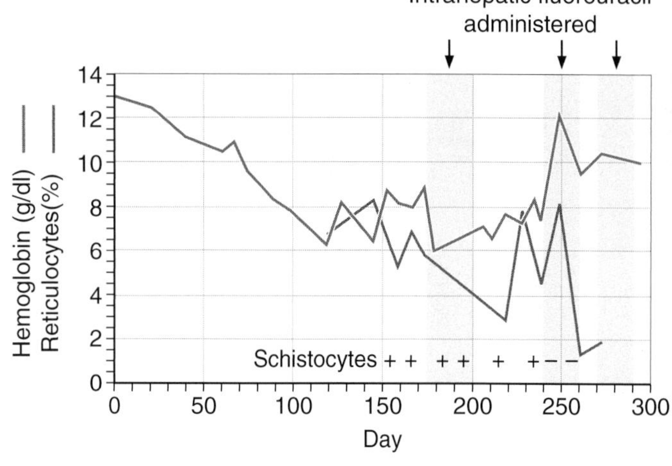

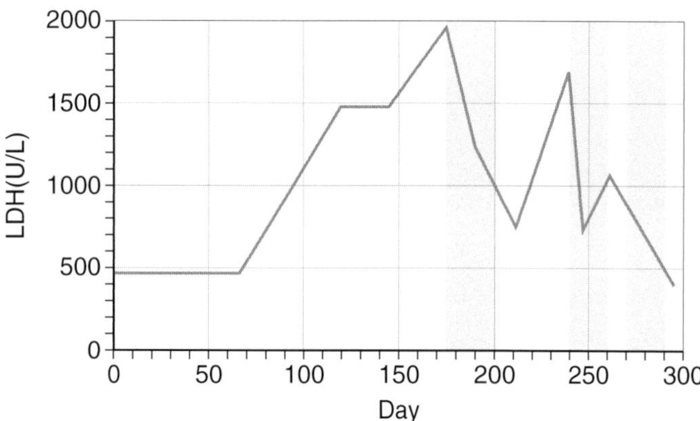

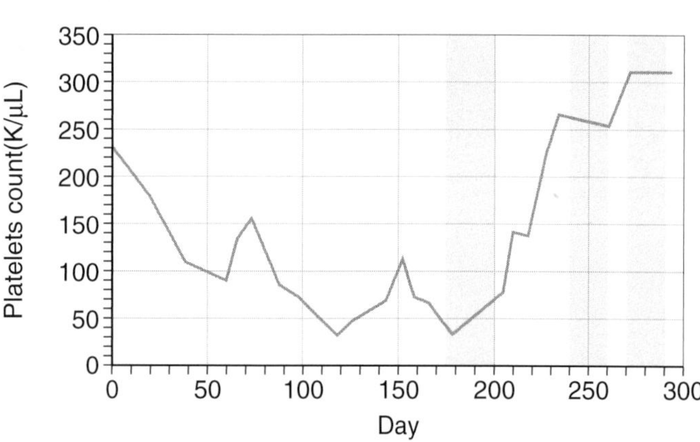

■ **Figure 26–7.** Clinical course of a patient with colon carcinoma and metastases isolated to the liver treated with intrahepatic infusions of fluorouracil as indicated in the top panel. Before treatment, the patient had developed progressive anemia and thrombocytopenia associated with a rise in reticulocyte count and LDH and the appearance of schistocytes in her peripheral blood. After the first fluorouracil infusion, the anemia stabilized and the platelet count began to rise. After subsequent infusions, all of the laboratory parameters returned to normal. (From Horne MK, Cooper B: Microangiopathic hemolytic anemia with metastatic adenocarcinoma: response to chemotherapy. South Med J 75:503–504, 1982. Copyright Lippincott Williams and Wilkins, used with permission.)

Laboratory Features

Anemia

The severity of the anemia caused by mechanical forces depends upon the rate of hemolysis and the regenerative capacity of the erythroid marrow. Both parts of this balance are heavily influenced by the underlying etiology of the hemolysis. An individual who is hemolyzing and is not iron deficient can accelerate red cell production six- to eightfold without becoming more than minimally anemic.[34,35] This degree of response is dependent upon a steady supply of iron being recycled from hemolyzed red cells. With chronic intravascular hemolysis, however, urinary iron loss can lead to iron deficiency and restrict the erythropoietic response.[17] This deficiency is reflected in a damped reticulocytosis and progressive anemia. If the underlying etiology of the hemolysis is neoplastic, inflammatory, or renal, the primary disease and its treatment (such as chemotherapy) may suppress the erythropoietic response and worsen the anemia.

Reticulocytosis

Reticulocyte counts are generally higher with hemolytic anemia than with anemia caused by hemorrhage because the lysing red cells provide a ready supply of iron for erythropoiesis, whereas after blood loss, iron must be mobilized from stores or absorbed from the diet, both slower processes.[35]

Although the reticulocyte count reflects the marrow output of young red cells, it is a complex parameter that requires interpretation. Reticulocytes are defined by their content of RNA, which is degraded over several days as the cells mature. In the absence of anemia, the peripheral blood contains predominantly mature reticulocytes with minimal RNA that is lost in about 24 hours. Therefore, the normal reticulocyte count represents the fraction of the red cell mass that is replaced each day, about 1%. In the presence of anemia, however, younger reticulocytes enter the circulation (sometimes referred to as "shift" cells).[36,37] Automated blood cell counting instruments, which detect RNA with fluorescent markers, designate these younger reticulocytes as the "high fluorescent" fraction. On a stained peripheral blood smear, they appear slightly gray and larger than average.[37] Therefore, the reticulocyte count (percentage or absolute) reflects two factors: the rate of new red cell production and the transit time of young red cells in the marrow. As anemia worsens, the transit time shortens, increasing the number of circulating reticulocytes and falsely suggesting that erythropoiesis has increased more markedly.

In an anemic patient with a healthy marrow, shift cells represent about half of the circulating reticulocytes. Because patients with chronic hemolysis are able to increase their red cell production six- to eightfold (greater than patients who must rely on dietary iron or mobilization from iron stores), they typically have reticulocyte counts approximately twice this value (12–16%) when they are minimally anemic.[34] If their red cell lifespan shortens to less than 15–20 days (about 15% of normal), they become more anemic because their daily maximum red cell output cannot completely replace the volume of red cells hemolyzed each day. Because young red cells tend to be more resistant to lysis than are older ones, older cells are preferentially lost and the reticulocytes increase in percentage but not in absolute numbers. The anemia progresses until the daily loss of red cells equals the marrow's capacity to replace them. Then a new equilibrium is reached at a lower red cell mass.

The level of reticulocytosis, therefore, cannot be used as a precise index of the severity of hemolysis. If a patient has hemolytic anemic and does not have a reticulocyte count of at least 15%, suppression of the erythropoietic response, as by iron deficiency, inflammation, or chemotherapy is likely. Identifying and removing such restraints should improve the anemia.

Red Cell Fragments

The hallmark of mechanical hemolysis is the red cell fragment identified on a peripheral blood smear (see Fig. 26–2). Although the fragments can have a variety of shapes, the most specific for mechanical hemolysis is the schistocyte or schizocyte ("cleft" cell), which has points. Unfortunately, schistocytes are not entirely specific for mechanical hemolysis. An occasional schistocyte can be found in the peripheral blood smears of patients with many different diseases, some as common as iron deficiency anemia (see Fig. 26–2*B*), and they can also be artifactual. However, in clinically significant mechanical hemolysis, the frequency of schistocytes is far greater than in other settings, appearing in most high-power fields, sometimes many per field. The fragments can be as small as platelets and may be misidentified as such by automated blood cell analyzers (see Fig. 26–2*A*). Because thrombocytopenia frequently accompanies mechanical hemolysis, visually inspecting a peripheral blood smear may be necessary to determine whether the reported platelet count has been inflated by microcytic red cell fragments.

Serum Markers

Intravascular hemolysis of any cause, including mechanical stress, introduces red cell cytoplasm into the plasma. The most commonly measured plasma constituent of red cell cytoplasm is lactate dehydrogenase (LDH). Because LDH clears so slowly, with a half-life of about 24 hours, it accumulates to high levels and is a relatively quantitative reflection of the degree of hemolysis.[38,39]

Of course, the most abundant constituent of red cell cytoplasm is hemoglobin. In plasma, free hemoglobin dissociates to dimers that rapidly bind to haptoglobin.[9–12] However, the amount of haptoglobin normally present in plasma can only bind approximately 0.5% of the whole blood content of hemoglobin. Furthermore, haptoglobin-hemoglobin complexes are cleared by the liver within several hours, and hemolysis does not stimulate haptoglobin synthesis (although inflammation does). As a consequence, plasma haptoglobin is easily depleted with even the smallest amount of hemolysis. A low haptoglobin may not reveal the true extent of the hemolytic process, but a normal plasma haptoglobin virtually excludes clinically significant hemolysis.

Once haptoglobin is depleted, hemoglobin dimers (relative molecular mass ~32,000) can circulate briefly and are cleared by renal glomerular filtration.[10] Up to a point, this hemoglobin is removed by renal tubular epithelial cells and metabolized to bilirubin and to hemosiderin, which can be found in the urinary sediment several days later, after the epithelial cells have sloughed (see Fig. 26–5). A hemoglobin load sufficiently high (>5 gm/day) will exceed the capacity of the tubular epithelium, and hemoglobinuria will result.

Hemoglobin that is not cleared renally becomes oxidized (methemoglobin) and dissociates into globin chains and metheme, which binds to hemopexin and albumin and is eventually cleared by hepatocytes.[9,10] Hemopexin and methemalbumin are rarely used clinically as diagnostic parameters.

Because red cell fragments are removed by macrophages, their hemoglobin content is metabolized to unconjugated bilirubin, which is often elevated in the plasma in states of mechanical hemolysis. The capacity of the liver to clear unconjugated bilirubin is so great that the red cell lifespan must be shortened by half or more before unconjugated bilirubin increases in the serum. The rate of conversion of heme to bilirubin by macrophages appears to be limited, so even with brisk hemolysis, the concentration of unconjugated bilirubin in the serum does not rise more that threefold above normal, to a limit of about 3 mg/dL.[40,41] Like serum haptoglobin levels, the unconjugated bilirubin concentration, although routinely available to clinicians, may not accurately reflect the extent of hemolysis.

Urine Hemosiderin and Hemoglobin

Hemosiderin can be detected by Prussian blue staining in the urinary sediment of virtually all patients with mechanical hemolysis (see Fig. 26–5). Because it is derived from hemoglobin metabolized in tubular epithelial cells, hemosiderin only appears in the urine when these cells slough. There is a lag of several days between the time hemoglobin dimers are filtered by glomeruli and when the iron of that hemoglobin appears in the urinary sediment. As mechanical hemolysis is usually chronic, hemosiderin is almost always present.

If the amount of hemoglobin passing through the renal tubules exceeds the epithelium metabolizing capacity, free hemoglobin dimers appear in the urine.

DIFFERENTIAL DIAGNOSIS

The diagnosis of mechanical hemolysis requires both evidence of intravascular red cell destruction (elevated serum LDH, urine hemosiderin) and the presence of red cell fragments in the peripheral blood. If red cell fragments are absent or rare, other forms of intravascular hemolysis (such as delayed transfusion reaction [see Chapter 99] and paroxysmal nocturnal hemoglobinuria [see Chapter 25]) should be considered. If fragments are seen on a peripheral smear but evidence of hemolysis is lacking, the fragments are nondiagnostic. In march hemoglobinuria, the incriminating evidence will be transient, although urine hemosiderin will not appear until a few days after the inciting exercise. With other causes of mechanical hemolysis, characteristic laboratory abnormalities persist (Fig. 26–8).

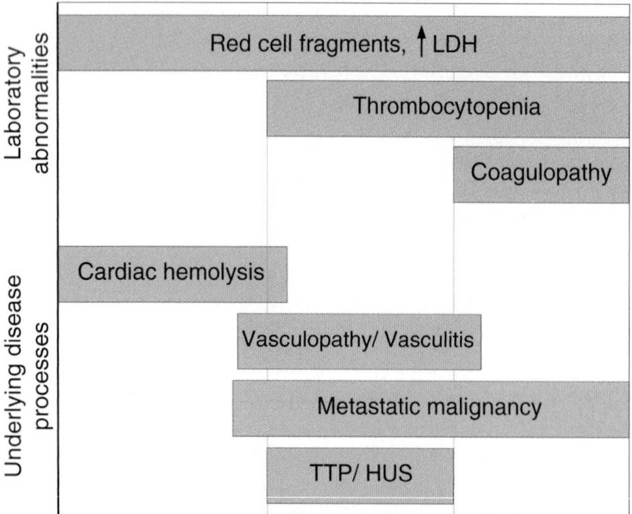

Figure 26–8. Typical laboratory abnormalities associated with the underlying disease processes that cause mechanical hemolysis.

Thrombocytopenia often accompanies mechanical hemolysis related to metastatic malignancy or vasculopathy but is only rarely associated with cardiac etiologies (see Fig. 26–7).[13–15,31,32] In the absence of an identified disease known to cause mechanical hemolysis, the additional presence of thrombocytopenia raises the possibility of TTP or HUS (see Chapter 62). Establishing the correct diagnosis can be difficult. A renal biopsy is helpful if it can be performed safely. Relatively mild renal dysfunction plus neurologic changes favor TTP; an assay for ADAMTS-13 may be diagnostic. With evidence of a coagulopathy, DIC must be considered, although establishing this mechanism rarely alters therapy, which should be directed at the underlying disease.

The ultimate cause of the hemolysis is usually not difficult to identify by standard clinical evaluation because mechanical hemolysis is typically a reflection of advanced disease. However, if hemolysis is the first sign of a malignancy or if the relationship of strenuous exercise to the history of dark urine is not appreciated, the primary diagnosis may be elusive.

TREATMENT

March hemoglobinuria usually does not need treatment, although changing exercise patterns and equipment (like shoes!) can be preventive. Otherwise, curative treatment of mechanical hemolysis requires reversing the underlying disease process. Hemolysis from cardiac sources may prompt surgery to repair a perivalvular leak or to place or replace a prosthetic valve. Metastatic malignancies and renal vasculopathy require aggressive treatment with chemotherapy or immunosuppressive drugs. Mechanical hemolysis secondary to TTP or HUS, for specific therapies for these syndromes are available (see Chapter 62).

SUPPORTIVE CARE AND LONG-TERM MANAGEMENT

Iron replacement may allow compensation for the hemolysis until definitive treatment is possible. An adequate supply of folic acid and vitamin B_{12} must also be assured. If there are complicating conditions such as renal insufficiency or chronic inflammatory diseases, adding erythropoietin to iron supplementation should be considered.[42] If necessary, patients should be supported with red cell transfusions. Allowing anemia related to cardiac pathology to progress to the point of tachycardia will accelerate the hemolysis because red cells are lysed with each heartbeat.

PROGNOSIS

The prognosis of mechanical hemolysis is closely linked to the course of the primary disease. In patients with advanced metastatic carcinoma, mechanical hemolysis is a sign of rapid disease progression. In contrast, therapeutic options are available for patients with hemolysis related to cardiac valve malfunction.

CURRENT CONTROVERSIES & FUTURE CONSIDERATIONS

Mechanical Hemolytic Anemia

- Controversies related to mechanical hemolysis generally arise from issues related to the primary underlying diseases.
- Optimal management of mechanical hemolysis can be difficult for individual patients: what level of anemia is tolerable, is transfusional support indicated, is a trial of erythropoietin worthwhile, and when more aggressive and potentially dangerous treatment of the underlying disease is warranted. Typical questions are the risk of cardiac surgery versus the diminished quality of life associated with transfusion dependence, or whether chemotherapy will worsen the anemia by suppressing erythropoiesis more than it suppresses a primary malignancy.

Suggested Readings*

Antman AH, Skarin AT, Mayer RJ, et al: Microangiopathic hemolytic anemia and cancer: a review. Medicine 58:377–384, 1979.

Brain MC, Dacie JV, Hourihane DO'B: Microangiopathic haemolytic anaemia: the possible role of vascular lesions in pathogenesis. Br J Haematol 8:358–374, 1962.

Brain MC, Azzopardi JG, Baker LRI, et al: Microangiopathic haemolytic anaemia and mucin-forming adenocarcinoma. Br J Haematol 18:183–193, 1970.

Hershko C: The fate of circulating haemoglobin. Br J Haematol 29:199–204, 1975.

Mecozzi G, Milano AD, De Carlo M, et al: Intravascular hemolysis in patients with new-generation prosthetic heart valves: a prospective study. J Thorac Cardiovasc Surg 123:550–556, 2002.

Full references for this chapter can be found on accompanying CD-ROM.

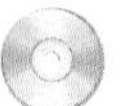

SECTION 3
Malignant and Proliferative Hematologic Diseases

CHAPTER 27
Leukemias: Diagnosis and Classifications

Konstanze Döhner, MD, Krzysztof Mrózek, MD, PhD, Hartmut Döhner, MD, and Clara D. Bloomfield, MD

KEY POINTS

Leukemias: Diagnosis and Classifications

- Morphologic review of bone marrow and/or blood smears, immunophenotyping, conventional cytogenetics, fluorescence in situ hybridization and molecular genetic techniques such as polymerase chain reaction (PCR) are the major tools in the diagnosis and classification of leukemias.
- The World Health Organization classification of hematopoietic neoplasms combines morphologic, immunophenotypic, genetic, and clinical features into a working nomenclature; it permits the definition of biologically homogeneous disease entities that have clinical relevance.
- Immunophenotyping by flow cytometry is informative for the diagnosis of distinct subtypes of acute and chronic leukemias.
- PCR monitoring of minimal residual disease during and after therapy is becoming more important to predict clinical outcome.
- Using modern molecular techniques, leukemia-associated gene mutations have been detected that are of prognostic importance and/or may lead to novel molecularly targeted therapies.

INTRODUCTION

Leukemias represent a heterogeneous group of malignant hematopoietic disorders that are categorized as acute myeloid leukemia (AML), acute lymphoblastic leukemia (ALL), chronic myelogenous leukemia (CML), and chronic lymphocytic leukemia (CLL). These entities differ with regard to epidemiology, biology, clinical course, and prognosis, and their etiology is still largely unknown. Exposure to chemical mutagens (e.g., alkylating agents, benzene) and ionizing radiation, as well as association with some constitutional disorders (e.g., Down syndrome, Fanconi's anemia) increases the risk of developing certain types of leukemia.[1]

Most of the leukemias exhibit chromosomal aberrations and/or gene mutations that alter normal gene function or expression and thus contribute to leukemic transformation. Moreover, cytogenetics and, increasingly, molecular genetics provide the most important prognostic information in these diseases.[2–4] Identification of genetic subsets has led to the application of tailored, and in a few instances molecularly targeted, therapies that have improved patient outcome. In AML, several cytogenetic abnormalities—t(8;21)(q22;q22), inv(16)(p13q22)/t(16;16)(p13;q22), t(15;17)(q22;q11~21), and balanced translocations involving band 11q23—are now part of the new World Health Organization (WHO) classification of AML.[5] As a consequence, cytogenetic and molecular genetic investigations have become an essential part of the routine diagnostic work-up of the leukemias.

Despite continuous improvements in cytogenetic methodology, however, varying proportions of the different leukemia types lack chromosome aberrations detectable by conventional cytogenetic analysis. In such karyotypically normal leukemias, molecular genetic analyses are increasingly useful for the identification of pathogenetically relevant genetic lesions that allow further leukemia subclassification and discrimination between prognostically different subsets of patients. Recently, DNA microarray–based gene expression profiling has been used to explore systematically the molecular variation underlying the biologic and clinical heterogeneity of hematopoietic malignancies.[6–16] Gene expression profiling of the acute leukemias has allowed a comprehensive classification that includes previously identified genetically defined subgroups and novel gene clusters of prognostic significance. Because of its complexity, this technique is not currently routinely used in diagnostics and prognostication of leukemias, but the novel insights it provides will likely contribute to the development of further molecularly targeted therapies.

ACUTE MYELOID LEUKEMIA

Diagnosis

AML is a clonal expansion of immature myeloid cells in the bone marrow, blood, or other organs. Standard in the diagnosis of AML is the cytologic examination of Wright-Giemsa– or May-Grünwald-Giemsa–stained blood and bone marrow smears by light microscopy, allowing reproducible classification by experienced morphologists in most of the cases (see Chapter 100). Until 1999, the most widely used AML classification was the French-American-British (FAB) classification that described the degree of differentiation and the lineage of leukemia based on predominantly morphologic criteria. The FAB classification also included cytochemical stains such as myeloperoxidase, nonspecific esterase, Sudan black B, and periodic acid–Schiff.[17] With the intention to link previous, predominantly morphologic classification systems with newly emerging scientific data, the current WHO classification of hematopoietic neoplasms was recently implemented.[5] This new classification comprises four major categories of AML (Table 27–1):

(i) *AML with Recurrent Genetic Abnormalities*: This group includes four entities, each characterized by the presence of balanced chromosome translocations/inversions and their resulting gene rearrangements: t(8;21) and *RUNX1/CBFA2T1*, inv(16)/t(16;16) and *CBFB/MYH11*, t(15;17) and *PML/RARA*, and various translocations involving chromosome band 11q23 that create fusions of the mixed lineage leukemia (*MLL*) gene with another gene located on the translocation partner chromosome (Figs. 27–1 and 27–2).

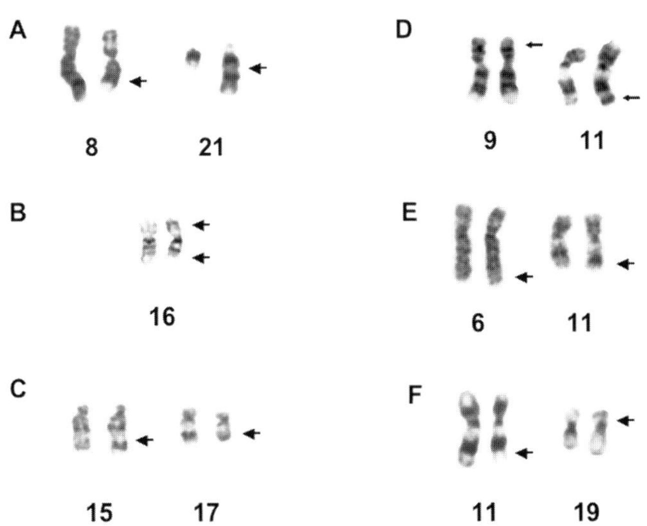

Figure 27–1. G-banded partial karyotypes demonstrating recurrent chromosome abnormalities whose presence is used to classify AML. ***A***, t(8;21)(q22;q22). ***B***, inv(16)(p13q22). ***C***, t(15;17)(q22;q12a~21). ***D–F***, The most frequent among more than 30 recurring translocations involving chromosome band 11q23 in AML: ***D***, t(9;11)(p22;q23); ***E***, t(6;11)(q27;q23); and ***F***, t(11;19)(q23;p13.1).

(ii) *AML with Multilineage Dysplasia*: This group of myeloid leukemias is characterized by dysplasia in two or more cell lineages, generally including megakaryocytes.

(iii) *AML, Therapy-Related*: These leukemias develop as a consequence of prior cytotoxic and/or radiation therapy (see Chapter 30). Two major forms can be distinguished, one arising after therapy with alkylating agents and/or radiation, and another developing after therapy with topoisomerase II inhibitors. The alkylating agent/radiation–related disorder usually develops with a latency of 5–6 years; chromosome abnormalities most often include loss of genetic material from 5q and/or 7q that frequently occur as part of a complex karyotype. The topoisomerase II inhibitor–related AML typically develops 2–3 years after exposure, and is frequently associated with the presence of a balanced translocation or

TABLE 27–1. WHO Classification of Acute Myeloid Leukemia

Acute Myeloid Leukemia with Recurrent Genetic Abnormalities

- Acute myeloid leukemia with t(8;21)(q22;q22) [*AML1(RUNX1)/ETO(CBFA2T1)*]
- Acute myeloid leukemia with abnormal bone marrow eosinophils and inv(16)(p13q22) or t(16;16)(p13;q22) (*CBFB/MYH11*)
- Acute promyelocytic leukemia with t(15;17)(q22;q11~21) (*PML/RARA*) and variants
- Acute myeloid leukemia with 11q23 (*MLL*) abnormalities

Acute Myeloid Leukemia with Multilineage Dysplasia

- Following a myelodysplastic syndrome (MDS)/myeloproliferative disease (MPD)
- Without antecedent MDS or MDS/MPD, but with dysplasia in at least 50% of cells in two or more myeloid lineages

Acute Myeloid Leukemia and Myelodysplastic Syndromes, Therapy-Related

- Alkylating agent/radiation–related type
- Topoisomerase II inhibitor–related type (some may be lymphoid)
- Other types

Acute Myeloid Leukemia Not Otherwise Categorized, classify as:

- Acute myeloid leukemia, minimally differentiated
- Acute myeloid leukemia without maturation
- Acute myeloid leukemia with maturation
- Acute myelomonocytic leukemia
- Acute monoblastic and monocytic leukemia
- Acute erythroid leukemias (erythroid/myeloid and pure erythroleukemia)
- Acute megakaryoblastic leukemia
- Acute basophilic leukemia
- Acute panmyelosis with myelofibrosis
- Myeloid sarcoma

Acute Leukemia of Ambiguous Lineage

- Undifferentiated acute leukemia
- Bilineal acute leukemia

Biphenotypic Acute Leukemia

From Jaffe ES, Harris NL, Stein H, Vardiman JW (eds): World Health Organization Classification of Tumours: Pathology and Genetics of Tumours of Haematopoietic and Lymphoid Tissues. Lyon: IARC Press, 2001, with permission.

inversion, most often involving band 11q23 and the *MLL* gene.

(iv) *AML Not Otherwise Categorized*: This group comprises cases not fulfilling the criteria of groups (i) to (iii); they are classified based on morphologic and cytochemical features in part patterned after the FAB classification.

In contrast to the FAB classification, the blast threshold in the blood or marrow required for the diagnosis of AML in the WHO classification has been reduced from 30% to 20%. However, in patients with t(8;21), inv(16)/t(16;16), and t(15;17), the diagnosis of AML can be made even if the percentage of marrow blasts is lower than 20%.[18]

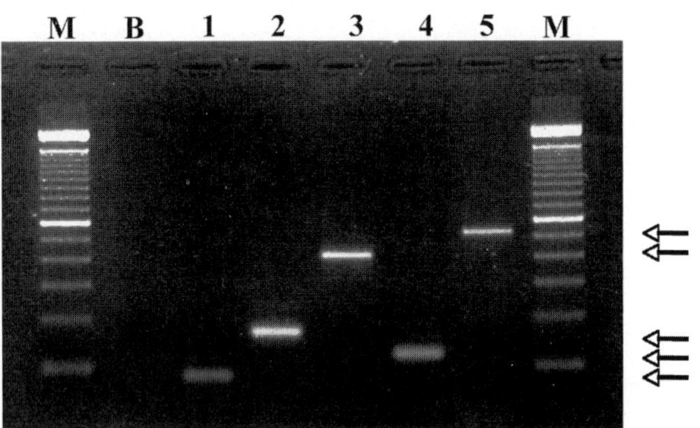

Figure 27–2. Diagnostic reverse transcriptase–polymerase chain reaction for the detection of the most common AML-associated gene fusions resulting from (i) a t(15;17) (sample no.1; s-form/82 bp); (ii) t(8;21) (sample no.2; 161 bp); (iii) inv(16) type A (sample no.3; 418 bp); (iv) inv(16) type D (sample no 4; 123 bp); and (v) t(9;11) (sample no. 5; 6A-fusion; 532 bp). Abbreviations: M, 100–base pair DNA ladder; B, blank control containing water instead of cDNA; 1–5, samples from five different AML patients. *Arrows* indicate the specific fusion product.

Immunophenotyping

The primary role of immunophenotypic analysis in AML is in distinguishing between AML and ALL in the minimally differentiated leukemias and in diagnosis of acute megakaryoblastic leukemia.[5] Minimally differentiated leukemias show no evidence of myeloid differentiation by morphology and cytochemistry, but by immunophenotyping there is expression of early hematopoietic-associated antigens such as CD34, CD38, and human lymphocyte antigen (HLA)-DR; myelomonocytic-associated antigens are usually negative or only weakly positive. Megakaryoblastic leukemias are characterized by expression of the platelet glycoproteins CD41 and/or CD61.

Cytogenetic and Molecular Diagnostics

Conventional cytogenetic analysis using chromosome banding techniques, mostly G-banding, is the "gold standard" in the genetic diagnosis of acute leukemias. A large number of recurrent balanced and unbalanced chromosome aberrations have been described in AML,[19] the more frequent of which are presented in Table 27–2.

TABLE 27–2. Frequent Chromosome Aberrations in Acute Myeloid Leukemia

Cytogenetic Abnormality	Genes Involved	Morphologic Association	Incidence*
Translocations/Inversions			
t(8;21)(q22;q22)	*RUNX1/CBFA2T1*	M2 with Auer rods	6%
inv(16)(p13q22) or t(16;16)(p13;q22)	*CBFB/MYH11*	M4Eo	7%
t(15;17)(q22;q11~21)	*PML/RARA*	M3/M3v	7%
t(9;11)(p22;q23)	*MLL/AF9*	M5	2%
t(6;11)(q27;q23)	*MLL/AF6*	M4 and M5	~1%
inv(3)(q21q26) or t(3;3)(q21;q26)	*EVI1/RPN1*	M1, M4, M6, M7?	~1%
t(6;9)(p23;q34)	*DEK/CAN*	M2, M4	~1%
Chromosomal Imbalances			
+8	?	M2, M4, and M5	9%
−7/7q−	?	No FAB preference	7%
−5/5q−	?	No FAB preference	7%
−17/17p−	*TP53*	No FAB preference	5%
−20/20q−	?	No FAB preference	3%
9q−	?	No FAB preference	3%
+22	?	M4, M4Eo	3%
+21	?	No FAB preference	2%
+13	?	M0, M1	2%
+11	*MLL*†	M1, M2	2%
Complex Karyotype‡			**10%**
Normal Karyotype			**44%**

*Frequency determined among 1311 patients with de novo AML enrolled in the Cancer and Leukemia Group B (CALGB) study 8461.[31]
†Partial tandem duplication of the *MLL* gene.
‡Defined as three or more chromosomal aberrations in the absence of t(8;21), inv(16)/t(16;16), t(15;17), or t(9;11).

Some of these abnormalities are associated with characteristic morphologic and presenting features and/or clinical outcome. The prevalence of major karyotypic groups in adult AML is depicted in Figure 27–3. It has been repeatedly demonstrated, in both retrospective and prospective studies, that karyotype is one of the most important prognostic factors for response to induction treatment, risk of relapse, and survival.[20–33] Currently, pretreatment cytogenetic findings are often categorized into three risk groups, favorable, intermediate, and adverse[27,28,31] (Fig. 27–4). The cytogenetic risk systems proposed by the three major collaborative studies[27,28,31] share many common features, but also differ in some aspects (Table 27–3). Nevertheless, results of cytogenetic

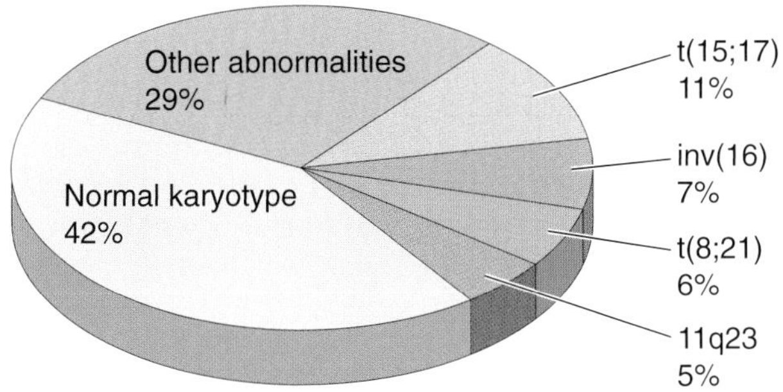

Figure 27–3. Frequency of major cytogenetic groups among 1561 adult patients with de novo AML enrolled in the Cancer and Leukemia Group B study 8461. The four cytogenetic abnormalities included in the WHO category (i), AML with recurrent genetic abnormalities, comprise 29% of cases.

TABLE 27–3. Risk Groups in Acute Myeloid Leukemia According to Cytogenetics

Risk Group	Karyotypic Feature*
Favorable	**t(8;21); inv(16)/t(16;16); t(15;17)**
Intermediate	**none (normal karyotype); −Y,** del(7q)[†]; del(9q)[†]; t(9;11)[‡]; del(11q)[‡]; isolated +8,[§] +11, +13, +21, del(20q)[‖]
Adverse	**complex karyotype; inv(3)/t(3;3); −7;** t(6;9)[¶]; t(6;11)[#]; t(11;19)(q23;p13.1)[#]; −5; del(5q)[**]

*__Bold type__ indicates abnormalities whose prognostic significance is agreed upon by major studies.[27,28,31]

†Classified as adverse by Southwest Oncology Group/Eastern Cooperative Oncology Group (SWOG/ECOG).[28]

‡Would be included in "abn 11q" category and classified as adverse by SWOG/ECOG.[28]

§Classified as adverse with respect to overall survival by Cancer and Leukemia Group B (CALGB).[31]

‖Would be included in "abn 20q" category and classified as adverse by SWOG/ECOG.[28]

¶Classified as intermediate by virtue of being "other structural" abnormality by Medical Research Council (MRC)[27] and as intermediate by CALGB (but only with respect to probability of attainment of complete remission).[31]

#Would be included in "abnormal 11q23" category and classified as intermediate by MRC[27] and as intermediate by CALGB (but only with respect to probability of attainment of complete remission)[27]

**Classified as intermediate with respect to probability of attainment of complete remission and survival by CALGB if not part of a complex karyotype.[31]

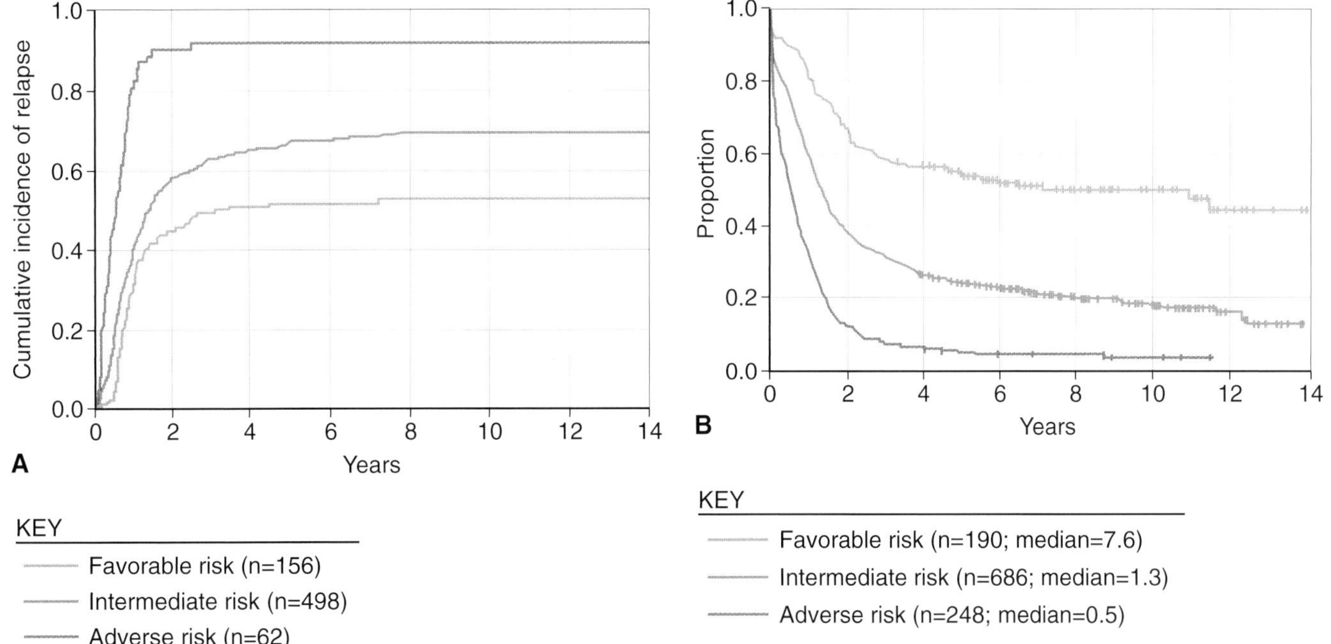

Figure 27–4. Comparison of cumulative incidence of relapse ($P < .001$) *(A)* and overall survival ($P < .001$) *(B)* of adult de novo AML patients categorized into favorable, intermediate, and adverse cytogenetic risk groups using the Cancer and Leukemia Group B (CALGB) criteria. (From Byrd JC, Mrózek K, Dodge RK, et al: Pretreatment cytogenetic abnormalities are predictive of induction success, cumulative incidence of relapse, and overall survival in adult patients with de novo acute myeloid leukemia: results from Cancer and Leukemia Group B [CALGB 8461]. Blood 100:4325–4336, 2002. © the American Society of Hematology.)

TABLE 27–4. Gene Mutations in AML with Normal Cytogenetics

Gene Involved	Genetic Mechanisms	Incidence
FLT3	Internal tandem duplication (ITD) and point mutations of the tyrosine kinase domain (TKD)	30–40%
CEBPA	Mostly loss-of-function mutations	10–15%
MLL	Partial tandem duplication (PTD)	8%

analyses at diagnosis are being used to stratify therapy.[34,35] Moreover, a recent study has demonstrated that the presence of karyotypically abnormal cells in the marrow on the first day of morphologically documented first complete remission following induction chemotherapy is an important adverse prognostic indicator in AML,[36] supporting the use of cytogenetic remission as a criterion of complete remission in AML.[37] Molecular cytogenetic (e.g., fluorescence in situ hybridization [FISH]) or molecular genetic (e.g., polymerase chain reaction [PCR]) techniques are of limited value in the initial diagnostic work-up if used as the only diagnostic test, but have been proposed for the diagnosis of recurrent translocations/inversions or for cases in which chromosome banding analysis fails.[38–40]

Approximately 40–50% of adult patients with AML lack microscopically visible chromosome aberrations. In this group of patients, recent molecular genetic studies have detected gene mutations that impact on prognosis (Table 27–4). The gene most frequently affected by mutations is the FMS-like tyrosine kinase 3 (*FLT3*), a member of the class 3 receptor tyrosine kinase family. Two types of activating *FLT3* mutations have been described in AML, internal tandem duplications of the gene that can be detected in 20–30% of younger adults with AML and, less frequently (7%), point mutations of D835 (single-letter amino acid code) within the *FLT3* tyrosine kinase domain.[41,42] A number of studies have demonstrated that *FLT3* internal tandem duplication is associated with a significantly inferior clinical outcome in younger adult[43–47] and pediatric AML patients,[48–50] with some studies demonstrating that the worst outcome is conferred by *FLT3* internal tandem duplication coupled with lack of a *FLT3* wild-type allele or a high *FLT3* mutant/wild-type allele ratio.[49–52]

A second gene affected by mutation is *CEBPA*, the gene coding for the CCAAT/enhancer binding protein α, a transcription factor involved in the regulation of myelopoiesis.[53] *CEBPA* mutations have been identified in approximately 15–20% of AML patients with normal cytogenetics, and the presence of a *CEBPA* mutation has been associated with a significantly better clinical outcome both in karyotypically normal patients[54] and in those classified in the intermediate prognostic category.[55,56] The partial tandem duplication of the *MLL* gene, which is frequently involved in chromosomal translocations, is found in approximately 5–10% of AML patients with normal cytogenetics. Several studies have demonstrated that the *MLL* partial tandem duplication is associated with a significantly shorter duration of complete remission[57,58] or relapse-free interval[59] in AML patients with a normal karyotype. In addition, recent studies have demonstrated that high expression of the brain and acute leukemia, cytoplasmic (*BAALC*) gene in the blood of cytogenetically normal AML patients adversely impacts outcome.[60–62]

Recently, DNA microarray–based gene expression profiling has been used in AML to identify molecular subgroups with distinct gene expression signatures. Three relatively large studies have found that gene expression profiling allows a comprehensive classification of AML that includes previously identified genetically defined subgroups and novel gene clusters of prognostic significance.[12,13,15]

PCR monitoring of minimal residual disease (MRD) during and after therapy has been used to predict clinical outcome in patients exhibiting specific fusion transcripts resulting from chromosomal translocations or inversions.[63–69] Real-time reverse transcriptase–PCR (RT-PCR) is a novel method that allows the identification of MRD by quantification of the chimeric transcripts. In acute promyelocytic leukemia expressing *PML/RARA*, real-time RT-PCR allows identification of patients who are at an increased risk of relapse and can receive salvage therapy early that may result in improved clinical outcome.[68,70] The prognostic value of MRD quantification for other AML-associated fusion transcripts remains to be determined.[71–73]

ACUTE LYMPHOBLASTIC LEUKEMIA

Diagnosis

ALL is a clonal expansion of immature lymphoid cells in the bone marrow, blood, thymus, and other lymphoid organs. In the new WHO classification, ALL is classified primarily based on immunophenotype, being subdivided into precursor B lymphoblastic leukemia/lymphoma, precursor T lymphoblastic leukemia/lymphoma, and a mature B-cell neoplasm, Burkitt's leukemia/lymphoma.[5] There is general consensus that the FAB distinction between FAB L1 and L2 is not helpful and should be abandoned.[74] Blasts of precursor B lymphoblastic leukemia are small to medium-sized with variable, mostly scant cytoplasm (L1 or L2 morphology in the FAB classification). Blasts of mature B-cell ALL (B-ALL) are medium-sized with deeply basophilic cytoplasm often containing abundant lipid vacuoles (L3 FAB type); usually there are many mitotic figures indicative of a high proliferation rate. Although considered one disease in the current WHO classification, clinicians often arbitrarily diagnose "lymphoblastic leukemia" in cases with more than 25% bone marrow blasts and "lymphoblastic lymphoma" when patients present with extensive nodal disease with a bone marrow blast count of less than 25%.

Immunophenotyping

As noted above, immunophenotyping is the foundation of current classification of ALL. It can also assist in ALL subclassification; further subgroups can be identified based on the stage of differentiation of the leukemic blasts (Table 27–5). Precursor B lymphoblastic leukemias are characterized by the expression of CD19 and/or CD79a and/or CD22; specific immunophenotypic subgroups of B precursor lymphoblastic leukemia include (1) pro–B-ALL (no additional differentiation markers); (2) common (c)-ALL (additional expression of CD10); and (3) pre–B-ALL (cyIgM$^+$).[75]

Mature B-ALL is characterized by expression of surface immunoglobulin M (sIgM), and cytoplasmic (cy) or surface (s) κ or λ light chains. T-lineage lymphoblastic leukemias are characterized by the expression of cyCD3 or sCD3. Specific immunophenotypic subgroups of T-lineage lymphoblastic leukemia include (1) pro–T-cell ALL (T-ALL) (CD7$^+$), (2) pre–T-ALL (CD2$^+$ and/or CD5$^+$ and/or CD8$^+$), (3) cortical T-ALL (CD1a), and (4) mature T-ALL (sCD3$^+$, CD1a$^-$). The immunophenotypic profile of ALL has been shown to have prognostic significance and it is used to stratify treatment.[76]

TABLE 27–5. Immunophenotypic Classification of Acute Lymphoblastic Leukemias*

Type	Criteria
B-lymphoid†	≥2 positive markers: CD19$^+$, CD79a$^+$, CD22$^+$
Pro–B-ALL	No other positive B-cell marker
Common ALL (c-ALL)	Additional CD10$^+$
Pre–B-ALL	Additional cytoplasmic IgM$^+$
Mature B-ALL	Cytoplasmic/membrane κ$^+$ or λ$^+$, membrane IgM$^+$
T-lymphoid‡	Cytoplasmic or membrane CD3$^+$
Pro–T-ALL	CD7$^+$
Pre–T-ALL	CD2$^+$/CD5$^+$/CD8$^+$
Cortical T-ALL	CD1a$^+$
Mature T-ALL	Membrane CD3$^+$ and CD1a$^-$
ALL with myeloid marker	Coexpression of 1–2 myeloid markers, no criteria for biphenotypic acute leukemia (see Table 27–6)

*Classification according to the European Group for the Immunophenotypical Characterization of Leukemias (EGIL).
†Usually terminal deoxynucleotidyl transferase (TdT)$^+$.
‡Usually TdT$^+$, HLA-DR$^-$, CD34$^-$.
From Bene MC, Castoldi G, Knapp W, et al: Proposals for the immunological classification of acute leukemias. Leukemia 9:1783–1786, 1995, with permission.

Criteria for the diagnosis of biphenotypic acute leukemias are given in Table 27–6. This category of acute leukemias is characterized by blasts that coexpress myeloid and T- or B-lineage–specific antigens or concurrent B- and T-lineage antigens.[5] Many markers are only lineage-associated and not specific, particularly in early hematopoietic cell development. Therefore, the coexpression of one or two cross-lineage antigens is not a sufficient criterion to diagnose biphenotypic leukemia; myeloid antigen–positive ALL and lymphoid antigen–positive AML are not uncommon and should be clearly distinguished from biphenotypic acute leukemias.

Cytogenetic and Molecular Diagnostics

In mature B-ALL, the translocation t(8;14)(q24;q32), or its variants, t(2;8)(p12;q24) and t(8;22)(q24;q11), are almost always found and are diagnostic. FISH can also be used for the diagnosis of the t(8;14).

B-lineage leukemias in adults are primarily characterized by the presence of recurrent chromosomal translocations[2,77] (Table 27–7). By far the most important is the t(9;22)(q34;q11.2), which is found in 25–30% of adult ALL cases (Fig. 27–5) and carries a poor prognosis in the absence of allogeneic stem cell transplantation (see Chapter 32). Other relatively common translocations involve band 11q23, with the t(4;11)(q21;q23) being the most common; all of them confer a relatively poor prognosis. In children with B-lineage ALL, recurring chromosomal translocations are seen in different proportions from adults (see Fig. 27–5) and ploidy status has been of greater prognostic significance. Traditionally, ploidy status has been assigned to patients lacking recurring cytogenetic abnormalities. Such cases have been considered hypodiploid (<46 chromosomes), low hyperdiploid (47–50 chromosomes), high hyperdiploid (>50 chromosomes), and diploid (46 normal chromosomes). Recurrent translocations include t(12;21)(p13;q22), t(9;22)(q34;q11.2), t(1;19)(q23;p13.3) and der(19)t(1;19)(q23;p13.3), t(4;11)(q21;q23), and t(11;19)(q23;p13.3). Translocation (12;21)(p13;q22), which is the most common chromosome aberration in childhood pre–B-ALL but rare in adults, is cryptic; that is, it cannot be discerned microscopically using banding techniques because it juxtaposes similarly banded

TABLE 27–6. Immunophenotypic Classification of Biphenotypic and Undifferentiated Acute Leukemias

Biphenotypic Acute Leukemia (BAL)†

Score*	B-Cell Lineage	T-Cell Lineage	Myeloid Lineage
2	CD79a‡, cyIgM, cyCD22	sCD3, cyCD3, TCRα/β	Myeloperoxidase, (Lysozyme)
1	CD10, CD19, CD20	CD2, CD5, CD8, CD10	CD117, CD13, CD33, CD65
0.5	TdT, CD24	TdT, CD7, CD1a	CD14, CD15, CD64

Undifferentiated Acute Leukemia

Not classified by the above criteria, usually CD34$^+$, HLA-DR$^+$, CD38$^+$, and CD7$^+$.

*Scoring system for markers proposed by the European Group for the Immunologic Classification of Leukemia (EGIL).[75]
†BAL is defined if score >2 for the myeloid lineage and >1 for the lymphoid lineage; each positive marker counts for the corresponding score.
‡CD79a may also be expressed in some cases of precursor T lymphoblastic leukemia/lymphoma.

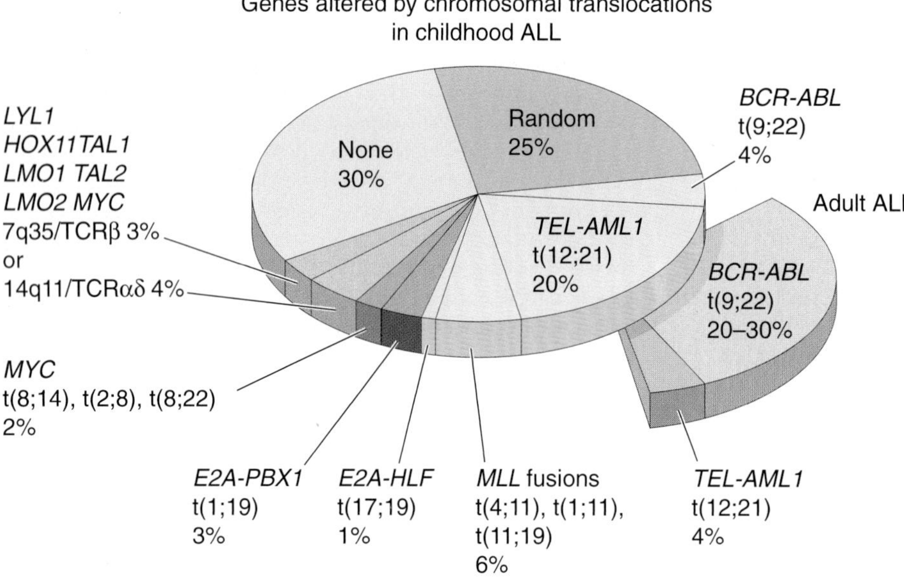

Figure 27–5. Distribution of translocation-generated fusion genes among the commonly recognized immunologic subtypes of ALL in children and adults. (Adapted from Look AT: Genes altered by chromosomal translocations in leukemias and lymphomas. *In* Vogelstein B, Kinzler KW [eds]: The Genetic Basis of Human Cancer. New York: McGraw-Hill, 1998, pp 109–141.)

TABLE 27–7. Frequent Chromosome Aberrations in Acute Lymphoblastic Leukemia

Abnormality	Genes Involved
B-Lineage Acute Lymphoblastic Leukemia	
Mature B-ALL	
t(8;14)(q24;q32)	*MYC/IGH*
t(2;8)(p12;q24)	*MYC/IGK*
t(8;22)(q24;q11)	*MYC/IGL*
B-Precursor ALL	
t(9;22)(q34;q11.2)	*BCR/ABL*
t(12;21)(p13;q22)	*ETV6/RUNX1*
t(4;11)(q21;q23)	*MLL/AF4*
t(1;19)(q23;p13.3)/der(19) t(1;19)(q23;p13.3)	*E2A/PBX1*
t(11;19)(q23;p13.3)	*MLL/ENL*
T-Lineage Acute Lymphoblastic Leukemia	
t(5;14)(q35;q32)	Overexpression of *TLX3 (HOX11L2)*
t(11;14)(p15;q11)	*LMO1 (RBTN1)/TCRD*
t(11;14)(p13;q11)	*LMO2/TCRD*
t(10;14)(q24;q11)	*TLX1 (HOX11)/TCRD*
t(7;10)(q35;q24)	*TLX1 (HOX11)/TCRB*
t(7;19)(q35;p13)	*TCRB/LYL1*

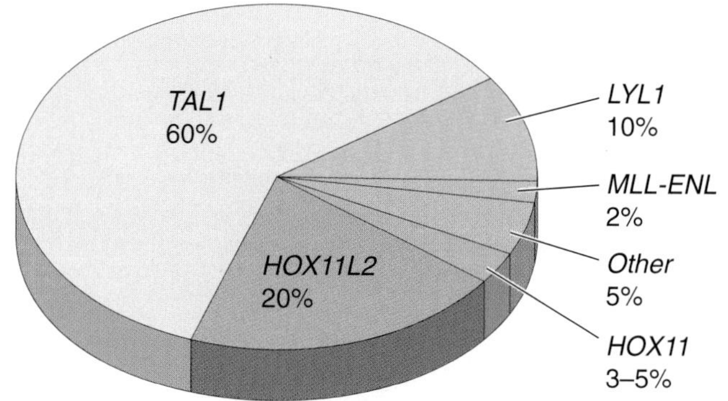

Figure 27–6. Distribution of transcription factor oncogenes among childhood T-cell ALL. (Courtesy of Drs. Adolfo A. Ferrando and A. Thomas Look, Dana-Farber Cancer Institute, Boston, MA.)

regions. It is readily detected using RT-PCR and/or FISH, as are t(9;22), t(11;19), and t(4;11).

As in AML, the pretreatment karyotype has been shown to be of great prognostic significance in both adult and childhood ALL.[78–85] High hyperdiploidy and the t(12;21) have been associated with good prognosis, whereas hypodiploidy, the t(4;11), and in particular the t(9;22) predict inferior outcome.[86–94]

Standard cytogenetics is of limited use in T-lineage ALL because most cases have a normal karyotype. Recently, molecular genetic techniques have allowed classification into multiple genetic subgroups that may be prognostically and eventually therapeutically relevant (Figs. 27–6 and 27–7). About one third of patients with T-lineage ALL harbor balanced translocations involving the T-cell receptor gene *TCR* α and δ loci at band 14q11, the β locus at 7q35, and the γ locus at 7p14-15, with various partner genes. These translocations usually lead to altered expression of hematopoietic transcription factors by juxtaposition to the regulatory elements of the T-cell receptor genes. The most common rearrangement involving one of the *TCR* loci in adult ALL is t(10;14)(q24;q11.2),[83,85] which results in overexpression of the *TLX1* (*HOX11*) gene at 10q24.[95] *TLX1* gene overexpression also occurs in patients without microscopically detectable t(10;14) or other aberrations involving 10q24, and both the t(10;14) and *TLX1* gene overexpression have been associated with a favorable clinical

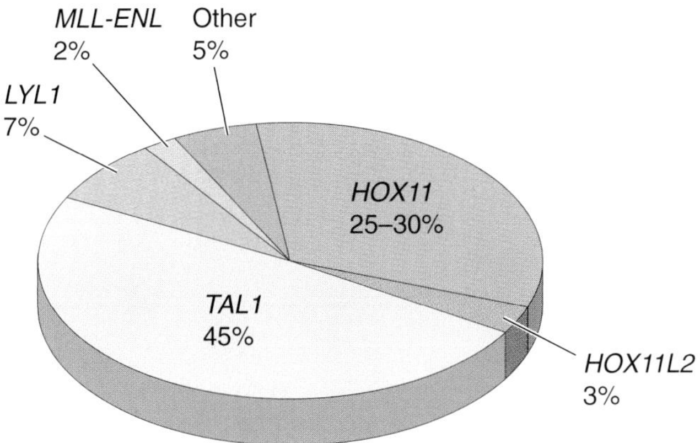

Figure 27–7. Distribution of transcription factor oncogenes among adult T-cell ALL. (Courtesy of Drs. Adolfo A. Ferrando and A. Thomas Look, Dana-Farber Cancer Institute, Boston, MA.)

outcome.[83,85,96,97] Another genetic event common in T-ALL (detected in 22–23% of pediatric and 13% of adult patients) is the overexpression of the *TLX3* (*HOX11L2*) gene at 5q35, which is most frequently, but not always, associated with a recently discovered cryptic t(5;14)(q35;q32) and its variants,[98] and has been associated with poor prognosis in some,[9,99] but not all,[100] studies.

DNA microarray–based gene expression profiling of leukemic blasts can accurately identify many known prognostic subtypes of ALL, including T-ALL, and ALL with *E2A-PBX1*, *TEL-AML1*, or *BCR-ABL* gene fusions or *MLL* rearrangements, and ALL with hyperdiploid karyotypes with more than 50 chromosomes.[9–11] In a further step toward developing gene expression profiling into a useful front-line diagnostic tool, new subtype discriminating genes have been identified, including novel markers that might provide new insights into the altered biology underlying ALL.[11] In a very recent study, genes that are differentially expressed in ALL cells with resistance to four antileukemic drugs were identified and the pattern of gene expression was related to the outcome of treatment.[14]

Recently, multiplex PCR assays have been used in ALL for the detection of clonally rearranged immunoglobulin and T-cell receptor genes. The MRD-based evaluation of initial response to front-line therapy has emerged as a highly relevant diagnostic tool, particularly in ALL of children and young adults, in whom the level of MRD has been shown to be an independent prognostic factor allowing a precise risk group classification.[101] Modern treatment protocols increasingly use this prognostic factor to tailor treatment.[102,103]

CHRONIC MYELOGENOUS LEUKEMIA

Diagnosis

CML is a myeloproliferative disease originating from an abnormal pluripotent hematopoietic stem cell. It is consistently associated with and diagnosed by the presence of the t(9;22)(q34;q11.2) or one of its variants and/or the *BCR-ABL* fusion gene. The natural course of the disease is characterized by an indolent chronic phase (CML-CP) followed by the aggressive stages, accelerated phase (CML-AP) and blast phase (CML-BP) (see Chapter 31). In CML-CP, there is marked leukocytosis (mostly >100 × 10^9/L) with a maturation shift toward precursor cells. There is absolute basophilia and in many cases also eosinophilia. The platelet counts are normal or increased and may exceed 1000 × 10^9/L; the hematocrit is normal or slightly decreased. Bone marrow trephine biopsy reveals marked hypercellularity with a maturation pattern of neutrophils and their precursor cells similar to that seen in the blood; the blast count is usually less than 5%. Other features may include smaller hypolobulated megakaryocytes, an increase in reticulin fibers, and the presence of pseudo-Gaucher cells and sea-blue histiocytes. The diagnosis of CML, accelerated or blast phase, is made when one or more of the criteria listed in Table 27–8 are present.

TABLE 27–8. Chronic Myelogenous Leukemia: Criteria for Accelerated and Blast Phase*

Accelerated Phase:
Blasts 10–19% of white blood cell counts in peripheral blood and/or nucleated bone marrow cells
Peripheral blood basophilia ≥20%
Persistent thrombocytopenia (<100 × 10^9/L) unrelated to therapy, or persistent thrombocytosis (>1000 × 10^9/L) unresponsive to therapy
Increasing spleen size and increasing white blood cell count unresponsive to therapy
Cytogenetic evidence of clonal evolution
Blast Phase:
Blasts ≥20% of peripheral blood white cells or of nucleated bone marrow cells
Extramedullary blast proliferation
Large foci or clusters of blasts in the bone marrow biopsy

*The diagnosis of accelerated or blast phase may be made when one or more of the above criteria are present.
From Jaffe ES, Harris NL, Stein H, Vardiman JW (eds): World Health Organization Classification of Tumours: Pathology and Genetics of Tumours of Haematopoietic and Lymphoid Tissues. Lyon: IARC Press, 2001, with permission.

Immunophenotyping

In CML, the role of immunophenotyping is limited. It is primarily performed in CML-AP and CML-BP to identify the lineage from which blasts are derived.

Cytogenetic and Molecular Diagnostics

The genetic hallmark of CML is the translocation t(9;22)(q34;q11.2), resulting in the creation of the Philadelphia chromosome (Ph). On the molecular level, this translocation fuses sequences of the *BCR* gene on chromosome 22 with sequences of the *ABL* gene on chromosome 9. In the majority of CML cases, the breakpoint occurs in the major breakpoint cluster region of the *BCR* gene, resulting in an abnormal fusion protein (p210) with increased tyrosine kinase activity.[104] The chromosomal translocation (including variant forms) is present in more than 95% of CML cases. In the remaining cases, the *BCR-ABL* fusion gene results from submicroscopic rearrangements and can be detected by molecular techniques.

CML-AP and CML-BP in most cases are characterized by the acquisition of additional chromosome abnormalities such as an extra der(22)t(9;22), trisomy 8, and isochromosome i(17q).[105]

Monitoring of residual disease by quantitative determination of the *BCR-ABL* transcript level using real-time RT-PCR has major clinical relevance. Significant reduction of *BCR-ABL* transcript levels following therapy with the specific tyrosine kinase inhibitor imatinib mesylate has been associated with a high probability of remaining progression-free (see Chapter 31). Moreover, the detection of the *BCR-ABL* fusion transcript after allogeneic stem cell transplantation predicts relapse and may guide the use of donor lymphocyte infusions or the use of imatinib.[106–109]

CHRONIC LYMPHOCYTIC LEUKEMIA

Diagnosis

B-cell CLL (B-CLL) is a lymphoproliferative disorder characterized by a progressive accumulation of long-lived, immune-incompetent, clonal B lymphocytes in the blood, bone marrow, and lymphoid tissues. Based on criteria established by the International Workshop on CLL[110] and the National Cancer Institute–sponsored Working Group Guidelines for CLL[111] CLL is diagnosed when there is a sustained and absolute lymphocytosis (>10 × 10^9/L), a bone marrow aspirate showing more than 30% lymphocytes, and a pattern of cell surface marker expression consistent with B-CLL. Morphologically, neoplastic cells are usually monomorphic small, round B lymphocytes, with a varying admixture of larger lymphocytes or prolymphocytes. In the case of nuclear irregularity, other subtypes of lymphoproliferative disorders should be considered.

Immunophenotyping

Immunophenotyping of leukemic cells is an important tool in the diagnosis of B-CLL. The clonal B cells are characterized by expression of CD19, CD5, and CD23; in contrast to other B-cell lymphomas, there is low expression of surface immunoglobulin and of CD79b. This typical immunophenotypic profile allows differential diagnosis from other lymphoproliferative disorders that also may present with a leukemic phase (Table 27–9). Flow cytometry is also being used to assess prognostic markers. High expression of CD38 has been associated with inferior prognosis[112–115]; more recently, the intracellular signaling molecule ZAP-70 has been shown to be a surrogate marker for the mutation status of the immunoglobulin genes (see next) and to have important prognostic significance.[116–118]

TABLE 27–9. Immunophenotype of B-Cell Chronic Lymphocytic Leukemia and Related B-Cell Lymphoproliferative Disorders

Surface Antigen	B-CLL	MCL	WM	FL
CD19	+	+	+	+
CD20	+	+	+	+
CD5	+	+	+/−	−
CD23	+	−	−	−
Cyclin D1	−	+	−	−
CD10	−	−	+/−	+
CD79b	+/−	+	+	+

Abbreviations: FL, follicular lymphoma; MCL, mantle cell lymphoma; WM, Waldenström's macroglobulinemia; +, positive; −, negative; +/−, weakly positive or negative.

TABLE 27–10. Incidence of Chromosomal Abnormalities Detected by Use of FISH in 325 Patients with Chronic Lymphocytic Leukemia

Aberration Frequency	No. of Patients(%)*
13q deletion	178 (55%)
11q deletion	58 (18%)
12q trisomy	53 (16%)
17p deletion	23 (7%)
6q deletion	21 (6%)
8q trisomy	16 (5%)
t(14q32)	14 (4%)
3q trisomy	9 (3%)
Clonal abnormalities	268 (82%)
Normal karyotype	57 (18%)

*One hundred seventy-five patients had one aberration, 67 had two aberrations, and 26 had more than two aberrations.
From Döhner H, Stilgenbauer S, Benner A, et al: Genomic aberrations and survival in chronic lymphocytic leukemia. N Engl J Med 343:1910–1916, 2000, with permission.

Cytogenetic and Molecular Diagnostics

Similar to the acute leukemias, in CLL, disease-associated genetic markers have become very important for classification and predicting prognosis. Molecular analysis has shown that there are two variants of CLL based on the mutation status of the variable segments of the immunoglobulin heavy chain genes (IgV_H): one variant with unmutated *VH* genes, thought to originate from pregerminal center cells (comprising approximately 40% of the cases), and another with mutated *VH* genes, thought to be derived from postgerminal center cells.[119–121] Most importantly, *VH* mutation status provides important prognostic information, with unmutated cases showing an unfavorable prognosis and cases with mutated *VH* genes associated with slow disease progression and long survival[112,122–124] (Fig. 27–8). Using FISH of interphase cell nuclei ("interphase cytogenetics") with a CLL-specific DNA probe set, cytogenetic abnormalities

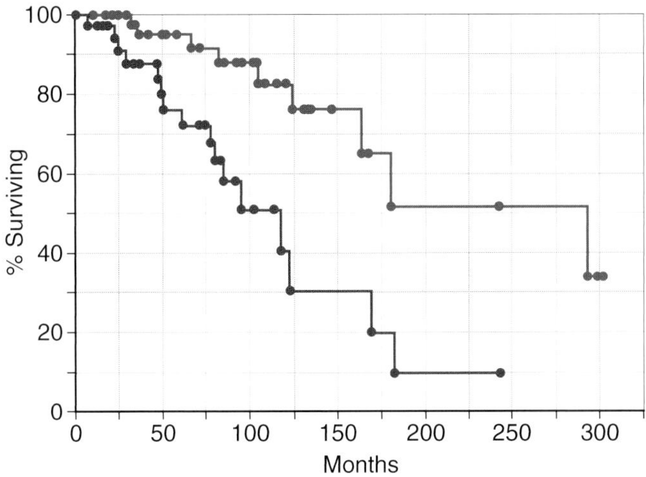

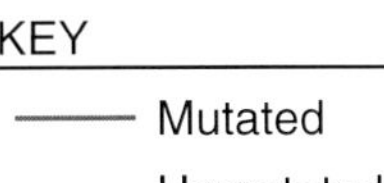

Figure 27–8. Estimated survival probabilities in CLL patients with mutated and unmutated immunoglobulin genes of CLL. Median survival for unmutated CLL: 117 months; median survival for mutated CLL: 293 months. The difference is significant at the *P* = .001 level (logrank test). (From Hamblin TJ, Davis Z, Gardiner A, et al: Unmutated Ig VH genes are associated with a more aggressive form of chronic lymphocytic leukemia. Blood 94:1848–1854, 1999, with permission.)

can now be detected in about 80% of CLL cases[125]; the most frequent aberrations are 13q deletion, 11q deletion, trisomy 12, and 17p deletion (Table 27–10). In part, these abnormalities have been associated with clinical characteristics (e.g., 11q deletion with extensive lymphadenopathy) or resistance to treatment (e.g., 17p deletion).[126–132] Most importantly, these abnormalities have also been shown to strongly predict for disease progression and survival (see Chapter 34) (Fig. 27–9). It is important to note that cytogenetic abnormalities and *VH* mutation status provide independent prognostic information.[123,124]

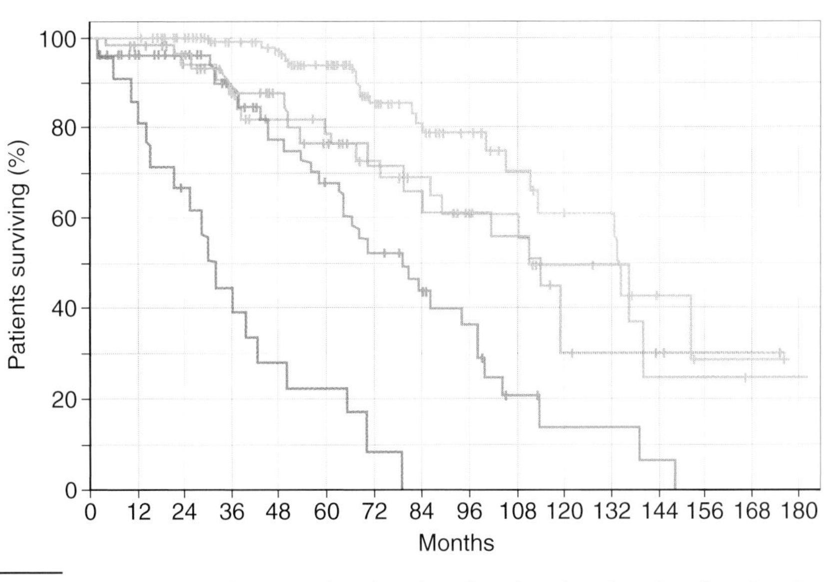

No. at risk																
17p deletion	23	18	13	8	5	4	1	0	0	0	0	0	0	0	0	0
11q deletion	56	53	47	43	33	27	20	15	10	4	2	2	1	0	0	0
12q trisomy	47	44	41	29	24	17	14	13	12	11	4	3	2	1	1	0
Normal	57	51	45	37	30	27	20	17	12	11	6	5	2	2	1	1
13q deletion as sole abnormality	117	117	106	91	80	63	45	36	24	16	12	11	3	1	1	0

Figure 27–9. Estimated survival probabilities in patients of five hierarchical genetic categories of CLL. The median survival times for the 17p deletion, 11q deletion, 12q trisomy, normal karyotype, and 13q deletion (as a single abnormality) groups were 32, 79, 114, 111, and 133 months, respectively. (From Döhner H, Stilgenbauer S, Benner A, et al: Genomic aberrations and survival in chronic lymphocytic leukemia. N Engl J Med 343:1910–1916, 2000, with permission.)

Suggested Readings*

Harrison CJ, Foroni L: Cytogenetics and molecular genetics of acute lymphoblastic leukemia. Rev Clin Exp Hematol 6:91–113, 2002.

Jaffe ES, Harris NL, Stein H, Vardiman JW (eds): World Health Organization Classification of Tumours: Pathology and Genetics of Tumours of Haematopoietic and Lymphoid Tissues. Lyon: IARC Press, 2001.

Mrózek K, Heinonen K, Bloomfield CD: Clinical importance of cytogenetics in acute myeloid leukaemia. Best Pract Res Clin Haematol 14:19–47, 2001.

Stilgenbauer S, Döhner H: Molecular genetics and its clinical relevance. Hematol Oncol Clin North Am 18:827–848, 2004.

Full references for this chapter can be found on accompanying CD-ROM.

This work was supported in part by grants from the National Cancer Institute, Bethesda, MD (5P30CA16058), and the Coleman Leukemia Research Fund to K.M. and C.D.B. and by grants from the Deutsche José Carreras Leukämie Stiftung (DJCLS-R00/18 and -R/4/26f) and from the Bundesministerium für Bildung und Forschung (Kompetenznetz „Akute und chronische Leukämien"; 01GI9981) to K.D. and H.D.

CHAPTER 28

ACUTE MYELOGENOUS LEUKEMIA

Elihu H. Estey, MD

KEY POINTS

Acute Myelogenous Leukemia

- There are two principal variants of AML:

  AML with balanced reciprocal chromosomal translocations or inversions—has a relatively favorable prognosis, occurs in 25% of cases, has a median age of 40 years, has an incidence that does not increase with age, and is not associated with antecedent hematologic disorder or cytotoxic therapy.

  AML with gain or loss of chromosomal material—has a poor prognosis, occurs in 75% of cases, has an incidence that increases with age (median age 65–70), and has a frequent history of cytotoxic therapy or myelodysplastic syndrome.

- At least two "hits" are required for development of AML. One hit is associated with activating mutations in receptor tyrosine kinases (*FLT3* internal tandem duplications or point mutations in *ras* or *kit*), providing a survival or proliferative advantage. The other involves transcription factor fusions that block hematopoietic differentiation and subsequent apoptosis.
- The prognosis of AML reflects both the treatment-related mortality rate and duration of remission. Covariates predicting treatment-related mortality include performance status, age, and organ function. Remission rate and duration are predicted by cytogenetic pattern, *FLT3* gene status, and type of presentation (de novo vs. antecedent hematologic disorder).
- Prognostic information should be used to develop a treatment plan unless life-threatening symptoms require immediate intervention.
- Stem cell transplantation (either allogeneic or autologous) in patients in first complete remission should be performed in the context of a clinical trial and be reserved for poor-prognosis patients.

INTRODUCTION

Acute myelogenous leukemia (AML) is the final common pathway of a finite number of mutational events in hematopoietic marrow-derived stem cells resulting in increased proliferation, decreased apoptosis, and failure to differentiate into red cells, granulocytes, monocytes, and platelets. Normal feedback loops maintaining homeostasis and normal interactions with marrow stroma are disrupted, leading to failure of normal blood cell production. Marrow failure ensues rapidly, leading to death. Cells with adherence properties can accumulate in lung or brain, with extreme hyperleukocytosis reducing blood flow and causing fatal organ failure. Figure 28–1 illustrates the development of AML.

EPIDEMIOLOGY AND RISK FACTORS

Like many cancers, AML is a disease of aging (see Chapter 33). Based on 1980 cases of leukemia reported to the Danish Cancer Registry during the 4-year period from 1973 to 1976, Brincker[1] estimated that the median age at diagnosis of AML was 64 years. Age has a particular impact on incidence for AML cases arising from prior myelodysplastic syndrome, those demonstrating trilineage dysplasia despite the absence of a history of myelodysplastic syndrome, and those with monosomies of chromosomes 5 and/or 7 (−5,−7) or deletions of the long arms of these chromosomes (5q−,7q−). In contrast, the incidence of the 25% of cases with chromosomal translocations, in particular inversion 16 [inv(16)] and translocations of chromosomes 8 and 21 [t(8;21)] and chromosomes 15 and 17 [t(15;17)], which typically present de novo and without dysplasia, is approximately constant with increasing age. Thus, there are two principal types of AML, one associated with the noted translocations or inversions and one with gains or loss of chromosomal material, often in complex patterns.[2]

Rare cases of congenital diseases associated with chromosome breakage or defective DNA repair (e.g., Fanconi's anemia) are at increased risk for development

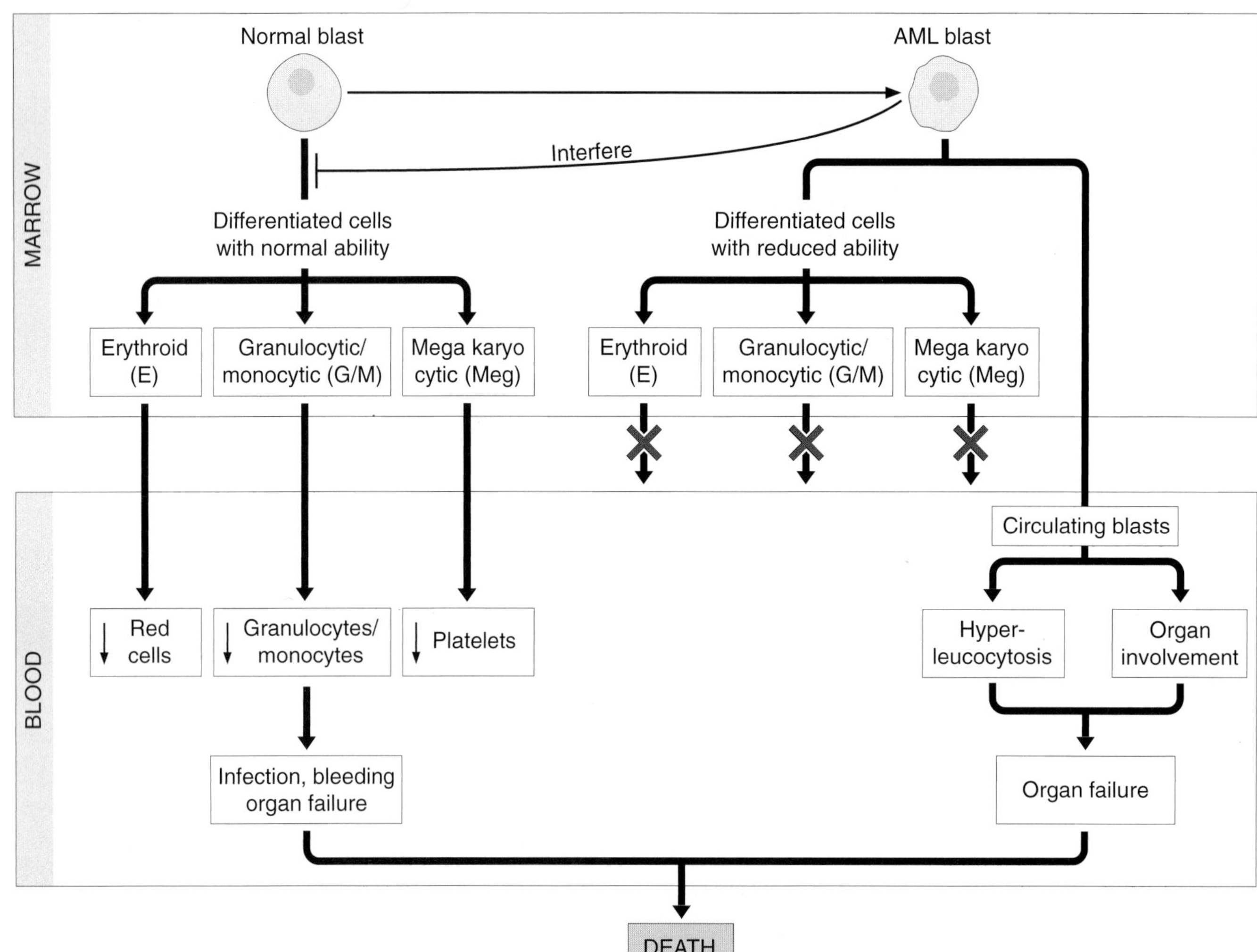

Figure 28–1. Pathophysiology of AML. Unknown events transform some normal blasts into AML blasts. The former are relatively incapable of maturing into normal granulocytes, red cells, and platelets. In addition, they decrease the ability of normal blasts to differentiate. The consequence is bone marrow failure. In addition, AML blasts are capable of escaping from marrow to blood and of infiltrating organs such as the lung or brain, thus also contributing to death.

of AML. These few instances support the general observation that maintenance of DNA is essential and point to needed research into acquired or polymorphic defects in the general population. Children with congenital neutropenia associated with a mutated granulocyte colony-stimulating factor (G-CSF) receptor (Kostmann's syndrome) are also at risk.[3] By far the greatest risk for AML, however, is associated with receipt of cytotoxic therapy (which itself induces both DNA damage and proliferative stress) for other conditions, generally cancers (see Chapter 104). When treatment for the primary process is successful, and patients are alive for many years, the latent risk becomes apparent. Examples include patients treated for breast cancer, lymphoma, and childhood acute lymphocytic leukemia. Such AML is called "secondary" or treatment-related AML.[4] Relative risks for AML in these patients may be as much as 50 times normal, with a peak cumulative incidence of 10%.

Secondary AML assumes two forms. Alkylating agent–associated AML occurs within 5–10 years and becomes rare thereafter. Abnormalities of chromosomes 5 and/or 7 are common. Topoisomerase II inhibitor–associated AML occurs with a latency of less than 5 years and is seen after use of drugs such as anthracyclines and epipodophyllotoxins. Translocations involving the long arm of chromosome 11 (11q) are characteristic of these secondary AMLs (Table 28–1). Environmental exposures causing DNA damage and mutations that are associated with an increased risk of leukemia include benzene, pesticides, and other carcinogens found in cigarettes.[5,6]

Because most patients given alkylating agents or exposed to benzene do not develop AML, other factors including genetic predisposition likely play a role. Monozygotic twins are more prone to develop AML than dizygotic twins. Acute promyelocytic leukemia (APL; discussed in depth in Chapter 30) is more frequent in Hispanics[7]; for example, APL comprises 30% of AML in Peru versus 5% in the United States, and Mexican Americans are more prone to develop APL than other AMLs.[8] Polymorphisms in genes that encode enzymes that metabolize carcinogens may also contribute (Table 28–2). Examples include NADP(H) quinine oxidoreductase

TABLE 28–1. Cytogenetic Abnormalities by Patient Type: M. D. Anderson, 1980–2004

	Age < 70 yr, No Prior Chemotherapy	Age > 69 yr, No Prior Chemotherapy	Prior Chemotherapy (Median Age 59 yr)
Patients	2022	572	342
Abnormalities of chromosomes 5 and/or 7	16%	26%	42%
Inversion 16 or translocations (15;17) or (8;21)	17%	4%	8%
Other abnormalities	24%	26%	29%
No abnormality or insufficient	43%	44%	21%

TABLE 28–2. Effect of Genetic Polymorphisms on Development of AML

Gene	Polymorphism	Effect	Predisposes To	Comment	Reference
NQO1	Cysteine to threonine at nucleotide 609	Lowers NQO1 activity	Secondary AML, particularly with chromosome 5 and/or 7 abnormalities (−5/−7)	15% of −5/−7 patients had 2 mutant alleles, 38% 1 mutant allele; expected frequencies 5% and 34% ($P = .002$)	9
			De novo AML, particularly with inv(16)	Odds ratio for developing inv(16) if had 1 or 2 (vs 0) mutant alleles was 8.13	10
CYP1A1	Isoleucine to valine at amino acid 462	Increases inducibility with resultant accumulation of toxic metabolites	N-*ras* mutations	2.36 odds ratio if had 1 or 2 mutant alleles (95% CI 1.01–5.53); no effect on *FLT3* internal tandem duplications	10
			Poor-risk cytogenetic abnormalities: −5/−7 or deletion of long arm of chromosome 3 [del(3q)]	15.94 odds ratio if had 1 or 2 mutant alleles	11

Abbreviations: CI, confidence interval; CYP1A1, cytochrome P-450 isotype 1A1; NQO1, NADP(H) quinine oxidoreductase.

(*NQO1*) and cytochrome P-450 genes such as *CYP1A1*.[9–11] Defining these polymorphisms and reducing exposures in high-risk groups is a priority.

PATHOPHYSIOLOGY

It is becoming increasingly apparent that AML has a multistep pathogenesis, and an evolving clinical process.

Antecedent Hematologic Disorders

Approximately 40% of patients with AML have a documented abnormality in blood counts for at least 1 month prior to presentation (unpublished M. D. Anderson data). The antecedent hematologic disorder is usually a myelodysplastic syndrome, itself caused by a stem cell–damaging process causing mutation, translocation, or the like, that has remained stable for some time. Evidence for this hypothesis comes from study of patients with a familial platelet disorder that is characterized by thrombopenia and myelodysplasia.[12] Affected individuals have an *AML1/ETO* fusion gene, in which *AML1* (also known as *RUNX1*) is inappropriately juxtaposed to *ETO*, as described later with respect to t(8;21). However, familial platelet disorder patients do not develop AML unless additional cytogenetic aberrations develop.[12] The frequency of activating mutations increases during evolution of the hematologic abnormalities. Shih and colleagues[13] found that the frequency of internal tandem duplications (ITDs) in the *FMS*-like tyrosine kinase (*FLT3*) gene and of N-*ras* mutations increased during progression from myelodysplastic syndrome to AML. *FLT3* ITDs were more frequent in the paired samples at the AML stage (3/70 vs. 10/70) as were N-*ras* mutations (5/70 vs. 15/70).

Transcription Factor Fusions as Inhibitors of Normal Differentiation

Balanced reciprocal chromosomal translocations, or functionally equivalent inversions, are found in 25% of AML patients under age 60. There are at least 25–30 such translocations, further defined in Chapter 27. Chief among them are (p11;q22)(inv16), t(8;21)(q22;q22), and t(15;17)(q22;q11). These translocations affect transcription factors and can be classified into a few subgroups according to the particular transcription factor fusions that result[14] (Table 28–3). A prototype example are translocations involving core-binding factor (CBF). CBF is a transcription factor that contains α and β subunits;

TABLE 28–3. Transcription Factor Fusions in Human Leukemias

Translocation	Fusion Gene
Core-Binding Factor (*CBF*)	
t(8;21)(q22;q22)	*AMLI/ETO*
t(3;21)(q26;q22)	*AMLI/EVII*
inv(16)(p11;q22)	*CBFβ/SMMHC*
Retinoic Acid Receptor-α (*RARα*)	
t(15;17)(q22;q11)	*PML/RARα*
t(5;17)(q31;q11)	*NPM/RARα*
t(11;17)(p13;q11)	*PLZF/RARα*
***HOX* Family Members**	
t(7;11)(p15;p15)	*NUP98/HOXA9*
t(2;11)(q31;q15)	*NUP98/HOXD13*
t(12;13)(p13;q12)	*TEL/CDX2*
***ETS* Family Members**	
t(12;22)(p13;q11)	*MNI/TEL*
t(16;21)(p11;q22)	*TLS/ERG*

From Gilliland DG, Griffin JD: The roles of *FLT3* in hematopoiesis and leukemia. Blood 100:1532–1542, 2002, with permission.

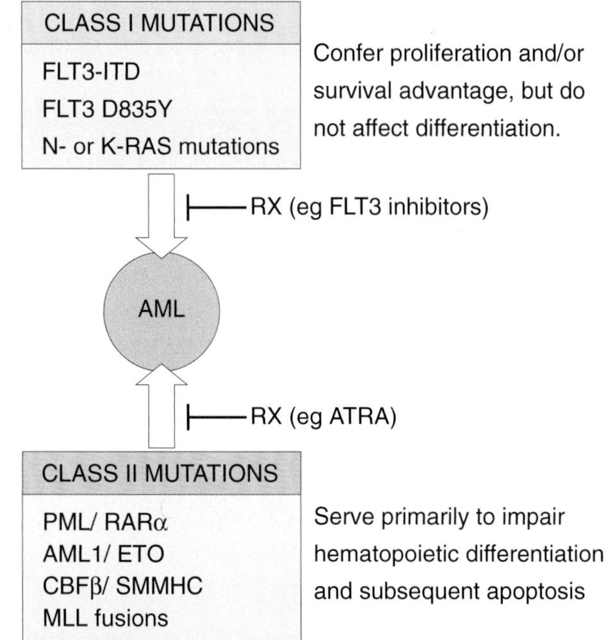

Figure 28–2. It has been hypothesized that two types of mutations act in concert to produce AML. Hence, treatment should encompass (at least) two therapies designed to reverse the effects of these mutations. (See Downing[122] for details.)

CBF-α is also called AML-1. CBF regulates expression of various genes important in normal hematopoietic differentiation; included are genes for cytokines and cytokine receptors. Indeed, mouse models in which both *AML1* alleles are "knocked out" lack definitive hematopoiesis and undergo early embryonic death. The t(8;21) translocation and the other translocations involving *AML1* depicted in Table 28–3 result in disruption of *AML1*, for example, by forming *AML1/ETO* in the case of t(8;21). The AML-1/ETO fusion protein acts as a "dominant negative" inhibitor of the normal *AML1* gene because ETO recruits corepressors, including histone deacetylases, to CBF promoters, a process confirmed by *AML/ETO* "knock-in" mouse models.[14] AML-1/ETO also inhibits the promoter for the *C/EBPα* gene, resulting in suppressed expression of C/EBP-α, a transcription factor crucial for granulocyte differentiation.[15] The effect of inv(16) or t(16;16) is similar to that of t(8;21), but with involvement of the CBF-β subunit of CBF rather than the CBF-α (AML-1) subunit. For this reason, t(8;21), inv(16), and t(16;16) are frequently considered together as CBF AML.

An analogous picture of transcription factor fusions and dominant negative inhibition of normal promoters occurs with APL[16,17] and is covered in Chapter 30. Other corepressors involved are members of the homeobox (HOX) and ETS families (see Table 28–3).

FLT3 Internal Tandem Duplications and *ras* Mutations Convey a Survival or Proliferative Advantage

FLT-3 is a receptor tyrosine kinase and a member of a family that includes the platelet-derived growth factor receptor and c-Kit.[18] The FLT-3 ligand stimulates proliferation of AML blasts synergistically with cytokines such as G-CSF or granulocyte-macrophage colony-stimulating factor. These findings suggest that FLT-3 plays a role in survival and proliferation of AML blasts; its downstream effectors are being identified. Ten percent to 30% of patients with AML have ITDs in the juxtamembrane domain of *FLT3;* ITDs are the most common genetic aberration in AML, are disproportionately frequent in patients with t(15;17) or a normal karyotype, are very infrequent in patients with abnormalities of chromosomes 5 and/or 7, and appear to confer a poor prognosis with conventional therapy, particularly when both alleles are affected.[19–20] A smaller proportion of patients (<5%) have mutations in the activation loop of *FLT3,* and some patients appear to have high levels of *FLT3* transcripts without an ITD or mutation; these patients also appear to have a poor prognosis.[21] Both ITDs and activation loop mutations are thought to result in loss of FLT-3 autoinhibition. As a result, FLT-3 kinase is constitutively activated, providing a proliferative or survival advantage. N- or K-*ras* mutations occur in less than 10% of patients and have had no consistent effect on prognosis. Like *FLT3* aberrations, *ras* mutations are also thought to confer a survival or proliferative advantage to the affected blasts. *FLT3* ITD or *ras* mutations alone may not be sufficient, because mouse models of these processes develop only a myeloproliferative syndrome, not AML.[18]

Two-Hit Model for Development of AML

The two-hit model suggests that (at least) two types of mutations must be present for AML to develop[18] (Fig. 28–2; see Table 28–3). "Class I" mutations, which include *FLT3* ITDs, *FLT3* activating loop mutations, c-*kit* mutations, and N- or K-*ras* mutations, convey a survival or proliferative advantage. "Class II" mutations impair differentiation, thus inhibiting apoptosis. Mouse models of individual mutations show synergy in leukemogenesis when combined.[22] Infrequently, patients have mutations of only a single gene, such as *FLT3* and *ras* or inv(16), t(8;21), t(15;17) and *MLL* fusions (*MLL* is an upstream effector of *HOX* gene expression). In these cases it is postulated that a second, currently cryptic, genetic lesion is also present. Thirty percent of patients with APL have *FLT3* ITDs (class I) in addition to *PML/RAR* ITDs (class II).[19]

Role of Epigenetics

Epigenetics refers to the presence, sometimes perpetuated by clonal inheritance, of changes in gene expression without genetic changes. Epigenetic phenomena have the same functional effects as mutations and are mediated through DNA methylation and histone modification attracting histone deacetylases that inhibit gene expression. In mammals, DNA methylation affects cytosine, but only when it is part of a CpG dinucleotide. Abnormal methylation of promoter CpG "islands" silences gene expression in malignant cells. Recently, it was found that epigenetic silencing may also occur with histone H3 lysine 9 methylation.[23]

Epigenetic silencing associated with promoter methylation occurs in AML.[24] This includes genes involved in cell cycle regulation (p15 and p16, methylated in 30–90% of cases) and apoptosis (DAP kinase, methylated in 40% of cases). Younger patients with a high degree of methylation at multiple loci have an unexpectedly poor outcome despite the absence of chromosomal abnormalities,[24] whereas in other settings an improved survival may occur.[25]

Proteolytic Processing

MLL fusion genes generated as a consequence of translocations involving 11q are thought to contribute to development of AML through dysregulated *HOX* gene expression.[26] Hsieh and coworkers have identified a novel protease, taspase 1, that cleaves MLL and is required for *HOX* gene expression.[27] Assuming taspase 1 cleavage sites are preserved in the *MLL* fusions, a taspase 1 inhibitor might impair expression of selected *HOX* genes and have a role in therapy of AML.

PML/RAR-α can undergo cleavage by neutrophil elastase expressed in promyelocytes. Mice deficient in this protease do not develop APL after introduction of PML/RAR-α.[28] This may occur with other AML fusion proteins as well (see Table 28–3).

CLINICAL FEATURES AND DIAGNOSIS

As indicated by the word "leukemia" ("white blood"), AML was first recognized because of the tremendous excess in white blood cell count seen in some patients with the disease. However, most patients with AML present with low or normal white blood cell counts and seek medical attention because of such anemia-related symptoms as fatigue, weakness, or dyspnea on exertion. Presentation with bleeding or infection is considerably rarer. Bleeding, particularly in the presence of a low white blood cell count, should bring to mind the possibility of APL, which frequently requires urgent treatment. Most AML patient present with an abnormal blood count and symptoms; less than 5% of cases are asymptomatic. The physical examination should focus on detecting evidence of infection, in particular fever and/or bleeding (petechiae, bruises), because administration of antibiotics and platelet transfusions is principally governed by such observations. Lymphadenopathy and splenomegaly may also be present.

Both blood smear and marrow analysis, as discussed in Chapter 27, demonstrate an excess of blasts. These blasts can be shown by histochemical stains (e.g., peroxidase or nonspecific esterase) or by immunophenotyping (e.g., positive for CD33 or CD13) to be myeloid in origin. In some cases, the diagnosis can be made based on an excess (e.g., >5–10%) of myeloblasts in the peripheral blood. Indeed, in cases with greater than 10,000 circulating blasts, analyses of cytogenetic and *FLT3* status can be successfully done using peripheral blood, but a bone marrow aspirate and biopsy provide more accurate information.[29] In addition, marrow cellularity and cytogenetic analysis should be routine if the possibility of AML is entertained. Other essential components of the initial evaluation are serum chemistries (particularly creatinine, uric acid, and bilirubin), coagulation tests, chest radiograph, electrocardiogram, and, in patients under age 70–75, human lymphocyte antigen (HLA) typing of the patient and siblings, bearing in mind the possibility of allogeneic stem cell transplantation (SCT). Note that a high blast count can give rise to spurious hypoxia, hypoglycemia, and hyperkalemia.

DIFFERENTIAL DIAGNOSIS

In general, the diagnosis of AML is straightforward given that blasts or abnormal promyelocytes are readily apparent in blood or marrow and can be easily shown to be myeloid in origin. In a few instances there is a departure from this pattern:

1. *"Dry tap"*—An inaspirable marrow is more likely in patients with the acute megakaryocytic version of AML (M7 in the French-American-British [FAB] classification system)[30,31] because of the degree of fibrosis. Blasts are positive for CD41 or show platelet peroxidase positivity on electron microscopy.
2. *Excess of monocytes or erythroid cells*—The presence of greater than 80% monocytes is considered diagnostic of acute monocytic leukemia (FAB M5b). However, greater than 50% normoblasts and pronormoblasts suggests erythroleukemia (FAB M6).
3. *Negative histochemistry and surface markers*—Patients whose blasts show no evidence of myeloid or lymphoid differentiation have acute undifferentiated leukemia and are treated as having AML, FAB type

MO. Point mutations in the *AML1* gene have been found in 25% of these cases.[32] These patients have a poor prognosis.

Distinction from Myelodysplastic Syndrome

The FAB system uses 30% blasts as the minimal diagnostic criterion for AML,[30] whereas the World Health Organization system sets the threshold at 20%.[33] Patients below these cutoffs but with excess blasts (>5%) have myelodysplastic syndrome. However, the decision to treat a patient as having AML rather than myelodysplastic syndrome should rest at least as much on the clinical as on the morphologic picture, and may have similar outcome.[34,35]

Natural History

Historical data suggest that untreated AML has a median survival of 6 months.[36] Moreover, trials comparing supportive care with chemotherapy show worse survival and similar morbidity in the supportive care group.[37] Nonetheless, some older patients with untreated AML, a good performance status, and a low white blood cell count can survive up to 2 years after diagnosis, but there are no good predictors of this group. Thus, emphasis should be placed on treatment of all patients with AML who are younger than age 70–75 and have a good performance status.

TREATMENT

Conventional Treatment

For the past 30 years, conventional treatment of AML has been based on combinations of anthracyclines and cytosine arabinoside (ara-C) designed to induce marrow hypoplasia, leading to restoration of normal blood counts. Conventional remission induction therapy consists of a combination of an anthracycline such as daunorubicin at 45–60 mg/m^2 daily on days 1–3 (or, interchangeably, idarubicin at 12 mg/m^2 on days 1–3) and ara-C given by continuous infusion at 100–200 mg/m^2 daily on days 1–7; this combination is called "3+7." Subsequent management of the patient is illustrated in Figure 28–3.

Therapy of AML is traditionally divided into remission induction and postremission phases. A complete remission reflects successful reduction in the blast count and restoration of hematopoiesis. Complete remission is essentially defined by a marrow with less than 5% blasts and sufficient functionality to produce platelet and neutrophil counts greater than 100,000/mm^3 and 1000/mm^3 respectively.[38] Once complete remission is maintained for 3 years, the risk of relapse declines markedly to only 5–10%, at which time the patient can be considered "potentially cured."[39] Patients who achieve complete remission, even if not cured, live longer proportionate to the time spent in complete remission.[36] Various less stringent response criteria ("minor response," "hematologic improvement") have been proposed. Such responses have had much less effect on prolonging survival than has complete remission[40] (Fig. 28–4).

Prognostic Factors and Their Use in Planning Treatment

Conventional therapy produces a complete remission rate of about 60% and a median complete remission duration of approximately 1 year. Median survival time is about the same. Approximately 10–15% of patients are alive in remission 3 years after beginning treatment ("potentially cured").[39] However, the heterogeneity in AML and prognostic features leads to complete remission rates in subgroups that range from less than 30% to greater than 90%, with less than 5% to greater than 60–70% of patients potentially cured. This variability makes it inadvisable to speak of "the outcome" of treatment for AML.

Patients with AML fail to be cured either because treatment is too toxic, leading to treatment-related mortality, or because the disease is resistant to treatment, leading to failure to achieve complete remission or, more commonly, only a brief complete remission. Treatment-related mortality should be limited to death in the first 3 weeks of treatment. Thereafter, most deaths are related to persistent disease, often with profound myelosuppression.

Despite the difficulties in separating treatment-related mortality and resistance, the prognostic factors that predict for these outcomes can be distinguished (Table 28–4). These include a Zubrod performance status of 3–4,[41] increasing age,[42] abnormal organ function, and prognostically unfavorable cytogenetics. Inherited polymorphisms in genes that metabolize carcinogens and chemotherapeutic agents or function in repair of DNA damage are also likely to be important. African American males (although not females) have shorter survival than whites, which also suggests additional genetic factors.[43]

Pretreatment cytogenetic status is the principal covariate predicting resistance to conventional therapy[44–48] (Table 28–5). Patients are typically divided into better,

TABLE 28–4. Prognostic Factors Following Administration of Conventional Therapy

	Predictors of Treatment-Related Mortality	Predictors of Resistance to Treatment
Established	Performance status Age Organ function Serum albumin	Cytogenetics Type of presentation: de novo vs. secondary or after antecedent hematologic disorder Status of *FLT3* gene Presence of multidrug resistance (MDR) protein *MLL* gene duplications
Less well established	Inherited polymorphisms in genes concerned with metabolism of carcinogens	*C/EBPα* gene mutations Expression of *BAALC* gene Inherited polymorphisms in carcinogen-metabolizing or DNA repair genes

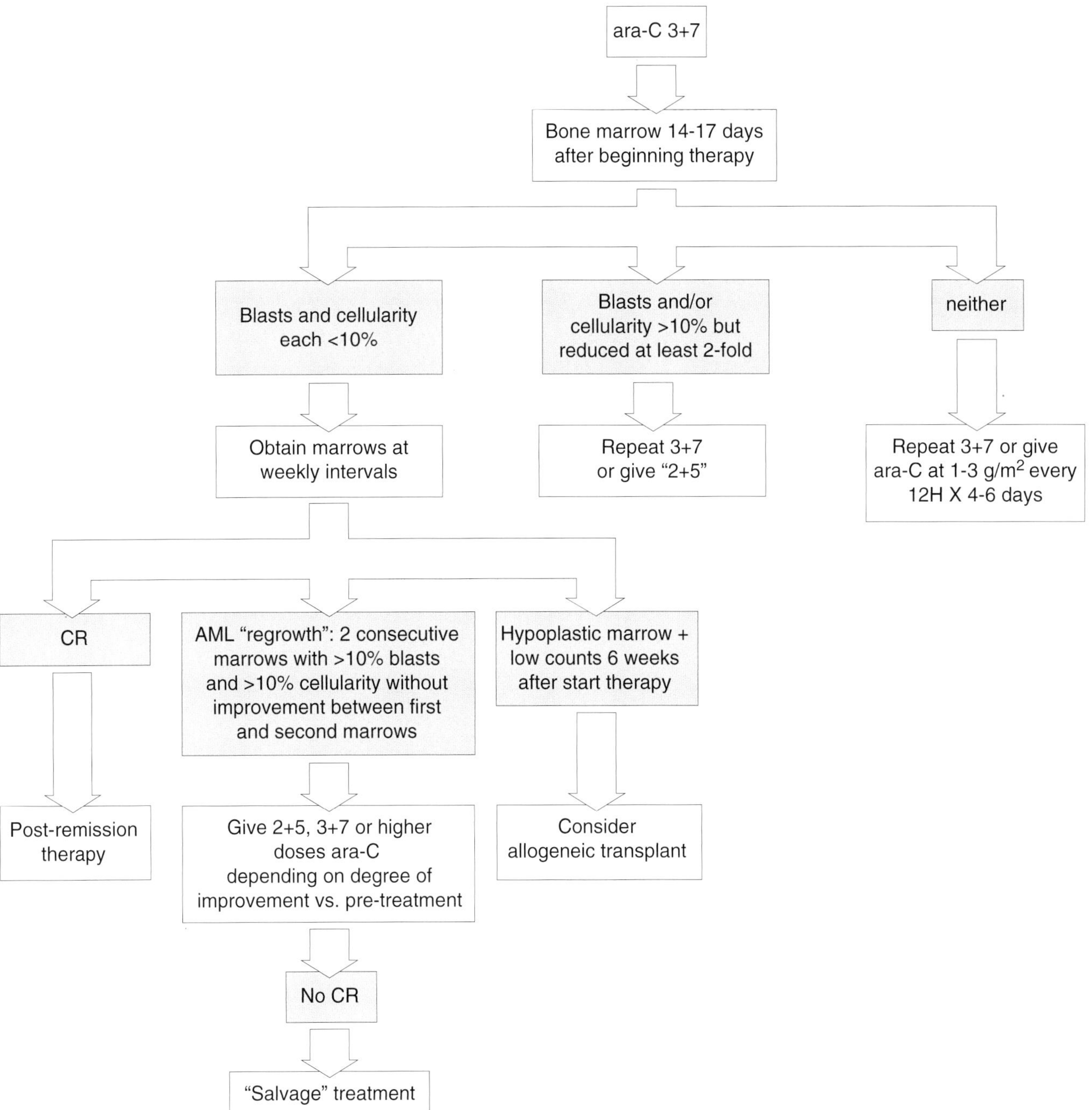

Figure 28–3. Standard management of remission induction for AML.

intermediate, and worse groups. The better group consists of patients with CBF AML, as described earlier. The most commonly occurring worse prognosis abnormalities are monosomies of chromosomes 5 and/or 7(–5,–7) or deletions of the long arms of these chromosomes (5q–,7q–); henceforth this group is referred to as "–5/–7" (see Table 28–1). These abnormalities generally occur in a complex pattern with multiple clonal abnormalities.

Currently technology using polymerase chain reaction rather than karyotype to diagnose abnormalities has been controversial, with the Cancer and Leukemia Group B (CALGB) finding only infrequent abnormalities[49] and the Medical Research Council (MRC) finding more common abnormalities, in particular 31 of 84 patients with inv(16) or t(8;21).[50,51] For the moment, cytogenetic analysis is standard.[52]

Prior myelodysplastic syndrome and –5/–7 abnormalities appear to predict resistance.[34,53] Similarly, in patients with a normal karyotype,[19,21,54,55] the presence of *FLT3* ITDs, mutations, and high levels of *FLT3* transcripts[22] are independent predictors of a higher relapse rate. Increased P-glycoprotein (MDR-1) increases efflux of anthracyclines, particularly in older patients, and increases resistance to induction therapy.[55–57] In contrast, duplications in the *MLL* gene, which are present in 5–10% of patients with a normal karyotype, appear to have rel-

TABLE 28–5. Effect of Predictors of Therapeutic Resistance on Outcome with Conventional Therapy

Predictor	CR Rate	Long-Term CR Rate	Reference
Cytogenetics:			44–48
Inv(16), t(8;21)	80–95%	≥50%	
−5/−7, abnormal 3q, 11q	30–50%	<5%	
Other karyotypes and normal	50–80%	10–25%	
De novo presentation	50–80%	<10% to 50%	34,54
History abnormal counts, secondary AML	40–70%	<10% to 20%	
Wild-type *FLT3* (age <60)	85%	55%	19 (also see 54,55)
FLT3 ITD (age <60)	80%	35%	56 (also see 57)
MDR negative (age >55)	60%	Depends on cytogenetics, type of presentation, *FLT3* status	
MDR positive (age >55)	30%		
Patients age <60 with normal karyotype:			59 (also see 58)
Without *MLL* gene duplications	89%	40%	
With *MLL* gene duplications	78%	<5%	

Abbreviation: CR, complete remission.

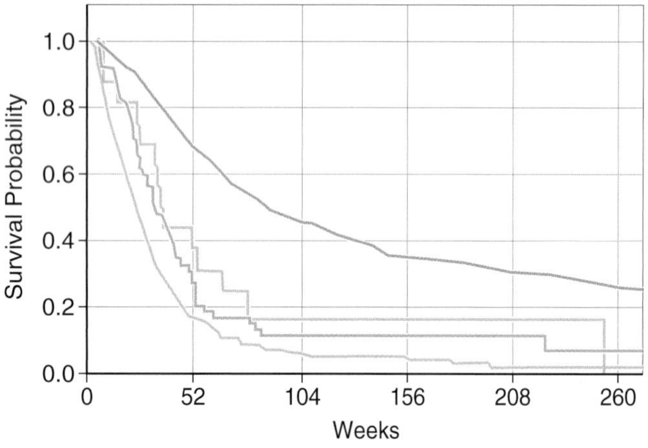

KEY

	Total	Fail	Subset
—	946	636	CR in 1 course
—	184	66	>5% blasts
—	64	53	<5% blasts, no CRp
—	17	14	CRp

Figure 28–4. M. D. Anderson data showing effect of type of response on survival time dated from complete remission (CR) date (946 patients) or date when patient was declared resistant (no CR, 265 patients) to initial induction therapy. Seventeen of the 265 resistant patients had a "CRp" designation; that is, they met all criteria for CR but their platelet count remained less than 100,000/mm^3, although they did not require platelet transfusions. Another 64 of the 265 had less than 5% marrow blasts at resistance date, but did not meet criteria for CRp, and 184 had greater than 5% marrow blasts at resistance date. Results were not affected by differences in times to CR, CRp, less than 5% marrow blasts, or greater than 5% marrow blasts. (See de Lima and colleagues[39] for details.)

atively little effect on achievement of complete remission, but shorten remission duration.[58,59]

Table 28–6 indicates important prognostic information that can guide therapy. There are three fundamental treatment options: no therapy other than transfusions and antibiotics, conventional therapy, and investigational therapy. The "no treatment" option is viable only in patients in whom the likelihood of treatment-related mortality is similar to or greater than the likelihood of complete remission and for whom investigational therapy is not an option (see Table 28–4).

TABLE 28–6. Prognostic Information to be Obtained at Diagnosis

Mandatory	Suggested
Cytogenetics (better vs. intermediate vs. worse)	Presence of MDR-1 protein
Age (<60 vs. >59)	*MLL* gene status (duplicated vs. normal)
Zubrod performance status (0–2 vs. 3–4)	
Serum bilirubin and creatinine (<1.6 vs. >1.5)	
Abnormal blood count for >1 month (yes vs. no)	
Secondary AML (yes vs. no)	
FLT3 gene status (ITD or mutation vs. normal)	

Usually therapeutic decisions in AML revolve around whether a patient should receive conventional or investigational therapy. Conventional treatment in patients age 60+ is associated with a mortality rate of 30% or greater by 10 weeks. Many patients can wait 2–4 weeks before beginning treatment to allow cytogenetic and *FLT3* analyses that can guide treatment toward that most likely to benefit the patient.

Eventually, mathematical predictive models may be used. However, current recommendations focus on specific groups of AML patients. Figure 28–5 depicts survival in three groups following induction therapy: (1) inv(16), t(16;16), or t(8;21) (i.e., CBF AML); (2) non–CBF AML in patients age 60+ years ("older patients"); and (3) non–CBF AML in patients younger than 60 ("younger patients"). Similar results by group were obtained with idarubicin + ara-C or analogous regimens (fludarabine + ara-C ± idarubicin; topotecan + ara-C ± cyclophosphamide).[60] Within each of the latter two groups, out-

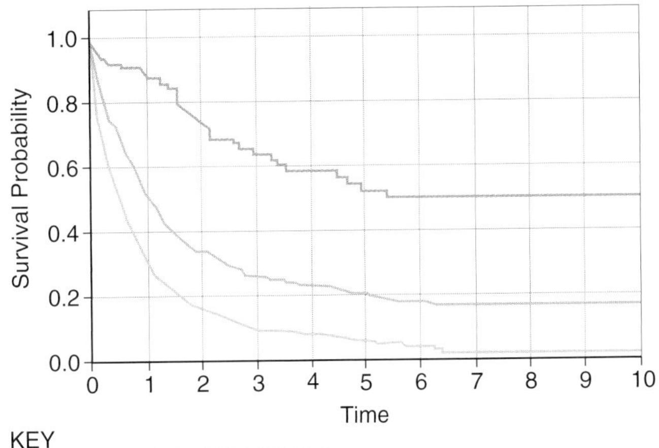

Figure 28–5. Survival from start of treatment for three different groups (M. D. Anderson data).

comes can also be stratified by adverse risk factors, including worse prognosis cytogenetics (see Table 28–5), presence of a *FLT3* ITD or mutation, Zubrod performance status greater than 2, an antecedent hematologic disorder, secondary AML, serum bilirubin or creatinine each greater than 1.6 mg/dL, or MDR positivity.

CBF AML

Patients with inv(16), t(8;21), or the much rarer t(16;16) comprise less than 10% of unselected cases. Approximately 85% are under age 60. Although frequently associated with FAB subtype M4EO, 40% of the 112 M. D. Anderson cases of inv(16) seen in the past 25 years have had less than 5% marrow eosinophils. Similarly, although t(8;21) AML is most often associated with FAB subtype M2, 30% of the 94 cases of t(8;21) AML were not. Treatment including high-dose (2–3 gm/m^2 per dose) or intermediate-dose (1–2 gm/m^2 per dose) ara-C either as induction or consolidation therapy cures greater than 50% of patients under age 60 (see Fig. 28–5).[61] Virtually all relapses are observed within 5 years. [The cumulative incidence of relapse 8 years from complete remission date, corresponding to the median follow-up time, is 21 ± 10% in patients with t(8;21) and 43 ± 10% in patients with inv(16). In contrast, the cumulative incidence of relapse in patients given one course of high-dose ara-C is 64 ± 9% for t(8;21) and 70 ± 11% for inv(16).[62]] A slightly different regimen used by the MRC[44] involves standard induction therapy followed by two courses of ara-C at 1 gm/m^2 daily for 5 courses plus an anthracycline. Survival and sustained remission rates were similar to the CALGB results: 30% relapse at 5 years among 122 t(8;21) patients and 42% among 57 inv(16) patients. Several groups have noted that survival is superior in inv(16) patients. This superiority reflects the frequent ability to induce multiple complete remissions in inv(16) AML.

Thus, in these variants, neither SCT (allogeneic or autologous) nor investigational regimens are commonly used. The rare cases of t(16;16) have a prognosis similar to cases with inv(16), and patients with deletion 16q [del(16q)] have prognoses more reminiscent of those seen in normal-karyotype AML than in patients with inv(16); these observations may reflect the association between t(16;16), but not del(16q), and disruption of CBF.

The principal prognostic covariate in t(8;21) AML following treatment with high-dose or intermediate-dose ara-C is the initial white blood cell count.[63] Similarly, age less than 35 versus greater than 35 is the chief predictor of prognosis in inv(16) AML,[64] with relapse-free survival probabilities at 3 years of 67% versus 30%. After accounting for these prognostic covariates, outcome in both t(8;21) and inv(16) AML was unaffected by dose of ara-C (1 gm/m^2 vs. 3 gm/m^2) or use of SCT. Other genetic changes may also affect prognosis, including fusion transcripts [*AML1/ETO* for t(8;21), *CBFβ/MYH11* for inv(16)][65,66] and mutations in the c-Kit tyrosine kinase.[67]

For high-risk patients, investigational approaches including fludarabine (30 mg/m^2 daily on days 1–5) and ara-C (2 gm/m^2 daily on days 1–5) may be reasonable.[68] After induction, three postremission courses of ara-C (2 gm/m^2 every 12 hours on days 1, 3, and 5) are included. Other agents, including histone deacetylase inhibitors, are in early clinical trials. Figure 28–6 provides a suggested treatment algorithm for patients with CBF AML.

AML in Older Patients (Age ≥ 60 Years)

Three important features of AML in older patients (age > 55–60) are the high rate of treatment-related mortality, the low complete remission rate, and the high relapse rate in patients who survive initial treatment. Thus, 32% of the 1006 patients age 60+ treated at M. D. Anderson since 1991—excluding the less than 5% of older patients with t(8;21), inv(16), or APL—died within 10 weeks of beginning induction chemotherapy (treatment-related mortality). This time roughly corresponds to the time needed to evaluate two courses of chemotherapy, with 5% of the deaths occurring in patients in complete remission. The complete remission rate was 47%.[69] Furthermore, only 42% of patients age 55+ are given treatment with curative intent,[70] and the proportion referred to academic centers for such treatment may also be relatively low.

The data in Table 28–7 should be discussed with patients to help them decide whether to receive conventional rather than investigational therapy. Not all clinical trials provide better results, so a fully informed patient is essential. For example, a trial in which patients age 60+ were randomized to receive 3+7 etoposide with or without the MDR-1 inhibitor PSC8333 was terminated early because of excess treatment-related mortality and morbidity in the PSC833 arm, despite dose reductions in daunorubicin and etoposide designed to reduce treatment-related mortality.[71] Conventional therapy may thus be optimal in the better prognosis subset of older patients.[72] Others, such as those with worse prognosis

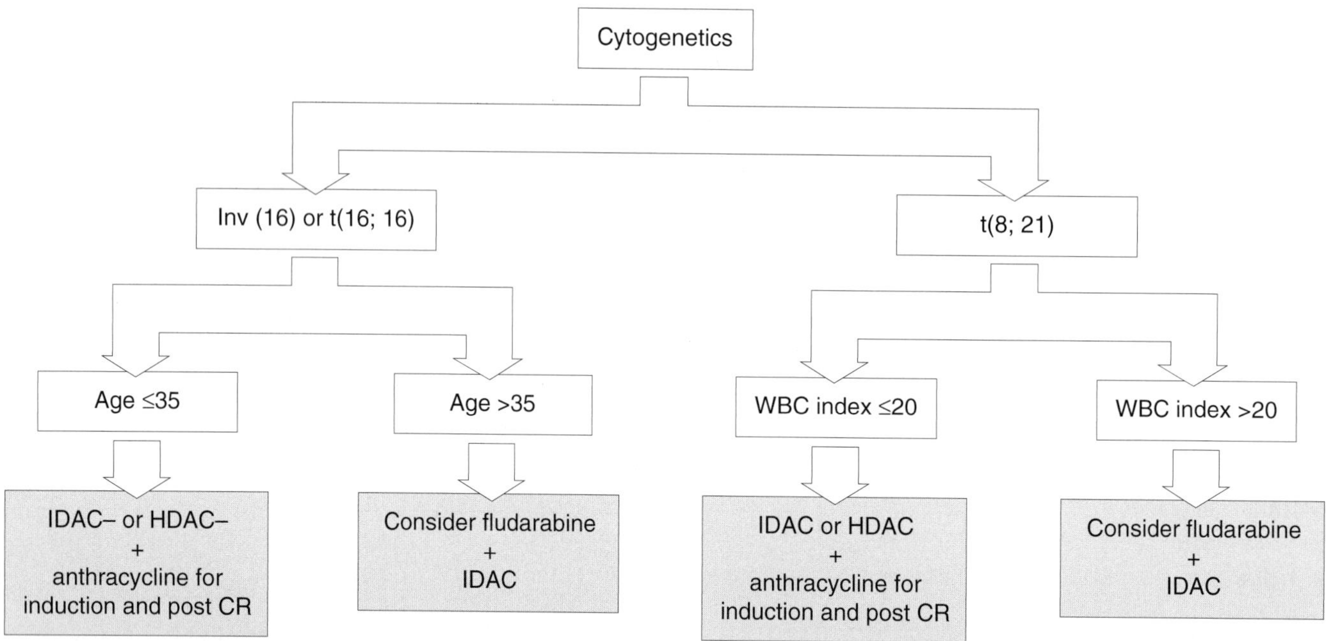

Figure 28–6. Suggested management of patients with inv(16), t(16;16), or t(8;21). The white blood cell (WBC) index is the initial WBC count × initial % marrow blasts/100. (See Byrd and colleagues[62] and Nguyen and coworkers[63] for details.)

TABLE 28–7. Probabilities of Event-Free Survival (EFS) and Survival in Patients Age 60+

	All Patients (n = 1006)		Better Prognosis Patients (n = 199)		Worse Prognosis Patients (n = 807)	
Months from Start of Therapy	**EFS Probability (i.e., Alive in CR)**	**Survival Probability**	**EFS Probability**	**Survival Probability**	**EFS Probability**	**Survival Probability**
6	28%	50%	50%	65%	23%	46%
12	16%	30%	32%	46%	13%	26%
24	9%	16%	18%	32%	7%	11%
36	6%	10%	10%	21%	5%	7%

Abbreviation: CR, complete remission.

cytogenetics, a *FLT3* ITD or mutation, or poor performance status[72], should opt for trials of new agents; this recommendation is supported by the National Cooperative Cancer Network (NCCN), a consortium of academic centers.[73]

Current Approaches to Investigational Therapy

"Targeted" Therapies

Targeted therapies are those with a defined target thought to be relatively specific to AML cells. Examples include the farnesyl transferase inhibitor tipifarnib (R115777),[74] originally developed as a Ras inhibitor because farnesylation is a critical step in Ras processing; the FLT-3 inhibitors PKC412,[75,76] CEP701,[77] and SU5416[78]; inhibitors (e.g., PTK787[79]) of other receptor tyrosine kinases; the histone deacetylase inhibitors SAHA and depsipeptide; and the demethylating agent decitabine.[80] Early studies suggest that targeted therapies are less likely to produce treatment-related mortality and morbidity than is chemotherapy, with which they are thus contrasted. However, these studies also suggest that complete remission rates may be lower with chemotherapy than targeted therapy, although targeted therapy can produce "minor responses." Whether complete remission is requisite for a prolongation in survival with targeted therapy, as it is with chemotherapy,[40] is unknown, although results with R115777 suggest that minor responses may be considerably more useful than no response.[74] However, because survival appears similar with the targeted therapies tested to date and with chemotherapy[76] (E. Estey and J. Karp, unpublished data), there is interest in combinations of targeted therapy with other targeted therapies, or with chemotherapy. An example of the latter is low-dose ara-C (e.g., 20 mg twice daily for 10 days every 28 days). It is quite possible that low-dose ara-C will produce less treatment-related mortality than regimens such as 3 + 7. Data from the MRC suggest that low-dose ara-C is superior to hydroxyurea in prolonging survival in older patients with AML (A. Burnett, personal communication). Hence various combinations of targeted therapy and low-dose ara-C have been proposed. It should be emphasized that, to date, there has been no necessary correlation between the pretreatment status of the supposed target as measured in patient cells and patients' response to the targeted therapy,[74,76] highlighting the difficulty in rationally assigning patients to targeted therapies.

Chemotherapy

It is plausible that new drugs (clofarabine, VNP, triapene), although potentially associated with treatment-related mortality rates similar to those of older drugs, may have more anti-AML effect.[81,82] In principle, these new drugs could be combined with older drugs (e.g., clofarabine + ara-C + idarubicin) or with targeted therapy. Reasons for using new chemotherapy with or without targeted therapy, rather than targeted therapy plus drugs such as low-dose ara-C, as initial therapy include the possibility that only the former will produce complete remission, that complete remission will remain the crucial surrogate for survival, and that, given the natural history of AML in the elderly, unsuccessful use of targeted therapy plus low-dose ara-C as initial therapy will compromise probability of response to the newer chemotherapy.

Figure 28–7 provides a treatment algorithm for older patients.

AML in Younger Patients (Age < 60 Years)

Patients with No Adverse Risk Factors

The complete remission rate among 306 such patients treated at M. D. Anderson since 1991 was 76% and the 10-week mortality (treatment-related mortality) rate only 8% (Table 28–8). These results were produced by treatments containing ara-C at 1–2 gm/m^2 daily for 4–5 days (intermediate-dose ara-C) with either idarubicin, fludarabine, or topotecan.[61] Further support for the use of higher doses of ara-C during induction comes from a meta-analysis of all randomized trials comparing high-dose (2–3 gm/m^2 per dose) and standard dose (100–200 mg/m^2 per dose) ara-C during induction.[83] This analysis indicated that high-dose ara-C (1) improved median and 4-year relapse-free survival and 4-year survival, (2) had no effect on induction results or median survival, (3) led to more frequent infections and central nervous system toxicity, and (4) remained inadequately assessed in patients age 60 and older. Support for use of higher doses of ara-C during postremission therapy comes from a CALGB trial[61] randomizing patients in complete remission to four courses of ara-C at either (1) 3 gm/m^2 every 12 hours on days 1, 3, and 5; (2) 400 mg/m^2 daily on days 1 through 5 by continuous infusion; or (3) 100 mg/m^2 daily on days 1 through 5 by continuous infusion. Following completion of ara-C, patients received four more 3+7-like courses. With more than 8 years of follow-up in younger patients without adverse risk features (but also without CBF AML), the 3-gm/m^2 and the 400-mg/m^2 doses were equivalent and superior to the 100-mg/m^2 ara-C dose, respectively.

Other investigational treatment schedules have been explored. The CALGB, for example, has reported that

TABLE 28–8. Probabilities of Event-Free Survival (EFS) and Survival in Patients Under Age 60

	Better Prognosis Patients ($n = 306$)		Worse Prognosis Patients ($n = 537$)	
Months from Start of Therapy	**EFS Probability**	**Survival Probability**	**EFS Probability**	**Survival Probability**
6	59%	83%	34%	62%
12	43%	66%	20%	42%
24	26%	47%	13%	25%
36	20%	37%	9%	19%

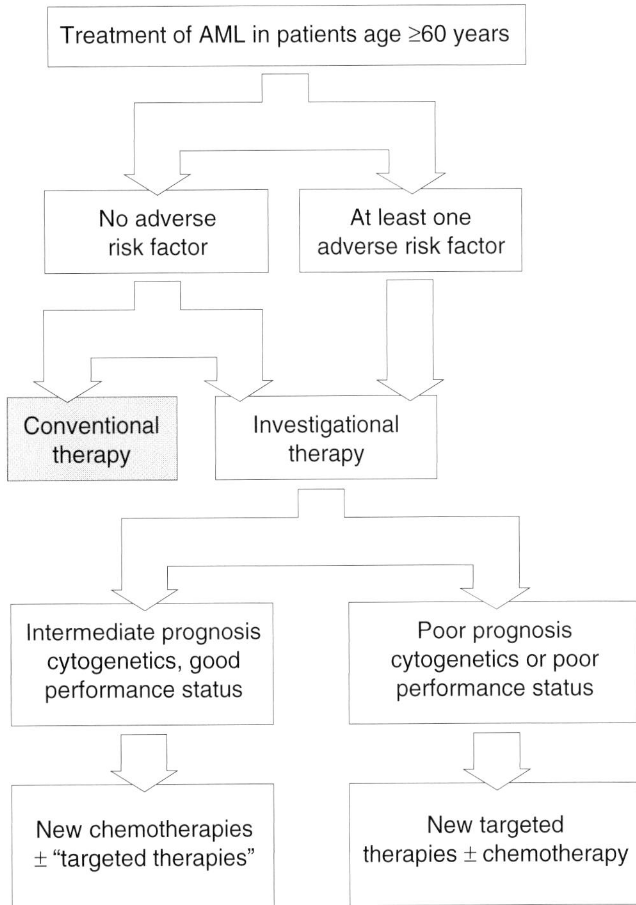

Figure 28–7. Suggested management of AML in older patients. Patients with elevated bilirubin or creatinine can be considered functionally equivalent to those with poor performance status.

patients under age 60 tolerate daunorubicin doses of 90 mg/m^2 daily for 3 days in combination with ara-C at 100 mg/m^2 daily for 7 days and etoposide 100 mg/m^2 daily for 3 days.[84] A French trial[85,86] randomized 600 patients under age 65 among (1) 3+7, using a daunorubicin dose of 80 mg/m^2 daily for 3 days and an ara-C dose of 200 mg/m^2 daily for 7 days, following which a second course began once response to the first course was known (no earlier than day 20); (2) "double induction," in which a second course of chemotherapy (ara-C 1 gm/m^2 daily for 3 days, mitoxantrone 12 mg/m^2 daily for 2 days) began on day 20 regardless of whether the marrow was hypocellular on that day; or (3) "timed-sequential induction," in which the same second course was administered on days 8–10 again regardless of marrow status. Rates of complete remission (76%) and treatment-related mortality (10%) were similar in each arm. However, in patients under age 50, relapse-free survival was longer in the timed-sequential induction arm, although this did not translate into improved survival. Considerable research into postremission treatment is ongoing, including the use of *FLT1* inhibitors and the PR-1 vaccine.[87]

Patients with Adverse Risk Factor(s)

Patients with at least one adverse risk factor have a worse prognosis, and in the M. D. Anderson experience have a treatment-related mortality rate of 24% and a complete remission rate of 52% (see Tables 28–7 and 28–8).

Stem Cell Transplant

The role of autologous and allogeneic transplant for acute leukemias is reviewed in Chapters 94 and 95. Extensive analyses have shown modest but persistent benefits of SCT in appropriate patients.[88–93] However, in no trial does the group assigned to either allo-SCT or auto-SCT have longer survival.[91,93–95] These studies demonstrate decreased relapse rates with allo-SCT and, less strikingly, with auto-SCT. Despite an increase in treatment-related mortality, particularly with allo-SCT, the reduced frequency of relapse more than compensates for the increased frequency of death in complete remission. Using cytogenetics to prognosticate,[93] investigators found a trend for patients with inv(16) or t(8;21) to live longer if assigned to chemotherapy rather than allo-SCT, and patients less than 35 years of age lived longer if presenting with AML containing prognostically intermediate karyotypes. Outcome was poor regardless of treatment modality in patients with a poor-prognosis karyotype.[91,93,96] Even in SCT patients, relapse-free survival in patients transplanted in second complete remission is influenced by length of the first chemotherapy-maintained complete remission.[97] No benefit is seen with SCT in patients with *FLT3* mutations.[98] In short, there is no compelling evidence to recommend that patients in first complete remission receive conventional SCT using HLA-compatible sibling donors.[99] Furthermore, prior to SCT, administration of consolidation therapy does not improve outcome.[100]

TABLE 28–9. Complete Remission (CR) Rates by Duration of First CR in Patients Given IDAC- or HDAC-Containing Regimens for First Salvage at M. D. Anderson, 1991–2004*

Duration of First CR (mo)	Patients	CR (%)
0 (primary refractory)	119	22 (18)
0–6	84	16 (19)
6.1–12	124	27 (22)
>12	133	76 (57)

*APL excluded.
Abbreviations: HDAC, high-dose ara-C; IDAC, intermediate-dose ara-C.

New investigational approaches to transplantation may alter these recommendations. For instance, the role of minitransplants,[94,101–103] the use of intravenous rather than oral busulfan to overcome the erratic pharmacology of the latter,[104] the role of anti-CD45 radiolabeled antibodies,[105] and use of alternative donors (e.g., unrelated cord blood)[106] are all being studied.

Therapy of Relapsed/Refractory AML

Recurrence of AML occurs in most newly diagnosed patients who attain complete remission, and, on average, 20% of patients never enter initial complete remission ("primary refractory"). The most important predictor of outcome in these patients following "salvage" is length of first complete remission, considering primary refractory patients as having a first complete remission duration of 0 (Table 28–9).[107,108] Probabilities of remaining alive in (second) complete remission at 1, 2, and 3 years for the 133 patients with first complete remission duration of greater than 1 year are 38%, 27%, and 24%, and the corresponding survival probabilities are 61%, 25%, and 20%, somewhat better than the average for untreated patients (see Tables 28–7 and 28–8). Because karyotype impacts survival in relapsing patients to the same extent as in de novo patients,[109] the intensity of treatment should consider prognosis. Allo-SCT or auto-SCT should be considered. An allo-SCT should not be delayed until second complete remission, although such delay often occurs in practice for reasons of logistics or because of a high circulating blast count. If an allo-SCT cannot be performed as soon as relapse is recognized, re-induction therapy should include higher dose ara-C. In contrast, if an allo-SCT was given in first complete remission, emphasis might be placed on high-dose ara-C for re-induction and in second complete remission, or, if a second allo-SCT is performed, a different donor might be employed. Complete remission rates less than 25% in patients with first complete remission duration of less than 1 year (see Table 28–9) and worse survival probabilities suggest little benefit from conventional high-dose or intermediate-dose ara-C regimens, whereas a significant long-term survival can be obtained with allo-SCT, which includes patients under 60 with good performance status and organ function who lived at least 3 months after relapse date.

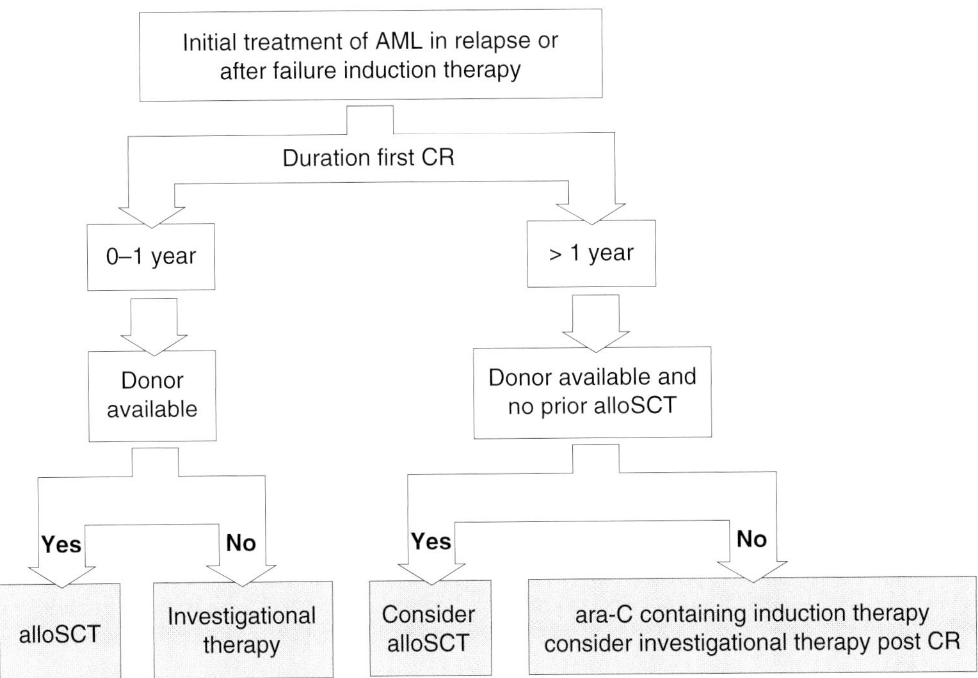

Figure 28–8. Suggested management of patients about to receive first treatment for AML in first relapse or AML that has not responded to initial induction therapy.

If a HLA-matched sibling donor cannot be identified, patients with first complete remission duration of less than 1 year should consider an unrelated SCT (unrelated matched donor or an umbilical cord transplant) or use of investigational agents and agents such as gemtuzumab ozogamycin (GO, Mylotarg),[110] which is approved for use as therapy for untreated AML in older patients.[111] Figure 28–8 provides an algorithm for initial treatment of patients with relapsed/refractory AML.[112] Patients who fail such treatment are prime candidates for investigational therapies.

Emergency Treatment

Although a full characterization of the AML is appropriate to guide therapy in most patients, there are circumstances that dictate emergency treatment:

1. White counts in excess of 50,000/mm^3 or a rapidly rising white count can lead to leukostasis in the lung or brain and thrombosis. Although hydroxyurea and leukapheresis are often used in these circumstances, initiation of an ara-C–containing therapy is more effective given the questionable ability of the former two modalities to eliminate AML in tissues.[113]
2. Dyspnea accompanied by bilateral, symmetrical densities on chest radiograph suggests leukemic infiltration of the lung, particularly if the white blood cell count exceeds 10,000/mm^3 or is rapidly rising, or if the blasts show monocytic features or are CD14, CD64, or CD56 positive.[114] Rapid induction is indicated in this case as well.
3. The well-known risk of fatal hemorrhage associated with APL (FAB M3) prompts the need for urgent treatment (see Chapter 30).
4. Disseminated intravascular coagulation can, rarely, be a feature of AML subtypes other than M3. FAB M5 is notable in this regard.

Treatment should be based on age and performance status. Older patients (age ≥ 60 years) or those with a poor performance status (Zubrod 3–4) should receive 3+7 (see Fig. 28–3). Younger patients with better performance status should receive daunorubicin (60–90 mg/m^2 daily on days 1, 2, and 3) and intermediate-dose ara-C (e.g., 1–2 gm/m^2 daily on days 1–5) or high-dose ara-C (2–3 gm/m^2 every 12 hours on days 1, 3, and 5). Subsequent planning should be based on cytogenetics, *FLT3* gene status, and the like (see Table 28–6).

SUPPORTIVE CARE

Neutropenia and dysfunctional neutrophil function require use of broad-spectrum antibiotic and antifungal agents.[115] A number of studies show the value of prophylaxis with fluconazole[116] or itraconazole[117] during remission induction. Once fever develops, antibiotics can be used as indicated in Figure 28–9. Of note, voriconazole has been suggested to be more effective than amphotericin in treatment of *Aspergillus*.[118]

Numerous studies of granulocyte transfusions have shown benefit, but they should also be considered in older patients and "sicker" younger patients under the following circumstances: (1) pneumonia documented by chest radiograph or chest computed tomography scan,[119] (2) sepsis, and (3) a fever of unknown origin that fails to respond to 3 days of antibiotics. Granulocytes come from donors (relatives or friends) given G-CSF 1 day prior to each of three to four donations per donor. Rarely, respiratory deterioration after granulocyte transfusion can

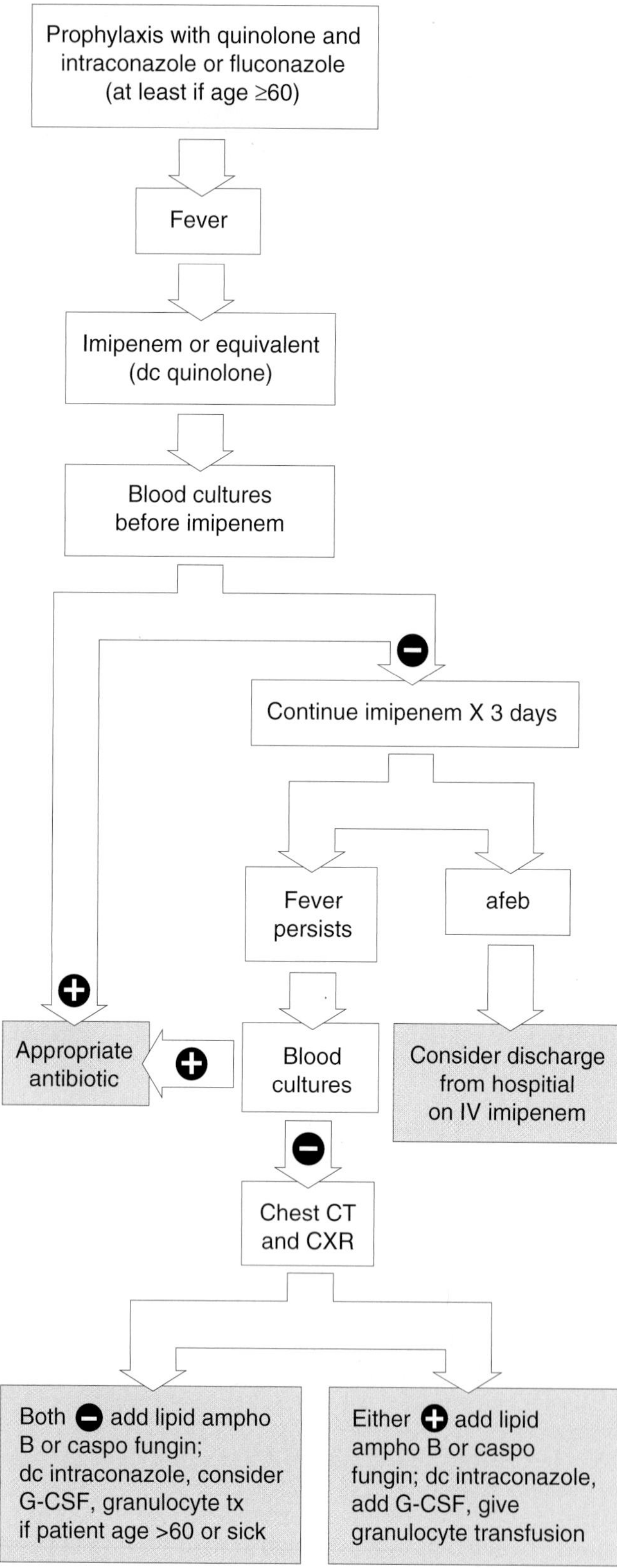

■ **Figure 28–9.** Suggested management of patients with AML and fever with no source obvious on initial physical examination excluding fever within 4 hours of a transfusion or during administration of chemotherapy, in particular ara-C.

occur, although granulocyte migration to the site of infection can give rise to transient deterioration in the chest radiograph despite clinical stability or improvement. G-CSF is also regularly given to patients with documented infection as well as those with severe neutropenia. At many centers, G-CSF is discontinued if no benefit is seen in 3–4 days.

A platelet count less than 10,000/mm^3, or a hemoglobin less than 8.0 gm/dL, triggers transfusions. These values, however, must be considered in clinical context (see Chapter 30). A patient who is bleeding should receive transfusions even if the platelet count is greater than 50,000/mm^3, as should a patient with ischemic heart disease with a hemoglobin of 9–10.0 gm/dL; in contrast, young asymptomatic patients may tolerate hemoglobins of 7.0 gm/dL, particularly if anemia is long-standing. Patients whose platelet count fails to rise after transfusion should only receive transfusions for bleeding or confounding risk such as hypertension, to avoid exacerbating alloimmunization. A randomized trial indicated that in-line filtration of platelet products provides equal benefit from single-donor and pooled random donor platelet sources.[120]

Fluid overload is common during induction therapy both from tumor lysis and from intravenous fluid administration. In some instances, this is viewed as "diffuse alveolar hemorrhage" when diuresis is indicated. Rather, blood seen in bronchial fluid is most often due to inflammation, not hemorrhage.

Neutropenia Precaution Practices

Hospitalization

Although hospitalization is common during induction therapy, in certain parts of the country, routine hospitalization during induction or postremission therapy is discouraged to avoid exposure to hospital infections.[121] If hospitalized, patients should be treated in HEPA-filtered or laminar airflow spaces.

Masks

Commonly, hospital units for patients with hematologic malignancies use neutropenic precautions, including the use of masks. Because bacteria and fungi, rather than viruses, are the typical causes of infection,[115] and most are part of the patient flora, it is unclear whether masks are beneficial; therefore, their use varies across the United States.

Diet

Although fresh fruits and vegetables harbor both bacteria and fungi, their contribution to infection is unclear. They are restricted in many hospitals, but not in all. Likewise, flowers and plants are restricted, although careful studies are lacking on their transmission of infectious agents to patients.

CURRENT CONTROVERSIES & FUTURE CONSIDERATIONS

Acute Myelogenous Leukemia

- Will identification of inherited polymorphisms and gene expression profiles allow "individualization" of therapy in patients with AML based on prognosis and drug metabolism.
- To what extent are epigenetic factors contributory to the etiology or prognosis of AML?
- Is minimal residual disease important to the prognosis of AML?
- What are the most effective therapies for older patients with AML, and will these therapies prolong life?
- What are the best models for drug development in AML, particularly the newer targeted therapies used alone and in combination with conventional agents?
- Will conventional precautionary practices (e.g., avoidance of fresh fruits, vegetables, and flowers; wearing masks; hospitalization during periods of neutropenia) be supported by quantitative evidence?

Suggested Readings*

Bloomfield CD, Lawrence D, Byrd JC, et al: Frequency of prolonged remission after high-dose cytarabine intensification in AML varies by cytogenetic subtype. Cancer Res 58:4173–4179, 1998.

Cheson BD, Bennett JM, Kopecky KJ, et al, for the International Working Group for Diagnosis, Standardization of Response Criteria, Treatment Outcomes, and Reporting Standards for Therapeutic Trials in Acute Myeloid Leukemia: Revised recommendations of the International Working Group for Diagnosis, Standardization of Response Criteria, Treatment Outcomes, and Reporting Standards for Therapeutic Trials in Acute Myeloid Leukemia. J Clin Oncol 21:4642–4649, 2003.

Estey E: How I treat older patients with AML. Blood 96:1670–1673, 2000.

Gilliland DG, Griffin JD: The roles of *FLT3* in hematopoiesis and leukemia. Blood 100:1532–1542, 2002.

Grimwade D, Walker H, Harrison G, et al: The predictive value of hierarchical cytogenetic classification in older adults with AML: analysis of 1,065 patients entered into the MRC AML 11 trial. Blood 98:1312–1320, 2001.

Full references for this chapter can be found on accompanying CD-ROM. 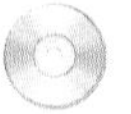

CHAPTER 29

Secondary Myelodysplasia/ Acute Myeloid Leukemia

Carolyn A. Felix, MD

KEY POINTS

Secondary Myelodysplasia/Acute Myeloid Leukemia

- The two broad classes of chemotherapy associated with secondary leukemia and myelodysplasia are alkylating agents and topoisomerase II inhibitors.
- Although most patients receive multimodality treatment and/or combination chemotherapy, the forms of leukemia associated with these agents generally are distinct.
- Alkylating agent–related leukemias have a longer latency; cumulative dose, other treatment factors, and host factors including age and genetic factors influence susceptibility.
- Treatment factors, including cumulative dose and schedule, that may influence the risk of leukemias after topoisomerase II inhibitors are more controversial, but the risk has been higher with particular agents and schedules, and genetic variation in drug-metabolizing enzymes is important.
- Secondary leukemia of both forms is an important complication of autologous hematopoietic stem cell transplantation.
- Cytogenetic features of alkylating agent–related leukemias are complete or partial deletions of chromosomes 5 and 7 and complex, unbalanced numerical and structural cytogenetic abnormalities.
- Putative critical tumor suppressor gene(s) at chromosomes 5q and 7q remain unknown.
- Balanced chromosomal translocations are the primary molecular alterations in leukemias related to topoisomerase II inhibitors, the most common of which involve the *MLL* gene at chromosome band 11q23.
- Alkylating agent–related leukemias typically present with antecedent myelodysplasia, whereas leukemias associated with topoisomerase II inhibitors have heterogeneous presentations characteristic of the underlying translocations—both can be insidious.
- Cytogenetics is an important prognostic factor.
- Most cases of secondary leukemia are resistant to current treatment strategies, but intensive regimens including hematopoietic stem cell transplantation, if feasible based on prior treatment, have been more successful.

INTRODUCTION

About 7% of long-term primary cancer survivors develop second cancers.[1] Second cancers are "secondary" when there are identifiable epidemiologic exposure-disease relationships. Certain individuals are genetically predisposed to developing second cancers, including secondary cancers following particular exposures. The clinical exposures associated with specific secondary cancers are cytotoxic chemotherapy drugs and therapeutic radiation. Leukemias and myelodysplasia (MDS) represent a small fraction of secondary cancers overall (Fig. 29–1) and are linked mainly to chemotherapy exposures. Two broad classes of cytotoxic chemotherapy drugs are associated with secondary leukemia and myelodysplasia: alkylating agents and topoisomerase II inhibitors.[2–4] In contrast, therapeutic radiation has been linked mainly to secondary solid tumors, which are the more common secondary cancers,[5–11] as well as to some cases of leukemia.[12,13] Cytotoxic chemotherapy drugs have been implicated in acute myeloid leukemia (AML) of all morphologic subtypes, myelodysplasia, acute lymphoblastic leukemia, and chronic myelogenous leukemia (reviewed in Felix[4,14]). The majority of patients who develop secondary leukemia/myelodysplasia (60% in one large series) have not received chemotherapy alone,[15] and chemotherapy regimens are likely to contain alkylating agents and topoisomerase II inhibitors.[15] Nonetheless, two major forms of secondary leukemia attributed to alkylating agents or topoisomerase II inhibitors have been recognizable. There are many more reports of chemotherapy-related leukemias in adults than in children[15,16]; however, leukemia has become an increasingly important complication of cytotoxic chemotherapy in children because children are more likely to survive after primary cancer treatment than are adults.[2,17]

EPIDEMIOLOGY AND RISK FACTORS

Alkylating Agent-Related Leukemias

Incidence and Risk

The types of alkylating agents used in anticancer treatment are listed in Table 29–1.[18–20] Alkylating agents are not only cytotoxic but also leukemogenic by virtue of alkylation, the formation of covalent bonds between alkyl groups (i.e., saturated carbon atoms) in the drugs and cellular biomolecules.[18] Oxygen and nitrogen atoms of the DNA bases are targets for alkylation. The first report of alkylating agent–related AML/MDS was in 1970.[21] Virtually all alkylating agents carry some risk of secondary AML/MDS.[15,22] Depending on the specific alkylating agents, the regimens in which they are administered, and the primary cancers (Table 29–2), cumulative risks in adults followed for 4–11 years have ranged from 2% to greater than 20%.[23] Although increasing age at the start of treatment is an important risk factor,[24] dose-intensive pediatric sarcoma regimens have been associated with a similar high incidence.[25] The peak incidence of alkylating agent–related leukemia after Hodgkin's disease occurs at 6 years from the first exposure with a range from 2 to 12 years, after which there is a plateau.[24]

Cumulative alkylating agent dose is a primary determinant of risk, but the different alkylating agents are not equally leukemogenic.[26] The alkylating agent score, which incorporates the number of different alkylating agents given and duration of the treatment, was predictive of risk in pediatric patients with Hodgkin's disease.[27] Melphalan is a more potent leukemogen than cyclophosphamide.[28–30] Regimens with alkylating agents and radiation are more leukemogenic than radiation therapy alone.[24,30,31] Splenectomy for Hodgkin's disease has been implicated in an increased risk of alkylating agent–related acute myeloid leukemia.[32,33]

Cisplatin has been used for anticancer treatment since 1969, but it took more than 2 decades for the leukemia risk to be recognized because of the use of platinum analogues in combination regimens. In a case-control study of women with ovarian cancer who received cisplatin or carboplatin, there was a fourfold increased risk,[34] and platinum analogue–based testicular cancer treatment carries a significant, dose-dependent risk.[35] In children, leukemias with monosomies of chromosomes 5 and 7, characteristic of alkylating agent–related leukemias, have

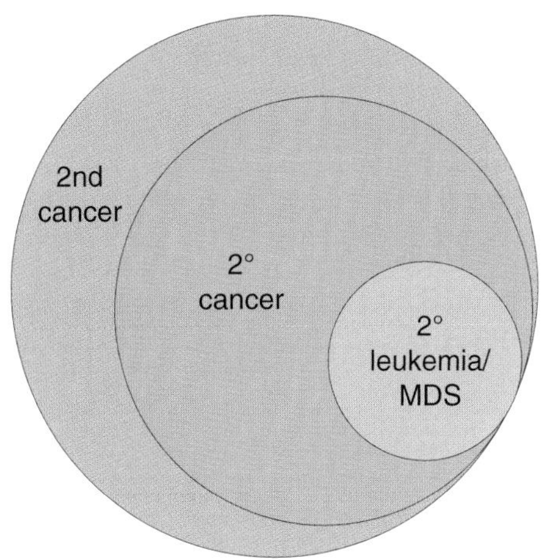

Figure 29–1. Diagram of relationship of secondary leukemia/myelodysplasia to secondary cancers and second cancers overall.

TABLE 29–1. Classification and Features of Alkylating Agents Used in Anticancer Treatment Associated with Secondary Leukemia[18–20,39,400]

Class	Agents	Features
1. Bifunctional	Nitrogen mustards	Form covalent bonds with bases in DNA
	Mechlorethamine	Can cause interstrand crosslinks, which defines bifunctionality
	Mechlorethamine analogues	Form carcinogenic O-6-methylguanine residues
	Melphalan	Can bridge two guanine molecules at N-7 positions
	Chlorambucil	
	Cyclophosphamide	
	Ifosfamide	
	Aziridines	
	Thiotepa	
	Alkyl alkane sulfonates	
	Busulfan	
	Nitrosoureas	
	BCNU (carmustine)	
2. Nonclassic	Procarbazine	Lack bifunctionality
	Dacarbazine	Contain N-methyl groups and form covalent bonds with DNA upon activation
	Temozolomide	
	Hexamethylmelamine	
3. Platinum analogues	Cisplatin	Contain transition metal platinum atom, which forms strong covalent bonds with DNA
	Carboplatin	Form intrastrand N-7-alkyl adducts on adjacent deoxyguanosines or deoxyguanosine and deoxyadenosine
		Form monoadducts and interstrand crosslinks less often

TABLE 29–2. Risk Factors for Alkylating Agent–Related AML/MDS

Treatment Factors	Specific alkylating agent	
	Cumulative dose	
	Chemotherapy regimen (number of alkylating agents used, duration of treatment, intensity of treatment, other leukemogenic drugs)	
	Therapeutic radiation	
	Splenectomy	
	Autologous stem cell transplantation	
Host Factors	Age	
	Primary disease	
	Germline mutations in tumor suppressor genes	*NF1* *TP53*
	Genetic variation in genes encoding DNA damage recognition and repair proteins	*XRCC1* *hMSH2* *XPD*
	Genetic variation in drug-metabolizing enzymes	*CYP3A4* **CYP2D6* **CYP2C19* *GSTT1* *GSTP1* **GSTM1* *NQO1*

Asterisk indicates that polymorphism does not track with any one form of secondary AML/MDS.

been diagnosed after chemotherapy including platinum analogues.[36–38] Platinum analogues also may potentiate the leukemogenicity of topoisomerase II inhibitors such as doxorubicin or etoposide.[39–43]

Alkylating agents are widely used in antecedent conventional chemotherapy and myeloablative conditioning regimens in patients receiving autologous stem cell transplantation, which has a substantial risk of secondary AML/MDS. The risk in this population increases with cumulative alkylating agent dose, age, duration of prior chemotherapy, prior radiation therapy, use of radiation therapy in the conditioning regimen, and repeated transplantations.[44–48] Most often the posttransplant leukemias are characterized by complex numerical and structural karyotypic abnormalities, including loss of chromosomes 5 and 7, the hallmark features of alkylating agent–related acute myeloid leukemia.[47,49,50] The risk is higher after autologous transplantation of peripheral blood stem cells harvested after priming with chemotherapy and cytokines than after bone marrow transplantation without priming.[44,46,47] The commonly early occurrence of the leukemias following autologous stem cell transplantation (often within 12 months) has suggested that the prior chemotherapy and events preceding transplantation are the primary determinants of risk.[47] Detection of the leukemia-associated cytogenetic abnormalities by fluorescent in situ hybridization before the myeloablative conditioning in 9 of 12 cases of posttransplantation myelodysplasia has suggested that the prior chemotherapy caused at least the initial damage.[51] However, the preparative myeloablative chemotherapy and total-body irradiation used for transplantation may contribute to the risk.[47] Whether posttransplantation AML/MDS develops from cells in the infused autograft or from cells in the patient is unknown,[46] but fluorescent in situ hybridization has not detected the chromosomal aberrations in peripheral blood–derived autografts used for transplantation.[52]

Genetic Predisposition

Individuals with germline mutations in certain tumor suppressor genes are genetically predisposed to AML/MDS following alkylating agent treatment. Germline mutations in the *NF1* tumor suppressor gene that activate the Ras signal transduction pathway are associated with an increased risk of myelodysplasia with monosomy 7 after alkylating agent treatment.[53–57]

The p53 protein is central to the cellular DNA damage response pathway. Germline mutations in the p53 tumor suppressor gene have been associated with MDS/AML following alkylating agent treatment[37,38,58] even without a family history of the Li-Fraumeni syndrome.[58] Young children with primary rhabdomyosarcoma are a high-risk population because 23% have germline p53 mutations without a family history of cancer.[59] Germline p53 mutations have been detected in young children with treatment-related MDS/AML characterized by chromosome 5 and 7 deletions after rhabdomyosarcoma treatment.[58,60] Germline p53 mutations are also present in about 3% of children with osteosarcoma without first-degree relatives with cancer.[37,61] The occurrence of secondary acute myeloid leukemia with abnormalities of chromosomes 5, 7, and 17 suggests that alkylating agent–exposed patients with osteosarcoma harboring germline p53 mutations are also at an increased risk.[37,38] The complex numerical and structural karyotypic abnormalities in alkylating agent–related leukemias associated with germline p53 mutations, typically including loss of chromosomes 5, 7, and 17p, are consistent with the genomic instability that accompanies loss of wild-type p53.[37,38,58] The leukemias also may be characterized by segmental jumping translocations in which multiple, intact, amplified copies of oncogenes such as *ABL* or *MLL* are dispersed extrachromosomally and throughout the genome.[60,62,63] Germline p53 mutations contribute to this form of genomic instability when DNA-damaging agents are administered.[60,64,65]

Genetic variation in cellular proteins that recognize and repair alkylating agent–induced DNA damage can modulate the risk, an example of which is the *XRCC1* gene product involved in base-excision repair and repair of single-strand breaks.[66] Reduced DNA repair capacity from a polymorphism in this gene may protect against leukemia, although chemotherapy exposures were not specified.[66] Microsatellite instability is found in a large proportion of adult cases of treatment-related AML/MDS (94%).[67] A polymorphism in the *hMSH2* mismatch repair gene was significantly overrepresented in cases of acute myeloid leukemia following exposures to agents that alkylate at the O-6 position of guanine and was associated with microsatellite instability, possibly suggesting that the *hMSH2* polymorphism predisposes to alkylating agent–related acute myeloid leukemia by inducing mismatch repair mutations.[68] Genetic variation in the *XPD* (xeroderma pigmentosum group D) gene encoding a DNA helicase in the nucleotide excision repair pathway may protect against myeloid cell death after alkylating agent treatment and has been implicated in the predisposition to this form of acute myeloid leukemia.[69]

The risk of secondary AML/MDS is further modulated by genetic variations in phase I and phase II drug metabolism pathways. Phase I metabolism by cytochrome P-450 (CYP) enzymes converts several anticancer drugs to reactive, electrophilic, water-soluble intermediates that can damage DNA.[70,71] Glutathione-*S*-transferases (GSTs), *N*-acetyltransferases, epoxide hydrolases, and sulfotransferases are phase II inactivation and detoxification enzymes.[70–73]

A polymorphism *(CYP3A4-V)* in the nifedipine-specific response element (NFSE) in the *CYP3A4* promoter was examined as a risk factor for treatment-related leukemia[74] because CYP3A is involved in the metabolism of alkylating agents (cyclophosphamide, ifosfamide) and topoisomerase II inhibitors (etoposide, teniposide).[75,76] Although most treatment-related leukemias in the study had chromosome band 11q23 translocations typical of topoisomerase II inhibitor–related cases, several treatment-related leukemias without such translocations also were examined.[74] A significant deficit of this polymorphism was observed for all treatment-related leukemias compared to de novo cases, suggesting that the relationship of *CYP3A4* genotype with alkylating agent–related leukemias should be studied further.[74] The wild-type *CYP3A4* promoter genotype *(CYP3A4-W)* was significantly associated with epipodophyllotoxin-related cases.[74] The A-to-G transition polymorphism in the NFSE, later named the *CYP3A4*1B* allele, was found to track with *CYP3AP1*1, CYP3A5*1,* and other *CYP3A* genotypes,[77] indicating the need to further evaluate *CYP3A* genotypes in secondary leukemia risk.

Slow metabolizer variants of the *CYP2D6* and *CYP2C19* genes have been linked to an increased risk of secondary leukemias with chromosomal abnormalities, but not specifically to either alkylating agent or topoisomerase II inhibitor–related cases.[78]

An increased risk of myelodysplasia was identified in adults with the *GSTT1*-null genotype,[79] predicting that this polymorphism would prove to be a predisposing factor in alkylating agent–related myelodysplasia.[79] In a Japanese population it was confirmed that individuals with the *GSTT1*-null genotype are at increased risk for treatment-related myelodysplasia.[80] In a large British study the frequencies of *GSTM1*- and *GSTT1*-null genotypes were increased in de novo and treatment-related acute myeloid leukemia.[81] A *GSTP1* polymorphism was specifically associated with treatment-related leukemias characterized by complex karyotypes and chromosome 5q and 7q deletions, and there was exposure to alkylating agents in most patients where data on chemotherapy exposures were available.[81] Reactive metabolites of several alkylating agents are GSTP1 substrates.[81]

The enzyme NAD(P)H:quinone oxidoreductase 1 detoxifies simple quinones and their derivatives and protects cells against oxidative stress.[82–85] An inactivating C609T polymorphism is significantly overrepresented in treatment-related leukemias, especially cases with chromosome 5 and/or 7 abnormalities.[86,87]

DNA Topoisomerase II Inhibitor-Related Leukemias

Incidence and Risk

The other distinct form of secondary leukemia surfaced in the late 1980s, coincident with widespread usage of epipodophyllotoxins.[41,42,88–107] Secker-Walker and colleagues observed acute lymphoblastic leukemia with the t(4;11) translocation complicating neuroblastoma therapy with doxorubicin and teniposide in 1985.[108] In 1987, Ratain and associates implicated the etoposide in combination chemotherapy for non–small-cell lung cancer in the development of secondary leukemia with monoblastic features.[109]

Topoisomerase II is an essential cellular enzyme that relaxes supercoiled DNA by transient cleavage and religation of the double helix. Each subunit of the enzyme homodimer forms a short-lived covalent bond with the phosphate residue of the base 3′ to the site of cleavage, introducing four-base staggered nicks into both strands of the DNA. The enzyme-DNA cleavage intermediate is called the cleavage complex.[110] Agents targeting topoisomerase II act via either or both of two broad mechanisms. In the first mechanism, the drug converts topoisomerase II into a cellular toxin by stabilization of the cleavage complex, either by decreasing the reverse rate of religation or increasing the forward rate of cleavage, both of which increase cleavage complexes.[110,111] Drugs that disrupt the cleavage-religation reaction in this manner are called topoisomerase II "poisons" because the resulting DNA strand breaks can initiate apoptosis or promote illegitimate recombination.[111] The second broad mechanism involves true catalytic inhibition of enzymatic function.[112,113] Anticancer drugs associated with this form of leukemia are topoisomerase II poisons, but some have mixed activities of poisons and catalytic inhibitors of the enzyme (Table 29–3).[111,114,115]

Despite the risk of leukemia, etoposide is among the most widely used, highly efficacious anticancer drugs.[110,111] Teniposide previously was used for pedia-

TABLE 29–3. Classification and Features of DNA Topoisomerase II–Targeted Anticancer Drugs[110,111,114,115,401]

Type	Agents	Features
Nonintercalative	Epipodophyllotoxins	Natural plant alkaloids
	Etoposide	Enzymatic poisons
	Teniposide (not currently in use)	Decrease religation rate
Mixed groove binders/ intercalators	Anthracyclines	Mixed enzymatic poisons/catalytic inhibitors
	Daunorubicin	
	Doxorubicin	
	4-Epi-doxorubicin	Decrease religation rate
	Anthracenedione	Enzymatic poison
	Mitoxantrone	
	Dactinomycin	Dual topoisomerase I and II poison/ catalytic inhibitor

tric acute lymphoblastic leukemia[88,96] and solid tumors,[116] and lung cancer in adults.[117–121] The protocols associated with the highest 6-year cumulative risks of acute myeloid leukemia, 12.4% and 12.3%, administered teniposide on weekly and twice-weekly schedules.[88] Intercalating agents that disrupt the topoisomerase II cleavage-religation reaction (see Table 29–3) also have been implicated in leukemogenesis, including daunorubicin, doxorubicin, 4-epi-doxorubicin, mitoxantrone, and dactinomycin.[94,108,122–132] The European APL Group recently found an increasing incidence of therapy-related acute promyelocytic leukemia with greater usage of mitoxantrone and anthracyclines for breast cancer and reported that 22% of APL cases are therapy-related.[133] Intensive, high-dose epirubicin-containing regimens for breast cancer also are associated with a significantly increased risk.[134]

Chemotherapy targeting topoisomerase II is administered in multiagent regimens with additional leukemogenic drugs, and certain primary diseases may confer some risk for leukogenesis.[135] Therefore, the International Agency for Research on Cancer (IARC) concluded that there is "limited evidence" for the carcinogenicity of etoposide alone and that etoposide "probably" is carcinogenic in humans,[135] despite over 150 case reports[135] and many cohort studies suggesting that etoposide is leukemogenic.[42,43,88,91,97,103,109,136–140] Based on cohort studies on patients with gonadal tumors,[42,43,103,107,139,140] the IARC concluded that there is "sufficient" evidence in humans for the carcinogenicity of etoposide in combination with cisplatin and bleomycin.[135]

The median latency from exposure to epipodophyllotoxin-related leukemia is 24–30 months,[2,141] but the latency has been up to 10 years.[142,143] The overall incidence following epipodophyllotoxin-containing regimens is about 2–3%.[144] The National Cancer Institute Cancer Therapy Evaluation Program monitored the occurrence of leukemia in 12 clinical trials administering low (<1500 mg/m^2), moderate (1500–2999 mg/m^2), or high (≥3000 mg/m^2) epipodophyllotoxin total doses. Respective calculated cumulative 6-year rates of 3.2%, 0.7%, and 2.2% indicated lack of a dose-response effect, suggesting other primary risk factors in the context of multiagent regimens[144] (Table 29–4). However, in a recent case-control study of treatment-related leukemia after pediatric solid tumors in which etoposide total doses in many cases were greater than 6 gm/m^2, cumulative etoposide and anthracyclines doses both affected risk.[145] Schedule may be a determinant of risk.[144,145] Intermittent weekly or twice-weekly epipodophyllotoxin schedules for primary acute lymphoblastic leukemia used commonly in the past were associated with incidences of 5.9% and 12%.[88,91] Schedule alterations and substitution of other agents for epipodophyllotoxins reduced but did not eliminate the risk following primary acute lymphoblastic leukemia.[91,146,147] Oral etoposide administration on a semicontinuous schedule (3 days/wk for 3 weeks in a row every 4 weeks) or a continuous schedule (21 consecutive days out of 28 days) may be associated with a higher risk, but effects of schedule versus dose could not be separated because most of these patients received greater than 6 gm/m^2 of etoposide.[145]

TABLE 29–4. Risk Factors for DNA Topoisomerase II Inhibitor–Related Leukemia

Treatment Factors	Specific DNA topoisomerase II inhibitor	
	Intermittent weekly or twice-weekly schedules	
	Cumulative dose (>6 gm/m^2 etoposide)?	
	Semicontinuous/continuous etoposide schedules?	
	Chemotherapy regimen (intensity of treatment, other leukemogenic drugs)	
	Therapeutic radiation	
	Preceding L-asparaginase	
	Preceding antimetabolite	
	G-CSF	
	Autologous stem cell collection after priming with etoposide	
Host Factors	Ethnicity	
	Primary disease	
	Genetic variation in drug-metabolizing enzymes	*CYP3A4* TPMT
	Other polymorphism	*MLL* trinucleotide repeat

One cohort study of patients with primary acute lymphoblastic leukemia suggested that L-asparaginase administration during the preceding week potentiates the leukemogenicity of epipodophyllotoxins.[148] Methotrexate and mercaptopurine administration preceding epipodophyllotoxin also may increase the risk.[91,137,146] An excess of this form of secondary leukemia has been reported among Hispanic patients.[91,149,150] Acute myeloid leukemia also occurs after Langerhans cell histiocytosis therapy with epipodophyllotoxins; the independent association between Langerhans cell histiocytosis and malignancies has suggested a contribution of primary disease to risk.[151–154] The incidence following pediatric solid tumor regimens generally has been lower than with certain acute lymphoblastic leukemia treatment protocols.[89,155] However, an excess risk has been reported in patients with primary Hodgkin's disease or osteosarcoma.[145] More intensive solid tumor regimens are associated with a greater risk.[127,128] It has been suggested that, in pediatric sarcoma regimens, it is the combination of intercalating topoisomerase II inhibitors with alkylating agents and irradiation that increases risk.[125] Leukemia is a complication of autologous stem cell transplantation, as described earlier.[44,46,47] In patients with lymphomas, a 12.3-fold increased risk was observed when the autologous stem cells were collected after priming with etoposide; the leukemias had characteristic translocations of topoisomerase II inhibitor–exposed cases.[155]

Granulocyte colony-stimulating factor (G-CSF) can induce leukemia cell growth in vitro.[156] When patients on two consecutive St. Jude's acute lymphoblastic leukemia protocols were examined altogether and children receiving radiation were excluded, the incidence of treatment-related leukemia was higher in patients who received G-CSF, and the majority of cases had translocations of chromosome band 11q23.[156]

Recently, pediatric and adult cases of MDS/AML with hallmark cytogenetic features of alkylating agent–related cases have emerged after administration of all-*trans* retinoic acid and anthracyclines, mitoxantrone, or etoposide for primary acute promyelocytic leukemia.[157–161] The incidence in one series was 6.5%.[161] These cases raised questions about whether topoisomerase II inhibitors can cause myelodysplasia similar to alkylating agent treatment or whether the MDS/AML represents leukemia relapse with an unrelated clone.[157–162]

The t(15;17) and inv(16) occur in leukemias following topoisomerase II inhibitors as well as after radiation only,[16,163] suggesting that heterogeneous exposures may create a risk for treatment-related leukemias with balanced translocations.

Genetic Predisposition

CYP3A4 converts epipodophyllotoxin to a catechol metabolite that is readily oxidized to a quinone.[164–166] When the *CYP3A4* promoter NFSE polymorphism[167] was evaluated in pediatric patients exposed to one or more anticancer drugs metabolized by CYP3A, the wild-type genotype increased, and heterozygous or homozygous variant genotypes decreased, the risk of epipodophyllotoxin-related leukemias with *MLL* translocations.[74] This *CYP3A4* promoter genotype-leukemia association was validated in a study of Israeli adults[168]; but was not observed in pediatric patients who developed treatment-related acute myeloid leukemia following primary acute lymphoblastic leukemia therapy containing etoposide or teniposide.[169] The wild-type (AA) genotype at the *CYP3A4* promoter NFSE is associated with lower etoposide clearance in whites.[170] It is plausible that the *CYP3A4* genotype modulates susceptibility to this form of leukemia because epipodophyllotoxins and their metabolites are genotoxins.[171–173] Furthermore, etoposide catechol, the major etoposide metabolite, is detectable in the plasma of patients receiving treatment with etoposide,[174–176] and patients receiving multiple-day bolus doses are exposed to higher concentrations of etoposide catechol with successive days of treatment.[174,177]

Etoposide catechol is formed primarily through CYP3A4 metabolism,[166,178] but little is known about the relative importance of CYP3A5 in etoposide metabolism.[77] In primary hepatocytes in culture, etoposide at high concentrations induces only modest increases in CYP3A5 messenger RNA and protein[178] and slight increases in CYP3A4 messenger RNA.[178] Alternatively, because ifosfamide induces CYP3A4 in primary cultured hepatocytes,[179] combined drug administration may contribute to increased etoposide catechol formation by CYP3A4.[177] Prednisone also induces etoposide clearance and affects catechol formation.[170] Consistent with the polygenetically determined metabolism of most chemotherapeutic drugs,[70–72] *MDR1, CYP3A5, UGT1A1* (UDP-glucuronyltransferase 1A1), and *VDR* (vitamin D receptor) genetic polymorphisms affect etoposide disposition further.[170] Relationships of these polymorphisms to the risk of secondary leukemia have not been addressed. There also are racial differences in effects of specific genotypes on etoposide disposition.[170]

In contrast to leukemias following alkylating agent treatment, *GSTT1-* and *GSTM1*-null genotypes are not predisposing factors to epipodophyllotoxin-related leukemia following primary acute lymphoblastic leukemia.[180]

The gene encoding thiopurine-*S*-methyltransferase (TPMT), which inactivates thiopurines, is also polymorphic.[181,182] The use of etoposide with thiopurines uncovered TPMT deficiency as a possible risk factor for this form of leukemia when a trend toward lower TPMT activity was found among children with primary acute lymphoblastic leukemia who developed treatment-related acute myeloid leukemia following a regimen containing etoposide in induction and maintenance.[175]

An association has also been suggested between topoisomerase II inhibitor–related acute myeloid leukemia in adults and a polymorphism at a trinucleotide (GAA) repeat tract within an Alu sequence in intron 6 in the *MLL* breakpoint cluster region.[183]

PATHOPHYSIOLOGY

Although the chromosomal and molecular aberrations in treatment-related leukemias reflect prior therapy with distinct classes of cytotoxic drugs, 85–90% of cases have chromosomal aberrations that occur in primary leukemias and myelodysplasia.[184]

Cytogenetic and Molecular Alterations in Alkylating Agent-Related Leukemias

The archetypal cytogenetic features of alkylating agent–related leukemias are complete or partial deletions of chromosomes 5 and 7 and complex, unbalanced numerical and structural cytogenetic abnormalities.[23] Deletions of critical tumor suppressor genes at chromosomes 5q and 7q are believed to underlie their pathogenesis; however, the specific genes important in leukemia pathogenesis in these regions are unknown. Potential chromosome 5q and 7q regions of involvement derive from de novo and treatment-related cases.

Deletions of Chromosome 7 or 7q

Chromosome 7 aberrations, present in 50% of cases of treatment-related AML/MDS,[185] are the most commonly observed changes in leukemias following alkylating agent treatment.[184] More than 80% of cases of MDS/AML with 7q deletions have allelic loss of the entire region from chromosome 7q22 to 7q31. Rare cases with allelic loss at 7q31 and 7q22 loci but retention of sequences between these loci, or submicroscopic allele imbalance for a different distal locus, potentially indicate multiple critical genes on chromosome 7q.[186] Examples of candidate genes that have been evaluated on chromosome 7q include *hDMP1* (cyclin D–binding Myb-like protein) at chromosome band 7q21,[187] and *MLL5*[188] and *PIK3CG* at chromosome band 7q22.[189]

Deletions of Chromosome 5 or 5q

The second most common cytogenetic abnormality in alkylating agent–related MDS/AML is −5/del(5q).[184] del(5)(q13q33) and del(5)(q13q35) are major subsets of

5q deletions.[190] Translocations or paracentric inversions involving 5q11 to 5q13 also are observed.[190] A deleted region in a 2.0-Mb interval at 5q13.1 was identified in a subset of cases of MDS/AML.[190] The del(5q) is often a covert unbalanced translocation.[184] Breakpoints of the 5q deletion vary greatly, but many hematopoiesis genes localize to chromosome 5q.[185,191] The *IRF1, IL5, CDC25C, IL3, GMCSF, EGR1, FMS,* and *MCSF1R* genes are at chromosome band 5q31.[185] Cases of MDS/AML often have simultaneous hemizygous deletions of the *PURA* and *PURB* genes, at chromosome bands 5q31.1 and 7p13, respectively.[192] The *SSBP2* gene encoding a sequence-specific single-stranded DNA-binding protein is a candidate gene at chromosome band 5q13.3.[193] Co-segregating deletions of chromosome 5q13.3 and *TP53* at chromosome 17p13 have suggested functional cooperativity between loss of a putative tumor suppressor gene at chromosome 5q13.3 and loss of p53.[194]

Other Molecular Alterations

Accompanying *RAS* oncogene mutations occur in a significant proportion of cases of alkylating agent–related leukemia.[195–197] In one series of cases of treatment-related AML/MDS with deletions of chromosomes 5 and 7, the incidence of K-*ras* and N-*ras* mutations overall was 9%, but the incidence in the cases with monosomy 7 or del(7q) was 19%.[197]

TP53 mutations have been detected in 27% of unselected adult cases of treatment-related AML/MDS, the majority of which followed alkylating agent treatment.[198] *TP53* mutations were identified in AML/MDS following multiagent ovarian cancer therapy, often including platinum analogues[199]; the propensity for G-to-A transitions possibly suggested specific DNA damage from these agents.[199] *MLL* gene amplification in the form of segmental jumping translocations also was identified as a recurrent abnormality in alkylating agent-related leukemias with *TP53* mutations.[200]

Hypermethylation causing inactivation of the p15 *(INK4B)* and p16 *(INK4A)* cell-cycle regulatory genes occurs in a large proportion of therapy-related AML/MDS.[201] p15 hypermethylation, which occurs more often, is significantly associated with −7/del(7q).[201]

Pedersen-Bjergaard proposed two subgroups of alkylating agent–related leukemias.[184] The first subgroup includes cases with −7/del(7q) without chromosome 5 abnormalities. The −7/del(7q) abnormalities may be present in only subclones of the cells, and these leukemias may contain additional aberrations such as t(3;21), *RAS* mutations, and p15 promoter methylation, but usually not *TP53* mutations.[184] The second subgroup includes cases with −5/del(5q), which represent primary alterations and not subclone evolution.[184] Additional aberrations including −7/del(7q) and unidentified marker chromosomes may be acquired, and *TP53* mutations are common.[184] Duplication or amplification/segmental jumping translocation of the unrearranged *MLL* gene is a recurrent abnormality in this subgroup and is associated with *TP53* mutations.[184,200]

Gene expression profiling experiments validated the distinct subgroups of cases with −7/del(7q) without chromosome 5 involvement and cases with −5/del(5q).[184,202] Cases with −5/del(5q) and complex karyotypes exhibited higher expression of cyclin A2 *(CCNA2)*, cyclin E2 *(CCNE2)*, *CDC2*, the checkpoint gene *BUB1*, *MYC*, and the Myc-regulated gene CDC28 protein kinase 2 *(CKS2)*, as well as loss of expression of the IFN consensus sequence-binding protein *(ICSBP)* gene and reduced expression of chromosome 5 genes such as *APC*.[202] The second subgroup with −7 or simple karyotypes without −5/del(5q) was characterized by downregulation of the *TAL1*, *GATA1*, and *EKLF* hematopoietic transcription factor genes, and *FLT3* (FMS-like tyrosine kinase 3) and *BCL2* upregulation.[202]

Somatic *AML1* point mutations that would affect DNA binding of core-binding factor β have been identified in 38% of cases of therapy-related AML/MDS following alkylating agent treatment with or without local radiation.[203] Hypermethylation of the *DAP* gene results in loss of function of DAP (death-associated protein) kinase, which positively regulates apoptosis, in 50% of treatment-related AML/MDS following alkylating agent treatment.[204]

Cytogenetic and Molecular Alterations in DNA Topoisomerase II Inhibitor-Related Leukemias

Balanced Chromosomal Translocations

Balanced chromosomal translocations are the primary molecular alterations in leukemias related to topoisomerase II inhibitors.[184,205] Translocations of an 8.3-kb breakpoint cluster region between exons 5 and 11 of the 100-kb *MLL* gene at chromosome band 11q23 occur most often.[206–210] The de novo counterpart of treatment-related leukemias with *MLL* translocations are the acute lymphoblastic and myeloid leukemias of infants, which have similar translocations.[211] Virtually all of the other balanced translocations observed in de novo acute myeloid leukemia including t(8;21) and its variants,[43,89,125,131,212–219] t(15;17),[124,133,144,163,220–223] inv(16) and t(16;16),[141,163,212,213,222,224] t(8;16),[213] t(9;22),[225] and heterogeneous translocations disrupting *NUP98* at chromosome band 11p15,[226–234] also can occur. The distribution of balanced translocations in 511 cases of treatment-related leukemia from a recent International Workshop is summarized in Figure 29–2.

MLL, MLL Fusion Proteins, and Leukemogenesis

The *MLL* (Mixed-Lineage Leukemia; Myeloid Lymphoid Leukemia) gene encodes a large, complex oncoprotein that regulates transcription[235–240] (Fig. 29–3). *MLL* was also named *HRX* and *Htrx1* because of its regional amino acid similarity to the *Drosophila* trithorax *(trx)* gene[236,238,241] (Fig. 29–4*A*). MLL maintains *HOX* gene expression early during mammalian skeletal, craniofacial, and neural development and hematopoiesis.[242–244]

Functional motifs of MLL are summarized in Figure 29–4*A*. Constructs comprising MLL AT hook motifs have been shown to promote p21 and p27 upregulation, cell cycle arrest, and monocyte differentiation.[245] The subnuclear localization of MLL is directed by the amino-

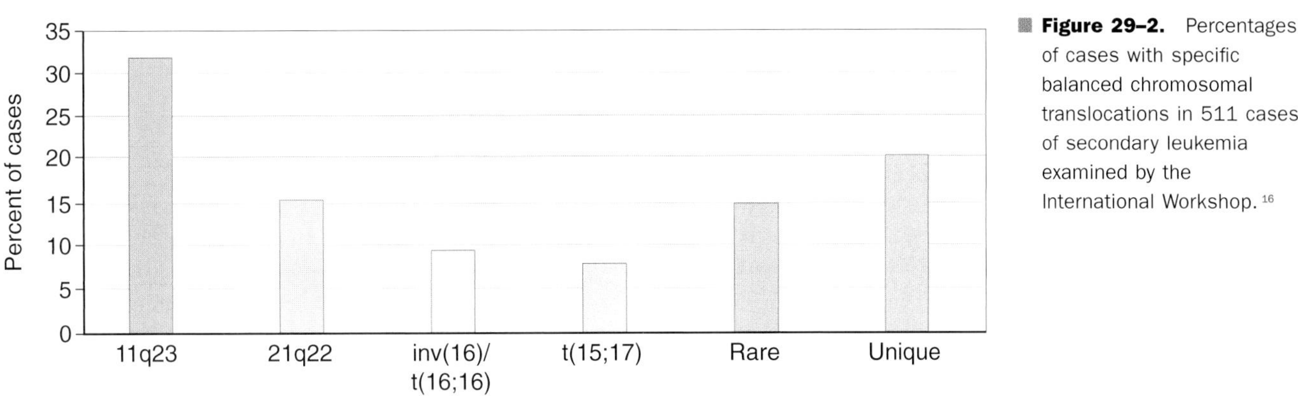

Figure 29–2. Percentages of cases with specific balanced chromosomal translocations in 511 cases of secondary leukemia examined by the International Workshop.[16]

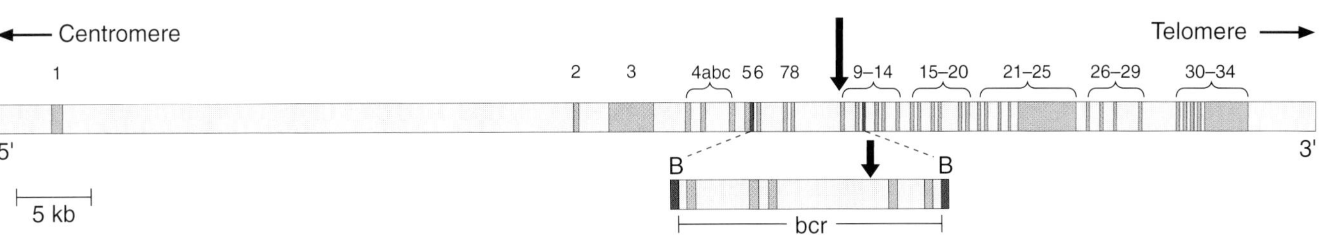

Figure 29–3. Genomic organization of *MLL* gene at chromosome band 11q23. *Bam*HI sites (indicated by *B*) define the breakpoint cluster region (bcr). *Arrow* indicates area between bcr coordinates 6587 to 6606 3′ in intron 8 where multiple cloned translocation breakpoints in cases of secondary leukemia have been localized, which is consistent with a translocation breakpoint hotspot.[278,335,336,397] (Adapted from Rasio D, Schichman SA, Negrini M, et al: Complete exon structure of the *ALL1* gene. Cancer Res 56:1766–1769, 1996.)

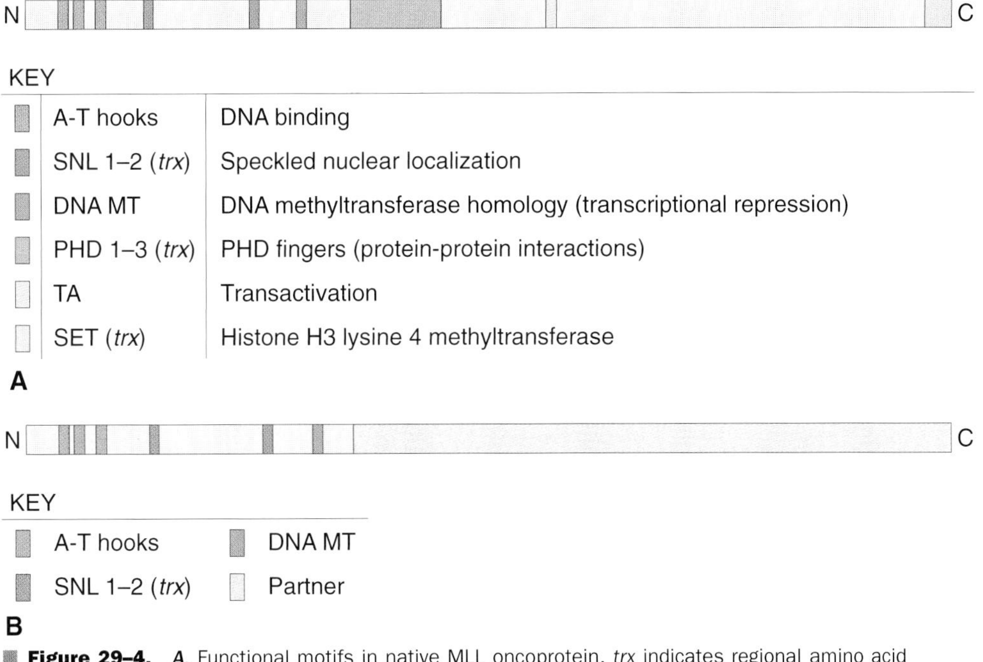

Figure 29–4. *A,* Functional motifs in native MLL oncoprotein. *trx* indicates regional amino acid homology to *Drosophila* trithorax. Functions of domains are listed.[241,246,248,398,399] *B,* Functional motifs in MLL fusion proteins produced from the 5′-*MLL*–partner gene-3′ rearrangement on the der(11) chromosome. The MLL PHDs (plant homeodomains), the transactivation domain, and the SET domain are replaced by the carboxyl terminus of the partner protein. (Adapted from Ayton PM, Cleary ML: Molecular mechanisms of leukemogenesis mediated by MLL fusion proteins. Oncogene 20:5695–5707, 2001.)

terminal SNL motifs.[241] The MT domain is part of a transcriptional repression region.[241–245] The PHD mediates MLL homodimerization and protein-protein interactions, including binding to a nuclear cyclophilin, which modulates target gene expression.[246] The SET domain interacts with the SWI/SNF chromatin remodeling complex, which activates transcription.[247] Consistent with its role in epigenetic gene regulation, the SET domain has specific histone H3 lysine 4–specific methyltransferase activity that regulates *HOX* promoters.[248] MLL exists in a large macromolecular protein complex that is involved in the remodeling, acetylation, deacetylation, and methylation of nucleosomes and histones.[249] Menin, the product of the *MEN1* tumor suppressor gene, is a newly identified MLL-associated protein that forms complexes with not only native MLL but also MLL fusion proteins.[250] Taspase 1 cleaves MLL into an amino- terminal fragment with transcriptional repression properties and a carboxy-terminal fragment with transcriptional activation properties, which associate in the large macromolecular protein complex.[251,252] MLL proteolytic cleavage and association of its amino- and carboxy-terminal fragments is critical for proper nuclear sublocalization and proper *HOX* gene regulation.[252]

MLL translocations involve more than 40 partner genes that encode diverse partner proteins[253–257] (Table 29–5). Many MLL partner proteins have structural motifs of nuclear transcription factors,[237,238,258–266] transcriptional regulatory proteins,[267–270] or other nuclear proteins.[271–273] Others are cytoplasmic proteins[129,142,143,274–290] or proteins in different cellular locations.[291–296] Included in the partner genes is *MLL* itself; *MLL* self-fusions result in partial tandem duplications of several more 5′ exons.[132,263,297] The most common *MLL* partner genes are *AF4, ENL,* and *AF9.*[298] Only a subset of the partner genes is involved in acute lymphoblastic leukemia; the partner genes in acute myeloid leukemia are more diverse. Several partner genes indicated in Table 29–5[129,142,143,261,267,268,270,276,286,299] were first discovered in treatment-related leukemias and some but not all of these recur in de novo cases. Conversely, several *MLL* partner genes in de novo leukemias recur as partner genes in treatment-related cases.[126,132,300,301] Of interest, the MLL partner proteins AF4 and AF9 interact with each other.[302]

A few of the *MLL* partner genes are members of the same gene families, as also shown in Table 29–5[255,256,260,285,287–290,303,304] Others encode proteins with otherwise similar functions[261,266,305,306]; however, there is no unifying functional relationship between the many partner proteins.

Fusion proteins from the der(11) transcripts of *MLL* translocations (Fig. 29–4*B*) have been shown to transform hematopoietic progenitors and bring about leukemia in mice.[255,307–312] The Taspase 1 proteolytic cleavage site is lacking from the fusion proteins, and the fusion proteins cannot interact with the MLL carboxyl terminus.[251,252] The murine models suggest that transcriptional activation may be a key function of nuclear MLL partner proteins.[241,306,313] The role of cytoplasmic MLL partner proteins may involve forced MLL dimerization or oligomerization.[314]

Altered *HOX* expression appears to be a common pathway in *MLL* fusion protein leukemias regardless of the partner gene (Fig. 29–5).[250,315–319] Both *HOXA9* and the HOX coregulator gene *MEIS1* are overexpressed in leukemias of patients with *MLL* translocations.[316] Depending on the partner gene and the murine model, the altered *HOX* expression is essential for leukemogenesis

TABLE 29–5. MLL Partner Proteins

Nuclear Proteins	Cytoplasmic Proteins	Cell Membrane Proteins
Transcription Factors	AF1p	AF6
LAF-4	AF1q	CALM
AF4	**AF3p21**	LARG
AF5α	**GMPS**	GPHN
AF5q31	**LPP**	MYO1F
AF6q21	GRAF	
AF9	CDK6	**ER/Golgi Apparatus Protein**
AF10	FBP17	Alkaline ceramidase
MLL	ABI-1	
AF17	CBL	
ENL	MPFYVE	**Ribosome Protein**
AFX	GAS7	RPS3
Transcriptional Regulators	**MSF**	
CBP	LASP1	
ELL	EEN	
p300	hCDCrel	
Nuclear Proteins of Unknown Function	SEPTIN6	
LCX		
AF15q14		

Partner proteins highlighted in the same colors are encoded by genes in the same family. Boxes in bold indicate corresponding partner genes discovered in treatment-related leukemias.

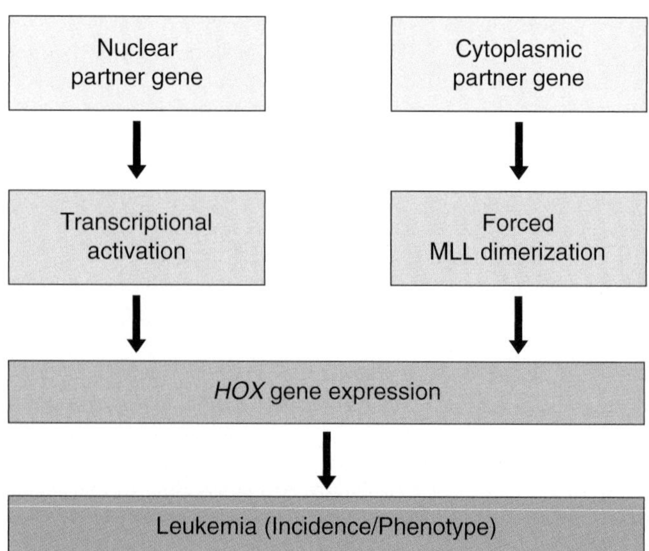

■ **Figure 29–5.** Model for common pathway to MLL leukemogenesis by diverse fusions with nuclear and cytoplasmic partner genes through altered *HOX* expression.[250]

or may influence the leukemia phenotype, latency and penetrance.[315,317–319]

Latency to leukemia in the murine models has suggested that secondary alterations may be important in MLL oncoprotein leukemogenesis in addition to the translocations.[241,255] Unlike in alkylator-induced leukemias, *TP53* mutations are not observed in leukemias associated with topoisomerase II inhibitors.[58] Overexpression of *FLT3* and *FLT3* mutations have emerged as important secondary alterations in leukemias with *MLL* translocations and tandem duplications,[316,320–323] although treatment-related cases have not been studied comprehensively. *FLT3* internal tandem duplication mutations also are especially common in acute promyelocytic leukemia with the t(15;17), but mostly de novo cases were examined.[324]

Timeline of Acquisition of MLL Translocations Relative to Treatment

In pediatric cases of treatment-related acute myeloid leukemia following primary neuroblastoma[129] or primary acute lymphoblastic leukemia,[325] the *MLL* translocation was absent in the bone marrow at primary cancer diagnosis but emerged during the treatment, suggesting that treatment caused and did not select for a preexisting translocation. In *MLL*-rearranged infant leukemias, the translocation is a somatic, in utero event and the latency is short (from some time in pregnancy to leukemia diagnosis in the infant).[285,326,327] However, de novo *MLL*-rearranged leukemias in older children generally are not traceable to birth,[328] which also is consistent with a causative role of topoisomerase II inhibitors in the translocations. Nonetheless, *MLL* translocations can be present early during anticancer treatment at low cumulative doses of these agents.[129]

DNA Damage and Repair Mechanisms

There is new experimental evidence in a human primary CD34$^+$ cell model that etoposide induces a full spectrum of *MLL* rearrangements that remain stable after clonal expansion, resembling those associated with secondary leukemias in patients.[329] These results provide additional evidence for a direct causal relationship between topoisomerase II inhibitors and the translocations.

The association of topoisomerase II–targeted chemotherapy with leukemias has suggested that the translocations are a consequence of repair of drug-induced topoisomerase II–mediated damage (reviewed by Felix and others[3,330–332]). Early Southern blot analyses of adult treatment-related leukemias suggested a biased distribution of *MLL* genomic breakpoints 3′ in the breakpoint cluster region and disruption of a scaffold attachment region containing a putative topoisomerase II site.[333] There is heterogeneity in *MLL* translocation breakpoint distribution in the breakpoint cluster region in treatment-related leukemias in children, but a hotspot region in intron 8 that is 3′ in the breakpoint cluster region has emerged from the molecular cloning of *MLL* genomic breakpoint junctions[126,129,132,267,278,300,334–336] (see Fig. 29–3). In cases in which both genomic breakpoint junctions have been characterized, the sequences reveal precise or near-precise interchromosomal DNA recombinations with gains or losses of no or, more often, a few bases.[129,278,300,334–336] The relatively precise interchromosomal DNA recombinations are consistent with the processing of four-base staggered double-stranded breaks from topoisomerase II cleavage.[278,334,336] In treatment-related cases of acute lymphoblastic leukemia with t(4;11)[334] or acute myeloid leukemia with t(9;11),[336] the translocation breakpoints in *MLL* and its partner gene were reciprocally cleaved by topoisomerase II in vitro, and functional, drug-induced topoisomerase II cleavage sites could be resolved to form the breakpoint junctions.[334,336] Etoposide as well as its genotoxic catechol and quinone metabolites increase topoisomerase II cleavage complexes at or near *MLL* translocation breakpoints.[173,334,336]

These data favor the model in which topoisomerase II mediates the chromosomal breakage leading to *MLL* translocations in topoisomerase II inhibitor–related leukemias.[336] However, an alternative mechanism has been proposed whereby apoptotic nucleolytic cleavage damages *MLL*.[337–339] Recently it was shown that mitoxantrone induces topoisomerase II cleavage at a translocation breakpoint hotspot in the *PML* gene in treatment-related acute promyelocytic leukemia where there was clinical exposure to this agent,[340] consistent with a translocation mechanism in which the DNA damage is a consequence of topoisomerase II cleavage.[340]

In treatment-related and de novo leukemias with *MLL* translocations alike, microhomologies of several overlapping bases at or near the translocation breakpoints in *MLL* and partner genes have suggested DNA damage resolution by the repair mechanism of nonhomologous end-joining (NHEJ).[129,278,285,300,334,336,341–344] The recently reported t(9;11) translocation in a case of treatment-related acute myeloid leukemia, which occurred without the gain or loss of any bases, suggested direct repair of topoisomerase II cleavage sites by the precise NHEJ mechanism.[336,345] More often, DNA double-stranded breaks from mutagenic agents cannot be repaired directly, and some limited processing is required for NHEJ to ensue,[345] which is consistent with several small deletions[129,278] and a templated single-base insertion[334] at various *MLL* breakpoint junctions in other treatment-related cases. Recombinations of Alu sequences frequently are involved in *MLL* tandem duplications.[346]

CLINICAL FEATURES AND DIAGNOSIS

Although chemotherapy is used in multiagent, multimodality contexts, secondary MDS/AML attributed to alkylating agents and topoisomerase II inhibitors are generally recognizable as distinctive clinical syndromes.[15,22,91,228,347] Alkylating agent–related leukemias typically present with antecedent myelodysplasia, and have a long latency and the archetypal cytogenetic abnormalities described at length earlier. Figure 29–6 shows the bone marrow from a patient with secondary myelodysplasia in which the morphology was

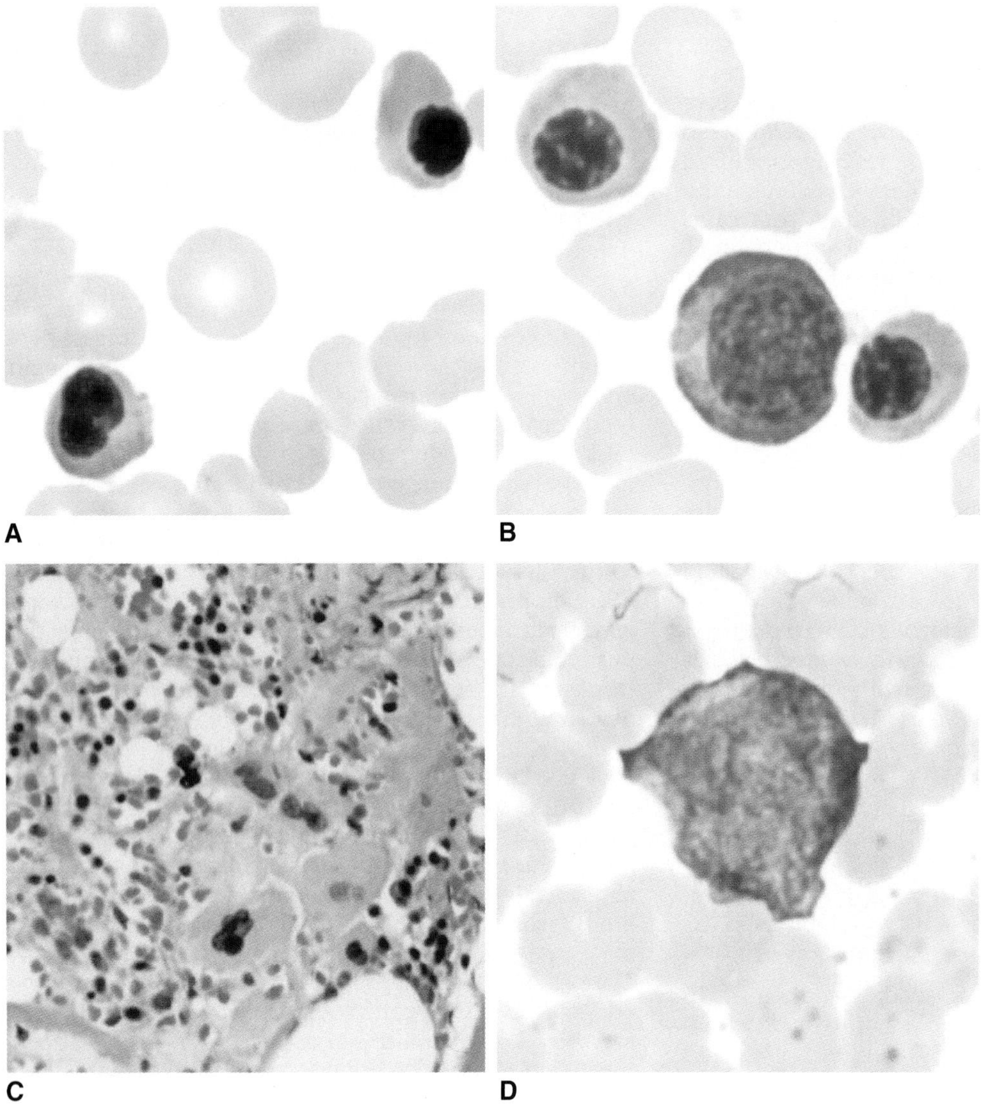

Figure 29–6. Example of refractory anemia with excess blasts in transition. ***A,*** Orthochromatic normoblasts with nuclear irregularities. ***B,*** Two normoblasts with maturation asynchrony. Nuclei are polychromatic but the cytoplasm is orthochromatic. ***C,*** Hypolobated megakaryocytes with clustering. ***D,*** Increased blasts were seen similar to that shown, approximately 5–8% of the marrow cellularity. (Courtesy of John Choi, MD.)

consistent with refractory anemia with excess blasts in transition.

Leukemias associated with topoisomerase II inhibitors have heterogeneous presentations, which are characteristic of the underlying chromosomal translocations. Epipodophyllotoxin-related leukemias with *MLL* translocations usually are myelomonocytic (FAB M4) or monoblastic (FAB M5) variants of acute myeloid leukemia,[348,349] but also can present as other acute myeloid leukemia subtypes, myelodysplasia, or acute lymphoblastic leukemia.[91,228,347] Figure 29–7 shows the diagnostic bone marrow and immunohistochemical special stains in a case of secondary acute myeloid leukemia with FAB M5 morphology. At least to some degree, the lineage and morphologic heterogeneity in *MLL*-rearranged leukemias are influenced by the partner gene. Cases with t(4;11) fusing *MLL* with *AF4* present as acute lymphoblastic leukemia.[132,278,300,334,350] Cases with t(11;16) fusing *MLL* with *CBP* (CREB binding protein) present as myelodysplasia.[267,268,299,351]

The archetypal presentation of cases with t(8;21) is FAB M2 acute myeloid leukemia[43,89,125,131,212–219] but variant *AML1 (CBFA2)* translocations have heterogeneous morphologic MDS/AML presentations.[218] The t(15;17) is associated with FAB M3 acute promyelocytic leukemia.[124,133,144,163,212,220–223,352] Cases with inv(16) and t(16;16) present as myelomonocytic leukemias with eosinophilia (FAB M4eo).[141,163,212,213,222,224] Typically the t(8;16) is associated with FAB M4 morphology and the leukemia exhibits erythrophagocytosis as a prominent feature.[213] The t(9;22) is associated with chronic myelogenous leukemia, acute myeloid leukemia, or acute lymphoblastic leukemia presentations.[225]

In a study comparing clinical presentations in 24 children with treatment-related MDS/AML to 960 de novo pediatric cases, patients with treatment-related MDS/AML were significantly older at diagnosis, had lower white blood cell counts, were more likely to have myelodysplasia, and were less likely to have hepatomegaly, splenomegaly, or hepatosplenomegaly.[150] In addition, the treatment-related leukemias exhibited classic acute myeloid leukemia translocations less often than the de novo cases.[150]

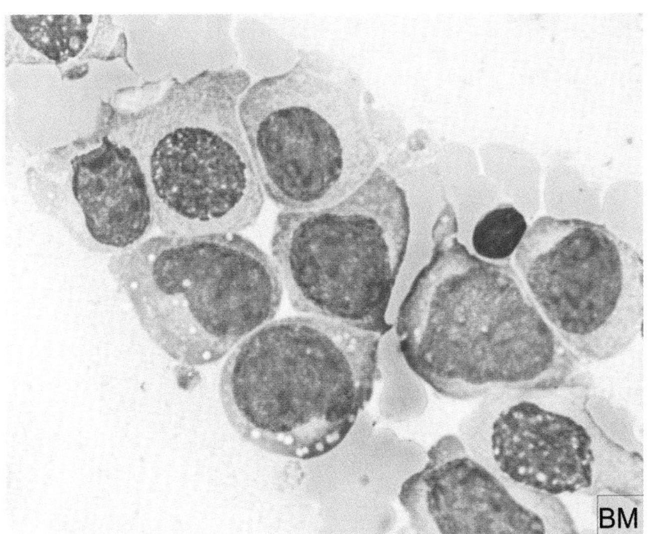

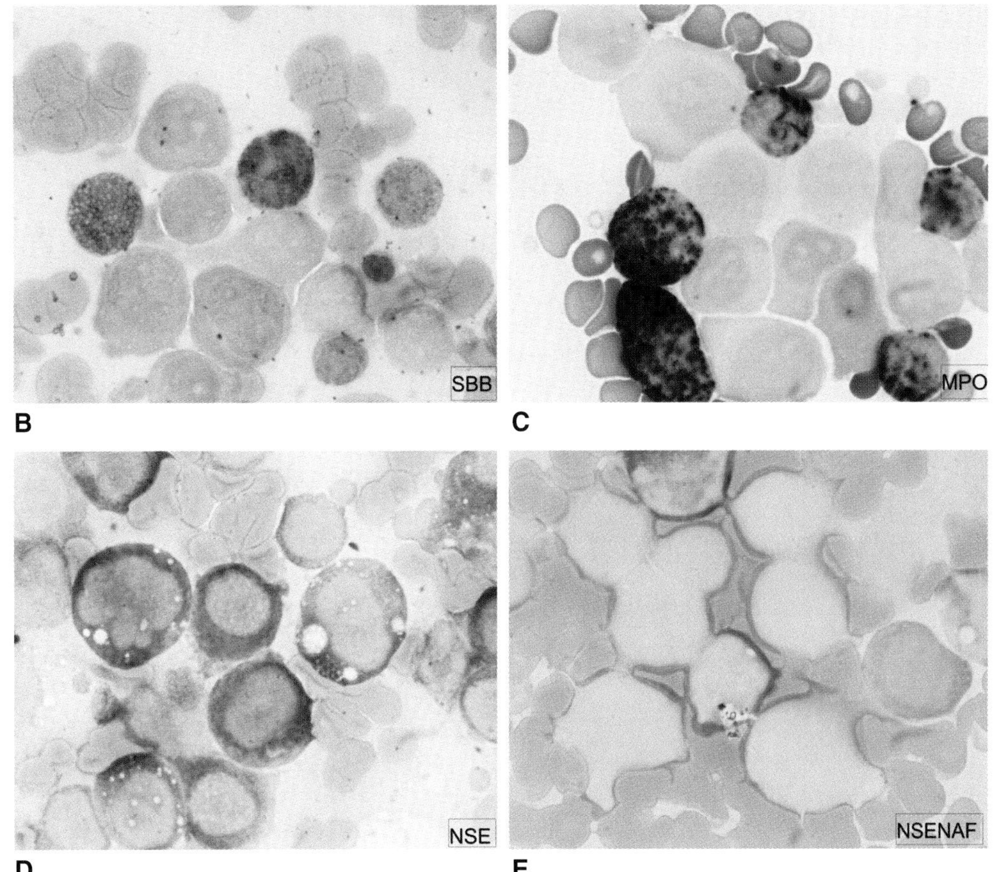

Figure 29–7. Example of diagnostic bone marrow (**A**) and immunohistochemical special stains (**B–E**) in case of secondary acute myeloid leukemia with FAB M5 morphology typical of myeloid leukemias with *MLL* translocations. (Courtesy of John Choi, MD.)

DIFFERENTIAL DIAGNOSIS

If the differential diagnosis is carefully considered, it may be possible to recognize a preleukemic phase in the early stage of the secondary leukemia incidentally during the routine laboratory testing performed for the primary cancer follow-up.[184] However, the peripheral blood cytopenias and monocytosis that may be harbingers of leukemia[129] can also masquerade as routine effects of treatment. It is important to distinguish cytopenias associated with preleukemia from chemotherapy-induced bone marrow suppression, especially if the cytopenias are persistent. Secondary leukemia should be considered in the differential diagnosis when refractory cytopenias emerge during or after chemotherapy. Infectious causes (e.g., viral) and other drug-related causes of suppression of the marrow should also be considered. The monocytosis that occurs regularly during recovery of the bone marrow after chemotherapy must also be distinguished from an emergent leukemia clone with myelomono-

TREATMENT ALGORITHM FOR SECONDARY LEUKEMIA

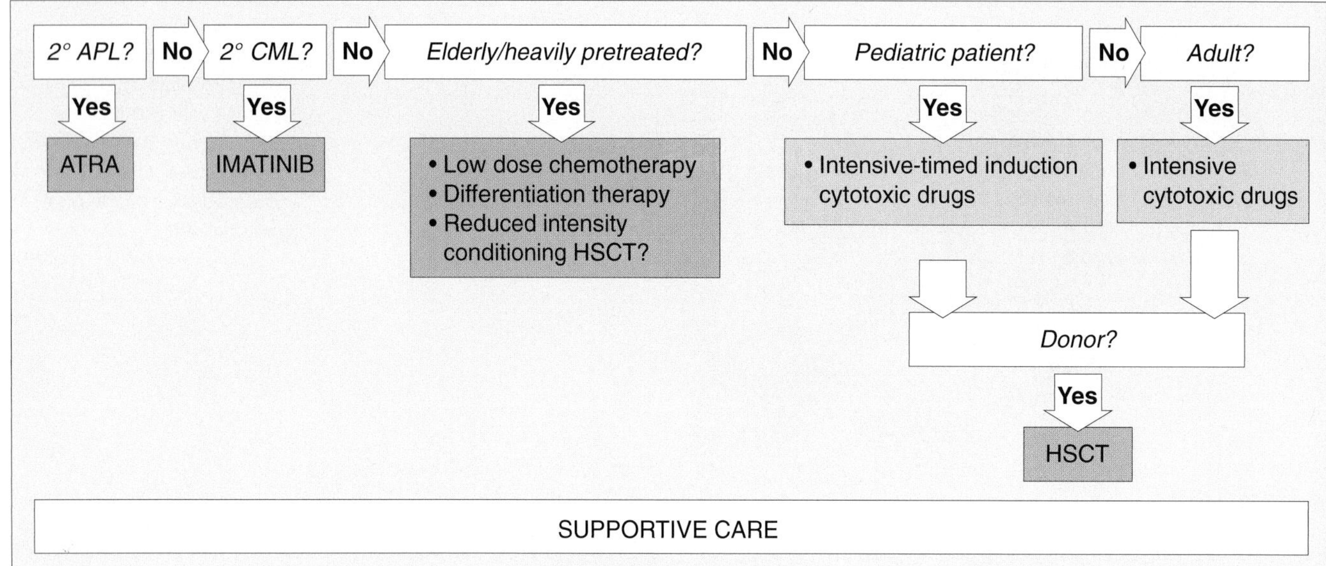

Figure 29–8. Treatment algorithm for secondary leukemia.

cytic/monoblastic features.[129] Many cases of treatment-related AML/MDS present with high percentages of marrow blasts enabling FAB classification[184] and a straightforward leukemia diagnosis. However, a heightened awareness of this treatment complication is essential because the secondary leukemia/myelodysplasia presentation can be much more subtle. Especially after autologous stem cell transplantation, rather than high percentages of marrow blasts, the only evidence of leukemia may be refractory cytopenias accompanied by clonal cytogenetic abnormalities.[47] Absent of clonal cytogenetic abnormalities, immunophenotypic evidence of occult leukemia[353] should be searched for to make the diagnosis.

TREATMENT

The therapeutic possibilities for secondary leukemias and myelodysplasia include cytotoxic chemotherapy, hematopoietic stem cell transplantation, differentiating agents, palliation/supportive care, and targeted therapeutics as well as combinations of these different strategies[16,124,147,184,210,354–365] (Fig. 29–8). Although the general lack of clinical trials or series of uniformly treated patients with secondary leukemias has confounded a systematic evaluation of efficacy of these treatments,[150,366] it has become clear in both adults and children with secondary AML/MDS that intensive therapy is most advantageous. However, the feasibility of administering further intensive antileukemia therapy is determined in large part by the prior primary cancer treatment.[150] It also is well recognized that secondary leukemias are generally less responsive to either cytotoxic chemotherapy or hematopoietic stem cell transplantation than de novo cases.

Cytotoxic Chemotherapy and Hematopoietic Stem Cell Transplantation

Early results in patients with Hodgkin's disease who developed treatment-related acute myeloid leukemia demonstrated not only some successes with hematopoietic stem cell transplantation in younger patients transplanted in remission, but also substantial mortality from the complications.[367,368] A mean complete remission rate of 30.7% and a mean 2-year disease-free survival of 19% were observed with allogeneic bone marrow transplantation in one retrospective series of adults.[360] Depending on the regimens, recent studies have reported long-term disease-free survival rates for allogeneic stem cell transplantation of treatment-related AML/MDS approximating about 30%.[369,370] Patients less than 35 years old with treatment-related acute myeloid leukemia can also benefit from allogeneic transplantation using a human lymphocyte antigen–matched unrelated donor.[371]

The International Workshop on therapy-related AML/MDS described earlier examined outcome data retrospectively in a heterogeneously treated, largely adult population.[16] An overall survival advantage was observed in patients undergoing intensive therapy with hematopoietic stem cell transplantation (n = 67) compared to intensive therapy without transplantation (n = 289). The median survival was 15 months (95% confidence interval [CI], 10.3–30.9 months) and the 5-year survival was 26.7% with transplantation, compared to a median survival of 10 months (95% CI, 8.0–12.0 months) and a 5-year survival of 16.2% without transplantation. Chromosome 5 and/or 7 abnormalities were associated with a median survival of 7 months (95% CI, 6.0–9.9 months) and overall survival rates at 1, 2, and 5 years of 28.5%, 12.5%, and 3.2%, respectively. The median survival was 10 months (95% CI, 8.0–12.0 months), with overall survival rates at 1, 2, and 5 years of 42.6%, 42.6%, and 19.3%, respectively, in cases without these abnormalities.

Most cases of treatment-related MDS/AML in the pediatric population also are resistant to current treatment strategies.[147,150,210] Long-term survival rates were 10–20% in two retrospective pediatric reviews of epipodophyllotoxin-related acute myeloid leukemia, and the few survivors generally underwent allogeneic bone marrow transplantation.[147,210] The 3-year disease-free survival was 19% in a retrospective study of allogeneic bone marrow transplantation for pediatric treatment-related MDS/AML following primary acute lymphoblastic leukemia.[372] In another retrospective study of allogeneic bone marrow transplantation for treatment-related MDS/AML in children, the 2-year disease-free survival was 24% (95% CI, 5–53%).[373] In the Children's Cancer Group 2891 study, patients were randomly assigned to standard-timing or intensive-timing induction therapy with dexamethasone, cytarabine, thioguanine, etoposide, and daunorubicin, with or without G-CSF. The 50% induction rate in 24 patients with treatment-related MDS/AML was significantly worse than the 72% induction rate in those in patients with treatment-related MDS/AML who received de novo disease.[150] However, disease-free survival was similar (45% vs. 53%) if induction was achieved.[150] Moreover, respective overall long-term survival rates in patients with treatment-related MDS/AML who received standard-timing versus intensive-timing induction were 0% and 32%, suggesting that intensive-timing induction can improve the outcome.[150]

Hematopoietic Stem Cell Transplantation with Reduced-Intensity or No Conditioning

Reduced-intensity conditioning for hematopoietic stem cell transplantation is another approach that may prove beneficial.[374,375] Durable remissions and potential graft-versus-leukemia effects have been described in adults with de novo or treatment-related AML/MDS, using the strategy of reduced-intensity conditioning with hematopoietic stem cell transplantation as consolidation therapy in first remission; results were especially promising for three patients with treatment-related AML/MDS included in the study.[375] In pediatric de novo myelodysplasia, it is possible to perform allogeneic bone marrow transplantation without conditioning in at least in some cases.[376]

Low-Dose Chemotherapy and Differentiating Agents

In elderly or heavily pretreated patients, intensive chemotherapy and hematopoietic stem cell transplantation are not feasible. Low-dose melphalan is an option that has been used successfully in some cases.[377] Use of low-dose cytarabine as a differentiating agent has been associated with significant mortality from myelosuppression and short overall survival (about 3 months), comparable to supportive care.[378] Other differentiating agents used for myelodysplasia are arsenic trioxide, the combined differentiating agents all-*trans* retinoic acid and erythropoietin, or G-CSF and erythropoietin,[363–365] but efficacy in treatment-related myelodysplasia remains to be determined.

Azacitidine is a cytotoxic drug that also induces differentiation at low doses, possibly through DNA methyltransferase inhibition or multifactorial mechanisms.[379] Findings of hypermethylation of specific genes in treatment-related myelodysplasia[201,204] have suggested a potential role for demethylating agents in the therapy of treatment-related AML/MDS. In a randomized trial of azacitidine versus supportive care for myelodysplasia, which also included patients with secondary myelodysplasia, azacitidine treatment was associated with clinical responses in 60% of patients (7% complete remission, 16% partial remission, 37% improved), prolonged time to leukemia transformation, and prolonged survival.[379] There are also encouraging data suggesting that 5-aza-2′-deoxycytidine can result in clinical responses in treatment-related AML/MDS.[380]

Molecularly Targeted Treatments

Molecularly targeted approaches for secondary leukemias are especially attractive and are being actively sought because of the poor treatment outcomes and toxicities associated with intensive chemotherapy and hematopoietic stem cell transplantation. All-*trans* retinoic acid is the first example of a useful targeted agent for the subset of patients with de novo or treatment-related acute promyelocytic leukemia.[124] The tyrosine kinase inhibitor imatinib mesylate is now routinely used for newly diagnosed BCR-ABL$^+$ chronic myelogenous leukemia and may enable reduction in conditioning intensity before hematopoietic stem cell transplantation.[381] Imatinib also has been tested in BCR-ABL$^+$ acute lymphoblastic leukemia.[382,383] Although unstudied, imatinib may prove important in BCR-ABL$^+$ treatment-related leukemias, especially in heavily pretreated patients. In addition, imatinib targets other tyrosine kinases, and complete remission was achieved using imatinib for a case of refractory c-Kit$^+$ secondary acute myeloid leukemia.[384]

Promising preclinical data have shown sensitivity of *MLL*-rearranged leukemias with *FLT3* mutations to FLT-3 tryosine kinase inhibitors.[320,323,385] Leukemia-specific fusion proteins from chromosomal translocations disrupting various transcription factors are other molecular targets for potential future leukemia-specific drugs.[386] Approaches for targeting messenger RNA with antisense, ribozymes or RNA interference may prove useful for the chromosomal translocations that create leukemia-specific fusion transcripts.[387–391]

Supportive Care

Supportive care, including blood product support and the management of infections, is an important adjunct to all of the definitive therapies for secondary leukemias that are currently in use. Until recently, supportive care alone with antibiotics and transfusions was considered standard care for high-risk myelodysplasia, including secondary myelodysplasia, because of the high mortality from bone marrow failure and leukemia transformation.[379] However, in the randomized trial of azacitidine versus supportive care described previously, azacitidine proved the superior treatment option, with improvement not only in response rates and survival times but also in the quality of life for this population.[379]

PROGNOSIS

Treatment factors are critical determinants of prognosis in the secondary leukemias, as described previously, with the most favorable outcomes achieved in patients in whom intensive therapies are feasible. Disease factors are other determinants of prognosis. The subsets of alkylating agent–related leukemias with −7/del(7q) without chromosome 5 abnormalities may have different outcomes than the cases with −5/del(5q) and unbalanced chromosome 5 translocations.[184] Leukemias with chromosome 5 abnormalities and their associated molecular aberrations, especially p53 loss of heterozygosity, are uniformly associated with an extremely poor prognosis.[184] In contrast, patients with treatment-related myelodysplasia with −7 as the sole abnormality without excess blasts may have prolonged survival, although the outcome usually is unfavorable.[184] A subset of children with −7/del(7q) treatment-related myelodysplasia achieve spontaneous hematologic and cytogenetic improvement without any therapy, but the factors associated with this clinical outcome are uncertain.[392,393] Observations of transient monosomy 7 myelodysplasia after primary cancer regimens including G-CSF administration have suggested that observation is appropriate in this setting.[361]

Treatment-related leukemias with *MLL* translocations are associated with a grave prognosis, with significantly shorter median survival than leukemias with chromosome band 21q22 abnormalities, inv(16), or t(15;17).[16] Patients with treatment-related leukemias characterized by t(8;21), inv(16), and t(15;17) respond more favorably to therapy, similar to de novo cases with the same translocations.[124,213,224,368,394] In analyses conducted using gene expression profiling, cases of acute myeloid leukemia with the t(8;21), inv(16), or t(15;17) clustered into unique, genetically defined, favorable prognostic subgroups.[395,396]

CURRENT CONTROVERSIES & FUTURE CONSIDERATIONS

Secondary Myelodysplasia/Acute Myeloid Leukemia

- What are the critical tumor suppressor genes at chromosome 5q and 7q?
- What is the role of chemotherapy dose and schedule in topoisomerase II inhibitor–related cases?
- Should large-scale pharmacogenomic profiling and screening for germline tumor suppressor gene mutations and mutations in critical DNA repair proteins be implemented to identify individuals at highest risk?
- What are the best host-specific and disease-specific biomarkers to predict this treatment complication?
- Is it feasible to individualize primary cancer therapy without compromising efficacy to reduce the risk?
- Will molecularly targeted agents ultimately change the generally dismal outcome?

Suggested Readings*

Blayney DW, Longo DL, Young RC, et al: Decreasing risk of leukemia with prolonged follow-up after chemotherapy and radiotherapy for Hodgkin's disease. N Engl J Med 316:710–714, 1987.

Mistry AR, Felix CA, Whitmarsh RJ, et al: DNA topoisomerase II in therapy-related acute promyelocytic leukemia. N Engl J Med 252:1529–1538, 2005.

Pedersen-Bjergaard J, Andersen MK, Christiansen DH, Nerlov C: Genetic pathways in therapy-related myelodysplasia and acute myeloid leukemia. Blood 99:1909–1912, 2002.

Ratain MJ, Kaminer LS, Bitran JD, et al: Acute nonlymphocytic leukemia following etoposide and cisplatin combination chemotherapy for advanced non-small-cell carcinoma of the lung. Blood 70:1412–1417, 1987.

Rowley JD, Olney HJ: International workshop on the relationship of prior therapy to balanced chromosome aberrations in therapy-related myelodysplastic syndromes and acute leukemia: overview report. Genes Chromosomes Cancer 33:331–345, 2002.

Smith MA, Rubenstein L, Anderson JR, et al: Secondary leukemia or myelodysplastic syndrome after treatment with epipodophyllotoxins. J Clin Oncol 17:569–577, 1999.

Full references for this chapter can be found on accompanying CD-ROM.

CHAPTER 30

ACUTE PROMYELOCYTIC LEUKEMIA

Martin S. Tallman, MD, Simrit Parmar, MD, and LoAnn C. Peterson, MD

KEY POINTS

Acute Promyelocytic Leukemia

Diagnosis

- The t(15;17) translocation leading to the PML/RARα fusion protein represents the genetic identity of acute promyelocytic leukemia (APL).
- There is no increase in incidence with age.
- Patients present with easy bruising, petechial hemorrhages, and mucosal bleeding, including gingival bleeding, epistaxis, and conjunctival hemorrhages.
- Pancytopenia is common, although some patients, especially those with the microgranular variant, may present with leukocytosis.
- Circulating abnormal promyelocytes with numerous coarse cytoplasmic azurophilic granules with multiple, frequently with intertwined Auer rods.
- Flow cytometry frequently shows $CD13^+$, $CD33^+$, $CD45RA^+$, and $CD117^+$. Cells are typically negative for CD34, HLA-DR, and CD11b.
- Poor prognostic factors include white blood cell count greater than 10,000/μL, platelet count less than 40,000/μL, age 55–60 years or greater, and CD56 overexpression.

Treatment

- Anthracyclines and all-*trans* retinoic acid (ATRA) are the mainstays of induction therapy.
- Coagulopathy at presentation or during induction is a cause of early death.
- The treatment of therapy-related APL should be similar to that of de novo APL.
- Concurrent therapy with ATRA and chemotherapy is better than therapy with either agent alone.
- Retinoic acid syndrome, a cardiorespiratory distress syndrome, usually occurs between the second day and third week of treatment with ATRA. This is usually treatable with early administration of high-dose corticosteroid therapy.
- Reverse transcriptase–polymerase chain reaction (RT-PCR) is a powerful tool for assessment of response to treatment. Therapy should be initiated at the time of molecular relapse, confirmed by RT-PCR alone.
- Arsenic trioxide is the treatment of choice for relapsed APL.
- Prolonged heart rate–corrected Q-T interval and APL differentiation syndrome are the most common drug-related toxicities seen with arsenic trioxide.
- Stem cell transplantation should be offered to patients in second complete remission.

INTRODUCTION

Acute promyelocytic leukemia (APL) is a distinct subtype of acute myeloid leukemia (AML), identified by the French-American-British classification as AML M3 and associated with the chromosomal translocation t(15;17).[1] APL was first described in 1957 in three patients with "a very rapid fatal course of only a few weeks' duration, a white blood cell picture dominated by promyelocytes, and a severe bleeding tendency due to fibrinolysis and thrombocytopenia."[2,3] The French-American-British classification was established in 1976.[4] APL has unique molecular genetic changes, a typical clinical presentation, a high complete remission rate with anthracyclines, and prolonged long-term survival in response to differentiation therapy with all-*trans* retinoic acid (ATRA). Patients frequently present with easy bruising, leukopenia, circu-

TABLE 30–1. Pathogenesis of Coagulopathy in APL

Mechanism	Putative Mediators
DIC	Tissue factor
	Cancer procoagulant
	Cytokines (IL-1, TNF)
Fibrinolysis	tPA, uPA, PAI-1
	Annexin
Proteolysis	Elastases (targets include fibrinogen and vWF)

Abbreviations: IL-1, interleukin-1; PAI-1, plasminogen activator inhibitor-1; TNF, tumor necrosis factor; tPA, tissue-type plasminogen activator; uPA, urokinase; vWF, von Willebrand factor.

lating promyelocytes, and thrombocytopenia and anemia. Life-threatening coagulopathy, manifested by disseminated intravascular coagulation (DIC), hyperfibrinolysis, or both, is often aggravated by chemotherapy (Table 30–1). Elevated levels of fibrin D-dimer, prothrombin fragment 1.2, thrombin-antithrombin complex, and fibrinopeptide A indicate the presence of DIC.[5] Historically, there has been a high early death rate as a result of bleeding. The diagnosis of APL is established by the presence of a balanced reciprocal translocation between chromosomes 15 and 17, t(15;17)(q22;q21), which leads to formation of two fusion genes, promyelocytic leukemia/retinoic acid receptor α (*PML-RARA*) and *RARA-PML,* the former being considered to play a crucial role in leukemogenesis.[6,7] Before 1986, at daunorubicin doses of 150–210 mg/m^2, complete remission rates of 60–68% were achieved[8–13] with a median survival duration ranging from 13 to 25 months.[14] With the introduction of ATRA in 1987 as a differentiating agent[15] and arsenic trioxide (ATO) in 1992 as an inducer of both apoptosis and differentiation,[16] marked improvement has occurred in the outcome of patients with both de novo and relapsed APL.[17–30] Historically, this disease was once characterized as the most rapidly fatal human leukemia. Now, APL is the most frequently curable leukemia in adults.

EPIDEMIOLOGY AND RISK FACTORS

Incidence

APL accounts for approximately 10–15% of all U.S. and European patients with AML.[1,31] However, the incidence is as high as 32% in some areas of China[32] and 46% among AML patients of Hispanic origin.[33] Using data from large studies from the United States and Europe with a total of 4639 AML patients, 500 patients (10.8%) had APL.[14,34–39] Among a total of 3229 AML patients registered in all clinical trials of the Italian cooperative group GIMEMA, 335 patients were classified as APL (10.4%).[40,41] Unlike other types of AML, there appears to be no significant rise in the incidence of APL with age after age 20.[42,43]

A higher frequency of APL among patients of Hispanic origin (originating in Latin America, i.e., from Mexico or Central or South America) with AML was observed in Los Angeles County.[44] Of 80 AML Hispanic patients at the University of Southern California Medical Center, 37.5% had APL compared to only 6.5% of non-Hispanic patients with AML.[33] In a larger population-based survey of AML patients in the entire county of Los Angeles, 24.3% of Hispanic patients had APL compared with 8.3% of non-Hispanic patients.[33] Subsequent reports from Peru,[45] Mexico,[46] and Texas[47] support this observation, although its origins remain unclear. The population distribution of the breakpoint sites in the *PML* gene at the 16;17 translocation in all patients with APL from Europe[27,48–51] and the United States[52,53] is 50–55% for *bcr1,* 8–20% for *bcr2,* and 27–49% for *bcr3*. However, the rate of *bcr1* is 75% among Hispanic patients,[54] suggesting a genetic predisposition.

Etiologic Factors

Environmental Risk Factors

No environmental and/or occupational risk factors have been identified for APL. Two reports from China have shown that exposure to bimolane (a drug used for the treatment of psoriasis) is associated with APL.[55,56] However, a causal relationship remains to be established.

Therapy-Related APL

The incidence of therapy-related APL ranges between 1.7% and 5.8%[57] (see Chapter 29). The median time from chemotherapy exposure to the onset of APL generally ranges between 25 and 36 months, with no preleukemic phase.[57–59] In a large retrospective analysis of 106 patients, those treated for breast cancer or lymphoma were most commonly affected.[57] No significant differences were found in karyotypic abnormalities or the type of *PML-RARA* fusion in the two cohorts. Secondary APL patients were characterized by a predominance of females ($P < .003$), 71% of whom had a primary malignancy of the reproductive tract, as well as higher median age ($P < .05$) and worse performance status ($P < .005$) compared to de novo cases.[58,59] Treatment outcome of the primary disease was not a risk factor.[58,59] In the GIMEMA experience, treatment outcome for primary and secondary APL was similar: the complete remission, 4-year event-free survival, and 4-year overall survival rates are 97% and 93%, 65% and 68%, and 85% and 78% in the secondary and de novo APL groups, respectively.[58] Thus, the approach to therapy for de novo and therapy-related APL should be similar.[58]

MOLECULAR PATHOGENESIS

PML/RARα

The t(15;17) translocation represents the genetic identity of APL.[60–62] The balanced reciprocal translocation involves fusion of the *RARA* gene present on chromosome 17 to the *PML* gene on chromosome 15, generating PML/RARα chimeric protein.[60–62] The PML-RARα

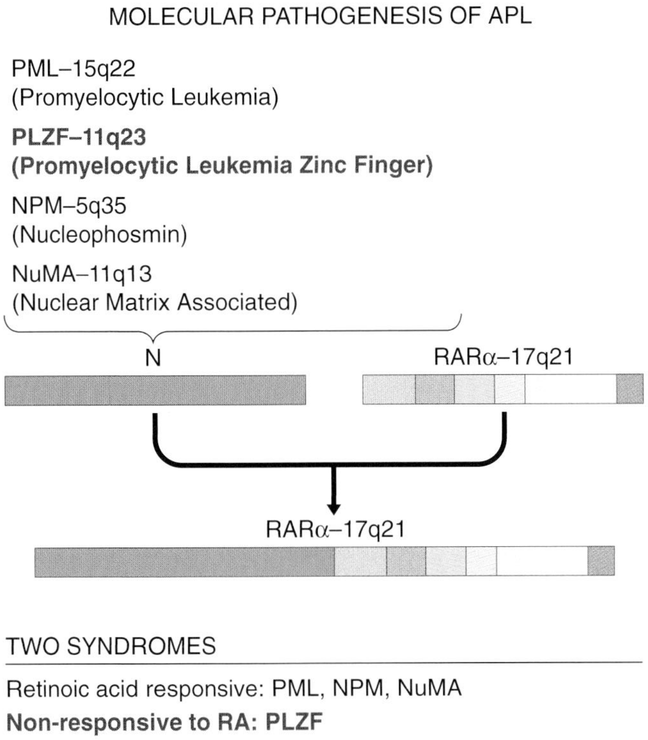

MOLECULAR PATHOGENESIS OF APL

PML–15q22
(Promyelocytic Leukemia)

PLZF–11q23
(Promyelocytic Leukemia Zinc Finger)

NPM–5q35
(Nucleophosmin)

NuMA–11q13
(Nuclear Matrix Associated)

N

RARα–17q21

RARα–17q21

TWO SYNDROMES

Retinoic acid responsive: PML, NPM, NuMA
Non-responsive to RA: PLZF

Figure 30–1. Molecular pathogenesis of APL. The four chromosomal translocations associated with APL result in fusion proteins in which the B through F domains of RARα, including the DNA-binding and ligand-binding domains of protein, are linked through the carboxyl terminus to four different nuclear proteins containing self-association domains. (From Melnick A, Licht JD: Deconstructing a disease: RARalpha, its fusion partners, and their roles in the pathogenesis of acute promyelocytic leukemia. Blood 93:3167–3215, 1999, with permission.)

fusion protein not only constitutes the molecular signature of APL, but also contributes to its pathogenesis by disrupting the wild-type function of both *RARA* and *PML* genes[60–66] (Fig. 30–1). The PML-RARα fusion gene product always contains the same regions of RARα, including the nuclear receptor DNA and ligand-binding domains, whereas the amino-terminal PML sequences show patient-to-patient variability determined by the translocation breakpoint within the *PML* gene and by alternative exon splicing.[51] There are three breakpoint clusters within the *PML* gene: intron 3 (*bcr3,* or short form), exon 6 (*bcr2,* or long form), and intron 6 (*bcr1,* or short form). The mechanism by which these breakpoints are determined is not known. The generation of PML-RARα has several effects.[62,67] First, PML-RARα forms homodimers that recruit two corepressor molecules, SMRT and N-coR, more tightly as compared to the RAR-RXR heterodimer formed by the wild-type RARα. These corepressors are part of a multiprotein complex that includes histone deacetylases (HDACs). Deacetylation of histones alters the conformation of chromatin and its accessibility to the transcriptional machinery, resulting in transcriptional silencing. This may be the basis of the block of myeloid differentiation at the promyelocyte level. Treatment with ATRA leads to dissociation of the PML-RARα-HDAC-mSin3-NcoR-repressor complex and recruitment of coactivators (NcoA-1/SRC-1, CBP/p300, p/CIP, and ACTR), resulting in transcriptional activation of sensitive genes[62,67,68] (Fig. 30–2*A*). Furthermore, the PML-RARα oncoprotein possesses the same binding affinity to retinoic acid–responsive elements as wild-type RARα, which leads to dominant-negative silencing of RAR-RXR-mediated transcription.[62–64,69] Whereas wild-type RARα and signal transducer and activator of transcription 1α (STAT1α) synergistically stimulate transcription from an interferon response element–containing reporter, PML-RARα does not. This suggests that the cross-talk between interferon and retinoid signaling may be defective in APL.[62]

In addition to transcriptional repression of retinoid nuclear receptor functions, PML-RARα also inhibits the tumor suppressor and proapoptotic functions of PML, conferring the leukemic blasts a proliferative and survival advantage.[65,66] Even though the PML-RARα oncoprotein retains the major functional domains of the *PML* gene, its normal physiologic functions are inhibited.[65,66] Such an inactivation of the *PML* gene involves its displacement from the well-studied nuclear organelle called the PML nuclear body or oncogenic domains, which are normally distributed as discrete nuclear speckles (10–20 in number), into hundreds of indistinct micropunctate subnuclear domains seen in APL.[65,66,70] The disruption of nuclear bodies relocalizes PML and thereby limits its inherent capacity to interact with other PML oncogenic domain coinhabitants and transcriptional modulators, such as p53, DAXX, SUMO-1, Sp 100, Sp 140, CBP, DAXX, and Rb.[65,66,70] Although the role of nuclear bodies in transcriptional regulation is still under investigation, both ATRA and ATO treatment of APL blasts restores the structure of nuclear bodies.[62,68,71–73] However, the pathogenic significance of nuclear body disruption is challenged by its lack of occurrence in non-PML/RARα subtypes of APL and also by in vitro results obtained by transfecting a mutant form of PML/RARα into leukemic cells.[74] Such a transfection of mutated fusion protein lacking the coiled-coiled moiety of the *PML* gene results in myeloid differentiation block in the absence of nuclear body disruption in leukemic cells.[74] The results indicate that the disruption of nuclear bodies is not the most critical change necessary to induce a maturation arrest in APL blasts and that additional mechanisms are involved in its pathogenesis.

The critical role of PML-RARα in the pathogenesis of APL and thus as an oncoprotein has been supported by the generation of transgenic mouse models of the disease.[75,76] In all these models, a significant delay in onset of leukemia suggests that a second, as yet uncharacterized, genetic hit is required for transformation. When the transgenic mice were crossed with PML-null mice, leukemia developed at an accelerated rate, supporting the growth-suppressive effect of PML.[77] Furthermore, consistent with this notion that other pathways may contribute to the leukemogenesis, constitutively active forms of the Fms-like tyrosine kinase 3 (FLT3) receptor are seen in 37% of APL cases,[78,79] particularly those with elevated white blood cell (WBC) count. When mutant FLT3 is transduced into the marrow of *PML/RARA*-expressing

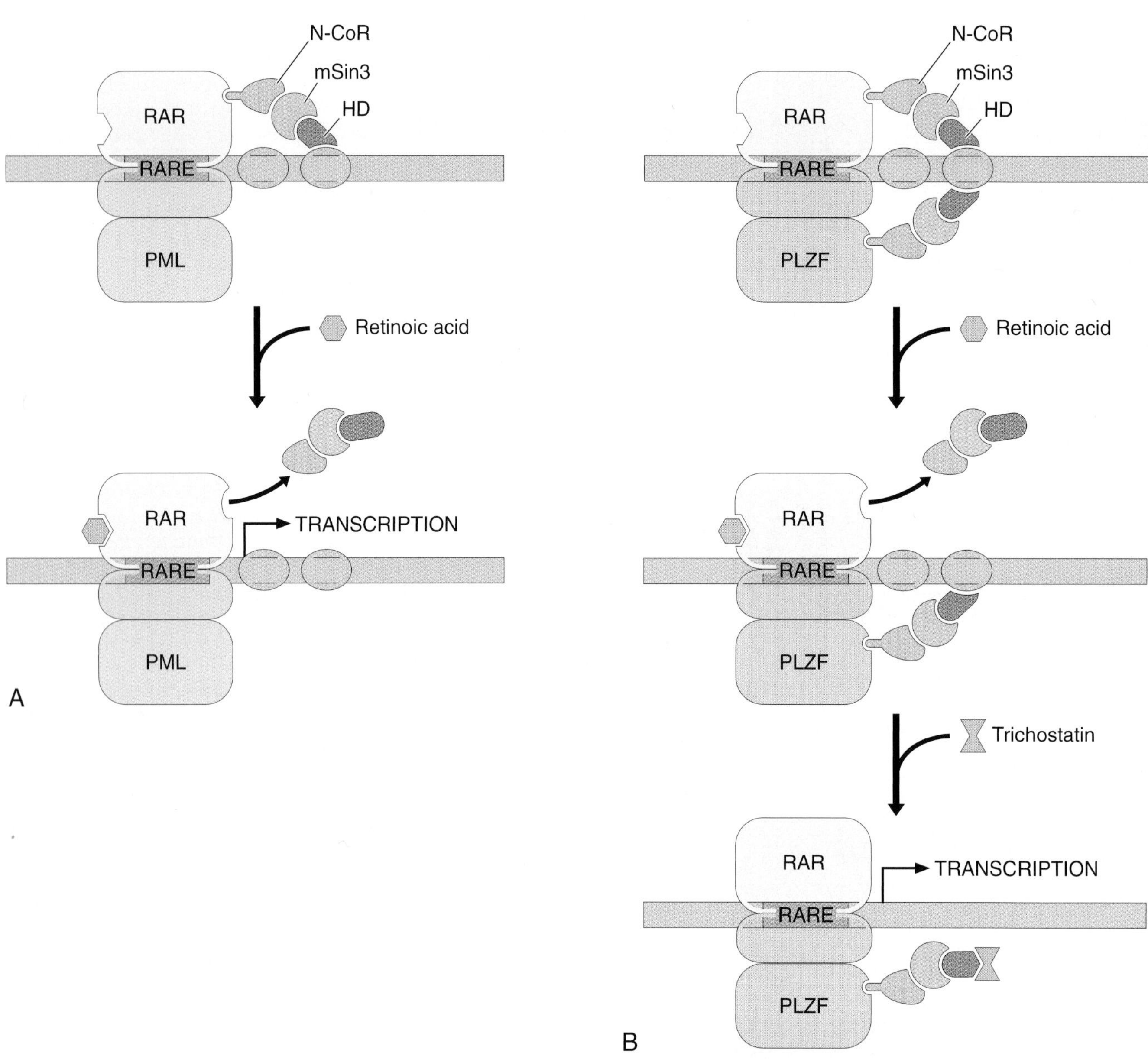

■ **Figure 30–2.** *A,* A model for the interactions of APL fusion proteins with the N-CoR-mSin3-histone deacetylase (HD) complex. DNA-bound PML/RARα interacts with N-CoR (or SMRT) and recruits the mSin3-HD complex, decreasing histone acetylation and producing repressive chromatin organization and transcriptional regression. Retinoic acid (RA) induces dissociation of the N-CoR-mSin3-HD complex, recruitment of coactivators with histone acetyltransferase activity (not shown), increased levels of histone acetylation, chromatin remodeling, and transcriptional activation. *B,* PLZF/RARα has two N-CoR binding sites that, even in the presence of RA, recruit the N-CoR-mSin3-HD complex and maintain transcription repression. (From Grignani F, De Matteis S, Nervi C, et al: Fusion proteins of the retinoic acid receptor-alpha recruit histone deacetylase in promyelocytic leukaemia. Nature 391:815–818, 1998, with permission.)

mice, APL develops with a short latent period, emphasizing the multistep nature of the disease.[80]

Other RARα Fusion Partner Proteins

Even though in 98% of cases the t(15;17) translocation is the predominant genetic abnormality, a promyelocytic leukemia zinc finger (PLZF)/RARα fusion gene product resulting from reciprocal translocation of t(11;17)(q23;q21) has been described in 0.8% of APL cases.[81] Patients with this finding present with phenotypic features similar to APL (Fig. 30–2*B*). In other patients, the *PML* gene of the X/RARα chimera is substituted by other transcription factors such as nuclear mitotic apparatus (t(11;17)(q13;q21)), nucleophosmin (t(5;17)(q35;q21)), or STAT5B (17q21.3-q23).[62,82,83] APL patients bearing the PLZF/RARα and STAT5B/RARα translocations are highly resistant to the differentiating effects of ATRA therapy[62,82,83] because the fusion protein recruits corepressors through both the RARα and PLZF moieties, wherein ATRA treatment cannot release all the HDAC-corepressor complex bound to the basal transcriptional machinery.[62,82] HDAC inhibitors reverse the resistance of PLZF-RARα transcriptional repression to retinoid-based differentiating therapy and are currently being tested in humans.[68,74]

FLT3 Mutation in APL

FLT3/internal tandem duplication (ITD) mutations occur in 35–39% of patients with APL[84,85] associated with leukocytosis.[86] A study of 107 APL patients identified 20 patients with FLT3/ITD and 20 patients with Asp835 mutation.[87] The microgranular variant (M3v) form of leukemia was found to be associated with a higher frequency of only ITD ($P = .002$). There was no significant difference in complete remission, overall survival, or event-free survival between patients with or without FLT3 mutations. There is emerging evidence that SU11657, a tyrosine kinase inhibitor that targets FLT3, cooperates with ATRA to cause regression of APL in a transgenic mouse model.[88]

Effect of ATRA

In addition to activating the transcription of repressed target genes,[75] ATRA treatment of APL blasts leads to caspase-mediated degradation of the PML/RARα chimeric protein.[89] ATRA appears to regulate the antiproliferative actions of this protein in APL by activating signaling pathways that may or may not be nuclear receptor mediated.[90]

CLINICAL FEATURES

Symptoms and Signs

In general, patients present with profound hemorrhagic manifestations, including hemoptysis, hematuria, vaginal bleeding, melena, hematemesis, and pulmonary and intracranial bleeding. Easy bruising, petechial hemorrhages, and prolonged bleeding from skin injuries are common. Mucosal bleeding may include gingival bleeding, epistaxis, and conjunctival hemorrhages (Fig. 30–3*A* and *B*). Occasionally, patients present with bleeding from gastrointestinal, genitourinary, bronchopulmonary, or central nervous system locations (Fig. 30–3*C*) or from splenic and renal infarcts (Fig. 30–3*D* and *E*).

DIAGNOSIS

Laboratory Findings

The leukocyte count in APL is typically decreased, but 20% of patients present with leukocytosis. Patients with micrognanular APL more commonly present with leukocytosis. Anemia and thrombocytopenia are present in most cases, and the thrombocytopenia is often severe (<50,000/μL). DIC is common, with decreased fibrinogen, elevated fibrin degradation products, and prominent microangiopathy. Nucleated red cells are absent because erythropoiesis is depressed.

Blood and Bone Marrow

The peripheral blood almost always shows circulating abnormal promyelocytes, although their numbers vary and may be low. The bone marrow is hypercellular, and the dominant cells in the bone marrow are abnormal promyelocytes that comprise approximately 30–100% of the bone marrow cells (Fig. 30–4). In classic hypergranular APL, numerous coarse azurophilic granules in the cytoplasm characterize the neoplastic cells. The nuclear contour varies and may be bilobed, folded, or reniform. Occasionally the heavy azurophilic granules within the cytoplasm obscure the nuclear outlines.[91] Auer rods, often multiple and intertwined, are common (Fig. 30–5); myeloblasts are infrequent. Cytochemical stains show that the abnormal promyelocytes are intensely positive for myeloperoxidase; they may also be weakly positive for nonspecific esterase. Some granules contain histamine and can induce hyperhistamintemia.[92]

Microgranular (hypogranular) APL represents about 20% of cases of APL[93–96] (Fig. 30–6). The granules are submicroscopic in size (not visible by light microscopy). In these cases, the leukemic cells often exhibit bilobed or folded nuclei, and may be confused with acute monocytic leukemia. Often, at least some of the abnormal promyelocytes contain visible abundant granules and/or multiple Auer rods, and are strongly myeloperoxidase positive.

Immunophenotype

The leukemic promyelocytes from patients with APL and the t(15;17) translocation have a characteristic, although not diagnostic, immunophenotype. The leukemic promyelocytes express CD33 and CD13. CD34 and HLA-DR are typically absent or expressed on only a subset of the leukemic cells.[97–99] More mature myeloid antigens such as CD14,[100] CD15,[101] and CD11b[100] are weakly expressed or absent. c-Kit (stem cell factor receptor, CD117) is expressed by a high percentage of APL cases[102,103] as is CD45RA.[104] CD2 and CD9 are frequently coexpressed.

Elevated CD34 and CD2 expression is seen in the microgranular APL variant.[105–107] Furthermore, increased expression of neural adhesion molecule (CD56 antigen), associated with poor clinical outcome, is found in S-form cells.[108,109]

Molecular Diagnosis of APL

The detection of the fusion gene transcript PML/RARα by the reverse transcriptase–polymerase chain reaction (RT-PCR) technique is a specific molecular marker of APL.[110–112] Detection of PML/RARα predicts responsiveness to ATRA,[99,111,113] particularly when morphologic and cytogenetic studies are inconclusive.[114–118] For the prompt initiation of ATRA-containing therapy, RT-PCR

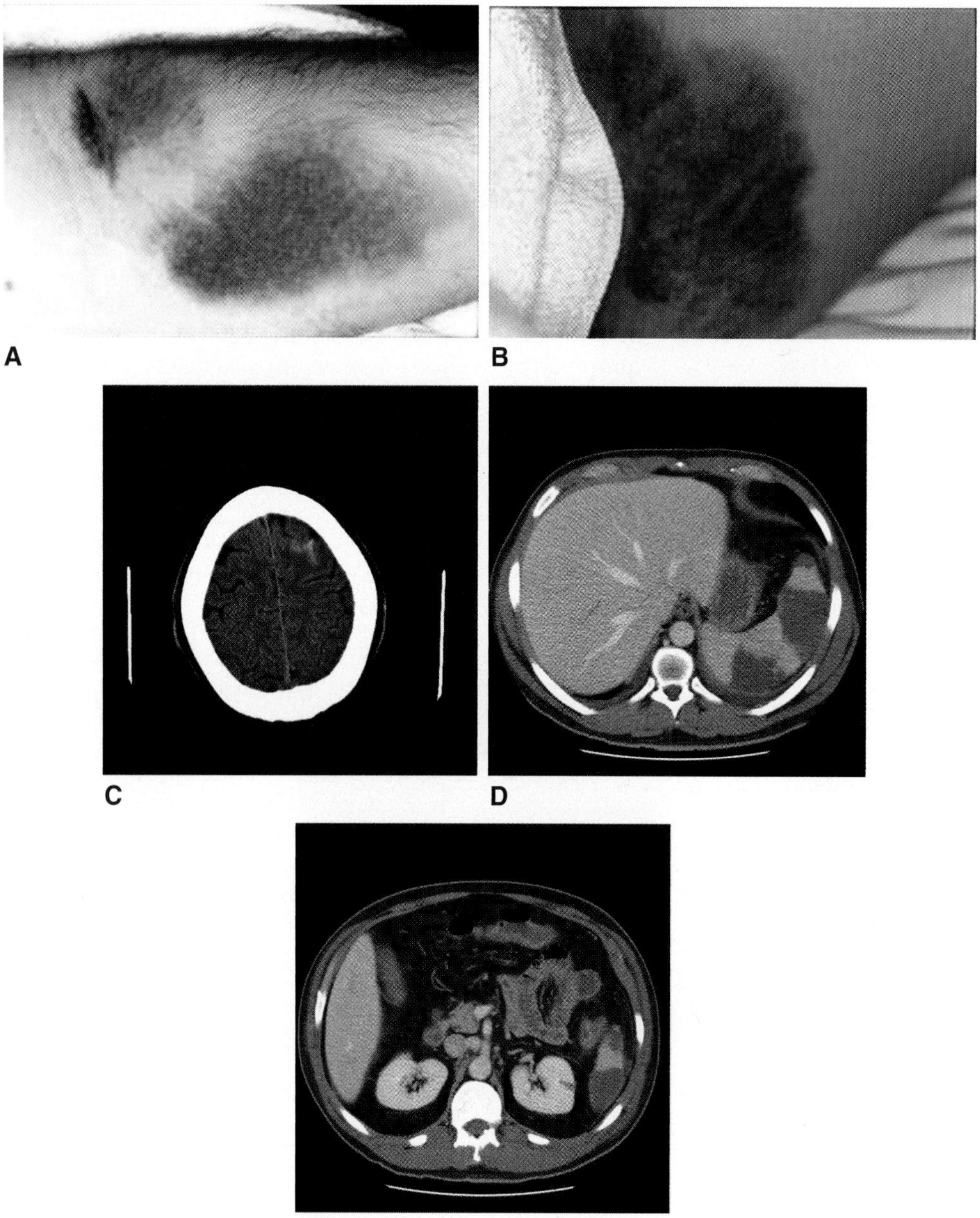

Figure 30–3. Different clinical manifestations of the coagulopathy in newly diagnosed APL patients. ***A,*** Arm bruising. ***B,*** Ecchymosis on thigh. ***C,*** Subarachnoid hemorrhage. ***D,*** Splenic infarctions. ***E,*** Renal infarctions.

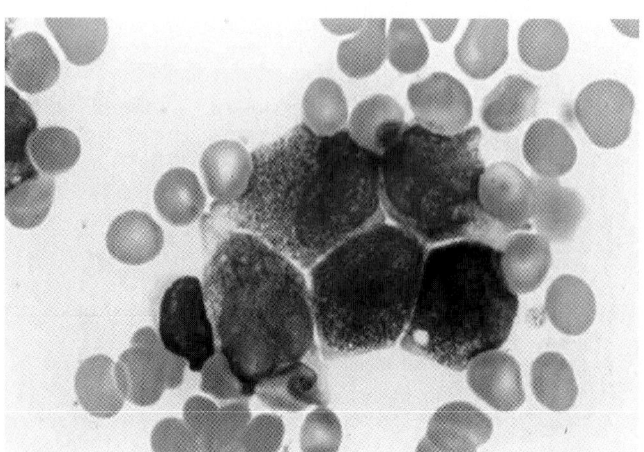

Figure 30–4. Several abnormal hypergranular promyelocytes in bone marrow aspirate from a patient with APL.

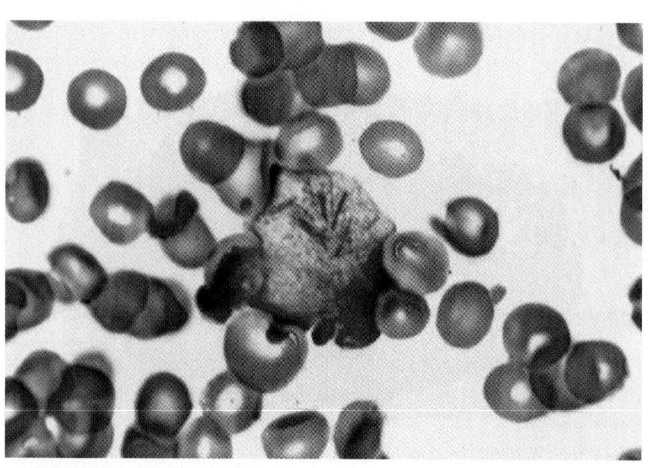

Figure 30–5. Multiple Auer rods in the cytoplasm of this cell in a bone marrow aspirate from a patient with APL. The cell is damaged, making the Auer rods easier to see.

provides more rapid diagnosis than fluorescent in situ hybridization analysis; however, the latter is equally specific.[99,113] PG-M3 monoclonal antibody directed against the amino-terminal portion of PML produces a characteristic pattern known as PML nuclear bodies.[117–120] These nuclear bodies are disrupted in APL cells that bear the t(15;17), from the normal speckled to a microgranular pattern. This technique is particularly useful in the diagnosis of the microgranular variant of APL (M3V).[121]

TREATMENT

Induction Therapy

Anthracyclines and retinoic acid are the mainstays of induction therapy for patients with APL (Table 30–2). The observation of the exquisite sensitivity of APL to daunorubicin, originally reported by Bernard and colleagues[8] in 1973, was confirmed by other European groups in the 1980s and was extended to other anthracyclines, with a complete remission rate of 55–90% and 50–65% relapse, resulting in a 30–40% survival at 2 years.[10,12,122] Unlike other AML subtypes, anthracyclines are able to induce long-lasting remissions when given as single agents in induction therapy for APL, perhaps because of the absence of the multidrug resistance glycoprotein p170.[123–125] A dramatic response to treatment with oral ATRA in APL patients was initially noted by investigators in Shanghai in 1988[17] and subsequently confirmed by other groups.[21,22] Figure 30–7 shows changes in the morphology of the bone marrow aspirate in a patient with APL treated with ATRA at day 0, 12, and 37. Despite initial high complete remission rates, remissions induced with ATRA monotherapy are short lived, prompting the inclusion of conventional chemotherapy in the initial treatment.[20,22,126] Furthermore, some patients treated with ATRA alone develop a rapid increase in WBC count that in some, but not all, patients is associated with the retinoic acid syndrome (RAS).[22,49,127,128]

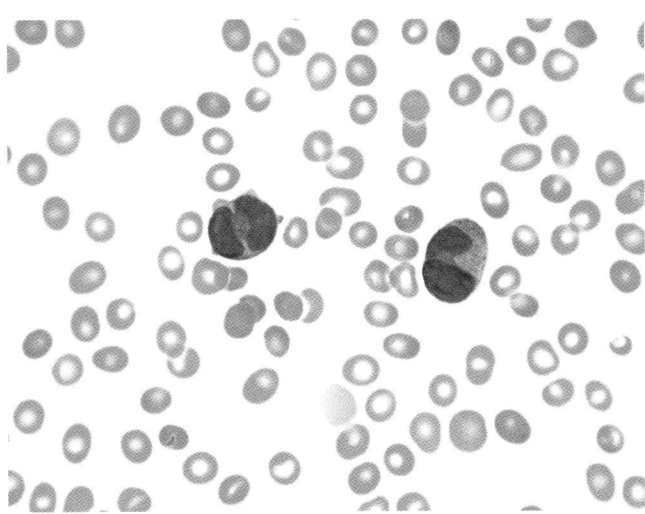

■ **Figure 30–6.** Blood smear from a patient presenting with microgranular APL. The leukocyte count was elevated. Note the characteristic bilobed nucleoli of these leukemic cells.

A prospective randomized trial conducted by the European APL group shows that concurrent ATRA plus chemotherapy leads to a better outcome as compared to sequential treatment.[30] The event-free survival at 2 years is 84% in the concurrent arm compared to 77% in the sequential arm. This difference is attributable to a significant decrease in the risk of relapse at 2 years (6% in the concurrent arm vs. 16% in the sequential arm; P = 0.04).[129] Late relapses are uncommon with chemotherapy treatment.[129] Initial treatment with a combination of ATRA and chemotherapy has the benefit of possibly reducing the incidence of RAS from approximately 25% with ATRA alone[127,128] to 10%.[13,130,131]

Role of Cytarabine

The role of cytarabine as part of initial induction therapy has been questioned. Two retrospective comparisons and a prospective study showed no difference in the complete remission rate between the patients treated with daunorubicin alone and those treated with daunorubicin

TABLE 30–2. Results of Recent Trials of ATRA Plus Chemotherapy in Newly Diagnosed APL

Group	Year	Randomized	No. of Patients	CR Rate (%)	Outcome
Wang et al.[206]	1992	No	400	75	NA
Wang et al.[206]	1995	No	423*	NA	5-yr OS, 18–71%
Soignet et al.[26]	1997	No	73	89	5-yr DFS, 67%
Tallman et al.[25]	1997	Yes†	346	69–72	3-yr DFS, 32–67%
Estey et al.[132]	1997	No	43	77	1.5-yr DFS, 80%
Asou et al.[172]	1998	No	196	88	4-yr DFS, 62%
Avvisati[207]	1998	No	480	95	4-yr DFS, 75%
Burnett et al.[168]	1999	Yes‡	239	70–87	4-yr OS, 52–71%
Fenaux et al.[30]	1999	Yes§	413	90–95	2-yr EFS, 77–84%
Sanz et al.[130]	1999	No	123	89	2-yr DFS, 92%

*ATRA versus chemotherapy versus ATRA + chemotherapy (two protocols).
†ATRA versus chemotherapy.
‡Short (5-day) course of ATRA prior to chemotherapy versus extended ATRA begun with chemotherapy.
§ATRA given simultaneously with versus after chemotherapy.
Abbreviations: ATRA, all-*trans*-retinoic acid; CR, complete remission; DFS, disease-free survival; EFS, event-free survival; NA, not available; OS, overall survival.

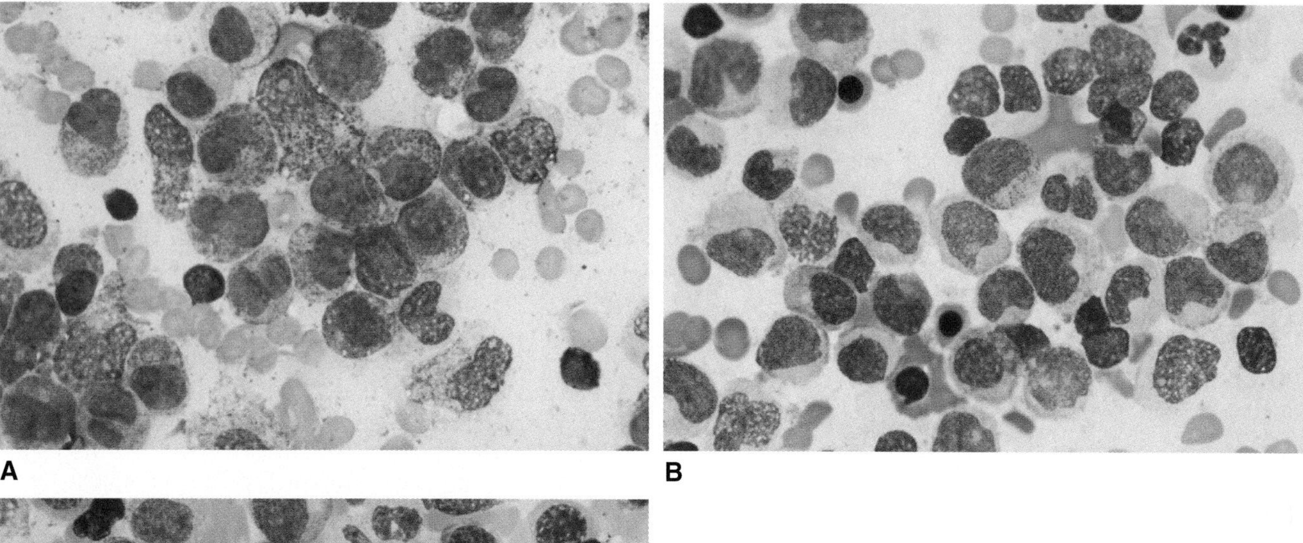

A B

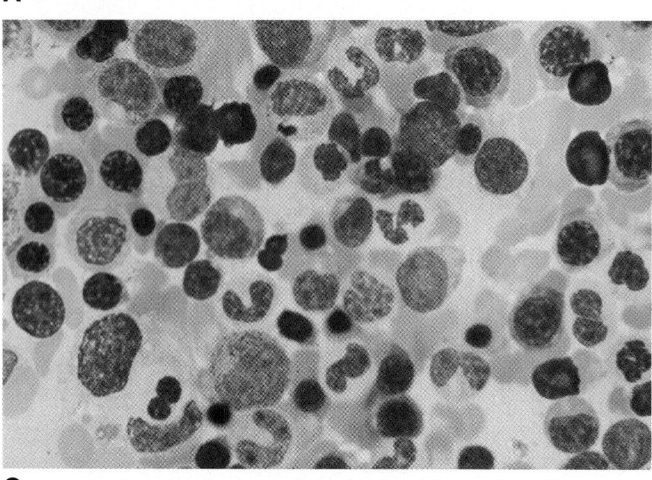

C

■ **Figure 30–7.** Changes in the morphology of the bone marrow aspirate in a patient with APL treated with ATRA. ***A,*** Day 0: Pretreatment bone marrow. ***B,*** Day 12: Maturing myeloid and metamyelocytes. ***C,*** Day 37: Complete hematopoietic differentiation with maturation of all lineages.

in combination with cytarabine.[10,11,13,132] Thus, cytarabine is not an important agent in APL.

Role of Monoclonal Antibodies

Estey and associates[133] reported the role of gemtuzumab ozogamicin, an anti-CD33 monoclonal antibody chemically linked to calicheamicin, a potent cytotoxic agent. Nineteen patients with newly diagnosed APL were treated with ATRA in combination with gemtuzumab ozogamicin. Complete remission was achieved in 14 of 16 patients (88%; 95% confidence interval, 62–98%) given gemtuzumab ozogamicin and ATRA without idarubicin. Jiang and coworkers reported a possible benefit in relapse-free survival when gemtuzumab ozogamicin is included with ATRA in the induction regimen with or without idarubicin.[134] Prolonged hematologic and molecular remission after monotherapy with gemtuzumab ozogamicin given at the time of the third relapse has been reported.[135] However, randomized studies are needed.

Arsenic Trioxide for APL

In a study of 10 pediatric patients, a 90% complete remission rate was achieved with ATO as a single agent, with minimal short-term complications and no relapse during 24 months of follow-up.[136] In another larger study of 63 patients, a complete remission rate of 81% was reported when ATO was used as a single agent.[137] One randomized study of 61 patients with APL utilized three treatment groups, ATRA, ATO, and the combination of ATRA and ATO.[138] Although complete remission rates in all the three groups were high (≥90%), the time to achieve complete remission and the relapse rate were most favorable in the combination group.

Special Considerations during Induction

Impact of ATRA on the Coagulopathy

The coagulopathy associated with APL is a complex disorder (see Table 30–1).[5,139–141] Before the introduction of ATRA, fatal hemorrhages were a major cause of failure. Since then, a number of studies have confirmed that ATRA improves the hemostatic laboratory parameters and bleeding complications.[97,139,142] ATRA-induced remission is accompanied by prompt improvement of the coagulopathy.[21,98] An analysis of the trial carried out by the GIMEMA group compared the coagulopathy and transfusion requirements in patients treated with ATRA and a historical control population. ATRA led to a significant

TABLE 30–3. Comparison of Incidence and Outcome of Retinoic Acid Syndrome

Study	Year	No. of Patients	Induction	Incidence (%)	Mortality (%) with RAS	Mortality (%) due to RAS
Fenaux et al.[30]	1999	413	ATRA ± Chemo	15	8	1
Frankel et al.[152]	1994	78	ATRA	27	29	8
Tallman et al.[25]	1997	172	ATRA	26	5	1
Asou et al.[172]	1998	196	ATRA ± Chemo	6	9	0.5
Firkin et al.[161]	1999	87	ATRA + Steroids	16	21	3
Avvisati[207]	1998	480	ATRA + Chemo	9	4	0.4
Sanz et al.[130]	1999	123	ATRA + Chemo	6	17	0.8

Abbreviations: ATRA, all-*trans* retinoic acid; Chemo, chemotherapy; RAS, retinoic acid syndrome.

reduction of early mortality, fatal and nonfatal bleeding, days with platelet count less than 20 × 10^3/μL, days with fibrinogen less than 100 mg/dL, and platelet and red blood cell consumption.[143] A number of laboratory studies have confirmed the decrease or normalization of clotting and fibrinolytic markers during the first or second week of therapy with ATRA and reduced proteolysis of the von Willebrand factor.[144–147] In vitro ATRA treatment of the NB4 cell line, expressing the characteristic t(15;17) translocation, is associated with loss of expression of circulating procoagulant[148] and decreased expression of tissue factor.[149] Studies show that the reduction in profibrinolytic parameters is more complete than the reduction in procoagulant parameters,[146,150] which may explain the observation that some patients develop thrombosis during ATRA exposure. The effect of ATRA on endothelial cells counteracts the downregulation of thrombomodulin and inhibits the tumor necrosis factor-α– and interleukin-1β–mediated release of tissue factor[150] and protects the endothelium against the prothrombotic potential of these cytokines. Other effects of ATRA include improved endothelial cell fibrinolytic function, upregulation of integrins, downregulation of cathepsin G expression by the APL cells, and differential regulation of adhesion molecules on the blast cells.[147] Treatment with ATRA reverses the excessive annexin II–mediated fibrinolytic activity of leukemic promyelocytes by blocking transcription of the annexin II gene.[151]

Retinoic Acid Syndrome

The major toxicity of ATRA is RAS, a cardiorespiratory distress syndrome manifested by fever, weight gain, respiratory distress, interstitial pulmonary infiltrates, pleural and pericardial effusion, episodic hypotension, and acute renal failure.[152,153] Usually this syndrome occurs between the second day and the third week of treatment. This has been shown in some, but not all, studies to be more common among patients who present with a high WBC count or develop rapid leukocytosis. Its relationship with increased rate of extramedullary relapse, particularly in the central nervous system, remains unclear.[154–158] This syndrome is not caused by leukostasis as seen in other subtypes of AML, in which leukemic blasts obstruct the microcirculation, but rather is due to interstitial infiltration of maturing leukocytes. If not promptly recognized and treated, RAS can lead to death from progressive hypoxemia and multiorgan failure. In earlier experiences before the recognition of this syndrome, 30% of patients with RAS died.[127] In the North American Intergroup study, in which ATRA was administered alone before chemotherapy, the incidence of RAS was 26%; with early recognition, the mortality was reduced to 5% with prompt administration of dexamethasone.[25,128] Chemotherapy after initial treatment with ATRA appears to decrease the incidence of the syndrome (Table 30–3).[30,159] Wiley and Firkin[160] treated 19 patients with ATRA alone and added prophylaxis with prednisone 75 mg/day in 12 patients whose WBC count rose above 10 × 10^9/μL. Pulmonary toxicity was seen in only two patients, associated with increase in WBC count, and these patients subsequently received chemotherapy. Other studies confirm the benefit of prednisone or dexamethasone[153,161,162] in reduction of mortality. If RAS is severe, it is prudent to discontinue ATRA until symptoms resolve. Then ATRA may be continued under the coverage of steroids.

There are several proposed pathophysiologic mechanisms for RAS. The plasma free serine protease activity of cathepsin G, which is known to enhance capillary permeability, is stimulated in patients treated with ATRA.[163] ATRA also causes increased expression of lymphocyte function–associated antigen-1 and other cellular adhesion molecules, resulting in increased binding to epithelium.[164,165] Interleukin-1β, tumor necrosis factor-α, and interleukin-6, which are known to promote leukocyte activation, may play a role in the clinical features of hypotension and pulmonary infiltrates.[166]

Postremission Therapy

Consolidation Chemotherapy

Recent data from the PETHEMA group[167] show that treatment with ATRA in combination with anthracyclines in consolidation therapy leads to an overall reduction in the relapse rate from 20.1% to 8.7% (P = .004). In intermediate-risk patients, as determined by an elevated WBC count (≥10,000/μL) and platelet count (>40,000/μL), this rate decreased from 14.0% to 2.5% (P = .006). This improved antileukemic efficacy also translated into significantly better disease-free survival and overall survival.

Three trials have included high-dose (1–3 gm/m^2) cytarabine in consolidation.[25,168,169] In most studies, consolidation chemotherapy includes an anthracycline-based regimen. The North American Intergroup Study administered one cycle of daunorubicin 45 mg/m^2/day for 3 days and standard-dose cytarabine 100 mg/m^2/day for 7 days as a first consolidation course, followed by high-dose cytarabine 2 gm/m^2 twice daily for 4 days with daunorubicin 45 mg/m^2/day for 2 days.[25] The long-term follow-up of this study confirms that 5-year disease-free survival and overall survival were longer with ATRA than with daunorubicin for induction (69% vs. 29% and 69% vs. 45%, respectively). Based on both induction and maintenance randomizations, the 5-year disease-free survival is 16% for patients randomized to daunorubicin and observation, 47% for daunorubicin and ATRA, 55% for ATRA and observation, and 74% for ATRA and ATRA[170] (Fig. 30–8). Emerging data suggest little, if any, role for cytarabine in consolidation.[168–172] In a prospective study conducted by the PETHEMA group,[167] omission of cytarabine from both induction and consolidation therapy resulted in an initial complete remission rate of 90% with a molecular response of 95% at the end of consolidation therapy and a 3-year overall survival of 78–85%.[167] It has become routine to administer at least two cycles of postremission therapy with ATRA and an anthracycline-containing regimen.[173]

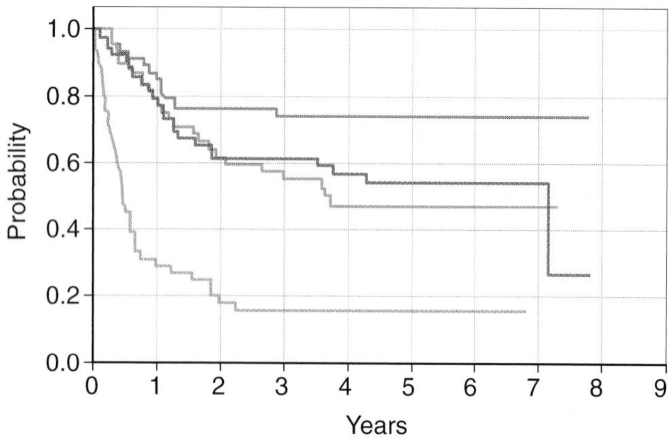

KEY

GROUP	TIME INTERVAL (YEARS) 0–2	2–4	4–6	6–8
DA/ATRA	18/50	6/28	0/18	0/8
DA/Obs	40/51	1/8	0/6	0/2
ATRA/ATRA	11/49	1/34	0/26	0/9
ATRA/Obs	20/54	2/32	1/24	1/12

EVENTS/AT RISK

Figure 30–8. North American Intergroup Study follow-up data on patients treated with daunorubicin versus ATRA. (From Tallman M, Andersen J, Schiffer C, et al: All-trans retinoic acid in acute promyelocytic leukemia: long-term outcome and prognostic factor analysis from the North American Intergroup protocol. Blood 100:4298–4302, 2002, with permission.)

Maintenance Therapy

There appears to an important role for maintenance therapy, which includes ATRA alternating with low-dose chemotherapy, in APL patients who achieve complete remission. This is particularly true in patients at a high risk of relapse, such as those presenting with a high WBC count (≥10,000/μL) and older adults (>60 years)[29] (Table 30–4). In the North American Intergroup study, patients in complete remission after two courses of consolidation therapy were assigned to receive either maintenance treatment with ATRA at standard doses or observation alone. The 3-year disease-free survival was 75% in patients receiving ATRA compared to 60% in patients without any maintenance therapy, and 18% in patients who received induction with chemotherapy alone followed by observation.[25] The European APL 93 trial randomly assigned patients in complete remission to ATRA in standard doses for 15 days every 3 months, 6-mercaptopurine (6-MP) 90 mg/m^2/day plus methotrexate (MTX) 15 mg/m^2/wk, the combination of ATRA and 6-MP/MTX in these dosages, or observation.[30] An additive effect of the two maintenance treatments was seen with a 2-year relapse rate of 7.4% and 2-year event-free survival and overall survival of 93%. Benefit was greater in patients presenting with elevated WBC counts ($P = 0.003$). Currently, maintenance treatment with ATRA in combination with 6-MP and MTX is the standard of care in APL patients in complete remission after consolidation therapy. However, no added benefit of maintenance therapy was seen in patients who were molecularly negative for PML/RARα at the end of three courses of intensive consolidation therapy.[174] A suggested treatment strategy for patients with APL is provided in Table 30–5.

TABLE 30–4. Maintenance Therapy in APL

Study	Year	No. of Patients	Maintenance	Relapse Rate (%)
Fenaux et al.[30]	1999	63	ATRA	20
		64	ATRA + CT	9
		67	Observation	32
Tallman et al.[25]	1997	94	ATRA	32
		105	Observation	57
Sanz et al.[167]	2004	378	ATRA + CT	7.5

Abbreviations: ATRA, all-*trans* retinoic acid; CT, chemotherapy.

Role of Minimal Disease Monitoring

Apart from its value in diagnosis, the technique of RT-PCR offers a powerful tool for sensitive assessment of response to treatment.[99,111,113] Several prospective studies have evaluated the significance of sequential RT-PCR analysis.[27,130,168,175] After completion of consolidation, 90–95% of patients tested RT-PCR negative.[27,130,168] Detection of residual disease at the end of consolidation therapy or thereafter predicts increased risk of relapse.[168,175,176] Fourteen patients received salvage therapy with ATRA plus idarubicin at the time of molecular relapse and had a 2-year Kaplan-Meier survival estimate of 92%.[176] This study appears to justify the initiation of treatment at the time of molecular relapse as determined by RT-PCR, which should be confirmed in at least two separate bone marrow samples before initiating salvage therapy.[175] However, the major difference in the outcome curves occurred very early. A current limitation is failure to quantitate the amount of residual disease precisely.[177] The RT-PCR technique holds considerable promise of providing adequate quantitative standardization and therefore may promote more objective evaluation of residual APL. In 22 patients evaluated for conversion of positive RT-PCR assays, 11 (50%) became RT-PCR negative after HuM195 treatment without additional therapy.[178]

Relapse

Approximately 10–20% of patients receiving initial treatment with ATRA plus chemotherapy will eventually develop hematologic relapse.[167] Second complete remission can be achieved with ATRA if the last exposure occurred greater than 6–12 months before relapse, but long-term remission duration with ATRA alone is rare.[179,180]

TABLE 30–5. Suggested Treatment Strategy for APL

Induction	ATRA + anthracycline-based chemotherapy
Consolidation	Anthracycline-based chemotherapy to molecular negativity
Maintenance	ATRA ± low-dose chemotherapy for 1–2 yr
Molecular Monitoring	RT-PCR from PB every 3–6 mo for 2–3 yr
Relapse	Arsenic, then ASCT (allogeneic if RT-PCR is positive) (Consider prophylactic IT therapy)

Abbreviations: ASCT, autologous stem cell transplant; ATRA, all-*trans* retinoic acid; IT, intrathecal; PB, peripheral blood; RT-PCR, reverse transcriptase–polymerase chain reaction.

Arsenic Trioxide

Investigators from China first reported a role of ATO in relapsed and refractory APL,[16,181,182] and this has been confirmed in Europe and the United States.[29,183] In the multicenter U.S. trial of 40 patients with relapsed APL, a complete remission rate of 85% and a high complete molecular remission rate of 78% were observed after two courses of ATO (Table 30–6). The 2-year relapse-free and overall survival estimates for the combined trials are 49% and 63%, respectively.[183] Currently, ATO is considered the treatment of choice for patients with relapsed disease, particularly in patients exposed to ATRA in the last 12 months. This should be followed by consolidation and maintenance as noted previously. The best choice of therapy in second relapse is unclear, mainly because of the small number of patients included in studies.

ATO-Related Toxicities

The most common drug-related toxicities with ATO are hyperleukocytosis (WBC count ≥10,000/μL), APL differentiation syndrome, and prolonged Q-T interval. Prolongation of the heart rate–corrected Q-T interval has very rarely led to torsade de pointes, a potentially fatal cardiac arrhythmia. The degree of prolongation was found to be higher in men (P = .053) and in patients with hypokalemia but was not associated with age.[184] Patients taking concomitant medications known to prolong the Q-T interval are also predisposed to this complication when treated with ATO (P = .01). The U.S. Food and Drug Administration recommendations for safe administration of ATO are listed in Table 30–7.

APL differentiation syndrome in response to ATO treatment is reminiscent of RAS associated with ATRA. Manifestations include fluid retention, pulmonary infiltrates and/or pleural effusions, dyspnea, myalgias, arthralgias, fever, and weight gain.[185] Similar to RAS, APL differentiation syndrome is managed effectively by a short course of corticosteroids (e.g., oral or intravenous dexamethasone 10 mg twice daily for 3–5 days beginning with the first sign or symptom).[153] In a study of 26 patients with

TABLE 30–6. Use of Arsenic Trioxide (ATO) in APL

Study	Year	As Compound	Status of Disease	No. of Patients	CR Rate (%)
Sun et al.[16]	1992	Ailing-1	De novo + relapsed	32	65.6
Huang[208]	1995	Composite Indigo Naturalis tablets	De novo + relapsed	60	98.0
Zhang et al.[181]	1996	ATO	De novo	30	73.3
			Relapsed	42	52.4
Shen[28]	1997	ATO	Relapsed	10	90.0
Soignet et al.[29]	1998	ATO	Relapsed + refractory	12	92.0
Niu et al.[182]	1999	ATO	De novo	11	72.7
			Relapsed	47	85.1
Soignet et al.[209]	1999	ATO	Relapsed + refractory	40	85.0

TABLE 30–7. U.S. Food and Drug Administration Recommendations for Safe Administration of Arsenic Trioxide

Before Starting Arsenic Trioxide Therapy
Obtain electrolyte abnormalities
Correct preexisting electrolyte abnormalities
If Q-Tc interval is >500 msec:
Institute corrective measures
Reassess Q-Tc before starting therapy
Discontinue (whenever possible) concurrent medications known to prolong the Q-Tc interval
During Arsenic Trioxide Therapy
Maintain:
Potassium concentration above 4 mEq/dL
Magnesium concentration above 1.8 mg/dL
Obtain serial ECGs
Hospitalize patient and place on cardiac telemetry if:
Absolute Q-T interval >500 msec *or*
Patient has any symptoms such as syncope or palpitations

Abbreviations: ECGs, electrocardiograms; Q-Tc, heart rate–corrected Q-T interval.

relapsed/refractory APL treated with ATO, 33% developed APL differentiation syndrome,[186] and the syndrome was more common in patients with leukocytosis.

Role of Stem Cell Transplantation

Despite the high probability of achieving a second remission with ATO, relapsed patients appear to benefit from autologous (auto) or allogeneic (allo) hematopoietic stem cell transplantation (SCT).[187] Older studies of patients treated without ATRA or ATO reported a relapse rate of 64% and a transplant-related mortality of 40% in patients undergoing allo-SCT and a relapse rate of 54% and a transplant-related mortality of 23% in patients undergoing auto-SCT in second complete remission.[188,189] The same study group reported a 16% relapse rate and a transplant-related mortality of 4% in 45 patients after auto-SCT.[190] Prolonged clinical and molecular remissions have been obtained in patients undergoing SCT even in the presence of initial RT-PCR–positive results for PML/RARα.[191,192] In a small series of poor-prognosis APL patients undergoing allo-SCT, actuarial probabilities at 10 years of overall survival, disease-free survival, and relapse in the entire group of 17 patients were 53%, 46%, and 33%, respectively.[193] The relatively good outcome and low transplant-related mortality are features that support the use of auto-SCT in APL patients in second or more complete remission, whereas allo-SCT should be considered in patients who have any evidence of persistent disease following ATO.

PROGNOSIS

Unfavorable prognostic factors in newly diagnosed APL include older age and elevated WBC count.[168,172] Early death resulting from hemorrhage is the major adverse event.[180,194,195] Independently, WBC count greater than 20,000/μL[170] or 10,000/μL[196,197] and a platelet count of less than 40,000/μL[198] correlate with increased relapse risk. Based on combined data from a study by the GIMEMA and PETHEMA groups, patients can be segregated into low (WBC count <10,000/μL and platelet count >40,000/μL), intermediate (WBC count <10,000/μL and platelet count <40,000/μL), and high (WBC count >10,000/μL) risk groups, each with a distinctive relapse-free survival curve ($P < .0001$).[198]

Mutations in FLT3/ITD are present in 32% of APL patients[199]; their presence is associated with leukocytosis and poor disease-free survival and overall survival in AML.[79,85,200] Neither the PML/RAR isoform subtype[201] nor other cytogenetic abnormalities appear to be uniformly recognized prognostic factors.[202–205] The slow kinetics of molecular remission and persistence of or conversion to RT-PCR positivity for PML-RARα after consolidation have been correlated with increased risk of hematologic relapse.[168] Finally, the expression of the antigen identified by CD56 has been associated with poor prognosis in patients with APL.[108,109] Expression of CD2 has been associated with a high complete remission rate and improved event-free survival independent of the WBC count and inclusion of ATRA in induction.[107]

The introduction of ATRA as targeted therapy for APL has remarkably improved the long-term outcome of this disease. Once one of the most fatal malignancies, APL now is curable in approximately 75–85% of patients. Chemotherapy with anthracyclines remains critically important in the management of APL, because most patients relapse with ATRA alone. Maintenance therapy appears to have a unique role in the achievement of long-term remission in many patients. Early death in approximately 10% of patients as a result of hemorrhage and disease relapse in approximately 10–20% continue to be the main obstacles to cure in APL.

CURRENT CONTROVERSIES & FUTURE CONSIDERATIONS

Acute Promyelocytic Leukemia

- Optimal early treatment for the coagulopathy in APL
- Omission of cytarabine in initial induction and consolidation therapy
- Treatment for patients in second complete remission
- Role of intrathecal chemotherapy in relapsed APL
- Prognostic influence of additional cytogenetic abnormalities
- Best induction therapy for patients with cardiac disease who cannot receive anthracyclines
- Potential role of arsenic trioxide in induction therapy

Suggested Readings*

de Botton S, Chevret S, Coiteux V, et al: Early onset of chemotherapy can reduce the incidence of ATRA syndrome in newly diagnosed acute promyelocytic leukemia (APL) with low white blood cell counts: results from APL 93 trial. Leukemia 17:339–342, 2003.

Fenaux P, Chastang C, Chevret S, et al: A randomized comparison of all transretinoic acid (ATRA) followed by chemotherapy and ATRA plus chemotherapy and the role of maintenance therapy in newly diagnosed acute promyelocytic leukemia. The European APL Group. Blood 94:1192–1200, 1999.

Melnick A, Licht JD: Deconstructing a disease: RARalpha, its fusion partners, and their roles in the pathogenesis of acute promyelocytic leukemia. Blood 93:3167–3215, 1999.

Sanz MA, Lo Coco F, Martin G, et al: Definition of relapse risk and role of nonanthracycline drugs for consolidation in patients with acute promyelocytic leukemia: a joint study of the PETHEMA and GIMEMA cooperative groups. Blood 96:1247–1253, 2000.

Soignet SL, Frankel SR, Douer D, et al: United States multicenter study of arsenic trioxide in relapsed acute promyelocytic leukemia. J Clin Oncol 19:3852–3860, 2001.

Tallman M, Lefebvre P, Baine R, et al: Effects of all-trans retinoic acid or chemotherapy on the molecular regulation of systemic blood coagulation and fibrinolysis in patients with acute promyelocytic leukemia. J Thromb Haemost 2004 (in press).

Tallman MS, Andersen JW, Schiffer CA, et al: All-trans-retinoic acid in acute promyelocytic leukemia. N Engl J Med 337:1021–1028, 1997.

Full references for this chapter can be found on accompanying CD-ROM.

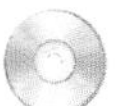

CHAPTER 31

Chronic Myeloid Leukemia

John M. Goldman, DM, FRCP, FRCPath

> **KEY POINTS**
>
> **Chronic Myeloid Leukemia**
>
> - Chronic myeloid leukemia (CML) has an annual incidence of about 1.3 per 100,000 population.
> - The disease usually starts in the chronic phase and progresses spontaneously after some years to a more advanced phase (accelerated or blastic phases).
> - CML starts in a single pluripotential stem cell.
> - All leukemia cells have a specific cytogenetic abnormality, the Philadelphia chromosome (designated Ph or 22q−).
> - The Ph chromosome carries a *BCR/ABL* fusion gene.
> - Allogeneic stem cell transplantation performed in the chronic phase can eradicate the leukemia, but the procedure remains hazardous.
> - Imatinib mesylate induces complete cytogenetic remissions in 70–80% of previously untreated patients.

INTRODUCTION

Chronic myeloid leukemia (CML), in the past referred to as "chronic granulocytic leukemia," "chronic myelocytic leukemia," or "chronic myelogenous leukemia," was in the 1840s probably the first of the leukemias to be recognized.[1-3] The pivotal discovery in 1960 that leukemia cells of patients with CML had a specific and consistent cytogenetic abnormality,[4] the Philadelphia (Ph) chromosome, initiated decades of productive laboratory research that yielded a detailed cellular and molecular characterization of CML and a targeted drug therapy, the tyrosine kinase inhibitor imatinib. Today CML is understood to be due to acquisition in a single hematopoietic stem cell of a specific molecular abnormality, the *BCR/ABL* fusion gene, arising from the Ph chromosome, which confers on that cell and its clonal progeny a proliferative advantage over their normal counterparts.[5] The resulting massive expansion of myeloid cells produces the associated clinical features.[6,7]

There are three sequential clinical phases of CML (Table 31–1). The disease usually presents in an indolent or chronic phase that responds well to a variety of different therapeutic approaches. Historically, after a median interval of about 4 years, there is "spontaneous" progression to an accelerated phase and subsequently to a phase of blastic transformation (also referred to as blastic crisis); some patients proceed directly from chronic phase to blast phase.[8,9] Together the accelerated and blastic phases are often referred to as "advanced-phase" CML. Occasionally advanced phase is characterized by myelofibrosis or osteomyelofibrosis rather than blastic cell proliferation. Survival after onset of the accelerated phase ranges from 6 months to 2 years, but the median survival of patients in blastic phase is less than 6 months.

EPIDEMIOLOGY

CML appears to have a consistent annual incidence in all countries for which adequate data exist, about 1.3 per 100,000 population, and is slightly more common in males than in females.[10] The median age of onset is about 55 years, and increases with age. CML is exceedingly rare in younger persons but does occasionally occur in children and even in neonates. A few families have been described with two or more members affected by CML. An association with specific human leukocyte antigen (HLA) types has been described but not confirmed.[11,12] The only known predisposing cause is exposure to high doses of ionizing radiation; CML has been diagnosed in persons who survived atomic bombs exploded in Japan in 1945[13] and patients successfully treated with radiotherapy for ankylosing spondylitis or malignant conditions.[14,15]

PATHOPHYSIOLOGY

Cytogenetics

Nowell and Hungerford at the Wistar Institute in Philadelphia discovered that the leukemia cells from patients with CML contained a G-group chromosome with a foreshortened long arm[16]; this abnormal chro-

TABLE 31–1. Definitions of Phases of CML

WHO Criteria	IBMTR Criteria
Chronic Phase	
Ability to reduce spleen size and restore and maintain "normal" blood count with appropriate therapy	Not specifically defined
Accelerated Phase—one or more of the following:	
Blasts 10–19% of WBCs in peripheral blood and/or of nucleated bone marrow cells	Blasts 10–19% in blood or marrow
Peripheral blood basophils ≥20%	Peripheral blood basophils ≥20%
Persistent thrombocytopenia (<100 × 10^9/L) unrelated to therapy, or persistent thrombocytosis (>1000 × 10^9/L) unresponsive to therapy	Persistent thrombocytopenia (<100 × 10^9/L) unrelated to therapy
Increasing spleen size and increasing WBC count unresponsive to therapy	Persistent thrombocytosis (>1000 × 10^9/L) unresponsive to therapy
Cytogenetic evidence of clonal evolution	
Blastic Phase—one or more of the following:	
Blasts >20%	
Extramedullary blast cell proliferation	
Large foci or clusters of blasts in the bone marrow biopsy	

Abbreviations: IBMTR, International Bone Marrow Transplant Registry; WBC, white blood cell; WHO, World Health Organization.

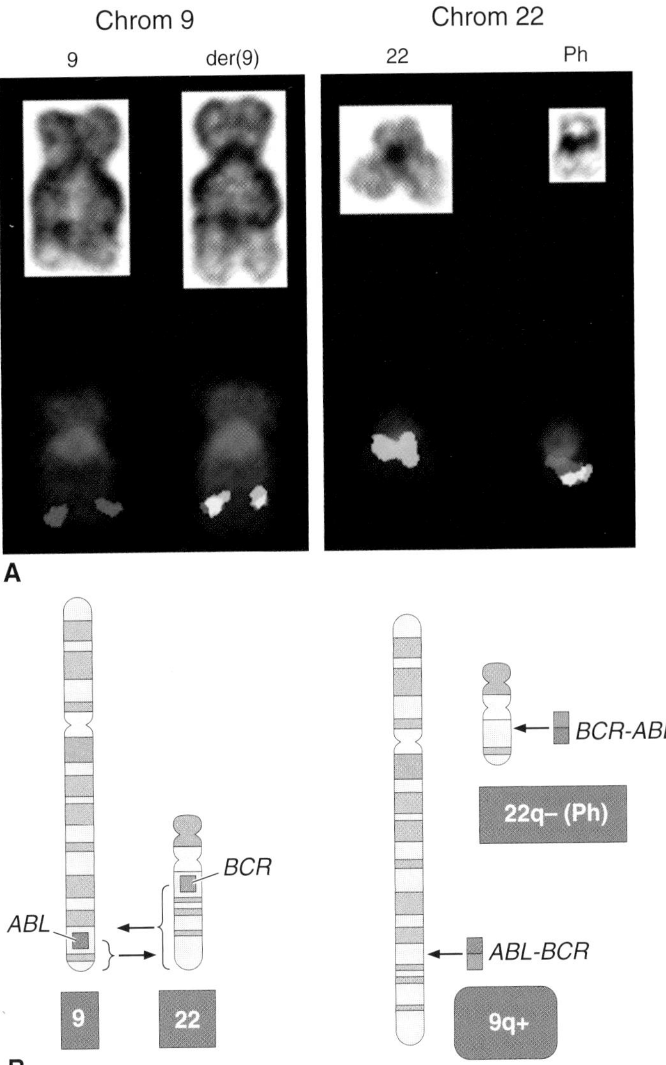

Figure 31–1. *A,* Chromosomes 9q+ and 22q–. The *upper left panel* shows a normal chromosome 9 and an abnormal chromosome 9 with extra material on the long arm [9q+ or der(9)]; the *upper right panel* shows a normal chromosome 22 followed by an abnormal chromosome 22 with loss of material from the long arm (22q– or Ph). The *lower panel* shows the corresponding chromosomes subjected to fluorescent in situ hybridization to locate the positions of the *ABL (red)* and *BCR (green)* genes, respectively. The normal chromosome 9 shows two red signals and the normal chromosome 22 shows two green signals. The Ph chromosome shows both red and green signals and a yellow signal where the red and green overlap, consistent with the presence of a *BCR/ABL* fusion gene; the 9q+ also shows both red and green signals with a yellow signal where the red and green overlap, consistent with the presence of a reciprocal *ABL/BCR* fusion gene. *B,* The Ph chromosome. *Left,* Schematic representation of one normal 9 and one normal 22 chromosome showing position of the *ABL* gene at 9q34 and the *BCR* gene at 22q11. The Ph translocation involves reciprocal balanced exchange of genetic between the long arms of both chromosomes, indicated by the *arrows. Right,* The derivative 9q+ (Ph chromosome) and 22q– resulting from the translocation. Note the positions of the *BCR/ABL* fusion gene on 22q– and the reciprocal *ABL/BCR* fusion gene on 9q+.

mosome was subsequently categorized as one of the two number 22 chromosomes and designated the Philadelphia chromosome. In 1973, Rowley reported that the long arm one of the number 9 chromosomes was elongated in CML cells and suggested that the Ph chromosome arose as a result of a reciprocal translocation involving chromosomes 9 and 22[17]; further analysis identified the translocation as t(9;22)(q34;q11) (Fig. 31–1). In most newly diagnosed patients, the Ph chromosome is found in all or almost all cells of the granulocytic, erythroid, and megakaryocytic series, as well as in dendritic cells. It is present in some B lymphocytes and a small proportion of T lymphocytes but not in marrow fibroblasts or in other tissues.[18]

The Ph chromosome is found in about 90% of patients with the clinical manifestations of CML; about 10% of patients have morphologically normal-appearing 9 and 22 chromosomes in marrow metaphases and are therefore classified as having Ph chromosome–negative CML.[19-21] This group is heterogeneous. Some have molecular evidence of CML—40% have an "occult" *BCR/ABL* fusion gene in chromosome 22, identified by fluorescent in situ hybridization with fluorochrome-labeled probes for *BCR* and *ABL* genes—whereas the remaining patients have no identifiable cytogenetic or molecular lesions. Finally, a small group appears to have another myeloproliferative process, with clonal cytogenetic abnormalities involving t(5;12) or t(8;13).

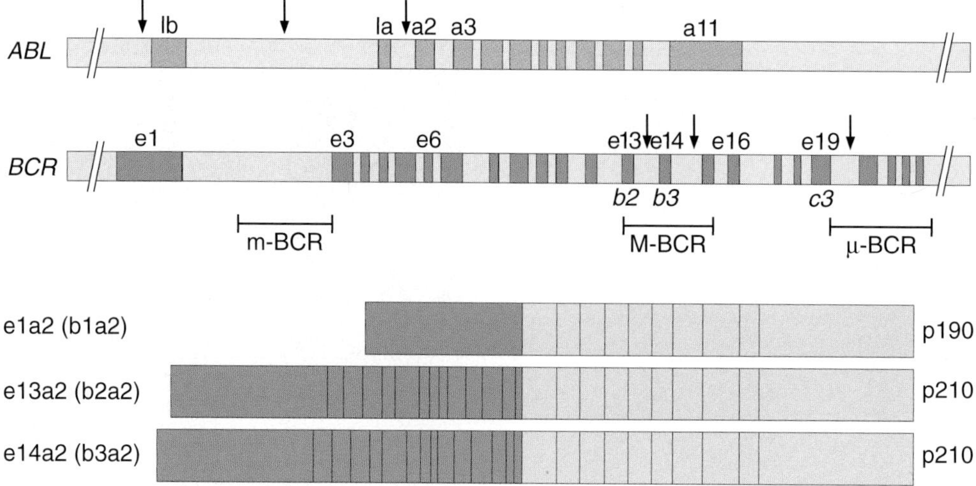

Figure 31–2. The normal *ABL* and *BCR* genes and the three different fusion transcripts encoded by the *BCR-ABL* fusion genes. Diagram of the *ABL* and *BCR* genes *(top)* with the three principal mRNA transcripts resulting from the *BCR/ABL* fusion gene *(bottom)*. Genes: *ABL* and *BCR* exons are shown as *pink* and *blue boxes*, respectively. *ABL* exons are numbered according to current practice. *BCR* exons are numbered according to the revised system, with earlier nomenclature shown below in italics. *Vertical arrows* show the various intronic positions where the break in each gene usually occurs. Note that in CML the *ABL* break occurs most commonly between exons Ia and a2; the *BCR* break occurs usually either between exons e13 and e14, giving a e13a2 mRNA junction, or between exons e14 and e15, giving a e14a2 junction. e1a2 mRNA junctions are found predominantly in Ph-positive acute lymphoblastic leukemia and the e19a2 junction in Ph-positive chronic neutrophilic leukemia.

Molecular Features

The molecular basis of the Ph translocation was elucidated in the 1980s[22–26] (Fig. 31–2). The translocation involves the *ABL* gene located on the long arm of chromosome 9 and the *BCR* gene located on the long arm of chromosome 22. The centromeric portion of the *BCR* gene recombines with the telomeric portion of the *ABL* gene (together with the remaining telomeric portion of 9q) to form the *BCR/ABL* fusion gene on chromosome 22, and the centromeric portion of the *ABL* gene recombines with the telomeric portion of the *BCR* gene (together with all telomeric DNA) to form an *ABL/BCR* fusion gene on the 9q+ chromosome.

The precise function of neither of these normal genes is well defined. The *ABL* gene is ubiquitously expressed in normal human tissues and may control entry into the cell cycle at defined checkpoints; it may also facilitate apoptosis in radiation-damaged cells. The Abl protein contains a number of distinct domains, one of which is a kinase that, under tight regulation, can catalyze the phosphorylation of itself and other proteins on tyrosine residues. The normal *BCR* gene may control the oxidative burst in activated neutrophils. In CML, the *BCR/ABL* gene is expressed in all leukemia cells as a 7.8-kb messenger RNA (mRNA) and an oncoprotein with a molecular mass of 210 kDa, usually referred to as $p210^{BCR\text{-}ABL}$.

In both the *ABL* and *BCR* genes, the breakpoints are always intronic, but the precise position varies in different patients.[27] The *ABL* breakpoints may occur almost anywhere over 7.8 kb in the intron upstream of *ABL* exon 2, and the *BCR* break is usually in the intron between exons e13 and e14 or in the intron between exons e14 and e15. Thus mRNA resulting from the fusion genes has either an e13a2 junction (previously referred to as b2a2) or an e14a2 junction (previously referred to as b3a2). About 40% of patients have the former junction and 55% have the latter; 5–10% of patients express mRNAs with both junctions. Very rare patients have an e19a2 mRNA junction that expresses an oncoprotein of 230 kDa molecular mass.[28] About one third of patients with Ph chromosome–positive acute lymphoblastic leukemia have a CML-type mRNA junction, whereas the remainder have an e1a2 junction and a p190 oncoprotein.

The mechanism by which the activated tyrosine kinase in the Bcr/Abl oncoprotein results in the clinical features of CML is still poorly understood. The juxtaposition of Bcr sequences upstream of the Abl kinase domain releases the Abl kinase from its normal tight regulation and results in aberrant phosphorylation of a wide variety of cytoplasmic proteins. As a result, there is a block in a physiologic apoptotic mechanism involving myeloid progenitors and decreased adherence to marrow stroma that allows CML progenitors to escape normal inhibitory regulation. The mediators of these processes are the Bcr/Abl-activated signal transduction pathways involving RAS, phosphatidylinositol 3-kinase and AKT, and STAT 5.[29]

The Bcr/Abl-positive CML progenitor and stem cells are unduly susceptible to spontaneous acquisition of additional genetic and cytogenetic changes, a character-

TABLE 31–2. Molecular and Cytogenetic Features of Blastic Disease*

Nonrandom Cytogenetic Changes	Genes That May Be Involved in Some Patients
+Ph	*p53*
+8	*p16*
iso-17q	*EVI1*
−19	*RAS*
	LYN
	RB
	MYC

*Any of the acquired abnormalities listed may be present in individual patients in established blastic transformation; however, some patients have no detectable cytogenetic or molecular changes in addition to the Ph chromosome and the *BCR/ABL* fusion gene.

istic referred to as genomic instability. A common manifestation of this process is cytogenetic "evolution" identified during the chronic phase or at the onset of advanced-phase disease; some of these changes are common (+8, iso-17q, and a second Ph chromosome), but other apparently random changes are frequent as well (Table 31–2). Blastic phase is probably due at least in part to de novo activation of a number of oncogenes other than *BCR/ABL*; mutations and deletions in *p53*, *p16*, *RB*, *MYC*, *EVI1*, and other known oncogenes are described but no consistent pattern has yet emerged.

CLINICAL AND HEMATOLOGIC FEATURES

Chronic-Phase Disease

Clinical Features

Perhaps one half of patients present with symptoms attributable to splenomegaly, hemorrhage, or anemia, but many are diagnosed only as a result of routine blood tests performed as part of medical examinations or screening for other reasons. Symptoms when present may include lethargy, loss of energy, shortness of breath on exertion, weight loss, and hemorrhage from various sites. Increased sweating is characteristic.[30,31] Spontaneous bruising or unexplained bleeding from gums, intestinal tract, or urinary tract is relatively common. There may be visual disturbances. Fever and lymphadenopathy can occur but are rare in chronic-phase CML. The patient may have severe pain or discomfort in the splenic area, often associated with splenic infarction, or have noticed a lump or mass in the left upper abdomen. Visual disturbances may be due to retinal hemorrhages. Sudden hearing loss is a rare symptom. Patients may present with features of gout or priapism, both of which are also rare.

Fifty percent to 70% of patients have splenomegaly at diagnosis. The spleen varies from just palpable to massive enlargement that occupies all the left side of the abdomen and extends also into the right iliac fossa. The liver is frequently also enlarged but with a soft edge that may be difficult to define. There may be no other abnormal findings. Ecchymoses of varying sizes and ages may be present, forming discolored subcutaneous lumps. Some patients have asymptomatic retinal hemorrhages. Very high leukocyte counts may produce features of leukostasis with retinal vein engorgement and respiratory insufficiency.[32]

Hematologic Values

Patients with splenomegaly are usually anemic, whereas the hemoglobin concentration may be normal in patients with early disease (Fig. 31–3). The leukocyte count at diagnosis is usually between 20 and 200 × 10^9/L, but the diagnosis of CML can be established in patients with persistent leukocytosis in the range of 12 to 20 × 10^9/L. Occasionally patients present with leukocyte numbers above 200 × 10^9/L, very rarely above 500 × 10^9/L. The smear shows a full spectrum of cells in the granulocyte series ranging from blast forms to mature neutrophils with peaks of myelocytes and neutrophils. The *percentage* of blast cells is related to the *absolute number* of leukocytes, but percentages higher than 12 suggest that the patient may already have entered the accelerated or early blastic phase. The percentage of eosinophils and basophils is increased, and indeed the absence of basophilia casts doubt on the diagnosis. Absolute numbers of lymphocytes and monocytes are slightly increased, but both are reduced as percentages in the differential count. Platelet numbers are usually high (in the range of 300 to 600 × 10^9/L) but may be normal or even reduced. Occasional nucleated red cells are present in the circulation in some patients. The alkaline phosphatase content of the neutrophil cytoplasm is diminished or absent. Bcr/Abl transcripts can be demonstrated in the blood with ease using the reverse transcriptase–polymerase chain reaction.

Examination of the bone marrow by aspiration or trephine biopsy is not strictly necessary to confirm the diagnosis of CML but is usually performed in order to assess the degree of marrow fibrosis, for cytogenetic analysis, and to exclude occult transformation. The marrow aspirate may show multiple small hypercellular fragments or may be so hypercellular that discrete fragments cannot easily be discerned. The aspirate smear trails show a cellular composition resembling that of CML blood. The blast cells in chronic phase number 2–12%. Eosinophils and basophils are usually prominent. Megakaryocytes are small, hypolobated, and very numerous. Gaucher-like cells may be present. The marrow biopsy shows complete loss of fat spaces with dense hypercellularity. The reticulin content may be normal or modestly increased.

Prediction of Duration of Survival at Time of Diagnosis

Many attempts have been made to predict the duration of survival for an individual patient who presents with chronic-phase disease (Table 31–3), but all of these must now be questioned because of the new therapeutic options, and all patients with CML should be treated

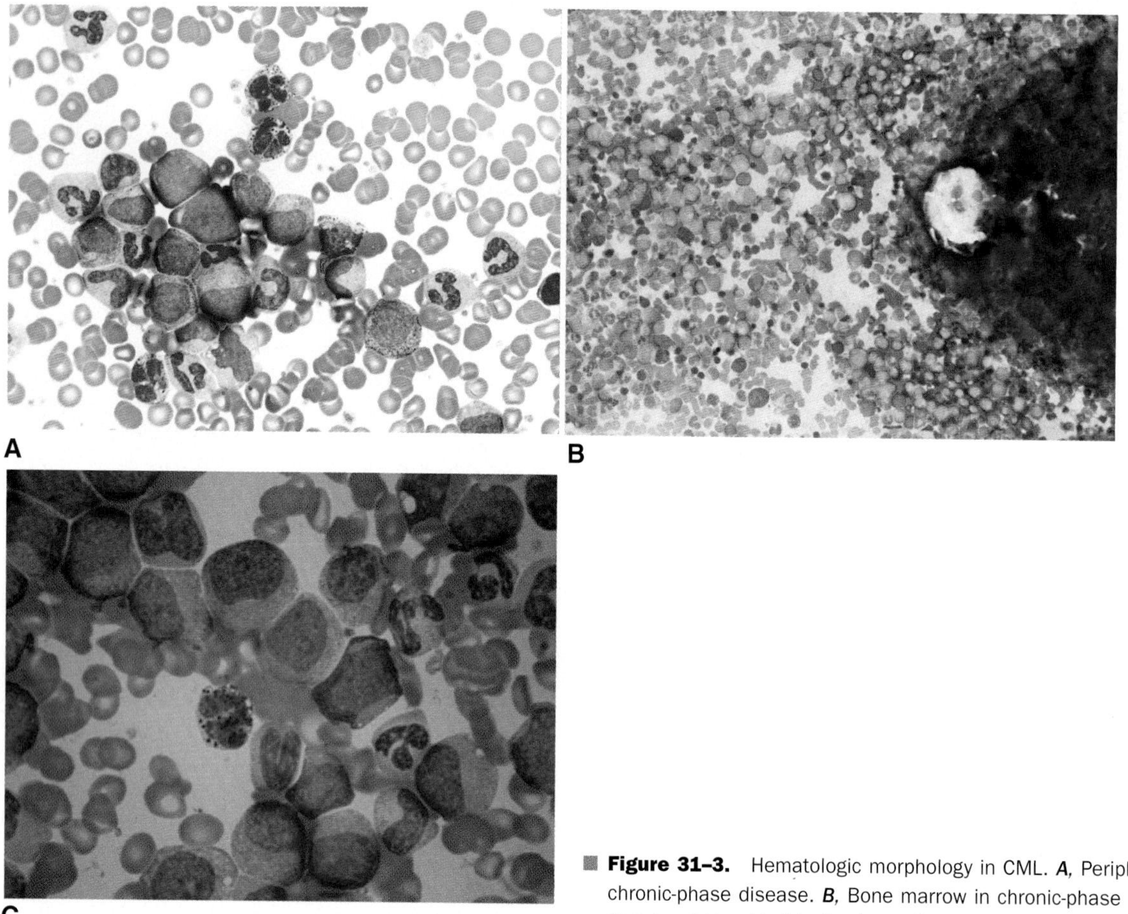

A

B

C

Figure 31–3. Hematologic morphology in CML. *A,* Peripheral blood in chronic-phase disease. *B,* Bone marrow in chronic-phase disease. *C,* Peripheral blood in blastic-phase disease.

TABLE 31–3. Prognostic (Risk) Scores in Newly Diagnosed Chronic-Phase CML*

Sokal (1984)[33]	Hasford (European) (1998)[34]
Basis for Calculating the Prognostic Scores	
Age (yr)	Age (yr)
Platelet count ($\times 10^9$/L)	Platelet count ($\times 10^9$/L)
Spleen size (cm below costal margin)	Spleen size (cm below costal margin)
Blasts in blood (%)	Blasts in blood (%)
	Eosinophils in blood (%)
	Basophils in blood (%)
Definitions of Risk Groups (Median Survivals from Diagnosis)	
Low: <0.8 (60 mo)	Low: <780 (98 mo)
Intermediate: 0.8–1.2 (45 mo)	Intermediate: 781–1480 (65 mo)
High: >1.2 (30 mo)	High: >1481 (42 mo)
Based On:	
Patients treated predominantly with busulfan	Patients treated predominantly with interferon alfa

*The actual scores for individual patients may be calculated by reference to the equations available on the Internet
(Sokal: *http://www.nrbg.ncl.ac.uk/cgi-bin/cml/sokal.pl;*
European: *http://www.pharmacoepi.de/dmlscore.html*).

promptly. The system devised by Sokal and colleagues in 1984[33] is still most commonly used and allows patients to be categorized as high risk, intermediate risk, and low risk (Fig. 31–4).[34,35]

Advanced-Phase Disease

Clinical Features

The clinical features associated with advanced disease are variable.[36,37] In some cases, the patient is initially entirely asymptomatic and the diagnosis is based entirely on blood and marrow findings. In others, the patient may develop fevers, excessive sweating, anorexia and weight loss, or bone pain. Rarely, there are localized single or multiple lytic lesions of bone. Occasionally, patients present with generalized lymphadenopathy; node biopsy shows infiltration with blast cells that may be myeloid or lymphoid. Localized skin infiltrates may be seen. Discrete masses of immature leukemia cells can develop at almost any site, sometimes referred to as "chloromas" or "granulocytic sarcomas." Patients with lymphoid blast cells in the blood and marrow also may have involvement of the cerebrospinal fluid, or central nervous system leukemia may be recognized only later.

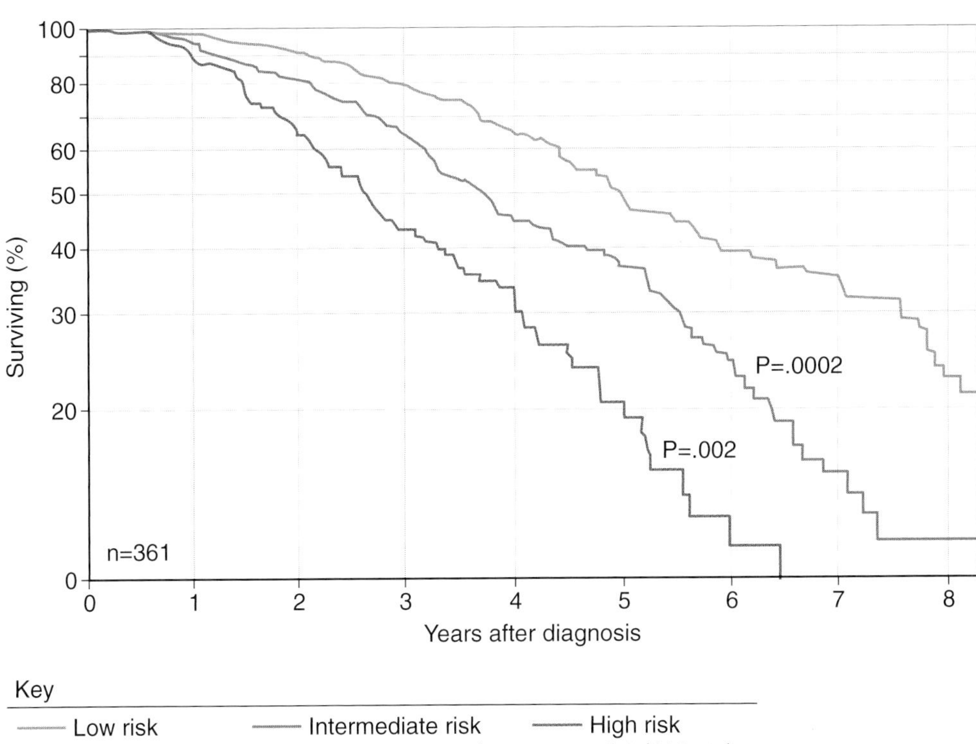

Figure 31–4. Survival from diagnosis for a group of 361 patients treated predominantly with busulfan classified as low risk, intermediate risk, and high risk according to criteria established by Sokal et al.[33] Note the log scale on the *y* axis. (See Table 31–3 for more detail.)

Hematologic Values

The hematologic picture in accelerated-phase disease also vary. It may differ little from chronic-phase CML, but blast cell numbers may be increased disproportionately. There may be anemia in the presence of a normal leukocyte count. Platelet numbers may be greatly increased ($>1000 \times 10^9$/L) or reduced ($<100 \times 10^9$/L) unrelated to treatment. Marrow morphology is no longer consistent with chronic-phase disease, often with increased numbers of blast cells and/or increased fibrosis. Blastic transformation is defined by the presence of more than 30% blasts or blasts plus promyelocytes in the blood or marrow,[9,36] but frequently blast cell numbers in both sites exceed 80%. Blast morphology is very variable. About 70% of patients have blasts classifiable generally as myeloid that resemble the cells that characterize acute myeloid leukemia. Such cells may be predominantly myeloblastic, monoblastic, erythroblastic, or megakaryoblastic, and blast cells of different lineages frequently coexist.[38] More accurate definition is provided by cytochemical and immunophenotypic characterization. About 20% of patients have lymphoid blast cells; these may resemble the FAB-L1 cells that typify childhood acute lymphocytic leukemia or, more commonly, have an L2 appearance. Immunophenotyping shows the typical membrane markers of a precursor B-cell acute lymphocytic leukemia, CD10 (CALLA) and CD19 positivity, and enzymatic assay may show nuclear positivity for terminal deoxynucleotidyl transferase.[39,40] Molecular studies show clonal rearrangement of immunoglobulin genes and sometimes also of T-cell receptor genes. The remaining 10% of blast cell transformations have mixed myeloid and lymphoid characteristics.

Biochemical Changes

Biochemical changes in CML are nonspecific. The serum uric acid level may be elevated, the lactate dehydrogenase level is usually raised, and the serum vitamin B_{12} level and B_{12} binding capacity are greatly increased as a result of raised levels of transcobalamin I. Very rarely, serum potassium may be spuriously high as a result of leakage of intracellular potassium from platelets or, less commonly, from leukocytes after phlebotomy. In such cases, the potassium level in freshly drawn citrated blood is usually normal; the electrocardiogram shows no evidence of hyperkalemic effects. In blastic transformation, the serum uric acid level may be raised, sometimes substantially, and tests of liver function are usually moderately abnormal. Hypercalcemia is present occasionally, usually due to bone destruction; very rarely, may be attributable to a parathormone-like substance high serum calcium produced ectopically by the blast cells.

TREATMENT

Chronic-Phase Disease

In the past CML was regarded as inexorably fatal, but the management of the newly diagnosed chronic-phase patient has altered dramatically in recent years[41]: the leukemia can in some cases be eradicated by stem cell transplantation (SCT), and drug trials of imatinib suggest the possibility of substantial prolongation of life compared with previous medical therapies. For most patients, the first treatment will be imatinib or the combination of imatinib with another agent in a research trial. When to proceed to SCT, particularly for younger patients, is now an active area of research. Because SCT should be considered, all siblings and other family members should be HLA typed. The issue of gonadal function is important, and men who have not completed their families should be offered semen cryopreservation; the possible adverse effects of treatment on pregnancy should be discussed with women of childbearing age. Some centers will collect and cryopreserve peripheral blood stem cells for autografting that may be desirable at a later stage in the disease.

Chemotherapy

Many different agents have been used to treat CML. Some of these, together with newer drugs now under evaluation, are listed in Table 31–4.

Imatinib Mesylate

The single most important agent for chronic-phase disease is imatinib mesylate. Imatinib mesylate (Gleevec or Glivec; previously known as STI571) is an Abl tyrosine kinase inhibitor that entered clinical trials in 1998. Initial studies showed that it controlled the clinical and hematologic features of CML already resistant to interferon alfa and also induced major or complete cytogenetic responses in over 50% of patients.[42,43] Though the molecule has little structural resemblance to ATP, it is thought to act by blocking access for ATP to the ATP-binding pocket of the kinase domain of the Bcr/Abl oncoprotein thereby preventing the enzyme from phosphorylating downstream effector molecules. In subsequent clinical trials, the drug was compared prospectively with the combination of interferon alfa and cytarabine, which had until then been regarded as the best initial treatment for newly diagnosed patients. Imatinib, administered orally at a dose of 400 mg/day, resulted in a 74% complete cytogenetic remission rate compared with 14% in those receiving interferon alfa and cytarabine[44] (Fig. 31–5). Progression-free survival was significantly better in the imatinib-treated cohort (97.2% vs. 90.3%; $P < .001$). Studies in which early results with imatinib were compared with historical control patients treated predominantly with interferon suggest a major survival benefit,[45,46] results so impressive that randomized trials without imatinib are unlikely. With higher doses of imatinib, such as 600 or 800 mg daily, hematologic and cytogenetic responses occur more rapidly than with 400 mg/day, but the survival advantage of these more aggressive regimens is not yet established.

Toxicities of imatinib include nausea, headache, cutaneous eruptions, and fluid retention. Abnormalities of liver chemistry occur in some cases, and very rare patients have sustained significant liver damage. A minority of patients experience some degree of cytopenia, particularly when there is long-standing disease or marrow fibrosis; neutropenia can be treated effectively with granulocyte colony-stimulating factor, but thrombocytopenia

TABLE 31–4. Agents Used to Treat Chronic-Phase CML

In the Past	Present	Experimental
^{32}P	Imatinib	BMS-354825 (Dasatinib)
		AMN107
Busulfan	Interferon alfa	Decitabine
Melphalan	Hydroxyurea	Homoharringtonine
Dibromomannitol	Imatinib with other agents	Arsenic trioxide
Cytarabine		Adaphostin
		17-Allylaminogeldanamycin (17-AAG)

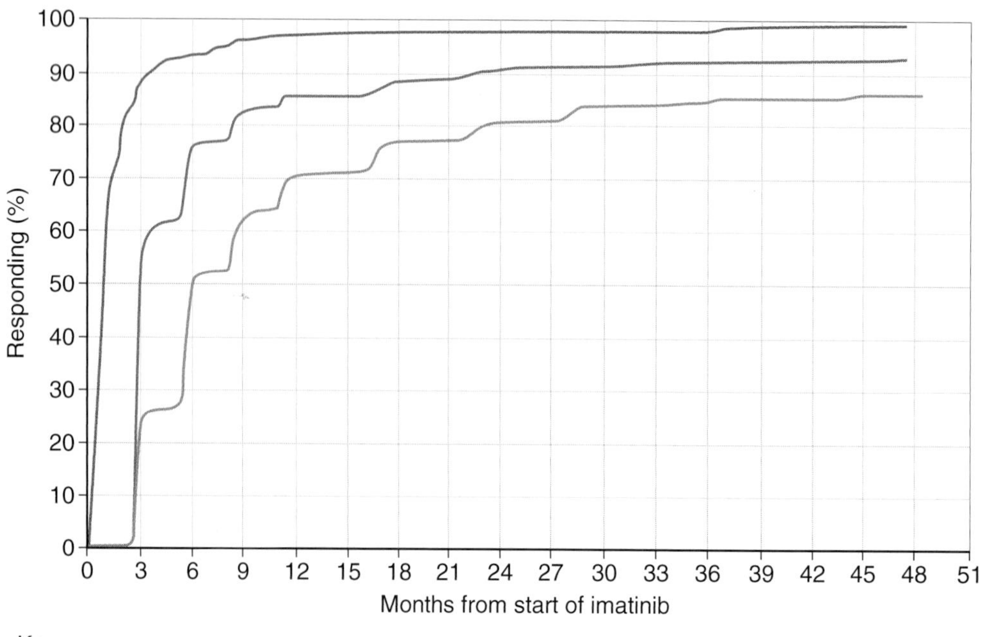

Figure 31–5. Estimated response to imatinib in previously untreated patients. Newly diagnosed patients with CML in chronic phase entered into the IRIS study received imatinib at 400 mg daily. At 42 months from start of treatment, the estimated incidence of complete hematologic response was 98% (95% confidence interval [CI], 96–100%), that of major cytogenetic response was 91% (95% CI 88–94%), and that of complete cytogenetic response was 84% (95% CI 81–88%). (The steps in the curves for cytogenetic data reflect the study design which called for examination of bone marrow cytogenetics at 3-month intervals.)

may necessitate temporarily interrupting treatment, which is generally preferable to merely reducing dosage.

Patients who respond to treatment can reliably be monitored by serial cytogenetic and molecular studies.[35,47,48] The majority of patients should achieve Ph-negative status within 3–6 months of starting imatinib; this can be verified by routine bone marrow cytogenetics or fluorescent in situ hybridization studies designed to identify the *BCR/ABL* gene in peripheral blood leukocytes. Thereafter, molecular monitoring depends on a reverse transcriptase–polymerase chain reaction assay to identify and quantitate low levels of Bcr/Abl transcripts in the peripheral blood or bone marrow. A quantitative reverse transcriptase–polymerase chain reaction assay should have a sensitivity of $1:10^5$ or $1:10^6$. About one third of patients treated with imatinib achieve very low levels of Bcr/Abl transcripts, and in about 5% the transcripts are undetectable.[35] Such patients have much better progression-free survival than those with a lesser degree of transcript number reduction or who remain 100% Ph chromosome positive. Patients who fail to respond to imatinib or who lose their response are probably candidates for alternative therapies including SCT (Table 31–5).

The molecular mechanisms underlying acquired resistance to imatinib have been partially defined.[49,50] In some cases, patients who initially respond to imatinib and then lose their response can be shown to overexpress $p210^{BCR\text{-}ABL}$. In other cases of acquired resistance, there is clonal expansion of a Ph-positive clone with a point mutation in the Abl kinase domain, leading to an amino acid substitution that apparently prevents binding of imatinib but leaves intact the capacity of the kinase to transmit the leukemogenic signal[51] (Fig. 31–6). Point mutations in the phosphate-binding (P-loop) domain of the Abl kinase also are associated with resistance to imatinib and an increased propensity for progression to advanced-phase disease.[52]

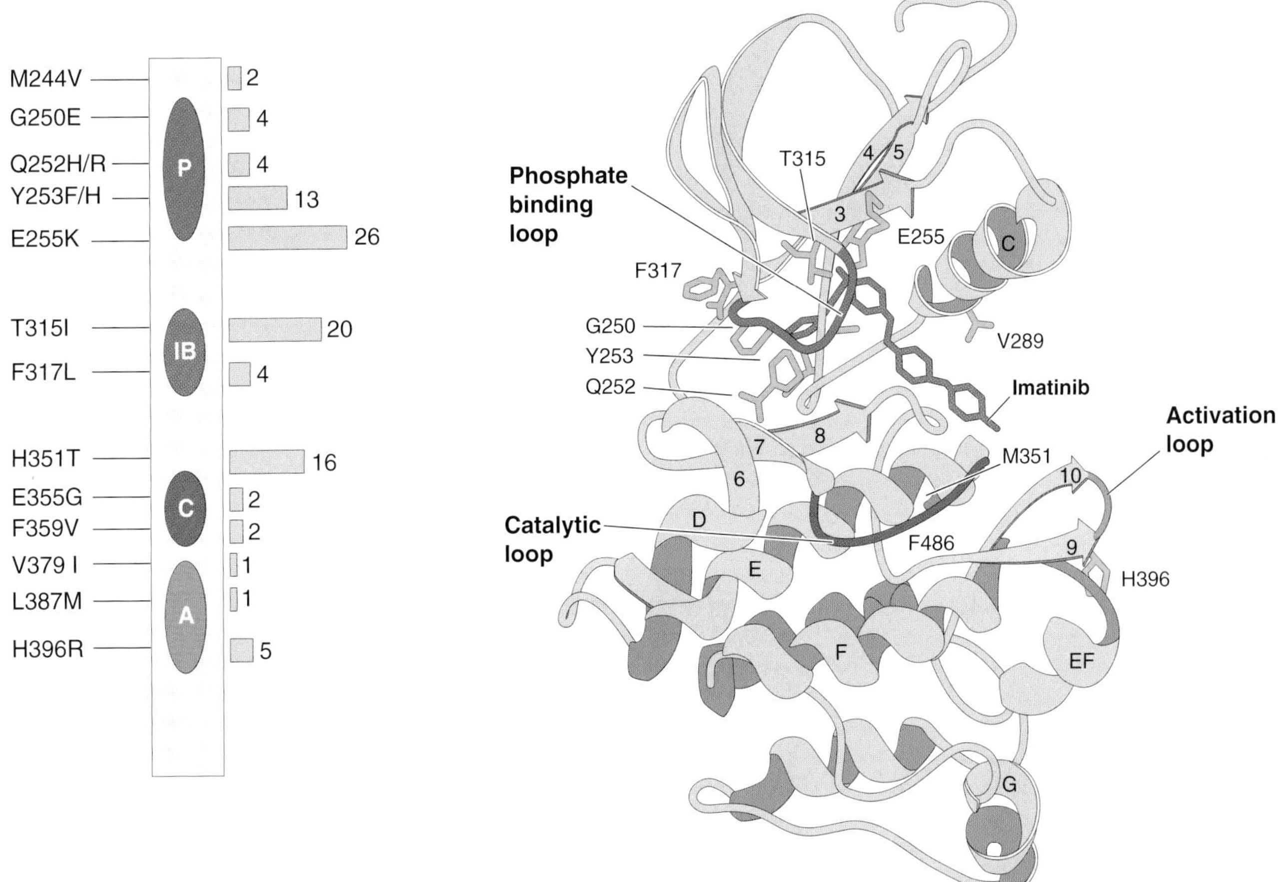

■ **Figure 31–6.** The Abl kinase domain and the principal CML mutations. *Right,* Schematic view of the crystal structure of the Abl kinase domain (amino acids 240–500) showing the relative positions of the adenosine triphosphate binding (P) loop *(brown)*, the activation (A) loop *(green)*, and the catalytic (C) loop *(red)*. Imatinib is shown *(purple)* in contact with the P-loop and extending into an area designated the imatinib-binding (IB) domain. *Left,* A scheme showing the position of mutations identified in 100 different CML patients with varying degrees of resistance to imatinib. The amino acid substitutions are shown to the left and the number of patients with the respective mutation to the right. (From Tauchi T, Ohyashiki K: Leuk Res 28[Suppl 1]:S39–S45, 2004, with permission; based on data compiled from Shah NP, Nicoll JM, Nagar B, et al: Multiple BCR-ABL kinase domain mutations confer polyclonal resistance to the tyrosine kinase inhibitor imatinib [STI571] in chronic phase and blast crisis chronic myeloid leukemia. Cancer Cell 2:117, 2002; and Druker BJ: Semin Hematol 40:50, 2003.)

TABLE 31–5. Possible Criteria to Define Loss of Response to Imatinib Used as a Single Agent

Loss of response to imatinib is defined by any one of the following:

1. Recurrent signs or hematological features of chronic-phase disease
2. Increasing level of Ph-positive marrow metaphases or Bcr/Abl-positive cells identified in the peripheral blood by FISH*
3. Increasing number of Bcr/Abl transcripts in the blood in a patient previously in complete cytogenetic remission

*The finding of an increasing proportion of Ph-positive cells bearing a Bcr/Abl kinase domain mutation by fluorescent in situ hybridization (FISH) may be regarded as evidence of imatinib resistance.

Interferon Alfa

Interferon alfa is one of a series of related glycoproteins of biologic origin with antiviral and antiproliferative properties. It has historical importance in the treatment of CML but is used far less now because of the availability of Abl kinase inhibitors. Studies in the early 1980s showed that interferon alfa could reduce the leukocyte count and reverse all features of CML in 70–80% of patients.[53,54] Moreover, 5–15% of patients achieved major reduction in the percentage of Ph-positive marrow metaphases with restoration of Ph-negative (putatively normal) hematopoiesis.[55] When compared with hydroxyurea, interferon alfa offered a survival advantage that was maximal for those who achieved complete cytogenetic remissions.[56,57] These observations meant that interferon alfa replaced hydroxyurea and busulfan in the 1990s as primary treatment for CML in chronic phase.[58,59]

Interferon alfa is administered by subcutaneous injection at daily doses of 3–5 MU/m^2 without clear dose response.[60] Almost all patients experience fevers, shivers, muscle aches, and general flu-like features on starting the drug; these usually persist 2–3 weeks but may be alleviated by acetaminophen. A significant minority of patients cannot tolerate the drug due to lethargy, malaise, anorexia, weight loss, depression and other affective disorders, or alopecia. Autoimmune syndromes, such as thyrotoxicosis, may occur.

Hydroxyurea

Hydroxyurea also has a traditional role in the treatment of CML and is undoubtedly the simplest drug to use in chronic phase. Hydroxyurea is a ribonucleotide reductase inhibitor that targets relatively mature myeloid progenitors in proliferative cycle. Its pharmacologic action is rapid and readily reversible. Treatment for patients in chronic phase begins at 1.0–2.0 gm daily by mouth. The leukocyte count falls within days and the spleen reduces in size, but treatment is palliative because reversion to normal cytogenetics is rare. Side effects include nausea, diarrhea, and abdominal pain. Some patients suffer ulcers of the buccal mucosa. Skin rashes are seen, and leg ulcers occur very occasionally. Most patients develop megaloblastic changes in the marrow and macrocytosis in the blood. The drug may also be useful in patients unable to tolerate or who develop resistance to imatinib.

Busulfan

Busulfan (1,4-dimethanesulfonyloxybutane), a polyfunctional alkylating agent, was the mainstay of treatment for CML from 1960 through 1980[61–63] but is now infrequently used (except as conditioning before SCT procedures). It targets a relatively primitive stem cell, and the effects of administration persist for weeks after stopping the drug. Treatment was conventionally started with 8 mg daily by mouth, and the dosage was reduced as the leukocyte count began to fall. Dose reduction or drug cessation before the leukocyte count fell below 20×10^9/L was essential because profound and prolonged leukopenia might otherwise be produced. Patients who achieved normal leukocyte counts could then be maintained with daily doses between 0.5 and 2.0 mg/day. Overdosage induced severe marrow failure, often irreversible. Toxicities included inevitable gonadal failure (amenorrhea and azoospermia). Other and permanent effects included cutaneous pigmentation, pulmonary fibrosis, cataract formation, and a wasting syndrome resembling hypoadrenalism.

Drug Combinations

Attempts have been made to improve the results of imatinib used as a single agent at standard dose (400 mg/daily) or at higher doses (600 or 800 mg/day).[64] Relatively small numbers of patients have been treated with imatinib in combination with interferon alfa,[65] cytarabine, and arsenic trioxide. None of these combinations provides a higher response rate than does imatinib alone, but long term survival data are not yet available.

Newer Approaches Under Development

Although early results with imatinib as a single agent are extremely promising, current efforts aim to improve the rate of complete cytogenetic response and possibly also to prolong survival. Combining imatinib with other effective anti-CML agents is an obvious option, as mentioned previously. A variety of new agents designed to inhibit the Abl kinase are now entering phase I/II clinical trials. AMN107 is a chemically modified version of imatinib that inhibits some of the Ph-positive clones with Abl kinase domain mutations that are resistant to imatinib. BMS-354825 (dasatinib) differs from imatinib in that they it can inhibit the kinase function of both the Abl oncogene and the Src protein; it too inhibits proliferation of cells with Abl mutations associated with imatinib resistance.[66] Such new agents are proving useful for patients who develop imatinib resistance; they may also be useful for treating newly diagnosed CML in combination with imatinib.

The observation that a graft-versus-leukemia effect plays a major role in eradication of leukemia cells after allogeneic SCT[67,68] provoked interest in the role of immunotherapy for CML in chronic phase. Vaccination with peptides derived from the Bcr/Abl oncoprotein shows early promise.[69–71] Other possible vaccines are based on the role of Pr-3, WT1, and elastase as possible targets for a graft-versus-leukemia effect.[72,73]

Stem Cell Transplantation

Allogeneic SCT

Allogeneic stem cell transplantation (allo-SCT) was first used to treat patients with CML in chronic phase in the early 1980s,[74–77] and it became rapidly evident that with engraftment many patients recovered normal hematopoiesis, with the disappearance of both their leukemia and Ph-chromosome. The majority of patients alive and free of disease at 5 years post-SCT are likely to remain so indefinitely, satisfying an operational definition of "cure"[78,79] (Fig. 31–7; see also Chapter 94). In general, the allograft procedure for patients with CML is similar to those adopted for other forms of leukemia (see Chapter 94). HLA-identical sibling donors are preferable to HLA-matched unrelated donors. The pretransplantation conditioning comprises the combination of cyclophosphamide and total-body irradiation, though cyclophosphamide and busulfan have recently gained popularity.[80] For patients in chronic phase, the source of stem cells is usually bone marrow rather than peripheral blood,[81] and graft-versus-host disease prophylaxis is conventionally cyclosporine and methotrexate. Various approaches to T-cell depletion have been tested but they invariably increase the risk of relapse.[82,83]

In the absence of an HLA-identical sibling donor, many patients have been transplanted with hematopoietic stem cells collected from HLA-mismatched family members or phenotypically HLA-matched unrelated volunteer donors.[84-87] Small numbers of adult patients have been allografted with stem cells from umbilical cords of unrelated neonates. In general, these transplants have been less successful than matched sibling donor procedures, but, with improving methods of HLA typing and prevention of infection after transplantation, results of alternative donor transplants should improve.

A retrospective analysis of a large database of CML patients treated by allografting compiled for the European Group for Blood and Marrow Transplantation (EBMT) identified five important variables that predicted the probability of survival for a given donor/recipient combination[88] (Table 31–6, Fig. 31–8). Very similar findings were reported subsequently by the International Bone Marrow Transplant Registry in Wisconsin.[89] The relevant factors are patient age, disease phase, disease duration, donor-recipient histocompatibility, and donor/recipient gender combination. The probability of survival for a given patient can be estimated with reasonable confidence, and may range from a low of 10% to a high of 60–70%. However, individual transplant centers have

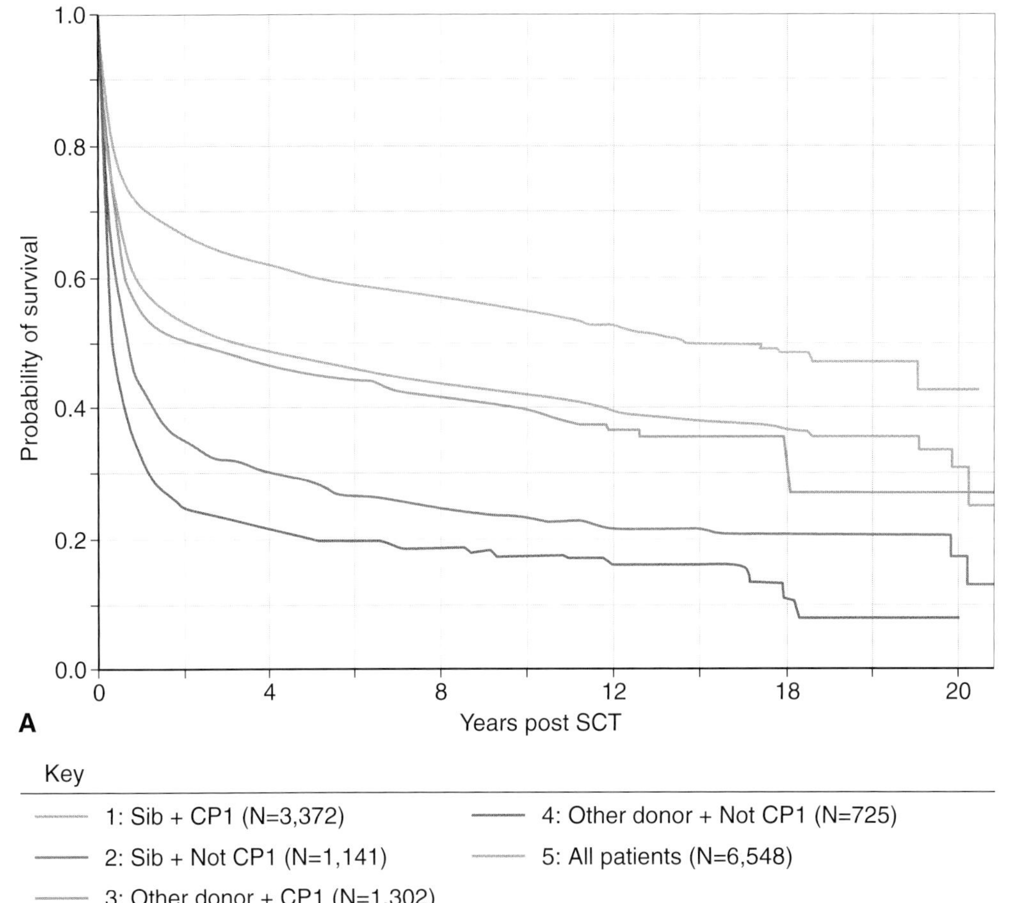

Figure 31–7. Probability of *(A)* survival and *(B)* relapse after allogeneic stem cell transplantation for CML according to phase of disease at transplantation and type of HLA match with donor. Abbreviations: CP1, patients in original chronic phase; Not CP1, patients in advanced phase and patients who progressed to advanced phase but were restored to chronic phase before transplantation; SCT, stem cell transplantation; Sib, HLA-identical sibling donor. (Data provided by the Center for International Blood and Marrow Transplant Research in Milwaukee, Wisconsin.)

Figure continued on following page

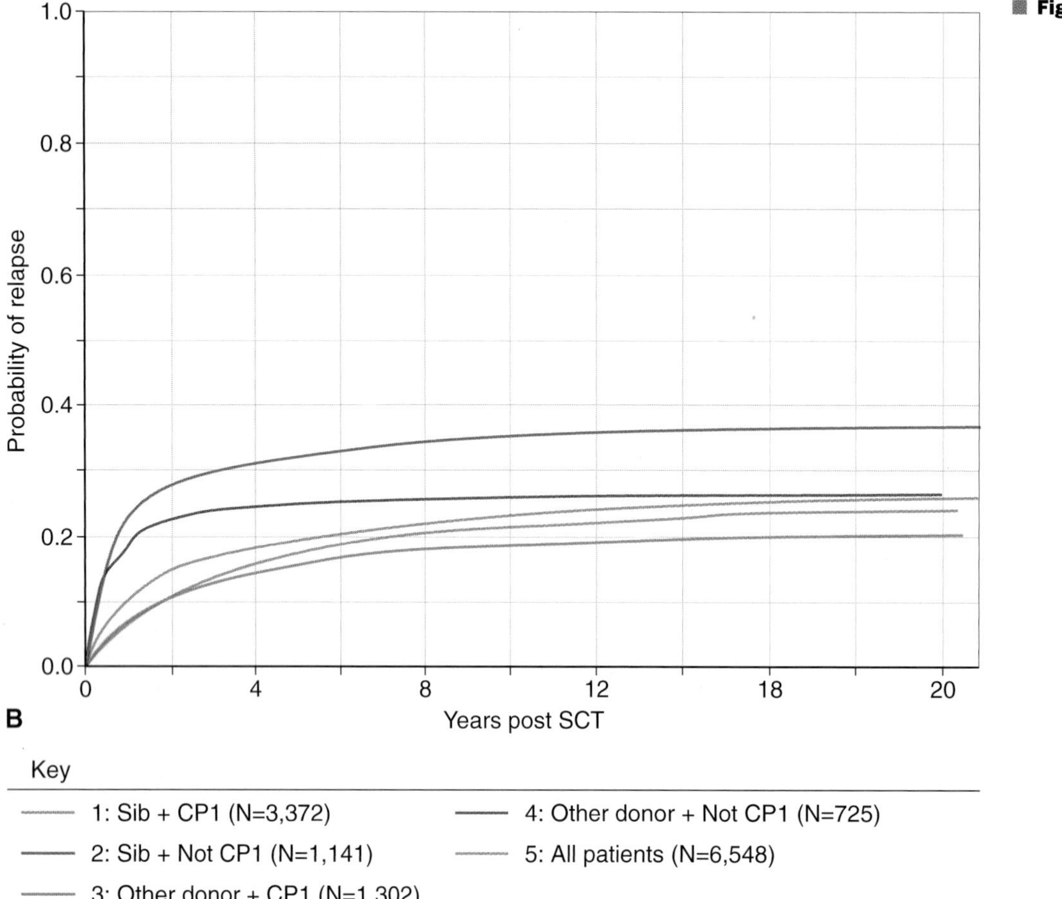

Figure 31–7, cont'd

TABLE 31–6. Criteria Used to Define the (Gratwohl) Risk Score*

Factor	Points
Age (yr):	
<20	0
20–40	1
>40	2
Donor/recipient HLA compatibility:	
HLA-identical sibling	0
Alternative donor	1
Phase of CML:	
Chronic	0
Accelerated	1
Blastic	2
Duration of disease:	
<1 year	0
1 year or more	1
Donor compatibility:	
Male patient with female donor	0
Any other gender combination	1

*Based on analysis of patients in the European Group for Blood and Marrow Transplantation (EBMT) register. *Note:* With this scoring system, the minimum possible score is 0 and the maximum is 7.

reported results very much superior to those that might be predicted from this analysis.

Transplant-related mortality after allo-SCT for CML may be due to graft-versus-host disease, opportunistic infection, veno-occlusive disease of the liver, or other causes. Efforts to reduce the risk of graft-versus-host disease, such as depletion of T cells from the donor inoculum, have usually been accompanied by an increased risk of leukemia relapse. In the absence of T-cell depletion, the probability of relapse within the first 2 years after transplantation ranges between 10% and 30%. For patients alive and free of leukemia 5 years post-SCT, the annual risk of relapse thereafter is 1–2%. Relapses as late as 16 years post-SCT are described, and therefore patients are monitored indefinitely either by routine marrow cytogenetics or, more conveniently, by regular quantitative polymerase chain reaction for Bcr/Abl transcripts.

Relapse of leukemia after allo-SCT, indicated by the persistence or reappearance of Ph-positive metaphases in the bone marrow or a rising level of Bcr/Abl transcripts, requires additional therapy. Donor lymphocyte infusions, whereby lymphocytes collected from the original transplant donor are transfused to the patient, can induce complete remissions[90,91] and produce a graft-versus-leukemia effect without causing graft-versus-host disease.[92–94] In patients who were transplanted prior to the introduction of imatinib, introduction of this drug to treat relapse may be useful.[95,96]

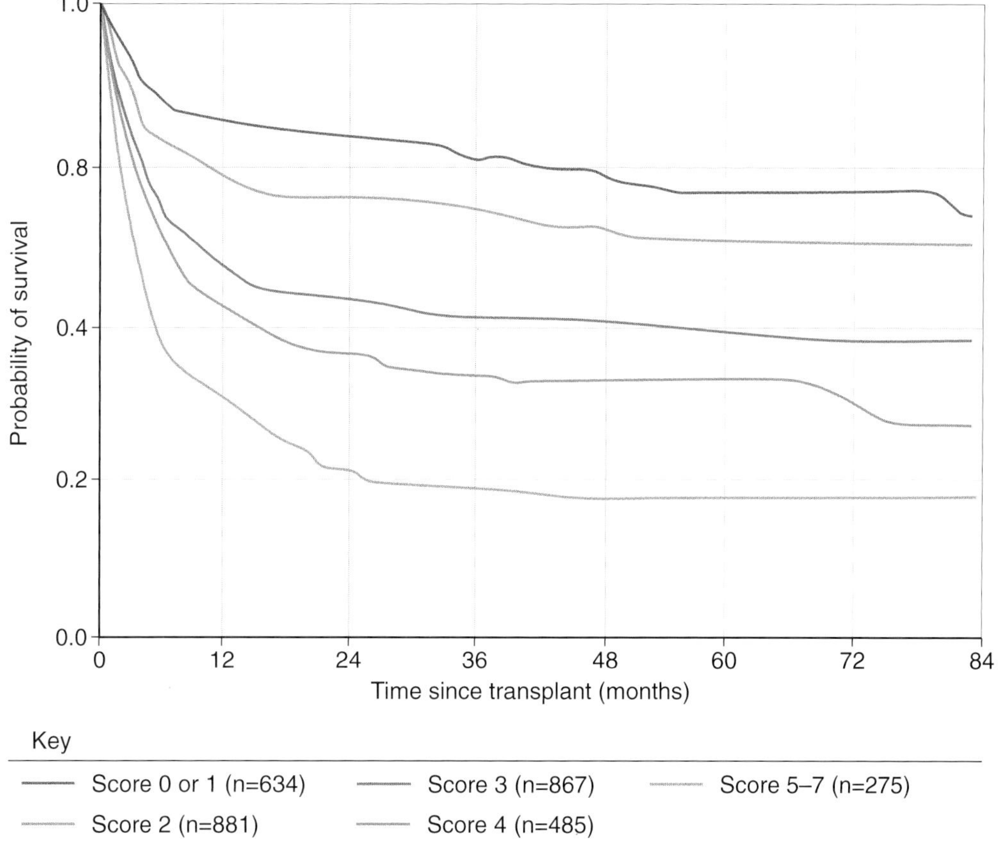

Figure 31–8. Overall survival in a cohort of 3143 patients reported to the European Group for Blood and Marrow Transplantation according to EBMT risk score (see Table 31–6 for details).

The realization that the graft-versus-leukemia effect played a crucial role in the eradication of CML after allo-SCT led to the idea that the intensity of chemotherapy or of chemoradiotherapy could be substantially reduced by reliance on the capacity of the donor lymphoid cells to eradicate the leukemia. Such transplants have been referred to variously as "nonmyeloablative," "reduced intensity conditioning" or "mini-transplants"; different conditioning schedules have been used.[97] The risk of transplant-related mortality appears to be lower than with a conventional conditioning,[98,99] but it is still too early to draw firm conclusions about the capacity of such transplants to "cure" CML.

Autologous SCT

Early in the course of CML, leukemia stem cells coexist with normal stem cells. Clinical studies of autologous SCT conducted with such mixed populations of stem cells have been inconclusive.[100,101] Of greater interest is the attempt to treat patients with high-dose chemotherapy (busulfan), followed by marrow rescue with stem cells that are predominantly or entirely Ph negative. Cells can be collected from the peripheral blood in the recovery phase after administration of high-dose chemotherapy, such as the mini-ICE combination (idarubicin, cytarabine, and etoposide) followed by administration of granulocyte colony-stimulating factor.[102,103] This type of autologous SCT has led to durable Ph-negative hematopoiesis in some patients, but whether they gain a survival benefit is not established.

Advanced-Phase Disease

Chemotherapy

It is difficult to make general statements about the optimal management of patients with advanced-phase disease because the features of acceleration are so very varied. Some patients can be managed merely with a minor alteration in their cytotoxic drug regimen. Some respond to imatinib if they have not previously received this drug.[104] Patients already on imatinib who progress to accelerated phase may still obtain benefit from hydroxyurea or busulfan. Enlarged spleens can be removed. Red cell transfusions relieve symptoms when anemia predominates. Disease moving toward overt blastic transformation may respond to appropriate cytotoxic drug combinations. Allogeneic SCT should be considered for younger patients with suitable donors.

Established blastic transformation may be treated with combinations of cytotoxic drugs in the hope of prolonging life, but cure can no longer be a realistic objec-

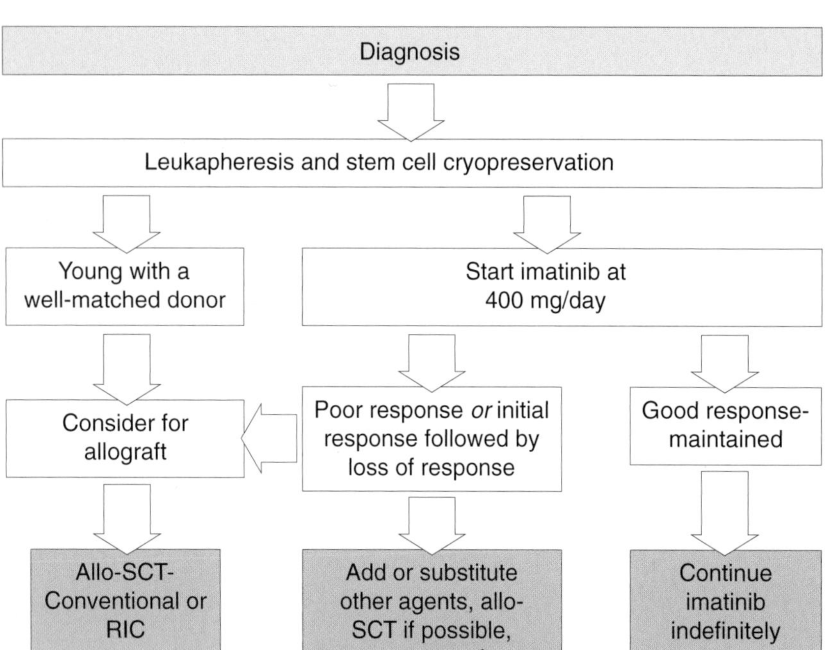

Figure 31–9. Treatment scheme for new CML patient. *Notes:* The initial use of imatinib at 600 or 800 mg/day may prove more effective than 400 mg/day. There is currently debate as to whether any newly diagnosed patient (other than one with a syngeneic identical twin) should be offered initial treatment by allogeneic stem cell transplantation (allo-SCT). There is also uncertainty as to whether transplant is best performed with conventional or with reduced intensity conditioning (RIC). The role of autografting is not established.

tive.[105,106] Imatinib may be remarkably effective in controlling the clinical and hematologic features of CML in blastic phase, but the effect is short lived[107] and the drug should be used as a prelude to more effective therapy. Conversely, it is not unreasonable to adopt a palliative approach involving a relatively innocuous drug such as hydroxyurea at higher dosage to restrain blast cell numbers and thus maintain the patient at home for as long as possible. Myeloid transformation can be treated with drugs appropriate to the induction of remission in acute myeloid leukemia, daunorubicin and cytosine arabinoside with or without etoposide. The blast cells will be reduced substantially in most cases, but numbers usually increase again within 3–6 weeks. Perhaps 20% of patients are restored to apparent chronic-phase disease for 3–6 months, a very small minority, probably less than 10%, may achieve substantial degrees of Ph-negative hematopoiesis (more likely in patients who entered blastic transformation soon after diagnosis).

Patients in lymphoid transformation may be treated with drugs applicable to the management of adult acute lymphoblastic leukemia (prednisolone, vincristine, daunorubicin, and methotrexate with or without L-asparaginase). More than 50% will be restored to a second chronic phase, status which can be maintained with daily 6-mercaptopurine and weekly methotrexate or SCT. Because leukemia involving the central nervous system is relatively common in responding patients, those who achieve a second chronic phase should receive neuroprophylaxis with intrathecal methotrexate weekly for 6 consecutive weeks. The administration of cranial irradiation is probably excessive. Some patients treated for lymphoid transformation of CML sustain long periods of apparent remission.

Stem Cell Transplantation

Allogeneic SCT using HLA-matched sibling donors can be performed in accelerated-phase CML[108]; the probability of leukemia-free survival at 5 years is 30–50%. SCT performed in overt blastic transformation nearly always fails. The mortality resulting from graft-versus-host disease is extremely high, and the probability of relapse in those who survive the transplant procedure is very considerable. The probability of survival at 5 years is consequently 0–10%.

THERAPEUTIC DECISIONS IN CML

Until recently it was conventional to offer allo-SCT to all newly diagnosed patients under the age of 45 or 50 years who had suitable transplant donors, but the advent of imatinib has fundamentally altered this approach[109,110] (Fig. 31–9). Most hematologists now recommend starting all newly diagnosed patients on imatinib as a single agent or on imatinib in combination with other suitable agents. Some however believe that there is a small subset of newly diagnosed patients who are unquestionably eligible for allo-SCT as primary therapy. To identify this subset, one might use the EBMT scoring system to identify a subgroup of patients with a relatively low risk of transplant-related mortality and then adjust the criteria for this subgroup in accordance with the Sokal risk score, which identifies patients with relatively good or poor estimated survivals with nontransplant therapy. Along these lines many pediatricians believe that initial treatment by SCT is still the best approach for managing children with CML. In the absence of clear data defining that subgroup of patients who should receive SCT as initial therapy, the clinician must take into account the patient's own desire (or reluctance) to proceed to allo-SCT soon after diagnosis.

SCT remains the treatment of choice in patients failing imatinib, but newer agents may alter even this perspective. At present, the criteria for assessing failure cannot be defined with any certainty, but the patient who fails to achieve hematologic control within 3 months or a reasonable level of Ph chromosome negativity within 6–12 months may be less likely to obtain survival benefit from imatinib (see Table 31–5) and should be offered allo-SCT.

VARIANTS OF CHRONIC MYELOID LEUKEMIA

Chronic Myelomonocytic Leukemia

This is a rare condition that affects predominantly elderly men but is found at all ages (see Chapter 31). Although included in the French-American-British classification of the myelodysplastic syndromes, it is probably better regarded as a discrete entity. The patient may present with features of anemia or hemorrhage. The spleen is typically enlarged and thus the clinical picture superficially resembles CML. The blood and marrow are, however, quite different. Marrow cells lack a Ph chromosome. Blood monocytosis is prominent, and monocyte numbers may be as high as 50×10^9/L. Thrombocytopenia is common. Basophilia and eosinophilia are absent. Dysplastic changes are usually present in the granulocyte and erythroid series.

Very rare patients have been described with a chronic myelomonocytic leukemia–like blood picture associated with consistent cytogenetic abnormalities in their leukemia cells other than t(9;22). Most have either a t(5;12) associated with fusion of the *TEL* (*ETV6*) and *PDGFRB* genes or a t(8;13) associated with fusion of the *ZNF198* and *FGFR1* genes. *PDGFRB* and *FGFR1* are both receptor tyrosine kinases, and their activation by fusion with a partner gene suggests a mechanism of leukemogenesis analogous to that seen in Bcr/Abl-positive CML. The t(5;12) and t(8;13) leukemias are both characterized by prominent eosinophilia, but basophilia is usually absent. The t(5;12) leukemias respond extremely well to low doses of imatinib; the t(8;13) leukemias do not and are clinically much more aggressive.

Chronic Neutrophilic Leukemia

This exceedingly rare disorder is usually diagnosed incidentally. The patient has a raised blood neutrophil count without immature granulocytes nor basophilia or eosinophilia. The neutrophil alkaline phosphatase level is usually high. The marrow is hypercellular but cytogenetic studies are normal. The diagnosis is based largely on exclusion of other identifiable causes for the leukocytosis. Most patients have no symptoms referable to the neutrophilia and no physical signs, although some have minor degrees of splenomegaly. Treatment often is not required.

CURRENT CONTROVERSIES & FUTURE CONSIDERATIONS

Chronic Myeloid Leukemia

- What signal transduction pathways are critical in linking the activated Bcr/Abl kinase in the cytoplasm to nuclear events?
- What is the molecular explanation for the genomic instability that predisposes to progression of disease from chronic to advanced phase?
- What is the basis of the graft-versus-leukemia effect? Can it be exploited outside the context of a conventional transplant?
- Can imatinib alone eradicate leukemia in any patient?
- What is the basis of acquired resistance to imatinib? Will the new generation of tyrosine kinase inhibitors prove better than imatinib?
- What are the indications for allogeneic stem cell transplantation today?

Suggested Readings*

Barrett AJ: Allogeneic stem cell transplantation for chronic myeloid leukemia. Semin Hematol 40:59–71, 2003.

Carella AM, Beltrami G, Corsetti MT: Autografting in chronic myeloid leukemia. Semin Hematol 40:72–86, 2003.

Druker BJ, Talpaz M, Resta DJ, et al: Efficacy and safety of a specific inhibit of the BCR-ABL tyrosine kinase in chronic myeloid leukemia. N Engl J Med 344:1031–1037, 2001.

Goldman JM, Druker B: Chronic myeloid leukemia: current treatment options. Blood 98:2039–2042, 2001.

Goldman JM, Melo JV: Chronic myeloid leukemia—advances in biology and new approaches to treatment. N Engl J Med 349:1449–1462, 2003.

Gratwohl A, Hermans J, Goldman JM, et al: Risk assessment for patients with chronic myeloid leukaemia before allogeneic bone marrow transplantation. Lancet 352:1087–1092, 1998.

Guilhot F, Chastang C, Michallet M, et al: Interferon alfa-2b combined with cytarabine versus interferon alone in chronic myelogenous leukemia. N Engl J Med 337:223–229, 1997.

Hasford J, Pfirrmann M, Hehlmann R, et al: A new prognostic score for survival of patients with chronic myeloid leukemia treated with interferon alfa. Writing Committee for the Collaborative CML Prognostic Factors Project Group. J Natl Cancer Inst 90:850–858, 1998.

Hughes TP, Kaeda J, Branford S, et al: Frequency of major molecular responses to imatinib or interferon alfa plus cytarabine in newly diagnosed chronic myeloid leukemia. N Engl J Med 349:1421–1430, 2003.

Jaffe ES, Harris NL, Stein H, Vardiman JW (Eds): World Health Organisation Classification of Tumours—Tumours of the Haematopoietic and Lymphoid Tissues. Lyon: IARC Press, 2001, pp 20–26.

Melo JV: The molecular biology of chronic myeloid leukaemia. Leukemia 10:751–756, 1996.

Mughal TI, Yong A, Szydlo R, et al: Molecular studies in patients with chronic myeloid leukaemia in remission 5 years after allogeneic stem cell transplant define the risk of subsequent relapse. Br J Haematol 115:569–574, 2001.

O'Brien SG, Guilhot F, Larson RA, et al: Imatinib compared with interferon and low dose cytarabine for newly diagnosed chronic-phase chronic myeloid leukemia. N Engl J Med 348:994–1004, 2003.

Sawyers CL: Chronic myeloid leukemia. N Engl J Med 340: 1330–1340, 1999.

Shah NP, Tran C, Lee FY, et al: Overcoming imatinib resistance with a novel ABL kinase inhibitor. Science 305:399–401, 2004.

Sokal JE, Cox EB, Baccarani M, et al: Prognostic discrimination in 'good risk' chronic granulocytic leukemia. Blood 63: 789–799, 1984.

Full references for this chapter can be found on accompanying CD-ROM.

CHAPTER 32

Acute Lymphoblastic Leukemia

Raul C. Ribeiro, MD, and Ching-Hon Pui, MD

KEY POINTS

Acute Lymphoblastic Leukemia

Diagnosis

- Abnormalities of at least two hematopoietic lineages are typically present at the diagnosis of acute lymphoblastic leukemia (ALL). However, many nonmalignant processes can cause abnormalities of one or more hematopoietic lineages.
- Isolated thrombocytopenia is not an initial manifestation of ALL and is more likely to be immune mediated.
- Bone pain and inflammatory joint changes accompanied by minimal changes in blood counts are relatively common in pediatric ALL. Some patients may present with normal blood counts. This constellation of signs and symptoms can be confused with rheumatologic disorders. Bone marrow examination establishes the correct diagnosis.
- Not uncommonly, severe pancytopenia is the main presenting feature of ALL. Rarely, hypereosinophilia can be the predominant feature in ALL or precedes the diagnosis of ALL.

Treatment

- The intensity of treatment is tailored to specific clinical and biologic factors at the time of diagnosis and to the response to early therapy.
- Central nervous system (CNS) leukemia can be eradicated or prevented by intrathecal medications in conjunction with effective systemic chemotherapy. Irradiation of the CNS is rarely used in the management of ALL.
- Hematopoietic stem cell transplantation has a limited role in the management of newly diagnosed ALL. Patients who have the *BCR/ABL* fusion gene or have high levels of minimal residual disease after remission induction chemotherapy may benefit from this procedure during first complete remission.

Supported in part by grant CA-21765 from the National Institutes of Health (U.S. Department of Health and Human Services), a Center for Excellence grant from the State of Tennessee, and the American Lebanese Syrian Associated Charities (ALSAC). C. H. Pui is the American Cancer Society F. M. Kirby Clinical Research Professor.

INTRODUCTION

Leukemia results from the malignant transformation of one of a variety of hematopoietic cells at some point in its myeloid or lymphoid differentiation (Table 32–1; see also Chapters 28, 31, 33, and 34). The lymphoid system undergoes an extraordinary remodeling and expansion process during childhood and adolescence; therefore, it is not surprising that acute lymphoblastic leukemia (ALL) is the most common pediatric leukemia and is relatively infrequent in adults. The typical patient with ALL is between the ages of 3 and 5 years and has previously been well, with a relatively short history of pallor, an increased bleeding tendency (ecchymoses and petechiae), and fever. Physical examination may reveal hepatosplenomegaly and generalized lymph node enlargement. The peripheral blood findings are variable but generally show abnormality of two or more hematopoietic lineages. However, the clinical and laboratory manifestations of ALL can vary markedly. In most cases of childhood ALL, the bone marrow is completely replaced by leukemic lymphoblasts.

EPIDEMIOLOGY, RISK FACTORS, AND PATHOPHYSIOLOGY

Incidence

Sixty percent of the approximately 4000 cases of ALL diagnosed annually in the United States occur in individuals younger than 20 years of age.[1] Twelve percent of all cases of leukemia diagnosed in the United States are ALL; it is the most common malignancy diagnosed in patients younger than 15 years, accounting for 23% of all cancers and 76% of all leukemias in this age group. The age-specific incidence pattern is bimodal. The first peak occurs between ages 2 and 4 years; rates then fall during later childhood, adolescence, and young adulthood. A second, smaller incidence peak is noted during the sixth decade (Fig. 32–1).[2,3] The peak incidence between ages 2 and 4 years is much lower in black children (45 cases per 1 million population) than in white children (120 cases per million) in the United States. Among children younger than 15 years, the male/female ratio is 1.2:1, but among children between ages 15 and 19 years it is 2:1. International variation in the incidence of both ALL and

TABLE 32–1. Distribution of Human Leukemias by Age at Time of Diagnosis

	Percent of Total by Age (yr)				
Type of Leukemia	**<20**	**20–44**	**45–64**	**65–84**	**>85**
Acute lymphoblastic leukemia	63.9	15.4	10.8	8.4	1.5
Chronic lymphocytic leukemia	0.0	2.6	27.9	57.0	12.5
Acute myeloid leukemia	6.1	14.5	23.3	47.6	8.5
Chronic myeloid leukemia	2.2	19.2	26.2	42.3	10.1
Others	3.4	10.1	23.2	46.5	16.8

Source: Surveillance, Epidemiology and End Results (SEER) Program.[2]

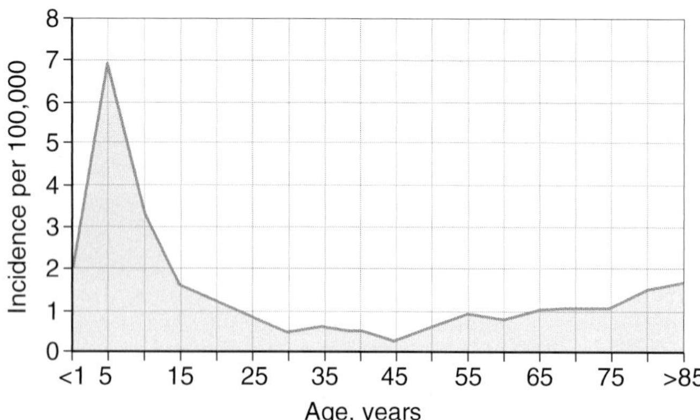

Figure 32–1. Age-specific incidence of acute lymphoblastic leukemia.

non-Hodgkin's lymphoma has been reported.[4,5] ALL occurs with greater frequency in Northern and Western Europe, North America, and Oceania than in Asia and Africa.[6] In Europe, the highest rate of ALL is found in Denmark.[7]

Risk Factors and Mechanisms of ALL

The causes of ALL remain elusive. Most patients with ALL do not have predisposing factors or constitutional abnormalities. An increased risk of ALL has been associated with Down syndrome,[8,9] neurofibromatosis,[10] Shwachman syndrome,[11] Bloom syndrome,[12] Li-Fraumeni syndrome,[13] ataxia-telangiectasia,[14,15] and Klinefelter's syndrome.[16] Children with Down syndrome have a risk of leukemia 10–30 times that of other children. Remarkably, children with Down syndrome who are less than 3 years of age have a 400 times greater risk of acute megakaryoblastic leukemia than do other children. ALL occurs at an older age in children with Down syndrome and is usually B-cell precursor ALL without the specific chromosomal translocations commonly associated with ALL.[17] Diseases associated with increased chromosomal fragility, including ataxia-telangiectasia, Nijmegen breakage syndrome, and Bloom syndrome, are associated with an increased risk of ALL.[18] Patients with ataxia-telangiectasia have a 70 times greater risk of ALL (particularly of the T-cell phenotype) than do others.[14] The *ATM* (ataxia-telangiectasia mutated) gene encodes a 350-kDa protein that regulates several genes involved in the repair of double-stranded DNA breaks and in regulation of the cell cycle and apoptosis. Somatic and germline *ATM* gene mutations have been reported in sporadic T-cell ALL.[19]

Environmental exposure to various agents has been implicated in the development of ALL. Prenatal exposure to diagnostic x-rays confers a slightly increased risk of ALL.[20] There is a weak association between exposure to nuclear fallout, to occupational, natural terrestrial, or cosmic ionizing radiation, and to therapeutic radiation and ALL. Other factors associated with an increased predisposition to leukemia include pesticide exposure, parental cigarette smoking before or during pregnancy, maternal alcohol consumption during pregnancy, and increased consumption of dietary nitrites or water contaminated with trichloroethylene.[3] Recent studies have suggested that genetic polymorphisms of xenobiotic-metabolizing enzymes may interact with environmental, dietary, maternal, and other external factors to predispose to the development of ALL.[21–23] Interestingly, variants of methylenetetrahydrofolate reductase have been linked to a decreased risk of ALL in adults[24] and children.[25] Folate supplementation may decrease the risk of ALL in children.[26]

Studies in twins have shown that, when an identical twin develops leukemia with the t(4;11)/*MLL/AF4*, the other twin will almost certainly develop leukemia with the same fusion gene within weeks or a few months. In contrast, there is a lower concordance rate in identical twins with hyperdiploid or B-cell precursor ALL that has the *TEL/AML1* fusion. These data are consistent with clinical epidemiologic observations that, when an identical twin develops leukemia within the first year of life, the likelihood that the other twin will develop ALL approaches 100%. The rate of leukemia in an identical twin is much smaller when the other twin develops leukemia after the first year of life. However, not all ALL-specific fusion genes develop in utero. For example, the t(1;19)/*E2A/PBX1* fusion gene has a postnatal origin in most cases[27] (Fig. 32–2). Although inactivating mutations or deletions of *RB* are rare in ALL, epigenetic silencing of the RB pathway occurs in cases of childhood and adult T-cell ALL and in a small proportion of childhood B-lineage ALL.[28,29] Likewise, components of the p53 pathway are sometimes altered in ALL.[30,31]

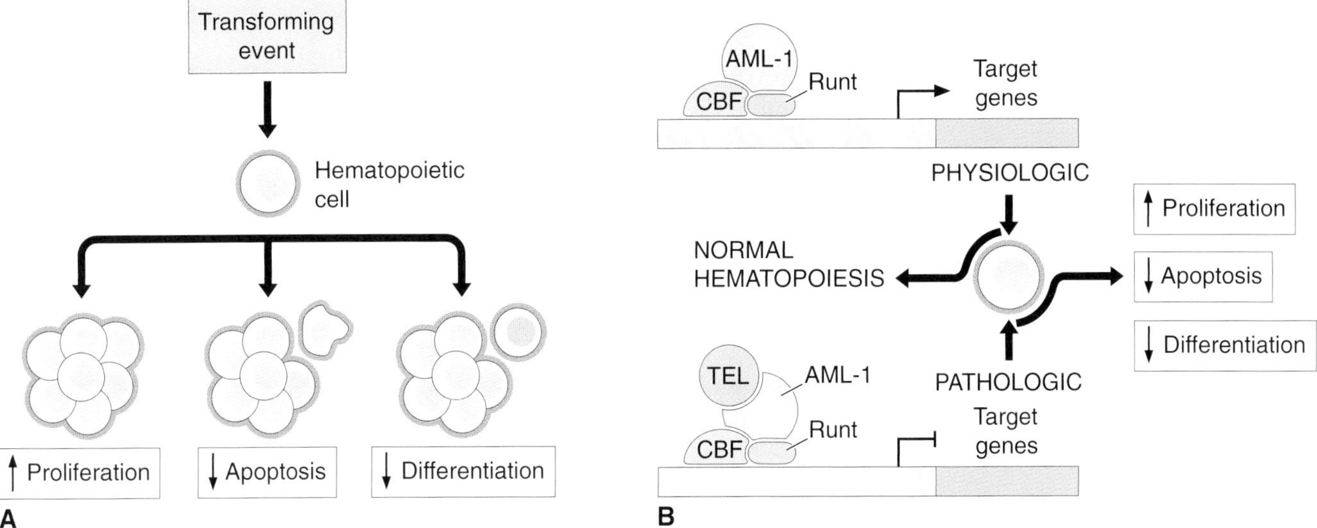

Figure 32–2. Pathogenesis of leukemia. *A,* Leukemic transforming events in hematopoietic stem cells result in increased clonal cell proliferation and decreased differentiation and apoptosis. *B,* Disruption of genes that encode subunits of core-binding factor (CBF), a multimeric transcription factor complex involved in the regulation of hematopoiesis, is considered to be pivotal in leukemogenesis. AML-1 is the DNA-binding subunit of CBF and other transcriptional coactivators. In acute lymphoblastic leukemia, the function of CBF is repressed by the chimeric TEL/AML protein (found in about 22% of cases of childhood leukemia) encoded by the translocated *TEL* (chromosome 12) and *AML1* (chromosome 21) genes.

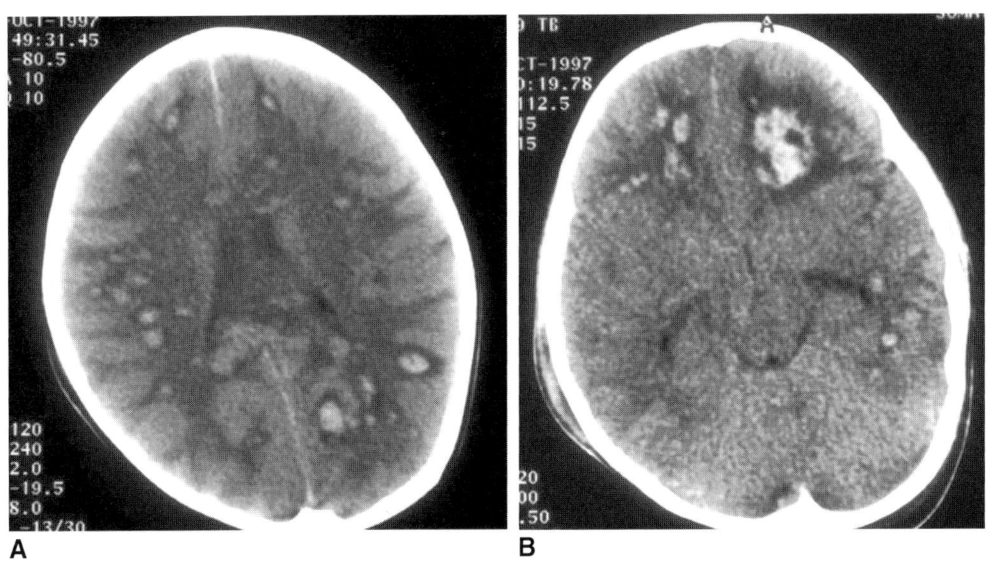

Figure 32–3. *A,* Axial computed tomography scans of the brain in a child with newly diagnosed acute lymphoblastic leukemia and hyperleukocytosis reveal multiple bilateral hemorrhagic lesions. These lesions typically involve only the white matter. *B,* The same patient had a large hemorrhagic lesion in the frontal region with associated vasogenic edema.

CLINICAL FEATURES, DIAGNOSIS, AND CLASSIFICATION

Signs and Symptoms

The signs and symptoms of ALL may develop abruptly or insidiously.[32–37] In older patients, cardiovascular manifestations of anemia, such as dyspnea, angina, and dizziness, may be the predominant initial features.[36] Fever resulting from infection or, more commonly, proinflammatory cytokines is one of the most common signs, occurring in about 60% of patients. Pallor, fatigue, lethargy, petechiae, ecchymosis, and bone pain are also common. Bone pain and arthralgia, especially in children, are very common presenting features of ALL.[38] Marrow necrosis, another cause of severe bone pain and tenderness, occurs in rare cases. Arthralgia and bone pain are less severe in adults. Occasionally, intracranial hemorrhage caused by leukostasis can be the first manifestation of leukemia (Fig. 32–3). Patients with marked leukocytosis (white blood cell count > 400×10^9/L) are at high risk of this complication.[39] Physical examination frequently reveals pallor, petechiae, and ecchymoses. Enlargement of the liver, spleen, and lymph nodes is the most common extramedullary manifestation of ALL; the organomegaly is more pronounced in children than in adults (Table 32–2). About 10% of children and 15% of adults with ALL, usually of the T-cell immunophenotype,

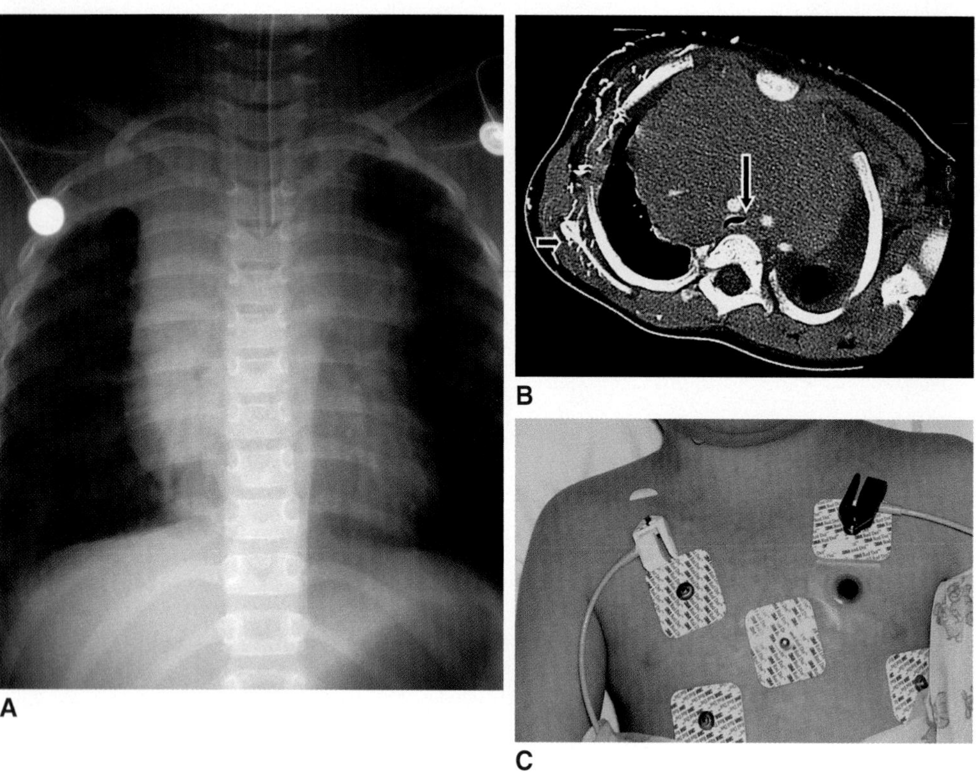

Figure 32–4. *A,* Chest radiograph of a 10-year-old boy with acute lymphoblastic leukemia shows a large mediastinal mass. *B,* Computed tomography shows narrowing of the trachea caused by mechanical compression of the mediastinal mass *(long arrow)*, a left pleural effusion, and increased collateral circulation *(short arrow)*. *C,* Signs of superior vena cava syndrome include edema of the neck and increased collateral circulation in the chest.

TABLE 32–2. Selected Presenting Clinical and Laboratory Features of ALL

Feature	Percentage of Total	
	Children	**Adults**
Physical Examination		
Fever	50–60	35–55
Bleeding	40–50	30–35
Bone or joint pain	20–30	20–30
Marked adenopathy	15–20	10–15
Hepatomegaly	50–60	30–35
Splenomegaly	50–60	50–60
Testicular enlargement	1	<1
Laboratory Findings		
Leukocyte count ($\times 10^9$/L)		
<10	50	40
>100	10	15
Hemoglobin concentration		
<8	50	30
>10	20	50
Platelet count ($\times 10^9$/L)		
<50	50	50
>100	30	25
More than 90% blast cells in bone marrow	80	70
Mediastinal mass	10	15
CNS leukemia	3	10

present with a large anterior mediastinal mass (Fig. 32–4*A* and *B*), sometimes accompanied by pleural effusions and superior vena cava syndrome (Fig. 32–4*C*).[40] Mediastinal involvement is a medical emergency, and early management should avoid general anesthesia.

Central nervous system (CNS) (meningeal) involvement is generally asymptomatic at diagnosis but may be associated with cranial nerve palsy, commonly of the seventh cranial nerve. Ophthalmologic examination may reveal papilledema and, occasionally, leukemic infiltration of the optic nerve, retina, iris, cornea, or conjunctiva. Rarely, leukemic infiltration of the orbit may cause proptosis. Spinal cord compression by an extramedullary deposit of leukemia cells is a rare finding at presentation but requires immediate attention to avoid irreversible neurologic damage. Clinically detected painless testicular enlargement occurs in about 2% of male patients, generally in infants or in patients with T-cell leukemia and hyperleukocytosis (Fig. 32–5). Other uncommon presenting features include subcutaneous nodules (leukemia cutis), enlarged parotid glands (Mikulicz's syndrome), and priapism.

Laboratory and Radiographic Findings

Presenting white blood cell counts range from 0.1 to 1500 $\times 10^9$/L (median, 10–12 $\times 10^9$/L). Hyperleukocytosis (>100 $\times 10^9$/L) is seen in fewer than 20% of patients (see Table 32–2). Neutropenia is a common finding; a neutrophil count less than 0.5 $\times 10^9$/L is found in 20–40% of patients and is associated with a high risk of bacterial infection. Hypereosinophilia, which can cause fever, coughing, wheezing, and congestive heart failure, may precede the diagnosis of ALL by several months.[41] A specific chromosomal genetic abnormality, the t(5;14)(q31;q32), which results in activation of the *IL3* gene, is thought to play a role in leukemogenesis and hypereosinophilia in

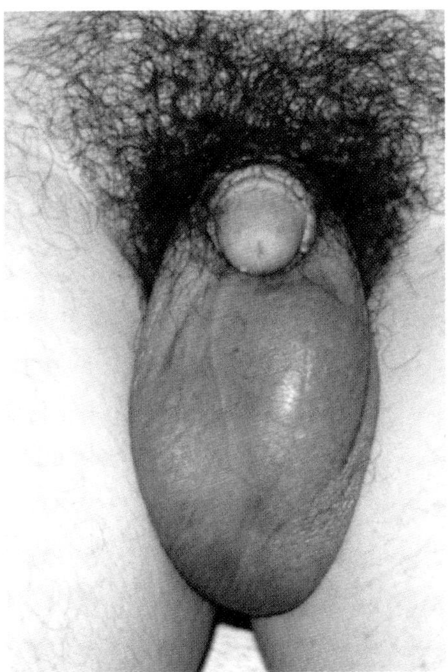

Figure 32–5. Left testicular enlargement in a patient with newly diagnosed T-cell acute lymphoblastic leukemia.

these cases.[42] Thrombocytopenia is a very common finding in ALL.

Coagulation parameters are usually normal and the plasma fibrinogen concentration tends to be elevated, reflecting a systemic inflammatory response. Mild coagulopathy with slightly increased prothrombin and partial thromboplastin times and a low fibrinogen concentration can be seen in about 3% of cases.[36,43] Rarely, disseminated intravascular coagulation has been associated with pre–B-cell ALL and the t(17;19)(q22;p13) chromosomal abnormality.[44]

Serum lactate dehydrogenase activity is increased in most patients with ALL.[45] Leukemic involvement of the kidneys can be associated with increased serum concentration of creatinine, urea nitrogen, uric acid, and phosphorus. Hypercalcemia, which is observed in less than 1% of patients with ALL, results from release by the leukemic cells of parathyroid hormone–related peptide or other cytokines and from leukemic infiltration of the bone.[46] Elevated serum transaminase activity, reflecting liver dysfunction, occurs in 10–20% of patients with ALL but is usually mild and has little clinical or prognostic importance.[32]

Chest radiography is required to identify a mediastinal mass or pleural effusion. Skeletal involvement, which occurs in about 50% of patients with ALL, is seen radiographically as metaphyseal bands, periosteal reactions, osteolytic lesions, osteosclerosis, and osteopenia sometimes leading to vertebral collapse.[47]

Central Nervous System

Lumbar puncture and examination of the cerebrospinal fluid are integral components of the initial evaluation of a child with ALL. Leukemic blast cells can be identified in the cerebrospinal fluid of as many as one third of pediatric patients at diagnosis,[48] but only 2–3% of patients have overt CNS leukemia, with 5 or more blasts per microliter of cerebrospinal fluid in the presence of cranial nerve palsy. The presence of leukemic cells in cytocentrifuge preparations of cerebrospinal fluid predicts an increased risk of CNS relapse[49] and requires more intensive intrathecal therapy.[50] Although this diagnosis can be confounded by a traumatic lumbar puncture,[51,52] the current practice at St. Jude Children's Research Hospital is to give intrathecal therapy to all pediatric ALL patients at diagnostic lumbar puncture. Maneuvers to avoid a traumatic tap may impact survival.[50,53]

Bone Marrow

Although the bone marrow is completely replaced by lymphoblasts in about 85% of cases of childhood ALL, a finding of 25% or more blast cells is required for the diagnosis of leukemia. In most cases, the lymphoblasts tend to be relatively small with scant, light blue cytoplasm; a round, slightly indented nucleus; fine to slightly coarse and clumped chromatin; and inconspicuous nucleoli.[54] In other cases, the lymphoblasts are larger, with conspicuous nucleoli and moderate amounts of cytoplasm. Lymphoblasts in some cases can contain azurophilic cytoplasmic granules similar to those observed in myeloid leukemias, although these granules (which are mitochondria) stain positively with Sudan black B and not with myeloperoxidase stain.[55] In mature B-cell leukemia (Burkitt's leukemia), the lymphoblasts are characterized by intensely basophilic cytoplasm, regular cellular features, prominent nucleoli, and cytoplasmic vacuolation. Cytochemical stains (Sudan black and stains for myeloperoxidase and the nonspecific esterases, including α-naphthylbutyrate and α-naphthylacetate esterase) separate lymphoid from myeloid, monocytic, and megakaryocytic leukemias. ALL blast cells are negative for myeloperoxidase activity.

Immunophenotypic characterization of blast cells identifies B-lineage cells (CD19, cytoplasmic CD79a), T-lineage cells (CD7, cytoplasmic CD3), and myeloid cells (CD13, CD33, cytoplasmic myeloperoxidase).[56] Cases of B- and T-cell precursor ALL can be also subdivided into CD10-positive (so-called common ALL antigen) and CD10-negative ALL[57,58]; CD10-positive cases generally have more favorable outcome than CD10-negative cases (Table 32–3). Myeloid-associated markers may be expressed on lymphoblasts but are not prognostic factors.[37,59]

Genetic Findings

Specific numeric or structural genetic abnormalities can be detected in about 75% of adult and pediatric leukemias (Fig. 32–6).[21,56,60–64] Submicroscopic genetic alterations, such as the *TEL/AML1* fusion, *AML1* amplification, and deletions of tumor suppressor genes, are not detected by standard karyotyping procedures.[21,65,66] The most common methods used to evaluate genetic changes

TABLE 32–3. Selected Features of Immunologically Defined Subtypes of ALL

Subtype	Useful Markers	Associated Features
B Cell	CD10, CD19, CD22, CD79, cIg, sIgμ	Most common immunophenotype of pediatric and adult ALL
Pre-pre–B cell	CD10⁻, cIg⁻, sIgμ⁻	Infants and adults, high leukocyte count, CNS leukemia, DNA index of 1, *MLL* rearrangement, poor prognosis
Early pre-B cell	CD10⁺, cIg⁻, sIgμ⁻	Most common type of pediatric (65%) and adult (52%) ALL, low leukocyte count, DNA index >1.16, *TEL/AML1* fusion, favorable prognosis
Pre-B cell	CD10±, cIg⁺, sIgμ⁻	Black race, high leukocyte count, DNA index 1, *E2A/PBX1* fusion, favorable prognosis with intensive chemotherapy
Mature B cell	CD10±, sIgμ⁺, CD22⁺, sIgκ⁺ or sIgλ⁺	Common extramedullary involvement (abdomen, kidneys, CNS), male preponderance, favorable prognosis with intensive chemotherapy program
T Cell	CD7, cCD3, CD2, CD1, CD10, CD4, CD8	Male predominance, more common in young adult (18%) than pediatric (12%) ALL, mediastinal masses, high leukocyte count
Pre-thymic T cell	CD34⁺,CD8⁻, CD4⁻, CD3⁻, CD10⁻	High levels of *BCL* and *LYL1* gene expression, unfavorable prognosis
Early cortical T cell	CD8⁺, CD4⁺, CD1⁺, CD10⁺, CD3^low	About 30% and 10% of adult and pediatric T-cell ALL, respectively; overexpression of *HOX11* gene, favorable prognosis
Late cortical T cell	CD8⁺, CD4⁺, CD3^high, CD2⁺, CD10⁻	Expression of antiapoptotic molecules (BCL2A1), unfavorable prognosis

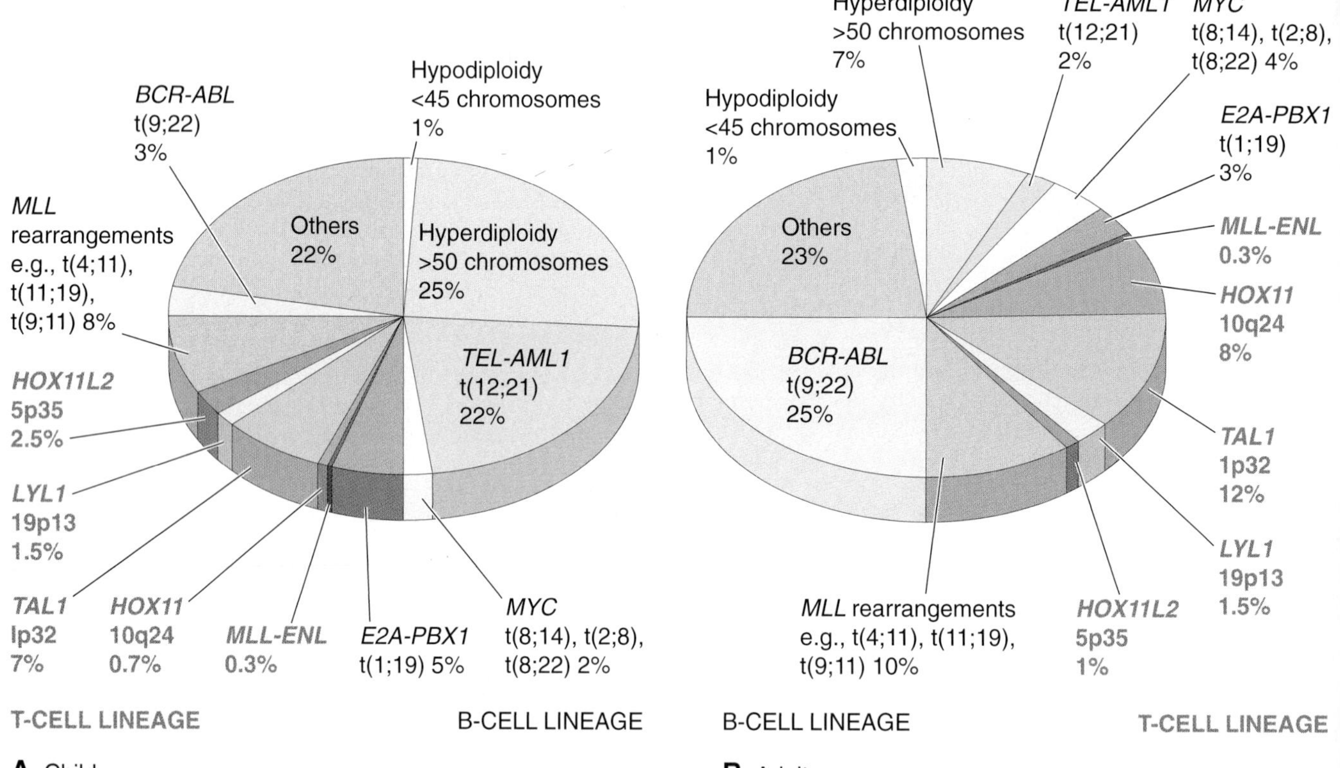

Figure 32–6. Distribution and frequency of genetic abnormalities in acute lymphoblastic leukemia cells in children *(A)* and adults *(B)*.

in ALL are fluorescent in situ hybridization and reverse transcriptase–polymerase chain reaction assays.

More recently, gene expression profiling has added a new dimension to the study of ALL. For example, this method has been used to further classify T-cell ALL into several distinct genetic subgroups: *HOX11L2*, *LYL1* plus *LMO2*, *TAL1* plus *LMO1* or *LMO2*, *HOX11*, and *MLL/ENL*; the last two subgroups are associated with a favorable outcome.[60,61] Analysis of numerical chromosome changes, which can be detected by flow cytometry or karyotyping, has identified two groups—hyperdiploidy (>50 chromosomes) and hypodiploidy (<45 chromosomes)—that are associated with favorable and unfavorable prognosis, respectively.[67–71]

Differential Diagnosis

Childhood ALL can mimic several nonmalignant and malignant diseases, including immune thrombocytopenic purpura with petechiae, ecchymoses, and bleeding[72]; aplastic anemia presenting with pancytopenia and hypoplastic bone marrow; and infectious mononucleosis and other viral illnesses. There are rare cases of pancytopenia and hypocellular bone marrow followed by a period of spontaneous hematopoietic recovery preceding clinical ALL.

Because patients with ALL may present with migratory arthralgias, which can be confused with rheumatoid arthritis, a complete blood count should be obtained. A bone marrow examination may be indicated prior to glucocorticoid or methotrexate treatment for presumed pediatric rheumatic diseases. In children, ALL should also be distinguished from small round cell tumors that involve the bone marrow, including neuroblastoma, rhabdomyosarcoma, and retinoblastoma.

Prognostic Factors

Among patients with B-cell precursor ALL, those of ages between 1 and 10 years and a presenting leukocyte count less than 50 × 10^9/L have standard risk of relapse,[73] whereas others are classified as being at high risk.[32] Genetic changes contribute to risk of poor response and relapse. Hyperdiploidy (>50 chromosomes) or *TEL/AML1* fusion gene is associated with excellent outcome.[21]

In T-cell ALL, *HOX11* overexpression or the *MLL/ENL* fusion gene has a favorable prognosis.[60,74] Some subtypes of ALL, such as ALL with any 11q23 chromosomal abnormality in infants or ALL with the Philadelphia chromosome, generally have a dismal outcome.[75,76] Cumulative prognostic scores incorporate T-cell, mature B-cell, or B-cell precursor status and genetic classification to prospectively assign 45–50% of children with ALL to receive antimetabolite-based therapy, 45% to receive more intensive and potentially toxic therapy, and about 5% to receive hematopoietic stem cell transplantation (HSCT). About 10–20% of patients in any of these prognostic categories still experience relapse.

Pharmacodynamic and pharmacogenomic factors that affect drug efficacy also contribute to prognosis (Fig. 32–7).[76–81] There is considerable variation in the absorption, metabolism, and systemic clearance of antileukemia agents that is impacted by concomitant medications. Administration of anticonvulsants such as phenytoin, phenobarbital, or carbamazepine induces production of cytochrome P-450 enzymes, which can accelerate the metabolism of antileukemia agents and reduce systemic exposure to these drugs.[82] Patients who have homozygous or heterozygous deficiency of thiopurine methyltransferase, the enzyme that inactivates mercaptopurine, tend to have more severe neutropenia during maintenance therapy and more favorable outcome, but are at increased risk of irradiation-associated brain tumors and secondary myeloid leukemia, probably because their systemic exposure to mercaptopurine is higher.[83–86] Moreover, the absence of both alleles of the *GSTM1* or *GSTT1* and the *GSTP1* Val105/Val105 genes have been associated with a lower risk of relapse, perhaps because of the reduced metabolism and clearance of cytotoxic chemotherapy.[87] Thus, drug delivery, metabolism, and exposure combined with pharmacogenomics impact on patient prognosis.

Another approach to prognosis is assessment of early response and minimal residual disease, both of which impact outcome.[88,89] Minimal residual disease measurements of rare leukemic cells by flow-cytometric detection or polymerase chain reaction analysis of clonal genotypic markers provide a degree of sensitivity and specificity that is not possible with morphologic assessment.[90–93] Patients in immunologic or molecular remission (defined as <0.01% leukemic blasts) on completion of 6-week induction therapy have a significantly better outcome than others.[90,91] Remarkably, patients whose residual disease is reduced to 0.01% or less after only 2 weeks of remission induction appear to have an exceptionally good treatment outcome (Fig. 32–8).[94,95] Conversely, the

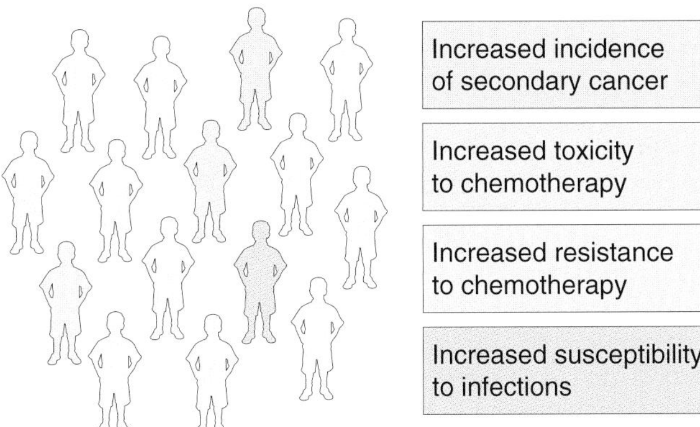

Figure 32–7. Adverse effects of antileukemia treatment are influenced by polymorphisms in genes that encode enzymes that are involved in drug metabolism.

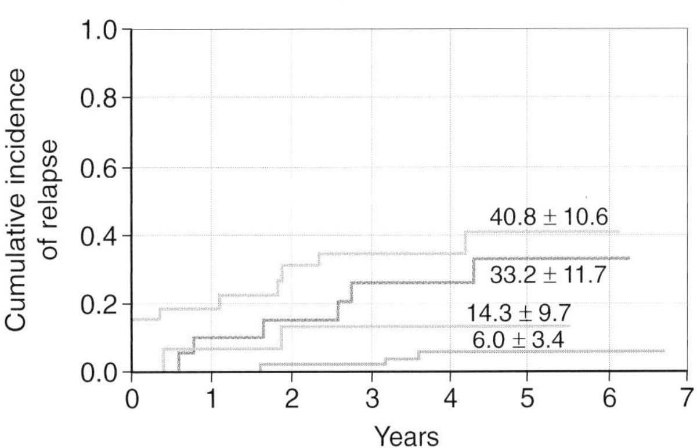

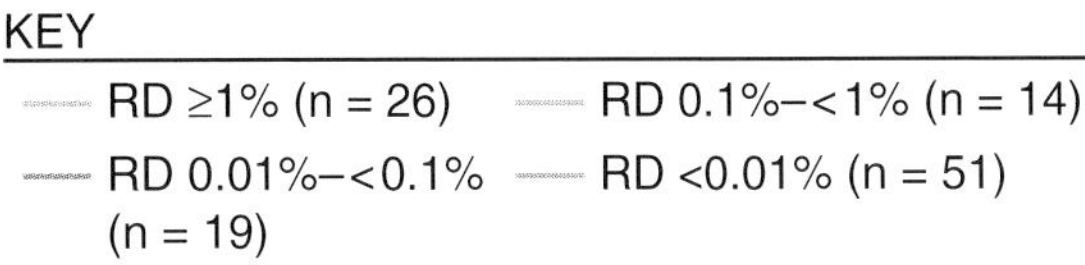

Figure 32–8. The cumulative incidence of relapse in children with acute lymphoblastic leukemia is correlated with the proportion of leukemia cells remaining in the bone marrow after 2–3 weeks of remission induction therapy. A level of residual disease (RD) less than 0.01% in the bone marrow is associated with an exceptionally low risk of relapse.

presence of residual disease at levels of 0.1% or greater 4 months after remission induction was associated with an estimated 70% cumulative risk of relapse.[96,97] Prognostic factor analysis of ALL may improve further with the use of gene expression profiling.[98–100] This technology may offer better predictive value than current techniques.

TREATMENT

Primary Therapy

Risk-adapted therapy that incorporates ALL heterogeneity and patient tolerance has been a major advance in the management of ALL.[21] Thus, recent large ALL trials result in similar overall outcomes. These trials incorporate consensus principles of therapy: combination agents for induction and a different set of agents for maintenance, using regimens with prolonged duration of treatment; and careful attention to early treatment of the CNS to prevent CNS recurrence.[101–104] Finally, it is generally accepted that, in infants, mature B-cell (Burkitt's) leukemia and possibly leukemia with the t(4;11) genetic abnormality should be treated differently from progenitor B- and T-cell leukemias.

Treatment for leukemias that arise from the B-cell precursors and the T-cell lineage consists of three parts: remission induction (early therapy), intensification (consolidation), and prolonged continuation (maintenance) therapy. CNS-directed therapy usually overlaps the treatment phases during the first year. Cases of pediatric ALL are typically divided into three prognostic categories—standard risk, high risk, and very high risk. Adult cases are generally divided into two risk groups.[105,106] The U. S. Children's Oncology Group has proposed addition of a very-low-risk category for children with an exceptionally good prognosis.[107,108]

Induction of Remission

The initial goal in the treatment of childhood ALL is to reduce the leukemia burden sufficiently to allow normal bone marrow function, which theoretically reflects a reduction from 10^{12} to 10^{10} leukemic cells. A combination of glucocorticoid (prednisone, prednisolone, or dexamethasone), vincristine, and L-asparaginase is typically used, and it induces remission within 4–6 weeks in about 95% of cases. A fourth drug, usually an anthracycline, is commonly incorporated into this early phase of therapy, particularly for adults, adolescents, and children at high risk of relapse.[105–107]

L-Asparaginase dose intensity improves pediatric ALL outcomes.[109] Three preparations of L-asparaginase derived from *Escherichia coli*, each with a different pharmacokinetic profile, are currently available and should be dosed based on predicted half-life.[110] Elspar (Merck, USA) has a shorter half-life (1.28 ± 0.35 [standard deviation] days) than does Leunase (Kyowa Hacco Kogyo, Japan) or the polyethylene glycol–conjugated pegaspargase (Merck, USA; 5.73 ± 3.24 days).[111–113] L-Asparaginase derived from *Erwinia chrysanthemi* has a half-life of 0.65 ± 0.13 days.[114–117] All asparaginases are administered intramuscularly to lessen the potential for severe hypersensitivity reaction. Pegaspargase is usually administered at a dosage of 2500 IU/m^2 two weeks apart for newly diagnosed ALL. The dosage of the native *E. coli* L-asparaginase preparations ranges from 6000 to 10,000 IU/m^2, administered two to three times per week for 6–12 doses. The development of antibodies to asparaginase can also interfere with the potency of available preparations.[118] Elspar is administered three times per week to all newly diagnosed patients. Patients who have residual disease at the midpoint of induction therapy receive an additional three doses. However, a delay of several weeks in L-asparaginase administration to the postremission period as consolidation therapy does not reduce the likelihood of complete remission or event-free survival and is associated with fewer thrombotic complications.[119,120]

After receiving prednisone, vincristine, L-asparaginase, and daunorubicin, most patients have no evidence of leukemia in standard microscopic ("morphologic") bone marrow studies. These patients receive "reinforcement" therapy consisting of various agents, including cyclophosphamide, 6-mercaptopurine, and cytarabine. If necessary, this phase can be delayed until fever or extreme neutropenia improves.

Consolidation and Re-induction (Delayed Intensification) Therapy

After bone marrow function is restored, patients in complete remission are candidates for a consolidation phase and one or two courses of re-induction therapy. Between these treatment phases, patients receive weekly non-myeloablative chemotherapy. Consolidation and intensification of therapy are widely accepted as essential components of the overall treatment of ALL.[121] These treatment components are sequentially delivered over the 3–6 months immediately after induction chemotherapy. This approach is unlike that of the myeloablative chemotherapy used after remission induction for acute myeloid leukemia. Consolidation therapy uses high doses of multiple agents not given during the induction phase. Re-induction consists essentially of the readministration of the induction-regimen drugs. The re-induction phase is also referred to as delayed intensification (either single or double).

Regimens commonly used for childhood ALL consolidation include high-dose methotrexate with or without mercaptopurine[81,121]; high-dose L-asparaginase given for an extended period[122,123]; or a combination of dexamethasone, vincristine, L-asparaginase, and doxorubicin followed by thioguanine, cytarabine, and cyclophosphamide.[121,124] This phase of therapy has improved outcome of patients with both low- and high-risk ALL.[125] Postremission therapy with L-asparaginase and doxorubicin was associated with an improved outcome in patients with T-cell leukemia.[123,126] Similarly, very high-dose (5 g/m^2) methotrexate has also been shown to improve outcome in T-cell ALL.[121,127,128] This observation is consistent with data showing that a high plasma concentration of methotrexate is required to produce a therapeutic intracellular concentration of active methotrexate metabolites in T-lineage blast cells.[67,129] Moreover, certain subtypes of B-lineage ALL blast cells, such as those that harbor either the *TEL/AML1* or *E2A/PBX1* fusion gene, accumulate methotrexate polyglutamates at a significantly lower level than blast cells with hyperdiploidy or other genetic abnormalities,[130] necessitating higher doses of methotrexate.

The Children's Cancer Group reported that double delayed intensification was more effective than single intensification in preventing ALL relapse for intermediate-risk cases with prior early response.[131] The addition of pulses of vincristine and prednisone after single delayed intensification therapy was less effective than double intensification, suggesting that the benefit of double delayed intensification was due either to increased dose intensity of other agents such as asparaginase or anthracycline or to the timing or scheduling of the intensification regimen. The data also suggest that prednisone and vincristine pulses may not be needed after delayed intensification.

In adult ALL, early intensification with high-dose cytarabine and daunomycin—a regimen typically used for acute myeloid leukemia—did not result in better outcome in a randomized study.[132,133] In another randomized trial, the outcome of patients receiving a 4-month intensification phase that included methotrexate, cytarabine, thioguanine, cyclophosphamide, and L-asparaginase was similar to that of patients receiving a 1-month intensification regimen consisting of cyclophosphamide and L-asparaginase.[134] However, several nonrandomized studies strongly suggest that early intensive consolidation therapy confers a benefit, especially in young adults.[135–137] Subtypes of adult ALL may benefit from the combination of cyclophosphamide and cytarabine, and patients with standard-risk and high-risk ALL could benefit from high-dose cytarabine.[135,136] Moreover, patients with Philadelphia chromosome–positive or *BCR/ABL*–positive ALL appear to benefit from additional treatment with imatinib mesylate (Gleevec), which may be used during remission induction and continuing in the other phases of postremission therapy.[138,139] Another example is the excellent results of two German multicenter trials featuring high-dose cytarabine, mitoxantrone, and allogeneic HSCT in cases bearing the t(4;11).[140]

Maintenance Therapy

Maintenance therapy continues for 2.5–3 years after remission induction therapy. Maintenance therapy is essential to cure ALL, although the mechanisms by which it works are poorly understood. It is possible that the remaining clonogenic leukemia cells are suppressed indefinitely (eliminated) as a result of modulation of the hematopoietic system by continual exposure to nonmyeloablative chemotherapy. The drugs and schedules used during this phase have evolved over 4 decades and are largely based on empirical evidence. Because some findings suggest that 3 years of maintenance chemotherapy benefits boys but not girls,[141–143] the current St. Jude study assigns girls to a total of 2.5 years of chemotherapy and boys to 3 years. Reduction of the duration of maintenance chemotherapy resulted in an increased rate of relapse,[144,145] although two thirds of the patients could apparently be cured with only 12 months of treatment.[146] Postremission treatment given for only 5–10 months was associated with a poor outcome in two adult ALL trials.[133,147]

Daily oral mercaptopurine, preferably taken at night on an empty stomach, and weekly doses of parenteral methotrexate constitute the framework of maintenance chemotherapy. Mercaptopurine is more effective when given orally each day than when given intravenously once a week.[123,148–151] The combination of mercaptopurine and methotrexate should not be withheld because of occasional increases in hepatic enzyme activity; these abnormalities are usually reversible and have no clinical significance.[152] Outcome appears to be improved when the dosages of mercaptopurine and methotrexate are adjusted on the basis of intracellular concentration of their active metabolites and on neutrophil counts.[83,144,153–155] Although mercaptopurine dose intensity has been associated with prognosis in ALL,[83] frequent monitoring is necessary to avoid severe neutropenia, which can reduce overall dose intensity by requiring long delays in chemotherapy. The clinical tolerance of mercaptopurine depends on the function of thiopurine *S*-methyltransferase, an enzyme that catalyzes the *S*-methylation (inactivation) of mercaptopurine and is encoded by several autosomal codominant alleles with diverse activity. Approximately 1 in 300 individuals inherits homozygous inactive alleles of thiopurine *S*-methyltransferase and 1 in 10 is heterozygotic. In these cases, standard doses of mercaptopurine can cause severe hematologic side effects, and thus the daily dose is reduced to as little as 5–10% of the standard dose.[156] Heterozygotic patients have intermediate enzyme activity[86] resulting in a spectrum of tolerance to mercaptopurine. To avoid prolonged myelosuppression, the dosage should be adjusted according to the level of enzyme activity, intracellular thioguanine nucleotide level, and absolute neutrophil count.[86,157] Patients with intermediate enzyme deficiency tolerate mercaptopurine well with only moderately reduced dosage. Although these patients appear to have excellent ALL cure rates, they are at higher risk of therapy-related leukemia and irradiation-related brain tumor than their counterparts with the homozygous wild-type phenotype,[85,158] and such patients should be carefully monitored once identified.[159] These observations have fueled interest in examining inherited genetic polymorphisms that affect drug metabolism and disposition.[21,77,79]

Hematopoietic Stem Cell Transplantation

Indications for HSCT during first remission of ALL continue to evolve (see Chapter 94). In general, HSCT is contemplated when a subtype of ALL is expected to have a successful response rate of 30% or less with chemotherapy alone. Philadelphia chromosome–positive or *BCR/ABL*–positive ALL has a very poor prognosis when treated with chemotherapy alone, and patients with this cytogenetic abnormality benefit from allogeneic HSCT from a matched related donor during first complete remission. Indications for allogeneic HSCT in this subtype of ALL may change as *ABL* protein kinase inhibitors are incorporated into the treatment armamentarium.[160] Regardless of the leukemia genotype, patients who have a poor initial response to induction therapy are commonly considered for allogeneic HSCT during first remission.[76,106,161–163] Allogeneic HSCT has also been studied in adult ALL; long-term event-free survival rates range from 30% to 40% with chemotherapy alone and from 40% to 60% with allogeneic HSCT.[106,161,164,165] Allogeneic HSCT appeared to improve the outcome of adults with the t(4;11) translocation[140] but not that of children with the same genotype.[162,163,166] The indications for transplantation during first remission should be reevaluated as chemotherapy and transplantation continue to improve.

CNS-Directed Therapy

The CNS is involved at the time of diagnosis of ALL in about 3–5% of patients. Overt CNS leukemia at the time of diagnosis is usually associated with age less than 1 year, the presence of T-cell markers, a hypodiploid karyotype, presence of the Philadelphia or *BCR/ABL* genetic abnormality, and very high white blood cell counts. These features increase the risk of CNS relapse.[50] The CNS appears to be a "sanctuary" for leukemia cells, and effective ALL treatment requires presymptomatic CNS-directed therapy.

In the mid-1960s, St. Jude investigators demonstrated that 24 Gy of radiotherapy delivered to the cranium and 15 Gy to the spine reduced the rate of CNS relapse from 50% to 5%.[104] A subsequent study showed that intrathecally administered methotrexate could replace craniospinal radiotherapy in patients with intermediate-risk ALL.[167] Because substantial toxicity, including second cancer, neurocognitive deficits, endocrinopathy, and psychosocial dysfunction, is associated with CNS irradiation,[168] several modifications have yielded the following consensus: (1) the dose and field of irradiation can be reduced when appropriate intrathecal and systemic therapies are provided[121]; (2) radiation therapy can be eliminated completely for patients with low-risk ALL[150]; (3) preventive CNS-directed therapy is not necessary beyond 1 year after complete remission; (4) intensive intrathecal therapy alone prevents CNS leukemia in more than 80% of children with ALL[50,169]; and (5) in high-risk cases, the radiation dose can be reduced to 12 Gy without increasing the risk of CNS relapse, provided that effective systemic chemotherapy is used.[121] Several technical elements are crucial in pediatric CNS-directed therapy. First, the introduction of leukemia cells into the CNS by a traumatic lumbar puncture adversely affects outcome,[52,53] and only experienced clinicians should perform the lumbar puncture with drug administration. Platelets are administered to patients with thrombocytopenia to increase the platelet count to approximately 100×10^9/L. Second, CNS-directed therapy is intensified in patients at high risk of CNS leukemia (i.e., Philadelphia chromosome–positive or *BCR/ABL*–positive ALL, hypodiploid karyotype, leukemic cells in the cerebrospinal fluid) and in patients who experience traumatic lumbar puncture.[51,52] Last, to allow even distribution of intrathecal medications throughout the CNS, patients should remain in a prone position for 30 minutes or longer after the procedure.

Salvage Therapy (Partial Responses and Relapse)

Traditionally, relapse has been defined as the detection of leukemic cells at any site in the body after a complete morphologic and clinical remission is achieved.[170] The mechanisms of late relapse are still unknown. In some cases with the *TEL/AML1* fusion gene, molecular studies suggest a strong clonal relatedness between the leukemia cells studied at diagnosis and at relapse. These data provide evidence that, in at least some cases of childhood ALL, a preleukemic clone persists during remission, and subsequent relapse reflects the emergence of a new subclone (created by additional, independent genetic events) from that pool of leukemia progenitor cells.[171,172]

Bone marrow is the most common site of relapse in ALL. CNS and testicular relapses have decreased substantially in most contemporary childhood ALL treatment programs.[123,173,174] Rarer extramedullary relapse sites include the skin, eye, ear, ovary, uterus, bone, muscle, tonsil, kidney, mediastinum, pleura, and paranasal sinus.[175] Clinical and laboratory features of bone marrow relapse include fever, bone pain, pallor, petechiae, enlargement of the liver or spleen, anemia, leukocytosis, leukopenia, and thrombocytopenia. Persistent pancytopenia in patients who have previously been tolerating chemotherapy well may be the first sign of marrow relapse. Most CNS relapses are asymptomatic: leukemic cells are usually observed during surveillance examination of the cerebrospinal fluid, before the onset of signs and symptoms. Occasionally, patients who experience CNS relapse will have signs and symptoms of increased intracranial pressure or cranial nerve palsy. Rarely, leukemia infiltration of the hypothalamus results in hyperphagia, obesity, and behavior abnormalities (hypothalamic obesity syndrome).[176] Patients who have testicular relapse usually present with painless testicular enlargement that is most often unilateral.

Hematologic relapse is associated with poor outcome, particularly in patients who experience relapse while on therapy or after a short initial remission, who have T-cell immunophenotype or the Philadelphia chromosome or *BCR/ABL* genetic abnormality, or who have an isolated hematologic relapse.[177–181] Relapse after a first remission of more than 30 months (late relapse), isolated extramedullary relapse, or presence of the *TEL/AML1* fusion gene is associated with a greater likelihood of a second, durable remission.[182] Approximately 50% of patients who have late relapses have a prolonged second remission, compared to fewer than 10% of those who have early relapse.[177,178,183] The treatment used to obtain a second remission usually includes a combination of dexamethasone, vincristine, L-asparaginase, anthracycline, etoposide, high-dose cytarabine, and high-dose methotrexate.[184] For patients with high-risk disease features, matched-related donor allogeneic HSCT is the treatment of choice if a second remission is achieved.[185–189] A matched unrelated donor or suitable cord blood are acceptable alternatives for patients who do not have histocompatible related donors.[190–194] Autologous transplantation offers no advantage over chemotherapy for patients who are not candidates for allogeneic HSCT.[195,196] Details of current approaches to transplantation for leukemia are outlined in Chapters 94 and 95.

Extramedullary relapse is usually an isolated relapse in the CNS or testicles. However, leukemia cells are frequently detected in the bone marrow by minimal residual disease studies.[197,198] Therefore, extramedullary relapse is considered a systemic disease and is managed with intensive systemic therapy. For children with an isolated CNS relapse, the efficacy of salvage therapy depends partly on whether the relapse occurs during or after completion of treatment and partly on whether CNS irradiation was used. Treatment with intensive systemic and intrathecal chemotherapy and CNS irradiation is associated with long-term second remissions in about 50% of patients who did not receive previous CNS radiotherapy and who were off treatment at the time of relapse.[199,200] Cranial radiotherapy is mandatory in these cases. There is controversy about the timing of delivery of cranial irradiation; systemic and intrathecal treatment for 4–6 months before definitive radiotherapy appears to be associated with better long-term disease control. Intrathecal treatment should not be given after cranial radiotherapy because of an increased risk of neurotoxicity. Because of the high rate of success of salvage therapy for patients with isolated CNS relapse, HSCT is not recommended.

Patients who experience relapse after CNS irradiation have a particularly poor prognosis.[199–201] Similarly, adults with isolated CNS relapse have a dismal outcome. HSCT has been used in the management of these high-risk cases.[196,201] However, it has not been conclusively determined whether autologous or allogeneic transplantation is more advantageous than intensive chemotherapy.

Isolated testicular relapse has become very uncommon with current treatment regimens. Because of this rarity, the outcome of retrieval treatment has been studied only in patients who received less intensive chemotherapy regimens prior to testicular relapse. Two thirds of patients with late testicular recurrence can be cured with this approach.[202–205] Testicular irradiation was avoided by administering high-dose methotrexate in one study,[206] but the efficacy of this method remains to be determined. In rare instances of biopsy-proven unilateral testicular relapse, some investigators advocate orchiectomy of the involved testis without irradiation of the "uninvolved" testis, in an attempt to preserve testicular function. Orchiectomy has also been considered for patients who have a testicular relapse after HSCT.[207] The optimal treatment and the prognosis of patients who have relapses at unusual extramedullary sites are unclear. However, the same principles that apply to the clinical management of CNS or testicular relapse would probably apply to this subgroup.

SUPPORTIVE CARE AND LONG-TERM MANAGEMENT

Management of supportive care elements of induction therapy and transplantation are outlined in Chapters 90, 96, and 97. Information on the long-term side effects of treatment is provided in Chapter 34.

Hyperleukocytosis

White blood cell counts approaching 400×10^9/L at the time of diagnosis of ALL can be associated with leukostasis syndrome.[39] Neurologic and pulmonary signs and symptoms predominate in leukostasis syndrome and include dizziness, blurred vision, tinnitus, ataxia, confusion, somnolence, stupor, coma, tachypnea, dyspnea, pulmonary infiltrates, and progression to frank respiratory failure. Transfusion of packed red blood cells should be delayed until the leukocyte count is reduced in cases of extreme hyperleukocytosis. Either leukapheresis or exchange transfusion (in small children) can be used.[208,209] Modification of induction therapy with low-dose glucocorticoids or adding vincristine or cyclophosphamide (in cases of B-cell ALL) reduces cell burden in most cases.

Metabolic Complications

Tumor lysis syndrome with hyperuricemia, hyperphosphatemia, hypocalcemia, hyperkalemia, and azotemia may occur even without treatment or may follow initial induction therapy (Fig. 32–9). Administration of fluids at a daily rate of 2–3 L/m^2 dilutes intravascular solutes such as urates and phosphates, increases renal blood flow and glomerular filtration, and flushes precipitated solutes from the renal tubules. Hemodialysis is sometimes necessary to correct the metabolic complications. The availability of recombinant urate oxidase (rasburicase) has dramatically facilitated the prevention and management of hyperuricemia in patients with lymphoproliferative diseases.[210] Gentle chemotherapy, when used in conjunction with hyperhydration and urate oxidase, has virtually eliminated the need for hemodialysis in patients with B-cell ALL.[211]

Hyperglycemia develops in 10% of children during induction therapy with prednisone, vincristine, and L-asparaginase.[212] Risk factors for glucose intolerance include adolescent age, obesity, a family history of diabetes mellitus, Down syndrome,[212] and high-dose glucocorticoids. Insulin resistance caused by glucocorticoids, and decreased insulin production in response to hyperglycemia and downregulation of insulin receptors by L-asparaginase, have been implicated in the pathogenesis of this complication.

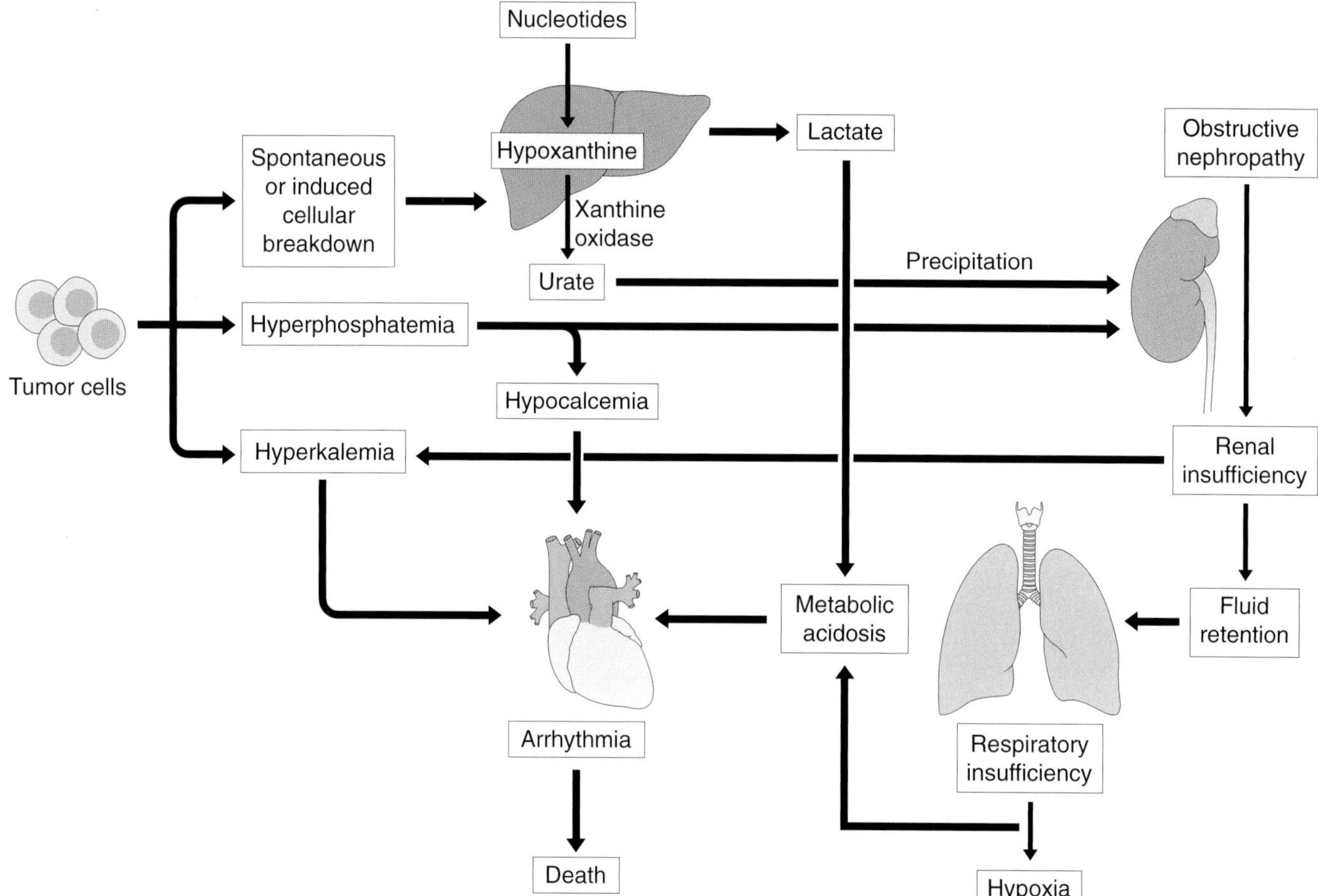

Figure 32–9. Pathogenesis of tumor lysis syndrome.

Hemorrhagic Complications

Thrombocytopenia is common in ALL of childhood. Rarely, devastating intracranial or pulmonary bleeding is the chief finding at presentation. High leukocyte counts (i.e., >400 × 10^9/L) may also be responsible.[39] Disseminated intravascular coagulation or coagulopathy resulting from hepatic dysfunction is rare.[36] Bleeding after L-asparaginase may occur with hypofibrinogenemia.

A hypercoagulable state is relatively common during induction treatment that includes L-asparaginase and a glucocorticoid.[112,213,214] As many as 5% of patients may experience vascular thromboembolic phenomena leading to cerebral and/or peripheral vein thrombosis.[215] Any vessel may be affected, but morbidity is greater when the CNS is involved. Cerebral thrombosis should be distinguished by magnetic resonance imaging or computed tomography from lesions caused by reversible ischemic events (occipital-parietal encephalopathy), which are usually associated with acute hypertension.[113,216] Occasionally, cerebral thrombosis may not become apparent by diagnostic imaging until a few days after the onset of symptoms and signs. The mechanism of thromboembolism has not been elucidated. L-Asparaginase is usually deleted from induction therapy and low-molecular-weight and heparin is used to treat these patients.

Long-Term Side Effects of Treatment

Although leukemia relapse continues to be the most common adverse event in children treated for ALL, patients are also at risk of treatment-related morbidities.[168,217,218] Common late side effects associated with antileukemic therapy are summarized in Table 32–4. Use of systemic and intrathecal methotrexate increases the frequency of neurotoxicity.[111,219,220] Use of glucocorticoids has been associated with osteonecrosis.[221–223] Risk factors for osteonecrosis include female sex, age greater than 10 years at diagnosis, and genetic polymorphisms in the vitamin D receptor.[224] Altered mineral metabolism and bone mineral density are observed at diagnosis of childhood ALL, during therapy, and in long-term survivors, especially those who received high cumulative doses of glucocorticoid or methotrexate or who had cranial irradiation.[225,226] These patients are at risk of bone fractures, although the relationship between fractures and bone mass parameters has not been conclusively established.[227] Early detection of osteopenic changes and the introduction of therapy should prevent fractures.

Anthracyclines can produce severe cardiomyopathy.[228,229] CNS irradiation given in combination with systemic and intrathecal chemotherapy to prevent or treat meningeal leukemia is associated with several late neu-

TABLE 32–4. Late Side Effects of Chemotherapy Agents Used in the Treatment of ALL

Treatment	Late Complications
Prednisone (or prednisolone), dexamethasone	Avascular necrosis of bone, osteopenia, growth retardation
Anthracycline	Cardiomyopathy (caused by a high cumulative dose)
Mercaptopurine	Osteoporosis (caused by long-term use), acute myeloid leukemia, and possibly irradiation-induced CNS tumors in patients with thiopurine methyltransferase deficiency
Methotrexate	Leukoencephalopathy, osteopenia (caused by long-term use), cognitive deficits
Epipodophyllotoxins	Acute myeloid leukemia
Cytarabine	Decreased fertility (caused by a high cumulative dose)
Cyclophosphamide	Bladder cancer or acute myeloid leukemia (rare), decreased fertility (due to a high cumulative dose)
Intrathecal methotrexate, cytarabine, hydrocortisone	Encephalopathy or myelopathy (caused by a high cumulative dose)
Brain irradiation	Seizure, mineralizing microangiopathy, hypothalamic dysfunction (growth hormone deficiency), thyroid dysfunction, obesity, osteopenia, brain tumor, basal cell carcinoma, parotid gland carcinoma, hair loss, cataract (rare), dental abnormalities

CURRENT CONTROVERSIES & FUTURE CONSIDERATIONS

Acute Lymphoblastic Leukemia

- Gene expression profiling and proteomics studies to elucidate mechanisms of leukemogenesis and leukemic cell drug resistance.
- Individualized therapy based on leukemic cell genetics, and host pharmacokinetic, pharmacodynamic, and pharmacogenetic characteristics, as well as early treatment response as determined by the level of minimal residual leukemia.
- Developing therapy targeted against gene or cellular pathways responsible for leukemic cell transformation, proliferation, and survival.
- International collaboration to study the biology of specific subtypes of leukemia and to investigate the proper treatment approach accordingly.

rocognitive deficits, and endocrine abnormalities that can lead to obesity, short stature, precocious puberty, and osteoporosis have been well documented.[57] Female sex and young age are risk factors for these complications.

Growth velocity is reduced during therapy of ALL. Patients who receive chemotherapy alone usually recover their growth velocity and reach their constitutional height potential after treatment is completed, although hypothalamic dysfunction may occur.[230] Patients who are treated with 18–24 Gy of cranial irradiation generally have a reduced final adult height. The effect of radiation on growth hormone secretion depends on the radiation dose-volume that affects the hypothalamic-pituitary axis.[231]

Malignant brain tumors and secondary acute myeloid leukemia are among the most serious complications of ALL treatment. Factors that predispose to brain neoplasms include cranial irradiation in children 6 years of age or younger and intensive use of antimetabolites before and during cranial irradiation.[85,232] The median latency period for high-grade and low-grade glioma is 9 years and 20 years, respectively.[168,232] The development of secondary acute myeloid leukemia is associated with treatment with the epipodophyllotoxins.[233,234] The long-term survival rate of patients with this complication is dismal, even with allogeneic stem cell transplantation.[233]

Suggested Readings*

Arico M, Valsecchi MG, Camitta B, et al: Outcome of treatment in children with Philadelphia chromosome-positive acute lymphoblastic leukemia. N Engl J Med 342:998–1006, 2000.

Burger B, Zimmermann M, Mann G, et al: Diagnostic cerebrospinal fluid examination in children with acute lymphoblastic leukemia: significance of low leukocyte counts with blasts or traumatic lumbar puncture. J Clin Oncol 21:184–188, 2003.

Campana D: Minimal residual disease studies in acute leukemia. Am J Clin Pathol 122 Suppl:S47–S57, 2004.

Evans WE, McLeod HL: Pharmacogenomics–drug disposition, drug targets, and side effects. N Engl J Med 348:538–549, 2003.

Ferrando AA, Look AT: Gene expression profiling in T-cell acute lymphoblastic leukemia. Semin Hematol 40:274–280, 2003.

Ferrando AA, Neuberg DS, Dodge RK, et al: Prognostic importance of TLX1 (HOX11) oncogene expression in adults with T-cell acute lymphoblastic leukaemia. Lancet 363:535–536, 2004.

Holleman A, Cheok MH, den Boer ML, et al: Gene-expression patterns in drug-resistant acute lymphoblastic leukemia cells and response to treatment. N Engl J Med 351:533–542, 2004.

Ito C, Kumagai M, Manabe A, et al: Hyperdiploid acute lymphoblastic leukemia with 51 to 65 chromosomes: a distinct biological entity with a marked propensity to undergo apoptosis. Blood 93:315–320, 1999.

Mandel K, Atkinson S, Barr RD, Pencharz P: Skeletal morbidity in childhood acute lymphoblastic leukemia. J Clin Oncol 22:1215–1221, 2004.

Pui CH, Relling MV, Downing JR: Acute lymphoblastic leukemia. N Engl J Med 350:1535–1548, 2004.

Pui CH, Schrappe M, Ribeiro RC, Niemeyer CM: Childhood and adolescent lymphoid and myeloid leukemia. Hematology (Am Soc Hematol Educ Program) 18–45, 2004.

Relling MV, Hancock ML, Rivera GK, et al: Mercaptopurine therapy intolerance and heterozygosity at the thiopurine S-methyltransferase gene locus. J Natl Cancer Inst 91:2001–2008, 1999.

Skibola CF, Smith MT, Kane E, et al: Polymorphisms in the methylenetetrahydrofolate reductase gene are associated with susceptibility to acute leukemia in adults. Proc Natl Acad Sci U S A 96: 12810–12815, 1999.

Full references for this chapter can be found on accompanying CD-ROM.

CHAPTER 33

Pediatric Leukemias

Alan S. Wayne, MD

KEY POINTS

Pediatric Leukemias

- Leukemia is the most common pediatric malignancy. Acute lymphoblastic leukemia accounts for the majority of cases, but the incidence ratio of leukemia subtype varies with age.
- A number of congenital and acquired conditions predispose to leukemia in pediatrics; however, usually no such underlying disorder is identified.
- The most common presenting symptoms and signs are nonspecific, thus the differential diagnosis includes a broad array of systemic conditions. However, diagnosis is usually readily confirmed by analysis of the peripheral blood and/or bone marrow.
- Treatment, which is specific to the leukemia subtype and risk-adapted based on clinicopathologic prognostic features, leads to cure for the majority of individuals.
- Aggressive age-specific supportive care is critical to successful outcome, as is long-term monitoring for disease- and treatment-associated late effects.

INTRODUCTION

Leukemia is the most common pediatric cancer diagnosis (Fig. 33–1).[1] Acute lymphoblastic leukemia (ALL) accounts for about 75%, and acute myeloid leukemia (AML) for about 20%, of pediatric leukemias. Chronic myeloid leukemia (CML) and juvenile myelomonocytic leukemia (JMML) are infrequent[2,3] (Fig. 33–2). Despite substantial therapeutic advances, malignancy represents the leading cause of death from disease in children and adolescents (Fig. 33–3) and leukemia is the most common cause of cancer-related mortality (Fig. 33–4).[4] Many aspects of leukemia are common across age groups, and the reader is referred to other chapters in this text for extensive reviews of diagnosis and classification of ALL, AML, and CML. The purpose of this chapter is to highlight unique features of leukemia in childhood and adolescence.

EPIDEMIOLOGY AND RISK FACTORS

The incidence of leukemia in pediatric age groups in the United States has increased modestly over the past 2 decades[5] (Fig. 33–5). Age-specific incidence rates range from approximately 1 in 10,000 to 1 in 50,000 children under the age of 20 years (see Fig. 33–2). Leukemia accounts for about one half of all cancer in 2- to 3-year-olds. The peak incidence of ALL is between the ages of 2 and 9 years, whereas the age-specific incidence of AML is relatively stable throughout childhood and adolescence. Toddlers and school-age children have a 10- to 15-fold preponderance of ALL, whereas older adolescents have a nearly equal likelihood of developing ALL or AML (see Fig. 33–2). Infants less than 1 year of age are most likely to develop acute leukemia involving the mixed-lineage leukemia gene (*MLL*) at the 11q23 locus, or less commonly JMML.[6–9] JMML makes up about 2% of leukemia cases and 25% of myelodysplastic syndrome cases in childhood, three quarters of which occur in children under 3 years of age. Philadelphia chromosome (Ph^1) CML accounts for approximately 10% of leukemia cases in older adolescents.[10]

A variety of conditions predispose to childhood leukemia, although in most cases there is not an underlying disorder (Table 33–1). Trisomy 21, the most common disorder that predisposes to leukemia, confers a 10- to 20-fold increased risk of ALL and a 500-fold risk of megakaryocytic AML.[11,12] Patients with Fanconi's anemia have a greater than 50% lifetime risk of developing AML or myelodysplastic syndrome.[13] Individuals with neurofibromatosis type 1 have a high incidence of JMML, accounting for 10–25% of cases of this rare leukemia.[14] Siblings of children with leukemia have a two- to fourfold increased risk of developing leukemia.[15] There is strong monozygotic twin concordance (25% overall), especially in infants[16] (Fig. 33–6).

There are geographic and ethnic variations in the incidence of leukemia subtypes in children (Fig. 33–7).[9,17,18] For example, reported rates of ALL range from a low of 9 per 1 million population in Kuwait to 47 per 1 million in Costa Rica, and selective underrepresentation of B-precursor ALL has been noted in specific populations in Africa, the Middle East, and South America. ALL is more common in industrialized nations, and the emergence of childhood peak incidences early during the industrialization timeline suggests environmental contributors, although few such factors have been clearly implicated (see Table 33–1).[9]

PATHOPHYSIOLOGY

Infectious agents may play a role in leukemogenesis. Human T-lymphotrophic virus type 1 is pathogenic in the development of adult T-cell leukemia, which is rarely encountered in children except with infection early in life.[19,20] Epstein-Barr virus is implicated in a minority of cases of mature B-cell ALL. Late exposure to common viruses has been postulated to contribute to the high incidence of ALL in school-aged children in industrialized nations.[17,21–23]

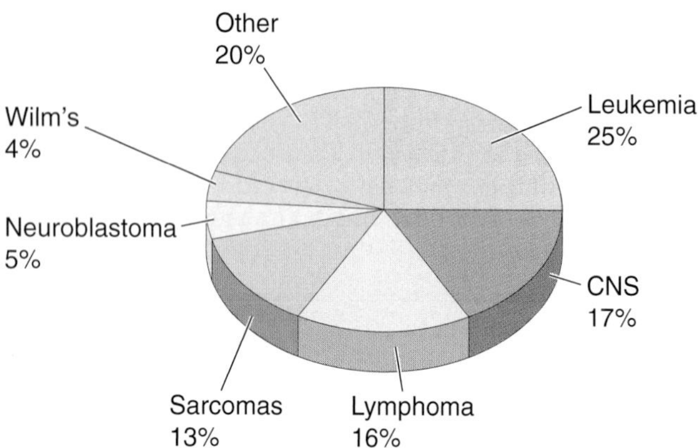

Figure 33–1. Distribution of cancer types in children. Data from National Cancer Institute Surveillance, Epidemiology and End Results (SEER) Program, 1975–1995, for children less than 20 years of age.[1]

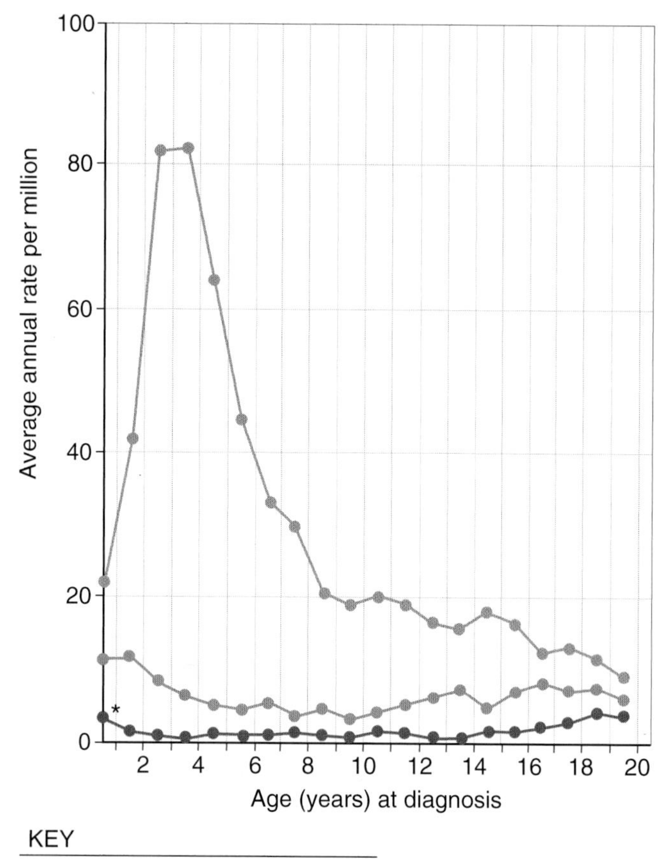

Figure 33–2. Age-specific incidence rates of leukemia. Data from National Cancer Institute SEER Program, 1976–1994.[3] CML peak in first year of life ("*") likely represents misclassified cases of JMML.

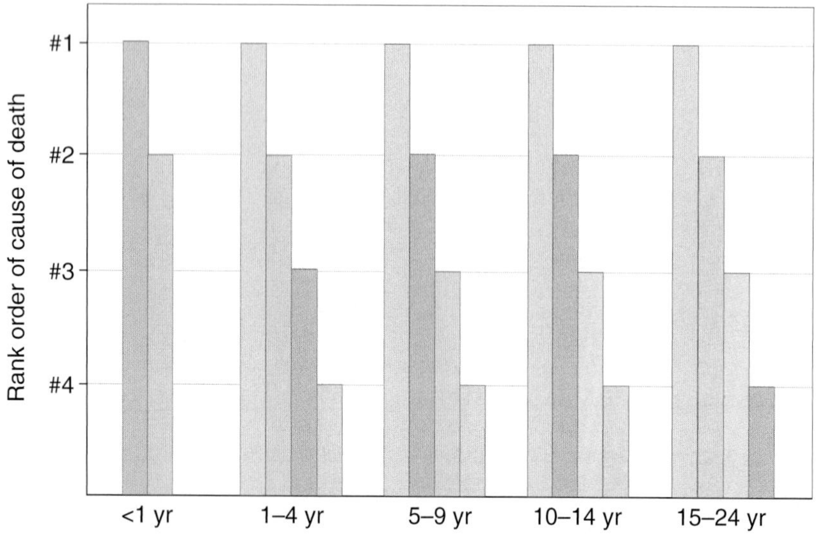

Figure 33–3. Leading causes of death by age. Data from National Center for Health Statistics, 1990 (*www.cdc.gov/nchs/nvss.htm*).

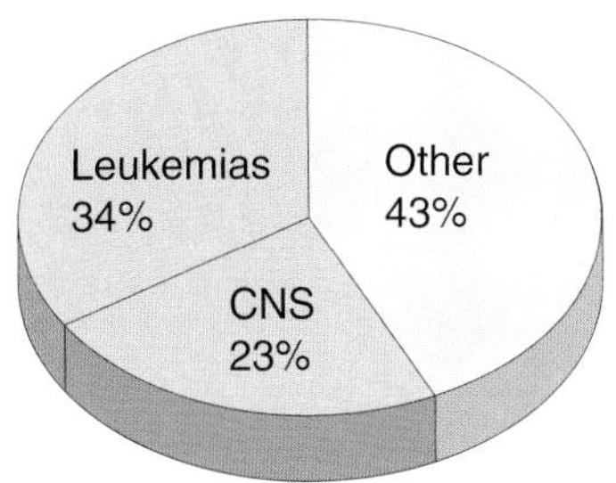

Figure 33–4. Distribution of cancer-associated mortality in children. Data from National Cancer Institute SEER Program, 1995, for children less than 20 years of age.[4]

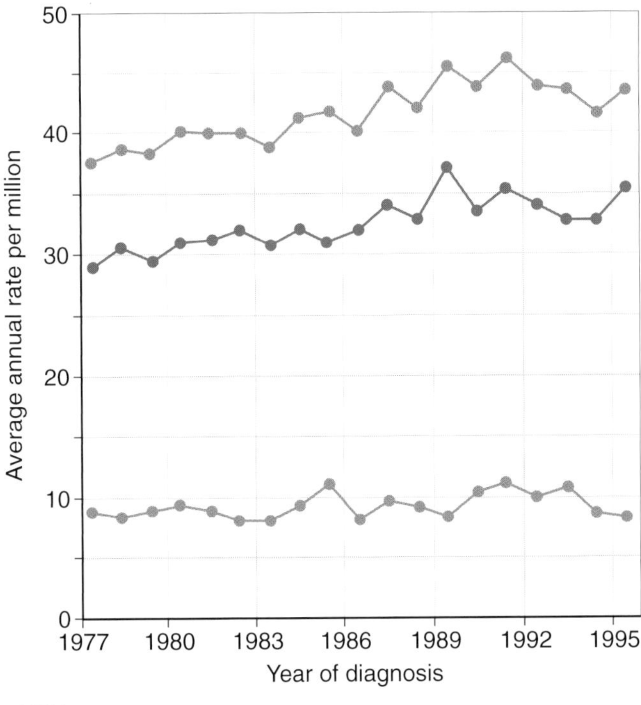

Figure 33–5. Incidence rates of leukemia in children, age-adjusted to 1970 U.S. standard population. Data from National Cancer Institute SEER Program, 1977–1995, for children less than 15 years of age.[3]

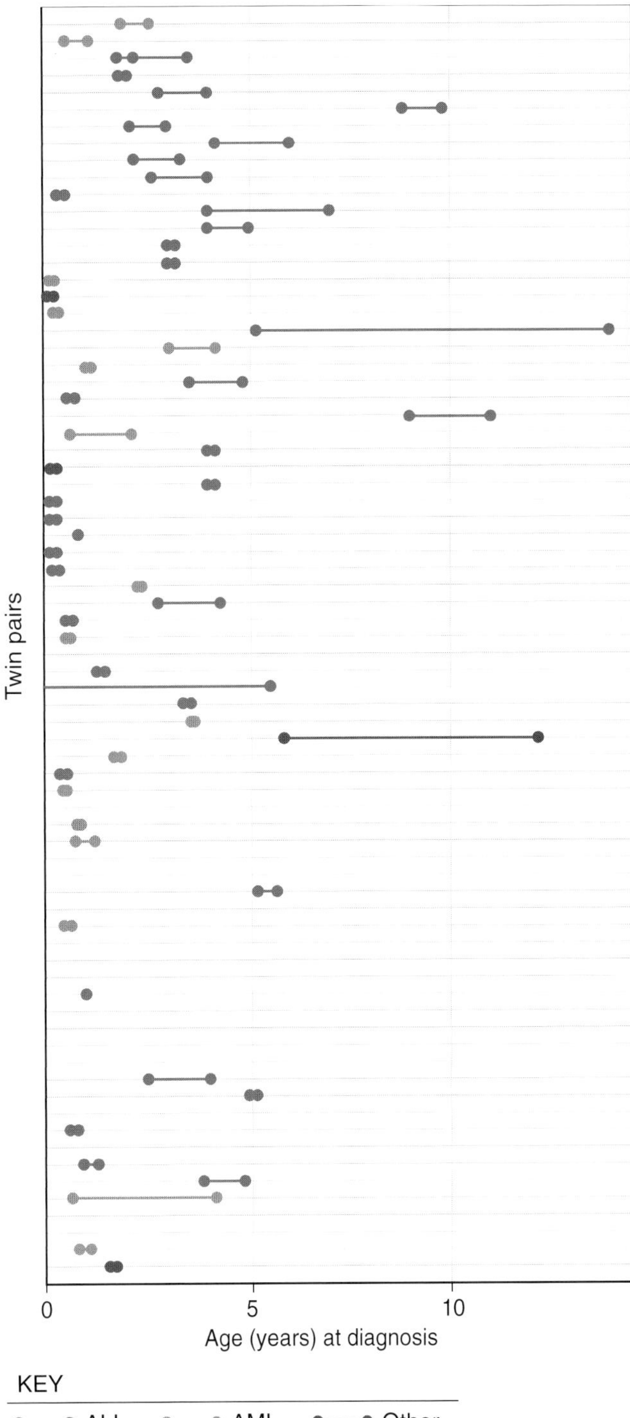

Figure 33–6. Concordant acute leukemia in monozygotic twins. Rows represent individual twin pairs. (Modified from Greaves MF, Maia AT, Wiemels JL, Ford AM: Leukemia in twins: lessons in natural history. Blood 102:2321–2333, 2003.)

The majority of children with leukemia have secondary chromosomal abnormalities in the malignant cells, including translocations and/or aneuploidy.[24–28] The genes involved in recurrent translocations are commonly transcription factors or coactivators expressed in hematopoietic tissues.[29,30] In some cases of ALL and AML, these translocations have been shown to be prenatal in origin.[31,32] Studies in monozygotic twin pairs with concordant leukemia show a wide range in the latency period to leukemia diagnosis, and most pairs develop the same leukemia subtype and possibly the identical clone[16] (see Fig. 33–6). Prolonged latency that in some cases exceeds 5 years, and the observation that approximately 1% of normal cord blood samples harbor the t(12;21) (*TEL/AML1*) translocation in $CD10^+$ lymphoid precursors, support a "two-hit" model of leukemogenesis.[33] Prenatal exposure to environmental factors, such as DNA topoisomerase II inhibitors in food, has been postulated to initiate infant leukemia associated with *MLL* rearrangements.[34]

TABLE 33–1. Epidemiologic Features of Pediatric Leukemia in the United States

	ALL	AML	JMML
Male : female	1.3 : 1 overall 4 : 1 T-ALL	1 : 1	2 : 1
Race	White : black 2 : 1	Hispanic increased risk	
Predisposing conditions	Trisomy 21 (15-fold risk) Neurofibromatosis type 1 Chromosomal breakage and immunodeficiency disorders (e.g., ataxia-telangiectasia, Bloom syndrome, Shwachman-Diamond syndrome, hyperimmunoglobulin M syndrome, hypogammaglobulinemia) Li-Fraumeni syndrome Langerhans cell histiocytosis Klinefelter's syndrome Increasing maternal age	Trisomy 21 (50-fold risk AML, 500-fold risk megakaryoblastic) Chromosomal breakage and immunodeficiency disorders (e.g., Fanconi's anemia [15,000-fold risk], Bloom syndrome, ataxia-telangiectasia, Shwachman-Diamond syndrome, Kostmann's syndrome) Klinefelter's syndrome Neurofibromatosis type 1 Aplastic anemia treated with immunosuppression Paroxysmal nocturnal hemoglobinuria Myelodysplastic syndrome Familial monosomy 7	Neurofibromatosis type 1 (500-fold risk) Noonan syndrome Monosomy 7
Environmental factors	Radiation	Topoisomerase II inhibitors Alkylating agents Radiation	

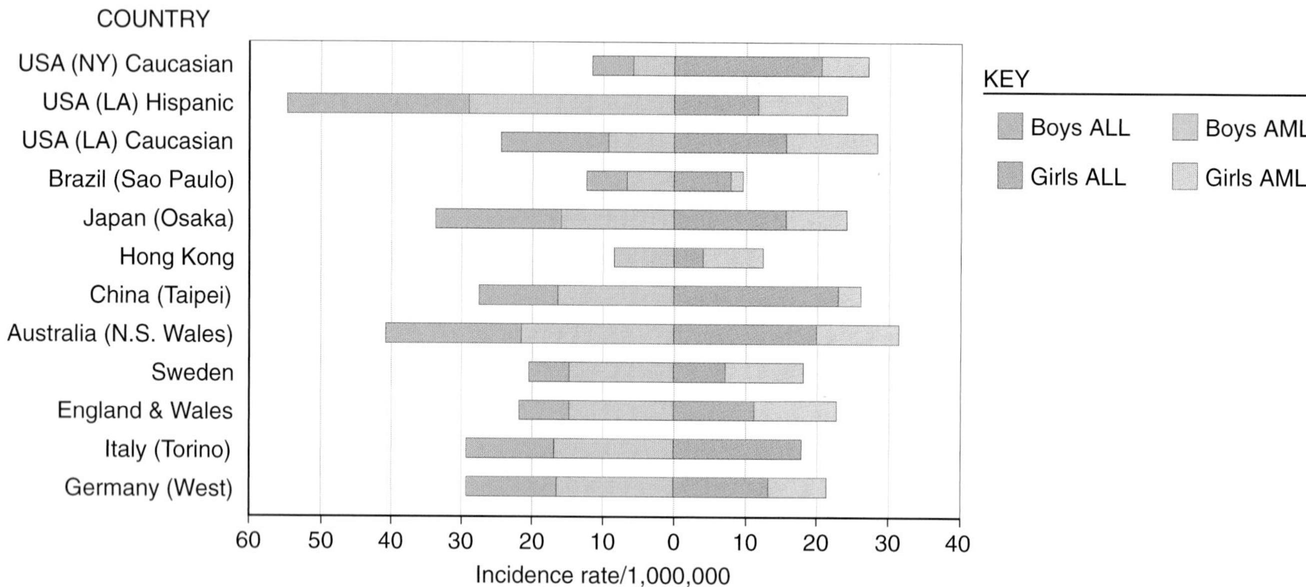

Figure 33–7. Geographic variation of leukemia incidence in infants. Data represent cases of leukemia in infants less than 1 year of age at diagnosis per 1 million live births as reported by international cancer surveillance programs primarily from 1970 through 1980. Abbreviations: LA, Los Angeles; NY, New York City. (Modified from Ross JA, Davies SM, Potter JD, et al: Epidemiology of childhood leukemia with a focus on infants. Epidemiol Rev 16:243–272, 1994.)

Approximately one third of patients with JMML have cytogenetic abnormalities, predominantly monosomy 7. Activating *ras* mutations are found in 25% of patients. Notably, deficiency in the *NF1* gene product (neurofibromin) leads to constitutive activation of *ras* in another 25% of patients with JMML. Finally, one third of patients have mutations in the *PTPN11* gene that result in amplification of signaling through SHP-2, which is also seen in patients with Noonan's syndrome. The consequence of mutations in the *ras*, *NF1*, or *PTPN11* pathways is dysregulation of granulocyte-macrophage colony-stimulating factor signaling via Ras and phosphatidylinositol 3′-kinase[14] (Fig. 33–8). In vitro blood and bone marrow cultures from patients with JMML show spontaneous granulocyte-macrophage colony-forming units and hypersensitivity to granulocyte-macrophage colony-stimulating factor.[35]

GATA1 mutations have been implicated in the pathophysiology of megakaryoblastic AML and transient myeloproliferative disorder associated with trisomy 21.[36,37]

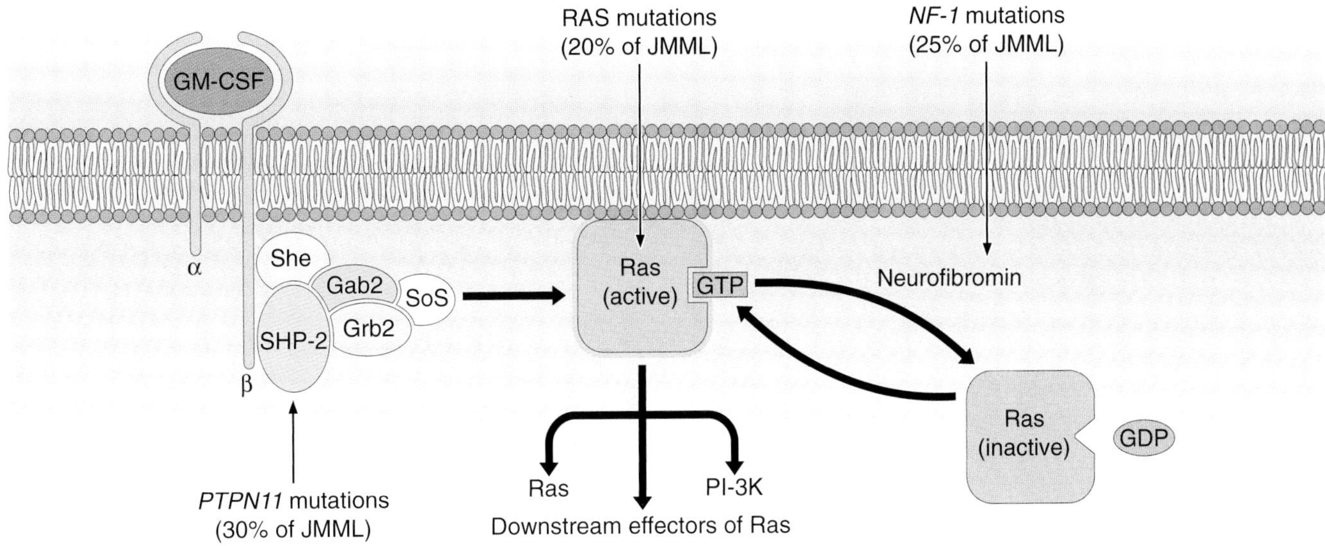

Figure 33–8. Altered granulocyte-macrophage colony-stimulating factor pathway in the pathophysiology of JMML. Abbreviations: GDP, guanosine diphosphate; GM-CSF, granulocyte-macrophage colony-stimulating factor; GTP, guanosine triphosphate; see text for other abbreviations. (Modified from Emanuel PD: Juvenile myelomonocytic leukemia. Curr Hematol Rep 3:203–209, 2004.)

CLINICAL FEATURES AND DIAGNOSIS

Clinical Features

Children with leukemia usually present with signs and symptoms of infiltration of the bone marrow, liver, spleen, and/or lymph nodes, although almost any organ can be affected. Marrow involvement leads to peripheral blood findings of cytopenias and/or circulating blasts. Central nervous system involvement occurs in 2–30% of children with ALL and AML. This is most commonly manifested by the asymptomatic finding of blasts in the cerebrospinal fluid, but can include cranial neuropathy, intracranial hypertension, infarction, and hemorrhage. Although occult infiltration of the testes can be found in up to 25% of boys with ALL at diagnosis, overt involvement marked by painless testicular enlargement is uncommon in ALL and rare in AML. T-cell ALL frequently presents with bulky adenopathy, mediastinal mass, and/or pleural effusion. Intestinal intussusception, usually ileocecal, resulting from Peyer's patch infiltration is almost always confined to mature B-cell ALL. Skin infiltration, or leukemia cutis, is most commonly associated with AML and monocytic differentiation, as are extramedullary masses, or chloromas, which are seen in approximately 10% of patients with AML.

Infants with ALL and MLL rearrangements have a unique phenotype that is characterized by hyperleukocytosis, absence of CD10 expression, myeloid antigen (CD15) coexpression, and poor prognosis.[6,38] Gene expression profiling supports the designation of infant acute mixed-lineage leukemia as a distinct biologic subtype.[39]

JMML, an entity formerly known as juvenile chronic myelogenous leukemia, has distinctive clinical and laboratory features (Table 33–2; see Box 33–1 later).[14,40,41]

TABLE 33–2. Common Presenting Features of JMML

Clinical
Boys (60%)
Age <5 yr (95%)
Hepatosplenomegaly (100%)
Upper respiratory and other infections (50%)
Hemorrhage (50%)
Skin rash (60%): xanthogranulomatous, myelomonocytic infiltrates, café au lait spots
Pulmonary infiltrates
Features of neurofibromatosis type 1 (15%)
Peripheral Blood
Leukocytosis
Anemia
Thrombocytopenia
Immature granulocytes and monocytes
Blasts <5%
Bone Marrow
Hypercellular
Myeloid and monocytic precursor expansion
Blasts <20%

Ten percent of infants with trisomy 21 develop a transient myeloproliferative disorder. Although transient myeloproliferative disorder is sometimes referred to as "transient leukemia," 20% of such infants require chemotherapy to manage life-threatening consequences of blast infiltration, and up to one third go on to develop AML in the first few years of life.[42]

Laboratory Features

Laboratory abnormalities are often noted on routine studies performed as part of the work-up for presenting signs and symptoms. Essential initial screening studies for an individual with suspected leukemia are detailed in Table 33–3. Hyperleukocytosis (white blood cell count > 50,000/µL) can be seen with all subtypes of leukemia, but it is most commonly associated with T-cell ALL, AML with monoblastic differentiation, JMML, and infants with *MLL* rearrangements. Isolated thrombocytopenia is uncommon in ALL and AML. Severe thrombocytopenia out of proportion to marrow blast infiltration is often seen in JMML (see Table 33–2).

Diagnostic Confirmation and Classification

Abnormal results on screening laboratory evaluation (see Table 33–3), especially cytopenias or leukocytosis, should lead to close inspection of the peripheral blood smear. If leukemia is suspected, further evaluation is required to confirm or refute the diagnosis as rapidly as possible (Table 33–4). Bone marrow examination should be employed early in the diagnostic evaluation of suspected leukemia. Diagnosis is usually readily confirmed by analysis of the peripheral blood and/or bone marrow. Routine hematopathologic staining, immunohistochemistry, flow cytometry, and cytogenetics are used to further define the subtype and identify prognostic factors. Leukemia subtype should be classified according to the World Health Organization system. As in adults, the majority of children and adolescents with ALL have a precursor B-cell (pre-B) phenotype, whereas T-cell ALL accounts for 10–15% and mature B-cell ALL less than 5% (Fig. 33–9). The predominant AML phenotypes in pediatric patients are t(8;21), inv(16)(p13q22), AML without maturation, AML with maturation, and myelomonocytic, although infants are more likely to have 11q23-associated mixed-lineage, monoblastic/monocytic and megakaryoblastic subtypes (Fig. 33–10).[27,43,44] Erythroid leukemia is distinctly uncommon in children.[45] Certain cytogenetic abnormalities are not apparent on routine karyotyping and thus molecular testing may be required, most notably

TABLE 33–3. Initial Screening Studies for Suspected Leukemia

Test	Findings
Complete blood count	Cytopenia(s), leukocytosis
Peripheral blood smear	Blasts, immature forms
Chemistry panel	↑ LDH, ↑ uric acid, ↑ transaminases
Coagulation studies	↑ PT, ↑ PTT, disseminated intravascular coagulation
Chest radiograph	Mediastinal mass, pleural effusion, adenopathy
Oxygen saturation	Hypoxemia

Abbreviations: LDH, lactate dehydrogenase; PT, prothrombin time; PTT, partial thromboplastin time.

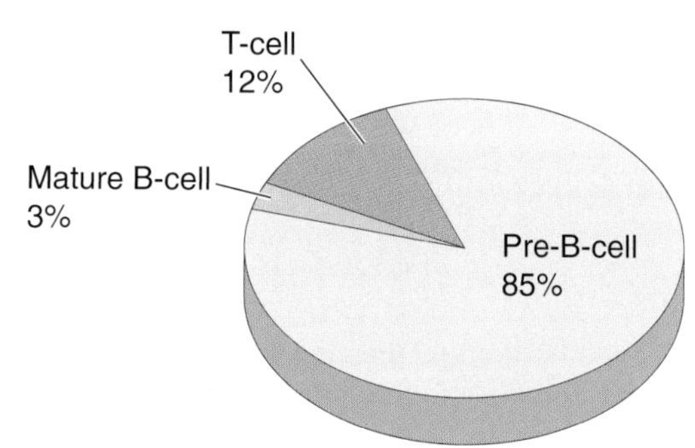

Figure 33–9. Approximate frequency of ALL phenotypes in children.

TABLE 33–4. Confirmatory Studies for Suspected Leukemia

Test	Findings	Notes
Bone marrow aspirate	Diagnostic confirmation of leukemia	May not be needed if prominent blasts on peripheral blood or pleural fluid.
Flow cytometry	Blast phenotype determination	Performed on marrow, blood, or pleural fluid blasts.
Cytogenetics, standard and/or molecular techniques	Subtype-specific translocations and/or aneuploidy	Performed on marrow, blood, or pleural fluid blasts.
Immunohistochemistry	Lineage-specific markers	Largely replaced by flow-cytometric analysis.
Chest CT scan		Should be performed for large mediastinal mass or suspected SVC syndrome, or airway compromise.
Brain CT or MRI		Should be performed for neurologic signs or symptoms or suspected leukostasis.
Spine MRI		Should be performed for signs or symptoms of spinal cord compression.
Spinal tap with cell count and cytologic analysis of centrifuged pellet ("cytospin")	Blasts in the cerebrospinal fluid	To minimize the risk of traumatic introduction of blasts, lumbar puncture should be performed by an experienced practitioner, and when possible, *after* diagnostic confirmation of leukemia so that intrathecal chemotherapy can be administered with the first spinal tap (ALL and AML only).
Ophthalmologic exam		For suspected ocular involvement
Peripheral blood or bone marrow CFU-GM	Spontaneous proliferation, GM-CSF hypersensitivity	JMML only
Hemoglobin electrophoresis	↑ Hemoglobin F	JMML only

Abbreviations: CFU-GM, granulocyte-macrophage colony-forming units; CT, computed tomography; GM-CSF, granulocyte-macrophage colony-stimulating factor; MRI, magnetic resonance imaging; SVC, superior vena cava.

for t(12;21), found in approximately 25% of childhood ALL. Lumbar puncture is required to evaluate for meningeal leukemia in ALL and AML. The diagnostic criteria for JMML are listed in Box 33–1.

Emergent Presentations

There are a number of emergent presentations that require immediate recognition and intervention in order to preserve organ function (Table 33–5). Anesthesia or sedation should be avoided in children with suspected airway compromise, and the least invasive procedure possible should be employed in the initial diagnostic evaluation.

DIFFERENTIAL DIAGNOSIS

Leukemia commonly presents with relatively nonspecific systemic symptoms. Consequently, the differential diagnosis may include a variety of chronic, subacute, and acute fulminant pediatric conditions associated with musculoskeletal pain, fever, malaise, hepatosplenomegaly, adenopathy, cytopenias, or bleeding (Box 33–2).

TREATMENT

General Recommendations

Pediatric cancers are relatively uncommon in comparison to adult malignancies. Treatment of leukemia should be stratified based on diagnostic subtype and clinicopathologic features using regimens that have been systematically developed via pediatric cooperative group clinical trials. Age-appropriate supportive care is critically important to a successful outcome. Consideration should also be given to the potential adverse effects on developing organs. For all of these reasons, it is recommended that children and adolescents with leukemia be treated at centers with pediatric oncology expertise.

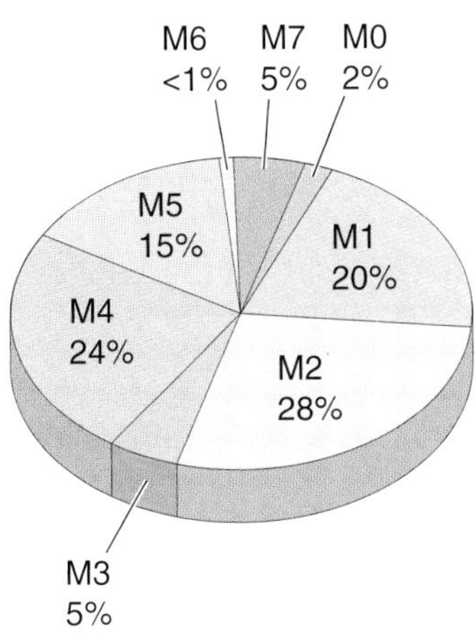

Figure 33–10. Approximate frequency of AML subtypes in children according to French-American-British (FAB) classification system.

Box 33–1. World Health Organization Diagnostic Criteria for JMML

Peripheral blood monocyte count >1000/μL
Blasts + promonocytes <20% of peripheral white blood cells and bone marrow nucleated cells
Philadelphia chromosome negative
At least two of the following:
- White blood cell count >10,000/μL
- Immature granulocytes in peripheral blood
- Clonal cytogenetic abnormality (e.g., monosomy 7)
- In vitro hypersensitivity of myeloid progenitors to granulocyte-macrophage colony-stimulating factor
- Hemoglobin F increased for age

TABLE 33–5. Emergent Presentations of Leukemia

Emergent Presentation	Intervention	Highest Risk
Leukostasis	Oxygen, leukapheresis, platelet and/or fresh frozen plasma transfusion to reduce risk of central nervous system hemorrhage	Varies with degree of hyperleukocytosis by subtype: AML ≥ 100,000/μL; ALL ≥ 400,000/μL; Rare in CML, JMML
Neutropenia with fever or infection	Broad-spectrum intravenous antibiotics	
Thrombocytopenia	Platelet transfusion	
Disseminated intravascular coagulation	Fresh frozen plasma, cryoprecipitate	Acute promyelocytic leukemia
Tumor lysis syndrome	Intravenous hydration, allopurinol or rasburicase, electrolyte correction	Mature B-ALL (Burkitt)
Airway obstruction	Oxygen, corticosteroids	T-ALL
Superior vena cava syndrome	Corticosteroids	T-ALL
Pericardial tamponade	Pericardiocentesis, corticosteroids	T-ALL
Intussusception	Surgical decompression	Mature B-ALL (Burkitt)
Central nervous system symptoms	Corticosteroids and/or radiation	
Ocular involvement	Radiation	
Spinal cord compression	Corticosteroids and/or radiation	

Box 33–2. Differential Diagnosis of Leukemia in Pediatrics

- Autoimmune disorders
  - Crohn's disease
  - Evans's syndrome
  - Juvenile rheumatoid arthritis (Still's disease)
- Bone marrow failure syndromes
  - Acquired aplastic anemia
  - Congenital marrow failure syndromes
- Fever of unknown origin
- Gastrointestinal conditions
  - Intussusception
  - Portal hypertension
- Hemoglobinopathies
  - β-Thalassemia
  - Sickle cell disease
- Hypereosinophilia
- Immunodeficiency
  - Hyperimmunoglobulin M syndrome
  - Leukocyte adhesion defect
- Infection
  - Cytomegalovirus, other "TORCH" infections
  - Epstein-Barr virus
  - Ehrlichiosis
  - Enteric fever
  - Gingivitis
  - Histoplasmosis
  - Human herpesvirus 6
  - Human immunodeficiency virus
  - Leishmaniasis
  - Lyme disease (i.e., *Borrelia burgdorferi*)
  - Osteomyelitis
  - Pertussis
  - Rocky Mountain spotted fever
  - Septic arthritis
- Leukemoid reaction
- Lymphoproliferative disorders
  - Autoimmune lymphoproliferative syndrome
  - Hemophagocytic lymphohistiocytosis—familial or acquired
  - Posttransplantation lymphoproliferative syndrome
  - X-linked lymphoproliferative syndrome (Duncan's syndrome)
- Metabolic disorders
  - Ascorbic acid deficiency (scurvy)
  - Inborn errors of metabolism (i.e., storage diseases)
  - Juvenile pernicious anemia
- Malignancy
  - Lymphoma
  - Myelodysplastic syndrome
  - Myelofibrosis
  - Neuroblastoma, metastatic
  - Retinoblastoma
  - Sarcoma, metastatic
- Musculoskeletal conditions
  - Osteopetrosis
  - Trauma
- Sarcoidosis
- Transient myeloproliferative disorder of Down syndrome

Dosing

Chemotherapy for pediatric patients is usually dosed according to body surface area. However, to decrease the risk of severe toxicity in infants under 1 year of age, certain agents should be dosed on a weight (per kilogram) basis. Intrathecal chemotherapy is dosed according to age, which is the primary determinant of cerebrospinal fluid volume.[46]

Treatment Regimens

Therapy should be instituted as soon as possible, especially in the setting of acute leukemia. The general approach to treatment of childhood ALL is standard worldwide.[29,47] The initial management of pediatric AML is also fairly similar,[24,48] although there is disagreement about the role for allogeneic hematopoietic stem cell transplantation for children who have human lymphocyte antigen (HLA)–matched sibling donors. The only curative approach for JMML is allogeneic stem cell transplantation. Transplantation is also routinely employed for CML, although the availability of imatinib mesylate has raised questions about the optimal timing of such treatment (Table 33–6).

Acute Lymphocytic Leukemia

Approximately 80% of children with ALL will be cured with combination chemotherapy. Treatment for B-precursor and T-cell ALL is stratified based on phenotype and prognostic factors (Table 33–7)[49,50] and consists of induction, consolidation/intensification/re-induction, central nervous system sterilization, and maintenance for a total of 2–3 years.[51–58] Those with mature B-cell phenotype should be treated as per Burkitt's lymphoma regimens, which most commonly employ dose- and sequence-intensive, short-course combination chemotherapy.[59–61] In light of the excellent treatment results, many current-era clinical trials include modifications designed to decrease toxicity for children with lower risk features.

The intensity of therapy is tailored according to the risk of relapse. Age, white blood cell count, central nervous system involvement, DNA index, and phenotype are used for the initial risk group determination.[49] The risk group assignment is subsequently adjusted based on cytogenetics and response to induction, the latter of which is defined by morphologic blast reduction in peripheral blood or bone marrow and/or minimal residual disease determination by flow cytometry or polymerase chain reaction amplification.[62] Initial remission induction therapy consists of three to five drugs given as a 28-day cycle.[51–58] Refer to these references for treatment regimens. This is followed by multiple consolidation/intensification/re-induction cycles and then by prolonged maintenance therapy. Central nervous system prophylactic treatment is integrated throughout all phases of therapy. In order to reduce long-term neurotoxicity, recent trials have replaced prophylactic cranial irradiation with central nervous system–directed chemotherapy for most patients.[63–65] Intensive intrathecal chemotherapy in combination with systemic agents that penetrate the cerebrospinal fluid, most notably dexamethasone and high-dose methotrexate, provides excellent prophylaxis. To minimize the risk of meningeal contamination associated with traumatic lumbar puncture, initial diagnostic spinal taps should be performed by clinicians experienced in the procedure, after correction of thrombocytopenia and coagulopathy, and with intrathecal chemotherapy administration.[66,67] Boys with overt testes involvement require bilateral testicular irradiation.

In comparison to chemotherapy, relapse rates are lower after allogeneic stem cell transplantation; however, treatment-related mortality rates are increased.[68] Thus, stem cell transplantation is rarely employed for children with ALL in first complete remission except for those with "ultra-high-risk" features such as induction failure and t(9;22).[69]

TABLE 33–6. General Approach to Treatment of Pediatric Leukemia

Leukemia Type	Treatment Approach
ALL	Risk-directed Treatment phases (excluding mature B-cell): Induction Consolidation/intensification/re-induction Maintenance Central nervous system treatment Mature B-ALL: as per Burkitt's lymphoma regimens
AML	Treatment phases (excluding promyelocytic): Induction Consolidation/intensification Central nervous system treatment ? Matched-sibling stem cell transplantation in first remission Promyelocytic: Include all-*trans* retinoic acid during induction and maintenance
JMML	13-*cis*-retinoic acid Allogeneic stem cell transplantation
CML	Imatinib mesylate Allogeneic stem cell transplantation

Acute Myeloid Leukemia

Components of standard AML treatment regimens include induction, consolidation, and central nervous system sterilization. The use of all-*trans* retinoic acid during induction and maintenance for acute promyelocytic leukemia leads to improved results (~80% disease-free survival) in that subtype.[70,71] Young children with AML and Down syndrome also have excellent outcomes despite the use of less intensive regimens.[72,73] The outcome for other subgroups is poor, and only about 50–75% of children with AML are cured. Thus, despite the identification of prognostic factors (Table 33–8),[74–77] stratified treatment approaches are less commonly employed in AML than in ALL.[78] The primary aim of most pediatric AML trials remains to try to improve disease-free survival rates through increased treatment intensity.

Approximately 75–90% of pediatric patients with AML will achieve a complete remission after initial induction with regimens that commonly consist of cytarabine (Ara-C) and anthracyclines with or without additional agents.[78–85] Augmentation of induction improves disease-free survival rates even in the absence of increases in complete remission rates.[86] Chemotherapy dose escalation ("dose intensity")[78,85] and treatment interval compression ("intensive timing")[84] have been successfully utilized in this regard. Postremission consolidation is critical, and high-dose Ara-C is commonly used in combi-

TABLE 33–7. Prognostic Factors in Childhood B-Precursor ALL

	"Lower" or "Standard" Risk Factors	"Higher" Risk Factors
Age (yr)	1–9	≥10 <1
White blood cell count (/μL)	<50,000	≥50,000
Central nervous system involvement	Negative	Positive
Chromosomes	t(12;21), Double or triple trisomy 4/10/17	11q23, t(1;19), t(9;22)
DNA index	≥1.16	<1.16 <1.0 >1.78
Initial treatment response	Rapid	Slow Induction failure

TABLE 33–8. Prognostic Factors in Childhood AML

	"Lower" Risk Factors	"Higher" Risk Factors
Age (yr)	≥1	<1
White blood cell count (/μL)	<100,000	≥100,000
Central nervous system involvement	Negative	Positive
Cytogenetics	Trisomy 21, t(15;17), t(8;21), inv(16)	*Flt3* internal tandem duplications, 11q23, t(9;22), −7, −5, secondary
FAB subtype	M1, M2, M3, M4eo	Infant M4/5, M6, M7
Initial treatment response	Rapid	Slow Induction failure

TABLE 33–9. Disease-Free Survival Rates in Clinical Studies of Postremission Therapy for Childhood AML

Study	Allogeneic Stem Cell Transplantation (%)	Chemotherapy (%)	Autologous Stem Cell Transplantation (%)	Median Follow-Up (yr)
AML-80[93]	43	31		6
AIEOP LAM-87[91]	51*	27	21	5
CCG-213[96]	54*	37		5
CCG-251[95]	45*	32		8
POG-8821[90]	52*	36	38	3
MRC AML-10[79]	61*	46	68†	7
AML BFM-93[78]	64	61		5
CCG-2891[92]	55*	47	42	8
LAME-89/91[80,81]	72*	48		6

*P ≤ .05 allogeneic versus others.
†P ≤ .05 autologous versus chemotherapy.

nation with other agents for two to three cycles.[78,79,83,85–88] Randomized trials of standard consolidation regimens versus high-dose chemotherapy with autologous stem cell rescue have shown mixed results[79,89–92] (Table 33–9). Although relapse rates are lower with autologous rescue, treatment-associated mortality is increased. Allogeneic stem cell transplantation is commonly employed in first complete remission for pediatric patients who have HLA-matched sibling donors. There have been multiple "genetic randomization" studies in which individuals with HLA-matched sibling donors were assigned to transplantation. Allogeneic stem cell transplantation is associated with lower relapse rates and higher disease-free survival rates in comparison to chemotherapy alone or followed by high-dose therapy with autologous rescue[79,89–96] which many patients have sustained remission and improved quality of life[97] (Fig. 33–11; see Table 33–9). These associated benefits may be off-set by transplant-related morbidity and mortality, which increase with advancing age.[79,98–101] Consequently, there is debate as to whether transplantation should be employed in first complete remission versus second complete remission for children with matched sibling donors.[101–103] Despite the fact that children tolerate AML therapy better than adults, supportive care remains essential and may be the major determinant in survival. Reported toxic mortality rates with pediatric regimens range from 3% to 14%.[83,104] Intrathecal Ara-C is most commonly used for central nervous system sterilization for pediatric patients with AML.[48,105,106]

Juvenile Myelomonocytic Leukemia

JMML is usually resistant to therapy and rapidly progressive, with a median survival of approximately 7 months. Fifty percent of patients with JMML respond to treatment with 13-*cis*-retinoic acid.[107] Chemotherapy may transiently reduce disease burden. However, stem cell transplantation represents the only curative option for this aggressive disorder, although disease-free survival rates are less than 50% even with transplantation.[108–110]

Chronic Myeloid Leukemia

Studies with imatinib mesylate in pediatric CML are limited, and allogeneic stem cell transplantation is the only therapy that has been shown to be curative. Disease-free survival rates are inversely related to age and exceed 80% for young children with matched sibling donors. Outcome is best when transplant is performed in first chronic phase and with a shorter diagnosis-transplant interval. Transplant-related mortality is low in pediatric

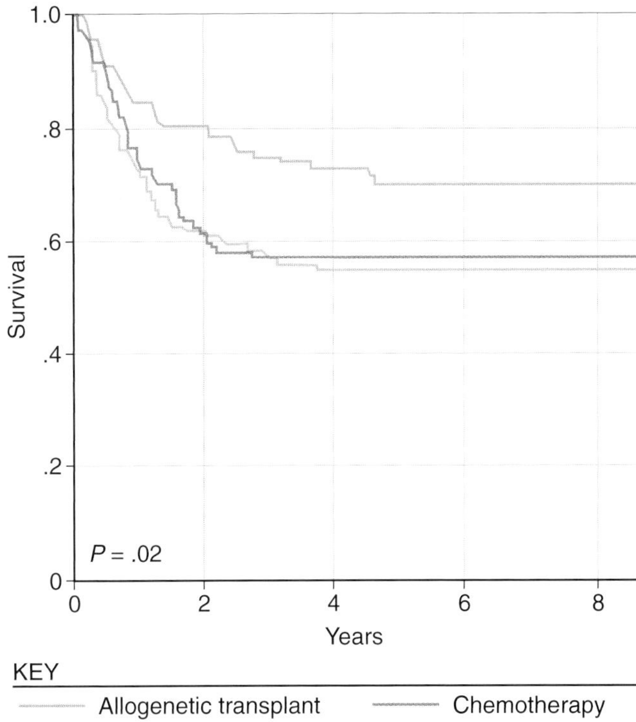

Figure 33–11. Postremission therapy for pediatric AML. Data from patients randomized to intensive-timing induction in Children's Cancer Group Study #2891, the largest published three-armed trial of postremission therapy for pediatric AML.[92] Subjects with HLA-matched sibling donors were assigned to allogeneic stem cell transplantation (n = 113). All others were randomized between autologous transplant (n = 115) versus chemotherapy alone (n = 108). Data represent actuarial survival at 8 years from first remission.

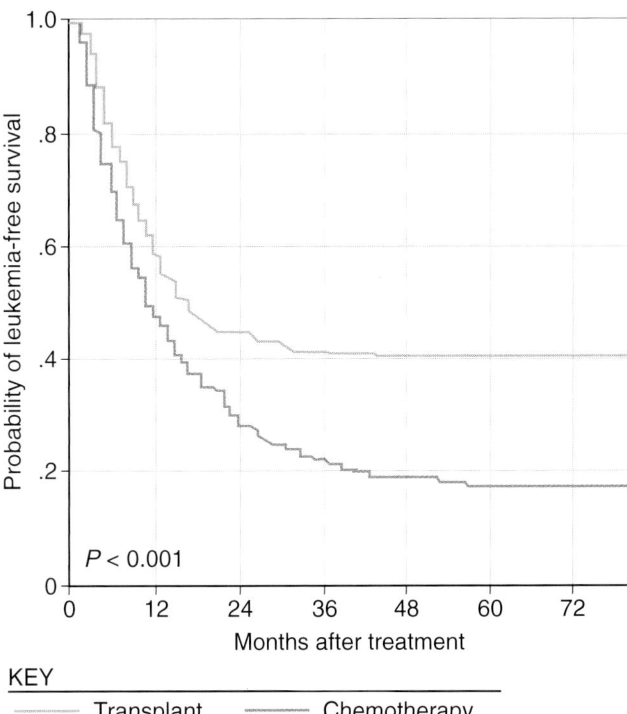

Figure 33–12. Matched sibling donor stem cell transplantation versus chemotherapy for relapsed pediatric ALL. Matched-pair analysis (n = 255 pairs) of patients with ALL in second remission from Pediatric Oncology Group and International Bone Marrow Transplant Registry databases.[68] Data represent disease-free survival at 5 years from second remission.

patients, thus matched unrelated donor stem cell transplantation is usually recommended for those who lack sibling donors.[111–113] Transplantation is clearly indicated for those who develop accelerated- or blastic-phase disease, preferably after a second chronic phase is achieved.[114] For patients started on imatinib mesylate, a number of criteria for consideration of stem cell transplantation have been proposed, including loss of therapeutic response and failure to achieve a complete hematologic response by 3 months or a substantial cytogenetic response by 3–6 months of treatment.[111,115] Even if stem cell transplantation is not planned for initial treatment, donor availability and transplant options should be considered soon after diagnosis for all children with CML.

Management of Relapse

Allogeneic stem cell transplantation in second complete remission using a related or unrelated donor is usually recommended for children with ALL and AML who sustain a bone marrow relapse. Allogenic stem cell transplantation confers a relapse-free survival advantage over chemotherapy alone, in part because of an allogeneic effect[68,116] (Fig. 33–12). Curative salvage can be achieved with chemotherapy alone in approximately 30% of patients with ALL[117] and 10–30% of those with AML.[81,118,119] Durable disease-free survival is more likely when first complete remission duration exceeds 12 months and when initial treatment was with a standard-risk regimen. Up to 50% of children with ALL who sustain an isolated extramedullary relapse can be cured with chemotherapy and radiation.[120]

Stem Cell Transplantation

In comparison to adults, children with leukemia have decreased transplant-related mortality and improved survival after allogeneic stem cell transplantation[121,122] (Fig. 33–13). As detailed earlier, this has led to the application of stem cell transplantation as a curative approach for all subtypes of pediatric leukemia.

SUPPORTIVE CARE AND LONG-TERM MANAGEMENT

Aggressive monitoring and supportive care are essential to prevent or manage complications of leukemia and treatment during all phases of therapy. Many of these are common to adult and pediatric populations, although there are a variety of age-specific considerations.

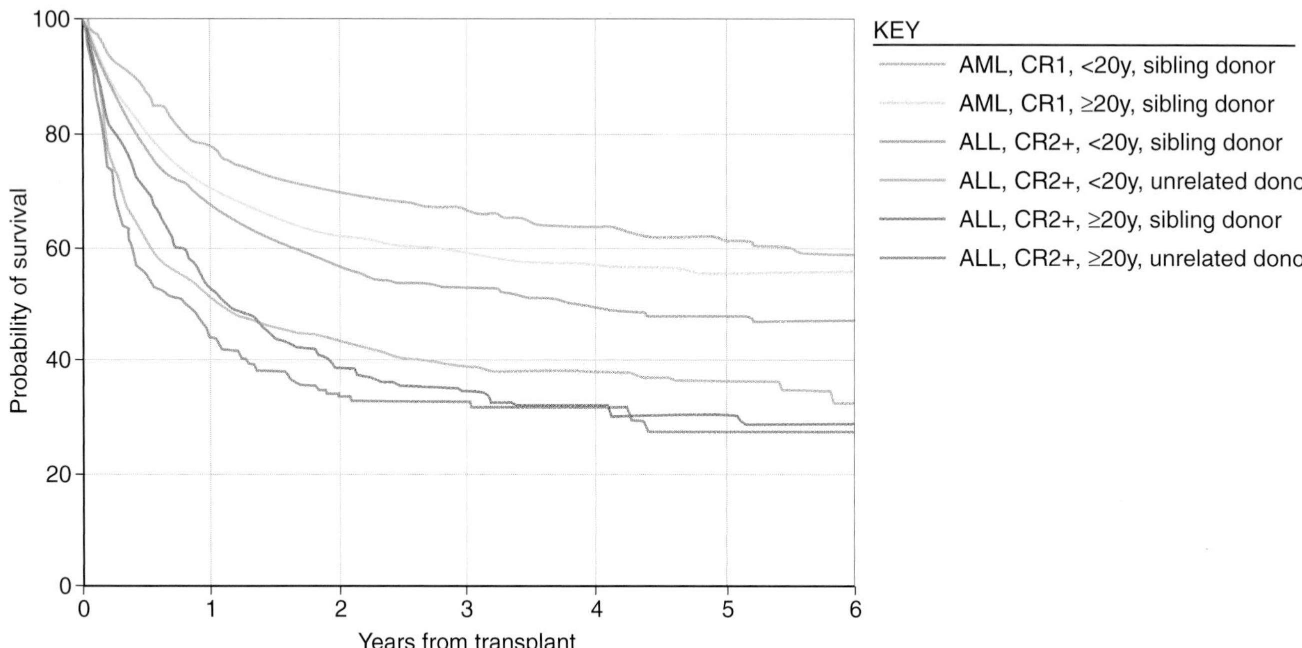

Figure 33–13. Age-related survival after allogeneic stem cell transplantation. Data from International Bone Marrow Transplant Registry and Autologous Blood and Marrow Transplant Registry for transplants performed between 1996 and 2001 for AML in first remission ($n = 3187$) and ALL in second remission ($n = 2318$).[122] Data represent probability of survival at 3 years from transplant.

Tumor Lysis Syndrome

Those children with high tumor burden and rapid cell turnover, most notably those with ALL and AML with hyperleukocytosis and mature B-ALL (Burkitt), are at highest risk for tumor lysis syndrome. Close monitoring of metabolic and renal function is required during initiation of therapy. Tumor lysis precautions should be started as soon as possible after diagnosis and at least 12 hours prior to the start of induction (Box 33–3).

Transfusion Support

Transfusions are commonly required during therapy for pediatric leukemia. Indications vary with the specific clinical situation, and dosing should be based on blood volume and weight (Box 33–4). Concomitant anemia partially offsets the hyperviscosity associated with hyperleukocytosis. Thus, red cell transfusion should be avoided whenever possible in that setting. Until the blast count is reduced, the hemoglobin and hematocrit should be increased slowly and to the minimum level necessary to alleviate symptoms of anemia using small-aliquot transfusion. To prevent bleeding, platelet counts should routinely be maintained above 10,000/µL. Levels above that are recommended for infants, patients with hemorrhage, prior to invasive procedures such as lumbar puncture, and to reduce the risk of central nervous system hemorrhage associated with leukostasis.[123]

Platelets and red cells should be leukodepleted to decrease the risk of febrile reactions, HLA alloimmunization with subsequent platelet refractoriness, and cytomegalovirus transmission, although cytomegalovirus-seronegative blood products may offer advantage in

Box 33–3. Tumor Lysis Syndrome Prophylaxis

Allopurinol

Urate oxidase (rasburicase) is an alternative for management of extreme hyperuricemia.

Hydration

Intravenous fluids at a rate of >2 times maintenance (>120 mL/m^2/hr) should be adjusted to maintain urine specific gravity <1.010 and normal urine output. Potassium should be avoided because of the risk of hyperkalemia.

Alkalinization

To decrease the risk of uric acid nephropathy, urine may be alkalinized with sodium bicarbonate for patients with hyperuricemia. *Caution:* It is recommended that the urine pH be maintained between 6.5 and 7.5 because a high pH is associated with hypoxanthine crystallization. In addition, alkalinization should be avoided in the setting of hyperphosphatemia because of the risk of calcium/phosphate precipitation.

Laboratory Studies

Frequent serial monitoring should include serum potassium, phosphorus, calcium, creatinine, and uric acid during initiation of induction.

Box 33–4. Pediatric Transfusions

Total Blood Volume

(Nomograms that estimate TBV based on height and weight can also be used.)
Infant: 100 mL/kg
Child: 80 mL/kg

Packed Red Blood Cells

Indication: Manage or prevent symptomatic anemia
Threshold for prophylactic transfusion:
Standard risk factors: Hematocrit 20–25%
Caution: Avoid red cell transfusion in setting of hyperleukocytosis to reduce risk of hyperviscosity.
Dose: Calculated to raise the hematocrit to a desired level:

$$\text{Volume of packed cells required (mL)} = (HCT_d - HCT_i) \times TBV/HCT_{PRBCs}$$

Platelets

Indication: Manage or prevent bleeding resulting from thrombocytopenia
Threshold for prophylactic transfusion (platelet count):
Standard risk: 10,000/μL
Additional bleeding risk cofactors or invasive procedures: 50,000–100,000/μL
Dose: 0.1 U/kg → 50,000/μL

Fresh Frozen Plasma

Indication: Manage or prevent bleeding resulting from coagulopathy
Dose: 10 mL/kg → 20% activity

Cryoprecipitate

Indication: Manage or prevent bleeding resulting from hypofibrinogenemia
Dose: 0.2 U/kg → 135 mg/dL

Abbreviations: HCT_d, desired hematocrit; HCT_i, initial hematocrit; HCT_{PRBCs}, hematocrit of packed red blood cells (varies by institution); TBV, total blood volume.

TABLE 33–10. Unique Transfusion-Associated Risks in Pediatrics

Complication	Product Manipulation	Notes
Volume overload	Small aliquot Volume reduced	Infants, young children, and those with large transfusion requirements are at greatest risk. Consider multiple aliquots from single units to decrease donor exposure.
Cytomegalovirus (CMV) infection	CMV negative (or leukodepleted)	Most pediatric patients are CMV negative.
Graft-versus-host disease	Irradiated	Children with possible underlying immunodeficiency and with severe immunosuppression (e.g., post–stem cell transplantation) are at greatest risk.

regard to the latter.[124–126] Single-donor (i.e., apheresis) platelets are recommended to reduce donor exposure and associated risks, including HLA alloimmunization and septic reactions.[127] Pediatric patients are at increased risk for certain additional transfusion-related risks, and specialized blood products should be employed to minimize these (Table 33–10).

Infection Prophylaxis

Aggressive infection surveillance, prophylaxis, and treatment are essential throughout all phases of leukemia therapy. There are a number of age-specific infectious issues to be considered. As with chemotherapy, antibiotics should be dosed by weight or body surface area. All patients require *Pneumocystis carinii* pneumonia prophylaxis. The standard regimen is trimethoprim (TMP)/sulfamethoxazole (SMX) at a dose of 75 mg TMP/m^2/dose (maximum 160 mg TMP) twice a day orally three times per week. An alternative regimen should be substituted for patients with allergy or myelosuppression associated with TMP/SMX. Routine childhood immunizations should not be administered during leukemia therapy, and resumption of vaccination should commence at least 3 months after completion of treatment. Live vaccines are generally contraindicated, and household contacts (e.g., siblings) should not be given live oral polio vaccine.[128–131] Varicella vaccination should be considered for those children without prior chickenpox infection or immunization after remission is achieved. Nonimmune individuals should receive varicella zoster immune globulin within 3–4 days of exposure to varicella, including attenuated postvaccination illness. Children undergoing treatment for ALL commonly develop hypogammaglobulinemia. Immunoglobulin G levels should be assayed for those with recurrent infections, and, if low, intravenous immunoglobulin supplementation is recommended at a dose of approximately 500 mg/kg every 4 weeks as needed to maintain an immunoglobulin G level greater than 500 mg/dL.

Procedures

A central element of care is the management and prevention of pain and anxiety associated with the multitude of required procedures. Central venous catheters are recommended for most children to facilitate repeated venipuncture and improve safety and tolerability of chemotherapy administration. Conscious sedation or anesthesia is recommended for bone marrow aspirations and spinal taps. To minimize associated risks, attempts should be made to perform needed procedures under

TABLE 33–11. Common Late Effects of Pediatric Leukemia

Late Effect	Contributing Factors	Prevention	Management
Cardiomyopathy	Anthracyclines Cardiac irradiation	Monitor left ventricular function Limit cumulative anthracycline dose to <400 mg/m^2 Employ dexrazoxane Cardiac shielding	Afterload reduction Inotropic agents
Neurocognitive dysfunction	Cranial and total-body irradiation Specific chemotherapy agents, including intrathecal and high-dose methotrexate and cytarabine	Eliminate or dose-reduce radiation	Specialized educational program Neurodevelopmental assistance
Endocrinopathies	Craniospinal and total-body irradiation Alkylating agents	Eliminate or dose-reduce radiation	Hormone replacement Infertility treatment
Osteonecrosis	Corticosteroids	Limit corticosteroid dose and duration	Analgesics Joint replacement
Secondary malignancy	Radiation Alkylating agents, epidophyllotoxins, antimetabolites	Avoid or dose-reduce specific agents	Early detection and specific therapy

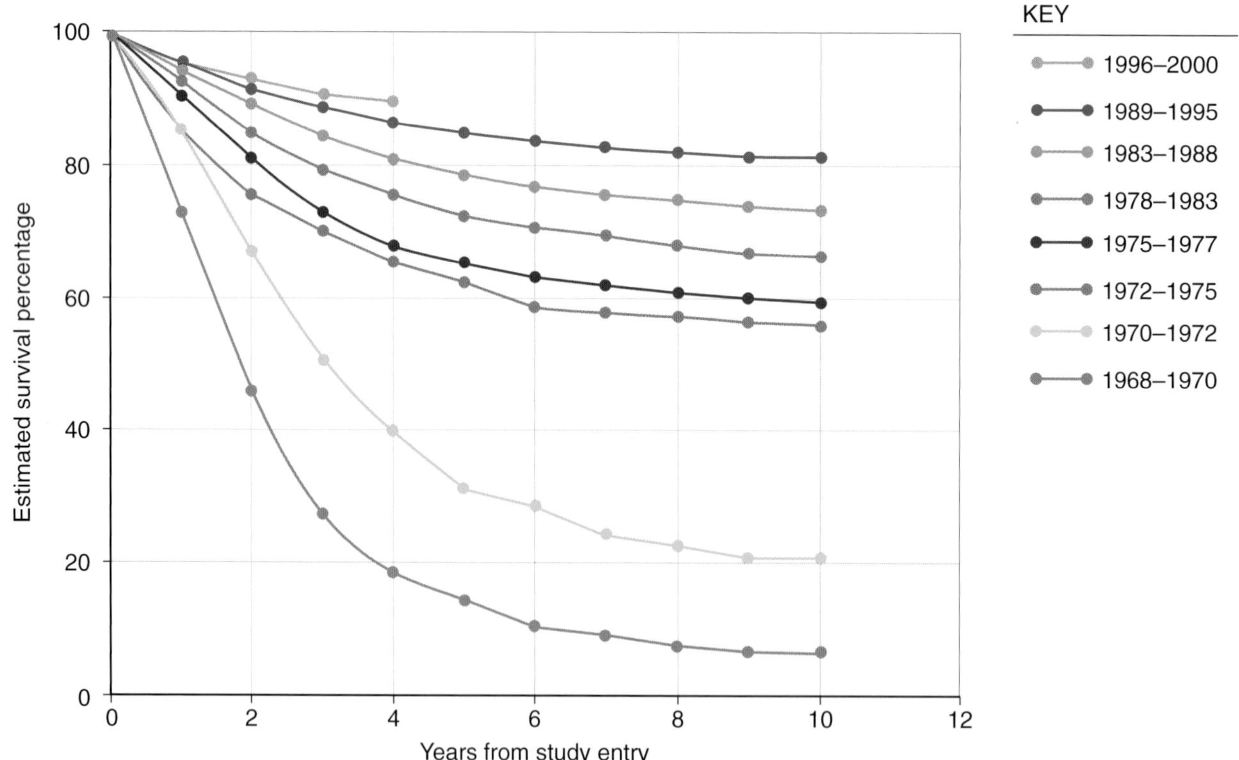

■ **Figure 33–14.** Survival by study era in pediatric ALL. (Data from Children's Oncology Group, provided courtesy of G.H. Reaman and H. Sather.)

the same sedation/anesthesia when feasible. For example, after the initial diagnosis of leukemia is confirmed, it is common to coordinate central venous catheter placement, bone marrow aspiration for any additional needed studies, and initial lumbar puncture for diagnosis and intrathecal chemotherapy administration (for ALL and AML only).

Psychosocial Support

The diagnosis and treatment of pediatric cancer has significant impact not only on the affected child, but also on siblings, parents, and other family members. Temporary home schooling may be required to overcome medically required absenteeism. At the same time, it is important to try to prevent social isolation, which is a multifactorial phenomenon commonly associated with pediatric cancer diagnosis and treatment. Disease-related educational programs for classmates and teachers may facilitate school reentry.[132] Long-term psychosocial consequences of treatment may require ongoing support into adult life.

Late Effects

Many survivors of childhood leukemia have substantial sequelae of underlying disease and its treatment[133,134] (Table 33–11). Long-term follow-up is critical to monitor for disease recurrence, treatment-associated toxicity, and secondary malignancy.

PROGNOSIS

There have been steady improvements in the treatment of pediatric leukemias due in part to global participation in cooperative group clinical trials and advances in supportive care.[135] Progress has been greatest in the setting of ALL[47] (Fig. 33–14), although outcome is dependent on prognostic factors and varies within risk groups based on differences in chemotherapy bioavailability, compliance, and pharmacogenetics.[136–139] The outlook for children with AML is slowly improving, and more than 50% achieve long-term disease-free survival.[48] The prognosis for those with JMML remains poor at this time.[14] Children with CML have high cure rates with allogeneic stem cell transplantation.[140]

CURRENT CONTROVERSIES & FUTURE CONSIDERATIONS

Pediatric Leukemias

- Despite great progress in the development of curative treatment for leukemia, many children and adolescents around the globe do not have access to the most effective therapies. Efforts are needed to make curative treatment available to all children.[141]
- With improvements in leukemia-free survival rates, the consequences of treatment have become clear.[97,133,134] Equally efficacious but less toxic regimens are needed to improve the quality of life for survivors. In an attempt to reduce long-term neurotoxicity in ALL, cranial irradiation has been reduced or eliminated for most patients. The impact on central nervous system relapse rates and neurocognitive outcome has yet to be fully defined.[63,64,142]
- Studies with newly developed targeted therapies are being conducted in specific leukemia subtypes, including the Bcr/Abl tyrosine kinase inhibitor imatinib mesylate (Ph[1] leukemia), FLT-3 inhibitors (ALL, AML), farnesyltransferase inhibitors (JMML), and monoclonal antibody–based agents (ALL, AML). The optimal way to combine these agents with standard therapy must be defined.[143,144]
- Novel technologies have the potential to advance our understanding of the biology of leukemia, which should foster the development of new therapies and preventative strategies.[39,145] Recently, gene expression analysis has been shown to be predictive of treatment response and outcome in lymphoid and myeloid leukemias.[146–151] Proteomic analysis might be utilized to increase the sensitivity of detection of disease and treatment toxicities, which in turn might facilitate earlier intervention.[145,152]
- Methods to augment antileukemia immune responses, both in the autologous and the allogeneic settings, are being developed and hold promise for patients of all ages.[153–156]

Suggested Readings*

Bennett C, Hsu K, Look AT: Myeloid leukemia, myelodysplasia, and myeloproliferative disease in children. *In* Nathan DG, Orkin SH, Ginsburg D, Look AT (eds): Nathan and Oski's Hematology of Infancy and Childhood (ed 6). Philadelphia: WB Saunders, 2003, pp 1167–1209.

Emanuel PD: Juvenile myelomonocytic leukemia. Curr Hematol Rep 3:203–209, 2004.

Goldman JM, Marin D: Management decisions in chronic myeloid leukemia. Semin Hematol 40:97–103, 2003.

Golub TR, Arceci RJ: Acute myelogenous leukemia. *In* Pizzo PA, Poplack DG (eds): Principles and Practice of Pediatric Oncology (ed 4). Philadelphia: Lippincott Williams & Wilkins, 2002, pp 545–589.

Margolin JF, Steuber CP, Poplack DG: Acute lymphoblastic leukemia. *In* Pizzo PA, Poplack DG (eds): Principles and Practice of Pediatric Oncology (ed 4). Philadelphia: Lippincott Williams & Wilkins, 2002, pp 489–544.

Pui C-H (ed): Childhood Leukemias. New York: Cambridge University Press, 1999.

Pui C-H, Rellins MV, Downing JR: Acute lymphoblastic leukemia. N Engl J Med 350:1535–1548, 2004.

Reis LAG, Smith MA, Gurney JG, et al (eds): Cancer Incidence and Survival Among Children and Adolescents: United States SEER Program 1975–1995 (NIH Publ. No. 99-4649). Bethesda, MD: National Cancer Institute, 1999. (Available at: *http://www-seer.ims.nci.nih.gov*)

Silverman LB, Sallan SE: Acute lymphoblastic leukemia. *In* Nathan DG, Orkin SH, Ginsburg D, Look AT (eds): Nathan and Oski's Hematology of Infancy and Childhood (ed 6). Philadelphia: WB Saunders, 2003, pp 1135–1166.

CHAPTER 34

Chronic Lymphocytic Leukemia

Michael R. Grever, MD, Amy S. Gewirtz, MD, and John C. Byrd, MD

KEY POINTS

Chronic Lymphocytic Leukemia

Diagnosis

- Peripheral absolute lymphocytosis greater than 5000/μL that may show small lymphoid cells of uniform size and condensed nuclei is diagnostic of chronic lymphocytic leukemia (CLL).
- The diagnosis also must differentiate CLL from other chronic lymphoid malignancies: prolymphocytic leukemia, which shows extreme lymphocytosis with prominent nucleoli; and mantle cell lymphoma, a homogeneous population of small lymphoid cells with irregular nuclear contour and inconspicuous nucleoli. Mantle cell lymphoma may present with "blastic" changes and an aggressive clinical course.
- A monoclonal population of leukemic cells in CLL shows a characteristic immunophenotype consisting of $CD5^+CD19^+$ $CD23^+$ and weak CD20 positivity.

Clinical Manifestations

- Fatigue
- Bone marrow failure (anemia, thrombocytopenia, neutropenia)
- Infection
- Autoimmune complications
- Lymphadenopathy, splenomegaly, or bulk tumor progression
- Transformation to aggressive hematologic malignant disease

Prognosis

- Clinical prognostic features include clinical stage (either Rai or Binet system) and bone marrow pattern of lymphoid infiltration.
- Laboratory findings predictive of prognosis include immunoglobulin mutational status, fluorescent in situ hybridization analysis for cytogenetic subsets, CD38 expression, p53 mutational status or gene deletion, and ZAP-70 expression.

INTRODUCTION

Chronic lymphocytic leukemia (CLL) is the most common form of adult leukemia in the Western hemisphere. CLL, a chronic malignant disease characterized by a multitude of clinical features, was initially described as an accumulative disorder of abnormal lymphocytes.[1] In his original description, Dameshek displayed insight into the pathobiologic basis for this disease. CLL is a distinct neoplastic disorder of $CD5^+$ B cells that have difficulty in undergoing apoptosis. Many of the molecular entities that appear to be responsible for inhibiting induction of apoptosis in these leukemic cells are centered on the Bcl-2 family of antiapoptotic proteins.[2] Over the past decade, increasing molecular differences observed in leukemic cells derived from these patients explain the enormous diversity in clinical course experienced by these patients.[3–6]

Recently, investigators have claimed that CLL is really two disease entities that can be separated by the mutational status of the immunoglobulin variable region (Ig V) gene.[7,8] In the normal maturation of the B cell, the Ig V gene undergoes a specific rearrangement that provides for the potential diversity of response in immunoglobulin protein synthesis responding to antigenic stimuli. Patients who have a mutated Ig V gene detected in their leukemic B cells subsequent to this rearrangement have a favorable prognosis, and those who harbor an unmutated Ig V gene in their malignant cells have a much more aggressive clinical course.

In fact, a plethora of new molecular observations are associated with a variable prognosis in specific subsets of patients.[9–15] CLL is a complex malignant disease process. Although the basic biologic defect reflects difficulty in undergoing apoptosis, there is a clear-cut element of disordered lymphoproliferation as well.[16,17] The majority of leukemic cells obtained from these patients are locked in "G_0" and are not engaged in cell division. Yet, an important subset of the leukemic cells does proliferate, contributing to the ultimate progressive increase in tumor burden.

Management of this disease requires thorough knowledge of the new prognostic subsets, understanding of the biologic abnormalities underpinning the disease, and knowing the therapeutic strategies for controlling the disease. In the following sections, we provide an updated understanding of the classification of the specific forms of this disease, and the selection of treatment intended to provide long-term disease control. Although this is currently an incurable disease, vigorous research in experimental therapeutics hopefully will change the outcome for these patients.

EPIDEMIOLOGY

Interesting differences exist between CLL and the other forms of adult leukemia. CLL does not occur with the same prevalence in all parts of the globe.[18,19] In the Western hemisphere, this form of chronic leukemia actually is more prevalent. Patients are diagnosed with CLL more often in the United States and Europe than in the Far East. In populations immigrating to the United States from Asian countries, the frequency of the diagnosis does not change. There have been associations linking CLL to farming and to chemical agents used in agriculture.[20–22] Furthermore, there has been a recent association of CLL and exposure to Agent Orange during the Vietnam era.[23,24] CLL is one type of leukemia that has not been associated with radiation exposure.[25,26]

Families have recently been identified with a definite proclivity for developing this disease.[27] In particular, patients with CLL have a remarkable increased risk for others in the family to be diagnosed with this disease. It is estimated in some populations that 5–10% of the cases of CLL may be associated with the familial form of the disease.[27,28] Efforts are underway to characterize the molecular differences between those afflicted with familial forms of CLL and those who develop spontaneous disease. In some cases, there has been a tendency for earlier onset of symptoms in patients with the familial form of the disease.

CLL is more frequent in males (i.e., about a 1.5- to 1.8-times increased incidence in men over women).[28–30] It is diagnosed in about 10,000–15,000 new cases per year in the United States. The median age at diagnosis is approximately 66 years old, but at least 20% of patients are less than 55 years of age. Although there does not appear to be a difference in clinical outcome for those developing the disease early in life, it will ultimately have an impact on the survival of those who are younger than 50 at the time of diagnosis. Older patients may actually die from other causes, or they may succumb to the consequences of this disease. Unfortunately, the majority of patients will die from the disease or its many complications.

Recently, monoclonal $CD5^+$ B lymphocytes have been observed in otherwise healthy adults. B cells with an immunophenotype very close to that observed in CLL have been identified in family members of patients who have this form of chronic leukemia. This observation raises the possibility that the patients harboring the monoclonal cells have an entity reminiscent of monoclonal gammopathy of undetermined significance in myeloma.[27,31–33] The long-term follow-up of these patients will ultimately provide a better understanding of the natural history of this phenomenon.

PATHOPHYSIOLOGY

Origin and Progression of the Leukemia

The transforming event to neoplasia occurs in a common lymphocyte precursor cell (CLP).[34] In utero, all fetal B cells are $CD5^+$. This proportion of cells markedly declines in number after birth. The CLP cell undergoes change resulting in a monoclonal population of B cells with a characteristic antigenic expression pattern. The leukemic cells are identified by $CD5^+CD19^+CD23^+$ features. Furthermore, specific subsets of these cells have other characteristic features that have a major impact on the clinical course of the disease. These cells either have a mutation involving the Ig V gene regions or they are identical to germline cells being classified as unmutated. Although the leukemic cells have difficulty in undergoing apoptosis related to the expression of specific antiapoptotic proteins (e.g., Bcl-2, Mcl-1, etc.), there is also a proliferative compartment resulting in an overproduction of the malignant cells.

Circulating malignant B cells are frequently seen in this disease, and most organs are infiltrated with these cells. Accumulation of the cells within the bone marrow results in ultimate progressive infiltration.[18,28,29,34] It is speculated that the microenvironment within the bone marrow or lymph nodes contributes to the progressive increase in tumor burden. The bone marrow pattern initially may be interstitial, and then will develop nodular infiltrates that are nontrabecular. As the disease burden progresses, the bone marrow will become diffusely infiltrated, resulting in anemia, thrombocytopenia, and neutropenia.

Complications of Leukemia: From Dysfunctional Immunity to Bulk Disease and Subsequent Neoplastic Transformation to Aggressive Disease

Early on, CLL has been associated with autoimmune phenomena involving cellular elements of the blood-forming organs. Interesting autoimmune complications can involve other tissues as well (e.g., paraneoplastic pemphigus involves the oral and bronchial mucosal cells).[35–39] The initial autoimmune complications can involve polyclonal antibodies directed against normal tissue, reflecting a profound dysfunction of the normal immune effector cells in these patients from the very beginning of the disease.[40] T-cell compartmental defects are present before chemotherapy, and may be more disrupted following use of specific therapies (e.g., fludarabine, Campath monoclonal antibody directed against CD52).[41–44]

Bulk disease can involve almost any organ, but widespread lymph node involvement including both the liver and spleen are targeted. Although progressive increase in tumor burden in lymph nodes and related structures can cause symptoms, many features of this disease are not correlated with bulk disease. Excessive fatigue may be related to anemia, but often is overwhelming even in the absence of a decrease in hemoglobin. The autoimmune complications may be the presenting manifestations of the disease, and can be troublesome to relate directly to CLL at an early stage of the illness. For example, patients may present with autoimmune thrombocytopenia that is initially thought to be idiopathic (i.e., immune thrombocytopenic purpura). Follow-up or extensive investigation may reveal a very small, but characteristic, CLL cell population in the circulation. Finally, some patients may present with recurrent infections and hypogammaglobulinemia at various stages in the course of the disease. Thus, normal immune cell function is disordered early in the course of the leukemia. It is important to realize that the autoimmune complications do not necessarily track with the bulk of disease in nodes and organs, and thus require specific treatment.

As the disease progresses, the genetic abnormalities may become substantially more complex. Patients may develop abnormalities of specific chromosomes (e.g., the deletion 17p−) or a mutation in p53, both of which confer a worse prognosis.[45] Malignant progression of the disease may be associated with an increasing number of prolymphocytes (prolymphocytic transformation of the CLL), or a frank Richter's transformation to a highly resistant large-cell lymphoma may dominate.[29,46,47] In fact, approximately 5–10% of patients with CLL will have a highly malignant transformation to a more aggressive lymphoid neoplastic disease as the terminal event.

In order to adequately follow patients with this disease, it is mandatory that the physician recognize the protean manifestations of the disease resulting from basic pathophysiologic deficits that are an integral part of this malignant disease. These patients have abnormalities of their immune system resulting in either infectious or secondary malignancies. For instance, patients with CLL have a significantly increased risk of basal cell and squamous cell cutaneous carcinomas. Paradoxically, they may have serious complications resulting from an overly vigorous, poorly controlled autoimmune process. The disease can invade retroperitoneal structures, lymph nodes, the spleen, and the liver. The bone marrow is frequently informative, either showing reduction in normal hematopoietic production or reflecting autoimmune complications ranging from absent red cell precursors (e.g., pure red cell aplasia either from autoimmune inhibition of normal red cell production or from concomitant parvoviral infection) to excessive numbers of megakaryocytes associated with antibody destruction of platelets.

CLINICAL FEATURES AND DIAGNOSIS

Confirming the Diagnosis

Many patients have no symptoms at the time of the diagnosis, but are diagnosed as having CLL on the basis of an abnormal laboratory test. Fatigue is the most common complaint of those presenting with symptoms, but they may also present with enlarged lymph nodes. The common clinical features of this disease are listed in Table 34–1.

The diagnostic work-up reveals an absolute lymphocytosis (>5000/μL), and the circulating leukemic cells are confirmed to be monoclonal by immunoglobulin staining. Although the diagnosis of CLL is suggested upon review of the peripheral blood smear consisting of small lymphocytes, confirmation of a monoclonal population of abnormal lymphocytes by flow cytometry is absolutely required. In fact, the diagnosis can be made by demonstrating a monoclonal population of leukemic cells bearing the characteristic immunophenotype of $CD5^{+}CD19^{+}CD23^{+}$ and weak CD20 positivity. In addition, CD79b and FMC7 are frequently weak to negative. Surface immunoglobulin is characteristically weakly positive as well.[28,49]

TABLE 34–1. Clinical Features of Chronic Lymphocytic Leukemia

Symptoms and Signs
No symptoms or signs of disease (30–50% of patients at presentation)
Fatigue (most common symptom either with or without anemia)
Organ enlargement (lymph nodes, splenomegaly, hepatomegaly)
Fever, night sweats, or weight loss
Complications
Frequent infections (most common cause of serious morbidity & death)
Dysregulated immune system (e.g., Evans's syndrome, hemolytic anemia & immune thrombocytopenia, paraneoplastic pemphigus, pure red cell aplasia)
Secondary malignancies
Transformation to high-grade hematologic malignancy (e.g., Richter's syndrome with large-cell lymphoma, CLL/prolymphocytic transformation)
Laboratory Features
Absolute lymphocytosis (>5000/μL)
Monoclonal population of lymphoid cells (either κ or λ light chains)
Hypogammaglobulinemia (about 60% of patients)
Bone marrow > 30% lymphoid cells on aspirate; biopsy will show nodular, interstitial or diffuse pattern of infiltration

Because there are no specific karyotypic abnormalities that are diagnostic of CLL, fluorescent in situ hybridization (FISH) studies can be useful in distinguishing other lymphoid malignancies that may masquerade as CLL. Specifically, FISH results showing t(14;18)(q32;q21) would be consistent with follicular lymphoma in a leukemic phase or t(11;14)(q13;q23) would be diagnostic of mantle cell lymphoma. Either of these clinical entities could be confused with CLL if the review of the peripheral smear was the sole diagnostic study performed.[28,50] Therefore, it is essential to immunophenotype the monoclonal cells, and to order FISH studies in some cases to establish the correct diagnosis.

Morphologic features of CLL reveal cells that are small, with scant cytoplasm and distinctive nuclear chromatin clumping or condensation; more than 10% lymphoid cells with nucleoli suggests the diagnosis of a prolymphocytic transformation from CLL. A diagnosis of primary de novo prolymphocytic leukemia can be suspected by review of the peripheral blood smear if the patient has more than 55% prolymphocytes associated with a high peripheral blood count and splenomegaly.[51] Nuclear clefts or other unusual cytologic features (e.g., lymphoplasmacytoid appearance) suggest an alternative diagnosis of lymphoid

TABLE 34–2. Diseases Mimicking CLL: Distinguishing Laboratory Features

Disease	Immunophenotype	FISH & Other Features*
CLL[†]	CD5$^+$, CD19$^+$, CD23$^+$, CD20^{+dim}, sIg^{+dim}, FMC7$^-$, CD79b weak or neg	del(13q14), del(11q22.3), del(17p13.1), or del(6q21). Trisomy 12q13 or normal
Mantle cell lymphoma	CD5$^+$, CD20$^{+bright}$, sIg$^{+bright}$, CD23$^-$, cyclin D1$^+$	t(11;14)(q13;q32)
PLL	CD5$^+$ (or neg), FMC7$^+$, sIg$^{+bright}$	t(11;14)(q13;q32), del(17p13.1) High peripheral lymphoid cell counts
HCL	CD5$^-$, CD11c$^{+bright}$, CD25$^+$, CD103$^+$, HML-1$^+$, B-ly7$^+$	No consistent cytogenetic abnormality. Low peripheral white cell count with absolute monocytopenia
HCL-V	Same as HCL except CD25$^-$	No consistent cytogenetic abnormality. High peripheral lymphoid cell counts; lymphoid cells have projections; may see monocytes
SLVL	CD5$^-$ (some +), CD11c+ (50% cases), CD25+ (25% cases); however, if CD25$^+$, usually neg for CD11c/103	del(13q14), trisomy 3. Splenomegaly common. Peripheral smear shows cells with projections
FCC lymphoma/leukemia	CD5$^-$, CD10$^+$, CD20$^+$	t(14;18)(q32;q21) Peripheral blood smear shows lymphoid cells with scant cytoplasm & nuclear clefts (buttock cells), bone marrow shows paratrabecular lymphoid infiltrates

*Fluorescent in situ hybridization showing the characteristic chromosomal abnormalities often observed in lymphoid malignancies.
†No cytogenetic abnormality is diagnostic for CLL, but the presence of the t(11;14) or cyclin D1 protein expression usually is diagnostic for mantle cell lymphoma.
Abbreviations: CLL, chronic lymphocytic leukemia; FCC, follicular center cell lymphoma/leukemia; HCL, hairy cell leukemia; HCL-V, hairy cell leukemia, variant form; PLL, prolymphocytic lymphoma; sIg, surface immunoglobulin expression; SLVL, splenic lymphoma with villous lymphocytes.

malignancy that can be further confirmed by flow cytometric immunophenotypic staining and FISH analysis. Immunophenotyping of peripheral blood is sensitive, and may also be used to identify minimal residual disease following effective therapy of CLL.[28] Furthermore, a small number of "normal" individuals have been identified with a monoclonal population of circulating cells with a CLL immunophenotype. This entity has been recognized in families of patients with CLL, and has been termed *monoclonal B-cell lymphocytosis*.[52] In Table 34–2, the distinguishing laboratory features of B-cell CLL are displayed in comparison with other diseases that mimic the clinical presentation of this disease.

Predicting the Prognosis from Laboratory Studies

Because the diagnosis of CLL can actually be established with peripheral blood studies confirming the presence of a characteristic monoclonal B-cell lymphocytosis, the use of additional laboratory studies may predict the clinical course and prognosis of the disease. Demonstration of additional markers by three-color flow cytometry (e.g., CD38 positivity in >20% of the circulating abnormal cells that also are CD5$^+$/CD19$^+$) identifies a patient with poorer prognosis.[27] Initially, it was proposed that demonstration of CD38 positivity identified the population of CLL patients who also were characterized as having the unmutated form of the Ig V_H gene.[7] Patients with an unmutated Ig V_H have a more aggressive course; however, demonstration of CD38 positivity has not been confirmed to identify the population of patients with unmutated Ig V_H gene.[53] Therefore, investigation of both CD38 positivity by flow cytometry and Ig V_H mutational status provides useful information regarding the projected aggressiveness of the clinical course.

Multiple studies from different laboratories have now confirmed the adverse prognostic significance of showing that the leukemic cells either express CD38 positivity or have an unmutated form of the Ig V_H gene.[7,8,54–56] The analysis of mutational status of the Ig V_H gene is more time consuming, but demonstration that there is hypermutation of the rearranged V_H gene paradoxically confers a better overall prognosis for disease course, response to therapy, and disease-free survival.[29]

Extensive work with FISH probes has also showed that more than 80% of patients with CLL have a cytogenetic abnormality.[15,50] Dohner and colleagues have established a hierarchy of abnormalities, with 17p–, 11q–, trisomy 12, normal cytogenetics, and 13q– representing progressively more favorable prognoses.[15] Furthermore, CLL patients with 6q– have more bulk disease, and may require therapy earlier than the other patient subsets.[57,58] Standard cytogenetics have been routinely attempted in many patients with this disease, but have been less informative considering that many of the leukemic cells arrested in G_0 are unlikely to undergo mitosis even in response to mitogens.

Recently, expression of ZAP-70 protein by Western analysis in leukemic cells from patients with CLL has been strongly correlated with Ig V_H mutational status.[9] There has been controversy when various methods are utilized to characterize the ZAP-70 expression, and this has been complicated by the expression of this protein

Box 34–1. Prognostic Features in Chronic Lymphocytic Leukemia

Classic Clinical Staging Systems

- Modified Rai or Binet Systems
- Bone marrow pattern of lymphoid cell infiltration (diffuse worse than nodular/interstitial)
- Increased number of prolymphocytes in peripheral blood
- Increased serum markers reflecting disease burden (lactate dehydrogenase, β_2-microglobulin, soluble CD23, and thymidine kinase)
- Lymphocyte doubling time (<6–12 months)

Additional Prognostic Features

- Chromosomal abnormalities: del(17p13.1); del (11q22.3); trisomy 12q13; normal cytogenetics, and del(13q14)

Mutation or deletion p53 gene

- High percentage of lymphoid cells positive for CD38 expression (should gate on CD5, CD19, and CD20 populations)
- Mutational status of Ig V_H genes (unmutated worse than mutated)
- ZAP-70 protein expression high in CLL cells (research test not yet validated by commercial laboratories)

A high-risk patient would have the following profile: unmutated Ig V_H gene; FISH demonstration of cells with either 17p deletion or 11q23 deletion; and cells highly positive for CD38 expression or for ZAP-70 protein expression. Because of the inability of different laboratories to reproduce similar results for ZAP-70 expression, this should not be used for clinical decision making in patients with CLL.

on normal T and natural killer cells.[59] Despite these caveats, several studies have confirmed that increased expression of ZAP-70 in peripheral blood mononuclear cells is associated with a worse outcome.[9–11] One study has associated increased expression of ZAP-70 protein with those patients having the cytogenetic categories with the worst prognosis (e.g., 6q−, 17p− or a mutation of p53, and 11q−).[10] Thus, there are many new molecular parameters that can be incorporated into an assessment of the prognosis of patients with CLL. In Box 34–1, the studies that have been identified to have prognostic significance for patients with CLL are outlined.

Demonstration that p53 protein in leukemic cells is abnormal has been correlated with outcome and response to standard therapy.[60] Patients harboring a deletion of 17p (by FISH) may have an absence of this protein that is critical for inducing apoptosis following therapy.[61,62] Furthermore, denaturing gradient gel electrophoresis analysis can identify patients with a potential mutation of the p53 gene that can be confirmed by DNA sequence analysis of exons 5 through 9.[62] Single-stranded conformational polymorphism or other techniques may also be utilized in segregating those patients that may have such a mutation in p53. Although analysis of p53 is not currently readily available in most clinical laboratories, increasing evidence supporting the importance of many of these prognostic studies is growing. Supplementation of the older clinical staging systems (e.g., Rai or Binet system) with modern molecular profiling will become increasing integrated into therapeutic decision making for this disease in the near future.[29]

Classic Clinical Staging Systems of Rai and Binet

For at least a quarter of a century, patients who were diagnosed with CLL were staged according to the clinical staging criteria published by Drs. Rai and Binet. Both systems were based on extent of bulk disease and bone marrow involvement, with either anemia or thrombocytopenia being associated with the worst projected clinical outcomes.[64,65] Dr. Rai's classification was used more frequently in North America, and was revised in an effort to simplify the system.[66] Dr. Binet's classification was used more often in Europe, and both are clinically quite useful at the time of initial diagnosis. Considering that many patients are now diagnosed earlier with the increasing use of flow cytometry, the older classifications would identify many new patients with either stages I or II, A or B. The newer molecular studies will hopefully enable accurate risk stratification for patients at an earlier stage of the disease process. As treatments improve, this assignment based on risk may identify a group of patients who would benefit from experimental therapies at an earlier time point. Studies are under discussion to develop an optimal strategy for utilizing these newer prognostic tools for improving patient outcomes.

Bone Marrow Biopsy and Aspiration

A bone marrow biopsy and aspirate are not required to establish the diagnosis of CLL. Although prognostic information may be obtained in conjunction with this invasive study, it may be best to perform the biopsy and aspirate before initiating therapy rather than simply as a component of the diagnostic work-up.[31] Many studies in the past have correlated a diffuse pattern of involvement with a worst prognosis.[29] Certainly, interstitial or nodular leukemic involvement of the marrow may be associated with a better overall prognosis.

In contrast, performance of a bone marrow examination before initiating therapy for the CLL is very valuable. For example, anemia is a common reason for initiating therapy. Multiple mechanisms potentially are responsible for anemia in the setting of this disease. Patients with anemia should be approached in a very basic manner to define whether the reduction in hemoglobin is related to decreased production or increased peripheral destruction. In many situations, there may be simultaneous causes for anemia. Prior to starting therapy, the patient should have a reticulocyte count and an examination of the peripheral blood smear. In a patient with an elevated reticulocyte count, the observation of spherocytes prompts a Coombs test to search for the presence of autoimmune destruction of red blood cells. If an increased destruction of red cells is suggested, then appropriate immune suppression is initiated.[37] Furthermore, a bone marrow examination may reveal a concomitant increase in the number of megakaryocytes. This finding should raise consideration of simultaneous autoimmune destruction of platelets, and the diagnosis of Evans's syndrome, in these patients.[37]

The bone marrow biopsy permits an assessment of bone marrow cellularity at baseline before starting therapy with chemotherapeutic agents. Considering the impact of combined therapy with fludarabine and other cytotoxic chemotherapy, a cumulative effect on bone marrow cellularity becomes an important component for monitoring the number of planned courses of therapy.[67,68] Understanding the status of bone marrow iron stores and fibrosis can also be important in predicting the tolerability of chemotherapy. Patients have been identified either with underlying myelodysplasia or myelofibrosis as the predominant cause for anemia in the setting of CLL, in whom the leukemia was not the sole cause for the reduction in peripheral blood counts.[67,70,71] In those patients, the reduction in hemoglobin and platelets could be made worse by assuming that the reduced counts were simply related to progressive infiltration with leukemic cells. Finally, patients with CLL are also subject to pure red cell aplasia secondary either to autoimmune impairment of red cell production or to infection with B19 parvovirus.[37,72,73] Failure to understand the underlying mechanism for bone marrow failure can result in clinical deterioration if chemotherapy is inappropriately initiated as a therapeutic choice. Therapeutic approaches to treating parvoviral infection with intravenous immunoglobulin have resulted in hematologic improvement in those patients whose red cell aplasia was a result of this viral infection. The process of using a bone marrow examination to identify the underlying pathogenesis for deterioration in blood counts is a wise investment in therapeutic planning for patients with this disease.

In performing a diagnostic bone marrow aspiration and biopsy before initiating therapy, it may be necessary to plan for additional studies (e.g., culture of the marrow or flow cytometry) depending upon the clinical situation. In changing therapy or re-initiating therapy following a hiatus from prior therapy, it is wise to consider a follow-up bone marrow examination before making major changes in therapy. Many patients have experienced severe bone marrow hypoplasia as a result of the initial chemotherapy, and this information becomes critically important before embarking upon a new course of therapy with new therapy that may further reduce the bone marrow function.

DIFFERENTIAL DIAGNOSIS

Establishing the diagnosis of B-cell CLL requires review of a peripheral blood smear in conjunction with flow cytometric immunophenotyping. In addition, documentation of a restricted monoclonal population of B-cells expressing predominantly either λ or κ light chains is essential.[28,31,49] The characteristic immunophenotypic profile identified in Table 34–2 can be supplemented by FISH studies to demonstrate that cytogenetic abnormalities consistent with CLL are also present. There is no specific cytogenetic abnormality that will permit an unequivocal diagnosis of CLL alone. Several of the entities listed in Table 34–2 may mimic the clinical and laboratory presentation of CLL. In Figure 34–1, the morphology of CLL is presented along with examples of both mantle cell lymphoma and prolymphocytic leukemia as two entities that could be confused with CLL. It is critically important to identify whether the patient has true CLL or one of the diverse forms of lymphoid malignancy that could masquerade as this disease. The projected adverse outcome and necessary therapy for the other diseases mandate that they be distinguished from CLL.

In individual cases, there may be difficulty in finally deciding whether a patient has a blastic form of mantle cell leukemia or CLL. Identification of the characteristic t(11;14) translocation by FISH probe or the finding of cyclin D1 expression in an abnormal lymphoid infiltrate would be consistent with a diagnosis of mantle cell lymphoma in a leukemic phase, and this distinction would markedly change the projected outcome and therapeutic approach. A decision as to whether a patient has CLL, CLL in transformation to prolymphocytic leukemia, or true prolymphocytic leukemia makes a huge difference with respect to projected survival and response to therapy.

In general, the observation of greater than 55% prolymphocytes on a peripheral blood smear of a newly diagnosed patient favors a diagnosis of de novo B-cell prolymphocytic leukemia.[51] B-cell prolymphocytic leukemia is characterized by large cells often displaying a single prominent nucleolus. This aggressive disease presents with a very high white blood cell count, massive splenomegaly, and very little peripheral adenopathy. The leukemic cells from a patient with B-cell prolymphocytic leukemia may be negative for CD5 and positive for FMC7 and CD22, thus distinguishing them from B-cell CLL.[74]

Two additional forms of leukemia may be confused with CLL. Both splenic lymphoma with villous lymphocytes (SLVL) and the rare variant form of hairy cell leukemia (HCL-V) may present with elevated white blood cell counts associated with circulating lymphoid-appearing cells.[49] Typical hairy cell leukemia usually presents with a low peripheral blood count and pancytopenia.[75–77] Patients with typical hairy cell leukemia have circulating cells with hair-like projections and absolute monocytopenia.[28] In contrast, in both SLVL and HCL-V, the malig-

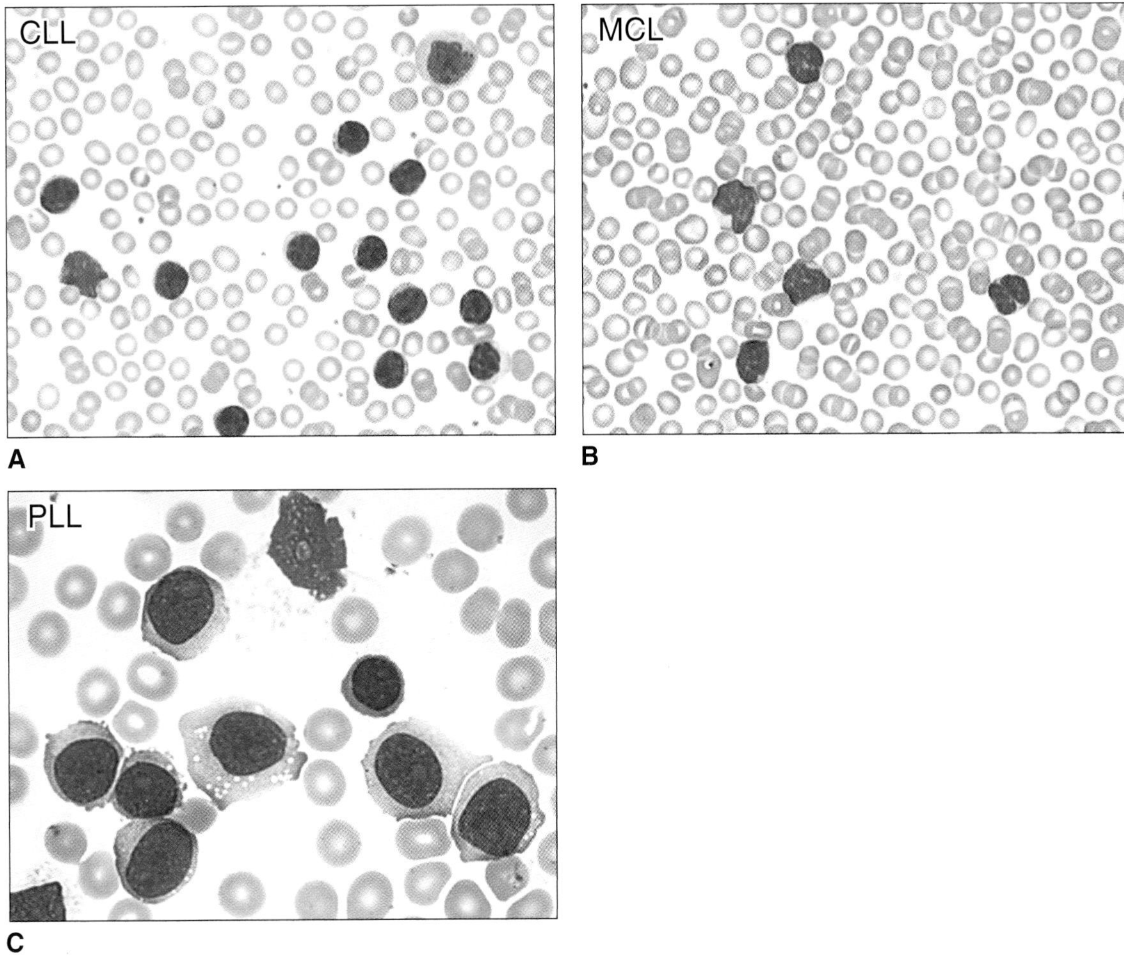

Figure 34–1. Distinguishing CLL from mantle cell lymphoma and prolymphocytic leukemia: the peripheral blood smear.

nant cell will have cytoplasmic projections but the immunophenotype is clearly different from that of true hairy cell leukemia. With typical hairy cell leukemia, the malignant cells have the characteristic immunophenotype: $CD5^{-}CD11c^{+}CD25^{+}CD103^{+}$. In SLVL, the malignant cell is usually $CD5^{-}$, but may be positive in a minority of cases.[78] The cells may be confused with hairy cell leukemia and be positive for CD11c and CD25. However, most of the $CD25^{+}$ cells do not coexpress CD11c and CD103. Finally, patients harboring HCL-V may present with a high peripheral white blood cell count with cells that are lymphoid in appearance and have a nucleolus. The cells are bright for $CD11c^{+}$, but are negative for CD5 and CD25. Therapeutic options for SLVL are quite different than for CLL, and HCL-V does not respond well to therapy. In particular, the response is far less gratifying than for typical hairy cell leukemia.[79]

Follicular center cell lymphoma with a leukemic phase is associated with circulating lymphoid cells that are $CD5^{-}$, and may be $CD10^{+}$.[49] Presenting clinical features of this indolent lymphoma may masquerade as CLL, and thus it is important to include this entity in the differential diagnosis as well. The obvious reason for specifically identifying the diagnosis of CLL apart from these other entities relates directly to the very practical need to define optimal therapy and prognosis.

TREATMENT

As shown in Box 34–2, the general indications used in making a decision to treat involve both clinical judgment and experience. Presently, the treatment available for CLL is not curative. Consequently, there should be a thoughtful reason and plan identified for those patients who will be subjected to the multiple risks associated with treatment. Patients are usually required to be symptomatic from the leukemia before instituting therapy. In general, the development of either anemia or progressive thrombocytopenia is an indication for starting therapy.[48] It is extremely important to understand the underlying pathologic mechanisms responsible for either anemia or thrombocytopenia. Defining whether the predominant mechanism is either decreased production or increased peripheral destruction is essential in selecting the optimal therapeutic approach.

If the anemia or thrombocytopenia reflects increasing bone marrow infiltration, then selection of effective chemotherapy is appropriate. If the mechanism for lowered counts is related to autoimmune destruction of the cellular elements, then effective immunosuppressive therapy with either prednisone (e.g., 1 mg/kg/day) or another agent (e.g., cyclosporine) is required.[37]

Box 34–2. Therapy of CLL: Making the Decision of "When to Treat"

Asymptomatic Patients with Low-Stage Disease

Observation with routine physical examinations and serial blood studies

Symptomatic Patients Who Should Be Considered for Treatment

- Systemic symptoms: weight loss, fever, night sweats, and extreme fatigue related to disease
- Bulky disease: massive or rapidly progressive splenomegaly or lymphadenopathy
- High proliferative features (e.g., LDT* < 6 months)
- Progressive bone marrow failure (e.g., anemia with hemoglobin < 11 gm/dL; or thrombocytopenia with platelets <100,000/μL)
- Autoimmune phenomena (i.e., unresponsive to adequate trial with steroids)
- Lymphocyte count in excess of certain numbers depending upon clinical judgment (e.g., >300,000/μL)[†]

*LDT, lymphocyte doubling time.

[†]Some patients have had serious consequences of leukostasis with extremely high peripheral counts, but these data are somewhat anecdotal. Initiation of treatment in patients with very high absolute lymphocyte counts depends upon clinical judgment of the physician considering the patient's risks for vascular compromise (e.g., either pulmonary or central nervous system symptoms). Frequently, there are other reasons for considering initiation of therapy in patients with extremely high lymphocyte counts.

In patients with rapid lymphocyte doubling times, therapy should be contemplated. Patients whose absolute lymphocyte count doubles in less than 6 months usually will require therapy reflecting an increasing leukemic burden.[48] These patients often will develop a simultaneous progressive increase in lymphadenopathy or organomegaly (i.e., splenomegaly), and the laboratory surveillance of increasing absolute lymphocyte count will generally precede the other more ominous findings of decreasing blood counts or discomfort associated with increasing bulk disease. In fact, either symptomatic lymphadenopathy or organomegaly is also an indication to initiate systemic therapy.[31,80,81] Patients often experience symptoms of night sweats, low-grade fever, and increasing fatigue as the disease enters a phase requiring therapy.

Many physicians and their patients focus intently on the absolute lymphocyte count. Certainly, these counts will fluctuate, and patients need to be reassured that minor changes should not be cause for alarm. Many patients have a gradual, but progressive increase in the absolute lymphocyte count. Although hyperleukocytosis is clearly harmful in acute leukemia, patients will usually tolerate counts in the 100,000 range quite well. There may be other concomitant laboratory abnormalities requiring therapy in those patients whose white blood cell count is now at the 100,000/μL level. Specifically, some of these patients may require therapy related directly to anemia or progressive thrombocytopenia. However, some patients with CLL do indeed experience serious consequences when the absolute lymphocyte count exceeds a certain level. Although that level has not been rigorously defined, patients whose white count exceeds 300,000–500,000/μL have developed symptoms of vascular compromise (e.g., pulmonary leukostasis, priapism, or stroke).[82] Therefore, the physician's clinical judgment must be exercised when deciding upon therapy based solely on the absolute lymphocyte count.

In selection of therapy, many factors must be considered. In older patients requiring control of bulk disease or progressive elevation of their counts, the use of either chlorambucil or cyclophosphamide has been effective.[31,83] For initial therapy, these agents usually produce partial remissions and not complete responses. In 1988, Grever and colleagues reported that fludarabine was useful in achieving responses in heavily treated patients.[84] Subsequently, a large multi-institutional prospective randomized study demonstrated that front-line use of fludarabine (25 mg/m^2/day for 5 days every month for 4–6 months) was associated with a higher complete response rate and some improvement in time to re-treatment compared to chlorambucil.[85] Additional comparative studies showed that fludarabine was more effective than combination chemotherapy in the same clinical setting. Consequently, many physicians now employ fludarabine as front-line therapy.

Several studies show that combined therapy using either fludarabine and simultaneous Rituxan or fludarabine and cyclophosphamide produce a higher complete response rate than fludarabine alone.[68,86–88] Byrd and colleagues showed that the combined use of fludarabine and Rituxan was superior to the serial use of fludarabine followed by Rituxan.[89,90] The triple combination of fludarabine, cyclophosphamide, and Rituxan produced the highest complete response rate yet.[87] However, this study needs to be confirmed before this combination becomes the standard of care considering the serious toxicity encountered with these agents. There are suggestions that the time to treatment failure is prolonged while a higher number of patients achieve a complete response.

Consequently, investigations continue to define newer therapies that may be effective in dealing with specific forms of CLL that are resistant to the purine analogue combinations (e.g., fludarabine, cyclophosphamide, and Rituxan). Campath, a monoclonal antibody directed against CD52, has been effective in reducing residual bone marrow involvement following standard chemotherapy. It is encouraging that this agent can be effective in patients who have an abnormality in the p53 protein within the leukemic cell clone.[91] It is disappointing that this agent is less effective in patients with resistant bulky disease, and that there are serious immunosuppressive consequences following the administration of Campath.

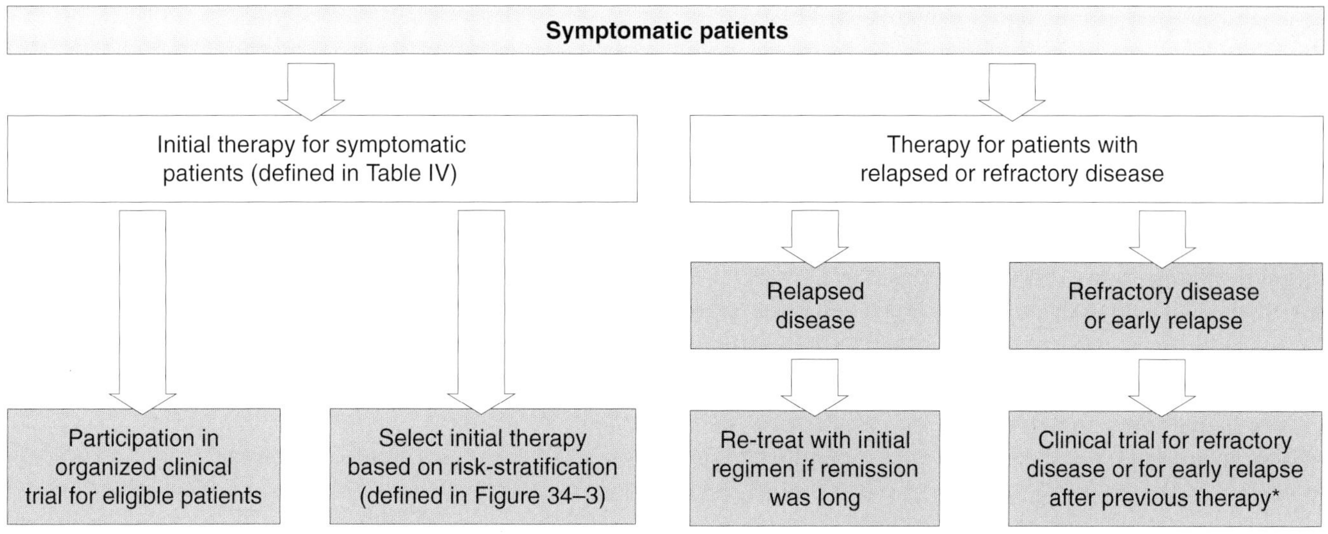

*Consider prior to clinical findings (eg. patients with bulky disease do not respond well to Alemtuzumab, or patients with mutations or deletion of p53 will not likely respond with a durable remission to Fludarabine alone).

Figure 34–2. Making a current therapeutic decision for all patients with CLL.

Another exciting new agent, Flavopiridol, is under early investigation in patients with refractory disease.[92] It is encouraging that this agent also is effective irrespective of the status of the p53 protein in the leukemic cells. Although this drug can produce an overall 42% response rate in heavily treated patients, there are major challenges associated with the administration of this agent, which is still under active development. Based upon a pharmacologically designed schedule for drug administration, Flavopiridol has produced fatal tumor cell lysis in a small number of patients. Encouraging results have evolved as extensive preparation for managing aggressive tumor lysis has been effective in protecting these patients. Furthermore, the responses observed are quite durable, and have occurred in those patients predicted to be nonresponders (i.e., patients with deletions in 17p and/or mutations in p53).[93] More work will clearly be required before this agent can be incorporated into the normal therapeutic strategy. However, it could provide a hopeful approach for increasing the number of patients achieving a complete remission following standard induction chemotherapy. In Figure 34–2, a schematic approach in recommending current therapeutic intervention for all patients with CLL is outlined.

Bone marrow transplantation using either allogeneic or autologous stem cell sources has been pursued in limited locations since the late 1980s.[94] In the majority of successful cases, patients have been younger. Although the incidence of graft-versus-host disease (GVHD) may be less than anticipated, there is still a high mortality associated with this approach. The lower than anticipated incidence of GVHD may relate to the extensive prior use of fludarabine in treating these patients.

Fludarabine is now being explored as an integral part of the immunosuppressive preparation for receiving an allogeneic transplant.[95] As a potent immunosuppressive agent, there appears to be a direct impact of this agent on the frequency of severe GVHD in patients with previously treated CLL. This phenomenon still requires explanation. Studies have been reported showing that several purine nucleoside analogues (including pentostatin) may reduce the severity of GVHD subsequent to transplantation.[96] Many older patients have been previously excluded from the trials of stem cell transplantation, so the full impact of this approach for those with this disease will require much more work.

SUPPORTIVE CARE AND LONG-TERM MANAGEMENT

Dealing with Risks and Prevention of Infection

The major complications associated with this disease are related to infection, autoimmunity, and secondary malignancies. The underlying cause of increased risk for infection is complex. Patients with this disease are often neutropenic and have progressive hypogammaglobulinemia.[31,97] There are intrinsic abnormalities of the immune effector cells at the time of diagnosis, and the treatment of the disease further impairs normal immune cell function in these patients.[31]

The most frequent infectious organisms are bacterial, often reflecting those pathogens that rely on immunoglobulin for effective infection control. Thus, *Streptococcus pneumoniae*, *Staphylococcus aureus*, and *Haemophilus influenzae* complicate mucosal surface infectious sites.[98] Pneumonia and sinusitis are frequently encountered. In addition, gram-negative bacterial infections can complicate urinary tract infections. *Escherichia coli*, *Klebsiella pneumoniae*, and *Pseudomonas aeruginosa* may be involved. Infection in general needs to be addressed promptly, and treatment may need to be extended in duration depending upon clinical features of the illness. Patients who are neutropenic may require treatment for a longer period of time than those with normal hematologic parameters.

Despite the difficulty in mounting a vigorous immune response to vaccines, patients should be offered an annual "flu shot."[31,98] In addition, these patients should receive Pneumovax to reduce the risk of a fatal pneumonia.[31] These vaccinations should be initiated as early in the course of the illness as possible, because the immune responsiveness of the patients will decline with time.[98] Patients may benefit from administration of intravenous immunoglobulin on a monthly basis, but this intervention has been more beneficial for those with frequent moderate infections rather than in preventing life-threatening infections. Administration of intravenous gamma globulin is both expensive and inconvenient, and consequently its use should be fully justified by the previous clinical course of the patient.

Patients with CLL are more vulnerable to atypical infectious organisms. Viral infections may be more dangerous in these patients, and those who have been treated with chemotherapy or antibody therapy may be particularly at risk of serious viral infection.[31] For example, patients developing varicella-zoster should be promptly and aggressively treated with antiviral therapy. In patients who have had prior therapy with fludarabine or alemtuzumab, cytomegalovirus should be considered in the presence of fever. Aggressive diagnostic studies to confirm a cytomegalovirus infection should be pursued if it is suspected. Subsequently, initiation of specific antiviral therapy should be instituted when the suspicion is high.

Opportunistic organisms may be more problematic in those patients who have previously received a purine nucleoside analogue in combination with additional agents. Furthermore, it is critically important to remember that the T-cell defect that follows a purine nucleoside analogue may persist for a year or more.[99,100] Therefore, patients who have received a purine nucleoside analogue (e.g., fludarabine) and then are treated with combined chemotherapy, steroids, or other immunosuppressive therapy are candidates for prophylaxis for both viral diseases and *Pneumocystis jiroveci (P. carinii)*. Therefore, many of these patients require prophylactic sulfamethoxazole/trimethoprim (or a substitute if sensitive to sulfa) and acyclovir.[101] Many opportunities exist for further defining the optimal regimen of antibacterial or other agents in these patients. Duration of such therapy is currently based upon clinical judgment, and evidence-based decisions would obviously be better. It is possible to at least monitor the recovery of T-cell numbers, but the functional assessment of their effectiveness is not yet routinely achievable.

The use of granulocyte colony-stimulating factor as adjunctive therapy in actively infected patients may be justified for overwhelming bacterial or fungal infections. Many of the patients who are most at risk for infection following myelosuppressive chemotherapy are compromised with respect to their ability to respond to these agents because of reduced normal bone marrow function. The combined use of fludarabine and cyclophosphamide appears to have a marked effect on the functional reserve of the bone marrow. This effect is often cumulative, and it is recommended that serial bone marrow biopsies be considered for those patients receiving more than 4–6 months of combined therapy to avoid severe depletion of bone marrow reserve. In patients receiving combinations of these agents, granulocyte colony-stimulating factor is often included as part of the regimen.[86,102]

The causes for anemia in patients with CLL are quite complex. For this reason, it is important to understand the basic mechanism(s) underlying each individual case. Consequently, a bone marrow biopsy with aspiration, including an iron stain, may be useful prior to initiating therapy for the leukemia. Establishing the basic cause of the anemia is essential for effective therapy. For example, patients with an associated iron deficiency anemia will also require a meticulous search for occult gastrointestinal bleeding. Considering the increased risk for common solid tumor malignancies in this patient population, strict adherence to principles of understanding the underlying mechanisms for symptoms and signs becomes paramount.[31]

In patients with acquired autoimmune hemolytic anemia, it is often advisable to control the active hemolysis with immunosuppressive therapy before initiating chemotherapy.[37] In this same group of individuals, autoimmune destruction of platelets may require an adequate course of immunosuppressive therapy. A common error involves premature discontinuation of immunosuppressive therapy with relapse of increased peripheral destruction. Although it is important to avoid undue immunosuppression, it is equally important to taper the doses of steroids following successful control of the destructive process.

Immunosuppressive therapy may be required for pure red cell aplasia that occurs in a subset of these patients. It is also important to search for parvoviral infection as an underlying cause of the anemia in those patients who have a picture compatible with red cell aplasia. Often, parvovirus is suspected when a marked paucity of red blood cell precursors is accompanied by occasional giant pronormoblasts.[103] Careful review of the bone marrow by the treating hematologist is frequently very insightful, because many reports are simply returned with a statement indicating massive involvement of the bone marrow with CLL.

In patients who appear to have increased peripheral destruction of platelets, antiplatelet antibodies may be helpful. However, close inspection of the bone marrow to assess the megakaryocytic mass will be very helpful in evaluating the underlying basis for thrombocytopenia. Careful surveillance for evidence of immune destruction of all cellular elements is essential for those patients being treated with purine nucleoside analogues. For example, patients have developed a very aggressive autoimmune destructive process involving either red cells or platelets while receiving these agents. In fact, patients have also been observed to develop an autoimmune neutropenia associated with delayed granulocyte recovery following fludarabine.[104] Several of these patients have been reported to show a maturational arrest, often at the myelocyte stage, with delayed granulocyte recovery that can be quite prolonged.

Role of the Internist

Prompt and meticulous attention to prevention and treatment of infection in the patient population with CLL is mandatory. If access to the hematologist is limited, each patient should have a well-informed general internist who is readily accessible. In addition, this physician should ensure that there is meticulous surveillance for secondary malignancies.[105–107] Patients should be strongly encouraged to discontinue smoking, and to maintain the usual activities recommended for early diagnosis (e.g., colonoscopy, mammography, routine skin inspection for cutaneous malignancies). Careful observation of symptoms such as increasing fatigue or weight loss should be vigorously pursued. In 5–10% of patients with CLL, there will be a malignant transformation to a more aggressive lymphoma.[46] Patients with weight loss, night sweats, and increasing adenopathy should be considered for biopsy of suspicious tissue to ensure that Richter's transformation has not occurred. Standard chemotherapy for CLL is usually not effective in the management of these patients with aggressive malignant transformation. Thus, therapeutic decisions will be based upon accurate diagnostic identification of the histopathology in specific malignant transformed sites. Patient participation in ongoing research protocols will hopefully improve this grave situation.

An equally important component of supportive care includes dealing with the patient and family concerns associated with a life-threatening chronic disease. Most patients are reassured by an honest, caring physician who takes adequate time to explain changing laboratory parameters. Patients have increasing access to information on the Internet, and often come prepared to ask sophisticated questions relating to prognosis and treatment. In selecting the newer molecular prognostic studies for the individual patient, it will be important to assess the patient's preparedness to deal with the data. If the patient clearly wants this information, it is important to be responsive. However, it is important to understand the patient whose chronic disease will be complicated immensely by the nonjudicious disclosure of information predicting a poor prognosis when little can be done currently to change the course of the illness.

Attention to anxiety in patients and those who care for them is paramount. The diagnosis of this disease may adversely impact on job opportunities and many of life's decisions. The importance of being an informed and concerned listener is matched by the need to attend urgently to the physical dangers associated with the disease (e.g., infection, immunosuppression, and progressive bulk disease).

PROGNOSIS

In assessing a new patient, it is advisable to utilize the standard clinical staging systems outlined here in combination with the newer molecular studies listed in Box 34–1. Although we have decades of data to validate the outcome of patients assigned to specific stages of the disease (e.g., using modified Rai staging or Binet's system), extensive data will soon emerge to further refine the prognostic information evolving from the newer studies. In addition, it will continue to be advisable to obtain a bone marrow aspiration and biopsy before initiating therapy for CLL because this will yield important information about mechanisms of abnormal laboratory studies as well as providing useful information about prognosis. However, it is not currently necessary to obtain a bone marrow study at the time of initial diagnosis unless therapy is being considered.

In Figure 34–3, a proposed strategy for incorporating clinical and molecular studies is presented to enhance the utilization of the prognostic data to plan a course of action for the individual patient. Improvement in therapy will result from diligence and persistence in conducting well-designed clinical trials. Consequently, the natural history of this incurable malignant disease may yield better outcomes following improvement in therapy similar to the encouraging story observed over the past 2 decades for hairy cell leukemia. The introduction of the purine nucleoside analogues enabled the achievement of a substantial number of complete remissions, and this accomplishment has had a very favorable impact on the outcome of the disease for those patients.

HAIRY CELL LEUKEMIA: A SUCCESS STORY

Approximately four and a half decades ago, Bouroncle and colleagues described the clinical manifestations of a relatively rare hematologic disorder initially termed *leukemic reticuloendotheliosis.*[76] This malignant disease, later called hairy cell leukemia, had a marked male predominance, and was most often observed in elderly patients. The presenting symptoms and clinical signs were most often attributable to bone marrow failure and infection. Patients often had neutropenia and an absolute monocytopenia. Impaired immunity resulted in very severe opportunistic infections complicating the course of a fatal disease that responded very poorly to existing chemotherapy. Most patients had splenectomy as the sole therapeutic approach, resulting in transient improvement in hematologic parameters. Following decades of attempts to improve therapy, there was little to offer the patient with progressive disease.[78] In the mid-1980s, the median survival was still approximately 4–5 years.

Early observations by Spiers and colleagues in 1984 showed that patients could achieve a complete remission with a novel inhibitor of adenosine deaminase (pentostatin).[108] Others had observed responses with this agent in patients with CLL, and had also confirmed these original responses in hairy cell leukemia. In fact, Kraut and colleagues reported that low-dose pentostatin (deoxycoformycin) induced complete remissions in over 90% of patients with hairy cell leukemia.[109] In 1990, Piro and colleagues reported that 11 of 12 patients with hairy cell leukemia achieved a complete remission with another purine nucleoside analogue (cladribine or 2-chlorodeoxyadenosine).[110] Thus, two new highly effective agents completely changed the ability to treat patients with this fatal form of chronic leukemia.

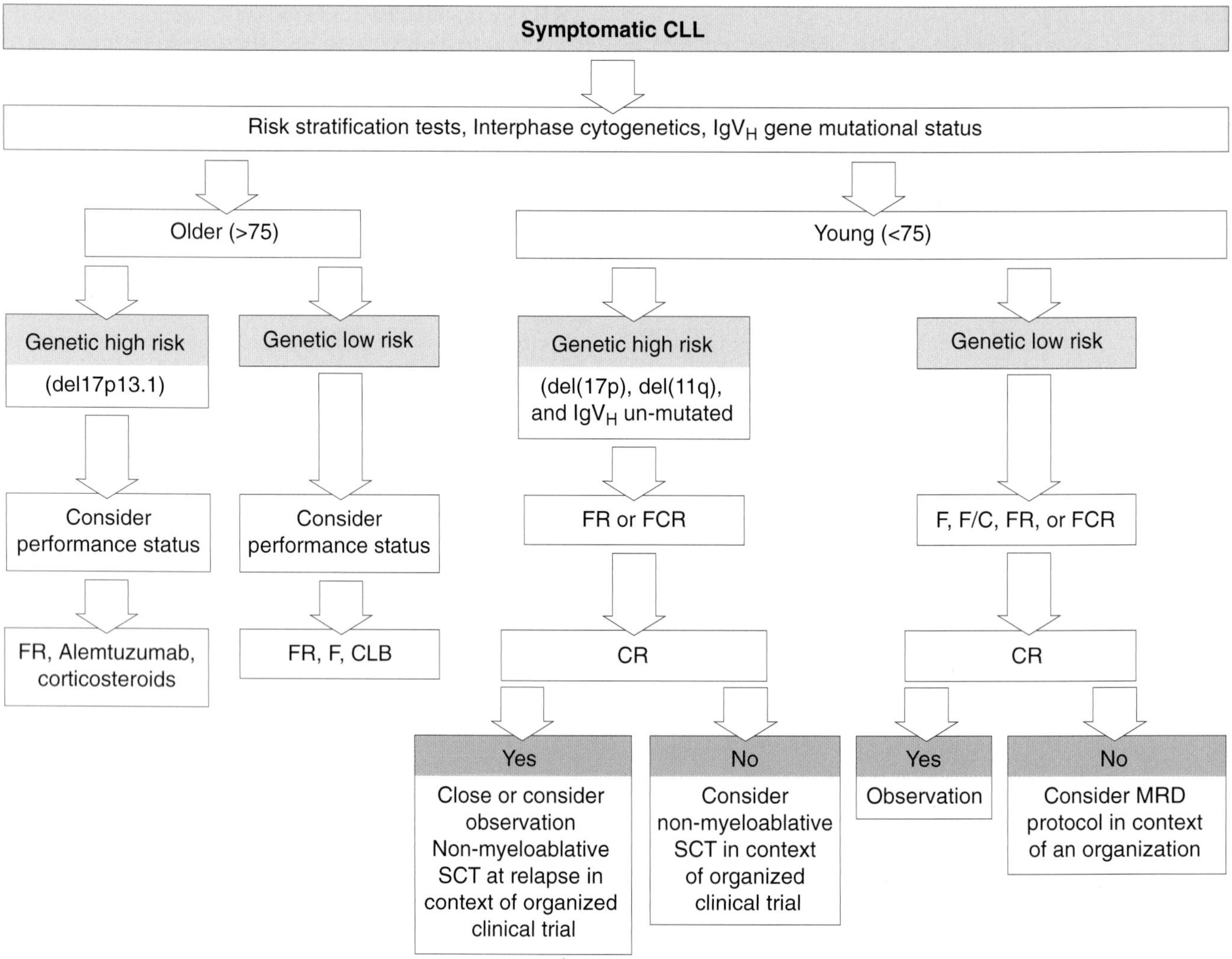

KEY

F = Fludarabine
FC = Fludarabine plus Cyclophosphamide
FR = Fludarabine plus Rituximab
FCR = Fludarabine plus Cyclophosphamide and Rituximab
CLB = Chlorambucil
MRD = Minimal residual disease
SCT = Stem cell transplant

Figure 34–3. Incorporating clinical and laboratory facts to establish the prognosis and plan of action for patients with CLL.

Long-term follow-up of patients with hairy cell leukemia treated with either pentostatin or cladribine have produced outstanding results. Most patients who achieved a complete remission are long-term survivors.[111–113] Patients who have successfully achieved a complete remission may live as long as those who are age-matched controls. In those patients with a complete clinical remission who are carefully examined, residual hairy cell leukemia can be found. In patients who show progression of disease, repeat therapy with the initial purine nucleoside has resulted in successful remission. In those patients who failed to respond, recent evidence has shown variable responses to rituximab.[114,115] New therapeutic strategies for patients with hairy cell leukemia need to be pursued. Some investigators have shown that CD52 expression occurs,[116] and this raises the question of the potential for using the monoclonal antibody Campath-1H in this setting. Considering the impaired immune system associated with the underlying disease and the complications resulting from prior exposure to purine nucleoside analogues, the use of this agent will need to be carefully monitored because of the risk of infection. All of these considerations focus upon the need to continue clinical research in an effort to continuously improve our treatment for these chronic forms of leukemia. Certainly, the substantial advancements made in treating hairy cell leukemia should provide encouragement to both patients with CLL and their physicians that similar progress will be made in this disease as well.[78]

Current Controversies & Future Considerations

Chronic Lymphocytic Leukemia

- Clinical investigations are being designed to employ molecular and clinical prognostic parameters to guide risk-stratified therapeutic decisions.
- Validation of prognostic parameters with clinical response to therapy and outcomes will be required.
- Clinical trials to explore early intervention for patients with high-risk CLL will require careful follow-up and promising new therapies.
- New drug discovery and development efforts to circumvent mechanisms of resistance are needed.
- Exploration of novel therapies to enhance the achievement of molecular remissions will need to be carefully pursued within the context of organized clinical trials.
- New therapeutic strategies with less intrinsic immune suppression are needed.

Suggested Readings*

Byrd JC, Peterson BL, Morrison VA, et al: Randomized Phase 2 study of fludarabine with concurrent versus sequential treatment with rituximab in symptomatic, untreated patients with B-cell chronic lymphocytic leukemia: results from Cancer and Leukemia Group B 9712 (CALGB 9712). Blood 101:6–14, 2003.

Byrd JC, Rai KR, Sausville EA, Grever MR: Old and new therapies in chronic lymphocytic leukemia: now is the time for a reassessment of therapeutic goals. Semin Oncol 25:65–74, 1998.

Chiorazzi N, Rai KR, Ferrarini M: Mechanisms of Disease: Chronic lymphocytic leukemia. N Engl J Med 352:804–815, 2005.

Diehl L, Ketchum L: Autoimmune disease and chronic lymphocytic leukemia: autoimmune hemolytic anemia, pure red cell aplasia, and autoimmune thrombocytopenia. Semin Oncol 25:80–97, 1998.

Dohner H, Stilgenbauer S, Benner A, et al: Genomic aberrations and survival in chronic lymphocytic leukemia. N Engl J Med 343:1910–1916, 2000.

Full references for this chapter can be found on accompanying CD-ROM.

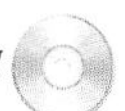

CHAPTER 35

Hairy Cell Leukemia

J. C. Cawley, MBChB, MD, PhD, FRCP, FRCPath, F Med Sci

KEY POINTS

Hairy Cell Leukemia

Diagnosis

- Pancytopenia and isolated splenomegaly in the absence of liver disease suggest hairy cell leukemia.
- Identification of typical hairy cells in the blood makes the diagnosis.
- Demonstration of tartrate-resistant isoenzyme 5 of acid phosphatase (TRAP) in hairy cells, a typical malignant-cell immunophenotype, and a fibrotic-infiltrated marrow confirm the diagnosis.
- Differential diagnosis includes variant-form hairy cell leukemia, splenic lymphoma with villous lymphocytes, and other marginal zone proliferations.

Treatment

- Asymptomatic patients without significant cytopenias should be left untreated.
- Symptomatic patients with significant cytopenias need therapy.
- Purine analogues are the first-line drugs.
- Chlorodeoxyadenosine and deoxycoformycin are comparably effective.
- Rituximab is now second-line therapy.

INTRODUCTION

Definition

Hairy-cell leukemia is a clonal proliferation of pathognomonic hairy cells that infiltrate the red pulp of the spleen and the bone marrow, and causing the splenomegaly and peripheral cytopenias so distinctive of the disease.

History

Although the disease may have been described earlier, it was the report of Bouroncle, Wiseman, and Doan in 1958 that clearly established hairy cell leukemia as a distinct entity (at the time called leukemic reticuloendotheliosis). For years, the disease attracted attention because of uncertainty about the nature of the diagnostic hairy cells, now clearly identified as mature B cells. More recently, the sensitivity of hairy cell leukemia to interferon and nucleosides generated further interest. Currently, the major issues are the precise nature of the malignant cells, the underlying oncogenic event(s), and the treatment of patients resistant to nucleoside therapy.

EPIDEMIOLOGY AND RISK FACTORS

The incidence of hairy cell leukemia is similar in Europe and the United States, about 3 cases per 1 million population per year. The mean age at presentation is approximately 50 years, with no marked difference between men and women. The male/female ratio is approximately 4:1. Hairy cell leukemia occurs in many different ethnic groups and has a very wide geographic distribution. However, typical hairy cell leukemia is rare in Japan.

A number of possible environment risks have been identified in epidemiologic studies, including exposures to benzene, agricultural chemicals, and radiation.[1] However, none of these associations is particularly convincing, and the cause of the disease remains unknown.

Fifteen patients with familial hairy cell leukemia have now been described.[2,3] There is no strong association with any specific human lymphocyte antigen type, and the significance of these rare familial cases is difficult to assess.

PATHOPHYSIOLOGY

The malignant hairy cell is central to the pathophysiology of hairy cell leukemia. The hairy cell is a form of highly activated clonal memory B cell[4,5] (Table 35–1). Microarray analysis has shown that hairy cells have the gene signature of memory cells,[5] a conclusion consistent with earlier observation that hairy cells are often class-switched[6] and immunoglobulin V_H hypermutated.[7]

The specific oncogenic event(s) in hairy cell leukemia is(are) still unknown but are likely to be, at least partly, responsible for the cells' highly activated phenotype. There is no consistent karyotypic abnormality, although a wide range of nonspecific chromosome findings have been described; changes in 5q may be important. Mutations of *p53* and *BCL6* occur in approximately one third of cases but they are of unclear functional significance. Cyclin D1 (PRAD-1) is overexpressed for reasons other than 11 : 14 translocation.

The signals responsible for the activation of hairy cells, now partially characterized, have a dual origin. Some originate from microenvironmental stimuli such as cytokines, but these are in turn influenced by constitutive signals arising from the oncogenic event. Truly constitutively active signals include ERK 1/2 and the Rho GTPases Rac and Cdc42. Active ERK has been shown to be important in hairy cell survival,[8] and the active Rho GTPases play an important role in the in vitro persistence of the distinctive surface ruffles and microvilli of hairy cells.[9] The intrinsically activated state of hairy cells is likely to be responsible for most if not all of the distinctive and unusual properties of hairy cells that determine the specific pathologic features of the disease. Thus, intrinsically activated hairy cell integrins and other adhesion receptors determine many of the distinctive homing characteristics of hairy cells (Table 35–2).

In addition to direct communication with the microenvironment by adhesion receptors, there is also a mutual interaction between hairy cells and other resident tissue cells mediated by cytokines. Several cytokines have now been implicated in the pathogenesis of hairy cell leukemia,[4] among which fibroblast growth factor and tumor necrosis factor are particularly important. Autocrine fibroblast growth factor stimulates hairy cells to produce and secrete fibronectin, which is responsible, at least in part, for the distinctive fibrosis of hairy cell leukemia.[10–12] Autocrine tumor necrosis factor has been shown to promote the survival of hairy cells.[4]

Other Cell Types

Direct bone marrow invasion damages hematopoiesis and contributes to pancytopenia. Both monocytes and dendritic cells are virtually absent from peripheral blood, and the mechanism remains unclear. Functional abnormalities of T cells, especially after nucleoside therapy, contribute to immunosuppression. Defects in hemopoietic cells, monocytes/dendritic cells, and T cells all contribute to defective immunity in hairy cell leukemia.

In the spleen and liver, hairy cells associate with and replace endothelial cells lining the splenic and hepatic sinusoids. The association with endothelial cells is responsible for the distinctive infiltration of splenic red pulp and hepatic sinusoids and for the formation of pathognomonic pseudosinuses. Before nucleoside therapy, the absolute number of circulating T cells is relatively normal, as is the CD4:CD8 ratio. However, these T cells are often abnormal[13] and they show a skewed and

TABLE 35–1. Immunophenotypic Features of Hairy Cells

Antigen Expressed	Comment
Strong light-chain–restricted surface immunoglobulin (Ig)	Multiple heavy-chain isotypes are expressed, indicating class switching has taken place. IgG3 subtype is most frequent.
CD19 CD20 CD40 FMC7	Markers of mature, but not terminally differentiated, B cells.
CD22 CD25* CD72 CD154	Activation markers.
CD11c CD103	Hairy cell "restricted" and therefore of diagnostic value.
CD27	Marker of memory cells.
CD95	Engagement by Fas ligand does not induce apoptosis.

*CD25 positivity, together with expression of CD11c and CD103 and the absence of CD5, distinguishes hairy cell leukemia from hairy cell leukemia–like disorders and chronic lymphocytic leukemia variants.

TABLE 35–2. Adhesion Receptor Expression by Hairy Cells (HCs)

Adhesion Receptor	Comment
Integrins (CD)	
$\alpha_4\beta_1$ (41d/29)	Highly expressed. Involved in binding to matrix (FN) & other cells (VCAM-1, CD106).
$\alpha_5\beta_1$ (49e/29)	Highly expressed. Involved in binding to, and assembly of, FN matrix.
$\alpha_v\beta_1$ (51/29)	Weakly expressed. Function in HCs unclear.
$\alpha_L\beta_2$ (11a/18)	Little or no expression.
$\alpha_M\beta_2$ (11b/18)	Weakly expressed. Function in HCs unclear.
$\alpha_x\beta_2$ (11c/18)	Highly expressed and diagnostically important. Receptor for a number of ligands, including ICAM-1 (CD54), but function in HCs unclear.
$\alpha_v\beta_3$ (51/61)	Receptor for vitronectin and PECAM-1 (CD31). Important in HC motility.
$\alpha_e\beta_7$ (103/β_7)	Highly expressed and diagnostically important. Receptor for E-cadherin, but function in HCL not clear.
Other Adhesion Receptors	
CD44	Highly expressed together with V_3 isoform. HC receptor for hyaluronan.
L-selectin (62L)	Little or no expression. Shed on cell activation.

Abbreviations: FN, fibronectin; HCL, hairy cell leukemia; ICAM-1, intercellular adhesion molecule-1; VCAM-1, vascular cell adhesion molecule-1; PECAM-1, platelet/endothelial cell adhesion molecule-1.

restricted expression of T-cell receptor of Vβ-chain families.[14] This altered expression may represent a T-cell reaction to tumor antigens[14] and may further aggravate the associated immunodeficiency of the disease.

CLINICAL FEATURES AND DIAGNOSIS

Symptoms and Signs

History

Nonspecific symptoms such as weakness, weight loss, and dyspnea are the most common complaints (Fig. 35–1). Symptoms attributable to neutropenia-associated infection and thrombocytopenic bleeding lead to presentation in most remaining patients.

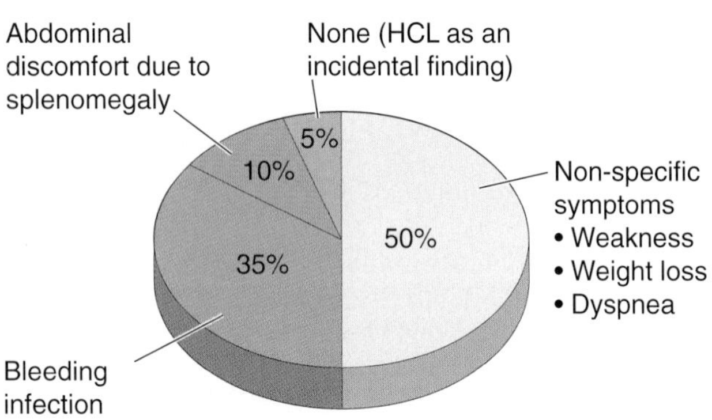

Figure 35–1. Clinical presentations in hairy cell leukemia.

Physical Examination

Splenomegaly is by far the most constant physical finding and is present in about 80% of patients. Hepatomegaly is much less frequent and, when present (in ~40%), is usually modest. Usually, there is no palpable lymphadenopathy, but imaging may reveal some para-aortic node enlargement (Fig. 35–2*A*). Substantial upper abdominal lymphadenopathy, detectable by computed tomography scanning, occurs in up to 15% of patients during the course of the illness (Fig. 35–2*B*). The cells infiltrating these enlarged nodes often appear larger and more primitive than typical hairy cells, and this complication may represent disease transformation, analogous to the evolution of other low-grade lymphomas such as follicular center cell lymphoma.

Infections and Fevers

Historically, infections were a major cause of morbidity and mortality, with acute bacterial infections related to severe neutropenia and opportunistic infections secondary to the more general cellular immune defect present in hairy cell leukemia. Since the introduction of effective treatments, infections occur much less frequently.

Persistent fever, especially after therapy, can be a diagnostic challenge (Table 35–3).

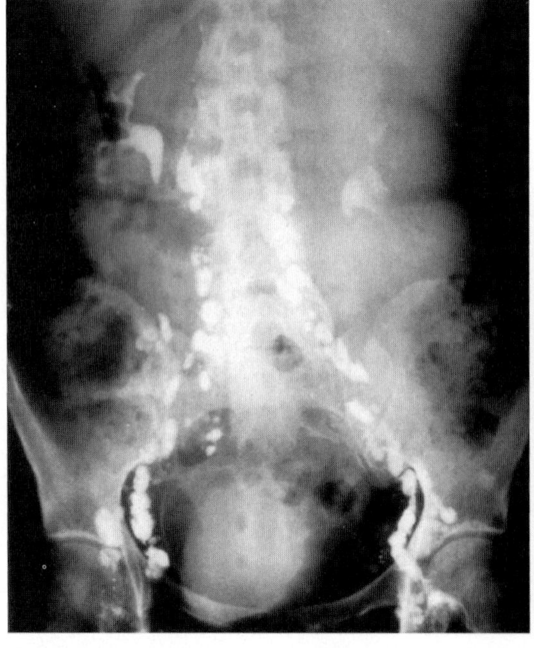

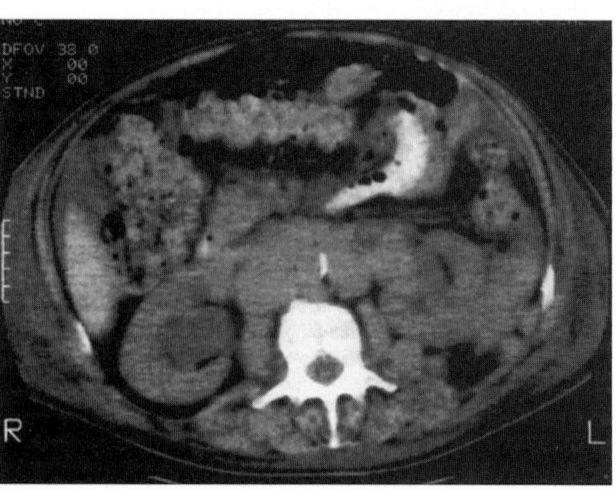

A B

Figure 35–2. *A,* Para-aortic lymphadenopathy in hairy cell leukemia. Lymphangiography is no longer indicated in the disease, but this radiograph demonstrates the modest enlargement of para-aortic lymph nodes (LN), which are often seen in the absence of peripheral node enlargement. *B,* Major upper abdominal LN enlargement. A substantial nodal prevertebral mass is seen. Development of this complication is a form of high-grade transformation, and infiltrating hairy cells are larger than those present in the chronic phase of the disease.

Second Malignancy

Second tumors now represent a major cause of death in the disease. Many different types of cancer, both hematologic and nonhematologic, occur, possibly as a consequence of longer survival with effective therapy.

Diagnosis

The diagnosis of hairy cell leukemia depends on a combination of findings (Table 35–4).

TABLE 35–3. Causes of Fever in Hairy Cell Leukemia

Vasculitic syndrome
Chlorodeoxyadenosine treatment
Infection:
Gram-negative bacterial infections
Legionella
Atypical mycobacterial infection
Listeria
Toxoplasmosis
Fungal (especially *Aspergillus*)

TABLE 35–4. Diagnosis of Hairy Cell Leukemia

- Pancytopenia and splenomegaly in the absence of liver disease raise suspicion
- Pathognomonic TRAP-positive HCs in PB
- Characteristic HC immunophenotype ($CD11c^+$, $CD25^+$, and $CD103^+$ clonal B cells)
- Diagnostic marrow: typical infiltrate with halo appearance and diffuse reticulin fibrosis

Abbreviations: HC, hairy cell; PB, peripheral blood; TRAP, tartrate-resistant isoenzyme 5 of acid phosphatase.

Laboratory Findings

Morphology

On the blood smear, the hairy cell is larger than most lymphocytes (15–30 μ) and is usually readily recognized by the presence of irregular fine cytoplasmic projections at its periphery (Fig. 35–3*A*). The eccentric nucleus is round or oval but may be indented, and nuclear chromatin is finely dispersed, although nucleoli are not conspicuous. The cytoplasm is relatively abundant and has a pale slate-blue color.

Cytochemistry

The nature of the hairy cells is confirmed by testing for tartrate-resistant isoenzyme 5 of acid phosphatase (TRAP).[15] This isoenzyme is relatively specific for hairy cells and is readily demonstrated in a simple cytochemical reaction performed in the presence of tartrate. Strong reactivity is observed in at least a proportion of the hairy cells (Fig. 35–3*B*).

Ultrastructure

At the ultrastructural level, scanning electron microscopy shows that the surface projections are composed of distinctive ruffles and finger-like microvilli[16] (Fig. 35–4*A*). On transmission electron microscopy, surface projections together with a cytoplasm containing abundant pinocytotic vesicles and abundant mitochondria and occasional strands of rough endoplasmic reticulum are distinctive features (Fig. 35–4*B*). Characteristic ribosome-lamellar complexes of unknown function occur in approximately 50% of cases[17,18] and in from less than 1% to almost 100% of the cells in an individual patient[18] (Fig. 35–5).

Blood

Anemia, leukopenia, and thrombocytopenia are characteristic of hairy cell leukemia at presentation, and pan-

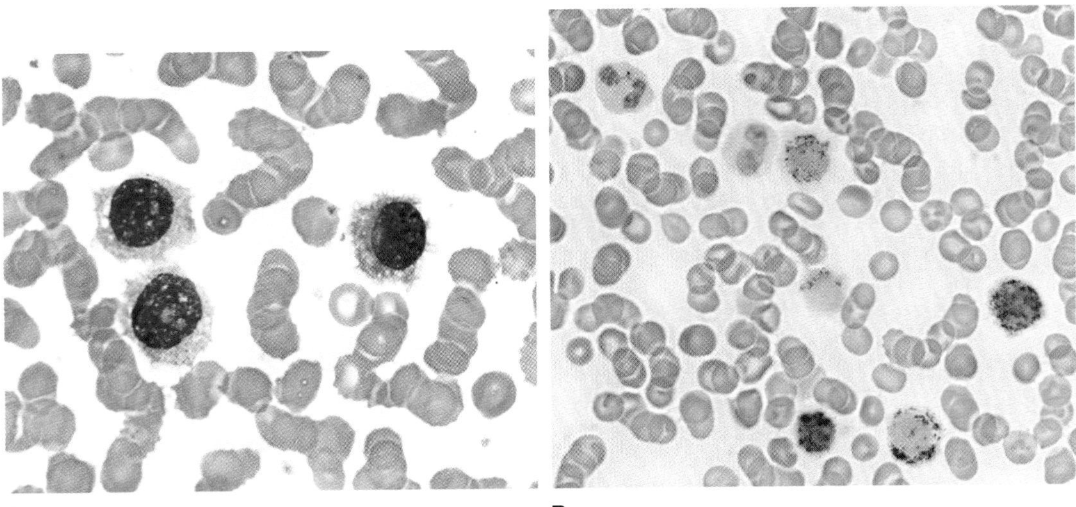

Figure 35–3. *A*, Circulating hairy cells. *B*, Tartrate-resistance isoenzyme 5 of acid phosphatase (TRAP) positivity in hairy cells. Note that the hairy cells contain strong overall enzyme activity, while the nearby neutrophils contain little or no reactivity.

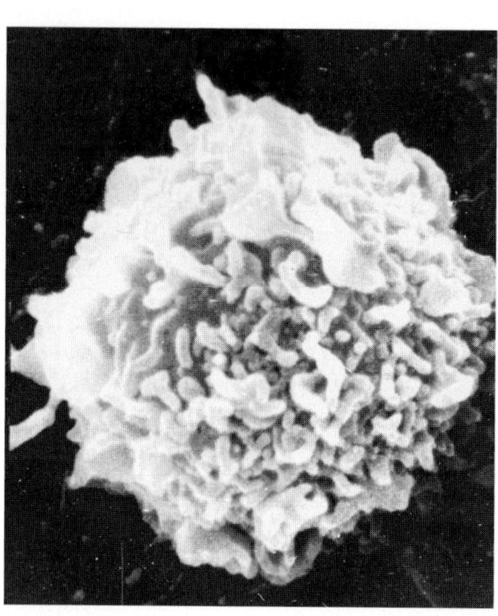
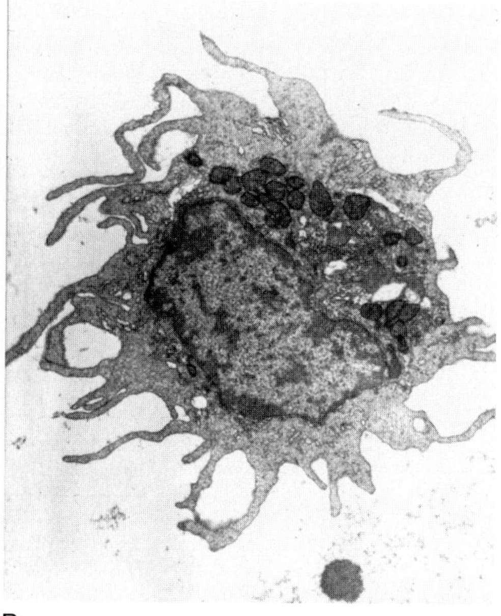

■ **Figure 35–4.** *A,* Scanning electron micrograph of a hairy cell. Note the distinctive mixture of surface ruffles and microvilli. *B,* Transmission electron micrograph of a hairy cell. The surface ruffles and microvilli are especially well demonstrated.

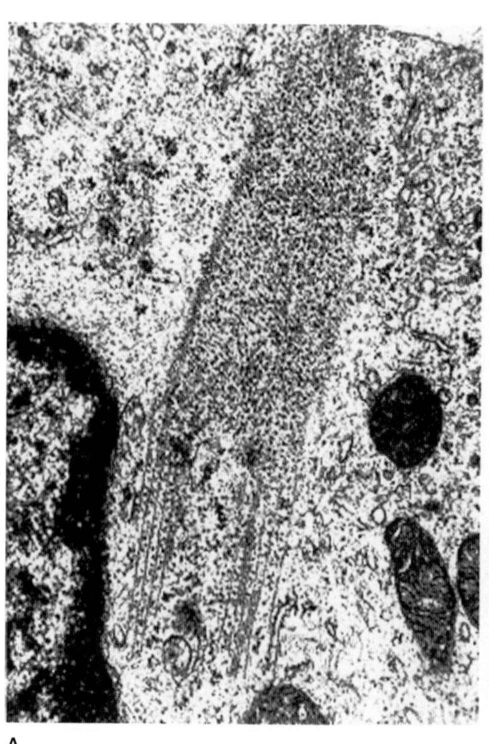
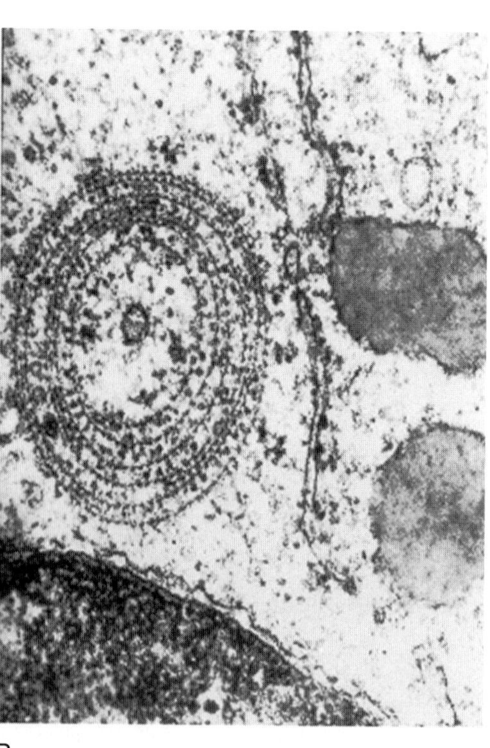

■ **Figure 35–5.** Ribosome-lamellar (R-L) complexes. *A,* An R-L complex sectioned partly longitudinally *(left)*; on the *right* the complex is cut obliquely. *B,* An R-L complex in transverse section. R-L complexes sometimes can be faintly seen in Romanowsky-stained cells, where they occupy up to about 50% of the diameter of the hairy cell.

cytopenia is observed in around 70% of patients. The most variable parameter is the leukocyte count.

Anemia

There is usually moderate anemia (mean, ~10 gm/dL) and the mean cell volume is either normal or slightly elevated. The etiology of anemia is multifactorial: impaired marrow function, splenic pooling, reduced red cell survival, and an increased plasma volume all contribute.

Leukocytes

Neutropenia and a profound monocytopenia are nearly always present in active disease; both are probably the result of either direct or indirect suppression of the bone marrow by infiltrating hairy cells. The percentage of morphologically recognizable hairy cells varies from almost none to 100% but in general increases with the white blood cell count.

Platelets

Thrombocytopenia is present in more than 80% of patients, as a result of both splenic sequestration and suppressed production of defective platelets.

Bone Marrow

The bone marrow is not aspirable in about half of cases, likely as a result of the increased stromal reticulin fibers characteristic of the disease.[19] The trephine biopsy is almost invariably abnormal, showing diffuse infiltration by hairy cells, which are often surrounded by a clear zone, forming a "halo" appearance (Fig. 35–6*A*). Granulopoiesis and monocytopoiesis are reduced, and erythropoiesis is relatively spared. Areas of hairy cell infiltration are accompanied by fine diffuse reticulin fibrosis, visualized in silver-stained sections. Fibronectin is a major component of this fibrosis and is produced by the hairy cells themselves; stromal fibroblasts are inconspicuous (Fig. 35–6*B*).[10]

Spleen and Liver

Splenectomy and/or liver biopsy are rarely required for diagnosis. If examined, both the spleen and liver are consistently infiltrated by hairy cells in distinctive and diagnostic patterns. In the spleen, hairy cells home to and expand the red pulp, so that the residual white pulp becomes progressively obliterated. In the red pulp, hairy cells replace endothelial cells lining the sinusoids and as a result form splenic "pseudosinuses," diagnostic of hairy cell leukemia (Fig. 35–6*C*).[20] These pseudosinuses contribute to the splenic red cell pooling that is characteristic of the disease.[21] In the liver, hairy cells infiltrate both the portal tracts and hepatic sinusoids (Fig. 35–6*D*).[22] In the portal tracts, the infiltration is diffuse and associated with reticulin fibrosis, but the general architecture of the liver remains intact and there is usually no biliary obstruction or derangement of liver function tests. In the sinusoids, the hairy cells may lie free within the lumen or in close association with the endothelium and adjacent hepatocytes.[23]

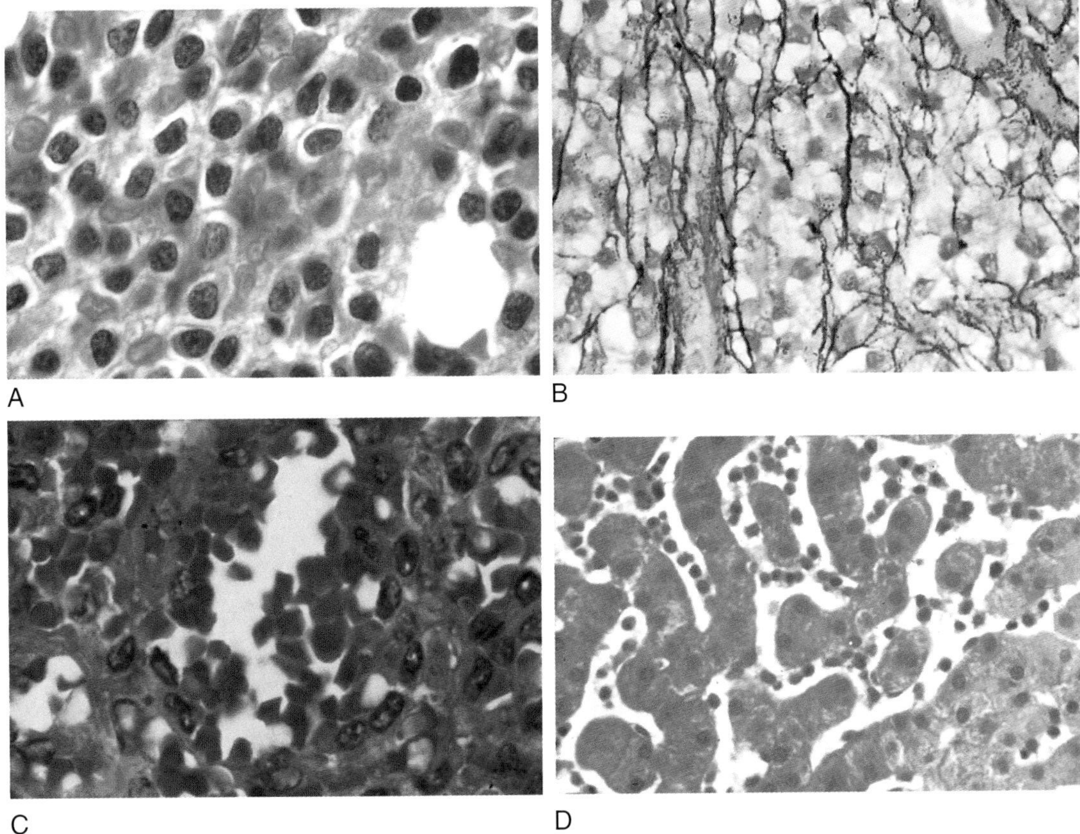

Figure 35–6. ***A,*** Infiltrated bone marrow. Note the pale areas surrounding many of the hairy cells, imparting the so-called halo appearance. ***B,*** Bone marrow fibrosis in hairy cell leukemia. Note the fine fibrosis observed in silver-stained material. Fibronectin is a major component of this fibrosis and is produced by the hairy cells themselves rather than by stromal fibroblasts. ***C,*** Splenic pseudosinus. These structures are formed as a result of hairy cells replacing the endothelial cells lining the red-pulp sinuses. Pseudosinuses are responsible for the major splenic red cell pooling that can be observed in the disease. ***D,*** Hepatic infiltration in hairy cell leukemia. The hairy cells either lie free in the hepatic sinusoids or replace the endothelial cells lining the sinusoids. The portal tracts (not shown) are often heavily infiltrated with hairy cells that are associated with fibrosis; nevertheless, hepatic function is usually preserved.

TABLE 35–5. Clinical Features of Hairy Cell Leukemia–like Disorders

Feature	HCL-V	SLVL	Marginal Zone Proliferations Involving Blood
Abnormal cells	Smaller than typical HCs with a higher nuclear/cytoplasmic ratio. Hairs less prominent than in HCs. Clumped nuclear chromatin.	Smaller than HCs, but bigger than the cells of HCL-V. Cytoplasm less abundant than that of HCs and often polarized, with hairs located at the poles of the cell.	Resemble HCs in size and abundant cytoplasm, but hairs not as conspicuous. Nucleus lacks the fine, ground-glass chromatin of HCs.
WBC count	Grossly elevated	Usually not markedly elevated	Usually not markedly elevated
BM function/findings	No monocytopenia. Other cytopenias usually not marked. Fibrosis not prominent; no halos.	No monocytopenia. Marrow function well preserved. Fibrosis not prominent; no halos.	No monocytopenia. Marrow function well preserved. Infiltration is paratrabecular. Fibrosis not prominent.
TRAP	Weak or absent	Usually present, but is usually low to moderate and in only a minority of cells	Negative
Immunophenotype	Usually lacks CD25 & CD103	Usually lacks CD25 & CD103	Usually lacks CD25 & CD103
Other features		IgM paraproteinemia often present (60%)	LN involvement may be conspicuous when appearances = monocytoid B-cell lymphoma.

Abbreviations: BM, bone marrow; HCL-V, variant-form hairy cell leukemia; HCs, hairy cells; IgM, immunoglobulin M; LN, lymph node; SLVL, splenic lymphoma with villous lymphocytes; TRAP, tartrate-resistant isoenzyme 5 of acid phosphatase; WBC, white blood cell.

DIFFERENTIAL DIAGNOSIS

The diagnosis is usually straightforward. Diagnostic difficulties can arise in two circumstances: first, when few or no typical hairy cells are present in the blood; and second, when the clinical or pathologic presentation is atypical. In very leukopenic patients, hairy cells may be inconspicuous in the peripheral blood, but abnormal cells are usually easily found in buffy-coat preparations or in the bone marrow.

When clinical or pathologic features are atypical, the problem is differentiating typical hairy cell leukemia from other hairy cell leukemia–like disorders[24–27] (Table 35–5). The most important feature is the malignant cell itself, which, although variably "hairy," is readily distinguishable from the typical hairy cell.

TREATMENT

Hairy cell leukemia is unique among chronic lymphoproliferative disorders in being extremely sensitive to interferon alfa and nucleosides. In the absence of adhesion, interferon alfa kills hairy cells by sensitizing them to the apoptotic effects of autocrine tumor necrosis factor.[28] Apoptosis likely is a consequence of the intrinsic activation in hairy cells of the proapoptotic p38 and JNK mitogen-activated protein kinases (these kinases are not activated in chronic lymphocytic leukemia cells, which are resistant to interferon-induced killing under identical conditions).[29] It is still unclear why hairy cells are so susceptible to nucleosides.

Because therapy of hairy cell leukemia is associated with significant toxicity, treatment should be delayed until the patient becomes definitely symptomatic or cytopenic. Individual physicians often decide what constitutes "significant" cytopenia(s), but neutrophil counts less than 1×10^9/L, hemoglobin less than 10 gm/dL, and platelet counts less than 100×10^9/L have been suggested as appropriate levels to prompt treatment.[30]

TABLE 35–6. Therapeutic Responses to Nucleosides and Interferon Alfa

	dCF	CdA	IFN Alfa
CR (%)	72–87	50–91	5–32
PR (%)	4–15	7–37	52–70
Overall response rate (%)	>85	>85	70–80
DFS at around 5 yr (%)	~50–90	~70–90	~20–30

Abbreviations: CdA, chlorodeoxyadenosine; CR, complete remission; dCF, deoxycoformycin; DFS, disease-free survival; IFN, interferon; PR, partial remission.

Nucleoside Analogues

Purine analogues (nucleosides) are the treatment of choice. Both chlorodeoxyadenosine (CdA) and deoxycoformycin (dCF) have been extensively used and are of comparable efficacy (Table 35–6). The efficacy of dCF was first recognized in 1984, and CdA was introduced a little later. Nucleosides produce more rapid and complete remissions than does interferon, and the latter agent is now rarely employed.

Normally, intracellular levels of nucleosides are controlled by adenosine deaminase (ADA) in a unique degradation pathway. In this pathway, purine analogues, including deoxyadenosine nucleosides, accumulate and are phosphorylated to nucleotides by deoxycytidine kinase (dCK). dCK is the rate-limiting enzyme, generating deoxynucleoside triphosphates that are incorporated into DNA. This pathway is especially important in lymphocytes, which contain particularly high levels of dCK and low levels of phosphatase. When there is marked DNA catabolism or when deoxyadenosine is present at high levels in the circulation, dCK has the potential to produce high levels of toxic deoxyadenosine triphosphate within lymphocytes. Normally, the lymphocyte is protected from this potential toxicity by ADA, which metabolizes deoxyadenosine to deoxyinosine and eventually to uric acid. Both dCF and CdA disrupt the normal salvage pathway for purine nucleosides. dCF inhibits ADA, and CdA is an analogue of deoxyadenosine, which is resistant to breakdown by ADA. Therefore, the nucleotide derivatives of both CdA and dCF selectively accumulate within lymphocytes, where they are either directly toxic or become incorporated into and damage DNA.[30,31] It is unclear why hairy cells are so much more sensitive to these toxic metabolites than are normal and other malignant lymphocytes.

Which drug to give first is a matter of patient/physician preference. There is no major cross-resistance between CdA and dCF and, when a patient relapses after one agent, the other nucleoside can be administered (Fig. 35–7).

CdA (Cladribine, Leustat)

CdA has been utilized in hairy cell leukemia in various doses and by different routes[30]; the optimal method has not been established by direct comparisons of the alternatives. Most used is a continuous infusion over 7 days (0.09 mg/kg/day, or 3.6 mg/m^2/day, both in 500 mL 0.9% saline). Administered in this way, the agent causes marked marrow suppression and a high incidence of fevers (~40%, mostly culture negative[30]). Therefore, it may be better to infuse the drug intermittently (0.15 mg/kg weekly for 6 weeks); this regimen is equally efficacious and has reduced toxicity.[32]

dCF (Pentostatin, Nipent)

As with CdA, dCF also has been administered in different regimens.[33] The usual dose is 4 mg/m^2 intravenously every 2 weeks until complete remission; starting at half-dose in frail or very cytopenic patients is reasonable. Because of its renal metabolism, the manufacturer recommends that the drug should not be given when the creatinine clearance is less than 60 mL/min; at creatinine clearances between 50 and 60 mL/min, it is probably safe to administer the agent at half-dose (2 mg/m^2). The creatinine clearance should be measured in all patients before administration of dCF; if less than 50 mL/min, CdA would be the preferred alternative (Table 35–7). As with CdA, marrow suppression is the major toxicity of dCF. In addition, photosensitivity is a notable side effect, and patients should avoid direct exposure to sunlight.

TABLE 35–7. Issue Concerns in Nucleoside Therapy

Issue	Comment
Renal function	Creatinine clearance should be measured; dCF should not be given if <50 mL/m^2
Transfusion-associated GVHD	All cellular blood products should be irradiated
Immunosuppression	Long-term cotrimoxazole probably sensible

Abbreviations: dCF, deoxycoformycin; GVHD, graft-versus-host disease.

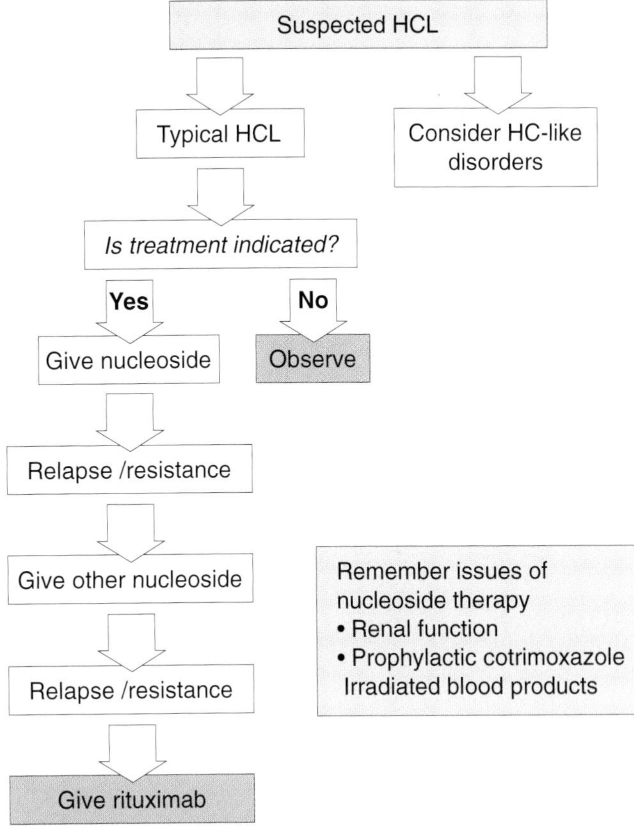

Figure 35–7. Management strategy in hairy cell leukemia.

Treatment-Related Toxicity

Nucleoside analogues produce profound depletion of CD4 T cells. Although opportunistic infections are uncommon, *Pneumocystis* prophylaxis (cotrimoxazole 480 mg/day) is advisable until about 6 months after discontinuation of nucleoside therapy.

Granulocyte colony-stimulating factor (G-CSF) shortens the period of neutropenia following nucleoside administration and increases the median nadir of the neutrophil count, but these effects do not translate into clinical benefit in terms of numbers of febrile episodes. Therefore, routine use of G-CSF is not recommended.[34] In life-threatening infections or when there is other evidence of neutropenia-associated opportunistic infection, G-CSF may be utilized to increase the neutrophil count.

Because of the immunosuppression associated with nucleoside therapy, infusion of blood products can occasionally result in transfusion-associated graft-versus-host disease and fatal aplastic anemia. All blood and platelets must be irradiated before administration to the patient who has received nucleoside analogues.[35]

Rituximab (Chimeric Anti-CD20 Monoclonal Antibody)

Hairy cells express high levels of CD20, and it is therefore not surprising that rituximab is active in the disease.[36] Because nucleosides are so effective, rituximab should be reserved for patients who are refractory to them or who have relapsed shortly after sequentially receiving both nucleosides. In such cases, the response rate to anti-CD20 monoclonal antibody is 80%, with a complete remission rate of approximately 50%.[36] However, responses are less complete in patients who are refractory to nucleosides than in those who have simply relapsed after dCF/CdA. Rituximab has minimal toxicity. The usual course is 375 mg/m^2 weekly for 8 weeks.[36]

Other Treatments

Interferon Alfa

In 1984, the first report of the efficacy of interferon alfa in hairy cell leukemia attracted much interest[37] and, for a period, this drug replaced splenectomy as the principal treatment.[38] However, interferon alfa is clearly less effective than are the nucleoside analogues and has a less rapid onset of action (see Table 35–6). Interferon alfa should no longer be used as first-line treatment; it can have activity in patients who have relapsed after nucleosides, but the response rate is low and the responses less complete and durable than those achieved with rituximab. Interferon alfa currently is indicated only for hairy cell leukemia refractory to both nucleoside and rituximab therapies.

Recombinant Immunotoxins

Two such agents with activity in hairy cell leukemia have recently been developed.[39,40] Both are chimeric proteins in which the Fv portion of monoclonal antibodies reactive against either CD22 or CD25 has been fused to a fragment of *Pseudomonas* exotoxin A. The anti-CD22 immunotoxin is currently entering Phase II testing in hairy cell leukemia and is not yet widely available.[40]

Older Treatments

Before the introduction of interferon alfa, splenectomy and chlorambucil were mainstays of treatment. Both produced clear and sustained benefit in some patients[41,42] but are now rarely, if ever, used.

Treatment of Hairy Cell Leukemia-like Disorders

Many patients with splenic lymphoma with villous lymphocytes and related marginal zone proliferations are not symptomatic nor seriously cytopenic, so they do not require treatment. When therapy is indicated, both splenectomy[43] and fludarabine[44] are effective, clinical circumstances and patient/physician preferences dictating which to use first. Nodal forms of marginal zone lymphoma should be treated like other low-grade lymphomas.

In variant-form hairy cell leukemia requiring treatment, splenectomy is preferred.[45] Most variant-form hairy cell leukemia is resistant to interferon alfa. Nucleosides have some activity (~50% partial response rate), but are much less effective than in typical hairy cell leukemia HCL.[46]

Early in the course of hairy cell leukemia, neutropenic fevers should be treated as in other hematologic malignancies. Later, when the disease becomes refractory to nucleosides, the need for supportive care becomes similar to that required in other refractory or transformed low-grade non-Hodgkin's lymphomas.

PROGNOSIS

Before the introduction of nucleosides, survival in hairy cell leukemia was very variable, with a median of about 50 months. With the use of nucleosides, approximately 95% of patients survive 5 years,[47] and approximately 80% are still alive at 10 years.[48] Five- and 10-year relapse-free survival rates are of the order of 80% and 65%, respectively.[48]

CURRENT CONTROVERSIES & FUTURE CONSIDERATIONS

Hairy Cell Leukemia

- Certain aspects of the pathophysiology of hairy cell leukemia (specific expression of TRAP) remain unexplained.
- The primary oncogenic event responsible for the intrinsic activation of hairy cell leukemia is unknown.
- Treatment of patients who are resistant to nucleosides/rituximab/interferon alfa remains difficult, but immunotoxins currently under development may be useful.

Suggested Readings*

Baker PK, Pettitt AR, Slupsky JR, et al: Response of hairy cells to IFN-alpha involves induction of apoptosis through autocrine TNF-alpha and protection by adhesion. Blood 100:647–653, 2002.

Basso K, Liso A, Tiacci E, et al: Gene expression profiling of hairy cell leukemia reveals a phenotype related to memory B cells with altered expression of chemokine and adhesion receptors. J Exp Med 199:59–68, 2004.

Burthem J, Cawley JC: Hairy-Cell Leukaemia. London: Springer-Verlag, 1996.

Saven A, Beutler E (eds): Hairy-cell leukaemia. Best Pract Res Clin Haematol 16(1), 2003.

Tallman MS, Polliack A (eds): Hairy Cell Leukemia. London: Harwood, 2000.

Full references for this chapter can be found on accompanying CD-ROM.

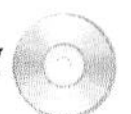

CHAPTER 36

Polycythemia Vera and Essential Thrombocythemia

Xylina T. Gregg, MD, and Josef T. Prchal, MD

KEY POINTS

Polycythemia Vera and Essential Thrombocythemia

Diagnosis

- An elevated or high-normal erythropoietin level is useful to exclude polycythemia vera in nonphlebotomized patients.
- An elevated red cell volume may be useful to confirm polycythemia in patients with borderline elevations of hematocrit.
- Essential thrombocythemia is a diagnosis of exclusion.
- Patients with a clinical diagnosis of essential thrombocythemia but polyclonal hematopoiesis have a low incidence of thrombohemorrhagic events.
- When polycythemia or thrombocytosis is present in children or there is a family history of polycythemia or thrombocytosis, causes other than polycythemia vera or essential thrombocythemia should be considered.

Treatment

- Treatment is indicated for polycythemia vera or essential thrombocythemia patients with a prior history of thrombosis or age greater than 60 years.
- Patients with "spent phase" should be considered for nonmyeloablative stem cell transplantation.
- Aspirin therapy is effective in relieving erythromelalgia and other symptoms of microvascular occlusion and may reduce thrombotic complications in polycythemia vera, but it is contraindicated in patients with a history of bleeding or a platelet count greater than 1,000,000/μL.

INTRODUCTION

Polycythemia vera and essential thrombocythemia are chronic myeloproliferative disorders (MPDs), a disease category that includes idiopathic myelofibrosis and chronic myelogenous leukemia (CML). MPDs are characterized by clonal proliferation of myeloid blood cells, that is, granulocytes, red cells, and platelets. Although polycythemia vera is clinically distinguished by an elevated red cell mass and essential thrombocythemia by elevated platelets, there may be considerable overlap in the clinical features of these disorders. Only CML has a specific marker, the Philadelphia chromosome (see Chapter 31), and diagnosis of the other MPDs is made for the most part on clinical criteria. A recent genetic analysis observed common loss of homozygosity on chromosome 9p and mutations and polymorphisms of the Janus kinase 2 (JAK2) gene[37d] in each of the three disorders other than CML. Thus, polycythemia vera, essential thrombocythemia, and idiopathic myelofibrosis may at times be difficult to distinguish from each other or from reactive processes.

POLYCYTHEMIA VERA

Epidemiology and Risk Factors

Polycythemia vera occurs in all age groups, but is uncommon in children and young adults. The median age at diagnosis is 60.[1,2] The incidence is slightly higher in men (2.8 cases per 100,000 population vs. 1.3 per 100,000 in women).[3] Most cases of polycythemia vera are sporadic, but there are rare familial cases.[4] However, because there is no specific diagnostic test for polycythemia vera, some familial cases diagnosed as "polycythemia vera" may in fact be due to other inherited causes of polycythemia. For example, some patients with primary familial and congenital polycythemia (PFCP) have splenomegaly and in vitro erythroid progenitor characteristics of polycythemia vera and may fulfill the clinical criteria of polycythemia vera; some of these patients have been inappropriately treated with ^{32}P or chemotherapy.[5] Similarly, a significant proportion of Chuvash polycythemia patients have also been misdiagnosed as having polycythemia vera and treated with chemotherapy.[6] There are no clearly identified risk factors for development of polycythemia vera.

Pathophysiology

Clonality

Polycythemia vera results from an acquired mutation in a pluripotent hematopoietic progenitor cell. Clonality studies based on the phenomenon of X-inactivation have shown that red cells, granulocytes, platelets, monocytes, and B lymphocytes are all part of the clone.[7,8] The majority of T lymphocytes and natural killer cells are polyclonal, but a small proportion of these cells are also derived from the polycythemia vera clone[9]; this polyclonality is presumed to be due to the presence of long-lived normal T cells that preceded the development of the clone.

Erythroid Progenitor Assays

Erythropoietin is the principal regulator of erythropoiesis. Variable levels of erythropoietin are required at the different stages of erythroid maturation.[10] Erythropoietin is most important for terminal maturation of erythroid cells at the level of the erythroid colony-forming units during normal adult erythropoiesis. However, polycythemia vera erythroid progenitors exhibit "erythropoietin independence," which refers to spontaneous erythroid colony formation in vitro when the progenitors are grown in media without exogenously added erythropoietin, but in the presence of serum[11] (Fig. 36–1). This formation of endogenous erythroid colonies (EEC) is dependent on minute quantities of insulin-like growth factor-I (IGF-I) present in the serum or other lipid-containing substances. When rigorous serum-free conditions are used, erythroid burst-forming units from patients with polycythemia vera show normal sensitivity to erythropoietin but markedly increased sensitivity to IGF-I.[12] However, some of the published data on the influence of IGF-I on erythropoiesis must be interpreted with caution. Mutations of the erythropoietin receptor (*EPOR*) leading to increased sensitivity to erythropoietin are a demonstrated cause of PFCP,[13] and the central role of erythropoietin hypersensitivity in the pathogenesis of this disease has been shown using native PFCP progenitors, transfected cells, and an animal PFCP model.[14] Nevertheless, when examined in rigorous serum-free conditions,[15] neither PFCP nor polycythemia vera erythroid burst-forming units were hypersensitive to erythropoietin, but both were hypersensitive to IGF-I. These data demonstrate that, although studies in rigorous serum-free conditions teach us valuable lessons about the control of erythropoiesis, they do not simulate in vivo situations where cells are exposed to multiple cytokines. Furthermore, these data suggest shortcomings of serum free assays and point to likely "cross-talk" of cytokine receptors occurring under more physiologic conditions.

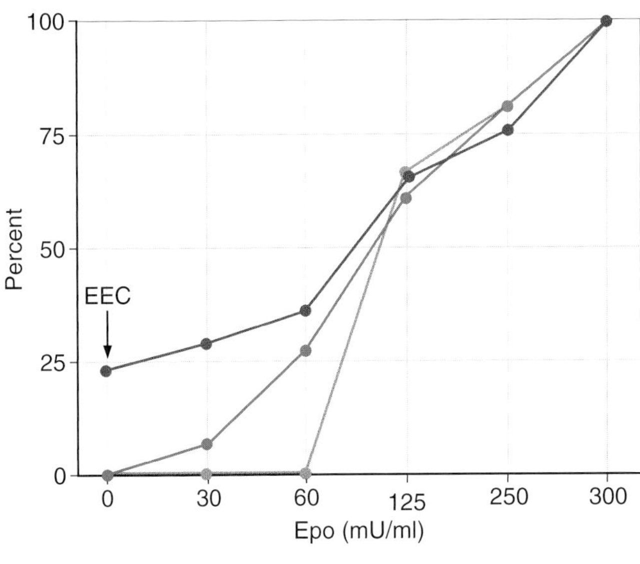

Figure 36–1. Endogenous erythroid colony formation in polycythemia vera from plated erythroid progenitors at different erythropoietin (Epo) concentrations. Abbreviations: EEC, endogenous erythroid colonies; PV, polycythemia vera; PFCP, primary familial and congenital polycythemia.

Molecular Studies in Polycythemia Vera

The molecular defect resulting in polycythemia vera is unknown. Mutations in the *EPOR* gene have not been found in this disorder,[13,16,17] and expression of EPOR, affinity of erythropoietin for EpoR, and number of EPORs on erythroid progenitors are normal.[18,19] However, variant expression of an alternatively spliced form of the EpoR has been described in polycythemia vera. Normal erythroid progenitor cells express two transcripts of the *EPOR*, one full length (*EPOR-F*) and one truncated (*EPOR-T*). The EpoR-T has a dominant negative function against EpoR-F, and *EPOR-T* messenger RNA (mRNA) is markedly decreased in polycythemia vera, which theoretically might explain the erythropoietin hypersensitivity seen in this disease.[20]

Abnormalities in cell signaling may be a final common pathway resulting in the characteristic features of polycythemia vera. Overexpression of *bcl*-xL, an inhibitor of apoptosis,[21] and decreased levels of the thrombopoietin receptor c-Mpl[22,23] have been observed in polycythemia vera, but neither of these findings is specific for the disorder. Abnormalities of STAT3,[24] SHP-1 phosphatase,[25] protein tyrosine phosphatase activity,[26] protein kinase C,[27] IGF-I receptor,[28] p16/p14 negative control elements of the cell cycle,[29] and tumor suppressor gene H19[30] have all been reported in polycythemia vera patients, but mutations of these genes have not been found, and some of these data have been challenged by other investigators.[5]

Increased levels of mRNA for polycythemia rubra vera 1 (PRV-1) receptor (a member of the urokinase plasminogen activator receptor superfamily) in peripheral blood granulocytes have been described in patients with polycythemia vera.[31] However, PRV-1 does not play a role in the pathogenesis of polycythemia vera, because the PRV-1 gene is not mutated in polycythemia vera and no differences were found in mRNA levels in erythroid progenitors of polycythemia vera, reactive polycythemia, and normal controls,[32,33] nor are there any differences in the protein level of PRV-1.[33] In addition, this observed increase of PRV-1 granulocyte mRNA is not specific for polycythemia vera; it is also found in patients with essential thrombocythemia, idiopathic myelofibrosis, and congenital MPDs and in some normal persons.[34–37]

The potentially most important discovery thus far in the molecular biology of polycythemia vera was made in late 2004 by Vainchenker's group, who reported that the majority of polycythemia vera patients are heterozygous for a single nucleotide somatic mutation in the JAK2 kinase (*JAK2V617F*) gene, a tyrosine kinase that is normally activated via the erythropoietin-EPOR axis and stimulates erythropoiesis by controlling proliferation, apoptosis, and erythroid differentiation.[37a,37b] The presence of this mutation in most polycythemia vera patients was subsequently confirmed by others.[37c–37f] The exact function of this mutation remains to be determined. Although an acquired heterozygous mutation would be expected to be "dominant"; i.e., that it would override the effect of a normal JAK2 allele, surprisingly, when mutated and wild-type *JAK2* genes were simultaneously introduced into hematopoietic cell lines, the polycythemia vera phenotype was not reproduced.[37b] It should be noted that a different conclusion was drawn by other investigators using a biochemical approach.[37e,37f] Both *JAK2* alleles are mutated in 30% of polycythemia vera patients via a previously described phenomenon, uniparental disomy,[9] which causes loss of heterozygosity usually by duplication of the portion of the chromosome bearing the mutated *JAK2*.

However, several observations suggest that *JAK2V617F* is neither pathognomonic nor specific for polycythemia vera. Approximately 20% of polycythemia vera patients with classical EEC and the full polycythemia vera phenotype do not have this mutation.[37b] A significant proportion of patients with idiopathic myelofibrosis and essential thrombocythemia also have this mutation, suggesting that it is not specific to polycythemia vera.[37b–37f] Other data indicate that this mutation is not even specific to myeloproliferative disorders. The Mayo clinic group found that patients with myelodysplastic syndrome and some patients with chronic myelomonocytic and neutrophilic leukemias have *JAK2V617F*.[37g] The MD Anderson group confirmed these findings and also found this mutation in Ph-negative chronic myelogenous leukemia and megakaryocytic leukemia, but in only 5 of 10 acute leukemia patients with antecedent polycythemia vera.[37h]

Clinical Features

Symptoms

Many cases of polycythemia vera are detected incidentally on routine complete blood counts done for unrelated reasons in asymptomatic patients. Symptomatic patients may present with various nonspecific complaints, including dizziness, weakness, headaches, visual disturbances, paresthesias, and sweats.[1] Pruritus, especially after bathing, may be very troublesome, but the pathologic basis for the pruritus remains unknown.[38]

Erythromelalgia is a syndrome of painful, reddened, erythematous digits that is associated with thrombocytosis and characteristically responds rapidly (within hours) to low-dose aspirin therapy (81 mg).[39] This syndrome occurs in approximately 3% of polycythemia vera patients[40]; its pathogenesis is unknown but may involve platelet-mediated endothelial cell injury. Secondary gout may occur as a result of increased uric acid from high cell turnover. Polycythemia vera patients are at increased risk for hemorrhage, primarily gastrointestinal bleeding. An extremely high platelet count and the use of antiplatelet drugs are risk factors for bleeding complications.[41] There is also an increased frequency of other gastrointestinal problems, including epigastric pain and peptic ulcer.

Physical Examination

Palpable splenomegaly and facial plethora are the most frequent physical findings, occurring in approximately two thirds of patients in the Polycythemia Vera Study Group (PVSG) studies.[1] However, as more cases are detected incidentally and at an earlier stage, these abnormalities may be noted less commonly and the physical examination may be unremarkable.

Laboratory Findings

In addition to polycythemia, thrombocytosis and granulocytosis also occur. In the initial PVSG study, 60% of patients had platelet counts greater than 400,000/μL and 40% had leukocyte counts greater than 12,000/L.[1] Extreme thrombocytosis (>1,000,000/μL) is not uncommon. Hyperuricemia, resulting from increased cell turnover, was present in 55% of the PVSG study patients.[1]

Thrombosis

Thrombosis is the presenting manifestation of polycythemia vera in 20% of patients[2] and is the leading cause of mortality in polycythemia vera[2,41,42] (Table 36–1). Both arterial and venous thrombotic events occur and include cerebrovascular accident, myocardial infarction, peripheral arterial thrombosis, deep venous thrombosis, and pulmonary embolism.[2,42] Erythromelalgia is a unique thrombosis-related syndrome characterized by painful, reddened digits caused by ischemia resulting from microvascular occlusion and that may progress to frank necrosis and gangrene. Thrombosis may also occur at unusual sites, such as the portal, splenic or mesenteric, or hepatic (Budd-Chiari syndrome) veins. The diagnosis of polycythemia vera should always be considered in patients presenting with these unusual thromboses, even in the absence of polycythemia. The demonstration of EEC in erythroid colony cultures may identify some of these patients with unsuspected polycythemia vera.[43–46] In one report of 20 patients with idiopathic Budd-Chiari syndrome, 16 had EEC, although only 2 had an overt myeloproliferative disorder.[45] The incidence of thrombosis is highest in the 12 months prior to diagnosis and the first few years after diagnosis and then appears to decline.[2,42]

TABLE 36–1. Causes of Death in Polycythemia Vera

	PVSG[42]		GISP[2]		ECLAP[41]	
Cause of Death	*n*	**(%)**	*n*	**(%)**	*n*	**(%)**
Thrombosis	64	(29.2%)	71	(37.0%)	67	(40.8%)
Hematologic malignancy	51	(23.3%)*	28	(14.6%)†	21	(12.8%)†
Other malignancy	35	(16.0%)	29	(15.1%)	32	(19.5%)
Hemorrhage	15	(6.8%)	5	(2.6%)	7	(4.3%)
Myelofibrosis/"spent phase"	7	(3.2%)	4	(2.1%)	1	(0.6%)
Myelodysplasia	NR	NR	1	(0.5%)	NR	NR
Other	47	(21.5%)	54	(28.1%)	36	(22.0%)
TOTAL	219	(100%)	192	(100%)	164	(100%)

*Includes leukemia and lymphoma.
†Acute leukemia only.
Abbreviations: ECLAP, European Collaboration on Low-Dose Aspirin in Polycythemia Vera; GISP, Gruppo Italiano Studio Policitemia; NR, not reported; PVSG, Polycythemia Vera Study Group.

Risk Factors

The major predictors of thrombosis are a prior history of thrombotic event and age greater than 70 years.[2,42] In a retrospective Italian study of 1213 patients with polycythemia vera, there were 2.8 thrombotic events per 100 patients per year in the group ages 40–59 years compared to 5.1 events per 100 patients per year in those older than 70 years.[2]

In the PVSG-01 trial, which randomized patients to phlebotomy alone versus phlebotomy plus chlorambucil or ^{32}P, the incidence of thrombosis was greatest in the phlebotomy alone arm, although the risk seemed limited to the first 3 years of therapy.[42] Neither the hematocrit nor the platelet count at the time of thrombosis was statistically different from that in patients without thrombotic events; however, hematocrits greater than 52% and platelet counts greater than 1,500,000/μL were rarely seen.

The underlying mechanisms causing thrombosis are not fully known. Pearson and Wetherley-Mein[47] reported an increased incidence of thrombotic episodes in those polycythemia vera patients with higher hematocrits. There was a trend to increased thrombosis with platelet counts greater than 400,000, but this was not statistically significant. Based on these findings, the recommendation to maintain the hematocrit of these patients at 45% or less evolved. However, the hematocrit is unlikely to be the only factor causing thrombosis. Patients with polycythemia of high altitude or resulting from heart disease have thrombotic complications far less than those seen in polycythemia vera. When 100 cyanotic patients with congenital heart disease were observed for a total of 748 patient-years, no patient with polycythemia developed cerebral arterial thrombosis.[48] Large studies of patients with Eisenmenger syndrome[49] and other cyanotic heart diseases[50] also raised caution against routine phlebotomy for asymptomatic elevation of hematocrit. Although mice are not people, transgenic mice with extreme polycythemia (hematocrit 85%) caused by constitutive overexpression of erythropoietin did not develop the expected thrombotic complications.[51]

Other Modifiers of Thrombosis

Because platelets and white blood cells are also part of the polycythemia vera clone, a role for these cells can be hypothesized, and abnormalities of endothelial cells or coagulation proteins may be other contributing factors. Polycythemia vera patients have increased platelet thromboxane A_2 production, which stimulates platelet aggregation.[52] Other described abnormalities in polycythemia vera patients that might contribute to a prothrombotic state include decreased levels of proteins C and S and antithrombin III,[25,53] decreased fibrinolytic activity,[54] activation of coagulation proteins by clonal polycythemia vera neutrophils,[55] decreased platelet response to the inhibitor prostaglandin D_2,[56] and abnormal in vivo activation of leukocytes, platelets, and endothelial cells.[52,55,57]

Non–polycythemia vera–related factors, including hereditary conditions, could potentially contribute to thrombotic events. In a prospective study, the PI^{A2} polymorphism of the platelet glycoprotein (GP) IIIa was associated with an increased risk of arterial thrombosis in polycythemia vera patients.[58] However, polymorphisms of GPIb and GPIa, or the presence of the prothrombin G20210A mutation or factor V Leiden mutation did not correlate with thrombohemorrhagic events.[58]

Aspirin

The use of high-dose aspirin (300 mg three times a day) in combination with dipyridamole (75 mg three times a day) in polycythemia vera patients caused unacceptable hemorrhagic side effects without decreasing thrombotic events.[42] However, others[52] argued that lower dose aspirin (100 mg/day or less) sufficiently inhibits thromboxane A_2 generation without inhibition of prostacyclin (which prevents platelet endothelial adhesion), thus potentially improving the risk/benefit ratio of aspirin therapy in polycythemia vera. This led to the large prospective multicenter ECLAP study (European Collaboration on Low-Dose Aspirin in Polycythemia Vera), which showed that daily low-dose aspirin reduced the

TABLE 36–2. PVSG Criteria for the Diagnosis of Polycythemia Vera

	Major Criteria		Minor Criteria
A1	Increased RBC mass Male: ≥36 mL/kg Female: ≥32 mL/kg	B1	Thrombocytosis (platelet count > 400,000/μL)
A2	Normal arterial O_2 saturation (≥92%)	B2	Leukocytosis (WBC count > 12,000/μL)
A3	Splenomegaly (palpable)	B3	Increased leukocyte alkaline phosphatase* (>100)
		B4	Increased serum vitamin B_{12}/binders* (B_{12} > 900 pg/mL) (Unbound B_{12} binding capacity > 2200 pg/mL)

Diagnosis is virtually certain if all three major criteria *or* A1 + A2 + any two minor criteria are present.
*Not specific for PV; see text.
Abbreviations: RBC, red blood cell; WBC, white blood cell.

number of nonfatal arterial and venous thromboses, albeit by a small amount, with only minor risk of bleeding.[59] Because most of the thrombotic complications were not prevented, this study suggests that only a minor fraction of thromboses are attributable to platelets, and the mechanism of the majority of thrombotic complications in polycythemia vera remains unexplained.

Postpolycythemic Myeloid Metaplasia

Postpolycythemic myeloid metaplasia, or "spent phase," is characterized by a progressive decrease in erythrocyte production, increasing splenomegaly, and myelofibrosis. Thrombocytopenia and anemia are common, and the peripheral blood examination shows leukoerythroblastic features. It is difficult, and often impossible, to distinguish this stage of polycythemia vera from idiopathic myelofibrosis unless a preceding history of polycythemia is known. The extent to which chemotherapy or ^{32}P therapy may influence the development of the spent phase is not defined, but this syndrome is clearly one aspect of the natural history of polycythemia vera.[60]

Acute Leukemia

Acute leukemia, usually myeloid, is another fatal complication of polycythemia vera. The ECLAP observational study of 1638 patients reported a 6.3 relative risk of developing leukemia 10 years after the diagnosis of polycythemia vera.[41] In the PVSG-01 randomized trial, the incidence of acute leukemia at 18 years of follow-up was 1.5% in the phlebotomy-only arm, 10% in the ^{32}P arm, and 13% in the chlorambucil arm.[60] The contribution of other myelosuppressive therapies to the development of leukemia remains controversial.

Development of the spent phase is associated with an increased risk of leukemic transformation. In the PVSG-01 study, the incidence of acute leukemia was 23.7% versus 7.1% in patients with and without myelofibrosis, respectively.[42]

Diagnosis

The diagnosis may be straightforward in patients who present with classic findings of polycythemia, thrombocytosis, leukocytosis, and splenomegaly. However, many patients present at earlier stages, and the lack of a single specific diagnostic test for polycythemia vera makes diagnosing this disease sometimes challenging. The PVSG criteria for the diagnosis of polycythemia vera (Table 36–2) were developed in the late 1960s to rapidly diagnose patients "within two office visits" for possible enrollment in clinical trials.[42] These criteria were widely adopted into clinical practice because of the lack of a satisfactory alternative. These criteria identify a relatively homogeneous population of polycythemia vera patients; however, not all patients with the disorder will fulfill the PVSG requirements. Some of the criteria (leukocyte alkaline phosphatase, vitamin B_{12} levels) are nonspecific and not useful in modern hematology practice, whereas newer techniques and tests may be more helpful. Therefore, other diagnostic algorithms have been proposed that incorporate subsequently described features of polycythemia vera. The World Health Organization criteria[61] are shown in Table 36–3; others have been proposed.[62–64] However, none of these is in wide use.

TABLE 36–3. World Health Organization Criteria for the Diagnosis of PV

Elevated RBC mass without obvious secondary cause		
	AND	
One of the following	*OR*	**Two of the following**
Splenomegaly		Platelet count > 400,000/μL
Karyotypic abnormality other than t(9;22)		WBC count > 12,000/μL
Endogenous erythroid colony formation		Bone marrow showing panmyelosis
		Low serum EPO

Abbreviations: EPO, erythropoietin; RBC, red blood cell; WBC, white blood cell.

Red Cell Mass Studies

Red cell mass studies are used to distinguish absolute polycythemia from relative or "spurious" polycythemia. Ideally, the red cell volume and plasma volume should be measured separately. Although it is common practice to measure one parameter and calculate the other based on the hematocrit, this technique is subject to error.[65–67] Unfortunately, the ^{131}I-labeled albumin necessary to measure the plasma volume is at the time of this writing no longer commercially available.

It may not be necessary to measure red cell mass in all patients. In one report,[68] a hematocrit greater than 60% in males and greater than 55% in females was almost always associated with true polycythemia. Others[69] have reached a similar conclusion.

Bone Marrow

The bone marrow in polycythemia vera is usually hypercellular with hyperplasia of the myeloid lineages, and the majority of the specimens have absent iron stores.[70] Although some workers have described specific morphologic features in the bone marrow of patients with polycythemia vera,[71–73] the morphologic criteria suggested for the definitive diagnosis of polycythemia vera have not been validated for inter- and intraobserver reproducibility. Thus, the value of the bone marrow in the diagnosis of polycythemia vera and the other MPDs remains controversial, because there are no proven unique histopathologic features.

The most useful finding from a bone marrow examination may be an abnormal karyotype, but this is present in fewer than 20% of polycythemia vera patients at diagnosis.[74,75] The frequency of chromosomal abnormalities increases with duration of disease and is 70–80% in patients with myelofibrosis or leukemic transformation.[74] The most frequent chromosomal abnormalities are various 9p abnormalities, 20q−, 13q−, and trisomy 9 and 8, but many other nonrandom abnormalities occur and none is specific for polycythemia vera.[74–78] A recent study identified mutations in JAK2 in chromosome 9p, often accompanied by loss of homozygosity.[37d] This has been observed in a large proportion of patients with polycythemia vera (65%), essential thrombocytosis (23%), and idiopathic myelofibrosis (57%), providing a clear molecular link to their etiology. The most common mutation was *V617F*, common to each disease. This mutation increases the proliferation and survival of hematopoietic progenitor cells.[37d] Patients with this mutation in JAK2 had a longer duration of disease and a higher complication rate including fibrosis, hemorrhage, and thrombosis.[37d] Increased marrow reticulin or fibrosis may be present at diagnosis, but does not appear to predict the chance of developing spent phase.[66]

Erythropoietin Levels

Polycythemia vera erythroid progenitors grow in the absence of exogenously added erythropoietin (erythropoietin independence), and serum erythropoietin levels are low in polycythemia vera patients (Fig. 36–2). Older erythropoietin assays were too insensitive to detect subnormal levels of erythropoietin, but using improved technology, several studies have documented serum erythropoietin levels below the normal reference range in patients with polycythemia vera.[79–83] Erythropoietin levels remain low even after phlebotomy,[83] which increases erythropoietin levels in normal individuals.

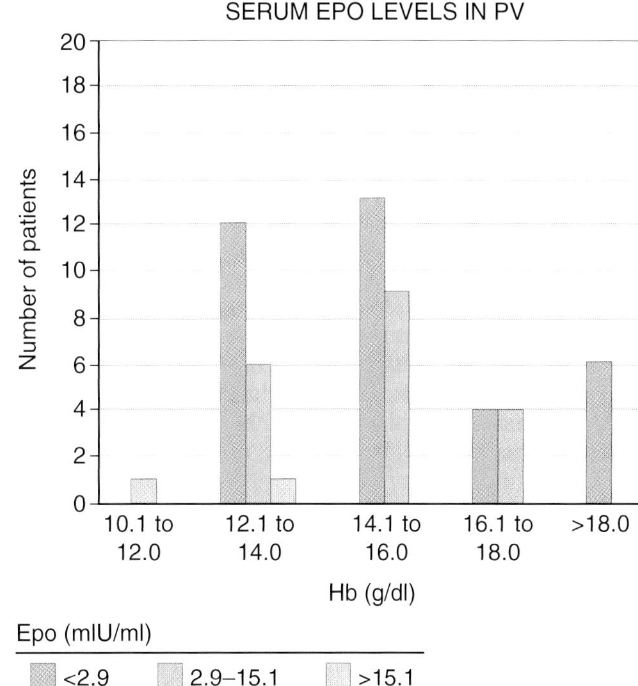

Figure 36–2. Serum erythropoietin (Epo) values at various hemoglobin (Hb) levels in treated and untreated polycythemia vera patients. (From Messinezy M, Westwood N, El-Hemaidi I, et al: Serum erythropoietin values in erythrocytoses and in primary thrombocythaemia. Br J Haematol 117:47–53, 2002, with permission.)

Patients with secondary polycythemia usually have normal to elevated erythropoietin levels, although considerable overlap exists in the range of erythropoietin levels between patients with polycythemia vera and those with secondary polycythemia.[79,82] Although an elevated erythropoietin level generally excludes the diagnosis of polycythemia vera, a low erythropoietin level is not pathognomonic of the disorder because patients with PFCP have as low or lower erythropoietin levels.[5,84]

Erythroid Colony Cultures

Detection of EEC in cultures of bone marrow or peripheral blood may be the most specific test for polycythemia vera[5,85] (see Fig. 36–1). In one study, all patients with polycythemia vera but none with secondary or other causes of polycythemia had EEC.[86] Rare EEC may at times be observed in PFCP and in Chuvash polycythemia, but unlike the EEC of polycythemia vera, these are abrogated by pretreatment with erythropoietin and EPOR-blocking antibodies.[87,88]

In experienced hands, demonstration of EEC is a specific and sensitive means for detecting polycythemia vera and may be useful in diagnosing patients with unusual presentations such as Budd-Chiari syndrome[43–46] or isolated thrombocytosis.[89] There are many modifications of this assay, and its execution requires considerable experience. Its main limitations are the laborious, expensive technique and lack of commercial availability.

Tests of Potential Diagnostic Utility

The use of other diagnostic assays is being investigated. Thrombopoietin, a potent stimulator of platelet production, is produced at a constant rate, and its levels are regulated by binding to its receptor, c-Mpl. Levels of c-Mpl on platelets and megakaryocytes have been shown to be decreased in patients with polycythemia vera,[22] which should lead to increased circulating thrombopoietin levels. The major limitations of an assay of c-Mpl levels in the diagnosis of polycythemia vera are its difficulty and nonspecificity. Increased expression of *bcl*-xL, an antiapoptotic gene, in polycythemia vera erythroid progenitors has been reported,[21] but this is not specific for polycythemia vera either.

Recently, increased mRNA levels of PRV-1 have been reported in polycythemia vera granulocytes but not their progenitors.[33] The exact function of PRV-1 in normal hematopoiesis is unclear and likely plays no significant role in polycythemia vera pathophysiology, because there are no differences in the amount of this protein between normal and polycythemia vera progenitors. However, it may be a useful diagnostic marker of the disease; depending on the report, between 80% and 100% of polycythemia vera patients have increased granulocyte PRV-1 mRNA. However, elevated levels are also seen after granulocyte colony-stimulating factor therapy and other nonspecific stimuli, and PRV-1 mRNA levels cannot reliably discriminate polycythemia vera from congenital polycythemias and various thrombocythemic states.[35,36]

Differential Diagnosis

The differential diagnosis lies in distinguishing polycythemia vera from other causes of polycythemia (Table 36–4 and Fig. 36–3) and occasionally from the other MPDs. Relative polycythemia may be suspected in patients taking diuretics, smokers, or obese patients. If available, a red cell mass study can distinguish relative from absolute polycythemia. Hypoxia, often smoking-related, is a common cause of secondary polycythemia. Intermittent hypoxia, such as with sleep apnea, can also result in polycythemia, but patients may have normal oxygen saturations. If this diagnosis is suspected, sleep studies or other specialized tests may be necessary to document hypoxia. Carboxyhemoglobinemia is another mechanism by which smoking causes polycythemia; this can be measured in arterial blood gas analyses. Familial causes of polycythemia have been misdiagnosed as polycythemia vera; unfortunately a number of these patients were inappropriately treated with ^{32}P and other chemotherapeutic agents. Familial polycythemia may be suspected if there is an autosomal dominant family history; however, autosomal recessive familial polycythemias also occur and these may not have a family history. A history of polycythemia since childhood or young adulthood may be an important clue.

Some patients present with extreme thrombocytosis and normal hematocrit and are initially diagnosed as having essential thrombocythemia, but over a period of time eventually develop the full polycythemia vera phenotype. Demonstration of EEC may be useful in identifying these cases of "latent" polycythemia vera.[89]

TABLE 36–4. Differential Diagnosis of Polycythemia

Acquired
Primary
Polycythemia vera
Secondary
Hypoxemia
Chronic lung disease
Sleep apnea
Right-to-left cardiac shunts
High altitude
Autonomous erythropoietin production
Hepatocellular carcinoma
Renal cell carcinoma
Cerebellar hemangioblastoma
Pheochromocytoma
Parathyroid carcinoma
Meningioma
Uterine leiomyoma
Polycystic kidney disease
Following renal transplantation (probable abnormal angiotensin II signaling)
Carbon monoxide exposure (carboxyhemoglobinemia)
Smokers
Environmental
Cobalt exposure
Androgens/anabolic steroids
Exogenous erythropoietin administration ("Epo doping")
Hereditary
Primary
Primary familial and congenital polycythemia
Erythropoietin receptor mutations
Unknown gene mutations
High-oxygen-affinity hemoglobins
2,3-biphosphoglycerate deficiency
Mixed Primary and Secondary
Chuvash polycythemia

Treatment

The treatment of polycythemia vera is largely based on the results of three trials conducted by the PVSG study group in the United States and from European cooperative trials (Tables 36–5 and 36–6). Commonly used therapies can be categorized into four main categories: red cell mass reduction (phlebotomy), antiplatelet therapy, cytoreductive therapy, and interferon alfa (IFN), whose mechanism of action is unknown. Therapies directed at elimination of the abnormal clone (i.e., bone marrow transplant) are primarily investigational.

Phlebotomy

Phlebotomy is a mainstay of treatment of polycythemia vera. The goal is to maintain the hematocrit within the normal range; although a value of 45% is often quoted,[66,90] this is not derived from prospective studies. It is also unknown if a lower target hematocrit is required in women, as some have suggested.[66] The advantage to

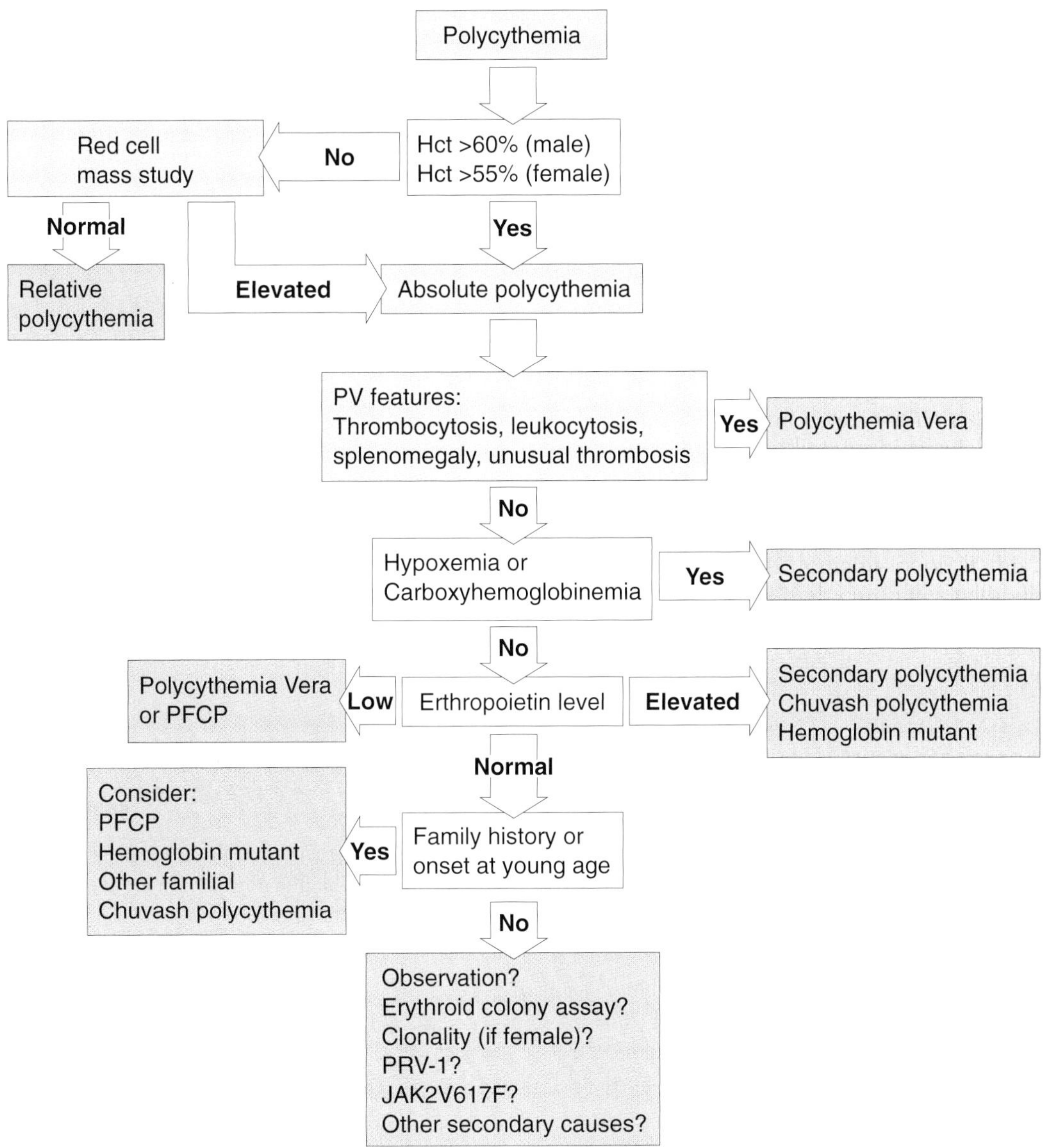

Figure 36–3. Diagnostic algorithm for polycythemia vera (PV). Abbreviations: PFCP, primary familial and congenital polycythemia; PRV-1, polycythemia rubra vera 1 (increased mRNA levels in PV neutrophils; see text). The role of JAK-2 mutation *(JAK2V617F)* in the differential diagnosis of polycythemia vera remains to be established.

phlebotomy is a rapid, effective reduction in red cell mass; the disadvantages are the inconvenience and the potential for increase in thrombotic episodes, although this risk appears to be limited to the first 3 years of therapy.

Cytoreductive Therapy

Alkylating Agents

The alkylating agents, including chlorambucil, busulfan, and pipobroman, are an effective means of controlling white blood cell count and platelet count in addition to contributing to control of the red cell mass, but concern about potential leukemogenicity has limited their use in modern hematology practice. In the PSVG-01 study, which randomized patients to phlebotomy alone, phlebotomy plus ^{32}P, or phlebotomy plus chlorambucil, overall survival was the poorest in the chlorambucil-treated arm because of the increased frequency of hematologic malignancies. Acute leukemia accounted for the majority of the hematologic malignancies, but non-Hodgkin's lymphoma also occurred; this complication appears to be unique to chlorambucil.[42] The incidence of gastrointestinal cancers and skin cancers was also increased in the chlorambucil-treated patients.

The contribution of the other alkylating agents to leukemia development is less clear. A randomized trial comparing pipobroman, an agent used in Europe but not available in the United States, to hydroxyurea reported a 10% risk of leukemia development at 13 years, which was not statistically different between the two arms.[91] A

TABLE 36–5. Clinical Trials in Polycythemia Vera

Trial	Design	Number Enrolled	Results
PSVG-01	Phlebotomy alone vs. phlebotomy + ^{32}P vs. phlebotomy + chlorambucil	431	Phlebotomy arm had more thrombotic events in first 3 yr. More leukemia in ^{32}P and chlorambucil arms. Survival statistically inferior with chlorambucil.
PVSG-05	^{32}P vs. aspirin (300 mg 3 times daily) + dipyridamole (75 mg 3 times daily)	178	Increased bleeding with aspirin (7% vs. 0%), especially if platelet count > 930,000/μL. Increased thrombosis with aspirin. Combined death, thrombosis, and hemorrhage in aspirin arm 8 times higher than in ^{32}P arm.
PVSG-08	Phase II (efficacy) trial of hydroxyurea	51	Hydroxyurea-treated patients had decreased thrombosis compared to phlebotomy-only arm of PSVG-01. Leukemia development not statistically different from phlebotomy alone historical control.
French Polycythemia Study Group	Hydroxyurea vs. pipobroman in patients < age 65	292	Increased myelofibrosis with hydroxyurea (17% vs. 2.1%). No difference in overall survival, thrombosis, or leukemic conversion.
French Polycythemia Study Group	^{32}P alone vs. ^{32}P followed by hydroxyurea in patients > age 65	461	Trend to increased leukemia with hydroxyurea, but not statistically significant. No difference in thrombosis, myelofibrosis, or overall survival.
EORTC	^{32}P vs. busulfan	293	Decreased thrombosis and improved overall survival (70% vs. 55% at 10 yr) with busulfan. Overall survival increased in busulfan arm.
ECLAP	Aspirin 100 mg/day vs. placebo	518	Decrease in nonfatal thrombotic events with aspirin. No difference in major hemorrhagic events.

TABLE 36–6. Risk-Adjusted Treatment Options for Polycythemia Vera

Risk Category	Criteria	Treatment	Comments
Low	Age < 60 yr *and* No thrombosis	Phlebotomy ± aspirin 100 mg/day if no contraindications*	
High	Age > 60 yr *or* Prior thrombosis	Hydroxyurea	Proven reduction in thrombosis in clinical trial.
		Phlebotomy	To control hematocrit.
		Anagrelide	If recurrent thrombosis and persistent thrombocytosis, or hydroxyurea undesired.
		Interferon alfa	Consider in younger patients, painful splenomegaly, intractable pruritus.
		± Aspirin 100 mg/day if no contraindications*	

*Contraindications to aspirin include prior bleeding history, platelet count > 1,000,000/μL, concurrent anagrelide use.

single-arm study of 163 patients treated with pipobroman reported a 5% incidence of leukemia in the first 10 years,[92] and a retrospective study of 65 patients treated with busulfan alone found a 3% incidence of leukemia.[93] A European Organization for Research on Treatment of Cancer (EORTC) trial compared busulfan to ^{32}P and found slightly improved survival with busulfan.[94,95]

Hydroxyurea

Hydroxyurea is effective therapy for controlling the erythrocyte, leukocyte, and platelet counts, and decreased the risk of thrombosis during the first few years of therapy when compared to a historical cohort treated with phlebotomy alone.[42] The main disadvantage is the need for continuous therapy, because the blood counts rebound if the drug is stopped. The risk of leukemogenesis is controversial; studies have either shown no increase in risk or a non–statistically significant increase in risk of acute leukemia.[91,96–102]

Radioactive Phosphorus

Radioactive phosphorus (^{32}P) has the advantage of infrequent administration but the disadvantages of increased risk of leukemia and spent phase. The long-standing control of peripheral blood counts with a single dose and proven reduction of thrombotic complications are attractive options for selected patients. Thus, ^{32}P may still have an occasional role in the treatment of elderly patients who are unable to travel for frequent medical visits.

Anagrelide

Anagrelide is effective in controlling thrombocytosis in the majority of patients with MPDs, including polycythemia vera.[103] Side effects include headache, diarrhea, fluid retention, and tachycardia; most symptoms improve with continued therapy.

Interferon Alfa

IFN inhibits the in vitro proliferation of hematopoietic stem cells, although the mechanism by which it does so is unknown. IFN suppresses in vitro erythroid, myeloid, and megakaryocytic colony growth of polycythemia vera progenitors.[104–106] More recent evidence suggests that IFN can stimulate humoral and cell-mediated immunity against the polycythemia vera clone.[107] Furthermore, the release of transforming growth factor-β and platelet-derived growth factor from abnormal megakaryocytes is hypothesized to be a factor in bone marrow fibrosis, and it is theorized that IFN might decrease or prevent marrow fibrosis by its action on megakaryocytic progenitors, although this remains to be proven. Thus, by acting at the level of the pluripotent stem cell, IFN has the potential to directly affect the malignant clone in polycythemia vera and has been shown to be beneficial in treatment. In clinical trials, IFN in doses ranging from 3 to 35 million IU/week reduced the frequency of phlebotomies by 82% and eliminated phlebotomy in 50%.[108] Spleen size was reduced in 77% of patients and pruritus was controlled in 81%. Leukocytosis and thrombocytosis also improved. The remissions induced by IFN may persist after discontinuation of the drug.[109]

Evidence that IFN has some effect on the malignant clone is supported by documentation of cytogenetic remissions in polycythemia vera patients with a chromosomal abnormality[110–113] and demonstration of reversion of granulocytes and platelets from clonal to polyclonal.[36] IFN is the only agent reported so far with these effects on the polycythemia vera clone.

Unlike many prior therapies for polycythemia vera, IFN has no known mutagenic or teratogenic effects. The main disadvantages to IFN therapy are its expense, the inconvenience of subcutaneous administration, and its often intolerable side effects. In one study, 21% of patients withdrew from therapy because of side effects,[108] which include flulike symptoms, myalgias, arthralgias, asthenia, depression, peripheral neuropathy, hepatotoxicity, and renal toxicity.

Antiplatelet Therapy

In the PVSG-05 study, high-dose aspirin (900 mg/day) in addition to the antiplatelet agent dipyridamole (225 mg/day) was compared to ^{32}P therapy. The aspirin arm was associated with significant increase in gastrointestinal bleeding without improvement in thrombosis.[42]

However, low-dose aspirin has fewer side effects and may be beneficial in reducing thrombosis. Thromboxane A_2 generation by platelets is increased in polycythemia vera patients, and thus thromboxane-mediated platelet activation may be an important factor in thrombosis in these patients. Low-dose aspirin selectively inhibits thromboxane formation and has been shown to reduce major thrombotic events in patients with acute coronary syndromes, who also have significant increases in thromboxane synthesis.[114–116] The ECLAP study randomized 518 polycythemia vera patients without a clear indication or contraindication to aspirin therapy to aspirin 100 mg/day or placebo.[59] The median age at enrollment was 60 years; only approximately 10% of patients in each arm had a prior history of thrombosis. There was a statistically significant reduction in nonfatal thrombotic events in the aspirin-treated group, with no increase in major hemorrhagic episodes. Thus, low-dose aspirin is a reasonable consideration in polycythemia vera patients without a contraindication to this therapy.

Bone Marrow Transplantation

The largest report on the use of bone marrow transplantation is from Seattle, which describes 12 patients with polycythemia vera and 13 with essential thrombocythemia who received allogeneic (16 related, 9 unrelated) marrow or peripheral blood stem cell transplant.[117] All patients had advanced disease with either myelofibrosis and cytopenias or transformation to acute leukemia or myelodysplastic syndrome. The age range was 18–60 years. There were nine transplant-related deaths, seven of whom had acute leukemia or myelodysplastic syndrome. However, at a median follow-up of 41 months (range, 5–116 months) posttransplant, 16 patients were alive and 14 were in continued unmaintained remission. These data suggest that allogeneic transplantation may be feasible and effective for a select group of patients. Because polycythemia vera primarily affects older people, most patients are not realistic candidates for allogeneic transplantation; thus nonmyeloablative transplantation is being actively explored. The limited amount of data on allogeneic nonmyeloablative transplant in idiopathic myelofibrosis are encouraging,[118,119] although it remains to be shown if these results will also apply to high-risk polycythemia vera.

Imatinib Mesylate

Imatinib mesylate is a small-molecule drug that inhibits tyrosine kinases. Although developed to inhibit the Bcr-Abl tyrosine kinase associated with CML, it has similar inhibitory activity against stem cell factor receptor (c-Kit) and platelet-derived growth factor receptor.[120–122] In addition to its efficacy in CML, imatinib has activity in idiopathic hypereosinophilic syndrome[120] and gastrointestinal stromal tumors.[123] An imatinib-sensitive tyrosine phosphoprotein has been identified in some polycythemia vera leukocytes.[124] Case reports have shown some clinical benefit of imatinib in polycythemia vera patients, primarily in reducing phlebotomy requirements.[125–127] Additional studies are needed to determine the potential role of imatinib in polycythemia vera.

Supportive Care and Long-Term Management

Pruritus

Pruritus is a characteristic feature of polycythemia vera and may be present in up to 48% of patients.[38] Often difficult to control, pruritus may be the factor most negatively affecting quality of life in polycythemia vera patients. Although it classically and frequently is aggravated by a hot bath, the cause of pruritus is unknown. Histamine release is a postulated mechanism, but the data to support histamine or mast cell contribution to pruritus are conflicting.[128–131] Treatment of pruritus is often frustrating. Phlebotomy has no benefit. Therapies that have been tried with varying degrees of success include antihistamines (H_1 and H_2 receptor blockers)[38,132] and aspirin.[133] IFN is effective, but has substantial other toxicities.[108] Selective serotonin reuptake inhibitors (paroxetine, fluoxetine) significantly relieved pruritus in 8 of 10 studied patients.[134] Narrow-band ultraviolet B phototherapy was also effective in a small study of 10 patients.[135]

Erythromelalgia

Erythromelalgia is a clinical syndrome of painful burning sensation and erythema of the hands and feet. It is not specific to polycythemia vera or other MPDs, and in one series of 168 patients with erythromelalgia, only 15 had an MPD.[136] It is frequently associated with elevated platelet counts, and a role for transient thrombotic occlusion by platelet aggregates has been proposed.[137] It usually responds rapidly and completely to aspirin 81 mg,[39] but some patients may require cytoreductive[138] or IFN[139,140] therapy to control their symptoms.

Postpolycythemic Myelofibrosis

Management of patients in the spent phase is largely supportive, with transfusions as needed for symptoms. Treatment with erythropoietin for anemia and androgens for anemia and thrombocytopenia occasionally results in clinical benefit, and steroids may relieve constitutional symptoms.[41] Hydroxyurea, busulfan, and IFN may decrease the rate of progression of splenomegaly. The role of splenectomy is controversial, but potential benefits include red cell transfusion independence and relief of pain and abdominal discomfort in those patients with recurrent painful splenic infarcts.[141] However, a large Mayo Clinic series pointed to a significant mortality and morbidity of splenectomy in this polycythemia vera subgroup.[142]

Other therapies are being explored in the treatment of myelofibrosis. Thalidomide may ameliorate anemia, thrombocytopenia, and splenomegaly; unfortunately, side effects are common.[41] Nonmyeloablative stem cell transplantation has shown promise,[118] and other agents that may modify the disease are also under investigation.[41]

Prognosis

The median survival of treated patients in the PVSG trials ranged from 9 to 13.5 years.[60,143] Others have suggested a much longer life expectancy, including one study in which the survival of polycythemia vera patients was similar to that of a control group.[144] Nevertheless, most studies agree there is some excess mortality attributable to complications of polycythemia vera. In a retrospective Italian study of 1213 polycythemia vera patients, the median duration of survival was more than 15 years.[2] However, the age- and sex-standardized mortality rate for these patients was 1.7 times that of the general Italian population. Another study showed that even patients younger than 50 years had increased mortality compared to the general population, although their median survival was 23 years.[145]

ESSENTIAL THROMBOCYTHEMIA

Epidemiology and Risk Factors

Essential thrombocythemia is a less common disorder than polycythemia vera, with only one case of essential thrombocythemia for every four polycythemia vera cases.[146] The true incidence is difficult to determine because of the lack of large epidemiologic studies. In Olmsted County, Minnesota, the incidence was 2.53 per 100,000 population[146]; in Denmark, the incidence was lower at 0.59 per 100,000.[147] However, the incidence appears to have increased with the advent of automated platelet counting.[147] Many studies have shown a slight female predominance.[146–149] The average age at diagnosis is 60,[147–149] but there is a separate peak in young females. Of all the chronic MPDs, essential thrombocythemia has the highest proportion of young female patients affected.[34,150–152] Essential thrombocythemia is an extremely rare occurrence in childhood.[153,154]

Frequently misdiagnosed as essential thrombocythemia, familial thrombocythemias are inherited disorders caused by germline mutations that are typically inherited in an autosomal dominant fashion. Several molecular defects have been identified, including several 5′ mutations of the thrombopoietin gene resulting in more efficient translation of thrombopoietin mRNA[155] and mutations of the thrombopoietin receptor,[156] but in other families the causative gene mutation remains to be found.[157]

Pathophysiology

The cause of essential thrombocythemia is unknown. Mutations of the thrombopoietin receptor (c-Mpl) have not been identified.[158,159] Expression of c-Mpl is decreased on platelets in essential thrombocythemia,[160] and thrombopoietin levels are inappropriately normal or elevated.[161,162] However, these findings are not specific for essential thrombocythemia.[35] Recently, loss of homozygosity at chromosome 9p has been identified in some patients.[37d] In 23% of patients with essential thrombocytosis, a mutation was seen. As noted above, this mutation results in a hematopoietic progenitor cell proliferation and cell survival advantage.

Clonality studies using X-chromosome inactivation patterns have shown that the erythrocytes, granulocytes, and platelets are derived from a single clone.[163] Some studies have reported polyclonal hematopoiesis in patients with a clinical diagnosis of essential thrombocythemia.[164] However, thrombotic events appear to occur primarily or exclusively in those patients with monoclonal hematopoiesis.[164–166] This observation suggests that those patients with polyclonal hematopoiesis have a biologically separate disease, although clinically indistinguishable, from classic essential thrombocythemia. Some reports[161,164] also describe clonal platelets without clonality of other myeloid cells, a finding difficult to reconcile with the origin of essential thrombocythemia from a pluripotent hematopoietic progenitor; however, technical differences in the clonality assays used may account for some of these discrepancies.[36]

Abnormal responses of megakaryocytic and erythroid progenitors to erythropoietin and thrombopoietin have been reported; one of the more promising assays described increased sensitivity of megakaryocytic progenitors to thrombopoietin in serum free cultures.[167] However, the specificity and universal applicability of these assays have not yet been established.

Clinical Features and Diagnosis

Symptoms

Patients may present with thrombotic and/or hemorrhagic symptoms. However, with the implementation of automated platelet counting, many asymptomatic patients are detected incidentally on a complete blood count.[147]

Physical Examination

Mild splenomegaly may be present in up to 40% of patients.[168,169] Otherwise, the physical examination is usually unremarkable.

Laboratory Findings

An unexplained and sustained elevation of the platelet count is the defining feature of essential thrombocythemia, whereas the white blood cell count and hemoglobin are normal. The level of thrombocytosis required for a diagnosis of essential thrombocythemia is arbitrary and differs among investigators. The PVSG established a platelet count greater than 600,000/μL for diagnosis and required a platelet count greater than 1,000,000/μL for patients entering therapeutic protocols. Others[170] have used platelet counts of greater than 450,000/μL as their criteria.

Pseudohyperkalemia and pseudohypoxemia may occur in patients with extreme thrombocytosis.

Thrombosis

The frequency of thrombosis at the time of diagnosis varies among studies, with a range of 9–84%.[152] However, these studies were uncontrolled, did not include the same patient populations, and used widely different definitions of major and minor thrombotic events. In the only controlled study, the risk of thrombotic events was 6.6% per patient-year in patients with essential thrombocythemia versus 1.2% per patient-year in 200 patients with monoclonal gammopathy of undetermined significance.[171]

Thrombosis occurs both in large vessels and in the microvasculature. Arterial thrombosis is more common than venous.[172] Neurologic symptoms resulting from cerebrovascular ischemia are common, occurring in 25% of patients.[173] Symptoms are often transient, and include headache, dizziness, paresthesias, visual disturbances, and transient ischemic attacks.[174–176]

Microvascular occlusions in the digits cause pain, distal extremity gangrene, and erythromelalgia.[39] Myocardial infarction or angina may occur, and some of these patients have normal coronary arteries.[177–179] Deep venous thrombosis of the lower extremities and pulmonary embolism are the most common venous thrombotic events.[180] Unusual sites of thrombosis, such as the hepatic or portal vein, are more commonly seen in polycythemia vera, but also occur in patients with essential thrombocythemia.[181]

The only clearly established risk factors for development of thrombosis are a history of prior thrombotic event and age greater than 60 years.[171,182] Comorbid conditions such as smoking, diabetes mellitus, hyperlipidemia, and hypertension did not influence the incidence of thrombosis in one study.[171] Other studies reported that hypercholesterolemia and smoking were associated with increased risk for thrombosis.[183,184] However, all of these studies are limited by their retrospective design.

The degree of elevation of the platelet count does not appear to affect the risk for thrombosis. Thrombotic complications have been reported in essential thrombocythemia patients even with platelet counts between 400,000 and 600,000/μL.[185] Although a positive correlation between the platelet count and thromboses has not been established, lowering the platelet count with cytoreductive therapy clearly decreases the incidence of thrombosis.[171,186]

Hemorrhage

Bleeding symptoms are usually minor and generally affect mucosal membranes, gastrointestinal tract, and skin.[187] The incidence rate of major hemorrhagic complications in essential thrombocythemia patients was 0.33% per patient-year.[171] Extreme elevations in platelet count (>1,500,000/μL) and the use of aspirin or nonsteroidal anti-inflammatory drugs increase the risk for bleeding.[172] The hemorrhagic manifestations in patients with platelet counts greater than 1,500,000/μL appear to be due to an acquired von Willebrand syndrome.[188] Von Willebrand factor antigen levels are normal, but ristocetin cofactor activity is decreased and there is an absence of large and intermediate von Willebrand factor multimers, simulating type II von Willebrand disease.

Acute Leukemia and Myelofibrosis

Acute leukemia is a well-described complication of essential thrombocythemia.[189] The contribution of cytoreductive therapy to the development of leukemia is unclear; however, leukemic transformation in the absence of any previous therapy has been docu-

TABLE 36–7. Criteria for the Diagnosis of Essential Thrombocythemia*

Sustained elevation of platelet count (>600,000/μL)
Mutation in JAK2
Exclude causes of reactive thrombosis:
- Infection
- Collagen vascular disease (antinuclear antibody, rheumatoid factor)
- Inflammation (normal C-reactive peptide and sedimentation rate)
- Iron deficiency (normal iron stores or stainable iron on bone marrow aspirate)
- Malignancy
- Hemolytic anemia
- Other causes of reactive thrombosis: splenectomy, etc.

Exclude other clonal hematologic disorders:
- Chronic myelogenous leukemia (no Philadelphia chromosome or *bcr-abl* gene rearrangement)
- Polycythemia vera (normal red blood cell mass or hemoglobin < 18 gm/dL)
- Myelofibrosis (bone marrow fibrosis < 1/3 involvement)
- Myelodysplasia (no typical cytogenetic abnormalities, e.g., 5q–)

Megakaryocyte hyperplasia with atypical megakaryocytes and megakaryocyte clustering on bone marrow aspirate and biopsy (*controversial*)

*Considerations in the differential diagnosis of essential thrombocythemia, with suggested tests in parentheses.

TABLE 36–8. Causes of Thrombocytosis

Diagnosis	Platelet count >500,000/μL (732 Patients)		Platelet count > 1,000,000/μL (280 Patients)	
	N	(%)	*N*	(%)
Myeloproliferative Disorders	89	(12.3%)	38	(13.6%)
ET	40	(5.5%)	11	(3.9%)
CML	24	(3.3%)	16	(5.8%)
PV	18	(2.5%)	5	(1.8%)
Myelofibrosis	4	(0.6%)	2	(0.7%)
Unclassified	3	(0.4%)	4	(1.4%)
Reactive Thrombocytosis	620	(84.6%)	231	(82.5%)
Tissue damage	269	(36.7%)	32	(11.4%)
Infection	154	(21.0%)	72	(25.7%)
Malignancy	85	(11.6%)	33	(11.8%)
Chronic inflammatory disorders	65	(8.9%)	21	(7.5%)
Postsplenectomy	12	(1.6%)	43	(15.4%)
Other	35	(4.8%)	30	(10.7%)
Unknown Etiology	23	(3.1%)	11	(3.9%)

Data from 732 inpatients and outpatients with platelet count of greater than 500,000/μL and 280 hospitalized patients with platelet count greater than 1,000,000/μL. Modified from Griesshammer et al.[192] and Buss et al.[193]
Abbreviations: CML, chronic myelogenous leukemia; ET, essential thrombocythemia; PV, polycythemia vera.

mented.[190,191] The risk of developing myelofibrosis is approximately 0.9% per year.[152]

Diagnosis

Differential Diagnosis

Essential thrombocythemia is a diagnosis of exclusion, because there is no specific marker or test for this disorder. Secondary or reactive causes of thrombocytosis as well as the other MPDs must be considered and excluded before a diagnosis of essential thrombocythemia can be made. Many lists of diagnostic criteria have been published; however, they are all arbitrary (see Table 36–7 for an example).

Reactive causes account for the majority of cases of thrombocytosis[192,193] (Table 36–8). The degree of thrombocytosis is not useful in distinguishing reactive from primary thrombocythemia.[192,194] In a study of 280 hospitalized patients with extreme thrombocytosis, 82% had reactive causes.[193] Most patients with reactive thrombocytosis do not have bleeding or thrombotic complications.[192,194]

Diagnostic Tests

Appropriate clinical evaluation and laboratory tests should be performed to exclude causes of reactive thrombosis and other hematologic disorders (see Table 36–7).

The role of bone marrow studies in the diagnosis of essential thrombocythemia has not been definitively established, and it seems to be more commonly performed in Europe than in the United States. Although some have described specific bone marrow morphologic abnormalities,[195] these features have not been validated by blinded objective analyses. Indications for a bone marrow analysis may include suspected myelodysplastic syndrome or idiopathic myelofibrosis, or concern for transformation to leukemia, myelodysplastic syndrome, or spent phase in established essential thrombocythemia patients. A bone marrow study may also be necessary to evaluate for t(9;22) (or *bcr-abl*) and 5q–, because some patients with CML or myelodysplastic syndrome with 5q– have been mistaken for those with essential thrombocythemia. Measurement of serum thrombopoietin levels is not useful, because elevated thrombopoietin levels have been described in both reactive thrombocytosis and essential thrombocythemia.[196] Erythroid colony cultures to determine the presence of EEC may be helpful to distinguish cases of polycythemia vera that present with thrombocytosis and normal hematocrit.[166]

Treatment

Treatment recommendations are limited by the lack of available rigorous scientific data in essential thrombocythemia. Most recommendations are made based on the opinion of expert clinicians; risk-adjusted guidelines for therapy have been proposed[152,197] (see Table 36–9 for an example).

Observation

Observation without therapy may be appropriate for selected groups of patients. In a prospective study,

TABLE 36–9. Risk-Adjusted Treatment Options for Essential Thrombocythemia

Risk Category	Criteria	Treatment
Low	Age < 60 yr *and* Platelet count < 1,500,000/μL *and* No thrombosis	Observation
Intermediate	Neither high nor low	Observation *or* Hydroxyurea or anagrelide* or IFN†
High	Age > 60 yr *or* Prior thrombosis	Hydroxyurea or anagrelide or IFN

*Hydroxyurea preferred for patients greater than age 60; anagrelide preferred for patients less than age 60.
†IFN is used in pregnant women and is another option for younger patients.
Abbreviation: IFN, interferon alfa.

patients younger than age 60 with no prior history of thrombosis and with platelet counts less than 1,500,000/μL did not have an increased incidence of thrombosis compared to the control group.[198] Other observational studies of this "low-risk" population also noted low rates of thrombohemorrhagic events.[199] However, not all agree with this recommendation.[200–202]

Hydroxyurea

Hydroxyurea is a nonalkylating agent that causes cytoreduction of all the myeloid blood cells and has been shown to be efficacious in controlling the platelet count in the majority of essential thrombocythemia patients.[171,186] In a randomized trial in high-risk patients (age >60 or prior history of thrombosis), hydroxyurea significantly reduced thrombotic events compared to the control group (3.6% vs. 24%)[186]; however, there was no difference in survival at a median follow-up of 73 months.[152]

The main concern about the use of hydroxyurea is potential leukemogenicity. Some studies have suggested an increased risk of leukemia development, particularly with the sequential use of hydroxyurea and alkylating agents,[203–205] but others have not shown an increase in leukemia.[206] However, most of these studies are uncontrolled and there has been no randomized trial sufficiently powered to detect a significant risk of leukemic transformation with hydroxyurea therapy.

Anagrelide

Anagrelide reduces platelet formation by an unknown mechanism and controls thrombocytosis in essential thrombocythemia, myelofibrosis, CML, and polycythemia vera. The usual starting dose is 0.5 mg four times daily, titrated up by 0.5 mg weekly as needed. A reduction in platelet count may occur within 1 week. Many trials[103,207–211] have demonstrated the effectiveness of anagrelide in reducing the platelet count, although none was randomized. In a review of 442 essential thrombocythemia patients treated in various trials, the overall response rate was 93%.[152] Fourteen percent of patients withdrew as a result of side effects, mostly headache, fluid retention, tachycardia, and diarrhea. Anemia may also develop; a greater than 3-gm/dL decrease in the hemoglobin occurred in 24% of patients on long-term anagrelide therapy.[212] No increase in leukemic transformation has been reported.[213]

In contrast to hydroxyurea, there are no data indicating that anagrelide reduces the risk of thrombosis. In a study of 35 patients younger than 50 years treated with anagrelide for a median of 10.8 years, a complete response (defined as a platelet count <450,000/μL) occurred in 74%.[212] However, 20% had thrombotic episodes and 20% had major hemorrhagic events; all of these events occurred at platelet counts greater than 400,000/μL.

Interferon Alfa

IFN reduces the platelet count to less than 600,000/μL in 90% of patients within 3 months.[214] The average starting dose is 3–5 million units daily. The drawback to IFN is its significant toxicity; in a review of 273 essential thrombocythemia patients, 25% withdrew from therapy.[214] However, IFN may be appropriate in pregnant women and high-risk women of childbearing age because of its lack of teratogenicity. Additionally, no increased risk for leukemia development has been reported.

Antiplatelet Therapy

Aspirin is very effective therapy for the palliation of erythromelalgia and other symptoms resulting from microvascular occlusion.[215,216] The contribution of aspirin to reducing major thrombotic events in essential thrombocythemia is unknown, although the ECLAP study[59] showed a slight but statistically significant reduction in thrombosis with the use of low-dose aspirin in polycythemia vera patients. Aspirin therapy increases the risk for bleeding, and most hemorrhagic events have been reported in patients with platelet counts greater than 1,000,000/μL[215,217]; aspirin should be used judiciously in these patients.

Plateletpheresis

Plateletpheresis is effective in lowering the platelet count in patients with life-threatening thrombosis or hemorrhage.[218] Cytoreductive therapy should be simultaneously instituted because plateletpheresis is an ineffective long-term therapy.

Management in Pregnancy

Essential thrombocythemia has the highest proportion of young female patients of all the MPDs; thus, pregnancy is not an uncommon occurrence. The management of pregnant patients with essential thrombocythemia is a challenge because thrombosis is the main complication of this disorder and is accentuated by the prothrombotic state of pregnancy. In a review of 155 pregnancies in 86 women with essential thrombocythemia, only 59% resulted in a live birth.[150] First-trimester abortion was seen in 31% of pregnancies; the main cause was placental infarction. Maternal thrombotic or hemorrhagic complications were infrequent but were more common than in normal pregnancy. Nevertheless, pregnancy did not appear to adversely affect the course and prognosis of essential thrombocythemia.

A large review of pooled outcome data from 461 pregnancies in women with essential thrombocythemia reached similar conclusions.[152] There was no correlation between the platelet count and pregnancy outcome. Therapy impact was difficult to evaluate because management of essential thrombocythemia pregnancies was heterogeneous. A benefit for aspirin therapy was suggested, because 79 of 106 patients treated with aspirin had successful pregnancies, compared with only 80 of 145 patients not receiving aspirin. However, there was no direct evidence for the efficacy of aspirin.

The benefit of heparin during pregnancy has not been established, but heparin may have a role in selected cases. An Italian consensus panel[152] recommended that women with essential thrombocythemia and a history of thrombosis should receive heparin at prophylactic doses during the third trimester, and those women with either a peripheral or a placental thrombotic episode during pregnancy should receive low-molecular-weight heparin at therapeutic doses.

If cytoreductive therapy is necessary during pregnancy, IFN is the drug of choice. The Italian panel suggested the following indications for platelet-lowering therapy: a history of major thrombosis or major bleeding, platelet count greater than 1,000,000/μL, familial thrombophilia, or cardiovascular risk factors. Anagrelide is not recommended in pregnancy because of its ability to cross the placenta and uncertainty about its teratogenic potential. Hydroxyurea is also not recommended during pregnancy; however, no malformations and only one stillbirth (in a women who had eclampsia) were reported in 15 infants born to women who were treated with hydroxyurea at conception and/or during pregnancy.[152]

Prognosis

Several studies have reported a decreased life expectancy in essential thrombocythemia patients compared to the general population.[144,147,202,219,220] However, one study of 74 females less than 50 years old found that the incidence of life-threatening thrombosis or hemorrhage and leukemic development was low and that overall survival was similar to that of an age- and sex-matched control population.[199]

CURRENT CONTROVERSIES & FUTURE CONSIDERATIONS

Polycythemia Vera and Essential Thrombocythemia

- What is the optimal hematocrit for polycythemia vera patients?
- When should myelosuppressive therapy be used in polycythemia vera?
- What are the best diagnostic tests for polycythemia vera?
- When should low- and intermediate-risk essential thrombocythemia be treated?
- What is the molecular basis of polycythemia vera and essential thrombocythemia?

Suggested Readings*

Barbui T, Barosi G, Grossi A, et al: Practice guidelines for the therapy of essential thrombocythemia. A statement from the Italian Society of Hematology, the Italian Society of Experimental Hematology and the Italian Group for Bone Marrow Transplantation. Haematologica 89:215–232, 2004.

Cortelazzo S, Finazzi G, Ruggeri M, et al: Hydroxyurea for patients with essential thrombocythemia and a high risk of thrombosis. N Engl J Med 17:1132–1136, 1995.

James C, Ugo V, Le Couedic JP, et al: A unique clonal JAK2 mutation leading to constitutive signalling causes polycythaemia vera. Nature 434:1144–1148, 2005.

Kralovics R, Buser A, Teo S, et al: Comparison of molecular markers in a cohort of patients with chronic myeloproliferative disorders. Blood 102:1869–1871, 2003.

Kralovics R, Passamonti F, Buser AS, et al: A gain-of-function mutation of JAK2 in myeloproliferative disorders. N Engl J Med 352:1779–1790, 2005.

Landolfi R, Marchioli R, Kutti J, et al: Efficacy and safety of low-dose aspirin in polycythemia vera. N Engl J Med 350:114–124, 2004.

Prchal JT: Polycythemia vera and other primary polycythemias. Curr Opin Hematol 2:112–116, 2005.

Full references for this chapter can be found on accompanying CD-ROM.

CHAPTER 37

Myelofibrosis with Myeloid Metaplasia

Ayalew Tefferi, MD

KEY POINTS

Myelofibrosis with Myeloid Metaplasia

Diagnosis

- Myelofibrosis with myeloid metaplasia (MMM) should be suspected in the presence of marked splenomegaly and/or myelophthisis (leukoerythroblastic blood smear).
- Neither splenomegaly nor myelophthisis are specific for either MMM or bone marrow fibrosis in general.
- The differential diagnosis of bone marrow fibrosis should include MMM, chronic myeloid leukemia, myelodysplastic syndrome, other atypical myeloproliferative disorders, acute leukemia, lymphoma, hairy cell leukemia, metastatic cancer, autoimmune diseases, hyperparathyroidism, and infections.
- Bone marrow examination for suspected MMM should be accompanied by cytogenetic studies of either the bone marrow or peripheral blood.

Treatment

- Drug therapy has not been shown either to cure the disease or to prolong life in MMM. It is used for palliative purposes and to that effect alleviates anemia and splenomegaly in a subset of patients.
- Effective drugs in the treatment of MMM include androgen preparations, corticosteroids, erythropoietin, thalidomide, and hydroxyurea.
- Splenectomy is indicated for the management of drug-refractory, symptomatic splenomegaly, symptomatic portal hypertension, high red blood cell transfusion requirement, and severe constitutional symptoms and cachexia.
- Involved-field, low-dose irradiation is effective in the treatment of nonhepatosplenic extramedullary hematopoiesis.
- Allogenic blood stem cell therapy provides a viable treatment option for young patients with high-risk disease.

INTRODUCTION

Myelofibrosis with myeloid metaplasia (MMM), also known as idiopathic myelofibrosis, presents either de novo (agnogenic myeloid metaplasia) or in the setting of either polycythemia vera (postpolycythemic myeloid metaplasia) or essential thrombocythemia (postthrombocythemic myeloid metaplasia) at a rate of 10–20% after 15–20 years of follow-up[1,2] (see Chapter 36). The clinical phenotype includes progressive anemia, massive splenomegaly, hepatosplenic as well as nonhepatosplenic extramedullary hematopoiesis (EMH), and a leukoerythroblastic blood smear.[3] Patients with MMM experience both shortened survival (median of 5–7 years)[4,5] and a quality of life that is often compromised by frequent red blood cell transfusions, a markedly enlarged spleen, and profound constitutional symptoms.[6] Causes of death in MMM include leukemic transformation, which occurs in 8–23% of patients in the first 10 years after diagnosis.[7,8]

Disease Classification

MMM was first described in 1879[9] and is currently classified as a myeloproliferative disorder (MPD). The term *"myeloproliferative disorder"* was first coined by Dameshek in 1951 to emphasize the clinicopathologic interrelationship between MMM (then referred to as idiopathic or "agnogenic" myeloid metaplasia), chronic myeloid leukemia (CML; then referred to as chronic granulocytic leukemia), essential thrombocythemia (then referred to as megakaryocytic leukemia), polycythemia vera, and erythroleukemia (Di Guglielmo's syndrome).[10] Between 1967 and 1981, Fialkow and colleagues showed that the "myeloproliferative disorders" are also biologically interrelated on the basis of being clonal stem cell disorders with involvement of both myeloid and lymphoid lineage.[11–18] Several other myeloid entities, including myelodysplastic syndrome (MDS) and atypical MPD, have since been shown to display clinicopathologic as well as biologic attributes that distinguish them as chronic myeloid disorders. This and other[19] developments in the

TABLE 37–1. A Semi-molecular Classification of Chronic Myeloid Disorders

1. **Myelodysplastic Syndrome**
2. **Myeloproliferative Disorders**
   a. **Classic Myeloproliferative Disorders**
      i. **Molecularly-defined**
         1. Chronic myeloid leukemia *(Bcr/Abl⁺)*
      ii. **Clinicopathologically-assigned**
         (Bcr/Abl⁻ and frequently associated with JAK2^{V617F} mutation)
         1. Essential Thrombocythemia
         2. Polycythemia Vera
         3. Myelofibrosis with Myeloid Metaplasia
   b. **Atypical Myeloproliferative Disorders**
      i. **Molecularly-defined**
         1. PDGFRA-rearranged Eosinophilic/Mast Cell Disorders (e.g., *FIP1L1-PDGFRA)*
         2. *PDGFRB*-rearranged Eosinophilic Disorders (e.g., *TEL/ETV6-PDGFRB*)
         3. Systemic Mastocytosis Associated with *c-kit* Mutation (e.g., *c-kit*^{D816V})
         4. *8p11* Myeloproliferative Syndrome (e.g., *ZNF198/FIM/RAMP-FGFR1*)
      ii. **Clinicopathologically-assigned**
         (infrequently associated with JAK2^{V617F} mutation)
         1. Chronic Neutrophilic Leukemia
         2. Chronic Eosinophilic Leukemia, Molecularly Not Defined
         3. Hypereosinophilic Syndrome
         4. Chronic Basophilic Leukemia
         5. Chronic Myelomonocytic Leukemia
         6. Juvenile Myelomonocytic Leukemia (associated with recurrent mutations of RAS signaling pathway molecules including *PTPN11* and *NF1*)
         7. Systemic Mastocytosis, Molecularly Not Defined
         8. Unclassified Myeloproliferative Disorder

field have led to the consideration of new classification systems that continue to rely on the original concept laid down by Dameshek[3] (Table 37–1).

EPIDEMIOLOGY

Population-based studies have reported varying incidence figures for MMM ranging from 0.4 to 1.5 per 100,000 population.[20–24] As is the case with most other myeloid malignancies, disease incidence increases with age, although childhood occurrence is rare.[23,25] A higher incidence of MMM and related MPD, compared to other ethnic groups, has been suggested in persons of Jewish ancestry and especially in those of Ashkenazi origin.[26] The median age at diagnosis is greater than 60 years, with a male/female ratio of 1.2 : 1.6.[4,7,24] A large Mayo Clinic database of patients with MMM reveals a quarter of the patients to be more than 70 years of age and only 5% under age 40 years. In two other large series of patients with MMM consisting of 323 cases, only 9 patients (2.8%) were age 30 years or less.[27] This partly explains the rarity of concomitant MMM and pregnancy.[28] In general, there is no hard evidence that links MMM with environmental toxins, although associations have been suggested for benzene and other industrial solvents, Thorotrast injections, and radiation accidents.[29–33]

PATHOGENESIS

Clonal Studies

Clonality in MPDs, including MMM, has been extensively addressed by the utilization of clonal assays that are based on allelic polymorphisms (when they exist, thus making a given patient heterozygous or "informative") between the paternally and maternally derived X chromosomes in females. The difference in X chromosome inactivation pattern between "normal" and "clonal" cell populations may be demonstrated in informative females at either the DNA level (based on methylation differences between active and inactive genes),[34] or post-DNA level (based on the fact that RNA and enzyme expression is restricted to the active chromosome).[35–37]

One of the X-chromosome—based clonal assays involves glucose-6-phosphate dehydrogenase isoenzyme analysis. As early as the 1970s and 1980s, the use of such assays suggested that patients with MPDs, including essential thrombocythemia,[18] polycythemia vera,[13] and MMM,[16] have clonal hematopoiesis that originates at the stem cell level and may involve both myeloid and B-lymphoid lineage.[38] This early observation has been supported by more recent investigations using X-linked DNA[39,40] and transcript[36] analysis in informative females. Most recently, a combination of immunomagnetic cell separation technique and interphase cytogenetics was used to directly demonstrate clonal involvement of both B and T lymphocytes, as well as myeloid, erythroid, and megakaryocyte precursors, in MMM.[41]

Cytogenetic and Other Genetic Studies

Despite the abundant evidence for clonal hematopoiesis in MMM, the nature of the disease-causing genetic mutation remains elusive. Recurrent cytogenetic abnormalities that are seen in approximately 50% of chemotherapy-naive patients with MMM include del(20q11;q13), del(13q12;q22), trisomy 8, trisomy 9, t(1;7), del(12p11;p13), monosomy or long arm deletions involving chromosome 7, and trisomy 1q.[5,42] However, the individual lesions occur in only the minority of patients and none is specific to MMM. Furthermore, the application of molecular cytogenetic studies by fluorescent in situ hybridization did not disclose additional, karyotypically occult, structural lesions.[43]

Other pathogenesis-targeted studies in MMM at the genetic level have included mutation screening for type III receptor tyrosine kinases (c-Kit, c-Fms, FLT-3)[44] and genome-wide scanning for loss of heterozygosity.[45] The results from such studies have been largely unrevealing despite the identification of frequent (20–43%) loss-of-heterozygosity sites involving chromosomes 1p, 1q, 2p, 3q, and 3p.[45] In contrast, gene expression studies have suggested a more consistent alteration of gene function, including both downregulation (e.g., *RARB2,* located at 3p24; *BCL1,* located at 11q13; *cdc2,* located at 10q21) and upregulation (e.g., *HMGA2,* located at 12q13-q15; *FKBP51,* located at 6p21; *GATA2,* located at 3q21; *JUNB,* located at 19p13.2) in MMM-derived CD34 cells.[45–48] Other studies have suggested that the JAK/STAT pathway is involved and STAT5 is constitutively activated in both CD34 cells and megakaryocytes from patients with MMM.[49] Recently, mutations of JAK2 have been described as discussed in Chapter 36.

Pathogenesis of the Bone Marrow Stromal Reaction in MMM

In addition to clonal myeloproliferation, the bone marrow in MMM displays excess collagen fibrosis, new bone formation, and angiogenesis.[50,51] The demonstration of polyclonal fibroblast proliferation as well as alterations in both cellular and extracellular levels of various fibrogenic and angiogenic cytokines (e.g., platelet-derived growth factor [PDGF], transforming growth factor-β [TGF-β], basic fibroblast growth factor, vascular endothelial growth factor) has been the basis for the current assumption that the bone marrow stromal aberration in MMM is reactive and mediated by nosogenic cytokines derived from clonal megakaryocytes and monocytes[52–54] (Fig. 37–1).

The possible pathogenetic role of megakaryocyte-derived cytokines in the stromal reaction that accompanies MMM was further suggested by the demonstration of thrombopoietin (TPO)-induced MMM-like disorder in mice (megakaryocytic hyperplasia, myelofibrosis, anemia, extramedullary hematopoiesis).[55] However, in humans with MMM, there is no evidence of either excess TPO production[56–58] or a genetic mutation involving the genes for TPO or its receptor (c-Mpl).[56,59] Specifically, neither TPO nor c-Mpl appear to be essential for endogenous megakaryocyte growth in human MMM.[56] However, MMM megakaryocytes from both the experimental and human disease models display decreased surface expression of c-Mpl,[60] and this might result in decreased clearance of TPO and increased concentration of local TPO, which might contribute to further megakaryocyte and other cell proliferation as well as stimulation of production of other cytokines (see Fig. 37–1).[61]

An alternative explanation for the proliferation of bone marrow megakaryocytes in MMM was suggested by a recent report involving mice that are mutant for the GATA-1 transcription factor.[62] Such mice underexpress GATA-1 and, over time, develop an MMM-like phenotype with megakaryocytic hyperplasia, myelofibrosis, anemia, and extramedullary hematopoiesis. This is consistent with the role of GATA-1 in erythroid and megakaryocyte maturation, and acquired GATA-1 mutations have been reported in Down syndrome—associated transient myeloproliferative disorder and megakaryoblastic leukemia.[63,64] However, in human MMM, there is so far

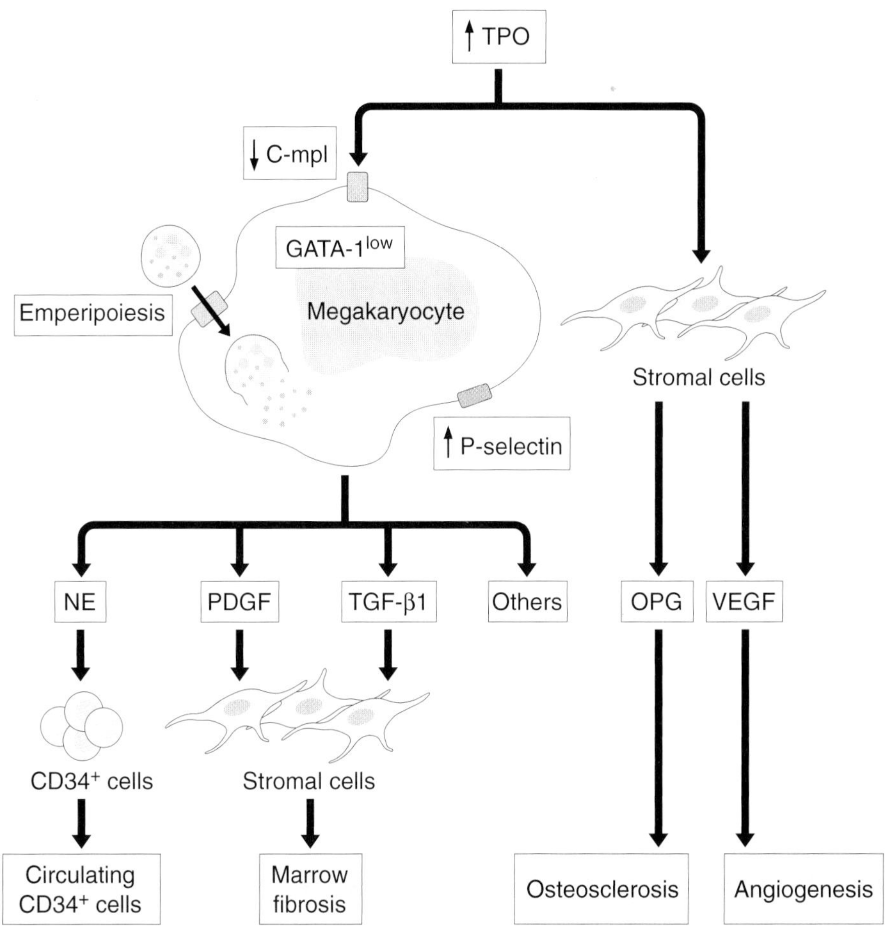

Figure 37–1. Pathogenetic mechanisms in myelofibrosis with myeloid metaplasia (MMM). In mice, either thrombopoietin (TPO) overexposure or intrinsic GATA-1 underexpression results in megakaryocyte proliferation and the MMM phenotype. Megakaryocytes in such mice as well as in human MMM underexpress the TPO receptor (Mpl). This in turn leads to decreased TPO clearance and local TPO excess that might enhance megakaryocyte accumulation as well as stimulate cytokine production. Abnormal release of transforming growth factor-β (TGF-β), platelet-derived growth factor (PDGF), and neutrophil elastase (NE) might result from pathologic interaction between MMM megakaryocytes and neutrophils. These and other cytokines, including vascular endothelial growth factor (VEGF) and osteoprotegerin (OPG), might contribute to several components of the stromal reaction in MMM.

no evidence of either similar mutations or underexpression of GATA-1.[65]

In TPO-induced murine MMM, both myelofibrosis (via hematopoietic stem cell—derived TGF-β1) and osteosclerosis (via stroma-derived osteoprotegerin) have been directly linked to specific cytokines.[66,67] In contrast, the evidence that links various cytokines, including TGF-β1, PDGF, basic fibroblast growth factor, vascular endothelial growth factor, and tissue inhibitors of matrix metalloproteinases, to human MMM-associated bone marrow fibrosis as well as angiogenesis has been circumstantial at best.[68] Nevertheless, tissue abundance of these cytokines might result from pathologic interaction of megakaryocytes and neutrophils (emperipolesis) that is induced by increased expression of P-selectin by the former (see Fig. 37–1).[69] Similarly, neutrophil-derived elastase and other enzymes might contribute to the abnormal peripheral blood egress of myeloid progenitors in MMM.[70,71]

CLINICAL FEATURES AND DIAGNOSIS

Signs and Symptoms

Splenomegaly and Other Manifestations of Extramedullary Hematopoiesis

The prominent clinical feature in MMM is marked splenomegaly, which is secondary to EMH (Fig. 37–2). Information from a large clinical database from the Mayo Clinic reveals that the spleen is palpable in approximately 80% of the patients at diagnosis (median distance from the left costal margin = 8 cm; range, 1–27 cm). Some patients may experience splenic infarcts with severe pain that may be referred to the left shoulder.[72] EMH also occurs in the liver, which is often enlarged as well; lymph nodes (1–7% incidence of palpable lymphadenopathy); and other nonhepatosplenic tissue, including the pleura (effusion), peritoneum (ascites), lung (interstitial process), and paraspinal and epidural spaces (spinal cord and nerve root compression).[73–75] Diagnostic tests for

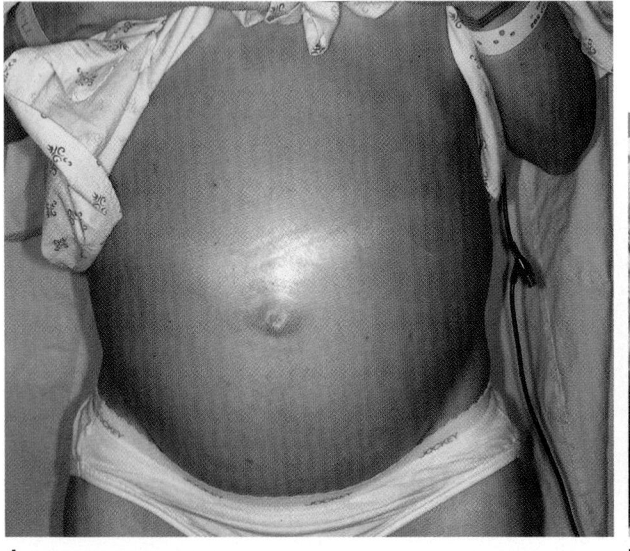

A

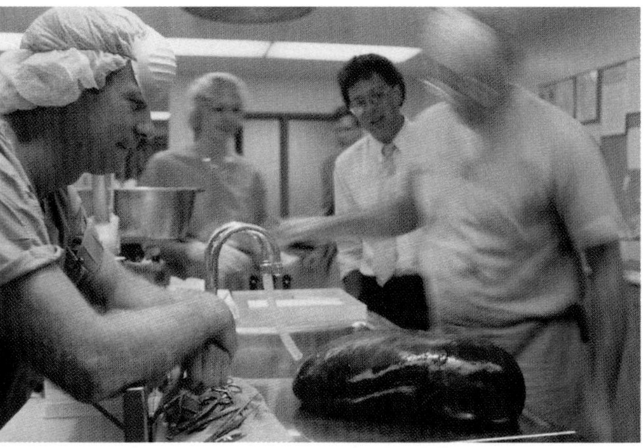

B

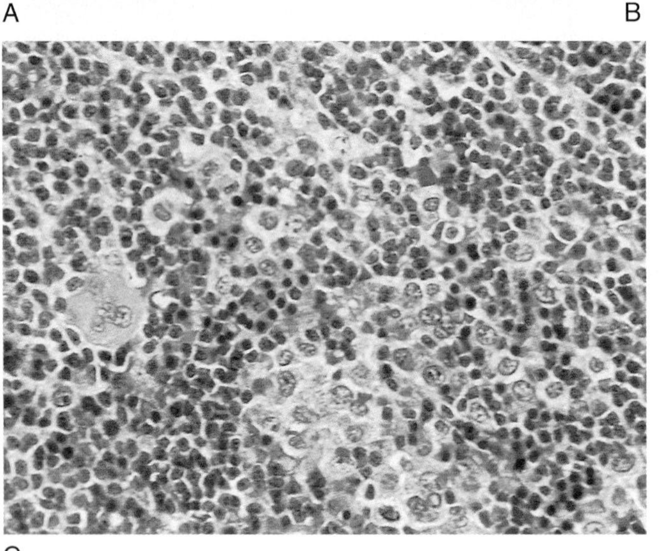

C

Figure 37–2. *A*, Massive splenomegaly in a patient with MMM. *B*, Surgically removed spleen in myelofibrosis. *C*, Histology showing extramedullary hematopoiesis.

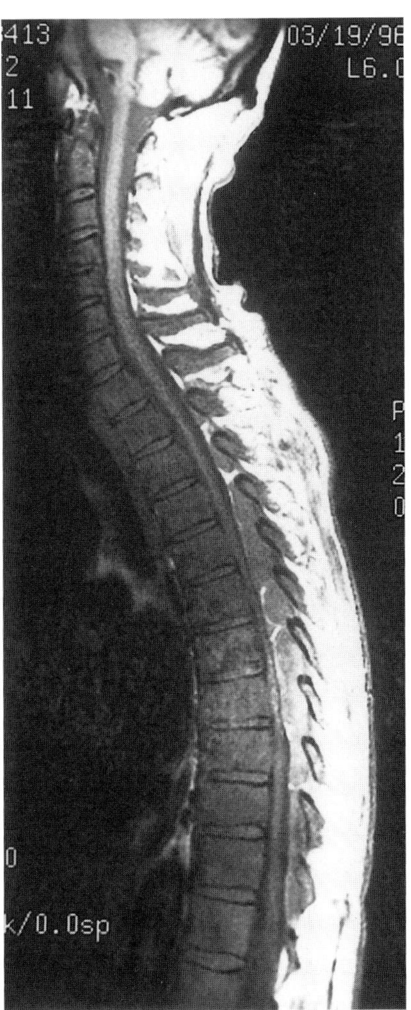

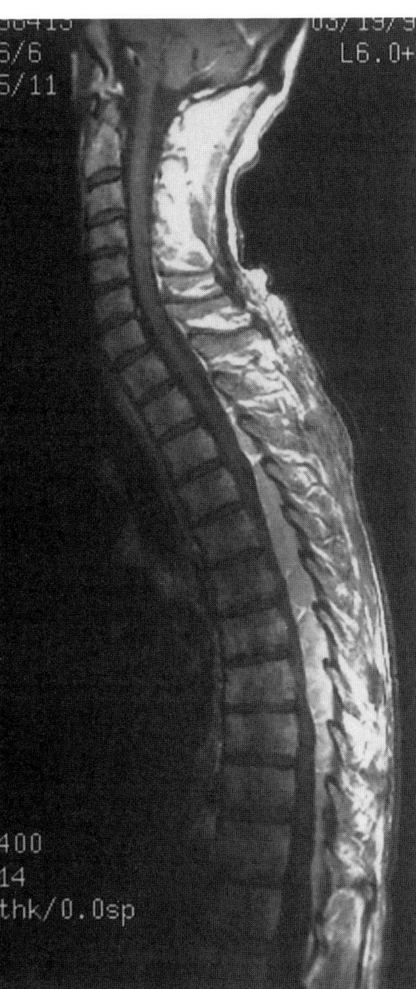

Figure 37–3. Extramedullary hematopoiesis involving the thoracic spinal canal, with cord compression from T5 to T8 (MRI).

EMH include tissue biopsy, cytologic analysis (a transudate with megakaryocytes and granulocyte precursors), a technetium sulfur colloid scan, computed tomography, and spinal magnetic resonance imaging (Fig. 37–3).

Constitutional and Other Symptoms

Splenomegaly in MMM is often associated with mechanical discomfort, early satiety (30–44% incidence), profound fatigue (50–63%), anorexia, weight loss (7–25%), night sweats and low-grade fever (5–17%), abnormal bowel movement, and portal hypertension.[73,74,76] Other clinical manifestations of MMM include peripheral edema, bone pain, arthralgias, uric acid nephropathy, and gout. In addition, a minority of patients might experience pulmonary hypertension, congestive heart failure, thrombohemorrhagic complications, and recurrent infection.[73,77]

Leukemic Transformation and Other Causes of Death

The reported incidence of transformation into acute leukemia in MMM ranges from 8% to 23% in the first decade of the disease and causes approximately 15% of deaths in MMM patients.[7,73,76] In a retrospective analysis of 91 such patients, all the events typed as acute myeloid leukemia (AML), with all French-American-British subtypes represented except AML M3.[78] Almost all the patients (98%) died of the particular complication at a median of 2.6 months (range, 0–24.2 months) from time of leukemic transformation. The overall results of induction chemotherapy were similar to those of supportive care alone, although a subset of patients so treated (41%) transiently reverted to the chronic phase of the disease.[78] Other causes of death in MMM include infections (26–29%), bleeding (11–22%), heart failure (7–15%), liver failure (3–8%), solid tumor (3%), respiratory failure (3%), and portal hypertension (6%).[7,76]

Laboratory Findings

Approximately 50% of patients with MMM present with a hemoglobin level of less than 10 gm/dL, and the anemia is severe enough to require transfusions in 20%.[4,74,76] However, up to 30% of the patients may not be anemic at the time of initial diagnosis.[4] The causes of anemia in MMM include ineffective hematopoiesis, the replacement of normal hematopoietic tissue with collagen fibrosis, and hypersplenism. Other diagnostic features of MMM

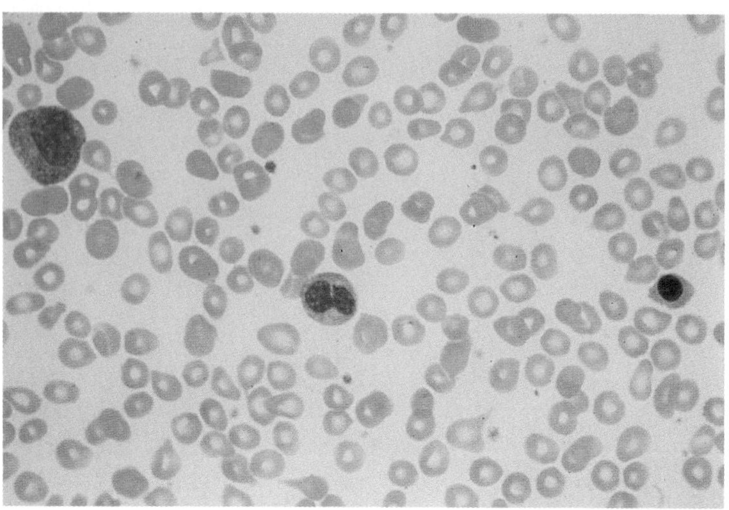

Figure 37–4. Peripheral blood smear in myelofibrosis showing a leukoerythroblastic picture: dacryocytes, nucleated red cells, and immature granulocytes.

include leukocytosis (41–49% incidence), leukopenia (7–22%), thrombocytosis (13–31%), thrombocytopenia (21–37%), the presence of circulating myeloblasts (33–53%), increased serum levels of lactate dehydrogenase (83%), and low cholesterol levels (32%).[4,73,74,76] Leukocytosis at the time of diagnosis may exceed 30,000/μL in 11% of the patients.[4]

Diagnosis

Clinical features that warrant consideration of MMM in the differential diagnosis include myelophthisis and marked splenomegaly. Myelophthisis refers to the presence, on peripheral blood smear, of nucleated red blood cells, left-shifted granulocytes (metamyelocytes, myelocytes, promyelocytes, myeloblasts), and teardrop-shaped erythrocytes (dacryocytes) (Fig. 37–4). Myelophthisis is almost always present at diagnosis. In contrast, although the incidence of palpable spleen in MMM is traditionally reported to be more than 95%,[7,73,79] earlier diagnosis made possible by the increased frequency of routine blood testing has resulted in an increased percentage of patients diagnosed before their spleen becomes palpably enlarged.[80] Hepatosplenomegaly in MMM is secondary to EMH.

It is underscored that both marked splenomegaly and myelophthisis are relatively nonspecific and can accompany other disorders. Massive splenomegaly is also a characteristic feature of CML, lymphoma, hairy cell leukemia, hyperreactive malarial splenomegaly, kala-azar (visceral leishmaniasis), Gaucher's disease, splenic cystic lymphangiomatosis, systemic lupus erythematosus, and sarcoidosis.[81] Similarly, myelophthisis might accompany other bone marrow—infiltrating processes, including metastatic cancer,[82,83] lymphoma,[84] and infections.[85]

Bone Marrow Histology

The bone marrow in patients with MMM is not easily aspirated (dry tap), and this makes it difficult to accurately assess morphology as well as obtain adequate samples for cytogenetic analysis. The usual findings in the core biopsy include atypical megakaryocyte hyperplasia, a stranded appearance that is consistent with collagen fibrosis, osteosclerosis, and intrasinusoidal hematopoiesis (Fig. 37–5*A*). The degree of fibrosis may be better estimated by the use of either a reticulin (silver impregnation) or trichrome stain (Fig. 37–5*B*). In a variant of the disease that is referred to as "cellular phase" MMM, the bone marrow is devoid of obvious fibrosis and instead displays florid cellularity with intense megakaryocytic dysplasia and clustering (Fig. 37–5*C*).

Bone marrow fibrosis is not specific to MMM and could also occur in the setting of other hematologic as well as nonhematologic disorders (Table 37–2). In this regard, it should be noted that nonmalignant reactive bone marrow fibrosis is rare and includes a variety of causes outlined and referenced in Table 37–2. However, bone marrow fibrosis not infrequently accompanies metastatic cancer involving the bone marrow,[86] CML,[87] MDS,[88] systemic mastocytosis,[89] chronic eosinophilic leukemia,[90] and hairy cell leukemia.[91] Bone marrow morphologic examination combined with immunohistochemistry and cytogenetic studies should clarify the diagnosis in most instances with the exception of MDS with fibrosis (MDS-f), the bone marrow features of which might be difficult to distinguish from those of MMM. The latter diagnosis requires the demonstration of dysplasia in two or more cell lineages, including the erythroid lineage. The presence of ringed sideroblasts per se is not adequate to distinguish MDS-f from MMM.[92]

Immunohistochemistry

The use of immunohistochemical stains and cytogenetic studies provides additional information that is helpful to distinguish MMM from other myeloid malignancies associated with fibrosis. In this regard, CD34 immunoperoxidase staining of the bone marrow biopsy is helpful in determining an estimate of the marrow blast percentage. Because megakaryoblasts typically do not stain with *anti*-CD34, CD61 staining may also be useful in supporting a suspected diagnosis of megakaryocytic leukemia (AML M7). The latter is sometimes referred to as acute myelofi-

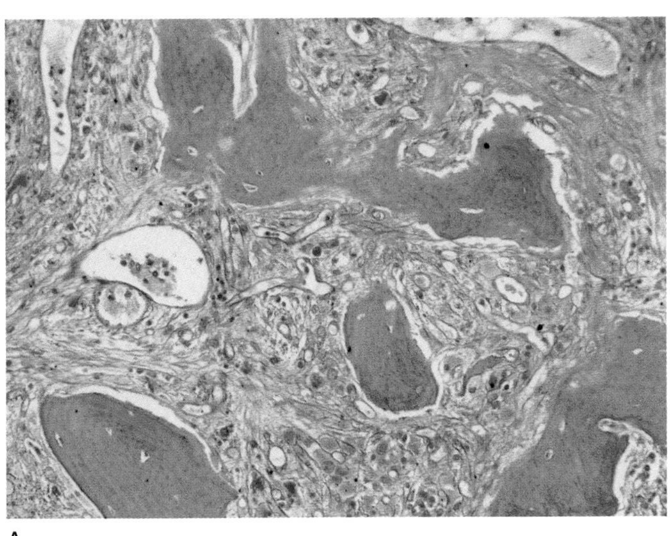

A

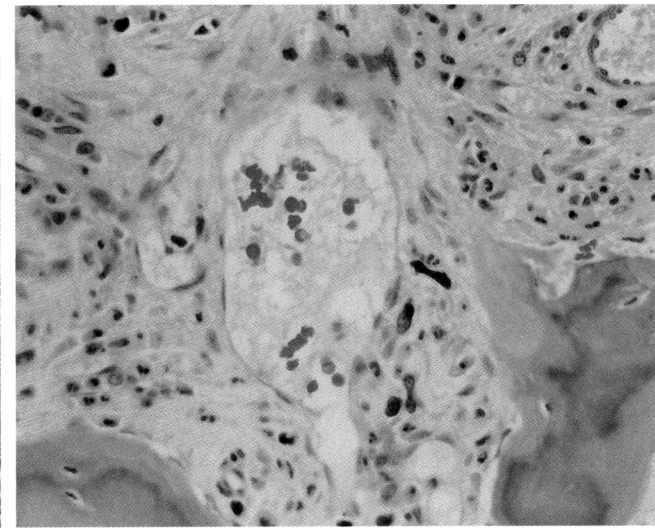

B

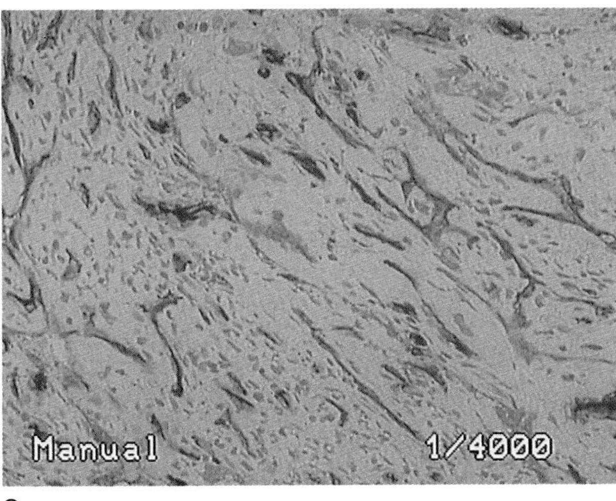

C

Figure 37–5. Bone marrow histology in myelofibrosis showing megakaryocytic hyperplasia and dysplasia (*A;* reticulin stain) and collagen fibrosis (*B;* hematoxylin and eosin stain). *C,* Bone marrow angiogenesis.

TABLE 37–2. Causes of Bone Marrow Fibrosis

Hematologic Disorders		
Myeloid Disorders	**Lymphoid Disorders**	**Nonhematologic Disorders**
Myelofibrosis with myeloid metaplasia [3]	Hairy cell leukemia[91]	Metastatic cancer [186]
Chronic myeloid leukemia [175]	Hodgkin's lymphoma[183]	Autoimmune myelofibrosis [187]
Myelodysplastic syndrome [92]	Non-Hodgkin's lymphoma[184]	Systemic lupus erythematosus [188]
Chronic myelomonocytic leukemia [176]	Multiple myeloma[185]	Kala-azar (leishmaniasis) [189]
Chronic eosinophilic leukemia [177]		Tuberculosis [190]
Systemic mastocytosis [178]		Paget's disease [191]
Acute megakaryocytic leukemia [179]		HIV infection [192]
Other acute myeloid leukemias [180]		Vitamin D–deficient rickets [193]
Acute lymphocytic leukemia [181]		Renal osteodystrophy [194]
Acute myelofibrosis [93]		Hyperparathyroidism [195]
Malignant histiocytosis [182]		Gray platelet syndrome [196]
		Familial infantile myelofibrosis [197]

Abbreviation: HIV, human immunodeficiency virus.

brosis and is characterized by severe constitutional symptoms, a nonpalpable spleen, pancytopenia, and the presence of circulating blasts. However, some cases of acute myelofibrosis are not classifiable as acute megakaryocytic leukemia.[93] In general, patients with acute myelofibrosis present with severe constitutional symptoms, circulating blasts, and no splenomegaly.

Cytogenetics

Cytogenetic studies in MMM carry both diagnostic and prognostic value.[5] If the bone marrow aspirate is inadequate for cytogenetic analysis, then the test should be performed on the peripheral blood because of the presence of an increased progenitor cell pool.[94] The possibility of CML is further pursued by performing a peripheral blood fluorescent in situ hybridization assay for *bcr/abl*.[95] At diagnosis, approximately one third to one half of patients with MMM display karyotypic abnormalities, including del(20q11;q13), del(13q12;q22), trisomy 8, trisomy 9, and t(1;7), each occurring in 10–20% of cases.[5,7] Although none of these cytogenetic markers carries diagnostic specificity, the detection of an expected versus unexpected cytogenetic profile serves as an additional piece of information during the process of making a working diagnosis.

Risk Stratification for Prognosis and Treatment

Large retrospective studies in MMM report an overall median survival that ranges from 3.5 to 10 years.[4,7,73,76] Factors that have been associated with inferior survival include anemia (hemoglobin <10 gm/dL),[4,7,73,76,79] constitutional symptoms,[7,76] circulating blasts (≥1–3%),[4,7,76] leukocytosis (>30,000/μL),[4,7] leukopenia (<3000/μL),[4,7] age greater than 60 years,[4,7,73,74,76,79] male sex,[4,7] thrombocytopenia (<100,000/μL),[4,7] the percentage of immature myeloid cells,[74,79] hepatomegaly,[4] weight loss,[4] abnormal karyotype (+8, 12p–),[4,5,42] and markedly increased lactate dehydrogenase.[76] Among these, a hemoglobin level of less than 10 gm/dL, constitutional symptoms, circulating blasts, and extreme ranges of leukocyte counts were the factors that usually maintained prognostic value on multivariate analysis. In addition, more recent studies have suggested a possible prognostic value for the degree of bone marrow angiogenesis[51] and peripheral blood CD34 count.[71] In comparison, in most studies, survival was not affected by the spleen size[4]; bone marrow histology, including degree of myelofibrosis and osteosclerosis[4,5,73,76]; or therapeutic modalities used.[4]

A number of prognostic scoring systems have been proposed in order to risk stratify patients with MMM. In a large Japanese study of 336 patients, the presence of a hemoglobin level of 10 gm/dL or greater, a platelet count of 100,000/μL or greater, and less than 3% circulating blasts predicted a median survival of approximately 15 years.[7] Median survival dropped to 5 years otherwise. These findings were somewhat similar to those of a Spanish study with a prediction of 15-year median survival in young patients with a hemoglobin level of 10 gm/dL or greater in the absence of either constitutional symptoms or circulating blasts.[96] When patients of all ages were considered, the latter study suggested a median survival of more than 8 years in "low-risk" patients and less than 2 years in "high-risk" patients.[76]

An Italian study identified low (age <45 years, hemoglobin level >13 gm/dL, *and* <24% immature myeloid cells) intermediate (age >45 years *or* >24% immature myeloid cells *or* hemoglobin <13 gm/dL), and high (age >45 years *and* hemoglobin <13 gm/dL *and* >21% immature myeloid cells) risk groups with median survivals of greater than 20 years, 12 years, and 5.5 years, respectively.[79] Similarly, another Italian study found a hemoglobin of greater than 10 gm/dL and less than 10% immature myeloid cells to predict a median survival of approximately 7 years.[74] A French study suggested a median survival of only 1 year for patients who displayed both a hemoglobin level of less than 10 gm/dL and either leukocytosis (white blood cell count >30,000/μL) or leukopenia (white blood cell count < 4000/μL).[4] In the absence of these adverse factors, median survival was estimated at 8 years.[4] Based on these and other observations, it is possible to formulate a risk category for most patients with MMM that might assist in treatment decision making (Table 37–3).

MANAGEMENT

It is important to recognize the fact that the majority of patients with MMM are diagnosed after their 60th birthday and might not be suitable candidates for allogeneic hematopoietic stem cell transplantation (AHSCT). However, conventional drug therapy might provide

TABLE 37–3. Risk Stratification in Myelofibrosis with Myeloid Metaplasia*

Risk Category	Hemoglobin < 10 gm/dL	Constitutional Symptoms	Circulating Blasts ≥ 3%	WBC > 30 × 10^9/L or < 4 × 10^9/L
Low	No	No	No	No
Intermediate	Presence of one of the above adverse feature			
High	Presence of two or more of the above adverse features			

*Expected median survival is greater than 10 years in low-risk, 5–10 years in intermediate-risk, and less than 5 years in high-risk disease.

palliation in terms of both anemia and splenomegaly. Similarly, both splenectomy and involved-field irradiation have a defined palliative role in the treatment of MMM. Investigational therapy in MMM includes both experimental drug therapy and AHSCT.

Conventional Treatment in Myelofibrosis

Drugs

Androgen preparations (e.g., oral fluoxymesterone 10 mg twice daily), corticosteroids (e.g., oral prednisone 30 mg/day), and erythropoietin (e.g., 40,000 units subcutaneously once weekly) are used as first-line therapy for alleviation of anemia.[3,97–103] An approximate 30% response rate with median remission duration of 1 year is expected from the use of one or more of these treatment modalities. Similarly, danazol (600–800 mg/day) has been reported to be effective therapy for both anemia and thrombocytopenia in some patients with MMM and could be considered as a second-line therapeutic option.[104]

Symptomatic splenomegaly is initially treated with hydroxyurea (e.g., starting dose of 500 mg 2 or 3 times daily).[105] Patients vary in their response to hydroxyurea therapy, and adverse drug effects include worsening of anemia and thrombocytopenia as well as mucocutaneous ulcers. Other cytoreductive drugs that might be considered either prior to splenectomy or in those patients who are poor surgical candidates include intravenous cladribine (5 mg/m^2/day in a 2-hour infusion for 5 consecutive days, to be repeated for four to six monthly cycles),[106] oral melphalan (2.5 mg 3 times weekly),[107] oral busulfan (2–6 mg/day with close monitoring of blood counts),[108,109] and intravenous daunorubicin (50 mg/m^2 weekly for 4–8 weeks). Obviously, cytoreductive therapy should be accompanied with adequate hydration and use of allopurinol, and left ventricular function should be assessed prior to the use of daunorubicin. In my experience, interferon alfa therapy has had limited value in alleviating anemia associated with MMM.[110–115]

Splenectomy

Splenectomy is indicated in the presence of drug-refractory splenic pain and/or discomfort, high red blood cell transfusion requirements, and symptomatic portal hypertension.[116] The procedure provides symptomatic relief for the majority of patients and durable anemia response in 25% of the patients. However, splenectomy might not benefit patients with severe thrombocytopenia. Operative mortality is approximately 9%, and 25% of patients may experience postsplenectomy thrombocytosis and progressive hepatomegaly. Portal-systemic shunt surgery may be performed in conjunction with splenectomy for the treatment of symptomatic portal hypertension.[117] The experience from my institution suggests that postsplenectomy occurrence of leukemic transformation in MMM represents the natural progression of the disease and not the result of the specific treatment modality.[116,118]

Radiation Therapy

Involved-field radiation therapy works best for nonhepatosplenic EMH[75,119] but has limited value in controlling symptomatic enlargement of the spleen and liver.[120,121] Splenic irradiation is given in a total dose of 100–500 cGy in 5–10 fractions. The procedure is associated with a more than 10% mortality rate from consequences of cytopenia, and the benefit (reduction of spleen size) is often transient (median response duration is 6 months). In contrast, low-dose irradiation is effective for the treatment of paraspinal/epidural EMH (1000 cGy in 5–10 fractions) as well as EMH resulting in pleural and peritoneal effusions (100–500 cGy in 5–10 fractions).[75] Symptomatic pulmonary hypertension that is not secondary to a thromboembolic process has been associated with MMM and is believed to arise from diffuse pulmonary EMH.[77] Diagnosis is confirmed by technetium-99 m sulfur colloid scintigraphy, which shows diffuse pulmonary uptake, and treatment with single-fraction (100 cGy) whole-lung irradiation has been shown to be effective.[119]

Investigational Drug Therapy in Myelofibrosis

Over the last decade, my group at the Mayo Clinic has explored experimental drug therapy that was intended to interfere with cytokines that are believed to mediate the bone marrow fibrosis and angiogenesis in MMM. In this regard, the drugs that were shown to be clinically ineffective include imatinib mesylate (inhibits PDGF receptor—associated tyrosine kinase activity),[122] interferon alfa (nonspecific myelosuppressive agent),[115] anagrelide (interferes with terminal differentiation of megakaryocytes and platelet production),[123] pirfenidone (impairs fibroblast proliferation and collagen synthesis),[124] and suramin (inhibits TGF-β binding on fibroblasts).[125] In contrast, the drugs that showed promise of activity include thalidomide (has antiangiogenic activity and also inhibits tumor necrosis factor-α [TNF-α] production)[126,127] and etanercept (a soluble TNF-α receptor that produced a 60% response rate in constitutional symptoms).[128]

Thalidomide

The demonstration of florid bone marrow angiogenesis in MMM[51] encouraged the development of several small pilot studies that evaluated the therapeutic value of thalidomide either alone[126,127,129–135] or in combination with other drugs[136,137] in MMM. Studies that involved 10 or more patients have demonstrated a response rate of 20–62% in anemia, 25–80% in thrombocytopenia, and 7–30% in splenomegaly.[127,129,131,132,134,135] Information from these studies indicates that low-dose thalidomide (50 mg/day) was as effective as higher doses (200 mg/day or more) and that the addition of prednisone to the lower dose schedule improves drug tolerance and may enhance the erythropoietic activity of the drug.[129,136] Long-term analysis of thalidomide-based drug therapy suggests a durable response in a quarter of the patients, including some in whom the drug was discontinued.[138] Unusual thalidomide drug effects in MMM, all reversible, include extreme leukocytosis and thrombocytosis.

The mechanism of action of thalidomide in MMM is currently unknown. A longer follow-up is necessary to confirm the currently observed lack of drug-induced reversal in bone marrow microvessel density.[138] Both angiogenesis and TNF-α have been implicated in the pathogenesis of MMM, and the latter might be particularly detrimental to effective erythropoiesis.[51,139] It is therefore possible that the drug promotes effective erythropoiesis through its either anti-TNF or antiangiogenesis activity. Alternatively, thalidomide may facilitate effective hematopoiesis through its immunomodulatory properties. Thalidomide costimulates T-lymphocyte proliferation,[140] inducing T_H2 cytokine (interleukin-4 and interleukin-5) but not T_H1 cytokine (interferon-γ) production.[141] Interleukin-4 synergizes with stem cell factor and other cytokines to enhance effective hematopoiesis,[142,143] whereas both interferon-γ and TNF-α effect the opposite, possibly by promoting programmed cell death.[144] Finally, unlike the case in multiple myeloma,[145,146] thalidomide-associated thrombosis was observed in only one patient.

Etanercept

In the only clinical trial that used etanercept (25 mg subcutaneously twice weekly) in MMM, 3 of 20 evaluable patients (15%) had a hemoglobin response and an impressive 60% response rate was documented in terms of constitutional symptoms, including fatigue, weight loss, and night sweats.[128] Other than injection site reactions, which occurred in 20% of the patients, other side effects were infrequent and included severe and reversible pancytopenia in one patient. Etanercept is a soluble TNF receptor that might involve a mechanism of action similar to that of thalidomide.

Imatinib Mesylate

The rationale for imatinib mesylate use in MMM has centered around its inhibition of PDGF-mediated signaling, which, along with other cytokines such as TGF-β and basic fibroblast growth factor, is implicated in the pathogenesis of the bone marrow stromal reaction.[3] In patients with CML, the significant regression of bone marrow fibrosis[147] and neoangiogenesis[148] with imatinib therapy was associated with histologic normalization of the bone marrow, consistent with the widespread view that myelofibrosis in chronic MPDs is a reactive process that is mediated by cytokines, which are derived from one or more of the clonally involved myeloid cells. Reversal of myelofibrosis with imatinib therapy has similarly been reported for patients with *FIP1L1-PDGFRA*—positive eosinophilic disorder.[90] To date, however, the results of imatinib therapy in MMM have not been impressive.

In one study,[122] 16 of 23 MMM patients (70%) treated at the 400-mg/day dose level needed to have treatment withheld because of toxicity. Only 11 patients (48%), including those in whom treatment could be restarted at the 200-mg/day dose level, were able to complete 3 months of therapy. Although none experienced a response in anemia, 11 patients (all with a baseline platelet count of >10^5/μL) had a greater than 50% increase in the platelet count, and 2 patients had a greater than 50% decrease in spleen size. In another study of 18 MMM patients treated at the 400-mg/day dose level,[149] 4 had complete resolution of splenomegaly, and 3 had improvement of anemia or thrombocytopenia alone. Fourteen of the total 18 patients discontinued treatment after a median of 15 weeks as a result of either toxicity, or absent or transient response. Other studies have confirmed the limited activity of imatinib in reducing bone marrow fibrosis in MMM and the high frequency of drug toxicity, whereas the results on benefit were mixed.[150–153]

Allogeneic Stem Cell Transplantation in Myelofibrosis

Treatment with AHSCT, either myeloablative[154–156] or reduced-intensity conditioning,[157,158] is directed at eradicating the mutant MMM clone. However, the particular treatment modality is risky in terms of both death and morbidity, and is not applicable to the majority of patients with MMM.[159] The three largest studies regarding myeloablative AHSCT (both related and matched unrelated) total 147 patients among them.[155,156,160] In general, engraftment was not a problem, with more than 80% of patients achieving safe neutrophil counts by day 30.[160] However, transplant-related death and morbidity were not trivial, resulting in a 5-year survival of only 14% for patients over age 44 years in one study[160] and a 2-year overall survival of 41% in another study.[156] In the most favorable of the three studies, 20 of the 56 patients had died within 3 years of the transplant and the reported incidence of chronic graft-versus-host disease was 59% at a median follow-up period of only 2.8 years.[155]

In general, transplantation outcome in younger patients was encouraging in all three of these studies, with projected 5-year survival rates of above 60%, and clinical as well as histologic remissions were documented in the surviving patients.[155,160] Furthermore, because transplant outcome was significantly better in good-prognosis patients compared to the outcome in poor-prognosis patients, it has been argued that the window of opportunity for cure is lost by delaying transplantation until the disease progresses. However, it is important to recognize the fact that transplantation-age patients with good-prognosis MMM can expect a median survival of 15 years or more and do not have to contend with transplant-associated risk of death and/or chronic graft-versus-host disease.[96]

For these reasons, AHSCT, either myeloablative or reduced-intensity conditioning, is not recommended for the patient whose life expectancy is estimated to exceed 10 years (Fig. 37–6). In contrast, it is reasonable to consider AHSCT in patients less than 60 years of age in whom a survival of less than 5 years can be reliably predicted.[4,96] The transplant treatment decision is particularly difficult in those patients with an expected survival of 5–10 years, and for such patients, as well as those over

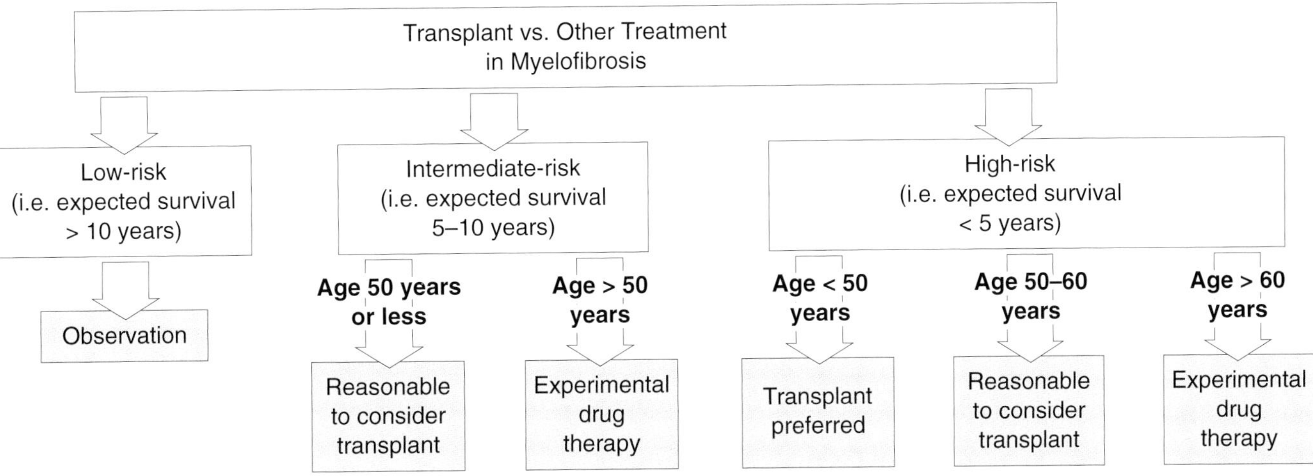

Figure 37–6. Transplantation decision making in myelofibrosis with myeloid metaplasia.

age 60 years, experimental drug trials offer an attractive alternative.

In regard to reduced-intensity AHSCT, a preliminary report from a multicenter study of 20 patients (median age 50 years) with MMM, including 5 who experienced leukemic transformation, 1-year treatment-related mortality, relapse rate, and survival were of 37%, 36%, and 54%, respectively. However, when reduced-intensity AHSCT was performed before transformation, 1-year survival increased to 77%.[161] A limited number of other studies, consisting of fewer than six study patients each, support the feasibility of reduced-intensity AHSCT in terms of engraftment, attainment of full donor chimerism, and ability to induce both clinical and pathologic remissions.[157] However, a longer follow-up period as well as a larger sample size is needed to clearly define the durability of full donor chimerism, long-term relapse rate, and quality of life. Such information is critical because the potential beneficiaries of reduced-intensity AHSCT are the subset of patients with good-prognosis disease. Finally, AHSCT has been shown to be feasible in MMM and of potential value in disease palliation in terms of anemia and splenomegaly.[162]

CONCLUDING REMARKS

Approximately 30 years ago, Murray N. Silverstein prepared a monograph that described the natural history of MMM as well as palliative treatment modalities, including the use of androgen preparations, corticosteroids, alkylating agents, radiation therapy, and splenectomy.[97] Little has since been accomplished in terms of therapy, although both AHSCT[154] and thalidomide drug therapy[126] are now considered effective in a subset of patients. Rational treatment approaches await elucidation of the underlying pathogenetic mechanisms of both clonal myeloproliferation and bone marrow stromal reaction in MMM. In this regard, recent studies have suggested a potential pathogenetic role for bone marrow angiogenesis,[51] TGF-β,[66] osteoprotegerin,[67] and GATA-1[62] in MMM, and such information, although unlikely to reveal the disease-causing molecular events, should guide selection of experimental drugs that warrant therapeutic testing.

CURRENT CONTROVERSIES & FUTURE CONSIDERATIONS

Myelofibrosis with Myeloid Metaplasia

- Adequately sized clinical trials with long follow-up durations are direly needed to clarify the role of allogeneic blood cell therapy in MMM.
- Rational drug therapy in MMM awaits elucidation of the underlying pathogenetic mechanisms.
- Additional Phase I and Phase II studies are key in identifying drugs with antidisease activity in MMM, but the time currently is not ripe for Phase III studies.
- Does the new finding of JAK2 mutations common to MMM, polycythemia vera, and essential thrombocytosis (see Chapter 36) indicate an underlying common pathogenesis and will this lead to common treatments.

Suggested Readings*

Barosi G, Grossi A, Comotti B, et al: Safety and efficacy of thalidomide in patients with myelofibrosis with myeloid metaplasia. Br J Haematol 114:78–83, 2001.

Cervantes F, Alvarez-Larran A, Talarn C, et al: Myelofibrosis with myeloid metaplasia following essential thrombocythaemia: actuarial probability, presenting characteristics and evolution in a series of 195 patients. Br J Haematol 118:786–790, 2002.

Cervantes F, Pereira A, Esteve J, et al: Identification of "short-lived" and "long-lived" patients at presentation of idiopathic myelofibrosis. Br J Haematol 97:635–640, 1997.

Mesa RA, Steensma DP, Pardanani A, et al: A Phase 2 trial of combination low-dose thalidomide and prednisone for the treatment of myelofibrosis with myeloid metaplasia. Blood 101:2534–2541, 2003.

Okamura T, Kinukawa N, Niho Y, Mizoguchi H: Primary chronic myelofibrosis: clinical and prognostic evaluation in 336 Japanese patients. Int J Hematol 73:194–198, 2001.

Tefferi A: Myelofibrosis with myeloid metaplasia. N Engl J Med 342:1255–1265, 2000.

Full references for this chapter can be found on accompanying CD-ROM.

CHAPTER 38
EOSINOPHILIC LEUKEMIA

Barbara J. Bain, MBBS, FRACP, FRCPath

KEY POINTS

Hypereosinophilia

- There are many causes of hypereosinophilia, among which chronic eosinophilic leukemia is relatively uncommon.
- Eosinophilic leukemia is a clonal neoplastic condition resulting from mutation of a multipotent myeloid stem cell or progenitor cell or, less often, from mutation of a pluripotent lymphoid-myeloid stem cell.
- The diagnosis of eosinophilic leukemia requires either evidence of clonality or the presence of features indicative of neoplasia.
- The causes of idiopathic hypereosinophilic syndrome are unknown, and it is a diagnosis of exclusion.

INTRODUCTION

The term *eosinophilic leukemia* refers to a leukemia with predominantly eosinophilic differentiation. Most such leukemias represent a clonal expansion originating in a multipotent myeloid stem cell or progenitor cell, with the neoplastic clone also including cells of myeloid lineages other than eosinophils. Less often, eosinophilic leukemia results from a mutation in a pluripotent lymphoid-myeloid stem cell; in these cases, although eosinophilia is the predominant hematologic feature, the leukemic clone includes cells of T lineage or, less often, B lineage. Eosinophilic leukemia can be either acute or chronic but, if unspecified, the term should be taken to mean chronic eosinophilic leukemia. Eosinophilic leukemia must be distinguished both from reactive eosinophilia and from the idiopathic hypereosinophilic syndrome (HES). The latter condition is, by definition, of unknown origin. Conventionally, the diagnosis of idiopathic HES requires the presence of sustained inexplicable eosinophilia with resultant tissue damage.[1,2]

Chronic eosinophilic leukemia is a chronic myeloproliferative disorder with predominantly eosinophilic differentiation. It is closely related to "chronic myelomonocytic leukemia with eosinophilia" and to "atypical chronic myeloid leukemia with eosinophilia." The distinction between these three closely related groups of disorders is, to some extent, arbitrary, because patients with the same cytogenetic or molecular genetic abnormality can present with a variety of hematologic features. The diagnosis of eosinophilic leukemia can be difficult because not all patients have clear evidence of the true nature of the condition. Sometimes the diagnosis can only be made in retrospect when a patient categorized as having idiopathic HES suffers a transforming event (acute myeloid leukemia [AML] or granulocytic [myeloid] sarcoma) or develops signs of a clonal cytogenetic abnormality.[3] Either of these events provides circumstantial evidence that the initially idiopathic condition was actually neoplastic, with a further mutation in a cell of the neoplastic clone having led to disease evolution. Acute transformation may occur many years after presentation with eosinophilia, an interval as long as 24 years having been observed.[4]

Definition

The World Health Organization (WHO) has proposed criteria for the diagnosis of eosinophilic leukemia.[5] It is required that there be an eosinophil count of more than 1.5×10^9/L, increased bone marrow eosinophils, and less than 20% blast cells in both blood and marrow. Diagnoses of AML, myelodysplastic syndrome, and other myeloproliferative disorders, including Philadelphia chromosome (Ph)–positive/*BCR-ABL*–positive chronic myeloid leukemia must be excluded. Although the WHO publication does not specifically say so, it may be inferred that myelodysplastic/myeloproliferative disorders (overlap syndromes) should also be excluded. In addition, there must be either (1) cytogenetic or molecular genetic evidence of clonality or (2) an increase of blast cells in the blood to more than 2% or an increase in bone marrow blast cells to between 5% and 19%.

EPIDEMIOLOGY AND RISK FACTORS

Eosinophilic leukemia is rare and occurs at all ages. It is considerably more common in men than in women, at least in part because two of the cytogenetic/molecular genetic entities that can present as eosinophilic leukemia are considerably more common in men. Occasional cases

TABLE 38–1. Important Cytogenetic/Molecular Genetic Entities That Can Present as Eosinophilic Leukemia

Cytogenetic/Molecular Genetic Entity	Hematologic Presentation
FIP1L1-PDGFRA fusion	Chronic eosinophilic leukemia, possibly with increased mast cells
The 8p11 syndrome	Chronic eosinophilic leukemia, acute myeloid leukemia or myeloid sarcoma, T-cell lineage acute lymphoblastic leukemia, B-cell lineage acute lymphoblastic leukemia
Myeloproliferative disorder with t(5;12)(q33;p13) or other rearrangement of *PDGFRB* (the 5q33 syndrome)	Chronic eosinophilic leukemia, atypical chronic myeloid leukemia (with or without eosinophilia), chronic myelomonocytic leukemia (with or without eosinophilia)

follow exposure to leukemogenic drugs, but, in general, the cause is unknown.

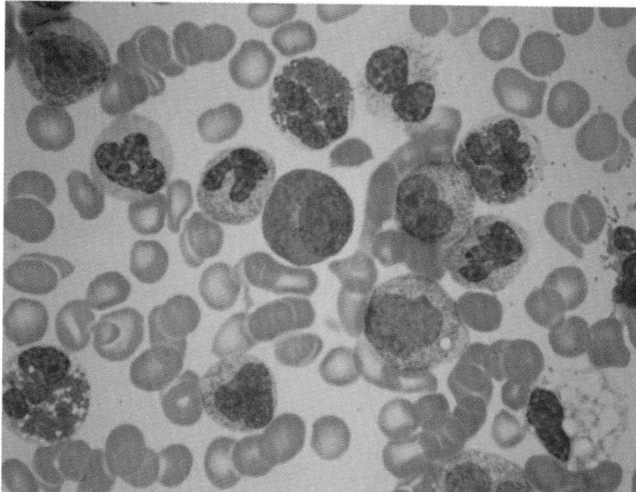

Figure 38–1. Peripheral blood film in a patient with chronic eosinophilic leukemia associated with a *FIP1L1-PDGFRA* fusion gene showing greatly increased numbers of cells of neutrophil and eosinophil lineages.

PATHOGENETIC CLASSIFICATION OF EOSINOPHILIC LEUKEMIA

A number of entities have now been defined on the basis of cytogenetic or molecular genetic abnormalities that usually or sometimes have the hematologic features of chronic eosinophilic leukemia. Because of the major prognostic and therapeutic significance of some of these entities, the subclassification of chronic eosinophilic leukemia has now become important. It is the genetic abnormality that determines the nature of the disorder, and these conditions are best defined primarily on the basis of the genetic abnormality rather than on whether or not the patient meets the criteria for eosinophilic leukemia (e.g., the criteria for chronic myelomonocytic leukemia with eosinophilia or atypical chronic myeloid leukemia with eosinophilia). Often the genetic abnormality involves a gene encoding a tyrosine kinase involved in intracellular signaling pathways.[6] The most important of these syndromes are summarized in Table 38–1[7] and are described here in more detail.

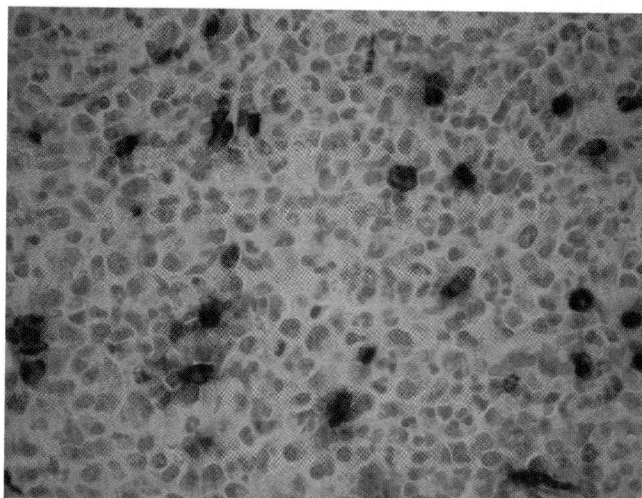

Figure 38–2. Bone marrow trephine biopsy section, showing increased but dispersed mast cells, identified by immunohistochemistry for mast cell tryptase, in a patient with a *FIP1L1-PDGFRA* fusion gene.

Chronic Eosinophilic Leukemia with *FIP1L1-PDGFRA* Fusion

A significant proportion of patients with otherwise unexplained sustained eosinophilia can now be demonstrated to have a *FIP1L1-PDGFRA* fusion gene as the result of a cryptic deletion of chromosome 4.[8,9] Cytogenetic analysis is often normal, but sometimes there is either an abnormality of chromosome 4 or an unrelated chromosome abnormality. This condition is more common in males. There are often "myeloproliferative" feature such as hepatomegaly, splenomegaly, a hypercellular bone marrow, increased peripheral blood neutrophils and precursors (Fig. 38–1), or an increased serum vitamin B_{12} concentration. Bone marrow mast cells and serum tryptase may be increased[10–12] (Fig. 38–2).

Another fusion gene involving *PDGFRA*, *BCR-PDGFRA*, has been described in two patients with chronic myeloid leukemia.[13] In one of these patients there was a marked increase of eosinophils in the bone marrow and in the other there was prominent peripheral blood eosinophilia (total white cell count 101 × 10^9/L with 22% eosinophils). Transformation to T-lymphoblastic lymphoma occurred in the second patient. Imatinib (see below) was not administered to either of these patients.

8p11 Syndrome

The term *8p11 syndrome* was coined to describe a group of three conditions involving the same or a similar breakpoint on chromosome 8.[14] It is now known that all

TABLE 38–2. Cytogenetic Abnormalities That May Give Rise to *FGFR1* Rearrangements and the 8p11 Syndrome

Cytogenetic Abnormality	Molecular Abnormality	Reference
t(8;13)(p12;q12)	*ZNF198-FGFR1*	15
t(6;8)(q27;p12)	*FOP-FGFR1*	16
t(8;9)(p12;q33)	*CEP110-FGFR1*	17
t(8;17)(p11;q25)	*TIAF1-FGFR1**	18
t(8;19)(p12;q13.3)	*HERVK-FGFR1**	19
t(8;22)(p11;q11)	*BCR-FGFR1*	20
ins(12;8)(p11;?p11p22)	*GEMS-FGFR1**	18

*Single cases.

TABLE 38–3. Myeloproliferative Disorders with t(5;12)(q33;p13) or Other Cytogenetic Event Resulting in *PDGFRB* Rearrangement—the 5q33 Syndrome

Cytogenetic Abnormality	Molecular Abnormality	Reference
t(5;12)(q33;p13)	*ETV6-PDGFRB**	27
t(1;5)(q23;q33)	*PDE4DIP-PDGFRB**	28
t(5;7)(q33;q11.2)†	*HIP1-PDGFRB*	29
t(5;10)(q33;q21)‡	*H4/D10S170-PDGFRB*	30–32
t(5;17)(q33;p13)†	*RAB5-PDGFRB**	33

*Imatinib responsiveness has been demonstrated.
†Single cases.
‡Two cases.

involve the *FGFR1* gene,[15] and the syndrome has been expanded to include other rare rearrangements of the same gene (Table 38–2).[16–21] The 8p11 syndrome occurs over a wide age range (3–84 years, median age 32 years).[14] There is a slight male predominance. This syndrome has some analogies with Ph-positive chronic myeloid leukemia in that the mutation occurs in a pluripotent lymphoid-myeloid stem cell. Some patients present with chronic eosinophilic or other myeloid leukemia and subsequently suffer an acute transformation, which may be myeloid, T lymphoblastic, or, least often, B lymphoblastic.[22–26] The myeloid transformation may be to AML but is quite often to myeloid sarcoma. Other patients present with acute leukemia, a presentation that can be regarded as analogous either to Ph-positive acute myeloid or acute lymphoblastic leukemia or to presentation of Ph-positive chronic myeloid leukemia already in blast transformation. If remission occurs, there can be reversion to a chronic phase of the disease. The relevant cytogenetic abnormality is demonstrable in all phases of the disease, including during presentation as chronic eosinophilic leukemia. The cytogenetic abnormality is present in myeloblasts, T lymphoblasts, and B lymphoblasts.

The 8p11 syndrome has a poor prognosis, with many patients either presenting with acute leukemia or suffering acute transformation within 1–2 years.

Eosinophilic and Related Chronic Myeloid Leukemias with t(5;12)–the 5q33 Syndrome

Eosinophilic leukemia and related chronic myeloid leukemias with eosinophilia are recognized in association with t(5;12)(q33;p13), a chromosomal rearrangement that gives rise to a *ETV6-PDGFRB* fusion gene[27] (Fig. 38–3). Variant translocations also involving rearrangement of the *PDGFRB* gene at 5q33 give rise to similar types of chronic myeloid leukemia, so, by analogy with the 8p11 syndrome, this group of disorders could be designated the 5q33 syndrome (Table 38–3).[27–33] In this syndrome the relevant mutation occurs in a multipotent myeloid stem cell. The disease occurs at all ages (8–80 years, with a median of 42 years) and shows an unexplained striking male predominance.[34]

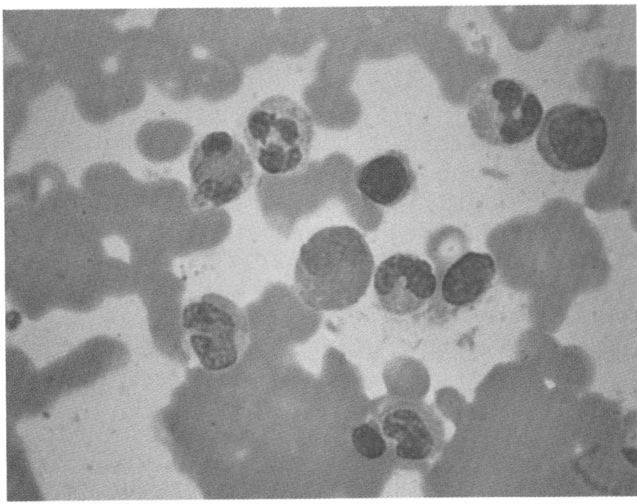

Figure 38–3. Bone marrow aspirate in a patient with t(5;12)(q33;p13).

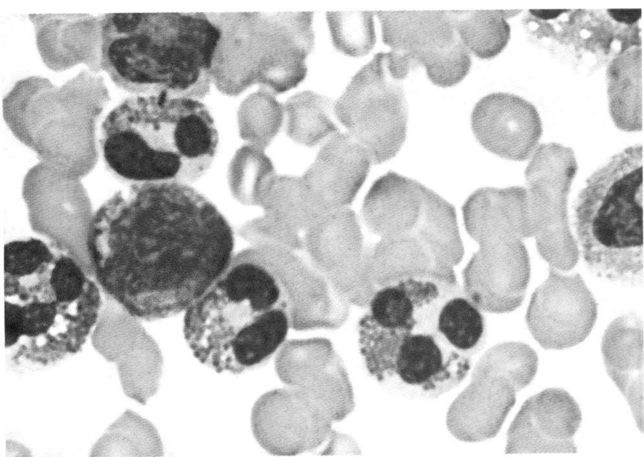

Figure 38–4. Chronic eosinophilic leukemia associated with trisomy 10.

TABLE 38–4. Criteria for the Diagnosis of Chronic Eosinophilic Leukemia in a Patient with Sustained Unexplained Eosinophilia

	Nature of Evidence of a Neoplastic Condition	Conclusive Evidence	Strong Supporting Evidence
Criteria permitting diagnosis at presentation	Clinical evidence		Hepatomegaly, splenomegaly
	Hematologic evidence	Increased percentage of blast cells, including myeloid sarcoma	Anemia, high serum vitamin B_{12} concentration
	Cytogenetic evidence	Clonal cytogenetic abnormality demonstrated in eosinophils or of type previously reported in eosinophilic leukemia	Clonal cytogenetic abnormality in myeloid cells
	Molecular genetic evidence	Molecular genetic abnormality demonstrated in eosinophils or of type previously reported in eosinophilic leukemia	Clonal molecular genetic abnormality in myeloid cells; very skewed expression of X-chromosome genes
Criteria permitting diagnosis only in retrospect	Hematologic evidence	Transformation to AML or development of myeloid sarcoma	
	Cytogenetic evidence	Development of a clonal cytogenetic abnormality	

PATHOPHYSIOLOGY

The clinicopathologic features of eosinophilic leukemia may include those characteristic of any chronic myeloid leukemia, being the result of the proliferation of leukemic cells in the bone marrow, liver, and spleen. Other clinicopathologic features are the result of the release of inflammatory mediators from eosinophils. Such inflammatory mediators may be released in the bloodstream or within infiltrated tissues. Among tissues damaged, cardiac damage is often prominent, with damage to the pericardium, myocardium, and endocardium. Thrombosis on damaged valves can give rise to embolic phenomena. The peripheral and central nervous systems are also susceptible to inflammatory mediator damage. Vasculitis can occur.

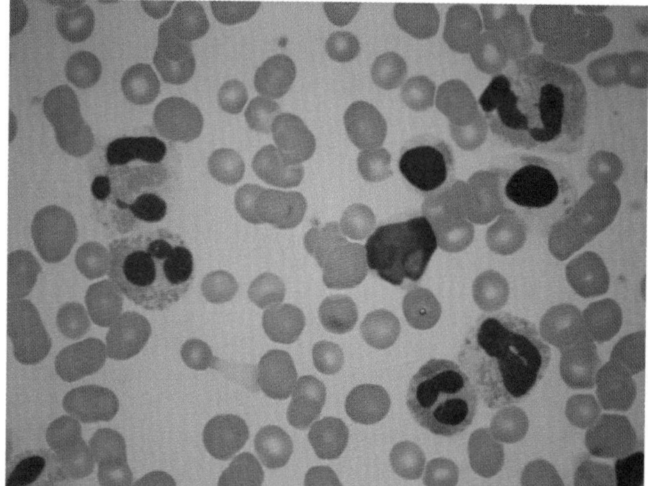

Figure 38–5. Reactive eosinophilia in a patient with B-cell lineage acute lymphoblastic leukemia.

CLINICAL FEATURES AND DIAGNOSIS

The diagnosis of eosinophilic leukemia requires the presence of significant eosinophilia plus clinical, hematologic, cytogenetic, or molecular genetic evidence that the disorder is leukemic in nature (Table 38–4). If there is clear cytogenetic/molecular genetic evidence of clonality of myeloid cells of if myeloblasts are increased (Fig. 38–4), there is no need for the eosinophilia to be sustained for any arbitrary period of time before the diagnosis is made. In fact, delay in diagnosis should be avoided because progressive tissue damage can occur. In the absence of genetic evidence of clonality, a significant increase in blast cells again provides firm grounds for the diagnosis. Other evidence supporting a diagnosis of leukemia may be found but is less definitive, and, in these circumstances, exclusion of alternative diagnoses becomes more important.

In patients with increased blast cells or a clonal cytogenetic/molecular genetic abnormality, there is no need to search for alternative causes of eosinophilia. However, the assessment of an individual patient should proceed in a logical manner, so that the diagnostic procedures most likely to result in a definitive diagnosis are performed first. The clinical history is important, both for assessing the possible cause of eosinophilia and for indicating the likelihood of relevant tissue damage. The clinical assessment should be comprehensive and should include a travel history and history of drug exposure and of any apparent adverse reactions to drugs. Cardiac and respiratory symptoms should be specifically sought. Physical examination should likewise be comprehensive. Organs and systems of particular relevance include the liver, spleen, lymph nodes, skin (infiltration or vasculitis), heart, lungs, and central and peripheral nervous systems. A blood count, blood film, and careful differential count should be a very early part of the assessment, with the hematologist looking specifically for blast cells (either lymphoblasts or myeloblasts), immature granulocytes, monocytes, lymphoma cells, and dysplastic features in any lineage (Figs. 38–5 and 38–6). Eosinophils may be cytologically abnormal in reactive eosinophilia, so that features such as degranulation, vacuolation, hyperlobation, and hypolobation are not very useful in the differential diagnosis. However, degranulation and the often-associated vacuolation should be noted because they tend to correlate with tissue damage from release of inflammatory mediators.

The results of this initial clinical and hematologic assessment may provide clues to the diagnosis and indicate the next procedure to be performed. Thus, a history of travel to endemic regions, with or without pulmonary infiltration, might indicate the need for exclusion of parasitic infection. Apparent skin infiltration, lymphadenopathy, or lymphocytosis would be an indication for skin biopsy, lymph node biopsy, or immunophenotypic analysis of peripheral blood or other lymphocytes. This might include an extended analysis for expression of a limited repertoire of T-cell receptor variable region genes, indicative of a clonal population.[35,36] Immunophenotypic analysis might be supplemented by molecular analysis for T-cell receptor rearrangement.

In patients in whom the history, physical examination, and preliminary investigations do not provide any other clues to the underlying diagnosis, a bone marrow aspirate, trephine biopsy, and cytogenetic analysis should be performed without delay. The trephine biopsy sometimes reveals systemic mastocytosis or lymphomatous infiltration. Because of the major therapeutic implications, a specific test for the *FIP1L1-PDGFRA* fusion gene should be performed and rearrangement of the *PDGFRB* gene should also be sought. Fluorescent in situ hybridization for the *CHIC2* gene, deleted when there is *FIP1L1-PDGFRA* fusion, is a useful technique for the presumptive identification of this fusion gene.[37] Reverse transcriptase–polymerase chain reaction can also be used.

The diagnostic algorithm will differ, according to the clinical history and physical findings (Figs. 38–7 and 38–8).

Figure 38–6. Reactive eosinophilia in a patient who had been administered interleukin 3.

DIFFERENTIAL DIAGNOSIS

Reactive Eosinophilia

In some patients the diagnosis of reactive eosinophilia is readily made. This is so for some patients with parasitic infections, some with cancer-associated eosinophilia, and most with allergic reactions to drugs. In other patients, the underlying cause, and therefore the nature of the condition, is very difficult to elucidate. Occult causes of hypereosinophilia include lymphoma and other neoplasms. Hodgkin's disease can be associated with prominent eosinophilia, but the disease itself is rarely occult when standard diagnostic procedures are applied. However, in non-Hodgkin's lymphoma (NHL), particularly NHL of T-cell lineage, the eosinophilia may be the dominant manifestation of the disease with the lymphoma itself being quite difficult to detect. Skin infiltration and lymphocytosis are clear indications to investigate for underlying NHL. In otherwise unexplained hypereosinophilia, investigations directed at identifying an

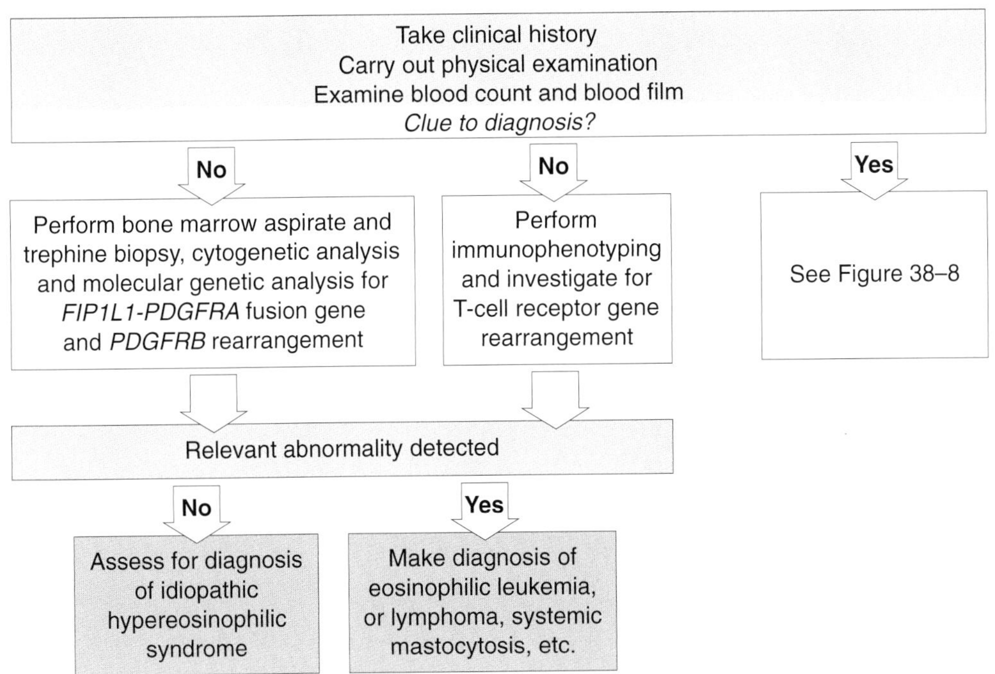

Figure 38–7. Diagnostic algorithm when initial assessment provides no clue to the diagnosis.

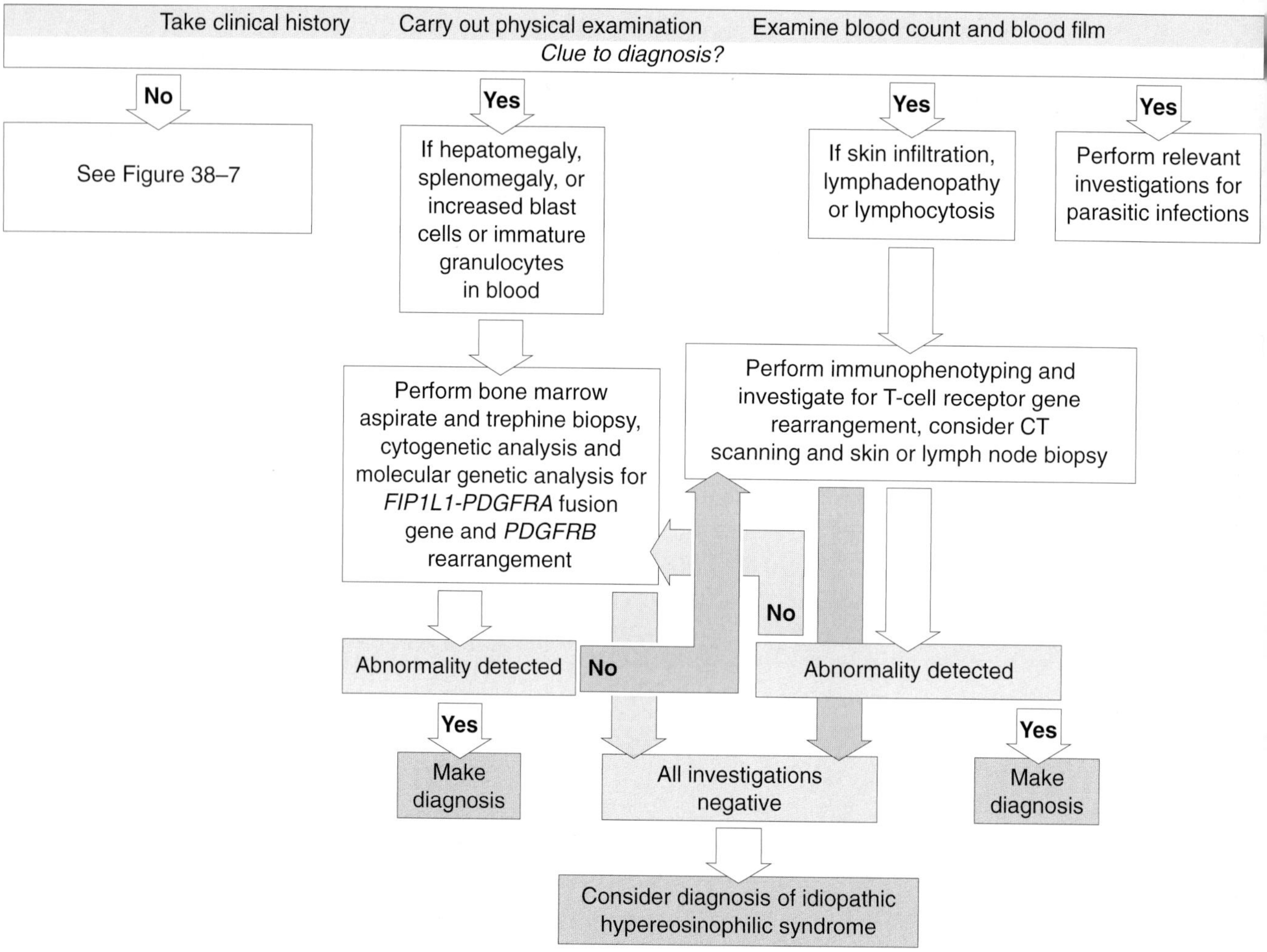

Take clinical history | Carry out physical examination | Examine blood count and blood film
Clue to diagnosis?

No → See Figure 38–7

Yes → If hepatomegaly, splenomegaly, or increased blast cells or immature granulocytes in blood → Perform bone marrow aspirate and trephine biopsy, cytogenetic analysis and molecular genetic analysis for *FIP1L1-PDGFRA* fusion gene and *PDGFRB* rearrangement → Abnormality detected → Yes → Make diagnosis; No → Perform immunophenotyping and investigate for T-cell receptor gene rearrangement, consider CT scanning and skin or lymph node biopsy / All investigations negative

Yes → If skin infiltration, lymphadenopathy or lymphocytosis → Perform immunophenotyping and investigate for T-cell receptor gene rearrangement, consider CT scanning and skin or lymph node biopsy → Abnormality detected → Yes → Make diagnosis; No → Perform bone marrow aspirate and trephine biopsy… / All investigations negative

Yes → Perform relevant investigations for parasitic infections

All investigations negative → Consider diagnosis of idiopathic hypereosinophilic syndrome

Figure 38–8. Diagnostic algorithm when initial assessment provides a clue to the diagnosis.

underlying NHL should also be done, despite the lack of any clinical or laboratory features suggesting this diagnosis. In the absence of any identifiable lymphadenopathy or skin infiltration, immunophenotyping of peripheral blood lymphocytes and DNA analysis for the detection of T-cell receptor gene rearrangement are indicated.

Acute Eosinophilic Leukemia

The term *acute eosinophilic leukemia* indicates an AML with predominantly eosinophilic differentiation. If using the French-American-British (FAB) classification,[38] such a case would have at least 30% bone marrow blast cells and differentiation would be predominantly eosinophilic; the FAB category would be M2 AML, because there would be sufficient granulocytic differentiation to satisfy the criteria for this category. It is common for the designation "M2Eo" to be used for such cases, although this is not a FAB designation. Some patients with M2Eo AML with extremely high eosinophil counts[39,40] have been found to have t(8;21)(q22;q22), a category of leukemia in which a lesser degree of maturation to eosinophils is common. Another cytogenetic/molecular genetic category of AML in which there is a greater or lesser degree

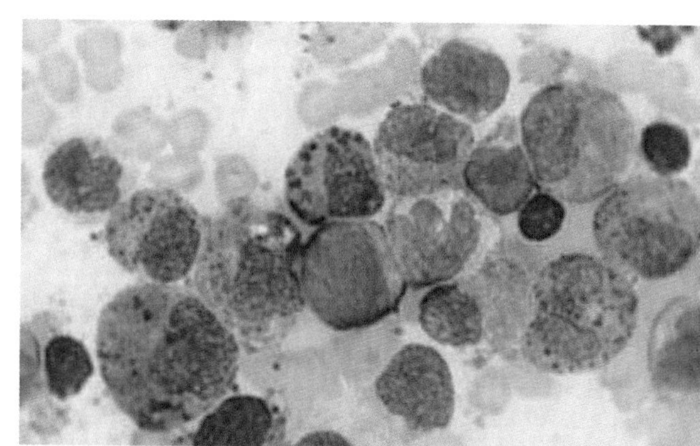

Figure 38–9. Acute myeloid leukemia associated with inv(16)(p13q22).

of eosinophilic maturation is that associated with inv(16)(p13q22) or t(16;16)(p13;q22) with formation of a *CBFB-MYH11* fusion gene (Fig. 38–9). Such leukemias can fall into various FAB categories of AML but are most often M4 AML (acute myelomonocytic leukemia) with prominent eosinophilic differentiation, commonly referred to as "M4Eo." Such cases would not generally be referred to as acute eosinophilic leukemia because there is usually also prominent monocytic differentiation, although this designation would be appropriate for the minority of patients with predominantly eosinophilic differentiation. There are occasional other patients with acute eosinophilic leukemia with miscellaneous karyotypic abnormalities. Among these, one rare but recurring abnormality is t(10;14)(p14;q21).[41,42]

In the WHO classification, a minimum of 20% bone marrow or peripheral blood blasts is required for a case to be categorized as AML.[43] There is no specific category for eosinophilic leukemia (although there is a category for acute basophilic leukemia). Occasional patients have acute eosinophilic leukemia that is therapy related, and such cases would be assigned to that WHO category. Cases of acute eosinophilic leukemia that are found to have t(8;21), inv(16), or t(16;16) would be assigned to the WHO category of AML with recurrent genetic abnormalities. Any other cases of acute eosinophilic leukemia are likely to be assigned to the WHO category "acute myeloid leukemia not otherwise categorized, acute myeloid leukemia with maturation"—a category similar, but certainly not identical, to the FAB M2 category.

However it is defined, acute eosinophilic leukemia is characterized by increased bone marrow blast cells and predominant eosinophilic differentiation. There is usually, but not always, peripheral blood eosinophilia, and the eosinophils may be cytologically abnormal with hypogranularity, cytoplasmic vacuolation, and hyperlobated or hypolobated nuclei. They may also show cytochemical abnormalities, aberrant positivity for chloroacetate esterase having been described in patients with inv(16) or t(16;16). The bone marrow, in addition to blast cells, shows promyelocytes of eosinophil lineage, eosinophil myelocytes, and eosinophils. Eosinophil promyelocytes have primary granules that are azurophilic in their staining characteristics; in addition, there are often some basophilic granules and some eosinophilic granules, the latter permitting the lineage to be recognized. The granules with basophilic staining characteristics are early eosinophil granules, conveniently referred to as "pro-eosinophilic" granules to avoid any possibility of confusing them with the granules of basophils.

Dead eosinophils give rise to Charcot-Leyden crystals (Fig. 38–10), which are seen free in tissues and sometimes also seen within intact eosinophils. Charcot-Leyden crystals are particularly prominent if there has been bone marrow necrosis.

Making a distinction between acute and chronic eosinophilic leukemia is generally straightforward, being based on the percentage of blast cells present. However, it should be noted that, in any patient found to have t(8;21), inv(16), or t(16;16), the diagnosis is acute rather than chronic eosinophilic leukemia, regardless of the blast percentage.

Idiopathic Hypereosinophilic Syndrome

This condition was first defined by Chusid and colleagues nearly 30 years ago as a condition in which there was unexplained eosinophilia (eosinophil count > 1.5×10^9/L) persisting for at least 6 months and leading to tissue damage.[1] The requirement for the eosinophilia to persist and remain unexplained for 6 months served to exclude examples of reactive eosinophilia in which an explanation emerged during this time. The requirement for tissue damage, such as cardiac damage, would appear to be less important because there is likely to be a phase of this disease that precedes tissue damage. Such patients can be regarded as having chronic idiopathic eosinophilia, with the recognition that they may well have the same spectrum of underlying disorders as those with idiopathic HES. The WHO classification is based on these well-established criteria, but the criteria have been expanded in light of more recent discoveries.[5] There must be (1) persistent eosinophilia, with the eosinophil count being at least 1.5×10^9/L; (2) no explanation for the eosinophilia; (3) no aberrant cytokine-secreting T-cell population; (4) less than 5% bone marrow blast cells and no more than 2% peripheral blood blast cells; and (5) no clonal cytogenetic or genetic abnormality or any other evidence that the eosinophils are clonal.

Some patients with idiopathic HES survive only a short time, dying as a result of cardiac or other damage resulting from the release of eosinophil granule contents. It appears likely that this group includes at least some patients who do actually have eosinophilic leukemia but in whom death occurs before a defining transformation event permits the diagnosis to be made.

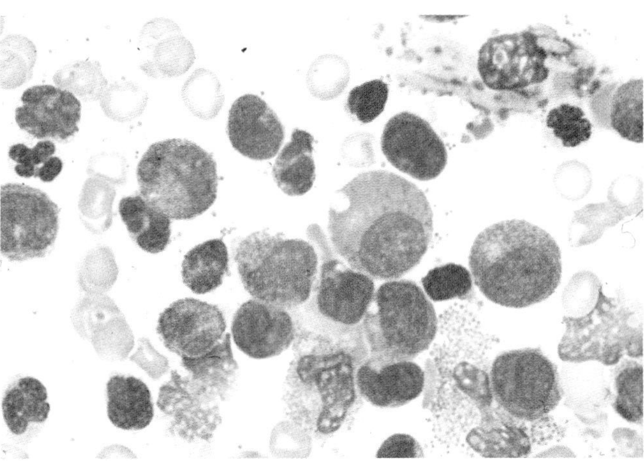

Figure 38–10. Bone marrow aspirate from a patient with acute myeloid leukemia associated with t(8;21)(q22;q22) with increased bone marrow eosinophils, showing Charcot-Leyden crystals (top right).

Systemic Mastocytosis

Chronic eosinophilic leukemia associated with *FIP1L1-PDGFRA* fusion must be distinguished from systemic mastocytosis. Both conditions can have eosinophilla, increased serum tryptase and bone marrow mast cell infiltration. However systemic mastocytosis is associated with a *KIT* mutation and is generally resistant to imatinib.

TREATMENT

Chronic Eosinophilic Leukemia

The correct management of chronic eosinophilic leukemia requires that the underlying genetic abnormality be defined so that molecularly targeted therapy can be applied, when relevant.

Imatinib has shown a remarkable efficacy in patients with the *FIP1L1-PDGFRA* fusion gene. The mechanism of action is inhibition of tyrosine phosphorylation of the FIP1L1-PDGFRA protein and its downstream target, STAT5.[8,21,37] The disease is responsive to lower imatinib doses than are conventionally used in Ph-positive chronic myeloid leukemia (e.g., 100 mg/day), but it is possible that elimination of minimal residual disease will require higher doses, comparable to those used in Ph-positive disease. Complete molecular remissions have been reported.[44] Early initiation of treatment is critical because some patients have responded to imatinib but have nevertheless died of cardiac complications of the hypereosinophilia. Acute cardiac failure can occur soon after starting treatment and may be corticosteroid responsive.[45,46] A trial of imatinib therapy is also clearly indicated in any patients identified with *BCR-PDGFRA* fusion.

Imatinib has also been found to be efficacious in the 5q33 syndrome and is indicated in all patients with rearrangement of the platelet-derived growth factor receptor β (*PDGFRB*) gene. Efficacy has been shown in patients with *ETV6-PDGFRB*, *PDE4DIP-PDGFRB*, *RAB5-PDGFRB*, and other undefined *PDGFRB* rearrangements.[28,33,47] One patient has been reported who responded to interferon alfa,[48] but this would no longer be the treatment of choice.

There is as yet no specific therapy applicable to the 8p11 syndrome. One patient was reported to have had a transient response to interferon.[49] The prognosis is so poor that stem cell transplantation should be considered. By analogy with Ph-positive chronic myeloid leukemia, it seems preferable that this should be done while the disease is still in chronic phase.

There is no clear best option for patients with miscellaneous cytogenetic or molecular genetic abnormalities or with no detectable abnormality. Hydroxyurea (now known as hydroxycarbamide), with or without corticosteroids, gives some control of the disease. Interferon has been useful in some patients, with complete cytogenetic remission sometimes occurring.[50–52]

The Idiopathic Hypereosinophilic Syndrome

Traditionally, idiopathic HES has been treated with hydroxyurea, sometimes supplemented by corticosteroids or vincristine. Alemtuzumab (CD52 monoclonal antibody) was of benefit in a single patient.[53] Imatinib responses have occurred in several patients who were demonstrated *not* to have a *FIP1L1-PDGFRA* fusion gene, although the disease was generally less responsive than chronic eosinophilic leukemia with *FIP1L1-PDGFRA*. This suggests that, in some patients with idiopathic disease, there may be activation of a tyrosine kinase resembling PDGFRA or PDGFRB.[54]

CURRENT CONTROVERSIES & FUTURE CONSIDERATIONS

Hypereosinophilia

- The discovery of the *FIP1L1-PDGFRA* fusion gene has revealed the nature of a significant proportion of cases of hypereosinophilia that would previously have been idiopathic. However there remain idiopathic cases, the true nature of which requires elucidation.
- The relationship between systemic mastocytosis and a condition characterized by hypereosinophilia, bone marrow mast cell infiltration and *FIP1L1-PDGFRA* fusion is becoming clearer. Current evidence suggests that the latter condition should NOT be regarded as a form of systemic mastocytosis.
- Stem cell transplantation is currently the only effective treatment for the 8p11 syndrome. It may be anticipated that a therapeutic approach directed at the molecular abnormality will lead to safer and equally effective treatment.

Suggested Readings*

Bain BJ: Cytogenetic and molecular genetic aspects of eosinophilic leukaemia. Br J Haematol 122:173–179, 2003.

Bain BJ: On overview of translocation-related oncogenesis in the chronic myeloid leukaemias. Acta Haematol 107:57–63, 2002.

Bain B, Pierre R, Imbert M, et al: Chronic eosinophilic leukemia and the hypereosinophilic syndrome. *In* Jaffe ES, Harris NL, Stein H, Vardiman JW (eds): World Health Organization Classification of Tumours: Pathology and Genetics of Tumours of Haematopoietic and Lymphoid Tissues. Lyon: IARC Press, 2001, pp 29–31.

Cools J, DeAngelo DJ, Gotlib J, et al: A tyrosine kinase created by the fusion of the *PDGFRA* and *FIP1L1* genes as a therapeutic target of imatinib in idiopathic hypereosinophilic syndrome. N Engl J Med 348:1201–1214, 2003.

Simon HU, Plötz SG, Dummer R, et al: Abnormal clones of interleukin-5-producing T cells in idiopathic eosinophilia. N Engl J Med 341:1112–1120, 1999.

CHAPTER 39
BIOLOGY OF LYMPHOID MALIGNANCY

Laurence de Leval, MD, PhD, and Nancy Lee Harris, MD

KEY POINTS

Biology of Lymphoid Malignancy

- The improved molecular and pathologic characteristics of lymphoid malignancies has lead to both clustered and detailed sub-classification of these disorders.
- Lymphoid malignancies can now be accurately classified, providing important prognostic information and therapeutic direction.
- Lymphoid malignancies arise from chromosomal rearrangements, viral infection and oncogenes activation.
- Lymphoid malignancies arise as clonal expansion of specific differentiation phenotypes of lymphoid cells from the most "stem-like" to the most differentiated.
- Newer classifications of mantle cell, NK cell, anaplastic large cell lymphomas, and the subclassification of Hodgkin's lymphomas into "classical" and "nodular lymphocyte predominance" better organize these disorders along their pathogenesis, and prognosis.
- Newer treatments, especially antibody therapy and targeted therapeutics necessitate an appreciation of these detailed distinct diseases within the group of lymphoid malignancies.

INTRODUCTION

Lymphoid neoplasms encompass a large group of clonal lymphoid proliferations with different clinical presentations, pathologic features, and biologic behavior. Among these, Hodgkin's lymphoma is segregated from all other forms, which constitute a heterogeneous group referred to as non-Hodgkin's lymphoma. In the United States, lymphomas currently represent about 5% of all cancers and are the fifth most common cancers. It is estimated that about 61,000 new lymphoma cases are diagnosed yearly in the United States, including approximately 7000 cases of Hodgkin's lymphoma and 54,000 cases of non-Hodgkin's lymphoma. For both forms of lymphomas, incidence is higher among men than women and is higher for whites than African Americans and other ethnic groups (Fig. 39–1*A* and *B*). There has been little variation in the incidence of Hodgkin's lymphoma over the past decades (see Fig. 39–1*A*), and the mortality rate has significantly decreased as a result of improvements in the treatment (Fig. 39–1*C*). In contrast, both the incidence and the mortality attributed to non-Hodgkin's lymphoma have increased, with the incidence rate nearly doubling since the early 1970s, then stabilizing in the past 5 years (Fig. 39–1*B* and *D*). The increase in incidence has affected all types of non-Hodgkin's lymphoma, especially aggressive diseases and those occurring in extranodal locations. Although a substantial proportion of the increase is attributable to the human immunodeficiency virus (HIV) epidemic, significant increases have been observed in non–HIV-related cases as well, in all age groups.[1] The reasons for this increasing incidence of non-Hodgkin's lymphoma are poorly understood, but may reflect improved diagnostic techniques, wider administration of immunosuppressive therapies, and association with various infectious agents. Even after accounting for these, there remains a significant unexplained increase in incidence. Postulated risk factors include a familial predisposition, a genetic susceptibility to non-Hodgkin's lymphoma, lifestyle factors, and environmental or occupational exposures.[2,3]

Worldwide, lymphomas are more common in developed countries with the highest incidence in the United States and in Europe. These diseases are much less frequent in China, and have an intermediate rate of incidence in South America, Africa, and Japan.

PRINCIPLES OF LYMPHOMA CLASSIFICATION

The Kiel Classification and the Working Formulation

Few areas in pathology have evoked as much controversy as the classification of lymphomas. Many classifications have been proposed over the past 30–40 years. From the 1980s through the early 1990s, two lymphoma

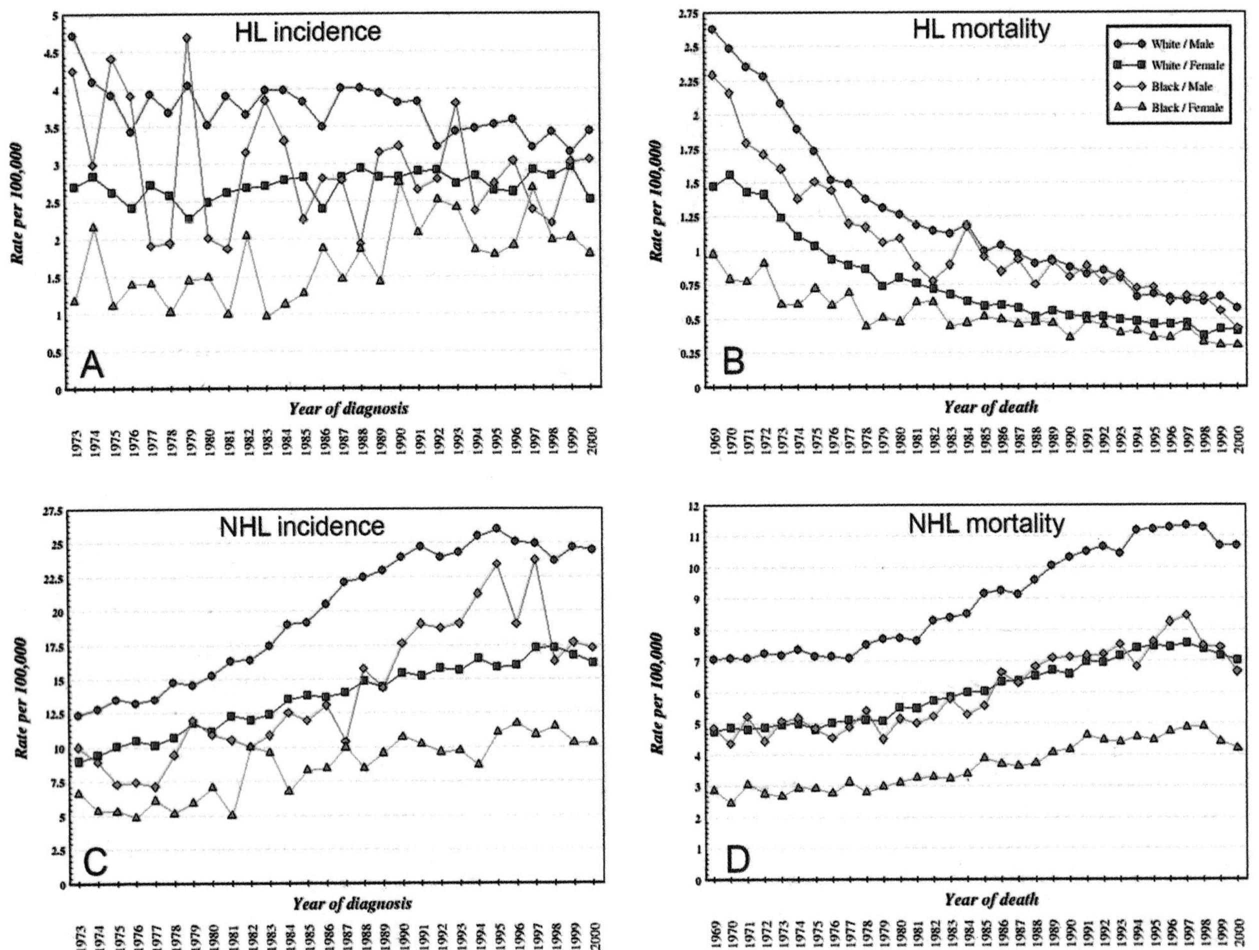

Figure 39–1. Incidence (*A* and *C*) and mortality rate (*B* and *D*) trends of Hodgkin's lymphoma (HL) and non-Hodgkin's lymphomas (NHL) in the United States over the 1973–2000 period. Data from the SEER Program and the National Center for Health Statistics (*http://seer.cancer.gov*).

classifications were used in different parts of the world. The Kiel Classification[4,5] developed by Karl Lennert in Germany came to be widely used in Europe; in this approach, primarily intended for classification of nodal diseases, lymphomas were classified according to a hypothetical scheme of B- and T-lymphocyte differentiation, and the nomenclature reflected the putative normal counterpart of the neoplastic cells. In contrast, the Working Formulation for clinical usage was widely used in the United States.[6] In this scheme, non-Hodgkin's lymphomas were divided on clinical grounds into three prognostic groups: low, intermediate and high grade. Within each group, classification was based purely on morphologic criteria, in particular the nodular versus diffuse growth pattern and the size of the tumor cells (small versus large versus mixed small and large).

This lack of consensus on lymphoma classification and terminology caused problems for both pathologists and clinicians, and caused difficulty in interpreting published studies. In addition, in the 1980s and 1990s, many new disease entities were described (e.g., mantle cell lymphoma and extranodal marginal zone lymphoma) that were not included in either classification, leading to confusion among both pathologists and oncologists about which were "real" diseases that they should be recognizing in daily practice. Finally, the introduction of the new techniques of immunophenotyping and molecular genetic analysis led to confusion about what, if anything, should be the modern "gold standard" for defining disease entities.

The Revised European-American Classification of Lymphoid Neoplasms

In the early 1990s, the International Lymphoma Study Group (ILSG), a group of approximately 20 hematopathologists from the United States, Europe, and Asia, adopted a new approach to lymphoma classification, in which all available information—morphology, immunophenotype, genetic features, and clinical features—was used to define a disease entity. The importance of each of these features differs among the disease entities, and there is no one gold standard for defining all diseases. The consensus list of well-defined disease entities was published in 1994 as the Revised European-American Classification of Lymphoid Neoplasms (REAL) scheme.[7] Although its initial publication elicited considerable controversy,[8] experience over the years has shown that it can be reproducibly applied by most pathologists and that the entities described have distinctive clinical features, making it a useful and practical classification.[9,10]

The World Health Organization Classification of Neoplasms of the Hematopoietic and Lymphoid Tissues

Recently, under the auspices of the World Health Organization (WHO), members of the European and American hematopathology societies collaborated on a comprehensive classification of all hematopoietic and lymphoid neoplasms, published as a monograph in 2001.[11] The WHO classification, an updated form of the REAL proposal, represents the first true international consensus on the classification of hematologic malignancies and is currently widely used worldwide by both pathologists and clinicians.

Categories of Lymphoid Neoplasms

The WHO classification of lymphoid neoplasms (Table 39–1) recognizes three major categories that can be defined based on a combination of morphology and cell lineage: B-cell neoplasms, T-cell and natural killer (NK)-cell neoplasms, and Hodgkin's lymphoma. Both lymphomas and lymphoid leukemias are included in this classification, because both solid and circulating phases are present in many lymphoid neoplasms, and distinction between them is artificial. Thus, B-cell chronic lymphocytic leukemia and B-cell small lymphocytic lymphoma are simply different manifestations of the same neoplasm, as are lymphoblastic lymphomas and acute lymphoid leukemias, and Burkitt's lymphoma and Burkitt's cell leukemia.

Biologic Basis for Classification of Lymphoid Neoplasms

Lymphomas derive from B cells, T cells, or NK cells at various stages of differentiation and possess many features of their normal counterparts. These features—including normal genetic events, gene expression, immunophenotype, morphology, homing patterns, and proliferation fraction—in large part dictate the clinical behavior of these diseases. Thus, understanding the normal counterpart of neoplastic cells can provide a useful framework for understanding the biology of the lymphomas (Fig. 39–2).

Two major categories of lymphoid neoplasms are recognized: precursor (lymphoblastic) neoplasms, corresponding to the earliest stages of differentiation, and peripheral or mature neoplasms, corresponding to later stages of differentiation. Lymphoblastic neoplasms tend to be more common in children, who have large pools of precursor cells, whereas those neoplasms corresponding to mature effector cells tend to be seen more often in adults; for example, plasma cell myeloma is common in older adults with large pools of post–germinal center antigen-exposed plasma cells, as is mycosis fungoides, which is a neoplasm derived from effector $CD4^+$ T cells. Tumors corresponding to proliferating normal cells such as lymphoblasts or centroblasts are likely to be rapidly

TABLE 39–1. The WHO Classification of Lymphoid Neoplasms (2001)

B-Cell Neoplasms

Precursor B-Cell Neoplasms

Precursor B-lymphoblastic leukemia/lymphoma (precursor B-cell acute lymphoblastic leukemia) (B-ALL)

Mature (Peripheral) B-Cell Neoplasms

Predominantly Disseminated

Chronic lymphocytic leukemia/B-cell small lymphocytic lymphoma (CLL/SLL)
B-cell prolymphocytic leukemia (B-PLL)
Lymphoplasmacytic lymphoma (LPL)
Splenic marginal zone B-cell lymphoma (splenic lymphoma with villous lymphocytes) (SMZL)
Hairy cell leukemia (HCL)
Plasma cell myeloma/plasmacytoma

Primary Extranodal

Extranodal marginal zone B-cell lymphoma of mucosa-associated lymphoid tissue (MALT)

Predominantly Nodal

Nodal marginal zone B-cell lymphoma (MZL)
Follicular lymphoma (FL)
Mantle cell lymphoma (MCL)
Diffuse large B-cell lymphoma (DLBCL)
  Mediastinal (thymic) large B-cell lymphoma (MLBCL)
  Intravascular large B-cell lymphoma (IVL)
  Primary effusion lymphoma (PEL)
Burkitt's lymphoma/leukemia (BL)
Lymphomatoid granulomatosis (LyG)

T- and NK-Cell Neoplasms

Precursor T- and NK-Cell Neoplasms

Precursor T-lymphoblastic leukemia/lymphoma (precursor T-cell acute lymphoblastic leukemia) (T-ALL)
Blastoid NK-cell lymphoma

Mature (Peripheral) T-Cell Neoplasms

Predominantly Disseminated

T-cell prolymphocytic leukemia (T-PLL)
T-cell large granular lymphocytic leukemia (T-LGL)
Aggressive NK-cell leukemia
Adult T-cell lymphoma/leukemia (HTLV-1+) (ATLL)

Primary Extranodal

Extranodal NK/T-cell lymphoma, nasal type
Enteropathy-type T-cell lymphoma (ETCL)
Hepatosplenic T-cell lymphoma
Subcutaneous panniculitis-like T-cell lymphoma (SPTCL)
Mycosis fungoides/Sézary syndrome (MF)
Primary cutaneous anaplastic large-cell lymphoma (ALCL)

Predominantly Nodal

Peripheral T-cell lymphoma, not otherwise specified (PTCL-NOS)
Angioimmunoblastic T-cell lymphoma (AITCL)
Primary systemic anaplastic large-cell lymphoma (ALCL)

Hodgkin's Lymphoma

Nodular Lymphocyte Predominant Hodgkin's Lymphoma (NLPHL)

Classical Hodgkin Lymphoma (cHL)

Nodular sclerosis classical Hodgkin's lymphoma (grades 1 and 2) (NSHL)
Mixed cellularity classical Hodgkin's lymphoma (MCHL)
Lymphocyte-rich classical Hodgkin's lymphoma (LRHL)
Lymphocyte-depleted classical Hodgkin's lymphoma (LDHL)

Adapted from Jaffe ES, Harris NL, Stein H, et al (eds): Pathology and Genetics: Neoplasms of the Haematopoietic and Lymphoid Tissues. Lyon: IARC Press, 2001.

growing and clinically aggressive, whereas those that correspond to resting stages, such as small lymphocytic lymphoma/chronic lymphocytic leukemia, are more likely to be indolent. Lymphoid neoplasms also reflect their normal counterpart in their growth and homing pattern: tumors of bone marrow–derived precursors become acute leukemias and those of marrow-homing plasma cells become multiple myeloma; tumors derived from cells of mucosa-associated lymphoid tissue (MALT) tend to involve such sites; and follicular lymphoma cells derived from germinal center centroblasts and centrocytes populate the follicles of lymphoid tissues throughout the body.

Grading and Prognostic Groups

Over 30 distinct entities are listed in the WHO classification of lymphoid neoplasms. These diseases are in most cases unrelated to one another, that is, we can no longer talk about "lymphoma" or "non-Hodgkin lymphoma" as a single disease with a range of histologic grades and clinical aggressiveness. One of the corollaries of defining

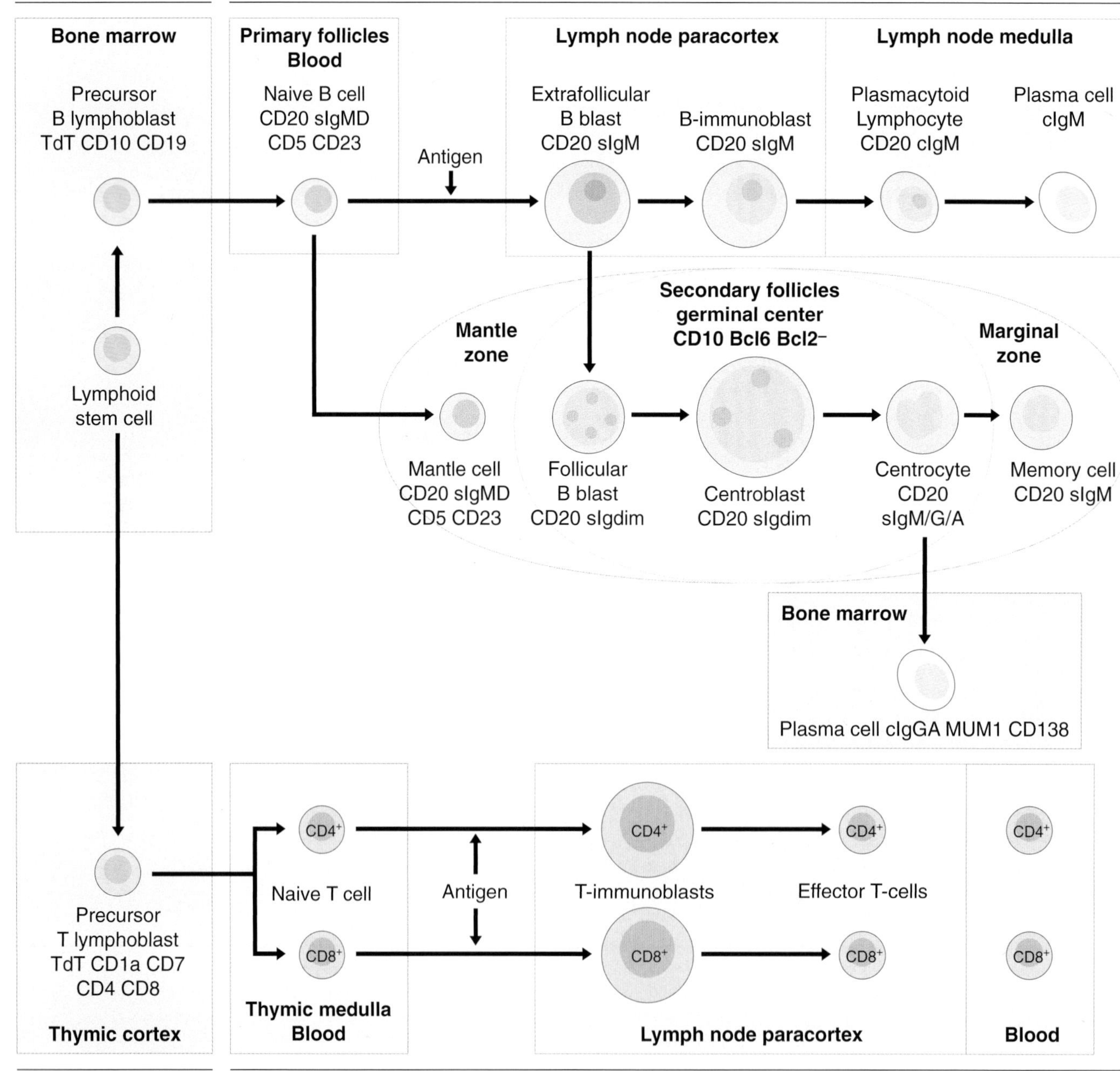

distinct lymphoma entities is that it is neither possible nor helpful to sort them according to histologic grade or clinical aggressiveness. For example, although it is true that many lymphomas composed of relatively small cells with a low proliferation fraction have a generally indolent course, at least one of them—mantle cell lymphoma—is rather aggressive. In addition, each has a distinctive set of presenting features and, often, different treatments (e.g., hairy cell leukemia vs. B-chronic lymphocytic leukemia vs. MALT lymphoma). Several of the lymphomas that we can now recognize have within themselves a range of histologic grade (number of large cells or proliferation fraction) and clinical aggressiveness (e.g., follicular lymphoma and mantle cell lymphoma). Thus, histologic grade should be applied within a disease entity, not across the whole range of lymphoid neoplasms. In practice, treatment of a specific patient is determined not by which broad "prognostic group" the lymphoma falls into, but by the specific histologic type of lymphoma, with the addition of grade within the tumor type, if applicable, and clinical features such stage, age, performance status, and the International Prognostic Index.[12]

Organization of the WHO Classification of Lymphoid Neoplasms

Because of the impracticality of arranging the list of B and T/NK-cell lymphoid neoplasms according to prognostic groups, the WHO classification lists them first according to differentiation stage and secondarily according to predominant clinical presentation (see Table 39–1). Three broad categories of clinical presentation are recognized: predominantly disseminated diseases that often involve bone marrow and may be leukemic, primary extranodal lymphomas, and predominantly nodal diseases that are often disseminated and may also involve extranodal sites. This approach is intended for convenience and ease of learning only, by placing diseases that are likely to resemble one another both clinically and histologically in proximity to one another in the list and in a text. It also has some biologic relevance, because there appear to be important biologic differences between primary nodal and primary extranodal lymphomas, particularly in the T/NK-cell diseases. However, any principle of sorting these neoplasms is artificial, and the list can be regrouped in different ways for different purposes.

PATHOPHYSIOLOGY OF NON-HODGKIN'S LYMPHOMA

Genetic Alterations

Analogous to most human cancers, the genetic lesions involved in non-Hodgkin's lymphoma include the activation of proto-oncogenes and the disruption of tumor suppressor genes.[13] The type and nature of genetic aberrations associated with hematologic malignancies and solid tumors are in part different. In contrast to many carcinomas that display random genomic instability, the genome of lymphoma cells is relatively stable and lymphomas generally lack defects in DNA mismatch repair genes that cause microsatellite instability.[14] Lymphoma karyotypes are characterized by few—occasionally single—recurrent nonrandom chromosomal abnormalities. Historically, karyotypic analysis of non-Hodgkin's lymphoma metaphases has represented the major clue toward the identification and cloning of most abnormalities in non-Hodgkin's lymphoma, and several cellular oncogenes and tumor suppressor genes have been identified in association with some of the more common chromosome translocations that characterize lymphoid malignancies.[15–17]

Figure 39–2. Hypothetical scheme of T-cell and B-cell lymphocyte differentiation. Each stage occurs at a specific anatomic site and architectural location within each lymphoid organ, and is characterized by changes in surface antigen expression. There are two major phases of differentiation: an antigen-independent phase occurring in the primary lymphoid organs (bone marrow and thymus) and an antigen-dependent phase occurring in the secondary lymphoid organs (lymph nodes, spleen, mucosa-associated lymphoid tissue [MALT]). A postulated common lymphoid stem cell gives rise to both B- and T-cell lines. The early stages are stem cells and lymphoblasts (precursor T and B cells), which are self-renewing. Antigen-independent differentiation results in mature, naive T and B cells that are capable of responding to antigen that binds to their surface antigen receptors (T-cell receptor [TCR] and B-cell receptor [BCR] or surface immunoglobulin [sIg], respectively). Naive B cells are found in the blood and in primary follicles and mantle zones of secondary follicles. Naive T cells are found in the blood, in the thymic medulla, and also in the paracortex of lymph nodes. Upon exposure to antigen, the naive lymphocyte undergoes "blast transformation" and becomes a large, proliferating cell, which gives rise to progeny that are antigen-specific effector or memory cells.

Antigen-dependent B-cell differentiation may occur along two pathways. In T-cell–independent reactions there is an immunoblastic paracortical reaction leading to the generation of short-lived immunoglobulin (Ig)M–secreting plasma cells migrating to the lymph node medulla. The germinal center reaction is the hallmark of T-cell–dependent responses. B-cell blasts activated in the paracortex upon antigen encounter migrate to the center of a primary follicle, proliferate, and differentiate into centroblasts that further mature to centrocytes. In the germinal center, B cells undergo somatic mutations of the variable (V) region of the immunoglobulin V genes and class switching of the immunoglobulin heavy chain (IgH) gene, allowing for expression of IgG, IgA, or IgE. Only cells with favorable immunoglobulin V gene mutations (i.e., those resulting in a higher affinity of the BCR for the antigen) are positively selected and survive. These centrocytes may then differentiate to effector cells (usually IgG- or IgA-secreting plasma cells) homing to the bone marrow or to memory cells, which may collect into a marginal zone. Antigen-dependent T-cell differentiation occurs in the paracortex of the lymph node and results in expanded clones of effector $CD4^+$ and $CD8^+$ T cells (helper and cytotoxic, respectively) and memory cells that may pass into the blood.

Abbreviations: CD, cluster of differentiation; sIg, surface immunoglobulin expression; cIg, cytoplasmic immunoglobulin expression; TdT, terminal deoxynucleotidyl transferase.

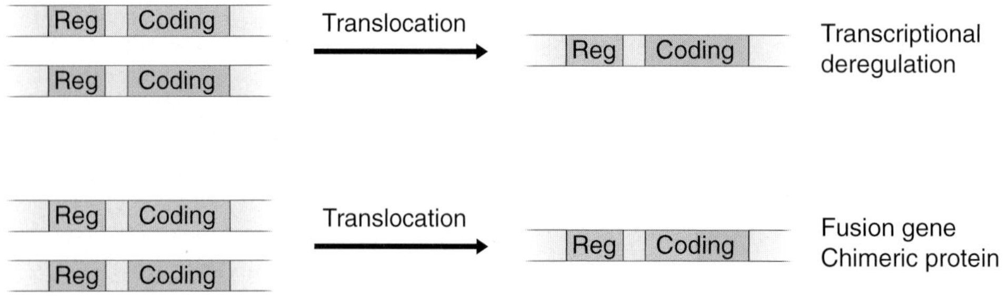

Reg | Coding
Reg | Coding
Translocation
Reg | Coding
Transcriptional deregulation

Reg | Coding
Reg | Coding
Translocation
Reg | Coding
Fusion gene
Chimeric protein

Figure 39–3. Types of chromosomal translocations found in lymphoid neoplasms.

Proto-oncogenes

Chromosomal Translocations

Chromosomal translocations represent the main mechanism of proto-oncogene activation in non-Hodgkin's lymphoma. Each of these translocations is preferentially associated with a specific subtype of lymphoma (Table 39–2).[18,19] The most common translocations involved in lymphoid neoplasms place a gene that is normally silent in resting cells under the influence of a promotor associated with either an immunoglobulin (Ig) or T-cell receptor (*TCR*) gene, resulting in deregulated expression of the gene and giving the cell either a growth or a survival advantage (Fig. 39–3, upper panel). Examples include the t(8;14)(q24;q32) in Burkitt's lymphoma, which places the *c-myc* gene under the immunoglobulin heavy chain promotor[18]; the t(14;18)(q32;q32) of follicular lymphoma, which places the *bcl*-2 gene on chromosome 18 under the immunoglobulin promotor[15,17,20]; and the t(11;14)(q13;q32) in mantle cell lymphoma, which places the cyclin D1 gene (associated with the *bcl*-1 breakpoint) on chromosome 11 under the immunoglobulin promotor.[16,21] In some lymphoid neoplasms, a chromosomal translocation results in a fusion of two genes, resulting in a chimeric protein that may be either abnormally activated or inactivated (see Fig. 39–3, lower panel). Examples include the translocations involving the *ALK* (anaplastic lymphoma kinase) gene on 2p23 with various partner genes in anaplastic large-cell lymphoma,[22–26] resulting in fusion proteins with a conserved kinase activity and with the ability to self-associate in a ligand-independent fashion, thus being constitutively active.[22] Another example is the t(11;18)(q21;q21) in MALT lymphoma, which produces an API-2/MALT-1 fusion protein.[27] This mechanism of oncogenic rearrangement by fusion proto-oncogene activation is more commonly encountered in myeloid neoplasms and some precursor lymphoblastic leukemias.

The translocations can be detected by fluorescence in-situ hybridization (FISH) or polymerase chain reaction (PCR),[28,29] or by using a reverse transcriptase technique to detect RNA produced by an altered or fused gene (RT-PCR).[30] In many cases, the translocation results in overexpression of a protein that can be detected by immunohistochemistry, eliminating the need for genetic studies. Examples of this are the expression of cyclin D1 because of the t(11;14) in mantle cell lymphoma, Bcl-2 because of the t(14;18) in follicular lymphoma, and ALK-1 because of the t(2;5) and variants in anaplastic large-cell lymphoma. To the extent to which specific histologic subtypes and/or prognostic groups of lymphomas are associated with specific gene rearrangements, detection of these rearrangements is useful in the characterization of lymphomas (see Table 39–2). The PCR technique can be used to detect disseminated, residual, or recurrent lymphoma on very small biopsy specimens, or in the blood.[31,32] Finally, studies of the function of the translocated oncogenes are providing clues to the mechanisms of oncogenesis.

Molecular Processes Modifying the Genes Encoding the Antibody Molecules

Somatic hypermutation, a process that introduces point mutations and occasional small deletions or duplications at a very high rate into DNA sequences of immunoglobulin V_H and V_L gene regions (variable regions of the heavy and light chains of immunoglobulin genes) of germinal center B cells, has been recently evidenced as another mechanism involved in lymphomagenesis. Somatic hypermutation in normal germinal center B cells is not restricted to immunoglobulin V genes but also targets the 5′ sequences of the *bcl*-6 gene, a proto-oncogene expressed at high levels by germinal center B cells acting as a transcription repressor essential to the germinal center reaction, as well as in the *FAS* gene.[33–35] Some of these mutations may be selected during lymphomagenesis for their activity in deregulating *bcl*-6 gene expression.[33,36,37] In a large proportion of diffuse large B-cell lymphomas, an aberrant hypermutation activity may target multiple loci, including the 5′ untranslated or coding sequences of several other proto-oncogenes, including *c-myc*. Interestingly, the hypermutable genes are susceptible to chromosomal translocations in the same region, consistent with a role for hypermutation in generating translocations by DNA double-stranded breaks. Thus, by mutating multiple genes, and possibly by favoring chromosomal translocations, aberrant hypermutation may represent a major contributor to lymphomagenesis.[38]

Class switch recombination also occurs in the germinal center B cells and results in the replacement of an expressed heavy chain constant-region gene by a downstream constant-region gene. This is done by a recombination event that deletes DNA between repeated sequences ("switch regions") located upstream of the constant-region genes involved.[39] The DNA breaks that are induced during class switch recombination coincide with the sites of chromosomal translocations in certain lymphoid malignancies, comprising many of those asso-

TABLE 39–2. Genetic Abnormalities in Lymphoid Neoplasms

Proto-oncogenes Gene*	Chromosomal Translocation		Biologic Function	Lymphoma
alk			Anaplastic lymphoma kinase = tyrosine kinase	
	t(2;5)(p23;q35)†	NPM/ALK†	Nucleophosmin-ALK fusion	Anaplastic large-cell lymphoma (75%)‡ Diffuse large B-cell lymphoma, ALK+ (rare)
	t(1;2)(q21;p23)†	TPM 3/ALK†	Tropomyosin 3–ALK fusion	Anaplastic large-cell lymphoma (15%)‡
	t(2;17)(p23;q23)†	CLTC/ALK†	Clathrin heavy chain–ALK fusion	Anaplastic large-cell lymphoma (2%)‡ Diffuse large B-cell lymphoma, ALK+
	t(2;3)(p23;q21)†	TFG/ALK†	TRK-fused gene–ALK fusion	Anaplastic large-cell lymphoma (2%)‡
	inv(2) (p23;q35)†	ATIC/ALK†	ATIC enzyme–ALK fusion	Anaplastic large-cell lymphoma (2%)‡
bcl-1	t(11;14)(q13;q32)	Bcl-1/IgH	Cell cycle regulator	Mantle cell lymphoma (all) Hairy cell leukemia (some) Multiple myeloma (15%)
bcl-2	t(14;18)(q32;q21)	Bcl-2/IgH	Negative regulator of apoptosis	Follicular lymphoma (90%)
	t(2;18)(q11;q21)	Bcl-2/Igκ		Diffuse large B-cell lymphoma (20%)
	t(18;22)(q21;q11)	Bcl-2/Igλ		
bcl-3	t(14;19)(q32;q13)	Bcl-3/IgH	NF-κB subunit	B-CLL/SLL (rare)
*bcl-6**	t(3;14)(q27;q32)	Bcl-6/IgH	Transcriptional repressor necessary for germinal center formation	Diffuse large B-cell lymphoma (30%)
	der(3)(q27)	Bcl-6/var		
bcl-10	t(1;14)(p22;q32)		Activator of the NF-κB pathway	MALT lymphoma (<5%)
FGFR3	t(4;14)(p16;q32)	FGFR-3/IgH	Receptor to fibroblast growth factor	Multiple myeloma (15%)
c-maf	t(14;16)(p16;q32)	c-Maf/IgH	Transcription factor	Multiple myeloma (5%)
MALT1	t(14;18)(q32;q21)	MALT-1/IgH	Paracaspase, binds to Bcl-10	MALT lymphoma (18%) (other than gastrointestinal & pulmonary)
	t(11;18)(q21;q21)†	API-2/MALT-1†	Fusion protein, increases NF-κB activity	MALT lymphoma (50%)
*c-myc**	t(8;14)(q24;q32)	c-Myc/IgH	Transcription factor regulating cell proliferation	Burkitt's lymphoma (30–100%)
	t(2;8)(p11;q24)	c-Myc/Igκ		Diffuse large B-cell lymphoma (10%)
	t(8;22)(q24;q11)	c-Myc/Igλ		
	t(8;14)(q24;q11)	c-Myc/TCR-β		Precursor T-lymphoblastic lymphoma
MUM1 (IRF4)	t(6;14)(p25;q32)	MUM-1/IgH	Transcription factor involved in plasma cell differentiation	Multiple myeloma (rare)
pax-5	t(9;14)(p13;q32)	PAX-5/IgH	Transcription factor regulating B cell proliferation & differentiation	Lymphoplasmacytic lymphoma (rare) Multiple myeloma (rare)

Tumor Suppressor Genes

Gene*	Mechanism of Inactivation	Biologic Function	Lymphoma
ATM	Point mutation; deletion	Protein kinase, maintains genomic stability	Mantle cell lymphoma
*FAS**	Point mutation	Membrane receptor transducing apoptotic signal	HL and NHL
p53	Point mutation; deletion	Transcription factor, maintains DNA integrity	B-CLL, Burkitt's lymphoma, ATLL Transformed follicular and mantle cell lymphomas
p16	Deletion; hypermethylation	Cell cycle regulator (cdk inhibitor)	Transformed NHL
p21	Deletion	Cell cycle regulator (cdk inhibitor)	Transformed NHL

Chromosomal Additions and Deletions

Chromosomal Abnormalities	Genes Involved	Lymphomas
Isochromosome 7q	Unknown	Hepatosplenic γ/δ T-cell lymphoma
Trisomy 3	Unknown	MALT lymphomas Some splenic and nodal marginal zone lymphomas
Trisomy 12	Unknown	B-CLL (30%)
Trisomy 18	Unknown	Some marginal zone lymphomas
del(6q)	Unknown	B-cell lymphomas (10–40%)
del(13q)	Unknown	B-CLL (25%)

*Genes altered by somatic hypermutations in lymphoma.
†Translocations leading to fusion genes and chimeric proteins.
‡Percentages are expressed in reference to anaplastic large-cell lymphomas expressing ALK protein.
Abbreviations: ATLL, adult T-cell lymphoma/leukemia; B-CLL/SLL, B-cell chronic lymphocytic leukemia/small lymphocytic lymphoma; cdk, cyclin-dependent kinase; HL, Hodgkin's lymphoma; MALT, mucosa-associated lymphoid tissue; NF-κB, nuclear factor-κB; NHL, non-Hodgkin's lymphoma.

ciated with sporadic Burkitt's lymphoma and multiple myeloma.[40,41]

Proto-oncogene Amplification

Gene amplification is another mechanism of gene activation. This mechanism is rather frequently involved in non-Hodgkin's lymphoma, in particular in diffuse large B-cell lymphoma.[42] For example, *rel, myc, bcl*-2, and *mdm*-2 are among the proto-oncogenes that are amplified in subsets of diffuse large B-cell lymphoma.[43,44] Detection of gene amplification is facilitated by the use of conventional or microarray-based comparative genomic hybridization,[45] FISH techniques, and Southern blotting.

Tumor Suppressor Genes[13,46]

The tumor suppressor genes most frequently involved in the pathogenesis of non-Hodgkin's lymphoma are represented by p53, p16, *RB1* (retinoblastoma-like 1), and *ATM* (ataxia-telangiectasia mutated). Inactivation of tumor suppressor genes often appears as a secondary event associated with lymphoma evolution or transformation, rather than a primary genetic abnormality. The mechanisms of inactivation include point mutations, gross deletions, and hypermethylation; inactivation usually occurs through deletion of one allele and nonsense/missense mutation or hypermethylation of the other.

The CD95 (*FAS*) gene, which is involved in the control of apoptosis, was recently proposed as a tumor suppressor gene.[47] Inherited mutations of the *FAS* gene lead to autoimmune lymphoproliferative syndrome and predispose to B-cell lymphoma.[48] Somatic mutations of the *FAS* gene impairing the transduction of the apoptosis signal are found at variable frequencies (overall 15%) in a variety of lymphomas and may be acquired by somatic hypermutation as a side effect of the germinal center reaction.[35]

Other Chromosomal Changes

Various other recurrent chromosomal abnormalities are described in non-Hodgkin's lymphoma, including chromosomal deletions and additions. Chromosomal deletions frequently involve the long arms of chromosome 6 (6q21-6q23 and 6q25-6q27)[49,50] and chromosome 13 (13q14, frequently deleted in chronic lymphocytic leukemia/small lymphocytic lymphoma).[51] These chromosomal regions presumably represent tumor suppressor loci, but candidate genes have so far not yet been identified.

Infectious Agents

A variety of infectious agents have been identified as either linked to or truly causative of lymphomas. Among viruses, the Epstein-Barr virus (EBV) is associated with the largest variety of lymphoproliferations. In addition to being found in a proportion of classical Hodgkin's lymphoma, EBV is present in nearly 100% of endemic Burkitt's lymphoma[52] and in 40% of sporadic and HIV-associated cases,[53,54] is detected in virtually all cases of extranodal nasal-type T/NK-cell lymphoma,[55] and is clearly implicated in the pathogenesis of lymphoproliferations occurring in the setting of immunodeficiency. The Kaposi sarcoma–associated herpesvirus (formerly called human herpesvirus 8) is another herpesvirus more recently found in association with lymphoproliferations (primary effusion lymphoma[56] and the lymphomas associated with multicentric Castleman's disease in HIV-infected individuals[57]).

The human T-cell leukemia virus type 1 (HTLV-1) is causally linked to adult T-cell leukemia/lymphoma, a disease endemic in Japan and in the Caribbean area.[58] The cumulative lifetime risk for development of adult T-cell lymphoma/leukemia among seropositive individuals is higher in males than in females and overall less than 5%,[59] indicating the necessity for additional events for overt development of malignancy. Clonally integrated HTLV-1 is found in all cases. The p40 tax viral protein leads to transcriptional activation of many genes in infected lymphocytes.

Several reports document an association between hepatitis C virus (HCV) and splenic lymphoma with villous lymphocytes,[60] and type II cryoglobulinemia. Treatment of patients with HCV and cryoglobulinemia or splenic marginal zone lymphoma with interferon to reduce the viral load has been associated with regression of the lymphoma.[61–63] HCV infection has also been documented in lymphomas without cryoglobulinemias, especially MALT lymphomas of the salivary glands and liver, two common sites of viral infection.[64] The pathogenic mechanism underlying B-cell expansion is still an open question. HCV has B-cell lymphotropism and viral proteins have indeed been detected in lymphoma tissues,[65] but it is an RNA virus, which cannot integrate into the genome. It is not clear at this point whether HCV has transforming properties or whether these neoplasms are antigen-driven, a hypothesis favored by the finding of a certain sequence similarity between the immunoglobulin sequences of HCV-associated lymphoproliferations and anti-HCV antibodies, and the demonstration of ongoing somatic mutations in some HCV-associated lymphoproliferations.[66,67]

Bacteria, or at least immune responses to bacteria, have also been implicated in the pathogenesis of extranodal B-cell marginal zone lymphoma of the MALT type. The most convincing and best documented example is that of gastric MALT lymphoma arising in association with *Helicobacter pylori* infection. Several strands of evidence indicate that gastric MALT lymphoma arises from acquired MALT induced by *H. pylori* infection.[68] In early stages of MALT lymphoma, MALT lymphoma cells preserve B-cell properties and their growth may be driven by antigenic stimulation. Lymphoma growth in vitro is dependent on the presence of T cells activated with *H. pylori* antigens, and antibiotic treatment causes regression of the lymphoma in many patients.[69–71] In later stages of gastric MALT lymphoma, acquisition of genetic abnormalities, such as t(11;18)(q21,q21) or t(1;14)(p22;q32), is associated with tumor escape from its growth dependency.[72]

Similarly, *Borrelia burgdorferi* has been implicated in the pathogenesis of cutaneous MALT lymphoma.[73,74] Intestinal MALT lymphoma associated with immunoproliferative small intestinal disease/α chain disease has been associated with mixed bacterial infections and more recently with *Campylobacter jejuni* infection.[75–77] Development of pyothorax-related lymphoma, strongly associated with EBV infection, is closely related to antecedent *Mycobacterium tuberculosis* infection.[78,79]

Immunologic Status

An abnormality of the immune system—either immune deficiency or autoimmune disease—is a major risk factor for the development of lymphomas, especially of B-cell type.[11] Although evidence of immune system abnormalities is lacking in most patients with lymphomas, immunodeficient patients have a markedly increased risk of developing a lymphoproliferative disorder. The major forms of immunodeficiency currently encountered include HIV infection, iatrogenic posttransplantation immunosuppression, and primary immune deficiencies. Patients with some autoimmune diseases are at increased risk of extranodal MALT-type lymphoma, for example, salivary gland lymphoma in patients with Sjögren's disease[80–82] or thyroid lymphoma in patients with Hashimoto's thyroiditis.[83–85] Patients with celiac disease are at risk of enteropathy-associated T-cell lymphoma.[86]

TABLE 39–3. Frequency of B- and T/NK-Cell Lymphomas*

Diagnosis	% of Total Cases
Diffuse large B-cell lymphoma	30.6
Follicular lymphoma	22.1
MALT lymphoma	7.6
Peripheral T-cell lymphoma	7.0
Peripheral T-cell lymphoma, NOS	3.7
Extranodal T/NK-cell lymphoma	1.4
Angioimmunoblastic	1.2
All others	0.7
CLL/SLL	6.7
Mantle cell lymphoma	6
Mediastinal large B-cell lymphoma	2.4
Anaplastic large-cell lymphoma	2.4
Burkitt's lymphoma	2.5
Nodal marginal zone lymphoma	1.8
Precursor T-lymphoblastic lymphoma	1.7
Lymphoplasmacytic lymphoma	1.2
Other types†	8.0

*These percentages were established on the basis of the review of more than 1300 diagnostic biopsies collected in five study centers around the world, which did not include areas where human T-cell leukemia virus type 1 is endemic.

†Includes categories representing less than 1% of total cases.

Abbreviations: CLL/SLL, chronic lymphocytic leukemia/small lymphocytic lymphoma; MALT, mucosa-associated lymphoid tissue; NOS, not otherwise specified.

From: A clinical evaluation of the International Lymphoma Study Group classification of non-Hodgkin's lymphoma. The Non-Hodgkin's Lymphoma Classification Project. Blood 89:3909–3918, 1997.

MATURE B-CELL NEOPLASMS

Mature B-cell neoplasms comprise over 80% of non-Hodgkin's lymphomas[9] (Table 39–3). The most common types are diffuse large B-cell lymphoma and follicular lymphoma, which together account for more than half of all non-Hodgkin's lymphomas.

Historically, the relationship between normal B-cell subpopulations and categories of lymphomas has been assessed by a combination of morphology and immunophenotype. In the last decade, analysis of somatic mutations in the rearranged immunoglobulin genes of lymphoid malignancies has emerged as an interesting tool to studying the cellular origin of the tumors because distinct patterns have been evidenced in different lymphoma categories. Although the presence of somatic hypermutations has usually been taken as the hallmark of germinal center B-cells and their descendants,[39] this concept has been recently challenged by novel data indicating the possibility of somatic hypermutations outside the germinal center.[87,88] Analysis of the pattern of somatic hypermutations may indicate whether these occurred as a result of antigen selection. The presence of intraclonal variation within lymphoid neoplasms is taken as indicative of ongoing mutations, and therefore a relationship to the germinal center.

In the past few years, the use of genomic-scale gene expression profiling (complementary DNA and oligonucleotide-based DNA microarrays) has brought new insight into the relationship of B-cell malignancies to normal stages of B-cell differentiation and activation.[89] Different stages of normal B-cell differentiation, including naive and memory blood cells, germinal center cells, and mitogenically activated blood B cells, are characterized by distinct gene expression signatures. Distinct lymphoid malignancies are also characterized by distinct gene expression signatures, resembling those of different subsets of normal B cells. The "molecular classes" of lymphoid malignancies, defined on the basis of their gene expression signatures, largely overlap with the currently defined lymphoma categories, thereby confirming the rationale of the principles used for classification.[90–92] In addition, this approach has been found useful for the identification of "molecular subclasses" within certain defined clinicopathologic categories. For example, gene expression profiling of diffuse large B-cell lymphoma—the single largest and most heterogeneous category of B-cell lymphoma—has identified distinct molecular subgroups that are clinically relevant.[90,91] Gene expression profiling also has generated data that are relevant to our understanding of certain subtypes of uncertain origin, for example, mediastinal large B-cell lymphoma, found to resemble Hodgkin cells, and hairy cell leukemia, found to resemble memory B cells.[93–95]

Figure 39–4 illustrates the model of histogenesis and pathogenesis of B-cell neoplasms, and Table 39–4 summarizes the phenotypic, genetic, and molecular features of the most common mature B-cell neoplasms.

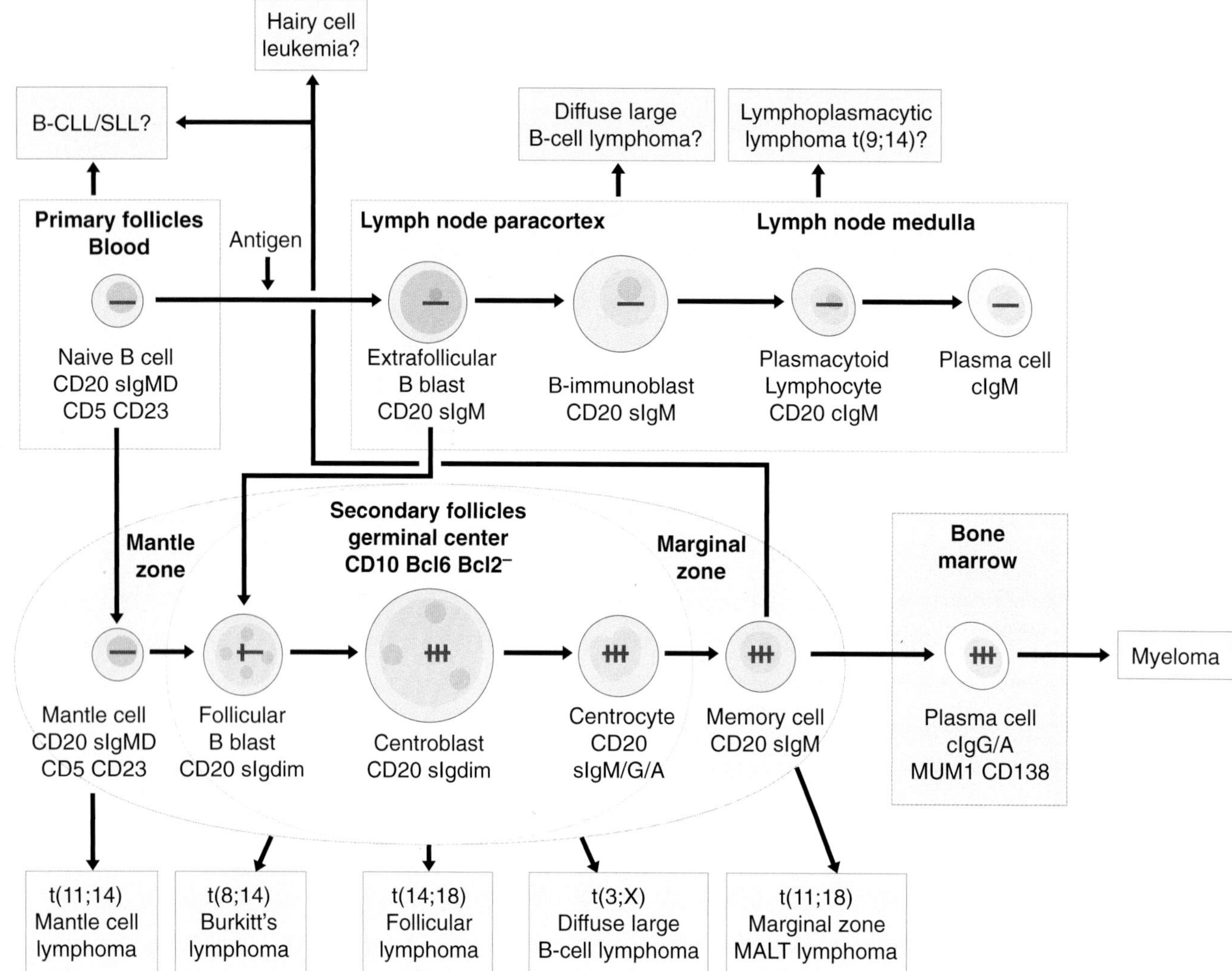

Figure 39–4. Histogenetic and pathogenetic model of mature B-cell neoplasms. The follicular (T-cell–dependent) and extrafollicular pathways of normal B-cell differentiation are represented. Rearranged immunoglobulin heavy chain genes are symbolized with a horizontal bar in the nucleus, and somatic mutations in the immunoglobulin V region are symbolized with vertical lines. The most common types of mature B-cell neoplasms are linked to their putative normal counterparts. The genetic lesion most frequently associated with each lymphoma category is also indicated.

Predominantly Disseminated B-Cell Neoplasms

Chronic Lymphocytic Leukemia/Small Lymphocytic Lymphoma

B-cell chronic lymphocytic leukemia comprises 90% of chronic lymphoid leukemias; nonleukemic B-cell small lymphocytic lymphoma accounts for less than 5% of non-Hodgkin's lymphomas. Most of these patients will ultimately develop marrow and blood infiltration. The clinical course is usually indolent, with an overall median survival of 10–12 years. Transformation to a high-grade lymphoma (Richter's syndrome, usually a diffuse large B-cell lymphoma, or occasionally lymphoproliferations resembling Hodgkin's lymphoma) occurs in approximately 3% of the cases.[96,97] Some cases are clonally related to the preexisting chronic lymphocytic leukemia and others represent second clonally unrelated malignancies.[98,99]

The lymph node infiltrate of chronic lymphocytic leukemia/small lymphocytic lymphoma is composed predominantly of small lymphocytes with round condensed nuclei,[100] admixed with fewer than 5% larger lymphoid cells (prolymphocytes and paraimmunoblasts), usually clustered in pseudofollicles (Fig. 39–5*A*). Cases with increased prolymphocytes (5–55%) may have a worse prognosis. Chronic lymphocytic leukemia cells are positive for B-cell–associated antigens, although CD20 may be very weak, have faint surface IgM with coexpression of IgD in most cases, typically express both CD5 and CD23 as well as CD43, and are negative for cyclin D1.[101] About 50% of cases have abnormal karyotypes.[102] Trisomy 12 correlates with atypical histology and an aggressive clinical course, and abnormalities of 13q (mostly interstitial deletions) are associated with long survival.[103–107] Inactivation of p53 is associated with a poor prognosis.[107]

TABLE 39–4. Immunohistologic and Genetic Features of Common Mature B-Cell Neoplasms

	Immunohistologic Features										Ig Genes*			Gene Expression Profile†
Neoplasm	**sIg**	**cIg**	**CD5**	**CD10**	**Bcl-6**	**Bcl-2**	**CD23**	**CD43**	**Cyclin D1**	**Genetic Abnormality**	**R**	**M**	**O**	
B-SLL/CLL	+	−/+	+	−	−	+	+	+	−	trisomy 12; del 13q	+	+60% −40%	− −	Memory B cell
LPL	+	+	−	−	−	+	−	+/−	−	t(9;14); *pax*-5 del 6(q23)	+	+	−	Not known
HCL	+	−	−	−	−	+	−	+	+/−	None known	+	+	−	Memory B cell
Myeloma	−	+	−	−/+	−	+	−	−/+	−/+	t(1;14); *bcl*-1 t(4;14); *FGFR3* t(14;16); c-*maf* t(6;14); cyclin D3	+	+	−	Plasma cells
SMZL	+	−/+	−	−	−	+	−	−	−	del 7q	+	+60% −40%	+/− −	Not known
MALT	+	+/−	−	−	−	+	−/+	−/+	−	trisomy 3 t(11;18)	+	+	+	Not known
FL	+	−	−	+/−	+	+/−	−/+	−/+	−	t(14;18); *bcl*-2	+	+	+	GC-like
MCL	+	−	+	−	−/+	+	−	+	+	t(11;14); *bcl*-1	+	−/+ (rare)	−	Naive B cell
DLBCL	+/−	−/+	−	−/+	+/−	+/−	NA	−/+	−	3q; *bcl*-6 t(14;18), *bcl*-2 t(8;14); c-*myc*	+	+	+/−	GC-like (50%) ABC-like (30%) Type 3(20%)
MLBCL	−/+	−	−	−/+	+/−	+/−	−/+	−	−	9p 2p amplifications	+	+	−	"Hodgkin-like"
BL	+	−	−	+	+	−	−	−	−	t(8;14); c-*myc*	+	+	−	GC-like

*R, rearranged Ig genes; M, somatic hypermutations in the V regions; O, ongoing mutations.
†ABC, activated B-cell; GC, germinal center; Type 3, a gene expression profile distinct from both GC-like and ABC-like.
For abbreviations of neoplasms, see Table 39–1.

Immunoglobulin heavy and light chain genes are rearranged. About 60% of the cases have immunoglobulin variable-region mutations. Patients with immunoglobulin-unmutated chronic lymphocytic leukemia tend to have a more advanced clinical stage at presentation and shorter median survival in comparison to those with immunoglobulin-mutated chronic lymphocytic leukemia (8–10 years vs. 15–25 years).[107–109] Expression of CD38 has been reported to be associated with a worse prognosis and has been proposed as surrogate marker for immunoglobulin V_H mutations, but this is controversial.[107,108,110,111] In contrast, expression of ZAP-70, which may be ascertained by flow cytometry, RT-PCR, or immunohistochemical assays, has been recently shown to be a reliable marker of immunoglobulin V_H mutations and prognosis.[112,113] Trisomy 12 tends to occur in unmutated cases, whereas normal karyotypes and 13q deletions occur more often in mutated cases.[104]

The cellular origin of chronic lymphocytic leukemia is uncertain. The expression of CD5 was initially taken to suggest that chronic lymphocytic leukemia originates from recirculating $CD5^+CD23^+$-naive B cells.[114] The identification of mutated cases has led to the hypothesis that a fraction may derive from a germinal center–experienced B cell, possibly a memory cell.[109,115] By gene expression profiling, both mutated and unmutated chronic lymphocytic leukemia display a gene expression signature that is related to the profile of memory B cells, suggesting an origin from memory B cells in most cases.[92]

B-Cell Prolymphocytic Leukemia

This extremely rare disease (<1% of B-cell leukemias) is a malignancy of B-prolymphocytes (medium-sized, round lymphoid cells with a single, prominent nucleolus) affecting blood, bone marrow, and spleen.[11] Patients typically present with very high white blood counts ($>100 \times 10^9$). Cases of transformed chronic lymphocytic leukemia and chronic lymphocytic leukemia with increased prolymphocytes are by definition excluded. A significant proportion of the cases diagnosed in the past as B-cell prolymphocytic leukemia by morphology and immunophenotype harbor the t(11;14)(q13;q32) translocation and/or cyclin D1 staining and are currently classified as leukemic mantle cell lymphoma.[116] The median survival in a series of 35 patients was 65 months.[117]

Lymphoplasmacytic Lymphoma (±Waldenström's Macroglobulinemia)

Lymphoplasmacytic lymphoma is a rare lymphoma occurring in older adults. The tumor consists of a diffuse proliferation of small lymphocytes, plasmacytoid lymphocytes, and plasma cells, with variable numbers of immunoblasts, usually involving bone marrow, peripheral blood, lymph nodes, and spleen. Plasmacytoid variants of other lymphomas have to be excluded. A monoclonal serum paraprotein of IgM type, with or without hyperviscosity syndrome (Waldenström's macroglobulinemia) is present in most patients[118]; the paraprotein may have autoantibody or cryoglobulin activity. Cases with mixed cryoglobulinemia may be related to HCV infection. Similar to chronic lymphocytic

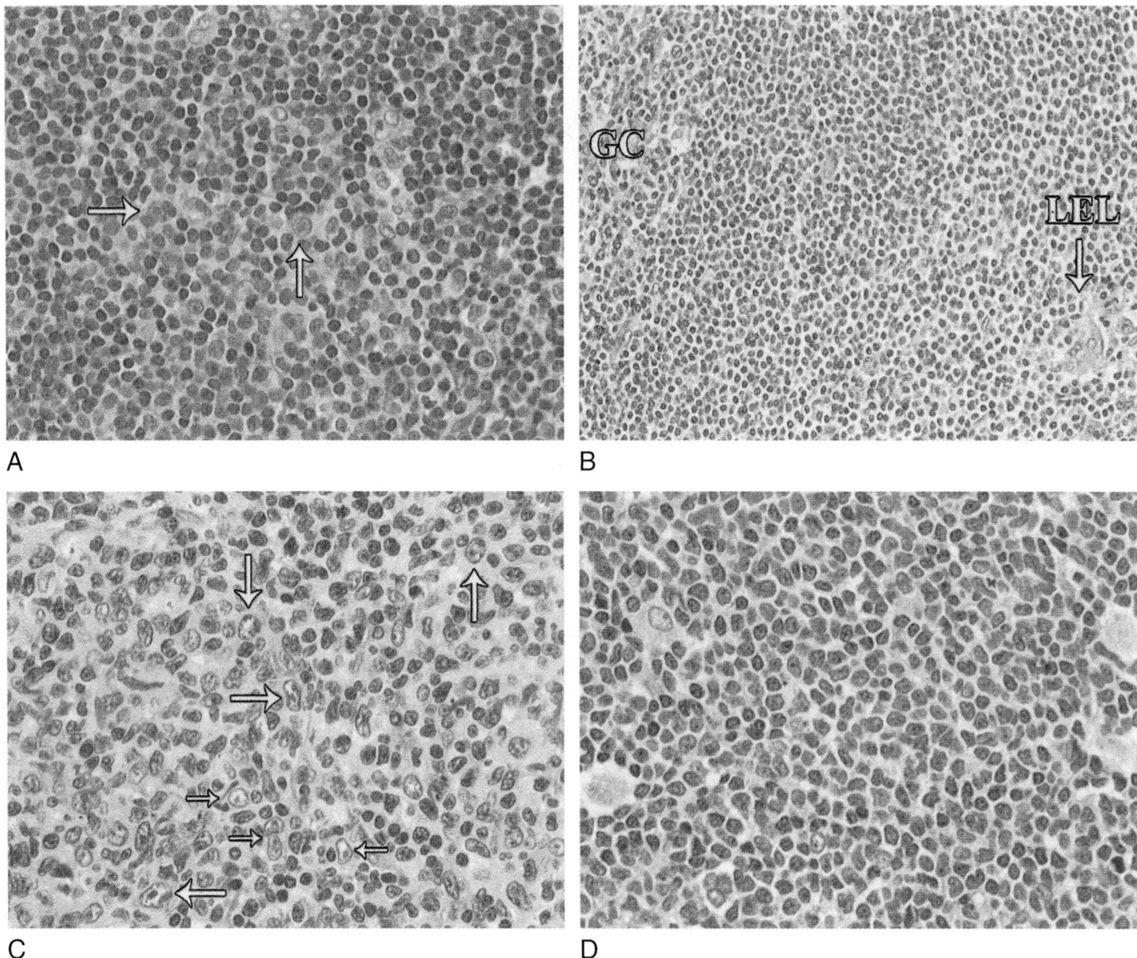

Figure 39–5. Common small B-cell lymphomas. ***A,*** B-cell small lymphocytic lymphoma/chronic lymphocytic leukemia, consisting of a diffuse infiltrate of small lymphocytes with scattered prolymphocytes and paraimmunoblasts *(arrows)*. ***B,*** Extranodal marginal zone lymphoma (MALT lymphoma) of the stomach, showing infiltration of the lamina propria by small lymphocytes with irregular nuclei and moderate amounts of clear cytoplasm with destructive infiltration of gastric glands (lymphoepithelial lesion, LEL). A residual germinal center (GC) is seen on the left. ***C,*** Follicular lymphoma consisting of an admixture of centrocytes (small cleaved cells) and centroblasts (large noncleaved cells) *(long arrows)*; nuclei of follicular dendritic cells can also be recognized *(short arrows)*. ***D,*** Mantle cell lymphoma, consisting of an infiltrate of small lymphoid cells with irregular nuclei; scattered histiocytes with abundant eosinophilic cytoplasm are also present.

leukemia, the clinical course of lymphoplasmacytic lymphoma is usually indolent.[9]

The cells have surface and cytoplasmic (some cells) immunoglobulin, usually of IgM type, and usually lack IgD. They strongly express B-cell–associated antigens (CD19, CD20, CD22, CD79a) and are $CD5^-CD10^-Bcl\text{-}6^-$ $Bcl\text{-}2^+cyclin\ D1^-CD23^-CD43^{+/-}$.[101,119]

Translocation t(9;14)(p13;q32) and rearrangement of the *PAX5* gene has been reported in occasional cases; most patients in these series lacked paraproteinemia.[120–122] *PAX5* encodes a nuclear transcription factor, B-cell–specific activator protein, that is involved in the regulation of several B-cell–specific genes and the control of B-cell development.[123] A high frequency of 6q deletions (42% of the cases) has been reported among a series of 74 patients with Waldenström's macroglobulinemia, none of whom carried a t(9;14) translocation.[124]

Immunoglobulin heavy and light chain genes are rearranged, and variable-region genes show somatic mutations with lack of intraclonal variation, and no evidence of isotype-switch transcript.[125,126] Lymphoplasmacytic lymphoma is thought to derive from a peripheral B lymphocyte stimulated to differentiate to a plasma cell, possibly corresponding to the primary immune response to antigen, or from a post–germinal center cell that has undergone somatic mutation but not heavy chain class switch.

Hairy Cell Leukemia

Hairy cell leukemia is a neoplasm of small B-lymphoid cells with an oval nucleus and abundant cytoplasm with "hairy" projections in the bone marrow and peripheral blood, diffusely infiltrating bone marrow and splenic red pulp. The cells strongly express CD103, CD22, and CD11c.

Plasma Cell Myeloma

Plasma cell myeloma is a clonal proliferation of immunoglobulin-secreting, terminally differentiated B cells. Patients typically present with osteolytic lesions and a serum monoclonal immunoglobulin. The bone marrow contains greater than 10% plasma cells (usually >30%), which are distributed in clusters and sheets in biopsy specimens. The plasma cells contain monotypic immunoglobulin of IgG, IgA, or less often, IgD or IgE type; 10% have light chains only. They typically lack CD19 and CD20, variably express CD45, and express CD38, MUM-1, and CD138. Myeloma cells are usually strongly positive for CD56, a feature that may be useful in the differential diagnosis from monoclonal gammopathy of unknown significance and reactive plasmacytosis.[127,128] Immunoglobulin heavy and light chain genes are rearranged and show variable-region mutations consistent with post–germinal center cells.[129] Cytogenetic abnormalities are common and are typically complex; several recurrent translocations have been described (see Table 39–3). Cases with t(11;14) are cyclin D1^{+}. The prognosis depends on the clinical stage at diagnosis. Median survival is about 3 years. The 10% of patients with plasmablastic or other atypical morphologies have a worse prognosis.

Splenic Marginal Zone Lymphoma, ± Villous Lymphocytes (Splenic Lymphoma with Villous Lymphocytes)[11,130,131]

Splenic marginal zone lymphoma accounts for only 1–2% percent of chronic lymphoid leukemias found on bone marrow examination, but up to 25% of low-grade B-cell neoplasms in splenectomy specimens.[132–134] Patients typically present with splenomegaly and lymphocytosis, usually without peripheral lymphadenopathy, and may have circulating neoplastic cells with short "villous" projections, and a small M component.[135] Extranodal sites are not typically involved, and, despite the "marginal zone" name, this disease appears to be completely distinct from MALT lymphoma. The course is extremely indolent, and splenectomy may be followed by prolonged remission.

In the spleen, the neoplastic cells of splenic marginal zone lymphoma/splenic lymphoma with villous lymphocytes occupy both the mantle and marginal zones of the splenic white pulp[136,137]; those in the marginal zone have somewhat dispersed chromatin and abundant, pale cytoplasm, resembling marginal zone cells, and are admixed with centroblasts and immunoblasts. The red pulp, splenic hilar lymph nodes,[138] and bone marrow are also often involved. Splenic marginal zone lymphoma cells express IgM, IgD, and B-cell antigens (CD19, CD20, CD22) but typically lack CD5, CD10, CD43, CD23, Bcl-6, cyclin D1, CD11c, and CD25, and are usually positive for Bcl-2.[132,139–141]

Cytogenetic studies have shown several recurrent chromosomal abnormalities. However, 7q21-32 allelic loss or translocations involving this region, detected in up to 40% of the cases, appear to be characteristic of splenic marginal zone lymphoma.[130,142–145] Abnormalities at 7q may induce dysregulation of the *CDK6* gene.[146] Trisomy 3, found in nodal and extranodal marginal zone lymphoma, has also been reported in a variable proportion of cytogenetically abnormal splenic marginal zone lymphoma.[130,147,148] The t(11;18)(q21;q21) translocation found in MALT lymphomas has not been reported in splenic marginal zone lymphoma.

The molecular genetic features are heterogeneous. Some cases (30–50%) show no significant mutations in their immunoglobulin V_H gene regions, whereas others (50–70%) are characterized by a high degree of somatic mutation with or without evidence of antigen selection and with ongoing mutations in some cases.[149–153] In one series, unmutated cases had more frequent 7q31 deletions and an adverse clinical course.[152] The putative cell of origin is uncertain. Mutated cases may arise from a post–germinal center, memory B cell of splenic type.

Extranodal Marginal Zone B-Cell Lymphoma of MALT Type

MALT lymphoma, the third most common type of B-cell lymphoma, occurs in organs that normally lack organized lymphoid tissue. Fifty percent involve the gastrointestinal tract, and they comprise almost 50% of all gastric lymphomas.[154] They also represent 40–60% of lymphomas in other glandular epithelial tissues, such as the ocular adnexa, thyroid, lung, breast, and salivary gland[155–159]; skin or soft tissue may also be the primary site. There is a broad age range[9,160] and a slight female preponderance.[101] The majority of patients present with localized (stage I or II) extranodal disease. The bone marrow is involved in 15–30%; the frequency of marrow involvement differs according to the primary site. "Acquired MALT" secondary to autoimmune disease, in particular Sjögren's syndrome or Hashimoto's thyroiditis, or to infection, such as *H. pylori* gastritis, in these sites is thought to be the substrate for lymphoma development[161] (see previous section on infectious agents). MALT lymphomas run an indolent natural course. Localized MALT lymphomas of the stomach that do not respond to antibiotics, and those occurring in other sites, may be cured with local treatment, typically radiation.[158,162–164] Dissemination or recurrence may occur; these are often in other localized extranodal sites, with long disease-free intervals.[159,165,166]

MALT lymphoma reproduces the morphologic features of normal MALT, with a polymorphous infiltrate of small lymphocytes, marginal zone (centrocyte-like) B cells, and plasma cells, admixed with scattered blastic cells, occupying the marginal zone of reactive follicles and in some cases "colonizing" and disrupting these follicles.[86,167,168] In epithelial tissues, neoplastic cells typically infiltrate the epithelium, forming so-called lymphoepithelial lesions (Fig. 39–5*B*).[167] Marginal zone lymphoma of MALT type is by definition a low-grade lymphoma histologically, that is, a lymphoma composed predominantly of small cells. When clusters or sheets of blasts are present, a separate diagnosis of large B-cell lymphoma is made and these cases are associated with a worse prognosis. MALT lymphoma cells express surface immunoglobulin (sIg) (M > G > A), lack IgD, and may show plasmacytoid differentiation (40% of the cases). They express B-cell–associated antigens (CD19, CD20, CD22, CD79a) and lack CD5, CD10, Bcl-6, and cyclin D1.[101,136]

The most common numerical chromosomal abnormality is trisomy 3, present in about 60% of cases, but this is not specific for this lymphoma type.[169,170] Three recurrent translocations have been reported in MALT lymphomas (see Table 39–2). The t(1;14)(p22;q32), which was first described,[169] is in fact rarely seen (<5% MALT cases)[171]; it causes overexpression of the *bcl*-10 gene.[172] The second recurrent translocation, t(11;18)(q21;q21), is seen in 25–40% of gastric MALT lymphoma cases and a similar proportion of pulmonary cases.[173,174] However, the frequency of this translocation in other MALT lymphomatosis much lower and it is not present in either salivary gland or thyroid MALT lymphomas. The t(11;18)(q21;q21) translocation is associated with a fusion of the *API2* and *MALT1* genes, with MALT-1 being part of the same signaling pathway as Bcl-10.[27] The third described translocation in MALT lymphomas, t(14;18)(q32;q21), also leads to deregulated expression of the *MALT1* gene.[175] This translocation is typically seen in MALT lymphomas other than gastric or pulmonary MALT lymphomas; its overall prevalence is around 20% of all MALT lymphomas. Although downstream targets of *bcl-10/MALT1* alterations are unclear, the current evidence suggests that they operate through activation of the nuclear factor-κB (NF-κB).[72,170]

The t(11;18)(q21;q21) is a marker for cases of gastric MALT lymphomas that are at a more advanced stage and that will not respond to *H. pylori* eradication.[72,176,177] It can be detected by RT-PCR or FISH if routine cytogenetics are not available. The t(11;18) is often the only cytogenetic abnormality, whereas t(11;18)-negative cases often have aneuploidy characterized by trisomy of chromosomes 18, 3, and 7 and/or 11.[178] In addition, cases with the t(11;18) are less likely to undergo transformation to high-grade lymphoma. Thus, there appear to be two pathways of lymphomagenesis in gastric MALT lymphomas: one that acquires the t(11;18) early in development, becomes independent of *H. pylori* for growth, but is genetically stable; and another that remains dependent on *H. pylori* for a longer period, becomes genetically unstable, and acquires sequential genetic abnormalities, ultimately transforming to diffuse large B-cell lymphoma if untreated.

Immunoglobulin genes of MALT lymphoma are rearranged, and the variable region has a high degree of somatic mutation with a pattern suggestive of antigen selection as well as intraclonal diversity indicating ongoing mutations.[179,180] MALT lymphoma is thought to derive from a post–germinal center B memory cell.

Predominantly Nodal B-Cell Lymphomas

Nodal Marginal Zone B-Cell Lymphoma

Nodal marginal zone lymphoma is a primary nodal B-cell lymphoma that morphologically resembles nodal involvement by marginal zone lymphoma of MALT type or splenic type, but without evidence of extranodal or splenic disease.[11] This diagnosis should not be made in a patient with known risk factors for MALT lymphoma. Two morphologic types have been described: cases that resemble MALT lymphoma and are IgD$^-$, and cases that more closely resemble splenic marginal zone lymphoma and are IgD$^+$.[181] The disease is relatively indolent but, unlike MALT lymphoma, probably not curable.[182]

Follicular Lymphoma

Follicular lymphoma, the second most common lymphoma in the United States, affects predominantly older adults, with a slight female predominance.[9,10] It is a neoplasm of follicular center B cells composed of a mixture of centrocytes and centroblasts, which has at least a partially follicular pattern (Fig. 39–5*C*). Both cytology and pattern vary from case to case. Histologic grading along a three-grade scale (1, 2, and 3a) is based on the abundance of centroblasts by microscopic counting.[11,183] Rarely, follicular lymphoma consists almost entirely of centroblasts (grade 3b).[11] Follicular lymphoma cells are usually sIg$^+$ (IgM > IgG > IgA). The tumor cells express pan-B-cell–associated antigens, and are usually CD10$^+$Bcl-6$^+$Bcl-2$^+$CD5$^-$CD23$^{-/+}$CD43$^-$ (most cases).[184–189] Tightly organized meshworks of follicular dendritic cells are present in follicular areas.[190,191] Most patients have widespread disease at diagnosis, but the clinical course is generally indolent (median survivals in excess of 8 years). Histologic grading is predictive of outcome, with grades 1 and 2 cases having a median survival of 7–8 years, which is unaffected by aggressive therapy, and grade 3 cases having a shorter median survival, which is significantly improved by treatment with anthracycline-containing regimens.[192,193] Some studies have suggested that the presence of diffuse areas is associated with a worse prognosis.[194,195] The presence of a diffuse component in a grade 3 follicular lymphoma is classified as diffuse large B-cell lymphoma; these cases are associated with an inferior survival that is similar to the survival of patients with diffuse large B-cell lymphoma.[196]

Translocation t(14;18)(q32;q21) and *bcl*-2 gene rearrangement with consequent Bcl-2 protein overexpression are present in the majority of the cases (85–90%).[15,17,19,197] Overexpression of Bcl-2 protein results in inhibition of apoptosis, thought to be a critical pathogenetic event in the development of follicular lymphoma[20]; however, a small proportion of follicular lymphomas do not have *bcl*-2 gene rearrangement and do not express Bcl-2, and *bcl*-2 rearrangements have been occasionally detected in the peripheral blood of healthy individuals,[198] suggesting that other factors are involved in follicular lymphoma development. Abnormalities of 3q27 and/or *bcl*-6 rearrangement are found in about 15% of the cases, and 5′ mutations of the *bcl*-6 gene are found in approximately 40%.[34] Translocations of *bcl*-2 and *bcl*-6 appear to be two mutually exclusive events.[199]

Immunoglobulin heavy and light chain genes are rearranged, with extensive and ongoing somatic mutations, similar to normal germinal center cells and consistent with a germinal center derivation.[200,201]

Mantle Cell Lymphoma

Mantle cell lymphoma is a disease of older adults with a marked male predominance (75%).[9] The majority (70%) of patients are in stage IV at diagnosis; sites involved include lymph nodes, spleen, Waldeyer's ring, bone marrow (>60%), blood (up to 50%), and the gastrointestinal tract (lymphomatous polyposis).[202] The median overall survival in most series is 3 years, with no plateau in the curve.[203,204]

Mantle cell lymphoma is typically composed of monomorphous small to medium-sized lymphoid cells, with slightly irregular or "cleaved," nuclei that may have a diffuse, nodular, mantle zone, or mixed pattern in lymph nodes (Fig. 39–5*D*). The blastoid variant, composed of cells resembling either lymphoblasts or large cleaved cells and showing a high mitotic rate, has been reported in some studies to be more aggressive.[9,204–209] Mantle cell lymphoma cells express strong sIgM and IgD (often of λ light chain type), and B-cell–associated antigens; most coexpress CD5, and CD43, and usually lack CD23, CD10, and Bcl-6.[204,207] Nuclear cyclin D1 protein is present in virtually all cases and is the gold standard for the diagnosis.[210–214]

A t(11;14)(q13;q32) in the majority of the cases results in rearrangement of the *bcl*-1 locus and overexpression the cyclin D1 gene, which encodes a protein involved in the regulation of the cell cycle transition between the G_1 and the S phase and is not normally expressed in lymphoid cells.[211,212,215–218] It is believed that cyclin D1 overexpression in mantle cell lymphoma promotes tumorigenesis by increasing cell proliferation; however, the pathogenetic role of cyclin D1 has not been proven.[219] Other mechanisms deregulating the cell cycle have been identified. Most cases show loss of p27 as a result of increased degradation.[220] Hypermethylation and inactivation of p16,[221] as well as p53 mutations,[222] are commonly found in association with blastoid variants.[222–224] In a large-scale gene expression study, an index based upon the level of expression of 20 genes involved in cell proliferation was able to discriminate four groups of patients with different overall survival.[214]

Immunoglobulin heavy and light chain genes are rearranged and lack somatic mutations in most cases, indicating a pre–germinal center stage of differentiation, consistent with an origin from naive B cells.[225,226]

Diffuse Large B-Cell Lymphoma

Diffuse large B-cell lymphoma, the most common type of lymphoma, encompasses marked biologic heterogeneity. It may occur de novo or as a high-grade transformation of a small B-cell lymphoma. Median age at presentation is in the seventh decade, but may occur at any age. Patients typically present with a rapidly enlarging mass, with B symptoms in one third of the cases.[9,10] About 50% have localized disease involving nodal or, in up to 40% of the cases, various extranodal sites. Overall, long-term survival is less than 50%.[11,227] The International Prognostic Index[228] stratifies patients into risk groups and is predictive of outcome.

In its usual form, diffuse large B-cell lymphoma is a diffuse proliferation of large lymphoid cells that may be classified as centroblastic (80% of the cases), immunoblastic (10% of the cases, more common among immunosuppressed patients), or centroblastic-polymorphous (with features intermediate between centroblastic and immunoblastic)[11,229] (Fig. 39–6*A* and *B*). Immunoblast-rich tumors have been found to have a worse prognosis in several studies; however, there is currently no consensus on the usefulness of histologic subtyping.[10,230–233] Bone marrow involvement in diffuse large B-cell lymphoma, seen in about 15% of the cases, may appear either as a large-cell infiltrate or, slightly more often, as an infiltrate of small atypical B cells—so-called discordant marrow involvement[234]; the latter is not associated with a worse prognosis than cases without marrow involvement.[235]

Diffuse large B-cell lymphomas express CD45, one or more B-cell–associated antigens (CD19, CD20, CD22, CD79a), and often surface immunoglobulin. Therapy of B-cell lymphoma with chimeric antibodies against CD20 can result in the loss of CD20 antigen expression.[236] About 10% of de novo diffuse large B-cell lymphomas (i.e., excluding Richter's syndrome) express CD5.[237–242] $CD5^+$ diffuse large B-cell lymphomas are reported to occur in elderly women, with a predilection for extranodal involvement, especially bone marrow and spleen,[238,239] and to be associated with shorter survival in comparison with $CD5^-$ tumors[240,243] but this remains controversial.[244] Bcl-2 protein expression is found in 30–60% of diffuse large B-cell lymphomas.[245–248] Whereas *bcl*-2 translocation at diagnosis has no prognostic significance,[249,250] several large-scale clinical trials have pointed toward an association between Bcl-2 expression and decreased disease-free or overall survival.[249,251–256] Approximately 70% express Bcl-6 protein,[185,247,256–261] and this has been found in several studies to be associated with a better prognosis,[260,262] a finding not confirmed by others.[256] Approximately one third express CD10, usually together with Bcl-6, a combined phenotype referred to as "germinal center–like"[240,255,258,259,261,263–265] that has been found to be associated with the presence of the t(14;18) translocation in some studies, indicating a possible origin of these tumors in germinal center–derived cells or transformed follicular lymphomas,[256,258,263,266–268] and associated with a better prognosis in several clinical series, but possibly predisposing to late relapses.[269]

Many cases exhibit complex karyotypes. The most frequent recurrent cytogenetic abnormalities are rearrangements of *bcl*-6 at the 3q27 locus in about 30% of the cases, which is of uncertain prognostic significance.[270–277] In addition, *bcl*-6 is the target of somatic mutations in its 5′ untranslated region in 70% of the cases.[278,279] Translocation of the *bcl*-2 gene occurs in 20–30% of cases,[203,280] often associated with disseminated disease. For both *bcl*-2 and *bcl*-6, there is no direct correlation between gene rearrangement and protein expression, with many cases lacking the cytogenetic abnormality but having protein expression. The c-*myc* gene is rearranged in about 10% of the cases.[19,275] Mutations in the p53 gene (correlated

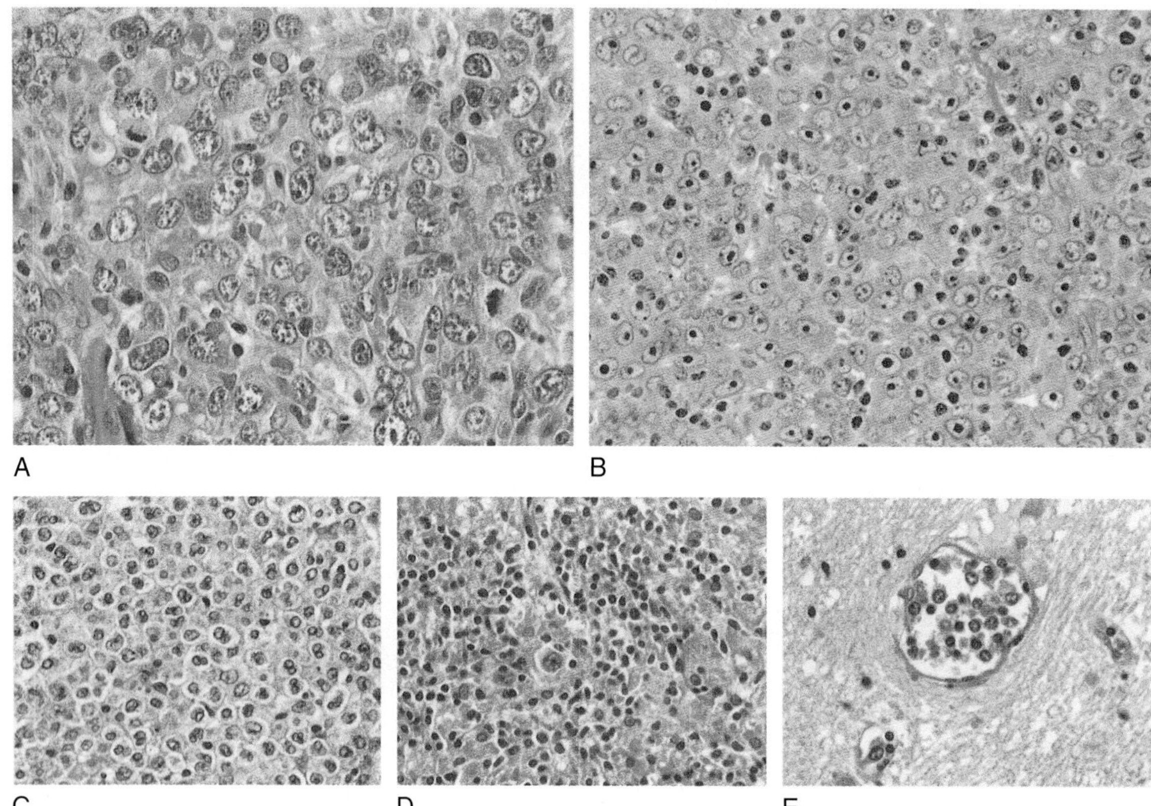

Figure 39–6. Diffuse large B-cell lymphoma. The most common subtypes are centroblastic *(A)*, composed of centroblast-like cells (large lymphoid cells with one to three peripheral nucleoli), and immunoblastic *(B)*, composed of immunoblast-like cells (large lymphoid cells with a single central nucleolus and a moderate amount of basophilic cytoplasm). Primary mediastinal large B-cell lymphoma *(C)* often comprises large lymphoid cells with clear cytoplasm and lobated nuclei. In the T-cell/histiocyte-rich variant *(D)*, large neoplastic B cells are scarce, scattered among a reactive background composed of histiocytes and non-neoplastic small T cells. Intravascular lymphoma *(E)* consists of an intravascular proliferation of large neoplastic B cells and often involves the central nervous system.

with a $p53^+/p21^-$ immunophenotype) are detected in about 20% of diffuse large B-cell lymphomas[281–283] and are associated with clinical drug resistance[284,285] and poor outcome.[282,283,285,286] Immunoglobulin genes are rearranged and most have somatic mutations in the variable-region genes,[287,288] often with ongoing mutations,[39,289] consistent with a germinal center or post–germinal center derivation.

Recently, evaluation of gene expression profiles by complementary DNA microarray techniques identified three molecularly distinct forms of diffuse large B-cell lymphoma: a germinal center-like form characterized by the expression of genes normally expressed by germinal center B cells, an activated B-cell–like form characterized by the expression of genes normally induced during in vitro activation of peripheral blood B cells, and type 3 diffuse large B-cell lymphoma.[90,290] Patients with germinal center–like diffuse large B-cell lymphomas had better outcomes than those with activated B-cell–like and type 3 diffuse large B-cell lymphomas.[90,290]

Diffuse Large B-Cell Lymphoma Variants

In the *T-cell/histiocyte–rich* variant of diffuse large B-cell lymphoma, there are fewer than 10% large neoplastic B cells scattered in a background of non-neoplastic T cells with or without histiocytes (Fig. 39–6*D*). The tumor cells may resemble neoplastic cells of Hodgkin's lymphoma.[291] T-cell/histiocyte–rich diffuse large B-cell lymphoma usually presents with advanced-stage disease with nodal, splenic,[292] and bone marrow involvement. Immunophenotypic studies are essential to distinguish this variant from peripheral T-cell lymphoma and Hodgkin's lymphoma (especially the nodular lymphocyte predominance type[293,294]). Neoplastic cells are thought to derive from a progenitor cell of germinal center origin.[291,295] It is unclear whether outcome of the T-cell/histiocyte–rich variant is worse than that of "usual" diffuse large B-cell lymphoma.[296,297]

The *anaplastic variant* is composed of large pleomorphic cells, forming cohesive sheets with a sinusoidal pattern of growth.[11] Many cases express CD30 but are negative for ALK expression and are biologically unrelated to anaplastic large-cell lymphoma of T-cell derivation.[298]

The *plasmablastic variant* was initially described as a tumor occurring in the oral cavity in HIV-infected patients,[299] but since then similar lesions have been reported in other anatomic sites[300] as well as in non–HIV^+

individuals.[301] The tumor cells are immunoblastic in morphology, with or without plasmacytoid differentiation, are negative for CD45 and CD20, may be positive for CD79a, and are positive forVS38c and CD138. EBV is detected in the majority of HIV-associated cases.[301]

Diffuse large B-cell lymphoma with expression of ALK was initially described by Delsol and colleagues[302] as composed of large immunoblast-like tumors expressing ALK, epithelial membrane antigen (EMA), VS38c, CD138, and cytoplasmic IgA, lacking expression of CD20 and CD30, and weakly positive for CD45. These cases, lacking the t(2;5) translocation associated with anaplastic large-cell lymphoma of T-cell type, were originally thought to express full-length ALK. However, further analysis of these and several similar cases showed that they contained ALK fused to clathrin as a consequence of t(2;17)(p23;q23) translocation, one of the variant translocations seen in anaplastic large-cell lymphoma.[303–305] Recently, a few cases of diffuse large B-cell lymphoma with plasmablastic morphology expressing the NMP-ALK fusion as a consequence of a t(2;5)(p23;q35) have also been reported.[306,307]

Mediastinal (Thymic) Large B-Cell Lymphoma

Mediastinal large B-cell lymphoma comprises 7% of large B-cell lymphomas and 2.4% of all non-Hodgkin's lymphomas.[9,10] This lymphoma tends to occur in young patients (median age of about 35 years), and affects women more commonly than men. Patients present with an anterior mediastinal mass originating in the thymus, with symptoms related to local invasion.[308–310] Relapses tend to occur in distant extranodal sites such as the central nervous system and the gastrointestinal tract. Current cure rates are similar to those for other large-cell lymphomas of similar stage.[309,311]

Mediastinal large B-cell lymphoma is cytologically heterogeneous, but clear cells, multilobated nuclei, and compartmentalizing sclerosis are common features (Fig. 39–6*C*). The neoplastic cells express the B-cell antigens CD19, CD20, and CD79a but frequently lack surface immunoglobulin, despite expression of the appropriate transcription factors,[312] and have defective expression of human lymphocyte antigen class I and/or class II molecules.[313,314] A proportion of cases also express CD30. Some cases are positive for CD10 expression; Bcl-6 staining is found in more than half of the cases.[261,312] Most cases are Bcl-2^+.

The genetic and molecular features of mediastinal large B-cell lymphoma support the concept that this is a pathogenetically distinct subtype of diffuse large B-cell lymphoma. Mediastinal large B-cell lymphomas exhibit several characteristic genetic abnormalities, including gains at 9p and 2p, and the associated *JAK2* and *rel* loci, but they lack *bcl-2* or *bcl-6* gene rearrangements.[315–317] Overexpression of the *MAL* gene has been identified in about 70% of primary mediastinal large B-cell lymphomas and is not found in diffuse large B-cell lymphomas arising in other sites.[318,319] The gene expression profile of mediastinal large B-cell lymphoma differs from that of other diffuse large B-cell lymphomas and partly overlaps with that of classical Hodgkin's lymphoma cell lines,[94,95] also supporting the hypothesis that there may be some pathogenic overlap between mediastinal large B-cell lymphoma and some forms of Hodgkin's lymphoma ("gray zone" lymphomas).

Mediastinal large B-cell lymphoma has been postulated to derive from medullary thymic B cells.[320] The tumor cells in the majority of the cases carry Bcl-6 mutations[312] and isotype-switched immunoglobulin genes with a high load of somatic mutations without evidence of ongoing mutations,[321] suggesting an origin from germinal center–experienced B cell.

Intravascular Large B-Cell Lymphoma

This extremely rare subtype consists of a disseminated intravascular proliferation of large B cells, involving small blood vessels, without an obvious extravascular tumor mass or leukemia[322] (Fig. 39–6*E*). It may be associated with defective expression of homing receptors.[323] The central nervous system, kidneys, lungs, and skin are commonly involved. Patients present with symptoms related to organ dysfunction secondary to vascular occlusion. Many reported cases were diagnosed at autopsy. If a timely diagnosis is made, long-term survival appears to be possible.[324]

Primary Effusion Lymphoma

This rare and aggressive disease originally identified in acquired immunodeficiency syndrome patients, may also occur in other clinical settings.[325,326] Patients present with effusions in serous cavities, generally with no formation of tumor masses. Primary effusion lymphoma is composed of large, often pleomorphic cells. They are usually CD45^+ but lack expression of B-cell antigens and surface immunoglobulin and are often positive for MUM-1 and CD138 as well as CD30.[327] The tumor cells are characteristically infected by the Kaposi sarcoma–associated herpesvirus, and most cases are co-infected with EBV.[56,328] Immunoglobulin genes are clonally rearranged and carry somatic mutations in their variable region. The gene expression profile of primary effusion lymphoma shows features intermediate between those of immunoblasts and plasma cells, suggesting a plasmablastic derivation.[329]

Large B-Cell Lymphoma, Lymphomatoid Granulomatosis Type

This is an EBV$^+$ large B-cell lymphoma with a T-cell–rich background.[330–333] Patients typically present with extranodal disease, most commonly involving the lungs, central nervous system, and/or kidneys. Evidence of past or present immunosuppression may be found. Morphologically, lymphomatoid granulomatosis may resemble nasal-type NK/T-cell lymphoma, but there is no biologic and little clinical overlap between the two entities. Lymphomatoid granulomatosis is graded (1 to 3) according to the number of large B cells. The lower grade cases are not typically treated as lymphoma; grade 3 cases fulfill the criteria for large B-cell lymphoma in a T-cell–rich background, and may be clinically aggressive.[334]

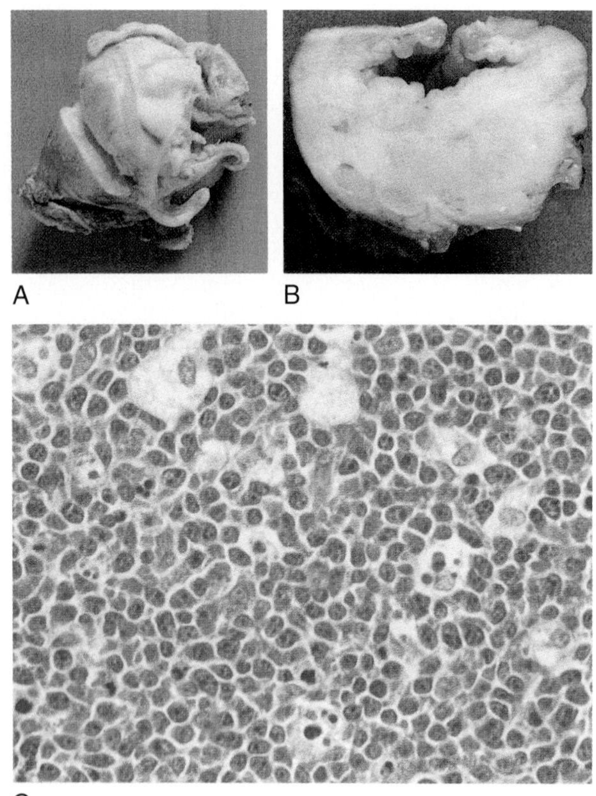

Figure 39–7. Burkitt's lymphoma, sporadic type, in a European child, forming a large ileocecal mass (***A*** and ***B***). The tumor is composed of medium-sized cells with a high mitotic rate with scattered tingible body macrophages, imparting a so-called starry-sky appearance (***C***).

Burkitt's Lymphoma

Three distinct forms of Burkitt's lymphoma are recognized: endemic Burkitt's lymphoma (primarily found in Africa), sporadic Burkitt's lymphoma (comprising 30% of pediatric lymphomas in the United States), and immunodeficiency-associated Burkitt's lymphoma (most often affecting HIV^{+} patients).[335] In all groups, the majority of patients are male. Patients present with rapidly growing tumor masses. In endemic cases, the jaws and other facial bones are often involved. In sporadic cases, the majority present with abdominal tumors[336] (Fig. 39–7*A* and *B*). Immunodeficiency-related cases more often involve lymph nodes, and both these and sporadic cases may present as acute leukemia. Burkitt's lymphoma is highly aggressive but potentially curable. Intensive chemotherapy results in cure rates of up to 90%, although survival is lower in patients with higher stage disease and is lower in adults than in children.[337,338]

Burkitt's lymphoma cells are monomorphic, medium-sized cells with round nuclei, multiple nucleoli, and basophilic cytoplasm. There is a very high rate of proliferation, and a "starry-sky" pattern is imparted by macrophages that have ingested apoptotic tumor cells (Fig. 39–7*C*). Some cases may have larger cells or an admixture of immunoblast-like cells, and there is morphologic overlap with diffuse large B-cell lymphoma. These borderline cases are designated "atypical Burkitt's lymphoma" or "Burkitt-like," provided that *c-myc* rearrangement can be demonstrated or that the proliferation fraction of viable cells (Ki67 labeling) is at least 99%.[339,340]

Burkitt's lymphoma cells express sIgM and B-cell–associated antigens (CD19, CD20, CD22, CD79a), as well as CD10 and Bcl-6; they lack CD5, Bcl-2, and CD23.[341] Immunoglobulin heavy and light chain genes are rearranged, with somatic mutations in most cases, consistent with their putative derivation from early follicular blasts.[342–344] Most cases have a translocation of *c-myc* from chromosome 8q to either the immunoglobulin heavy chain region on chromosome 14q [t(8;14)(q24;q32)] or light chain loci on 2q [t(2;8)] or 22q [t(8;22)]. Other genetic alterations include p53 mutations, found in 30% of the cases,[345] and alteration of the putative tumor suppressor gene retinoblastoma-like 2 (*RB2*) in endemic cases.[346] Virtually all endemic cases contain EBV genomes,[54] as do 25–40% of sporadic and immunodeficiency-associated cases.[53] In EBV-positive cases, the tumor cells contain a clonal viral episomal genome, and display a type I latency program of gene expression (EBV-encoded small RNAs [EBERS] and EBV nuclear antigen 1 [*EBNA1*] expression).[347] The exact role of EBV in the pathogenesis of Burkitt's lymphoma is not understood.

MATURE T/NK-CELL NEOPLASMS

Neoplasms of mature (peripheral) T and NK cells are uncommon, comprising less than 10% of non-Hodgkin's lymphomas worldwide (see Table 39–3). The rarity and the complexity of these tumors lead to difficulty in establishing simple and straightforward classification.

In B-cell neoplasms, there is usually a good correlation between morphology, phenotype, genetic alterations, and well-defined clinical entities. In that regard, T/NK-cell neoplasms are strikingly different. First, many distinct T/NK-cell diseases have a broad range of cellular composition, from pleomorphic small cells to anaplastic large cells, meaning that morphology is not a reliable basis for defining disease entities. A second problem is that immunophenotypic and genetic features have proven less useful in classification of T-cell than B-cell malignancies. Many distinct diseases lack distinct immunophenotypes, many antigens are expressed in more than one neoplasm, and there is variability of immunophenotype both among cases of a given entity and within a given case over time. Finally, although genetic abnormalities may eventually be helpful in diagnosis and classification, the genetics of many of these diseases are largely unknown. In contrast to B-cell lymphomas, there are no convenient markers of monoclonality, although the presence of an aberrant immunophenotype may point toward a diagnosis of malignancy.[348] Therefore, molecular genetic studies, most commonly PCR studies for detection of rearrangement of the *TCR* genes, are generally required in order to evaluate the clonality of a T-cell proliferative process.[349,350]

Thus, defining entities in the T/NK-cell systems often requires additional information. The most important

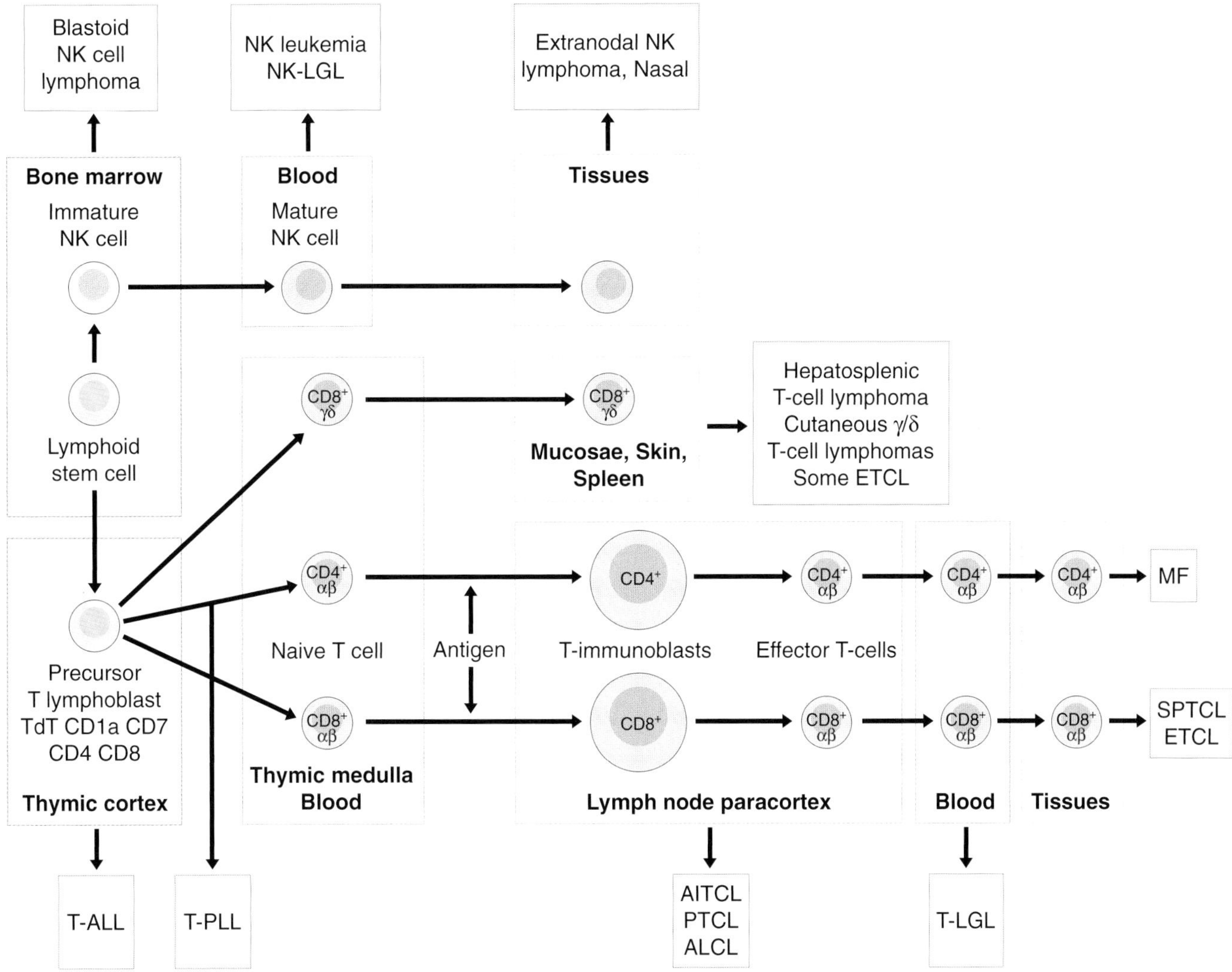

Figure 39–8. Schematic representation of T-cell and NK-cell differentiation with their postulated neoplastic counterparts. Antigen-independent stages of T-cell differentiation occur in the bone marrow and thymus; the corresponding tumor is precursor T-lymphoblastic lymphoma/leukemia (T-ALL). Mature naive (virgin) T cells, either $CD4^+$ or $CD8^+$, are found in the thymic medulla, in the circulation, and in the paracortex of lymph nodes; some may give rise to cases of T-cell prolymphocytic leukemia (T-PLL) and some to peripheral T-cell lymphomas. Antigen-dependent reaction occurs in the paracortex of lymph nodes, and many peripheral T-cell lymphomas (peripheral T-cell lymphomas not otherwise specified [PTCL-NOS]; angioimmunoblastic T-cell lymphoma [AITL]; anaplastic large-cell lymphoma [ALCL]) appear to correspond to proliferating peripheral T cells. From the immunoblastic reaction come antigen-specific T cells of either CD4 or CD8 type, as well as memory cells, that may recirculate and home to peripheral tissues. Some cases of peripheral T-cell lymphomas are thought to correspond to effector T cells. Mycosis fungoides (MF) corresponds to a mature, effector $CD4^+$ T cell, T-cell large granular lymphocyte leukemia (T-LGL) to a mature effector $CD8^+$ cell, and many extranodal T-cell lymphomas to cytotoxic T cells. γ/δ T cells are usually $CD8^+$; they constitute a minority of circulating T cells and have a predilection for homing to the spleen, skin, and mucosae. These cells are thought to give rise to most cases of hepatosplenic T-cell lymphomas as well as some enteropathy-associated T-cell lymphomas (ETCL) and a subset of cutaneous T-cell lymphomas.

Natural killer (NK) cells appear to derive from a common progenitor with T cells. Immature NK cells are thought to be the precursor to blastoid NK-cell lymphoma/leukemia. Some types of large granular lymphocytic (LGL) leukemia and extranodal T/NK-cell lymphoma appear to correspond to mature NK cells.

appears to be location: nodal versus extranodal presentation may be more important than either cellular morphology or immunophenotype in defining the disease entity. Other important morphologic features include architecture, vascularization, and the presence of non-lymphoid cells such as histiocytes and dendritic cells. The presence of some viruses (EBV, HTLV-1) is also a key feature in defining some entities. Finally, other clinical features such as age, sex, ethnicity, and history of celiac disease are also important.

Mature T/NK-cell lymphomas manifest the immunophenotypic features of post-thymic T lymphocytes or mature NK cells (Fig. 39–8). T cells are genetically characterized by functional rearrangement of the *TCR* genes, and, based on the structure of the TCR, two classes of T cells are recognized: α/β and γ/δ.[351] Both express CD3, which is composed of γ, δ, and ε chains. γ/δ T cells are $CD4^-CD8^-$ or $CD4^-CD8^+$; they comprise less than 5% of T cells and show a restricted distribution mainly to the epithelia, where they are involved in mucosal immunity, and to the red pulp of the spleen.[352] α/β T cells are divided into $CD4^+$ (mainly T helper cells, with a T_H1 or T_H2 profile of cytokine secretion) and $CD8^+$ (mainly cytotoxic) subsets. NK cells are distinguished by the absence of *TCR* rearrangement and membrane TCR expression.[351,353] NK cells share some markers with T cells because they can express CD2, CD7, CD43, CD45RO, and cytoplasmic (but not surface) CD3 (ε chain). NK cells are usually $CD4^-CD8^-$ but may be $CD8^+$, and they express one or several of the "NK-associated" antigens (CD11b, CD16, CD56, CD57), none of which, except maybe CD16, is entirely specific because they can also be expressed by some T cells.[354] Both NK cells and cytotoxic T cells express cytotoxic proteins, including perforin, granzyme B, and T-cell intracellular antigen-1.[355,356]

Leukemic or Disseminated T/NK-Cell Neoplasms

These include T-cell prolymphocytic leukemia,[357–359] T-cell large granular lymphocyte leukemia,[360,361] aggressive NK-cell leukemia, NK-cell large granular lymphocyte leukemia,[362] and adult T-cell leukemia/lymphoma.[363] Their main features are summarized in Table 39–5.

Extranodal T/NK-Cell Neoplasms[364]

Most extranodal T/NK-cell neoplasms have a cytotoxic phenotype, which may predispose to apoptosis of tumor cells and bystander reactive cells. The three major categories are nasal, intestinal, and subcutaneous panniculitis-like. Many extranodal T/NK-cell neoplasms are associated with EBV (Fig. 39–9*A* to *D*); the association is site-dependent and shows geographic variation. Tumors resembling any of the three prototypes may occur in a variety of extranodal sites (Table 39–6). Extranodal T/NK-cell lymphomas occur at increased frequency in the setting of immune suppression, especially after organ transplantation.

Extranodal NK/T-Cell Lymphoma, Nasal-Type (Formerly Angiocentric Lymphoma)

This disease, rare in the United States and Europe, is more common in Asia. It presents in children or adults as an extranodal mass, typically as a midfacial palatal or nasal destructive tumor.[365–369] Tumor cells are characterized by a broad morphologic spectrum,[365,369] and may be admixed with a reactive infiltrate; thus early lesions may be misdiagnosed as inflammatory. Tumor cells often display angioinvasion; extensive necrosis is frequent and can make diagnosis difficult. The neoplastic cells in most cases have an NK phenotype, with constant expression of CD56 antigen and of cytotoxic granule proteins,[370] and have no *TCR* gene rearrangement. Virtually all cases

TABLE 39–5. Features of Disseminated/Leukemic Mature T/NK-Cell Neoplasms

Neoplasm*	Morphology	Immunophenotype†	Cytotoxic Granules‡	TCR§	Virus	Genetic Abnormality	*TCR* Genes‖	Clinical Course
T-PLL	Prolymphocytes Small lymphocytes	$sCD3^+CD5^+CD7^+$ $CD4^+CD8^-$ (60%) $CD4^+CD8^+$ (25%) $CD4^-CD8^+$ (15%)	−	α/β	−	inv14(q11;q32) trisomy 8q del(12p13) del(11q23)	R	Progressive Survival <1 year
T-LGL	Large granular lymphocytes	$sCD3^+CD5^+CD7^-$ $CD4^-CD8^+$ $CD16^+CD56^-CD57^+$	+	α/β (γ/δ)	−	None known	R	Indolent
NK-LGL	Large granular lymphocytes	$sCD3^-CD5^-CD7^-$ $CD4^-CD8^{-/+}$ $CD16^+CD56^+CD57^+$	+	−	−		G	Indolent
Aggressive NK cell leukemia	Cells similar to but larger than large granular lymphocytes	$sCD3^-CD5^-CD7^-$ $CD4^-CD8^-$ $CD16^{+/-}CD56^+CD57^-$	+	−	EBV		G	Aggressive to fulminant
ATLL	Flower cells	$sCD3^+CD5^+CD7^-$ $CD4^+CD8^-$ (most) $CD30^{-/+}$	−	α/β	HTLV-1		R	Acute and lymphomatous: aggressive Chronic and smoldering: protracted course

*T-PLL, T-cell prolymphocytic leukemia; T-LGL, T-cell large granular lymphocytic leukemia; NK-LGL, NK-cell large granular lymphocytic leukemia; ATLL, adult T-cell leukemia/lymphoma.

†+/−, >50% positive; −/+, <50% positive.

‡Cytotoxic granules = T-cell intracellular antigen-1, perforin, and/or granzyme.

§*TCR*, T-cell receptor gene.

‖G, germline; R, rearranged.

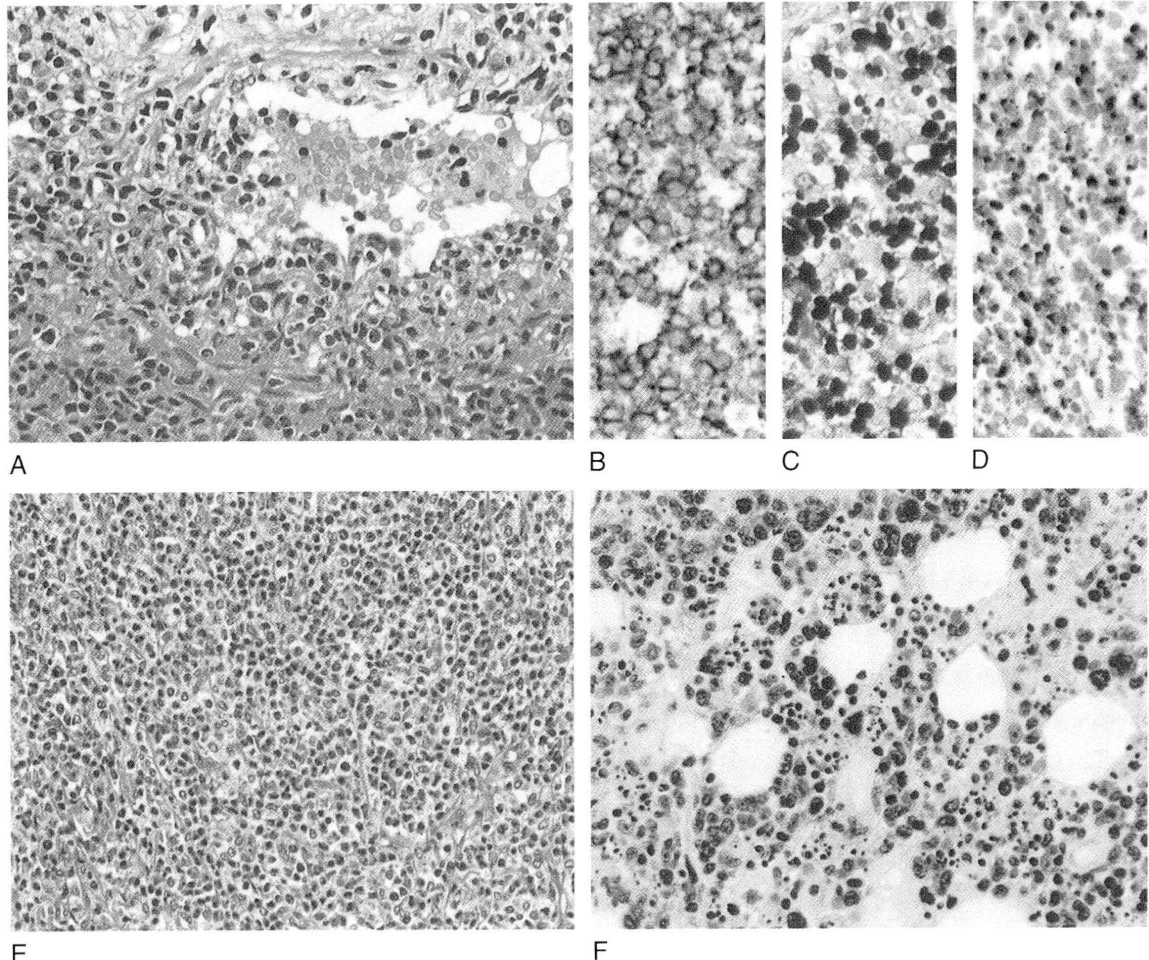

■ **Figure 39–9.** Extranodal T/NK-cell lymphomas. ***A,*** Nasal NK/T-cell lymphoma composed of an infiltrate of medium-sized pleomorphic cells invading a blood vessel wall. ***B–D,*** Neoplastic cells are uniformly positive for CD56 ***(B)***, are positive for Epstein-Barr virus–associated RNA (EBER) (in situ hybridization) ***(C)***, and strongly express cytotoxic proteins such as T-cell intracellular antigen-1 (TIA-1) ***(D)***. ***E,*** Enteropathy-associated T-cell lymphoma showing an eosinophil-rich infiltrate of medium-sized atypical lymphoid cells. ***F,*** Subcutaneous panniculitis-like T-cell lymphoma showing a dense interstitial infiltrate of atypical lymphoid cells in the subcutaneous fat, with rimming of individual fat cells by the lymphoma cells.

are positive for EBV.[371,372] The clinical course is typically aggressive, with relapses in other extranodal sites.[371,373–376] Hemophagocytic syndromes are a classical clinical complication, likely related to EBV.[374,376]

Enteropathy-Type T-Cell Lymphoma

This is an intestinal lymphoma that occurs in association with celiac disease in adults who typically have a rather brief history of gluten-sensitive enteropathy. Early treatment of celiac disease appears to eliminate the risk of lymphoma. It may also occur as the initial event in a patient found to have villous atrophy in the resected intestine. Some patients without evidence of enteropathy have either anti-gliadin antibodies or the typical human lymphocyte antigen type of patients with celiac disease, or both.[377–379] Enteropathy-type T-cell lymphoma commonly occurs in the jejunum, as single or multiple ulcerated lesions.[380] Presentation as an acute abdominal emergency is common.[381] The tumors are cytologically variable, and there is often a prominent infiltrate of eosinophils (Fig. 39–9*E*). There are often increased intraepithelial T cells in the adjacent mucosa, with or without villous atrophy.[382] The tumor cells, thought to derive from intestinal intraepithelial T cells, are usually $sCD3^{+}CD5^{-}CD7^{+}CD4^{-}CD8^{-/+}$ and contain cytotoxic proteins.[383–385] CD30 may be positive in some cells.[386] The *TCR* genes are clonally rearranged.[387] The course is aggressive and prognosis is poor.

Early lesions (ulcerative jejunitis) may show mucosal ulceration with only scattered atypical cells and numerous reactive histiocytes, without formation of large masses[388]; these lesions are nonetheless clonal. Clonal *TCR* gene rearrangements have also been found in cases of celiac disease unresponsive to a gluten-free diet (refractory sprue), suggesting that these cases may represent low-grade intraepithelial T-cell lymphoma (epitheliotropic lymphoma).[389]

TABLE 39–6. Immunohistologic and Genetic Features of Common Mature T/NK-Cell Neoplasms with Predominantly Extranodal or Nodal Presentation*

Neoplasm	CD3 S;C	CD5	CD7	CD4	CD8	CD30	TCR†	NK (16; 56)	Cytotoxic Granules‡	EBV	Genetic Abnormality	*TCR* Gene§
Predominantly Extranodal												
NK/T-cell lymphoma, nasal type	–;+	–	–/+	–	–	–/+	–	NA; +	+	++	p53 alterations Del(6q) Del(13q)	G
ETCL	+	–	+	–	+/–	+/–	α/β >> γ/δ	–	+	–	None known	R
Hepatosplenic T-cell lymphoma	+	–	+	–	–	–	γ/δ > α/β	+; –/+	+	–	Iso 7q	R
SPTCL	+	+	+	–	+	–/+	α/β	–	+	–	None known	R
Mycosis fungoides	+	+	–/+	+	–	–	α/β	–	–	–	None known	R
Cutaneous ALCL	+	+/–	+/–	+/–	–	++	α/β	–	–/+	–	None known	R
Predominantly Nodal												
PTCL-NOS	+/–	+/–	+/–	+/–	–/+	–/+	α/β > γ/δ	–/+	–/+	–/+	inv 14; complex	R
AITCL	+	+	+	+/–	–/+	–	α/β	–	NA	+/–	Trisomy 3 Trisomy 5	R
ALCL	+/–	+/–	NA	–/+	–/+	++	α/β	–	+	–	t(2;5); NPM/ALK	R

*+, >90% positive; ++, strongly positive in all cases; +/–, >50% positive; –/+, <50% positive; –, <10% positive; NA = not available.
†*TCR*, T-cell receptor gene.
‡Cytotoxic granules = T-cell intracellular antigen-1, perforin, and/or granzyme.
§G, germline; R, rearranged.
For abbreviations of neoplasms, see Table 39–1.

Hepatosplenic T-Cell Lymphoma

Patients are predominantly young adult males presenting with marked hepatosplenomegaly and thrombocytopenia.[390,391] Several cases have been reported in immunosuppressed allograft recipients.[392,393] This lymphoma consists of a proliferation of medium-size lymphoid cells within the sinusoids of the splenic red pulp, liver, and bone marrow.[394] Patients typically respond to treatment but relapse with refractory disease, and median survival is less than 2 years.[395,396] The cells are $CD2^+CD3^+CD5^-CD4^-CD8^-CD16^+CD56^{+/-}$; most cases express the γ/δ receptor and have a nonactivated cytotoxic phenotype (T-cell intracellular antigen-1 positive, granzyme negative).[396–399] Some cases may have the α/β *TCR* phenotype. The *TCR* genes are rearranged. The tumor cells are EBV negative. Isochromosome 7q has been documented in many cases of both γ/δ and α/β type.[400–403]

Subcutaneous Panniculitis-like T-Cell Lymphoma

Subcutaneous panniculitis-like T-cell lymphoma is a cytotoxic T-cell lymphoma usually derived from α/β $CD8^+$ T cells (less often $CD4^+$ or γ/δ T cells) that preferentially infiltrates the subcutaneous adipose tissue, resembling panniculitis. It is composed of atypical lymphoid cells of various sizes, usually with round or slightly irregular, hyperchromatic nuclei, often with marked tumor necrosis and karyorrhexis (Fig. 39–9*F*). The disease may present in an indolent fashion but typically becomes aggressive; patients may respond to aggressive therapy.[404–406] Hematophagocytic syndromes are common, although the tumor is EBV^-.

Mycosis Fungoides

Mycosis fungoides is a mature T-cell lymphoma of adults presenting in the skin with patches/plaques and composed of epidermotropic small to medium-sized T cells with cerebriform nuclei.[407] Tumor cells are $CD2^+CD3^+TCR\alpha\beta^+CD5^+CD7^{-/+}$. Most cases are $CD4^+$.[408] The *TCR* genes are clonally rearranged.[409] The disease has an indolent course with progression from patches to plaques and eventually tumors. Long-term remissions can be obtained in the early stages.

Primary Cutaneous Anaplastic Large-Cell Lymphoma

Primary cutaneous anaplastic large-cell lymphoma affects predominantly older adults and is rare in children. The cytologic features are similar to those of systemic anaplastic large-cell lymphoma. The neoplastic cells express T-cell antigens and CD30, and are usually $CD4^+$. Unlike systemic anaplastic large-cell lymphoma, most cutaneous cases are negative for ALK and EMA.[410,411] The *TCR* genes are clonally rearranged. The t(2;5) is typically absent, and its presence should raise the concern that the tumor is a cutaneous manifestation of systemic anaplastic large-cell lymphoma.[412] The prognosis is favorable.

There is morphologic and clinical overlap with lymphomatoid papulosis, and, in a given case, the pathologist may not be able to distinguish between these two entities without a clinical history (chronic relapsing, healing lesions vs. progressive growth); thus, the histologic diagnosis "$CD30^+$ cutaneous lymphoproliferative disorder" may be made if clinical data are lacking.

Nodal T/NK-Cell Neoplasms

Peripheral T-Cell Lymphoma, Unspecified

This heterogeneous category encompasses mature T-cell lymphomas not fulfilling the specific criteria as for being categorized as one of the other defined recognizable subtypes. These account for about half of all mature T-cell lymphomas (see Table 39–3). The median age of patients with unspecified peripheral T-cell lymphoma is in the seventh decade, and 65% of the patients have stage IV disease.[9] Presentation is usually nodal, but any site may be affected. Blood eosinophilia, pruritus, and hemophagocytic syndromes may occur.[413] Unspecified peripheral T-cell lymphomas typically contain a mixture of small and large atypical cells. The presence of cells with clear cytoplasm, increased vascularization, and eosinophilia are frequent features (Fig. 39–10*A*).[414–416] Admixed epithelioid histiocytes may be numerous (lymphoepithelioid variant, or Lennert's, lymphoma).[417] T-cell–associated antigens are variably expressed ($CD3^{+/-}CD2^{+/-}CD5^{+/-}CD7^{-/+}$) (see Table 39–6); aberrant phenotypes characterized by loss of one or more of these is common. Most cases are $CD4^{+}CD8^{-}$ and are usually noncytotoxic.[418] The *TCR* genes are usually rearranged.[419,420] EBV is usually absent in the tumor cells. No specific cytogenetic or oncogene abnormality has been reported, although complex karyotypes are common in cases with larger cells. The clinical course is aggressive, and relapses are more common than in large B-cell lymphoma.[421–423] This lymphoma subtype has one of the lowest overall and failure-free survival rates.[9,10]

Angioimmunoblastic T-Cell Lymphoma

This is one of the most common peripheral T-cell lymphomas encountered in Western countries.[229] Angioim-

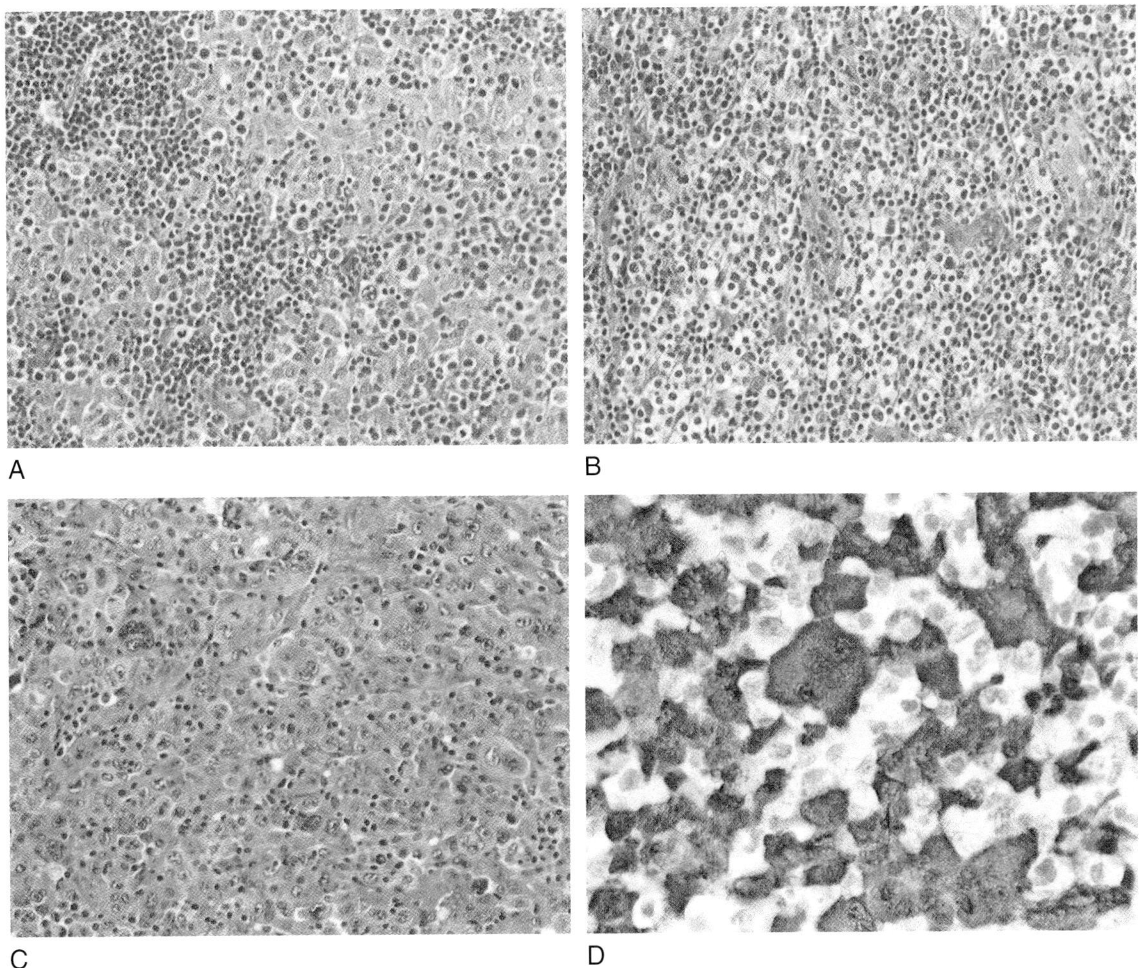

Figure 39–10. Nodal T-cell lymphomas. ***A,*** Peripheral T-cell lymphoma, not otherwise specified, is composed of medium-sized and large cells with pleomorphic, irregular nuclei; this case also displays a prominent histiocytic infiltrate and mild eosinophilia. ***B,*** Angioimmunoblastic T-cell lymphoma shows prominent vascularization and a neoplastic infiltrate composed of medium-sized atypical cells with clear cytoplasm. ***C,*** Anaplastic large-cell lymphoma involving a lymph node composed of large pleomorphic cells. ***D,*** In this case associated with a t(2;5) translocation, neoplastic cells showed strong nuclear and cytoplasmic immunoreactivity for ALK protein.

munoblastic T-cell lymphoma is clinically distinctive: patients typically have generalized lymphadenopathy, fever, weight loss, skin rash, polyclonal hypergammaglobulinemia,[424] and susceptibility to infections. Distinctive pathologic features of angioimmunoblastic T-cell lymphoma include prominent arborizing vascularization, perivascular proliferation of follicular dendritic cells ($CD21^+$),[229] and the presence of EBV-positive B-cell immunoblasts. Three overlapping histologic patterns with hyperplastic follicles, with depleted follicles, or without follicles have been described.[425] The lymphoid cells are a mixture of small lymphocytes, immunoblasts, plasma cells, and medium-sized cells with round nuclei and clear cytoplasm (Fig. 39–10*B*). Tumor cells express T-cell–associated antigens and usually CD4 with aberrant coexpression of CD10.[425,426] The *TCR* genes are rearranged in 75%; IgH gene rearrangement is detected in 10%, corresponding to expanded EBV^+ B-cell clones.[427–430] Trisomy 3 and/or 5 may occur.[431] The course is moderately aggressive, with occasional spontaneous remissions, and is not reliably predicted by the histologic appearance. Median survivals range from 15 to 24 months, and its curability has not been well established. Some patients develop a secondary EBV^+ large B-cell lymphoma.

Anaplastic Large-Cell Lymphoma

Anaplastic large-cell lymphoma represents about 2% of all lymphomas, but about 10% of childhood lymphomas and 50% of large-cell pediatric lymphomas.[229,432,433] Primary systemic anaplastic large-cell lymphoma may involve lymph nodes or extranodal sites, including the skin, but is not localized to the skin; it has a bimodal age distribution in children and adults. The tumor cells are large with round or pleomorphic, often horseshoe-shaped or multiple nuclei with multiple or single prominent nucleoli, and abundant cytoplasm (Fig. 39–10*C*). The so-called hallmark cell has an eccentric nucleus and a prominent, eosinophilic Golgi region.[434] The growth is cohesive and often sinusoidal in lymph nodes.[435] Lymphohistiocytic and small-cell variants have been described.[436,437] The tumor cells are uniformly strongly positive for CD30, and usually express EMA and cytotoxic granule proteins.[438,439] By molecular analysis, anaplastic large-cell lymphoma can usually be shown to be of T-cell origin; however, many cases have lost expression of many of the T-cell–associated antigens. About 80% of the cases are characterized by a translocation involving the *ALK* gene on chromosome 2p23, most commonly a t(2;5)(p23;q35),[440,441] which results in a fusion with the nucleophosmin gene (*NPM*) on chromosome 5, but variant translocations have also been identified (see Table 39–3). Cases with *ALK* translocations have ALK protein expression detectable by immunohistochemistry (Fig. 39–10*D*),[442] and have a better prognosis than ALK-negative cases. Pediatric cases are more likely to be ALK^+ than adult cases.[410,443] Anaplastic large-cell lymphoma in children is characterized by frequent high stage but a good response to therapy with excellent overall survival.[432,433,441] In adults, the tumor is aggressive but potentially curable, similar to other aggressive lymphomas.[444]

HODGKIN'S LYMPHOMA

Hodgkin's lymphoma differs from most other malignant tumors in its unique cellular composition: a minority of neoplastic cells (Hodgkin and Reed-Sternberg [H-RS] cells and their variants) in a background of non-neoplastic reactive cells. The clinical features and responses to treatment of Hodgkin's lymphoma differ dramatically from those of most so-called non-Hodgkin's lymphomas, suggesting that a specific immunologic reaction is important not only in the definition but also in the clinical behavior of this disease. Two major types of Hodgkin's lymphoma are recognized, based on morphology, immunophenotype, and clinical features: nodular lymphocyte predominance Hodgkin's lymphoma and classical Hodgkin's lymphoma (Table 39–7; see also Table 39–1).[11]

Nodular Lymphocyte Predominance Hodgkin's Lymphoma

Nodular lymphocyte predominance Hodgkin's lymphoma accounts for about 5% of the cases of Hodgkin's lymphoma.[445] The median age is in the mid-30s, but cases may be seen both in children and in the elderly. The male : female ratio is 3 : 1 or greater. Nodular lymphocyte predominance Hodgkin's lymphoma usually involves peripheral lymph nodes, with sparing of the mediastinum. About 80% of the patients in most series are stage I or II at the time of the diagnosis, but rare patients may present with stage III or IV disease, with a concomitantly worse prognosis.[446] Over 90% of the patients have a complete response to therapy, and 90% are alive at 10 years. Both late and multiple relapses are more common than in other types of Hodgkin's lymphoma; however, these are usually isolated nodal recurrences, and are not associated with poor survival.[447–450] The cause of death is often non-Hodgkin's lymphoma, other cancers, or complications of treatment, rather than Hodgkin's lymphoma.[446] Patients with nodular lymphocyte predominance Hodgkin's lymphoma have a low (3–6%) rate of progression to diffuse large B-cell lymphoma.[451–454] In the reported cases, the prognosis of these patients appears to be significantly better than that for patients with usual diffuse large B-cell lymphoma, and patients who respond to treatment may later relapse with only nodular lymphocyte predominance Hodgkin's lymphoma.[452]

Lymphocyte predominance Hodgkin's lymphoma by definition has at least a partially nodular growth pattern (Fig. 39–11*A*); diffuse areas are present in a minority of the cases, and it is controversial whether purely diffuse cases exist.[445] The Reed-Sternberg cell variants have vesicular, polylobated nuclei and distinct but small, usually peripheral nucleoli and have been designated L&H cells (lymphocytic and/or histiocytic of Lukes and Butler) or "popcorn" cells, because of the resemblance of their nuclei to an exploded kernel of corn (Fig. 39–11*B*).[455] The background is predominantly lymphocytes; clusters of epithelioid histiocytes may be numerous, and plasma cells, eosinophils, and neutrophils are rarely seen and, if present, are not numerous.[456] Occa-

TABLE 39–7. Distinctive Features of Nodular Lymphocyte Predominance Hodgkin's Lymphoma (NLPHL) and Classic Hodgkin's Lymphoma (CHL)

	NLPHL	CHL
Clinical Features		
Frequency	5–10% of all Hodgkin's lymphoma	90–95% of all Hodgkin's lymphoma
Sex ratio	Striking male predominance	Roughly equally affects both sexes
Age	Unimodal distribution (30–50 yr)	Bimodal distribution
Involvement	Cervical, axillary, or inguinal nodes; mediastinal involvement exceptional	Often involves cervical nodes; mediastinal involvement frequent
Stage	Usually localized	Majority localized
Pathologic Features		
Histologic pattern	Nodular ± diffuse	Diffuse or nodular
Neoplastic cells		
Morphology	Lymphohistiocytic cells (L&H cells)	Hodgkin and Reed-Sternberg cells (H-RS cells)
Immunophenotype	$CD45^+$	$CD45^-$
	$CD20^+$	$CD20^{-/+}$
	$CD30^-$	$CD30^+$
	$CD15^-$	$CD15^+$
	Bcl-6^+	Bcl-$6^{-/+}$
Reactive background		
Small B cells	Numerous	Scarce
Small T cells	Variable numbers	Numerous
$CD57^+$ cells	Numerous	Less numerous than in NLPHL
$CD21^+$ FDC	+	−/+
Eosinophils	Absent	Present
EBV Association	No	40–50%
Genetic Features		
Rearranged Ig genes	Yes	Yes
Mutated	Yes	Yes
Ongoing mutations	Frequent	Rare
Crippling mutations	Rarely	25% of cases
Cell of origin	Antigen-selected germinal center B cell	Preapoptotic germinal center B cell
bcl-6 rearrangements	In about 50% of cases	No

Abbreviations: FDC, follicular dendritic cells; Ig, immunoglobulin.

sional sclerosis may cause some cases to resemble nodular sclerosis Hodgkin's lymphoma.

The tumor cells are $CD45^+$, express B-cell–associated antigens (CD19, 20, 22, 79a) but lack CD15 and CD30, and are usually strongly positive for Bcl-6 (Fig. 39–11*D* and *E*).[457] The background lymphocytes in the nodules are a mixture of polyclonal B cells with a mantle zone phenotype (IgM^+ and IgD^+), and numerous T cells, many of which are $CD57^+$, similar to the T cells in normal and progressively transformed germinal centers.[458] T cells typically surround the neoplastic B cells, forming rings.[459,460] A prominent concentric meshwork of follicular dendritic cells is present within the nodules (Fig. 39–11*C*).[461]

Classical Hodgkin's Lymphoma

Classical Hodgkin's lymphoma is defined by the presence of classical, diagnostic Reed-Sternberg cells with the immunophenotype of classical Hodgkin's lymphoma ($CD15^+CD30^+$, T- and B-cell–associated antigens usually negative). Classical Hodgkin's lymphoma is divided into four subtypes: nodular sclerosis, mixed cellularity, lymphocyte-depleted, and lymphocyte-rich. Nodular sclerosis Hodgkin's lymphoma is the most common subtype in developed countries (60–80% in most series) (Fig. 39–11*F*). It is most common in adolescents and young adults, but can occur at any age; females equal or exceed males. The mediastinum and other supradiaphragmatic sites are commonly involved. Mixed cellularity Hodgkin's lymphoma comprises 15–30% of Hodgkin's lymphoma cases in most series; it may be seen at any age, and lacks the early adult peak of nodular sclerosis Hodgkin's lymphoma (Fig. 39–11*G*). Involvement of the mediastinum is less common than in nodular sclerosis Hodgkin's lymphoma, and abdominal lymph node and splenic involvement are more common. Lymphocyte-depleted Hodgkin's lymphoma is the least common variant of Hodgkin's lymphoma, comprising less than 1% of the cases in recent reports. It is most common in older people, in HIV^+ individuals,[462,463] and in nonindustrialized countries. Lymphocyte-depleted Hodgkin's lymphoma frequently presents with abdominal lymphadenopathy and spleen, liver, and bone marrow involvement, without peripheral lymphadenopathy. The stage is usually advanced at diagnosis; however, response

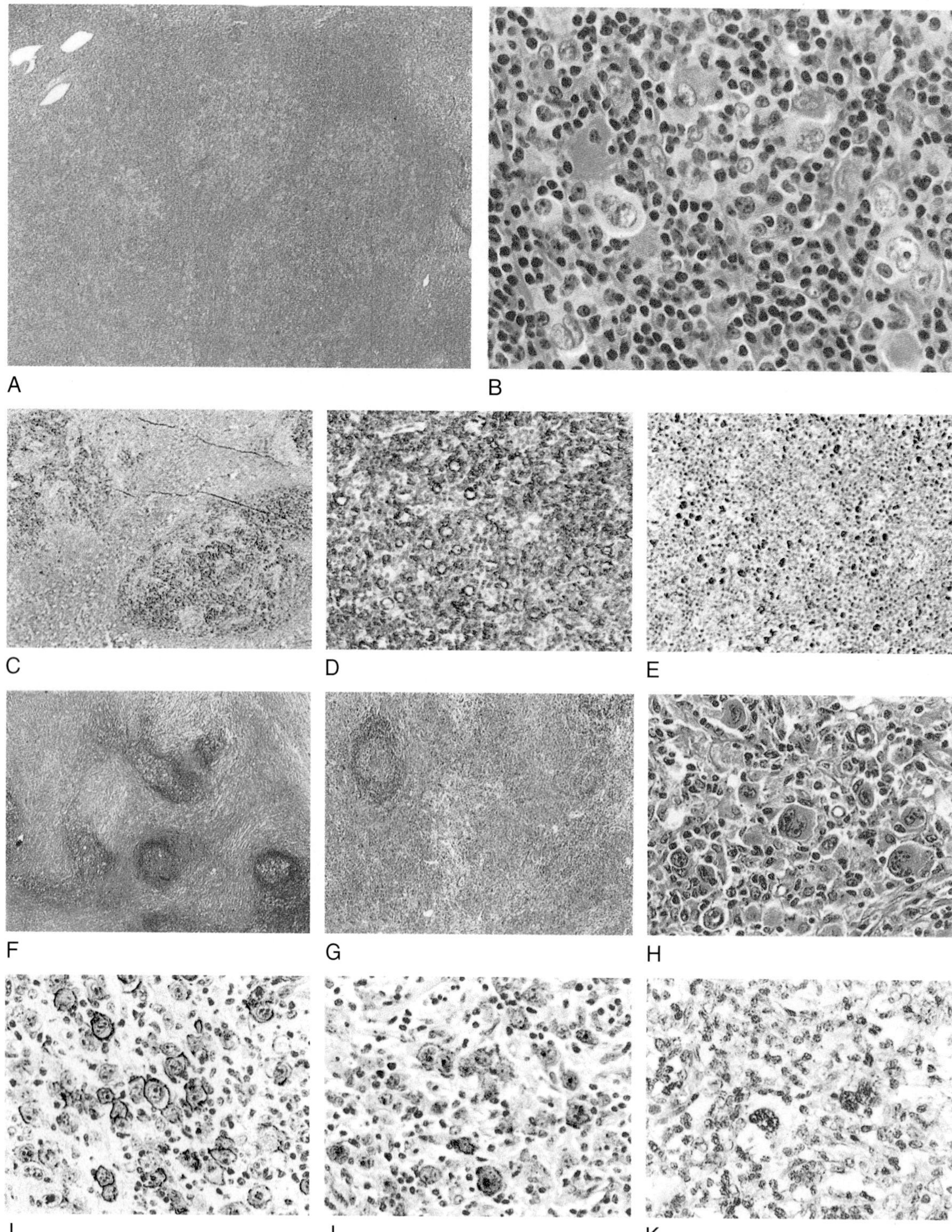

Figure 39–11. Hodgkin's lymphoma. ***A–E,*** Nodular lymphocyte predominance Hodgkin's lymphoma. ***A,*** Low magnification showing large nodules effacing the nodal architecture. ***B,*** High magnification showing large mononucleated and multilobulated "popcorn" cells in a background of reactive histiocytes and small lymphocytes. ***C,*** The nodules are associated with a meshwork of $CD21^+$ follicular dendritic cells. ***D,*** Immunoperoxidase staining for CD20 showing strong positivity of the large neoplastic cells and small B lymphocytes in the background. ***E,*** Immunoperoxidase staining for Bcl-6 showing positivity of the neoplastic cells.

F–K, Classical Hodgkin's lymphoma. ***F,*** Nodular sclerosis type, showing cellular nodules separated by fibrous bands. ***G,*** Mixed cellularity type, showing an interfollicular infiltrate. ***H,*** Classical Reed-Sternberg cells in a mixed reactive background. ***I,*** Immunoperoxidase staining for CD30, showing membrane and focally paranuclear Golgi region staining of Reed-Sternberg cells. ***J,*** Immunoperoxidase staining for CD15, showing membrane and focally paranuclear Golgi region staining of Reed-Sternberg cells. ***K,*** In situ hybridization showing positivity of Reed-Sternberg cells for Epstein-Barr virus RNA (EBER).

to treatment is reported not to differ from that of other subtypes.[464] Lymphocyte-rich classical Hodgkin's lymphoma comprised 6% of 1959 cases of Hodgkin's lymphoma in a recent study, similar in frequency to nodular lymphocyte predominance Hodgkin's lymphoma.[465] The clinical features at presentation seem to be intermediate between those of nodular lymphocyte predominance Hodgkin's lymphoma and classic Hodgkin's lymphoma. Similar to nodular lymphocyte predominance Hodgkin's lymphoma, patients had early-stage disease and lacked bulky disease or B symptoms; like both nodular lymphocyte predominance and mixed cellularity Hodgkin's lymphoma, and in contrast to nodular sclerosis Hodgkin's lymphoma, they lacked mediastinal disease and had a predominance of males; and like mixed cellularity Hodgkin's lymphoma, they had an older median age than either nodular lymphocyte predominance or nodular sclerosis Hodgkin's lymphoma.

Classical Hodgkin's lymphoma is subclassified according to the cellular composition of the background infiltrate. Nodular sclerosis Hodgkin's lymphoma has at least a partially nodular pattern, with fibrous bands separating the nodules. The characteristic cell is the lacunar type Reed-Sternberg cell, with multilobated nuclei, small nucleoli, and abundant, pale cytoplasm that retracts in formalin-fixed sections, producing an empty space, or lacuna. Diagnostic Reed-Sternberg cells are also present, but may be rare. In mixed cellularity Hodgkin's lymphoma, the infiltrate is usually diffuse or at most vaguely nodular, without band-forming sclerosis, although fine interstitial fibrosis may be present. Reed-Sternberg cells of the classical, diagnostic type and mononuclear variants are present (Fig. 39–11*H*). Diagnostic Reed-Sternberg cells are large cells with bilobed, double, or multiple nuclei, with a large, eosinophilic, inclusion-like nucleolus in at least two lobes or nuclei. The infiltrate in both nodular sclerosis and mixed cellularity Hodgkin's lymphomas typically contains lymphocytes, epithelioid histiocytes, eosinophils, and plasma cells. The infiltrate in lymphocyte-depleted Hodgkin's lymphoma is diffuse and often appears hypocellular as a result of the presence of diffuse fibrosis and necrosis; there are large numbers of classical Reed-Sternberg cells and bizarre "sarcomatous" variants, with a paucity of other inflammatory cells. Confluent sheets of Reed-Sternberg cells and variants may occur and rarely predominate ("reticular" variant or "Hodgkin's sarcoma").[455,462] Prior to the availability of immunophenotyping studies, many cases diagnosed as lymphocyte-depleted Hodgkin's lymphoma were in reality cases of large B-cell lymphoma or T-cell lymphomas, often of the anaplastic large-cell lymphoma type.[466,467] The term *lymphocyte-rich classical Hodgkin's lymphoma* is used for cases of Hodgkin's lymphoma with Reed-Sternberg cells of classical type, both by morphology and immunophenotype, with a background infiltrate that consists predominantly of lymphocytes, with rare or no eosinophils. The pattern may be diffuse or nodular, resembling nodular lymphocyte predominance Hodgkin's lymphoma.[465,468,469] Thus, cases of lymphocyte-rich classical Hodgkin's lymphoma may require immunophenotyping for differential diagnosis.

The British National Lymphoma Investigation (BNLI) developed a system for grading nodular sclerosis Hodgkin's lymphoma (grades 1 and 2), based on the number and atypia of the Reed-Sternberg cells in the nodules.[470] About 80% of the cases in most series are grade 1 and 20% are grade 2. Recent results from American and European centers have had conflicting results, showing either no influence on outcome, or a significantly worse outcome for nodular sclerosis grade 2 patients.[471–473]

In 75–80% of the cases of classical Hodgkin's lymphoma, the tumor cells are $CD15^{+}CD30^{+}$ (Fig. 39–11*I* and *J*). CD45 is typically absent. Expression of B-cell antigens occurs in 5–50%, usually only weakly and in a minority of the cells.[474,475] In contrast to nodular lymphocyte predominance Hodgkin's lymphoma, the Reed-Sternberg cells of most cases of classical Hodgkin's lymphoma lack the nuclear Bcl-6 protein.[476] One study found that cases that lacked CD15 but expressed CD30 had a significantly worse freedom from relapse and overall survival than $CD15^{+}$ cases. The background lymphocytes in classical Hodgkin's lymphoma are predominantly $CD4^{+}$ T cells, but in nodular areas of nodular sclerosis or lymphocyte-rich classical Hodgkin's lymphoma, the background lymphocytes are B cells, similar to lymphocyte predominance Hodgkin's lymphoma, and meshworks of follicular dendritic cells are seen with antibodies to CD21 or CD35. In EBV^{+} cases, the tumor cells express EBV-encoded small RNAs and EBV latent membrane protein (LMP) but not EBV nuclear antigen-2 (EBNA-2) (Fig. 39–11*K*).

Pathogenesis of Hodgkin's Lymphoma

Cellular Origin of Neoplastic Cells in Hodgkin's Lymphoma

It is now clear that neoplastic cells in virtually all cases of classical as well as nodular lymphocyte predominance Hodgkin's lymphoma represent clonal populations of transformed germinal center B cells[477] (Fig. 39–12). This was established by amplification of clonal rearranged immunoglobulin genes bearing somatic hypermutations from single H-RS cells isolated by micromanipulation from primary Hodgkin's lymphoma biopsy specimens.[478–482] In lymphocyte predominance Hodgkin's lymphoma, the lymphohistiocytic (L&H) tumor cells show intraclonal V gene diversity, indicating ongoing mutations, and thus are probably derived from antigen-selected germinal center B cells. In contrast, in classical Hodgkin's lymphoma, the H-RS cells often have "crippled" mutations rendering originally functional immunoglobulin rearrangements nonfunctional, suggesting that they are derived from negatively selected "preapoptotic" germinal center B cells that are destined to undergo apoptosis but rescued by some transforming event.[477,483]

In rare cases of classical Hodgkin's lymphoma, H-RS cells carry clonal *TCR* rearrangements, indicating the rare occurrence of the disease as a T-cell lymphoma.[484,485]

Although the genetic findings have a strong impact on our understanding of the biology of Hodgkin's lym-

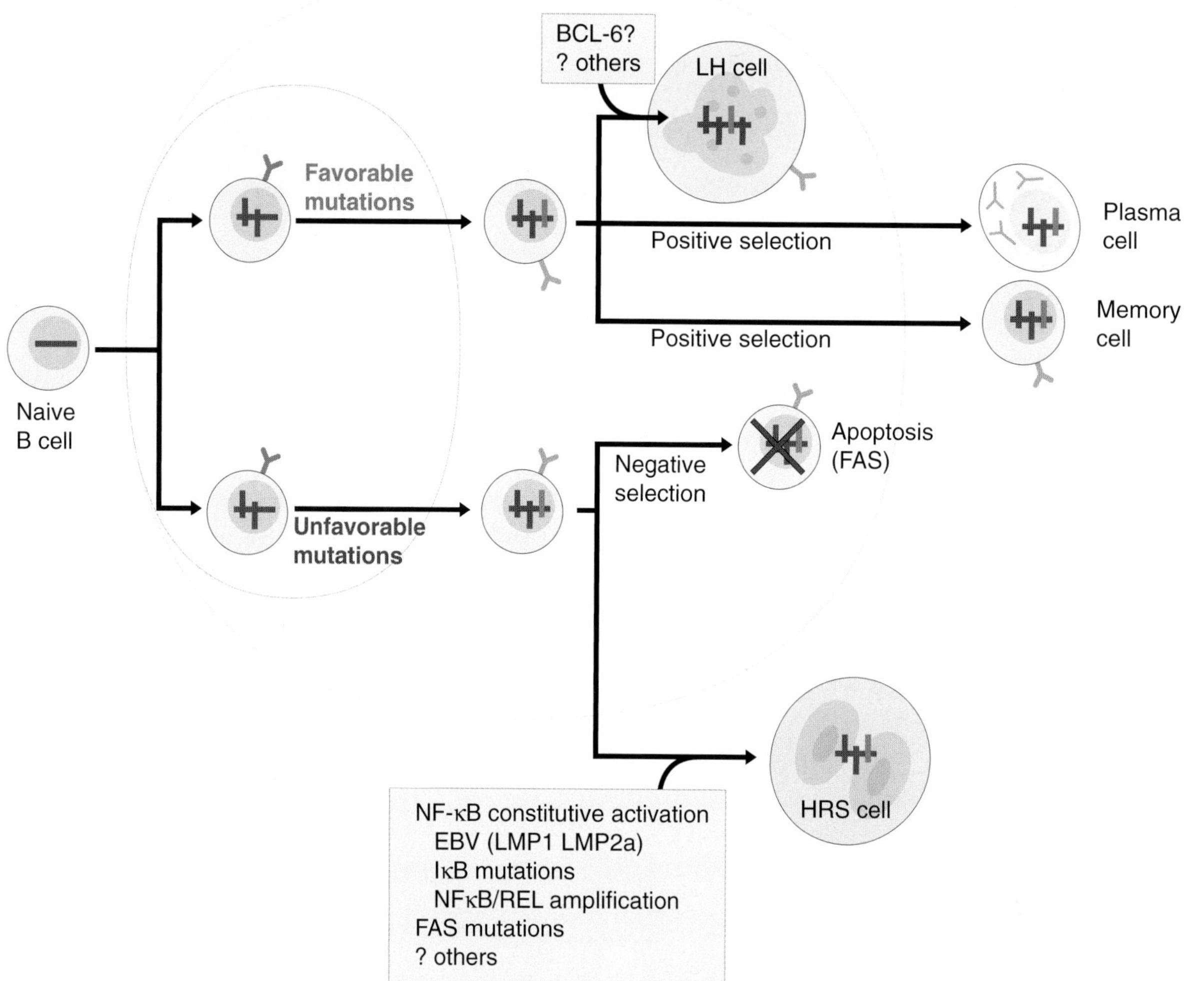

Figure 39–12. Pathogenic model of Hodgkin's lymphoma. Both nodular lymphocyte predominance Hodgkin's lymphoma (NLPHL) and classical Hodgkin's lymphoma (cHL) represent in most instances clonal proliferations of transformed germinal center B cells. Rearranged immunoglobulin heavy chain gene is symbolized with a horizontal bar in the nucleus, and somatic mutations in the immunoglobulin V region are symbolized with vertical lines. Abbreviations: HRS, Hodgkin and Reed-Sternberg cells of cHL; L&H cell, lymphocytic and histiocytic cell of NLPHL.

phoma, many other features of H-RS and L&H cells are not yet understood.

Mechanisms Involved in the Survival of H-RS Progenitors in Classical Hodgkin's Lymphoma

In the germinal center stage of B-cell differentiation, there is strong selection for cells presenting high-affinity B-cell receptor (BCR). However, the malignant cell clones in classical Hodgkin's lymphoma arise in the absence of selection for antigen. Moreover, a characteristic feature of H-RS in classical Hodgkin's lymphoma is the lack of expression of surface immunoglobulin, resulting from alterations in the immunoglobulin genes that prevent their expression and/or dysregulation of the immunoglobulin transcription machinery.[486,487] Because the BCR complex provides important survival signals to developing B cells, absence of immunoglobulin expression could put H-RS cells at a survival disadvantage.

There is growing evidence that the transcription factor NF-κB plays a major role as the central effector of malignant transformation. Most cases of classical Hodgkin's lymphoma are indeed characterized by a constitutive activation of the NF-κB transcription factor,[488,489] and inactivation of this factor in vitro induces massive apoptosis of H-RS–derived cell lines.[488] In a quiescent state, NF-κB is retained in the cytoplasm by aggregation with IκB proteins, especially IκBα; after stimulating signaling, these become phosphorylated, dissociate from NF-κB, and release it into the nucleus. NF-κB has a central role in inflammatory responses by upregulation of a proproliferative and antiapoptotic gene expression program in lymphocytes. Thus, constitutive NF-κB activation may provide H-RS cells with self-sufficiency in growth signals to become disconnected from regulatory interactions with their environment. In addition, other activational transcription signals have been found to be active in classical Hodgkin's lymphoma, including different STAT (signal transducer and activator of transcription) proteins and AP1.[490–492]

Another way by which H-RS cells may escape apoptosis is by acquiring resistance to FAS-mediated apoptotic machinery normally operating in the germinal center. Experimental data have shown that H-RS–derived cell lines are resistant to FAS-mediated apoptosis,[493] and H-RS cells in classical Hodgkin's lymphoma tissues show constitutive expression of c-FLIP (a strong physiologic inhibitor of FAS-mediated apoptosis).[494]

Contribution of EBV Infection to Oncogenesis in Classical Hodgkin's Lymphoma

Various findings are suggestive of EBV being an environmental factor contributing to oncogenesis in classical Hodgkin's lymphoma. EBV is detected in H-RS cells of classical Hodgkin's lymphoma in about 40–50% of the cases, with the highest frequency in mixed cellularity subtype cases. Infected H-RS cells exhibit a type II program of latent infection with expression of EBV nuclear antigens (EBNA), latent membrane protein (LMP)-1, and LMP-2a.[347] LMP-1 is known to have oncogenic potential by triggering Bcl-2 expression and activating NF-κB via the CD40 cell-signaling pathway, allowing cells to evade apoptotic mechanisms. LMP-2a shuts down BCR signaling but to some extent mimics the BCR signaling itself, thereby providing important prosurvival signals to B cells. Thus, it is hypothesized that the expression of LMP-1 and LMP-2a by EBV^+ H-RS cells is a key pathogenic event in EBV^+ classical Hodgkin's lymphoma, enabling the preapoptotic progenitor to survive negative selection; the acquisition of further changes may then lead to clonal expansion. However, the role of EBV in pathogenesis is still not clear, because the EBV^- cases have the same phenotype and no other viruses have been detected.

Specific Genetic Changes That May Underlie the Clonal Expansion of H-RS Clones

Cytogenetic studies in Hodgkin's lymphoma are limited when compared to those in non-Hodgkin's lymphoma; there are intrinsic problems in obtaining metaphase chromosomes in Hodgkin's lymphoma, and a limited number of abnormal karyotypes have been reported until now.[495,496] H-RS cells are characterized by a high degree of chromosomal instability with predominance of hyperdiploid complex karyotypes, and frequently harbor recurrent numerical and structural aberrations as detected by classical cytogenetics and FISH analysis, but so far no specific cytogenetic marker has been identified. Comparative genomic hybridization indicates typical genetic patterns in Hodgkin's lymphoma, with recurrent gains and losses of distinct chromosomal regions.[497] In some instances, candidate genes possibly involved in the malignant transformation of H-RS and L&H cells have been characterized. For example, amplifications of the *NFkB/rel* locus at 2p13-16 has been demonstrated in a substantial proportion of the cases, which may cause constitutional activation of the NF-κB pathway.[498–500] *JAK2* and *mdm-2* are two other genes that were found to be amplified in certain cases.

At the molecular genetic level, mutations in candidate oncogenes or tumor suppressor genes have been found in some cases. Deleterious mutations in the *IκBα* gene have been detected in a subset of EBV-negative classical Hodgkin's lymphoma,[501,502] adding weight to the concept of *IκBα* mutations as central transforming events in classical Hodgkin's lymphoma in the absence of EBV. Mutations of the p53 tumor suppressor gene appear to be a rare event in H-RS cells.[503] *FAS* gene mutations in the functional death domain occur only in rare cases of classical Hodgkin's lymphoma, but may in these cases be involved in the pathogenesis of the disease.[504]

Role of Cytokines and Chemokines in Classical Hodgkin's Lymphoma

In classical Hodgkin's lymphoma tissues, accumulation of reactive cells occurs in response to a variety of factors secreted by H-RS cells, mostly T_H2 cytokines and chemokines, including interleukin (IL)-4, IL-5, tumor necrosis factor-α, granulocyte-macrophage colony-stimulating factor, and TARC (for review, see Skinnider and Mak[505]). Of these, IL-5 expression correlates with tissular eosinophilia.[506] The chemokine TARC may be responsible for the predominance of T_H2 cells in the infiltrate.[507] The expression of T_H2 cytokines and chemokines also contributes to a local suppression of T_H1 cells involved in the cellular immune response. H-RS cells are characterized by membrane expression of several receptors of the tumor necrosis factor receptor superfamily (in particular CD30 and CD40); these receptors may in turn be activated by their corresponding ligands expressed by reactive cells (i.e., CD30 ligand on eosinophils and CD40 ligand on T cells), with the signaling cascade eventually resulting in NF-κB activation. Constitutive expression of IL-13 by H-RS cells provides another autocrine survival signal via STAT-6 activation.[491,508]

Mechanisms of Transformation in Nodular Lymphocyte Predominance Hodgkin's Lymphoma

In accordance with their distinct clinical and pathologic features, classical Hodgkin's lymphoma and nodular lymphocyte predominance Hodgkin's lymphoma also differ in their pathogenetic mechanisms. For example, EBV is virtually never detected in L&H cells of nodular lymphocyte predominance Hodgkin's lymphoma. At the genetic level, L&H cells are, similarly to H-RS cells, characterized by chromosomal instability, and comparative genomic hybridization studies have shown evidence of recurrent chromosomal imbalances. A recent study reports a high frequency of *bcl-6* rearrangements in nodular lymphocyte predominance Hodgkin's lymphoma (about half of the cases) but not in classical Hodgkin's lymphoma (none of the cases tested), suggesting that genomic rearrangements of this oncogene may play a role in the initiation of nodular lymphocyte predominance Hodgkin's lymphoma and reinforcing the concept of two distinct categories of Hodgkin's lymphoma.[509]

CURRENT CONTROVERSIES & FUTURE CONSIDERATIONS

Biology of Lymphoid Malignancy

- Lymphoid neoplasms are a diverse group of tumors arising from cells of the immune system. The normal counterpart of many but not all of these tumors can be recognized.
- With available techniques, a large number of clinically and biologically distinct tumors can be defined; in daily practice, fewer than 10 of these make up the majority of the cases seen by clinicians and pathologists.
- New genetic data are enhancing our ability to define clinically relevant subsets of heterogeneous groups such as diffuse large B-cell lymphomas.
- Recognizing distinct diseases is important for future progress in understanding the pathogenesis of diseases and in defining optimal therapies.

Suggested Readings*

Alizadeh AA, Eisen MB, Davis RE, et al: Distinct types of diffuse large B-cell lymphoma identified by gene expression profiling. Nature 403:503–511, 2000.

Du MQ, Isaccson PG: Gastric MALT lymphoma: from aetiology to treatment. Lancet Oncol 3:97–104, 2002.

Jaffe ES, Harris NL, Vardiman, Stein H (eds): Pathology and Genetics: Neoplasms of the Haematopoietic and Lymphoid Tissues. Lyon: IARC Press, 2001.

Kuppers R, Klein U, Hansmann ML, et al: Cellular origin of human B-cell lymphomas. N Engl J Med 341:1520–1529, 1999.

Full references for this chapter can be found on accompanying CD-ROM.

CHAPTER 40

Hodgkin's Lymphoma

Beate Klimm, MD, Karolin Behringer, MD, Henning Bredenfeld, MD, and Volker Diehl, MD

KEY POINTS

Hodgkin's Lymphoma

Diagnosis

- Hodgkin's lymphoma should always be proven by excisional biopsy, which is sent to an expert pathologist for initial diagnosis.
- Accurate staging procedures and risk factor assessment are indispensable for an adequate stage- and risk-adapted therapy.
- Patients with Hodgkin's lymphoma should preferably be enrolled into clinical trials.

Treatment

- In most centers, patients with early-stage favorable or early-stage unfavorable Hodgkin's lymphoma are treated with combined-modality strategies, including two to six cycles of polychemotherapy (e.g., ABVD) followed by radiotherapy to the involved field. The treatment for advanced stages consists of more cycles or more intensive regimens plus radiotherapy to possible residual masses.
- For patients relapsing after combined-modality treatment or patients with primary progressive disease, a high-dose chemotherapy regimen plus autologous stem cell transplantation still offers a definite chance of cure.
- In addition to excellent cure rates, modern treatment strategies also aim at reducing therapy-induced acute and long-term toxicities without loss of efficacy.

INTRODUCTION

Hodgkin's lymphoma, earlier called Hodgkin's disease, is one of the neoplastic diseases of the lymphatic tissue and was named after Thomas Hodgkin, who first described the disease in 1832.[1] It can basically be distinguished from other types of malignant lymphoma by presenting characteristic types of tumor cells, called Hodgkin and Reed-Sternberg (H-RS) cells, in a background of non-neoplastic cells such as lymphocytes, histiocytes, neutrophils, eosinophils, and monocytes.[2,3] The histologic subclassification of Hodgkin's lymphoma considers both the morphology and immunophenotype of the H-RS cells and the composition of the cellular background. The World Health Organization classification differentiates between the classic form of Hodgkin's lymphoma, with $CD30^+$ H-RS cells, and the nodular lymphocyte–predominant form of Hodgkin's lymphoma (NLPHL), with $CD20^+$ lymphocytic and histiocytic cells (Table 40–1).[4]

Early in the disease process, Hodgkin's lymphoma is typically restricted to the lymph nodes. However, lymphatic structures are often exceeded with progression of disease, which then results in organ involvement, mainly of the bone marrow, liver, or lungs. Without an effective therapy, the classic form of Hodgkin's lymphoma is fatal.

EPIDEMIOLOGY AND RISK FACTORS

Incidence

In Europe and the United States, the annual incidence of Hodgkin's lymphoma is about 2–3 per 100,000 persons at risk, and has stayed almost constant over the last decades.[5] As a result of great clinical progress in recent years, the mortality simultaneously improved significantly, particularly in the 1990s, from previous rates above 2 to a current mortality rate of about 0.5.[6]

Age and Histologic Distribution

In industrialized countries, the onset of Hodgkin's lymphoma has historically shown two peaks, one in the third decade and a second peak for patients older than 50 years. However, in more recent data, the second peak seems to disappear, because many large B-cell lymphomas of that age group were mistaken for the lymphocyte-depleted Hodgkin's lymphoma subtype in the past.[7] Slightly more men than women develop Hodgkin's lymphoma (1.4 : 1). Four of five men and three of four women develop Hodgkin's lymphoma prior to the age

TABLE 40–1. World Health Organization Classification of Hodgkin's Lymphoma

WHO Classification	Frequency
Classical Hodgkin's lymphoma	
Nodular sclerosis Hodgkin's lymphoma (grades 1 and 2)	60–70%
Mixed-cellularity Hodgkin's lymphoma	20–30%
Lymphocyte-rich classic Hodgkin's lymphoma	3–5%
Lymphocyte-depleted Hodgkin's lymphoma	0.8–1%
Nodular lymphocyte–predominant Hodgkin's lymphoma	3–5%

Adapted from Harris NL, Jaffe ES, Diebold J, et al: The World Health Organization classification of neoplastic diseases of the hematopoietic and lymphoid tissues. Report of the Clinical Advisory Committee meeting, Airlie House, Virginia, November, 1997. Ann Oncol 10:1419–1432, 1999.

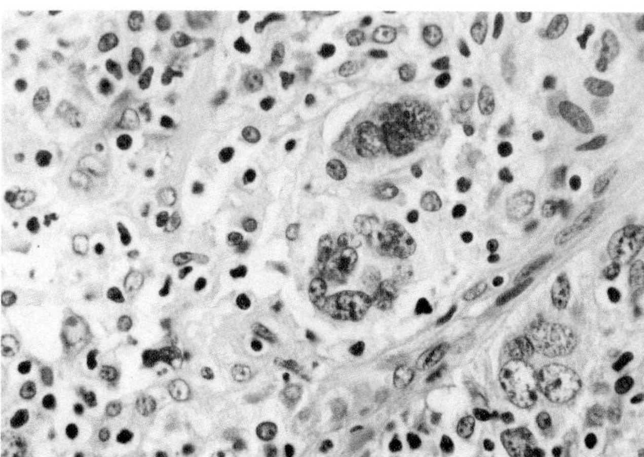

Figure 40–1. Histology of an affected lymph node. Staining reveals the typical giant mono- and multinucleated Hodgkin and Reed-Sternberg (H-RS) cells.

of 60, which is very early compared to most other malignancies.[8] The most common nodular-sclerosing subtype is notably expressed among young adults, whereas the frequency of the mixed-cellularity subtype increases with age. Other subtypes are diagnosed rather seldom in Western countries.[9]

Environmental Risk Factors

There is a noteworthy difference in the onset of Hodgkin's lymphoma between developing and industrialized countries. In developing countries, the disorder usually appears during childhood and the incidence decreases with age, whereas in industrialized countries, the first peak is viewed in young adulthood. Furthermore, in economically developed countries, the early occurrence of Hodgkin's lymphoma is often related to high maternal education, early birth order, low number of siblings and playmates, and single-family dwellings.[10,11]

An involvement of viral infections (e.g., Epstein-Barr virus [EBV]) in the pathogenesis of Hodgkin's lymphoma was suggested by several studies. Patients with a medical history of mononucleosis are at higher risk for development of Hodgkin's lymphoma.[12,13] In about 50% of cases of classic Hodgkin's lymphoma in industrialized countries, EBV DNA is present in the H-RS cells, predominantly in the mixed-cellularity subtype.[14] In contrast, underprivileged patients as well as patients from developing countries show EBV-positive H-RS cells in about 90% of cases.[15–17]

Genetic Factors

Genetic components seem to contribute to the appearance of Hodgkin's lymphoma, because family members are at a three- to ninefold increased risk of developing the same disease.[18,19] The analysis of monozygotic twin pairs, and the remarkable incidence with which both twins are affected, strongly support the idea of Hodgkin's lymphoma as a disorder involving a genetic imbalance.[20] However, no specific mechanism or genetic aberration has been identified so far, and familial Hodgkin's lymphoma appears to play only a role in a small subset of Hodgkin's lymphoma patients.

PATHOPHYSIOLOGY

For a long time, Hodgkin's lymphoma was considered as an infectious disease, as indicated by its former name, "lymphogranulomatosis." The giant mono- and multinucleated H-RS cells (Fig. 40–1) typically account for less than 1% of the affected tissue in classic Hodgkin's lymphoma, which made systematic analyses difficult in the past. The detection of their malignant clonal origin in microdissected cells by polymerase chain reaction was demonstrated only recently.[21] H-RS cells are derived from germinal-center B cells in more than 90% of cases[22]; however, in a small group of patients, the H-RS cells exhibit T-cell characteristics.[23]

In classic Hodgkin's lymphoma, immunophenotyping has demonstrated that H-RS cells stain positive for CD15 in about 80% and for CD30 in about 90% of cases. The activation of B-cell antigens has only been reported in a few cases.[24] In contrast, in NLPHL the lymphocytic and histiocytic cells are scattered in the nodular structures and are usually $CD45^+$. They express B-cell–associated antigens as CD20 in 98% of cases, but also express CD19, CD22, CD79a, and EMA; however, they lack CD15 and CD30.

Despite enormous efforts and progress in basic research, many key questions concerning transforming events and pathways, oncogenic viruses, and the exact mechanism(s) by which H-RS cells resist apoptosis in the germinal center still remain unanswered. Some reports suggest that nuclear factor-κB is a central effector of malignant transformation in classic Hodgkin's lymphoma by downregulation of an antiapoptotic signaling network.[25,26] Also, *LMP1* as an EBV-encoded gene may induce tumorigenesis in triggering nuclear factor-κB activation.[27]

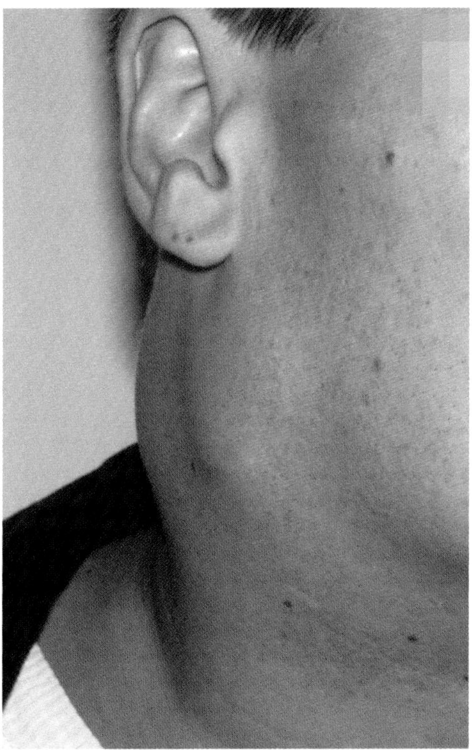

■ **Figure 40–2.** Cervical lymph node swelling in a young male with newly diagnosed Hodgkin's lymphoma.

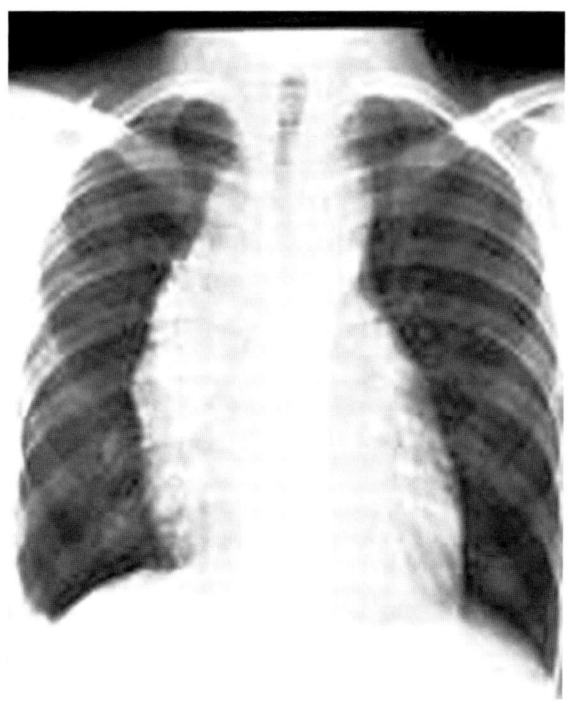

■ **Figure 40–3.** Intrathoracic involvement of Hodgkin's lymphoma: a mediastinal mass detected by chest radiograph.

CLINICAL FEATURES AND DIAGNOSIS

Symptoms and Signs

Usually, indolent swellings that are localized in the cervical or supraclavicular region in 60–70% of the cases are noticed, but axillary or inguinal lymph nodes are also often observed (Fig. 40–2). Almost two thirds of patients with newly diagnosed classic Hodgkin's lymphoma have radiographic evidence of intrathoracic involvement (Fig. 40–3). Symptoms caused by a large mediastinal mass include feeling of pressure, cough, venous congestion, or even dyspnea owing to tracheal compression or pericardial or pleural effusions. Hepato- or splenomegaly can indicate hepatic or splenic involvement, but affected organs can also present at normal size. In advanced stages, adjacent regions such as lung, pericardium, chest wall, or bone can be invaded, and patients sometimes suffer from osseous pain or neurologic or endocrinologic symptoms. The frequency of involvement of anatomic sites with disease in untreated patients is shown in Table 40–2. Compared to classic Hodgkin's lymphoma, NLPHL normally begins as a localized, slowly growing, and very benign entity with participation of only one peripheral nodal region, most often a cervical, axillary, or inguinal lymph node.

About 40% of patients, especially those with initial abdominal involvement or advanced-stage disease, demonstrate systemic symptoms called B symptoms, including fever greater than 38°C, nighttime sweating, and weight loss greater than 10% within the previous 6 months. Other symptoms comprise pain at the site of nodal involvement shortly after drinking alcohol, pruritus, and fatigue.

TABLE 40–2. Anatomic Sites of Disease Involved in Untreated Patients with Hodgkin's Lymphoma

Anatomic Site	Involvement (%)
Waldeyer's ring	1–2
Cervical nodes	60–70
Axillary nodes	30–35
Mediastinum	50–60
Hilar nodes	15–35
Para-aortic nodes	30–40
Iliac nodes	15–20
Mesenteric nodes	1–4
Inguinal nodes	8–15
Spleen	30–35
Liver	2–6
Bone marrow	1–4
Total extranodal	10–15

Modified from Gupta RK, Gospodarowicz MK, Lister TA: Clinical evaluation and staging of Hodgkin's disease. *In* Mauch PM, Armitage JO, Diehl V, et al (eds): Hodgkin's Disease. Philadelphia: Lippincott Williams & Wilkins, 1999, Chapter 15.

Physical Examination

The physical examination should include a thorough inspection and palpation of possibly involved nodal regions, as well as examination of the abdomen, the liver and spleen, and the spine and a thoracic auscultation.

Histology

An excisional biopsy of a suspicious lymph node should be performed to confirm the initial diagnosis of Hodgkin's lymphoma. Enough material should be extracted for diagnosis; however, "spacious debulking" to reduce tumor mass does not influence prognosis of Hodgkin's lymphoma. The assessment of bone marrow is important for disease staging and for establishing a baseline evaluation of normal bone marrow prior to therapy.

Laboratory Findings

Laboratory diagnostics are necessary to assess serologic risk factors and to check organ function to assess the feasibility of the therapy regimen. They should include differential blood counts, erythrocyte sedimentation rate, coagulation values, and levels of transaminases, alkaline phosphatase, γ-glutamyltransferase, lactate dehydrogenase, bilirubin, glucose, creatinine clearance, urea, uric acid, total protein, albumin, and thyroid-stimulating hormone. Also, tests should be performed to detect EBV, human immunodeficiency virus, and hepatitis B and C viruses.

Staging

Staging procedures have become less invasive in recent years. Nowadays, clinical staging methods include chest radiography; abdominal sonography; computed tomographic scans of the neck, thorax, abdomen and pelvis; bone marrow biopsy and aspiration; and bone marrow and/or skeletal radionuclide imaging. In some selected cases, additional procedures such as magnetic resonance imaging, positron emission tomography, or a liver biopsy may be indicated. Pathologic staging procedures such as laparotomy or splenectomy to assess occult infradiaphragmatic disease are no longer carried out routinely because of the severe side effects accompanying these procedures (i.e., overwhelming postsplenectomy infection [OPSI syndrome], a bacterial sepsis that occurs after splenectomy). Also, pathologic staging is no longer needed because better imaging techniques are available and because systemic chemotherapy is currently given to the majority of patients in early stages.

The extent of Hodgkin's lymphoma at diagnosis is described according to the Ann Arbor classification (devised at the Ann Arbor Conference in 1971).[28] The presence of clinical (e.g., B symptoms, bulky disease), biologic (e.g., age, gender), and serologic (e.g., high erythrocyte sedimentation rate) risk factors further discriminates the prognosis of Hodgkin's lymphoma patients, and these factors help to tailor risk-adapted modern therapy. The Cotswold classification, which was proposed during a meeting in Cotswold, England, in 1989, is the latest modification of the Ann Arbor classification. The Cotswold classification supplements the Ann Arbor classification with additional information on prognostic clinical, biologic, and laboratory factors: the number and location of anatomic sites involved, and the presence of bulky nodal disease, extranodal extension of disease, and subdiaphragmatic involvement (Table 40–3).[29]

DIFFERENTIAL DIAGNOSIS

The differential diagnosis of Hodgkin's lymphoma includes all types of benign or malignant lymph node

TABLE 40–3. The Cotswold Staging Classification for Hodgkin's Lymphoma

Cotswold Staging Classification	
Stage I	Involvement of a single lymph node region or lymphoid structure (e.g., spleen, thymus, Waldeyer's ring) or involvement of a single extralymphatic site (IE)
Stage II	Involvement of two or more lymph node regions on the same side of the diaphragm; localized contiguous involvement of only one extranodal organ or site and lymph node region(s) on the same side of the diaphragm (IIE).
	The number of anatomic regions involved should be indicated by a subscript (e.g., II_3)
Stage III	Involvement of lymph node regions on both sides of the diaphragm (III), which may also be accompanied by involvement of the spleen (IIIS) or by localized contiguous involvement of only one extranodal organ site (IIIE), or both (IIISE)
	III_1 With or without involvement of splenic, hilar, celiac, or portal nodes
	III_2 With involvement of para-aortic, iliac, and mesenteric nodes
Stage IV	Diffuse or disseminated involvement of one or more extranodal organs or tissues, with or without associated lymph node involvement
Designations Applicable to Any Disease Stage	
A	No symptoms
B	Fever (temperature > 38°C), drenching night sweats, unexplained loss of 10% of body weight within the preceding 6 mo
X	Bulky disease (a widening of the mediastinum by > one third of the presence of a nodal mass with a maximal dimension > 10 cm)
E	Involvement of a single extranodal site that is contiguous or proximal to the known nodal site
CS	Clinical stage
PS	Pathologic stage (as determined by laparotomy)

Modified from Lister T, Crowther D, Sutcliffe S, et al: Report of a committee convened to discuss the evaluation and staging of patients with Hodgkin's disease: Cotswold meeting. J Clin Oncol 7:1630–1636, 1989.

swelling caused by other types of lymphoma or cancer or by infectious or reactive diseases (Table 40–4). Hodgkin's lymphoma is exclusively diagnosed by a pathologist by analyzing samples that were extracted from affected tissue by biopsy (fine-needle puncture mostly offers insufficient material to specify the diagnosis). Sometimes the differential diagnosis between Hodgkin's lymphoma and certain types of non-Hodgkin's lymphoma can be very challenging. In particular, the borderline between diffuse large B-cell lymphoma and NLPHL can pose difficulties, as can the distinction between T-cell/histiocyte-rich large B-cell lymphoma and mixed-cellularity Hodgkin's lymphoma or NLPHL, and between large B-cell lymphoma, anaplastic $CD30^+$ type, and lymphocyte-depleted variants of Hodgkin's lymphoma (Fig. 40–4).

TREATMENT

Choice of Treatment

In patients with Hodgkin's lymphoma, the treatment decision is made according to stage and risk factor pattern. Unlike the situation in non-Hodgkin's lymphoma, the histologic subtype—except in the lymphocyte-predominant type—does not guide the treatment decision. Patients are usually assigned either to a group with anatomically localized disease, which is called early-stage Hodgkin's lymphoma or to a group with anatomically more disseminated disease, which is called advanced-stage Hodgkin's lymphoma. Risk factors discriminate between an early-stage favorable group, which includes patients in stage I or II without risk factors, and an early-stage unfavorable (or intermediate) group, which comprises those in stage I or II with certain risk factors (Table 40–5). Stage III and IV patients are generally allocated to the advanced-stage risk group.

The recognized stages and risk factors differ slightly among the various countries and study groups in Europe and the United States, but have become comparable in principle. Typically, the clinically most relevant prognostic factors for stratifying patients are the stage of

TABLE 40–4. Differential Diagnosis of Hodgkin's Lymphoma

Other lymphatic neoplasms (e.g., non-Hodgkin's lymphoma)
Metastases of other solid tumors
Lymphadenopathy of infectious origin
Bacterial (e.g., purulent or tuberculous manifestations)
Viral (e.g., EBV [infectious mononucleosis], HIV, CMV)
Fungal (e.g., coccidioidomycosis)
Parasitic (e.g., toxoplasmosis)
Lymphadenopathy of reactive origin
Sarcoidosis
Diseases of the soft tissues
Diseases of the skin
Medications (e.g., diphenylhydantoin)

Abbreviations: CMV, cytomegalovirus; EBV, Epstein-Barr virus; HIV, human immunodeficiency virus.

HODGKIN'S LYMPHOMA: DIFFERENTIAL DIAGNOSIS

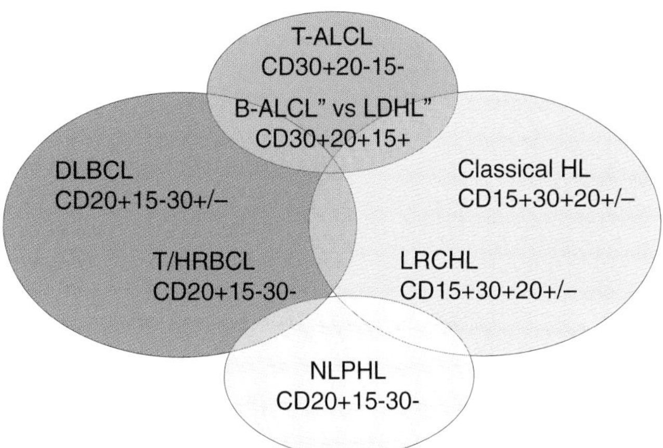

Figure 40–4. Differential diagnosis of Hodgkin's lymphoma (HL). There is morphologic overlap between classic HL, lymphocyte-rich classic HL (LRCHL), nodular lymphocyte-predominant HL (NLPHL), lymphocyte-depleted HL (LDHL), T-cell–rich/histiocyte-rich large B-cell lymphoma (T/HRBCL), B-cell anaplastic large-cell lymphoma (B-ALCL), and T-cell anaplastic large-cell lymphoma (T-ALCL). Immunophenotyping can be useful in the differential diagnosis.

TABLE 40–5. Definition of Treatment Groups According to the EORTC/GELA and GHSG

Treatment Group	EORTC/GELA	GHSG
Early-stage favorable	CS I–II without risk factors (supradiaphragmatic)	CS I–II without risk factors
Early-stage unfavorable (intermediate)	CS I–II with ≥1 risk factor (supradiaphragmatic)	CS I, CSIIA with ≥1 risk factor; CS IIB with risk factors C/D but without risk factors A/B
Advanced stage	CS III–IV	CS IIB with risk factors A/B CS III–IV
Risk factors (RF)	A: Large mediastinal mass B: Age ≥ 50 yr C: Elevated ESR* D: ≥4 involved regions	A: Large mediastinal mass B: Extranodal disease C: Elevated ESR* D: ≥3 involved regions

*Erythrocyte sedimentation rate 50 mm/hr or greater without or 30 mm/hr or greater with B symptoms.
Abbreviations: EORTC, European Organization for Research and Treatment of Cancer; GELA, Groupe d'Études des Lymphomes de l'Adulte; GHSG, German Hodgkin Lymphoma Study Group.

TABLE 40–6. Polychemotherapy Regimens Used in the Treatment of Hodgkin's Lymphoma

Seldom/Formerly Used Regimens	Drug Combination				Reference
MOPP	Mechlorethamine, Oncovin (vincristine), procarbazine, prednisone				58,59,60
COPP	Cyclophosphamide, Oncovin (vincristine), procarbazine, prednisone				52,57,65
LOPP	Leukeran (chlorambucil), Oncovin (vincristine), procarbazine, prednisone				61
EBVP	Epirubicin, bleomycin, vinblastine, prednisone				45
VAPEC-B	Vincristine, Adriamycin (doxorubicin), prednisolone, etoposide, cyclophosphamide, bleomycin				69
ChlVPP/EVA	Chlorambucil, vinblastine, procarbazine, prednisolone, etoposide, vincristine, Adriamycin (doxorubicin)				69
MEC	Mechlorethamine, CCNU (lomustine), vindesine, Alkeran (melphalan), prednisone, epidoxorubicin, vincristine, procarbazine, vinblastine, bleomycin				70
IMEP	Ifosfamide, methotrexate, etoposide, prednisone				52,65
Commonly Used Regimens	**Drug Combination**	**Dose (mg/m²)**	**Route**	**Schedule (days)**	**Reference**
ABVD/ABV/AVD/AV (Cycle length: 28 days)	Adriamycin (doxorubicin)	25	IV	1 + 15	49,53
	Bleomycin	10	IV	1 + 15	
	Vinblastine	6	IV	1 + 15	
	Dacarbazine	375	IV	1 + 15	
BEACOPP baseline/escalated (Cycle length 21 days)		Baseline/escalated			57,71,72,73
	Bleomycin	10	IV	8	
	Etoposide	100/200	IV	1–3	
	Adriamycin (doxorubicin)	25/35	IV	1	
	Cyclophosphamide	650/1250	IV	1	
	Oncovin (vincristine)	1.4 (max. 2mg)	IV	8	
	Procarbazine	100	PO	1–7	
	Prednisone	40	PO	1–14	
	G-CSF (for escalated regimen)			From day 8	
BEACOPP-14	Like BEACOPP baseline but with a cycle length of only 14 days (Prednisone 80 mg/m² days 1–7; G-CSF from day 8)				
Stanford V (12 wk)*	Mechlorethamine	6	IV	Wk 1, 5, 9	68
	Adriamycin (doxorubicin)	25	IV	Wk 1, 3, 5, 7, 9, 11	
	Vinblastine	6	IV	Wk 1, 3, 5, 7, 9, 11	
	Vincristine	1.4 (max. 2mg)	IV	Wk 2, 4, 6, 8, 10, 12	
	Bleomycin	5	IV	Wk 2, 4, 6, 8, 10, 12	
	Etoposide	60 × 2	IV	Wk 3, 7, 11	
	Prednisone	40	PO	Wk 1–10, every 2 days	
	G-CSF			After dose reduction or delay	

*Dose reductions for patients over 50.
Abbreviation: G-CSF, granulocyte colony-stimulating factor.

disease and the presence of systemic B symptoms. Great tumor burden (e.g., bulk >10 cm or mediastinal mass one third of the thoracic diameter or more) has been accepted as an unfavorable factor by most groups.

In the United States, patients are typically treated in accordance with the classifications of early stages (I to IIA or IIB) and advanced stages (I to IIB with bulky disease or III to IVA or IVB). Additionally, the Canada Clinical Trial Group and the Eastern Cooperative Oncology Group (ECOG) subdivide early-stage Hodgkin's lymphoma into a low- and a high-risk group. The low-risk category comprises patients less than 40 years of age with NLPHL or nodular sclerosing histology with an erythrocyte sedimentation rate less than 50 mm/hr and the involvement of three or fewer nodal regions, whereas the high-risk category includes all other stage I and II patients, excluding those with bulky disease (>10 cm). In Europe, The European Organization for Research and Treatment of Cancer (EORTC), the Groupe d'Études des Lymphomes de l'Adulte (GELA), and the German Hodgkin Lymphoma Study Group (GHSG) have assigned patients in early stages (I and II) to favorable or unfavorable (or intermediate) groups depending on the risk factors listed in Table 40–5.

The drug combinations of all chemotherapy regimens mentioned in the following discussion are identified in Table 40–6.

Early-Stage Favorable Hodgkin's Lymphoma

History

During the past years, treatment strategies for early-stage favorable Hodgkin's lymphoma have strikingly changed. For a long time, extended-field irradiation to all initially

TABLE 40–7. Selected Trials for Early-Stage Favorable Hodgkin's Lymphoma

Trial*	Therapy Regimen†	# Pts.	Outcome‡	Ref.
SWOG #9133	A. 3 cycles AV + STLI (36–40 Gy)	165	FFTF 94%; SV 98% (3 yr)	42
	B. STLI (36–40 Gy)	161	FFTF 81%; SV 96% (3 yr)	
Stanford V (CSI–IIA)	8 wk Stanford V + modified IF RT (30 Gy)	65	FFP 94.6%; SV 96.6% (16 mo; estimated for 3 yr)	43
Milan 1990–97	A. 4 cycles ABVD + STLI	65	FFP 97%; SV 93% (5 yr)	44
	B. 4 cycles ABVD + IF RT	68	FFP 97%; SV 93% (5 yr)	
EORTC/GELA H7F	A. 6 cycles EBVP + IF RT (36 Gy)	168	RFS 90%; SV 98% (5 yr)	45
	B. STNI	165	RFS 81%; SV 95% (5 yr)	
EORTC/GELA H8F	A. 3 cycles MOPP/ABV + IF RT (36 Gy)	271	RFS 99%; SV 99% (4 yr)	46
	B. STNI	272	RFS 80%; SV 95% (4 yr)	
EORTC/GELA H9F	A. 6 cycles EBVP + IF RT (36 Gy)		Ongoing trial	47
	B. 6 cycles EBVP + IF RT (20 Gy)		Arm C (no RT) closed because of high relapse rate	
	C. 6 cycles EBVP			
GHSG HD7	A. EF RT 30 Gy (40 Gy IF RT)	305	FFTF 75%; SV 94% (5 yr)	48
	B. 2 cycles ABVD + EF RT 30 Gy (40 Gy IF RT)	312	FFTF 91%; SV 94% (5 yr)	
GHSG HD10	A. 4 cycles ABVD + IF RT (30 Gy)		No final results	
	B. 4 cycles ABVD + IF RT (20 Gy)		2-yr follow-up: FFTF 96.6%; SV 98.5%	
	C. 2 cycles ABVD + IF RT (30 Gy)			
	D. 2 cycles ABVD + IF RT (20 Gy)			
GHSG HD13	A. 2 cycles ABVD + IF RT (30 Gy)		Ongoing trial	
	B. 2 cycles ABV + IF RT (30 Gy)			
	C. 2 cycles AVD + IF RT (30 Gy)			
	D. 2 cycles AV + IF RT (30 Gy)			

*EORTC, European Organization for Research and Treatment of Cancer, GELA, Groupe d'Études des Lymphomes de l'Adulte; GHSG, German Hodgkin Lymphoma Study Group; SWOG, Southwest Oncology Group.

†EF RT, extended-field radiotherapy; IF RT, involved-field radiotherapy; STLI, subtotal lymphoid irradiation; STNI, subtotal nodal irradiation. Drug combinations of chemotherapy regimens are listed in Table 40–6.

‡FFTF, freedom from treatment failure; FFP, freedom from progression; RFS, relapse-free survival; SV, overall survival.

Modified from Diehl V, Stein H, Hummel M, et al: Hodgkin's lymphoma: biology and treatment strategies for primary, refractory, and relapsed disease. Hematology (Am Soc Hematol Educ Program) 225–472, 2003.

involved and adjacent lymph node regions was regarded as standard treatment. As a sole treatment modality, extended-field radiotherapy was primarily administered to a total dose of 40 Gy. Kaplan demonstrated a close relationship between radiation dose and cure rates up to 40 Gy, above which toxicity becomes excessive.[30] Over the next 30 years, therapy evolved as research showed the advantages of combination chemotherapy prior to radiotherapy, resulting in a dramatic drop in 10-year risk of failure.[31,32] The introduction of involved-field radiotherapy, restricted to initially involved lymph node regions, became possible when irradiation was combined with prior short-duration chemotherapy for control of occult lesions. However, longer follow-up of patients who underwent extended-field irradiation revealed significant late sequelae as competing causes of deaths. Long-term treatment–related events included subsequent death from heart disease,[33,34] pulmonary dysfunction,[35] thyroid disease,[36] and secondary malignancies.[37–40] When radiotherapy alone was given, a superior outcome was proven for patients treated with the extended-field technique compared with the involved-field technique.[32] Other results demonstrated a superior overall survival after extended-field radiotherapy compared to MOPP chemotherapy alone; patients relapsing after irradiation alone were more likely to achieve a second complete remission.[41]

Trials

Many randomized studies confirmed the superiority of combined-modality treatment versus radiotherapy alone. Further clinical trials were conducted to analyze radiation fields and doses and determine the optimal chemotherapy regimen in early favorable stages (Table 40–7).

The Southwest Oncology Group demonstrated that patients treated with combined-modality therapy consisting of three cycles of doxorubicin and vinblastine followed by subtotal lymphoid irradiation (STLI) had a markedly superior outcome in terms of freedom from treatment failure than those only receiving STLI.[42] Other studies from Milan and Stanford revealed that STLI can be effectively replaced by involved-field radiotherapy after short-duration chemotherapy (ABVD or Stanford V), while maintaining high freedom from progression and high survival rates.[43,44] The EORTC-GELA group demonstrated that combined-modality therapy with either six cycles of EBVP (H7F trial) or three cycles of MOPP/ABV (H8F trial) followed by involved-field radiotherapy yielded a significant better event-free survival than subtotal nodal irradiation alone.[45,46] The aim of the ongoing H9F trial was to evaluate a dose reduction of radiotherapy (36 Gy vs. 20 Gy vs. no radiotherapy) after administering six cycles of EBVP. However, the arm without radiotherapy had to be closed because of numerous relapses.[47] In the GHSG, a combined-modality approach was first established by the HD7 trial, in which two cycles of ABVD plus extended-field radiotherapy was shown to be superior to extended-field radiotherapy alone in terms of freedom from treatment failure.[48] Overall survival was equal in both arms because of a very effective salvage treatment. The HD10 trial was then performed to study a possible reduction of chemotherapy (two vs. four cycles of ABVD) or involved-field radiotherapy (20 vs. 30 Gy). Interim results after 2 years suggest no differences in treatment results either between the number of cycles of chemotherapy or between the different doses of radiotherapy applied. Because improvement of treatment results for early favorable stages may realistically have reached its limits, the aim of the ongoing HD13 trial is to omit certain chemotherapeutic drugs because of their toxicity profile, hopefully without loss of efficacy. Currently, patients are randomized to two cycles of ABVD, ABV, AVD, or AV followed by 30-Gy involved-field radiotherapy.

Standard Treatment

Most centers and groups in Europe and the United States have accepted combined-modality treatment, consisting of two to four cycles of chemotherapy (e.g., ABVD) followed by involved-field radiotherapy as standard treatment for early favorable stages. The only exception is NLPHL subtype stage IA without any risk factors. Taking into account the favorable prognosis, the EORTC and the GHSG currently recommend treatment with 30-Gy involved-field radiation only after careful staging for stage IA NLPHL.

Early-Stage Unfavorable (Intermediate-Stage) Hodgkin's Lymphoma

History

For the early-stage unfavorable (or intermediate) category of Hodgkin's lymphoma, a combined-modality treatment strategy was established much earlier than for early-stage favorable disease. However, there was a strong desire to define the best therapy regimen. On the one hand, a detoxification of therapy could be attained by reducing the radiation dose and field size. On the other hand, the aim was to improve the efficacy of chemotherapy by altering the type of drugs and the number of cycles, without compromising the effect by inducing severe toxicities. In the 1960s, MOPP- or COPP-like regimens were predominantly used. The ABVD regimen was first introduced and described by Bonnadonna and associates in 1975.[49] Alternating or hybridization of this ABVD regimen with a MOPP- or COPP-like regimen did not achieve superior outcome compared with ABVD alone.[50–52] Currently four cycles of ABVD are considered the standard chemotherapy regimen in the treatment of early-stage unfavorable Hodgkin's lymphoma. This consensus basically emerged from studies for advanced-stage Hodgkin's lymphoma: ABVD alone was shown to be equally effective and less myelotoxic than alternating MOPP + ABVD, and both were superior to MOPP alone in the treatment of advanced stages.[53]

Trials

Radiotherapy to the extended field has been superseded by involved-field treatment, a change that does not compromise the efficacy of treatment (Table 40–8). A cooperative study compared six cycles of MOPP sandwiched around 40 Gy of radiotherapy applied with either the involved-field or extended-field technique. Results from 173 patients reported no difference in terms of disease-free survival or overall survival.[54] An Italian study headed by the Milan group entered 140 patients with early favorable (see Table 40–7) and unfavorable stages into a randomized trial comparing STLI with involved-field radiotherapy after four cycles of ABVD. Treatment outcome was similar in both arms. The largest trial investigating this issue was performed by the GHSG (HD8 trial). A total of 1204 patients were randomly assigned to two alternating cycles of COPP/ABVD plus radiotherapy using either the extended-field or the involved-field technique. Final results at 5 years did not reveal any differences in terms of response, freedom from treatment failure, or overall survival between the two treatment arms; however, more acute toxicities from radiotherapy, and a tendency for more long-term toxicities, were reported in the extended-field radiotherapy arm.[55] In the H8U trial, the EORTC compared six cycles of MOPP/ABV + 36-Gy involved-field radiotherapy with four cycles of MOPP/ABV + 36-Gy involved-field radiotherapy and four cycles of MOPP/ABV + STLI. Again, there was no difference among the arms, including the different types of radiotherapy given, in terms of response rates, failure-free survival, or overall survival.[56]

Despite the excellent results obtained by ABVD + radiotherapy, about 15% of patients with early-stage unfavorable disease still relapse within the first 5 years and another 5% or so still suffer from primary progressive disease. Thus, ongoing trials are analyzing combined-modality protocols comparing ABVD with more intense, novel regimens that were previously used for the treatment of advanced stages. The EORTC trial H9U as well as the recently closed GHSG trial HD11 compared four cycles of ABVD with four cycles of BEACOPP baseline regimen, and a current ECOG trial (E2496) is evaluating the role of the Stanford V chemotherapy regimen. In addition, two large trials (EORTC H8U and H9U) are currently analyzing whether four cycles of combined-modality treatment are as effective as six cycles. The ongoing HD14 trial of the GHSG is administering the BEACOPP escalated regimen, which was shown to be very effective in the treatment of advanced-stage Hodgkin's lymphoma, to patients with early-stage unfavorable disease.[57]

Standard Treatment

Currently, the "gold standard" for patients in early unfavorable stages is a combined-modality treatment with four (to six) courses of effective chemotherapy, typically ABVD, followed by radiotherapy with 30 Gy to the involved field.

TABLE 40–8. Selected Trials for Early-Stage Unfavorable/Intermediate Stage Hodgkin's Lymphoma

Trial*	Therapy Regimen†	# Pts.	Outcome‡	Ref.
EORTC/GELA H7U	A. 6 cycles EBVP + IF RT (36 Gy)	160	RFS 68%; SV 82% (6 yr)	47
	B. MOPP/ABV + IF RT	156	RFS 90%; SV 89% (6 yr)	
EORTC/GELA H8U	A. 6 cycles MOPP/ABV + IF RT (36 Gy)	335	RFS 94%; SV 90% (4 yr)	47,56
	B. 4 cycles MOPP/ABV + IF RT (36 Gy)	333	RFS 95%; SV 95% (4 yr)	
	C. 4 cycles MOPP/ABV + STNI	327	RFS 96%; SV 93% (4 yr)	
EORTC/GELA H9U	A. 6 cycles ABVD + IF RT		Ongoing trial	47
	B. 4 cycles ABVD + IF RT			
	C. 4 cycles BEACOPP + IF RT			
SWOG/ECOG #2496	A. 6 cycles ABVD + IF RT (36 Gy) to bulk (>5 cm)		Ongoing trial	
	B. 12 wk Stanford V + IF RT (36 Gy) to bulk (>5 cm)			
GHSG HD8	A. 2 cycles COPP + ABVD + EF RT (30 Gy) + bulk (10 Gy)	532	FFTF 86%; SV 91% (5 yr)	55
	B. 2 cycles COPP + ABVD + IF RT (30 Gy) + bulk (10 Gy)	532	FFTF 84%; SV 92% (5 yr)	
GHSG HD11	A. 4 cycles ABVD + IF RT (30 Gy)		No final results	
	B. 4 cycles ABVD + IF RT (20 Gy)		2-yr follow-up: FFTF 97.4%; SV 89.9%	
	C. 4 cycles BEACOPP baseline + IF RT (30 Gy)			
	D. 4 cycles BEACOPP baseline + IF RT (20 Gy)			
GHSG HD14	A. 4 cycles ABVD + IF RT (30 Gy)		Ongoing trial	
	B. 2 cycles BEACOPP escalated + 2 ABVD + IF RT (30 Gy)			

*ECOG, Eastern Cooperative Oncology Group; EORTC, European Organization for Research and Treatment of Cancer; GELA, Groupe d'Études des Lymphomes de l'Adulte; GHSG, German Hodgkin Lymphoma Study Group; SWOG, Southwest Oncology Group.
†EF RT, extended-field radiotherapy; IF RT, involved-field radiotherapy; STNI, subtotal nodal irradiation. Drug combinations of chemotherapy regimens are listed in Table 40–6.
‡FFTF, freedom from treatment failure; RFS, relapse-free survival; SV, overall survival.
Modified from Diehl V, Stein H, Hummel M, et al: Hodgkin's lymphoma: biology and treatment strategies for primary, refractory, and relapsed disease. Hematology (Am Soc Hematol Educ Program) 225–472, 2003.

Advanced-Stage Hodgkin's Lymphoma

History and Current Trials

The first polychemotherapy regimen that was applied for advanced stages of Hodgkin's lymphoma by de Vita and colleagues at the National Cancer Institute was a combination of drugs called MOPP.[58–60] For the first time, cure rates of about 50% were achieved. The same regimen with cyclophosphamide (COPP) or Leukeran (LOPP) instead of mechlorethamine presented similar efficacy.[61] The ABVD regimen showed the advantage of inducing fewer acute toxicities, particular concerning sterility, compared to MOPP.[62,63] Large multicenter trials proved the superiority of ABVD and alternating MOPP + ABVD versus MOPP alone.[53,64] Hybrid regimens such as MOPP/ABV were demonstrated to be as effective as alternating MOPP + ABVD.[50] Alternating more substances (e.g., COPP/ABV/IMEP versus COPP/ABVD) did not result in better outcome, either.[65] However, results from a randomized comparison of ABVD and MOPP/ABV hybrid showed a greater incidence of acute toxicity, myelodysplastic syndrome, and leukemia with MOPP/ABV.[51] Thus, ABVD is considered the accepted standard against which all new combinations have to be compared.

The New Generation of Regimens

Long-term follow-up of over 15 years shows a progression-free survival of about 50% and an overall survival of about 65% for patients in advanced stages treated with ABVD.[66] Different study groups have made attempts to improve these rates by developing new regimens with additional drugs such as etoposide and by employing dose intensification, which became possible with the availability of colony-stimulating factors and modern antibiotics. The seven-drug regimen known as Stanford V was shown to be effective in a Phase II trial of 142 patients, with a 5-year freedom from progression of 89% and an overall survival rate of 96% at a median of 5.4 years.[67,68] The Manchester group developed the VAPEC-B and the ChlVPP/EVA regimens and demonstrated a significantly superior outcome with ChlVPP/EVA compared to VAPEC-B in a trial with 282 patients.[69] An Italian intergroup trial pointed at better failure-free survival rates for MEC and ABVD versus Stanford V after 3 years.[70] The GHSG first developed the BEACOPP baseline regimen on the basis of the earlier COPP/ABVD regimen, without vinblastine and dacarbazine but with addition of etoposide and given in a 22-day cycle. After confirming the feasibility of the regimen, the dosage was increased from the amount used in the baseline regimen to that used in the escalated BEACOPP regimen.[71–73] Results from a large randomized multicenter trial comparing the COPP/ABVD, BEACOPP baseline, and BEACOPP escalated regimens provided the proof of concept. For 1195 patients, the 5-year rates of freedom from treatment failure were 69% in the COPP/ABVD group, 76% in the BEACOPP baseline group, and 87% in the BEACOPP escalated group. The overall survival rates were 83%, 88%, and 91%, respectively.[57] However, BEACOPP is associated with a higher rate of toxic effects compared to ABVD, including hematologic toxicities, sterility, and the occurrence of late effects such as acute myeloid leukemia and myelodysplastic syndrome, the latter mainly associated with etoposide.[74,75] For both the ABVD and the BEACOPP regimens, especially when combined with radiotherapy, pulmonary toxicity can be quite severe, requiring discontinuation of bleomycin because of respiratory impairment or even failure.

A recently initiated EORTC global trial (#20012) was designed to ascertain whether escalated BEACOPP is superior to ABVD by comparing eight cycles of ABVD with four cycles of BEACOPP escalated plus four courses of BEACOPP baseline.[47] A further intensification of induction therapy of high-risk patients by replacing the second four of eight cycles of ABVD with high-dose therapy and autologous stem cell transplantation did not result in better outcome compared with conventional treatment after 5 years.[76]

Role of Radiotherapy

The benefit of consolidating radiotherapy in the treatment of advanced stages of Hodgkin's lymphoma is not definitively certain, but irradiation contributes to late toxicities, especially solid tumors, including breast, lung, gastrointestinal, urogenital, bone, and soft tissue cancer.[77–79] The risk of second cancer significantly increases with younger age at first treatment.[37,38,80] Recent results provide evidence that particularly the risk of breast cancer strongly depends on the age at first treatment, on the hormonal status, and on the radiation dose given.[81] The relative risk of breast and lung cancer greatly increases with increasing radiation field size.[39,40] Therefore, trials currently evaluate the value of radiotherapy after successful chemotherapy for advanced Hodgkin's lymphoma. The EORTC recently demonstrated that irradiation did not improve outcome in patients who had already achieved a complete remission after six to eight cycles of MOPP/ABV.[82] Results of the recently terminated HD12 trial and the ongoing HD15 trial of the GHSG will help to shed some light on this emotionally charged topic. In the HD15 trial, the effectiveness of chemotherapy with or without radiotherapy is being tested by only applying 30-Gy radiotherapy to residual tumor masses of more than 2.5 cm that are positron emission tomography positive. Several controlled trials were also evaluated by a meta-analysis comparing combined-modality approaches versus chemotherapy alone. Results pointed at equal rates of tumor control and even better rates of overall survival in patients treated only with chemotherapy.[83]

Standard Treatment

In many centers, ABVD plus application of consolidating radiotherapy to residual disease is considered the gold standard for patients with advanced-stage Hodgkin's lymphoma. However, the question about the optimal chemotherapy combination for advanced stages is not yet fully answered. In spite of higher toxicities, the GHSG recommends the BEACOPP escalated regimen because of its significant better outcome rates at 5 years, at least for high-risk patients with more than two risk factors according to the International Prognostic Score (Table 40–9).[84] Longer follow-up periods will further elucidate the balance between the initial response rates and long-term side effects of the different regimens.

TABLE 40–9. International Prognostic Score Factors*

Serum albumin < 4 gm/dL
Hemoglobin < 10.5 gm/dL
Male sex
Age of 45 yr or older
Stage IV disease (according to the Ann Arbor classification)
Leukocytosis (at least 15,000/mm³)
Lymphocytopenia (<600/mm³ or <8% of white cell count, or both)

*For advanced stages, a number of adverse prognostic factors present at diagnosis were analyzed by the International Prognostic Score (IPS). The seven factors listed were significant in the final Cox regression model (relative risk: 1.26–1.49; *P* value: <.001 to <.011).

Patients with two or more of these factors have worse prognosis without more intense treatment.

Adapted from Hasenclever D, Diehl V: A prognostic score for advanced Hodgkin's disease. International Prognostic Factors Project on Advanced Hodgkin's Disease. N Engl J Med 339:1506–1514, 1998.

Relapsed or Refractory Hodgkin's Lymphoma

Patients with relapsed Hodgkin's lymphoma basically have a fair chance for permanent cure with salvage therapy. This salvage therapy can consist of salvage radiotherapy, conventional salvage chemotherapy, antibody treatment in selected cases, or high-dose chemotherapy followed by autologous stem cell transplantation. The choice of therapy depends on a diversity of factors, including initial stage and histology of disease, initial treatment, time since end of treatment, and stage and site of relapse as well as patient age, general condition, and concomitant disease. Therefore, it is important to consult an experienced hemato-oncologist or hematology center before deciding on the treatment strategy. In addition, a complete staging should always be performed, as for initial disease. Also, relapse should be histologically confirmed and a secondary non-Hodgkin's lymphoma should be excluded.[85]

Patients who relapse after initial radiotherapy for early-stage disease often achieve long-lasting remissions with conventional chemotherapy. However, patients relapsing after initial chemotherapy most often require a special salvage regimen such as high-dose therapy with peripheral blood stem cell transplantation (PBSCT). The introduction of PBSCT and growth factors, such as granulocyte colony-stimulating factor, has allowed higher doses of drugs in more effective and aggressive regimens (e.g., BEAM). The strategy has been shown to produce 30–65% long-term disease-free survival in selected patients with refractory and relapsed Hodgkin's lymphoma.[86–89]

Furthermore, two randomized trials that acknowledge the superiority of high-dose chemotherapy plus PBSCT were published. In a trial conducted by the British National Lymphoma Investigation (BNLI), patients with relapsed or refractory Hodgkin's lymphoma receiving high-dose BEAM with autologous stem cell transplantation fared significantly better than those treated with conventional-dose mini-BEAM, resulting in a 3-year event-free survival of 53% versus 10%.[90] In the HD-R1 trial of the GHSG, chemosensitive patients who relapsed after chemotherapy were randomized to four cycles of Dexa-BEAM or two cycles of Dexa-BEAM followed by BEAM and PBSCT. Final results demonstrated a higher rate of freedom from treatment failure in the transplanted group (55% vs. 34%), whereas overall survival did not differ significantly.[91]

The success of a high-dose chemotherapy regimen followed by PBSCT is not only dependent upon prognostic factors such as tumor burden or chemosensitivity. A prognostic score based on treatment outcome of patients with relapsed Hodgkin's lymphoma also defined the time to relapse, the clinical stage at relapse, and the presence of anemia as independent risk factors.[92] The DHAP regimen was shown to be very effective in reducing tumor mass prior to high-dose therapy.[93] Currently, the HD-R2 trial of the GSHG and EORTC for patients with relapsed Hodgkin's lymphoma is evaluating the role of additional sequential therapy with high-dose single drugs (cyclophosphamide, methotrexate/vincristine, and etoposide) prior to BEAM and PBSCT.[94]

Allogeneic stem cell transplantation is not considered a standard treatment in patients with relapsed Hodgkin's lymphoma so far, basically because of high rates of transplantation-associated mortality. However, most observations include multiple pretreated patients in poor medical condition with an unfavorable risk profile. The alternative of a "mini-allogeneic transplant" with reduced nonmyeloablative conditioning prior to transplantation shows much lower mortality rates, but is still experimental.[95,96]

Experimental Treatment Approaches

Experimental approaches in the treatment of Hodgkin's lymphoma include passive immunotherapy with antibody-based regimens for specific targeting of malignant cells and active immunotherapy with modulation of cellular response by cytokines, tumor vaccines, or gene transfer. Currently the anti-CD20 antibody rituximab is available for treatment of NLPHL at diagnosis or relapse, but the follow-up of studies is still short.[97,98] The use of human monoclonal anti-CD30 antibody is currently being tested for patients with $CD30^+$ refractory lymphoma.[99,100]

SUPPORTIVE CARE AND LONG-TERM MANAGEMENT

Palliative Treatment

Depending on the number and character of relapses, previous therapies, the patient's age, and the presence of concomitant disease, clinicians should carefully evaluate whether a curative or a palliative approach is chosen. A palliative regimen can still achieve satisfactory abatement of pain and disorders, improve general condition, and lead to partial, sometimes long-lasting, remissions. A promising alternative is monotherapy with gemcitabine, vinorelbine, vinblastine, idarubicin, or etoposide. These drugs can be used alone or potentially combined with corticosteroids. In a Phase II study, gemcitabine proved to be a suitable and well-tolerated substance, even for patients with multiple relapses.[101] Efforts are underway to incorporate gemcitabine into regimens for untreated Hodgkin's lymphoma; however, the combination of gemcitabine and bleomycin frequently leads to severe pulmonary toxicity and should therefore be avoided.[102,103]

Follow-up

During the follow-up period for Hodgkin's lymphoma patients, attention should be paid to some crucial points. First, more than two thirds of relapses occur within 2.5 years and more than 90% within 5 years after initial treatment. Thus, the patient should be given a schedule for

TABLE 40–10. Information for Patients Concerning Follow-up Examinations*

Examination Time Point	1st Year			2nd–4th Year	5th Year Onward
	Month 3	Month 6	Month 12	Every 6 Months	Annually
Physical examination	X	X	X	X	X
Case history	X	X	X	X	X
Laboratory tests					
Blood count and differential distribution	X	X	X	X	X
ESR, CRP	X	X	X	X	X
TSH	X	X	X	X	X
CT† (if PR)	X†		X		
Chest radiograph (if no CT)	X		X	X‡	X
Lung function			X		
Abdominal ultrasound	X		X	X	X

*Modified from the current GHSG trial protocol for the first-line treatment of advanced-stage Hodgkin's lymphoma (HD 15).
†Further CT scans are recommended according to findings in final restaging and follow-up.
‡Imaging examinations annually.
Abbreviations: CRP, C-reactive protein; CT, computed tomography; ESR, erythrocyte sedimentation rate; PR, partial remission; TSH, thyroid-stimulating hormone.

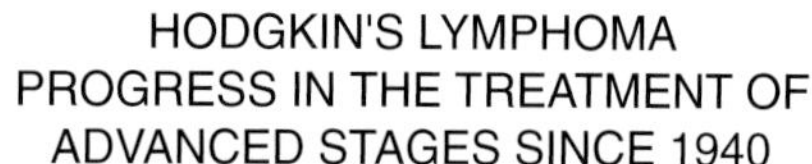

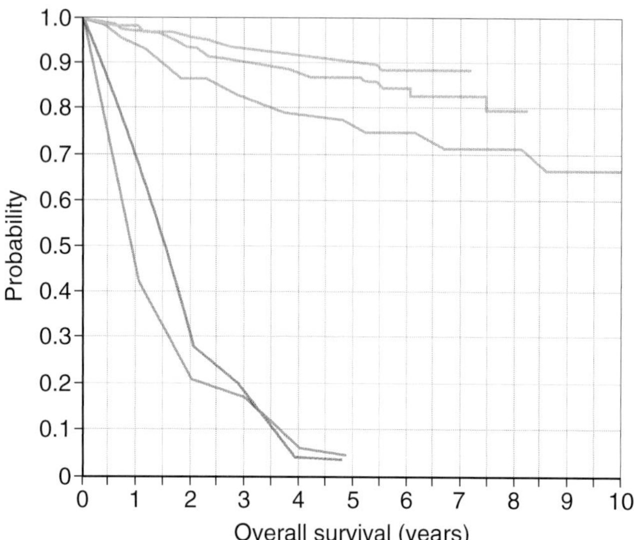

KEY

- No treatment (1940)
- Only alkykating agents (1965)
- COPP + ABVD (1988-93)
- BEACOPP baseline (1993-98)
- BEACOPP escalated (1993-98)

Figure 40–5. Progress in the treatment of advanced stages of Hodgkin's lymphoma during the last century. (Adapted from Diehl V, Re D, Josting A: Hodgkin's disease: clinical manifestations, staging, and therapy. *In* Hoffmann R, et al [eds]: Hematology: Basic Principles and Practice [ed 4]. in press; modified from data gathered by de Vita, including data from GHSG trials.)

follow-up visits and examinations (Table 40–10). Second, a number of long-term toxic effects related to treatment of Hodgkin's lymphoma can occur. They include such minor disorders as endocrine dysfunction, long-term immunosuppression, and viral infections. Serious impairments consist of lung fibrosis from bleomycin and/or irradiation,[35,104,105] myocardial damage from anthracyclines and/or irradiation,[34,106] sterility,[107–109] growth abnormalities in children, opportunistic infections, psychological and psychosocial problems, and fatigue.[110] Potentially fatal effects comprise the OPSI syndrome after splenectomy or spleen irradiation and secondary neoplasms. Acute myeloid leukemia and/or myelodysplastic syndrome are mostly observed within the first 3–5 years and secondary non-Hodgkin's lymphoma mainly at 5–15 years after initial treatment.[74,77,85,111] Solid tumors—as mentioned in the section on radiotherapy for advanced-stage Hodgkin's lymphoma—can also occur decades after initial treatment and sometimes even as multiple tumors.

PROGNOSIS

Hodgkin's lymphoma has become highly curable over the past decades because of effective and risk-adapted chemo- and radiotherapy. Clinical trials achieved 5-year rates of freedom from treatment failure of more than 90% for early favorable and more than 80% for early unfavorable and advanced stages. Five-year overall survival rates were about 85–90%.[48,55,57] Prior to the introduction of effective polychemotherapy for advanced stages, when no treatment or only alkylating agents were given, all patients died within the first 5 years (Fig. 40–5). For patients with relapsed Hodgkin's lymphoma, outcome rates were significantly improved with the use of high-dose therapy and PBSCT (freedom from treatment failure of 55% and overall survival of 71% for patients with chemosensitive relapse).[91]

Despite all the clinical progress, the prognosis is worse for some patients who cannot be treated with a curative approach at diagnosis or who relapse owing to age, concomitant disease, or organ impairment. Furthermore, a small proportion of patients show primary refractory disease and, thus far, specific markers are missing that can predict such unfavorable courses of disease at diagnosis. In the future, hopefully biologic or genetic markers may discriminate high-risk patients, for whom more intensive regimens may be appropriate.

CURRENT CONTROVERSIES & FUTURE CONSIDERATIONS

Hodgkin's Lymphoma

- The optimal number of chemotherapy cycles, the type of drugs, and the dose and field of radiotherapy in early favorable and early unfavorable stages must be determined.
- There is a need to define the best therapy scheme for advanced stages and to evaluate the role of radiotherapy after successful chemotherapy.
- Research must identify predictive values for refractory or very unfavorable courses of Hodgkin's lymphoma.

Suggested Readings*

Bonadonna G, Zucali R, Monfardini S, et al: Combination chemotherapy of Hodgkin's disease with Adriamycin, bleomycin, vinblastine, and imidazole carboxamide versus MOPP. Cancer 36:252–259, 1975.

Connors JM: Current clinical trials for advanced Hodgkin's lymphoma in North America: history, design and rationale. Ann Oncol 13(Suppl 1):92–95, 2002.

Diehl V, Franklin J, Pfreundschuh M, et al: Standard and increased-dose BEACOPP chemotherapy compared with COPP-ABVD for advanced Hodgkin's disease. N Engl J Med 348:2386–2395, 2003.

Diehl V, Stein H, Hummel M, et al: Hodgkin's lymphoma: biology and treatment strategies for primary, refractory, and relapsed disease. Hematology (Am Soc Hematol Educ Program) 225–472, 2003.

Horning SJ, Hoppe RT, Breslin S, et al: Stanford V and radiotherapy for locally extensive and advanced Hodgkin's disease: mature results of a prospective clinical trial. J Clin Oncol 20:630–637, 2002.

Raemaekers J, Kluin-Nelemans H, Teodorovic I, et al: The achievements of the EORTC Lymphoma Group. European Organisation for Research and Treatment of Cancer. Eur J Cancer 38(Suppl 4):S107–S113, 2002.

Schmitz N, Pfistner B, Sextro M, et al: Aggressive conventional chemotherapy compared with high-dose chemotherapy with autologous haemopoietic stem-cell transplantation for relapsed chemosensitive Hodgkin's disease: a randomised trial. Lancet 359:2065–2071, 2002.

Full references for this chapter can be found on accompanying CD-ROM. 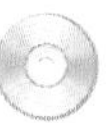

CHAPTER 41

Cutaneous Lymphoma

Sean Whittaker, MD, FRCP, Richard Edelson, MD, Lindy P. Fox, MD, and Robin Russell-Jones, MA, FRCP, FRCPath

KEY POINTS

Cutaneous Lymphoma

- In the skin, primary cutaneous T-cell lymphomas (CTCLs) are more common than B-cell lymphomas, and mycosis fungoides is the most common form of CTCL.
- Mycosis fungoides is a clonal proliferation of mature $CD4^+$ helper/inducer T cells with a marked homing capacity for the upper dermis and epidermis. Histopathologically, it is defined by intraepidermal collections of malignant lymphocytes adhering to Langerhans cells in formations known as "Pautrier microabscesses," which collectively represent the predominant skin sites of proliferation of the neoplastic cells.
- Sézary syndrome, considered the leukemic variant of CTCL, is distinguished from erythrodermic CTCL by the degree of blood involvement. Both must be distinguished from pseudo–Sézary syndrome, a benign disorder associated with erythroderma and the presence of "activated" T lymphocytes in the peripheral blood.
- Although no disease-specific translocations have been identified, CTCL is characterized by high rates of genomic instability at both the chromosomal and the nucleotide level and inactivation of genes involved in the control of apoptosis and the cell cycle through both mutation and hypermethylation. Both Sézary syndrome and mycosis fungoides show a similar pattern of genomic abnormalities, suggesting that they are part of the same disease spectrum.
- Cutaneous lymphoid hyperplasia, or lymphocytoma cutis, a benign, usually reactive, condition that carries a favorable prognosis, is often difficult to differentiate from neoplastic cutaneous infiltrates with similar histologic features.
- B-cell lymphomas presenting in the skin should be classified either as a cutaneous manifestation of a systemic B-cell lymphoma or as an extranodal B-cell lymphoma (marginal zone lymphoma, diffuse large B-cell lymphoma, or primary cutaneous follicle center lymphoma) if complete staging investigations reveal no evidence of systemic disease.
- The prognosis of primary cutaneous diffuse large B-cell lymphoma varies widely, and Bcl-2 positivity may be a more important prognostic indicator than location on the leg.

INTRODUCTION

In 1975, demonstration that the great majority of lymphoid infiltrates associated with the skin were of T-cell type led to the introduction of the term *cutaneous T-cell lymphoma* (CTCL).[1] Subsequently, different subsets both of CTCL and of primary cutaneous B-cell lymphomas were identified.[2] Mycosis fungoides is the most common of the CTCL subsets, but other subsets with clearly identifiable clinicopathologic features and varying prognoses have also been described. Current classifications of cutaneous lymphomas are based on clinical, pathologic, immunopathologic, molecular, and cytogenetic findings[3,4] all of which have a critical influence on therapeutic approach. A critical observation has been the realization that lymphomas with a similar pathology arising in different organs carry very different prognoses. It is also now clear that primary cutaneous B-cell lymphoma, not as rare as once believed, represents approximately one third of all primary cutaneous lymphomas.[2] The European Organisation for Research and Treatment of Cancer (EORTC) classified primary cutaneous lymphomas in 1997.[3–5] The recent World Health Organization (WHO) classification has encompassed most of the EORTC primary cutaneous lymphoma categories with the exception of distinct cutaneous B-cell lymphomas[5] (Table 41–1). A consensus EORTC-WHO classification of cutaneous lymphomas (Table 41–2) has been published recently.[6]

EPIDEMIOLOGY AND RISK FACTORS

Given the initial presentation of CTCL in the skin, an etiologic role for occupational or environmental exposure was suggested early on. Case-control studies investigating this theory have reported conflicting results and, thus, no consistent support for such factors has been documented.[7–9] The increased incidence of CTCL in African Americans, the frequent presentation in whites in sun-protected body regions, and the brisk responses to ultraviolet (UV) therapy have collectively raised the possibility that UV exposure plays an apparently protective role in CTCL. However, identification of B-wavelength (UVB)–specific mutations in the tumor suppressor gene *p53* indicates that, in at least some patients, DNA damage

TABLE 41–1. EORTC Classification for Cutaneous Lymphomas with Equivalent Entities in REAL and WHO Classifications

REAL	EORTC	WHO
Mycosis fungoides Sézary syndrome	**Indolent**	Mycosis fungoides
	Mycosis fungoides (MF)	Variants: follicular mucinosis Pagetoid reticulosis
	MF + follicular mucinosis Pagetoid reticulosis	
Peripheral T-cell lymphoma	Large-cell CTCL, CD30$^+$ Anaplastic Pleomorphic Immunoblastic	Primary cutaneous anaplastic large-cell lymphoma Peripheral T-cell lymphoma
	Lymphomatoid papulosis	Lymphomatoid papulosis (T-cell proliferation of uncertain malignant potential)
	Aggressive	
	Sézary syndrome Large-cell CTCL CD30$^-$ negative	Sézary syndrome Peripheral T-cell lymphoma
	Provisional	
	Granulomatous slack skin	MF variant
	CTCL-pleomorphic small/medium	Peripheral T-cell lymphoma
Provisional entity: Subcutaneous panniculitis–like T-cell lymphoma	Subcutaneous panniculitis–like T-cell lymphoma	Subcutaneous panniculitis–like T-cell lymphoma

TABLE 41–2. WHO-EORTC Classification of Cutaneous Lymphomas

Cutaneous T-Cell and Natural Killer (NK) Cell Lymphomas

Mycosis fungoides
Mycosis fungoides variants and subtypes
  Folliculotropic mycosis fungoides
  Pagetoid reticulosis
  Granulomatous slack skin
Sézary syndrome
Adult T-cell leukemia/lymphoma
Primary cutaneous CD30$^+$ lymphoproliferative disorders
  Primary cutaneous anaplastic large-cell lymphoma
  Lymphomatoid papulosis
Subcutaneous panniculitis–like T-cell lymphoma (α/β)
Extranodal NK/T-cell lymphoma, nasal type
Primary cutaneous peripheral T-cell lymphoma, unspecified
  Primary cutaneous aggressive epidermotropic CD8$^+$ T-cell lymphoma (provisional)
  Cutaneous γ/δ T-cell lymphoma (provisional)
  Primary cutaneous CD4$^+$ small/medium-sized pleomorphic T-cell lymphoma (provisional)

Cutaneous B-Cell Lymphomas

Primary cutaneous marginal zone B-cell lymphoma
Primary cutaneous follicle center lymphoma
Primary cutaneous diffuse large B-cell lymphoma, leg type
Primary cutaneous diffuse large B-cell lymphoma, other
  Intravascular large B-cell lymphoma

Precursor Hematologic Neoplasm

CD4$^+$/CD56$^+$ hematodermic neoplasm (blastic NK cell lymphoma)

From Willemze R, Jaffe ES, Burg G, et al: WHO-EORTC classification for cutaneous lymphomas. Blood 105:3768–3785, 2005.

resulting from this UV radiation may accelerate aggressive subclone formation. Other potential genetic factors that may also contribute to the pathogenesis of CTCL are under investigation.[10–12]

Clinical and pathologic similarities to cutaneous involvement in adult T-cell lymphoma has led to an intensive search for human T-lymphotrophic virus type 1 (HTLV-1) and related viruses in mycosis fungoides. However, extensive investigations have failed to conclusively implicate any of the currently recognized HTLV-associated viruses.[13–17] Likewise, the prevalence in endemic areas of southwestern Japan, the Caribbean, and southeastern United States of HTLV-1–associated T-cell lymphoma/leukemia, whose malignant cells exhibit the same lymphocyte phenotype and epidermotropism of CTCL cells, has suggested that another retrovirus may be causative of CTCL.[18,19] Thus far, no direct evidence of this association has been reported. Even if one is found, it will likely be only one contributory factor.

A high incidence of second malignancies, notably nonmelanoma skin cancer and small-cell lung cancer, has been reported in both mycosis fungoides[9,20] and Sézary syndrome.[21] Other types of lymphoma/leukemia and Hodgkin's lymphoma have also been described in association with mycosis fungoides and Sézary syndrome.[22–24] In addition, there is an increased incidence of lymphomas and leukemias in relatives of mycosis fungoides patients.[11]

Apart from Epstein-Barr virus infection in patients who are immunosuppressed, the etiology of primary cutaneous B-cell lymphomas is unknown. The development of immunocytomas in patients with acrodermatitis chronica atrophicans has led to speculation about the role of chronic antigen stimulation by *Borrelia burgdorferi* leading to neoplastic transformation of cutaneous B cells. The detection of *Borrelia* DNA in some cutaneous lesions of immunocytomas and marginal zone B-cell lymphomas using polymerase chain reaction has provided support for this role, but the frequency of positivity varies considerably in different geographic regions, with positive results in Central Europe and Scotland[25–29] but no evidence of an association in the United States.[7]

PATHOPHYSIOLOGY

The majority of cutaneous lymphomas are clonal proliferations[28,29] of mature CD4$^+$ helper/inducer T cells[30,31] with a marked homing capacity for the papillary dermis and epidermis. Because the cells of origin are skin-tropic "cutaneous T cells," various presentations of this category of cutaneous lymphomas (which includes mycosis fungoides and Sézary syndrome) have been grouped together as "cutaneous T-cell lymphoma." The homing to skin by CTCL cells, and probably normal "cutaneous T cells," appears to be mediated in part by the surface glycoprotein cutaneous lymphoid antigen.[32,33] Transient binding of CTCL cell cutaneous lymphoid antigen to E-selectin on endothelial cells enhances CTCL cell adherence to the walls of cutaneous venules, thereby facilitating their exit from the circulation and into the skin, while transiting the upper dermis (Fig. 41–1).

The pathognomonic microscopic feature of CTCL is its distinctive epidermotropism of malignant cells[34] (Fig. 41–2) in the form of "Pautrier microabscesses." After entering the epidermis, CTCL cells interact with Langerhans cells, the skin-based dendritic antigen-presenting cells. The Pautrier microabscesses (composed almost exclusively of malignant CTCL cells adhering to Langerhans cells[35]) and smaller foci of intraepidermal CTCL cells are the principal proliferative skin sites for CTCL cells.[36] Dendritic cells stimulate CTCL proliferation via contact between the dendritic cell class II major histocompatibility complexes and the clone-specific CTCL T-cell receptor (TCR) for antigen (Fig. 41–3).[37,38] The level of CTCL proliferation stimulated in this manner is profound. Only immature dendritic cells can support this CTCL cell proliferation, and the CTCL cells themselves significantly slow maturation of dendritic cells. Once the dendritic cells mature, the CTCL cells become apoptotic and die.

CTCL can be broadly divided into two major stages, earlier stage disease in which the malignant cells are only able to proliferate in the skin and a advanced stage disease in which the malignant cells can proliferate in visceral organs. The clinical distinction between these two stages can be challenging because the malignancy arises from recirculatory T cells, which normally percolate between the blood, skin, and lymphatics. Therefore, merely finding small numbers of CTCL cells in those sites is insufficient, in the absence of histologic or clinical evidence of extracutaneous collections of cells, to identify a functionally metastatic state. Yet, in the advanced stages of the malignancy, the CTCL subclones do develop the capacity to replicate outside of the skin, without signaling from Langerhans cells. At that stage, the clinical presentation may not be separable from peripheral T-cell lymphoma with skin involvement.

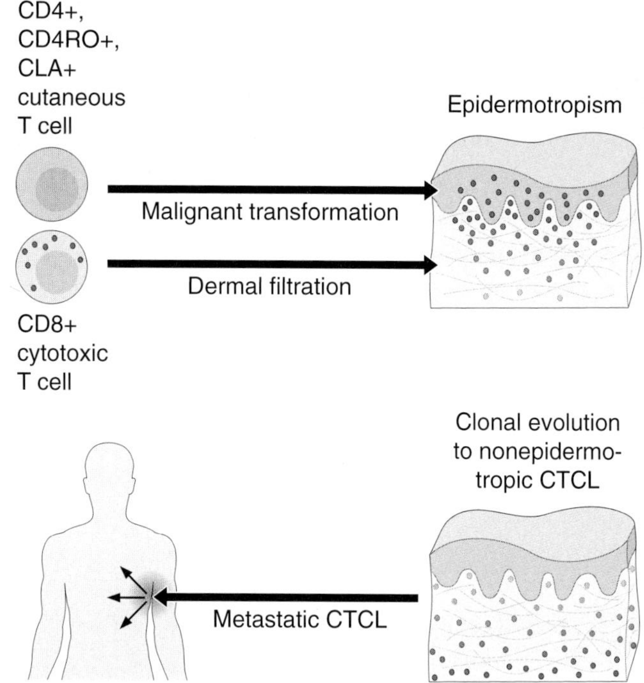

Figure 41–1. CTCL evolves from a distinct subset of normal T cells, referred to as "cutaneous T cells" because of their propensity to percolate through the skin, seeking invading pathogens or tumor antigens, and ordinarily comprising approximately 20% of the circulating T-cell pool. These CD4$^+$ (helper/inducer) and CD45RO45$^+$ (memory) T cells also display cutaneous lymphoid antigen (CLA), which, through its binding to E-selectin on dermal endothelial cells, enhances the capacity of these T cells to adhere to dermal capillaries and then exit into the surrounding tissue. Cutaneous T cells can clonally transform into CTCL cells, which retain the capacity to localize in the skin and collect in the epidermis. The dermal infiltrate in early plaque-stage CTCL contains significant numbers of CD8$^+$ putatively anti-CTCL defensive cells. As subclones of progressively more aggressive malignant cells evolve, the epidermotropism is progressively lost and invasive cutaneous tumors form. Probably at least in part because of the production of the T-cell–suppressive cytokine interleukin-10 (IL-10) by the CTCL cells, the tumors are composed almost entirely of malignant T cells, without a significant local host response. At this stage, the cells acquire the capacity to disseminate widely and form visceral tumors. Although visceral collections can cause organ failure, death most commonly results from systemic immunosuppression, perhaps secondary to massive quantities of IL-10 produced by the CTCL cells, and resultant opportunistic infections.

Epidermotropic CTCL plaques are clinical manifestations of a mixture of infiltrating CTCL and normal reactive T cells, whereas tumors are composed mostly of malignant cells. In early plaques, normal T cells dominate the dermal infiltrate and most of the CTCL cells are in the epidermis.[39] The clinician must therefore be aware that clinical resolution does not always equate with histologic clearance.

Tissue compartmentalization is responsible for a major part of CTCL distribution. Just as normal "cutaneous T

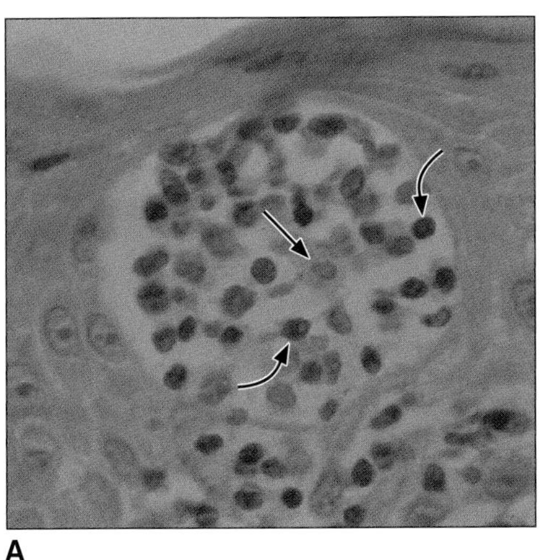

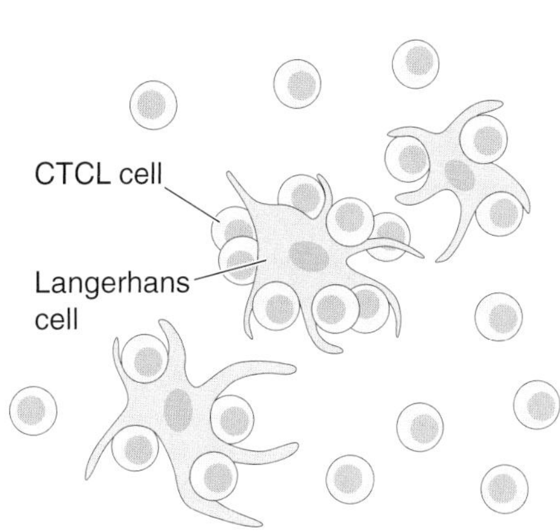

Figure 41–2. Hematoxylin and eosin–stained section of CTCL plaque. ***A,*** Intraepidermal collections of malignant T cells are pathognomonic of cutaneous T-cell lymphoma in the early epidermotropic phase. These "Pautrier microabscesses" have been shown by immuno-electron microscopy to be composed of malignant T cells *(curved arrows)* adherent to stellate Langerhans cells *(straight arrow).* ***B,*** Drawing of CTCL cell adherence to central Langerhans cell.

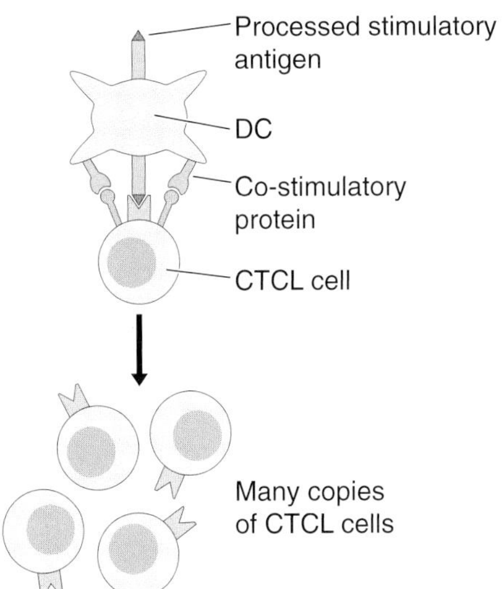

Figure 41–3. Stimulation of CTCL cell proliferation by Langerhans cells. Laboratory data suggest that proliferation of CTCL cells in these intraepidermal locations is driven by engagement of Langerhans cell class II major histocompatibility complexes with the clonal T-cell receptors of the CTCL cells. In vitro, interruption of this dynamic interaction by selective monoclonal antibodies prevents proliferation of the CTCL cells and leads to their death. Therefore, it has been suggested that as-yet unidentified antigens presented to the CTCL cells by Langerhans cells may be at the core of the pathogenesis of this lymphoma.

cells" avoid the bone marrow and home to the perifollicular regions of lymph nodes during their circulation through the body, so do CTCL cells. It is therefore uncommon, even with significant blood involvement, for CTCL cells to infiltrate the bone marrow and directly suppress hematopoiesis, whereas it is common for lymphoid follicles to be retained even where there is early CTCL nodal involvement.

CLINICAL FEATURES, CLASSIFICATION, AND DIAGNOSIS

Mycosis Fungoides

Mycosis fungoides, a low-grade form of CTCL derived from α/β lymphocytes with a mature T helper cell phenotype, represents a proliferation of small to medium-sized pleomorphic cells with cerebriform nuclei. Mycosis fungoides cells are usually CD2, CD3, and CD4 positive and express cutaneous lymphoid antigen.[32] Childhood cases may exhibit a cytotoxic phenotype, a feature that does not appear to be associated with a worse prognosis.[40]

Mycosis fungoides is an indolent disease process with extremely variable clinical manifestations (Figs. 41–4 through 41–6). Nonspecific skin changes, often misdiagnosed as eczema or psoriasis, may precede the diagnosis of mycosis fungoides by many years. Even when the diagnosis is suspected clinically, the initial histology may be nondiagnostic. Repeat histology with molecular analysis may be required before the diagnosis can be established with certainty. Close liaison between the clinician and a pathologist with expertise in skin lymphoma cannot be overemphasized.

The prognosis in mycosis fungoides is determined by the extent of the skin involvement, the type of cutaneous lesions, and the presence of nodal or visceral disease.[41] The tumor-node-metastasis (TNM) classification and a clinical staging system are shown in Tables 41–3 and 41–4.[42] Proper management of mycosis fungoides depends upon a detailed knowledge of the protean clinical manifestations and pathologic features of this disease, features that may not be adequately reflected in this staging system. For example, patients with stage IB disease with lesions involving more than 10% of the skin surface have a 10-year survival rate of 95% if the lesions are patches or thin plaques versus 65% if thick plaques are present as well.[43]

The histopathologic changes of mycosis fungoides mirror the spectrum of disease seen clinically. In patch- or plaque-stage disease, there is a mixed perivascular or bandlike dermal infiltrate containing a variable propor-

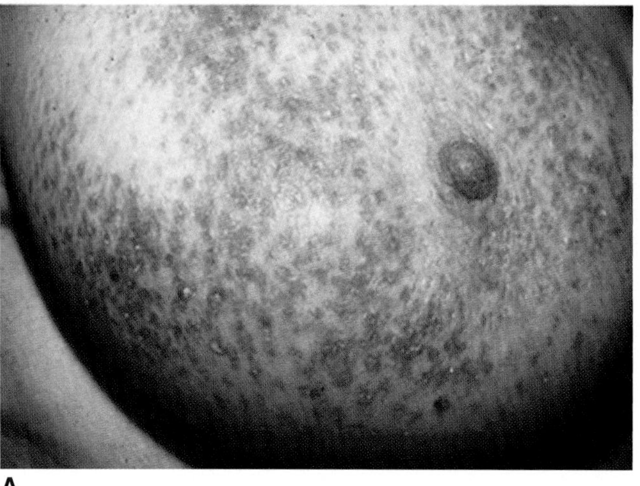

A

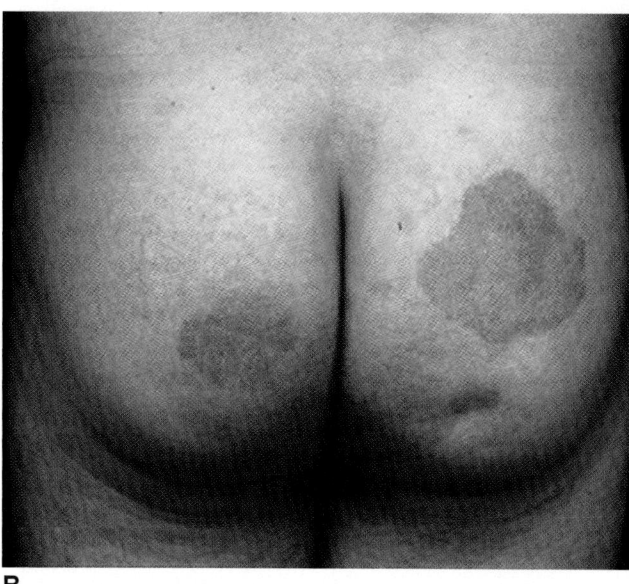

B

■ **Figure 41–4.** Clinical appearance of early mycosis fungoides. ***A,*** Poikilodermatous patch on the breast showing telangiectasia and epidermal atrophy. ***B,*** Thin plaques of irregular outline on nonexposed sites.

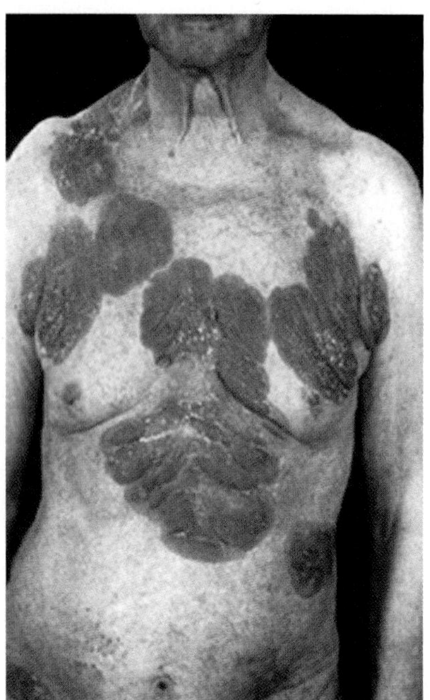

■ **Figure 41–5.** Thick plaque–stage CTCL. These lesions are well demarcated and more infiltrated than those depicted in Figure 41–4*B*.

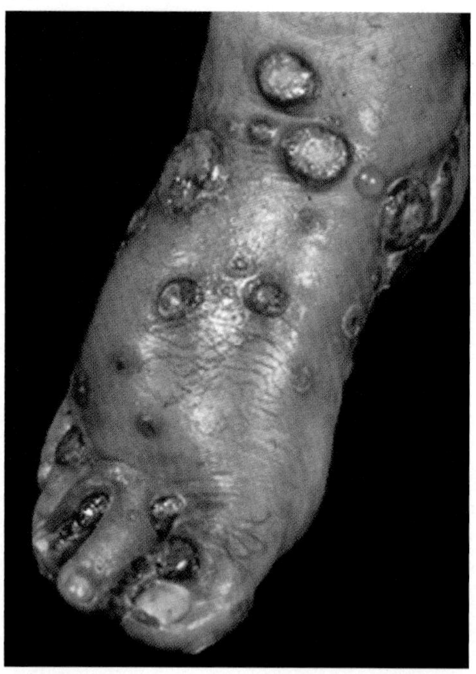

■ **Figure 41–6.** Tumor-stage CTCL. Multiple, exophytic, eroded nodules on the foot.

tion of pleomorphic cells with irregular nuclei (Fig. 41–7). Typically there is involvement of the epidermis by infiltrating neoplastic lymphocytes as single cells (epidermotropism), collections of atypical cells (Pautrier microabscesses), or colonization of the basal cell layer by a line of neoplastic cells ("string of pearls").[44] In early cases, the proportion of neoplastic cells in the dermis is low and can be difficult to distinguish from the background inflammatory cells. Although there is no immunophenotypic marker that reliably identifies mycosis fungoides, the majority of epidermotropic cells are $CD4^+$, and may demonstrate loss of CD7.[45] In situations in which there is diagnostic uncertainty, molecular analysis of lesional skin may demonstrate a clone of T cells. If doubt remains, repeat biopsies after an interval of some months may establish the correct diagnosis.

In tumor-stage disease, the proportion of neoplastic cells increases, the dermis is occupied by a diffuse infiltrate extending into the deep reticular dermis, and epidermotropism may be lost. Large-cell transformation can occur and is associated with a worse prognosis.[46] Transformed lymphocytes may be pleomorphic, anaplastic, or immunoblastic and may demonstrate CD30 positivity, but these features do not seem to carry any independent prognostic significance.[47] Aberrant immunophenotypes with loss of pan–T-cell antigens are commonly encountered in tumor-stage mycosis fungoides. By this stage, the disease has lost many of its distinguishing histologic characteristics and may resemble a cutaneous peripheral T-cell lymphoma.

TABLE 41–3. TNM Classification of Mycosis Fungoides/Sézary Syndrome

Cutaneous Involvement (T)	
T_0	Lesions clinically and/or histologically suspicious but not diagnostic
T_1	Patches/plaques involving less than 10% of skin
T_2	Patches/plaques involving more than 10% of skin
T_3	Tumors present
T_4	Erythroderma
Lymph Nodes (N)	
N_0	Clinically and pathologically normal
N_1	Palpable; pathologically not involved
N_2	Clinically nonpalpable; pathologically mycosis fungoides
N_3	Clinically enlarged; pathologically mycosis fungoides
Viscera (M)	
M_0	No visceral spread
M_1	Visceral spread present
Peripheral Blood (B)	
B_0	<5% atypical circulating mononuclear cells
B_1	>5% atypical circulating mononuclear cells

TABLE 41–4. Staging System for Mycosis Fungoides/Sézary Syndrome Related to TNM Classification

Stage	T	N	M
IA	T_1	N_0	M_0
IB	T_2	N_0	M_0
IIA	T_{1-2}	N_1	M_0
IIB	T_3	N_{0-1}	M_0
III	T_4	N_{0-1}	M_0
IVA	T_{1-4}	N_{2-3}	M_0
IVB	T_{1-4}	N_{0-3}	M_1

Peripheral lymph node enlargement is commonly encountered in mycosis fungoides and often reflects a reactive proliferation of the skin-associated lymphoid tissue. In the TNM classification, clinically enlarged nodes are classified as N_1 if they are dermatopathic and N_3 if they are lymphomatous, but more refined systems have been proposed.[48] The prognostic value of lymph node staging is improved with molecular analysis, because the presence of a T-cell clone worsens the prognosis in patients with dermatopathic or early lymph node involvement.[49]

The WHO accepts three clinicopathologic variants of mycosis fungoides: follicular mucinosis, pagetoid reticulosis, and granulomatous slack skin. In follicular mucinosis, patients present with infiltrated plaques showing alopecia on the head and neck. Although lesions typical of patch or plaque mycosis fungoides often coexist, the prognosis of follicular mucinosis is closer to that of tumor-stage mycosis fungoides.[50] Follicular mucinosis is distinguished histologically by a perifollicular infiltrate, degeneration of the follicular epithelium with formation of mucin, and infiltration of the follicular epithelium by pilotropic atypical lymphocytes. The atypical lymphocytes in follicular mucinosis exhibit the same cytology and immunostaining properties as those in typical cases of mycosis fungoides. TCR gene analysis will often reveal a T-cell clone. Although a benign variant of follicular mucinosis is recognized, this is a diagnosis of exclusion,[51] and long-term follow-up is required.

Pagetoid reticulosis, or Woringer-Kolopp disease, is characterized by a solitary hyperkeratotic plaque located on an acral site.[52] Histology exhibits a markedly epidermotropic infiltrate of medium-sized pleomorphic cells with a pericellular halo. Some cases are derived from γ/δ T cells, and the immunophenotype is variable.[53,54] A disseminated form, Ketron-Goodman disease, carries a poor prognosis.[55]

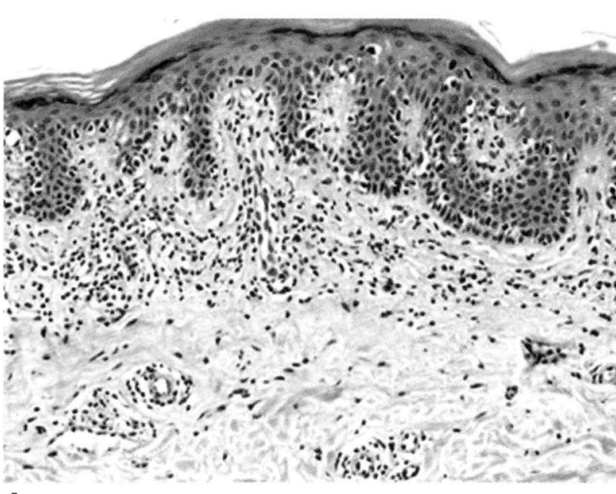
A

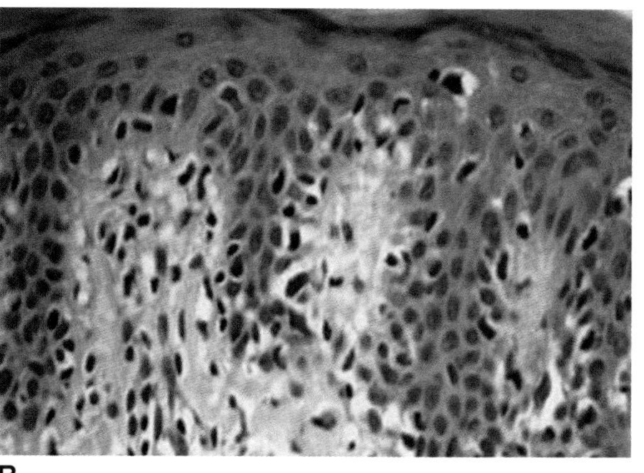
B

Figure 41–7. Histology of patch/thin plaque–stage mycosis fungoides (hematoxylin and eosin staining). ***A,*** Medium-power photomicrograph shows a bandlike and perivascular infiltrate of lymphoid cells with moderate acanthosis. ***B,*** High-power photomicrograph shows atypical pleomorphic cells with hyperchromatic angulated nuclei and peripheral halos distributed along the basal-cell layer and scattered within the epidermis.

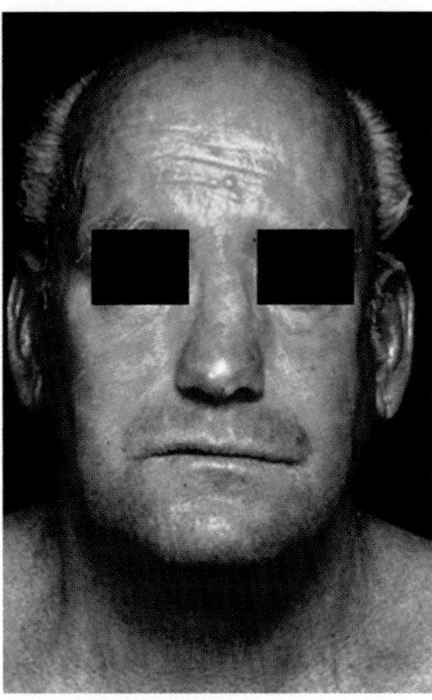

A

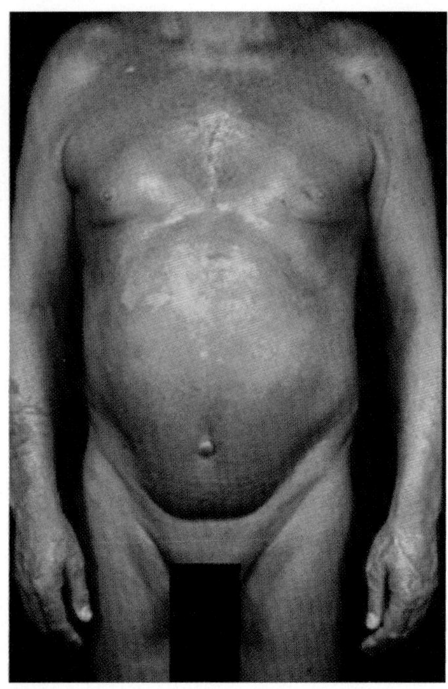

B

Figure 41–8. Erythroderma caused by Sézary syndrome. Note loss of body hair, generalized erythema, and inguinal lymphadenopathy.

Excessively rare, granulomatous slack skin is normally preceded by mycosis fungoides–type patches with an infiltrate of T lymphocytes and small-cell cytology. The characteristic features are pendulous skinfolds at flexural sites such as the groin or axillae.[56] Histologically, one observes mammoth giant cells scattered within the reticular dermis. TCR gene rearrangement studies have confirmed a T-cell origin for this condition.[56]

Sézary Syndrome

Sézary syndrome is characterized by erythroderma, lymphadenopathy, and neoplastic T lymphocytes in the peripheral blood (Figs. 41–8 and 41–9). Pruritus is usually severe. The erythroderma is often infiltrative and may be associated with hair loss, nail dystrophy and lichenification. As in mycosis fungoides, lymphadenopathy usually involves skin-associated lymphoid tissue. Sézary syndrome carries a poor prognosis, with a median survival of 2–4 years.[57] It usually arises de novo but can develop in the context of a patient with mycosis fungoides who becomes erythrodermic. Because Sézary cells exhibit the same morphologic and immunophenotypic features as mycosis fungoides cells, Sézary syndrome is distinguished from erythrodermic mycosis fungoides only by the degree of blood involvement. However, because erythrodermic mycosis fungoides represents a spectrum, any attempt to distinguish Sézary syndrome from cases that show a lesser degree of hematologic involvement is necessarily arbitrary. The EORTC hematologic criteria for diagnosing Sézary syndrome include a CD4:CD8 ratio greater than 10 and a peripheral blood T-cell clone.[3] Patients thus defined have a poor prognosis, with a median survival of only 2 years. Russell-Jones and Whittaker proposed 5% circulating Sézary cells combined with the evidence of a clonal population in the peripheral blood.[58] This defines a lower tumor burden with a median survival of 45 months.[59]

Because there is no consensus on an exact definition of Sézary syndrome, an alternative approach is to develop a staging system that incorporates both lymph node status and hematologic stage. A hematologic staging system comprising five categories, H0 to H4, showed an increase in disease-specific death rate for each category, with the most significant change occurring at H2, defined by 5% Sézary cells with a T-cell clone demonstrated by polymerase chain reaction, or a T-cell clone demonstrated by Southern blot analysis only.[60] The need for a hematologic histologic staging system has also been recognized by the International Society for Cutaneous Lymphoma (ISCL) and is currently being tested in a larger multicenter study under the auspices of the ISCL.[61]

Another challenge in diagnosing Sézary syndrome is the identification of a neoplastic T-cell population in the peripheral blood. Not all cases of Sézary syndrome exhibit large cells. Small and medium-sized variants exist and may be difficult to distinguish from inflammatory skin conditions that generate reactive lymphocytes.[62] Strict diagnostic criteria are therefore needed to distinguish genuine cases of cutaneous T-cell lymphoma/leukemia from pseudo–Sézary syndrome (Fig. 41–10). An abnormal population of circulating T cells can be demonstrated by cytogenetic methods, an aberrant phenotype on fluorescence-activated cell sorter analysis, loss of the CD26 antigen, or clonality by TCR gene analysis.[59,63] If suspected cases of Sézary syndrome demonstrate none of the above criteria, then a definitive diagnosis should not be made.

Despite some differences, the histologic changes in Sézary syndrome are not dissimilar to those described in

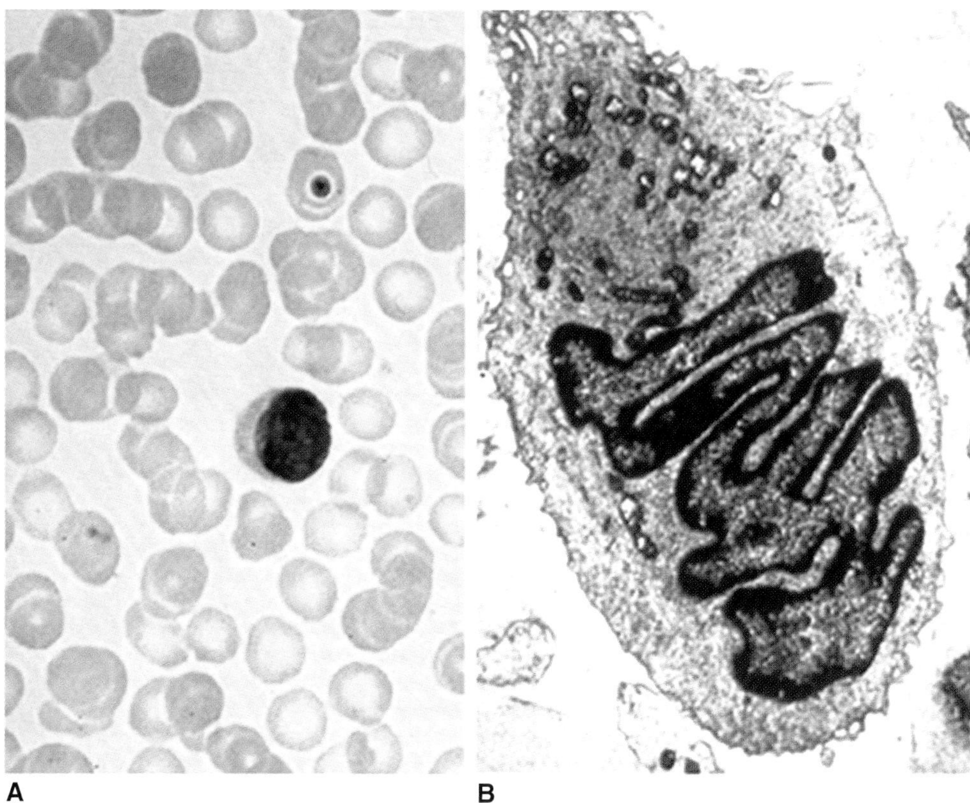

Figure 41–9. Morphology of Sézary cells. *A*, Atypical mononuclear cells on a peripheral blood smear. *B*, Cerebriform nucleus visualized on an ultrathin section.

mycosis fungoides. A bandlike dermal infiltrate containing numerous atypical lymphocytes is characteristic. Epidermotropism is a more variable feature, and the size of Sézary cells varies in the skin, as it does in the blood. Patients with small circulating Sézary cells may only show minimal atypia histologically, and in this situation a definitive diagnosis of erythrodermic CTCL cannot be made on histologic criteria alone. Where doubt remains, TCR gene analysis is a reliable and reproducible method of identifying a clonal T-cell population in the skin. The presence of an identical clone in both skin and blood lends strong support to a diagnosis of erythrodermic CTCL.[64]

CD30$^+$ Cutaneous Lymphoproliferative Disorders

Lymphomatoid Papulosis

Lymphomatoid papulosis is a cutaneous lymphoproliferative disorder of uncertain malignant potential. Ten percent of cases are associated with a second lymphoma, including mycosis fungoides, Hodgkin's lymphoma, or primary cutaneous anaplastic large-cell lymphoma (PCALCL). In cases of lymphomatoid papulosis associated with mycosis fungoides, the same T-cell clone can be demonstrated in both types of lesions.[65,66] Clinically, lymphomatoid papulosis is characterized by recurrent eruptions consisting of crops of papules and nodules that typically ulcerate and then heal over a period of 4–6 weeks. Histologically, there is a wedge-shaped polymorphous infiltrate containing a mixture of larger atypical cells. In lymphomatoid papulosis type A, these cells are CD30 positive and resemble anaplastic cells. In type B, there are medium-sized CD30$^-$ cells with cerebriform nuclei resembling mycosis fungoides cells. Lymphomatoid papulosis in association with mycosis fungoides may be of type A, type B, or a mixed pattern.[66] Reports that T-cell clones are present only in type B or mixed variants,[67] coupled with findings that the CD30$^+$ large anaplastic cells in lesions of lymphomatoid papulosis are polyclonal,[68] raise the possibility that the CD30$^+$ cells of type A are reactive rather than neoplastic and may account for the benign nature of this disorder.

Primary Cutaneous Anaplastic Large-Cell Lymphoma

PCALCL is characterized by single or grouped nodules that are larger, fewer in number, and more persistent than those in lymphomatoid papulosis. Multifocal disease occurs in approximately 20% of cases, and ulceration is common. PCALCL carries a favorable prognosis with a 5-year survival of over 90%. Patients with involvement of regional lymph nodes also have a favorable prognosis, but such cases must be distinguished from systemic anaplastic large-cell lymphoma with cutaneous involvement.[69] PCALCL occurring in patients with human immunodeficiency virus infection or post–organ transplantation immunosuppression carries a poor prognosis.[70]

Histologically, PCALCL is characterized by a diffuse infiltrate of large anaplastic cells occupying the reticular dermis with ulceration, no epidermotropism, and a background of inflammatory cells. Unlike in lymphomatoid papulosis, the anaplastic cells are arranged in sheets

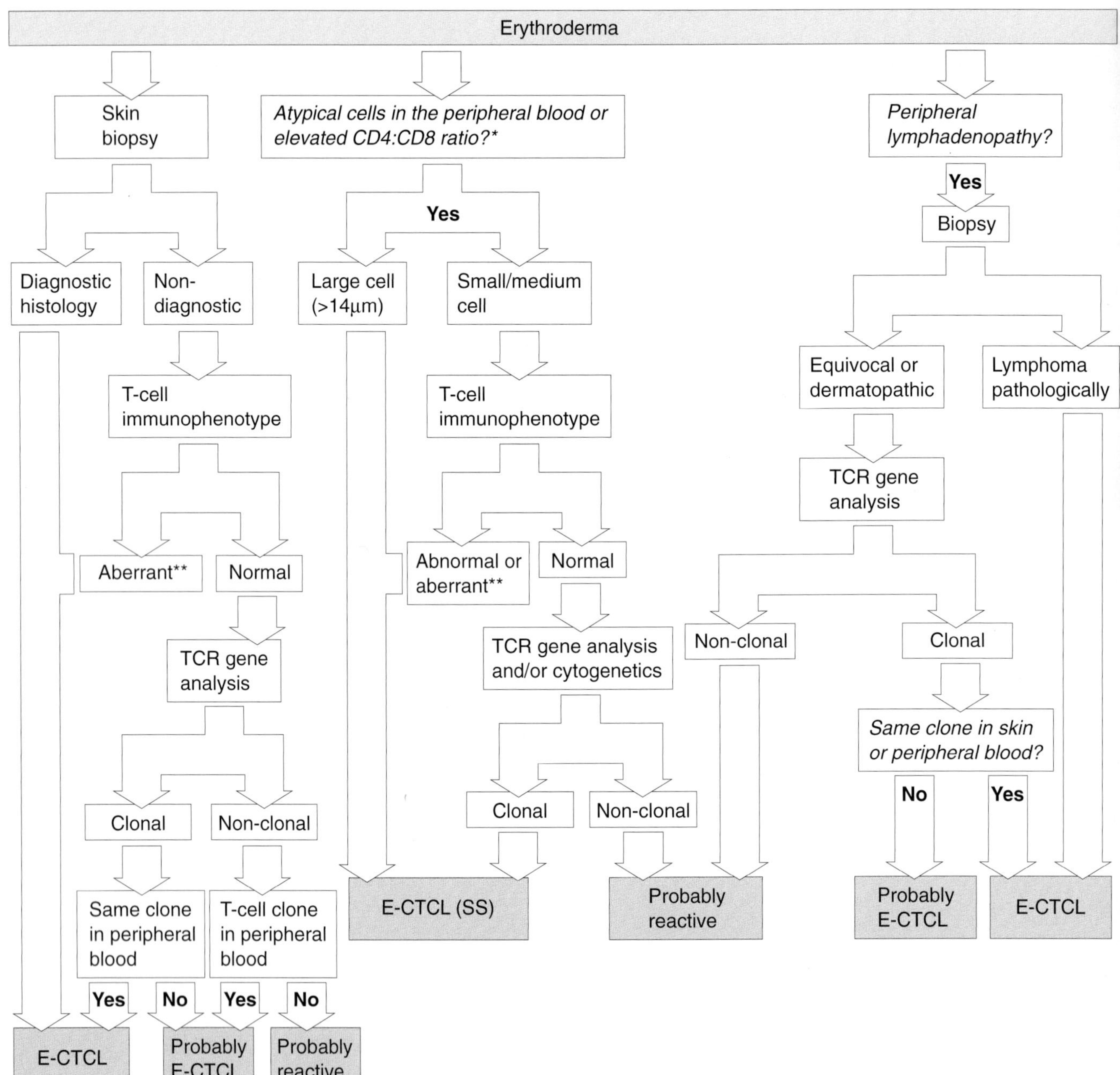

Figure 41–10. Algorithm for the evaluation and diagnosis of erythroderma caused by cutaneous T-cell lymphoma (E-CTCL) versus "reactive" causes of erythroderma. (Redrawn from Russell-Jones R: Diagnosing erythrodermic cutaneous T-cell lymphoma. Br J Dermatol 2005 [in press]).

*A CD4:CD8 ratio greater than 10 or an absolute Sézary count of 1×10^9/L has been proposed as a diagnostic criterion for Sézary syndrome, but this algorithm requires additional immunophenotypic or genotypic data. Even so, a Sézary count $>1 \times 10^9$/L or a CD4:CD8 ratio greater than 10 increases the probability of neoplasia, and separates Sézary syndrome from E-CTCL with lesser degree of blood involvement.

**Abnormal T-cell immunophenotype = an increased population of $CD4^+$ cells that are CD26 negative (>30%). Aberrant T-cell immunophenotype = loss of pan–T-cell markers such as CD2, CD3, or CD5, and/or double-negative T cells (CD4 and CD8 negative).

rather than singly or in clusters and comprise more than 80% of the infiltrate. The neoplastic cells are ALK-1 negative but usually retain T-cell markers such as CD2 or CD3. Most cases also express cytotoxic granules such as TIA-1 or granzyme B,[71] and a T-cell derivation can be confirmed by TCR gene analysis. Unlike $CD30^+$ B-cell lymphomas, PCALCL is not associated with Epstein-Barr virus. Careful clinicopathologic correlation is mandatory to distinguish $CD30^+$ transformed mycosis fungoides from another $CD30^+$ lymphoproliferative disorder such as lymphomatoid papulosis or PCALCL, because the prognosis is very different in these different situations.

Subcutaneous Panniculitis–like T-Cell Lymphoma

Subcutaneous panniculitis–like T-cell lymphoma is derived from cytotoxic T cells and preferentially involves the subcutaneous tissue.[72] Two subtypes are recognized: those derived from α/β cells and those derived from γ/δ cells. The latter group more commonly involves the dermis or epidermis as well as the subcutis, is associated with the hemophagocytic syndrome, and carries a worse prognosis.[73,74] Clinically, this lymphoma presents as single or multiple subcutaneous nodules that occasionally ulcerate. The characteristic histologic feature is a lobular panniculitis with neoplastic cells rimming the fat spaces. The condition must be distinguished from inflammatory panniculitides.[75] The majority of cases derived from α/β cells, in which case the cytotoxic T cells show a mature cytotoxic phenotype (CD2, CD3, and CD8 positive) and express the cytotoxic granules TIA-1, granzyme B, and perforin. Cases derived from γ/δ cells are CD8 negative and CD56 positive, and in the new WHO-EORTC classification these lesions are classified separately from the α/β type (see Table 41–2). Neither subset is Epstein-Barr virus associated. TCR gene analysis confirms a clonal T-cell disorder in both types.

Blastic Natural Killer Cell Lymphoma

According to the WHO classification, this is a cutaneous lymphoma of uncertain histogenesis,[76] though a derivation from plasmacytoid dendritic cell has been suggested.[77] It usually presents with widely disseminated purplish plaques and nodules. Histologically, there is a monomorphic infiltrate of medium-sized cells with finely dispersed chromatin. Pseudo-rosetting around blood vessels is a characteristic feature. Although the cells are CD4 and CD56 positive, they do not normally express cytotoxic granule proteins, pan–T-cell markers, or myelomonocytic markers such as CD68, CD33, or myeloperoxidase. TCR gene analysis does not show evidence of a TCR gene rearrangement.[78] The prognosis is poor because systemic involvement and poor response to chemotherapy are characteristic.

Cutaneous B-Cell Lymphomas

Major differences exist between the EORTC and WHO classifications of cutaneous B-cell lymphomas.[79] B-cell lymphomas presenting in the skin should be classified either as a cutaneous manifestation of a systemic B-cell lymphoma or as an extranodal B-cell lymphoma if complete staging investigations reveal no evidence of systemic disease. Although any systemic B-cell lymphoma can involve the skin, primary cutaneous B-cell lymphomas are limited to marginal zone lymphoma (MZL), diffuse large B-cell lymphoma (DLBCL), and primary cutaneous follicle center lymphoma. Realizing that cutaneous extranodal lymphomas do not inevitably become systemic avoids the inappropriate administration of chemotherapy for an indolent disease process with an excellent prognosis.

Cutaneous Lymphoid Hyperplasia (Lymphocytoma Cutis)

The elements of a normal reactive lymph node follicle—a well-formed germinal center, tingible body macrophages, a well-defined mantle zone, and a surrounding infiltrate of polyclonal B cells, T cells, histiocytes, eosinophils, and occasional blasts—can be reproduced in the skin. Known as cutaneous lymphoid hyperplasia or lymphocytoma cutis, these lesions can be seen in association with insect bite reactions, scabies, drug reactions, *Borrelia* infection, tattoo reactions, and vaccinations. It is often difficult to differentiate these benign lesions from neoplastic infiltrates in the setting of nodular skin lesions with the indicated histologic features arising in the absence of known precipitating factors. In addition, the classical method of distinguishing between a reactive and neoplastic B-cell infiltrate by means of light chain typing is technically difficult in skin.

Cutaneous Marginal Zone Lymphoma

MZLs arise from B lymphocytes normally located outside of the mantle zone, but also induce germinal center formation (best visualized using a follicular dendritic cell marker such as CD21). Tumor cells in MZL may show a centrocytic, plasmacytoid, or monocytoid cytology.[80] Although light chain typing can aid in differentiating lymphocytoma cutis from MZL, not all MZLs show plasmacytoid differentiation. In addition, although the neoplastic cells in MZL are CD20, CD79a, and Bcl-2 positive and CD5, CD10, and Bcl-6 negative, these immunostains do not distinguish neoplastic cells from normal marginal zone B lymphocytes. In difficult cases, morphologic criteria can be helpful. For example, a MZL can be diagnosed if there is a monomorphic infiltrate with an appropriate immunophenotype. However, if the infiltrate is polymorphous and light chain typing is noncontributory, the diagnosis cannot be established with certainty. In this situation, immunoglobulin gene analysis is helpful because the demonstration of clonality provides presumptive evidence of neoplasia. It is important to note that the only study to examine outcome in relation to clonality in cases of suspected cases of MZL did not demonstrate any significant differences in clinical behavior or prognosis.[81]

Cutaneous Follicle Center Cell Lymphoma and DLBCL

There is considerable confusion about the concept of primary cutaneous follicle center lymphoma. In lymph nodes, neoplastic follicles contain a mixture of centrocytes and centroblasts. The neoplastic cells are of B-cell origin (CD20 and CD79a positive) and express germinal center cell markers (CD10 and Bcl-6) but, unlike normal follicle center cells, are Bcl-2 positive.[82] This often reflects the presence of a t(14;18) translocation with upregulation of Bcl-2 expression. When a nodal follicular lymphoma presents in the skin, it may lose some of its follicular architecture but retains the characteristic immunoprofile and cytogenetic changes. Complete staging investigations for follicular lymphomas presenting in the skin should therefore include a whole-body computed tomography scan and bone marrow examination with molecular analysis of the aspirate. If these demonstrate systemic disease, then the patient should be treated as such.

More difficult to define are primary cutaneous B-cell lymphomas that either show a follicular architecture or are derived from both centrocytes and centroblasts but lack a follicular growth pattern. Although controversial, it seems that most of these cases are Bcl-2 negative and lack the t(14;18) translocation.[83-86] The relationship to nodal follicular lymphoma is uncertain, but, because the prognosis is excellent, these patients should be treated with skin-directed radiotherapy rather than chemotherapy.

In the WHO classification, cutaneous follicle center lymphomas are recognized as a variant of follicular lymphoma and exhibit the same immunoprofile as reactive germinal centers. In contrast, the EORTC use a broader definition of "primary cutaneous follicle center cell lymphoma (FCC lymphoma)" and includes in this category all cases of primary cutaneous DLBCLs that arise at any site on the body other than the leg (Fig. 41–11). The rationale behind this categorization is that DLBCLs arising on the leg appear to carry a worse prognosis than those arising at other anatomic sites (5-year survival of 57% vs. 95%, respectively).[87] Of note, most primary cutaneous DLBCLs on the leg are Bcl-2 positive. Bcl-2 is known to be indicative of a poor prognosis in DLBCL at extracutaneous sites,[88] and data from a multicenter French study demonstrate that this applies to the skin as well.[89] Thus, Bcl-2 was shown to be of prognostic significance in cutaneous DLBCL, whereas anatomic location on the leg did not survive multivariate analysis. Despite these observations, the concept of primary cutaneous DLBCL, leg type, has been retained in the new joint EORTC-WHO classification.[6]

TREATMENT

A proposed treatment algorithm based on stage of mycosis fungoides/Sézary syndrome is presented in Table 41–5, and salient aspects of specific therapeutic regimens are discussed in detail in the following text.

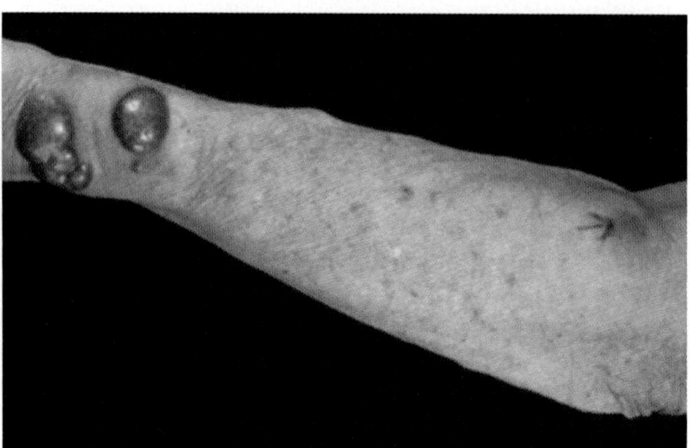

Figure 41–11. Exophytic nonulcerated nodules of diffuse large B-cell lymphoma.

Topical Therapy in Mycosis Fungoides

Topical Mechlorethamine (Nitrogen Mustard)

Mechlorethamine is an effective topical therapy for early mycosis fungoides (patches/thin plaques). Retrospective reviews have reported complete response rates of 51–80% in stage IA, 26–68% in stage IB, 61% in stage IIA, and 22–60% in stage III disease.[90-92] Duration of response varies, but cures are possible in some stage IA disease. Adverse effects of topical mechlorethamine include an irritant dermatitis, contact hypersensitivity (40%), and secondary nonmelanoma cutaneous malignancies.

Topical Carmustine (BCNU)

A retrospective review of topical BCNU therapy revealed complete responses of 86% in stage IA, 47% in stage IB, 55% stage in IIA, 17% in stage IIB, 21% in stage III, and 0% in stage IV disease.[93] Median time to complete response was 11.5 weeks. Alternate-day or daily treatment with BCNU in dilute alcohol or ointment can be used. Total doses should not exceed 600 mg per course, and repeated courses may be required. Contact hypersensitivity is uncommon (10%), but bone marrow suppression is common (30%) and requires monitoring of blood counts.

Topical Corticosteroids

Potent topical corticosteroids (class I) can induce clinical remissions in early-stage disease, but the duration of response is unknown.[94]

Topical Retinoids

The U.S. Food and Drug Administration (FDA) has approved 1% bexarotene (Targretin) gel for the treatment of stage IA/IB disease. A Phase III open study of 1% bexarotene gel in stage IA/IB/IIA disease showed a response rate of 44%, with four patients (8%) showing a complete response.[95] Median duration of treatment was 165 days, with a relapse rate of 32%. Irritant contact dermatitis occurred in 12% of patients.

Topical Peldesine (BCX-34)

Peldesine inhibits purine nucleoside phosphorylase, which is involved in purine degradation within lymphocytes. A randomized controlled trial that compared topical peldesine with a placebo (vehicle control) in 90 patients with stage IA/IB mycosis fungoides showed partial or complete clinical responses in 28% of peldesine-treated patients and 24% of placebo-treated patients (P = .677).[96] Although no significant benefit was apparent, this is the only published placebo-controlled trial in CTCL, the results of which suggest a high placebo therapeutic response of topical therapy in early-stage mycosis fungoides.

TABLE 41–5. Treatment Algorithm—Mycosis Fungoides/Sézary Syndrome

Stage	First Line	Second Line	Experimental	Not Suitable
IA	SDT/No therapy	SDT/No therapy	Bexarotene gel	Chemotherapy
IB	SDT	Interferon alfa + PUVA TSEB therapy	Denileukin diftitox Bexarotene	Chemotherapy
IIA	SDT	Interferon alfa + PUVA TSEB therapy	Denileukin diftitox Bexarotene	Chemotherapy
IIB	Radiotherapy/TSEB therapy Chemotherapy	Interferon alfa Denileukin diftitox Bexarotene	Autologous PBSCT Miniallograft	Cyclosporine
III	PUVA ± interferon alfa ECP ± interferon alfa Methotrexate	TSEB therapy Bexarotene Denileukin diftitox Chemotherapy Alemtuzumab	Autologous PBSCT Miniallograft	Cyclosporine
IVA	Radiotherapy/TSEB therapy Chemotherapy	Interferon alfa Denileukin diftitox Alemtuzumab	Autologous PBSCT Miniallograft	Cyclosporine
IVB	Radiotherapy Chemotherapy	Palliative therapy	Miniallograft	

Abbreviations: ECP, extracorporeal photopheresis; PBSCT, peripheral blood stem cell transplant; PUVA, psoralen plus A-wavelength ultraviolet photochemotherapy; SDT, skin-directed therapy; TSEB, total skin electron beam.

Phototherapy in Mycosis Fungoides/Sézary Syndrome

PUVA (psoralen plus A-wavelength ultraviolet) photochemotherapy and broadband UVB, narrowband UVB, and high-dose UVA1 phototherapy have been used with benefit in mycosis fungoides.[97–99] There have been no adequate comparative studies of different phototherapy modalities or regimens in CTCL. PUVA is an ideal therapy for stage IB/IIA disease intolerant of or failing to respond to topical therapies. Treatment schedules usually include 2–3 weekly treatments until disease clearance or best partial response. PUVA induces response rates of 79–88% in stage IA and 52–59% in stage IB disease with variable response durations.[100] Flexural sites often fail to respond completely. There is no significant response in tumor-stage (IIB) disease. Maintenance therapy is rarely effective at preventing relapse.[27] The main adverse effect is the development of nonmelanoma skin cancer, the risk of which increases when the total number of PUVA sessions exceeds 200 or a total cumulative dose exceeds 1200 J/cm^2. Although PUVA is one of the most effective therapies for patients with early-stage mycosis fungoides, there are no data to establish if PUVA can improve overall survival.

Immunotherapy in Mycosis Fungoides/Sézary Syndrome

Immunotherapy in CTCL is intended to enhance antitumor host immune responses by promoting the generation of cytotoxic T cells and type 1 T helper cell cytokine responses. Studies of interferon-alfa have shown overall response rates of 45–74% with complete responses of 10–27%.[101–102] Various dosage schedules have shown that response rates are higher with larger doses[101] and in early (IB/IIA, 88%) compared to late (III/IV, 63%) stages of disease.[102] Combined interferon-alfa and retinoids produce response rates similar to those of interferon-alfa alone and are not recommended.[103] Cyclosporine is not recommended in CTCL because it has been associated with rapid disease progression.[104] Trials evaluating the utility of interferon gamma and interleukin-2 and -12 have shown promise in the application of immunotherapy to the treatment of CTCL.[105–107]

Extracorporeal Photopheresis

Extracorporeal photopheresis (ECP) is licensed by the FDA for the treatment of CTCL. Randomized controlled trials of ECP are required to assess effects on disease-free and overall survival. Several studies suggest that total baseline Sézary count is an important predictor of response, but data on baseline CD8 counts are conflicting.[108,109] Overall survival data have been reported in four studies of ECP in erythrodermic disease, with median survivals of 39–100 months from diagnosis.[110–113] A systematic review of response rates in erythrodermic disease (stage III/IVA) with ECP has shown overall responses of 35–71% with complete responses of 14–26%.[114] More difficult to interpret are studies that have involved small patient numbers, earlier stages of disease, and various concurrent therapies. Two recent randomized crossover studies have demonstrated that ECP is of equivalent efficacy to oral methotrexate in patients with erythrodermic CTCL, but inferior to PUVA in stage IB mycosis fungoides, even for patients who exhibit a peripheral blood T-cell clone.[115,116]

Systemic Retinoids in Mycosis Fungoides/Sézary Syndrome

Etretinate/Acitretin/Isotretinoin

A systematic review of open studies of oral retinoids in mycosis fungoides and Sézary syndrome showed an overall mean response rate of 58% and a complete response rate of 19%, with a median duration of response of 3–13 months.[117] A nonrandomized study in mycosis fungoides and Sézary syndrome comparing 13-*cis*-retinoic acid with etretinate showed similar efficacy and toxicity.[118] Although acitretin and etretinate have some efficacy in early stages of mycosis fungoides, they are probably less effective than PUVA or interferon-alfa.

Bexarotene

Bexarotene, a novel retinoid that binds to the retinoid X receptor, has both antiproliferative and proapoptotic properties. The most effective tolerated oral dose is 300 mg/m^2/day, although responses improve with higher doses. Side effects are transient, reversible, and generally mild, but most patients while on therapy require treatment for hyperlipidemia and central (hypothalamic) hypothyroidism. At 300 mg/m^2/day, response rates of 54% in early-stage disease (IA/IB/IIA)[119] and 45% in advanced mycosis fungoides (stage IIB-IVB) and notable reductions in pruritus in stage III disease[120] were noted. Comparative studies and data on disease-free and overall survival are needed.

Combination Regimens Involving Photochemotherapy and Systemic Therapies

Several studies have attempted to evaluate and compare the efficacy of combination therapies such as PUVA/interferon-alfa and PUVA/acitretin. Results vary, but it appears that combination therapy may be useful in patients with resistant early-stage mycosis fungoides and Sézary syndrome, with a possible decrease in cumulative dose, increase in responsiveness, and increase in duration of response with certain combinations.[121–124]

Toxin and Antibody Therapies in Mycosis Fungoides/Sézary Syndrome

Denileukin Diftitox (Diphtheria IL-2 Fusion Toxin, DAB$_{389}$-IL-2, Ontak)

Denileukin diftitox, a diphtheria toxin and interleukin 2 fusion protein, has completed Phase I/II studies and received provisional FDA approval for the treatment of resistant or recurrent CTCL. Phase III studies of 71 heavily pretreated patients with stage IB to IVA mycosis fungoides, and more than 20% CD25$^+$ lymphocytes, showed an overall response rate of 30% and a complete response rate of 10%.[125] The median duration of response was 6.9 months. The optimally tolerated dose (18 μg/kg/day) is given intravenously for 5 days and repeated every 21 days for four to eight cycles. Adverse effects include flulike symptoms, acute infusion-related hypersensitivity, vascular leak syndrome, and transient elevations of hepatic enzymes. Myelosuppression is rare.

Antibody Therapies

Humanized chimeric anti-CD4 monoclonal antibody, alemtuzumab (CAMPATH-1H; humanized anti-CD52), fully humanized anti-CD4 antibody, and radiolabeled anti-CD5 antibody have also been used in mycosis fungoides with variable and often short-lived partial responses.[126–129]

Radiotherapy in Mycosis Fungoides/Sézary Syndrome

Superficial Radiotherapy

Individual thick plaques, eroded plaques, or tumors of CTCL can be treated successfully with fractionated low-dose superficial orthovoltage radiotherapy.[130] Large tumors may be treated by electrons, the choice of energy being dependent on tumor size and thickness. Radiotherapy is often used with PUVA.[131] Treatment is palliative except for solitary localized disease for which "cure" is possible. High-dose fractionation regimens for individual lesions should be avoided in mycosis fungoides, not only because complete response rates are similar to those for low-dose regimens, but also to reserve the option of treating recurrent disease adjacent to previously treated areas.

Total Skin Electron Beam Therapy

A systematic review of open, uncontrolled, and mostly retrospective studies of total skin electron beam (TSEB) therapy as monotherapy in CTCL showed that responses are stage dependent, with complete responses of 96% in stage IA, IB, and IIA disease; 36% in stage IIB disease; and 60% in erythrodermic (stage III) disease. High relapse rates indicate that TSEB therapy is not curative even in early-stage mycosis fungoides.[132] Greater skin surface dose and higher energy are associated with a higher rate of complete response, with 5-year relapse-free survivals of 10–23%.[132] A retrospective study of erythrodermic disease showed a complete response rate of 60%, 26% progression-free survival at 5 years, and overall median survival of 3.4 years.[133] Patients with stage III disease did better than those with significant nodal or hematologic (stage IVA/IVB) disease. Longer response duration was noted for those who received more than 20 Gy (4–9 MeV).

A randomized clinical trial comparing TSEB therapy and multiagent chemotherapy with sequential topical therapy revealed a higher complete response rate in the TSEB/chemotherapy group, but there was no significant difference in disease-free or overall survival.[134] A retrospective study comparing TSEB therapy alone and TSEB therapy followed by ECP in erythrodermic CTCL reported an overall complete response rate of 73% after TSEB therapy, with a 3-year disease-free survival of 49% with TSEB therapy alone (overall survival, 63%) and of 81% with TSEB therapy followed by ECP (overall survival, 88%).[135]

TSEB therapy should be reserved for those who fail first- and second-line therapies.[136] Adverse effects include radiation-induced secondary cutaneous malignancies, telangiectasia, pigmentation, anhidrosis, pruritus, alopecia, and xerosis. Although TSEB therapy is usually given only once in a lifetime, several reports have documented additional courses and noted a decrease in both the total doses tolerated and duration of response with subsequent courses.[137,138] Consensus EORTC recommendations have been published to optimize the efficacy of TSEB therapy in CTCL.[139]

Chemotherapy in Mycosis Fungoides/Sézary Syndrome

Single-Agent Chemotherapy Regimens

Although the lack of controlled studies makes interpretation difficult, single-agent regimens may have similar efficacy to, but lower toxicity than, combination regimens and therefore may be preferable as palliative therapy in late stages of mycosis fungoides and Sézary syndrome.[117]

Methotrexate

A retrospective report of low-dose methotrexate in erythrodermic CTCL (stage III/IVA) (where a majority [62%] of patients satisfied criteria for Sézary syndrome) has shown a 41% complete remission rate with an overall response of 58%.[131,140] Median freedom from treatment failure and overall survival were 31 months and 8.4 years, respectively.

Purine Analogues

Because they exert a selective lymphocytotoxic effect independent of cell division, purine analogues such as deoxycoformycin, 2-chlorodeoxyadenosine, and fludarabine are attractive therapeutic candidates for CTCL. Although efficacy in CTCL is moderate and response durations may be short, most reported patients were heavily pretreated and relatively chemoresistant. Patients with Sézary syndrome appear to respond better than those with late stages of mycosis fungoides.[117,141–145]

Gemcitabine

A Phase II prospective trial of the pyrimidine antimetabolite gemcitabine in 44 previously treated patients with CTCL (30 patients with stage IIB/III mycosis fungoides) reported partial responses of 59% and complete responses of 12%, with a median duration of 10 and 15 months, respectively.[146]

Doxorubicin

An open study of pegylated liposomal doxorubicin (20 mg/m^2 monthly to maximum of 400 mg or eight cycles) in 10 patients with various stages of mycosis fungoides revealed a complete response in 6 and a partial response in 2 patients, with a median response duration of 15 months.[147]

Combination Chemotherapy

Despite short response durations, late stages of CTCL (IIB-IVB) require treatment with systemic chemotherapy. A systematic review of all systemic chemotherapy in mycosis fungoides/Sézary syndrome showed an overall response rate of 81% in 331 patients treated with various combination regimens, with a complete response rate of 38% and response duration of 5–41 months. No cures were documented for patients with late stages of disease (IIB-IVB).[117] Recent prospective, nonrandomized studies of multiagent chemotherapy regimens have revealed similar overall response rates.[148,149]

Myeloablative Chemotherapy with Stem Cell Transplantation

High-dose chemotherapy with TSEB therapy and/or total-body irradiation followed by autologous bone marrow transplantation in six mycosis fungoides patients with advanced disease revealed five complete clinical responses with disease relapse in three patients within 100 days.[150] The other patients were disease free at almost 2 years posttransplantation. High-dose chemotherapy combined with either TSEB therapy or total-body irradiation and followed by autologous peripheral blood stem cell transplantation in nine patients with stage IIB/IVA mycosis fungoides revealed complete responses in eight patients and durable clinical responses in four patients, with a median disease-free survival of 11 months.[151] Isolated case reports of high-dose chemotherapy with total-body irradiation followed by allogeneic bone marrow or stem cell transplantation have shown long-term complete remissions in both stage IIB mycosis fungoides and Sézary syndrome.[152,153] To date, there are no data to indicate if this approach affects disease-free or overall survival, and controlled trials are needed.

Treatment of Primary Cutaneous T-Cell Lymphoma Variants

Because the primary cutaneous CD30$^+$ T-cell lymphomas represent a spectrum of disease with an excellent prognosis, skin-directed therapy is indicated.[69] Lymphomatoid papulosis is radiosensitive. PUVA and low-dose methotrexate can prevent recurrent lesions,[69,154] and high-dose chemotherapy is *not* indicated. Skin-directed treatment of PCALCL is also appropriate unless patients develop very extensive cutaneous involvement or systemic disease.[69]

Primary cutaneous T-cell lymphomas, such as CD30$^-$ large-cell pleomorphic, anaplastic, and immunoblastic variants, have a poor prognosis. When disease is restricted to the skin, radiotherapy may be indicated, but systemic dissemination requiring multiagent chemotherapy is likely. Extranasal (cutaneous) natural killer–like/T-cell lymphoma and blastic natural killer cell lymphoma both have a poor prognosis, as does the γ/δ subtype of subcutaneous panniculitis–like T-cell lymphoma. These categories of CTCL invariably require systemic chemotherapy.

Treatment of Primary Cutaneous B-Cell Lymphomas

Primary cutaneous MZL has an excellent prognosis. Although radiotherapy is often appropriate, other patients may simply be observed.[155] Interferon alfa may be effective either systemically or intralesionally.[156] In cases associated with *Borrelia burgdorferi,* antibiotic therapy is appropriate.[156] In cases of primary cutaneous follicle center cell lymphoma, superficial radiotherapy is the treatment of choice. Solitary lesions may be treated with excision and subsequent radiotherapy to reduce the risk of local recurrence. In rare cases with very extensive cutaneous disease or systemic involvement, single-agent treatment with chlorambucil or combination chemotherapy may be indicated.[155,157,158] Primary cutaneous DLBCL occurring as a solitary tumor may be treated with radiotherapy, but in most other patients chemotherapy is also required, especially for multifocal disease and tumors showing Bcl-2 positivity.[159] The role of rituximab has yet to be determined, although intralesional administration may be effective.[160–162]

PROGNOSIS

Prognostic data for mycosis fungoides/Sézary syndrome based on the TNM and clinical staging system are presented in Table 41–6. Multivariate analysis has established that age at onset (>60 years), skin stage, and the presence of nodal (stage IVA) or visceral (stage IVB) disease are independent prognostic factors in mycosis fungoides.[163–167] A patient's life expectancy is not adversely affected in stage IA disease, with a 5- and 15-year disease-specific survival rate of 100% and 98%, respectively.[41] The disease-specific survival for each stage of mycosis fungoides is depicted in Table 41–6.[168,169] Of note, patients with thick plaques or folliculotropic disease may have a worse prognosis than expected for the stage of disease.[50,170] The presence of a peripheral blood T-cell clone identical to that in skin may also indicate which patients with early-stage disease are likely to develop disease progression.[171] The development of lymph node disease (stage IVA) has a significant impact on prognosis.[48] Sézary syndrome patients have a poor prognosis, with an overall median survival of 32 months from time of diagnosis.[172] In erythrodermic CTCL, peripheral nodal disease is the most important prognostic factor, although the peripheral blood tumor burden is also very close to significance.[60]

Primary cutaneous $CD30^+$ lymphoproliferative disorders have an excellent prognosis. Only 10% of patients with lymphomatoid papulosis develop an associated lymphoma. Primary cutaneous $CD30^+$ large-cell lymphomas have a 90% 5-year disease-specific survival. Patients with loco-regional disease may have a worse prognosis.[69]

TABLE 41–6. Published Prognostic Data in Mycosis Fungoides/Sézary Syndrome

	IA	IB	IIA	IIB	III	IVA	IVB	Overall	Reference	N	Median FU (yr)
OS at 5 yr	99%	86% (75%)	49%	65%		40%	0%	80%	van Doorn*	309	5.2
	100%	84%		52%	57%				Zackheim†	489	4.7
	97%	72%		40%	41%	27%**	27%**	68%	Kim‡	525	5.5
						15%	15%		Coninck§	112	
OS at 10 yr	84%	61% (21%)	49%	27%		20%	0%	57%	van Doorn	309	5.2
	100%	67%		39%	41%				Zackheim	489	4.7
						5%	5%		Coninck	112	
	88%	55%		26%	24%			53%	Kim	525	5.5
DSS at 5 yr	100%	96% (81%)	68%	80%		40%	0%	89%	van Doorn	309	5.2
	100%	95%	84%	56%	65%	30%**	30%**	81%	Kim	525	5.5
DSS at 10 yr	97%	83% (36%)	68%	42%		20%	0%	75%	van Doorn	309	5.2
DSS at 15 yr	98%	85%	71%	32%	49%	14%**	14%**		Kim	525	5.5
Median survival	NR	12.1 yr		3.3 yr	4.0 yr			11.4 yr	Kim	525	5.5
						13 mo	13 mo		Coninck	546	
DP at 5 yr	4%	21%	65%	32%		70%	100%		van Doorn	309	5.2
	10%	22%		56%	48%				Kim	525	5.5
DP at 10 yr	10%	39%	65%	60%		70%	100%		van Doorn	309	5.2
	13%	32%		72%	57%				Kim	525	5.5
DP at 20 yr	0%	10%		36%	41%				Coninck	546	
	16%	40%		81%	78%				Kim	525	5.5

All actuarial survival curves calculated according to the Kaplan-Meier method and based on stage at diagnosis.

*In the 2000 study by van Doorn and colleagues [168] (and in a subsequent publication by van Doorn [50]), the presence of follicular mucinosis was an independent poor prognostic feature possibly related to depth of infiltrate in patients with stage IB disease (DSS of 81% and 36% and OS of 75% and 21% at 5 and 10 years, respectively). A lack of a complete response to initial therapy, as well as increasing clinical stage and the presence of extracutaneous disease, was also associated with a poor outcome ($P < .001$) in a multivariate analysis. A different staging system was used in this study (based on Hamminga and colleagues [164]), but, for the purposes of this table, the staging has been altered to be consistent. Only 3 patients had stage IVB disease and only 18 patients each had stages IIA and IVA disease. Therefore, the results for these stages must be interpreted cautiously.

†In the 1999 study by Zackheim and colleagues [43], black patients had a relatively more advanced stage of disease than white patients. The TNM classification was used in this study. Lymph node stage had an unfavorable impact on survival, but this trend did not reach significance for each individual T stage because of a lack of sufficient power (an estimated 1700 subjects required), and stage IIA/IVA patients were not designated separately. Similar considerations apply to peripheral blood involvement. The finding of similar outcomes for patients with stage IIB (T_3) and III (T_4) disease is consistent with other studies, but this might reflect a lack of lymph node staging data included in this study.

‡In the 2003 study by Kim and colleagues [41], the median survival for stage IA patients was not reached at 32.5 years. **The OS and DSS figures were based on stage IV disease, with no distinction made between stage IVA and IVB. This is a recent retrospective study, but some of the data have previously been published based on different stages of disease.

§The 2001 study by Coninck and colleagues [169], included 112 patients with extracutaneous disease at presentation or with progression and 434 patients with only cutaneous disease, giving the 546 patients listed in the table for median survival and disease progression.

Abbreviations: DP, disease progression; DSS, disease-specific survival; NR, not reached; OS, overall survival.

CURRENT CONTROVERSIES & FUTURE CONSIDERATIONS

Cutaneous Lymphomas

- What are the appropriate criteria for the diagnosis of early mycosis fungoides?
- Our current staging system for mycosis fungoides, although useful in many regards, is inherently flawed because stage III has a better prognosis than stage IIB. Should the staging of mycosis fungoides be extended to include hematologic stage and pathologic features such as large-cell transformation or p53 positivity?
- Should erythrodermic CTCL be classified separately from mycosis fungoides, and then staged depending upon the degree of blood as well as lymph node involvement?
- Is genomic instability primary or secondary? Do genomic abnormalities carry prognostic significance?
- Are the immunosuppression and resulting opportunistic infections of advanced CTCL caused by physical displacement of normal T cells by malignant cells, by systemic effects of CTCL-produced cytokines (i.e., IL-10), or by broad-based T-cell suppression by the CTCL regulatory cells (CTCL T-regs)?
- Should evidence of clonality in the peripheral blood be an absolute requirement for the diagnosis of Sézary syndrome?
- Should subcutaneous panniculitis–like T-cell lymphoma of γ/δ derivation be classified with other γ/δ T-cell lymphomas, or should it be regarded as a more aggressive variant of subcutaneous T-cell lymphoma of α/β derivation?
- What is the cell of origin for blastic natural killer cell lymphoma? Is it a $CD4^+$ plasmacytoid dendritic cell?
- Early mycosis fungoides is treated with skin-directed therapy such as topical chemotherapy and phototherapy, but does this affect prognosis, and should therapy be intermittent, alternating, or continuous?
- Do topical therapies have their impact directly on the skin-homing malignant T cells or through inhibition of the stimulatory impact of Langerhans cells on CTCL cell proliferation?
- Should vaccination therapy for advanced mycosis fungoides involving TCR idiotypes be abandoned because of the difficulty of sequencing the TCR genes individually for each patient?
- Does cutaneous lymphoid hyperplasia exist on the spectrum of B-cell lymphomas or should it be considered a separate and benign entity?
- Is primary cutaneous follicle center cell lymphoma a separate entity from nodal follicular lymphoma and diffuse large B-cell lymphoma?
- Should the concept of "leg-type diffuse large B-cell lymphoma" be abandoned in favor of prognostic factors such as Bcl-2 positivity that are known to be biologically relevant?

The prognosis for primary cutaneous MZL is excellent, with an estimated 5-year survival of 98–100%.[173–175] The estimated 5-year survival of patients with primary cutaneous follicle center cell lymphoma is 94–97%.[176] Primary cutaneous DLBCL has a variable prognosis, with lesions arising on the leg having a worse prognosis than histologically similar lesions elsewhere. A 5-year survival of 58% is provided by the Dutch data.[87] However, the poor prognosis in this group is at least partly linked to the tumor cell cytology and expression of Bcl-2.[89,177]

Suggested Readings*

Berger CL, Hanlon D, Kanada D, et al: The growth of cutaneous T-cell lymphoma is stimulated by immature dendritic cells. Blood 99:2929–2939, 2002.

Beylot-Barry M, Sibaud V, Thiebaut R, et al: Evidence that an identical T cell clone in skin and peripheral blood lymphocytes is an independent prognostic factor in primary cutaneous T cell lymphomas. J Invest Dermatol 117:920–926, 2001.

Edelson R, Berger C, Gasparro F, et al: Treatment of cutaneous T-cell lymphoma by extracorporeal photochemotherapy. N Engl J Med 316:297–303, 1987.

Grange F, Petrella T, Beylot-Barry M, et al: Bcl-2 protein expression is the strongest independent prognostic factor of survival in primary cutaneous large B-cell lymphomas. Blood 103:3662–3668, 2004.

Kim YH, Liu HL, Mraz-Gernhard S, et al: Long-term outcome of 525 patients with mycosis fungoides and Sezary syndrome: clinical prognostic factors and risk for disease progression. Arch Dermatol 139:857–866, 2003.

Vergier B, de Muret A, Beylot-Barry M, et al: Transformation of mycosis fungoides: clinicopathological and prognostic features of 45 cases. French Study Group of Cutaneous Lymphomas. Blood 95:2212–2218, 2000.

Vonderheid E, Bernengo M, Burg G, et al, for the ISCL: Update on erythrodermic cutaneous T-cell lymphoma: report of the International Society for Cutaneous Lymphomas. J Am Acad Dermatol 46:95–106, 2002.

Whittaker SJ, Marsden JR, Spittle M, Russell Jones R: Joint British Association of Dermatologists and U.K. Cutaneous Lymphoma Group guidelines for the management of primary cutaneous T-cell lymphomas. Br J Dermatol 149:1095–1107, 2003.

Willemze R, Jaffe ES, Burg G, et al: WHO-EORTC classification for cutaneous lymphomas. Blood 105:3768–3785, 2005.

Zackheim HS, Amin S, Kashani-Sabet M, McMillan A: Prognosis in cutaneous T-cell lymphoma by skin stage: long-term survival in 489 patients. J Am Acad Dermatol 40:418–425, 1999.

CHAPTER 42

Primary and Secondary Central Nervous System Lymphomas in Immunocompetent and Human Immunodeficiency Virus–Positive Patients

Lauren E. Abrey, MD, and Andrés J. M. Ferreri, MD

KEY POINTS

Primary and Secondary Central Nervous System Lymphomas in Immunocompetent and Human Immunodeficiency Virus–Positive Patients

- Primary central nervous system lymphoma (PCNSL) occurs predominantly in individuals over 50 years of age. Rapid clinical onset with nonspecific neurologic deficits occurs in about 50% of cases; the frontal lobe is often involved, so personality changes are frequent.
- Radiographic characteristics include an isointense lesion on the pre-gadolinium T1-weighted magnetic resonance image localized in the periventricular regions with intense and homogeneous enhancement after contrast administration.
- Diffuse large B-cell lymphomas constitute 75–90% of cases.
- Staging procedures currently used for aggressive non-Hodgkin's lymphoma are strongly recommended.
- Prognostic factors include patient age, performance status, serum lactate dehydrogenase level, cerebrospinal fluid protein concentration, and involvement of deep structures of the brain.
- Standard treatment consists of high-dose methotrexate–based chemotherapy followed by whole-brain radiotherapy. This strategy produces a 2-year overall survival of 65–80%. The optimal methotrexate schedule appears to be an initial rapid administration followed by a 3- to 6-hour infusion.
- Ocular irradiation should be included in the treatment of patients with ocular lymphoma.
- Salvage therapy may be attempted for patients with recurrent or refractory PCNSL.
- Secondary central nervous system (CNS) lymphoma is a devastating complication of non-Hodgkin's lymphoma. High-risk patients with Burkitt's lymphoma, aggressive T-cell lymphoma, and high International Prognostic Index score diffuse large B-cell lymphoma should receive prophylactic therapy in an effort to prevent CNS dissemination.
- The advent of highly active antiretroviral therapy has both decreased the incidence and improved the prognosis for patients with acquired immunodeficiency virus–related PCNSL. These patients should be treated with aggressive antiviral therapies in addition to methotrexate-based chemotherapy.

PRIMARY CENTRAL NERVOUS SYSTEM LYMPHOMA IN IMMUNOCOMPETENT PATIENTS

Epidemiology and Risk Factors

Primary central nervous system lymphoma (PCNSL) comprises only 4% of all primary brain tumors and less than 1% of extranodal non-Hodgkin's lymphomas.[1] However, the incidence has increased in the last several decades in both immunodeficient[2] and immunocompetent individuals.[3] A recent epidemiologic study showed that the incidence of PCNSL has tripled in the healthy population.[4,5] This increase is not attributable to improvements in diagnostic techniques and continues to be unex-

TABLE 42–1. Comparison of Clinical, Radiologic, and Histologic Features of PCNSL in Immunocompetent and Immunodeficient Patients

	Immunocompetent Patients	Immunodeficient Patients
Epidemiology	Increasing	Decreasing since HAART
Pathogenesis	Unknown	EBV infection, c-*myc* translocation
Male : female ratio	1.4 : 1	7.4 : 1
Median age (yr)	55–60	30
Duration of symptoms to diagnosis (mo)	2–3	1–2
Clinical presentation	Focal deficits (>50%)	Mental status changes (>50%)
MRI	Iso- or hyperdense (90%) Enhancement (95%)	Iso- or hyperdense (90%) Enhancement (90%)
Number of lesions	Solitary (60–70%)	Multiple (>50%)
CSF cytology	Performed: 65% Positive: 10–25%	Performed: <5% Positive: 25%
Histology	DLCL: 75–85% T cell: 2%	DLCL: 75% Small noncleaved: 25% T cell: <1%
EBV genomic DNA	Rare	Positive
Survival (mo)	RT alone: 12–18 CTM: 25–45 None: 3	RT alone: 3 CTM: 10–12 None: <1

Abbreviations: CSF, cerebrospinal fluid; CTM, combined-treatment modality; DLCL, diffuse large-cell lymphoma; EBV, Epstein-Barr virus; HAART, highly active antiretroviral therapy; MRI, magnetic resonance imaging; RT, radiotherapy.

Updated from Ferreri AJ, Reni M, Villa E: Primary central nervous system lymphoma in immunocompetent patients. Cancer Treat Rev 21:415–446, 1995.

plained. If the incidence continues to increase at this rate over the next decade, PCNSL will become the most frequent brain neoplasm.

There are significant differences between PCNSL in immunocompetent and immunocompromised patients (Table 42–1). The relationship between PCNSL and immunosuppression of viral,[6–8] iatrogenic,[2,9,10] or congenital[2,11] origin is well known. Whereas Epstein-Barr virus infection and the translocation of proto-oncogene c-*myc* result in the proliferation of malignant lymphocytes in human immunodeficiency virus (HIV) patients,[12–14] the pathogenesis of PCNSL in apparently immunocompetent patients remains unknown. The fact that PCNSL predominantly occurs in the elderly suggests a possible reduction in immunologic vigilance, particularly of T lymphocytes. The proliferation of B lymphocytes produced by chromosomal abnormalities or viral stimulation might give rise to the development of a monoclonal lymphoma as a result of the lack of suppressive activity of T-cells.[15] This proliferation may be particularly facilitated in the extranodal areas with peculiar immunologic characteristics, such as the central nervous system (CNS).[7]

In contrast to other non-Hodgkin's lymphomas, there is no evidence of a hereditary pathogenesis of PCNSL. However, PCNSL as second neoplasm has been reported by several authors.[16–18] This phenomenon may be explained by a genetic predisposition or a carcinogenic effect of the antineoplastic therapy administered to the initial tumor.

Pathophysiology and Pathogenesis

The large majority of PCNSLs in immunocompetent patients are Epstein-Barr virus–negative diffuse large B-cell lymphomas; T-cell PCNSLs are rare (1–2%).[19] Rare forms are represented by marginal zone lymphomas, intravascular large B-cell lymphomas (Fig. 42–1), anaplastic large-cell lymphomas (Fig. 42–2), and Hodgkin's lymphoma.[20–22] In the majority of cases, a vasocentric proliferation with infiltration of the cerebral parenchyma among the involved vessels, and the multiplication of the basal membranes of the blood vessels encased by the neoplasm, may be observed. Because lymphocyte migration into the CNS depends on a selective interaction of the lymphocytic adhesion molecules with the vascular endothelium of the CNS, this might explain the typical perivascular localization and vasocentric proliferation of PCNSL.[23] A reactive perivascular T-cell infiltration is observed in 30% of cases (Fig. 42–3).

Data obtained from experiments of gene expression profiling have demonstrated a germinal-center origin for PCNSL. Mutations of *bcl-6* have been found in 50% of PCNSLs of immunocompetent patients, and expression of the Bcl-6 protein has been found in 100% of all investigated lymphomas.[24] Bcl-6 has been recently reported as a favorable predictor of survival in PCNSL.[25] Molecular studies show an intermediate to high frequency of somatic mutations (~13%) among the clonally rearranged immunoglobulin H genes.[26,27] This significantly exceeds the average mutation frequency of normal B-cells, which is 5–6%, and those found in other lymphoma entities. Analysis of V-region genes demonstrates a biased use of V_H; the V_H4-34 gene segment of the V_H4 family has been found to be preferentially used. Intraclonal nucleotide heterogeneity was observed, indicating that the V_H genes are still under the influence of the somatic hypermutation mechanism. On further analysis, the ratio of replacement to silent mutations (R/S ratio) showed evidence for the preservation of a functional immunoglobulin structure and functional antibody.

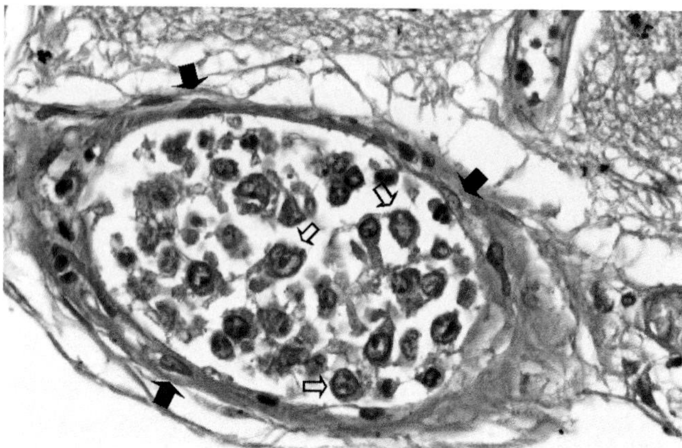

Figure 42–1. Intravascular lymphoma of the brain (hematoxylin and eosin staining). The growth of neoplastic large cells *(open arrows)* occurs exclusively within the blood vessel lumen (endothelial cells; *full arrows*). (Courtesy of Maurilio Ponzoni, MD, Department of Pathology, San Raffaele H Scientific Institute, Milan, Italy.)

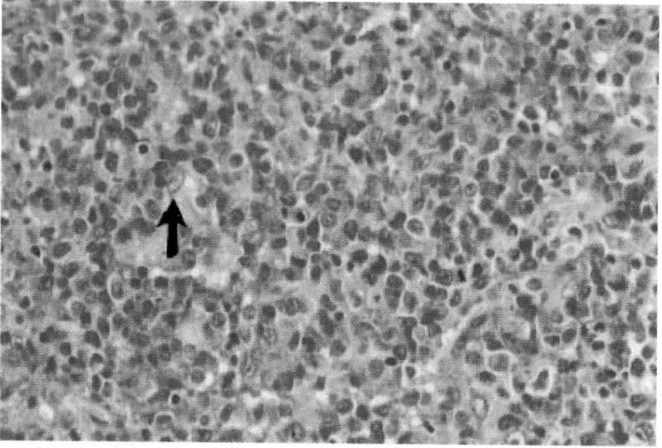

A

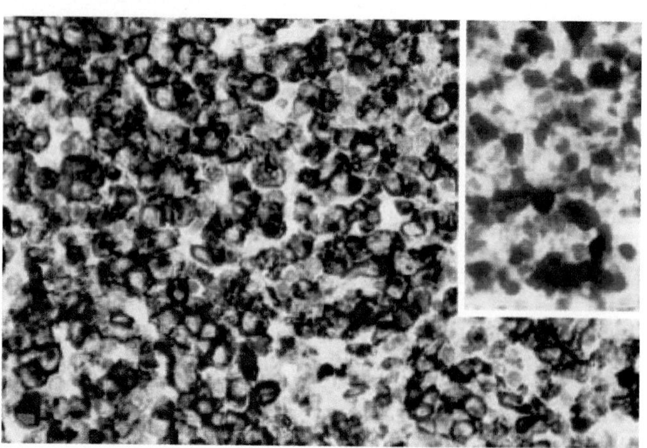

B

Figure 42–2. A case of primary brain CD30$^+$, ALK1$^+$ anaplastic large-cell lymphoma ("alkoma") with a combination of uncommon variants. ***A,*** The neoplastic population is composed of medium to large cells. A monocyte is indicated by an *arrow* in order to illustrate the overall smaller size of lymphomatous cells (hematoxylin & eosin staining; ×400). ***B,*** Lymphoma cells are strongly and diffusely reactive for CD30 molecule. *Inset* (top right) shows intense nuclear reactivity for ALK-1 protein (×400).

TABLE 42–2. Patient Characteristics in a Retrospective Multicenter Series of 378 Immunocompetent Patients with PCNSL

Age	
Median	61 yr
Range	14–85
Age >70 yr	14%
Male : female ratio	1.4 : 1
Performance status (ECOG score)	
0–1	35%
2–3	50%
4	15%
Prior cancer	4%
Histology	
Indolent	5%
Diffuse large B-cell lymphoma	60%
Highly aggressive	15%
Unclassified	20%
T-cell phenotype	2%
Elevated serum LDH level	35%
Intraocular disease	13%
Positive CSF cytology examination	16%
High CSF protein concentration	61%
Multiple lesions	34%
Involvement of deep structures of the brain*	36%

*Refers to basal ganglia and/or brainstem and/or cerebellum.
Abbreviations: CSF, cerebrospinal fluid; ECOG, Eastern Cooperative Oncology Group; LDH, lactate dehydrogenase.
From Hochberg FH, Miller DC: Primary central nervous system lymphoma. J Neurosurg 68:835–853, 1988, with permission.

Among genes involved in cell cycle regulation, p16^{INK4a} deletion and methylation have been observed in 50% and 66% of PCNSL, respectively; hypermethylation or deletion of p14^{ARF} has been detected in 56% of cases. Concomitant deletions of both occur in a third of PCNSLs, and are paralleled by loss of expression at the protein level. The expression of apoptosis-related genes, such as Bcl-2 family proteins BAX and BCL-X, is not increased in PCNSLs of immunocompetent patients.[28] The biologic and prognostic relevance of these features is far from being completely understood because only small, single-institution series are available.

Clinical Features

PCNSL occurs in all age groups but mostly in individuals over 50 years of age, with a slight predominance in males (Table 42–2). Performance status (ECOG score) is 2 or better in 70% of cases.[19] Clinical onset is acute to subacute, with most patients having symptoms for 1–3 months prior to diagnosis. Nonspecific focal neurologic deficits and personality changes are the presenting symptoms in about 50% of the cases; headaches (56%) and signs of intracranial hypertension, such as nausea (35%), vomiting (11%), and papilledema (32%), are also frequent.[29] Generalized seizures, brainstem or cerebellar dysfunction, or extrapyramidal syndromes are uncommon.[30–32] Occasional patients will present with symptoms of ocular or leptomeningeal involvement. Ocular lymphoma typically presents as a nonspecific monocular uveitis with floaters or visual blurring. Leptomeningeal

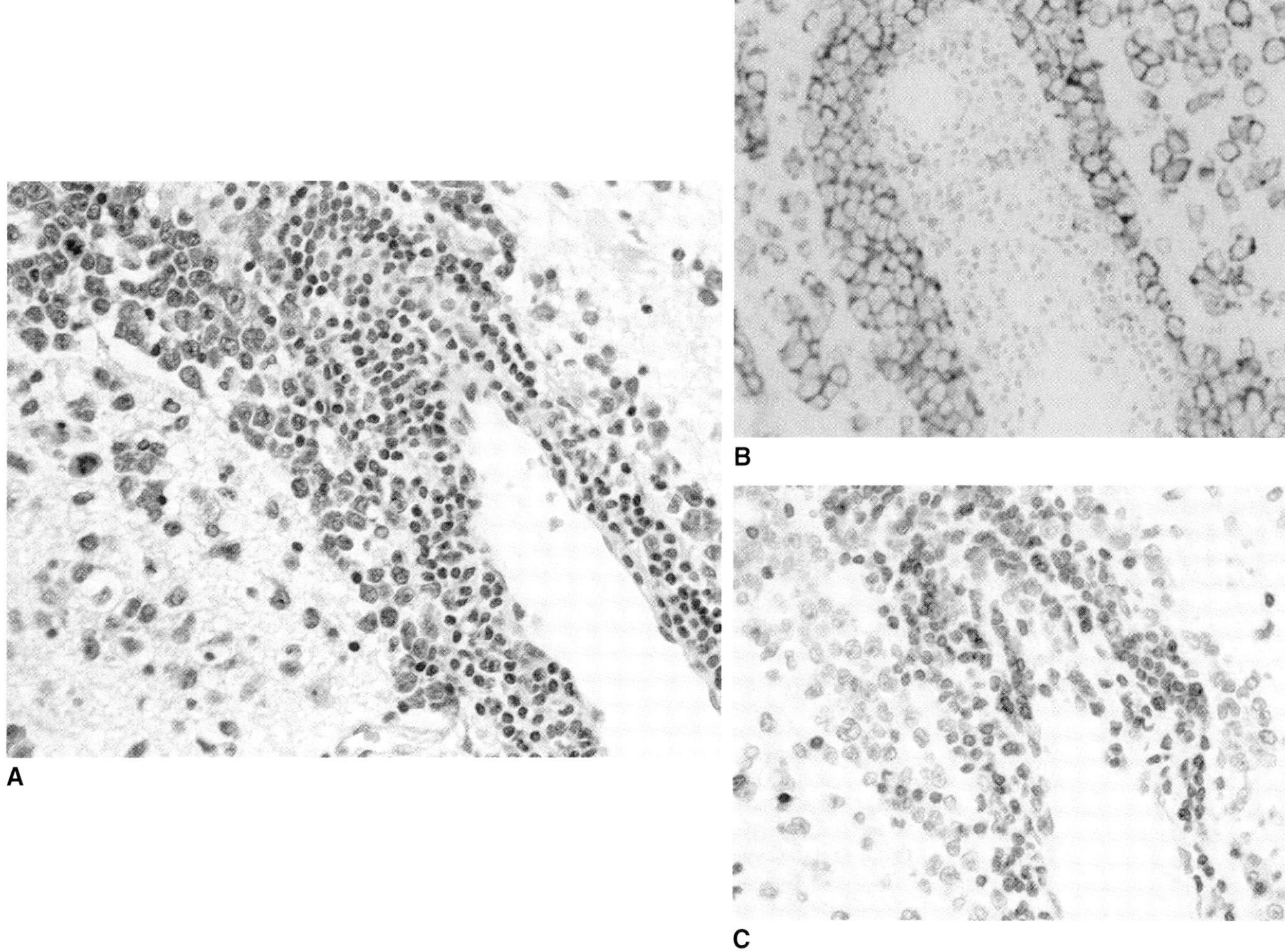

Figure 42–3. Diffuse large B-cell lymphoma of the brain. ***A***, Diffuse perivascular proliferation of neoplastic large cells with infiltration of surrounding cerebral parenchyma. Smaller cells densely infiltrating the perivascular space—that is, the space between the vascular wall and neoplastic large cells—are observed in 30% of PCNSLs. Conversely to neoplastic large cells, which are CD20$^+$ ***(B)***, small cells are reactive T lymphocytes, with CD20$^-$ ***(B)***, CD3$^+$ ***(C)*** pattern. (Courtesy of Dr. Maurilio Ponzoni, Department of Pathology, San Raffaele H Scientific Institute, Milan, Italy.)

dissemination may result in radiculopathy, mental status changes, or increased intracranial pressure. Systemic symptoms are present in 2% of cases.[19]

Localization

PCNSLs can arise in the brain parenchyma, the eye, the leptomeninges, and the spinal cord (Fig. 42–4). In the majority of cases, PCNSL presents as a single lesion, deeply localized, usually in the periventricular regions infiltrating the corpus callosum and the basal ganglia, and with variable perilesional edema (Fig. 42–5). Multiple lesions are observed in 30–40% of cases[19] (Fig. 42–6). Sometimes the neoplasm symmetrically infiltrates both the cerebral hemispheres via the corpus callosum, giving origin to the typical radiographic "butterfly" image. Only 10–15% of the lesions are in the infratentorial fossa (Fig. 42–7).

PCNSL tends to infiltrate the subependymal tissues, disseminating through the cerebrospinal fluid (CSF) to the meninges.[33] Primary leptomeningeal lymphoma in the absence of a parenchymal mass represents less than 10% of the cases; however, malignant lymphocytes can be detected in the CSF of 15–20% of PCNSL patients.[19,34] An autopsy study demonstrating meningeal involvement in 100% of the cases[35] suggests that leptomeningeal dissemination is underestimated with current methods. In 5–20% of cases, PCNSL involves the eyes.[19,34] Because the eye is an extension of the CNS, its involvement is not considered a systemic dissemination, even if bilateral. The involvement of both eyes occurs in almost 80% of the cases.[19,34] The neoplastic cells can infiltrate the vitreous humour, the retina, the choroid, and, less frequently, the optic nerve.[36] Spinal cord involvement is rare.

Imaging

Although pathognomonic radiologic patterns of PCNSL do not exist,[13,36,37] computed tomography scanning and magnetic resonance imaging (MRI) may suggest the diagnosis. Gadolinium-enhanced MRI is the optimal imaging modality. Most lesions are supratentorial and periven-

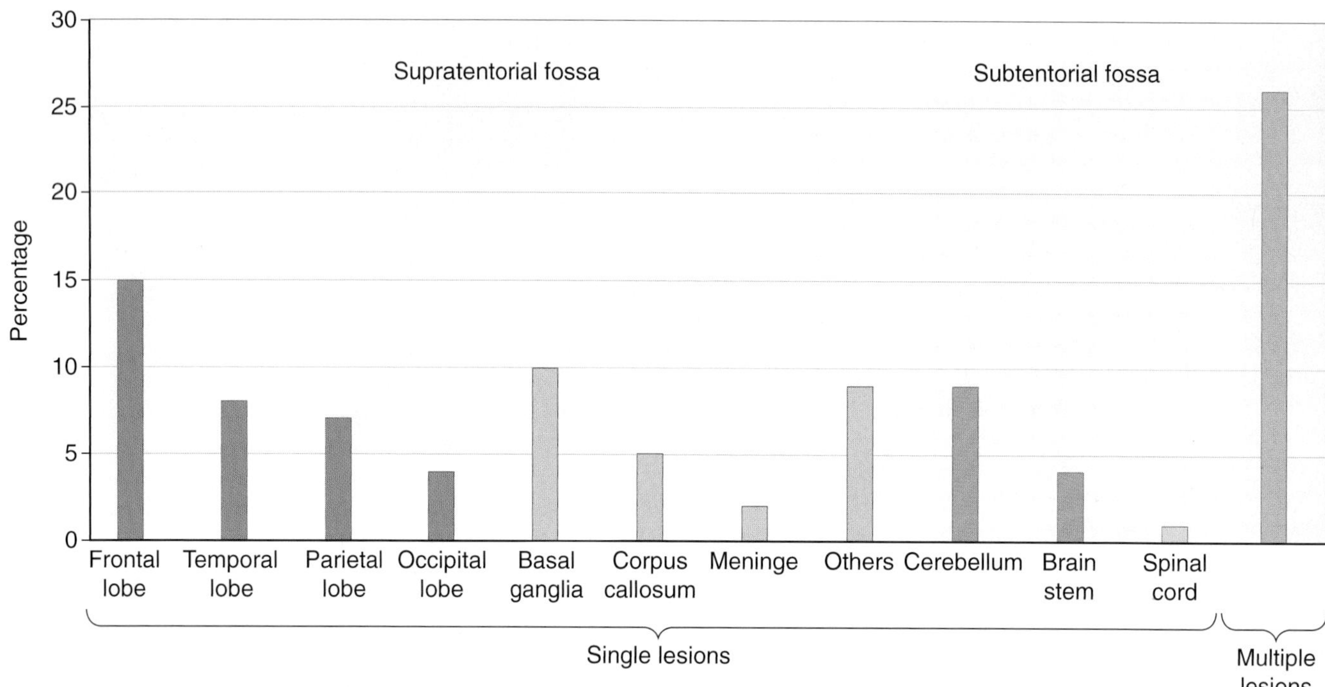

Figure 42–4. Distribution of sites of disease in PCNSL in immunocompetent patients. In cases with single lesions, the frontal lobe is the most common site of disease.

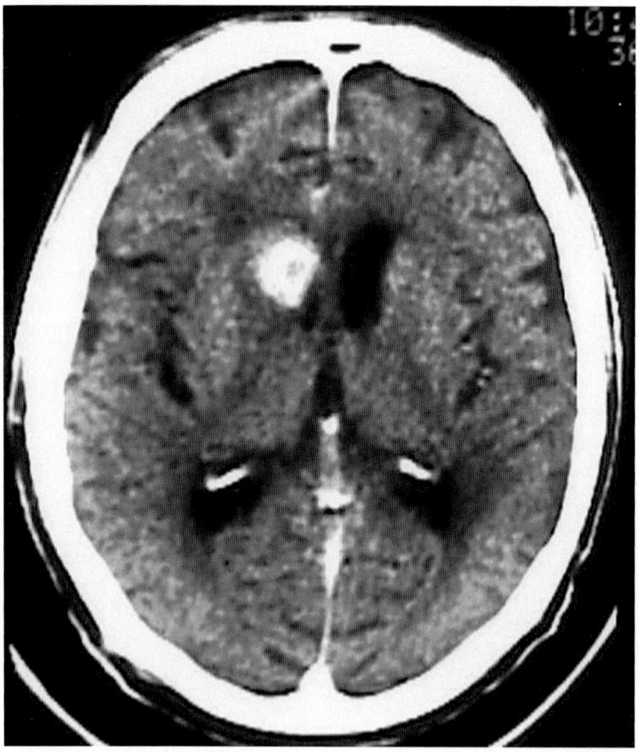

Figure 42–5. Contrast-enhanced computed tomography scan of PCNSL presenting as a poorly delimited, single lesion, localized in the right periventricular regions and infiltrating the corpus callosum and basal ganglia.

tricular, often involving deep structures such as the corpus callosum and basal ganglia. Lesions may be hypo- or hyperintense on precontrast T1-weighted imaging. Contrast administration results in intense and homogeneous enhancement[38–40] (Fig. 42–8); only about 12% of lesions are nonenhancing.[34] Peritumoral edema and local mass effect is often less than expected with intracranial lesions of other etiologies. Calcification, hemorrhage, or cyst formation is rare. In some cases, a diffuse infiltration of the white matter accompanied by a slight enhancement can be observed.

N-isopropyl-*p*-[^{123}I]iodoamphetamine single-photon emission computed tomography (^{123}I-IMP SPECT) and ^{18}fluorodeoxyglucose positron emission tomography (FDG-PET) may be useful diagnostic modalities in PCNSL. In a series of 96 patients with brain tumors, including 11 PCNSL patients, ^{123}I-IMP SPECT showed an increased accumulation on delayed images in PCNSL, while a decreased accumulation was observed in all other brain tumors.[41] An IMP index of greater than 1 on early (15-minute), delayed (6-hour), and extra-delayed (24-hour) ^{123}I-IMP SPECT images has been observed in 40%, 70%, and 90% of PCNSL patients, respectively, whereas the IMP index is less than 1 on any image of both malignant gliomas and meningioma.[41] The high ^{123}I-IMP retention on SPECT images is regarded as characteristic of PCNSL and may be more useful for diagnosis of this tumor than is ^{123}I-IMP uptake on a single SPECT image.[41] FDG-PET has excellent sensitivity in the detection of systemic non-Hodgkin's lymphoma and PCNSL, and the latter has been shown to have a high cell density and metabolic rate that make it possible to discriminate it from normal brain and other high-grade brain tumors on PET imaging.

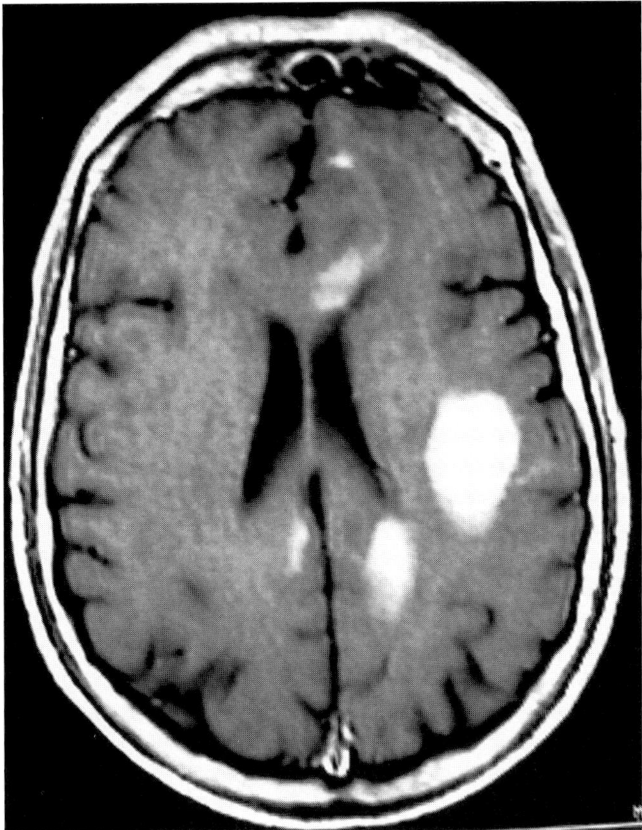

Figure 42–6. PCNSL presents as multiple lesions in 30–40% of cases in immunocompetent patients. Brain metastases from extracranial tumor are the main differential diagnosis in these patients.

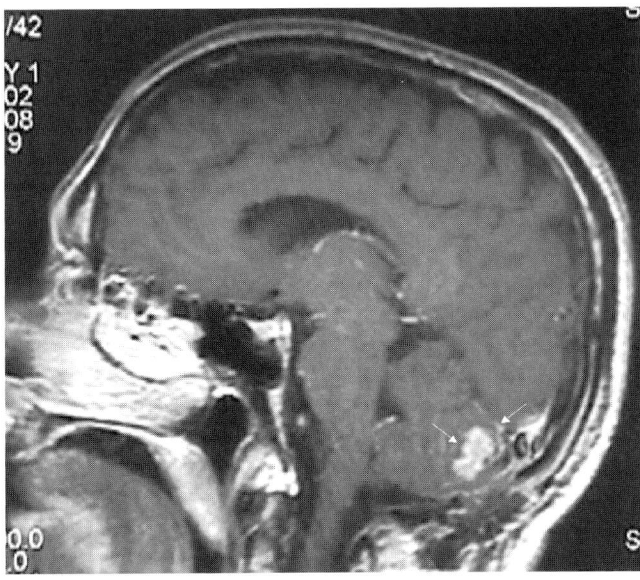

Figure 42–7. Single-lesion PCNSL of the posterior fossa *(arrows)*. Lesions of the infratentorial region are present in less than 15% of cases.

TABLE 42–3. Staging Procedures and Pretreatment Evaluation

Staging Procedures
Whole-brain MRI
CSF evaluation: cytology, cell count, total protein
Ophthalmologic evaluation (including slit-lamp examination)
Thorax and abdomen CT scan
Bone marrow aspirate and biopsy
Testicular ultrasonography (elderly males)
Pretreatment Evaluation
Performance status
Physical and neurologic examination
Biochemical serum profile
Baseline neuropsychiatric tests
Renal and hepatic functionality tests (creatinine clearance)
HIV evaluation
Serum lactate dehydrogenase level

Abbreviations: CSF, cerebrospinal fluid; CT, computed tomography; HIV, human immunodeficiency virus; MRI, magnetic resonance imaging.

Staging and Pretreatment Evaluation

PCNSL requires a complete staging work-up, including physical examination, routine blood studies, total-body computed tomography scan, slit-lamp examination and indirect ophthalmoscopy, CSF cytology and biochemical examination, and bone marrow biopsy; testicular ultrasonography should be considered in older men (Table 42–3).[42,43] The presence of systemic lymphoma during staging work-up or within 2 months of diagnosis has been observed in 5% of PCNSL patients.[42] Incomplete staging of patients in prospective PCNSL trials produces unreliable conclusions.[44]

Ocular involvement is symptomatic in up to 20% of cases at the time of diagnosis, but an additional 6% can be detected during the ophthalmologic examination as a part of the staging.[16] Therefore, a detailed ophthalmologic examination, including study of the uvea, the choroid, and the retina with slit-lamp and indirect ophthalmoscopy, is necessary. Suspicion of vitreal infiltration should be confirmed by vitrectomy.

CSF protein concentration is increased in 65–85% of cases with diffuse meningeal infiltration.[19,35,45,46] CSF cytology may allow diagnosis of PCNSL in patients who cannot be biopsied. Moreover, a positive CSF cytology has potential prognostic and therapeutic implications. Unfortunately, it is not possible to identify lymphomatous cells in every case and sometimes not even in the presence of an extensive meningeal infiltration.[31] Immunohistochemical analysis of the κ and λ chains and polymerase chain reaction studies may improve the diagnostic yield of CSF samples.[47,48] Although most PCNSLs have a B-cell phenotype,[49–51] these neoplasms are associated with a polyclonal proliferation of reactive T lymphocytes in greater than 50% of cases. Therefore, the study of both clonogenicity and immunophenotype may differentiate the reactive or neoplastic character of lymphocytic pleocytosis.[52] Finally, in some cases, the use of electronic microscopy could facilitate the definitive diagnosis.[53]

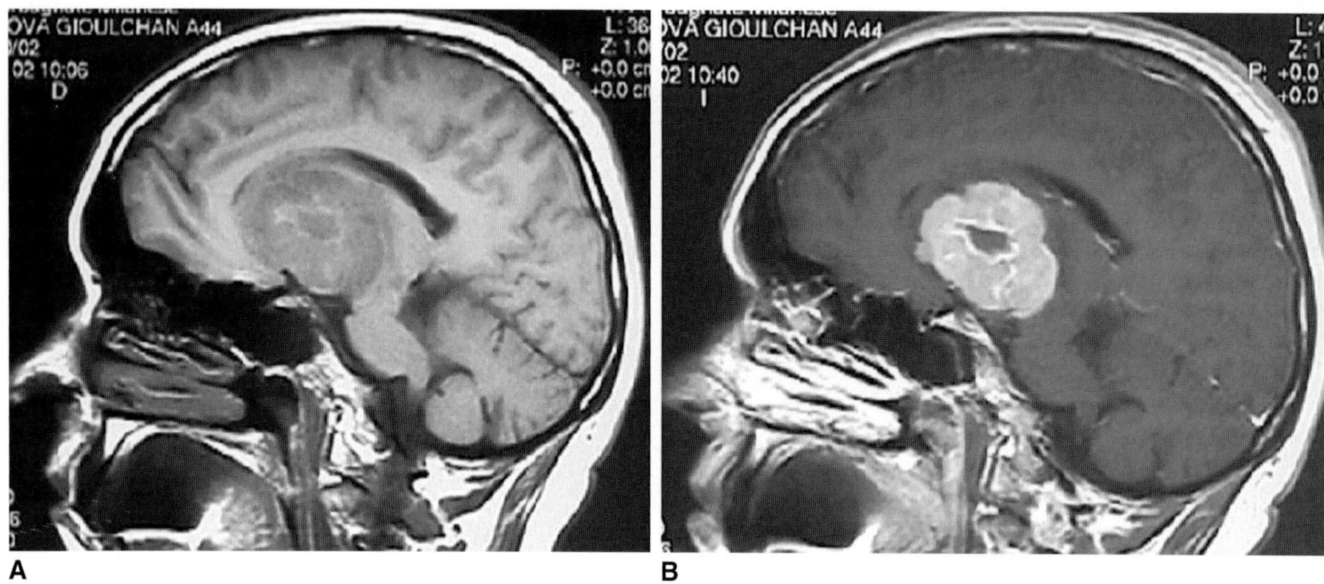

■ **Figure 42–8.** *A*, Isointense lesion infiltrating basal ganglia and lateral ventricles in pre–contrast infusion MRI. *B*, Enhanced lesion after gadolinium infusion.

Treatment

The optimal treatment of PCNSL requires a multidisciplinary approach. If neuroimaging suggests the possibility of PCNSL, then a biopsy is the most appropriate surgical approach. In contrast to most other primary brain tumors, aggressive surgical resection does not improve survival and may result in neurologic deterioration, and therefore should be avoided. In addition, corticosteroids, which are routinely started in any patient with a new intracranial mass, have a potent oncolytic effect, causing tumor cell lysis and radiographic regression in up to 40% of patients.[54–56] The onset of action is quite rapid, with marked reduction in tumor size within 24–48 hours. Therefore, steroids should be withheld in any patient with a presumptive diagnosis of PCNSL until stereotactic biopsy has been performed. Both radiotherapy and chemotherapy are used as the definitive treatment for PCNSL and are discussed in detail in this section (Table 42–4).

Radiotherapy

PCNSL is a radiosensitive tumor, and whole-brain radiotherapy (WBRT) has been the standard treatment for many years, with median survivals ranging from 10 to 18 months.[57,58] WBRT is necessary because of the diffuse infiltrative nature of PCNSL; attempts to treat with focal brain radiotherapy have resulted in high rates of recurrences within and outside of the irradiated port.[59] Although microscopic CSF dissemination is common, more extensive craniospinal radiotherapy does not confer additional survival benefit.[18,60] Furthermore, craniospinal radiotherapy is associated with significant morbidity, limiting the ability to administer adjuvant chemotherapy.

The optimal dose of WBRT is controversial, but the results of several studies suggest a dose between 40 and 50 Gy. Pollack and colleagues reported improved long-term survival in patients treated with 40–50 Gy as compared with those who received less than 40 Gy.[36] Murray and coworkers reported a 5-year survival rate of 42.3% for patients receiving 50 Gy or more compared with 12.8% for those treated with less than 50 Gy.[46] However, WBRT doses greater than 50 Gy are associated with an increased risk of treatment-related neurotoxicity.[61] A prospective Radiation Therapy Oncology Group (RTOG) study of 40-Gy WBRT followed by a 20-Gy focal boost demonstrated a radiographic response in 62% and a complete response rate in 19%.[62] The addition of a boost did not improve local tumor control or survival. A more recent RTOG study failed to show a clear benefit in terms of disease control or reduced neurotoxicity when hyperfractionated radiotherapy was used.[63] Therefore, the best current recommendation is to treat patients with 40–50 Gy WBRT.

Primary Chemotherapy

The use of chemotherapy has significantly improved the outcome of patients with PCNSL. Similar to systemic non-Hodgkin's lymphoma, PCNSL is a chemosensitive tumor; however, the standard agents used to treat non-Hodgkin's lymphoma are not effective in PCNSL because of their inability to penetrate the blood-brain barrier (BBB). Several studies have examined the role of preradiotherapy CHOP/CHOD (cyclophosphamide, doxorubicin, vincristine, and prednisone/dexamethasone) or MACOP-B (low-dose methotrexate, doxorubicin, cyclophosphamide, vincristine, prednisone, and bleomycin) and found survival to be similar to WBRT alone at 8–16 months.[60,64,65] Although many patients have an initial radiographic response, most relapse after two to three cycles. This may be explained by PET studies that demonstrate normalization of the disrupted BBB 3 to 4 weeks after initial chemotherapy, suggesting that the

TABLE 42–4. Various Treatment Regimens for PCNSL

Reference	Regimen*	*N*	CRch	CRall	CR + PRch	CR + PRall	OS (mo)	PFS (mo)
Chemotherapy with WBRT								
163	CHOP vs. none	53	—		—			22v. 10, ns
65	CHOP, A	50	—	33%	—	63%	10.4	6.7
170	CHOD/BVAM	57	62–64%	68–77%	70–77%	68–81%	40	
70	MPV, IT, A	52	56%	87%	90%	94%	60	nr
63	MPV, IV, A	102	58%	—	94%	—	37	24
171	M	46	—	82%	—	95%	33	65% (at 24 mo)
55	M, A	31	—	87%	78%	93%	42.5	41
172	MBVP, IT	52	33%	69%		81% or 77%	46	—
Chemotherapy Alone								
173	M, L, P, MP, IT	50	42%	—	48%	—	14.3	6.8
174	M	25	52%	—	74%	—	nr	12.8
91	M, T, V, D, IT	14	79%	—	100%	—	nr	16.5
175	M, V, I, C, A, IV	65	61%		71%		50	—
176	M	37	30%	—	35%	—	—	13.7 (11 CR only)
73	M, A, BEAM	28			57%		nr	5.6 (EFS)
72	M+, BBBD	74	65%		68%		41	
WBRT Alone								
177	None	41		39%		63%	11.6	

*Regimens include the following: A, cytarabine (Ara-C); BBBD, blood-brain barrier disruption; BEAM, carmustine, etoposide, cytarabine, melphalan; BVAM, carmustine, vincristine, cytarabine, methotrexate; C, cyclophosphamide; CHOD, cyclophosphamide, doxorubicin, vincristine, dexamethasone; CHOP, cyclophosphamide, doxorubicin, vincristine, prednisone; D, dexamethasone; I, ifosfamide; IT, intrathecal administration; IV, intraventricular administration; L, lomustine (CCNU); M, methotrexate; MBVP, methotrexate, teniposide, carmustine, methylprednisolone; MP, methylprednisolone; MPV, methotrexate, procarbazine, vincristine; P, procarbazine; T, thiotepa; V, vinca alkaloids.

Abbreviations: CRall, complete remission with all treatment; CRch, complete remission with chemotherapy; EFS, event-free survival; nr, no response; ns, not significant; OS, overall survival; PFS, progression-free survival; PRall, partial remission with all treatment; PRch, partial remission with chemotherapy.

bulky tumor not protected by the BBB responds, but microscopic tumor is not adequately treated and progresses.[66]

High-dose methotrexate (HD-MTX) is the most active agent in the treatment of PCNSL. Whereas standard-dose methotrexate does not cross the BBB, doses of 1 gm/m^2 or greater result in tumoricidal levels in the brain parenchyma, and doses of 3.5 gm/m^2 or greater yield tumoricidal levels in the CSF. Therefore, most treatment regimens incorporate HD-MTX (1–8 gm/m^2) alone or in combination with other chemotherapeutic agents followed by WBRT. This combined-modality approach has resulted in response rates approaching 100% and median survivals ranging between 30 and 60 months.[67–69] The issues that remain unresolved are whether to give methotrexate alone or in combination with other chemotherapeutic agents, and what are the optimal administration schedule and dose of methotrexate.

Chemotherapy Alone

There has been increasing interest in using chemotherapy alone in order to minimize the neurotoxicity that has been observed by many investigators when using HD-MTX in combination with WBRT.[70] One approach has been to employ hyperosmolar agents to disrupt the BBB, followed by intra-arterial methotrexate.[71,72] This technique results in overall response and survival rates similar to those with the combined-modality approach; however, this is a procedurally intensive treatment administered under general anesthesia monthly over 1 year. Careful neuropsychological testing of this patient cohort has been performed and indicates that patients in remission do not develop delayed neurotoxicity.

Other strategies to enhance the efficacy of chemotherapy, in an effort to replace the benefit of radiotherapy, have included consolidation myeloablative chemotherapy with autologous stem cell support, and maintenance cycles of HD-MTX.[73,74] To date, both of these approaches have demonstrated efficacy and feasibility in Phase II trials; however, further study is necessary to validate and optimize these results.

It is possible to treat older patients with standard methotrexate-based chemotherapy alone with an overall survival similar to a combination of methotrexate-based chemotherapy and WBRT.[70] However, patients treated with chemotherapy alone may be more likely to relapse, and patients who receive WBRT are more likely to develop delayed neurotoxicity. More importantly, older patients are able to tolerate aggressive chemotherapy without an increase in acute morbidity. Clinically, these patients often improve during chemotherapy, with resolution of neurocognitive deficits and improvement in performance status.

Intrathecal Chemotherapy

The role of intrathecal chemotherapy in the treatment of PCNSL is controversial. Many studies have included the routine use of intrathecal methotrexate for all patients irrespective of the results of cytologic studies. This strategy is supported by the fact that leptomeningeal dissemination is seen in 20–100% of patients and elevated CSF protein levels are associated with a poor prognosis.[75,76] Furthermore, the experience in systemic lymphoma and leukemia clearly supports the use of intrathecal chemotherapy to prevent or eradicate leptomeningeal disease. However, it is possible to achieve tumoricidal CSF levels of methotrexate with rapid systemic administration of doses of $3 gm/m^2$ or greater,[77] and two separate studies have failed to identify a clear survival or disease control benefit in patients treated with intrathecal drugs, including patients with positive CSF cytology.[19,33]

New Strategies

The use of monoclonal antibody therapy has significantly altered the treatment and outcome for patients with systemic non-Hodgkin's lymphoma; therefore, this strategy is being actively explored in the treatment of PCNSL. Theoretically, an intact BBB would limit the passage of molecules the size of monoclonal antibodies, and prevent the attainment of therapeutic levels. However, there is evidence that the BBB is permeable in PCNSL and disrupted in proportion to the degree of gadolinium enhancement visualized on MRI scan; PCNSL typically has dense uniform contrast enhancement on MRI. Furthermore, PET studies document a permeable BBB in PCNSL and pathologic evaluation of PCNSL vessels demonstrates a porous endothelial lining.

Rituximab, a monoclonal antibody to CD20, has shown evidence of antitumor activity in case reports of PCNSL and is actively being incorporated into several clinical trials. Radiolabeled monoclonal antibodies provide a unique opportunity to quantify the delivery of these potentially therapeutic molecules as well as a possible mechanism to deliver low-energy targeted radiation that may be less toxic.

Salvage Therapy

Salvage treatment will be necessary in 5–10% of patients with refractory disease, and up to 50% who ultimately relapse.[63,78] Median survival for patients with recurrent or refractory disease without treatment is 2 months, but salvage treatment may substantially improve survival.[79] Unfortunately, the optimal salvage regimen has not been defined and a variety of possible strategies have been reported. Radiotherapy may be used at recurrence in patients who have not received radiotherapy, but neurotoxicity remains a concern.[78,80,81] Therefore, salvage chemotherapy is often used in an effort to improve disease control while preserving quality of life.[81–84]

Intensive chemotherapy with hematopoietic stem cell rescue was used in a series of 22 patients with promising results. An objective response was seen in 82% and the overall 3-year survival was 64%; however, five of seven patients older than 60 years died from treatment complications.[82] Six of seven patients (86%) with recurrent or refractory PCNSL had an objective response to PCV (procarbazine, lomustine [CCNU], and vincristine), with a progression-free survival of more than 1 year in four patients.[83] More than one third of patients treated with etoposide, ifosfamide, and cytarabine at relapse achieved an objective response and were progression free at 1 year. However, this regimen has a high risk of neutropenic fever.[84] Re-induction with HD-MTX resulted in a response in approximately 50% of patients, with a median progression-free survival of 10 months; eight patients achieved a response following radiotherapy.[81] Salvage treatment with topotecan has a similar objective response rate of four of seven patients (57%); grade 3–4 neutropenia was seen in all patients.[85] A Phase II study of temozolomide salvage therapy resulted in an objective response rate of 24% (95% confidence interval, 11–45%), with a median progression-free survival of more than 6 months in complete responders.[86] Rituximab has also been administered as a single agent in refractory PCNSL with reported clinical and radiographic response.[87–90]

The choice of the optimal salvage strategy at this time should take into consideration the patient's age, performance status, site of relapse, and prior therapy. Potential toxicity is especially important for older patients who comprise the majority of those who relapse, because they are often unable to tolerate aggressive salvage regimens and are at the highest risk for treatment-related neurotoxicity.

Intraocular Lymphoma

Intraocular lymphoma can occur in isolation (primary ocular lymphoma) or as a component of more extensive PCNSL. The malignant lymphocytes involve the vitreous or retina and spare the orbital cavity. Patients typically present with floaters and blurred vision and are often misdiagnosed as having a benign ophthalmologic condition. Patients treated for isolated ocular lymphoma have an 80% risk of developing cerebral involvement up to 10 years or more after initial diagnosis and therefore merit meticulous long-term follow-up.

There is no standard treatment approach to isolated ocular lymphoma. Ocular lymphoma is exquisitely sensitive to corticosteroids (including topical ophthalmic preparations) and focal radiotherapy. Systemic administration of methotrexate and cytarabine can yield therapeutic levels of drug in the intraocular fluids, and clinical responses have been documented; however, relapse is common.[91–93] Direct intravitreal administration of chemotherapy is a valid therapeutic alternative.

In PCNSL patients with a component of ocular lymphoma, the posterior two thirds of the globe should be irradiated to a dose of 36–40 Gy. Treatment planning should take into account both intracranial and ocular disease to eliminate overlapping fields and to minimize any toxicity to the optic nerve and retina. Radiotherapy will effectively control ocular lymphoma and improve visual acuity, but ocular relapse may occur. Patients with recurrent visual symptoms require careful reevaluation to differentiate between recurrent ocular lymphoma and secondary radiotherapy-related toxicity, including epithe-

TABLE 42–5. Possible Prognostic Factors

Patient-Related Factors
Age
Performance status
Tumor-Related Factors
Serum lactate dehydrogenase level
Cerebrospinal fluid protein concentration
Histology
Reactive perivascular T-cell infiltrate
bcl-6 expression
Duration of symptoms
Number of lesions
Infratentorial lesions
Involvement of deep regions of the brain
Treatment-Related Factors
Response to steroids
Use of primary chemotherapy
Use of high-dose methotrexate

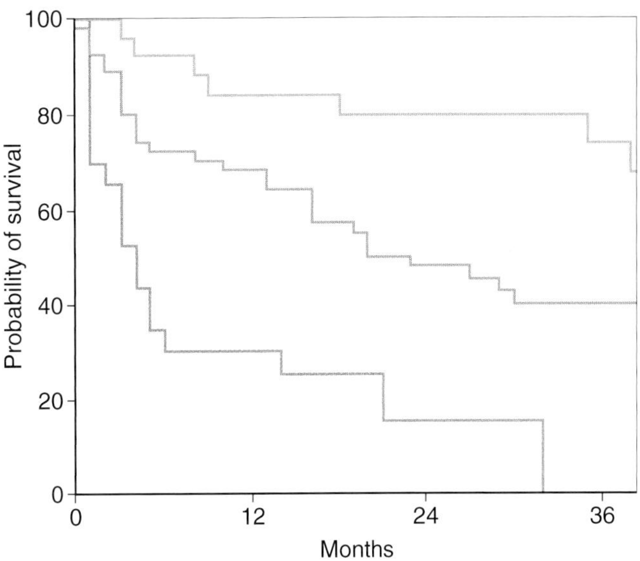

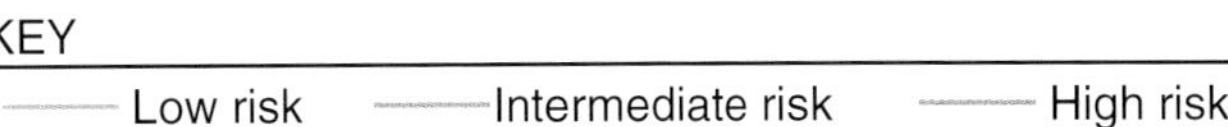

Figure 42–9. Survival curves for PCNSL patients grouped according to the International Extranodal Lymphoma Study Group prognostic score. Patients with 0–1 (low risk), 2–3 (intermediate risk), or 4–5 (high risk) unfavorable features have a 2-year survival of 80 ± 8%, 48 ± 7%, and 15 ± 7% ($P < .00001$), respectively. (From Ferreri AJ, Blay J-Y, Reni M, et al: A prognostic scoring system for primary central nervous system lymphomas: the International Extranodal Lymphoma Study Group Experience. J Clin Oncol 21:266–272, 2003, with permission.)

lioid keratopathy, posterior cataracts, retinopathy, and optic neuropathy.[94]

Prognostic Factors

The majority of prospective trials and large retrospective series have identified age and performance status as the most important prognostic variables; however, multiple other variables have been proposed as possible prognostic factors in PCNSL (Table 42–5). The use of the International Prognostic Index (IPI) did not distinguish risk groups in PCNSL. In a study of 378 immunocompetent patients with PCNSL, age, performance status, serum lactate dehydrogenase level, CSF protein concentration, and the involvement of deep structures of the brain were found to be independent predictors of response and survival.[75] These variables were then used to develop a prognostic scoring system that distinguishes three different risk groups based on the presence of none or one, two or three, or four or five unfavorable features[75] (Fig. 42–9). If validated in further studies, the International Extranodal Lymphoma Study Group scoring system may result in the application of risk-adjusted therapeutic strategies. Other histopathologic, biologic, and molecular markers with potential prognostic value are currently under investigation.[95] Among others, tumors with Bcl-6 protein expression have been associated with improved survival in one series of 33 PCNSL cases (101 months vs. 14.7 months; $P = .002$).[25] The presence of a reactive perivascular T-cell infiltrate has also been reported as a positive prognostic factor.[95]

Future Perspectives

A number of fundamental clinical and biologic challenges have to be addressed in future PCNSL studies (Table 42–6). The biologic relevance of abnormalities in genes involved in cell cycle regulation, as well as the role of specific biologic risk factors, deserves to be investigated in larger series. The development of PCNSL animal models will allow us to address some biologic and therapeutic issues,[96] such as the imaging of lymphoma dissemination to the CNS and the molecular mechanisms that govern CNS dissemination. This approach could contribute to the development of novel experimental therapies and new methodologies for early diagnosis of oculocerebral lymphoma. Finally, the immune responsiveness of the CNS to malignant lymphoma, and the role for the adhesion molecules lymphocyte function–associated antigen-1 and intercellular adhesion molecule-1 in lymphoma cell infiltration, remain among the most exciting investigational aspects in PCNSL.

A more extensive and coordinated multidisciplinary cooperation will become an important strategy to address some of the fundamental clinical and biologic research questions for PCNSL.[97,98] This is particularly relevant in the field of therapeutic management, where several questions remain unanswered. This strategy will allow us to identify the best methotrexate-based chemotherapy regimen for newly diagnosed PCNSL, the most effective administration schedule for HD-MTX, new active drugs, and the best treatment for meningeal and ocular involvement. The role of consolidation WBRT as well as the optimal radiation dose and schedule should be defined.

TABLE 42–6. Fundamental Challenges to be Addressed in Future PCNSL Studies

Molecular and Pathologic Issues

The origin of PCNSL cells
The role of the CNS as an immunologically privileged organ
The regulated neuroimmune network where the CNS is integrated
The blood-brain barrier characteristics and tumor accessibility
The biologic relevance of abnormalities in genes involved in cell cycle regulation
The role of specific biologic risk factors
The prognostic role of biologic and molecular markers
Issues addressable by using animal models

Three-Dimensional Imaging of Lymphoma Dissemination to the CNS

Molecular mechanisms that govern CNS dissemination
Development of novel experimental therapies
New methodology for early diagnosis of oculocerebral lymphoma
Immune responsiveness of the eye and brain to malignant lymphoma
Targeting genes to the brain and eyes
Role for the adhesion molecules LFA-1 and ICAM-1 in lymphoma cell infiltration

Therapeutic Issues

What is the best methotrexate-based chemotherapy regimen for newly diagnosed PCNSL?
What is the best administration schedule (dose, infusion, timing) for HD-MTX?
What is the best treatment for meningeal lymphoma?
Is intrathecal chemotherapy necessary for all patients with PCNSL?
Is WBRT necessary for all patients with PCNSL?
Have the optimal dose and schedule of WBRT been defined?
What is the best treatment for ocular involvement in patients with PCNSL?
What is the optimal salvage treatment for progressive or relapsed PCNSL?
What is the role for BBBD? What therapy should be associated with BBBD?
What patients could obtain benefit from high-dose chemotherapy supported by autologous stem cell transplantation? What are the optimal induction and high-dose chemotherapy regimens?

Abbreviations: BBBD, blood-brain barrier disruption; ICAM-1, intercellular adhesion molecule-1; LFA-1, lymphocyte function–associated antigen-1.

TABLE 42–7. Variables Associated with an Increased Risk for CNS Recurrence in Non-Hodgkin's Lymphoma

Advanced disease[99,101,106,178]
Peripheral blood involvement[179]
Bone marrow infiltration[99,100,180]
Systemic symptoms[178]
Increased serum levels of lactate dehydrogenase[101,104]
High International Prognostic Index score[103,105]
Highly aggressive lymphoma histotypes[101]
Involvement of more than one extranodal site[103]
Testicular lymphoma[178,179,181,182]
Breast lymphoma[183]
Involvement of gastrointestinal tract[178]
Lymphoma of the paranasal sinus[178]
Lymphoma of the epidural soft tissues[184]

SECONDARY CNS LYMPHOMAS IN IMMUNOCOMPETENT PATIENTS

Risk Factors

CNS relapse is a devastating and almost uniformly fatal complication of non-Hodgkin's lymphoma and other aggressive hematologic malignancies. The risk of CNS relapse ranges between 5% and 30% in all non-Hodgkin's lymphoma subtypes,[99,100] with a cumulative risk of CNS relapse at 4 years of 17%.[101] Overall, CNS recurrence is observed in less than 3% of indolent lymphomas, 5% of aggressive lymphomas (diffuse large B-cell and peripheral T-cell lymphomas), and 24% of Burkitt's and lymphoblastic lymphomas.[102] The analysis of risk factors for CNS relapse in non-Hodgkin's lymphoma is limited by differences in the definition criteria and retrospective nature of reported studies. Some authors have chosen to exclusively analyze patients with CNS disease as the initial site of recurrence,[103] whereas others have included patients with CNS relapse at any time.[101] Nevertheless, several variables, including advanced disease, increased serum levels of lactate dehydrogenase, certain extranodal sites of disease, and highly aggressive lymphoma histologies, have been associated with an increased risk for CNS recurrence in non-Hodgkin's lymphoma (Table 42–7).[101,104]

Nearly 5% of patients with large B-cell lymphoma develop CNS recurrence, with an actuarial risk at 1 year after diagnosis of 4.5%.[103] This risk can be reduced to less than 2% if patients are treated with chemotherapy that includes intrathecal and systemic HD-MTX.[105] The interval between non-Hodgkin's lymphoma diagnosis and CNS recurrence ranges from 0 to 44 months, with a median of 3 to 6 months, but only 4% of CNS relapses occur later than 1 year from lymphoma diagnosis.[103,106] In 20% of cases, CNS recurrence is concurrent with early systemic progression, but, in 30% of cases, it precedes systemic progression by up to 6 months. Isolated CNS recurrence has been observed in 5% of patients with aggressive lymphomas treated without intrathecal chemotherapy.[106] The outcome, whether the recurrence is leptomeningeal or parenchymal, is disappointing, with all patients having died within 2 years from CNS progression.[106]

Among several variables tested for risk of CNS relapse, the involvement of more than one extranodal site and an increased serum level of lactate dehydrogenase have been proposed as independent predictors of CNS recurrence in aggressive lymphomas.[103,105] Patients displaying both of these unfavorable features have an actuarial risk for CNS recurrence of almost 20% at 1 year.[103] The IPI score has been proposed as an independent predictor of risk of CNS recurrence in patients treated with both conventional chemotherapy and autologous stem cell transplantation.[103,105] The risk is increased for patients with a high IPI score, but CNS recurrence occurs in all the IPI risk groups.

Prophylaxis of CNS Relapse

Given the high morbidity and mortality associated with CNS dissemination of non-Hodgkin's lymphoma, a prophylactic strategy, analogous to that employed successfully for acute lymphoblastic leukemia, is indicated. However, the incidence of CNS recurrence in non-

Hodgkin's lymphoma is not sufficiently high to warrant the use of CNS prophylaxis in all patients.

In highly aggressive lymphomas, such as Burkitt's or lymphoblastic lymphomas, the 5-year CNS recurrence rate was substantially higher among patients who did not receive CNS prophylaxis (32–78%) in comparison to patients who did (19%).[102,107–110] This wide variation may be explained, in part, by the variable proportion of T-cell lymphoblastic lymphoma patients within the study cohorts. Similar to T-cell acute lymphoblastic leukemia, patients with T-cell lymphoblastic lymphoma may have a higher risk for CNS relapse.[110] The inclusion of CNS-directed prophylaxis led to substantial reduction in CNS relapse rates in lymphoblastic lymphoma patients: 0–36% with intrathecal chemotherapy alone,[109,111,112] 3–21% with intrathecal chemotherapy and cranial irradiation,[109,111,113,114] and less than 5% with early intrathecal chemotherapy, cranial irradiation, and systemic HD-MTX and high-dose cytarabine.[18,29,33] As a consequence, patients with Burkitt's and lymphoblastic lymphomas now receive intrathecal chemotherapy, systemic HD-MTX or high-dose cytarabine, and cranial irradiation as prophylaxis. The combination of all three strategies resulted in the lowest incidence of isolated or combined CNS relapses (1–12%).[109,115,116]

For aggressive lymphomas, predominantly diffuse large B-cell lymphoma and peripheral T-cell lymphoma, CNS prophylaxis is currently used in 10–15% of cases[103]; however, there is still no uniformity of practice, which reflects the complexity of the situation and the fact that the published data are open to differing interpretations. The identification of patient subgroups for which CNS prophylaxis may be of benefit is therefore important. Prophylaxis may reduce the risk of CNS relapse in patients with a high IPI score, particularly those with a high serum lactate dehydrogenase level, involvement of more than one extranodal site, testicular lymphoma, or paranasal sinus involvement. All these subgroups of patients should be assessed for CNS involvement at diagnosis (history, neurologic examination, MRI, and lumbar puncture). Intrathecal chemotherapy and the addition of systemic HD-MTX or high-dose cytarabine to conventional chemotherapy reduce the CNS relapse rate and appear to be as effective as and less toxic than cranial irradiation.[117] A trial of 708 adults ages 61–69 years with at least one adverse IPI feature compared a relatively intense chemotherapy program, incorporating both intrathecal methotrexate and consolidation with systemic methotrexate, ifosfamide, and cytosine arabinoside, with the standard CHOP regimen.[118] The frequency of CNS recurrence was significantly lower in the experimental arm (8 vs. 25; $P = .003$).[118] These results have confirmed an earlier analysis suggesting that the outcome of patients receiving CNS prophylaxis in the form of intrathecal and intravenous methotrexate was better than that of matched historical controls.[104]

Treatment of CNS Disease

In a large proportion of cases, CNS relapse is accompanied by or soon followed by systemic relapse, and the patient's outcome is determined equally by the control of systemic and CNS disease, even in patients with isolated CNS recurrence.[119] Therefore, treatment should be directed at the entire craniospinal axis, and should also provide control of systemic disease. Systemic high-dose chemotherapy is the most effective strategy that meets these requirements. Similar to PCNSL, the choice of drugs is based on the ability to cross the BBB and antilymphoma activity. Most of the first-line combinations against secondary CNS lymphoma contain HD-MTX and/or high-dose cytarabine. Even if the most effective administration schedules for these drugs in secondary CNS lymphomas remain to be defined, adequate doses allow the achievement of therapeutic drug concentrations in the CSF and brain parenchyma. Because most lymphoma patients with an increased risk of CNS relapse are treated with these drugs as first-line treatment, systemic chemotherapy could be troublesome as a result of the limited number of drugs able to cross the BBB. Some anecdotal experience with cisplatin-based regimens has been reported,[103] and allogeneic or autologous transplantation may prove beneficial for selected patients.[120,121] Patients with leptomeningeal involvement without focal neurologic deficits are usually treated with intrathecal chemotherapy (methotrexate, cytarabine, and hydrocortisone) twice a week, using an Ommaya reservoir.[103] Although this strategy invariably results in a decrease in the percentage of tumor cells in the CSF, symptomatic improvement occurs in less than 20% of cases.[103] A slow-release formulation of cytarabine injected once every 2 weeks produces a higher response rate and a better quality of life relative to that produced by free cytarabine injected twice a week.[122] Patients with focal neurologic deficits or intraparenchymal lesions in the brain, cranial nerves, or spinal cord are commonly treated with radiation therapy, which results in symptomatic improvement in more than 65% of cases. However, response is transient, and progression of CNS disease or systemic dissemination is the rule.[103]

High-Dose Chemotherapy with Autologous and Allogeneic Transplantation

Some reports conclude that 20–40% of adults with non-Hodgkin's lymphoma and CNS disease can achieve durable remissions after high-dose chemotherapy and autologous transplantation, primarily patients with highly aggressive lymphomas in first remission at the time of transplantation.[120,121,123–129] Attempts to transplant adults with hematologic malignancies and active CNS disease have had disappointing results. In adults with highly aggressive lymphoma, the presence of CNS disease before autologous transplantation, but not present at transplant, does not adversely affect outcome, whereas active CNS disease has been associated with a progression-free survival of 9% at 71 months.[120] Therefore, the best recommendation would be to limit the use of autologous or allogeneic transplantation to those patients whose CNS disease is in remission.

Conditioning regimens are not specifically designed for patients with CNS disease. Ideally, drugs should be chosen on the basis of antilymphoma activity and capacity to cross the BBB. Total-body irradiation is highly immunosuppressive, has good antitumor activity, and is not affected by the BBB. However, this strategy is associated with an increased risk of severe neurotoxicity, especially when combined with intrathecal chemotherapy or systemic HD-MTX or cytarabine.[130,131] Combinations of busulfan and cyclophosphamide are good alternatives to total-body irradiation. At appropriate doses, busulfan is able to cross the BBB[132]; data regarding CNS penetration of cyclophosphamide are conflicting.[133] These drugs, with or without thiotepa, can be curative in children with highly aggressive lymphomas and CNS involvement, but risk of severe neurotoxicity is high in previously irradiated patients.[121,134] Some lymphoma patients with CNS involvement have been treated with nitrosourea-based conditioning regimens, obtaining a 5-year progression-free survival similar to those obtained with total-body irradiation–containing regimens (20% vs. 42%; $P = .3$).[120] Novel conditioning combinations need to be investigated considering the disappointing results with this strategy.

High-Dose Chemotherapy with Allogeneic Transplantation

There is some evidence to suggest that allogeneic transplantation is superior to autologous transplantation for the prevention or treatment of CNS recurrence in highly aggressive lymphomas and acute lymphoblastic leukemia in both children and adults.[124,135] Moreover, consolidation with allogeneic bone marrow transplantation is associated with significantly improved outcome in children with early CNS recurrence of acute lymphoblastic leukemia.[135] Conversely, it is conceivable that graft-versus-lymphoma effects may extend to the CNS and contribute to eradication of CNS disease.[136–139] However, survival benefit with this strategy is obscured by increased treatment-related mortality.[120] Moreover, the real impact of allogeneic transplantation in CNS recurrence is difficult to define considering the interpretation bias related to the effect of immunosuppressive therapy used for prevention or treatment of graft-versus-host disease.

CNS INVOLVEMENT IN HIV-RELATED LYMPHOMAS

Risk Factors

Low CD4 count (<50 cells/µL) and high peripheral HIV viral load are the most significant risk factors for the development of PCNSL. The incidence in patients with CD4 counts less than 50 cells/µL is 20-fold higher than those with counts greater than 350 cells/µL. More than half of patients will have had an acquired immunodeficiency syndrome (AIDS)–defining illness prior to the development of PCNSL, offering additional indirect evidence that immune function must be significantly impaired before PCNSL arises.[140,141] There is no evidence that the route of HIV transmission is an independent risk factor for PCNSL.[142,143] Similar to the HIV-negative population, no established occupational, chemical, or environmental causes exist.[144]

Approximately 50% of HIV-positive patients with systemic non-Hodgkin's lymphoma will develop leptomeningeal dissemination. Therefore, a staging lumbar puncture for CSF cytology is recommended in all patients, and CNS prophylaxis should be considered. Elevated plasma levels of Epstein-Barr virus DNA may be useful to predict subsequent development of leptomeningeal lymphoma.[145]

Pathophysiology

The malignant lymphocytes seen in PCNSL tend to be distributed along vascular channels as perivascular cuffs. They are of B-cell origin, display large-cell and immunoblastic histologies, and uniformly exhibit Epstein-Barr virus–associated DNA. Small noncleaved-cell, mixed large- and small-cell, and T-cell lymphomas are rare. Virtually all AIDS-related PCNSLs are associated with Epstein-Barr virus infection. Latent infection induces an activated B-cell state, and these cells have the potential to become neoplastic. Expression of several Epstein-Barr virus proteins, including latent membrane protein-1, triggers several oncogenic signaling pathways, probably through *bcl-6* mutations or *c-myc* translocations. Current hypotheses propose that the B-cells proliferate uncontrollably in the absence of effective cellular immunity, resulting in tumor formation in AIDS patients and others with immunodeficiencies.[146,147]

Clinical Features and Diagnosis

AIDS-related PCNSL patients are typically younger at diagnosis than those with non–AIDS-related PCNSL, with a median age of 37 versus 60 years. The most common presenting symptoms are altered mentation, focal neurologic deficits, increased intracranial pressure, and seizures. Although these findings are similar to those seen in immunocompetent patients, the incidence of seizures is higher in AIDS-related PCNSL.

AIDS-related PCNSL is an aggressive disease, and multiple CNS compartments may contain active tumor, including the brain parenchyma, leptomeninges, spinal cord, and eye. The newly diagnosed patient requires a careful evaluation to define the extent of neurologic disease as well as an evaluation to exclude systemic lymphoma. Furthermore, one must take into account the possibility that an HIV-positive patient with PCNSL may have other coincident CNS pathologies such as toxoplasmosis. Leptomeningeal lymphoma often presents with vague cognitive change, but patients may have signs of increased intracranial pressure or multifocal neurologic deficits. All newly diagnosed patients should have a lumbar puncture for cytology. Worsening visual acuity or floaters are suggestive of ocular lymphoma with involvement of the vitreous, uvea, or retina. Because asymptomatic ocular lymphoma and concomitant HIV-related ocular pathology are common, detailed ophthalmologic evaluation including slit-lamp examination should be performed in all newly diagnosed PCNSL patients. Vitrectomy may be used to confirm the diagnosis, although prior corticosteroid treatment may cause false-negative results. Patients rarely present with spinal cord involvement, but spinal cord signs can herald relapsing disease. Gadolinium-enhanced MRI of the spine is warranted in any patient with neurologic findings referable to the spinal cord or cauda equina. A computed tomography scan of the chest, abdomen, and pelvis or a body PET scan should be done to exclude systemic disease.

Imaging

AIDS-related PCNSL has a distinct MRI appearance as compared with non–AIDS-related PCNSL. PCNSL lesions in immunocompetent patients are usually unifocal and periventricular and may involve the corpus callosum. AIDS-related PCNSL lesions are heterogeneous, are often peripheral or cortically based, rarely involve the corpus callosum, and are usually multifocal.[2,148,149] Gradient echo planar sequences often reveal subacute and asymptomatic hemorrhage in AIDS-related PCNSL but have no clinical significance.[150–152] The dense, uniform contrast enhancement typical of non–AIDS-related PCNSL is uncommon in AIDS-related PCNSL lesions,[153,154] which generally show ring enhancement with central necrosis.[141,151,155–157] This radiographic picture of ring enhancement is also typical for cerebral toxoplasmosis and may be seen with cerebral abscesses and progressive multifocal leukoencephalopathy, emphasizing that radiographic appearance alone is not diagnostic of AIDS-related PCNSL.

Newer imaging technologies may be useful to distinguish PCNSL from opportunistic infections. FDG-PET studies can guide stereotactic biopsy to the most metabolically active portion of the tumor, and the finding of a PET-avid lesion is suggestive of malignancy as opposed to infection. However, because other CNS malignancies are reported in the HIV population, this finding should not be considered diagnostic of PCNSL. Relatively high uptake signal on thallium-201 SPECT studies suggests neoplasia, whereas low uptake is consistent with infection. Given the variety of diseases indistinguishable by imaging, SPECT data alone should probably not be used to establish a diagnosis or to determine treatment.[158] However, a study looking at the accuracy of diagnosing AIDS-related PCNSL using a combination of thallium SPECT scanning and CSF examination for Epstein-Barr virus found 100% sensitivity and a 100% false-negative rate. Therefore, biopsy could reasonably be avoided in those patients with increased thallium uptake on SPECT scanning and a positive CSF sample for Epstein-Barr virus DNA; in all other patients, a brain biopsy is required for diagnosis.[159] A study of magnetic resonance spectroscopy evaluation of multiple lesions of different etiologies found that all lesions had similar spectra. Although this may be explained in part by the presence of necrosis, it suggests that magnetic resonance spectroscopy lacks the specificity needed for a diagnostic imaging tool.[160]

Treatment

Because the profoundly immunocompromised are at greatest risk of AIDS-related PCNSL, these patients have a much worse prognosis than non-AIDS patients. They tolerate cytotoxic chemotherapies poorly and develop more infectious complications. Bone marrow toxicity and a high rate of opportunistic infections frequently complicate treatment regimens. Before antiretroviral therapy, the mean survival was 1 to 2 months without treatment. WBRT improved overall survival to 3 to 4 months.[2,161]

Since the advent of highly active antiretroviral therapy (HAART), the incidence of AIDS-related PCNSL has decreased and the ability to deliver adequate chemotherapy to those HIV-positive patients who develop PCNSL has dramatically improved. Many investigators report that HAART improves survival even without chemotherapy, suggesting improved outcome resulting from immune system recovery.[162] Although data remain scarce, several small institutional studies have published median survivals approaching or exceeding 1 year in patients receiving HAART with or without other specific antitumor therapy.[163,164] This is in contrast to earlier data that indicated only 10% of patients survived 1 year.

Therefore, HIV-positive patients with newly diagnosed PCNSL should be started on HAART (or have their HAART regimen optimized) and on appropriate prophylaxis for opportunistic infections. It is possible that this approach will be adequate in patients who are retroviral drug naive. However, most patients will require additional specific antitumor therapy. Given the likelihood that WBRT may exacerbate or accelerate the risk of HIV-related dementia, it seems most appropriate to initiate therapy with methotrexate-based chemotherapy, similar to the approach in immunocompetent patients. Jacomet and colleagues treated 15 individuals with AIDS-related PCNSL with HD-MTX ($3\,gm/m^2$ every 14 days for six cycles).[165] With a mean CD4 count of 30 cells/μL and a median Karnofsky performance status of 50, the complete response rate was 50%, with a median survival of 10 months. Tosi and associates evaluated oral zidovudine (2, 4, and $6\,mg/m^2$) and intravenous methotrexate at 1 gm/m^2 (moderate dose) plus leucovorin rescue weekly for three to six cycles. In 29 patients with a median CD4 count of 133 cells/μL, 46% had a complete response and the median survival was 12 months.[166]

New Strategies

In addition to treating the AIDS-related PCNSL population with strategies similar to those used in the immunocompetent population, it may be appropriate to explore aggressive or targeted antiviral strategies.[167] Given the fact that nearly 100% of AIDS-related PCNSL is Epstein-Barr virus positive, strategies that directly target Epstein-Barr virus or causative viruses such as human herpesvirus 8 may be effective. A small series of patients treated with parenteral zidovudine (1.6 gm twice daily), ganciclovir (5 mg/kg twice daily), and interleukin-2 (2 million units twice daily) produced an excellent response in four of

CURRENT CONTROVERSIES & FUTURE CONSIDERATIONS

Primary and Secondary Central Nervous System Lymphomas in Immunocompetent and Human Immunodeficiency Virus–Positive Patients

PCNSL

- What is the optimal dose of systemic methotrexate?
- Are multiagent methotrexate-based chemotherapy regimens superior to single-agent methotrexate?
- Does intrathecal methotrexate contribute to disease control, survival, or neurotoxicity?
- Is it reasonable to defer or eliminate WBRT? In which subpopulations?
- What is the optimal therapy for leptomeningeal lymphoma? Ocular lymphoma?
- What is the best approach to salvage therapy?
- Is treatment-related neurotoxicity related primarily to WBRT? What is the contribution, if any, of HD-MTX?

Secondary CNS Lymphoma

- Which groups of non-Hodgkin's lymphoma patients should always receive prophylactic CNS treatment?
- What is the optimal therapy of CNS dissemination of PCNSL?
- Should patients with any history of CNS dissemination be offered myeloablative chemotherapy with either autologous or allogeneic stem cell support?

AIDS-Related PCNSL

- How much does the use of HAART impact the incidence and prognosis of AIDS-related PCNSL?
- What is the optimal therapy for patients with AIDS-related PCNSL?
- Given the high rates of HIV-related dementia, should WBRT be routinely deferred in these patients?

five patients.[168] Future studies will use a regimen of induction intravenous zidovudine, ganciclovir, and interleukin-2 followed by maintenance subcutaneous interleukin-2 and oral ganciclovir.

Suggested Readings*

DeAngelis LM, Seiferheld W, Schold SC, et al: Combination chemotherapy and radiotherapy for primary central nervous system lymphoma: Radiation Therapy Oncology Group Study 93-10. J Clin Oncol 20:4643–4648, 2002.

Ferreri AJ, Abrey LE, Blay JY, et al: Summary statement on primary central nervous system lymphomas from the Eighth International Conference on Malignant Lymphoma, Lugano, Switzerland, June 12 to 15, 2002. J Clin Oncol 21:2407–2414, 2003.

Roychowdhury S, Peng R, Baiocchi RA, et al: Experimental treatment of Epstein-Barr virus-associated primary central nervous system lymphoma. Cancer Res 63:965–971, 2003.

van Besien K, Ha CS, Murphy S, et al: Risk factors, treatment, and outcome of central nervous system recurrence in adults with intermediate-grade and immunoblastic lymphoma. Blood 91:1178–1184, 1998.

Full references for this chapter can be found on accompanying CD-ROM.

CHAPTER 43

Non-Hodgkin's Lymphoma

Omer N. Koç, MD, and Wyndham H. Wilson, MD, PhD

KEY POINTS

Non-Hodgkin's Lymphomas

Diagnosis

- Enlarged lymph nodes and related symptoms constitute the most common presentation.
- Neoplastic cells are monoclonal populations of B (85%) or T (15%) lymphocytes. Immunohistochemistry, karyotyping, and/or molecular characterization are necessary for diagnosis. Importantly, inflammatory and infectious diseases may mimic lymphoma.
- 18-Fluoro-2-deoxyglucose positron emission tomography scans are highly sensitive and specific for staging at presentation and at treatment completion.
- Clinical and molecular features are useful for clinical prognosis.

Biology

- Most lymphoma subtypes are not associated with a characteristic chromosomal translocation.
- Molecular profiling is defining a new lymphoma taxonomy and method of prognostication and identifying therapeutic targets.

Treatment

- Lymphomas are treatment responsive, but outcome is predominantly influenced by the histologic and molecular subtype.
- Indolent lymphomas are usually incurable and are managed with observation or treatment based on the clinical setting.
- Aggressive lymphomas are potentially curable but require proper diagnosis and optimal treatment.
- Anti-CD20 antibody therapy has significantly improved treatment outcome in B-cell lymphomas.
- Relapsed patients may achieve additional benefit with autologous and/or allogeneic stem cell transplantation.

INTRODUCTION

The term *non-Hodgkin's lymphoma* denotes a number of distinct neoplastic disorders of the lymphoid system with overlapping pathologic and clinical features (Table 43–1). Non-Hodgkin's lymphoma is characterized by a monoclonal expansion of lymphoid cells. The genotype and phenotype of malignant cells for any given type of lymphoid malignancy can now be traced to a specific stage in physiologic lymphoid maturation, and the majority of non-Hodgkin's lymphomas arise from germinal center B lymphocytes (Table 43–2). The precise characterization of the origin of a neoplastic transformation will lead to a molecular classification of non-Hodgkin's lymphoma.

MECHANISMS OF LYMPHOMAGENESIS

At a molecular level, the genetic lesions identified in lymphomas include oncogene activation or loss of tumor suppressor genes caused by chromosomal translocation, deletion, or mutation, or by introduction of exogenous viral genomes into the human chromosome. Distinguishing immunologic and genetic features, presumably reflecting disease biology, have been identified for many lymphoma subtypes and are incorporated into the World Health Organization classification. However, what is absent is an adequate understanding of the "ripple effect" of these genetic abnormalities on the cellular gene expression.

The genetic hallmark of follicular lymphoma, the most common indolent lymphoma subtype, is the t(14;18)(q32;q21) translocation with rearrangement of the *bcl*-2 gene, present in 80–90% of cases, and overexpression of the Bcl-2 gene product (Table 43–3).[1,2] Inhibition of apoptosis by Bcl-2, which occurs in normal germinal center cells, appears to play an important role in lymphomagenesis.[1,3] However, constitutive Bcl-2 expression is not necessarily required for survival, because it may be turned off in follicular lymphoma cells that have undergone aggressive transformation.[4] The role of p53 mutation/deletion observed in some transformed follicular lymphomas is also uncertain, although loss of p53 function is associated with decreased apoptosis and clinical drug resistance.[5,6]

TABLE 43–1. World Health Organization Classification of Lymphomas

B-Cell Neoplasms

Precursor B-Cell

Precursor B-lymphoblastic leukemia/lymphoma

Mature B-Cell

Chronic lymphocytic leukemia/small lymphocytic lymphoma
Lymphoplasmacytic lymphoma
Splenic marginal zone lymphoma
Extranodal marginal zone B-cell lymphoma of mucosa-associated lymphoid tissue (MALT lymphoma)
Nodal marginal zone B-cell lymphoma
Follicular lymphoma
Mantle cell lymphoma
Diffuse large B-cell lymphoma
  Mediastinal (thymic) large B-cell lymphoma
  Intravascular large B-cell lymphoma
  Primary effusion lymphoma
Burkitt's lymphoma/leukemia

B-Cell Proliferations of Uncertain Malignant Potential

Lymphomatoid granulomatosis
Posttransplantation lymphoproliferative disorder, polymorphic

T-Cell and NK-Cell Neoplasms

Precursor T-Cell

Precursor T-lymphoblastic leukemia/lymphoma
Blastic NK-cell lymphoma

Mature T-Cell and NK-Cell

Adult T-cell leukemia/lymphoma
Extranodal NK/T-cell lymphoma, nasal type
Enteropathy-type T-cell lymphoma
Hepatosplenic T-cell lymphoma
Subcutaneous panniculitis-like T-cell lymphoma
Mycosis fungoides
Sézary syndrome
Primary cutaneous anaplastic large-cell lymphoma
Peripheral T-cell lymphoma, unspecified
Angioimmunoblastic T-cell lymphoma
Anaplastic large-cell lymphoma

From Jaffe ES, Harris NL, Diebold J, Muller-Hermelink HK: World Health Organization classification of neoplastic diseases of the hematopoietic and lymphoid tissues: a progress report. Am J Clin Pathol 111:S8–S12, 1999.

Among aggressive lymphomas, diffuse large B-cell lymphoma is the most common type, comprising a third of all lymphomas,[7] but contains multiple disease entities as indicated by its variable clinical presentation, natural history, morphologic variants, and molecular characteristics.[8] The diverse morphologic variants of diffuse large B-cell lymphoma, which include centroblastic, immunoblastic, T-cell/histiocyte–rich, and anaplastic types, have some known molecular correlates.[8] Other diffuse large B-cell lymphoma subtypes are also distinct, such as primary mediastinal B-cell lymphoma and intravascular large B-cell lymphoma.[8] Likewise, large-cell "transformation" of an indolent B-cell lymphoma/leukemia, a relatively common occurrence, involves pathways of lymphomagenesis distinct from de novo diffuse large B-cell lymphoma.[9]

Within diffuse large B-cell lymphoma, a common molecular abnormality observed in over half of cases involves the deregulation of *bcl*-6, either through promoter substitution or by multiple, often biallelic mutation clustering in its 5′ noncoding region[10] (see Table 43–3). Bcl-6 protein functions as a transcription factor that binds a specific DNA sequence and represses transcription from linked promoters. It is important in the normal functioning of the germinal center B cells and is required for germinal center cell formation during the antigen-driven immune response.[11] Diffuse large B-cell lymphomas with high expression of Bcl-6 are usually of germinal center B-cell origin and of good prognosis.[12,13] Overexpression of Bcl-2 is present in 24–55% of cases.[14,15] Interestingly, only 14–17% of these cases were found to harbor a *bcl*-2 gene rearrangement from the t(14;18) translocation, indicating variable molecular mechanisms of Bcl-2 overexpression. Paradoxically, overexpression of the Bcl-2 protein but not the *bcl*-2 gene rearrangement is associated with decreased survival, suggesting that the antiapoptotic effect of the Bcl-2 protein is not the important determinant of outcome.[14,15] Other molecular findings in diffuse large B-cell lymphoma include mutation of the p53 gene in approximately 20% of cases; this has also been associated with decreased survival and drug resistance, presumably through its antiapoptotic effects.[5,16] Specific immunophenotypic and genotypic features have also been associated with the primary mediastinal B-cell lymphoma subtype of diffuse large B-cell lymphoma, such as overexpression of the *MAL* gene, a finding that supports a unique biologic heritage for this disease.[8,17,18]

Mantle cell lymphoma is considerably less common than diffuse large B-cell lymphoma and only relatively recently was recognized as a distinct disease entity[8] (see Table 43–3). Virtually all cases contain the t(11;14)(q13;q32) translocation between the immunoglobulin heavy chain and the cyclin D1 (*PRAD1*, *bcl*-1) genes.[19] Deregulation of *bcl*-1 leads to overexpression of its gene product, cyclin-D1, which promotes progression from G_1 to S of the cell cycle.[20] Unlike diffuse large B-cell lymphoma, most mantle cell lymphoma patients are incurable and have a relatively short median survival of 3–5 years.[21]

EPIDEMIOLOGY AND RISK FACTORS

The age-adjusted incidence of non-Hodgkin's lymphoma rose rapidly in the United States between the 1970s and mid-1990s, with some stabilization since 1995; in 1997, there were approximately 55,000 new cases of non-Hodgkin's lymphoma diagnosed in the United States (Fig. 43–1*A*). The lifetime probability of developing non-Hodgkin's lymphoma is 2.1% (1 in 48) for males and 1.76% (1 in 57) for females.[22] These are diseases of older patients, occurring at a median age of 65 years, and dramatically increase in incidence with age (Fig. 43–1*B*).

The rapid increase in the incidence of non-Hodgkin's lymphoma in the United States is not fully understood but is multifactorial. Although some of the increase may be technical, such as improved diagnosis, diseases such

TABLE 43–2. Lymphoma Subtypes and B-cell Stages of Differentiation

	B Cells	Immunoglobulin Genes	Somatic Mutations	Ig Protein	Marker	Corresponding Lymphoma	
Foreign antigen independent ↓	Stem cell	Germline	None	None	CD34		Bone marrow ↓
	Pro-B cell*	Germline	None	None	CD19, CD79a, BSAP, CD34, CD10, TdT		
	Pre-B cell†	IgH rearrangement μ chain (cytoplasm)	None	Igμ	CD19, CD45R, CD79a, BSAP, CD34, CD10, TdT	B-LBL/ALL	
	Immature B cell	IgL/IgH$^-$ rearrangements IgM (membrane)	None	IgM (membrane)	CD19, CD20, CD45R, CD79a, CD10, BSAP		
Foreign antigen dependent ↓	Mature naive B cell	IgH/L rearrangements IgM and IgD (membrane)	None	IgM/IgD	CD19, CD20, CD45R, CD79a, BSAP, CD5	B-CLL, MCL	Peripheral lymphoid tissue
	Germinal center (CB and CC)	IgH/L rearrangements Class switch	Introduction of somatic mutations	Ig (minimal or absent)	CD19, CD20, CD45R, CD79a, BSAP, CD10, Bcl-6	BL, FL, LPHL, DLBCL, cHL‡	
	Memory B	IgH/L rearrangements	Somatic mutations	IgM	CD19, CD20, CD45R, CD79a BSAP	MZL, B-CLL	
Terminal differentiation	Plasma cell	IgH/L rearrangements	Somatic mutations	IgG > IgA > IgD	CD38, Vs38c, MUM-1, CD138	Plasmacytoma/ myeloma	

*There is a developmental stage between the pro-B-cell and the pre-B cell for which no universally accepted term exists. Terms previously used are "pre-pre-B" and "common B-cell precursor." This intermediate cellular stage most commonly gives rise to B-LBL/ALL.

†For a detailed description of the Ig gene rearrangement events, early and late pre-B cells are distinguished.

‡The relationship to germinal center cells can only be determined by molecular biologic investigations, because the phenotype of the tumor cells is completely changed following the malignant transformation.

Abbreviations: B-CLL, B-cell chronic lymphocytic leukemia; BL, Burkitt's lymphoma; B-LBL/ALL, B-cell lymphoblastic lymphoma/precursor B-lymphoblastic leukemia/lymphoma; CB, centroblasts; CC, centrocytes; cHL, classical Hodgkin's lymphoma; DLBCL, diffuse large B-cell lymphoma; FL, follicle center lymphoma; Ig, immunoglobulin; LPHL, lymphocyte predominant Hodgkin's lymphoma; MCL, mantle cell lymphoma; MZL, marginal zone B-cell lymphoma; TdT, terminal deoxynucleotidyl transferase.

Modified from Stein H, Coupland SE, Hummel M: Genetic events and gene expression in B-cell differentiation. Hematology (Am Soc Hematol Educ Program) 194–200, 2001.

TABLE 43–3. Genetic Features of Non-Hodgkin's Lymphoma (NHL) Subtypes

NHL Histologic Type	Translocation	% of Cases Affected	Proto-oncogene Involved	Mechanism of Proto-oncogene Activation	Proto-oncogene Function
Lymphoplasmacytic lymphoma	t(9;14)(p13;q32)	50	*PAX5*	Transcriptional deregulation	Transcription factor regulating B-cell proliferation and differentiation
Follicular lymphoma	t(14;18)(q32;q21) t(2;18)(p11;q21) t(18;22)(q21;q11)	90	*bcl*-2	Transcriptional deregulation	Negative regulator of apoptosis
Mantle cell lymphoma	t(11;14)(q13;q32)	70	*bcl*-1/cyclin D1	Transcriptional deregulation	Cell cycle regulator
MALT lymphoma	t(11;18)(q21;q21) t(1;14)(p22;q32)	50 Rare	*API2/MLT* *bcl*-10	Fusion protein Transcriptional deregulation	*API2* has antiapoptotic activity Antiapoptosis (?)
Diffuse large B-cell lymphoma	der(3)(q27)	35	*bcl*-6	Transcriptional deregulation	Transcriptional repressor required for GC formation
Burkitt's lymphoma	t(8;14)(q24;q32) t(2;8)(p11;q24) t(8;22)(q24;q11)	80 15 5	*c-myc*	Transcriptional deregulation	Transcription factor regulating cell proliferation and growth
Anaplastic large T-cell lymphoma	t(2;5)(p23;q35)	60	*NPM/ALK*	Fusion protein	*ALK* is a tyrosine kinase

Modified from Pasqualucci L, Dalla-Favera R: Molecular pathogenesis of non-Hodgkin's lymphoma. Hematology (Am Soc Hematol Educ Program) 200–205, 2001.

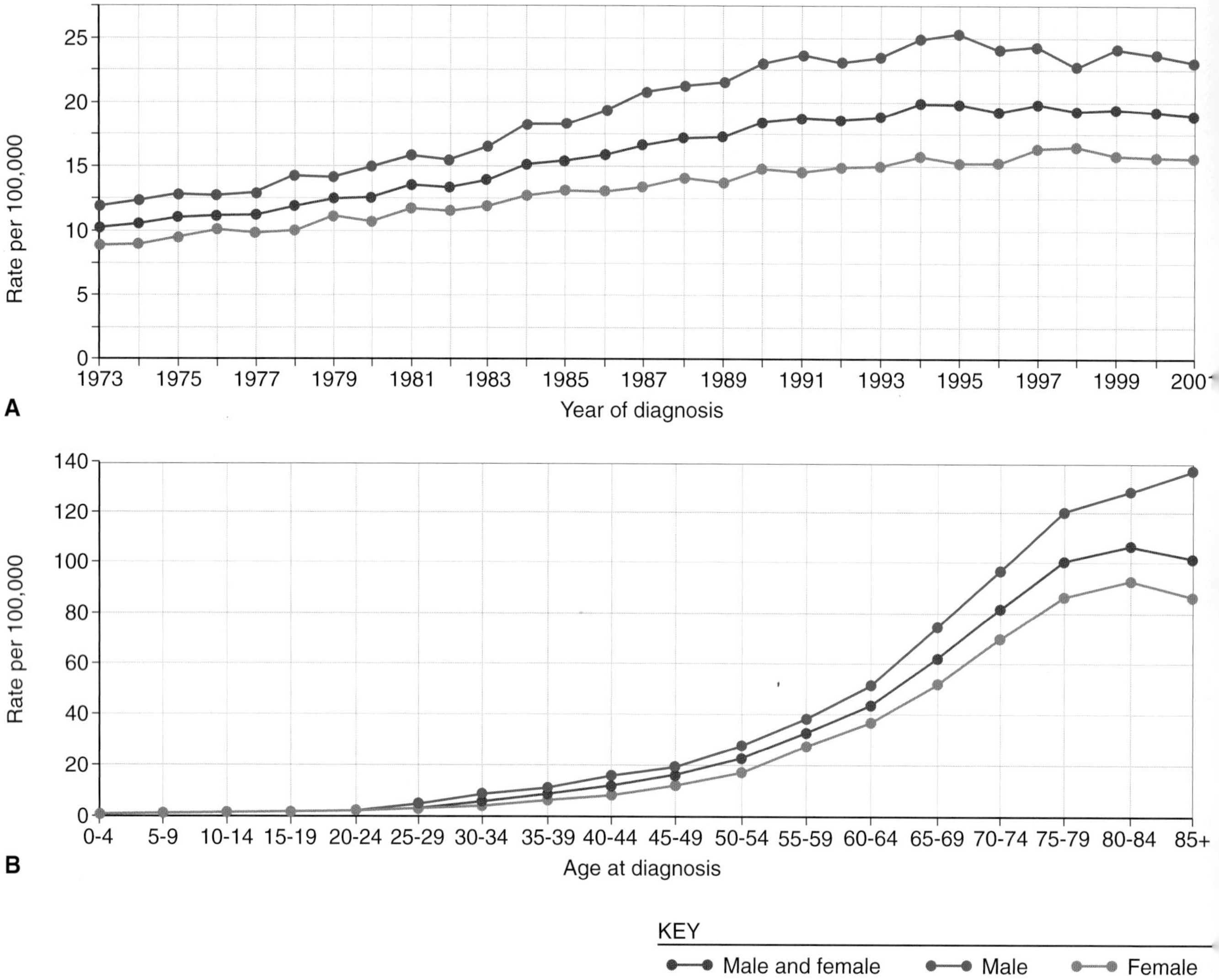

Figure 43–1. *A,* Age-adjusted rate of non-Hodgkin's lymphoma in males, females, and combined. Data are shown for each year between 1973 and 2001. *B,* Rate of non-Hodgkin's lymphoma in males, females, and combined according to age. Data from the SEER Program (*http://www.seer.cancer.gov*).

as human immunodeficiency virus (HIV) are clearly associated with an increased incidence of B-cell lymphomas. Other viruses, such as Epstein-Barr virus (EBV), hepatitis C virus, and human T-lymphotrophic virus type 1 are also associated with B- and T-cell lymphomas (Table 43–4).[23] Immunosuppressive drugs for allogeneic transplantation and immunologic diseases also increase the risk of lymphoma, as do a number of man-made environmental toxins.

The incidence of non-Hodgkin's lymphoma in the United States is greater than that in many other countries. The most striking difference has been observed in follicular lymphomas, which have been encountered less frequently in Asia. Recent epidemiologic studies linked blood transfusions, use of aspirin and other nonsteroidal anti-inflammatory drugs, and dark-colored hair dyes with up to twofold increases in relative risk of non-Hodgkin's lymphoma.[24–26]

CLINICAL FEATURES AND DIAGNOSIS

Clinical Presentation

Non-Hodgkin's lymphoma presents with enlarged lymph nodes. It can have a variable clinical presentation ranging from asymptomatic lymphadenopathy to severe organ compromise, such as airway obstruction or intestinal obstruction in aggressive lymphomas. A minority of patients may have systemic symptoms related to excess metabolism and inflammatory molecules produced either directly by lymphoma cells or by host tissues. These symptoms include malaise, fatigue, loss of appetite, weight loss, night sweats, intermittent fevers, and itching especially after bathing.

In an analysis of 1283 newly diagnosed patients with non-Hodgkin's lymphoma, 58% of the patients had advanced (stage III or IV) disease and 32% had bone marrow involvement (Table 43–5).[27] Thirty-one percent

TABLE 43–4. Infectious Etiologies of Lymphomas

Infectious Agent	Lymphoma Subtype	Mechanism and Potential Role of Infectious Agent	Other Factors
EBV	Burkitt's lymphoma	C-Myc activation; serves as cofactor	Malaria-induced immunosuppression
	Posttransplantation lymphoproliferative diseases	EBV; direct activation	Immunocompromised hosts
	Hodgkin's disease	Unknown; may cooperate with mechanisms of lymphomagenesis	Mixed cellularity, lymphocyte-depleted subtypes; AIDS-related Hodgkin's lymphoma
	Nasal angiocentric lymphoma	EBV; likely cofactor	More common in Asia
HTLV-1	Adult T-cell leukemia and lymphoma	HTLV-1; direct role	Possibly genetic or environmental factors
KSHV	Primary effusion B-cell lymphoma	KSHV; likely cofactor	May cooperate with EBV in AIDS
	Castleman's disease (plasma-cell variant)	KSHV; may be direct	Associated with AIDS
Hepatitis C	B-cell lymphomas	Immune stimulation of B cells; indirect effect	Chronic active infection
Helicobacter pylori	Extranodal marginal zone B-cell lymphoma (MALT) of the stomach	Activation of T cells by *H. pylori* antigens	Gastric ulcer

Abbreviations: AIDS, acquired immunodeficiency syndrome; EBV, Epstein-Barr virus; HTLV-1, human T-lymphotrophic virus type 1; KSHV, Kaposi's sarcoma-associated herpesvirus; MALT, mucosa-associated lymphoid tissue.

TABLE 43–5. Staging Classification of Lymphoma

Stage	Ann Arbor Classification	Cotswold Modification[50]
I	Involvement of a single lymph node region (I) or of a single extralymphatic organ or site (I_E)	Involvement of a single lymph node region or lymphoid structure
II	Involvement of two or more lymph node regions on the same side of the diaphragm alone (II) or with involvement of limited, contiguous extralymphatic organ or tissue (II_E)	Involvement of two or more lymph node regions on the same side of the diaphragm (the mediastinum is considered a single site, whereas the hilar lymph nodes are considered bilaterally); the number of anatomic sites should be indicated by a subscript (e.g., II_3)
III	Involvement of lymph node regions on both sides of the diaphragm (III), which may include the spleen (III_S); a limited, contiguous extralymphatic organ or site (III_E); or both (III_{ES})	Involvement of lymph node regions on both sides of the diaphragm: III_1 (with or without involvement of splenic hilar, celiac, or portal nodes) and III_2 (with involvement of para-aortic, iliac, and mesenteric nodes)
IV	Multiple or disseminated foci of involvement of one or more extralymphatic organs or tissues, with or without lymphatic involvement	Involvement of one or more extranodal sites in addition to a site for which the designation E has been used

*All cases are subclassified to indicate the absence (A) or presence (B) of the systemic symptoms of significant fever (>38.0°C [100.4°F]), night sweats, and unexplained weight loss exceeding 10% of normal body weight within the previous 6 months. The clinical stage (CS) denotes the stage as determined by all diagnostic examinations and a single diagnostic biopsy only. In the Ann Arbor classification, the term *pathologic stage* (PS) is used if a second biopsy of any kind has been obtained, whether negative or positive. In the Cotswold modification, the PS is determined by laparotomy; X designates bulky disease (widening of the mediastinum by more than one third or the presence of a nodal mass with a maximal dimension greater than 10 cm).

of these patients had involvement of two or more extranodal sites, commonly soft tissues of the upper aerodigestive track, paranasal sinuses, stomach and intestine, thyroid, testes, bone, and skin. The central nervous system can be involved exclusively or as a part of disseminated disease. Clinical signs and symptoms of extranodal lymphoma can vary greatly and can mimic any other malignancy or inflammatory or infectious diseases.

Prognostic Factors

The clinical prognostic factors in aggressive lymphomas were analyzed in 2031 newly diagnosed patients.[28] The following parameters were associated with a worse outcome: age over 60 years, Ann Arbor stage III or IV, serum lactate dehydrogenase above normal, Eastern Cooperative Oncology Group performance status of 2 or greater, and involvement of two or more extranodal sites. A clinical prognostic model known as the International Prognostic Index (IPI) was developed using these five factors (Table 43–6). In the IPI, one point is allocated for the presence of each parameter, and in the study, the 5-year survival rates were 73%, 51%, 43%, and 26% for scores of 0–1, 2, 3, and 4–5, respectively.[28] Based on this model, the IPI is commonly used for assessment of clinical prognosis and for treatment stratification in research protocols. Recently, a validated prognostic index based

TABLE 43–6. Prognostic Indexes for Lymphoma

International Prognostic Index for Aggressive Lymphomas (IPI)[28]

Prognostic Score	Frequency (%)	Progression-Free Survival at 5 yr (%)	5-yr Survival (%)
0	7	84	89
1	22	77	90
2	29	67	81
3	23	60	78
4	12	51	61
≥5	7	42	56

Follicular Lymphoma International Prognostic Index (FLIPI)[197]

Number of Risk Factors	% of Patients	10-yr Survival (%)
0–1: Low risk	36	71
2: Intermediate risk	37	51
≥3: Poor risk	27	36

on the IPI was developed for follicular lymphoma[29] (see Table 43–6). Age, stage, and serum lactate dehydrogenase, in addition to hemoglobin level and number of nodal areas, were used as parameters in this Follicular Lymphoma International Prognostic Index (FLIPI). These correlates reliably predicted survival.

The factors comprising the IPI and FLIPI are surrogates for biologic features. Several biological markers have been evaluated and correlate with prognosis, particularly in diffuse large B-cell lymphoma. These include Bcl-2, Bcl-6, and MUM-1.[30–34] Several studies have identified Bcl-2 expression as a marker of poor outcome. Wilson and colleagues[35] determined that the monoclonal antibody rituximab may overcome Bcl-2–associated chemotherapy resistance in untreated diffuse large B-cell lymphoma, and this finding was subsequently validated by the Groupe d'Études des Lymphomes de l'Adulte (GELA) group in a randomized study.[36]

Molecular profiling is a relatively new and powerful technique that has yielded a new taxonomy and molecular predictors of clinical outcome in several lymphoma subtypes.[37–40] With this technique, the differential transcription of genes into messenger RNA, which depend on a multiplicity of factors including cell lineage, differentiation, and intracellular pathways, can be assessed. Until isolated tumor cells are analyzed, the composite gene expression profile also includes infiltrative cells of the tumor microenvironment. Ultimately, these profiles should be related to protein expression to infer specific functionality of the observed changes. Molecular profiling of hundreds of diffuse large B-cell lymphoma cases suggested it can be divided into a subtype derived from a germinal center B cell, termed a *germinal center B cell–like* (GCB) diffuse large B-cell lymphoma, and a subtype derived from an activated post–germinal center B cell, termed *activated B cell–like* (ABC) diffuse large B-cell lymphoma. Genes associated with GCB diffuse large B-cell lymphoma included known markers of germinal center differentiation such as CD10 and the *bcl-6* gene, which may be translocated or mutated in diffuse large B-cell lymphoma, as well as numerous new genes (Fig. 43–2*A*).[10] In contrast, most genes that defined ABC diffuse large B-cell lymphoma were not expressed by normal germinal center B cells, but instead were induced during in vitro activation of peripheral B cells such as cyclin D2 and CD44.[41,42] These results suggest that the GCB and ABC diffuse large B-cell lymphoma subtypes are derived from B cells at different stages of differentiation and are pathogenetically distinct.

If this new taxonomy defines true diffuse large B-cell lymphoma subtypes, one would also predict that it should have clinical prognostic value. Because all biopsies analyzed in this study were de novo diffuse large B-cell lymphoma and came from untreated patients who then received doxorubicin-based chemotherapy, it was possible to correlate survival and the diffuse large B-cell lymphoma subtype.[43,44] This analysis revealed a statistically significant difference in overall survival at 5 years of 59% in the GCB and 31% in the ABC subtype of diffuse large B-cell lymphoma (Fig. 43–2*B*). Furthermore, these subgroups were also statistically significant within each of the prognostic subgroups identified by the IPI, indicating that this index and molecular profiling identify different features that influence survival. These results led to a larger study by Rosenwald and associates in which samples from 240 patients with diffuse large B-cell lymphoma were analyzed by molecular profiling and for the presence of genomic abnormalities.[38] This larger study reconfirmed the validity of the ABC and GCB taxonomy, and identified a third group, termed *type 3*, that did not highly express the genes associated with the former subtypes and does not appear to be a distinct diffuse large B-cell lymphoma subtype. Using a supervised approach of the gene expression profiles from these cases, a molecular prognostic predictor was developed for diffuse large B-cell lymphoma (Fig. 43–2*C*).[38] The final model combined four expression signatures—the GCB signature (favorable), the major histocompatibility complex class II signature (favorable), the lymph node signature (favorable), and the proliferation signature (unfavorable)—with expression of the bone morphogenetic protein-6 (*BMP6*) gene (unfavorable). To estimate survival outcome, each diffuse large B-cell lymphoma case is assigned a score calculated from the weighted sum of these components and ranked in quartiles according to their scores (see Fig. 43–2*C*). This model successfully predicted survival risk and was independent of the IPI.

Mantle cell lymphoma, although relatively uncommon, is both aggressive and incurable, with a median survival of 3–4 years.[21] To help gain insights into its pathogenesis with the aims of identifying new therapeutic targets and of predicting survival outcome, a study of 101 cases was undertaken.[40] A supervised approach to discover genes associated with survival found that 58% of the predictor genes were associated with cellular proliferation, with higher expression of this signature being associated with worse overall survival (Fig. 43–3*A*). By using a quantitative measure of tumor cell proliferation, a predictive model was developed that subdivided patients into quartiles with median survival times of 0.8, 2.3, 3.3, and 6.7 years (Fig. 43–3*B*).

To help gain further insight into the clinical heterogeneity of follicular lymphoma, molecular profiling of 191 samples was performed using an Affymetrix U133

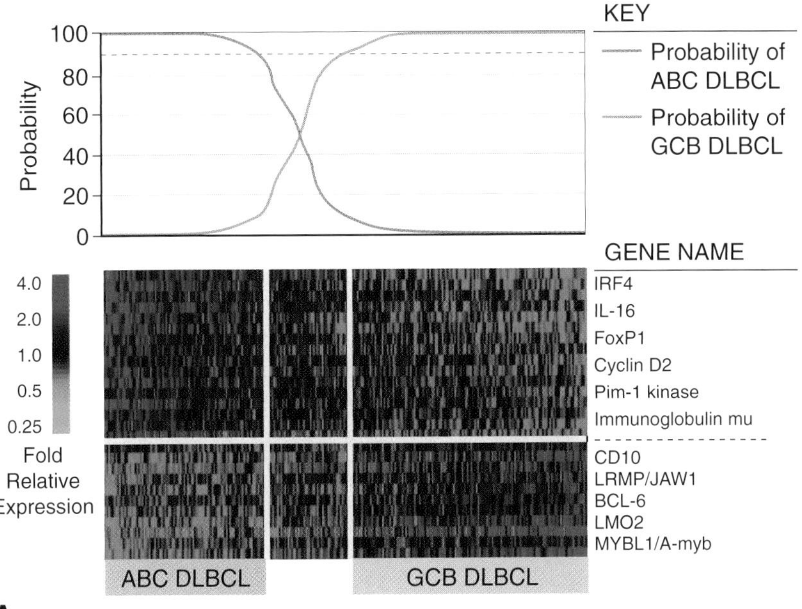

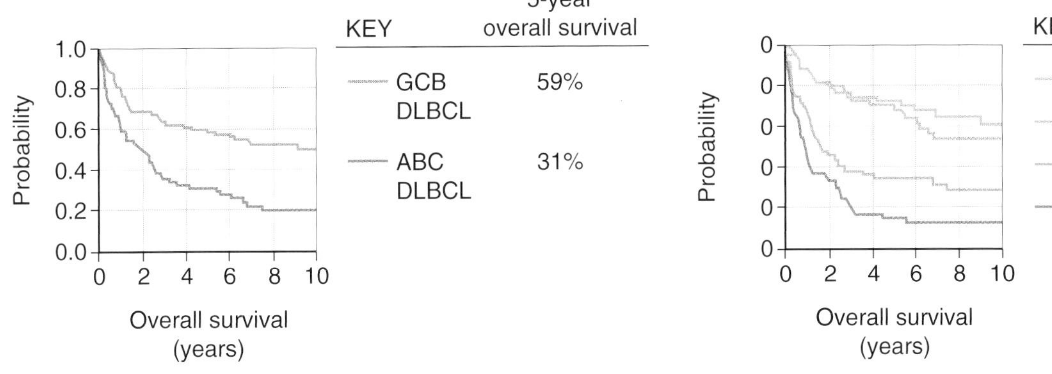

Figure 43–2. Diagnosis of diffuse large B-cell lymphoma (DLBCL) subtypes by gene expression and development of a molecular outcome predictor in previously untreated patients with DLBCL following chemotherapy. ***A,*** The expression levels of 27 genes from the subgroup predictor in 274 DLBCL samples are shown according to the color scale at the *left.* Six named genes that showed increased expression in either the ABC or GCB subgroups are shown at the *right.* The likelihood that a DLBCL sample belongs to the ABC or GCB subgroup is shown on *top* and arranged by probability. ***B,*** Kaplan-Meier estimates of overall survival according to GCB or ABC DLBCL subtype. ***C,*** Kaplan-Meier estimates of overall survival according to the molecular outcome predictor for each quartile.

microarray and a molecular predictor of survival was developed.[45] Overall, 81 predictor genes were identified, which appeared to reflect tumor-infiltrating immune cells in the tumor mass and B-cell differentiation genes, and these were used to construct a predictive model. This study showed for the first time that genes associated with different tumor-infiltrating immune cells, which were divided into immune response-1 (IR-1) and -2 (IR-2) signatures, were the important molecular determinants of clinical outcome. The molecular model divided patients into quartiles based on their relative expression of the IR-1 and IR-2 signatures, and yielded median survivals of 3.9 and greater than 15 years at the highest and lowest quartiles, respectively. Importantly, the model could stratify patient survival even within the IPI good risk category. These findings suggest that the immune microenvironment plays an important role in the clinical heterogeneity of follicular lymphoma, possibly in its capacity to regulate follicular lymphoma cell replication and death.

Diagnosis and Staging

During the evaluation of lymphadenopathy, a history of potentially causative factors such as prior malignancy, chemotherapy or radiation treatment, and/or an autoimmune or immunodeficiency disease should be sought. A detailed physical examination should be performed with special attention to lymph node regions. The most important diagnostic test is a partial or complete excisional surgical biopsy. Needle biopsies are highly discouraged.

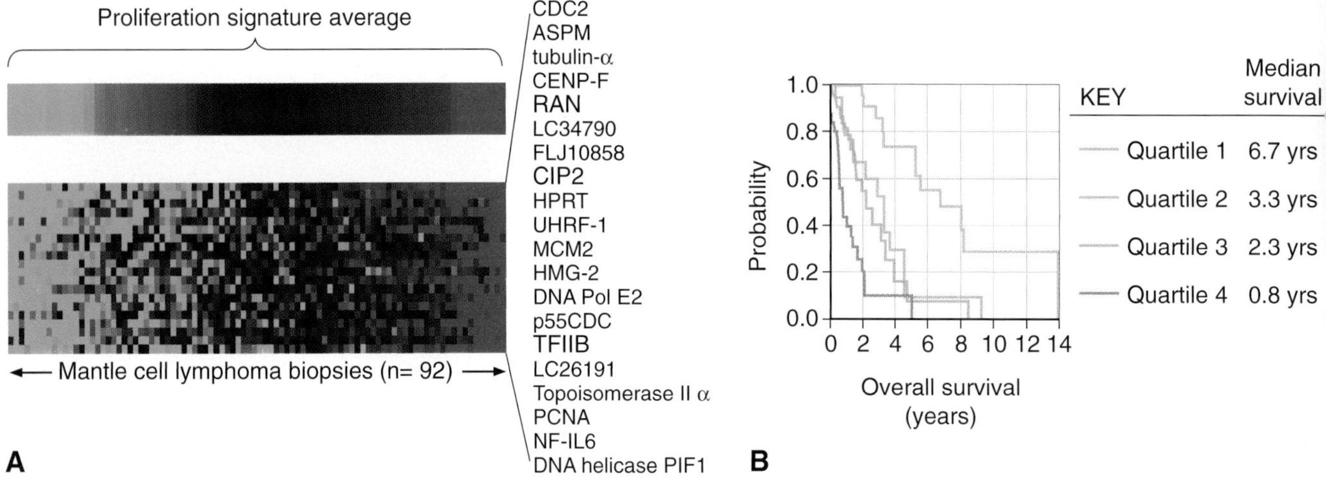

Figure 43–3. Gene expression-based predictor of survival in mantle cell lymphoma. ***A***, Expression of 20 proliferation signature genes used to compute the proliferation signature average. Cases are ordered according to their proliferation signature average. The color scale depicts a fourfold range in gene expression. ***B***, Kaplan-Meier estimates of overall survival according to the molecular outcome predictor for each quartile. Only the proliferation signature contributed to the outcome prediction.

Laboratory studies should include a complete blood count, serum chemistry (including lactate dehydrogenase level) assay, and HIV and hepatitis serology tests. An abnormally elevated lactate dehydrogenase has important prognostic implications.[46] Potential infectious etiologies for lymphoma should be assessed as indicated and include HIV, EBV, hepatitis C virus, *Helicobacter pylori*, human T-lymphotrophic virus type 1, *Borrelia burgdorferi*, human herpesvirus 8, *Campylobacter jejuni*, and *Chlamydia psittaci* (see Table 43–4). Serum protein electrophoresis with immunoglobulin quantification should be performed when indicated, as in Waldenström's macroglobulinemia. This test may detect a monoclonal paraprotein, which can be monitored for disease response, as well as immunoglobulin deficiency, which may accompany these diseases and predispose to opportunistic infections.

Imaging studies should include a chest radiograph and computed tomography of the chest, abdomen, and pelvis (with intravenous contrast if possible). The need for additional imaging studies, including magnetic resonance imaging and positron emission tomography (PET) scanning depends on the clinical presentation and sites of disease. Evaluation of the head by either computed tomography or magnetic resonance imaging is undertaken if central nervous system disease is highly suspected.

The incidence of bone marrow involvement varies according to histology but can approach 70% in indolent B-cell lymphoma.[47] Bone marrow assay is a standard investigation that should be routinely undertaken at diagnosis. Patients at high risk of central nervous system disease should undergo a lumbar puncture at diagnosis with evaluation of the cerebrospinal fluid. Certain histologic subtypes and clinical paradigms are associated with a higher risk of central nervous system disease.[48] Flow cytometric analysis of cerebrospinal fluid should be undertaken in addition to cytologic evaluation.[49]

The Ann Arbor staging system of non-Hodgkin's lymphoma (see Table 43–5) has been superseded by the IPI score but helps define the extent of disease.[50]

Radiologic Evaluation

Computed tomography scanning remains the key imaging modality during the initial evaluation and staging of patient's with non-Hodgkin's lymphoma and in evaluating response to therapy. 18-Fluoro-2-deoxyglucose (FDG)-PET provides sensitive functional imaging of lymphomas as well (Fig. 43–4). A retrospective evaluation of 172 patients with various histologies of lymphoma found that 98–100% of diffuse large B-cell, mantle cell, and follicular lymphomas were detectable by FDG-PET.[51] However, detection frequencies were below 70% for patients with marginal zone and peripheral T-cell lymphomas. FDG-PET has a higher sensitivity and specificity for detecting nodal and extranodal disease compared to conventional radiographic modalities.

Findings of FDG-PET scans obtained after therapy have been shown to have prognostic value. In one study, 26 of 93 scans were positive for residual disease.[52] All 26 of these patients relapsed, with a median progression-free survival of only 73 days. In contrast, only 11 of 67 patients with normal PET scans after chemotherapy relapsed, with a median progression-free survival of 404 days. Furthermore, early restaging with FDG-PET was of prognostic value.[53] Seventy patients with aggressive non-Hodgkin's lymphoma underwent FDG-PET scanning at mid-treatment. Thirty-three patients had persistent abnormal PET scan and none of these patients achieved durable complete remission, whereas 31 of 37 patients with negative PET scans remained in complete remission long term. Mid-treatment PET scan was a stronger prognostic predictor for both progression-free and overall survival than was the IPI.

FDG-PET at diagnosis

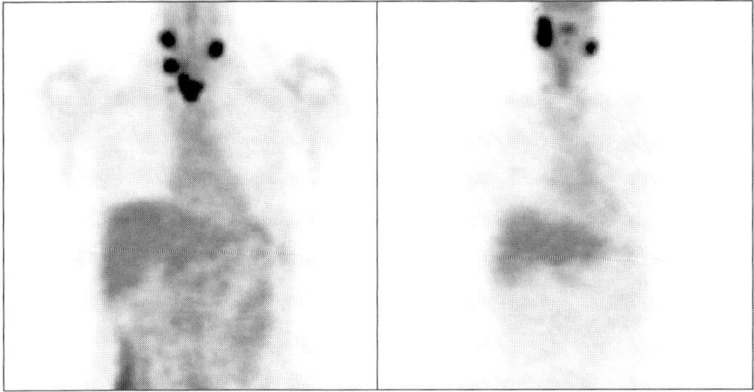

FDG-PET 2 months later after 3 cycles of R-CHOP

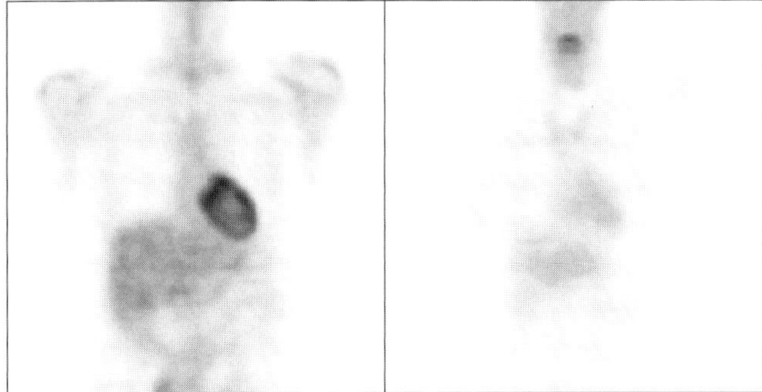

Figure 43–4. FDG-PET scan before and after treatment with R-CHOP. Resolution of cervical and upper mediastinal disease is shown.

MANAGEMENT OF INDOLENT LYMPHOMA

Indolent lymphomas are incurable chronic diseases that require intermittent therapy to control clinical signs and symptoms. Effective treatments provide long-term complete or partial remissions. Furthermore, intensive treatments, such as allogeneic stem cell transplantation (SCT), are currently being investigated as potentially curative therapy. Because treatment of asymptomatic patients has not been shown to result in improved survival, a delay in initiating treatment is often reasonable. Most clinicians initiate therapy for symptomatic patients with bulky disease, diffuse bone marrow infiltration resulting in abnormal blood counts, threatened organ function, and rapid tumor growth.

Most indolent lymphomas are of follicular histology (25% of all non-Hodgkin's lymphomas). Although three grades based on the number of centroblasts per high-power field are identified, only grade 3b is considered more aggressive and may be biologically related to de novo diffuse large B-cell lymphoma. Small lymphocytic lymphoma closely resembles chronic lymphocytic leukemia, as does lymphoplasmacytic lymphoma. Other indolent histologies include marginal zone and mucosa-associated lymphoid tissue (MALT) lymphoma, which are treated similar to follicular lymphomas. Three risk groups have been defined based on clinical characteristics as expressed by the FLIPI (see Table 43–6).

Early-Stage Disease

Some follicular lymphoma patients have stage I or II disease with no convincing evidence of systemic spread. Radiotherapy alone has been widely used for this patient population, with median survival times close to 15 years and a substantial number of patients remaining alive 20 years after therapy. It is, however, not clear if these patients have to be treated immediately or if their treatment could be deferred. A retrospective analysis of 43 patients with stage I or II follicular lymphoma who did not receive any therapy revealed that 63% did not require therapy during the median follow-up of 86 months.[54] Remaining patients required therapy in a median of 22 months. This study suggests that, in selected early-stage follicular lymphoma patients, treatment can be safely deferred. An aggressive strategy of prolonged combination chemotherapy followed by involved-field radiation therapy[55] was associated with a 10-year time to treatment failure of 76% and overall survival of 82% in early stage follicular lymphoma. However, high risk of secondary malignancies dampen enthusiasm for this approach.

Asymptomatic Advanced-Stage Disease

Relatively small randomized trials have investigated the long-term outcome of asymptomatic patients promptly treated with single-agent or combination chemotherapy versus those closely monitored without active therapy (Table 43–7). A study from the National Cancer Institute of 104 patients randomized 44 to watch-and-wait status and 45 to aggressive combination chemotherapy with the ProMace-MOPP regimen, followed by total nodal irradiation.[56] An additional 15 patients were symptomatic and received immediate treatment. As expected, disease-free survival was superior with treatment, but overall survival was similar in both groups, with 83% and 84% survival at a median follow-up of 4 years. Four patients (10%) in the combined-modality therapy group developed myelodysplasia. In a long-term study that included 309 patients with asymptomatic advanced-stage, low-grade non-Hodgkin's lymphoma from the United Kingdom,[57] 158 patients were randomized to receive oral chlorambucil 10 mg day and 151 were observed. With a median follow-up of 16 years, the overall survival was similar in both groups (5.9 years for chlorambucil, 6.7 years for observation). Approximately 20% of the patients in the observation arm did not require therapy during 10 years of follow-up, including 40% of those who were 70 years of age or older.

Initial Treatment of Symptomatic Advanced-Stage Disease

The choice of initial therapy for patients with indolent lymphoma with symptomatic disease can be difficult and should be tailored to the patient and disease characteristics (see Table 43–7). Patients with high disease burden and disabling symptoms should be treated more aggressively with multiagent regimens. If the disease is slowly progressing and gradually becoming symptomatic, starting with less toxic therapy and gradually escalating

TABLE 43–7. Treatment Regimens and Outcome for Indolent Lymphoma

Patient Group	Therapy*	Response Rates (%)	Complete Response (%)	Median Survival†	References
Asymptomatic	Observation	–	–	6–7 years (OS)	56,57
	Chlorambucil	–	–	6–7 yr (OS)	
Symptomatic	CVP ± R	60–80	10–40	3–5 yr (PFS)	59–63
	CHOP ± R	90–100	40–80	5–7 yr (PFS)	
	FND ± R	90–100	70–90	5–7 yr (PFS)	
	R ± Maintenance R	60–75	15–40	2–3 yr (PFS)	
Relapsed	Rituximab	40–60	10–20	8–24 mo (PFS)	81–84
	Radioimmunotherapy	65–80	15–50	8–24 mo (PFS)	86–89
	Chemotherapy	60–90	15–40	12–24 mo (PFS)	80

*CHOP, cyclophosphamide, doxorubicin (Adriamycin), vincristine, prednisone; CVP, cyclophosphamide, vincristine, prednisone; FND, fludarabine, mitoxantrone and dexamethasone; R, rituximab.
†OS, overall survival; PFS, progression-free survival.

the intensity of the treatments may be an acceptable approach.

Numerous single and combined chemotherapy agents can be used to achieve partial or complete responses in patients with indolent lymphoma (see Table 43–7). Single-agent chlorambucil or cyclophosphamide with or without prednisone, commonly used in the past, has good response rates albeit rarely complete. More aggressive combination chemotherapy has higher complete remission rates, but overall survival is not necessarily impacted. In a study of 259 patients with stage III or IV low-grade non-Hodgkin's lymphoma randomized to oral chlorambucil/prednisone versus cyclophosphamide, doxorubicin, vincristine, and prednisone (CHOP), the response rate was higher with CHOP (36% vs. 60%) but there was no survival difference (46 vs. 52 months).[58] Importantly, there is no plateau on the survival curve for the treatment of low-grade lymphomas, with a survival median of 6.9 years.[59]

Anti-CD20 monoclonal antibody (rituximab) has significantly improved the treatment of indolent B-cell lymphomas. In 41 untreated patients with indolent lymphoma, rituximab yielded an overall response rate of 64%, with 15% complete response, and 77% were progression free at 12 months.[60,61] Rituximab induction followed by maintenance was tested as a first-line treatment in 62 patients with follicular lymphoma, grades 1 and 2, and small lymphocytic lymphoma.[62] The overall response rate was 47%, with stable disease in the remaining patients. Further improved responses occur with maintenance therapy, with a median progression-free survival of 34 months. Protracted or "maintenance" rituximab in newly diagnosed or relapsed or refractory follicular lymphoma is also beneficial, with response rates of 67% in untreated patients versus 46% in previously treated patients[63] and prolonged median event-free survival of 23 months in the maintenance group compared to 12 months in the observation group.

The addition of rituximab to combination chemotherapy also improves response rate and duration. Six cycles of CHOP and rituximab (R-CHOP) resulted in an overall response rate of 95%, of which 55% were complete, and the median progression-free survival was 82.3 months.[64] Some patients achieved molecular remissions by t(14;18) polymerase chain reaction analysis.[65] In a randomized trial of cyclophosphamide, vincristine, and prednisone with or without rituximab, the combination was clearly superior in both the response rates and durations.[66] In a randomized study involving cyclophosphamide, vincristine, and prednisone, addition of maintenance rituximab[67] improved progression-free survival (4.5 years vs. 2.5 years in the no-maintenance group), and the effectiveness of rituximab was confirmed in another trial evaluating rituximab maintenance with either fludarabine and mitoxantrone or CHOP.[68]

Immunoglobulin G fragment-C (Fc) receptor polymorphisms are associated with different rituximab response rates.[69] The Fc portion of the antibody is involved in binding to a specific receptor and mediates an antibody-dependent cellular cytotoxicity reaction. Polymorphisms of the receptors to this fragment result in higher affinity to the antibody with corresponding enhancement of the antibody-dependent cellular cytotoxicity. The valine/valine polymorphism at amino acid 158 in FCγ receptor 3A (15% of the patients), and the histidine/histidine polymorphism at amino acid 131 of FCγ receptor 2A (25% of the patients) were independently associated with freedom from progression after rituximab.

A number of other immunologic approaches have also been tested, including interferon and idiotype vaccine. Although some of the interferon studies have shown improved survival in follicular lymphoma, other studies have been negative.[70,71] Eleven patients with chemotherapy-induced first clinical remission who had persistent polymerase chain reaction–detectable tumor cells in blood were given anti-idiotype vaccination and developed humeral and cellular responses.[72] Eight of 11 patients converted to molecular remission, which was sustained long term after vaccination. Other idiotype vaccine studies have also shown regression of follicular lymphoma following idiotype vaccines.[73] Because of these promising results, several randomized studies of idiotype vaccine have been instituted.

There are subtypes of indolent lymphomas that require unique therapy. Splenic lymphoma with villous lymphocytes is a special subset with splenomegaly and clonal expansion of B-cells with villous projections in blood. Splenectomy may be initial therapy. In patients with chronic hepatitis C virus infection and splenic lymphoma with villous lymphocytes, treatment with interferon alfa, alone or in combination with the antiviral agent ribavirin, was associated with clearance of hepatitis C virus RNA and regression of lymphoma (in seven of nine patients).[74] Importantly, hepatitis C virus–negative patients did not respond to this therapy.

Advanced MALT lymphomas can be effectively treated with regimens described for follicular lymphoma. Localized gastric MALT associated with *Helicobacter pylori* should be treated with antibiotics unless tumor cells have t(11;18), which predicts poor response to antibiotic therapy[75] (see Table 43–3). Approximately 70% of the cases of stage I_E gastric MALT regress following eradication of *H. pylori* with antibiotics.[76] Patients with localized disease and persistent lymphoma despite antibiotics can be effectively treated with radiotherapy. Other common sites of MALT lymphoma include the salivary glands, lungs, and ocular adnexa. Rituximab is an active agent in MALT lymphomas.[77] In patients thus treated, overall responses were 73%, with 44% complete remissions.

Relapsed Disease

Patients who had benefit from initial therapy can be re-treated with the same agents, although alternative regimens can be chosen.[78] There are multiple active treatments for relapsed patients (see Table 43–7). One active regimen is the combination of fludarabine, mitoxantrone, and dexamethasone.[79,80] In a Phase II trial of 51 patients with relapsed or refractory low-grade lymphoma, overall and complete response rates were 94% and 47%, respectively, with a 14-month median failure-free survival.[80]

Rituximab has been extensively investigated in patients with relapsed indolent lymphoma (see Table 43–7). One hundred sixty-six patients were given rituximab 375 mg/m^2 weekly for four doses and 48% responded with a 13-month median time to progression.[81] Other studies show that rituximab[82] can also be used in re-treatment of patients who relapsed after previously rituximab therapy.[83] An overall response rate of 40% is seen, even in patients with bulky disease (greater than 10 cm), although most responses are only partial.[84]

To enhance the activity of anti-CD20 antibody therapy, murine forms have been conjugated to iodine-131 and yttrium-90. Both of these agents are commercially available, iodine-131 tositumomab (Bexxar) and ibritumomab tiuxetan (Zevalin). Iodine-131 tositumomab was tested in 60 patients with low-grade or transformed B-cell non-Hodgkin's lymphoma.[85,86] The response rate was 65%, with a median duration of response of 6.5 months. Among 22% of patients who achieved complete remission, the response duration was over 47 months. Four patients developed secondary myelodysplasia.[87] Ibritumomab tiuxetan was tested in patients who had no objective response to rituximab or progressed within 6 months after rituximab.[88] Among 54 patients with follicular lymphoma, 74% responded (15% complete) and the median time to progression was 6.8 months. Delayed grade 4 neutropenia developed in 35% of the patients. Ibritumomab tiuxetan compared to rituximab was also tested in a randomized controlled trial in patients with relapsed, refractory, or transformed follicular lymphoma.[89] Ibritumomab tiuxetan had a higher overall response rate of 80% versus 56% with rituximab, and a complete response rate of 30% versus 16%, respectively.

Stem Cell Transplantation in Indolent Lymphoma

High-dose therapy with autologous hematopoietic stem cell support for indolent lymphoma has been tested in a variety of clinical settings, including (1) as a consolidation therapy in first partial or complete remission,[90–92] (2) in relapse,[93–97] and (3) in transformed lymphoma[98,99] (Table 43–8). Details of this modality are presented in Chapter 95. In a study of 92 untreated patients with advanced follicular lymphoma, 87% received high-dose chemotherapy and autologous SCT without purging,[91] with 4-year overall and disease-free survival rates of 84% and 67%, respectively. The GELA study group presented similar results,[100] with a statistically significant improvement in 7-year overall survival of 86% in the SCT arm versus 74% in the interferon arm.

A number of groups have investigated autologous transplantation in relapsed disease.[93–97] A large study reported a 42% disease-free and 66% overall survival at 8 years after antibody-purged autologous bone marrow transplantation.[93] The patients, whose bone marrow was successfully purged, had significantly better outcomes, although marrow free of non-Hodgkin's lymphoma may only be a surrogate marker for lower disease burden.[93] Autologous transplantation in transformed indolent lym-

TABLE 43–8. Transplantation for Indolent Lymphomas

Patient Group	Graft	OS	DFS	References
Initial diagnosis	Autologous	>80% at 7 yr	50–70% at 7 yr	90,91,100
Relapsed	Autologous	50–60% at 5 yr	35–45% at 5 yr	93,95,96
	Allogeneic	50% at 5 yr	80% at 5 yr	96,101,102
Transformed	Autologous	40–50% at 5 yr	30–35% at 5 yr	98,99

Abbreviations: DFS, disease-free survival; OS, overall survival.

TABLE 43–9. Treatment Regimens for Aggressive Lymphomas

Patient Group	Therapy*	Patient Group†	Complete Response (%)	Overall Response (%)	Survival End Points‡	References
Initial diagnosis	R-CHOP	All IPI and age ≥60 yr	76		EFS 57% at 2 yr	109
	ACVBP	Low IPI and age ≥18 yr	86	–	EFS 65% at 5 yr	198
	DA-EPOCH-R	All IPI and age ≥18 yr	94	–	PFS 82% at 28 mo	122
	CHOEP	Good prognosis (low LDH) and age 18–60 yr	88	–	EFS 69% at 5 yr	118
	CHOP-14	All IPI and age >60 yr	76	–	EFS 44% at 5 yr	117
Relapsed	DHAP	Recurrent lymphoma	31	26.5	OS 25% at 2 yr	172
	ESHAP	Recurrent lymphoma	37	33	OS 31% at 3 yr	199
	DA-EPOCH	Relapsed DLBCL	36	34	OS 30% at 6 yr	78
	R-ICE	Relapsed DLBCL	53	35	–	173

*ACVBP, doxorubicin, cyclophosphamide, vindesine, bleomycin, and prednisone; CHOEP, cyclophosphamide, doxorubicin, vincristine, etoposide, and dexamethasone; CHOP, cyclophosphamide, doxorubicin, vincristine, and dexamethasone; CHOP-14, 14-day dose-intensified CHOP; DA, dose-adjusted; DHAP, cisplatin, high-dose ara-C, and dexamethasone; EPOCH, etoposide, vincristine, doxorubicin, cyclophosphamide, and prednisone; ESHAP, etoposide, methylprednisolone, and ara-C with cisplatin; ICE, ifosfamide, carboplatin, and etoposide; R, rituximab.
†DLBCL, diffuse large B-cell lymphoma; IPI, International Prognostic Index; LDH, lactate dehydrogenase.
‡EFS, event-free survival; OS, overall survival; PFS, progression-free survival.

phomas has a reported 5-year overall survival of 51% and progression-free survival of 30%.[98]

Because indolent lymphomas are essentially incurable with standard or high-dose therapy, several groups have investigated allogeneic transplantation based on the hypothesis that the graft-versus-lymphoma effect may eradicate residual disease.[101] A series of 113 patients with advanced indolent lymphoma reported by the International Bone Marrow Transplant Registry were treated with allogeneic transplantation, with an overall and disease-free survival rate of 49% at 3 years with only 16% recurrences, all within 2 years; however, treatment-related mortality was 40%.[102]

To reduce the toxicity of allogeneic transplantation, nonmyeloablative allogeneic transplantation has been studied (see also Chapter 94). This approach was tested in 20 patients with indolent and aggressive lymphoma, including five cases of mantle cell lymphoma.[103] At 25 months' median follow-up, the estimated 3-year progression-free survival was 95%. Matched unrelated donor bone marrow transplantation[104] resulted in an overall survival rate of 50% at 3 years but with 33% treatment-related mortality. Clinical trials with larger numbers of patients and longer follow-up, as well as randomized study designs, are necessary to establish the role of allogeneic transplantation.

MANAGEMENT OF AGGRESSIVE LYMPHOMAS

Diffuse large B-cell lymphoma, Burkitt's lymphoma, and mantle cell lymphoma are the most common aggressive lymphomas.[40]

Diffuse Large B-Cell Lymphoma

Diffuse large B-cell lymphoma is the most prevalent lymphoma subtype, comprising 30–40% of all lympomas.[8] Although the median age at diagnosis is in the seventh decade, this subtype affects children and adults of all ages. There are several morphologic variants that include centroblastic, immunoblastic, T-cell/histiocyte–rich, and anaplastic, and molecular profiling is further refining this taxonomy.[8,38,39] Diffuse large B-cell lymphoma can arise de novo or from the histologic transformation of indolent lymphomas. Patients may present with nodal or extranodal disease and localized or disseminated disease. Diffuse large B-cell lymphoma can arise in any organ, and thus different clinical behaviors and natural histories are seen in certain subtypes, such as primary mediastinal B-cell lymphoma, which arises in the mediastinum.

Systemic chemotherapy is the mainstay of treatment for diffuse large B-cell lymphoma (Table 43–9). Radiation alone is associated with high recurrence rates.[105] In early-stage disease (I/II), there is some controversy as to whether radiation adds benefit to chemotherapy. Based on randomized studies of chemotherapy versus combined-modality therapy that showed an advantage for combined-modality treatment, this became the standard. However, longer follow-up of these studies showed a convergence of the overall survival curves and reopened the debate.[106,107] Doxorubicin, cyclophosphamide, vindesine, bleomycin, and prednisone (ACVBP) showed statistical superior outcomes versus CHOP followed by radiotherapy.[108] Furthermore, R-CHOP is more effective than CHOP alone in early-stage disease.[109] However, treatment of primary mediastinal diffuse large B-cell lymphoma may require chemotherapy followed by radiation. In a study of 50 patients with untreated primary mediastinal diffuse large B-cell lymphoma who received low-dose methotrexate, doxorubicin, cyclophosphamide, vincristine, prednisone, and bleomycin followed by radiation, 66% had a persistently positive gallium scan after the chemotherapy alone,[110] but this percentage fell to 19% after radiation consolidation. In other smaller studies of patients with primary mediastinal diffuse large B-cell lymphoma utilizing dose-adjusted etoposide, vincristine, doxorubicin, cyclophosphamide, and prednisone (DA-EPOCH), progression-free and overall survival rates were 68% and 79%, respectively, with negative gallium scans at the end of treatment.[30] Addition of rituximab improved progression-free and overall survival to 93% and 100%, respectively, in another small study.[111] These results suggest that radiation may not be needed in most early-stage patients and its use should be carefully balanced against long-term side effects such as secondary cancers.[112]

The chemotherapy "standard" for diffuse large B-cell lymphoma is in flux (see Table 43–9). In the early 1990s, a randomized trial comparing four major regimens established CHOP as the standard, based on equivalent efficacy to the other more toxic and/or costly regimens.[113] Unfortunately, only one third of patients achieve long-term event-free survival with CHOP, leaving much room for improvement.[109,113–115] A randomized comparison of ACVBP, a high-dose CHOP variant, and standard CHOP in 708 patients ages 61–69 years with aggressive lymphoma and at least one adverse prognostic factor in the age-adjusted IPI[115] found that the ACVBP and CHOP groups had event-free survival rates of 39% and 29% (P = .005) and overall survival rates of 46% and 38% (P = .036), respectively, showing an improved outcome for ACVBP. Both arms had a similar rate of complete remission, with 58% in the ACVBP group and 56% in the CHOP group. However, long-term benefit of ACVBP was due to a lower rate of central nervous system progression in the ACVBP arm (P = .004). In patients with a low IPI score, ACVBP appears equivalent to methotrexate with bleomycin, cyclophosphamide, and etoposide.[116] The German Lymphoma Study Group recently reported the preliminary results of a four-arm comparison of 14- and 21-day CHOP and CHOP with etoposide in younger and older (>60 years) patients with untreated aggressive lymphomas.[117,118] In younger patients with low-risk disease, the addition of etoposide improved overall survival from 74% to 88%. However, in older patients, CHOP time intensification (i.e., 14-day CHOP compared to 21-day CHOP) was associated with an improved survival (54% vs. 45%, respectively). A looming question is the absence of an obvious biologic basis for the different findings in older and younger patients.

Recent studies suggest that rituximab may increase the efficacy of chemotherapy. A randomized study of CHOP versus R-CHOP was performed in 197 patients 60 years of age or older with diffuse large B-cell lymphoma.[109] Patients who received R-CHOP had a higher rate of complete remission compared to CHOP alone (76% vs. 63%, respectively). With a median follow-up of 2 years, the event-free survival rates of R-CHOP and CHOP were 57% and 38%, and at 3 years they were approximately 51% and 38%, respectively. Addition of maintenance rituximab in patients 60 years of age and older with diffuse large B-cell lymphoma is not yet proven, but initial analysis shows benefits.[119] Hence, R-CHOP has become the de facto new standard for diffuse large B-cell lymphoma, although longer follow-up will be needed to accurately assess the impact of rituximab.

To help overcome drug resistance, a DA-EPOCH regimen for diffuse large B-cell lymphoma[30,35,111,120] was developed based on principles of drug action and pharmacodynamics.[121] In a Phase II study of 50 untreated patients with advanced diffuse large B-cell lymphoma, 92% achieved complete remission and, at the median follow-up of 62 months, 70% were progression-free.[30] To help overcome resistance associated with Bcl-2, a Phase II study of DA-EPOCH with rituximab[120] in 77 untreated diffuse large B-cell lymphoma patients revealed a progression-free survival of 82% at a median 28 months of follow-up,[122] with an improved response in patients with Bcl-2–positive tumors with the ABC subtype of diffuse large B-cell lymphoma.[36]

Studies continue to evaluate initial treatment of aggressive diffuse large B-cell lymphoma with high-dose chemotherapy and autologous transplantation, but this combination is not proven to be more efficacious than conventional chemotherapy.[123–125] Now that standard treatment employs rituximab, the conclusions from these trials are further confounded.

Burkitt's Lymphoma

Burkitt's lymphoma is the most aggressive lymphoma and accounts for 3–5% of all lymphomas. Pathologically, Burkitt's lymphoma is characterized by an extremely high growth fraction and spontaneous cell death. Phenotypically, Burkitt's lymphoma cells are $CD20^+$ and $CD10^+$, and terminal deoxynucleotidyl transferase is rarely expressed, consistent with a germinal center origin.[126] Endemic Burkitt's lymphoma in Africa is virtually always associated with infection by EBV in the first 2 decades of life and often involves the jaw, orbit, paraspinal regions, mesentery, and gonads.[127,128] In contrast, sporadic Burkitt's lymphoma in Western countries involves EBV in 20% of cases, commonly presents in the abdomen, and rarely involves the jaw.[129–131] When bulky or disseminated disease is present, central nervous system involvement may be seen. Rare cases present as acute leukemia and are usually referred to as the L3 subtype of acute lymphoblastic leukemia within the French-American-British (FAB) classification. In adults, Burkitt's lymphoma (<1% of adult non-Hodgkin's lymphomas) is frequently associated with HIV infection.

The high proliferation rate of Burkitt's lymphoma led to the use of dose-intensive treatment with a short cycle time to theoretically minimize tumor regrowth between cycles.[132,133] These regimens employed multiple drugs, typically administered in alternating combinations. The high rate of central nervous system spread also led to the standard use of central nervous system prophylaxis.[127] A variety of high-intensity, short-duration regimens have achieved durable remissions in from 47% to 84% of patients.[134–137] These include the French LMB and German Berlin-Frankfurt-Munster protocols and the National Cancer Institute CODOX-M/IVAC regimen. All of these regimens share similar features regarding choice of agents, short cycle length, and central nervous system prophylaxis. Although most Burkitt's lymphoma occurs in children, Magrath and colleagues showed that adults and children have a similar disease outcome when treated with the same regimen,[132] although adults experience increased treatment-related deaths.[132,138] In a more recent study of 22 patients, the progression-free survival was 68% with a median follow-up of 29 months.[138] In an ongoing National Cancer Institute study, DA-EPOCH with rituximab (DA-EPOCH-R) in untreated adult Burkitt's lymphoma is well tolerated and effective for adult Burkitt's lymphoma.[30,31]

Mantle Cell Lymphoma

Mantle cell lymphoma originates from CD5-positive mantle zone B-cells. It occurs at a median age of approximately 60 years and has a male predominance.[8] Most patients present with advanced-stage disease, and the median survival is 3 years.[139] The t(11;14) translocation is seen in almost all cases, with expression of the cyclin D1 (*bcl*-1) gene product.

Mantle cell lymphoma responds to chemotherapy, but responses are generally temporary and the disease is usually incurable. Depending upon the clinical circumstances, treatment strategies may range from observation to aggressive treatment. The Hyper-CVAD (cyclophosphamide, vincristine, doxorubicin, and dexamethasone) regimen has demonstrated good efficacy.[140,141] In a Phase II study of 45 patients, 25 of whom were untreated, 94% responded with 38% complete remissions,[141] an improvement over a historical cohort of patients who received CHOP. Combining Hyper-CVAD with rituximab improved outcomes, with 89% of patients achieving a complete remission and 90% remaining failure-free at 2 years.[142] Use of CHOP-R for mantle cell lymphoma resulted in a 48% achieved complete remission rate, but median progression-free survival was only 16.6 months.[143] The DA-EPOCH-R regimen has also been used, with a complete response rate of 93% in untreated mantle cell lymphoma.[144]

Several groups have investigated the role of high-dose chemotherapy and autologous SCT in mantle cell lymphoma. In general, results are mixed and autologous transplantation cannot be considered standard; in particular, outcomes have been poor for relapsed patients.[145] A report from the European Blood and Bone Marrow Transplant and Autologous Blood and Marrow Transplant Registries described 195 patients who underwent autologous transplantation for mantle cell lymphoma.[146] Five-year overall survival and progression-free survival rates were 50% and 33%, respectively.

Nonmyeloablative allogeneic SCT has also been tested in recurrent mantle cell lymphoma.[147] In a heavily pretreated group of 18 patients, 17 achieved complete remission and only 3 patients progressed after a median follow-up of 26 months. Event-free survival at 3 years was 82%. These are encouraging results and suggest the presence of a graft-versus-lymphoma effect.

A proteasome inhibitor, bortezomib, appears to have significant activity in relapsed refractory mantle cell lymphoma.[148,149] Preliminary data from a Phase II trial with 25 mantle cell lymphoma patients treated with twice-weekly bortezomib reported an overall response rate of 52%, with five complete remissions and a median response duration of 5.7 months.[149]

Acquired Immunodeficiency Syndrome–Related Lymphoma

Rates of lymphoma are markedly increased in the setting of HIV infection, with a 1000-fold higher incidence of Burkitt's lymphoma and 400-fold higher incidence of diffuse large B-cell lymphoma.[8,150] Specific subtypes such as primary effusion lymphoma and plasmablastic lymphoma are mostly seen in the setting of HIV infection and carry a poor prognosis. With the advent of highly active antiretroviral therapy (HAART) and improved survival, it is important to approach these lymphomas with curative intent.[151] Systemic chemotherapy has included regimens such as CHOP, but its efficacy has been disappointing and its toxicity high compared to results in HIV-negative lymphoma.[152] One great controversy in the treatment of acquired immunodeficiency syndrome–related lymphoma has been whether or not to suspend HAART therapy during chemotherapy. HAART potentially enhances the cytotoxicity of chemotherapy drugs, which may increase clinical toxicity, necessitating chemotherapy drug dose reduction and thus compromising curability. One approach that has been investigated is to suspend HAART during chemotherapy with prompt resumption after completing all treatment. The infusional regimen EPOCH, with HAART suspension, demonstrated 74% complete remission and 72% overall survival at a median follow-up of 53 months.[31] Importantly, following successful treatment, the CD4 cell counts and HIV viral loads returned to pretreatment levels or improved above these levels. Currently, the AIDS Malignancy Consortium is testing EPOCH in a randomized trial.

EBV-Associated Lymphoproliferative Disorders

There are several lymphoproliferative disorders that are associated with EBV.[153,154] Posttransplantation lymphoproliferative disorder usually occurs following solid organ transplantation.[154] This entity encompasses a broad spectrum of diseases with varying degrees of clinical aggressiveness. It is usually initially treated by withdrawal of chronic immunosuppression and/or rituximab.[154] However, chemotherapy may be required in aggressive cases and/or those that are resistant to immunosuppression withdrawal and rituximab. Chronic methotrexate for autoimmune disorders such as rheumatoid arthritis is also associated with an increased incidence of EBV^+ lymphoproliferative disorders.[155] Of interest, a recent report suggests that methotrexate may be permissive for EBV reactivation in chronically infected B cells.[156] Lymphomatoid granulomatosis is a rare but increasingly recognized EBV^+ lymphoproliferative disorder that mostly involves extranodal sites.[153] Low pathologic grades of lymphomatoid granulomatosis are very sensitive to interferon alfa, whereas higher grades require chemotherapy.[157]

T/NK-Cell Lymphoma

T/NK-cell lymphomas comprise around 15% of all lymphomas and are distributed over at least 14 subtypes.[8]

As such, most subtypes are relatively rare and not well studied from a biologic or clinical perspective. These tumors are derived from a mature T-cell and are classified by name or as a peripheral T-cell, unspecified, and as a group may be termed *peripheral T-cell lymphomas*. In general, however, diseases such as anaplastic large-cell lymphoma, adult T-cell lymphoma, natural killer (NK)-cell lymphomas, and cutaneous lymphomas are not included in this designation. With the exception of cutaneous T-cell lymphoma, which is discussed in Chapter 41, T/NK-cell lymphomas are typically aggressive. Of course, there is significant clinical and biologic heterogeneity.[131] A survival analysis highlighted the poor outcome of peripheral T-cell lymphomas compared to diffuse large B-cell lymphomas or anaplastic large-cell lymphomas.[3] In these patients, outcome was dependent on the IPI score. Only 15% of patients had low IPI score and of these only 27% were alive without disease at 5 years. In contrast, irrespective of IPI score, over 80% of patients with anaplastic large-cell lymphoma were alive at 5 years, highlighting the excellent prognosis of this subgroup.

Three large series have reported the clinical outcome of patients with T-cell lymphoma, many of whom received CHOP-based treatment.[158–160] These cases comprised peripheral T-cell lymphomas, unspecified, in 49–66% of cases, anaplastic large-cell lymphoma in 15–21% of cases, and angioimmunoblastic T-cell lymphoma in 12–24% of cases. The complete remission rate for all T-cell cases varied from 49% to 65%, and in all series, anaplastic large-cell lymphoma cases had a favorable outcome. IPI score was predictive of outcome, with a 5-year survival of 60–80% in low (0–1), 20% in intermediate (2–3), and 0% in high (4–5) IPI score patients.[161]

The poor outcome of peripheral T-cell lymphomas has prompted investigation for more effective agents and treatment approaches. Purine analogues have shown activity, with response rates of 25–60%, but like other therapies are rarely curative.[162] Monoclonal antibody treatment with alemtuzumab, which binds the CD52 antigen, has also shown activity, with 36% response in a small series of heavily pretreated patients.[163] Several combination studies of alemtuzumab- and doxorubicin-based chemotherapy are currently ongoing. Other novel agents with activity include denileukin diftitox and depsipeptide, but these have not been well studied.[164–166] Autologous SCT has also shown a poor outcome in peripheral T-cell lymphomas. In a study of 37 patients from Finland, 43% had progressed with a median follow-up of 2 years.[167] Patients with anaplastic large-cell lymphoma had a significant better outcome than those with peripheral T-cell lymphoma, with an overall survival of 85% versus 35%, respectively. Because of the possibility of a graft-versus-lymphoma effect, clinical trials of allogeneic SCT in peripheral T-cell lymphoma are ongoing.[168]

Salvage of Relapsed Aggressive Lymphomas

Relapsed aggressive lymphomas require combination chemotherapy for adequate disease control. Patients with chemotherapy-sensitive disease have the best outcome with autologous SCT.[123] However, patients with chemotherapy-resistant disease should be considered for experimental treatments, such as allogeneic SCT.[169] Some relapsed patients with local disease may be salvaged with radiation therapy. Examples include primary mediastinal diffuse large B-cell lymphoma, which can remain local even at relapse, and posttransplantation lymphoproliferative disorders, which may have an isolated resistant EBV clone following combination chemotherapy.[170]

Chemotherapy

There are a variety of active salvage chemotherapy regimens for relapsed or refractory diffuse large B-cell lymphoma (see Table 43–9).[171–175] Platinum-containing regimens, such as etoposide, methylprednisolone, and ara-C with cisplatin (ESHAP) and ifosfamide, carboplatin, and etoposide (ICE), are currently among the most widely used salvage treatments.[173,175,176] In patients with aggressive de novo lymphoma, which may be potentially curable, ESHAP yielded complete responses in 26% and 3-year overall survival was 31%. Although it is common to avoids agents used during induction when relapse occurs, this may not be optimal.[38,177] Rather, salvage regimens developed around the most active front-line agents show high activity.[78] For instance, using EPOCH chemotherapy in patients who had failed or relapsed after receiving similar drugs on a bolus schedule[78] resulted in a 70% response rate with 36% complete remissions and a median overall survival of 12.6 months. Rituximab may add to efficacy. The addition of rituximab to the ICE regimen (R-ICE) significantly increased the rate of complete remission from 27 to 53%, respectively.[173]

Stem Cell Transplantation

Multiple studies have established the utility of autologous SCT for relapsed aggressive lymphomas (Table 43–10)[178,179] (see also Chapter 95). Although some results are impressive, the evolution of treatment options makes direct comparison with current treatments difficult. For instance, one trial used cisplatin with high-dose ara-C and

TABLE 43–10. Transplantation for Aggressive Lymphomas

Patient Group	Graft	Survival	References
High risk (CR/PR1)	Autologous	65–75% OS at 5yr	124,125,186–189,200–202
Sensitive relapse	Autologous	40–50% DFS at 5yr	178–180
Primary refractory	Autologous	30–40% DFS at 3yr	181,182

Abbreviations: CR/PR1, first complete or partial remission; DFS, disease-free survival; OS, overall survival.

dexamethasone (DHAP) salvage chemotherapy and randomized 109 responders to receive four more cycles of DHAP or high-dose chemotherapy and autologous SCT.[180] With a median follow-up of 63 months, the 5-year event-free survival rates with and without SCT were 46% and 12%, respectively. Autologous SCT has also been tested in patients with primary refractory lymphoma and has yielded overall and event-free survivals of 40–50% and 30–40%, respectively.[181,182] Patients who achieve a partial response to front-line chemotherapy fare better with SCT, with 73% overall and progression-free survival rate.[183] Studies suggest that newer salvage regimens such as R-ICE and DA-EPOCH-R are more active than DHAP.[120,173] It must be noted that, because current front-line regimens are more effective, patients who fail today have relatively more resistant tumors compared to patients in older studies.[30,35,109,111,122] However, improvements in autologous SCT are also being investigated, such as the use of rituximab and iodine-131 tositumomab radioimmunotherapy.[184,185] In one study of rituximab following transplantation for relapsed lymphoma, the 2-year event-free and overall survival rates were 83% and 88%, respectively.[185]

Multiple studies have explored the role of autologous SCT for front-line treatment of high-risk patients, with mixed results.[186–189] In considering autologous SCT, one has to consider late toxicities, which include secondary myelodysplasia or leukemia. In a case-control study of 2739 patients who received autologous SCT, 56 patients were identified with myelodysplasia or leukemia.[190] The risk of myelodysplasia/acute myeloid leukemia was associated with the intensity of pretransplantation chemotherapy, particularly with nitrogen mustard and chlorambucil, and with total-body irradiation at 13.2 Gy but not lower doses.

PRECURSOR B- AND T-CELL LYMPHOMA

Precursor B-lymphoblastic and T-lymphoblastic lymphomas are highly aggressive diseases.[8] These are rare forms of lymphoma that can have primarily nodal or leukemic presentations and are classified as either precursor B-lymphoblastic and T-lymphoblastic lymphomas or acute lymphoblastic leukemia. Precursor B-lymphoblastic and T-lymphoblastic lymphoma typically presents in the mediastinum and often involves the meningeal space. It is more prevalent in young males and some 80% have a T-cell phenotype. A variety of regimens have been used for treatment, including ACVBP, CHOP-based chemotherapy, and SCT stem cell transplantation. The GELA recently report their cumulative results on 92 patients treated with ACVBP followed by consolidation with a different standard-dose or high-dose regimen. With a median follow-up of 34 months, the 5-year projected overall and event-free survivals were 32% and 22%, respectively.[191] Although other studies have reported somewhat higher overall survivals of 50–56% at 3 years with similar approaches, differences in patient characteristics likely account for much of the variation.[192–194] These studies highlight the need for aggressive treatment of these diseases.

NOVEL AGENTS

Success of anti-CD20 antibody therapy in B-cell lymphomas has let to the development of antibodies to different B-cell targets. In a Phase I/II trial, humanized anti-CD22 antibody was tested in 55 patients with recurrent indolent non-Hodgkin's lymphoma.[195] Overall, nine patients (18%) achieved an objective response, including three complete responses. The CD22 molecule was also targeted with an antibody conjugated to a chemotherapeutic agent. CMC-544, an immunoconjugate of calicheamicin targeted to CD22, was shown to be cytotoxic against CD22-positive B-cell lymphoma lines in xenografts.[196] Other antibodies targeting CD80, CD30, CD4, and CD23 molecules are also under development. A large number of compounds that interfere with molecules involved in receptor signaling, cell survival, and antiapoptosis are being tested and include proteasome inhibitors, Bcl-2 antisense molecules, and protein kinase C and mTOR inhibitors.

COMPLICATIONS OF TREATMENT

The successful treatment of non-Hodgkin's lymphoma may be associated with late complications. Many of these complications may not become evident for 5–20 years, making long-term follow-up essential. Major complications include infertility, anthracycline-related cardiotoxicity, bleomycin- or radiation-induced pulmonary complications, hypothyroidism, and, most importantly, secondary malignancies. Use of alkylating agents and topoisomerase inhibitors is associated with significantly increased risk of myelodysplastic syndrome and acute myeloid leukemia. The risk appears to be directly related to the cumulative dose and increases with age. Radiation therapy can significantly increase the risk of secondary tumors in areas of primary therapy and scatter. Young women are at risk for breast cancer after radiotherapy to the chest. There is significantly increased risk of lung cancer in smokers following chest radiotherapy.

A general guideline for follow-up of patients after completion of therapy involves visits every 3 month for 2 years, then every 6 months for 3 years, and then annually. During these visits, examination of the lymph node areas, abdomen, thyroid, and skin is important. Routine laboratory studies with blood counts, liver function tests, and lactate dehydrogenase levels should be performed. Patients with disease in the chest can be followed with chest radiographs. Thyroid-stimulating hormone level should be monitored annually in patients who had neck radiotherapy. Mammography for women should start 10 years after diagnosis of lymphoma or at age 40, whichever comes first. Patients should be immunized against influenza yearly, and pneumococcal immunization should be provided every 6 years.

Routine use of computed tomography and PET scans in asymptomatic patients for detecting early relapsed disease is controversial. There are no studies to indicate that such an approach improves outcome. Furthermore, most studies indicate that patients with relapse are readily detected as a result of signs and symptoms of the disease during scheduled or unscheduled visits. Therefore, site-

CURRENT CONTROVERSIES & FUTURE CONSIDERATIONS

Non-Hodgkin's Lymphoma

- Advances in the development of prognostic biomarkers and targeted therapy will allow individualized therapy of non-Hodgkin's lymphoma patients in the future.
- The optimal timing and type of initial therapy for indolent non-Hodgkin's lymphoma remains controversial, although recent studies suggest that rituximab-based combination chemotherapy may prolong survival. Molecular profiling can aid in therapeutic decisions by accurately predicting natural history and novel therapeutic targets.
- Idiotype vaccination is a promising strategy for indolent non-Hodgkin's lymphoma, but its therapeutic role will depend on the results of several randomized studies that have yet to be reported and/or completed.
- New molecular targets, such as proteasome degradation pathway and nuclear factor-κB have been identified in non-Hodgkin's lymphoma. Along with targeted monoclonal antibodies, small molecular inhibitors are likely to increase effectiveness and decrease toxicity of lymphoma therapy.
- The role and timing of autologous and/or allogeneic stem cell transplantation remains controversial in indolent lymphomas, including mantle cell lymphoma. Clinical trials with biologic correlates are likely to identify subpopulations of patients who may benefit from these treatments.

directed imaging modality should be used based on symptoms, clinical examination findings, and results of the routine blood work. The role of sensitive detection techniques such as PET scanning should be prospectively studied to determine if such detection can improve the outcome in asymptomatic patients with relapsed disease.

Suggested Readings*

A predictive model for aggressive non-Hodgkin's lymphoma. The International Non-Hodgkin's Lymphoma Prognostic Factors Project. N Engl J Med 329:987–994, 1993.

Coiffier B, Lepage E, Briere J, et al: CHOP chemotherapy plus rituximab compared with CHOP alone in elderly patients with diffuse large-B-cell lymphoma. N Engl J Med 346:235–242, 2002.

Dave SS, Wright G, Tan B, et al: Prediction of survival in follicular lymphoma based on molecular features of tumor-infiltrating immune cells. N Engl J Med 351:2159–2169, 2004.

Rosenwald A, Wright G, Chan WC, et al: The use of molecular profiling to predict survival after chemotherapy for diffuse large-B-cell lymphoma. N Engl J Med 346:1937–1947, 2002.

Solal-Celigny P, Roy P, Colombat P, et al: Follicular Lymphoma International Prognostic Index. Blood 104:1258–1265, 2004.

****Full references for this chapter can be found on accompanying CD-ROM.***

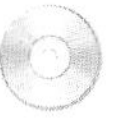

CHAPTER 44

Human Immunodeficiency Virus Type 1– and Human T-Lymphotropic Virus Type 1–Associated Lymphomas

Scot C. Remick, MD, and William J. Harrington, Jr., MD

KEY POINTS

Human Immunodeficiency Virus Type 1– and Human T-Lymphotropic Virus Type 1–Associated Lymphomas

HIV-1–Related Non-Hodgkin's Lymphoma

Diagnosis

- Heightened clinical suspicion is warranted in all cases that present with clinical signs and symptoms of immunodeficiency (e.g., unexplained fever, wasting, mucocutaneous candidiasis, and especially extranodal sites of disease involvement).
- The clinician must seek identifiable risk behaviors for acquisition of human immunodeficiency virus (HIV) infection.
- Non-Hodgkin's lymphoma must be considered in the differential diagnosis in known HIV-infected patients with fever of unknown origin.
- Thorough clinical staging (body computed tomography [CT] or magnetic resonance imaging [MRI] and consideration of positron emission tomography scanning) and biopsy confirmation (e.g., nodal or extranodal tissue, bone marrow, cerebrospinal fluid analysis [generally in all cases]) is essential.

Treatment

- Given routine use of more potent antiretroviral therapy (highly active antiretroviral therapy [HAART] regimens), overall prognosis is improved. In all instances, referral to and participation in clinical trials is to be encouraged. In the absence of a trial, the current standard of care warrants the use of full-dose anthracycline-based combination (e.g., CHOP) chemotherapy.
- Infusional anthracycline-based chemotherapy regimens (e.g., CDE and EPOCH) yield the highest complete response rates and have the longest survival, but definitive comparative trials of bolus versus infusional strategies have not been conducted.
- In select patients with advanced acquired immunodeficiency syndrome (AIDS), poor performance status, and other poor-risk clinical features, it may be prudent and appropriate to treat with dose-modified chemotherapy (e.g., generally 50% dose reduction).
- The use of rituximab in B-cell, CD20-positive AIDS-related non-Hodgkin's lymphoma must be considered investigational; its use restricted to the clinical trial setting.
- All patients are best managed with concurrent colony-stimulating factor support and prophylaxis for *Pneumocystis* pneumonia.
- In selected patients with extensive tumor burden and/or rapid evolution of disease, aggressive hydration and electrolyte management are necessary. Central nervous system (CNS) prophylaxis may be restricted to certain clinical settings as well (i.e., in those patients with high-grade tumor histology, bone marrow or testicular involvement, or disease involvement of the head and neck, paranasal sinuses, and/or epidural areas that may invade the CNS).
- It is generally advisable to continue/prescribe antiretroviral therapy with chemotherapy, though preliminary experience with planned interruption of antiretroviral therapy with infusional EPOCH chemotherapy has not had untoward effects.

HTLV-1–Associated Lymphomas

Diagnosis

- Heightened clinical suspicion is warranted in patients who present with cutaneous lesions and/or hypercalcemia.
- Patients are generally from human T-lymphotropic virus type 1 (HTLV-1)–endemic areas.

- Differential diagnosis includes cutaneous T-cell lymphoma (HTLV-1 negative) and Sézary's syndrome. T-cell subset analysis may be helpful because the CD4 lymphocyte count is generally elevated.
- CT or MRI imaging, bone marrow biopsy, and immunophenotyping of the tumor must be done. HTLV-1 serology must also be performed to differentiate adult T-cell leukemia/lymphoma (ATL) from other T-cell lymphomas.

Treatment

- Standard chemotherapy regimens for the acute and lymphoma forms of ATL have produced very poor results but may be used initially to treat life-threatening metabolic complications such as hypercalcemia.
- Patients with the chronic or smoldering forms of ATL probably should not be treated with combination chemotherapy (because of immunosuppressive effects) but may benefit from biologic response modifiers such as azidothymidine and interferon alfa, anti–interleukin-2 receptor (anti-Tac) antibodies, or milder agents (oral etoposide).
- Patients with any form of ATL should be referred to a clinical trial whenever possible. Limited experience suggests that, in some cases, allogeneic bone marrow transplant may be curative.
- Arsenic trioxide alone or in combination with interferon alfa and inhibitors of nuclear factor-κB may have clinical activity in ATL.

INTRODUCTION

Human retroviruses, primarily human T-lymphotropic virus type I (HTLV-1) and human immunodeficiency virus type 1 (HIV-1, formerly known as human T-cell lymphotropic virus type III or lymphadenopathy-associated virus), are important viral pathogens. HTLV-I was identified in 1980, three years prior to the onset of the acquired immunodeficiency syndrome (AIDS) epidemic.[1,2] HTLV-1 is a transforming retrovirus directly linked to adult T-cell leukemia and other T-cell lymphoproliferative tumors,[3] which are prevalent in Japan. Endemic HTLV-1 infection has been described in other regions of the world. Since the inception of the AIDS epidemic in 1981, it was recognized that the incidence of central nervous system (CNS) lymphoma and subsequently B-cell or indeterminate phenotype non-Hodgkin's lymphoma was markedly increased in HIV-infected individuals. HIV-1 was identified in 1984 as the causative agent of HIV infection and AIDS.[4,5] It is not an oncogenic or transforming virus, but the development of lymphoma is multifactorial and clearly associated with the profound cellular immunodeficiency that evolves with progressive HIV infection. With improvements in the primary management of HIV infection and emergence of more potent antiretroviral regimens, the incidence of lymphoma is diminishing in regions of the world where there is greater access to these highly active antiretroviral therapy (HAART) regimens.[6] In other parts of the world with the greatest burden of HIV infection and less access to HAART, such as sub-Saharan Africa, B-cell tumors are emerging as more common causes of morbidity and mortality.[6]

It is especially important to emphasize at the outset that, with the evolution of antiretroviral therapy, the natural history of AIDS-related non-Hodgkin's lymphoma is highly dynamic. It is important to reconcile the natural history and therapeutic interventions reported for lymphoma in this setting in the context of current antiretroviral therapy. Taken together, the lymphoproliferative diseases characteristic of both HIV-1 and HTLV-1 infection (Table 44–1) are infrequent but important malignancies in the spectrum of human lymphoproliferative disorders encountered in clinical practice.

HIV-1-RELATED NON-HODGKIN'S LYMPHOMA

Epidemiology and Risk Factors

It was recognized early on in the AIDS epidemic that the risk of developing lymphoma was over 100-fold greater in HIV-infected patients. Approximately 5–10% of HIV-infected patients are destined to develop lymphoma, and in 3% of patients lymphoma is the AIDS-defining illness.[7] The risk of developing lymphoma steadily increases with duration of HIV infection and advancing immunosuppression. What is paradoxical is that prospects for increased survival are enhanced by HAART; however, long-term survivors of HIV infection may remain at increased risk for the development of lymphoma.[8–14] This scenario is reminiscent of the experience in patients undergoing solid organ transplantation, in whom there is a 0.04% to 0.3% per annum increased risk of developing lymphoma because of iatrogenic immunosuppression.

With the emergence of the HAART therapeutic era in the Western world starting in 1996, an initial sharp decline in the incidence of AIDS-related primary CNS lymphoma was observed.[15–22] By 2000, the incidence of systemic AIDS-related non-Hodgkin's lymphoma was observed to decline as well in regions of the world where there was access to HAART regimens. These observations could be explained in part by short-term improvement in immune function attributed to HAART. The occurrence of CNS lymphoma is more closely linked to immunodeficiency than is systemic lymphoma, which may explain the disparity in declining incidence rates of CNS versus systemic disease. Conversely, despite a dramatic increase in the incidence of Kaposi's sarcoma coincident with the AIDS epidemic in parts of Africa, a corresponding increase in the incidence of lymphoma over the first 15 years of the epidemic was not observed. It appeared that the risk of AIDS-related lymphoma in developing countries was much lower than in developed countries, though underascertainment and earlier death from competing mortality among other infectious diseases or AIDS-related complications could explain this observation. By 1999, the incidence of AIDS-related non-Hodgkin's lymphoma had statistically significantly increased. Age-standardized incidence rates per 100,000 persons were 7.4 in males and 5.7 in females in Uganda. Similar reports

TABLE 44–1. Salient Biologic and Clinical Features of AIDS (HIV-1)–Related and HTLV-1–Related Lymphoproliferative Diseases

	HIV-1	HTLV-1
Incidence	Western world: decreasing; likely lifelong risk Developing world: increasing	Remains rare though endemic patterns of disease
Pathology		
Tumor grade	Low, <5% Intermediate, 75% High, 25%	Intermediate/high, 100%
Tumor clonality	Usually monoclonal	Clonal
Molecular markers	*bcl*-6	Increased soluble IL-2R, $CD25^+$, $CD4^+$
Associated viruses		
EBV	CNS lymphoma, 100% Systemic lymphoma, 30–50%	HTLV-1 in all cases
HHV-8	PEL, 100% (PEL-EBV, 90%); KS link to immunoblastic lymphoma	
Extranodal disease		
At presentation	Very common	Very common
Bone marrow	25%	25% or greater
CNS disease	<5%	Unknown
Treatment		
Primary CNS lymphoma	Radiation; likely combined modality for good-risk patients	—
Systemic lymphoma	Standard-dose chemotherapy; infusional regimens likely more active	Allogeneic BM transplant may be curative; systemic chemotherapy
Under investigation	Role of rituximab Sequencing of antiretroviral therapy Immune reconstitution	Arsenic trioxide/IFN alfa Anti-CD25 antibodies
Median survival		
Primary CNS lymphoma	Advanced AIDS and poor risk, 2–3 mo; likely improved in HAART era, >20% 1-yr survival	—
Systemic lymphoma	Poor risk, 7–8 mo; improved in HAART era, 30–40% long-term survival with no adverse risk factors	6 mo to 1 yr

Abbreviations: AIDS, acquired immunodeficiency syndrome; BM, bone marrow; CNS, central nervous system; EBV, Epstein-Barr virus; HAART, highly active antiretroviral therapy; HHV-8, human herpesvirus 8; IFN, interferon; IL-2R, interleukin-2 receptor; KS, Kaposi's sarcoma; PEL, primary effusion lymphoma.

of increased risk of non-Hodgkin's lymphoma in Kenya and other parts of Africa in HIV-infected individuals are emerging as well. Adult Burkitt's lymphoma has been increasingly observed in the backdrop of HIV infection in contrast to the endemic pattern of disease, which afflicts young children. CNS lymphoma is rarely encountered in Africa, which is likely attributable to both limited diagnostic capability and death from other AIDS-related illnesses.

Pathophysiology

The pathogenesis of lymphoma in the setting of underlying HIV infection is complex. There is likely an interaction between host factors—such as accompanying progressive immunodeficiency, which is the hallmark of untreated HIV infection—and molecular and genetic alterations, which may occur de novo or result from co-infection with Epstein-Barr virus (EBV) or human herpesvirus 8 (Table 44–2).[23–30] Progressive immune suppression, chronic antigen stimulation, and resultant B-cell proliferation—initially polyclonal and proceeding to oligoclonal and monoclonal lymphoid expansion—are important for lymphomagenesis.[31] Associated immune activation and dysregulation of cytokine modulatory pathways (especially interleukin-6 and interleukin-10), altered *bcl*-6, p53, and c-*myc* oncogene expression, and coexisting viral infection(s) have all been implicated in the pathogenesis of lymphoma in this setting as well.[32–36] A proposed molecular and histogenic model of AIDS lymphoma pathogenesis identifies four major pathways (Fig. 44–1).[37,38] In the first, Burkitt's lymphoma is characterized by mild immunodeficiency, germinal center–derived B cells, multiple genetic lesions, and a highly proliferative tumor. Large-cell (centroblasts) and immunoblastic (immunoblasts) lymphoma, associated with intermediate immunodeficiency, are composed of post–germinal center B cells, which can be distinguished on the basis of *bcl*-6 expression (large cell) and *LMP1* expression (immunoblastic). Primary CNS lymphoma can be considered a variant of immunoblastic lymphoma with severe immunodeficiency and ubiquitous association with EBV infection. Finally, a fourth pathway is AIDS-associated primary effusion lymphoma, caused by human herpesvirus 8 infection and frequently associated with EBV infection as well, which is discussed more fully in Chapter 45.[39]

Clinical Features and Diagnosis

It was recognized early into the AIDS epidemic that the clinical course of AIDS-related non-Hodgkin's lymphoma

TABLE 44–2. Immunologic, Molecular, and Virologic Pathogenic Determinants of AIDS-Related Lymphoma

	Burkitt's/Burkitt-like	Large Cell (Centroblasts)	Immunoblastic (Immunoblasts)	Primary CNS Lymphoma
CD4 lymphocyte count	Usually normal to mild decrease	Decreased	Decreased	<50/μL
Relationship to germinal center	Germinal center B cells	Germinal center B cells	Post–germinal center B cells	Post–germinal center B cells
Histogenic profile	Ki67⁺ (very high proliferative index)	Bcl-6⁺/MUM-1⁻/CD138⁻	Bcl-6⁻/MUM-1⁺/CD138⁺	Bcl-6⁻/MUM-1⁺/CD138⁺
Molecular markers				
c-myc	>65–100%	30%	(—)	(—)
LMP1	(—)	(—)	65–75%	90%
p53	50–60%	Rare	Rare	No data
EBV infection	30–50%	30%	>90%	100%

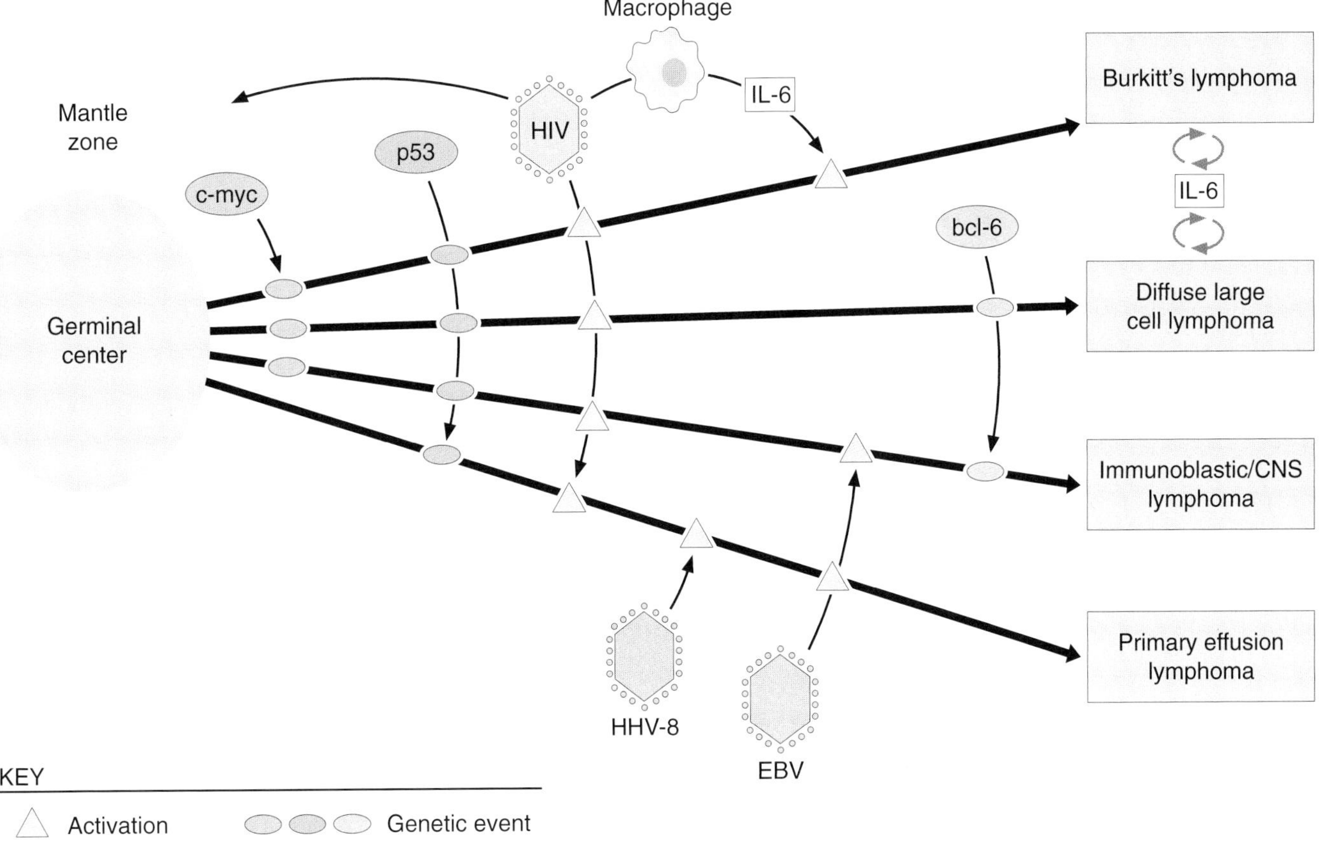

Figure 44–1. Schema outlining the pathogenesis of AIDS-related non-Hodgkin's lymphoma.

was much more aggressive than the course of this disease in patients without HIV infection.[40–46] In general, AIDS-related non-Hodgkin's lymphoma is characterized by higher grade (40–60%), extranodal disease (80%) (Fig. 44–2), advanced clinical stage (60–70%); and shortened survival (median, 7–8 months) when compared with lymphomas in HIV-seronegative patients.[47,48] At the time of clinical presentation prior to the HAART era, the median CD4 lymphocyte count was 100 cells/μL.[46] In the HAART era, patients are less immune suppressed, with median CD4 lymphocyte counts ranging between 150 and 200 cells/μL.[49–52] In addition, the incidence of leptomeningeal involvement at diagnosis and over the course of disease appears to be declining as well. This could be attributable to the altered natural history of underlying HIV infection in the HAART era and perhaps less predominance of high-grade histologies (offset by increase in intermediate-grade large-cell lymphoma).[48,53–55] There remains a clear male predominance in AIDS lymphoma in the United States, but in other regions

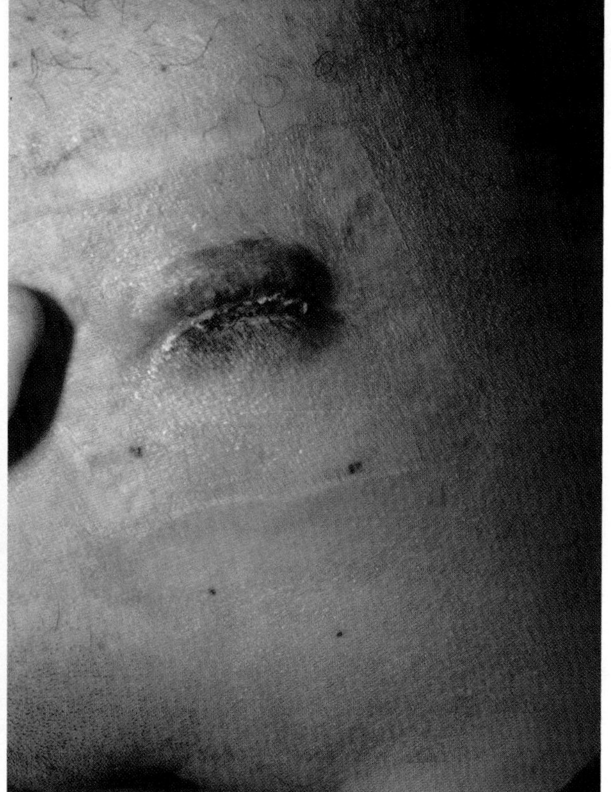

Figure 44–2. *A,* HIV-infected patient presenting in the pre-HAART era with extensive extranodal disease of the neck; biopsy confirmed a malignant lymphoma of the large cell type. ***B,*** Follow-up after four cycles of dose-modified CHOP combination chemotherapy demonstrating complete resolution of tumor mass.

of the world most affected by the epidemic, such as sub-Saharan Africa, there is nearly an equal distribution of cases in men and women. This is reflective of the predominant heterosexual transmission of HIV infection in developing countries.

Diagnosis of AIDS-related non-Hodgkin's lymphoma is established by pathologic confirmation of malignant lymphoma in biopsy material of involved lymph node(s), bone marrow, or other extranodal site(s). Although tissue diagnosis of AIDS-related CNS lymphoma is encouraged given the modestly improved outcome in the HAART era, this diagnosis also can be established by detection of EBV DNA in cerebrospinal fluid employing polymerase chain reaction techniques.[56–60] An algorithm for the diagnostic approach to HIV-infected patients with focal brain lesions is outlined in Figure 44–3.

Differential Diagnosis

In an HIV-infected patient, the primary differential diagnosis of peripheral lymphadenopathy is malignant lymphoma versus an infectious etiology and consideration of another neoplasm, such as Kaposi's sarcoma. Common infectious causes of lymphadenopathy include mycobacterial disease, sexually transmitted diseases, and mycotic infections, especially in areas or regions of the world where these conditions are prevalent (or endemic).[61] These entities are usually reconciled on appropriate work-up and review of biopsy material. Although this may seem straightforward, often biopsies of peripheral lymph nodes, extranodal masses, or bone marrow may not be collected or processed properly, which leads to delays in establishing a diagnosis. Circumstances such as inappropriate staining for assorted pathogens, improper collection and submission of specimens using sterile technique, and/or lack of retrieval of fresh tumor tissue for im-portant diagnostic flow cytometry and other molecular studies may limit the diagnostic yield of any given biopsy. Consequently, a diagnosis may not be entertained because of an incomplete initial pathologic work-up of submitted tissue. This is overcome by heightened clinical suspicion of underlying HIV infection and close communication between the clinician, surgeon, or other physician obtaining the tissue and the pathologist prior to the biopsy.

A common presentation in patients with advanced HIV infection is fever of unknown origin. In this instance, a diligent evaluation of the patient to include consideration of an underlying lymphoma is appropriate, with thorough physical examination, radiographic studies to guide diagnostic intervention(s), and/or consideration of bone marrow aspiration and biopsy for diagnosis and culture. An isolated and marked elevation in serum lactate dehy-

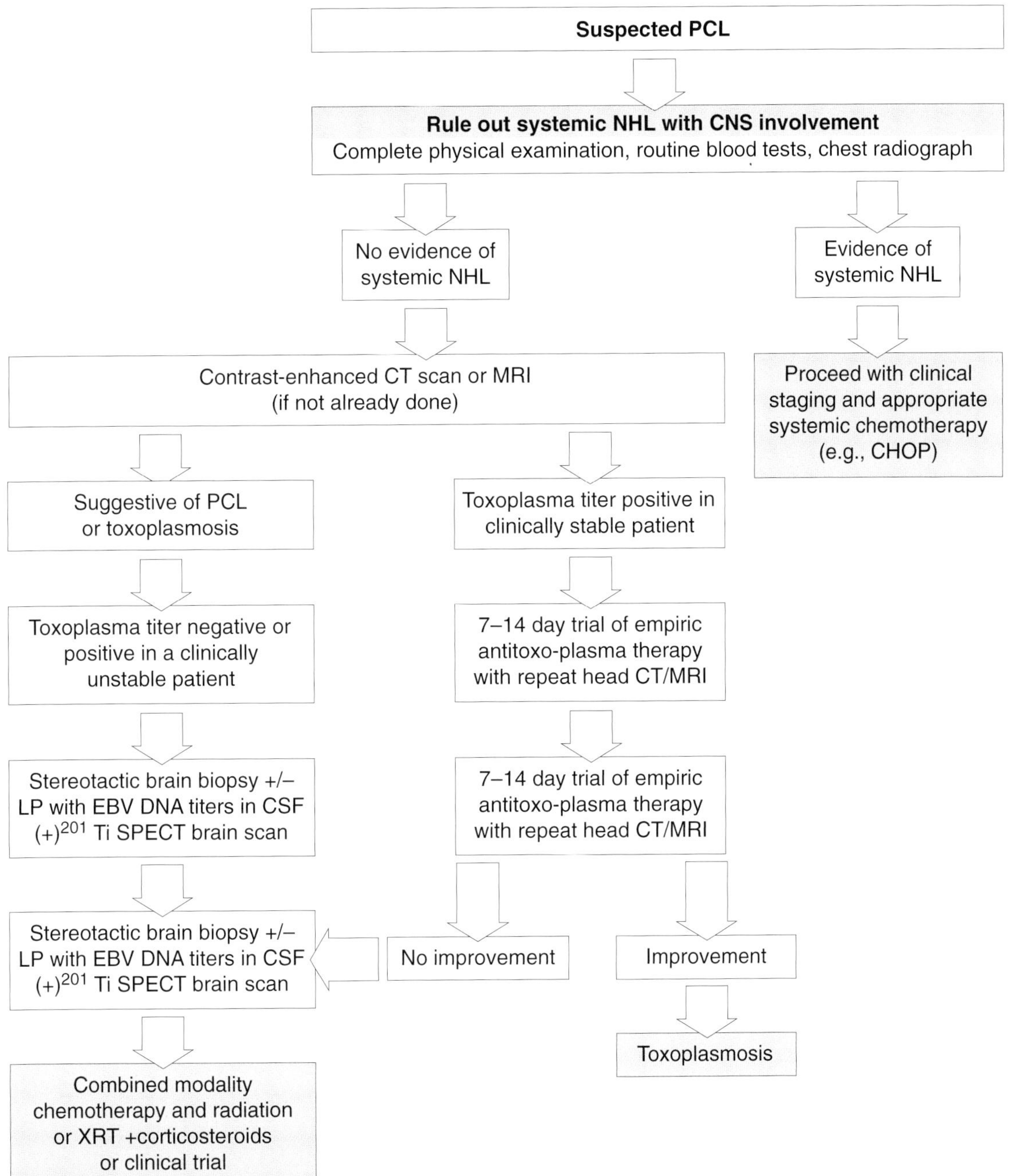

Figure 44–3. Algorithm for the diagnostic approach to HIV-infected patients with focal brain lesions.

drogenase in relation to other serum transaminases may also be suggestive of an underlying lymphoproliferative disorder.

For HIV-infected patients presenting with an isolated CNS mass lesion, the differential diagnosis of primary CNS lymphoma is invariably suspected when the CD4 lymphocyte count is less than 50 cells/μL. Given this scenario, the differential diagnosis of a space-occupying CNS mass lesion is broad and includes toxoplasmosis, which may be on the decline as a result of HAART and widespread use of trimethoprim-sulfamethoxazole prophylaxis.[62] Progressive multifocal encephalopathy, fungal and bacterial abscess, tuberculosis, gummatous lesions, infarct, and glioma can also present as focal lesions. Radiographic features are nonspecific, and, given improved outcomes with antiretroviral therapy and better clinical status of many patients at presentation, aggressive diagnostic evaluation leading to biopsy is appropriate.[63–65] This tumor is always associated with EBV virus infection, which is of considerable diagnostic importance as alluded to earlier (see Fig. 44–3).[63,66–68]

Treatment

At the outset of the AIDS epidemic, more aggressive and dose-intensive combination chemotherapy regimens were explored secondary to the more virulent clinical course of AIDS lymphoma. Early results were dismal, regimens were poorly tolerated, and there was a trend toward shortened survival.[69] More traditional and dose-modified combination chemotherapy regimens (e.g., m-BACOD) were evaluated in conjunction with antiretroviral therapy, incorporation of colony-stimulating factors, and use of various CNS prophylaxis strategies because of the proclivity of AIDS lymphoma to disseminate or relapse in this site.[70,71] Over the first 15 years of the epidemic, complete responses ranged between 20% and 60%, with median survival duration of between 4 and 7 months.[72–74] The largest randomized trial ever conducted in AIDS-related lymphoma in the pre-HAART era (ACTG 142, by the AIDS Clinical Trials Group) employed standard-dose versus low-dose m-BACOD (dose-modified bleomycin doxorubicin, lomustine, vincristine, and methotrexate).[71]

Presently, with the availability of improved antiretroviral therapy, prophylaxis, and supportive treatment for opportunistic infections in patients with advanced AIDS, we are returning to traditional (full-dose) chemotherapy approaches similar to those used in the non–HIV-infected lymphoma patient (e.g., CHOP combination chemotherapy [AIDS Malignancy Consortium AMC 005 study]).[70,75,76] Encouraging results have been obtained with infusional anthracycline-based combination chemotherapy regimens such as CDE (Eastern Cooperative Oncology Group protocol E1494)[77–82] and EPOCH[83] (Table 44–3). The best clinical results to date have been reported by investigators at the National Cancer Institute, with a complete response rate of 74% and disease-free and overall survival of 92% and 60%, respectively, at 53 months median follow-up.[83] What is also intriguing about this study is the strategy of suspension of antiretroviral therapy over the course of chemotherapy to avoid increased risk of drug-drug interactions and potential for increased toxicity, and to enhance overall patient compliance. Furthermore, the chemotherapy was dose-adjusted on the basis of CD4 lymphocyte count in an attempt to individualize therapy. Although this strategy of suspending antiretroviral therapy did not result in adverse clinical outcome (i.e., HIV-1 viral load and CD4 lymphocyte counts returned to baseline by 3 and 12 months, respectively),

TABLE 44–3. Recently Reported Chemotherapy Regimens for Treatment of AIDS-Related Non-Hodgkin's Lymphoma in the United States

	m/CHOP (AMC 005 Study, 2001)	EPOCH (NCI Study, 2003)	CDE (ECOG E1494 Study, 2004)
Number of centers	Multicenter	Single center	Multicenter
Number of patients	40 (mCHOP) 23 (full dose)	39	43 (pre-HAART era) 55 (HAART era)
Drugs			
Cyclophosphamide	375* or 750 mg/m² IV day 1	187* (CD4 <100/µL) or 375 mg/m² (CD4 ≥100/µL) IV day 5; dose-adjusted thereafter†	200 mg/m²/day CIV days 1–4 (96 hr)
Doxorubicin	25* or 50 mg/m² IV day 1	10 mg/m²/day CIV days 1–4 (96 hr)	12.5 mg/m²/day CIV days 1–4 (96 hr)
Vincristine	1.4 mg/m² (2.0 mg maximum dose)	0.4 mg/m²/day CIV days 1–4 (96 hr); dose not capped	—
Prednisone	100 mg PO days 1–5	60 mg/m²/day PO days 1–5	—
Etoposide	—	50 mg/m²/day CIV days 1–4 (96 hr)‡	60 mg/m²/day CIV days 1–4 (96 hr)§
Filgrastim (G-CSF)	300 µg (<70 kg) or 480 µg (>70 kg) SQ days 4–13 full-dose	5 µg/kg/day SQ day 6 until ANC >5000/µL past nadir	5 µg/kg/day SQ day 5 until ANC >10,000/µL past nadir
CNS prophylaxis	Physician discretion (IT cytarabine 50 mg weekly ×4 recommended)	Yes (last 17 patients)	Recommended high-grade histology; bone marrow involvement, or disease invading epidural sites
Schedule	Every 3 wk for 2 cycles beyond CR minimum of 4 cycles	Every 3 wk for a total of 6 cycles	Every 4 wk for 2 cycles beyond CR up to 8 total cycles
Median CD4 count/µL	Full-dose: 122/µL mCHOP: 138/µL	198/µL	Pre-HAART era: 90/µL HAART era: 227/µL
CR rate	48% full-dose 30% mCHOP (nonrandomized study)	74%	45%
Survival (median)			
Progression free	Full-dose: not reached mCHOP: median CR duration 9 mo	73% at 53 mo	Pre-HAART era: 6.0 mo HAART era: 8.1 mo
Overall	Not reported	60% at 53 mo	Pre-HAART era: 6.8 mo HAART era: 13.7 mo (Combined 2-yr survival rate: 43%)

*Dose-modified dosage for agent.

†Dose-adjusted as follows beyond cycle 1: if nadir ANC greater than 500/µL, increase dose by 187 mg/m² above previous cycle to maximum cyclophosphamide dose 750 mg/m²; for nadir ANC less than 500/µL or platelets less than 25,000/µL, decrease dose 187 mg/m² below previous cycle.

‡Etoposide, doxorubicin, and vincristine can be admixed in the same intravenous solution.

§Cyclophosphamide and doxorubicin admixed in same bag of intravenous fluid and administered via a central line; etoposide diluted in a separate liter of intravenous fluid and infused separately centrally or peripherally.

Abbreviations: AMC, AIDS Malignancy Consortium; ANC, absolute neutrophil count; CDE, infusional cyclophosphamide, doxorubicin, and etoposide; CIV, continuous intravenous infusion; CR, complete response; ECOG, Eastern Cooperative Oncology Group; EPOCH, infusional etoposide, prednisone, vincristine, cyclophosphamide, and doxorubicin; G-CSF, granulocyte colony-stimulating factor; HAART, highly active antiretroviral therapy; IT, intrathecal; m/CHOP, dose-modified and full-dose CHOP (cyclophosphamide, doxorubicin, vincristine, and prednisone); NCI, National Cancer Institute; SQ, subcutaneous.

it must be considered investigational and requires a larger, multicenter clinical trial. New biologic and cellular therapies are also being developed that are based on disease pathogenesis and mechanistic principles.[84–88] In this regard, it is important to comment on the potential enhanced toxicity of adding rituximab to CHOP chemotherapy that has recently been reported in a large multicenter trial conducted by the AIDS Malignancy Consortium. In this study (AMC 010), the addition of rituximab to standard-dose CHOP led to increased infectious complications and deaths attributable to sepsis.[89] It is possible that delayed recovery of humoral immunity could contribute to this increased risk of life-threatening bacterial infections in HIV-infected patients.

For patients with CNS lymphoma, radiation therapy has been the primary treatment modality. Combined chemotherapy and radiation therapy or systemic combination chemotherapy regimens tailored to penetrate the CNS appear to improve survival (approximately 3 years) in HIV-seronegative patients and are now preferred over radiation therapy alone in this setting. For selected AIDS patients this approach may be appropriate. There is, however, very limited published clinical experience with these approaches because of the marked decline in incidence of this tumor. Because EBV infection is ubiquitous in AIDS-related primary CNS lymphoma, investigational antiviral and cellular therapies (targeting EBV) are being studied.[90–95]

In summary, chemotherapy continues to evolve coincident with improvements in the underlying management of HIV infection, and participation in clinical trials must be encouraged (see Table 44–3).[86,96–98] Infusion-based chemotherapy regimens appear to be more active and yield improved survival compared with bolus-administered regimens. Full-dose standard chemotherapy such as CHOP may also be appropriate. Comparative trials, however, have not been done. The use of rituximab must be restricted to the clinical trial setting. Dose modification (approximately 50% of myelosuppressive drugs in a regimen) may be appropriate in selected patients with advanced AIDS, poor performance status, or poor end-organ function, including bone marrow reserve, and in those patients with serious comorbidities at the time of lymphoma diagnosis.

Supportive Care and Long-Term Management

Table 44–4 outlines supportive care measures suitable for patients with AIDS-related lymphoma. In the majority of instances, it is prudent to administer concomitant colony-stimulating factor support to blunt the neutropenia associated with cytotoxic chemotherapy in HIV-infected patients with lymphoma. In this regard, granulocyte colony-stimulating factor may be preferable to granulocyte-monocyte colony-stimulating factor, which in vitro

TABLE 44–4. Suggested Supportive Care Guidelines for Managing Patients with AIDS-Related Non-Hodgkin's Lymphoma

Supportive Care Indication	Therapeutic Intervention
Generally Recommended for All Patients	
Bone marrow support: colony-stimulating factors	
Filgrastim (G-CSF) or	5–10 µg/kg SQ 24 hr after chemotherapy, daily beyond ANC recovery
Sargramostim (GM-CSF)	250 µg/m² SQ daily as above (usually given concurrently with antiretroviral therapy)
Primary prophylaxis	
Pneumocystis pneumonia: trimethoprim-sulfamethoxazole	Double-strength tablet PO daily or alternatively 3 times a week
Oral mucocutaneous candidiasis: fluconazole	100 mg PO daily
Mycobacterium avium complex: azithromycin	1200 mg PO weekly (usually when CD4 lymphocyte count <50 cells/µL)
Antiretroviral therapy	Generally administered concurrently; avoid myelosuppressive zidovudine; interruption of ARV therapy—consider clinical trial; with conventional-dose chemotherapy regimens with cyclophosphamide and doxorubicin, no dose adjustment necessary with concurrent protease inhibitors. Follow NIH guidelines (see Yeni et al.[103])
Consider in Selected Patients	
Bone marrow support	
Erythropoietin *or*	40,000–60,000 units SQ every week
Darbepoetin	200 µg SQ every 2 wk
Other opportunistic infection/secondary infection prophylaxis	See USPHS/IDSA Prevention of Opportunistic Infections Working Group[104]
Leptomeningeal prophylaxis	(For patients with high-grade histology; bone marrow or testicular involvement; and bulky disease in head & neck, paranasal sinus, epidural areas)
Methotrexate *or*	10 mg IT + leucovorin 50 mg PO q6h × 4 doses weekly × 4
Cytosine arabinoside	50 mg IT weekly × 4
Tumor lysis	(For patients with high-grade and highly proliferative tumors—aggressive hydration, alkalinization of urine, and fluid and electrolyte monitoring)
Allopurinol	600 mg PO × 1 dose; then 300 mg daily (generally cycle 1)

Abbreviations: ANC, absolute neutrophil count; ARV, antiretroviral; G-CSF, granulocyte colony-stimulating factor; GM-CSF, granulocyte-macrophage colony-stimulating factor; IT, intrathecal; NIH, National Institutes of Health; PO, by mouth; SQ, subcutaneous.

increases HIV replication.[99] The clinical significance of this increase is not well defined, because in many instances antiretroviral therapy is also administered concurrently with chemotherapy.[100–103] Early experience with the nonmyelosuppressive nucleoside analogue didanosine and more active HAART regimens are suggestive of bone marrow–sparing effects with infusional CDE and CHOP chemotherapy. It is not presently standard practice to withhold antiretroviral therapy during chemotherapy, though preliminary success with this strategy has been published using EPOCH infusional chemotherapy. The rationale for this technique was mentioned earlier, and strong consideration should be given to referring patients to clinical trials to address this question. Generally, all AIDS patients treated with cytotoxic chemotherapy should receive *Pneumocystis* pneumonia prophylaxis regardless of CD4 lymphocyte counts, which can decline rapidly with anticancer therapy. Other prophylactic measures can be individualized depending on CD4 lymphocyte count and opportunistic infection profile for a given patient.[104] For patients with highly proliferative and bulky disease (usually high-grade lymphoma), aggressive hydration, prophylaxis for hyperuricemia, and careful monitoring of fluid and electrolyte balance are crucial to minimize risk of tumor lysis syndrome over the initial several days following institution of chemotherapy. CNS prophylaxis of the leptomeninges can be achieved in a variety of ways, but is usually reserved for patients at risk for CNS dissemination.[105] These patients are those with high-grade histology, bone marrow or testicular involvement, and bulky lesions particularly of the head and neck, paranasal sinus, and epidural areas that may invade the CNS.

Upon completion of chemotherapy, efforts should be directed at maintaining appropriate antiretroviral therapy and monitoring improvement in CD4 lymphocyte counts, with opportunistic infection prophylaxis discontinued when CD4 counts exceed 200 cells/μL. Patients are generally seen at 2- to 4-month intervals following the first 2 years of treatment. For patients with good risk factors, there are tangible prospects for long-term freedom from progression and possible cure. The attendant lifelong risk by virtue of underlying immunosuppression for either new or late relapse lymphoma requires that these patients be followed diligently.

Prognosis

Age greater than 35 years, history of injection drug use as the mode of acquisition of HIV infection, stage III or IV disease, and CD4 lymphocyte counts less than 100/μL were identified as independent adverse prognostic factors in patients with AIDS-related non-Hodgkin's lymphoma treated with m-BACOD in the pre-HAART era.[106,107] During the nucleoside analogue (pre-HAART) era, approximately 10–20% of patients could be cured or, more appropriately, survive free from progression of their lymphoma. In patients with none of these adverse prognostic features, up to 30% survived 3 years. As improvements in antiretroviral therapy have been achieved, a corresponding increase in survival has been observed in patients with AIDS-related lymphoma as well, with nearly 40–50% of patients surviving with long-term freedom from progression. The longest reported survival for patients with AIDS-related lymphoma, who received EPOCH, is 60% at 53 months. There are limited reports on the utility of the International Prognostic Index in AIDS-related non-Hodgkin's lymphoma, for which a meta-analysis is planned.[108–110] What is also emerging in several studies is the impact HAART therapy has on improved clinical outcomes.[90,111–114] It is possible that treatment of HIV infection may be as important as selection of the chemotherapy regimen for patients with AIDS-related lymphoma.

HTLV-1–ASSOCIATED NEOPLASMS

Epidemiology and Risk Factors

Between 10 and 20 million people worldwide are infected with HTLV-1.[115] This retrovirus was first identified in 1980 in a cell line derived from a patient with cutaneous T-cell lymphoma, and it is the first retrovirus shown to be associated with human disease.[115,116] HTLV-1 is a member of the genus *Deltaretrovirus*. Its RNA genome of 9032 nucleotides contains *gag*, *pol*, and *env* genes typical of retroviruses. HTLV-1 differs from leukemia viruses of animal origin in that it carries no typical oncogene but rather a 3′ terminal sequence called pX. This region encodes several proteins, including Tax, Rex, and p12, by alternating reading frames and spliced messages (Fig. 44–4).[115] Although there are many HTLV-1 carriers, only about 1–5% of those infected develop adult T-cell leukemia/lymphoma (ATL). An even smaller percentage (approximately 1%) develops the demyelinating neurologic disease tropical spastic paraparesis (TSP), which was first linked to HTLV-1 in 1985.[116,117] The pathogenic processes that lead to the development of these two diseases in a minority of carriers remain largely unclear, although a great deal has been learned about the epidemiology of the virus. HTLV-1 is endemic in the southern islands of Japan, the Caribbean basin, certain regions of Brazil, Colombia, central Africa, Indonesia, and Iran (Fig. 44–5).[118–121]

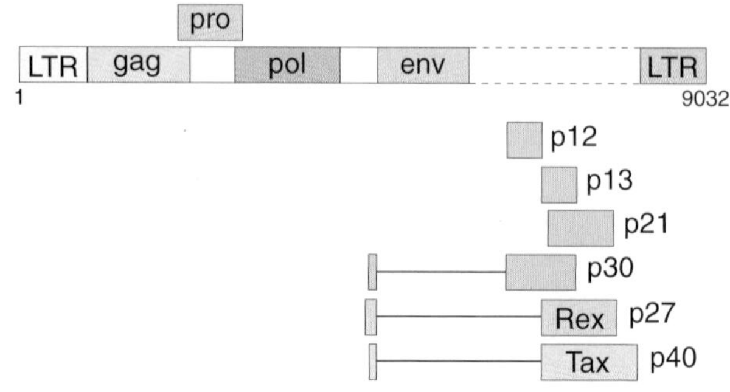

Figure 44–4. Schematic of the HTLV-1 provirus. Messenger RNAs encoded by the pX region are shown below.

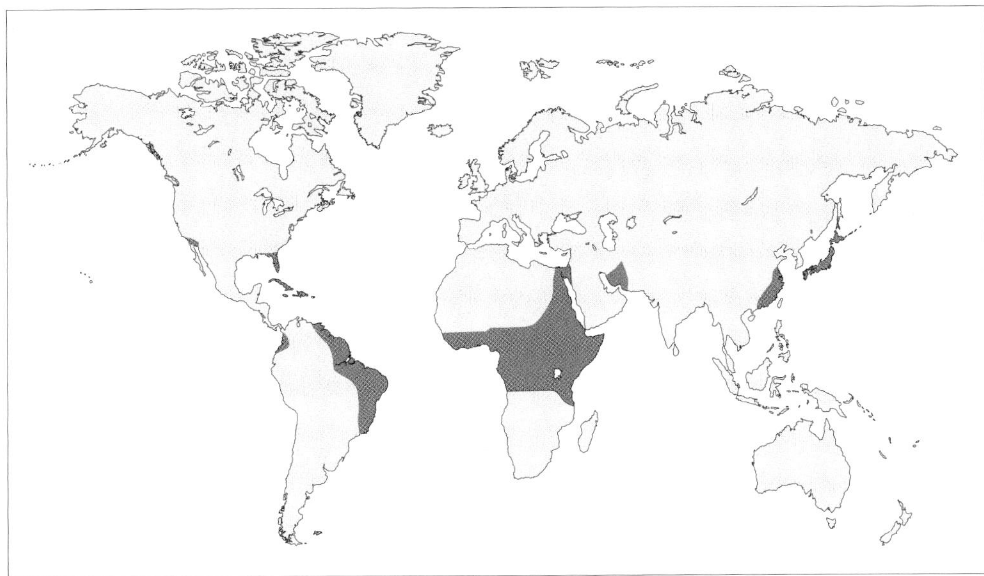

Figure 44–5. Shaded areas represent geographic regions where HTLV-1 is endemic.

HTLV-1 is transmitted vertically (transplacentally or via breast milk), sexually, or parenterally. Viral transmission appears to occur solely through the transfer of HTLV-1–infected lymphocytes. Therefore, as opposed to HIV-1, the risk of transmission by noncellular blood products such as fresh or frozen plasma is minimal.[118,122–128] Also in contrast to HIV-1, sequence variation among different geographic isolates of HTLV-1 is quite limited. Studies to detect viral strains that are clearly either leukemogenic or neuropathic have been mostly inconclusive, although some data suggest that variations in the Tax sequence may be associated with either ATL or TSP. In addition, certain human lymphocyte antigen (HLA) alleles have been linked to the development of ATL, whereas others may predispose carriers to TSP.[129,130] The route of infection may influence the evolution of HTLV-1–associated disease. Most, if not all, cases of ATL are thought to occur after a prolonged latency period of 40–50 years following vertical transmission, whereas parenteral exposure, particularly via blood transfusion, favors development of TSP.[126,127] HTLV-1 can infect a variety of cell types, including B lymphocytes, dendritic cells, and fibroblasts, although it only transforms helper T cells. The provirus load in asymptomatic carriers fluctuates within a relatively narrow amplitude but may reach very high levels (estimated at 5% of all peripheral blood mononuclear cells) in patients with TSP.[119,127] Two recent publications have shed light on how the virus gains entry and spreads from cell to cell. Upon contact with an uninfected cell, cytoskeletal polarization occurs in the infected cell and HTLV-1 core (Gag proteins) and genome complexes accumulate at the junction with the uninfected cell and are transferred to the uninfected cell through the "immunologic synapse" (Fig. 44–6).[131] This finding may explain why cell free blood products do not efficiently transmit HTLV-1. The identity of the HTLV-1 envelope receptor that the virus uses to initially gain entry into cells has also been elusive. Recently a group of French investigators have demonstrated that the ubiquitous vertebrate glucose transporter GLUT-I is a receptor for HTLV-1.[132]

Pathophysiology

The study of events that lead to the evolution of ATL has been exceedingly difficult because of the relatively low incidence in HTLV-1 carriers and the prolonged latency period between infection and onset of disease. Most research on the oncogenic properties of HTLV-1 has focused on the viral transactivator Tax. Tax induces the expression of a variety of viral genes through the viral long terminal repeat as well as cellular genes through interactions with pleotropic transcription factors such as nuclear factor-κB (NF-κB), CREB, SR-F, and AP-1 (Fig. 44–7).[133–136] Tax-mediated activation of NF-κB results in the upregulation of many genes involved in proliferation, cell cycle activation, and resistance to apoptosis, such as those for interleukin-2 and interleukin-2 receptor (IL-2R), Bcl-xL, and interleukin-6.[135] In addition, Tax can repress certain DNA repair and tumor suppressor genes such as DNA polymerase β and, indirectly, p53 through inhibition of recruitment of CREB binding protein.[134,135] Tax also inhibits transforming growth factor-β (TGF-β) signaling, possibly enabling HTLV-1–infected T cells to escape TGF-β–mediated suppression.[137] Although Tax stimulates proliferation of HTLV-1–infected cells in vitro, it is also a major target of cytotoxic T cells in vivo.[138] These findings suggest that immune surveillance plays an important role in the elimination of cells that carry the provirus and prevents the development of ATL in most carriers. One prospective study demonstrated that anti-Tax antibodies were detected in low titers for up to 10 years among HTLV-1 carriers who eventually developed ATL.[139] Tax can immortalize T cells in vitro, and transgenic mice expressing the Tax gene under the control of

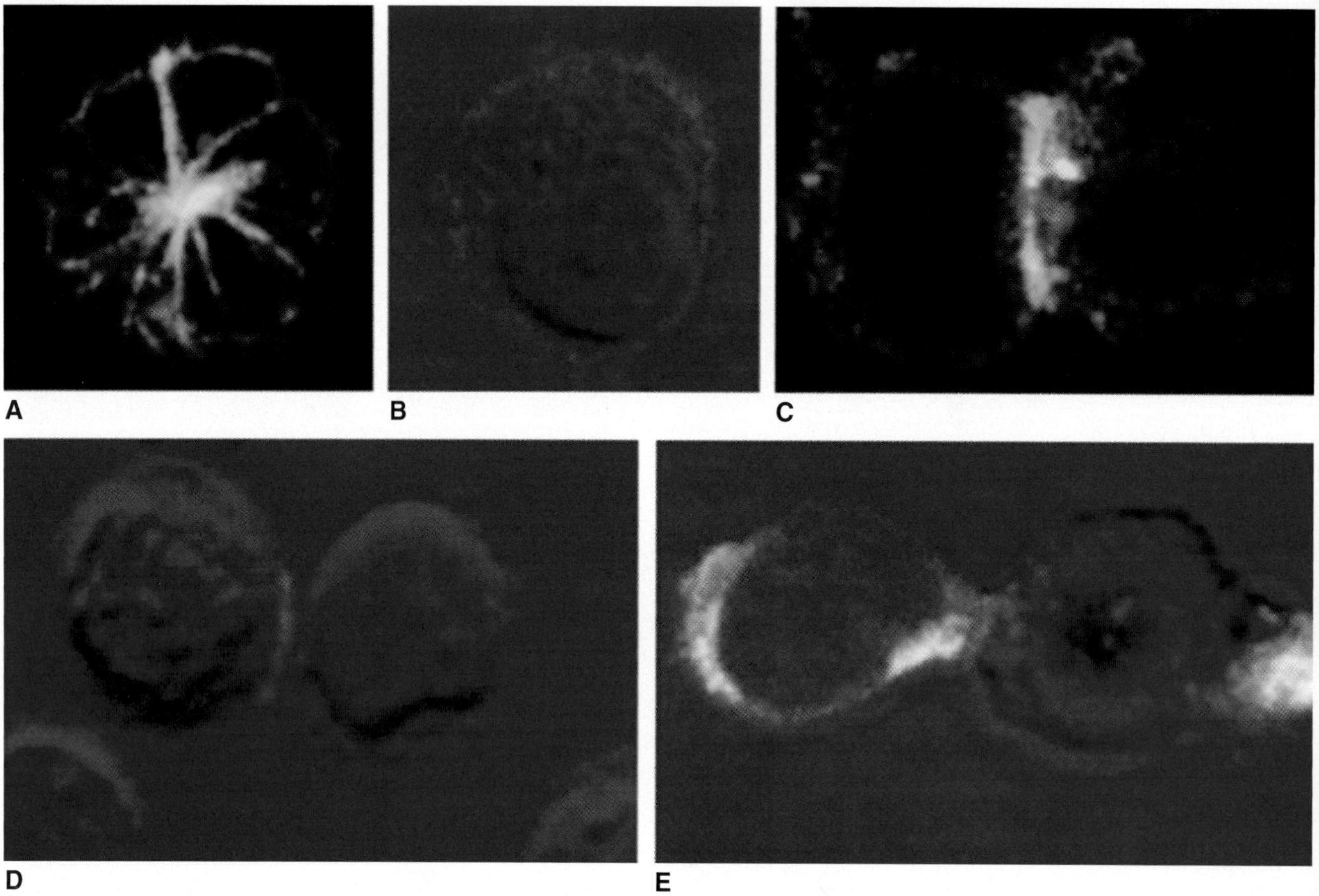

A B C D E

■ **Figure 44–6.** Organization of HTLV-1 proteins and host cell proteins in the viral synapse. Isolated lymphocytes naturally infected with HTLV-1 express the Gag protein, shown in *red (A),* and the Env protein, also shown in *red (B),* in an unpolarized manner. Contact with another cell induces polarization of the HTLV-1 Gag protein *(D)* within 40 minutes, and transfer to the other cell *(E)* within 2 hours. The polarized Gag protein *(red)* frequently accumulates at the intercellular contact in the center of a ring of talin *(green)* *(C)*, which resembles the appearance of the immune or immunological synapse. (Reprinted with permission from Igakura T, Stinchcombe JC, Goon PK, et al: Spread of HTLV-I between lymphocytes by virus-induced polarization of the cytoskeleyton. Science 299:1713–1716, 2003. Copyright 2003 AAAS.)

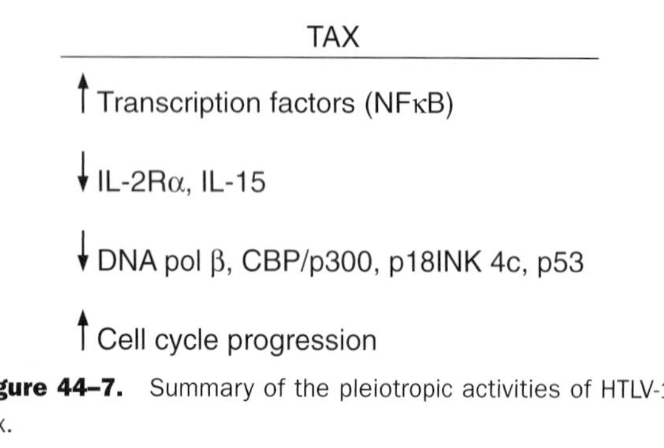

■ **Figure 44–7.** Summary of the pleiotropic activities of HTLV-1 Tax.

a variety of promoters develop mesenchymal tumors, neurofibrosarcomas, and mammary adenomas but not an ATL-like syndrome.[140–144]

The p12 protein appears to be important in establishing optimal viral infectivity. p12 reportedly binds to the cytoplasmic domain of the IL-2R β chain and increases transcriptional activities of signal transducers and activators of transcription.[145] Rex regulates nuclear cytoplasmic transport of viral messenger RNA.[146] p30 is a negative regulatory protein that binds to the spliced messenger RNA that encodes Tax and Rex, thereby inhibiting virus expression.[147]

Clinical Features and Diagnosis

ATL may present in a variety of forms. Four distinct subtypes have been described: acute, smoldering, chronic, and lymphomatous. Lymphomatous ATL usually presents with disseminated organ involvement, including hepatosplenomegaly, lytic bone lesions, and hypercalcemia, with few circulating leukemic cells. Acute ATL is characterized predominantly by leukemia, marrow infiltration, and frequently hypercalcemia. CNS involvement is common in these subtypes.[148,149] The median survival of these two ATL subtypes is around 6 months to 1 year, with a 5-year survival of less than 5%.[148–150]

Smoldering ATL is characterized by leukocytosis and cutaneous involvement, and chronic ATL typically manifests as leukemia with adenopathy but without hypercalcemia or CNS involvement. These subtypes may have a relatively indolent course, although an increasing

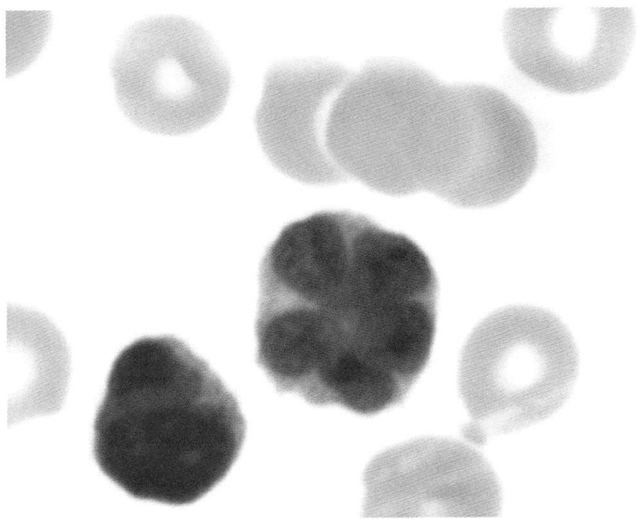

Figure 44–8. Photomicrograph of an ATL cell, which demonstrates a characteristic multilobed "cloverleaf" nucleus.

leukocytic count and an elevated level of expression of proliferation markers may herald progression to acute ATL.[151–153]

ATL cells have a striking morphology, with convoluted or cerebriform nuclei reminiscent of Sézary cells seen in HTLV-1 mature cutaneous T-cell lymphomas (Fig. 44–8). These cells typically express T-cell markers CD2, CD3, CD4, and CD5 and activation antigens HLA-DP, HLA-DQ, and HLA-DR and the interleukin-2 α chain receptor CD25. Variant subtypes ($CD4^-CD8^+$ and $CD4^-CD8^-$) have been described.[153,154]

There are no specific chromosomal abnormalities associated with ATL. Abnormalities of chromosomes 6 and 14 and trisomy 3 and 7 have been described. Seropositivity for HTLV-1 (although seronegative cases have been described) in conjunction with the above-mentioned clinical characteristics generally confirms the diagnosis, and assays with newer generation Western blots distinguish between HTLV-1 and HTLV-2. Analysis by Southern blot with an HTLV-1–specific probe that demonstrates mono- or oligoclonal integration of the provirus in DNA derived from tumor tissue is absolute proof of ATL, although this is rarely applied in most clinical settings.[153,154] There are some data suggesting that certain findings (high serum-soluble IL-2R, mutations of CD95, absence of detectable CD4 or CD8 surface antigens, or defective proviral integration) may predict more aggressive or refractory disease.[155–157]

Differential Diagnosis

The differential diagnosis of ATL requires the exclusion of cutaneous T-cell lymphoma (CTCL), which is not associated with HTLV-1. Acute ATL presents with a very elevated leukocyte count, usually 50,000–100,000 cells/μL or greater, which is rarely seen in CTCL. Both types of tumors may exhibit circulating cerebriform lymphocytes that express mature (CD-4) T-cell markers. ATL is easily distinguished from CTCL through serologic testing. Pautrier microabscesses, once thought to be pathognomonic of CTCL, may also be seen in cutaneous ATL.[158,159] Because lymphomatous ATL may present as any one of several histologic subtypes, including diffuse, mixed, and large-cell immunoblastic lymphoma, diagnosis may be more difficult. All patients with aggressive $CD4^+$ T-cell lymphomas should be screened for HTLV-1 antibodies. Almost all patients with ATL are either from, or ancestrally linked to, HTLV-1 endemic areas.[150,153] It is important to remember that African Americans may have ancestral ties to these regions and may have acquired the virus through vertical transmission from an asymptomatic carrier. As opposed to lymphoblastic lymphoma, ATL rarely presents with a mediastinal mass. As in the case of HIV-related lymphoma, ATL patients are profoundly immunocompromised, and concomitant opportunistic infections such as *Pneumocystis jiroveci* pneumonia or disseminated *Strongyloides* are very common.

Treatment

Therapy for ATL, particularly the acute and lymphomatous types, is disappointing. In a large published series of over 800 Japanese patients treated with a variety of chemotherapeutic regimens, the median survival was 6.2 and 10.2 months, respectively, for acute and lymphomatous ATL.[160] Most of the large clinical trials conducted in Japan have employed a variety of aggressive non-Hodgkin lymphoma and acute lymphoblastic leukemia regimens. With some of the most intensive regimens, complete response rates of 40% or more have been reported. Unfortunately these were invariably short lived and resulted in little increase in survival.[160] Resistance to chemotherapy in acute and lymphomatous ATL may be related to adverse molecular features such as P-glycoprotein overexpression and p53 mutations.[161,162] More recent approaches to therapy have employed deoxycoformycin and irinotecan; however, little benefit was apparent.[163–166]

Allogeneic bone marrow transplantation has been successful in a number of ATL patients, although severe immunodeficiency resulting from both the underlying disease and preparatory regimens is a significant problem.[166] A trial of high-dose chemotherapy and autologous bone marrow transplantation had disappointing results, with no long-term survivors.[167]

Targeted therapy using conjugated and unconjugated anti-Tac monoclonal antibodies has produced several complete and partial remissions in ATL patients. This approach may be promising, especially if combined with other targeted therapies.[168,169] Two independent Phase II trials of azidothymidine (AZT) and interferon (IFN) alfa for ATL were published in 1995. A high response rate was noted, and, although most patients relapsed, several had prolonged responses.[170,171] Another Phase II study that employed higher dose AZT (1 gm daily) and IFN alfa (9 million units daily) produced an even higher response rate, particularly among acute ATL patients.[172] We have recently begun to use high-dose parenteral AZT (1.5 gm twice daily) and IFN alfa (5–10 million units twice daily) as an induction regimen in leukemic ATL, followed by maintenance oral AZT and subcutaneous IFN alfa. Among six patients treated, there have been three survivors (duration, 8 months to 3 years). Interestingly, despite regression of their disease, DNA hybridization studies performed on peripheral blood mononuclear cells continued to detect T-cell receptor rearrangements (Ramos and colleagues, unpublished data). Therefore, AZT and IFN alfa are likely to suppress rather than eliminate the malignant clone.

Recently, investigators have explored the use of arsenic trioxide (As_2O_3) in combination with IFN alfa in ATL. Interestingly, in vitro studies demonstrated that As_2O_3 inhibited the expression of the viral transactivator Tax in HTLV-1–infected cells.[173] A clinical trial is underway that hopefully will determine whether this combination holds promise for ATL. ATL, like other viral-mediated lymphoproliferative diseases, is dependent upon constitutive expression of NF-κB. Recent studies of both As_2O_3/IFN and another inhibitor of NF-κB, Bay-11, suggest that inhibition of this transcription factor may be a promising therapeutic approach for ATL.[174,175]

The milder forms of ATL have a much more indolent course, and patients frequently present with a prolonged history of cutaneous involvement. Immediate treatment, especially with aggressive chemotherapy regimens, is probably unwarranted and may exacerbate underlying immune deficiency. Oral etoposide, anti–IL-2R antibodies, or AZT and IFN alfa therapy are likely to produce results superior to high-dose chemotherapy.

More effective therapy for ATL is clearly needed. Development of new strategies is limited by the lack of an animal model that develops an ATL-like disease, the inability to establish long-term cell cultures, and the inherent difficulty of early detection. The use of severe combined immune deficient mice inoculated with primary ATL cells to test novel agents may be a useful strategy. Such an approach was recently used to demonstrate activity of anti-CD52.[176] Clinical trials to test novel agents, alone or in combination, should be designed to include geographic areas outside the United States or Europe where HTLV-1–related diseases are prevalent.

Supportive Care and Long-Term Management

Unfortunately, long-term management of ATL patients is a very rare occurrence. For those who have responded

CURRENT CONTROVERSIES & FUTURE CONSIDERATIONS

Human Immunodeficiency Virus Type 1– and Human T-Lymphotropic Virus Type 1–Associated Lymphomas

HIV-1–Related Non-Hodgkin's Lymphoma

- The optimal chemotherapy approach remains to be determined, but infusional strategies may yield higher complete response rates, prolonged freedom from progression, and better survival. Enrollment in clinical trials must be encouraged.
- The role of rituximab must be defined for the subset of patients with B-cell, CD20$^+$ lymphoma, because observations from recent clinical trials are suggestive of increased risk of infectious complications and possible adverse outcome. This is not akin to the clinical experience in de novo or HIV seronegative/indeterminate non-Hodgkin's lymphoma, for which rituximab has improved outcomes. The reason for this may be more pronounced and sustained effects on humoral immunity in HIV-infected patients.
- The use of concurrent antiretroviral therapy with systemic anticancer therapy is generally regarded as the current standard of care. Experience with infusional EPOCH chemotherapy, in which planned suspension or interruption of antiretroviral therapy did not appear to adversely affect outcome, may have practical advantages. Chief among these is avoidance of polypharmacy, with fewer drug-drug interactions and less drug toxicity, as well as enhanced compliance. The optimal sequencing of antiretroviral therapy with anticancer treatment is under investigation.
- The role of peripheral blood stem cell and nonmyeloablative bone marrow transplantation strategies as salvage therapy for relapsed patients is under investigation and is appropriate given the improved outcomes observed with more efficacious antiretroviral regimens. This approach may also provide insight into immune reconstitution.
- It is important to prospectively identify clinical, biologic, and molecular prognostic factors, which ultimately will guide the selection of therapy and improve the therapeutic outcome for patients with AIDS-related non-Hodgkin's lymphoma.

HTLV-1–Associated Lymphomas

- Cytotoxic chemotherapy may induce brief remission in ATL but is virtually never curative.
- Smoldering or chronic ATL may be amenable to biologic response modifiers, so early recognition of these forms of ATL is important.
- As yet, there is no reliable predictive assay to determine whether an HTLV-1 carrier will develop ATL.
- ATL patients are profoundly immunocompromised and prone to opportunistic infections. For as yet undefined reasons, these patients seem to be uniquely at risk for disseminated *Strongyloides*.

to AZT and IFN alfa, treatment should be continued indefinitely because we and others have documented rapid recurrence in patients who have been taken off these agents. As is the case for HIV-related lymphoma, patients undergoing chemotherapy for ATL often require colony-stimulating factor support. Patients with smoldering ATL, if not treated with biologic response modifiers as mentioned previously, require close monitoring for evidence of development of acute or lymphomatous ATL. Examination of cutaneous lesions and T-cell subset analysis should be performed frequently. Patients with smoldering or chronic ATL often succumb to opportunistic infections.

Prognosis

The prognosis for the aggressive forms of ATL remains poor. Although most patients respond to a variety of therapies, the duration of response is almost invariably short and survival of greater than a year is rare. Detection of elevated levels of soluble IL-2R, mutations in CD95, and atypical phenotypic variants in ATL patients may indicate an even worse prognosis. Patients with smoldering ATL may have an indolent course and a long survival and probably should be treated with milder therapy if at all.

Suggested Readings*

Carbone A: Emerging pathways in the development of AIDS-related lymphomas. Lancet Oncol 4:22–29, 2003.

Gill PS, Harrington W Jr, Kaplan MH, et al: Treatment of adult T-cell leukemia-lymphoma with a combination of interferon alfa and zidovudine. N Engl J Med 332:1744–1748, 1995.

Kaplan LD, Straus DJ, Testa MA, et al, for the National Institute of Allergy and Infectious Diseases AIDS Clinical Trials Group: Low-dose compared with standard-dose m-BACOD chemotherapy for non-Hodgkin's lymphoma associated with human immunodeficiency virus infection. N Engl J Med 336:1641–1648, 1997.

Little RF, Pittaluga S, Grant N, et al: Highly effective treatment of acquired immunodeficiency syndrome related lymphoma with dose-adjusted EPOCH: impact of antiretroviral therapy suspension and tumor biology. Blood 101:4653–4659, 2003.

Otieno MW, Banura C, Katongole-Mbidde E, et al: Therapeutic challenges of AIDS-related non-Hodgkin's lymphoma in the United States and East Africa. J Natl Cancer Inst 94:718–732, 2002.

Poiesz BJ, Ruscetti FW, Gazdar AF, et al: Detection and isolation of type C retrovirus particles from fresh and cultured lymphocytes of a patient with cutaneous T-cell lymphoma. Proc Natl Acad Sci U S A 77:7415–7419, 1980.

Ratner L, Lee J, Tang S, et al, for the AIDS Malignancy Consortium: Chemotherapy for human immunodeficiency virus-associated non-Hodgkin's lymphoma in combination with highly active antiretroviral therapy. J Clin Oncol 19:2171–2178, 2001.

Scadden DT: AIDS-related malignancies. Annu Rev Med 54:265–303, 2003.

Shimoyama M: Diagnostic criteria and classification of clinical subtypes of adult T-cell leukaemia-lymphoma: a report from the Lymphoma Study Group (1984–87). Br J Haematol 79:428–437, 1991.

Sparano JA, Lee S, Chen MG, et al: Phase II trial of infusional cyclophosphamide, doxorubicin, and etoposide in patients with human immunodeficiency virus-associated non-Hodgkin's lymphoma: an Eastern Cooperative Oncology Group trial (E1494). J Clin Oncol 22:1491–1500, 2004.

Full references for this chapter can be found on accompanying CD-ROM.

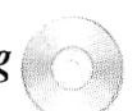

CHAPTER 45

Epstein-Barr Virus–Related and Kaposi's Sarcoma–Associated Herpesvirus–Related Neoplasms

Giovanna Tosato, MD, Richard F. Little, MD, MPH, and Robert Yarchoan, MD

KEY POINTS

Epstein-Barr Virus–Related and Kaposi's Sarcoma–Associated Herpesvirus–Related Neoplasms

Diagnosis

- Most of these diseases are much more common in patients with severe immunosuppression, especially from acquired immunodeficiency syndrome.
- Many of these diseases have distinctive epidemiologic patterns. Those caused by Kaposi's sarcoma–associated herpesvirus (KSHV) generally follow the distribution of KSHV infection. Epstein-Barr virus–associated nasopharyngeal carcinoma and gastric carcinoma are more frequent in Asia.
- Viral gene expression profiling is important in the diagnosis of a number of these diseases, including posttransplantation lymphoproliferative disease, Kaposi's sarcoma, and primary effusion lymphoma.

Treatment

- Treatment of the underlying immunosuppression is important in the therapy for a number of these diseases, especially those in which clonal malignant transformation has not taken place (such as posttransplantation lymphoproliferative disease and Kaposi's sarcoma).
- Standard treatment for a number of these diseases, such as lymphoid granulomatosis, multicentric Castleman's disease, and primary effusion lymphoma, has not been established.

INTRODUCTION

Two gammaherpesviruses, Epstein-Barr virus (EBV) and Kaposi's sarcoma–associated herpesvirus (KSHV), are associated with a variety of neoplasms (Table 45–1). A number of these tumors preferentially affect immunodeficient individuals, but others develop in people with normal immune systems. The biology of these viruses and certain nonmalignant diseases caused by them are described in Chapters 74 and 75. In this chapter, we focus on the tumors caused by or associated with these herpesviruses. This has been an area of intense research in the last 2 decades, and in fact the discovery of KSHV as a new virus in 1994 has led to an enhanced appreciation for the key role of viruses in tumors arising in immunodeficient patients.

EBV-ASSOCIATED TUMORS

Posttransplantation Lymphoproliferative Disease

Posttransplantation lymphoproliferative disease (PTLD) represents a manifestation of unrestrained proliferation of lymphocytes latently infected with EBV. It is observed in a proportion of EBV-infected transplant recipients who are profoundly T-cell immunodeficient as a result of immunosuppressive regimens used in the setting of transplantation.

Epidemiology and Risk Factors

The frequency of PTLD varies depending on the type of transplant. PTLD occurs in 1–2% of kidney transplants, 0.5–10% of bone marrow or stem cell transplants, 2–15% of liver transplants, 2–15% of heart transplants, and 10–20% of lung transplants.[1,2] The incidence of PTLD increases in transplant recipients who undergo primary EBV infection, in those who develop cytomegalovirus infection after transplantation, and in recipients of T-cell–depleted or human lymphocyte antigen–mismatched bone marrow transplants.[3-5] The risk for development of PTLD is related primarily to the degree and duration of immunosuppression; anti-CD3 antibodies (OKT3) alone or in combination with other drugs have been identified as a risk factor in some studies.[4-6] The interval from transplantation to the development of PTLD is variable, but most cases are diagnosed within the first 6 months following transplantation.[7] Occasionally, PTLD is diagnosed years after the transplantation.

Pathogenesis

Primary infection with EBV, which is followed by a long-lasting persistence of EBV-infected B lymphocytes, is associated with seroconversion and the development of a long-lasting specific T-cell immunity (see Chapter 74).

TABLE 45–1. Malignant and Hyperproliferative Diseases Associated with EBV and KSHV Infection

Disease	Viral Association	Association Frequency
Posttransplantation lymphoproliferative disease	EBV	100%
Burkitt's lymphoma*		
Endemic	EBV	>95%
Sporadic	EBV	<30%
AIDS-associated	EBV	20–50%
CNS AIDS lymphoma	EBV	100%
Hodgkin's disease		
HIV-associated	EBV	>80%
Not HIV associated	EBV	40–60%
Nasopharyngeal carcinoma	EBV	>95%
Hemophagocytic lymphohistiocytosis	EBV	>50%
Lymphomatoid granulomatosis	EBV	>95%
Kaposi's sarcoma	KSHV	100%
Multicentric Castleman's disease		
HIV-associated	KSHV	>90%
Not HIV associated	KSHV	~50%
Primary effusion lymphoma	KSHV	100%
	EBV	>80%

*See Table 45–3 for other HIV-associated systemic lymphomas.
Abbreviations: AIDS, acquired immunodeficiency syndrome; CNS, central nervous system; HIV, human immunodeficiency virus.

EBV-immune T lymphocytes are responsible for preventing the outgrowth of EBV-infected cells (Fig. 45–1).[8,9] PTLD is a reflection of unrestrained proliferation of EBV-infected B lymphocytes in patients without adequate T-cell immunity against the virus.[8,10] The EBV-infected cells are usually of recipient origin, except in the case of stem cell transplants, in which they are usually of donor origin, and they are often polyclonal.[4] Tissues affected with PTLD show expression of all five EBV latency proteins and the EBV-encoded RNAs[1] (Table 45–2).

Clinical Features and Diagnosis

Patients with PTLD present with a variety of symptoms ranging from infectious mononucleosis–like manifestations (see Chapter 74) to symptoms derived from mass lesions in the gastrointestinal tract, liver, kidney, lung, or other organs. In children, the site of the lesion is most frequently abdominal (64%), less frequently involving the thorax (50%), head and neck (25%), or brain (6%).[5] The transplanted organ is often the site of PTLD; this is believed to be due to accumulation of inflammatory cells as well as the cytokines and chemokines they produce.[1,4] Many patients with PTLD display abnormally elevated levels of cell-associated EBV in the circulation compared to transplant recipients without PTLD.[1,11] The diagnosis of PTLD is based upon histologic features compatible with those of a lymphoproliferative disease in which a substantial proportion of the cells are EBV infected as determined by staining for EBV DNA, EBV-encoded RNAs, or EBV proteins.[12,13] Distinct histologic subtypes have been identified ranging from infectious mononucleosis–like lesions to large-cell lymphoma or Burkitt-like lesions (Fig. 45–2).[13-15]

Treatment

Therapy of PTLD is designed to reduce T-cell immunosuppression and the number of EBV-infected B cells, but no standardized approach currently exists. When possible, immunosuppressive drugs are suspended or their dosage reduced to allow reconstitution of EBV-immune T cells without loss of the graft.[11] Localized lesions, particularly those in the gastrointestinal tract, are often resected.[5] Radiotherapy is often used for central nervous system (CNS) disease.[5] Treatment with anti-CD20 monoclonal antibody (rituximab) has been effective at induc-

TABLE 45–2. EBV Genes Expressed in EBV-Positive Malignancies

Disease	*EBNA1*	*EBNA2*	*EBNA3*	*LMP1*	*LMP2*	EBERs
PTLD	+	+	+	+	+	+
Burkitt's lymphoma	+	–	–	–	–	+
AR-PCNS lymphoma	+	+	+	+	+	+
Hodgkin's disease	+	–	–	+	+	+
NPC	+	–	–	+	+	+
Gastric carcinoma	+	–	–	–	+	+

Abbreviations: AR-PCNS, AIDS-related primary central nervous system lymphoma; EBERs, EBV-encoded RNAs; NPC, nasopharyngeal carcinoma; PTLD, posttransplantation lymphoproliferative disease.

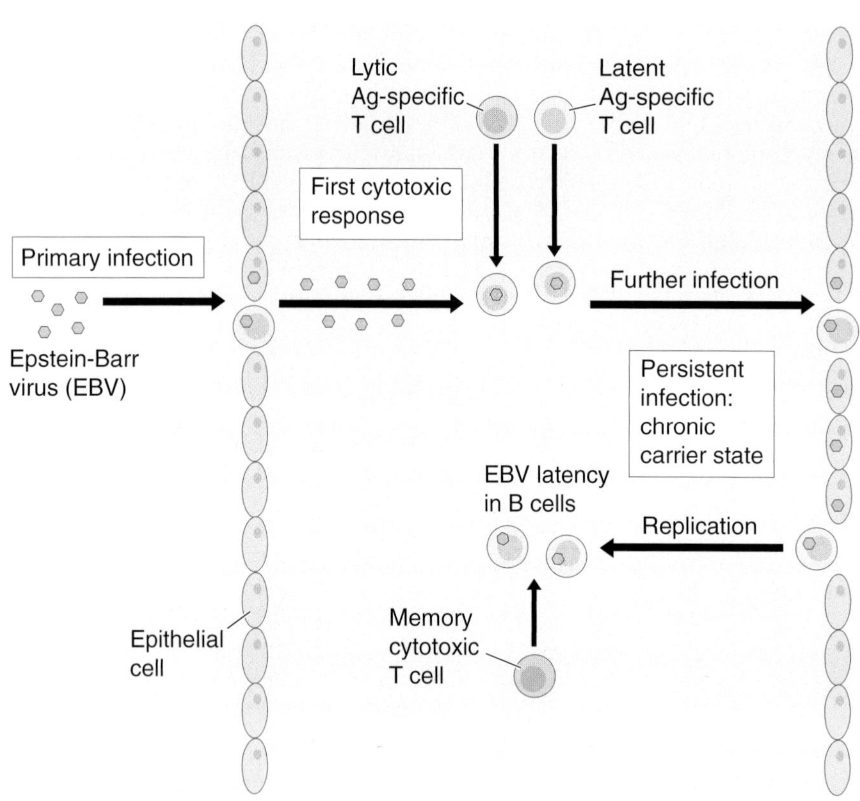

Figure 45–1. Schematic representation of EBV–B-cell interactions and T-cell immunity directed at EBV-infected cells.

ing complete remissions.[5,16,17] Remissions have also been achieved with low-dose chemotherapy with, for example, cyclophosphamide (600 mg/m^2) for 1 day and prednisone (2 mg/kg/day) for 5 days administered every 3 weeks for six cycles.[5,18] Other treatment regimens with cyclophosphamide, doxorubicin, vincristine, and prednisone have also been successful.[4] Adoptive immunotherapy with infusion of EBV-immune T cells from the recipient, from a donor matched with the recipient, or from the donor of the graft (if the PTLD is of donor origin) has been helpful in some cases.[19] Use of interferon alfa with reduced immunosuppression has been reported to achieve complete responses, but may be associated with a risk of graft rejection.[4] Although antiviral agents are ineffective against cells latently infected with EBV, such as those present in PTLD, prophylaxis with acyclovir or ganciclovir used at the time of transplantation has shown some evidence of effectiveness in uncontrolled studies.[20,21]

Prognosis

Overall prognosis of PTLD is difficult to establish, given the availability of few controlled studies, use of different therapies, limited numbers of patients, and short follow-ups. Overall estimates of 40–70% mortality have been reported after solid organ transplantation.[22] Use of anti-CD20 antibodies was reported to achieve 50–65% complete remission, and the 1-year survival was reported at 50%.[17] Predictors of poor response to anti-CD20 treatment include multivisceral involvement, late-onset PTLD (>1 year after transplant), and CNS disease.[23]

Burkitt's Lymphoma

Burkitt's lymphoma is a form of undifferentiated B-cell lymphoma characterized histologically by a monomorphous population of cells with many mitotic figures and apoptotic cells. A "starry sky" appearance is often present, reflecting macrophage ingestion of apoptotic cells. Karyotypic changes involving translocation of the c-*myc* oncogene (located on chromosome 8) to chromosome 14, 22, or 2, and associated c-Myc deregulation, characterize Burkitt's lymphoma. Chapters 39 and 43 present descriptions of lymphoma biology and of other non-Hodgkin's lymphomas (NHLs), respectively.

Virtually all Burkitt's lymphomas occurring in equatorial Africa are EBV positive, but only 20–80% of Burkitt's lymphomas outside the endemic region are infected with the virus.[24] In United States, 20% of all Burkitt's lymphomas are EBV infected. Among human immunodeficiency virus (HIV)–associated lymphomas, Burkitt's lymphoma accounts for about 30% of all lymphomas.[25–27] Acquired immunodeficiency syndrome (AIDS)–associated Burkitt's lymphomas are EBV positive in 30–50% of cases.[27]

Malaria, which is endemic in equatorial Africa and can stimulate B-cell growth and reduce T- and natural killer (NK) cell responses, has been considered a risk factor for the development of endemic Burkitt's lymphoma, but its contribution remains unclear.[28] A pathogenetic role of EBV in endemic Burkitt's lymphoma has been suspected for some time but still remains undefined.[28,29] Among the EBV latency genes, only *EBNA1* and occasionally low levels of *LMP2* are expressed in endemic Burkitt's lym-

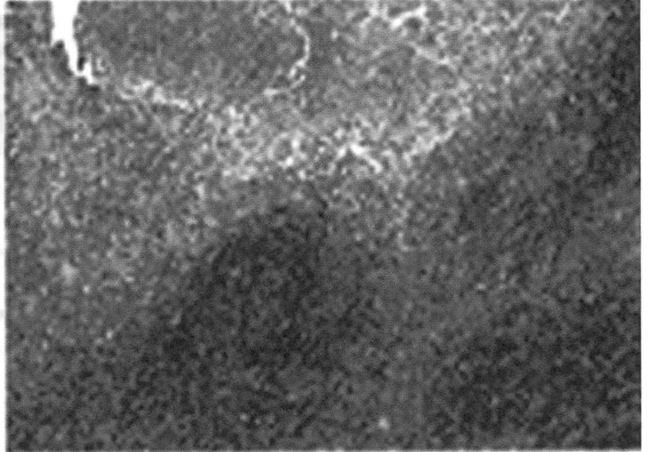

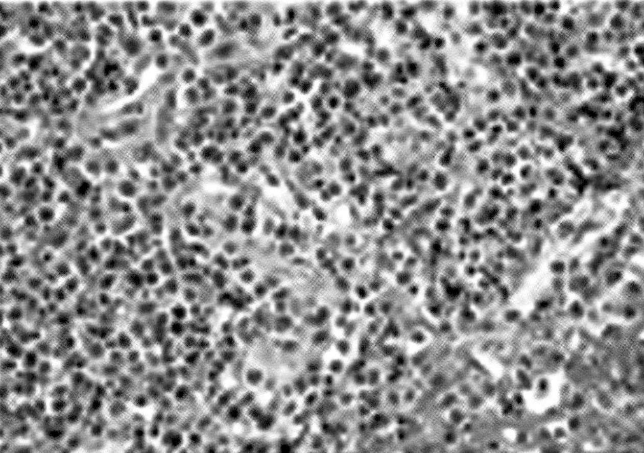

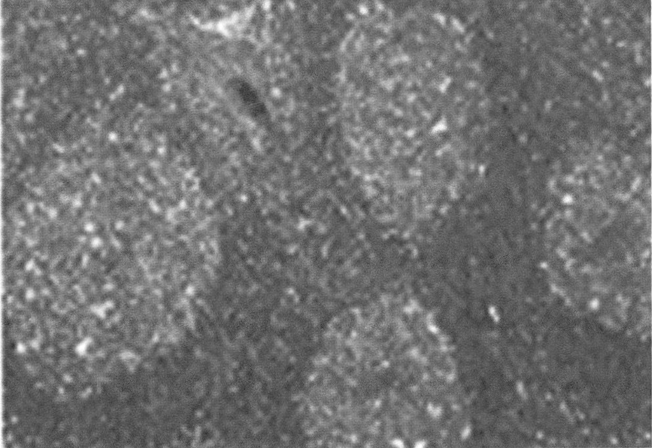

Figure 45–2. Hematoxylin and eosin staining of lymph nodes representative of EBV-induced infectious mononucleosis, posttransplantation lymphoproliferative disease, and lymphoid hyperplasia. (Modified from Teruya-Feldstein J, Jaffe ES, Burd PR, et al: The role of Mig, the monokine induced by interferon-gamma, and IP-10, the interferon-gamma-inducible protein-10, in tissue necrosis and vascular damage associated with Epstein-Barr virus-positive lymphoproliferative disease. Blood 90:4099–4105, 1997, with permission.)

phoma tissues (see Table 45–2).[29–31] Burkitt's lymphoma cells are resistant to T-cell killing because of reduced or absent expression of EBNA-3 protein, surface adhesion molecules, peptide transporters associated with antigen presentation, and human lymphocyte antigen class I molecules.[32,33]

Endemic Burkitt's lymphoma peaks in children between 5 and 10 years old, has a 2:1 male/female ratio, and in about 50% of cases involves the jaw in association with the developing molar tooth buds. The second most frequent location of endemic Burkitt's lymphoma is the abdomen (Fig. 45–3).[28,34] The diagnosis of Burkitt's lymphoma is based upon characteristic histologic features comprising a monotonous infiltration of B lymphocytes expressing the cell surface markers CD19 and CD20, a very high growth rate fraction with nearly 100% of cells positive for the proliferation-associated Ki-67 marker, and a starry sky pattern. Establishing cytogenetic evidence of c-*myc* oncogene (on chromosome 8) translocation to chromosomes 14, 22, or 2 is recommended.[34] EBV infection is documented by detection of EBV-related DNA, EBV RNA, or EBV proteins in the majority of tumor cells. Information on detailed staging and treatment is presented in Chapter 43. Recent studies in children show an overall 6-year event-free survival rate of 89%, reaching 100% in patients classified as stage I.[35]

Peripheral AIDS-Related NHL

HIV-infected patients are at increased risk for systemic NHL, and a substantial percentage of these tumors are EBV associated. The CD4 counts of HIV-infected patients influence the risk that they will develop NHL, the tumor type, and the likelihood that the tumor will be EBV associated (Table 45–3).[36–39] With regard to EBV involvement, about 20–50% of the AIDS-associated Burkitt's lymphomas and 30% or less of the AIDS-associated diffuse large B-cell lymphoma centroblastic variant that typically develop in patients with high CD4 counts are EBV associated. However, 80% or more of AIDS-related diffuse large B-cell immunoblastic lymphomas that typically develop in patients with low CD4 counts are EBV associated.[38] Many of these tumors express the full spectrum of EBV latency genes.

Since the introduction of highly active antiretroviral therapy (HAART) as standard HIV care, there has been improved survival in AIDS-related NHL. The use of HAART has also been associated with a shift in tumor types, with a decreased proportion of lymphomas with unfavorable prognostic features, and this is likely attributable to improvement in immune function.[37] Diffuse large B-cell immunoblastic lymphomas, which are most often associated with advanced HIV disease, have decreased the most in incidence, whereas the incidence of tumors associated with relatively well-preserved immune function has been stable.[40] It is noteworthy that AIDS-related NHL incidence within any given CD4 stratum has been unaffected by HAART.[37] The preponderance of tumors seen in the HAART era are those associated with better prognosis, and this certainly contributes to the improved survival in the HAART era. This

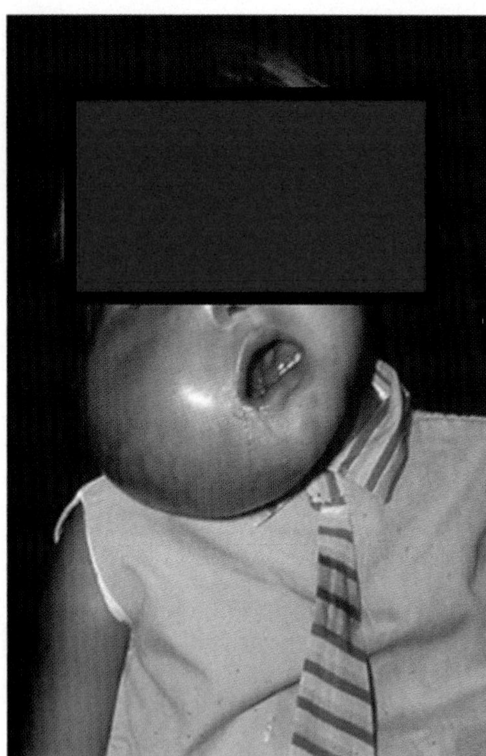
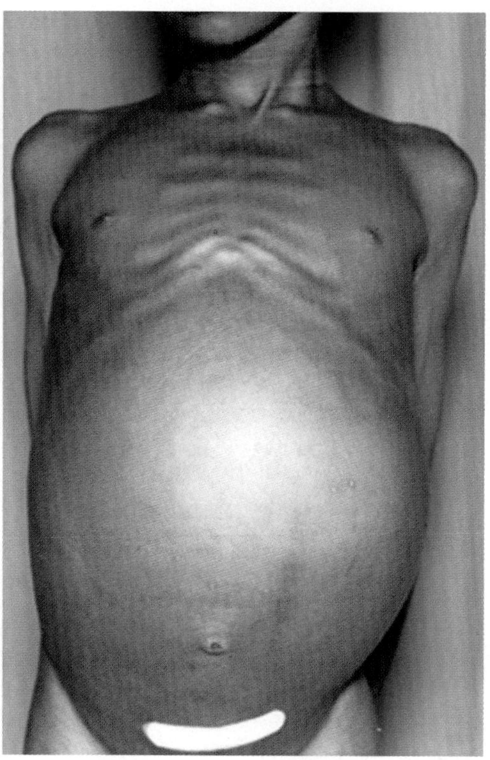

Figure 45–3. Patient with Burkitt's lymphoma involving the jaw and the abdomen. (Courtesy of Dr. K. Bathia.)

TABLE 45–3. EBV and Immunologic Associations in HIV-Associated Lymphomas

Disease	Approx. % of ARL	EBV %	CD4 Cells
Hodgkin's lymphoma	5	>80	Often well preserved
Burkitt's and Burkitt-like lymphoma	30–40	20–50	Often well preserved
Plasmacytoid	20	50–70	Often well preserved
Systemic DLBCL			
Centroblastic	25	30	Often well preserved
Immunoblastic	10	90	Usually <50/μL
PBLOC	<10	70	Usually <50/μL
Primary effusion lymphoma*	<4	>80*	Usually <200/μL
PCNSL	10–20	Nearly 100	Almost always <50/μL

*100% of PELs are associated with KSHV.
Abbreviations: ARL, AIDS-related lymphomas; DLBCL, diffuse large B-cell lymphoma; PBLOC, plasmablastic lymphoma of the oral cavity; PCNSL, primary central nervous system lymphoma.

shift may also provide some insight toward explaining the long-standing observation that the primary prognostic determinant in AIDS-related NHL is the CD4 cell count.[41] More detailed information on NHL and on AIDS-associated lymphomas is found in Chapters 43 and 44, respectively.

Primary Central Nervous System Lymphoma

Primary central nervous system lymphomas (PCNSLs) developing in immunocompetent patients rarely are associated with EBV. However, PCNSLs that arise in patients with immunodeficiency are often EBV associated, and this association is almost universal in patients with AIDS[42] (Table 45–4). Most such AIDS-related PCNSLs develop in patients with CD4 counts under 50 cells/μL in the peripheral blood. Two main types of AIDS-related PCNSL are recognized, with different morphology, latency antigen expression, and histiogenic origin (Table 45–5).

The association of AIDS-related PCNSL with EBV has been the underpinning for a major diagnostic advance. Until recently, the diagnosis of these tumors in AIDS patients with CNS masses involved brain biopsy; alternatively, the tumors were presumptively diagnosed in patients who failed a 2- to 3-week trial of antitoxoplasmosis therapy. Several subsequent studies have shown that, in AIDS patients with focal CNS lesions, the combination of positive thallium-201 single-photon emission computed tomography of the brain and EBV DNA polymerase chain reaction in cerebrospinal fluid can be highly selective and sensitive for the diagnosis of AIDS-related PCNSL.[43,44] These studies revealed that, if both of these tests were positive, the diagnosis of PCNSL was almost certain. If both tests were negative, the negative predictive value for lymphoma was essentially 100%. These findings allow the earlier initiation of therapy for PCNSL and the avoidance of the potential morbidity of brain biopsy. It should be noted, however, that most of these data were derived before the development of HAART, and two recent reports raise concerns that EBV polymerase chain reaction and nuclear medicine studies may not be as specific in patients receiving HAART as previously established.[45,46] Clinicians should keep alert for further developments in this area.

Prior to the availability of HAART, the median survival of patients with AIDS-related PCNSL was generally less than 4 months.[47] The standard treatment was radiotherapy of the brain and treatment of the underlying HIV infection.[48] With effective HAART, the prognosis may be substantially better for many patients, with many surviving longer than 1–2 years. As patients' survival with AIDS-related PCNSL improves, lessons from the treatment of non–AIDS-related PCNSL may prove informative. Fifty percent or more of those non-AIDS patients with PCNSL treated with whole-brain radiotherapy can develop neurocognitive defects affecting quality of life and impairing longer term survival prospects.[49] Those treated with high-dose methotrexate–based chemotherapy regimens, however, do not appear to suffer the late neurotoxicity that is frequently associated with radiotherapy to the brain.[49] Given with leucovorin rescue, methotrexate can be administered without immunosuppressive effects, and such a strategy may prove useful in AIDS-related PCNSL, at least among those patients with HAART-sensitive HIV. Strategies to limit toxicity by deferring radiotherapy in favor of chemotherapy may be developed so that therapy modification could be made early based on tumor markers, such as EBV, rather than on morbid decline, but these are areas of potential research interest and not at this time recommendations for standard clinical approaches.

Additionally, the presence of EBV in AIDS-related PCNSL may be exploitable both as a disease marker and therapeutically. Cerebrospinal fluid EBV burden appears to decrease with effective PCNSL treatment, and may be potentially useful as an index of treatment effect.[50] Also, several meaningful tumor responses were observed in a small pilot study utilizing the antiviral drugs zidovudine and ganciclovir in combination with interleukin-2.[51]

TABLE 45–4. Comparison of Clinical and Viral Features of AIDS and Non–AIDS-Related PCNSL

	HIV +	HIV −
% Primary brain tumors as NHL	>95	3.5
% of all NHL	20%	1–2%
Male/female ratio	9:1	3:2
Age of peak incidence	Any age: CD4 cell dependent	≥6th decade
EBV association	100%	Rare

HIV-Associated Hodgkin's Lymphoma

Hodgkin's lymphoma, though not AIDS defining, occurs with increased frequency in HIV-infected patients, and in this setting is EBV associated in 80–100% of cases.[52] By contrast, in HIV-negative patients approximately 30% of cases of Hodgkin's lymphoma are EBV related, and usually in association with the mixed-cellularity histologic subtype.[53–55] Of interest, even though HIV-associated Hodgkin's lymphoma is EBV associated, it tends to occur at relatively well-preserved CD4 cell counts, underscoring the functional immune defects that can belie the absolute CD4 cell count in HIV disease. HIV-infected individuals with EBV-associated Hodgkin's lymphoma often have a relatively poor prognosis as compared to young, otherwise healthy adults with EBV-associated Hodgkin's lymphoma.[56] The reader is referred to a broad discussion of Hodgkin's lymphoma in Chapter 40.

TABLE 45–5. Comparison of EBV Association, Latency Expression, and Histiogenic Origin in AIDS and Non–AIDS-Related PCNSL

HIV	Morphology	EBV	LMP-1	BCL-6	BCL-2	Histiogenic Origin
+	Immunoblastic plasmacytoid	+	+	−	+	Non-GC B cell
+	Large noncleaved cell	+	−	+	−	GC B cell
−	Large noncleaved cell	−	−	+	−	GC B cell

Abbreviation: GC, germinal center.

From Rosenwald A, Wright G, Chan WC, et al: The use of molecular profiling to predict survival after chemotherapy for diffuse large-B-cell lymphoma. N Engl J Med 346:1937–1947, 2002.

EBV-Associated T/NK Cell Lymphoproliferative Diseases

EBV-associated T/NK cell lymphoproliferative diseases represent rare and almost always fatal diseases characterized by EBV infection of T and/or NK cells that are observed predominantly in East Asians. They comprise three entities: hemophagocytic lymphohistiocytosis, T-cell lymphoma, and NK cell lymphoma. It is currently unclear how T and NK cells become infected with EBV because these cells are resistant to EBV infection in vitro, and disease pathogenesis is unclear. It is hypothesized that, unlike B cells, T and NK cells infected with EBV may be poor inducers of T-cell immunity to the virus, allowing outgrowth of virally infected cells.[57]

Hemophagocytic Lymphohistiocytosis

Hemophagocytic lymphohistiocytosis presents as an acute severe illness with high and persistent fever, CNS symptoms, hepatosplenomegaly, severe cytopenia, and coagulopathy with hypofibrinogenemia.[58,59] An additional diagnostic feature is hypertriglyceridemia. The T cells in this illness are infected with EBV. The severe systemic manifestations are attributed to release of cytokines, including tumor necrosis factor-α.[58,60] Different tissues, including the bone marrow and lymph nodes, show histologic evidence of macrophage phagocytosis,[61,62] and are infiltrated with EBV-infected T lymphocytes, mostly CD45RO$^+$ and CD8$^+$ cells[63] (Fig. 45–4). Treatment has been directed at reducing the number of EBV-infected T cells, macrophage activation, and cytokine levels by use of chemotherapy, corticosteroids, and plasmapheresis.[64,65]

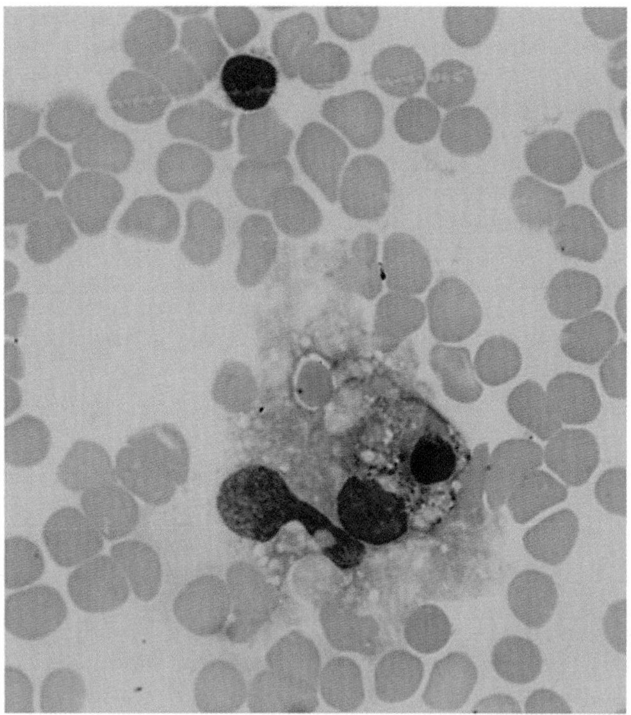

A

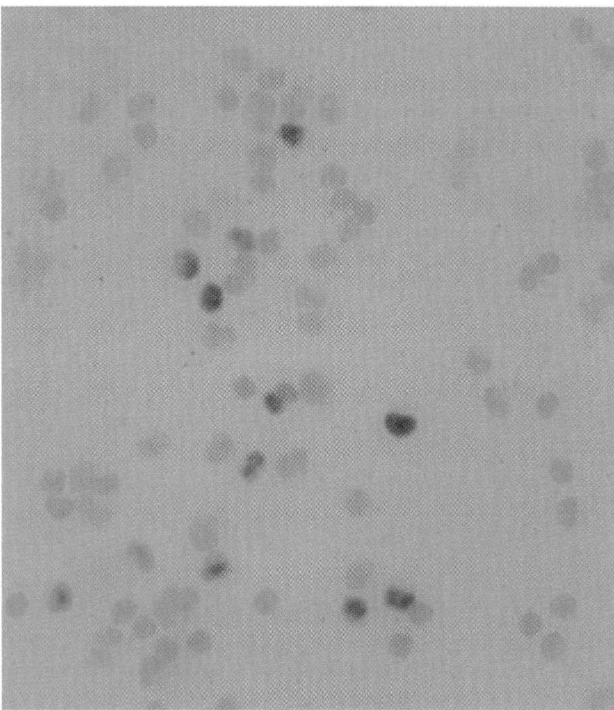

B

Figure 45–4. EBV-associated hemophagocytic lymphohistiocytosis. ***A,*** Histiocytic phagocytosis. ***B,*** EBV-encoded RNA–positive cells in the bone marrow. (Courtesy of Dr. H. Kanegane.)

EBV-Positive T-Cell Lymphoma

EBV-positive T-cell lymphoma is associated with chronic active EBV infection (see Chapter 74). Most forms are nodal T-cell lymphomas and contain monoclonal EBV DNA.[66–68] Most lymphomas have a CD4$^+$ T-cell phenotype, but EBV infection may extend to other lymphocytes, particularly in advanced stages of the disease (Fig. 45–5).[66,68,69] Most of these lymphomas have been refractory to chemotherapy, and allogeneic bone marrow transplants have been performed with limited success.[70]

EBV-Positive NK Cell Lymphomas

Nasal and nasal-type EBV-positive NK cell lymphomas represent the second most frequent extranodal lymphoma among Chinese in Hong Kong, and are not uncommon in Asia and in South and Central America.[57,61] They present as a form of nasal destructive disease, often extending to the palate and sometimes to the larynx and the upper respiratory and digestive tracts.[71] Erythema of the skin and orbital swelling are often present. Histologically, these tissues display prominent zonal necrosis and infiltration with atypical cells, identified as NK cells infected with EBV, mixed with a prominent inflammatory infiltrate; there is also evidence of vascular damage.[72] Initial disease remissions are usually achieved with local

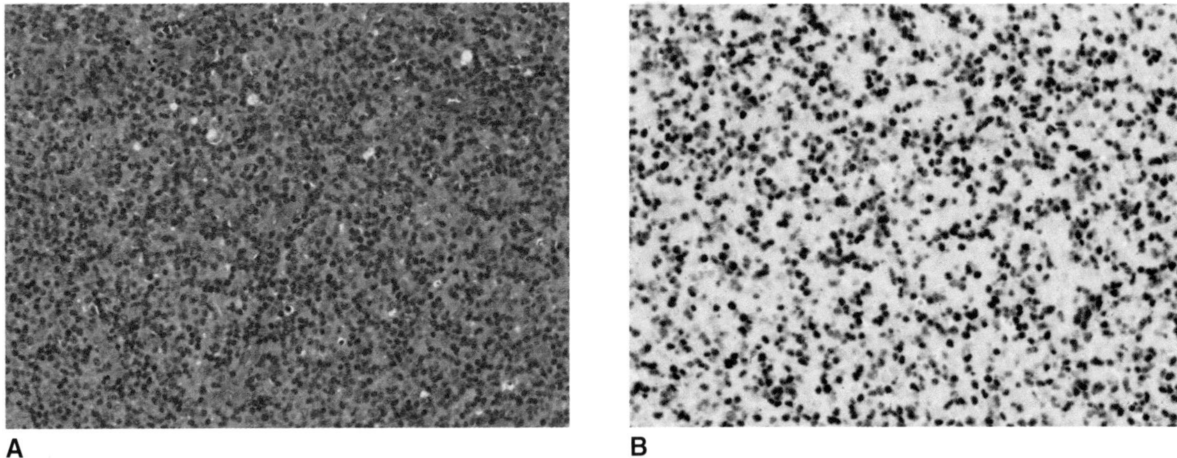

Figure 45–5. Nodal EBV-positive lymphoma in a patient with chronic EBV infection. *A*, Typical histology. *B*, EBV-encoded RNA staining. (Courtesy of Dr. H. Kanegane.)

irradiation and/or chemotherapy, but the disease is almost always fatal.[57]

Nasopharyngeal Carcinoma

Epidemiology and Risk Factors

Nasopharyngeal carcinoma is a type of epithelial head and neck cancer that occurs endemically in southern China, where it represents the third most common malignancy among men.[73] Nasopharyngeal carcinoma occurs sporadically in the West. Virtually all nasopharyngeal carcinomas from endemic regions and most nasopharyngeal carcinomas from nonendemic regions are EBV infected.[74] The geographic pattern of incidence suggests participation of genetic and environmental factors, such as consumption of salted fish and other preserved foods containing nitrosamines.[73,75]

Pathogenesis

EBV can replicate in the epithelial cells lining the oropharyngeal cavity and in the parotid gland during EBV-induced infectious mononucleosis, and EBV is commonly detected in the saliva from healthy EBV-seropositive individuals. However, latent EBV infection is not detected in normal epithelial cells.[76–79] Nasopharyngeal carcinoma tissues are latently infected with EBV and show transcription of EBV-encoded RNAs; the genes encoding EBNA-1, LMP-1, and LMP-2; and several *Bam*HI-A fragments.[74] Nasopharyngeal carcinoma tissues and some premalignant lesions contain clonal EBV, suggesting that EBV infection is an early event in the development of the malignancy and that the tumor represents a monoclonal expansion of a single cell.[74,80] Preinvasive lesions and normal nasopharyngeal epithelium from high-risk individuals have displayed characteristic chromosome deletions at a high frequency, suggesting that early genetic lesions may predispose cells to EBV infection or allow for EBV latency (Fig. 45–6).[73,81,82]

Diagnosis

Methods for early detection of nasopharyngeal carcinoma include measurement of immunoglobulin A antibodies against EBV viral capsid antigen[83,84] and detection of circulating EBV DNA. Rising immunoglobulin A antibody titers to EBV viral capsid antigen and levels of EBV DNA have been shown to correlate with the presence of nasopharyngeal carcinoma and to be useful markers in high-risk regions.[85] Cervical lymphadenopathy is the most common manifestation, followed by nasal, aural, and neurologic symptoms.[86] The diagnosis is histologic. Based on the degree of cell differentiation, three histologic types are distinguished: type I, keratinizing squamous cell carcinoma; type II, nonkeratinizing squamous cell carcinoma; and type III, undifferentiated carcinoma.[73,87] Current methods of disease staging[86] incorporate all major prognostic parameters.

Treatment and Prognosis

Standard treatment of nasopharyngeal carcinoma includes local radiotherapy alone or with concurrent administration of cisplatin.[86] With radiotherapy alone, the overall survival at 10 years is 85% for localized nasopharyngeal carcinoma without regional lymph node involvement and without distant metastases (stages I and II), and 55% in more advanced stages (II and IV) of disease.[88] Local recurrence and metastatic disease are usually treated with a combination of cisplatin and 5-fluorouracil. Use of antibodies directed at the epidermal growth factor receptor, which is expressed on nasopharyngeal carcinoma, in conjunction with cisplatin has yielded promising early results in clinical trials.[86] The median survival for patients with metastatic disease is approximately 9 months.[86,89]

Gastric Carcinoma

EBV-positive gastric carcinomas represent a distinct group of carcinomas characterized by EBV infection of

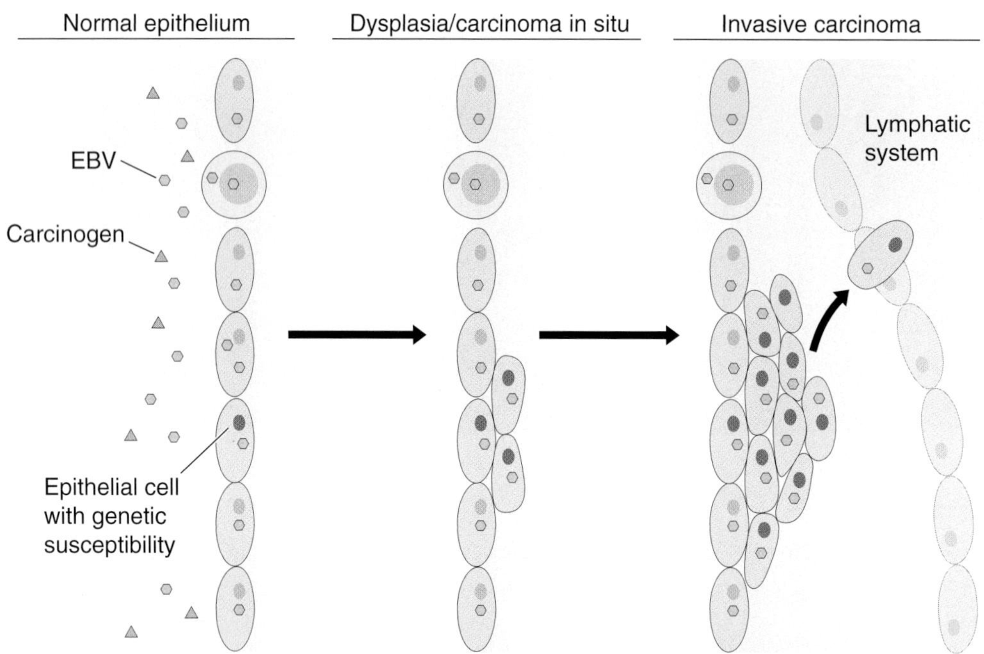

Figure 45–6. Schematic representation of multistep carcinogenesis of nasopharyngeal carcinoma.

almost all tumor cells.[90–92] Approximately 10% of all gastric carcinomas worldwide, and 80% of the rare lymphoepithelioma type, are EBV infected.[91,92] Compared to all gastric carcinomas, EBV-positive tumors occur more frequently in males, affect a somewhat younger population, localize preferentially to the proximal stomach, belong to the histologic tubular type in about 50% of cases, and display less lymph node involvement.[91,92] *Helicobacter pylori* infection, which induces a chronic gastritis and mucosal atrophy, is linked to the development of gastric carcinoma,[93] but there is no difference in *H. pylori* infection between EBV-positive and EBV-negative tumors.[94] The role of EBV in the pathogenesis of EBV-positive gastric carcinoma is currently unclear.[91,92] Normal gastric mucosa is EBV negative,[95] but some dysplastic lesions of the gastric mucosa were found to be EBV positive and monoclonal virus was isolated from several tumors.[91] EBV-encoded RNAs, the latency genes *EBNA1* and *LMP1,* and transcripts from the *Bam*HI-A region are expressed in these carcinomas (see Table 45–2).[91,96]

The diagnosis of EBV-positive gastric carcinoma is based upon the identification of EBV infection in tissues with gastric carcinoma, and surgical treatment follows the guidelines for other gastric carcinomas. The cancer-related survival rate was reported to be significantly higher in patients with EBV-positive gastric carcinomas as opposed to EBV-negative gastric carcinomas, whereas the overall survival (~25% at 10 years) was not different.[92]

Lymphomatoid Granulomatosis

This is a rare lymphoproliferative disease characterized by EBV infection of B cells, a prominent reactive T-cell infiltrate, tissue necrosis, and often a characteristic perivascular localization.[97–99] The nodular mass lesions more frequently involve the lung, kidney, liver, and brain.[97] The pathogenesis of the disease is unclear, except that a proportion of patients may have an underlying immunodeficiency and that certain chemokines induced by the EBV-infected B cells participate in causing the vascular-based tissue necrosis.[100,101] The pattern of EBV gene expression is currently unknown. The natural history of the disease is variable and ranges from that of a benign process to an aggressive form of large-cell lymphoma.[98] Accordingly, some patients are untreated and others are treated with various chemotherapeutic regimens.[98]

EBV-Associated Leiomyosarcomas

These are exceedingly rare smooth muscle tumors described in immunocompromised solid organ transplant recipients, patients (especially children) with AIDS, and patients with congenital immunodeficiencies.[102–106] The pattern of EBV gene expression has been reported to include all EBV latency genes,[103] but the role of EBV in the pathogenesis of this malignancy is undefined. Some of these tumors have been treated surgically, others with chemotherapy or irradiation. Surgical removal of the lesions was curative in two cases,[105,107] whereas the other patients died, but it is unclear to what extent the underlying condition (AIDS, solid organ transplant) and its complications contributed to the outcome.

KSHV-RELATED TUMORS

The epidemiology of Kaposi's sarcoma during the initial years of the AIDS epidemic, and in particular its higher incidence in men who have sex with men than injection drug users, provided strong evidence that an agent other that HIV was involved in the pathogenesis of this disorder. However, the search for this factor was unsuccessful until 1994, when Patrick Moore, Yuan Chang, and colleagues identified a new gammaherpesvirus in a Kaposi's sarcoma lesion.[108] This virus, which is called either Kaposi's sarcoma–associated herpesvirus or human herpesvirus 8, was subsequently found to also be the etiologic agent for primary effusion lymphoma (PEL) and for many cases of multicentric Castleman's disease (MCD) (see Table 45–1).[109,110] Primary KSHV infection in children can cause a febrile illness associated with a maculopapular skin rash,[111] but many such infections appear to be clinically silent. There was one report suggesting that KSHV was associated with multiple myeloma, but this was not confirmed in a number of subsequent studies.[112] Also, there was a recent report linking KSHV to certain cases of pulmonary hypertension,[113] but the significance of this association is uncertain at this time.

Kaposi's Sarcoma

Epidemiology and Risk Factors

Kaposi's sarcoma is a multicentric, angioproliferative tumor that most frequently involves the skin (Fig. 45–7). It was originally described by Moritz Kaposi in 1872 as an indolent tumor developing in elderly men.[114] A sudden increase in Kaposi's sarcoma among young gay men in certain coastal cities in the United States was one of the earliest indications of the AIDS epidemic, and Kaposi's sarcoma has been the most frequent HIV-associated tumor. There are several epidemiologically distinct forms of Kaposi's sarcoma: a classic form most commonly arising in elderly men in countries bordering the Mediterranean Sea; a more aggressive endemic form developing in both men and women in Africa; the epidemic form associated with HIV infection; a form observed in HIV-negative gay men; and a form developing in transplant recipients. It is now known that all forms are manifestations of the same disease and all are caused by KSHV infection.[115–119] Moreover, the prevalence of Kaposi's sarcoma roughly parallels the prevalence of KSHV in different populations around the world.

In the absence of immunosuppression, only about 1 in 400 to 1 in 1500 KSHV-infected individuals develop Kaposi's sarcoma. However, as many as one in two patients co-infected with HIV and KSHV will develop Kaposi's sarcoma.[118,120–122] Among HIV-infected individuals, Kaposi's sarcoma is much more common in men who have sex with men than in those in other risk groups. Although KSHV can be detected in blood and occasionally in semen, it can most readily be found in saliva, and this appears to be the main mode of spread from one individual to another.[123,124]

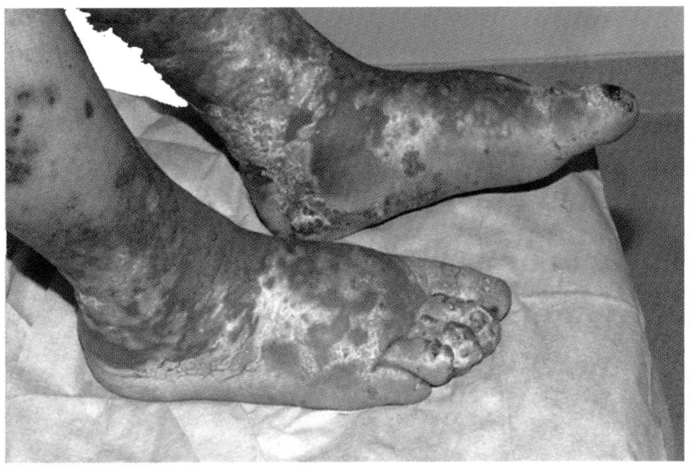

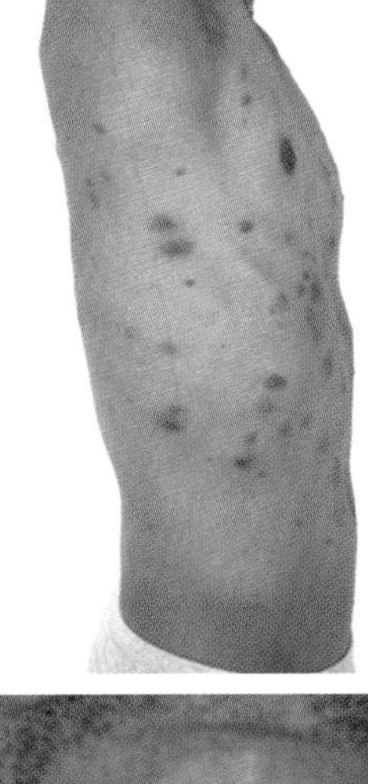

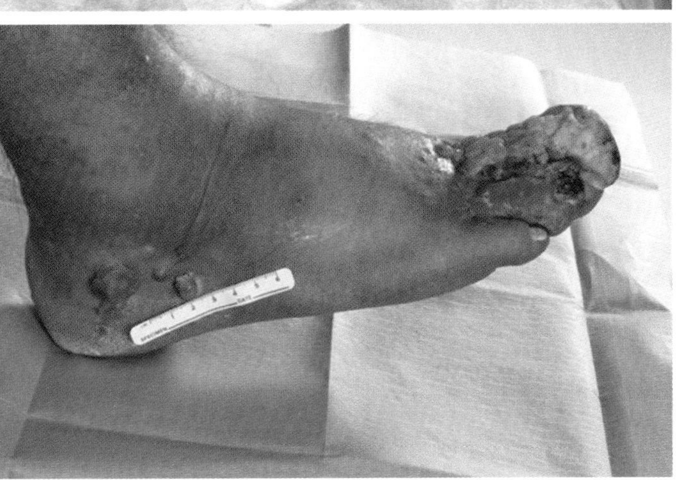

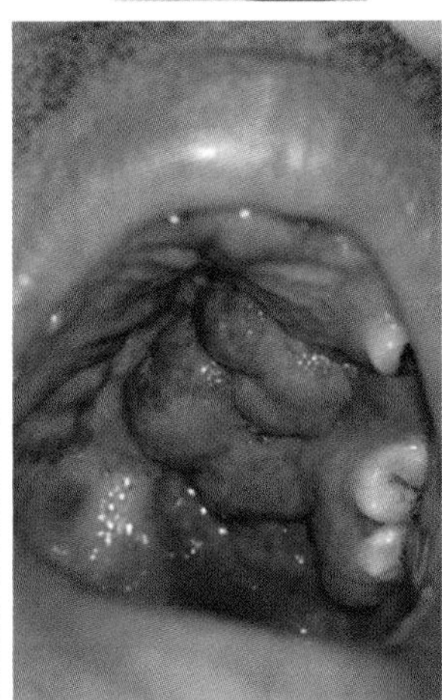

Figure 45–7. Kaposi's sarcoma (KS) in the era of HAART. Shown are photos of KS involving the feet *(left upper and lower panels)*, skin *(right upper panel)*, and upper palate *(right lower panel)*.

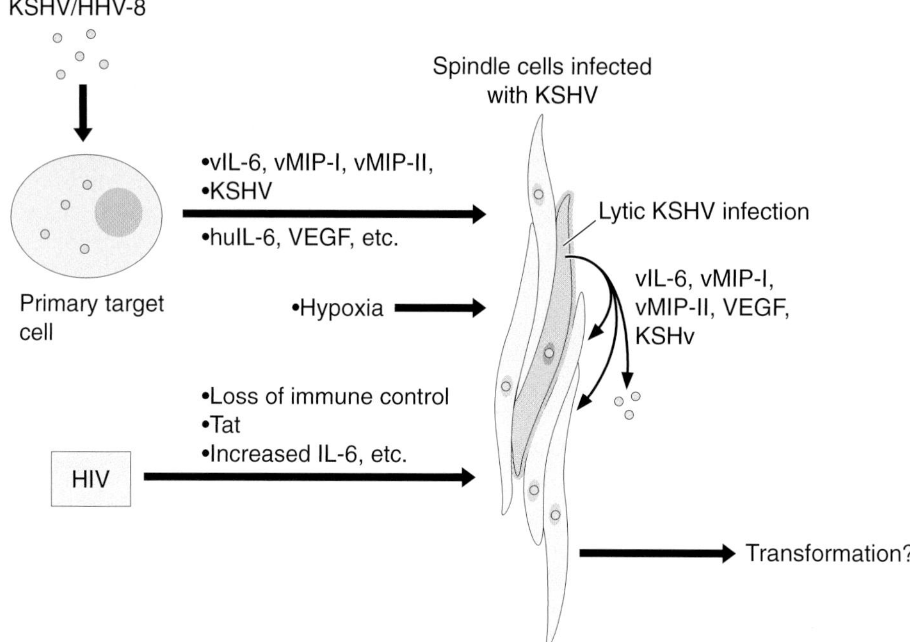

Figure 45–8. Proposed model for the pathogenesis of Kaposi's sarcoma. In this model, a circulating KSHV-infected cell, perhaps a B cell or monocyte, infects an endothelial spindle cell precursor with KSHV. This infected cell becomes a spindle cell and proliferates in response to a number of factors, including KSHV-encoded factors (such as viral interleukin-6 [IL-6] and macrophage inflammatory proteins MIP-1, MIP-2, and MIP-3) and cellular factors induced by KSHV (such as cellular vascular endothelial growth factor [VEGF] and IL-6). Lytic KSHV infection in a minority of the spindle cells (which can be augmented by hypoxia) contributes to the process. HIV contributes through immunosuppression and immune dysregulation (with increased IL-6 and other cytokines). Also, HIV Tat protein may aid in infection of endothelial cells by KSHV. It is possible that transformation of the lesion may occur late in the disease process.

Pathogenesis

The lesions of Kaposi's sarcoma are characterized by spindle cells that are believed to be of lymphatic endothelial cell origin.[125,126] Most of the spindle cells in Kaposi's sarcoma lesions contain KSHV in a latent form, and detection of KSHV-encoded latency-associated nuclear antigen can be useful in making the pathologic diagnosis of Kaposi's sarcoma.[127] At any given time, a minority of Kaposi's sarcoma spindle cells are undergoing KSHV lytic infection (Fig. 45–8). KSHV encodes for a number of factors with direct or indirect angiogenic properties, and it is believed that these factors play a major role in the pathogenesis of Kaposi's sarcoma. Among the factors with direct angiogenic activity are viral analogues of interleukin-6 (viral IL-6) and three macrophage inflammatory proteins (viral MIP-1, MIP-2, and MIP-3).[128–130] In addition, KSHV encodes for a constitutively active G protein–coupled receptor that activates hypoxia inducible factor and induces the secretion of vascular endothelial growth factor and other proangiogenic factors.[131,132]

The genes for the factors noted previously are for the most part expressed during the early stages of lytic replication and can in turn promote the growth of spindle cells. Thus, it appears that production of proangiogenic and related factors by the few cells undergoing lytic KSHV replication plays a major role in the pathogenesis of Kaposi's sarcoma. There is recent evidence that hypoxia can induce KSHV replication and specifically activate certain lytic genes,[133,134] and this may explain why Kaposi's sarcoma preferentially develops in areas of the body with a relatively poor blood supply (such as the feet). It is unclear at this time whether Kaposi's sarcoma is a polyclonal hyperproliferative condition, or whether clonal tumor expansion occurs in some patients.[135,136] It is possible that clonal transformation occurs only in the more advanced stages of the disease.

In patients infected with KSHV, HIV is a substantial risk factor promoting the development of Kaposi's sarcoma. Some of the reasons for this association include HIV-induced immunodeficiency, HIV-associated immunologic dysregulation with an increase in IL-6 and related cytokines, spindle cell growth induced by HIV Tat protein, and enhanced KSHV cell entry induced by Tat.[137–140] With the widespread use of HAART in Western countries, there has been a decrease in the incidence of HIV-associated Kaposi's sarcoma.[141,142]

Staging and Treatment

With regard to the staging of Kaposi's sarcoma, it is important to remember that this is a multicentric disease

TABLE 45–6. Staging Classifications for HIV-Associated Kaposi's Sarcoma*

	Good Risk (0)	Poor Risk (1)
Tumor (T)	Confined to skin and/or lymph nodes, and/or oral disease confined to the palate.	Tumor-associated edema or ulceration; extensive oral Kaposi's sarcoma (KS); gastrointestinal KS; or KS in other non-nodal viscera.
Immune system (I)	CD4 cells ≥150 μL	CD4 cells <150 μL
Systemic illness (S)	No history of opportunistic infection or thrush; no B symptoms (unexplained fever, night sweats, >10% involuntary weight loss; or diarrhea) persisting for more than 2 wk; Karnofsky performance status ≥70	History of opportunistic infections and/or thrush; B symptoms present; Karnofsky performance status <70; other HIV-related illnesses (e.g., neurologic disease, lymphoma).

*Schema based on Krown et al. [143] and Nasti et al. [144] In the ACTG criteria, patients are scored separately on the three criteria (e.g., $T_1I_0S_1$) and considered poor risk overall if they are poor risk in any of the criteria. The original classification called for a CD4 cutoff of 200 cells/μL, but this was later revised to 150 cells/μL. It was recently proposed by Nasti et al. [144] that the CD4 count is not of independent prognostic value in the era of HAART and that patients are poor risk overall if they are T_1S_1.

and that the existence of multiple lesions does not mean that the disease has metastasized. A classification system developed by the AIDS Clinical Trials Group (ACTG) for HIV-associated Kaposi's sarcoma classifies patients as good or poor risk based on their extent of tumor, the status of their immune system, and the degree of systemic illness[143] (Table 45–6). Patients were categorized as good risk or poor risk in each of the categories, and patients who were poor risk in any category were deemed poor risk. It has been suggested recently that the CD4 count does not independently confer prognostic information and that the system should be revised so that only patients who are poor risk in both the tumor and systemic illness categories are termed poor risk overall.[144] Both systems are currently in use today. Because Kaposi's sarcoma is a multicentric disease, it has been a challenge to define tumor responses to therapy. Many investigators use systems based on that of the ACTG, in which a complete response is defined as the absence of all tumor tissue and a partial response as a 50% decrease in the total number of lesions, the total area of several "marker" lesions, the number of nodular lesions, or the size of measurable visceral disease in the absence of disease progression.[145]

For patients with HIV-associated Kaposi's sarcoma, it has also been observed that effective treatment of the underlying HIV infection with HAART can induce remission of Kaposi's sarcoma in as many as 20–40% of patients.[146–148] Remissions are most likely to occur in patients who have not previously received antiretroviral therapy, who have good-risk Kaposi's sarcoma, and who have a good-risk HIV viral load and good immunologic response to HAART. A recent study found that patients with advanced Kaposi's sarcoma who are already on HAART are very unlikely to respond to antiretroviral therapy alone.[149]

There is no evidence that patients with Kaposi's sarcoma can be "cured" with any available therapy or that achieving a complete response prevents disease recurrence. The goal of therapy in Kaposi's sarcoma is thus to achieve long-term control with acceptable toxicity. All patients with HIV-associated Kaposi's sarcoma should be treated with effective antiretroviral therapy, and in some cases this may be sufficient. For those patients needing additional specific Kaposi's sarcoma therapy, this should be given along with HAART whenever possible. Patients with a few local lesions may be treated with any of a variety of approaches, including local radiation therapy, electron beam therapy, cryotherapy, photodynamic therapy, or intralesional chemotherapy.[118,150–156] Surgical excision is rarely worthwhile, and there is even evidence that Kaposi's sarcoma may develop in wound edges.[157] HIV-infected patients often develop excessive toxicity from radiotherapy, especially in mucosal surfaces, and lower doses than usual are recommended. Topical 9-*cis*-retinoic acid (alitretinoin gel) is approved for treatment of cutaneous Kaposi's sarcoma, but can cause local inflammation and skin lightening.[158] Systemic interferon alfa is approved for Kaposi's sarcoma and has been found to be most effective in patients with over 100–150 CD4 cells/μL and disease confined to the skin.[159,160] However, its use must be weighed against the systemic toxicities, including fever, malaise, and occasional depression.

Patients with more advanced Kaposi's sarcoma are generally treated with cytotoxic chemotherapy. It is impossible to give clear-cut guidelines for the use of such therapy in Kaposi's sarcoma, and the decision must be individualized based on the extent of disease and the degree to which it distresses the patient. Some disease characteristics that would lead to a consideration of cytotoxic therapy include extensive disease, painful lesions, Kaposi's sarcoma–associated edema or effusions, visceral disease, or unsightly disease. A number of cytotoxic agents have been found to be effective in Kaposi's sarcoma, including the vinca alkaloids, bleomycin, and the anthracyclines.[161,162] Most physicians with expertise in treating Kaposi's sarcoma now consider pegylated liposomal doxorubicin (Doxil) or liposomal daunorubicin (DaunoXome) as first-line therapy.[163–165] These approaches have in general replaced combination chemotherapy approaches for patients with advanced Kaposi's sarcoma because of equivalent activity but lower toxicity. Paclitaxel has been found to have substantial activity in patients with advanced Kaposi's sarcoma or who have failed anthracyclines, and it is now approved by the U.S. Food and Drug Administration for the latter indication.[166,167]

A problem with such therapies, however, is that they can have cumulative toxicity, especially in patients with underlying immunodeficiency from HIV disease. There is thus an interest in developing pathogenesis-based approaches. Antiherpes drugs have been considered, and there is evidence that ganciclovir can reduce the incidence of Kaposi's sarcoma in patients with advanced AIDS.[168] There are also a few case reports describing regression of Kaposi's sarcoma with antiherpes drugs.[169] However, a small trial of cidofovir failed to show any tumor responses,[170] and the available information at this time would argue against the use of antiherpes treatment for established Kaposi's sarcoma. The lesions of Kaposi's sarcoma are highly vascular, and in fact it is intralesional and extravasated blood that gives the lesions their typical purplish hue. Over the past few years, several antiangiogenic approaches have been tested. Thalidomide (which has both antiangiogenic and immunomodulatory activity) was shown in uncontrolled trials to have activity, but its use was accompanied by substantial toxicity.[171,172] Recently, two other agents with antiangiogenic effects, Col-3 and interleukin-12, were shown to induce Kaposi's sarcoma tumor responses.[173,174] The next few years are likely to see continued research in antiangiogenic approaches to Kaposi's sarcoma therapy.

Primary Effusion Lymphoma

KSHV causes two malignant or hyperproliferative conditions in which the target cell is a B cell: PEL and MCD. PEL is a lymphoma that develops in effusions in the pleura, peritoneum, or other body cavities, usually without an associated tumor mass (Fig. 45–9). Although such tumors had been described in the literature before the discovery of KSHV,[175] PEL was defined as a distinct clinical entity only when the association of this unusual tumor with KSHV was appreciated.[109,176,177] Some cases of PEL are infected with KSHV alone, but over 80% are co-infected with EBV.[109,176] PEL is usually seen in HIV-infected patients with fewer than 200 circulating CD4 cells/μL, and many patients have preexisting Kaposi's sarcoma. Although it is often considered a rare tumor, PEL may be underdiagnosed; in a recent study from Italy, it was found to comprise about 4% of cases of NHL in AIDS.[178]

The tumors exhibit a distinctive morphology with features of anaplastic and large-cell lymphoma.[109,176,177] They usually do not express B-cell surface antigens, but most cases show clonal rearrangement of immunoglobulin genes indicating a B-cell origin of the tumors.[179] PEL cells generally express CD45 and one or more activation-associated antigens. KSHV exists in a latent form, although there is often limited lytic gene expression.[180–182] There is evidence that secretion of viral IL-6, interleukin-10, and vascular endothelial growth factor by PEL cells contributes to the pathogenesis of this unusual tumor.[130,183]

Classic PEL tumors are characterized by their lack of solid tumor masses. However, they can sometimes invade tissues late in the course of the disease.[109,176] Also, KSHV can sometimes cause solid immunoblastic lymphomas that resemble PEL histologically and may or may not be associated with effusions.[184] There is no standard therapy for PEL.[178] Many cases are treated with antilymphoma chemotherapy regimens, but the outcome is often poor and, even when responses are achieved, many patients relapse. In a recent single-institution study, the median survival was 6 months.[178]

Multicentric Castleman's Disease

MCD is a rare systemic lymphoproliferative disease in which a prominent clinical feature is constitutional symptomatology related to cytokine overproduction. In patients with HIV infection, almost all MCD cases are associated with KSHV, whereas in HIV-negative cases,

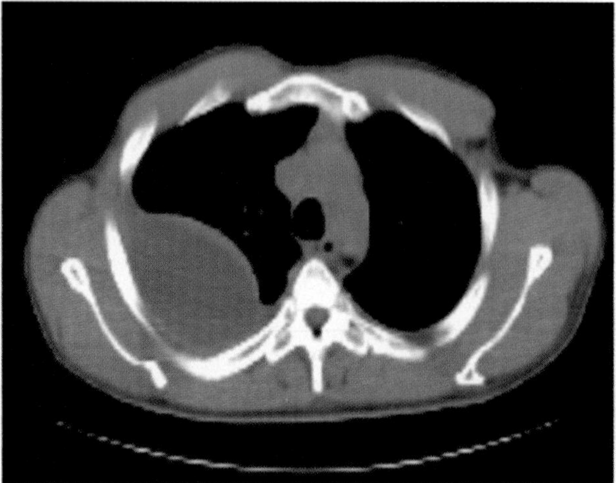

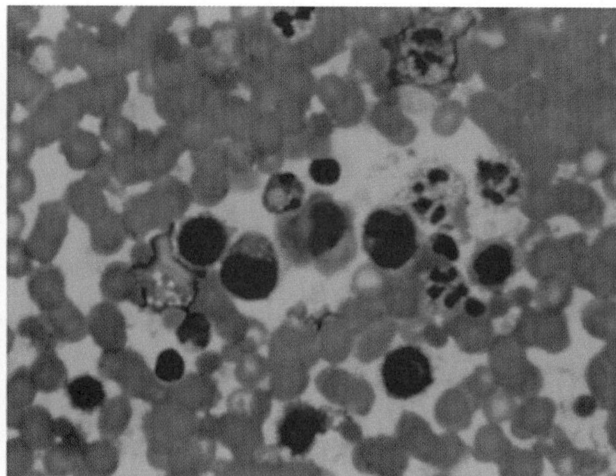

Figure 45–9. *Left,* Chest computed tomography scan of a patient with PEL, showing extensive pulmonary effusion. *Right,* Hematoxylin and eosin–stained pleural fluid cell block section of PEL effusion. The cells exhibit cytomorphologic features that appear to bridge large-cell immunoblastic lymphoma and anaplastic large-cell lymphoma.

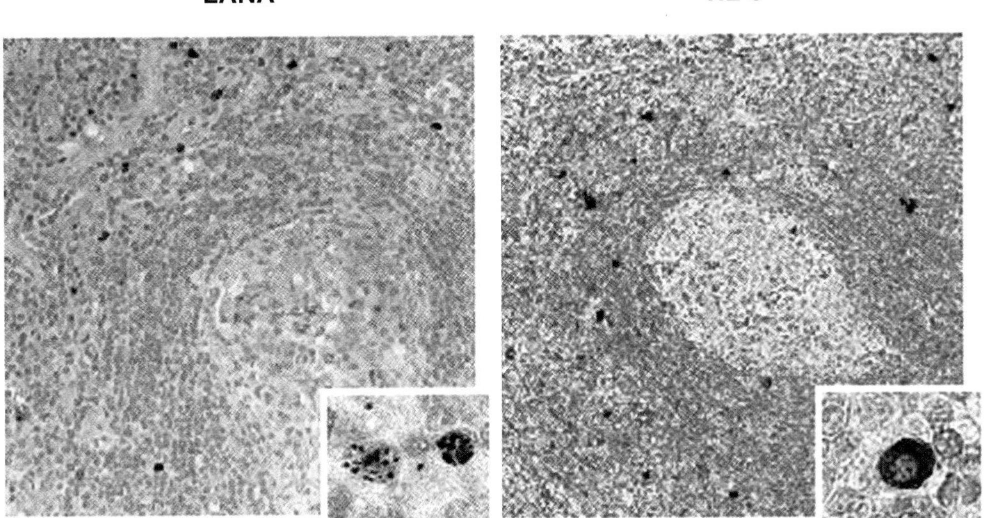

Figure 45–10. Photomicrograph of a lymph node involved with HIV-associated multicentric Castleman's disease stained with KSHV latency-associated nuclear antigen (LANA), a latent antigen *(left)*, and KSHV viral IL-6, a lytic antigen *(right)*. *Insets* show details of a representative cell at higher magnification. As can be seen, most KSHV-infected cells express both latent and lytic antigens, including viral IL-6, the cause of much of the symptomatology of this disease. (Adapted from Aoki Y, Tosato G, Fonville TW, Pittaluga S: Serum viral interleukin-6 in AIDS-related multicentric Castleman disease. Blood 97:2526–2527, 2001, with permission.)

about 40% are related to KSHV.[185] MCD can occur in hyaline vascular and plasma cell histologic types, and KSHV-associated MCD most often resembles the plasma cell type.[186] The histology is often characterized by small hyalinized germinal centers surrounded by layers of small lymphocytes. Immunohistochemical staining shows a number of plasmablasts expressing KSHV latency-associated nuclear antigen; although polyclonal, almost all of these cells usually express immunoglobulin M λ chain.[187,188] Interestingly, KSHV-infected cells in MCD frequently show expression of KSHV viral IL-6 and other lytic KSHV genes (Fig. 45–10).[180,181,189]

Clinically, MCD is characterized by recurrent high fevers, constitutional symptoms, hepatosplenomegaly, and lymphadenopathy.[186] The patients often have cytopenias, hepatic dysfunction, and renal dysfunction. C-reactive protein levels are frequently elevated.[190] Research studies have shown that these patients often have high serum levels of viral and/or cellular IL-6, and this is believed to be responsible for many of the features of the disease.[182,191,192] MCD patients may also have Kaposi's sarcoma, and a number go on to develop NHL.

There have been few prospective studies of this condition, and there is no defined therapy. The median survival is approximately 2.5 years. In small pilot studies, antibodies to IL-6 or the IL-6 receptor were found to give symptomatic relief and a reduction of lymphadenopathy.[193,194] Much of the remaining clinical literature consists of case reports, and a problem in evaluating such studies is that the disease can spontaneously wax and wane. Among the therapies that have been reported to be beneficial in one or more cases are single-agent vinblastine, interferon alfa, and multiagent lymphoma chemotherapy. Ganciclovir therapy has recently been reported to have activity in three cases.[195] As we learn more about the pathogenesis of this condition, it is possible that other therapies based on an understanding of disease pathogenesis will be developed.

CURRENT CONTROVERSIES & FUTURE CONSIDERATIONS

Epstein-Barr Virus–Related and Kaposi's Sarcoma–Associated Herpesvirus–Related Neoplasms

- What is the role of these herpesviruses in the pathogenesis of the tumors that develop in the absence T-cell immunodeficiency, such as endemic Burkitt's lymphoma, nasopharyngeal carcinoma, or T-cell or NK cell lymphomas?
- Can we devise therapies for these diseases that target or exploit the presence of the oncogenic virus?
- What is the specific therapeutic role of HAART during the treatment for AIDS-associated NHL with curative intent?
- Can we devise strategies, based on parameters related to the oncogenic virus, to assess the risk of these tumors developing in immunosuppressed patients, and develop strategies to prevent their occurrence?

Suggested Readings*

Antman K, Chang Y: Kaposi's sarcoma. N Engl J Med 342:1027–1038, 2000.

Boshoff C, Weiss R: AIDS-related malignancies. Nat Rev Cancer 2:373–382, 2002.

Lo KW, To KF, Huang DP: Focus on nasopharyngeal carcinoma. Cancer Cell 5:423–428, 2004.

Straus SE, Cohen JI, Tosato G, Meyer J: Epstein-Barr virus infections: biology pathogenesis, and management. Ann Intern Med 118:45–48, 1993.

Young NS, Beris P (eds): Herpesviruses in hematology. Semin Hematol 40:105–171, 2003.

Full references for this chapter can be found on accompanying CD-ROM.

CHAPTER 46

CRYOGLOBULINEMIA

Clodoveo Ferri, MD, Anna Linda Zignego, MD, and Stefano A. Pileri, MD

KEY POINTS

Cryoglobulinemia

- The presence in the serum of one or more immunoglobulins that reversibly precipitate at temperatures below 37°C is termed *cryoglobulinemia.*

Diagnosis and Differential Diagnosis

- Cryoglobulinemia type I, composed of single monoclonal immunoglobulin (Ig), represents a paraprotein generally associated with hematologic disorders (lymphoplasmacytic lymphoma/Waldenström's macroglobulinemia, multiple myeloma, etc.). It is per se asymptomatic, with the exception of possible hyperviscosity syndrome.
- Mixed cryoglobulinemia, type II (polyclonal IgG-monoclonal IgM) or type III (polyclonal IgG-polyclonal IgM), is an immune complex–mediated systemic vasculitis (leukocytoclastic vasculitis) involving the small vessels.
- Mixed cryoglobulinemia may be secondary to various immunologic, hematologic, and infectious diseases, or it can represent a distinct disorder, "essential" mixed cryoglobulinemia. Since the causative role of hepatitis C virus (HCV) has been definitely established, the term *essential* is now used to refer to only a small percentage of patients.
- There are no diagnostic criteria for mixed cryoglobulinemia. Classification criteria include serum mixed cryoglobulins, hypocomplementemia (low C4), leukocytoclastic vasculitis, a typical clinical triad (purpura, weakness, arthralgias), and multiple organ involvement (liver, kidney, peripheral nerves; widespread vasculitis; neoplastic disorders, mainly B-cell lymphomas).
- Mixed cryoglobulinemia may share various clinicoserologic features with different immunologic/neoplastic diseases—in particular other systemic vasculitides, Sjögren's syndrome, autoimmune hepatitis, and B-cell lymphomas.

Treatment

- Treatment of cryoglobulinemia type I is mainly directed to the underlying disorders.
- Treatment of mixed cryoglobulinemia syndrome is particularly challenging because of its complex etiopathogenesis, including HCV infection and autoimmune and lymphoproliferative alterations. The disease can be treated at three different levels by means of etiologic, pathogenetic, and/or symptomatic therapies.
- An attempt to eradicate the HCV infection (interferon ± ribavirin) should be made in all patients with HCV-related mixed cryoglobulinemia, particularly in those with active hepatitis.
- The immunosuppressors (cyclophosphamide or rituximab), alone or in combination with high-dose steroids and/or plasma exchange, can be usefully employed in mixed cryoglobulinemia patients with severe/active complications (glomerulonephritis, widespread vasculitis, sensorimotor neuropathy).
- Symptomatic therapy includes low- to medium-dose steroids, plasma exchange, and a low-antigen-content diet.
- Asymptomatic mixed cryoglobulinemia patients do not need any treatment, and mild manifestations generally require only symptomatic therapies (low-dose steroids, low-antigen-content diet).

Prognosis

- Mixed cryoglobulinemia patients have a significantly reduced life expectancy compared to the general population. Poor prognostic factors are patient age greater than 60 years at the time of diagnosis, male gender, and renal involvement.
- Careful clinical monitoring of mixed cryoglobulinemia patients is mandatory, with particular attention to neoplastic complications (B-cell lymphomas, hepatocellular carcinoma, and thyroid cancer).

INTRODUCTION

Definition

Cryoglobulinemia is defined as the presence in the serum of one (monoclonal cryoimmunoglobulinemia) or more (mixed cryoglobulinemia) immunoglobulins (Igs), which

TABLE 46–1. Classification of Cryoglobulins

	Type I Cryoglobulinemia	Type II Mixed Cryoglobulinemia	Type II–III Mixed Cryoglobulinemia	Type III Mixed Cryoglobulinemia
Composition/ biologic characteristics	Single monoclonal Ig (IgG, A, M) or Bence-Jones proteins Self-aggregation through Fc fragment of Ig	Monoclonal component (usually IgM) Polyclonal Ig (mainly IgG) predominant, cross idiotype WA mRF (IgM)* Aggregation through RF and Fc portion of IgG	Oligoclonal IgM component Polyclonal Ig (mainly IgG) predominant, cross idiotype WA mRF (IgM) Aggregation through RF and Fc portion of IgG	Polyclonal mixed Ig (all isotypes) RF activity of one polyclonal component (usually IgM) Aggregation through RF and Fc portion of IgG
Pathologic characteristics	Tissue histologic alterations of underlying disorder	Leukocytoclastic vasculitis B-lymphocyte expansion and tissue B-cell infiltrates	Leukocytoclastic vasculitis B-lymphocyte expansion and tissue B-cell infiltrates	Leukocytoclastic vasculitis B-lymphocyte expansion and tissue B-cell infiltrates
Underlying diseases	Lymphoproliferative disorders: multiple myeloma, Waldenström's macroglobulinemia CLL, B-cell NHL	"Essential" or secondary to infections (HCV, others) Autoimmune/ lymphoproliferative disorders	"Essential" or secondary to infections (HCV, others) Autoimmune/ lymphoproliferative disorders	"Essential" or secondary to infections (HCV, other viruses, bacterial, fungal, parasitic) Autoimmune disorders
Clinical manifestations	Hemorheologic disturbances Acrocyanosis, gangrene, Raynaud's phenomenon Occlusive vasculopathy	Purpura, arthralgias, weakness Systemic IC vasculitis Complicating B-cell NHL	Purpura, arthralgias, weakness Systemic IC vasculitis Complicating B-cell NHL	Purpura, arthralgias, weakness Systemic IC vasculitis

*For information on WA monoclonal rheumatoid factors (mRF) see Gorevic and Frangione,[3] Abel et al.,[16] and Knight and Agnello.[36]
Abbreviations: CLL, chronic lymphocytic leukemia; HCV, hepatitis C virus; IC, immune complex; Ig, immunoglobulin; NHL, non-Hodgkin's lymphoma; RF, rheumatoid factor.

precipitate at temperatures below 37°C and redissolve on rewarming.[1–6] This is an in vitro phenomenon; the intimate mechanism(s) of cryoprecipitation still remain obscure. It could be secondary to intrinsic characteristics of mono- or polyclonal immunoglobulin components, or it may be caused by the interaction among single components of the cryoprecipitate.[1–6]

Classification

Cryoglobulinemia is traditionally classified into three subgroups[4]: type I, composed of single monoclonal immunoglobulin, usually a paraprotein; and type II and type III mixed cryoglobulinemias, immune complexes composed of polyclonal IgGs (the autoantigens) and mono- or polyclonal IgMs, respectively. The IgMs are the corresponding autoantibodies with rheumatoid factor activity (Table 46–1). Cryoglobulinemia type I is found mainly in patients with overt lymphoid tumors (i.e., lymphoplasmacytic lymphoma/Waldenström's macroglobulinemia, multiple myeloma, etc.)[2–6] (see Table 46–1); it is generally asymptomatic, but in a few cases can be complicated by hyperviscosity syndrome. Mixed cryoglobulinemia types II and III can be associated with various infectious, immunologic, or neoplastic diseases.[2–6] Cryoprecipitates are analyzed by immunoelectrophoresis, immunofixation, immunoblotting, or two-dimensional polyacrylamide gel electrophoresis. Type II–III mixed cryoglobulinemia may be composed of oligoclonal IgMs or polyclonal immunoglobulins.[7] The composition of this particular serologic subset seems to reflect the most recent molecular studies showing the presence of oligoclonal B-lymphocyte proliferation in liver and bone marrow biopsies in the majority of patients with type II mixed cryoglobulinemia.[8,9]

Variable amounts of circulating mixed cryoglobulins are commonly detected in a great number of infectious, immunologic, or neoplastic disorders.[2–6] Mixed cryoglobulinemia, first described in 1966 as "essential" but now known to be associated with hepatitis C virus (HCV) infection, represents a distinct disorder[5] and presents with a typical clinical triad—purpura, arthralgias, and weakness—and frequent multiple organ involvement (Fig. 46–1; see Table 46–2 later).[2–6]

EPIDEMIOLOGY AND RISK FACTORS

The prevalence of mixed cryoglobulinemia presents great geographic heterogeneity, being more common in Southern Europe than in Northern Europe or Northern America. The disease is considered to be a relatively rare disorder; however, as yet there are no adequate epidemiologic studies regarding its overall prevalence. Mixed cryoglobulinemia syndrome affects predominantly women (female/male ratio = 3.7:1), and the disease onset varies between the fourth and sixth decades[10] (see Table 46–2 later).

Environmental Factors

Although chronic hepatitis may be observed in patients with mixed cryoglobulinemia,[2,3,6,11,12] hepatitis B virus (HBV), potentially involved in another systemic vasculitis, i.e., the polyarteritis nodosa,[13] is a causative factor of mixed cryoglobulinemia in fewer than 5% of individ-

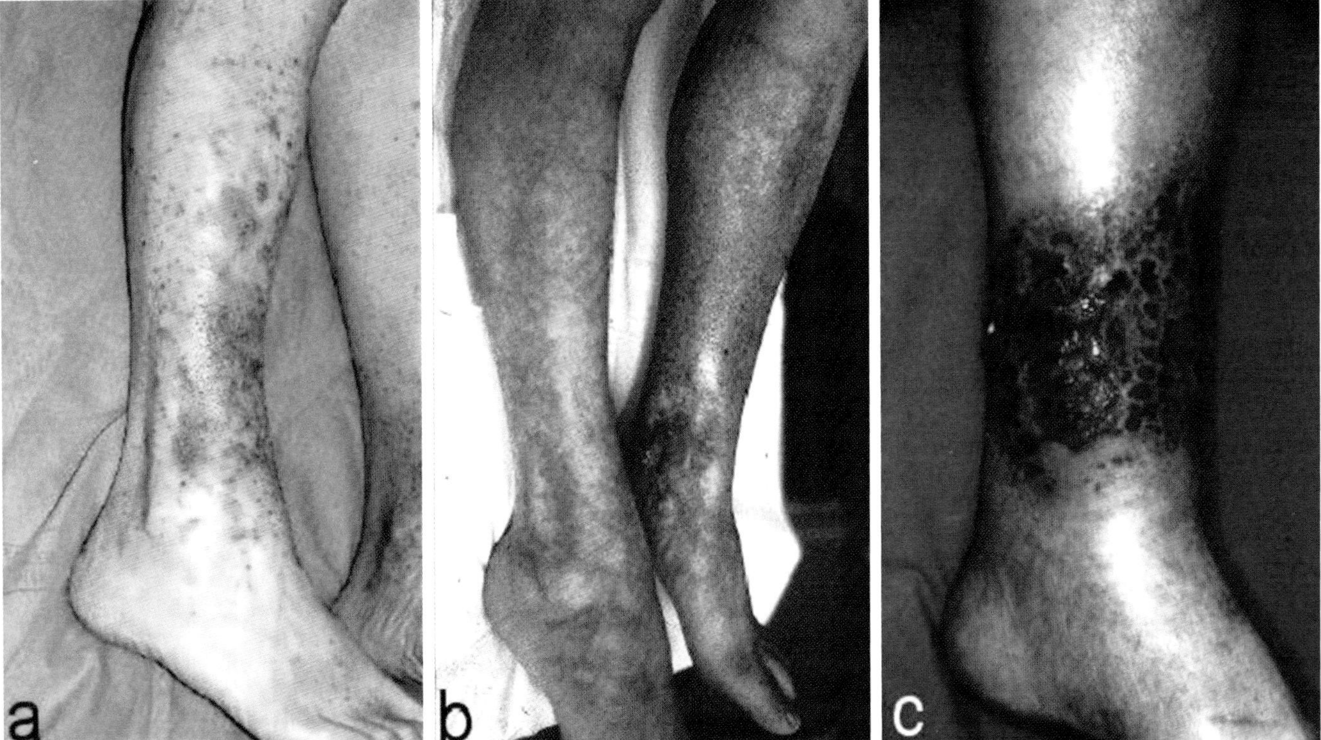

Figure 46–1. Cutaneous cryoglobulinemic vasculitis. *A,* Recent onset, palpable purpura on the legs with both isolated and confluent purpuric lesions. *B,* Ochreous coloration of the skin with stocking distribution caused by chronic hemosiderin deposits in a patient with mixed cryoglobulinemia of 15 years' duration; a residual perimalleolar scar is seen on the left leg from a healed vasculitic ulcer. *C,* Large and torpid ulcer on the left leg with diffuse hyperpigmentation of the surrounding skin.

uals.[6] Conversely, epidemiologic studies suggest an important role for HCV in the pathogenesis of mixed cryoglobulinemia[14–18] because the prevalence of serum anti-HCV antibodies varies from 70% to 100% of individuals.[17] HCV RNA is often markedly concentrated (1000-fold) in the cryoprecipitates,[16] and direct involvement of HCV antigens may occur in immune complex–mediated cryoglobulinemic vasculitis.[6,19,20]

Genetic Factors

The low incidence of mixed cryoglobulinemia in HCV-infected individuals[21,22] suggests other environmental, geographic, and/or genetic factors.[6,23]

PATHOPHYSIOLOGY

Small Vessel Systemic Vasculitis

The histopathologic hallmark of mixed cryoglobulinemia is the leukocytoclastic vasculitis (Fig. 46–2) of small vessels, including arterioles, capillaries, and venules,[2,3,6,18,20] as a result of vessel deposition of circulating immune complexes, mainly the cryoglobulins, and complement. It is a necrotizing vasculitis characterized by extensive fibrinoid necrosis of the vessel wall with permeation of the wall by disintegrating neutrophils. The consequence of vasculitis is the ischemic organ damage responsible for different clinical manifestations of mixed cryoglobulinemia syndrome (Fig. 46–3): skin purpura and ulcers (see Fig. 46–1), peripheral neuropathy, glomerulonephritis, lung alveolitis, endocrine disorders, and diffuse vasculitis (see Table 46–2 later).[2,3,6]

B-Cell Proliferation

Whereas the immune complex–mediated vasculitis is the final step of this complex process, unregulated B-lymphocyte expansion,[3] perhaps resulting from HCV infection, may initiate the process. The B cell population may expand as an immune response to HCV, but B cells may also be infected and proliferate, leading to a high frequency of HCV RNA–positive lymphocytes in peripheral blood and bone marrow of cryoglobulinemic patients.[24–26] In addition, cross-reactive autoantibodies directed to both HCV antigens and antigens of the host may contribute to the syndrome.[6,23] In type II mixed cryoglobulinemia complicated by B-cell non-Hodgkin's lymphoma (B-NHL), the analysis of lymph node sections showed that viral proteins were detectable in the cytoplasm of lymphoid cells in the lymph node cortex or in the tumoral tissue, whereas frankly anaplastic cells were negative. These findings suggest that, in patients with type II mixed cryoglobulinemia, the B-cell infection precedes tumoral transformation.[27]

The exact malignant transformation potential of HCV is not clear, because it is a nonintegrating RNA tumor virus. Although the action of viral proteins is likely,[28] major effects on intracellular signaling transduction pathways have not been identified.[29] Likewise, co-infection by HCV and other lymphotropic viruses does not appear etiologic,[30,31] even though in vitro studies showed that Epstein-Barr virus nuclear antigen 1 is able to enhance HCV replication.[32] Laboratory investigations in HCV-positive type II MC suggest the importance of a chronic stimulation of the B-cell by HCV epitopes; in this context, some B-cell subpopulations with favorable and/or dominant genetic characteristics will emerge.[6,23,33,34] This hypothesis recalls the pathogenetic role of *Helicobacter pylori* in MALT lymphoma of the stomach, for which different evolutive phases are requested.[6]

HCV E2 protein binds CD81 (a tetraspannin on the surface of B cells), and this may amplify the physiological polyclonal stimulation of the B-cell compartment induced by HCV infection.[35] Most cases of HCV-related lymphoproliferation have t(14;18) translocation or *bcl*-2 rearrangement, present in up to 85% of cases of type II mixed cryoglobulinemia.[37,38] The antiviral treatment generally utilized for HCV-related liver diseases might also play a role in prevention of the development of mixed cryoglobulinemia and probably of different B-cell lymphoproliferative disorders.[38,39] Thus, malignant transformation as well as clonal proliferation appears to be a multistep process (Fig. 46–4).

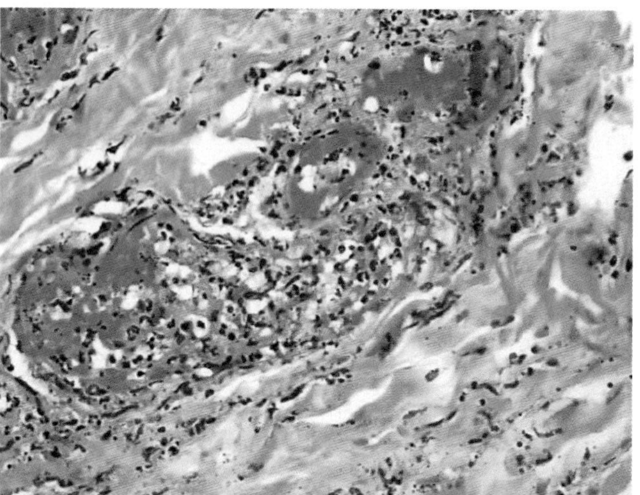

Figure 46–2. Severe necrotizing leukocytoclastic vasculitis: extensive fibrinoid necrosis of the vessel wall with permeation of the wall by disintegrating neutrophils. Leukocytoclastic vasculitis is secondary to the vessel deposition of circulating immune complexes, mainly the cryoglobulins, and complement.

Histopathologic Alterations

The B-cell lymphoma observed in patients with type II mixed cryoglobulinemia[6,23] may be a diffuse large B-cell lymphoma (observed in 40–50% of cases), marginal-zone lymphoma (extranodal, nodal, or splenic), or, more rarely, B-cell chronic lymphocytic leukemia and lymphoplasmacytic lymphoma (Fig. 46–5).[40–42] These lower grade indolent lymphomas are also termed *monotypic lymphoproliferative disorders of undetermined significance* (MLDUS).[1,23,42] Of interest, type II mixed cryoglobulinemia–related MLDUS has its highest incidence in the same geographic areas where about 30% of "idiopathic" B-cell lymphoma patients also display HCV positivity, and where an increased prevalence of HCV genotype 2a/c has been observed in both mixed cryoglobulinemia and B-cell lymphoma.[23,43]

Type II mixed cryoglobulinemia–associated MLDUS presents two main pathologic patterns: B-cell chronic lymphocytic leukemia–like and lymphoplasmacytic lymphoma–like[23] (see Fig. 46–5). The former latter is characterized by CD79a$^+$ CD5$^+$ CD23$^+$ lymphoid infiltrates in the liver and bone marrow, which consist of small lymphocytes, prolymphocytes, and paraimmunoblasts and show moderate immunoglobulin expression with monotypic restriction on immunohistochemistry studies.[44] Infiltrates tend to remain unmodified in the bone marrow and may undergo spontaneous regression in the liver in

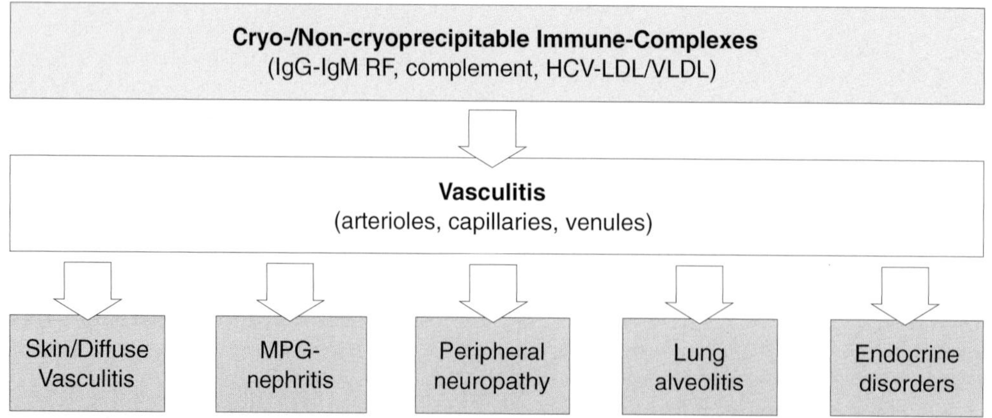

Figure 46–3. Cryoglobulinemic vasculitis involving small vessels (arterioles, capillaries, and venules) is secondary to the vessel deposition of circulating immune complexes, mainly the cryoglobulins, and complement. Cryoprecipitates may also include concentrated HCV virions along with low-density and very-low-density lipoproteins. Vasculitic lesions are responsible for damage to various organs.

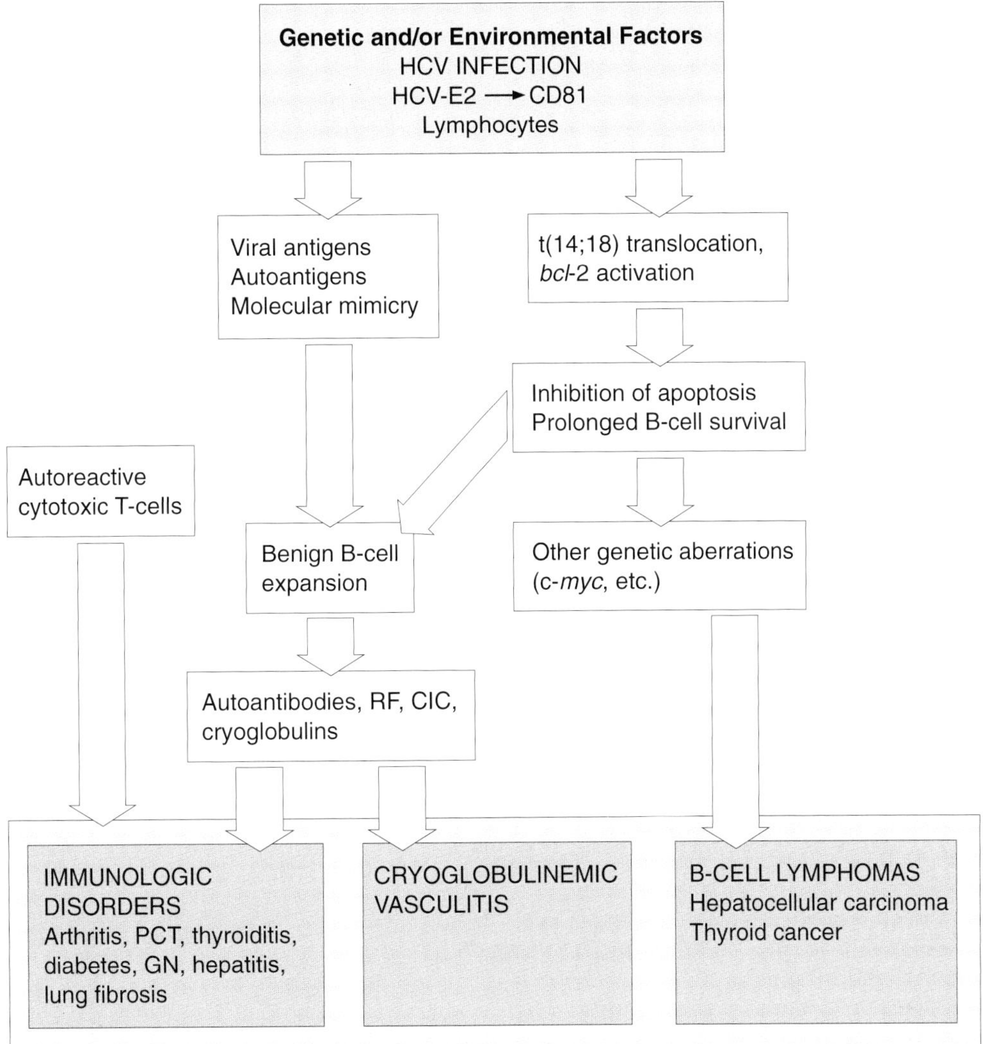

Figure 46–4. Etiopathogenesis of mixed cryoglobulinemia (MC) and other HCV-related disorders. HCV infection may exert a chronic stimulus on the immune system. The consequence is a benign B-cell lymphoproliferation producing a variety of autoantibodies, including rheumatoid factor (RF), cryoprecipitable immune complexes (CIC), and non-cryoprecipitable immune complexes. These serologic alterations may explain, at least in part, the appearance of various organ-specific and non–organ-specific immunologic disorders, including MC syndrome. The t(14;18) translocation, frequently found in MC patients, leads to the activation of *bcl*-2 proto-oncogene, which is responsible for prolonged B-cell survival. Other genetic aberrations are necessary for the development of frank B-cell lymphomas and other malignancies in a minority of cases. Abbreviations: GN, glomerulonephritis; PCT, porphyria cutanea tarda.

Interestingly, there is a clinicoserologic and pathologic overlap among different HCV-related diseases; MC syndrome represents a crossroad between autoimmune and neoplastic disorders.

cases of cirrhotic evolution.[42] Notably, regression of lymphoid infiltrates in the bone marrow has been observed following interferon therapy and clearance of the virus.[45] The high frequency of immunocytic morphology reported by others (for a comprehensive review of the topic see reference 23) likely reflects the different terminologies used through time. A critical review of the reports in the literature reveals that most of the Ic-like proliferations of the past were identified by applying the cytologic criteria of the Updated Kiel Classification,[46] which differ from those of the presently used REAL/WHO Classification.[44,47] In any case, the few cases still classifiable as LPL/Ic-like MLDUS are sustained by a $CD79a^+/CD5^-/CD23^{-/+}$ population, which consists of small lymphocytes, lymphoplasmacytoid elements, and plasma cells and expresses cytoplasmic monotypic Ig at high levels. Molecular analysis of immunoglobulin V_H region polymerase chain reaction in 35 portal lymphoid infiltrates from 11 HCV-positive patients (7 with and 4 without type II cryoglobulinemia) showed a single band in 21 infiltrates, two bands in 10, and 3 bands in 4.[8] Likewise, the pattern of B-cell expansion in

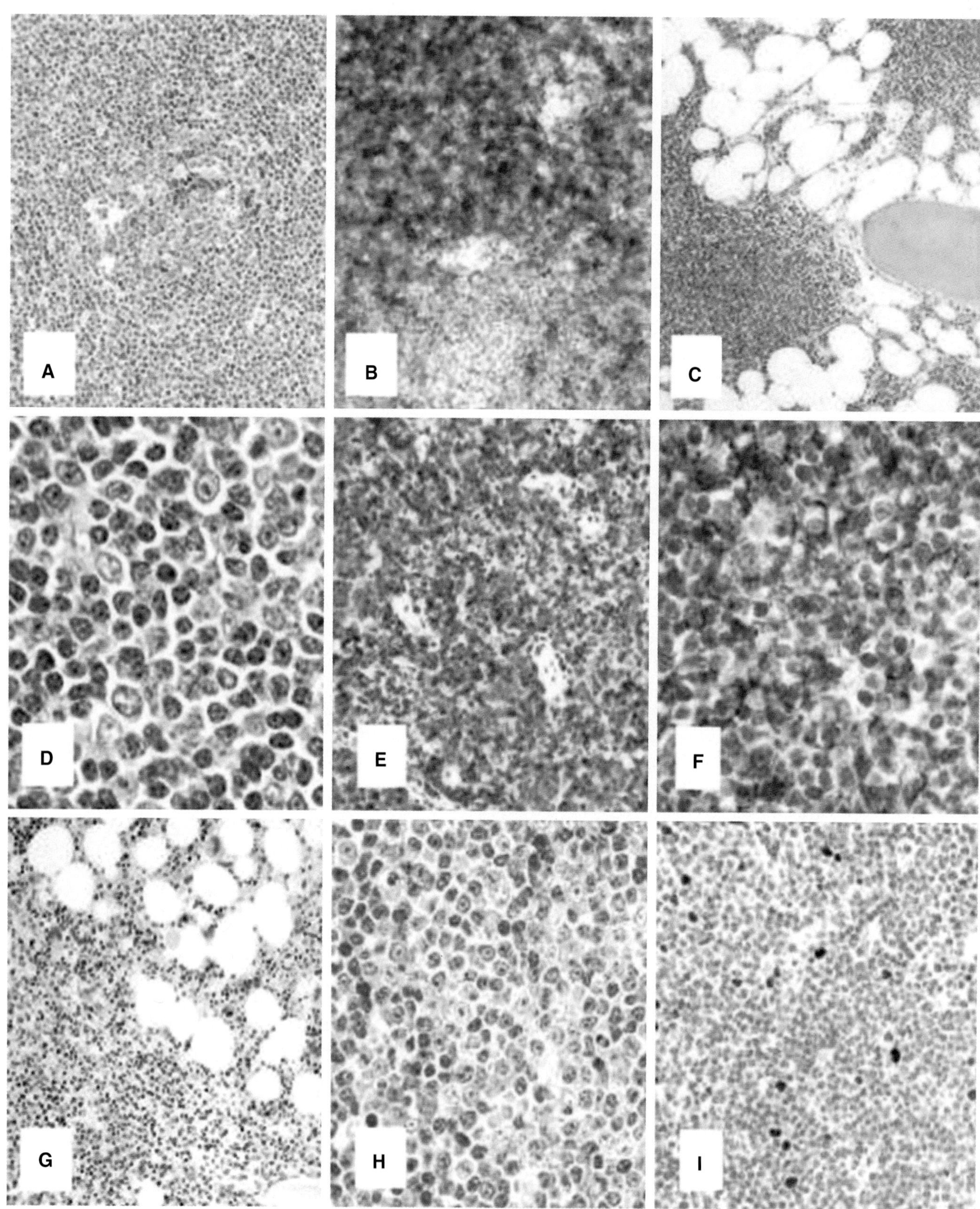
A
B
C
D
E
F
G
H
I

12 of 15 bone marrow biopsies from HCV-positive patients with type II mixed cryoglobulinemia was oligoclonal.[9]

CLINICAL FEATURES AND DIAGNOSIS

Symptom and Signs

Table 46–2 shows the main demographic, clinical, serologic, and virologic features observed in a large Italian mixed cryoglobulinemia patient series,[10] which substantially reflect the characteristics of other reported series.[6,10,16]

Cutaneous manifestations of mixed cryoglobulinemia are the most frequent symptoms of the disease. Orthostatic purpura is usually intermittent, and the dimension and dissemination of skin lesions vary widely, from sporadic, isolated petechiae to severe vasculitic lesions, often complicated by torpid ulcers of the legs and malleolar areas (see Fig. 46–1). Two thirds of patients have ochreous coloration on the legs.

Mixed cryoglobulinemia patients commonly report arthralgias and a mild, nonerosive oligoarthritis, which is often sensitive to low doses of steroids with or without hydroxychloroquine.[6,10,55–57] These patients also complain of xerostomia and xerophthalmia; however, only a few cases meet the current criteria for the classification of primary Sjögren's syndrome.[6,10] Peripheral neuropathy, more often presenting as mild sensory neuritis, is a frequent complication of the mixed cryoglobulinemia[6,10,58]; it is secondary to vasculitis of the vasa nervorum or direct autoimmune nerve injury, or both.[6,1055,58,59] Usually, patients complain of paresthesias with painful and/or burning sensations in the lower limbs, often with nocturnal exacerbation. Central nervous system involvement with dysarthria and hemiplegia is rare and often difficult to distinguish from the most common atherosclerotic manifestations.[6,10]

Overt chronic hepatitis progressing to cirrhosis can be observed at any time during the natural history of the disease. In some individuals, especially in combination with renal involvement, chronic hepatitis becomes a life-threatening complication. On the whole, the clinical course is less severe than that of patients with HCV-related chronic hepatitis without mixed cryoglobulinemia syndrome.[6,10] Similarly, hepatocellular carcinoma is uncommon.[6,10,60] Membranoproliferative glomerulonephritis type I is a common and severe complication caused by cryoglobulinemic nephropathy.[2,6,10]

Widespread vasculitis involving medium to small arteries, capillaries, and venules with multiple organ involvement is observed in a minority of patients.[2,6,10,20]

TABLE 46–2. Demographic, Clinical, Serologic, and Virologic Features of 210 Mixed Cryoglobulinemia Patients

Demographic Features	
Female/male ratio	3.7:1
Mean age at disease onset (yr)	53 ± 11.6
Mean age at diagnosis (yr)	56.4 ± 11.2
Mean disease duration (yr)	10.5 ± 7.3
Clinical Features	
Purpura	98%
Weakness	100%
Arthralgias	98%
Arthritis	7%
Raynaud's phenomenon	48%
Sicca syndrome	53%
Skin ulcers	22%
Peripheral neuropathy	80%
Liver involvement	77%
Renal involvement	30%
Lung involvement	2%
Diffuse vasculitis	6.2%
Hyperviscosity syndrome	0.5%
B-cell lymphoma	10%
Hepatocellular carcinoma	3.3%
Thyroid cancer	1%
Serologic Features	
MC type II/type III ratio	2
Cryocrit (%)	4.4 ± 11.7
Rheumatoid factor	98%
C4 (mg/dL) (nv 20–60)	11 ± 7.7
C3 (mg/dL) (nv 90–180)	100 ± 28
Autoantibodies*	56%
Virologic Features	
Anti-HCV Ab ± HCV RNA	92%
Anti-HBV Ab	42%
HBsAg	9%

*Autoantibodies: antinuclear, antimitochondrial, and/or anti–smooth muscle antibodies.

Abbreviations: Ab, antibody; HBsAg, hepatitis B surface antigen; HBV, hepatitis B virus; HCV, hepatitis C virus; MC, mixed cryoglobulinemia; nv, normal values.

From Ferri C, Sebastiani M, Giuggioli D, et al: Mixed cryoglobulinemia: demographic, clinical, and serological features, and survival in 231 patients. Semin Arthritis Rheum 33:355–374, 2004.

Figure 46–5. Histopathologic findings of B-cell lymphoproliferation in mixed cryoglobulinemia patients. ***A,*** Nodal marginal-zone lymphoma detected in an HCV-positive patient with mixed cryoglobulinemia. Note the residual germinal center in the middle part of the field. (Giemsa staining, × 150.) ***B,*** In the same patient, there is strong expression of the IRTA-1 gene product. Marginal-zone B cells characteristically express the IRTA-1 gene. Note the unstained residual germinal center. (Alkaline phosphatase–antialkaline phosphatase [APAAP] labeling technique, Gill's hematoxylin counterstaining, × 150.) ***C,*** Lymphoid nodules in the bone marrow biopsy of an HCV-positive cryoglobulinemic patient. (Hematoxylin and eosin staining, × 50.) ***D,*** On cytologic grounds, the nodules correspond to B-cell chronic lymphocytic leukemia–like MLDUS. (Giemsa staining, × 500.) ***E,*** The same cells express CD5. (APAAP labeling technique, Gill's hematoxylin counterstaining, × 150.) ***F,*** CD23 positivity is also appreciated. (APAAP labeling technique, Gill's hematoxylin counterstaining, × 400.) ***G,*** An immune complex–like infiltrate in the bone marrow of an HCV-positive cryoglobulinemic patient. (Giemsa staining, × 75.) ***H,*** Cytologic details at higher magnification. Note the features of plasmacytoid/plasmacytic differentiation. (Giemsa staining, × 400.) ***I,*** The lymphoid infiltrate has a very low proliferative activity, as shown by the Ki-67 marking. (APAAP labeling technique, Gill's hematoxylin counterstaining, × 200.)

Abdominal pain, simulating an acute abdomen, is the presenting symptom of intestinal vasculitis. A timely diagnosis and high-dose steroid treatment are necessary for this life-threatening complication.[6,10] In addition, interstitial lung disease may occur,[61–66] with subclinical alveolitis, as demonstrated by means of bronchoalveolar lavage in unselected mixed cryoglobulinemia patient series.[6,10,66] In rare cases, this generally mild manifestation may lead to clinically evident interstitial lung fibrosis.[61,62,64]

Some endocrine gland dysfunction can be observed in a significantly higher number of mixed cryoglobulinemia patients compared with age- and sex-matched controls—in particular, diabetes mellitus type 2 and thyroid and gonadal dysfunction.[6,10,67–73] Diabetes mellitus may represent a frequent complication of HCV infection, with or without cryoglobulinemia.[69–73] This manifestation shows a peculiar phenotype: patients with HCV-positive diabetes were leaner than controls, and had significantly lower total cholesterol and systolic and diastolic blood pressure compared to HCV-negative diabetics.[69] Transient hyperthyroidism can be observed in patients undergoing interferon treatment,[6,10] and hypothyroidism, often subclinical, and erectile dysfunction are detectable in a significant number of mixed cryoglobulinemia patients.[68]

Hyperviscosity syndrome resulting from high levels of serum cryoglobulins is rare.[74] Hemolytic complement activity is almost invariably depressed, showing the typical pattern of low or undetectable C4 and normal or relatively normal C3 serum levels. Of interest, an in vitro consumption of complement can be observed as a result of the anticomplement activity of some cryoimmunoglobulins.[2,3,6,10] The level of circulating cryoglobulins rarely correlates with the mixed cryoglobulinemia features.

One or more serum autoantibodies, more frequently low-titer antinuclear (diffuse pattern), antimitochondrial, or anti–smooth muscle, can be detected in over half of patients without any relationship with other clinicoserologic parameters. Serum anti-HCV antibodies, almost invariably associated with HCV RNA, are detectable in the large majority of mixed cryoglobulinemia patients.[6,10,15] Conversely, markers of HBV infection can be detected in over one third of patients, often associated with HCV infection; isolated ongoing HBV infection is rare.[6,10,15]

History

The most common (>50%) mixed cryoglobulinemia clinical pattern is a mild, slowly progressive disorder with a relatively good prognosis and survival.[10] In over one third of patients, usually after a long-term follow-up period, severe multiorgan involvement may develop.[10] Renal and/or liver failure, more often associated with cardiovascular complications, especially in male patients, is the most common cause of death.[10] In a limited but significant percentage (10–15%) of cases, the mixed cryoglobulinemia is complicated by a malignancy, generally as a late manifestation.[6,10,23]

Physical Examination

In most cases the presence of typical palpable purpura or areas of ochreous coloration on the legs (see Fig. 46–1) is sufficient to suspect the diagnosis of mixed cryoglobulinemia. The neurologic evaluation should assess peripheral sensory neuropathy or motor involvement.[58] Peripheral edema, ascites, and arterial hypertension are important symptoms of liver and/or kidney involvement. Spleen or lymph node enlargement, or both, as well as constitutional symptoms (fever, fatigue, etc.) may indicate the presence of malignant lymphomas.[10]

Diagnosis

Diagnosis of mixed cryoglobulinemia syndrome may be anticipated by the presence of skin vasculitis, hepatitis, nephritis, or peripheral neuropathy, but the detection of circulating mixed cryoglobulins is essential. In some patients, repeated cryoglobulin determinations may be necessary because cryoprecipitable immune complex levels vary over time.[6] To avoid artifact, blood sampling, clotting, and serum separation by centrifugation should be always carried out at 37°C, and the cryocrit determination and cryoglobulin characterization at 4°C, both immediately and at a later time point (Fig. 46–6). Moreover, cryocrit determinations should be done on blood samples without anticoagulation to avoid false-positive results caused by cryofibrinogen. Generally, the analysis of cryoprecipitate is carried out by means of immunoelectrophoresis or immunofixation, or by more sensitive methodologies such as immunoblotting or two-dimensional polyacrylamide gel electrophoresis.[6,7,75] Preliminary criteria proposed for the classification of mixed cryoglobulinemia are noted in Table 46–3.

TABLE 46–3. Proposed Criteria for the Classification of Mixed Cryoglobulinemia Patients

	Serologic	Pathologic	Clinical
Major	Mixed cryoglobulins Low C4	Leukocytoclastic vasculitis	Purpura
Minor	Rheumatoid factor⁺ HCV⁺ HBV⁺	Clonal B-cell infiltrates (liver and/or bone marrow)	Chronic hepatitis MPGN Peripheral neuropathy Skin ulcers

"Definite" Mixed Cryoglobulinemia Syndrome:

a) Serum mixed cryoglobulins (± low C4) + purpura + leukocytoclastic vasculitis
b) Serum mixed cryoglobulins (± low C4) + 2 minor clinical symptoms + 2 minor serologic/pathologic findings

"Essential" or "Secondary" Mixed Cryoglobulinemia:

Absence or presence of well-known disorders (infectious, immunologic, or neoplastic)

Abbreviations: HCV⁺ or HBV⁺, markers of hepatitis C virus or hepatitis B virus infection (anti-HCV ± HCV RNA, HBV DNA, or hepatitis B surface antigen); MPGN, membranoproliferative glomerulonephritis.

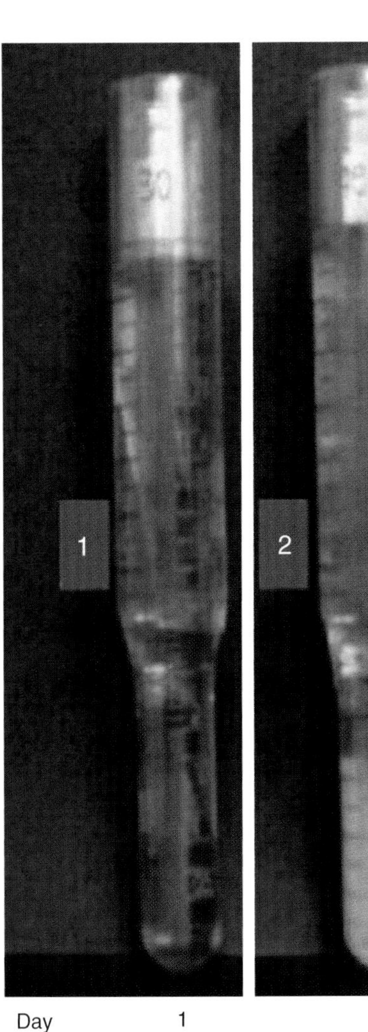

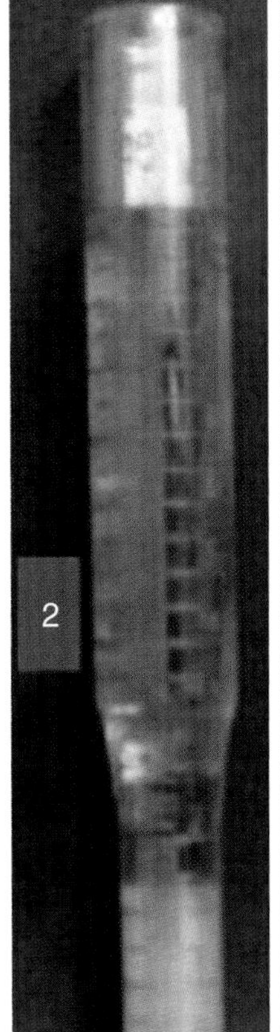

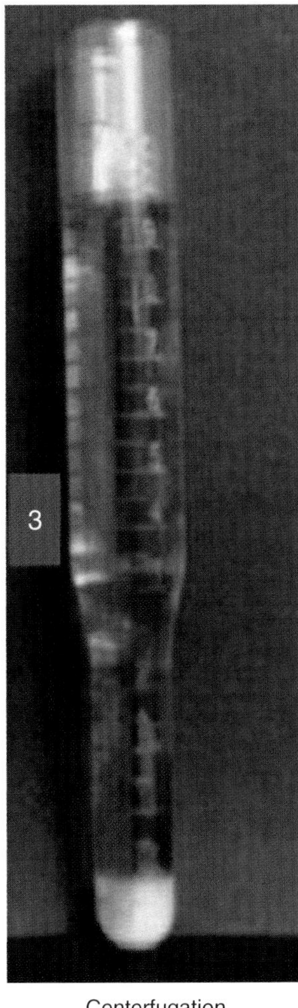

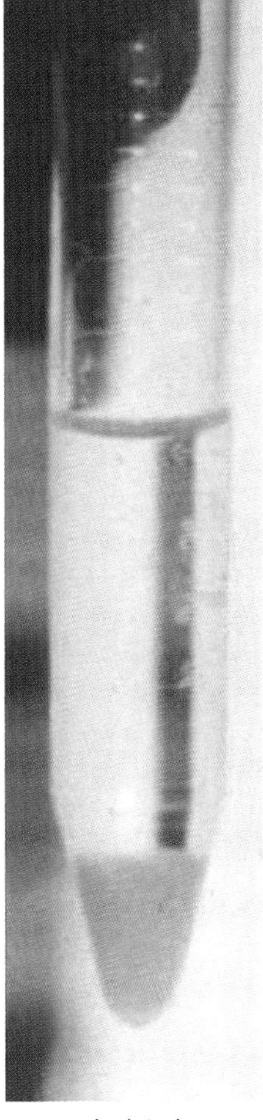

Figure 46–6. Cryoglobulin detection. Serum sample of a patient with mixed cryoglobulinemia syndrome, from left to right:

- Serum immediately after isolation by centrifugation of blood sample at 37°C.
- Presence of whitish cryoimmunoprecipitate in the serum stored at +4°C for 7 days.
- Packed cryoglobulins after serum centrifugation at +4°C and 1400 r.p.m.; the corresponding cryocrit is 5% (i.e., percentage of packed cryoglobulins with respect to total serum in graduated Wintrobe tube [(0.5/10 mL]).
- Isolated and washed cryoglobulins after centrifugation at +4°C in polysaline buffer.

DIFFERENTIAL DIAGNOSIS

Mixed cryoglobulinemia is classified among the systemic vasculitides, in the subgroup of small vessel vasculitides, which also includes cutaneous leukocytoclastic vasculitis and Henoch-Schönlein purpura.[10]

Differential diagnosis from other systemic vasculitides is quite easy if serologic markers (cryoglobulinemia, specific autoantibodies, and complement profile) and histopathologic patterns (different alterations and size of involved vessels) are correctly evaluated. Mixed cryoglobulinemia and Sjögren's syndrome may share various symptoms: xerostomia, xerophthalmia, arthralgias, purpura, serum cryoglobulins and rheumatoid factor, and the possible complication with B-NHL.[57,76] Histopathologic alterations of salivary glands and specific autoantibodies (anti-RoSSA/LaSSB) of Sjögren's syndrome[76] are rarely found in mixed cryoglobulinemia patients; conversely, HCV infection, cutaneous leukocytoclastic vasculitis, and visceral organ involvement (renal, liver) are seldom recorded in primary Sjögren's syndrome. However, in some patients the differential diagnosis may be very difficult; it might be appropriate to classify these cases as mixed cryoglobulinemia/Sjögren's overlap syndrome.

Patients with autoimmune hepatitis may present with low amounts of serum cryoglobulins, HCV positivity, and some extrahepatic manifestations, such as thyroiditis, sicca syndrome, and arthritis.[77,78] High-titer autoantibodies (antinuclear, anti–smooth muscle, anti-LKM1) are more often detectable in autoimmune hepatitis, whereas leukocytoclastic vasculitis and complications such as membranoproliferative glomerulonephritis are typically found in mixed cryoglobulinemia patients.[10] B-NHL complicating HCV-related mixed cryoglobulinemia can be confused with some idiopathic B-NHL cases showing clinicoserologic findings of mixed cryoglobulinemia (see Fig. 46–4).

TREATMENT

Type I cryoglobulinemia shows a variable clinical course and prognosis depending on the underlying disease, which may vary from benign monoclonal gammopathy of undetermined significance to malignant B-cell neoplasias; consequently, the treatment is mainly directed to these disorders.[6] However, hyperviscosity syndrome caused by the large amounts of circulating cryoglobulins may require plasma exchange treatment.

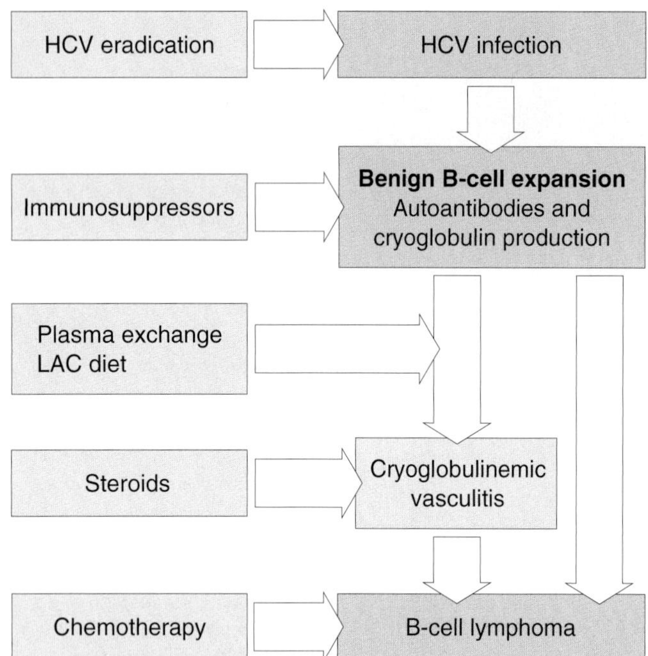

■ **Figure 46–7.** The cascade of events leading from HCV infection to mixed cryoglobulinemia (MC) syndrome *(right)* dictates that a correct therapeutic approach to MC should include etiologic, pathogenetic, and symptomatic therapies (*left;* see text). Abbreviation: LAC, low-antigen-content.

Treatment of Mixed Cryoglobulinemia Syndrome

Eradication of HCV

Because HCV represents the triggering factor of the disease and may also exert a chronic stimulus on the immune system (Fig. 46–7; see also Fig. 46–4), an attempt at HCV eradication should be made in all cases of HCV-associated mixed cryoglobulinemia.[79–83] Interferon therapy leads to clinical improvement, mirrored by inhibition of HCV replication and regression of indolent lymphoid infiltrates in bone marrow.[84] Therapy with interferon alfa/ribavirin may induce the regression of t(14;18)-bearing B-cell clones in HCV-positive patients.[39] However, HCV eradication is usually obtained in only a minority of treated patients; moreover, the clinical usefulness of antiviral treatment is often transient and may trigger or severely worsen the peripheral sensorimotor neuropathy or other immune-mediated processes.[6,10,85–90] Because there are no predictive parameters available for this harmful complication, interferon therapy should be carefully administered to patients with severe peripheral neuropathy. Rheumatoid-like polyarthritis, thyroid disorders, and erectile dysfunction may complicate interferon alfa therapy in patients with hepatitis C or mixed cryoglobulinemia.[6,10,79] Thus, although interferon alfa can be effective, its side effect profile makes its use complex[6,10,79,90,91] even when combined with ribavirin.[92–94] The possible immunomodulating effect of alpha-interferon can explain its efficacy on clinical symptoms also in HCV-negative MC patients.[95] Ultimately, a vaccine against HCV might eradicate mixed cryoglobulinemia.[96]

Immunosuppressive Treatment

Cyclophosphamide (1–2 mg/kg PO daily) is employed for the most severe, life-threatening complications of mixed cryoglobulinemia.[6,10,79] A short time course (2–3 months) of cyclophosphamide, in association with high-dose steroids and/or plasma exchange, may be effective in treating active or rapidly progressive glomerulonephritis, recent-onset sensorimotor neuropathy, or widespread vasculitis.[2,6,10,79] However, cyclophosphamide does not affect the progression of HCV infection or liver disease.

Rituximab, a monoclonal chimeric antibody that binds to the B-cell surface antigen CD20, has been usefully employed in some patients with HCV-positive mixed cryoglobulinemia.[97,98] Although these patients improved, an increase in serum HCV RNA was observed. This suggests that a combination of monoclonal anti-CD20 antibody and antiviral agents might be indicated.[99]

Corticosteroids and Plasma Exchange

Corticosteroids, alone or in association with plasma exchange and/or immunosuppressors, may be useful in patients with HCV-related mixed cryoglobulinemia who have failed to respond to interferon alfa, when this drug is contraindicated, or in the presence of severe, rapidly progressive disease. Both traditional and double-filtration plasma exchange are able to achieve a dramatic reduction of circulating immune complex levels, including the cryoglobulins, as well as a reduction in the viral loading.[6,10,79] Plasma exchange is useful in mixed cryoglobulinemia patients with severe manifestations, especially active cryoglobulinemic nephropathy.[6,10,79] The beneficial effect of these interventions may be improved by addition of oral cyclophosphamide at doses of 50–100 mg/day for 4–8 weeks. This drug can prevent the rebound phenomena observed after the plasmapheresis discontinuation. A low-antigen-content diet has been employed in some immune complex–mediated disorders.[6,10,100,101] In mixed cryoglobulinemia patients, this particular dietetic treatment can improve the serum clearance of immune complexes by restoring the activity of a reticuloendothelial system overloaded by large amounts of circulating cryoglobulins.[100]

Therapeutic Strategy

Treatment of mixed cryoglobulinemia should be tailored for the single patient, according to the severity of clinical symptoms[6,10,79] (Fig. 46–8). During the asymptomatic phase no intervention is indicated. Early manifestations may respond to low-dose steroids. Pegylated interferon alfa/ribavirin should be used in any patient with active manifestations. Life-threatening vasculitic manifestations must be promptly treated with a combined therapy of plasma exchange, high-dose steroids, and immunosuppressors. Treatment of B-cell malignancy complicating HCV-positive mixed cryoglobulinemia must be monitored

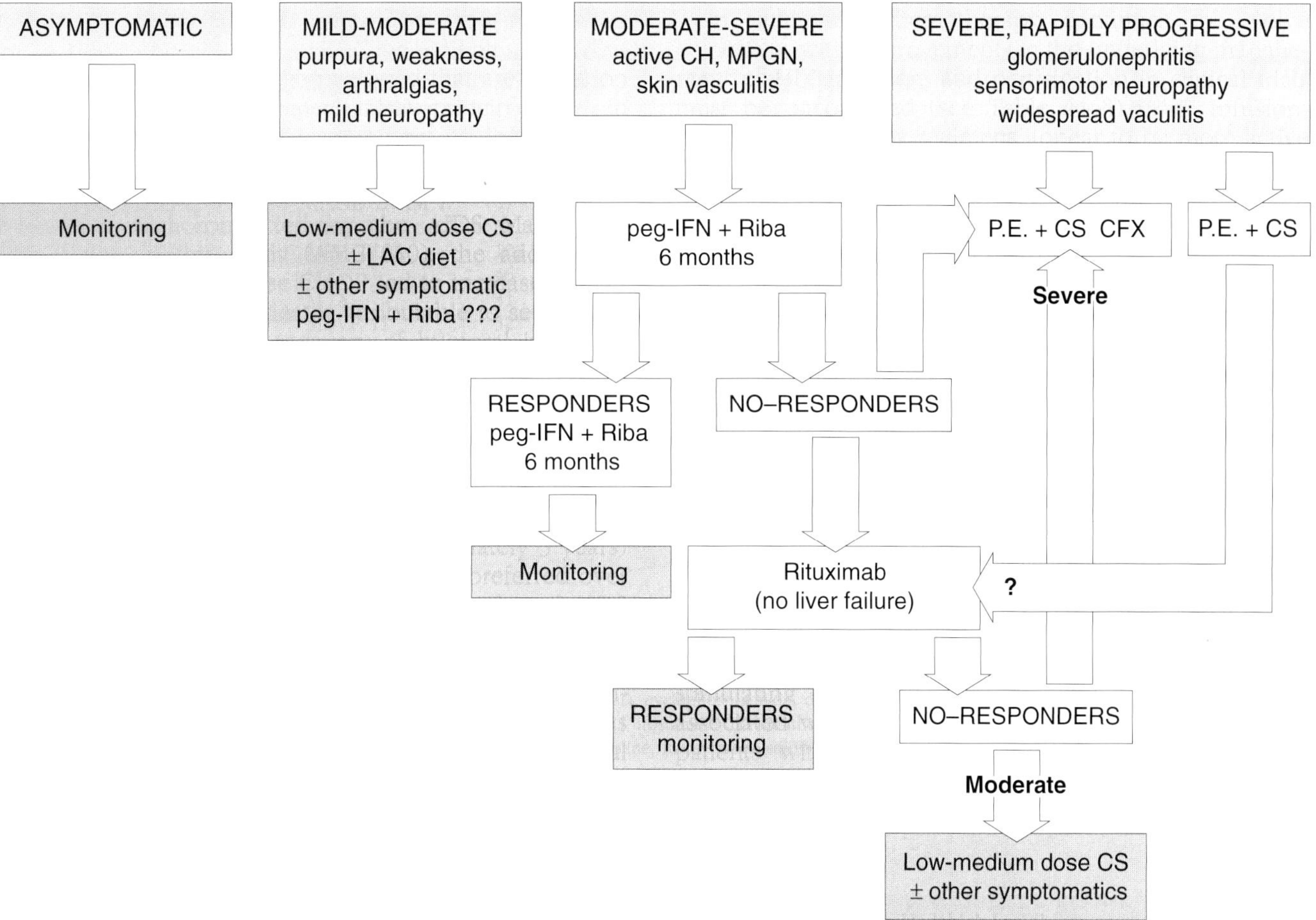

Figure 46–8. Therapeutic strategy in mixed cryoglobulinemia patients according to different prognostic subsets (see text). Abbreviations: CFX, cyclophosphamide; CH, chronic hepatitis; CS, corticosteroids; IFN, interferon alfa; LAC, low-antigen-content; MPGN, membranoproliferative glomerulonephritis; P.E., plasma exchange; Riba, ribavirin.

Current Controversies & Future Considerations

Cryoglobulinemia

- HCV infection is the triggering factor in the majority of mixed cryoglobulinemia patients; this association varies widely among patient populations from different geographic areas. Which are the potential genetic and environmental cofactors responsible for this epidemiologic heterogeneity?
- Which are the causative factors involved in HCV-negative mixed cryoglobulinemia patients?
- Because HCV may exert its pathogenetic role only indirectly, which are the actual viral and host factors involved in the pathogenesis of mixed cryoglobulinemia syndrome?
- Does the malignancy represent an evolutionary stage of the indolent B-cell expansion? Or is it an ex novo complication?
- Which are the actual pathogenetic mechanisms involved in the carcinogenesis (lymphoma, papillary thyroid cancer) complicating the mixed cryoglobulinemia?
- In some patients, the differential diagnosis between mixed cryoglobulinemia and other diseases, namely Sjögren's syndrome, autoimmune hepatitis, other systemic vasculitides, and B-cell neoplasias, is quite difficult. Therefore, the development of validated diagnostic criteria for mixed cryoglobulinemia syndrome would be opportune.
- Antiviral therapy with interferon ± ribavirin is useful in about one fourth of mixed cryoglobulinemia patients; the definition of parameters predictive for its efficacy and tolerability could be decisive for the therapeutic strategy.
- The greater usefulness of sequential versus combined therapy with antivirals (interferon ± ribavirin) and immunosuppressors (cyclophosphamide or rituximab) should be evaluated by means of controlled trials in the near future.

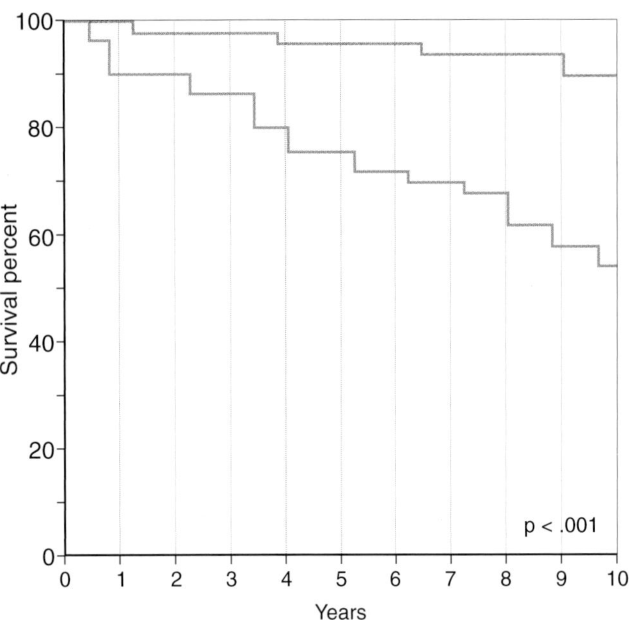

Figure 46–9. Cumulative 10-year survival rate of 231 mixed cryoglobulinemia patients compared to age- and sex-matched cohort from the Italian general population.

carefully because combining antilymphoma therapy with interferon for HCV increases the potential for toxicity as a result of liver and/or kidney disease.

SUPPORTIVE CARE AND LONG-TERM MANAGEMENT

Mixed cryoglobulinemia is a chronic disease, and late appearance of end-organ complications can occur. Atherosclerotic changes may complicate immune-mediated vascular damage. Steroid treatment may induce diabetes,[69] further exacerbating vascular disease. Cryoglobulinemia may be responsible for hemorheologic alterations, which may favor the appearance of vasculitic ulcers on the lower limbs,[74] exacerbated by venous insufficiency. Vascular manifestations, often associated with paresthesias resulting from peripheral sensory neuropathy, may lead to inadvertent trauma to the lower extremities. Finally, osteoporosis may represent another important complication of mixed cryoglobulinemia in women and in elderly men undergoing long-term treatment with steroids.

PROGNOSIS

Mixed cryoglobulinemia patients have a significantly reduced life expectancy[10] (Fig. 46–9). The most common causes of mortality are glomerulonephritis with renal failure, severe hepatitis complicated by cirrhosis, diffuse vasculitis, and malignancies (10–15% of cases; B-NHL, hepatocellular carcinoma, and papillary thyroid cancer).[10] Overall survival is similar in patients with type II and type III disease regardless of the presence of HCV infection.[10]

Suggested Readings*

Abel G, Zhang QX, Agnello V: Hepatitis C virus infection in type II mixed cryoglobulinemia. Arthritis Rheum 36:1341–1349, 1993.

Ferri C, Pileri S, Zignego AL: Hepatitis C virus, B-cell disorders, and non-Hodgkin's lymphoma. *In* Goedert JJ (ed): Infectious Causes of Cancer: Targets for Intervention. Totowa, NJ: Humana Press, 2000, pp 349–368.

Ferri C, Sebastiani M, Giuggioli D, et al: Mixed cryoglobulinemia: demographic, clinical, and serological features, and survival in 231 patients. Semin Arthritis Rheum 33:355–374, 2004.

Ferri C, Zignego AL, Pileri SA: Cryoglobulins. J Clin Pathol 55:4–13, 2002.

Gorevic PD, Frangione B: Mixed cryoglobulinemia cross-reactive idiotypes: implication for relationship of MC to rheumatic and lymphoproliferative diseases. Semin Hematol 28:79–94, 1991.

Full references for this chapter can be found on accompanying CD-ROM.

CHAPTER 47

Multiple Myeloma and Related Diseases

A. Keith Stewart, MBChB, FRCPC, MRCP, and Joseph Mikhael, MD, FRCPC

KEY POINTS

Multiple Myeloma

- Myeloma is a clinically heterogeneous disease defined by genetically variable subsets.
- Therapy is tailored by age.
- Younger patients benefit from high-dose melphalan and stem cell transplantation.
- Novel therapeutic agents, including thalidomide, bortezomib, and Revlimid, are now available or in clinical trials.
- Comprehensive care requires supportive therapy for anemia, renal failure, bone disease, and infection risk and appreciation of potential emergent conditions (e.g., hypercalcemia, cord compression, deep venous thrombosis).

INTRODUCTION

Multiple myeloma is a malignancy of terminally differentiated plasma cells initiated by the malignant transformation of a B lymphocyte during immunoglobulin heavy chain gene rearrangement. These plasma cells (Fig. 47–1) typically produce an immunoglobulin, also referred to as a monoclonal protein (M protein) (Fig. 47–2), which can be detected in blood, urine, or both. Multiple myeloma arises as part of a multistep pathogenesis that begins with the relatively common monoclonal gammopathy of unknown significance (MGUS) and terminates with the marrow failure and extramedullary disease that frequently now characterizes the end stages of disease. Furthermore, once developed the disease of multiple myeloma is heterogenous in clinical features, molecular basis, and prognosis.

EPIDEMIOLOGY

The annual incidence of multiple myeloma is approximately 4 per 100,000 and comprises approximately 1% of all malignant disease and 10% of hematologic malignancies. The incidence of multiple myeloma does not appear to be increasing, and previous suggestions that it may be rising are now attributed to more sensitive diagnostics, an aging population, and wider screening.

The median age of patients is 66 years, with less than 3% of patients diagnosed under the age of 40. Myeloma has a slight male predominance for unknown reasons and is nearly twice as common in black populations as in whites. The lowest incidence occurs in Asian populations, although myeloma does occur in all races and geographic locations.

The 1973–1998 Surveillance, Epidemiology, and End Results (SEER) program[1] tracked survival rates of all cancers, and indicated 5-, 10-, and 20-year survivals for multiple myeloma of 31%, 10%, and 4%, respectively. A recent Mayo Clinic series[2] demonstrated that median duration of survival of patients did not differ among patients according to the year of diagnosis (e.g., 1985–1987, 1988–1990, 1991–1994, and 1995–1998), although it may be expected that recent advances in therapy will by now have overcome this statistic.

RISK FACTORS

The etiology of multiple myeloma is unknown. Many possible causes have been implicated, including genetic, environmental, and infectious factors. A genetic predisposition is suggested because of the increased incidence among African patients, along with several reports of family clusters of myeloma. In the Mayo Clinic series[2] of over 1000 patients, a family history of cancer in first-degree relatives was found in 42%. At least one report[3] has linked familial mutation in *p16/CNDK4* with both melanoma and myeloma.

Exposure to radiation has been associated with the development of myeloma. This is based on an increased incidence in atomic bomb survivors, radiation workers, and patients previously treated with radiation.[4] Various chemicals have also been linked to myeloma, including benzene and other organic solvents, herbicides, and insecticides. However, the size of these studies is small

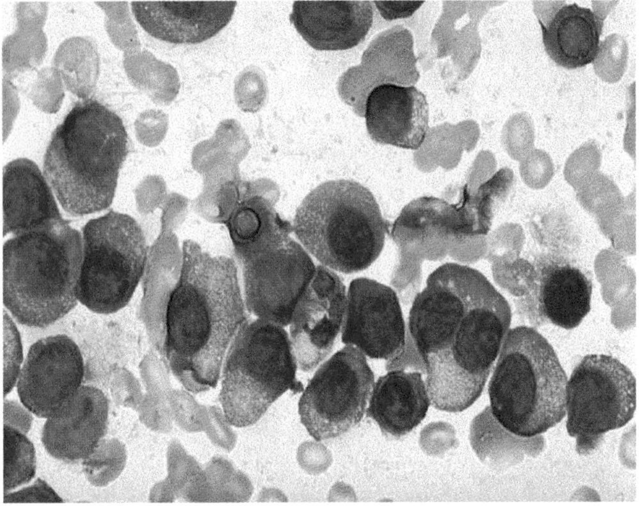

Figure 47–1. Multiple myeloma plasma cells.

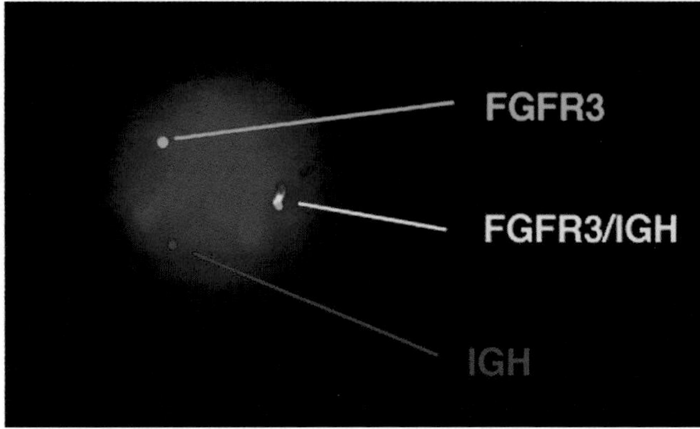

Figure 47–3. Multiple myeloma arises from immunoglobulin heavy chain translocations in 50% switch regions of patients. Shown here is a t(4;14) detected by fluorescence in situ hybridization which accounts for 15% of patients.

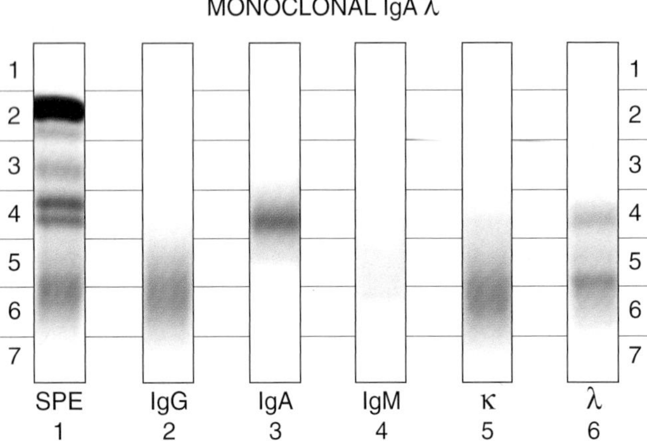

Figure 47–2. Monoclonal protein.

for each of these risk factors, and the data for chemical exposure are not complete.[5]

No definitive evidence has emerged for an infectious pathogenesis of multiple myeloma. Human herpesvirus 8 has been associated with Kaposi's sarcoma; it has also been linked to myeloma by one study but generally refuted by others,[6–8] and the presence of human herpesvirus 8 in myeloma patients appears similar to that of the general population.

PATHOPHYSIOLOGY

The clinical disease of multiple myeloma arises from malignant transformation of a late-stage B cell. Although the seminal event has yet to be categorically defined, it is apparent that illegitimate switch recombination of partner oncogenes into the immunoglobulin heavy chain (IgH) are one of the earliest definable genetic events.[9] Interestingly, only 50% of myelomas appear to harbor an IgH translocation. These translocations primarily involve partner oncogenes cyclin D1, cyclin D2, fibroblast growth factor receptor-3 (Fig. 47–3), c-*maf* and *maf*-B. The remaining 50% of patients appear to frequently exhibit cytogenetic hyperdiploidy and to upregulate the cell cycle control genes cyclin D1 and D2 through an as-yet unknown mechanism. The net result of these genetic abnormalities is the development and propagation of a clonal population of B cells within the bone marrow secreting a monoclonal protein that is the hallmark of myeloma and its forebears. Up to 3% of the general population in their eighth decade can harbor a monoclonal protein in their serum but often have no other associated illness. Thus, secondary events must transpire and create the malignant phenotype of multiple myeloma, which occurs at a frequency of 1.5% of patients with MGUS each year. These secondary events are not well defined, but mutation of kinases such as fibroblast growth factor receptor-3, deletions of chromosomes 13, upregulation of c-*myc*, and mutations of *ras* are some notable contributors.[10]

Further genetic analysis has revealed that such genetic features are of prognostic significance. For example, myeloma patients who harbor a t(4;14) or t(14;16) IgH translocation appear to have a particularly poor prognosis, whereas patients with a t(11;14) IgH translocation appear to do rather well. Similarly, genetic deletions involving chromosome 13 appear to impart a very poor prognosis, particularly when such abnormalities are detected by conventional cytogenetics.[11]

Having sustained a secondary event, the malignant plasma cells that characterize myeloma begin to proliferate in the bone marrow microenvironment, producing monoclonal proteins and causing osteolytic bone disease. The slow accumulation of these malignant cells gradually results in the characteristic clinical features of myeloma of anemia, bone resorption, hypercalcemia, renal failure, and immunodeficiency.

Having established itself, myeloma is dependent on a number of microenvironment features, including the bone marrow stroma itself and the cytokines interleukin-6 and insulin-like growth factor-1,[12] although the bone disease that arises in myeloma patients appears to be mediated in part by Rank ligand/osteoprotegerin or, as has been more recently suggested,[13] by the Wnt signaling antagonist Dickkopf1 (DKK1). Much remains to be learned about the molecular pathophysiologic basis of

TABLE 47–1. Clinical Features of Multiple Myeloma

Skeletal	"Punched-out" lytic bone lesions (skull, long bones common) Generalized osteoporosis Pathologic fractures and bone pain
Renal	Renal dysfunction caused by light chain toxicity and/or deposition, hypercalcemia, or amyloid deposition
Hematologic	Cytopenias (anemia common) caused by plasma cell infiltration of bone marrow, renal failure, or anemia of chronic disease Bleeding tendency—mostly caused by interference with coagulation by M protein or thrombocytopenia from marrow infiltration Hyperviscosity syndrome—visual changes, headache, confusion, bleeding, coma, "sausage veins" on funduscopy
Neurologic	Cord compression from vertebral collapse and/or plasmacytoma Mental changes (may be due to hyperviscosity, hypercalcemia) Peripheral neuropathy caused by M protein, amyloidosis, or drug treatment side effects
Metabolic	Hypercalcemia—confusion, polyuria, polydipsia, constipation, weakness, fatigue
Immunologic	Predisposition to recurrent infections as a result of suppression and dysfunction of normal immunoglobulins or neutropenia from chemotherapy

multiple myeloma. That said, advances have already been made that promise the early introduction of targeted therapies and superior prognostic indicators.

CLINICAL FEATURES

Signs and Symptoms

Characteristic clinical features of multiple myeloma are anemia, renal failure, bony lesions with pathologic fractures and associated pain, hypercalcemia, and recurrent infections (Table 47–1). These features may result directly from mass accumulations of plasma cells in tissues (plasmacytomas) or indirectly from effects of the M protein and/or cytokines secreted by plasma cells. Many patients, however, will present with asymptomatic anemia or monoclonal gammopathy discovered on incidental laboratory testing.

Laboratory Features

The vast majority (~95%) of patients with myeloma will have a serum M protein measurable by serum protein electrophoresis and/or a urine M protein with excreted light chains (Bence Jones protein) detectable by electrophoresis of a 24-hour urine collection. The heavy and light chain components of the M protein can be identified by immunoelectrophoresis or immunofixation. The most common immunoglobulin subtype is IgG (60%), followed by IgA (20%), light chains alone (10%), and less commonly IgD, IgE, and IgM (<5%). In approximately 5% of patients, no M protein in either serum or urine can be detected, although recently use of a free light chain assay with greater sensitivity has reduced this number further. A bone marrow aspirate and biopsy will show an increase of plasma cells (>10%) that often have immature morphologic features. Other characteristic but less specific laboratory findings include a normocytic, normochromic anemia; rouleaux ("stacked coin" appearance) of red blood cells on peripheral film analysis; and an elevated sedimentation rate. Presence of one of these nonspecific findings that is not otherwise explained clinically should trigger an investigation for multiple myeloma (Table 47–2).

TABLE 47–2. Investigations in Multiple Myeloma

Serum protein electrophoresis
24-hour urine collection for total protein quantitation
Immunoelectrophoresis or immunofixation of serum and urine
CBC with differential and reticulocyte counts
Serum creatinine, calcium, uric acid, electrolytes, lactate dehydrogenase, alkaline phosphatase
Bone marrow aspirate and biopsy for plasma cell percentage, cytogenetics, and molecular diagnostics recommended
Skeletal survey
If indicated: Biopsy of soft tissue masses
If available: β_2-microglobulin, C-reactive protein, plasma cell labeling index
If hyperviscosity is suspected: serum viscosity
If clinically indicated: cryoglobulins, MRI or CT of affected areas, staining for amyloidosis, bone densitometry

Abbreviations: CBC, complete blood count; CT, computed tomography; MRI, magnetic resonance imaging.

Radiologic Findings

A skeletal survey, which includes plain radiographs of the skull, ribs, spine, pelvis, shoulders, and long bones of the limbs, is used to identify osteopenia, or the typical "punched-out" lesions, of myeloma (Fig. 47–4). Because myeloma lesions are osteolytic in nature, a bone scan, which best detects osteoblastic lesions, is not generally useful. Computed tomography or magnetic resonance imaging (MRI) may be used to delineate plasmacytomas, particularly in areas of cord compression requiring urgent treatment. MRI scanning of the spine is sensitive in detecting patchy plasma cell involvement of the bone marrow and may be used for this purpose when a skeletal survey is negative but the index of suspicion for myeloma is high. MRI is becoming more common as treatment options improve and careful staging becomes more important. Although positron emission tomography can detect plasmacytomas, its use as a diagnostic tool is only now being explored. Bone densitometry is frequently employed to monitor osteoporosis.

DIAGNOSIS

The diagnosis of multiple myeloma requires a greater than 10% bone marrow plasmacytosis plus one of the following:

- A serum M protein by electrophoresis
- A urine M protein by electrophoresis
- Lytic bone lesions or generalized osteoporosis seen on skeletal survey
- Presence of a soft tissue plasmacytoma

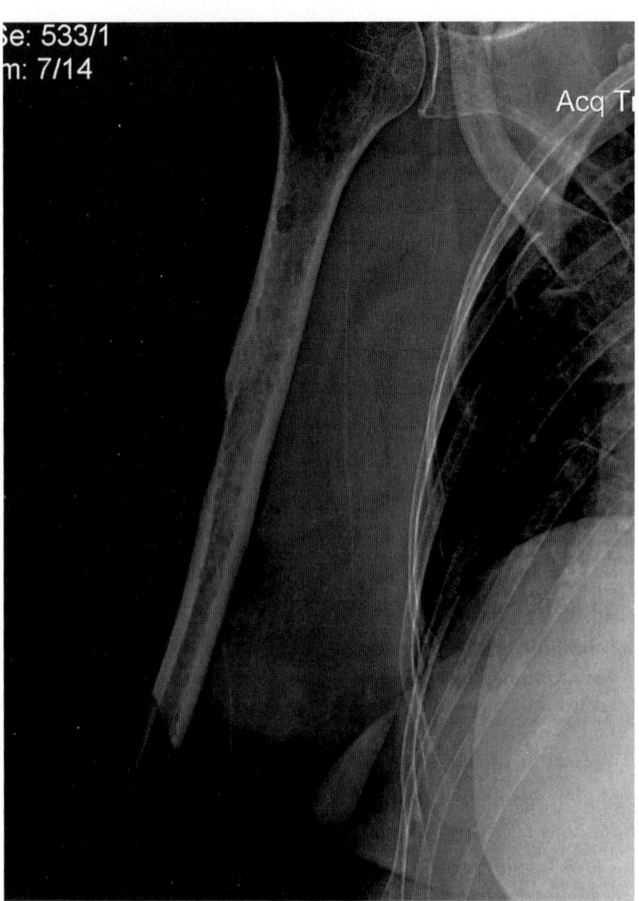

Figure 47–4. Radiograph showing typical osteopenia and lytic bone disease of multiple myeloma.

Asymptomatic patients with less than 10% bone marrow plasmacytosis, a low concentration of M protein in urine or blood, and absent bone lesions or cytopenias have an MGUS (Fig. 47–5) (see Chapter 48). MGUS may be difficult to distinguish from smoldering or early-stage myeloma. Features that may help to support a diagnosis of myeloma include reciprocal depression of the normal immunoglobulin levels, high paraprotein concentration (>30 gm/L in serum or 1 gm/day urinary M protein), and abnormal plasma cell morphology (e.g., immature forms, multinuclearity).

Patients with greater than 10% bone marrow plasmacytosis without bone lesions or other clinical manifestations of myeloma are considered to have smoldering myeloma. Although neither MGUS nor smoldering myeloma requires immediate therapy, it is nevertheless important to distinguish between the two because prognoses differ.

Amyloidosis is a primary disease but can present as a complication of myeloma whereby amyloid fibrils composed of components of the M protein deposit in tissues and cause organ dysfunction (see Chapter 51). This disorder should be suspected in myeloma patients with progressive neuropathy, cardiac dysfunction with hypotension, enlarged tongue, swollen joints, hepatomegaly, or nephrotic syndrome. A needle biopsy of involved tissue for special staining is most likely to yield a diagnosis, but, if involved tissue is inaccessible, blind abdominal fat pad needle aspirates may be helpful.

TREATMENT

Although there are many treatment options for patients with multiple myeloma, there is presently no cure for the disease. The disease may remain indolent for years in many patients, particularly in those with low levels of M protein (<30 gm/L) and absent bony lesions. Because there is no evidence that early treatment pro-

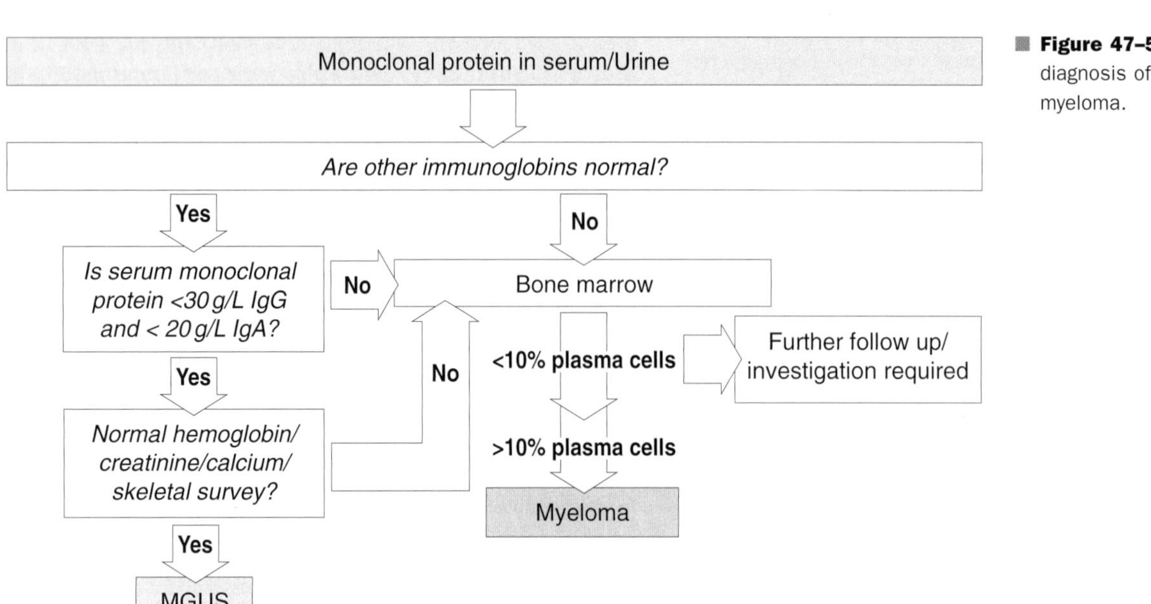

Figure 47–5. Differential diagnosis of multiple myeloma.

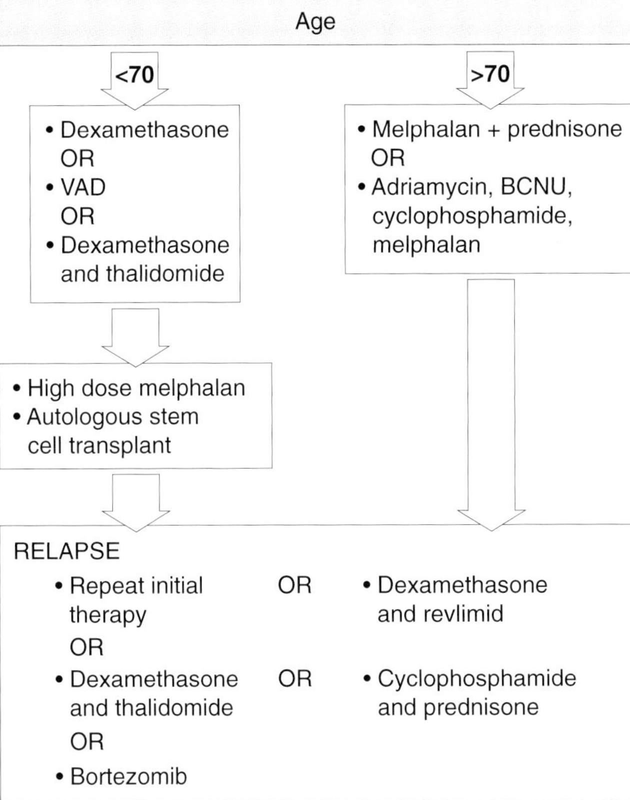

Figure 47–6. Because myeloma is a systemic disorder from the onset, the primary treatment modality is chemotherapy.

longs survival, therapy should be reserved for patients with symptoms. Those with smoldering myeloma should not be treated except in a clinical trial. Treatment should be initiated, however, in patients with impending complications (such as bony lytic lesions predisposing to pathologic fractures) even if they are not yet symptomatic. Because myeloma is a systemic disorder from the onset, the primary treatment modality is chemotherapy.

Induction Chemotherapy

It is important that therapies be chosen that reflect a myeloma patient's candidacy for high-dose melphalan with stem cell support, because therapies vary widely for younger, healthier patients who pursue an aggressive intervention versus elderly, less well, or disinclined patients who choose a more conservative approach (Fig. 47–6). Indeed, it is recommended that all myeloma patients be considered for clinical trials, because this disease remains incurable and newer therapeutic agents and a better understanding of molecular events triggering the disease have ushered in an era of risk-adapted therapy.

Conservative Regimens

For elderly patients or those who either do not want or cannot tolerate aggressive therapy, various oral chemotherapy regimens may be used, although these are rapidly being supplanted by newer agents. Traditionally, MP (oral melphalan [Alkeran] 9 mg/m^2 and prednisone 100 mg daily for 4 days given at 4- to 6-week intervals) has been most frequently used. Because melphalan has erratic gastrointestinal absorption, it should be given in the morning on an empty stomach, and doses must be titrated to the midcycle blood counts. A nadir of mild neutropenia (1000–1500 cells/λL) and/or thrombocytopenia (<100,000 cells/μL) is recommended to ensure maximal efficacy. Severe cytopenias requiring cycle delays or transfusion support should be avoided by reducing the dose of melphalan by 2- to 4-mg/day decrements. Treatment is continued until maximal reduction in the M protein has occurred and a plateau reached for a minimum of 2 months (approximately 1 year of treatment). At this point, maintenance therapy should begin because two large randomized studies[14] have now demonstrated benefit to maintenance with prednisone (50 mg orally on alternate days) or dexamethasone 40 mg for 4 days each month. Cyclophosphamide (Cytoxan) at doses of 400–500 mg orally weekly can be used in place of melphalan in selected patients. Cyclophosphamide is less likely to suppress thrombopoiesis and, unlike melphalan, has less myelosuppressive potentiation in renal failure. It is often administered in conjunction with prednisone 100 mg orally on alternate days.

Using the standard MP regimen, 50–60% of patients will respond with a greater than 50% drop in M protein, but fewer than 5% will attain a complete remission (complete clearing of M protein in the bone marrow and no other evidence of disease). Median overall survival is 3–4 years. Advantages to this regimen include ease of administration and minimal toxicity. Unfortunately, alkylating agents such as melphalan predispose to late development of myelodysplasia and leukemia. A major disadvantage is damage to the stem cell pool required for later high-dose therapy support.

Adding thalidomide to MP has been shown[15] to increase response rates to 90% and complete responses to greater than 20%; however, the incidence of complications, including deep venous thrombosis, is high. Randomized trials now underway may result in a new recommendation for routine use of thalidomide in newly diagnosed elderly patients.

Novel Therapies

Recently a number of novel therapies have emerged which have changed the landscape for myeloma therapy. They are discussed briefly here.

Bortezomib (Velcade)

Bortezomib is a novel agent which inhibits the cellular proteasome—a function on which late stage B cells seem particularly dependant. In part, this efficacy is based on the dependence of plasma cells on NF-κB and proteolytic degradation of its inhibitor, IF-κB. Bortezomib blocks proteolysis of IFκB, allowing IFκB to bind NFκB, thereby blocking signaling from NFκB. This reduces IL-6 production and limiting the proliferative signal to malignant plasma cells. In initial studies, bortezomib had its greatest single agent efficacy against myeloma. Treatment is by twice weekly injection of 1.3 mg/m^2 on a 3 week schedule, followed by a weekly schedule after 5–8 cycles of treatment. Phase II clinical studies in relapsed or refractory myeloma showed an overall 35% response rate. A subsequent phase III clinical trial comparing bortezomib with high-dose dexamethasone in relapsed patients was associated with significant improvement in 1-year survival and overall survival for bortezomib versus dexamethasone and was associated with a 41% reduction in risk of death.[16] This is the first and largest randomized study demonstrating a survival advantage in relapsed/refractory myeloma. Bortezomib is also now being evaluated as a front-line therapy with overall response rates of ~40% as a single agent and 75–80% with high complete and near complete response rates of up to 32% in combination therapy. Other studies are employing a combination of thalidomide and bortezomib, although the efficacy of this combination is not established. Painful neuropathy, nausea, diarrhea and cytopenias are notable toxicities. Despite this toxicity profile, it may be the most effective agent introduced in the past 10 years for myeloma.

Thalidomide

Thalidomide is highly active against myeloma with 30% of refractory patients responding to single agent therapy. In combination with corticosteroids, response rates are ~65%. Although initially tested in advanced disease, it is now used across the entire spectrum of disease. First employed for its anti-angiogenic properties the exact mechanism of action in myeloma is unknown, although inhibition of *wnt* signaling has recently been implicated. The usual starting dose is 50 to 100 mg with a target dose of 200 mg by mouth daily, therapy is usually indefinite until progression. Common side effects include constipation, sedation, sensory peripheral neuropathy and deep venous thrombosis. The latter is most troubling and routine anticoagulants are recommended when used in combination with other drugs particularly in newly diagnosed patients.

Lenalidomide (Revlimid)

Lenalidomide is chemically similar to thalidomide and has recently completed clinical trials and is under regulatory review.[16a] It has activity in thalidomide failures and has a different side effect profile including myelosuppression, muscle cramps and venous thrombosis. In initial clinical trials, single agent response rates of ~35% are observed and in combination with corticosteroids, response rates of ~65% in relapsed disease and 90% in newly diagnosed disease are noteworthy.[16b] Interim results of Phase III trials, which compared lenalidomide and dexamethasone with dexamethasone alone, showed that the combination significantly delayed time to disease progression. Median time to progression for the North American trial was 60 weeks versus 20 weeks for the dexamethasone alone arm.

Aggressive Regimens

In younger patients, multidrug regimens using combinations of melphalan, vincristine, anthracyclines, BCNU, cyclophosphamide, and prednisone or dexamethasone have an extensive track record and often produce a faster onset of action than MP; thus, these may be useful in patients with high tumor loads and acute renal failure. The most common of these regimens is VAD (intravenous vincristine [Oncovin] 0.4 mg, doxorubicin [Adriamycin] 9 mg/m^2 by continuous infusion, and oral dexamethasone [Decadron] 20 mg/m^2 daily for 4 days starting on days 1, 9, and 17 of each month). VAD is easily administered and well tolerated, and has minimal myelosuppressive effect. Combination chemotherapy regimens such as VAD do not, however, improve response rates or survival over standard MP. Nevertheless, they have gained in popularity particularly for use in induction prior to high-dose therapy and autologous stem cell transplantation.

Dexamethasone, when used as a single agent (usually given in a dosing schedule similar to that for VAD), is also effective in treatment of myeloma. Although unproven, it is generally considered as effective as VAD. Complications such as osteoporosis, avascular necrosis of bone, diabetes, cataracts, hypertension, and recurrent infections may limit long-term use. Again, some of these combinations are also being superseded by newer agents in ongoing clinical trials.

Relapse After Conventional Chemotherapy

Generally within 1–2 years of discontinuation of therapy, disease will recur. Half of those patients who have relapsed after a first course of MP will respond to reinstitution of MP starting at previously effective doses. Development of drug resistance and cumulative myelosuppression, however, will eventually limit repeated cycles. At this point, a switch to dexamethasone alone or in combination with thalidomide may be efficacious. The latter is particularly useful in patients with cytopenias and in those reluctant to continue intravenous therapy. In a large randomized trial,[17] bortezomib has recently been shown to confer a disease-free and overall survival benefit in relapsed patients when compared to dexamethasone alone. Revlimid has also recently been shown to be active in large phase III clinical trials and will soon be available. If recurrence is localized to a single bony lesion, palliative localized radiation as a single agent may be appropriate.

High-Dose Melphalan with Autologous Stem Cell Support

Use of high-dose melphalan with stem cell support is presently the standard of care in patients with symptomatic myeloma under age 70 years.[18] In preparation for high-dose therapy, patients generally first receive four to six cycles of conventional chemotherapy for induction. Induction regimens as described previously using nonalkylating agents (e.g., VAD, dexamethasone and thalidomide, or dexamethasone alone) are specifically chosen to avoid damage to stem cells. High-dose melphalan (Alkeran) (200 mg/m^2) is the most common transplant regimen used. Mortality from transplant toxicity is low at 1–3%, hence it is relatively safe. In a landmark randomized trial[19] in myeloma patients under age 65, the transplant procedure led to improved overall survival of 52% at 5 years versus 12% in patients treated with conventional chemotherapy alone. Unfortunately, most patients following transplantation will continue to have evidence of the disease and all will eventually relapse. Another approach is to intensify high-dose therapy with double (or tandem) transplants,[20] which in some but not all studies has proven to be of further benefit, particularly to patients not obtaining a complete remission after the first round of high-dose therapy. Maintenance therapies with various agents (e.g., interferon alfa, steroids, thalidomide, Revlimid, and combination chemotherapy) following high-dose therapy have been used in clinical trials attempting to improve on these results. No study has yet confirmed a role for maintenance therapy in this setting, but several large trials are nearing completion.

Relapse After High-Dose Therapy and Autologous Transplantation

There is no clear standard of treatment following relapse after high-dose therapy and autologous transplantation. Patients are generally reinduced with bortezomib, dexamethasone, and/or thalidomide, but repeat autotransplantation, allotransplantation, and experimental agents such as Revlimid are under investigation. Other options include use of cyclophosphamide and prednisone, which is well tolerated in this setting, or entry into a clinical trial.

Allogeneic Transplantation

An allogeneic transplantation uses stem cells obtained from a human lymphocyte antigen–matched donor, usually a sibling, rather than the patient's own cells for regenerating the bone marrow. There is some, albeit limited, evidence that an immunologic reaction mounted by the infused donor lymphocytes against the patient's myeloma cells (graft-versus-myeloma response) can help control the disease. This proposed reaction is comparable to that proven in leukemia patients undergoing allogeneic transplantation (graft-versus-leukemia response). Allotransplantation in myeloma can lead to significant reduction in tumor mass with high response rates (complete remissions of approximately 40%). Unfortunately, deaths from toxic reactions are common (>20%), and this mode of treatment is infrequently utilized. Miniallogeneic transplantation has recently been proposed as a solution and is under intense investigation; however, early results have suggested that graft-versus-host disease remains a significant problem and durable responses are few. Allogeneic transplantation should therefore be reserved for clinical trials.

Refractory Myeloma

Nowadays patients will progress through use of alkylating agents (high or conventional dose), high-dose corticosteroids, thalidomide, and bortezomib before being declared refractory. Median survivals of 5–6 years are the norm in younger patients. However, because cures are rare, most patients are ultimately identified as refractory to conventional agents and most will receive all active agents in some sequence. Having exhausted these options, patients may still qualify for one of numerous investigational therapies as part of a clinical trial, including targeted small molecule approaches, monoclonal antibodies, or targeted radiotherapies. Clinical trials should be actively pursued in this population because there is no consensus for optimal management.

PROGNOSIS

Traditionally the prognosis for multiple myeloma has been defined by the stage of disease at the time it is diagnosed. Patients diagnosed with MGUS generally have a benign course, with only 1.5% of patients per year going on to develop clinical myeloma. A further 15–20% of such patients will develop lymphoma or other hematologic malignancies over a 10-year period. In contrast, patients diagnosed with smoldering myeloma will usually go on to develop clinically demonstrable myeloma within 2–3 years of diagnosis. Various prognostic features of smoldering myeloma can be used to predict which patients are more likely to progress.

Patients with active myeloma treated with conventional low-dose alkylating agent therapies have a median survival of 3–4 years, with only 5% of patients living 10 years. Recently use of maintenance steroids and thalidomide and the introduction of Revlimid, Velcade, and better supportive care may have improved this generalized prognosis. For younger patients, particularly those able to undergo high-dose melphalan therapy with peripheral blood stem cell support, median survivals are now generally in the range of 5–6 years, with up to 25% of patients living 10 years. The recent introduction of thalidomide and bortezomib along with improved supportive care measures may already have changed this natural history.

Prognostic Staging Systems

An important caveat to these numbers is that not all myeloma is created equal, and there are some patients with poor genetic risk features who have very poor outcomes even with aggressive therapy, whereas there are other patients with good genetic or other prognostic features who have superior outcomes that may well be independent of the type or aggressiveness of therapy provided. Although the field is moving quickly, recent prognostic staging systems that have been developed promise to simplify the stratification of myeloma patients into specific groups suitable for targeted approaches to therapy. As an example, using traditional measures such as the β_2-microglobulin and albumin levels, the Myeloma International Staging System can separate myeloma patients using a simple algorithm into low-, intermediate-, and high-risk populations.[21] Such clinically driven staging systems will likely be replaced over the next 5 years with more powerful and specific genetics-based prognostic criteria. For example, there is already evidence that a combination of chromosome translocation status and expression level of cyclin D can group patients into prognostically significant categories (see later). Indeed, it is recommended that all patients have conventional cytogenetics and chromosome translocation status by fluorescent in situ hybridization or reverse transcriptase–polymerase chain reaction assessed at diagnosis. Gene expression profiling also promises to provide a powerful prognostic tool.

Genetic-Based Prognosis and Risk-Adapted Therapy

Recently, a rational gene expression profile-based prognostic schema[22] has used a combination of the IgH translocation and expression of cyclin D to define five distinct populations of myeloma patients with unique prognoses and the potential for highly targeted therapeutic intervention. With these developments in mind, it is timely to address the role of molecular genetic testing in the clinical management of myeloma. Sufficient information is now available to result in a strong recommendation for the adoption of routine molecular genetic testing in myeloma patients. Specifically, three independent studies[23–25] involving close to 500 patients have identified a poor prognosis associated with the presence of IgH translocations with the exception of t(11;14), which appears to have a neutral or perhaps favorable prognostic influence. Because therapies targeting at least one of these translocations (the t(4;14) translocation) will soon be in clinical trials, it is now strongly recommended that all newly diagnosed myeloma patients be tested for t(4;14), t(11;14), and t(11;16). Similarly, numerous studies have determined that the presence of any metaphase abnormalities by conventional cytogenetics will confer a poor prognosis—most particularly the deletion of chromosome 13.[26] Thus it is also recommended that all patients have conventional cytogenetics performed on their bone marrow samples. A recent study[27] has also demonstrated that the deletion of chromosome 17 (perhaps implicating *p53*) also confirms a poor prognosis in myeloma patients undergoing autologous stem cell transplantation; thus when possible, analysis for a deletion of *p53* should also be included in the molecular diagnostic work-up. The detection of t(4;14), t(14;16), deletion of chromosome 13 on metaphase analysis, and deletion of *p53* by fluorescent in situ hybridization will help define high-risk prognostic groups who do not generally benefit from stem cell transplantation and should be steered toward more investigational therapies soon after diagnosis. Alternatively, patients lacking these poor risk factors are likely to benefit from a high-dose melphalan–based approach.

SUPPORTIVE CARE

Along with specific therapy directed at myeloma cells, the management of a patient with myeloma must include aggressive supportive care. Areas that must be addressed include anemia, bony disease, hypercalcemia, renal insufficiency, infection, and the hyperviscosity syndrome.

Anemia

The majority of patients with multiple myeloma who undergo treatment will have anemia that will require intervention. Although their specific myeloma therapy will ultimately improve their anemia, a more rapid intervention is usually required. Often the use of blood transfusions cannot be avoided in patients with critical hemoglobin levels. However, the use of erythropoietin therapy has significantly altered transfusion practices in myeloma.

Erythropoietin has now been studied in randomized, placebo-controlled trials demonstrating its ability to increase hemoglobin levels and reduce transfusion requirements.[28] Furthermore, it has been shown to significantly improve patients' quality of life. Recently the American Society of Hematology and the American Society of Clinical Oncology have published guidelines on the management of anemia.[29]

Bony Disease

The majority of patients with myeloma also have bony involvement; if not lytic lesions or fractures, they will likely have osteopenia. Imaging with MRI may even identify more involvement of the disease than initially suspected on screening investigations. Patients should be initially screened by means of a skeletal survey looking at the skull, spine, pelvis, humeri, and femora.[30] The radiographs should be repeated at 6-month intervals or sooner if pain develops. Plain radiographs are superior to technetium bone scans in identifying lesions in myeloma.

More severe complications can arise as a result of the bony disease in myeloma. Lytic lesions can give rise to fractures (especially in vertebrae or long bones). In the case of long bones, surgical intervention with fixation may be necessary for fracture prophylaxis. Bony pain should be well controlled with analgesia. Although patients should avoid activity that may be traumatic, exercise will enhance bone strengthening.

Radiation may be effective locally in the control of bony pain. It should be limited to patients with severe pain and whose bony disease is localized, thus allowing for focused radiation. Extensive radiation may compromise bone marrow function and should be avoided.

The mainstay of therapy for myeloma patients with bony disease is the use of bisphosphonates. They have been demonstrated to reduce the number of skeletal events, including pathologic fracture, the need for radiation or surgery, and spinal cord compression. The American Society of Clinical Oncology clinical practice guidelines for the use of bisphosphonates in multiple myeloma were published in 2002.[31] It was recommended that either pamidronate (90 mg by intravenous infusion given over 2 hours) or zoledronic acid (one 4-mg intravenous infusion given over 15 minutes) be given every 3–4 weeks in patients with multiple myeloma who have one or more lytic lesions on radiographs. Bisphosphonates should also be given to patients with severe osteopenia. Most patients who have tolerated the drug well will remain on it indefinitely. Recently, however, both avascular necrosis of the jaw and chronic renal dysfunction have been recognized as complications of chronic use, and long-term use will need to be balanced against these potential risks.

Another means of dealing with the severe bony sequelae of myeloma is surgical intervention. Vertebroplasty involves percutaneously injecting bone cement under fluoroscopic guidance into a collapsed vertebral body. Kyphoplasty is a technique that involves the introduction of inflatable bone tamps into the vertebral body that will restore its original height. The remaining cavity can then be filled with bone cement to ensure stability of the process. These procedures can lead to less pain and increased overall patient functioning.[32]

Spinal cord compression from an extramedullary plasmacytoma should be suspected in patients with severe back pain, weakness, or paresthesias of the lower extremities, or bladder or bowel dysfunction or incontinence. MRI or computed tomographic myelography of the entire spine must be performed immediately if this complication is suspected, because immediate institution of therapy is critical. Urgent radiation with concomitant dexamethasone is primary therapy. Surgical decompression is rare, but may be necessary if neurologic deficits increase with radiation and medical treatment.

Hypercalcemia

Hypercalcemia occurs in approximately 10–15% of patients with myeloma at diagnosis. It is mostly due to increased osteoclastic activity resulting from factors such as macrophage inflammatory protein 1-alpha, lymphotoxin and interleukin-6. Patients with hypercalcemia may present with no symptoms, may have evidence of volume contraction, may have renal insufficiency, or may even present in coma. Treatment consists of aggressive hydration with isotonic saline and, depending on the extent of renal insufficiency, the use of a bisphosphonate.

Renal Insufficiency

Renal insufficiency occurs in approximately one third of patients with myeloma. Multiple mechanisms may mediate its presence, including cast nephropathy, hypercalcemia, myeloma therapy, infection, light chain deposition disease, and amyloidosis. Therapy involves identifying and treating the underlying cause. This usually involves hydration and, in some cases, plasmapheresis for acute renal failure. Recent randomized trials, however, have suggested that pheresis is futile in this population. Patients who develop end-stage renal disease can be treated with hemodialysis or peritoneal dialysis. Although the presence of renal insufficiency may increase treatment-related mortality, it is not an indication to withhold aggressive therapy.

Infection

Infections are more prevalent in patients with myeloma because of their immunocompromised state. Rapid treatment of suspected or confirmed infections should be initiated. Prompt treatment of bacterial infection is essential in patients with multiple myeloma. Immunization with pneumococcal and influenzal vaccines may be helpful although antibody responses are suboptimal.[33] Prophylactic bactrim or a quinolone antibiotic is recommended during induction therapy.

Hyperviscosity Syndrome

Hyperviscosity syndrome is a rare occurrence in myeloma. However, when it does occur, it is characterized by oral or nasal bleeding, blurred vision, neurologic symptoms, and heart failure.[34] Serum viscosity measurements may not correlate well with symptoms or the clinical findings. Plasmapheresis promptly relieves the symptoms and should be performed regardless of the viscosity level if the patient is symptomatic.

MYELOMA VARIANTS

Monoclonal Gammopathy of Unknown Significance

Patients with MGUS have less than 10% bone marrow plasmacytosis, a low concentration of M protein in urine or blood, and absent bone lesions or cytopenias and are asymptomatic (see Chapter 48). The frequency of MGUS increases with age, affecting 5% of individuals over age 70 and 10% over age 80. One third will ultimately progress to either myeloma, lymphoma, or macroglobulinemia over 15 years (conversion rate, 1–2%/year). Patients with MGUS, therefore, should have their M protein levels monitored initially every 3–6 months and then, if there is no progression, yearly. No treatment is needed unless progression is noted.

Isolated Plasmacytoma of Bone

Patients with a solitary lytic bone lesion do not have bone marrow plasmacytosis and are otherwise asymptomatic. The diagnosis is made on needle biopsy of the bone lesion itself. Half of the patients will have a detectable serum M protein that usually resolves with radiation therapy. Local radiation to the lesion (35–45 Gy) will lead to a greater than 50% survival over 10 years, significantly better than in myeloma. Two thirds of patients, however, will eventually progress to myeloma and require systemic treatment. There is no evidence to date that initiating chemotherapy early at the solitary bone lesion stage changes the rate of conversion to myeloma.

Extramedullary Plasmacytoma

Plasmacytomas may also present as soft tissue tumors most commonly in tonsils, nasopharynx, and paranasal sinuses, without evidence of bony disease or marrow plasma cell infiltration. As with solitary bone plasmacytomas, radiotherapy is the primary mode of therapy. A wider radiation field than with bone plasmacytomas is

used, however, because the pattern of spread is via regional lymph nodes. Surgical resection can also be used but should be followed by adjunctive radiotherapy. An associated serum M protein found in one third of patients usually disappears with adequate treatment. Persistence or a recurrence of a previously resolved M protein should warn of disease progression. Myeloma will eventually develop over 15 years in approximately 20% of patients, at which point systemic chemotherapy is indicated.

POEMS Syndrome

Patients with POEMS syndrome have an osteosclerotic myeloma (versus osteolytic in typical myeloma) with any one or more of the following:

- P—demyelinating polyneuropathy
- O—organomegaly: hepatosplenomegaly, lymphadenopathy
- E—endocrinopathy: hypogonadism, hypothyroidism
- M—M protein in blood or urine
- S—skin abnormalities: hyperpigmentation, hypertrichosis

Bone marrow plasmacytosis is usually less than 5%. Renal failure and hypercalcemia are rare. Survival for patients with POEMS (median 96 months) appears improved over that for myeloma patients (median 30 months). Treatment is anecdotal, with responses reported to standard melphalan and prednisone, radiotherapy, steroids alone, and plasmapheresis. Plasmapheresis has been utilized to decrease the M protein presumed to cause neuropathy, but responses are variable and usually transient.

CURRENT CONTROVERSIES & FUTURE CONSIDERATIONS

Multiple Myeloma

- Induction therapy: Add thalidomide, Revlimid, or bortezomib to front-line treatment?
- One or two transplants: Early tandem transplant or delayed second transplant?
- Optimal salvage therapy: Bortezomib/thalidomide versus cyclophosphamide + prednisone (balance of convenience, efficacy, toxicity, and cost)? Single-agent or combination therapy?
- Risk-adapted therapy: Use of risk-adapted approach? Use of gene expression profiling?
- Targeted therapy: Therapeutic decisions by molecular targets (e.g., fibroblast growth factor receptor-3)?

Suggested Readings*

Attal M, Harousseau J-L, Facon T, et al: Single versus double autologous stem-cell transplantation for multiple myeloma. N Engl J Med 349:2495–2502, 2003.

Barlogie B, Shaughnessy J, Tricot G, et al: Treatment of multiple myeloma. Blood 103:20–32, 2004.

Berenson JR, Hillner BE, Kyle RA, et al: American Society of Clinical Oncology clinical practice guidelines: the role of bisphosphonates in multiple myeloma. J Clin Oncol 20:3719–3736, 2002.

Dammaco F, Castoldi G, Rodjer S: Efficacy of epoetin alfa in the treatment of anaemia of multiple myeloma. Br J Haematol 113:172–179, 2001.

Kuehl WM, Bergsagel PL: Multiple myeloma: evolving genetic events and host interactions. Nat Rev Cancer 2:175–187, 2002.

Kyle RA, Therneau TM, Rajkumar SV, et al: A long-term study of prognosis in monoclonal gammopathy of undetermined significance. N Engl J Med 346:564–569, 2002.

Myeloma Trialists' Collaborative Group: Combination chemotherapy versus melphalan plus prednisone as treatment for multiple myeloma: an overview of 6,633 patients from 27 randomized trials. J Clin Oncol 16:3832–3842, 1998.

Richardson P, Barlogie B, Berenson J, et al: A Phase 2 study of bortezomib in relapsed, refractory myeloma. N Engl J Med 348:2609–2617, 2003.

Singhal S, Mehta J, Desikan R, et al: Antitumor activity of thalidomide in refractory multiple myeloma. N Engl J Med 341:1565–1571, 1999.

***Full references for this chapter can be found on accompanying CD-ROM.**

CHAPTER 48

MONOCLONAL GAMMOPATHY OF UNDETERMINED SIGNIFICANCE

Roger G. Owen, MB BCh, MD, MRCP, MRCPath

KEY POINTS

Monoclonal Gammopathy of Undetermined Significance

- Monoclonal immunoglobulins are frequently found in the sera of apparently normal individuals, and their incidence increases with age.
- Monoclonal immunoglobulins may indicate underlying myeloma or a lymphoproliferative disorder, but the majority of patients are asymptomatic and have no evidence of such disease. This is termed *monoclonal gammopathy of undetermined significance* (MGUS). For IgG, IgA, and IgM, monoclonal protein is <30 gm/L.
- The plasma cells in MGUS have many of the phenotypic and genotypic features of myeloma plasma cells but, despite this, the overall rate of progression to symptomatic disease is relatively low at approximately 1% per annum.
- The vast majority of patients with MGUS are asymptomatic, but a minority have symptoms and signs attributable to the physicochemical properties of their monoclonal protein. These features include amyloidosis and light chain deposition disease, adult-acquired Fanconi's syndrome, cryoglobulinemia, and autoimmune phenomena such as peripheral neuropathy and cold agglutinin disease.
- No specific treatment is required in MGUS, although careful clinical and laboratory evaluation is required at presentation in order to exclude underlying myeloma or lymphoproliferative disorder.

INTRODUCTION

Monoclonal immunoglobulins are frequently found in the sera of apparently normal individuals, and their incidence shows a progressive increase with age.[1–3] Their presence may indicate underlying multiple myeloma or a lymphoproliferative disorder such as Waldenström's macroglobulinemia, but the majority of patients have no evidence of these disorders. Monoclonal gammopathy of undetermined significance (MGUS) therefore refers to the presence of monoclonal immunoglobulin in the serum and/or urine without the clinical and laboratory features of multiple myeloma, Waldenström's macroglobulinemia, or another lymphoproliferative disorder.[4] The great majority of patients with MGUS are entirely asymptomatic, although there is a low but definite risk of progression, estimated to be approximately 1% per annum.[5–18]

EPIDEMIOLOGY AND RISK FACTORS

Several large population-based studies have demonstrated that up to 0.5% of adults have monoclonal immunoglobulins demonstrable in their sera. The incidence shows a progressive increase with age such that 1% of those age 50 years and above and 3% of those over 70 years of age will have monoclonal immunoglobulins.[1–3,19–21]

In most published series there is a slight male predominance, but this has no clinical relevance. Racial differences have been demonstrated, and the incidence of MGUS appears higher in black Americans than in age-matched whites, whereas it may be lower in Japanese individuals.[21–24] Despite these apparent racial differences, MGUS has been widely described in the United States, Western Europe, Scandinavia, Africa, India, Australasia, and the Far East.[1–3,5–34] Systematic comparative studies have not been performed, however, and there are no clear data on the influence of geography and ethnicity on the overall incidence of MGUS or its progression.

The cause of MGUS is unknown. Some epidemiologic studies have suggested a possible etiologic role for tobacco smoking and occupational exposure to asbestos, fertilizers, mineral oils, petroleum, and radiation.[35,36] However, given the high prevalence of MGUS, these studies have generally been small and have lacked the statistical power to make valid conclusions. There are no known genetic risk factors, but a number of small studies have described the familial occurrence of MGUS, although this appears to be rare and as yet no candidate genes have been identified.[37–39]

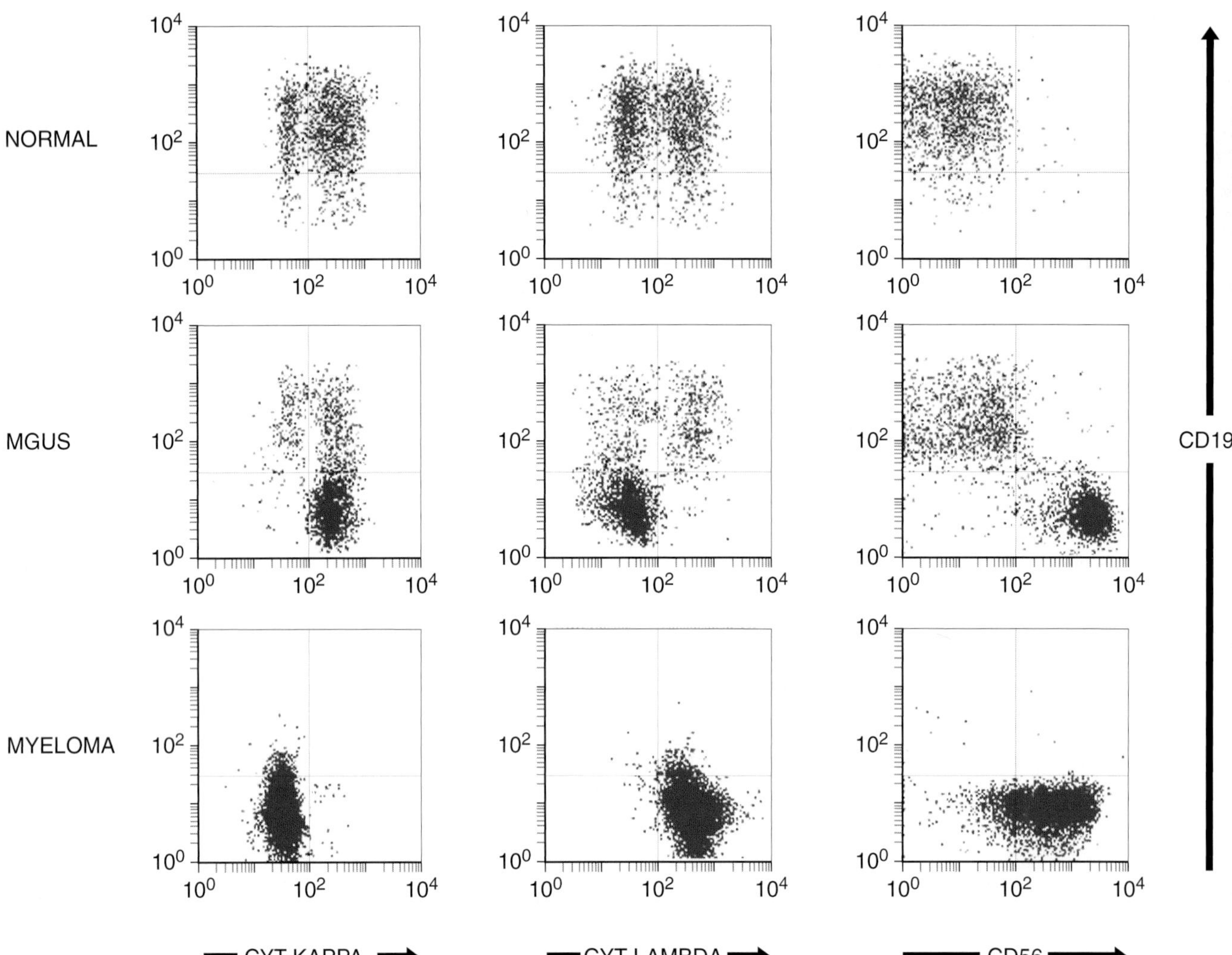

Figure 48–1. Flow cytometric evaluation of bone marrow plasma cells using CD19 and CD56. *Top,* Normal bone marrow plasma cells, which are CD19$^+$ CD56$^-$ and polyclonal with regard to immunoglobulin light chain expression. *Bottom,* The pattern seen in patients with established myeloma. Plasma cells have a neoplastic phenotype (CD19$^-$ CD56$^+$ in this case) and appear to be λ light chain restricted. *Middle,* The pattern typically seen in MGUS. A population of neoplastic plasma cells (CD19$^-$ CD56$^+$ and colored *red*) are evident that are clonal by virtue of κ light chain restriction. Normal plasma cells (CD19$^+$ CD56$^-$) are also present, but these appear polyclonal.

PATHOPHYSIOLOGY

Considerable advances have been made in our understanding of the underlying biology of MGUS. This has largely occurred as a direct result of an improved understanding of the complex biology of multiple myeloma (see Chapter 47). It is becoming increasingly clear that the plasma cells of patients with IgG and IgA MGUS share many of the phenotypic and genotypic features seen in multiple myeloma plasma cells. The underlying biology of IgM MGUS, however, is far less clear.

Immunophenotypic Studies

The immunophenotype of myeloma plasma cells differs considerably from that of normal bone marrow plasma cells. Normal and neoplastic plasma cells differ in their scatter characteristics in that the latter have higher forward and side scatter. Neoplastic plasma cells are also characterized by loss of CD19, weaker expression of CD27, CD37, CD38, and CD45, and aberrant expression of CD56, CD117, and CD126.[40–53] These differences allow the identification of both normal and neoplastic plasma cell populations within the same specimen (Fig. 48–1). In this regard, CD19 and CD56 are the most discriminatory markers; normal plasma cells are consistently CD19$^+$ CD56$^-$, whereas neoplastic plasma cells may be CD19$^-$ CD56$^+$ (65% of cases), CD19$^-$ CD56$^-$ (30% of cases), or CD19$^+$ CD56$^+$ (5% of cases).[40–45] Cases of myeloma with an apparently normal phenotype have been described but these appear to be very rare.[54,55] Flow cytometry studies in MGUS have demonstrated that distinct populations of neoplastic plasma cells are evident in up to 90% of cases, and they comprise a median of 0.6% of bone marrow leukocytes. This population is monoclonal by immunoglobulin light restriction and polymerase chain reaction but also appears to be aneuploid in a significant proportion of cases.[40–45] Multiple

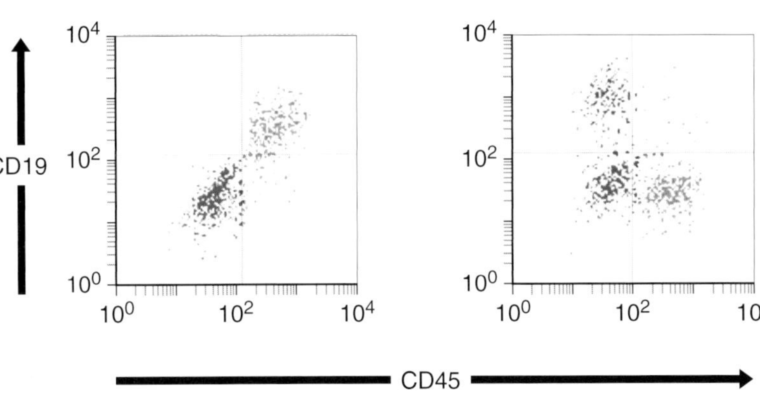

Figure 48–2. Multiple plasma cell populations in a patient with MGUS. In this example, two distinct populations of neoplastic plasma cells (CD19⁻ CD56⁺ and CD19⁻ CD56⁻, *red*) are identified in addition to a population of normal CD19⁺ CD56⁻ plasma cells *(green)*.

distinct neoplastic populations may also coexist within the same patient (Fig. 48–2). Flow cytometric evaluation of plasma cell populations using CD19 and CD56 is useful in the diagnostic setting and appears to be predictive of outcome (see later).[56]

Genotypic Studies

Conventional cytogenetic analysis is rarely if ever abnormal in MGUS, which is due to the low level of bone marrow infiltration and the low proliferative capacity of the clonal plasma cells. Fluorescence in situ hybridization (FISH) combined with immunofluorescence staining for cytoplasmic immunoglobulin allows for karyotypic assessment even when minimal numbers of plasma cells are present.[57] Such studies have clearly demonstrated that MGUS plasma cells harbor complex karyotypic abnormalities. Studies using a variety of centromeric probes have demonstrated that aneuploidy, and in particular hyperdiploidy, is common occurring in up to 70% of patients at presentation.[58–62] FISH studies on flow-sorted cells have demonstrated that the chromosomal changes are confined to those plasma cells with an aberrant phenotype.[61] The pattern of whole chromosome gains is very similar to that seen in multiple myeloma, with trisomies of chromosomes 3, 7, 9, and 11 being particularly common (Fig. 48–3). It is also clear from these studies that several related subclones may exist within the same patient and that the acquisition of new abnormalities occurs over time but does not necessarily correlate with transformation to multiple myeloma.[58,59,61]

Translocations involving the immunoglobulin heavy chain (IgH) locus at 14q32 are characteristically found in myeloma; they are demonstrable in the vast majority of cell lines and in up to 60% of patient specimens. These translocations, which are thought to arise through errors in isotype switch recombination, involve a number of partner chromosomes, including 11q13, 4p16, 16q23, and 6p25, which deregulate cyclin D1, *FGFR3*, c-*maf*, and *MUM1*, respectively.[63] Several FISH studies have also demonstrated that 14q32 translocations are evident in a significant proportion of patients with MGUS[64–67] (see Fig. 48–3). Such translocations occur in up to 50% of patients, and the spectrum of translocations seen is broadly similar to that seen in patients with myeloma. In addition, the deregulation of cyclin D1 and *FGFR3* has also been demonstrated in MGUS patients with the t(11;14) and t(4;14), respectively, suggesting that the functional consequence of these translocations is similar in MGUS and myeloma.[64,65,68] In addition to IgH translocations, Fonseca and colleagues have described a number of patients with translocations involving the Igλ locus,[65] which have also been described in myeloma cell lines and patient samples.[69–71]

Loss of chromosome 13 material is a further common finding in myeloma and appears to confer an adverse outcome in this setting.[72–74] These abnormalities, however, are also observed in up to 50% of MGUS patients and appear, in a manner similar to myeloma, to consist of large deletions of the long arm or loss of the whole chromosome[61,65–67,72,73,75,76] (see Fig. 48–3). Chromosome 13 abnormalities appear to be significantly associated with the t(4;14), a pattern that is also well described in myeloma.[77–80]

A number of studies have demonstrated the presence of hyperdiploidy, IgH translocations, and abnormalities of chromosome 13 in patients with primary amyloidosis,[81–83] confirming a common pathogenetic basis for MGUS, primary amyloidosis (see Chapter 51), and multiple myeloma (see Chapter 47). The cytogenetic studies published to date in MGUS are summarized in Table 48–1.

Pathogenesis of IgM MGUS

The underlying pathogenetic mechanisms seen in IgG and IgA MGUS are likely to be very different from those seen in IgM MGUS given the fact that the latter rarely, if ever, progresses to multiple myeloma. There are no data regarding the cytogenetic abnormalities seen in IgM MGUS. However, 14q32 translocations and abnormalities of chromosome 13 do not appear to be a feature of Waldenström's macroglobulinemia, although a significant proportion of patients appear to have deletion of chromosome 6q.[84–88] It remains to be seen whether the clonal cells in IgM MGUS will be characterized by these features.

Gene Expression Profiling

Further insights into the biology of MGUS have been gained recently with the use of gene expression profil-

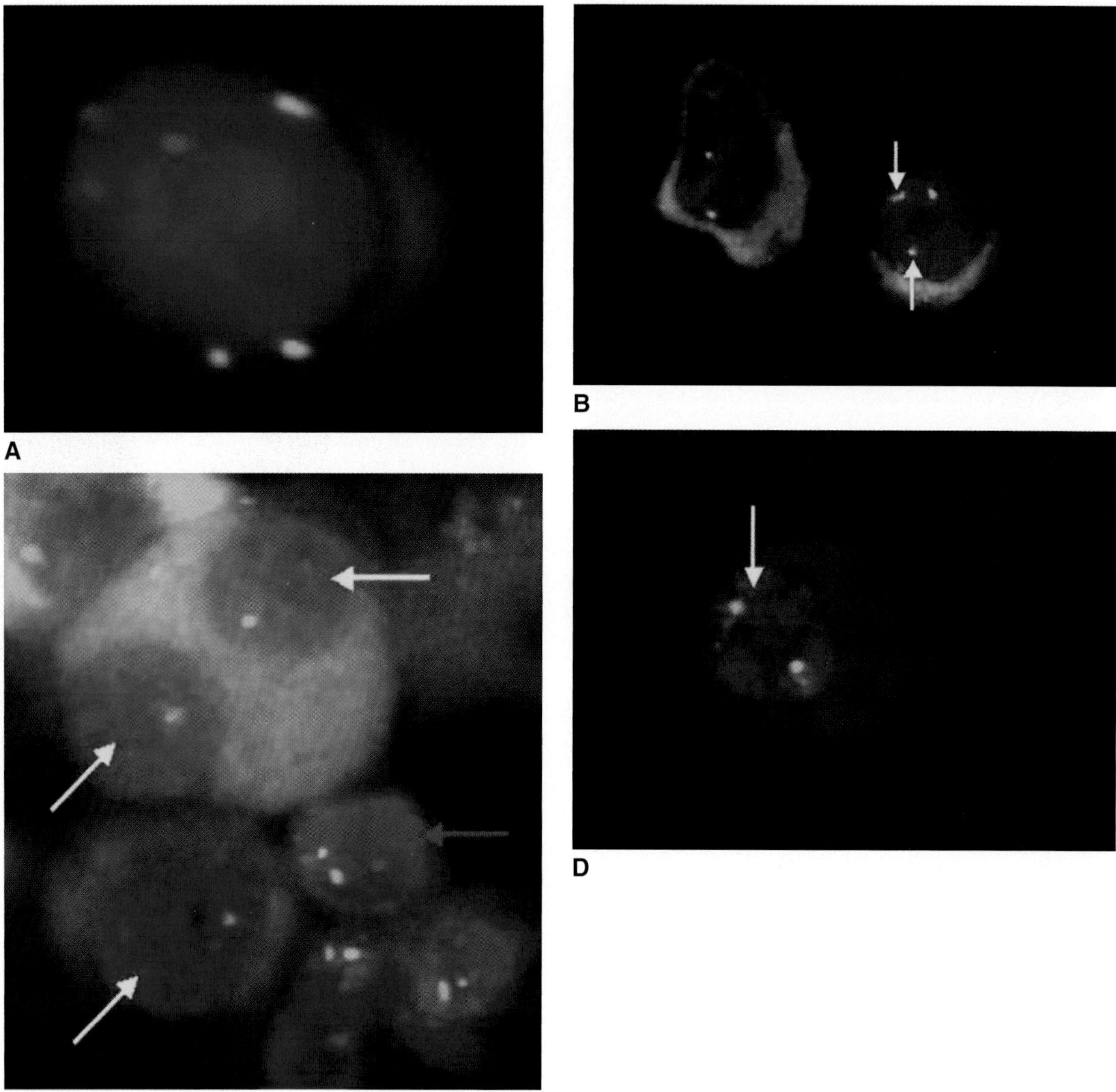

Figure 48–3. Cytogenetic abnormalities in MGUS plasma cells. Hyperdiploidy, IgH translocations, and monosomy 13/deletion 13q are demonstrable in a significant proportion of patients. ***A,*** The presence of both trisomy 3 and trisomy 11 in the same plasma cell. ***B,*** The presence of the t(11;14). IgH probes (labeled *green*) and cyclin D1 probes (labeled *red*) are used in this analysis. A normal cell containing two discrete signals for both IgH and cyclin D1 is shown to the left. The cell to the right is a plasma cell containing a t(11;14) indicated by the presence of two fusion signals *(yellow arrows)*. ***C*** and ***D,*** Abnormalities of chromosome 13 using 13q14 probes (labeled *red*) and 13q34 probes (labeled *green*). ***C,*** The presence of monosomy 13 in two plasma cells, one of which is a large binucleate form. Monosomy 13 is indicated in these cells by loss of both 13q14 and 13q34 signals, which is highlighted by the *yellow arrows*. A normal cell containing two 13q14 signals and two 13q34 signals is highlighted by the *red arrow*. ***D,*** A plasma cell with two 13q34 *(green)* signals but a single 13q14 *(red)* single, indicative of deletion 13q14.

ing, which can be used to determine the expression of large numbers of genes. Davies and coworkers[89] found that the gene expression profile of MGUS plasma cells was very similar to that of myeloma plasma cells but differed considerably from that of normal plasma cells. This analysis did, however, identify 74 genes differentially expressed in MGUS plasma cells compared to myeloma, including some involved in cell growth, signal transduction, and intracellular transport.[89] Further studies with this technology should help elucidate the key genetic events in the transformation of MGUS.

CLINICAL FEATURES

The vast majority of MGUS patients will by definition have no symptoms or clinical signs. However, a minority will have clinical features that are directly attributable

TABLE 48–1. Fluorescence In Situ Hybridization Studies in MGUS*

	Hyperdiploidy	14q32 Translocations	Deletion 13q/Monosomy 13
Zandecki et al.[58]	12/28 (43%)	ND	ND
Zandecki et al.[59]	13/19 (68%)	ND	ND
Lloveras et al.[60]	8/35 (23%)	ND	ND
Rasillo et al.[61]	17/30 (57%)	ND	6/30 (21%)
Drach et al.[62]	19/36 (53%)	ND	ND
Miura et al.[64]	ND	7/13 (54%)	ND
Fonseca et al.[65]	ND	27/59 (46%)	24/48 (50%)
Avet-Loiseau et al.[66,67]	ND	36/79 (46%)	16/79 (20%)
Konigsberg et al.[75]	ND	ND	13/29 (45%)
Bernasconi et al.[76]	ND	ND	5/18 (28%)

*Hyperdiploidy, translocations involving the IgH locus at 14q32, and deletion/monosomy of chromosome 13 are demonstrable in a significant proportion of patients with MGUS.
Abbreviation: ND, not detected.

to the physicochemical properties of their monoclonal proteins.

Immunoglobulin Deposition Diseases

In some individuals, monoclonal immunoglobulins or, more commonly, fragments of monoclonal light chains have the propensity for tissue deposition. Primary amyloidosis is the most common and best characterized manifestation of this process. Patients may present with cardiac failure, nephrotic syndrome, malabsorption, carpal tunnel syndrome, and peripheral and autonomic neuropathies. These features occur as a result of the extracellular deposition of amyloid fibrils consisting of the amino termini of clonal immunoglobulin light chains in these tissues. The propensity for monoclonal proteins to form amyloid deposits and their tissue tropism are largely determined by the immunoglobulin light chain genes used; λ light chains predominate, and specific λ variable region genes are associated with different patterns of tissue tropism.[90] Primary amyloidosis is discussed in detail in Chapter 51.

Nonamyloid immunoglobulin deposition is a rare complication of monoclonal gammopathy.[91–101] Such deposits lack the structural and staining properties of amyloid in that they tend to form granular rather than fibrillar deposits and are typically noncongophilic. These deposits usually consist of monoclonal light chains or light chain fragments, producing a condition known as light chain deposition disease. Less commonly, deposits may consist of heavy chain determinants (heavy chain deposition disease) or both light and heavy chain determinants (light and heavy chain deposition disease). Renal involvement is the most common clinical feature and patients may present with nephrotic syndrome or progressive renal failure. Cardiac involvement resulting in congestive cardiac failure and arrhythmias, peripheral neuropathy, and hepatic involvement is also frequently seen. The underlying pathologic mechanism in light chain deposition disease has many similarities to primary amyloidosis. In light chain deposition disease, κ light chains are the rule and there appears to be restricted use of specific κ variable region genes. Sequence analysis also demonstrates the presence of mutations, which generate hydrophobic residues resulting in a partially unfolded and insoluble protein.[91,95,96,101] In heavy chain deposition disease, the monoclonal heavy chain appears to be truncated as a result of deletion of the C_H1 domain, although it would appear that variable region mutations are also required for tissue deposition.[97–99]

Adult-acquired Fanconi's syndrome has some features in common with light chain deposition disease. In this disorder, monoclonal immunoglobulin light chains, predominantly of κ type, deposit and crystallize in proximal renal tubular cells, resulting in the urinary loss of amino acids, glucose, phosphate, and uric acid. The main clinical features are metabolic disturbances, bone disease, and renal failure.[102] The underlying pathologic mechanism is very similar to light chain deposition disease in that there is a restricted use of specific κ variable region genes, which are resistant to proteolysis as a consequence of hydrophobic or nonpolar residues generated by the somatic hypermutation process.[103–105]

Cryoglobulins

Monoclonal immunoglobulins may also act as cryoglobulins, that is, they precipitate at temperatures below 37°C and redissolve on warming.[106] Type I cryoglobulins consist of monoclonal immunoglobulin only, whereas type II cryoglobulins generally consist of a complex of polyclonal IgG and a monoclonal immunoglobulin, usually IgM κ with rheumatoid factor activity. The latter is typically associated with hepatitis C virus infection, and the monoclonal component appears to have a distinct pattern of heavy and light chain variable region gene usage.[107] Type I cryoglobulins are frequently asymptomatic, whereas type II cryoglobulins are classically associated with skin purpura, arthralgia, Raynaud's phenomenon, and vasculitis affecting the skin, kidneys, liver, and peripheral nerves.[106] Cryoglobulinemia is discussed in detail in Chapter 46.

Autoimmune Phenomena

In a proportion of patients, the monoclonal immunoglobulin has autoantibody specificity, which may result in a variety of autoimmune phenomena.[108–110] These are primarily associated with monoclonal proteins of IgM type.

Peripheral neuropathies occur in 5–10% of patients with IgM monoclonal proteins and are frequently associated with autoantibody activity directed against a variety of neural antigens, including myelin-associated glycoprotein, sulfatide, and gangliosides such as GalNac-GD_{1a}, GM_1, GM_2, and GD_{1b}. The autoantibody specificity, to a certain extent, determines the clinical phenotype and electrophysiologic findings.[108,109,111–113] Peripheral neuropathies are also encountered in patients with IgG and IgA monoclonal proteins, but evidence for a clear pathologic role is generally lacking. They are more likely to represent coincidental findings in patients who might otherwise be diagnosed with chronic inflammatory demyelinating polyneuropathy.[114–116]

In cold agglutinin disease, the monoclonal protein is almost invariably of IgM κ type and has autoantibody specificity directed against I or i blood group antigens. The affinity of the autoantibody is temperature dependent such that antibody binding seldom occurs at body temperature but occurs as the temperature falls. The classic clinical features are therefore acrocyanosis, Raynaud's phenomenon, and episodic cold-induced hemolysis. Sequence analysis has also been informative in cold agglutinin disease, because the heavy chain variable region is almost always encoded by the V_H4–34 gene segment.[117,118]

Rarely, patients may present with a bleeding tendency that may be due to either autoantibody specificity directed against platelet antigens (resulting in immune thrombocytopenia) or the von Willebrand factor protein.[119–124] Acquired angioedema, myasthenia gravis, and glomerulonephritis have all been described in patients with monoclonal immunoglobulins that possess autoantibody activity directed against C1 esterase inhibitor, cholinesterase receptor, and the glomerular basement membrane, respectively.[109,125–129] It must be noted, however, that the presence of an autoimmune disorder in a patient with MGUS does not necessarily imply a pathogenic role for the monoclonal protein. Coincidental polyclonal autoantibodies can also occur, which can complicate the clinical assessment.[130–133]

DIAGNOSIS AND DIFFERENTIAL DIAGNOSIS

Serum protein electrophoresis should be performed in all patients in whom multiple myeloma, primary amyloidosis, or a B-cell lymphoproliferative disorder is suspected. Agarose gel electrophoresis is the method of choice[134]; monoclonal immunoglobulins appear as a distinct band on the electrophoresis gel or as a narrow peak on the densitometer tracing, usually within the γ or β region. Immunofixation using specific antisera is then required to determine the heavy chain isotype and light chain class (Fig. 48–4).

Ideally, all patients with monoclonal proteins detectable in their sera should be referred for evaluation at a specialist center. The main purpose of this is to identify those patients with an underlying disorder such as myeloma but also those rare MGUS patients who have clinical features attributable to the properties of their monoclonal protein. It is crucial to consider the heavy chain isotype when assessing patients with monoclonal gammopathy. Patients with IgG or IgA proteins may have underlying myeloma or, less commonly, primary amyloidosis, solitary plasmacytoma, or a B-cell lymphoproliferative disorder.[134] IgM proteins, in contrast, are most commonly associated with an underlying lymphoproliferative disorder, usually Waldenström's macroglobulinemia, whereas primary amyloidosis appears uncommon and IgM myeloma exceedingly rare.[135–137] These differences are reflected in the different diagnostic criteria utilized for IgG/IgA MGUS and IgM MGUS, which are detailed in Tables 48–2 and 48–3, respectively.[4,138]

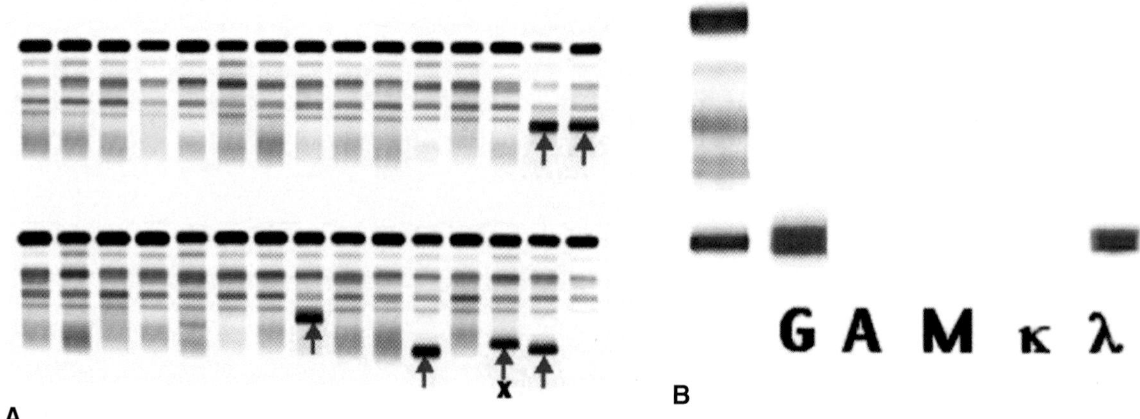

■ **Figure 48–4.** Serum protein electrophoresis and immunofixation. *A,* Agarose gel electrophoresis; monoclonal immunoglobulins of varying electrophoretic mobility are indicated. *B,* Immunofixation performed on sample X confirms the presence of an IgG λ monoclonal protein.

TABLE 48–2. Diagnostic Criteria for IgG/IgA MGUS

IgG and IgA monoclonal protein <30 gm/L
Bone marrow plasma cells <10%*
No evidence of myeloma-related end-organ or tissue impairment†
No clinical or laboratory evidence of other B-cell lymphoproliferative disorders

*Bone marrow aspirate smears should be both particulate and cellular. A trephine biopsy should be obtained in all cases and should demonstrate minimal/low-level plasma cell infiltration.
†Myeloma-related end-organ or tissue impairment is defined by any of the following: anemia, hypercalcemia, renal impairment, bone disease, symptomatic hyperviscosity, amyloidosis, or recurrent bacterial infections.[4]

TABLE 48–3. Diagnostic Criteria for IgM MGUS

IgM monoclonal protein <30 gm/L
No evidence of bone marrow infiltration by lymphoma
No constitutional symptoms, cytopenia, or organomegaly

Bone Marrow Assessment

Bone marrow examination is essential in all patients with a circulating monoclonal protein. The presence of anemia, renal insufficiency, hypercalcemia, and bone pain all suggest underlying myeloma, whereas the presence of anemia, constitutional symptoms, palpable adenopathy and splenomegaly, and peripheral blood lymphocytosis may indicate an underlying lymphoproliferative disorder. Primary amyloidosis (and the nonamyloid immunoglobulin deposition disorders) should be considered in those patients with significant proteinuria/nephrotic syndrome, congestive heart failure, carpal tunnel syndrome, malabsorption, and orthostatic hypotension. The presence of immune paresis and urinary light chain excretion is not indicative of underlying myeloma, however, because they are both demonstrable in up to 30–40% of patients with MGUS.[134] Monoclonal proteins consisting of immunoglobulin light chains only and those of IgD type are similarly no longer considered to be diagnostic of underlying myeloma.[139–141]

The interpretation of the bone marrow examination in asymptomatic patients is more debatable. Some experts suggest that bone marrow examination need only be performed in those patients with monoclonal protein concentrations of 20 gm/L or greater.[134] This approach to investigation is based upon the assumption that the concentration of monoclonal protein is predictive of the underlying pathologic diagnosis. This is only partly true because, although the concentration of monoclonal protein rarely if ever exceeds 30 gm/L in MGUS, it is not uncommon for patients with an underlying disorder to have concentrations of less than 30 gm/L. This is particularly relevant to those patients with IgM monoclonal proteins because the majority of patients with Waldenström's macroglobulinemia and other lymphoproliferative disorders have serum concentrations of considerably less than 30 gm/L.[110,136]

MGUS can only be definitively diagnosed if the bone marrow shows no evidence of myeloma or a B-cell lymphoproliferative disorder. IgG and IgA MGUS may be diagnosed if there are less than 10% plasma cells on an adequate marrow aspirate smear and minimal plasma cell infiltration on the trephine biopsy and no evidence of a B-cell lymphoproliferative disorder.[4] IgM MGUS may be diagnosed if there is no evidence of bone marrow infiltration by a B-cell lymphoproliferative disorder.[138] It is good practice to obtain a trephine biopsy in all cases because this provides a better assessment of the extent of bone marrow infiltration than even the best quality aspirate smears. An adequate trephine biopsy (at least 1 cm in length) also ensures that a diagnosis can be reliably made even when the bone marrow aspirate specimen is of poor quality.

Immunophenotypic Studies

Flow cytometry is a useful adjunct to morphologic assessment in these patients and is routinely performed in many hematopathology laboratories. Neoplastic plasma cells may be differentiated from their normal counterparts by virtue of the loss of CD19 and/or the expression of CD56, because normal plasma cells are consistently $CD19^+$ and $CD56^-$. In addition, a plasma cell clonality can be estimated by clustered surface expression of either λ or κ restriction (see Fig. 48–1). Normal plasma cells are rarely, if ever, detected in patients with established myeloma but they are present in up to 60% of patients with MGUS[40–45] (see Fig. 48–1). The relative proportion of normal and neoplastic plasma cells in MGUS varies considerably from patient to patient. In approximately 40% of cases, neoplastic plasma cells are present exclusively, and careful assessment of the extent of infiltration is required in these cases. Flow cytometry may also be used to assess bone marrow aspirate specimens for the presence of clonal B cells. This is particularly relevant to those patients with IgM monoclonal proteins, in whom Waldenström's macroglobulinemia or other lymphoproliferative disorders are the main differential diagnoses.

In a minority of patients, immunohistochemistry on the trephine biopsy sections may be required to complete the diagnostic bone marrow assessment. CD138 as well as λ and κ chain immunostaining is very useful to determine the extent of plasma cell infiltration, and CD20 immunostaining may be used to exclude bone marrow infiltration by a B-cell lymphoproliferative disorder.[142]

Because of the pleotropic presentation of patients with a circulating monoclonal immunoglobulin, a normal bone marrow assessment does not exclude a diagnosis of primary amyloidosis or solitary plasmacytoma. It should be noted that small populations of neoplastic plasma cells are demonstrable in the bone marrow specimens of the majority of patients with these conditions.[143] Similarly, careful clinical and laboratory assessment is required to determine whether there is any evidence of pathology attributable to the physicochemical properties of the monoclonal protein, such as cold agglutinin disease and peripheral neuropathy. Additional laboratory investigations will be determined by the clinical assessment in these patients. A diagnostic algorithm for patients

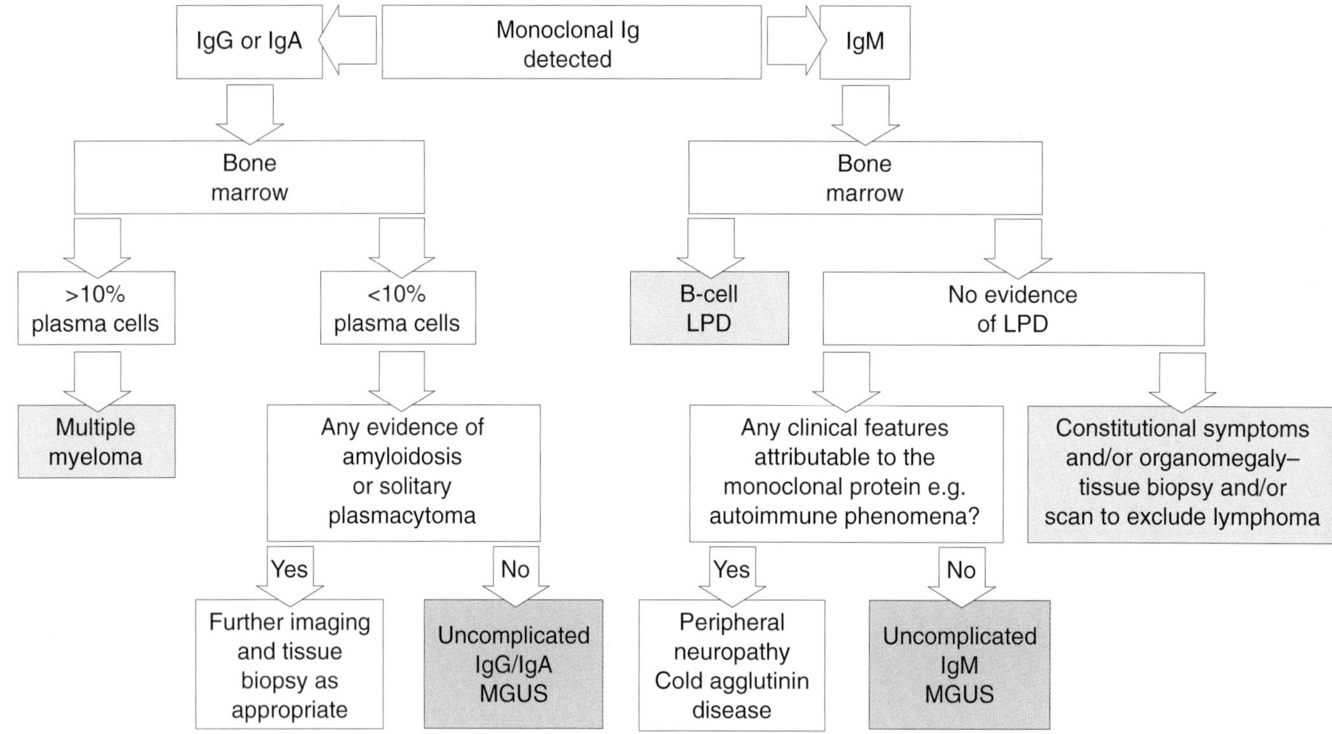

Figure 48–5. Diagnostic algorithm for MGUS.

presenting with monoclonal immunoglobulins is outlined in Figure 48–5.

TREATMENT

The vast majority of patients with MGUS do not require any specific therapeutic intervention. Those rare patients who present with clinical features attributable to their monoclonal protein often present difficult therapeutic challenges. However, there are a number of key points to consider when assessing the treatment options for such patients. First, there is generally no relationship between the presence of an underlying lymphoproliferative disorder or concentration of monoclonal immunoglobulin and severity of symptoms. In fact, the converse may often be true because severe symptoms can occur at very low concentrations and the monoclonal immunoglobulin may only be detectable by sensitive methods such as immunofixation or serum free light chain assay. Second, a significant proportion of patients with these disorders may not require specific cytoreductive therapy; their symptoms may be alleviated with symptomatic measures. Chemotherapy approaches may be appropriate in some patients although response rates vary considerably, in part because it is often difficult to establish a clear etiologic role for the monoclonal immunoglobulin in the clinical disease.

Immunoglobulin Deposition Diseases

Patients with nonamyloid monoclonal immunoglobulin deposition present considerable therapeutic problems. Myeloma therapy regimens such as melphalan and prednisolone and anthracycline-containing combinations such as VAD (vincristine, adriamycin, and dexamethasone) have been employed with some success in patients with nonamyloid immunoglobulin deposition diseases[91,92] (see Chapter 51). This approach may not be applicable to all patients because a significant proportion present with irreversible single organ involvement, typically end-stage renal failure or cardiac failure. Solid organ transplantation may be an approach in these patients, although monoclonal immunoglobulin will inevitably deposit in the transplanted organs over time. Autologous stem cell transplantation is also an attractive approach because it may be that clinically meaningful responses only occur in the context of a complete serologic response. This approach is widely used in primary amyloidosis[144] and may be applicable to those patients with nonamyloid deposition diseases who have potentially reversible multisystem involvement. It may also have a role as an adjunct to solid organ transplantation in those patients with irreversible single-organ damage.

Adult-acquired Fanconi's syndrome should not be considered in this way. The prognosis is generally good, and the disease is usually adequately controlled with supplements of calcium, phosphate, and vitamin D. Cytotoxics are not indicated and only expose the patient to unnecessary risks of infection and secondary leukemia.[102]

Autoimmune Phenomena

Patients who present with autoimmune phenomena frequently gain benefit from relatively simple symptomatic measures. Patients with peripheral neuropathies may benefit from simple analgesics, agents such as gabapentin, and the provision of physical therapy and aids, and those with cold agglutinin disease learn to avoid the cold.[145,146] Acquired von Willebrand's disease is typically treated with intravenous immunoglobulin, but recombinant factor VIIa may also be used in the setting of an acute bleeding episode.[120–124,147,149] Patients with acquired C1 esterase inhibitor deficiency may benefit from antifibrinolytic agents, and factor concentrate is available for acute episodes of angioedema, although the dose required is significantly higher than that used for patients with congenital deficiency.[125,126,149]

Cytotoxic treatment may be considered in a proportion of patients with IgM-associated demyelinating peripheral neuropathy. However, only limited published data are available on the activity of alkylating agents, purine analogues, and rituximab in this setting, and the results are generally disappointing.[146,150–153] These results likely reflect in part the low rate of complete responses seen with these agents. It may therefore be appropriate, at least in some patients with progressive disabling neuropathy, to increase the intensity of treatment with the aim of achieving a complete serologic response. Autologous stem cell transplantation may therefore have a role in a limited number of patients.[154] Rituximab appears to be effective in patients with symptomatic cold agglutinin disease, although there are also published data on the efficacy of alkylating agents and purine analogues.[155–158]

PROGNOSIS AND LONG-TERM MANAGEMENT

Progression Risk

The risk of progression to symptomatic disease in MGUS is approximately 1% per annum. In arguably the definitive long-term study, 1384 patients from southeastern Minnesota were observed for a median of 15.4 years and a total of 11,009 person-years. The overall risk of progression was 12%, 25%, and 30% at 10, 20, and 30 years, respectively. The relative risk of progression to multiple myeloma, primary amyloidosis, Waldenström's macroglobulinemia, and plasmacytoma was 25, 8.4, 46, and 8.5, respectively.[5] These data are broadly corroborated by a number of similar studies published by groups from Spain, Italy, Iceland, Denmark, Greece, and the Netherlands,[7–16] which are detailed in Table 48–4.

In the Minnesota study, the most significant factor associated with risk of progression was the concentration of monoclonal immunoglobulin. There was a progressive increase in risk with increased concentration such that the risk of progression at 10 years was 6%, 7%, 11%, 20%, 24%, and 34% for those patients with initial concentrations of 5 gm/L or less, 6–10 gm/L, 11–15 gm/L, 16–20 gm/L, 21–25 gm/L, and 26–30 gm/L, respectively.[5] The concentration of monoclonal immunoglobulin was also significantly associated with progression in several other studies.[8,14] In the Minnesota analysis, heavy chain isotype was also significantly associated with risk of progression. This appeared greater for those patients with IgA and IgM monoclonal proteins, whereas the risk of progression was greater for those patients with IgA bands in studies from Spain, Denmark, and Iceland.[10,14,15] Several studies have suggested that the presence of urinary free light chains and reduction in normal polyclonal immunoglobulins are also predictive of progression.[7,8,14] The prognostic relevance of cytogenetic changes is unclear. However, it is intriguing to note that abnormalities that appear to confer a poor outcome in patients with established myeloma, such as the t(4;14) and chromosome 13 abnormalities, do not as yet appear to predict progression in patients with MGUS.

Progression Risk in IgM MGUS

The majority of published studies assessing risk of progression in MGUS consider all patients with asymptomatic monoclonal proteins as a single group. This is not entirely appropriate because the spectrum of progression is largely determined by the heavy chain isotype. Patients with IgG and IgA MGUS will progress to multiple myeloma, primary amyloidosis, and rarely solitary plasmacytoma and lymphoproliferative disorders.[134] In contrast, patients with IgM MGUS primarily evolve to Waldenström's macroglobulinemia and other lymphoproliferative disorders; they rarely, if ever, progress to myeloma and primary amyloidosis is also rare.[135–137] A limited number of studies have assessed the progression risk exclusively in patients with IgM monoclonal proteins. In an additional analysis, 213 patients from southeastern Minnesota with IgM MGUS were observed for a median of 6.3 years and a total of 1567 person-years; the cumulative incidence of progression was 10%, 18%, and 24% at 5, 10, and 15 years, respectively. The relative risk of progression to Waldenström's macroglobulinemia, chronic lymphocytic leukemia, and other lymphoproliferative disorders was 262, 14.8, and 5.7, respectively.[6] These data are broadly corroborated by a number of similar studies published by groups from Spain, Italy, and Denmark,[14,17,18] which are detailed in Table 48–5. The concentration of monoclonal immunoglobulin was again significantly associated with the risk of progression. In the study of Kyle and associates, the risk of progression at 10 years was 14%, 13%, 26%, 34%, and 41% for those patients with initial concentrations of 5 gm/L or less, 6–10 gm/L, 11–15 gm/L, 16–20 gm/L, and 21–25 gm/L, respectively.[6]

Overall Survival

The outcome of patients who develop myeloma, Waldenström's macroglobulinemia, or other lymphoproliferative disorders following a documented diagnosis of MGUS is unclear. The limited available data suggest that the outcome is not substantially different from that of patients who present with de novo disease.[7,159,160]

There are considerable published data on the risk of progression to symptomatic disease in MGUS (see Table 48–4). It must be noted that the overall rate of progression is low at approximately 1% per annum, and the majority of patients will ultimately die of unrelated causes. However, a number of studies have demonstrated

TABLE 48–4. Follow-up Studies in MGUS

Study Location	Median Follow-up	No. of Patients	Risk of Progression*	Risk Factors Associated with Progression
Minnesota [5]	15.4 yr	1384	12% at 10 yr 25% at 20 yr 30% at 30 yr	Concentration† IgA and IgM
Italy [8]	70 mo	335	6.8% at 70 mo	BMPC >5% Concentration† ULC Immune paresis Age >70 yr
Netherlands [9]	6.75 yr	88	9.1% at 5 yr 21.3% at 10 yr 38% at 15 yr 48.3 at 20 yr	BMPC >2% κ Light chain
Denmark [14]	4.9 yr	1247	7.7% at 5 yr 13% at 10 yr 18.3% at 15 yr	IgA Immune paresis Female sex Age <70 yr Concentration†
Spain [10]	56 mo	128	8.5% at 5 yr 19.2% at 10 yr	IgA
Italy [16]	11.5 yr	263	6.1% at 5 yr 15.4% at 10 yr 31.3% at 20 yr	NS
Spain [11]	37.8 mo	397	4.5% at 5 yr 15% at 10 yr 26% at 15 yr	NS
Iceland [15]	6 yr	504	10% at 6 yr	IgA
Italy [7]	65 mo	1231	14% at 10 yr 30% at 15 yr	BMPC >5% ULC Immune paresis ESR
Netherlands [12]	NS	334	11% at 14 yr	κ Light chain
Greece [13]	71 mo	63	3% at 71 mo	NS

*The overall rate of progression in MGUS is approximately 1% per annum.
†Serum concentration of monoclonal immunoglobulin.
Abbreviations: BMPC, bone marrow plasma cells; ESR, erythrocyte sedimentation rate; NS, not stated; ULC, urinary light chain excretion.

TABLE 48–5. Follow-up Studies in IgM MGUS

Study Location	Median Follow-up	No. of Patients	Risk of Progression	Risk Factors Associated with Progression
Minnesota [6]	6.3 yr	213	10% at 5 yr 18% at 10 yr 24% at 15 yr	Concentration* Albumin
Italy [17]	49 mo	452	8% at 5 yr 21% at 10 yr	Concentration* Hemoglobin PB lymphocytosis
Denmark [14]	4.9 yr	231	RR 17.2	Concentration* Age <70 yr Female sex
Spain [18]	5 yr	52	13.3% at 10 yr 27.7% at 20 yr	BMPC >5% BML >20%

*Serum concentration of monoclonal immunoglobulin.
Abbreviations: BML, bone marrow lymphocytes; BMPC, bone marrow plasma cells; PB, peripheral blood; RR, relative risk.

that overall survival in patients with MGUS appears to be inferior to that of the control population. Kyle and associates[5] found that the median survival of MGUS patients was significantly shorter than that of age- and sex-matched controls (8.1 vs. 11.8 years); similarly, Gregersen and colleagues found that MGUS patients had a standardized mortality ratio of 2.1 when compared to the control population.[161] This difference is in part attributable to the excess mortality associated with the development of symptomatic disease, although some studies have demonstrated an excess of nonhematologic cancers, ischemic heart disease, and bacteremia.[161–163] This difference does not necessarily imply a causal association and is more likely to reflect a selection bias, because patients with these disorders are more likely to have serum protein electrophoresis performed.

Long-Term Management

The risk of progression to symptomatic disease requiring therapy is considered the main rationale for long-term follow-up in patients with MGUS.[5,134] Following the completion of initial staging investigations, most experts advocate review on at least an annual basis. It is assumed that such follow-up will allow earlier intervention with consequent reduction in morbidity and improvement in survival.[159] There must be some doubt over the validity of this approach because progression occurs abruptly in many patients and may not be associated with a preceding rise in concentration of monoclonal immunoglobulin.[134,160,164–166] A more systematic approach to risk assessment and follow-up is required. It is intriguing that, although karyotypic abnormalities appear common in MGUS, they do not as yet appear to predict progression despite the fact that many of these abnormalities confer a poor outcome in patients with established myeloma. A potential approach to identifying those patients at high risk of progression would be to identify those patients with occult evidence of end-organ impairment such as bone disease. A number of studies have demonstrated that a proportion of MGUS patients have evidence of increased bone resorption, although it remains to be seen whether these abnormalities predict progression.[167–169]

An alternative approach would be to identify those patients in whom the risk of progression is negligible. These patients may be reassured and discharged from long-term follow-up while the remaining patients may be monitored in a more systematic and meaningful manner. Baldini and coworkers suggested that those patients with a monoclonal immunoglobulin concentration of less than 15 gm/L without immune paresis and urinary light chain excretion and less than 5% bone marrow plasma cells had a very low risk of progression.[8] Similarly, Van de Donk and colleagues suggested that a monoclonal immunoglobulin concentration of less than 10 gm/L and a bone marrow plasmacytosis of less than 2% defined very-good-risk disease.[9] Identifying low-risk patients by virtue of the phenotypic and genotypic characteristics of their plasma cells is an attractive approach. In this regard, it is unclear whether the absence of clonal karyotypic abnormalities predicts for a very low incidence of progression. Flow cytometric studies may be helpful in this context, because the preservation of a population of phenotypically normal plasma cells appears to be associated with a negligible risk of progression.[56] Gene expression profiling may ultimately identify the key genetic events associated with progression, which should facilitate the development of a more systematic approach to risk assessment.[89]

CURRENT CONTROVERSIES & FUTURE CONSIDERATIONS

Monoclonal Gammopathy of Undetermined Significance

- Although considerable advances have been made in our understanding of the pathobiology of MGUS, the mechanisms underlying transformation remain unclear. Insights into this transition may be achieved with the use of gene expression profiling, particularly if paired samples from the same patient can be analyzed.
- It is to be hoped that a greater understanding of the pathobiology of MGUS will allow for a more detailed and systematic approach to the initial investigation of patients. Assessing bone marrow plasma cells for the presence or absence of the key genetic events associated with progression may more accurately define those patients at high risk of progression.
- Trials of innovative and experimental therapies may be appropriate in well-defined groups of patients with "high-risk MGUS."
- Detailed clinical and laboratory evaluation of patients should not be used only to define those at high risk of progression. Identifying those with a negligible risk is also very worthwhile because these patients may be spared the uncertainty and worry of long-term follow-up.
- Treatment of the clinical syndromes attributed to the properties of the monoclonal immunoglobulin remains unsatisfactory. High-dose therapy with stem cell transplantation support is conceptually attractive but as yet unproven. Trials of agents such as thalidomide and its immunomodulatory analogues and the proteasome inhibitor bortezomib may be applicable to some patients.

Suggested Readings*

Davies FE, Dring AM, Li C, et al: Insights into the multistep transformation of MGUS to myeloma using microarray expression analysis. Blood 102:4504–4511, 2003.

Fonseca R, Bailey RJ, Ahmann GJ, et al: Genomic abnormalities in monoclonal gammopathies of undetermined significance. Blood 100:1417–1424, 2002.

The International Myeloma Working Group: Criteria for the classification of monoclonal gammopathies, multiple myeloma and related disorders: a report of the International Myeloma Working Group. Br J Haematol 121:749–757, 2003.

Kyle RA, Therneau TM, Rajkumar SV, et al: A long-term study of prognosis in monoclonal gammopathy of undetermined significance. N Engl J Med 346:564–569, 2002.

Kyle RA, Therneau TM, Rajkumar SV, et al: Long-term follow-up of IgM monoclonal gammopathy of undetermined significance. Blood 102:3759–3764, 2003.

Owen RG, Treon SP, Al-Katib A, et al: Clinicopathological definition of Waldenstrom's macroglobulinemia: consensus panel recommendations from the Second International Workshop on Waldenstrom's Macroglobulinemia. Semin Oncol 30:110–115, 2003.

Full references for this chapter can be found on accompanying CD-ROM.

CHAPTER 49

WALDENSTRÖM'S MACROGLOBULINEMIA

Dimitrios Tzachanis, MD, PhD, Robin M. Joyce, MD, and Lowell Schnipper, MD

KEY POINTS

Waldenström's Macroglobulinemia

- Waldenström's macroglobulinemia is a clinicopathologic entity of elevated monoclonal IgM in patients with underlying lymphoplasmacytic lymphoma.
- Signs and symptoms may include anemia, hyperviscosity, cold agglutinins, cryoglobulinemia, bleeding diathesis, and amyloidosis.
- Hyperviscosity should be promptly diagnosed and treated in patients with symptoms and serum viscosity greater than 4 cP.
- Differential diagnosis includes monoclonal gammopathy of undetermined significance, multiple myeloma, lymphoplasmacytic lymphoma, and other lymphomas with increased immunoglobulin IgM.
- Alkylating agents, purine analogues, and rituximab are all transiently effective as treatment, and maximal response may be delayed for many months. High-dose chemotherapy with autologous bone marrow transplant should be considered in suitable patients.

INTRODUCTION

Jan Gosta Waldenström's (1906–1996) contributions to hematology are significant. He introduced the distinction of monoclonal versus polyclonal gammopathy and was the first to describe monoclonal gammopathy of undetermined significance and distinguish it from clinically significant multiple myeloma.[1] In 1944, he described two patients with oronasal bleeding, lymphadenopathy, anemia, thrombocytopenia, elevated erythrocyte sedimentation rate, and bone marrow infiltration by lymphoid cells.[2] He noticed the poor quality of their peripheral blood and bone marrow smears and was able to demonstrate a very high serum viscosity in both of them. More importantly, he noted the presence in their serum of a high-molecular-weight homogeneous globulin. Based on his observations, he proposed the existence of a distinct clinical syndrome with the previously mentioned features, which he contrasted with multiple myeloma based on the absence of osteolytic lesions and the lymphocytic rather than plasmacytic bone marrow infiltration. Waldenström's high-molecular-weight globulin was later identified as monoclonal immunoglobulin (Ig) M. Waldenström's initial description remains characteristic of the classic clinical and laboratory abnormalities of Waldenström's macroglobulinemia.

Diagnostic Criteria

There is no universally accepted definition for Waldenström's macroglobulinemia. Most authors use this term to describe the chronic lymphoproliferative disorder characterized by the presence of lymphoplasmacytic lymphoma in the bone marrow and/or lymph nodes associated with a monoclonal serum IgM paraprotein. However, others mean by *Waldenström's macroglobulinemia* the clinical syndrome caused by the presence in the serum of monoclonal IgM paraprotein regardless of the underlying pathologic diagnosis.

In the Revised European/American Lymphoma (REAL) and World Health Organization (WHO) classification systems, Waldenström's macroglobulinemia is recognized as a clinical syndrome most commonly (but not exclusively) associated with the distinct disease entity "lymphoplasmacytic lymphoma."[3,4] In 2002, the faculty of the Second International Workshop on Waldenström's Macroglobulinemia proposed a clinicopathologic definition.[5] Waldenström's macroglobulinemia was defined as a B-cell lymphoproliferative disorder characterized primarily by bone marrow infiltration with a predominantly intertrabecular pattern along with demonstration of an

IgM monoclonal gammopathy. The underlying pathologic diagnosis is considered to be lymphoplasmacytic lymphoma. This is defined by the REAL and WHO criteria as a tumor of small lymphocytes showing evidence of plasmacytoid/plasma cell differentiation without any of the clinical, morphologic, or immunophenotypic features of other lymphoproliferative disorders. Based on this definition, the term *Waldenström's macroglobulinemia* does not apply to IgG- or IgA-secreting lymphoplasmacytic lymphomas. Additionally, the demonstration of an IgM monoclonal protein is not sufficient for the diagnosis of Waldenström's macroglobulinemia because this can be seen in other low-grade B-cell lymphoproliferative disorders, in multiple myeloma, and in monoclonal gammopathy of undetermined significance as well.

EPIDEMIOLOGY AND RISK FACTORS

Waldenström's macroglobulinemia is a rare disease that most commonly affects elderly Caucasian men.[6] The median age at diagnosis is 72 years. It accounts for about 2% of the hematologic malignancies.[7] In the United States there are 3.4 new cases per 1 million men and 1.7 per 1 million women every year.[8] The incidence rate rises sharply with age to become 36.3 for men over the age of 75. This rate is about the same as that for hairy cell leukemia and about 20 times less than that for multiple myeloma.[8] Waldenström's macroglobulinemia is much more common among Caucasians, in contrast to multiple myeloma, which appears more frequently in African Americans.[6,8]

A familial form of Waldenström's macroglobulinemia has been described. So far 12 families with a high number of Waldenström's macroglobulinemia cases have been reported.[9] The patients are usually younger and more frequently male than in the sporadic form of the disease, and there is a high prevalence of IgM monoclonal gammopathy in their first-degree relatives.[9] The existence of a familial form of Waldenström's macroglobulinemia suggests a possible pathogenetic role for genetic factors.

PATHOPHYSIOLOGY

The malignant clone in Waldenström's macroglobulinemia seems to be derived from the transformation of a post–germinal center B cell that has undergone somatic mutation but not isotype switching (Fig. 49–1). In B-cell–derived tumors, variable region (V) gene analysis can reveal the stage of B-cell maturation where the malignant transformation has occurred.[10] V_H genes in Waldenström's macroglobulinemia were found to have extensive somatic mutations with no intraclonal variation.[11–14] This observation suggests a postgerminal origin for the malignant clone in Waldenström's macroglobulinemia. The transformation to a malignant clone occurs prior to isotype switching, because tumor-derived isotype switch variants are not detected. The hypermutated V_H status suggests that the Waldenström's macroglobulinemia clone might be derived from memory cells, but most tumor cells lack the characteristic memory cell marker CD27.[14]

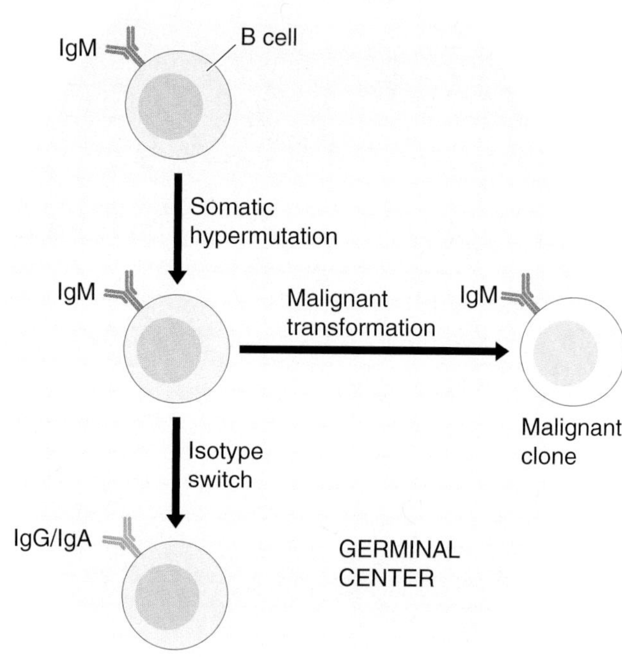

Figure 49–1. B-cell maturation and proposed site of malignant transformation of cell in Waldenström's macroglobulinemia.

Little is known about the pathogenetics of Waldenström's macroglobulinemia. When the malignant B cells are cultured in vitro, they differentiate into monoclonal IgM-secreting plasma cells.[15] This differentiation seems to be at least partially depended on autocrine interleukin-6[15] and it can be inhibited by retinoic acid and by the interferons α and γ.[16,17] Waldenström's macroglobulinemia cells were found to express abnormal variants of the membrane protein hyaluronan synthase that synthesizes the extracellular matrix protein hyaluronan.[18] This may be a mechanism that regulates cell migration or protects the malignant cells from the immune system. In contrast to multiple myeloma, the dysregulation of apoptosis in Waldenström's macroglobulinemia is not regulated by nuclear factor-κB.[19] Some studies suggested a pathogenetic role for the Kaposi's sarcoma–associated herpesvirus/human herpesvirus 8[20]; however, other studies did not confirm the presence of human herpesvirus 8 in the bone marrow of patients with Waldenström's macroglobulinemia.[21] The observation that the deletion of the long arm of chromosome 6 is frequently present in Waldenström's macroglobulinemia cells has prompted a search for putative tumor suppressor genes.[22] Microarray gene profiling and proteomic experiments are currently being conducted.

CLINICAL FEATURES AND DIAGNOSIS

The most common presenting symptoms of Waldenström's macroglobulinemia are fatigue, hyperviscosity, weight loss, fever and night sweats, bleeding, and neurologic symptoms such as peripheral neuropathy; a significant proportion of the patients are asymptomatic (Table 49–1).[23,24] The clinical manifestations of Waldenström's macroglobulinemia can be divided into those related to direct tumor infiltration and those related to the circulating macroglobulin.

Tumor infiltration of the bone marrow by lymphoplasmacytic lymphoma is present in all cases of Waldenström's macroglobulinemia. Depending on the degree of the marrow infiltration, patients may have normal counts, a mild anemia, or even severe pancytopenia.[23,25] Lymphadenopathy, splenomegaly, or hepatomegaly is not uncommon at presentation.[26] Rarely, patients with Waldenström's macroglobulinemia might have tumor infiltration of the lung, kidney, gut, or skin. Osteolytic lesions are not seen (Box 49–1).

IgM is a very-high-molecular-weight pentameric protein and it is mostly confined in the intravascular space. Therefore, even a relatively small increase in the circulating IgM concentration can induce a significant rise in the serum viscosity. In addition, IgM facilitates erythrocyte rouleaux formation, which further increases the plasma viscosity. Clinically, high serum viscosity is associated mainly with neurologic symptoms such as blurry vision, headaches, diplopia, and ataxia.[25,27] Marked hyperviscosity can lead to vision loss, mental status changes, and coma. In addition, patients may develop fatigue, mucocutaneous bleeding, and cardiac failure. About a third of the patients with Waldenström's macroglobulinemia present with symptoms related to hyperviscosity.[23] Funduscopic abnormalities are common in patients with the hyperviscosity syndrome. The classic finding is the "sausage link" appearance of the fundus resulting from the presence of segmented and dilated retinal veins. Retinal hemorrhages and exudates and papilledema are also common. Symptoms related to hyperviscosity usually appear when the serum viscosity rises to more than 4 centipoise (cP). Most patients with a serum viscosity higher than 5 cP will be symptomatic.[28] In these cases, the serum IgM concentration is always above 3 gm/dL.[25]

Cryoglobulins undergo reversible precipitation at low temperatures (~4°C). Type I cryoglobulins consist of monoclonal IgM and can be detected in up to 20% of patients with Waldenström's macroglobulinemia, but less than 5% of patients will have symptoms.[29] Patients with cryoglobulinemia may develop Raynaud's phenomenon, palpable purpura, arthralgias, or glomerulonephritis.

Cold agglutinin disease can develop if the monoclonal IgM protein behaves as an antibody that reacts with erythrocyte antigens at low temperatures, and is observed

Box 49–1. Main Clinical Features of Waldenström's Macroglobulinemia

- Clinical features may be related to either disease burden or paraprotein.
- Bone marrow infiltration is present in all cases and may be manifested by a range of symptoms from mild anemia to severe pancytopenia.
- Splenomegaly and hepatomegaly are common even at presentation.
- Osteolytic bone lesions are not present.
- Lymphadenopathy is not a common initial presentation.

TABLE 49–1. Clinical Features of Waldenström's Macroglobulinemia

Feature	Signs and Symptoms	Etiology	Frequency
Hyperviscosity	Fatigue, blurred vision, vision loss, retinal vein hemorrhage, ataxia, dyspnea, coma, "sausage link" retinal veins	Elevated IgM (>3 gm/dL) and/or serum viscosity >4 cP	30%
Cryoglobulinemia	Raynaud's phenomenon, palpable purpura, arthralgia, glomerulonephritis	Reversible precipitation of type I cryoglobulins at <4°C	20% laboratory finding 5% symptomatic
Cold agglutinin	Mild, chronic hemolysis; agglutinin may occur on cold areas of the body, leading to acrocyanosis, livedo reticularis, and Raynaud's phenomenon	IgM reacts with erythrocyte membrane at low temperature	10%
Sensorimotor polyneuropathy	Distal polyneuropathy, mononeuritis multiplex, symmetrical sensory polyneuropathy, autonomic neuropathy	Cryoglobulins produce ischemic or inflammatory mononeuritis multiplex via inflammation of vasa nervorum or direct neural involvement Amyloid deposition in endoneural vessels	10%
Amyloidosis	Cardiomyopathy, malabsorption, macroglossia, bleeding diathesis	Primary AL-λ light chain Amyloid-associated protein (AA)	Uncommon Very Rare
Schnitzler's syndrome	Erythematous urticarial skin lesions	IgM deposits, vasculitis from IgM deposition	Rare
Skin	Firm, flesh-colored papules	IgM deposition	Rare
Gastrointestinal	Steatorrhea	IgM deposition in lamina propria	Rare
Acquired von Willebrand's disease	Bleeding (mucosal)	IgM against von Willebrand's factor	Rare

in about 10% of patients with Waldenström's macroglobulinemia.[25,29] The hemolysis is usually mild and chronic. The erythrocytes tend to agglutinate in the colder areas of the body's circulation and the patients develop acrocyanosis, livedo reticularis, and Raynaud's phenomenon.

A significant proportion of patients with Waldenström's macroglobulinemia (about 10%) have a chronic sensorimotor peripheral neuropathy.[29–32] In approximately half of these patients the monoclonal IgM reacts with myelin-associated glycoprotein.[33,34] The nerve conduction studies and the sural nerve biopsies in these patients show demyelination, and the cerebrospinal fluid protein level is elevated. In some other patients with neuropathy, the monoclonal IgM reacts with various gangliosides on the peripheral nerves.[35,36] Cryoglobulinemia in patients with Waldenström's macroglobulinemia can cause a distal symmetrical polyneuropathy or a mononeuropathy multiplex via inflammation and ischemia.[37] Amyloid deposition in the nerve or endoneural vessels can also cause a polyneuropathy in the form of a symmetrical sensorimotor peripheral neuropathy or autonomic neuropathy.[38] About 5% of patients with peripheral neuropathy have a monoclonal gammopathy. Therefore, protein electrophoresis should be part of the initial work-up in all patients with unexplained peripheral neuropathy (Box 49–2).

Amyloidosis is a relatively uncommon complication of Waldenström's macroglobulinemia (see Chapter 51). In most cases, it is of the primary (AL) type and the amyloid deposit consists of a λ light chain. Rarely, it can be of the nonimmunoglobulin amyloid-associated protein (AA) type. Cardiac, renal, hepatic, and pulmonary involvement can occur and negatively affect the patients' survival, because most patients with amyloidosis will succumb to cardiac failure rather than to the underlying lymphoma.[38]

In contrast to multiple myeloma (see Chapter 47), renal insufficiency is unusual in Waldenström's macroglobulinemia. When it occurs, it is usually secondary to direct kidney infiltration by the lymphoplasmacytic lymphoma, amyloid deposition, or cryoglobulinemia. Cast nephropathy from light chain deposition is rare. Nephrotic syndrome and glomerulonephritis can develop and are usually secondary to amyloidosis or cryoglobulinemia, respectively.[39,40]

The intraepidermal deposition of IgM can cause firm, translucent, flesh-colored papules.[41] An erythematous urticarial skin vasculitis associated with monoclonal IgM has been described and is known as Schnitzler's syndrome.[42,43] In addition, the lymphoplasmacytic cells in Waldenström's macroglobulinemia may directly infiltrate the skin and produce macular or papulonodular lesions.

In rare cases, patients with Waldenström's macroglobulinemia may develop diarrhea, steatorrhea, and malabsorption secondary to IgM deposition in the lamina propria of the gastrointestinal tract or to direct infiltration by the lymphoplasmacytic cells.[44]

The most common hematologic abnormality in Waldenström's macroglobulinemia is a normochromic, normocytic anemia (Box 49–3). In more advanced cases, pancytopenia is observed. The most characteristic finding on the peripheral blood smear is rouleaux formation.

Box 49–2. Evaluation of Patient with Suspected Waldenström's Macroglobulinemia

- Trephine bone marrow biopsy
- Bone marrow aspirate—with morphologic and flow cytometric evaluation
- Serum protein electrophoresis (not nephelometry)
- Urine protein electrophoresis
- Computed tomography scan of torso to evaluate for lymphadenopathy and organomegaly
- Quantitative measurement of IgG, IgM, and IgA
- Ophthalmologic examination
- Partial thromboplastin time (PTT)
- Complete blood count with differential
- Serum creatinine
- Serum lactate dehydrogenase
- Serum viscosity
- Skeletal radiographs to include long bones and skull to evaluate for osteolytic lesions
- Cryoglobulins
- Cold agglutinin

Lymphocytosis and monocytosis are common. The erythrocyte sedimentation rate is usually markedly elevated. The β_2-microglobulin level is elevated in about 50% of the patients.[23]

Patients with hyperviscosity and bleeding diathesis will have a prolonged thrombin time, prolonged bleeding time, and abnormal platelet aggregation studies.[45] In rare cases, the monoclonal IgM reacts with von Willebrand factor and patients develop acquired von Willebrand's disease.[46] Idiopathic thrombocytopenic purpura can also develop in Waldenström's macroglobulinemia.[47]

Serum protein electrophoresis reveals a characteristic sharp, narrow spike of monoclonal IgM in the gamma region. Reciprocal reductions in IgG and IgA may be present but not as commonly as in multiple myeloma. In most cases, the monoclonal IgM is of the κ light chain type. Urine protein electrophoresis is usually normal.

PROGNOSTIC FACTORS AND TREATMENT INDICATIONS

Waldenström's macroglobulinemia is an incurable and slow-growing disease. Frequently patients die of unrelated causes. The median survival of patients is 5 years,

Box 49–3. Laboratory Findings

- Normochromic, normocytic anemia
- Pancytopenia
- Lymphocytosis
- Monocytosis
- Rouleaux
- Markedly elevated erythrocyte sedimentation rate
- Elevation of β_2-microglobulin
- Prolonged bleeding time (occasionally)
- Prolonged partial thromboplastin time (occasionally)
- Abnormal platelet aggregation (occasionally)
- Serum protein electrophoresis with sharp, narrow spike of monoclonal IgM (most often κ); remainder of protein electrophoresis often normal
- Urine protein electrophoresis is most often normal

Box 49–4. Supportive Care Measures

- Plasma exchange for hyperviscosity
- Prophylaxis against *Pneumocystis jiroveci* pneumonia if more than four to six cycles of purine analogues are used and CD4 count is less than 200 cells/μL
- Prevention of varicella-zoster infection or prompt treatment to prevent dissemination
- Prompt treatment of bacterial infections, particularly with encapsulated organisms
- Irradiation of all cellular blood components
- Evaluation for coagulation disorder
- Supplementation of IgG with intravenous immunoglobulin in patients with profound hypogammaglobulinemia (IgG < 500 mg/dL) and history of severe infection

and at least 20% of patients live for more than 10 years.[23,26] Many patients remain stable for years. Therefore, asymptomatic patients should not be treated regardless of the level of IgM or the degree of bone marrow infiltration. Prognostic factors associated with poor survival have been described.[48–50] These can help identify the asymptomatic patients who will need treatment in the near future. The degree of anemia and the presence of pancytopenia are significantly associated with poor survival. High β_2-microglobulin is another negative prognostic factor. The older the age at diagnosis, the worse is the prognosis, even after correction for the normal age-related mortality.

Treatment is generally recommended for patients with disease-related complaints such as fatigue, weight loss, fever, night sweats, the hyperviscosity syndrome, amyloidosis, symptomatic cryoglobulinemia, neuropathy, nephropathy, bulky adenopathy, or organomegaly, a hemoglobin level of less than 10 gm/dL or a platelet count of less than 100 × 10^9/L.[51] For asymptomatic patients, close follow-up every 3–6 months is recommended.[51]

TREATMENT

Figure 49–2 presents a treatment algorithm for Waldenström's macroglobulinemia, and Box 49–4 lists supportive care measures. Plasmapheresis is mainly used for the treatment of the hyperviscosity syndrome, but patients with symptomatic peripheral neuropathy or cryoglobulinemia also may benefit from a rapid reduction in the level of circulating IgM. Because 80% of the total IgM is intravascular, a single plasma exchange can result in significant and prolonged reduction of the IgM level and the serum viscosity.[25,52] Patients who present with the hyperviscosity syndrome and anemia should not be transfused before plasmapheresis, because blood transfusions raise the viscosity. Plasmapheresis is a short-term treatment and should be combined with systemic therapy.

Chemotherapy

First-line systemic therapy options include alkylating agents (mainly chlorambucil), the nucleoside analogues cladribine and fludarabine, and the monoclonal antibody rituximab. There are no prospective, double-blind, randomized trials comparing these agents against each other as first-line treatment. It should also be taken into account that various authors use different definitions of Waldenström's macroglobulinemia and different response criteria (Box 49–5).

For the treatment of refractory or relapsed disease, there is no standard of care. For patients who had a durable (>1-year) initial response to first-line therapy, use of the same agent is reasonable.[53] Otherwise one of the alternative first-line agents can be used. In patients who are candidates for an autologous stem cell transplantation, exposure to stem cell–toxic agents such as alkylating agents and purine analogues should be minimized.[54]

The alkylating agent chlorambucil is frequently used as first-line treatment for Waldenström's macroglobulinemia (Table 49–2). Kyle and colleagues showed in a prospective randomized trial that daily (at 0.1 mg/kg/day) and intermittent (at 0.3 mg/kg/day for 7 days every 6 weeks) chlorambucil were equally effective and resulting in a 68% response rate and 5.4-year median sur-

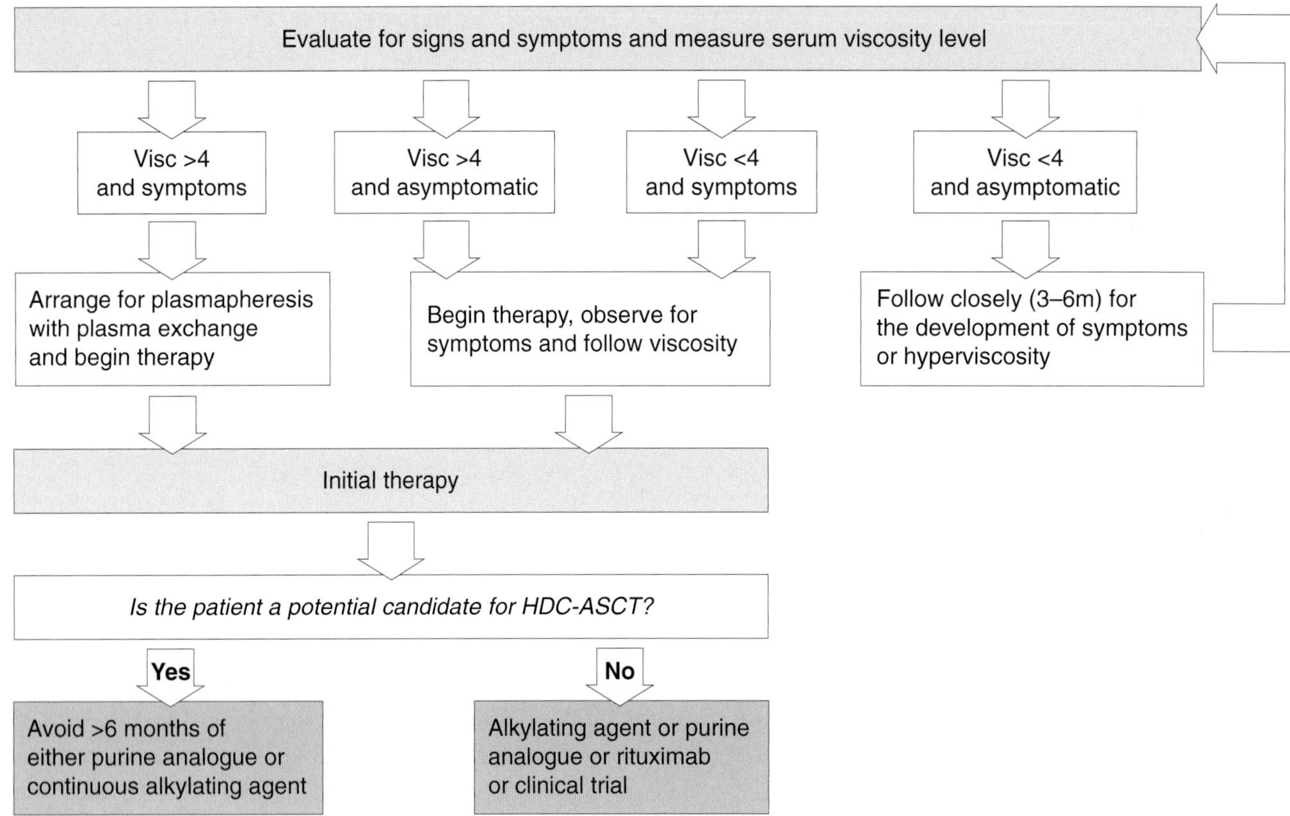

Figure 49–2. Treatment algorithm for Waldenström's macroglobulinemia.

Box 49–5. Uniform Response Criteria from Second International Workshop on Waldenström's Macroglobulinemia

- Total IgM level does not correlate with disease burden among patients.
- IgM measurement is useful to follow in a particular patient.
- Cold agglutinin and cryoglobulins may affect determination of IgM levels; therefore, if present, serum IgM level should be measured under warm conditions.
- IgM monoclonal protein levels as determined by electrophoresis may be used as a determinant of disease response.
- Decrease in lymph node and splenic size may lag behind IgM measurements. The converse may also occur.
- Response may be slow, particularly with purine analogues. Patients should be followed until best overall response.

Complete Response

- Complete disappearance of serum and urine monoclonal IgM by immunofixation
- Resolution of adenopathy and organomegaly
- No signs and symptoms directly attributable to Waldenström's macroglobulinemia
- Absence of malignant cells by bone marrow histologic evaluation

Partial Response

- ≥50% and reduction in serum IgM on serum protein electrophoresis
- ≥50% improvement in bulky adenopathy and organomegaly on computed tomography scan
- No new signs or symptoms or other evidence of disease

Progressive Disease

- >25% increase in serum IgM from lowest attained response, confirmed on second evaluation or progression of disease related symptoms

From Weber D, Treon SP, Emmanouilides C, et al: Uniform response criteria in Waldenström's macroglobulinemia: consensus panel recommendations from the Second International Workshop on Waldenström's Macroglobulinemia. Semin Oncol 30:127–131, 2003.

TABLE 49–2. Representative Samples of Chemotherapy Regimens

Drug	Dosage
Chlorambucil	0.1 mg/kg/day or 0.3 mg/kg/day × 7 days every 6 wk
Fludarabine	25–30 mg/m² daily × 5 days every 4 wk for 4–8 cycles
Cladribine	0.1 mg/kg/day CIV × 7 days or 0.12 mg/kg bolus IV × 5 days or 1.5 mg/m² SC q8h × 7 days
Rituximab	375 mg/m² IV every 4 wk Q wk for 4 wk

Abbreviations: CIV, continuous intravenous infusion; IV, intravenous; SC, subcutaneous.

vival.[55] Responses can be slow, and the authors made the point that patients should be treated for at least 6 months before abandoning chlorambucil. The combination of chlorambucil and prednisone is associated with a response rate and median survival similar to those of single-agent chlorambucil.[23,29] The corticosteroids though may be useful in patients with autoimmune phenomena or cryoglobulinemia.[25]

Alkylating agents have also been used in combination regimens as first-line treatment. Case et al. treated 33 patients with the M-2 protocol (carmustine [BCNU], cyclophosphamide, vincristine, melphalan, and prednisone) and reported a response rate of 82% and an actuarial survival projection at 10 years of 58%.[56] Dimopoulos and Alexanian treated 20 patients with CHOP (cyclophosphamide, doxorubicin, vincristine, and prednisone) and reported a response rate of 65% and a median survival of 7.3 years.[29] The median survival did not reach statistical significance when it was retrospectively compared to the combination of chlorambucil and prednisone. In the same study, 16 patients treated with CVP (cyclophosphamide, vincristine, and prednisone) had a response rate of 44% and a median survival of 3 years.[29] Garcia-Sanz et al., in another retrospective analysis of 217 cases, reported a lower response rate and median survival associated with the use of CVP compared to single-agent chlorambucil.[23] The oral combination of melphalan, cyclophosphamide, and prednisone produced a response rate of 74% in 34 patients reported by Petrucci and colleagues.[57] These authors did not report the response duration.

The nucleoside analogues that have been used in the first-line treatment of Waldenström's macroglobulinemia are fludarabine and cladribine. Both these agents can cause T-cell immunodeficiency and myelosuppression. When used as first-line treatment, they are associated with response and overall survival rates that are similar to those associated with the alkylating agents. None of these purine analogues has proven to be superior to the others. Foran and coworkers reported a 79% response rate in 19 patients treated with fludarabine as first-line therapy (at 25 mg/m²/day for 5 days every 4 weeks until maximum response plus two further consolidation cycles).[58] An intergroup trial from the United States administered fludarabine (at 30 mg/m²/day for 5 days every 4 weeks for four to eight cycles) to 118 previously untreated patients and reported an "at least 50% reduction in tumor mass" in 33% of patients and a median progression-free survival of 42 months.[50] Fludarabine has also been used in the treatment of refractory or relapsed disease with response rates that range between 11% and 50%.[50,59–63] A French multicenter randomized study found fludarabine to produce a higher response rate and a longer event-free survival than CAP (cyclophosphamide, doxorubicin and prednisone) in 92 patients treated in first relapse after treatment with alkylating agents.[62]

Cladribine can be administered either as a continuous infusion at 0.1 mg/kg/day for 7 days,[64,65] as a bolus infusion at 0.12 mg/kg/day over 2 hours for 5 days,[66] or even as a subcutaneous bolus injection (0.5 mg/kg over 5 days[67] or 1.5 mg/m² every 8 hours for 7 days[64]). Two or three monthly courses are usually given. Weber and associates reported a 73% response rate and a median survival of 73 months in 16 previously untreated patients treated with continuous-infusion cladribine.[64] Other authors have reported a similar response rate in first-line treatment with either bolus or continuous-infusion cladribine and a response rate ranging between 14% and 53% for patients with relapsed or refractory disease.[65,68–71]

The malignant cells in Waldenström's macroglobulinemia strongly express CD20, which is the target of the monoclonal antibody rituximab. Rituximab may be preferred as the initial treatment in patients who are candidates for stem cell transplantation because it is not toxic to stem cells, in contrast to the alkylating agents and the nucleoside analogues.[54] Dimopoulos et al. treated 17 previously untreated patients with rituximab and reported a 35% response rate and a 47% stable disease rate.[72] In another study, this same group reported a response rate to rituximab that was 40% in 15 previously untreated and 50% in 12 pretreated patients.[73] The effectiveness of rituximab in the relapsed setting was also shown by Treon and coworkers, who in a retrospective study of 30 patients treated with rituximab after zero to six prior regimens reported a 27% partial response, a 33% "minor" response rate, and a 30% stable disease rate.[74] Rituximab can be administered at a dose of 375 mg/m² every week for 4 or 8 weeks.[75] Alternatively, patients have received two monthly cycles of weekly treatment at 375 mg/m² given 3 months apart.[72] A transient increase in serum IgM can be observed after initiation of treatment with rituximab and is not indicative of treatment failure, but may be secondary to enhanced plasmacytic differentiation of the tumor cells.[73] Clinical responses to rituximab may occur several months after the initiation of treatment.[73]

Treatment of Relapsed or Refractory Disease

High-dose chemotherapy followed by an autologous stem cell transplantation seems to be very effective for the treatment of refractory or relapsed disease in patients who can tolerate the high treatment-related toxicity.[76–81] In a retrospective multicenter study, Tournilhac et al. reported a response rate of 95% in 19 heavily pretreated patients who underwent an autologous transplantation.[79]

Their treatment-related mortality rate was 6%.[79] However, this treatment modality has not been widely used because of the advanced age of most of the patients and the indolent course of the disease. Some investigators recommend consideration of high-dose chemotherapy in eligible patients with primary refractory disease, relapsing disease, or complicating amyloidosis.[54]

Allogeneic transplantation is considered experimental in Waldenström's macroglobulinemia. The great majority of the patients are not good candidates for this treatment modality because they are of advanced age and have slow-growing disease. Tournilhac et al. reported a treatment-related mortality rate of 40% in 10 patients treated with allogeneic transplantation, although their median age was only 46 years.[79] In this study, all 10 allografts derived from full-matched sibling donors. One patient underwent a nonmyeloablative conditioning regimen and the other transplants were conventional. Allogeneic transplantation has been associated with long-term responses and even with a curative potential via an immunologic mechanism.[79–83] Therefore, young, healthy patients with macroglobulinemia should be considered for an allogeneic transplantation in the appropriate clinical and research setting.[54]

Other options for patients with relapsed or refractory disease include the use of thalidomide and interferon alfa. Thalidomide has been used either alone or in combination with dexamethasone and clarithromycin.[84–87] Dimopoulos et al. reported a response to thalidomide in 3 of 10 previously untreated and 2 of 10 previously treated patients.[86] See Chapter 47 for a more detailed description of early clinical trials with these agents as well as bortezomib. All have efficacy in the relapsed setting although there have been insufficient patients to conduct clinical trials with all of these agents. Interferon alfa and interferon gamma have been found to have some activity in patients with Waldenström's macroglobulinemia, but the data are too limited to draw any safe conclusions regarding the use of these agents in macroglobulinemic patients.[88–91] Other agents currently under investigation in the relapsed/refractory setting are the proteasome inhibitor bortezomib, the anti-CD52 antibody alemtuzumab, and the radioactively labeled anti-CD20 antibody yttrium-90 ibritumomab tiuxetan; the combination of rituximab and thalidomide is being studied as a first-line treatment.

CURRENT CONTROVERSIES & FUTURE CONSIDERATIONS

Waldenström's Macroglobulinemia

- Appropriate method to evaluate and follow patients with suspected hyperviscosity
- The use of multiagent combination chemotherapy over sequential single-agent chemotherapy
- Duration of treatment, particularly in light of delayed responses
- Frequency and mechanism of follow-up (computed tomography scan, IgM levels, serum protein electrophoresis, viscosity?)
- The role of nonmyeloablative allogeneic stem cell transplantation
- New agents under investigation: thalidomide, CC5013 (thalidomide analogue), various combinations with rituximab, and bortezomib

Suggested Readings*

Anagnostopoulos A, Aleman A, Giralt S: Autologous and allogeneic stem cell transplantation in Waldenstrom's macroglobulinemia: review of the literature and future directions. Semin Oncol 30:286–290, 2003.

Dimopoulos MA, Alexanian R: Waldenstrom's macroglobulinemia. Blood 83:1452–1459, 1994.

Dimopoulos MA, Panayiotidis P, Moulopoulos LA, et al: Waldenstrom's macroglobulinemia: clinical features, complications, and management. J Clin Oncol 18:214–226, 2000.

Gertz MA, Anagnostopoulos A, Anderson K, et al: Treatment recommendations in Waldenstrom's macroglobulinemia: consensus panel recommendations from the Second International Workshop on Waldenstrom's Macroglobulinemia. Semin Oncol 30:121–126, 2003.

Kyle RA, Garton JP: The spectrum of IgM monoclonal gammopathy in 430 cases. Mayo Clin Proc 62:719–731, 1987.

Leblond V, Levy V, Maloisel F, et al: Multicenter, randomized comparative trial of fludarabine and the combination of cyclophosphamide-doxorubicin-prednisone in 92 patients with Waldenstrom macroglobulinemia in first relapse or with primary refractory disease. Blood 98:2640–2644, 2001.

Owen RG, Johnson SA, Morgan GJ: Waldenstrom's macroglobulinaemia: laboratory diagnosis and treatment. Hematol Oncol 18:41–49, 2000.

Owen RG, Treon SP, Al-Katib A, et al: Clinicopathological definition of Waldenstrom's macroglobulinemia: consensus panel recommendations from the Second International Workshop on Waldenstrom's Macroglobulinemia. Semin Oncol 30:110–115, 2003.

Treon SP, Agus DB, Link B, et al: CD20-directed antibody-mediated immunotherapy induces responses and facilitates hematologic recovery in patients with Waldenstrom's macroglobulinemia. J Immunother 24:272–279, 2001.

Waldenström J: Incipient myelomatosis or "essential" hyperglobulinemia with fibrinogenopenia—a new syndrome? Acta Med Scand 117:216, 1944.

Full references for this chapter can be found on accompanying CD-ROM.

CHAPTER 50

HISTIOCYTOSIS

Robert J. Arceci, MD, PhD

KEY POINTS

Langerhans Cell Histiocytosis

- Langerhans cell histiocytosis (LCH) is a clonal, myeloproliferative disorder of immature Langerhans cells with variable clinical behavior.
- Diagnosis is made by biopsy of an involved site.
- Although some forms of LCH may be limited and self-resolving, others may be progressive and fatal.
- Systemic chemotherapy will significantly improve the outcome for patients with multisystem LCH.
- Recurrent disease is common in patients with multisystem disease.
- A poor response to the initial 6–12 weeks of treatment portends a very poor prognosis.
- Adverse long-term sequelae are common and may include endocrinologic, skeletal, dental, liver, lung, neurocognitive, and neurodegenerative problems.

Hemophagocytic Lymphohistiocytosis

- Hemophagocytic lymphohistiocytosis (HLH) is due to an immune deficiency of cytolytic T-lymphocyte or natural killer cell functions that regulate macrophage responses.
- HLH may be primary (inherited) or secondary, resulting from associated infections or malignancy.
- The diagnosis of HLH is based on clinical, laboratory, and genetic criteria.
- Some patients present with initial central nervous system signs and symptoms.
- Prompt treatment with immunochemotherapeutic approaches is critical.
- The only known curative treatment for primary HLH is allogeneic bone marrow transplantation.
- Genetic counseling is critical for families with primary HLH.
- Long-term follow-up is required for patients with HLH.

INTRODUCTION

The histiocytoses are a diverse group of heterogeneous disorders that primarily involve cells of the mononuclear phagocytic system. The generic and historic term *histiocyte* derives from the Latin *histion*, meaning "little web," and *kytos*, meaning "cell." A histiocyte is thus a resident tissue (meaning "web") mononuclear phagocyte.

Biologically Based Classification of the Histiocytoses

Although the two main types of histiocytes, namely dendritic cells and macrophages, are derived from a common hematopoietic progenitor cell, they can be distinguished by differences in their morphology, lineage-distinctive markers, and function. Dendritic (from the Greek *dendros*, referring to the cells' treelike arborization) cells, and particularly Langerhans cells, are the principal antigen-presenting cells responsible for stimulating primary T-lymphocyte responses. They are especially important in host immunity to virus as well as tumor or self antigens. They are weakly phagocytic but express high levels of major histocompatibility complex class I and II antigens as well as T-lymphocyte costimulatory cell surface receptors. Langerhans cells are most commonly located in the skin and in mucous membrane as well as in lymphoid tissues. When activated by antigen, they migrate from their primary location along lymphatic channels to parafollicular regions of lymph nodes, where they interact and stimulate antigen-specific T lymphocytes. In addition to activating T lymphocytes, Langerhans cells are capable of secreting a variety of important inflammatory cytokines, which in turn contribute to mounting immune responses. In contrast, macrophages (from the Greek referring to "large eaters") play important roles in innate immunity through the phagocytosis of large particulate antigens, including bacteria. Following ingestion of these antigens, macrophages process and then display pieces of them on their cell surface in order to stimulate T-lymphocyte responses. Macrophages are primarily located in lymphoid tissues as well as in most organs, where they assume tissue-specific characteristics, such as the Kupffer cells in the liver. Similar to Langerhans cells, macrophages are also potent producers of immune and inflammatory cytokine-soluble mediators that act to attract lymphocytes, eosinophils, neutrophils, and other mononuclear phagocytes. In such an "inflammatory" microenvironment, macrophages often become multinucleated giant cells as well as nonspecifically ingesting red cells (erythrophagocytosis) or other hematopoietically cellular elements (hemophagocytosis). Of note, although Langerhans cells and macrophages are potent stimulators of lymphocytes, there are specific subsets of T lymphocytes that in turn suppress macrophage activation and proliferation in order to contain and eventually turn off immune responses.

In part based on the above-noted biologic distinctions between the types of cells that are primarily responsible for or play a major role in the pathogenesis of the specific disorders, the histiocytoses were separated in 1985 into three major classes. These historical classifications included

I—The Langerhans cell histiocytoses, which included the historical eponyms of eosinophilic granuloma, Hand-Schüller-Christian disease and Abt-Letterer-Siwe disease

II—The non–Langerhans cell histiocytoses, which included primary and secondary hemophagocytic lymphohistiocytoses as well as macrophage activation syndromes

III—Malignant histiocytoses, including disorders such as monocytic leukemia and rare malignant tumors of the mononuclear phagocytic system

A more recent refinement of this classification system takes into account the more general categories of dendritic and non-dendritic cell disorders. Thus, the current classification includes (Table 50–1)

I—Histologically nonmalignant proliferative dendritic cell disorders, including Langerhans cell histiocytosis (LCH) and juvenile xanthogranulomatous disease

II—T-lymphocyte/macrophage activation syndromes associated with immune deficiency, malignancies, and infections, including primary or inherited hemophagocytic lymphohistiocytosis (HLH); secondary HLH, associated most frequently with certain viral infections, cancer, or immunosuppressive therapy; and the reactive disorder known as "sinus histiocytosis with massive lymphadenopathy" (Rosai-Dorfman disease)

III—Malignant disorders of the mononuclear phagocytic system, including monocytic leukemia and malignant dendritic cell– or macrophage-derived malignancies

TABLE 50–1. Current Classification of Histiocytic Disorders

I. Histologically nonmalignant, dendritic cell proliferative disorders
 A. Langerhans cell histiocytosis
 B. Juvenile xanthogranulomatous disease
II. T-lymphocyte/macrophage activation disorders (immune reactive disorders)
 A. Hemophagocytic syndromes associated with immune deficiency
  Primary or familial hemophagocytic lymphohistiocytosis
  Chédiak-Higashi syndrome
  Griscelli syndrome
  X-linked lymphoproliferative syndrome
 B. Hemophagocytic syndromes associated with infection
  Secondary or nonfamilial hemophagocytic lymphohistiocytosis
   Infection-associated hemophagocytic syndrome
 C. Hemophagocytic syndromes associated with malignancy
  Malignancy-associated hemophagocytic syndrome
 D. Sinus histiocytosis with massive lymphadenopathy (Rosai-Dorfman disease)
 E. Solitary histiocytoma (macrophage phenotype)
 F. Multicentric reticulohistiocytosis (frequently associated with arthritis)
 G. Generalized eruptive histiocytoma
III. Malignant disorders
 A. Monocytic leukemia (French-American-British classification: M5)
 B. Malignant monocytic cell neoplasm
 C. Malignant dendritic cell neoplasm
 D. Malignant macrophage cell neoplasm

The accurate diagnosis and classification of the histiocytic disorders is of critical importance in terms of performing the proper staging work-up, selection of appropriate treatment, evaluation of responses, and follow-up, as well as patient and family counseling. This chapter focuses on the most frequently encountered disorders, namely LCH and HLH.

LANGERHANS CELL HISTIOCYTOSIS

Epidemiology

The estimated incidence of LCH has been reported to be between 4 and 8 patients per million children. There may be as many cases in adults as well. Rare instances of familial cases have been reported, particularly in identical twins but also in fraternal twins and parent/child combinations.

Pathophysiology

Although the cause of LCH remains unknown, the disease has been demonstrated to be a clonal proliferation of immature and abnormal Langerhans cells, which further display DNA microsatellite instability and characteristic regions of chromosome loss and gain. The cytokine environment, which contributes to the local

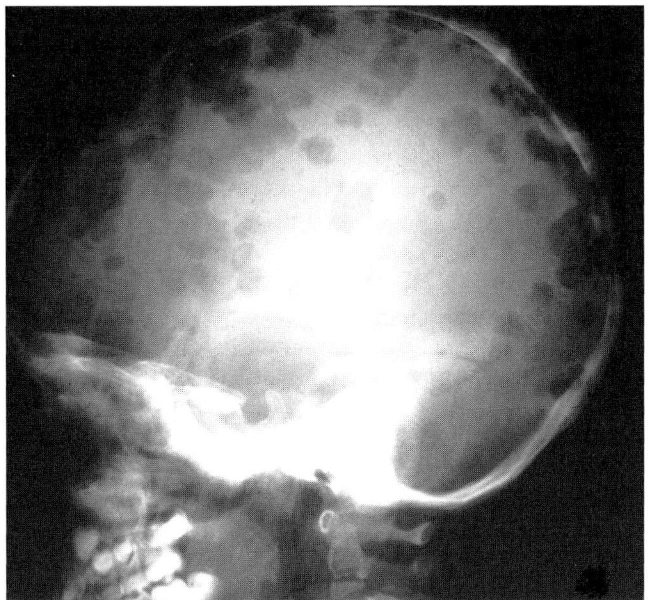

■ **Figure 50–1.** X-ray of a child with LCH showing multiple lytic lesions involving the skull.

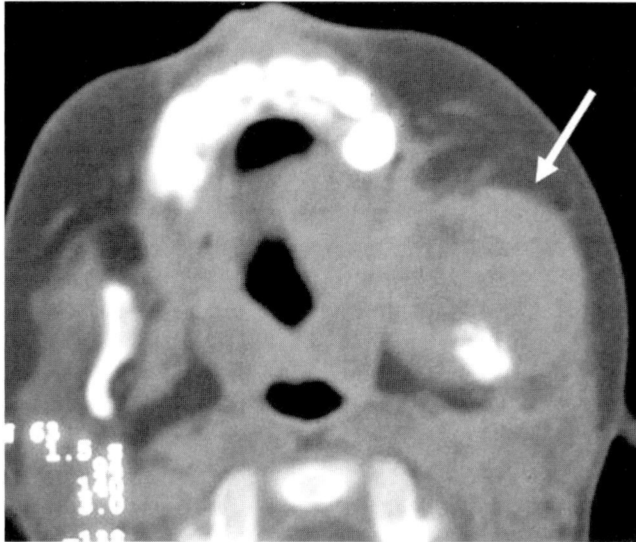

■ **Figure 50–2.** MRI examination of a child with a large, erosive, soft tissue lesion of LCH involving the mandible.

and systemic pathophysiology of LCH, is a result of the activity of the Langerhans cells, lymphocytes, and macrophages. There have been no consistent immunologic abnormalities identified in patients with LCH, suggesting, along with the previous information, that the Langerhans cell is the primary cell responsible for LCH.

Clinical Features and Diagnosis

Presenting Features

The clinical presentation of LCH can occur at any age and can be quite variable, with nearly every organ being at some risk of involvement. In addition, in some patients, the disease may be self-limited and resolve spontaneously, whereas in other individuals, LCH can be relentlessly progressive and fatal.

The historical eponyms of eosinophilic granuloma (usually unifocal LCH), Hand-Schüller-Christian disease (skull lesions, exophthalmos, and diabetes insipidus or, more typically, multifocal involvement), and Abt-Letterer-Siwe disease (systemic LCH) all describe various presentations of a disease that is pathologically similar. Eosinophilic granuloma usually presents as a solitary lesion of bone associated with pain and swelling. Although the calvarium is most commonly affected (Fig. 50–1), other sites include the mandible (Fig. 50–2), long bones, ribs, scapulae, and vertebrae. The small bones of the hands and feet are usually spared. Lesions appear as "punched-out" holes and sometimes have sclerotic edges as observed by plain radiograph. Vertebrae plana often presents with back pain, and radiographic examination shows a collapsed vertebral body. Magnetic resonance imaging may also show a soft tissue component that can rarely lead to spinal cord compression. Multifocal bone involvement and eczematoid skin rash, usually involving

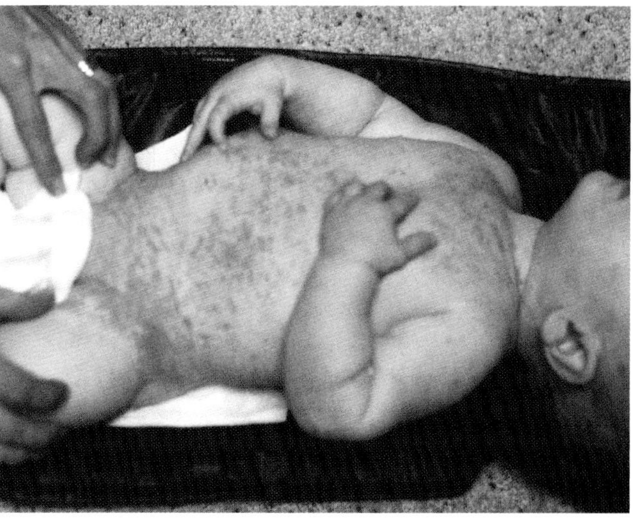

■ **Figure 50–3.** A typical demonstration of diffuse skin involvement in an infant with LCH.

the scalp, axilla, and groin, are characteristic of LCH in the young child, but also can appear in adults of any age (Figs. 50–3 and 50–4). The oral cavity is commonly involved as well as lymph nodes.

Lung, liver, and brain involvement can also occur and should be carefully considered in the work-up. The acute changes observed in the lung include the development of micronodular infiltrative disease, cyst formation, and pneumothoraces. Acute liver involvement includes elevated transaminases, and increased bilirubin that can proceed to sclerosing cholangitis.

The most common type of brain involvement is diabetes insipidus, which may occur at any time before or during the course of the disease. LCH can also present with extensive, systemic involvement characterized by rash, gum disease, hepatosplenomegaly, bone lesions, gastrointestinal involvement, and pancytopenia resulting

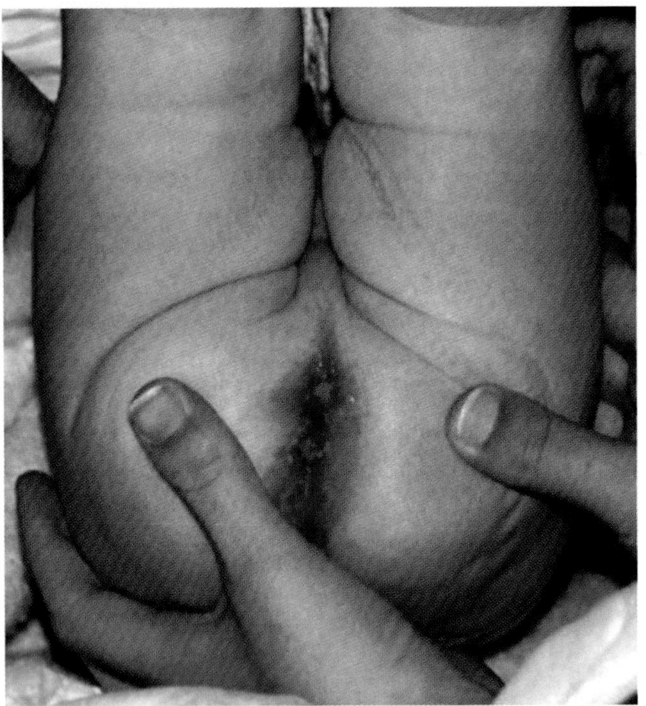

■ **Figure 50–4.** Perianal skin involvement of LCH in an infant.

from splenic sequestration as well as bone marrow replacement by histiocytes. This most severe presentation of LCH most commonly occurs in infants, who may present with failure to thrive. Progression from disease that has limited involvement to severe, systemic disease is rare.

Diagnosis

The diagnosis of LCH should always be based on a biopsy of involved tissue. The histologic appearance should include characteristic Langerhans cells, which are typically rounded and have pale cytoplasm and folded nuclei. These cells should stain positive for expression of the surface antigen CD1a and the cytoplasmic marker S100. There is also a mixed cellular infiltrate comprising lymphocytes, eosinophils, neutrophils, macrophages, and sometimes multinucleated giant cells. The most easily accessible site should be used for biopsy. This usually means the skin or gums, but sometimes lymph nodes and bone lesions must be biopsied to make the diagnosis.

Determination of Extent of Disease

Once a diagnosis has been made by biopsy of an involved site, the extent of disease should be determined in order to determine the type of treatment that will be most useful and the likely outcome. There is no completely agreed-upon standard work-up for patients with LCH, in part because of the variable clinical presentation and course different patients may follow.

A complete blood count and differential, as well as liver and kidney function tests, should be done in all patients to assess systemic involvement of these organs. Although the estimated sedimentation rate often correlates with the extent and activity of disease, it is nonspecific and fluctuates similar to other acute-phase reactants, such as fibrinogen and C-reactive protein. A urinalysis with specific gravity should be done to establish that the patient does not have diabetes insipidus. However, if there is any question of a patient having diabetes insipidus, then a proper water deprivation test should be performed to document serum and urine osmolality as well as antidiuretic hormone levels. A chest radiograph should be obtained as baseline as a means of detecting clinically silent disease such as bullous cysts. Magnetic resonance imaging of the brain with gadolinium contrast is more frequently being recommended at the time of diagnosis in order to establish baseline findings, especially in terms of the hypothalamus and pituitary region but also other areas of central nervous system (CNS) involvement. This is especially true in patients with lesions of the skull bones, such as sphenoid, temporal, and mastoid bones, which are considered to be "CNS risk" lesions and are associated with an increased incidence of subsequent brain adverse sequelae.

Most patients should have a skeletal survey and a technetium bone scan because these two studies are complementary, with the former detecting primarily active and older healed lesions and the latter better at detecting very early lesions. These studies may also be useful in following the response of patients to therapy, but both plain radiographs and bone scans may remain abnormal for months after initial presentation. Additional diagnostic tests, such as bronchoscopy or chest computed tomography, lumbar puncture, endocrinologic work-up, bone marrow aspirate and biopsy, or gastrointestinal biopsy, should be done only when there is clinical evidence for organ involvement or dysfunction.

Differential Diagnosis

The differential diagnosis may include skin disorders such as eczema, malignant bone tumors, and immunodeficiency disorders as well as leukemias, lymphomas, and disseminated solid tumors such as neuroblastoma or sarcomas. In addition, LCH may sometimes appear in patients with other disorders, particularly those with lymphoid malignancies, further complicated the differential diagnosis.

Treatment

Management of Patients with Limited LCH

Limited disease localized to the skin can be observed for regression. If the disease does not regress and is problematic, it can usually be effectively treated with topical steroids, or, in more refractory cases, with the use of topical tacrolimus, nitrogen mustard, or PUVA (psoralen plus ultraviolet A light). Patients with isolated bone lesions (eosinophilic granuloma) often only require curettage of the lesion. Extensive surgery should not be done to accomplish a complete resection if that will involve potential adverse long-term problems. Curettage is usually sufficient to eradicate the disease, although recurrence at the same site can occur. The subsequent development of other skeletal lesions should not require more surgery or biopsy. If such a lesion is relatively asymptomatic, then it may need no treatment and may regress on its own over a period of weeks to months. Lesions that cause significant pain, but do not threaten vital structures and are not in "risk" sites, can be effectively treated with local injection of corticosteroids or with oral nonsteroidal anti-inflammatory agents such as indomethacin or ibuprofen over several weeks. When isolated lesions threaten organ function or cosmetic appearance, they may require immediate intervention with relatively low-dose (usually between 400 and 800 cGy) radiation.

Management of Patients with Multisystem LCH

The AIEOP-CNR-HX 83 and the DAL-HX 83/90 trials, using such agents as vinblastine and etoposide in conjunction with prednisone, achieved 60–90% complete response rates depending on the extent of involvement patients presented. The rate of complete response was greater in patients with multifocal bone disease than in patients with extensive organ involvement and/or dysfunction. Overall survival was greater than 90% for patients without organ dysfunction and approximately 45–65% for patients with extensive disease involvement and organ dysfunction. The recurrence rate was also highest in patients with more extensive disease involvement. The first international cooperative group study, LCH-I, was a prospective, randomized trial that compared the response and outcome for patients treated with prednisone plus either vinblastine or etoposide (VP-16). This study showed that there was no difference in response rate or outcome for patients randomized to receive vinblastine compared to those who received etoposide during the first 6 weeks of therapy. The response of patients after 6 to 12 weeks of therapy was predictive of overall survival. In addition, patients who were 2 years of age or older and who did not have pulmonary, hepatosplenic, or hematopoietic involvement had a response rate of about 90% and an overall survival of 100%.

A comparison of the results from the DAL-HX 83/90 study to those of the LCH-I study suggested that the more aggressive therapeutic approach of DAL-HX 83/90 had resulted in a lower recurrence rate as well as a lower rate of diabetes insipidus. The LCH-II study was thus designed to test in a randomized fashion whether high-risk patients with multisystem LCH benefit from more aggressive treatment with VP-16, vinblastine, and a corticosteroid compared to only vinblastine plus a corticosteroid. The outcome results of this trial have not yet been officially reported. The current LCH-III study is examining whether the addition of intermediate-dose methotrexate to prednisone and vinblastine during initial therapy and low-dose methotrexate during continuation therapy improves outcome for multisystem "risk" patients (Table 50–2).

These studies have shown that a subset of patients require very minimal therapeutic interventions, whereas other patients clearly benefit from systemic treatment. Whether more aggressive multiagent therapy is the optimal approach or whether maintenance therapy significantly reduces the risk of significant, recurrent disease requires further study. More effective chemotherapeutic regimens have decreased the role of radiation therapy, which now should only be used in patients with lesions that could cause acute organ damage.

TABLE 50–2. Treatment Stratification of Patients on LCH-III Study

Group I: Multisystem "Risk" Patients (eligible for randomization)	Involvement of one or more risk organs (hematopoietic system, liver, lungs, or spleen)
Group II: Multisystem "Low-Risk" Patients (not eligible for randomization)	Multiple organs involved but without involvement of "risk" organs
Group III: Single-System "Multifocal Bone Disease" and Localized "Special Site" Involvement	Multifocal bone disease (i.e., lesions in 2 or more different bones) Localized special site involvement (e.g., "CNS-risk" lesions with intracranial soft tissue extension or vertebral lesions with intraspinal soft tissue extension)

Adapted from Histiocyte Society LCH-III study.

Treatment of Recurrent LCH

Patients with recurrent disease often respond to the same drugs with which they initially were treated and showed response. However, for patients with progressive disease while on therapy, alternative approaches are required. Different approaches have included immunomodulatory therapies as well as alternative cytolytic agents. The responses to immunosuppressive agents, such as cyclosporin A or antithymocyte immunoglobulin, have been anecdotal and, at best, transient. Several studies using 2-chlorodeoxyadenosine (2-CdA; cladribine), including an international Phase II trial, have shown remissions in over a third of patients. Some patients with refractory disease have responded to the synergistic combination of cladribine plus cytosine arabinoside, a regimen with proven benefit in patients with relapsed acute myelogenous leukemia. Hematopoietic stem cell transplantation has also been successfully utilized in patients with refractory disease, with variable results and significant treatment-related toxicity. Nonmyeloablative bone marrow transplantation is now being tested to try to reduce treatment-related morbidity and mortality. Targeted immunotherapy, for example, with anti-CD52 antibodies (Campath) and anti-CD1a antibodies, is an interesting approach but not yet fully tested in clinical trials. The application of inhibitors of activated cytokine receptors and their downstream signal transduction pathways is also likely to be a future area of important investigation. Strategies for prevention and/or treatment of progressive fibrosis of the lung, sclerosing cholangitis, and fibrosis of the liver as well as a neurodegenerative pattern of CNS involvement have not been developed and need further work.

Supportive Care and Long-Term Management

Over half the patients with multisystem and/or relapsing disease will have significant late effects. These sequelae commonly include orthopedic problems (including arthritis), hearing loss, and dental abnormalities. CNS problems include diabetes insipidus, and approximately half of these patients will develop panhypopituitarism. As patients have been followed for longer periods of time, an increasing number of them have been noted to develop neurocognitive deficits and psychological problems as well as neurologic complications characterized by a distinctive neurodegenerative pattern of CNS involvement. Patients who develop pulmonary or hepatic fibrosis may progress such that organ transplantation is required. Patients with LCH appear to have a lifelong susceptibility of increased risk of pulmonary disease associated with cigarette smoking. The development of secondary malignancies has also been reported in patients with LCH. Similar to survivors of childhood cancer, patients with LCH require long-term follow-up by a multidisciplinary health care team with knowledge of LCH.

Prognosis

Patients with limited involvement of LCH usually have an excellent prognosis and may not require systemic therapy, whereas patients with multifocal skeletal lesions, refractory skin disease, or other organ involvement will usually significantly benefit from systemic treatment. Although this latter group of patients has an excellent overall survival, these patients also have a significantly high incidence of disease recurrence and adverse long-term sequelae. The prognosis for patients with systemic disease and organ dysfunction who do not show a good response to the first 6–12 weeks of treatment is a poor survival of approximately 20%.

Communication and Counseling

Patients and parents need to be made aware of the potential short- and long-term complications of having multisystem LCH. For those patients with lack of response following 6–12 weeks of initial therapy, the prognosis is quite poor. Patients should be told that recurrent disease may be a lifelong issue in some cases, but that these recurrences are usually not life-threatening. Exceptions to this include the development of significant liver and/or pulmonary disease associated with fibrosis and organ failure. To this end, hepatic toxins should be avoided and patients should be strongly counseled never to smoke. Finally, patients need to be followed closely for long-term endocrinologic, neurocognitive, psychological, and neurodegenerative signs and symptoms.

Pitfalls

The diagnosis and treatment of patients with LCH is exceedingly challenging. The first pitfall to avoid is not making the correct diagnosis because one does not include LCH as part of the differential diagnosis of more common disorders such as malignancies, immune deficiencies, and different forms of cancer. Biopsy is required for diagnosis, but the anatomic site that is biopsied should always be the one associated with the least morbidity. For instance, it makes little sense to biopsy a skull lesion when a skin or oral lesion can be more easily biopsied.

Once a diagnosis is made, the proper approach to treatment needs to be initiated. For some patients, the disease may be self-resolving and thus may not require therapeutic intervention. Unfortunately, there is no definitive test to predict which patients will have disease that self-resolves and which will have disease that progresses. Close follow-up is therefore required to assure that treatment can be initiated as soon as it becomes clear that the disease is not self-resolving. The use of radiation therapy should not be considered unless a vital organ is being threatened (because of the increased risk of secondary malignancies). Performing surgery on a recurrent lesion when less invasive therapeutic approaches would be helpful should be avoided. The lack of recognition of pulmonary fibrosis, sclerosing cholangitis, and neurodegenerative disease as part of the spectrum of clinical manifestations of LCH is a significant pitfall and has resulted in delays in diagnosis and therapy, even if that therapy is only supportive care.

HEMOPHAGOCYTIC LYMPHOHISTIOCYTOSIS

Epidemiology

Primary HLH is most commonly an autosomal inherited disorder that has been estimated to affect approximately 1.2 children per 1 million children per year. Consanguinity is commonly observed in these families. Also of note is that, although primary HLH most typically affects infants and very young children, some adolescent cases have been documented based on the finding of characteristic mutations of known causative genes. Nearly all adults with HLH will have the secondary form.

Pathophysiology

Although the HLH syndromes usually are the result of an immune deficit and/or dysregulatory defect, the common final pathway is the proliferation of lymphocytes and, particularly, hemophagocytic macrophages (Fig. 50–5). HLH may be inherited (primary) or acquired (secondary). Several genetic causes have been described that give rise to inherited syndromes that result in HLH (Table 50–3). A wide variety of associated etiologies have been reported to be in part responsible for secondary HLH, which historically have been referred to as either infection-associated hemophagocytic syndrome (IAHS), viral-associated hemophagocytic syndrome (VAHS), or malignancy-associated hemophagocytic syndrome (MAHS).

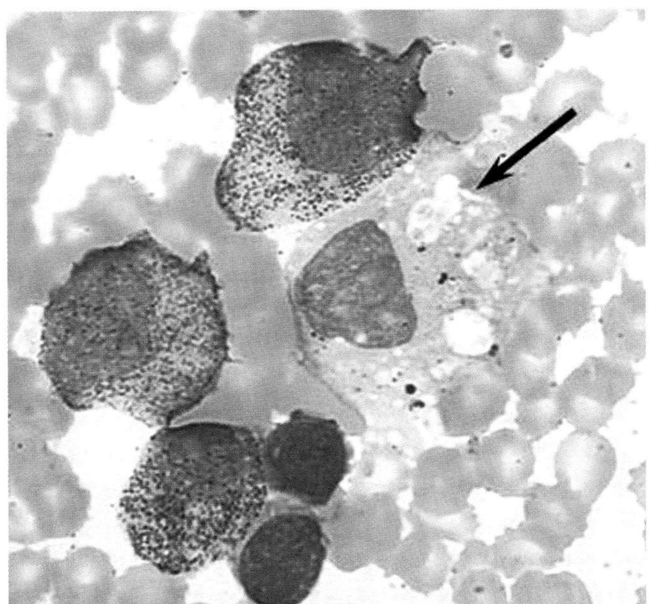

Figure 50–5. An example of hemophagocytosis observed in cases of HLH.

TABLE 50–3. T-Cell/Macrophage Activation Syndromes

Disorder	Inheritance	Gene Defect
Chédiak-Higashi syndrome	AR	LYST
Griscelli syndrome	AR	Myonin Va
XLP	X	SAP
HLH	AR	Perforin, MUNC13-4 Syntaxin

Abbreviations: AR, autosomal recessive; X, X-linked; XLP, X-linked lymphoproliferative disease.

Adapted from Arceci RJ: The histiocytoses: the fall of the Tower of Babel. Eur J Cancer 35:747–767, 1999; discussion Eur J Cancer 35:767–769, 1999.

Decreased numbers of defective natural killer (NK) cells or cytolytic T lymphocytes are fundamental to the initiation and pathophysiology of the HLH disorders. This deficiency or lack of cytolytic regulation of macrophage activity is believed to lead to extensive macrophage activation, proliferation and hemophagocytosis along with systemic hypercytokinemia. The increased cytokine production involves excess production of a variety of inflammatory cytokines, including interleukin (IL)-2, IL-6, IL-10, IL-12, tumor necrosis factor-α, and interferon-γ. The infiltrative lesions of such syndromes are characterized by the presence of nonclonal accumulations of activated macrophages and lymphocytes along with hemophagocytosis. The function of most organs, but particularly the liver, spleen, lymph nodes, bone marrow, and CNS, can be adversely affected as a result of such lymphohistiocytic infiltrates and the hypercytokinemia. Whether they are due to an inherited or acquired immune deficiency, a variety of infectious agents, notably viruses such as Epstein-Barr virus and cytomegalovirus, can trigger or exacerbate these disorders.

Clinical Features and Diagnosis

Presenting Features

Patients with primary HLH commonly present at less than 1 year of age, whereas secondary HLH usually presents at older ages. Patients most commonly present with fever, hepatosplenomegaly, and sometimes lymphadenopathy, with skin rash characterized as eczematoid on the scalp or maculopapular on the torso. Pulmonary involvement resulting from lung lymphohistiocytic infiltrates as well as the effects of hypercytokinemia leading to capillary leak can present with tachypnea and poor oxygenation. Pancytopenia secondary to hepatosplenomegaly and/or bone marrow infiltration with hemophagocytic macrophages may lead to pallor, increased bruising, and increased susceptibility to infection. In infants, failure to thrive is a common finding. Some infants present with CNS involvement, most commonly manifested by the occurrence of seizures and/or hydrocephalus.

A complete blood count and differential will demonstrate cytopenias and often pancytopenia. Hyperferritinemia and increased serum CD25 (IL-2 receptor) levels are surrogate markers of the inflammatory response. Other features include hypertriglyceridemia, believed to be secondary to cytokine downregulation of lipoprotein lipase activity, and hypofibrinoginemia, possibly secondary to macrophage activity as well as a consumptive coagulopathy that is observed in these patients. Elevated liver transaminases and increased serum bilirubin occur as a result of hepatic dysfunction secondary to hypercytokinemia as well as lymphohistiocytic infiltration. Hemophagocytosis can be observed in any organ, but characteristically is found in the bone marrow, liver, and spleen. Several bone marrow samples may be needed before hemophagocytosis is detected. When there is CNS involvement, the cerebrospinal fluid shows a mononuclear pleocytosis. Immunologic studies will show decreased or absent NK cell activity, although NK cell numbers may not be decreased. Brain magnetic resonance imaging may show infiltrative disease as well as involvement of the leptomeninges and hydrocephalus. The identification of specific infections or concomitant cancer, especially lymphoid malignancies and particularly cutaneous T-cell lymphoma or γ/δ T-cell lymphomas, should be pursued.

Diagnosis

The diagnosis of HLH is based on clinical, laboratory, and pathologic criteria and, more recently, the identification of mutations in specific genes (Table 50–4). In 1991, the Histiocyte Society published consensus criteria to guide in the diagnosis of HLH. Five criteria were required: fever, hepatosplenomegaly, at least two cytopenias, hypertriglyceridemia and/or hypofibrinoginemia, and hemophagocytosis. Subsequently, additional criteria were added: hyperferritinemia, low or absent NK cell activity, and elevated CD25 levels. Thus, current diagnostic criteria require five of the eight criteria or the identification of specific gene mutations or the presence of familial disease.

Differential Diagnosis

The differential diagnosis for HLH includes infection-associated, viral-associated, and malignancy-associated hemophagocytic syndromes and other macrophage activation disorders such as those associated with rheumatic disorders. Other disorders that can present with HLH-like signs and symptoms include X-linked lymphoproliferative syndrome, Chédiak-Higashi syndrome in its accelerated phase, and Griscelli syndrome (silver hair and immunodeficiency syndrome). It is also important to rule LCH. Of note, there have been cases of LCH occurring at the same time as HLH, possibly secondary to infection and/or immunodeficiency associated with treatment for the LCH.

TABLE 50–4. Diagnostic Criteria for Hemophagocytic Lymphohistiocytosis (HLH)*

Clinical

Fever
Hepatosplenomegaly

Laboratory

Hematologic

Cytopenias (≥2 of 3 lineages in peripheral blood)
Hemophagocytosis

Serum Values

Hypertriglyceridemia (fasting triglyceride levels ≥2 mmol/L or ≥3 SD above normal)
Hypofibrinogenemia (≤1.5 gm/L or ≤3 SD below normal)
Hyperferritinemia

Immunologic

Low or absent NK function
Elevated soluble CD25 serum levels

Additional

Molecular demonstration of known gene mutation
Presence of familial disease

*Diagnosis requires five of the eight clinical and laboratory criteria or the identification of specific gene mutations or presence of familial disease.
Abbreviation: SD, standard deviation.

Treatment and Prognosis

HLH is usually rapidly fatal without prompt initiation of effective treatment. Optimal initial therapy should include a combination of cytotoxic and immunosuppressive agents in order to obtain a complete remission. The Histiocyte Society HLH-94 and HLH-2004 international trials have successfully combined the use of VP-16, high-dose steroids, and cyclosporin A. When patients have CNS involvement, intrathecal methotrexate is recommended. Although this type of combination therapy is quite effective at achieving disease remission, the only truly curative treatment for primary HLH is allogeneic bone marrow transplantation, giving a 3-year overall survival of approximately 50% when combined with initial chemoimmunosuppressive treatment. For patients who undergo bone marrow transplantation, the 3-year probability of survival is approximately 60%. The prognosis is worse for patients who undergo transplantation with evidence of active disease, but this is not a contraindication to transplantation.

Patients with severe and/or persistent secondary HLH should be treated with initial therapy as recommended by the HLH-94/HLH-2004 clinical trials, including VP-16, high-dose steroids, and cyclosporin A. If viral- or malignancy-associated etiologies are identified, then specific therapies should be initiated for them. Patients who achieve a complete remission of their disease after the initial 8 weeks of treatment can be observed off therapy and may not require prolonged continuation therapy. However, when patients with secondary HLH show recurrence and/or progression, they may also require allogeneic bone marrow transplantation (Fig. 50–6). In cases of mild, secondary HLH, less intensive therapy can be tried, such as a course of corticosteroids or intravenous gamma globulin.

Supportive Care and Long-Term Management

Long-term adverse sequelae may include a variety of bone marrow transplantation–associated problems, such as growth abnormalities, sexual maturation and fertility issues, and secondary malignancies and the conse-

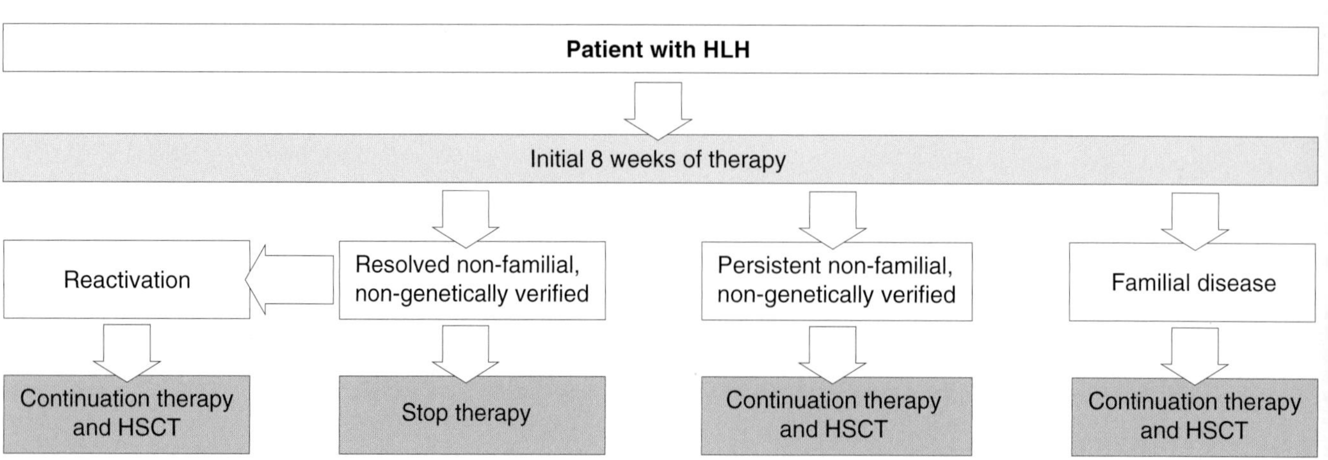

Figure 50–6. Treatment algorithm for patients with HLH as recommended by the HLH 2004 International Histiocyte Society Protocol.

quences of graft-versus-host disease. Neurocognitive, psychological, and neurologic problems (e.g., seizures) may develop as a result of HLH involvement as well as bone marrow transplantation. In addition, secondary leukemias may result from VP-16 exposure. Long-term follow-up is critical for these patients.

Communication and Counseling

Patients and families must be informed of the gravity of the diagnosis of HLH and given an overview of the treatment, including the possible need for bone marrow transplantation with its long-term adverse sequelae. In addition, it is critical to provide genetic counseling for cases of primary HLH. At the current time, no approved prenatal diagnostic test is available.

Pitfalls

The prompt and accurate diagnosis of HLH, along with the rapid initiation of appropriate treatment, is extremely important. In many cases, the diagnosis and treatment of these patients should be considered a medical emergency. Failure to pursue a complete diagnostic work-up promptly may lead to a delay in therapy and poor outcome. It is also critical to always take a good family history to determine consanguinity or if other individuals in the family have had similar disorders, even those family members who might have died from unknown causes during infancy.

Current Controversies & Future Directions

Histiocytosis

- Determining the etiology of LCH: neoplasia? immune dysregulation? something in between?
- Improving therapy and outcome for patients with refractory and/or progressive LCH
- Reducing the frequency of disease recurrence and late complications of LCH, including lung, liver, and CNS involvement
- Defining additional genetic causes for HLH and how they can be used for early diagnosis and genetic counseling as well as possibly future therapies
- Development of new treatment approaches to improve the approximately 50% survival plateau currently achieved

Suggested Readings

Arceci RJ: The histiocytoses: the fall of the Tower of Babel. Eur J Cancer 35:747–767, 1999; discussion Eur J Cancer 35:767–769, 1999.

Arceci RJ, Longley BJ, Emanuel PD: Atypical cellular disorders. Hematology (Am Soc Hematol Educ Program) 297–314, 2002.

Arico M, Nichols K, Whitlock JA, et al: Familial clustering of Langerhans cell histiocytosis. Br J Haematol 107:883–888, 1999.

Egeler RM, Neglia JP, Arico M, et al: Acute leukemia in association with Langerhans cell histiocytosis. Med Pediatr Oncol 23:81–85, 1994.

Egeler RM, Neglia JP, Puccetti DM, et al: Association of Langerhans cell histiocytosis with malignant neoplasms. Cancer 71:865–873, 1993.

Feldmann J, Callebaut I, Raposo G, et al: S. Munc13-4 is essential for cytolytic granules fusion and is mutated in a form of familial hemophagocytic lymphohistiocytosis (FHL3). Cell 115:461–473, 2003.

Henter JI: Biology and treatment of familial hemophagocytic lymphohistiocytosis: importance of perforin in lymphocyte-mediated cytotoxicity and triggering of apoptosis. Med Pediatr Oncol 38:305–309, 2002.

Henter JI, Arico M, Elinder G, et al: Familial hemophagocytic lymphohistiocytosis: primary hemophagocytic lymphohistiocytosis. Hematol Oncol Clin North Am 12:417–433, 1998.

Henter JI, Samuelsson-Horne A, Arico M, et al: Treatment of hemophagocytic lymphohistiocytosis with HLH-94 immunochemotherapy and bone marrow transplantation. Blood 100:2367–2373, 2002.

Laman JD, Leenen PJ, Annels NE, et al: Langerhans-cell histiocytosis "insight into DC biology". Trends Immunol 24:190–196, 2003.

Nanduri VR, Bareille P, Pritchard J, Stanhope R: Growth and endocrine disorders in multisystem Langerhans' cell histiocytosis. Clin Endocrinol (Oxf) 53:509–515, 2000.

Nanduri VR, Lillywhite L, Chapman C, et al: Cognitive outcome of long-term survivors of multisystem Langerhans cell histiocytosis: a single-institution, cross-sectional study. J Clin Oncol 21:2961–2967, 2003.

Stepp SE, Dufourcq-Lagelouse R, Le Deist F, et al: Perforin gene defects in familial hemophagocytic lymphohistiocytosis. Science 286: 1957–1959, 1999.

CHAPTER 51
AMYLOIDOSIS

Raymond L. Comenzo, MD

KEY POINTS

Amyloidosis

- There are different types of amyloidosis, but the vast majority of cases with systemic multiorgan disease and monoclonal gammopathies are light chain amyloidosis (AL).
- Tissue biopsy is paramount for making the diagnosis, and abdominal fat pad aspirate is adequate in the majority of cases.
- The majority of systemic AL patients have elevated free serum immunoglobulin light chains by the new free light chain assay, and the free light chains represent the fibril precursor protein.
- The serum markers of myocardial injury (troponins, brain natriuretic peptide) are useful markers of amyloid cardiac involvement and prognosis.
- Autologous stem cell transplantation is effective therapy for AL patients with fewer than two major organs involved and limited cardiac involvement, and results in significant improvement in 60% of AL patients with peripheral nervous systemic and autonomic involvement.
- Amyloid patients should be treated in clinical trials whenever possible.

INTRODUCTION

Definition

Amyloidosis results from the formation of insoluble fibrillar protein deposits in tissues, impairing the function of critical organs, often fatally. In tissue sections stained with hematoxylin-eosin, amyloid appears as amorphous, hyaline, and eosinophilic, whereas, with Congo red staining in polarized light, what was amorphous and eosinophilic changes to apple-green, punctate, and streaky.[1] The term *amyloid* was coined by the pathologist Virchow in 1854 to describe deposits seen in postmortem liver that were thought to be starch or cellulose because they had an affinity for iodine.[2] Amyloid derives from abnormal precursor subunit proteins that self-assemble, assume a predominantly β-sheet secondary structure, and form fibrillar deposits associated with other proteins such as amyloid P component, apolipoprotein E, and the vitamin K–dependent coagulation factors.[3–7]

Amyloidosis is a disease of protein misfolding or misconformation, based on a large body of experimental evidence indicating that the various fibril precursor subunit proteins are intrinsically amyloid-forming.[7] The fibril precursor subunit proteins for the different types of amyloidosis are listed in Table 51–1, and include hereditary variants, secondary (or AA) variants, and variants related to B-cell disorders, the focus of this chapter.[8] Immunoglobulin light chain (AL) amyloidosis is both a disorder of protein conformation cum deposition and a clonal B-cell disorder.[9,10] The list of organs and tissues potentially affected by amyloid deposition is extensive. Rare hereditary variants can affect the cornea and cerebral vasculature; pancreatic islet cells in type 2 diabetes can be affected by amyloid deposits derived from an islet polypeptide. There are both localized and systemic forms of AL amyloidosis; the etiology of localized forms is not always clear but usually relates to local accretions of clonal B cells (plasma cells or lymphoma cells) secreting amyloid-forming light chains.[10]

Systemic AL Amyloidosis

Systemic AL amyloidosis has been called primary systemic amyloidosis.[11,12] It is the most common form of the disease and until recently was viewed as untreatable and fatal. In addition to involvement of major viscera, AL amyloidosis also frequently involves the soft tissues, joints, endocrine organs (notably the thyroid) and vasculature. There is a poorly understood organ tropism to AL amyloidosis; patients tend to present with a dominant

TABLE 51–1. Types of Amyloidosis

Type	Fibril Precursor Protein	Clinical Syndrome
AL, AH	Immunoglobulin light or heavy chain	Localized, primary systemic
ATTR	Mutant transthyretin	Hereditary
AA	Serum amyloid A (prealbumin)	Secondary
AApoA1	Apolipoprotein A1	Familial amyloidotic polyneuropathy (FAP, Iowa)
AGel	Gelsolin	FAP (Finnish)
Aβ2m	β_2-Microglobulin	Dialysis associated
AFib	Fibrinogen A α chain	Renal amyloid, hypertension

symptomatic involved organ early in the course of disease.

EPIDEMIOLOGY

The epidemiology of amyloidosis is difficult to define. In the United States, it is a rare disorder with an age-adjusted incidence estimated to be 5.1–12.8 per million person-years, resulting in approximately 1275–3200 new cases a year, an incidence in the range of chronic myelogenous leukemia or Hodgkin's lymphoma.[11] AL amyloidosis appears to be more common in men, but the difference may be due to self-selection and referral bias. At diagnosis, only 10% of patients are less than 50 years old; over half of patients newly diagnosed with AL amyloidosis are between 50 and 70 years old.[12] Although the AL plasma cell clone is usually not malignant, survival without treatment is poor because of progressive organ failure.[12] Less than 5% of AL patients survive 10 years from diagnosis.[13,14] The time from onset of symptoms to the diagnosis of AL amyloidosis varies depending on the dominant symptomatic organ system. In patients presenting with congestive heart failure or nephrotic syndrome, symptoms usually have been present for a median of 3 months.[12] Patients with neuropathy or slowly progressive hepatomegaly may be symptomatic for a year prior to diagnosis.

Other rare forms of AL amyloidosis include hereditary amyloidosis caused by mutations in proteins such as fibrinogen Aα and apolipoprotein A1.[15–18] From 1999 to 2004 at Memorial Sloan-Kettering, there were 240 patients with amyloidosis, 4 of whom (1.6%) had hereditary variants (2 with Met30 and two with Ala60). The incidence of these other hereditary forms of amyloidosis is also not known, but these variants are very rare. Secondary amyloidosis can also occur in association with familial Mediterranean fever and, rarely, with sarcoidosis or Hodgkin's lymphoma.

PATHOPHYSIOLOGY

The fibril precursor protein for amyloid caused by B-cell disorders is usually a monoclonal free immunoglobulin (Ig) light chain[19,20] and may be associated with non-Hodgkin's lymphoma, particularly lymphoplasmacytic and mucosal-associated lymphoid tissue lymphomas, and Waldenström's macroglobulinemia. Localized disease of the larynx, tracheobronchial tree, duodenum, or bladder usually does not progress to systemic AL amyloidosis but carries a variable long-term prognosis.[21]

Comparing AL amyloidosis to hereditary variants, one confronts a paradox. Because AL is an acquired disorder, it is perplexing that AL patients become symptomatic and can deteriorate rapidly, whereas the clinical tempo of hereditary variants appears more indolent despite lifelong presence of the fibril precursor protein. The degree to which such free immunoglobulin light chain species can cause cellular damage and symptoms of disease independent of actual tissue deposits is an emerging and controversial area.

Immunoglobulin Light Chains

The variable region of immunoglobulin light chains is globular and rich in αβ strands, and disproportionately made in plasma cells.[22–28] The effects of primary structure on the conformations of immunoglobulin light chains appears to be the basis for amyloid.[29,30] Uncommon amino acid substitutions in critical residues may affect the stability and interactive properties of misfolded or partially folded light chains.[30] Such intermediate forms may be prone to self-assemble aberrantly.[31–33] Over time, these filaments either form thicker units or grow by extension as soluble light chain monomers or stack one upon another.[30,34] In contrast, in some hereditary transthyretin (TTR) variants, single-point mutations in the primary sequence result in dissociation of the TTR tetramer; the monomers are variably unstable, and filaments and fibrils form as the abnormal monomers self-assemble.

Another major constituent of amyloid deposits is the plasma glycoprotein serum amyloid P component (SAP), one of the pentraxin family of proteins.[35] SAP may be a pathologic chaperone for amyloid fibrils; it employs a calcium-dependent binding mechanism in its interactions with amyloid fibrils, and fibrils studded with SAP molecules in vitro are better protected from phagocytosis and proteolytic degradation.[36] In addition, the interactions between AL light chains and other passenger constituents of amyloid deposits, such as glycosaminoglycans, may also stabilize filament and fibril formation and enhance the resistance of AL deposits to proteolysis.[37]

Clonal Plasma Cells and Immunoglobulin V_L Genes

In the majority of patients with AL amyloidosis, free monoclonal light chains and minimal bone marrow plasmacytosis are detected, often in association with suppression of noninvolved immunoglobulin production.[9] Sixty percent of patients have marrow biopsies showing 10% or fewer clonal plasma cells.[11] The levels of monoclonal protein and the plasma cell infiltrates in the marrow do not increase over time, as is the case in multiple myeloma. The clones that cause AL amyloidosis are distinctly different from myeloma clones with respect to their repertoire of immunoglobulin light chain variable region germline (Ig V_L) genes but similar in that their immunoglobulin genes are highly mutated (i.e., antigen-driven or post–germinal center clones) and surprisingly similar to myeloma clones with respect to their cytogenetics.[38–45]

The repertoire of Ig V_L genes in AL amyloidosis is skewed, unlike that in myeloma, which is similar to the normal expressed repertoire.[41,42] The basis for this pattern of gene utilization is unknown. Nearly half of all AL clones employ one of three immunoglobulin λ V_L genes, the 2a2 (λII), the 3r (λIII), and 6a (λVI) germline donors. AL clones using genes derived from the 3r germline donor have a significantly higher divergence from the germline sequence than those using the 6a donor.[46,47] Interestingly, cytogenetic abnormalities commonly seen in myeloma clones are also found in AL amyloidosis. Aneuploidy is common, with trisomies of chromosomes 7, 9, 11, 15, and 18 seen in a significant fraction of cases. Immunoglobulin heavy chain translocations of chromosome 14, including t(4;14), are common and abnormalities of chromosome 13 frequent in AL amyloidosis.[44,45]

Organ Tropism

One of the curious hallmarks of AL amyloidosis is the variety of organs that may be symptomatically involved.[9,11] A third of patients present with dominant renal amyloidosis in the form of nephrotic syndrome. The association between the 6a germline gene and initial presentation with renal amyloid has been shown in three laboratories with three different cohorts of patients. The 2a2 and 3r germline donors are associated with multisystem disease involving the heart, and patients with Vκ clones were more likely to have dominant hepatic involvement. The basis for the tropism remains obscure, as is the mechanism by which misfolded light chain proteins cause progressive organ dysfunction and clinical disease at a tempo more rapid than that seen in hereditary variants of amyloidosis.

CLINICAL FEATURES

The common symptoms of systemic AL amyloidosis are fatigue, weight loss, and decreased libido; the diagnosis, however, is rarely made until patients manifest symptoms of specific organ dysfunction[9,11,48] (Table 51–2). The diagnosis requires biopsy material from the abdominal fat or rectum revealing amyloid deposits in blood vessels, because the vasculature of virtually every organ system except the central nervous system is usually involved. If the index of suspicion is high, biopsy of dysfunctioning organs should be obtained and electron microscopic preparations requested in order to distinguish AL amyloidosis from light chain deposition disease.

Renal Involvement

Nephrotic syndrome without hypertension or progressive renal failure is common. Signs and symptoms are peripheral edema, "frothy" urine, low serum albumin, and elevated cholesterol. Many patients are asymptomatic, but half will have daily proteinuria of 10 gm or more. Anasarca and massive proteinuria with hypoalbuminemia but normal serum creatinine and blood urea nitrogen concentrations are less common. Volume depletion can cause salt craving orthostasis mimicking autonomic neuropathy.[49]

TABLE 51–2. Noninvasive Criteria for Amyloid-Related Major Organ Involvement*

Heart
Echocardiogram showing increased mean ventricular wall thickness and thickened valves with no history of hypertension or valvular heart disease
Electrocardiogram showing unexplained low voltage
New York Heart Association Functional Capacity Class II or higher without ischemic heart disease
Kidneys
Twenty-four-hour albuminuria greater than 500 mg/dL
Liver/GI Tract
Right upper quadrant discomfort
Early satiety
Hepatomegaly
Elevated alkaline phosphatase and γ-glutamyltranspeptidase
Peripheral Nervous System
Lower extremity sensory or polyneuropathy
Impotence, diarrhea or constipation
Orthostatic hypotension

*Although a positive biopsy remains the gold standard for organ involvement per se, patients may have biopsies showing amyloid in the liver or gastrointestinal tract, for example, without symptoms or signs of organ dysfunction.

Cardiac Involvement

A third of AL patients have dominant symptomatic cardiac involvement at diagnosis and often present with symptoms of right-sided heart dysfunction such as dyspnea on exertion, congestive hepatopathy, and lower extremity edema. Early in the course of disease, left ventricular function is preserved despite ventricular thickening resulting from amyloid. On examination, findings may include prominent jugular venous distention and a right-sided third heart sound. Coronary angiography usually shows minimal coronary artery disease. Patients with diastolic heart failure without hypertension but with low systolic blood pressures (e.g., <110 mm Hg) should be considered for endomyocardial biopsies to enable earlier diagnosis.

As cardiac amyloid advances, the heart walls thicken (to >15 mm) and become noncompliant, causing a restrictive cardiomyopathy. Diminished cardiac output is exacerbated by an increased heart rate. Even low doses of cardioselective β-antagonists or calcium channel blockers can be useful but risk frank congestive heart failure. Atrial thrombi may be present even in sinus rhythm, and the occurrence of atrial fibrillation is associated with a high risk of thromboembolism.[50] Other manifestations include symptomatic bradycardia or micturition syncope, sudden cardiac death,[51] and conduction disturbances and other arrhythmias, as well as sinus arrest and atrioventricular block. The efficacy of antiarrhythmic agents or implanted defibrillators has not yet been defined.

The most practical and informative method for assessing cardiac amyloid remains the echocardiogram, with findings of concentric ventricular hypertrophy with thickening of the posterior wall and septum in diastole, mimicking that seen with hypertensive heart disease or hypertrophic cardiomyopathy.[52] Unlike the electrocardiograms of patients with bona fide ventricular hypertrophy, though, the electrocardiograms of patients with cardiac amyloid often show extremely low voltage with left-axis deviation and a pseudoinfarct pattern.

Markers of Myocyte Injury

AL amyloidosis is a disease in which heart involvement is prevalent at diagnosis and, therefore, chemical markers of myocyte injury are likely to be useful in screening. Indeed, brain natriuretic peptide (BNP), amino-terminal (NT)-proBNP, and the troponins have been shown to be useful screening and prognostic markers of AL cardiac involvement.[53,54] In the initial studies of NT-proBNP, the presence of levels greater than 152 pg/mL was associated with significantly poorer overall survival (Fig. 51–1*A*).[53] Troponin levels also provide useful information for staging patients at diagnosis and a staging system has been devised using both NT-proBNP and troponin C.[54] The preliminary data strongly suggest that patients with abnormal elevations of both BNP and troponin have a very poor prognosis; although these tests provide elegance in staging, whether they add anything to the traditional evaluation of patients with advanced cardiac amyloid remains to be determined. In 32 consecutive newly diagnosed patients enrolled in a Phase II trial, median baseline troponin levels were significantly higher in cardiac patients, 0.09 (range, 0–0.61) versus 0 (0–0.12) in other patients ($P < .05$), and this was also the case for BNP levels, 918 (234–3450) versus 74.5 (37.5–413) ($P < .01$).[55] Figures 51–1*B* and *C* demonstrate how BNP can decrease in cardiac amyloid patients when the fibril precursor free light chain (FLC) is reduced with therapy, indicating that these markers will likely provide a more sensitive, convenient, and useful tool for clinical assessment than echocardiography, for example.

Liver and Gastrointestinal Involvement

Patients present with symptomatic hepatic or gastrointestinal amyloid 25% of the time.[56] Patients may complain of early satiety, weight loss, nausea, dyspepsia, and right upper quadrant fullness or discomfort. Malabsorption, pseudo-obstruction, and frank rectal bleeding are rare.[57,58] Gastrointestinal symptoms may also be a function of autonomic neuropathy interfering with gastric motility. Amyloid deposits in the bowel may be focal or diffuse. Enlargement of the tongue (macroglossia) can make eating and drinking difficult and can have significant dental, cosmetic, and psychological sequelae. Airway obstruction and sleep apnea rarely occur. Spontaneous bowel perforation and splenic or hepatic rupture resulting from amyloid are not common but can occur and require aggressive surgical management.[57]

Peripheral and Autonomic Neuropathy

AL patients present with peripheral neuropathy 20% of the time. Patients usually have a symmetrical lower extremity neuropathy with dysesthesias, as opposed to the asymmetrical picture seen in chronic inflammatory demyelinating polyneuropathies.[59] Sensory neuropathy usually has a distal-to-proximal and symmetrical pattern, and motor neuropathy is less common. Autonomic dysfunction is common and associated with symptoms such as orthostatic hypotension, impotence, chronic dysgeusia and nausea, and constipation or diarrhea. Isolated profound postural hypotension can occur without concomitant tachycardia because of cardiac dysautonomia and the heart's inability to respond appropriately. The co-occurrence of orthostatic hypotension and cardiac failure or nephrotic syndrome limits the use of angiotensin-converting enzyme inhibitors and some other drugs because they may exacerbate hypotension.

Connective tissue, skin, muscles, the respiratory tract, and the genitourinary system are among the other organ systems that can be involved with amyloid. A history of carpal tunnel syndrome may precede the disease by a year or more, and an erosive arthritis may occur, sometimes mistaken for psoriatic arthritis. Periorbital ecchymoses ("raccoon eyes") are pathognomonic for AL amyloidosis and are seen in one fifth of patients.[9]

DIAGNOSIS AND DIFFERENTIAL DIAGNOSIS

Tissue Biopsy

The diagnosis of AL amyloidosis should be considered in patients with low-level monoclonal gammopathies who are sicker than they should be and in patients with progressive unexplained neuropathy, autonomic dysfunction, or diastolic cardiac failure. Patients with hereditary amyloidosis often present with the latter findings. Patients with systemic AL amyloidosis also often have constitutional symptoms, proteinuria and edema, peripheral polyneuropathy, and symptomatic noninfectious hepatomegaly. The critical steps in diagnosis are thinking of amyloidosis and obtaining a tissue biopsy.

Occasionally the diagnosis is missed despite obtaining tissue because deposits are not easily appreciated with hematoxylin-eosin and neither the primary physician nor the pathologist requests Congo red staining. In the majority of cases, a tissue diagnosis can be established by Congo red staining of abdominal fat or rectal biopsy tissue; biopsy of an involved organ should be pursued if abdominal fat and rectal biopsies are unrevealing.[60–62] The differential diagnosis includes light chain deposition

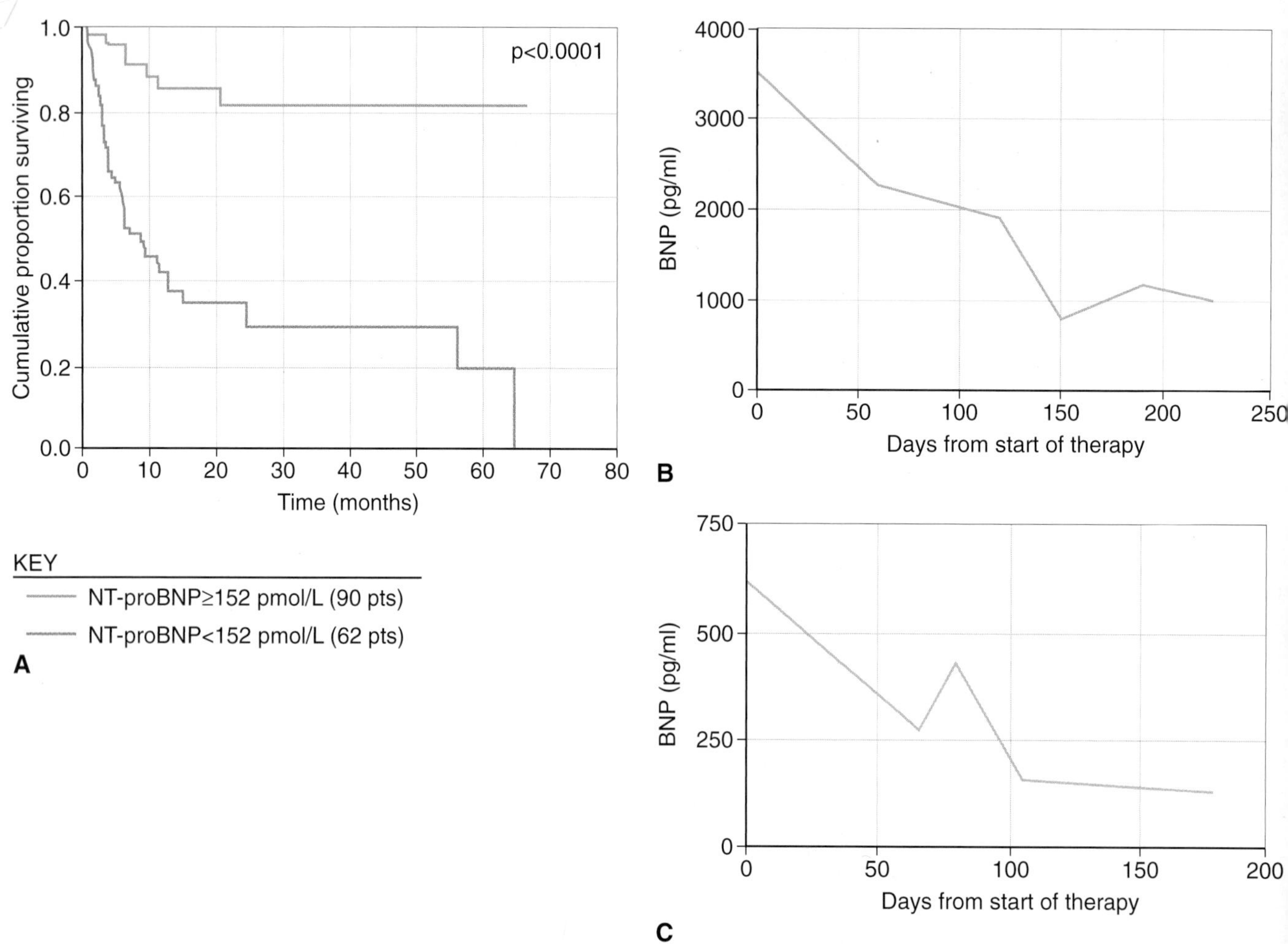

Figure 51–1. *A,* This Kaplan-Meier survival plot shows that newly diagnosed AL amyloidosis patients with elevated NT-proBNP levels (>152 pmol/mL) have significantly poorer survival than those with levels below that value. Elevated NT-proBNP is associated with amyloid heart involvement, a known deleterious prognostic factor. (From Palladini G, Campana C, Klersy C, et al: Serum N-terminal pro–brain natriuretic peptide is a sensitive marker of myocardial dysfunction in AL amyloidosis. Circulation 107:2440–2445, 2003, with permission). *B,* The BNP in this 42-year-old man with cardiac amyloid was over 3000 pg/mL prior to stem cell transplantation (SCT). As the pathologic free λ light chain levels dropped from 160 to 15 mg/dL, the BNP gradually declined over the 6-month period post-SCT. There was no change in the echocardiogram but there was an improvement in clinical status. *C,* The BNP in this 52-year-old woman with multiple myeloma and cardiac amyloidosis was over 600 pg/mL prior to oral therapy with melphalan and dexamethasone. As the pathologic free λ light chain level dropped from 94 mg/dL to normal, the BNP declined as well. There was no change on the echocardiogram, but the patient had improvement in both tachycardia (resolved) and her clinical status.

disease and neuropathy associated with monoclonal gammopathy (nonamyloid). Electron microscopy may be necessary to distinguish these possibilities.

Free Light Chains

The recent availability of a reliable and highly sensitive serum FLC assay has significantly changed the way that patients with AL amyloidosis and nonsecretory myeloma are diagnosed and monitored during therapy.[63–67] Historically, 5–10% of AL patients presented with no evidence by immunofixation of a monoclonal gammopathy, although careful inspection of immunohistochemically stained marrow specimens would allow one to infer the presence of clonal disease in some instances. In a study of 18 patients with AL amyloidosis and negative serum and urine immunofixation studies, two thirds were found to have abnormal serum FLC concentrations.[65] These results are particularly striking because the FLC assay is quantitative, unlike immunofixation studies, and in some cases may be more sensitive than immunofixation for the presence of clonal FLCs.

A series of FLC values in newly diagnosed patients with amyloidosis is depicted in Figure 51–2. Examples of how the FLC level is useful for monitoring patients in therapy are shown in Figure 51–3; stable declines after treatment of greater than 50% from baseline values have been shown retrospectively to be associated with prolonged survival.[66,67]

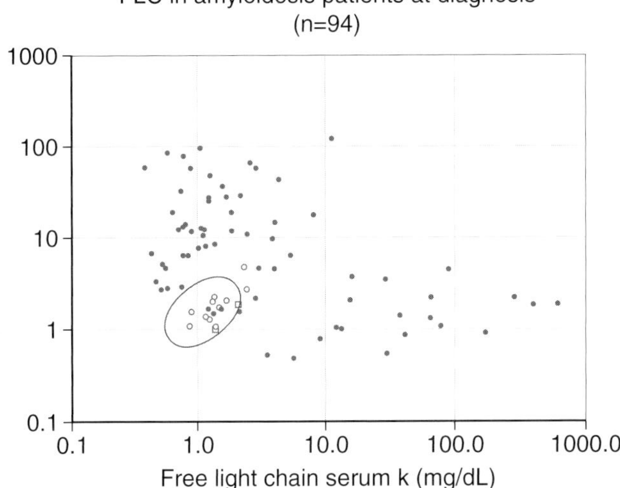

Figure 51–2. Serum free light chain (FLC) levels in 94 patients with newly diagnosed amyloidosis. The axes are logarithmic. The *dark circles* represent values in those with systemic AL ($n = 76$), the *open circles* those with localized AL ($n = 14$), and the *open squares* those with hereditary amyloidosis ($n = 4$). Patients were seen at Memorial Sloan-Kettering between May 2002 and May 2004. The *oval* depicts the normal range.

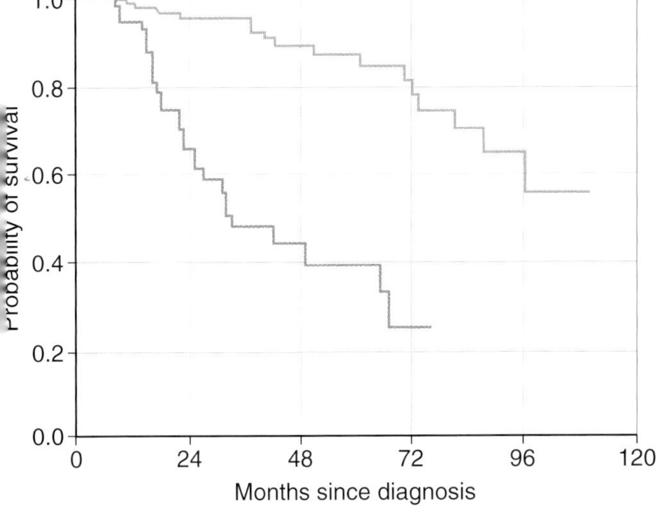

Figure 51–3. Kaplan-Meier estimate of survival in 137 patients with systemic AL amyloidosis treated after initial assessment. Eighty-six patients (63%) had a greater than 50% fall in the concentration of the amyloidogenic free light chain as the result of treatment. Their survival was significantly greater than those whose free light chain concentration fell by less than 50% after completing chemotherapy ($P < .0001$). (From Lachmann HJ, Gallimore R, Gillmore JD, et al: Outcome in systemic AL amyloidosis in relation to changes in concentration of circulating free immunoglobulin light chains following chemotherapy. Br J Haematol 122:78–84, 2003, with permission).

Amyloid Scans

As noted earlier, SAP is a normal serum protein that specifically binds to all types of amyloid fibrils. When SAP is labeled with ^{123}I, it can be used for whole-body scintigraphic imaging to confirm the presence of amyloid.[68,69] Bone marrow involvement and heterogeneous organ involvement are much more characteristic of AL amyloidosis than of other types. Until the use of such scans becomes more commonplace, however, amyloid involvement is best diagnosed noninvasively following the parameters noted in Table 51–2.

Clinical Evaluation

In addition to plasma cell disease testing, a standard clinical evaluation should include detailed history and physical examination. Family history is also important because of the pattern of polyneuropathy and untimely death associated with many mutant TTR variants of hereditary amyloidosis. Additional standard studies include a complete blood count, coagulation screen (prothrombin time by International Normalized Ratio), renal and hepatic blood chemistries, BNP or NT-proBNP, troponin, a 24-hour urine collection for total protein, chest radiograph, electrocardiogram, and echocardiogram. Chest radiography may show prominent vascular markings and pleural effusions, the latter associated with left-heart failure or nephrotic syndrome with hypoalbuminemia. In patients with relevant findings, a gastric emptying scan, nerve conduction studies, and pulmonary function tests may be useful.

The peripheral blood picture is usually normal and anemia rare; if present, it may be due to amyloidosis associated with myeloma, chronic gastrointestinal bleeding and consequent iron loss, massive marrow deposits of amyloid, or renal dysfunction causing inappropriately low erythropoietin levels. Elevated prothrombin times or prolonged activated partial thromboplastin times occur with the presence of thrombin inhibitors (about 30% of patients) or factor X deficiency (about 5% of patients).[70,71] The latter is usually associated with hepatosplenic amyloidosis. In patients with hepatic involvement, abnormal liver function tests are often limited to an elevated alkaline phosphatase. A rising bilirubin level is a poor prognostic sign and usually a preterminal event.

Misdiagnosis of AL Amyloidosis

There are a number of clinical situations that may mimic AL amyloidosis. In black patients, particularly those over the age of 60, the concern of misdiagnosing AL amyloidosis is raised because of the increased frequency of both hereditary amyloid and monoclonal gammopathy of undetermined significance.[72,73] It is important to keep in mind that monoclonal gammopathy of undetermined significance is found in 5% of normal individuals over the age of 70.[73] In patients with hypertension, renal amyloidosis, and low-level monoclonal proteins, the concern is warranted based on a recent report of patients with the fibrinogen A α chain variant of hereditary amyloid and low-level monoclonal proteins being misdiagnosed and undergoing dose-intensive chemotherapy and autologous stem cell transplantation (SCT).[74] In elderly patients with monoclonal gammopathy and senile cardiac amyloid, there is no apparent reason to treat. Finally, patients presenting with peripheral nervous system involvement only and a monoclonal plasma cell disorder may have one of the mutant TTR variants.[9]

TREATMENT

Cytoreductive Therapy

The primary approach to therapy is to reduce the production of the amyloidogenic light chain by reducing the clonal plasma cell population. The ultimate aim is to achieve a complete hematologic response with negative immunofixation studies and significant (>50%) reduction in the pathologic FLC level, ideally with normalization of both light chain levels.

The same therapeutic approaches used for multiple myeloma have been used to treat AL amyloidosis; those supported by clinical trials are delineated in Table 51–3. There have been several Phase III clinical trials showing the benefit of cytoreductive oral therapy with melphalan and prednisone (MP), and numerous Phase II trials showing the benefit of intravenous high-dose melphalan with autologous SCT.[75–83] Other regimens such as single-agent dexamethasone and VBMCP (vincristine, BCNU, melphalan, cyclophosphamide, and prednisone) have also been examined in clinical trials.[84–87]

The conundrum of therapy is that a less toxic treatment that works too gradually will be ineffective because death may occur before the FLCs have been reduced, and an aggressive therapy designed to work quickly will likely be too toxic for patients with extensive visceral involvement. Hence, the initial determination is whether the patient is eligible for SCT based on extent of organ involvement and age and disease progression.

Overall median survival with MP is prolonged from 12 to 18 months in placebo-controlled trials[75–77]; however, responders did survive significantly longer than non-responders (median 89 vs. 14 months).[75] Patients with nephrotic syndrome fared better than those with cardiac involvement, of whom only 15–20% responded. Risks include a 20% risk of myelodysplasia that may lead to secondary leukemia.[88] Only about 5% of patients treated with alkylating agents survived for 10 years or more.[14] VAD (vincristine, doxorubicin, and dexamethasone) induces remission in 70% of patients with myeloma with a rapid response and with maximum response reached after 2 or 3 months in most patients. However, patients with amyloid are likely more vulnerable than myeloma patients to some of the side effects of this regimen, including ileus, neuropathy, fluid retention, and cardiac toxicity. Dexamethasone alone (40 mg/day for 4 consecutive days on days 1–4, 9–12, and 17–20 of a 30-day cycle) produces hematologic responses in 30% of patients.[84]

Recently a combination of oral melphalan and dexamethasone (MelDex) was shown in a Phase II clinical trial (n = 46) for patients ineligible for SCT to be effective and well tolerated.[86] Overall and complete hematologic response rates were 67% and 33%, with 4% treatment-related mortality. Median survival in responders had not been reached at 2 years. Another recent cooperative group Phase II trial (n = 93) showed that initial pulse dexamethasone followed by lower dose dexamethasone maintenance and interferon alfa (DexIFN) likely provides a benefit.[85] Overall survival at 2 years was 60% and median survival was 31 months in this cohort of patients, only 25% of whom were eligible for SCT by standard criteria. Hematologic response rate was over 50%, with 24% complete hematologic responses and 45% organ responses in those evaluable. Both of these approaches compare favorably with MP.

Autologous Stem Cell Transplantation

In the mid 1990s, clinical trials were conducted using dose-intensive intravenous melphalan and autologous hematopoietic SCT to treat AL amyloidosis.[78–81] SCT reversed or arrested the organ disease in nearly two thirds of surviving patients at numerous centers, and amyloid scintiscans demonstrated resorption of AL deposits after the reduction or elimination of the clonal plasma cell disorder that is their root cause.[81] As the production of light chain is halted, and once the patient has recovered from SCT, the organ disease, performance status, and quality of life may improve in the first year post-SCT.[89,90]

However, the long-term efficacy of SCT in AL amyloidosis is still evolving and controversial.[83,91–94] Overall survival data from three series of patients treated with SCT at single centers are shown in Table 51–4. In the largest single-center series, median survival over an 8 year period of patients undergoing SCT was 4.5 years.[93] In

TABLE 51–3. Landmark Clinical Trials in Systemic AL Amyloidosis

Reference	Phase	Therapy	Two-Year Survival	Hematologic Complete Response Rate, % (*N*)	Organ Response Rate, % (*N*)
75	III	Pulse melphalan & prednisone	<50%	<5%	NA
78	II	SCT (Mel 200)	68%	62 (13)	67 (11)
80	II	SCT (Mel 140 + TBI/Mel 200)	NA	30 (6)	60 (12)
85	II	DexIFN	60%	24 (13)	45 (33)
86	II	MelDex	NA	33 (15)	48 (22)

TABLE 51–4. Single-center Overall Survival Data with SCT

Reference	Patients	TRM (N (%))	Survival
94	66	9 (14%)	70% at 2 years
93	312	49 (16%)	Median 4.6 years
113	94	4 (4%)	81% at 2 years

TRM = treatment-related mortality, including deaths in mobilization and within 100 days of transplant.

addition, treatment-related deaths within 100 days was between 20% and 39%, making SCT in this population particularly morbid.[78–81,92] Despite this, a recent SCT trial restricted to those newly diagnosed patients identified a 20% peri-transplant mortality.[82] Patient selection has became more of a priority, as is reflected in the recent summary data shown in Table 51–4.[93,94]

Issues Arising from Clinical Trials of AL Amyloidosis with Cytoreductive Therapy and SCT

Treatment-Related Mortality and Clinical Trial Design

The extent of amyloid organ involvement clearly accounts for much of the treatment-related mortality. Patients with two or fewer organ systems involved have significantly superior 100-day survival (81%, or 25 of 31 patients) compared to those with more than two systems involved (25%, or 4 of 12 patients; $P < .01$, Fisher's exact test).[78,79] Similar results can be appreciated in an examination of the multicenter studies reported.[81,95] Death results from a range of causes, all related to limited visceral and vascular reserve, including cardiac arrhythmias, intractable vascular collapse and hypotension, multiorgan failure, and gastrointestinal bleeding. Toxic responses to transplantation occur more frequently in patients with amyloidosis than in those who receive transplants for other indications.

Treatment-related morbidity in SCT for AL amyloidosis is also a function of the dose of intravenous melphalan, as indicated by the lower-grade toxicities experienced by SCT patients treated with 100 as opposed to 200 mg/ m^2 of melphalan.[78,79] Grade 2 to 4 gastrointestinal toxicity with 200 mg/m^2 of melphalan occurs nearly 40% of the time, and is much less common in patients treated with 100 or 140 mg/m^2. Gastrointestinal bleeding has been a significant cause of early mortality with SCT.[96] Gastrointestinal bleeding particularly is unusual after autologous transplantation and in greater frequency and severity is unique to patients with AL amyloidosis. If amyloid extensively infiltrates the submucosa of the stomach or lower tract, the potential for severe mucositis with hemorrhage clearly must be anticipated, while neuropathic compromise of the enteric plexus often results in atony, persistent posttransplantation nausea, and failure to thrive. For these reasons, pretransplantation planning and peritransplantation supportive care become essential. Recommendations with respect to peritransplantation management have recently been described in detail and include a complete assessment of coagulation status.[91]

A recently reported randomized prospective Phase II clinical trial aptly depicts the outcomes with SCT in new patients.[82] Importantly, unlike the overall experiences described in Table 51–4, all patients enrolled in the trial were within 12 months of diagnosis and untreated. These results, therefore, are most relevant to newly diagnosed patients and are shown in Figure 51–4. One hundred patients were stratified based on organ involvement and time from diagnosis, and randomized to receive SCT either as initial therapy (Arm 1) or after two cycles of oral melphalan and prednisone (Arm 2). The end points were survival and hematologic and organ responses. The overall peritransplantation (100-day) treatment-related mortality was 27%, and 12% of patients died in association with stem cell mobilization and collection. There were no significant differences between the two arms with respect to overall survival at a median of 4 years' follow-up. At 5 years post-SCT, the overall survival was 50% for Arm 1 and 39% for Arm 2. The complete hematologic response rates were 21% and 17% (intention-to-treat), and 42% of patients achieved a clinical improvement in amyloid disease at 1 year.

Fewer patients received SCT in Arm 2 because of disease progression during oral MP. Hence, newly diagnosed patients with AL amyloidosis eligible for SCT did not benefit from initial treatment with oral MP, and there was a survival disadvantage for patients with cardiac involvement if SCT was delayed by initial oral chemotherapy.[97] For patients with two or fewer major organs involved and for those without cardiac involvement, median survival had not been reached at a median of 4 years' follow-up. For those with more than two organs involved, median survivals in the two arms were 9.3 and 5.2 months. At this time, it is reasonable to consider SCT for patients with one or two organs involved and those with uncomplicated cardiac disease. Furthermore, the dose of intravenous melphalan should be attenuated based on age and organ involvement, a risk-adapted approach based on the dose-related differences in toxicity observed in clinical trials (at 100 and 200 mg/m^2 of intravenous melphalan) and on age-related differences in survival.[91]

Continued efforts to treat AL amyloidosis with SCT will depend on clinical trials that evaluate approaches designed to make SCT less morbid or to answer specific questions of interest. A provocative single-center tandem transplant Phase II trial has been reported in which 35 patients were enrolled, 28 of whom were eligible for tandem transplant based on stem cell collections.[98] Fifteen (54%) achieved a complete hematologic response after the first SCT (melphalan 200 mg/m^2), with one treatment-related death. Nine of the 12 patients who failed to achieve complete response proceeded to receive a second SCT (melphalan 140 mg/m^2) with one treatment-related death. Overall, 18 patients achieved complete response, with two treatment-related deaths; whether achievement of complete response after tandem transplant in this disease translates into extended survival remains to be seen.

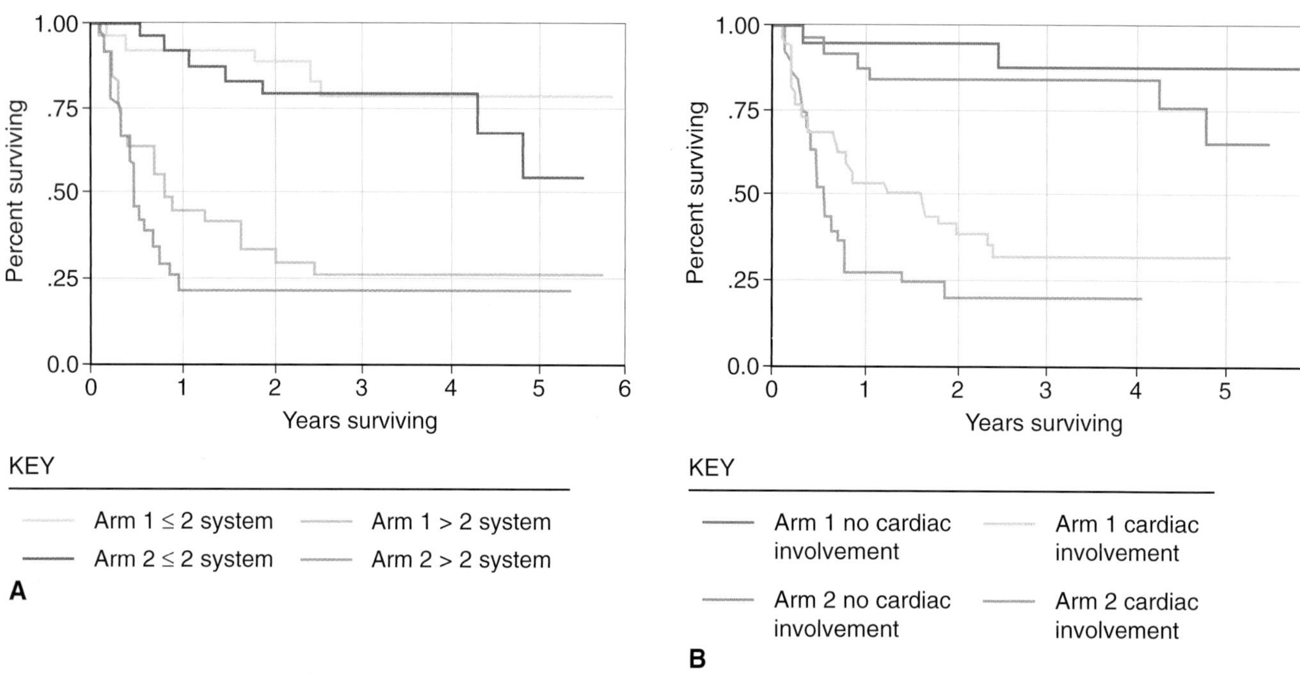

Figure 51–4. Shown are Kaplan-Meier survival curves for 100 newly diagnosed untreated patients with AL amyloidosis enrolled in a Phase II clinical trial in which they were randomized to receive immediate stem cell transplantation (Arm 1) or stem cell transplantation after two cycles of melphalan and prednisone (Arm 2). ***A***, Survival in both arms was significantly impacted by the number of organs involved. ***B***, Survival was also worse in both arms for patients with cardiac involvement.

Monitoring Response to Therapy

In clinical trials for patients with AL amyloidosis, the primary end point should remain survival from time of diagnosis. It will not benefit AL patients if a treatment stops the disease but the process of disease reversal causes sudden death, for instance, because of intractable cardiac arrhythmias. The design of novel Phase II trials should therefore include explicit criteria of treatment-related mortality and stopping rules. Moreover, in Phase III trials the end point of overall survival should remain a primary one.

In addition to survival, patients may benefit from improved organ function. Organ responses have been based on noninvasive testing and have usually been described as improved, stable, or worsened. Biopsy-based criteria do not exist, and amyloid scans, though likely useful to monitor response, are of limited availability.[68,99] For patients with cardiac involvement, a response is defined as a decrease of 2 mm or more in mean left ventricular wall thickness for those with baseline wall thickness greater than 11 mm, or a decrease of two classes in their New York Heart Association classification (i.e., from III to I). For patients with renal involvement, a response is defined as a 50% decrease in daily proteinuria without progressive renal insufficiency, and for those with hepatic involvement a response is a decrease in liver span of 2 cm or more with a concomitant decrease of alkaline phosphatase by 50%. For patients with neuropathic involvement, a response is defined as normalization of orthostatic vital signs and symptoms, and resolution of gastric atony and of abnormal findings on neurologic examination.

Scoring the response of the clonal plasma cell disease to therapy has recently become more challenging as a result of the availability of the FLC assay.[63-65] Immunofixation remains the "gold standard," hence the definition of a complete hematologic response remains negative immunofixation electrophoresis of serum and urine. It is now reasonably obvious that the resolution of amyloid disease in AL patients after therapy is a function of at least two variables: the serum FLC concentration and the amyloidogenicity of the FLC. As a rule of thumb, reductions of the FLC that exceed 50% of baseline are likely to lead to improvements in amyloid disease and prolonged survival.[65]

Evaluation of hematologic response in AL amyloidosis has been based on myeloma response criteria, and recently more or less on the so-called Blade criteria.[100] When the clonal plasma disease becomes undetectable by immunofixation and marrow plasma cells and other elements normalize by immunostaining for plasma cell antigens, the patient has had a complete response. Patients achieving at least a 50% reduction in baseline serologic measures of plasma cell activity (M spike, quantitative immunoglobulin) are considered partial responders (Table 51–5).

Solid Organ Transplantation

The use of solid organ transplantation (liver, heart, and kidney) in patients with AL amyloidosis is frequently deemed inappropriate because of the likely accumulation of amyloid in the grafted organ. Liver transplant, in contrast, is a therapy of choice for hereditary amyloido-

TABLE 51–5. A Risk-Adapted Approach to SCT for AL Amyloidosis

Good Risk (Any Age; All Criteria Met)
No cardiac involvement
Only 1 or 2 major organs involved among kidneys, liver/gastrointestinal tract, peripheral nervous system
Creatinine clearance >51 mL/min
Intermediate risk (Age < 71)
1 or 2 organs involved
May have compensated cardiac involvement
May have renal involvement with creatinine clearance <51 mL/min
Poor Risk (Either Criteria)
More than 2 major organs involved
Advanced cardiac amyloid

sis and has even led to the use of "domino" grafts in which the otherwise normal mutant TTR–producing liver is used as an allograft.[101–103] This situation is slowly changing. In the past decade a number of AL patients have successfully undergone cardiac allograft and then SCT; the feasibility of this approach is established and a Phase II trial needs to be performed to demonstrate safety and efficacy in a systematic fashion.[104–106] Renal transplantation has also been shown to be effective, and renal allografts survive for lengthy periods in many recipients especially after SCT.[107] Renal failure requiring dialysis develops in about a third of patients after 2 years despite standard oral therapy but only in about 10% of patients after dose-intensive therapy with stem cell support.[90,108]

New Approaches

Chemotherapeutic approaches to AL amyloidosis treat the disease by cytoreduction of the clonal plasma cells and the fibril precursor protein. It is on that basis that clinical trials of such agents as thalidomide, Revlimid (a thalidomide analogue), and bortezomib are being conducted or planned. New and different approaches under investigation attempt to mobilize or inhibit amyloid deposition, and include amyloid-reactive antibodies and a competitive inhibitor of SAP binding to amyloid fibrils.[104–106] The development of amyloid-reactive antibodies was based on the premise that an immune reaction to amyloid deposits might help to stimulate fibril disassembly.[109–111] Amyloid tumors formed in the skin of healthy mice resolved within several weeks after the generation of antiamyloid antibodies that recognized antigenic determinants on AL amyloid fibrils. The therapeutic potential of this approach was demonstrated by developing antiamyloid murine antibodies to treat mice that had human amyloid tumors. "Amyloidolysis" occurred in treated but not untreated animals. The antibody localized within the amyloid tumors and caused rapid resorption of this material by neutrophils. The manufacture of a chimeric antibody is currently complete and clinical trials will begin in the near future.

Several investigators have identified inhibitors of amyloid fibril formation. In the murine model for AA amyloidosis, small-molecule anionic sulfates and sulfonates have been shown to inhibit fibril formation and lead to resorption.[112] Also, the effects of SAP on amyloid fibrils have been evaluated in numerous ways; for example, mice with targeted deletion of the SAP gene showed reduced inducibility of AA amyloidosis, and the displacement of SAP enhanced proteolysis. Hence, it is reasonable to suggest that SAP might be a useful therapeutic target.[69] Although preliminary results were encouraging, the current status of SAP inhibitors as agents for reversing AL amyloidosis remains under study.[111]

PROGNOSIS

Survival remains the primary end point for patients and for clinical investigators. SCT for AL amyloidosis is effective in younger patients and safe for those with limited disease; hopefully, the risk-adapted approach will optimize benefit and limit mortality.[91,113] Patients diagnosed today with AL amyloidosis with heart involvement still can expect limited survival, and those diagnosed with

CURRENT CONTROVERSIES & FUTURE CONSIDERATIONS

Amyloidosis

- Because AL patients improve so dramatically with elimination of circulating free light chains (precursor protein), the issue of toxicity of light chain forms, perhaps misfolded or partially aggregated species, is open to question.
- Others believe, however, that the amyloid deposits are the primary cause of the observed pathology.
- Given the limited repertoire of immunoglobulin light chain genes involved in AL amyloidosis, are AL plasma cells responding to a limited number of antigens and if so, can these be identified?
- Will monoclonal antibody therapy directed toward AL plasma cells for AL amyloidosis be able to reverse the disease?
- The next generation of clinical trials for AL patients needing salvage therapy will involve new drugs such as bortezomib and thalidomide analogues, although the toxicity is anticipated to be high and clear-cut stopping rules will be needed.
- The next generation of clinical trials for newly diagnosed AL patients will include Phase III trials for autologous SCT and Phase II trials seeking to combine active regimens such as MelDex with SCT.

renal involvement only can expect survival in excess of 5 years after SCT. In addition, the promise of modified dexamethasone-based regimens (MelDex, DexIFN) combined with the logic of risk-adapted melphalan dosing in SCT may provide the basis for clinical trials that combine both approaches. Finally, it is most encouraging that new drugs to mobilize amyloid from organs are just about to enter clinical trials. These agents may eliminate the supply of fibril precursor protein light chains, inhibit their self-assembly, and enhance resorption of deposits.

Suggested Readings*

Comenzo RL, Gertz MA: Autologous stem cell transplantation for primary systemic amyloidosis. Blood 99:4276–4282, 2002.

Dispenzieri A, Gertz MA, Kyle RA, et al: Prognostication of survival using cardiac troponins and N-terminal pro-brain natriuretic peptide in patients with primary systemic amyloidosis undergoing peripheral blood stem cell transplant. Blood 104:1881–1887, 2004.

Falk RH, Comenzo RL, Skinner M: The systemic amyloidoses. N Engl J Med 337:898–909, 1997.

Kyle R, Gertz M, Greipp P, et al: A trial of three regimens for primary amyloidosis: colchicine alone, melphalan and prednisolone, and melphalan, prednisolone and colchicine. N Engl J Med 336 1202–1207, 1997.

Lachmann HJ, Booth DR, Booth SE, et al: Misdiagnosis of hereditary amyloidosis as AL (primary) amyloidosis. N Engl J Med 346 1786–1791, 2002.

Lachmann HJ, Gallimore R, Gillmore JD, et al: Outcome in systemic AL amyloidosis in relation to changes in concentration of circulating free immunoglobulin light chains following chemotherapy Br J Haematol 122:78–84, 2003.

Merlini G, Bellotti V: Molecular mechanisms of amyloidosis. N Engl J Med 349:583–596, 2003.

Palladini G, Campana C, Klersy C, et al: Serum N-terminal pro-brain natriuretic peptide is a sensitive marker of myocardial dysfunction in AL amyloidosis. Circulation 107:2440–2445, 2003.

Sanchorawala V, Wright DG, Seldin DC, et al: High-dose intravenous melphalan and autologous stem cell transplantation as initial therapy or following two cycles of oral therapy for the treatment of AL amyloidosis: results of a randomized prospective trial. Bone Marrow Transplantation 33:381–388, 2004.

Skinner M, Sanchorawala V, Seldin DC, et al: High-dose melphalan and autologous stem-cell transplantation in patients with AL amyloidosis: an 8-year study. Ann Intern Med 140:85–93, 2004.

Full references for this chapter can be found on accompanying CD-ROM.

CHAPTER 52

Mastocytosis

Melody C. Carter, MD, and Dean D. Metcalfe, MD

> **KEY POINTS**
>
> **Mastocytosis**
>
> - Age of onset of mastocytosis ranges from birth to adulthood.
> - Diagnosis is by tissue biopsy, usually of the skin or bone marrow.
> - Presentation may be cutaneous, systemic, or both.
> - The incidence of allergic disease is similar to that in the general population.
> - Most often mastocytosis is associated with a somatic mutation of the c-*kit* gene.

INTRODUCTION

Since the first description of the cutaneous manifestations of mastocytosis by Nettleship and Tay in 1869,[1] recognition has grown that mastocytosis is heterogeneous in manifestations and prognosis. The term *mastocytosis* was first coined by Sézary in 1936.[2] However, discoveries regarding the molecular and cellular mechanisms in the last 10 years have been instrumental in developing contemporary approaches in understanding the etiology, diagnosis, and therapy of mastocytosis.

Mastocytosis is a disease characterized by the presence of excessive numbers of mast cells in the skin and internal organs, such as the bone marrow, gastrointestinal tract, lymph nodes, liver, and spleen. Symptoms related to mast cell degranulation are frequently observed in all categories of mastocytosis. These may include episodic pruritus, blister formation, flushing, dyspepsia, diarrhea, abdominal pain, musculoskeletal pain, and hypotension. In addition, some patients may have an associated non–mast-cell clonal hematologic disorder, whose clinical presentation will reflect that of this associated disorder.

Depending on the mast cell burden and the extent of the tissue involvement, the disease may present with a number of varied clinical manifestations. On the benign end of the spectrum is pediatric-onset mastocytosis limited to skin. Patients are typically diagnosed with urticaria pigmentosa skin lesions within the first 6 months of life and experience regression or improvement of the skin lesions by the time they reach puberty. Conversely, patients with adult-onset mastocytosis generally have evidence of systemic mastocytosis, defined by involvement of an organ system other than skin. Systemic mastocytosis in most cases in adults appears to be a persistent or progressive clonal disorder of the mast cell progenitor and to be associated with activating mutations in c-*kit,* the gene that codes for Kit, the receptor for stem cell factor (SCF). Systemic mastocytosis can follow a benign or indolent course, or it may be associated with life-threatening hematologic disorders. The correct diagnosis of mastocytosis and classification of the disease variant are important for an accurate prognosis and selection of therapy.

EPIDEMIOLOGY AND RISK FACTORS

Prevalence

Mastocytosis is an unusual disease, with an estimated 20,000–30,000 affected individuals in the United States. It is approximately equally distributed among males and females. Mastocytosis is not associated with an increased prevalence of atopy, although mast cells are a key effector cell in allergic inflammation.

Genetic Factors

Mastocytosis in adults appears to be frequently associated with somatic mutations at codon 816 of c-*kit*. However, mastocytosis in most cases does not appear to be an inherited disorder. Urticaria pigmentosa in some children has been associated with mutations in codon 816 of c-*kit,* sometimes with evidence of systemic disease. An inactivating mutation at position 839 has been described in some children with urticaria pigmentosa.

Familial inheritance has been reported in approximately 50 families since the mid-1880s.[3] In those families, less than half of the kindreds reviewed had more than one generation affected.[3] A case of familial telangiectasia macularis eruptiva perstans (TMEP) affecting three generations, with onset during childhood, has been

TABLE 52–1. Selected Mast Cell Mediators

Mediators	Biologic Effects	Possible Consequences
Preformed		
Histamine	Vasodilation, increased vascular permeability, gastric hypersecretion, bronchoconstriction	Hypotension, flushing, urticaria, abdominal pain (peptic, colic), diarrhea, malabsorption
Heparin	Anticoagulant, inhibition of platelet aggregation	Prolonged bleeding time
Tryptase	Endothelial cell activation, fibrinogen cleavage, mitogenic for smooth muscle cells	Osteoporosis/osteopenia
Chymase	Converts angiotensin I to II, remodeling, lipoprotein degradation	Hypertension
Newly Synthesized		
Leukotrienes	Increased vascular permeability, bronchoconstriction, vasoconstriction	Bronchospasm, hypotension
Prostaglandins	Vasodilatation, bronchoconstriction	Flushing, urticaria
Cytokines		
SCF	Growth and survival of mast cells	Mast cell hyperplasia
TNF-α	Activation of vascular endothelial cells, cachexia, fatigue	Weight loss, fatigue
TGF-β	Fibrosis	Fibrosis
IL-5	Eosinophil growth factor	Eosinophilia
IL-6	Growth and survival of mast cells	Fever, bone pain, osteoporosis/osteopenia
IL-16	Lymphocyte accumulation	Focal aggregates

Abbreviations: IL, interleukin; SCF, stem cell factor; TGF-β, transforming growth factor-β; TNF-α, tumor necrosis factor-α.

reported. Similarly, an inherited form of deafness was seen in two siblings with mastocytosis with clinical features similar to the familial form of the disease. Familial mastocytosis does not appear to be associated with a mutation at codon 816 in c-*kit*.

PATHOPHYSIOLOGY

Mast cells have been traditionally recognized in terms of their effector role in the genesis of allergic disease. Following immunoglobulin E–mediated activation, mast cells release preformed mediators such as histamine, generate lipid-derived substances such as leukotrienes, and synthesize and release growth factors and cytokines (Table 52–1). This knowledge, taken together with the presence of mast cells in lymphoid tissues, along nerves and blood vessels, and throughout connective tissues, as well as within tissues that interface with the outside environment (i.e., the skin and the gastrointestinal tract), facilitates the formulation of hypotheses about their function. Current evidence supports a role for mast cells in host defense against microorganisms and a regulatory function in both the T_H1 and T_H2 T helper–type inflammatory response. Mast cells may also stimulate connective tissue repair and maintain the vasculature.

Hematologic Origin

Mast cells are derived from CD34$^+$Kit$^+$CD13$^+$ hematopoietic cell progenitors.[4–9] SCF, a general hematopoietic growth factor, is essential for mast cell proliferation and survival. Terminal differentiation of mast cells occurs in vascularized tissues under the influence of SCF, plus additional cytokines including interleukin IL-6, IL-9, and nerve growth factor. Once in tissues, mast cells typically do not undergo further proliferation.

Mast Cell Distribution

Mast cells containing tryptase (MC_T) are found in mucosal tissues. MC_T mast cells may be found in proximity to T2 T helper cells. MC_T are increased in allergic and parasitic diseases and decreased in human immunodeficiency virus–infected individuals.[10] The other mast cell phenotype contains both tryptase and chymase (MC_{TC}) and is the predominant mast cell found in the skin and connective tissues. MC_{TC} also expresses carboxypeptidase and cathepsin G. Increased numbers of MC_{TC} are found in fibrotic diseases.[11,12]

Kit and c-*kit* Mutations

Kit (Fig. 52–1) is a type III tyrosine kinase receptor found on the surface of mast cells that regulates cell proliferation and differentiation. Kit is dimerized by SCF and initiates signal transduction. Kit consists of three domains: an extracellular region composed of five immunoglobulin-like motifs (the first three of which bind SCF), a single short transmembrane region, and a cytoplasmic region. The cytoplasmic region of the protein includes the kinase domain, which is divided into an adenosine triphosphate (ATP)–binding region and a phosphotransferase region.

Kit is encoded by the proto-oncogene c-*kit* located on human chromosome 4. Several mutations have been identified in mastocytosis, the most common being a substitution of valine (V) for aspartate (D) at codon 816 (D816V). Tyrosine (Y) may also be substituted for aspartate (D816Y).[13,14] These mutations give rise to SCF-

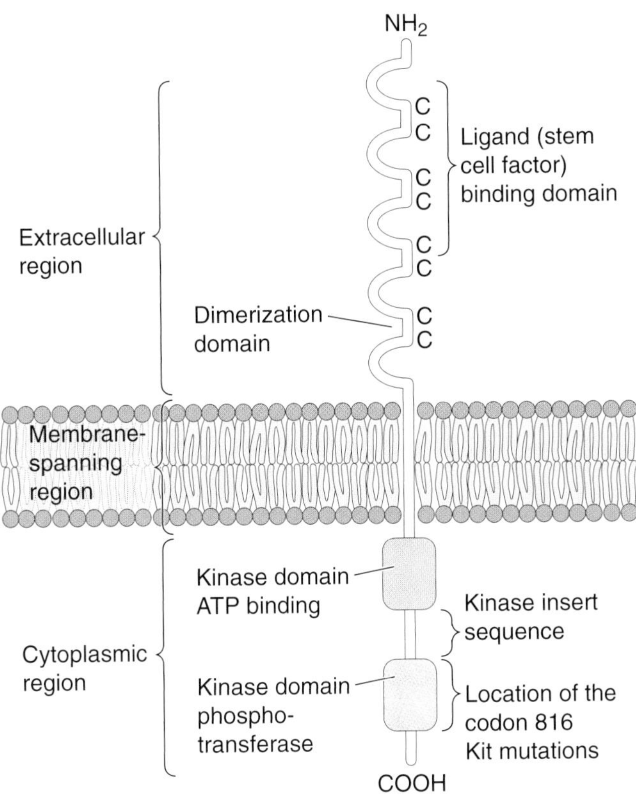

Figure 52–1. Schematic of Kit molecule (CD 117).

independent activation of Kit. The consequence is believed to be continued cell division and/or survival that result in mast cell hyperplasia. A novel germline mutation has been recently identified in *c-kit* located within the sequence that codes for the transmembrane region of Kit.[15] A polymorphism in the gene for the IL-4 receptor α chain resulting in increased activity increases the apoptosis of mast cells and is associated with less aggressive disease.[16,17] Bone marrow cells of patients with mastocytosis have been found to express the antiapoptotic protein Bcl-x.[18]

Mast Cell Mediators

Many of the symptoms of mastocytosis are the result of an increase in release of preformed inflammatory mediators stored in mast cell granules and newly formed inflammatory mediators produced following mast cell activation (see Table 52–1). Preformed mediators include histamine, proteoglycans such as heparin, and tumor necrosis factor-α. Newly formed mediators, which are derived from arachidonic acid, include the sulfidopeptide leukotrienes and prostaglandin D_2. Also synthesized and released are specific cytokines and chemokines. Histamine is one of the primary mediators, contributing to pruritus, increased vascular permeability, and vascular instability. Histamine also contributes to gastric hypersecretion and subsequent peptic ulceration.[19] Flushing and hypotension may be the result of a systemic vasodepressor effect caused by mediators including histamine.

IL-6 is produced by inflammatory cells, such as monocytes, macrophages, mast cells, activated T cells, fibroblasts, and neutrophils. IL-6 has been found to be highly expressed by keratinocytes in psoriatic skin.[20] IL-6 in the presence of SCF may help prevent mast cell apoptosis.[21] Levels of IL-6 are elevated in the plasma of patients with systemic mastocytosis and correlate with plasma tryptase levels and with dermal mast cell numbers.[22,23]

CLINICAL FEATURES AND DIAGNOSIS

Classification

Mastocytosis is not a single well-defined disorder but rather a spectrum of diseases characterized by abnormal growth and accumulation of mast cells. Although all classes of the disease have been seen across a wide age range, the majority of cases demonstrate a bimodal distribution of disease presentation. Sixty-five percent of patients are diagnosed with pediatric-onset disease[24] appearing as early as birth, with the remainder demonstrating an adult-onset pattern with disease usually occurring after the fourth decade.

Mastocytosis is divided into distinct variants on the basis of clinical presentation, pathologic findings, and prognosis (Table 52–2). Patients in the cutaneous and indolent categories have a good prognosis. Children present predominately with cutaneous disease. Most adult patients with mastocytosis present with indolent systemic mastocytosis and may have one or more of the more common findings: flushing, syncope, cutaneous disease, peptic ulcer disease, malabsorption, bone marrow mast cell aggregates, skeletal abnormalities, hepatosplenomegaly, and mild abdominal lymphadenopathy. In most cases, patients with indolent disease gradually accrue more mast cells as symptoms progress. Such patients are managed successfully for decades using medications that provide symptomatic relief.

The second most common form of disease in adults is systemic mastocytosis with an associated hematologic non–mast cell disorder (SM-AHNMD). This variant is associated with hematologic disorders such as myelodysplastic disease with attendant bone marrow and peripheral blood abnormalities. A third category of patients with mastocytosis present with enlarged liver, spleen, and lymph nodes and often peripheral eosinophilia and are categorized as having aggressive systemic mastocytosis. The disease course is rapid. The fourth category, mast cell leukemia, is rare and is characterized by the presence of malignant mast cells in the peripheral blood, which by definition must constitute greater than 10% of the nucleated cells.[25] Mast cell sarcoma is an extremely rare form of mastocytosis that has only been documented in a limited number of cases.[26–28] The disease is defined by a local destructive (sarcoma-like) growth of a tumor consisting of highly atypical mast cells, similar in morphology to those seen in mast cell leukemia.

The symptoms of mastocytosis are often secondary to the release of preformed inflammatory mediators stored

TABLE 52–2. World Health Organization (WHO) Classification of Mastocytosis*

Variant Term	Abbreviation	Subvariants
Cutaneous mastocytosis	CM	Urticaria pigmentosa (UP) Maculopapular CM (MPCM) Diffuse CM (DCM) Mastocytoma of skin
Indolent systemic mastocytosis	ISM	Smoldering SM Isolated bone marrow mastocytosis
Systemic mastocytosis with an associated clonal hematologic non–mast cell lineage disease	SM-AHNMD	SM-AML SM-MDS SM-MPD SM-CMML SM-NHL
Aggressive systemic mastocytosis	ASM	
Mast cell leukemia	MCL	Aleukemic MCL
Mast cell sarcoma		
Extracutaneous mastocytoma		

*For details of the WHO classification of mastocytosis, see Valent and colleagues.[56,79]

TABLE 52–3. Diagnostic Criteria for Systemic Mastocytosis*

Major

Multifocal dense infiltrates of mast cells in bone marrow and/or other extracutaneous organs

Minor

1. More than 25% of the mast cells in bone marrow aspirate smears or tissue biopsy sections are spindle shaped or display atypical morphology
2. Detection of a codon 816 c-*kit* point mutation in blood, bone marrow, or lesional tissue
3. Mast cells in bone marrow, blood, or other lesional tissue expressing CD25 or CD2
4. Baseline total tryptase level of greater than 20 ng/mL

*The major and one minor or three minor criteria are needed. For more details, see Valent and colleagues.[56,79]

in mast cell granules, and newly formed inflammatory mediators produced following mast cell activation, that vary with the intensity of the attack (see Table 52–1). These include flushing, pruritus, dyspnea, paresthesias, warmth, nausea, vomiting, diarrhea, abdominal pain, vascular instability, headache, palpitations, light-headedness, and syncope. Attacks may be followed by lethargy that may last for several hours. Inability to concentrate, memory impairment, irritability, and personality changes have also been reported in some patients.

Pruritus (88%) is reported to be the most frequent symptom experienced by patients with bone marrow–proven mastocytosis, followed by gastrointestinal symptoms (80%) and flushing (43%).[19] Abdominal pain was the most common gastrointestinal symptom, followed by diarrhea, nausea, and vomiting. In some patients, attacks may be precipitated by physical stimuli such as heat, cold, pressure, alcohol, and certain medications (e.g., opiates, aspirin). Although uncommon, radiocontrast agents, venoms, and estrogens are reported as additional triggers.

Diagnosis

The diagnosis of mastocytosis is suspected by clinical presentation and established by histopathologic examination of an involved tissue, particularly the bone marrow. Additional studies such as a serum tryptase, bone scintography, gastrointestinal imaging, computed tomography, and endoscopy, may also be appropriate based on presenting complaints. A neuropsychiatric consult may also be helpful. Histamine metabolites are usually elevated in a 24-hour urine specimen in patients with mastocytosis.[29–31] The test, however, appears to be neither more sensitive nor more specific than measurement of serum total tryptase.[32]

The bone marrow is the most useful biopsy site to establish the pathologic diagnosis of systemic disease. Major and minor disease-defining criteria are listed in Table 52–3. Flow-cytometric immunophenotyping of bone marrow mast cells in patients with systemic disease will help to define the disease when these cells are $CD2^+$ and $CD25^+$.[33] Measurements of soluble Kit and soluble IL-2 receptor α chain (sCD25) may also be useful in selecting those patients who should be considered for a bone marrow biopsy, and in the documentation of disease progression.[34]

The most common clinical finding in patients with mastocytosis is the presence of typical skin lesions of urticaria pigmentosa, which appear as fixed, dark red-brown macules or papules. Darier's sign is the local whealing of such a lesion when rubbed or scratched. Other rare forms of cutaneous mastocytosis include mastocytoma, diffuse cutaneous mastocytosis, and TMEP.

Pediatric Versus Adult Mastocytosis

For most pediatric-onset cases, the first sign of disease appears before 6 months of age in the form of lesions of urticaria pigmentosa (Fig. 52–2), with resolution during adolescence.[24] Urticaria pigmentosa lesions in adult-onset mastocytosis (Fig. 52–3) tend to persist, and the overall course of disease is more complex. The systemic involvement seen in adult-onset disease is observed less commonly in children.[35] The majority of pediatric patients appear to lack the Asp816Val and Asp816Tyr activating mutations often found in adults. A Gly839Lys mutation has been found in skin lesions of some pediatric patients with mastocytosis.[36]

Cutaneous Mastocytosis

In one study of 112 patients with cutaneous disease, the mean number of years with the disease was 4, 11, and 20.5 years for those with a solitary lesion, multiple lesions at birth or appearing in early childhood, and multiple

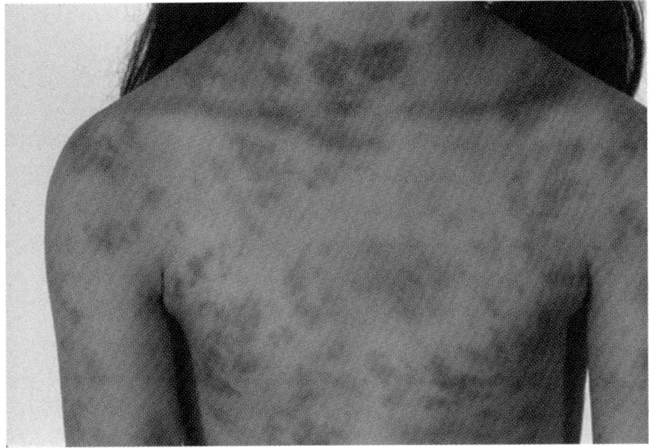

Figure 52–2. Child with urticaria pigmentosa. Both large and small pigmented lesions are visible.

lesions appearing after childhood, respectively.[37] Solitary mastocytomas either were noted at birth or developed within a median time of 1 week. Such mastocytomas consisted of collections of mature mast cells and appeared as macules, plaques, or nodules (Fig. 52–4). Irritation of a mastocytoma lesion may cause systemic symptoms such as flushing.

Urticaria pigmentosa is observed in more than 90% of adult patients with indolent systemic mastocytosis and less than 50% of adults with an associated hematologic disorder or other aggressive forms of the disease. Urticaria pigmentosa has been reported in identical and fraternal twins and two sets of triplets,[38–44] including some twins who were discordant.[45–47] The lesions of urticaria pigmentosa tend to be concentrated on the trunk, although they may affect all areas of skin, including the mucous membranes. The face and scalp are less affected, particularly in older children and adults. The palms and soles tend to remain free of lesions. Lesions usually spare areas exposed to sun or are more subtle in these areas. The biopsy of a urticaria pigmentosa lesion reveals extensive dermal mast cell infiltrates and accumulation of melanin pigment in the epidermis and in macrophages (Fig. 52–5). Infants and young children with urticaria pigmentosa may experience idiopathic bullous eruptions or have such bullous eruptions in association with infections or following routine immunizations.[35,48]

Diffuse cutaneous mastocytosis (Fig. 52–6) is diagnosed almost exclusively in infants, although it may persist into adult life.[49] It is characterized by a diffuse infiltration of the dermis by mast cells with the phenotypic expression of thickened skin with a peau d'orange appearance and/or a reddish brown discoloration. Lesions characteristic of urticaria pigmentosa may also be present. Dermographism and hemorrhagic blistering are common. Patients with diffuse cutaneous mastocytosis appear to be at increased risk for flushing, hypotension, shock, and death.[50] Diarrhea and other gastrointestinal manifestations may be present.[51] Children with diffuse cutaneous mastocytosis generally experience improvement in the skin texture with time.

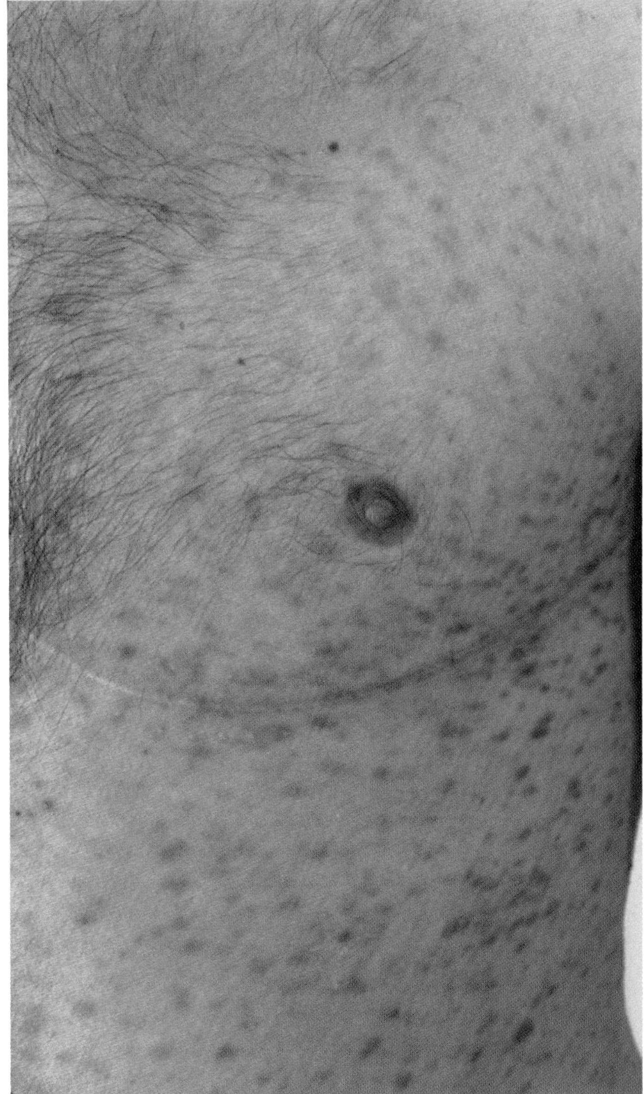

Figure 52–3. Adult with urticaria pigmentosa. Lesions are small, reddish brown macules and papules.

TMEP is a rare form of mastocytosis seen predominately in adults. The lesions are red-brown, telangiectatic, small macules with an irregular border. The occurrence of Darier's sign and pruritus is variable, and blisters are not features of this disease. The biopsy reveals increased numbers of perivascular mast cells.

Systemic Mastocytosis

Systemic mastocytosis is characterized by increased mast cell density involving organs other than the skin. The criteria for the diagnosis are outlined in Table 52–3.[52–54]

Classic bone marrow lesions are seen on microscopic examination of a bone marrow biopsy (Fig. 52–7), while the aspirate mast cells show abnormal morphology (Fig. 52–8). The bone marrow lesions are disseminated, often peritrabecular foci comprising mast cell aggregates with associated T and B lymphocytes and eosinophils.[55] Focal lesions may show a central core of lymphocytes surrounded by mast cells, with eosinophils at the margins of the lesions. Hypercellularity or abnormal myeloid maturation patterns have been associated with a less favorable outcome.[56,57] Bone marrow mast cells may also be identified and characterized using multiparametric flow cytometry[33] for the CD2 and CD25 antigens. Cytogenetic studies also reveal chromosomal aberrations,[58] suggesting a genetic instability of the hematopoietic cells in mastocytosis.[58]

Hepatic and splenic involvement has been reported to occur frequently in patients with all variants of systemic disease.[59] The most common liver abnormality is an elevated serum alkaline phosphatase, which must be distinguished from that released from bone. Transaminases may also be elevated. The most serious complications of liver involvement in mastocytosis are portal hypertension and ascites, which result from mast cell infiltration, fibrosis, and an associated venopathy.

Bone marrow infiltration with mast cells may induce bone changes that produce radiographically detectable lesions in up to 70% of patients[53] and associated abnormalities on bone scan.[60] The most commonly reported abnormalities are diffuse, poorly demarcated, sclerotic, and lucent areas involving the axial skeleton.[61] Back pain secondary to osteoporosis with vertebral compression fractures may be a presenting feature of systemic mastocytosis.[62]

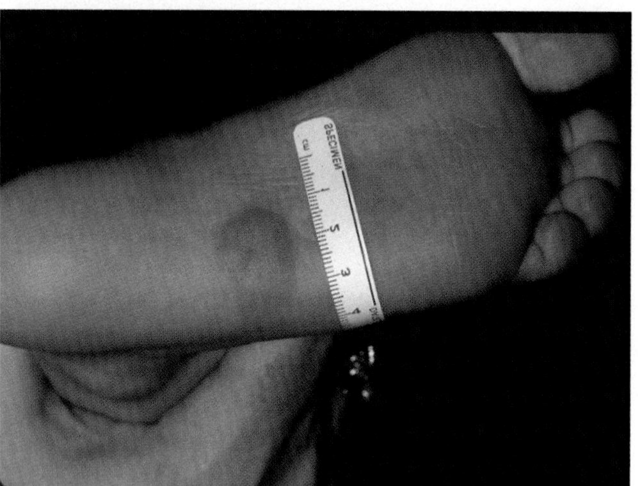

■ **Figure 52–4.** Mastocytoma on the sole of a 3-year-old child.

Indolent Systemic Mastocytosis

The majority of adult patients with mastocytosis present with the indolent variant of the disease. It is characterized by extracutaneous mast cell hyperplasia with or without cutaneous involvement, although most cases present with urticaria pigmentosa.[53] Symptoms result from mediator-related mast cell degranulation and are typically the presenting medical problem.[63–65] The bone marrow is affected in indolent systemic mastocytosis and is characterized by multifocal collections of mast cells.[66,67] The infiltration grade is low. Mast cell infiltrates may also be detected in the liver, spleen, and gastrointestinal tract.[68–72] Clonal mast cells often have the c-*kit* mutation D816V.[13,36,73–76] The serum tryptase concentration is usually elevated,[77,78] even in isolated bone marrow mastocytosis.[79]

Smoldering mastocytosis is another subvariant of indolent systemic mastocytosis.[57,80–83] There is extension of the clonal disease process to several myeloid lineages. These patients have extension bone marrow infiltration, discrete signs of myelodysplasia or myeloproliferation, and palpable organomegaly (hepato-, spleno-, or lymphadenopathy).[57,79–83] The c-*kit* mutation D816V is usually detected in bone marrow cells as well as other myeloid cells.[57,80–83]

SM-AHNMD and Aggressive Systemic Mastocytosis

Up to one third of adults with systemic mastocytosis develop a concurrent hematologic abnormality such as a myeloproliferative disease or myelodysplastic syn-

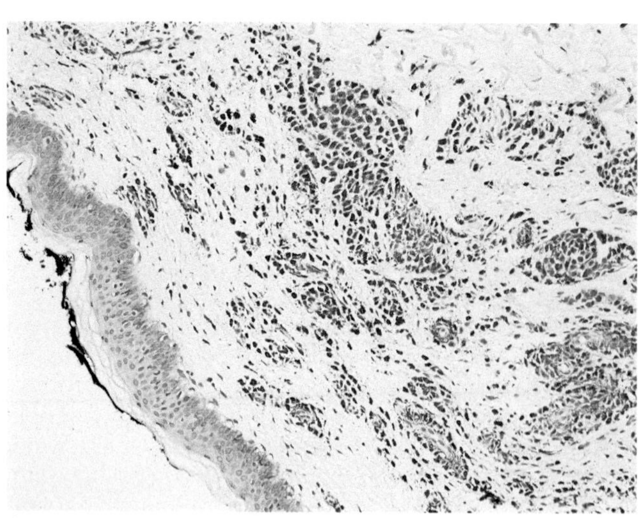

A

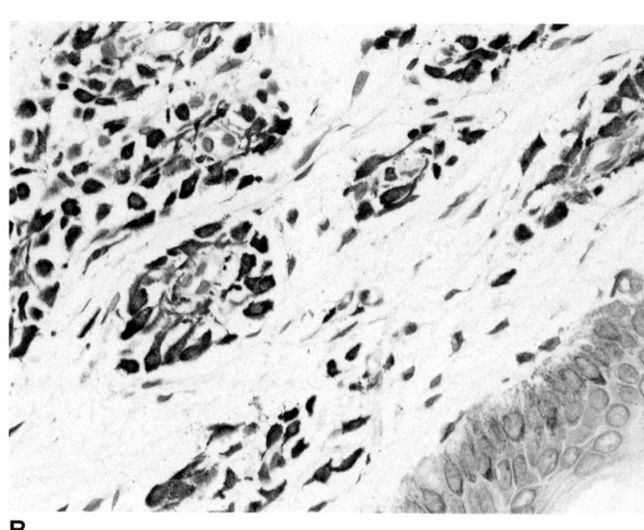

B

■ **Figure 52–5.** Histopathology of urticaria pigmentosa. The pattern of mast cell distribution in the skin may range from scattered and diffuse to a more clustered pattern. Toluidine blue stain at 10 × magnification *(A)* and at 40 × magnification *(B)* demonstrates mast cells with fine blue-purple granules in their cytoplasm.

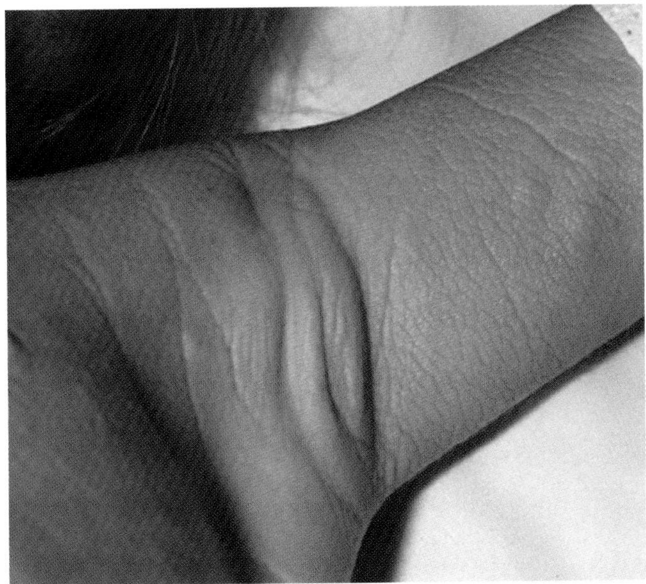

■ **Figure 52–6.** Child with diffuse cutaneous mastocytosis.

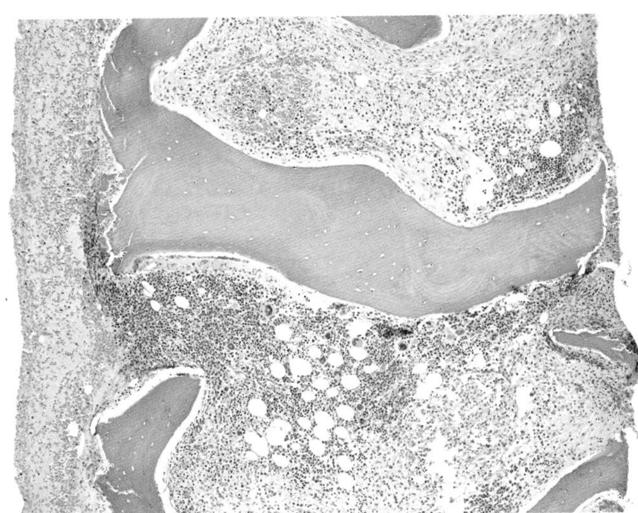

■ **Figure 52–7.** Bone marrow from an adult patient with systemic indolent mastocytosis (hematoxylin and eosin stain, ×5). Classical bone marrow lesions seen in mastocytosis may be adjacent to bone. Lesions are composed of mast cells admixed with lymphocytes and eosinophils.

drome[52,54,79,84–86] or, less commonly, non-Hodgkin's lymphoma.[72,84,87] Aggressive systemic mastocytosis is characterized by organopathy resulting from pathologic infiltration of the liver, bone marrow, spleen, lymph nodes, or gastrointestinal tract by neoplastic mast cells.[79,88–92] The histology of the bone marrow in aggressive systemic mastocytosis shows a variable degree of infiltration.[93] A significant percentage (>20%) of mast cells exhibit bi- or multilobed nuclei (high-grade morphology).[79,93] Metachromatic blasts may also be detected. However, mast cells usually comprise less than 20% of the nucleated cells in the bone marrow smears. The

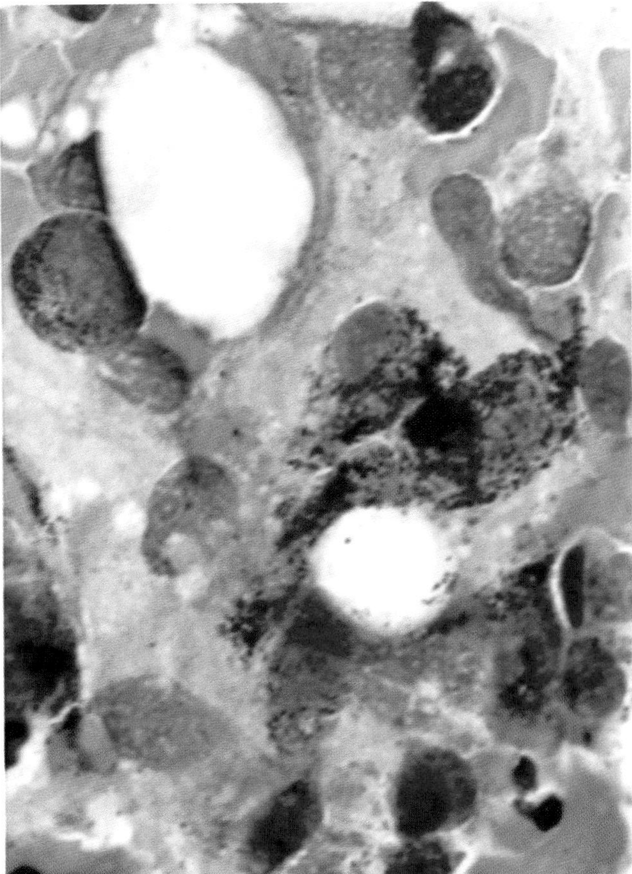

■ **Figure 52–8.** Morphologic abnormality in bone marrow mast cell in systemic mastocytosis.

blood count may reveal cytopenias, leukocytosis, eosinophilia, or monocytosis.[88–91] Liver enzymes and liver function parameters are often abnormal. Osteolysis may be indicated by elevated levels of serum calcium and alkaline phosphatase, as well as an elevated lactate dehydrogenase. The D816V mutation may be identified in some cases,[94,95] indicating overlap between aggressive systemic mastocytosis, SM-AHNMD, and smoldering indolent systemic mastocytosis.[96]

Mast Cell Leukemia

Mast cell leukemia is characterized by high-grade (malignant) peripheral mast cells and/or bone marrow infiltration. Mast cell leukemia is defined by a triad: (1) criteria for the diagnosis of systemic mastocytosis are present, (2) mast cells comprise 20% or more of all nucleated cells in bone marrow smears, and (3) there is multiorgan failure. Cutaneous lesions are absent. The bone marrow typically demonstrates diffuse infiltration with neoplastic immature mast cells accompanied by anemia and thrombocytopenia.[25,79,97] A severe coagulation disorder manifested by signs of consumption, loss of clotting factors, a decrease in platelets, and hyperfibrinolysis, develops with severe bleeding in the gastrointestinal tract. In most cases, multiorgan failure, including bone marrow failure, develops over weeks to months.[98–103]

Mast Cell Sarcoma

Mast cell sarcoma is characterized by a destructive growth of highly atypical mast cells. Tumors may be located at different organ sites than are associated with other forms of systemic disease. These sites include the larynx, ascending colon, and an intracranial site.[27,28,104] Secondary generalization with involvement of visceral organs and hematopoietic tissues has been reported.[27,28,104] Cell atypia in mast cell sarcoma is extensive and comparable to high-grade cytologic abnormalities found in mast cell leukemia.

Extracutaneous Mastocytoma

Not to be confused with mast cell sarcoma, an extracutaneous mastocytoma is a localized benign tumor consisting of mature tissue mast cells. There is no systemic involvement. In contrast to mastocytoma of the skin, mastocytomas in extracutaneous organs are very rare. Thus far, extracutaneous mastocytomas have been primarily detected in the lungs.[105,106] Important differentiating features of extracutaneous mastocytosis in contrast to mast cell sarcoma are the lack of an aggressive and destructive growth pattern and low-grade cytology.

Pregnancy

Mast cells are known to have estrogen and progesterone receptors, so they are present in the myometrium with pregnancy, and appear to affect the second stage of labor.[107–110] A review of eight women during 11 pregnancies indicated that all of the women had a diagnosis of indolent systemic mastocytosis. Medication during pregnancy consisted of H_1 and H_2 antihistamines. In two cases, urticaria pigmentosa lesions increased postpartum. There were no life-threatening manifestations of mastocytosis. None of the children developed urticaria pigmentosa or systemic mastocytosis during the period of observance.[111]

DIFFERENTIAL DIAGNOSIS

Children with cutaneous mastocytosis present with a spectrum of findings from solitary or multiple mastocytomas to urticaria pigmentosa or diffuse cutaneous mastocytosis. Blistering, if present, must be differentiated from other bullous diseases of children. Thus, the differential diagnosis of cutaneous mastocytosis should exclude (1) bullous impetigo and (2) chronic bullous disorders of childhood. Occasionally, skin biopsies from patients with atopic dermatitis lesions have been misdiagnosed as urticaria pigmentosa because of an increase of mast cells observed in eczema. The clinical presentation helps delineate between the two disorders. Substantial heterogeneity in clinical presentation may be observed in patients with adult-onset disease. In systemic mastocytosis, clinical presentation may or may not include cutaneous manifestations, organomegaly and/or impairment of organ function, and an indolent or aggressive course. It is important to differentiate systemic mastocytosis from other diagnoses (Table 52–4).

TABLE 52–4. Differential Diagnoses to be Considered When Systemic Mastocytosis Is Suspected

Benign cutaneous flushing
Idiopathic anaphylaxis
Carcinoid syndrome
Mast cell hyperplasia (underlying conditions, including parasitic infections, tumors)
Myelomastocytic leukemia, myelomastocytic cell spread in myelodysplastic syndromes
Tryptase-positive acute myeloid leukemia
Kit-positive acute myeloid leukemia with aberrant expression of CD2 (FAB AML-M4eo)
Acute myeloid leukemia with aberrant expression of *c-kit* point mutation (Asp-816-Val)
Chronic myeloid leukemia with accumulation of tryptase-positive cells
Idiopathic myelofibrosis with focal accumulation of mast cells
Acute or chronic basophilic leukemia with increase in mast cells
Immunocytoma with reactive focal increase in bone marrow mast cells

TREATMENT

Management of patients within all categories of mastocytosis includes (1) careful counseling of patients in addition to parents in pediatric cases, and of care providers; (2) avoidance of factors triggering disease exacerbation; (3) treatment of acute episodes of systemic hypotension; (4) treatment of chronic symptoms; and, if indicated, (5) an attempt to treat organ infiltration by mast cells and any associated hematologic abnormality.

Symptomatic

The treatment of mastocytosis is focused on symptomatic therapy. H_1 antihistamines such as hydroxyzine, diphenhydramine, and cetirizine are used to control tone and permeability of the vascular bed, and H_2 antihistamines such as ranitidine and proton pump inhibitors such as omeprazole are useful to manage gastric acid secretion.[112] Anticholinergics may be useful in controlling diarrhea.[113] Aspirin has been used to mitigate flushing, tachycardia, and syncope. Antileukotrienes appear to demonstrate a variable response in controlling symptoms of flushing, diarrhea, and abdominal cramping.[114–117] Studies have reported that oral cromolyn at reasonably high doses decreases abdominal complaints and may be beneficial in decreasing bone pain and headaches and improving cognitive abilities.[114,118–121] Malabsorption and ascites may be relieved by the administration of glucocorticoids.[90] In the latter instance, therapeutic doses of oral glucocorticoids may be considered for 10–20 days, with a gradual taper to 15–20 mg every other day.[122,123] Patients with ascites who develop concomitant portal hypertension represent a management challenge that is associated with a poor prognosis.[124]

Cutaneous Disease

Topical glucocorticoids have been shown to be efficacious in the treatment of urticaria pigmentosa lesions, although effects are time limited. In children with bullous formation, skin management should be focused on prevention of infection and body fluid homeostasis. Bullae usually heal without scarring, although postinflammatory hyperpigmentation may result. The lesions of TMEP tend to be unresponsive to conventional therapies.[125–130] In limited studies, laser therapy has been useful in some patients.[127,129]

There is a subset of children with mastocytomas who develop systemic symptoms caused by the release of mast cell mediators. In this circumstance, surgical excision should be considered.[131,132] An alternate approach involves injection of the mastocytoma with glucocorticoids to induce involution of the lesion.[133]

Systemic Disease

Systemic Hypotension

Systemic hypotension has been seen in all categories of mastocytosis.[134–137] Acute therapy includes intramuscular epinephrine and support of hemodynamic function. Patients and care providers should be prepared to use an auto-injector (Epi-Pen/Epi-Pen Jr.) for emergent situations. Wearing a medical alert device is also recommended.

Immunomodulation

Drug Treatments

Based on in vitro studies,[138,139] response to treatment of systemic forms of mastocytosis with interferon alfa, often with glucocorticoids, is varied.[140–149] Interferon alfa-2b was not found to affect the extent of mast cell infiltration of the bone marrow,[148–150] but some patients with systemic disease respond.[151–154] The current recommendation is to restrict use of interferon alfa to patients with high mast cell burden or with severe side effects, such as collapse of vertebral bodies associated with severe osteoporosis.[154]

Case reports of the successful use of cladribine (2-chlorodeoxyadenosine), a purine nucleoside analogue, in inducing clinical remissions in patients with more aggressive forms of mastocytosis suggest continued evolution in attempts to treat this disease.[154,155]

Imatinib is a tyrosine kinase inhibitor that inhibits the kinase activity of Kit. It has been shown to suppress proliferation of an HMC-1 human mast cell line carrying the wild-type codon at 816 but not the mutated 816 codon.[156] This compound has been reported to dramatically decrease the bone marrow mast cell burden, serum tryptase level, and clinical symptoms in a patient with a novel mutation (F522C) in the transmembrane region of Kit.[18] Imatinib has been reported to result in histologic or clinical responses in 5 of 12 patients with mastocytosis.[157] Although these patients were reported to lack a codon 816 or juxtamembrane mutations, it is not clear whether they had any distinguishing histopathologic changes in their bone marrow mast cells or carried other c-*kit* mutations.

Splenectomy

Splenectomy has been used in the management of patients with aggressive systemic mastocytosis or SM-AHNMD.[158–162] Massive splenomegaly, especially if associated with hypersplenism[160] or portal hypertension, may be an indication for splenectomy. In these patients, splenectomy decreases the mast cell burden and ameliorates pancytopenia. Nevertheless, it should be considered as a high-risk surgical procedure, in part because some patients with aggressive systemic mastocytosis have impaired liver function.

SUPPORTIVE CARE AND LONG-TERM MANAGEMENT

Counseling of Patients and Providers

Complete information about mastocytosis, including guidelines for avoidance of triggering factors (Table 52–5) and risks associated with systemic hypotension, should be given to the patients and/or their parents (in cases of affected children). Information given to doctors and other care providers may additionally include information on premedication for general anesthesia and on radiographic studies with contrast media, and on avoidance and treatment of hymenoptera sting anaphylaxis in patients at risk.

General Anesthesia and Mastocytosis

It is known that some drugs used in general anesthesia may induce mast cell mediator release.[163–165] The exact

TABLE 52–5. Possible Physical Stimuli and Pharmacologic Agents That May Trigger Mast Cell Mediator Release

Immunologic Stimuli
Venoms (immunoglobulin E–mediated bee, snake venom)*
Polymers (dextran, gelatin)
Complement-derived anaphylatoxins
Biologic peptides (substance P, somatostatin)
Nonimmunologic Stimuli
Physical stimuli (heat, cold, friction, sunlight)
Drugs: aspirin and other NSAIDS,†,‡ thiamine, alcohol, narcotics,† polymixin B, radiographic dyes, and some drugs used in general anesthesia (inductors and muscle relaxants)
Emotional factors
Stress, anxiety
Miscellaneous§

*Venom immunotherapy has been used safely and successfully in selected patients with mastocytosis and venom sensitivity.[130]

†Patient responses vary; these factors appear to be a problem is less than 10% of patients.

‡Aspirin and other nonsteroidal anti-inflammatory drugs (NSAIDs) may induce mast cell degranulation in some patients and may be safely used at therapeutic doses in other patients.

§Triggers such as foods, environmental allergens, and other factors that are inciting agents in specific individuals should be avoided.

Data from Longley and colleagues,[14] Lerno and colleagues,[174] Metcalfe,[185] Goins,[190] Stellato and colleagues,[191] Oude Elberink and colleagues,[192] Peachell and Morcos,[194] Alto and Clarcq,[195] and Teuber and Vogt.[196]

CURRENT CONTROVERSIES & FUTURE CONSIDERATIONS

Mastocytosis

- There are well-documented cases of adverse reactions to anesthetics, hymenoptera venom, radiocontrast dyes, and analgesics. However, the majority of patients with mastocytosis have not had major events relating to these categories.
- The approach to patients with mastocytosis should be with the utmost caution and preparedness for emergent situations.
- There is no specific treatment modality that is curative for mastocytosis. Targeting of the constitutive kinase activity of mutated Kit in systemic mastocytosis has attracted more attention, as low-molecular-weight inhibitors of signal transduction become available for clinical use. Targeting Kit may also be of value when larger studies are conducted with imatinib.
- Bone marrow transplantation may be promising in patients with severe disease and specific subtypes.

incidence of complications in general anesthesia in mastocytosis patients is not known, and there appears to be a great variability in patient response. Despite this, general anesthesia is generally considered to be a procedure with higher risk of adverse events in patients with mastocytosis. Severe reactions, including systemic hypotension, anaphylactoid reactions, and coagulopathy, even resulting in death, have been reported.[163–173] This is particularly important in patients with a history of allergic or adverse reactions and known sensitivities, such as those with a history of adverse reactions to general anesthesia.[174–181] Samples to determine serum tryptase levels[182,183] may be obtained and blood coagulation parameters should be monitored preoperatively and during anesthesia if suspected mast cell degranulation events occur. The primary objective in the treatment of all clinical forms of mastocytosis is to prevent release of mast cell mediators and to block their effects to control the symptoms and signs of the disease.[14,63,181,184–189]

PROGNOSIS

Cutaneous mastocytomas in children usually disappear with time. Patients with more benign or indolent forms of adult-onset disease may live relatively normal lives with proper medical control of their symptoms. Other patients have aggressive forms of mastocytosis and a much less optimistic prognosis. Among patients with adult-onset mastocytosis, the best prognosis is achieved by those with indolent systemic mastocytosis. Rarely does this form progress to a more severe pattern, such as SM-AHNMD or aggressive systemic mastocytosis. Prognosis of SM-AHNMD depends on the prognosis of the associated hematologic non–mast cell disease. In aggressive systemic mastocytosis, the life expectancy is usually a few years. Mast cell leukemia and mast cell sarcoma have the worst prognosis, with average life expectancies of 6–12 months.

Suggested Readings*

Akin C, Kirshenbaum AS, Semere T, et al: Analysis of the surface expression of c-*kit* and occurrence of the c-*kit* Asp816Val activating mutation in T cells, B cells, and myelomonocytic cells in patients with mastocytosis. Exp Hematol 28:140–147, 2000.

Carter MC, Metcalfe DD: Paediatric mastocytosis. Arch Dis Child 86:315–319, 2002.

Valent P, Akin C, Sperr WR, et al: Diagnosis and treatment of systemic mastocytosis: state of the art. Br J Haematol 122:695–717, 2003.

Valent P, Akin C, Sperr WR, et al: Mast cell proliferative disorders: current view on variants recognized by the World Health Organization. Hematol Oncol Clin North Am 17:1227–1241, 2003.

Worobec A: Treatment of systemic mast cell disorders. Hematol Oncol Clin North Am 14:659–687, 2000.

Full references for this chapter can be found on accompanying CD-ROM.

CHAPTER 53

DISEASES OF THE SPLEEN

Alan Lichtin, MD, and James R. Cook, MD, PhD

KEY POINTS

Diseases of the Spleen

Diagnosis

- A myriad of disorders can present with problems related to the spleen, reflecting either hypersplenism or hyposplenism.
- One must have a fundamental understanding of the histology and function of white pulp and red pulp.
- One can determine the level of function of the spleen by analyzing the peripheral blood smear, particularly with attention to Howell-Jolly bodies or circulating malignant cells (especially in lymphoma cases).
- Increasing use of laparoscopic splenectomy has made certain diagnoses more difficult for pathologists.

Treatment

- The treatment of any disorder related to spleen over- or underactivity depends upon the underlying disorder.
- When the spleen is a site of infection, antibiotics or antifungals can clear splenic infections.
- Splenic artery embolization can accomplish the same outcome as a splenectomy in selected cases.
- In certain lymphomas, splenectomy may be the only treatment necessary for durable remission to occur.
- The convalescence after a laparoscopic splenectomy is usually much shorter and easier for the patient, compared to the more traditional open splenectomy.

INTRODUCTION

Before approaching the diseases of the spleen, one must first understand the anatomy and function of the normal spleen. There are several excellent textbooks about the spleen, and a deeper explanation of issues related to the spleen may be found in them.[1,2,2a]

The spleen resides in the left upper quadrant and is fed by the splenic artery. Splenic venous outflow is into the portal circulation. The splenic vein courses just posterior to the pancreas. Approximately 10% of individuals possess smaller, accessory spleens. Additional nodules of splenic tissue may also grow as implants on serosal surfaces following traumatic rupture, a process known as splenosis.

Embryologically, the spleen arises entirely from mesoderm. In the fifth week of gestation, there is a condensation of mesenchymal cells in the dorsal wall of the abdomen. In the fourth month of fetal life, lymphocytes appear. B cells predominate throughout fetal life and are present by the 13th week. The red and white pulp are apparent after the 24th week. In fetal life, the spleen is a site of hematopoiesis, along with the liver. Hematopoiesis in the spleen peaks at around the 18th week, at which time the bone marrow begins to take over that role.[3]

Anatomy

The normal spleen is covered by a thin, fibrous capsule. Because of the relatively delicate nature of this capsule, traumatic rupture of the spleen is more common than rupture of other abdominal organs. Similarly, needle biopsy of the spleen is more hazardous than biopsy of other intra-abdominal organs, such as the liver, which is encased within a thicker capsule.

The splenic artery courses into the spleen through the hilum and divides into branches that pierce into the substance of the spleen. The largest of these arterial branches are called central arteries, and the more distal ones are known as trabecular arteries. The trabecular arteries compartmentalize the spleen into sinus units. Trabecular arteries also branch off from the internal surface of the splenic capsule. These central and trabecular arteries feed into areas called the white pulp.

White Pulp

Surrounding the central and trabecular arteries are cylindrical areas of lymphocytes, predominately T lymphocytes, with some macrophages and plasma cells. Especially around the central arteries, these areas are called the periarterial lymphoid sheath. Because of the large number of lymphocytes present, these regions appear grossly as white nodules on the cut surface of the spleen, giving rise to the term *white pulp* (Fig. 53–1).

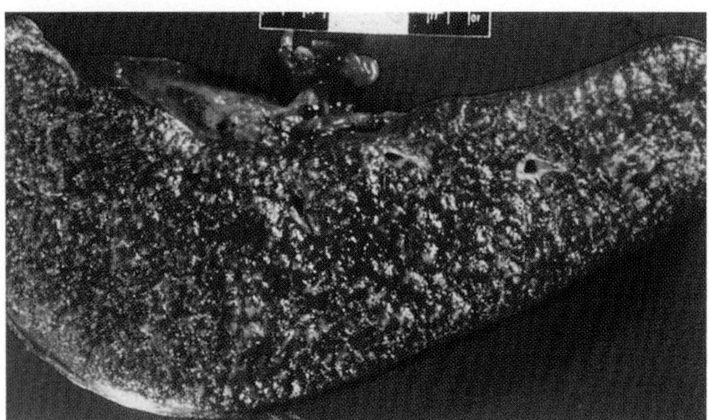

Figure 53–1. Gross appearance of the spleen. The white pulp appears as punctate, pale white areas on the cut surface of the spleen, and the red pulp appears as a homogeneous maroon color. The white pulp is somewhat prominent in this spleen, removed from a patient with rheumatoid arthritis.

Arising within this lymphoid sheath are lymphoid follicles, which are predominantly composed of B cells. Primary follicles consist of small lymphocytes with scant cytoplasm. Because antigens are presented into the spleen, the white pulp can expand and the follicles can develop distinct zones of lymphocytes (Figs. 53–2*A* and 53–3*A*). Some follicles will develop a pale, central area known as the germinal center, which is the site of B-cell antigen recognition. The germinal center is surrounded by a dark rim of predominantly small lymphocytes, mostly B cells, called the mantle zone. Between the mantle zone and the red pulp, a pale rim of lymphocytes known as the marginal zone is present. Marginal zones may also be observed around some primary follicles. The marginal zone is where the arterial supply begins to terminate and is believed to be the initial location for antigens to be trapped and processed.

Red Pulp

The red pulp of the spleen is a unique bed of vascular sinuses separated by splenic cords, known as the cords of Billroth (Figs. 53–2*B* and 53–3*B*). These sinuses are the terminal sites of arterial flow, beyond the white pulp (penicilliary arterioles). These vascular sinuses are where blood is filtered. The cells lining the sinus walls are elongated endothelial cells and are not bound to each other by tight junctions. There is no continuous basement membrane. Rather, there is a discontinuous grid of basement membrane that encircles the sinus, called ring fibers. Macrophages reside outside of these sinuses and cytoplasmic projections from macrophages surround the sinus. The ring fibers are anchored in position by the dendritic processes of these macrophages.

There are two routes that arterial blood can take on the way to splenic venules and then veins: an "open" system and a "closed" system. The open system drains slowly, whereas the closed system is more rapid. The open, or slow, system is where the gradual filtration of blood occurs. In the closed system, there is direct passage of blood from arteriole to capillary to a venule and then a vein. More of the blood pursues the closed route compared to the open circuit. Even so, during a typical day, the entire blood volume does traverse the filtration beds of the splenic cords, where it is exposed to the phagocytic macrophages so closely aligned to the cords. This is where blood is filtered and where senescent red blood cells (RBCs) are destroyed. It is also where damaged RBCs are culled from the circulation. RBCs are forced to undergo extreme deformation as they pass through the splenic cords into the sinusoids. When red cells are more rigid, as in cytoskeletal disorders (e.g., hereditary splenocytosis), they are unable to traverse these sinuses without being trapped and phagocytized by macrophages. The splenic macrophages also "pit" the red cells, during which inclusions such as Heinz bodies (e.g., as seen in unstable hemoglobin disorders, or in enzymopathies such as glucose-6-phosphate dehydrogenase deficiency) are excised without leading to the destruction of the red cell. The macrophages also remove particulate matter from the circulation, including bacteria and abnormal macromolecules produced in some metabolic disorders, such as lysosomal storage diseases (e.g., Gaucher's disease).

Roles of the Spleen

There are four major roles of the spleen: filtration, immunologic, storage, and hematopoietic.

Filtration

The filtration role is subdivided into (1) culling; (2) pitting; (3) erythroclasis (a term indicating destruction of red cells into fragments); and (4) bacterial or particulate removal. Culling may be physiologic or pathologic. The normal spleen destroys senescent RBCs, which is a physiologic, normal process. However, if red cells are abnormally rigid, as in hereditary splenocytosis, then the red cells are culled because of this pathologic condition. When such a pathologic condition occurs, one may also find other cytopenias. Pitting involves the removal of small intracellular inclusions, such as nuclear material (Howell-Jolly bodies, as are seen in the peripheral smear of asplenic patients) or denatured hemoglobin (Heinz bodies). *Erythroclasis* is an older term for the splitting of red cells into fragments that return to the circulation. These fragmented red cells are cleared during subsequent passage through the spleen. This may be seen in autoimmune hemolysis, thalassemias, and hemoglobinopathies, especially sickle cell disease. The spleen may directly filter or remove bacteria from the circulation. This filtration role of the spleen coincides with its immunologic role (see the next section).

Immunologic

The lymphoid part of the spleen, mostly white pulp, traps and processes antigens. Once these antigens are trapped and processed, cytokines and antibodies are formed and then released into the venous blood and enter the portal circulation.

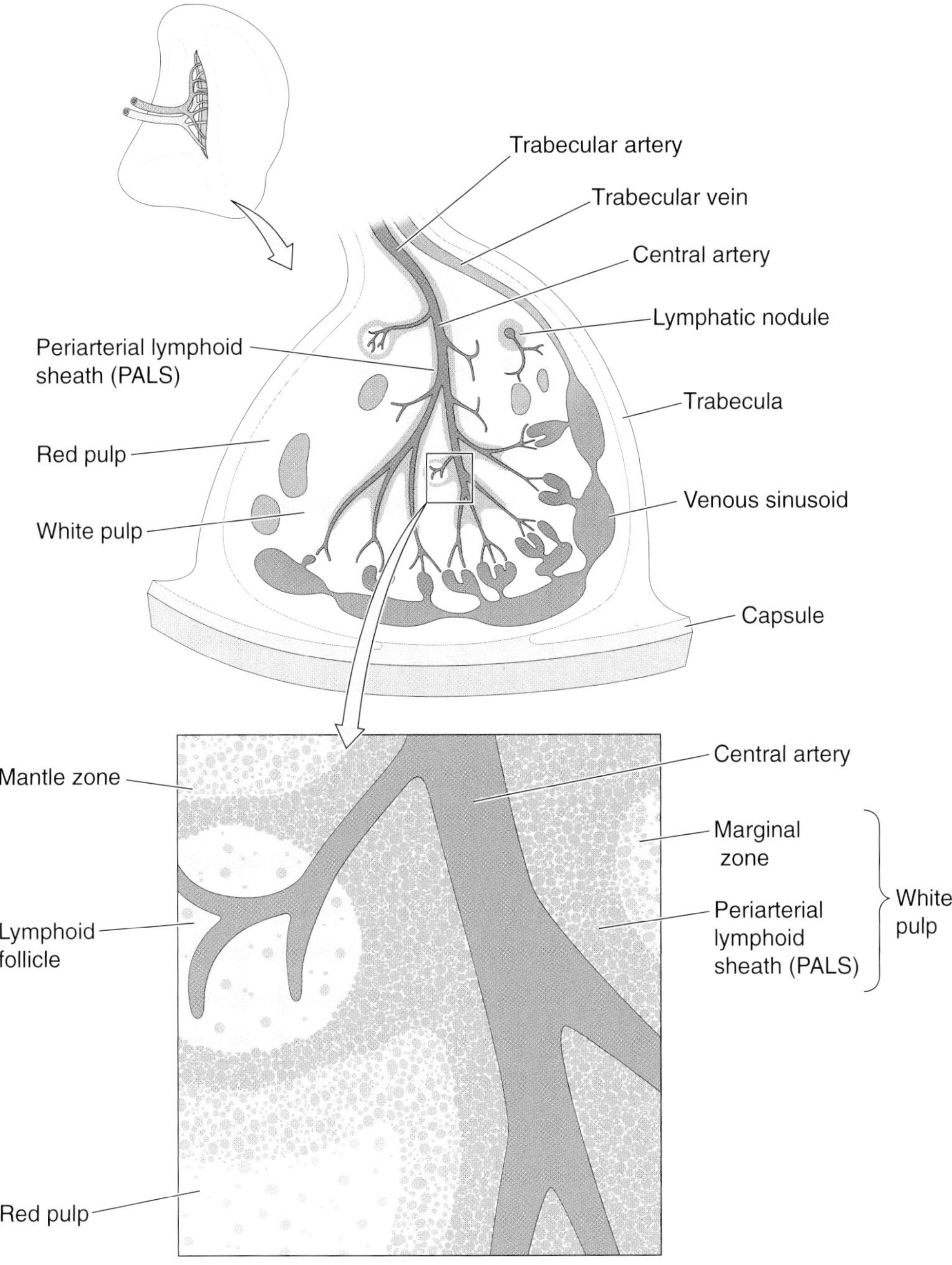

Figure 53–2. Schematic diagrams of normal red pulp *(A)* and white pulp *(B)*. *Figure continued on following page*

Only 1% of splenectomized patients are prone to fulminant sepsis with encapsulated organisms, predominantly *Streptococcus pneumoniae*.[4] Why this percentage is so low is puzzling, but must relate to the fact that there is redundancy within the lymphoid system. Splenectomized people do have slightly lower antigen-specific immunoglobulin M production and a marginal drop in immunoglobulin G levels.

Lymphocytes are also transformed and proliferate in response to antigens. White pulp expansion can occur during viral infections, particularly with Epstein-Barr virus, and in autoimmune disorders, especially rheumatoid arthritis. Indeed, splenomegaly is a hallmark of Felty's syndrome (triad of neutropenia, splenomegaly, and rheumatoid arthritis).

Storage

In dogs, the spleen can be a storage site for red cells. The fibrous capsule of the spleen in the dog can contract and, during hypovolemic shock, this reservoir of red cells helps to reconstitute the blood volume. However, in humans, the spleen only holds 20–40 mL of red cells. In contrast to erythrocytes, however, the red pulp of the human spleen holds about one third of the body platelet mass. A large number of granulocytes are also held within the spleen. When the spleen enlarges, the red pulp cords widen and there is prolonged exposure of all cells to the hostile environment within the red pulp. This leads to a greater degree of macrophage phagocytosis and cell counts drop.

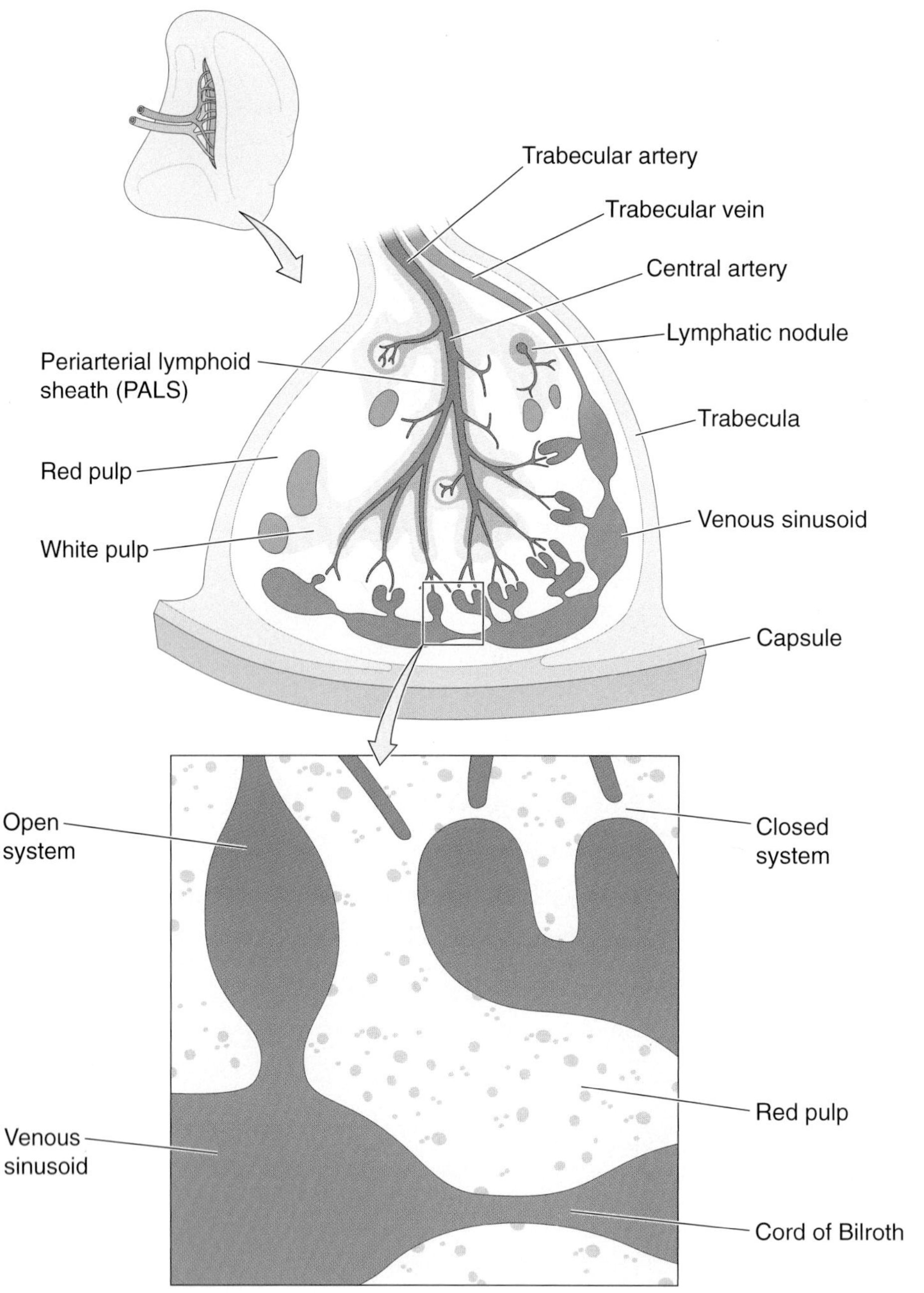

■ **Figure 53–2, cont'd**

Hematopoietic

The ability of the spleen to mimic marrow function is what constitutes its hematopoietic function. The most remarkable setting for this is in patients with myelofibrosis, for whom splenomegaly can become massive. Extramedullary hematopoiesis is seen histologically in these spleens (Fig. 53–4).

EPIDEMIOLOGY AND RISK FACTORS

These terms are not entirely conducive to a review of diseases of the spleen. However, one should be aware that enlargement of the spleen to the point of being palpable on physical examination occurs in 3% of the normal population.

Congenital absence of the spleen is very rare, and occurs in conjunction with cardiovascular and pulmonary anomalies or in infants with situs inversus. Congenital hypoplasia of the spleen is seen in patients with Fanconi's anemia. A sign of hypofunction of the spleen is the presence of Howell-Jolly bodies on the peripheral smear. When RBCs enter the red pulp, they are "pitted," as mentioned earlier. During this process, inclusions are removed from the red cells. These inclusions include remnants of nuclear material (Howell-Jolly bodies), denatured hemoglobin (Heinz bodies), intracellular parasites such as malaria, or siderotic granules

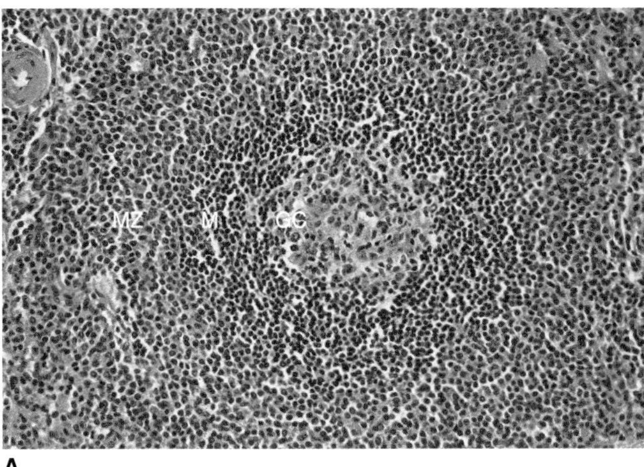

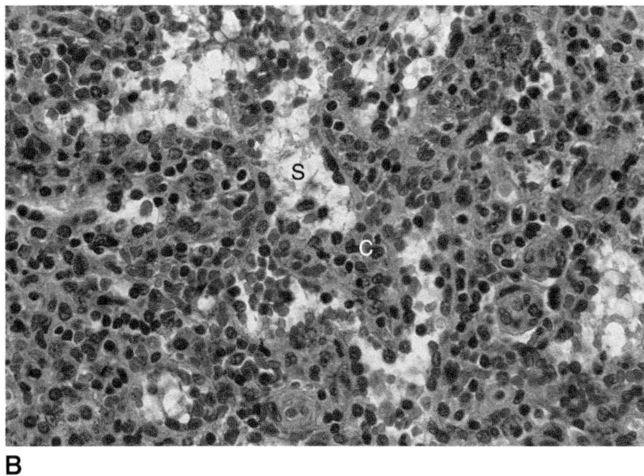

Figure 53–3. *A,* Normal white pulp nodule. A central germinal center (GC) is present, surrounded by a rim of small, darkly staining lymphocytes known as the mantle zone (M) and an outer, pale-staining rim of lymphocytes known as the marginal zone (MZ). ***B,*** Normal red pulp. The red pulp consists of the splenic sinus (S), containing numerous red cells and other peripheral blood elements, separated by cords (C) containing histiocytes, stromal cells, and lymphocytes.

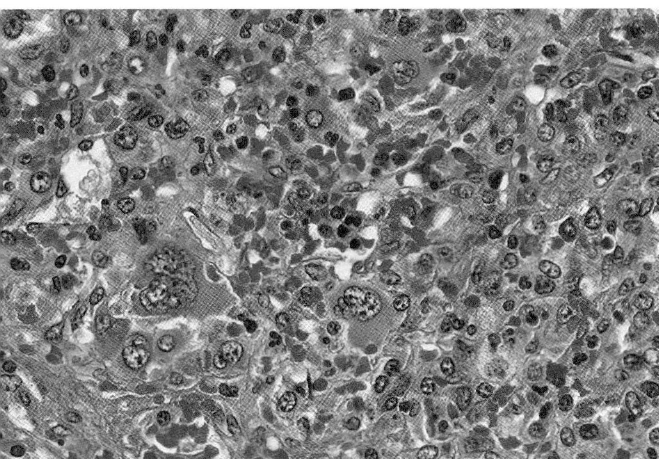

Figure 53–4. Extramedullary hematopoiesis within the spleen. This spleen, removed from a patient with long-standing myelofibrosis, weighed over 10 pounds and demonstrated extensive extramedullary hematopoiesis.

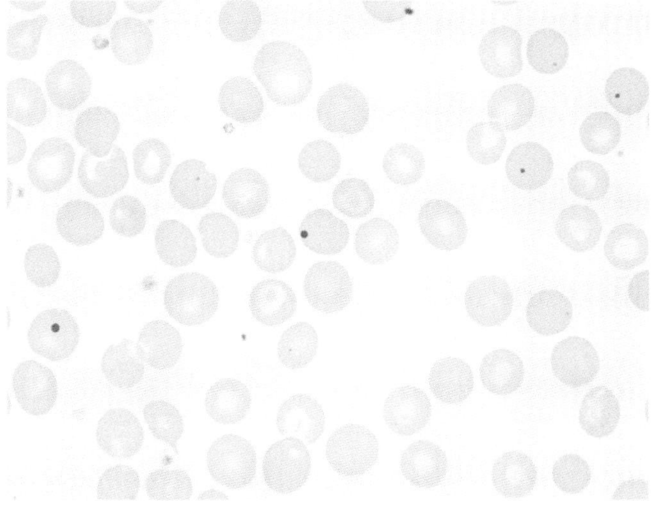

Figure 53–5. Peripheral smear findings indicative of hyposplenism. Numerous Howell-Jolly bodies are present, and there is poikilocytosis with target cells. (Wright-Giemsa stain.)

(Pappenheimer bodies). Newborns may have Howell-Jolly bodies because of the relative immaturity of the red pulp.

Traumatic rupture of the spleen occurs when there is enough blunt trauma to induce a tear in the splenic capsule. This clinical scenario occurs more frequently in individuals who have this risk, such as those involved with contact sports or those having vehicular accidents, and tends to occur more frequently in individuals whose spleen is enlarged, as in infectious mononucleosis. Individuals with underlying splenomegaly, especially secondary to infectious mononucleosis, have a higher risk for splenic rupture. Splenic rupture has been rarely observed in patients receiving granulocyte colony-stimulating factor and in patients with chronic myelogenous leukemia receiving imatinib mesylate.

PATHOPHYSIOLOGY

Problems with the spleen can be divided into those conditions in which the spleen does not function well enough (hyposplenism) and those in which the spleen is too functional (hypersplenism). If the spleen enlarges, it can either be hypofunctioning or hyperfunctioning. Generally, if the spleen shrinks, it becomes hypofunctional.

Individuals who have hyposplenism or asplenia (congenital or postsplenectomy) have Howell-Jolly bodies and Pappenheimer bodies on peripheral smear. There is also poikilocytosis with target cells and acanthocytes (Fig. 53–5). All of these latter cells reflect the loss of spleen function of removing deformed RBCs. Most normal individuals develop a slight granulocytosis and thrombocytosis after splenectomy, but, curiously, they do not

TABLE 53–1. Conditions Associated with Hyposplenism

Congenital

Hypoplasia

Fanconi's anemia
Immunodeficiencies
  Bruton's disease
  Severe combined immunodeficiency
  Immunoglobulin A deficiency
  DiGeorge syndrome
  Agammaglobulinemia

Asplenia

Acquired

Illnesses in Which the Spleen Becomes Atrophic

Sickle cell anemia
Subacute bacterial endocarditis
Embolic disease
Celiac disease[5]
Other malabsorption states
Radiation exposure/chemotherapy
Systemic lupus erythematosus
Other autoimmune disorders
Human immunodeficiency virus infection
Pernicious anemia

Surgical Removal of the Spleen

Enlarged but Hypofunctional Spleen

Myeloproliferative disorders
  Polycythemia vera
  Essential thrombocythemia
  Chronic idiopathic myelofibrosis
Infiltrating diseases
  Amyloidosis
  Leukemias
  Lymphomas
  Multiple myeloma
  Sarcoidosis
Malabsorption
Infectious mononucleosis
Miliary tuberculosis

become polycythemic. Table 53–1 presents a list of hyposplenic conditions.

Table 53–2 lists those disorders for which the spleen becomes overactive (hypersplenism). These individuals tend to have anemia, neutropenia, or thrombocytopenia, yet lack the red cell changes of hyposplenism (i.e., no Howell-Jolly or Pappenheimer bodies). It should be noted that some disorders, such as autoimmune diseases, appear on both the hyposplenism list and the hypersplenism list. This is because, in some individuals, there is more of an effect on spleen function, usually early in the onset of the disease, leading to Howell-Jolly bodies. Over time, there might be such an expansion of the lymphoid compartments within the white pulp that hypersplenism becomes predominant and causes cytopenias to occur.

CLINICAL FEATURES AND DIAGNOSIS

Clinical Features of Splenic Disease

Palpable splenomegaly, especially progressive, usually denotes some abnormality within the spleen. Most

TABLE 53–2. Conditions Associated with Hypersplenism

Liver disease, especially cirrhosis
Portal vein thrombus
Splenic vein thrombus
Autoimmune diseases
Granulomatous disease
Lysosomal storage diseases
  Gaucher's disease
  Niemann-Pick disease
Myeloproliferative disorders
Hemoglobinopathies
  Sickle cell disease variants, e.g., Sickle-C
Thalassemias
Lymphomas
Leukemias
  Chronic lymphocytic leukemia
  Hairy cell leukemia
  Lymphoplasmacytic lymphoma/Waldenström's macroglobulinemia

patients have no pain from this, but those with myeloproliferative disorders often have discomfort. This might be from small infarctions over time or it might be secondary to capsular distention. Patients with splenomegaly often complain of early satiety. As food enters the stomach and distends it, the stomach abuts against the enlarged spleen and the sensation of hunger is aborted.

Cirrhotic patients have many stigmata of this condition, and their palmar erythema, spider telangiectasias, asterixis, jaundice, and susceptibility to infection overshadow the splenomegaly symptomatically. The cytopenias associated with cirrhosis and hypersplenism contribute to the morbidity of this condition. Especially prominent is thrombocytopenia, because these patients already have a coagulopathy with underproduction of clotting factors (except factor VIII). Once they start bleeding, as when an esophageal varix ruptures, lack of an adequate platelet count contributes to bleeding.

The clinical presentation of splenic disease is dependent upon the underlying disease. Patients with acute leukemia usually come to medical attention because of problems with their blood counts, as opposed to a problem with the spleen. Tuberculosis or human immunodeficiency virus patients will have night sweats and weight loss before a complaint referable to the spleen is registered.

Infarction of the Spleen

Several conditions may cause part of the spleen to have inadequate oxygen delivery, leading to a splenic infarct. The larger the spleen becomes in a patient with a myeloproliferative disorder, the greater tendency for infarction. These are usually distal within the spleen, causing a wedge-shaped area of underperfusion, commonly approaching the splenic capsule. Pain in the left upper quadrant and fever are common presenting features. This tendency to infarction is less common in the large spleens of lymphoma or acute leukemia patients.

Embolic events to the spleen, such as those seen in infective endocarditis, atheroemboli, or from left atrial clots (as seen in atrial fibrillation) can also cause wedge-shaped infarctions with pain in the left upper quadrant.

Individuals with hemoglobinopathies, particularly homozygous sickle cell anemia, can have chronic, small infarctions leading to a shrunken nubbin of a spleen—the so-called autoinfarction. Individuals with sickle cell trait may develop massive spleen infarction if they engage in severe exertional exercise (military recruits undergoing arduous training exercises, or marathon runners) or if they are placed in sudden decompression in an airplane.

Infections of the Spleen

A septic embolus from a valve affected by endocarditis can cause a splenic abscess. Bacteremia itself can lead to focal deposits of bacterial infection in the spleen, but this is not typical. Usually some anatomic defect, such as a prior infarct, may become secondarily infected.

Fungal diseases can target the spleen. Severely immunocompromised, heavily treated chemotherapy patients, such as acute leukemia patients in their nadir, can develop hepatosplenic candidiasis. Hallmark features of this condition include elevated alkaline phosphatase levels, shaking chills, and high fevers. Long-term use of antifungals and a return of polymorphonuclear leukocyte counts can clear this life-threatening infection. Disseminated histoplasmosis can affect the spleen either in a diffuse or a nodular fashion. Many otherwise healthy individuals have calcified nodules in their spleens, seen on computed tomography scans, that are sequelae of previous fungal illness.

The classic viral infection that causes splenomegaly and expansion of the white pulp is infectious mononucleosis. Malarial infection is a common cause of splenomegaly in malaria-prone regions.

Diagnosis of Splenic Disease

Besides abnormalities on physical examination, much information can be derived regarding splenic function by obtaining a complete blood count and reviewing the peripheral smear. Careful review of red cell morphology, looking for Howell-Jolly bodies, is essential for diagnosing conditions of hyposplenism.

Radiographic imaging of the spleen is very helpful. In obese subjects, feeling the spleen size is difficult. Even in thin individuals, it is difficult to be certain of spleen size in those with strong abdominal wall musculature. Ultrasound can help determine spleen size and whether there are cysts in the spleen. Computed tomography is a standard method for determining spleen size. Often, in cases of portal hypertension or in portal or splenic vein thrombosis, the radiologist can indicate these findings. The nuclear medicine liver-spleen scan with single-photon emission tomography imaging can corroborate the computed tomography findings if secondary hypersplenism is occurring.[6]

Flow-cytometric analysis of the peripheral blood can be useful in documenting the presence of leukemia or lymphoma. However, lymphomas can be present in

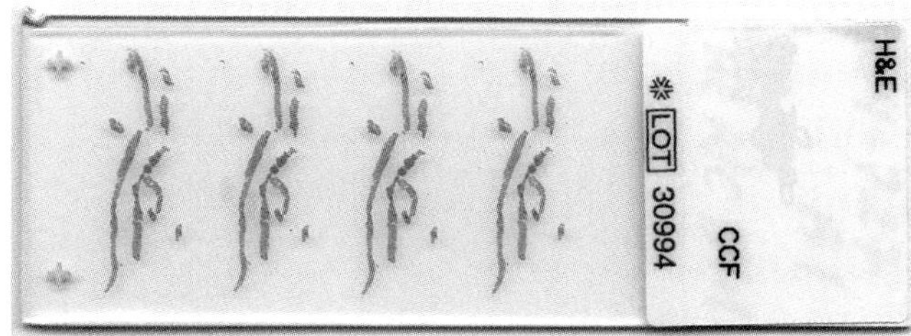

A

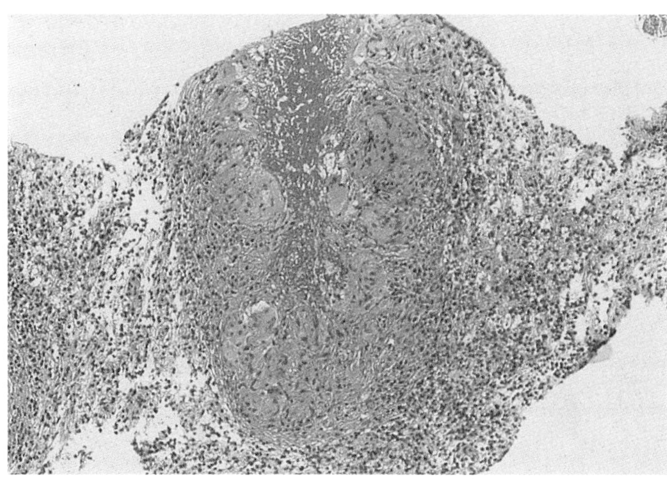

B

Figure 53–6. *A*, Needle biopsy of the spleen in a patient with confluent splenic masses. ***B***, Extensive granulomatous inflammation was present, consistent with mycobacterial disease.

spleen and marrow without detectable circulating malignant lymphocytes. In such settings, an examination of the bone marrow may be helpful. Finding marrow involvement by non-Hodgkin's lymphoma or, more rarely, involvement by Hodgkin's disease may eliminate the need for splenectomy. Some interventional radiologists can perform needle biopsies of the spleen (Fig. 53–6), but this can lead to hemorrhage and emergent splenectomy. Ultimately, especially in some splenic-based lymphomas such as splenic lymphoma with villous lymphocytes, one must perform a splenectomy to make a definitive diagnosis (Fig. 53–7).

DIFFERENTIAL DIAGNOSIS

Figure 53–8 presents the differential diagnosis of splenomegaly.

TREATMENT

The treatment of hypo- or hypersplenism will depend upon the underlying cause. Infections need appropriate antibiotics. Cancers need proper chemotherapy. Symptomatic Gaucher's disease patients need enzyme replacement therapy. Autoimmune diseases need their immune-modifying agents.

There are some conditions for which splenectomy plays a therapeutic role. For example, historically, hairy

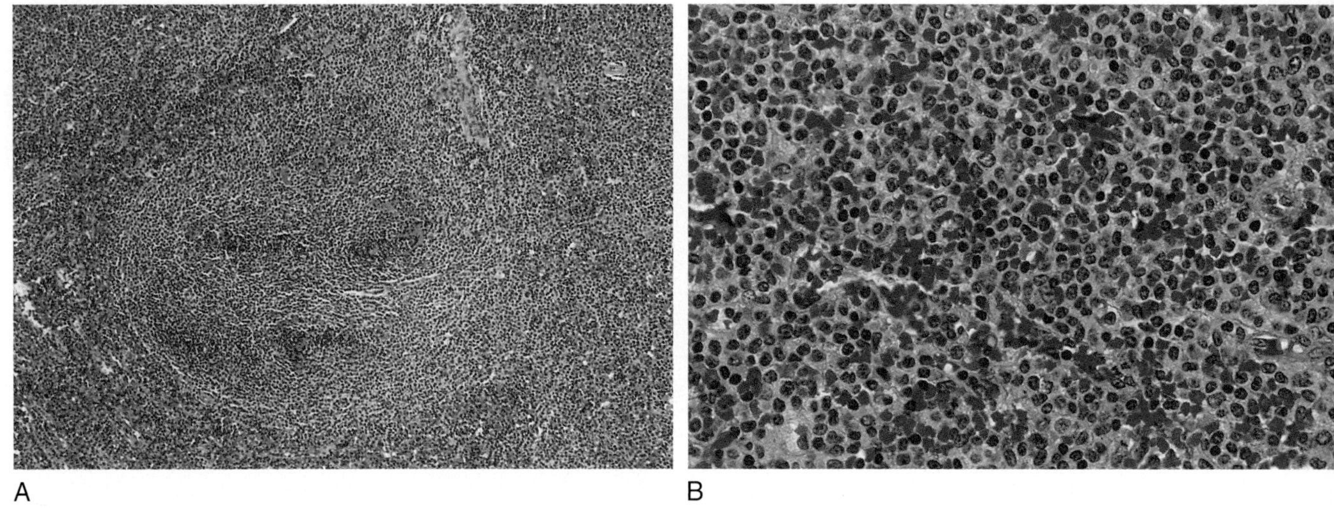

Figure 53–7. Splenectomy may be required for definitive diagnosis of splenic leukemias and lymphomas. ***A,*** Expanded white pulp nodule in a case of splenic marginal zone lymphoma. ***B,*** Extensive red pulp infiltrate in a case of hairy cell leukemia. In each case, peripheral blood flow cytometry identified neoplastic B cells, but a specific diagnosis could not be established until splenectomy was performed, allowing for assessment of the growth pattern within the spleen.

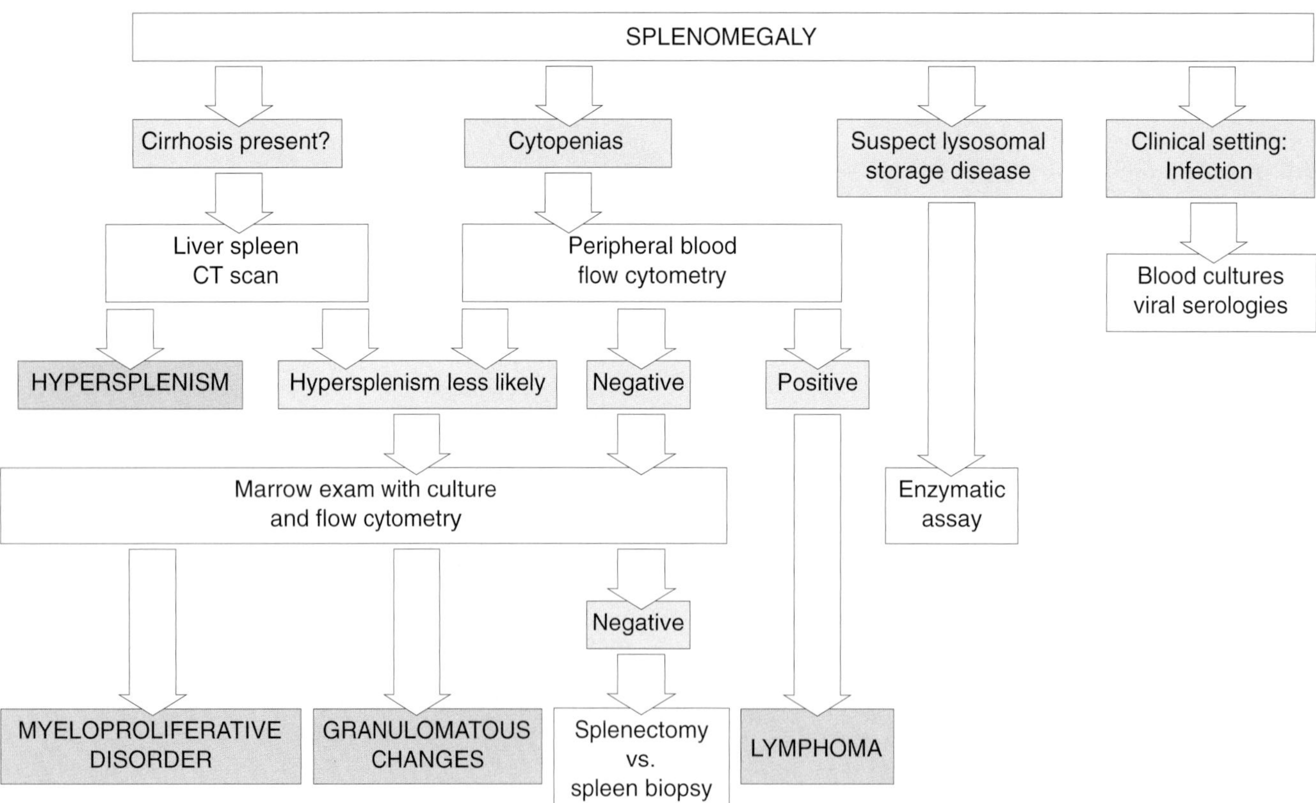

Figure 53–8. Differential diagnosis of splenomegaly.

cell leukemia was treated with splenectomy. The marrow neoplasia persisted, but blood counts would often normalize for years, even decades. Sixty percent of patients with steroid-refractory immune thrombocytopenic purpura and about half the patients with autoimmune hemolysis benefit from splenectomy and can maintain normal platelet or RBC counts for the duration of their lives. Individuals with RBC cytoskeletal defects such as hereditary spherocytosis benefit from splenectomy. Jaundice improves, hemoglobin rises, and patients feel better because the red cell survival increases by removing the red pulp macrophages. Painful splenomegaly in myeloproliferative disorders, especially chronic myeloid leukemia, and myelodysplasia, can be ameliorated with low doses of radiation therapy to the spleen, or with splenectomy.

Unfortunately, for cirrhotic patients who have portal hypertension with cytopenias, there are limited options. Splenectomy does benefit some of these patients, but surgeons often do not want to subject these patients to the bleeding risks. Also, among patients who are candidates for liver transplantation, the splenectomized patients tend to clot off the portal vein, which interferes with a successful transplantation. Platelet transfusions do not predictably raise the platelet count, even transiently, secondary to overactive macrophage clearing in the enlarged spleen. Transjugular intrahepatic portosystemic shunt placement and distal splenorenal shunting may improve platelet counts.

Other, less utilized treatments for splenomegaly are dearterilization[7] or embolization, either using coils or gel foam.[8] This tends to be very painful, but may have a role for an individual who is not a surgical candidate. Some surgeons have explored partial splenectomy as a way to preserve some degree of spleen function while removing the bulk of the spleen.

There is a 1% risk of fulminant pneumococcal (or other encapsulated bacteria) sepsis for individuals who have a splenectomy. This is more common if the splenectomy occurs in the childhood years. Presplenectomy immunization for pneumococcus, *Haemophilus influenzae*, and meningococcus may reduce this risk. Persons who have had a splenectomy should seek immediate medical attention if they feel suddenly, dramatically ill. Initiating early antibiotics after obtaining appropriate cultures can be life-saving for a septic splenectomized patient.

SUPPORTIVE CARE AND LONG-TERM MANAGEMENT

As with treatment, the underlying disease will dictate supportive care and long-term management. Splenomegaly that is associated with an underlying infection will recede with the eradication of the infection. Splenomegaly associated with a myeloproliferative disorder for which curative treatments are available, such as chronic myeloid leukemia (after allogeneic bone marrow transplantation) will resolve the spleen enlargement. Sometimes there is splenic hypofunction after allogeneic bone marrow transplantation.[9] However, for patients with polycythemia vera who enter the spent phase or patients with progressive myelofibrosis, the outlook for resolution of the splenomegaly is bleak. As these patients endure the progressive worsening of these states, the splenomegaly can be a major source of morbidity. Splenectomy can temporarily help, but perioperative morbidity (infections, clotting or bleeding) and mortality are high. Radiation therapy, in low doses, does provide palliative relief for painful splenomegaly in this setting.[10]

CURRENT CONTROVERSIES & FUTURE CONSIDERATIONS

Diseases of the Spleen

- Percutaneous biopsy of splenic lesions can be done; however the risks are greater than with other organs. The skill of the person performing the biopsy should be kept in mind by a physician ordering the biopsy.
- The appropriate management of a cirrhotic patient with hypersplenism who has thrombocytopenia and requires surgery is difficult. Whether there may be a role for hemostatic agents such as recombinant factor VII is unresolved in this setting.
- The patient who has hypersplenism and is bleeding from thrombocytopenia presents a challenge. Platelet transfusions tend to be ineffective to maintain a durable rise in platelet count. Surgeons typically do not like to perform splenectomies in this setting because of the bleeding risk and because of high portal pressures.
- For patients with congenital membrane cytoskeletal disorders, the timing of splenectomy is controversial. If severe anemia occurs with the need for transfusion on a frequent basis, splenectomy is certainly indicated.

Suggested Readings*

Boulder AJ: The Spleen. London: Chapman & Hall, 1990.
Wilkens BS: The spleen. Br J Haematol 117:265, 2002.
Wolf BC, Neiman RS: Disorders of the Spleen. Philadelphia: WB Saunders, 1989.

Full references for this chapter can be found on accompanying CD-ROM.

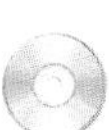

SECTION 4
INHERITED AND ACQUIRED METABOLIC BLOOD DISEASES

CHAPTER 54
PORPHYRIAS

Shigeru Sassa, MD, PhD

KEY POINTS

Porphyrias

Diagnosis

- Porphyrias are due to deficiencies of enzymes in the heme biosynthetic pathway. In most cases the enzymatic deficiency is inherited, but some cases also occur as acquired deficiencies.
- Porphyrias can be classified either as (1) erythropoietic porphyrias, such as congenital erythropoietic porphyria (CEP), hepatoerythropoietic porphyria, and erythropoietic protoporphyria; (2) acute hepatic porphyrias, such as δ-aminolevulinate dehydratase (ALAD) porphyria, acute intermittent porphyria (AIP), hereditary coproporphyria, and variegate porphyria; or (3) chronic hepatic porphyria, such as porphyria cutanea tarda (PCT).
- Both erythropoietic protoporphyria and chronic hepatic porphyria present with cutaneous photosensitivity, but they are not associated with neurologic symptoms. In contrast, acute hepatic porphyrias are characterized by neurologic symptoms. Some of them (e.g., hereditary coproporphyria and variegate porphyria) may additionally have skin photosensitivity.
- All of the heme pathway intermediates are potentially toxic. Their overproduction causes the characteristic neurovisceral and/or photosensitizing symptoms.
- Solubility determines the excretion pattern of the metabolites. Water-soluble precursors and porphyrins are excreted mainly in the urine (δ-aminolevulinic acid [ALA], porphobilinogen, and uroporphyrin), lipid-soluble protoporphyrin is excreted mainly in the feces, and coproporphyrin, which has intermediate solubility, is excreted in both.
- Porphyrins produce free radicals when exposed to ultraviolet light (~400 nm). As a result, skin damage ensues in the light-exposed areas.
- Porphyrin precursors (e.g., ALA and porphobilinogen) are associated with neurologic symptoms of acute hepatic porphyrias, though the pathogenetic mechanism remains unclear.
- During an acute attack of acute hepatic porphyria, δ-aminolevulinate synthase 1 (ALAS1), the hepatic isoform of the first enzyme in the heme biosynthetic pathway, is induced. ALAS1 formation in normal hepatocytes is repressed by feedback inhibition by the final product, heme. Supplementation of heme by intravenous infusion can correct the metabolic defect in acute hepatic porphyrias.
- There is significant interaction between the primary gene defect in the heme biosynthetic pathway and environmental factors for ALAS1 induction. Demonstration of porphyrin precursors is essential for porphyrias with neurologic symptoms, such as ALAD porphyria, AIP, hereditary coproporphyria, and variegate porphyria, whereas porphyrin analysis is helpful for porphyrias with skin photosensitivity, such as CEP, erythropoietic protoporphyria, hepatoerythropoietic porphyria, hereditary coproporphyria, and variegate porphyria.

Treatment

- Acute attacks of acute hepatic porphyrias (e.g., ALAD porphyria, AIP, hereditary coproporphyria, and variegate porphyria) should be treated similarly by (1) avoiding the precipitating factors, (2) providing sufficient amounts of calories as carbohydrates (glucose infusion), and (3) intravenous infusion of hematin. Recognition and avoidance of precipitating events is the first key part of the treatment program for porphyria.
- Hemolytic anemia in CEP and hepatoerythropoietic porphyria may be treated by blood transfusion.
- Cutaneous photosensitivity of erythropoietic protoporphyria may be treated by oral β-carotene therapy, and that of PCT by phlebotomy or by oral chloroquine administration.

This work was supported in part by grants from the U.S. Public Health Service (DK32890) and The American Porphyria Foundation.

INTRODUCTION

Definition

The porphyrias are uncommon, complex, and fascinating metabolic conditions, caused by deficiencies in the activities of the enzymes of the heme biosynthetic pathway. Patients with symptomatic porphyria, particularly with acute crisis of hepatic porphyria, can suffer greatly, and, in rare cases, may die. Although congenital hepatic and erythropoietic porphyrias are inherited, similar porphyrias may also occur as acquired diseases. In addition, not all gene carriers of inherited porphyrias develop clinical disease, and there is a significant interplay between the primary gene defect and the secondary acquired or environmental factors. Thus porphyrias, particularly acute hepatic porphyrias, are the best model for pharmacogenetics in which gene-environment interaction can be studied.

The enzyme deficiencies can be either partial or nearly complete depending on the types of genetic mutations. As a result, various porphyrins, such as uro-, copro-, and protoporphyrin, and their precursors, such as δ-aminolevulinic acid (ALA) and porphobilinogen, are produced in excess, accumulate in tissues and are excreted in urine and/or stool. Two cardinal symptoms of the porphyrias are cutaneous photosensitivity and neurologic disturbances. Molecular analysis of gene defects has demonstrated that there are multiple and heterogeneous mutations in each porphyria.

Classification and Screening

Porphyrias can be classified either as (1) erythropoietic porphyrias, such as congenital erythropoietic porphyria (CEP), hepatoerythropoietic porphyria, and erythropoietic protoporphyria; (2) acute hepatic porphyrias, such as δ-aminolevulinate dehydratase (ALAD) porphyria, acute intermittent porphyria (AIP), hereditary coproporphyria, and variegate porphyria; or (3) chronic hepatic porphyria, such as porphyria cutanea tarda (PCT) (Fig. 54–1). Demonstration of porphyrin precursors is essential for porphyrias with neurologic symptoms, such as ALAD porphyria, AIP, hereditary coproporphyria, and variegate porphyria, whereas porphyrin analysis is helpful for porphyrias with skin photosensitivity, such as CEP, erythropoietic protoporphyria, hepatoerythropoietic porphyria, hereditary coproporphyria, and variegate porphyria (Fig. 54–2).

The Heme Biosynthetic Pathway

The enzymatic and intermediate steps in the heme biosynthetic pathway are illustrated in Figure 54–3. The two major organs involved in heme synthesis are the bone marrow and the liver. In the bone marrow, heme is made in erythroblasts and reticulocytes, which contain mitochondria. Circulating erythrocytes are incapable of forming heme because they lack mitochondria, though cytosolic enzymes in the heme biosynthetic pathway are present. The first intermediate of the heme biosynthetic pathway is ALA, a five-carbon aminoketone that is formed by the condensation of glycine and succinyl coenzyme A. Two molecules of ALA are combined to form the monopyrrole porphobilinogen; four molecules of porphobilinogen are then combined to form uroporphyrinogen, a cyclic tetrapyrrole. Uroporphyrinogen III is converted to coproporphyrinogen III, then to protoporphyrinogen IX, and subsequently to protoporphyrin IX. Finally, ferrous ion is inserted into protoporphyrin IX to form heme. Protoporphyrin IX is the immediate precursor of the various hemes and also of the chlorophylls. Information on enzyme proteins and genes for heme pathway enzymes is summarized in Table 54–1.

TABLE 54–1. Enzymes and Genes for Heme Biosynthesis

					Genome	
Enzyme	**Gene symbol**	**Chromosomal location**	**cDNA (bp)**	**Protein (aa)**	**Size (kb)**	**Organization***
δ-Aminolevulinate synthase						
Housekeeping	*ALAS1*	3p21.1	2199	640	17	11 exons
Erythroid-specific	*ALAS2*	Xp11.21	1937	587	22	11 exons
δ-Aminolevulinate dehydratase	*ALAD*	9q34				13 exons
Housekeeping			1149	330	15.9	Exons 1A + 2–12
Erythroid-specific			1154	330		Exon 1B + 2–12
Porphobilinogen deaminase	*PBGD*	11q23.3			11	15 exons
Housekeeping			1086	361		Exons 1 + 3–15
Erythroid-specific			1035	344		Exons 2–15
Uroporphyrinogen III synthase	*UROS*	10q25.2–q26.3			34	10 exons
Housekeeping			1296	265		Exon 1 + 2B-10
Erythroid-specific			1216	265		Exon 2A + 2B-10
Uroporphyrinogen decarboxylase	*UROD*	1p34	1104	367	3	10 exons
Coproporphyrinogen oxidase	*CPO*	3q12	1062	354	14	7 exons
Protoporphyrinogen oxidase	*PPO*	1q23	1431	477	5.5	13 exons
Ferrochelatase	*FeC*	18q21.3	1269	423	45	11 exons

*Number of exons and those encoding housekeeping and erythroid-specific forms.

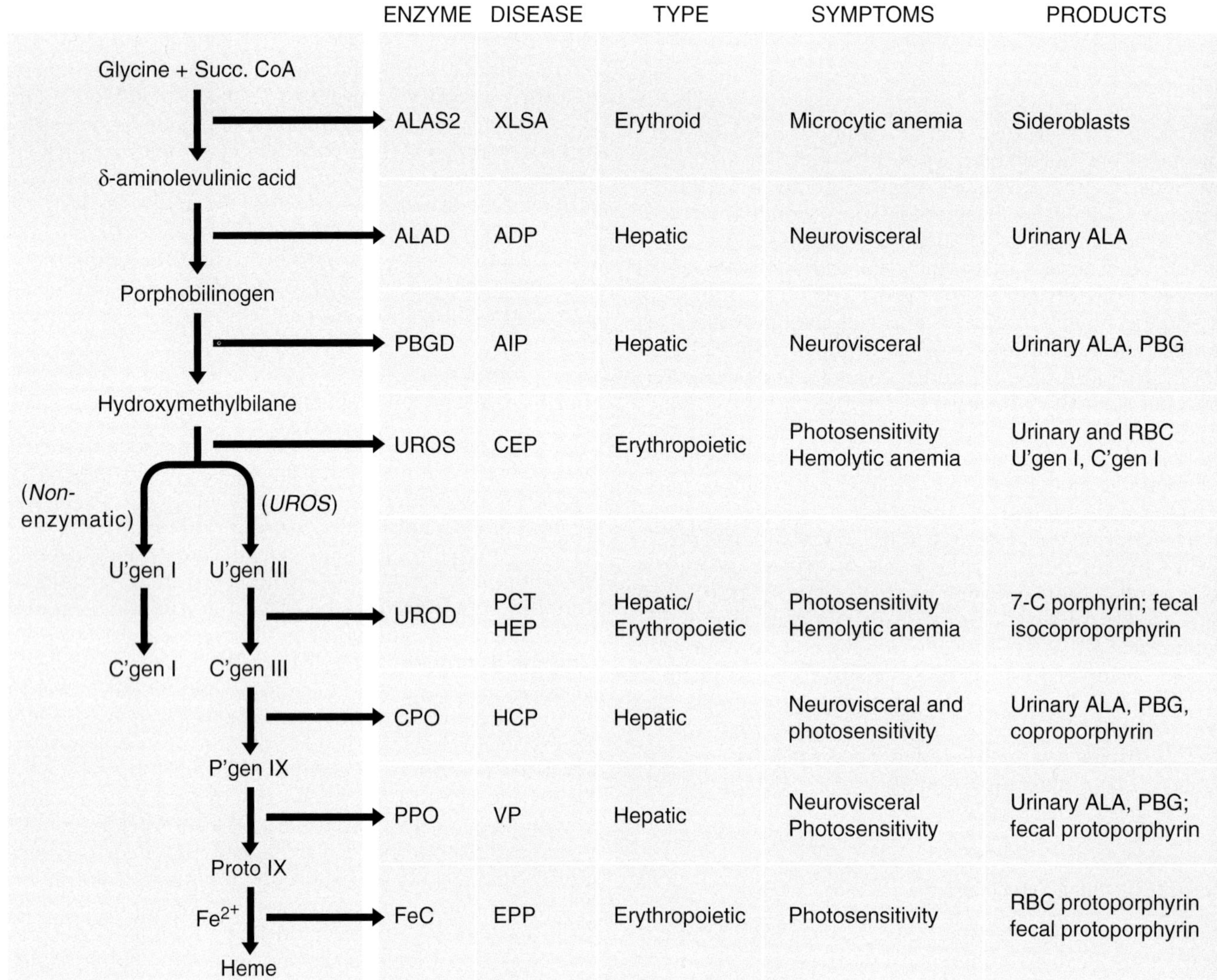

Figure 54–1. Classification of porphyrias. Enzymatic defects, associated diseases, major symptoms, and principal accumulation products are shown. The δ-aminolevulinate synthase 2 (ALAS2) defect is responsible for X-linked sideroblastic anemia but is not associated with any porphyria, because the enzymatic defect blocks production of δ-aminolevulinic acid (ALA), the obligatory precursor for porphyrin formation. δ-Aminolevulinate dehydratase (ALAD) porphyria and acute intermittent porphyria are accompanied by acute hepatic porphyria but not by photocutaneous porphyria, because their enzymatic defects do not result in an increase in porphyrin synthesis. Enzymatic defects beyond uroporphyrinogen III cosynthase (UROS) are all associated with photocutaneous porphyrias, because they produce excessive amounts of various porphyrins. Hereditary coproporphyria and variegate porphyria are additionally associated with acute hepatic porphyria. Abbreviations: CoA, coenzyme A; Copro, coproporphyrin; Isocopro, isocoproporphyrin; Proto, protoporphyrin; Uro, uroporphyrin. (Redrawn from Sassa S, Shibahara S: Disorders of heme production and catabolism. *In* Handin RI, Lux SE, Stossel TP [eds]: Blood: Principles and Practice of Hematology [ed 2]. Philadelphia: Lippincott Williams & Wilkins, 2003, pp 1435–1501.)

Excretion Patterns of Porphyrins and Precursors

The porphyrin precursors are excreted in urine and/or feces depending upon their solubility in aqueous and nonaqueous solvents, which is directly attributable to the number of carboxyl groups in each porphyrin molecule (Table 54–2).[1] Those porphyrias that have neurovisceral complaints are associated with increased excretion of ALA and/or porphobilinogen. For example, there is marked elevation of urinary ALA excretion in ALAD porphyria, and there is increased excretion of both ALA and porphobilinogen in AIP, hereditary coproporphyria, and variegate porphyria.

Porphyrias involving excess production of uroporphyrin, such as CEP, hepatoerythropoietic porphyria, and PCT, can be diagnosed by a urine collection because the porphyrins produced in excess are all water soluble and excreted into the urine. Uroporphyrin in urine may also be increased in AIP, in part because of nonenzymatic cyclization of porphobilinogen to uroporphyrin I upon storage of urine. Variegate porphyria and erythropoietic protoporphyria are both associated with overproduction

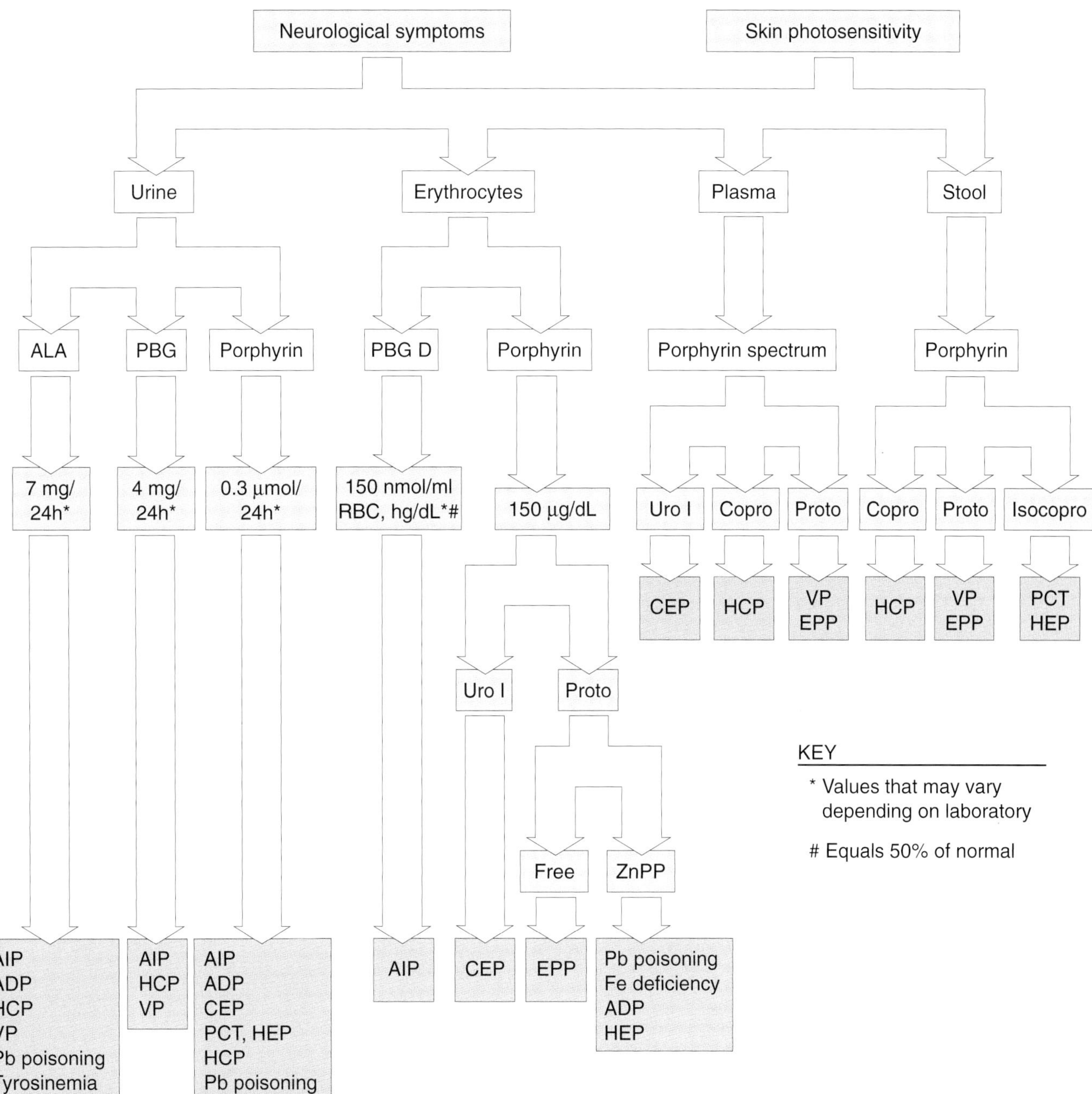

Figure 54–2. Screening strategy for porphyrias. Demonstration of porphyrin precursors such as ALA and/or porphobilinogen is essential for acute hepatic porphyrias such as ALAD porphyria, AIP, hereditary coproporphyria and variegate porphyria, which have accompanying neurologic symptoms. Porphyrin analysis is helpful for porphyrias with cutaneous photosensitivity, such as CEP, erythropoietic protoporphyria, and hepatoerythropoietic porphyria. (Redrawn from Sassa S: Understanding the porphyrias. *In* Rose BD [ed]: UpToDate. Wellesley, MA: UpToDate, 2001.)

of protoporphyrin, which is virtually insoluble in water but soluble in lipids. Thus, these disorders are best diagnosed through fecal collection of porphyrins, or by plasma porphyrin analysis. Because of its intermediate solubility, coproporphyrin is excreted in urine and stool and also found in plasma. Thus, increased amounts of coproporphyrin are found in all these body fluids in an acute attack of hereditary coproporphyria (see Table 54–2).

EPIDEMIOLOGY

Epidemiology is markedly different for each porphyria. A recent review identified 34 cases of CEP, 5 cases of hepatoerythropoietic porphyria, 154 cases of erythropoietic protoporphyria, 1 case of ALAD porphyria, 188 cases of AIP, 37 cases of hereditary coproporphyria, 54 cases of variegate porphyria, 51 cases of acute hepatic porphyria with uncertain classification, and 303 cases of PCT among a total of 827 cases of porphyrias reported.[2]

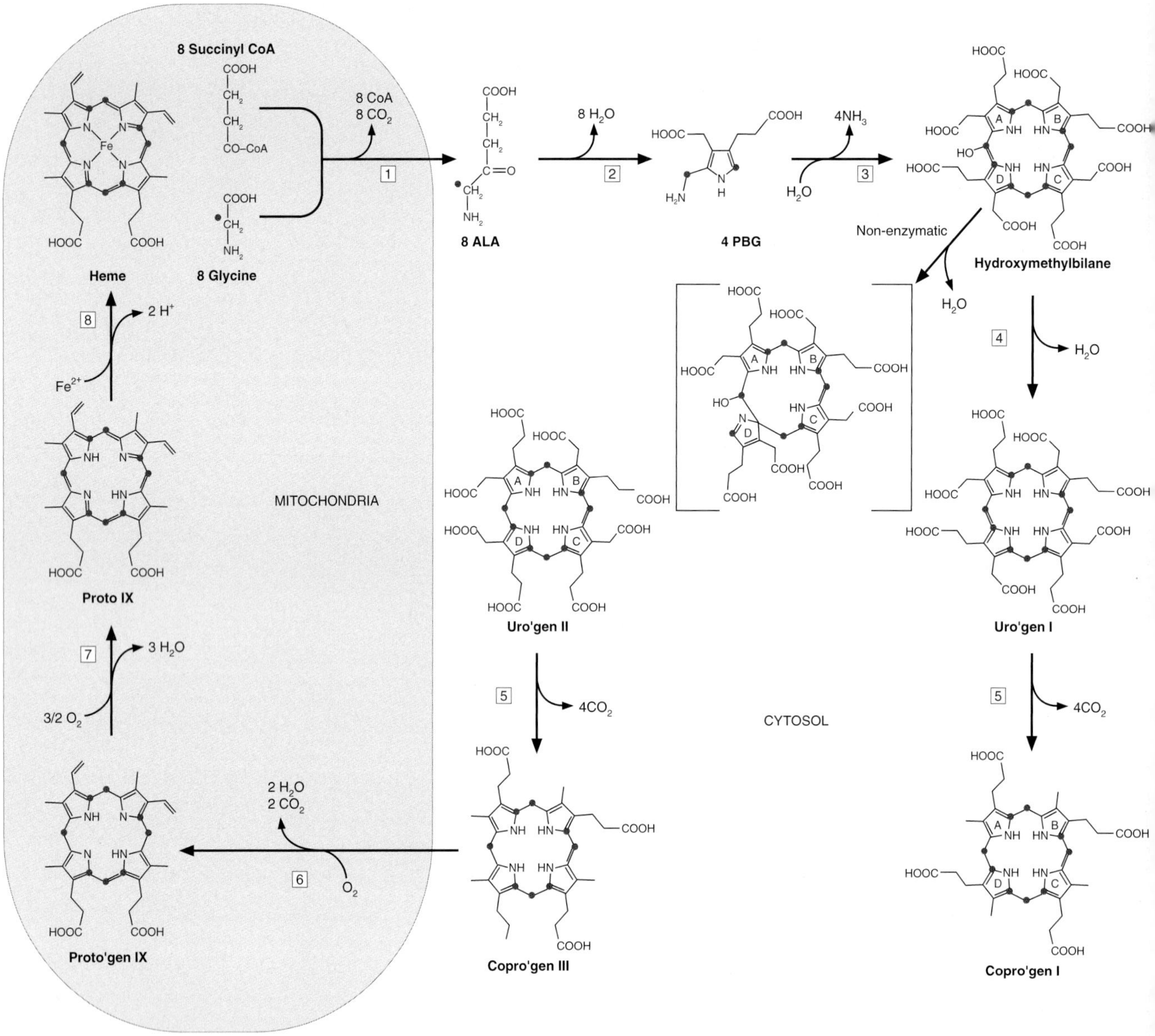

■ **Figure 54–3.** Enzymes and intermediates of the heme biosynthetic pathway. Step 1: ALAS. Step 2: ALAD. Step 3: PBGD. Step 4: UROS. Step 5: UROD. Step 6: CPO. Step 7: PPO. Step 8: Ferrochelatase. The carbon atom that is derived from the α carbon of glycine is shown as a *bold dot.* The structure that is denoted by the brackets after step 4 is the presumed intermediate whose pyrrole ring D becomes rearranged to yield uroporphyrinogen III. At step 7, 1 mole of oxygen is consumed per 1 mole of water produced. Abbreviation: CoA, coenzyme A.

ERYTHROPOIETIC PORPHYRIAS

Porphyrins in red cells can cause photosensitive erythrocyte lysis, resulting in hemolytic anemia in CEP and hepatoerythropoietic porphyria. Neonatal hemolytic anemia was also observed in the homozygous variant known as harderoporphyria.[3] In contrast, erythropoietic protoporphyria, a heterozygous disease in which photosensitivity is much milder than that seen in CEP and hepatoerythropoietic porphyria, rarely has an accompanying hemolytic anemia. Hemolytic anemia is also rarely seen in two other conditions of protoporphyrinemia, iron deficiency anemia and lead poisoning, because protoporphyrin in these conditions is chelated with zinc and tightly bound with the heme pocket in hemoglobin.[4] The effect of lifelong anemia in CEP or hepatoerythropoietic porphyria may lead to compensatory expansion of erythroid marrow, as in β-thalassemia major, which may result in pathologic fractures, vertebral compression or collapse, and shortness of stature. The hemolysis is also associated with varying degrees of splenomegaly and the production of pigment-laden gallstones.

Congenital Erythropoietic Porphyria

CEP is an erythropoietic porphyria inherited in an autosomal recessive fashion and causes photosensitivity

TABLE 54–2. Routes of Excretion of Heme Pathway Intermediates

Intermediate	ALA Equivalent	Number of Carboxyl (COOH) Groups	COOH/ALA Ratio	Excretion
ALA	1	1	1	Urine
Porphobilinogen	2	2	1	Urine
Uroporphyrin	8	8	1	Urine
Coproporphyrin	8	4	0.5	Urine, stool, plasma
Protoporphyrin	8	2	0.25	Bile, stool, plasma
Heme	8	2	0.25	Bile, stool, plasma

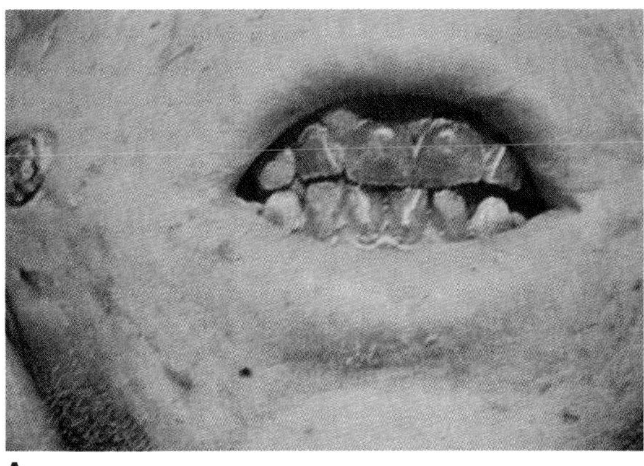

A

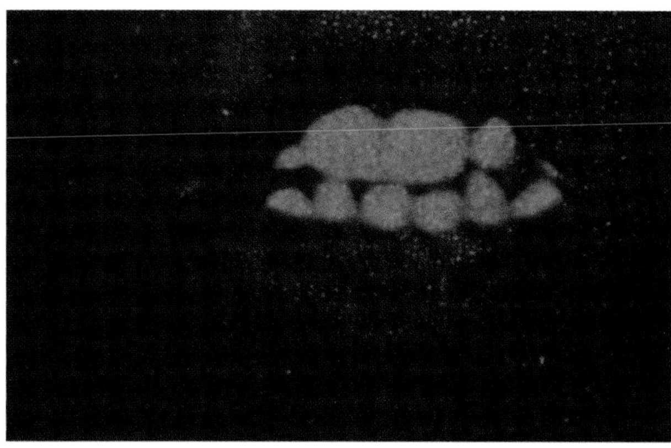

B

Figure 54–4. Erythrodontia in CEP. *A,* Normal view. Note the brownish discoloration of teeth by uroporphyrin deposition, the atrophic changes in the lip at the corner of mouth, the deformed healing of erosion on the right cheek, and the pigmentation and discoloration of the skin. *B,* Fluorescent view. When visualized under ultraviolet light, the teeth show intense fluorescence as a result of uroporphyrin deposition.

disorders. The primary abnormality is an almost complete absence of uroporphyrinogen III cosynthase (UROS) activity, which results in massive accumulation and excretion of uroporphyrin I and coproporphyrin I.

Pathophysiology

Mild to severe hemolysis is accompanied by anisocytosis, poikilocytosis, polychromasia, basophilic stippling, reticulocytosis, increased nucleated red cells, absence of haptoglobin, increased unconjugated bilirubin, increased fecal urobilinogen, and increased plasma iron turnover. Secondary splenomegaly, developing in response to the increased removal of damaged red cells from the circulation, may contribute to the anemia, and may also result in leukopenia and thrombocytopenia (i.e., hypersplenism). Splenectomy may reduce the need for transfusions, although signs of ineffective erythropoiesis may continue.

Severe cutaneous photosensitivity usually begins in early infancy manifested by increased friability and blistering of the epidermis on the hands and face and other sun-exposed areas. Hypertrichosis of the face and extremities is often prominent. Sunlight, other sources of ultraviolet light, and minor skin trauma increase the severity of the cutaneous manifestations (Fig. 54–4).

Molecular Pathology

To date, a variety of mutations that cause CEP have been identified in the *UROS* gene. The majority of patients with CEP are heteroallelic (i.e., compound heterozygous) for the *UROS* mutations. The most common mutation, C73R, was found in about 33% of the studied alleles. The next most common mutations were L4F and T228M (7% and 6%, respectively).

Clinical Findings

The major debilitating clinical features in patients with CEP are severe cutaneous photosensitivity and anemia. However, the age at onset and clinical severity of CEP are highly variable, ranging from nonimmune hydrops fetalis caused by severe hemolytic anemia in utero to milder and later onset forms, which have only cutaneous lesions in adult life. In most cases severe photosensitivity has developed soon after birth. Pink or red-brown staining of diapers as a result of markedly increased urinary porphyrins may be the first clue to the disease. A number of factors lead to the phenotypic variability in CEP, including (1) the amount of residual UROS activity, (2) the resultant degree of hemolysis and consequent stimulation of erythropoiesis, and (3) exposure to ultraviolet light. Therefore, as in other porphyrias, an interplay between environmental factors and the deficient enzyme activity is important for clinical expression of the disease. Overall life expectancy may be markedly diminished in more severely affected patients because of hematologic complications and an increased risk of infection.

The large amounts of isomer I porphyrinogens that accumulate in bone marrow erythroid precursors (especially normoblasts and reticulocytes) and erythrocytes undergo auto-oxidation to the corresponding porphyrins, causing hemolysis and ineffective erythropoiesis. They are also deposited in tissues and bones, cause cutaneous photosensitivity, and are excreted in large amounts in urine and feces. Photosensitivity occurs because these porphyrins are photocatalytic compounds. Exposure of the skin to sunlight and other sources of long-wave ultraviolet light results in blistering and vesicle formation and increased friability of the skin. Hemolysis is almost always present, but may not be accompanied by anemia if erythroid hyperplasia is sufficient to compensate for the increased rate of erythrocyte destruction. This degree of compensation may vary over time such that, as an example, anemia may be exacerbated during episodes of infection.

Diagnosis

CEP should be suspected when severe photosensitivity begins in infancy or childhood, and porphyrins are markedly increased in both erythrocytes and urine. Pink to dark reddish urine or staining of the diaper noted shortly after birth may be the first clue to the diagnosis. In some cases the disease is less severe and presents in adult life with a hemolytic anemia or skin lesions suggestive of PCT. Full characterization of porphyrin patterns by a research laboratory to confirm a deficiency of UROS and to determine the nature of the underlying mutation is indicated to confirm a diagnosis of CEP.

If heterozygous parents have had a child with this disease, the disease can be detected in utero in future pregnancies by one or more of the following: (1) red-brown discoloration and increased porphyrins (especially uroporphyrin I) in amniotic fluid[5]; (2) measurement of UROS activity in cultured amniotic fluid cells[6]; and (3) direct detection of *UROS* mutations in cultured amniotic cells.[7]

Differential Diagnosis

The differential diagnosis of CEP includes the other porphyrias with cutaneous symptoms, such as hepatoerythropoietic porphyria, PCT, variegate porphyria, hereditary coproporphyria, and erythropoietic protoporphyria. Hepatoerythropoietic porphyria is clinically similar to CEP but is distinguishable by the predominance of protoporphyrin (complexed with zinc) in red cells and isocoproporphyrin in stool.

Homozygous forms of other porphyrias such as variegate porphyria and hereditary coproporphyria may also be associated with photosensitivity in childhood and increased erythrocyte zinc protoporphyrin. In contrast to CEP, increased urinary concentrations of ALA and porphobilinogen are found during acute attacks in both variegate porphyria and hereditary coproporphyria. Variegate porphyria may be further differentiated by the presence of increased protoporphyrin in plasma and stool, and hereditary coproporphyria is characterized by increases in coproporphyrin in plasma, urine, and stool. Harderoporphyria, a homozygous variant of hereditary coproporphyria, is associated with symptoms similar to CEP, including neonatal hemolytic anemia. Erythropoietic protoporphyria is readily distinguished by a predominance of free protoporphyrin in erythrocytes and normal urinary porphyrins.

Treatment

Treatment of CEP involves three main components: (1) protection from sunlight and ultraviolet light exposure, (2) meticulous skin care, and (3) red cell transfusions and other hematologic supportive care. Bacterial infections that complicate cutaneous blisters require timely treatment. Repeated red cell transfusions can suppress erythropoiesis, thereby decreasing overall porphyrin production and resulting in reduced porphyrin levels, with a consequent reduction in photosensitivity and hemolysis.[8] Such therapy is most likely to be successful if the hematocrit is maintained at levels above 32% and deferoxamine is administered to reduce the resulting iron overload.

Other therapeutic interventions in CEP include (1) treatment with hydroxyurea to reduce bone marrow porphyrin synthesis,[9] (2) splenectomy to reduce transfusion requirements in patients with hypersplenism,[8] and (3) oral charcoal treatment to facilitate fecal excretion of porphyrins.[10] Heme infusion therapy, which is effective for treatment of the acute hepatic porphyrias, may not be effective in CEP. Chloroquine treatment, which is known to be beneficial in PCT, has not been useful in CEP.

Allogeneic bone marrow transplantation has proved curative for patients with CEP; to date four patients have been transplanted.[11–14] Successful marrow transplantation resulted in marked reduction of the photosensitivity and porphyrin levels. The success of bone marrow transplantation provides the rationale for hematopoietic stem cell gene therapy for CEP. Efforts are underway to develop retroviral-mediated transduction of hematopoietic stem cells for treatment of patients with CEP.

Hepatoerythropoietic Porphyria

Hepatoerythropoietic porphyria is a rare form of porphyria that is due to a homozygous, or compound heterozygous, deficiency of uroporphyrinogen decarboxylase (UROD). Only 20 cases of hepatoerythropoietic porphyria have been reported.

Clinical Findings

Hepatoerythropoietic porphyria resembles CEP clinically and usually presents in infancy or childhood with red urine, blistering skin lesions, hypertrichosis, and scarring. Sclerodermoid skin changes may be prominent. Erythrocyte porphyrins are increased, but they are predominantly type III isomers.

Hemolytic anemia is often present, and associated with splenomegaly. The biochemical findings in hepatoerythropoietic porphyria resemble those that are observed in PCT, and include predominant accumulation and excretion of uroporphyrin, heptacarboxylate porphyrin, and isocoproporphyrins. Erythrocyte zinc-protoporphyrin complex concentration is increased in hepatoerythropoietic porphyria.

Diagnosis

Severe cutaneous photosensitivity and hemolytic anemia suggest hepatoerythropoietic porphyria or CEP. Unlike CEP, hepatoerythropoietic porphyria is associated with predominant accumulation and excretion of type III uroporphyrin, heptacarboxylate porphyrin, and isocoproporphyrins. Erythrocyte zinc-protoporphyrin complex concentration is also increased.

Treatment

Treatment includes protection from sunlight, skin care, and blood transfusion. There is no evidence of iron overload in hepatoerythropoietic porphyria, and, unlike in PCT, phlebotomy is not beneficial.

Erythropoietic Protoporphyria

Erythropoietic protoporphyria is characterized by a partial deficiency of ferrochelatase activity, and is inherited in an autosomal dominant manner. Cutaneous photosensitivity characteristically begins in childhood, but there is no neurologic involvement. This is the most common erythropoietic porphyria. It has been described mostly in whites but does occur in other races, including blacks.

Pathophysiology

It has been proposed that (1) a mutant allele (M) and the C → T transition (N_T) in *trans* are both necessary for the expression of erythropoietic protoporphyria; and that (2) the N_T allele probably reduces ferrochelatase activity, compared with the ferrochelatase allele without the 23C → T transition (N_C); but (3) the N_T allele alone is not sufficient to bring about erythropoietic protoporphyria, even in its homozygous state. Thus, ferrochelatase activity in patients can be defined as M-N_T, that in silent gene carriers as M-N_C, and that in normal controls as N_C-N_C, N_C-N_T, or N_T-N_T (increasingly reduced ferrochelatase activity). This model appears to account for (1) why normal controls have a wide range of ferrochelatase activity, (2) why silent gene carriers have higher ferrochelatase activity than patients, and (3) why patients with erythropoietic protoporphyria have less than 50% of normal ferrochelatase activity.

Molecular analysis of ferrochelatase mutations has revealed missense mutations, splicing abnormalities, intragenic deletions, and possible nonsense mutations associated with functional deficiency of ferrochelatase. Among them, exon skipping is the most predominant.

Pathogenesis

Bone marrow reticulocytes are thought to be the primary source of the excess protoporphyrin that accumulates in tissues and is excreted in feces in erythropoietic protoporphyria. Bone marrow fluorescence is almost entirely in reticulocytes rather than nucleated erythroid cells. Unlike other conditions associated with increased erythrocyte protoporphyrin, erythrocyte protoporphyrin in erythropoietic protoporphyria is free and not complexed with zinc. Protoporphyrin is markedly increased in erythrocytes (Fig. 54–5) and plasma, and excreted in stool.

Clinical Findings

Cutaneous photosensitivity begins in childhood, affects sun-exposed areas such as the face and dorsum of the hands, and is generally worse in spring and summer. Common symptoms, including itching, painful erythema,

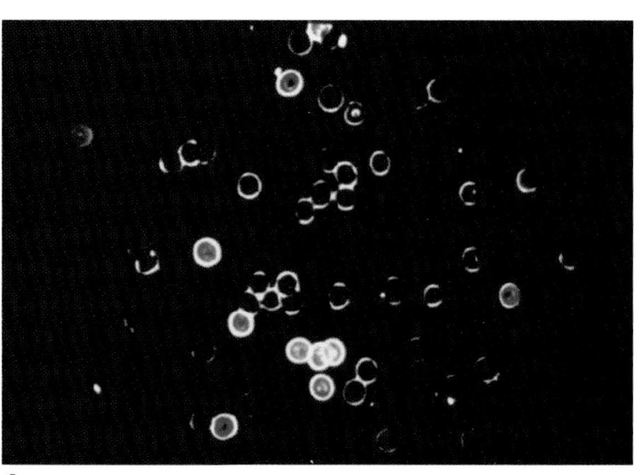

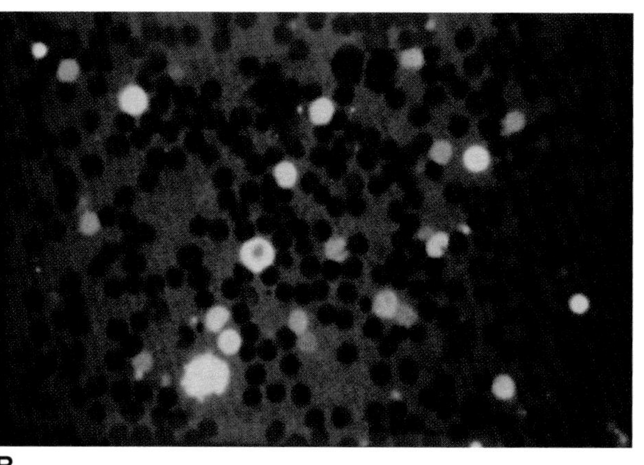

A B

Figure 54–5. Fluorocytes in erythropoietic protoporphyria. ***A***, Peripheral blood smear. Some erythrocytes show red fluorescence as a result of a large amount of protoporphyrin, but others do not. ***B***, Bone marrow smear. Some erythroblasts show red fluorescence as a result of a large amount of protoporphyrin, but others do not. Dimorphic distribution of fluorocytes in blood and of fluoroblasts in the bone marrow is a characteristic feature of erythropoietic protoporphyria.

and swelling, can develop within minutes of sun exposure. Diffuse edema of the skin in sun-exposed areas may resemble angioneurotic edema. On occasion, burning and itching can occur without obvious skin damage. Petechiae and purpuric lesions may occur. Skin lichenification, leathery pseudovesicles, and nail changes can be pronounced. Pigment changes and severe scarring are unusual. Vesicles and bullae are uncommon. Deformities of facial features and digits, which are common in CEP, hepatoerythropoietic porphyria, and PCT, do not occur in erythropoietic protoporphyria. Increased fragility and hirsutism are also not characteristic of this disease. Unlike in CEP, the teeth are not fluorescent in erythropoietic protoporphyria.

Mild anemia with hypochromia and microcytosis or mild anemia with reticulocytosis is sometimes noted in erythropoietic protoporphyria. Iron accumulation in erythroblasts and ring sideroblasts occur in some erythropoietic protoporphyria patients. The risk of biliary stones seems to be increased, and the stones contain protoporphyrin. Liver failure occurs in a minority of patients, but, if it occurs, it is associated with a poor prognosis.

Treatment

Oral administration of β-carotene is useful for treating erythropoietic protoporphyria. β-Carotene doses of 120–180 mg daily in adults are usually required to maintain serum carotene levels in the recommended range of 600–800 μg/dL, but doses up to 300 mg daily may be needed. Cholestyramine and other porphyrin absorbents such as activated charcoal may be helpful. Other therapeutic options include red blood cell transfusions, exchange transfusion, and intravenous hematin to suppress erythroid and hepatic protoporphyrin production, as well as liver transplantation. Although liver transplantation can be temporary beneficial, the new liver is susceptible to protoporphyrin-induced damage.

ACUTE HEPATIC PORPHYRIAS

The most common neurovisceral complaints in acute hepatic porphyrias are multifactorial:

1. Excess amounts of porphobilinogen or ALA may cause neurotoxicity.
2. Increased ALA concentrations in the brain may inhibit γ-aminobutyric acid release.
3. Heme deficiency may result in degenerative changes in the central nervous system.
4. Decreased heme synthesis in the liver results in decreased activity of hepatic tryptophan pyrrolase, increasing levels of brain tryptophan, and increased turnover of 5-hydroxytryptamine, a neurotransmitter.
5. ALA increases lipid peroxidation, and ALA-mediated lipid peroxidation may underscore the acute crisis of porphyria.

ALAD Porphyria

ALAD porphyria is rare. Only five cases have been molecularly confirmed: three German males, one Swedish baby boy, and one elderly Belgian man. It is an autosomal recessive disorder resulting from a homozygous deficiency of ALAD; the biochemical findings are listed in Table 54–3. Subjects heterozygous for ALAD deficiency are asymptomatic, but may be at risk for developing ALAD porphyria when exposed to environmental chemicals or toxins that further inhibit ALAD activity.

Acute Intermittent Porphyria

AIP is due to inherited (autosomal dominant) mutations in the porphobilinogen deaminase (*PBGD*) gene. The prevalence of AIP in the United States is thought to be 5–10 per 100,000. It is more common in northern European countries such as Sweden (60–100 per 100,000), Britain, and Ireland. More than 170 mutations of the *PBGD* gene have been described in AIP.

Pathophysiology

AIP patients can be classified into three subtypes. In type I (CRIM-negative) patients, PBGD activity and protein are reduced by approximately 50% in all tissues of patients. The mutations are either single base substitutions, or single base deletions resulting in a single amino acid substitution, or in truncated proteins produced by either splicing defects or frameshift mutations. In type II (without erythrocyte PBGD deficiency) patients, the defect is restricted to nonerythroid cells. Type III (CRIM-positive) patients are characterized by decreased PBGD activity with the presence of a structurally abnormal protein. The same PBGD defect is found in all tissues.

Pathogenesis

A mouse model in which PBGD deficiency was induced by gene targeting was developed recently.[15] These animals display impaired motor function, ataxia, increased levels of ALA in plasma and brain, and decreased heme saturation of liver tryptophan pyrrolase.

An inherited deficiency of PBGD is not in itself sufficient to cause clinical expression of AIP, because perhaps 90% of individuals who inherit a deficiency of PBGD never develop porphyric symptoms. Clinical expression is prompted by a number of precipitating factors (Fig. 54–6).

Drugs

Drugs that precipitate acute attacks of AIP include barbiturates and sulfonamide antibiotics (Table 54–4). Other implicated drugs can be found on a dedicated website at *http://www.uq.edu.au/porphyria/*. However, knowledge about the safety of many drugs and other over-the-counter preparations in acute porphyrias is incomplete. Most drugs that exacerbate AIP porphyria have the capacity to induce δ-aminolevulinate synthase (ALAS) activity in the liver. This process is closely associated with the induction of cytochrome P-450 enzymes, a process that increases the demand for hepatic heme synthesis.

TABLE 54–3. Biochemical Findings in Five Patients with ALAD Porphyria

Patient	German B [24,25]	German H [24,25]	Swedish [26]	Belgian [27,28]	German X [29]
Sex	Male	Male	Male	Male	Male
Age of Onset	15	15	At birth	63	17
Clinical Course	Moderate	Moderate	Severe	Mild	Mild
Laboratory Findings (%)*					
Plasma					
ALA	—	—	—	1155	—
Porphobilinogen	—	—	—	Normal	—
Coproporphyrin	300	167	—	—	—
Protoporphyrin	127	327	—	—	—
Urine					
ALA	2449	2373	8150	794	3192
Porphobilinogen	238	200	447	Normal	600
Uroporphyrin	361	224	—	888	294
Coproporphyrin	5380	4698	—	2987	7568
Total porphyrin	—	—	7247	—	—
Stool					
Coproporphyrin	Normal	Normal	284	285	—
Protoporphyrin	Normal	Normal	Normal	300	—
Erythrocyte					
Protoporphyrin (ZnPP)	3192	3164	663	408	543
Erythrocyte enzymes					
ALAD activity	0	1	1	1	8
Activation by dithiothreitol	None	None	None	None	None
Activation by Zn^{2+}	None	None	None	None	None
PBGD activity	Normal	Normal	Normal	Normal	Normal

*Upper limit of normal = 100%.
Abbreviations: ZnPP, zinc-protoporphyrin complex; –, not determined.

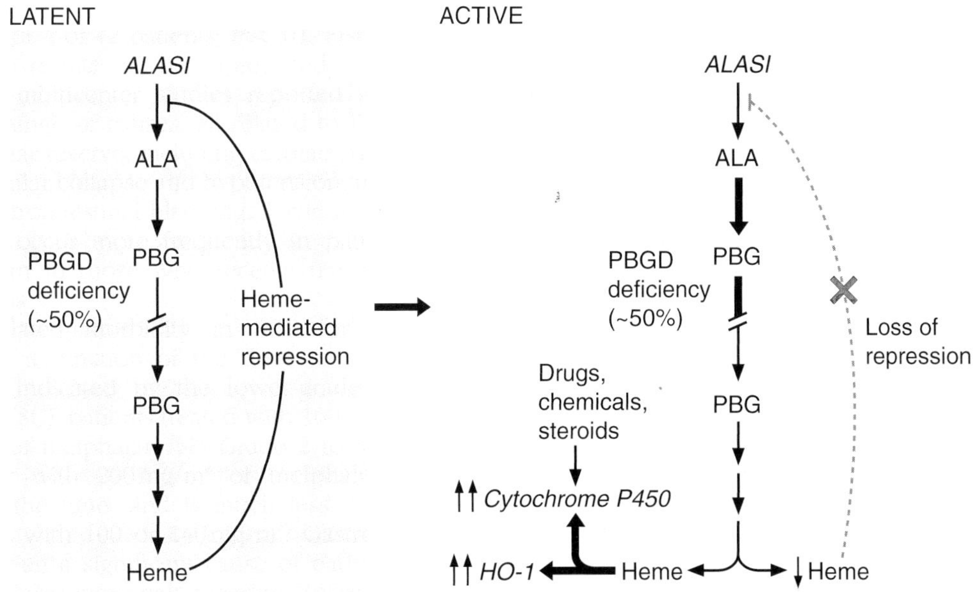

Figure 54–6. Enzymatic block in latent and active AIP patients, and loss of heme-mediated repression of ALAS1 during acute attacks, are shown when the disease is made clinically manifest by precipitating factors. Latent gene carriers of PBGD deficiency are clinically unaffected because there is heme-mediated repression of ALAS1, even in the presence of an approximately 50% decrease in PBGD activity. However, these subjects can be induced into acute attacks with increased ALAS1 expression when exposed to drugs, chemicals, steroids, or fasting, which are mediated by increased heme utilization for cytochrome P-450 synthesis, or facilitated heme breakdown by HO-1 induction.

TABLE 54–4. Categories of Safe and Unsafe Drugs in the Acute Porphyrias*

Unsafe	Potentially Unsafe	Probably Safe	Safe
ACE inhibitors (especially enalapril)	Alfadolone acetate	Adrenaline	Acetaminophen (paracetamol)
	Alfaxolone	Amitriptyline	
Antipyrine (phenazone)	Alkylating agents (cyclophosphamide,	Azathioprine	Acetazolamide
Aminopyrine (amidopyrine)	ifosfamide, busulphan, altretamine	Chloramphenicol	Allopurinol
Aminoglutethimide	[hexamethylmelamine, dacarbazine,	Cisapride	Amiloride
Barbiturates	chlorambucil, and melphalan may	Colchicine	Aspirin
N-Butylscopolammonium bromide	be safer])	Cyclosporin	Atropine
		Cytarabine	Bethanidine
Calcium channel blockers (especially	Benzodiazepines	Dicumarol	Bromides
nifedipine)	Captopril	Chloroquine	Bumetanide
Carbamazepine	Cephalosporins	Digoxin	Chloral hydrate
Chlorpropamide	Chlordiazepoxide	Daunorubicin	Cimetidine
Danazol	Clonidine	Doxazosin	Corticosteroids
Dapsone	Diazepam	Estrogens (natural/	Coumarins
Diclofenac	Diltiazem	endogenous)	Fluoxetine
Enalapril	Colistin	Ibuprofen	Gabapentin
Diphenylhydantoin	Dacarbazine	Imipramine	Gentamicin
Ethosuximide	Diphenhydramine	Indomethacin	Guanethidine
Ergot preparations	EDTA	Labetalol	Insulin
Ethchlorvynol	Etomidate	Lithium	Narcotic analgesics
Ethinamate	Estrogens (synthetic)	Losartan	Ofloxacin
Felbamate	Erythromycin	Methenamine	Penicillin and derivatives
Glutethimide	5-Fluorouracil	Methylphenidate	Phenothiazines
Griseofulvin	Gold compounds	Naproxen	Propranolol
Ketoconazole	Fluroxene	Neostigmine	Streptomycin
Lamotrigine	Heavy metals	Nortriptyline	Succinylcholine
Mephenytoin	Hydralazine	Nitrous oxide	Tetracycline
Metoclopramide	Hyoscine	Penicillamine	
Meprobamate	Iron chelators (deferoxamine, EDTA)	Procaine	
Methyprylon		Propanidid	
Nefazodone	Ketamine	Propofol	
Nifedipine	Lisinopril	Propoxyphene	
Novobiocin	Mefenamic acid	Rauwolfia alkaloids	
Phenylbutazone	Mifepristone (RU-486)	6-Thioguanine	
Primidone	Methyldopa	Thiouracils	
Pargyline	Metyrapone	Thyroxine	
	Mitotane		
Progesterone & progestins	Nalidixic acid	Tricyclic antidepressants	
Rifampin	Nikethamide		
Succinimides	Nitrazepam	Tubocurarine	
Sulfasalazine	Nitrofurantoin	Vigabatrin	
Sulfonamide antibiotics	*o,p'*-DDD	Vitamin B	
Sulfonmethane (Sulfonal) &	Pentazocine	Vitamin C	
sulfonethylmethane (Trional)	Phenoxybenzamine		
Sulfonylureas	Procarbazine		
Trimethadione	Pyrazinamide		
Valproic acid	Spironolactone		
Tranylcypromine	Theophylline		
	Tiagabine		
	Tramadol		
	Tricyclic antidepressants		
	Troglitazone		

Abbreviations: ACE, angiotensin-converting enzyme; DDD, dichlorodiphenyldichloroethane; EDTA, ethylenediaminetetraacetic acid.
From Anderson KE, Sassa S, Bishop DF, et al: Disorders of heme biosynthesis: X-linked sideroblastic anemia and the porphyrias. *In* Scriver CR, Beaudet AL, Sly WS, et al (eds): The Metabolic and Molecular Bases of Inherited Disease. New York: McGraw-Hill, 2001, pp 2991–3062, with permission.

Nutritional Factors

Reduced energy intake, usually instituted in an effort to lose weight, commonly contributes to attacks of acute porphyria. Thus, even brief periods of starvation during weight reduction, postoperative periods, or intercurrent illness should be avoided. Starvation in animals induces HO-1 activity, which can lead to depletion of regulatory hepatic heme pools and contribute to ALAS induction. Glucose and other forms of carbohydrate are effective in treating acute attacks of porphyria, although the precise mechanism by which glucose suppresses hepatic levels of ALAS is not known.

Smoking

Chemicals in tobacco smoke, such as polycyclic aromatic hydrocarbons, are known inducers of hepatic cytochrome P-450 enzymes and heme synthesis. An association between cigarette smoking and repeated attacks of porphyria was found in a survey of 144 patients with AIP in Britain. As a result, smoking cessation may have particular health benefits in patients with acute porphyrias.

Infections, Surgery, and Stress

Attacks of porphyria may develop during intercurrent infections and other illnesses, after major surgery, and during periods of psychological stress. Most of these conditions are known to increase hepatic HO-1 activity.

Clinical Findings

AIP is more common in women than in men, and very rare in children. Symptoms may appear at or anytime after puberty. The major clinical manifestations of AIP, including abdominal pain and other neurovisceral and circulatory disturbances, are due to effects on the nervous system. Neurologic and visceral symptoms are almost always intermittent and usually occur in acute attacks that develop over a few hours or days. The disease can be disabling but is only occasionally fatal. Abdominal pain has been reported in 85–95% of cases, followed by tachycardia (80%). Abdominal pain is usually severe, steady, and poorly localized but may be cramping. A variety of mental symptoms, pain in the limbs, head, neck, or chest, muscle weakness, and sensory loss can occur. Weakness most commonly begins in the proximal muscles and more often in the arms than in the legs.

The course of the neurologic manifestations of acute porphyria is highly variable. Sudden death may occur, presumably as a result of cardiac arrhythmia. Acute attacks of porphyria may resolve quite rapidly. The disease may be complicated by electrolyte abnormalities. Hyponatremia is common during acute attacks, and may help to suggest the diagnosis. This is sometimes due to the syndrome of inappropriate antidiuretic hormone secretion. The urine is often dark red in color (Fig. 54–7).

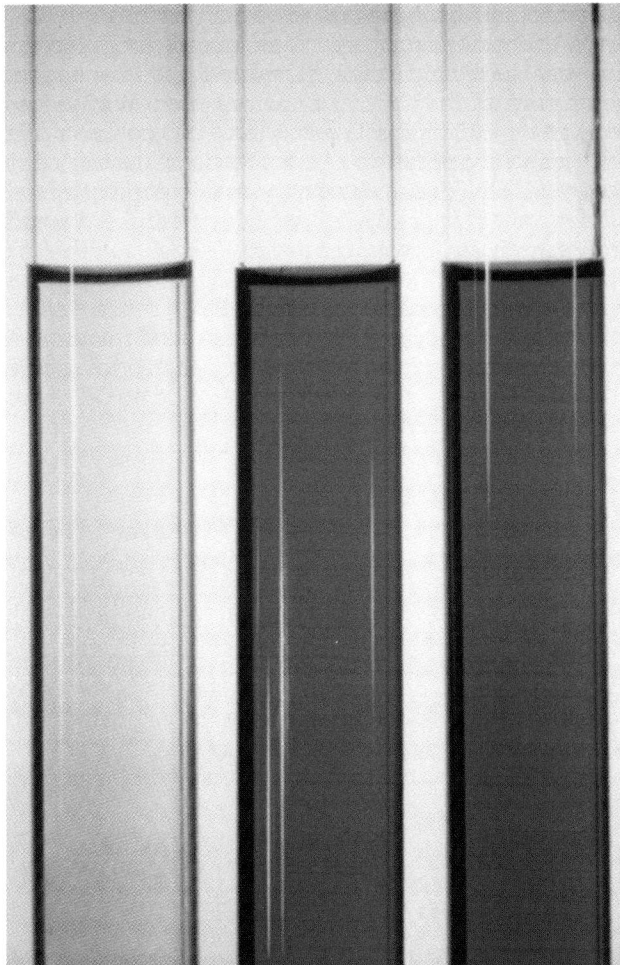

Figure 54–7. Color of urine of AIP patient. *Left,* Normal urine. *Center,* AIP urine. *Right,* Red wine that has been diluted with water. The urine of AIP patients is often referred to as "port-wine red" because of its color, which is due to the presence of porphobilin.

Diagnosis

Diagnosis can be established by the demonstration of reduced PBGD activity in erythrocytes (about 50% of normal) in type I and type III AIP patients. Type II AIP patients show normal PBGD activity in erythrocytes but have reduced PBGD activity in nonerythroid cells such as fibroblasts or lymphocytes. Patients with the clinically expressed disease excrete increased amounts of ALA and porphobilinogen in the urine, and often even during clinical remission. During an acute attack of AIP, there are further massive increases in excretion of these precursors (ALA, 25–100 mg/day; porphobilinogen, 50–200 mg/day) (see Fig. 54–2). Elevated levels of urinary ALA may additionally be seen in ALAD porphyria, hereditary coproporphyria, and variegate porphyria, and elevated levels of both ALA and porphobilinogen may be seen in hereditary coproporphyria and variegate porphyria.

Treatment

The treatment of acute attack is essentially the same for AIP, ALAD porphyria, hereditary coproporphyria, and variegate porphyria. Intravenous administration of carbohydrate (as dextrose) should be given to provide a minimum of 300 gm of carbohydrate per day. If available, the use of intravenous hematin (e.g., Normosang) is the treatment of choice; this curtails urinary excretion of ALA and porphobilinogen, thus mitigating acute attacks and perhaps the severity of neuropathy. It can be obtained from Orphan Europe (UK) Ltd, 32 Bell Street, Henley-on-Thames, Oxfordshire RG9 2BH, United Kingdom (telephone: 01491 414333; Fax: 01491 414443). In one case report, liver transplantation reduced urinary porphyrin precursor excretion to normal.[16]

As supportive treatment between attacks, it is important to maintain adequate nutritional intake, to avoid drugs known to exacerbate porphyria, and to treat other conditions (e.g., starvation, intermittent diseases, or infections). Nasal or subcutaneous administration of a long-acting agonist of luteinizing hormone–releasing hormone inhibits ovulation and greatly reduces the incidence of perimenstrual attacks of AIP in such women.[17] Pain, which is invariably present and severe, can be treated with frequent regular doses of narcotic analgesics.

Hereditary Coproporphyria

Hereditary coproporphyria is an autosomal dominant hepatic porphyria caused by a deficiency of coproporphyrinogen oxidase (CPO) activity. Symptoms are identical to those of AIP, except that it is sometimes also accompanied by cutaneous photosensitivity. Hereditary coproporphyria is much less frequent than AIP and variegate porphyria.[18]

Molecular Pathology

Molecular analysis of several families with hereditary coproporphyria, including the homozygous dominant form and the harderoporphyria variant, has revealed a variety of mutations in the *CPO* gene. These include missense, nonsense, and splice-site defects, as well as insertions and deletions.[19]

Clinical Findings

Hereditary coproporphyria usually presents with symptoms identical to AIP. Additionally, photosensitivity similar to that in PCT sometimes occurs. In a series of 53 cases of hereditary coproporphyria in Germany, the incidence of abdominal pain, neurologic symptoms, psychiatric symptoms, cardiovascular symptoms, and skin symptoms was 89%, 33%, 28%, 25%, and 14%, respectively.[18] The disease is latent before puberty, and symptoms are more common in adult women than men. This porphyria is exacerbated by many of the same factors that precipitate attacks in AIP, including barbiturates and other drugs, as well as endogenous or exogenous steroid hormones. Symptoms can occur in association with the menstrual cycle. Fasting, a risk factor for induction of both ALAS1 and HO-1, has also been shown to decrease hepatic CPO activity in pigs. The risk of hepatocellular carcinoma may be increased in this porphyria, as in AIP and variegate porphyria. A few homozygous cases of hereditary coproporphyria, with cutaneous lesions beginning in early childhood, have been reported.

The most prominent biochemical feature of hereditary coproporphyria is a marked increase in urinary and fecal coproporphyrin, predominantly isomer type III, with levels typically 10–200 times those of controls.[19] Urinary ALA, porphobilinogen, and uroporphyrin are also increased during acute attacks.

Treatment

Treatment of acute attacks of hereditary coproporphyria is identical to the treatment of AIP.

Variegate Porphyria

Variegate porphyria is an autosomal dominant acute hepatic porphyria caused by a deficiency in activity of protoporphyrinogen oxidase (PPO), the penultimate enzyme in the heme biosynthetic pathway. The disease is termed *variegate* because it can present either with neurologic manifestations, cutaneous photosensitivity, or both. It is also called porphyria variegata, protocoproporphyria, and South African genetic porphyria.

In most countries this porphyria is less commonly recognized than AIP. In contrast, variegate porphyria is very common in whites in South Africa, where it was first reported in 1945.[20] As many as 20,000 South Africans may carry this mutation, which is now found to be an R59W mutation of the *PPO* gene.

Clinical Findings

The acute attack is identical to that seen in AIP, and may include abdominal pain, tachycardia, vomiting, constipation, hypertension, neuropathy, back pain, confusion, bulbar paralysis, psychiatric symptoms, fever, urinary frequency, and dysuria. Hyponatremia with evidence of sodium depletion or inappropriate secretion of antidiuretic hormone can occur during acute attacks. Attacks of variegate porphyria are generally milder than those of AIP, and recurrent attacks are less common. Cutaneous photosensitivity is more common than in hereditary coproporphyria. Skin manifestations generally occur, and are usually of longer duration. They are very similar to those seen in PCT and hereditary coproporphyria, and include increased fragility, vesicles, bullae, erosions, milia, hyperpigmentation, and hypertrichosis of sun-exposed areas. Photosensitivity may be less commonly associated with variegate porphyria in northern countries, where sunlight is less intense.[21]

Fecal protoporphyrin and coproporphyrin and urinary coproporphyrin are markedly increased when variegate porphyria is clinically active. Urinary ALA, porphobilinogen, and uroporphyrin are increased during acute attacks but may be normal or only slightly increased during remission. Plasma porphyrin is commonly increased, and is a dicarboxylate porphyrin tightly bound to plasma proteins. Biliary porphyrins are also increased in variegate porphyria, and the risk of gallstones, which contain protoporphyrin, may be increased. The X porphyrin fraction (ether–acetic acid–insoluble porphyrins extractable from feces by urea-Triton) is increased in variegate porphyria. Rare homozygous variegate porphyria patients have markedly increased levels of erythrocyte zinc-protoporphyrin complex.[22]

Treatment

Treatment of acute attacks of variegate porphyria is identical to the treatment of AIP.

CHRONIC HEPATIC PORPHYRIA

Patients with chronic hepatic porphyria, such as PCT, have significant chronic cutaneous photosensitivity but not neurologic symptoms. The skin of patients with all types of cutaneous porphyrias (CEP, hepatoerythropoietic porphyria, PCT, variegate porphyria, and erythropoietic protoporphyria) is maximally sensitive to light near 400 nm, corresponding to the Soret band, the narrow peak absorption maximum characteristic of all porphyrins. When porphyrins absorb light of this wavelength, they enter an excited energy state. This energy is released as fluorescence and by the formation of singlet oxygen and other oxygen radicals that can result in tissue damage. This may then be accompanied by lipid peroxidation, oxidation of amino acids, and cross-linking of proteins in cell membranes.[23]

Petechiae and purpuric lesions may occur. Skin lichenification, leathery pseudovesicles, and nail changes can be pronounced. Chronic blistering lesions may develop; the fluid-filled vesicles rupture easily and the denuded areas become crusted and heal slowly; secondary infection is common. Previous areas of blisters may appear atrophic or brownish. Facial hypertrichosis, scarring, and hyperpigmentation may result.

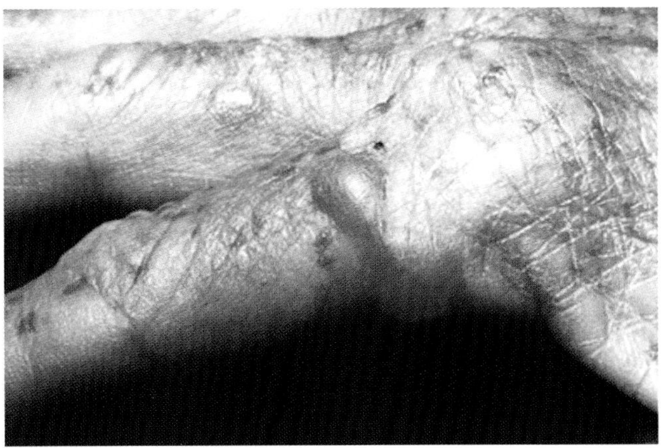

Figure 54–8. Vesicles and erosions are visible on the dorsum of the hand in a patient with PCT. (Courtesy of Jean-François Dufour, MD. From Sassa S: Porphyria cutanea tarda, hepatoerythropoietic porphyria, and toxic porphyria. *In* Rose BD [ed]: UpToDate. Wellesley, MA: UpToDate, 2001.)

Porphyria Cutanea Tarda

PCT is due to a profound deficiency of uroporphyrinogen decarboxylase activity in the liver. It is also called symptomatic porphyria, porphyria cutanea tarda symptomatica, or idiosyncratic porphyria.

Pathophysiology

PCT has been classified into three subtypes. Type I has decreased hepatic UROD activity but normal erythrocyte UROD activity, and is found in sporadic fashion without family history. Type II has decreased UROD activity both in red cells and in liver, and occurs as more than one case in a family. Type III is similar to type II with respect to familial occurrence, but erythrocyte UROD activity is normal. In contrast to PCT, hepatoerythropoietic porphyria is due to homozygous, or compound heterozygous, mutations of the *UROD* gene, and presents clinically as an entirely different disorder.

Clinical Findings

Chronic blistering lesions develop on sun-exposed areas of skin (Fig. 54–8). The fluid-filled vesicles rupture easily, and the denuded areas become crusted and heal slowly. Secondary infection can occur. Previous areas of blisters may appear atrophic or brownish. Facial hypertrichosis and hyperpigmentation are also common. Identification and avoidance of precipitating factors, especially alcohol, is important. All types of PCT respond readily to repeated phlebotomy. PCT can also be treated with chloroquine or hydroxychloroquine (administered in a very-low-dosage regimen).

Porphyrins accumulate in large amounts in the liver, and are increased in plasma. Uroporphyrin and heptacarboxylporphyrin are predominantly increased in urine. Multiple factors can contribute to inactivation or inhibition of hepatic UROD in this disease, probably by an iron-dependent oxidative mechanism, including alcohol, hepatitis C infection, estrogen, human immunodeficiency virus, smoking, and factors that increase hepatic iron content, such as mutations of the *HFE* gene. Liver biopsy frequently shows hemosiderosis, and serum iron and ferritin concentrations are increased. Patients often develop cirrhosis, and may occasionally develop hepatoma.

Urinary porphyrin excretion is markedly increased. There is no increase in ALA or porphobilinogen in this disorder. Fecal isocoproporphyrin is the biochemical stigmata of the disease, and its detection establishes the diagnosis. Isocoproporphyrin III is formed from dehydroisocoproporphyrinogen III, which is normally a minor product but can accumulate from pentacarboxylate porphyrinogen III if UROD activity is reduced.

Treatment

In type I PCT, the identification and avoidance of precipitating factors is the first line of treatment. Avoiding alcohol may improve symptoms. Phlebotomy will reduce urinary porphyrin concentration and body iron stores. Chloroquine is thought to chelate porphyrins to facilitate their water solubility, increasing excretion into urine. The efficacy of chloroquine therapy may be similar to that of phlebotomy, and combined therapy may diminish the incidence of side effects.

CURRENT CONTROVERSIES & FUTURE CONSIDERATIONS

Porphyrias

- The pathogenetic mechanism of neurologic symptoms remains unknown.
- Is molecular diagnosis useful for screening porphyrias? If the defective gene were identified in the proband, such information would be useful for screening gene carriers in the family.
- Is gene therapy possible in the near future? It is most likely to be attempted first in homozygous porphyrias, such as CEP, and may offer a great promise. In contrast, gene therapy for autosomal dominant forms of porphyria is a more complex problem, because treatment should be targeted to bring the derepressed ALAS1 in check. However, with the advent of new technology (e.g., siRNA for ALAS1), such treatment may also be possible in the future.
- What is the impact of porphyria gene defects in environmental medicine? Hepatic porphyrias represent the best model of pharmacogenetic disorders, and significant gene-environment interaction can be unraveled through studies in the acutely ill patients as well as in latent gene carriers. Latent gene carriers of acute hepatic porphyrias may represent a population that may be supersensitive to drugs, chemicals, or metals that interfere with heme biosynthesis.

Suggested Readings*

Anderson KE, Sassa S, Bishop DF, Desnick RJ: Disorders of heme biosynthesis: X-linked sideroblastic anemia and the porphyrias. *In* Scriver CR, Beaudet AL, Sly WS, Valle D (eds): The Metabolic & Molecular Bases of Inherited Disease. New York: McGraw-Hill, 2001, p 2991.

Sassa S: Diagnosis and therapy of acute intermittent porphyria. Blood Rev 10:53–58, 1996.

Sassa S: Understanding the porphyrias. *In* Rose BD (ed): UpToDate. Wellesley, MA: UpToDate, 2001.

Full references for this chapter can be found on accompanying CD-ROM.

CHAPTER 55
Sideroblastic Anemias

Mario Cazzola, MD, and Rosangela Invernizzi, MD

KEY POINTS

Sideroblastic Anemias

Diagnosis

- Males with hereditary X-linked sideroblastic anemia (XLSA) may present in the first two decades of life with anemia, or later with either anemia and/or symptoms and signs of parenchymal iron overload. Occasional patients, both men and women, may be diagnosed with this constitutional disease late in life.
- Distinctive features of XLSA are microcytic anemia with hypochromic red cells, increased red cell distribution width, and parenchymal iron overload.
- Patients with acquired refractory anemia with ring sideroblasts (RARS) have a median age at presentation of about 65 years. The isolated anemia is typically macrocytic; leukocyte and platelet counts are normal at diagnosis, and most patients have some evidence of iron overload, as indicated by increased serum iron, transferrin saturation, and serum ferritin.
- Bone marrow examination is crucial to the diagnosis in showing dyserythropoiesis and 15% or more ring sideroblasts. After Prussian blue staining, ring sideroblasts are identified as immature red cells in which 10 or more blue granules representing iron-loaded mitochondria form a ring around the nucleus.
- XLSA is caused by mutations in the erythroid-specific δ-aminolevulinate synthase gene (*ALAS2*). DNA or reticulocyte RNA should be tested for *ALAS2* mutations, in patients and family members irrespective of sex and age.

Treatment

- Management of XLSA involves treatment of anemia, prevention and reversal of iron overload, family studies to identify additional at-risk individuals, and genetic counseling.
- Most patients with XLSA are to some extent responsive to pyridoxine; the initial dosage is 75–150 mg/day.
- In XLSA, response to pyridoxine is greatly influenced by body iron status, and iron overload may suppress pyridoxine responsiveness. Reversal of iron overload by phlebotomy can result in higher hemoglobin concentrations during pyridoxine supplementation.
- Most patients with iron overload can safely undergo mild phlebotomy programs under pyridoxine supplementation.
- Supportive therapy is the only treatment currently available for patients with RARS.
- Patients with RARS with a regular need for blood transfusion should receive iron chelation therapy with desferrioxamine.

INTRODUCTION

The sideroblastic anemias are a heterogeneous group of inherited and acquired disorders characterized by anemia of varying severity and the presence of ring sideroblasts in the bone marrow.[1–3] Ring sideroblasts are erythroblasts with iron-loaded mitochondria, visualized on Prussian blue staining as a perinuclear ring of blue granules.

The history of sideroblastic anemia[2] starts in 1945, when Cooley, the same Detroit pediatric-hematologist who first described thalassemia in the 1920s, reported a family with microcytic anemia different from Mediterranean anemia.[4] This novel condition was later defined as X-linked sideroblastic anemia (XLSA), and its molecular basis was identified 50 years later by Cotter and coworkers.[5] Dacie and Doniach[6] described iron-positive granules in erythrocytes in 1947, and 10 years later French investigators[7] showed that these granules were iron-loaded mitochondria on electron microscopy. The sideroblastic bone marrow was first described in patients with refractory acquired anemia.[8] The term *sideroblastic anemia*, used to define inherited and acquired conditions with ring sideroblasts, was introduced in 1965.[9]

CLASSIFICATION AND EPIDEMIOLOGY

The sideroblastic anemias are classified as hereditary or acquired, as listed in Table 55–1. The most common of

TABLE 55–1. Classification of the Sideroblastic Anemias

Category	OMIM and Molecular Basis	Main Clinical Manifestation(s)
Hereditary Sideroblastic Anemias		
X-linked sideroblastic anemia (XLSA)	OMIM 301300; mutations in the erythroid-specific ALA synthase gene (*ALAS2*)	Anemia, iron overload
X-linked sideroblastic anemia with cerebellar ataxia (XLSA/A)	OMIM 301310; mutations in the *ABC7* gene (OMIM 300135)	Nonprogressive cerebellar ataxia
Mitochondrial myopathy, lactic acidosis, and sideroblastic anemia (MLASA)	OMIM 600462; autosomal recessive disorder caused by mutations in the *PUS1* gene (OMIM 608109)	Mitochondrial myopathy, lactic acidosis
Pearson's marrow-pancreas syndrome (sideroblastic anemia with vacuolization of marrow precursors and exocrine pancreatic dysfunction)	OMIM 557000; multiple deletions of mitochondrial DNA.	Exocrine pancreatic dysfunction
Acquired Sideroblastic Anemias		
Myelodysplastic syndrome (refractory anemia with ring sideroblasts [RARS]; refractory cytopenia with multilineage dysplasia and ring sideroblasts [RCMD-RS])	Point mutations in mitochondrial DNA in occasional patients	Anemia, pancytopenia
Myelodysplastic/myeloproliferative disorders with ring sideroblasts		Anemia, thrombocytosis
Ethanol-induced sideroblastic anemia		Anemia
Drug-induced sideroblastic anemia (chloramphenicol, isoniazid)		Anemia

the inherited forms is XLSA (Online Mendelian Inheritance in Man [OMIM] 301300), which is caused by mutations in the erythroid-specific δ-aminolevulinate synthase 2 gene (*ALAS2*). Fewer than 50 unrelated XLSA families have been reported to date. Other inherited sideroblastic anemias are rarer, and occasional cases of autosomal dominant and autosomal recessive sideroblastic anemia have not been characterized molecularly.

The most common acquired sideroblastic anemia is a myelodysplastic syndrome defined as refractory anemia with ring sideroblasts (RARS) (see Chapter 15). Myelodysplastic syndromes are frequent hematologic disorders: the crude incidence is about 5 per 100,000 population per year, and about 40 per 100,000 per year in individuals over 70 years of age.[10] Thus, refractory anemia with ring sideroblasts, which represents about one fourth of the myelodysplastic syndromes, is a relatively common hematologic disease of the elderly (see Chapter 73).

PATHOPHYSIOLOGY

Because of the heterogeneity of sideroblastic anemias, different pathophysiologic mechanisms operate in these conditions. Ring sideroblasts, increased mitochondrial ferritin, ineffective erythropoiesis, and iron loading are consistent features of all these syndromes.

Ferritin Sideroblasts and Ring Sideroblasts

Most of the iron used in erythroblasts for hemoglobin synthesis derives from transferrin internalized on the transferrin receptor (Fig. 55–1).[11] The excess iron is stored in ferritin molecules that partially aggregate, producing hemosiderin within specific endosomes called siderosomes. These iron-loaded endosomes are stained by the Perls' reaction (Prussian blue staining) in about one third of normal immature red cells, and erythroblasts with a few blue granules scattered in the cytoplasm are defined as "ferritin sideroblasts" (Fig. 55–2*A*). The number and size of ferritin sideroblasts typically increase in iron-loading anemias, such as thalassemia intermedia, and more generally whenever the iron supply to the erythroid marrow exceeds the amount required for hemoglobin synthesis (Fig. 55–2*B*).

After Prussian blue staining, the "ring sideroblasts" are identified as immature red cells in which 10 or more blue granules, representing iron-loaded mitochondria, form a ring around the nucleus (Fig. 55–2*C*). Ring sideroblasts differ from ferritin sideroblasts in two features (Fig. 55–2*D*): (1) Perls' reaction–positive granules tend to form a ring surrounding the nucleus, and (2) more important, the stained granules are iron-loaded mitochondria rather than cytoplasmic siderosomes containing ferritin and hemosiderin.

Mitochondrial Ferritin

Mitochondrial ferritin is a novel ferritin encoded by an intronless gene on chromosome 5q23.1.[12] The protein is synthesized as a precursor of about 30 kDa and targeted to mitochondria by a leader sequence of 60 amino acids, which is proteolytically removed inside the mitochondria. Mitochondrial ferritin has ferroxidase activity and is therefore likely to sequester potentially harmful free iron.[13] This protein has a very restricted tissue expression (erythroid cells, testis) and does not seem to be an obligatory intermediate in transfer of free iron to heme and other iron compounds in mitochondria. However, its level increases dramatically in sideroblastic anemia when heme synthesis is disrupted (Fig. 55–2*E*).[14]

Ineffective Erythropoiesis

A common mechanism of anemia is ineffective erythropoiesis, the premature death or apoptosis of immature

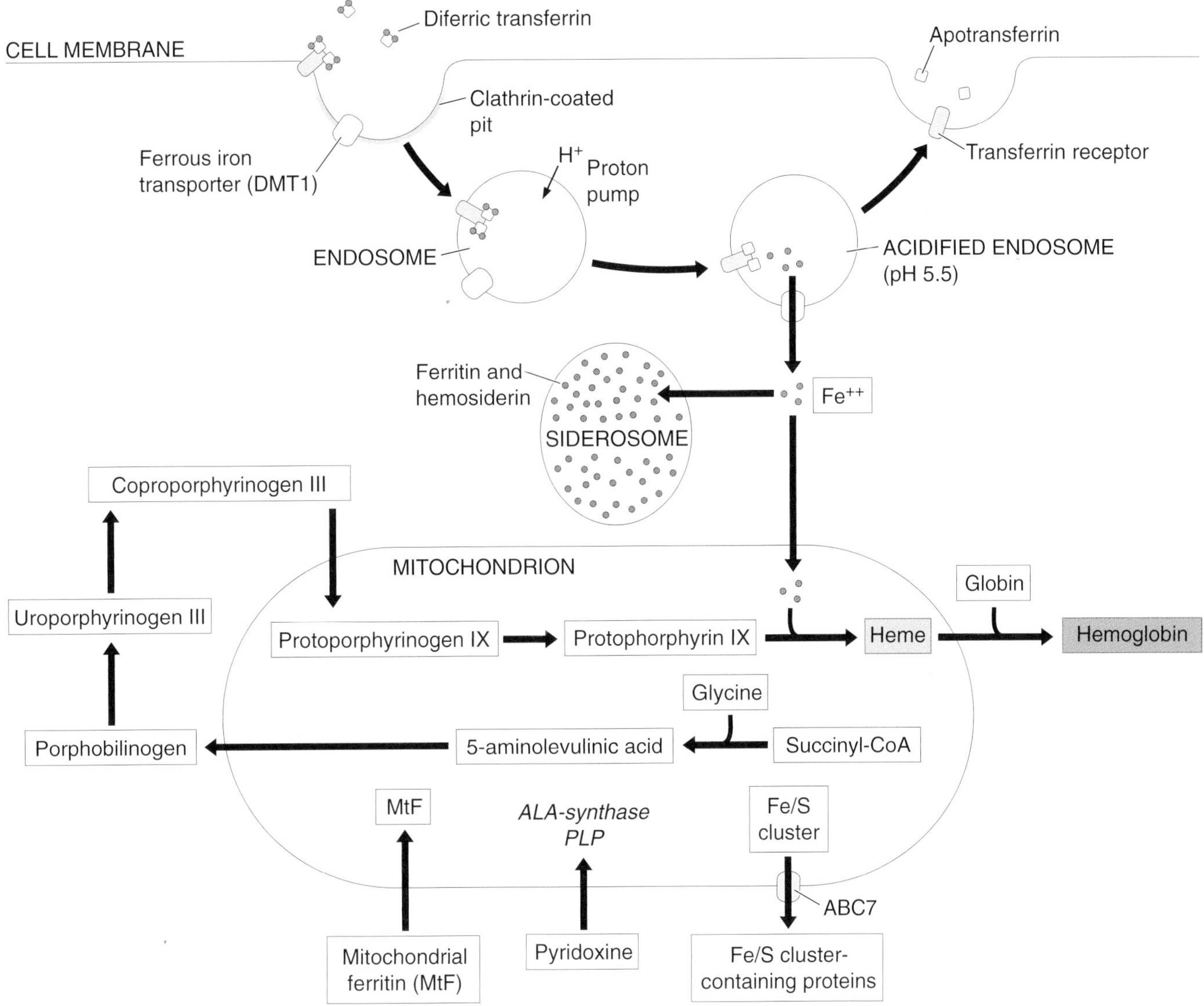

Figure 55–1. Cellular iron metabolism and hemoglobin synthesis in erythroid precursors. Iron procurement by mammalian cells is a typical pathway of receptor-mediated endocytosis. The transferrin receptor on the cell surface binds iron-loaded (diferric) transferrin with high affinity, and a transferrin-receptor complex is formed. A number of these complexes cluster in plasma membrane coated pits, enter the cell via coated vesicles, and move to endosomes, where the acidic pH induces iron release. Iron atoms are utilized for cellular functions and, when present in excess, are stored in ferritin molecules within specialized endosomes called siderosomes. After iron release, the transferrin-receptor complex is cycled back to the cell surface, and transferrin is released from the receptor to the plasma as apotransferrin.

In erythroid precursors, most of the iron is utilized for hemoglobin synthesis. The mitochondrion is primarily responsible for the synthesis of protoporphyrin and heme. Protoporphyrin synthesis begins and ends within the mitochondria after a transient shift to cytoplasm. The initial and limiting step is the formation of 5-aminolevulinic acid (ALA) from glycine and succinyl coenzyme A, which is mediated by erythroid ALA synthase (ALAS; EC 2.3.1.37, encoded by the erythroid-specific *ALAS2* gene). The ALAS2 protein is a pyridoxal 5′-phosphate (PLP)–dependent enzyme: PLP binding to the enzyme is crucial for its stability and catalytic activity. In humans, PLP derives from the pyridoxine absorbed from the gut. The final reaction of heme biosynthesis involves combination of ferrous iron with protoporphyrin IX and is mediated by ferrochelatase.

ABC7 is a "half-type" ATP binding cassette transporter of crucial importance for the maturation of cytosolic iron-sulfur (Fe/S) cluster–containing proteins, and is likely responsible for the transport out of mitochondria of Fe/S clusters destined for the cytosol.

Mitochondrial ferritin (MtF) is encoded by a nuclear gene and synthesized as a precursor that is targeted to mitochondria by a leader sequence. This leader is proteolytically removed inside the mitochondria and the resulting subunit forms typical ferritin shells. MtF is not an obligatory intermediate in transfer of free iron to heme and other iron compounds in mitochondria. Its level increases dramatically in sideroblastic anemia when heme synthesis is disrupted and mitochondrial iron overload occurs.

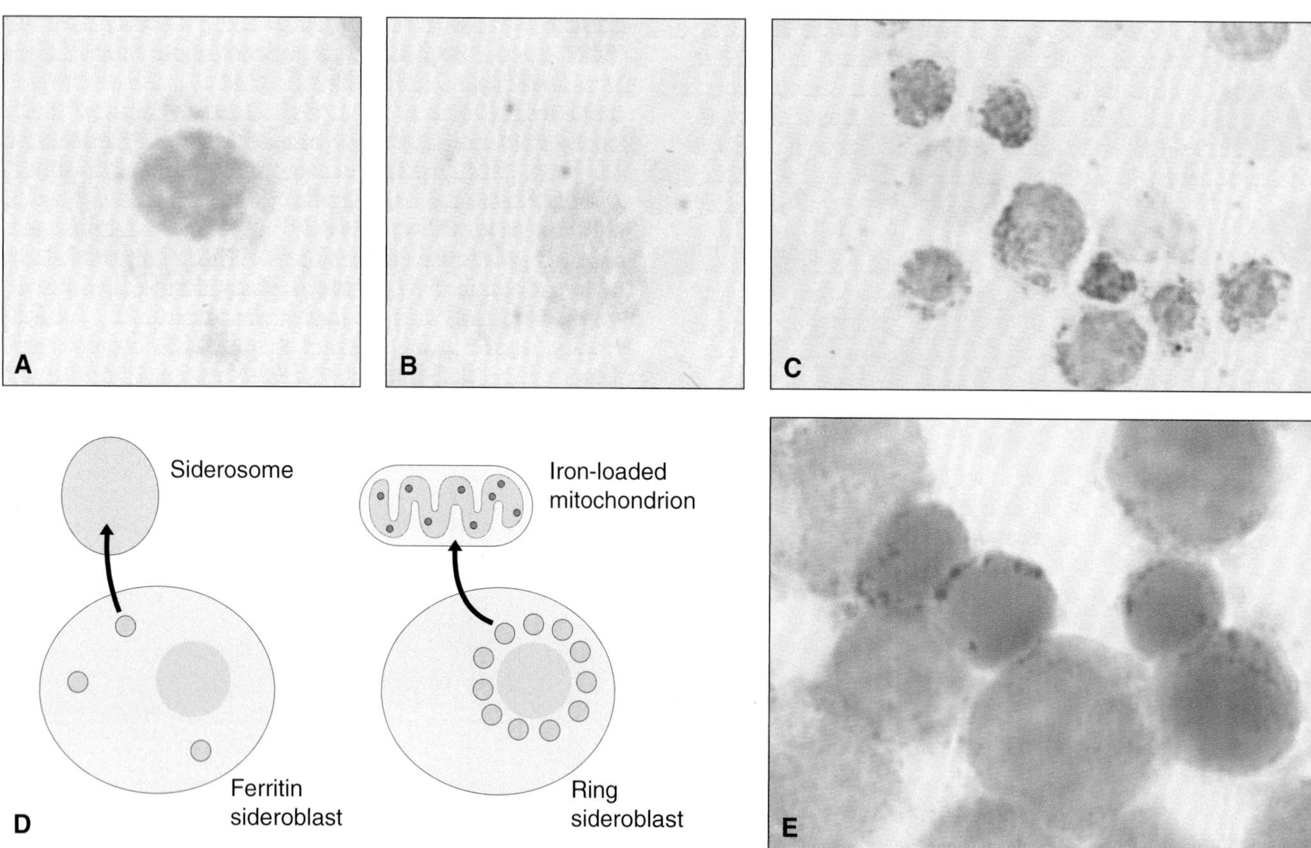

Figure 55–2. Ferritin sideroblasts and ring sideroblasts. ***A–C,*** Perls' Prussian blue–stained bone marrow (Perls' reaction, × 1250). ***A,*** Bone marrow smear from a healthy control shows ferritin sideroblast with few (4–5) small iron-containing granules. ***B,*** Bone marrow smear from a patient with iron overload shows ferritin sideroblast with more numerous (about 9) and rather large granules, diffusely scattered in the cytoplasm. ***C,*** Bone marrow smear from a patient with sideroblastic anemia shows ring sideroblasts with many granules (≥10) surrounding at least one third of the circumference of the nucleus. ***D,*** Schematic representation of ferritin and ring sideroblasts. ***E,*** Bone marrow smear from a patient with sideroblastic anemia (immunoalkaline phosphatase staining for mitochondrial ferritin, × 1250). Many erythroblasts are positive for mitochondrial ferritin (MtF), which appears as granules ringing the nucleus. This pattern is similar to that observed with the Perls' reaction ***(C)*** and consistent with mitochondrial localization of MtF.

nucleated red cells in the bone marrow, likely caused by mitochondrial iron overload.[15] Ineffective erythropoiesis represents the major factor responsible for anemia in XLSA. Patients have erythroid hyperplasia of the bone marrow but reticulocyte counts that are inappropriately low for the degree of anemia.[16] The pathogenesis of anemia is more complex in refractory anemia with ring sideroblasts, wherein variable combinations of ineffective erythropoiesis and reduced proliferative activity of erythroid cells are responsible for the defective red cell production.[17]

Abnormalities in mean cell volume (MCV) are common in sideroblastic anemias; two opposite patterns can be recognized. As a result of defective heme synthesis, XLSA is typically associated with impaired hemoglobin synthesis and in turn with microcytic (MCV < 80 fL), hypochromic (mean cell hemoglobin < 27 pg) red blood cells. By contrast, refractory anemia with ring sideroblasts is associated with red blood cell macrocytosis (MCV > 100 fL).

Iron Loading

Congenital anemias caused by ineffective erythropoiesis, such as XLSA, are associated with excessive iron absorption and progressive iron loading.[18] The degree of anemia is a poor predictor of iron loading, which correlates better with erythroid marrow activity. The mechanism by which erythroid marrow expansion induces a positive iron balance is unknown, but some components of the erythroid marrow must mediate the message between expanded erythropoiesis and increased intestinal iron absorption. Inactivation of hepcidin production by the liver may be responsible for excessive intestinal absorption in these patients.[19]

Parenchymal iron loading is less clinically relevant in patients with refractory anemia with ring sideroblasts because of shorter disease duration and less ineffective erythropoiesis in the acquired condition. However, RARS patients may present with iron overload, and in all individuals with a regular need for blood transfusion, secondary hemochromatosis ultimately occurs.

X-LINKED CONGENITAL SIDEROBLASTIC ANEMIA

XLSA is caused by missense mutations in the erythroid-specific gene *ALAS2* that result in deficient activity of the erythroid-specific form of the mitochondrial enzyme 5-aminolevulinate synthase (ALAS2; E.C. 2.3.1.37).[20,21] The housekeeping gene *ALAS1* is expressed at low levels in all tissues; the erythroid-specific gene *ALAS2* is expressed at high levels in erythroid precursors. Human *ALAS2* maps on chromosome Xp11.21, spans about 22kb, and consists of 11 exons of varying sizes.[21] Hemoglobin synthesis requires a coordinated production of heme molecules and globin chains (see Fig. 55–1 and Chapter 2). The *ALAS2* promoter contains putative binding sites for the transcription factors GATA-1 and NF-E2, which also play crucial roles in the erythroid-specific activation of globin genes.[22] Although *ALAS2* is primarily regulated at the transcriptional level, its expression is also modulated translationally, as synthesis of the *ALAS2* messenger RNA is dependent on an adequate iron supply.[23]

The erythroid-specific isoform of ALAS (X-chromosome–encoded ALAS2 protein) catalyzes the rate-limiting step in heme biosynthesis and provides the large quantity of heme required by erythroid cells for hemoglobin production (see Fig. 55–1). The ALAS2 protein is a pyridoxal 5′-phosphate (PLP)–dependent enzyme, and PLP binding to the enzyme is required for stability and catalytic activity.[21] As a mitochondrion enzyme, the ALAS2 protein must transit from the cytosol to the mitochondrial matrix, and this transport is likely important for regulation of its levels in the mitochondrial space.

Molecular Pathogenesis

There are now over 30 mutations in *ALAS2* described in more than 30 XLSA kindreds.[24–27] All but one of these mutations are single-base substitutions, which appear to be clustered with respect to gene structure within the region of the enzyme conserved in prokaryotes, encoded by exons 5–11. Altered substrate interaction, reduced affinity for PLP, lower apoenzyme stability, or inappropriate/ absent mitochondrial processing may all account for defective ALAS2 enzyme activity in bone marrow erythroblasts in XLSA.[21] A promoter mutation in *ALAS2* causing XLSA has been recently described[27]; this mutation occurred in or near three different putative transcription factor–binding sites and resulted in dramatic decreases in messenger RNA *ALAS2* level and protein activity.

Defective ALAS2 enzyme activity in bone marrow erythroid cells leads to insufficient protoporphyrin IX synthesis, mitochondrial iron overload, and intramedullary death of red cell precursors. Most but not all XLSA patients are, to a variable extent, responsive to pyridoxine, which is metabolized to PLP.

Almost all XLSA patients are hemizygous males. Most heterozygous females have only minor red cell abnormalities (in particular, an increased red cell distribution width [RDW]) but no clinical signs, because immature red cells expressing the normal ALAS2 are sufficient to sustain a normal level of red cell production. As in any X-linked disorder, the clinical phenotype of female carriers may be influenced by the pattern of X-chromosome inactivation (or lyonization). The adult female is a mosaic of two cell populations, one expressing the genes on the maternal X chromosome and the other expressing those on the paternal X chromosome. The distribution of the active parental X chromosome lies between 50:50 and 80:20 for most females. However, a small percentage of women are highly skewed: more than 80% of their cells express the alleles from one parental X chromosome. A few XLSA female heterozygotes may therefore preferentially express the mutant allele in erythroid cells and are anemic.[26,28] Different genetic and acquired mechanisms may lead to a skewed pattern of X-chromosome inactivation in females and represent causes of disease in women heterozygous for mutant X-chromosomal genes.

Clinical Features

Hematologic Findings and Body Iron Status

Affected males may present in the first two decades of life with anemia, or later with either anemia or evidence of parenchymal iron overload. Occasional patients do not become symptomatic until late in life. Phenotypic expression of XLSA varies considerably in males and is partly related to the type of *ALAS2* mutation.[24]

Anemia is microcytic (MCV < 80fL, generally between 60 and 70fL) and hypochromic (mean cell hemoglobin < 27pg), and is characterized by elevated values for RDW (>14%) (Table 55–2). The reticulocyte count is inadequately low for the degree of anemia (<3% and <150 × 10^9/L), excluding peripheral hemolysis as a major factor leading to anemia. The peripheral blood smear shows anisopoikilocytosis with hypochromic microcytes (Fig. 55–3*A*). Almost all patients with XLSA have evidence of iron loading at clinical onset, and symptoms of parenchymal iron overload can be the first manifestation of disease in middle-aged men (see Table 55–2). Bone marrow examination is of crucial diagnostic importance in showing dyserythropoiesis and ring sideroblasts (Fig. 55–3*B* and *C*).

Sideroblasts: Peculiar Clinical Issues

Coinheritance of Genetic Hemochromatosis as a Factor Worsening Parenchymal Iron Overload in XLSA

A major complication of XLSA is increased iron absorption and secondary iron overload. Although erythroid marrow expansion and ineffective erythropoiesis are central, additional abnormalities in iron absorption may further contribute to iron loading in individual patients with XLSA. HFE-related genetic hemochromatosis (OMIM 235200) is a common cause of increased iron absorption from the gut (see Chapter 56). The frequency of *HFE* C282Y allele is about 0.05 in white populations, and thus XLSA patients have a real possibility of also being *HFE* C282Y heterozygotes. Although the presence of the *HFE* C282Y gene is not required for iron loading to occur in XLSA patients, a significantly higher frequency of

TABLE 55–2. Hematologic Data from Representative Patients with XLSA

Parameter	14-Year-Old Boy	38-Year-Old Man	50-Year-Old Man	64-Year-Old Woman*
Hb (gm/dL)	8.1	7.6	9.4	5.2
MCV (fL)	65	64	67	74
MCH	20.3	19.2	19.1	23.8
Reticulocyte count ($\times 10^9$/L)	40	48	39	na
RDW (%)	na	30.9	29.5	22.5
Serum iron (μg/dL)	173	180	241	na
Serum ferritin (ng/mL)	383	859	6084	3954
Initial diagnosis	Heterozygous β-thalassemia	Myelodysplastic syndrome	Genetic hemochromatosis	Myelodysplastic syndrome
ALAS2 mutation/a mino acid change	G1236A/C395Y	G1731A/R560H	G1407A/R452H	G1236A/C395Y
Response to pyridoxine, average Hb (gm/dL)	14.6	9.6	13.4	12.3

*Grandmother of the 14-year-old boy.

Abbreviations: Hb, hemoglobin; MCH, mean cell hemoglobin; MCV, mean cell volume; na, not available; RDW, red cell distribution width.

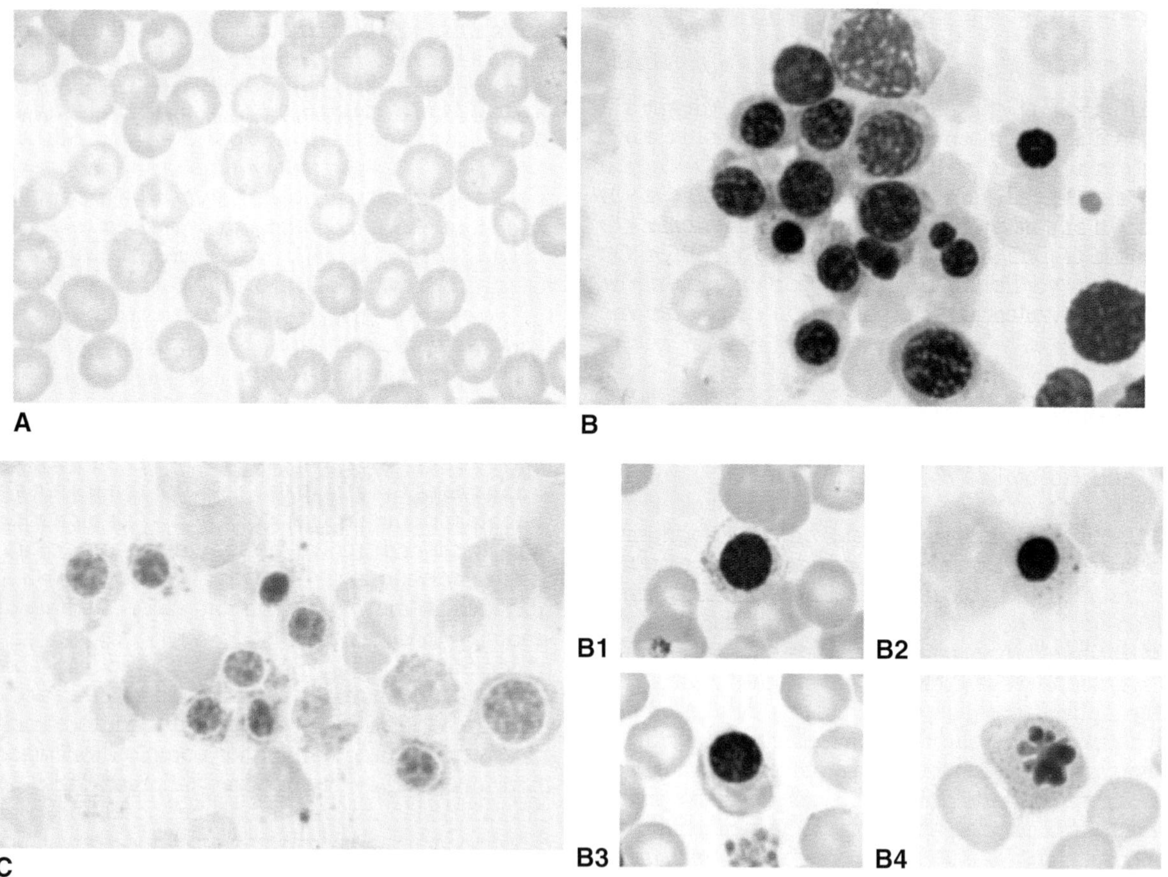

■ **Figure 55–3.** Peripheral blood and bone marrow smears from a patient with X-linked sideroblastic anemia. ***A,*** Peripheral blood smear showing anisopoikilocytosis with hypochromic microcytes and some target cells (May-Grünwald-Giemsa [MGG] staining, × 1250). ***B,*** Bone marrow smear showing erythroid hyperplasia with predominance of small late erythroblasts. Erythroblasts are small; cytoplasm is often incompletely hemoglobinized with occasional Pappenheimer bodies. (MGG, × 1250.) *B1–B4,* Bone marrow smear showing erythroid hyperplasia with predominance of small late erythroblasts. Small late dystrophic erythroblasts showing vacuolation, defective hemoglobinization, ill-defined edges, heavily granulated cytoplasm, and nuclear lobulation. (MGG, × 1250.) ***C,*** Bone marrow smear. Most late erythroid cells are ring sideroblasts with numerous (>10) positive granules disposed in a ring surrounding a third or more of the circumference of the nucleus. (Perls' reaction, × 1250.)

coinheritance of the mutant allele C282Y has been found in unrelated XLSA hemizygotes, implicating a role for coinheritance of *HFE* alleles in the expression of this disorder.[24] XLSA patients with the *HFE* C282Y mutation have more elevated serum ferritin levels than do those with no mutation. The 50-year-old man with severe iron overload reported in Table 55–2 was heterozygous for the *HFE* C282Y mutation: he was initially diagnosed with genetic hemochromatosis and only later found to have pyridoxine-responsive XLSA.

Late-Onset XLSA

Both anemia and iron overload may be associated with no or such mild manifestations that a diagnosis is ultimately made in an elderly individual.[28] Late-onset XLSA also has been occasionally described in heterozygous women who preferentially express the mutant allele in erythroid cells. In one elderly woman who presented with an apparently acquired sideroblastic anemia (see Table 55–2), molecular analysis revealed heterozygosity for a missense mutation in the *ALAS2* gene, and only the mutated gene in her reticulocytes. All analyzable women in her family showed skewed X-chromosome inactivation in leukocytes, indicating a hereditary condition associated with unbalanced lyonization. Because the preferentially active X-chromosome carried the mutant *ALAS2* allele, skewing exaggerated with aging worsened the genetic condition and abolished the normal *ALAS2* allele expression in the patient. About 3 of 10 female carriers of X-linked recessive disorders are expected to develop skewed hematopoiesis over time; skewing also may become extreme in those women whose lyonization is already unbalanced on a genetic basis, leading to development of clinical manifestations and mimicking an acquired condition.

Variable Penetrance and Phenotypic Expression of XLSA

Phenotypic expression of XLSA varies considerably in males and is partly related to the specific *ALAS2* mutation. In addition, modifying genes such as those for genetic hemochromatosis may significantly exacerbate XLSA in hemizygous males.

In a 38-year-old man who presented with microcytic anemia and iron overload, molecular analysis of *ALAS2* showed a 1731G→A mutation, predicting an R560H amino acid change (see Table 55–2).[25] A 36-year-old brother was hemizygous for this mutation and expressed the mutated *ALAS2* messenger RNA in his reticulocytes, but he had almost no phenotypic expression. All five heterozygous females from this family, including the three daughters of the nonanemic hemizygous male, showed marginally increased RDW. Thus, phenotypic expression can be absent in hemizygous males. Genetic counseling should rely on gene-based diagnosis.

Diagnosis and Genetic Counseling

The distinctive features of XLSA are microcytic anemia with hypochromic red cells, increased RDW, and laboratory evidence of parenchymal iron overload. Bone marrow aspiration and Perls' staining are required to demonstrate ring sideroblasts, and the genetic nature of the disease is established through mutation detection (Fig. 55–4).

Mutations can be detected in either genomic DNA or complementary DNA derived from the RNA of reticulocytes. Any subject who is suspected of having XLSA or belongs to a family with XLSA should have DNA or reticulocyte RNA tested for *ALAS2* mutations, irrespective of sex and age. DNA-based diagnosis facilitates testing of other family members. Although heterozygous women show some degrees of anisopoikilocytosis and marginally elevated RDW values, these criteria cannot be relied upon for routine diagnosis; genetic counseling requires that a diagnosis of the carrier state be made in the DNA.

Treatment

Management of XLSA involves treatment of anemia, prevention and treatment of iron overload, family studies to identify additional at-risk individuals, and genetic counseling.

Pyridoxine Supplementation

Most patients with XLSA are to some extent responsive to pyridoxine, which is metabolized to PLP, the cofactor for the ALAS2 enzyme. Every patient with XLSA should be treated with vitamin B_6. There is no consensus on the optimal daily dose, but available evidence indicates that 75–150 mg/day are effective in improving anemia in nearly all responsive patients. The lower dose (75 mg/day) should be used in younger and smaller patients, and the higher dose (150 mg/day) in larger patients, in those with regular physical activity, and in the elderly. Most patients show a complete or partial improvement in hemoglobin level: any significant increase in hemoglobin during pyridoxine therapy categorizes a patient as responsive. Small or equivocal increase in hemoglobin with treatment can be related to the drug by repeated observations or withdrawing and restarting the vitamin. Although the hemoglobin level can normalize, MCV, mean cell hemoglobin, and RDW improve but remain abnormal in all patients.

Response to pyridoxine supplementation is greatly influenced by body iron status: iron overload may suppress pyridoxine responsiveness. Reversal of hemochromatosis by phlebotomy generally results in higher hemoglobin concentrations during pyridoxine supplementation (Fig. 55–5). Therefore, combined phlebotomy (see later) and pyridoxine supplementation should be employed in the management of XLSA patients with refractory anemia and iron overload.

Some patients with XLSA are unresponsive to pyridoxine. Pyridoxine-refractory XLSA is due to mutations resulting in a reduction in the amount of functional mitochondrial enzyme, whereas pyridoxine-responsive XLSA is caused by mutations producing a reduction in stability and/or enzymatic activity of the functional enzyme.[21]

After a response, daily dosages at 37.5–75 mg should then be assessed to determine the lowest dose needed to maintain an adequate hemoglobin level. Dosages up to 300 mg/day should be employed in unresponsive or

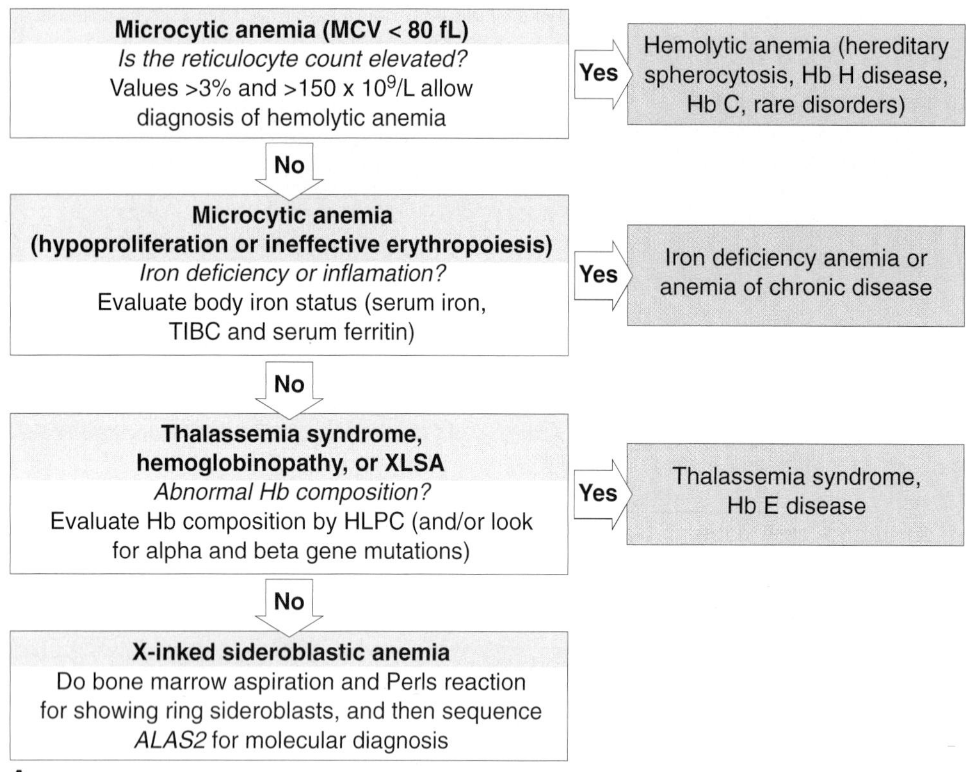

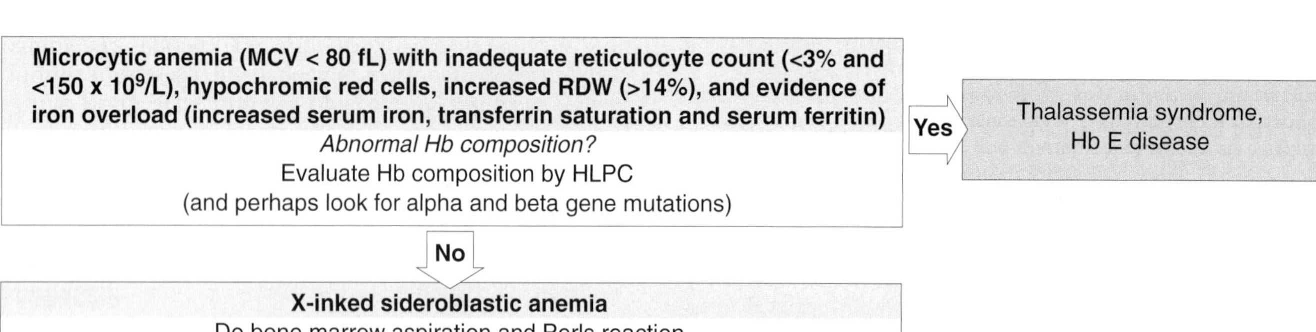

Figure 55–4. Diagnostic algorithm for X-linked sideroblastic anemia. *A*, Differential diagnosis of microcytic anemia. *B*, Differential diagnosis of microcytic anemia with inappropriately low reticulocyte count (<3% and < 150×10^9/L), hypochromic red cells, increased RDW (>14%), and evidence of parenchymal iron overload (increased serum iron, transferrin saturation, and serum ferritin).

partially responsive patients, but higher amounts should be avoided because they may cause peripheral sensory neuropathy. Careful monitoring of neurologic status is recommended in all treated patients.

Treatment of Iron Overload

The cause of death in XLSA patients is now secondary to the toxic effects of progressive iron overload resulting from sustained iron absorption and/or blood transfusions. Preventing and treating iron overload is therefore crucial.

Most patients with iron overload can safely undergo mild phlebotomy programs during pyridoxine supplementation: venesections (250–350 mL each, or 4–5 mL/kg body weight) can be performed every 2 weeks without any significant decline in hemoglobin level. There is generally a distinct elevation in hemoglobin once serum ferritin becomes normal (see Fig. 55–5). In patients with marginally elevated iron stores, iron overload can be avoided by two to three phlebotomies per year.

Severely anemic patients cannot undergo phlebotomy, and they require subcutaneous administration of desferrioxamine for treatment of iron overload. Doses of about

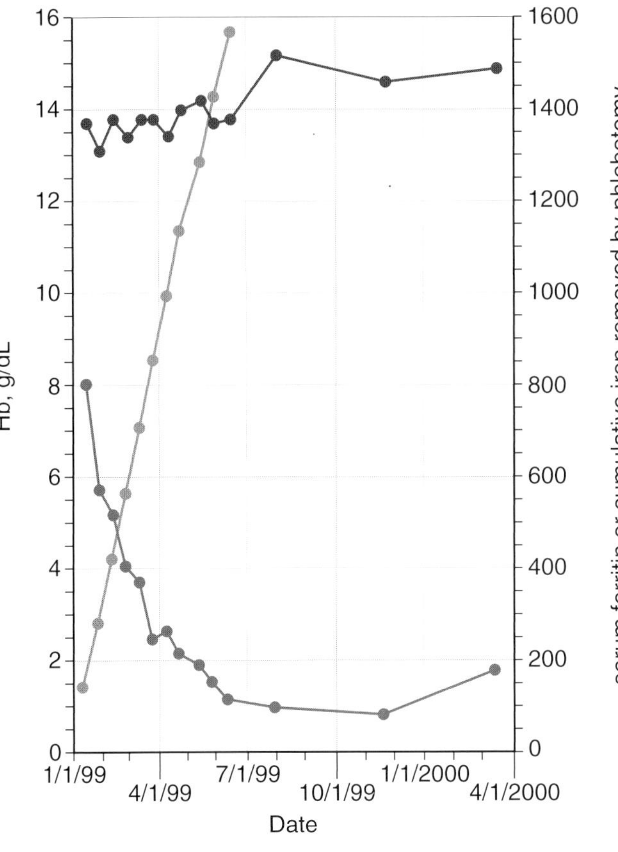

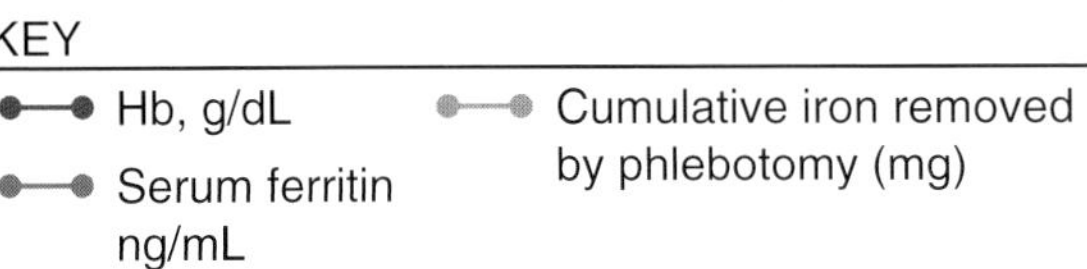

Figure 55–5. Phlebotomy in an XLSA patient. About 1.6 gm of iron was removed through venesections over a 6-month period under pyridoxine supplementation. The phlebotomy program (on average, 250 mL every 2 weeks) was easily performed, without significant decreases in hemoglobin level. Normalization of body iron stores resulted in higher hemoglobin levels. Despite the correction of anemia with pyridoxine, erythropoiesis remained expanded and led to iron loading (final part of serum ferritin time course), indicating the need for periodic preventive phlebotomies.

30–40 mg/kg/day should be administered, either by subcutaneous continuous infusion through a battery-operated portable pump (8 hr/day) or by twice-daily subcutaneous bolus injections (1 gm every 12 hours).

X-LINKED SIDEROBLASTIC ANEMIA ASSOCIATED WITH CEREBELLAR ATAXIA

XLSA associated with cerebellar ataxia (XLSA/A; OMIM 301310) is characterized by neurologic manifestations early in infancy with impaired gross motor and cognitive development.[29–31] Cerebellar ataxia is accompanied by selective cerebellar hypoplasia on computed tomography and does not worsen with age.

The severity of anemia varies considerably among the few families reported.[29–31] Patients have microcytic, hypochromic red cells with raised erythrocyte protoporphyrin levels, increased RDW values, and ring sideroblasts in the bone marrow. The anemia does not respond to pyridoxine, and body iron status is generally normal. This XLSA differs clinically from the classical XLSA (OMIM 301300), which does not have neurologic manifestations, is associated with iron overload, and is generally at least partially responsive to pyridoxine.

XLSA/A was mapped to Xq13 by linkage analysis[32] and then shown to be caused by missense mutations in the human *ABC7* gene, which encodes a "half-type" ATP binding cassette (ABC) transporter.[33,34] The ABC7 protein is a functional orthologue of Atm1p, which is important in the maturation of cytosolic iron-sulfur Fe-S cluster–containing proteins in yeast.[35,36] *ABC7* mutations result in impaired maturation of cytosolic Fe-S cluster-containing proteins.[30] Although the precise transport function of ABC7 is not certain, available evidence suggests a role in the transport out of mitochondria of Fe-S clusters destined for the cytosol (see Fig. 55–1).

The mechanism responsible for sideroblastic anemia is unclear because neither ALAS nor ferrochelatase activity is defective. Mitochondrial iron overload is likely caused by defects in transport function of ABC7, but why disruption in the export of Fe-S clusters or their precursors should prevent incorporation of iron into heme is unknown. In contrast to the anemia, cerebellar ataxia is always clinically relevant, so that *ABC7* mutations should be considered in any unexplained X-linked ataxia, even in the absence of hematologic abnormalities.

MITOCHONDRIAL MYOPATHY, LACTIC ACIDOSIS, AND SIDEROBLASTIC ANEMIA

Mitochondrial myopathy, lactic acidosis, and sideroblastic anemia (MLASA; OMIM 600462) is a rare autosomal recessive disorder of oxidative phosphorylation and iron metabolism. Hallmark features include progressive exercise intolerance during childhood, onset of sideroblastic anemia around adolescence, basal lactic acidemia, and mitochondrial myopathy.[37]

Linkage analysis and homozygosity testing of families with MLASA localized the candidate region on chromosome 12q24.33.[38] Subsequent studies identified a homozygous missense mutation in the pseudouridine synthase 1 gene (*PUS1*) in all patients with MLASA from these families.[39] Pseudouridylation of mitochondrial transfer RNAs would be responsible for mitochondrial myopathy and sideroblastic anemia.[40]

PEARSON'S MARROW-PANCREAS SYNDROME

Pearson's marrow-pancreas syndrome is a rare congenital disorder characterized mainly by exocrine pancreatic insufficiency and refractory sideroblastic anemia with vacuolization of marrow precursors.[41] There are many variants: patients may show pancytopenia, lactic acido-

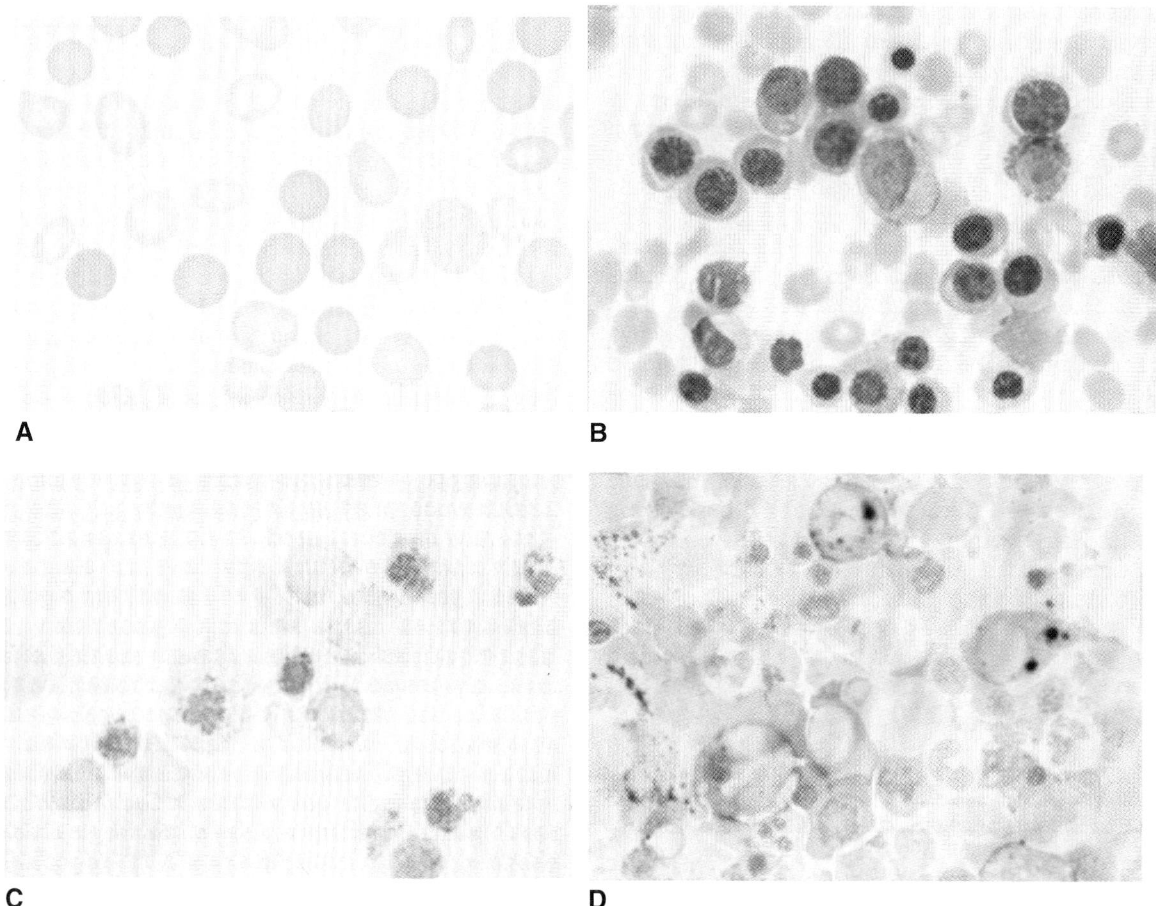

Figure 55–6. Acquired refractory anemia with ring sideroblasts (myelodysplastic syndrome). ***A***, Dimorphic peripheral blood film with a population of hypochromic microcytes and a population of normochromic macrocytes (May-Grünwald-Giemsa [MGG] staining, × 1250). ***B***, Bone marrow smear showing erythroid hyperplasia with predominant early and intermediate forms and macromegaloblastoid changes. The rare granulocytic cells look normal. (MGG, × 1250.) ***C***, Bone marrow smear showing erythroblasts with numerous granules positive to Perls' reaction disposed in perinuclear rings (ring sideroblasts). Siderotic granules are present also in very immature erythroid cells, whereas in hereditary and secondary sideroblastic anemias they are only in late erythroblasts. *Bottom,* A siderocyte. (Prussian blue staining, × 1250.) ***D***, Bone marrow smear stained for Perls' reaction showing numerous hemosiderin-laden macrophages. Iron overload is consequent both on ineffective erythropoiesis and on red cell transfusions. (Prussian blue staining, × 1250.)

sis, progressive muscle weakness, cataract, and other rare manifestations.[42]

Pearson's syndrome is caused by large mitochondrial DNA (mtDNA) deletions.[43–45] Single deletions of mtDNA are sporadic events normally occurring in isolated members of a family. Large deletions have been associated with three major clinical conditions: Pearson's syndrome, Kearns-Sayre syndrome (OMIM 530000),[46–49] and progressive external ophthalmoplegia (OMIM 550000).[50,51] Genetic-clinical correlations suggest that the type and extent of mtDNA deletions determine the clinical phenotype, but the pathogenesis of mitochondrial iron overload is unclear.

MYELODYSPLASTIC SYNDROMES

Myelodysplastic syndromes are discussed in Chapter 15. The World Health Organization (WHO) classification[52] of these disorders includes two conditions with ring sideroblasts: RARS and refractory cytopenia with multilineage dysplasia and ring sideroblasts (RCMD-RS).

Refractory Anemia with Ring Sideroblasts

RARS is characterized by isolated anemia, erythroid dysplasia only, less than 5% blasts and 15% or more ring sideroblasts in the bone marrow (Fig. 55–6).[52] The median age at onset is about 65 years.[53] Anemia is macrocytic (MCV > 100 fL) in most, and the reticulocyte count is in the normal range, reflecting an inappropriately low red cell output for the degree of anemia. Leukocyte and platelet counts are generally normal at presentation. Typically there is some evidence of iron overload, as indicated by increased serum iron, transferrin saturation, and serum ferritin.

Most patients with RARS do not have cytogenetic abnormalities; trisomy 8 and del(5q) are reported in some individuals.[54,55] Point mutations of mtDNA in pure acquired sideroblastic anemia[56,57] are of uncertain significance, and may reflect only limited clonality among hematopoietic stem cells.[58–60]

The natural history of RARS is characterized by an initial phase of erythroid hyperplasia and ineffective erythropoiesis, which is usually stable for many years but in a proportion of patients may be followed by a phase of marrow failure, with or without the later emergence of leukemic blasts.[53,61,62] RARS patients with no need for blood transfusion are very likely to be long survivors; those who become transfusion-dependent are at risk of death from the complications of secondary hemochromatosis. Nevertheless, median overall survival is greater than 5 years.

Refractory Cytopenia with Multilineage Dysplasia and Ring Sideroblasts

RCMD-RS is characterized by bicytopenia or pancytopenia with no or rare blasts and no Auer rods in the peripheral blood, and 1 × 10^9/L or fewer monocytes. Bone marrow examination shows dysplasia in 10% or more of cells in two or more myeloid cell lines, less than 5%

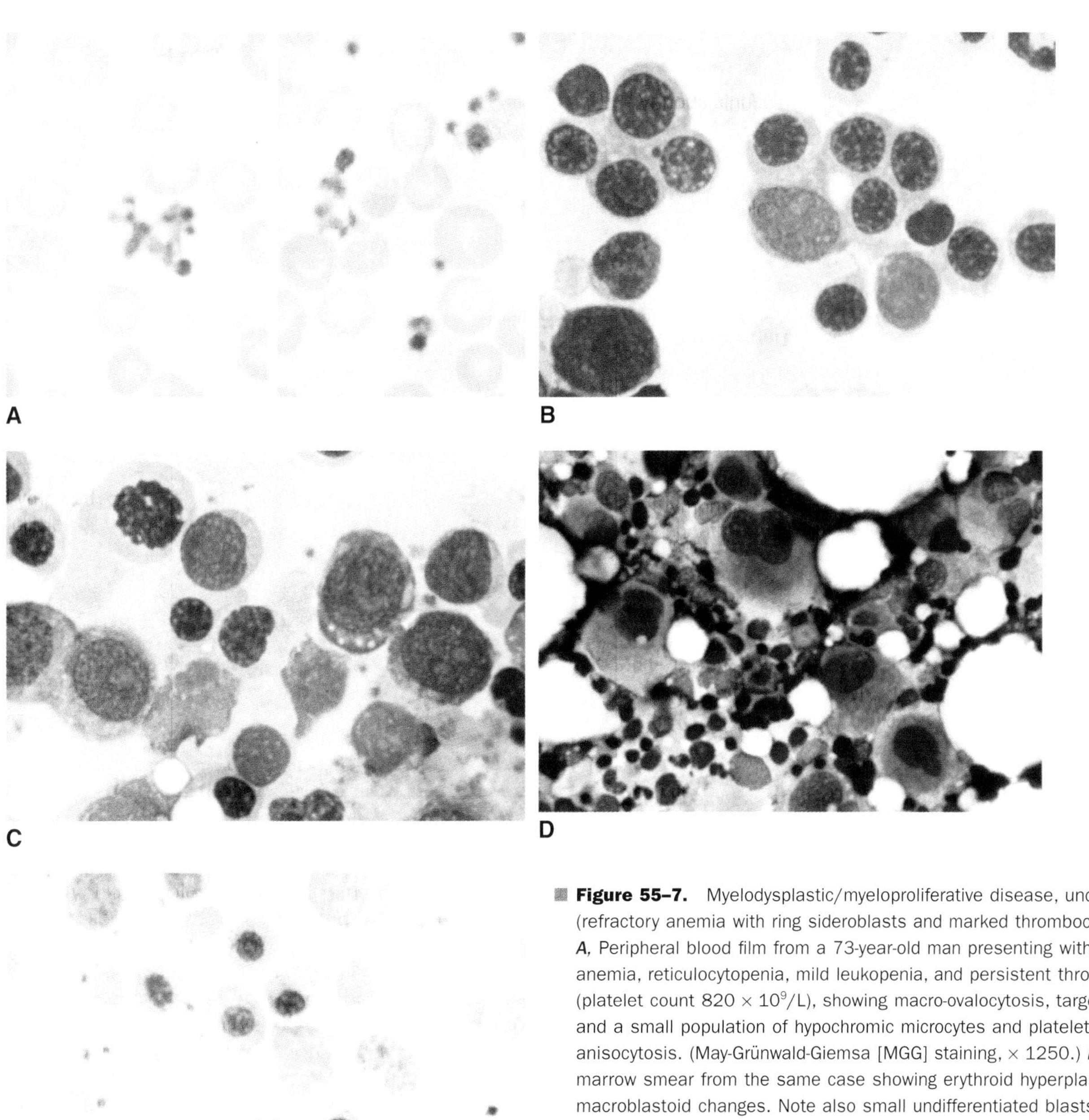

Figure 55–7. Myelodysplastic/myeloproliferative disease, unclassifiable (refractory anemia with ring sideroblasts and marked thrombocytosis). ***A,*** Peripheral blood film from a 73-year-old man presenting with macrocytic anemia, reticulocytopenia, mild leukopenia, and persistent thrombocytosis (platelet count 820 × 10^9/L), showing macro-ovalocytosis, target cells, and a small population of hypochromic microcytes and platelet anisocytosis. (May-Grünwald-Giemsa [MGG] staining, × 1250.) ***B,*** Bone marrow smear from the same case showing erythroid hyperplasia with macroblastoid changes. Note also small undifferentiated blasts. (MGG, × 1250.) ***C,*** Bone marrow smear showing proerythroblasts with vacuolated cytoplasm. *Top,* Atypical mitosis in a polychromatic erythroblast (MGG, × 1250). ***D,*** Bone marrow smear showing numerous dysplastic, often clustered, megakaryocytes (MGG, × 500). ***E,*** The same bone marrow specimen stained by Perls' reaction shows numerous ring sideroblasts and increased iron stores (Prussian blue staining, × 1250).

CURRENT CONTROVERSIES & FUTURE CONSIDERATIONS

Sideroblastic Anemias

- Mitochondrial ferritin is overexpressed in both hereditary and acquired sideroblastic anemias but the responsible mechanisms are not clear. The defective ALAS2 activity in bone marrow erythroblasts of patients with XLSA results in insufficient protoporphyrin IX synthesis and massive amounts of iron accumulate in the mitochondria; however, how transcription of the nuclear gene for mitochondrial ferritin is enhanced is unknown. Mitochondrial ferritin might be antiapoptotic and protect immature red cells against the adverse effects of mitochondrial iron overload.
- Flow cytometry immunophenotypic evaluation of mitochondrial ferritin might become a clinically useful diagnostic tool for sideroblastic anemias.
- Most patients with RARS do not show any cytogenetic abnormality. It is currently unknown whether these patients have point mutations in genes controlling mitochondrial iron metabolism.
- Regular iron chelation therapy with desferrioxamine may reduce red blood transfusion requirements and improve the degree of anemia in patients with RARS. However, the mechanism underlying these effects is not known. These findings require confirmation in prospective clinical trials.
- Oral iron chelators would be useful in the treatment of patients with sideroblastic anemia.

blasts, no Auer rods, and 15% or more ring sideroblasts in the bone marrow. In contrast to RARS, patients with RCMD-RS have a higher risk of death from bone marrow failure or evolution to leukemia, and a significantly lower overall survival, less than 5 years.[62]

Myelodysplastic/Myeloproliferative Disorders with Ring Sideroblasts

Refractory anemia with ring sideroblasts and marked thrombocytosis[63] is a rare myelodysplastic/myeloproliferative disease, unclassified in the WHO classification (Fig. 55–7).

Treatment of Acquired Refractory Sideroblastic Anemia

Several treatments have been proposed over several decades but few have met evidence-based criteria of efficacy.[64] Supportive therapy with blood products and conservative measures are instituted once a cytopenia becomes symptomatic. With regular transfusions of red blood cells, iron overload is inevitable (see Chapter 56). One unit of blood (400 mL) contains about 200 mg of iron, so that the annual burden is 2–4 gm. Although transfusion iron is primarily taken up by reticuloendothelial cells, it is later redistributed to parenchymal cells, at a rate proportional to erythroid proliferation and plasma iron turnover. When the body iron load exceeds 100–200 mg/kg, secondary hemochromatosis leads to liver disease, diabetes mellitus, and eventually heart failure. Any patient with an average life expectancy of more than 4 years who has received at least 30 blood transfusions or whose serum ferritin is greater than 1000 ng/mL should be treated with subcutaneous desferrioxamine, 30–40 mg/kg daily for 5 days a week. Long-term desferrioxamine iron chelation therapy is effective in retarding and even reversing organ damage caused by transfusion iron overload. Regular iron chelation therapy may occasionally reduce red blood transfusion requirements and improve the degree of anemia.

Suggested Readings*

Cazzola M, Barosi G, Bergamaschi G, et al: Iron loading in congenital dyserythropoietic anaemias and congenital sideroblastic anaemias. Br J Haematol 54:649–654, 1983.

Cazzola M, Barosi G, Gobbi PG, et al: Natural history of idiopathic refractory sideroblastic anemia. Blood 71:305–312, 1988.

Cazzola M, Invernizzi R, Bergamaschi G, et al: Mitochondrial ferritin expression in erythroid cells from patients with sideroblastic anemia. Blood 101:1996–2000, 2003.

Cotter PD, May A, Li L, et al: Four new mutations in the erythroid-specific 5-aminolevulinate synthase (*ALAS2*) gene causing X-linked sideroblastic anemia: increased pyridoxine responsiveness after removal of iron overload by phlebotomy and coinheritance of hereditary hemochromatosis. Blood 93:1757–1769, 1999.

Fleming MD: The genetics of inherited sideroblastic anemias. Semin Hematol 39:270–281, 2002.

May A, Bishop DF: The molecular biology and pyridoxine responsiveness of X-linked sideroblastic anaemia. Haematologica 83:56–70, 1998.

***Full references for this chapter can be found on accompanying CD-ROM.**

CHAPTER 56

IRON OVERLOAD

Gary M. Brittenham, MD

KEY POINTS

Iron Overload

Diagnosis

- Hereditary *HFE*-associated hemochromatosis is the most common form of inherited iron overload, affecting about 1 in 400 individuals in the U.S. population.
- Early diagnosis of homozygotes for hereditary *HFE*-associated hemochromatosis, followed by phlebotomy to remove excess iron, can prevent the later development of liver disease (with cirrhosis and hepatocellular carcinoma), cardiomyopathy, diabetes mellitus, and hypogonadism and promote a normal life expectancy.
- Genetic screening is recommended for all first-degree relatives of homozygotes for hereditary *HFE*-associated hemochromatosis.
- Early diagnosis of juvenile hemochromatosis, presenting before 20 or 30 years of age as cardiomyopathy, diabetes mellitus, and hypogonadism, can be life-saving.
- The combination of plasma transferrin saturation and plasma ferritin concentration is the best phenotypic screening test for all types of systemic iron overload.

Treatment

- The goal of treatment in all systemic iron overload is the *prevention* of accumulation of excessive body iron or, if a substantial body iron burden is already present at diagnosis, *rapid removal* of the excess.
- Phlebotomy provides a simple, safe, and effective treatment for hereditary and juvenile hemochromatosis and for most other forms of primary iron overload (except aceruloplasminemia).
- Iron-chelating therapy with subcutaneous or intravenous deferoxamine effectively removes iron when phlebotomy is not possible, such as in patients with transfusion-dependent refractory anemias (thalassemia major, sickle cell disease), with many iron-loading anemias (sideroblastic, myelodysplastic anemia), and with aceruloplasminemia.
- Most patients with iron overload require lifelong maintenance therapy to keep the body iron at normal or near-normal levels.

INTRODUCTION

Iron is an essential element required by every human cell to sustain metabolic function and to provide for growth and proliferation. Iron can serve as a carrier for oxygen and electrons and as a catalyst for oxygenation, hydroxylation, and other critical metabolic processes, in part because of its ability to reversibly and readily cycle between the ferrous (Fe^{+2}) and ferric (Fe^{+3}) oxidation states. The very reactivity that is metabolically useful also makes iron potentially dangerous. Ionic iron can participate in reactions to produce free radical and other reactive species, which in turn can damage cellular constituents. Normally, reserves of iron are deposited in cells throughout the body in the soluble storage protein ferritin and its insoluble derivative hemosiderin. Ferritin and hemosiderin sequester iron in a comparatively nontoxic form while keeping the metal ready for prompt mobilization when needed. If too much iron accumulates—iron overload—and exceeds the body's capacity for safe transport and storage, iron toxicity may produce widespread organ damage and death.

Definition

Iron overload is the general term used to describe an excess in total body iron. Humans lack any effective mechanisms to excrete surplus iron. As a consequence, the amount of iron within the body is physiologically controlled by meticulous regulation of iron absorption. Iron stores and absorption are reciprocally related so that, as stores decline, absorption increases. Normally, iron exchange with the environment is extremely restricted, with less than 0.05% of the total body iron acquired or lost each day. Iron overload develops in conditions that alter or bypass the normal control of body iron content by regulation of intestinal iron absorption. A classification of iron overload is provided in Table 56–1, which lists systemic disorders (both primary and secondary), perinatal forms, and diseases characterized by focal deposition of iron in excessive amounts.

EPIDEMIOLOGY AND RISK FACTORS

Globally, both genetic and environmental factors determine the types and prevalences of iron overload. In pop-

TABLE 56–1. Causes of Iron Overload

Primary Iron Overload

Hereditary hemochromatosis
- *HFE*-associated (OMIM* type 1: mutations in gene *HFE*)
- Non–HFE-associated
- –*TfR2*-associated (OMIM* type 3: mutations in gene for transferrin receptor 2)

Juvenile hemochromatosis (OMIM* type 2)
- *HJV*-associated (OMIM* type 2A: mutations in gene for hemojuvelin)
- *HAMP*-associated (OMIM* type 2B: mutations in gene for hepcidin)

Autosomal dominant hemochromatosis
- *SLC40A1*-associated (OMIM type 4: mutations in gene for ferroportin)
- Ferritin H-subunit messenger RNA A49U mutation–associated

Atransferrinemia

Aceruloplasminemia

Secondary Iron Overload

Iron-loading anemias (refractory; with erythroid hyperplasia and ineffective erythropoiesis)

Parenteral iron overload
- Transfusional iron overload
- Inadvertent iron overload from therapeutic injections

African dietary iron overload

Medicinal iron ingestion

Chronic liver disease

Porphyria cutanea tarda

Insulin resistance–associated hepatic iron overload

Perinatal Iron Overload

Neonatal hemochromatosis

Hereditary tyrosinemia (hypermethionemia)

Cerebrohepatorenal syndrome (Zellweger syndrome)

GRACILE (Fellman) syndrome

Focal Deposition of Iron

Renal hemosiderosis

Idiopathic pulmonary hemosiderosis

Associated with neurologic abnormalities
- Pantothenate kinase–associated neurodegeneration (formerly Hallervorden-Spatz disease)
- Neuroferritinopathy
- Friedreich's ataxia

*OMIM: For reference, this table lists the types of hemochromatosis as classified in OMIM (McKusick-Nathans Institute for Genetic Medicine, Johns Hopkins University, Baltimore, MD) and the National Center for Biotechnology Information database (National Library of Medicine, Bethesda, MD; available at: *http://www.ncbi.nlm.nih.gov/omim/*).

ulations of northern European ancestry, a genetic disorder, the homozygous state for hereditary (*HFE*-associated) hemochromatosis, is the most common type of iron overload[1–3] (Fig. 56–1). In an area bordering the Mediterranean and stretching from Southwest Asia and the Indian subcontinent to Southeast Asia, the most common types of iron overload are those associated with the iron-loading anemias and transfusion-dependent disorders such as the thalassemias and related hemoglobinopathies[4] (Fig. 56–2). In sub-Saharan Africa, dietary iron overload associated with consumption of iron-rich brewed beverages is a common problem that may also have a genetic component.[5] In the United States, the homozygous state for hereditary *HFE*-associated hemochromatosis is the most prevalent type of iron overload disorder, with homozygosity for the mutation in about 0.26% of the total population or in approximately 1 in 385 individuals.[6] In addition, iron overload develops in patients with iron-loading anemias or chronically transfused disorders, including aplastic, sideroblastic, and myelodysplastic anemias, thalassemia major and intermedia, congenital and acquired refractory anemia, and sickle cell anemia when red blood cell transfusion is used for prevention of stroke or other complications. Autosomal dominant hemochromatosis has been reported in a variety of ethnic groups, but data on its global distribution and prevalence are not yet available.[7] Otherwise, except for hereditary *HFE*-associated hemochromatosis, the remaining types of primary iron overload, the various forms of perinatal iron overload,[8] and the syndromes associated with localized deposits of iron all seem to be uncommon or rare disorders.[9]

Genetic Considerations

The gene that is mutated in most individuals with hereditary hemochromatosis, *HFE*, was first identified in 1996.[10] Since then, remarkable progress in discovering other genes involved in iron metabolism has revealed an unanticipated range of genetic heterogeneity and phenotypic variability in iron overload. At present, the recognition of genes involved in iron metabolism has outpaced our understanding of their specific roles. Despite knowledge of critical genes and gene products involved in the absorption, transfer, transport, and distribution of iron (Table 56–2), a detailed account of the molecular basis for regulation of iron metabolism remains elusive.[11]

A form of primary iron overload, the autosomal recessive disorder hereditary hemochromatosis due to mutations in *HFE*, is the most common genetically determined type of iron overload, accounting for 90% or more of cases in populations of northern European origin.[1] Patients typically present with organ dysfunction (liver disease, endocrinopathies, cardiomyopathy, arthritis, skin pigmentation) in the fourth or fifth decade of life. Although much less common, clinically identical forms of iron overload occur without mutations in *HFE*. Among these patients, a subset has a rare autosomal recessive disorder associated with mutations in *TfR2*, the gene for transferrin receptor 2[12,13] (hereditary hemochromatosis, *TfR2*-associated). The remainder of patients, in whom *HFE* and *TfR2* are normal, seem likely to have mutations in still unidentified genes involved in iron metabolism. Patients with the rare autosomal recessive disorder juvenile hemochromatosis have a pattern of iron loading like that in *HFE*-associated hemochromatosis, but they can present in the second decade of life[14,15] with cardiomyopathy, hypogonadism, or both. Most cases seem to be due to mutations in *HJV*, the gene for hemojuvelin, but a small number have mutations in *HAMP*, the gene for hepcidin.[16] Autosomal dominant hemochromatosis caused by mutations in *SLC40A1*, the gene for ferroportin, has been described in a variety of population groups.[7,17–20] An autosomal dominant pattern of inheritance has also been identified in a single family with a

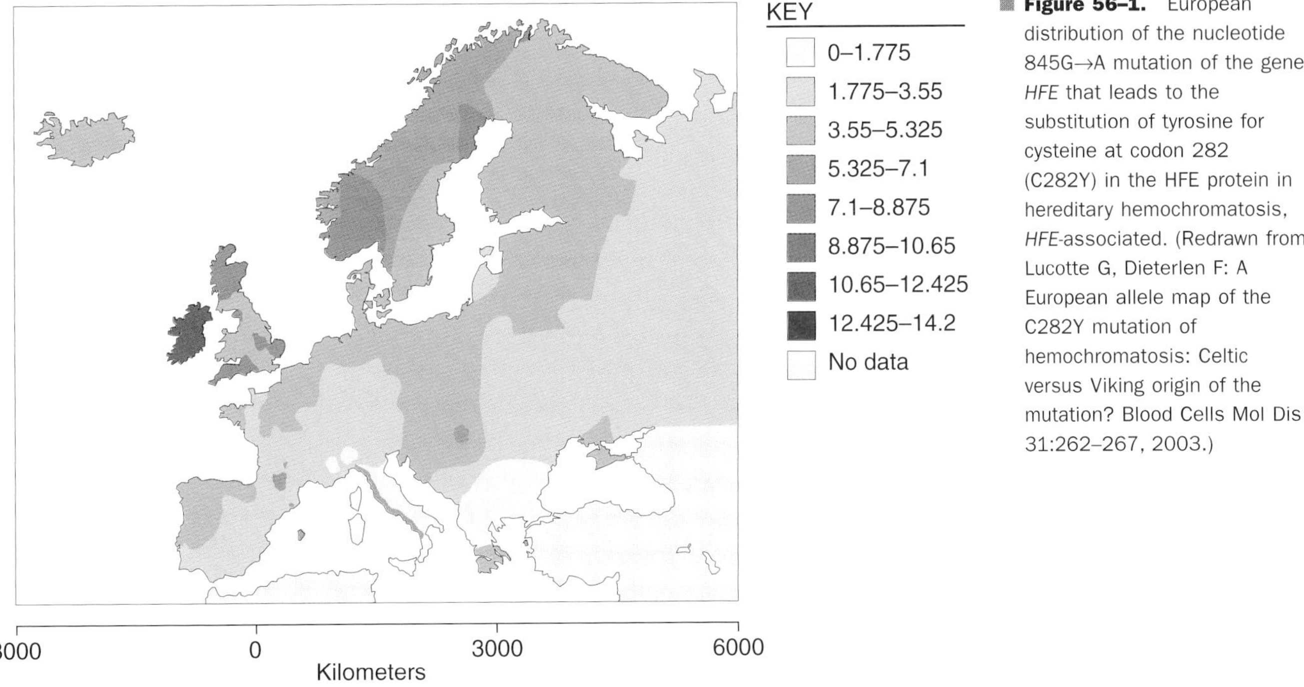

Figure 56–1. European distribution of the nucleotide 845G→A mutation of the gene *HFE* that leads to the substitution of tyrosine for cysteine at codon 282 (C282Y) in the HFE protein in hereditary hemochromatosis, *HFE*-associated. (Redrawn from Lucotte G, Dieterlen F: A European allele map of the C282Y mutation of hemochromatosis: Celtic versus Viking origin of the mutation? Blood Cells Mol Dis 31:262–267, 2003.)

TABLE 56–2. Selected Genes Involved in Iron Metabolism

Gene	Chromosomal Location	Protein Product	Function
TF	3q21	Transferrin	Iron-binding transport protein in plasma and extracellular fluid
TfR	3q29	Transferrin receptor	Receptor-mediated endocytosis of ferric transferrin
TfR2	7q22	Transferrin receptor 2	Unknown but seems to have a regulatory role in iron metabolism; receptor-mediated endocytosis of ferric transferrin
FTH	11q12-q13	Ferritin H subunit	Iron storage; H subunit has ferroxidase activity, L subunit catalyzes iron core formation
FTL	19q13.3-q13.4	Ferritin L subunit	
IRP1	9p22-p13	Iron regulatory proteins 1 and 2	Coordinate translational regulation of transferrin receptor and ferritin synthesis
IRP2	15		
HAMP	19q13	Hepcidin	Circulating antimicrobial peptide secreted by hepatocytes that decreases enterocyte and macrophage iron release
HFE	6p21.3	HFE	Unknown but seems to have a regulatory role in iron metabolism; the HFE/β_2-microglobulin heterodimer binds transferrin receptor
DCYTB		Dcytb (Duodenal cytochrome *b*)	Intestinal brush-border membrane ferric reductase; provides ferrous iron for uptake by DMT1
SLC11A2	12q13	DMT1 (Divalent metal transporter 1)	Iron transport from gastrointestinal lumen into enterocyte and from endosome to cytosol
SLC40A1	2q32	Ferroportin	Iron export from enterocytes, macrophages, and hepatocytes
CP	3q23-q24	Ceruloplasmin	Serum ferroxidase; required for iron efflux from macrophages and hepatocytes
HEPH	Xq11-q12	Hephaestin	Membrane-bound ceruloplasmin homologue for iron efflux from enterocytes

mutation in the gene for the iron-responsive element of the H subunit of ferritin.[21] Atransferrinemia and aceruloplasminemia are rare autosomal recessive disorders with distinctive syndromes of iron overload caused by mutations in *TF* and *CP*, the genes for transferrin[22] and ceruloplasmin, respectively.[23–25]

Secondary iron overload develops in many disorders with a genetic origin or component, including some of the iron-loading anemias, a number of the refractory anemias that require chronic red blood cell transfusion, porphyria cutanea tarda, and some inherited types of chronic liver disease.[26,27] Genetic factors may influence the development of African dietary iron overload[5] and possibly also susceptibility to iron accumulation with prolonged medicinal iron ingestion. A genetic basis has been established for many of the disparate disorders leading to perinatal iron loading[8] or to focal deposition of iron.[28]

The clinical severity of iron overload is affected by environmental, genetic, and other factors that modulate the quantitative extent of excess iron accumulation, iron

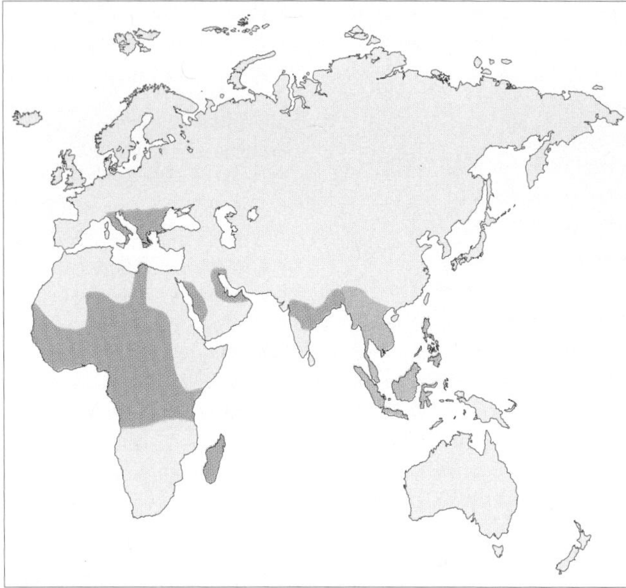

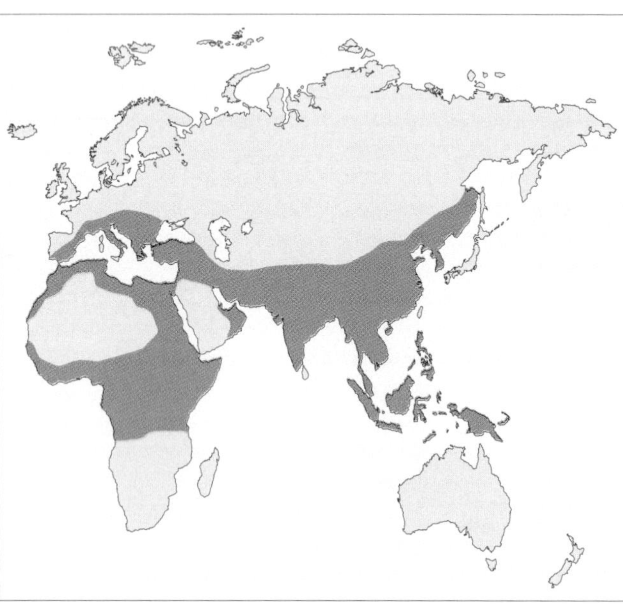

Figure 56–2. Global distribution of hemoglobins E and S *(upper panel)* and of α- and β-thalassemia *(lower panel)*. (Redrawn from Weatherall DJ, Clegg JB: Inherited haemoglobin disorders: an increasing global health problem. Bull World Health Organ 79:704–712, 2001.)

toxicity, or both (Fig. 56–3). Age and gender are important; in hereditary *HFE*-associated hemochromatosis, marked iron overload develops earlier in men than in women. Iron stores tend to be decreased by blood donation, physiologic blood losses (menstruation, pregnancy), pathologic blood loss, and malabsorption. Iron accumulation will be hastened by higher dietary iron intake, ingestion intake of therapeutic or supplemental iron, parenteral iron administration, and transfusion of red blood cells. Iron toxicity is accentuated by excessive alcohol intake, by nonalcoholic steatohepatitis, by viral hepatitis, and likely by large amounts of ascorbic acid.[29,30]

PATHOPHYSIOLOGY

The precise mechanisms by which iron injures cells and tissues are not known, but lipid peroxidation of membrane lipids in subcellular organelles, iron-induced lysosomal disruption, or both may be involved.[31] Twin studies suggest that still-unidentified genes profoundly influence iron accumulation and toxicity.[32] Nonetheless, the *magnitude of the body iron burden* is a primary determinant of toxicity in both primary and secondary iron overload. The greater the extent of iron excess, the greater the risk of clinical complications.[29,30,33] The *partition of the body iron burden between parenchymal and reticuloendothelial sites* is another key factor in iron toxicity. Iron deposits appear more hazardous in parenchymal cells and more benign in reticuloendothelial macrophages. For example, with equivalent body iron burdens, the greater parenchymal iron deposition found with hereditary *HFE*-associated hemochromatosis is likely to be more harmful than is the primarily reticuloendothelial accumulation of autosomal dominant (ferroportin-associated) hemochromatosis.[7,34] The *rate of iron accumulation* seems to be another critical determinant of toxicity. Consider patients with *HFE*-associated and juvenile hemochromatosis with similar magnitudes and patterns of iron accumulation: the former group would typically present in the fourth or fifth decade of life with liver disease, diabetes, and arthritis, whereas the latter may develop severe cardiomyopathy and hypogonadism by the second or third decade.[8,14,15] *Non–transferrin-bound plasma iron*, a heterogeneous pool of iron in the circulation that is not bound to the physiologic iron transporter transferrin, has been identified as a principal source of the abnormal tissue distribution of iron that develops with chronic iron overload.[35,36] Non–transferrin-bound plasma iron is rapidly taken up by hepatocytes in the liver, the major iron storage organ, perhaps through the divalent metal transporter 1 (DMT1; see Table 56–2)[37] and other pathways that remain poorly characterized. Non–transferrin-bound plasma iron also gains entry into cardiomyocytes, pancreatic β cells, and anterior pituitary cells specifically using L-type voltage-dependent Ca^{2+} channels not found in hepatocytes.[38] These distinct patterns of uptake of non–transferrin-bound plasma iron may contribute to the different patterns of iron loading in the liver compared to the heart and endocrine organs in iron overload. The *functional separation of the central nervous system, the testes, and the fetus* from the systemic circulation is a further factor influencing iron toxicity. Because these tissues cannot acquire iron directly from plasma transferrin,[28,39] iron must be taken up from the systemic circulation by barrier cells and then transported across the blood-brain and blood-cerebrospinal barrier into the brain interstitial and cerebrospinal fluids, across the blood-testis barrier,

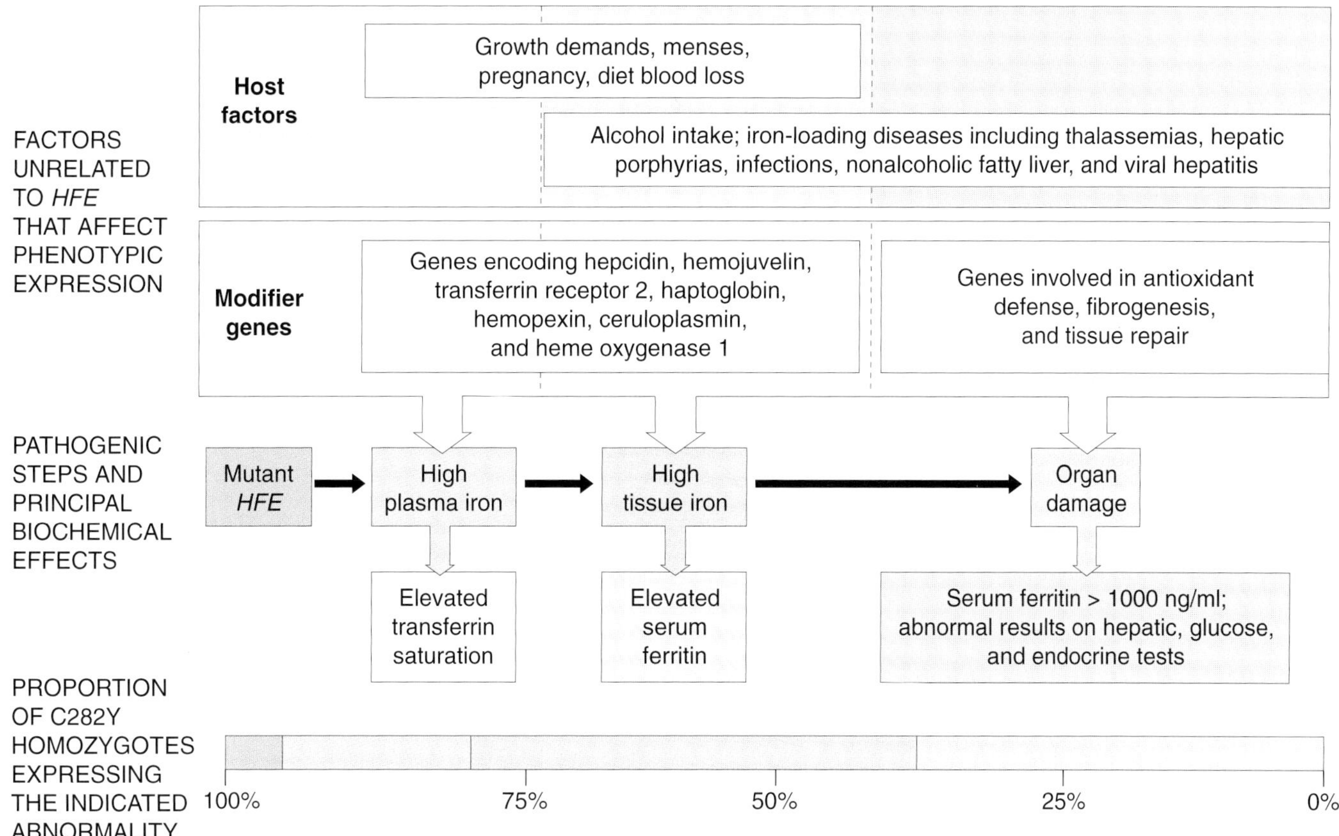

Figure 56–3. Diagrammatic representation of factors that influence the clinical expression of iron overload in individuals homozygous for the C282Y mutation in *HFE*-associated hereditary hemochromatosis. Host, environmental, and genetic factors interact to determine clinical expression. As shown in the top panel, progression may be retarded by decreases in iron accumulation as a consequence of growth, menstrual blood loss, pregnancy, low dietary intake, or blood loss. Progression may be accelerated by excessive alcohol intake, other iron-loading conditions, and liver disease. Other "modifier" genes also influence the expression; for example, severe iron loading is found in C282Y homozygotes who are also heterozygous for mutations in *HAMP*, the gene for hepcidin. In most individuals homozygous for the C282Y mutation, the plasma iron and transferrin saturation are increased. In a proportion of these, iron progressively accumulates in the liver and other tissues and, in some, reaches levels that lead to organ damage that may eventually be lethal. (Redrawn from Pietrangelo A: Hereditary hemochromatosis—a new look at an old disease. N Engl J Med 350:2383–2397, 2004.)

and from the placenta to the fetus. Disorders affecting the proteins responsible for iron supply to these compartments have distinctive manifestations.

CLINICAL FEATURES

The clinical complications of systemic iron overload usually develop only with substantial iron excess. In an adult male, of the roughly 4 gm of iron in the body as a whole, most is in functional compartments (in hemoglobin, myoglobin, heme, and nonheme enzymes), with less than 1 gm held as storage iron. With systemic iron overload, the amounts of iron in functional pools change little; the excess iron accumulates principally as storage iron. Moderate to severe iron overload, with an increase in body iron stores to 5–30 gm of iron or more, may develop with any of the types of primary iron overload. Among secondary forms of iron overload, iron accumulation of this magnitude is generally restricted to the iron-loading anemias (such as sideroblastic and myelodysplastic anemias and thalassemia intermedia) and chronically transfused refractory anemias[26,27] (such as thalassemia major, aplastic anemia, and sickle cell disease) and to African dietary iron overload.[5] Other forms of systemic iron overload generally have less than 5 gm of excess iron, although even this amount may function as a toxic cofactor (as in viral hepatitis, alcoholic liver disease, and nonalcoholic steatohepatitis).[30] Specific patterns of neurologic signs and symptoms occur in patients with aceruloplasminemia,[25,40,41] pantothenate kinase–associated neurodegeneration,[42] Friedreich's ataxia,[43] and neuroferritinopathy[44] that reflect the distribution of the excess iron in the brain and central nervous system.

Systemic Iron Overload

Early in the course of systemic parenchymal iron loading, before the amount of excess iron reaches the level required to produce tissue injury, patients are often entirely asymptomatic and may come to attention only because of abnormal laboratory results. With continued iron accumulation, they eventually develop symptoms of the underlying organ damage and may present with any of the characteristic manifestations of parenchymal iron deposition: liver disease, diabetes mellitus, gonadal insufficiency and other endocrine disorders, cardiac dysfunction, arthropathy, and increased skin pigmentation.[30,45,46]

Distinctive features of iron toxicity develop in specific organ systems. Liver disease is the most common complication of systemic iron overload, with the progressive development of hepatomegaly, functional abnormalities, fibrosis leading to cirrhosis, and, ultimately, a greatly increased risk of hepatocellular carcinoma.[3,30] Diabetes mellitus is another frequent adverse consequence of iron overload,[47] with the accompanying risks of almost all its secondary manifestations, including vascular disease, nephropathy, neuropathy, and retinopathy. Other endocrine abnormalities occur in pituitary and end-organ function.[3] During the second decade of life, both growth and sexual maturation may be retarded in untreated patients with juvenile hemochromatosis[14,15] or transfusional iron overload.[29,48] Iron-induced cardiomyopathy with heart failure, arrhythmias, or both, may be lethal in all varieties of systemic parenchymal iron overload. Cardiac disease often leads to the diagnosis in young patients with juvenile hemochromatosis[15] and is the most frequent cause of death in patients with transfusional iron overload.[29,48] Increased skin pigmentation occurs with all types of systemic iron overload. Chondrocalcinosis and other forms of arthropathy may be early manifestations of hereditary hemochromatosis[45,47] and also develop in other types of systemic parenchymal iron overload. Patients with transfusional and other forms of iron overload also may have an increased susceptibility to infections with certain organisms because of the increased availability of iron,[49] including *Vibrio vulnificus*, *Listeria monocytogenes*, *Yersinia enterocolitica*, *Escherichia coli*, *Candida* species, and *Mycobacterium tuberculosis*.[49–52]

Primary Iron Overload

The genetic characteristics and clinical features of the disorders responsible for primary iron overload are summarized in Table 56–3 and typical patterns of hepatic iron deposition are shown in Figure 56–4. The pattern of cardiac iron deposition found in the explanted heart of a patient with hereditary hemochromatosis is shown in Figure 56–5.

Hereditary Hemochromatosis

Patients with the clinical phenotype of hereditary hemochromatosis have inappropriately increased dietary iron absorption in conjunction with inability of reticuloendothelial macrophages to retain iron.[3] These abnormalities initially manifest as an increase in the plasma iron and transferrin saturation and subsequently by a chronic progressive accumulation of storage iron in the liver, heart, pancreas and other endocrine organs. Organ damage may not appear clinically until the fourth or fifth decade of life, when body iron stores have typically increased from the normal range of 1 gm or less to 15–20 gm or more.[53] The iron excess eventually produces liver and heart disease, diabetes mellitus, hypogonadism, arthritis, and skin pigmentation.

In populations of European ancestry, from 64% to 100% of cases clinically diagnosed as hereditary hemochromatosis are due to mutations in *HFE* and are classified as hereditary hemochromatosis, *HFE*-associated.[1] Most of those affected are homozygotes for a single-base mutation that leads to substitution of cysteine by tyrosine at position 282 in the HFE protein (designated as C282Y). The remainder of cases are "compound" heterozygotes for C282Y and either the mutation identified as H63D or, less commonly, that termed S65C.[54,55] The molecular mechanisms that underlie the effects of these mutations in *HFE* are not known but may involve hepcidin, the humoral antimicrobial peptide secreted by the liver which acts to decrease both intestinal iron absorption and the release of iron by macrophages[2,56–58] (see Table 56–2). Patients with hereditary hemochromatosis seem unable to increase hepcidin expression appropriately as body iron stores enlarge.[59] The availability of genetic testing for *HFE* mutations has made possible assessment of the penetrance of this form of hereditary hemochromatosis. Large studies have suggested that the penetrance is low[60,61]; one of these concluded that their "best estimate is that less than 1% of homozygotes develop frank clinical hemochromatosis."[61] This interpretation has been challenged,[62] and the outcome of further epidemiologic investigations, such as the Hemochromatosis and Iron Overload Screening (HEIRS) study[63] (see later), will be needed to resolve the issue. Other studies have suggested that at least some of the variability is the product of other genetic modifiers: homozygotes for the C282Y mutation in *HFE* who are also heterozygotes for a mutation in *HAMP*, the gene for hepcidin, have greater iron loading and more severe phenotypic expression.[64,65]

The rare patients who are homozygous for mutations in the gene for transferrin receptor 2, classified as hereditary hemochromatosis, *TfR2*-associated, are clinically indistinguishable from those with the *HFE*-associated form.[12,66,67] This phenotypic similarity suggests that these two proteins may act through a common mechanism regulating iron absorption by enterocytes and iron recycling by reticuloendothelial macrophages. Still other patients have been identified who share the clinical phenotype of hereditary hemochromatosis but do not have detectable mutations in either *HFE* nor *TfR2*. Clarification of the underlying genetic basis for these cases will likely identify other components involved in the regulation of dietary iron absorption and reticuloendothelial iron release.

Juvenile Hemochromatosis

Patients with the rare autosomal recessive disorder juvenile hemochromatosis have an accelerated rate of iron accumulation, estimated to be three to four times greater than that in *HFE*-associated disease.[68] The pattern of organ iron accumulation seems identical with that found in hereditary *HFE*-associated hemochromatosis, but severe iron overload develops much more rapidly.

TABLE 56–3. Genetic Disorders Associated with Iron Overload

Disorder	Gene Affected	Inheritance	Prevalence	Sites of Increased Iron Deposition	Biochemical Expression	Clinical Manifestations
Hereditary hemochromatosis				Parenchymal iron deposition in liver, heart, and endocrine organs	Variable; increased transferrin saturation in 1st–2nd decade followed by increased plasma ferritin	Liver disease, arthritis, diabetes, hypogonadism, cardiomyopathy, skin pigmentation; presenting in 4th–5th decade
HFE-associated [OMIM type 1]	*HFE*	Autosomal recessive	Common in populations of northern European ancestry			
TfR2-associated [OMIM type 3]	*TfR2*	Autosomal recessive	Rare			
Juvenile hemochromatosis				Parenchymal iron deposition in liver, heart, and endocrine organs	Increased transferrin saturation and plasma ferritin in 1st-2nd decade	Cardiomyopathy, hypogonadism, mild liver disease, presenting in 2nd–3rd decade
HJV-associated [OMIM type 2A]	*HJV*	Autosomal recessive	Rare			
HAMP-associated [OMIM type 2B]	*HAMP*	Autosomal recessive	Rare			
Autosomal dominant hemochromatosis				Reticuloendothelial iron deposition in liver, spleen, and bone marrow; may have late hepatocellular accumulation	Increased plasma ferritin in 1st decade; transferrin saturation low or normal until late in course	Mild fibrotic liver disease with mild or minimal anemia; may progress to hepatocellular involvement in 4th or 5th decade
SLC40A1-associated (ferroportin disease) [OMIM type 4]	*SLC40A1**	Autosomal dominant	Widespread with overall prevalence not yet determined			
H-ferritin IRE-associated	*FTH*	Autosomal dominant	Rare			
Atransferrinemia (hypotransferrinemia)	*TF*	Autosomal recessive	Rare	Parenchymal iron deposition in liver, heart, and endocrine organs; no iron in bone marrow, spleen	Plasma transferrin absent at birth; increased plasma ferritin	Transfusion-dependent iron deficiency anemia, growth retardation, poor survival without therapy
Aceruloplasminemia (hypotransferrinemia)	*CP*	Autosomal recessive	Rare	Marked iron accumulation in basal ganglia, liver, and pancreas	Low transferrin saturation; increased plasma ferritin	Progressive neurodegeneration of the retina and basal ganglia; diabetes

*Solute carrier family 40 (iron-regulated transporter), member 1.
Abbreviation: IRE, iron-responsive element.

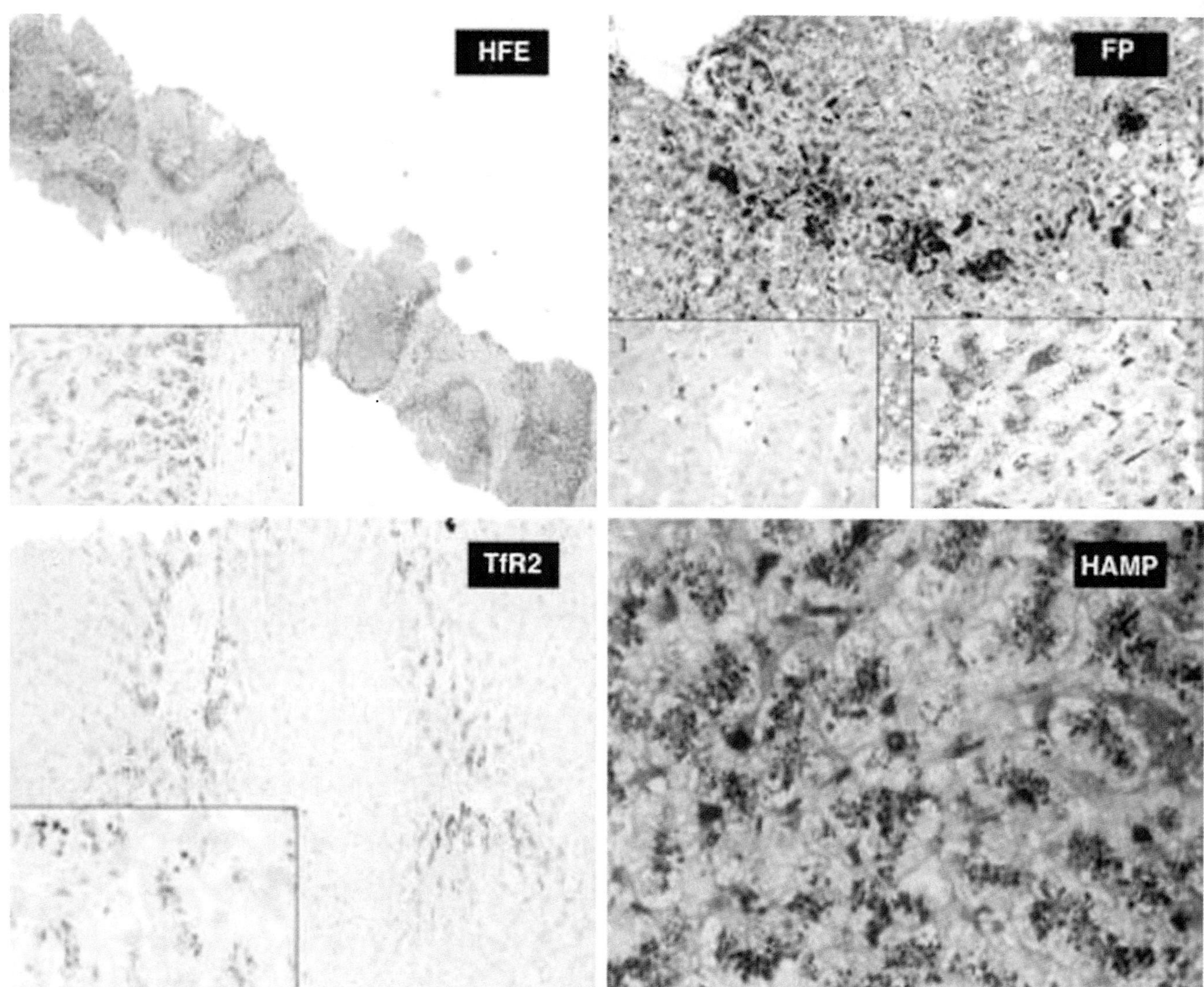

■ **Figure 56–4.** Patterns of iron deposition in primary iron-overload disorders (Perls' Prussian blue stain). ***A,*** Hereditary hemochromatosis, *HFE*-associated, with cirrhosis. *Inset,* iron deposits in hepatocytes. ***B,*** Autosomal dominant hemochromatosis, *SLC40A1*-associated (ferroportin disease), with advanced-stage disease. *Left inset panel,* early-stage disease with iron deposition predominantly in Kupffer cells. *Right inset panel,* late-stage disease with iron accumulation in both Kupffer cells and hepatocytes. ***C,*** Hereditary (*TfR2*-associated) hemochromatosis with periportal iron deposition. *Inset,* iron deposits in hepatocytes. ***D,*** Juvenile hemochromatosis, type 2B (*HAMP*-associated), with massive panlobular iron distribution. (From Pietrangelo A: Non-HFE hemochromatosis. Hepatology 39:21–29, 2004, with permission.)

Patients present symptomatically in the second or third decade[14,15] with hypogonadotrophic hypogonadism, diabetes mellitus, and cardiomyopathy, which may be lethal. A small proportion of patients (juvenile hemochromatosis, *HAMP*-associated) have been found to be homozygous for null mutations in *HAMP*,[16,69] the gene for hepcidin, but most (juvenile hemochromatosis, *HJV*-associated) are homozygous for mutations in *HJV*,[70–72] the gene encoding hemojuvelin, a protein of unknown function that may modulate hepcidin expression. The two forms of juvenile hemochromatosis are phenotypically indistinguishable, with the rapid accumulation of iron as a consequence of a complete loss of the capacity for hepcidin-mediated control of intestinal iron absorption.[2]

Autosomal Dominant Hemochromatosis

The distinguishing feature of autosomal dominant hemochromatosis resulting from mutations in *SLC40A1*, the gene for ferroportin, is predominantly reticuloendothelial iron overload.[17,18] Ferroportin is the protein responsible for the export of iron from macrophages involved in recycling iron derived from aged red blood cells, from enterocytes, and from hepatocytes. With a decrease in ferroportin activity, iron is retained within reticuloendothelial macrophages in the liver and spleen, and to a lesser degree by enterocytes and hepatocytes. Early in the course of this disorder, the plasma iron and transferrin saturation are low or normal but the plasma ferritin concentrations are increased, even during the first

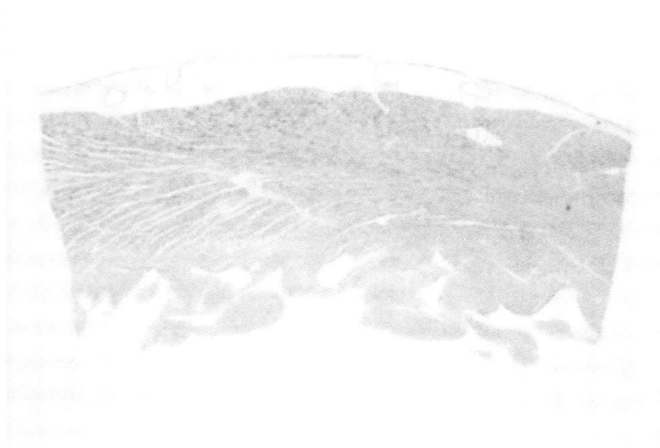

Figure 56–5. Lateral left ventricular myocardium, stained with Prussian blue for iron, from the explanted heart of a 36-year-old woman with hereditary hemochromatosis who received a cardiac transplant for heart failure. Extensive myocardial iron deposition is noted, with greater intensity of iron deposition near the epicardium. (From Schofield RS, Aranda JM Jr, Hill JA, Streiff R: Cardiac transplantation in a patient with hereditary hemochromatosis: role of adjunctive phlebotomy and erythropoietin. J Heart Lung Transplant 20:696–698, 2001, with permission.)

decade of life. With some mutations, initial reticuloendothelial iron deposition is eventually followed by parenchymal iron loading that is associated with hepatic fibrosis, diabetes, hypogonadism, arthritis, and cardiomyopathy.[7,34] Other ferroportin mutations apparently produce solely reticuloendothelial iron overload that is devoid of clinical manifestations and may not require treatment.[20,34] Because of impaired iron supply from macrophages, patients with mutations in the gene for ferroportin may have a reduced tolerance for phlebotomy and become anemic with therapy.[7]

Atransferrinemia

Atransferrinemia (hypotransferrinemia) is a very rare autosomal recessive disorder in which plasma transferrin is absent or extremely low.[22] Patients present with a severe hypochromic, microcytic anemia at birth, and die unless given transferrin infusions or blood transfusions. Iron absorption is increased, but the absorbed iron circulates as non–transferrin-bound plasma iron and is physiologically unable to enter developing erythroid precursors through transferrin receptors. The circulating non–transferrin-bound plasma iron is progressively deposited in the liver, pancreas, heart, and other parenchymal tissues, but iron is scant or absent in the bone marrow and spleen,[22,73,74] providing dramatic evidence of the importance of non–transferrin-bound plasma iron as a source of iron uptake by parenchymal tissues in both primary and secondary forms of iron overload.[36]

Aceruloplasminemia

Aceruloplasminemia (hypoceruloplasminemia) is a recently recognized, rare autosomal recessive disorder in which plasma ceruloplasmin is greatly decreased or absent.[23–25,41] Although ceruloplasmin contains 95% of the copper found in the plasma, the apparent role of this plasma protein is to catalyze the oxidation of ferrous to ferric iron, a prerequisite for iron binding by apotransferrin. In the absence of this ferroxidase activity, the egress of iron from cells is impaired.[75] The plasma iron and iron saturation are low, the plasma ferritin elevated, and a mild normochromic, normocytic anemia is often present. Patients usually present in the fourth or fifth decade of life with a triad of diabetes mellitus, progressive neurologic disease (dementia, dysarthria, and dystonia), and retinal degeneration.[23–25,41] Striking iron accumulation is evident in the liver, pancreas, and brain with smaller amounts of excess iron found in the spleen, heart, kidney, thyroid, and retina. Liver damage and fibrosis do not develop despite hepatic iron accumulations of the magnitude found in hereditary hemochromatosis.[25,40]

Secondary Iron Overload

Moderate or severe secondary iron overload generally develops only with the iron-loading anemias, transfusional iron overload, and African dietary iron overload.[30] The extent of iron accumulation is usually more modest in the remaining conditions associated with secondary iron overload (see Table 56–1).

Iron-Loading Anemias

Iron-loading anemias are refractory anemias in which excessive absorption of dietary iron may lead to severe iron overload[26,27,76–78]: thalassemia major and intermedia, hemoglobin E/β-thalassemia, congenital dyserythropoietic anemia, pyruvate kinase deficiency, and a variety of sideroblastic, myelodysplastic, and other anemias associated with blocks in the incorporation of iron into hemoglobin. The molecular basis for iron loading is unknown, but these disorders are distinguished by the combination of erythroid hyperplasia with ineffective erythropoiesis, and hepcidin regulation may be involved.[11] Patients may develop massive iron overload of the magnitude and with the complications found in hereditary hemochromatosis, including liver disease, diabetes mellitus, endocrine disorders, and cardiac dysfunction.[26,27,76,77] Severe iron overload may develop in patients with hemoglobin concentrations that are near normal because the risk of iron loading is determined not by the severity of the anemia but rather by the extent of ineffective erythropoiesis.[76]

Transfusional Iron Overload

Transfusional iron overload is the consequence of repeated administration of red blood cells to patients with chronic refractory anemia.[4,29,48] Transfusional iron loading begins in infancy in patients with severe congenital anemias such as thalassemia major and the Blackfan-Diamond syndrome, or later in life with acquired transfusion dependency as with aplastic anemia, pure red cell aplasia, and hypoplastic or myelodysplastic disorders. If the pathophysiology of the underlying disorder includes the combination of ineffective erythropoiesis and erythroid hyperplasia, increased absorption may also contribute to the iron burden. Sufficient numbers of transfusions administered to patients with sickle cell anemia, sickle cell/β-thalassemia or other sickling syndromes for prevention of recurrent complications such as stroke, severe infections, and incapacitating painful crises will also produce severe iron overload and the related complications.[79] The iron derived from transfused red blood cells initially accumulates in reticuloendothelial macrophages, but eventually parenchymal iron deposition develops with its attendant complications of liver disease, diabetes mellitus, and endocrine dysfunction; cardiac disease remains the most common cause of death in patients with thalassemia major and related disorders.[80]

African Dietary Iron Overload

African dietary iron overload is a distinct iron-loading disorder that is prevalent in sub-Saharan Africa in association with greatly increased dietary iron intake from a traditional fermented beverage of high iron content.[5,81,82] Iron burdens are quantitatively comparable to those in hereditary hemochromatosis and lead to liver disease with cirrhosis and hepatoma, pancreatic disease with diabetes mellitus, endocrine disorders, and cardiomyopathy.[5] Severe iron overload has also been documented in American patients of African ancestry.[83,84] A possible genetic component is not due to mutations in *HFE*. Recently, a common polymorphic mutation (Q248H) in *SLC40A1*, the gene for ferroportin, has been identified in populations of African ancestry, which may be associated with mild anemia and a tendency to iron loading.[85] Mutations in the gene for ferroportin, in combinations with other genetic conditions (such as thalassemia trait) or environmental factors (such as a high dietary iron content), may lead to iron overload.

Other Conditions with Secondary Iron Overload

Chronic liver disease with increased absorption of dietary iron may be associated with mild iron overload.[30] The *HFE* gene is not responsible. The cause of the increased absorption is unknown, but alcohol-induced folate and sideroblastic abnormalities with ineffective erythropoiesis and hyperferremia have been suggested as etiologic factors.[86] Quantitatively, the increase in body storage iron is mild, typically only 2–4 gm, with the excess stored in the liver in Kupffer cells rather than in hepatocytes. Nonetheless, the excess can have adverse effects. In alcoholic cirrhosis, the higher the liver iron, the shorter the survival.[87]

Porphyria cutanea tarda (Chapter 54) is the most common human porphyria. The liver produces excessive amounts of photosensitizing porphyrins which circulate to the skin and produce photosensitivity. Most patients have mild hepatic iron overload, and clinical and biochemical remission typically follow iron depletion by phlebotomy.[88] In patients of European origin, *HFE* mutations are common and may contribute to the pathogenesis of both the familial and sporadic forms of the disorder.[88,89] The mechanism for iron loading in patients without mutations in *HFE* is unknown.

Insulin resistance–associated hepatic iron overload is a recently described syndrome of iron overload in which the combination of an increased plasma ferritin with a normal transferrin saturation is found in association with glucose or lipid metabolic abnormalities.[90–93] The iron overload is typically mild or moderate and there is no evidence of familial transmission. Histologically, a mixed pattern of iron deposits in hepatocytes and sinusoidal cells is distinct from that of *HFE*-associated hemochromatosis.[94] The clinical value of phlebotomy to remove the modest iron excess in these patients is under study.[91,92,95,96]

Medicinal iron ingestion can increase body iron stores in patients with iron-loading disorders, especially iron-loading anemias. The effect of orally administered iron on body iron stores in individuals without genetic abnormalities affecting iron absorption is uncertain. Case reports have documented iron accumulation in patients who have taken medicinal iron for extended periods,[97] but the possible role of an unrecognized genetic disorder associated with iron loading in these individuals cannot be excluded.

Parenteral iron overload is sometimes inadvertently produced by repeated injections of parenteral iron preparations to treat anemias unresponsive to iron therapy, as in patients on chronic hemodialysis.[98]

Perinatal Iron Overload

Clinical features of perinatal iron overload develop in some rare or uncommon metabolic disorders in the newborn in whom the regulation of fetal or maternal-fetal iron balance is disrupted.[8,99,100] In some instances, severe hypotransferrinemia resulting from intrauterine liver disease is responsible. Neonatal (or perinatal) hemochromatosis is a diverse collection of disorders associated with severe congenital hepatic disease and deposits of iron in the liver, pancreas, heart, and other extrahepatic sites, with evidence of autosomal recessive inheritance in some cases.[99] In hereditary tyrosinemia (hypermethioninemia), moderate iron deposition is restricted to the liver, which is typically cirrhotic; renal abnormalities and hyperplasia of the pancreatic islet cells are also present.[101,102] The cerebrohepatorenal syndrome, or Zellweger syndrome, is a fatal disorder with an autosomal recessive mode of inheritance, characterized by abnormal facies, hypotonia, and polycystic kidneys. Parenchymal iron deposits are found in the liver, spleen, kidneys, and lungs.[103] The GRACILE (or Fellman) syndrome[104] is a newly described lethal neonatal disorder with autosomal recessive inheritance reported in Finnish families that includes hypotransferrinemia and hepatic iron deposition.

Focal Deposition of Iron

Clinical features of focal deposition of iron in other rare disorders are found in association with various patterns of localized iron deposition.[26,28] In idiopathic pulmonary hemosiderosis, repeated episodes of alveolar hemorrhage are followed by the uptake and sequestration of iron in pulmonary macrophages.[105] This excess iron is not available for use elsewhere, and iron stores in the liver and bone marrow may be decreased or absent. In conditions with chronic hemoglobinuria, renal hemosiderosis may develop and, in some cases, can cause renal failure.[106] Finally, remarkable progress is being made in understanding disorders with specific patterns of brain iron deposition in association with neurologic abnormalities,[28,107] including Friedreich's ataxia,[43] pantothenate kinase–associated neurodegeneration[42] (formerly Hallervorden-Spatz disease), and neuroferritinopathy.[44]

DIAGNOSIS

History

Patients with systemic iron overload may (1) be free of any indications of an underlying disorder; (2) present with nonspecific complaints such as fatigue, abdominal pain, or arthralgias; or (3) have symptoms suggesting iron-induced organ dysfunction, including chronic liver disease, cardiomyopathy, diabetes mellitus, sexual dysfunction, amenorrhea, and infertility. Specific attention should be paid to factors that could modify the body iron burden, such as use of dietary supplements, medicinal oral or parenteral iron administration, blood donation, pregnancies, and menstrual blood loss. In addition, details should be sought with respect to diabetes, obesity and hyperlipidemia, malabsorption, alcohol consumption, liver disease, porphyria cutanea tarda, risk factors for viral hepatitis, medications (including herbal or alternative agents), occupational exposure, and the family history of illnesses, including cataract and autoimmune disorders.

Physical Examination

The complete examination is performed with awareness of the vulnerable organ systems—the liver, heart, endocrine organs, joints, and skin—and should include careful neurologic assessment. No physical sign or combination of signs is pathognomonic of iron overload. Findings may range from the entirely unremarkable to the classical triad of "bronzed cirrhosis with diabetes," with palpable hepatomegaly and diffuse increased skin pigmentation ranging from slate gray to brown that develops in patients with advanced disease. "Reverse freckling," small pigment-free areas scattered over a distinctive slate-gray skin, suggests massive iron excess. A "painful handshake," resulting from arthritis of the second and third metacarpophalangeal joints, should raise the possibility of a diagnosis of primary iron overload.[45] More generally, arthropathy is an often-misdiagnosed manifestation of hereditary hemochromatosis and may be the presenting feature of the disease, especially arthritis affecting the wrists and knees. Physical signs should be sought of cataract, diabetes and its complications, heart disease, liver disease, and hypogonadism. With aceruloplasminemia, retinopathy, cerebellar ataxia, and extrapyramidal signs may be present. Patients with secondary iron overload may show evidence of the underlying disorder.

Laboratory Findings

A diagnostic algorithm for laboratory testing and pathologic evaluation of patients for primary iron overload is shown in Figure 56–6. After the full history and physical examination, clinical laboratory evaluation should include detailed assessment of liver function, including hepatitis serology, and a complete blood count, including an automated reticulocyte count. In some circumstances, bone marrow examination or measurement of plasma haptoglobin, plasma transferrin receptor, plasma ceruloplasmin, or urinary porphyrins may be helpful in the differential diagnosis (see later). Liver biopsy almost always allows definitive assessment of systemic iron overload and, if needed, should include quantitative measurement of the nonheme iron concentration, histopathologic examination of the distribution and pattern of iron accumulation in hepatocytes and Kupffer cells, and evaluation of the extent of tissue injury, with staging of any fibrosis. Additional clinical and laboratory studies should seek evidence of the complications of excess iron: testing for diabetes mellitus, evaluation of hormonal function, cardiac examination, joint and bone radiographs, and, especially if cirrhosis is present, screening for hepatocellular carcinoma.[3,30,45]

For specific evaluation for primary iron overload, a combination of phenotypic and genotypic methods is advisable. Phenotypic assessment alone can give biochemical indications of iron loading in patients with primary iron overload but will not identify all who are genetically at risk.[61] Genotypic screening for the C282Y and H63D mutations in *HFE* identifies most individuals who are at risk for developing *HFE*-associated hemochromatosis, especially in populations of predominantly northern European ancestry, but gives no information about the presence or magnitude of iron overload and will not identify other mutations associated with iron loading in populations of other ethnic backgrounds.[5,108,109] Measurement of the fasting plasma transferrin saturation is generally the best method for initial phenotypic evaluation,[1,3,45,110,111] with a persistent value of 45% or greater being the usual threshold for further investigation.[1,112] Apart from inflammation, infection, liver disease, malignancy, and other confounding conditions, plasma ferritin concentrations above the reference level for gender and age provide a biochemical indicator of possible iron overload.[30] In the absence of complicating factors, most patients with systemic iron overload will have an increased plasma transferrin saturation, plasma ferritin concentration, or both.[111]

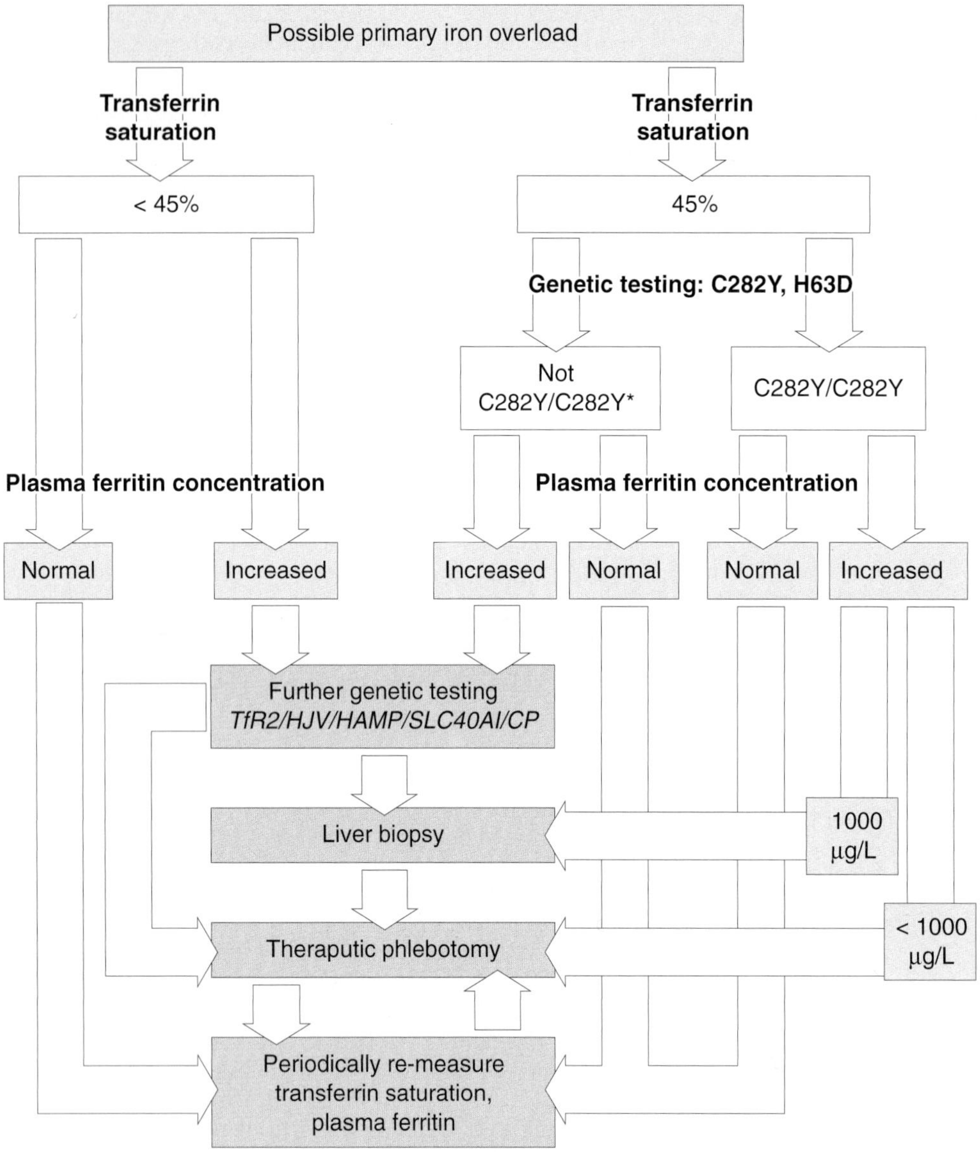

Possible primary iron overload

Transferrin saturation

Transferrin saturation

< 45%

45%

Genetic testing: C282Y, H63D

Not C282Y/C282Y*

C282Y/C282Y

Plasma ferritin concentration

Plasma ferritin concentration

Normal

Increased

Increased

Normal

Normal

Increased

Further genetic testing *TfR2/HJV/HAMP/SLC40AI/CP*

Liver biopsy

1000 μg/L

Theraputic phlebotomy

< 1000 μg/L

Periodically re-measure transferrin saturation, plasma ferritin

*Not C282Y/C282Y: i.e., genetic testing finds C282Y/H63D, C282Y/wt, H63D/H63D, H63D/wt,wt/wt, with wt = "wild type" or normal gene

Figure 56–6. Algorithm for the diagnosis of primary iron overload.

Patients with a plasma transferrin saturation of less than 45% and a plasma ferritin concentration within the laboratory reference range are unlikely to have primary iron overload; they need no further immediate evaluation but may be advised to undergo periodic reassessment (see Fig. 56–6). If the plasma transferrin saturation is 45% or greater but the plasma ferritin concentration is within the reference range, a clinically significant increase in body iron is unlikely, but both the plasma transferrin saturation and plasma ferritin concentration should be reexamined regularly. Patients who are homozygous for the C282Y mutation in *HFE* with a plasma ferritin concentration that is increased but less than 1000 μg/L are presumed to have iron loading, and therapeutic phlebotomy ordinarily should begin promptly. The risk of cirrhosis is slight and liver biopsy is not needed.[113] By contrast, patients who are homozygous for the C282Y mutation in *HFE* with a plasma ferritin of 1000 μg/L or greater have a substantial risk of cirrhosis, and hepatic biopsy is recommended for *prognosis*. Therapeutic phlebotomy should begin immediately.[53] Patients with a plasma transferrin saturation of 45% or greater and an increased plasma ferritin concentration who are not homozygous for the C282Y mutation should be considered for additional genetic testing of known genes associated with iron-related disorders, if available (such as for mutations in *TfR2*, *HAMP*, *HJV*, *SLC40A1*, and *CP*). If these additional genetic studies are unrevealing or unavailable, then hepatic biopsy is recommended for *diagnosis*.[3] The results of liver biopsy will almost always clarify the diagnosis and indicate the need for therapeutic intervention. Patients with a plasma transferrin saturation of less than 45% together with a plasma ferritin concentration increased above the laboratory reference range should have a measurement of plasma ceruloplasmin and further genetic testing for mutations in *CP* and *SLC40A1*. They should be carefully evaluated for confounding conditions (see later), including secondary iron overload[26,27] and hereditary hyperferritinemia with cataract.[112]

The diagnostic algorithm shown in Figure 56–6 is intended as a rational approach to diagnostic evaluation for primary iron overload with our current state of knowledge. The algorithm will need refinement as more genes and mutations affecting iron homeostasis are identified, as improved methods for genetic testing become available that allow simultaneous testing for multiple mutations in a variety of genes,[114,115] as methods for the noninvasive measurement of tissue iron are more generally accessible, and as the results of the HEIRS study (a prospective examination of approaches to screening and diagnosis of iron overload in a multiethnic, primary care–based sample of more than 100,000 adults[63]) are published.

In secondary iron overload, the underlying diagnosis will usually be obvious and assessment of the severity of iron overload is most important. Although the plasma ferritin is the most convenient indirect measure of the extent of iron accumulation, its interpretation is often complicated by the conditions that influence its concentration independently of body iron, including acute or chronic infection or inflammation, liver disease, hemolysis, ineffective erythropoiesis, and malignancy. Until noninvasive methods for measurement of tissue iron become more generally available, liver biopsy remains the most reliable clinical means for assessing the extent of systemic iron overload.[30]

DIFFERENTIAL DIAGNOSIS

The disorders comprising primary iron overload are rare or less common causes of common conditions: liver disease, heart disease, diabetes mellitus, arthritis, and hypogonadism. With individuals who present symptomatically, overlooking iron overload in the initial differential diagnosis is often the major obstacle to identifying the underlying disease. Two readily available laboratory tests, the plasma transferrin saturation and the plasma ferritin, are effective screening tools[45,47,116,117] that, together with the approach outlined in Figure 56–6, will usually lead to the correct diagnosis. With individuals who are asymptomatic, the goal is early detection to permit effective treatment that will prevent or arrest the development of complications. In the absence of confounding factors, the plasma transferrin saturation and the plasma ferritin detect the majority with iron loading. A proportion of individuals who are homozygous for the C282Y *HFE* mutation do not have elevations of either plasma transferrin saturation or plasma ferritin, and they can be identified only by genetic testing.[61] Their risk of iron loading is still uncertain,[118] and periodic reexamination of their plasma transferrin saturation and the plasma ferritin seems prudent.

An increased plasma ferritin concentration without an elevated transferrin saturation or evidence of iron overload may be due to hereditary hyperferritinemia with cataract, a recently identified autosomal dominant disorder in which affected family members present with early-onset bilateral nuclear cataracts and moderately elevated plasma ferritin concentrations resulting from increased concentrations of L-ferritin.[119,120] Plasma transferrin saturation is normal or low, body iron stores are not increased, and no hematologic or biochemical abnormalities are apparent. Mutations in the gene for the iron-responsive element in L-ferritin messenger RNA[121] are responsible; the only physical sign appears to be bilateral cataract.[120]

With iron-loading anemias, patients with only slight or mild anemia may develop severe iron overload. The risk of iron loading is determined by the extent of ineffective erythropoiesis and of erythroid marrow hyperplasia; these may be evaluated either morphologically with bone marrow examination or by measurement of the plasma transferrin receptor concentration.[76,122] With insulin resistance–associated hepatic iron overload, the plasma ferritin concentration often overestimates the actual increase in the hepatic iron concentration.[90,95,123] Porphyria cutanea tarda (Chapter 54) can be diagnosed by measurement of urinary porphyrins; in some populations, *HFE* mutations are relatively common in affected individuals.[88,89,124,125] The source of the iron overload in patients with transfusional iron loading is obvious, but accurate determination of the number of transfusions that patients have received is often surprisingly difficult. The various causes of perinatal iron overload are clearly distinguished by clinical and pathologic findings.[8,99,100] The diagnosis of idiopathic pulmonary hemosiderosis should be considered whenever iron deficiency anemia develops with coexisting pulmonary abnormalities.[105,126] Previously, demonstration of iron deposits in the brains of patients with Friedreich's ataxia,[43,107] pantothenate kinase–associated neurodegeneration[42] (formerly Hallervorden-Spatz disease), and neuroferritinopathy[44] was possible only at autopsy, but magnetic resonance imaging now provides a means of detecting localized brain iron during life.[33]

TREATMENT

General recommendations for treatment of iron overload are summarized in Box 56–1, but detailed accounts of regimens for specific forms of iron overload should guide therapy in individual patients. The primary goal of treatment of disorders of iron overload is prevention of accumulation of excessive body iron or, if the diagnosis of an iron-loading disorder is made only after a substantial body iron burden has accumulated, rapid removal of the excess. When possible, phlebotomy is the treatment of choice for iron overload and should begin promptly as soon as the diagnosis is established.[53] For most patients, phlebotomy should remove 500 mL of blood, containing 200–250 mg of iron, once weekly, until storage iron is depleted.[30] The regimen should be individualized; for patients with autosomal dominant hemochromatosis[7] or iron-loading anemia,[26] smaller amounts of blood will need to be withdrawn weekly, whereas for heavily loaded patients with hereditary hemochromatosis, a more

Box 56–1. Treatment of Iron Overload

Goal of Treatment

Prevention of accumulation of excessive body iron, or, if a substantial body iron burden is already present at diagnosis, rapid removal of the excess followed by lifelong maintenance therapy to keep body iron stores at normal or near-normal amounts.

Phlebotomy Therapy

Begin immediately after diagnosis to minimize exposure to toxic accumulations of iron.

- Rate of iron depletion should be individualized with respect to tolerance, diagnosis, and body iron burden to provide safe, effective, and rapid removal of excess iron.
  - *Hereditary, juvenile hemochromatosis:* Remove 500 mL blood once or twice weekly.
  - *Autosomal dominant hemochromatosis, iron-loading anemia, African dietary iron overload, porphyria cutanea tarda:* Reductions in amount or frequency of phlebotomy, or both, may be needed for individual patients.
- Measure hemoglobin or hematocrit before each phlebotomy; measure plasma ferritin after removal of each gram of iron.
- Continue phlebotomy until storage iron is depleted.
- Begin lifelong maintenance phlebotomy therapy to keep plasma ferritin less than 50 gm/L.

Iron-Chelating Therapy

Requires subcutaneous or intravenous infusion with small portable syringe pump.

- For iron removal when phlebotomy is not possible: patients with transfusion-dependent refractory anemias, many iron-loading anemias, aceruloplasminemia, and the rare patients with hereditary hemochromatosis in whom phlebotomy is not feasible
- Adjust dose of deferoxamine to magnitude of body iron load, best assessed by liver iron concentration; ordinarily, maximum dose is 50 mg deferoxamine/kg body weight/day
- Monitor growth, bone development, visual and auditory function

vigorous program of twice-weekly phlebotomy can be used. In a patient with porphyria cutanea tarda, the excess body iron will be removed after a few weeks of phlebotomy,[127] whereas in hereditary hemochromatosis with an initial body iron burden of 30 gm, removal of the excess iron may require 2 years or more.[30,53,124] Although prospective, controlled studies are lacking, patients with the modest iron overload that may develop with chronic liver disease do not seem to benefit from reduction of the iron load, and phlebotomy is generally not recommended.

For transfusion-dependent refractory anemias, most patients with iron-loading anemias, in aceruloplasminemia, and for the rare cases with hereditary hemochromatosis in whom phlebotomy is not possible, treatment with the iron chelator deferoxamine is the only means of preventing or removing toxic accumulations of iron.[29,48] In hereditary hemochromatosis with cardiac failure, phlebotomy and iron-chelating therapy may be combined. Because orally administered deferoxamine is not effectively absorbed, the chelator must be given by subcutaneous or intravenous infusion with a small portable syringe pump, ideally over 8–12 hours each day. Despite the rigors of this regimen, regular chelation therapy with deferoxamine can remove tissue iron, prevent organ damage, and prolong survival[128,129] and it provides the best available therapy for transfusional iron overload.

SUPPORTIVE CARE AND LONG-TERM MANAGEMENT

In patients with iron overload treated by phlebotomy, the rapid removal of excess iron should be followed by lifelong maintenance therapy to keep body iron stores within the normal range.[3,53] In some patients, phlebotomy of 500 mL of blood is needed as often as every 3–4 months, but others can be controlled within the normal range with much less frequent removal of blood. The best guide to the needed frequency of phlebotomy is the plasma ferritin level; a goal of a plasma ferritin less than 50 μg/L has been recommended.[30,45] In the United States, blood centers now can accept patients with hereditary hemochromatosis as regular donors with fewer restrictions than previously, a recent policy change that will help simplify maintenance phlebotomy.[130–132]

In iron overload treated by iron-chelating therapy, administration of ascorbic acid can enhance deferoxamine-induced iron excretion but carries the risk of an internal redistribution of iron from relatively benign storage sites in macrophages to a potentially toxic pool in parenchymal cells. Although the evidence is circumstantial, large doses of ascorbic acid should be regarded as hazardous in patients with iron overload.[29,48] Ascorbate supplementation is probably not needed if the diet includes ascorbate-rich foods. Deferoxamine is a generally safe and nontoxic drug in the iron-loaded patient, but systemic complications have been reported, including allergic anaphylactoid reactions, infections, visual abnormalities and auditory dysfunction, and growth retardation. The risk of many of these complications may be minimized by adjusting the deferoxamine dose to the magnitude of the body iron load.[133]

CURRENT CONTROVERSIES & FUTURE CONSIDERATIONS

Iron Overload

- What is the optimal strategy for screening to permit early phlebotomy therapy to prevent iron-related morbidity and mortality in homozygotes for hereditary *HFE*-associated hemochromatosis? Because the homozygous genotype is common and phlebotomy provides a simple, effective, and inexpensive therapy, *HFE*-associated hemochromatosis is ideal for screening. At present, uncertainty about the penetrance of the disease and concerns about privacy and the social and psychological consequences have engendered controversy over the best approach to screening.
- Improved methods allowing simultaneous testing for multiple mutations in a variety of genes should speed and simplify testing for genetic disorders leading to iron overload.
- Noninvasive means of measuring tissue iron, using magnetic susceptometry, magnetic resonance imaging, and other approaches, should replace liver biopsy for many purposes and allow monitoring of iron deposition and removal in other vulnerable organs.
- Continued progress in identifying the genes and proteins involved in iron metabolism should provide new insights into its regulation and lead to new diagnostic and therapeutic approaches not only to iron overload but also to other conditions, such as the anemia of chronic disorders.
- New, orally active iron-chelating agents, now in clinical trials, promise to revolutionize the treatment of iron overload that cannot be managed by phlebotomy.

PROGNOSIS

If patients with forms of iron overload managed by phlebotomy are diagnosed and treated before organ damage has developed, almost all the complications of iron excess can be prevented and life expectancy is normal.[53] Even if some tissue injury is already present at the time of diagnosis, phlebotomy prevents further progression in many disease manifestations and may produce improvement in some.[3] Hepatic function recovers, fibrosis is arrested and may even regress, and cardiac function can sometimes return to normal. Lightening of skin pigmentation usually begins early during phlebotomy. By contrast, only slight or no improvement is found for diabetes mellitus and other endocrine abnormalities. Arthritis typically shows little change and sometimes even progresses despite phlebotomy.[45] In hereditary hemochromatosis, if either diabetes or cirrhosis of the liver is present at diagnosis, life expectancy is diminished despite successful phlebotomy therapy.[53] Cirrhosis increases the risk of hepatocellular carcinoma by more than 200-fold.[53] In patients with iron overload who cannot be treated by phlebotomy, control of body iron with iron-chelating therapy is effective in improving the prognosis. The hepatic iron concentration can be decreased, hepatic function restored, growth and sexual maturation improved, and the risk of cardiac disease and early death diminished.[29,48]

Suggested Readings*

Bomford A: Genetics of haemochromatosis. Lancet 360:1673–1681, 2002.

Brittenham GM, Badman DG: Noninvasive measurement of iron: report of an NIDDK workshop. Blood 101:15–19, 2003.

Hentze MW, Muckenthaler MU, Andrews NC: Balancing acts: molecular control of mammalian iron metabolism. Cell 117:285–297, 2004.

Pietrangelo A: Hereditary hemochromatosis—a new look at an old disease. N Engl J Med 350:2383–2397, 2004.

Porter JB: Practical management of iron overload. Br J Haematol 115:239–252, 2001.

Full references for this chapter can be found on accompanying CD-ROM. 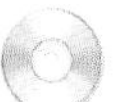

CHAPTER 57

Chronic Granulomatous Disease

Harry L. Malech, MD

KEY POINTS

Chronic Granulomatous Disease

Epidemiology

- The frequency of chronic granulomatous disease is about 1 : 200,000.
- About 75% of patients have the X-linked form of chronic granulomatous disease.
- Yearly mortality nationwide is about 5% for X-linked chronic granulomatous disease and 3% for p47phox-deficient autosomal recessive chronic granulomatous disease, but recent experience from centers specializing in the care of chronic granulomatous disease suggest that the current mortality is lower and may be under 3% and 1%, respectively. This suggests that dissemination of information about optimum prophylaxis and infection management can improve the outcome of morbidity and mortality at other centers.

Diagnosis

- The dihydrorhodamine flow cytometry assay appears to be more accurate than the nitroblue tetrazolium dye test at making the diagnosis of chronic granulomatous disease and can provide additional information.
- The diagnosis of chronic granulomatous disease should be confirmed with the quantitative ferricytochrome C superoxide assay.
- Western blot assays can be used to confirm or determine which, if any, of the four oxidase components are missing, providing information about genotype. DNA genomic sequencing to delineate mutations is required in some cases in order to make the final determination of genotype.

Presentation

- Soft tissue infection or osteomyelitis with *Serratia* is the most common presentation of chronic granulomatous disease in infants (<1 year old).
- Lung, lymph node, bone, or skin infection with *Burkholderia* bacterial species, *Nocardia,* or *Aspergillus* is a common presentation leading to the diagnosis of chronic granulomatous disease in older children or adults.
- Despite an overall decrease in *Staphylococcus aureus* infections in chronic granulomatous disease patients taking co-trimoxazole prophylaxis, this organism is responsible for more than 90% of liver abscesses in these patients.
- Unexplained partial gastric outlet obstruction or unexplained ureteral or bladder outlet obstruction without stone in a child may be the first presentation of chronic granulomatous disease.
- Chronic granulomatous disease patients can have a syndrome indistinguishable from Crohn's disease, and 20% of all patients have gastrointestinal granuloma problems, which may including chronic abdominal pain, esophageal dysmotility or stricture, gastrointestinal obstruction, and/or chronic colitis with bloody diarrhea.

Management

- Daily oral trimethoprim-sulfamethoxazole reduces infection frequency by 70% (ciprofloxacin or extended-spectrum oral cephalosporin may used as an alternate in sulfa-allergic patients) where the goal is to prevent *Serratia, Burkholderia,* and *Staphylococcus* infections.
- In children over 1 year of age, daily oral itraconazole 100–300 mg/day (4–5 mg/kg) reduces the incidence of deep fungal infection and is well tolerated. Administration with acidic cola beverages markedly increases absorption. Note that the liquid preparations of itraconazole used in children do not require food for absorption and potency is 9 : 5 relative to the pill form of itraconazole.
- Interferon gamma 50 μg/m^2 administered subcutaneously 3 days per week prophylactically reduces the frequency of severe infection over 70%, but cost, the requirement for injection, and side effects in some individuals (fever, malaise, headache, trouble with mental concentration tasks, and nightmares) reduce the number of patients who might benefit from using this treatment.

- Patients with chronic granulomatous disease should strictly avoid exposure to garden mulch, manure, digging, and construction sites. Over 50% of pan-lobular miliary inhalational fungal pneumonias can be directly related to proximity to spreading of garden mulch.
- Patients with high frequency of life-threatening infections who have a fully human lymphocyte antigen–matched sibling should be considered for bone marrow transplantation.
- Twenty percent of chronic granulomatous disease patients have chronic inflammatory bowel disease that in many cases is indistinguishable from Crohn's disease but may manifest as only chronic abdominal pain. About 10% of patients have one or more episodes of acute bladder and/or ureteral obstruction. Acute granuloma exacerbations of these types are best treated with 0.5–1 mg/kg prednisone tapered over 6 weeks, but about 30% of patients require indefinite maintenance with alternate-day oral prednisone (0.1–0.2 mg/kg) to prevent recurrence (prophylactic steroids).

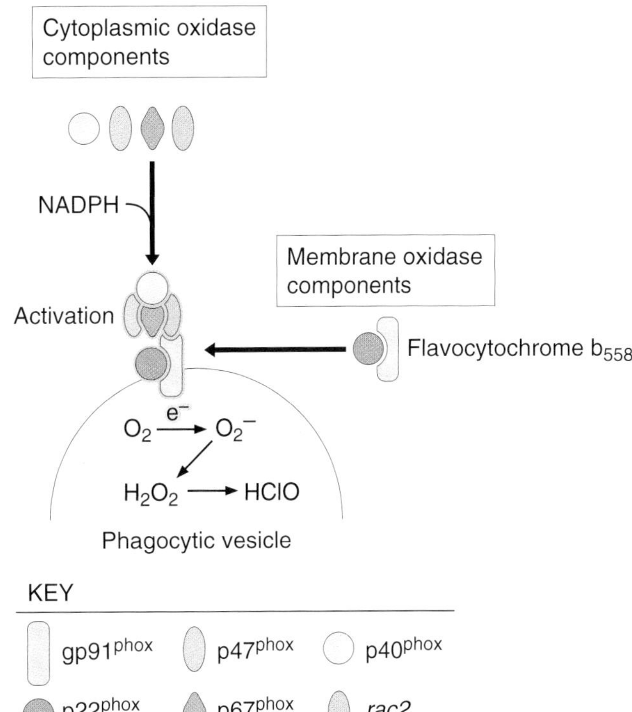

Figure 57–1. The enzymatically active phagocyte NADPH oxidase (phox) is composed of six separate protein subunits and requires assembly from both transmembrane components and the cytoplasm, which are recruited to the forming phagocytic vesicle by activation of the phagocytic cell.

INTRODUCTION

Chronic granulomatous disease is an inherited immune deficiency characterized by recurrent bacterial and fungal infections of lungs, liver, lymph nodes, bones, and skin. Patients also have both micro- and macrogranulomas (accumulations of cells associated with inflammation) that may impair organ function.[1–3] The neutrophils, monocytes, and eosinophils of patients with chronic granulomatous disease fail to produce microbicidal superoxide and hydrogen peroxide. The phagocyte NADPH oxidase (phox) responsible for superoxide production in these cells is composed of six protein subunits[4–23] (Fig. 57–1). The gp91phox subunit in association with the p22phox subunit comprises cytochrome b_{558}, a transmembrane protein containing binding sites for NADPH, flavin, and heme. In resting cells, most cytochrome b_{558} is present in small intracellular membrane vesicles. In the resting cells, the other four subunits are found in the cytoplasm. Of these, most of the cytoplasmic p47phox, p67phox, and p40phox exist bound together as a high-molecular-weight complex. The final component of the oxidase is the Rac-2, which is a GTPase of the Rho subfamily of the Rac superfamily of small GTP-binding proteins.[24] When phagocytes are activated, as when they engulf a microorganism, intracellular signaling events occur that result in fusion of the vesicles containing the cytochrome b_{558} with the forming phagosome and the translocation of the cytoplasmic subunits of the oxidase to the phagosome membrane, where they bind to the intracellular domains of the cytochrome b_{558} subunits. This results in electron flow from NADPH to molecular oxygen to produce superoxide.[25] Chronic granulomatous disease results when one of the subunits of the oxidase is either missing or defective, and either the assembly process fails or the complex does not transfer electrons.

EPIDEMIOLOGY AND RISK FACTORS

It is known from the patient registries of chronic granulomatous disease from several countries that the frequency is about 1 in 200,000 in the general population. In the registry in the United States, about 75% of patients have the X-linked form of chronic granulomatous disease, which involves mutations of the gp91phox gene present on the X chromosome. About 20% of patients have autosomal recessive chronic granulomatous disease resulting from mutations in the p47phox gene present on chromosome 7. Three percent and 2% of patients, respectively, have autosomal recessive disease resulting from mutations in either p67phox (chromosome 1) or p22phox (chromosome 16). Registry survival data indicates that patients with X-linked chronic granulomatous disease have a higher rate of infections and higher mortality (about 3–5% rate of death per year) than the p47phox-deficient autosomal recessive patients (about a 1–2% rate of death per year)[26–31] (Fig. 57–2). Although an extraordinarily rare immune deficiency/recurrent infection syndrome associated with an inherited abnormality of Rac-2 (a heterozygous dominant-negative effect mutation) has been described, the disease phenotype does not resemble chronic granulomatous disease (there are no granulomas) and the primary defect at the cellular level is a defect in neutrophil movement with only a mild defect in oxidase activity.[32–37] No patient with a disease process attributed to a primary deficiency of the p40phox subunit of the oxidase has been reported.

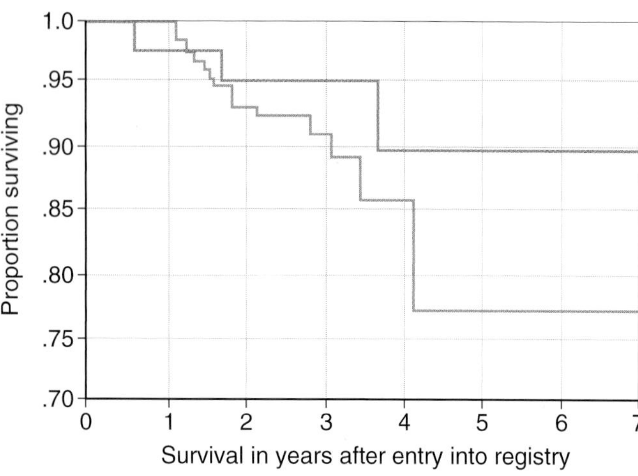

Figure 57–2. Chronic granulomatous disease survival data.

The mean age at diagnosis of X-linked chronic granulomatous disease is about 3 years of age, whereas male and female autosomal recessive patients are on average not diagnosed until over 7 or 8 years of age, respectively. Some patients, particularly those with p47phox autosomal recessive chronic granulomatous disease, may reach adulthood without a diagnosis being made.[26–31] Thus, an adult without a known predisposing factor who has a type of infection that is unusual in the general population, but typical of chronic granulomatous disease (e.g., *Burkholderia cepacia* or other *Burkholderia* species pneumonia, *Aspergillus* pneumonia, staphylococcal liver abscess, *Serratia marcescens* soft tissue or bone infection), should have specific testing for chronic granulomatous disease.[38–42]

CLINICAL FEATURES AND DIAGNOSIS

Clinical Presentations

An often fatal first presentation of p47phox-deficient autosomal recessive chronic granulomatous disease in teenagers or adults is an inhalation-related acute miliary aspergillosis that shares many of the features of allergic bronchopulmonary aspergillosis (ABPA). Although both syndromes may occur following an acute exposure to aerosolized *Aspergillus* spores (spreading garden mulch is the most common exposure), and are associated with patchy or miliary pulmonary infiltrates and a hypoxia that is very responsive to steroid administration, ABPA does not require systemic antifungal therapy, whereas the inhalation-related acute miliary aspergillosis infection in a patient with chronic granulomatous disease will initially appear to respond to steroids alone, but will then progress to death of the patient without administration of systemic antifungal antibiotics (agents with potent anti-*Aspergillus* activity that include voriconazole, candidacidins, intravenous itraconazole, and amphotericin B preparations, but not fluconazole). The diagnosis and treatment of this syndrome are discussed in more detail later.

Soft tissue infection or osteomyelitis with *Serratia* is the most common presentation in infants (<1 year old). Lung, lymph node, bone, or skin infection with *Burkholderia* bacterial species, *Nocardia*, or *Aspergillus* is a common presentation leading to the diagnosis of chronic granulomatous disease in older children or adults.[38–42] Liver abscess with *Staphylococcus aureus* is a less common initial presentation.[43] Patients with chronic granulomatous disease are more susceptible than normal to tuberculosis, and, in countries with a high endemic rate of tuberculosis (e.g., India and China), a severe infection with tuberculosis may be the presenting infection in a child with chronic granulomatous disease. In countries with a low endemic incidence of tuberculosis, such as western Europe, the United States, and Japan, tuberculosis in patients with chronic granulomatous disease is uncommon. However, the microgranulomas associated with chronic granulomatous disease can at times be similar enough to those seen in tuberculosis that many patients, before their diagnosis of chronic granulomatous disease is discovered, may be told that they have a "culture-negative" tuberculosis and are actually treated for it. Later, when the diagnosis of chronic granulomatous disease is made, their medical records continue to carry a diagnosis of tuberculosis, but in most cases a review of their old records suggests that this was a misdiagnosis.

Although other presentations are common with chronic granulomatous disease, these other presentations do not in themselves usually lead to this diagnosis. Chronic granulomatous disease may be associated with unexplained partial gastric outlet obstruction or unexplained ureteral or bladder outlet obstruction without stone in a child. A large bladder granuloma can present as a "pseudotumor" (mistakenly misdiagnosed as a cancer until histology shows granuloma formation).[44] Chronic granulomatous disease is a rare cause of a syndrome indistinguishable from Crohn's disease; in fact, at some time in their lives at least 20% of patients with chronic granulomatous disease have gastrointestinal granuloma problems that may include chronic abdominal pain and/or bloody diarrhea. In some cases, such as older teenagers or young adults with the p47phox autosomal recessive form of chronic granulomatous disease, who have a lower incidence of infections than do patients with the X-linked form, the lower gastrointestinal colitis may be their primary or only problem.[45,46]

Diagnostic Testing

The dihydrorhodamine flow cytometry assay is the most accurate and useful diagnostic test for chronic granulomatous disease, though the nitroblue tetrazolium dye slide test is still widely used.[47,48] One problem with the nitroblue tetrazolium test is that this is a manual visual scoring test, and some patients with the p47phox-deficient or mild variant forms of X-linked chronic granulomatous disease may partially develop staining in the test, which is misinterpreted as normal. This leads to missed diagnoses and delayed proper treatment of these patients. The dihydrorhodamine flow cytometry assay is thus the preferred test because intermediate levels of subnormal production of oxidants characteristic of the autosomal recessive or variant forms of chronic granulomatous disease can be recognized (Fig. 57–3). If possible, diagnosis should be confirmed with the quantitative ferricytochrome C superoxide assay in specialized laboratories. In addition, specialized laboratories can perform Western blot assays to determine which, if any, oxidase components are missing (Fig. 57–4). Although the combination of these tests (including testing of maternal blood to detect the mosaicism seen in X-linked chronic granulomatous disease carriers; see Fig. 57–3*A*) usually confirms the genetic type of chronic granulomatous disease, in some cases DNA sequencing must be done in order to make the final determination of genotype.[49,51] Genotype testing of all patients might seem desirable in all cases, but it is only available in specialized research laboratories. Fortunately, it is necessary only for prenatal genetic counseling and research purposes, and generally it is not necessary to determine the genetic subtype or the actual mutation for the proper medical management of chronic granulomatous disease.

CLINICAL MANAGEMENT

Prophylaxis and Maneuvers for Infection Prevention

Based on several clinical studies, chronic granulomatous disease patients in the United States are routinely placed on a prophylactic infection prevention regimen[51,53] consisting of the following medications:

1. Daily oral trimethoprim-sulfamethoxazole (co-trimoxazole: about 4.6 mg/kg/day trimethoprim and 22.8 mg/kg/day sulfamethoxazole for bacterial prophylaxis)
2. Daily oral itraconazole (about 4–5 mg/kg/day for fungal prophylaxis)
3. Three-times-weekly subcutaneous injections of recombinant interferon gamma (50 $\mu g/m^2$ surface area)

In 1989–1990, a large international double-blind study (126 chronic granulomatous disease patients participated in the United States and Europe) of interferon gamma demonstrated that prophylaxis with this immune hormone reduces infection rates by more than 70%, and the Food and Drug Administration (FDA) approved prophylactic use of recombinant interferon gamma in patients with chronic granulomatous disease.[53] Despite this, controversy remains among some physicians about its use, primarily because this medicine is very costly, it requires injections, it does have some side effects (see later) and its mechanism of action leading to infection reduction has not been elucidated. For these reasons, some physicians have considered triaging patients such that only those with a history of many recurrent infections receive interferon gamma. However, most chronic granulomatous disease specialists recommend that all patients be offered the opportunity to receive interferon gamma prophylaxis.[53–57] Interferon gamma does not cure chronic granulomatous disease and does not even improve the oxidase activity of neutrophils in most patients, but its action to decrease infection probably relates to heightened surveillance function of the patient's immune system overall. As one example of such an effect, interferon gamma increases the numbers and activity of receptors on neutrophils for the Fc portion of gamma globulin, but this is only one of many effects.[58–60] The "cost" for this global increase in immune activity is that interferon gamma can have side effects that include transient low-grade fever, as well as headaches and general malaise, but these effects often can be relieved by acetaminophen. A question often raised is whether a patient with chronic granulomatous disease who is not on prophylactic interferon gamma should be started on gamma interferon as part of the treatment for an acute systemic bacterial or fungal infection. There are no clinical trials or animal studies to support or refute the use of interferon gamma as part of the treatment of an acute infection in a patient with chronic granulomatous disease, though there are anecdotal reports purporting to observe a positive effect. Because natural levels of interferon gamma are elevated already in the setting of acute infections, and because interferon gamma will synergistically increase the febrile response to infection and also exacerbate hemodynamic instability following major surgery, our approach has been to actually cease the administration of prophylactic interferon gamma in the setting of high fever or in the perioperative period of major surgery associated with an acute infection.

Although the source or precipitating event for most infections in patients with chronic granulomatous disease is unknown, there are some situations that are known to be high risk for developing inhalational fungal pneumonias. Patients with chronic granulomatous disease are cautioned to avoid sites where there is spreading or handling of manure or where furrowing or digging of the soil is occurring. Patients should also avoid construction sites. Over 50% of pan-lobular inhalation-related acute miliary fungal pneumonias in patients with chronic granulomatous disease can be directly related to proximity to spreading of garden mulch. In the United States, the overall mortality would be significantly reduced by the simple measure of keeping patients with chronic granulomatous disease from being present when garden mulch is being applied. Once on the ground and well settled, the mulch is not a risk unless kicking or raking again results in aerosolization.

Infection Diagnosis and Treatment

Infections in chronic granulomatous disease patients may have a variety of presentations.[38–43,61,62] Infections *may or may not* be associated with fever, neutrophilia, high erythrocyte sedimentation rate (ESR), or high C-reactive protein. Malaise may be the only symptom, so it is important to pay attention to a patient or a patient's parent who insists that the patient does not feel well or has pain

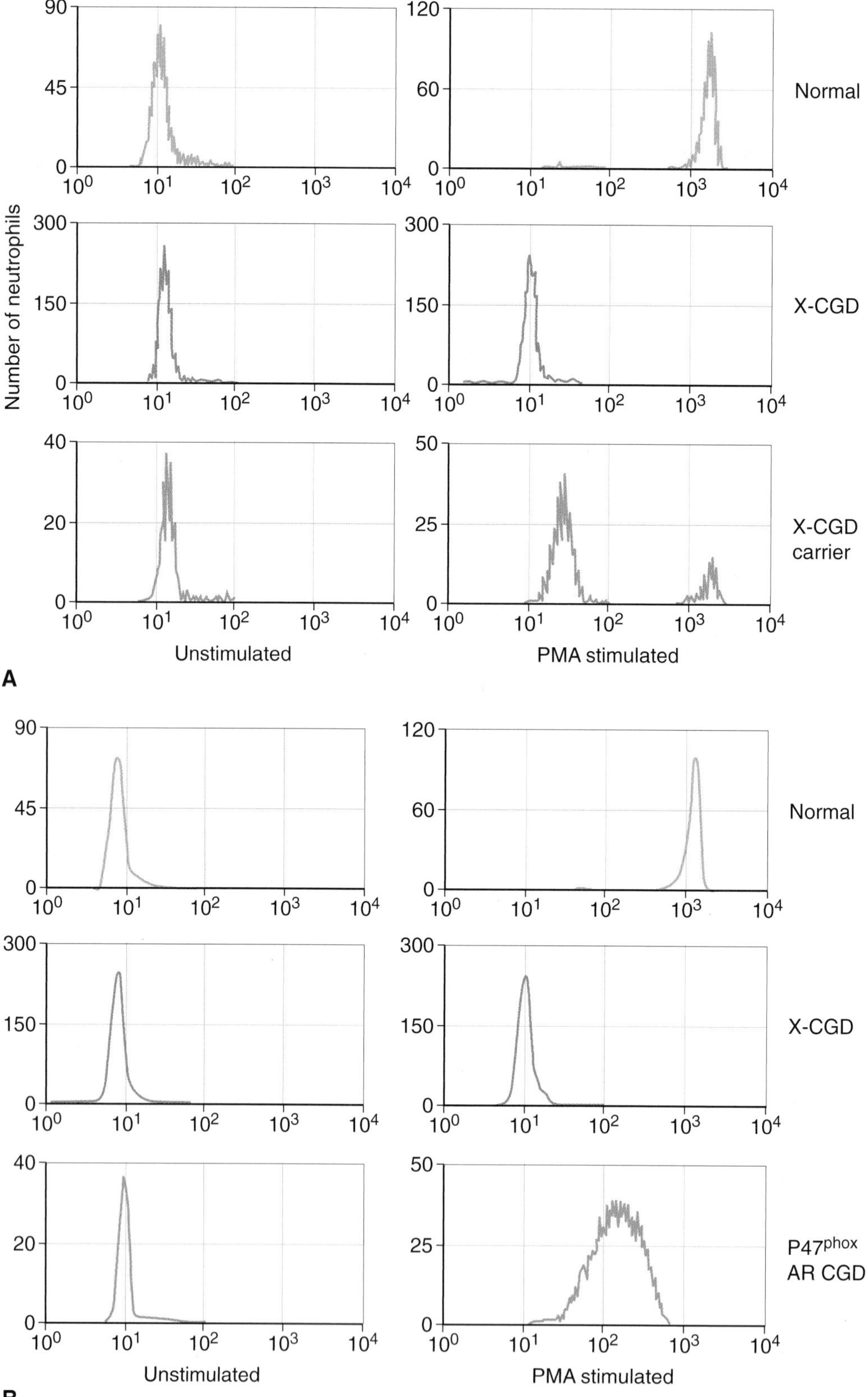

Figure 57–3. *A,* Dihydrorhodamine (DHR) assay demonstrating low fluorescence of stimulated neutrophils from a patient with X-linked chronic granulomatous disease (middle right panel of ***A***) compared to normal (top right panel of ***A***); two peaks seen in female carriers of X-linked chronic granulomatous disease (lower right panel of ***A***). ***B,*** DHR assay comparing the almost total failure to increase fluorescence following stimulation of neutrophils from a patient with X-linked chronic granulomatous disease (middle right panel of ***B***) should be contrasted with the characteristic "broad" peak of increased but subnormal fluorescence typical of stimulated neutrophils from a patient with the autosomal recessive p47phox-deficient form of chronic granulomatous disease (lower right panel of ***B***). (Adapted from Vowells SJ, Fleisher TA, Sekhsaria S, et al: Genotype dependent variability in flow cytometric evaluation of NADPH oxidase function in patients with chronic granulomatous disease. J Pediatr 128:104, 1996.)

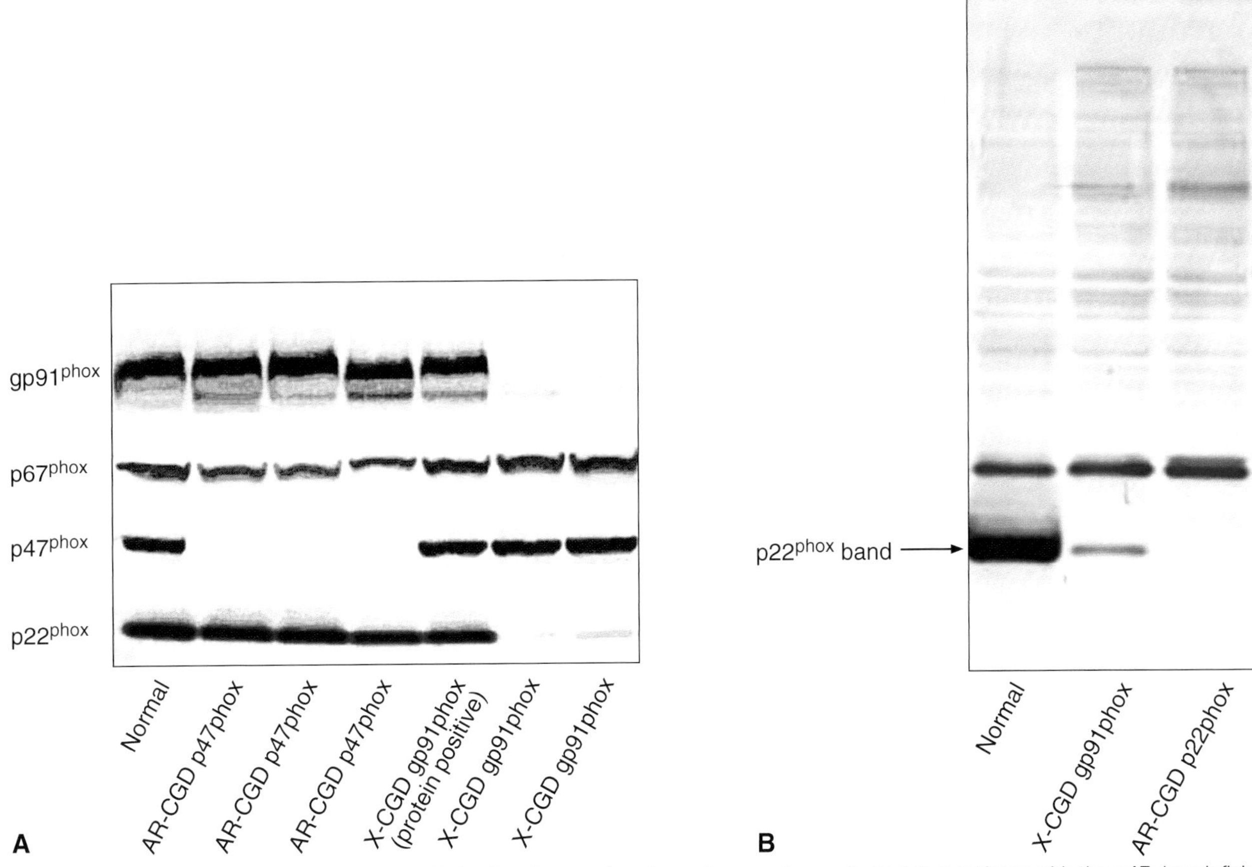

Figure 57–4. *A*, Western blot of neutrophils in chronic granulomatous disease demonstrating that patients with the p47phox-deficient autosomal recessive form typically have no detectable p47phox protein. Most patients with X-linked chronic granulomatous disease lack detectable gp91phox, but some patients express normal amounts of a nonfunctional gp91phox protein (gp91phox protein–positive X-linked chronic granulomatous disease). *B*, Western blot of neutrophils in chronic granulomatous disease demonstrating decreased p22 expression in the X-linked form and absence of p22 expression in the p22phox-deficient autosomal recessive form.

in the chest or other location, even where no fever or high white blood cell count is detected. We particularly have been impressed with young children who seem active and happy with apparently normal physical examination, but with the parent insisting something is just not right, who turn out to have a significant pneumonia on computed tomography scan. Fungal infection (50% of chronic granulomatous disease infections), including pneumonia, is indolent, often presenting with only malaise and no fever or neutrophilia (or even as only an incidental finding of a small lung infiltrate on routine x-ray at routine biannual exam). Although *Aspergillus* is most common, other fungal infections are seen.[61] However, high fever is more common in *Nocardia, Serratia,* or *Burkholderia* bacterial species infections and may also be part of the presentation of inhalation-related acute miliary fungal pneumonias.[38–43,61,62] Note that pneumonia in young chronic granulomatous disease patients may present as abdominal pain, so all patients presenting with abdominal pain should also have a computed tomography scan of the chest. It should be noted that intravenous contrast administration is not needed and not helpful for chest computed tomography in patients with chronic granulomatous disease. We find that the ESR and C-reactive protein are both useful tests in assessing infection or response to treatment (we prefer the ESR). Although not absolutely diagnostic (they can at times be normal with some infections), the ESR or C-reactive protein are more often abnormal in the presence of infection than is the white blood cell count, and they may be particularly helpful in indolent fungal infections in which no fever or leukocytosis is present.

In following large numbers of chronic granulomatous disease patients at the National Institutes of Health (NIH), we find that, where infection is suspected, chest and liver computed tomography scans (or other computer imaging, such as magnetic resonance imaging or positron emission tomography) are high-yield and cost-effective procedures. Many early infections are not seen on a regular chest x-ray that are easily apparent on computed tomography of the chest. Early diagnosis can result in the ability to treat an infection completely in the outpatient setting and avoid the increased cost and inconvenience of hospitalization. We do in some cases try empirical oral antibiotic treatment (see later) for very small lung infiltrates. However, for significant lung infiltrates or other large, deep organ infections, tissue diagnosis for histology and culture is important for patients with chronic granulomatous disease because of the potential for fungus infection, and because 20% of pneumonias are mixed infections (fungus and *Nocardia* or *Burkholderia* species are most common). At the NIH, transthoracic needle biopsy under computed tomography or fluoroscopy guidance yields a higher diagnostic rate (80%) than bronchoscopy (40%), particularly for fungus infection.[63] We find that many fungi do not grow and that cytopathology and microbiology support with special fungal stains or fluorescence wet mount stains are essential (Fig. 57–5). Usually the cytopathology technician is available to immediately handle needle biopsy specimens that are obtained under computed tomography or fluoroscopy guidance. This is important because several needle passes may be needed before tissue with granulomas is obtained, as determined by quick stain of a small portion of the material that has been placed on a slide from the needle. In dividing the needle biopsy material for cytology or microbiology studies, it is essential that the cytology lab receives a significant portion of actual pieces of tissue. Diagnosis of fungal or nocardial pneumonia is a reason to do a bone scan and head computed tomography, because chest wall (rib) and vertebral extension or distant metastasis of infection to bone is common, and lung nocardial infection can be associated with silent brain abscess.

Forty percent to 50% of serious deep tissue infections in patients with chronic granulomatous disease are fungal. Seventy percent to 80% of fungal infections are with *Aspergillus* species. We have shown that *Aspergillus nidulans* is associated with higher rates of bone involvement and higher mortality than *Aspergillus fumigatus*.[64] Non-*Aspergillus* infections include a wide variety of molds and yeasts (e.g. *Paecilomyces*,[61] *Candida glabrata* or *Candida parapsilosis*, and others). Special note should be made of the fact that that *Paecilomyces* is often misclassified as *Penicillium* and ignored by a microbiology lab, but *Paecilomyces* is an etiologic agent of significant infections in chronic granulomatous disease patients. Again, as noted earlier, 10–20% of fungal infections are mixed (another fungus, *Nocardia* species, or *Burkholderia cepacia* or *Burkholderia gladioli*).

Fifty percent of pneumonias in patients with chronic granulomatous disease are fungal pneumonias. We have noted two different types of fungal pneumonia (Box 57–1). The most common is a nodular/segmental pneumonia in which one or more nodules occur or lung segments are involved that show up on x-ray or computed tomography scan of the chest as a dense infiltrate with surrounding normal lung tissue (Fig. 57–6). The usual presentation for such a pneumonia is as an indolent process in which malaise and fever appear slowly over several weeks. In some cases there may be no fever and just a cough or mild chest pain. Predisposing events are usually not determined. The other type of fungal infection can be termed reticulomiliary (Fig. 57–7). Often there is a predisposing history in the previous 2 weeks of

Box 57–1. Types of Fungal Pneumonias in Patients with Chronic Granulomatous Disease

Miliary/Pan-lobular (Less Common)

- Rapid onset (days)

Severe shortness of breath

- Pan-lobular miliary infiltrate
- Causative event often identified (e.g., spreading garden mulch)
- Occasionally fatal misdiagnosis: *Aspergillus* hypersensitivity pneumonia

Nodular/Segmental (More Common)

- Slow onset (weeks)
- None to medium fever ± cough ± chest pain
- Discrete dense infiltrates
- Causative event rarely identified

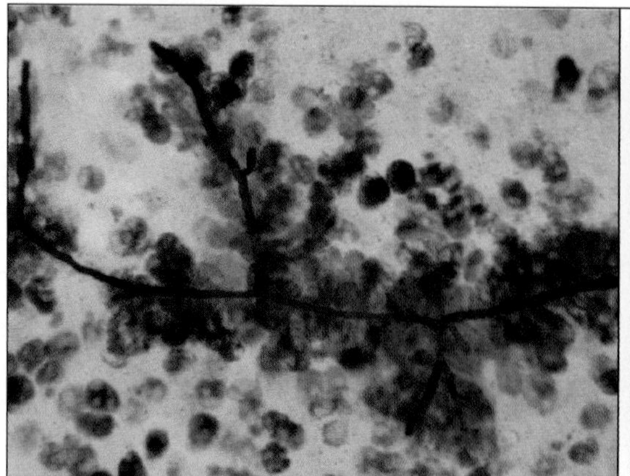
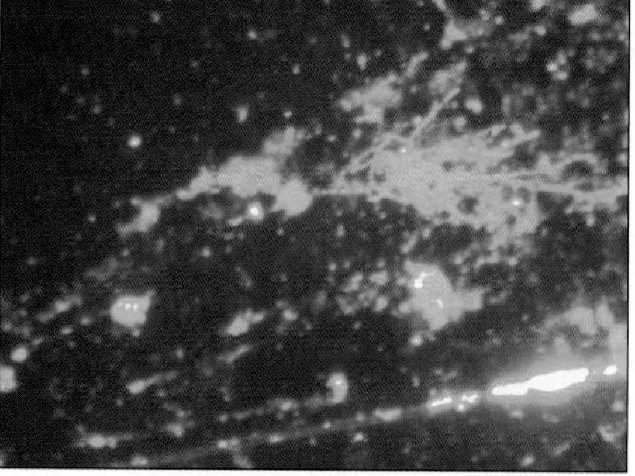

Figure 57–5. Specimens from transthoracic needle biopsy showing fungal hyphae (silver stain) at the *left* and *Nocardia* (fluorescence stain) at the *right*.

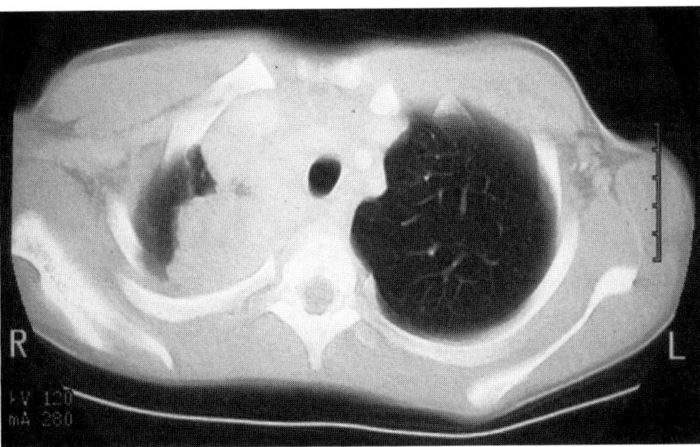

Figure 57–6. Large nodular *Aspergillus fumigatus* pneumonia infiltrate at the apex of the right lung. The presentation of this pneumonia was subacute with normal white blood cells count, moderately elevated ESR, and no fever. The patient complained of malaise and chest pain.

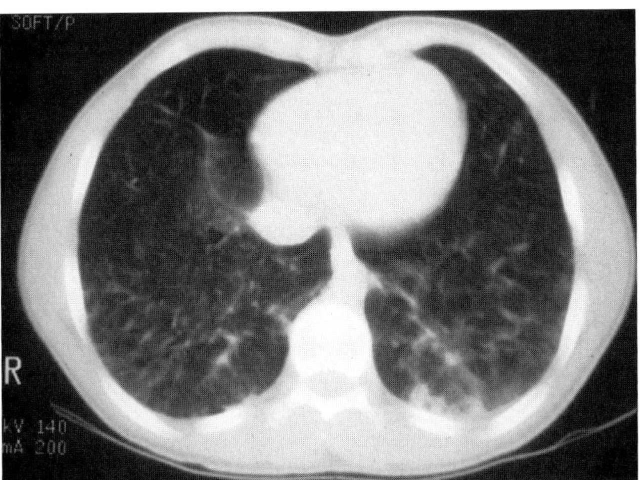

Figure 57–7. Reticulomiliary inhalational *Aspergillus fumigatus* fungal pneumonia. A chest x-ray was read as "normal," but the computed tomography scan is abnormal and the patient had severe hypoxia.

intense exposure to gardening mulch, digging in the soil, handling manure, or working on a construction project. The presentation is often that of relatively acute onset of shortness of breath and high fever. Early in the process, a regular chest x-ray may appear normal, but a computed tomography scan will often reveal pan-lobular reticulomiliary densities. As the process progresses, these infiltrates will enlarge and coalesce. At the same time, the patient may have a low blood oxygen saturation out of proportion to what might be expected from the extent of disease seen on the computed tomography scan. This type of presentation in a patient with chronic granulomatous disease should be considered a medical emergency requiring immediate attention.

Because *Aspergillus* is often isolated from either bronchoscopy or transthoracic needle biopsy, this syndrome can be confused with that of the *Aspergillus* hypersensitivity pneumonitis, also known as ABPA. This conclusion is a grave error that can lead to death of the patient if potent antifungal therapy active against *Aspergillus* is not administered. Like ABPA, part of the treatment must be with high-dose steroids that are necessary to achieve adequate oxygenation, which is impaired by the pan-lobular exuberant inflammatory granulomatous reaction associated with chronic granulomatous disease. However, unlike ABPA, these patients also must be treated promptly and aggressively with antifungal agents such as the new antibiotic voriconazole or the not yet FDA-approved agent posaconazole,[65] both of which have very potent oral activity against *Aspergillus,* to avoid the high mortality associated with this syndrome. Inhalational pneumonias often have multiple organisms, and treatment should include coverage for *Nocardia* and *Burkholderia* species. Occasionally, this type of pneumonia may be seen from only a bacterial etiology, so diagnostic studies to determine etiology are important.

After pneumonias, liver abscesses are the second most common severe deep tissue infection of patients with chronic granulomatous disease.[43] In patients who are reliably taking their prophylactic medications, infections with *S. aureus* at sites other than the liver are not common, yet in almost 90% of liver abscesses, *S. aureus* is the causative agent. The pathophysiologic basis for this empirical observation is unclear, and it should not be assumed that a patient presenting with staphylococcus liver abscess has been negligent about taking prophylactic trimethoprim-sulfamethoxazole. In patients with chronic granulomatous disease, liver abscess is complicated by exuberant granuloma formation with a major fibrotic component. Thus, most liver abscesses are not a collection of pus surrounded by a capsule, but instead are a solid fibrotic mass studded with microabscesses and granulomas (Fig. 57–8). Although needle biopsy can sometimes make the microbiologic diagnosis, this explains why rarely is more than a scant amount of pus drained from the site, and why simple drainage is not a therapeutic option. Very prolonged antibiotic treatment (many months) can sterilize relatively small liver abscesses of this type, but larger abscesses require surgical extirpation of the fibrotic mass of microabscesses. Without surgery for such solid microabscessed lesions, cure is difficult and relapse rates are high. On an experimental basis in patients who for a variety of reasons cannot have surgery, but whose abscesses have failed to respond to many months of medical therapy, we have at NIH been testing the potential of needle-guided radiofrequency heat ablation methods developed to treat cancers to also ablate these medically refractory fibrogranulomatous staphylococcal liver abscesses in chronic granulomatous disease patients. This appears to have worked in three patients treated this way at NIH, though it is too early to determine if this currently experimental approach has the potential to replace surgical extirpation.

Management of Granuloma-Related Complications

In addition to infections, patients with chronic granulomatous disease also suffer from problems related to granuloma formation.[66–79] Of note is that 50% of patients have recurrent episodes of gastrointestinal granuloma formation (chronic abdominal discomfort, intermittent vom-

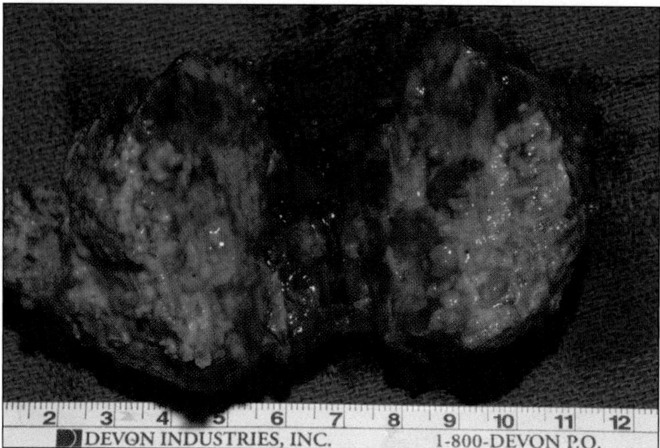

Figure 57–8. Surgically excised liver abscess. "Botryomycotic" semisolid mass is most common; this cannot be "drained" by percutaneous needle aspirate, and responds best to surgical removal.

iting, and even frank obstruction), and 20% have actual inflammatory bowel disease (manifested by chronic diarrhea and/or rectal abscess, fissure, or fistulas). Also, about 10% of chronic granulomatous disease patients have one or more episodes of acute bladder and/or ureteral obstruction. It is important to be aware that young male patients with chronic granulomatous disease who suddenly complain that they have pain or other acute problems with urination probably have a granuloma of the bladder at the urethral outlet. These patients should not be instrumented, but instead should have an ultrasound examination to confirm the presence of the granuloma and should immediately be placed on high-dose steroids. We have seen patients given a high dose of oral prednisone (1–2 mg/kg) have significant improvement of urinary symptoms overnight or even in a few hours. We treat acute granuloma exacerbations of the bowel or urinary tract with 0.5–1 mg/kg prednisone for the first week and then taper over 6 weeks, but about 30% of our patients require indefinite maintenance with alternate-day oral prednisone (0.1–0.2 mg/kg every other day) to prevent recurrence (prophylactic steroids). Curiously, in some patients with chronic granulomatous disease, a permanent maintenance dose of prednisone given every other day that might appear to be homeopathic (1–2 mg oral prednisone every other day in a 25-kg child or 5 mg every other day in a 60-kg adult) may control granuloma-related symptoms of the gastrointestinal tract (chronic abdominal pain or diarrhea) that reappear if the steroid is stopped.

CONTROVERSIAL OR EXPERIMENTAL THERAPIES

Bone Marrow Transplantation

Allogeneic bone marrow or other hematopoietic stem cell transplantation represents the only current treatment capable of permanently curing chronic granulomatous disease by replacing the oxidase-deficient neutrophils, monocytes, and tissue macrophages with donor cells produced from marrow that have normal oxidase activity.[80–86] As noted earlier, the outlook for survival and long periods of normal infection-free living for chronic granulomatous disease patients has greatly improved and continues to improve. This has resulted from effective prophylactic regimens (trimethoprim-sulfamethoxazole, itraconazole, interferon gamma, low-dose alternate-day steroids where necessary for granuloma control); aggressive approaches to infection diagnosis (computed tomography, magnetic resonance imaging, needle biopsy); improvements in antibiotics (particularly the availability of voriconazole, a potent oral antifungal alternative to intravenous amphotericin B, and linezolid, a potent oral anti-staphylococcal agent); and early recognition of specific types of infections and granuloma/inflammation syndromes and the proper treatment of these problems. However, significant improvements have also occurred in bone marrow transplantation, which include better molecular matching of donor to recipient, improved agents and methods for marrow and immune suppression conditioning, improvements in agents and methods to detect and treat transplant-associated infection, and improvements in agents and methods to prevent or treat acute and chronic graft-versus-host disease. Thus, the risk-benefit ratio of allogeneic stem cell transplantation for chronic granulomatous disease is changing, and currently it is difficult to make blanket statements about the role of allogeneic stem cell transplantation in the management of chronic granulomatous disease.

Chronic granulomatous disease patients most at risk are those with the completely oxidase-negative X-linked form, and that subset of patients of any genetic sub-type who have a sustained history of recurrent life-threatening infections. The lowest morbidity and mortality from allogeneic stem cell transplantation is seen in children with a fully human lymphocyte antigen–matched sibling donor. Thus, a consensus is beginning to emerge that chronic granulomatous disease patients at highest risk who have such a donor should be considered for allogeneic transplantation. Although experimental nonablative marrow conditioning regimens can reduce morbidity and make possible the consideration of transplantation in a chronic granulomatous disease patient who has an incurable and otherwise fatal infection, experimental nonablative conditioning regimens have been reported to be associated with a significantly higher rate of graft failure, particularly in children. Therefore, in a patient with chronic granulomatous disease considered for matched sibling donor transplantation who is not actively infected at the time of transplantation, the current consensus appears to favor more conventional marrow conditioning regimens. There may be a place for matched unrelated transplants, including unrelated cord blood transplants, in a specific patient based on infection history, but such transplants carry significantly higher risk of morbidity, mortality, and graft failure, and must be considered experimental.

Gene Therapy

There is active research into the potential of gene therapy for chronic granulomatous disease, and some clinical trials have been conducted. Until very recently, approaches to gene therapy have resulted in full correction of the oxidase activity in far less than 0.5% of circulating neutrophils, with the effect lasting only several months when ex vivo stem cell gene therapy was used in a setting where there was no bone marrow preparative conditioning.[87–91] However, recent improvements in the efficiency of gene transfer vectors, and the application of marrow conditioning to enhance engraftment of gene-corrected stem cells, have resulted in an improved outcome in a recently reported trial of gene therapy for chronic granulomatous disease using a busulphan conditioning regimen.[92] In gene therapy trials for another immune deficiency (X-linked severe combined immune deficiency resulting from mutations in the interleukin-2 receptor γ chain), the appearance of lymphocytic leukemias in three of eight patients with X-linked severe combined immune deficiency whose immune systems were restored by gene therapy raised a cautionary note regarding the potential risks of insertional oncogenesis from retrovirus-mediated gene therapy. However, it may be possible to use insulators or other approaches to mitigate the effects of insertional mutagenesis on surrounding genes, and investigators in the field continue to work on the development of gene therapy for chronic granulomatous disease.

CURRENT CONTROVERSIES & FUTURE CONSIDERATIONS

Chronic Granulomatous Disease

- Should all patients with chronic granulomatous disease be treated with prophylactic interferon gamma, or only patients with many frequent recurrent infections? The only randomized double-blind study suggests that all patients may benefit but does not address relative benefit of relatively "healthy" versus "chronically ill" chronic granulomatous disease patients.
- Do patients with chronic granulomatous disease have an increased frequency of defined autoimmune disorders (Crohn's disease, rheumatoid arthritis, sarcoid, etc.) that complicate the underlying granuloma formation specific to the disease (i.e., is chronic granulomatous disease a risk factor in development of autoimmune disorders)?
- Should all patients with X-linked chronic granulomatous disease who have complete absence of oxidase activity and who also have a human lymphocyte antigen–matched sibling be offered a hematopoietic stem cell transplant? Should such transplantation involve fully ablative conditioning, or reduced-intensity (subablative) conditioning, or be nonablative (so-called minitransplant)?
- Can safe and effective gene therapy for chronic granulomatous disease be developed? This will likely require improved vectors and also the use of some level of conditioning with a stem cell–active regimen (low-dose busulfan or low-dose radiation).

Suggested Readings*

Abati A, Cajigas A, Holland SM, Solomon D: Chronic granulomatous disease of childhood: respiratory cytology. Diagn Cytopathol 15:98, 1996.

Chin TW, Stiehm ER, Falloon J, Gallin JI: Corticosteroids in treatment of obstructive lesions of chronic granulomatous disease. J Pediatr 111:349, 1987.

Gallin JI, Alling DW, Malech HL, et al: Itraconazole prophylaxis for fungal infections in chronic granulomatous disease of childhood. N Engl J Med 348:2416, 2003.

Horwitz ME, Barrett AJ, Brown MR, et al: Treatment of chronic granulomatous disease with nonmyeloablative conditioning and a T-cell-depleted hematopoietic allograft. N Engl J Med 344:881, 2001.

Jirapongsananuruk O, Malech HL, Kuhns DB, et al: Diagnostic paradigm for evaluation of male patients with chronic granulomatous disease, based on the dihydrorhodamine 123 assay. J Allergy Clin Immunol 111:374, 2003.

Johnston RB Jr: Clinical aspects of chronic granulomatous disease. Curr Opin Hematol 8:17, 2001.

Kis E, Verebely T, Meszner Z: Inflammatory pseudotumor of the bladder in chronic granulomatous disease. Pediatr Nephrol 17:220, 2002.

Klempner MS, Malech HL: Phagocytes: normal and abnormal neutrophil host defenses. *In* Gorbach SL, Bartlett JG, Blacklow NR (eds): Infectious Diseases (ed 3). Philadelphia: Lippincott Williams & Wilkins, 2003, pp 14–39.

Lublin M, Bartlett DL, Danforth DN, et al: Hepatic abscess in patients with chronic granulomatous disease. Ann Surg 235:383, 2002.

Malech HL: Progress in gene therapy for chronic granulomatous disease. J Infect Dis 179(Suppl 2):S318, 1999.

Malech HL, Maples PB, Whiting-Theobald N, et al: Prolonged production of NADPH oxidase-corrected granulocytes following gene therapy of chronic granulomatous disease. Proc Natl Acad Sci U S A 94:12133, 1997.

Marciano BE, Rosenzweig SD, Kleiner DE, et al: Gastrointestinal involvement in chronic granulomatous disease. Pediatrics 114:462–468, 2004.

Margolis DM, Melnick DA, Alling DW, Gallin JI: Trimethoprim-sulfamethoxazole prophylaxis in the management of chronic granulomatous disease. J Infect Dis 162:723, 1990.

Segal BH, Leto TL, Gallin JI, et al: Genetic, biochemical, and clinical features of chronic granulomatous disease. Medicine (Baltimore) 79:170–200, 2000.

Seger RA, Gungor T, Belohradsky BH, et al: Treatment of chronic granulomatous disease with myeloablative conditioning and an unmodified hemopoietic allograft: a survey of the European experience, 1985–2000. Blood 100:4344, 2002.

Winkelstein JA, Marino MC, Johnston RB Jr, et al: Chronic granulomatous disease: report on a national registry of 368 patients. Medicine (Baltimore) 79:155–169, 2000.

**Full references for this chapter can be found on accompanying CD-ROM.*

CHAPTER 58

Autoimmune Lymphoproliferative Syndrome

V. Koneti Rao, MD, and Stephen E. Straus, MD

KEY POINTS

Autoimmune Lymphoproliferative Syndrome

- Autoimmune lymphoproliferative syndrome (ALPS) is associated with mutations that impair the activity of lymphocyte apoptosis proteins.
- Mutations in the gene encoding the apoptosis signaling protein Fas underlie most cases of ALPS.
- ALPS often manifests as the most common childhood hematologic disorder, immune thrombocytopenic purpura.
- Clinical features of ALPS include childhood-onset chronic lymphadenopathy, hepatosplenomegaly, and autoimmune cytopenias.
- Patients with ALPS who have Fas mutations also have a significantly increased risk of lymphoma.

INTRODUCTION

Autoimmune lymphoproliferative syndrome (ALPS) is an inherited genetic disease in which a failure of apoptotic mechanisms that help to maintain normal lymphocyte homeostasis leads to accumulation of lymphoid mass and persistence of autoreactive cells.[1,2] Chronic nonmalignant lymphadenopathy and splenomegaly in young children with recurring autoimmune cytopenias are the typical constellation of clinical features of ALPS, first described by Canale and Smith in 1967.[3] With the discovery of its cellular and molecular bases, ALPS is understood now to represent a discrete and novel syndrome, characterized clinically by early childhood onset of prominent nonmalignant lymphadenopathy and hepatosplenomegaly, autoimmune cytopenias, and by an increased risk of lymphoma. Mutations in genes that regulate lymphocyte survival are etiologic in most cases.

EPIDEMIOLOGY AND RISK FACTORS

ALPS has been reported from all parts of the globe among every racial and ethnic group, of 300 patients published worldwide, 200 are enrolled as subjects in studies at the Clinical Center of the National Institutes of Health (NIH). Because of its variable disease manifestations, often presenting with overlapping clinical symptoms common to other hematologic disorders, ALPS must often be underdiagnosed. Many patients have multiple affected family members, because the mutations in apoptosis pathway genes associated with ALPS are inherited in an autosomal dominant fashion.

MOLECULAR PATHOGENESIS AND PATHOPHYSIOLOGY

Molecular Mechanism of Apoptosis

Apoptosis was originally observed as a morphologic feature of programmed cell death characterized by nuclear pyknosis. The term is now widely used to describe cells' innate ability to self-destruct through a series of molecular events in death effector pathways, leading to an orderly demise and eventual phagocytosis of cellular remains. Apoptosis is distinct from cellular necrosis, because it avoids unwarranted inflammation or tissue damage. In 2002, Brenner, Horvitz, and Sulston received the Nobel Prize in Medicine and Physiology for their seminal studies leading to identification of genes regulating programmed cell death in the nematode *Caenorhabditis elegans*. The biologic significance of these genes is underscored by their conservation in mammalian evolution. The core death program in the nematode, as in humans, involves activation of a proteolytic cascade of self-cleaving initiator and effector caspases, a class of cysteine proteases that share cysteine-aspartate residues, similar to the zymogens found in the coagulation and complement activation pathways.

Apoptosis can be triggered by any of several death effector molecules that activate caspases, either through receptor-ligand interactions at the cell surface (the extrinsic pathway) or by induction of enzymes in mitochondria (the intrinsic pathway). Induction of apoptosis from the plasma membrane is mediated by binding of specific ligands to proteins in the tumor necrosis factor receptor superfamily (TNFRSF), leading to their aggregation and recruitment of cytoplasmic adapter molecules. In the case of Fas (Apo-1/CD95/TNFRSF-6), the best studied of all apoptosis effector molecules, the binding of Fas ligand (FasL) or agonistic antibodies to Fas triggers trimerization and rapid recruitment to a domain in the cytoplasmic portion of Fas termed the *death domain* (DD) of the homologous region of the cytoplasmic adaptor protein, Fas-associated death domain protein (FADD). This is followed by the recruitment of procaspase 8 or 10 through the interaction of death-effector domains in the amino termini of FADD and the procaspases. The resulting Fas/FADD/caspase complex is termed the *death-inducing signaling complex* (DISC)[4,5] because its formation culminates in apoptosis of cells that express Fas (Fig. 58–1). The mitochondrial pathway is initiated by DNA damage or growth factor deprivation and dysregulation of members of the p53 and Bcl-2 family of proteins, leading to mitochondrial permeabilization and release of apoptogenic factors such as cytochrome *c*, supramolecular activation complex, and granzyme B into the cytosol, triggering caspase activation and apoptosome complex formation. To date, ALPS has only been associated with defects in the receptor-mediated apoptosis pathway.

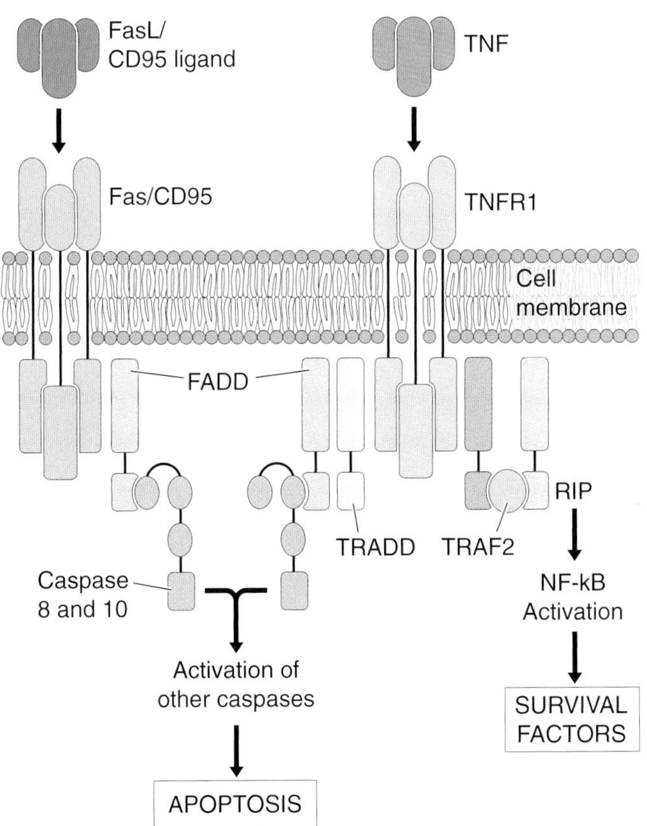

Figure 58–1. Induction of apoptosis from the plasma membrane is mediated by binding of specific ligands to proteins in the tumor necrosis factor receptor superfamily (TNFRSF), leading to their aggregation and recruitment of cytoplasmic adapter molecules.

Apoptosis in Immune Surveillance

Cellular systems with a high intrinsic proliferation capacity and cell turnover in the body, such as hematopoietic cells, have elegant physiologic mechanisms to regulate the rates of both cell proliferation and cell death and thus to maintain homeostasis of a population of cells as a whole. For cells of the immune system, apoptosis plays a key role in the termination of redundant immune responses by eliminating unnecessary effector cells through negative selection to avoid autoimmunity and tissue damage. In general, T cells that are able to mount an immune response against antigen peptides bound to major histocompatibility complex molecules undergo positive selection to ensure a repertoire of cells that are capable of responding to foreign antigens. Strongly self-reactive lymphocytes are removed from the repertoire by negative selection before they become fully mature and might initiate damaging autoimmune reactions, and immunologic tolerance is established to ubiquitous self antigens. The default fate of developing lymphocytes, in the absence of any signal received from the antigen receptor on the cell surface, is death. The vast majority of developing lymphocytes die either before emerging from the central lymphoid organs or before maturing in the peripheral lymphoid organs. The small fraction of lymphocytes that survive to form the mature lymphocyte population express a large repertoire of receptors capable of responding to a virtually unlimited variety of nonself antigens.

MRL/lpr$^{-/-}$ Murine Model of ALPS

Mature lymphocytes undergo a life cycle of activation and immune effector responses followed by apoptosis triggered primarily by Fas, which is highly expressed on activated B and T lymphocytes. The essential role that Fas exerts in maintaining lymphocyte homeostasis and peripheral immune tolerance to prevent autoimmunity was first elucidated by studies in Fas-deficient MRL/lpr$^{-/-}$ mice. Mice homozygous for Fas mutations develop hypergammaglobulinemia, glomerulonephritis, massive lymphadenopathy, and expansion of an unusual population of T-cell receptor α/β cells that are negative for both CD4 and CD8, otherwise known as double-negative T cells.[6–8]

Fas Dysregulation

The pivotal role of Fas protein in maintaining immune homeostasis in humans was revealed by the recognition and characterization of ALPS. In contrast to the homozygous recessive murine *lpr* mutations, most humans with ALPS have heterozygous Fas mutations that act in an autosomal dominant fashion (Fig. 58–2). In vitro studies showed that mutant Fas protein inhibits the function of normal Fas protein in humans, resulting in diminished Fas-mediated apoptosis and the accumulation of the activated lymphocytes that manifest as aberrant lymphoproliferation and autoimmunity.[9,10] ALPS presents in early childhood with lymphadenopathy, splenomegaly, and

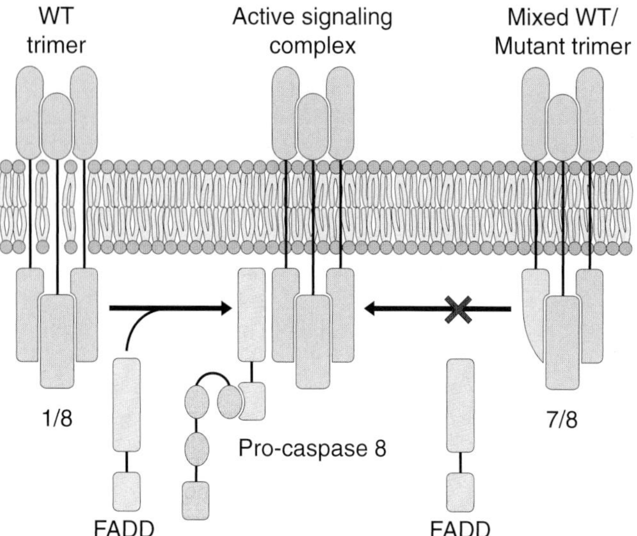

Figure 58–2. For Fas (Apo-1/CD95/TNFRSF-6), the best studied of all apoptosis effector molecules, the binding of Fas ligand (FasL) or agonistic antibodies to Fas triggers trimerization and rapid recruitment to a domain in the cytoplasmic portion of Fas termed the *death domain* (DD) of the homologous region of the cytoplasmic adaptor protein, Fas-associated death domain protein (FADD). In vitro studies showed that mutant Fas protein inhibits the function of normal Fas protein in humans, resulting in diminished Fas-mediated apoptosis and the accumulation of the activated lymphocytes that manifest as aberrant lymphoproliferation and autoimmunity.

autoimmune cytopenias. There is a significantly increased risk of lymphomas, indicating that receptor-mediated apoptosis pathways also serve to delete aberrant clones of lymphocytes with oncogenic potential (Fig. 58–3). The *TNFRSF6* gene may be a tumor suppressor gene because it is silenced in many sporadic tumors.[11,12] Somatic mutations of the *TNFRSF6* gene (coding Fas protein) occur in a fraction of childhood Hodgkin's lymphoma cases and may favor the escape of the precursor of the Reed-Sternberg clone from apoptosis. In one report, 20% of B-cell lymphomas derived from (post) germinal center B cells possess somatic mutations in exon 9 of Fas, which encodes its pivotal intracellular death domain.

Though autosomal dominant transmission of heterozygous germline mutations in the *TNFRSF6* (Fas) gene alone account for some 75% of all ALPS cases, occasional patients with homozygous mutations have been described as having a very severe disease phenotype.[13] There is also a small subset of patients with phenotypic features of ALPS associated with somatic mutations in intracellular regions of Fas in isolates of circulating double-negative T cells.[14,15]

CLINICAL FEATURES AND DIAGNOSIS

Case Definition and Classification

Diagnostic criteria for ALPS include chronic, nonmalignant lymphadenopathy and/or splenomegaly persisting for at least 6 months; defective (less than half-normal) Fas-mediated lymphocyte apoptosis as assayed in vitro; and

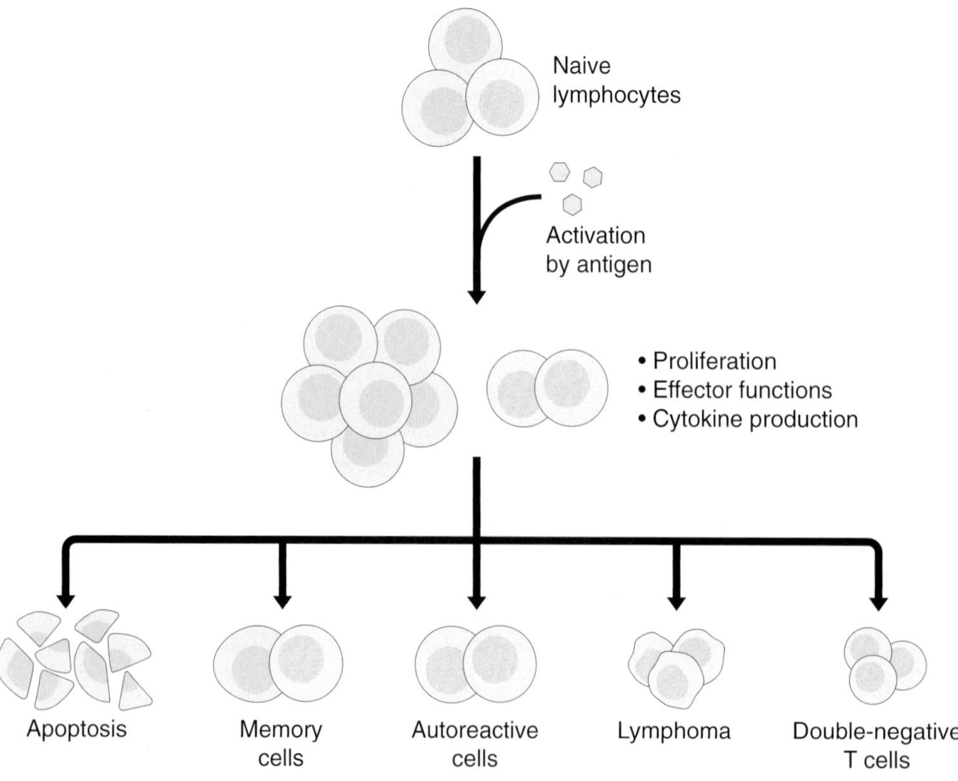

Figure 58–3. Survival advantage and effects of lymphocytes with Fas mutations. Normal lymphocyte homeostasis depends on maintaining a balance between the expansion of naive cells and their elimination by apoptosis, with a small minority of the cells that are generated after stimulation persisting as memory lymphocytes. Somatic mutations in a fraction of naïve cells *(brown)* lead to their persistence as double-negative T cells, premalignant cells, and autoreactive cells that can mediate autoimmune responses. (From Puck JM, Straus SE: Somatic mutations—not just for cancer anymore [Perspective]. N Engl J Med 351:1388–1390, 2004, with permission.)

elevated (≥1% or ≥ 20/μL) circulating double-negative T cells[1,2] (Table 58–1).

ALPS is currently classified as ALPS type Ia and Ib when the patient carries mutations in the genes encoding Fas or FasL, respectively (Table 58–2). Patients with ALPS type II possess mutations in genes for caspase 8 or 10, and patients in whom no mutation has as yet been identified are classified as ALPS type III.[16–18] The clinical and laboratory features of ALPS do not differ markedly between patients in whom mutations have been identified and those without identifiable mutations[1,2] (Table 58–3).

Clinical Manifestations and Natural History

Enlargement of the lymph nodes and spleen in children with ALPS may be massive and distort anatomic landmarks, or be more modest and best identified by computed tomographic scanning or ultrasound imaging[2,21] (Fig. 58–4). Regardless of extent, lymphadenopathy persists for years in almost all patients.

Cytopenias contribute to multiple episodes of pallor and icterus associated with hemolytic anemia, spontaneous bruises and mucocutaneous hemorrhages, and bacterial infection associated with neutropenia. Nonhematologic autoimmune diseases reported in association with ALPS include Guillain-Barré syndrome, glomerulonephritis, uveitis, and autoimmune liver disease.[1,19] As patients undergo long-term evaluation, the potential for multiple autoimmune diseases involving different organ systems in a single patient with ALPS is increasingly recognized.

The median age of initial presentation with florid lymphadenopathy and splenomegaly is about 24 months. Adenopathy and splenomegaly may decrease in extent through adolescence. Similarly, clinical manifestations of refractory, chronic cytopenias are most severe in childhood, so that 50% of patients require a splenectomy; however, symptoms related to cytopenias may occur at any age. Asplenic ALPS patients require special vigilance against sepsis caused by pneumococcal bacteremia, which can be fatal.

Assessment of relatives of ALPS probands with Fas or caspase 10 mutations usually identifies a parent, a sibling, or a more distant relative with identical heterozygous mutations. Many such family members manifest few if

TABLE 58–1. Criteria for the Diagnosis of ALPS

Required Features

Chronic nonmalignant lymphadenopathy and/or splenomegaly
Increase in circulating T cells that are $CD4^-CD8^-$ and express the α/β T-cell receptor above the normal range of 0.1–0.9% of lymphocytes (absolute counts of 2–17)
Demonstration of defective antigen-induced lymphocyte apoptosis on in vitro culture

Supporting Features

Family history of autoimmune lymphoproliferative syndrome
Typical findings on histopathologic analysis of lymph node or splenic tissue
Mutations of genes encoding Fas or related apoptosis signaling proteins

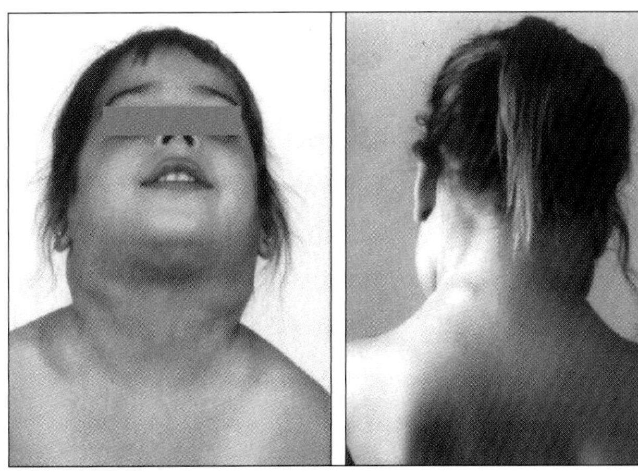

Figure 58–4. Visible lymphadenopathy in a typical child with ALPS.

TABLE 58–2. Gene Defects in ALPS Cases*

ALPS Type	Defective Gene	Protein	Percent of ALPS Cases
Ia	*TNFRSF6*	Fas, major transmembrane receptor for apoptosis in lymphocytes	74
Ia, somatic mutant	*TNFRSF6* (hematopoietic cell defect)	Same as type Ia	Unknown
Ib	*TNFSF6*	Fas ligand	<1
IIa	*CASP10*	Caspase 10, intracellular apoptosis pathway protease	~2
IIb	*CASP8*	Caspase 8, intracellular apoptosis pathway protease	<1
III†	Unknown	Unknown	24

*The percentages of ALPS cases are based on the 178 cases in a series studied at the National Institutes of Health. *TNFRSF6* denotes tumor necrosis factor receptor superfamily member 6, and *TNFSF6* tumor necrosis factor superfamily member 6.
†A subgroup of ALPS type III may be Ia, somatic mutant.[15]

TABLE 58–3. Clinical Features in 79 Patients with Autoimmune Lymphoproliferative Syndrome*

Sex	Female, N = 43	Male, N = 36
Race	White, 69 Black, 6	Other, 4
Median age at presentation (range)	2 yr (birth–15 yr)	

Clinical Manifestation in Patients	*n* (%)
Lymphoproliferative disease	79 (100)
Splenomegaly	75 (95)
Lymphadenopathy	76 (96)
Hepatomegaly	57 (72)
Lymphoma	7 (9)
Autoantibodies†	64 (81)
Autoimmune disease	37 (47)
Hemolytic anemia‡	23 (29)
Idiopathic thrombocytopenic purpura	18 (23)
Neutropenia	15 (19)
Glomerulonephritis	2 (3)
Optic neuritis or uveitis	2 (3)
Guillain-Barré syndrome	1 (1)
Primary biliary cirrhosis	1 (1)
Coagulopathy/factor VIII inhibitor	1 (1)

Modified From Sneller MC, Dale JK, Straus SE: Autoimmune lymphoproliferative syndrome. Curr Opin Rheumatol 15:417–421, 2003.
*Data compiled from probands and relatives with autoimmune lymphoproliferative syndrome (47 discrete families).
†Thirty patients had one or more autoantibodies but no autoimmunity disease.
‡Direct Coombs test was positive for both immunoglobulin G and C3d in all patients with hemolytic anemia.

any clinical features of ALPS, even if they share similar in vitro apoptosis defects. Elevation in double-negative T cell numbers is typically not present in the absence of the clinical stigmata of ALPS. The likelihood that an individual who carries a Fas mutation will manifest ALPS appears to depend on several factors, only some of which are known. Mutations involving the intracellular death domain of the Fas molecule are much more likely than mutations in extracellular domain mutations to cause manifest ALPS features, and they have a more severe clinical phenotype.[20]

ALPS patients with germline mutation of the intracellular domain of Fas have a greatly increased (14- to 51-fold) risk of developing non-Hodgkin's and Hodgkin's lymphoma,[22,23] underscoring the critical role played by receptor-mediated apoptosis in eliminating proliferating lymphocytes with oncogenic potential. Among the cohort of 200 patients enrolled at the NIH Clinical Center, 11 have developed lymphomas (6 Hodgkin's and 5 B-cell non-Hodgkin's), with a median age at presentation with lymphoma of 17 years (range 2–50 years).

Laboratory Findings

Markers of Autoimmune Disease

The most common autoantibodies detected in ALPS are directed against red blood cells and detected by the Coombs direct antiglobulin test. Overt autoimmune cytopenias may include autoimmune hemolytic anemia, thrombocytopenia, and neutropenia.[2] Other features of ALPS are hypergammaglobulinemia and the presence of multiple circulating autoantibodies,[24–26] including immunoglobulins directed against platelets and neutrophils. Potentially pathogenic autoantibodies are seen often in the absence of overt autoimmune disease.

Associated Abnormalities of Peripheral Blood, Bone Marrow, and Lymph Nodes

Eosinophilia and monocytosis are frequent in ALPS.[27] A bone marrow aspirate showing some degree of dyserythropoiesis[28] and depletion of iron stores is not uncommon. Lymphocyte dysregulation in ALPS is revealed by an elevated percentage of double-negative ($CD3^+$ $CD4^-$ $CD8^-$) T cells in peripheral blood,[29] bone marrow, and lymphoid tissues (Fig. 58–5). Patients with ALPS also have a skewed T_H2-type immune response, one manifestation of which is elevated interleukin-10 plasma levels.[30]

In Vitro Apoptosis Defect

All patients with ALPS, by definition, exhibit defective lymphocyte apoptosis, which must be assayed in vitro by specialized laboratories using peripheral blood lymphocytes cultured in the presence of interleukin-2 for a few days and stimulated with phytohemagglutinin. Apoptosis is induced by a monoclonal antibody that binds to activated Fas on the cell surface; the majority of cells from normal controls are killed, whereas lymphocytes from patients with ALPS are relatively spared.[31]

Diagnosis

The complex presentation of generalized adenopathy, splenomegaly, and autoimmune cytopenias in childhood is a diagnostic challenge, because these clinical and laboratory features overlap those with other pediatric hematologic disorders, including lymphoma, hereditary spherocytosis, Evans's syndrome,[32] and Rosai-Dorfman disease.[33] The first step in management is to establish the diagnosis. The diagnostic criteria for ALPS were provided earlier. A lymph node biopsy may be appropriate: defective lymphocyte apoptosis produces a characteristic pathologic picture of reactive follicular hyperplasia and sometimes marked paracortical expansion with immunoblasts and plasma cells on microscopic section. Often a combination of follicular hyperplasia and paracortical expansion by a mixed infiltrate containing double-negative T cells, a feature unique to ALPS, helps differentiate this syndrome from other benign and malignant lymphoproliferative lesions[34] (Fig. 58–6). Assuming that another disease is not revealed by a biopsy, the diagnosis of ALPS requires laboratory evaluation of the proband and relevant family members, by immunophenotyping of peripheral blood for enumeration of double-negative T cells and in vitro apoptosis assay, as well as detailed molecular genetic analysis for mutations in

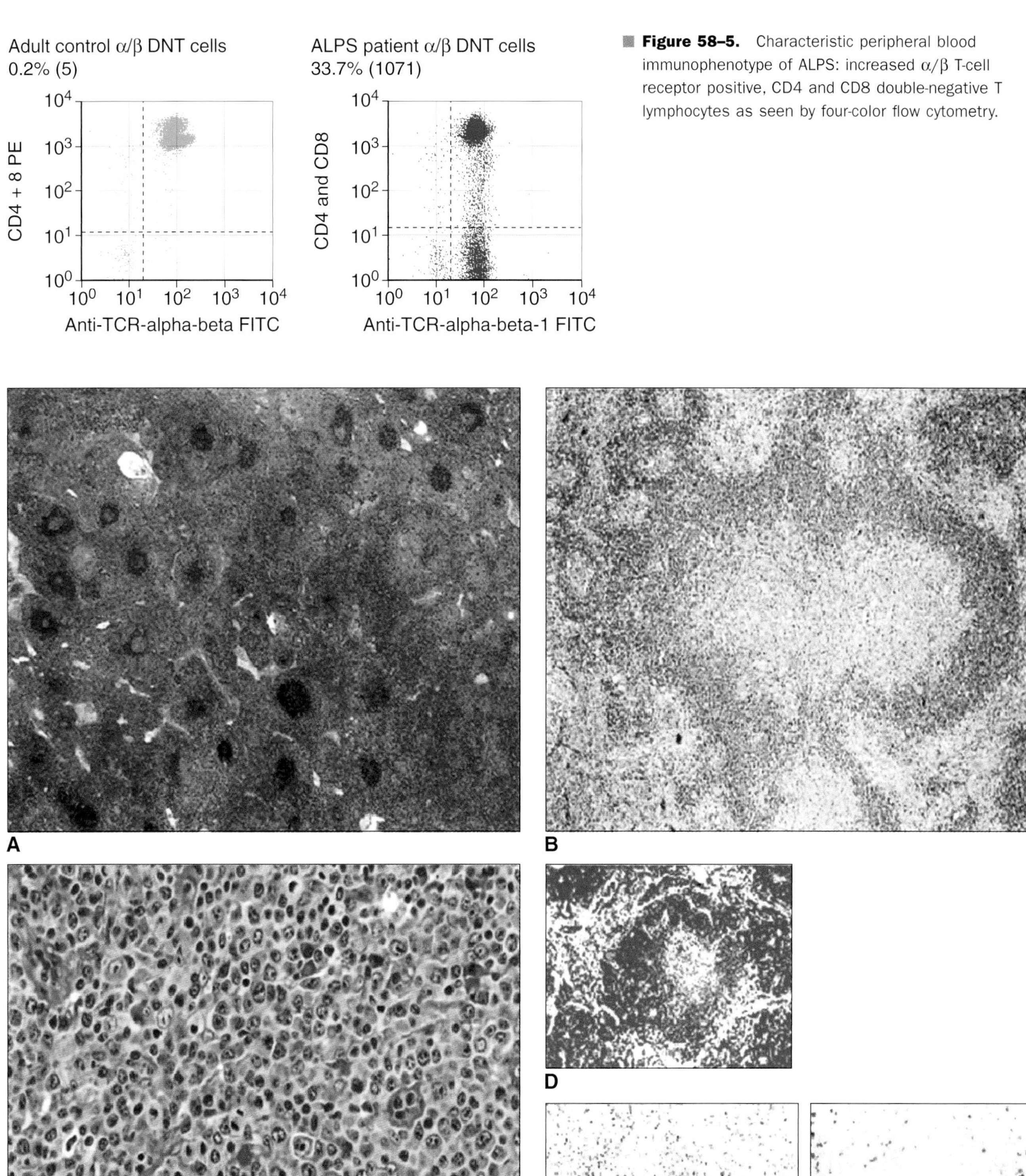

Figure 58–5. Characteristic peripheral blood immunophenotype of ALPS: increased α/β T-cell receptor positive, CD4 and CD8 double-negative T lymphocytes as seen by four-color flow cytometry.

Figure 58–6. Histopathology of lymph nodes in ALPS. ***A***, The paracortex is markedly expanded by lymphocytes with pale pink cytoplasm. Primary and secondary follicles are numerous. Some follicles show regressive changes *(upper right)*. (Hematoxylin and eosin [H&E]; original magnification, ×100.) ***B***, Progressive transformation of germinal centers was a focal but relatively frequent finding. (H&E; original magnification, ×200.) ***C***, The paracortex is populated by lymphocytes, plasma cells, and immunoblasts. Note frequent mitotic figures. (H&E; original magnification, ×600.) ***D–F***, Lymph node demonstrates paracortical expansion by $CD3^+$ double-negative T cells. Immunoperoxidase stains (ABC immunoperoxidase technique, hematoxylin counterstain; original magnification, ×200) performed in paraffin sections demonstrate expansion of interfollicular regions by $CD3^+$ T cells ***(D)*** that are largely $CD4^-$ ***(E)*** and $CD8^-$ ***(F)***. Most $CD4^+$ cells are within germinal centers.

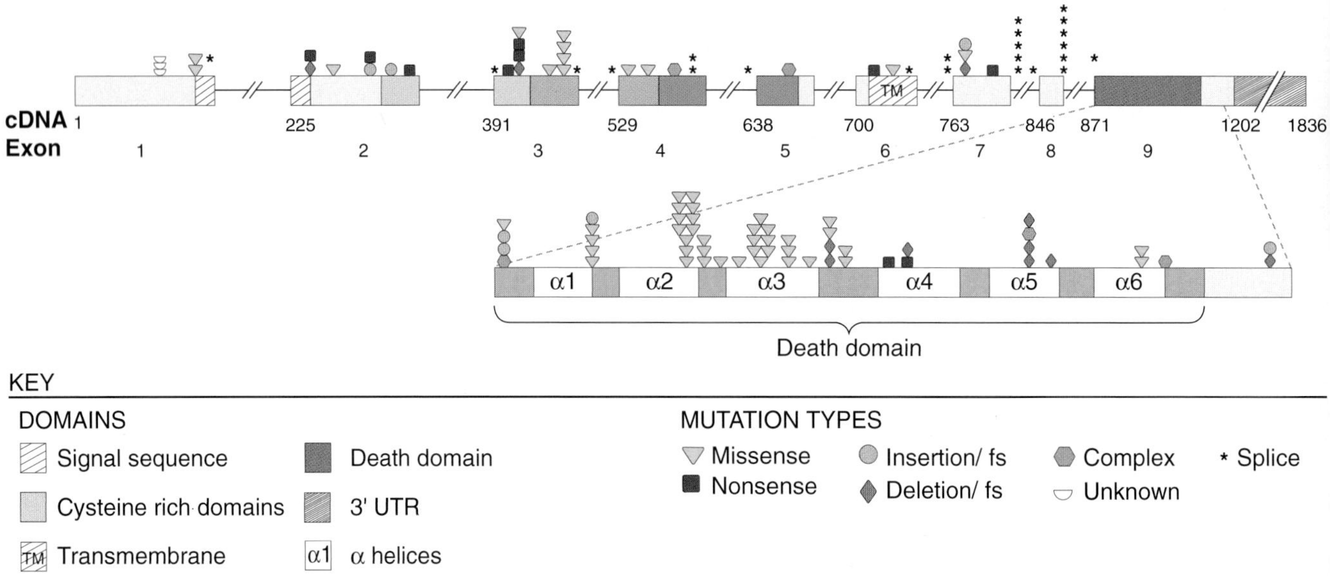

■ **Figure 58–7.** Reported Fas (*TNFRSF6*) mutations causing ALPS, showing distribution of the mutations along the nine exons of the gene. (Data from *http://research.nhgri.nih.gov/ALPS/*)

apoptosis pathway genes implicated in ALPS: Fas, FasL, caspase 10, and caspase 8 (Fig. 58–7).

TREATMENT

Once the diagnosis is confirmed, formal genetic assessment and counseling of the proband and the extended family are important, both to define the degree of disease penetrance and to educate relatives about the immediate and long-term risks of ALPS. The parents of affected children with ALPS must be advised of the need to seek timely help for any systemic symptoms or the onset of significant cytopenias, as well as unexpected fluctuations in lymph node and spleen size. They are also made aware of the implication of the underlying risk of lymphomas in those with an abnormal intracellular domain of the Fas protein and the morbidity associated with asplenia (Fig. 58–8).

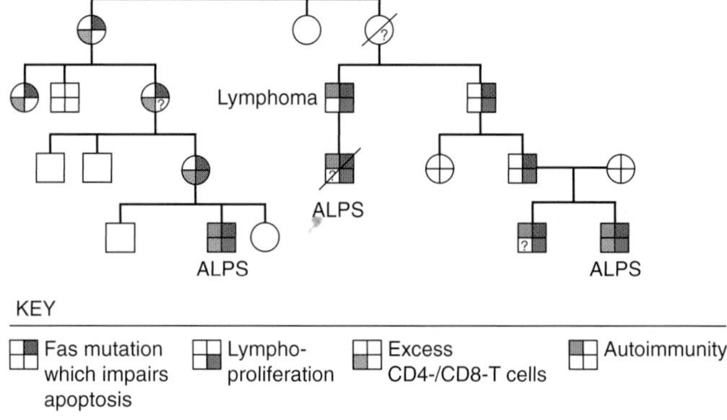

■ **Figure 58–8.** Pedigree tree in a typical ALPS type Ia patient.

Management of Lymphoproliferation and Hypersplenism

Although massive adenopathy in growing children can incite considerable anxiety and may be socially isolating, treatment is not specifically indicated to reduce lymph node size for cosmetic reasons alone. Neither corticosteroids nor immunosuppressive drugs such as azathioprine, cyclosporine, or mycophenolate mofetil consistently shrink the spleen or lymph nodes in patients with ALPS. The use of Fansidar for *Pneumocystis jiroveci (P. carinii)* prophylaxis was reported in a small series of patients with ALPS and ALPS-like conditions to be associated with reductions in lymphoproliferation[35]; however, our experience with this drug as well as its active component, pyrimethamine, failed to show regression of adenopathy or splenomegaly.

Approximately half of the 200 ALPS patients being studied at the NIH Clinical Center have had a splenectomy in order to manage recurring and chronic cytopenias, nearly 75% of whom achieved long-term remission. However, five asplenic ALPS patients have had fatal opportunistic infections and many others have developed pneumococcal sepsis. Thus, splenectomy should be avoided unless it is the only remaining measure to control chronic, refractory, life-threatening cytopenias. Spleen-guards made of fiberglass have been used with some success in some active children, allowing them to participate in activities at a reduced risk of splenic rupture.

Asplenia Care in ALPS Patients

All asplenic ALPS patients should receive long-term antibiotic prophylaxis against pneumococcal sepsis using penicillin V or fluoroquinolones. Many ALPS patients seem unable to produce or maintain antibodies directed against polysaccharide antigens following vaccination. General recommendations include use of an alert bracelet noting that the patient is asplenic, antibiotic prophylaxis and periodic surveillance, and reimmunization if needed, against pneumococci using both 7-valent Prevnar and 23-valent Pneumovax.[36]

ALPS-Related Cytopenias

The initial management of ALPS-related autoimmune cytopenias (autoimmune hemolytic anemia, immune thrombocytopenic purpura, autoimmune neutropenia) is similar to that used for cytopenias in other patient populations. In patients with severe thrombocytopenia and/or autoimmune hemolytic anemia, high-dose pulsed therapy with methylprednisolone (5–30 mg/kg × 1–2 days) followed by low-dose prednisone (1–2 mg/kg) maintenance oral therapy to be tapered slowly over months may be helpful. Intravenous immunoglobulin, 1–2 gm/kg, concomitant with pulsed-dose methylprednisolone, may benefit some patients with severe autoimmune hemolytic anemia by abrogating antibody-mediated red cell destruction and allowing sustained packed red blood cell transfusion support for severe anemia. Some ALPS patients with chronic neutropenia and associated infections benefit from daily, to as infrequently as thrice weekly, low-dose granulocyte colony-stimulating factor (1–2 μg/kg SC).

There is a single case report of successful treatment of cytopenias with combined Rituximab and vincristine in a patient with ALPS.[37] Rituximab (375 mg/m^2/wk × 4), used for refractory, chronic cytopenias in five ALPS patients in our cohort, led to durable responses in two. Some patients, especially those with massive splenomegaly and hypersplenism, may be refractory to standard drug regimens and packed red blood cell transfusions and require ongoing chronic, long-term immunosuppression. Our initial experience in 13 patients finds that mycophenolate mofetil (600 mg/m^2 given twice daily) is an effective corticosteroid-sparing agent in most cases. Mycophenolate mofetil may allow splenectomy to be avoided or postponed in young ALPS patients.[38]

Surveillance for Lymphoma

Chronic adenopathy in ALPS fluctuates in extent over time, which can create the concern of evolving lymphoma if one or more nodes enlarge unusually. ALPS patients need close observation with serial computed tomography scans, and they frequently undergo repeated biopsies. Most ALPS patients with lymphoma have responded to conventional multiagent chemotherapy and radiation. They present additional diagnostic challenges once therapy is discontinued because ALPS-associated adenopathy recurs and must be distinguished from relapsing lymphoma. Noninvasive tests are desirable in ALPS to help determine if a biopsy is warranted and which of many enlarged nodes will likely yield informative tissue. Positron emission tomography (PET) using [^{18}F] fluoro-2-deoxy-D-glucose (FDG) uptake, as measure of cellular glucose metabolism, has become standard in the staging and follow-up evaluation of cancers, including lymphomas.[39,40] Formal, prospective studies exploring the potential value of whole-body FDG-PET scan to determine whether qualitative or quantitative FDG local-

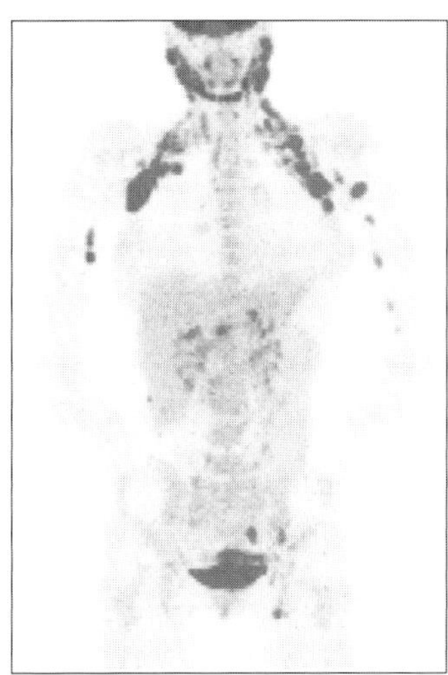

Figure 58–9. Representative FDG-PET scan in a patient with ALPS type Ia showing significant generalized lymphadenopathy in this asplenic patient. Research protocol to define PET "signature" in ALPS in order to develop noninvasive method of identifying emergence of lymphoma in ALPS patients is being undertaken at the NIH Clinical Center.

TABLE 58–4. Clinical History of a Representative ALPS Ia Patient (YOB: 1956)

1958	Splenomegaly, adenopathy, hepatomegaly, and thrombocytopenia. Treated with methotrexate, 6-mercaptopurine, and prednisone for lymphosarcoma.
1969	Lymph node biopsy showing paracortical lymphoid hyperplasia (Canale-Smith syndrome).
1974–1978	Autoimmune hemolytic anemia (hemoglobin 2.0). Underwent splenectomy.
1988–1989	Immune thrombocytopenic purpura. Thrombocytopenia responded to prednisone
1994	*Postpartum fever. Liver abscess. Progressed to more fevers, night sweats, fatigue, weight loss. Diagnosed with Hodgkin's lymphoma, mixed cellularity, stage IIIB. Treated with ABVD and mantle radiation.
1998	Admission for epistaxis, platelet count 3000. Treated with steroids, WinRho.
1999	Platelets 5000, bleeding gums, petechiae. Treated with WinRho, vincristine. Developed secondary vincristine neuropathy.
2001	Relapsed Hodgkin's lymphoma. Treated with ESHAP × 6 cycles.
2002	Computed tomography (CT) scan showed right pelvic mass markedly reduced in size (20 cm), no new nodes. Positron emission tomography (PET) showed uptake at supraclavicular neck, increase activity superior to bladder in left iliac region. No palpable nodes. No constitutional symptoms.
2003–2005	Ongoing evaluation at NIH Clinical Center ALPS clinic every 3 months by CT and PET scans for recurrent adenopathy. Biopsy negative for recurrent lymphoma.

*Her son (YOB 1994) also has ALPS with associated visible adenopathy and splenomegaly.

CURRENT CONTROVERSIES & FUTURE CONSIDERATIONS

Autoimmune Lymphoproliferative Syndrome

- ALPS is the first autoimmune disease whose genetic basis has been defined. Similar molecular mechanisms might underlie related syndromes.
- ALPS illustrates the importance of apoptosis in remodeling the lymphocyte repertoire and deleting autoreactive cells and cells with oncogenic potential.
- Novel therapeutic interventions are necessary to control the lymphoproliferative process in patients with ALPS who have chronic lymphadenopathy and splenomegaly and are at increased risk of lymphoma.
- Studies are underway to assess the utility of the MRL/$lpr^{-/-}$ mouse model for preclinical evaluation of various therapeutic agents to enhance apoptosis in the lymphocytes with germline Fas mutation.
- In ALPS patients, long-term control of lymphoproliferation without using immunosuppression is desirable.
- Controlling autoimmune cytopenias in ALPS by inhibiting lymphocyte proliferation may also prevent lymphoma transformation in individuals at elevated risk because of intracellular Fas mutations.

ization can differentiate ALPS patients with benign, albeit prominent, adenopathy from those with ALPS-associated lymphomas are in progress (Fig. 58–9).

Allogenic Bone Marrow Transplantation

Very few patients with ALPS are so ill from their cytopenias and resistant to conventional immunosuppressive treatment as to justify allogenic bone marrow transplantation. Nevertheless, stem cell transplantation has been successful in ALPS.[41,42] Chronic cytopenias of most ALPS patients improve with age, and the short- and long-term risks of allogenic stem cell transplantation need to be balanced against the severity and refractory nature of the chronic cytopenia- and/or lymphoproliferation-related morbidity of an individual with ALPS. A sibling donor must be free from a known mutation in an apoptosis pathway gene. Mortality resulting from matched unrelated donor–derived allogenic bone marrow transplantation is too high (35–45%) to warrant the procedure for the vast majority of patients with a chronic disease like ALPS who have a near-normal life expectancy. Alternative donor–derived stem cell transplantation should be reserved for those ALPS patients with a severe phenotype,[43,44] such as that associated with the rare occurrence of a homozygous Fas mutation.

PROGNOSIS

The major determinants of morbidity and mortality in ALPS depend on the severity of the autoimmune disease, hypersplenism and asplenia-related sepsis, and the development of lymphoma. The overall prognosis in ALPS is good. However, those patients at risk of developing lymphomas need surveillance over the course of many years, mainly by monitoring of their adenopathy (Table 58–4).

Suggested Readings*

Canale VC, Smith CH: Chronic lymphadenopathy simulating malignant lymphoma. J Pediatr 70:891–899, 1967.

Cohen PL, Eisenberg RA: *lpr* and *gld*: single gene models of systemic autoimmunity and lymphoproliferative disease. Annu Rev Immunol 9:243–269, 1991.

Debatin K, Stahne K, Fulda S, et al: Apoptosis in hematological disorders. Semin Cancer Biol 13:149–158, 2003.

Holzelova E, Vonarbourg C, Stolzenberg MC, et al: Autoimmune lymphoproliferative syndrome with somatic Fas mutations. N Engl J Med 351:1409–1418, 2004.

Lenardo MJ: Introduction: the molecular regulation of lymphocyte apoptosis. Semin Immunol 9:1–5, 1997.

Puck JM, Straus SE: Somatic mutations—not just for cancer anymore (Perspective). N Engl J Med 351:1388–1390, 2004.

Rieux-Laucat F, Blachere S, Danielan S, et al: Lymphoproliferative syndrome with autoimmunity: a possible genetic basis for dominant expression of the clinical manifestations. Blood 94:2575–2582, 1999.

Sneller MC, Dale JK, Straus SE: Autoimmune lymphoproliferative syndrome. Curr Opin Rheumatol 15:417–421, 2003.

Sneller MC, Wang J, Dale JK, et al: Clinical, immunologic, and genetic features of an autoimmune lymphoproliferative syndrome associated with abnormal lymphocyte apoptosis. Blood 89:1341–1348, 1997.

Straus SE, Jaffe ES, Puck JM, et al: The development of lymphomas in families with autoimmune lymphoproliferative syndrome (ALPS) with germline Fas mutations and defective lymphocyte apoptosis. Blood 98:194–200, 2001.

Full references for this chapter can be found on accompanying CD-ROM.

SECTION 5
DISEASES OF ALTERED COAGULATION

CHAPTER 59

INHERITED AND ACQUIRED DISORDERS OF PLATELET FUNCTION

Joel S. Bennett, MD

KEY POINTS

Inherited Platelet Disorders

- Patients with platelet function abnormalities present with mucocutaneous bleeding rather than the hematomas characteristic of patients with coagulation disorders such as hemophilia.
- Inherited disorders of platelet function, although uncommon to rare, can cause serious bleeding.
- The Bernard-Soulier syndrome, caused by the inability of platelets to adhere to subendothelial von Willebrand factor (vWF), results from deficiency or dysfunction of a platelet receptor for vWF, the glycoprotein (GP) Ib-IX-V complex, and is associated with macrothrombocytopenia as well.
- In Glanzmann thrombasthenia, platelets are unable to aggregate because of deficiency or dysfunction of the integrin $\alpha_{IIb}\beta_3$ (GPIIb/IIIa), a receptor for fibrinogen and vWF on activated platelets.
- Disorders of platelet secretion can be due to the absence of a specific class of platelet granule or to biochemical abnormalities that impair granule exocytosis.

Acquired Platelet Disorders

- Acquired disorders of platelet function are relatively common and are generally mild, but can cause serious bleeding in the presence of another disorder of hemostasis.
- Medications are the most common cause of acquired platelet dysfunction; a few medications prolong the bleeding time and cause or exacerbate bleeding, more prolong the bleeding time without inducing bleeding, and many more only affect platelet function ex vivo or in vitro.
- Of medications that affect platelet function, only aspirin, the thienopyridines, and the GPIIb/IIIa ($\alpha_{IIb}\beta_3$) antagonists substantially impair clinical hemostasis.
- Acquired platelet dysfunction can be responsible for bleeding in patients with renal failure or with antiplatelet antibodies, and after cardiopulmonary bypass.
- Platelet function is frequently abnormal in patients with chronic myeloproliferative disorders and can be impaired by the monoclonal proteins that are produced in the plasma cell dyscrasias.

INTRODUCTION

The differential diagnosis for a patient with bleeding symptoms, a normal platelet count, normal screening tests of coagulation, and a prolonged bleeding time consists of acquired and inherited disorders of platelet function and von Willebrand disease. von Willebrand disease is discussed in Chapter 64; this chapter discusses patients whose bleeding symptoms are specifically due to disorders of platelet function.

Platelets are responsible for primary hemostasis in arteries and in the microcirculation. Because of the demanding flow conditions in these vascular beds, platelets have evolved mechanisms that enable them to slow sufficiently to adhere to sites of vascular damage and then form hemostatic plugs that resist the shear forces of flowing blood (Fig. 59–1). Patients with platelet function abnormalities present with mucocutaneous bleeding (petechiae, excessive bruising, epistaxis, menorrhagia) rather than the hematomas characteristic of patients with coagulation disorders such as hemophilia. Disorders of platelet function can be either inherited or acquired. Although the former are uncommon to rare, they can cause serious bleeding; the latter are relatively common and are generally mild.

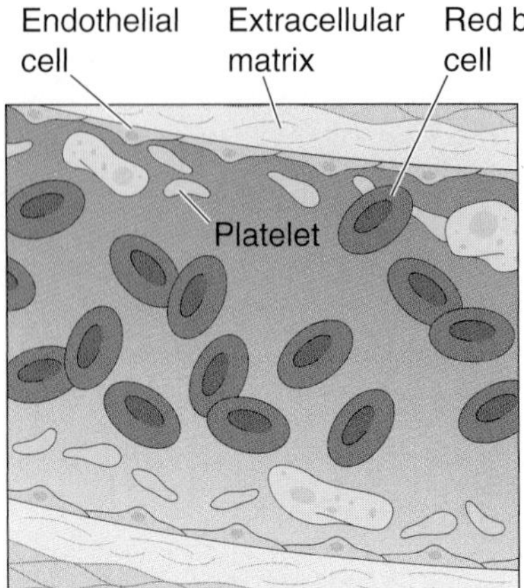

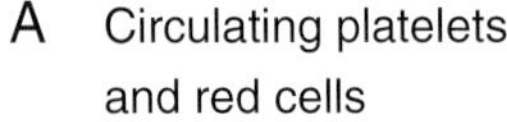

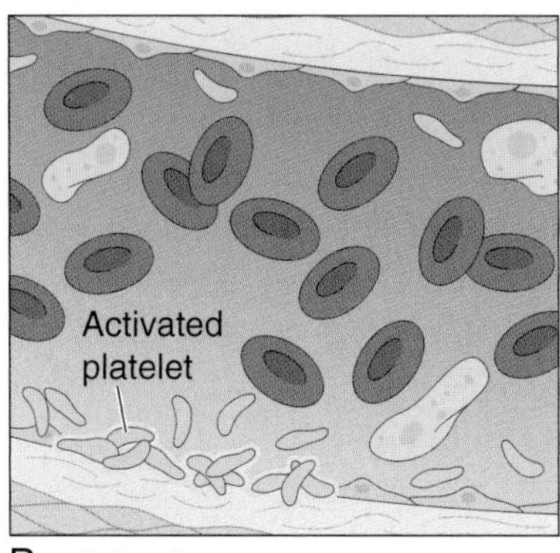

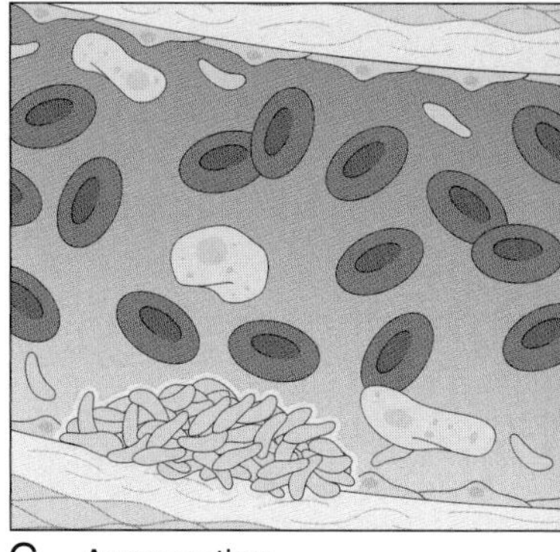

Figure 59–1. Stages of platelet function. ***A***, Platelets are pushed to the periphery of the column of blood by circulating red cells, facilitating their ability to adhere to breaks in the vascular endothelium. ***B***, When platelets encounter a break in the endothelium, they adhere to components of the exposed subendothelial connective tissue. ***C***, Activated platelets aggregate upon the layer of adherent platelets to form a stable hemostatic plug. (Adapted from Bennett JS: Mechanisms of platelet adhesion and aggregation: an update. Hosp Pract 27:124–140, 1992, with permission.)

INHERITED DISORDERS OF PLATELET FUNCTION

It is convenient for clinical and conceptual purposes to subdivide inherited platelet function disorders into disorders of platelet adhesion, aggregation, secretion, and procoagulant activity.

Platelet Adhesion

Platelets circulate in a nonreactive state, maintained in part by endothelial cell–derived nitric oxide and prostacyclin, until they encounter a break in the vascular endothelium. Platelets then tether to collagen, fibronectin, laminin, and von Willebrand factor (vWF) in exposed subendothelial connective tissue via specific cell surface receptors and translocate along the damaged surface.[1] Collagen is a particularly important subendothelial component in this regard because it is not only a substrate for platelet adhesion, but an agonist for platelet aggregation and a binding site for vWF as well.[2]

Bernard-Soulier Syndrome

Platelets must translocate on collagen-bound vWF in blood vessels where the shear rate is high to form a hemostatic plug. In 1948, Bernard and Soulier described a bleeding syndrome characterized by a markedly prolonged bleeding time, very large platelets, and thrombocytopenia.[3] This rare disorder, given the eponym Bernard-Soulier syndrome, is due to the inability of platelets to adhere to subendothelial vWF and results from deficiency or dysfunction of a platelet receptor for vWF, the glycoprotein (GP) Ib-IX-V (GPIb-IX-V) complex.[4]

Pathophysiology

GPIb-IX-V is a noncovalent complex of 165,000 molecular weight (MW) GPIb, 20,000 MW GPIX, and 82,000 MW GPV.[5–7] GPIb itself is a disulfide-linked heterodimer of 143,000 MW GPIbα and 22,000 MW GPIbβ.[8] Each protein is a member of the leucine-rich repeat motif superfamily[9]: GPIbα contains 8 leucine-rich repeats, GPIbβ and GPIX contain 1 each, and GPV contains 15. A crystal structure of GPIbα bound to vWF has revealed that leucine-rich repeats 1 and 5–8 of GPIbα bind tightly to the A1 domain of vWF[10] (Fig. 59–2). There are approximately 25,000 copies of GPIb and GPIX on the platelet surface, but only half as many copies of GPV, suggesting that each GPIb-IX-V complex contains two GPIb and two GPIX molecules and one molecule of GPV. The assembly of GPIb-IX-V complexes is most efficient when cells coexpress GPIbα, GPIbβ, and GPIX,[11] explaining why mutations in either of these proteins impairs GPIb-IX-V expression. GPV is not required for GPIb-IX-V expression[12]; why it is missing from Bernard-Soulier syndrome platelets is not known.

Although vWF is a normal component of plasma, it cannot bind spontaneously to GPIb-IX-V. However, incubating platelets with the antibiotic ristocetin or the snake venom protein botrocetin in vitro induces vWF binding to GPIb-IX-V.[13,14] It is likely that there are physiologic equivalents of ristocetin and botrocetin, but their identity is uncertain. One possibility is that vWF in the subendothelial connective tissue can bind to GPIb-IX-V, whereas vWF in plasma cannot.[15] It is also possible that shear stress is the agent that induces vWF binding to GPIb-IX-V.[16]

Genetics

At least 36 mutations responsible for Bernard-Soulier syndrome have been identified, 17 involving the gene for GPIbα, 11 the gene for GPIbβ, and 8 the gene for GPIX. All but two are missense mutations, frameshifts, and premature stop codons.

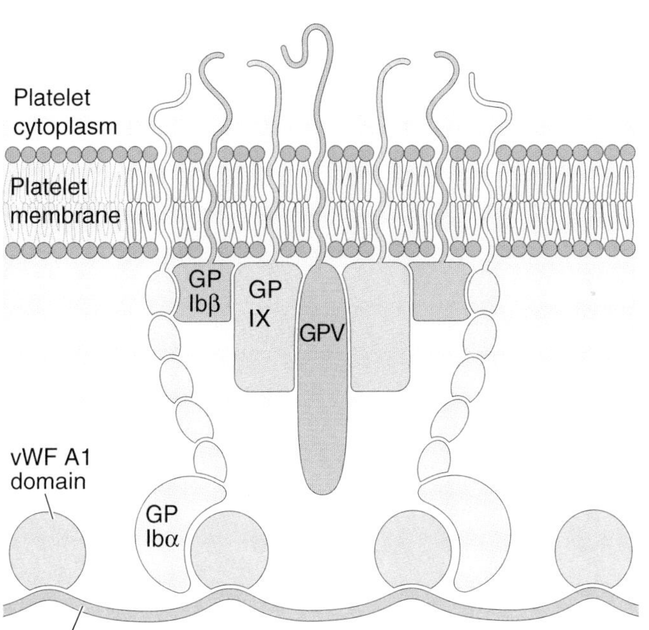

Figure 59–2. Diagram of platelet GPIb-IX-V complex bound to the A1 domain of vWF. Each GPIb-IX-V complex is thought to consist of two GPIb molecules, two GPIX molecules, and one GPV molecule. In the presence of high shear, the A1 domain of subendothelial vWF is able to bind to a domain composed of leucine-rich repeats 1 and 5–8 that is located in the amino-terminal portion of GPIbα.

Clinical Features

Bernard-Soulier syndrome is an autosomal recessive disorder that presents in infancy or childhood with the mucocutaneous bleeding characteristic of platelet dysfunction.[5] Most patients are also thrombocytopenic and have bleeding times prolonged to greater than 20 minutes. In addition, Bernard-Soulier syndrome platelets are large: 30–80% have a mean diameter greater than 3.5 μm on stained peripheral blood smears compared to the diameter of normal platelets, which ranges from 1.5 to 3.0 μm.[17] Although the severity of hemorrhage in Bernard-Soulier syndrome varies, it can be severe, requiring frequent transfusion and the suppression of menses.

Diagnosis

When Bernard-Soulier syndrome is suspected on clinical grounds, it can be confirmed by showing that platelets are unable to agglutinate in the presence of ristocetin or botrocetin when vWF is present. Bernard-Soulier syndrome platelets aggregate normally in response to conventional aggregating agonists such as ADP and collagen.

Differential Diagnosis

Other disorders associated with large platelets and thrombocytopenia, listed in Table 59–1, can be differentiated from Bernard-Soulier syndrome because the platelets in these disorders agglutinate in the presence of ristocetin. These disorders include the autosomal dominant May-Hegglin and Sebastian syndromes, in which Döhle body–like inclusions are present in leukocytes, and the Fechtner and Epstein syndromes, in which patients also suffer from hereditary nephritis, cataracts, and sensorineural deafness.[18] Each of the syndromes results from mutations in the *MYH9* gene encoding nonmuscle myosin heavy chain IIA (see Chapter 7). Platelet function in the syndromes is normal; if bleeding occurs, it is usually due to thrombocytopenia. Large platelets and thrombocytopenia are also seen in the gray platelet syndrome as a result of platelet α-granule deficiency[19]; the Montreal platelet syndrome, associated with spontaneous platelet aggregation at pH 7.4[20]; and Mediterranean macrothrombocytopenia, resulting from a putative difference in platelet count and size between northern and southern Europeans.[20]

TABLE 59–1. Disorders Characterized by Large Platelets and Thrombocytopenia

Disorder	Etiology
Bernard-Soulier syndrome	GPIb-IX-V deficiency
May-Hegglin syndrome	*MYH9* mutations
Sebastian syndrome	*MYH9* mutations
Epstein's syndrome	*MYH9* mutations
Fechtner syndrome	*MYH9* mutations
Gray platelet syndrome	Platelet α-granule deficiency
Montreal platelet syndrome	Unknown
Mediterranean macrothrombocytopenia	Unknown
Autoimmune thrombocytopenia (ITP)	Antiplatelet autoantibodies

Abbreviation: ITP, immune thrombocytopenic purpura.

Although antibodies against GPIb-IX-V can be detected in patients with idiopathic thrombocytopenic purpura,[21] bleeding in these patients is almost always due to thrombocytopenia. However, acquired Bernard-Soulier syndrome has been reported in lymphoproliferative disorders and myelodysplasia.[22] In platelet-type von Willebrand disease, mutations within the vWF-binding domain of GPIbα permit spontaneous vWF binding to GPIbα.[10]

Treatment

Platelet transfusions are usually required to treat bleeding in patients with Bernard-Soulier syndrome (Table 59–2). Hormonal therapy is effective in managing menorrhagia. Desmopressin acetate (DDAVP) (see later) has been reported to shorten the bleeding time in these individuals, but its effectiveness for bleeding has not been reported.[23] Recombinant factor VIIa has been used successfully to treat epistaxis in several children with Bernard-Soulier syndrome, but its general utility remains to be determined.[24] Two severely affected sisters were successfully treated by hematopoietic stem cell transplantation.[24,25]

Collagen Receptor Deficiency

A number of proteins on platelets can bind to collagen, but only GPVI and $\alpha_2\beta_1$ are required for this interac-

TABLE 59–2. Treatment of Inherited Platelet Disorders

Disorder	Platelet Transfusion	DDAVP	Corticosteroids	Recombinant Factor VIIa
Bernard-Soulier syndrome	TC	?	N	Y
Glanzmann's thrombasthenia	TC	N	N	Y
Gray platelet syndrome	TC	?	NIA	NIA
δ-Granule deficiency	Y	TC	?	?
Aspirin-like secretion defects	Y	TC	Y	NIA
Scott syndrome	Y	N	N	NIA

Modified from Bennett JS: Hereditary disorders of platelet function. *In* Hoffman R, Benz EJ Jr, Shattil SJ, et al (eds): Hematology, Basic Principles and Practice (ed 4). Philadelphia: Elsevier, 2005, pp 2327–2345.
Abbreviations: DDAVP, desmopressin; N, no; NIA, no information available; TC, treatment of choice; Y, yes; ?, possibly effective.

tion.[26,27] GPVI, a 62,000 MW member of the immunoglobulin gene superfamily, is noncovalently associated with the F_c receptor γ chain.[28,29] $\alpha_2\beta_1$ is a widely-expressed integrin whose α subunit contains a collagen-binding I domain that is homologous to the A1 domain of vWF.[30,31] In a current model of platelet adhesion, platelet tethering to vWF by GPIb-IX-V enables GPVI to bind to collagen and initiate intraplatelet signaling.[32] These signals enhance $\alpha_2\beta_1$ binding to collagen, resulting in shear-resistant platelet adhesion.

Clinical Features

Several patients with mild mucocutaneous bleeding have been reported whose platelets fail to aggregate when exposed to collagen and adhere poorly to collagen-coated surfaces.[33,34] In most cases, these platelets lack either GPVI or $\alpha_2\beta_1$, but in two cases, anti-GPVI antibodies were present.[35]

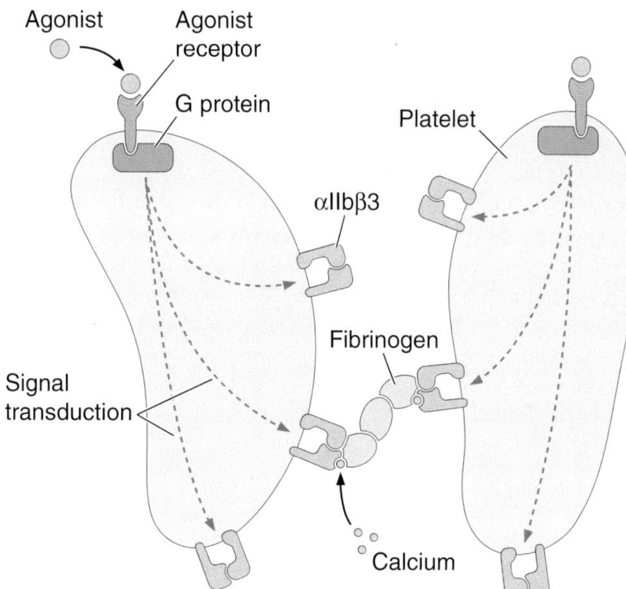

Figure 59–3. Mechanism of platelet aggregation. Agonist binding to receptors on the platelet surface initiates signal transduction pathways that convert the integrin $\alpha_{IIb}\beta_3$ from its inactive to its active conformation. Then, in the presence of divalent cations such as Ca^{2+}, fibrinogen binds to active $\alpha_{IIb}\beta_3$ on adjacent platelets, cross-linking the platelets into aggregates. (Adapted from Bennett JS: Mechanisms of platelet adhesion and aggregation: an update. Hosp Pract 27:124–140, 1992, with permission.)

Platelet Aggregation

The formation of a shear-resistant platelet plug requires platelet aggregation mediated by the integrin $\alpha_{IIb}\beta_3$ (GPIIb/IIIa).[36] $\alpha_{IIb}\beta_3$ mediates platelet aggregation by binding macromolecular ligands such as fibrinogen and vWF to cross-link adjacent platelets (Fig. 59–3).[37–39] Although circulating platelets express approximately 80,000 copies of $\alpha_{IIb}\beta_3$ on their surface,[40] $\alpha_{IIb}\beta_3$ is unable to bind ligands until it is converted to its active conformation by platelet agonists such as ADP and thrombin.[37]

Glanzmann's Thrombasthenia

The inherited absence of platelet aggregation was described by Glanzmann in 1918 and was subsequently named Glanzmann's thrombasthenia.[41] Glanzmann's thrombasthenia is due to deficiency or dysfunction of $\alpha_{IIb}\beta_3$.[42] Consequently, Glanzmann's thrombasthenia platelets are unable to bind sufficient amounts of fibrinogen or vWF to aggregate.

Pathophysiology

$\alpha_{IIb}\beta_3$ is a calcium-dependent heterodimer.[43] α_{IIb} itself is a disulfide-linked dimer of a 125,000 MW heavy chain ($\alpha_{IIb}\alpha$) that binds to β_3 and a 23,000 MW light chain ($\alpha_{IIb}\beta$) that anchors α_{IIb} in the platelet membrane.[44] β_3 is a single-chain cysteine-rich protein containing 28 disulfide bonds.[45] The $\alpha_{IIb}\beta_3$ heterodimer is assembled from α_{IIb} and β_3 subunits in the endoplasmic reticulum. In the absence of heterodimer formation, each subunit is retained in the endoplasmic reticulum and eventually degraded.[46] Nonetheless, successful heterodimer assembly does not guarantee $\alpha_{IIb}\beta_3$ expression on the platelet surface because mutations that perturb the conformation of assembled heterodimers also cause endoplasmic reticulum retention.[47]

In addition to activating $\alpha_{IIb}\beta_3$, platelet stimulation causes the α_{IIb} and β_3 cytoplasmic tails to associate with the platelet cytoskeleton,[48] enabling the force of cytoskeletal contraction to be transmitted to the fibrin clot, which results in clot retraction. Active $\alpha_{IIb}\beta_3$ also promotes platelet spreading on subendothelial connective tissue by binding to vWF and fibronectin.[49]

Genetics

Glanzmann's thrombasthenia is an autosomal recessive disorder with disease clusters in populations where consanguinity is common.[50] Glanzmann's thrombasthenia has been subclassified into three types: type I, in which platelets contain less than 5% of the normal amount of $\alpha_{IIb}\beta_3$ and clot retraction and α-granule fibrinogen are absent; type II, in which platelets contain 10–20% of the normal amount of $\alpha_{IIb}\beta_3$, clot retraction is decreased, and α-granule fibrinogen is present; and "variant" disease, in which the platelet content of $\alpha_{IIb}\beta_3$ is 50% of normal or greater and there is a qualitative $\alpha_{IIb}\beta_3$ abnormality.[50]

At least 34 different α_{IIb} and 29 different β_3 mutations have been identified in patients with Glanzmann's thrombasthenia. Of these, 57% result in type I, 30% in type II, and 13% in variant disease. About half of the mutations have been large and small gene deletions, splicing abnormalities, and nonsense mutations. Of 33 missense mutations, the majority perturb $\alpha_{IIb}\beta_3$ folding, but six have produced "variant" Glanzmann's thrombasthenia by impairing fibrinogen binding to $\alpha_{IIb}\beta_3$ or preventing $\alpha_{IIb}\beta_3$ activation.

Clinical Features

Glanzmann's thrombasthenia typically presents in neonates and infants with mucocutaneous bleeding, occasionally following circumcision.[50] Bleeding in Glanzmann's thrombasthenia generally results from situations that would also cause bleeding in a normal individual. Thus, purpura, epistaxis, and menorrhagia are frequent. Bleeding at menarche may be severe, and childbirth presents a severe hemostatic stress. Serious bleeding may follow trauma or surgery in patients not transfused with normal platelets. The apparent decline in the severity of Glanzmann's thrombasthenia with age is likely due to a decrease in the incidence of conditions such as epistaxis with aging.

Diagnosis

Glanzmann's thrombasthenia is a rare disorder, but should be considered in a patient with a lifelong history of mucocutaneous bleeding. Complete absence of macroscopic platelet aggregation is diagnostic. In addition, Glanzmann's thrombasthenia platelets are unable to support normal clot retraction and the fibrinogen content of their α-granules is reduced or absent. The latter occurs because megakaryocytes do not synthesize fibrinogen, but deposit it in their α-granules via $\alpha_{IIb}\beta_3$-mediated endocytosis of plasma fibrinogen.[51]

Differential Diagnosis

The failure of stimulated platelets to aggregate differentiates Glanzmann's thrombasthenia from other disorders of platelet adhesion and secretion. Rarely, acquired syndromes mimic inherited Glanzmann's thrombasthenia. Autoantibodies against $\alpha_{IIb}\beta_3$ are present frequently in patients with immune thrombocytopenic purpura, but antibodies that induce a Glanzmann's thrombasthenia–like state are unusual. However, acquired Glanzmann's thrombasthenia has been reported in multiple myeloma. In congenital afibrinogenemia, lack of plasma fibrinogen can prolong the bleeding time and impair ex vivo platelet aggregation.

Treatment

Bleeding in patients with Glanzmann's thrombasthenia requires platelet transfusion (see Table 59–2). Human lymphocyte antigen–matched platelets should be used to lessen the chance of platelet alloimmunization. Protein A–Sepharose immunoadsorption has been reported to restore the efficacy of transfused platelets when this occurs.[52] Hormonal therapy is useful in controlling menorrhagia, and the use of fibrinolytic inhibitors such as ε-aminocaproic acid or tranexamic acid can be helpful in controlling bleeding after dental extraction. There is one report that DDAVP can shorten the bleeding time in Glanzmann's thrombasthenia and improve hemostasis during minor dental surgery.[53] Infusions of recombinant factor VIIa have been reported to be efficacious, particularly in patients who have developed $\alpha_{IIb}\beta_3$ alloantibodies.[25] Two severely affected children were successfully treated by bone marrow transplantation.[54,55]

Platelet Secretion

Platelets contain four types of granules (α-granules, dense or δ-granules, lysosomes, and microperoxisomes) whose contents are secreted when platelets are stimulated.[56] Although the function of many platelet secretion products is unclear, secretion disorders frequently result in mild to moderate bleeding,[57] confirming that secretion is necessary for normal hemostasis.

α-Granule Deficiency (Gray Platelet Syndrome)

There are approximately 50 α-granules in platelets containing a variety of proteins, some of which are specific for platelets (platelet factor 4, β-thromboglobulin, platelet-derived growth factor, and thrombospondin) and others that are also present in plasma (fibrinogen, vWF, albumin, coagulation factor V, immunoglobulin G, fibronectin, and a number of protease inhibitors).[58] The α-granule membrane also contains some of the same proteins present in the platelet plasma membrane ($\alpha_{IIb}\beta_3$ and GPIb-IX-V) and others that are granule-specific (P-selectin and osteonectin).[59,60] These proteins are translocated to the platelet surface during platelet secretion. Inherited α-granule deficiency (gray platelet syndrome) was described by Raccuglia in 1971 as a rare disorder resulting from the specific absence of morphologically recognizable α-granules in the platelets of affected individuals.[19]

Pathophysiology

Gray platelet syndrome megakaryocytes and platelets contain vacuoles and small α-granule precursors that stain for vWF and fibrinogen.[61] Other types of platelet granules are present in normal numbers. This suggests that the abnormality in gray platelet syndrome is an inability to target proteins to α-granule precursors. The inability to package platelet-derived growth factor in α-granules allows it to leak from megakaryocytes, perhaps accounting for the bone marrow fibrosis seen in gray platelet syndrome.[62]

Genetics

Gray platelet syndrome appears to be an autosomal disease.[63] A disorder resembling gray platelet syndrome is present in the Wistar Furth rat and is inherited in an autosomal recessive fashion.[64]

Clinical Features

Gray platelet syndrome patients present with a lifelong history of mild to moderate mucocutaneous bleeding and have variably prolonged bleeding times, moderate thrombocytopenia (25,000–150,000/μL), and reticulin fibrosis of the bone marrow.[63,65] Their platelets are large and gray in appearance on stained blood smears. Agonist-stimulated platelet aggregation is usually normal, but the platelet content of platelet factor 4, β-thromboglobulin, fibrinogen, vWF, factor V, fibronectin, and thrombospondin is markedly decreased, whereas the platelet factor 4 and β-thromboglobulin concentrations in plasma are normal or elevated.[65]

Differential Diagnosis

Decreased α-granule contents occur in factor V Quebec, in which the unexplained ectopic expression of urokinase in α-granules results in the degradation of many α-granule proteins and produces a moderately severe bleeding disorder accompanied by mild thrombocytopenia.[66,67]

Treatment

Severe bleeding episodes may require the transfusion of normal platelets (see Table 59–2). DDAVP (see later) shortened the bleeding time in one patient and was used as prophylaxis for a dental extraction.[68]

Dense Granule Deficiency (δ-Storage Pool Disease)

Platelets contain three to six δ-granules that are storage sites for ADP, ATP, calcium, pyrophosphate, and serotonin.[69] Platelet δ-granules are related to a group of lysosome-related granules including melanosomes, neutrophil azurophilic granules, and the basophilic granules of basophils and mast cells.[70] Moreover, the δ-granule membrane contains CD63 (granulophysin), which corresponds to the melanoma-associated antigen ME491, the lysosomal membrane protein-1 (LIMP-1), and the lysosomal membrane–associated protein-3 (LAMP-3).[70] The membrane also contains P-selectin, GPIb, and $\alpha_{IIb}\beta_3$.[71] δ-Granule deficiency is a heterogeneous group of disorders that can be subdivided into deficiency states associated with albinism and those in otherwise normal individuals.

Pathophysiology

The biogenesis of δ-granules in megakaryocytes is poorly understood. However, δ-granule deficiency occurs in tyrosinase-positive albinism in humans, pigment dilution syndromes in mice and rats, and as part of a Chédiak-Higashi–like syndrome in cattle, cats, mink, foxes, and killer whales, implying that that the biogenesis of dense granules, melanosomes, and lysosomes is related. The mechanism by which dense granules accumulate ATP and ADP is also not known.

Genetics

Hermansky-Pudlak syndrome (HPS) and Chédiak-Higashi syndrome (CHS) are autosomal recessive disorders. Phenotypes similar to HPS have been identified in 14 genetically distinct mouse strains; seven of the affected murine genes have also been detected in human HPS. Prototypical HPS or HPS-1 is a rare disease worldwide, but it occurs with a frequency of 1 in 1800 in northwest Puerto Rico.[72] Besides albinism, HPS-1 patients suffer from decreased visual acuity, nystagmus, granulomatous colitis, and a fatal form of pulmonary fibrosis.[73,74] The phenotypic expression of the six other HPS mutations in humans varies from mild to severe.[70] CHS results from mutations in the gene *CHS1*, an orthologue of the murine *bg* gene, mutated in the beige mouse.[75,76] *CHS1* mutations that prevent synthesis of the full-length CHS1 protein are associated with a severe fatal childhood form of CHS, whereas missense mutations are associated with a milder clinical course, less frequent infections, and survival into adolescence and adulthood.[77]

Clinical Features

Patients with δ-granule deficiency present with mild to moderate mucocutaneous bleeding. Platelet counts and platelet morphology are usually normal and bleeding times are usually, but not always, prolonged.[57] In most patients, platelet aggregometry reveals absence of second-wave aggregation when platelets are stimulated by ADP, epinephrine, and low concentrations of collagen, but responses to high collagen concentrations may be normal.[78,79] Serotonin uptake into δ-granule–deficient platelets is normal, but their steady-state serotonin content is decreased because serotonin storage sites are absent.[80] Moreover, because the pool of ADP located in the δ-granules is absent, the ATP:ADP ratio of δ-granule–deficient platelets is 3.0 or greater, whereas the ratio in normal platelets is less than 2.5. The altered ATP:ADP ratio can be used for the diagnosis of δ-granule deficiency.[57]

Differential Diagnosis

δ-Granule deficiency has been reported in patients with the Wiskott-Aldrich syndrome/X-linked thrombocytopenia,[81] the syndrome of thrombocytopenia with absent radii,[82] Ehlers-Danlos syndrome,[83] and osteogenesis imperfecta.[84] It is associated with albinism in HPS (oculocutaneous tyrosinase-positive albinism, platelet dense granule deficiency, and ceroid-like inclusions in cells of the reticuloendothelial system)[70] and CHS (partial oculocutaneous albinism, frequent pyogenic infections, and giant lysosomal granules in cells of hematologic and nonhematologic origin).[85] In HPS and CHS, there is a quantitative deficiency of δ-granules. In δ-storage pool disease in nonalbinos, the number of δ-granule precursors is normal or nearly normal, suggesting that the problem is an inability to package δ-granule contents. In some nonalbinos, δ-granule deficiency is associated with a variable deficiency of α-granules (αδ-storage pool disease).[86]

Treatment

Bleeding in patients with δ-granule disease can be controlled by platelet transfusion (see Table 59–2). This is seldom necessary because other methods to improve hemostasis are available.

Bleeding can be controlled using DDAVP, a vasopressin analogue whose pressor effects are substantially less than its antidiuretic effects.[87] DDAVP releases high-molecular-weight vWF multimers and tissue plasminogen activator from endothelial cells.[53] Released vWF accounts for the beneficial effect of DDAVP in some forms of von Willebrand disease, but the mechanism by which DDAVP shortens the bleeding time and improves hemostasis in patients with δ-granule deficiency is uncertain.

DDAVP is administered intravenously at a dose of 0.3 μg/kg over 15–30 min (maximum dose 20 μg).[53] The drug can also be given intranasally or subcutaneously.[53,88] Shortening of the bleeding time occurs within 30–60 minutes and can persist for up to 4 hours. The drug can be given repeatedly at 12- to 24-hour intervals, but tachyphylaxis occurs. Side effects of DDAVP, discussed in detail in Chapters 63 and 64, are uncommon and mild.[53]

Prednisone at doses of 20–50 mg for 3–4 days has been reported to improve hemostasis in a variety of patients with inherited platelet disorders.[89] Bleeding time shortening occurs within 3 days and can persist for up to 3–7 days after the prednisone is stopped. There are also reports suggesting that recombinant factor VIIa can be effective in managing bleeding in patients with δ-granule deficiency.[25]

Bone marrow transplantation reverses the immunologic and hemostatic manifestations of CHS,[90] but surviving patients later develop neurologic deficits.[85] The drug pirfenidone, an antifibrotic agent, may slow the progression of fatal pulmonary fibrosis in patients with HPS.[91]

Aspirin-like Secretion Disorders

Inherited mutations that perturb the biochemistry of platelet secretion can result in impaired platelet function that resembles the antiplatelet effects of aspirin.

Pathophysiology

These disorders represent a heterogeneous collection of uncommon biochemical abnormalities. Abnormalities have been reported in platelet arachidonic acid metabolism[92] and in platelet responsiveness to endogenous and exogenous thromboxane A_2[93] and to the calcium ionophores A23187 and ionomycin.[94] A notable patient whose platelets responded poorly to multiple agonists was found to have decreased membrane GTPase activity as a result of decreased expression of the G-protein subunit Gαq.[95] Several patients have been reported whose platelets respond poorly to ADP because of mutations in the Gαi-coupled ADP receptor $P2Y_{12}$.[96]

Genetics

Because most patients have been reported in individual case reports, it has not been possible to determine their mode of inheritance.

Clinical Features

In addition to mucocutaneous bleeding, the bleeding time of patients with this type of secretion abnormality is usually prolonged. However, when it is normal or only slightly prolonged, it may become markedly prolonged after the patient has ingested aspirin.[97]

Treatment

The approach to treatment in patients with these disorders is identical to that for patients with δ-granule deficiency (see Table 59–2).

Platelet Procoagulant Activity

The "tenase" and "prothrombinase" complexes that activate coagulation factors X and prothrombin, respectively, assemble on the surface of activated platelets. Isolated deficiency of platelet procoagulant activity is exceedingly rare. In addition to the one well-studied patient after whom the disorder is named (Scott syndrome),[98] three additional patients have been reported[99,100] and a recessive disorder identical to Scott syndrome has been reported in German shepherd dogs.[101]

Clinical Features and Pathophysiology

The index case presented with spontaneous hematomas as well as bleeding after surgical and dental procedures, a pattern suggestive of a coagulation rather than a platelet disorder.[98] Nonetheless, prothrombin and partial thromboplastin times were normal, as were bleeding times and platelet function studies. However, serum prothrombin times were short, indicating that there was decreased prothrombin consumption during blood clotting. This suggested that tenase and prothrombinase assembly on the platelet surface might be defective, a possibility that was confirmed by finding impaired factor X activation in the presence of platelets[102] as well as a decreased number of platelet-binding sites for factor Xa.[98] Furthermore, there was decreased agonist-stimulated exposure of anionic phospholipid on the platelet surface,[103] implying that there was a defect in the mechanism responsible for the loss of membrane asymmetry after platelet stimulation.

ACQUIRED DISORDERS OF PLATELET FUNCTION

Whereas the inherited disorders of platelet function are rare, acquired disorders of platelet function are relatively common. However, they are usually asymptomatic or mild. Nonetheless, they can be of substantial clinical importance when they are engrafted upon another hemostatic abnormality. Acquired platelet disorders can be subclassified into those attributed to medications, to systemic illnesses, and to hematologic disorders.

Medications Affecting Platelet Function

Medications are the most common causes of acquired platelet dysfunction. A few medications prolong the bleeding time and cause or exacerbate bleeding, a number of others prolong the bleeding time without inducing bleeding, and many more only affect platelet function ex vivo or in vitro (Table 59–3). Drugs that result in thrombocytopenia are discussed in Chapter 61.

Nonsteroidal Anti-inflammatory Drugs

Aspirin

Acetylsalicylic acid (aspirin) transfers its acetyl group to serine 529 of the enzyme prostaglandin endoperoxide H synthase, also known as cyclooxygenase, and irreversibly inactivates the enzyme.[104] Of three cyclooxygenase isoforms, platelets only express cyclooxygenase-1.[105] Inactivation of cyclooxygenase-1 prevents the conversion of the arachidonic acid released from platelet membrane phospholipids to prostaglandin endoperoxides and the subsequent conversion of the endoperoxides to thromboxane A_2 by thromboxane synthase. Accordingly, platelet responses to ADP, epinephrine, arachidonic acid, and low concentrations of collagen and thrombin that depend on thromboxane A_2 synthesis are impaired. However, responses to high concentrations of collagen or thrombin are not affected.[106,107]

Aspirin also acetylates cyclooxygenase in endothelial cells, preventing the synthesis of prostacyclin (prostaglandin I_2 [PGI_2]), a potent vasodilator and platelet inhibitor.[108] Nonetheless, aspirin prolongs the bleeding time of normal individuals, although not necessarily into the abnormal range, indicating that its effect on platelets predominates.

Platelet prostaglandin synthesis is almost completely inhibited by a single 160-mg dose of aspirin or by 30 mg taken daily for 7–10 days.[105] In normal individuals, the effect of aspirin on the bleeding time is slight and requires that greater than 95% of the cyclooxygenase-1 in the circulating platelets be inhibited.[109] The bleeding time generally remains prolonged for 1–4 days after

TABLE 59–3. Selected Medications That Cause Platelet Dysfunction[1]

Drug	Affects Ex Vivo Platelet Function	Increases Bleeding Time	Increases Risk of Bleeding
Aspirin[2]	++	++	++
Other NSAIDs (e.g., sulfinpyrazone, indomethacin, ibuprofen, sulindac, naproxen, piroxicam, tolmetin, zomepirac)	+	+[3]	+/–[4]
High-dose penicillins and related antibiotics (cephalosporins)	+	+	+/–[4]
Thienopyridines (ticlopidine, clopidogrel)[2]	++	++	++
GPIIb/IIIa antagonists (abciximab, tirofiban, eptifibatide)[2]	++	++	++
PGI_2 analogues (prostacyclin, iloprost)	+	+	–
Phosphodiesterase inhibitors (dipyridamole, cilostazol)	+	?[5]	–
Heparin	+	+	+[6]
Plasminogen activators	+	?	+[7]
Nitric oxide, nitroglycerin, nitroprusside	+	+	–
Calcium channel blockers	+ (high doses)	–	–
β-Blockers (propranolol)	+	–	–
Volume expanders (dextran, hydroxyethyl starch)	+	+	+/–
Tricyclic antidepressants	+	–	–
Phenothiazines	+	–	–
Local and general anesthetics (lidocaine, tetracaine, cocaine, halothane)	+	+/–[8]	–
Antihistamines (diphenhydramine, chlorpheniramine, mepyramine)	+	–	–
Radiographic contrast agents	+	+/–[8]	–
Cyclosporin A	+	–	–
Chemotherapeutic agents (mithramycin, daunomycin, BCNU)	+	+	–

[1]Medicines commonly encountered in clinical practice.
[2]Regularly affects platelet function, prolongs bleeding time, and predisposes to excessive bleeding.
[3]Can cause transient bleeding time prolongation.
[4]Can exacerbate bleeding in presence of another hemostatic defect.
[5]Data not available.
[6]Bleeding the result of the anticoagulant effect of heparin.
[7]Bleeding the result of the fibrinolytic activity of plasmin.
[8]+/–, Observed on occasion.
Abbreviations: NSAIDs, nonsteroidal anti-inflammatory drugs; PGI_2, prostaglandin I_2; +, Yes; ++, well-established complication; –, no.

aspirin has been discontinued, but platelet aggregation tests may be abnormal for up to a week until inhibited platelets are replaced.[110]

Aspirin has little effect on hemostasis in normal individuals, but there was a slight, insignificant increase in hemorrhagic strokes among physicians who took aspirin as primary prophylaxis against myocardial infarction.[111] Whether aspirin increases surgical bleeding is not clear, but it is safe to perform epidural and spinal anesthesia in patients who have ingested aspirin.[112] However, aspirin can markedly prolong the bleeding time and precipitate hemorrhage in individuals with preexisting hemostatic abnormalities.

Other Nonsteroidal Anti-inflammatory Drugs

Drugs such as ibuprofen and naproxen reversibly inhibit cyclooxygenase enzymes. Their effect is usually short lasting (<4 hours),[113] although the effect of piroxicam may last for days because of its prolonged half-life.[114] These drugs may also transiently prolong the bleeding time,[115] but this is usually of no clinical significance.

Antibiotics

High doses of most penicillins can cause a prolongation of the bleeding time[116] and can reduce platelet aggregation, secretion, and ristocetin-induced platelet agglutination.[117] This effect is maximal after 1–3 days of administration and may persist for several days after the antibiotic is stopped. Although clinically significant bleeding can occur, it is far less common than prolongation of the bleeding time.[118] Patients with coexisting hemostatic defects may be more prone to this complication. However, this is an uncommon and unpredictable complication of penicillin administration and should only be considered as a cause for bleeding in the appropriate setting. A similar pattern of platelet dysfunction has been reported with some cephalosporins and related antibiotics.[119]

Thienopyridines

The thienopyridines ticlopidine and clopidogrel are prodrugs whose metabolites bind irreversibly to the platelet ADP receptor $P2Y_{12}$.[120] Thus, they inhibit ADP-dependent platelet responses, and both drugs prolong the bleeding time. Although an effect of these drugs on platelet function can be measured within 24–48 hours of the first dose, it is not maximal for 4–6 days because it is dependent on drug metabolism.[121,122] However, a loading dose of clopidogrel can shorten the time required for its maximal antiplatelet effect.[123] The effect of these drugs on platelet function may persist for 4–10 days after the drugs have been discontinued.[124]

The thienopyridines have potentially serious hematologic side effects, including neutropenia and, less commonly, aplastic anemia and thrombocytopenia.[121,125] In addition, thrombotic thrombocytopenic purpura has been reported in approximately 1 in 5000 patients treated with ticlopidine.[126] Although thrombotic thrombocytopenic purpura has also been reported in patients receiving clopidogrel, its incidence appears to be substantially less.[127]

$\alpha_{IIb}\beta_3$ (GPIIb/IIIa) Antagonists

The $\alpha_{IIb}\beta_3$ antagonists are used in the treatment of ischemic coronary artery disease.[128] Three antagonists—abciximab, eptifibatide, and tirofiban—have been approved for this purpose.[128] Abciximab is a chimeric human-murine Fab fragment of the anti-$\alpha_{IIb}\beta_3$ monoclonal antibody 7E3, eptifibatide is a cyclic heptapeptide based on the snake venom disintegrin barbourin, and tirofiban is an arginine-glycine–aspartic acid–based peptidomimetic analogue of tyrosine.[129] As predicted from the phenotype of patients with Glanzmann's thrombasthenia, these drugs can predispose to bleeding. Platelet transfusions can reverse the $\alpha_{IIb}\beta_3$ inhibition induced by abciximab. It is less clear that platelet transfusion can reverse the effects of the other $\alpha_{IIb}\beta_3$ antagonists, but these drugs have short half-lives when renal and hepatic function are normal. Nevertheless, when excessive bleeding requires intervention, platelet transfusion should be tried to decrease the concentration of platelet-bound drug.

Thrombocytopenia occurring within 24 hours of drug administration has also been observed in a small number of patients.[130] The pathogenesis of the thrombocytopenia is uncertain, but it may be related to the presence of preexisting anti-$\alpha_{IIb}\beta_3$ antibodies that recognize epitopes on $\alpha_{IIb}\beta_3$ exposed by antagonist binding.[131] The thrombocytopenia usually reverses readily when the drug is stopped, but it can be reversed by platelet transfusion if clinically indicated. Thrombocytopenia in patients receiving these drugs must be differentiated from pseudothrombocytopenia caused by drug-induced platelet clumping ex vivo[132] from heparin-induced thrombocytopenia, and from other causes of thrombocytopenia depending on the clinical circumstances.

Medications That Increase Platelet Cyclic AMP

Dipyridamole, a pyrimidopyrimidine derivative, inhibits cyclic nucleotide phosphodiesterase, increasing the platelet concentration of cyclic AMP. It may also inhibit the breakdown of cyclic GMP, potentiating the inhibitory effect of nitric oxide on platelets. Although dipyridamole inhibits platelet function in vitro, its clinical utility has been controversial, perhaps because of the limited bioavailability of older formulations.[133] Intravenous infusions of prostaglandin E_1, PGI_2, or stable PGI_2 analogues stimulate platelet adenylyl cyclase, increasing platelet cyclic AMP.[134] However, the clinical utility of these agents is limited by their short half-life and side effects that include peripheral vasodilation.[135] Cilostazol, a phosphodiesterase III inhibitor, is used for the treatment of peripheral vascular disease.[136] Nitric oxide and organic nitrates such as nitroglycerin inhibit platelet function in vitro by activating guanylyl cyclase and increasing platelet concentrations of cyclic GMP.[137] High concentrations of caffeine and theophylline inhibit platelet phosphodiesterases in vitro.

Anticoagulants and Fibrinolytic Agents

Heparin functions as an anticoagulant by activating the protease inhibitor antithrombin. It may also impair platelet function by preventing thrombin generation and by binding to the heparin-binding domain of vWF.[138,139] Conversely, heparin can enhance ex vivo platelet aggregation by binding to specific receptors on the platelet surface.[140] Whether this latter property of heparin contributes to type I heparin-induced thrombocytopenia is not known.[141]

High concentrations of plasmin-generated fibrin(ogen) degradation products inhibit ex vivo platelet aggregation by competing with intact fibrinogen for binding to $\alpha_{IIb}\beta_3$.[142] Plasmin itself inhibits platelet arachidonic acid metabolism,[143] impairs the interaction of platelets with vWF by enzymatically degrading GPIb,[144] and causes the disaggregation of platelet aggregates by cleaving the fibrinogen that holds them together.[145] It is uncertain whether any of these effects contribute to the bleeding that can complicate fibrinolytic therapy.

Drugs That Affect the Cardiovascular System

Nitroprusside,[146] nitroglycerine,[147] and propranolol[148] decrease platelet aggregation and secretion ex vivo, as can inhaled nitric oxide. High concentrations of calcium channel blockers such as verapamil, nifedipine, and diltiazem inhibit ex vivo platelet aggregation, but therapeutic doses have no effect on the bleeding time.[149,150] High concentrations of quinidine can cause a mild prolongation of the bleeding time and can potentiate the effect of aspirin.[151]

Dextran infusions impair platelet function in vivo, but curiously are without effect when added to platelet-rich plasma.[152] Although hydroxyethyl starch is generally safe, it may prolong the bleeding time and predispose to hemorrhage when administered in doses exceeding 20 mL/kg of a 6% solution.[153]

Miscellaneous Agents

A number of drugs, including antidepressants,[154] phenothiozines,[155] general anesthetics,[156] cocaine,[157] and heroin,[158] perturb platelet function in vitro, but the clinical significance of these effects is doubtful. Similarly, chemotherapeutic agents such as mithramycin, daunorubicin, BCNU, cisplatin, and cyclophosphamide, used alone or in combination, have been reported to impair in vitro and ex vivo platelet function,[159–161] as have antihistamines,[162] the serotonin antagonist ketanserin,[163] and radiographic contrast agents.[164] Cyclosporin A has been reported to enhance ADP-stimulated platelet aggregation in vitro, but may impair platelet aggregation ex vivo.[165]

Platelet Dysfunction Associated with Systemic Disorders

Uremia

Historically, uremia was a frequent cause of spontaneous bleeding, but with the advent of dialysis, the frequency of hemorrhage in patients with renal failure has decreased substantially.[166] Nonetheless, abnormal platelet function in uremia remains an issue because it may contribute to bleeding after surgery or trauma and in conjunction with anatomic lesions of the gastrointestinal tract.[167] Additional discussion of this topic can be found in Chapter 83.

TABLE 59–4. Factors Responsible for Platelet Dysfunction in Uremia

Factor	Biochemical or Physiologic Basis
Renal failure–associated anemia	Defective platelet adhesion
Impaired platelet adhesion to vWF	Impaired vWF binding to GPIb-IX-V
Defective platelet activation	Reduced agonist-induced calcium release Impaired arachidonic acid metabolism Decreased δ-granule ADP Increased platelet cyclic AMP content Presence of small dialyzable platelet activation inhibitors (guanidinosuccinic and phenolic acids)
Increased nitric oxide synthesis	Upregulation of L-arginine transport into platelets Guanidinosuccinic acid may mimic the effect of nitric oxide

Pathogenesis

Factors responsible for the defective function of uremic platelets are listed in Table 59–4. Chronic renal failure can also be associated with mild thrombocytopenia resulting from diminished marrow production and decreased platelet survival.[168] When thrombocytopenia is present in this setting, one must also consider other possibilities, including medications that can cause both thrombocytopenia and renal failure and systemic diseases such as multiple myeloma, systemic vasculitis, thrombotic thrombocytopenic purpura/hemolytic-uremic syndrome, eclampsia, and renal allograft rejection.

Clinical Features

Hemorrhage in patients with renal failure most often involves the skin and the gastrointestinal and genitourinary tracts. Gastrointestinal hemorrhage is usually associated with an anatomic lesion, most commonly angiodysplasia and peptic ulceration.[167] Small perirenal hematomas are common after kidney biopsy in patients with renal failure, but gross hematuria is uncommon.[169] Severe bleeding after biopsy is usually due to needle lacerations of the kidney or spleen, anomalous vessels, heparin anticoagulation, or the presence of renal amyloid. The bleeding time is frequently prolonged in patients with renal failure. Nonetheless, the presence of a prolonged bleeding time should not be used as an indicator of hemorrhagic risk.[170,171]

Treatment

Abnormal platelet aggregation and a prolonged bleeding time are common in uremia, but they are not, by themselves, indications for therapeutic intervention. Nonetheless, there are a number of interventions that

TABLE 59–5. Modalities Available to Treat Abnormal Hemostasis in Uremia

Modality	Comments
Dialysis	Hemo- and peritoneal dialysis are equally effective.
Increase in hematocrit	Goal is to increase hematocrit to 27–32% using transfusion or preferably recombinant erythropoietin to facilitate platelet adhesion.
DDAVP	Treatment of choice for acute situations when dialysis is not effective.
Conjugated estrogen	Several days are required for their effect to be seen.
Cryoprecipitate	Inconsistent results argue against routine use.

can either partially or completely correct a prolonged bleeding time and may also improve clinical hemostasis (Table 59–5).

1. Intensive dialysis shortens the bleeding time and reverses a bleeding diathesis in many, but not all, patients.[172] Peritoneal dialysis and hemodialysis are equally effective.[173] If a patient undergoing dialysis bleeds, it may be worthwhile to increase the intensity of dialysis.
2. Increasing the hematocrit to 27–32% by red cell transfusion[174] or recombinant erythropoietin[175] can shorten the bleeding time and may diminish clinical bleeding as well.
3. DDAVP has been reported to shorten the bleeding time in 50–75% of patients with uremia.[176] If dialysis is not effective, DDAVP is the treatment of choice for uremic bleeding, particularly if only a short-term effect is required.
4. Conjugated estrogens shorten the bleeding time in most, but not all, uremic patients.[177] They are administered at a dose of 0.6 mg/kg intravenously for 5 days. Shortening of the bleeding time occurs within 72 hours of the first dose, the maximal effect is observed at 5–7 days, and the effect can persist for up to 14 days.
5. Infusions of cryoprecipitate have been reported to shorten the bleeding time in uremic patients and to ameliorate bleeding,[178] but these effects are not consistent, arguing against the routine use of cryoprecipitate for uremic bleeding.

Antiplatelet Antibodies

Pathogenesis

The mechanism by which auto- or alloantibodies impair platelet function is not usually apparent; in several cases, antibody binding to specific platelet glycoproteins such as $\alpha_{IIb}\beta_3$, GPIb-IX-V, $\alpha_2\beta_1$, and GPVI has been responsible.[179] In most cases, the functional consequences of antibody binding are obscured by bleeding caused by thrombocytopenia.

Clinical Features

Antibody binding to platelets occurs in several pathologic conditions, including immune thrombocytopenic purpura, systemic lupus erythematosus, and platelet alloimmunization, and often results in thrombocytopenia as a result of decreased platelet survival. Concomitant platelet dysfunction should be suspected in a patient with immune thrombocytopenic purpura or systemic lupus erythematosus who has mucocutaneous bleeding at a platelet count not ordinarily associated with bleeding (i.e., platelet counts > 30,000–40,000/μL).[180] Platelet dysfunction resulting from platelet-bound autoantibody has also been described in individuals, usually women, with normal platelet counts and "easy bruising."[181]

TABLE 59–6. Cardiopulmonary Bypass–Induced Platelet Dysfunction

Qualitative Platelet Defects	Potential Causes
Prolonged bleeding time	Hypothermia
Impaired ex vivo agonist-stimulated platelet aggregation	Platelet contact with fibrinogen-coated synthetic surfaces and the blood-air interface
Decreased ristocetin-induced platelet agglutination	Cardiotomy suction
α- and δ-granule deficiency	Platelet exposure to traces of thrombin, plasmin, ADP, and complement
Enhanced release of soluble CD40 ligand; enhanced generation of platelet microparticles	Effect of drugs administered before or during bypass: heparin, aspirin, GPIIb/IIIa antagonists, protamine

Cardiopulmonary Bypass

Approximately 5% of patients undergoing extracorporeal bypass experience excessive postoperative bleeding. Roughly half of these cases are due to surgical causes, and much of the remainder result from thrombocytopenia, platelet dysfunction, and hyperfibrinolysis.[182]

Clinical Features

Thrombocytopenia is a consistent feature of bypass. Platelet counts usually decrease to approximately 50% of presurgical levels, and thrombocytopenia may persist for several days.[182] The bypass circuit also induces defects in platelet function. The nature of these defects and their pathogenesis are listed in Table 59–6. The severity of the functional abnormalities correlates with the duration of bypass,[183] but they generally resolve within 2–24 hours.[182] When hyperfibrinolysis occurs, it is likely due to thrombus formation in the pericardial cavity, followed by local and systemic fibrinolysis.[184]

Treatment

If excessive nonsurgical bleeding occurs after cardiopulmonary bypass, the patient is not hypothermic, and administered heparin has been fully reversed, use of pharmacologic agents and judicious transfusions of platelets, cryoprecipitate, fresh frozen plasma, and red blood cells is appropriate.

A number of maneuvers have been tried to reduce the hemostatic abnormalities associated with bypass. These include coating the artificial surfaces of bypass devices with heparin,[185] using centrifugal rather than roller pumps,[186] performing coronary artery surgery without bypass,[187] and using pharmacologic agents.[188] Infusions of prostaglandin E_1, PGI_2, or stable PGI_2 analogues have been tried in animal models and humans, but have not shown overall benefit, in part because of significant toxicity, including hypotension.[135] When excessive postoperative blood loss occurs in association with a prolonged bleeding time, it may or may not respond to DDAVP.[189] Recombinant factor VIIa has also been used successfully to treat uncontrolled postoperative bleeding.[190] Inhibition of fibrinolysis using aprotinin, ε-aminocaproic acid, and tranexamic acid can reduce mediastinal blood loss and transfusion requirements. When aprotinin is used, it is started preoperatively and continued for the duration of surgery.[191] It has also been applied topically to the pericardium to inhibit local fibrinolysis.[192]

Miscellaneous Disorders

Platelet dysfunction occurs in chronic liver disease. However, the existence of a platelet function defect specific for liver disease is unlikely.[193] When bleeding occurs in liver disease, its cause is usually multifactorial, including decreased coagulation factor production, fibrinolysis, dysfibrinogenemia, disseminated intravascular coagulation, and thrombocytopenia caused by hypersplenism and thrombopoietin deficiency. Disseminated intravascular coagulation can be associated with reduced platelet aggregation and acquired storage pool deficiency.[194] The elevated levels of fibrin(ogen) degradation products and low fibrinogen levels in disseminated intravascular coagulation may also contribute to defective platelet function.[142] These factors are discussed at greater length in Chapter 84.

Platelet Dysfunction Associated with Hematologic Diseases

Chronic Myeloproliferative Disorders

Pathogenesis

Factors that contribute to the hemostatic abnormalities in the myeloproliferative disorders include:

1. Increased whole-blood viscosity in polycythemia vera.[195]
2. Abnormalities of platelet structure and function. When viewed by light or electron microscopy, platelets from patients with these disorders may be larger or smaller than normal, and may be abnormally shaped, and there may be decreased numbers of storage granules.[196] In addition, a myriad of biochemical abnormalities, have been detected in these platelets. One notable abnormality is the absence of a primary wave of aggregation in response to epinephrine; this abnormality has been used diagnostically.[197] Conversely, spontaneous platelet aggregation has been reported in essential thrombocythemia,[198] as has increased thromboxane A_2 synthesis.[199] Despite these biochemical abnormalities, bleeding times are prolonged in only a minority of patients and do not correlate with a propensity for hemorrhage or thrombosis.[200]
3. Elevated platelet counts. The contribution of an elevated platelet count per se to the risk of hemorrhage and thrombosis is uncertain, and the risk of these events cannot be confidently predicted from the degree of thrombocytosis.[197]
4. Leukocyte and/or endothelial dysfunction may contribute to the thrombotic phenotype in some individuals, perhaps via leukocyte-platelet and leukocyte–endothelial cell interactions.[197]

Clinical Features

Both bleeding and thrombosis contribute to the morbidity and mortality of patients suffering from the myeloproliferative disorders polycythemia vera, essential thrombocythemia, myelofibrosis with myeloid metaplasia, and chronic myelogenous leukemia.[197,201,202] Most symptomatic patients experience either bleeding or thrombosis; however, some experience both during the course of their disease. Bleeding usually involves the skin or mucous membranes. Thrombosis can be arterial or venous and may occur in unusual locations such as the hepatic, portal, and mesenteric circulations. Thus, myeloproliferative disorders account for a substantial proportion of patients with Budd-Chiari syndrome (hepatic vein thrombosis) and portal vein thrombosis.[203] Patients with essential thrombocythemia may experience ischemia and necrosis of the fingers and toes as a result of digital artery thrombosis, microvascular occlusion in the coronary circulation, and transient neurologic symptoms resulting from cerebrovascular occlusion.[204] A syndrome of redness and burning pain in the extremities, termed erythromelalgia, is associated with essential thrombocythemia and polycythemia vera.[205,206] Vascular complications are more likely to occur in patients older than 60 and in patients with other risk factors for vascular disease. An acquired form of von Willebrand disease can occur in individuals with chronic myelogenous leukemia and other myeloproliferative syndromes.[207]

Treatment

Therapy should be considered for symptomatic patients, for patients over 60 years of age, and for individuals about to undergo surgery.[208] Treatment includes correction of polycythemia and platelet count reduction to less than 400,000/mm^3, either by plateletpheresis or cytoreductive agents.[209]

Cytoreductive agents include hydroxyurea, interferon alfa, and anagrelide. Anagrelide, an imidazoquinazolin, is thought to decrease platelet counts by specifically impairing megakaryocyte maturation.[210] It has little effect on red and white cell counts and is not known to be leukemogenic. Whether it decreases the incidence of thrombosis or hemorrhage is not known. Ten percent to 20% of patients taking anagrelide experience neurologic, gastrointestinal, and cardiac side effects, in particular fluid retention, necessitating discontinuation of the drug.

Low-dose aspirin may be useful in patients with essential thrombocythemia and thrombosis, particularly in those with erythromelalgia and/or digital and cerebrovascular ischemia.[205] A recent double-blind, placebo-controlled study of patients with polycythemia vera suggested that daily low-dose aspirin can reduce the risk of nonfatal arterial/venous cardiovascular events, although overall and cardiovascular mortality were not significantly reduced.[211] However, aspirin can exacerbate or induce a bleeding tendency in patients with these disorders and should be used judiciously.

In pregnant patients, interferon alfa has been recommended if platelet cytoreduction is required, and aspirin is useful for microvascular symptoms. Heparin at conventional doses is recommended for prophylaxis and treatment of venous thrombosis.

Leukemias and Myelodysplastic Syndrome

By far the most frequent cause of bleeding in these diseases is thrombocytopenia, but abnormal platelet function has also been described. In myeloid leukemias and myelodysplasia, decreased agonist-stimulated platelet aggregation and secretion have been observed, as has decreased platelet procoagulant activity.[212,213] These functional abnormalities may be due to acquired storage pool deficiency or a defect in platelet signal transduction and are intrinsic to the platelets. The platelet function abnormalities reported in patients with lymphoid leukemias are less likely to be due to the leukemic process.[212] Acquired von Willebrand disease has been reported in association with hairy cell leukemia.[214]

Plasma Cell Dyscrasias

Pathogenesis

Platelet dysfunction in plasma cell dyscrasias likely occurs when the associated monoclonal paraprotein interacts nonspecifically with the platelet surface. Thus, platelet dysfunction is more common when the paraprotein concentration is high.[215] In addition, specific interactions between monoclonal proteins and platelet receptors such as $\alpha_{IIb}\beta_3$ have been described.[216] Multiple myeloma, monoclonal gammopathy of undetermined significance, and chronic lymphocytic leukemia can also cause an acquired form of von Willebrand disease (see later).

Clinical Features

These diseases can interfere with normal hemostasis in a number of ways, including thrombocytopenia, hyperviscosity, and amyloidosis with or without acquired factor X deficiency. Platelet dysfunction has been observed in patients with multiple myeloma, macroglobulinemia, and monoclonal gammopathy of undetermined significance.[217] Furthermore, the bleeding time in these patients can be prolonged, even in the absence of clinical bleeding.

Treatment

Because platelet dysfunction results from high concentrations of paraprotein, cytoreductive therapy to reduce protein production should be considered.[218] Plasmapheresis can control bleeding by reducing the level of protein and can be life-saving during acute bleeds.[219] Cryoprecipitate, DDAVP, high-dose intravenous gamma globulin and/or plasmapheresis may be transiently effective in patients with acquired von Willebrand disease.

Acquired von Willebrand Disease

Clinical Features

An acquired form of von Willebrand disease can occur in patients with multiple myeloma, macroglobulinemia, low-grade non-Hodgkin's lymphoma, chronic lymphocytic leukemia, and the myeloproliferative disorders, as well as in patients with autoimmune disorders.[220] In patients with these diseases, mucocutaneous bleeding with or without the presence of a prolonged bleeding time should raise suspicion of this possibility. In patients with hematologic diseases, a specific anti-vWF antibody is present, whereas in autoimmune disorders, anti-vWF antibodies may be part of a generalized autoimmune response.[221] The presence of a vWF inhibitor may or may not be detectable in the laboratory depending on whether the antibody neutralizes vWF function or simply leads to accelerated vWF clearance.

Treatment

Treatment includes DDAVP,[222] vWF-containing factor VIII concentrates,[223] or high-dose intravenous immunoglobulin.[224] The latter has been most efficacious in patients with lymphoproliferative disorders or monoclonal immunoglobulins.[221] Treatment of the underlying disease is only sometimes helpful.[225]

CURRENT CONTROVERSIES & FUTURE CONSIDERATIONS

Inherited and Acquired Platelet Disorders

- Investigation into the basis for inherited and acquired disorders of platelet function has provided a framework for much of our current knowledge of platelet biochemistry and physiology. Conversely, as the latter disciplines progress, we will develop a better understanding of these disorders and how to manage their clinical consequences. At the present time, therapeutic intervention is non-specific and in many cases, only partially effective. Whether recombinant Factor VIIa represents a universal and effective therapy for the hemorrhage the results from these disorders should become clear in the near future.

Suggested Readings*

Bennett JS: Novel platelet inhibitors. Annu Rev Med 52:161–184, 2001.

George JN, Caen JP, Nurden AT: Glanzmann thrombasthenia: the spectrum of clinical disease. Blood 75:1383–1395, 1990.

Huizing M, Boissy RE, Gahl WA: Hermansky-Pudlak syndrome: vesicle formation from yeast to man. Pigment Cell Res 15:405–419, 2002.

Lopez JA, Andrews RK, Afshar-Kharghan V, et al: Bernard-Soulier syndrome. Blood 91:4397–4418, 1998.

Patrono C: Aspirin as an antiplatelet drug. N Engl J Med 330:1287–1294, 1994.

Full references for this chapter can be found on accompanying CD-ROM.

CHAPTER 60

Immune, Posttransfusional, and Neonatal Thrombocytopenia

David K. Jin, MD, PhD, and James B. Bussel, MD

KEY POINTS

Immune Thrombocytopenic Purpura

Diagnosis

- Establish the diagnosis of immune thrombocytopenic purpura (ITP) by identifying the thrombocytopenia, then ruling out other causes of thrombocytopenia.
- Key elements to evaluate in ITP include the patient's history, family history, physical examination, complete blood count, medications, and peripheral blood smear.
- Expected physical signs include mucocutaneous bleeding, petechiae, purpura, and easy bruising.
- Negative physical signs are hepatosplenomegaly, lymphadenopathy, signs of malignancies, and abnormal radiographs.
- Response to ITP-specific treatment is the "gold standard" confirmation of diagnosis.
- In both children and adults, there is a significant tendency to improvement over time (i.e., 1 year), so management after initial treatment should be restricted to nontoxic treatments pending spontaneous improvement or the decision that the ITP is persistent.

Treatment

- Consider comorbidities and lifestyle of patients with ITP in assessing the risks and benefits of initial treatment.
- Standard practice is to initiate oral prednisone to support the platelet count in a safe range until a remission occurs; duration of therapy is controversial.
- Other therapeutic options include intravenous immunoglobulin (IVIG), high-dose oral dexamethasone, anti-D, anti-CD20 monoclonal antibody, and splenectomy.
- Combining treatments such as IVIG, intravenous steroids, intravenous anti-D (in Rh^+, Coombs' test–negative patients), and even intravenous vincristine is useful to acutely increase the platelet count in refractory patients (or to suggest another diagnosis in nonresponders).
- For chronic refractory ITP, anti-CD20 monoclonal antibody, cyclophosphamide, vincristine, azathioprine, mycophenolate mofetil, cyclosporin, danazol, and possibly thrombopoietic agents can be considered.
- Overrestriction of activities such as sports or travel is common and should be avoided.

IMMUNE THROMBOCYTOPENIC PURPURA

Introduction

Immune thrombocytopenic purpura (ITP; idiopathic thrombocytopenic purpura) is an acquired autoimmune disorder characterized by a low platelet count and mucocutaneous bleeding.[1,2] The clinical criteria of ITP include isolated, often severe thrombocytopenia with otherwise normal blood counts and unremarkable findings from the peripheral blood smear and physical examination along with no apparent etiologic cause of thrombocytopenia. In children, ITP is in general an acute disease that often improves within several weeks and resolves within several months. In contrast, ITP in adult patients is a more persistent disease. Serologic testing is generally not of diagnostic or prognostic value and has no apparent role in routine evaluation or management at this time. The typical patient with ITP presents with petechiae and ecchymoses; more serious bleeding includes epistaxis, hematochezia, hematuria, and, rarely, life-threatening intracranial hemorrhage (ICH). This definition for ITP is particularly useful for pediatric outpatients who are otherwise completely well. It is less applicable for complicated cases in hospitalized adults who are concomitantly on several medications for a number of comorbid conditions.

Epidemiology and Risk Factors

Incidence

ITP is considered a common acquired bleeding disorder. From a Scandinavian survey that used a platelet count cutoff at 50,000/μL, the annual incidence of ITP in adults was estimated to be 32 per 1 million population per year.[3] This survey included only symptomatic adults with ITP. However, if incidental cases of ITP in asymptomatic adults are also considered, the incidence rate could be as high as 55 per million per year. Data in children are more limited. Other more limited estimates are similar (i.e., 66 per million).

Age and Geographic Distribution

Epidemiologic data derived from reported case series have shown that the peak age in children with ITP is 2–4 years, with both genders equally affected. A female preponderance begins in adolescence and continues into adulthood; approximately 70% of adult ITP cases are women, and 72% of these women are less than 40 years of age. However, the study from Denmark suggested that the incidence of ITP increased in the elderly, in whom there was no gender predominance,[3] and the traditional view of ITP as primarily a disease in young women is debatable because a recent population-based cohort study from the Northern Health Region of England showed no significant gender difference in this disease.[4]

Pathophysiology

The pathogenesis of ITP is presumed to be accelerated platelet destruction via specific autoantibodies in the great majority of cases. Recent work has suggested that these antibodies may also inhibit megakaryocytes,[5,6] adding reduced platelet production to the peripheral destruction to help explain the severe thrombocytopenia. Whether or not this is the explanation, information acquired from a number of sources all suggest that platelet production is often decreased and that this is a key component of the thrombocytopenia. However, these platelet- and megakaryocyte-reactive antibodies are not demonstrable in all patients, and assays for antiplatelet antibodies have not yet proven to be important for management decisions. An alternative mechanism, T-cell–mediated cytotoxicity, has been postulated for patients not demonstrating autoantibodies.[7,8] It is very possible that cytotoxic T cells targeted, for example, to glycoprotein (GP) IIb/IIIa contribute to immune platelet destruction even when antiplatelet antibodies are present. An overview of pathogenesis of ITP is illustrated in Figure 60–1.

T-Cell–Mediated Cytotoxicity

Olsson and colleagues[8] have recently demonstrated that $CD3^+$ T lymphocytes isolated from ITP patients had increased expression of cytotoxic genes, including those for Apo-1/Fas, granzyme A, granzyme B, and perforin, together with genes involved in the T-cell response, such as those for interferon-γ and interleukin-2 receptor, as compared with control subjects. These genes were upregulated whether or not the patient was in remission, but only patients in remission upregulated the *Kir* genes. These data are consistent with a pathophysiology including T-cell–mediated cytotoxicity as a plausible mechanism for platelet destruction in ITP.

Helicobacter pylori and Hepatitis C

The link between *Helicobacter pylori* and ITP remains controversial. A recent report by Franceschi and associates has demonstrated cross-reactivity between anti–cytotoxin-associated gene A (anti-CagA) antibodies and human platelet antigens in patients with active ITP, leading to reduced platelet survival.[9] Their serologic data support a temporal association between the disappearance of anti-CagA antibodies in the serum and improvement of ITP after eradication of *H. pylori*. However, the identity of the cross-reacting platelet antigens, their population prevalence, and the pathogenicity of different strains of *H. pylori* remain unknown. Accelerated consumption via interaction with von Willebrand factor has also been postulated. In a prospective study, Michel and coworkers could not confirm that *H. pylori* is not involved in either the initiation or the perpetuation of ITP because the prevalence of *H. pylori* infection in the ITP cohort was low and eradication of *H. pylori* did not positively influence the clinical course of the ITP in any of the 14 patients.[10] More than 20 reports exist on the topic, and no consensus has been reached.

The relationship between hepatitis C and thrombocytopenia has been much less well studied than has that between *H. pylori* and ITP. Certain patients, however, have responded to suppression or eradication of hepatitis C with substantial improvement in their platelet counts, and steroid use may have adverse consequences in these patients. Acutely, however, initiation of interferon treatment may further lower the platelet count and can result in serious hemorrhage. In this regard, human immunodeficiency virus (HIV) infection has the clearest direct relationship to thrombocytopenia. In greater than 75% of non–end-stage HIV-infected patients with thrombocytopenia, reducing the viral load to undetectable level will result in a substantial platelet increase.

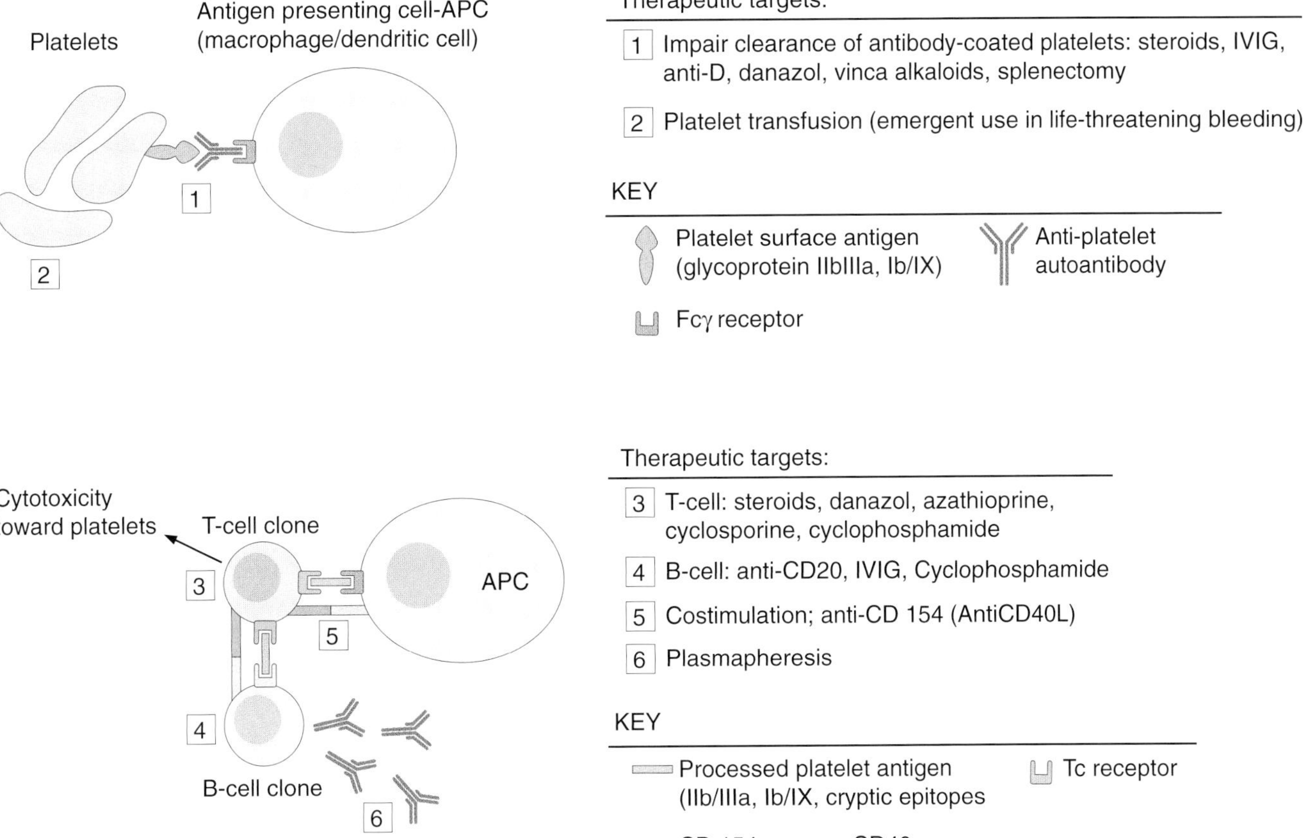

Figure 60–1. Pathogenesis and therapeutic targets for immune thrombocytopenic purpura.

Chemokine-Induced Mobilization of Megakaryocytic Progenitors

Avecilla and colleagues[11] recently demonstrated complete restoration of platelet counts in severely thrombocytopenic thrombopoietin- or thrombopoietin receptor (c-Mpl)–deficient mice after administration of chemokines such as stromal-derived factor-1 or fibroblast growth factor-4. These data suggest that chemokines may modulate mobilization of megakaryocytic progenitor cells from the marrow osteoblastic/endosteal niche to the vascular niche, and thus increase the platelet count in the peripheral circulation. Neither plasma levels nor the marrow localization of chemokines in ITP patients has been investigated; therefore, the role of chemokines in ITP remains elusive. However, in view of the importance of platelet production in ITP, this area could be of considerable importance.

Clinical Features

The clinical presentation of ITP has a high degree of variability. Onset of the disease may be acute or insidious. The practice of routinely reporting a platelet count with all requests for blood counts has resulted in the increased identification of asymptomatic mild thrombocytopenia, thereby extending the clinical spectrum of ITP. Furthermore, it has increased the detection of adult patients with ITP whose platelet counts decrease steadily over months to years. This in turn may revise views of the pathophysiology of ITP, which typically are based on an acute development of thrombocytopenia rather than slow progression over months to years.[12] The bleeding manifestations of thrombocytopenia in ITP are classically described as mucocutaneous, to distinguish them from the delayed, slowly evolving visceral hematomas characteristic of coagulation disorders such as hemophilia. The spectrum of bleeding tendency in symptomatic patients ranges from major hemorrhage to scattered petechiae and easy bruising. In general, petechiae and ecchymoses (i.e., wet purpura) are expected symptoms in ITP. Epistaxis, gingival bleeding, and menorrhagia are also relatively common but typically mild, whereas overt gastrointestinal bleeding, macroscopic hematuria, and ICH are, fortunately, rare. The extent of bleeding in ITP patients varies with age. Older patients with ITP appear to have more frequent severe bleeding, such as gastrointestinal hemorrhage and ICH,[13] possibly because of comorbid conditions such as hypertension. In the United States, a recent 3-year survey of children with ITP yielded approximately five de novo cases of ICH per year (manuscript in preparation). This confirmed clinical wisdom that two factors, bleeding beyond petechiae and ecchymoses, and head trauma, each suggested that more serious bleeding might occur.

TABLE 60–1. Differential Diagnosis of Thrombocytopenia

Drug-induced thrombocytopenia
Posttransfusion purpura
Thrombotic thrombocytopenic purpura
Hemolytic-uremic syndrome
Gestational thrombocytopenia
Chronic disseminated intravascular coagulopathy
Myelodysplasia (myelodysplastic syndrome)
Congenital or acquired amegakaryocytic thrombocytopenia
Inherited thrombocytopenias (e.g., von Willebrand disease type 2B, Wiskott-Aldrich syndrome/X-linked thrombocytopenia, and the *MYH9* mutation–associated family [May-Hegglin syndrome, Fanconi's anemia, Bernard-Soulier syndrome, thrombocytopenia with absent radius syndrome, trisomies 13 or 18])

Diagnosis

History and Physical Examination

Essentially, the diagnosis of ITP is established by identifying the thrombocytopenia, and then ruling out other causes of thrombocytopenia (Table 60–1). The key elements in the initial evaluation include the patient's history, the physical examination, complete blood count, and examination of the peripheral blood smear. The history should be explored for other etiologies of thrombocytopenia, including other diseases and drug use, symptoms of systemic illness, and findings consistent with inherited thrombocytopenia, such as family history of thrombocytopenia, renal failure, high-tone hearing loss, or immunodeficiency. A family history of other autoimmune diseases such as thyroiditis supports the likelihood of ITP.

Physical examination should not reveal hepatosplenomegaly, lymphadenopathy, or any other signs of malignancy, and the radiographs should be normal. Signs of mucocutaneous bleeding and findings consistent with unrelated comorbid conditions are expected.

Laboratory Findings

Traditionally, the diagnosis of ITP is considered when there is an isolated, usually severe thrombocytopenia on the complete blood count. Secondary ITP (i.e., associated with chronic lymphocytic leukemia and with Evans's syndrome) can be seen with abnormalities of white cells and red cells, respectively. ITP with a mild microcytic anemia can occur either with thalassemia trait or with iron deficiency. Examination of the peripheral blood smear may show the presence of giant platelets (Fig. 60–2). However, it is essential to exclude in vitro platelet clumping that can cause a falsely low platelet count (secondary to ethylenediaminetetraacetic acid–dependent agglutinins) and to ensure that there are no abnormalities of the white and red blood cells. Cold-dependent platelet agglutinins and autoantibodies that induce "rosetting" of platelets around neutrophils and/or monocytes can also cause pseudothrombocytopenia. Examination of the peripheral blood smear may also provide evidence of other causes of true thrombocytopenia, such as the

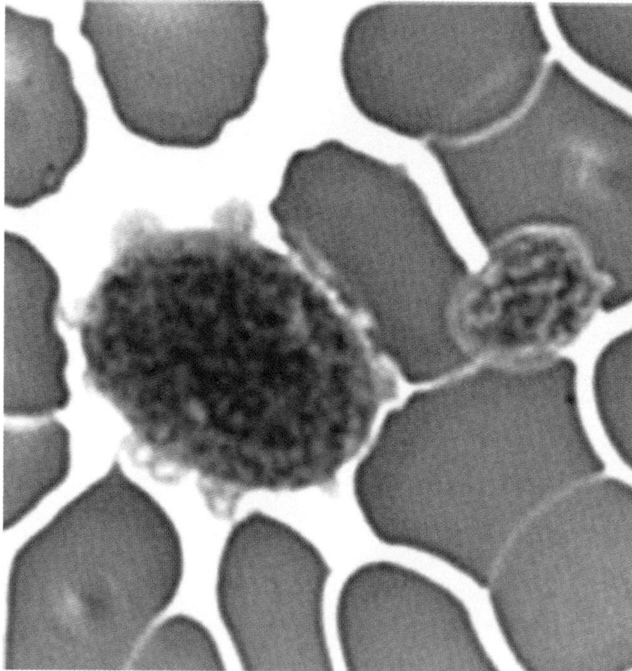

■ **Figure 60–2.** Blood smear shows presence of giant platelets.

presence of schistocytes in thrombotic thrombocytopenic purpura/hemolytic-uremic syndrome; the presence of hemolytic anemia and renal failure also distinguish these disorders from ITP. Finally, if the platelets are too small (Wiskott-Aldrich syndrome) or too large (Bernard-Soulier syndrome, syndromes associated with *MYH9* mutations), then these nonimmune thrombocytopenias need to be considered (see Chapters 7 and 59). Tests for antiplatelet antibodies are not helpful. Most important is a thorough history taking to rule out drug-induced thrombocytopenia, including that caused by over-the-counter drugs, vitamins, dietary supplements (especially quinine), or herbal remedies. Testing for drug-induced thrombocytopenia is possible but subject to false negatives if, for example, a drug metabolite is involved rather than the drug itself.

Bone marrow aspiration and biopsy are generally not required in most patients with suspected ITP. However, it is recommended in patients over 50–60 years of age even with isolated thrombocytopenia to rule out myelodysplastic syndrome. The latter is associated with dyspoiesis (abnormal megakaryocytes and with hypercellularity). Failure to respond to ITP treatment, and any suspicious findings (i.e., anemia, leuko- or neutropenia, or splenomegaly), warrant a bone marrow examination as well. In a typical bone marrow examination of an ITP patient, the marrow is normocellular with normal erythropoiesis and myelopoiesis. Megakaryocytes appear normal or slightly increased in number, generally with a shift to more immature forms with hypoploidy.

A presumptive diagnosis of ITP is made when the history, physical examination, complete blood count, peripheral blood smear, and bone marrow examination (if performed) all suggest ITP and do not suggest other etiologies for the patient's isolated thrombocytopenia.

Depending upon the history and physical examination, additional tests in ITP patients beyond a complete blood count, including differential and reticulocyte counts, may include HIV testing in patients with risk factors, hepatitis C and *H. pylori* testing, immunoglobulin levels to detect hypogammaglobulinemia and selective immunoglobulin (Ig)A deficiency, antinuclear antibodies, blood type and direct antiglobulin (Coombs') test to determine both suitability for anti-D therapy and the presence of Evans's syndrome, lupus anticoagulant testing, and thyroid function tests.

Treatment

Initial Management

There is no accepted threshold platelet count that defines a universally accepted indication for initial treatment, especially in children. In adults, a platelet count less than 20,000/μL is generally considered a minimum for treatment. The primary goal is not to achieve a normal platelet count, but rather to prevent bleeding. It is important to consider comorbidities and lifestyle of patients with ITP in assessing the risks and benefits of initial treatment. There are very limited data concerning the effectiveness of different therapies for ITP on long-term outcomes, other than for rituximab (Rituxan) and splenectomy. This consideration is often initially neglected because even in adults there is an important tendency to spontaneous improvement.

Oral Prednisone

In adults, the standard practice is to initiate treatment with oral prednisone at 1 mg/kg body weight per day. The goal is to support the platelet count in a safe range until a remission occurs. The duration of initial prednisone treatment is determined by the platelet count response; there is no consensus about the appropriate duration of treatment nor how to institute a tapering of the dose. A commonly applied schedule is to taper and discontinue prednisone over 4–8 weeks after achieving a normal platelet count. The response rates to oral prednisone range from 50% to 75%, with most cases of positive clinical responses occurring within the first 1–2 weeks of treatment but a percentage of responses taking longer. The incidence rates of continuous remission range from less than 5% to over 30%, depending on the duration of ITP and duration of follow-up. Most responding adults will have recurrence of thrombocytopenia when prednisone is being tapered or after it is discontinued. In one series, 39% percent of adult patients treated with oral prednisone had a complete remission; however, only half of these patients showed a sustained complete remission lasting more than 6 months after the maintenance prednisone was discontinued, indicating that further treatment is needed.[14]

High-Dose Oral Dexamethasone

In a prospective study of adult ITP patients, Cheng and coworkers[15] recently reported a 4-day course of high-dose oral dexamethasone (40 mg/day) as an effective initial therapy. There was an initial response in 106 of the 125 eligible patients (85%), with platelet counts increased by at least 20,000/μL by day 3 of treatment, and the mean platelet count was 101,400 ± 53,200/μL at 1 week after the initiation of treatment. Among the patients with initial response, 50% had a sustained response with platelet counts of more than 50,000/μL and required no further treatment during 2–5 years of follow-up. The remaining 53 patients with relapse (at a median time of 45 days) all responded to a second 4-day course of oral dexamethasone. Treatment was well tolerated and there was no discontinuation of treatment as a result of intolerable side effects in this study. A prior study using this regimen demonstrated lasting effects in chronic refractory ITP but it could not be confirmed in follow-up studies,[16,17] and most clinicians think there is a low rate of lasting efficacy when high-dose dexamethasone is used in patients with long-standing ITP. High-dose dexamethasone may result in lasting responses in newly diagnosed patients. However, it should be used cautiously, and additional confirmatory studies will be needed before this protocol can be recommended as treatment of ITP at or near diagnosis.

Intravenous Anti-D

Anti-D (WinRho) consists of immunoglobulin that is hyperimmune, with a high titer of IgG that binds to the erythrocyte D antigen; it is only effective in Rh-positive patients and primarily in those who have not undergone splenectomy. A positive direct antiglobulin test appears to aggravate the risk of hemolysis and is a relative contraindication. The mechanism is based on the immune-mediated clearance of the sensitized erythrocytes that occupy the Fc receptors in the reticuloendothelial system, thereby minimizing removal of antibody-coated platelets. The standard regimen for anti-D is 50–75 μg/kg body weight per day, with the 75 μg/kg dose leading to overnight platelet increases in 70% or more of both adults and children.[18] The response rate to anti-D in one series was about 70%, with the increase in platelet count lasting more than 21 days in 50% of the responders.[19] It has been recently shown by Cooper and associates that FcγRIIa and FcγRIIIa polymorphisms correlate with cytokine levels and platelet increments in response to anti-D, implicating a different modulatory role for anti-D as compared to intravenous immunoglobulin (IVIG).[20] A part of the mechanism presumably involves cytokine release consequent to Fc receptor interaction with the Fc piece of IgG on agglutinated red cells, but this remains to be confirmed.[20,21]

Intravenous Immunoglobulin

A standard regimen with IVIG (1 gm/kg body weight per day for 1–3 consecutive days) in conjunction with prednisone or dexamethasone is used in patients with ITP at diagnosis to treat internal bleeding, when the platelet count remains below 5000/μL despite treatment for several days with steroids, or when extensive purpura, including wet purpura, are present. Approximately 80%

of patients will show initial clinical response; however, sustained remission is infrequent. Preparation for surgery in which a near-normal platelet count is required (i.e., cardiothoracic or orthopedic) and in refractory patients in whom the platelet count falls to less than 10,000/µL with bleeding symptoms are other settings for the use of IVIG. In the latter, as with initial therapy with IVIG in which prednisone is started, another treatment (danazol, azathioprine, rituximab) whose mechanism of effect is slower in onset but whose effects are intended to be long lasting needs to be used concomitantly. The cost of IVIG is considerable. Complications such as renal failure, thrombosis, and pulmonary insufficiency may occur, although these are infrequent; the first can be minimized by choice of preparation of IVIG and/or using sterile water as a diluent instead of saline. The most common reaction is headache, which can be severe enough to include cerebrospinal fluid pleocytosis (aseptic meningitis). Rarely, anaphylactic reactions may occur in patients with history of congenital IgA deficiency, although IgA-depleted IVIG may be selected for use in these patients; this is *not* an issue in panhypogammaglobulinemic patients.

Splenectomy

Decisions about splenectomy depend on the severity of ITP, the patient's response to and tolerance of steroids and other treatments, and the patient's preferences regarding surgery.[22] As many as one half of hematologists recommend splenectomy within 1–6 months if more than 10 mg of prednisone per day is required to maintain the platelet count above 30,000/µL. In adult patients with ITP, it remains controversial as to whether to perform splenectomy 1–3 months from diagnosis if there is no sustained response to steroids, or to wait for at least 1 year before deciding to proceed to surgery; patients increasingly prefer the latter approach. Data on the use of intravenous anti-D and with rituximab suggest that at least one third to more than one half of patients who relapse as prednisone is tapered may nonetheless be able to avoid splenectomy.[23,24] Some clinicians may also choose to try danazol or, rarely, azathioprine. If selected, splenectomy should be performed laparoscopically if possible. There does not appear to be an excess incidence of accessory spleens in such cases, and the postoperative morbidity is clearly less. The long-term outcome (i.e., at 20–30 years following surgery) remains unknown other than the fact that the maintenance of clinical remission is approximately 60%.[25] Overwhelming sepsis can be minimized by patient education and repeated administration of Pneumovax at 5-year intervals.

Children

Approximately 80% of children with ITP spontaneously improve within 6–12 months from the time of diagnosis. Therefore, treatments such as IVIG 0.5–1 g/kg, intravenous anti-D 50–75 µg/kg, and prednisone 1–4 mg/kg are administered as needed to transiently support the platelet count until spontaneous improvement is attained. Exactly how much treatment is needed and in whom are debated, with the only consensus being that signs and symptoms of bleeding beyond petechiae and ecchymoses warrant treatment. Otherwise, certain centers also use a platelet count (i.e., 10,000–30,000/µL) as the threshold for treatment, whereas others do not and treat only for bleeding. In essentially all centers, when platelet counts stabilize at more than 20,000–30,000/µL, no further treatment is generally required. If the patient remains refractory to initial treatment, the only intervention proven to be curative is splenectomy, although data on rituximab are promising.[26] The consensus is to wait at least 1 year from the time of diagnosis and until the patient is older than age 5, in an attempt to preserve the immunologic functions of the spleen through this period. Furthermore, there should be a "reason" (i.e., toxicity of other treatment, bleeding, poor compliance, etc.) to recommend surgery. In children, the cure rate is thought to be higher than in adults (75–80%), although long-term follow-up data are lacking.

Management for Chronic Refractory ITP

Treatment of patients, almost all adults, who have undergone and failed to respond to splenectomy is controversial and entirely lacking controlled data. Two recent publications[27,28] both document an important morbidity and especially mortality in patients with very low platelet counts despite splenectomy. The most promising, novel treatment is anti-CD20 monoclonal antibody (rituximab), which transiently depletes normal B cells and has led to apparent cures in as many as 30% of refractory patients.[29] Further studies are required. Other treatments such as low-dose intravenous chemotherapy (cyclophosphamide and vincristine), and oral agents such as azathioprine, mycophenolate mofetil, cyclosporin, and danazol have been explored in pilot series. No treatment, other than anti-CD20 monoclonal antibody and possibly repeated intravenous IV cyclophosphamide, has been demonstrated to have a significant cure rate, defined as the platelet count remaining elevated even when the medication is discontinued. Experimental treatments with very preliminary data include autologous bone marrow transplantation[30] and recombinant thrombopoietin/thrombopoietin-mimetic agents; the latter appear especially promising because of their potentially universal applicability; their novel mechanism of action, which would permit them to be combined with other treatments; and their apparent lack of toxicity. A proposed treatment algorithm for chronic refractory ITP is shown in Figure 60–3.

Special Circumstances: Pregnancy

Because ITP may often occur in younger women of child-bearing age, pregnancy in a woman with ITP is not infrequent. Management considerations need to be separated between the mother and the fetus/neonate. The mother is actually far less well studied than is the child. IVIG and

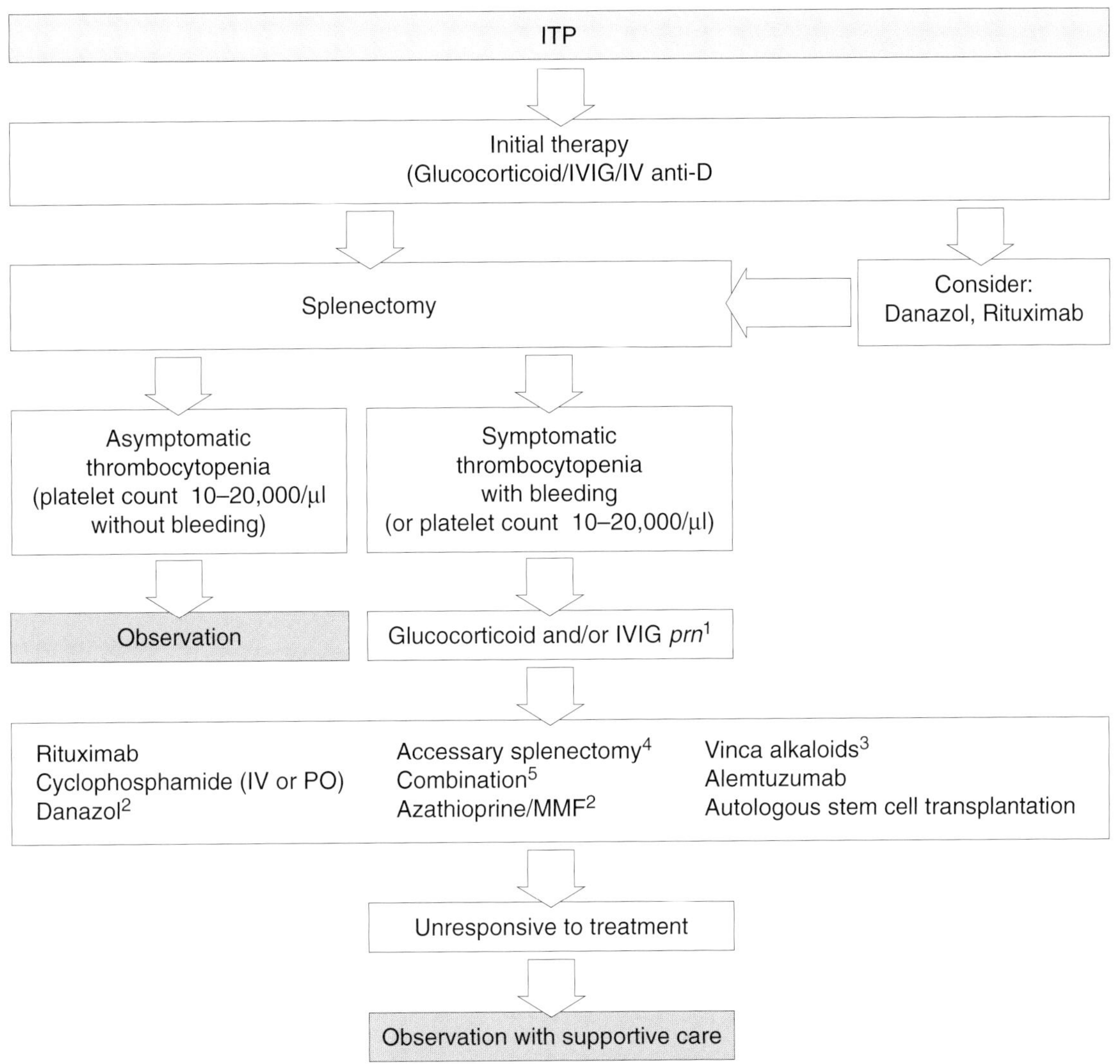

Figure 60–3. Treatment algorithm for chronic ITP. Notes: [1]Short term management to support the platelet count and avoid bleeding.[2]Better in combination than used alone. [3]Only as part of combination therapy (efficacy too low and toxicity too high to use as single-agent treatment). [4]Only with response to initial splenectomy lasting 2 or more years. [5]Cyclophosphamide, vincristine, and prednisone or IVIG, methylprednisolone, vincristine, danazol, and azathioprine.

prednisone are the primary treatments of ITP, but intravenous anti-D has recently been shown to be safe and effective as well. Splenectomy is reserved for the second trimester in the most difficult cases. In general, a maternal platelet count of 20,000–30,000/μL is sufficient throughout the pregnancy both for the mother to avoid bleeding, as in the nonpregnant state, and also to prevent hemorrhagic miscarriage. At the time of delivery, it is considered desirable to achieve a platelet count of 50,000/μL, and anesthesiologists often require counts of 80,000/μL for an epidural. For a scheduled delivery, IVIG or intravenous anti-D is often helpful. For the mother who is delivering spontaneously, a daily dose of prednisone, usually a minimum of 20 mg/day, and judicious use of other agents will mostly be sufficient. It has become clear that there is no need to perform an elective cesarean section for the sake of the fetus. The consensus is that delivery should be according to obstetric indications. There are no clear data on how the pregnancy will affect the ITP; an unknown but probably small fraction of women will worsen during the pregnancy. A fraction of women with ITP will also develop their ITP at the end of the pregnancy.

It is thought that, just as the risk of hemorrhagic morbidity and mortality in the mother is very low, the same is true for the fetus and newborn. One study documented fetal thrombocytopenia as early as 21 weeks of gestation,[31] but fetal blood sampling is not used because the

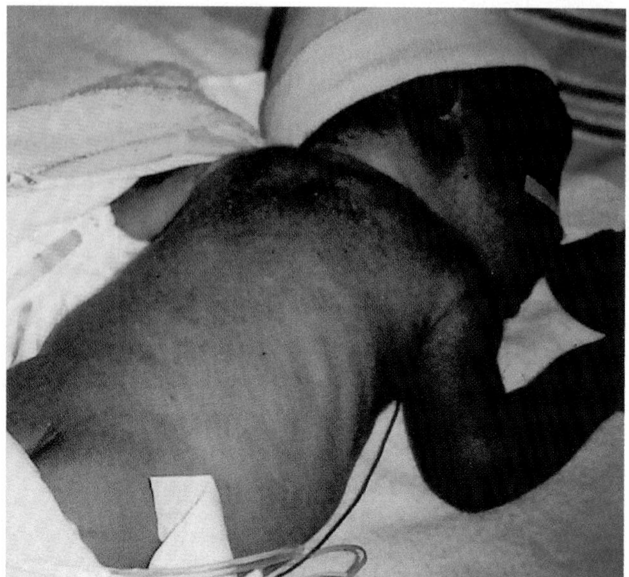

Figure 60–4. Diffuse petechiae on the back of an infant with neonatal alloimmune thrombocytopenia. (Courtesy of Patrick Gallagher, MD.)

small but important risk of the procedure is believed to outweigh the benefit of knowing the exact count. Overall, as many as 40% of neonates of mothers with ITP may be born with mild thrombocytopenia, but only approximately 10% will have platelet counts less than 50,000/μL and only 5% will have counts less than 20,000/μL. A crucial issue that muddies the data is that, unlike babies with alloimmune thrombocytopenia (AIT) (Fig. 60–4), infants of mothers with ITP are often born with adequate platelet counts but have the counts fall to low levels 1–3 days after birth. Thus the exact numbers exhibiting a certain count depend upon how long counts are followed. The very low rate of ICH (~1%), which is not very different in frequency from that of normal newborns, may reflect the fact that platelet counts may be adequate at delivery, although they may decline in the days following delivery. There is no evidence that breast-feeding by mothers with ITP affects the infant's platelet count.

Prognosis, Supportive Care, and Long-Term Management

The overall outcome of children and adults with ITP is good, and the long-term outcome is generally favorable even without splenectomy.[14] Nonetheless, episodes of serious bleeding, especially ICH, can occur and seem in general to be preventable by the maintenance of a minimal but adequate platelet count (i.e., >20,000–30,000/μL). Therefore, in the beginning (i.e., the first year of disease), treatment as required is appropriate and will allow patients to improve spontaneously. If there is not an acute response to single treatments, combinations of treatments will likely be useful. Failure to respond to IVIG + intravenous steroids + intravenous anti-D + vincristine, all administered on the same day, is suggestive of another disease (i.e., a nonimmune form of thrombocytopenia such as myelodysplastic syndrome or marrow failure, such as aplastic anemia or amegakaryocytic thrombocytopenia). If there is response to treatment but continued requirement for it, it is important not to give too much prednisone for too long (the exact amount and duration are undefined, with a high degree of individual variability). Monitoring bone density for osteoporosis and periodic slit-lamp examinations to check for the early development of cataracts are important in these patients. Treatments such as repeated infusion with intravenous anti-D, rituximab, splenectomy, or an oral medication such as danazol or azathioprine (provided that the liver function tests are normal) are all appropriate for the patient who does not improve. If the patient fails to improve despite these measures and requires continued treatment, then the experimental treatments indicated earlier may be appropriate. Confirmation of diagnosis is only achieved by response, albeit transient, to the acute treatments (IVIG, intravenous anti-D, and to a lesser extent steroids). It is very difficult to distinguish a patient with the most severe ITP, one who does not respond even transiently to any treatment, from a patient with severe thrombocytopenia from another cause, such as myelodysplastic syndrome, if the latter condition is not evident on testing such as a bone marrow aspirate and biopsy.

Supportive care consists of monitoring for toxicities of treatment such as decreased vitamin D and calcium levels, with institution of alendronate (Fosamax) if needed. Agents that may be of use, although they are not anticipated to alter the platelet count, include aminocaproic acid (Amicar), especially for mouth and nose bleeding; oral contraceptive agents or medroxyprogesterone acetate (Depo-Provera) for heavy menses; and iron to prevent development of iron deficiency anemia.

Issues in Diagnosis and Treatment

A number of issues are yet to be resolved in the diagnosis and treatment of ITP. The major issue that involves both children and adults is the determination of treatment: who needs it and what should be used. Certain patients clearly require an urgent increase in the platelet count if it is too low: those with ongoing bleeding beyond petechiae and ecchymoses, a (especially recent) history of severe bleeding, major head trauma, and ingestion of aspirin or other nonsteroidal anti-inflammatory agents that have antiplatelet effects (e.g., on cyclooxygenase inhibitor). For other ITP patients, when to treat and with what is more difficult to determine. Studies on this topic or on bleeding tendencies would be useful. Similarly, the long-term effects of acutely administered treatments such as dexamethasone or rituximab need confirmatory studies. Better analysis of mechanism of treatment effects would allow more rational choice of combinations. Similarly, studies of individual patients could allow better prediction of response to specific treatments and also characterization of patients more rationally according to their pathophysiology. In this regard, a simple testing panel that would be specific for ITP (i.e., a platelet antibody test) would be extremely helpful for clarifying the diagnosis.

POSTTRANSFUSION PURPURA

Posttransfusion purpura (PTP) is a rare complication of blood transfusion characterized by severe thrombocytopenia, usually occurring 1–2 weeks after transfusion. PTP has an estimated frequency of 1 in 50,000 transfusions and is associated with a recall alloimmune response against one of the human platelet antigens (HPAs). The human platelet antigen-1 (HPA-1; Zw) system is localized on platelet GPIIIa or the β_3 integrin. The two alleles differ by a single nucleotide polymorphism, represented by leucine (HPA-1a; Zw1^a) and proline (HPA-1b; Zw1^b) at amino acid position 33 of the GPIIIa of the GPIIb/IIIa complex.[32] The pathogenesis of PTP is still unknown, but there are two proposed mechanisms. One states that HPA-1/anti–HPA-1 immune complexes mediate the destruction of autologous platelets. The other plausible mechanism assumes a transient loss of tolerance for self during the stimulation with alloantigen, resulting in formation of platelet autoantibodies or pan-reactive platelet antibodies.

PTP typically occurs in HPA-1b–homozygous (HPA-1a–negative) multiparous women after receiving blood or blood components from an HPA-1a–positive donor (98% of the white populations are HPA-1a negative). This causes in vivo destruction of the patient's HPA-1a–negative platelets, leading to profound thrombocytopenia. PTP is often characterized by severe bleeding associated with a definite risk of fatal hemorrhage. Most patients with PTP have spontaneous recovery within 7–35 days. Remission can be accelerated by plasmapheresis, corticosteroids, and high-dose IVIG.[33-36] Approximately 1 in 350 pregnant women form HPA-1a antibodies. In some HPA-1a–alloimmunized women, blood transfusion may precipitate an episode of PTP.

NEONATAL THROMBOCYTOPENIA

This disease entity can be divided between nonimmune thrombocytopenia and immune thrombocytopenia. Nonimmune thrombocytopenia has many causes (sepsis, viral infection, asphyxia, thrombosis, liver disease, etc). It has several characteristics: (1) the platelet count is low but not very low; (2) there is usually little bleeding; (3) the neonate is usually premature and sick; and (4) treatment involves platelet transfusions, administered as needed. The latter may depend on (in addition to the degree of bleeding) the birth weight, Apgar scores, and presence or absence of an intraventricular hemorrhage. Immune thrombocytopenia has been extensively studied in the past 20 years and occurs in approximately 1 in 500–1000 deliveries. Significant neonatal thrombocytopenia as a result of maternal ITP is very infrequent (see earlier); far more common is AIT (see Fig. 60–4). Pl^{A1} or HPA-1a is the platelet antigen most commonly involved, but an increasing number of antigens have been discovered. At least 15 antigens are now known to be involved in cases of AIT. Screening of all pregnancies is under investigation but is not likely to be universally instituted in the near future. As many as 10–20% of all cases will suffer an ICH as a result of the thrombocytopenia; more importantly, more than half of these hemorrhages will occur prenatally as a result of fetal thrombocytopenia.

The diagnosis of AIT is based upon the severity of the thrombocytopenia (platelet count <50,000/µL on the first day of life), the absence of another explanation for the thrombocytopenia, *or* a familial history of transient neonatal thrombocytopenia. The presence or absence of a response to random platelets is surprisingly unhelpful in making the diagnosis. Similarly, 40% of 107 cases of fetal thrombocytopenia had platelet counts of 20,000/µL or less before 25 weeks of gestation, so even very premature infants may be severely affected by AIT.[37] Rarely, other diagnoses may need to be considered. These include amegakaryocytic thrombocytopenia (either idiopathic or with absent radii) or trisomies 13 and 18. Treatment after birth optimally is matched platelets. These can either come from the mother or from a matched, unrelated donor; the latter has been proposed to be a Pl^{A1-}, Br a$^-$ donor so that the platelets will be suitable for more than 90% of recognized cases even before any typing is performed. IVIG and/or random platelet transfusions can be administered in addition or if matched platelets are not available. The urgency and extent of treatment depend upon the platelet count and the presence or absence of an ICH; the threat of the latter mandates that an imaging study (ultrasound, computed tomography, or magnetic resonance imaging) be performed as soon after birth as possible. There is now extensive experience with antenatal treatment in the subsequent pregnancy, in which therapy is administered to the mother to increase the fetal platelet count and avoid (antenatal) ICH. Because both AIT and autoimmune thrombocytopenia are due to maternal transplacentally transferred antibody, the thrombocytopenia typically spontaneously improves within 1–4 weeks.

CURRENT CONTROVERSIES & FUTURE CONSIDERATIONS

Immune Thrombocytopenic Purpura

- What is the real natural history of ITP, especially in adults? How many people will spontaneously improve, when, and why?
- New diagnostic tests and approaches need to be developed.
- A better way to define who needs treatment should be developed, including risk of bleeding and not just the platelet count.
- How often is platelet production decreased, and how does it affect treatment response?
- Pharmacogenomics needs to be expanded and made accessible so responsiveness to individual treatments can be better predicted.

Suggested Readings*

Avecilla ST, Hattori K, Heissig B, et al: Chemokine-mediated interaction of hematopoietic progenitors with the bone marrow vascular niche is required for thrombopoiesis. Nat Med 10:64–71, 2004.

Cines DB, Blanchette VS: Immune thrombocytopenic purpura. N Engl J Med 346:995–1008, 2002.

Cines DB, Bussel JB: How I Treat ITP. Blood 2005 (in press).

McMillan R, Wang L, Tomer A, et al: Suppression of in vitro megakaryocyte production by antiplatelet autoantibodies from adult patients with chronic ITP. Blood 103:1364–1369, 2004.

Olsson B, Andersson PO, Jernas M, et al: T-cell-mediated cytotoxicity toward platelets in chronic idiopathic thrombocytopenic purpura. Nat Med 9:1123–1124, 2003.

Full references for this chapter can be found on accompanying CD-ROM.

CHAPTER 61

Drug-Induced Thrombocytopenia

James N. George, MD

KEY POINTS

Drug-Induced Thrombocytopenia

- Drug-induced thrombocytopenia is a common cause of sudden, severe, and symptomatic thrombocytopenia in normal people.
- Thrombocytopenia may be caused by many drugs; it also can be caused by foods and herbal remedies.
- The frequency of drug-induced thrombocytopenia increases with age, probably related to the many medications that most older people take.
- Drug-induced thrombocytopenia is often initially diagnosed as immune thrombocytopenic purpura (ITP).
- Recognition of the drug etiology for thrombocytopenia is essential to avoid unnecessary treatments for ITP and to prevent recurrence.
- The documentation of a drug (or herbal remedy or food) as the etiology for thrombocytopenia can be determined by clinical criteria or by laboratory demonstration of drug-dependent antibodies.
- Drug-induced thrombocytopenia most often occurs after several weeks of continuous exposure to the drug, or after longer periods of intermittent use.
- Thrombocytopenia caused by platelet glycoprotein (GP)IIb/IIIa-blocking drugs, used for interventional cardiology procedures, is distinct because it can occur immediately following the initial exposure to the drug, mediated by naturally occurring antibodies to conformation-dependent epitopes on GPIIb/IIIa.

INTRODUCTION

Drug-induced thrombocytopenia is an important clinical problem because it can present as sudden, unexpected thrombocytopenia in a previously asymptomatic person. Drug-induced thrombocytopenia can be severe and can cause major bleeding and death from bleeding.[1,2] Often the initial diagnosis is immune thrombocytopenic purpura (ITP); unless the drug etiology is recognized, this incorrect diagnosis will lead to inappropriate treatment.[3] A drug etiology for the thrombocytopenia may not be apparent because patients may consider medications or herbal remedies that they take infrequently and that they regulate themselves as not relevant to their bleeding symptoms, and therefore they may not report them to their physician (Fig. 61–1).[4–6] The frequency of drug-induced thrombocytopenia increases with advancing age,[1,7] probably related to the increasing drug use among older persons.[8] A recent study of Medicare enrollees demonstrated that 90% of enrollees took at least one medicine per week; 12% took 10 or more different medications each week.[8]

Quinine was the first drug to be reported as a cause of thrombocytopenia, 140 years ago,[9] and may currently be the most common cause of drug-induced thrombocytopenia. In this original report,[9] four patients were described who developed acute purpura and bleeding following administration of quinine; symptoms resolved within several days of discontinuing quinine. These patients introduced the disorder of drug-induced thrombocytopenia to the medical literature and illustrate the clinical problem described in this chapter. Quinine is also important because studies that have characterized drug-dependent antibodies have most often focused on quinine-dependent antiplatelet antibodies.

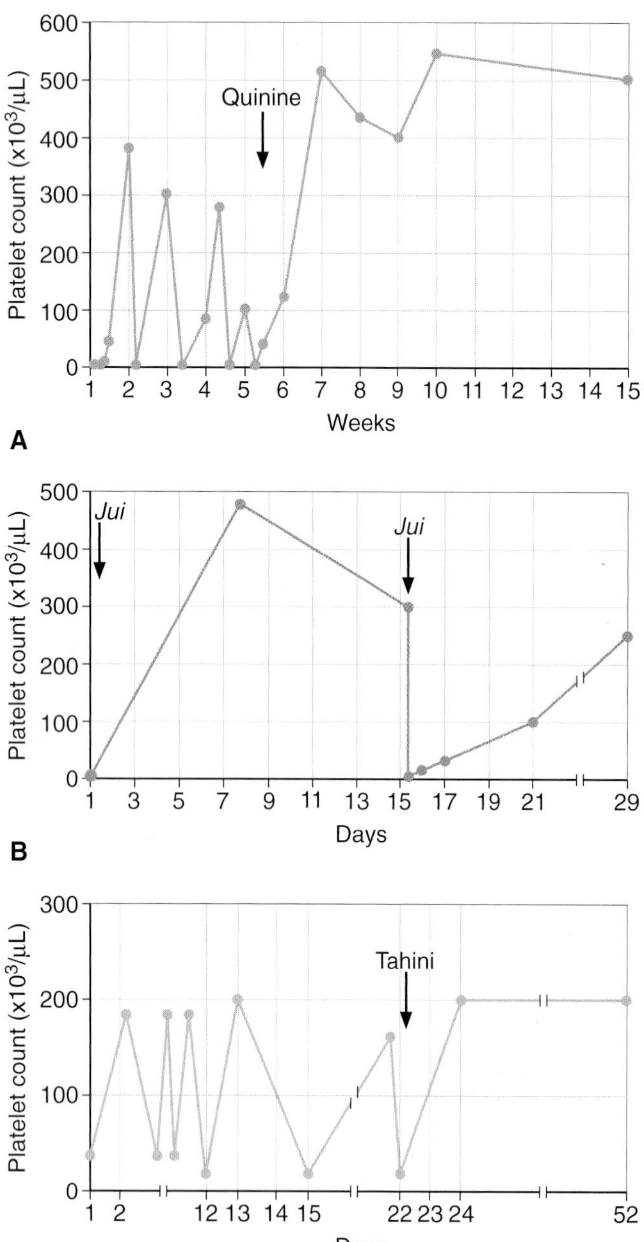

Figure 61–1. Patient A, Quinine-induced thrombocytopenia. A 68-year-old white man had ITP requiring a splenectomy 7 years previously, with a subsequent complete remission. He was taking no medications at that time, specifically no quinine. Then he had multiple acute recurrent episodes of severe and symptomatic thrombocytopenia that were assumed to be recurrent ITP. He was told to stop all his medications; insulin was substituted for an oral hypoglycemic agent. Although he said he was only taking insulin for his diabetes and prednisone for his ITP, in fact he continued to take quinine intermittently until this was recognized by explicit questions. He had assumed that quinine was harmless. After completely stopping quinine, he has been well for 5 years.[4] The *arrow* marks the thrombocytopenic episode that immediately followed documented quinine ingestion; quinine ingestion was assumed to cause the previous thrombocytopenic episodes. **Patient B,** Jui-induced thrombocytopenia. A 51-year-old Japanese woman was admitted with a platelet count of 16,000/µL and a presumed diagnosis of ITP. Her platelet count resolved without treatment, and this observation led to more inquiry about her drugs. She had taken Jui, a traditional Chinese herbal remedy, for several days before each annual health examination in the past 3 years. With informed consent, she was rechallenged with Jui, supplied as a tea bag infused in 600 mL of water. Following ingestion of the tea, her platelet count fell from 305,000/µL to 2000/µL within hours, accompanied by the appearance of petechiae. She was treated with oral prednisone, intravenous immunoglobulin, and a platelet transfusion; the platelet count recovered within 2 weeks.[5] **Patient C,** Tahini-induced thrombocytopenia. A 28-year-old woman was admitted with diffuse petechiae and a platelet count of 37,000/µL. Her platelet count recovered spontaneously, but over the next 3 months it fluctuated between 30,000/µL and 180,000/µL. When she had a platelet count of 18,000/µL, she was treated with prednisone but thrombocytopenia recurred with a platelet count of 6000/µL 13 days later, while she was still on prednisone. The patient herself had noted a temporal relation between the consumption of tahini (pulped sesame seeds, the principal ingredient of the traditional Middle Eastern food hummus) and the occurrence of thrombocytopenia. With informed consent, 200 mg of tahini was given orally and her platelet count fell from 161,000/µL to 34,000/µL within 1 day, recovering to 189,000/µL 9 days later.[6] The *arrow* marks the thrombocytopenic episode that immediately followed documented tahini ingestion; tahini ingestion was assumed to cause the previous thrombocytopenic episodes.

There are multiple mechanisms by which drugs may cause thrombocytopenia, both immune and nonimmune. This chapter focuses on immune-mediated thrombocytopenias because, among patients with unexpected thrombocytopenia, they are more common and more difficult to recognize. Comprehensive descriptions of drug-induced marrow suppression, drug suppression of megakaryocytopoiesis, and varieties of nonimmune drug-induced platelet destruction are presented in recent reviews.[10,11]

EPIDEMIOLOGY

Although the frequency of drug-induced thrombocytopenia is consistently reported to be approximately 1 case per 100,000 population per year (Table 61–1), these estimates, based on data from hospitalized patients or reports to registries, may be underestimates. Evidence for under-recognition is that many patients subsequently recognized to have drug-induced thrombocytopenia are often initially diagnosed and treated for ITP. In a cohort of 273 patients with a clinical diagnosis of ITP, 18 (7%) were subsequently recognized to have drug hypersensitivity as the etiology for their thrombocytopenia.[3] Several of these patients had had a splenectomy before drug-induced thrombocytopenia was recognized.[3] These 18 patients were recognized over 7 years in a region with a population of 3 million. Therefore, the incidence of initially unrecognized drug-induced thrombocytopenia in this region was at least 0.1 per 100,000 population per year.

TABLE 61–1. Drugs Most Commonly Associated with Thrombocytopenia Assessed by Different Methods of Patient Identification

	Study					
	Böttiger*	**Pedersen-Bjergaard†**	**Danielson‡**	**Kaufman§**	**Neylon‖**	**George¶**
Country	Sweden	Denmark	United States	United States	United Kingdom	Worldwide
Years	1966–1970	1968–1991	1972–1981	1983–1991	1993–1999	1865–2004
Method	Reports to Swedish Adverse Reaction Committee	Reports to Danish Committee on Adverse Drug Reactions	Hospital records, Puget Sound Group Health Cooperative	Hospital records, case control study	Cohort of patients with initial diagnosis of ITP	All English-language published case reports
Frequency	1/100,000 per yr	1/100,000 per yr	0.6/100,000 per yr	1.8/100,000 per yr	0.1/100,000 per yr misdiagnosed as ITP	Not applicable
Most common drugs	Quinidine Quinine Thiazides Chlorthalidone Furosemide Phenylbutazone Oxyphenbutazone Indomethacin Carbimazole Diphenylhydantoin	Gold sodium thiomalate Trimethoprim-sulfamethoxazole Quinidine Valproic acid Penicillamine Carbamazepine Ibuprofen Indomethacin Quinine Naproxen	Quinidine Quinine Sulfamethoxazole	Aspirin Quinidine Quinine Acetaminophen Digoxin Dipyridamole Trimethoprim-sulfamethoxazole Hydrochlorothiazide Propranolol Atenolol	Quinine Trimethoprim-sulfamethoxazole Thiazides	Quinidine Quinine Acyclovir Trimethoprim-sulfamethoxazole Rifampin *Para*-aminosalicylic acid Acetaminophen Cimetidine Danazol Methyldopa

*In a series of three papers,[7,12,13] Böttiger and colleagues analyzed patients with thrombocytopenia in Sweden, focusing on drug-induced thrombocytopenia. Data were reports received by the Swedish Adverse Drug Reaction Committee.

†Pedersen-Bjergaard and colleagues reported on the frequency, clinical characteristics, and drug-specific characteristics of thrombocytopenia caused by noncytotoxic drugs in a series of articles from 1996 to 1998.[14–16] Drug-induced thrombocytopenia was identified by voluntary reports from hospital doctors and general practitioners to the Danish Committee on Adverse Drug Reactions.

‡Danielson and colleagues[17] identified all patients who were members of the Group Health Cooperative of the Puget Sound who were discharged from the hospital over a period of 10 years (1972–1981) with diagnoses of drug-induced disorders. Thrombocytopenia was one of the disorders studied.

§Kauffman and colleagues performed a case-control study in Eastern Massachusetts, Rhode Island, and Philadelphia, identifying all patients who were admitted to the hospitals with severe and symptomatic thrombocytopenia and who had a rapid and complete recovery.[18] Sixty-two cases were identified and the drugs these patients had taken in the previous week were compared to the drugs taken in the previous week by 2625 hospitalized control patients, who were selected on the basis of same age and sex and according to diagnosis-independent antecedent drug use.

‖Neylon and associates[3] studied a cohort of adults with a new diagnosis of ITP in the Northern Health Region of England from 1993 to 1999. Data presented in this table are on 18 patients whose initial diagnosis was ITP but who were subsequently discovered to have drug-induced thrombocytopenia.

¶George and colleagues have systematically identified and analyzed all case reports of drug-induced thrombocytopenia, beginning with the initial report of quinine-induced thrombocytopenia in 1865 and continuing through August 2004.[1,19,20,20a] The complete data from these analyses are available on the Platelets on the Internet website (*http://moon.ouhsc.edu/jgeorge*).

Recognition of drug-induced thrombocytopenia is inevitably even more difficult in a patient who has a previously well-documented diagnosis of ITP, confirmed by persistent thrombocytopenia in the absence of any drugs or other potential etiologies. For example, the patient with quinine-induced thrombocytopenia in Figure 61–1 had had well-documented ITP 10 years previously, when he had not taken quinine or any other medications, and the recurrent episodes of acute, severe thrombocytopenia 10 years later were initially and appropriately considered to be caused by recurrent ITP.[4]

Many drugs have been reported to cause thrombocytopenia. The extensive lists in many publications are often too long and too uncritical to be helpful. The criteria for inclusion of drugs on these lists are often not described and may not be based on strong evidence. Commonly used drugs are listed together with drugs that are no longer used; drugs commonly reported to cause thrombocytopenia are listed together with drugs that have only been rarely reported to cause thrombocytopenia. Even these extensive lists may be incomplete. Descriptions of drug-induced thrombocytopenia are usually restricted to drugs approved by agencies such as the U.S. Food and Drug Administration (FDA) and listed in sources such as the American Hospital Formulary Service.[1] However, the steadily growing use of herbal remedies and other alternative and complementary medicines[21] is increasing the potential for drug-induced thrombocytopenia caused by nonformulary agents.

Documentation of thrombocytopenia caused by herbal remedies remains uncommon. This may be the result of lack of recognition but may also result from the difficulty of establishing definite evidence for a causal relationship to a specific compound because the composition of herbal remedies is often undocumented and uncertain.[21] However, clear examples of a definite causal relationship exist, such as the report of a patient with repeated, profound thrombocytopenia caused by a traditional Chinese herbal medicine, Jui[5] (see Fig. 61–1). The difficulty in determining the exact etiology for the thrombocytopenia is illustrated by Jui, which is a commercial name for a product that contains multiple different herbs.[5]

Foods may also cause acute and severe thrombocytopenia, and they also are not included in most descriptions of drug-induced thrombocytopenia. As with herbal remedies, published reports are uncommon, but one well-documented case report describes recurrent severe thrombocytopenia caused by tahini (pulped sesame seeds), the principal ingredient of the traditional Middle Eastern food hummus[6] (see Fig. 61–1). These examples illustrate the potential for an increased occurrence and recognition of drug/food/herbal remedy–induced thrombocytopenia.

Documentation of Causality

The etiology of drug-induced thrombocytopenia can be established in multiple ways (Table 61–2). In addition to systematically analyzing individual case reports with the algorithm illustrated in Figure 61–2, data from randomized controlled clinical trials can establish definite evidence for a causal relationship between a drug and thrombocytopenia. This has been the method that has documented the common occurrence of thrombocytopenia caused by the platelet glycoprotein (GP)IIb/IIIa blockers used in interventional cardiology.[22] Case-control studies can also provide strong evidence that a drug is causally related to thrombocytopenia.[18]

In addition to these clinical criteria, laboratory studies can demonstrate drug-dependent antiplatelet antibodies (Fig. 61–3), providing an additional method to document that a drug is the etiology for thrombocytopenia. However, laboratory documentation is possible only in a minority of patients because

1. Tests for demonstrating drug-dependent antibodies are not routinely available; they are accurately and reproducibly performed only in specialized research laboratories.
2. Available methods vary in their sensitivity to detect responsible drug-dependent antibodies (see discussion of assay methodology later).
3. The distinction between a "positive" and "negative" test may be arbitrary.
4. Some drugs that cause thrombocytopenia are relatively insoluble in water and are therefore difficult to incorporate into in vitro assays.
5. A metabolite formed in vivo, rather than the primary drug, can be the sensitizing agent and therefore tests using the primary drug may be negative.[23]

TABLE 61–2. Criteria for Documentation of a Drug as the Etiology of Thrombocytopenia

Clinical Criteria
Individual case reports*
Randomized controlled clinical trials†
Epidemiology‡
Laboratory Criteria
Demonstration of drug-dependent antiplatelet antibodies§

*The systematic evaluation of individual published case reports is illustrated in Figure 61–2.
†Randomized controlled clinical trials have identified GPIIb/IIIa-blocking agents as a cause for thrombocytopenia.[20]
‡Epidemiology studies are described in Table 61–1.
§Methods for demonstration of drug-dependent antiplatelet antibodies are described in the text and illustrated in Figure 61–3.

Relative Risk

Although the variety of agents that can cause thrombocytopenia is vast, relatively few drugs are among the most common causes of drug-induced thrombocytopenia in most studies. Table 61–1 lists the most common drugs determined by six different studies using different methodologies. Although there are some differences among the drugs listed in these studies, more important is the presence of several drugs, such as quinine and trimethoprim-sulfamethoxazole, on multiple lists. The differences among drugs implicated as a cause of thrombocytopenia may be related to the different perspectives of the studies. Two of the studies described in Table 61–1 were reports to committees responsible for surveillance of adverse drug reactions in Sweden and Denmark[7,12–16]; the most common drugs in their reports are similar. One study reported an analysis of hospital records that included a diagnosis of drug-induced thrombocytopenia[17]; the three drugs documented for causing thrombocytopenia in more than one patient are similar to the drugs reported to Swedish and Danish authorities.

A different approach was used by Kaufman and colleagues,[18] who surveyed hospital records for patients with thrombocytopenia who had an acute onset and a rapid recovery (see Table 61–1). The use of all drugs in the previous week by these patients was compared to the drug use of hospitalized control subjects. In this case-control study, the frequent documentation of quinidine, quinine, and trimethoprim-sulfamethoxazole was similar to the results with other methods. However, two of the most common drugs associated with acute and reversible thrombocytopenia, aspirin and dipyridamole, are not on of the lists in any of the other studies presented in Table 61–1. There have been only two case reports of aspirin-induced thrombocytopenia, one with probable and one with possible evidence for a causal relation to thrombocytopenia; there has never been a case report with probable or definite evidence linking dipyridamole to thrombocytopenia (*http://moon.ouhsc.edu/jgeorge*).[1,19,20,20a] Although the case-control methodology may have identified aspirin and dipyridamole inaccurately, it is perhaps more likely that agents as common as aspirin are overlooked and not recognized as a potential etiology for acute thrombocytopenia.

The perspective of Neylon and coworkers[3] is important because this study focused on patients diagnosed with ITP (see Table 61–1). The 18 patients in this cohort who had drug-induced thrombocytopenia were not recognized until their "ITP" recurred in spite of treatment.

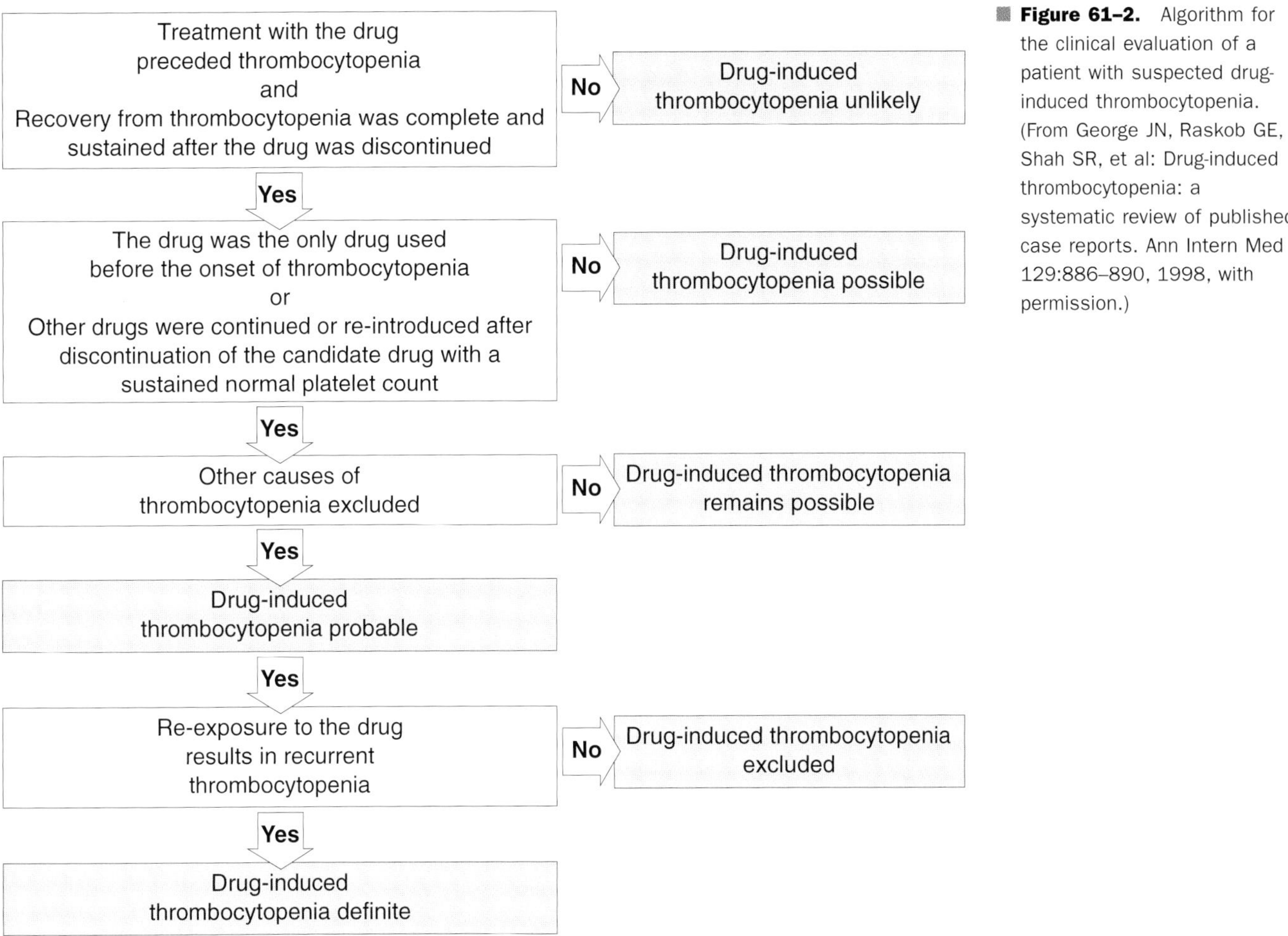

Figure 61–2. Algorithm for the clinical evaluation of a patient with suspected drug-induced thrombocytopenia. (From George JN, Raskob GE, Shah SR, et al: Drug-induced thrombocytopenia: a systematic review of published case reports. Ann Intern Med 129:886–890, 1998, with permission.)

Then a more detailed history revealed the drug-induced etiology; in two patients the etiology was quinine in tonic water. This perspective emphasizes the importance of persistent vigilance to identify potential alternative etiologies for thrombocytopenia.

To better understand the relative risks of the many drugs associated with thrombocytopenia, my colleagues and I have systematically reviewed all English-language published case reports describing drug-induced thrombocytopenia (see Table 61–1).[1,19,20,20a] Through August 2004, 964 articles containing 1316 patient case reports describing thrombocytopenia related to 281 drugs have been systematically analyzed.[1,19,20] We developed a methodology for establishing levels of certainty using four criteria to evaluate case reports of patients with suspected drug-induced thrombocytopenia (see Fig. 61–2). This algorithm illustrates the sequential approach to establishing the causal relationship between a drug and thrombocytopenia. The initial criterion is self-evident, that treatment with the drug preceded thrombocytopenia and recovery from thrombocytopenia was complete and sustained after the drug was discontinued. The most difficult criterion to assess in many reports is the documentation that the drug was the only drug used before the onset of thrombocytopenia or that other drugs were continued or reintroduced after discontinuation of the candidate drug, with a sustained normal platelet count. It is also often difficult to exclude other potential causes of thrombocytopenia, the third criterion. In patients who are hospitalized with complex illnesses, this may not be possible. The final criterion represents the definite proof or rejection of the drug-induced etiology, but may not always be appropriate: documentation of recurrent thrombocytopenia with readministration of the drug. Although readministration of a suspected drug may not be appropriate because of perceived risk, it may be critical if the drug is commonly accessible and future exposure may be inevitable, for example, with drugs such as with acetaminophen. Examples of the importance and also the risks of readministration are illustrated in Figure 61–1 for Jui[5] and tahini.[6] Most often, this rechallenge has already occurred because the patient has taken the agent on multiple occasions with recurrence of symptomatic purpura (see Fig. 61–1).

Using these criteria (see Fig. 61–2), 60 of the 281 reported drugs had definite evidence, based on recurrence of thrombocytopenia with re-administration of the drug. Twenty-four additional drugs had two or more reports with probable evidence, also establishing the validity of their causal relationship to thrombocytopenia. Fifty-five of these 84 drugs that continue to be commonly used are listed in Table 61–3.

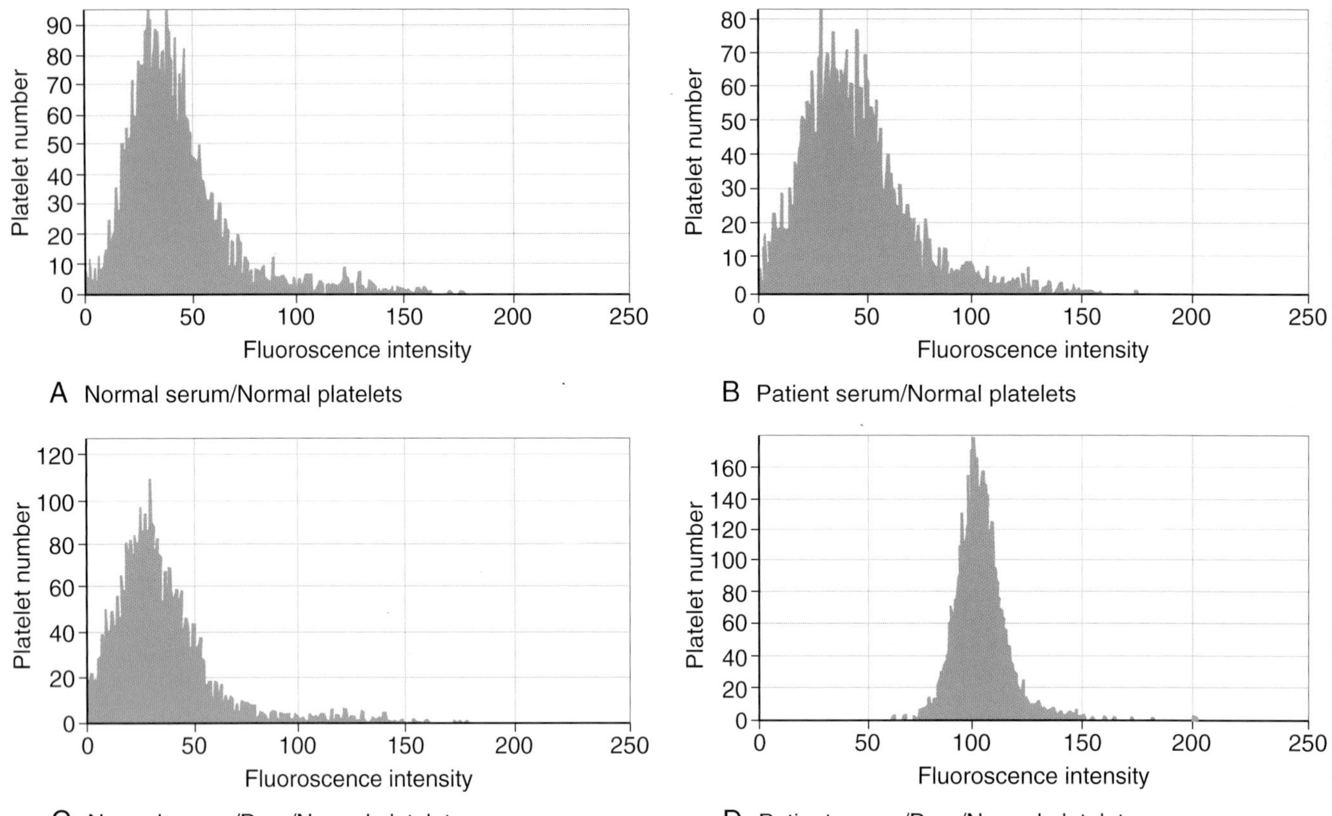

Figure 61–3. Flow cytometry documentation of a drug-dependent antibody. Binding of immunoglobulin (Ig)G drug-dependent antibodies to platelets in the presence of the sensitizing drug is demonstrated by subsequent binding of fluorescein-tagged anti–human IgG. The increased fluorescence is demonstrated by the shift to the right in ***D***, demonstrating the reaction of patient serum in the presence of the drug. In the absence of continual presence of the drug, drug-dependent antibodies do not bind to normal platelets ***(B)***. Normal serum, which does not contain drug-dependent antibodies ***(A*** and ***C)***, deposits no IgG on the platelet surface, even in the presence of the drug.

PATHOPHYSIOLOGY

Typical Drug-Dependent Antibodies

Drug-dependent antibodies are an unusual class of antibodies that react with specific epitopes on platelet surface glycoproteins only in the presence of soluble drug. Many drugs are capable of inducing these antibodies but, for unknown reasons, certain classes of drugs, such as quinine and sulfonamides, are much more common. Early descriptions of drug-dependent antibodies described them as haptens and postulated that the sensitizing drug was covalently linked to a platelet membrane protein, forming the new antigen. However, most reactions between drugs and platelets are weak and reversible, and drug-dependent antibodies typically do not recognize drug-treated platelets when the soluble drug is not present. A possible exception may occur in patients treated with large doses of penicillin, which can bind covalently to proteins by means of its β-lactam structure.[24] This is not consistent with a classical hapten reaction. Another previous postulate was that antibodies formed to the soluble drug, creating immune complexes that reacted with platelet Fc receptors. When these immune complex reactions were first hypothesized, the platelet was described as an "innocent bystander," a term that still persists in spite of evidence that this hypothesis is incorrect. The immune complex hypothesis was excluded by the demonstration that drug-dependent antibodies bound to their target antigens by their Fab, rather than their Fc, domain.[25,26]

The mechanism for drug-dependent antibody formation is a result of the sensitizing drug reacting noncovalently with one or more platelet membrane glycoproteins to create a target epitope, typically composed of both the drug and adjacent peptide residues (Fig. 61–4*A*). Many drugs that can cause thrombocytopenia are amphipathic and are normally transported in plasma bound to hydrophobic sites on albumin.[27,28] Therefore, it has been postulated that these drugs react with hydrophobic domains on platelet surface glycoproteins. The result of drug binding to the platelet surface glycoprotein is a change in protein conformation, and this conformational change reveals a new immunogenic site. The epitope may consist of structural features of both the drug and adjacent peptide residues,[29] or the conformational change induced by drug binding may create an epitope distant from the drug, composed only of a newly revealed sequence on the surface protein.

Epitopes for drug-dependent antibodies have been identified on multiple major platelet surface glycoproteins

TABLE 61–3. Drugs Causing Thrombocytopenia, Supported by Patient Case Reports with Level 1 (Definite) Evidence or Level II (Probable) Clinical Evidence

Drug (Brand Name)	Patient Case Reports	
	Definite Evidence	Probable Evidence
Abciximab (ReoPro)	0	3
Acetaminophen (Tylenol, Panadol, and others)	4	4
Acetazolamide (Diamox)	0	2
Acyclovir (Zovirax)	2	14
Alprenolol (Aptin)	1	0
Aminosalicylic acid (Asacol, Canasa, Pentasa, and Rowasa)	3	1
Amiodarone (Cordarone)	2	0
Amphotericin B (Amphocin, Fungizone)	2	1
Ampicillin (Omnipen, Totacillin)	2	2
Amrinone (Inocor)	1	0
Atorvastatin (Lipitor)	1	0
Captopril (Capoten)	1	2
Carbamazepine (Tegretol)	2	1
Cephalothin (Keflin)	1	0
Chlorpromazine (Thorazine)	1	0
Chlorpropamide (Diabinese)	3	2
Cimetidine (Tagamet)	1	6
Clidinium bromide/chlordiazepoxide (Librax, Quarzan, and others)	0	2
Danazol (Danocrine)	3	4
Deferoxamine (Desferal)	1	0
Diatrizoate meglumine (Urografin)	1	2
Diatrizoate meglumine/diatrizoate sodium (Hypaque Meglumine)	2	0
Diazepam (Valium)	1	0
Diclofenac (Cataflam and Voltaren)	2	2
Diethylstilbestrol (Stilphostrol)	1	0
Digoxin (Lanoxin)	3	0
Ethambutol (Myambutol)	1	2
Fluconazole (Diflucan)	0	2
Haloperidol (Haldol)	1	0
Hydrochlorothiazide (Aquazide-H, Esidrix, and others)	1	2
Ibuprofen (Motrin)	2	2
Indinavir (Crixivan)	2	0
Interferon	0	6
Interferon alfa (Roferon-A and Intron A)	1	5
Iopanoic acid (Telepaque)	1	1
Isoniazid (Nydrazid)	1	0
Isotretinoin (Accutane, Amnesteem, Claravis)	1	1
Jui (Chinese herbal medicine)	1	0
Levamisole (Ergamisol)	2	0
Lithium (Lithonate, Eskalith, and others)	1	0
Live Attenuated Measles Vaccine (Morbilvax and Rimevax)	1	2
Lotrafiban	0	5
Measles, Mumps, Rubella Vaccine (M-M-R II)	1	1
Minoxidil (Loniten)	1	0
Naphazoline (Privine, Vasocon-A)	1	0
Naproxen (Naprosyn, Naproxen)	0	4
Nitroglycerine (Nitrogard, Nitroglyn)	1	0
Octreotide (Sandostatin)	1	0
Oxyphenbutazone (Tandearil and Oxalid)	2	2
Pentoxifylline (Trental, Pentoxifylline)	1	0
Phenytoin (Dilantin)	2	2
Piperacillin (Pipracil)	1	0
Procainamide (Pronestyl)	0	2
Quinine (Quinamm, Quindan, and others)	10	12
Ranitidine (Zantac)	1	2
Recombinant Hepatitis B Vaccine (Comvax, Engerix-B, Pediarix, Recombivax HB, and Twinrix)	0	2
Rifampin (Rifadin, Rimactane)	6	5
Roxifiban (Klerval)	0	2
RPR 109891	0	3
Simvastatin (Zocor)	0	2
Sulfapyridine	0	2
Sulfasalazine (Azulfidine)	1	2
Sulfathiazole (Sulfathiazole, Sulfacetamide, Benzoylsulfanilamide)	1	1
Sulfisoxazole (Gantrisin)	1	4
Sulindac (Clinoril)	0	2
Tamoxifen (Nolvadex)	2	0
Tiagabine (Gabitril)	1	0
Ticlopidine (Ticlid and Ticlopidine)	0	3
Tolmetin (Tolectin)	1	1
Trimethoprim/sulfamethoxazole (Bactrim, Septra, and others)	3	12
Valproate (Depacon)	1	3
Vancomycin (Vancoled)	2	3

Drugs with at least one report with definite evidence, or two separate reports with probable evidence, are presented, based on the analysis illustrated in Figure 61–2 and described in our publications[1,19,20,20a] and on our website (*http://moon.oubsc.edu/jgeorge*). Drugs that are currently not used, or used only infrequently, have been deleted from this list.

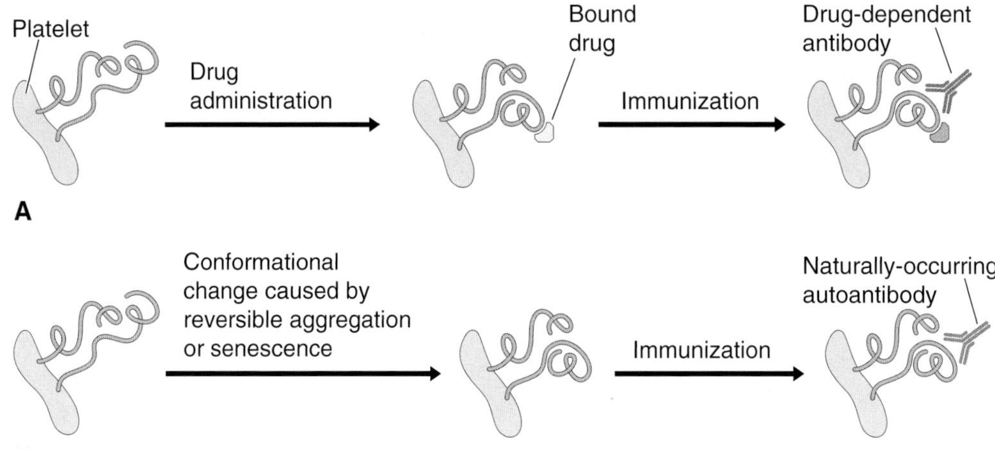

Figure 61–4. *A,* Schematic representation of drug-dependent antibody binding to platelet surface glycoproteins. The diagram illustrates the change in conformation of the platelet surface protein upon binding of a drug, which may cause immunization with development of a drug-dependent antibody to a newly revealed sequence on the glycoprotein. The drug-dependent antibody may bind only to peptide sequences on the platelet glycoprotein, or may bind to an epitope sharing glycoprotein sequences with structural components of the drug at the binding site. ***B,*** Schematic representation of the development of naturally occurring antiplatelet antibodies. The diagram illustrates a hypothetical conformational change that may be caused by reversible platelet aggregation or senescence and could stimulate the development of naturally occurring autoantibodies against newly revealed peptide sequences. The presence of these naturally occurring antibodies may be an explanation for the development of severe drug-induced thrombocytopenia with GPIIb/IIIa-blocking agents immediately following initial exposure. This naturally occurring alteration of GPIIb/IIIa may also explain why normal people may have naturally occurring antibodies that cause platelet agglutination when glycoprotein GPIIb/IIIa is conformationally altered by EDTA, the anticoagulant use for routine blood counts.

TABLE 61–4. Localization of Epitopes for Drug-Dependent Antibodies on Platelet Surface Glycoproteins*

Glycoprotein	Epitope	Drug	Reference
Ib-IX-V complex	Ibα, amino acids 283–293	Quinine	30
	IX, Arg_{110}, Gln_{115}	Quinine	31
		Rifampin	32
		Ranitidine	33
	V	Gold	34
IIb/IIIa	IIIa, amino acids 50–66	Quinine	35
	IIb/IIIa, requires intact complex	Sulfamethoxazole, sulfisoxazole	23
PECAM-1	second immunoglobulin homology domain	Carbimazole, quinidine	36

*Drug-dependent antibodies can react with multiple platelet surface glycoproteins, but often only with restricted epitopes that are common to multiple different drugs.
Abbreviation: PECAM-1, platelet/endothelial cell adhesion molecule-1.

(Table 61–4). A common epitope for drug-dependent antibodies is on the GPIX component of the GPIb-V-IX complex.[31–33] Several different drug-dependent antibodies, isolated from patients with acute severe thrombocytopenia caused by quinine, rifampin, and ranitidine, all react with a common site on GPIX.[31–33] Other specific sites that have been identified as targets of drug-dependent antibodies are described in Table 61–4. Two or more distinct drug-dependent antibodies, each recognizing a different target, may be present in the same patient.[37,38] Further molecular characterization of the epitopes recognized by drug-dependent antibodies may help to resolve the questions of how drugs promote binding of these antibodies to their targets and cause platelet destruction, and why certain individuals are susceptible to the formation of drug-dependent antibodies.

Thrombocytopenia Caused by GPIIb/IIIa-Blocking Agents

Acute thrombocytopenia caused by the new class of antithrombotic agents that block the fibrinogen receptor

TABLE 61–5. Distinct Characteristics of Typical Drug-Induced Thrombocytopenia and Thrombocytopenia Caused by GPIIb/IIIa-Blocking Agents*

Clinical Characteristic	Typical Drug-Induced Thrombocytopenia	GPIIb/IIIa-Blocking Agent–Induced Thrombocytopenia
Drugs	Most drugs listed in Table 61–3	Most GPIIb/IIIa blockers.
Frequency	Rare, even with the most commonly reported drugs	1% of patients with many drugs. Frequency may be up to 5% with approved intravenous agents and 13% with investigational oral agents.[39]
Occurrence of thrombocytopenia	Exposure required for sensitization; median length of exposure, 21 days[15]	May occur immediately following initial exposure. With continuous oral administration, half occur immediately, half at about 14 days.[40] May also cause pseudothrombocytopenia.
Drug-dependent antibody	In some patients, antibodies may have specificity for multiple surface glycoproteins	Conformation-dependent epitopes on GPIIb/IIIa. Naturally occurring drug-dependent antibodies related to the occurrence of thrombocytopenia are present in 4% of subjects.[40]

*Distinct characteristics of thrombocytopenia caused by GPIIb/IIIa-blocking agents are compared to characteristics of thrombocytopenia caused by other drugs.

on GPIIb/IIIa has important clinical characteristics distinctive from other drug-induced thrombocytopenias (Table 61–5). These agents are designed to mimic the arginine-glycine–aspartic acid site in fibrinogen that is the ligand recognized by GPIIb/IIIa. Therefore, they inhibit fibrinogen binding to platelets and thereby inhibit platelet aggregation. Early in the development of these drugs, it was noted that acute, severe thrombocytopenia may occur immediately following the first exposure.[41–43] Therefore, it was apparent that the drug-induced thrombocytopenia caused by this class of agents was related to preexisting, naturally occurring antibodies. This is distinct from typical drug-induced thrombocytopenia, which requires a period of sensitization to develop drug-dependent antibodies, typically several weeks of continuous or intermittent drug administration. GPIIb/IIIa-blocking agents induce conformational changes in GPIIb/IIIa when they bind to platelets and, as expected, the antibodies dependent on this class of agents react with epitopes on ligand-occupied GPIIb/IIIa.[41–43]

The frequency of occurrence of drug-induced severe thrombocytopenia caused by GPIIb/IIIa–blocking agents is much greater than that for any other drug or class of drugs. For example, current clinical trials with abciximab have documented an immediate occurrence of severe thrombocytopenia in 1% of patients.[22] Other reports document even higher frequencies with approved intravenous agents, up to 5%,[44] and with oral agents given continuously for several weeks, the frequency of thrombocytopenia may be as high as 13%.[39] Tests for drug-dependent antibodies in patients who have not received GPIIb/IIIa-blocking agents have been developed to screen patients prior to the initial administration.[40] As with all tests for drug-dependent antiplatelet antibodies, the definition of a "positive" test is empirical. In one study, roxifiban-dependent antiplatelet antibodies were identified in 4% of patients prior to drug administration. The clinical importance of this observation was confirmed when the frequency of roxifiban-induced thrombocytopenia decreased from 2.0% to 0.2% when patients with preexisting roxifiban-dependent antibodies were excluded from the clinical trials.[40]

Naturally occurring autoantibodies to GPIIb/IIIa may occur because of conformational changes induced by reversible platelet aggregation or by platelet senescence (Fig. 61–4*B*). These naturally occurring autoantibodies can cause platelet agglutination and thereby cause pseudothrombocytopenia in routine blood samples collected in the anticoagulant ethylenediaminetetraacetic acid (EDTA). These EDTA-dependent platelet agglutinins are a common example of naturally occurring autoantibodies to conformation changes in GPIIb/IIIa.[45,46] It is assumed that the epitope for EDTA-dependent platelet agglutinins is created by calcium chelation in the EDTA-anticoagulated sample, resulting in dissociation of the GPIIb and GPIIIa subunits. The frequency of pseudothrombocytopenia caused by EDTA-dependent platelet agglutinins has been consistently documented to be about 0.1% of the population in multiple large surveys.[47–52] Naturally occurring autoantibodies to platelets are, of course, not unique; many normal people have low titers of multiple naturally occurring autoantibodies, such as antinuclear antibodies and cold agglutinins.

The observations on EDTA-platelet agglutinins provide a precedent for the occurrence of preexisting, naturally occurring antibodies that may cause thrombocytopenia when a conformational change in GPIIb/IIIa is induced by a GPIIb/IIIa-blocking agent.[40] A link between these two phenomena, thrombocytopenia caused by GPIIb/IIIa-blocking agents and pseudothrombocytopenia caused by platelet agglutination in the presence of EDTA, is that the GPIIb/IIIa–blocking agents can also cause EDTA-dependent pseudothrombocytopenia.[52–55] In one of the early studies of abciximab, 4 of 21 patients developed pseudothrombocytopenia following intravenous infusion of abciximab.[56] These patients did not have EDTA-induced platelet agglutination in their preinfusion blood samples; therefore, the EDTA-dependent platelet agglutinins in these patients required the presence of abciximab on the platelet surface, probably causing an additional conformational change in GPIIb/IIIa.[56]

Currently approved GPIIb/IIIa-blocking agents are given by intravenous infusions for brief periods. Other

GPIIb/IIIa-blocking agents have been developed that can be administered orally for prolonged treatment durations. With the oral agents, acute thrombocytopenia can develop after 2 weeks of administration,[41,43] similar to the occurrence following sensitization in typical drug-induced thrombocytopenia.

CLINICAL FEATURES AND DIAGNOSIS

When a patient has recurrent episodes of acute severe thrombocytopenia, an etiology related to a drug, herbal remedy, or food must be assumed to be the cause and the history must be pursued until the etiologic agent is identified.

The clinical steps for establishing the diagnosis of drug-induced thrombocytopenia are illustrated in Figure 61–2. The key to clinical diagnosis is an explicit history. Simply asking patients what medications they take is not sufficient. Patients will often not describe medicines that they regulate themselves and take only occasionally, with the innocent assumption that their physician is only interested in regularly prescribed medications. Patients will also not describe herbal remedies or over-the-counter medications without explicit questions. Quinine must be specifically sought in the history, not only in medications but also in quinine-containing beverages such as tonic water and Schweppes Bitter Lemon. The amount of quinine required to trigger severe thrombocytopenia is easily achieved by the quinine concentration in these beverages, and acute thrombocytopenia caused by exposure to quinine in beverages has been repeatedly documented.[57–63] Quinine tablets have been the familiar remedy for nocturnal leg cramps for over 60 years,[64] and leg cramps are a very common problem. In response to the question, "Have you had trouble with cramps in your calves and feet at night?", 276 (56%) of 490 outpatients surveyed at the Denver Veterans Administration Medical Center reported that they had; one fourth of these patients reported daily leg cramps.[65] Because of the absence of data to support the safety and efficacy of quinine, the FDA banned over-the-counter marketing of quinine in 1994.[66] The following year, the FDA notified manufacturers that prescription quinine could no longer carry "nocturnal leg cramps" as an indication for therapy on approved labeling.[66] In spite of the restriction on quinine sales, its use continues to be nearly universal among people with regular leg cramps. A variety of quinine-containing products are marketed in general merchandise stores as well as nutrition centers.[4] These products are widely discussed among people seeking information about remedies for leg cramps in Internet "chat rooms."[4]

The occurrence of acute thrombocytopenia caused by a drug that has been taken regularly for many months or years is uncommon. In our review, the time of drug ingestion before the initial occurrence of thrombocytopenia in patients who had definite evidence for the drug etiology ranged from less than 1 day to 3 years, with a median of 14 days.[1]

The onset of drug-induced thrombocytopenia is often accompanied by systemic symptoms of flushing, with a feeling of warmth, and often also chills. Bleeding manifestations are the typical mucocutaneous symptoms characteristic of severe thrombocytopenia. Major bleeding is often reported in association with severe drug-induced thrombocytopenia; fatal bleeding has also been reported.[2]

Drug-dependent antibodies can be demonstrated by flow cytometry,[23,67] as illustrated in Figure 61–3. Multiple other methods have been developed to identify drug-dependent antibodies. Other common techniques are enzyme-linked immunosorbent assay using immobilized platelet glycoproteins as targets,[67,68] and monoclonal antibody–specific immobilization of platelet antigens (MAIPA) assays.[30,36] Different assays have varying sensitivities for different patients and different drugs.[69] The inconsistency of identification is a limitation of the laboratory diagnosis. The dilution of serum required for flow cytometry assays may cause this technique to be less sensitive than the MAIPA method.[31] The use of undiluted serum in flow cytometry may cause nonspecific binding of immunoglobulin to the platelet surface even in the absence of the drug. The inconsistency of documentation of drug-dependent antibodies by different techniques[69] may be related to low binding affinity of the drug for platelets, low binding affinity of the drug-dependent antibodies to their antigen, or low antigen site density on the platelet surface. In these assays, it is critical that the drug be present at all stages at a concentration that will assure a high molar ratio of drug to antibody. For some drugs that are poorly water soluble, additional techniques to achieve drug solubility are required.

TREATMENT

The only necessary and appropriate treatment is withdrawal of the provoking drug, herbal remedy, or food. Multiple studies have documented prompt and complete recovery within 1–2 weeks of withdrawal of the drug.[1,15,69] However, because the occurrence of acute,

CURRENT CONTROVERSIES & FUTURE CONSIDERATIONS

Drug-Induced Thrombocytopenia

- What is the actual frequency of thrombocytopenia as an adverse reaction to herbal remedies and foods, as well as to approved drugs?
- How can tests for drug-dependent antibodies be standardized for routine clinical use?
- What are the mechanisms for development of naturally occurring antibodies to GPIIb/IIIa?
- How can tests for naturally occurring antibodies to platelet GPIIb/IIIa be used clinically to avoid acute thrombocytopenia following initial exposure to GPIIb/IIIa-blocking agents?

severe thrombocytopenia can never be clearly distinguished from ITP, prednisone is nearly always given at the conventional dose of 1 mg/kg in addition to withdrawing the suspected drug.[15] The difference between prednisone use in a patient with suspected drug-induced thrombocytopenia and its use in patients with suspected ITP is that, when a drug-induced etiology is suspected, the prednisone can be discontinued abruptly as the platelet count recovers. Prompt sustained recovery of the platelet count following discontinuation of prednisone further supports the diagnosis of drug-induced thrombocytopenia, because ITP in adults characteristically has a prolonged course requiring more prolonged immunosuppressive treatment.

Suggested Readings*

Drugs That Cause Thrombocytopenia

George JN: Database for drug-induced thrombocytopenia. *In* Platelets on the Internet. Hematology/Oncology Section, Department of Medicine, University of Oklahoma Health Sciences Center. Available at: *http://moon.ouhsc.edu/jgeorge*, 2005.

George JN, Raskob GE, Shah SR, et al: Drug-induced thrombocytopenia: a systematic review of published case reports. Ann Intern Med 129:886–890, 1998.

Rizvi MA, Kojouri K, George JN: Drug-induced thrombocytopenia: an updated systematic review. Ann Intern Med 134:346, 2001.

Foods, Beverages, and Herbal Remedies That Cause Thrombocytopenia

Arnold J, Ouwehand WH, Smith G, Cohen H: A young women with petechiae. Lancet 352:618, 1998.

Azuno Y, Yaga K, Sasayama T, Kimoto K: Thrombocytopenia induced by Jui, a traditional Chinese herbal medicine. Lancet 354:304–305, 1999.

Brasic JR: Quinine-induced thrombocytopenia in a 64-year-old man who consumed tonic water to relieve nocturnal leg cramps. Mayo Clin Proc 76:863–864, 2001.

Thrombocytopenia Caused by Platelet GP IIb-IIIa Blocking Agents

Brassard JA, Curtis BR, Cooper RA, et al: Acute thrombocytopenia in patients treated with the oral glycoprotein IIb/IIIa inhibitors xemilofiban and orbofiban: evidence for an immune etiology. Thromb Haemost 88:892–897, 2002.

Seiffert D, Stern AM, Ebling W, et al: Prospective testing for drug-dependent antibodies reduces the incidence of thrombocytopenia observed with the small molecule glycoprotein IIb/IIIa antagonist roxifiban: implications for the etiology of thrombocytopenia. Blood 101:58–63, 2003.

Molecular Mechanisms of Drug-Dependent Antibody Formation

Asvadi P, Ahmadi Z, Chong BH: Drug-induced thrombocytopenia: localization of the binding site of GPIX-specific quinine-dependent antibodies. Blood 102:1670–1677, 2003.

Peterson JA, Nyree CE, Newman PJ, Aster RH: A site involving the "hybrid" and PSI homology domains of GPIIIa (β-integrin subunit) is a common target for antibodies associated with quinine-induced immune thrombocytopenia. Blood 101:937–942, 2003.

Full references for this chapter can be found on accompanying CD-ROM.

CHAPTER 62

Thrombotic Thrombocytopenic Purpura and Hemolytic-Uremic Syndrome

X. Long Zheng, MD, PhD, and J. Evan Sadler, MD, PhD

KEY POINTS

Thrombotic Thrombocytopenic Purpura and Hemolytic-Uremic Syndrome

Diagnosis

- Profound thrombocytopenia, hemolytic anemia, fragmentation of red blood cells, markedly elevated serum lactate dehydrogenase level in the presence or absence of neurologic symptoms, and renal dysfunctions are sufficient for diagnosis of thrombotic thrombocytopenic purpura (TTP).
- If underlying etiologies, including drugs, sepsis, disseminated intravascular coagulation, hematopoietic stem cell transplantation, disseminated malignancy, and pregnancy, are evident, the diagnosis of nonidiopathic TTP should be made.

Treatment

- Once the presumptive diagnosis is made, plasma exchange should be initiated immediately. If plasma exchange is not available, plasma infusion should be started.
- All patients should be treated with corticosteroids in conjunction with plasma exchange.
- For patients who are resistant to plasma exchange, adjunctive immunosuppressive therapies, including vincristine, splenectomy, cyclophosphamide, and rituximab, should be considered.

INTRODUCTION

Thrombotic thrombocytopenic purpura (TTP), first described by Eli Moschcowitz in 1924,[1] is a severe microvascular occlusive thrombotic microangiopathy. The hallmark of TTP is systemic platelet clumping that leads to organ ischemia, profound thrombocytopenia, and fragmentation of red blood cells.[2–4] The onset is often dramatic and life-threatening, requiring immediate treatment with plasma infusion or plasma exchange. If left untreated, the mortality rate is as high as 85–100%. Plasma exchange has reduced the mortality rate to between 10% and 30%.[5–13]

TTP includes at least three distinct entities: congenital TTP (also named Upshaw-Schülman syndrome), idiopathic TTP, and nonidiopathic TTP. Congenital TTP is caused by a hereditary deficiency of a metalloprotease that cleaves von Willebrand factor (vWF) in the plasma.[14–16] Idiopathic TTP can be caused by an acquired deficiency of the same vWF-cleaving metalloprotease resulting from autoantibodies that inhibit the protease activity.[13,17–19] Conditions that are associated with nonidiopathic TTP include hematopoietic progenitor cell transplantation (HPCT),[20,21] certain drugs,[22,23] malignancy,[24,25] and pregnancy.[26–28] These insults may directly injure endothelial cells, resulting in microvascular thrombosis independent of vWF-cleaving metalloprotease activity.

Hemolytic-uremic syndrome is a similar type of microvascular disease that occurs usually in children and causes pronounced renal failure. This syndrome was initially described by Gasser and colleagues in 1955.[29] Hemolytic-uremic syndrome can be divided into two types: diarrhea-positive hemolytic-uremic syndrome (D^+HUS) or “typical” hemolytic-uremic syndrome, and diarrhea-negative hemolytic-uremic syndrome (D^-HUS) or “atypical” hemolytic-uremic syndrome. D^+HUS constitutes 95% of the cases, occurring 4–5 days after a prodromal diarrhea, and mainly affects children.[30,31] D⁻HUS is relatively rare, developing without a precedent diarrheal symptom. D⁻HUS is heterogeneous, and is seen in both adults and children.[23,32–35] In adults, D⁻HUS may be quite difficult to distinguish from TTP on the basis of clinical symptoms and laboratory results because the two syndromes overlap significantly.[36–40] For example, patients diagnosed with TTP do have renal dysfunction with increased serum creatinine level, hematuria, and proteinuria.[12,13] Conversely, other patients diagnosed with hemolytic-uremic syndrome may develop neurologic symptoms.[12] Furthermore, some cases labeled hemolytic-uremic syndrome have been reported to respond to plasma exchange therapy.[12] Consequently, current criteria require only unexplained thrombocytopenia and microangiopathic hemolytic anemia for the diagnosis of TTP, and for the initiation of plasma exchange therapy.[12,13,41] In this chapter, all adults who meet the criteria of thrombocytopenia and microangiopathic hemolytic anemia, with or without neurologic symptoms and renal dysfunction, are described as having thrombotic thrombocytopenic purpura instead of "thrombotic thrombocytopenic purpura/hemolytic-uremic syndrome"[6,37] or "thrombotic microangiopathy,"[42,43] terms that have been used interchangeably in the literature. In children, however, hemolytic-uremic syndrome appears to be a distinct group of disorders caused either by *Escherichia coli* infection[30,44–49] or sometimes by complement dysregulation.[50–63] The therapy and prognosis of hemolytic-uremic syndrome in pediatric populations are quite different from those of adult TTP, and are discussed separately under "Hemolytic-Uremic Syndrome."

THROMBOTIC THROMBOCYTOPENIC PURPURA

Epidemiology

Incidence and Risk Factors

In the United States, one[64] to several thousand[3] new TTP cases are diagnosed annually, with an estimated incidence of approximately 3 per 1 million population per year[65] for idiopathic TTP. However, the incidence of nonidiopathic TTP may be much higher. TTP has been reported to occur in about 5–6% of patients with disseminated malignancy,[66] although signs of concurrent disseminated intravascular coagulation often are present, which make the diagnosis of TTP unsupportable. TTP has been associated with various adenocarcinomas,[67–69] breast cancer,[69,70] small-cell lung cancer,[71–73] squamous cell carcinomas,[74] thymoma, Hodgkin's disease,[75,76] and non-Hodgkin's lymphoma.[75,77,78] The incidence of diagnosed TTP following HPCT varies considerably, ranging from 0 to 74%,[38,79–82] with a median incidence of 7.9%.[38] This wide range of reported incidences probably reflects the use of different diagnostic criteria as well as other confounding HPCT-related complications that mimic the hematologic features of TTP.[38] Human immunodeficiency virus infection has been reported in association with TTP, with a rate of positivity of 1.4–30%[12,83] depending on the patient population. Women who are either pregnant or in the postpartum period make up 12–31% of TTP cases.[6,9,27,36,42,84,85] The estimated incidence of TTP in women with pregnancy is reported to be approximately 1 in 25,000 births,[86] and about three fourths of these patients present with symptoms in their third trimester or peripartum.[6,9,36,42,84] TTP also has rarely been reported to occur following bee stings,[87,88] dog bites,[89–91] and carbon monoxide poisoning.[89–91]

A long list of drugs, including quinine, mitomycin, cyclosporine, FK506, ticlopidine, and clopidogrel, can cause TTP.[22,23,92] The estimated incidence of TTP in patients who take ticlopidine,[93,94] a potent antiplatelet agent used to maintain patency after coronary artery stenting, is about 1 in 1600–5000 patients. For this reason and perhaps others, clopidogrel, another antiplatelet drug, has replaced ticlopidine as the agent of choice to combine with aspirin for patients undergoing arterial stenting.[95,96] The incidence of TTP is less with clopidogrel than with ticlopidine, and is estimated to be 1.2–27.8 per million.[97–100]

Age, Sex, and Geographic Distribution

TTP may occur in infants[101–103] and elderly individuals.[12,13] However, most patients with idiopathic TTP are young females in their fourth decade of life.[12,13,104–107] The female/male ratio in idiopathic TTP is 4:1[13] to 2:1.[5,12,84,108] However, the gender distribution in nonidiopathic TTP is almost equal.[12,13] No particular geographic distribution of cases has been observed for idiopathic or secondary TTP.

Genetic Factors

ADAMTS13 Gene Mutations

Congenital TTP is transmitted in an autosomal recessive pattern and is caused by defects of a vWF-cleaving metalloprotease that has now been identified as a member of the *ADAMTS* family, so named for the combination of *a disintegrin and metalloprotease with thrombospondin* type 1 repeats (Fig. 62–1). The human *ADAMTS13* gene is located on chromosome 9 q34.[14–16,109–111] ADAMTS13 is synthesized in the liver.[14–16,110–112] Various *ADAMTS13* mutations that affect ADAMTS13 protease activity have been identified in patients with congenital TTP (Fig. 62–1). Most patients are compound heterozygous, but a few homozygotes have been described.[16,113–117] All reported patients with congenital TTP and *ADAMTS13* gene mutations have had a severe deficiency (<5% of normal) of plasma ADAMTS13 activity.[16,109,113–119]

Other Factors

The factor V Leiden mutation was reported in one study to be associated with acquired TTP among patients with normal ADAMTS13 levels, with an odds ratio of 17.1:1.[120] The factor V Leiden mutation renders factor V resistant to cleavage by activated protein C, a potent anticoagu-

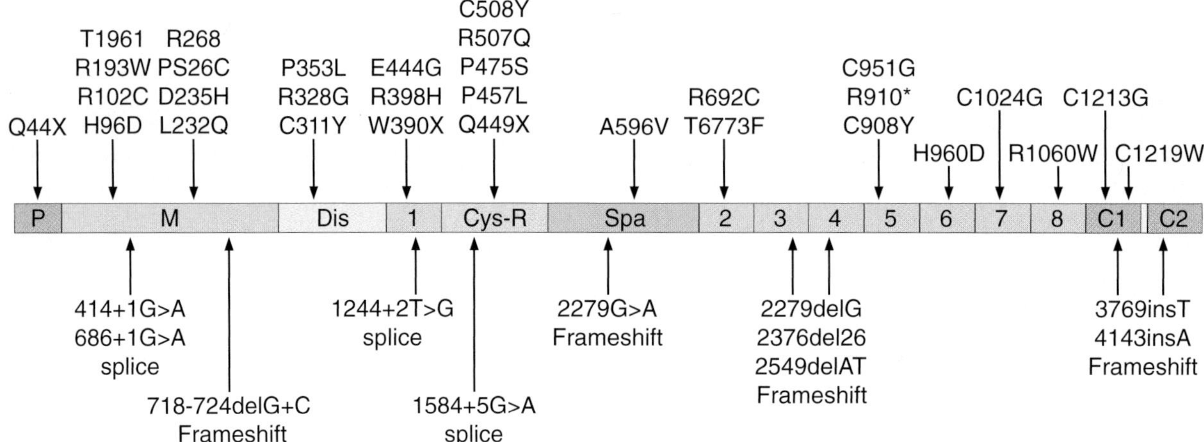

Figure 62–1. ADAMTS13 domain structure and the mutations identified in patients with congenital TTP. ADAMTS13 consists of a propeptide (P), a metalloprotease domain (M), and a disintegrin domain (Dis), followed by the first thrombospondin type 1 repeat (TSP1), a cysteine-rich domain (Cys-R), and a spacer domain (Spa). The carboxyl terminus of ADAMTS13 contains seven additional TSP1 repeats (2 to 8) and two CUB (*C*1r/C1s, *u*rinary epidermal growth factor, and *b*one morphogenetic protein) domains (C1 and C2). The missense or nonsense mutations are shown above the domain structure; the splice site and frameshift mutations are shown below.

lant that inactivates blood clotting factors V and VIII (see Chapter 67). Other potential genetic risk factors for arterial and venous thrombosis were not associated with TTP.[120] One study has reported that the class II human lymphocyte antigen DR53 protects against the development of TTP and confers a relative risk of 0.09 compared to the absence of DR53.[121]

Pathogenesis

Histologic Changes

The characteristic pathologic feature of TTP is a hyaline thrombus composed predominantly of platelets with a minimal amount of fibrin.[122–125] The thrombotic lesions are accompanied by localized endothelial cell proliferation and detachment. These occluding thrombi are found in capillaries and small arterioles in all tissues but most strikingly in the myocardium, with variable involvement of the kidney, pancreas, adrenal glands, and brain and relative sparing of pulmonary and hepatic vessels.[122–125] Immunohistochemistry showed that the platelet thrombi are rich in vWF[123,125] with little fibrinogen or fibrin; immunoglobulins and complement are often found in the thrombi as well.

Role of ADAMTS13

In healthy individuals, vWF multimers are secreted from endothelial cells, and may be cleaved by plasma ADAMTS13, possibly on the endothelial cell surface.[126] ADAMTS13 cleaves the Tyr^{842}-Met^{843} bond in the central A2 domain of vWF, producing the normal plasma vWF multimer distribution.[127,128] This cleavage prevents the persistence of the "unusually large" vWF multimers that otherwise may remain attached to the endothelial cell surface via interaction with P-selectin.[129] Congenital or acquired ADAMTS13 deficiency would lead to an accumulation of unusually large vWF multimers[129] that are very adhesive and can induce platelet aggregation (Fig. 62–2)[130] and microvascular thrombosis, the characteristic pathologic change of TTP.

Other Mechanisms

Other mechanisms have been proposed to contribute to the pathogenesis of TTP, but their role has not been established conclusively. These include endothelial cell activation[131] and cell death[132,133] caused by antibodies against endothelial cells or against glycoprotein IV (CD36) on the platelet and endothelial cell surface.[134,135] The activation and death of microvascular endothelial cells are associated with markedly increased plasma microparticles that are rich in tissue factor and procoagulant phospholipids.[132,136] These events could result in further endothelial activation, activation of coagulation via extrinsic pathway, platelet aggregation, and microvascular thrombosis.

Clinical Features

History

Patients with congenital TTP may have a history of jaundice with markedly elevated indirect bilirubin and low platelet counts soon after birth that was not explained by blood group ABO and Rh incompatibility.[103,137] Neurologic symptoms are present in about 60% of patients[7,8,13] and may include headache, confusion, aphasia, alterations of consciousness from lethargy to coma, hemiparesis, blindness, and seizures.[6,8,12,13,138] Because of low red blood cell and platelet counts, patients may present with weakness, fatigue, and mucocutaneous bleeding, including gum oozing, nose bleeding, easy bruising,

NORMAL

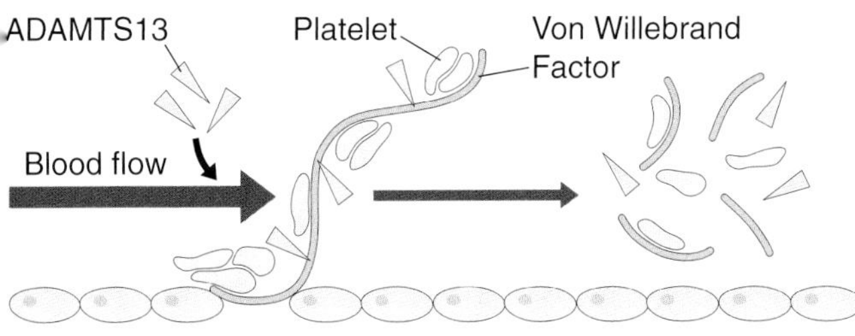

ADAMTS13 DEFICIENCY

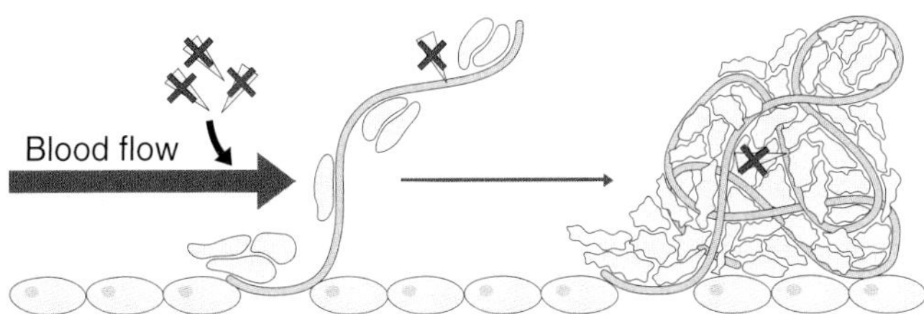

Figure 62–2. The proposed mechanism by which ADAMTS13 deficiency causes TTP. In healthy individuals *(upper panel)*, ADAMTS13 cleaves "unusually large" (UL)-vWF multimers on the endothelial cell surface and prevents an accumulation of UL-vWF multimers on the cell surface. In patients with ADAMTS13 deficiency *(lower panel)*, the UL-vWF multimers cannot be cleaved promptly, resulting in platelet aggregation and formation of microthrombi in small arteries, a characteristic pathologic change of TTP.

gastrointestinal bleeding, hematuria, excessive vaginal bleeding, and postpartum hemorrhage. One third of patients may have fever.[6,13,84,108] Eleven percent to 14% of patients may present with acute onset of abdominal discomfort, perhaps related to gastrointestinal ischemic events or to pancreatitis.[124,138]

Physical Examination

No constellation of signs is particularly characteristic of TTP. Patients may appear well or may be moribund. Physical examination may discover many findings that could be caused by platelet dysfunction, anemia, or diffuse microvascular thrombosis. For example, one may detect pallor, petechiae, and various abnormalities that usually cannot be explained by a single anatomic lesion. Patients may have abdominal pain and tenderness.[139–142]

Diagnosis

An algorithm for the diagnosis of TTP and/or hemolytic-uremic syndrome is presented in Figure 62–3.

Blood

In both idiopathic and nonidiopathic TTP, microangiopathic hemolytic anemia and thrombocytopenia are present in virtually all patients at presentation.[6,12,13] The most striking finding often is severe thrombocytopenia. The platelet count is usually less than 20×10^9/L.[6,12,13] Anemia is almost universal and may be extremely severe. In one large series, the median hemoglobin concentration was 8–9 gm/dL, and the hematocrit was approximately 28%.[13] Coagulation studies are usually normal or mildly abnormal, which helps to differentiate TTP from disseminated intravascular coagulation. The fibrinogen level is usually normal or elevated. Mildly elevated fibrinogen degradation products can be seen in up to 70% of patients,[143] as in other acutely ill patients. The hallmark of TTP is a microangiopathic blood picture with schistocytes, helmet cells, and similarly fragmented forms of red blood cells in the peripheral blood smear (Fig. 62–4). In a recent report, the mean percentage of schistocytes in patients with TTP was 8.4% (range, 1–18%) compared to 0.05% in healthy individuals.[144] Increased reticulocytes and occasionally nucleated red blood cells can be seen in the peripheral blood smear. Hemolysis may be manifested by increased serum indirect bilirubin, absent haptoglobin, and increased serum lactate dehydrogenase. Serum lactate dehydrogenase elevation may be caused by tissue ischemia from diffuse microvascular thrombosis, in addition to the mechanical destruction of erythrocytes.[145] Various degrees of renal dysfunction with increased serum creatinine may be seen.[6,7,12,13,108] Patients may also have microscopic hematuria and proteinuria. The direct antiglobulin (Coombs') test is almost always negative.

ADAMTS13 Activity and Inhibitors in Plasma

Plasma levels of ADAMTS13 activity in healthy adults range from 50% to 178% of the mean value.[106] The levels of ADAMTS13 activity are often moderately reduced in patients with liver disease, disseminated cancers,[146] and chronic metabolic and inflammatory conditions and in pregnant women and newborns.[147] However, rarely do the levels of ADAMTS13 activity decrease to less than 10% of normal in these conditions. In contrast, all patients with congenital TTP and most patients with acquired idiopathic TTP have a severe deficiency (<3–5% of normal) of plasma ADAMTS13 activity.[13,104–106,148] In patients with nonidiopathic TTP, the plasma levels of ADAMTS13 activity are usually normal or mildly reduced.[13,24,25] In pregnant women with HELLP (*h*emolytic anemia, *e*levated *l*iver enzyme, and *l*ow *p*latelets) syndrome, the ADAMTS13 level is only mildly reduced.[149]

Autoantibody inhibitors were reported initially in 65–95% of patients with idiopathic TTP and severe ADAMTS13 deficiency.[104,105] Subsequent studies have found a lower prevalence of inhibitors of 31% and 44%,[13,107] perhaps because the patient populations were less highly selected. Although inhibitors have been found in patients with nonidiopathic TTP, inhibitors have otherwise been detected almost exclusively in patients with idiopathic TTP.[12,13,104–107,150] TTP associated with ticlopidine, and possibly that associated with clopidogrel, represent interesting exceptions that are consistent with a drug-induced autoimmune disorder.

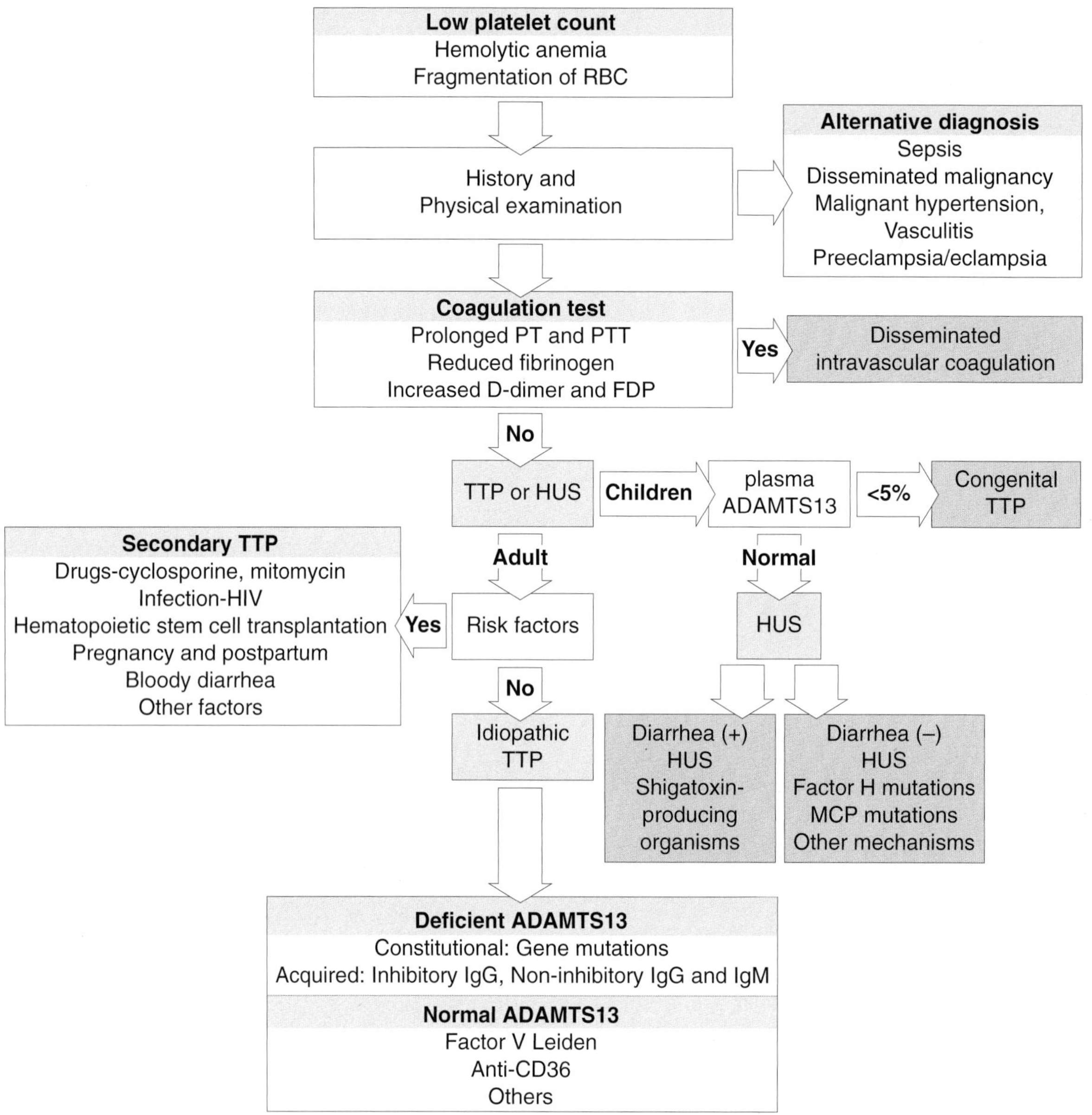

■ **Figure 62–3.** Algorithm for diagnosis of TTP and hemolytic-uremic syndrome.

ADAMTS13 inhibitors were detected in six of seven patients with ticlopidine-associated TTP,[18,94] and in two patients with clopidogrel-induced TTP.[151]

Bone Marrow

Examination of the bone marrow in TTP may show an increase in megakaryocytes, hyaline thrombi in small vessels, endothelial cell apoptosis, and erythrocyte fragmentation.[152] However, tissue biopsies are not necessary to make the diagnosis of TTP, nor are they recommended because of their low sensitivity.

Differential Diagnosis

It is important to differentiate congenital TTP from D$^-$ HUS in children, because plasma infusion is an efficacious and life-saving treatment for congenital TTP. Plasma ADAMTS13 activity should be checked for children with microangiopathic hemolytic anemia and jaundice who do not clearly have D$^+$HUS or another obvious cause of hemolysis.[103,153] Severe deficiency of ADAMTS13 favors a diagnosis of congenital TTP over atypical D$^-$HUS.[16,148] In adults, the clinical distinction between TTP and hemolytic-uremic syndrome can be very difficult. Many studies have shown that severe deficiency (<5% of normal) of ADAMTS13 activity with or without antibody inhibitors is very specific for the diagnosis of idiopathic TTP.[104,148,154] Several recent studies, however, have raised concerns about the variable sensitivity of ADAMTS13 testing, reporting that between 45% and 100% of patients with idiopathic TTP have severe ADAMTS13 deficiency.[12,13,104,107] Conversely, patients with nonidiopathic TTP have almost always normal or slightly reduced

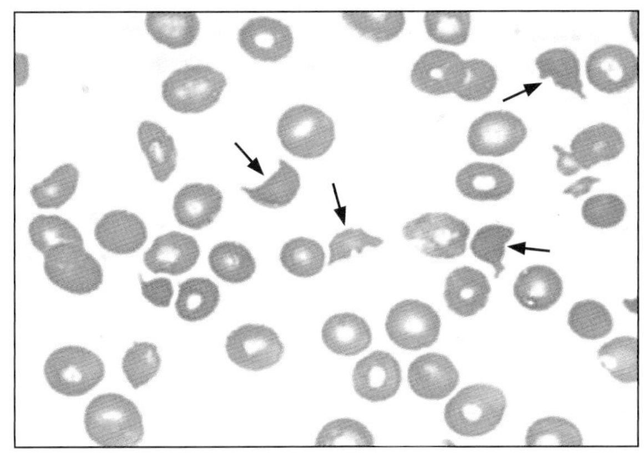

Figure 62–4. Red blood cell fragmentation (schistocytosis). The *arrows* indicate the fragmented red blood cells (schistocytes) in a peripheral blood smear from a 30-year-old man with recurrent TTP.

plasma levels of ADAMTS13; severe ADAMTS13 deficiency in nonidiopathic TTP is very uncommon.[12,13,20]

Thrombocytopenia and microangiopathic hemolytic anemia may occur in the following conditions: disseminated intravascular coagulation, preeclampsia, or eclampsia; the preeclampsia-associated HELLP syndrome; malignant hypertension; severe vasculitis; scleroderma with associated hypertension and renal failure; Evans's syndrome or a concurrent autoimmune thrombocytopenia and direct Coombs' test–positive autoimmune hemolysis; and malfunctioning prosthetic cardiac valves. Of these, the most frequently challenging diagnostic dilemma is between TTP and disseminated intravascular coagulation. Prolongation of the prothrombin time or partial thromboplastin time with a low fibrinogen level and elevated fibrin degradation products points to a diagnosis of disseminated intravascular coagulation (see Chapter 89). In addition, the percentage of schistocytes and the level of serum lactate dehydrogenase are generally lower in disseminated intravascular coagulation than in TTP.[155] In patients after HPCT, however, the evidence of microangiopathic changes on peripheral blood smear is not sufficient to establish a diagnosis of TTP; patients who have fragmentation of greater than 5% of red blood cells, accompanied by neurologic changes or renal dysfunction, should be considered to have post-HPCT TTP.[156,157]

Treatment

A detailed algorithm for the treatment of TTP is presented in Figure 62–5.

Congenital TTP

Congenital TTP caused by mutations in the *ADAMTS13* gene[16,113,115,116] can be reversed or prevented by the infusion of fresh frozen plasma or cryosupernatant, at a dose of 5–10 mL/kg body weight every 2–3 weeks.[103,153] The plasma half-life of the infused ADAMTS13 is about 2–3 days,[158] and an ADAMTS13 level of only about 5–10% of normal appears sufficient to prevent symptoms.[159,160] Recombinant ADAMTS13 metalloprotease has been expressed,[112,161,162] but currently is not available for the treatment of congenital TTP.

Idiopathic TTP

The mainstay of treatment of idiopathic TTP is daily therapeutic plasma exchange.[5–7,9,12,13,163,164] Plasma exchange was superior to plasma infusion in randomly controlled trials,[7,165] possibly because plasma exchange not only replenishes the deficient ADAMTS13, but also removes autoantibodies against ADAMTS13.[13,17,19,94,104,166] Plasma exchange should be initiated as early as the presumptive diagnosis is made. One to one and one half plasma volumes of fresh frozen plasma is typically administered daily[6–8,12,13,36] or occasionally twice daily.[36] Other than fresh frozen plasma, replacement fluids that have been used successfully include solvent/detergent-treated plasma[167,168] and cryosupernatant.[169,170] Cryosupernatant is theoretically attractive because it is depleted in large vWF multimers that might exacerbate ongoing platelet thrombus formation. A small randomized clinical trial showed that, when compared to fresh frozen plasma, cryosupernatant was not associated with a better outcome in adult idiopathic TTP,[171] although other reports suggest it may be more efficacious in some cases.[172] If plasma exchange is unavailable or must be delayed more than a few hours, then treatment with plasma infusion can be given as tolerated until plasma exchange is possible.

It is empirically recommended that daily plasma exchange should continue for a minimum of 2–3 days after achieving a complete remission,[6,13,173] which is defined by a normal neurologic status, platelet count, and serum lactate dehydrogenase, with a rising hemoglobin. The duration of plasma exchange therapy required to achieve remission is highly variable, ranging from 3 to more than 90 procedures.[7,12,13] Premature withdrawal of plasma exchange may be associated with prompt exacerbation of TTP in 18–86% of cases, necessitating the resumption of daily plasma exchange and addition of adjunctive therapies.[6,7,12,13,174] In an effort to minimize the risk of early relapse, plasma exchange procedures often are tapered rather than stopped abruptly, but this practice has not been validated by a clinical trial.

Intravenous methylprednisolone or oral prednisone, 2 mg/kg body weight daily, has been combined with daily plasma exchange in the initial treatment or as adjunctive treatment of TTP.[6,12,13,163] As yet, no trial has addressed whether such a combination approach is superior to plasma exchange alone. Autoantibodies against ADAMTS13 and perhaps other antigens contribute to the pathogenesis of idiopathic TTP, and cytokines released during inflammation lead to an increase in vWF levels that could exacerbate the disease. Therefore, combining the anti-inflammatory and immunosuppressive effects of corticosteroids with plasma exchange may be reasonable, as recommended by the British Society of Hematology.[175] The use of low-dose aspirin also has been recommended, based on a similar rationale.[175]

Experience with vincristine in the treatment of TTP is limited to case reports, and the evidence for efficacy is

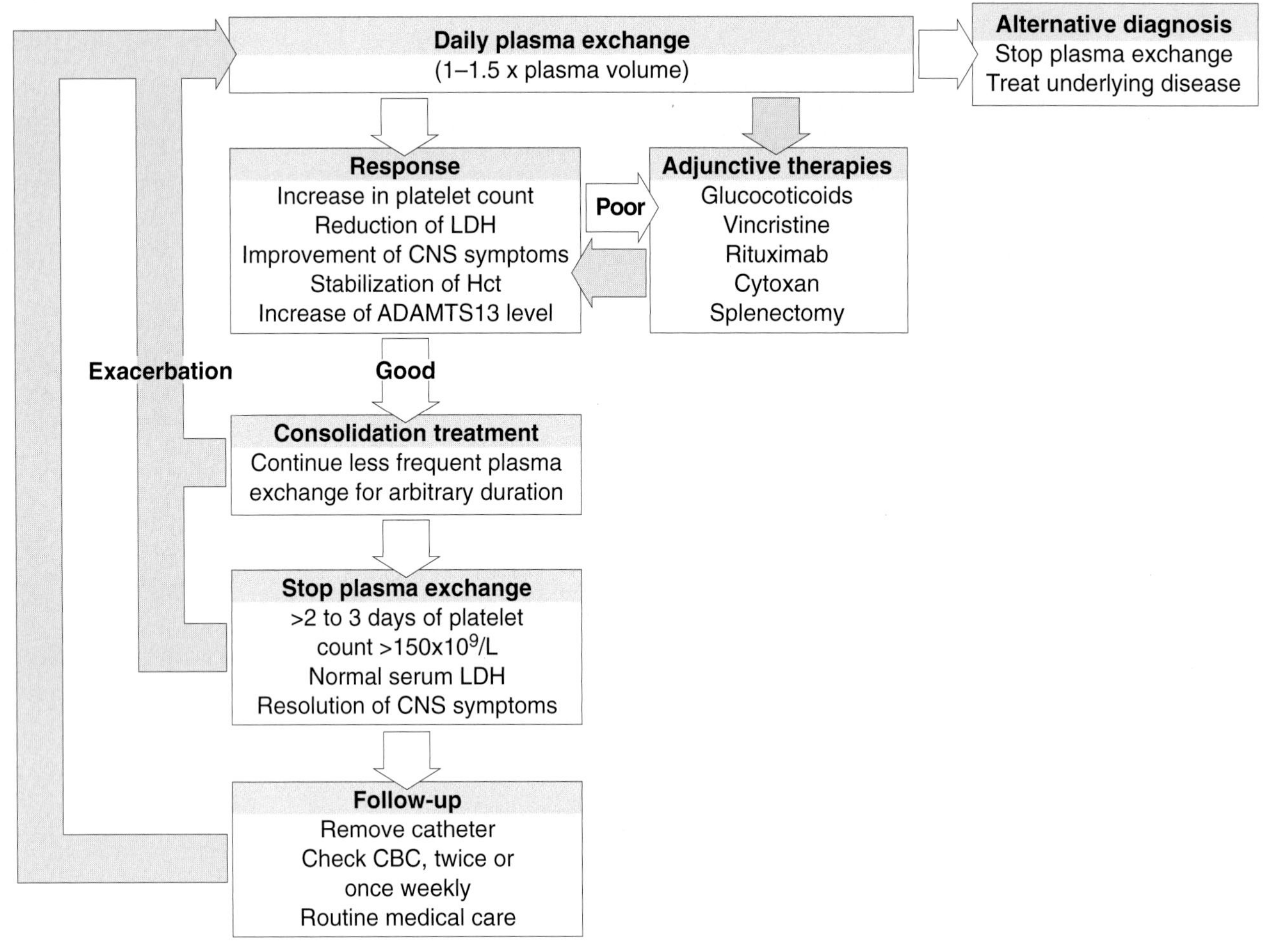

Figure 62–5. Algorithm for treatment of TTP.

inconclusive. Vincristine has been used mainly in patients who are resistant to plasma exchange,[176–178] typically at a dose of 1 mg intravenously repeated every 3–4 days for a total of four doses.[175] Higher doses have also been used.[179,180] A role for early administration of vincristine (within 3 days of presentation) has been advocated based on a small retrospective study.[181]

Immunosuppression with cyclophosphamide has been used for the treatment of TTP, particularly in patients with frequent relapses[182–184] and patients with a high titer of autoantibodies against ADAMTS13.[19] Cyclophosphamide has been combined with doxorubicin (Adriamycin), vincristine, and prednisone (CHOP)[185,186] or with rituximab[19] to treat recurrent TTP.

Cyclosporine is associated with an increased risk of microangiopathy after HPCT, but there are reports of its successful use to treat refractory TTP, with dosing to achieve trough serum levels of 200–300 μg/L.[19,187–189] The apparent efficacy of immunosuppression with cyclosporine is consistent with the current model of autoimmunity in idiopathic TTP. However, much remains unknown with regard to the optimal dose and duration of treatment, and the likelihood of response.

Rituximab, a chimeric anti-CD20 monoclonal antibody developed for the treatment of non-Hodgkin's lymphoma, has emerged as a promising treatment for autoimmune disorders.[190–193] Rituximab alone or in combination with other cytotoxic agents (such as vincristine or cyclophosphamide) can induce durable remissions in chronic relapsing TTP that is associated with ADAMTS13 inhibitors.[19,194–198] Rituximab typically is given at doses of 375 mg/m^2 body surface area, weekly, for either 4 or 8 weeks.[19,199] Patients usually respond clinically within 2–5 weeks after initiating rituximab therapy.[19,194,195,197–19]

Splenectomy has been combined with medical therapy for refractory TTP, and durable remission rates of 87–91% have been reported.[5,81] Retrospective studies have shown that, on average, about 7% of patients (ranging from 0 to 33%) with TTP receive splenectomy in addition to plasma exchange therapy.[173] The development of laparoscopic splenectomy has increased the safety of the procedure and reduced the postoperative recovery period for patients with TTP.[200–202] Splenectomy may result in a normalization of plasma ADAMTS13 activity and elimination of ADAMTS13 inhibitors,[203–205] suggesting that the spleen may be a major source of autoantibodies.

Prognosis

The etiology and underlying pathogenesis of TTP correlate with clinical response and mortality.[6–13,22,23,38,65,69,163,164,173,206–210] Patients with idiopathic TTP plus severe deficiency of ADAMTS13 activity respond more frequently to plasma exchange therapy and have lower mortality than patients with nonidiopathic TTP.[11–13] For example, the average mortality of patients with idiopathic and nonidiopathic TTP was about 18% and 54%, respectively, based on the data of two prospective studies.[12,13] Among patients with nonidiopathic TTP, a particularly high mortality rate was observed in post-HPCT patients, ranging from 43% to 100% with an average of 70% from eight studies published.[12,13,37,156,208,209,211,212] The high morality rate in post-HPCT TTP could reflect the severity of the underlying complications of HPCT.

The platelet count and serum lactate dehydrogenase level at day 3 after the initiation of daily plasma exchange are reported to predict response to therapy and survival.[213,214] In one study, the mean day 3 lactate dehydrogenase level for survivors was 364 U/L, versus 891 U/L for nonsurvivors ($P < .005$)[213]; the mean day 3 platelet count for survivors was 119 × 10^9/L, versus 46 × 10^9/L for nonsurvivors ($P < .005$). Similarly, a ratio of lactate dehydrogenase concentration before the third session to lactate dehydrogenase concentration before the first session (lactate dehydrogenase ratio) of less than 0.6 predicted a favorable outcome with a sensitivity of 0.96 and a specificity of 0.83.[214]

HEMOLYTIC-UREMIC SYNDROME

Hemolytic-uremic syndrome is a major cause of acute renal failure in early childhood. It is characterized by acute renal involvement, microangiopathic hemolytic anemia, and thrombocytopenia. Most cases are preceded by an episode of diarrhea that may be hemorrhagic, and these are referred to as D$^+$HUS. D$^+$HUS usually is caused by an enteric infection with Shiga toxin–producing *E. coli* (STEC).[30,31,48,215,216] *Escherichia coli* O157:H7 is the most frequently found serotype,[30,48,216–218] although other *E. coli* serotypes have been shown to cause hemolytic-uremic syndrome as well.[31,218,219] In children with D$^+$HUS, nearly 40% of patients require temporary dialysis, up to 20% develop serious extra renal events, and the mortality rate is 3–5% in the acute phase.[220,221] D$^-$HUS is less common, and is itself heterogeneous[63,222]: some cases are familial,[223] some have a recurring course,[224] some have a neonatal onset,[225] and some are related to infection with neuraminidase-producing microbes.[226–228] D$^-$HUS is generally associated with a greater morbidity and mortality than D$^+$HUS.[32,35,229,230] A subset of D$^-$HUS patients has been found to have dysregulation of the alternative complement pathway. For instance, mutations in the genes encoding factor H,[55,58,63,150,231–233] a soluble complement regulator, and membrane cofactor protein (MCP),[61,62] a transmembrane protein that is mainly expressed in the kidney, may be the primary underlying defects in some children with D$^-$HUS. Effective therapy for D$^-$HUS is largely unknown, and the overall mortality rate is approximately 26%.[234]

Epidemiology

Infection with Shiga Toxin–Producing Bacteria

Escherichia coli O157:H7 accounts for at least 60% of Shiga toxin–producing bacteria associated with D$^+$HUS in children[45] and occasionally in adults. The annual incidence of human infection with *E. coli* O157 has been reported to be at least 8 per 100,000 population in North America.[218] The clinical manifestations of *E. coli* O157 infection range from symptom-free carriage to nonbloody diarrhea, hemorrhagic colitis, hemolytic-uremic syndrome, and death. Over 70% of patients report bloody diarrhea in most series,[30,47,235] although a lower frequency has been reported in some outbreaks.[236] The percentage of cases with bloody diarrhea that progresses to hemolytic-uremic syndrome ranged from 3–7% in a series of sporadic cases[48,237] to between 20% and 30% in some outbreaks.[216,217,219,236] Hemolytic-uremic syndrome usually occurs 4–6 days after the onset of diarrhea.[217–219] Antibiotic treatment may increase the incidence of hemolytic-uremic syndrome in children.[238]

Other Shiga toxin–producing organisms, including *Shigella dysenteriae*,[239] *Citrobacter freundii*,[240] and additional *E. coli* serotypes (O26, O111, O145, O11, and O103),[35,241] can also cause diarrhea, hemorrhagic colitis, and hemolytic-uremic syndrome. In some countries, these non-O157 serotypes may be of greater clinical and public health importance than *E. coli* O157.[241]

Factor H Mutations

Approximately 10–20% of patients who have either familial or sporadic D$^-$HUS may have inherited factor H deficiency caused by mutations in the factor H gene.[57,61,62,232,233,242–244] None of the mutations were ever found in healthy control subjects. The factor H gene is located on chromosome 1; mutations are found throughout the gene but tend to cluster near the carboxyl terminus of factor H, an area important for binding both to anionic molecules and to complement C3b.[63,231] Almost all (approximately 94%) of the reported cases are heterozygotes in whom only one defective allele was found, and their serum levels of factor H may be normal, reduced in half, or even increased[58,63,232,233,245] as determined by enzyme immunoassay, depending on the location of the mutations. In a few cases, factor H gene mutations were identified on both alleles; the serum levels of both complement C3 and factor H in these cases may be extremely low (<5–10% of normal).[43,53–56,246] Homozygous or compound heterozygous deficiency of factor H is estimated to occur in approximately 1 in 400,000 white residents in the United States.[247]

Membrane Cofactor Protein Mutations

MCP (also known as CD46) is a widely expressed transmembrane complement regulator. Like factor H, MCP inhibits complement activation by regulating C3b deposition on targets.[60,248] In a subset of children with D$^-$HUS, mutations were identified on the *MCP* gene as a cause of the disease.[61,62] Both heterozygous and homozygous mutations of *MCP* have been detected and include small in-frame deletions, frameshifts with premature termination, and missense mutations resulting in either reduced expression of cell surface MCP or reduced binding activity toward complement C3b.[61,62]

Pathogenesis

Histology

Hemolytic-uremic syndrome preferentially involves the kidneys; vascular lesions occur infrequently in pancreas, brain, and adrenal glands and typically spare the myocardium.[124] The thrombi of hemolytic-uremic syndrome appear to be composed predominantly of fibrin with few platelets and little vWF.[124,249,250] These pathologic changes are quite different from those seen in TTP, in which platelets and vWF are major constituents of the lesions.[123,124] Endothelial cell damage is a hallmark of D$^+$HUS in children,[31] and endothelial cell swelling may be so extreme as to occlude the capillary lumen.[251] Dramatic destruction of the renal cortex may occur, and glomeruli show a range of changes that vary according to the age of the process and whether or not arterial changes are present. Glomerular thrombosis is characteristic, with an enlarged appearance that suggests capillary congestion rather than ischemia. Extension of thrombosis into the afferent arteriole is common.[252] Mesangial changes appear to be uncommon.[253] The tubules are often atrophic, may show necrosis, and frequently contain hyaline casts and red blood cells.[251] Fewer cases of D$^-$HUS have been studied histologically, so information about this heterogeneous disorder is relatively incomplete and generalization is difficult. However, the lesions appear to be distinct from those of D$^+$HUS or TTP, with substantial mesangial involvement and less glomerular thrombosis in D$^-$HUS.[253] Extensive arteriolar involvement has been reported to correlate with an adverse outcome.[229,253]

Shiga Toxin in D$^+$HUS

Humans are infected with *E. coli* O157 by ingestion of contaminated food or water. Most food-borne outbreaks have been traced to foods derived from cattle, especially ground meat and raw milk.[218,236,254] Unpasteurized fruits and juices account for a growing number of recognized outbreaks.[255,256] Waterborne outbreaks of *E. coli* O157 infection have occurred as a result of drinking[257] and swimming in unchlorinated water.[258] Person-to-person transmission has occurred in day care and residential care facilities.[44,259,260] *Escherichia coli* O157 may produce one or more Shiga toxins that consist of one A subunit and five B subunits. The B subunits bind to the glycosphingolipid globotriaosylceramide[2,30,232,261] on microvascular endothelial cells in brain and kidney, and on monocytes and platelets; the A unit is subsequently internalized and inhibits protein synthesis by removing a specific adenine base from the 28S ribosomal RNA subunit, leading to cell death.[30,261,262] Shiga toxin 1 also stimulates the release of tumor necrosis factor α, interleukin-1, interleukin-6, and interleukin-10 from monocytes and epithelial cells of renal glomeruli and tubules.[263–266] These cytokines can increase the expression of globotriaosylceramide on renal endothelial cells and increase the binding of Shiga toxin 1.[262,266,267] Shiga toxin 1 also can induce endothelial cells to secrete unusually large vWF multimers[268] and increase the expression of vitronectin ($\alpha_V\beta_3$ integrin) receptors, P-selectin, and platelet/endothelial cell adhesion molecule 1.[267] In addition, Shiga toxin 1 may activate platelets.[265] These events may directly or indirectly damage endothelial cells, which may potentiate renal microvascular thrombosis by promoting the activation of the blood coagulation cascade.[2]

Complement Dysregulation in D$^-$HUS

Low serum concentrations of complement C3 have been identified in some patients with D$^-$HUS.[50–52,269,270] Among such cases, a subset appear to be caused by mutations in either the factor H gene[61,233] or *MCP*.[61,62] Factor H is a 150-kDa soluble plasma protein consisting of 20 homologous "complement control protein" (CCP) modules. The CCP-1 to CCP-4 modules bind to intact complement component C3b, CCP-6 to CCP-10 bind to the C3c fragment within C3b, and CCP-16 to CCP-20 bind to the C3d fragment within C3b. CCP-20 also contains polyanionic or heparin-binding sites that may enable factor H to bind endothelial cells and protect against complement attack (Fig. 62–6).[59,150,231] MCP consists of four CCP modules followed by an *O*-glycosylated segment and a transmembrane domain. MCP appears to be expressed by all cells except erythrocytes, and it serves as a cofactor for plasma serine protease factor I in the degradation of C3b and C4b deposited on tissues. Mutation in the factor H gene or *MCP* can impair the regulation of complement activation through the alternative pathway.[60,62,232] This unchecked complement activation leads to the attachment of neutrophils and macrophages to endothelial cells, further cellular damage, and microvascular thrombosis (see Fig. 62–6).[60,62,232,271]

Clinical Features

An algorithm for the diagnosis of hemolytic-uremic syndrome is presented in Figure 62–3.

History and Physical Examination

D$^+$HUS

The initial symptoms of STEC infection follow an incubation period of approximately 3–5 days and typically include abdominal cramps and nonbloody diarrhea.[30] Approximately one third of patients develop hemorrhagic colitis, which probably results from Shiga toxin interaction with endothelial cells lining the microvasculature of the gut lamina propria.[31] Hemolytic-uremic syndrome occurs in approximately one tenth to one fourth of cases, approximately 1 week after the onset of diarrhea.[35,272,273] The mean age at onset of D$^+$HUS was 1.9 years, with a range from 1 month to 14.9 years in a series of 387 chil-

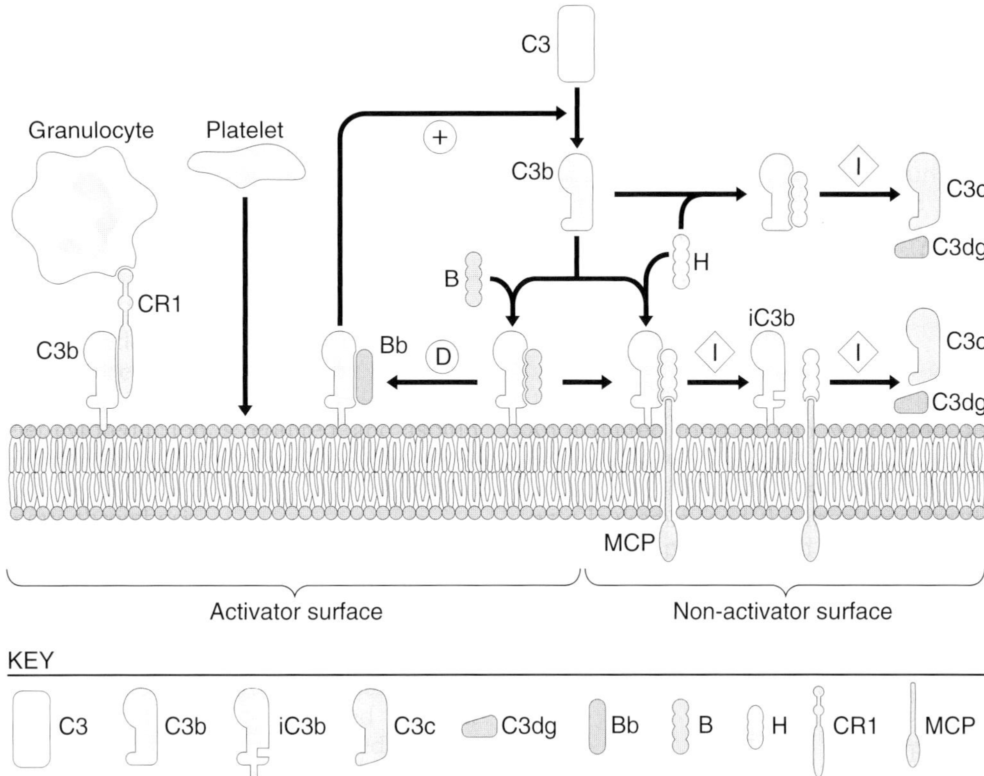

Figure 62–6. Mechanism of D⁻HUS caused by mutations in the genes for factor H and membrane cofactor protein (*MCP*). Endothelial cell injury allows complement activation via the alternative pathway on the endothelial cell surface. Complement C3b, which has bound to the activated surfaces, binds factor B and generates C3 convertase C3bBb, which drives an amplification loop (+) to produce more complement activation. Factor H and MCP bind to and accelerate the decay of C3b and C3bBb, the C3 convertase of the alternative pathway, and act as cofactors for protease factor I to cleave and to inactivate C3b. In factor H and MCP deficiency, increased complement activation through the amplification loop is favored.[60,294] (Adapted from Bonnardeaux A, Pichette V: Complement dysregulation in haemolytic uraemic syndrome. Lancet 362:1514–1515, 2003.)

dren; the sexes were affected equally.[35,272,273] Children with hemolytic-uremic syndrome are characterized by a combination of acute renal failure, anemia, thrombocytopenia and bleeding abnormalities, central nervous system disturbances, and cardiovascular changes. Renal manifestations include oliguria or anuria, microscopic hematuria, and sometimes gross hematuria. Manifestations of both anemia and a tendency to bleed include intense pallor, weakness, melena, hematemesis, hematuria, petechiae, and ecchymoses. Central nervous system disturbances include irritability, restlessness, tremors, and ataxia. Generalized convulsions have been observed.

D⁻HUS

In a series of 23 children with D⁻HUS, the mean age at onset was 5 years (range from 3 days to 13.8 years).[234] All patients presented with renal failure, anemia, and thrombocytopenia.[61,62,234,274] Many patients (approximately 90%) had hematuria and proteinuria; some were anuric at admission. Over half of the patients with D⁻HUS required dialysis.[234,275] Approximately 40–60% of children with D⁻HUS developed hypertension.[234,275] Cardiomyopathy and cerebral convulsions were also seen in children with D⁻HUS.[234,275] Infections may have been a triggering factor in about half of patients.[234] Neuraminidase-producing *Streptococcus pneumoniae* was the causative organism in several patients.[226,228,234]

Laboratory Findings

Elevated blood urea nitrogen and serum creatinine levels and hyperkalemia reflect acute renal failure. Acute microangiopathic hemolytic anemia and thrombocytopenia are characteristic of hemolytic-uremic syndrome, with increased serum lactate dehydrogenase and bilirubin levels. Red blood cell morphology is abnormal, with the presence of numerous schistocytes, helmet cells, burr cells, and various other fragmented cells; reticulocytes are often increased. Coombs' test is almost invariably negative. Neutrophilic leukocytosis is more frequently found in children with D⁺HUS.[238] Megakaryocytes in the marrow are usually present in normal numbers.

Both microbiologic and serologic assays of STEC infection should be pursued.[276] Stool should be collected to examine for the presence of free fecal Shiga toxin by cell culture assay[277] and streaked onto MacConkey agar for STEC isolation.[35] Serum samples may be collected immediately upon diagnosis of hemolytic-uremic syndrome and 2 weeks later to test for antibodies to the lipopolysaccharides of several major STEC serogroups (*E. coli* O157, O26, O103, O111, and O145) by enzyme-linked immunosorbent assay.[278,279]

Plasma ADAMTS13 activity is almost always normal in children with D⁺HUS,[148,250] but was reported in one series to be severely deficient in 26% of children with D⁻HUS.[148] This subset of children with D⁻HUS and severe ADAMTS13 deficiency represented a somewhat unusual presentation of congenital TTP or Upshaw-Schülman syndrome, which usually is not associated with profound renal failure.[103,113,148,280,281] Therefore, ADAMTS13 testing may be useful in children with D⁻HUS.[148] A fraction of patients with D⁻HUS and normal ADAMTS13 levels have mutations in factor H gene or *MCP*, and could benefit from appropriate testing.[61,23]

Treatment

D⁺HUS

Management of D⁺HUS in children remains supportive, requiring meticulous attention to fluid and electrolyte balance and nutrition, in addition to correction of severe anemia and control of hypertension, seizure, and azotemia.[282] Dialysis may be necessary in about 50% of cases; red blood cell transfusion is required in about 75% of cases. Adjunctive therapies such as transfusion of fresh frozen plasma, intravenous immunoglobulin, and plasma exchange have not proven to be effective in patients with *E. coli* O157 infection–associated hemolytic-uremic syndrome.[30]

Some treatments with a plausible theoretical rationale have been ineffective or harmful. For example, antibiotic treatment of children with *E. coli* O157:H7 infection appeared to increase the risk of hemolytic-uremic syndrome.[238] In a prospective cohort study, hemolytic-uremic syndrome developed in 5 of 9 children given antibiotics (56%), as compared with 5 of 62 children who were not given antibiotics (8%; $P < .001$).[238] Similarly, oral therapy with a Shiga toxin–binding agent such as Synsorb PK (Synsorb Biotech, Inc., Calgary, Alberta) failed to diminish the severity of D⁺HUS in a prospective, randomized, double-blind clinical trial.[283] The prevalence of death or serious extrarenal events was 18% and 20% in the experimental and placebo groups, respectively ($P = .86$).[283]

D⁻HUS

The underlying causes of D⁻HUS are heterogeneous, and no consistently effective therapy has been reported. Plasma infusion and exchange would seem to be a logical therapeutic approach for patients with factor H deficiency,[55,284] because normal fresh frozen plasma contains approximately 440 mg of functional factor H per liter.[55,284] Unfortunately, such treatment only transiently improved the hemolytic-uremic syndrome associated with factor H deficiency, and did not prevent progression to renal failure and dialysis.[32,285,286] The reported recurrence rate of D⁻HUS after renal transplantation ranges from 8% to 30% with graft loss.[287,288] In some cases, the outcome can be predicted based upon knowledge of the underlying cause of D⁻HUS, as discussed in the following section.

Prognosis

Among children infected with STEC, the severity of colitis and magnitude of leukocytosis appear to correlate with the likelihood that the infection will progress to hemolytic-uremic syndrome.[238] Once hemolytic-uremic syndrome develops, however, prognostic factors have been difficult to identify consistently. The following factors were reported to correlate with a poor prognosis in children with hemolytic-uremic syndrome: (1) oliguria greater than 14 days or anuria greater than 7 days[32]; (2) absence of diarrhea[35,289]; (3) high white blood cell count[275,282,290]; (4) hypertension[230,289]; (5) marked proteinuria[289]; (6) relapse or recurrence[289]; and (7) the presence of widespread and severe arteriolar changes on renal biopsy.[289] The prognostic value of diarrhea has been confirmed repeatedly, but that of most other factors has not.[35]

The mortality rate in children with typical D⁺HUS in the acute phase is approximately 3–5%.[282] A similar fraction of cases develops end-stage renal disease.[282] Barring reinfection with STEC, relapses of D⁺HUS do not occur, and the risk of recurrence after renal transplantation is close to zero. When it occurs in adults, particularly in the elderly, D⁺HUS has a much higher rate of death and long-term disability.[290]

The prognosis of D⁻HUS is much worse than that of D⁺HUS, with a mortality of 10%[35] to 22%[234] in two recent reports; end-stage renal disease developed in a further one fourth to one half of surviving patients.[35,275,285]

The risk of disease recurrence after renal transplantation in patients with D⁻HUS has ranged from 8%[288] to 16.6%,[287] but subgroups may be identified with a particularly bad or good prognosis. For example, almost all patients with D⁻HUS caused by factor H gene mutations have had recurrent disease after kidney transplantation, which is reasonable because factor H is synthesized mainly in the liver, so kidney transplantation does not correct the deficiency.[233,291,292] Combined liver and kidney transplantation was performed in one child with hemolytic-uremic syndrome and factor H deficiency, which restored a normal factor H level and was not followed by a recurrence of renal disease.[293] Conversely, the outcome of renal transplantation in patients with *MCP* mutations has been relatively favorable, with no disease recurrence in three patients.[61] MCP is a membrane-bound protein that is expressed throughout the normal kidney, and endogenous MCP in the transplanted organ presumably protects the kidney in the MCP-deficient recipient.

The clinical and laboratory criteria for the diagnosis of D⁺HUS are imperfect, and these limitations should be considered when assessing the prognosis of individual patients. A study of 276 Italian hemolytic-uremic syn-

CURRENT CONTROVERSIES & FUTURE CONSIDERATIONS

Thrombotic Thrombocytopenic Purpura and Hemolytic-Uremic Syndrome

- The differentiation of TTP and hemolytic-uremic syndrome is not always possible based on current clinical or laboratory criteria, so empirical treatment with plasma exchange should be strongly considered if the distinction is uncertain. Better criteria for diagnosis are needed.
- The underlying pathogenesis of nonidiopathic TTP remains elusive because its occurrence is independent of ADAMTS13 metalloprotease deficiency.
- The mortality of patients with nonidiopathic TTP is much higher than that of patients with idiopathic TTP and ADAMTS13 deficiency despite plasma exchange and other adjunctive therapies; the optimal treatment for this heterogeneous group of patients remains to be determined.
- For most children with D^-HUS, the underlying etiology is still not known. Factor H and MCP deficiencies account for only a small fraction of cases.
- The current therapies for D^-HUS in children are rarely effective. Plasma exchange has at best transient effect; relapse or recurrent disease is common.

drome patients found that approximately 68% had a history of diarrhea (D^+) as well as documented STEC infection ($STEC^+$). Among these patients, 65–76% of D^+STEC^+, D^+STEC^-, and D^-STEC^+ patients recovered normal renal function compared with only 34% of patients with D^-STEC^-,[35] suggesting that absence of prodromal diarrhea and lack of evidence of STEC infection were independently associated with a poor renal prognosis.

Suggested Readings*

Caprioli J, Castelletti F, Bucchioni S, et al: Complement factor H mutations and gene polymorphisms in haemolytic uraemic syndrome: the C-257T, the A2089G and the G2881T polymorphisms are strongly associated with the disease. Hum Mol Genet 12:3385–3395, 2003.

Furlan M, Robles R, Galbusera M, et al: von Willebrand factor-cleaving protease in thrombotic thrombocytopenic purpura and the hemolytic-uremic syndrome. N Engl J Med 339:1578–1584, 1998.

Levy GG, Nichols WC, Lian EC, et al: Mutations in a member of the *ADAMTS* gene family cause thrombotic thrombocytopenic purpura. Nature 413:488–494, 2001.

Richards A, Kemp EJ, Liszewski MK, et al: Mutations in human complement regulator, membrane cofactor protein (CD46), predispose to development of familial hemolytic uremic syndrome. Proc Natl Acad Sci U S A 100:12966–12971, 2003.

Tsai HM, Lian EC: Antibodies to von Willebrand factor-cleaving protease in acute thrombotic thrombocytopenic purpura. N Engl J Med 339:1585–1594, 1998.

Vesely SK, George JN, Lämmle B, et al: ADAMTS13 activity in thrombotic thrombocytopenic purpura-hemolytic uremic syndrome: relation to presenting features and clinical outcomes in a prospective cohort of 142 patients. Blood 102:60–68, 2003.

Zheng X, Chung D, Takayama TK, et al: Structure of von Willebrand factor-cleaving protease (ADAMTS13), a metalloprotease involved in thrombotic thrombocytopenic purpura. J Biol Chem 276:41059–41063, 2001.

Zheng X, Richard KM, Goodnough LT, Sadler JE: Effect of plasma exchange on plasma ADAMTS13 metalloprotease activity, inhibitor level, and clinical outcome in patients with idiopathic and non-idiopathic thrombotic thrombocytopenic purpura. Blood 103:4043–4049, 2004.

Full references for this chapter can be found on accompanying CD-ROM.

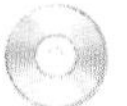

CHAPTER 63

The Hemophilias: Factor VIII and Factor IX Deficiencies

Margaret V. Ragni, MD, MPH

KEY POINTS

The Hemophilias: Factor VIII and IX Deficiencies

Clinical Diagnosis

- Hemophilia is an X-linked bleeding disorder; males are affected and females are carriers.
- Hemophilia is caused by a deficiency of coagulation factors VIII and IX (FVIII:C, FIX:C).
- Clinical features include bleeding with circumcision; spontaneous bleeding into joints (hemarthroses) and muscles (hematomas); spontaneous or traumatic intracranial, retroperitoneal, or genitourinary bleeding; traumatic bleeding; and postoperative bleeding.

Laboratory Diagnosis

- The activated partial thromboplastin time (aPTT) is prolonged and the aPTT 1 : 1 mix is normal.
- Hemophilia is classified by levels of FVIII:C or FIX:C, which are low, as severe (<0.01 U/mL; spontaneous, traumatic bleeding); moderate (0.01–0.04 U/mL; traumatic bleeding, rarely spontaneous); or mild (≥0.05 U/mL; infrequent traumatic bleeding).

Current Therapy and Indications

- Recombinant factor VIII or IX is used for prophylaxis before invasive procedures or surgery; for treatment of acute, recurrent joint bleeding; and for induction of immune tolerance to neutralize factor VIII and IX inhibitors.
- Recombinant factor VIIa is used for bypass therapy in the presence of hemophilia A and B inhibitors.
- DDAVP is the preferred treatment for mild hemophilia A.
- Hepatitis A and B vaccines are given to prevent infection with hepatitis A and B through transfusion.
- Amicar is used for oropharyngeal bleeding or before surgery.

Complications of Treatment

- The most common complications of treatment are inhibitor formation; central venous access device infection; allergic reactions; infection with hepatitis A, B, or C or human immunodeficiency virus (HIV); and co-infection with hepatitis C and HIV.
- Other transmissible diseases include parvovirus B19 and Creutzfeldt-Jakob disease.

INTRODUCTION

Although hemophilia is a rare disorder caused by deficient or defective factor (F) VIII or factor IX and characterized by bleeding into joints (hemarthroses) and muscles (hematomas), it has played and continues to play a dramatic role in history. As early as the second century AD, the Talmud described the X-linked inheritance, recommending that circumcision be avoided in families in which two boys had bled or died with the procedure[1]; this was later confirmed in the 1800s.[2,3] The early deaths from bleeding among tsars and kings of Russia, Spain, and Germany—the offspring of the most famous carrier, Queen Victoria—affected the course of history.[4] In this century, the dramatic deaths from hepatitis and acquired immunodeficiency syndrome in the hemophilia population provided unprecedented impetus to improve blood safety,[5,6] develop recombinant clotting factor concentrates, and initiate human immunodeficiency virus (HIV)$^+$ solid organ transplantation trials[7] and hemophilia gene transfer trials.[8] Finally, thrombosis, rare in hemophilia but a major killer in Western society, is being explored in hemophilia disease models.[9,10]

EPIDEMIOLOGY AND RISK FACTORS

Incidence

The incidence of hemophilia is 1 in 10,000 male births. Hemophilia A is nearly six times more common than hemophilia B, with the two forms accounting for 85% and 15% of those affected, respectively. The disease exhibits no racial predilection, with similar incidence for white, African American, and Hispanic American groups.[11,12]

Age and Geographic Distribution

The prevalence of hemophilia increases with age, peaking in the second and third decades, because individuals with mild disease, who account for one third of cases, have no spontaneous bleeding and, thus, are not diagnosed until they bleed after trauma or surgery later in life. Despite the mortality associated with HIV infection and acquired immunodeficiency syndrome, the number one cause of death in this population,[13,14] demographic models predict only minimal losses and minimal effect on the steady-state hemophilia population.[15] With treatment advances for HIV infection, hepatitis C is fast becoming a leading cause of death in this population.[13,14,16] Worldwide, the majority of individuals with hemophilia are likely never diagnosed, and, if they are, the high cost of clotting factor concentrates severely limits treatment of such individuals in developing countries.

PATHOPHYSIOLOGY

Hemostasis

Hemophilia is a disorder of "secondary hemostasis" in which there is a defect or deficiency in either factor VIII (hemophilia A) or factor IX (hemophilia B) in the intrinsic pathway (Table 63–1). In the sequence of events following vessel injury (Fig. 63–1*A*, *B*), the objective of secondary hemostasis is formation of a fibrin clot to seal the vessel injury and prevent further blood loss. Thus, the reason individuals with hemophilia bleed is that the fibrin clot they form is unstable, jelly-like, and ineffective, delaying secondary hemostasis.[17,18] When vessel injury occurs, von Willebrand factor (vWF) adheres to the damaged vascular endothelium and serves as a tissue glue to allow platelets to stick to the damaged vessel (platelet adhesion).[17] As platelets become activated, they begin to adhere to each other (platelet aggregation), and when this process becomes irreversible, ADP is released (the platelet release reaction), resulting in formation of the platelet plug, which further contracts and retracts through the action of thrombosthenin, the platelet actin-myosin–like protein[17] (see Fig. 63–1*A*). Platelet plug formation, or "primary hemostasis," results in rapid but only temporary cessation of bleeding. For durable hemostasis, a fibrin clot must form (secondary hemostasis). At the same time the platelet plug is forming, the extrinsic and intrinsic coagulation pathways become activated. The vascular endothelium, once injured, activates the coagulation system through two pathways: (1) damaged endothelium releases tissue factor (TF), which binds to factor VIIa, activating the extrinsic system; and (2) damaged endothelium activates factor XI through surface contact, activating the intrinsic system[17] (see Fig. 63–1*B*). Following activation of factor X, thrombin (factor IIa) is formed and, on the platelet phospholipid scaffolding, converts fibrinogen to fibrin. Following subsequent cross-linking by factor XIII, the fibrin fibrils form a stronger and more compact fibrin clot, thereby achieving secondary hemostasis[17] (see Fig. 63–1*B*). Once initiated by the TF-FVIIa complex, sustained clot formation through this "coagulation cascade" (see Fig. 63–1*C*) requires adequate factors VIII and IX.[18] This explains the typical delayed bleeding in patients with hemophilia. In summary, hemophilia is a disorder of secondary hemostasis in which there is a single clotting defect (deficiency of clotting factor VIII or IX) leading to a slow-forming, ineffective fibrin clot, which results in delayed spontaneous or traumatic bleeding.

TABLE 63–1. Primary Versus Secondary Hemostasis

	Primary Hemostasis	Secondary Hemostasis
Defects	Platelet plug formation	Fibrin clot formation
Disorders	von Willebrand disease	Hemophilia A, B
	Platelet disorders	Vitamin K deficiency
	Quantitative	Liver disease
	Qualitative	DIC
Bleeding symptoms	Mild, early, mucosal	Severe, late, body cavity

Abbreviation: DIC, disseminated intravascular coagulation.

Factors VIII and IX

Both factor VIII deficiency and factor IX deficiency are clinically indistinguishable X-linked disorders, caused by mutations in genes located on the long arm of the X chromosome (Xq27 and Xq28, respectively)[19] (Fig. 63–2*A*). The factor VIII gene is over 186 kilobases (kb) long and contains 26 exons, with a 9.0-kb factor VIII messenger RNA transcript that encodes the 2332–amino acid mature protein and a short signal sequence.[19] The FVIII protein contains three A, one B, and two C domains.[19] Following thrombin and factor Xa activation, the protein is cleaved into an amino-terminal heavy chain and a carboxy-terminal light chain, linked by calcium. The factor IX gene is 34 kb long and contains 8 exons, with a 2.8-kb factor IX messenger RNA transcript that encodes the 415–amino acid mature protein and short signal and propeptide sequences.[19] This FIX protein contains six domains, including one pro-sequence and one Gla domain, two epidermal growth factor, one activation peptide, and one catalytic domain, linked by disulfide bridges. The FVIII and FIX proteins are each synthesized in the liver and released into the plasma, where they circulate. Because factor VIII is large and subject to proteolytic activation in the plasma, it circulates bound to vWF, from which it is released following vessel injury. The cloning of factors VIII and IX[20,21] has led to the characterization of the molecular genetic defects causing hemophilia, enabling carrier detection and prenatal diagnosis, and the availability of recombinant factor, which has revolutionized hemophilia treatment.

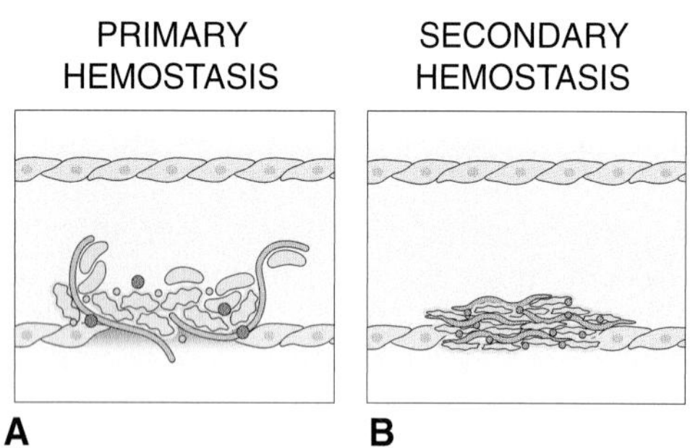

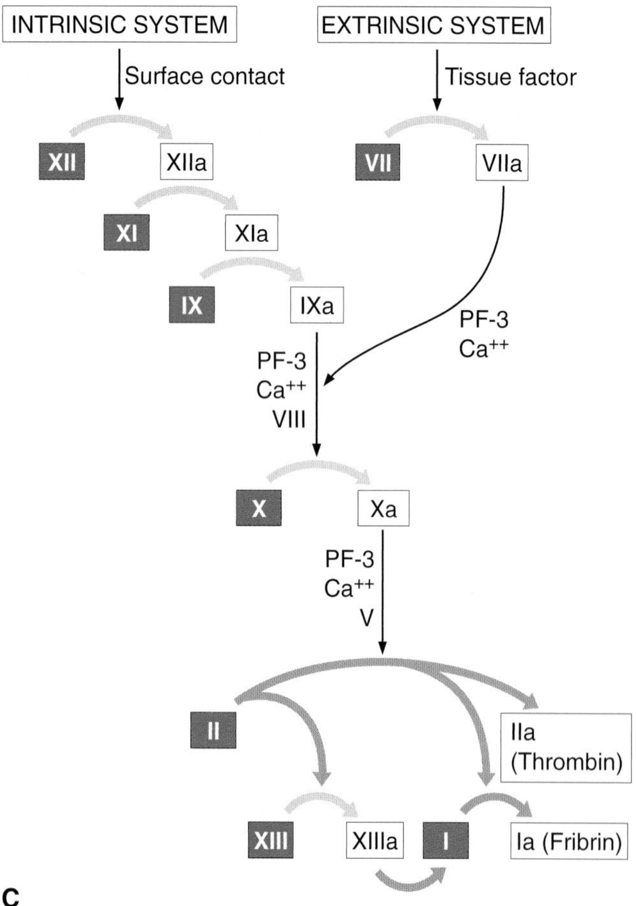

Genetic Mutations

Hemophilia is an X-linked, recessive congenital bleeding disorder, primarily affecting males and carried by females (Fig. 63–3). Rarely, the disease may occur in females, for example, when there is extreme lyonization, Turner's syndrome (XO), or double heterozygosity, such as when two hemophilia genes are inherited, one from a carrier mother and one from an affected father.[22–24] In approximately one third of cases, the disease arises with no previous family history, as a recent genetic mutation, as predicted by Haldane.[25] A wide diversity of molecular genetic mutations may cause hemophilia (Table 63–2), although in 20% or more of cases the defect may not be determined.[19,26] The majority of patients with severe hemophilia A (about 45%), or about 30% of patients overall, including moderate and mildly affected individuals, have a factor VIII intron 22 inversion mutation.[26] This mutation, which arises primarily in male germ cells, is caused by a flip of the single telomeric end of the X chromosome, which allows recombination between a sequence in intron 22 (Int22h region) of the factor VIII gene and an identical sequence (one of two such sequences) located 300 kb distal to the factor VIII gene at the telomeric end of the X chromosome (26b) (see Fig. 63–2*B*). The remaining mutations causing hemophilia A are point mutations, including missense and nonsense

Figure 63–1. *A,* Schema of primary hemostasis. When vessel injury occurs, Von Willebrand Factor adheres to the damaged vascular endothelium and serves as a tissue glue to allow platelets to stick to the damaged vessel. Platelets become activated, as small amounts of thrombin (a potent aggregating agent) are formed through activation of the coagulation system through interaction of tissue factor-VIIa with damaged vascular endothelium and surface contact (see ***C***). Activated platelets adhere to the damaged vascular endothelium, platelet adhesion, then begin to stick to each other, platelet aggregation, and the platelet release reaction occurs, with release of ADP. This series of events serves to allow temporary and early hemostasis through platelet plug formation. The plug becomes stronger and smaller through the action of thrombasthenin, the actin-myosin like protein, and stops the initial loss of blood. ***B,*** Schema of secondary hemostasis. The sequence of events following injury and initial formation of the platelet plug and activation of the coagulation cascade, include formation of fibrin fibrils on the platelet phospholipid surface, lending strength to the temporary platelet plug structure. Once fibrin becomes cross-linked with factor XIII, or fibrin stabilizing factor, the clot becomes stronger and secondary hemostasis is achieved. ***C,*** Coagulation cascade. When vessel injury occurs, as the tissue factor-VIIa complex is activated through damaged vascular endothelium, the extrinsic system is activated, with activation of factor X. The intrinsic system is activated through surface contact with factor XI, with subsequent activation of factors IX, VIII and subsequent activation of the common pathway, through factor X. This then activates factors V and II, with subsequent formation of thrombin (IIa) and subsequently fibrin (Ia). This series of linked coagulation reactions, the "coagulation cascade" occurs on the platelet phospholipid surface.

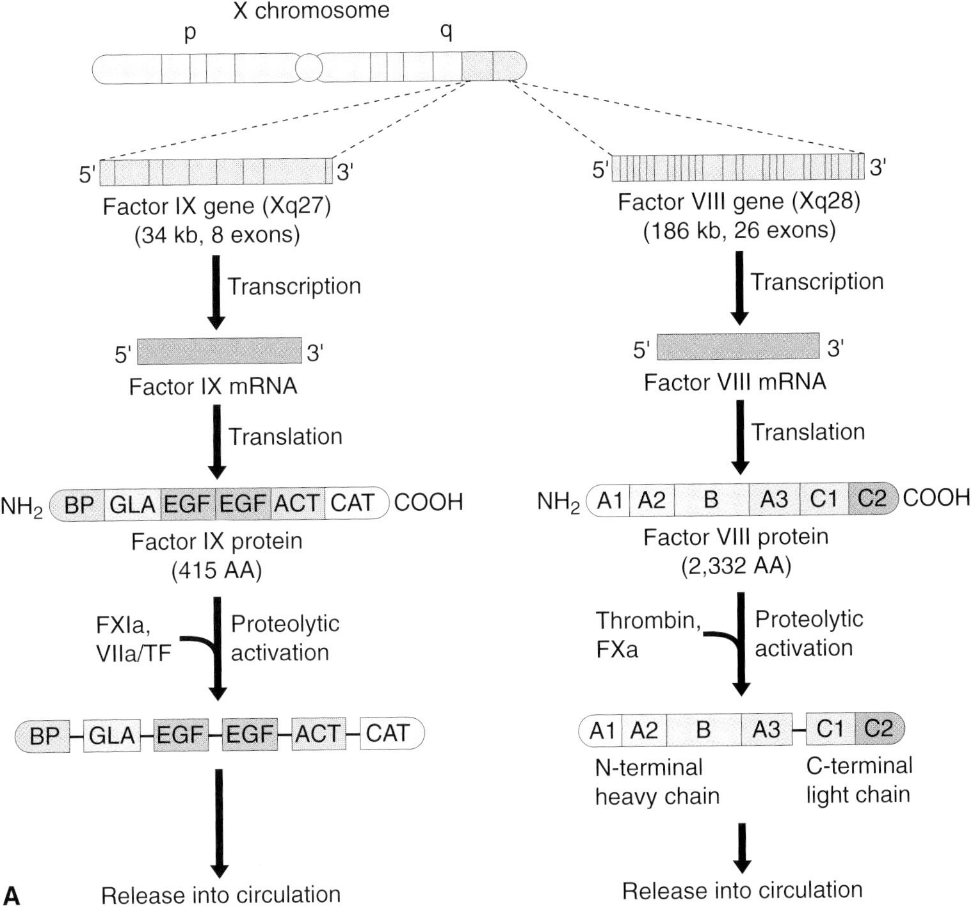

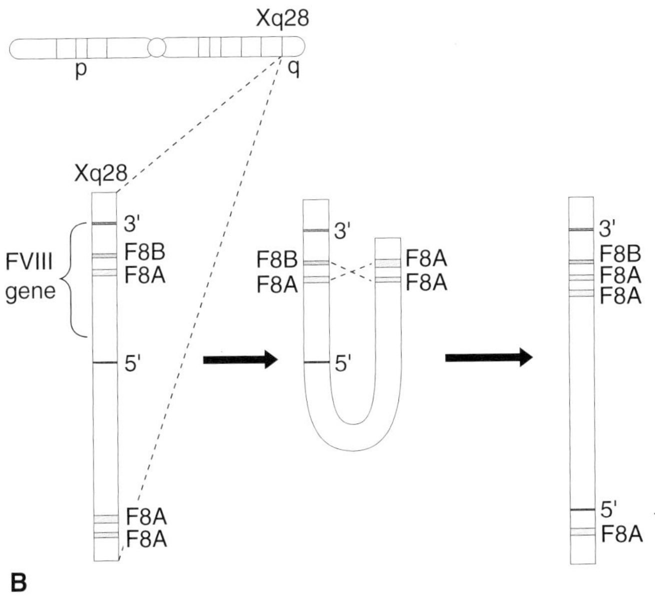

■ **Figure 63–2.** *A,* Factor VIII and IX from genes to messenger RNA to active protein. The factor VIII gene is over 186 kilobases (kb) long and contains 26 exons. The 9.0-kb factor VIII messenger RNA transcript encodes the 2332–amino acid protein that contains three A, one B, and two C domains. Following exposure to thrombin or factor Xa, the factor VIII protein is cleaved into an amino-terminal heavy chain and a carboxy-terminal light chain, linked by calcium. The factor IX gene is 34 kb long and contains 8 exons. The 2.8-kb factor IX messenger RNA transcript encodes a 415–amino acid protein that contains six domains, including one pro-sequence and one glutamic acid (GLA), two epidermal growth factor (EGF), one activation peptide (act), and one catalytic domain, linked by disulfide bridges. Proteolytic activation of factor VIII requires thrombin; factor XIa and tissue factor (TF)–factor VIIa activate factor IX. ***B,*** The factor VIII gene inversion mutation is the most common gene defect causing severe hemophilia A. This mutation is caused by recombination of a 9.6-kb sequence within intron 22 of the factor VIII gene (Int22h) and an almost identical sequence 300 kb distal to the factor VIII gene at the telomeric end of the X chromosome.

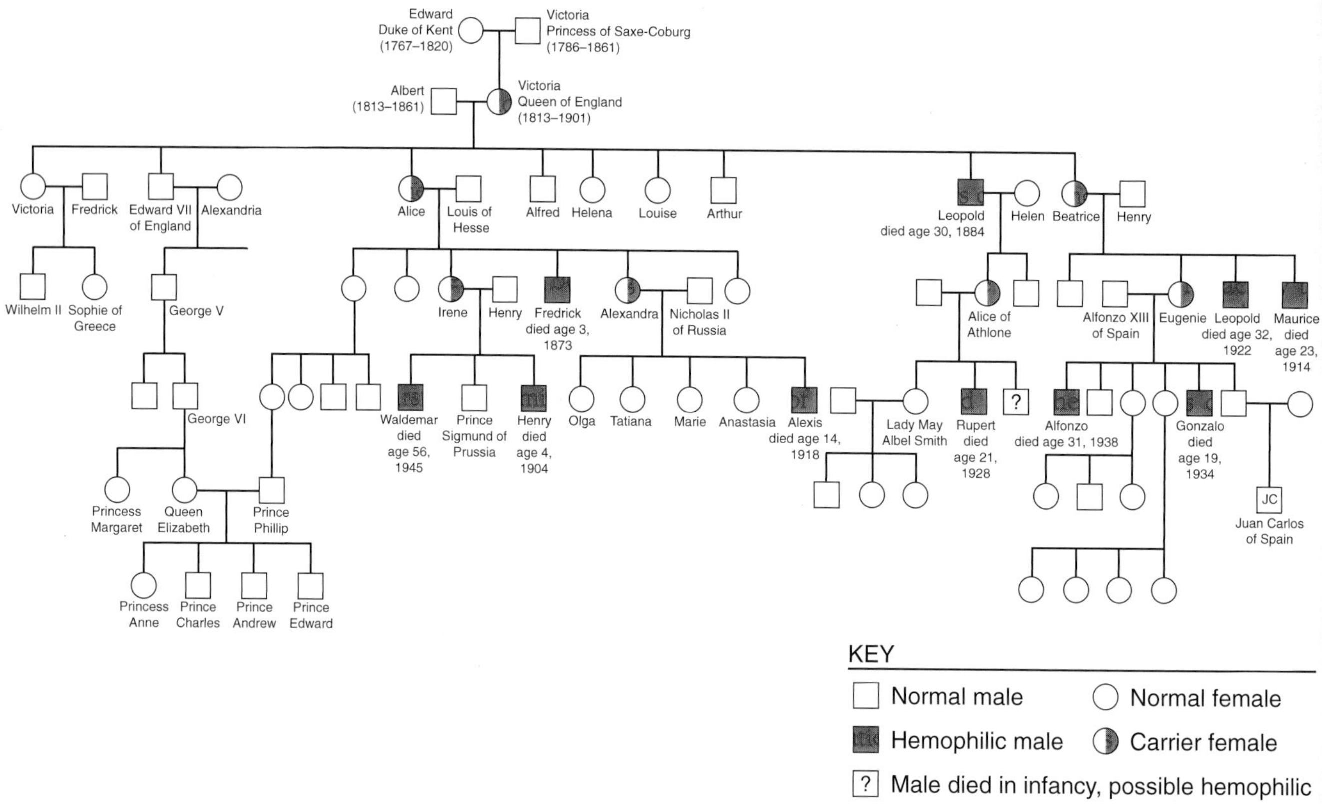

Figure 63–3. Pedigree of hemophilia: the royal genes of Queen Victoria. The inheritance of hemophilia is X-linked recessive: males are affected and females are carriers of the defective X gene. Queen Victoria was the most famous carrier, and her affected offspring sat on the thrones of Russia, Germany, and Spain. Their early deaths changed the course of history.

- First generation: Queen Victoria's son
  - Prince Leopold—died at age 30, in 1884
- Second generation: Queen Victoria's grandsons
  - Fred, son of Alice—died at age 3, in 1873
  - Leopold, son of Beatrice—died at age 32, in 1922
  - Maurice, son of Beatrice—died at age 23, in 1914
- Third generation: Queen Victoria's great-grandsons
  - Waldemar, son of Irene—died at age 56, in 1945
  - Henry, son of Irene—died at age 4, in 1904
  - Alexis, son of Alix—died at age 14, in 1918
  - Rupert, son of Alice of Athlone—died at age 21, in 1928
  - Alfonso, son of Eugenie—died at age 31, in 1938
  - Gonzalo, son of Eugenie—died at age 19, in 1934

TABLE 63–2. Mutations Causing Hemophilia

	Hemophilia A	Hemophilia B
Point mutations	70%	90%
Missense mutations		
Nonsense mutations		
Messenger RNA splice-site mutations		
Deletions	5–10%	5–10%
Whole gene deletions		
Partial gene deletions		
Microdeletions		
Insertions	<5%	<5%
Inversions/rearrangements	20%	<5%
Intron 22 inversion		

mutations or, less commonly, deletions or insertions. Among patients with hemophilia B, point mutations, including missense, nonsense, and messenger RNA splice-site mutations, are most common (see Table 63–2). Truncating mutations (e.g., large deletion and nonsense mutations) appear to be more common among patients who develop inhibitors to factor VIII or factor IX.[26] A database of mutations maintained for hemophilia A may be found at *http://europium.csc.mrc.ac.uk/webpages/main/main.htm*, and for hemophilia B at *http://www.kcl.ac.uk/ip/petergreen/haeBdatabase.html*.

CLINICAL FEATURES

The single most common clinical presentation in severe hemophilia, which accounts for 60% of cases, is circum-

TABLE 63–3. Clinical Manifestations in Hemophilia

Bleeding Symptoms in Hemophilia
Circumcision bleeding
Oral bleeding
Hemarthrosis
Hematoma
Postoperative bleeding
Hematuria
Retroperitoneal hematoma
Compartment syndrome
Psoas muscle hematoma
Intracranial hemorrhage

Bleeding Symptoms in Symptomatic Carriers
Oral, dental bleeding
Postpartum bleeding
Postoperative bleeding
Menorrhagia
Epistaxis

Factors Affecting Bleeding
Severity of factor VIII:C, IX:C deficiency
Presence of a second coagulation defect
  Type 1 von Willebrand disease
  Other coagulation disorder
  Thrombocytopenia (HIV, ITP, other)
Concomitant medication affecting coagulation, platelets
  NSAIDs
  ASA or ASA-containing medications
  Drug-induced thrombocytopenia

Abbreviations: ASA, acetylsalicylic acid; HIV, human immunodeficiency virus; ITP, immune thrombocytopenic purpura; NSAIDs, nonsteroidal anti-inflammatory drugs.

cision bleeding (Table 63–3). Other early symptoms of neonatal bleeding include subdural or periosteal bleeds following vacuum extraction delivery,[27] which is contraindicated when an infant with hemophilia is expected.[28] Within the first year of life, children with moderate or severe disease may present with mouth bleeding or frenulum hematomas, which may cause significant iron deficiency anemia from brisk blood loss. Defective jelly-like clots may form in the oral cavity, which must be removed in order for an effective clot to form with factor concentrate and antifibrinolytic therapy (see later). As the infant becomes mobile, hematomas (muscle bleeds) or hemarthroses (joint bleeds) begin to occur, with pain, swelling, and reduced range of motion.

Classical Manifestations of Hemophilia

The major clinical symptoms include hemarthroses of the knees, ankles, or elbows and hematomas, which may occur in body cavities, including the pelvis, retroperitoneum, neurovascular compartment, cranium, and spinal canal (Fig. 63–4; see also Table 63–3). Traumatic or postoperative/postprocedural bleeding may also occur. The severity of bleeding depends on the severity of disease. Patients with severe disease (factor VIII or IX level <0.01 U/mL) experience spontaneous and traumatic bleeding, usually three to four times per month. Those with moderate disease (factor VIII or IX level 0.01–0.04 U/mL) experience primarily traumatic bleeding, which occurs three to four times or so per year. Those with mild disease (factor VIII or IX level ≥0.05 U/mL) have no spontaneous bleeding and bleed infrequently, usually in association with trauma, surgery, or a complicating medication (e.g., aspirin, nonsteroidal anti-inflammatory drugs [NSAIDs]). Among mild patients, the presenting symptom may not occur until later in life, when trauma or surgery leads to uncontrolled bleeding and even transfusion. In contrast to acquired disorders of coagulation, hemophilia and other congenital coagulation disorders are characterized by chronic disability and require specialized, ongoing treatment and medical care. In fact, a distinct survival advantage has been shown for affected individuals whose care is provided at a specialized center (e.g., a hemophilia treatment center), where medical expertise is available.[29]

Joint Hemorrhage

Even before onset of a clinically recognizable joint bleed, affected individuals describe an initial sensation of warmth, tingling, or prickling in the joint. Over the course of minutes to hours, there is swelling and subsequent pain as the synovial lining is stretched by blood in the joint. When bleeding in a joint space (hemarthrosis) recurs, it leads to disruption of the synovial lining and inflammation (synovitis) and early disability. Proteolytic enzymes in the blood destroy local cartilage in the joint space, with subsequent loss of joint motion and ultimately loss of synovial lining, pain, and progressive disability. The frequent and recurrent nature of joint bleeding may lead to the development of chronic hemophilic arthropathy and orthopedic disability by the time a hemophilic is in his 20s or 30s. This may require aggressive factor treatment and early surgical intervention, resulting in high health care costs.[30] Joint aspiration is generally avoided in the management of acute hemarthroses because of the potential risk of infection and septic arthritis; however, aspiration may be helpful in pain management of the rare, exquisitely painful or morbidly swollen hemarthrosis.

Early in hemophilic joint disease, there may be subtle irregularities of the articular cartilage and small bone cysts visible on magnetic resonance imaging.[31] If bleeding recurs in the "target joint," and/or if treatment is inadequate or delayed, the synovial thickening may persist between bleeds, leading to synovial hypertrophy and effusion. A radiograph may show joint space narrowing (Fig. 63–5*A*) and magnetic resonance imaging may demonstrate evidence of synovial hyperplasia and hemosiderin deposition.[31,32] As the synovial lining thins, the contact of uncushioned bone on bone may lead to severe pain and disability and surgical intervention in the second or third decade of life (Fig. 63–5*B*), several decades before degenerative joint disease occurs in the general population.

With the introduction of prophylaxis in the form of clotting factor infusion three to four times weekly to prevent joint bleeds (Table 63–4), there has been a major

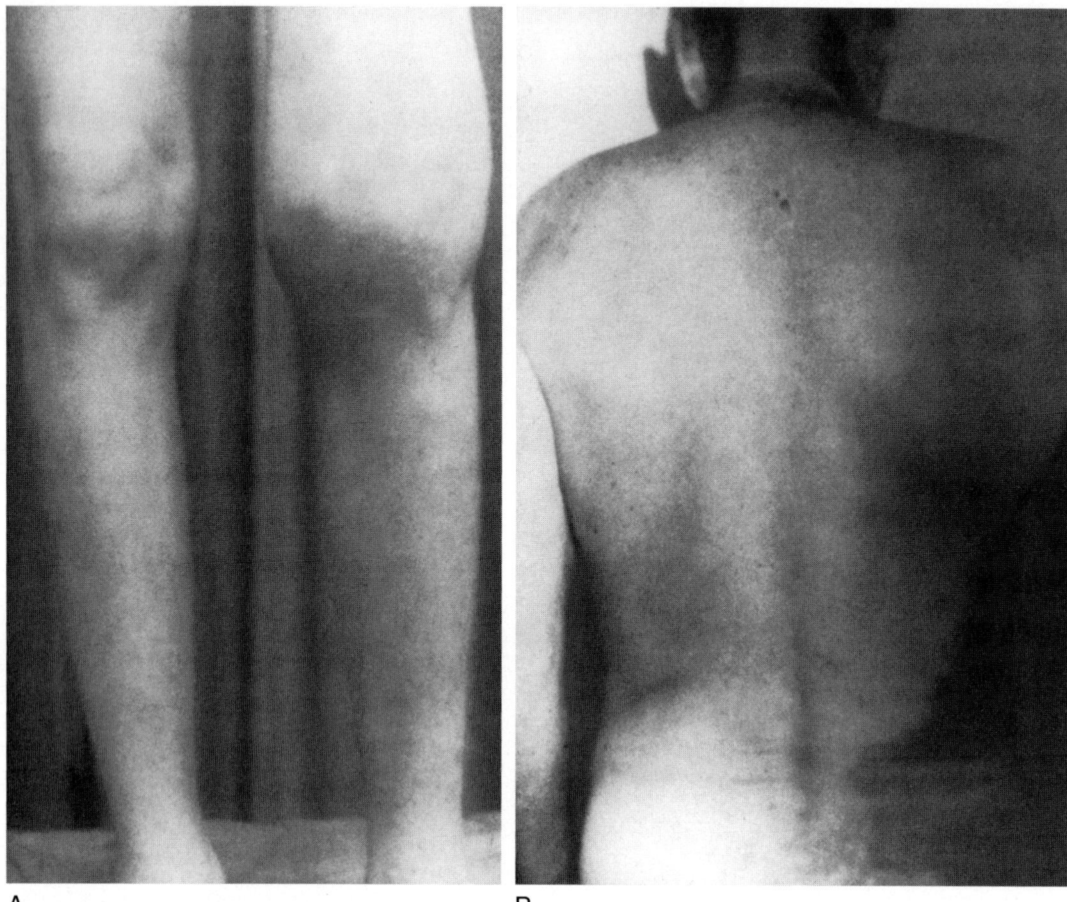

Figure 63–4. Common sites of bleeding in hemophilia. ***A,*** Left knee hemarthrosis in a young man with hemophilia A. There is severe swelling and bogginess of the blood-filled joint space, devoid of the usual landmarks and with associated warmth, pain, and reduced range of motion. ***B,*** Right posterior flank hematoma sustained after trauma in an elderly man with hemophilia A. On examination, there was significant swelling, warmth, discoloration, and pain. Laboratory findings included iron deficiency anemia.

TABLE 63–4. Prevalence of Prophylaxis in Hemophilia

Subjects	4553
Prophylaxis ≥ once/wk	50%
Prophylaxis ≥ 3 days/wk	30%
Indication for prophylaxis	
First joint bleed	38%
Target joint bleed	66%
Use of CVAD ≤ 5 yr of age	80%

From Blanchette VS, McCready M, Achonu C, et al: A survey of factor prophylaxis in boys with hemophilia followed in North American hemophilia treatment centers. Haemophilia 9(Suppl 1):19–26, 2003. Abbreviation: CVAD, central venous access device.

improvement in joint disease morbidity and outcomes. By maintaining a factor level of 1% or greater, spontaneous bleeding may be avoided and joint disease averted.[33,34] There is reduction in bleeding events overall, with improved range of motion, and reduction in the need for surgery (Box 63–1).[35–38] These advantages have come at a cost, however, both financial and medical. With prophylaxis, there is as much as a threefold increase in factor use over standard "reactive" treatment approach; every-other-day treatment comes to 15 treatments per month rather than the standard 4 or 5 per month, leading to higher cost.[39,40] Yet, aggressive factor replacement may not be sufficient to prevent all joint disease, and, for that reason, some advocate arthroscopic surgery[41] or radioactive synovectomy[42] once a child has developed a target joint. Because these are unresolved issues, a trial is being developed through the National Heart, Lung and Blood Institute Transfusion Medicine Hemostasis Clinical Network to compare prophylaxis versus arthroscopic or radionuclide synovectomy in early target-joint disease in children.

Symptomatic Carriers

Because hemophilia is an X-linked recessive disease, it occurs in rare cases in females who arise, for example, from a union of an affected male and a female carrier, such as in the Amish population through intermarriage.[24]

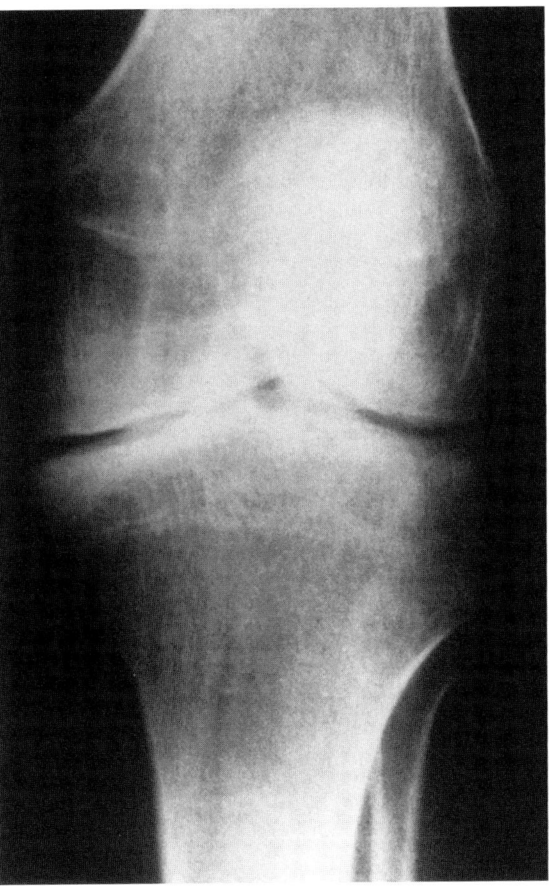

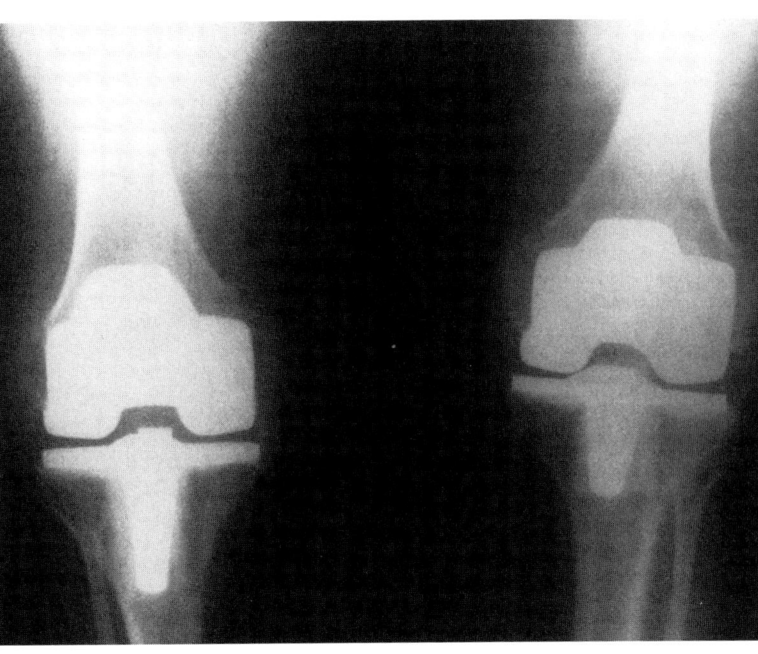

A B

Figure 63–5. Clinical and radiographic findings in hemophilia. *A*, Radiograph of chronic hemophilic arthropathy of the knee in a man with hemophilia A. There is joint space narrowing, loss of bone density near the joint, and subchondral cyst formation. *B*, Radiograph following bilateral knee arthroplastic surgery for chronic hemophilic arthropathy.

Box 63–1. Prophylaxis in the Prevention of Joint Disease in Hemophilia[35–38]

Potential Benefits of Prophylaxis

- Prevention of hemorrhages
- Prevention of loss of joint motion
- Prevention of arthropathy, progressive joint damage
- Prevention of musculoskeletal deformity
- Reduction in pain, disability
- Reduction in orthopedic surgery
- Reduction in hospital, emergency room visits
- Improvement in overall quality of life

Potential Risks of Prophylaxis

- High frequency of factor use
- High factor cost
- Infectious complications of venous access devices

Although generally asymptomatic, some carriers may become symptomatic, depending on the severity of the deficiency.[24] Studies in small Amish kindreds in Pennsylvania have found that postpartum bleeding and dental bleeding are the most common symptoms in symptomatic females, with the former requiring factor treatment[24] (see Table 63–3). They may also develop bruising, epistaxis, or hematomas, although, in contrast to women with other bleeding disorders, menorrhagia appears to be uncommon.[24] In general, it should be noted that the presence of a second coagulation defect may increase bleeding symptoms. For example, if a carrier female also has type 1 von Willebrand disease or an acquired coagulopathy, such as antibiotic-induced

TABLE 63–5. Differential Diagnosis of Hemophilia

Diagnosis	aPTT	aPTT 1:1Mix	PT	Closure Time	Bleeding Symptoms
Factor VIII, IX, XI deficiency	↑	nl	nl	nl	Yes
Factor XII deficiency	↑	nl	nl	nl	No
von Willebrand disease	↑	nl	nl	↑	Yes
Lupus anticoagulant	↑	↑	nl	nl	No
Acquired hemophilia (anti–factor VIII)	↑	↑	nl	nl	Yes
Heparin effect	↑	↑	nl	nl	±
Vitamin K deficiency	↑	nl	↑	nl	±
Liver disease	↑	nl	↑	±	±
Disseminated intravascular coagulation	↑	nl	↑	↑	Yes

Abbreviations: aPTT, activated partial thromboplastin time; nl, normal; PT, prothrombin time.

vitamin K deficiency or NSAID-induced platelet dysfunction (see Table 63–3), her bleeding tendency may be greater than expected. This underscores the importance of obtaining a past bleeding history, family history, and medication history to help determine the cause(s) of bleeding.

DIAGNOSIS AND DIFFERENTIAL DIAGNOSIS

Laboratory Diagnosis of Hemophilia

The diagnosis of hemophilia is based on factor assays of clot formation, specifically activated partial thromboplastin time (aPTT)–based one-stage clotting assays. Because factor VIII and factor IX are essential components of the intrinsic pathway (see Fig. 63–1*B* and *C*), when either factor is missing, the aPTT is prolonged. There is correction of the prolonged aPTT in a 1 : 1 mix, confirming a deficiency state: factor VIII deficiency (hemophilia A) or factor IX deficiency (hemophilia B). Generally, fibrin clot formation is normal and the aPTT is in the normal range when factor levels are greater than 30%, and spontaneous bleeding is generally uncommon when factor levels are greater than 5%.

Differential Diagnosis of Prolonged aPTT

Disorders of fibrin clot formation, or secondary hemostasis, include disorders of coagulation in which there is a defect or deficiency in one or more coagulation factors in the intrinsic or extrinsic pathways (Table 63–5). These may be congenital or acquired. Typically, congenital deficiencies affect a single clotting factor, whereas acquired deficiencies affect multiple factors (see Table 63–1). The deficiency of factor VIII or IX results in a prolonged aPTT, a measure of the time to form a fibrin clot in the intrinsic pathway (see Chapter 105). Thus, disorders considered in the differential diagnosis of a prolonged aPTT include specific *congenital* factor deficiencies in the intrinsic pathway, including factors XII and XI, prekallikrein, high-molecular-weight kininogen, and FVIII-vWF; and *acquired* disorders, including an acquired anticoagulant (blocking or specific). A prolonged aPTT with failure to correct in a 1 : 1 mix suggests the presence of an inhibitor, including the lupus anticoagulant, that is associated with clotting rather than bleeding, or specific inhibitors of coagulation, such as an acquired anti-FVIII inhibitor. The latter typically present as severe bleeding in an individual who never previously bled; this is typically either in the elderly or in the postpartum period. If the prothrombin time is also prolonged, other possibilities include vitamin K deficiency, heparin effect, liver disease, or disseminated intravascular coagulation (see Table 63–5).

TABLE 63–6. Treatment Products and Recommendations for Hemophilia

Recombinant clotting factor concentrates
Recombinant factor VIII concentrate
- Initial dose: 50 U/kg IV
- Maintenance dose: 25 U/kg IV
- Prophylaxis: 25 U/kg IV 3–4 days/week

Recombinant factor IX concentrate
- Initial dose: 75–100 U/kg IV
- Maintenance dose: 35–50 U/kg IV
- Prophylaxis: 35–50 U/kg 2–3 days/wk

Desmopressin
Intravenous (DDAVP): 0.3 μg/kg IV
Intranasal (Stimate)
- 150 μg in one nostril (weight <50 kg)
- 300 μg in one each nostril (weight ≥50 kg)

Amicar (aminocaproic acid): 50 mg/kg PO q6h
Hepatitis A and B vaccines

Abbreviations: IV, intravenously; PO, orally.

MANAGEMENT AND TREATMENT

Clotting Factor VIII and IX Concentrates

Treatment of bleeding symptoms in hemophilia has greatly improved from Rasputin's hypnotic spells to stop Prince Nicholas' hemarthroses[1] to the recombinant clotting factor concentrates, which enable correction of factor

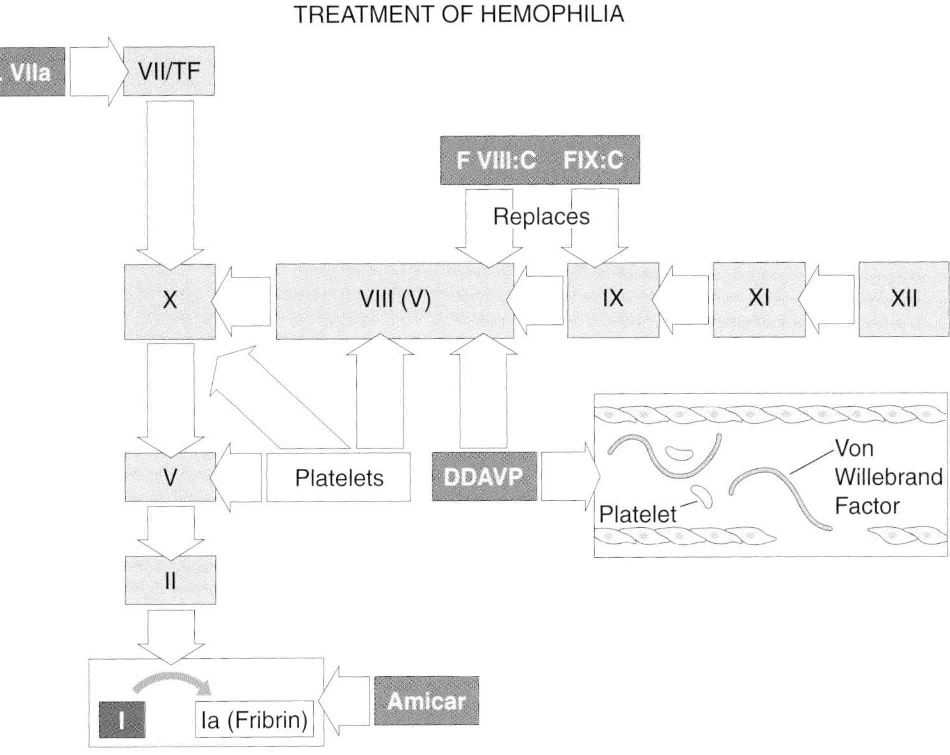

Figure 63–6. Hemophilia treatment. Site of action of the various treatment modalities for hemophilia A and B, including clotting factors VIII, IX, and VIIa, DDAVP, and Amicar (see text).

levels to normal within minutes by slow intravenous infusion and cessation or prevention of hemophilia bleeding (Table 63–6, Fig. 63–6). Standard factor VIII dosing is based on an expected 0.02-U/mL increase in plasma factor VIII for each 1 U/kg of factor VIII infused, and factor IX dosing is based on an expected 0.01-U/mL increase in plasma factor IX for each 1 U/kg of factor IX infused.[43] Maintenance dosing, such as that used following surgery or invasive procedures, is based on a plasma factor VIII half-life of 8–12 hours and a plasma factor IX half-life of 12–24 hours[43] (see Table 63–6). With the introduction of recombinant technology in the 1990s, an unprecedented level of treatment safety has been realized, with virtual elimination of HIV and hepatitis B and C risk. Recombinant products available include recombinant factor VIII,[44,45] recombinant factor IX,[46] and recombinant factor VIIa concentrates.[47] In general, to avoid bleeding complications, patients infuse themselves prophylactically before diagnostic procedures, before performing an activity such as basketball or skiing that is known to cause a bleed, or when circumstances may prevent a potentially needed treatment, such as just before travel. Although there is limited experience in symptomatic carriers or the rare affected female,[48] prevention of postpartum bleeding requires at least 3–4 days of factor.[24]

Surgical Management

Patients requiring surgery or invasive procedures should discontinue all NSAIDs at least 3 days before surgery and any platelet inhibitory drugs at least 1–2 weeks prior to surgery or procedures. In the patient undergoing surgery or a procedure, a dose of recombinant clotting factor calculated to achieve circulating levels of 100% (see Table 63–6) should be given immediately preoperatively, that is, within 5–10 minutes of the procedure. The aPTT may be monitored to establish effect quickly. Good communication between the hematologist managing the patient and the pharmacy, surgeon, and anesthesiologist is essential to assure availability of the product and verify the route, dose, and timing of the product to be given. If the patient has an inhibitor, an inhibitor titer should be assessed at least 1 week prior to surgery. Postoperatively, patients should be monitored for continuing bleeding by blood pressure, hemoglobin level, and/or brief clinical assessment to avoid bleeding complications, and treatment should be continued for up to 3 weeks postoperatively, depending on the procedure.

DDAVP, Amicar, and Other Agents

DDAVP (1-deamino-8-d-arginine vasopressin; desmopressin) is the drug of choice for treatment of mild hemophilia A.[49] It is given by intravenous or intranasal (Stimate) administration (Table 63–6, Figure 63–6). Because peak factor VIII levels achieved with the intranasal form are significantly lower than those by the intravenous route, the former is reserved for minor procedures. Side effects include tachycardia, headache, and flushing, which are caused by the vasodilatory effects of DDAVP,[49,50] and hyponatremia and volume overload, caused by the antidiuretic effect of DDAVP.[50,51] The latter, however, may be more common in children, and may be prevented by avoiding excessive fluid intake.[50,51] With repeated dosing, tachyphylaxis occurs as vWF stores are depleted.[51] Therefore, if additional treatment is required beyond three doses of DDAVP, recombinant factor VIII concentrate may be used. For oropharyngeal or genitourinary bleeding, the antifibrinolytic agents Amicar (ε-aminocaproic acid)[52] or tranexamic acid[53] may be given orally for 7–10 days, reducing factor use to the first 1 or 2 perioperative days. Amicar has been shown to be safe and effective in the treatment of bleeding in hemophilia A and B[52]; 8–10 glasses of water daily during treatment are recommended to avoid renal toxicity. All hemophilics should receive hepatitis A vaccine and hepatitis B vaccine, the former at 2 years of age or older and the latter beginning at birth, or at the time of diagnosis, per the current U.S. Public Health Service guidelines for individuals with bleeding disorders.[54,55] Cryoprecipitate is no longer recommended for treatment of hemophilia because this cold precipitate of plasma does not withstand inactivation procedures to prevent transmissible agent contamination.

COMPLICATIONS

Patients with hemophilia may suffer complications of the disease or its treatment. Historically, the complications of treatment have been nearly as severe as the disease itself and have accounted for the most common causes of death in hemophilia, including acquired immunodeficiency syndrome, the leading cause of death,[13,14] and hepatitis C liver disease, the second leading cause of death.[14,16] For most children born since the late 1980s, who have been treated with recombinant clotting factor concentrates, or plasma-derived concentrates manufactured with viral inactivation techniques, the risk of HIV and hepatitis C virus (HCV) infection is nearly zero, and lifespan approaches that for the general population. Thus, although the most significant complications of hemophilia continue to be those associated with complications of treatment, deaths from bleeding complications have been significantly reduced over the last century. However, for the patient who has no access to or is unable to afford any clotting factor, much less recombinant clotting factor, lifespan is shortened accordingly by death from bleeding complications.

Bleeding Complications of Hemophilia

The bleeding complications of hemophilia have been significantly reduced by clotting factor concentrates, and, with the continually improving safety of clotting factor concentrates, primarily relate to the complications of unrecognized or inadequately treated bleeding: orthopedic disability and bone destruction, pseudotumors, and neurologic sequelae, such as compartment syndromes. Among bleeding complications, central nervous system bleeding, although rare, is the most common bleeding cause of death. Drugs that inhibit platelets or coagulation factors may also lead to unusual or unexpected bleeding complications.

Orthopedic Bone Destruction

Occasionally, unresolved long-standing joint hemorrhage and chronic calcification related to chronic, unresolved hemorrhages may cause aggressive bone destruction, which may lead to pseudotumor formation.[56] The pseudotumor may present as a bony mass that enlarges despite treatment. Pathologically, the pseudotumor is an encapsulated collection of blood in bone that destroys bone. The bony erosion, if unchecked by aggressive factor treatment, may lead to joint instability, deformity, and gait disturbance. Despite high-dose, long-term daily factor replacement, resolution is difficult and may require surgical intervention, joint reconstruction, radiation therapy, or, rarely, amputation.[56]

Compartment Syndrome

Delayed or inadequate treatment may also result in the rare development of a compartment syndrome,[57] such as in the forearm or thigh at a site of a recent bleed. Although aggressive factor replacement may reduce the compartment pressure by stopping the bleeding, if treatment is delayed or bleeding uncontrolled, neurologic compromise may ensue, leading to numbness and weakness as the internal pressure of the compartment increases.[57] Compromise of the blood supply to the muscle and other tissues may lead to swelling and severe pain, requiring intravenous narcotics and fasciotomy of the compartment to relieve the condition.[57] Despite surgical release, compartment syndrome surgery may require skin grafting, and this may lead to possible lifelong scars and strictures, limiting motion, and potentially irreversible neurologic defects.

Neurologic Sequelae

Among patients with serious central nervous system bleeding, whether traumatic or spontaneous, paraplegia, retardation, or even death may result. To prevent lifelong devastating consequences, the importance of prophylactic factor infusion at the earliest sign of unexplained headache, vomiting, stiff neck, or unexplained change of consciousness cannot be overemphasized. Although uncommon, neurologic complications may go unrecognized, particularly in early infancy, when serious sequelae of bleeding occur following delivery.[27] Patients with inhibitors may be at greater risk for central nervous system bleeding and neurologic sequelae and death, likely related to their poor response to standard treatment.[58]

Life-Threatening Bleeding

Individuals with hemophilia, particularly those with severe disease, are at risk for spontaneous bleeding.[16,59] If treatment is delayed, the dose inadequate, an inhibitor present, the product unavailable, or the injury considered not severe enough to treat, significant morbidity or even mortality may result. A headache or head injury may be a life-threatening central nervous system bleed, or a backache or a muscle "pull," a retroperitoneal bleed. Errors in judgment, busy schedules, or the cost and bother of treatment may stand between life and permanent disability or death, and the lifelong risk of life-threatening bleeding remains a potential psychological burden and stress for individuals with hemophilia.

Drugs Inhibiting Hemostasis

Unexpected or prolonged bleeding in hemophilia may suggest a second coagulation defect, such as with aspirin, NSAIDs, or other platelet inhibitors (antibiotics) or anticoagulants. It is critical to take a medication history, especially of medications containing aspirin, and stop potentially offending agents, to limit bleeding complications. Encouraging patients to call to check on the safety of new medications may avoid future bleeding problems.

Complications of Treatment

The life expectancy of individuals with hemophilia has dramatically improved, from the early deaths of affected individuals in childhood and young adulthood in the 19th and early 20th century, as noted in the royal pedigree (see Fig. 63–3), to the achievement of a near-normal lifespan by the late 1970s with the introduction of clotting factor concentrates (see Table 63–6). However, this success was interrupted by the transmission of HIV and HCV through clotting factor concentrates, which became leading causes of death in the 1980s. With the introduction of viral inactivation techniques in the manufacture of concentrates in 1983–1985, the risk of HIV was virtually eliminated. Moreover, with the implementation of highly active antiretroviral therapy in 1996, survival has improved greatly, with many patients enjoying a normal lifespan. For those with HCV infection, the introduction of antiviral therapy has cleared the virus in many, resulting in rare deaths related to HCV infection alone. However, among those with HIV/HCV co-infection, some patients survive HIV disease only to die of HCV end-stage liver disease or require liver transplantation (see later). Despite an unprecedented level of safety and efficacy, there remain a number of complications of current replacement therapy. These include venous access device infection, inhibitor formation, allergic reactions, thrombosis, hepatitis, HIV/HCV co-infection, and transmissible agents (Box 63–2).

Venous Access Device Infection

Central venous access devices (CVADs) are widely used in 40–60% of children with hemophilia to infuse factor.[60–62] The leading complication of CVAD use is infection of the device, which occurs in up to 30% of patients at a median 3–4 years of age, typically within the first 4 months of use.[61,63] Furthermore, up to 50% show venographic evidence of thrombosis in central veins within 5 years of CVAD use,[64] the long-term significance of which is not known. CVAD infections are twice as likely in patients receiving factor concentrate to build immune tolerance than in those on prophylaxis.[61,65]

Box 63–2. Hemophilia Treatment: Considerations and Complications[157,158]

Considerations for Treatment

- Infectivity
- Immunogenicity
- Thrombogenicity
- Availability
- Affordability

Complications of Hemophilia Treatment

- Inhibitor formation
- Central venous access device infection
- Allergic reactions
- Thrombogenicity
- Hepatitis C
- HIV/HCV co-infection
- Transmissible agents

A number of factors may contribute to clot formation, including decreasing vessel size,[66] lower body weight,[67] frequent access,[61] and the thrombogenic plastic in the device.[68] This potential health risk is also a financial burden, averaging $8000 per episode per year.[39] Yet, the benefits of prophylaxis are believed to far outweigh the risk of CVAD complications, although some institutions switch to peripheral infusion as soon as tolerated.

Inhibitor Formation

One of the most difficult complications of hemophilia treatment is the formation of inhibitors to infused factor, estimated to occur in 15–25% of those with hemophilia A and 3–5% of those with hemophilia B[69,70] (Table 63–7). Inhibitors are alloantibodies directed at infused factor, unrelated to type or purity,[70,71] that render patients refractory to standard replacement therapy. Inhibitors typically occur after a median of 9 treatment days,[69–72] at a median age of 2 years,[69,71,72] and more commonly in those with severe disease[72,73] and African Americans, in whom the prevalence is twofold higher.[69] Clinically, inhibitors also appear to be frequently associated with central nervous system bleeding.[58] The preferential occurrence of inhibitors in patients with large deletions or nonsense mutations[74,75] suggests that factor VIII or factor IX gene-product expression is important in immune system recognition of self and non-self. The mechanism by which inhibitors interfere with coagula-

TABLE 63–7. Characteristics of Hemophilia Inhibitor Formation

Incidence	15–25% in hemophilia A 3–5% in hemophilia B
Characteristics	More common in severe disease, African Americans
Immune response	IgG4 alloantibody to infused factor VIII, IX
Mechanism	T-cell, B-cell response to foreign factor VIII, IX
Age at onset	Median 2 yr of age
Factor exposure	Median 9 exposures
Clinical symptoms	More frequent, severe bleeding; central nervous system bleed
Outcome	Higher morbidity, earlier deaths
Treatment	Ineffective, costly, complex
Tolerance induction	Relation to inhibitor duration, genotype

From Ragni MV: Inhibitor formation in African-Americans with hemophilia A [abstract no. 3606]. Blood 94:642a, 1999.

Box 63–3. Treatment Modalities for Hemophilia Inhibitors

- Hemostasis
  - Bypassing agents: FEIBA, APCC concentrates
  - Recombinant factor VIIa
  - High-dose factor VIII (limited to patients with very low titer)
  - Porcine factor VIII
- Development of tolerance to the inhibitor
  - Immune tolerance: recombinant factors VIII, IX

tion depends on the site of inhibition: for example, factor VIII inhibitors binding to residues 485–508 in the A2 heavy chain interfere with Xase activation[76–78]; those binding to residues 2303–2332 in the C2 light chain interfere with phospholipid binding,[79–81] and those binding to residues 1649–1689 in the B/A3 junction interfere with vWF binding.[82] Inhibitors are typically diagnosed when parents notice than an affected child is not responding to treatment or during routine screening by Bethesda assay (see Chapter 105). The goal of treatment is twofold: to eradicate the inhibitor and to manage acute bleeding episodes effectively (Box 63–3). Treatment of inhibitors is complex, costly,[39,40] and/or inadequate, including that with prothrombin complex concentrates,[83] activated factor IX complexes,[84,85] factor IX concentrates,[86] recombinant FVIIa,[87] and porcine FVIII,[88] and immunoadsorption.[89] Induction of immune tolerance by daily factor VIII (or IX)[90,91] to neutralize the inhibitor is costly, requires high-level compliance, and is complicated in some patients by anaphylaxis[92] or nephrotic syndrome.[93] Furthermore, the optimal dose and duration of factor to induce tolerance in inhibitor patients is not known. Thus, a European-U.S. Immune Tolerance Induction Study, comparing low- and high- dose induction, is underway in association with the International Society of Thrombosis and Haemostasis and the North American Hemophilia and Thrombosis Research Society.

Allergic Reactions

Clotting factor concentrates are protein-based products and, as such, their use is subject to allergic reactions.[92,93] Allergic reactions, although infrequently reported, appear more common with factor IX products, and may include rash, pruritus, fever, tachycardia, tachypnea, stomach or intestinal pain, nausea, vomiting, and diarrhea, or the development of anaphylaxis.[92,93] Despite the availability of a variety of drugs to reduce these symptoms, including anti-inflammatory agents, steroids, pressors, and intravenous fluids, the ultimate result may be that certain products must be avoided, or, if no other substitute exists, high-dose anti-inflammatory agents may be required prior to treatment. Allergic reactions appear to be associated with inhibitor formation, and, in the case of factor IX concentrate, may also be associated with the nephrotic syndrome.[72,92,93]

Thrombogenicity

Thrombosis is uncommon in individuals with a bleeding diathesis, although it may be associated with the use of clotting factor products, for example, plasma-derived factor IX concentrate, activated clotting factor products, and recombinant factor VIIa.[94–96] Risk factors for thrombosis in these settings are not known, although thrombotic events may occur after prolonged use and/or high doses of these products, postoperatively, or when catheters are placed to assist with infusion.[94–96] There is limited experience in the treatment of such complications, although a short course of anticoagulation with concomitant clotting factor replacement might be considered. Potential prevention measures might include limiting the duration of high-dose factor use, limiting the use of activated clotting factor concentrates, limiting the duration of peripheral catheter use, and mobilizing postoperative patients early.

Hepatitis C

HCV is the major cause of chronic hepatitis in individuals with hemophilia who were exposed to the virus through administration of older clotting factor concentrates[97,98]; chronic hepatitis C is a major cause of morbidity and the second leading cause of death in this group.[13,14,16] Unlike other risk groups for hepatitis, hemophilics were younger at HCV exposure[98] and were repeatedly exposed to multiple hepatitis viruses.[99–103] Over 90% of patients treated with plasma-derived clotting factor concentrates during the 1970s and 1980s became infected with HCV,[97,98,104] and nearly all were HCV RNA positive by polymerase chain reaction,[105] consistent with the detection of HCV in untreated clotting factor concentrates.[105] As a result, now 20+ years later,[106–108] over 80% of adults with hemophilia are infected with HCV,[109] and chronic liver disease remains a serious health problem. About 60% of HCV-infected hemophilics have intermittent liver function test elevations[97,98,104] and 25% or more have biopsy-documented cirrhosis.[110–113] Thus, although an unknown proportion of HCV-infected hemophilics may be at risk for end-stage liver disease, there are no noninvasive ways to predict this, and, if we could predict the outcome, hepatitis C treatment is not always effective (see later). Although liver biopsy is the best predictor of disease progression,[114] and despite the uncommon occurrence of bleeding complications,[115] even under factor coverage, few hemophilic patients undergo liver biopsies.[109]

HCV/HIV Co-Infection

Up to a decade after initial HCV infection,[106–108] primarily between 1982 and 1983, over 40% of hemophilic patients with HCV infection also became infected by HIV,[116,117] all of whom are now over 18 years of age.[109] Unfortunately, HIV has an adverse effect on HCV liver disease, leading to persistent HCV replication,[118] high HCV RNA viral load,[119,120] advanced fibrosis,[113] and rapid liver disease progression,[121,122] with high mortality.[14,123] In a study of 157 hemophilic men with chronic HCV infection, the relative risk of end-stage liver disease was 3.7-fold greater in HIV^+ than HIV^- patients.[14] Risk factors for liver disease progression in hemophilic men include age at HCV exposure, co-infection with hepatitis B surface antigen, co-infection with HIV, and alcohol.[14] The mechanism by which HIV leads to more rapid end-stage liver disease remains unknown, although the HIV-associated decline in $CD4^+$ T helper lymphocyte number and function, and defective $CD4^+$ proliferation and $CD4^+$ apoptosis,[124–126] may weaken the limited immune response to HCV infection. HIV is also known to upregulate cytokines,[126] including interleukin-6[127,128] and transforming growth factor-β,[129,130] that are secreted in response to liver injury and lead to liver cell damage, and thereby may cause liver disease progression.[131] Unfortunately, response to HCV antiviral therapy in hemophilia is poor, with a 30% response rate to standard interferon plus ribavirin antiviral therapy,[132] and even poorer responses among those with HCV/HIV co-infection.[133]

End-Stage Liver Disease

Despite advances in antiviral treatment of HIV infection, which has slowed disease progression and reduced mortality,[134] many hemophilic men are surviving HIV infection, only to succumb to progressive HCV liver disease.[4] For those who develop end-stage liver disease, HIV remains a contraindication to transplantation. A recent pilot study of liver transplantation in co-infected subjects with end-stage liver disease, the first of whom was a man with hemophilia,[135] found that survival in HIV^+ recipients is comparable to that in age- and race-matched HIV^- recipients (Table 63–8).[13] Thus, growing data support the

TABLE 63–8. End-Stage Liver Disease (ESLD) and Liver Transplantation

Etiology of HIV⁺ ESLD			
Hepatitis C virus infection	83%		
Other causes (hepatitis B virus infection, fulminant hepatic failure)	17%		
Epidemiology of HIV⁺ ESLD			
Hemophilic subjects	30%		
Nonhemophilic subjects	70%		
Survival After Liver Transplantation			
	12 Mo	**24 Mo**	**36 Mo**
HIV^-	87%	73%	73%
HIV^+	87%	82%	78%

Data from Ragni MV, Belle SH, Im K, et al: Survival in HIV-infected liver transplant recipients. J Infect Dis 188:1412–1420, 2003.

notion that HIV should no longer be a contraindication to transplantation. Furthermore, because survival after transplantation is independent of pretransplantation CD4 or HIV viral load, transplant candidates should not be excluded on the basis of their inability to tolerate highly active antiretroviral therapy.[13] A multicenter study of orthotopic liver transplantation in HIV, sponsored by the National Institute of Allergy and Infectious Diseases, should help confirm or refute these findings. Because end-stage liver disease may worsen unexpectedly, for example, as a result of poor tolerance of highly active antiretroviral therapy or bacterial infections associated with immune dysfunction of HIV and liver disease,[14] individuals with HIV infection and end-stage liver disease should undergo early evaluation, preferably at the first signs of end-stage liver disease.

Transmissible Agents

The availability of recombinant products devoid of human plasma, and elimination of the requirement for added albumin in their manufacture,[45] has virtually eliminated blood-borne transmission. Yet, to the extent that trace human plasma is present in clotting factor concentrates, there is the potential for transmission of other agents, such as nonenveloped viruses, hepatitis A,[99] parvovirus B19,[136] and Creutzfeldt-Jakob disease and variant Creutzfeldt-Jakob disease agents.[137–140] Neither studies of hemophilic men exposed to pooled plasma derivatives[137] nor studies of transfusion recipients exposed to products donated by individuals infected with variant Creutzfeldt-Jakob disease[138] have found evidence of exposure to either disease[137]; thus, the risk of transmission remains theoretical. Parvovirus B19, a small nonenveloped DNA virus that evades current viral inactivation techniques for plasma-derived products and is potentially transmitted through blood,[141,142] appears to be associated with no clinical sequelae among hemophilic patients.[136] Ultimately, prevention of potential known and unknown

Box 63–4. Hemophilia Gene Transfer

Goals of Hemophilia Gene Transfer

- Eliminate spontaneous bleeds
- Prevent chronic joint disease
- Reduce health care costs
- Avoid inconvenience of infusions
- Avoid transmissible disease risk
- Avoid blood product shortages
- Improve quality of life

Hemophilia Gene Transfer Trials

- Ex vivo plasmid factor VIII gene transfer into autologous fibroblasts[147,148]
- Intramuscular adeno-associated viral vector (AAV) factor IX gene transfer[144]
- Intravenous retroviral factor VIII gene transfer[143]
- Intrahepatic AAV factor IX gene transfer[145]
- Intravenous gutless adenoviral factor VIII gene transfer[146]
- Autologous fibroblasts exposed ex vivo to a retrovirus with hFIX minigene

Potential Risks of Hemophilia Gene Therapy

- Inhibitor formation
- Inflammatory response
- Hepatotoxicity
- Germline transmission
- Insertional mutagenesis
- Unforeseen risks

agent transmission to hemophilics through blood products depends on safeguards in place for the blood supply.

Prospects for Gene Transfer

The goal of gene transfer is safe, sustained production of factor VIII or IX. Because the factor VIII and IX genes have been cloned and outcome is measurable by standard coagulation assays, hemophilia is an ideal model disease for gene transfer (Box 63–4). By achieving an increase in factor VIII or IX to greater than 5%, spontaneous bleeding is averted and, thereby, most of the morbidity of the disease. Since 1999, a total of 46 subjects have been enrolled in six hemophilia gene transfer trials utilizing a variety of approaches, including retroviral vector,[143] adeno-associated viral vector,[144,145] and adenoviral vector[146] approaches; plasmid technology[147,148]; and gene mutation suppression.[149] Transient increases in factor VIII and IX levels observed in some subjects in these studies have given the first glimpse of efficacy, although none of these increases has been sustained. Adverse effects have been minor, such as local pain at a muscle injection site,[144] immunologic response to vector with liver dysfunction,[145] and transient liver toxicity with thrombocytopenia.[146] By understanding the mechanisms by which these events have occurred, vector design and target tissue may be optimized, and immunogenicity reduced or eliminated. Because hemophilia is not a lethal disease and treatment, although invasive, is safe and effective, the major goal, aside from effective gene transfer, is safe gene transfer.[8] Thus, those involved in the gene transfer effort will need to be vigilant for potential risks, including inhibitor formation,[150] allergic reactions,[151,152] hepatitis,[145,153] germline transfer,[154,155] and insertional mutagenesis.[156]

Current Controversies & Future Considerations

The Hemophilias: Factor VIII and IX Deficiencies

Current Controversies

- Prevention of joint bleeding: primary or secondary prophylaxis?
- Optimal treatment of target joints: prophylaxis or arthroscopic surgery?
- Management of inhibitors: low-dose versus high-dose immune tolerance induction; rituximab (Rituxan) in cases of refractory inhibitors
- Prevention of venous access device infection: recombinant tissue-type plasminogen activator

Future Considerations[159-185]

- Designer molecules: modifications to achieve higher specific activity, modifications to reduce immunogenicity
- Novel approach to induce tolerance: B- and T-cell co-receptor blockade, oral tolerance, DNA vaccination
- New approaches to gene transfer: RNA repair, circulating endothelial cells, hematopoietic stem cells

Suggested Readings*

Hoyer LW: Hemophilia A. N Engl J Med 330:39–47, 1994.

Leisner RJ, Khair K, Hann IM: The impact of prophylactic treatment on children with severe hemophilia. Br J Haematol 92:973–978, 1996.

Mannucci PM, Tuddenheim EGD: Medical progress: the hemophiliac—from royal genes to gene therapy. N Engl J Med 344:1773–1779, 2001.

Ragni MV: Hemophilia gene transfer: a plea for safety. Mol Ther 6:1–5, 2002.

Ragni MV: Transfusion transmitted disease: hepatitis C virus infection and liver transplantation. *In* Lee CA, Berntorp E, Hoots K (eds): Textbook of Haemophilia. Malden, MA: Blackwell Publishing, 2005, pp 207–213.

Schlesinger KW, Ragni MV: Safety of the new-generation recombinant clotting factor concentrates. Expert Opin Drug Safety 1:213–223, 2002.

Full references for this chapter can be found on accompanying CD-ROM.

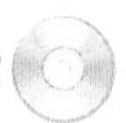

CHAPTER 64

Von Willebrand Disease

Elina Armstrong, MD, PhD, and Barbara A. Konkle, MD

KEY POINTS

Von Willebrand Disease

- Von Willebrand disease (VWD) is the most common congenital bleeding disorder in males and females.
- VWD predominantly affects the primary hemostatic response.
- Quantitative or qualitative defects of VWF are caused by a variety of mutations.
- Subtypes of VWD are classified as 1, 2A, 2B, 2M, 2N, and 3.
- VWD is characterized by mucocutaneous and postoperative bleeding manifestations, including epistaxis, bleeding after dental extractions, menorrhagia, and easy bruising.
- Diagnosis includes a detailed bleeding history, family history, and laboratory tests for VWF antigen, VWF activity, factor VIII activity, VWF multimer analysis, and ristocetin-induced platelet aggregation.
- Treatment is with DDAVP, FVIII/VWF concentrates, antifibrinolytic agents, and estrogen.

INTRODUCTION

Von Willebrand disease (VWD) is the most common inherited bleeding disorder, with a prevalence of approximately 1% when defined as decreased laboratory values of von Willebrand factor (VWF) levels.[1] Approximately one tenth of this group has clinical bleeding symptoms.[2] Clinically, VWD is characterized by mucocutaneous and postoperative bleeding of varying severity in both males and females. A variety of mutations in the VWF gene lead to a quantitative or qualitative deficiency of VWF, and there are also acquired forms of VWD.

Inherited VWD was first described in 1926 by Erik von Willebrand, a Finnish physician who reported an autosomal bleeding disorder in a family living on the Åland Islands, an archipelago between Sweden and Finland.[3–6] The family tree is shown in Figure 64–1. The proband was a 5-year-old girl who was severely affected with multiple bleeding episodes from the nose and lips and after tooth extractions. She bled to death at the age of 14 years during her fourth menstrual period. Nine of her 12 siblings were also affected, and 4 of them had died before age 4 of uncontrollable bleeding. Both of her parents had severe nosebleeds when younger, and several of her maternal aunts had had profuse menstrual bleeds. Von Willebrand named the disorder "hereditary pseudohemophilia" because he recognized the autosomal inheritance pattern in his study of 66 other family members (in contrast to the sex-linked recessive pattern seen in the hemophilias).

After an assay for factor VIII (FVIII) became available in the 1950s, it was demonstrated that patients with VWD had decreased plasma levels of factor VIII. Several reports described families with severe bleeding disorder characterized by factor VIII deficiency and a prolonged bleeding time. In the late 1950s and early 1960s, it was discovered that plasma concentrate could be used to correct the bleeding diathesis and that the mechanism involved another factor besides factor VIII, which stimulated release or synthesis of factor VIII and affected platelet adhesiveness. Von Willebrand factor was isolated and characterized in the 1970s.[5,7]

EPIDEMIOLOGY

It is estimated that approximately 1 in 1000 people have symptomatic VWD that requires specific treatment. Type 1 VWD represents approximately 70% of cases. Severe type 3 is estimated to have an incidence of approximately 3 cases per 1 million population.[8] A precise determination of prevalence cannot be made because of difficulties in the diagnosis of VWD. Type 1 VWD is inherited in an autosomal dominant fashion, but has variable expressivity and reduced penetrance, making diagnosis difficult. For example, up to 50% of obligate carriers of this most common type have been found to be asymptomatic in kindred studies.[9] These characteristics of type 1 VWD are likely due to other superimposed epigenetic factors, as well as environmental influences.

VWF is a large multimeric glycoprotein that circulates in plasma at a concentration of 0.5–1.0 mg/dL. Platelets contain approximately 15% of the quantity in plasma.[10] The level of VWF in plasma is influenced by several variables, including age, race, blood group, pregnancy, hormones, stress, and smoking. Genetic factors account for

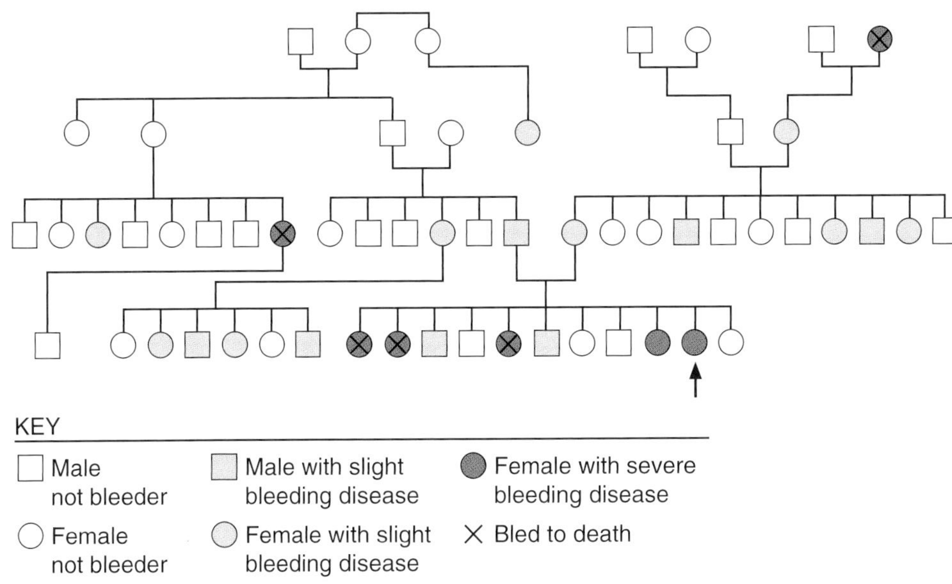

Figure 64–1. The pedigree of the first described family with VWD. The proband is indicated with an *arrow*. (Adapted from von Willebrand EA: Hereditär pseudohemofili. Finska Läkaresälskapets Handlingar 67:7–112, 1926.)

approximately 60% of the variation, with ABO blood group accounting for approximately 30% of this.[11] Individuals with blood group O have approximately 30% lower levels than blood groups A, B, and AB. The blood group AB is associated with the highest level. Significant linkage between VWF antigen and the ABO locus has been observed, and the H antigen has been suggested to mediate the ABO effect on plasma VWF concentration.[12,13] Race accounts for approximately 7% of genetic factors affecting VWF levels, because VWF levels have been observed to be significantly higher in the African American population compared to whites independent of blood group.[14,15]

Many patients found to have low VWF levels do not have bleeding symptoms, which often raises a dilemma regarding diagnosis. An alternative approach has been suggested in which mild to moderately low VWF levels would be considered a risk factor for bleeding rather than a disease.[2] Low VWF levels do not correlate well with clinical bleeding and thus asymptomatic people should not be screened for VWD.[16] It remains controversial whether a low VWF level without a bleeding history would identify a risk factor, rather than label a person with a diagnosis of VWD. This is further confounded by the need for a preoperative assessment and treatment plan in persons without past "at-risk" situations. Thus, decisions about treatment in these patients should be based on clinical criteria, including bleeding history, type of clinical situation, and other predisposing factors such as use of medications that inhibit platelet function.

PATHOPHYSIOLOGY

Von Willebrand Factor

The VWF gene is located in the distal short arm of chromosome 12. The gene of 178 kb in size is composed of 52 exons.[17,18] A partial nonfunctional duplication, VWF pseudogene, is present on chromosome 22 and includes exons that encode domains A1, A2, and A3[19] (Fig. 64–2).

The VWF protein is composed of homologous domains, which include three A domains, three B domains, two C domains, and four D domains with different functional properties (see Fig. 64–2). A1 contains binding sites for platelet glycoprotein (GP)Ib, heparin, collagen, and ristocetin; A2 contains the cleavage site for the VWF protease; and A3 contains a second binding site for collagen. Domain C1 contains a binding site for platelet GPIIb/IIIa and D′ as well as the contiguous part of D3 contain the binding site for factor VIII.[20–22]

VWF is synthesized in endothelial cells and megakaryocytes as a primary translation product of 2813 amino acids; it subsequently undergoes considerable processing, including dimerization and multimerization to very large forms.[23,24] The primary translation product contains a propeptide also known as von Willebrand antigen II.[25]

Dimers are produced in the endoplasmic reticulum early during processing of the protein by formation of disulfide bonds between the carboxy-terminal ends of the pro-VWF.[26] This is followed by the addition of carbohydrate residues and subsequent transportation to the Golgi apparatus, where dimers undergo further glycosylation and sulfation.[24,27] Multimers of a spectrum of sizes are formed by disulfide bond formation between the dimers. Some are exceedingly large, more than 20 million Da. Synthesis of VWF is regulated in part by hormones, because VWF production in endothelial cells has been shown to be increased by estrogen and thyroid hormone.[28,29]

Larger VWF multimers (as high as 10,000–20,000 kDa) are targeted to endothelial cytoplasmic storage granules, the Weibel-Palade bodies.[30,31] In platelets, VWF is stored in the α-granules.[32] Active secretion of the larger, most functional forms of VWF from the storage sites is triggered by a number of physiologic agonists, including α-adrenergic agonists such as epinephrine, thrombin, fibrin, and histamine, as well as after the administration of 1-deamino-8-D-arginine vasopressin (DDAVP).[33,34] This

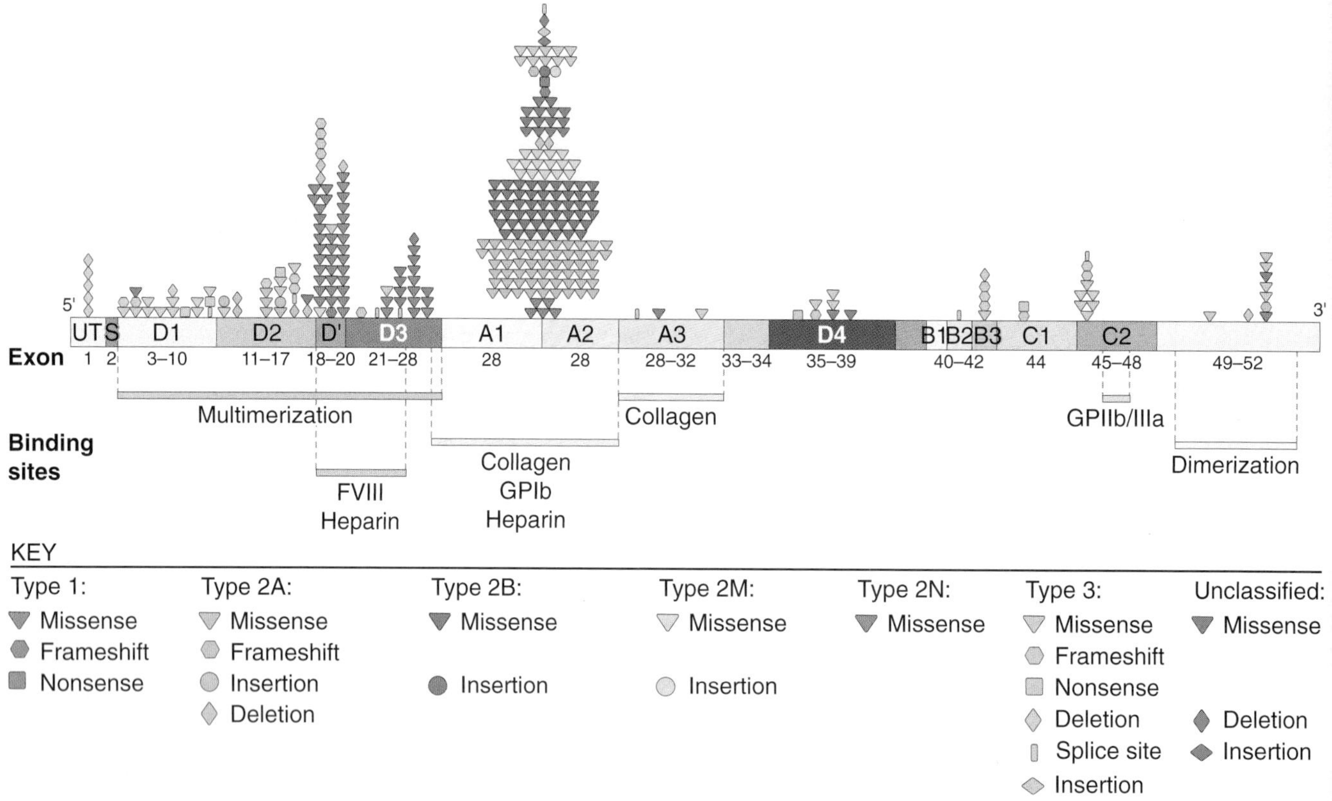

Figure 64–2. Schematic illustration of VWF protein structure with the functional domains and VWD mutations as reported in the VWD database (*www.Sheffield.ac.uk/vwf*). As shown, the majority of mutations have been identified in exon 28, mostly for type 2 VWD, resulting in defects in specific functional domains.

release results in larger multimers than those usually present in the circulation.[35] Processing of the unusually large multimers takes place in the plasma within about 4 hours by the VWF-cleaving protease, which converts the larger multimers into the slightly smaller forms normally seen in the circulation.[36,37] The complementary DNA sequence of this protein has been identified; the protein is a member of the ADAMTS family of metalloproteinases[38–40] (see Chapter 62). Deficiency of this protease is associated with thrombotic thrombocytopenic purpura.[41] Another protein, thrombospondin-1, has been shown to play a role in the processing of the unusually large multimers.[42] The normal half-life of circulating VWF is approximately 8–12 hours.

The larger multimers are well suited to act as bridging molecules between platelets and the injured vessel subendothelium as well as between platelets, because the repeated binding sites allow multiple interactions with both platelet receptors and subendothelial structures at sites of injury.[43] VWF circulates as flexible 2-nm-thick strands in a tangled coil configuration, which becomes more linear under conditions of high shear stress.[44] This conformation change exposes the binding sites in the A1 domain for the receptor GP1b-IX-V complex on the surface of platelets, which mediates platelet adhesion and aggregation under conditions of high shear (Fig. 64–3).[45,46] Activation of circulating VWF may occur as VWF binds to subendothelial structures exposed after endothelial damage, possibly immobilizing and exposing multiple VWF A1 domains toward the vessel lumen where platelets are present.[47] Activation may also occur when VWF is exposed to the high shear stresses that are present in small vessels, so the conformation of VWF changes from a globular form to a linear form in which the A1 domains are available for binding to the platelet GP1b-IX-V complex.[46] Platelets adhering to VWF become activated and express a functional GPIIb/IIIa receptor, which can interact with VWF. These interactions further induce irreversible binding of platelets to the subendothelium via the VWF and may also contribute to platelet aggregation, especially under high shear conditions.[48,49]

The mechanisms for VWF binding to the subendothelial connective tissue are not well defined. VWF binds to multiple types of collagen (types I, II, III, IV, V, and VI), but type VI collagen appears to be especially important.[50,51]

Another important function of VWF is that it acts as a carrier protein for factor VIII.[52] Factor VIII has a markedly shortened half-life unless it is bound to VWF in circulation, because VWF protects factor VIII from proteolytic inactivation by activated protein C and its cofactor, protein S. VWF binding to collagen induces a conformational change within the factor VIII–binding motif of VWF, lowering the affinity for factor VIII. After thrombin cleavage, activated factor VIII is released from VWF and serves as a cofactor in factor Xa production and subsequent thrombin generation. Low factor VIII con-

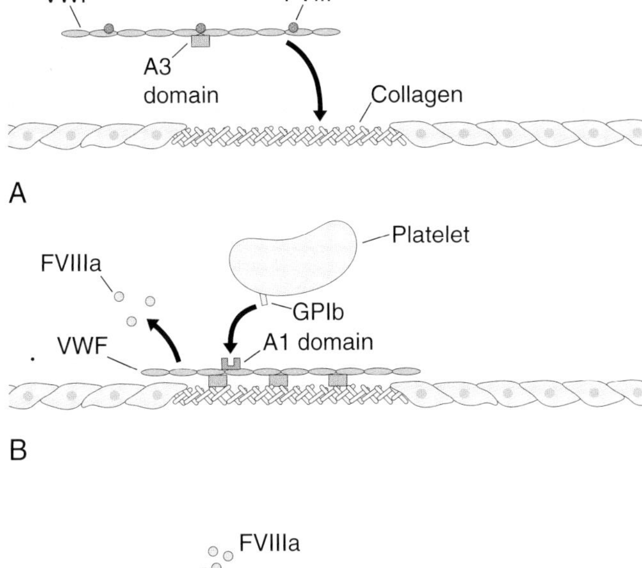

Figure 64–3. Functions of VWF in high-shear conditions. ***A,*** VWF multimer in circulation binds FVIII. At the site of vascular injury, VWF binds to exposed collagen present in the vessel wall via its A3 domain. ***B,*** Once VWF is bound to collagen, the A1 domain becomes exposed and the initial contact of platelets can take place via the interaction of the platelet receptor GPIb-IX-V complex and the A1 domain. VWF binding to collagen induces conformational change, which leads to release of factor VIII and its activation. ***C,*** Platelets become activated and further binding of VWF occurs between the GPIIb/IIIa receptor and the C2 domain of VWF, which mediates spreading of the platelet and firmer adhesion.

centration in patients with VWD results in a defect in fibrin clot formation in addition to VWF abnormalities that affect primary platelet plug formation.

Von Willebrand Disease

Inherited von Willebrand disease has been classified into three types based on clinical laboratory tests and genetic information about the mutations responsible for the disease[53] (Table 64–1). The inheritance is autosomal with variable expressivity and reduced penetrance. Types 1 and 3 result from quantitative deficiency, whereas type 2 is characterized by several qualitative abnormalities of VWF. A database of VWF mutations has been established by the International Society of Thrombosis and Haemostasis (ISTH) and is maintained by the University of Sheffield, UK (*www.Sheffield.ac.uk/vwf*). Over 300 mutations have been reported, and some of the specific mutations that result in VWD have been identified in areas of the gene that code for the known functional domains and would thus be expected to interfere with a particular function (see Fig. 64–2). A French VWD network has also reported several gene defects specific to type 2VWD.[54]

Type 1

The mutations causing type 1VWD are largely undefined. Only 14 gene defects were su bmitted to the ISTH registry as of June 2004; these include two small deletions, one nonsense mutation, and 11 missense mutations (*www.shef.ac.uk/vwf/SSCsummary.html*). It is possible that regulatory sequences outside of the VWF gene may be responsible for most cases of this disorder.[55] Two large studies of type 1VWD, one in Canada and one in Europe, are currently underway and have as goals to define mutations in type 1VWD (*www.shef.ac.uk/euvwd*).[56] Mutations producing decreased levels of VWF protein would result from decreased synthesis or increased clearance. One candidate mutation that has been reported in a few patients with type 1VWD is Cys386→Arg, located within the D3 domain of VWF.[57] This mutation affects cysteine residues and may modify disulfide bond formation between monomers, causing inhibition of multimer assembly and retention of mutant VWF within the cell as a result of defective pairing of the mutant subunit either with another abnormal monomer or with the normal monomer from the second (normal) allele.[58] Defects at other genetic loci may be important, such as a Tyr1584Cys variation in 10 of 70 Canadian families with type 1VWD, which appears to result in increased cellular retention of the VWF protein.[59]

Type 2A

Mutations located in the region encoding the A2 domain are primarily responsible for type 2A VWD.[20,54] These mutations are associated with a decrease in the hemostatically active high- and intermediate-molecular-weight multimers of VWF (Fig. 64–4). Some mutations cause a defect in the intracellular assembly and transport of normal VWF multimers, and others affect a normal cleavage site in VWF, resulting in increased susceptibility to proteolysis.[60–62] All but a few of these mutations occur within a 134–amino acid sequence (Gly742–Glu875) and one mutation, Arg834→Trp, accounts for almost one third of cases.[63,64] Recessive forms of type 2A are caused by mutations within the propeptide, resulting in impaired multimer formation, and by a Cys2011→Arg mutation, which prevents dimerization of VWF subunits.[65]

Type 2B

Four mutations causing type 2B disease occur within a 35–amino acid sequence and account for the majority of patients with this disease variant.[66] The abnormal VWF binds more readily to the platelet GPIb-IX-V receptor; thus, it represents a "gain-of-function" mutation.[67] The increase in binding of larger VWF multimers to platelets results in their loss from the circulation and in thrombocytopenia in some patients, as a result of clearance of the small platelet aggregates that are formed.[68] Type 2B VWD can be differentiated from type 2A by "increased"

TABLE 64–1. Classification of vWD

	Features				
vWD Classification	**Description**	**Inheritance**	**Laboratory Findings**	**Multimer Analysis**	**Prevalence**
Type 1	Partial quantitative deficiency of VWF Mild to moderate phenotype	Autosomal dominant	Parallel reductions in VWF antigen, VWF activity, and factor VIII	Normal distribution	70–80%
Type 2A	Qualitative VWF defect caused by missense mutations within the A2 domain Moderate to severe phenotype	Autosomal dominant	Reduced VWF activity–to-antigen ratio (<0.6)	Loss of mid-sized and highest molecular weight multimers	10–15%
Type 2B	Qualitative VWF defect caused by increased binding to platelet GPIb Moderate to severe phenotype	Autosomal dominant	Reduced VWF activity–to-antigen ratio (<0.6) Abnormal RIPA	Loss of highest molecular weight multimers as a result of binding to platelets and clearance	~5%
Type 2M	Qualitative defects in platelet-VWF interaction	Autosomal dominant	Reduced VWF activity–to-antigen ratio (<0.6)	Normal distribution	Rare
Type 2N	Qualitative defect results in decreased VWF binding of factor VIII Phenotype resembles moderate hemophilia A	Autosomal dominant	Reduced factor VIII level (2–10%)	Normal distribution	Rare
Type 3	Severe quantitative defect of VWF	Autosomal recessive	Marked reductions or absence in VWF levels Low factor VIII (5–10%)	Absent	Rare

Abbreviation: RIPA, ristocetin-induced platelet aggregation.

ristocetin-induced platelet aggregation test, wherein agglutination is present at lower concentrations of ristocetin than seen in normal subjects.

Type 2M

Type 2M VWD is a rare disorder with autosomal dominant inheritance characterized by reduced VWF function in spite of the presence of large multimers, which differentiates it from 2A VWD.[69] The ISTH registry reported 18 mutations causing the defect (*www.shef.ac.uk/euvwd*). The majority of the mutations are located in exon 28, which codes for the GPIb-IX-V–binding site of VWF protein.

Type 2N

Type 2N VWD (N for Normandy, France, where one of the first patients was described) is a rare disorder in which mutations affect the amino-terminus of the mature VWF molecule within the binding site for factor VIII, causing decreased binding to factor VIII.[54,70–72] The mutations occur in the D′ and D3 domains in several areas over the first 91 amino acids of the mature subunit.[73] Affected patients present with low levels of factor VIII (usually 5–15% of normal) as a result of proteolytic cleavage that is usually impeded by its binding to VWF of factor VIII.[74] In comparison to other forms of VWD, the platelet-related functions of VWF are not affected and VWF antigen and multimer patterns are normal. In order to result in a low plasma factor VIII, a type 2N mutation must be present on both alleles (recessive inheritance), or there must be a defect in one allele and another VWF defect on the second allele causing decreased synthesis.

Type 3

Type 3 VWD is a rare disease characterized by a marked decrease or absence of detectable VWF.[75] It is a homozygous or compound heterozygous disorder that can result from different genetic defects, including nonsense, missense, and frameshift mutations; partial or complete deletions; and nondeletion defects resulting in loss of VWF messenger RNA expression.[76,77] The most common identified mutation is a frameshift mutation in exon 18, which has been shown to be the molecular defect in the original family described by von Willebrand.[78]

Platelet-type VWD

This is a rare intrinsic platelet defect resulting from an abnormality caused by missense mutations in the platelet receptor GPIbα gene that result in more avid binding to normal VWF.[79–82] Similar to type 2B VWD, high-molecular-weight VWF multimers are cleared from the circulation with the bound platelets. This disorder is also called pseudo-VWD.[83,84]

CLINICAL FEATURES

Although low laboratory values are common, only a fraction of patients come to medical attention because of bleeding symptoms and are diagnosed as having VWD.

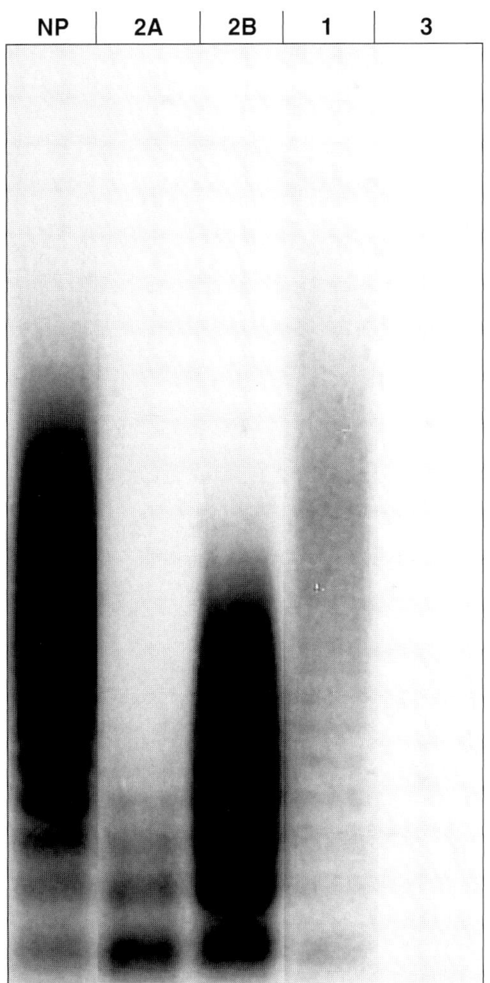

Figure 64–4. vWF multimer analysis. Multimers from plasma of patients with type 1, type 2A, type 2B, and type 3 VWD are shown compared to normal plasma (NP), as analyzed by agarose gel electrophoresis. Type 2A shows absence of high- and intermediate-molecular-weight multimers, and type 2B shows absence of the highest molecular weight multimers, whereas type 1 shows normal multimer distribution with reduced amounts and in type 3 multimers are absent.

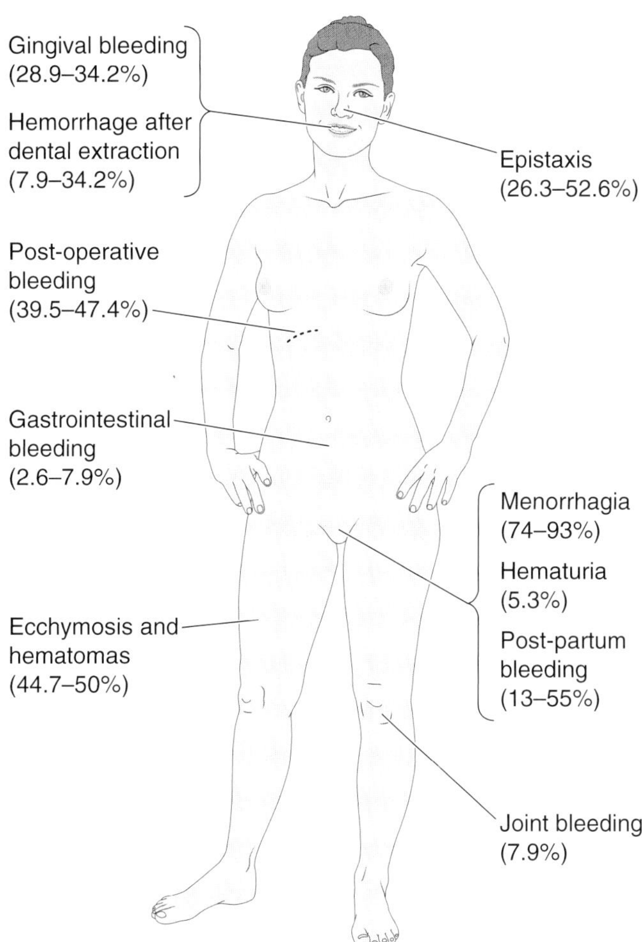

Figure 64–5. Clinical bleeding symptoms by type and frequency (%) in patients with type 1 VWD. (Data from Ragni and colleagues,[137] Kadir and colleagues,[85] Kouides and colleagues,[147] and Ziv O, Ragni M: Bleeding manifestations in males with von Willebrand disease. Haemophilia 10:162–168, 2004.)

This low incidence of bleeding is due to the mild nature of the disease in many patients and to the lack of bleeding challenges and/or lack of recognition of excessive bleeding (e.g., heavy menstrual bleeding) in others. Bleeding symptoms in VWD occur when VWF is decreased in the plasma or platelets, or when a qualitative defect in VWF impairs its functions. These abnormalities mostly affect the primary hemostatic response, resulting in clinical manifestations similar to those seen in other platelet disorders. Commonly seen are easy bruising, skin bleeding, and prolonged bleeding from mucosal surfaces (oropharyngeal, vaginal, and gastrointestinal) (Fig. 64–5).

Type 1 VWD is mostly associated with mild to moderate bleeding diatheses. A typical history in a patient with type 1 VWD includes epistaxis in childhood, lifelong easy bruising, and bleeding with dental extractions or other invasive dental procedures. Approximately 74% of women with VWD have a history of heavy menstrual bleeding[85] and may have bleeding during the peripartum period, often at or within hours of delivery and at 5–10 days after delivery; the bleeding can persist for weeks. Because bleeding from mucosal surfaces is the predominant symptom, patients may have undergone surgical procedures without excessive bleeding. In patients with mild VWD, the ingestion of aspirin or other antiplatelet medications can precipitate bleeding, which may not have otherwise occurred. Some patients remain asymptomatic, and are diagnosed during the course of screening studies because of a family member with VWD.

Bleeding manifestations are more serious and tend to occur earlier in life in patients with type 2 or type 3 VWD. These patients often have symptoms in infancy or when they begin to learn to crawl and walk, as bleeding occurs after the usual minor traumas. Eruption of teeth may also cause bleeding. Affected young women may have life-threatening hemorrhage with their first menstruations. Serious and often recurrent gastrointestinal bleeding can also occur, especially when associated with angiodysplasia.[86] Soft tissue, joint, and urinary bleeding resulting from factor VIII deficiency can occur when there is a marked reduction in plasma factor VIII.[71,87] This occurs in type 2N VWD with a defect in factor VIII binding, or in type 3 with extremely low or absent plasma VWF. Because of the recessive inheritance of type 3 VWD, the phenotype of the parents of these patients is usually a milder bleeding disorder if any.

DIAGNOSIS AND DIFFERENTIAL FEATURES

The patient's personal and family history of bleeding episodes is very important in diagnostic evaluation. Specific questions need to be directed to challenges such as invasive dental procedures, tonsillectomy, and other surgical procedures involving mucous membrane surfaces, as well as menstrual and peripartum bleeding. A negative history does not rule out the diagnosis in patients with a family history of VWD, and symptoms limited to bruising need to be interpreted with caution. There may be a history of excessive bruising or bleeding after the use of aspirin or nonsteroidal anti-inflammatory agents.

Because plasma VWF levels can be increased for physiologic reasons and because of the apparent overlap of VWF levels and nonspecific bleeding symptoms in normal subjects and patients with VWD, it may be difficult to establish the diagnosis of mild VWD. As has been noted, there is a continuum of VWF levels between normal subjects and patients with VWD.[2] The difficulty in distinguishing patients with mild disease from normal subjects is also compounded by the lack of correlation between bleeding symptoms and a specific level of VWF.

In patients with borderline laboratory results, the diagnostic testing should be repeated on two or three occasions, separated by 4–6 weeks, and available family members can be studied.[88] Knowledge of the patient's blood type may be helpful in some cases because normal individuals with type O blood have plasma levels of VWF that are 25–30% lower than those in type A, B, or AB individuals. With VWF levels below 50%, the bleeding tendency has been found to be the same regardless of the blood type, suggesting that the use of ABO-adjusted ranges for VWF levels may not be essential for diagnosis.[89] In individuals with type O blood and moderate reductions in plasma VWF, the presence or absence of a bleeding history and family studies are needed to confirm or exclude a diagnosis of VWD.[90]

A number of physiologic or disease states can influence plasma VWF and factor VIII levels, and must be taken into account when trying to establish a diagnosis of inherited VWD. As an example, thyroid hormone and estrogen promote VWF synthesis.[29] Deficiency of thyroid hormone reduces plasma VWF in both normal subjects and patients with VWD. Conversely, patients with mild VWD who take birth control pills or estrogen replacement therapy may increase their slightly low VWF levels into the normal range. In addition to normal individual variability, plasma VWF and factor VIII are acute-phase reactants, and their levels increase one to three times over baseline during exercise, adrenergic stimulation, inflammatory processes, and pregnancy.[91–94] As a result of this variability, normal ranges for most of these factors are extremely broad, usually in the range of 50–150%.

Laboratory Testing

The laboratory tests used to evaluate and screen for VWD are described in detail in Chapter 105 of this book. These include the prothrombin time, activated partial thromboplastin time, VWF antigen (VWF:Ag), VWF activity as ristocetin cofactor (VWF:RCo) or as collagen binding (VWF:CB) activity, and factor VIII activity (FVIII:C). The VWF levels may vary greatly on laboratory testing in the same subject at different time points.[95]

The bleeding time may be prolonged in VWD and can be helpful with differential diagnosis of platelet disorders. Although the bleeding time does not correlate well with any specific plasma VWF assay or bleeding symptoms, it may be helpful diagnostically if it is abnormal.[96] However, because of low sensitivity and specificity and dependence on the person performing the test, many practitioners have abandoned the use of this test. In general, bleeding time is not recommended as a preoperative screening test because it does not predict the likelihood of excessive bleeding during and after procedures in patients without an underlying bleeding disorder.[97]

Different methods have been developed to assess platelet and VWF function in an automated assay. The most widely studied and used is the PFA-100, where the time to clot formation of anticoagulated whole blood is assessed under flow on a membrane coated with collagen and either ADP (C/ADP) or epinephrine (C/EPI). The PFA-100 has been shown to have varying sensitivity to VWD depending on the subtype and VWF values, with more severely affected individuals more likely to have abnormal values. In use for diagnosis of VWD, Favaloro and colleagues reported a sensitivity of 96.7% (C/EPI) and 76.7% (C/ADP), a specificity of 69.2% (C/EPI) and 90.6% (C/ADP).[98] The value of this test as a screening assay to detect mild VWD, for which the diagnostic evaluation is most challenging, is unclear because false-negative results are seen.[99,100]

Systematic interpretation of the specific laboratory tests will guide the differentiation of the various VWD subtypes, as illustrated in Table 64–1 and by the diagnostic algorithm in Figure 64–6.

TREATMENT

The first step in treatment decisions is to establish an accurate and complete diagnosis of VWD. Because of the variability in bleeding symptoms, the VWD type needs to be considered in the setting of the patient's past bleeding history and response to treatment. In addition, information regarding other medical conditions and medications is needed. Patients should be instructed to avoid aspirin and other nonsteroidal anti-inflammatory drugs with cyclooxygenase-1 inhibitory activity that can

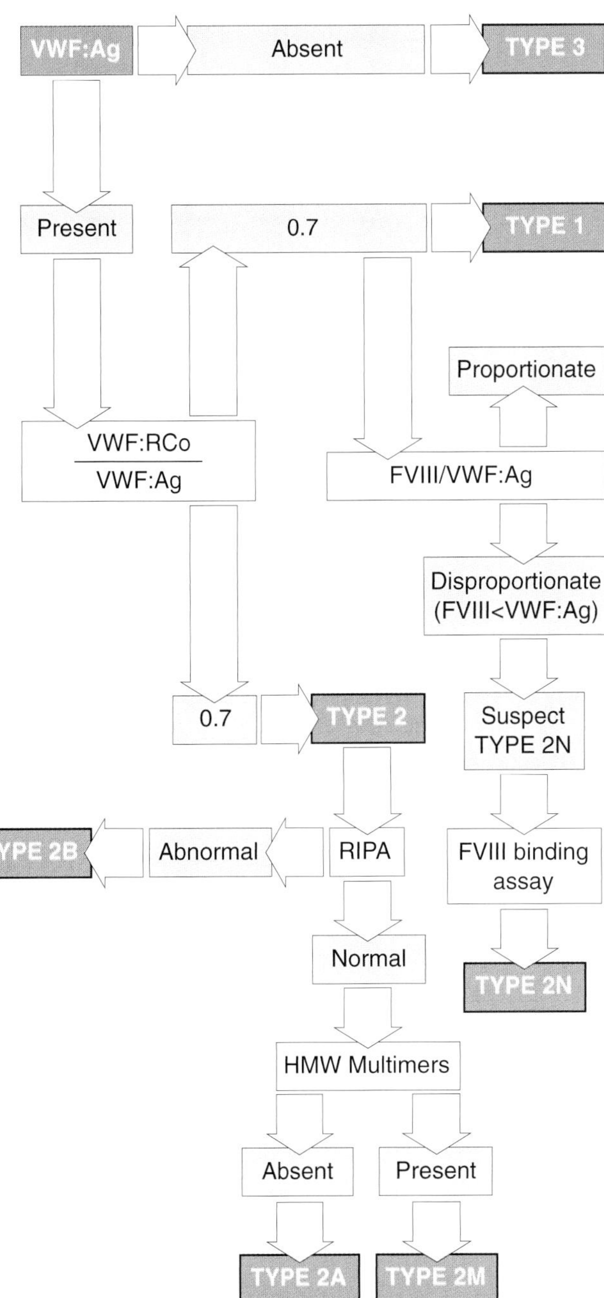

Figure 64–6. Schematic illustration of a diagnostic algorithm for differentiating various VWD subtypes by specific laboratory assays. (Adapted from Siboni SM, Ferrario M, Ferrera C [with the supervision of Federici AB and Mannucci PM]: Von Willebrand Disease, A Complex, Not Complicated Disorder. Milan, Italy: Pragma Editrice, 2002.)

aggravate bleeding symptoms. Rarely, correction of the platelet defect resulting from antiplatelet agents may have to be considered by administering platelet transfusion. DDAVP has been shown to accelerate correction of the in vitro platelet dysfunction induced by antiplatelet agents.[101]

The general goal of therapy in patients with VWD is to correct the dual defect of primary hemostasis and intrinsic coagulation reflected by low levels of VWF and factor VIII coagulant activity.[102,103] There are five classes of specific medications for the treatment of VWD. These include DDAVP, replacement therapy with FVIII/VWF-containing concentrates, antifibrinolytic agents, topical thrombin or fibrin sealant, and estrogen therapy in some settings in women (Table 64–2). Monitoring of the treatment is mostly clinical because there is no laboratory test for VWF that correlates well with bleeding symptoms.[96] In some cases, the VWF:RCo and FVIII levels may be helpful in monitoring response if available in a timely fashion.[104,105]

Desmopressin (DDAVP)

DDAVP, a synthetic analogue of the antidiuretic hormone, increases VWF and factor VIII levels presumably by promoting the release of VWF from endothelial cell storage sites.[34] DDAVP may also have other actions such as enhanced hemostasis in patients with platelet function defects. DDAVP can be administered intravenously, by subcutaneous injection, or by intranasal spray (Stimate). An increase in VWF and factor VIII levels is expected at approximately 30–60 minutes after intravenous infusion, and the effectiveness persists for 6–12 hours.[106] Hemostatic response has been reported with every 24-hour dosing, thus a repeat dose may be given every 12–24 hours.[107] Tachyphylaxis occurs after repeated administration, and, because of the persistent antidiuretic activity, water retention leading to serious hyponatremia can occur.[108,109] Intranasal therapy can be particularly convenient to control excessive menstrual bleeding,[110] frequent epistaxis, or bleeding related to minor surgery or tooth extraction. The peak effect with intranasal administration is at 2 hours.

DDAVP is effective in almost all patients with type 1VWD as well as with many patients with type 2A disease.[111] Although data are limited, DDAVP may also produce a good response in some patients with type 2M VWD.[112] A proportion of these patients with severe bleeding symptoms and marked prolongation of the bleeding time do not respond sufficiently to DDAVP.[113] Because of the variability in response, a trial infusion should be given in advance of a planned procedure to assess the response.[114] In contrast, patients with type 2B disease often have thrombocytopenia as a result of increased binding of the abnormal VWF to platelet GPIb and clearance from the circulation, which can worsen after treatment with DDAVP.[115] The reduction in platelet count is transient, usually normalizing within 2 hours.[116] DDAVP may be considered in type 2B disease with caution and only after a treatment trial has been conducted.[117] Patients with type 2N disease have VWF with impaired binding to factor VIII. An increase in this dysfunctional molecule will not lead to an increase in factor VIII levels, and thus DDAVP treatment is ineffective. DDAVP does not increase VWF levels in patients with type 3VWD because of a lack of VWF in the storage sites and is not recommended in this disorder.[118]

TABLE 64–2. Treatment of VWD

	Treatment				
vWD Type	**Minor Bleeding or Trauma***	**Low-Risk Procedure†**	**Major Bleeding or Trauma‡**	**High-Risk Surgery§**	**Menorrhagia**
Type 1	DDAVP	DDAVP	VWF concentrate (100% correction)	VWF concentrate (100% correction)	Estrogens DDAVP Antifibrinolytic
Type 2A	DDAVP VWF concentrate (50% correction)	DDAVP VWF concentrate	VWF concentrate (100% correction)	VWF concentrate (100% correction)	Estrogens DDAVP Antifibrinolytic
Type 2B	VWF concentrate (50% correction)	VWF concentrate	VWF concentrate (100% correction) Platelets	VWF concentrate (100% correction) Platelets	Estrogens Antifibrinolytic
Type 2M	DDAVP VWF concentrate (50% correction)	DDAVP VWF concentrate	VWF concentrate (100% correction)	VWF concentrate (100% correction)	Estrogens DDAVP Antifibrinolytic
Type 2N	VWF concentrate (50% correction)	VWF concentrate	VWF concentrate (100% correction)	VWF concentrate (100% correction)	Estrogens Antifibrinolytic VWF concentrate
Type 3	VWF concentrate (100% correction)	VWF concentrate	VWF concentrate (100% correction)	VWF concentrate (100% correction)	VWF concentrate Antifibrinolytic

*Epistaxis, mouth and gum bleeds, superficial lacerations, and skin bleeds.
†Dental cleaning, skin biopsy, vaccination, and local anesthesia injection.
‡Bleeding in the head, neck, throat, abdomen, pelvis, spine, iliopsoas, or hip; compartment bleeds; fractures or dislocations; deep lacerations; and serious trauma.
§Wisdom tooth extractions (when multiple or impacted); abdominal, thoracic, or spinal surgery; and neurosurgery.

VWF/FVIII Concentrates

Replacement therapy with VWF is indicated in the treatment of patients with types 3 and 2N VWD and in other subtypes with more severe phenotype. It is also indicated in some patients with type 1 VWD undergoing major procedures, in whom it is important that hemostasis be maintained for several days. VWF-containing factor replacement is also indicated in patients with type 1 VWD who have moderately low levels of VWF, in more serious bleeding situations, with major trauma or surgery, or when other measures fail (see Table 64–2). Several products are available that contain VWF in high concentration, including "intermediate-purity" plasma-derived VWF-containing factor VIII concentrates and more highly purified VWF concentrates. A recombinant VWF product is in development.[119] Unless there is no other option, treatment with cryoprecipitate is not recommended at the present time because of the potential risk of viral transmission.

One of the intermediate-purity factor VIII concentrates, Humate-P, is approved by the Food and Drug Administration for use in the United States for treatment of VWD. It is labeled with ristocetin cofactor activity units, and studies of its efficacy in patients with VWD have been published.[120–122] Two similar products, Alphanate Solvent-Detergent and Alphanate Solvent Detergent/Heat Treated, have been studied in a prospective trial, which documented efficacy of the concentrates in patients with VWD undergoing invasive procedures.[123] These products are not labeled for VWF activity units and have not been approved for this use in the United States.

Several other high-purity factor products are available in Europe. LFB-VWF, a very-high-purity VWF concentrate, is produced in France and contains a much higher ratio of VWF activity to factor VIII (approximately 10:1), compared to Humate-P (approximately 2.5:1).[124] Another concentrate, BPL-8Y, is manufactured in the United Kingdom and approved for use there.[125] Recombinant human VWF, which contains a full spectrum of multimers as well as adequate levels of VWF activity and antigen, has been produced in CHO cells. When tested in dogs with VWD, there was good recovery of VWF with the expected hemostatic effects.[126] Recombinant VWF has not yet been studied in humans.

Recommendations for replacement doses of VWF are empirical because no laboratory test adequately predicts the hemostatic effects. The dose given is also dependent upon the site and the degree of bleeding. In general, the goal is to maintain the activity of factor VIII and of VWF between 50% and 100% for 3–10 days for more serious bleeding or major surgery. The infusion of 40–60 IU/kg of ristocetin cofactor activity as labeled on these concentrates raises the plasma concentration to 50–100% (0.5–1.0 U/mL).[127,128] Patients with severe VWD who have mucous membrane bleeding, particularly gastrointestinal bleeding, may require higher replacement doses of VWF (80–100%). If bleeding in severe VWD is not controlled by VWF replacement therapy, patients may benefit from platelet transfusions.[129] The intermediate-purity factor VIII concentrates and higher purity VWF concentrates are pasteurized, dry-heat treated, or solvent-detergent treated to reduce the risk of transmission of viruses such as hepatitis viruses and human immunodeficiency virus. There appears to be a small risk of venous thromboembolism when intermediate-purity factor VIII concentrates are used in high doses as replacement therapy during perioperative periods or for gastrointestinal bleeding.[130] In some of these cases, a high factor VIII level (>200%) may have contributed to the thrombosis. Therefore, factor VIII concentrations should be followed on a daily basis to avoid levels in excess of 200%.[130]

Antifibrinolytic Agents

Antifibrinolytic therapy, including ε-aminocaproic acid (EACA; Amicar) and tranexamic acid (Cyclokapron), has been used to prevent dissolution of the hemostatic plug that is formed, particularly in mucous membrane areas. These drugs can be used as sole therapy in cases of mild bleeding or as an adjunct to other medications. Both drugs can be given orally or intravenously; however, the oral formulation of tranexamic acid is not available in the United States. For intravenous dosing, EACA can be given as a continuous infusion of 1 gm/hr, with a maximum dose of 24 gm/day. A loading dose of 4 gm given over an hour will hasten the effect. When given orally, antifibrinolytic agents must be given repeatedly over a 24-hour period because of their short half-lives (particularly EACA), and the dose must be adjusted in patients with renal insufficiency. EACA is usually given four times daily in a dose of 50–100 mg/kg (maximum 24 gm in 24 hours), and tranexamic acid is given two to three times daily in a dose of 15–25 mg/kg. When administered for epistaxis, dental procedures, or other similar procedures, the agents are given for periods varying from 3 to 7 days.[131] Antifibrinolytic medications are relatively contraindicated in upper urinary tract bleeding.

Topical agents are most often used for nasal or oral bleeding. These include micronized collagen (Avitene), fibrin sealant, and Gelfoam or Surgicel soaked in topical thrombin, which can be applied to local areas of bleeding.[132] Exposures to topical bovine thrombin carry a risk of antibody formation against bovine factor V that is present in the thrombin preparations, leading to bleeding complications because the antibodies can cross-react with human factor V.[133]

Recombinant FVIIa

Several authors have reported the successful use of recombinant factor VIIa in the treatment of patients with type 3 VWD who develop alloantibodies to VWF after receiving replacement therapy with VWF.[134,135] Factor VIIa bypasses the need for factor VIII and, for reasons not entirely understood, may also enhance platelet function in patients with intrinsic platelet disorders.[136,137]

WOMEN AND VWD

Management of Menorrhagia

Menorrhagia is the most common and often the initial symptom in women with VWD, many of whom have bleeding during and after delivery, with cesarean section, or with gynecologic procedures. Menorrhagia is evident at menarche in 60–93% of women with VWD, significantly influencing morbidity and quality of life, and the risk of postpartum hemorrhage is high in women with inherited bleeding disorders.[138–140] It is recommended that adolescents and adult women presenting with severe menorrhagia should be screened for VWD, and that hysterectomy should not be performed before consideration of bleeding disorders.[141] Women with VWD should be followed in hemophilia treatment centers to best coordinate their care.

The use of estrogen therapy for menorrhagia in patients with VWD was suggested by the incidental observation that three women with type 1 disease had significantly less bleeding and improved hemostasis when they took estrogen (either for oral contraception or prevention of menopausal symptoms).[142] Estrogen acts at least in part by increasing the synthesis of VWF,[28] but also by the physiologic effect on menstruation. Thus, higher estrogen-containing preparations are not necessarily more effective. DDAVP can be used in patients with type 1 and 2A VWD during the first days of the menstrual period; intranasal administration is often effective and convenient.[143–145] Antifibrinolytic agents have also been found effective.[146] In women without defined bleeding disorders, tranexamic acid has been documented to decrease menstrual blood flow by 45% when given as a 1-gm dose four times a day on days 1–4 of menstruation.[147] A lower dose may also be effective, and a combination of treatments may be needed because no single approach will be effective in all patients.[148]

VWD and Pregnancy

Treatment is not needed during pregnancy in the majority of women with VWD (see Fig. 64–7 for decision algorithm). During the second and third trimesters of pregnancy, there is decreased bleeding tendency as a result of an increase in the levels of VWF to two to three times baseline; however, the qualitative abnormalities in type 2 VWD will persist and thrombocytopenia in type 2B VWD may worsen.[149,150] Because the VWF concentration drops shortly after the delivery, the postpartum period is often associated with significant bleeding complications,[151,152] and primary or secondary postpartum hemorrhage may occur. The average time of onset for secondary hemorrhage in women with VWD is from 11 to 23 days postpartum. Thus, DDAVP or VWF replacement therapy may be required shortly after and/or sometime in the first 2–4 weeks after delivery. DDAVP may be problematic prior to delivery because it has a theoretical possibility of initiating contractions, although adverse effects of administering it just before delivery have not been reported.[152] In practice, VWD treatment with DDAVP prior to delivery is rarely indicated because levels usually normalize by the third trimester in women with type 1 disease. Therefore, the VWF levels should be checked before pregnancy and again at the third trimester, and, if still low, therapy for the delivery as well as postpartum would be indicated (see Fig. 64–7).

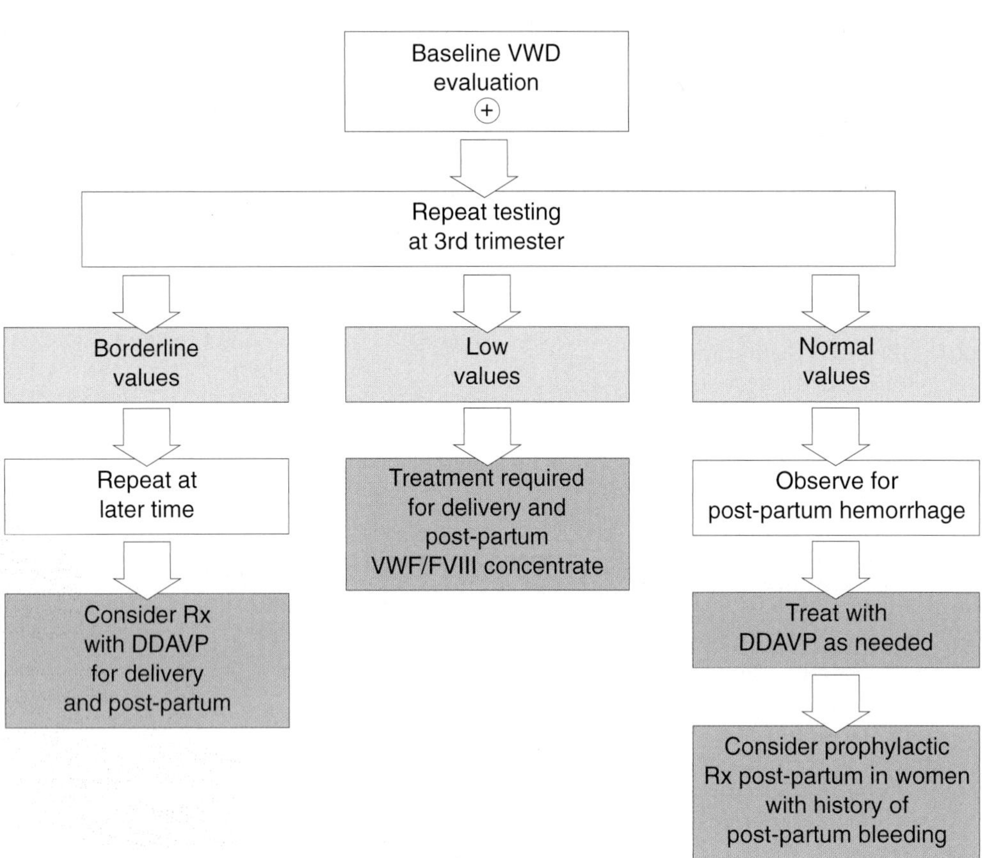

Figure 64–7. Schematic illustration of a treatment algorithm for VWD and pregnancy.

Knowledge of the woman's type of VWD, activity of factor VIII and VWF, response to DDAVP, and past bleeding episodes is useful for guiding peripartum therapy.[103]

For patients with low third-trimester VWF or factor VIII levels, an early anesthesia consultation should be obtained prior to the onset of labor to discuss options for regional anesthesia or analgesia. Low factor VIII appears to be the most important determinant of increased bleeding during delivery.[147] It is generally recommended that factor VIII levels be at or above 50% for a cesarean section.[153] Cesarean section should be reserved for the usual obstetric indications because the risk of fetal intraventricular hemorrhage caused by fetal VWD is rare.[154] In families with moderate and severe types of VWD, elective neonatal procedures (e.g., circumcision) should be delayed until the infant's VWD status had been determined.

ACQUIRED VON WILLEBRAND SYNDROME

Acquired VWD or von Willebrand syndrome is associated with a number of different disease states and is caused by several different pathophysiologic mechanisms.[155–157] These include antibody formation, proteolysis, binding to tumor cells with increased clearance, and decreased synthesis. Acquired VWD is most frequently described in patients with clonal lymphoproliferative and autoimmune diseases (e.g., systemic lupus erythematosus), some of whom have demonstrable antibodies to VWF.[158,159]

In some instances, plasma antibodies to VWF have been demonstrated by mixing studies of the suspect patient plasma and normal plasma, showing an inhibition of VWF in a functional assay, and by localization of the inhibitory activity to the immunoglobulin G fraction.[160,161] In a number of cases, the antibody is apparent only after warming of the patient's plasma to disrupt immune complexes.[162] In others, the antibody is functionally neutral but binds to VWF, causing increased clearance of VWF. The antibody may not be demonstrable in functional assays because much of it is cleared via immune complexes, but it can be demonstrated by enzyme-linked immunosorbent assay binding or immunoblotting. Analysis of the multimeric structure of the patient's VWF often shows a decrease in the high-molecular-weight multimers in both immune and nonimmune acquired VWD. This observation suggests that antibodies, if present, may have a higher affinity for the larger multimers and/or that the larger multimers may be more susceptible to degradation and clearance by either immune, proteolytic, or shear mechanisms.[163,164]

Nonimmune mechanisms have also been described in patients with acquired VWD:VWF may be adsorbed onto tumor cells (e.g., in Wilms' tumor, multiple myeloma, and Waldenström's macroglobulinemia).[165,166] VWF multimers may be degraded by proteolytic enzymes such as plasmin during accelerated fibrinolysis in decompensated cirrhosis, pancreatitis, and disseminated intravascular coagulation, or in patients receiving thrombolytic therapy. It may also be degraded by elastase-like enzymes derived from myeloid elements in myeloproliferative disorders.[167,168] High-molecular-weight VWF multimers may be reduced or absent from the plasma in patients with noncyanotic congenital heart disease, high-grade aortic stenosis, and angiodysplasia, perhaps as a result of binding of VWF and platelet adhesion and/or aggregation at sites of high shear forces. Although some of these patients may have a bleeding tendency, there does not appear to be increased bleeding in the majority.[164,169] VWF levels may be reduced in hypothyroidism. A small percentage of these patients have a bleeding diathesis, which can be reversed with thyroid replacement therapy.[170] Pharmacologic agents such as dextrans, hydroxyethyl starch, and valproic acid have been implicated as agents causing acquired VWD.[171–173]

An inverse relationship has been observed between platelet counts and large VWF multimers in many patients with myeloproliferative diseases, and it has been suggested that increasing numbers of platelets circulating in blood result in increased removal of large VWF multimers from plasma. The decrease in high-molecular-weight multimers may be responsible, at least in part, for the bleeding tendency seen in patients with thrombocytosis associated with myeloproliferative diseases. The relationship between increased platelet counts and decreased large VWF multimers has also been documented to occur in one study in patients with reactive thrombocytosis, but this remains controversial.[174,175]

Treatment of Acquired VWD

Treatment of acquired VWD depends in part upon the pathogenetic mechanism and the severity of bleeding symptoms.[176] Treatment of the underlying condition may result in VWF levels improving or returning to normal, and should be pursued in those cases in which treatment is feasible. Treatment of bleeding or prophylaxis for invasive procedures usually involves VWF-containing concentrates or DDAVP for minor bleeds or procedures.[152,176,177] The response to replacement therapy can be erratic and transient, especially in patients with circulating inhibitors of VWF and in patients with extremely low values. Thus, frequent monitoring of factor VIII and VWF levels during treatment is indicated.[177] Patients with circulating inhibitors will require higher doses of VWF, and the dose requirements may change if the factor is needed over several days or weeks. Antifibrinolytic therapy can be used for minor bleeding, for dental or other mucosal procedures, and in combination with other modalities.

High-dose intravenous immunoglobulin at a dose of 1 gm/kg/day for 2 days may restore normal VWF levels for several days and has been used in patients with acquired VWD associated with autoimmune disease or a monoclonal gammopathy. It acts at least in part by increasing the half-life of circulating VWF[178] and may be successful in patients who do not respond to DDAVP.[179] Recombinant factor VIIa may have some effectiveness in life-threatening situations.[180] Other treatments that are less often used include plasmapheresis, extracorporeal immunoadsorption, and immunosuppressive medications for the underlying disease (e.g., corticosteroids for systemic lupus erythematosus).[181] The treatment of underlying disorders is the goal, while bleeding symptoms should be managed with DDAVP, factor VIII/VWF concentrates and high-dose intravenous immunoglobulin depending on the nature of bleeding and responsiveness to treatment.

Current Controversies & Future Considerations

Von Willebrand Disease

- Mild decreases in VWF levels may be better viewed as a risk factor for bleeding than a disease.
- Genetic and environmental factors that modulate VWF levels are only partially defined.
- There is a poor correlation between VWF levels and bleeding symptoms; better predictors of bleeding risk are needed.
- Whether VWD protects from atherosclerotic cardiovascular disease or other thrombotic conditions is not known.
- The optimal dosing of plasma-derived VWF/FVIII concentrates for bleeding episodes and for prophylaxis has not been determined.
- Future treatment options include recombinant VWF product, which is under clinical development. In addition, interleukin-11 has been shown to increase plasma levels of factor VIII and VWF in preclinical studies.

Suggested Readings*

Mannucci PM: Treatment of von Willebrand's disease. N Engl J Med 351:683–694, 2004.

Rick ME, Walsh CE, Key NS: Congenital bleeding disorders. *In* Broudy VC, Prchal JT, Tricot GJ (eds): Hematology 2003, American Society of Hematology Education Program Book. Washington, DC: American Society of Hematology, 2003 , pp 559–574.

Roque H, Funai E, Lockwood CJ: von Willebrand disease and pregnancy. J Matern Fetal Med 9:257–266, 2000.

Sadler JE, Mannucci PM, Berntorp E, et al: Impact, diagnosis and treatment of von Willebrand disease. Thromb. Haemost. 84:160–174, 2000.

von Willebrand disease: a guideline from the UK Haemophilia Centre Doctors' Organization. Haemophilia 10:199–231, 2004.

Full references for this chapter can be found on accompanying CD-ROM.

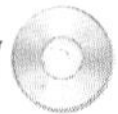

CHAPTER 65

Acquired Inhibitors to Clotting Factors

Sabah Sallah, MD, and Jean-Marie Saint-Remy, MD, PhD

KEY POINTS

Acquired Inhibitors to Clotting Factors

Diagnosis

- An inhibitor to factor VIII should be suspected in any patient presenting with spontaneous or posttraumatic soft tissue, skin, or any type of life-threatening hemorrhage. Patients almost always deny prior serious bleeding history.
- A prolonged activated partial thromboplastin time (aPTT) that does not correct in mixing studies with low or undetectable factor VIII level is diagnostic of an inhibitor. Although the lupus anticoagulant is often included in the differential diagnosis of a prolonged aPTT, it should be emphasized that patients with the lupus anticoagulant are much more likely to present with thrombotic rather than bleeding episodes. A baseline inhibitor titer against human and porcine factor VIII should be obtained in every newly diagnosed patient with inhibitor to factor VIII.
- An underlying malignancy is an increasingly recognized condition in patients with acquired hemophilia. However, extensive search for a malignancy, unless indicated by clinical examination, laboratory tests, and imaging studies obtained to assess or follow up the course of the patient with an acquired inhibitor, is not indicated at this time.

Management

- Administer intravenous fluids and red blood cells as required. Label the chart as acquired hemophilia and alert the staff against using aspirin, nonsteroidal anti-inflammatory drugs, antiplatelet agents, and heparin.
- In patients with severe hemorrhage (drop $\geq$ 2 gm/dL in hemoglobin or any critical bleed), administer 90 μg/kg recombinant activated factor VII (rFVIIa) and repeat every 3 hours. Porcine factor VIII (100 U/kg), if available, and factor VIII inhibitor bypassing activity (FEIBA; 75–100 U/kg) are both acceptable alternatives.
- In patients with less severe bleeding, administer either rFVIIa, porcine factor VIII, or FEIBA.
- Assess factor VIII level and Bethesda titer every 48 hours if possible until the acute bleeding episode is under control.
- Start prednisone with or without cyclophosphamide immediately and follow factor VIII level and Bethesda titer periodically.

ACQUIRED INHIBITORS AGAINST FACTOR VIII

Introduction

The term *acquired inhibitor* implies the spontaneous appearance of an autoantibody against a coagulation factor. The most common acquired inhibitors are by far those targeted against factor VIII. The formation of an inhibitor that interferes with factor VIII clotting activity leads to bleeding diathesis, prolonged activated partial thromboplastin time (aPTT), and low to undetectable plasma factor VIII activity. Because of the absence of past bleeding history, the condition is often referred to as acquired hemophilia. With the exception of postpartum inhibitors, the average age of the patients with acquired hemophilia is 61.5 years.[1–5] Another clinical feature that characterizes acquired hemophilia is the predominance of soft tissue hemorrhage in contrast to the hemarthroses most often observed in patients with congenital hemophilia.[2,3,5] Acquired hemophilia should be differentiated from disseminated intravascular coagulation (DIC) by the presence of prolonged aPTT that does not correct with mixing studies and the normal fibrinogen and D-dimer. Appropriate tests should be performed to rule out the presence of antiphospholipid antibodies.

Epidemiology and Associated Conditions

Incidence

Acquired hemophilia is a rare disease with an estimated incidence of 1 case in 500,000 to 1 million persons.[1,6,7] However, this figure should be approached with caution because of the relatively few large studies addressing the frequency of this disorder. Interestingly, antibodies against factor VIII were described in 17% of 500 plasma samples from healthy donors.[8] The titer of antibody in these healthy individuals ranged between 0.4 and 2.0 Bethesda units (BU), whereas the mean factor VIII level did not differ between those with and without the antibody.[8] The inhibitors in this case may be similar to other natural antibodies that are directed against several serum proteins and rarely lead to clinical complications. Overall, there is no clear gender or race predominance in patients diagnosed with acquired hemophilia.

Underlying Conditions

Traditionally, it has been thought that at least half of the patients with acquired hemophilia have no recognizable illness.[1] However, an increased number of individuals with acquired inhibitors to factor VIII and underlying cancer and other medical disorders have been reported in the past few years, causing a slight shift in the distribution of associated conditions (Table 65–1).[9–18] In a recent report, the most common malignancies diagnosed in patients with acquired hemophilia were prostate cancer, chronic lymphocytic leukemia, and lung cancer.[9] Approximately 50% of these patients had advanced or metastatic disease. Postpartum inhibitors to factor VIII usually appear within 3 months and as late as 12 months after delivery.[2,19–22] A small number of inhibitors have been diagnosed during the pregnancy period. Although all types of autoimmune disorders have been described in patients with acquired hemophilia, systemic lupus erythematosus appears to be the most commonly observed in this setting.[1–5] The formation of autoantibodies against factor VIII has been described after the administration of a host of medications, including penicillin, sulfa, phenytoin, ciprofloxacin, interferon alfa, and fludarabine.[1–5,23,24]

TABLE 65–1. Common Medical Conditions Encountered in Patients with Acquired Hemophilia

Associated Conditions	Percentage
Idiopathic	38
Malignancy	17.5
Autoimmune	15
Postpartum	10
Skin disease	4.5
Drug reaction	2
Others*	13

*Other conditions include chronic medical disorders such as asthma, hypertension, diabetes, and congestive heart failure. However, it is not certain whether these conditions are directly responsible for the appearance of the antibody.

It is not clear whether the underlying disorders reported in patients with acquired hemophilia are directly responsible for the appearance of the inhibitors. The presence of these autoantibodies may represent dysregulation of the immune systems, idiosyncratic reaction, or an epiphenomenon rather than a causal association.

Pathophysiology

Tolerance

Tolerance to self-proteins is established centrally in the thymus for T cells and in the bone marrow for B cells. However, this is not an on-off phenomenon, and the immune system has to find a compromise between maintaining the capacity to react to any foreign antigen it could encounter and reducing the risk of self protein recognition. A brief overview is presented of the mechanisms by which tolerance is established and maintained in the periphery, to help understand how and why tolerance can be broken, with special emphasis on coagulation factor VIII.

Central Tolerance

T cells are educated in the thymus, in which they are exposed to self-antigens. Such an exposure occurs in the form of complexes between stretches of amino acids bound to major histocompatibility complex (MHC) class II molecules. The source of self-antigen iszthreefold. First, soluble antigens are trapped for presentation by epithelial cells in the thymus medulla. Second, bone marrow–derived antigen-presenting cells (APCs) are known to migrate to the thymus for presentation of self-antigens to T cells. Third, local transcription of antigen occurs through activation of autoimmunity regulator.[25] In addition to these mechanisms, self-reactive T cells have a last chance to escape deletion by editing or revising their T-cell receptor (TCR), processes by which they can lose their capacity to react with self-antigen.

Obviously, antigens that are not presented by one of these mechanisms (e.g., because they are sequestered) do not elicit self-reactive T-cell elimination. However, such elimination requires sufficient TCR avidity; low-avidity T cells are not deleted. Furthermore, inefficient MHC class II presentation of the self-antigen will also allow T cells to escape deletion, as will presentation of an antigen isoform different from the physiologic one.

The thymus has another function, which is to select natural regulatory $CD4^+$ T cells, which are characterized by expression of glucocorticoid-induced tumor necrosis factor receptor–related protein and CD25. The selection of regulatory T cells depends on the activation of transcription factor Foxp3. The function of the thymus gradually disappears with age in humans. At birth, the peripheral pool of "educated" T cells is replenished, which stands in contrast with the situation in mouse.

B cells are sorted out for self-reactivity in the bone marrow. High-avidity recognition results in apoptosis. However, as many as 50% of self-reactive B cells can undergo B-cell receptor (BCR) editing, which affects both the heavy and the light chains. Unsuccessful editing leads to apoptosis, and B cells then transit to the spleen. Three populations can be distinguished. Follicular B cells are highly T-cell dependent for activation, somatic mutation, class switch recombination, and affinity maturation. Activation occurs via BCR engagement. This is the population of B cells that carries memory. In addition, two other populations of B cells have been described. Marginal-zone B cells are activated by BCR cross-linking and noncognate interaction with T cells, which is dispensable. B1 cells also require BCR cross-linking for activation and are fully independent of T-cell help. Interestingly, marginal-zone B cells and B1 cells are preferentially recruited when antigen is administered by the intravenous route.

Peripheral Tolerance

Figures 65–1 and 65–2 depict the main mechanisms by which tolerance is maintained in the periphery. For the sake of clarity, intrinsic and extrinsic mechanisms are separated. In Figure 65–1, mechanisms operating at the T- and B-cell levels are shown facing each other, illustrating what they have in common. These intrinsic mechanisms are mediated through the antigen-specific receptor, TCR or BCR.[26–28] Basic principles rely on simple rules: absent or too weak receptor recognition results in ignorance. Recognition in absence of sufficient costimulation drives T cells to anergy, which, in B cells, is obtained by either BCR destabilization[29] or interaction with negatively signaling receptors.[30] Specific lymphocyte deletion is the result of hyperstimulation. The capacity of B and T cells to edit or revise their antigen receptor in the periphery offers yet another mechanism by which unresponsiveness can be established.[31–33]

Extrinsic mechanisms deal with intervention of regulatory T cells,[34] either from the natural repertoire selected in the thymus, or from adaptation of T cells in the periphery. The number and characteristics of subpopulations of T cells endowed with regulatory properties are as yet not entirely defined and are a matter of current research.[35] Figure 65–2 provides an overview of the three main subsets of adaptive regulatory T cells as established today.[36] The role of dendritic cells has only recently emerged and is expected to evolve rapidly.[37] For the time being, two subsets of such cells have been functionally defined, as depicted in Figure 65–2.

Mechanisms Leading to Autoimmunity

The diagram presented in Figure 65–3 does not intend to review all possible mechanisms through which an autoimmune reaction could occur, but rather to provide a logical approach to understand how autoantibodies can be elicited to coagulation factors. As reviewed previously, a tolerance state results from equilibrium between APCs presenting self-peptides in a tolerogenic way and specific T cells kept in a state of unresponsiveness. Events that will disrupt this equilibrium at the APC and/or the T-cell level have the potential to trigger an autoimmune response. Genetic factors leading to predisposition to autoimmunity are not included in Figure 65–3. Potentially any gene regulating B-cell or T-cell activation could be involved. However, apart from the classical examples of single-gene deletion, such as Fas ligand deficiency, predisposition to autoimmunity most likely relies on complex interactions of numerous genes, which are far from being fully understood.

Characteristics of Factor VIII Autoantibodies

The factor VIII molecule consists of a large heterodimer made of a heavy and a light chain, as shown in Figure 65–4. Using mouse and human monoclonal antibodies, at least 10 nonoverlapping epitopes have been identified that are spread over the entire factor VIII molecule, with the exception of the B domain.

However, not all antibodies inhibit the function of factor VIII. Inhibitor antibodies recognize sites that are directly or indirectly involved in either factor VIII activation or factor VIII interaction with coagulation factors required for the formation of the tenase complex (factor IX, factor X, phospholipids). Inhibitor antibodies also frequently inhibit the binding of factor VIII to its chaperone protein, von Willebrand factor, thereby reducing factor VIII stability. At least some of the antibodies that recognize sites distant from functional epitopes could play a role in the clearance of the factor VIII molecule.

Autoantibodies to factor VIII can be observed in the general context of autoimmune diseases or as an unexpected occurrence in otherwise healthy individuals. Risk factors for autoimmunity are numerous and are described elsewhere.[38] Attempts to identify factors that underpin the susceptibility to inhibitor formation in healthy individuals have been scarce. Thus, MHC class II haplotypes are only loosely associated with such risk, possibly because of the large size of the factor VIII molecule and/or the promiscuous nature of T-cell epitopes.[39] Recently, a preferential recruitment of VH1 gene products in the formation of antibodies to the C2 domain has been described.[40] Whether this is linked to a yet to be defined genetic susceptibility, or to the physicochemical characteristics of antibodies carrying VH1 is still to be determined.

Autoantibodies to factor VIII appear late in life. They are thought to emerge from the activation of a small number of B-cell clones, but this is likely to vary according to the underlying disease, when present. Autoantibodies, like alloantibodies, usually belong to the immunoglobulin (Ig)G isotype, although monoclonal IgM and IgA autoantibodies have also been described.[41–43] The isotype determination of specific antibodies has demonstrated the large predominance of IgG4 antibodies with, in some cases, an accompanying IgG1. The same trend is observed with alloantibodies, although in this case IgG2 antibodies can also be found.

Inhibitors to factor VIII are subdivided into two categories depending upon the kinetics of factor VIII inactivation. Type I are high-affinity antibodies that completely inhibit factor VIII function in a dose-dependent manner, and type II antibodies follow a more complex mechanism, with only incomplete factor VIII inhibition,

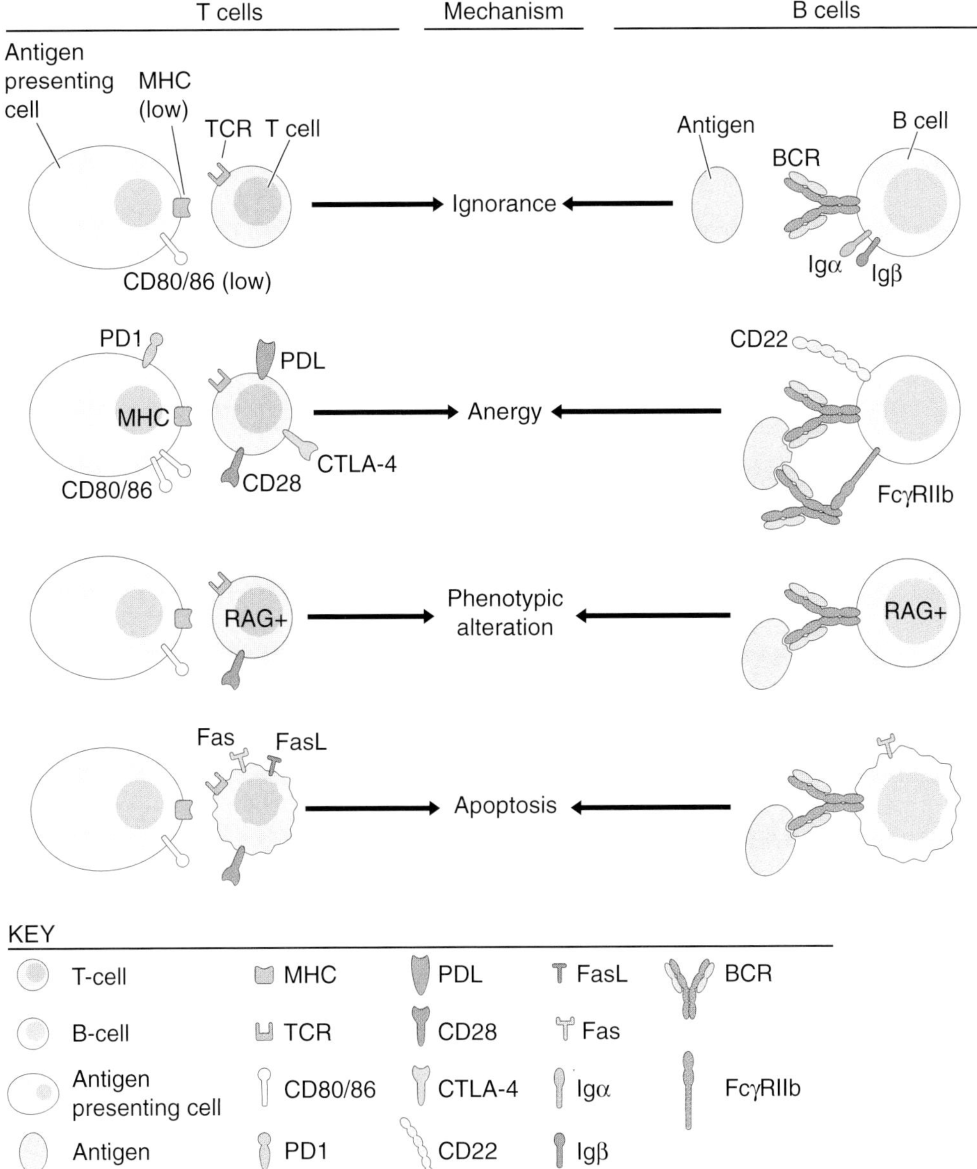

Figure 65–1. Intrinsic mechanisms of peripheral tolerance at the T- and B-cell level. *Left,* Autoreactive T cells are maintained in an unresponsive state or deleted in the periphery by a number of intrinsic mechanisms. Four non–mutually exclusive intrinsic mechanisms have been described:

1. *Ignorance:* T cells do not encounter antigen because of sequestration or are exposed to antigen at a concentration that is too low to trigger activation.
2. *Anergy:* T cells recognize antigen in the context of MHC class II determinants but without appropriate secondary signal costimulation or with secondary signaling through cytotoxic T-lymphocyte antigen-4 (CTLA-4) or PD-1.
3. *Phenotypic alteration:* T cells are activated but alter their phenotype toward a nonpathogenic one by changing the pattern of secreted cytokines (T_H1/T_H2 skewing), revising or editing TCRs through gene rearrangement, changing the avidity threshold required for activation, or altering chemokine receptors and trafficking.
4. *Apoptosis:* T cells upregulate surface Fas and FasL upon activation, which results in the cell committing suicide.

Right, Likewise, four non–mutually exclusive intrinsic mechanisms maintain peripheral B-cell unresponsiveness or delete self-reactive B cells:

1. *Ignorance:* Antigens with insufficient avidity or limited access to BCRs are ignored.
2. *Anergy:* B-cell activation is inhibited by signals transduced through CD22 and/or FCγRII binding or by BCR destabilization by low-affinity antigen.
3. *Phenotypic alteration:* BCR editing and revision occur in the periphery, altering antigen specificity and preventing deletion.
4. *Apoptosis:* Upregulation of Fas at the surface of activated B cells can result in deletion by FasL-bearing cells.

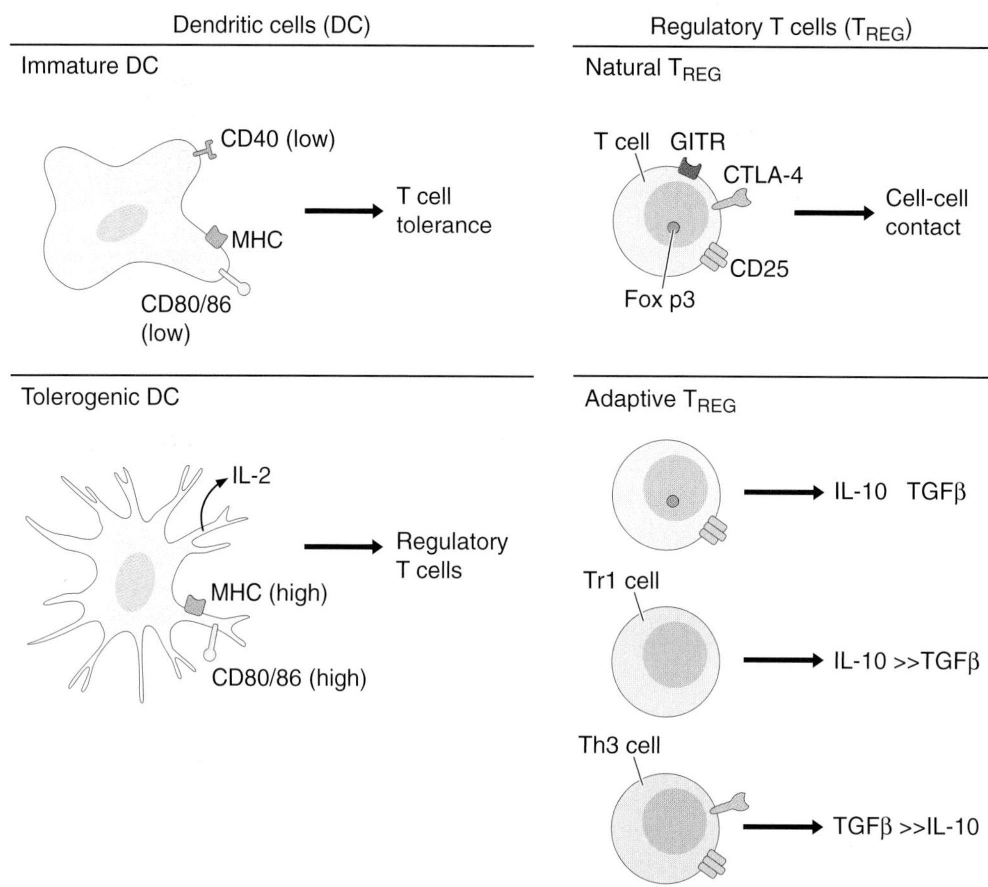

Figure 65–2. Extrinsic mechanisms of peripheral tolerance at the T-cell level. In addition to intrinsic mechanisms, tolerance can be induced in $CD4^+$ T cells by antigen-presenting cells and/or regulatory T cells:

1. Presentation of self-antigens by immature dendritic cells expressing low levels of costimulatory molecules, or by tolerogenic dendritic cells inducing regulatory T cells.
2. Natural regulatory T cells (Treg) are actively selected in the thymus; they are characterized by surface expression of CD25, cytotoxic T-lymphocyte antigen-4 (CTLA-4), and glucocorticoid-induced tumor necrosis factor receptor–related protein (GITR) and by activation of the transcription suppressor Fox p3. They regulate $CD4^+$ T cells by direct cell-cell contact and induction of tryptophan catabolism in target cells.
3. Different subsets of adaptive regulatory T cells have been described according to antigen dose, frequency, and route of administration. Adaptive $CD25^+$ Treg carry the phenotype $CTLA\text{-}4^-GITR^-$; they are generated by exposure to transforming growth factor-β (TGF-β) and exert their activity by secreting suppressive cytokines (interleukin [IL-10] and TGF-β) and by target cell lysis. Tr1 are induced in the presence of IL-10 and produce both TGF-β and IL-10. T_H3 cells are induced by oral administration of antigen and produce mainly TGF-β.

even when present in large molar excess[44] (see Fig. 65–3).

Localization of Inhibitor Epitopes

Major epitopes recognized by autoantibodies to factor VIII have been studied by immunoprecipitation,[45] and have been shown to be almost exclusively located within the A2 and C2 domains. This stands in contrast to alloantibodies, which also bind to epitopes located outside these two domains. More precisely, major epitopes of factor VIII are located toward the carboxy-terminal end of the C2 domain and/or at the amino-terminal end of the A2 domain.[45,46]

Mechanisms of Factor VIII Inhibition

One can easily understand how antibodies inhibit the function of factor VIII from the mere knowledge of the two major binding sites for autoantibodies on the factor VIII molecule. Thus, the C2 domain mediates the binding of factor VIII to both von Willebrand factor and phospholipids. The effect of antibody binding to the C2 domain has been studied in great detail[47] thanks to the elucidation of the crystal structure of a complex formed between the C2 domain and a human monoclonal antibody derived from a patient's B memory cell repertoire.[48] Single amino acid residue substitutions within the C2 domain have functionally confirmed the information gained from the structure. Although such investigations

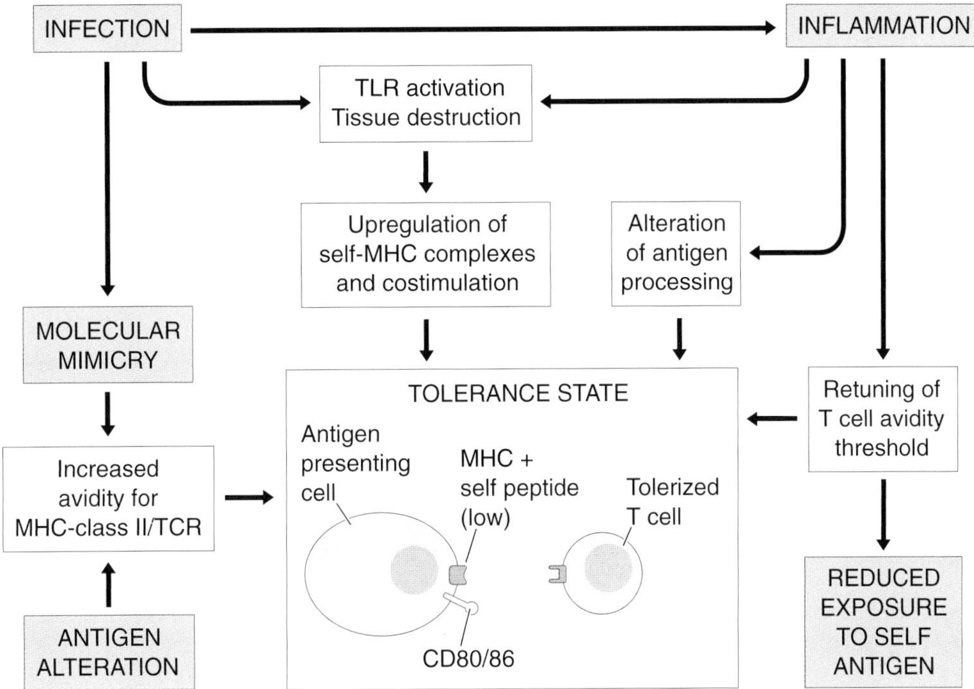

Figure 65–3. Mechanisms leading to autoimmunity. Autoreactive T cells can be activated in the periphery under various intricate circumstances as shown:

1. Infection can activate Toll-like receptors and result in tissue destruction, which will trigger a "danger" signal; this will lead to upregulation of both MHC class II complexes and costimulatory signals at the surface of APCs.
2. Inflammatory mediators increase surface receptors on APCs, but also lead to alteration of antigen processing by direct activation/inhibition of enzymes involved in early protein degradation. Such mediators have been shown to modify the T-cell affinity threshold.
3. Molecular mimicry leads to preactivation of T cells, together with other events associated with infection.
4. Alteration of antigen by side chain modification can lead to increased affinity for either MHC class II complexes or TCRs.
5. Reduced exposure to self-antigen can turn up the T-cell affinity threshold.

have not yet been carried out directly with autoantibodies, the functional behavior of autoantibodies to the C2 domain strongly suggests that epitopes recognized by auto- and alloantibodies are similar or located in close proximity.

Binding to the hydrophobic hairpin loops of the C2 domain results in inhibiting the binding of factor VIII to phospholipids, an essential step in the formation of the tenase complex. Binding to C2 also alters the binding of factor VIII to von Willebrand factor. In this case, however, the situation is rendered more complicated because of the multiple binding sites of von Willebrand factor onto the light chain. For instance, the acidic a3 region contains a binding site that acts cooperatively with the C2 domain for factor VIII binding. Type II inhibitors, a category to which most autoantibodies belong (see earlier), are deemed to compete with von Willebrand factor for the binding to factor VIII.

The second binding site for autoantibodies on the A2 domain immediately suggests that antibodies could accelerate the dissociation of the A2 domain from A1, to which it is bound noncovalently. The spontaneous dissociation of A2 is known to represent the major mechanism by which factor VIII is spontaneously inactivated. An additional mechanism of antibody-mediated factor VIII inactivation could be driven by interference with the binding of the A2 domain to factor IX.

Clinical Features and Diagnosis

Presentation

The clinical manifestations of patients with circulating anticoagulants to factor VIII are related to the severity and site of bleeding (Table 65–2). Although the presentation is usually sudden, some patients describe more gradual onset and recurrent or intermittent bleeding episodes such as hematuria or hemoptysis.[1–5,23,29] Patients may complain of fatigue, shortness of breath, epistaxis, easy bruising, or blood in stools. Difficulty swallowing or abdominal pain secondary to retropharyngeal or retroperitoneal hemorrhage, respectively, may be experienced by some patients. Occasionally, patients with acquired hemophilia complain of swelling of a limb associated with pain and numbness as a result of the development of a compartment syndrome.

CHARACTERISTICS OF AUTO-ANTI FACTOR VIII ANTIBODIES

A IgG subclasses and antibody binding sites to FVIII

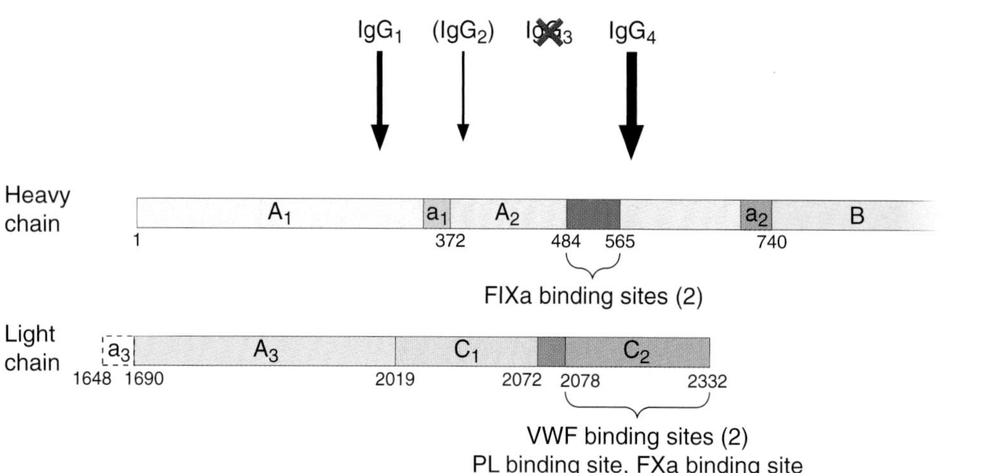

B Kinetics of binding

Type I (Alloantibodies)

Residual FVIII activity (%)

100
10
1

0 5 10 15 20

Antibody (μg/ml)

Type II (Alloantibodies and autoantibodies)

Residual FVIII activity (%)

100
10
1

0 5 10 15 20

Antibody (μg/ml)

C Mechanisms of FVIII neutralization

(1) Steric hindrance in tenase complex formation

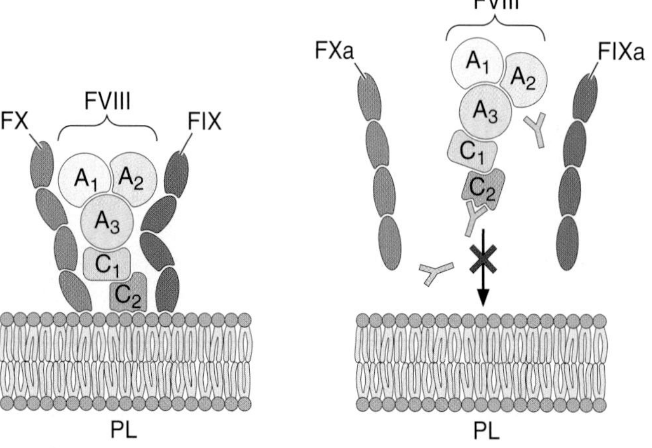

(2) Competition for vWF binding sites

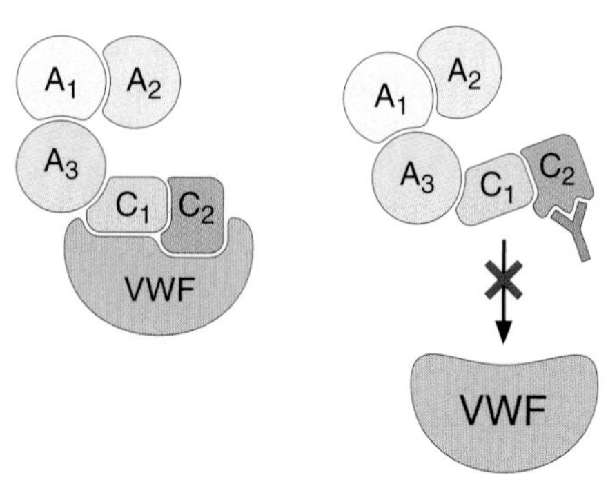

History and Physical Examination

The medical history of patients with acquired hemophilia may indicate the presence of known medical problems such as cancer, rheumatoid arthritis, asthma, or drug ingestion. Recent surgery or procedures such as dental extraction or bladder catheterization may be reported by some patients. Because the majority of patients with spontaneous autoantibodies against factor VIII are elderly, chronic diseases such as hypertension, diabetes, and congestive heart failure are quite common. Physical examination may reveal pallor, tachycardia, and hypotension. Ecchymoses are common on the torso, whereas soft tissue hemorrhage most often affects the abdominal and thigh areas. Bleeding at multiple sites, such as the skin and periorbital and gastrointestinal areas, has been reported in one fifth of the patients with acquired hemophilia.[1–6]

Diagnosis

The characteristic laboratory finding in patients with acquired hemophilia is a prolonged aPTT, normal prothrombin time (PT), and normal thrombin time.[4,7,50,51] The diagnostic approach for a prolonged aPTT is shown in Figure 65–5. Because binding and inactivation of factor VIII by the antibody is time and temperature dependent, a mixture of the patient's plasma with an equal volume of normal plasma should be incubated for 2 hours at 37° C.[4,7,51] An approach to the diagnosis of factor VIII inhibitors is depicted in Table 65–3. The aPTT, on mixture with normal plasma, will also remain prolonged in patients with the lupus anticoagulant. The dilute Russell's viper venom test and the hexagonal-phase phospholipids tests can rule out the presence of lupus anticoagulant. Assays of factors VIII, IX, XI, and XII at multiple dilutions of the patient's plasma mixed with normal plasma are important to confirm the specificity of the inhibitor. If the inhibitor is targeted against factor VIII, the factor level will remain low or undetectable no matter how much the patient's plasma is diluted.

TABLE 65–2. Common Sites of Bleeding Episodes in Patients with Acquired Hemophilia

Site of Hemorrhage	Percentage
Soft tissues	55
Hematuria	22
Gastrointestinal	9.6
Skin	8.5
Compartment syndrome	8.3
Postoperative	7.8
Retroperitoneal	6
Multiple sites	22

The Bethesda assay is used to quantify the inhibitor level in patients with acquired hemophilia.[52] However, the Bethesda assay may underestimate the in vivo potency of these inhibitors. Therefore, it is desirable to report the antibody titer calculated from the lowest dilution that yields 50% residual factor VIII activity after 2 hours' incubation.[2,7,51] Even with prolonged incubation, low-titer inhibitors may not be detected by the Bethesda method. To improve on reporting, the Nijmegen modification of the Bethesda assay was introduced in 1995.[53] In the modified Bethesda assay, the normal plasma is buffered with imidazole and the imidazole buffer in the control mixture is replaced with immunodepleted factor VIII–deficient plasma. This process avoids a pH shift that may cause loss of factor VIII activity unrelated to binding by the antibody.[53,54] There is no correlation between the inhibitor titer measured by the Bethesda unit and the degree of prolongation of the aPTT.[53,54] Despite these drawbacks, the Bethesda assay remains a useful tool for clinicians to determine the severity of acquired hemophilia and to follow the course of treatment. Cross-reactivity against porcine factor VIII can be assessed by replacing human factor VIII with porcine factor VIII in the Bethesda assay.[7] Measurement of the inhibitor titer against porcine factor VIII is important when considering the use of porcine concentrates for the treatment of acute bleeding episodes in patients with acquired hemophilia.

A cut-off level of 5–10 BU has been traditionally used to separate low from high inhibitor titer.[4,7] Although this distinction is more applicable to patients with congenital hemophilia and alloantibodies, the magnitude of inhibitor titer may be useful to determine the therapeutic approach

Figure 65–4. Characteristics of anti–factor VIII autoantibodies. Antibodies toward factor VIII belong to the IgG isotype. All subclasses are represented in alloantibodies, except IgG2, whereas in autoimmune hemophilia, IgG subclasses are restricted to IgG4 subclasses with, in some cases, IgG1.

The circulating factor VIII molecule consists of a heterodimer made of a heavy chain containing the A1 and A2 domains together with variable lengths of the B domain. This heavy chain is associated through a divalent cation-dependent to an 80-kDa light chain containing the A3, C1, and C2 domains. Immunoprecipitation assays have demonstrated that the majority of alloantibodies bind to the A2, A3, C1, and C2 domains, whereas autoantibodies bind only to epitopes located in the A2 and/or C2 domains.

Alloantibodies are defined as "type 1 inhibitors" when they completely inhibit factor VIII function following second-order kinetics or as "type 2 inhibitors" if the kinetics of binding follows a more complex mechanism by which factor VIII is not completely inhibited. Autoantibodies belong always to the type 2 category.

Two mechanisms of factor VIII activity inhibition have been described:

1. Antibody binding to the C2 domain of the factor VIII molecule induces a steric hindrance by which the binding of factor VIII to surface phospholipids, which is a crucial step in the formation of the tenase complex, is inhibited.
2. Autoantibodies can also interfere with the binding of factor VIII to von Willebrand factor, thereby reducing the half-life of circulating factor VIII.

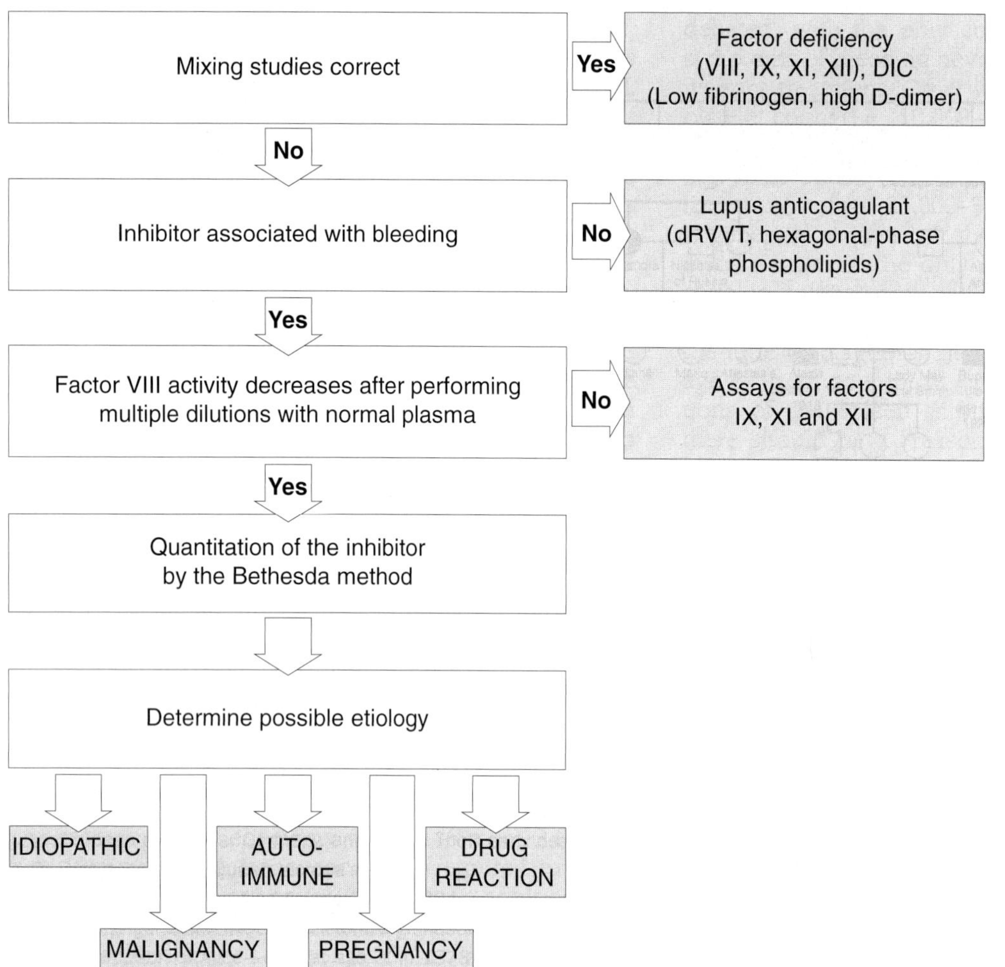

Figure 65–5. Diagnostic algorithm for a prolonged aPTT.

TABLE 65–3. An Approach to the Detection of Factor VIII Autoantibodies

History	No prior history of personal or familial bleeding tendency.
Presentation	Muscular or cutaneous hemorrhage is common, but soft tissue, retropharyngeal, or retroperitoneal bleeding episodes can be life-threatening.
Coagulation tests	Prolonged aPTT, normal PT, normal platelet count, and normal fibrinogen.
Mixing studies	The goal is to demonstrate whether the prolonged aPTT is due to factor deficiency or the presence of an inhibitor against factor VIII. Mixture of the patient's plasma with normal plasma will correct the prolonged aPTT in the presence of a factor deficiency, whereas the prolonged aPTT will not correct if an inhibitor is present in the patient's plasma. The aPTT should be performed on the mix immediately and again after incubation at 37°C for 1–2 hr. The latter step is important to reveal low-titer inhibitors that may not be detected on the immediate mixture.
Inhibitor specificity	Increasing dilutions of the patient's plasma are added to normal plasma and determination of the residual activity of clotting factors in normal plasma is performed. If the inhibitor is targeted against factor VIII, the factor will remain equally deficient in the factor VIII assay regardless of how much the patient's plasma is diluted. Assay of other factor levels (IX, XI, and XII) will be normal or even increased with serial dilution of the patient's plasma. Deficiency of factor XII, high-molecular-weight kininogen, or prekininogen does not lead to bleeding tendency.
Quantitation of the inhibitor	The Bethesda assay is the most universally acceptable method used to define the level of inhibitor against factor VIII. One Bethesda unit (BU) is the lowest dilution of the patient's plasma that yields 50% residual factor VIII activity in a mixture with pooled normal plasma incubated for 2 hr at 37°C. The Bethesda titer can be used as a rough guide to project the severity of hemorrhage and as a uniform measurement to follow after treatment and to compare levels among different patients. The Bethesda titer, however, should not be used to calculate the dose of the agent used for treatment.

TABLE 65–4. Comparison Between Auto- and Alloantibodies Against Factor VIII

	Autoantibody	Alloantibody
Incidence	Estimated at 1/500,000 of the general population	20% of patients with severe hemophilia
Age	61.5 yr (mean)	Usually young hemophiliacs
Prior bleeding history	None	Known factor VIII deficiency
Most common site of hemorrhage	Soft tissues	Joints
Type of antibody	IgG, commonly subtype IgG4	IgG, commonly subtype IgG4
Inhibitor response	Usually low responder	Usually high responder
Kinetics of inhibitor	Usually complex, type II	Linear, type I
Impact of inhibitor	Bleeding may be life-threatening	No increase in the frequency of bleeding, but the appearance of inhibitor complicates treatment

TABLE 65–5. Agents Used for the Management of Acute Bleeding Episodes in Patients with Acquired Hemophilia

	Dose	Response Rate (%)	Mortality (%)	Comments
Recombinant FVIIa [25]	90 μg/kg q2–3h	35/38 (92)	7.9	None of the pretreatment parameters predicted response.
FEIBA [45]	75–100 U/kg q8–12h	30/34 (88)	8.8	Responders were more likely to have less severe hemorrhage and lower inhibitor titer.
Porcine factor VIII [46]	Mean dose 84 U/kg	51/65 (78)	15	None of the pretreatment parameters predicted response.
Intravenous immunoglobulin [61]	1000 mg/kg × 2 days *or* 400 mg/kg × 5 day	6/16 (37.5)	6.25	Responders were more likely to have low inhibitor titer.

in nonhemophilic individuals as well. Unlike congenital hemophilia, the majority of patients with acquired inhibitors targeted to factor VIII do not develop an anamnestic response (i.e., increase in the antibody level after the infusion of factor VIII or bypassing agents).[55–57]

Differential Diagnosis

Congenital hemophilia can be differentiated from acquired inhibitors to factor VIII by the medical history of the patient. Comparison between the two conditions is shown in Table 65–4. Although patients with antiphospholipid antibodies are more likely to develop venous and/or arterial thrombotic episodes, an increased risk for hemorrhage may be manifested by some patients.[58] The majority of these patients have hypoprothrombinemia, thrombocytopenia,. or renal failure. Autoantibodies against factor IX or factor XI are rare and can be diagnosed by assays of these factors after mixing with normal plasma.[59–62] Acquired inhibitors to factor V are associated with prolongation of the aPTT and PT that does not correct with mixing studies.[63,64] Sepsis, recent surgery, or known malignancy can be identified in the vast majority of patients with DIC.[65,66] Bleeding or oozing from multiple sites is more common in DIC than in acquired inhibitors. However, the pattern of bleeding and the presence of possible underlying risk factors are not sufficient to distinguish between DIC and acquired hemophilia. Laboratory data in DIC typically reflect activation of the coagulation cascade manifested as low fibrinogen, high D-dimer, low antithrombin, and low platelet counts.[65,66] A prolonged aPTT in DIC usually corrects with mixing studies.

Treatment

Management of Acute Bleeding Episodes

The initial therapeutic approach to patients with spontaneous inhibitors to factor VIII is not different from any other type of bleeding diathesis. Supportive measures include the administration of intravenous fluids and transfusion of packed red blood cells as clinically required. Once the diagnosis is confirmed, the medical chart should be labeled as acquired hemophilia and intramuscular injections and medications such as aspirin, nonsteroidal anti-inflammatory drugs, antiplatelet agents, and heparin should be avoided. Specific treatment aimed at correcting the hemostatic defect by bypassing, overwhelming, or neutralizing the inhibitor should be administered. The products commonly used for treatment of the acute hemorrhagic episodes in acquired hemophilia are listed in Table 65–5.[67–72]

The hemostatic effect of recombinant activated factor VII (rFVIIa) involves binding with tissue factor expressed on the injured endothelium.[44,73,74] Subsequently, the tissue factor/rFVIIa complex activates factors X and IX, thereby bypassing the need for factor VIII for coagulation. Another important mechanism of action of rFVIIa appears to be related to the binding of rFVIIa to the surface of activated platelets, leading to the generation of thrombin.[75–78] Other bypassing agents include factor

TABLE 65–6. Agents Used for the Immunosuppression of Factor VIII Inhibitors

	Dose	Response Rate (%)	Time to Respond (wk)
Prednisone (P) + cyclophosphamide (C)[66]	P: 1 mg/kg/day × 3–9 wk C: 2 mg/kg/day × 6 wk	21/31 (68)	3–21
Factor VIII + cyclophosphamide (C), vincristine (V), prednisone (P) (administered every 3–4 wk)[67]	C: 500 mg IV day 1, then 200 mg days 2–5 V: 2 mg IV day 1 P: 100 mg/day × 5 days	11/12 (92)	6–12
2-Chlorodeoxyadenosine[73]	0.1 mg/kg continuous infusion × 7 days	6/6 (100)	19
Rituximab[74]	375 mg/m^2/wk × 4	4/4 (100)	3–12

VIII inhibitor bypassing activity (FEIBA) and AUTOPLEX.[55–57,69,79] These products contain variable amounts of deliberately activated vitamin K–dependent factors. Currently, there is no acceptable laboratory method to assess the response to rFVIIa or activated prothrombin complex concentrates. A thrombin generation assay has recently been proposed as a useful tool to monitor the bioavailability of FEIBA.[80]

Patients presenting with mild to moderate hemorrhage and low inhibitor titer can be treated with porcine factor VIII (75 U/kg every 8–12 hours),[69,70] FEIBA (75 U/kg every 8–12 hours),[55,69] or rFVIIa (90 µg/kg every 3 hours).[49,68] For patients with acquired hemophilia and severe bleeding episodes, rFVIIa (90 µg/kg every 3 hours),[49,68] porcine factor VIII (100 U/kg every 8–12 hours),[70,78] or FEIBA (75–100 U/kg every 8–12 hours) should be infused.[55,69] For patients with very high inhibitor titer (>100 BU), or those not responding initially to concentrate infusion, plasma exchange (1–1.5 volume) or immunoadsorption to reduce the inhibitor titer should be attempted.[81–84] A 10,000- to 15,000-U bolus of human factor VIII followed by a 1000-U/hr continuous infusion should be administered following these procedures.[68] If the inhibitor titer is not known, rFVIIa (90 µg/kg) should be immediately administered. The level of inhibitor against human or porcine factor VIII does not affect the response to rFVIIa. Patients with high inhibitor titer against porcine factor VIII may have lower response rate when using porcine factor VIII concentrates or FEIBA.[69–71] Anamnestic response to the infusion of FEIBA has been reported in patients with acquired inhibitor.[55] Intravenous immunoglobulin (IVIG) has been used with some success in patients with autoantibodies to factor VIII.[85,86] However, IVIG is usually administered following concentrates such as FEIBA or porcine factor VIII, or in conjunction with corticosteroids. Decrease in the inhibitor titer after IVIG may be delayed and temporary.[85] Treatment of the underlying condition, such as cancer or autoimmune disorder, may enhance the response to the different modalities used for the immediate management of the inhibitor.[9,10]

Clinical evaluation remains the best monitoring tool to follow patients with acquired hemophilia. In addition, hemoglobin level should be obtained at least on a daily basis during initial treatment, and it is advisable to repeat measurement of factor VIII and the Bethesda titer every 48 hours until signs of complete arrest of bleeding have been achieved. Subsequently, periodic evaluation of factor VIII activity and Bethesda titer should be performed. Baseline imaging studies to evaluate the bleeding site may be repeated as required. Thromboembolic complications have been reported in patients receiving rFVIIa or FEIBA; however, the incidence appears to be extremely low. Increase in D-dimers and DIC has been observed in a few patients after the administration of FEIBA.[67–69,87–89] Allergic or anaphylactic reactions may occasionally occur in patients treated with porcine factor VIII.[70]

Immunosuppression of the Inhibitor

Once the presence of an inhibitor against factor VIII is confirmed, immunosuppressive therapy aimed at the eradication of the inhibitor should be initiated immediately. The response rate when using immunosuppression is defined as complete disappearance of the inhibitor and increase in factor VIII activity. The time to achieve response varies with the modality used to treat the inhibitor (Table 65–6).[90–98] The most commonly used regimen is prednisone and cyclophosphamide.[90] This regimen should be continued for at least 3 weeks with weekly monitoring of the Bethesda titer. A reasonable goal to achieve when using corticosteroids is reduction of at least 50% of the inhibitor level by the end of the third week.[90] Otherwise, consideration should be given to an alternative treatment. The infusion of factor VIII at a dose of 50–100 U/kg followed by the administration of cyclophosphamide, vincristine, and prednisone for at least two to three cycles is an effective regimen for the long-term control of the antibody.[91] It is not clear whether the infusion of factor VIII is an essential requirement for a successful outcome from this regimen. Rituximab and 2-chlorodeoxyadenosine have been recently shown to be highly effective in the treatment of acquired hemophilia.[97,98] However, the experience with these agents is rather limited. Other treatment options used to control the production of the antibody include cyclosporine (100–200 mg daily) and azathioprine (2 mg/kg/day).[94] Patients receiving immunosuppressive therapy for acquired hemophilia should be monitored regularly with Bethesda titers and factor VIII levels and watched closely for any complications of such treatment.

Prognosis

A mortality rate of 22% resulting from hemorrhage or complications of treatment of the inhibitor was reported in earlier series.[1] However, lower mortality rates (<10%) have been observed in patients with acquired hemophilia in more recent series.[49,55,97,98] This may be due to better recognition of the disorder or availability of more products for the treatment of inhibitors. Overall, the prognosis of patients with acquired hemophilia appears to be somewhat related to the underlying condition that might have triggered the formation of the inhibitor. For example, the prognosis of inhibitors in postpartum women is excellent, with resolution of the inhibitor in more than 97% of patients following the administration of immunosuppressive therapy.[19,21] The persistence of the inhibitor in patients with cancer impacts adversely on the overall survival of these patients.[9] In one study, the overall survival rates of patients with cancer and persistent inhibitor versus those who achieved complete disappearance of the inhibitor were 17% and 75%, respectively.[9] A good response to treatment in this group of patients correlated with early-stage tumors and with a low inhibitor level at the time of diagnosis. Acquired hemophilia appearing after the administration of certain medications usually has a good response to treatment of the inhibitor provided the offending agent is discontinued.[23] The level of inhibitor titer and the severity of the hemorrhagic episode may influence the survival and long-term response of patients with acquired inhibitors to factor VIII.[69] However, it should be emphasized that the number of patients evaluated is too limited to provide predefined criteria to predict the course of inhibitors. Although spontaneous remission of the inhibitor has been reported in rare patients, the unpredictability of the course of illness requires the administration of immunosuppressive therapy and very close follow-up for all patients with acquired hemophilia.[6]

ACQUIRED INHIBITORS TO OTHER COAGULATION FACTORS

Inhibitors Against Factor V

The spontaneous development of inhibitors that neutralize the clotting activity of factor V is a rare occurrence. The majority of acquired inhibitors to factor V have been associated with the use of bovine thrombin in surgical procedures.[99] Bovine thrombin contains small amounts of factor V, and is usually mixed with fibrinogen to make fibrin glue, which is used as a local hemostatic plug. The inhibitor usually appears after a mean of 8.3 days following the application of bovine thrombin.[99] Other conditions that have been described in patients with acquired factor V antibodies include autoimmune disorders, pregnancy, cancer, and the administration of antibiotics.[100,101]

The clinical presentation of patients with factor V inhibitors ranges from asymptomatic to detection as part of a preoperative work-up to severe or fatal hemorrhagic episodes.[100–102] The laboratory evaluation reveals prolongation of the aPTT and PT, normal fibrinogen level, and normal thrombin time.[99,103] Mixing studies with normal plasma do not correct the prolonged aPTT and PT. Confirmation of the inhibitor is made by the finding of low to undetectable factor V levels in mixtures with normal plasma. The Bethesda assay can be modified to measure the inhibitor titer against factor V.

Because platelet factor V is usually protected from inactivation by the autoantibody, platelet transfusion may be used to treat the bleeding episodes in these patients.[104] Recombinant activated factor VII may be another therapeutic option to control the hemorrhagic events. Plasma exchange can be used to reduce the inhibitor titer in some patients with factor V inhibitors.[105] Although the course of factor V inhibitors is usually self-limited, immunosuppression using prednisone, cyclophosphamide, or cyclosporine should be attempted.[106] Recently, high-dose IVIG was used successfully for the treatment of two patients with acquired factor V inhibitors.[107]

Acquired Inhibitors to Factor XIII

Factor XIII covalently cross-links fibrin monomers to produce a stable clot. Acquired inhibitors to factor XIII are rare, but their presence may lead to severe or fatal hemorrhagic diathesis.[108] The patients are usually elderly, and a history of medication intake, such as isoniazid, penicillin, or procainamide, or an underlying autoimmune disorder was identified in a few case reports.[109,110] Most inhibitors to factor XIII are immunoglobulins of the IgG type.[111,112] Factor XIII inhibitors are subdivided into three types. Type I inhibitors interfere with the activation of the A_2B_2 subunits by thrombin; therefore, no factor XIIIa (A_2*) is formed. Type II inhibitors are targeted against the transamidating activity of A_2*, and type III inhibitors interfere with the reactivity of fibrin substrate with factor XIIIa.[112–115] Screening coagulation tests, including aPTT, PT, and bleeding time, are normal. Fibrinogen level and coagulation factor assays are within normal limits. The diagnosis is made by demonstrating the ability of 5 M urea or 1% monochloracetic acid to dissolve fibrin clots that have not been cross-linked. Plasma exchange can be used to treat the inhibitor.[115] Immunosuppressive therapy produces variable results.[112,116]

Acquired Inhibitors to Factors XI, X, VII, IX, and XII

Inhibitors against factor XI have been reported in patients with systemic lupus erythematosus, rheumatoid arthritis, and malignancy.[61,62] Ecchymoses, localized hematoma, and hematuria have been reported in patients with inhibitors to factor XI. Laboratory tests usually show a prolonged aPTT that does not correct with mixing studies and a low level of factor XI. Some patients with acquired inhibitors to factor XI may respond favorably to immunosuppressive therapy.[61] Control of a bleeding episode using rFVIIa was recently reported in a patient with antibody against factor XI.[117]

Inhibitors to factor X are IgG immunoglobulins that may interfere with the activation of factor X by the tissue factor/FVIIa or the FIXa/FVIIIa/phospholipids complexes.[118–120] Direct activation by Russell's viper venom may be inhibited as well. The presentation may be with mucosal bleeding, ecchymoses, or hematoma. Both the aPTT and PT are prolonged. Low plasma level of factor

X and demonstration of inhibitory activity in mixing studies is required for the diagnosis of anti–factor X inhibitors.

A related clinical condition may be encountered in the setting of amyloidosis, in which patients may exhibit severe factor X deficiency, which is due to adsorption of factor X to amyloid fibrils, particularly in the spleen.[121] Though technically not an inhibitor, and not associated with failure to correct the PT and aPTT on mixing studies, acquired factor X deficiency can be a challenging clinical problem in the 5% or so of amyloidosis patients who develop this complication. Splenectomy may result in improvement in coagulation and cessation of bleeding[122]; rFVIIa has successfully been used to provide hemostasis for the surgical procedure.[123]

Very few patients with acquired inhibitors to factor VII have been reported.[124–127] In one case, the inhibitor was an IgG immunoglobulin that interacted with the light chain of factor VII. In another patient, the antibody to factor VII led to severe intracranial hemorrhage.[127] A third patient with aplastic anemia was reported to have an autoantibody that did not interfere with the activity of factor VII.[126] An isolated prolongation of the PT that does not correct with mixing studies and a low level of factor VII are suggestive of the diagnosis of inhibitor. Recently, inhibitor formation against factor VII was reported in patients undergoing stem cell transplantation.[128] Treatment with plasma exchange should be considered in patients with hemorrhage. The use of rFVIIa in a dose that can overwhelm the antibody (30–90 μg/kg) may be considered to treat the bleeding episodes secondary to inhibitors to factor VII.

Inhibitors to factor IX are rare.[59,60] Interestingly, two young children without history of hemophilia have been diagnosed with anti–factor IX inhibitors.[59,60] High-dose IVIG and dexamethasone were used to suppress the inhibitor in one of these two patients.[35]

Acquired inhibitors against factor XII and other contact-phase proteins have been reported in patients receiving chlorpromazine and in liver disease.[129] The formation of inhibitors to factor XII causes asymptomatic prolongation of the aPTT that does not correct with mixing studies and a low level of plasma factor XII.

CURRENT CONTROVERSIES & FUTURE CONSIDERATIONS

Acquired Inhibitors to Clotting Factors

- The Bethesda assay, even with the Nijmegen modification, is acceptable but not ideal. The assay cannot be used to calculate the dose or determine the agent to be used in a particular patient. Also, the Bethesda method may underestimate the severity of some antibodies against factor VIII. There is no clear correlation between the level of the inhibitor and the course or prognosis of acquired hemophilia.
- The pattern of kinetics and behavior of autoimmune inhibitors is different from that encountered in patients with congenital hemophilia. Should we use the same cutoff level (5–10 BU) used to separate high inhibitor titer in acquired as in congenital hemophilia?
- Are clinical and imaging studies and follow-up of the hemoglobin level sufficient to monitor the treatment with bypassing agents?
- What is the duration of immunosuppression and what is the likelihood of recurrence using any specific agent?
- What are the best criteria to determine response and prognosis of patients with acquired hemophilia?

Suggested Readings*

Ananyeva NM, Lacroix-Desmazes S, Hauser CA, et al: Inhibitors in hemophilia A: mechanisms of inhibition, management and perspectives. Blood Coagul Fibrinolysis 15:109–124, 2004.

Feinstein DI, Green D, Federici AB, Goodnight SH: Diagnosis and management of patients with spontaneously acquired inhibitors of coagulation. *In* Proceedings of the American Society of Hematology. American Society of Hematology, 1999, pp 192–208.

Gilles JG, Arnout J, Vermylen J, et al: Anti-factor VIII antibodies of hemophiliac patients are frequently directed towards nonfunctional determinants and do not exhibit isotypic restriction. Blood 82:2452–2461, 1993.

Goodnow CC: Pathways for self tolerance and the treatment of autoimmune diseases. Lancet 357:2115–2121, 2001.

Kessler C, Garvey MB, Green D, et al (eds): Acquired Hemophilia. Princeton, NJ: Excerpta Medica, 1995.

Shevach EM: CD4+CD25+ suppressor T cells: more questions than answers. Nat Rev Immunol 2:389–400, 2002.

Walker LSK, Abbas AK: The enemy within: keeping self-reactive T cells at bay in the periphery. Nat Rev Immunol 2:11–19, 2002.

CHAPTER 66

Congenital Bleeding Disorders from Other Coagulation Protein Deficiencies

Arthur R. Thompson, MD, PhD

KEY POINTS

Congenital Bleeding Disorders from Other Coagulation Protein Deficiencies

- Rare bleeding disorders occur in all populations but, because they are often autosomal recessive, they are more frequent in populations with limited genetic diversity.
- Screening tests such as the activated partial thromboplastin and prothrombin times are often insensitive and may miss mild deficiencies of the clotting factors.
- Specific testing for rare congenital bleeding disorders should be undertaken when a history of excessive or prolonged bleeding is obtained and factors VIII and IX disorders as well as von Willebrand disease have been excluded.
- Treatment of rare bleeding disorders varies depending upon the availability of concentrates versus use of plasma, the concentration and survival of the deficient factor in plasma, and an at times poorly defined minimal level necessary for hemostasis.
- As with von Willebrand disease, the phenotypes of these autosomal disorders may be influenced by the type of bleeding and other predisposing or protective environmental or genetic factors.

INTRODUCTION

It is important to consider defects of other hemostatic proteins when a bleeding tendency is suggested by personal or family history but platelet disorders, hemophilias, and von Willebrand disease have been excluded. Although very uncommon to rare, bleeding disorders caused by deficiencies of other coagulation factors can be difficult to diagnose. Furthermore, as autosomal recessive disorders, their frequencies will depend upon the size of the gene pool in different populations. In some societies, children born from related parents are more frequent than in others; in other population groups, common defective genes exist as "founder" effects. Either of these conditions accounts for a higher frequency of a recessive disorder.

Of congenital bleeding tendencies caused by deficiencies other than factor VIII or IX or von Willebrand factor, factor XI is the most common, although its frequency varies considerably among populations. The other disorders generally are found in about 1–2 per million.[1,2] In a recent survey in which 56 hemophilia treatment centers in the United States and Canada participated,[2] the combined percentage of patients with rare bleeding disorders (other than factor XI deficiency) among those followed was 3.5%. This included some individuals who were asymptomatic despite low clotting factor activity levels and several mildly symptomatic heterozygous individuals. Homozygous subjects were defined operationally as those with under 20% clotting activities. Factor VII deficiency was most frequently encountered; those reported with factor X or XIII deficiency had the highest percentage of persons with more severe bleeding tendencies. Properties of the genes and proteins discussed in this chapter and their congenital bleeding tendencies are summarized in Table 66–1. The roles of these proteins in blood coagulation are highlighted in Figure 66–1.

Bleeding tendencies can be due to deficiencies of other coagulation factors because they are (1) important in thrombin generation, (2) affect clot structure (fibrino-

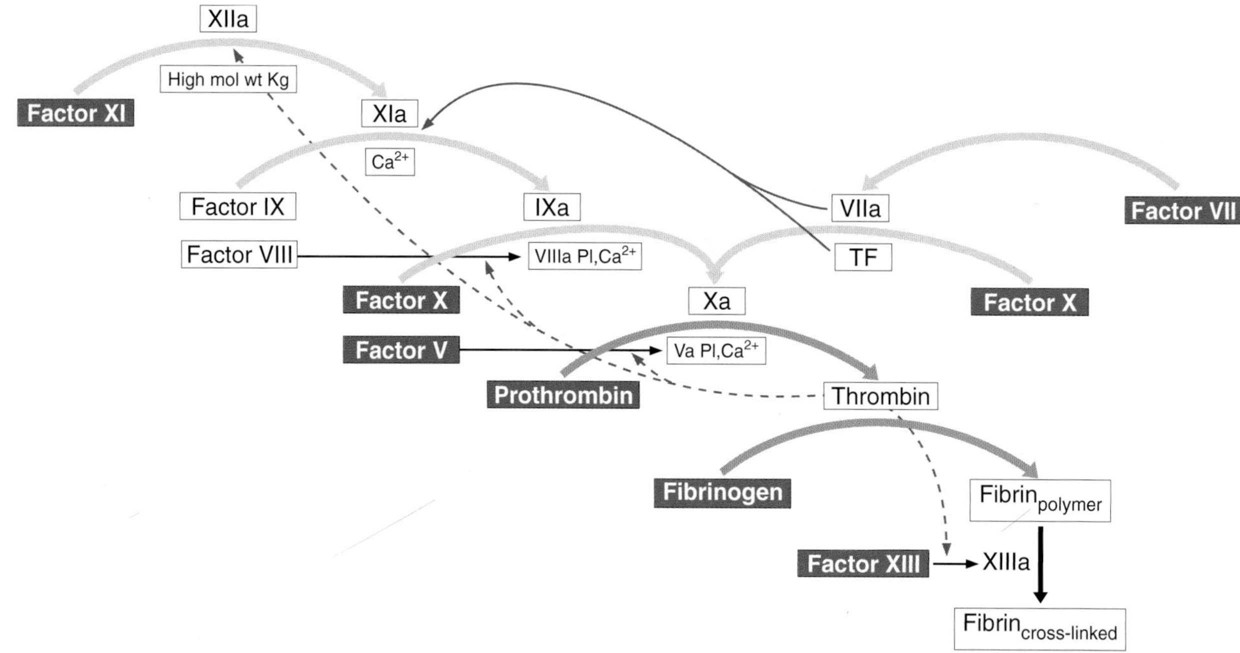

Figure 66–1. Roles of coagulation factors of which disorders produce rare bleeding tendencies. The clotting cascade is depicted with contact activation and initiation of intrinsic clotting in the *upper left* and the classic extrinsic system on the *upper right*. The seven factors considered in this chapter are indicated in *bold, midnight-blue boxes*. Reactions indicated by the *broad, curved, blue arrows* proceed by limited proteolysis by the responsible enzyme's trypsin-like serine protease domain. The enzyme is centered above and cofactors are centered below. Cross-linking of fibrin by factor XIIIa is indicated by the *vertical arrow (lower right)*. The darker shading of prothrombin conversion, fibrin formation, and cross-linking signifies reactants with significantly higher concentration in plasma than those involved in the earlier initiation or propagation steps. Coagulation in vivo predominantly results from an integrated pathway in which factor VIIa–tissue factor (TF) activates factor IX, as indicated by a *thin blue arrow*. Factor X activation begins the final common pathway. In addition to cleaving the A and B peptides to convert fibrinogen to fibrin, thrombin activates cofactors V and VIII, can convert factor XI to its active serine protease, XIa, and converts factor XIII to an active transglutaminase, XIIIa, that cross-links α and γ chains within the fibrin polymer. These latter steps are indicated by other reactions catalyzed by thrombin *(dashed blue arrows)*. Several combined deficiencies have been reported,[97] but of these, the only ones discussed in the text are those with a demonstrated common genetic defect, namely combined factors VII and X deficiency; deficiency of prothrombin and factors VII, IX, and X; and deficiency of factors V and VIII. Others can usually be attributed to chance co-occurrence or presence of both an acquired and an inherited defect.

gen or factor XIII), or (3) delay fibrinolysis. Neither cross-linking nor fibrinolytic abnormalities are detected in the common coagulation factor screening tests, so additional tests must be considered. Table 66–1 summarizes the characteristics of the coagulation factors considered in this chapter, including their genes, proteins, physiology, and deficiency states. If these other, uncommon to rare congenital coagulation factor deficiencies have been excluded, it is worth considering fibrinolytic disorders. A rapid lysis of clots can lead to a bleeding tendency that is very similar to a limited ability to form clots in response to a hemostatic challenge. Fibrinolytic disorders include homozygous or heterozygous α_2-antiplasmin deficiency,[3–5] plasmin activator inhibitor deficiency,[6,7] and excess tissue plasminogen activator.

Treatment or prevention of bleeding episodes in patients with rare bleeding disorders[1,8] depends upon the availability of a concentrate versus the need to use plasma, the recovery and survival of the infused deficient protein, and a minimum level necessary for hemostasis (see Table 66–1).

FACTOR XI DEFICIENCY

Background

In 1953, Rosenthal and colleagues[9] described a congenital bleeding tendency that, unlike the hemophilias, was associated with an autosomal recessive inheritance pattern. Furthermore, bleeding episodes were more responsive to therapy with plasma. Once this disorder could be distinguished by specific factor XI clotting activities, it became apparent that there was poor correlation between the risk of bleeding and the actual level.[10] Some individuals with undetectable levels, now known to be homozygous for a common nonsense genotype, are able to have normal hemostatic responses to major surgery or trauma, whereas others with levels equivalent to those of factor VIII or IX in mild hemophilias have prolonged oozing after even relatively minor trauma. Clinical deficiencies occur rarely in all populations and even animals. However, there is a high frequency of founder nonsense and missense mutations among persons of Ashkenazi Jewish descent.[11] Factor XI deficiency is thus the most commonly encountered of the rare bleeding disorders.

Pathophysiology

Factor XI is coded for by a gene on chromosome 4 and is probably synthesized in the liver. It remains to be established if small amounts can be synthesized by megakaryocytes.[12] Of note, factor XI knockout mice are normal without a detectable bleeding phenotype.[13] In vitro, factor XIa represents the contact activation product because it is activated by factor XIIa with high-molecular-weight kininogen. Deficiency of the latter two, or prekallikrein (a cofactor in factor XII activation), can prolong the activated partial thromboplastin time (aPTT) without any associated bleeding tendency.

In the aPTT, factor XIa cleaves the activation peptide from factor IX in a reaction requiring calcium, but not a lipid surface. The relevance of contact activation to coagulation in vivo has been questioned because factor IX is more readily activated by the factor VIIa–tissue factor complex of the "extrinsic system."[14] Alternatively, factor XI can be activated by thrombin,[15,16] such that the contact system is not required. Furthermore, factor XIa can activate factor IX more efficiently on the surface of activated platelets.[17] At this stage, it appears that there is a risk of abnormal bleeding, at least in some subjects with variably low levels of factor XI.

Genotyping has confirmed that the variable clinical phenotype correlates poorly with the severity of the defect and of the level of clotting activity or antigen present. Just over 10% of Ashkenazi Jewish persons are carriers. This is due to the high frequency of both a specific nonsense codon (Glu117 to stop) and a missense change (Phe283 to Leu).[11] Homozygotes with the nonsense mutation have undetectable factor XI levels (<1%), compound heterozygotes average 3% factor XI clotting activities, and individuals homozygous for the common missense change are somewhat higher, averaging 10%. Several families from the Basque population in Southern France have deficiency, and a different founder missense mutation (Cys38 to Arg) is responsible.[18] Among other populations, a variety of different genotypes have been described, much as in factor VIII or IX deficiency in different families with hemophilias A or B, respectively.

Factor XI circulates as a high-molecular-weight dimer and it is composed of 4 amino-terminal "apple" domains and a carboxy-terminal serine protease precursor or zymogen. On crystal structure, apple domains, which provide binding sites, form a "U"-shaped platform for the protease domain.[19] Once infused into a deficient patient, it has a high initial recovery and a long half-life or survival (see Table 66–1).

TABLE 66–1. Other Clotting Factors and Their Rare Bleeding Disorders

	Gene		Protein				Deficiency		
Clotting Factor	Chromosome*	Size (kb)	Molecular Weight (kDa)	Plasma Conc'n	$t_{1/2}$ (days)	Minimum for Hemostasis†	Knockout Mice	Frequency‡ (/10⁶)	Component Therapy
Factor XI	4q35	23	160‖	30 nM	3	0–20%	Normal	10	FFP (conc't)
Factor VII	13q34	13	50	10 nM	0.2	5–20%	Lethal	~1	r-VIIa; FFP
Factor X	13q34	27	55	170 nM	2	10–20%	Lethal	<1	IX conc't, FFP
Prothrombin	11p11	21	70	1.4 mM	2.5	10–20%	Lethal	<1	IX conc't, FFP
Factor V	1q24	80	330	20 nM	0.5	10–20%	Lethal	<1	FFP
Fibrinogen	4q31§	50	340‖	9 mM	4.5	0.5–1 mg/mL		<1	Cryoprecipitate
Aα		5.4	68				Bleeding		
Bβ		8	48						
γ		8.5	44						
Factor XIII			330‖	70 nM	10	5%		<1	FFP, conc't (cryo)
A subunit	6p25§	>160	75				Bleeding		r-conc't, platelets
B subunit	1q31§	28	80						

*Chromosomal localization as in Koeleman and colleagues.[98]

†Minimum level for normal hemostasis, an estimate and/or range as a percentage of average normal activity level.

‡Frequency is of clinically significant bleeding tendencies (varies among populations).

§Fibrinogen chains are coded for by a three-gene cluster, and factor XIII subunits, by separate genes.

‖Factor XI circulates as a disulfide-bonded dimer, and fibrinogen, as $(A\alpha/B\beta/\gamma)_2$; factor XIII circulates as A_2B_2 in plasma, but is A_2 in platelets.

Abbreviations: conc'n, plasma concentration; conc't, commercial concentrate, where IX conc't is intermediate-purity factor IX (containing factor X and prothrombin); FFP, fresh frozen plasma; r, recombinant; $t_{1/2}$, half-life in days.

Clinical Features

The diagnosis is usually suspected when a screening aPTT is prolonged and factor VIII and IX activities are normal. A specific factor XI clotting activity is obtained as a mixture of dilutions of the patient's citrated plasma into known, severely factor XI–deficient plasma and the times to clot after contact activation and recalcification are determined. Factor XI levels can also be assessed by immunologic testing, although those tests would not distinguish dysfunctional proteins and are of limited availability.

Brenner and associates[20] studied the bleeding tendencies in 45 families with factor XI deficiency in Israel. Of 26 members who either were homozygous for a common genotype or were compound heterozygotes, 58% had a positive history of abnormal bleeding. Of 46 heterozygous and 47 normal family members, the history was positive in 26% and 9%, respectively. When prolonged bleeding occurred, it was particularly common following operative procedures involving mucosal membranes, including the genitourinary tract; the risk was higher with lower factor XI clotting activities. Deficiency is found among women with menorrhagia, especially if onset was with menarche.[21,22] However, in most series there are some individuals with undetectable levels who have had normal hemostasis with major surgical challenges.

Among 38 factor XI–deficient patients in Iran, 18 had from less than 1% to 5% clotting activities and 20 were between 5% and 30%. Unlike the pattern in hemophilia A, bleeding episodes were similar in each group; just over half of each group had a history of abnormal postoperative bleeding without prior blood component therapy, for example.[23] There were no genotype data available for comparison with other series. Menorrhagia was reported in only 1 of the 13 women in Iran, and she was in the mild category. In another series, using a semiquantitative approach to menstrual blood loss, 59% of women with factor XI deficiency were identified as having menorrhagia.[21]

Treatment

Because of the high molecular weight and relatively long half-life of factor XI, treatment or prevention of bleeding is manageable with relatively low doses of plasma at infrequent intervals. Plasma-derived concentrates are prepared from large pools of human blood donors but have been treated with heat or solvent-detergent, methods very effective at killing any residual hepatitis B or C viruses or human immunodeficiency virus. One such product was available in the United Kingdom until the past few years; however, there was an associated thrombotic risk, particularly in older patients.[24] Adjunctive therapy including fibrin sealant and desmopressin has been used with variable success. A trial of tranexamic acid to reduce the bleeding from menorrhagia has been recommended.[21]

Of 21 Israeli patients who had received plasma therapy and were homozygous for the common nonsense genotype, 7 developed alloantibody inhibitors; 3 other patients with inhibitors were studied and also had this genotype and prior plasma exposure.[25] Because factor XI is present in platelets, platelet concentrates would theoretically be able to provide hemostasis, perhaps even in those patients who develop specific neutralizing antibodies or inhibitors to plasma factor XI. The usual approach to bleeding in patients with alloimmune inhibitors, however, is to try recombinant factor VIIa, or "bypassing" agents that are partially activated (e.g., low-purity factor IX concentrates).

CURRENT CONTROVERSIES & FUTURE CONSIDERATIONS

Factor XI Deficiency

- What accounts for the risk of bleeding among different patients or the same patient at different times? The genotype is predictive of in vitro factor XI clotting activity but there is poor correlation with bleeding risk, suggesting that other inherited or acquired influences on hemostasis affect the clinical phenotype to a much greater extent than in hemophilia A or B. It is possible in the future that a global measurement of thrombin generation or proteomic analysis of all hemostatic proteins may help predict bleeding risk.
- When or in whom should plasma be given prophylactically? Given an individual history of prolonged bleeding, prophylactic therapy is recommended prior to an invasive procedure to allow good initial hemostasis. "On demand" therapy after abnormal bleeding has occurred is more difficult to control. In the absence of a convincing history, even in "severe" deficiencies, a significant number of patients will not bleed with surgery, and the patient and his or her provider may elect to have a plan for receiving plasma if bleeding is encountered. The latter approach is more risky when surgery involves mucosal surfaces, including the genitourinary system, or involves an anatomic site where a hematoma could have dire consequences.

VITAMIN K-DEPENDENT FACTOR DISORDERS (OTHER THAN FACTOR IX DEFICIENCY, HEMOPHILIA B)

Factor VII Deficiency

Background

In 1951, Alexander and coworkers[26] described a family with an autosomal recessive bleeding disorder associated with a prolonged prothrombin time. This was subsequently referred to as factor VII deficiency. In such patients, tests of the intrinsic system clotting are normal and acquired deficiencies need to be excluded.

Pathophysiology

Factor VII is coded for by a gene on chromosome 13 and is synthesized by hepatocytes.[27] Of note, factor VII knockout mice appear to have developed normally at birth but die of perinatal hemorrhage.[28] Factor VIIa may circulate normally in trace levels; its initial activation event(s) is not known. With tissue factor, a transmembrane cofactor on monocytes or activated endothelium, factor VIIa rapidly converts factors IX and X from their zymogen precursors to active proteases. In plasma and especially in vivo, factor X activation is inhibited by tissue factor protease inhibitor such that, at relatively low concentrations of factor VIIa and, especially, tissue factor, factor VIIa predominantly activates factor IX and the intrinsic system.

Genotyping has revealed a variety of mutations within the factor VII gene, with a spectrum similar to that found in the more common hemophilia B.[27] Affected members are either homozygous (often when consanguinity is involved) or compound heterozygous. Of known polymorphisms, a common one specifying Gln substituted for Arg353 accounts for a quarter of the population variance; homozygous individuals may have activities in the 20–30% range but are asymptomatic despite variably prolonged prothrombin times.

Clinical Features

The diagnosis is suspected when a prothrombin time is prolonged but the activated partial thromboplastin time is normal. The bleeding tendencies in patients with congenitally low factor VII activities are quite variable. Of 28 Iranian and Italian patients with less than 2% clotting activities, recurrent mucosal bleeding was most prevalent, especially prolonged, recurrent epistaxis and, in women, menorrhagia.[29] Hemarthroses and deep muscle hematomas were less frequent than in patients with moderately severe hemophilia A or B. Nine patients underwent surgery without factor VII replacement therapy and only five had sufficient postoperative bleeding to require blood transfusions. A clinically severe phenotype is sometimes encountered, and fatal spontaneous intracranial hemorrhage has occurred in infancy. The factor VII clotting activity is somewhat more predictive of a clinically significant bleeding tendency than with factor XI; however, there are individuals who have from less than 1% to 52% activity in vitro who have a clinically mild bleeding tendency and others with as low as 4% who are asymptomatic. To some extent this variability is related to the genotype.[27]

Treatment

Fresh frozen plasma has been the standard therapy because low- to intermediate-purity factor IX concentrates made by adsorption to and elution from DEAE-substituted resins (all of those currently available) have considerably less factor VII than factors IX, X, and prothrombin activities. Hemostasis can often be achieved with lower volumes of plasma than required for hemophilia B, even though recoveries are similar to and the half-life of factor VII is considerably shorter than those of other vitamin K–dependent coagulation factors (see Table 66–1). The minimal level for normal hemostasis appears to be lower for factor VII than for factor IX. Major bleeding episodes are difficult to manage with plasma, however, because of the volumes required and the need for continual infusion. Recently, normal hemostasis has been achieved with doses of recombinant factor VIIa that are considerably lower than those used for bleeding in patients with hemophilia A or B and inhibitors.[30] By examining its effect in vivo, even lower doses are predicted to be hemostatic.[31] In one teen with severe deficiency, frequent target joint bleeding was decreased with twice-weekly prophylaxis and physical therapy; 12 hours after a dose of 80 μg/kg, there was still significant activity in a factor VII clotting assay.[32]

Factor X Deficiency

Background

Telfer and colleagues in the United Kingdom,[33] and Hougie and colleagues in North Carolina,[34] described patients with an autosomal recessive bleeding tendency that was associated with prolongations of both intrinsic and extrinsic system screening tests. This activity was adsorbed by salts of heavy metal ions similarly to factor IX in hemophilia B. It was shown to be another clotting protease zymogen and later named factor X.

Pathophysiology

Factor X is coded for by a gene on chromosome 13 that is within 3 kb of the gene for factor VII and is synthesized by hepatocytes. Factor X knockout mice die of neonatal hemorrhage[35]; prenatal transplantation of nondeficient fetal murine liver cells corrects or ameliorates the bleeding phenotype.[36] During clotting in vitro or coagulation in vivo, factor X is activated either extrinsically by factor VIIa–tissue factor or intrinsically by factor IXa–factor VIIIa on a lipid surface (see Fig. 66–1).

Genotyping has revealed a variety of mutations, with a spectrum similar to that found in the more common hemophilia B.[37] Affected members are either homozygous (often when consanguinity is involved) or compound heterozygous. Rarely, a large deletion or chromosomal rearrangement has accounted for combined deficiency of factors VII and X.

Clinical Features

The diagnosis is suspected when both the prothrombin time and the aPTT are prolonged and acquired deficiencies have been excluded. With some variants, extrinsic or intrinsic system activation of factor X may be less affected than activation by the protease in Russell's viper venom.[38] Thus the prolongation by intrinsic or extrinsic activation systems may be disproportionate, as would their respective screening tests.[39,40]

The severity of the bleeding tendency parallels the factor X clotting activity better than in factor VII deficiency, although milder deficiencies have a less predictable bleeding risk than do hemophilic patients with comparable clotting activities of factor VIII or IX. Compared to matched patients with hemophilia A, factor X–deficient patients had more frequent epistaxis and gastrointestinal bleeding but less in the oral cavity.[37] Among 18 Iranian patients with severe factor X deficiency, 7 had had prolonged oozing from their umbilical stump,[41] a feature distinct from the severe hemophilias. Of six Iranian women with less than 5% factor X clotting activities, four gave a history of menorrhagia. Increased fetal loss has also been observed.[41] Of 15 affected members of 13 unrelated Iranian families, the genotype correlated with the phenotype, with the one example of normal antigen in severe deficiency being lack of the propeptide cleavage site,[41] as found in the factor IX genes of several families with severe hemophilia B.[42]

Treatment

Fresh frozen plasma can usually provide normal hemostasis, but this may be difficult if the volume of colloid is too much for the patient to tolerate. Low- to intermediate-purity factor IX concentrates contain near-equivalent amounts of factors IX and X. Because they have undergone virucidal treatments, they are often preferred to fresh frozen plasma and can be used sparingly to reduce the risk of thrombosis.[37] Once infused, recovery of factor X is low, similar to that of factors VII and IX. However, factor X has a longer half-life than factor IX, of about 2 days. Furthermore, lower levels are usually sufficient for normal hemostasis (see Table 66–1). Four severely affected Irish infants were placed on early prophylactic treatments with factor IX concentrates after life-threatening, spontaneous bleeding episodes had occurred in two.[43]

Prothrombin Disorders

Background

Congenital hypoprothrombinemia was described by Josso and coworkers in 1962[44]; they subsequently confirmed the decrease in protein by immunologic assays. The presence of a dysfunctional prothrombin was described later.[45] Combined hypo-dysprothrombinemia has also been described and may be symptomatic.[46]

Pathophysiology

Prothrombin is coded for by a gene on chromosome 11 and is synthesized by hepatocytes. Prothrombin knockout mice either die as embryos or of neonatal hemorrhage by the first postnatal day; surviving embryos have characteristic yolk sac vasculature defects,[47,48] suggesting a developmental role of thrombin. Transgenic mice with liver-specific expression of prothrombin were created and crossed with prothrombin knockout mice. Of two lines recovered, one only corrected the embryonic lethality, whereas others survived with only a mild bleeding phenotype.[49] In the latter, the surviving mice had between 5% and 10% of the normal prothrombin levels circulating. These data predict that absolute deficiency is not compatible with fetal development, whereas trace levels may improve developmental defects but can be fatal with a very severe, early postnatal hemorrhagic disorder.

Genotyping patients has revealed a variety of mutations.[46] Affected members are either homozygous (often when consanguinity is involved) or compound heterozygous. In some cases of dysprothrombinemia, abnormalities of prothrombin activation as well as thrombin activity have been shown. An enzyme in *Echis carinatus* venom can directly activate prothrombin in the absence of cofactors and does not depend upon an intact Gla domain (which binds calcium and to a lipid surface); assays with this enzyme help distinguish some of the dysprothrombinemias.

Clinical Features

Among screening tests, the prothrombin and partial thromboplastin times are usually prolonged.[46] The thrombin time, however, is not affected because it depends upon addition of exogenous thrombin to plasma. A higher incidence in those of Latino ethnicity[2] may reflect a founder effect, as shown in persons of Puerto Rican descent.[50] The bleeding pattern depends upon the genotype, and the severity does correlate with the prothrombin clotting activity.[46] Although some patients have been reported as having less than 1% prothrombin clotting activity,[2] when they are examined with sensitive functional and immunologic assays, it is unclear if truly undetectable levels occur. To date, this is consistent with the embryonic lethality seen in knockout mice. Of 11 Iranian patients with hypoprothrombinemia and activity and antigenic levels between 2% and 10% of normal, spontaneous hemarthroses and deep muscle hematomas occurred as in the more severe hemophilias. In contrast to the hemophilias, two had had umbilical stump bleeding.[1] Epistaxis was common, although seldom severe, and women had menorrhagia. Heterozygous individuals average 50% activities and are usually asymptomatic.

Symptomatic dysprothrombinemia[45] is even less ? frequent than hypoprothrombinemia, and combined hypo-dysprothrombinemia has been described. Only three individuals were identified in the Iranian series of patients with rare bleeding disorders.[1] Among those with a bleeding tendency, activity levels are usually between 2% and 15%, with antigen levels from 50% to 100%.

Treatment

As is the case for Factor X, fresh frozen plasma can usually provide normal hemostasis, although the same constraints regarding volume of colloid apply. Low- to intermediate-purity factor IX concentrates contain large quantities of prothrombin. Because they have undergone virucidal treatments, they are often preferred to fresh frozen plasma and can be used sparingly to reduce the risk of thrombosis. Once infused, recovery of prothrombin is higher than that of the other vitamin K–dependent proteins because it is a larger protein. Prothrombin has a long half-life, nearly 3 days. Furthermore, lower levels are usually sufficient for normal hemostasis (see Table 66–1).

Combined Deficiency of Vitamin K-Dependent Proteins

Background

Rarely, a mild bleeding disorder is found due to a mild combined deficiency of all of the vitamin K–dependent proteins. This was first noted by McMillan and associates.[51] Its autosomal recessive inheritance suggested a defect in the vitamin K–dependent pathway; indeed, defects have recently been found in two enzymes responsible for vitamin K–dependent carboxylation of these factors.

Pathophysiology

The enzyme responsible for γ-carboxylation within the Gla domains of these proteins was isolated and mutations were found that are predicted to disrupt carboxylase activities in some, but not all, families with multiple deficiencies of the vitamin K–dependent proteins.[52,53] It has recently been found that deficiency of vitamin K oxide reductase, which reduces vitamin K back to its active form after oxidation during carboxylation, is another cause of multiple deficiencies of the vitamin K–dependent proteins.[54]

There are rare reports of combined factors VII and VIII or factors VII and V deficiencies (e.g., Acharya[2]). These need to be carefully evaluated to determine if they indeed reflect a true, single congenital defect versus an acquired or a combined acquired and congenital defect. This is particularly noteworthy because a mild deficiency of factor VII occurs early in liver disease or on a congenital basis when persons are homozygous for a common variant leading to levels lower than normal but still adequate for normal hemostasis. Indeed, there are no common structural features or synthetic or secretory pathways known for these proteins (as opposed to deficiencies of factors V and VIII; see later).

Clinical Features

Multiple defects of vitamin K–dependent hemostatic proteins lead to prolongation of both intrinsic (aPTT) and extrinsic (prothrombin time) screening tests. This is analogous to the acquired bleeding tendency caused by either vitamin K deficiency or antagonism, as with warfarin. When a bleeding tendency is present, symptoms are usually comparable to those of mild hemophilia B, with clotting activities of each protein between 10% and 20% of normal. Initial mutations described in the vitamin K epoxide reductase presented clinically as warfarin resistance.[54]

Treatment

Large, daily doses of oral vitamin K often ameliorate the bleeding tendency and partially correct the deficiencies, and may be sufficient to provide hemostatic levels of these coagulation factors. Fresh frozen plasma contains all the factors, and with mild deficiencies is often able to achieve hemostasis without volume overload. Currently available low-purity factor IX concentrates also contain factor X and prothrombin, but only small amounts of factor VII. They may be useful in the milder deficiencies because the patient's residual factor VII activity may be sufficient to achieve normal hemostasis. There may be a role for recombinant factor VIIa, especially in life-threatening bleeding episodes or to prepare patients for emergent surgery, although the currently reported experience is limited to patients on warfarin.[55]

CURRENT CONTROVERSIES & FUTURE CONSIDERATIONS

Vitamin K–Dependent Factor Disorders

- In addition to factor VII clotting activities, what influences the risk of bleeding? Is there a minimum level for hemostasis? The degree that correlations with genotype explain variability needs further analysis and data to evaluate for coexisting bleeding on thrombotic risk factors.
- For treatment of factor VII deficiency, what are the indications for and effectiveness of recombinant factor VIIa? Dosage may vary depending upon the presence of a dysfunctional protein that may compete with low levels of the activated species. Laboratory methods to assess response would help define optimal dosage amounts and frequency for hemostasis.
- For factor X deficiency, to what extent do differences in intrinsic, extrinsic, or venom activations occur? What are the genotype and clinical correlations? As a corollary, can heterozygosity for a dysfunctional protein produce a bleeding tendency? With so few patients available, it would be most helpful if a uniform set of assays and careful molecular and clinical data for each family were documented.
- For prothrombin, is completely deficient activity compatible with survival beyond neonatal life? Very sensitive functional and antigenic assays are required to address this.
- Are severe deficiencies of vitamin K–dependent carboxylase and/or oxide reductase compatible with life? Single- and double-knockout mice will be of interest and might determine if there are low levels of redundant systems for vitamin K–dependent carboxylation and, in addition, bone development where Gla proteins are also found.

FACTOR V DISORDERS

Factor V Deficiency

Background

Factor V deficiency is suspected when both the prothrombin time and aPTT are prolonged. It was first described by Owren and referred to as parahemophilia, a mild to severe bleeding tendency of autosomal recessive inheritance.[56] It occurs in about 1 per million population. In a series of 35 patients from Iran, 16 had undetectable levels (13 between 2% and 5% and 6 from 6% to 10% clotting activities) using an extrinsic system assay with rabbit brain thromboplastin.[57] Epistaxis, oral cavity bleeding, and menorrhagia were the most common spontaneous bleeding manifestations, although several patients experienced deep muscle hematomas and hemarthrosis. Abnormal bleeding was usually encountered after surgical procedures or deliveries, and those with lower factor V clotting activities tended to have more severe bleeding symptoms, including spontaneous neonatal intracranial bleeding.

Pathophysiology

Factor V is coded for by a gene on chromosome 1 and is synthesized in the liver and in megakaryocytes. Factor V participates in coagulation as the precursor to a cofactor (factor Va) in the prothrombinase complex. A model of human prothrombinase was created incorporating the crystal structure of part of factor Va, factor Vai.[58] The minimal level for normal hemostasis is usually around 15%. Complete gene knockout is lethal in mice,[59] although expression of trace levels led to survival in a transgenic model.[60] To date, only about 24 families with factor V deficiency have been genotyped. The variety of mutations is typified by a recent series including nine mutations in six European families, among whom four had compound heterozygosity and two were homozygous.[61] Factor V is also present in platelets. From mouse models, it appears that platelet factor V represents a distinct pool that is synthesized by the megakaryocyte but that the cofactor in the plasma compartment is sufficient to support prothrombinase.[62,63] Of the few families genotyped, null mutations predominate.[64]

Clinical Features

Among screening tests, the prothrombin and partial thromboplastin times should be prolonged, although there may be some variability in sensitivity with different reagents or instrumentation. A variety of bleeding symptoms are encountered; of 16 Iranian subjects with less than 1% factor V clotting activity, 2 had had spontaneous intracranial bleeding, and of 29 with less than 5%, half had epistaxis and half of the women had menorrhagia.[57] Mucosal bleeding, epistaxis, and oral cavity bleeding and prolonged bleeding associated with surgeries or post partum were fairly frequent in milder patients with 5–10% clotting activities. Among those with undetectable factor V clotting activity and a more severe phenotype, truncation mutations were predominant.[61]

Treatment

Currently there is no concentrate available containing factor V with the possible exception of platelets. The large size of the protein ensures a high intravascular recovery, especially compared with vitamin K–dependent proteins. Its half-life appears to be around 8–10 hours, although estimates vary from 3 to 30 hours. The minimum level for hemostasis is around 15%. Thus fresh frozen plasma has been the usual component for replacement therapy. One should follow postinfusion clotting activities and clinical responses. Alloantibody inhibitors have been encountered.[65]

Combined Factors V and VIII Deficiency

Background

An autosomal recessive, mild bleeding disorder involving deficiencies of factors V and VIII was described by Oeri and colleagues.[66] Combined deficiencies of these two clotting factors are usually comparable and, among some 100 families reported, activities have ranged from 4% to 30%, with most close to 15%. Immunoreactive levels are similarly reduced.[67]

Pathophysiology

Both factor V and factor VIII have a large B domain that is heavily glycosylated with Asn-linked high-mannose-containing carbohydrate chains. By positional cloning and family studies, especially in well-characterized Israeli families, it was found that one gene responsible for combined deficiency was on chromosome 18q21 and coded for an endoplasmic reticulum–Golgi intermediate compartment transport protein, ERGIC-53,[68] now referred to as LMAN-1 because of the high mannose content of proteins that bind to it. Of deficient families, 70% were found to have mutations in this intracellular transport protein and most specified a null phenotype.[69] Of 12 families with normal *LMAN1* genes and combined deficiency, 9 were found to be associated with a mutation in a gene named multiple coagulation factor deficiency type 2 (*MCFD2*) on chromosome 2p21.[70] The MCFD-2 protein turns out to be another transport protein that combines with LMAN-1 to facilitate the transfer of factors V and VIII to the Golgi apparatus for secretion.[70] Of the other three families, there is linkage to *MCFD2* in one but a genetic basis remains to be demonstrated; the other two may have been misclassified clinically.

Clinical Features

Combined deficiency of factors V and VIII should be considered if both the partial thromboplastin and prothrombin times are prolonged. The sensitivity of each screening test should be taken into account because, with some reagents and instrumentation, either the prothrombin time and/or the partial thromboplastin time may be within the upper normal range despite mild deficiencies of these factors. The bleeding tendencies (phenotypes) are usually mild, with clotting activities of factors V and VIII around 15% but occasionally as low as 4% and as high as 30%. Where examined, antigenic levels are comparable to the clotting activities. The bleeding tendency is similar to that in mild hemophilia A, namely excessive bleeding or prolonged oozing and delayed wound healing following trauma. Epistaxis and postextraction oral bleeding are common, as is menorrhagia and postpartum hemorrhage in women and postcircumcision bleeding in male infants.[71] Spontaneous intracranial hemorrhage has occurred in one subject and hemarthrosis in two (the latter with lower activity levels).

Treatment

Fresh frozen plasma will provide both of the deficient factors, as noted for factor V deficiency earlier. Where the factor V clotting activity is over 10–15%, factor VIII concentrates alone will often provide hemostasis, even for major surgical procedures. In one patient who underwent liver transplantation, a single dose of factor VIII was used preoperatively; within 4 hours, both plasma factors V and VIII clotting activities were normal, and levels were sustained in the normal range thereafter (A. R. Thompson, unpublished results, 1999).

CURRENT CONTROVERSIES & FUTURE CONSIDERATIONS

Factor V Disorders

- In addition to factor V clotting activity, what influences the risk of bleeding? What is the minimum level for normal hemostasis? The degree that the clinical phenotype correlates with the genotype will require genotyping more families.
- Does platelet factor V contribute to hemostasis? The evidence for megakaryocyte synthesis needs confirmation in animals other than mice.
- What is optimal treatment for factor V replacement? Dosing and frequency of plasma therapy should be examined on a larger number of patients and additional survival data in patients and animal models are needed to determine the degree of variability in clearance.
- For combined factors V and VIII deficiency, do levels or clinical phenotype correlate with the different deficiencies? What other proteins are involved in the intracellular transport pathway? Comparison of *LMAN1* with *MCFD2* knockout mice as well as double knockouts will be of interest.

FIBRINOGEN DISORDERS

Afibrinogenemia

Background

In 1920, Rabe and Saloman,[72] described a bleeding disorder in a 9-year-old boy whose parents were first cousins; furthermore, there was an absence of precipitate in the patient's plasma on heating or with $(NH_4)_2SO_4$, suggesting absence of fibrinogen. With more sensitive functional and immunologic assays, fibrinogen has been undetectable in over 200 families.[73,74]

Pathophysiology

The three fibrinogen genes occur as a cluster, Aα, Bβ, and γ, on chromosome 4. The protein is synthesized in liver and circulates as a major plasma protein that is a high-molecular-weight, disulfide-bonded dimer of the three chains $(A\alpha/B\beta/\gamma)_2$. When sufficient thrombin is generated, it removes fibrinopeptides A and B, generating fibrin monomers that polymerize into a gel or unstable clot.[75] This seals the site of injury in damaged blood vessels. The fibrinogen precursor also plays an important role in hemostasis by serving as a bridge to aggregate platelets that have been activated and expose specific binding sites on their surface.

Aα chain knockout mice appear normal at birth but have a bleeding tendency.[76] Although the Bβ and γ chains are synthesized, there are no detectable fragments that circulate in the Aα knockout mice. Neonatal or juvenile hemorrhagic complications are often fatal but their incidence is dependent upon the strain of mice homozygous for the disrupted Aα gene. Surviving females that become pregnant have fatal uterine bleeding initiated by fetal cell implantation.

In patients with afibrinogenemia that have been genotyped, the majority of mutations are null and occur in the Aα chain.[77] Exceptions are two missense mutations found in the Bβ chain. Homozygous and compound heterozygous individuals have been identified. In a database of 73 mutations associated with afibrinogenemia, 70% were in the Aα chain, 20% in the Bβ chain, and 10% in the γ chain.[78]

Clinical Features

Because fibrinogen provides the structural clot for kinetic assays, deficiency causes the prothrombin, partial thromboplastin, and thrombin times to all be prolonged. Furthermore, prolongation of the clotting time with reptilase (an enzyme from *Bothrops atrox*) is observed because this enzyme cleaves the A peptide of fibrinogen, producing a species that will polymerize into a clot. The bleeding time is often prolonged, as are platelet aggregations to common agonists, reflecting the importance of fibrinogen binding for platelet-platelet interactions and aggregation. Because fibrinogen is normally at one of the higher concentrations of plasma proteins and is a high-molecular-weight, asymmetrical species, the sedimentation rate is more rapid than normal with its deficiency. It seems reasonable that different genotypes, especially with missense mutations, have trace levels that may account for variable clinical presentation and the presence or absence of severe platelet dysfunction.[74]

The inheritance of afibrinogenemia is autosomal recessive and, although heterozygous parents and siblings frequently have hypofibrinogenemia, they are seldom symptomatic of any bleeding tendency. Severity is variable, with the most severe phenotypes experiencing umbilical stump and, in males, postcircumcision bleeding. Although serious bleeding episodes occur less frequently than in the severe hemophilias, some patients have prolonged oozing from simple skin scratches and abrasions. Menorrhagia is common, as are first-trimester spontaneous abortions. Spontaneous splenic ruptures have been reported, and several adult patients have had spontaneous intracranial hemorrhages.[73] Of 55 Iranian patients, 45 had had umbilical stump oozing, and 40 each experienced recurrent epistaxis, oral cavity bleeding, or muscle hematomas.[74] Hemarthroses occurred in 30 but were infrequent and usually associated with trauma. Only three had had intracranial bleeding; although ages ranged from 2 to 73 years, the median age was not provided. Of 20 affected Iranian women, 14 had menorrhagia.

Treatment

By ammonium sulfate fractionation, Cohn fraction I is rich in fibrinogen. Because it was frequently contaminated with viruses, its use was abandoned once cryoprecipitate was developed as a simple concentrate from small numbers of volunteer blood donors. Virally inactivated concentrates have been prepared in Japan and Europe. Because of the high recovery and long survival of fibrinogen (see Table 66–1), prophylaxis is usually feasible with weekly cryoprecipitate infusions.

Dysfibrinogenemia

Background

An abnormal fibrinogen was first documented by Imperato and Dettori.[79] Of over 300 reported, the majority of individuals were discovered incidentally and are asymptomatic. Among others, there may be a mild bleeding tendency or a risk of thrombosis.[80]

Pathophysiology

Because of the high concentration of fibrinogen in plasma and the frequency of discovery from screening tests, several abnormal fibrinogens have been identified; those that are near an amino terminus were characterized by direct amino acid sequencing. Frequently, an autosomal dominant inheritance is seen because the dysfunctional protein competes with the native fibrinogen in the kinetic tests. This also accounts for the detection of several variants that have no clinical significance. Symptomatic individuals are often compound heterozygotes for a mutation that decreases the secreted level and another that interferes with function, resulting in so-called hypo-dysfibrinogenemia. A current database[76] lists 230 families with known variants. Of the 55% with Aα chain variants, nearly half involve the thrombin cleavage site at Arg16. Of the 34% with γ chain variants, a third are in the codon for Arg275. These Arg codons contain a CpG dinucleotide and are thus "hot spots" for recurrent mutations. The carboxy-terminal portion of the γ chain is critical for end-to-end polymerization and also contains sites of dimerization by factor XIIIa. Indeed, several dysfibrinogenemic mutant residues modeled to the crystal structure may indirectly alter polymerization.[81] A variety of other kinetic effects are possible, including mutations that alter plasmin digestion or fibrinolysis; these would not necessarily prolong the thrombin time and may or may not be clinically significant.

Within the database, 21 reports (<10%) are listed as hypofibrinogenemia[78] with mutations scattered throughout the genes for each chain. Combined hypo-dysfibrinogenemia or results of actual levels, however, are not captured in this database.

Clinical Features

The hallmark of a dysfibrinogenemia is the low activity by a kinetic measure of fibrin generation, whereas the fibrinogen protein or antigen level is normal.[80] Especially where fibrinopeptide A cleavage is reduced or absent, the thrombin time is prolonged, as is the reptilase time. Of those patients with recurrent Arg16 Aα chain variants, 10 of 34 reported are listed as having a bleeding tendency and 5 others, a history of thrombosis. For those with Arg275 γ chain variants, the majority of the 23 patients for whom symptoms were recorded were asymptomatic; only 2 had a bleeding tendency and 4 others had a history of thrombosis.[78] Even when a bleeding tendency has been identified, other significant hemostatic defects have been carefully excluded only in a minority of cases. Thus in any patient with a mild bleeding tendency and dysfibrinogenemia or hypo-dysfibrinogenemia, the fibrinogen variant(s) may or may not be etiologic. A few cases have been reported of obstetric complications associated with an autosomal dominant abnormality of fibrinogen. A uterine wall hematoma was responsible for abruptio placenta in one woman who was otherwise asymptomatic, as were three affected males in her family.[82] It is possible that a thrombotic tendency could contribute to fetal loss in some women with a fibrinogen variant.

Treatment

When there is a bleeding tendency associated with dysfibrinogenemia or hypo-dysfibrinogenemia, the strategy is to increase the concentration of the native protein to offset the competition from the dysfunctional species. This is done with cryoprecipitate as a concentrated fibrinogen source, although the dose and frequency required are variable such that one likes to establish a treatment plan that works empirically for any given patient. It should also be borne in mind that bleeding may vary among different affected members of the same family, depending upon whether or not another hemostatic defect or risk profile is present. One Japanese woman who had lost four previous pregnancies received prophylactic fibrinogen concentrate three times per week and carried her fifth pregnancy to 29 weeks. At that point premature contractions and vaginal bleeding occurred, prompting cesarean section. Delivery was successful, although 5 units of blood were replaced despite a preoperative bolus of fibrinogen.[83] Another woman with hypo-dysfibrinogenemia and recurrent fetal loss also delivered a normal child after prophylactic fibrinogen.[84]

CURRENT CONTROVERSIES & FUTURE CONSIDERATIONS

Fibrinogen Disorders

- Do trace levels of fibrinogen protect against platelet dysfunction? More detail on phenotype-genotype correlations as well as more sensitive immunoassays will be necessary to resolve this.
- What is the minimum level for normal hemostasis during prophylactic therapy? In afibrinogenemia, it would also be helpful to know the level that would protect against spontaneous bleeding.
- Can one predict a bleeding phenotype among dysfibrinogenemias? Genotype-phenotype correlations and other hemostatic screening may help distinguish the more common asymptomatic variants.

FACTOR XIII DEFICIENCY

Background

Factor XIII was discovered by in vitro studies as a transglutaminase that cross-links fibrin to form an insoluble clot.[85] Sixteen years later, a congenital deficiency state was identified by Duckert and colleagues.[86] Although deficiency is rare, it should be considered when a congenital bleeding tendency is present or suspected and screening tests that depend upon fibrin polymerization, such as the prothrombin, partial thromboplastin, and thrombin, times are all normal.

Pathophysiology

Factor XIII circulates as a tetrameric protein with dimers of two subunits, A_2B_2, formed by noncovalent interactions. The genes for the A and B subunits are on chromosomes 6 and 1, respectively. Transglutaminase activity is provided by the A_2 dimer following cleavage of an amino-terminal activation peptide by thrombin. The B dimer stabilizes A_2 in circulation. Platelets have only A_2 dimers. Synthesis of the A subunits appears to occur in several tissues, including megakaryocytes, monocytes, and the placenta; the origin of circulating A_2 has not been established and contribution from liver has not been excluded. The B subunit appears to be synthesized in the liver.[87]

Mice with an A subunit gene knockout survive, but some die of neonatal hemorrhage.[88] Affected females that become pregnant develop vaginal bleeding and have spontaneous abortions as a result of massive placental hemorrhage.[88,89] A variety of missense, nonsense, frameshift, and splicing mutations have been identified in the factor XIII genes of affected individuals, including molecular modeling of A chain missense mutations to its crystal structure.[88,90] In symptomatic individuals, there is either homozygosity or compound heterozygosity for gene defects, only rarely with B subunit mutations[91] wherein a milder phenotype and platelet A_2 may be present.[90] Carriers have not been symptomatic. In a series of 10 unrelated Iranian subjects with clinically severe deficiency, homozygosity for a mutation in the A subunit gene was found in all, including two different frameshift genotypes and missense changes in the others.[92] One of the latter, Arg77 to His, was present in five of the families, suggesting a founder effect. A milder phenotype was present in one family homozygous for a splice junction genotype that is associated with trace levels of a normally spliced messenger RNA and, presumably, of functional protein in platelets and plasma.[93]

Clinical Features

Only approximately 5% levels of factor XIII are required for normal hemostasis; levels below this usually give a positive screening test in which fibrin clots from plasma samples solubilize when incubated with a denaturant such as urea. This is due to inadequate covalent cross-linking of the polymerized fibrin. Most of the patients described are severe, but it is difficult to distinguish low levels from absence of factor XIII. Also, for those on prophylaxis with monthly infusions, there is usually significant residual activity in trough samples. More sensitive functional and immunologic assays have been applied in some research settings, but are not widely available clinically. In the molecular correlation study of 10 Iranian subjects, it was noteworthy that all had at least half-normal levels of circulating B subunits on immunologic testing.[92]

Within different series, about 80% of subjects had had prolonged oozing from their umbilical stump, frequently requiring blood transfusion, 60% had easy bruisability, 50% had oral oozing or hemarthrosis, and 30% had at least one intracranial bleed.[92,94] Heavy menses have been noted in half of the women after menarche; one affected woman had had 13 miscarriages.[92] In addition, poor surgical wound healing with dehiscence and cheloid formation is often seen.

Treatment

There is sufficient factor XIII in infused normal plasma or cryoprecipitate to readily provide hemostatic levels.

Patients given platelet concentrates receive sufficient plasma as well. A plasma-derived concentrate prepared in Europe (originally purified from placental tissue) is more convenient and has been virally attenuated; it is used in several patients in the United States under an investigational drug status.[95] More recently, a recombinant A subunit has been developed and a Phase I trial in congenitally deficient patients looks promising.[96] Because of the large size and essentially complete intravascular recovery of factor XIII, as well as its long half-life in circulation (see Table 66–1), prophylaxis with monthly infusions is usually sufficient to prevent any abnormal bleeding episodes, even after trauma or surgery. Because clinically significant deficiency caused by an absent or abnormal B subunit rarely occurs, the response to a recombinant A_2 preparation is facilitated by stabilization from endogenous, circulating B dimers. A few cases of alloantibody inhibitors have been described.

Current Controversies & Future Considerations

Factor XIII Disorders

- Does the risk of spontaneous, life-threatening bleeding correlate with specific phenotypes? The presence of a milder phenotype with a given splicing genotype suggests that trace but undetectable levels of activity are protective. Additional genotype data on patients with similar phenotypes will be of great interest. More sensitive and specific functional assays are needed to detect trace levels and help predict a less severe phenotype.
- How important is platelet A_2 in hemostasis? It is possible that some genotypes with predominantly secretory defects may have residual activity from platelets but not in plasma. Additional studies on the platelets of individuals with null mutations in their B subunit genes as well as B subunit knockout mice would be of interest to determine if their platelet A_2 is normal and whether or not it will support hemostasis, at least under some circumstances. Trace levels of circulating A_2 might also account for a milder phenotype.

Suggested Readings*

Acharya SS, Coughlin A, DiMichele DM: Rare bleeding disorder registry: deficiency of factors II, V, VII, X, XIII, fibrinogen and dysfibrinogenemias. J Thromb Haemost 2:248–256, 2004.

Al-Mondhiry H, Ehmann WC: Congenital afibrinogenemia. Am J Hematol 46:343–347, 1994.

Anwar R, Miloszewski KJA: Factor XIII deficiency. Br J Haematol 107:468–484, 1999.

Bolton-Maggs PH, Perry DJ, Chalmers EA, et al: The rare coagulation disorders—review with guidelines for management from the United Kingdom Haemophilia Centre Doctors' Organisation. Haemophilia 10:593–628, 2004.

Mannucci PM, Duga S, Peyvandi F: Recessively inherited coagulation disorders. Blood 104:1243–1252, 2004.

Martinez J: Congenital dysfibrinogenemia. Curr Opin Hematol 4:357–363, 1997.

McVey JH, Boswell E, Mumford AD, et al: Factor VII deficiency and the FVII mutation database. Hum Mutat 17:3–17, 2001.

Montefusco MC, Duga S, Asselta R, et al: Clinical and molecular characterization of 6 patients affected by severe deficiency of coagulation factor V: broadening of the mutational spectrum of factor V gene and in vitro analysis of the newly identified missense mutations. Blood 102:3210–3216, 2003.

Saunders RE, O'Connell NM, Lee CA, et al: Factor XI deficiency database: An interactive web database of mutations, phenotypes and structural analysis tools. Hum Mutat 26:192–198, 2005. Also available at: http//www.FactorXI.org.

Stafford DW: The vitamin K cycle. J Thromb Haemost 3:1873–1878, 2005.

Uprichard J, Perry DJ: Factor X deficiency. Blood Rev 16:97–110, 2002.

**Full references for this chapter can be found on accompanying CD-ROM.*

CHAPTER 67

Inherited Thrombophilia

Marcel Levi, MD, PhD, and Saskia Middeldorp, MD, PhD

KEY POINTS

Inherited Thrombophilia

- (Recurrent) venous thrombosis may be due to inherited thrombophilia in 30–50% of patients.
- The annual risk of a first episode of thrombosis in patients with inherited thrombophilia is 0.5–2% per year.
- The risk of recurrent venous thromboembolism in patients with inherited thrombophilia and a previous episode of thrombosis is only slightly higher than in patients who have had thrombosis and do not have inherited thrombophilia.
- Acquired risk factors for venous thromboembolism (such as use of oral contraceptives) may considerably amplify the risk of thrombosis in patients with inherited thrombophilia.
- Management of inherited thrombophilia may, depending on the risk of the patient for recurrent thrombosis and bleeding complications, vary from lifelong anticoagulant treatment to no specific actions.

INTRODUCTION

Thrombophilia is defined as a disorder associated with an increased tendency to venous thromboembolism. Thrombophilia can be acquired, as in patients with cancer, or congenital, in which case a defect in the coagulation system is inherited. This chapter is limited to the various forms of inherited thrombophilia.

The first case of inherited thrombophilia was described in 1965 by Egeberg in a publication on a Norwegian family with a remarkable tendency to develop venous thrombosis, which was shown to be due to a deficiency of the physiologic anticoagulant antithrombin.[1] Since then, various forms of inherited thrombophilia have been identified and, in a large number of clinical studies, the relative and absolute risk for venous thromboembolism of each of these thrombophilic conditions has been studied.[2] A rough literature search in the PubMed database between 1966 and 2004 yields more than 15,000 publications on thrombophilia, of which the vast majority is related to inherited forms of this condition.

It is important to emphasize that thrombophilia is diagnosed on clinical grounds.[3] Major criteria are given in Table 67–1. The most common criteria for thrombophilia are recurrent venous thromboembolism, a family history of thrombosis, thrombosis with an unusual localization (Fig. 67–1), and thrombosis at young age, although the majority of patients with thrombophilia will have their first manifestation of thrombosis at a later age. In most patients with inherited thrombophilia, the tendency to venous thromboembolism is mild to moderate and can be easily controlled with antithrombotic agents. Defects leading to inherited thrombophilia may also cause clinical manifestations other than thrombosis, such as skin necrosis in patients with a protein C deficiency who are treated with vitamin K antagonists, or neonatal purpura fulminans in homozygous protein C deficiency (Fig. 67–2). Also, many thrombophilic disorders may cause an increased risk of pregnancy loss, preeclampsia, and the hemolysis, elevated liver enzymes, and low platelets (HELLP) syndrome of pregnancy.

Forms of Inherited Thrombophilia

Table 67–2 lists all inherited abnormalities with a certain associated increased risk of venous thromboembolism. In addition, Table 67–2 also lists a number of defects that have been reported to be associated with thrombophilia, but for which the evidence is equivocal. This is due to conflicting findings (e.g., factor XII deficiency),[4,5] a small numbers of patients studied so far (e.g., plasminogen deficiency, or decreased fibrinolysis resulting from defective release of plasminogen activators or increased levels of plasminogen activator inhibitor type 1),[6–8] or the fact that studies on the risk of thrombosis are ongoing (e.g., thrombomodulin mutations).[9]

The most frequently occurring established inherited thrombophilic defects are resistance to activated protein C caused by a point mutation in the gene for factor V (known as factor V Leiden or factor V:Q506; Fig. 67–3)

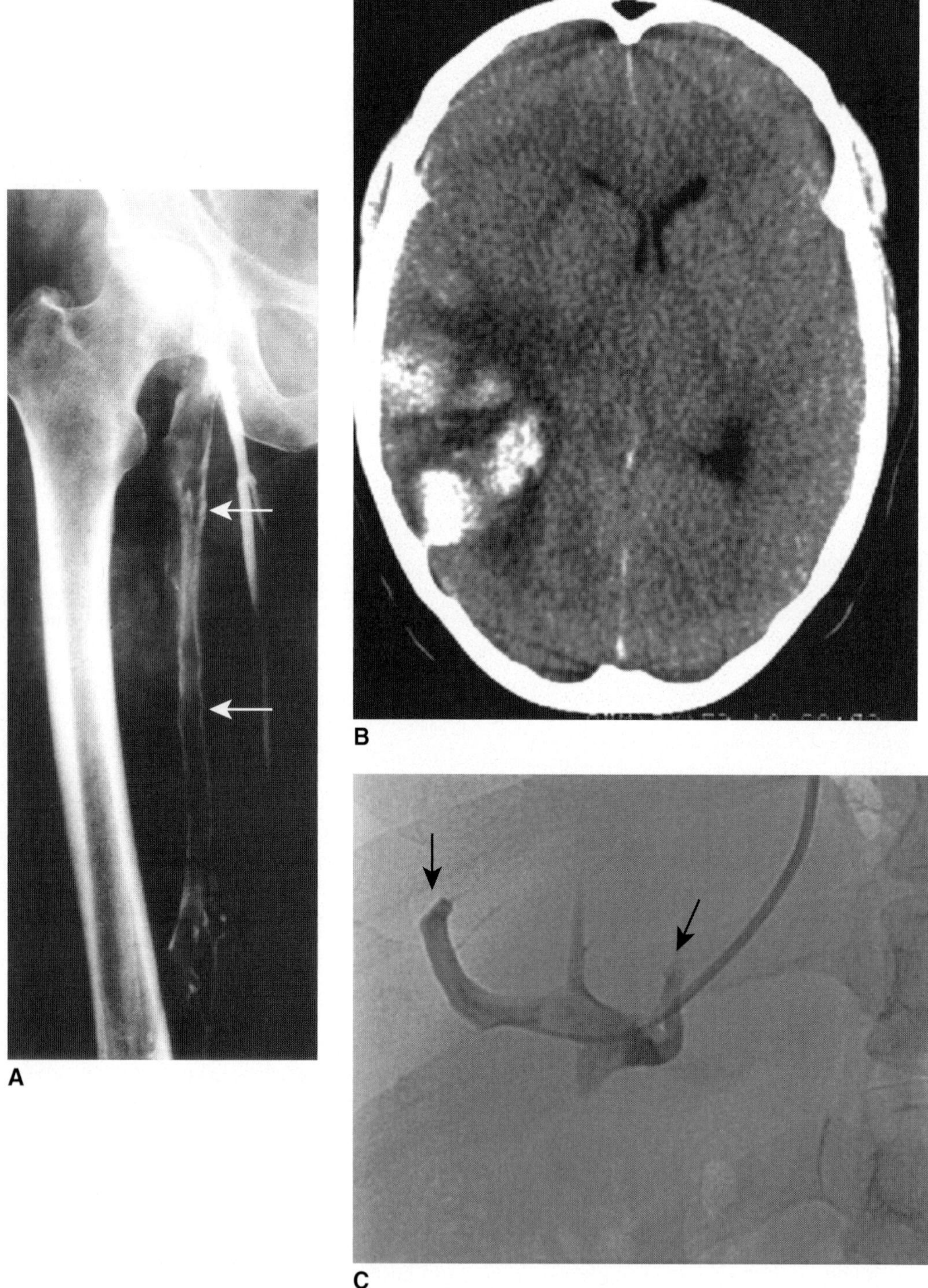

■ **Figure 67–1.** Examples of venous thrombosis that may occur in patients with inherited thrombophilia. *A,* Deep vein thrombosis of the lower extremity is the most common clinical manifestation of inherited thrombophilia. The *arrows* indicate contrast filling defects in the superficial femoral vein. Thrombosis may also occur at more unusual sites. *B,* Cerebral sinus vein thrombosis, as shown on computed tomography scan of the brain. *C,* Hepatic vein thrombosis in Budd-Chiari syndrome as shown by contrast venography; the *arrows* indicate blockages in the hepatic vein.

TABLE 67–1. Most Common Criteria for Thrombophilia

Recurrent venous thromboembolism
Thrombosis in an unusual site (cerebral sinuses, mesenteric, portal)
Venous thromboembolism at a young age
Family history of venous thromboembolism
Recurrent fetal loss
Preeclampsia, HELLP syndrome

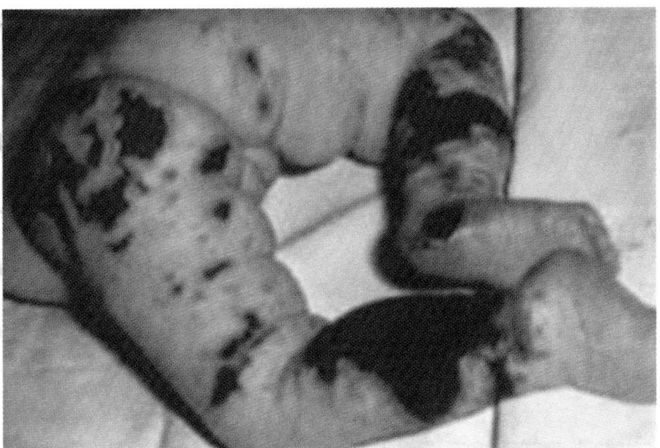

Figure 67–2. Purpura fulminans in a baby with homozygous protein C deficiency.

and a mutation in the prothrombin gene (prothrombin G20210A).[2,3] Antithrombin, protein C, and protein S deficiencies are relatively rare. Elevated levels of factor VIII have also been associated with an increased risk of venous thromboembolism. It seems that increased factor VIII levels are in part genetically determined, although the cause of the elevation in factor VIII is unknown. High levels of homocysteine can be caused by a homozygous mutation in methylenetetrahydrofolate reductase (MTHFR) and may therefore also be considered as a hereditary risk factor for thrombosis.[10] However, although hyperhomocystinemia is clearly associated with thrombosis, the etiologic role of the MTHFR mutation in thrombosis is less clear.[11,12] Therefore, we do not further discuss the MTHFR mutation in detail in this chapter.

EPIDEMIOLOGY

The reported prevalence of thrombophilia varies among different populations of patients with venous thromboembolism. Because of selection or diagnostic suspicion bias, a relatively high prevalence is found when series of patients with a suggestive family history or recurrent venous thromboembolism are studied by specialized laboratories; in contrast, a lower prevalence is established in consecutive, unselected patients (Table 67–3). In general, at present a laboratory abnormality can be detected in more than half of the patients with documented venous thromboembolism. Apart from patient selection, there are other factors influencing the prevalence of thrombophilia. The reported prevalence of

TABLE 67–2. Proven or Postulated Causes of Inherited Thrombophilia

Proven Causes	Postulated Causes*
Antithrombin deficiency	Plasminogen deficiency
Protein C deficiency	Increased histidine-rich glycoprotein
Protein S deficiency	Decreased plasminogen activator release
Factor V Leiden mutation (APC resistance)	Increased plasminogen activator inhibitor
Prothrombin G20210A mutation	Thrombomodulin mutations
Dysfibrinogenemia (rare)	Factor XII deficiency
Elevated factor VIII levels (etiology to be determined)	

*Postulated causes have not equivocally been proven in sound clinical studies or are under investigation.
Abbreviation: APC, activated protein C.

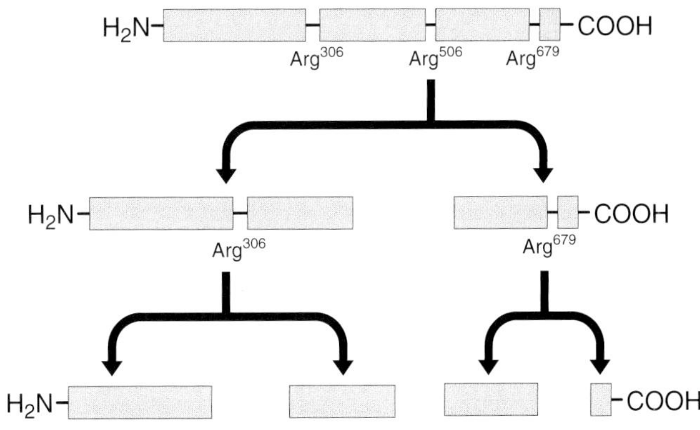

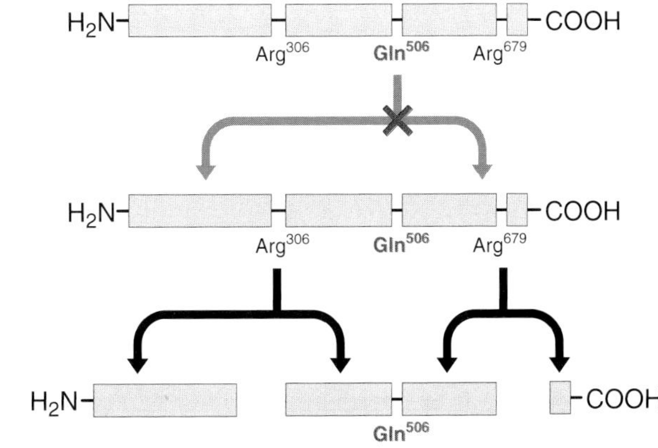

Figure 67–3. Schematic representation of the factor V Leiden mutation. At amino acid position 406, arginine (Arg) is replaced by glutamine (Gln), which makes the molecule less susceptible to cleavage by activated protein C at this site. Further cleavage of the factor V molecule at amino acid positions 306 and 679 can occur normally.

TABLE 67–3. Prevalence of an Inherited Thrombophilic Defect in Studies of Selected Series of Patients with Thrombosis (Recurrent Thrombosis, Positive Family History, etc.) and in Consecutive Patients with a First Episode of Venous Thrombosis

	Antithrombin Deficiency (%)	Protein C Deficiency (%)	Protein S Deficiency (%)	Factor V Leiden Mutation (%)	Prothrombin G20210A Mutation (%)	Increased Factor VIII Levels* (%)
Selected Series of Patients						
Gladson[118]	3.0	4.0	5.0	—	—	—
Ben-Tal[119]	7.5	5.6	2.8	—	—	—
Schattner[120]	3.3	3.3	3.3	28	—	—
Poort[121]	—	—	—	—	18	
O'Donnell[122]	—	—	—	—	—	17.3
Kraaijenhagen[93]	—	—	—	—	—	56.7
Consecutive Patients with Thrombosis						
Heijboer[123]	1.1	3.2	2.2	—	—	—
Pabinger[124]	2.8	2.5	1.3	—	—	—
Koster, Poort[121,125,126]	1.1	3.1	3.1	1	6.2	25
Cumming[127]	0.9	5.0	4.1	4.1	5.5	—
Brown[128]	—	—	—	5.9	5.0	—
Kraaijenhagen[93]	—	—	—	—	—	32.8

*Increased factor VIII levels are defined as >170%.

protein C or S deficiency can be influenced by differences in laboratory definition. The prevalence of the factor V Leiden and the prothrombin G20210A mutations varies in its geographic distribution.

In the general population, the prevalence of antithrombin deficiency is about 1:300 and the prevalence of protein C deficiency between 1:200 and 1:500, as documented by mass screening of blood donors.[13–15] [13–15] The prevalence of the factor V Leiden mutation and that of the prothrombin G20210A mutation vary in Europe between 2% and 7% and between 1% and 3%, respectively, whereas both mutations are rare in individuals of Asian or African descent (Fig. 67–4).[16–19]

PATHOPHYSIOLOGY

For most inherited thrombophilic disorders, there is a strong or at least moderate biologic plausibility that links the defect to the increased risk of venous thromboembolism. A deficiency of one of the physiologic anticoagulant proteins—antithrombin, protein C, or protein S—will theoretically lead to an imbalance in basal coagulation activation and thereby predispose to a prethrombotic state. This notion has in fact been confirmed in studies showing that a deficiency of one of these anticoagulant factors results in increased markers of thrombin generation.[20,21] The factor V Leiden mutation results in a decreased sensitivity of the mutated factor V for proteolytic degradation by activated protein C and thereby results in resistance to activated protein C (see Fig. 67–3). The prothrombin G20210A mutation results in (moderately) elevated prothrombin levels and may therefore lead to an increased prothrombotic tendency. A similar mechanism plays a role in the case of elevated factor VIII or XI levels. It should be mentioned, however, that from a biochemical perspective it is not crystal clear why increased levels of a clotting factor would lead to a more activated state of the coagulation system, and that additional, yet unidentified, mechanisms may play a role.

To establish a causal relationship between a thrombophilic laboratory abnormality and the occurrence of thrombosis, the observation that correction of the defect lowers the tendency to develop thrombosis would be helpful. Indeed, correction of decreased antithrombin or protein C levels has been shown to reverse the thrombotic risk (although this is not necessarily the treatment of choice in affected patients). Also, murine models of a targeted deletion of an anticoagulant protein (such as antithrombin or protein C) or targeted insertion of a prothrombotic mutation (such as factor V Leiden) result in a prothrombotic state.[22–24]

Clinical studies further confirm the association between thrombophilic defects in the coagulation system and the occurrence of venous thromboembolism. Such studies usually are designed as family studies (including affected and unaffected individuals), case-control studies, or prospective cohort studies. Numerous studies have assessed the relative risk of thrombosis in families with antithrombin, protein C, or protein S deficiency, or with the factor V Leiden or the prothrombin G20210A mutation.[3,25,26] The earlier studies in families with antithrombin, protein C, or protein S deficiency are likely to have overestimated the incidence of venous thromboembolism, because diagnostic confirmation of thromboembolism was often lacking and the diagnosis of previous episodes of venous thromboembolism was often made with knowledge of the deficiency status. This may have led to an overestimation of the prevalence of thrombosis, because it is well known that about two thirds of patients with clinical manifestations suggestive of venous thromboembolism do not have this diagnosis confirmed by objective tests. This contention is supported by the lower absolute and relative risks for venous throm-

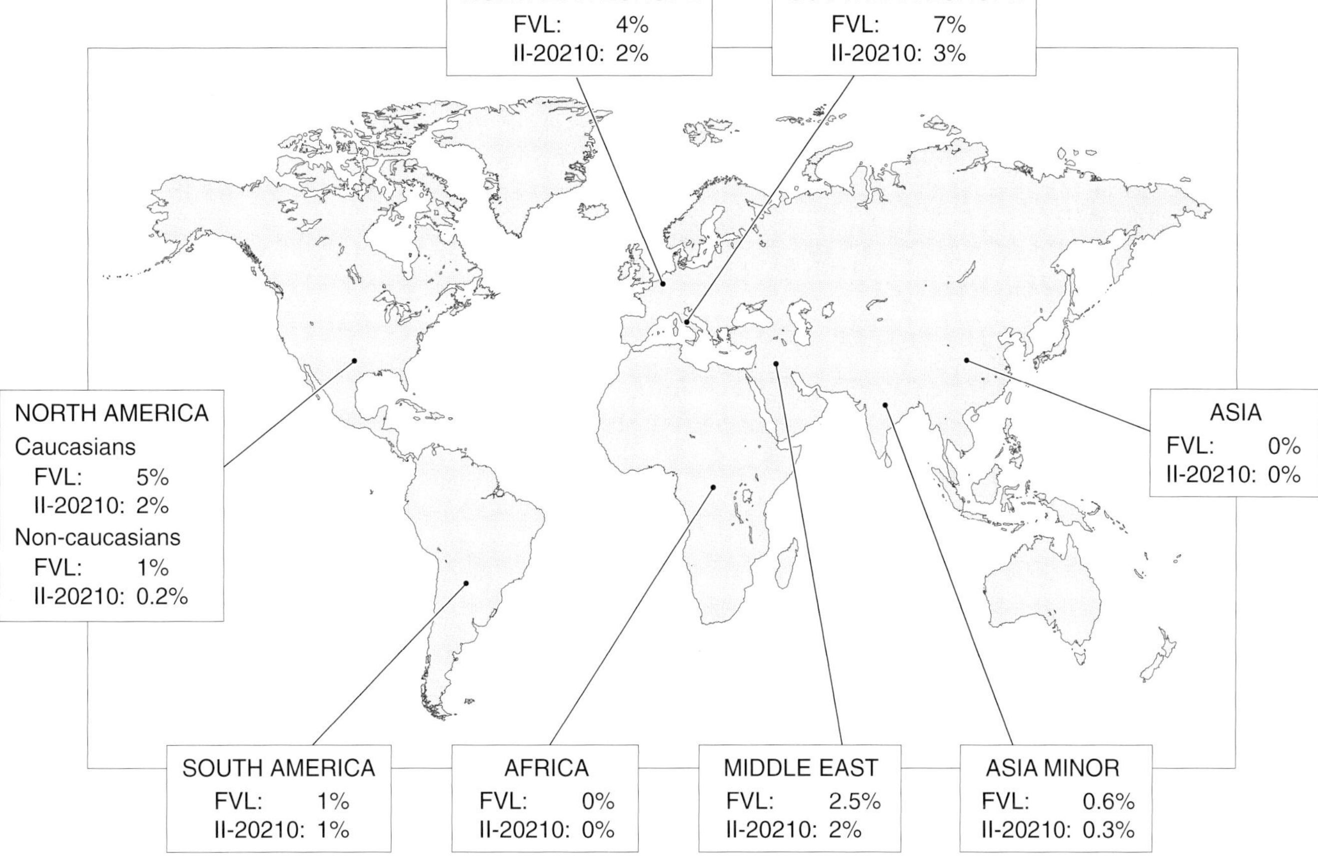

Figure 67–4. Geographic distribution of the prevalence of the two most common forms of inherited thrombophilia: the factor V Leiden (FVL) and the prothrombin G20210A (II-20210) mutation.

boembolism in carriers of antithrombin, protein C, and protein S deficiencies found in more recent studies.[2] The first family studies available for the prothrombin G20210A mutation show a similar outcome.[27–29] Finally, but importantly, a number of prospective cohort studies have now demonstrated that the incidence of venous thromboembolism in (asymptomatic) carriers of antithrombin, protein C, or protein S deficiency, as well as the factor V Leiden mutation, is higher than in the general population.[26,30,31]

CLINICAL FEATURES AND DIAGNOSIS

The classical clinical presentation of a thrombophilic defect is the development of venous thrombosis of the lower extremity and/or pulmonary embolism. Less commonly, patients may present with (recurrent episodes of) superficial thrombophlebitis or thrombosis at an unusual site, such as upper extremity thrombosis, thrombosis in the digestive tract (e.g., portal vein or mesenteric vein thrombosis), or cerebral sinus thrombosis. Patients with the most frequently occurring thrombophilic defects, the factor V Leiden and the prothrombin G20210A mutations, have in general a lower tendency to thrombosis than patients with a deficiency of antithrombin, protein C, or protein S (see later). Approximately half of the patients with a thrombophilic abnormality develop their first thromboembolism in a situation in which the risk of thrombosis is increased, such as in the puerperium, shortly after the initiation of oral contraceptive treatment, after trauma and/or immobilization, or in a postoperative state. Although thrombosis at a (relatively) young age is a criterion for thrombophilia, the vast majority of patients have their first thromboembolism in adulthood or even at an advanced age.[25] The theoretical concept underlying this clinical manifestation is that patients with thrombophilia have a prethrombotic state that is in itself insufficient to cause thrombosis but, when superimposed upon other risk factors for thrombosis (e.g., increasing age, or conditions known to increase the risk of thrombosis), may lead to the clinical event.

In general, antithrombin, protein C, and protein S deficiency and the factor V Leiden mutation do not appear to be strongly associated with a significantly increased risk of arterial thrombosis.[32] There are, however, some exceptions. Some case series have reported an association with arterial thrombosis, especially in children, and one case-control study among highly selected young women with acute myocardial infarction showed an association between the factor V Leiden mutation and the risk of myocardial infarction, especially when concomitant risk factors, such as smoking, were also present.[33–35] The prothrombin mutation has also been reported to be a

RR for major bleeding (columns); RR for VTE (rows)

RR for VTE	1.0	1.5	2.0	2.5	3.0	3.5	4.0	5.0	6.0	7.0
0.5	5	1	1	1	1	1	1	1	1	1
1.0	17	10	5	2	1	1	1	1	1	1
1.5	24	17	12	8	5	3	1	1	1	1
2.0	31	22	17	13	10	7	5	2	1	1
2.5	37	26	21	17	13	11	9	5	2	1
3.0	43	31	24	20	17	14	12	8	5	3
4.0	60	39	31	26	22	19	17	13	10	7
5.0	E	47	37	31	26	23	21	17	13	11
6.0	E	60	43	36	31	27	24	20	17	14
8.0	E	E	60	46	39	34	31	26	22	19

DETERMINATION OF THE OPTIMAL TREATMENT DURATION

1. Determine the relative risk for developing a recurrent VTE. In presence of 2 or more risk factors for recurrent VTE, the risk ratios should be multiplied.
2. Determine the risk for developing a major bleeding. In presence of 2 risk factors for major bleeding, the risk ratios should be multiplied.
3. The calculated RR's should be rounded down to the nearest stratum.
4. Read the corresponding treatment duration (in months) in the table.

FORMULA

$t = -14 \ln (0.39 \times (RR_{bleeding}/RR_{recurence}) - 1/12)$

RR FOR VTE		*95% CI*
Prothrombin mutation	1.4	(0.9–2.0)
Factor V Leiden	1.3	(1.0–1.7)
Elevated Factor VIII (>200IU/dl)	1.8	(1.0–3.3)
Prot C/S or ATIII deficiency	2.5	na
APLA	2.5	na
Hyperhomocysteinemia	2.5	na
Cancer*	2.0–4.0	na
Recurrent DVT	1.5	na
Secondary DVT	0.5	na
Multiply RR's for total score	....	....

RR FOR MAJOR BLEEDING		
Every 10 yr. above age of 40	1.5	(1.2–1.8)
Cancer	2.0	na
Multiply RR's for total score	....	....

KEY

RR=Relative risk

VTE=Venous thromboembolism

prot C=Protein C

prot S=Protein S

AT=Antithrombin

APLA=Antophospholipidantibodies

na=Not available

95%CI=95% confidence interval

E=Extended

*=RR=4.0 for pancreas, ovarian, lung and mucin secreting gastro-intestinal carcinoma. RR=2.0 for all other types of cancer

Figure 67–5. Proposed nomogram for determination of the optimal duration of anticoagulation in patients with venous thromboembolism. The relative risks (RR) for venous thromboembolism (VTE) and major bleeding are calculated using the table. Using the nomogram, the optimal duration is given in months. For example, a 70-year-old woman with a venous thrombosis after hip surgery (secondary thrombosis), who is otherwise healthy and has no thrombophilic risk factors, has a relative risk of 0.5 for thrombosis and a relative risk of 3.4 for bleeding (age is 3 × 10 years above 40 years), resulting in a treatment duration of 1 month. A 30-year-old man with recurrent idiopathic thrombosis and a persistent elevated factor VIII level has a relative risk for thrombosis of 1.8 (factor VIII) × 1.5 (recurrence) = 2.7 and a relative risk for bleeding of 1.0, resulting in a treatment duration of 37 months.

weak risk factor for myocardial infarction in selected young patients.[36,37] Recent meta-analyses show that, if there is any association between thrombophilic risk factors and arterial thrombosis, this relationship is very weak at best.[38,39]

As mentioned earlier, other clinical manifestations of thrombophilic abnormalities in the coagulation system are an increased risk of fetal loss, intrauterine growth retardation, or premature birth.[40–43] A plausible mechanism is placental (micro)vascular thrombosis, leading to infarction of the placenta and ensuing placental insufficiency. This hypothesis is supported by the observation that the risk of miscarriage is even further increased if both mother and fetus are carriers of factor V Leiden.[44] Other obstetric complications associated with thrombophilia are severe preeclampsia and the HELLP syndrome.[45–47]

Homozygous deficiency of protein C or S leads to purpura fulminans shortly after birth.[48] This is thought to be due to massive intravascular thrombosis of the skin vasculature. Similarly, patients with a protein C or S deficiency can develop skin necrosis when vitamin K antagonists are started, although this complication is quite rare.[49] Because proteins C and S have a relatively short half-life, these factors will drop relatively early after initiation of anti–vitamin K treatment (when the other vitamin K–dependent factors are still normal or only slightly decreased), resulting in a paradoxical net aggravation of the prethrombotic state.

Risk of Thrombosis in Thrombophilia

There is considerable variation in the relative risk for venous thromboembolism among the various forms of hereditary thrombophilia. In addition, the absolute risk of thrombosis is influenced by age and clinical circumstances (e.g., periods of immobilization, surgery, or pregnancy). Knowledge of both the absolute risk of venous thromboembolism in the untreated patient and the risk of bleeding with anticoagulants is required to make rational management decisions with respect to preventive strategies. Individualization of the duration of treatment based on this knowledge and using a decision model has been proposed.[50]

Table 67–4 lists the absolute risk of venous thromboembolism in carriers of thrombophilic defects. These figures are based on both retrospective and prospective studies. Retrospective studies are mostly studies in relatives of consecutive patients with various thrombophilic defects that compared the absolute incidence of venous thromboembolism in carriers and noncarriers.[26,27,51] These estimates may, however, be less reliable because (1) retrospective studies carry the risk of (unconscious) selection of patients and data, (2) the clinical diagnosis of thromboembolism was often not confirmed by objective tests, and (3) early deaths caused by fatal pulmonary events would not be accounted for. Prospective cohort studies of asymptomatic carriers of inherited thrombophilic defects are probably better suited to estimate the true incidence of thrombosis in thrombophilic patients.[30,31] As shown in Table 67–4, however, the differences between the retrospective and prospective studies are relatively small.

The risk of thromboembolism in individuals homozygous for thrombophilic defects, such as the prothrombin G20210A or the factor V Leiden mutation, is higher than in heterozygotes. Similarly, patients with a heterozygous mutation of one of these factors in combination with another thrombophilic abnormality (which is not uncommon in view of the relatively high frequency of the factor V Leiden and the prothrombin G20210A mutations) have a higher risk than patients with a single defect. For individuals homozygous for the factor V Leiden mutation, the relative risk for venous thromboembolism has been estimated to be as high as 80,[52] which does not exclude that homozygous individuals may remain asymptomatic throughout their lives.[53–55] Also, patients with a protein C deficiency more often experience thrombosis if they also carry a factor V Leiden mutation, compared to patients with a protein C deficiency alone.[56] A similar observation has been made in protein S–deficient families.[57,58] Finally, in a nested case-control study, the relative risk for idiopathic venous thromboembolism with either the factor V Leiden mutation or hyperhomocystinemia was approximately 3, whereas the combination of the two abnormalities was associated with a relative risk of 22.[59] Approximately half of the thromboembolic episodes in patients with inherited thrombophilic defects occur spontaneously. The risks of spontaneous venous thromboembolism are therefore approximately half of the figures given in Table 67–4.

Surgery, trauma, and prolonged immobilization are thought to be risk factors for venous thromboembolism in carriers of thrombophilic defects, although some studies show equivocal results.[60–62] Only a limited number of studies are available that have reported the risk of surgery-related venous thromboembolism in asymptomatic carriers. The estimated incidence of venous thromboembolism in relationship to high-risk situations is shown in Table 67–5.

Patients who use oral contraceptives or hormone replacement therapy have a higher risk of venous thromboembolism.[63–65] This risk is more pronounced in women with thrombophilia.[66,67] An estimation of the absolute risk of venous thromboembolism in women with thrombophilia who use oral contraceptives is shown in Table 67–6. Remarkably, a striking difference in the risk of venous thromboembolism during oral contraceptive use is observed in women with antithrombin, protein C, or protein S deficiency, compared to that observed in women with the factor V Leiden mutation (4% vs 0.7%

TABLE 67–4. Estimated Annual Incidence of a First Episode of Venous Thromboembolism in Carriers of Thrombophilic Defects

Age Group (yr)	Antithrombin Deficiency[26,32,129]	Protein C Deficiency[26,32]	Protein S Deficiency[26,32]	Factor V Leiden Mutation[31,51,60,130]	Prothrombin G20210A Mutation[27]
Prospective Studies: %/year (95% CI)					
All ages > 15					
All VTE	4.0 (1.3–8.8)	1.6 (0.5–3.5)	1.3 (0.4–3.0)	0.5 (0.13–1.3)	
Spontaneous VTE	1.6 (0.2–5.8)	1.0 (0.1–3.5)	0.4 (0–2.0)	0.25 (0.03–0.91)	
Retrospective Studies (%/year)					
Age < 15	0.1	0.1	0.2	0	
All ages > 15	1.0–2.9	1.0–3.0	1.0–3.1	0.3–0.5	0.46

Abbreviations: CI, confidence interval; VTE, venous thromboembolism.

TABLE 67–5. Incidence of Venous Thromboembolism (VTE) During an Episode of Surgery, Trauma, or Immobilization in Asymptomatic Carriers of Thrombophilic Defects

	Antithrombin, Protein C, or Protein S Deficiency	Factor V Leiden Mutation
Retrospective Studies [51,72]		
Total number of risk episodes	173	534
Number of VTE	14 (8%)	11 (2%)
Prospective Studies [26,30,31]		
Total number of risk episodes	31	69
No anticoagulant prophylaxis	16	40
Standard anticoagulant prophylaxis	15	29
Number of VTE	3 (10%)	1 (1.4%)

Note that, in the retrospective studies, different anticoagulant prophylaxis regimens were used, ranging from none to treatment with full-dose heparin or vitamin K antagonists.

TABLE 67–6. Estimated Incidence of Venous Thromboembolism During Oral Contraceptive Use in Asymptomatic Women with Thrombophilic Defects

	Antithrombin, Protein C, or Protein S Deficiency	Factor V Leiden Mutation
Retrospective Studies [51,72]		
Total number of years of OC use	117	722
Total number of VTE	5 (4.3%/yr)	5 (0.7%/yr)
Prospective Studies [26,31]		
Total number of years of OC use/number of women using OC	18/8	99/66
Total number of VTE	0 (0%/yr)	1 (1%/yr; 95% CI 0.0–5.5%)

Abbreviations: CI, confidence interval; OC, oral contraceptive; VTE, venous thromboembolism.

per year of oral contraceptive use). The prospective studies are in fact less informative because they are limited by sample size. No data are available on the absolute risk of venous thromboembolic disease for women with thrombophilia who are taking hormone replacement therapy.

During pregnancy, and in particular during the postpartum period, the risk of venous thromboembolism is increased.[68,69] A very high incidence of postpartum thromboembolic events has been reported in women with antithrombin deficiency (33%) and also for protein C and protein S deficiency (although the reported incidence in these patients seems somewhat lower).[70,71] However, these figures need to be interpreted with utmost caution and are likely to be overestimated because they were derived from case series in selected study populations and only a minority of the thromboembolic episodes were confirmed by objective tests. Moreover, the reported series included patients with previous thrombosis as well as asymptomatic carriers. There is a limited number of prospective studies on the incidence of thromboembolism in pregnant asymptomatic carriers of a thrombophilic defect (Table 67–7).[30,31,51,72,73]

TABLE 67–7. Estimated Incidence of Venous Thromboembolism (VTE) During Pregnancy and the Postpartum Period in Asymptomatic Women with Thrombophilic Defects

	Antithrombin, Protein C, or Protein S Deficiency: *N* (% of Pregnancies)	Factor V Leiden Mutation: *N* (% of Pregnancies)
Retrospective Studies [51,72,73]		
Total number of pregnancies	169	392
Total number of VTE	7 (4.1%)	8 (2.0%)
Number of VTE during pregnancy	2 (1.2%)	1/235 (0.4%)
Number of VTE in 6 weeks postpartum	5 (3.0%)	4/235 (1.7%)
Prospective Studies* [26,30,31]		
Total number of pregnancies	17	6
Total number of VTE	2 (12%)	0 (0%)
Number of VTE during pregnancy	0 (0%)	0 (0%)
Number of VTE in 6 weeks postpartum	2 (12%)	0 (0%)

*With use of different anticoagulant prophylaxis schedules, ranging from none to treatment with full-dose heparin in pregnancy and/or vitamin K antagonists in postpartum period.

Risk of Recurrent Thrombosis in Thrombophilia

The incidence of recurrent thrombosis after treatment with anticoagulants can be estimated from a substantial series of prospective studies. Analysis of these data reveals that the highest risk of recurrence is seen in patients with persistent risk factors (such as permanent immobilization or cancer) or in those who developed unprovoked ("idiopathic") thrombosis. In the first 2 years after the initial event, the risk of recurrent thrombosis in patients without thrombophilia can be estimated at 4.5% per year.[74–80] It should be mentioned that the risk of recurrent thromboembolism is highest after the acute episode and declines over time.[81–83] Also, a course of anticoagulants shorter than 6 months in patients with idiopathic venous thromboembolism will also result in a higher incidence of recurrences.[84–86]

There are many studies addressing the issue of whether patients with thrombophilia have a higher risk of recurrent venous thromboembolism (Table 67–8). Three retrospective studies have assessed the risk for recurrent thrombosis in patients with antithrombin, protein S, or protein C deficiency.[32,87,88] No prospective studies on the risk of recurrence in untreated patients

TABLE 67–8. Estimated Annual Incidence of a Recurrent Episode of Venous Thromboembolism in Carriers of Thrombophilic Defects

No Thrombophilic Defect	Antithrombin, Protein C, or Protein S Deficiency	Factor V Leiden Mutation	Prothrombin G20210A Mutation	Elevated Factor VIII Level (>200%)
Lindmarker[74]: 4.4%	Retrospective studies[32,87,88]: 7.3%	Lindmarker[74]: 4.4%	Lindmarker[74]: 4.0%	Kyrle[94]: 18.5%
Simioni[75]: 4.5%		Simioni[75]: 9.9%	Eichinger[79]: 6.0%	
Ridker[76]: 1.8%		Ridker[76]: 7.4%	de Stefano[91]: 6.5%	
Eichinger[89]: 6.0%		Eichinger[77]: 8.0%	Miles[92]: 8.7%	
Rintelen[78]: 5.0%		Rintelen[78]: 4.8%	Baglin[90]: 8.0%	
Eichinger[77]: 6.1%		Baglin[90]: 8.0%		
Kyrle[94]: 3.9%				
Baglin[90]: 7.0%				

with antithrombin, protein C, or protein S deficiency are available. Pooling the available data results in an estimated relative risk of 2.5 for a recurrent event in patients with a deficiency compared to patients without thrombophilia.[50] Carriers of the factor V Leiden mutation have been followed after a first episode of thrombosis in five prospective studies with a follow-up ranging from 1 to 6 years.[74–76,78,89,90] The results of almost all of these studies show that a heterozygous factor V Leiden mutation is only a weak risk factor for recurrent thrombosis in comparison to patients without this mutation. The calculated pooled odds ratio for the prospective studies, using the Mantel-Haenszel method, is 1.3 (95% confidence interval, 1.0–1.7).[50] Four studies have addressed the risk of recurrent thrombosis in heterozygous carriers of the prothrombin G20210A mutation. For this abnormality also, the risk of recurrent thrombosis is only slightly elevated in comparison to patients without the mutation (pooled odds ratio 1.4; 95% confidence interval, 0.9–2.0).[74,79,91,92] It should be mentioned, however, that the risk of recurrent thrombosis in patients who are homozygous for the factor V Leiden or the prothrombin G20210A mutation, or in patients with a combined thrombophilic defect, is much higher.[88] Studies reporting on the risk of recurrence in patients with increased factor VIII are rare. There are two studies demonstrating a dose-dependent relative risk for recurrent venous thromboembolism in patients with elevated factor VIII.[93,94] The odds ratio for the risk of recurrence in patients with factor VIII levels exceeding 200 IU/dL is 1.8 (95% confidence interval, 1.0–3.3).[50]

TREATMENT

It should be mentioned that straightforward management studies in asymptomatic thrombophilic subjects or patients with thrombosis and thrombophilia are rare, hence the recommended treatment strategies in these patients are based on the interpretation of studies assessing risk and the efficacy/safety ratio of various interventions. Absolute rather than relative risks are important in determining whether antithrombotic prophylaxis is warranted, and, if the risk of thrombosis is low, preventive strategies other than pharmacologic antithrombotic prophylaxis can be considered. The various strategies to prevent thrombosis in patients with thrombophilia are summarized in Table 67–9.

TABLE 67–9. Potential Preventive Strategies for Patients with Inherited Thrombophilia

Therapeutic-dose anticoagulation (e.g., vitamin K antagonists)
Prophylactic anticoagulation (e.g., low-dose [LMW] heparin)
Prophylactic anticoagulation during high-risk periods
No anticoagulation but avoid other prothrombotic stimuli (oral contraceptives, hormone replacement therapy)
No specific actions

Lifelong anticoagulant prophylaxis with vitamin K antagonists (targeted at an International Normalized Ratio of 2.0–3.0) is likely to be almost completely effective in preventing venous thromboembolism in patients with thrombophilia.[95,96] However, prolonged anticoagulation with vitamin K antagonists is associated with a high risk of major bleeding. The incidence of serious bleeding is about 2–3% per year, and the annual rates of life-threatening or fatal bleeding are 1.0% and 0.25%, respectively.[97,98] There are several risk factors for bleeding induced by vitamin K antagonists, such as increasing age, comorbid conditions, and the initial phase of anticoagulant treatment.[98,99] Other disadvantages associated with the prolonged use of vitamin K antagonists include the need for frequent laboratory monitoring and dose adjustments (despite the possibility to self-manage this treatment),[100] an impaired quality of life, and the need to avoid certain physical activities (e.g., sports).

Another strategy is the use of temporary prophylaxis in situations in which the risk of thrombosis in increased, such as during immobilization or postoperatively. This will potentially prevent half of all venous thromboembolic events in thrombophilic individuals. The most convenient way to achieve this prophylaxis is with low-dose subcutaneous low-molecular-weight (LMW) heparin once daily.[101] Although a formal prospective study is lacking, it may be assumed that this prophylaxis is as effective as thromboprophylaxis in high-risk situations in patients without thrombophilia.[87] The most important adverse effects of LMW heparin prophylaxis are bleeding (in 1–3% of patients)[102] and heparin-induced thrombocytopenia.[103] Another high-risk situation that may warrant antithrombotic prophylaxis is pregnancy and the postpartum period. In this situation, either low-dose or therapeutic-dose heparin may be considered. Nowadays, LMW heparin will be preferred in most situations. Alternatively, unfractionated heparin can be used; however, this carries the disadvantages of repeated subcutaneous injections daily, the risk of osteoporosis, and frequent laboratory monitoring and dose adjustments. Vitamin K antagonists are strictly contraindicated in the first trimester of pregnancy (because of their teratogenicity) and in the third trimester of pregnancy (because they will also cause anticoagulation of the fetus, which may cause intracerebral bleeding during birth). Retrospective studies in women with thrombophilic defects indicate that prophylaxis during pregnancy reduces the risk of thrombosis compared to historical controls not given prophylaxis.[104]

Withholding oral contraceptives and hormone replacement therapy is another preventive strategy in women with thrombophilia. There is ample information about the risks of thrombosis with oral contraceptive use in asymptomatic carriers with thrombophilia, but in those with a previous venous thromboembolic episode, the risk of recurrence is unknown. One approach is to discourage oral contraceptive use in all thrombophilic women, but it may be more appropriate to take into account whether alternative contraceptive strategies are acceptable for the patient. It is likely that discouraging oral contraceptives will increase the risk of unplanned pregnancies (which may then paradoxically increase the thrombotic risk), because oral contraceptives are associated with only a 0.1% risk of pregnancy per year, whereas alternative means of contraception have much higher risks.[105] The use of contraceptives containing progestogens only is probably not associated with an increased risk of venous thromboembolism, although there is one small study with conflicting results.[106] However, this form of contraception has other drawbacks, including the absence of menstruation in most women and the potential for increasing the risk of endometrial carcinoma. The decision to withhold or continue oral contraceptives in women with thrombophilia is ideally part of a counseling strategy, in which the various risks and alternatives are discussed between patient and doctor.

GUIDELINES FOR MANAGEMENT

Patients Who Have Never Had Thrombosis

The risk of thrombosis in patients with various forms of inherited thrombophilia is not equal, hence different management strategies may be employed based on the specific defect in a patient. In general, the risk of a first episode of thrombosis is lower in patients with heterozygosity for the factor V Leiden or the prothrombin G20210A mutation as compared with deficiencies of antithrombin, protein C, or protein S. Comparing the risk of a first episode of thrombosis for all forms of inherited thrombophilia (see Table 67–4) and the risks associated with prolonged anticoagulation, the use of anticoagulant treatment in asymptomatic carriers of a thrombophilic disorder cannot be advocated. However, because about 50% of patients will develop their first thrombosis in a situation known to be associated with a high risk of thrombosis, in such situations adequate anticoagulant prophylaxis is required. Because the risk of postoperative venous thromboembolism persists for a period of about 2–4 weeks after hospital discharge,[107,108] prolonged administration of anticoagulant prophylaxis may be justified in asymptomatic carriers of antithrombin, protein C, or protein S deficiency (see Table 67–5). The risk of postoperative thrombosis appears to be lower for asymptomatic individuals with the factor V Leiden or the prothrombin G20210A mutation, suggesting that a more vigorous approach than the routine perioperative prophylaxis is not indicated (see Table 67–5).

The optimal prophylactic approach to asymptomatic pregnant women with thrombophilia is uncertain, because management studies have not been performed. However, because the absolute risk of venous thromboembolism during pregnancy in asymptomatic women with any form of inherited thrombophilia is not very high (between 0.4% and 1.2%; see Table 67–7), clinical surveillance throughout pregnancy is appropriate for most women. In view of the higher thrombotic risk in the postpartum period (between 1.7% and 3%), treatment with oral anticoagulants or LMW heparin for 4–6 weeks after delivery should be considered. Heparin will not be excreted in breast milk, and breast-feeding is also possible in cases of vitamin K antagonist treatment by the mother, provided that the child is supplemented with vitamin K in doses that are normal for breast-fed children.

By consensus, oral contraceptives and hormone replacement therapy are in principle contraindicated in women with antithrombin, protein C, or protein S deficiency, because the annual risk of oral contraceptive–associated thromboembolism is approximately 4% (see Table 67–6). However, for asymptomatic women with the factor V Leiden mutation (and presumably also for those with the prothrombin G20210A mutation), the risk of thromboembolism is considerably lower (0.7%; see Table 67–6). Therefore, in such women a more balanced and patient-tailored approach should be followed. Discouraging oral contraceptive use would lower the annual risk of venous thromboembolism from approximately 7 to 2 per 1000 women, but might lead to an increase of a similar number of unplanned pregnancies if oral contraceptives are replaced by intrauterine devices or condoms. If oral contraceptives are used, levonorgestrel-containing pills (second generation) should be preferred, because they are associated with a 50% lower risk of thrombosis than oral contraceptives containing desogestrel or gestodene (third generation).[109–111]

Patients After a First or Recurrent Episode of Thrombosis

There is no difference in the treatment of an acute episode of venous thromboembolism between patients with and without thrombophilia. Initial treatment will consist of a short course of (LMW) heparin at a therapeutic dose and initiation of vitamin K antagonist treatment, aiming at an International Normalized Ratio of 2.0–3.0. The optimal duration of anticoagulant treatment in carriers of an inherited thrombophilic defect is a matter of debate. Because for the most frequently occurring forms of inherited thrombophilia, the risk of recurrence of thrombosis is only slightly higher than in patients without thrombophilia (see Table 67–8), many people advocate a similar duration of anticoagulation for a first episode of venous thromboembolism (i.e., 6–12 months in the case of idiopathic thrombosis). Alternatively, a somewhat longer treatment period may be considered, in particular in patients with a low risk of bleeding (e.g., younger patients without comorbidity). Ideally, the duration of treatment should be individualized, based on risk factors for recurrence and bleeding and on patient preference. A nomogram that can help with the determination of the optimal duration of anticoagulation is presented in Figure 67–5, but it should be stressed that this treatment algorithm needs prospective validation.[112] An alternative, somewhat simpler, approach is to stratify patients with inherited thrombophilia into three risk categories with respect to the chance of recurrence (Table 67–10). At lowest risk are those who had a single episode of venous thromboembolism associated with a well-defined reversible risk factor, such as surgery or pregnancy. At intermediate risk for recurrence are those who experienced their first venous thromboembolic episode spontaneously. At highest risk for recurrence are those who have had multiple spontaneous episodes and have a persistent risk factor, such as continued immobilization. Patients with more than one inherited thrombophilic defect or homozygosity for one defect are also considered to be at a higher risk for recurrence.[52,56,58,59] The lower the risk, the shorter the treatment duration (ranging from 3 to 6 months to lifelong treatment, as indicated in Table 67–10). These treatment guidelines are supported by two different decision analyses.[113,114] Obviously, it is fully justified to deviate from these treatment guidelines in specific circumstances. For example, if the first thrombosis occurred at an unusual but critical site (such as a cerebral sinus thrombosis) or is associated with serious long-term morbidity (such as a mesenteric vein thrombosis), prolonged anticoagulation may be justified.

After cessation of anticoagulant treatment in patients with thrombophilia who have experienced a thromboembolic event, special attention should be devoted to secondary prophylaxis in high-risk situations. Carriers of inherited thrombophilia who have experienced a venous thrombotic episode should receive routine prophylaxis with (LMW) heparin or vitamin K antagonists when they are exposed to risk situations such as surgery, trauma, or immobilization. Because it has been documented that the risk of venous thromboembolism remains increased for a period of approximately 2–4 weeks after major surgery, prolonged prophylaxis should be considered in symptomatic thrombophilic patients.[107,108] No management studies on the optimal prophylactic approach in pregnant women with thrombophilic defects and a history of venous thromboembolism are available. In view of the relatively high risk of recurrence during all trimesters of pregnancy, anticoagulant prophylaxis with (LMW) heparin should be considered throughout pregnancy. In studies in pregnant women (most without inherited thrombophilia) who received (LMW) heparin prophylaxis during pregnancy, recurrences were observed mostly in those who were treated with lower dosages.[115,116] Therefore, intermediate dosages (75–150 anti–factor Xa units/kg/day) or even therapeutic dosages that produce anti–factor Xa levels of at least 0.3 units/mL are probably indicated. Because the bioavailability and distribution volume of heparin may change in pregnancy, periodic measurement of the activated partial thromboplastin time (with use of unfractionated heparin) or anti–factor Xa plasma level (with use of LMW heparin) and, if required, adjustment of the heparin dose are advocated. LMW or unfractionated heparin should be discontinued 12 hours before delivery and restarted thereafter to avoid peripartum hemorrhage. Caution should be taken with the use of epidural or spinal anesthesia. The use of oral contraceptives and hormone replacement therapy is discouraged in women with inherited thrombophilic defects who have had venous thromboembolism. Premenopausal women should be counseled about alternative methods of contraception.

TABLE 67–10. Guidelines for Treatment of Venous Thromboembolism in Patients with Antithrombin, Protein C, or Protein S Deficiency, Factor V Leiden Mutation, or Prothrombin G20210A Mutation

Risk Category	Clinical Characteristics	Anticoagulant Therapy
Lowest	Provoked by a reversible risk factor	Initial treatment with IV heparin or SC LMWH Vitamin K antagonists for 3–6 mo
Intermediate	Spontaneous ("idiopathic" thrombosis)	Initial treatment with IV heparin or SC LMWH Vitamin K antagonists for up to 12 mo
Highest	Recurrent spontaneous venous thromboembolism Persistent risk factor (e.g., active cancer) Homozygous defects or combined defects	Initial treatment with IV heparin or SC LMWH Vitamin K antagonists for 12 mo to indefinitely

Abbreviations: IV, intravenous; LMWH, low-molecular-weight heparin; SC, subcutaneously.

SCREENING FOR THROMBOPHILIA IN PATIENTS WITH THROMBOSIS OR A FAMILY HISTORY OF THROMBOSIS

In about 30–50% of patients with a first episode of venous thromboembolism, an inherited thrombophilic defect may be detected. Because it is clear that half of the first thromboembolic episodes in patients with thrombophilia are not idiopathic, but occur in high-risk situations, and that many patients have their first episode later in life, it is usually very hard to predict the presence of thrombophilia on the basis of clinical findings. Because the identification of a thrombophilic defect is likely to result in an intensification of prophylaxis during high-risk situations and in an increase in the duration of oral anticoagulant after an episode of symptomatic thrombosis, it may be justified to screen all patients with venous thromboembolism for inherited thrombophilic defects.

A more difficult issue is that of the screening of asymptomatic family members of patients with inherited thrombophilia. Because antithrombin, protein C, or protein S deficiency, the factor V Leiden mutation, and the prothrombin G20210A mutation are transmitted as an autosomal dominant inheritance, half of the first-degree relatives will be carriers. In order to justify family screening, the benefits need to be balanced against the possible hazards of identifying asymptomatic individuals. Identification of an asymptomatic individual would probably lead to a more vigorous prophylactic approach during surgery, trauma, or immobilization, to the use of anticoagulants during the postpartum period, and to contraceptive counseling. These potential benefits should be weighed against the disadvantages of creating concern in asymptomatic individuals and to causing bleeding during prophylactic anticoagulation. Family screening is probably justified in cases of antithrombin, protein C, and protein S deficiency. However, whether the same is true for the factor V Leiden mutation or the prothrombin G20210A mutation is questionable and at present a matter of debate.[51,117]

Suggested Readings*

Middeldorp S, Buller HR, Prins MH, Hirsh J: Approach to the thrombophilic patient. *In* Colman RW, Hirsh J, Marder VJ, et al (eds): Hemostasis and Thrombosis: Basic Principles and Clinical Practice. Philadelphia: Lippincott Williams & Wilkins, 2001, pp 1085–1100.

Middeldorp S, Meinardi JR, Koopman MMW, et al: A prospective study of asymptomatic carriers of the factor V Leiden mutation to determine the incidence of venous thromboembolism. Ann Intern Med 135:322–327, 2001.

Ridker PM, Hennekens CH, Lindpaintner K, et al: Mutation in the gene coding for coagulation factor V and the risk of myocardial infarction, stroke, and venous thrombosis in apparently healthy men. N Engl J Med 332:912–917, 1995.

Rosendaal FR: Risk factors for venous thrombotic disease. Thromb Haemost 82:610–619, 1999.

Seligsohn U, Lubetsky A: Genetic susceptibility to venous thrombosis. N Engl J Med 344:1222–1231, 2001.

Full references for this chapter can be found on accompanying CD-ROM.

CURRENT CONTROVERSIES & FUTURE CONSIDERATIONS

Inherited Thrombophilia

- The usefulness of screening of asymptomatic family members of a patients with inherited thrombophilia and thrombosis is at present a matter of debate.
- It is not clear whether asymptomatic patients with inherited thrombophilia should in general be discouraged from using oral contraceptives.
- It is likely, although not yet definitively proven, that the management of a first episode of venous thromboembolism (including the duration of anticoagulation) in a patient with inherited thrombophilia is not different from the management of patients without inherited thrombophilia.

CHAPTER 68

Antiphospholipid Antibody Syndrome

Alice D. Ma, MD, and Robert A. S. Roubey, MD

KEY POINTS

Antiphospholipid Antibody Syndrome

- Antiphospholipid antibodies comprise a family of antibodies usually directed against phospholipid-binding proteins or complexes of these proteins coupled to phospholipids. Antiphospholipid antibodies are generally characterized as lupus anticoagulants or anticardiolipin antibodies. Lupus anticoagulants are detected functionally by their ability to prolong phospholipid-dependent clotting reactions, and anticardiolipin antibodies are detected by enzyme-linked immunosorbent assay.
- The antiphospholipid antibody syndrome is characterized by venous or arterial thrombosis, recurrent fetal loss, and thrombocytopenia in conjunction with the presence of antiphospholipid antibodies.
- Testing for antiphospholipid antibodies should be considered in any patient with unexpected or recurrent thrombosis, recurrent fetal loss, unexplained thrombocytopenia, or an unexpected prolongation of the activated partial thromboplastin time.
- Patients with thrombosis secondary to antiphospholipid antibodies are at high risk for recurrent thrombosis and generally require indefinite anticoagulation. Warfarin anticoagulation to a standard International Normalized Ratio target (2–3) is the standard of care.
- Women with recurrent miscarriages secondary to antiphospholipid antibodies have successfully carried pregnancies to term after treatment with heparin and aspirin.

INTRODUCTION

The antiphospholipid antibody syndrome (APS) defines a constellation of clinical symptoms, including venous and arterial thrombosis, recurrent pregnancy loss, and thrombocytopenia in association with autoantibodies having an apparent specificity for anionic phospholipids (Table 68–1).[1] Patients with APS may have systemic lupus erythematosus (SLE) or related autoimmune diseases, or the syndrome may occur in the absence of such diseases, in which case it is known as primary APS. A multicenter study suggested that there may be little or no fundamental difference between the primary and secondary syndromes.[2]

Terminology

Traditionally, antiphospholipid antibodies have been classified based upon the two types of clinical laboratory assays used to detect them (Table 68–2). First, antibodies that are detected by their ability to prolong certain in vitro, phospholipid-dependent coagulation reactions, such as the activated partial thromboplastin time (aPTT) are known as lupus anticoagulants. Second, antibodies that are detected in enzyme-linked immunosorbent assays (ELISAs) in which cardiolipin is immobilized on microtiter plates are known as anticardiolipin antibodies.

This classification and nomenclature are both confusing and inaccurate, because most autoantibodies associated with APS do not actually recognize anionic phospholipids. In patients with APS, the large majority of autoantibodies detected in lupus anticoagulant and anticardiolipin assays are directed against one or more phospholipid-binding plasma proteins and/or complexes of these proteins with phospholipids.[3] At this time, the best characterized autoantibodies with "anticardiolipin" and/or lupus anticoagulant activity are those directed against the plasma proteins β_2-glycoprotein I (β_2GPI)[4–10] and prothrombin.[11–18] Additionally, autoantibodies to other phospholipid-binding proteins (e.g., protein C and protein S),[19–21] not detectable in standard antiphospholipid antibody assays, may also be associated with APS. For ease of discussion, the terms *antiphospholipid antibodies* and *anticardiolipin antibodies* are used in this chapter, with the understanding that they do not accurately describe the antigenic specificities of the autoantibodies associated with APS.

EPIDEMIOLOGY

In cross-sectional studies, the prevalence of anticardiolipin antibodies in patients with SLE ranges from

TABLE 68–1. Preliminary Classification Criteria for Definite APS*

Clinical Criteria (at least 1 must be present)

1. Vascular thrombosis
   One or more clinical episodes of arterial, venous, or small vessel thrombosis in any tissue or organ, confirmed by imaging or Doppler studies, or histopathology (except for superficial venous thrombosis). For histopathologic confirmation, thrombosis should be present without significant evidence of inflammation in the vessel wall.
2. Pregnancy morbidity
   a. One or more unexplained deaths of a morphologically normal fetus at or beyond the 10th week of gestation, with normal fetal morphology documented by ultrasound or direct examination, *or*
   b. One or more premature births of a morphologically normal neonate at or before the 34th week of gestation because of severe preeclampsia or eclampsia, or severe placental insufficiency, *or*
   c. Three or more unexplained consecutive spontaneous abortions before the 10th week of gestation, with maternal anatomic or hormonal abnormalities and parental chromosomal causes excluded.

Laboratory Criteria (at least 1 must be present)

1. Anticardiolipin antibodies
   IgG and/or IgM isotype in blood, present in medium or high titer, on two or more occasions, at least 6 weeks apart, measured by a standardized ELISA for β_2GPI-dependent anticardiolipin antibodies.
2. Lupus anticoagulant
   Present in plasma, on two or more occasions at least 6 weeks apart, detected according to the guidelines of the International Society on Thrombosis and Haemostasis Scientific Standardization Subcommittee on Lupus Anticoagulants/Phospholipid-Dependent Antibodies[101]

*These classification criteria focus on the essential features of the syndrome, supported by prospective studies, in order to facilitate clinical studies. They are not designed for routine diagnostic use outside of such studies.

Abbreviations: ELISA, enzyme-linked immunosorbent assay; Ig, immunoglobulin; β_2GPI, β_2-glycoprotein I.

From Wilson WA, Gharavi AE, Koike T, et al: International consensus statement on preliminary classification criteria for definite antiphospholipid syndrome: report of an international workshop. Arthritis Rheum 42:1309–1311, 1999, with permission.

approximately 17% to 39%.[22] Lupus anticoagulants are present in 11–30%. Clinical manifestations of APS probably affect 30–50% of patients with these antibodies, or roughly 10–20% of lupus patients. The prevalence of primary APS is unknown. Retrospective studies have identified antiphospholipid antibodies in 5–30% of patients with a history of thrombosis but without SLE.[22-25] Ginsburg and colleagues[26] studied banked sera from a prospectively followed cohort of male physicians 40 years of age or older, without a prior history of thrombosis. Of 90 subjects who subsequently experienced an episode of deep venous thrombosis or pulmonary embolism over a 5-year period, 19 (21%) had IgG anticardiolipin antibody levels above the 95th percentile (>33 GPL units). No association with ischemic stroke was found, perhaps because of the study design and the age of the subjects. In contrast, data analyzed by Kittner and Gorelick indicate that antiphospholipid antibodies may account for approximately one third of new strokes in patients under the age of 50.[27] Recurrent idiopathic fetal losses in apparently healthy women are probably attributable to APS in 10–20% of cases.[28-30] The frequency of antiphospholipid antibodies in normal controls is approximately 2% (estimates range from 1% to 5%) and may increase with age.[22]

TABLE 68–2. Terminology for Antiphospholipid Antibodies

Term	Definition
Antiphospholipid antibodies	A family of antibodies that are directed against proteins such as β_2GPI or prothrombin, which bind to phospholipids. These antibodies are generally divided into two categories: the lupus anticoagulants and anticardiolipin antibodies.
Lupus anticoagulant	An antibody directed against phospholipid-binding proteins such as β_2GPI or prothrombin, which prolongs certain phospholipid-dependent clotting assays, such as the aPTT. These antibodies are detected functionally by their ability to prolong clotting assays in a phospholipid-dependent fashion.
Anticardiolipin antibodies	In patients with APS, these antibodies are usually directed against β_2GPI. These antibodies are detected by ELISA techniques using cardiolipin-coated plates and not by functional clotting assays.
Anti-β_2GPI antibodies	Antibodies detected in ELISA using purified human β_2GPI as the antigen.

Abbreviations: aPTT, activated partial thromboplastin time; β_2GPI, β_2-glycoprotein I; ELISA, enzyme-linked immunosorbent assay.

PATHOPHYSIOLOGY

Several general observations are compatible with the hypothesis that autoantibodies play a direct role in the pathogenesis of APS:

1. Unlike antinuclear autoantibodies, autoantibodies in APS target plasma proteins or components of cell surface membranes that are accessible to circulating antibodies.
2. A number of the antigens are involved in hemostasis.
3. Animal models of APS have been developed via passive transfer of immunoglobulins from patients with APS.[31–34]
4. The presence of antiphospholipid antibodies has been shown to precede the first episode of thrombosis, rather than develop as a sequela of a thrombotic event.[26]
5. The risk of developing clinical manifestations of APS correlates directly with the level of antiphospholipid antibodies.[26,35]

Autoantibody-Mediated Thrombosis: Potential Mechanisms

Thrombosis in patients with antiphospholipid antibodies may occur via the action of these autoantibodies on either the cellular or the humoral components of the coagulation and anticoagulant pathways. Antiphospholipid antibodies have been reported to have multiple effects on hemostatic reactions, including inhibiting the protein C pathway,[39,36–46] lowering levels of protein S,[47–51] inhibiting antithrombin activation,[52–54] enhancing the tenase complex,[55] and impairing fibrinolysis.[56–60]

Antiphospholipid antibodies also have many effects on the cellular components of hemostasis. There is increasing evidence that increased expression of tissue factor on circulating blood monocytes is an important mechanism of hypercoagulability in APS.[61–66] Anticardiolipin (anti-β_2GPI) antibodies from patient sera and patient-derived monoclonal anti-β_2GPI autoantibodies induce tissue factor expression on normal blood monocytes in vivo, and tissue factor expression is increased on monocytes from patients with IgG anticardiolipin antibodies and a history of thrombosis.

There are several mechanisms by which antiphospholipid antibodies may enhance the procoagulant activity of vascular endothelial cells.[67] Sera and IgG fractions from certain patients increase the expression of tissue factor,[68,69] the production of endothelin-1,[70] and the expression of the adhesion molecules E-selectin, vascular cell adhesion molecule-1, and intercellular adhesion molecule-1.[71–75] Additionally, there is some evidence that autoantibodies associated with APS inhibit production of endothelial cell prostacyclin (prostaglandin I_2), a potent vasodilator and platelet inhibitor.[76,77]

Several studies suggest that antiphospholipid antibodies induce platelet aggregation.[78–80] Monoclonal anti-β_2GPI antibodies bind to platelets in a β_2GPI-dependent fashion and lead to platelet activation in the presence of subthreshold concentrations of weak agonists.[81] There is also consistent evidence that antiphospholipid antibodies enhance platelet thromboxane A_2 production.[82–85]

Fetal Loss: Potential Mechanisms

Fetal losses related to APS are most likely due to hypoxia caused by insufficient uteroplacental blood flow.[31] Pathologic and physiologic findings include maternal spiral artery vasculopathy leading to placental infarction, chronic villitis, atherosis, a decreased number of syncytiovascular membranes, an increased number of syncytial knots, and fetal thrombi.[86–91] Placental infarction may result from decreased amounts of annexin A5 on the surface of placental villi of women with APS and recurrent fetal losses,[91–95] although normal amounts of placental annexin A5 have also been reported.[95,96]

Autoimmune Thrombocytopenia: Potential Mechanisms

Autoimmune thrombocytopenia is part of APS and thought to be due to the antiplatelet activity of a subset of these antibodies. Potential antigenic targets include β_2GPI bound to platelet membranes,[97] CD36,[98,99] and several major platelet membrane glycoproteins.[100]

CLINICAL FEATURES

A number of clinical scenarios may be attributable to the effect of antiphospholipid antibodies. These clinical features are protean and may be as innocuous as an asymptomatic prolongation of the aPTT or as devastating as catastrophic APS.

Prolongation of aPTT

Prolongation of the aPTT or other phospholipid-dependent clotting reactions is the hallmark of the lupus anticoagulant.[101] In general, this is found in asymptomatic patients who have had aPTTs determined for other reasons, such as preoperative evaluations. Patients and surgeons who are planning to operate on such patients can be reassured that these individuals are at no increased risk for bleeding. The only exceptions to this rule are the rare patients who have coexisting hypoprothrombinemia (discussed later in this section).

Thrombosis

Thrombotic events in nearly all sites of the vascular tree have been reported to occur in association with antiphospholipid antibodies. The deep and superficial veins of the lower extremity are the most common sites of venous thrombosis.[2,102,103] Deep venous thrombosis may be complicated by pulmonary embolism in up to half of cases.

Unlike many of the other hypercoagulable states, which are associated only with venous thromboses, antiphospholipid antibodies also lead to clots in the arterial system. Stroke is the most common form of arterial thrombosis seen in patients with antiphospholipid antibodies,[103–105] though myocardial infarctions and clots in other large and small arteries may also be seen.

Thrombosis may be the underlying disease process in a number of clinical events in patients with antiphospholipid antibodies. These include pregnancy loss (placental thrombosis and infarction),[86,87,106] renal dysfunction (thrombosis of intrarenal blood vessels),[107,108] cutaneous ulcers (thrombosis of dermal blood vessels),[109] certain forms of central nervous system disease (multi-infarct dementia),[110–112] and pulmonary hypertension (recurrent pulmonary emboli).[113]

Recurrent Pregnancy Loss

The presence of antiphospholipid antibodies in pregnant women is strongly associated with fetal deaths occurring from the late first trimester onward.[28,114] Spontaneous abortion occurring at less than 10 weeks' gestation is less well associated with antiphospholipid antibodies because of the high incidence of such losses in the general population.[115] In addition to fetal loss, antiphospholipid antibodies are also associated with an increased incidence of obstetric and postnatal complications, including preeclampsia, fetal distress, fetal growth impairment, and premature delivery, and with maternal thrombotic events in the postpartum period.[28,116] Most cases of fetal death related to antiphospholipid antibodies are preceded by fetal growth impairment and oligohydramnios.[115]

Thrombocytopenia

Thrombocytopenia in patients with SLE is associated with antiphospholipid antibodies. It occurs in nearly 40% of lupus patients with antiphospholipid antibodies and only 10% of patients without these antibodies.[117] Antiphospholipid antibodies are present in 70–80% of lupus patients with thrombocytopenia, and about 30% of patients with chronic autoimmune thrombocytopenia.[118] In patients with immune thrombocytopenia without other autoimmune disorders, antiphospholipid antibodies may be found in as many as 46%.[119,120]

In patients with APS, thrombocytopenia is usually moderate (platelet counts $> 50 \times 10^9$/L) and not associated with hemorrhage. Patients with antiphospholipid antibodies and low platelet counts are still at risk for thrombosis.[121]

Catastrophic APS

An acute syndrome of widespread, multiple vascular occlusions associated with antiphospholipid antibodies has been reported in at least 130 patients.[61,62,122,123] Common features include multiple vascular occlusive events presenting over a short period of time (days to weeks), usually affecting small vessels supplying organs (e.g., kidney, lungs, brain, heart, liver). Large vessel occlusions are less common than in typical APS. Recently, a registry of patients was established, and diagnostic criteria have been established and subsequently validated.[124,125] Most patients with catastrophic APS have a prior history of SLE, lupus-like disease, or primary APS. Previous symptoms and signs of APS are present in about half the reported cases. Apparent precipitating events, identifiable in about two thirds of cases, include infections, surgery, trauma, neoplasia, and withdrawal of anticoagulant medications. Catastrophic APS has a poor prognosis, with a fatality rate of nearly 50%. Major causes of death are cardiac (myocardial infarction, heart failure resulting from myocardial microthrombi, heart block) and pulmonary (acute respiratory distress syndrome, pulmonary embolism). A long-term outcome study of 58 catastrophic APS survivors found that 66% did well, without any further manifestations of APS (on anticoagulation) over an average follow-up period of 5–6 years.[126] Another 26% experienced further APS-related events, approximately a quarter of which were fatal. The remainder of patients did not develop further APS manifestations, but died either from complications of the initial catastrophic illness or from apparently unrelated causes.

Other Clinical Manifestations

Thrombotic Microangiopathy

Antiphospholipid antibodies have been reported in association with thrombotic microangiopathy.[108,127–137] This may be manifest only in the kidney or may be more systemic and be associated with a microangiopathic hemolytic anemia.

Hypoprothrombinemia

Hemorrhage in patients with antiphospholipid antibodies is rare and almost always due to either the presence of thrombocytopenia or the action of anti-prothrombin antibodies.[13,138–166] These antibodies do not interfere with prothrombin activity. Rather, they bind prothrombin and accelerate its clearance. The lupus anticoagulant/hypoprothrombinemia syndrome should be considered in patients with hemorrhage and prolonged prothrombin time and aPTT values. Although patients with strongly positive lupus anticoagulants can occasionally have a minimal prolongation of the prothrombin time, a value that is prolonged more than 2 or 3 seconds above normal in a patient with antiphospholipid antibodies should prompt measurement of prothrombin levels.

Valvular Heart Disease

Valvular heart disease is associated with the presence of antiphospholipid antibodies in patients with both SLE[167–169] and primary APS.[2,170,171] In particular, a number of patients have been reported with noninfective verrucous vegetations (Libman-Sacks endocarditis). Embolization of endocardial lesions may account for some of the cerebral ischemic events in these patients.[172–174]

Neurologic Syndromes

Cerebrovascular thrombosis and embolic stroke are the major neurologic manifestations of APS. Transient ischemic attack may also occur.[175] Nonstroke neurologic events that have been reported in patients with antiphospholipid antibodies include transverse myelitis,[176] Guillain-Barré syndrome, chorea,[177] migraine headache,[178] and syndromes resembling multiple sclerosis.[179,180] In a recent critical review of the literature, Chapman and colleagues concluded that none of these nonstroke conditions was definitely associated with antiphospholipid antibodies or APS.[112] In patients with SLE, the presence of consistently positive antiphospholipid antibodies was associated with cognitive impairment.[181]

Dermatologic Manifestations

Cutaneous ulcers, usually involving the lower extremities, have been reported in several series.[109,182,183] Livedo reticularis, a latticework of blue or red subcutaneous mottling, is often present in patients with antiphospholipid antibodies.[184] Certain patients with Sneddon's syndrome, the association of livedo reticularis and cerebrovascular disease, are recognized as having APS.[185,186] Skin necrosis has also been reported in association with antiphospholipid antibodies.[187,188]

Drug-Induced Antiphospholipid Antibodies

A number of medications, including chlorpromazine, hydralazine, phenytoin, and procainamide, may induce antiphospholipid antibodies.[143,189–192] Drug-induced antiphospholipid antibodies are often of the IgM isotype, and exhibit the same dependence upon β_2GPI as the autoimmune variety.[192,193] Thrombosis and thrombocytopenia have occurred in some patients with drug-induced antiphospholipid antibodies.[189,191]

Infection-Associated Antiphospholipid Antibodies

Lupus anticoagulants are frequently found in patients with bacterial infections.[194,195] Anticardiolipin antibodies may be found in patients with a variety of other infections, including human immunodeficiency virus,[196] adenovirus, rubella, varicella, syphilis, parvovirus,[197] and Lyme disease,[198] as well as those who have been vaccinated against smallpox.[199] Thrombosis is not seen at increased frequency in infected patients with antiphospholipid antibodies.

Antiphospholipid Antibodies in Children

As in adults, children with SLE who have antiphospholipid antibodies are at high risk for thrombosis, with a 54% thrombotic rate in such patients reported in one series.[200] It has been reported that up to one third of pediatric patients with thrombosis have circulating antiphospholipid antibodies, and that more than two thirds of children with cerebral ischemia have APS.[201] The prognosis and manifestations of children with thrombosis and antiphospholipid antibodies do not differ from those in adults.

However, in most children, antiphospholipid antibodies occur transiently after infections or vaccinations, and are generally without clinical sequelae.[202–204] Thus, in pediatric patients, antiphospholipid antibody testing must be repeated if clinical significance is to be attributed to them. At this time, prophylactic treatment of asymptomatic children with antiphospholipid antibodies cannot be advocated.

TABLE 68–3. Indications for Testing for the Presence of Antiphospholipid Antibodies

Prolongation of the aPTT
Unexplained venous thromboembolism
Deep venous thrombosis
Pulmonary embolism
Clots in other venous sites, such as cerebral sinus or mesenteric veins
Unexplained arterial thrombosis
Stroke or transient ischemic attacks in a young individual (<50 yr old)
Myocardial infarction in a young individual
Other arterial thrombosis
Recurrent fetal loss (especially after 10 weeks' gestation)
Thrombocytopenia (especially in a patient with systemic lupus erythematosus)
Catastrophic presentation with thromboses in multiple organs
Presence of systemic lupus erythematosus
Other clinical syndromes
Thrombotic microangiopathy (especially involving the kidney)
Other neurologic symptoms
Livedo reticularis
Cardiac valvular abnormalities

LABORATORY DIAGNOSIS

Patients with any of the above clinical scenarios should be considered for SLE testing. Additionally, in some centers all patients with SLE are screened for the presence of antiphospholipid antibodies as part of their serologic evaluation (Table 68–3).

Tests for both anticardiolipin antibodies and the lupus anticoagulant may need to be performed because the assays are discordant in up to 35% of patients with APS.[205] Although the strongest clinical associations have been established with IgG anticardiolipin antibodies, isolated IgM or IgA antibodies may be associated with the syndrome. *It should be strongly emphasized that the presence of antiphospholipid antibodies should be confirmed by repeating a positive test in 6–8 weeks* (Fig. 68–1).

Screening tests for the lupus anticoagulant include the dilute phospholipid aPTT, the dilute Russell's viper venom time, and the kaolin clotting time[101,206,207] (Fig. 68–2). These assays all use dilute concentrations of phospholipids to maximize the effect of any antiphospholipid antibodies present. Because each individual assay may be negative in up to 30% of patients, it is recommended that more than one test be performed to verify the presence of a lupus anticoagulant.[208] The combination of the dilute Russell's viper venom time and the dilute phospholipid aPTT was reported to have a sensitivity and specificity of 97% and 100%, respectively.[209]

If prolongation of one of these screening tests is observed, confirmation of a lupus anticoagulant requires (1) demonstration that prolongation of the screening test is due to an inhibitor rather than a factor deficiency (failure of the abnormal screening test to correct when patient plasma is mixed with normal plasma), and (2) demonstration of phospholipid dependence (the inverse relationship of phospholipid concentration to prolongation of the coagulation test). Phospholipid dependence may be demonstrated in an assay in which reduced phospholipid accentuates the anticoagulant activity (e.g., dilute phospholipid aPTT) or an assay in which excess phospholipid neutralizes the anticoagulant activity (e.g., platelet neutralization procedure, hexagonal-phase phospholipid neutralization procedure). It is important that platelets be completely removed from plasma before testing, or false-negative results can be obtained[210,211] (see Fig. 68–2).

Important strides have been made in the standardization of the anticardiolipin ELISA, including the establishment of positive standards for IgG, IgM, and IgA isotypes and corresponding GPL, MPL, and APL units.[212–214] Interlaboratory variation remains a problem, however.[215,216] In light of the importance of β_2GPI in the antigenic specificity of "anticardiolipin" autoantibodies, anti-β_2GPI ELISAs have been developed and are clinically available, though their role in clinical decision making has yet to be established.[6,8,10,217–220] Compared to anticardiolipin assays, anti-β_2GPI assays may be more specific for clinical manifestations of APS and may detect species-specific autoantibodies that recognize human, but not bovine, β_2GPI.[221] Further standardization efforts, interlaboratory comparisons, and prospective clinical studies will help define the role of anti-β_2GPI assays in clinical practice. Immunoassays for anti-prothrombin antibodies are also being evaluated.[12,14,17,18,142,222,223]

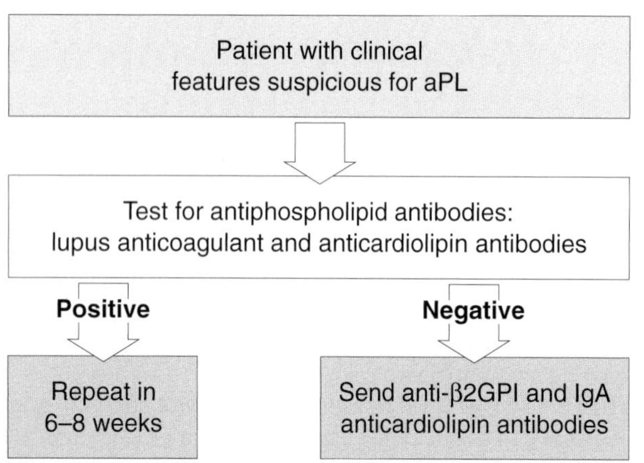

Figure 68–1. Diagnostic algorithm for antiphospholipid testing.

DIFFERENTIAL DIAGNOSIS

Patients with thrombosis should also be evaluated for hereditary and acquired hypercoagulable conditions other than APS. Similarly, patients with a history of pregnancy losses should be evaluated by an obstetrician who specializes in high-risk pregnancies to determine if there is an obstetric cause for the failed pregnancies. Other medical conditions, including thyroid disease and diabetes mellitus, should also be excluded.

The differential diagnosis of catastrophic APS syndrome typically includes lupus vasculitis, disseminated intravascular coagulopathy, and thrombotic thrombocytopenic purpura.

Patients with prolongations of the aPTT should also be evaluated for clotting factor deficiencies. Generally, mixing normal plasma 1 : 1 with patient plasma should substantially correct the aPTT prolongation if there is a clotting factor deficiency. For medicolegal reasons, prior to surgery, it may be advisable to measure levels of appropriate clotting factors such as factors VIII, IX, and

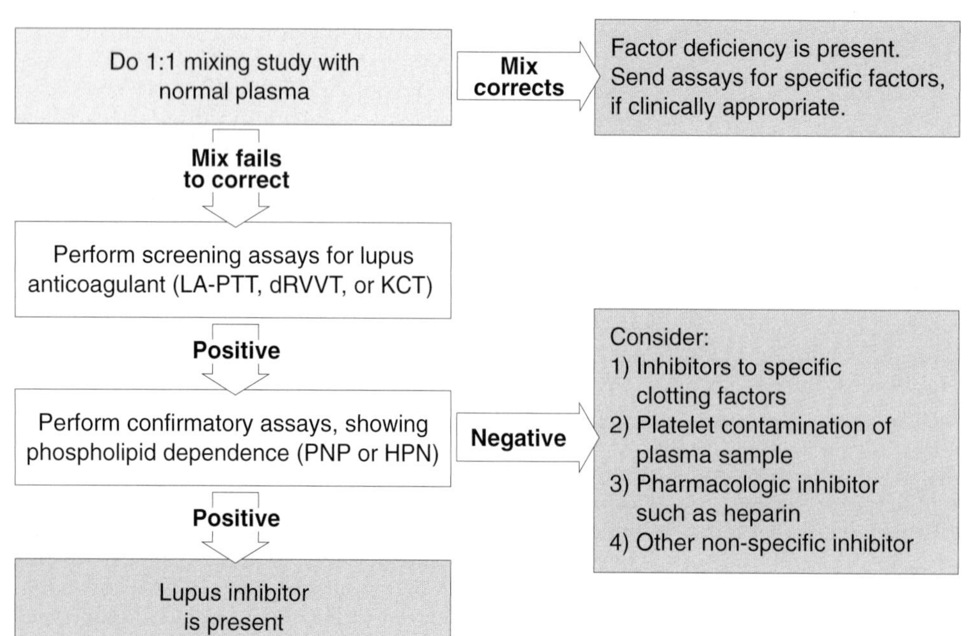

Figure 68–2. Diagnostic algorithm for evaluation of prolonged aPTT. Abbreviations: dRVVT, dilute Russell's viper venom time; HPN, hexagonal-phase phospholipid neutralization procedure; KCT, kaolin clotting time; LA-PTT, dilute phospholipid aPTT; PNP, platelet neutralization procedure.

XI. Patients with specific inhibitors to factor VIII may be confused with patients with the lupus anticoagulant. However, in the former case, serial dilutions of patient plasma will not lead to an apparent increase in the factor VIII activity. Additionally, patients with a factor VIII inhibitor will not show correction of the prolonged aPTT with addition of exogenous phospholipid, that is, there is no phospholipid dependence of their prolonged aPTT.

TREATMENT

The risks associated with moderate to high levels of antiphospholipid antibodies may be substantial. The relative risk of deep venous thrombosis, pulmonary embolism, or stroke (age < 50) is in the range of 7–8.[26,27] There are few controlled therapeutic trials in APS, and treatment remains largely empirical. A number of principles have emerged from retrospective studies and case reports that offer the clinician some guidance. Because the manifestations of patients with antiphospholipid antibodies encompass many specialties (hematology, rheumatology, obstetrics, neurology, nephrology, and pathology), it is important that the care provided to these patients be interdisciplinary and collaborative.

Thrombosis

Patients with a history of arterial or venous thrombosis and significant levels of antiphospholipid antibodies have a high risk for recurrent thrombosis.[224–227] Following immediate therapy with heparin, warfarin anticoagulation is required to prevent recurrent thrombotic events.[224–226] Retrospective studies suggested that a relatively high level of anticoagulation, that is, an International Normalized Ratio (INR) greater than 3.0, is necessary.[224,226,227] A recent randomized controlled trial, however, found that high-intensity warfarin (target INR, 3.1–4.0) was not superior to moderate-intensity warfarin (target INR, 2.0–3.0).[228] Indefinite anticoagulation may be necessary.[225] Given the risks of such treatment, the decision regarding long-term anticoagulation should be individualized and numerous factors should be considered, including the level of antiphospholipid antibodies, the type of thrombotic event, the temporal distance from the event, and the age and reliability of the patient. In certain patients, autoantibodies may interfere with accurate determination of the INR, requiring other tests to assess the level of anticoagulation.[229,230]

Pregnancy Loss

Treatment to prevent pregnancy loss and morbidity should be considered for women with moderate to high levels of antiphospholipid antibodies and a history of one or more otherwise unexplained fetal deaths (>10 weeks' gestation) or spontaneous abortions. Currently, most experts recommend treatment with heparin and low-dose aspirin.[28,231–233] A regimen of prednisone and aspirin appears to be equally efficacious but is associated with a higher frequency of adverse side effects, including infection, preeclampsia, gestational diabetes, and osteonecrosis.[234] With treatment, successful pregnancy rates of 70–80% are reported.[231,232]

It is advisable for women with APS who are considering pregnancy to have preconception consultations with their obstetrician and rheumatologist and/or hematologist. Low-dose aspirin is often initiated (or continued) at this time. Treatment with heparin is begun as soon as pregnancy is diagnosed, usually at 5–7 weeks' gestation. Either unfractionated or low-molecular-weight heparin (enoxaparin, dalteparin) may be used. For women without a history of thrombosis, a typical regimen is subcutaneous heparin, 5000–10,000 units every 12 hours, and aspirin, 81 mg daily. The lower dose of heparin appears to be equally efficacious.[231,235] For women with prior thrombosis, higher doses of heparin are recommended. Specific heparin regimens for prevention of APS-related pregnancy loss have recently been reviewed.[28] Heparin is withheld at the time of delivery, and then reinstituted for 4–6 weeks after delivery, because of the risk of thrombosis in the postpartum period. Intravenous immunoglobulin therapy is an option if heparin and prednisone fail,[236–238] although a small randomized controlled trial did not show an increased benefit of intravenous immunoglobulin over heparin and aspirin.[239]

Women with low levels of antiphospholipid antibodies and recurrent pregnancy loss may not require treatment. A randomized controlled trial, in which a majority of subjects had low antibody titers, observed successful pregnancy rates of 80–85% in patients receiving low-dose aspirin or placebo.[240]

Thrombocytopenia

Modest thrombocytopenia (platelet counts ~ 50×10^9/L) usually does not require treatment. Patients with lower platelet counts or those who have hemorrhage may require treatment with corticosteroids or other immunosuppressant therapy.[241] The presence of antiphospholipid antibodies does not usually impact the clinical response to therapy of patients with immune thrombocytopenia. Most patients with immune thrombocytopenia and antiphospholipid antibodies who have resolution of thrombocytopenia after treatment still show elevated levels of antiphospholipid antibodies.

Catastrophic APS

Most patients with catastrophic APS have received a combination of therapies, including anticoagulants, corticosteroids, plasmapheresis, cyclophosphamide, and intravenous immunoglobulin.[122,123] Anticoagulation appears to be particularly useful; survival was 62% in patients receiving anticoagulation versus 23% in those who were not anticoagulated.[122] In individual refractory cases, plasmapheresis[242–244] and defibrotide[245] have each been useful.

CURRENT CONTROVERSIES & FUTURE CONSIDERATIONS

Antiphospholipid Antibody Syndrome

Antiphospholipid Testing

- What is the role of protein-based immunoassays such as anti β_2GPI or anti-prothrombin assays in clinical decision making?

Antiphospholipid Therapy

- What is the role of specific immunomodulatory therapy (e.g., the β_2GPI-specific B-cell toleragen)?
- If antiphospholipid antibody titers disappear, is it acceptable to stop therapy?
- What is the role of alternative therapeutic approaches, such as the use of statins to treat APS?
- What is the proper treatment for the asymptomatic patient? Is aspirin alone either effective or sufficient in these patients?

Prognosis

- Are levels of antiphospholipid antibodies stable over time?
- Are the levels of antiphospholipid antibodies quantitatively associated with risk of thrombosis?
- Are there specific biomarkers that predict which patients with antiphospholipid antibodies are at highest risk for thrombosis?
- Are antiphospholipid antibodies associated with other biologic processes, such as accelerated atherosclerosis?

Asymptomatic Patients

The issue of the prophylactic treatment of individuals with antiphospholipid antibodies but without a history of thrombosis typically arises in three situations: patients with SLE found to have antiphospholipid antibodies on routine screening, women with a diagnosis of APS based on pregnancy morbidity, and individuals discovered to have a lupus anticoagulant during coagulation screening.[246] Low-dose aspirin is generally recommended in these situations.[246–248] Hydroxychloroquine may also be useful in patients with antiphospholipid antibodies and SLE.[248,249]

Suggested Readings*

Asherson RA, Cervera R, de Groot PG, et al: Catastrophic antiphospholipid syndrome: international consensus statement on classification criteria and treatment guidelines. Lupus 12:530–534, 2003.

Chapman J, Rand JH, Brey RL, et al: Non-stroke neurological syndromes associated with antiphospholipid antibodies: evaluation of clinical and experimental studies. Lupus 12:514–517, 2003.

Crowther MA, Ginsberg JS, Julian J, et al: A comparison of two intensities of warfarin for the prevention of recurrent thrombosis in patients with the antiphospholipid antibody syndrome. N Engl J Med 349:1133–1138, 2003.

Derksen RH, Khamashta MA, Branch DW: Management of the obstetric antiphospholipid syndrome. Arthritis Rheum 50:1028–1039, 2004.

Levine JS, Branch DW, Rauch J: The antiphospholipid syndrome. N Engl J Med 346:752–763, 2002.

Wilson WA, Gharavi AE, Koike T, et al: International consensus statement on preliminary classification criteria for definite antiphospholipid syndrome: report of an international workshop. Arthritis Rheum 42:1309–1311, 1999.

***Full references for this chapter can be found on accompanying CD-ROM.**

CHAPTER 69

HEPARIN-INDUCED THROMBOCYTOPENIA

Theodore E. Warkentin, MD, Mortimer Poncz, MD, and Douglas B. Cines, MD

KEY POINTS

Heparin-Induced Thrombocytopenia

Diagnosis

- Clinical suspicion of heparin-induced thrombocytopenia (HIT) is based upon the *4 T's:*
  - *T*hrombocytopenia: a platelet count fall of greater than 50% (usual nadir, 20–150 × 10^9/L)
  - *T*iming of thrombocytopenia (consistent with heparin-induced immunization)
  - *T*hrombosis or other sequelae (skin lesions, acute systemic reaction after intravenous heparin bolus, decompensated disseminated intravascular coagulation)
  - o*T*her explanation(s) for thrombocytopenia lacking
- Investigation for HIT antibodies can be accomplished with one or more assays:
  - Platelet factor 4/polyanion enzyme immunoassays
  - Washed platelet activation assays
  - Platelet-rich plasma platelet activation assays
- HIT antibody assays must be interpreted in the context of pretest probability.
- Duplex ultrasonography for lower limb deep venous thrombosis should be performed when HIT is strongly suspected.

Treatment

- The initial treatment of HIT is to transition the patient from heparin to an alternative, nonheparin anticoagulant.
- Alternative anticoagulants include lepirudin and argatroban (as well as bivalirudin, danaparoid, and fondaparinux in some jurisdictions).
- It is best to avoid/postpone the use of warfarin (or to administer vitamin K if warfarin was already started).
- In addition, prophylactic platelet transfusions should be avoided.

INTRODUCTION

Heparin-induced thrombocytopenia (HIT) can be defined as any clinical event best explained by platelet-activating, platelet factor 4 (PF4)–heparin-reactive antibodies ("HIT antibodies") in a patient who is receiving, or who has recently received, unfractionated heparin or low-molecular-weight (LMW) heparin.[1] Thrombocytopenia is the most common feature of HIT, and occurs in at least 95% of patients. Most patients with HIT develop thrombosis, either venous or arterial (or both). Occasionally, other sequelae arise, such as heparin-induced skin lesions or acute systemic reactions after intravenous bolus administration.

EPIDEMIOLOGY AND RISK FACTORS

Incidence

Unfractionated heparin is by far the most common cause of immune thrombocytopenia (Fig. 69–1).[2] The frequency of HIT varies from negligible levels to about 5%, depending on several factors, especially type of heparin, type of patient population, and duration of heparin therapy (Table 69–1).[3] Women may be more likely to develop HIT because they generate higher antibody levels.[4] The intensity of platelet count monitoring influences the frequency with which isolated HIT (no associated thrombosis) is detected, and the availability of appropriate assays for HIT antibodies determines to what extent HIT is reliably distinguished from other thrombocytopenic disorders. HIT can complicate a patient's first course of heparin, or may occur during repeat use in which previous exposure(s) had been uneventful.[5]

Genetic Factors

No genetic risk factors, including human leukocyte antigens (HLA),[6] have been defined. The influence of a platelet Fc receptor Arg/His-131 polymorphism is controversial.[7–11] Even patients with a previous history of HIT are not at substantially increased risk of developing

TABLE 69–1. Factors Influencing Incidence of HIT

Heparin preparation: bovine lung unfractionated heparin > porcine intestinal unfractionated heparin > (porcine-derived) LMW heparin
Patient population: postoperative > medical > obstetric patients/children/neonates
Duration of heparin: progressive increase in frequency as heparin continues from 5 to 14 days
Gender: female > male (1.5–2.0:1)
Intensity of platelet count monitoring
Laboratory testing for HIT antibodies

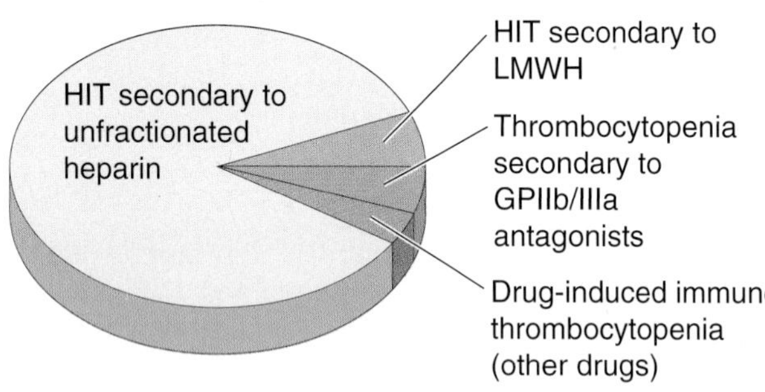

Figure 69–1. Relative frequencies of drug-induced immune thrombocytopenic syndromes.

recurrent HIT antibodies,[5,12] at least in certain clinical settings (although deliberate heparin reexposure is usually restricted to special situations; see "Heparin Reexposure" later).

PATHOPHYSIOLOGY

Figure 69–2 summarizes the pathophysiology of HIT. In brief, antibodies of the immunoglobulin (Ig) G class triggered by heparin activate platelets, and contribute to activation of endothelium and monocytes, resulting in a "hypercoagulability state" (increased thrombin generation[13]) that is prothrombotic (odds ratio for thrombosis, 20–40).[14]

PF4-Heparin Complexes

The antigen(s) of HIT reside not on heparin itself but rather on one or more neoepitopes on platelet factor 4 when it is complexed with heparin.[15–18] Platelet factor 4 is a 70–amino acid (7780-Da), cationic, platelet-specific member of the CXC subfamily of chemokines, and is stored within platelet α-granules. Four platelet factor 4 molecules self-associate to form compact tetramers of globular structure (~31,000 Da). The "nonspecific" role of heparin is illustrated by the observation that a syndrome identical to HIT can be caused by nonheparin polyanions such as pentosan polysulfate and polysulfated chondroitin sulfate.[19–22] Polyvinyl sulfonate also promotes platelet factor 4 neoepitope formation, forming the basis for a commercial enzyme immunoassay for HIT antibodies.[23]

Platelet Activation

The immune response is polyspecific, that is, antibodies are directed against multiple PF4/heparin neoepitopes. However, not all antibodies triggered by heparin use cause clinical HIT.[24–26] Titer and platelet-activating properties of the IgG class antibodies correlate with risk of HIT.[27–29]

Platelet activation is mediated by the platelet FcγIIa receptors.[30,31] The following sequence of events has been proposed.[32] First, heparin causes release of small amounts of platelet factor 4 from platelets by nonimmunologic mechanisms; the resulting PF4-heparin complexes bind to platelets via heparin. (Alternatively, heparin could bind to platelet factor 4 released during physiologic or pathologic platelet activation, e.g., normal platelet turnover or surgery, respectively.[33]) In immunized patients, the HIT IgG recognizes the platelet-bound PF4-heparin complexes. Subsequently, the Fc moieties of the PF4-heparin-IgG immune complexes engage the platelet FcγIIa receptors. Further platelet activation by HIT IgG occurs even though heparin remains in considerable molar excess to platelet factor 4. This suggests that the platelet surface microenvironment helps to achieve the necessary stoichiometric PF4:heparin relationship (1:1–2:1) as platelet factor 4 is increasingly released during progressive platelet activation. Thus, PF4-heparin-IgG immune complexes likely arise in situ on platelet surfaces, rather than forming first in plasma.

The average resting platelet expresses approximately 1000 copies of FcγIIa receptors. Upon activation resulting from receptor clustering induced by HIT IgG,[34] receptor numbers increase rapidly.[35,36] Adenosine diphosphate potentiates platelet activation by HIT IgG,[37] suggesting that partial platelet activation lowers the threshold for platelet activation by HIT IgG, perhaps explaining the predominance of HIT in postoperative patients.

Platelet activation by HIT IgG leads to formation of procoagulant, platelet-derived microparticles.[38–40] Elevated P-selectin levels on circulating platelets,[41] and increased levels of platelet-derived microparticles,[38] indicate that in vivo platelet activation occurs in HIT.

Endothelial and Monocyte Activation

Heparan sulfate is an endothelial cell surface glycosaminoglycan that is less sulfated than heparin and binds platelet factor 4 with lower affinity. Nevertheless, antibodies of both IgG and IgM class recognize platelet factor 4 bound to endothelial heparan sulfate, leading to speculation that high levels of platelet factor 4 during acute HIT could focus immunoinjury to the endothelium.[42] In vitro, HIT antibodies stimulate endothelial cells to produce tissue factor,[43,44] although it remains unclear to what extent this process requires costimulatory effects of activated platelets,[45,46] or occurs in vivo.[47] The presence of signal-transducing Fc receptors within endothelial cells of the superficial dermal vascular plexus[48] could help explain the pathogenesis of heparin-induced skin lesions.

Two reports[49,50] suggest that HIT IgG can activate monocytes in the presence of platelet factor 4, leading

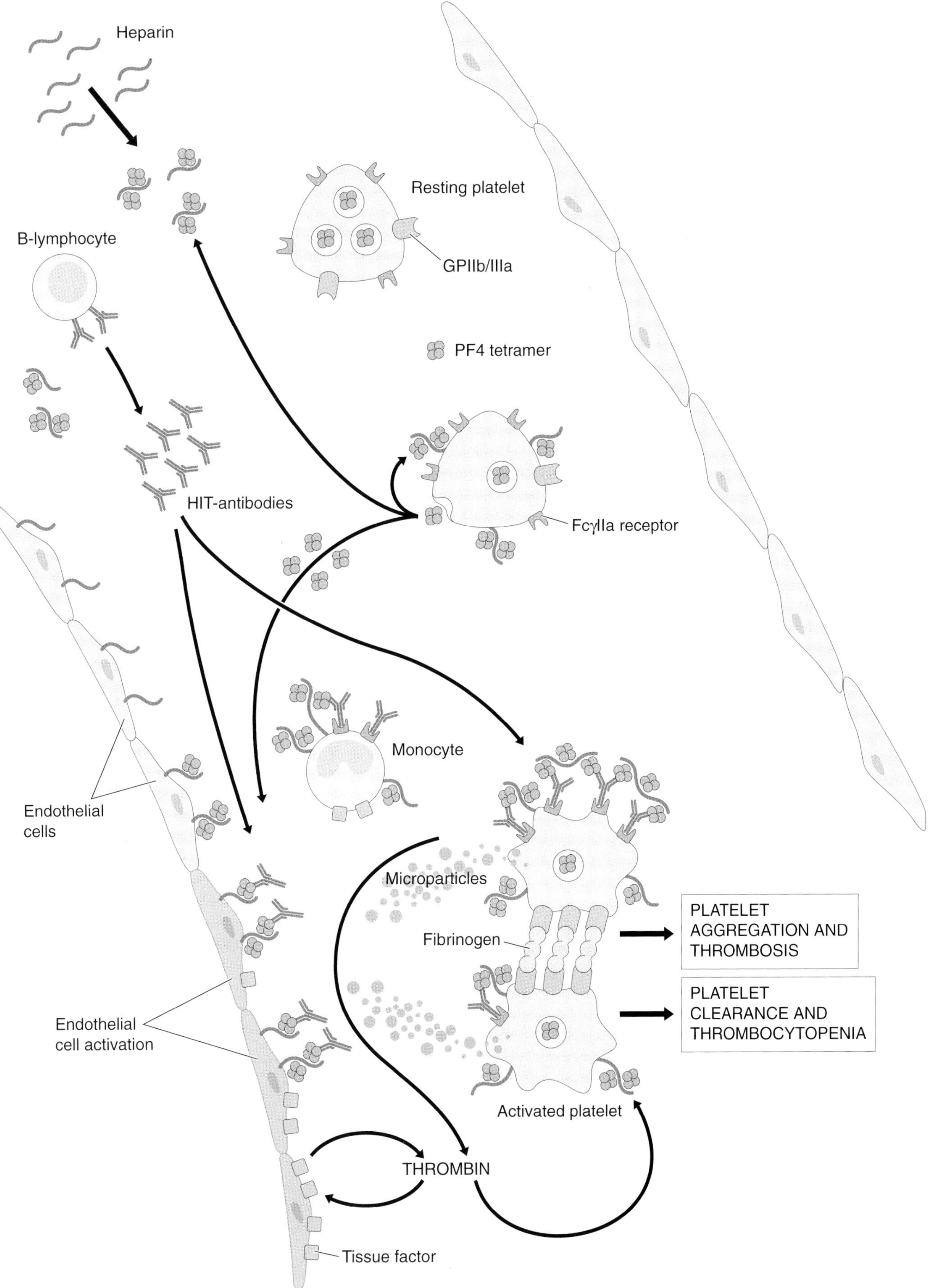

Figure 69–2. Pathophysiology of HIT. See text (Pathophysiology) for details.

to tissue factor expression and procoagulant activity. Heparin is not needed for platelet factor 4 to bind to monocytes, which express surface proteoglycans.

Thrombin Generation

Greatly increased levels of plasma thrombin-antithrombin complexes in HIT patients indicate that considerable thrombin is generated in vivo.[8] Increased thrombin generation is a general feature of hypercoagulability disorders with increased risk for venous thrombosis.

Animal Model

Reilly and investigators[51] have developed an animal model that recapitulates key clinical and laboratory features of HIT. These workers developed double-transgenic FcγRIIA/hPF4 mice, that is, mice expressing human FcγRIIa and human platelet factor 4 (mice lack platelet Fcγ receptors, and murine platelet factor 4 is not recognized by most HIT antibodies). When these mice are treated with an HIT-mimicking murine monoclonal antibody that recognizes the human PF4-heparin complex,[52] and then given heparin, severe thrombocytopenia and fibrin-rich thrombi in multiple organs result.

CLINICAL FEATURES AND DIAGNOSIS

Clinical Features

Thrombocytopenia

Table 69–2 lists the clinical features that suggest a diagnosis of HIT. The typical presentation is a large platelet count fall (50% or greater) that occurs during the day 5 to day 10 "window" after beginning heparin (first day of heparin = day 0) (Fig. 69–3).[5,25,26] Sometimes, the platelet count falls abruptly when a repeat course of heparin is begun (or the heparin dose is increased). Such rapid-onset HIT occurs in patients exposed to heparin within the past few weeks or months (usually within 30 days).[5,53] The association between rapid-onset HIT and recent heparin exposure is explained by the usual *transience* of HIT antibodies.[5] Rarely, thrombocytopenia and

TABLE 69–2. Clinical Features of HIT

Thrombocytopenia

Definition: Platelet count fall (usually >50%) in an appropriate temporal relationship to heparin therapy that is not more readily explained by another disorder.

Timing:

- *Typical-onset HIT:* platelets begin to fall usually 5–10 days after an immunizing exposure to heparin (most often, intraoperative or perioperative heparin).
- *Rapid-onset HIT:* an abrupt platelet count fall can occur when heparin is given to a patient who already has HIT antibodies resulting from a recent exposure.

Recovery after stopping heparin: variable, median 4 days to platelet count rise to >150 × 10^9/L; but 10% of patients take more than a week to recover.

Thrombosis

Venous thrombosis: deep venous thrombosis > pulmonary embolism > adrenal vein thrombosis (causing adrenal hemorrhagic infarction) > cerebral venous thrombosis > other visceral venous thrombosis

Arterial thrombosis: limb artery thrombosis > thrombotic stroke > myocardial infarction > mesenteric artery thrombosis > thrombosis in other arteries

Microvascular thrombosis: either secondary to coumarin (e.g., warfarin-induced venous limb gangrene or "classic" warfarin-induced skin necrosis) or disseminated intravascular coagulation (DIC) alone

Intracardiac thrombosis: intra-atrial or intraventricular thrombi

Heparin-Induced Skin Lesions (at Heparin Injection Sites)

Erythematous plaques
Skin necrosis

Acute Systemic Reactions

One or more of the following beginning 5–30 min after an intravenous unfractionated heparin bolus:

- *Inflammatory:* chills, rigors, fever, flushing
- *Cardiorespiratory:* tachycardia, hypertension, tachypnea, dyspnea, chest pain or tightness, cardiopulmonary arrest
- *Gastrointestinal:* nausea, vomiting, large-volume diarrhea
- *Neurologic:* headache, transient global amnesia

Decompensated DIC

One or more of the following (in the absence of another explanation):

- Prothrombin time (International Normalized Ratio) increase
- Fibrinogen decrease
- Microangiopathic blood film (see also Fig. 69–5)
- Circulating normoblasts (rare)

Preserved Hemostasis

Petechiae and other clinical evidence of thrombocytopenic bleeding are generally not present in HIT, even when severe thrombocytopenia is present.

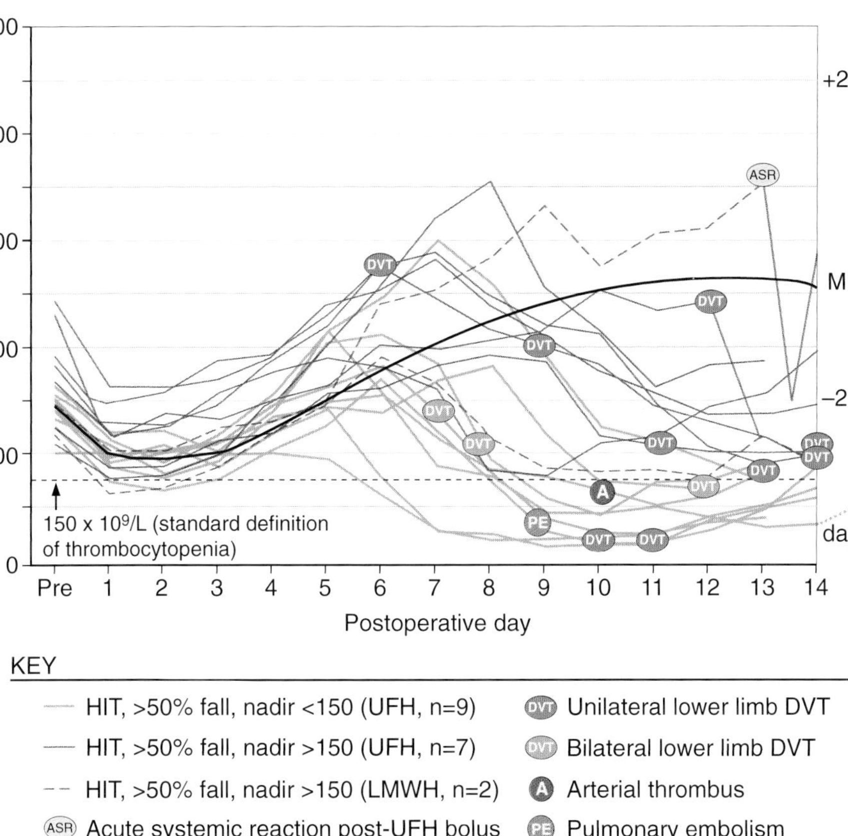

Figure 69–3. HIT in postoperative patients: typical timing of onset of thrombocytopenia. Eighteen patients with HIT were identified in a large clinical trial of unfractionated heparin and LMW heparin use after hip replacement surgery.[25,26] Thirteen of the 18 patients developed one or more thrombotic events. (See also Figure 69–8, which shows the "iceberg model" constructed from the data obtained from this clinical trial.) The light blue shaded area indicates the mean (±2 standard deviations) platelet count range in patients who did not form HIT antibodies.

thrombosis begin several days after all heparin has been stopped (delayed-onset HIT)[54–56]; typically, laboratory testing for HIT antibodies yields strong positive results.[54]

Despite the marked platelet count declines usually seen in HIT, severe thrombocytopenia (platelet count < 20×10^9/L) is uncommon. The median platelet count nadir is about 50–60 × 10^9/L (Fig. 69–4).[1,57] Examination of the blood film may reveal microangiopathic changes (red cell fragments, normoblasts) in the minority of patients who have overt disseminated intravascular coagulation (DIC) (Fig. 69–5).[57] In general, marked leukocytosis and severe "toxic" white cells suggest an alternative diagnosis, although these features may be seen in severe HIT.

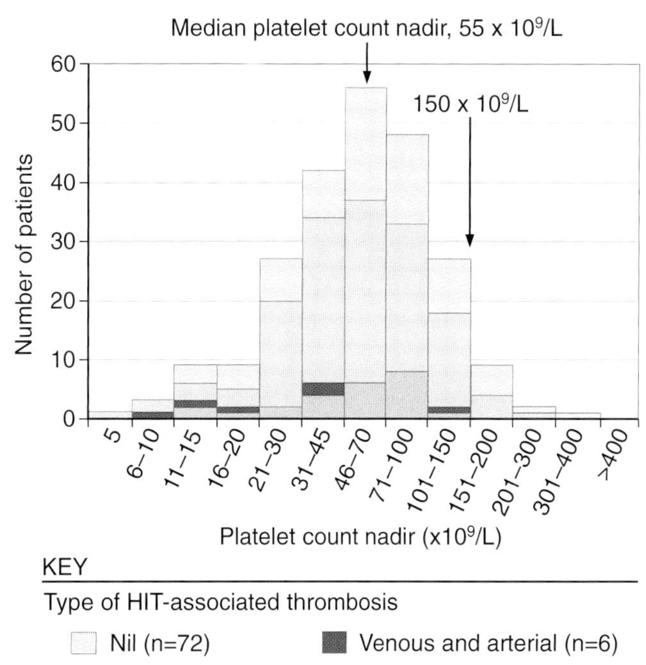

Figure 69–4. Platelet count nadirs and thrombosis: predominance of venous thrombosis. (From Warkentin TE: Heparin-induced thrombocytopenia: pathogenesis and management. Br J Haematol 121:535–555, 2003, with permission.)

Thrombosis

Thrombosis is a common complication of HIT, occurring in more than half the patients identified in prospective[1,2,58] and retrospective studies.[1,59–62] Figure 69–4 illustrates the relation between platelet count nadirs and presence of thrombosis. Venous thrombosis predominates,[1,61,62] although cardiac and vascular surgery patients with HIT more often develop arterial thrombosis.[60] Pulmonary embolism is the most common life-threatening thrombotic complication.

Limb Ischemic Syndromes

About 5–15% of HIT patients require limb amputation. There are two main causes of limb ischemia. The "classic" explanation is large artery occlusion(s) by platelet-rich

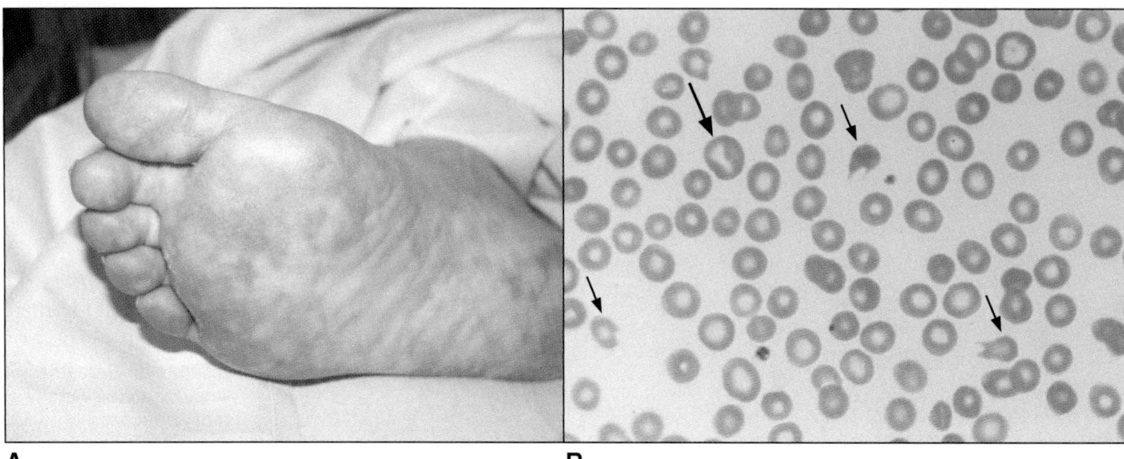

■ **Figure 69–5.** Foot ischemia despite palpable pedal pulses secondary to HIT-associated DIC. ***A,*** Ischemic foot. ***B,*** Blood film. Microangiopathic hemolysis is indicated by the thrombocytopenia, red cell fragments *(thin arrows)*, and polychromasia *(thick arrow)*. (From Warkentin TE: Clinical picture of heparin-induced thrombocytopenia. *In* Warkentin TE, Greinacher A [eds]: Heparin-Induced Thrombocytopenia [ed 3]. New York: Marcel Dekker, 2004, pp 53–106, with permission.)

"white clots,"[63] with absent pulse(s), usually necessitating surgical thrombectomy.[64,65]

The other limb ischemic syndrome is *venous limb gangrene*, usually associated with warfarin therapy.[8,66–69] Typically, acral (distal extremity) necrosis occurs in a limb (or limbs) with deep venous thrombosis, with palpable (or Doppler-identifiable) arteries. A diagnostic clue is a supratherapeutic International Normalized Ratio (INR; usually >3.5) during warfarin therapy, which results from very low factor VII levels that parallel concomitant severe reduction in protein C activity.[8,70] Rarely, decompensated DIC in HIT is complicated by limb ischemia caused by microvascular thrombosis in the absence of warfarin (see Fig. 69–5).[57]

Adrenal Hemorrhagic Necrosis

Unilateral or bilateral adrenal hemorrhagic necrosis secondary to adrenal vein thrombosis is a rare but well-described complication of HIT.[57,71,72] Bilateral adrenal hemorrhage typically presents as refractory hypotension with or without abdominal pain.

Heparin-Induced Skin Lesions

About 10–20% of patients who develop HIT while receiving subcutaneous unfractionated heparin or LMW heparin evince erythematous plaques or skin necrosis at the injection sites (Fig. 69–6).[57,73,74] The platelet count fall can be minor, despite the presence of dramatic skin lesions with strongly positive HIT antibodies. Arterial thrombosis may be associated with heparin-induced skin lesions.[75]

Acute Systemic Reactions

In a minority of patients with HIT antibodies, administration of an intravenous unfractionated heparin bolus leads to abrupt onset of signs and symptoms suggesting acute inflammation, cardiorespiratory compromise, neurologic events, or other unusual complications (see Table 69–2).[57,76,77] Typically, reactions begin 5–30 minutes after the bolus. The platelet count usually falls abruptly by at least 30%.

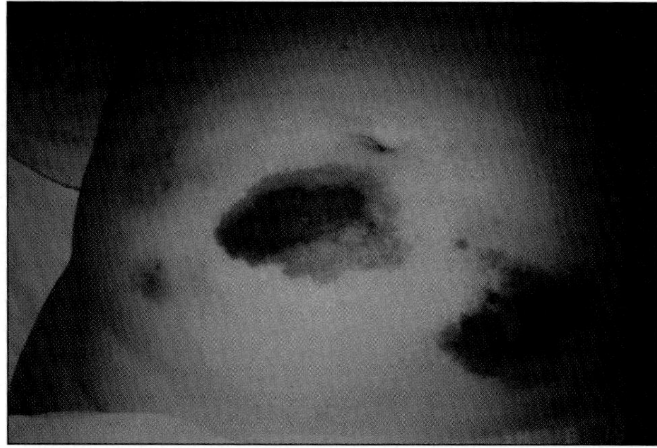

■ **Figure 69–6.** Heparin-induced skin lesions. Skin necrosis occurred at heparin injection sites. (From Warkentin TE: Heparin-induced skin lesions. Br J Haematol 92:494–497, 1996, with permission.)

Disseminated Intravascular Coagulation

Although most patients with HIT have laboratory evidence of increased thrombin generation,[8] only 10–15% have overt (decompensated) DIC (e.g., an elevated INR, low fibrinogen, and/or microangiopathic blood film).[57]

Laboratory Testing for HIT Antibodies

HIT antibodies can be detected using two types of assays: platelet activation assays and PF4/polyanion enzyme

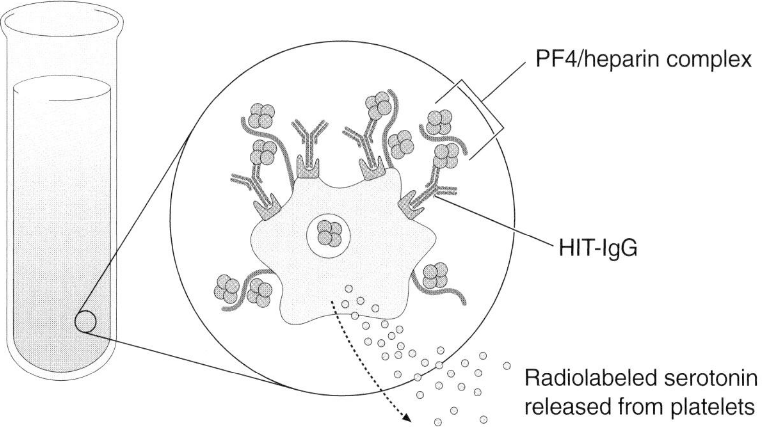

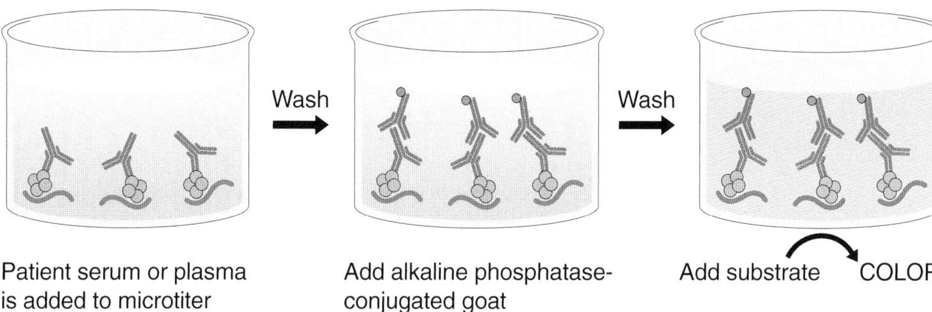

Figure 69–7. Laboratory tests for HIT antibodies: platelet activation assay and solid-phase PF4/polyanion enzyme immunoassay.

immunoassay ("antigen") assays (Fig. 69–7). Platelet activation assays using washed platelets (e.g., platelet serotonin release assay,[78,79] heparin-induced platelet activation assay[80–82]) have excellent operating characteristics (sensitivity-specificity tradeoff) when performed by experienced laboratories.[29,83,84] In contrast, conventional platelet aggregometry (using citrated "platelet-rich plasma") is less sensitive[81] and less specific[85] than washed platelet assays. One of us (D.B.C.) employs platelet-rich plasma to detect serotonin release with acceptable results,[86] but this has not been formally compared with other platelet activation assays.

Antigen assays are performed more often than platelet activation assays. Besides detecting HIT antibodies of the IgG class, two commercial solid-phase enzyme immunoassays also detect PF4/polyanion-reactive antibodies of the IgM and IgA classes,[23] which likely compromises diagnostic specificity.[83,87] Because washed platelet activation assays and PF4/polyanion antigen assays are very sensitive for detecting pathogenic HIT antibodies, negative testing using a blood sample obtained during acute thrombocytopenia essentially rules out a diagnosis of HIT.[88] Rare cases of patients with antibodies to other heparin-binding proteins, (e.g., interleukin-8 or neutrophil activating peptide-2) have been reported, often with an atypical presentation.[89,90] These patients usually have a negative enzyme immunoassay but a positive platelet activation assay.

The magnitude of a positive test result is useful when considering a diagnosis of HIT.[84,91] For example, subclinical seroconversion is common after cardiac surgery, so a weak-positive enzyme immunoassay (e.g., OD < 1.0) does not strongly support the diagnosis of HIT. In contrast, a patient with an unusual clinical profile, such as delayed onset of thrombocytopenia and thrombosis, but who tests strongly positive for HIT antibodies (e.g., > 90% serotonin release; OD > 2.0), likely has HIT.

Iceberg Model of HIT

Prospective studies reveal that only a minority of patients who form PF4/polyanion-reactive antibodies develop HIT.[24–26] Antigen assays are more likely than washed platelet activation assays to detect clinically insignificant antibodies.[29] Moreover, thrombotic complications tend to occur in patients who have a major platelet count fall that coincides with formation of platelet-activating IgG antibodies, whereas no increase in thrombosis rate is seen among antibody-positive patients whose platelet

Frequency of HIT and HIT antibodies after orthopedic surgery

Event	UFH (n=332)	LMWH (n=333)	P value
HIT-thrombosis (HIT-T)	3.6%	0.3%	<0.001
HIT (>50% platelet fall)	4.8%	0.6%	<0.001
Platelet-activating IgG antibodies (positive SRA)	9.9%	2.9%	0.010
Anti-PF4/heparin IgG antibodies (positive EIA)	15.6%	6.5%	0.011

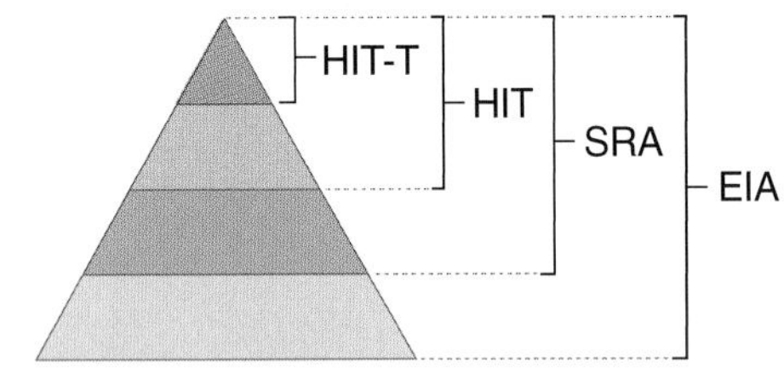

Figure 69–8. Iceberg model of HIT. The data shown represent frequencies of HIT-associated thrombosis, HIT (>50% platelet count fall), and seroconversion by platelet serotonin release assay and PF4/heparin enzyme immunoassay reported in a large clinical trial [25,26] of unfractionated heparin and LMW heparin given following orthopedic surgery.

count does not fall.[25,26] These concepts are illustrated in the "iceberg model" of HIT (Fig. 69–8). Figuratively speaking, the iceberg is "larger" (higher frequency of HIT antibody formation) and has greater "buoyancy" (higher breakthrough of clinical HIT) in patients treated with unfractionated heparin compared with LMW heparin.[3]

DIFFERENTIAL DIAGNOSIS

HIT should be considered in patients who develop thrombocytopenia and/or thrombosis during (or soon after stopping) heparin therapy. HIT should also be considered when such a patient presents to the emergency department following a recent hospitalization (delayed-onset HIT).[54–56]

Physicians can formulate a pretest probability of HIT based upon the magnitude and timing of the platelet count fall, the presence of thrombosis or other potential sequelae of HIT, and the presence of other explanations for thrombocytopenia, based upon the history, physical examination, and review of laboratory tests (e.g., peripheral blood film, DIC tests) (Fig. 69–9).[46] Especially when there is intermediate or high likelihood of HIT, diagnostic testing for HIT antibodies should be performed, although treatment decisions usually must be made before results become available. Duplex ultrasonography of the lower limbs is advised, because about half of HIT patients have subclinical deep venous thrombosis.[92]

The likelihood of HIT varies in different clinical situations. For example, HIT is unlikely within the first 4 postoperative days after cardiac surgery, even if heparin had been given during the preoperative period. The explanation is that thrombocytopenia secondary to hemodilution at cardiac surgery is universal, whereas significant immunization triggered by unfractionated heparin given to a preoperative (medical) patient is relatively unlikely (<1%). In contrast, a postoperative cardiac surgery patient whose platelet count has been rising between postoperative days 2 and 4, but who then develops an abrupt 50% or greater drop in platelet count between days 4 and 10, would have a pretest probability that is either intermediate or high, depending upon whether another plausible explanation for thrombocytopenia could be identified.

Besides perioperative hemodilution, other common causes of thrombocytopenia among hospitalized patients receiving unfractionated heparin include sepsis and multiorgan system failure. Disorders that can strongly mimic HIT on clinical grounds ("pseudo-HIT"[93]) include adenocarcinoma-associated DIC with venous and/or arterial thrombosis,[70] pulmonary embolism with DIC,[94] diabetic ketoacidosis with arterial thrombosis, antiphospholipid syndrome, septicemia with purpura fulminans, and endocarditis with septic embolization. Posttransfusion purpura, which presents as severe thrombocytopenia 5–10 days after blood transfusion, can be confused with HIT when both blood products and heparin were given perioperatively.[95] However, posttransfusion purpura usually causes severe thrombocytopenia and bleeding, whereas HIT typically evinces moderate thrombocytopenia without bleeding. Severe thrombocytopenia beginning abruptly after blood transfusion can be caused by platelet-reactive alloantibodies within donor blood (passive alloimmune thrombocytopenia).[96]

Hospitalized patients on heparin are usually receiving other drugs. However, drug-induced immune thrombocytopenia (other than HIT) is rare,[2] and typically causes severe thrombocytopenia (platelet count $< 20 \times 10^9$/L) with bleeding.[57] Implicated drugs include quinine, quinidine, vancomycin, sulfa antibiotics, and platelet glycoprotein (GP)IIb/IIIa antagonists (see Chapter 61).

A special situation is severe thrombocytopenia of abrupt onset soon after percutaneous coronary intervention. Although potential explanations include rapid-onset HIT or immune thrombocytopenia secondary to the iodinated contrast agent, the most likely cause is a platelet GPIIb/IIIa antagonist (abciximab, tirofiban, or eptifibatide).[97–99] These drugs cause abrupt, severe thrombocytopenia in 0.2–1% of patients even in the absence of previous drug exposure, because they potentiate reactivity of naturally occurring anti-GPIIb/IIIa antibodies. Giving an anticoagulant to such a patient because of an erroneous diagnosis of HIT could pose a high bleeding risk.

Microangiopathic hemolytic disorders can usually be distinguished from HIT on clinical grounds. However, because HIT sometimes presents in a "delayed" fashion and/or with prominent DIC (including microangiopathic blood film), confusion with postoperative thrombotic thrombocytopenic purpura could occur.[100,101]

Suspicion of HIT based upon the 4T's	Score	2	1	0
Thrombocytopenia	☐	>50% platelet fall to nadir ≥20	nadir 10-19, or 30-50% platelet fall	nadir <10, or <30% platelet fall
Timing of onset of platelet fall or thrombosis	☐	day 5-10, or ≤day 1 with recent heparin (within past 30 days)	>day 10 or timing unclear; or ≤day 1 with recent heparin (past 30-100 days)	day ≤4 (no recent heparin)
Thrombosis or other sequelae	☐	proven thrombosis, skin necrosis, or acute systemic reaction	progressive or recurrent thrombosis, or erythematous skin lesions	none
o**T**her cause(s) of platelet fall	☐	none evident	possible	definite
Total pre-test probability score	☐	periodic reassessment as new information can change pre-test probability (e.g., positive blood cultures)		

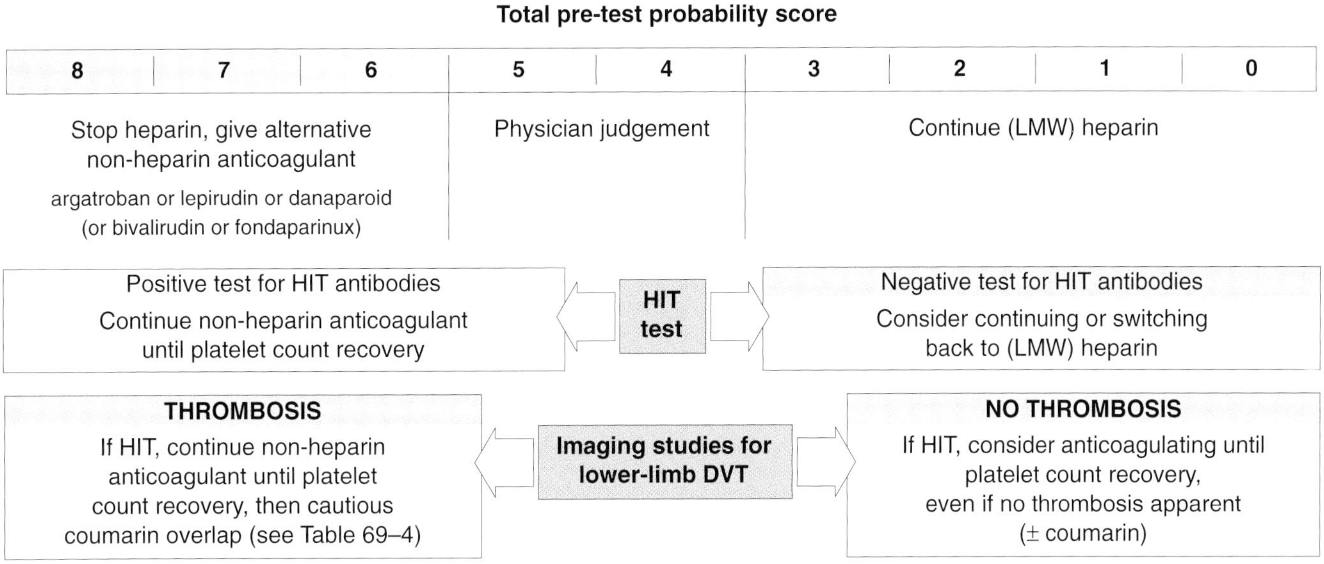

Total pre-test probability score

8	7	6	5	4	3	2	1	0
Stop heparin, give alternative non-heparin anticoagulant argatroban or lepirudin or danaparoid (or bivalirudin or fondaparinux)			Physician judgement		Continue (LMW) heparin			

Positive test for HIT antibodies
Continue non-heparin anticoagulant until platelet count recovery

HIT test

Negative test for HIT antibodies
Consider continuing or switching back to (LMW) heparin

THROMBOSIS
If HIT, continue non-heparin anticoagulant until platelet count recovery, then cautious coumarin overlap (see Table 69–4)

Imaging studies for lower-limb DVT

NO THROMBOSIS
If HIT, consider anticoagulating until platelet count recovery, even if no thrombosis apparent (± coumarin)

Figure 69–9. Differential diagnosis algorithm with approach to treatment. (Modified from Warkentin TE, Aird WC, Rand JH: Platelet-endothelial interactions: sepsis, HIT, and antiphospholipid syndrome. Hematology [Am Soc Hematol Educ Program] 497–519, 2003.)

TREATMENT

Discontinuation of Heparin

It is intuitive that outcomes might be improved if heparin is stopped because of suspicion for HIT raised by thrombocytopenia in the absence of thrombosis ("isolated HIT"). However, thrombotic events often occur despite heparin cessation (10% at 2 days; 30–40% at 10 days; 50% at 30 days; sudden thrombotic death, 5%).[59,60,102–104] In theory, discontinuing heparin could transiently *increase* hypercoagulability in HIT. Thus, prompt transition from heparin to an alternative anticoagulant is advised in most situations when HIT is strongly suspected.

Caveat: Dangers of Coumarin

Coumarin (e.g., warfarin) is ineffective or even deleterious among patients with HIT.[8,59,66–69] In particular, about 5–15% of patients with HIT-associated deep venous thrombosis develop venous limb gangrene because of a profound disturbance in procoagulant-anticoagulant balance: HIT contributes to increased thrombin generation, whereas warfarin leads to rapid depletion of protein C natural anticoagulant, especially in patients with overt DIC. Reversing coumarin (with oral or, preferably, intravenous vitamin K) should be considered in a patient who already is undergoing vitamin K antagonism when HIT is recognized.[105] Besides reducing the risk of coumarin necrosis, this lessens the risk of underdosing the alternative anticoagulant, because monitoring is usually performed using the activated partial thromboplastin time (aPTT), which is prolonged by coumarin.

TABLE 69–3. Alternative Anticoagulants for Treating HIT: Main Characteristics

Drug	Structure and function	Usual Starting Dose*	Usual Half-Life	Elimination	Adverse Events (Selected List) and Other Comments
Lepirudin	Bivalent DTI (hirudin)	(±0.4 mg/kg); 0.15 mg/kg/hr IV infusion (0.10 mg/kg/hr for isolated HIT)[†]	80 min	Predominant renal	Bleeding; post–IV bolus anaphylaxis
Bivalirudin	Bivalent DTI (hirudin analogue)	0.15 mg/kg/hr IV infusion	25–35 min	Enzymic (80%); renal (20%)	Bleeding
Argatroban	Univalent DTI (arginine derivative)	2 μg/kg/min IV infusion	40–50 min	Predominant hepatobiliary	Bleeding; prolongs INR more than the bivalent DTIs (complicates coumarin overlap)
Danaparoid	Mixture of GAGs with predominant anti-FXa activity	2250 U bolus[‡]; 400 U/hr × 4 hr; then 300 U/hr × 4 hr; then continue at 200 U/hr	25 hr (anti-FXa activity)	Partial renal	Bleeding; weak in vitro cross-reactivity against HIT antibodies seen in 15–40% of patient sera, usually without clinical significance; withdrawn from U.S. market (2002)
Fondaparinux	AT-binding pentasaccharide (indirect thrombin inhibitor)	? 7.5 mg SC qd (dosing not established)	17 hr (anti-FXa activity)	Partial renal	Cross-reactivity against HIT antibodies is absent; minimal experience, and thus effective dose in HIT is unknown

Agents indicated in **bold** are approved to treat HIT in at least one country.

*Lepirudin, bivalirudin, and argatroban are usually monitored by the aPTT. Lepirudin and argatroban dosing must be reduced substantially in patients with renal and hepatic dysfunction, respectively. Bivalirudin, danaparoid, and fondaparinux dosing should be reduced somewhat in patients with renal dysfunction.

[†]Suggested dose adjustments (% of original IV infusion rate) for renal insufficiency: serum creatinine 1.6–2.0 mg/dL (141–177 μmol/L), 50%; serum creatinine 2.1–3.0 mg/dL (178–265 μmol/L), 25%; serum creatinine, 3.1–6.0 mg/dL (266–530 μmol/L), 10%; serum creatinine >6.0 mg/dL (>530 μmol/L): 0.005 mg/kg/hr.[108]

[‡]Higher and lower initial boluses are appropriate in patients weighing >75 kg and <60 kg, respectively.

Abbreviations: AT, antithrombin; DTI, direct thrombin inhibitor; FXa, factor Xa; GAGs, glycosaminoglycans; IV, intravenous; qd, once daily; SC, subcutaneous.

Alternative Anticoagulants

Table 69–3 lists agents appropriate for the treatment of HIT. Lepirudin (Refludan), argatroban (Argatroban [U.S. trademark], Novastan [non-U.S. trademark]), and danaparoid (Orgaran) are approved in certain jurisdictions for treating HIT, whereas bivalirudin (Angiomax) and fondaparinux (Arixtra) are not approved for this indication, but show promise in small, uncontrolled studies.[105] Danaparoid was withdrawn from the U.S. market in 2002.

Both agents currently approved to treat HIT in the United States (lepirudin and argatroban) are *direct thrombin inhibitors* (DTIs), and were studied using a prospective cohort design with historical controls.[102–104] Only danaparoid was evaluated for HIT in a randomized trial (against dextran).[106]

Lepirudin is usually monitored by the aPTT, with the usual target range being 1.5–2.5 times baseline patient (or mean laboratory) aPTT. Bleeding resulting from drug accumulation is not uncommon, especially in the elderly (who may have unrecognized renal dysfunction). Another problem is post–intravenous bolus anaphylaxis, which occurs in about 1 in 625 patients reexposed to lepirudin.[107] To reduce these complications, recommendations[105,108] include the following:

1. Determine a standard curve using normal plasma "spiked" with lepirudin so as to determine the aPTT range that corresponds to therapeutic concentrations (about 0.6–1.4 μg/mL).
2. When thrombosis is not immediately life- or limb-threatening, avoid the initial intravenous lepirudin bolus, starting instead with intravenous infusion at 0.15 mg/kg/hr (assuming normal renal function).
3. For isolated HIT, start with a lower infusion rate (0.10 mg/kg/hr), and aim for a lower aPTT therapeutic range (1.5–2.0 times baseline).
4. Perform several aPTT assessments at 4- to 6-hour intervals during the first day to ensure that drug accumulation is not occurring because of unrecognized renal dysfunction.
5. Reduce lepirudin dosing according to renal function (see footnote † in Table 69–3).

Although IgG antihirudin antibodies are commonly generated in patients who receive this foreign polypeptide,[109,110] related adverse events are infrequent.

Argatroban is usually started at 2 μg/kg/min (only 0.5 μg/kg/min when hepatic dysfunction is suspected), and monitored by aPTT (usual target range, 1.5–3 times baseline aPTT). An important issue is prolongation of the INR by argatroban, which is more marked than with lepirudin and bivalirudin.[111–113] This poses problems during DTI-coumarin overlap. Our experience suggests it is reasonable to initiate argatroban at lower doses (e.g., 0.5 μg/kg/min) in patients in intensive care units, because some have marked increase in the aPTT despite no apparent hepatobiliary dysfunction.

In jurisdictions such as Canada and the European Union, danaparoid is another treatment option (see Table 69–3).[114] There is controversy as to whether prophylactic-dose danaparoid (750 U two or three times daily) is effective in patients with HIT.[115,116] In general, the therapeutic-dose regimen should be used if HIT is strongly suspected.[105] The low-dose danaparoid regimen is appropriate for patients in whom HIT is considered to be unlikely, but the physician prefers to prescribe an agent other than unfractionated heparin or LMW heparin. Whether prophylactic-dose fondaparinux (2.5 mg subcutaneously daily) will emerge as a similar option remains to be seen.

TABLE 69–4. Recommendations for Avoiding Coumarin-Induced Venous Limb Gangrene and Skin Necrosis Syndromes in Patients with HIT

1. In a patient who has already begun receiving coumarin when acute HIT is recognized, reverse coumarin anticoagulation with intravenous or oral vitamin K.
2. Delay coumarin anticoagulation until the platelet count has recovered to *at least* 100×10^9/L (preferably, 150×10^9/L).
3. Begin coumarin only in low, maintenance doses (e.g., initial dose ≤5 mg warfarin).
4. Administer coumarin only during overlapping alternative anticoagulation (minimum, 5-day overlap).
5. Do not stop the alternative anticoagulant until the platelet count has normalized and reached a stable plateau, with at least the last 2 days in the target therapeutic range.

DTI-Coumarin Overlap

The overlap between DTI and coumarin therapy in patients with HIT poses a risk for venous limb gangrene.[67,68] This is because initiation (or continuation) of coumarin during acute HIT, and premature discontinuation (or underdosing) of DTI, can produce the conditions for procoagulant-anticoagulant imbalance characteristic of this syndrome. Table 69–4 lists recommendations to minimize risk of this complication.[105]

New Thrombosis, Limb Amputation, and Death

Table 69–5 summarizes prospective studies of three anticoagulants used to treat HIT-associated thrombosis,[102,103,104,117,118] or to prevent thrombosis in isolated HIT.[102,103,118,119] The absolute risk of new thrombosis in the later trials ranged from 5% to 13%, representing a relative risk reduction of 62% (argatroban) and 78% (lepirudin) compared with historical controls. However, the amputation (5–15%) and mortality (10–20%) rates suggest that preventing new or progressive thrombosis might not avert loss of limb or life if thrombosis is advanced when therapy is begun. Results are better in isolated HIT, with absolute risk of new thrombosis ranging from 3% to 8%.

TABLE 69–5. HIT Treatment Outcomes of Alternate Anticoagulation

Study, Year	Regimen	*N*	Mean Days of Alternative Anticoagulant	% HIT-Antibody Positive	New Thrombosis Rate (RRR*)	Amputation Rate (RRR*)	Composite End Point (RRR*)	Major Bleed (% per Day Alternative Anticoagulant Given)†
HIT-Associated Thrombosis								
HAT-1/2, 2000[104]	Lep: 0.4 mg/kg bolus + 0.15 mg/kg/hr	113	13.3	100%	10.1 (63%)	6.5% (38%)	21.3% (55%)	1.4%
HAT-3, 2004[117]	Lep: bolus + 0.15 mg/kg/hr	98	14.0	100%	6.1% (78%)	5.1% (51%)	21.5% (55%)	1.5%
DMP, 2003[118]	Lep: bolus + 0.15 mg/kg/hr	496	12.1	77%	5.2% (NA)	5.8% (NA)	21.9%	0.45%
Arg-911, 2001[102]	Arg: 2 μg/kg/min	144	5.9	65%	19.4% (35%)	11.8% (−8%)	43.8% (22%)	1.9%
Arg-915, 2003[103]	Arg: 2 μg/kg/min	229	7.1	NA	13.1% (62%)	14.8% (−36%)	41.5% (27%)	0.9%
RCT vs. dextran, 2001[106]	Danap: bolus + infusion 200 U/hr	25	6‡	83%	12.0% (77%)	NA	20.0% (62%)	0%
Isolated HIT								
HAT1–3, 2002[119]	Lep: 0.10 mg/kg/hr	111	13.5	100%	2.7% (NA)§	2.7% (NA)§	9.0% (NA)§	1.1%§
DMP, 2002[118]	Lep: 0.10 mg/kg/hr	612	11.0	66%	2.1% (NA)‖	1.3% (NA)‖	≥15.7% (NA)‖	0.5%‖
Arg-911, 2001[102]	Arg: 2 μg/kg/min	160	5.9	65%	8.1% (64%)	1.9% (5%)	25.6% (34%)	0.6%
Arg-915, 2003[103]	Arg: 2 μg/kg/min	189	5.1	NA	5.8% (75%)	4.2% (−45%)	28.0 (28%)	1.0%

*RRR (relative risk reduction, expressed as percent) compared with historical controls (not shown).
†Calculated by dividing major bleed rate by number of mean days of alternative anticoagulant given.
‡Median (data provided by Dr. Harry Magnani, Organon NV).
§Data limited to on-treatment observation period.
‖Data limited to on-treatment observation period + 1 day.
Abbreviations: Arg, argatroban; DMP, drug monitoring program (postmarketing study); Danap, danaparoid; HAT, heparin-associated thrombocytopenia (prospective lepirudin study); Lep, lepirudin; NA, not available; RCT, randomized controlled trial.

The risk of major bleeding ranges from 1% to 2% per day of therapy with DTIs (see Table 69–5). Furthermore, no antidotes exist. Thus, selecting the appropriate drug, careful monitoring, and dose adjustments are important.

Cardiac Surgery in HIT Patients

Management of the patient with previous or acute HIT who requires cardiac surgery has been reviewed.[105,120] Repeat heparin exposure during surgery is recommended when HIT antibodies are no longer detectable (preferably, using one or two sensitive assays such as the serotonin release assay and enzyme immunoassay). Our experience suggests that a patient who tests weakly positive by enzyme immunoassay (<0.750 units) but who has a negative serotonin release assay also can receive heparin safely. Although the risk of rapidly generating pathogenic HIT antibodies appears low, it is prudent to restrict heparin use to the operation itself, and to use alternative anticoagulants for pre- and postoperative anticoagulation. Patients with recent HIT whose platelet count has recovered, but who still have detectable HIT antibodies ("subacute HIT"), are at risk for developing rapid-onset HIT upon heparin reexposure, unless the activation assay is negative and the enzyme immunoassay only weakly positive.

In patients with (sub)acute HIT who require urgent cardiac surgery, success is reported using an alternative anticoagulant (e.g., lepirudin[121,122] or bivalirudin[123]) during cardiopulmonary bypass. The largest study of lepirudin for cardiopulmonary bypass in patients with acute or previous HIT reported thrombosis-free survival in 54 of 57 patients (95%).[121] Bivalirudin has theoretical advantages over lepirudin, including a shorter half-life and predominantly nonrenal metabolism; it shows promise even for routine (non-HIT) cardiopulmonary bypass.[124] Combining unfractionated heparin with epoprostenol (prostacyclin analogue)[125,126] or tirofiban (platelet GPIIb/IIIa antagonist)[127] is another possible option.

Significantly lower doses of anticoagulation (about one half to one third) are required for "off-pump" cardiac surgery, and should be considered in appropriate patients.[120,128,129] Recently, bivalirudin compared favorably against unfractionated heparin (with protamine reversal) in a randomized trial for "off-pump" heart surgery in non-HIT patients.[130]

Vascular Surgery

Thromboembolectomy can be appropriate in patients with platelet-rich "white clots" occluding major limb arteries.[64] In contrast, surgery (including fasciotomy) is usually ineffective in patients with venous limb ischemia or gangrene; in contrast, aggresive anticoagulation plus intravenous vitamin K (to reverse vitamin K antagonism) may be beneficial.[131] Intraoperative anticoagulation using lepirudin,[132,133] argatroban,[134,135] and danaparoid[114] has been reported in this clinical situation in which usual anticoagulation with unfractionated heparin is contraindicated.

Hemodialysis in HIT Patients

Several approaches for managing nonheparin anticoagulation in hemodialysis HIT patients have been reported.[136] These include argatroban (either 2 μg/kg/min intravenously begun 4 hours predialysis; or a 100- to 250-μg/kg intravenous bolus at the start of dialysis, followed by 2 μg/kg/min intravenously adjusted by aPTT or activated clotting time[136,137]) and lepirudin (0.1-mg/kg bolus at start of dialysis; or 0.005 mg/kg/hr by intravenous infusion, e.g., for continuous venovenous hemofiltration, adjusted by aPTT[136]).

SUPPORTIVE CARE AND LONG-TERM MANAGEMENT

Unlike most other hypercoagulability disorders, HIT is a self-limited illness. Thus, ongoing supportive care and long-term management issues, if any, often involve sequelae of HIT-associated thrombosis, such as physical therapies for limb loss or residual deficits after a stroke. Indeed, in some situations, repeat exposure to heparin is appropriate.

Heparin Reexposure

HIT antibodies are usually transient,[5] and do not recur quickly (if at all) in antibody-negative former HIT patients reexposed to heparin.[5,7] However, deliberate reexposure to heparin is usually restricted to patients with an important indication for heparin and when alternative anticoagulants have limitations (e.g., cardiac or vascular surgery).[105,120]

CURRENT CONTROVERSIES & FUTURE CONSIDERATIONS

Heparin-Induced Thrombocytopenia

- Can HIT be avoided or reduced by substituting unfractionated heparin with LMW heparin or other anticoagulants?
- What is the diagnostic role of rapid-turnaround PF4/heparin enzyme immunoassays?
- What is the predictive value of clinical scores or algorithms for diagnosing HIT?
- Research is needed toward optimizing dosing and monitoring of DTIs.
- The efficacy and safety of alternative anticoagulant approaches for HIT (e.g., bivalirudin, fondaparinux) need to be determined.
- What is the frequency and clinical impact of HIT in children?

PROGNOSIS

The prognosis usually reflects the nature of any thrombotic complications, the severity of the HIT itself, and the presence of concomitant comorbidities. Thrombosis is often the initial presenting feature of HIT, and thus the onset of an early severe thrombotic event (or events) may limit the chance for a favorable outcome, even with otherwise appropriate therapy. Therapy likely reduces the risk of thrombotic death,[102,103] but does not affect death from other causes.

Suggested Readings*

Greinacher A, Eichler P, Lubenow N, et al: Heparin-induced thrombocytopenia with thromboembolic complications: meta-analysis of two prospective trials to assess the value of parenteral treatment with lepirudin and its therapeutic aPTT range. Blood 96:846–851, 2000.

Li ZQ, Liu W, Park KS, et al: Defining a second epitope for heparin-induced thrombocytopenia/thrombosis antibodies using KKO, a murine HIT-like monoclonal antibody. Blood 99:1230–1236, 2002.

Reilly MP, Taylor SM, Hartman NK, et al: Heparin-induced thrombocytopenia/thrombosis in a transgenic mouse model requires human platelet factor 4 and platelet activation through FcγRIIA. Blood 98:2442–2447, 2001.

Srinivasan AF, Rice L, Bartholomew JR, et al: Warfarin-induced skin necrosis and venous limb gangrene in the setting of heparin-induced thrombocytopenia. Arch Intern Med 164:66–70, 2004.

Visentin GP, Moghaddam M, Beery SE, et al: Heparin is not required for detection of antibodies associated with heparin-induced thrombocytopenia/thrombosis. J Lab Clin Med 138:22–31, 2001.

Warkentin TE, Levine MN, Hirsh J, et al: Heparin-induced thrombocytopenia in patients treated with low-molecular-weight heparin or unfractionated heparin. N Engl J Med 332:1330–1335, 1995.

Warkentin TE, Elavathil LJ, Hayward CPM, et al: The pathogenesis of venous limb gangrene associated with heparin-induced thrombocytopenia. Ann Intern Med 127:804–812, 1997.

Warkentin TE, Kelton JG: Temporal aspects of heparin-induced thrombocytopenia. N Engl J Med 344:1286–1292, 2001.

Warkentin TE, Greinacher A: Heparin-induced thrombocytopenia and cardiac surgery. Ann Thorac Surg 76:2121–2131, 2003.

Warkentin TE, Greinacher A: Heparin-induced thrombocytopenia: recognition, treatment, and prevention. The Seventh ACCP Conference on Antithrombotic and Thrombolytic Therapy. Chest 126 (3 Suppl):311S–337S, 2004.

Full references for this chapter can be found on accompanying CD-ROM.

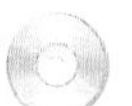

PART III

Consultative Hematology

CHAPTER 70

HEMATOLOGIC COMPLICATIONS OF PREGNANCY

Robert S. Siegel, MD, Khaled El-Shami, MD, PhD, and Kimberly Perez, MD

KEY POINTS

Hematologic Complications of Pregnancy

Anemias

- Anemia is the most common complication of pregnancy.
- The red cell mass increases by 20–30% and the plasma volume increases by 40–50%, resulting in a physiologic dilutional anemia characterized by normal mean corpuscular volume and mean corpuscular hemoglobin concentration.
- The iron requirement of pregnancy is 680–1000 mg. Insufficient iron supplementation is a frequent problem among women with poor prenatal care and may result in iron deficiency anemia.

Thrombocytopenias

- Thrombocytopenia is a common complication of pregnancy; the key to optimal management is identification of the etiology.
- Likely causes include gestational thrombocytopenia, which requires no therapy; immune thrombocytopenic purpura, human immunodeficiency virus infection, and systemic lupus erythematosus, which usually require therapy; and preeclampsia, HELLP syndrome, and thrombotic thrombocytopenic purpura (TTP)/hemolytic-uremic syndrome, which mandate immediate delivery.
- Patients with TTP/hemolytic-uremic syndrome must also be treated with immediate and daily plasmapheresis.

Inherited Bleeding Disorders

- Von Willebrand disease is the most common inherited bleeding disorder, affecting up to 1% of the population.
- Seventy percent of cases are type 1, usually a mild bleeding disorder, but all suspected patients should be evaluated in order to establish which subtype is present (type 1 to type 3). This analysis has both prognostic and important therapeutic implications.

Thrombosis

- There is a five- to sixfold increased risk of developing deep venous thrombosis (DVT) during pregnancy and in the postpartum period. Venous thromboembolism occurs in approximately 1 in 1000 pregnancies.
- DVT risk is increased in the presence of inherited or acquired thrombophilia. Inherited problems include antithrombin III deficiency, protein C and protein S deficiencies, factor V Leiden mutation, and prothrombin gene mutation.
- Acquired problems that can cause thrombophilia include obesity, age greater than 35 years, hyperemesis, immobilization, history of DVT, thrombosis, recent surgery, major trauma, ovarian hyperstimulation syndrome, antiphospholipid antibody syndrome, malignant disease, myeloproliferative disorders, and cesarean section.
- DVT can often be prevented in thrombophilic states or effectively treated during pregnancy. Most commonly, such patients can safely receive a low-molecular-weight heparin before delivery and warfarin for 6 weeks postpartum.

INTRODUCTION

Obstetricians often request consultation while caring for women who are pregnant and have developed a serious hematologic disorder. The request may come at any stage of pregnancy and often relates to problems that have not been previously evaluated. The purpose of this chapter is to review the most common hematologic complications of pregnancy and discuss their evaluation, diagnosis, and therapy. It includes sections devoted to anemia, thrombocytopenia and other bleeding disorders, and thromboembolic disease.

ANEMIAS

Iron Deficiency Anemia

Anemia is the most common complication of pregnancy.[1] Under normal circumstances, the red cell mass increases 20–30% during gestation, but the plasma volume increases by 40–50%, resulting in a net reduction in hemoglobin and hematocrit. By the end of pregnancy, women normally maintain a hemoglobin of 10–11 gm/dL and a hematocrit of 30–34%. Whereas hemoglobin and hematocrit progressively drop during the second and third trimesters, the mean corpuscular volume and mean corpuscular hemoglobin concentration remain unchanged. These latter features are important in differentiating the physiologic dilutional anemia of pregnancy from iron deficiency anemia, in which both mean corpuscular volume and mean corpuscular hemoglobin concentration are decreased (see Chapter 17).

The total additional iron requirement of a 40-week pregnancy is 680–1000 mg, almost half of which is in response to the expanding red cell mass.[1–4] Before regular iron supplementation was utilized for normal pregnancy, women were commonly iron deficient, often profoundly so. The diagnosis of iron deficiency is based on finding a microcytic, hypochromic anemia that is accompanied by a low serum ferritin, a low serum iron, a high total iron-binding capacity and a low serum iron/total iron-binding capacity ratio, typically less than 16%. An increase in total iron-binding capacity can be seen in 15% of pregnant women in the absence of iron deficiency.[5,6] The correlation between low serum ferritin and the absence of stainable bone marrow iron is about 75%, and the specificity of low serum ferritin for absent marrow iron is 98%.[7] The red blood cell count, hemoglobin, and hematocrit are all proportionately low, and examination of the peripheral blood smear reveals a low reticulocyte count. As in nonpregnant patients, the gold standard for iron deficiency remains the stainable bone marrow iron,[8–11] although bone marrow aspiration is rarely indicated to diagnose iron deficiency anemia during pregnancy. Hypochromic, microcytic anemias with a mean corpuscular volume less than 80 fL must be distinguished from the thalassemias.

Clinical manifestations of early iron deficiency anemia are usually mild, and the diagnosis is made during a routine complete blood count. More significant anemias are associated with tachycardia and cause symptoms such as fatigue and weakness. Problems specifically related to iron deficiency anemia include pica, cheilosis, and koilonychia.

All pregnant women should be offered iron supplementation in order to avoid depletion of iron stores. A dose of 60–120 mg/day of elemental iron is considered appropriate.[12,13] The rare patient who does not tolerate oral iron or has impaired iron absorption can be offered parenteral iron therapy.[14]

Macrocytic (Folate and Vitamin B_{12} Deficiency) Anemias

The folic acid requirement increases with the duration of pregnancy because of the increased need for this essential cofactor in nucleic acid synthesis. Folate that is stored primarily in the liver is usually sufficient for about 6 weeks. The daily folate requirement in the nonpregnant state is about 50 µg, but increases fourfold during gestation.[15] Women carrying multiple fetuses and those recovering from infection or hemolysis have further increased folate requirements. As is the case with other nutrients, the fetus is able to accumulate adequate folate even when the mother is deficient. Severe folate deficiency not only causes anemia in the mother, but also neural tube defects in the fetus.[16]

Macrocytic anemia, with a mean corpuscular volume of greater than 100 fL, suggests either reticulocytosis, megaloblastic anemia, alcohol toxicity, hypothyroidism, medication effect, or liver disease. Megaloblastic anemia is the most common cause of macrocytic anemia and is usually a consequence of folate or vitamin B_{12} deficiency in nonpregnant states. When megaloblastic anemia is noted, serum B_{12}, serum folate, and red blood cell folate levels should be checked. Examination of the blood smear often reveals dimorphic populations of red blood cells, hypersegmented neutrophils, and large platelets. The expected elevation in mean corpuscular volume associated with megaloblastic anemia could be offset by concomitant iron deficiency, leading to a combined nutritional anemia with normocytic indices.[17]

Vitamin B_{12} deficiency is rarely seen in pregnant patients. Because the folate requirement increases 5- to 10-fold by the third trimester, folic acid has been added to regular prenatal vitamins; most prenatal vitamins contain 0.8 mg of folate in addition to iron, and should preclude both iron and folate deficiency.[18] Women with significant hemoglobinopathies, those on anticonvulsants, or women with multiple gestations may require more than 1 mg of folate daily. After starting therapy in a folate-deficient pregnant woman, an increased reticulocyte count can be seen within 3 days and the hematocrit level can rise as much as 1% daily.

Sickle Cell Disease in Pregnancy

Women at risk for sickle cell disease should be screened for the disease. Its presence is easily diagnosed through the use of hemoglobin electrophoresis. Women testing positive for sickle cell trait (hemoglobin AS) generally have 35–45% hemoglobin S, are usually asymptomatic, and have no increased risk for poor perinatal outcome, except for an increased incidence of pyelonephritis.[19]

Although maternal mortality is uncommon in hemoglobin SS patients, there is considerable maternal morbidity.[20–22] Pregnant women with hemoglobin SS suffer a 50–70% incidence of infection,[22] with most of the infections affecting the urinary tract. Pulmonary infection with pneumococcal species, *Mycoplasma*, *Haemophilus*, and *Salmonella* is also common. Infections should be vigorously sought and promptly treated. Painful crises are more common during pregnancy, in part because of the increased infection risk.[23] Pregnancy-induced hypertension complicates approximately one third of pregnancies in women with sickle cell disease.

Pregnancies in hemoglobin SS patients are also associated with higher incidence of poor perinatal outcomes.[23] The rate of spontaneous abortions is estimated to be as high as 19–35%[24] and that of low birth weights 41–46%.[22,24] Approximately 30% of infants born to mothers with sickle cell disease have birth weights below 2500 gm,[25] and a multicenter study reported that 21% of infants born to mothers with sickle cell disease were small for gestational age.[23] Stillbirth rates of 8–10% have also been reported.[24,26]

Although the management of pregnant sickle cell disease patients should be individualized, there are guidelines that should be followed. Good antenatal care is important, as is early recognition of any organ dysfunction and its prompt management. Because sickle cell disease causes chronic hemolysis and triggers reticulocytosis even in the nonpregnant state, adequate folate supplementation is important to avoid a hypoproliferative megaloblastic crisis. Although many sickle cell patients are iron overloaded because of previous transfusions, others require iron supplementation to avoid iron deficiency.

The prophylactic use of exchange transfusions throughout pregnancy is not supported by the medical literature,[27,28] but they can be used in patients with recurring crises and persistent anemia, and possibly in the weeks prior to delivery. During delivery, maintaining adequate hydration, oxygenation, and good pain control are all essential.

Immune Hemolytic Anemias in Pregnancy

The classification and treatment of immune hemolytic anemias in pregnancy are the same as those seen in the nonpregnant state (see Chapter 24). In evaluating hemolytic anemia associated with pregnancy, one must immediately rule out offending medications that could trigger either immune-mediated hemolysis or hemolysis resulting from glucose-6-phosphate dehydrogenase deficiency.[29] Otherwise the assessment of hemolysis is similar to what would be done in nonpregnant states. Idiopathic hemolytic anemia that resolves with delivery may have been mild HELLP (microangiopathic hemolysis, elevated liver enzymes, and low platelets) syndrome or preeclampsia.

THROMBOCYTOPENIAS

Thrombocytopenia is the most common hematologic complication of pregnancy. Identifying the cause of pregnancy-associated thrombocytopenia is of paramount importance because each condition is managed differently and is associated with distinct maternal and/or fetal complications (Table 70–1).

TABLE 70–1. Pregnancy-Associated Thrombocytopenia

Gestational thrombocytopenia
Preeclampsia/HELLP syndrome
Immune thrombocytopenic purpura
Human immunodeficiency virus infection
Systemic lupus erythematosus and other vasculitides
Thrombotic thrombocytopenic purpura/hemolytic-uremic syndrome

Gestational Thrombocytopenia

The widespread use of automated blood counts has resulted in an increasingly common diagnosis of thrombocytopenia (platelet counts of <150,000/μL) in an otherwise healthy pregnant woman.[30] Gestational thrombocytopenia occurs in 7% of all pregnancies and typically presents with a platelet count of 100,000–150,000/μL (occasionally as low as 70,000/μL) that is not associated with an underlying medical disorder. It does not precede or follow pregnancy and is not associated with fetal thrombocytopenia.[31,32]

Gestational thrombocytopenia is mainly a dilutional phenomenon associated with increased plasma volume during pregnancy, although some investigators believe that decreased platelet survival may have a secondary role. Pregnant women with gestational thrombocytopenia should receive routine prenatal care through delivery.[33]

Immune Thrombocytopenic Purpura

Immune thrombocytopenic purpura (ITP) is a diagnosis that can be made only after other plausible causes are excluded. Specifically, one must rule out thrombocytopenia resulting from medications or other immune diseases such as systemic lupus erythematosus, preeclampsia, and HELLP syndrome. Other less common causes that should be considered are viral infection, including human immunodeficiency virus disease, and rarely a lymphoproliferative disease such as chronic lymphocyte leukemia. The peripheral smear should always be reviewed to rule out spurious thrombocytopenia. Bone marrow disease should be considered when evaluating profoundly thrombocytopenic pregnant women.

Patients with pregnancy-associated ITP typically have platelet counts that are lower than those seen in gestational thrombocytopenia.[30] The diagnosis is suggested when the patient does not fit into one of the other categories for thrombocytopenia and has been diagnosed with preexisting ITP, either in a nonpregnant state or during a previous pregnancy.

Although one needs to be concerned about the mother's platelet count, the primary focus of attention is the possibility of fetal thrombocytopenia. In an 11-year retrospective analysis of obstetric patients with ITP,[34] 32% of mothers required therapy, including corticosteroids and intravenous immunoglobulin. In patients who had previously suffered from ITP during pregnancy, the fetal platelet count in the second pregnancy was predicted by the platelet count of the first infant at birth. Among 115 babies born to ITP mothers, 5 had platelet counts between 20,000/μL and 49,000/μL and 6 had platelet counts below 20,000/μL. There was no association between the maternal and infant platelet counts. There were two fetal deaths in this study. The first was stillborn to a mother who had a platelet count greater than 100,000/μL during her pregnancy. In the second, a mother with ITP and a history of splenectomy had a platelet count of less than 50,000/μL. She had received intravenous immunoglobulin with a platelet response to greater than 300,000/μL at 26 weeks. The fetus was stillborn at 27 weeks.

One frustrating aspect of managing pregnancy-associated ITP is the inability to easily evaluate neonatal thrombocytopenia. Scalp vein sampling at the beginning of delivery is not a reliable or timely means for quantifying an infant's platelet count. Percutaneous umbilical cord blood sampling will allow an accurate determination of the fetal platelet count but is associated with a 2–5% risk of fetal loss.[35] Most investigators do *not* advocate the use of percutaneous umbilical cord blood sampling in the management of maternal ITP.

When maternal platelet counts drop to below 20,000/μL, prednisone and intravenous immunoglobulin are used to minimize bleeding. Cesarean sections are often utilized, although there is no evidence that the fetal loss rate or morbidity is improved. Splenectomy, when necessary, can be performed optimally during the second trimester. Following delivery, both the maternal and fetal platelet counts will rise. The neonatal platelet count may worsen for several days before it improves.

In summary, among patients with pregnancy-associated ITP, the overall fetal loss rate is 1–2%. Fetal loss appears to be unavoidable, and bleeding problems are uncommon and not associated with the maternal platelet count. Presently there is no established system for predicting neonatal thrombocytopenia. Infants at highest risk are those born to mothers with prior pregnancies in which severe fetal thrombocytopenia had occurred. Some investigators also believe that mothers with ITP who have had splenectomy and are chronically thrombocytopenic are also at higher risk for delivering thrombocytopenic infants.

Preeclampsia/HELLP Syndrome

Preeclampsia affects 5–15% of all pregnancies and refers to the development of hypertension and proteinuria, usually late in the third trimester. The risk is highest among primigravidas, and platelet counts are often subnormal in women with this syndrome. Severe thrombocytopenia with platelet counts below 50,000/μL occurs in less than 5% of cases. The likelihood of severe thrombocytopenia increases proportionately with the severity of preeclampsia. Recovery of the platelet count above 100,000/μL is typically seen within 3 days of delivery.[36]

The diagnosis of preeclampsia is made after ruling out HELLP syndrome and other causes of microangiopathic hemolytic anemia, including thrombotic thrombocytopenic purpura (TTP), hemolytic-uremic syndrome, and disseminated intravascular coagulation. The principal therapy for preeclampsia is prompt delivery. Symptoms and signs, including thrombocytopenia, typically resolve in subsequent days and weeks.

HELLP syndrome patients suffer from nausea, malaise, and abdominal pain and typically have platelet counts that are less than 100,000/μL. Such patients can develop HELLP syndrome independently, but preeclampsia evolves into HELLP syndrome in approximately 12% of patients. The primary therapy for HELLP syndrome is also prompt delivery. The platelet count and liver function studies begin a trend toward normal values within 4 days of delivery.[37] Infants born to mothers with preeclampsia and HELLP syndrome are not at risk for severe thrombocytopenia. Plasma exchange and dexamethasone therapy (at a dose of 6mg every 6 hours) may be helpful in severe postpartum HELLP syndrome.[38,39]

Thrombocytopenic Purpura/Hemolytic-Uremic Syndrome

There is an association between TTP/hemolytic-uremic syndrome and pregnancy that is poorly understood. TTP is characterized by a pentad of signs that include microangiopathic hemolytic anemia, fever, renal failure, neurologic abnormalities, and thrombocytopenia (see Chapter 62). The complete pentad occurs in less than 40% of patients, but 75% exhibit the triad of microangiopathic hemolytic anemia, thrombocytopenia, and some form of neurologic abnormality. Distinguishing TTP from preeclampsia, eclampsia, and the HELLP syndrome during pregnancy or in the postpartum period may be difficult.

The underlying pathophysiology for many TTP patients has been defined.[40–43] Von Willebrand factor (vWF) is produced by the endothelial cells and exists as large multimers in normal plasma. Under normal circumstances, the multimers are cleaved into smaller, normal-sized vWF proteins by a metalloproteinase known as ADAMTS13. When ADAMTS13 is absent or present in diminished quantities, there is an accumulation of large vWF multimers, which leads to increased platelet aggregation and platelet clumping.[40,43] In the familial type of TTP, ADAMTS13 activity was absent in six patients with inherited TTP and in 20 of 24 patients with nonfamilial disease.[43] In the acquired form, autoantibodies are the cause of diminished ADAMTS13 activity. Although the test is commercially available, therapy with daily plasma exchange should be initiated at the first sign of possible TTP.

The treatment of a pregnant woman with TTP in the third trimester includes plasma exchange and delivery as soon as possible. Plasma exchange remains the standard of care for treating postpartum mothers who have developed this disease.[44]

Neonatal Alloimmune Thrombocytopenia

Neonatal alloimmune thrombocytopenia can develop when the fetus inherits paternal platelet antigens that are not present in the mother. Fetal thrombocytopenia occurs when maternal isoantibodies cross the placenta and bind fetal platelets, marking them for removal by the reticuloendothelial system. The most common antigens include human platelet antigens HPA-1a and HPA-5b. Women who are at highest risk are those who are related to other women with neonatal alloimmune thrombocytopenia or had a prior pregnancy complicated by this disorder (see Chapter 60). The diagnosis should be considered when a healthy mother gives birth to an otherwise well infant with a profoundly low platelet count. Subsequent pregnancies tend to be more affected than the first. The most severe complication is fetal intracranial bleeding, 10–50% of which occurs in utero. Therapy of infants born with a profoundly low platelet count prominently includes the infusion of washed maternal platelets. Antenatal therapy includes the use of intravenous immunoglobulin, prednisone, and early delivery using cesarean section.[45]

INHERITED BLEEDING DISORDERS

Nonthrombocytopenic bleeding disorders can be divided among von Willebrand disease and, less commonly, other factor deficiencies. In a normal pregnancy, concentrations of factor VIII, vWF, factor VII, factor X, and fibrinogen rise continuously throughout pregnancy, and concentrations of plasminogen activator inhibitors decrease. Conversely, factors II, IX, and XII change minimally over the course of a normal pregnancy.

von Willebrand Disease

Von Willebrand disease is the most common inherited coagulation factor deficiency and affects up to 1% of the population[46,47] (see Chapter 64). Type 1 von Willebrand disease is autosomal dominant, comprises 70% of all cases, and typically causes only mild bleeding, even in the nonpregnant state. Type 2 is usually an autosomal dominant mutation and can be divided into four categories: 2A, 2B, 2M, and 2N. Together they account for about 20–25% of all von Willebrand patients. Type 3 is an autosomal recessive disorder and results in very low or undetectable levels of vWF. It is responsible for the most significant bleeding complications and accounts for approximately 5% of all cases.

Classical type 1 von Willebrand disease often presents as mild menstrual bleeding in the prepregnant state. By the time of delivery, the vWF levels have increased fourfold over those of the prepregnant state. The need for intervention at delivery is directly related to the vWF level, which should be determined at 36 weeks of gestation. By the time of delivery, patients should have vWF levels of at least 50 IU/dL in order to minimize bleeding risks.[48] DDAVP (desmopressin) is rarely necessary before delivery but may be useful in the postpartum state when vWF levels fall rapidly and hemorrhage becomes a higher risk.

Type 2A von Willebrand disease is a disorder that occurs because of a mutant vWF gene that is associated with a reduction in plasma vWF antigen, vWF activity, and ristocetin cofactor levels. Bleeding severity is related to the level of normal circulating vWF. DDAVP can be successfully used, particularly in the immediate post delivery period for not greater than 4 days. The response to DDAVP in type 2A disease is usually not as pronounced as in type 1. Most type 1 and 2A patients have safe von Willebrand factor levels at the time of delivery without intervention.[48–51]

Type 2B disease is due to mutations that result in an increased affinity of the von Willebrand molecule for platelet membrane glycoprotein Ib. As the vWF factor level rises during pregnancy, thrombocytopenia may develop and worsen because of platelet aggregation.[52] Type 2M disease is a rare autosomal dominant disorder with reduced vWF function in the presence of large vWF multimers. Type 2N disease is a rare syndrome in which there is reduced binding of vWF to glycoprotein Ib. These patients often have significant bleeding and present with a constellation of symptoms and signs that are more suggestive of hemophilia A. Multimer fractions are normal and platelets are unaffected. This disorder must be suspected in women (nonpregnant state or pregnant) who are found to have low factor VIII levels.

Type 3 disease is the least common but most severe form of the disease.[47] Patients suffer from an absence of the von Willebrand antigen and activity. vWF levels do not rise during the course of pregnancy in patients with type 3 disease, and, consequently, such patients are at risk for bleeding throughout gestation. The ristocetin cofactor level is the most important variable in determining the risk for postpartum bleeding. Such women also have an increased rate of first-trimester bleeding, although there is no increase in spontaneous abortion rates.

Patients with significant type 2B, 2M, 2N, or 3 von Willebrand disease should not receive DDAVP, but rather should be given factor replacement until the vWF level rises to 50 IU/dL. During a major bleeding episode, factor replacement should be given, such as Humate-P at a dose of 40–60 IU/kg every 8–12 hours for 3 days. The ristocetin cofactor level should be maintained at 50 IU/dL (see Chapter 64). Subsequently, patients may receive 50 IU/kg daily for approximately 7 days of therapy.[52–55]

Other Factor Deficiencies

Other inherited factor deficiencies rarely can cause bleeding problems. Both hemophilia A (factor VIII deficiency) and hemophilia B (factor IX deficiency) are X-linked recessive defects. Up to 20% of female carriers may have bleeding complications. Typically, hemophilia carriers have factor levels ranging from 50 to 150 IU/dL, and those patients with factor levels below 30 IU/dL are at risk for bleeding. Factor VIII carriers rarely have such low levels that they require therapy in late pregnancy. The uncommon patient with low factor VIII levels may benefit from DDAVP, or she can be treated with recombinant factor VIII for 3–4 days.[52,53] Factor IX levels usually do not increase during pregnancy. When hemophilia B patients have factor IX levels below 50 IU/dL, they require therapy in the form of recombinant factor IX concentrate for a total of 3–4 days at delivery.[52,53]

Factor XI deficiency is most common in the Ashkenazi Jewish population, where its heterozygous frequency is about 1 in 12. Such patients tend not to have spontaneous hemorrhage, but may bleed heavily during surgery, including cesarean section. Treatment for factor XI deficiency is fresh frozen plasma.[48]

THROMBOSIS

A woman carries a five- to sixfold increased risk of developing deep venous thrombosis (DVT) during pregnancy and for 6–8 weeks postpartum. Venous thromboembolism occurs in about 1 in 1000 pregnancies.[56,57] Most symptomatic DVT occurs later in the pregnancy and often is located in the left iliac vein, a consequence of compression of the left iliac vein by the right iliac artery and ovarian artery.[58,59] Iliac DVT often results in pulmonary embolization.

In considering the pathogenesis of venous thrombi occurring in normal pregnancies, it is important to recall Virchow's triad, which includes stasis, endothelial damage, and hypercoagulability. Lower extremity *stasis* occurs in most pregnancies when venous blood flow is thought to be reduced by 50% by the end of the second trimester, with the nadir at 36 weeks. Normal blood flow is restored after delivery. *Endothelial damage* occurs in the pelvic vessels during either normal vaginal delivery or cesarean section. *Hypercoagulability* occurs as a consequence of increased coagulation factors, including factor VIII; protein C and protein S deficiencies; and impaired fibrinolysis with increased plasminogen activator inhibitors 1 and 2. Physiologically, such changes provide protection against the hemostatic challenge imposed by delivery.

Thrombophilia defines an inherited or acquired condition in which single or multiple abnormalities increase the risk of thromboembolic disease (Fig. 70–1). Inherited problems include antithrombin III deficiency, protein C and protein S deficiencies, factor V Leiden mutation, prothrombin gene mutation G20210A, and MTHFR gene mutation. Inherited thrombophilia is present in 15% of Western populations and is found in 50% of patients who develop venous thromboembolism during pregnancy. The level of risk is dependent upon the severity of the underlying thrombophilic effects, history of thrombotic events, and additional risk factors, such as diabetes mellitus or obesity. Acquired risk factors that increase the risk of DVT in pregnancy include obesity (particularly weight >80 kg), age greater than 35 years, hyperemesis, immobilization, a history of thrombosis, recent surgery, major trauma, ovarian hyperstimulation syndrome, antiphospholipid antibody syndrome, malignant disease, myeloproliferative disorders, and cesarean section.[60]

Ovarian hyperstimulation syndrome results from the use of high-dose hormones utilized to trigger ovulation. In this setting, there is an increased risk of DVT,[61] particularly after a treatment cycle that results in pregnancy. Prophylaxis is indicated for high-risk women. Estradiol levels greater than 10 times normal increase the risk of DVT, as do polycystic ovaries. Thrombosis typically occurs between 7 and 10 weeks after treatment is begun. The mechanisms for thrombosis remain unclear, but DVT resulting from ovarian hyperstimulation syndrome often involves the internal jugular or neck veins, and can also be found in the upper extremities. About 25% of women suffering from thromboembolic disease associated with ovarian hyperstimulation syndrome develop arterial thrombi, including intracerebral occlusions[62] (see Fig. 70–1).

Management of DVT

Managing thrombophilic patients begins with identifying individuals who are at high risk. There is no evidence to support universal screening for inherited thrombophilia in all pregnant women. Screening should be performed in patients with a strong family history of DVT, and particularly those women who have had a prior episode of DVT in pregnant and nonpregnant states.

Among the most uncommon inherited venous thromboembolism risk factors, a quantitative deficiency in antithrombin III results in an odds ratio of 282 for having DVT compared to women with normal antithrombin III levels.[63] Women who have a qualitative antithrombin III problem have an odds ratio of 28 for a venous thromboembolism. The more common patients with prothrombin gene mutation and factor V Leiden (heterozygous) patients have an odds ratio of 4.4 and 4.5 respectively.[63] A different study shows that such patients have a relative risk for venous thromboembolism of 6.9 and 9.5, respectively.[64] Patients with protein C or protein S deficiency have a relative risk of 13.1.[65] Patients diagnosed with MTHFR C677T mutation (homozygous) have not been shown to have an increased risk of developing venous thromboembolism in pregnancy, perhaps because pregnant women are routinely placed on folate (Table 70–2). Patients with a history of venous thromboembolism have a recurrence rate of 10.9% per 100 patient-years during pregnancy and 3.7% per 100 patient-years after pregnancy.[66]

Treatment Guidelines

At present, there are no evidence based, mutually agreed-upon standards for venous thromboembolism prophylaxis in pregnant women.

Making the diagnosis of venous thromboembolism in pregnancy is similar to the process in nonpregnant states. Duplex ultrasonography should be employed to identify a DVT, although the procedure can be technically difficult in the later stages of pregnancy. If pulmonary embolism is suspected, patients should undergo a ventilation-perfusion scan or helical computed tomography. Limited venography is acceptable in pregnant patients if the study is limited to the waist and below.[67] Low D-dimer levels are helpful in ruling out a diagnosis of DVT. Making an accurate diagnosis is critical.

Table 70–3 shows treatment recommendations based on the 2004 American College of Chest Physicians conference on antithrombotic and thrombolytic therapy.[68] These recommendations vary according to patient history of venous thromboembolism, and include the use of anticoagulant drugs and heparin. Dose-adjusted unfractionated heparin can be given subcutaneously every 12 hours, such that a prothrombin time measured 6 hours after a dose is in the therapeutic range. Alternatively,

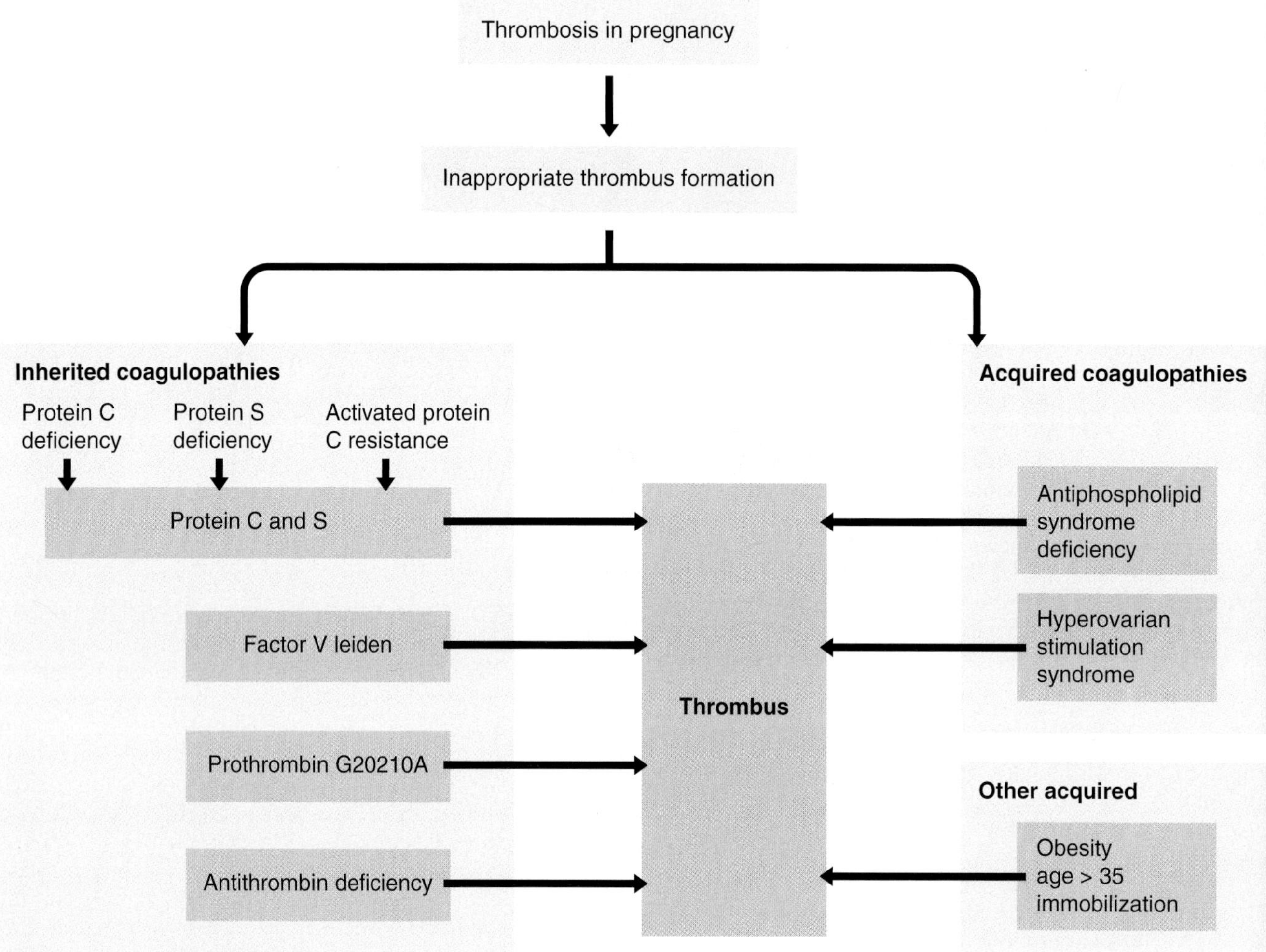

Figure 70–1. Inherited and acquired forms of thrombophilia in pregnancy.

TABLE 70–2. Risk of Venous Thromboembolism (VTE) in Pregnant Women with Inherited Forms of Thrombophilia

Thrombophilic Defect	Odds Ratio (95% CI) for VTE in Pregnancy*	Relative Risk (95% CI) for VTE in Pregnancy†	Relative Risk (95% CI) for VTE Postpartum‡
Type 1 (quantitative) antithrombin deficiency	282 (31–2532)	N/A	N/A
Type 2 (qualitative) antithrombin deficiency	28 (5.5–142)	N/A	N/A
Antithrombin deficiency (activity < 80%)	N/A	10.4 (2.2–62.5)	N/A
Factor V Leiden heterozygotes	4.5 (2.1–14.5)	6.9 (3.3–15.2)	8.7 (3.4–22.5)
Prothrombin G20210A	4.4 (1.2–16)	9.5 (2.1–66.7)	1.8 (0.6–5.4)
Any thrombophilia	N/A	N/A	9.0 (4.7–17.1)
Antithrombin, protein C, or protein S deficiency (not adjusted for parity)	N/A	N/A	13.1 (5.0–34.5)

Data from INATE.ORG (summary of published studies).

*Based on a retrospective study of 93,000 pregnancies for which odds ratios were calculated by screening women with VTE in pregnancy for thrombophilia and relating this to the known prevalence of these defects in the population.[63]

†Based on a study of 119 women with thromboembolism in pregnancy and 233 controls assessing for the presence of congenital thrombophilia. Relative risk was calculated after logistic regression to adjust for age, body mass index, use of oral contraceptives, protein C and S activity, factor V Leiden mutation, prothrombin gene G20210A mutation, MTHFR C677T mutation, and antithrombin activity.[64]

‡Based on a case-control study of 119 cases who had a first episode of objectively confirmed VTE in pregnancy or the puerperium and 232 controls. Relative risk was adjusted for parity, and there was no difference between relative risk in pregnancy or the puerperium.[65]

Abbreviations: CI, confidence interval; N/A, not available.

TABLE 70–3. Treatment Guidelines for Venous Thromboembolism (VTE) in Pregnancy

Thrombotic History/Thrombophilic Abnormality	Treat?	Therapy in Antepartum Period	Postpartum Therapy
VTE is diagnosed during pregnancy	Yes	Enoxaparin 1 mg/kg q12h (therapeutic anti-FXa) Dalteparin 100 IU/kg q12h (therapeutic anti-FXa) IV UFH as bolus, then UFH by CI × 5 days, then either dose-adjusted UFH or dose-adjusted LMWH Discontinue 24 hr before delivery	Therapeutically anticoagulate for 6 wk with LMWH, UFH, or warfarin
Patient has single previous VTE from temporary risk that is no longer present	No	None, surveillance only[69]	Therapeutically anticoagulate for 6 wk with LMWH, UFH, or warfarin
Patient has single previous VTE from prior pregnancy, estrogen therapy, or additional risks (e.g., obesity)	Yes	Enoxaparin 40 mg q24h Dalteparin 5000 U q24h	Therapeutically anticoagulate for 6 wks with LMWH, UFH, or warfarin
Patient has single previous idiopathic VTE or VTE associated with inherited form of thrombophilia and is not receiving anticoagulation	Yes	Enoxaparin 40 mg q24h Dalteparin 5000 U q24h *or* Intermediate-dose LMWH (Enoxaparin 40 mg q12h Dalteparin 5000 U q12h) *or* Minidose UFH (5000 U q12) *or* Moderate-dose UFH (adjusted to anti-Xa level of 0.1–0.3)	Therapeutically anticoagulate for 6 wk with LMWH, UFH, or warfarin
Patient has >2 episodes of VTE and/or is receiving long-term anticoagulation	Yes	LMWH given at therapeutic doses Enoxaparin 1 mg/kg q12h Dalteparin 100 IU/kg q12h UFH by CI or q12h (PTT is in therapeutic range)	Therapeutically anticoagulate for 6 wk with LMWH, UFH, or warfarin

Abbreviations: CI, continuous infusion; FXa, factor Xa; IV, intravenous; LMWH, low-molecular-weight heparin; PTT, prothrombin time; UFH, unfractionated heparin.
From Bates S, Greer IA, Hirsh J, Ginsberg J: Use of antithrombotic agents during pregnancy. Chest 126:627S–644S, 2004, with permission.

TABLE 70–4. Treatment Guidelines for Patients with Antiphospholipid Antibodies and Pregnancy Loss

Form of Thrombophilia	Obstetric History	Therapy
Positive APLA	Two or more pregnancy losses *or* One or more late pregnancy losses, preeclampsia, fetal growth retardation, or abruption	Aspirin plus mini- or moderate-dose UFH *or* Prophylactic LMWH
Congenital thrombophilia	Recurrent miscarriages Second- or third-trimester fetal loss Severe or recurrent preeclampsia or abruption	Prophylactic LMWH, minidose UFH Therapeutically anticoagulate for 6 wk postpartum with LMWH, UFH, or warfarin
APLA positive and a history of VTE		Adjusted-dose LMWH or UFH plus low-dose aspirin antepartum After delivery, resume oral anticoagulation
APLA positive, *no* prior history of VTE	These patients should still be considered at high risk for pregnancy loss	Surveillance *or* Prophylactic LMWH and/or low-dose aspirin (75–162 mg/day)

Abbreviations: APLA, antiphospholipid antibodies; LMWH, low-molecular-weight heparin; UFH, unfractionated heparin; VTE, venous thromboembolism.
From Bates S, Greer IA, Hirsh J, Ginsberg J: Use of antithrombotic agents during pregnancy. Chest 126:627S–644S, 2004, with permission.

therapeutic doses of a low-molecular-weight (LMW) heparin, adjusted for weight, can be administered once or (preferably) twice daily. LMW heparins have advantages over unfractionated heparin in pregnant women because

- LMW heparins cause less heparin-induced thrombocytopenia[70]
- LMW heparins have longer half-lives and a more predictable dose response[71]
- LMW heparins are less likely to cause osteoporosis after long-term use[72,73]

In the postpartum state, the patient with a DVT diagnosed during pregnancy should receive enoxaparin and dalteparin at the same therapeutic range or with warfarin, which should be monitored to ensure that the International Normalized Ratio is in the 2–3 range. If the patient is switched to warfarin, there should be a minimum 4-day overlap with LMW heparin or unfractionated heparin until the International Normalized Ratio becomes therapeutic. The use of an inferior vena cava filter is appropriate only if the patient has contraindications to therapeutic anticoagulation, including bleeding ulcers or malignant hypertension.

Thrombophilia and Pregnancy Complications and Loss

A recent meta-analysis has shown an association between fetal loss and factor V Leiden, activated protein C resistance, protein S deficiency, and the prothrombin gene mutation.[74] Consequently, women who have had recurrent pregnancy loss, a second-trimester miscarriage, or a history of intrauterine death or recurrent preeclampsia should be screened for thrombophilia.[68] Unfortunately, there has never been a study showing that anticoagulation will reduce the odds of fetal complications in this group of women. However, even without good randomized data, intervention with unfractionated heparin or LMW heparin is logical in view of the risks for venous thromboembolism in this population.

Antiphospholipid antibodies can occur in association with systemic lupus erythematosus, with certain drugs, or without explanation in an otherwise healthy individual.[75] Currently, there are compelling data that link the presence of antiphospholipid antibodies with increased risk of thrombosis[76] and pregnancy loss.[77–79] Women with recurrent pregnancy loss should be evaluated for the presence of antiphospholipid antibodies prior to the onset of a new pregnancy. Two randomized trials[80,81] have shown that the combination of aspirin and heparin can reduce the risk of fetal loss. Other trials have shown that LMW heparins are also effective.[82] One showed no difference between low-dose aspirin alone and low-dose aspirin with LMW heparin,[83] but a more recent study favored the use of enoxaparin.[84]

Recommendations for the treatment of women with antiphospholipid antibodies and a history of pregnancy loss are given in Table 70–4. Under any of the conditions described in Table 70–4, unfractionated heparin and LMW heparin are not secreted into breast milk and can be given to women who are nursing. There have been several reports that also confirm that warfarin does not cause an anticoagulant effect in the breast-fed infant.[85,86] Accordingly, both LMW heparins and warfarin appear safe in nursing mothers.

CURRENT CONTROVERSIES & FUTURE CONSIDERATIONS

Hematologic Complications of Pregnancy

- What is the role of prophylactic exchange transfusions in the final weeks of pregnancy in a woman with sickle cell disease?
- Is there a safe and reliable way to evaluate the platelet count of an infant being carried by a women with ITP?
- What is the optimal treatment approach for preventing DVT in high-risk women?
- What is the best means for preventing fetal loss in patients with antiphospholipid antibody syndrome?

Suggested Readings*

Bates S, Greer IA, Hirsh J, Ginsberg J: Use of antithrombotic agents during pregnancy. Chest 126:627S–644S, 2004.

Greer IA: Thrombosis in pregnancy: maternal and fetal issues. Lancet 353:1258–1265, 1999.

Mannucci PM: Treatment of von Willebrand's disease. N Engl J Med 351:683–694, 2004.

Serjeant GR, Loy SS, Crowther M, et al: Outcome of pregnancy in homozygous sickle cell disease. Obstet Gynecol 103:1278–1285, 2004.

Webert KE, Mittal R, Sigouin C, et al: A retrospective 11 year analysis of obstetric patients with idiopathic thrombocytopenic purpura. Blood 102:4306–4311, 2003.

****Full references for this chapter can be found on accompanying CD-ROM.***

CHAPTER 71

Hematology of the Newborn

Patrick G. Gallagher, MD

> **KEY POINTS**
>
> **Hematology of the Newborn**
>
> ***Diagnosis***
>
> - The differential diagnosis of neonatal anemia includes entities unique to the fetus and newborn. Investigation of the anemic neonate includes detailed pregnancy, labor, and delivery history and placental examination.
> - Many inherited coagulation deficiencies first present in the neonatal period, necessitating a high index of suspicion when evaluating the bleeding infant.
> - Acquired risk factors, such as perinatal asphyxia, sepsis, and central venous catheters, are more common than inherited thrombotic predisposition in sick neonates with thromboses.
> - Neonatal neutropenia may be transient, such as when associated with infection or maternal hypertension, or may be the initial manifestation of an inherited leukocyte abnormality.
>
> ***Treatment***
>
> - Red cell transfusions are required in many inherited erythrocyte disorders because of sluggish marrow response to erythropoietic stress in the first year of life.
> - Prenatal management and treatment of Rh hemolytic disease of the newborn has reduced neonatal morbidity from this disorder.
> - Vitamin K deficiency bleeding in the infant can be successfully prevented with either intramuscular or oral vitamin K.
> - Neonatal alloimmune thrombocytopenia has been treated with washed maternal platelets, human platelet antigen HPA-1a and -5b–negative platelets, intravenous immunoglobulin, and corticosteroids.
> - Severe neonatal hemorrhage caused by suspected coagulation factor deficiency is treated with fresh frozen plasma pending the diagnosis, after which the appropriate recombinant concentrate is administered.

HEMATOPOIESIS

Vertebrate hematopoiesis (see Chapter 1) begins in the yolk sac as early as 2 weeks' gestation, producing predominantly very large erythrocytes and some macrophages. By 6 weeks' gestation, the fetal liver becomes the primary site of hematopoiesis (Fig. 71–1). Erythroid cells, smaller than those produced in the yolk sac, begin to predominate and leukocytes and platelets are produced. By the end of the second trimester and after birth, the bone marrow is the predominant site of hematopoiesis and all cell lineages are formed.

Developmental Erythropoiesis

The switch from yolk sac erythropoiesis to the fetal liver is marked by production of smaller, mostly enucleate erythrocytes, the requirement for erythropoietin, and a gradual increase in hemoglobin concentration.[1–3] The average hemoglobin level at 10 weeks' gestation in 9 gm/dL, increasing to 11–12 gm/dL at 23 weeks, and 13–14 gm/dL by 30 weeks. By the beginning of the third trimester, hemoglobin stabilizes at levels slightly less than in the term neonate. During labor and delivery, hemoglobin may increase by 1–2 gm/dL from placental transfusion. After birth, decreased plasma volume leads to a peak in hemoglobin between 2 and 6 hours of life, stabilizing by 12 hours of age.

Fetal and neonatal erythrocytes differ from adult cells in many ways.[4] Composition of the two α-like globin chains and the two β-like globin chains that contribute to the hemoglobin tetramer varies during development (see Fig. 71–1).[5,6] During yolk sac erythropoiesis, the predominant hemoglobins are Gower 1 ($\zeta_2\varepsilon_2$), Gower 2 ($\alpha_2\varepsilon_2$), and Portland 1 ($\zeta_2\gamma_2$). The predominant hemoglobin during fetal life and at birth is fetal hemoglobin (Hb F; $\alpha_2\gamma_2$). Adult hemoglobin (Hb A; $\alpha_2\beta_2$) predominates by 6 months of age. Hemoglobin F–containing cells have a higher oxygen affinity and exhibit a rightward shift of the hemoglobin-oxygen dissociation curve (Fig. 71–2).[7] This benefits the fetus in utero, facilitating placental oxygen exchange from maternal blood to fetal erythrocytes. Hemoglobin F binds less strongly to 2,3-bisphosphoglycerate than Hb A, making it less susceptible to the reduction by 2,3-bisphosphoglycerate of hemoglobin's oxygen affinity.[7] Hemoglobin F denatures more

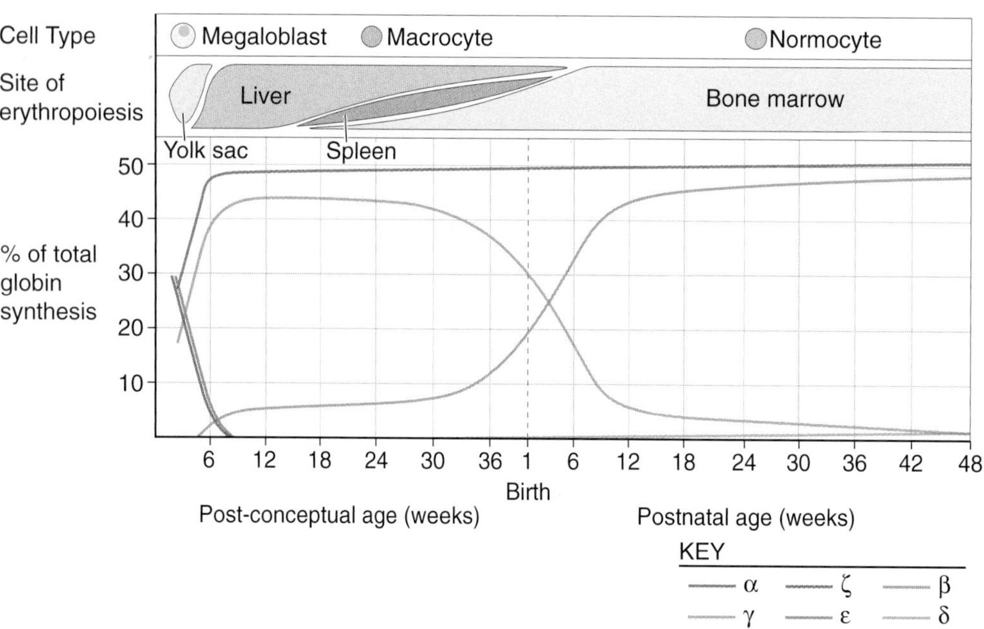

Figure 71–1. Schematic representation of the pattern of synthesis of the different globin chains at various stages of development, showing the sites of erythropoiesis, as well as the morphologic characteristics of the erythroid cells at different developmental stages. (Redrawn from Weatherall DJ, Clegg JB: The Thalassemia Syndromes [ed 3]. Oxford: Blackwell, 1981.)

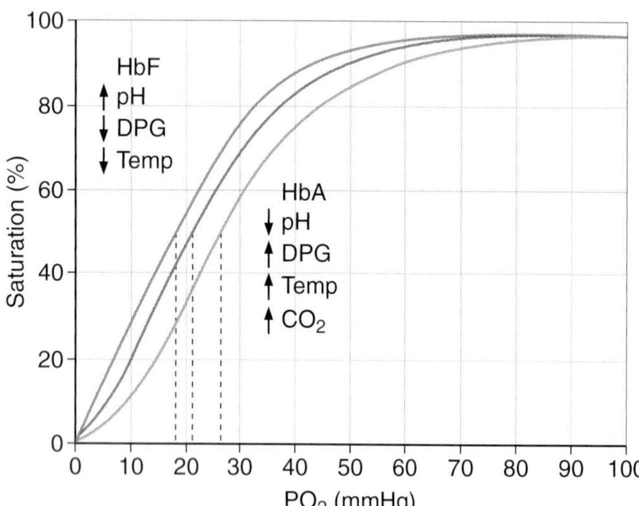

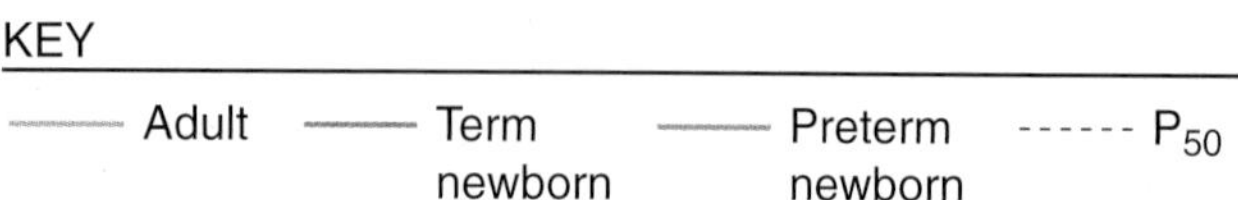

Figure 71–2. The oxygen dissociation curve of hemoglobin during different periods of development. The approximate P_{50} (i.e., oxygen tension at which the hemoglobin is 50% saturated) of adult blood is 27 mm Hg, that of a term newborn infant is 22 mm Hg, and that of a preterm newborn is 18 mm Hg. The heterotropic modifiers of hemoglobin function shown can increase (leftward shift) or decrease (rightward shift) hemoglobin oxygen affinity. (Redrawn from Bard H: Hemoglobin synthesis and metabolism during the neonatal period. *In* Christensen RD [ed]: Hematologic Problems of the Neonate. Philadelphia: WB Saunders, 2001, pp 365–388.)

readily than Hb A, damaging the membrane from within and shortening the red cell lifespan. Hemoglobin F is resistant to acid denaturation and is more soluble in strong phosphate buffers, the basis of the Kleihauer-Betke test.[8,9] Globin and heme biology are reviewed in Chapter 2.

Erythrocyte volume and size gradually decrease throughout gestation and after birth, resembling adult cells by 1 year of age.[10] The shape of fetal and neonatal erythrocytes is quite variable.[11] Acanthocytes, targets, and immature red blood cells are frequently found. Fetal and neonatal erythrocyte membranes exhibit increased deformability and increased monovalent cation permeability.[12] They have increased phospholipid and cholesterol per cell, resulting in a larger surface/volume ratio that renders them more osmotically resistant.[13,14] When performing osmotic fragility testing in a neonate to diagnose hereditary spherocytosis, a neonatal osmotic fragility curve should be used as control rather than an adult curve.[15] The expression of membrane surface receptors and antigens on neonatal erythrocytes varies from that in adult cells; for example, Lutheran, ABO, and I antigens are incompletely developed at birth, and others, such as Lewis, are absent. Neonatal erythrocytes have a more negative surface charge because of a higher sialic acid content, contributing to the decreased sedimentation rate observed in newborns.[16,17] Metabolic differences include increased production of glucose and ATP.[18] Several glycolytic enzymes have increased activity, and others, such as carbonic anhydrase and methemoglobin reductase, are reduced. Neonatal erythrocytes exhibit increased susceptibility to oxidant-induced damage, which may lead to glutathione instability, Heinz body formation, and methemoglobinemia.[19,20] These differences contribute to the decreased lifespan of the neonatal erythrocyte, 60–90 days in term infants and 35–50 days in preterm infants.[21]

TABLE 71–1. Normal Hematologic Values During the First Year of Life in Healthy Term Infants*

	Age (mo)						
n	0.5 (N = 232)	1 (N = 240)	2 (N = 241)	4 (N = 52)	6 (N = 52)	9 (N = 56)	12 (N = 56)
Hemoglobin (mean ± SE)	16.6 ± 0.11	13.9 ± 0.10	11.2 ± 0.06	12.2 ± 0.14	12.6 ± 0.10	12.7 ± 0.09	12.7 ± 0.09
−2 SD	13.4	10.7	9.4	10.3	11.1	11.4	11.3
Hematocrit (mean ± SE)	53 ± 0.4	44 ± 0.3	35 ± 0.2	38 ± 0.4	36 ± 0.3	36 ± 0.3	37 ± 0.3
−2 SD	41	33	28	32	31	32	33
RBC count (mean ± SE)	4.9 ± 0.03	4.3 ± 0.03	3.7 ± 0.02	4.3 ± 0.06	4.7 ± 0.05	4.7 ± 0.04	4.7 ± 0.04
−2 SD to +2 SD	3.9–5.9	3.3–5.3	3.1–4.3	3.5–5.1	3.9–5.5	4.0–5.3	4.1–5.3
MCH (mean ± SE)	33.6 ± 0.1	32.5 ± 0.1	30.4 ± 0.1	28.6 ± 0.2	26.8 ± 0.2	27.3 ± 0.2	26.8 ± 0.2
−2 SD	30	29	27	25	24	25	24
MCV (mean ± SE)	105.3 ± 0.6	101.3 ± 0.3	94.8 ± 0.3	86.7 ± 0.8	76.3 ± 0.6	77.7 ± 0.5	77.7 ± 0.5
−2 SD	88	91	84	76	68	70	71
MCHC (mean ± SE)	314 ± 1.1	318 ± 1.2	318 ± 1.1	327 ± 2.7	350 ± 1.7	349 ± 1.6	343 ± 1.5
−2 SD	281	281	283	288	327	324	321

*These values were obtained from a selected group of 256 healthy term infants followed at the Helsinki University Central Hospital who were receiving continuous iron supplementation and who had normal values for transferrin saturation and serum ferritin. Values at the ages of 0.5, 1, and 2 months were obtained from the entire group, and those at the later ages were obtained from the iron-supplemented infant group after exclusion of iron deficiency.
Abbreviations: MCH, mean corpuscular hemoglobin; MCHC, mean corpuscular hemoglobin concentration; MCV, mean corpuscular volume; RBC, red blood cell; SD, standard deviation; SE, standard error of the mean.
From Saarinen UM, Slimes MA: Developmental changes in red blood cell counts, and indices of infants after exclusion of iron deficiency by laboratory criteria and continuous iron supplementation. J Pediatr 92:412–416, 1978, with permission.

Erythropoiesis decreases at birth and hemoglobin falls, gradually reaching a nadir of approximately 11 gm/dL in healthy term infants at 8 weeks of life before erythropoiesis increases and the hemoglobin rises. This process is called physiologic anemia (Table 71–1).[22] These infants are asymptomatic, and this process appears to be a normal adaptation of the switch from intrauterine to extrauterine life.

NEONATAL ANEMIA

The differential diagnosis of nonphysiologic neonatal anemia is extensive and includes not only many of the causes of anemia seen in older patients, but also many unique to the fetus and newborn associated with pregnancy, labor, and delivery (Table 71–2).[15,23,24] Classifying anemia into categories of erythrocyte loss, including hemorrhage and hemolysis, and inadequate erythrocyte production provides a useful framework for the evaluation, diagnosis, and treatment of the anemic neonate. An algorithm for the evaluation of the anemic neonate is shown in Figure 71–3.

Erythrocyte Loss

Hemorrhage

In utero hemorrhage resulting in fetomaternal bleeding is typically via a transplacental route.[25] Associated conditions include placental abruption, placenta previa, vasa previa, and twin-twin transfusion (see Table 71–2). Spontaneous in utero hemorrhage (e.g., intracranial hemorrhage in a thrombocytopenic fetus) or hemorrhage after in utero trauma (e.g., after amniocentesis) is uncommon. Various placental lesions may lead to fetoplacental and fetomaternal hemorrhage.[26]

Fetal erythrocytes can be detected in the maternal circulation using various techniques,[27] but the most clinically useful test is the Kleihauer-Betke method.[9] In this method, Hb A is denatured and eluted from smears of adult red cells with an acid solution, leaving behind largely empty red cell membranes. Hemoglobin F resists denaturation and elution, so fetal cells stain darkly. Evaluation of the acid-treated maternal smear can give a quantitative estimate of the amount of fetal blood lost into the maternal circulation (2400 times the ratio of fetal/maternal cells observed = 1 mL of fetal blood). Kleihauer-Betke testing is invalid in conditions that elevate maternal Hb F levels (e.g., hemoglobinopathies) and in ABO incompatibility, in which removal of fetal cells from the maternal circulation by maternal anti-A or anti-B antibodies can lead to a false-negative result.

Most spontaneous fetomaternal hemorrhage occurs during labor and delivery.[25] Placental abruption, vasa previa, umbilical cord laceration, and nuchal cord may be associated with intrapartum hemorrhage.[28–31] Intrapartum trauma, particularly cranial trauma, can also lead to neonatal anemia. Trauma to the scalp, skull, or intracranial structures can result from traction applied manually, by forceps, or by vacuum-assist devices.[15] Adrenal, hepatic, and splenic hemorrhages have also been described.

Postpartum hemorrhage may be due to abnormalities of hemostasis, including congenital and acquired factor deficiencies and acquired and inherited platelet abnormalities (see later). Anemia frequently occurs in hospitalized neonates, particularly preterm infants, as a result of phlebotomy. Gastric and intestinal ulceration may also cause anemia.

TABLE 71–2. Differential Diagnosis of Neonatal Anemia

Excessive Erythrocyte Loss

Hemorrhage

Prenatal Hemorrhage

Transplacental hemorrhage
- Fetomaternal hemorrhage
- Abruptio placentae
- Placenta previa
- Vasa previa
- Velamentous insertion of umbilical cord
- Twin-twin transfusion

Traumatic fetal hemorrhage
- Maternal trauma
- Amniocentesis
- Cordocentesis

Placental lesions
- Chorioangioma
- Hematoma
- Hemangioma
- Choriocarcinoma

Other causes of fetal hemorrhage
- Intracranial bleeding
- Gastrointestinal bleeding

Intrapartum Hemorrhage

Placenta
- Abnormalities of placentation listed above
- Surgical laceration (e.g., incision of anterior placenta or cord at delivery)

Umbilical vessels
- Rupture of normal cord
- Rupture of abnormal cord
  - Aneurysm
  - Varix
  - Cyst
  - Funisitis with weakened vessels
  - Short cord
- Cord entrapment (e.g., by forceps)
- Tight nuchal cord
- Occult cord prolapse

Intrapartum neonatal trauma
- Cranial hemorrhage, including subgaleal, subarachnoid, and intraventricular hemorrhage
- Cephalohematoma
- Splenic rupture
- Adrenal hemorrhage
- Liver laceration
- Retroperitoneal hemorrhage

Postpartum Hemorrhage

Intracranial bleeding in the very-low-birth-weight infant

Gastric or intestinal ulceration

Hemorrhage from vascular malformation

Coagulation factor deficiency

Iatrogenic causes
- Phlebotomy
- Tracheal mucosal tear during endotracheal intubation
- Posterior pharyngeal tears during laryngoscopy or orogastric tube placement
- Vessel perforation during umbilical catheterization
- Intercostal vessel laceration during thoracostomy tube placement
- Gastric rupture from overdistention or orogastric tube placement
- Pulmonary hemorrhage during ventilation
- Bladder mucosal tear during catheterization
- Surgical wounds

Hemolysis

Extrinsic Hemolysis

Isoimmunization
- Rh sensitization
- ABO
- Others (e.g., Duffy, Kell, Lewis)
- Maternal autoimmune disorders
- Maternal medication use

Microangiopathic anemias
- Disseminated intravascular coagulation
  - Sepsis
  - Congenital infection—TORCHES, malaria

Vascular-related causes
- Kasabach-Merritt syndrome
- Renal artery
- Large vessel thrombosis
- Severe aortic coarctation
- Arteriovenous malformation

Oxidant exposure

Other
- Galactosemia
- Prolonged or recurrent acidosis

Intrinsic Hemolysis

Enzymopathies
- Hexose monophosphate shunt abnormality (e.g., G6PD deficiency)
- Embden-Meyerhof defect (glycolysis) (e.g., pyruvate kinase deficiency)
- Others

Red blood cell membrane defects
- Hereditary spherocytosis
- Hereditary elliptocytosis & related disorders
- Hereditary stomatocytosis

Hemoglobinopathies
- α-Thalassemia syndromes
- β-Globin cluster deletions
- Unstable hemoglobins

Erythrocyte Underproduction

Genetic Syndromes

Diamond-Blackfan syndrome

Congenital dyserythropoietic anemia

X-linked familial dyserythropoietic anemia

Fanconi's anemia

Schwachman syndrome

Pearson's syndrome

Aase syndrome

Bone Marrow Replacement Syndrome

Congenital leukemia

Transient myeloproliferative disorder—Down syndrome

Osteopetrosis

Infectious Suppression

Viral—parvovirus B19, cytomegalovirus, rubella, herpes simplex & Coxsackie B

Protozoal—toxoplasmosis

Overwhelming bacterial infection

Other

Maternal deficiencies (usually nutritional or genetic, e.g., transcobalamin II deficiency) leading to neonatal anemia—iron, folate, and B_{12}

Medications administered to mother or neonate

"Late" hyporegenerative anemia of Rh, Kell disease

From Gallagher PG: Neonatal anemia in blood. *In* Handin RI, Lux SE, Stossel TP (eds): Principles and Practice of Hematology (ed 2). Philadelphia: JB Lippincott, 2003, pp 1951–1976, with permission.)

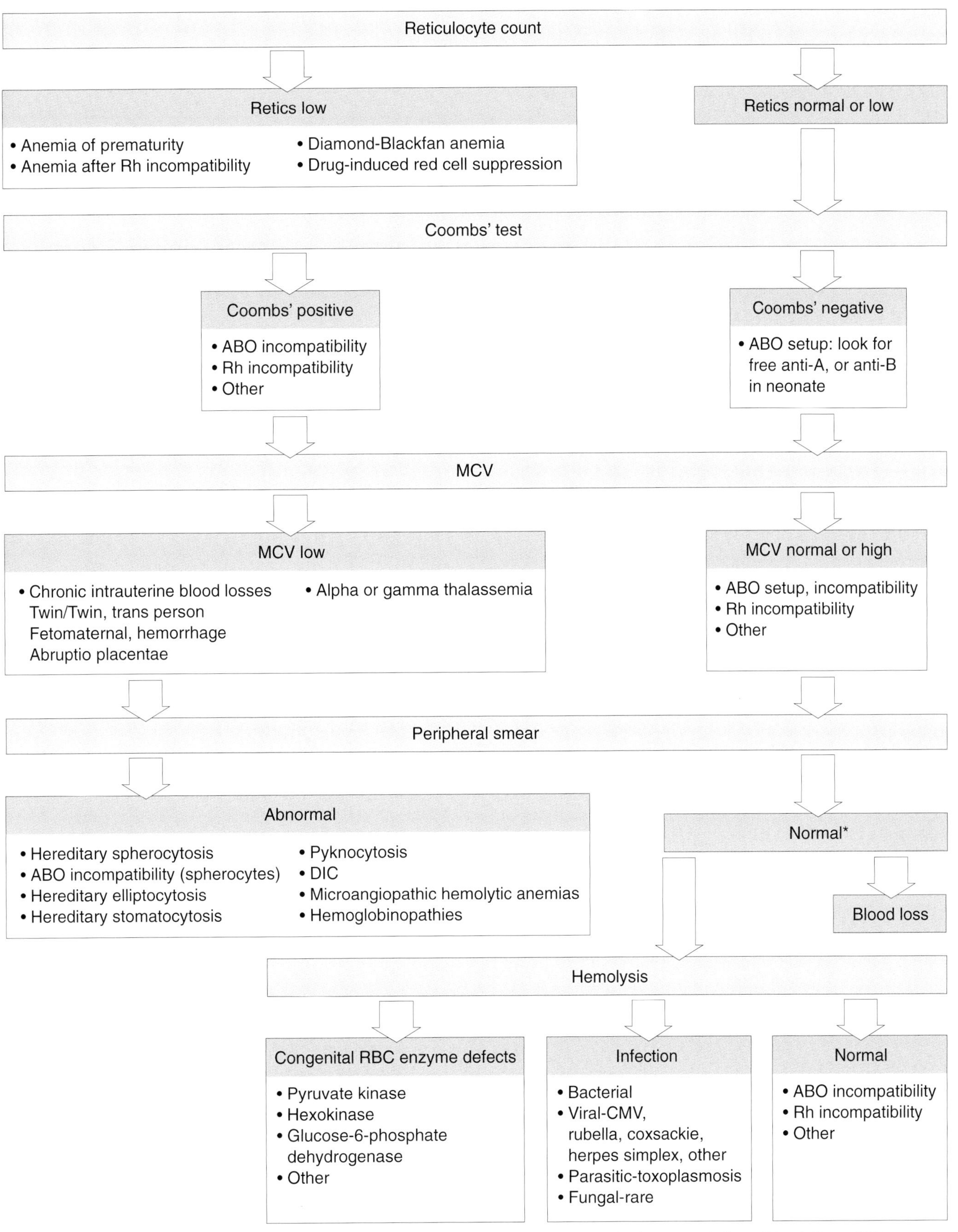

Figure 71–3. Evaluation of neonatal anemia. An *asterisk* indicates a smear with no predominant morphology. Abbreviations: CMV, cytomegalovirus; DIC, disseminated intravascular coagulation; MCV, mean corpuscular volume. (Redrawn from Nathan DA, Oski F: Hematology of Infancy and Childhood. Philadelphia: WB Saunders, 1993.)

Hemolysis

Hemolysis—extrinsic, intrinsic, or both—is common in the fetus and neonate (see Table 71–2). Many of the causes of hemolysis are reviewed in other chapters; aspects of several of these disorders specific to the neonate are discussed here.

Extrinsic Hemolysis

BLOOD GROUP INCOMPATIBILITY. Immune-mediated hemolytic anemia caused by blood group incompatibility is the most common cause of neonatal hemolytic anemia. Fetal erythrocytes cross the placenta, immunizing the mother with fetal antigens not present on her erythrocytes. Maternally derived alloantibody directed against the offending fetal erythrocyte antigen crosses the placenta and coats and destroys antigen-bearing fetal erythrocytes. ABO incompatibility is the most common picture observed in practice. In the past, Rh incompatibility was the most common and most severe cause of immune-mediated hemolytic anemia, also known as hemolytic disease of the newborn. Changes in clinical practice, including routine administration of anti-D immune globulin to at-risk women; advances in perinatal medicine, including amniocentesis, ultrasound with Doppler, and in utero transfusion therapy; and advances in neonatal critical care have considerably lessened the impact of this disease.

Rh Disease. For years, hemolytic disease of the fetus and newborn resulting from Rh disease was one of the major causes of perinatal death.[32,33] Delivery of erythrocytes that express Rh(D) antigen by blood transfusion or transplacental hemorrhage into the circulation of a mother who lacks the D antigen begins the Rh alloimmunization process. After the primary exposure to the Rh(D) antigen, repeat exposure leads to rapid production of anti-D immunoglobulin (Ig)G antibodies, which cross the placenta and attach to Rh antigen on fetal erythrocytes. Antibody-coated erythrocytes form rosettes on macrophages in the fetal reticuloendothelial system, particularly in the spleen, and they are removed from the circulation. This leads to anemia, accelerating fetal erythropoiesis in the liver, spleen, and bone marrow and, in severe cases, at extramedullary sites. Hemolysis also liberates heme, which is ultimately metabolized into bilirubin and cleared by the placenta.[34] Thus hyperbilirubinemia is a risk only for the delivered newborn.

The degree of Rh sensitization correlates with clinical severity and is directly related to the scale of the maternal antigen exposure and the number of exposures, worsening with each subsequent pregnancy.[33] Positive or rising antibody titers alert the obstetrician to the need for increased surveillance of an Rh-sensitized pregnancy.[35] In addition to serial antibody titers, the course of an Rh-sensitized pregnancy can be followed in a number of ways.[36,37] One of these is by frequent ultrasound to assess fetal well-being, detect hepatosplenomegaly or hydrops fetalis, and assess the degree of anemia by Doppler studies.[38] Moderate and severe anemia can reliably be detected noninvasively by Doppler ultrasound via an increase in the peak velocity of systolic blood flow in the middle cerebral artery.[39,40] Fetal blood sampling to assess the severity of fetal anemia has benefit in some situations. The development of hepatomegaly, splenomegaly, and abnormal middle cerebral artery flow velocities, or the appearance of hydrops fetalis, indicates a worsening prognosis and the need for in utero fetal transfusion or delivery if the infant is at or near term.

The clinical severity in Rh alloimmunization is variable.[41] In severe cases, there is in utero fetal demise or death shortly after birth from circulatory failure. Severely affected infants, many hydropic, require vigorous resuscitation with mechanical ventilation; treatment of heart failure; correction of anemia, hypoglycemia, and electrolyte abnormalities; diuresis; and phototherapy.[41–43] When the infant is stable, exchange transfusion may be needed for treatment of anemia, hyperbilirubinemia, or both. Less severely affected infants typically require phototherapy with or without red cell transfusion. Laboratory studies demonstrate a strongly positive direct antiglobulin test. Anemia is variable, and the blood smear shows polychromasia and nucleated red blood cells (erythroblastosis). Indirect hyperbilirubinemia is very common. Direct hyperbilirubinemia may develop in severe cases as a result of inspissated bile. Thrombocytopenia and neutropenia are common.[44]

The incidence, severity, and associated morbidity and mortality of Rh disease have all decreased. Even hydropic infants now experience less than 20% mortality. Anti-D prophylaxis, in utero transfusions, and optimal phototherapy have markedly decreased the need for exchange transfusion. Bilirubin encephalopathy resulting from Rh disease is now uncommon. Efforts to prevent Rh sensitization by the administration of Rh immune globulin in the appropriate clinical setting are ongoing.

ABO Incompatibility. Anti-A and anti-B antibodies are normally found in the serum of mothers who are group A, B, and O. Unlike Rh incompatibility, these antibodies develop in response to a variety of antigens, such as bacteria, and do not require the passage of blood into the maternal circulation. In type A and B mothers, these "natural" antibodies are of the IgM class that does not cross the placenta. In type O mothers, they are of the IgG class; late in pregnancy or at delivery, these preformed maternal anti-A or anti-B IgG antibodies are transferred across the placenta. Hemolysis of fetal or neonatal cells occurs rapidly after splenic recognition and removal. Because immature erythrocytes incompletely express A and B antigen sites, the cells may not be completely destroyed, creating a microspherocyte. Because the antibodies are preformed, ABO incompatibility can affect the first pregnancy.

Infants with ABO incompatibility typically present with neonatal hyperbilirubinemia.[45] There is mild anemia, reticulocytosis, and microspherocytosis. The diagnosis is confirmed in mother-infant dyads with the appropriate blood groups and a positive direct antiglobulin test. Because the number of antigen-antibody complexes on neonatal erythrocytes is often decreased after splenic removal, the antiglobulin test may only be weakly positive or even negative.[46] When desired, anti-A or anti-B antibodies can usually be eluted from the infant's erythrocytes. Most cases require only treatment with

TABLE 71–3. Relative Strength of Antigens on Cord Cells and Antigens Implicated in Hemolytic Disease of the Newborn (HDN)

Antigen Strength	Blood Group System or Antigen	Caused HDN
I. Well developed at birth	MNSsU	Yes*
	Rh	Yes
	Kell	Yes
	Duffy	Yes
	Kidd	Yes
	Diego	Yes
	Dombrock	Yes (mild)
	Scianna	
	Gerbich	Yes (mild)
	En[a]	
	Yt[b]	
II. Present at birth, weaker than adult	ABH	Yes
	P	No[†]
	Lutheran	Yes
III. Very weak or absent at birth	Yt[a]	
	Vel	
	Lewis	
	I	No
	Sd[a]	No

*Anti-M is rarely a cause of HDN.
[†]Anti Tj[a] (anti-PP1P[k]) has caused HDN.
From Kline W: Chemistry of blood group antigens and antibodies in hemolytic disease of the newborn. *In* Bell C (ed): A Seminar on Perinatal Blood Banking. Washington, DC: American Association of Blood Banks, 1978, with permission.)

phototherapy, although exchange transfusion to treat severe hyperbilirubinemia or anemia is sometimes necessary.

Other Blood Group Incompatibilities. Other blood group incompatibilities have been reported to cause hemolytic disease of the newborn (Table 71–3). Kell antigen alloimmunization may lead to significant fetal and neonatal anemia.[47,48] Unlike Rh antigen, Kell antigen is expressed on early erythroid progenitor cells and leads to anemia from both hemolysis and suppression of fetal erythropoiesis.[49]

Infants with Rh or Kell alloimmunization may develop a "late" anemia at 1–3 months of age characterized by anemia with reticulocytopenia resulting from decreased erythrocyte production and/or continued destruction of reticulocytes by maternal antibody.[50–52] This late anemia is found in both infants who have received intrauterine transfusion and those who have not. Transfusion is occasionally required. Erythropoietin therapy has been disappointing.[52,53]

ANGIOPATHIC ANEMIAS. Disseminated intravascular coagulation (DIC) is a common cause of anemia in neonates, most frequently in association with infection, including sepsis, meningitis, and necrotizing enterocolitis.[54–56] Kasabach-Merritt syndrome is a local consumptive coagulopathy with hypofibrinogenemia, thrombocytopenia, and a microangiopathic anemia in association with vascular malformations that typically presents in the neonatal period.[57–59] The anemia and coagulopathy, which may be severe, improve with regression or removal of the tumor. Other causes of hemolysis, including oxidant hemolysis (an acute hemolytic event presumably related to the oxidant sensitivity of neonatal erythrocytes that is not always associated with a known enzymopathy or with congenital Heinz body anemia), are listed in Table 71–2.

Intrinsic Hemolysis

Inherited hemolytic disorders of the erythrocyte presenting in the fetus and newborn include abnormalities of membrane structure and function, metabolism, and hemoglobin. Hyperbilirubinemia requiring phototherapy in the first few days of life is common in these disorders, particularly membrane abnormalities and glucose-6-phosphate dehydrogenase (G6PD) deficiency. Coinheritance of the Gilbert syndrome *UDPGT1* gene polymorphism intensifies neonatal jaundice in neonates with inherited erythrocyte abnormalities and may lead to rapid increases in bilirubin levels, increasing the risk of kernicterus.[60,61]

ERYTHROCYTE MEMBRANE DISORDERS. Disorders of the erythrocyte membrane (see Chapter 22) frequently are manifest in the neonate, particularly hereditary spherocytosis and, less commonly, hereditary elliptocytosis and hereditary pyropoikilocytosis.[18] Hereditary spherocytosis may present with significant jaundice and symptomatic anemia in the first few days of life.[62,63] Phototherapy and transfusion are frequently required. Rarely, exchange transfusion is needed. Spherocytes are present in variable numbers, and are absent in up to a third of neonates with hereditary spherocytosis. In severe cases, morphology is bizarre with anisocytosis, poikilocytosis, and numerous dense, small spherocytes. The incubated osmotic fragility test has proven to be a reliable diagnostic test in the newborn period.[64] A positive osmotic fragility test is specific not for hereditary spherocytosis, but for any disorder with spherocytosis. Sometimes, spherocytosis resulting from alloimmunization may not be differentiated from hereditary spherocytosis even after detailed history, physical examination, and laboratory testing. Observation over the first few months to determine whether spherocytosis persists or resolves is required to clarify the diagnosis.

Neonates with hereditary spherocytosis may experience more significant hemolytic anemia than adults. The etiology of this observation appears to be multifactorial. The inability of Hb F to bind 2,3-bisphosphoglycerate leads to increased levels in the neonatal erythrocyte, destabilizing the membrane junctional complex and worsening hemolysis.[65] A shorter lifespan of the neonatal erythrocyte, and the sluggish response of the marrow to erythropoietic stress in the first year of life, also contribute to the anemia.[66]

Rarely, severe forms of hereditary elliptocytosis present in the neonatal period with hemolytic anemia and jaundice, requiring phototherapy and blood transfusion.[67–69] Typically, the hemolysis wanes by 1–2 years of age and the patient goes on to develop typical hereditary elliptocytosis. Hereditary pyropoikilocytosis is an uncommon variant of hereditary elliptocytosis notable for severe hemolysis with erythrocyte morphology reminiscent of that seen in thermal burns.[70,71] It occurs predominantly in patients of African descent. The blood smear shows elliptocytes, poikilocytes with fragmentation, pyknocytes, and microspherocytosis. The mean corpuscular volume is low (50–65 fL) and the osmotic fragility test is abnormal. Infants with hereditary pyropoikilocytosis tend to experience severe hemolysis and anemia that gradually improves, evolving toward typical hereditary elliptocytosis during the first years of life.[71]

ENZYMOPATHIES. Congenital nonspherocytic hemolytic anemia includes disorders not due to immune-mediated disturbances, defects of hemoglobin or the erythrocyte membrane, or other disorders. It is a heterogeneous group of disorders caused by a variety of metabolic abnormalities of the red blood cell, including enzymopathies of glucose, glutathione, and nucleotide metabolism. Clinical, biochemical, and genetic heterogeneity are common within individual enzymopathies. Hemolytic anemia can develop as a result of enzyme or antioxidant deficiency or as a result of impaired enzyme function.

Disorders of the hexose monophosphate shunt or glutathione metabolic pathways impair the ability of the erythrocyte to adequately respond to oxidant stress. In the normal red cell, reduced glutathione detoxifies intracellular oxidants. G6PD deficiency is the major disorder in this group (see Chapter 23). In G6PD deficiency, inadequate levels of reduced glutathione result from the inability to generate NADPH, releasing oxidants to damage the erythrocyte. Oxidation of the sulfhydryl groups of hemoglobin produces methemoglobin and intracellular precipitates of hemoglobin called Heinz bodies. Three clinical syndromes have been associated with G6PD deficiency—neonatal jaundice, acute hemolytic anemia after an oxidative stress, and congenital nonspherocytic hemolytic anemia—and all three have been observed in the neonatal period.[72]

In most cases of neonatal jaundice associated with G6PD deficiency, anemia is mild. However, the degree of hyperbilirubinemia is variable and it may be severe, resulting in kernicterus or even death. Typically, jaundice appears between the second and third day of life. Spikes in bilirubin levels may occur. In most cases, phototherapy is adequate therapy, but occasionally exchange transfusions are necessary.[73,74] The etiology of neonatal jaundice in G6PD deficiency is unknown, but decreased hepatic excretion of bilirubin and hemolysis have both been implicated. Neonatal jaundice is increased in G6PD-deficient infants with Gilbert syndrome.[61] Hemolysis after transfusion with G6PD-deficient erythrocytes has been reported in neonates, leading to the recommendation that, in endemic areas of G6PD deficiency, blood donors be screened for G6PD deficiency prior to neonatal transfusion.[75,76]

Defects of the Embden-Meyerhof pathway may present in the neonatal period (see Table 71–2). Pyruvate kinase deficiency, the most common abnormality of this pathway, usually presents in the neonatal period or early childhood with anemia and jaundice (see Chapter 23).[18] Severe cases have presented with severe anemia in utero or in the first days of life. Hyperbilirubinemia is common, and phototherapy or exchange transfusion may be required.[77,78]

HEMOGLOBIN DISORDERS. The differences in globin chain synthesis during development (see earlier) create the variation in the fetal and neonatal manifestations of α- and β-thalassemia. α-Globin is the main α-like globin in the fetus by 9 weeks' gestation (see Fig. 71–1), with only low levels of the major embryonic α-like hemoglobin, Hb Portland, present. Thus abnormalities of α-globin may lead to severe anemia in utero. In contrast, the switch from fetal to adult β-like globin chains (γ- to β-globin) is not complete until several months of life. Abnormalities of β-globin are typically ameliorated in early infancy by the sustained production of Hb F (see Chapter 21).

α-Globin Defects. The severity of the α-thalassemia syndromes is related to the numbers of functional α-globin genes present.[79] Deletion of a single α-globin gene results in an asymptomatic carrier state. Deletion of two α-globin genes results in α-thalassemia trait with marked microcytosis, hypochromia, and mild anemia. Deletion of three α-globin genes results in Hb H disease. Infants with Hb H disease exhibit a hypochromic, hemolytic anemia with microcytosis and erythrocyte fragmentation.[79,80] Hemoglobin electrophoresis demonstrates Hb H β_4 and Hb Barts. Hydrops fetalis has been described in cases of nondeletional Hb H disease.[81] When microcytosis with or without anemia is detected in a neonate, the differential diagnosis includes Hb H disease, acute-on-chronic fetomaternal hemorrhage, and α-thalassemia trait. Hemoglobin electrophoresis, Kleihauer-Betke testing, family history, and ethnic origin clarify the diagnosis.

Homozygous α-thalassemia is due to deletion of all four α-globin genes. This usually leads to death of the fetus in utero from severe hemolytic anemia, congestive heart failure, and hydrops fetalis.[79] The major hemoglobin present is a tetramer of unpaired non-α chains, γ_4 or Hb Barts. Survival of the homozygous fetus to late gestation or the newborn period depends on the presence and amount of Hb Portland. In the rare case in which the child is born alive, death from cardiopulmonary collapse usually occurs shortly after birth. Improvements in prenatal diagnosis, interventional obstetric practice, and neonatal critical care are beginning to produce some survivors of homozygous α-thalassemia.[80] In over a dozen cases, expectant pregnancy management with in utero transfusion therapy, followed by postnatal transfusion therapy with iron chelation, has led to survival.[82] Concerns about congenital malformations and potential long-term effects of prolonged intrauterine hypoxia exist.

β-Globin Defects. Structural variants of β-globin, including β-thalassemia and sickle cell disease, typically do not present in the neonatal period. Large deletions of the β-globin gene cluster lead to the phenotype of γδβ-thalassemia,[83] which may present as a hypochromic, hemolytic neonatal anemia with prominent normoblastosis. Over time, the anemia improves with peripheral blood smear morphology similar to β-thalassemia trait. Unstable hemoglobins, that is, those that exhibit higher susceptibility to oxidation or reduced solubility compared to normal (see Chapter 21), may present with neonatal jaundice and hemolytic anemia.[84,85]

Decreased Erythrocyte Production

Decreased erythrocyte production is an uncommon cause of neonatal anemia. The etiologies can be classified as genetic syndromes, bone marrow replacement syndromes, infectious suppression, or other rare causes (see Table 71–2).[15] The most common cause of hypoplastic anemia in the fetus and newborn is the result of infection with parvovirus B19 (see Chapter 76).[86] Maternal parvovirus infection during pregnancy can infect the fetus, leading to severe anemia, nonimmune hydrops fetalis, and death.[87] If fetal demise does not occur, anemia and hydrops fetalis may resolve. In utero blood transfusion has been successfully employed to treat anemic, infected fetuses. Detection of a hypoplastic or aplastic anemia in an anemic newborn should raise the suspicion of parvovirus infection, and appropriate diagnostic testing should be performed.

Nutritional causes of neonatal anemia are uncommon.[88] Iron deficiency anemia is typically found in infants who have experienced prenatal blood loss with concomitant loss of hemoglobin iron stores. Vitamin B_{12} or folate deficiencies are rare. Hypoplastic anemia has been observed in neonates born to mothers taking various medications.[89,90]

Anemia of Prematurity

The physiologic anemia exhibited by term infants is also seen in preterm infants. However, although mean cord hemoglobin levels do not vary significantly between preterm and term infants, the decline in hemoglobin concentration occurs earlier in preterm infants, at approximately 4–8 weeks of age, and the concentration drops to significantly lower levels, with the nadir varying inversely with gestational age.[91–93] Called the anemia of prematurity, this nonphysiologic state is characterized by normocytic, normochromic anemia, reticulocytopenia, bone marrow hypoplasia, and erythropoietin levels inappropriately low for the degree of anemia. The degree of anemia varies with the degree of prematurity, nutritional status and intake, chronologic age, and type and severity of underlying illness. The pathogenesis of the anemia of prematurity is multifactorial, including a blunted response to erythropoietin, less efficient oxygen sensing by the fetal liver compared to the kidney, shorter erythrocyte lifespan, and both greater clearance and shorter half-life of erythropoietin in preterm infants. Phlebotomy and transfusion of blood with Hb A, which further blunt the hypoxic stimulus for erythropoietin production, worsen the anemia. Whether infants become symptomatic from anemia of prematurity, if, when, and at what levels of hemoglobin transfusion is indicated, and if erythropoietin therapy should be prescribed, are controversial issues in the anemia of prematurity.[93–98]

POLYCYTHEMIA

Intrauterine life is relatively hypoxic, and the fetus compensates by increasing red cell mass to levels higher than later in life. Intrauterine red cell mass can be increased by a primary abnormality of the erythropoietin/hypoxia-sensing mechanism or other conditions that increase hypoxia, or by conditions that reduce plasma volume.

Neonatal polycythemia is typically defined by a peripheral venous hematocrit of greater than 65%.[99] The age of the neonate, the site and method of collection, and the method of analysis influence the hematocrit. Neonatal polycythemia can be caused by increased red cell mass, decreased plasma volume, or both. Primary causes include conditions associated with intrauterine hypoxia, such as uteroplacental insufficiency, and maternal conditions such as severe heart disease, diabetes, smoking, and preeclampsia.[100] Conditions associated with polycythemia include the trisomies (13, 18, and 21), Beckwith-Wiedemann syndrome, thyrotoxicosis, and congenital adrenal hyperplasia. Primary causes of polycythemia include abnormalities of the erythropoietin receptor. Secondary causes of polycythemia include delayed cord clamping at delivery, twin-twin transfusion, and maternal-fetal transfusion.

The clinical findings associated with neonatal polycythemia correlate better with blood viscosity than hematocrit, thus the term *neonatal polycythemia-hyperviscosity syndrome*.[99,101] In affected infants, clinical findings include plethora, alterations in tone and state, irritability, and feeding difficulties. Complications include congestive heart failure, seizures, thrombosis (including renal vein thrombosis, peripheral gangrene, or sinus thrombosis), necrotizing enterocolitis, and increased risk of long-term neurologic abnormalities.[102,103] Hypoglycemia, hypocalcemia, and thrombocytopenia may be detected. Partial (reduction) exchange transfusion, replacing whole blood with crystalloid, improves many of the immediate complications.[104,105]

DEVELOPMENTAL HEMOSTASIS

The balance between hemorrhage and thrombosis is a dynamic process in the neonate. Neonates have diminished capacity to generate thrombin, regulate clot formation, and lyse formed clot. This balance is easily disrupted because the neonate has a low reserve capacity, rapidly leading to dramatic clinical manifestations of ineffective hemostasis.[106]

Coagulation and fibrinolytic factors do not cross the placenta. Most are synthesized in the fetal liver, some as early as 10 weeks' gestation. Levels and activity of many coagulant proteins, including the vitamin K–dependent factors, factors XI and XII, prekallikrein, high-molecular-weight kininogen, antithrombin III, and heparin cofactor II, are low at birth and reach adult levels over the period of several weeks to months.[107] Others, including factors V, VIII, and XIII, are close to adult levels at birth. In the fibrinolytic system, plasminogen and α_2-antiplasmin are low at birth and levels of tissue-type plasminogen activator and plasminogen activator inhibitor are double the normal adult levels.[108] α_2-Macroglobulin, an inhibitor of various proteolytic enzymes, including thrombin and plasmin, is more than double the adult value. Thus diagnosis of inherited abnormalities of hemostasis may be difficult in the neonatal period.[109]

The Bleeding Neonate

Hemorrhage in the neonatal period manifests as oozing from the umbilical cord, bleeding from sites of trauma (e.g., venipuncture site or after circumcision), diffuse mucous membrane hemorrhage, hematuria, and intracranial or pulmonary hemorrhage. Although intracranial hemorrhage is much more common in preterm infants, it is not rare in term infants with hemostatic abnormalities, particularly after traumatic delivery. Bleeding into muscles or joints, common in children with hemophilia, is rare in the neonatal period.[110]

Evaluation of the bleeding neonate should include a thorough family history, including the type, severity, onset, frequency, and inheritance (e.g., autosomal or X-linked).[110,111] The maternal history, including review of the pregnancy, labor, and delivery, should be obtained. An assessment of whether the baby is well or sick, and whether conditions associated with bleeding are present, should be performed. Petechiae, ecchymoses, mucous membrane bleeding, abdominal mass, bruits, hemangiomas, and evidence of birth trauma should be sought on physical examination. Bleeding in an otherwise healthy, term neonate is typically due to deficiency of coagulation factors, vitamin K deficiency, or alloimmune thrombocytopenia (see later). In a bleeding sick neonate, sepsis, DIC, or liver disease should also be considered. An approach to the bleeding neonate is shown in Figure 71–4.

Initial diagnostic testing should include complete blood count, platelet count, prothrombin time, activated partial thromboplastin time (aPTT), fibrinogen, and thrombin time. A decreased platelet count in the well neonate should prompt a review of etiologies of thrombocytopenia (see below). A prolonged aPTT alone that corrects with 1 : 1 mixing with normal plasma suggests hemophilia A or B. A prolonged prothrombin time suggests hereditary factor VII deficiency. Prolonged prothrombin time (mild) and aPTT (moderate-severe) that do not correct with 1 : 1 mixing of normal plasma suggest heparin effect. This is common in neonates, because many have indwelling umbilical vascular catheters with heparin-containing infusate. Like the reptilase time, this does not differentiate catheter contamination from heparin overdose. Prolonged prothrombin time, aPTT, and thrombin time that correct with 1 : 1 mixing with normal plasma suggest afibrinogenemia or early liver disease. Abnormalities of all the screening tests suggest DIC or severe liver disease. Finally, when all the screening tests are normal in a bleeding neonate, the differential diagnosis includes deficiency of factor XIII, plasminogen activator inhibitor-1, or α_2-antiplasmin; von Willebrand disease; or a qualitative platelet defect.

Inherited Abnormalities of Hemostasis

As noted previously, values for coagulation factor levels are developmental/gestational age related and are lower in the fetus and newborn than the older child and adult. A critically ill newborn with bleeding caused by sepsis or liver disease may also have an underlying congenital factor deficiency. Diagnosis and management of these newborns is extremely difficult. Hemophilia A and B and von Willebrand disease comprise 80–85% of congenital, non–platelet-associated bleeding disorders. Qualitative or quantitative defects in fibrinogen, deficiency of prothrombin and factors V, VII, X, and XIII, and combined factors V and VIII comprise the remaining 15–20% (Table 71–4).[112] The reader is referred to Chapters 63, 64, 66, and 72 for discussion of these disorders.

Hemophilia

Hemophilia A (factor VIII deficiency, 80–85% of cases) and hemophilia B (factor IX deficiency, 15–20% of cases) are X-linked disorders that affect all racial groups.[113] Approximately one third to one half of hemophilia cases are diagnosed in the neonatal period after screening a known carrier mother or during evaluation of neonatal hemorrhage. In hemophilic neonates, hemorrhage occurs after circumcision (30%), intracranially (28%), at puncture sites (18%), in the scalp (14%), as umbilical hemorrhage (6%), and at other sites. Bleeding at multiple sites is common. Recognition that hemorrhage at these sites may be due to hemophilia is important in obtaining early diagnosis and providing prompt, effective therapy. Critically important to recognize is intracranial hemorrhage, which occurs in approximately 1–4% of neonates with hemophilia.[114–116] Extracranial bleeding in the scalp and subgaleal space may also occur.

Bleeding in an otherwise healthy term male neonate with a normal platelet count suggests the diagnosis of hemophilia. Family history is negative in 30% of infants, representing new mutations. Laboratory evaluation typically yields a prolonged aPTT. However, in very mild cases, the aPTT may be normal and the affected neonate still at risk of bleeding. The diagnosis of hemophilia A in the newborn period is usually straightforward because levels of factor VIII reach adult levels by midgestation. However, only severe cases of hemophilia B are diagnosed in the neonatal period because normal term males have factor IX activity as low as 15%. Retesting at 6–12 months of age is recommended when hemophilia B is suspected.

Prenatal diagnosis is possible via chorionic villus sampling, amniocentesis, or fetal blood sampling.[116] Early ultrasound to determine fetal gender can guide the diagnostic evaluation. When desired, preimplantation diagnosis can be performed. There is controversy over the safest mode of delivery of newborns of known hemophilia carriers or even newborns with prenatally diagnosed hemophilia. Cesarean section does not appear to eliminate the risk of neonatal hemorrhage. Avoidance of scalp electrodes and cranial manipulation with vacuum or forceps assist devices seems prudent. Male infants of hemophilia carriers should have factor assays performed on a cord blood sample obtained at delivery from a vein on the fetal side of the placenta or via venipuncture shortly after birth.[116]

Treatment is indicated in cases of severe hemorrhage. Fresh frozen plasma is administered pending the diagnosis. The appropriate recombinant plasma concentrate is provided when the diagnosis is known. Activated recombinant factor VIIa has been used as a low-volume

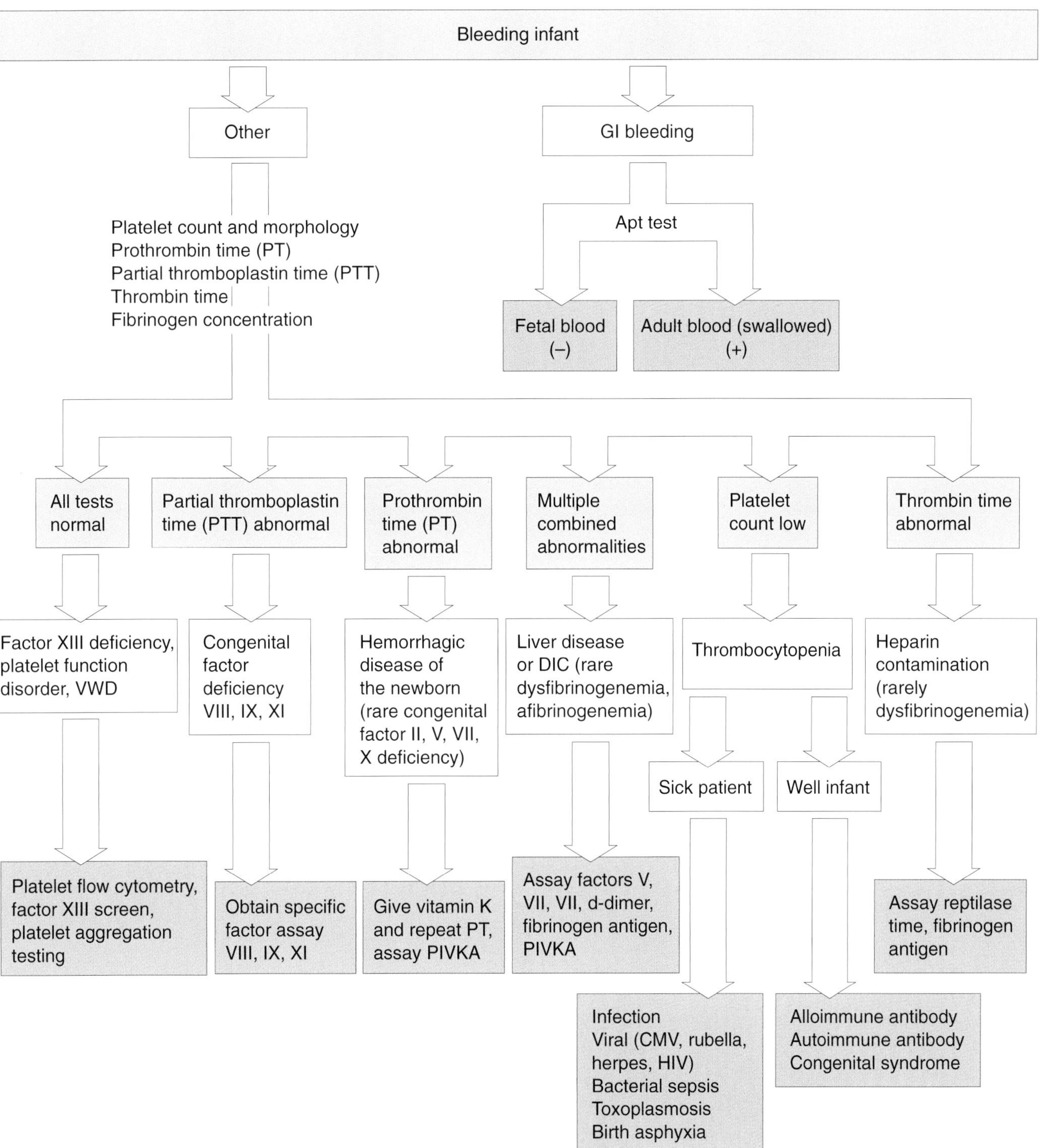

Figure 71–4. Evaluation of a bleeding newborn. (Redrawn from Hagstrom JN: Pathophysiology of bleeding disorders in the newborn. *In* Polin RA, Fox WW, Abman SH [eds]: Fetal and Neonatal Physiology [ed 3]. Philadelphia: WB Saunders, 2004, pp 1447–1460.)

therapeutic agent in the bleeding neonate with hemophilia.[117] Factor infusion should be provided prior to surgery or other invasive procedures.[118]

Von Willebrand Disease

Hemorrhage is uncommon in the fetus or newborn with von Willebrand disease.[119] However, cases of hemorrhage, including intracranial hemorrhage, have been reported.[120,121]

Acquired Abnormalities of Hemostasis

Acquired neonatal bleeding disorders include vitamin K deficiency, DIC, and bleeding during extracorporeal

TABLE 71–4. Congenital Coagulation Factor Deficiencies in the Newborn

	F VIII/IX	vWD	F XIII	F XI	F X	F VII	F V	F II	Fibrinogen
Incidence	1 in 5000 males (VIII), 1 in 30,000 males (IX)	1–2% of population	1 in 1,000,000	1 in 1,000,000	1 in 1,000,000	1 in 500,000	1 in 1,000,000	1 in 2,000,000	1 in 1,000,000
Inheritance	Sex-linked recessive	Autosomal recessive	Autosomal recessive	Autosomal recessive	Autosomal recessive	Autosomal recessive	Autosomal recessive	Autosomal recessive	Autosomal recessive
Bleeding Sites									
Total number reported	344	7	41	1	6	16	7	1	8
Intracranial	100	2	7		4	15	7 (2 prenatal)		1
Subgaleal/CepH	50	2	6		1	1			
Circumcision	101		1	1		1			2
Umbilical bleeding	23							1	
Puncture/hematoma	65	2	17		1	3	1		1
Other bleeds	23							1	
Tests									
PT	Normal	Normal	Normal	Normal	Prolonged	Prolonged	Prolonged	Prolonged	Prolonged
aPTT	Prolonged	Variable	Normal	Prolonged	Prolonged	Prolonged	Prolonged	Prolonged	Prolonged
Newborn factor level (day 0)	VIII 0.50–1.78 U/mL, IX 0.15–0.91 U/mL	0.50–287 U/mL	0.27–1.31 U/mL	0.10–0.66 U/mL	0.12–0.68 U/mL	0.5–1.78 U/mL	0.34–1.08 U/mL	0.26–0.70 U/mL	1.67–3.99 gm/L
Treatment									
Recombinant concentrate	Recombinant F VIII & F IX					Recombinant F VIIa			
Plasma-derived concentrate available	Yes	Yes	Yes			Recombinant F VIIa, PCC	Europe	PCC	Available in
Fresh frozen plasma	Yes		3 mL/kg every 4–6 wk (prophylaxis)	15 mL/kg, then 5 mL/kg every 24 hr	10–15 mL/kg, then 5–10 mL/kg every 24 hr	10 mL/kg every 6–12 hr Surgery 15–20 mL/kg then 3–6 mL/kg every 12 hr	15–20 mL/kg, then 5 mL/kg every 12–24 hr	15–20 mL/kg, then 3 mL/kg every 12–24 hr	
Cryoprecipitate (1 bag = 80 units F VIII and vWF, 200–300 mg fibrinogen)	1 bag/5 kg (hemophilia A only)	1 bag/5 kg	1 bag/10–20 kg every 3–4 wk (prophylaxis)						1 bag/5 kg, then 1 bag/15 kg daily

Abbreviations: aPTT, activated partial thromboplastin time; CepH, cephalohematoma; F, factor; PCC, prothrombin complex concentrates; PT, prothrombin time; vWD, von Willebrand disease; vWF, von Willebrand factor.

From Kulkarni R: Bleeding in the newborn. Pediatr Ann 30:548–568, 2001, with permission.

membrane oxygenation, after intraventricular hemorrhage of prematurity, and in patients with liver disease.[54–56]

Vitamin K Deficiency

Vitamin K is a necessary cofactor for the γ-carboxylation of the vitamin K–dependent coagulation factors (factor II, VII, IX, and X), which are critical for factor function. Vitamin K transmission across the placenta is poor, and newborn levels are significantly lower than maternal levels.[122,123] Vitamin K synthesized in the neonatal liver has a half-life of approximately 24 hours and, without supplementation, levels fall in the first few days of life. Formula-fed infants receive vitamin K both directly from the milk and from synthesis by intestinal flora. Breast-fed infants receive minimal amounts of vitamin K in breast milk and develop intestinal flora that do not synthesize vitamin K.

Vitamin K deficiency bleeding in infancy has been classified by time of onset into three categories: early, classic, and late.[123–126] Early vitamin K deficiency presents in the first 24 hours of life as "the bleeding neonate" (see earlier). It is associated with placental transfer of maternal medications, including some anticonvulsants, oral anticoagulants, antibiotics, and antituberculosis agents, that inhibit vitamin K activity in the newborn. Stopping offending medications and maternal vitamin K supplementation may prevent early disease. Classic and late vitamin K deficiency are described in detail in Chapter 72.

Disseminated Intravascular Coagulation

As in adults, the pathogenesis of DIC is poorly understood. In the bleeding neonate, transfusion support with fresh frozen plasma and platelets may be required. Cryoprecipitate may be given as a source of fibrinogen. However, high levels of factor VIII may be thrombogenic, an important consideration because some cases of neonatal DIC manifest bleeding and thrombosis. Resolution of the underlying medical condition leads to resolution of the DIC. If the underlying condition is expected to necessitate treatment for several days (e.g., the use of extracorporeal membrane oxygenation in severe sepsis) treatment with low-dose heparin has been advocated by some to reduce platelet and fibrinogen consumption.

Liver Disease

Severe liver disease may present like severe DIC. Synthesis of coagulation factors and thrombopoietin is decreased and there is consumption of coagulation factors and platelets. Thrombocytopenia is worsened by the presence of portal hypertension resulting from splenic sequestration.

Prothrombotic Disorders

Thrombotic complications are more common in neonates than other pediatric patients.[127,128] Advances in biomedical technology have been applied to more, and to more critically ill, neonates than ever before. Many of these neonates have associated risk factors for thrombosis, such as perinatal asphyxia, sepsis, necrotizing enterocolitis, respiratory distress syndrome, cardiac disease, polycythemia, renal disease, dehydration, diabetic mothers, and extracorporeal membrane oxygenation (Fig. 71–5).[129,130] Most also have the predisposing factor of an indwelling vascular catheter (up to 90% of cases of neonatal thrombosis are associated with a central venous catheter) with associated vascular injury, endothelial activation, and altered blood flow dynamics.[131] Developmental variations in coagulant and fibrinolytic protein levels and activity contribute to the thrombotic tendency.[130] Together, these conditions lead to elevated thrombin generation and subsequent thrombus formation.

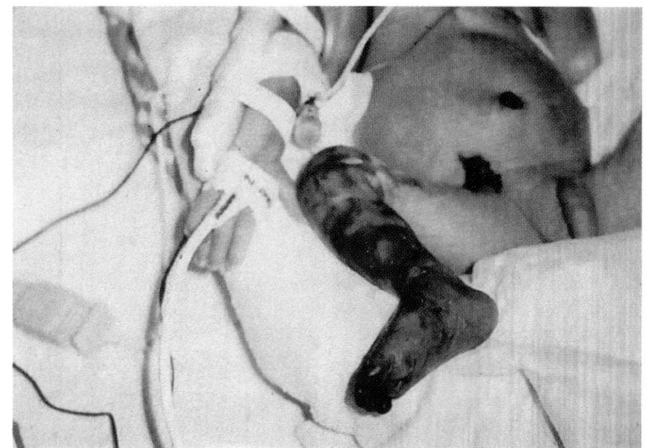

Figure 71–5. Septic thrombosis in the foot, leg, and inguinal region of an infant with *Staphylococcus aureus* bacteremia after removal of indwelling umbilical venous and arterial catheters.

Deficiency of protein C, protein S, or antithrombin III, mutations of coagulation factor V or II, and elevated lipoprotein(a) have been established as genetic risk factors for thromboembolic events in the neonatal period.[132] Homozygous protein C and protein S deficiency may present with purpura fulminans, severe DIC, and multiple, life-threatening thromboses.[133,134] Risk factors for thrombosis in adults, such as the factor V G1691A, the prothrombin G20210A, and the MTHFR C677T genotypes (see Chapter 67) have also been associated with neonatal thromboses, particularly with catheter-related thrombosis.[135,136]

Diagnosis and/or confirmation of thrombosis may be obtained by ultrasound with Doppler, venography, computed tomography, and magnetic resonance imaging.[137] Laboratory diagnosis of the hypercoagulable state relies on age-dependent reference values. Assays of protein C, protein S, antithrombin III, fasting homocysteine, and activated protein C resistance, and thrombotic genotyping as noted previously, should be performed 3–6 months after the thrombotic episode. The presence of lupus anticoagulant and anticardiolipin antibodies is typically sought in the mother.

Large, multicenter trials evaluating treatment of neonatal thromboembolism, including thrombolytic and anticoagulant therapy, are lacking.[127,137,138] Thus many treatment protocols are based on small clinical trials in neonates or adapted from guidelines of adult patient protocols.[128,137]

DEVELOPMENTAL THROMBOCYTOPOIESIS

The fetal platelet count is within the normal adult range by midgestation and increases linearly until term. Fetal and neonatal platelets differ biochemically and functionally from adult platelets.[139,140] Neonatal platelets exhibit decreased aggregation in response to a number of physiologic agonists, including epinephrine, ADP, collagen, thrombin, and thromboxane analogues. Delayed platelet shape change and granular release in response to agonists has been attributed to diminished calcium transport. P-selectin and glycoprotein (GP)IIb-IIIa and GPIb-IX complex expression are diminished after stimulation. Increased ristocetin-induced aggregation has been attributed to higher concentrations of von Willebrand factor and increased number/amount of functional high-molecular-weight von Willebrand factor multimers. Thrombopoietin, the major regulator of platelet homeostasis, appears at levels in the term neonate comparable to those found in adults, whereas median levels are lower in preterm infants. Cultured neonatal megakaryocyte progenitors exhibit a higher proliferative response to thrombopoietin than do adult progenitors.

Neonatal Thrombocytopenia

Thrombocytopenia is one of the most common hematologic abnormalities in neonatal intensive care unit patients. Up to one quarter of these patients exhibit thrombocytopenia during their hospitalization. Determining the cause of thrombocytopenia provides information on the likely clinical course, the severity, and the likelihood of hemorrhage. This is usually difficult because the etiology of thrombocytopenia is variable and it is often multifactorial (Table 71–5).[141] Neonatal platelet counts drop rapidly in response to hypoxia, acidosis, and infection. Neonatal thrombocytopenia is commonly associated with infection, both congenital and acquired, and it is associated with bacterial, viral, and fungal pathogens. The etiology of infection-associated thrombocytopenia is multifactorial because of increased destruction, decreased production, and, in some cases, DIC. Algorithms have been developed to evaluate thrombocytopenia based on onset, mechanism, or typical patterns of thrombocytopenia associated with specific disease processes.[142]

TABLE 71–5. Causes of Neonatal Thrombocytopenia

Increased Destruction

Maternally Associated

Common

Immune mediated
- Alloimmune neonatal thrombocytopenia
- Maternal autoimmune disorders (ITP, SLE)

Congenital infections

Uncommon

Maternal preeclampsia
Maternal drug use (such as quinidine, certain anticonvulsants, certain diuretics)
Rh disease
Placental abnormalities

Not Maternally Associated

Common

Infection
Perinatal asphyxia
- Meconium aspiration

Neonatal thrombosis (associated with indwelling catheters, coagulation abnormalities, and renal vein thromboses)

Uncommon

Respiratory distress syndrome
Congenital heart disease
Hemangiomas
Hypersplenism

Rare

Wiskott-Aldrich syndrome
Giant platelet syndromes (Bernard-Soulier, May-Hegglin, Mediterranean macrothrombocytopenia)
Von Willebrand disease type 2b
Inborn errors of metabolism

Decreased Production or Bone Marrow Replacement

Uncommon

Trisomy syndromes (13, 18)
Thrombocytopenia with absent radii

Rare

Amegakaryocytic thrombocytopenia
Fanconi's anemia, dyskeratosis congenita
Congenital leukemia
Neuroblastoma
Histiocytosis

Abbreviations: ITP, immune thrombocytopenic purpura; SLE, systemic lupus erythematosus.
From George D, Bussel JB: Neonatal thrombocytopenia. Semin Thromb Hemost 21:276–293, 1995, with permission.

Neonatal Alloimmune Thrombocytopenia

Neonatal alloimmune thrombocytopenia (NAIT) is the most common cause of severe thrombocytopenia in an otherwise well-appearing neonate in which maternal history is negative (see Chapter 60).[143,144] Prompt diagnosis and treatment are important to prevent hemorrhage, particularly intracranial hemorrhage.[145] NAIT is often compared to hemolytic disease of the newborn because the mother becomes sensitized to an allotype of a fetal platelet antigen inherited from the father. Maternal IgG alloantibodies cross the placenta and bind fetal platelets, marking them for removal by the reticuloendothelial system. In approximately 90% of cases, the parents are incompatible for human platelet antigens HPA-1a or -5b.[145,146]

Many infants with NAIT are asymptomatic or have only superficial petechiae or ecchymoses. Intracranial hemorrhage occurs in up to 10–20% of infants. Diagnosis is made by detecting maternal platelet-specific antibody and by parental platelet antigen typing. In some cases, maternal antibody may not be detected until later, necessitating repeat and/or additional testing. No correlation has been made between antibody titers or platelet isotypes and occurrence of NAIT.

Treatment is with antigen-negative platelets.[141] Transfusion of random platelets is futile because they are rapidly removed from the circulation. Transfusion of maternal platelets, after washing or plasma depletion to remove alloantibody, is effective. Some blood banks keep HPA-1a/5b–negative platelets on hand for cases of suspected NAIT. Intravenous immunoglobulin infusion and steroid administration are effective in the treatment of NAIT. Clinical severity and thrombocytopenia worsen with subsequent pregnancies. Occurrence of intracranial hemorrhage in the first infant predicts a worse prognosis in subsequent pregnancies. Antenatal treatment approaches include maternal intravenous immunoglobulin infusion with or without prednisone.

Autoimmune Thrombocytopenia

Less commonly than NAIT, neonatal thrombocytopenia is due to placental transfer of maternal autoantibodies that also cause maternal autoimmune disease such as idiopathic thrombocytopenic purpura (ITP), systemic lupus erythematosus, or hypothyroidism. In these cases, neonatal thrombocytopenia and the risk of hemorrhage is less than in NAIT.[147–149] ITP is probably the most common of these autoimmune disorders, complicating 1–2 per 1000 live births. Severe thrombocytopenia (<20,000/μL) is estimated to occur in 3% of neonates born to mothers with ITP.[150] Minor bleeding occurs in 3% and major bleeding occurs in 1% of these infants. A few cases of intracranial hemorrhage have been reported. The best predictor of severity of neonatal thrombocytopenia is a mother who has given birth to a previously affected neonate.[147,151] Unlike NAIT, there is no apparent benefit to maternal or fetal treatment during pregnancy.

After initial assessment by a platelet count from the umbilical cord at birth, serial counts should be obtained over the first week, because many infants born to mothers with ITP experience a nadir in platelet count over the first few days of life, probably related to increased endothelial cell function. Intravenous immune globulin or prednisone may be prescribed for infants with bleeding or severe thrombocytopenia. Platelet transfusions are typically not used because circulating antibodies react with all platelets.

Few data are available to guide decision making as to when platelet transfusion is indicated in the asymptomatic, thrombocytopenic neonate.[152,153] Recommendations have suggested transfusion at a level of 25,000–50,000/μL for well or stable neonates and 50,000–100,000/μL for sick or preterm infants. The roles of thrombopoietin or other factors, such as factor VIIa and interleukin-11, in the treatment of neonatal thrombocytopenia have yet to be elucidated.

Abnormalities of Platelet Function

Abnormalities of platelet function should be considered in neonates with petechiae, mucous membrane bleeding, or purpura and normal coagulation testing and platelet count. Acquired platelet dysfunction may occur after administration of agents to the mother or the infant (e.g., aspirin or indomethacin), or in patients with renal failure, liver disease, or dietary fatty acid deficiency and during treatment with extracorporeal membrane oxygenation. Rarely, bleeding caused by Glanzmann's thrombasthenia manifests in the neonatal period.[154]

LEUKOCYTE DISORDERS

Leukocytes are the major effector cells of the host response. Neutrophils circulate in the blood until they encounter signals for adhesion and movement. Mononuclear phagocytes (macrophages and monocytes) are cells resident in specific tissues (e.g., the spleen or lung) where they interact with lymphocytes to generate a local immune response. Myelopoiesis begins early in gestation, and at midtrimester, neutrophils exhibit some functional activity. At term, neutrophils still lack full functional capability. Neutrophil counts vary widely at birth, from 6000/mL to 26,000/mL, then fall after 12 hours of age to a level of approximately 5000/mL in the first week of life. Alterations in the number of circulating leukocytes may represent abnormal production or consumption, or both. Disorders of leukocyte function are reviewed in Chapter 57.

Leukopenia

A number of conditions have been associated with neonatal neutropenia (neutrophil count < 1500/mL).[155,156] Some of these disorders are transient (e.g., associated with maternal hypertension, infection, Rh disease, multiple gestation), and others are manifestations of inherited abnormalities (e.g., Kostmann's syndrome; see Chapter 13).[157,158] Similar to platelet disorders, neonatal isoimmune and autoimmune neutropenias have been described.[159,160] In most studies, neonatal neutropenia is the result of overwhelming sepsis, particularly in preterm infants, as a result of small marrow neutrophil storage pools. Immunotherapy with immunoglobulin and cytokines, particularly granulocyte and granulocyte-macrophage colony-stimulating factors, to augment neutrophil number and function has been attempted in septic, neutropenic neonates.[161–163] Large, randomized, multicenter clinical trials are lacking, and this therapy remains controversial.

Leukocytosis

The differential diagnosis of neonatal leukocytosis is similar to that in older patients, that is, reactive, leukemoid reaction, or leukemia but with variation. Many stressed or infected neonates present with neutropenia rather than neutrophilia. Leukemoid reactions in neonates are not rare, accounting for 1.3% of neonatal intensive care unit admissions in one report.[164,165] They are associated with antenatal maternal steroid administration, particularly in preterm infants. In one study, hyperviscosity was not observed.

CURRENT CONTROVERSIES & FUTURE CONSIDERATIONS

Hematology of the Newborn

- Rapid, DNA-based diagnostic testing will permit diagnosis of many inherited hematologic disorders in the perinatal period, facilitating management.
- Studies of neonatal erythropoiesis will reveal novel insights and treatment strategies for the anemia of prematurity.
- Development and refinement of noninvasive techniques to diagnose and expectantly manage the isoimmunized pregnancy will lead to further decreases in fetal and neonatal morbidity and mortality from this condition.
- Clinical trials will reveal optimal regimens for managing the pregnancy complicated by fetal platelet alloimmunization.
- Growth factors, alone or in combination, may prove to be of benefit in the treatment of neonatal anemia, thrombocytopenia, and/or neutropenia.

A leukemoid reaction or transient myeloproliferative disorder has been observed in some neonates with trisomy 21.[166] Life-threatening complications such as hydrops fetalis, liver failure, or cardiopulmonary involvement may occur. Most cases resolve spontaneously, but 20–30% of infants with transient myeloproliferative disorder/trisomy 21 develop acute megakaryocytic leukemia later in childhood. A truncation mutation of the transcription factor GATA-1 has been found in these patients (see Chapter 33).[167,168]

Leukemia is rare in the fetus or newborn even though it is the leading cause of neonatal death from neoplastic disease. Most patients have cutaneous findings, a high leukemic cell load, hepatosplenomegaly, and frequent central nervous system involvement.[169,170] Acute myeloid leukemia is three times as common as acute lymphocytic leukemia. Cytogenetic abnormalities occur in about two thirds of patients. Overall prognosis is poor with or without treatment, with an overall 3-year survival rate of approximately 25%. Death is typically due to infection and/or hemorrhage. There has been significant interest in elucidating the fetal origins of leukemia.[171]

Suggested Readings*

Bizzarro MJ, Colson E, Ehrenkranz RA: Differential diagnosis and management of anemia in the newborn. Pediatr Clin North Am 51:1087–1107, 2004.

Christensen RD, Calhoun DA, Rimsza LM: A practical approach to evaluating and treating neutropenia in the neonatal intensive care unit. Clin Perinatol 27:577–601, 2000.

Greenway A, Massicotte MP, Monagle P: Neonatal thrombosis and its treatment. Blood Rev 18:75–84, 2004.

Kulkarni R: Bleeding in the newborn. Pediatr Ann 30:548–556, 2001.

Pappas A, Delaney-Black V: Differential diagnosis and management of polycythemia. Pediatr Clin North Am 51:1063–1086, 2004.

Sola MC: Evaluation and treatment of severe and prolonged thrombocytopenia in neonates. Clin Perinatol 31:1–14, 2004.

Full references for this chapter can be found on accompanying CD-ROM.

CHAPTER 72

PEDIATRIC HEMATOLOGY

J. Paul Scott, MD, and Barbara Zieger, MD

KEY POINTS

Pediatric Hematology

- Hemoglobin is at the physiologic peak (17–19 gm/dL) at birth, declines to the physiologic nadir (9–10 gm/dL) at approximately 8–10 weeks of age, and reaches normal levels at 4–6 months of age.
- The total white blood cell count is elevated in normal infants (normal range: 13,000–38,000/mm^3 at day 1 of life, 5000–21,000/mm^3 at week 1) compared to older children and adults.
- The most common cause of anemia in children is iron deficiency resulting from inadequate intake; infants fed cow's milk, which is low in iron, are at particularly high risk.
- Sickle cell disease is the most common hemoglobinopathy of childhood. Most but not all children with the disease are identified in newborn screening programs. Common presenting manifestations include hand-foot syndrome, fever, splenic sequestration, and unexplained pain.
- Diamond-Blackfan anemia is a form of congenital red cell aplasia, and appears to be due to an abnormal response of the red cell precursors to erythropoietin.
- Neutropenia in infancy and childhood is usually transient and associated with viral infections.
- Consideration of the developmental differences in coagulation parameters from birth to puberty is important because these coagulation values are the basis for the diagnosis of congenital deficiencies.
- Bleeding symptoms in otherwise healthy infants are due to either congenital or acquired hemorrhagic disorders.
- Hemophilia A and B are the most commonly diagnosed congenital factor deficiencies during infancy.
- A patient with bleeding symptoms who is suspected of having vitamin K deficiency should be immediately administered vitamin K subcutaneously or intravenously.
- Compared to adults, the incidence of thromboembolic events is still rare in children.
- Neonates with homozygous protein C or protein S deficiency develop purpura fulminans within hours of birth.
- Central venous lines are the most common risk factor for thromboembolism in newborns and in children.

INTRODUCTION

Pediatric hematology involves the study of the interaction between the developmental biology of the growing child and congenital or acquired diseases that induce unique patterns of illness as the child ages. The unique characteristics of neonatal hematology were presented in Chapter 71. The transition from fetal to neonatal existence is responsible for major changes in the hematology, hemostasis, and immunology of the newborn. In Table 72–1, the characteristic changes in normal hematologic values of the newborn infant and growing child/adolescent are presented.[1] During the first 2 months of life, the hemoglobin that reached its physiologic peak at 17–19 gm/dL at birth declines to its "physiologic nadir." This is caused by the transition from the relatively low oxygen saturation sustained during fetal existence, which rapidly changes after birth when the child inspires room air and achieves normal neonatal blood oxygen saturation (>95%). The resultant marked increase in oxygen delivery to the kidney shuts down erythropoietin synthesis and neonatal red cell synthesis ceases. The hemoglobin gradually falls until levels sufficient to stimulate erythropoietin synthesis are attained. The hemoglobin level typically bottoms out around 9–10 gm/dL at 8–10 weeks of age, the so-called physiologic nadir. The rapidity of the fall in hemoglobin and depth of the nadir are accentuated in babies born prematurely ("anemia of prematurity"),[2,3] as shown in Figure 72–1. As the neonatal red blood cells age and are destroyed, the

TABLE 72–1. Normal Hematologic Values in Children

Age	Hemoglobin (gm/dL) Mean	Hemoglobin (gm/dL) −2 SD	MCV (fL) Mean	MCV (fL) −2 SD	MCH (pg) Mean	MCH (pg) −2 SD
1–3 days (capillary)	18.5	14.5	108	95	34	31
1 wk	17.5	13.5	107	95	34	28
2 wk	16.5	12.5	105	86	34	28
1 mo	14.0	10.0	104	85	34	28
2 mo	11.5	9.0	96	77	30	26
0.5–2 yr	12.0	10.5	78	70	27	23
2–6 yr	12.5	11.5	81	75	27	24
6–12 yr	13.5	11.5	86	77	29	25
12–18 yr						
Female	14.0	12.0	90	78	30	25
Male	14.5	13.0	88	78	30	25
18–49 yr						
Female	14.0	12.0	90	80	30	26
Male	15.5	13.5	90	80	30	26

Abbreviations: MCHC, mean corpuscular hemoglobin concentration; MCV, mean corpuscular volume; SD, standard deviation.
From Dallman PR: Blood and blood-forming tissues. *In* Rudolph A (ed): Pediatrics (ed 16). New York: Appleton-Century-Crofts, 1977, p 1111.

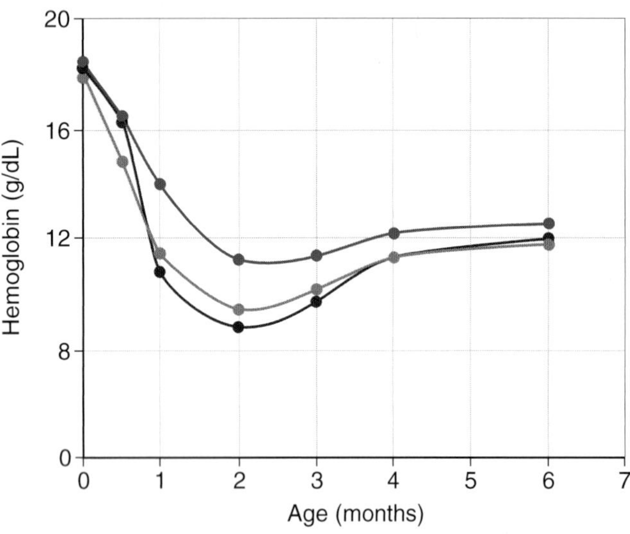

Figure 72–1. Graphic illustration of the effect of low birth weight (prematurity) on the "physiologic nadir" in infancy. (Data from Saarinen UM, Siimes MA: Developmental changes in red blood cell counts and indices in infants after exclusion of iron deficiency by laboratory criteria and continuous iron supplementation. J Pediatr 92:414, 1978; and Lundstrom U, Siimes MA, Dallman PR: At what age does iron supplementation become necessary in low birth weight infants? J Pediatr 91:882, 1977.)

hemoglobin falls until the kidney again senses insufficient oxygen delivery and resumes erythropoietin synthesis. The infant's hemoglobin then gradually increases during the first year of life. During fetal existence, hemoglobin F ($\alpha_2\gamma_2$) predominates. Around the time of birth,

TABLE 72–2. Reference Ranges for Leukocyte Counts in Children

Age	Total Leukocytes: Range	Neutrophils Range	Neutrophils %	Lymphocytes Range	Lymphocytes %
Day 1	13.0–38.0	6.0–28.0	68	2.0–11.0	24
1 wk	5.0–21.0	1.5–10.0	45	2.0–17.0	41
1 mo	5.0–19.5	1.0–9.0	35	2.5–16.5	56
1 yr	6.0–17.5	1.5–8.5	31	4.0–10.5	61
4 yr	5.5–15.5	1.5–8.5	42	2.0–8.0	50
16 yr	4.5–13.0	1.8–8.0	57	1.2–5.2	35

Adapted from Dallman PR: White blood cells. *In* Rudolph A (ed): Pediatrics (ed 16). New York: Appleton-Century-Crofts, 1977, p 1178.

β chain synthesis is switched on and γ chain synthesis switched off. Hemoglobin A ($\alpha_2\beta_2$) becomes the major hemoglobin by 4–6 months of age.[4] Thus, β chain disorders only become manifest after 4–6 months of age, whereas disorders of the α and γ chain may present in the neonatal period.

The characteristic changes in the white count and differential with age are shown in Table 72–2. In the newborn, the white count is typically elevated with a predominant left shift. By 1 month of age, the normal total white cell count has slightly declined and there is a shift to the right with a lymphocyte predominance. By age 4 years, the differential is about 50% mononuclear cells and 50% segmented cells.[5] As the child proceeds through adolescence, the differential count approaches that of an adult. It is striking that the upper limits of normal for white count and lymphocyte count in infancy are significantly higher than at any other time of life and markedly different from those of adolescents and adults. A knowledgeable clinician must recognize the marked age-dependent variation in normal values, lest a work-up be done on a patient whose values are normal for age. In the remainder of this chapter, specific common childhood hematologic complaints and their most common causes are discussed.

ANEMIA IN CHILDHOOD

Figure 72–2 presents an algorithm for the differential diagnosis of anemia in children using a combination of the reticulocyte count to assess the bone marrow response to anemia and the red blood cell hemoglobin (Hb) indices to characterize the type of anemia as microcytic, normocytic, or macrocytic.[6] Like all algorithms, this one presents a general approach to the differential diagnosis of anemia that must be adapted to the work-up of individual cases. The Reticulocyte Production Index (RPI) attempts to correct the reticulocyte count (retic ct) for the degree of anemia:

$$RPI = \text{retic ct} \times Hb_{observed}/Hb_{normal}$$

If there is extensive polychromasia on the smear, an additional correction factor should be used such that the RPI

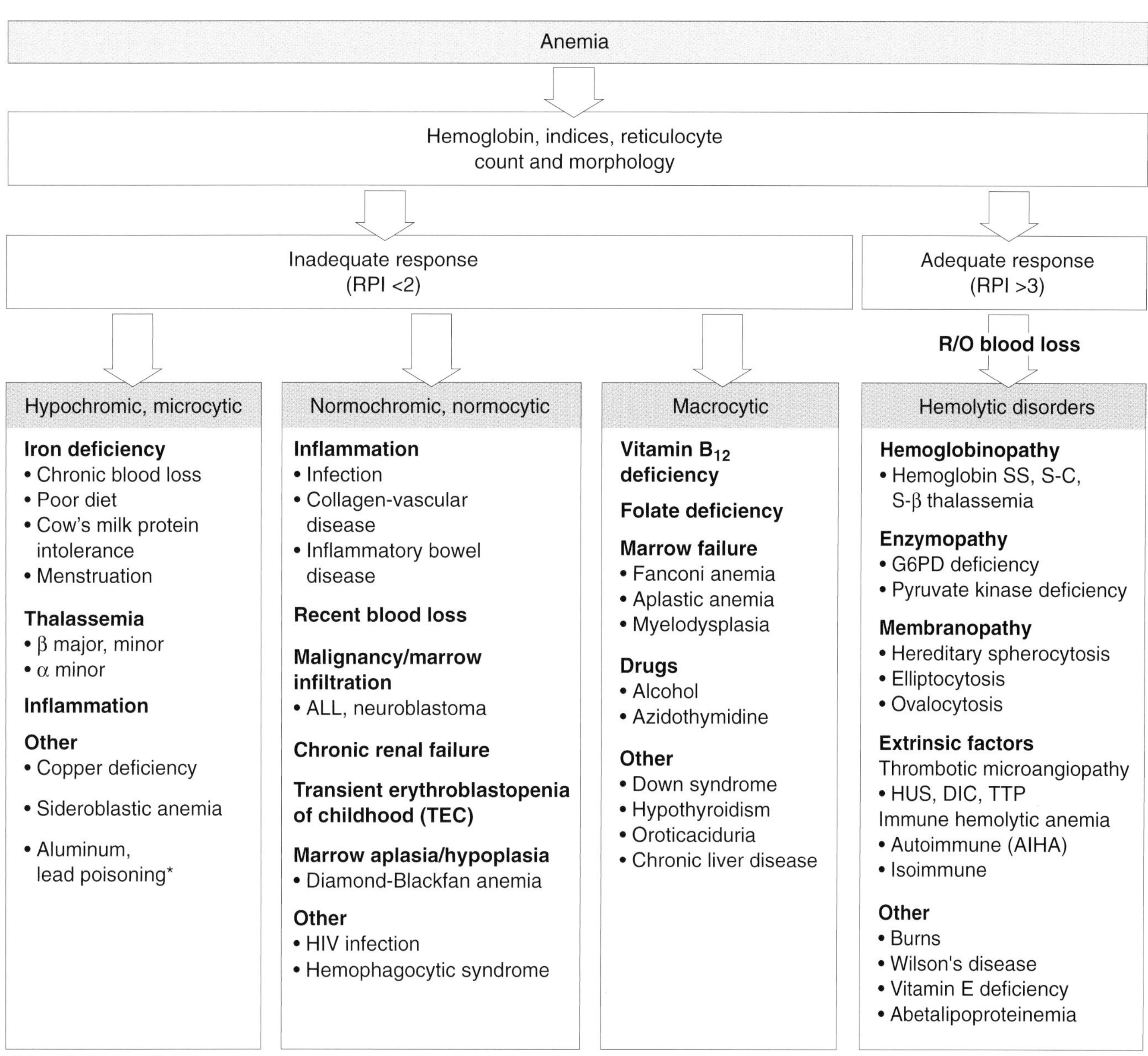

Figure 72–2. An algorithm for the differential diagnosis of anemia using the red cell indices and Reticulocyte Production Index to direct the work-up. (Adapted from Scott JP: Hematology. *In* Behrman RE, Kliegman RM [eds]: Nelson's Essentials of Pediatrics [ed 4]. Philadelphia: WB Saunders, 2002, p 612.)

should be multiplied by 0.5. Some recent automated red cell counters report an absolute reticulocyte number that should correct for the artifact caused by the degree of anemia.

Hypochromic, Microcytic Anemia in Childhood

Mild to moderate microcytic anemia is common in infancy.[7,8] The differential diagnosis of hypochromic, microcytic anemia in infancy is dominated by iron deficiency and the thalassemia minor syndromes (Table 72–3). Iron deficiency is the most common cause of anemia worldwide; tragically, this is a preventable problem.[9–12] The American Academy of Pediatrics recommends iron supplementation for breast-fed babies over 6 months of age or, alternatively, the use of an iron-containing formula for children who are bottle fed until 12 months of age.[13,14]

Infants represent a particularly high-risk population because of a coincidence of biologic vulnerability compounded by well-intentioned but knowledge-deficient parents. Infants fed cow's milk are at particularly high risk for iron deficiency anemia on the basis of two complicating factors. Cow's milk has a very low concentration of iron (0.7 mg/L).[10] In addition, a subset of babies fed a diet of cow's milk, particularly if done so prior to 1 year of age, develop intolerance to cow's milk protein,

TABLE 72–3. Findings in Hypochromic, Microcytic Anemia of Infancy

	Iron	Iron-Binding Capacity	Ferritin	Clues
IDA				
Mild	nl / ↓	nl / ↑	nl / ↓	↑RDW
Severe	↓↓	↑	↓↓	↓↓MCV
β-Thalassemia minor	nl	nl	nl	↑A_2, ↑F, ↑RBC, basophilic stippling
Anemia of inflammation	↓	↓	nl / ↑	Chronic illness

Abbreviations: A_2, Hemoglobin A_2; F, Hemoglobin F; IDA, iron deficiency anemia; MCV, mean corpuscular volume; RBC, red blood cells; RDW, red cell distribution width; ↑, increased; ↓, decreased; nl, normal.

resulting in gastrointestinal blood loss and sometimes a protein-losing enteropathy.[15] In these children, the history can be helpful if there is a clear-cut history of ingestion by the child of large volumes of milk and a poor intake of other foods. Inquiring how many bottles of milk the child drinks in a 24-hour period (not a day), and how often the parents buy milk, and how much, may be helpful. Despite the demonstrated efficacy of supplementation programs,[16] iron deficiency anemia remains common in children of lower socioeconomic status, especially in the Third World, probably because milk costs less than formula and is easier to use.[11,12,17]

Outside of infancy, the only other group of children who are particularly vulnerable to iron deficiency are menstruating teenage girls. The adolescent female's diet often provides inadequate iron to make up for menstrual blood loss.[18] In girls who are having excessive menstrual bleeding, there is often a delay in seeking medical care because the girl often does not know that the bleeding that she is experiencing is excessive. Iron deficiency in boys beyond infancy and in premenarchal girls implies blood loss. The most common site of blood loss is within the gastrointestinal tract, and a careful search for occult blood in the stool is necessary. A rare pediatric disorder, idiopathic pulmonary hemosiderosis—a syndrome of recurrent cough and pulmonary infiltrates perhaps related to milk protein intolerance—causes findings of iron deficiency anemia. Blood is lost into the lungs and iron is not recycled for use in erythroid synthesis, thus the patient essentially bleeds into the lungs, where the iron cannot be reutilized. The presence of hemosiderin-laden macrophages on bronchoalveolar lavage is diagnostic.[19]

The physical examination in a child with iron deficiency is often unremarkable. Most such children have normal growth and development. As the anemia becomes more severe, pallor develops so gradually that it is often not appreciated by the family. With severe iron deficiency, especially when associated with a protein-losing enteropathy, puffiness around the eyes and the extremities may be obvious. The stool should be examined for occult blood. Because iron is an essential element in enzymes and cytochromes, severe iron deficiency may cause neurologic changes, including apathy, irritability, and disinterest in the environment.[20] In addition to the hematologic manifestations of iron deficiency, there are data suggesting that iron deficiency can cause developmental problems, learning difficulties, and decreased energy.[20–23]

The work-up for iron deficiency depends on the severity of the disorder. For infants with a typical history of milk as the primary source of nutrition (milk babies) and with mild anemia, the best diagnostic test is the administration of 3–4 mg of elemental iron/kg/day and a recheck of the hemoglobin in 1–3 months, by which time the anemia should have corrected.[24] Common laboratory findings in iron deficiency are depicted in Table 72–3. In rare cases, it may be necessary to examine the bone marrow for iron stores to determine if a child with an ongoing inflammatory illness also has iron deficiency.

The treatment of iron deficiency is straightforward. Institution of iron replacement at a dose of 4–6 mg/kg/day of elemental iron promptly corrects any neurologic findings within 48 hours. By the end of the first week, a reticulocytosis should occur and correction of the anemia should occur at a rate of 1–2 gm/week, so that the hemoglobin should have returned to normal levels by 1 month following the diagnosis of iron deficiency. Iron stores will need to be built up over the next several months following normalization of the hemoglobin. Rarely in iron deficiency, the anemia is so severe as to require transfusion. In this situation, a transfusion of 5–10 mL/kg of packed red blood cells with the concomitant administration of furosemide as a diuretic is very effective in yielding a partial correction of the anemia. There is no need for further transfusion because the aim of transfusion is an improvement in perfusion of the brain and other vital organs.

The differential diagnosis of hypochromic, microcytic anemia includes the thalassemia minor syndromes: α-thalassemia minor, β-thalassemia minor, and hemoglobin E (see Chapter 21) as well as the anemia of inflammation.[25–27] Typical laboratory findings in iron deficiency, β-thalassemia minor, and anemia of inflammation are presented in Table 72–3. The ratio obtained by dividing the mean corpuscular volume by the red blood cell number (the "Mentzer index") often indicates whether thalassemia (ratio < 13) or iron deficiency is more likely.[28] The presence of either Bart hemoglobin (γ_4), indicating a form of α-thalassemia, or hemoglobin E may be detected on newborn hemoglobin screening in some states, leading to the diagnosis of these disorders. Newborn screening using biochemical methods cannot diagnose β-thalassemia trait.

Chronic Hemolytic Anemias in Children

Certain findings are common to most hemolytic anemias. To help organize the mechanisms causing the hemolytic anemias, the red cell has been often described as a "bag containing enzymes and hemoglobin." The most common disorder of the "bag" (membrane defect) is hereditary spherocytosis (HS). The most common enzyme defect is glucose-6-phosphate dehydrogenase (G6PD) deficiency and the most common hemoglobinopathy is sickle dell disease (SCD). The red cell traverses the circulation and thus may be damaged by external factors such as antibodies and toxins (Table 72–4). As noted in Chapter 71, hemolytic anemias, other than the β chain abnormalities, often present with unexplained, prolonged neonatal jaundice. As a cause of neonatal jaundice, hemolytic anemia is commonly undiagnosed because of the challenge of appropriately interpreting neonatal blood smears and the prevalence of physiologic jaundice. Congenital hemolytic anemia should be suspected in the circumstances of a neonate with severe jaundice, or falling hemoglobin, or persistent reticulocytosis.[29–31]

Hereditary Spherocytosis

In early infancy, severe HS may cause transfusion dependency, whereas moderate to mild HS may be asymptomatic or cause mild pallor and jaundice. Despite a normal hemoglobin at birth, infants with HS frequently require a transfusion for severe anemia between 4 and 8 weeks of age.[30] The protein defects underlying HS are discussed in depth in Chapter 22. Spherocytosis and other mild to moderate hemolytic anemias may cause unexplained splenomegaly that is only detected on a routine physical examination in an older child. Later in life, such children may develop recurrent abdominal pain in the right upper quadrant associated with gallstones. A family history of spherocytosis may be helpful because such patients often have a history of autosomal dominant anemia, jaundice, "hereditary splenectomy," and early gallbladder disease. Nevertheless, approximately 25% of HS patients have spontaneous mutations. Thus, a positive family history is helpful, but a negative history is not conclusive. The diagnosis of HS depends on the finding of spherocytes on the peripheral blood smear in conjunction with a negative direct antiglobulin test (Coombs test). The mean corpuscular hemoglobin concentration may be elevated in some cases, and an osmotic fragility test confirms the presence of spherocytes.[32,33] The hemolytic anemia of HS is cured by splenectomy. Some cases of HS have had an amelioration of their hemolytic anemia and maintenance of splenic function following partial splenectomy.[34]

G6PD Deficiency

The most common red cell enzymopathy is G6PD deficiency (see Chapter 23). There are two common forms of this X-linked disorder, polymorphic and sporadic. The so-called Mediterranean variant of G6PD deficiency causes a chronic, nonspherocytic hemolytic anemia. Children with the Mediterranean variant of G6PD may have jaundice in the neonatal period and chronic hemolysis with episodes of worsening anemia and increased jaundice, particularly with illness or ingestion of dietary substances such as fava beans.[35,36]

Sickle Cell Disease

The major hemoglobinopathy in children is SCD (Fig. 72–3*A*) In the modern era, newborn screening has revolutionized the care of children with SCD. In "the bad old days" prior to screening, these children presented with painful swollen hands and feet (hand-foot syndrome), fever caused by sepsis and/or meningitis, life-threatening anemia caused by massive splenic sequestration, or unexplained, persistent pain.[37] It is important to remember that, prior to 1970 in the United States, 30% of children with SCD died by age 4 of complications of the disease. Newborn screening accompanied by comprehensive care, careful parent education (anticipatory guidance), prophylactic penicillin, and increased medical vigilance have greatly improved survival for these children.[38,39] The mortality due to SCD in Wisconsin since the advent of newborn screening in 1988 is 0.51 per 100 patient-

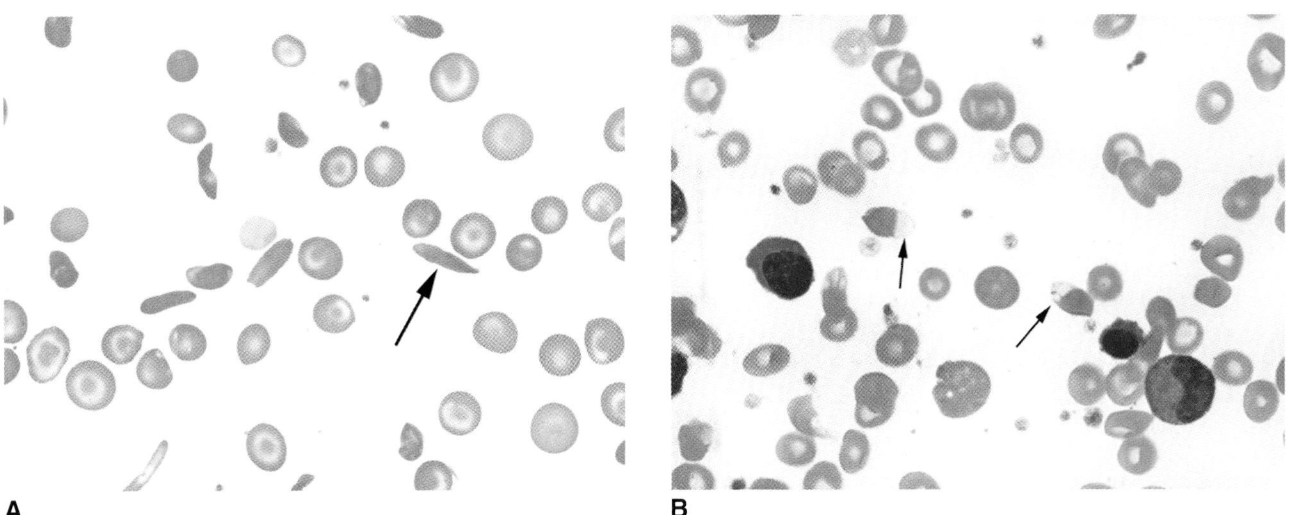

Figure 72–3. *A,* The peripheral blood smear of a child with sickle cell anemia (Hb SS). Note the target cells as well as the typical sickle forms. *B,* A smear from a child with G6PD deficiency. Note the characteristic "blister" cells, marked by the *arrow.* (Courtesy of B. A. Trost and J. P. Scott.)

TABLE 72–4. Differential Diagnosis of Common Causes of Hemolytic Anemia in Childhood

Chronic	Membrane defect: HS, elliptocytosis
	Enzymopathy: G6PD deficiency, PK deficiency
	Hemoglobinopathy: Hb SS, SC, S-β-thal
Acute onset	G6PD deficiency with oxidant exposure
	Autoimmune hemolytic anemia
	HUS/TTP, other thrombotic microangiopathies

Abbreviations: G6PD, glucose-6-phosphate dehydrogenase; Hb, hemoglobin; HS, hereditary spherocytosis; HUS/TTP, hemolytic-uremic syndrome/thrombotic thrombocytopenic purpura; PK, pyruvate kinase.

TABLE 72–5. Common Manifestations of Sickle Cell Disease

Age	Common Presentations
Infant	Hand-foot syndrome, fever (sepsis), splenic sequestration, unexplained pain
Child	Pain, acute chest syndrome (ACS), stroke, aplastic crisis, growth delay, poor school performance
Preteen/adolescent	Pain, priapism, ACS, delay in sexual maturation, avascular necrosis

years. Nevertheless, the pediatric hematologic consultant must be aware that there are states within the United States that do not screen for sickle cell, and that children of African descent born in countries that do not screen or those born on U.S. military bases overseas may not be diagnosed. Following diagnosis by newborn screening and confirmation of the precise hemoglobin phenotype (Hg SS, SC, S-β-thalassemia), the emphasis for pediatric hematologists is to deliver preventive care to the family and child with SCD. From the first visit to the comprehensive center, parents are counseled about the common childhood manifestations of SCD (Table 72–5) in an age-appropriate manner. Early appropriate education and intervention are the hallmarks of excellent care of children with SCD.

It remains unclear why some children with Hg SS disease have frequent life-threatening complications such as sequestration, stroke, and acute chest syndrome while others with an identical hemoglobin phenotype have relatively few complications. In a large collaborative cohort study, the presence of a low hemoglobin, elevated white count, and hand-foot syndrome in infants less than 1 year of age appeared to indicate a particularly high-risk group of children.[40] Two common pediatric disorders represent comorbidities that appear to contribute to the severity of SCD. Nighttime hypoxemia related to upper airway obstruction has been linked to an increased risk of stroke and pain crisis. Children with SCD should be carefully screened for symptoms and signs of upper airway obstruction resulting from enlarged tonsils and adenoids.[41,42] Asthma is very common among urban African Americans. Preliminary findings have linked asthma to an increased risk for acute chest syndrome and possibly stroke.[43–45] Thus, most children receiving therapy for acute chest syndrome are empirically treated with bronchodilators.[46] Both asthma and nighttime hypoxemia share a common theme: increased risk of hypoxemia is associated with more severe SCD.

As outlined in Chapter 20, the treatment of SCD is evolving. Hematopoietic stem cell transplantation has cured a number of children with SCD.[47] Hydroxyurea treatment appears to be effective in children with severe SCD as it is in adults, although there are no randomized, controlled trials in children demonstrating its efficacy.[48–50] Chronic transfusion therapy reduces the recurrence risk of stroke and decreases the frequency of both pain events and acute chest syndrome.[51] Recent investigations have focused on early detection and prevention of neurovascular complications of SCD.[52,53]

Childhood Acute Hemolytic Anemia

There are a limited group of disorders that commonly may trigger acute onset of hemolytic anemia in childhood. Each of the previously discussed congenital hemolytic disorders (see Table 72–4) may be exacerbated by infection, with a fall in hemoglobin and an increase in bilirubin, but review of the past history should point to chronicity of the process.

The history and physical findings in a child with acute hemolytic anemia are similar to those in an adult with this disorder, and include complaints of fatigue, headache, lethargy, pallor, jaundice, and dark urine. Because the onset of anemia is acute, there may be signs of cardiovascular instability, including tachycardia, hypotension, and poor peripheral perfusion. Patients with acute intravascular hemolysis may appear acutely ill and uncomfortable.[54] The peripheral blood smear is often crucial to indicate the proper diagnostic studies. The clinician should draw blood for typing and crossmatching immediately.

Autoimmune Hemolytic Anemia

Autoimmune hemolytic anemia (AIHA) in childhood often occurs following a viral illness with the sudden onset of hemolysis. The reticulocyte count may be low or mildly elevated.[55] There may be a large variation in the rapidity and severity of hemolysis. The patient who has evidence of acute hemolysis with a low reticulocyte count requires careful monitoring with frequent measurements of the hemoglobin because the child may rapidly decompensate. In AIHA the blood smear often shows spherocytes and rouleaux formation. Diagnosis of AIHA depends on detection of a positive direct or indirect antiglobulin test. The next key steps are to characterize the antibody and to institute treatment as discussed in detail in Chapter 24. About 80% of children with AIHA spontaneously remit over time.[56,57]

A-Variant G6PD Deficiency

In the United States, the most common form of G6PD deficiency (A-variant), present in 10% of African American males, causes production of an unstable enzyme. Thus, levels of G6PD fall as red cells age. When well, these individuals are not anemic and have no evidence of hemolysis. Following a severe bacterial infection, or after exposure to an oxidant drug (antimalarial), toxin (mothballs), or food (fava beans), these children may develop acute onset of hemolytic anemia, manifested by an acute drop in hemoglobin and the development of jaundice, hemoglobinuria, and hemoglobinemia.[58] There may be insufficient time for a reticulocyte response to anemia. The peripheral blood smear shows bite cells or blister cells (Fig. 72–3*B*). Thus, the G6PD level measured during a brisk reticulocytosis may be normal and levels may need to be rechecked when the child is well. The treatment of acute hemolytic episodes is to remove the offending oxidant if possible, and transfuse packed red blood cells for severe anemia.[35]

Hemolytic-Uremic Syndrome

The triad of microangiopathic hemolytic anemia, thrombocytopenia, and renal failure constitutes the hemolytic-uremic syndrome (HUS), a thrombotic microangiopathy. HUS typically presents with the acute onset of diarrhea, often bloody, secondary to a toxin produced by *Escherichia coli* 0157:H7.[59–61] Renal failure is the most serious complication of HUS, although hemolytic anemia and thrombocytopenia may be severe. The pathophysiology and treatment of HUS are discussed in detail in Chapter 62. Transfusion of platelets for thrombocytopenia in HUS is usually contraindicated.

Childhood Pure Red Cell Aplasia

Children with red cell aplasia usually present with the gradual onset of increasing pallor. The child may not seek medical care until the anemia is severe.[62–64] The differential diagnosis of the three most common childhood entities associated with red cell aplasia and some characteristic findings are presented in Table 72–6. Each of the three forms of red cell aplasia described here is commonly seen in early childhood. They are distinct from other marrow failure syndromes because the abnormality is limited to that of the red cell line. They are characterized by anemia, minimal or absent reticulocyte response, and virtual absence of red cell precursors in the marrow, as discussed in Chapter 12.

Diamond-Blackfan Anemia

Diamond-Blackfan anemia is a form of congenital red cell aplasia. Anemia is frequently present in the newborn. On clinical examination, some patients have associated congenital anomalies and small stature. Diamond-Blackfan anemia appears to be caused by an abnormal response of the red cell precursors to erythropoietin. Macrocytosis is present in about two thirds of the patients. Some patients have elevated levels of erythrocyte adenosine deaminase.[65–67] The molecular defects causing Diamond-Blackfan anemia have not been completely determined at this point. Initial treatment is packed red blood cell transfusion for severe anemia. About two thirds of patients will respond to corticosteroid therapy with an improvement in hemoglobin to near-normal levels. Some of these children can be managed with minimal doses of corticosteroid every other day, whereas others fail to respond to corticosteroids at any dose. Hematopoietic stem cell transplantation is curative.

Parvovirus B19 Infection

In children with an underlying hemolytic anemia, infection with parvovirus B19 causes acute red cell aplasia ("aplastic crisis"). The hemoglobin drops, often quickly, because the child is unable to compensate for the shortened red cell survival caused by the congenital hemolytic anemia.[68] Some such patients have mild hemolytic anemia that has eluded diagnosis for many years. Subtle clues, including a neonatal history of unexplained jaundice, a personal history of increased jaundice with acute infections (yellow eyes), or a family history of anemia, may point to the underlying hemolytic anemia.[69] Infection by parvovirus of red cell precursors in the marrow shuts down red cell synthesis completely. The reticulocyte count often approaches 0 (<0.1%). The smear may be particularly helpful in deducing that there is an underlying hemolytic process. Patients with a severe congenital hemolytic anemia, such as SCD, are at particular risk for severe complications, including stroke, associated with parvovirus-induced aplasia.

TABLE 72–6. Characteristic Findings in Common Red Cell Aplasia Syndromes of Childhood

	History	Physical Examination	Laboratory Findings
DBA	Anemia as newborn; age < 6 mo	Small stature, congenital anomalies	↑ MCV in majority
Aplastic crisis (parvovirus infection)	Neonatal jaundice, slapped cheeks, fever, rash	Jaundice, splenomegaly	Abnormal RBC morphology, ↑ bili, ↑ LDH
TEC	Age > 1 yr	Normal other than pallor, signs of anemia	Normal MCV, 60% neutropenic

Abbreviations: Bili, bilirubin; DBA, Diamond-Blackfan anemia; LDH, lactate dehydrogenase; MCV, mean corpuscular volume; RBC, red blood cell; TEC, transient erythroblastopenia of childhood; ↑, increased.

TABLE 72–7. Etiology of Splenomegaly in Childhood

	Specific Disorders
Acute	
Infection	Bacteria: SBE Virus: EBV, CMV Protozoa: Malaria, toxoplasmosis
Malignancy	ALL, lymphoma, histiocytosis syndrome
Chronic	
Hematologic	Hemolytic anemia, SCD, G6PD deficiency, HS, extramedullary hematopoiesis (thalassemia, myelofibrosis)
Congestive	Portal/splenic vein thrombosis Cirrhosis/hepatitis Congestive heart failure
Storage disorder	Niemann-Pick, Gaucher diseases
Cyst	Congenital or acquired
Inflammatory/autoimmune	SLE, sarcoidosis, rheumatoid arthritis, ALPS
Pseudo	Hyperinflation: Asthma

Abbreviations: ALL, acute lymphocytic leukemia; ALPS, autoimmune lymphoproliferative syndrome; CMV, cytomegalovirus; EBV, Epstein-Barr virus; G6PD, glucose-6-phosphate dehydrogenase; HS, hereditary spherocytosis; SBE, subacute bacterial endocarditis; SCD, sickle cell disease; SLE, systemic lupus erythematosus.

TABLE 72–8. Work-up of Child with Splenomegaly

Careful history and physical examination	
Laboratory tests	CBC, retic, smear, LDH, bili, liver enzyme, cultures, viral studies Doppler ultrasound Lysosomal enzyme studies* ANA* Bone marrow aspirate and biopsy* Liver biopsy*

*As indicated by initial evaluation.
Abbreviations: ANA, antinuclear antibodies; bili, bilirubin; CBC, complete blood count; LDH, lactate dehydrogenase; retic, reticulocyte count.

Transient Erythroblastopenia of Childhood

Transient erythroblastopenia of childhood (TEC) is a peculiar pediatric entity in which previously well young children develop gradual onset of anemia as a result of red cell aplasia. These children, usually older than 1 year, have a normal history and physical examination other than signs and symptoms of anemia.[70] There is neither evidence of hemolysis nor any past history suggestive of hemolytic disease. The complete blood count often shows severe anemia with a normal mean corpuscular volume and absent reticulocyte response. About 60% of cases have mild to moderate transient neutropenia at presentation.[71] The mechanism causing red cell aplasia in TEC is unknown. The treatment of TEC is transfusion of packed red blood cells to support the child with severe anemia and watchful waiting. It is rare for a child with TEC to require a second transfusion.

SPLENOMEGALY

Splenomegaly in children may present acutely or be a chronic finding depending on acuity of the process. The initial assessment of whether the onset of splenomegaly is acute depends heavily on whether the child has had regular well child visits and physical examinations. A differential diagnosis of common disorders causing splenomegaly in childhood is shown in Table 72–7.

In working up the patient for acute splenomegaly, there should be a careful search for systemic disease, usually an infectious or malignant disorder, as a cause. In the patient with chronic splenomegaly, clues include a history of preexisting hemolytic disease, liver disease, or the insertion of an umbilical venous catheter during the newborn period presenting years later with portal vein thrombosis–induced splenomegaly.[72–74] Consanguinity may be a clue for diagnosis of an underlying storage disease. Inflammatory diseases such as systemic lupus erythematosus or sarcoidosis should have characteristic clinical presentations. Physical examination for jaundice, pallor, hepatomegaly, lymphadenopathy, and signs of portal hypertension is indicated. The initial work-up for a child with splenomegaly is outlined in Table 72–8. For many children with acute onset of splenomegaly who appear well and have a normal complete blood count, the initial approach is often to wait a few weeks and reassess the patient because the most common cause is a preceding viral infection. A detailed discussion of disorders of the spleen is presented in Chapter 53.

COMMON LEUKOCYTE DISORDERS

Neutropenia in Infancy and Childhood

In early childhood, neutropenia is a common complication of viral infections and usually is transient. *Severe congenital neutropenia* and *cyclic neutropenia* are usually caused by a defect in the neutrophil elastase gene, as described in depth in Chapter 13. For many years, there had been an entity termed *chronic benign neutropenia of childhood.* In this disorder, children usually presented with common infections of infancy, including otitis, respiratory infections, and diarrhea, and were found to have a coincident neutropenia. Some children also had more characteristic skin and mucous membrane lesions typical of neutropenia, including recurrent fevers, mouth sores, and perianal infections. The prognosis was benign because the neutropenia usually resolved over time. Recent studies suggest that many such cases are due to the presence of autoantibodies directed against the neutrophil, so this disorder should be more appropriately termed *autoimmune neutropenia of infancy.*[75–78] The neutrophil count is often below $500/cm^3$. The diagnosis requires demonstration of antineutrophil antibodies. Children with autoimmune neutropenia have variable symptomatology and often are capable of mounting an adequate neutrophil response to acute infection. However, a subset of these children may need therapy with filgrastim for symptomatic infections. Usually this disorder remits spontaneously over the course of 1–3 years.

In contrast to the benign nature of autoimmune neutropenia, a subset of children with neutropenia present with signs and symptoms of recurrent infections. In addition to neutropenia, the work-up discloses that the child has hypogammaglobulinemia or a high level of immunoglobulin (Ig)M consistent with either common variable immune deficiency or hyper-IgM syndrome, both of which commonly have neutropenia during the course of the illness.[79,80] The treatment of these disorders is optimal management of the immune deficiency.

Childhood Lymphopenia

The most common cause of lymphopenia in children is clearly iatrogenic corticosteroid therapy for inflammatory disorders such as asthma. The differential diagnosis is relatively brief and requires attention to those disorders associated with immune deficiency. In the newborn period, severe lymphopenia is a good indicator of severe combined immunodeficiency. If lymphopenia is observed within the context of recurrent infections, the work-up should include a careful assessment of the child's cellular and humoral immune function, including quantitative and functional measures. One should measure not only the quantitative immunoglobulin levels but also functional antibody titers, as well as test to see if the child has a positive skin reaction to a common antigen such as *Candida*. In adolescents, the teen with lymphopenia should be evaluated for systemic lupus erythematosus, inflammatory bowel disease, and human immunodeficiency virus infection.[81,82]

Lymphocytosis

Lymphocytosis in children is usually viral in origin and can be seen with almost any virus. The mononucleosis syndromes caused by viruses of the Herpesviridae family cause a prominent lymphocytosis with "atypical" or "reactive" T lymphocytes (Fig. 72–4) that are directed against the Epstein-Barr virus–infected host B lymphocytes.[82,83] Pertussis in infants can trigger an impressive lymphocytosis, so the infant or older child who presents with paroxysms of cough (even if immunized) and an elevated total lymphocyte count should be tested for pertussis. A tuberculin skin test should also be done. In the older literature, there are reports of an entity termed *infectious lymphocytosis* wherein a marked lymphocytosis developed in a child with a viral illness. Over the past 20 years, there have been very few such reports, likely the result of increased sophistication in the diagnosis of viral illnesses. The diagnosis of lymphocytosis as a manifestation of lymphoid malignancies is presented in Chapter 33.

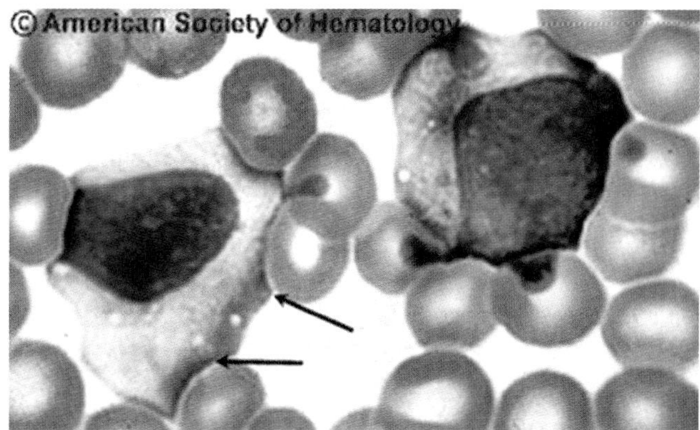

Figure 72–4. Characteristic lymphocytes from an adolescent with infectious mononucleosis. Note the large amount of cytoplasm and indentation of the lymphocyte cytoplasm by red cells *(arrows)*. (Reproduced with permission of American Society of Hematology Image Bank at http://www.ashimagebank.org/case.asp?case_id=100541&name=&subname=)

BLEEDING DISORDERS

Development of the Hemostatic System

From birth to puberty, the physiologic regulation of coagulation undergoes significant developmental changes. Table 72–9 shows a comparison of the coagulation parameters of healthy full-term infants with adult values,[84] and similar data are available for healthy premature infants.[85] These developmental differences in coagulation parameters can be caused by decreased synthesis of coagulation proteins,[86] accelerated clearance of these proteins[87] and/or consumption of components at the time of birth.

Fetal forms of some coagulation factors (such as factor XII, prekallikrein, factor VIII, and fibrinogen) have been described.[88,89] In addition, fetal forms of coagulation inhibitors (such as antithrombin III [AT III] and protein C) do exist.[90] It has been postulated that these fetal forms of coagulation factors and inhibitors have different functional activity.

Several authors have shown that von Willebrand factor (vWF) antigen (vWF:Ag) and vWF-collagen binding activity (vWF:CBA) are increased in newborns.[91] The increased level of vWF:CBA is explained by a higher level of active high-molecular-weight multimeric forms of vWF in this population.[92]

Thrombin generation is delayed and decreased in newborn plasma compared to adult plasma. The degree of impairment is comparable to that in plasma from adults receiving therapeutic doses of anticoagulants. This may explain the lower risk for thromboembolism in children.[93] Consideration of the developmental differences of coagulation factors is important because these coagulation values are the basis for the diagnosis of congenital deficiencies. In addition, plasminogen, tissue plasminogen activator, plasminogen activator inhibitor, α_2-antiplasmin, and histidine-rich glycoprotein, which

TABLE 72–9. Reference Values for Coagulation Tests in the Healthy Full-Term Infant During the First 6 Months of Life*

Coagulation Tests	Day 1	Day 5	Day 30	Day 90	Day 180	Adults
PT (sec)	**13.0 ± 1.43**	**12.4 ± 1.46**	**11.8 ± 1.25**	**11.9 ± 1.15**	**12.3 ± 0.79**	12.4 ± 0.78
aPTT (sec)	42.9 ± 5.80	42.6 ± 8.62	40.4 ± 7.42	**37.1 ± 6.52**	**35.5 ± 3.71**	33.5 ± 3.44
TCT (sec)	**23.5 ± 2.38**	23.1 ± 3.07	**24.3 ± 2.44**	**25.1 ± 2.32**	**25.5 ± 2.86**	25.0 ± 2.66
Factors†						
Fibrinogen (g/L)	**2.83 ± 0.58**	**3.12 ± 0.75**	**2.70 ± 0.54**	**2.43 ± 0.68**	**2.51 ± 0.68**	2.78 ± 0.61
II	0.48 ± 0.11	0.63 ± 0.15	0.68 ± 0.17	0.75 ± 0.15	0.88 ± 0.14	1.08 ± 0.19
V	0.72 ± 0.18	0.95 ± 0.25	0.98 ± 0.18	0.90 ± 0.21	0.91 ± 0.18	1.06 ± 0.22
VII	0.66 ± 0.19	0.89 ± 0.27	0.90 ± 0.24	0.91 ± 0.26	0.87 ± 0.20	1.05 ± 0.19
VIII	**1.00 ± 0.39**	**0.88 ± 0.33**	**0.91 ± 0.33**	**0.79 ± 0.23**	0.73 ± 0.18	0.99 ± 0.25
vWF	1.53 ± 0.67	1.40 ± 0.57	1.28 ± 0.59	1.18 ± 0.44	1.07 ± 0.45	0.92 ± 0.33
IX	0.53 ± 0.19	0.53 ± 0.19	0.51 ± 0.15	0.67 ± 0.23	0.86 ± 0.25	1.09 ± 0.27
X	0.40 ± 0.14	0.49 ± 0.15	0.59 ± 0.14	0.71 ± 0.18	0.78 ± 0.20	1.06 ± 0.23
XI	0.38 ± 0.14	0.55 ± 0.16	0.53 ± 0.13	0.69 ± 0.14	0.86 ± 0.24	0.97 ± 0.15
XII	0.53 ± 0.20	0.47 ± 0.18	0.49 ± 0.16	0.67 ± 0.21	0.77 ± 0.19	1.08 ± 0.28
PK	0.37 ± 0.16	0.48 ± 0.14	0.57 ± 0.17	0.73 ± 0.16	0.86 ± 0.15	1.12 ± 0.25
HK	0.54 ± 0.24	0.74 ± 0.28	**0.77 ± 0.22**	**0.82 ± 0.32**	**0.82 ± 0.23**	0.92 ± 0.22
XIII$_a$	0.79 ± 0.26	**0.94 ± 0.25**	**0.93 ± 0.27**	**1.04 ± 0.34**	**1.04 ± 0.29**	1.05 ± 0.25
XIII$_b$	0.76 ± 0.23	**1.06 ± 0.37**	**1.11 ± 0.36**	**1.16 ± 0.34**	**1.10 ± 0.30**	**0.97 ± 0.20**
AT III (U/mL)	0.63 ± 0.12	0.67 ± 0.13	0.78 ± 0.15	**0.97 ± 0.12**	**1.04 ± 0.10**	1.05 ± 0.13
β_2M (U/mL)	1.39 ± 0.22	1.48 ± 0.25	1.50 ± 0.22	1.76 ± 0.25	1.91 ± 0.21	0.86 ± 0.17
C_1E-INH (U/mL)	0.72 ± 0.18	**0.90 ± 0.15**	0.89 ± 0.21	1.15 ± 0.22	1.41 ± 0.26	1.01 ± 0.15
α_1AT (U/mL)	**0.93 ± 0.22**	**0.89 ± 0.21**	0.62 ± 0.13	0.72 ± 0.15	0.77 ± 0.15	0.93 ± 0.19
HC II (U/mL)	0.43 ± 0.25	0.48 ± 0.24	0.47 ± 0.20	0.72 ± 0.37	1.20 ± 0.35	0.96 ± 0.15
Protein C (U/mL)	0.35 ± 0.09	0.42 ± 0.11	0.43 ± 0.11	0.54 ± 0.13	0.59 ± 0.11	0.96 ± 0.16
Protein S (U/mL)	0.36 ± 0.12	0.50 ± 0.14	0.63 ± 0.15	**0.86 ± 0.16**	**0.87 ± 0.16**	0.92 ± 0.16

†All factors, except fibrinogen, are expressed as units per milliliter (U/mL), where pooled plasma contains 1.0 U/mL.

*All values are expressed as the mean ± 1 SD. Between 41 and 77 samples were assayed for each value for the newborn. Some measurements were skewed because of a disproportionate number of high values. The lower limits, which exclude the lower 2.5% of the population, have been given. All babies received vitamin K at birth. Values that are indistinguishable from those of adults (i.e., do not differ statistically from adult values) are listed in **bold** type.

Abbreviations: α_1AT, α_1-antitrypsin; aPTT, activated partial thromboplastin time; AT III, antithrombin III; β_2M, β_2-macroblobulin; C_1E-INH, C_1-esterase inhibitor; HC II, heparin cofactor II; HK, high-molecular-weight kininogen; PK, prekallikrein; PT, prothrombin time; TCT, thrombin clotting time; VII, factor VII procoagulant; vWF, von Willebrand factor.

From Andrew M, Paes B, Milner R, et al: Development of the human coagulation system in the full-term infant. Blood 70:165–172, 1987, with permission.

belong to the fibrinolytic system, are altered in newborns compared to adults.[94] In newborns, the capacity to generate plasmin is reduced.

Congenital Bleeding Disorders in Infants

Bleeding symptoms in otherwise healthy infants are due to either congenital or acquired hemorrhagic disorders. Hemophilia A (factor VIII deficiency) and hemophilia B (factor IX deficiency) can be diagnosed prenatally, through either examination of fetal DNA or examination of fetal coagulation factors (less frequently). In several case reports, prenatal diagnosis of deficiencies of factors V, VII, XIII, and vWF, or of platelet disorders, has been described.[95–98]

Characteristically, newborns with severe hemorrhagic disorders present with one or more bleeding symptoms such as bleeding in the scalp causing large cephalohematomas as a consequence of birth trauma, persistent bleeding from puncture sites, oozing from the umbilicus, and bleeding from incision wounds in the newborn that happen accidentally during cesarian section or after circumcision.[99] The risk of intracranial hemorrhage during infancy in patients with severe hemophilia A or B ranges from 1% to 4%.[100] Joint bleeding (characteristic for patients with severe hemophilia) does not usually occur during the neonatal period or during the first few months of life. Joint bleeds are observed frequently after the fifth to sixth month of life as soon as the young infant becomes more active. In older infants with hemophilia, hematomas, joint bleeds, and bleeding into the iliopsoas are described. Hemophilia A and B are the most commonly diagnosed congenital factor deficiencies during infancy (see Chapter 63). Because plasma concentrations of many coagulation proteins are reduced physiologically during the first weeks of life, in newborns the correct diagnosis of a congenital factor deficiency can present problems.

Three patterns of hemophilia A are distinguished: severe (factor VIII < 0.01 U/mL), moderate (0.01–0.05 U/mL), and mild (>0.06 U/mL) (see Chapter 63). Because the lower limit of normal for factor VIII is 0.50 U/mL, these forms of hemophilia A can be diagnosed at birth. In newborns, the severe and moderate forms of hemophilia B can be distinguished; however, for the mild forms of hemophilia B, repeated testing in later infancy may be necessary to confirm the diagnosis, because the lower limit of normal for factor IX at birth is approximately 0.15 U/mL.[84,85]

Because of the physiologic enhancement of vWF function during the first weeks of life, neonates with von Willebrand disease (vWD) rarely show bleeding symptoms. However, if the newborn presents with bleeding symptoms, specific assays for factor VIII and vWF should be performed to diagnose rarer forms of vWD with concomitant severe factor VIII deficiency. If the neonate presents with thrombocytopenia and bleeding symptoms, the newborn should be investigated for vWD type 2B. Thrombocytopenia and skin bleeding have been described in a neonate diagnosed with vWD type 2B.[101]

Rare congenital hemorrhagic disorders such as homozygous deficiencies of factors II, V, VII, X, XI, XII, prekallikrein, and high-molecular-weight kininogen can be diagnosed at birth because the plasma concentration of the corresponding coagulation factor is then reduced to less than 0.10 U/mL.[102] Patients with deficiencies of factor XII, high-molecular-weight kininogen, or prekallikrein do not generally present with bleeding symptoms. In children with homozygous factor XII deficiency who underwent tonsillectomy or adenoidectomy, no prolonged bleeding has been reported. However, in single patients with homozygous factor XII deficiency who underwent surgery involving the urogenital tract, postoperative bleeding occurred, most probably because of the high fibrinolytic activity in the urogenital tract.[103] Infants with homozygous factor VII or factor X deficiency can present with joint bleeding and severe hematomas.

Factor replacement with either fresh frozen plasma (FFP) or factor concentrates is used as therapy of deficiencies of factors II, V, VII, X, and XI. FFP is useful when the nature of the coagulopathy is unknown. Infusion of 10 mL/kg FFP increases the plasma concentration of a specific factor by approximately 0.10 U/mL in adults and older children. Depending on the situation (e.g., surgery, severe bleeding), the recovery of the specific coagulation factor should be measured after administration of the factor concentrate.

Newborns with inherited afibrinogenemia, hypofibrinogenemia, or dysfibrinogenemia in the homozygous state may present with bleeding symptoms (e.g., delayed umbilical bleeding) as described in neonates with homozygous factor XIII deficiency.[99,101] About 30% of patients with homozygous factor XIII deficiency develop a spontaneous intracranial hemorrhage during their lives. Either FFP or factor XIII concentrate is used as treatment.

Acquired Bleeding Disorders

Acquired bleeding disorders in otherwise healthy infants and children are due to either immune thrombocytopenia or vitamin K deficiency. In sick children, either liver failure or disseminated intravascular coagulation (DIC) can cause the bleeding symptoms.

Vitamin K Deficiency Bleeding

The vitamin K–dependent coagulation factors (II, VII, IX and X) are synthesized in the liver and stored there as inactive precursors (PIVKA, or proteins induced by vitamin K absence). Vitamin K induces the γ-carboxylation of these coagulation molecules and turns them into (zymogen) coagulation factors that are released into the blood. In the case of severe deficiency, the inactive forms of factors II, VII, IX, and X (decarboxylated factors) are released into the blood and can be detected there.

Three forms of vitamin K deficiency bleeding are distinguished. The rare early form of vitamin K deficiency occurs in breast-fed neonates within the first 24 hours of life. In some of these cases, the mother had received anticonvulsants, anticoagulants, rifampicin, or isoniazid without prophylactic treatment with vitamin K.[104] The classical form of vitamin K deficiency known as hemorrhagic disease of the newborn occurs between day 2 and day 7 of life in breast-fed, full-term newborns. Newborns and babies are at risk for developing vitamin K deficiency because breast milk does not contain sufficient vitamin K. After breast-feeding is stopped, vitamin K is absorbed together with the regular nutrition.

The late form (third form) of vitamin K deficiency occurs between weeks 2 and 8 and rarely after 3 months of life. The late form is often caused by low vitamin K content of the milk (almost exclusively in breast-fed infants), or by malabsorption of vitamin K (e.g., because of cholestasis, chronic diarrhea, cystic fibrosis, celiac disease, or intestine/colon resection) or other disorders such as α_1-antitrypsin deficiency and hepatitis.[104] Vitamin K deficiency develops slowly (symptoms often occur after 3–4 months) in children who receive parenteral nutrition. If the child is severely ill or receives antibiotics, the deficiency can develop faster. Vitamin K deficiency in children can cause gastrointestinal bleeding (hematemesis, melena), urogenital bleeding (hematuria), and intracranial or skin bleeding (Fig. 72–5). In addition, prolonged bleeding from puncture sites may be observed.

To establish a diagnosis of vitamin K deficiency, one first screens with the prothrombin time and the activated partial thromboplastin time (aPTT). The specific factor assays will show that factors II, VII, IX, and X are decreased. However, reduced levels of factor V (which is observed in liver failure) rule out vitamin K deficiency. A reduction of factor II activity and normal values for factor II concentration (antigen) indicate that the inactive form of factor II (PIVKA II) is higher than the active form and lead to the diagnosis of vitamin K deficiency. Low values of factor II activity combined with low values of factor II antigen are observed in diseases such as liver failure or hereditary factor II deficiency. Because factor VII has the shortest half-life (4–5 hours) of the vitamin K–dependent coagulation factors, factor VII activity declines first in vitamin K deficiency and in liver failure. In DIC, the prothrombin time is prolonged and thrombocytopenia and increased D-dimers are observed.

To prevent vitamin K deficiency, newborns receive prophylactic vitamin K. Depending on the country in which they reside and the condition of the newborn, vitamin K is administered either orally, intravenously, or intramuscularly. Most groups in the United States and Canada recommend a single dose of 0.5–1 mg intramuscularly. A meta-analysis reported that vitamin K prophylaxis intramuscularly was more effective than single-dose

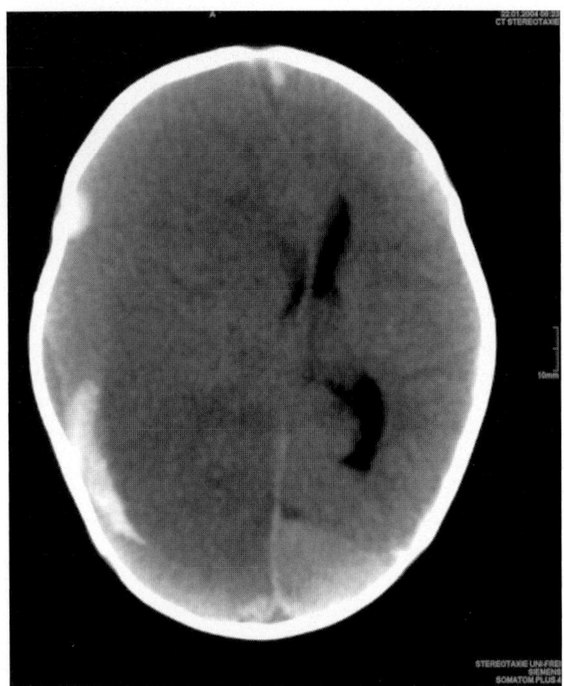

■ **Figure 72–5.** Vitamin K deficiency bleeding in a 7-week-old infant. Intracranial bleeding and edema on the right side and falx deviation are seen on computed tomography scan. (Courtesy of Dr. Moske, Department of Radiology, University of Freiburg.)

oral prophylaxis. However, multiple-dose oral prophylaxis may be a suitable alternative (used in Europe).[105] In Europe, if the newborn is premature or severely ill (shock or sepsis) or in cases of malabsorption of vitamin K, the vitamin K is given intravenously. In cases of vitamin K deficiency, oral administration of vitamin K shortens the prothrombin time within a few hours. In cases of malabsorption of vitamin K, parenteral administration is necessary. If the prothrombin time does not shorten after intravenous administration of vitamin K, liver failure must be considered.

A patient with bleeding symptoms who is suspected of having vitamin K deficiency should be immediately administered vitamin K subcutaneously or intravenously even before laboratory results confirm the diagnosis. Depending on the severity of bleeding, therapy with 10–20 mL/kg of FFP should be started in addition. The amount of plasma necessary to correct a severe vitamin K deficiency may result in volume overload. Therefore, in such life-threatening bleeding situations, a concentrate consisting of factors II, VII, IX, and X (prothrombin complex concentrate) can also be administered. Rarely, deficiency of all vitamin K–dependent factors results from mutations in the γ-glutamyl carboxylase gene[106] or the epoxide reductase gene.[107] Some of the patients show improved levels of active clotting factors after large doses of vitamin K.

Disseminated Intravascular Coagulation

DIC is an acquired coagulation disorder that is caused by various acute or chronic diseases.[108] Characteristically, a systemic intravascular coagulation process starts that causes thrombus formation in the microcirculation and then initiates fibrinolysis, causing an increased turnover of platelets and coagulation factors leading to an increased bleeding risk (see Chapter 89).

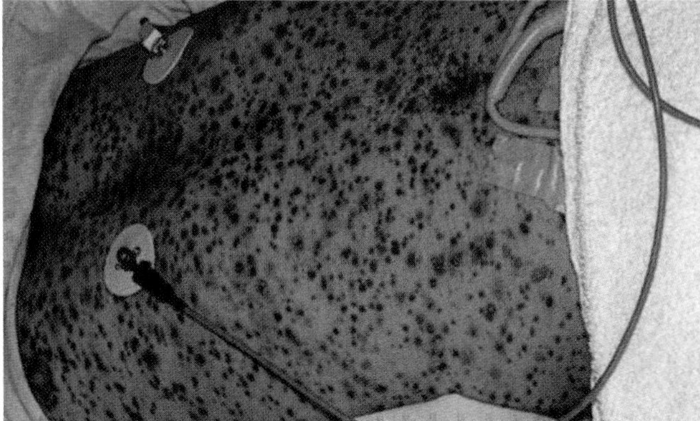

■ **Figure 72–6.** Skin lesions in a child with meningococcus sepsis and DIC. (Courtesy of Dr. Berner, Department for Children and Adolescents, University of Freiburg.)

DIC most often is caused by infection or sepsis (i.e., by infections with gram-negative bacteria or meningococcus) (Fig. 72–6). However, DIC can also develop in viral infections (e.g., varicella) and during or after extensive surgery and trauma. DIC has been reported in malignant diseases, in vascular disease, or during extracorporal membrane oxygenation. In premature newborns, DIC can also develop secondary to respiratory distress syndrome, hypothermia, and meconium or amniotic fluid aspiration syndromes.

The best prevention and treatment of DIC is early diagnosis and treatment of the underlying disease that causes the activation of coagulation and finally DIC. Besides low platelet counts, increased D-dimers, and prolonged prothrombin time and aPTT, reduced levels of protein C, protein S, and AT III are observed.

Other Disorders Associated with Bleeding Symptoms

Bleeding disorders have been described in newborns with cyanotic congenital heart disease[109,110] and liver disease. In addition, an increased risk of bleeding has been reported during or after cardiopulmonary bypass and during extracorporeal membrane oxygenation. These bleeding disorders are caused by reduced coagulation factors (because of hemodilution and consumption), activation of the fibrinolytic system, and quantitative and qualitative platelet defects.[111] The use of heparin (in cardiopulmonary bypass and extracorporal membrane oxygenation) increases the risk of bleeding.

Acquired Inhibitors in Coagulation

The diagnosis of "acquired inhibitors" can sometimes be difficult to establish because the clinical symptoms and the laboratory results can be very heterogeneous. Several groups of inhibitors are described.

Antiphospholipid Antibodies in Children

Antiphospholipid antibodies that occur during childhood are most frequently transient (see Chapter 68). These antibodies can develop after minor infections (mainly respiratory infections) and are usually discovered during preoperative screening (prolonged aPTT) in otherwise healthy children.[112] The etiology and pathology of these inhibitors remain unclear. They generally disappear after about 2–9 months; however, sometimes they can be detected for up to 3 years. No therapy has been described so far. These childhood-type antiphospholipid antibodies can cause bleeding if they are associated with hypoprothrombinemia or severe thrombocytopenia. In the literature, only a few children with these inhibitors have been reported to suffer from bleeding symptoms during or after surgery. If these childhood-type antiphospholipid antibodies are combined with protein C or S deficiency, they can lead to thromboembolic events.[113]

Inhibitors Against Single Coagulation Factors

During infancy, inhibitors against factor VIII or factor IX are described in patients with hemophilia A and B, respectively.[114] Usually these inhibitors develop in about 20–25% of patients with hemophilia A after about 9 exposure days (to exogenous factor VIII). Inhibitor antibodies occur in 1–3% of patients with severe hemophilia B. Characteristically, after administration of factor VIII or IX, respectively, the bleeding does not stop in these patients and the recovery of factor VIII or IX is insufficient. The work-up and management of inhibitors in patients with hemophilia are described in Chapters 63 and 105. Other acquired inhibitors against single coagulation factors are less frequent in children than in adults.

THROMBOTIC DISORDERS

The incidence of thrombotic events during infancy and childhood has continuously increased during the last decade. During the last 10 years, central venous lines (CVLs) and total parenteral nutrition, which increase thromboembolic risk, have been used more frequently. Compared to adults, the incidence of thromboembolic events such as deep venous thrombosis (DVT) and pulmonary embolism is still rare in children (40% vs. 5%, respectively). The Canadian Registry of Venous Thromboembolic Complications in Children reported an incidence of DVT/pulmonary embolism of 0.07 per 10,000 pediatric population and 5.3 per 10,000 hospital admissions.[115] The physiologic hemostatic system (decreased potential to generate thrombin compared to adults) is probably protective against thromboembolic disease. Several other factors (e.g., integrity of the vessel wall; no acquired thrombotic risk factors such as oral contraceptives, smoking, antiphospholipid antibodies) contribute to the low incidence of thrombosis in children. Most children with thrombosis suffer from a serious underlying disease such as congenital heart disease, nephrotic syndrome, cancer, trauma, surgery, or systemic lupus erythematosus.[115,116]

In the pediatric age group, infants less than 1 year of age and teenagers have the greatest risk for DVT/pulmonary embolism. CVLs are the most common risk factor for thromboembolism in newborns (>80%) and in children (>50%).[117] Because CVLs are placed in the upper venous system in children, most of the DVT in neonates and children occurs in the upper venous system and provides a source for pulmonary embolism.[118] CVLs in the upper venous system can cause chylothorax or eventual destruction of the upper venous system. The incidence of CVL-related thromboembolic events in children receiving long-term total parenteral nutrition varies from 1% based on clinical diagnosis, to 35% based on ventilation-perfusion scans or echocardiography, to 75% based on venography.[119] Eighteen percent of children who had a CVL in place for 48 hours developed a CVL-related DVT.[120] In children with acute lymphoblastic leukemia receiving asparaginase therapy, the incidence of DVT is 37% (proven by venography). Ultrasound technique missed about 80% of these clots in this study.[121]

To confirm the diagnosis, a venogram is the gold standard. However, in neonates and infants, frequent ultrasound is performed to diagnose the thromboembolic event. To detect pulmonary embolism, spiral computed tomography scan is recommended. Magnetic resonance imaging, magnetic resonance arteriography, and magnetic resonance venography are the best current methods to detect thromboembolic events.

Neonates

Clinically apparent thrombosis (excluding stroke) occurs in 2.4 per 1000 neonatal intensive care unit admissions.[122] The incidence of symptomatic thrombosis is 2.4–5.1 per 100,000 births.[122,123] Eighty percent of cases of renal vein thrombosis (RVT), the most common non–catheter-related venous thrombosis during infancy, occur in the first months of life.[122] In 75% of the cases, RVT is unilateral. In term infants, RVT often presents within the first days of life with hematuria (30% of the patients), proteinuria, a palpable abdominal mass, and thrombocytopenia. Infants of diabetic mothers are at higher risk to develop RVT because of polycythemia and increased platelet aggregability.

RVT has been described secondary to nephrotic syndrome, dehydration, fever, AT III deficiency, burns, and systemic lupus erythematosus in older children.[124] Using ultrasound techniques, the thrombus can be detected within the renal vein and possibly the inferior vena cava. Most important is an effective therapy of the predisposing cause of RVT. Dialysis will become necessary if the RVT occurs bilaterally. The use of anticoagulants or thrombolytic agents is highly controversial. Unfractionated heparin should be administered in the presence of unilateral RVT that extends into the inferior vena cava. Thrombolytic therapy may be considered in case of bilateral RVT and impending renal failure.[125]

Neonates with homozygous protein C or protein S deficiency develop purpura fulminans within hours of birth. Purpura fulminans is an acute, lethal syndrome that progresses rapidly. The neonate presents with hemor-

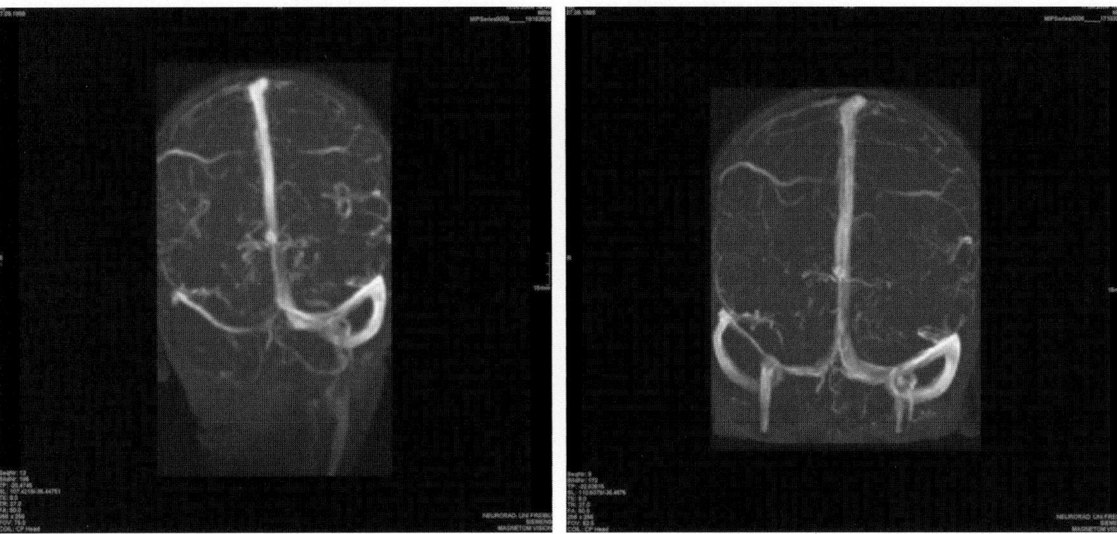

Figure 72–7. Sinovenous thrombosis in a child before and after heparin treatment as seen on magnetic resonance imaging scan. (Courtesy of Dr. Fisch, Department of Radiology, University of Freiburg.)

rhagic necrosis of the skin (due to dermal vascular thrombosis) and cerebral or ophthalmic damage. Early treatment with FFP (10–20 mL/kg every 12 hours) is necessary. As soon as the diagnosis of protein C deficiency is confirmed, protein C concentrate should be administered. Doses of protein C concentrate reported in the literature range from 20 to 60 U/kg. Replacement of protein C should be continued until the clinical lesions disappear (usually 6–8 weeks). Infants with homozygous protein C deficiency (and no detectable plasma concentration of protein C) require long-term treatment with oral anticoagulant therapy and intermittent protein C replacement with protein C concentrate. Some patients with homozygous protein C or S deficiency (with detectable plasma concentrations of protein C) have been treated with low-molecular-weight (LMW) heparin. Using LMW heparin avoids the risk of oral anticoagulant–induced skin necrosis and may reduce the risk of bleeding associated with high doses of oral anticoagulants.[126]

The incidence of sinovenous thrombosis in newborns is 41 per 100,000,[122] and in childhood is 0.67 per 100,000 (Fig. 72–7).[127] The incidence of neonatal arterial ischemic stroke is 28 per 100,000 live births, and the incidence in older children is 3.3 per 100,000 children per year.[128] Clinical symptoms of neonates with stroke are frequently lethargy and seizures.

Catheterization of the umbilical vessels bears a special thromboembolic risk for neonates. In up to 29% of neonates with umbilical venous catheters, thrombi have been detected radiographically.[129] As prophylactic therapy, continuous heparin infusion (3–5 U/hr) is administered through central lines in children.

Inherited Thrombotic Disorders

In most children, a combination of multiple risk factors causes thrombosis (Table 72–10). Injury to the endothelium (e.g., infectious vasculitis, vascular catheter) or dysregulation of coagulation (e.g., sepsis, congenital or acquired coagulation protein abnormality) can induce thrombosis. Typical for congenital prothrombotic conditions are a positive family history, early age of onset of thromboembolism, and recurrent thrombosis.

TABLE 72–10. Underlying Disorders or Other Predisposing Factors in Children with Venous Thrombosis or Pulmonary Embolism

Indwelling catheters
Surgery
Immobilization
Trauma, burns
Systemic lupus erythematosus
Infection
Tumor
Total parenteral nutrition
Disorder of hemostasis causing predisposition to thrombosis
Nephrotic syndrome
Estrogen use
Obesity
Ulcerative colitis
Immobilization
Heparin-induced thrombocytopenia
Polycythemia (infants of diabetic mothers)
Dehydration

Besides the most common inherited prothrombotic risk factors, such as protein C, protein S, and AT III deficiency, other prothrombotic conditions such as activated protein C resistance/factor V Leiden (FV-R506Q) and prothrombin G20210A polymorphism have been described.[130] Activated protein C resistance and prothrombin G20210A polymorphism have less impact on individual risk compared to protein C, protein S, and AT III deficiency; however, factor V Leiden and prothrombin G20210A occur with high frequency in certain populations and are therefore important. Activated protein C resistance (factor V Leiden) is due to a mutation in factor V (mutation of arginine-506 to glutamine-506) that makes the mutant form resistant to inactivation by normal activated protein C[131] (see Chapter 67).

Patients with dysfibrinogenemia can develop either bleeding symptoms (31% of cases) or thrombosis (11% of cases) depending on the kind of mutation.[132] Plasminogen deficiency or an increase of plasminogen activator inhibitor-1 can lead to an increased risk for thromboembolic events in adults.

A decreased activity of 5,10-methylenetetrahydrofolate reductase may cause an increased level of homocysteine, which is associated with a higher risk for arterial thrombosis (endothelial injury). The elevated level of homocysteine can result from a homozygous MTHFR mutation or from vitamin B_{12}, vitamin B_6, or folate deficiency.[133–135] Therefore, in such cases vitamin B_6, vitamin B_{12}, and folate levels should be measured; if reduced, they may be substituted.

Acquired Thrombotic Disorders

Lupus Anticoagulants

Lupus antibodies (anti-phospholipid antibodies) were so named because they were first described in patients with lupus erythematosus. They have since been identified in patients with other diseases (e.g., autoimmune disease, lymphoproliferative disease, infectious disease). These antibodies are not as frequently detected in children compared to adults. This group of autoantibodies are directed against phospholipid-protein complexes and cause a prolonged aPTT in phospholipid-dependent coagulation tests. Lupus antibodies (IgM and IgG antibodies) increase thromboembolic risk, especially in adults. Thrombosis has been reported in 5% of children with positive lupus antibodies. Characteristically, the aPTT is prolonged and several coagulation factors (VIII, IX, XI, and XII) are decreased as a result of a nonspecific inhibitory effect in the clotting assay. Additional tests (plasma exchange test, kaolin clotting time, and dilute Russell's viper venom time) are used to confirm the diagnosis (see Chapter 68).

Nephrotic Syndrome

In children with nephrotic syndrome, thromboembolic events do not develop as frequently as in adults (incidence 3.3% vs. 19.5–50%). The thromboembolic events were observed mainly during the first 3 months of diagnosis,[136] and are frequently associated with increased levels of factor VIII and fibrinogen and decreased levels of AT III and factor XII.

Thromboembolic Complications in Oncology Patients

Central venous catheters cause an increased thromboembolic risk in children with oncologic diseases. In addition, the thromboembolic risk increases if the tumor narrows blood vessels and changes blood velocity. Hormone therapy, cytostatic agents (e.g., L-asparaginase), and prednisone increase the thromboembolic risk even further.

In patients with bone marrow transplantation, veno-occlusive disease (VOD) is a dangerous complication. Characteristically, the children complain about pain in the upper abdomen and suffer from hepatomegaly, hyperbilirubinemia, and ascites. Several reasons for VOD have been discussed (low levels of protein C, protein S, and AT III or hypofibrinolysis, because plasminogen activator inhibitor-1 is increased in patients with bone marrow transplantation), but the etiology is not clear. The prophylactic use of heparin has been controversial. Attal and colleagues described a decrease in the incidence of VOD in patients who received continuous infusion of heparin (100 U/kg/day).[137] Defibrotide has been successfully used in the therapy of VOD.[138]

Oral Contraceptives

Oral contraceptives cause an increased risk of thrombosis (four times over baseline) because they lead to increased levels of vitamin K–dependent factors, factor VIII, and fibrinogen and decreased fibrinolytic activity.[139] This etiology must be considered in young women who present with thromboembolic disease.

Kawasaki Disease

Thrombotic complications during the acute phase of Kawasaki disease include medium and large vessel arteritis, arterial aneurysms, valvulitis, and myocarditis. The most severe complication is coronary artery aneurysm, which may cause stenosis or thrombosis and which will develop if initial treatment with aspirin was started too late or not initiated at all. Initial aspirin therapy consists of 80–100 mg/kg/day during the acute phase (up to 14 days as an anti-inflammatory agent), then in lower doses as an antiplatelet agent (3–5 mg/kg/day for 7 weeks or longer) to prevent coronary aneurysm thrombosis and infarction, which is the major cause of death in Kawasaki disease.[140,141] According to a meta-analysis, children treated with intravenous immunoglobulin and aspirin had a significantly lower incidence of coronary artery aneurysms than those treated with aspirin alone.[142]

Vascular Catheters

Symptomatic thrombotic complications in children occur most frequently (40%) from usage of arterial catheters or from cardiac catheterization via the femoral artery without prophylactic heparinization. Anticoagulation with heparin reduces the incidence of thromboembolism from 40% to 8%. Further heparin boluses are frequently used in prolonged procedures (>60 minutes).[143] Saxena and colleagues[144] reported that the administration of heparin 50 U/kg was equally efficacious as heparin 100 U/kg during cardiac catheterization.

Renal and Hepatic Artery Thrombosis

In children, renal artery thrombosis following kidney transplantation ranges from 0.2% to 3.5%. Young children especially are at risk to develop a renal artery thrombosis. Broyer and coworkers reported on prophylactic therapy with LMW heparin (0.4 mg/kg/every 12 hours for 21 days).[145,146] In a few patients with heparin-induced thrombocytopenia and kidney transplantation, hirudin (at a very low dose and under close monitoring) has been successfully used as prophylactic therapy.

Rela and associates[147] reported that the incidence of hepatic artery thrombosis following liver transplantation in children and adults, in their study, was 4.2%, and in children under 5 years of age the incidence was 11%. The prophylactic use of anticoagulants such as unfractionated heparin, LMW heparin, and aspirin is controversial.

Antithrombotic Treatment in Children

Standard Heparin

Standard heparin is widely used as an anticoagulant in children. In neonates, heparinization can be difficult because AT III is physiologically low at birth and can decrease even more in sick children. After an initial bolus of 75–100 U/kg of heparin (over 10 minutes), a maintenance dose of 28 U/kg/hr is administered in infants younger than 1 year, and 20 U/kg/hr is administered in children older than 1 year. The prolonged aPTT corresponds to an anti–factor Xa level of 0.3–0.7 U/mL. However, this laboratory test is not always available. Therefore, a prolongation of the aPTT to 2.0–2.5 times the control level (aPTT 60–85 sec) is considered to be adequate for therapeutic heparin levels.[148] The side effects of heparin are discussed in Chapters 88 and 69.

LMW Heparin

The recommended therapeutic dose for enoxaparin (LMW heparin) is 1.5 mg/kg subcutaneously every 12 hours for neonates and infants younger than 2 months, and 1 mg/kg subcutaneous every 12 hours for children older than 2 months. The recommended prophylactic dose for enoxaparin is 0.75 mg/kg subcutaneously every 12 hours for neonates and infants younger than 2 months, and 0.5 mg/kg subcutaneous every 12 hours for children older than 2 months. An advantages of LMW heparin is the twice-daily dosing, which can be facilitated by using a subcutaneous catheter for 1 week.[149]

Warfarin

The oral anticoagulant warfarin inhibits vitamin K, which is essential for synthesis of factors II, VII, IX, and X. Therefore, the sensitivity to warfarin is increased in the event of vitamin K deficiency, which may occur in breast-fed infants. Warfarin therapy, monitored by prothrombin time, is now reported as an International Normalized Ratio (INR), which makes the comparison of the patient's INR values when measured in different laboratories feasible.

Warfarin therapy can be initiated with a loading dose of 0.2 mg/kg (maximum 10 mg); then the dose needs to be adjusted to reach an INR of 2–3 (recommended therapeutic range). For children with prosthetic cardiac valves, the recommended INR is 2.5–3.5. Capillary whole-blood prothrombin time monitoring (providing an INR with a fingerstick sample of blood) provides excellent home management of warfarin anticoagulation therapy.[150] The complication of warfarin-induced skin necrosis (resulting from decreased protein C) can be prevented by starting the warfarin treatment under heparin therapy. Other complications of warfarin are increased bleeding risk and growth retardation. Depending on the severity of bleeding symptoms, vitamin K and/or prothrombin complex concentrate is administered to reverse bleeding.

Anticoagulant therapy after a thromboembolic event is dependent on the clinical situation.[151]

Thrombolytic Therapy

Commonly used thrombolytic agents in children are tissue plasminogen activator and urokinase. The relative risk/benefit ratio of thrombolytic therapy requires consideration on an individual basis. Fibrinogen levels should be measured frequently during thrombolytic therapy, because the risk of bleeding complications increases when fibrinogen levels fall below 100 mg/dL. Platelet counts should be above 100×10^9/L. The most common complication associated with the use of thrombolytic agents is hemorrhage. Significant bleeding should be treated by cessation of the thrombolytic agent as well as any other antithrombotic agents being administered concurrently.

CURRENT CONTROVERSIES & FUTURE CONSIDERATIONS

Pediatric Hematology

- How can we prevent iron deficiency anemia throughout all socioeconomic, ethnic, and racial groups?
- What is the optimal regimen for eradication of inhibitors in children with hemophilia?
- What are the underlying causes of warfarin resistance and sensitivity?
- Will recombinant Factor VIIa be useful in the management of platelet disorders? In the management of intracranial hemorrhage?
- Which child with SCD is at highest risk for stroke, acute chest syndrome, or other life threatening complications at an early age and thus should be a candidate for hematopoietic stem cell transplantation?
- Which child with autoimmune neutropenia should be treated with granulocyte colony-stimulating factor, and for how long?
- Can we develop more accurate, readily available testing for hereditary spherocytosis and other hemolytic anemias in the newborn?
- How can we better prevent thromboembolic events in neonates and in children with CVLs?

Suggested Readings*

American Academy of Pediatrics, Section on Hematology/Oncology and Committee on Genetics: Health supervision for children with sickle cell disease. Pediatrics 109:526–535, 2002.

Nathan D, Orkin S, Ginsburg D, Look A (eds): Hematology of Infancy and Childhood (ed 6). Philadelphia: WB Saunders, 2003, Chs 1, 2, 7, 10, 14, and 19.

Oski FA: Iron deficiency in infancy and childhood. N Engl J Med 329:190–193, 1993.

Segel GB, Hirsh MG, Feig SA: Managing anemia in a pediatric office practice: Part 1. Pediatr Rev 23:75–84, 2002, Part 2. Pediatr Rev 23:111–122, 2002.

Young SN, Alter BP (eds): Aplastic Anemia: Acquired and Inherited. Philadelphia: WB Saunders, 1994.

Full references for this chapter can be found on accompanying CD-ROM.

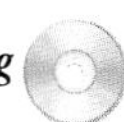

CHAPTER 73

GERIATRIC HEMATOLOGY

Nathan A. Berger, MD, and Daniel Rosenblum, MD, FACP

KEY POINTS

Geriatric Hematology

- Few abnormalities have been documented to be the result of age alone.
- Pathologic changes in the elderly are often the result of multiple interacting disorders.
- The assessment of an elderly individual with a hematologic disorder should include an evaluation of prognostic factors.
- Comorbidities and concomitant medications influence patient response to therapeutic regimens.
- Few therapeutic regimens have been systematically evaluated in the context of an aging population with comorbidities and concomitant medications.

INTRODUCTION

A comprehensive treatment of geriatric hematology is beyond the scope of a single textbook chapter because most of the disorders commonly seen by hematologists and described elsewhere in this textbook affect the geriatric population. Instead, this chapter is designed to present an expanded discussion of selected topics in hematology that have special importance to the geriatric population.

In 2003, the number of individuals over 65 in the United States was 35 million, a group representing 12% of the U.S. population and growing about eight times faster than the rest of the population. As the population ages, some hematologic diseases once considered rare have become common. As a consequence, the caseloads of anemia, acute myelogenous leukemia, myelodysplastic syndrome, venous thromboembolic disease, and nonvalvular atrial fibrillation now number over 5,000,000 in the United States. Hematologists are often called upon to recommend treatment for patients with these disorders, but evidence-based management is often unavailable in the older age groups because of a lack of adequate well-designed and well-controlled trials. The lack of evidence is a major reason for a chapter that deals with topics in geriatric hematology: it is a field ripe for exploration, burdened by beliefs not founded on careful scientific observation, and one to which clinical investigators are invited to pay increased attention. To support an evidence-based approach to medical management, regimens should be formally tested in the geriatric population, particularly those over 85 years of age, a group that will quintuple in size in the next four decades. Although many elderly individuals are healthy, health conscious, active, and productive, their hematologic needs are poorly defined. To provide adequate care will require special attention to the ways in which benign and pathologic changes affect the elderly.

A number of common precepts should be debunked. The belief that biologic changes such as anemia are part of the "normal aging process" is not based on careful studies. Rather, other factors that are more common in the elderly than in younger individuals are responsible for pathologic changes. In fact, anemia is not normally found in healthy elderly people. Some pathologic processes could be expected to worsen with the passage of time, but it is the duration of the process, not age, that results in the altered morbidity. Accumulation of genetic mutations may be a key factor as well. One cause of chromosomal change, telomeric shortening, is known to progress in susceptible individuals. The result is a process called "chromosomal aging." Shortened chromosomes are more susceptible to the sorts of genetic damage that could predispose to malignant change. It is not clear whether telomeric shortening is a hereditary or acquired disorder or, instead, a generalized manifestation of the "normal aging process." In any case, the resultant chromosomal changes are inhomogeneously distributed among individuals, with many elderly individuals having no significant karyotypic abnormalities.

A precise, uniformly accepted definition of the geriatric population has not been established. In preparing this chapter, we noted that many reports do not distinguish elderly subjects by means of objective criteria, but instead use an arbitrary age cutoff. Aging is a heterogeneous process. Frail elderly are prone to increased morbidity in contrast to their robust counterparts at the same age. Characteristics shown to have a greater influence on health than age include genetic predisposition, mutations, comorbidities, inactivity, and obesity. Investigators should stratify studies in aged individuals with these factors rather than use cohorts based on age alone. When formulating recommendations for elderly patients, hematologists should factor in functional status, mental performance characteristics, compliance patterns, personal economics, concomitant medications, alternative medicine usage, organ function, and disease-specific risk factors.

HEMATOLOGIC AND VASCULAR ASPECTS OF AGING

Normal Hematologic Values in the Elderly

In a recent literature search, longitudinal studies were absent from almost all discussions of age-associated trends in normal hematologic values (Table 73–1). Informal observations suggest that blood counts (hemoglobin, hematocrit, neutrophil count, lymphocyte count, and platelets) remain constant over decades in otherwise healthy aging seniors tested in the same laboratory. The onset of anemia in an elderly individual is invariably related to an identifiable pathologic process.

Red Blood Cells

Some investigators have maintained that mild anemia is normal for elderly individuals (hemoglobin <13 gm/dL in men, <12 gm/dL in women). So-called senile anemia was characterized as a mild, nonprogressive normochromic, normocytic anemia of obscure cause that lacked specific symptoms and did not respond to treatment.[1] In a recent report on centenarians,[2] among 14 men and 75 women, 6 of the men and 53 of the women had normal values (hemoglobin 13.9 ± 0.7 for men, 13.1 ± 0.8 for women), whereas anemia was diagnosed in 8 men (hemoglobin 11.8 ± 0.9) and 22 women (hemoglobin 10.5 ± 1.57). In this survey, all the anemic men and all but four of the anemic women had other known abnormalities that might have explained the anemia. Significantly, a majority of the subjects had normal values.

Platelets

Platelet counts do not change with age. Specific increases have been reported in β-thromboglobulin,[3] urine 2,3-dinor-thromboxane B_2, and von Willebrand factor; aggregation thresholds to ADP are lower[4] and the bleeding time is shorter.[5] In contrast, platelets from elderly subjects do not differ from platelets from younger subjects with respect to glycoprotein IIb/IIIa receptors, lipid peroxide, Na^+, K^+-ATPase activity, and sialic acid content.[6,7]

TABLE 73–1. Normal Hematologic Values in the Elderly*

Hemoglobin	Men ≥ 13 gm/dL Women ≥ 12 gm/dL
Platelets	≥150,000/μL
White blood cells	4500–10,000/μL
Coagulation factors	↑ Fibrinogen ↑ Factors V, VIII, and IX
Cytokines	↑ IL-6

*It is not established that age, by itself, is the cause of any changes in hematologic values.

Leukocytes

In a study in Italy and Germany of 148 subjects ranging from newborns to centenarians, there was no progressive change in leukocytes in subjects over 15 years old.[8] Specifically, total counts of leukocytes, lymphocytes, neutrophils, monocytes, eosinophils, and basophils remained constant.

Lymphocytes

The lymphocyte count does not decline with age. In a cohort study of individuals over 84 years old in Leiden, the Netherlands, a low lymphocyte count in subjects who were ill had no influence on short-term mortality. However, healthy elderly subjects with very low lymphocyte counts had an adverse prognosis. In 106 healthy subjects, a lymphocyte count in the lowest quartile was associated with a doubling of all-cause mortality during the following 2 years compared to subjects in the highest quartile. It is interesting that a 112-year-old individual in the Leiden study had a total lymphocyte count of $2.39 \times 10^9/L$, a value that placed her in the 93rd percentile of the study group.[9]

Lymphocyte function has been observed to change with age. Of particular interest are the findings of diminished natural killer cell activity,[10] increased $CD16^+$ lymphocytes, fluctuating CD95, and decrease $CD4^+$ lymphocytes. It is possible that the lymphocytes of the majority of individuals in their 70s and 80s are more susceptible to apoptosis when stimulated, thus accounting for the relatively poor secondary response to immune stimulation and apparent increased risk of infection in these individuals.

Although the cause of the altered membrane receptors in the lymphocytes of the aged remains unknown, it appears that studies of T-cell immune diseases, in particular those that affect the elderly, should take into account potential differences between normal, healthy elderly subjects and a younger normal, healthy population. Physiologic aging of lymphocytes, including changes in the surface receptors,[11] may account for immune differences common to elderly individuals. Loss of T-cell function has been imputed to thymic involution, a process that may continue until the sixth decade. Poor responsiveness to immunization in older individuals may be due to impaired T-cell function. In addition, bone marrow stem cells from older individuals have an impaired ability to differentiate into lymphocytes.[12]

A single randomized, placebo-controlled trial in elderly individuals provided evidence that vitamin and mineral supplementation resulted in a significant increase in immune responses as judged by CD4 T-cell percentage, natural killer cell activity, T-cell mitogenic response, and interleukin (IL)-2/IL-2 receptor expression as well as a reduced number of days of illness as a result of infection. In contrast, three other randomized, placebo-controlled studies of vitamin and mineral supplementation failed to show a benefit.[13] Although β-carotene supplementation in elderly male participants in the Harvard Physicians Health Study was associated with enhanced natural killer cell activity. However, β-carotene had no comparable effect on natural killer cell activity in younger men and may have had an adverse effect on the risk of lung cancer.[14]

Neutrophils

As mentioned previously, neutrophil numbers do not decline even with advanced age.[15] Di Lorenzio and colleagues reported a decline in superoxide in healthy nonagenarians compared to subjects in their 20s,[10] but this has no apparent clinical impact.

Coagulation Factors

Thrombotic disorders are a major cause of morbidity and mortality in the elderly. Age alone has not been proven to be the cause of the changes in any of a wide variety of coagulation factors that have been reported to be elevated in elderly individuals. Fibrinogen,[16] for example, has been shown to increase with age in several studies. Increased fibrinogen levels are correlated with an increased risk of cardiovascular events and increases in IL-6, which also has been reported to increase with age. Observers have described increases in factors V, VIII, and IX with age. In contrast, factors VII, X, and prothrombin were not shown to change. The mechanisms responsible for the changes in coagulation factor levels have not been identified.

Caution should be used in correlating age and coagulation factor levels, because factors such as lack of physical activity alone can cause levels to rise. A British study of older men reported that regular exercise reduced fibrinogen, plasma and blood viscosity, platelet count, coagulation factors VIII and IX, von Willebrand factor, D-dimer, tissue plasminogen activator (reflecting plasminogen activator inhibitor-1 levels), C-reactive protein, and white cell counts.[17] The effect of exercise on these factors was independent of a history of cardiovascular disease, smoking, and obesity. Weight loss reduced plasminogen activator inhibitor-1 levels in obese young men.[18] Thus, behavior, diet, and other factors may be the operative influence on changes in coagulation factors, rather than age alone.

Cytokines

A repeated finding in hematologic studies of aging is a rise in IL-6, a proinflammatory cytokine and a hematologic growth factor that stimulates B-cell production, T-cell activation, and thymocyte and platelet development. In one report, median IL-6 levels were 10 times higher in a group of centenarians than in a group of normal young adults. Increases in IL-6 could result from decreased androgen or estrogen production, a constant accompaniment of aging. The source of increased IL-6 production could be stimulated monocytes, fibroblasts, and endothelial cells, although the mechanism of stimulation is not clear. It could also be a byproduct of inflammation, because it is known to be made by macrophages, granulocytes, and lymphocytes. Increased IL-6 levels correlate with a variety of disorders, including inflammation and malignancy. It may be an important determinant of osteoporosis, depression, rheumatoid arthritis, B-cell neoplasias, and dementia. They induce C-reactive protein, haptoglobin, and fibrinogen. High levels of IL-6 are predictive of physical decline[19] and, along with C-reactive protein, of all-cause mortality in healthy elderly people.[20]

Vascular Changes

"Senescence" has been documented in the endothelium of the blood vessel wall. Plasma factors that contribute to endothelial senescence include tissue factor and factor VII, which initiate the coagulation cascade, as well as thrombomodulin, nitric oxide synthase, heparan sulfate–containing proteoglycans, tissue plasminogen activator, and plasminogen activator inhibitor-1. The signaling molecule, Ras can induce vascular senescence in vitro and in vivo.[21]

Bone Marrow Response

While blood cell counts and marrow cellularity may be normal, because the hematopoietic response to stress, chemotherapy, and hematopoietic growth factors appears blunted in patients over the age of 60. A variety of factors may account for this, including changes in the marrow microenvironment, altered cytokine production, and genetically defective marrow progenitor cells.[22]

ANEMIA IN THE ELDERLY

Risks Associated with Anemia

Anemia has a variable effect on mortality in elderly subjects (Box 73–1). In a Dutch study, anemia in apparently healthy people over 85 years old more than doubled the risk of mortality,[23] supporting the concept that the finding of unexplained anemia in older adults signifies masked pathology. Similar findings have been reported in other populations.[24] Anemic subjects had the highest mortality in every age group between 70 and 100. Subjects with the lowest hemoglobins had the highest mortality. Anemia predisposes to an increased risk from surgical procedures as well. Of note, the increased surgical risk associated with preoperative anemia is not reduced by preoperative transfusion.[25]

The genesis of anemia in the elderly is multifactorial and nonuniform.[26] An analysis by site of evaluation[27] revealed that hospital inpatients had a higher incidence of hematopathology than patients evaluated in a community outpatient setting. In contrast, nonhematologic causes of anemia, such as infection, were more prevalent in outpatients. Also, more cases of anemia were classified as "unexplained" in the outpatient setting. Some

Box 73–1. Anemia in the Elderly

- Not a normal finding
- Mortality doubled
- Secondary to
  - Organ failure (kidneys, liver)
  - Myelodysplasia
  - Bleeding
  - Medications
- Other factors
- Slow response to replacement therapy

of the unexplained anemia may have been due to renal failure and myelodysplastic syndrome (MDS) (see Chapter 15), which are likely to be underdiagnosed in elderly outpatients.

Causes of Anemia

Anemia is common in men and women over the age of 75, and is often associated with multiple specific morbidities. These include malignancy, renal failure, and gastrointestinal bleeding (Box 73–2). Hypothyroidism, occult gastrointestinal bleeding caused by benign or malignant disorders, malabsorption, myelosuppression, and idiosyncratic immune reactions should also be considered. Medications frequently cause anemia (Table 73–2). The list of medications often responsible for anemia includes nonsteroidal anti-inflammatory agents, proton pump inhibitors, cytotoxic agents, antibiotics, psychotropics, and cardiac medications. A variety of factors contribute to the retardation in marrow response, or "hematopoietic reserve,"[28] including impaired iron utilization associated with chronic disease states, chronic inflammatory diseases such as rheumatoid arthritis, and a reduced rate of growth of bone marrow stem cells.

Malignancy associated with blood loss is among the first considerations in patients referred for evaluation of anemia. It is important to exclude these diagnoses, even though they are relatively uncommon compared to the disorders mentioned previously, because of the potentially fatal implications. The incidence of colorectal cancer and pancreatic cancer rises steadily as people age, becoming the leading cause of fatal cancer in octogenarians. The familiar hallmarks—change in bowel habits and hematochezia—may be intermittent or absent. A rectal examination and flexible sigmoidoscopy may be negative. Iron deficiency associated with low ferritin levels is likely to develop within weeks of a slow, persistent blood loss. A colonoscopy or imaging study should be recommended in the belief that it is better to be overly cautious than neglectful, particularly since prompt management of localized cancer of the cecum is often curative. Anemia of obscure origin may be the first clue leading to the diagnosis of an occult malignancy such as myeloma, lymphoma, gastric cancer, and even nasopharyngeal cancer. Invasive tests may be required to establish a diagnosis. An aggressive approach to diagnosis can be justified by the possibility of finding a curable disease, such as a mucosa-associated lymphoid tissue (MALT) lymphoma (a gastrointestinal lymphoma associated with *Helicobacter pylori*) or cecal carcinoma, both of which should be addressed without delay.

MDS is relatively common among individuals over the age of 80. MDS is relatively subtle in its early stages and,

Box 73–2. Diagnosis of Anemia in the Elderly

- Trace development over time
- Evaluate underlying comorbidities (may be multiple):
  - Malignancy (especially gastrointestinal)
  - Inflammation
  - Kidney failure
  - Disease of the oral cavity
  - Liver failure
  - Poverty, inadequate diet, iron deficiency
  - Malabsorption
  - Alcoholism
  - Hypothyroidism
  - Bleeding
  - Surgical procedures
  - Primary disease of bone marrow
  - Medications (past and present) as a cause of bleeding, immune reaction, or marrow suppression
- Tailor treatment to etiology of anemia

TABLE 73–2. Examples of Medications Associated with Anemia

Class of Agent	Mechanism
Antibiotics	Myelosuppression Autoimmunity
Anticoagulants	Blood loss
Anti-inflammatories	Blood loss Myelosuppression
Cardiac medications	Myelosuppression Autoimmunity
Chemotherapy drugs	Myelosuppression
Proton pump inhibitors	Impaired iron absorption

as a consequence, is often overlooked. It is described in detail later in this chapter and in Chapter 15. It may be asymptomatic and associated with a chronic, steady anemia. Pancytopenia, if present, is an important clue. Evidence of ineffective erythropoiesis (high lactate dehydrogenase level, poikilocytosis, macrocytosis) can often be detected by examining the peripheral blood film.

Recent reports have emphasized a potential role of IL-6 in promoting anemia in elderly people. IL-6 suppresses erythropoiesis and the response of erythroid progenitor cells to erythropoietin. Hemodilution may also play a part because inflammatory conditions that produce a rapid rise in IL-6 may be associated with dramatic fluid retention, including an increase in plasma volume as great as 10–18%.

Evaluation of Anemia in the Elderly

The prevalence of anemia among the elderly imposes a need for efficient evaluation and effective management. Indeed, because multiple factors may be operative, it is helpful to remain open to additional possibilities even after a single cause of anemia has been established. Skilled consultants persist in the evaluation until plausible explanations are found, as illustrated in the following vignette.

A consultant saw an 80-year-old woman for anemia. The anemia was a slowly evolving, normocytic, normochromic anemia (hemoglobin 10.2 gm/dL) with no specific symptoms other than fatigue and lethargy. The woman had hypertension and arthritis, for which she took a β-blocker, a diuretic, and a nonsteroidal anti-inflammatory. Physical examination was nonrevealing. Stools were repeatedly negative for occult blood, and serum iron and transferrin saturation were in the low-normal range. An air-contrast barium enema and an upper gastrointestinal series were negative. Kidney function was marginal, with a creatinine of 2.4 mg/dL. Liver and thyroid function tests and a bone marrow aspirate were normal, and a direct antibody test was negative. The woman's anemia was slowly progressive; after 6 months, the hemoglobin was 9.1 gm/dL. Computed tomography scans of chest and abdomen were negative. Stool and serum iron studies were repeated: the stool occult blood test was positive, and the iron studies showed a low serum ferritin and transferrin saturation. A second air-contrast barium enema showed a nearly obstructing carcinoma of the transverse colon.

IRON DEFICIENCY AND IRON OVERLOAD

Of the common nutrients involved in regulation of hematopoiesis, iron is unique in that pathology may result from either deficiency or excess. The elderly are susceptible to both.

Iron Deficiency

Iron deficiency was present in 5% of the anemic and 8% of the nonanemic patients among 186 consecutive elderly subjects, median age 85, who were admitted to the geriatrics unit of a Swiss University Hospital, based on low serum iron and transferrin saturation in the absence of signs of inflammation or general malnutrition.[29] A low serum ferritin even without anemia should lead to a thorough investigation for gastrointestinal blood loss.[30] Therapy should be directed at the cause of iron loss. Supplemental iron therapy should be used to reconstitute iron stores. Oral iron therapy is the treatment of choice in the compliant older patient and is as efficient and rapid at restoring the hematocrit as parenteral iron therapy. Parenteral iron is recommended for patients unable or unwilling to take oral therapy and for subjects who fail to respond to an oral dose with a rise in transferrin saturation.

In the Swiss series,[29] 42% of the patients with anemia met criteria for generalized malnutrition, most characteristically associated with low values for serum albumin, cholinesterase, zinc, transferrin, and transferrin saturation. Another 14% of patients in the study were found to have anemia associated with inflammation as indicated by a high C-reactive protein level.

Iron Overload

Increased iron stores, as judged by serum ferritin levels, were prevalent in a group of elderly American subjects, 67–96 years old, who took supplemental iron or who consumed a diet rich in red meat and fruit. Iron stores were not increased in those who took vitamin C alone.[31] Little evidence of organ damage has been found in subjects given dietary iron supplementation in the absence of genetic abnormalities of iron homeostasis. Indeed, evidence has not established the existence of an age-related dysregulation of iron homeostasis.[31] Attention has been brought to the prevalence of hereditary hemochromatosis without symptomatic manifestations.[32,33] However, hereditary hemochromatosis has an insidious onset that may slowly lead to organ damage, so vigilance is in order in patients with asymptomatic iron overload.

Homozygosity for the gene responsible for hereditary hemochromatosis is estimated to be present in 0.5% of individuals of Northern European descent but may be clinically evident only in the elderly. Many patients with subclinical hemochromatosis are over 50 years old, and some are over 80. Using molecular biologic mutation analysis to screen large population samples, a study of more than 41,000 subjects identified the homozygous gene mutation most commonly found in hereditary hemochromatosis in 152 patients who had no greater prevalence of symptoms of hemochromatosis than did normal controls.[32]

Hereditary hemochromatosis and its associated tissue iron deposition can result in multisystem organ failure. Recent studies suggest, however, that asymptomatic adults in whom hereditary hemochromatosis is detected by genotyping are unlikely to develop clinically overt hemochromatosis or iron toxicity and are, therefore, unlikely to require therapeutic interventions to reduce iron stores.[32,33] Interventions to reduce iron stores should probably be reserved for symptomatic patients with elevated transferrin saturation, increased ferritin levels, and genotypic homozygous hemochromatosis and evidence of organ toxicity caused by iron. Asymptomatic patients should be observed on an annual basis for signs of progression to organ damage.

VITAMIN B_{12}-COBALAMIN AND FOLIC ACID DEFICIENCIES

Cobalamin deficiency is common in the elderly.[34,35] Elderly patients should undergo the same evaluation and management procedures for megaloblastic anemia caused by either cobalamin or folic acid deficiency as are used in younger individuals with deficiencies of these vitamins. However, as many as 12–25% of elderly subjects have been reported to have borderline cobalamin deficiency, sometimes accompanied by macrocytosis, with little or no anemia or other cytopenias. Of more consequence, neuropsychiatric disorders have been reported with borderline cobalamin deficiency and hallmark elevations of plasma methylmalonic acid and total homocysteine.[36–38] The borderline deficiency of cobalamin differs from pernicious anemia in that it is not associated with antibodies to intrinsic factor. Elderly subjects with borderline cobalamin deficiency have been reported to respond to oral administration of cobalamin at doses of 1000 μg/day with normalization of their mean corpuscular volume and methylmalonic acid level and improvement of some of their neuropsychiatric pathology, including cognitive performance and cerebral function, but not dementia.

Histamine H_2 receptor blockers and proton pump inhibitors interfere with absorption of dietary cyanocobalamin.[39] Elderly subjects on prolonged therapy with these agents have been noted to have vitamin B_{12} deficiency manifest as lowered vitamin B_{12} levels and elevated serum methylmalonic acid and homocysteine levels. The markers of vitamin B_{12} deficiency resolved when the elderly subjects were given 1000 μg of cyanocobalamin daily.

Poor nutrition and lack of leafy vegetables can give rise to folate deficiency with accompanying macrocytic anemia. Early myelodysplasia can also increase erythropoiesis, giving rise to an effective folate deficiency. Use of folate replacement in the management of anemia associated with myelodysplasia may avoid the need for transfusion or erythropoietin treatment.

HEMATOLOGIC DISORDERS ASSOCIATED WITH DRUGS, MECHANICAL DEVICES, AND ALTERNATIVE MEDICATIONS

Elderly subjects are more likely to be exposed to health-associated interventions than younger people. Some agents are of greater concern, however, such as alkylating agents, topoisomerase inhibitors, nonsteroidal anti-inflammatory drugs, certain classes of psychotropic medications (e.g., clozapine), cardiac antiarrhythmics (e.g., quinidine), propylthiouracil, some antibiotics and metabolic inhibitors, and cytotoxic agents. Use of these products should be preceded by effective patient education and prospective analysis of adverse events. Implanted devices in the arterial or venous circulation may be associated with thrombotic stimuli or microangiopathic hemolytic anemia. Patients with these devices should be appropriately monitored for anemia, thrombosis, thrombocytopenia, and changes in erythrocyte morphology.

The use of alternative medications by the elderly is on the rise in the United States.[40,41] Antiplatelet effects and interactions with anticoagulants are potential complications associated with the use of saw palmetto, gingko biloba, and St. John's wort. Yohimbine, an herbal remedy for erectile dysfunction, inhibits platelet aggregation.[42] Saw palmetto, which has been used for prostatism, can cause a reversible bleeding diathesis resulting in prolonged bleeding and intraoperative hemorrhage.[43]

Men may employ androgens for anabolic purposes, to stimulate libido, or to enhance sexual performance. Androgens increase erythropoiesis by stimulating sensitive bone marrow stem cells and by raising erythropoietin levels.[44] As a result, androgen users may develop an increased red cell mass. The erythrocytosis may be sufficient to induce symptoms suggestive of polycythemia vera, such as headache, pruritus, and weakness. Unlike polycythemia vera, however, androgen-induced erythropoiesis does not cause splenomegaly, a rise in leukocyte alkaline phosphatase, increased serum vitamin B_{12}–binding proteins, thrombocytosis, or leukocytosis. In addition, the erythrocytosis and the associated symptoms usually resolve after androgen stimulation is stopped.

DIRECT ANTIGLOBULIN TEST IN THE ELDERLY POPULATION

The elderly have been said to be at increased risk of having a positive direct antiglobulin test (DAT), which may indicate an age-related immune dysfunction. Autoimmune hemolytic anemia with a positive DAT may also occur. A positive DAT with or without anemia may be associated with a lymphoproliferative disorder, which, if present, is often the focus of evaluation and therapy. Two large series reported that the incidence of positive DATs in apparently healthy blood donors was between 1 in 7500 and 1 in 14,000.[45,46] Both series claimed that the incidence of positive DAT increases with age. However, neither series contained healthy patients over 65 who had a positive DAT. In the absence of compelling evidence that a positive DAT in older individuals is caused by physiologic immune dysfunction, a reasonable search for a malignant cause should be made.

BONE MARROW RESERVE AND TRANSPLANTATION

Alterations in bone marrow output as a function of aging have been variably ascribed to changes in hematopoietic regulatory growth factors, however, deficits, when they occur, can usually be bypassed by administration of hematopoietic growth factors.[46a] Age associated increases in the proinflammatory cytokine, IL-6, may contribute to development of anemia in older patients.[19,20,47] Proliferative capacity of hematopoietic stem cells may be sufficient to maintain normal hematologic status over several lifespans as evidenced by serial bone marrow transplants in experimental animals.[47a] However, hematopoietic stem cells from older human subjects have shown compromised proliferative capacity. Even so, the bone marrow of older people can maintain normal blood counts under normal conditions. Under abnormal conditions, the bone marrow reserves in the elderly may muster a limited response with delay in recovery of normal blood counts. Thus, elderly patients often do not respond with the brisk bone marrow proliferation seen in younger patients after typical stresses such as blood loss, recovery from acute infection, replacement of a missing nutrient, and the rebound associated with recovery from myelosuppressive chemotherapy. However, studies of the response to granulocyte colony-stimulating factor (G-CSF) in healthy young and old subjects show no significant age-related difference in dose response, marrow maturation, or increase in peripheral blood polymorphonuclear leukocyte count.[48] Nonetheless, the bone marrow stem cells of elderly individuals may be inadequate to support autologous transplantation.

Multiple studies have failed to show a significant difference between older and younger individuals who have cancer with respect to myelotoxicity after chemotherapy. Furthermore, comorbidities, common in the elderly, may compromise restoration of normal blood counts. For this reason, the National Cancer Center Network has recommended that older patients receiving myelosuppressive chemotherapy be given erythropoietin to correct anemia and G-CSF or granulocyte-macrophage colony-stimulating factor to hasten granulocyte count recovery.[49]

Replicative Senescence of Hematopoietic Stem Cells

Decay in functional numbers of hematopoietic stem cells after repeated divisions "replicative senescence" may be associated with a programmed cell death, as occurs in lymphocytes, an accumulation of acquired mutations, or both. Hematopoietic stem cells in humans and other species undergo age-associated shortening of chromosomal telomeres, an alteration that contributes to reduction in their long-term performance capacity.[50] In addition, these cells may develop a defect in DNA repair capacity that is progressive with age. For instance, mitogen-stimulated peripheral blood lymphocytes from subjects over 60 years were found to have a threefold increase in chromosomal translocations when compared to lymphocytes from subjects less than 40 years of age. Recent studies have detected a surprising level of multiple mutations in mitochondrial DNA of bone marrow and peripheral blood $CD34^+$ cells derived from healthy adult donors (a cohort age 54 and younger) compared to $CD34^+$ cells from umbilical cord blood.[51,52] The changes in nuclear and mitochondrial DNA may have a profound effect on myeloid function and replicative capacity, and a variety of hematologic abnormalities.

Hematopoietic Stem Cell Transplantation

Hematopoietic stem cell transplantation (HSCT) has frequently been reported to have higher rates of morbidity and mortality in older patients, limiting its use even as the incidence of most hematologic malignancies is increased in the elderly.[53] Unfavorable prognostic indicators for HSCT in leukemia are chromosomal abnormalities and expression of the multidrug resistance phenotype, both of which are more common in older individuals. Other factors that influence the outcome of HSCT include the type of transplant (autologous versus allogeneic), number of stem cells available for reconstitution, toxicity of the conditioning regimen, duration of neutropenia, presence of graft-versus-host disease (GVHD), and other comorbidities.[53] The use of G-CSF–mobilized peripheral blood hematopoietic stem cell $CD34^+$ cells has been associated with increased transplant success and reduction of morbidity and mortality following HSCT, in part as a result of more rapid recovery of granulocyte count and reduction of infectious compared to patients receiving bone marrow hematopoietic stem cells.

While there is an overall age associated decrease in peripheral blood hematopoietic stem cells,[53a] a wide range of individual variation has been shown so that some older subjects have decreased numbers of $CD34^+$ cells and others have levels equivalent to much younger subjects. Similar numbers of progenitors have been identified in G-CSF mobilized cells obtained from adults and children[54] and collection of sufficient $CD34^+$ cells can improve outcomes. Mortality in older patients with myeloma was reduced to 8% when two courses of high-dose chemotherapy each followed by autologous HSCT were used.[55] An increase in toxic deaths has been reported in older subjects exposed to conditioning regimens that included total-body irradiation. In contrast, chemotherapy conditioning regimens were not reported to increase toxic deaths in older individuals.[53]

Compared with the rates in younger individuals, the incidence of acute GVHD is moderately increased and chronic GVHD is markedly increased with age following allogeneic transplantation. Because the outcome of peripheral blood HSCT depends on management of GVHD, older patients who receive allogeneic transplants should be treated with aggressive preventive immunosuppressive regimens.

ACUTE MYELOGENOUS LEUKEMIA

The frequency of acute myelogenous leukemia (AML) rises with advancing age. In the 1980s, the median age of patients with AML was less than 62 years, with 54% of the patients being greater than 60 years old.[56] As the proportion of adults over 65 has increased, the median age of AML has shifted upward,[57,58] and is now over 64 years (Box 73–3). In the past, remission induction with chemotherapy was rarely attempted in older people because of a belief that it would be poorly tolerated and generally ineffective. Until recently, few studies of AML included subjects over 70. Since 1990, a large number of trials have been reported in subjects with eligibility criteria designed to include subjects more than 55 years old. The complete remission rates have been in the range of 50%, although many were of short duration. The prognosis of patients with AML is adversely influenced by

Box 73–3. Acute Myelogenous Leukemia in the Elderly

- Median age 64
- 7000 cases/U.S. population/year
- Prognostic factors predicting poor outcome:
  - Anemia
  - Unbalanced chromosomal translocations
  - Abnormal chromosome 5 or 7
  - High lactate dehydrogenase level
  - High white blood cell counts/blasts/neutropenia
  - Antecedent MDS
  - No complete remission after first course of therapy
  - Short complete remission
- Complete remission rate 40–50% for those admitted to trials (many otherwise eligible are excluded because of age alone)
- Treatment options:
  - High-dose cytarabine (25% neurotoxicity)
  - Gemtuzumab ozogamicin (deep venous thrombosis)
- Better prognosis with
  - Balanced chromosomal translocation
  - t(15;17), t(8;21), and inv(16)/t(16;16)
  - Younger age

antecedent chemotherapy with alkylating agents or a topoisomerase, hemorrhage, infection, poor performance status, and comorbidities. Prognostic factors clearly linked to a poor response rate include hemoglobin level, hypocellularity, abnormalities of chromosomes 5 and 7, complex chromosomal abnormalities, preexisting trilinear MDS, and comorbidities.[59,60] Multiple drug resistance (MDR1 positivity) is an additional risk factor that has been reported in about 70% of the acute leukemias of elderly people. Unfortunately, inhibition of the MDRI drug transporter increases the toxicity of chemotherapeutic agents, and does not improve remission rates.[60a] At present no improvement in survival has resulted from any of the interventions designed to improve outcome in older subjects with antecedent myelodysplasia, impaired drug clearance, and stem cells with decreased tolerance to myelosuppressive therapy.[61]

In reports from nine cooperative groups between 1985 and 1997, only about a third of subjects in the trials were over 60.[62] The data on elderly people with AML who received full doses of induction therapy consistently showed a complete remission rate of 40–50% with 17% two-year survival. Use of high-dose cytarabine in elderly adults has resulted in higher complete remission rates at a cost of a 25% mortality rate and unacceptable neurotoxicity.[63] Standard-dose cytarabine and full-dose daunorubicin (60 mg/m^2 for three courses) have improved the complete remission rate to 60% in some studies.[64] Use of myeloid growth factors[65–67] has been explored as a means of overcoming the susceptibility of elderly leukemic patients to infection and to produce an overall survival benefit. Although a benefit has been shown in some studies, no improvement in complete remission rate, early death, or overall survival has been reported.[68]

In 2000, the Food and Drug Administration approved gemtuzumab ozogamicin (GO, Mylotarg), a humanized monoclonal antibody directed to the CD33 antigen that is chemically conjugated to a potent toxin, calichemicin, for older adults in first relapse. It has activity against the majority of blasts in AML. When used alone gemtuzumab has been associated with a relatively high incidence of veno-occlusive disease.[69]

Acute promyelocytic leukemia differs from other leukemias. It has a good survival rate regardless of age.

MYELODYSPLASTIC SYNDROME

Myelodysplastic syndrome is a descriptive term comprising a group of disorders of hematopoietic maturation. The incidence[70] in elderly adults is close to 100/10^5, the same order of magnitude as colon carcinoma, and it is the most prevalent hematologic malignancy in patients over 75 (Box 73–4). Milder forms are likely to be underdiagnosed or to be ignored in the extremely aged because of its insidious onset and the presence of comorbidities. MDS is commonly subdivided according to the French-American-British classification into refractory anemia (RA), refractory anemia with ringed sideroblasts (RARS), refractory anemia with excess blasts (RAEB), and preleukemia(RAEB-t). The etiology of MDS is explored in Chapter 15 in this volume. The mechanism by which the elderly accumulate genetic mutations, whether repeated exposure or faulty repair mechanisms,[71] remains to be fully elucidated. Importantly, as many as a third of elderly people with AML have been reported to have antecedent MDS, which worsens the prognosis of AML.[72] Of those at risk, none had a greater risk of rapid onset of acute leukemia than elderly subjects with increased marrow blasts and adverse karyotypic characteristics. Milder forms of MDS are typified by subjects with trilinear dysplasia and chronic cytopenias but without an identified genetic mutation. In the more advanced forms of MDS, the disorder is characterized by clonality associated with a cytogenetic abnormality.[73] The risk of treatment-related MDS is increased in the elderly, often with a prolonged delay between exposure and the onset of MDS. Early forms of MDS are often underdiagnosed.

Patients with asymptomatic but progressive pancytopenia or progressive symptoms related to a cytopenia

Box 73-4. Myelodysplastic Syndrome in the Elderly

- Most common hematologic malignancy in the elderly
  - Affects $22/10^5$ per year over age 70
  - Affects $90/10^5$ per year over age 80
  - Compare with colon cancer ($360/10^5$ per year over age 75)
- Cause
  - Secondary to chemotherapy (alkylating agents), radiation therapy, benzene, other toxic products (50%)
  - Unknown (50%)
- Prognostic factors (IPPS)[97]:
  - Gradations of severity: RA, RARS, RAEB, RAEB-t
  - Karyotype abnormalities
    - Sometimes present
    - Del(q5), del(q20), −Y favorable
    - Complex, chromosome 7 unfavorable
  - Genetic mutations increase with time/age
- 20–30% progress to AML
- Most patients ultimately require transfusions as MDS progresses
- No general curative therapy
  - AML resistant to chemotherapy
  - Stem cell transplantation under study
  - Anti–thymocyte globulin toxic, relatively ineffective
  - No response to imatinib
  - 5-azacytidine recently approved

have received empirical therapy with folate, pyridoxine, danazol, and G-CSF with variable results. Patients with low erythropoietin levels and a moderate to severe anemia have been reported to benefit from therapy with erythropoietin; patients with low folate levels may improve with folic acid replacement.[74] If four doses of weekly erythropoietin fail to produce a rise in the patient's hemoglobin, a higher dose has been shown to be helpful in some patients and is currently being evaluated in clinical trials. However, if ineffective, the growth factor should be discontinued. The FDA recently approved 5-azacytidine for treatment of all subtypes of MDS. In a randomized, controlled trial the response rate (complete and partial) was 16% in the azacytidine arm.[75] Transfusion dependence (two units of packed red blood cells every 3 weeks) ultimately develops in the majority of individuals, although progression to transfusion dependency may not occur until after a prolonged period of stable or slowly progressive bone marrow dysfunction. Iron chelation therapy should be considered to treat or prevent iron overload in transfusion-dependent patients. Such patients accumulate approximately 0.25 gm of iron per unit transfused and develop a body burden of iron of 10–15 gm over 12–18 months of full-replacement transfusion. Severe complications of MDS obviate consideration of chelation therapy with desferotamine until newer oral agents are shown to be equally effective.

In general, patients with MDS who undergo transformation to AML do poorly. Early reports of clinical improvement[76] associated with anti–thymocyte globulin therapy for MDS prompted transient enthusiasm. Anti–thymocyte globulin has now been tested sufficiently to say that it is of limited value and highly toxic in elderly subjects (complete remission rate of 16%, with only 8% of 32 patients surviving over a year),[77] and at least one group has recommended against its use in unselected subjects with MDS.[78] Imatinib has been tested in a small group of subjects with MDS (n = 8) without clinical response.[79]

VENOUS THROMBOEMBOLIC DISEASE

The incidence of thrombotic events associated with venous thromboembolic disease increases a thousandfold between the ages of 40 and 75. In 75-year-olds, the reported risk has ranged from $100/10^5$ to $1000/10^5$ per year in various population groups. The risk continues to rise with each decade. The cause of the rise in thrombotic events is not altogether clear and may be tied to inactivity and other pathologic processes such as malignancy and inflammation that affect circulating levels of cytokines and coagulation factors, primary disorders of the vascular endothelium, or combinations of factors acting in concert (Boxes 73–5 and 73–6). A study in a Minnesota population compared risk factors in subjects who had a single episode of venous thromboembolism (VTE) with those in subjects who had never had a VTE.[80] The predominant risk factors were pathologic processes rather than age. In descending order, the major factors that increased the risk of VTE were recent surgery, trauma, hospital or nursing home confinement, presence of a malignant neoplasm with or without chemotherapy, central venous catheter or pacemaker placement, superficial vein thrombosis, and extremity paresis from neurologic disease. Four of the factors associated with an increased risk of VTE could be attributed to immobilization, five to irritation or disruption of veins, and six to hospitalization and/or an invasive procedure.

The decision to search for underlying pathology in a subject with a first episode of VTE is based on a careful

Box 73–5. Medical Conditions Associated with Increased Risk for Venous Thromboembolic Disease[98]

- Previous VTE
- Hypercoagulable state
- Paresis or paralysis of lower limb
- Neurologic disease that compromises mobility
- Malignancy (stomach, lung, pancreas, etc.)
- Recent myocardial infarction
- Congestive heart failure
- Severe chronic obstructive pulmonary disease
- Trauma
- Varicose veins
- Superficial vein thrombosis
- Severe infection
- Inflammatory bowel disease
- Obesity

Box 73–6. Iatrogenic Factors Associated with Increased Risk for Venous Thromboembolic Disease[98]

- Hospital or nursing home confinement
- Surgery
- Placement and presence of a central venous catheter or pacemaker
- Chemotherapy
- Hormone replacement therapy

survey of the history and physical examination and judgment about the potential risks and benefits of further evaluation and potential therapeutic interventions. However, malignancy should be considered in this setting because of its ominous implications. The malignancies most likely to cause VTE are cancer of the pancreas, lung, colon, gastrointestinal tract, and, occasionally, breast.[81]

Prevention of VTE should be strongly considered for patients at increased risk to reduce morbidity and mortality. Common risk conditions include postoperative recuperation from prosthetic hip or knee surgery, stroke, and trauma, and chronic conditions such as obesity, cancer, and lower extremity weakness. The risk of VTE is also increased in patients who have had a prior VTE; it is greatly increased in the first year and diminishes in subsequent years. A number of studies have shown a benefit in reduction of VTE in subjects at high risk when given prophylactic doses of unfractionated heparin (typically 5000 units three times daily) or low-molecular-weight (LMW) heparin (typically 40 mg daily). The incidence of VTE was reduced from 15% to 5% with LMW heparin therapy in a placebo-controlled trial in elderly subjects at risk because of medical problems.[82] Prophylaxis with low-dose unfractionated heparin or standard-dose LMW heparin is recommended by the Clinical Practice Committee of the American Geriatrics Society for elderly individuals with risk factors.[83] When warfarin is chosen as the oral anticoagulant, the therapeutic goal is an International Normalized Radio (INR) of 2.0–2.5, a range that optimally balances the antithrombotic benefits and the hemorrhagic risks. Long-term use of LMW heparin may be indicated depending on the nature of the risk and the duration of the comorbidity.

Box 73–7. Nonvalvular Atrial Fibrillation in the Elderly

- Risk of atrial fibrillation increases with age
- Risk of ischemic stroke increases with age in patients with atrial fibrillation
- Anticoagulation
  - Warfarin for patients at moderate or high risk
  - Aspirin for patients at low risk
  - Heparin not of benefit
- Dose-dependent lengthening of prothrombin time predicts risk
  - INR $\geq$ 2.0: effective protection
  - INR $\leq$ 1.8: no protection

ANTICOAGULATION FOR NONVALVULAR ATRIAL FIBRILLATION

The incidence of nonvalvular atrial fibrillation increases with age (Box 73–7), and in most instances requires judicious use of anticoagulation. In a 44-year study of healthy men, the annual incidence of atrial fibrillation was less than 0.5/1000 person-years at age 50, rising to 10/1,000 person-years by age 70.[84] In a British epidemiologic study, the incidence in people over age 65 was 4.7%.[85] By extrapolation from data applicable to current populations and the anticipated growth in the geriatric population, more than 5 million Americans will have atrial fibrillation by the year 2050. Over half of them will be over 80.

A variety of factors increase the risk of atrial fibrillation, including hypertension, coronary artery disease, congestive heart failure, cardiomyopathy, hyperthyroidism, alcohol, caffeine, certain medications, and cardiac inflammation. All are age related. Subjects with intermittent atrial fibrillation and those with sustained atrial fibrillation were at the same risk of ischemic stroke in a longitudinal cohort study,[86] with an annual risk of stroke of about 3.3% per year. Subjects with intermittent atrial fibrillation were more likely to be younger, female, and free of congestive heart failure. The chance of stroke rose to nearly 20% per year in the presence of multiple major risk factors such as left ventricular congestive heart failure, hypertension, increasing age, diabetes mellitus, and previous transient ischemic attack or ischemic stroke.

Several studies have analyzed risk factors of subsequent stroke. Two such studies, conducted by the Atrial Fibrillation Investigators and the Stroke Prevention in Atrial Fibrillation Investigators, evaluated patients 65 years and older who had nonvalvular atrial fibrillation and were not taking anticoagulant medication. By combining the data from these studies, a strong predictive model was developed that uses a scoring system known by its acronym as the CHADS2 index (representing the risk factors congestive heart failure, hypertension, age, diabetes mellitus, and stroke or transient ischemic attack).[87] The CHADS2 scoring system allows 1 point for each of the first four risk factors and 2 points for the last. A score of 0 is associated with an adjusted stroke rate of 1.9% per year, a score of 6 is associated with a risk of 18.2% per year. The Framingham study[88] identified increasing age, female gender, recent history of smoking, systolic hypertension, diabetes mellitus, myocardial infarction or congestive heart failure, heart murmur, and prior history of stroke or transient ischemic attack as risk factors for subsequent stroke. The latter model has been incorporated in a website (*http://www.nhlbi.nih.gov/about/framingham/stroke.htm*) that allows the user to enter patient data and derive a patient-specific prediction of the 5-year risk of stroke if the patient is not treated with anticoagulants.

Calculations of the risk of stroke are aimed at judging the value of stroke prevention. In at-risk patients, intervention is clearly warranted. A recent meta-analysis compared warfarin, aspirin, and placebo in various combinations and doses.[89] Conventional warfarin therapy was clearly effective in the meta-analysis, whereas aspirin therapy was of marginal value and low-dose warfarin with or without aspirin was of doubtful value. A significant increase in the risk of major bleeding was not observed in any of the trials. Several studies have confirmed the importance of using warfarin in doses sufficient to result in an INR of 2.0–3.0. Achievement of an INR of 2.0–3.0 reduced the risk of stroke by up to 50%, but the degree of benefit depended on the patient's risk factors. In contrast, the risk of stroke was increased by twofold in subjects treated with warfarin whose INR was less than 2.0, the resultant strokes were more likely to be severe, and the 30-day mortality was tripled.[90] Aspirin has a lower risk of major hemorrhage than warfarin[91] and may be adequate therapy in some instances. However, randomized trials comparing aspirin with warfarin in subjects with moderate to high risk of ischemic stroke have consistently shown warfarin to be superior[92] to aspirin. Nonetheless, all-cause 5-year mortality was not improved by treatment with warfarin for subjects at moderate to high risk because of the relatively high 5-year mortality associated with the patients' comorbidities.

Of note, hemorrhage is a major risk in patients who consume excessive amounts of alcohol, fall, or erratically take medications that enhance or inhibit the metabolism of warfarin. Observational data are lacking for predicting the risks in individuals over 80 years of age.[93] Prospective studies of the treatment of atrial fibrillation in subjects over 85 years old are needed.

Studies of alternatives to warfarin are underway. One of these alternative drugs, ximelagatran, an oral direct thrombin inhibitor, is the subject of two trials for prevention of ischemic stroke in older individuals, SPORTIF III and SPORTIF V.[94–96] In SPORTIF III, ximelagatran was compared to warfarin in 3410 subjects with atrial fibrillation and one or more risk factors for ischemic stroke. The risks of ischemic stroke, hemorrhagic stroke, and systemic embolism were comparable in both the ximelagatran (56/1703, or 3.3%) and the warfarin arms of the study. Major bleeding was not significantly different between the two groups. In SPORTIF V the results were

CURRENT CONTROVERSIES & FUTURE CONSIDERATIONS

Geriatric Hematology

- What, if any, are the biologic process that are specifically age-related? Do they include any of the following: immune function, coagulation, vascular endothelium, cell regeneration, or genetic function?
- Should all elderly people with aggressive diseases that lack effective therapeutic regimens be enrolled in clinical trials, or only those with the most favorable prognoses? Should chronologic age alone be used to determine trial eligibility?
- Given the rapid growth of the elderly population and its special needs with respect to hematologic diseases, should geriatric hematology be further developed as a discipline?

similar. Neither study showed a different result between the two treatment arms. Unlike warfarin, no monitoring is required for ximelagatran. However, ximelagatran requires twice daily dosing and may be associated with liver toxicity. Prospective analyses in older patients have yet to be published.

Suggested Readings*

Büchner T, Hiddemann W, Berdel W, et al: Acute myeloid leukemia: treatment over 60. Rev Clin Exp Hematol 6:46, 2002.

Desbiens NA: Deciding on anticoagulating the oldest old with atrial fibrillation: insights from cost-effectiveness analysis. J Am Geriatr Soc 50:863–869, 2002.

Izaks GJ, Westendorp RG, Knook DL: The definition of anemia in older persons. JAMA 281:1714, 1999.

Jacobs LG: Prophylactic anticoagulation for venous thromboembolic disease in geriatric patients. J Am Geriatr Soc 51:1472–1478, 2003.

Popplewell LL, Forman SJ: Is there an upper age limit for bone marrow transplantation? Bone Marrow Transplant 29:277–284, 2002.

Rothstein G: Disordered hematopoiesis and myelodysplasia in the elderly. J Am Geriatr Soc 51(3 Suppl):S22–S26, 2003.

Full references for this chapter can be found on accompanying CD-ROM.

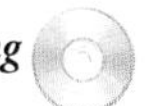

SECTION 2
INFECTIONS OF MARROW AND BLOOD

CHAPTER 74
EPSTEIN-BARR VIRUS

Jeffrey I. Cohen, MD

KEY POINTS

Epstein-Barr Virus

- Ninety-five percent of adults are infected with Epstein-Barr virus (EBV) and shed virus intermittently during life.
- Most of the symptoms of infectious mononucleosis are due to the T-cell response to the virus, rather than to EBV-infected B cells.
- EBV-infected proliferating B cells are restrained by cytotoxic T cells; impairment of cellular, not humoral, immunity is associated with uncontrolled proliferating virus-infected B cells.
- Acyclovir and other antivirals inhibit replication of viral DNA during lytic replication, but they have no effect on replication of EBV episomal DNA when latently infected cells proliferate. Antivirals are not effective for infectious mononucleosis.
- Corticosteroids reduce the T-cell response to infectious mononucleosis. Although they are useful to ameliorate severe symptoms (upper airway obstruction, severe hemolytic anemia), they are not routinely indicated in infectious mononucleosis because T cells are critical for the control of EBV-induced B-cell proliferation.

INTRODUCTION

Epstein-Barr virus (EBV) is a member of the *Herpesviridae* family, and, as with other viruses of this class, infection persists for life. Although most infections with EBV occur early in childhood and are asymptomatic or produce only nonspecific symptoms, EBV is a major cause of infectious mononucleosis. In rare patients, the virus causes chronic active EBV infection, or fatal mononucleosis as in patients with X-linked lymphoproliferative disease. EBV is associated with a number of B-cell and epithelial cell malignancies (see Chapter 45).

DESCRIPTION OF THE ORGANISM

Virus Biology

EBV is a member of the Gammaherpesvirinae subfamily.[1] The other human virus in this subfamily is human herpesvirus 8 (see Chapter 75). EBV virions consist of a lipid envelope, studded with glycoproteins, that surrounds a nucleocapsid, which in turn surrounds the linear viral DNA (Fig. 74–1).

EBV infection of B lymphocytes can result in two outcomes, latent or lytic infection. Latent infection is more common; in vitro the cells become transformed and can proliferate indefinitely. The major viral glycoprotein, gp350, on the surface of the virus binds to CD21 on the surface of B cells.[2] Another glycoprotein, gp42, along with gH and gL, binds to major histocompatibility complex class II molecules that serve as coreceptors of the virus on B cells.[3] The viral nucleocapsid is transported to the nucleus and the viral DNA enters the nucleus, where the linear EBV genome circularizes to form an episome that replicates when the cell divides. Latently infected B cells express a limited repertoire of viral proteins, and the viral genome is copied by the host cell DNA polymerase. Because acyclovir inhibits the viral DNA polymerase, but not the host cell polymerase, replication of the viral episome in latently infected cells is insensitive to acyclovir. Less frequently, virus infection of B cells can result in lytic infection. In this case the full complement of EBV proteins is expressed, virions are produced, and the cell dies. During lytic replication, the viral genome is copied by the viral DNA polymerase; therefore, this stage of replication is sensitive to the action of acyclovir. EBV infects epithelial cells through an unidentified receptor. Infection of epithelial cells results in lytic infection and death of the cell.[4]

Genes Expressed During Lytic Replication

The EBV genome encodes about 100 different gene products. The first genes expressed, the immediate-early genes, regulate viral gene expression, and one of their

TABLE 74–1. EBV Proteins That Modulate the Immune Response

Protein	Cellular Homologue	Function
LMP-1	CD40	Activates nuclear factor-κB, inhibits apoptosis
BZLF1	None	Inhibits interferon-γ activity
BHFR1	Bcl-2	Inhibits apoptosis
BALF1	Bcl-2	Regulates BHRF1
BARF1	CSF-1R	Inhibits interferon-α
BCRF1	IL-10	Inhibits interferon-γ and IL-12

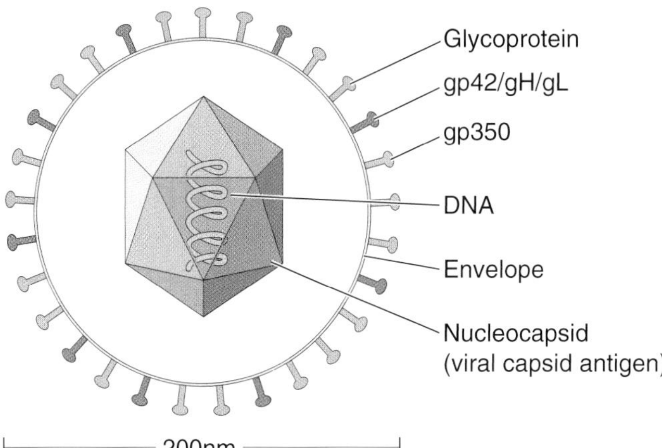

Figure 74–1. Structure of the Epstein-Barr virus. The virion consists of DNA, the nucleocapsid (which includes the viral capsid antigen), and the envelope (which contains glycoproteins). Glycoprotein 42 (gp42) is part of a trimolecular complex with gH and gL. The virion is approximately 200 nm in diameter.

protein products (BZLF1), inhibits the function of interferon-γ (Table 74–1).[5] The immediate-early phase is followed by early gene expression, which produces enzymes used for viral DNA replication, proteins that modulate apoptosis, and a soluble cytokine receptor. The viral enzymes include the viral thymidine kinase, which phosphorylates acyclovir, and the viral DNA polymerase, which is inhibited by acyclovir. EBV encodes two Bcl-2 homologues, one of which inhibits apoptosis.[6,7] The virus encodes a soluble colony-stimulating factor-1 receptor that inhibits production of interferon-α.[8] Several of the early proteins form a complex known as the early antigens; antibodies to these proteins are sometimes used in the diagnosis of EBV-associated disorders.

The late genes encode structural components of the virion, including the viral capsid antigen and the viral glycoproteins, as well as a viral cytokine. Measurement of antibody to viral capsid antigen is used in the diagnosis of acute infection. EBV produces several glycoproteins, including gp350 and gp42, that are critical for entry of the virus into B cells. EBV also encodes a homologue of interleukin-10, which functions as a growth factor for B cells and inhibits production of interferon-γ, which may reduce cytotoxic T-cell activity.[9]

TABLE 74–2. Selected EBV Genes Expressed During Latency

Gene	Activity	Comments
EBNA1	Episomal maintenance	Expressed in all EBV-associated diseases
EBNA2	Transactivator	
EBNA3	Regulates viral gene expression	Major target of virus-specific CTLs
LMP1	Transactivator, inhibits apoptosis	Viral oncogene, activates NF-κB
LMP2	Inhibits virus reactivation	
EBERs	Inhibit apoptosis	Used as a target for in situ hybridization

Abbreviations: CTLs, cytotoxic T lymphocytes; EBERs, EBV-encoded RNAs; NF-κB, nuclear factor-κB.

Genes Expressed During Latent Infection

Only 10 viral gene products are expressed in latently infected B cells (Table 74–2). These include EBV nuclear antigens (EBNAs), latent membrane proteins (LMPs), and EBV-encoded RNAs. Each of these genes is expressed in latently infected B cells in vitro, during infectious mononucleosis, and in EBV-associated lymphoproliferative disease that occurs after transplantation or in patients with human immunodeficiency virus infection. In other EBV-associated malignancies (Burkitt's lymphoma, Hodgkin's disease), different patterns of latent genes are expressed.[10] In contrast, latently infected B cells circulating in the periphery of healthy adults express only one of the EBNAs (EBNA-1), and only during cell division.[11]

EBNA-1 binds to a region on EBV DNA and allows the genome to replicate as an episome during cell division.[12] EBNA-2 upregulates the expression of a several viral and cellular genes.[13] The three EBNA-3 proteins regulate viral gene expression and are the predominant target of EBV-specific cytotoxic T cells.[14] LMP-1 is a functional homologue of CD40 in a constitutively activated form.[15] LMP-1 binds to tumor necrosis factor–associated factors to maintain activation of nuclear factor-κB, c-Jun amino-terminal kinase, and the p38 mitogen-associated protein kinase pathway, resulting in B-cell proliferation.[16] LMP-1 also acts as an oncogene, inhibits apoptosis, and upregulates expression of numerous cellular genes.[17,18] LMP-2 inhibits reactivation of virus from latency,[19] and the EBV-encoded RNAs have been shown to inhibit apoptosis in some studies.[20]

EPIDEMIOLOGY

Most persons are infected with EBV during childhood, and most infections during this time either are asymptomatic or result in nonspecific symptoms.[21] When infection is delayed until adolescence or young adulthood, EBV often results in infectious mononucleosis. Infectious mononucleosis is more frequent in industrialized countries, compared with developing countries: improved standards of hygiene delay onset of infection until after puberty.

EBV is usually spread by oral secretions during childhood. In adolescents or young adults, the virus is transmitted by kissing and possibly by sexual intercourse.[22] Infection also has been transmitted by blood transfusions or bone marrow transplantation.[23] EBV has been eradicated in some bone marrow transplant recipients, who have subsequently been reinfected with a new strain of the virus.[24]

Infectious mononucleosis occurs in males and females with an equal incidence. The incubation period of the disease is estimated to be about 5 weeks, with a range of 3–7 weeks.

INFECTIOUS MONONUCLEOSIS

Pathophysiology

EBV in humans is usually transmitted by virus-infected oral secretions. The virus infects oral epithelial cells, which subsequently infect B cells in the oropharynx, or B cells in the tonsil crypts may be infected directly (Fig. 74–2).[10,25] Infected B cells then traffic through the bloodstream to the lymph nodes, spleen, and other lymphoid organs. During acute infection, up to 1 in 10 to 1 in 100 B cells are infected with EBV. At this time, many B cells undergo lytic infection with production of virus particles; other B cells express the full repertoire of latent proteins, which results in B-cell proliferation. After recovery, the number of EBV-infected B cells remains at about 1 in 10^6 cells for life.[26] The latently infected B cells that circulate in the blood are memory B cells.[27] B cells that return to the oropharynx undergo lytic replication, resulting in shedding of the virus from the oropharynx.

Initial control of virus-infected B cells is due to the action of natural killer cells or human lymphocyte antigen (HLA) nonrestricted cytotoxic T cells.[28] During convalescence and later in life, EBV-specific cytotoxic T cells that recognize both latent and lytic viral antigens limit the proliferation of EBV-infected B cells.[29] Patients who are immunosuppressed with impaired cellular immunity often have greater numbers of EBV-infected B cells in their circulation and shed higher titers of virus in the saliva.

Clinical Features

Signs and Symptoms

Most patients with infectious mononucleosis present with sore throat, fever, and lymphadenopathy (Table 74–3).[30,31] Fever is most common in the first 2 weeks of the illness, but may persist for over 1 month; sore throat is more common during the first week of symptoms. Over

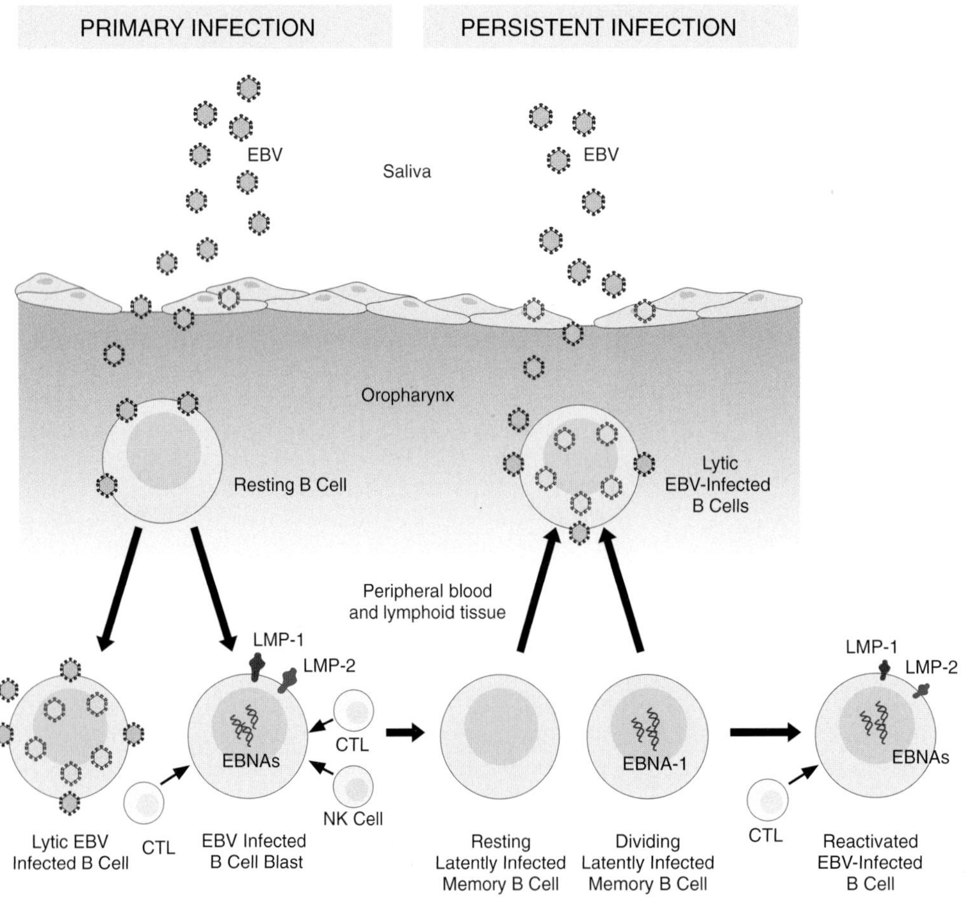

Figure 74–2. Pathogenesis of Epstein-Barr virus infection. (Adapted from Cohen JI: Epstein-Barr virus infection. N Engl J Med 343:481–492, 2000.)

TABLE 74–3. Signs and Symptoms of Infectious Mononucleosis

	Adults: Median (range)	Children: Median (range)
Symptoms		
Sore throat	75% (50–87%)	65% (45–75%)
Malaise	47% (42–76%)	24%
Headache	38% (22–67%)	ND
Abdominal pain, nausea, or vomiting	17% (5–25%)	18%
Chills	10% (9–11%)	ND
Signs		
Fever	98% (33–100%)	94% (90–98%)
Lymphadenopathy	95% (83–100%)	92% (83–94%)
Pharyngitis or tonsillitis	82% (74–91%)	44% (29–59%)
Splenomegaly	48% (40–64%)	50% (47–80%)
Hepatomegaly	12% (6–15%)	30% (28–60%)
Rash	8% (0–25%)	17% (8–34%)
Periorbital edema	5% (2–34%)	14%
Palatal enanthem	5% (3–13%)	ND
Jaundice	4% (2–10%)	4% (2–5%)

Abbreviation: ND, not determined.
Adapted from Cohen JI: Epstein-Barr virus infections, including infectious mononucleosis. *In* Braunwald E, Fauci AS, Kasper DL, et al (eds): Harrison's Principles of Internal Medicine (ed 5). New York: McGraw-Hill, 2001, pp 1109–1111.

one third of patients also note malaise, fatigue, and headache (often retro-orbital). Less frequent symptoms include myalgia, abdominal pain, anorexia, nausea, or vomiting. In most cases, symptoms last for 2–4 weeks.

Physical examination shows fever, lymphadenopathy, and pharyngitis in most patients (see Table 74–3). Lymphadenopathy and splenomegaly are more common during the first 2 weeks of the illness, and splenomegaly is more frequent in the second and third week. Lymphadenopathy usually affects the posterior cervical nodes, but generalized lymphadenopathy may be present. Lymph nodes are often tender and symmetrically involved, but they are not fixed in place. Pharyngitis is accompanied by tonsillar enlargement and an exudate. About half of patients have splenomegaly; other less frequent findings include hepatomegaly, a cutaneous eruption (Fig. 74–3*A*), and periorbital edema. The rash may be macular or papular. Treatment with antibiotics, especially ampicillin or cephalosporins, often induces a macular eruption in patients with infectious mononucleosis.

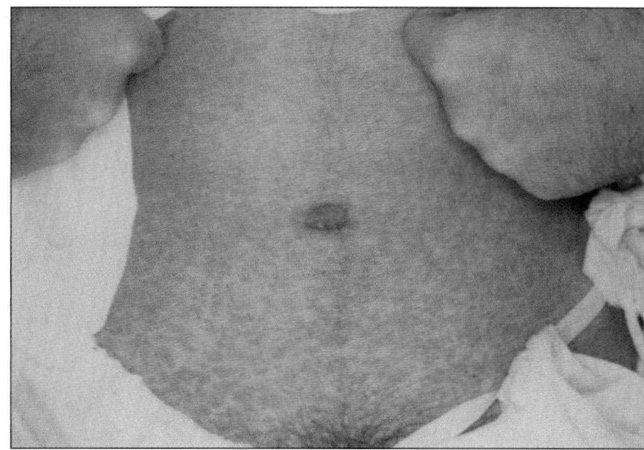

A

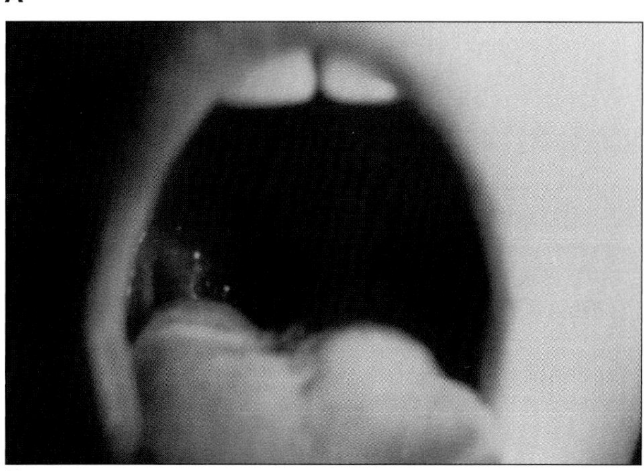

B

Figure 74–3. Physical findings with infectious mononucleosis. ***A,*** Rash. ***B,*** Enlarged tonsils. (From Cohen JI: Epstein-Barr virus infection. N Engl J Med 343:481–492, 2000.)

Complications

Severe complications of infectious mononucleosis are uncommon. Fatalities in individuals who are not immunocompromised are usually due to central nervous system involvement, splenic rupture, bacterial superinfection, or hepatic failure.

Most patients with infectious mononucleosis have a mild anemia for 1–2 months. About 2–3% of cases are complicated by autoimmune hemolytic anemia during the first 2 weeks of illness,[32] most are Coombs test positive and have cold agglutinins directed against the i antigen. Less frequent complications include pure red cell aplasia and aplastic anemia with pancytopenia. EBV has been detected in the bone marrow of some patients with acute infection and bone marrow failure.

Although low-grade thrombocytopenia is frequent in infectious mononucleosis, less than 0.5% of persons have severe thrombocytopenia during the first month.[33] Most cases resolve spontaneously and are likely due to consumption of platelets by an enlarged spleen, with or without antiplatelet antibodies. Less common complications include thrombocytopenic purpura, disseminated intravascular coagulation, and hemolytic-uremic syndrome.[34]

Most patients with infectious mononucleosis have only a low-grade neutropenia; however, severe neutropenia progressing to agranulocytosis has been reported.[35] Both antineutrophil antibodies and an absence of neutrophil precursors in the bone marrow can occur. EBV-associated hemophagocytosis is a rare complication of infectious mononucleosis.[36] Signs and symptoms include fever, hepatic dysfunction, pancytopenia, and hemorrhage. The bone marrow shows phagocytosis of nucleated red blood cells and platelets, and a massive increase in the number of histiocytes.

TABLE 74–4. Complications of Infectious Mononucleosis

Hematologic	Autoimmune hemolytic anemia, aplastic anemia, red blood cell aplasia, hemolytic-uremic syndrome, disseminated intravascular coagulation, thrombocytopenic purpura, agranulocytosis, hemophagocytic syndrome, splenic rupture
Central nervous system	Cerebellar ataxia, encephalitis, meningitis, meningoencephalitis, seizures, cranial neuropathy, Guillain-Barré syndrome, transverse myelitis, peripheral neuritis
Gastrointestinal	Jaundice, hepatic necrosis, hepatitis, pancreatitis
Cardiac	Myocarditis, complete heart block, pericarditis
Pulmonary	Interstitial pneumonitis, upper airway obstruction
Other	Vasculitis, cryoglobulinemia, nephritis, arthritis

TABLE 74–5. Laboratory Findings in Infectious Mononucleosis

Finding	Percentage of Patients
Lymphocytosis	100%
Atypical lymphocytes	100%
Leukocytosis	60–80%
Neutropenia	40–70%
Mild thrombocytopenia	30–50%
Leukopenia	10–20%
Elevated liver enzymes	60–100%
ALT, AST	50–75%
Alkaline phosphatase	80–95%
Bilirubin	30–50%

Abbreviations: ALT, alanine aminotransferase; AST, aspartate aminotransferase.

Splenic rupture occurs in less than 0.5% of cases of infectious mononucleosis.[37] This complication is more common at the end of the first month of illness, especially in males. Most patients have a favorable outcome. Upper airway obstruction may occur as a result of hypertrophy of lymphoid tissue (Fig. 74–3*B*) or edema and inflammation of the pharynx, epiglottis, or uvula. Patients may present with dyspnea, stridor, and dysphagia. Very rare persons with no obvious immune abnormality develop fulminant infectious mononucleosis and die. Other complications of infectious mononucleosis are listed in Table 74–4.

Laboratory Findings

The white blood cell count is often normal or slightly increased; leukocytosis may occur during the second week of illness (Table 74–5). A lymphocytosis is often present during the first week and reaches a peak in the second or third week,[38] up to 50–70% of the peripheral white blood cells are lymphocytes. Although there is a marked increase in the absolute number of T cells, there is a lesser rise in B-cell numbers. The increase in EBV-infected B cells and the T cells that proliferate in response to the B cells are responsible for the enlargement of lymphoid tissue during acute infection. An inverted CD4:CD8 ratio occurs as a result of both a reduction in CD4 cells and clonal expansions of CD8 cells. An increase in the number of natural killer cells and HLA-DR–positive cells also occurs. Low-grade neutropenia and thrombocytopenia are frequently noted. Over one third of the peripheral lymphocytes may be atypical (Fig. 74–4).[39,40] These cells have plasmacytoid features with abundant basophilic cytoplasm, vacuoles in the cytoplasm, and indented edges. Most atypical lymphocytes are CD8 cells; others are natural killer cells and B cells.

Liver function abnormalities are present in most cases, usually during the first 3 weeks of illness. The alkaline phosphatase is more elevated than is the serum transaminases, serum bilirubin is only mildly increased.

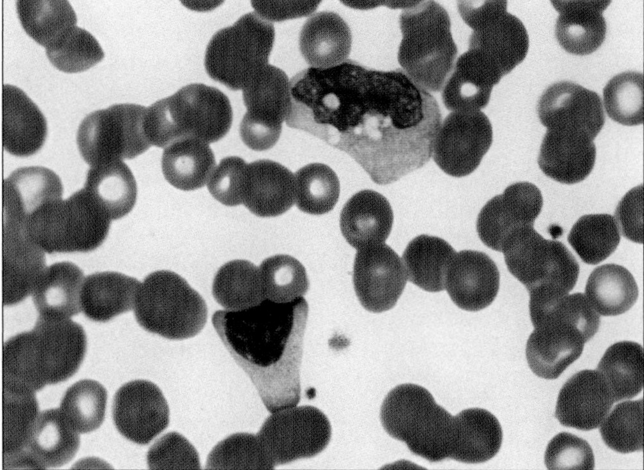

Figure 74–4. Atypical lymphocytes.

Diagnosis

Serologic Assays

The heterophile is the primary test in the diagnosis of infectious mononucleosis.[41] This assay measures antibodies in the serum that agglutinate beef, sheep, or horse erythrocytes after the serum has been absorbed with guinea pig kidney. While the heterophile test does not directly detect EBV proteins, it is highly sensitive and specific in persons who have signs and symptoms of infectious mononucleosis. Commercially available tests, such as the Monospot test, are easier to perform and are more sensitive than the classic heterophile test. The heterophile is usually positive at the onset of infectious mononucleosis and remains positive for 3 months after presentation of illness (Fig. 74–5). In some patients, the test may be positive for up to 9 months after onset of illness.

The combination of fever, sore throat, lymphadenopathy, atypical lymphocytes, and a heterophile titer of 40 or greater is diagnostic of EBV mononucleosis (Fig. 74–6). In some patients the heterophile test may be negative at the time of presentation, and repeated assessment 1–2 weeks later may be necessary. In younger

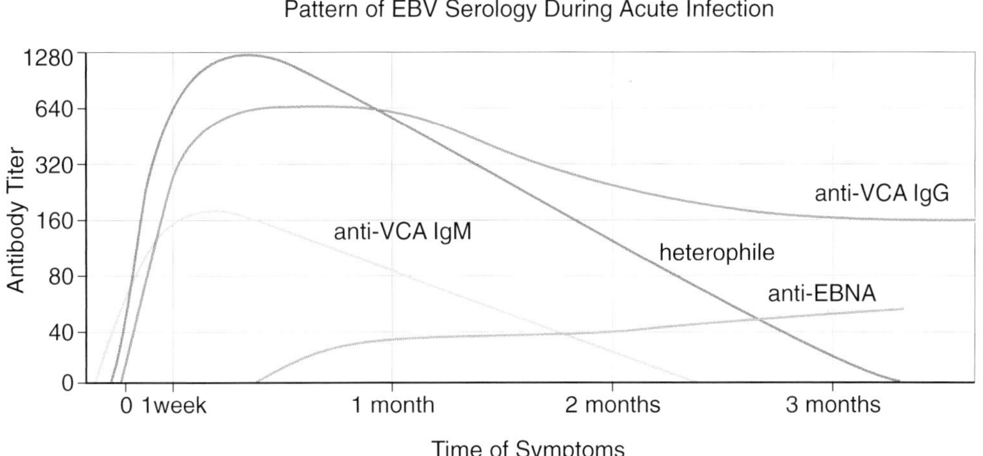

Figure 74–5. Patterns of EBV serology during acute infection.

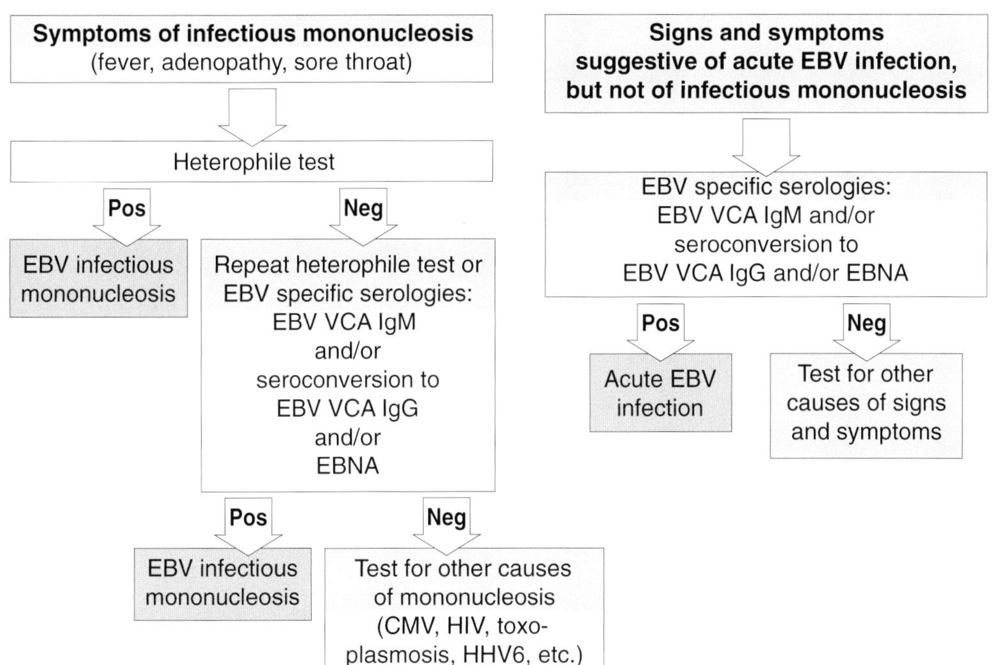

Figure 74–6. Algorithm for diagnosis of infectious mononucleosis.

children and in older adults, as well as persons without typical symptoms of infectious mononucleosis, the heterophile test may be negative and EBV-specific serologies may be required for diagnosis.

An EBV viral capsid antigen immunoglobulin (Ig)M titer of 1:10 or greater is the most useful EBV-specific assay for diagnosis of acute EBV infection, because the test remains positive for only 2 months after presentation. IgM antibody to EBV viral capsid antigen is present in more than 90% of persons at the onset of infectious mononucleosis. Seroconversion to a positive EBV viral capsid antigen IgG is occasionally useful for diagnosis of infectious mononucleosis, but, most patients have viral capsid antigen IgG at the time of presentation. A rise in viral capsid antigen IgG may occur with virus reactivation during immunodeficiency. EBV viral capsid antigen IgG persists for life.

Seroconversion to a positive EBNA antibody can be helpful for the diagnosis of infectious mononucleosis, because the EBNA antibody is usually not positive at the onset of illness. EBNA antibodies usually are detectable at 3–4 weeks after the onset of symptoms in nearly all patients with mononucleosis, and persist for life.

Although early antigen (EA) antibodies also appear at 3–4 weeks, and circulate for up to 6 months, they are present in only about 70% of patients with infectious mononucleosis. Antibodies to the early antigens are either restricted to the infected cell cytoplasm (EA-R) or diffusely present throughout the cells (EA-D). These antibodies are often detected with virus reactivation during immunodeficiency. EA-R antibodies may be present in patients with EBV-associated Burkitt's lymphoma. EA-D antibodies are detected in some patients with infectious mononucleosis, and in patients with EBV-associated nasopharyngeal carcinoma.

Molecular Assays

The polymerase chain reaction is used to measure levels of viral DNA in serum or in peripheral blood mononuclear cells. Viral DNA is detectable in the serum of persons with infectious mononucleosis and in patients with certain EBV malignancies.[42] Viral DNA is increased in peripheral blood mononuclear cells in autoimmune diseases (rheumatoid arthritis, systemic lupus erythematosus) and in patients with impaired cellular immunity (transplant recipients, acquired immunodeficiency syndrome patients). The level of viral DNA in blood has been used to monitor lymphoproliferative disease,[43] and detection of viral DNA in the cerebrospinal fluid has been predictive of central nervous system lymphoma in patients with acquired immunodeficiency syndrome.[44] In contrast, culture of EBV from body fluids is very time consuming and is generally not useful, as the virus is shed intermittently for life after acute infection.

Viral DNA is episomal in most EBV-associated malignancies. The viral genome contains a region that has variable numbers of repeats, but the number is fixed in a given cell. Analysis of the number of these repeats has been useful in the study of EBV-associated malignancies (Fig. 74–7).[45] When all of the cells have the same number of repeats, a single band is detected on Southern blotting, indicating that the tumor cells arose from a single EBV-infected cell and are therefore clonal for EBV. When clones originate from only a few cells, an oligoclonal process is present with a few bands detected on Southern blotting. In contrast, cells containing replicating EBV have both high-molecular-weight DNA (derived from viral episomes) and low-molecular-weight DNA (derived from linear viral genomes).

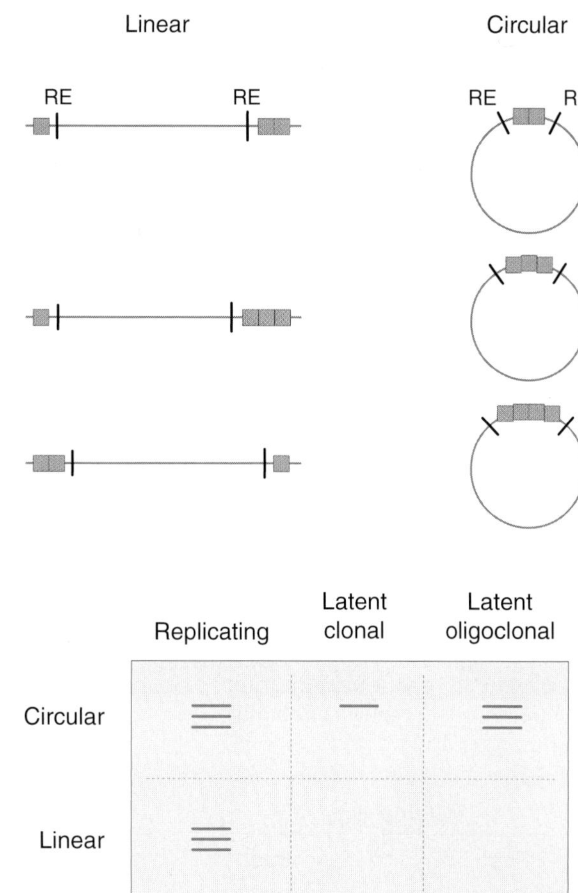

Figure 74–7. Southern blot to determine clonality and latent versus replicating virus. *Top,* Structure of the linear EBV genome (found in cells with replicating EBV DNA) and circular EBV genome (found in cells with latent and replicating viral DNA), with repeat regions *(boxes)* bounded by restriction endonuclease (RE) sites. *Bottom,* Southern blot of viral DNA isolated from cells with replicating EBV DNA and latent clonal or oligoclonal DNA. (Adapted from Katz BZ, Raab-Traub N, Miller G: Latent and replicating forms of Epstein-Barr virus DNA in lymphomas and lymphoproliferative disease. J Infect Dis 160:589–598, 1989.)

Pathology Assays

EBV infection, especially in virus-associated malignancies, can be diagnosed by finding viral nucleic acid or proteins in tissues. Because nearly all infected cells have a latent virus infection, assays to detect latent EBV RNA or proteins are used. The EBV-encoded RNAs are the most abundant viral RNAs and are detected by in situ hybridization[46] (Fig. 74–8*A*). LMP-1 and EBNA-2 (Fig. 74–8*B*) are frequently found in virus-infected cells.[47]

Differential Diagnosis

Although most cases of infectious mononucleosis are due to EBV, other infectious agents may also present with a similar syndrome. Cytomegalovirus is the most frequent cause of heterophile-negative infectious mononucleosis. Patients with cytomegalovirus infectious mononucleosis are older and present with a longer duration of fever than do those with EBV disease.[48] Sore throat, lymphadenopathy, and atypical lymphocytes are less frequent with cytomegalovirus than with EBV infectious mononucleosis. Acute human herpesvirus 6 infection can appear in adults similar to EBV infectious mononucleosis, but the number of atypical lymphocytes is usually more modest.[49] The human immunodeficiency virus acute retroviral syndrome may have a presentation similar to that of acute EBV, although lymphopenia, rash, aseptic meningitis, and diarrhea are more frequent in the former.[50] Acute toxoplasmosis may also present similar to EBV infectious mononucleosis; pharyngitis and splenomegaly are less common with toxoplasmosis. Other diseases that share some of the features of infectious mononucleosis are listed in Table 74–6.

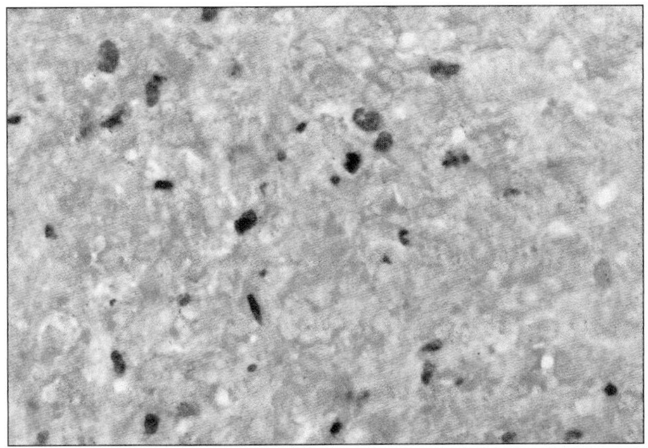

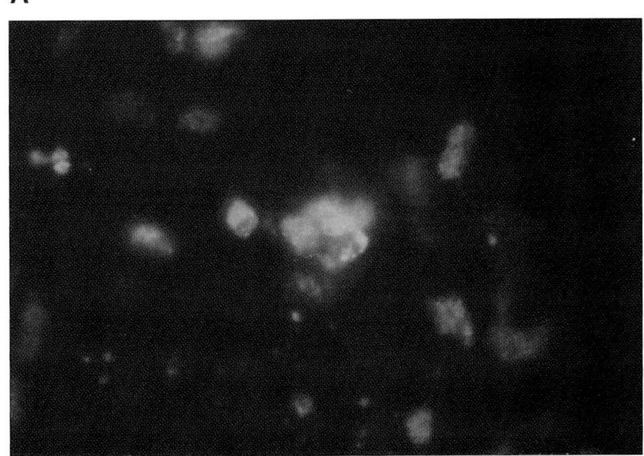

Figure 74–8. *A,* Detection of EBV-encoded RNA (EBER) in tissue by in situ hybridization. *B,* Detection of EBV nuclear antigen-2 (EBNA-2) in tissue by immunofluoresence.

TABLE 74–6. Differential Diagnosis of Infectious Mononucleosis

Disease	Fever	Sore Throat	Adenopathy	Atypical Lymphocytes
Cytomegalovirus	+	+/−	+/−	+
HHV-6	+	+	+	+
HIV	+	+	+	−
Toxoplasmosis	+	+/−	+	+/−
Viral hepatitis	+	−	+/−	+
Rubella	+	+/−	+	+/−
Bartonella	+	+/−	+	−
Drugs*	+	−	+	+/−
Lymphoma, leukemia	+	+	+	+

*Dilantin, sulfonamides.
Abbreviations: HHV-6, human herpesvirus 6; HIV, human immunodeficiency virus.

Treatment and Prevention

Most cases of infectious mononucleosis require no intervention or only symptomatic therapy (Fig. 74–9). Fever and headache can be treated with acetaminophen; nonsteroidal anti-inflammatory agents are effective to relieve myalgia and arthralgia. Excessive physical activity and contact sports should be avoided during the period of splenomegaly to reduce the likelihood of splenic rupture.

Pharyngeal exudates suggestive of streptococcal pharyngitis should be cultured; if β-hemolytic streptococci are isolated, penicillin, erythromycin, or azithromycin should be employed. Ampicillin and cephalosporins are contra-indicated because they frequently induce an exanthem in patients with infectious mononucleosis.

Corticosteroids are not necessary for the vast majority of cases of infectious mononucleosis. A number of clinical trials have been performed using corticosteroids for uncomplicated infectious mononucleosis; although some have shown a reduction in fever or pharyngitis, none has shown corticosteroids to be effective for reducing lymphadenopathy or splenomegaly, and they do not shorten the overall duration of disease.[51–57] In addition, corticosteroids have been associated with complications including bacterial superinfection, myocarditis, and encephalitis.[58,59] They may impair the cellular immune response to acute infection and alter the long-term equilibrium between the virus and the immune system. Thus, corticosteroids are not indicated for most cases of infectious mononucleosis.[60]

Corticosteroids are utilized in specific complications of infectious mononucleosis: impending upper airway obstruction as a result of lymphoid hypertrophy, severe autoimmune hemolytic anemia, and profound thrombocytopenia.[61,62] Prednisone is given at 1 mg/kg/day for 4 days and then is rapidly tapered over 7–10 days. Corticosteroids are used by some for EBV-associated myocarditis, pericarditis, or encephalitis.[60]

Acyclovir has been tested in clinical trials for EBV infectious mononucleosis.[63–67] Acyclovir did not have a significant effect on signs or symptoms of infectious mononucleosis, which are predominantly due to the cellular immune response to the virus. A meta-analysis of five randomized controlled trials of infectious mononucleosis treated with acyclovir or placebo showed no significant difference in clinical end points with acyclovir.[68] Although there was a significant reduction in virus shedding from the oropharynx with drug compared with placebo, 3 weeks after medical therapy was discontinued the difference was no longer significant. Acyclovir has no effect on latent virus in B cells.

A protocol combining both acyclovir and prednisone found no significant effect on the duration of symptoms.[68] Some authorities recommend acyclovir with corticosteroids when the latter are used to treat severe complications of infectious mononucleosis. In these settings, acyclovir is intended to limit virus replication that might increase in the presence of corticosteroids.

Almost all patients with infectious mononucleosis recover completely. Even when malaise and fatigue are prolonged for months, the long-term prognosis is excellent. Although most hematologic complications also ultimately resolve, severe thrombocytopenia or agranulocytosis can result in fatal hemorrhage or infection, respectively. Patients with aplastic anemia or hepatic necrosis often die from these conditions. Neurologic

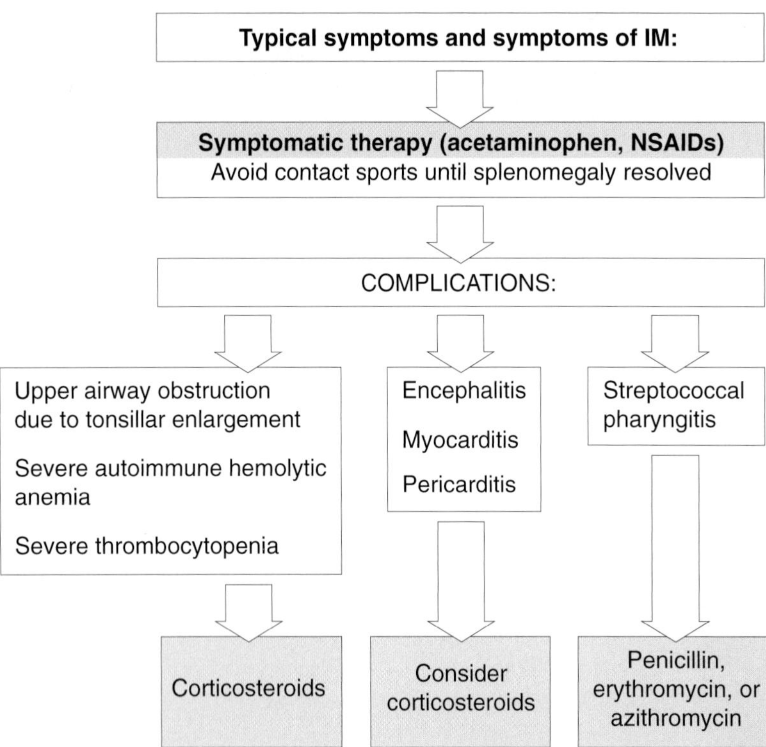

Figure 74–9. Algorithm for management of infectious mononucleosis.

problems also resolve, but EBV-associated encephalitis, cranial nerve palsies, or Guillain-Barré syndrome may produce neurologic residua.

Vaccines to prevent EBV are under development. A vaccine containing recombinant gp350 (the major envelope glycoprotein) was effective in preventing development of EBV lymphoma in primates that were challenged with high titers of EBV.[69] Adjuvant gp350 vaccines using alum or monophosphoryl lipid A are in current clinical trials in Europe. Another vaccine consisting of vaccinia virus expressing gp350 prevented EBV lymphomas in primates after challenge with EBV. This vaccine was given to nine seronegative children in China, and it induced neutralizing antibody responses and appeared to reduce the frequency of EBV infection in some recipients.[70] EBV peptide-based vaccines are also undergoing testing in Phase I clinical trials.[71]

X-LINKED LYMPHOPROLIFERATIVE DISEASE

X-linked lymphoproliferative disease (XLPD) is a rare genetic disorder in which previously healthy males develop severe, usually fatal disease after infection with EBV. Patients are also at higher risk of developing B-cell lymphomas even in the absence of EBV infection.

Clinical Features

Patients usually present with fulminant infectious mononucleosis (Table 74–7)[72] with multiorgan disease caused by infiltration of tissues with proliferating EBV-infected B cells, reactive T cells, and activated macrophages. Liver and bone marrow failure, resulting from destruction by infiltrating cells often accompanied by hemophagocytic syndrome, are frequent, and death is usually due to hemorrhage, hepatic encephalopathy, or infection. Those who survive acute infection with EBV often develop dysgammaglobulinemia with low IgG and elevated IgM and IgA levels.

TABLE 74–7. Clinical Manifestations of XLPD

Clinical Phenotype	Frequency	Survival Rates
Fatal infectious mononucleosis	58%	4%
Lymphoma (>90% B cell)*	30%	35%
Dysgammaglobulinemia (<IgG, >IgM)*	31%	55%
Aplastic anemia	3%	50%
Vasculitis, lymphomatoid granulomatosis	3%	29%

*These occur in some patients with XLPD and no exposure to EBV.
Adapted from Seemayer TA, Gross TG, Egeler RM, et al: X-linked lymphoproliferative disease: twenty-five years after the discovery. Pediatr Res 38:471–748, 1995.

Patients can present with B-cell lymphomas, even without preceding EBV infection. The lymphomas are often extranodal, and the small intestine is frequently involved. T-cell lymphomas are much less frequent. Other less common complications are shown in Table 74–7. Abnormalities in T-cell and natural killer cell funcion often occur, predisposing patients to opportunistic nfections.

Diagnosis

A familial history of fatal infectious mononucleosis in males is highly predictive of XLPD.[73] The gene responsible for the disease was recently identified and is termed *SAP* (SLAM-associated protein), *DSHP* (Duncan's syndrome human protein), or *SH2D1A* (SH2 domain 1A).[74–76] Nearly all boys with a familial history of fatal mononucleosis have a mutation in *SAP*, whereas sporadic cases usually have a normal *SAP* gene. *SAP* is expressed on the surface of T and natural killer cells and interacts with a number of other proteins, including SLAM on T cells and 2B4 and NTB-A on natural killer cells.[77] SAP inhibits SLAM-SLAM interactions on T cells, thereby inhibiting interferon-γ production.[78] SAP is important for the activity of 2B4 and NTB-A on the surface of natural killer cells; in the absence of SAP, natural killer cell cytotoxicity is impaired.[79,80] The markedly increased levels of interferon-γ and the impairment of natural killer cell activity in the absence of SAP may result in an unregulated T-cell response to EBV and allow proliferation of EBV-infected B cells, respectively.[81]

Treatment

Therapy for XLPD is usually ineffective.[82,83] Although antiviral drugs and cytotoxic chemotherapy are often used to limit lymphocyte-mediated destruction during fulminant mononucleosis, most patients die of acute EBV infection. Surviving patients who develop hypogammaglobulinemia are treated with infusions of immunoglobulin. Recently two patients with XLPD and primary EBV infection were treated with rituximab (anti-CD20 antibody) and both patients have survived for more than two years.[83a]

Because a vaccine for EBV is currently not available, many experts recommend that boys with XLPD who are not yet infected with EBV receive immunoglobulin infusions that contain neutralizing antibody to EBV. However, some boys have become infected with EBV and have died from mononucleosis despite immunoglobulin therapy. Bone marrow transplantation is the only method currently available to prevent the disease.

CHRONIC ACTIVE EBV INFECTION

Chronic active EBV infection is a very rare disorder in which infection with EBV results in a persistent, ongoing viral infection of one or more organ systems. The disease is more common in Asians and the prognosis is poor.

Clinical Features

Most patients with chronic active EBV infection present with persistent fever, lymphadenopathy, and splenomegaly (Table 74–8).[84] Thrombocytopenia, anemia, liver function abnormalities, and/or hypersensitivity to mosquito bites occur in one third or more of patients with chronic active EBV.

TABLE 74–8. Signs and Symptoms of Chronic Active EBV Infection

Sign or Symptom	Frequency
Fever	100%
Liver dysfunction	90%
Splenomegaly	90%
Lymphadenopathy	50%
Thrombocytopenia	50%
Anemia	48%
Hypersensitivity to mosquito bites	43%
Rash	28%
Hemophagocytic syndrome	21%
Coronary artery aneurysm	21%
Calcification of basal ganglia	18%
Oral ulcers	18%
Malignant lymphoma	16%
Interstitial pneumonia	12%
Central nervous system involvement	7%

From Kimura H, Hoshino Y, Kanegane H, et al: Clinical and virologic characteristics of chronic active Epstein-Barr virus infection. Blood 98:280–286, 2001, with permission.

A number of life-threatening complications occur in chronic active EBV infection. Patients with hemophagocytic syndrome present with fever and pancytopenia; examination of the liver, spleen, and/or bone marrow shows phagocytosis of erythrocytes and white blood cells. Levels of proinflammatory cytokines, including tumor necrosis factor-α and interferon-γ, are often elevated.[85,86] Although many patients initially have polyclonal gammopathy, they often have progressive loss of B cells and hypogammaglobulinemia. Cellular immune deficiencies, including low numbers of natural killer cells, lead to susceptibility to opportunistic, often fatal infections. Other complications of chronic active EBV infection are shown in Table 74–8.

Diagnosis

Chronic active EBV infection has been defined using three diagnostic criteria.[84,87] First, patients have a severe disease for 6 months or more with markedly elevated EBV serologies or have a chronic, progressive disease that began as a primary infection with EBV. Second, histology shows evidence of organ involvement such as hepatitis, interstitial pneumonitis, bone marrow hypoplasia, hemophagocytosis, lymphadenitis, or meningoencephalitis. Third, EBV DNA, RNA, or proteins are present in the affected tissues, or peripheral blood mononuclear cells show markedly elevated levels of EBV DNA. Patients must have no other immunocompromising condition. Although the cause of chronic active EBV infection is unknown, one patient was found to have mutations in both alleles of the perforin gene that impaired the normal processing of the protein and reduced cellular cytotoxicity.[88]

CURRENT CONTROVERSIES & FUTURE CONSIDERATIONS

Epstein-Barr Virus

- It is unknown why most infants and children are asymptomatic or have only mild symptoms with EBV, whereas adolescents and young adults so frequently present with infectious mononucleosis.
- Better treatments are needed for the severe complications of EBV that occur in otherwise normal persons.
- Why defects in the *SAP* gene result in inability to appropriately control infection with EBV, but not infections with other viruses must be established.
- Most patients with X-linked lymphoproliferative disease or chronic active EBV succumb during EBV infection. Therapy for EBV in immunologically impaired individuals is inadequate.
- A vaccine is needed to prevent EBV, especially in areas of the world where EBV-associated tumors (nasopharyngeal carcinoma, Burkitt's lymphoma) are common.

Treatment

Antiviral therapy is ineffective for chronic active EBV infection. Corticosteroids have provided temporary benefit, but the disease usually progresses. Other therapies, including cytotoxic agents (azathioprine, cyclophosphamide) and interferon-α or interferon-β, have had limited success, and long-term remissions are rare. Bone marrow transplantation[89] or infusion of EBV-specific cytotoxic T lymphocytes[90] has been effective in a small number of cases.

Suggested Readings*

Cohen JI: Epstein-Barr virus infection. N Engl J Med 343:481–492, 2000.

Rickinson AB, Kieff E: Epstein-Barr virus. *In* Knipe DM, Howley PM (eds): Fields Virology (ed 4). Philadelphia: Lippincott Williams & Wilkins, 2001, pp 2575–2627.

Schlossberg D (ed): Infectious mononucleosis (ed 2). New York: Springer-Verlag, 1989.

Straus SE, Cohen JI, Tosato G, Meier J: Epstein-Barr virus infections: biology, pathogenesis, and management. Ann Intern Med 118:45–48, 1993.

Thorley-Lawson DA: Epstein-Barr virus: exploiting the immune system. Nat Rev Immunol 1:75–82, 2001.

Full references for this chapter can be found on accompanying CD-ROM.

CHAPTER 75

Human Cytomegalovirus, Human Herpesvirus 8, and Other Herpesviruses

Jaroslaw P. Maciejewski, MD, PhD, Mario Luppi, MD, PhD, and Giuseppe Torelli, MD

KEY POINTS

Human Cytomegalovirus, Human Herpesvirus 8, and Other Herpesviruses

- Manifest cytomegalovirus diseases in immunologically normal host are rare.
- Cytomegalovirus is a common opportunistic pathogen after bone marrow transplantation.
- Cytomegalovirus infection can be associated with hematopoietic suppression of the graft and cytopenias.
- Monitoring for cytomegalovirus in blood is an effective measure to decrease morbidity and mortality. It allows for preemptive or prophylactic therapy depending on the risk.
- Risk factors for cytomegalovirus disease include T-cell depletion, placement of a seronegative transplant into a seronegative donor, and matched unrelated transplantation.
- Human herpesvirus 8 is the necessary etiologic agent of Kaposi's sarcoma and involved in primary effusion lymphoma and multicentric Castleman's disease/plasmablastic lymphoma mainly occurring in HIV infected subjects.
- Human herpesvirus 8 infection may be associated with the development of nonneoplastic manifestations in transplant patients.
- Human herpesvirus 8 may be transmitted with solid organ transplantation.
- Human herpesvirus 6 causes exanthem subitum in immuncompetent children and is an opportunistic pathogen in transplant patients.
- Human herpesvirus 6 infection should be investigated in transplant patients with encephalitis.

INTRODUCTION

Herpesviruses are large, enveloped, double-stranded DNA viruses that constitute an important group of human pathogens responsible for a variety of pathologies. In hematology, Epstein-Barr virus (EBV; see Chapter 74), human cytomegalovirus, and, as recently discovered, human herpesviruses 6, 7, and 8 play roles as opportunistic pathogens, causes of hematologic malignancies, or markers supporting the diagnosis of certain lymphomas. This chapter describes the roles of these herpesviruses in hematology.

HUMAN CYTOMEGALOVIRUS

Description of the Virus

Isolation of cytomegalovirus from salivary glands was simultaneously reported by Rowe and colleagues and Smith in 1956.[1,2] Because of the cytopathic effect that resulted in cell swelling and intranuclear inclusions, the virus was designated cytomegalovirus and the associated clinical syndrome was referred to as cytomegalic inclusion disease. The cytomegalovirus linear double-stranded genome (240 kb) is the largest of any herpesviruses. The DNA exists as four distinct isomers present in equimolar amounts, containing long and short unique sequences with both internal and terminal inverted repeats; the long and short unique sequences can invert in relationship to each other to create the four isomers. Electron micrographs of the virion show a pleomorphic lipid envelope with an electron-dense icosahedral core containing 162 capsomeres (Fig. 75–1).

Of importance for diagnostic procedures and the understanding of the pathophysiology of cytomegalovirus is its life cycle, characterized by the expres-

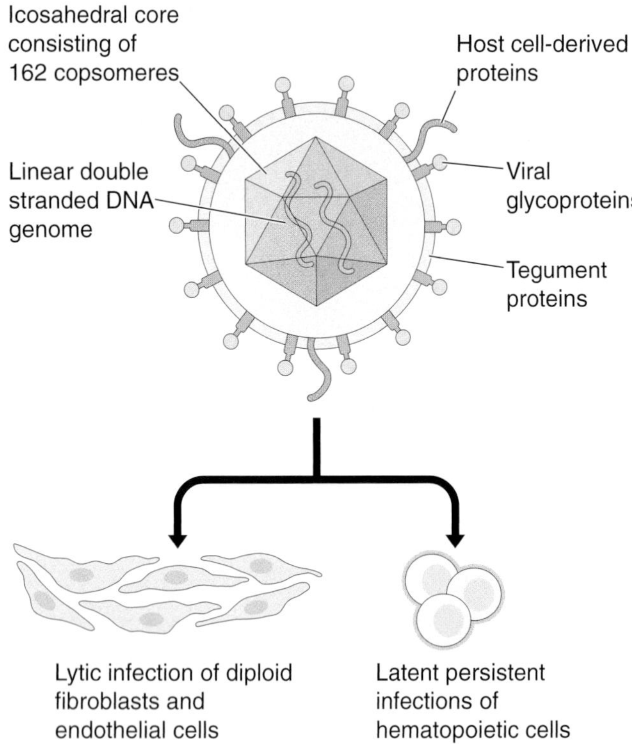

Figure 75–1. Biology of cytomegalovirus.

sion of immediate early (from 0 to 2 hours), early (<24 hours), and late (>24 hours) genes, which code for regulatory proteins, proteins associated with viral replication, and structural proteins (pp65, pp150 matrix proteins), respectively.[3–5] Cytomegalovirus can infect a variety of cells, including hematopoietic progenitor cells, granulocytes, lymphocytes, and macrophages, but productive infections appear to be restricted to endothelial cells and diploid fibroblasts, in which cytomegalovirus causes cell lysis. Productive infection releases large numbers of defective viral particles containing either no or a partial cytomegalovirus genome. In many cell types, cytomegalovirus results only in abortive infections, and in certain cells, such as hematopoietic progenitors and macrophages, cytomegalovirus causes a nonlytic latent infection responsible for the lifelong carrier status of individuals infected with this virus (see Fig. 75–1).

Epidemiology

Cytomegalovirus is endemic in the entire human population. Because in a normal host primary infection may be subclinical, the incidence of infection can be evaluated only by the presence of antiviral antibody; in the United States, the seropositivity rate approaches 50% and increases with age.[6] In developing countries, transmission and consequently seropositivity rates are much higher. Viremia (as detected by true virus isolation) appears to be far less prevalent and many be transient, but using polymerase chain reaction (PCR), cytomegalovirus DNA has been detected in as many as 98% of individuals over 50 years of age.[7,8] Cytomegalovirus can be transmitted orally, sexually, and parenterally. In blood, cytomegalovirus is mostly cell-associated, and rates of transmission by transfusion can be greatly reduced by the use of leukocyte-depleted blood products.[9,10] Even asymptomatic seropositive individuals may at times shed cytomegalovirus in urine and saliva. Cytomegalovirus can also be isolated from mother's milk.[11]

Pathophysiology

Infectious disease in the lungs, colon, or retina is characterized by cytopathic destruction of specific tissues resulting from a productive cytomegalovirus life cycle and release of infectious virus. Lytic infection is associated with cell death and damage to tissue integrity. The inflammatory reaction, with a release of various cytokines, contributes to the dysfunction of specialized cell types as well as to the histopathologic picture—these mechanisms are responsible for cytomegalovirus pneumonia and enteric or hepatic cytomegalovirus disease after bone marrow transplantation. Systemic consequences of cytomegalovirus disease may include cytokine-mediated inhibition of various organ functions, including of the bone marrow (see later). In addition, ganciclovir for therapy of cytomegalovirus infection is myelotoxic and itself can exacerbate the cytopenia, impairing recovery of hematopoietic stem cell function following stem cell transplantation.

The tropism of cytomegalovirus is broader than the cellular spectrum of cells supporting lytic cytomegalovirus infection, diploid fibroblasts and endothelial cells.[12–14] Most of the cell types susceptible to cytomegalovirus infection do not easily support viral replication. In blood, mononuclear phagocytes[15–17] as well as T or B lymphocytes[18–22] carry the genome of cytomegalovirus, which can, under suitable conditions, reactivate (see later).[16] Similar to mature blood cells, hematopoietic progenitor cells at various stages of differentiation[13,15,23,24] are susceptible to cytomegalovirus infection (see also later).

Interaction of Cytomegalovirus with Hematopoietic Cells

Cytomegalovirus can be found in the bone marrow after congenital infection without hematologic manifestations.[25] Cytomegalovirus has been often suspected in the impairment of bone marrow function, but a direct cytopathic effect on hematopoietic progenitor and stem cells is unlikely. Clinical effects of viral infection include delayed recovery of blood counts following hematopoietic stem cell transplant[26,27] and impaired immune reconstitution.[27] Several pathophysiologic mechanisms have been proposed for the hematologic consequences of cytomegalovirus infection[28] (Fig. 75–2).

In addition to hematopoietic progenitor cells, stromal elements constitute potential targets for cytomegalovirus.[29] Infection of stroma may be productive, resulting in lysis of the infected cells and release of infectious virus in the proximity of stem cells. Cellular responses, causing influx of lymphocytes and other immune cells secreting inhibitory cytokines, may further

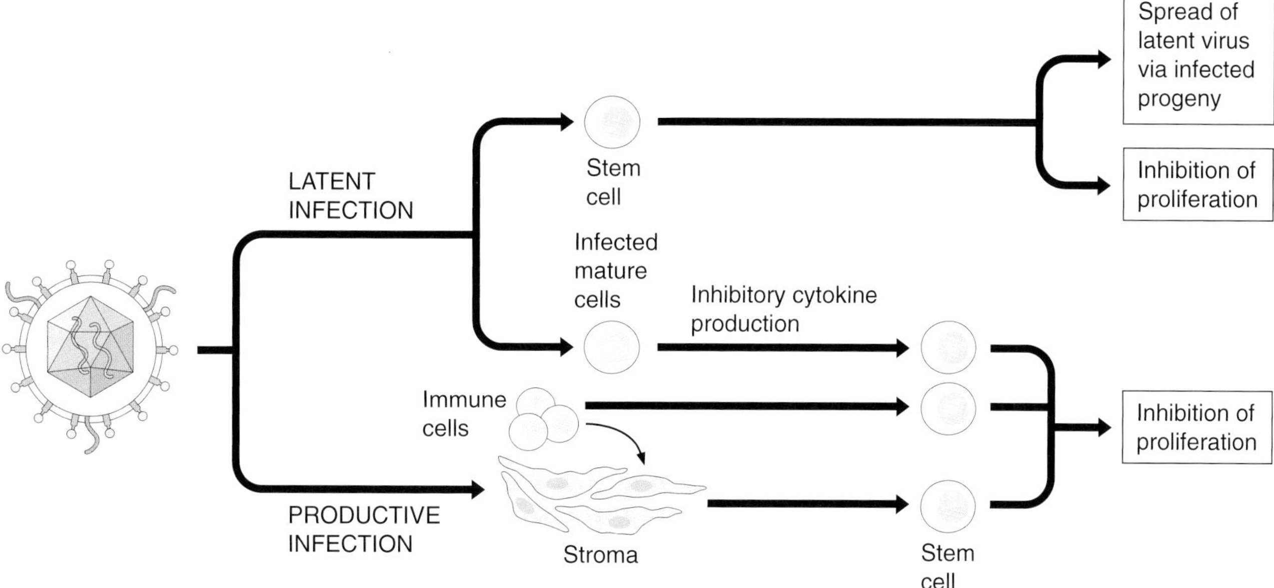

Figure 75–2. Hematopoietic effects of cytomegalovirus.

contribute to the inhibition of hematopoietic function. Infection of stromal cells can produce disturbances in cytokine and growth factor release. For example, selective impairment in granulocyte colony-stimulating factor production has been postulated for some strains of the virus.[29] Experimentally, in vitro challenge of unfractionated bone marrow cells with cytomegalovirus can inhibit colony formation, with dose-dependence.[13,15,30,31] The inhibition observed in tissue culture varies, especially between primary isolates and established laboratory strains.[29] In vitro challenge of purified CD34$^+$ cells with cytomegalovirus also decreases their colony-forming ability, suggesting a direct viral effect on hematopoietic progenitor and stem cells.[30,32,33] Infection of hematopoietic progenitor cells, including purified CD34$^+$ cells, by cytomegalovirus has been demonstrated in vitro and in vivo by a variety of methods, including experiments with recombinant cytomegalovirus strains engineered to express β-galactosidase that allows marking of infected cells.[32,34–36] Infected progenitor cells appeared to transmit virus to their progeny, including more mature myeloid cells[35,37,38] and megakaryocytes,[25,39] while cytomegalovirus infection along the erythroid maturation pathway was abortive.[32,35]

Latency

Cytomegalovirus persistence in the host despite intact immunity suggests a balance between latent and productive infections controlled by the cellular immune system. Minimally productive infection with little spread of the virus from cell to cell is very difficult to demonstrate experimentally but must underlie cytomegalovirus persistence. By analogy to EBV, cytomegalovirus is believed to persist in its latent form. Although viral proteins expressed during cytomegalovirus latency or those that may be needed for maintenance of the latent state have not been characterized, specific cytomegalovirus transcripts can be cloned from latently infected cells.[43,44] Lytic infection of fibroblast and endothelial cells precludes them as sites of cytomegalovirus latency. Infection of hematopoietic and other cells types does not result in productive viral infection, and experimental evidence supports their role in cytomegalovirus latency.[38,43,44] Latent infection of hematopoietic progenitors would explain the ability of virus to spread through the replication of infected cells.[37,45] Infectious virus has been recovered from macrophages generated by culture of monocytes from seropositive individuals.[16] The latent state of the virus provides protection from the immune system; conversely, certain cytokines may constitute signals for the initiation of the productive viral life cycle directly or through induction of cellular differentiation.[46]

Viral Targets of Immune Response

The cytomegalovirus genome encodes a variety of proteins; theoretically, all might be targeted by the humoral and cellular immune system. Antibodies generated during the immune response are specifically directed to envelope protein gB and tegument proteins pp65 and pp150, but some of the regulatory proteins, including immediate early antigen-1 (IEA-1 or pp72), can also generate an antibody response.

Cellular immune responses are much more complex. Cytotoxic T cells (CTLs) specific to pp65 expand after initial infection from a naive pool, and during reactivation from the memory cell pool; effector anti-pp65 CTLs likely reside within a CD57$^+$CD28$^-$ cell population. Expansion of individual cytomegalovirus-specific T-cell clones can be massive, and they may constitute 1–3% of the entire CD8 and or CD4 cell repertoire when measured by human lymphocyte antigen (HLA) tetramers or intracellular cytokine staining.[47–49] The proportion of pp65 tetramer–reactive CTLs is higher in seropositive individuals and can rise to 15% during cytomegalovirus reactivation.[48] Based on cytokine response following antigenic stimulation, the number of cytokine-producing effectors likely corresponding to cytomegalovirus-specific T cells was 10-fold higher in seropositive as compared to seronegative individuals.[50] T-cell receptor sequence analysis shows oligoclonality of cytomegalovirus-specific CTL responses, characterized by the presence of several expanded immunodominant T-cell clones.[51–55]

The most immunodominant cytomegalovirus target for the CD8 cellular immune response is matrix protein pp65,[56–59] and to lesser degree pp150,[57,59,60] but there are also measurable CTL responses to IEA-1 and gB.[56,61,62] However, gB- and IAE-1–specific CTLs, unlike those detected against matrix proteins, fail to lyse permissive fibroblasts infected with cytomegalovirus.[63] Specific peptides derived from pp65 and pp150 proteins that bind various HLA alleles have been identified.[47,49,56] HLA tetramers with peptides derived from pp65 allow for the quantitation of the specific CTL response in patients[47,49,56] (see also "Diagnostics").

Box 75–1. Clinical Manifestations of Cytomegalovirus Disease

Patients with Normal Immune System

- Subclinical infection/asymptomatic seroconversion
  - Latent carrier status
- Heterophil-negative infectious mononucleosis
- Cytomegalovirus hepatitis/subclinical hepatitis

Patients with Impaired Immune Responses

- Interstitial pneumonia (BMT)
- Graft failure/pancytopenia (BMT)
- Hepatitis
- Gastroenteric cytomegalovirus disease/cytomegalovirus colitis
- Hepatitis
- Asymptomatic persistent viruria/viremia
- Chorioretinitis (AIDS)

Congenital and Neonatal Infection

- Central nervous involvement
  - Inner ear infection/deafness
  - Mental retardation
- Pneumonia
- Gastroenteritis
- Generalized systemic infection
- Persistent infection of multiple organs with viremia/viruria
- Failure to thrive

Clinical Features of Cytomegalovirus Diseases

Cytomegalovirus causes a variety of pathologies, but in most instances infection of an immunocompetent host is subclinical and results in lifelong immunity that protects from cytomegalovirus reactivation. Primary infection is accompanied by viremia and viruria with subsequent immunoglobulin (Ig)M-to-IgG conversion. Occasionally, primary infection results in a cytomegalovirus mononucleosis–like syndrome: the clinical severity spectrum of this condition is wide. Another rare manifestation is cytomegalovirus hepatitis. Regardless of clinical symptoms, immunity to cytomegalovirus is not capable of totally eliminating the virus from the body, and the virus persists, likely in a latent form (see later). In some individuals, low IgM titers can be present for prolonged periods and are of no clinical relevance. Reactivation of virus may result in increase in IgG titer, but often only shedding of the virus without clinical symptoms is detectable. Infection with a different strain of cytomegalovirus can be associated with a recurrent IgM response.

In an immunocompromised host, cytomegalovirus causes a variety of life-threatening diseases (Box 75–1). The acquired immunodeficiency syndrome (AIDS) epidemic uncovered new, previously extremely rare manifestations of cytomegalovirus disease, especially retinitis and colitis. In AIDS, the degree of immunodeficiency correlates with the risk of CMV: CD4 cell numbers below 50/μL predict an extremely high risk of cytomegalovirus retinitis, whereas with CD4 counts above 100/μL of blood the likelihood of cytomegalovirus infection is low.[64] Similar correlations are likely true for the risk of cytomegalovirus disease following allogeneic stem cell transplant. More intense immunosuppression with newer drugs applied widely for a variety of conditions also has resulted in more common occurrence of cytomegalovirus infection outside the traditional presentations such as hematopoietic stem cell transplant or AIDS. Similarly, without developed immunity, unopposed cytomegalovirus infections cause severe birth defects (see Box 75–1). Infection resulting from the reactivation of virus during pregnancy results in less severe sequelae than does primary infection: both are difficult to establish on clinical grounds because, in most cases infection is subclinical. As with rubeola, infection early in the pregnancy is associated with more severe defects at birth.

The most important hematologic diseases caused by cytomegalovirus occur in the context of allogeneic hematopoietic stem cell transplant (see Box 75–1). In this setting, cytomegalovirus may be responsible for specific organ damage (see Chapter 94) as well as for delayed engraftment, likely resulting from inhibition of hematopoietic stem cell function. Cytomegalovirus also produces clinical disease in patients receiving immunosuppressive agents for the therapy of malignancies. Cytomegalovirus infection of transplant recipients may precipitate rejection, but discrimination of the primary event is difficult because suspicion of cytomegalovirus-induced graft rejection (graft-versus-host disease in transplant recipients) often results in institution of intense immunosuppression.

Occasional blood abnormalities associated with cytomegalovirus mononucleosis, which may prompt referral to the hematologist, are indistinguishable from those observed during EBV infection (see Chapter 74), including occurrence of large granular lymphocytes, lymphocytosis with greater than 10% atypical lymphocytes, liver enzyme abnormalities, splenomegaly, and leukopenia. Differentiation from EBV is provided by negativity for heterophil antibodies. Guillain-Barré syndrome may occur but is rare. Unlike in EBV mononucleosis, exudative pharyngitis and cervical adenitis are uncommon in cytomegalovirus mononucleosis.

Cytomegalovirus often has been implicated in suppression of bone marrow function, typically delayed engraftment or graft failure after transplant, as described above. Cytomegalovirus infection is often associated with depressed blood counts, but the primary and secondary causes (comorbidities, myelotoxic drugs) complicate the determination of whether bone marrow inhibition is directly due to viral infection. In addition to hematopoietic function, a decrease in the lymphocyte count as a consequence of cytomegalovirus infection is associated with significant mortality.[65] Association of specific genotypes of cytomegalovirus classified by variants of gB antigen was reported in aplastic anemia patients who underwent bone marrow transplantation[40,41]; the gB3 genotype was associated with graft failure, and that genotype was found to be more frequent in aplastic anemia patients.[42] There is little other evidence of cytomegalovirus as a significant etiologic agent of idiopathic aplastic anemia.

Diagnostics

Initial infection causes seroconversion, and the presence of antibodies indicates past cytomegalovirus exposure and a carrier status for latent cytomegalovirus. As with other viral infections, IgM positivity indicates recent infection and IgG positivity more remote infection. Cytomegalovirus IgM can persist, especially at low titers, and an increase in the IgM titer or reappearance of cytomegalovirus IgM may indicate reinfection with another strain or reactivation of latent virus.

Monitoring for cytomegalovirus viremia is effective in surveillance for virus and the basis for preemptive therapy.[66] Usually serial monitoring is instituted twice weekly and continued for the first 10 weeks posttransplantation. Cytomegalovirus viremia can be diagnosed by a variety of methods, including shell viral culture,[67] immunohistochemical detection of antigenemia,[68] and molecular assays such as various modifications of DNA and RNA PCR.[66,69,70] Immunohistochemical detection of antigenemia is a reliable technique performed on leukocyte smears; the level of viremia is expressed as number of cells positive for cytomegalovirus (as detected with an antibody usually directed against the IEA antigen) per high-power field. The test is rapidly performed. Recently molecular methods have gained wider application and now compete with traditional culture and histochemistry.[66,70] DNA PCR without quantitation can detect the presence of cytomegalovirus genome, but because of its high sensitivity, the results may not be informative in seropositive individuals. Cytomegalovirus DNA is strictly cell-associated, and blood leukocytes are used as a source of DNA for viral detection. The sensitivity and predictive value of the individual techniques used for viral detection have not been stringently compared.[69,71]

Quantitative PCR utilizing light-cycler technology is used for the detection of cytomegalovirus viremia and titer quantitation,[66] using either TaqMan probes (single-stranded DNA probes that release light upon degradation by Taq polymerase) or beacon probes (DNA probes that release light upon conformational change after hybridization to the internal segment of amplicons). Based on standard curves established with calibrated positive controls, the number of viral genome copies can be precisely determined and calculated.[72] Cytomegalovirus can be detected at levels as low as 1 and as high as 5×10^5 copies/mL, correlating well with the antigenemia measured per 2×10^5 leukocytes. Measurements can also be performed in plasma.[73]

Viremia may be asymptomatic, but an increase in viral titer may herald impending clinical manifestations. In many circumstances, clinical diagnosis of cytomegalovirus disease may be difficult, especially in the presence of graft-versus-host disease. Biopsy of affected tissues with immunohistochemical staining is often required to identify the etiology, but even histopathology results need to be assessed in the context of clinical symptomatology (Fig. 75–3).

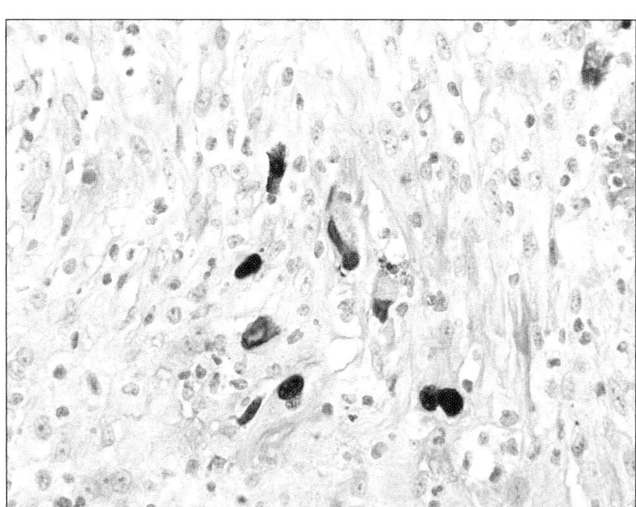

Figure 75–3. Detection of cytomegalovirus infection in tissues. Biopsy of an ulcerative lesion in colon mucosa infected with cytomegalovirus, with immediate early and early antigens stained brown by specific monoclonal antibody.

Measures of Risks and Susceptibility

The individual factors determining cytomegalovirus susceptibility have not been well characterized. The in vivo replication time of cytomegalovirus is short and highly influenced by the host immune response.[74] Despite relatively high percentages of cytomegalovirus-specific T cells present in normal seropositive individuals, only very profound immunodeficiency appears to predispose to cytomegalovirus diseases and relatively low numbers of lymphocytes are required to secure protection against cytomegalovirus. In AIDS, only a profound decrease in CD4 cells is associated with the risk of cytomegalovirus infection. Similarly, intense immunosuppression in aplastic anemia with antithymocyte globulin and cyclosporine, and highly immunosuppressive chemotherapy for solid tumors, do not appear to increase susceptibility to cytomegalovirus activation. Frequencies of CD8 cytomegalovirus-specific lymphocytes of 1–2 × 10^7/L of blood appear to correlate with protection from cytomegalovirus disease.[75,76] In addition, functional defects as well as predisposing lesions may determine the risk of infection and clinical manifestations.[77–79] For example, persisting antigenemia posttransplantation correlates with prior lymphocyte proliferation to cytomegalovirus,[80] and both lack of cytomegalovirus-specific T cell precursors as well as their functional impairment may predispose to cytomegalovirus disease.[81] After stem cell transplant, immaturity and the low diversity of the T-cell receptor repertoire of $CD4^+$ or $CD8^+$ cells may more subtly reflect the risk for cytomegalovirus and other viral infections.[82]

Anticytomegalovirus responses have been quantitated by a number of modern assays, including ELISPOT and other functional tests[52,58,83–86] and HLA tetramer technology.[49–51,81,84,87,88] In functional assays, T cells are stimulated in vitro and their activation measured by flow cytometry: both cytomegalovirus-specific $CD4^+$ and $CD8^+$ cells have been enumerated.[52,58,83–86] Antigen-stimulated cytokine ELISPOT is suitable to quantitate low numbers of cytomegalovirus-specific cells, whereas cytokine flow cytometry has a better dynamic range and also allows for phenotyping.[84]

HLA tetramer technology has made possible the rapid and sensitive quantification of peptide- and protein-specific lymphocytes. The list of known cytomegalovirus-derived peptides that can stimulate a T-cell response within a particular HLA restriction is increasing, and the initial restriction of this technique to HLA-A2 tetramers has been overcome by the ability to produce various classes of tetramers, including HLA-DR. Quantification of anticytomegalovirus pp65-restricted lymphocytes is a very sensitive method to evaluate anticytomegalovirus immune competence; after transplant, recovery of cytomegalovirus-specific CTLs inversely correlates with clinical cytomegalovirus reactivation or infection.[49,88] Antiviral T-cell responses, as identified by HLA tetramers, are very heterogeneous and polyclonal[55]; lymphocyte populations binding the tetramer-peptide complex differ regarding antigen affinity and functional capability, such as killing efficiency.

Therapy

Cytomegalovirus infections significantly contribute to mortality and morbidity after allogeneic stem cell transplantation. Traditionally, the risks and management strategies for patients with cytomegalovirus were defined by the serologic status of the donor and recipient. For example, cytomegalovirus-seropositive recipients of seronegative grafts have a high risk for cytomegalovirus disease, and seronegative donors should be used, if possible, for seronegative recipients.

The first principle of management of cytomegalovirus infections during transplantation is antiviral prophylaxis.[76,89–91] Ganciclovir has been most used as a preventive drug, especially in high-risk situations.[92–95] Acyclovir was effective in decreasing the incidence of cytomegalovirus disease when combined with preemptive ganciclovir treatment for viremia.[96] Valacyclovir moderately decreased the rate of cytomegalovirus infection in comparison to acyclovir.[97] Foscarnet is also useful for prophylaxis of high-risk patients. In general, preventive measures should be tailored to risk factors, including use of T-cell–depleted grafts, high-dose corticosteroids, and antithymocyte globulin and a high-risk serologic combination of donor and host. High risk patients may also require intense preemptive or prophylactic therapy, more frequent monitoring, and longer duration of therapy beyond clearance of the viremia (Box 75–2). Other measures of susceptibility to cytomegalovirus, such as pp65 tetramer technology, remain to be evaluated for their clinical value (see Box 75–2).

Hypoimmunoglobulinemia is frequent in stem cell transplant recipients, and administration of an immuno-

Box 75–2. Prevention of Cytomegalovirus Disease

Prevention of Exposure

- Leukodepletion of blood products
- Seronegative blood products
- Contact prevention for seronegative patients
  - Condoms
  - Avoiding contact with secretions

Prevention of Cytomegalovirus Manifestations

- Cytomegalovirus surveillance and preemptive therapy (ganciclovir therapy)
- Ganciclovir prophylaxis for patients at high risk for cytomegalovirus infections (see text)
- Preventive use of high-dose acyclovir/valacyclovir
- Intravenous immunoglobulin administration

Box 75–3. Therapy of Cytomegalovirus Disease after Stem Cell Transplant

Viremia in High-Risk Individuals

- Ganciclovir (1-week induction, for at least 3 weeks or until day 100 post-transplant *or* 2-week induction followed by maintenance until cytomegalovirus negativity [2 detections]) (see text)
- Addition of granulocyte colony-stimulating factor if neutropenia develops, *or* switch to foscarnet
- Foscarnet for neutropenic patients

Cytomegalovirus Disease

- High-dose ganciclovir
- High-dose foscarnet

globulin preparation may have a broader effect than its anticytomegalovirus activity. The impact of intravenous immunoglobulin on cytomegalovirus infection is less clear.[98] Hyperimmune cytomegalovirus IgG was not effective in prevention of cytomegalovirus infections.[99] Seronegative transplant recipients should receive leukodepleted blood from a seronegative donor.[100,101] Leukodepletion significantly reduces the risk of cytomegalovirus transmission by blood products.[9,10] The efficacy of filters has been confirmed by real-time assay for PCR cytomegalovirus.[102]

A major advance in the therapy of cytomegalovirus infection was the implementation of cytomegalovirus viremia monitoring that allows for initiation of early therapy, before the evolution to serious disease,[103,104] an approach called preemptive therapy (Box 75–3; see also Box 75–2). Preemptive therapy with ganciclovir has been introduced based on surveillance conducted using serial cytomegalovirus detection by any of the available methods, such as quantitative PCR.[95,105,106] Some investigators advocate short, low-dose preemptive ganciclovir therapy of viremic patients[107] in order to diminish ganciclovir myelotoxicity. Positive viral cultures prompt institution of ganciclovir therapy aimed at prevention of manifest cytomegalovirus disease.

Current antiviral agents for the therapy of manifest cytomegalovirus disease include ganciclovir and foscarnet. Cidofovir is a new anticytomegalovirus agent with moderate renal toxicity.[74,108] No definitive data are available on the efficacy of oral ganciclovir, but it appears to be a reasonable and well-tolerated alternative to intravenous ganciclovir prophylaxis.[14,109] Major toxicities may influence the choice of ganciclovir (myelosuppression) and foscarnet (nephrotoxicity) in specific clinical situations. Emergence of ganciclovir-resistant cytomegalovirus strains with mutations in the polymerase genes[110,111] is a serious clinical problem that may require the development of novel anticytomegalovirus antibiotics.

Cellular therapy of cytomegalovirus infection is a novel approach to cytomegalovirus disease.[112] Ex vivo expanded cytomegalovirus-specific T cells can be generated and infused at the time of cytomegalovirus disease. This strategy is extremely labor intensive and requires an individualized approach for ex vivo expansion. Nevertheless, preliminary experience of efficacy is promising. A number of vaccination strategies are in development and may translate to more generally effective preventive measures for individuals at risk for cytomegalovirus diseases.

HUMAN HERPESVIRUS 8

Description of the Virus

Human herpesvirus 8/Kaposi's sarcoma–associated herpesvirus was identified in 1994 from the Kaposi's sarcoma tissues of patients with AIDS (see Chapter 44).[113] Further epidemiologic and experimental studies indicated that human herpesvirus 8 was an essential etiologic agent involved in all clinical forms of Kaposi's sarcoma (classic, endemic, AIDS-related, and iatrogenic).[114–116] Human herpesvirus 8 is classified as a gammaherpesvirus, related to EBV and *Herpesvirus saimiri*. Like other herpesviruses, human herpesvirus 8 is a large, double-stranded DNA virus that replicates in the nucleus as a closed circular episome during latency but linearizes during virion packaging and replication. The human herpesvirus 8 viral genome is unique, compared with the genome of other human herpesviruses, because it contains genes associated either with the latent or the lytic phase of the viral cycle that are homologous to cellular genes involved in the control of the cell cycle and apoptosis.[114–116]

Epidemiology

Human herpesvirus 8 is not ubiquitous in the general population: seroprevalence rates are very low in the United Kingdom and United States and higher only in specific geographic areas, as in the Mediterranean and Africa, regions also with a high incidence of classic/endemic Kaposi's sarcoma. In nonendemic areas, human herpesvirus 8 is spread sexually, especially among homosexual men; human herpesvirus 8 seroprevalence rates are highest among men who report a large number of sexual partners or a history of sexually transmitted diseases. Nonsexual routes of transmission may be important in human herpesvirus 8–endemic areas, where infection is acquired early in childhood.[116] An independent association between human herpesvirus 8 infection with injection drug use may exist for women with or at risk for human immunodeficiency virus (HIV) infection, suggesting human herpesvirus 8 transmission through needle sharing.[117]

Infectious virus was detected in a North American blood donor,[118] but further studies have found no evidence of human herpesvirus 8 seroconversion among a small series of 32 recipients of transfused blood from human herpesvirus 8–seropositive donors.[119,120] Among children with sickle-cell anemia in Uganda, where human herpesvirus 8 infection is common in blood donors, blood transfusion has been found to be associated with a small risk of human herpesvirus 8 transmission, equivalent to the 1-year cumulative risk of infection from community sources.[121] Whether human herpesvirus 8 can be transmitted through transfusions of blood or blood derivatives remains unresolved. More data are available on the transmission of human herpesvirus 8 with grafts. In epidemiologic studies from the Cincinnati Transplant Tumor Registry and the Collaborative Transplantation Research Group of the Île de France, there was a higher incidence of Kaposi's sarcoma in kidney and liver allograft recipients, but a lower incidence in recipients of other solid organs, and Kaposi's sarcoma was rare among hematopoietic stem cell transplant patients.[122] The incidence of posttransplantation Kaposi's sarcoma varies among different ethnic groups, and is higher in those who are at increased risk for classic Kaposi's sarcoma and originate among endemic areas for human herpesvirus 8 infection.[116] Early studies suggested that posttransplantation Kaposi's sarcoma was primarily due to human herpesvirus 8 reactivation in endemic areas and to primary infection in nonendemic areas, but molecular tracing of the viral infection has shown that organ-related transmission is more common, accounting for about one third of the cases of posttransplantation Kaposi's sarcoma.[123–126]

Why is it that Kaposi's sarcoma is rare in marrow compared with solid organ transplants?[127] Elimination of a resident human herpesvirus 8 carrier state by myeloablation prior to BMT is possible, whereas immunosuppressive regimens used in patients receiving solid organ transplants do not destroy the cells harboring latent human herpesvirus 8, which may be reactivated (as occurs also for EBV).[128] Indeed, disseminated Kaposi's sarcoma has been successfully treated with an allogeneic marrow transplant in a 3-year-old HIV-negative child.[129] Alloreactivity in stem cell transplants also may be detrimental to Kaposi's sarcoma, so that graft-versus-leukemia effects may be protective against the emergence of the cancer. By molecular and immunohistochemical methods, human herpesvirus 8–infected neoplastic cells in the posttransplantation Kaposi's sarcoma lesions from five of eight renal transplant patients harbored genetic and/or antigenic markers of their matched donors[130] (Fig. 75–4). Similarly, posttransplantation lymphoproliferative diseases occurring in recipients of bone marrow grafts result from expansion of EBV-infected B cells of donor origin. The human herpesvirus 8 status of the graft donors and recipients could guide the proper use of human herpesvirus 8–positive allografts and prompt prophylactic/preemptive treatment of transplant recipients.

PATIENT

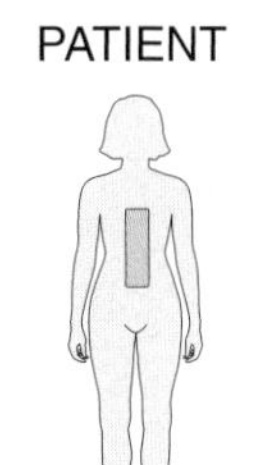

HLA A23; B45; B35; DR4; DR11; DR52–53; DQ2; DQ7

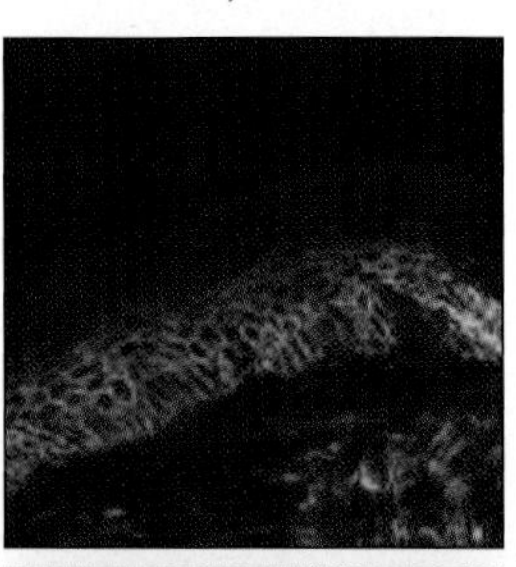

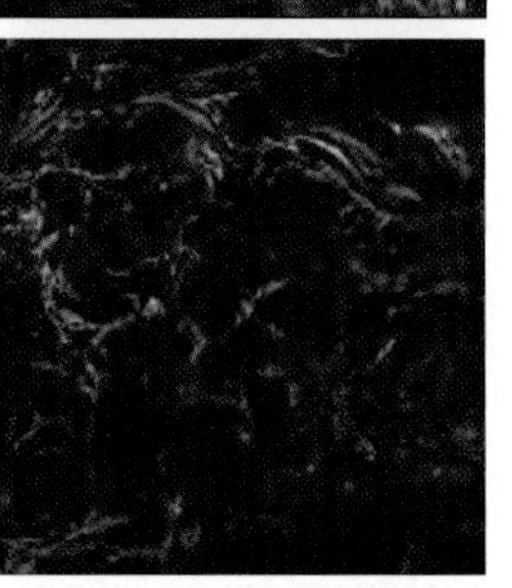

A HLA A23 + HLA A 30

DONOR

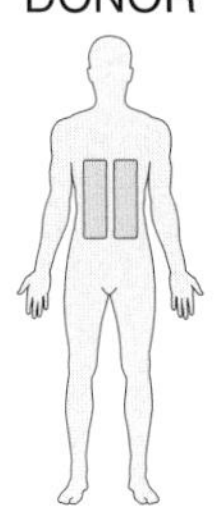

HLA A10; **A30**; B39; B44; DR7; DR11; DR52–53; DQ2; DQ7

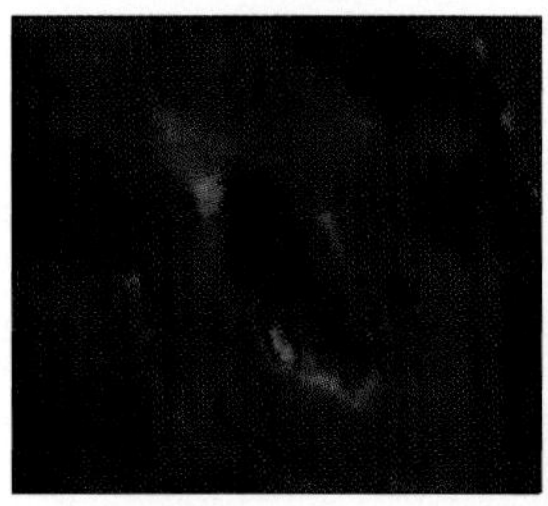

B HLA A 30 + LANA-1

Figure 75–4. Detection of donor and recipient HLA class I antigen as well as of human herpesvirus 8 latency-associated nuclear antigen-1 (LANA-1) in a Kaposi's sarcoma lesion of the skin from a renal transplant patient. ***A,*** Double immunofluorescence with antibodies against HLA-A23 and HLA-A24 *(green)* and against HLA-A30 and HLA-A31 *(red).* Whereas the epidermis and subepidermal vessels only express recipient HLA-A23 and HLA-A24 *(upper panel),* the tumor shows a prevalent expression of donor HLA-A30 and HLA-A31 in the endothelial cells *(lower panel).* (Magnification, × 300.) ***B,*** Double immunofluorescence with antibodies against HLA-A30 and HLA-A31 *(red)* and against HHV-8 LANA-1 *(green).* LANA-1 nuclear expression was detectable in neoplastic endothelial cells expressing the donor HLA-A30 and HLA-A31 antigen in the cytoplasm. (Magnification × 800.)

Pathophysiology

Human herpesvirus 8 can infect B lymphocytes in vitro but, unlike EBV, is not able to induce their immortalization.[131] Conversely, human herpesvirus 8 is capable of immortalizing endothelial cells in vitro in the presence of vascular endothelial growth factor.[132] Microvascular endothelial cells represent a mixed population of lymphatic endothelial cells and blood vascular endothelial cells, which are both susceptible to human herpesvirus 8 infection, although with different efficiencies, human herpesvirus 8 replicating better in lymphatic endothelial cells.[133] The gene expression profile of Kaposi's sarcoma neoplastic cells, as determined by microarray analysis, is closely related to that of lymphatic endothelial cells.[133]

Gene expression profiles of human herpesvirus 8–infected and uninfected lymphatic endothelial cells and blood vascular endothelial cells show that human herpesvirus 8 induces a transcriptional drift of both infected cell types, away from the pattern of uninfected populations and toward each other,[133] and Kaposi's sarcoma neoplastic spindle cells express both endothelial cell markers in vivo. Lymphatic reprogramming induced by human herpesvirus 8 infection in blood vascular endothelial cells is characterized by the downregulation of vascular genes and the induction of about 70% of the main lymphatic lineage-specific genes, including *PROX1*, a master gene that controls the embryonic development of the mammalian lymphatic system.[134] Angiopoietin-2 is among the lymphangiogenic molecules that are upregulated in lymphatic endothelial cells infected with human herpesvirus 8 in vitro, and its expression is detectable in Kaposi's sarcoma lesions in vivo; plasma levels are significantly higher in patients with AIDS-related Kaposi's sarcoma.[133] The $\alpha_3\beta_1$ integrin (CD49c/29) is an in vitro cellular receptor of the virus; $\alpha_3\beta_1$ integrin is abundantly expressed in endothelial cells, B cells, monocytes, and epithelial cells, the same target cells in which human herpesvirus 8 DNA and transcripts have been detected.[135]

Clinical Features of Human Herpesvirus 8 Diseases

Human herpesvirus 8 infection is associated with rare lymphoproliferative disorders—primary effusion lymphoma, multicentric Castleman's disease of plasma cell type, and plasmablastic lymphoma arising in the context of Castleman's disease—that mainly occur in HIV-infected individuals, often together with Kaposi's sarcoma (see Chapter 44).[136] In the general population, human herpesvirus 8 infection is rare in lymphoproliferative diseases other than primary effusion lymphoma or Castleman's disease; a suggested pathogenetic association between human herpesvirus 8 and multiple myeloma has not been confirmed.[136] Human herpesvirus 8 infection was concomitant with hepatitis C virus infection in one patient with plasma cell leukemia[137]; three cases of a germinotropic lymphoproliferative disorder occurred in association with both human herpesvirus 8 and EBV infections.[138] Human herpesvirus 8 DNA was detected in primary cerebral lymphoma in a woman who had received long-term corticosteroid therapy for uveitis.[139] EBV-negative, human herpesvirus 8–positive monoclonal, lymphoproliferative disease of polymorphic type in a human herpesvirus 8–seronegative man, 9 months after receiving a kidney from his HHV-8–seropositive father,[140] is consistent with lymphoproliferation secondary to iatrogenic immunosuppression. Nonmalignant plasmacytic proliferations have also been reported in two solid organ transplant patients.[141] Benign lymphadenopathy with germinal center hyperplasia and increased vascularity, in which human herpesvirus 8 DNA sequences were detected, has been reported in HIV-negative and HIV-positive young adults.[113,142] Well-documented human herpesvirus 8 primary infection in HIV-positive subjects is associated with fever, splenomegaly, and cervical lymphadenopathy, pathologically characterized by angiolymphoid hyperplasia.[143] Histologic features of florid follicular hyperplasia and increased vascularity, as are observed also in Castleman's disease, likely represent a distinct histologic pattern of lymphoid response induced by human herpesvirus 8 (Fig. 75–5). Lymphoproliferation characterized by persistent angiofollicular lymphadenopathy is induced in simian immunodeficiency virus–infected rhesus macaques, following infection with the simian homologue of human herpesvirus 8.[144]

As with other human herpesviruses, human herpesvirus 8 primary infection or reactivation may manifest as a variety of non-neoplastic pathologies. Human herpesvirus 8 DNA was detected in the lungs of HIV-negative and -positive patients with interstitial

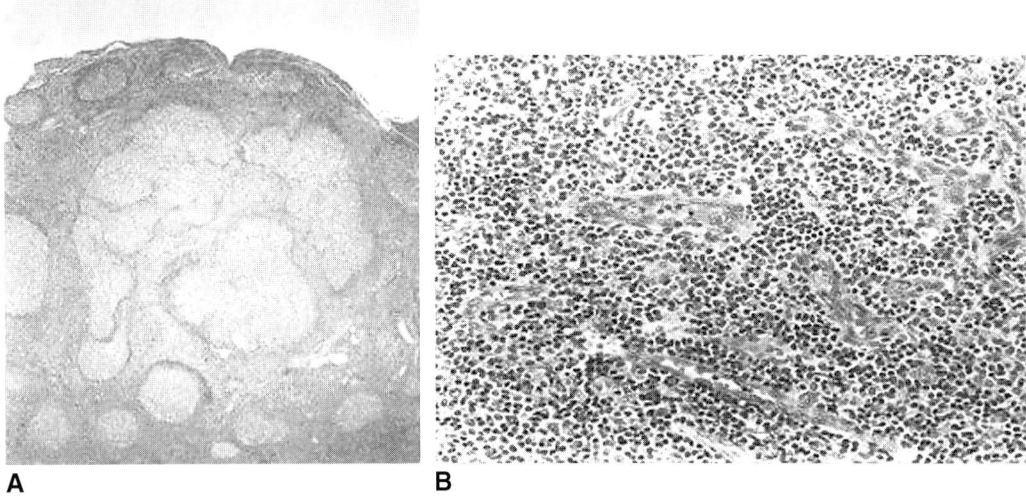

Figure 75–5. Histologic features of reactive lymphadenopathy positive for human herpesvirus 8. ***A,*** Germinal centers are enlarged and irregularly shaped, while mantle zones are partially lost (hematoxylin-eosin, original magnification × 20). ***B,*** Numerous small blood vessels are present in interfollicular areas (hematoxylin-eosin, original magnification × 200).

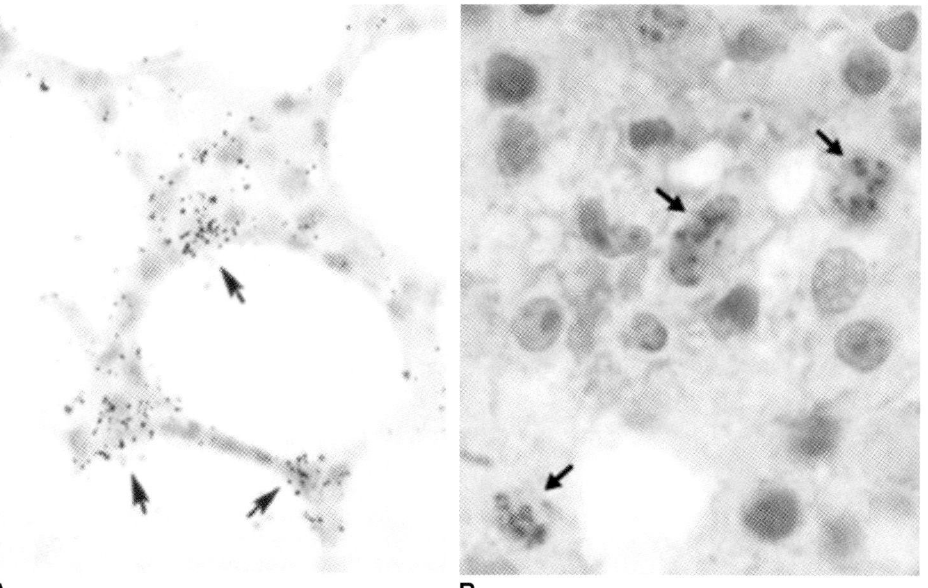

Figure 75–6. Localization of human herpesvirus 8 in the marrow cells of transplant patients with bone marrow failure associated with human herpesvirus 8 primary infection or reactivation. ***A,*** Detection of human herpesvirus 8–specific T0.7 RNA transcripts by in situ hybridization in the aplastic bone marrow of an autologous peripheral blood stem cell transplant patient (hematoxylin-eosin, original magnification × 300). ***B,*** Detection of human herpesvirus 8 LANA-1 by immunohistochemistry in the nuclei of bone marrow cells in the aplastic bone marrow of a renal transplant patient (hematoxylin, original magnification × 450).

pneumonitis.[145,146] Human herpesvirus 8 latency-associated nuclear antigen-1 (LANA-1) expression was observed in cells within the plexiform lesions of lung tissues from patients with primary pulmonary hypertension.[147] Fever, cutaneous rash, and hepatitis have been reported in a patient with non-Hodgkin lymphoma who had received autologous peripheral blood stem cells, resulting in human herpesvirus 8 reactivation.[148] Primary infection with human herpesvirus 8 was proven in two patients 4 months after kidney transplantation from the same human herpesvirus 8–seropositive cadaveric donor[125]: seroconversion and viremia coincided with development of a disseminated Kaposi's sarcoma in one case and with an acute syndrome of fever, splenomegaly, cytopenia, and marrow failure with plasmacytosis in the other. Human herpesvirus 8 reactivation was associated with fever and marrow aplasia with plasmacytosis in a patient with non-Hodgkin lymphoma after autologous peripheral blood stem cell transplantation; human herpesvirus 8 transcripts and LANA-1 were expressed in the few remaining immature myeloid progenitors (Fig. 75–6). Among herpesviruses, EBV also has been implicated in aplastic anemia,[149] and cytomegalovirus and human herpesvirus 6 are myelosuppressive in vitro and may delay platelet engraftment after transplantation (see above).[150,151] Bone marrow hypoplasia occurred in two patients who developed Kaposi's sarcoma after autologous stem cell transplantation[127]; in the setting of renal transplantation, human herpesvirus 8 primary infection produced marrow hemophagocytic syndrome, with peripheral pancytopenia, which resolved after antiviral treatment[152] (Fig. 75–7). Early descriptions of hematologic abnormalities in homosexual men with Kaposi's sarcoma, and in AIDS patients, included alterations in marrow cellularity and peripheral cytopenia.[153] Susceptibility of human fetal-derived mesenchymal stem cells to human herpesvirus 8 infection in culture suggests that these cells may have a role in the development of human herpesvirus 8–related pathology of the marrow.[154]

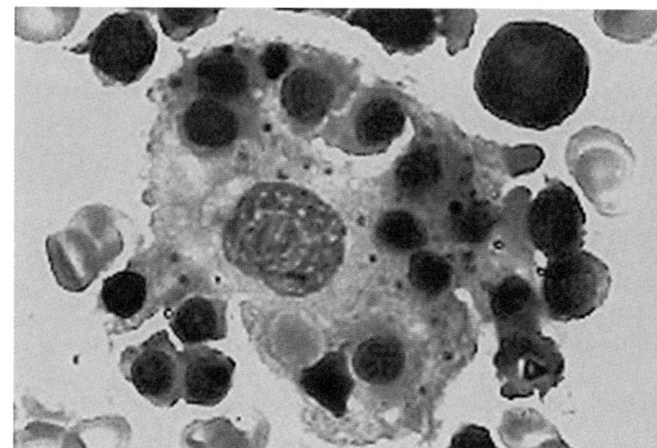

Figure 75–7. Bone marrow smear showing a macrophage containing numerous phagocytized normoblasts in a renal transplant patients with severe pancytopenia and hemophagocytosis after human herpesvirus 8 primary infection (May Grünwald Giemsa stain; magnification × 100).

The severity of human herpesvirus 8–associated illness in transplant patients is likely related to concurrent immunosuppression. Primary infection or reactivation of human herpesvirus 8 in immunocompetent subjects has milder consequences. Primary human herpesvirus 8 infection in five immunocompetent subjects led to mild, nonspecific symptoms and signs of diarrhea, fatigue, localized rash, and lymphadenopathy only.[155] Primary human herpesvirus 8 infection may cause a febrile maculopapular skin rash in immunocompetent children.[156] Human herpesvirus 8 DNA sequences in saliva suggest that oral secretion is the main mode of transmission in the pediatric age group.[156]

Although Kaposi's sarcoma is very rare after autologous and allogeneic hematopoietic stem cell transplantation, it may be responsible for subtle disease manifestations; the myelosuppressive effect of human herpesvirus 8 makes screening by a combination of serologic and molecular methods appropriate for clinical manifestations of a potentially infectious cause.[125,148]

Treatment

The efficacy of various antivirals against human herpesvirus 8 in vitro is controversial. Acyclovir is ineffective; ganciclovir, foscarnet, and cidofovir have been variably active in clinical reports.[152,157,158]

HUMAN HERPESVIRUS 6 AND HUMAN HERPESVIRUS 7

Description of the Pathogens

Human herpesvirus 6 was first isolated in 1986 from the peripheral blood mononuclear cells of patients with various lymphoproliferative disorders, some of whom were also infected with HIV.[159] Human herpesvirus 7 was first isolated in 1990 from the purified CD4 T cells of a healthy person, and 2 years later from a patient with chronic fatigue syndrome.[160,161] Like cytomegalovirus, both human herpesvirus 6 and human herpesvirus 7 are betaherpesviruses[162–165]; by direct DNA sequencing, human herpesviruses 6 and 7 are closely related. Human herpesviruses 6 and 7 lack the coding genes present in the short unique region of human cytomegalovirus,[166] an important genetic difference of uncertain pathogenic importance.

Two variants of human herpesvirus 6, A and B, have an overall nucleotide sequence identity of 90%.[165,167] Human herpesvirus 6 efficiently replicates in vitro and induces a cytopathic effect in CD4 T lymphocytes and in thymocytes in murine models.[168–170] Human herpesvirus 6 infects many types of hematopoietic cells, including CD8 T and B lymphocytes, natural killer cells, and monocytes/macrophages; for epithelial cells; and for neural cells.[168,171,172] Human herpesvirus 6 infection in vitro induces immunomodulatory effects as well as suppression of T-lymphocyte functions.[165,173] CD46 is a cellular receptor for both the human herpesvirus 6 A and B variants.[171] CD46 is a glycoprotein involved in the regulation of complement; its expression on the cell surface of all nucleated cells is consistent with the broad cellular tropism of human herpesvirus 6 in vitro.[174]

Human Herpesvirus 6 Epidemiology and Transmission

Human herpesvirus 6 is ubiquitous in humans throughout the world, with seroconversion occurring early in life.[175] Salivary contact is likely the vehicle for transmission, but intrauterine passage is also possible.[165,176] Human herpesvirus 6 can be transmitted by blood products and with bone marrow and solid organ transplantation.[165,176–178] Following primary infection, human herpesvirus 6 persists lifelong.

Pathophysiology

Virus persists in peripheral blood mononuclear cells, mainly in monocytes, although only rare cells are infected in healthy individuals, as shown by PCR testing.[179–181] Human herpesvirus 6 latency is unusual, because an extremely high viral load in the peripheral blood is accompanied by the integration of apparently the entire viral genome into host cell chromosomes[182,183]; it is likely human herpesvirus 6 can infect and integrate its genome into a very early self-renewing bone marrow precursor[184] (Fig. 75–8). Integrated viral genomes, longitudinally transmitted to differentiated cells without expression of the genes associated with the late phase of the viral cycle, would allow viral escape from cell-mediated immunity. Human herpesvirus 6 also may create a pool of infected bone marrow progenitors to serve as a reservoir of latent virus. Differentiation of maturing granulocytes permits expression of at least one late antigen in a small percentage of cells; virus released from latently infected granulocytes may be a source of human herpesvirus 6 dissemination and possibly lead to clinical disease.[184] The pattern of human herpesvirus 6 antigen expression is similar to that of human cytomegalovirus, which can infect myeloid progenitors in vitro and replicates and expresses specific genes on differentiation of monocytes to macrophages or in granulocytes.[185] Integration of human herpesvirus 6 genomes has been mapped to chromosome 17p13.3, chromosome 22q13, and chromosome 1q44 in different individuals affected with various lymphoproliferative disorders or immune diseases, such as multiple sclerosis.[183,186,187] Targeted integration may occur rarely in healthy subjects[188,189]; human herpesvirus 6 has been detected in blood but also in other somatic tissues, and the virus has been transmitted from parent to child in an integrated form.[188,189] Human herpesvirus 6, distinct from other herpesviruses, contains a gene homologous to the *rep* gene of adeno-associated virus, a DNA virus showing high integration specificity[190]; human telomere-like repeat sequences at both ends of the human herpesvirus 6 genome may relate to the integration site in chromosome 17p, which is also close to or within the telomere.[191] In addition to the bone marrow, the oropharynx/salivary glands, the epithelial mucosa of the female genital tract, and the brain tissue harbor viral genomes and represent reservoirs of virus in healthy individuals.[192–194]

Clinical Features of Human Herpesvirus 6 and 7 Diseases

Primary infection with human herpesvirus 6 variant B causes exanthem subitum (also known as sixth disease), a febrile illness often associated with seizures in young children.[195,196] No illness has been described following primary infection with variant A in immunocompetent individuals. In normal adults, primary infection with human herpesvirus 6 may cause an infectious mononucleosis–like syndrome, characterized by the presence in the peripheral blood of atypical CD4 lymphocytes expressing human herpesvirus 6 antigens.[197–199] Human herpesvirus 6 is an opportunistic pathogen after trans-

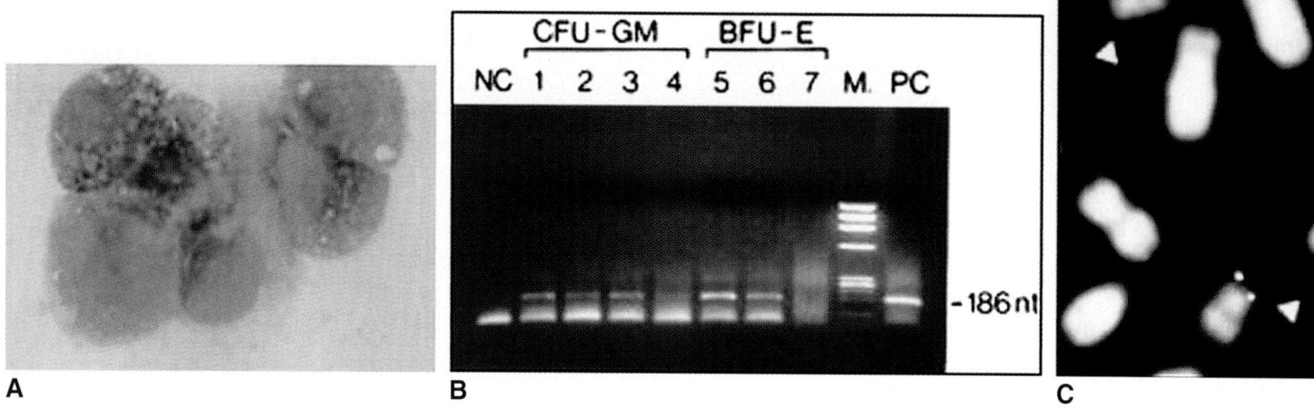

Figure 75–8. Integration of human herpesvirus 6 genome in the marrow cells. *A,* Bone marrow culture from a patient with a human herpesvirus 6 high-viral-load latency (May Grünwald Giemsa stain; magnification × 600). *B,* Ethidium bromide–stained gel agarose gel of representative human herpesvirus 6–positive colony-forming unit, granulocyte-macrophage (CFU-GM) (lanes 1 to 4) and burst-forming unit, erythroid (BFU-E) (lanes 5 and 6) colonies, as well as of one human herpesvirus 6–negative BFU colony (lane 7), from the patient, as determined by a polymerase chain reaction assay with primers derived from the ZVH14 sequence. Abbreviations: NC, HSB-2–uninfected DNA as a negative control; PC, human herpesvirus 6–infected HSB-2 cell line DNA as a positive control; M, molecular weight marker (Marker IX, Boehringer Mannheim). The length of the amplified product is indicated. *C,* Chromosome fluorescence in situ hybridization performed on metaphase chromosomes of cultured bone marrow from the patient, with the ZVB70 fragment of human herpesvirus 6 genome as the viral probe. A specific hybridization signal was detected on the terminal short arm of one chromosome 17 (17p13.3). Chromosomes 17 are indicated by *arrows.*

plantation.[197–199] The frequency of human herpesvirus 6 infection is 40–50% in bone marrow and peripheral blood stem cell transplant patients[176–178]; risk of infection is higher in allogeneic compared to autologous marrow and peripheral blood stem cell recipients, in patients transplanted for leukemia and lymphoma than for other diseases, and with treatment using anti-CD3 monoclonal antibody for the management of graft-versus-host disease.[200,201] Human herpesvirus 6 DNA is present at a higher copy number and for a longer period in cord blood stem cell than in bone marrow transplant or peripheral blood stem cell transplant patients.[202] In solid organ transplantation, the frequency of human herpesvirus 6 infection is 20–30%, but risk factors are not fully defined except for the use of OKT3 and antithymocyte globulin.[178,203,204] The timing of infection in transplant patients varies between 2 and 4 weeks in bone marrow, between 1 and 8 weeks in liver, and between 1 and 12 weeks in renal transplant patients (Fig. 75–9).[205] The clinical manifestations of human herpesvirus 6 primary infection and/or reactivation include fever and cutaneous eruptions,[206] bone marrow suppression,[146,207] thrombotic thrombocytopenic purpura,[208] encephalitis[201,204,209] (Fig. 75–10), and hepatitis[210]; most of these associations are anecdotal.[176,178,201,203] Observational studies have implicated infection with human herpesvirus 6, and human herpesvirus 7, as risk factors for cytomegalovirus disease.[211,212] With liver transplantation, human herpesvirus 6 viremia was associated with an eightfold higher risk of invasive fungal infection.[204]

Commercial rapid diagnostic assays are available for cytomegalovirus but not for human herpesvirus 6 (Tables 75–1 and 75–2). No randomized trials of the benefit of preventing or reducing the risk for human herpesvirus 6 replication have been conducted. Human herpesvirus 6 can be detected by PCR[213] when the virus is suspected: in cases of posttransplantation complications for which a viral etiology is suspected, and absent other common pathogens; and in cases of concomitant infections, but with clinical or pathologic features suggestive of human herpesvirus 6, such as acute marrow suppression and encephalitis. Ganciclovir and foscarnet have been employed empirically as therapy based on in vitro sensitivity of human herpesvirus 6 to these antivirals.[214]

TABLE 75–1. Diagnosis of Human Herpesvirus 6 Infection: Standard Methods

Method	Comments
Isolation of the virus	Time consuming
Serologic assay	Cross-reactions Insensitive in immunocompromised population Not a reliable indicator of active infection Useful for determination of seroprevalence
Biopsy specimen analysis	Useful in organ-specific syndromes by demonstrating cytopathic effects, although viral inclusions do not occur with human herpesvirus 6 infection
Immunohistochemical stain (p101; gp82)	Poor usefulness for early diagnosis and poor reliability for diagnosis of active infection
Alternative approach	Virus quantification provided by antigenemia assay

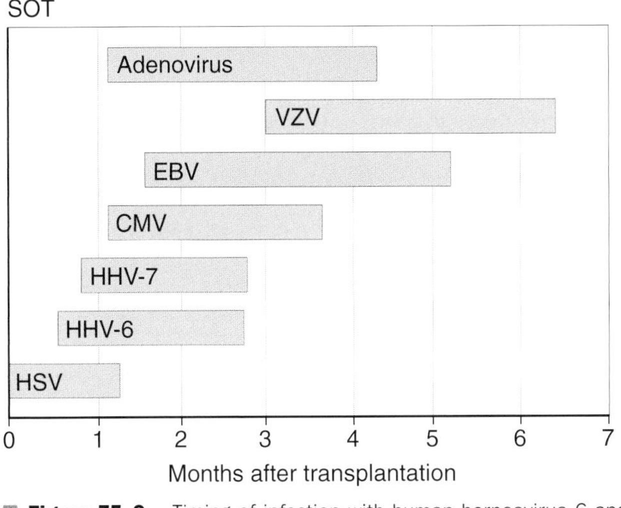

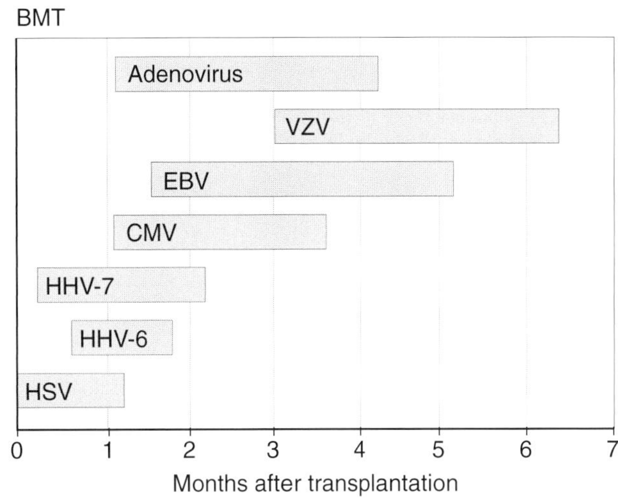

Figure 75–9. Timing of infection with human herpesvirus 6 and human herpesvirus 7 compared with that of other common viruses in solid organ transplant (SOT) and bone marrow transplant (BMT) patients.

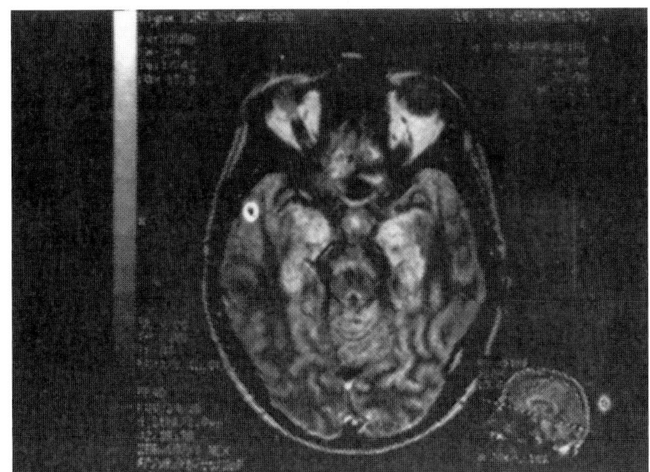

Figure 75–10. Proton density magnetic resonance imaging shows bilateral hyperintensity of the gray matter, involving the uncus and the anterior part of the parahippocampal gyrus, in a case of fatal human herpesvirus 6 encephalitis, occurring in a recipient of a T-cell–depleted peripheral blood stem cell transplant from a three-loci–mismatched related donor.

TABLE 75–2. Diagnosis of Human Herpesvirus 6 Infection: PCR-Based Methods

Method	Comments
Qualitative PCR	Insensitive at distinguishing latent from active infection
PCR of plasma PCR of cerebrospinal fluid	Fair reliability for diagnosis of active infection
Quantitative PCR	Sensitive, reproducible May detect strain-specific difference

Human herpesvirus 6 may be oncogenic, because specific viral genomic fragments transform animal and human cell lines in vitro.[215–217] Early serologic and molecular studies that suggested an association between herpesvirus 6 and lymphoma[218–222] have not been confirmed by in situ hybridization and immunohistochemistry.[223,224] Human herpesvirus 6 infection has been more consistently documented in sinus histiocytosis with massive lymphadenopathy, and expression of a human herpesvirus 6 protein in the late phase of the viral cycle is present in a significant proportion of the abnormal histiocytes, the hallmark of Rosai-Dorfman disease (Fig. 75–11).[224,225] Rosai-Dorfman disease may represent an exaggerated immunologic response to an infectious agent, pathophysiologically associated with herpesviruses in general, not only EBV but also human herpesvirus 6.[224,225] Human herpesvirus 6 gene expression has also been described in the neoplastic cells of a rare aggressive disorder, S-100 T-cell chronic lymphoproliferative disease.[226]

Human herpesvirus 7 can be isolated from the saliva of many healthy adults.[160,161,227] The virus replicates in vivo, at least in selected sites, without clinical consequences. Human herpesvirus 7 is tropic for CD4 T lymphocytes, and the glycoprotein CD4 is an essential component of its cellular membrane receptor.[228] Reciprocal interference between human herpesvirus 7 and HIV, which also uses CD4 as a receptor, occurs in vitro.[229] Human herpesvirus 7 reactivates latent human herpesvirus 6 genomes[230] in vitro; in stem cell transplant patients, a high human herpesvirus 7 load usually precedes the peak in human herpesvirus 6 viremia.[213]

Human herpesvirus 7 has not been clearly linked to any human disease. The virus has been implicated in clinical syndromes resembling exanthem subitum[231] and isolated from the peripheral blood of a Japanese child suffering from recurrent fever, hepatosplenomegaly, and pancytopenia, an illness clinically indistinguishable from chronic active EBV infection.[232] In most children, primary human herpesvirus 6 infection (occurring from 6 months

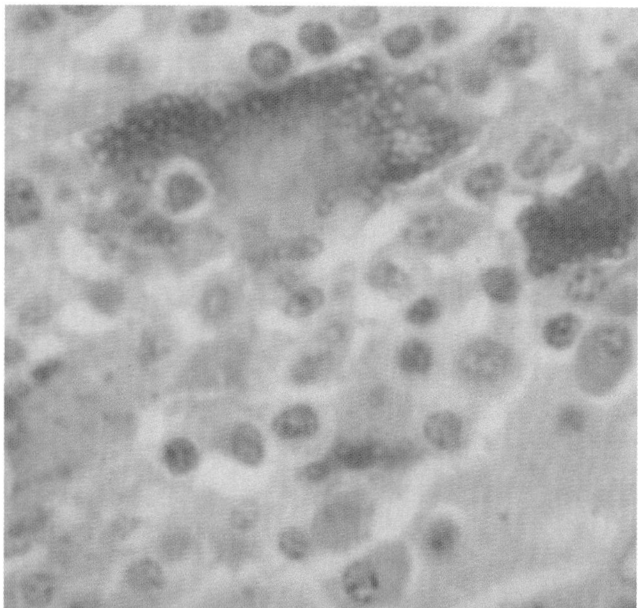

■ **Figure 75–11.** Abnormal histiocyte with emperipolesis in sinus histiocytosis with massive lymphadenopathy (Rosai-Dorfman disease), showing intense cytoplasmic expression of the lytic gp106 antigen of human herpesvirus 6 (immunoperoxidase method; × 400).

to 2 years of age) precedes primary human herpesvirus 7 infection (occurring from 2 years to 5 years of age).[177] In a few instances of stem cell transplantation, human herpesvirus 7 infection was linked to encephalitis and acute myelitis.[233,234] Human herpesvirus 7 together with human herpesvirus 6 appear to influence the severity of cytomegalovirus disease in all patients.[235,236]

CURRENT CONTROVERSIES & FUTURE CONSIDERATIONS

Human Cytomegalovirus, Human Herpesvirus 8, and Other Herpesviruses

- Are there hematologic syndromes other than cytomegalovirus-associated mononucleosis that are related to latent or productive cytomegalovirus infection?
- What is the anatomic site and mode of latency? Do hematopoietic progenitor and stem cells serve as a site of cytomegalovirus latency?
- Is there a causative relation between exacerbation of graft-versus-host disease and cytomegalovirus reactivation?
- Can latent cytomegalovirus be eradicated? Can cytomegalovirus vaccine be developed, and what would be the indication for vaccination?
- Why is Kaposi's sarcoma so rare in bone marrow/ peripheral blood stem cell transplant patients?
- Is human herpesvirus 8 transmissable with blood products?
- Is there any benefit in either preventing or reducing the risk for human herpesvirus 6 replication in transplant recipients?
- Does human herpesvirus 6 infection increase the risk for either cytomegalovirus or fungal infection in transplant patients?
- Does human herpesvirus 7 infection have any pathogenic potential?

Suggested Readings*

Cytomegalovirus

Boeckh M, Nichols WG: The impact of cytomegalovirus serostatus of donor and recipient before hematopoietic stem cell transplantation in the era of antiviral prophylaxis and preemptive therapy. Blood 103:2003–2008, 2004.

Clark DA, Emery VC, Griffiths PD: Cytomegalovirus, human herpesvirus-6, and human herpesvirus-7 in hematological patients. Semin Hematol 40:154–162, 2003.

Einsele H, Hebart H: CMV-specific immunotherapy. Hum Immunol 65:558–564, 2004.

Gandhi MK, Khanna R: Human cytomegalovirus: clinical aspects, immune regulation, and emerging treatments. Lancet Infect Dis 4:725–738, 2004.

Hewlett G, Hallenberger S, Rubsamen-Waigmann H: Antivirals against DNA viruses (hepatitis B and the herpes viruses). Curr Opin Pharmacol 4:453–464, 2004.

Human Herpesviruses 6, 7, and 8

Caserta MT, Mock DJ, Dewurst S: Human herpesvirus 6. Clin Infect Dis 33:829–833, 2001.

Schulz TF: Kaposi's sarcoma-associated herpesvirus (human herpesvirus 8): epidemiology and pathogenesis. J Antimicrob Chemother 45:15–27, 2000.

Wong SW, Bergquam EP, Swanson RM, et al: Induction of B cell hyperplasia in simian immunodeficiency virus-infected rhesus macaques with the simian homologue of Kaposi's sarcoma-associated herpesvirus. J Exp Med 190:827–840, 1999.

Full references for this chapter can be found on accompanying CD-ROM.

The contribution by Mario Luppi is dedicated to his wife Elena, his son Giacomo and to Antonio Romano, the neurosurgeon who has saved his life.

CHAPTER 76

Parvovirus B19

Kevin E. Brown, MD, and Neal S. Young, MD

KEY POINTS

Parvovirus B19

- B19 parvovirus, a small, nonenveloped DNA virus, is the etiologic agent of fifth disease, a common childhood exanthem, and of several hematologic diseases.
- Acute B19 parvovirus infection in an individual with underlying hemolytic disease causes transient aplastic crisis. Persistent infection in an immunodeficient host can lead to pure red cell aplasia. Infection of a second-trimester fetus may result in hydrops fetalis.
- The cellular receptor for B19 parvovirus is globoside or erythrocyte P antigen; expression of the receptor predominantly on erythroid cells explains the specificity of parvovirus for this lineage. Genetic absence of the receptor makes p antigen individuals not susceptible to parvovirus infection.
- Failure to produce neutralizing antibodies is the basis of parvovirus persistence; congenital (Nezelof syndrome), iatrogenic (cytotoxic and immunosuppressive drug therapies), and acquired immunodeficiencies are associated with red cell aplasia from this pathophysiology.
- Transient aplastic crisis only requires recognition and transfusion. Persistent B19 parvovirus infection responds to intravenous immunoglobulin infusions.

INTRODUCTION

Parvovirus B19 is the only member of the family *Parvoviridae* pathogenic in humans. B19 is now known to be the specific cause of several hematologic diseases amenable to treatment, and is even preventable. The virus was discovered in an asymptomatic blood donor, coded 19 in panel B, whose serum was being tested for hepatitis B and gave a false-positive result by counterimmunoelectrophoresis.[1] When the precipitin band was examined by electron microscopy, the nonenveloped 23-nm icosahedral virions were typical of the parvoviruses. Parvovirus B19 was first associated with human disease in 1981, when it was shown to be the cause of transient aplastic crisis (TAC) in sickle cell anemia,[2] and in 1983 its role in the etiology of fifth disease (erythema infectiosum) was established.[3] Chronic B19 infection causes severe pure red cell aplasia in immunosuppressed patients,[4,5] and fetal hydrops following maternal B19 infection in pregnancy.[6]

Classification

Parvoviruses are small nonenveloped viruses with a limited linear single-stranded DNA genome. Subfamilies and genera are divided based on their genome sequence, transcription map, and replication strategies (Table 76–1): the *Densovirinae* are viruses of insects and the *Parvovirinae* are viruses of vertebrates.[7] The genus *Parvovirus* contains a wide range of viruses of mammals and birds that can cause major diseases in their animal hosts, but no member of this family is known to infect humans. The genus *Dependovirus* includes many mammalian and avian species and at least nine different primate dependoviruses.[8] Adeno-associated viruses AAV-2, AAV-3, and AAV-5 are common human infections, and, although AAV DNA has been detected in some fetal abortion tissues,[9] none of the dependoviruses has been linked with disease in either humans or animals. Because of their apparent nonpathogenicity, AAVs are of great interest as viral vectors for gene therapy.

Parvovirus B19 is the first member and type species of the genus *Erythrovirus*, although closely related primate viruses have also been isolated from cynomolgus, rhesus, and pig-tailed macaques.[10,11] These erythroviruses share up to 60% homology with B19, with similar genome organization, erythroid tropism, and biologic behavior in their natural hosts.

Viral Properties

Parvovirus B19 virions are nonenveloped, 19- to 23-nm diameter, icosahedral viruses[12] (Fig. 76–1) encapsidating the single-stranded 5596-nucleotide DNA genome (equal amounts of plus and minus strands of DNA are packaged). The B19 genome has an internal coding sequence of 4830 nucleotides, flanked by identical terminal repeat

TABLE 76–1. Current Classification of the *Parvoviridae*

Subfamily	Genus	Species	Genotype
Densovirinae	*Brevidensovirus*		
	Densovirus		
	Iteravirus		
Parvovirinae	*Amdovirus*	Aleutian mink parvovirus	
	Bocavirus[†]	Bovine parvovirus	
	Dependovirus[†]	AAVs-1–9	Genotype 1
		Avian AAV	Genotype 2 (A6, Lali, VX)
	Erythrovirus[†]	B19 virus	Genotype 3 (V9)
		Simian parvovirus	
		Rhesus parvovirus	
	Parvovirus	MVM virus	
		Canine parvovirus	
		Feline panleukopenia virus	
		Porcine parvovirus	
		Rat parvovirus	
		*Goose parvovirus	
		*Muscovy duck parvovirus	

The International Committee on Taxonomy of Viruses originally classified B19 as a member of the autonomous parvovirus genus, but it was reclassified as the type member of the newly created *Erythrovirus* genus in 1993.
*The avian parvoviruses are currently included in the *Parvovirus* genus, but at the molecular level they are closer to the *Dependovirus* sequences.
[†]Genera contain human viruses.

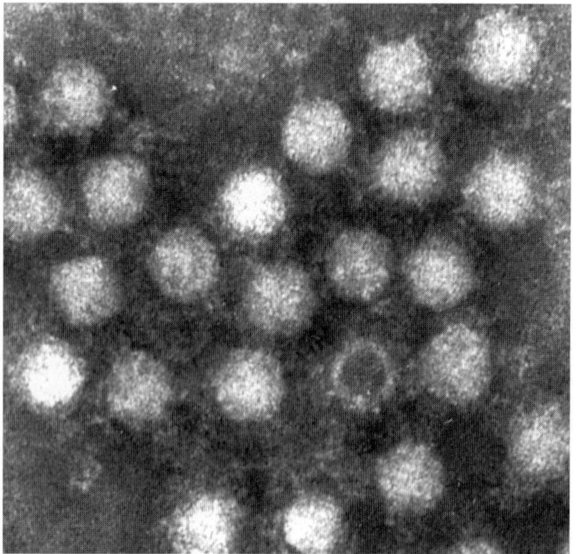

Figure 76–1. Electron micrograph showing parvovirus B19 particles in serum.

sequences at the 5′ and 3′ ends of 383 nucleotides that form an imperfect palindrome and hairpin structures, sufficiently long as to be visualized by electron microscopy.[13]

The viral genome is relatively well conserved, with approximately 5% sequence variation between genotype 1 isolates from different parts of the world and from different time periods.[14–16] Recently viral sequences from two additional B19 genotypes have been described,[17–20] of unclear significance; there is no clear correlation between viral sequence and disease manifestations.

The B19 genome has two large open reading frames and encodes three major proteins (Fig. 76–2). The large open reading frame on the left encodes a multifunctional nonstructural phosphoprotein, NS1. The protein upregulates its own promoter[21] and is required for viral replication and encapsidation of the viral genome within the virus. NS1 is cytotoxic, and induces cell cycle arrest[22] and caspase activation in infected cells.[23]

The large right-hand open reading frame encodes the capsid proteins; each virus consists of 60 capsid proteins (see Fig. 76–2). The major capsid protein, VP2, of 554 amino acids, makes up 95% of the capsid structure. The minor capsid protein, VP1, has an additional 227 amino acids at the amino terminus and contains the main neutralizing epitopes,[24] and a phospholipase motif[25] thought to be important for viral entry is localized to this unique region.

Parvoviruses are stable in lipid solvents (ether and chloroform), but they can be inactivated by formalin, oxidizing agents, and gamma irradiation. Transmission of parvovirus B19 by heat-treated blood products has been well documented.[26,27]

EPIDEMIOLOGY

Parvovirus B19 infection is common in childhood, and by the age of 15 years approximately 50% of children have acquired virus-specific immunoglobulin (Ig)G[28] (Fig. 76–3*A*). In temperate climates, most infections occur in the spring, and mini-epidemics occur at regular intervals several years apart (Fig. 76–3*B*). Secondary infection

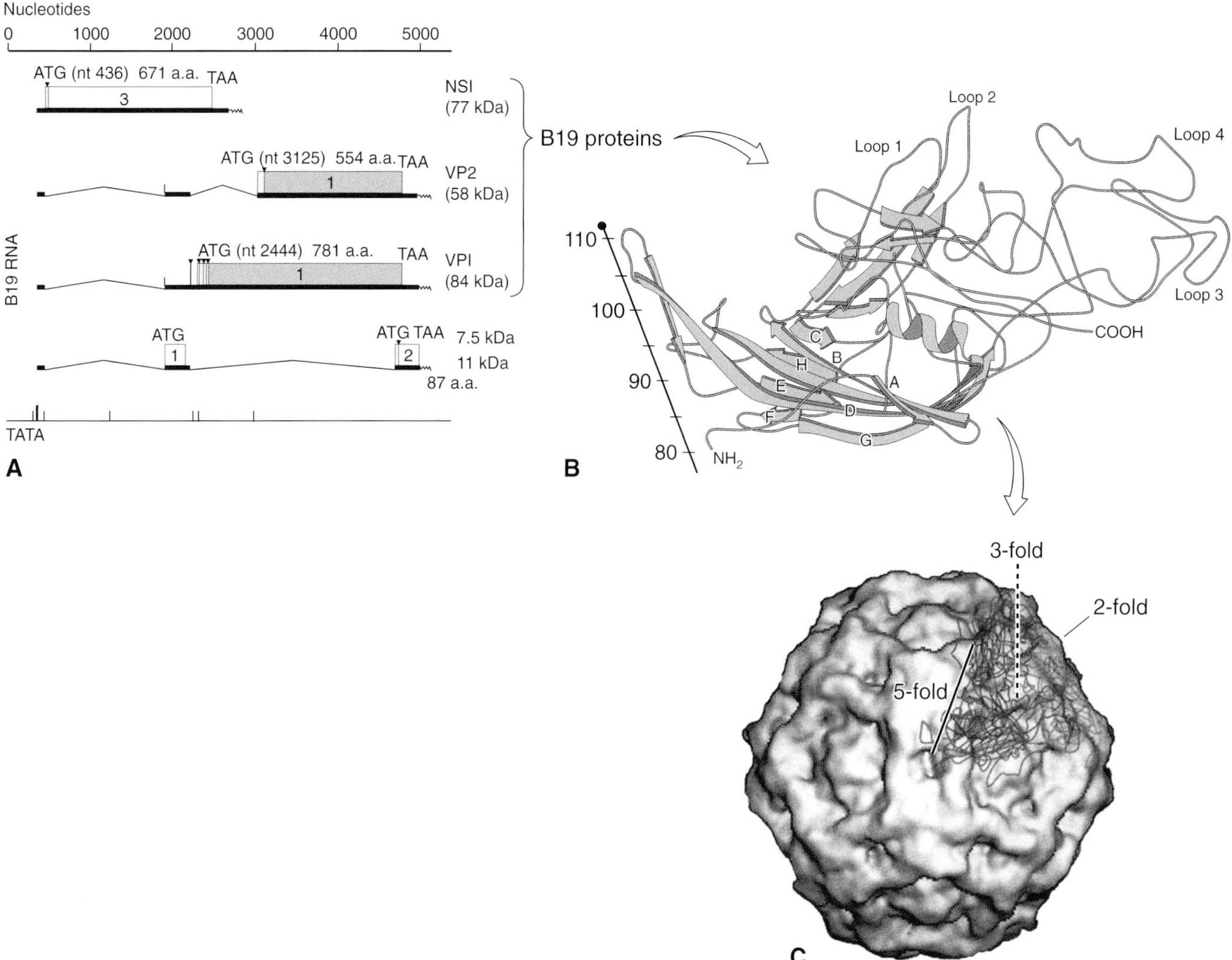

Figure 76–2. Transcription map *(A)*, ribbon diagram of capsid *(B)*, and cryo–electron micrograph of parvovirus particles showing position of VP2 capsid protein in virion structure *(C)*.

rates approach 50% in households,[29] and the virus spreads rapidly through families and in schools and other institutions. Transmission is predominantly by the respiratory route, probably by droplet spread, and is highest at the time of viremia and before the onset of rash or arthralgia.

Parvovirus B19 infections also can occur as a result of transfusion of blood or blood products,[26] most readily with pooled components, especially factor VIII and IX concentrates. Human parvovirus is highly resistant to temperatures below 100°C,[30] and solvent-detergent methods which inactive lipid-enveloped viruses are ineffective.[31,32] Since January 2002, the major producers of plasma-derived therapies in the United States have voluntarily instituted in-process control measures to help prevent the transmission of B19, with an aim of reducing the B19 viral load in therapeutic plasma products to the limit of less than 10^4 IU of B19 DNA/mL suggested by the Food and Drug Administration.[33]

PATHOPHYSIOLOGY

Parvovirus B19 Cellular Receptor and the P Blood Group System

The major cellular receptor for parvovirus B19 is globoside, a neutral glycosphingolipid found predominantly on erythroid cells or their progenitors, where it is known as the blood group P antigen.[34] The P blood group was discovered in 1927 by Landsteiner and Levine as part of studies to identify new human blood group antigens by immunizing rabbits with human erythrocytes. The P blood group system contains two common antigens, P_1 and P, and the rarer antigen, P^k. Bone marrow from rare individuals (<1:200,000) who do not have P on their erythrocytes—the blood group p phenotype (or Tja^-)—cannot be infected with parvovirus B19 in vitro, and, in seroprevalence studies, individuals with p phenotype

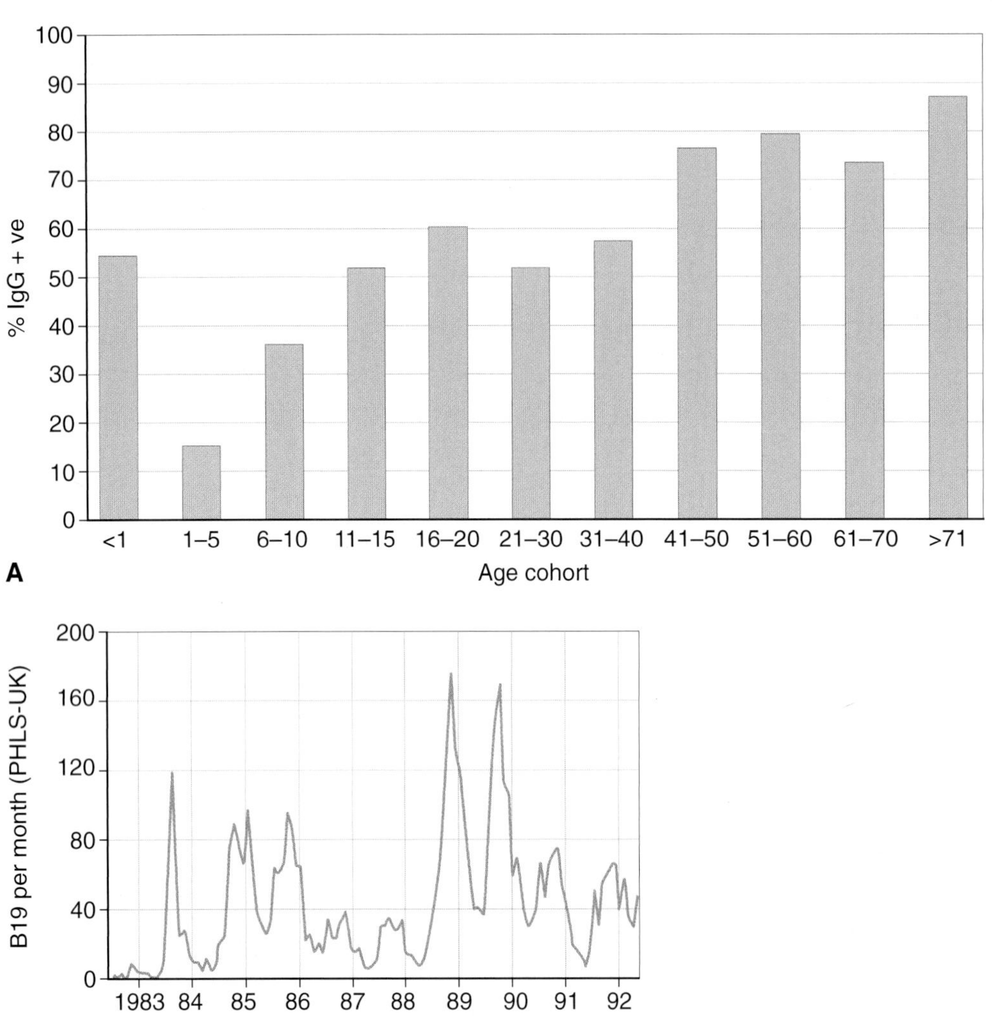

Figure 76–3. Epidemiology of parvovirus B19 infection. ***A,*** Prevalence of B19 IgG by age. ***B,*** Seasonal incidence of B19 infections as determined by B19 IgM positivity in a reference laboratory.

have no evidence of previous infection with parvovirus B19.[35]

Erythroid Tropism

Parvovirus B19, like all the autonomous parvoviruses, is dependent on mitotically active cells for its own replication. B19 also has a very narrow target cell range and can only be efficiently propagated in human erythroid progenitor cells (Fig. 76–4). The identification of the parvovirus B19 receptor as globoside in part explained this erythroid tropism. In human clonal progenitor studies, there is marked inhibition of erythroid colony formation by erythroid colony-forming units and erythroid burst-forming units, but no effect on granulocyte-macrophage colony-formation.[36] Susceptibility to parvovirus B19 increases with differentiation, and the pluripotent stem cell appears to be spared.[37] In erythroid progenitors, the virus is directly cytotoxic; expression of the parvovirus B19 NS protein induces cell death, and cells show the ultrastructural features typical of apoptosis.[38] Infected cultures are characterized by the presence of giant pronormoblasts or "lantern cells": early erythroid cells, 25–32 μm in diameter, with cytoplasmic vacuolization, immature chromatin, and large eosinophilic nuclear inclusion bodies (Fig. 76–5*A*). The light microscopic findings are also seen in the bone marrow of infected patients (Fig. 76–5*B*).

The tissue distribution of P antigen is consistent with the known tropism of B19, and, although other studies have confirmed that P antigen is required for B19 viral entry,[39] the P antigen receptor is clearly not the only mediator of permissivity.

In addition to erythroblasts and megakaryoblasts,[40] P antigen is also found on endothelial cells, which may be targets of viral infection and involved in the pathogenesis of transplacental transmission and the rash of fifth disease; on fetal myocardial cells; in the kidney[41]; in the placenta[42]; and on myeloblasts[43] and some B cells.[44] Parvoviral DNA can be detected in all these cells and tissue types, but it is unclear how efficiently the virus replicates, if it all, in nonerythroid tissues.

Immune Response to B19 Infection

In immunocompetent individuals, virus-specific IgM and IgG antibodies are made following experimental and natural B19 parvovirus infection (Fig. 76–6*A*). After

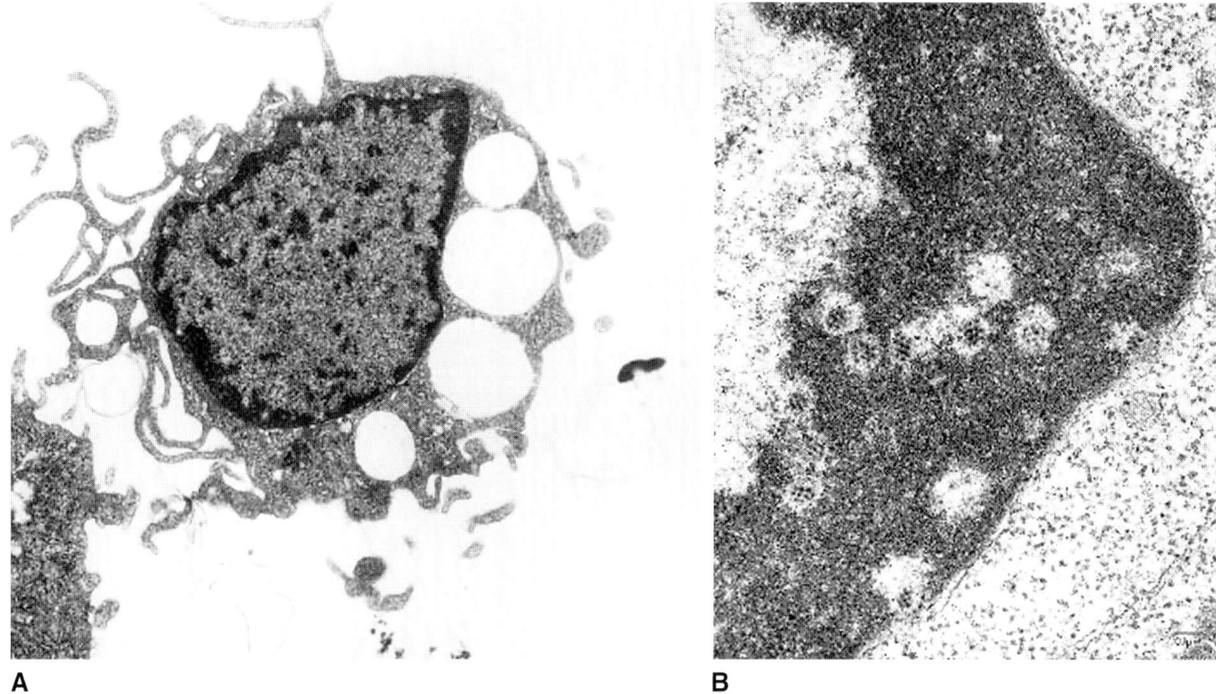

Figure 76–4. Electron micrographs showing parvovirus B19 in human erythroid progenitor cells infected in vitro. **A**, In this low power view, note the characteristic prominent vacuoles, pseudopod formation from the cytoplasm, and marginated chromatin in the nucleus. **B**, At higher magnification, lacunae within the nucleus contain crystalline arrays of parvovirus particles.

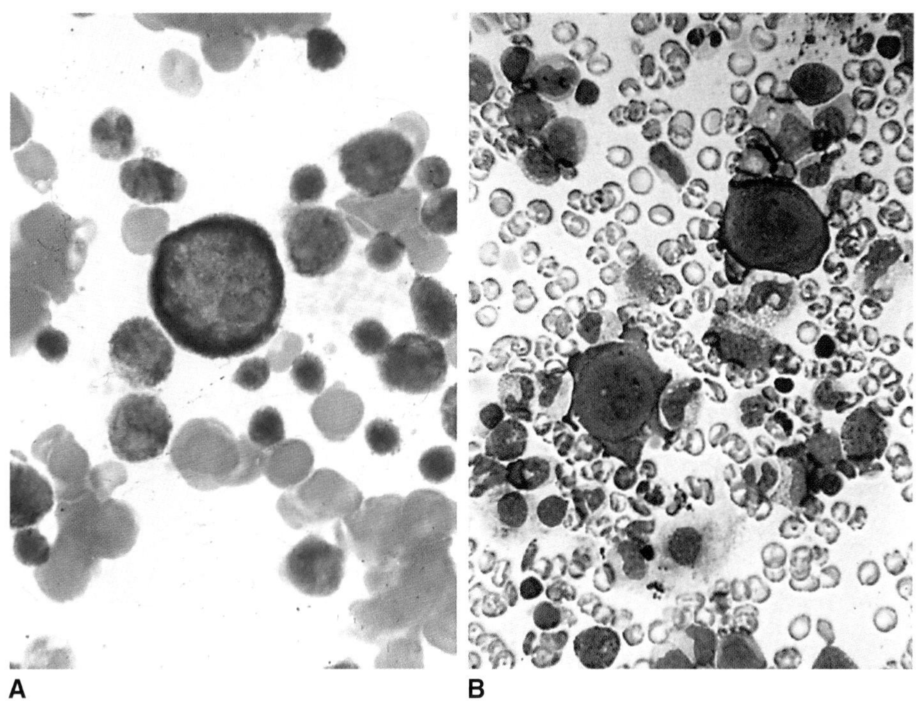

Figure 76–5. Hematologic changes secondary to infection with parvovirus B19. ***A***, Giant pronormoblast in marrow cells infected in vitro. ***B***, Lack of erythroid precursors in a persistently infected bone marrow.

intranasal inoculation, virus can first be detected at days 5–6 and peaks at days 8–9. IgM antibody to B19 appears about 10–14 days after infection and may be found in serum samples for several months after exposure. IgG antibody also appears about 2 weeks after infection; IgG persists for life and levels rise with reexposure. The early antibodies are directed against the major capsid protein (VP2), but, as the immune response matures, reactivity to the minor capsid protein (VP1) dominates. The immune response to VP1 appears to be critical for protective immunity: sera from patients with persistent B19 infection typically have antibody to VP2 but not to VP1.[45]

The humoral arm dominates the immune response to B19, because recovery from infection correlates with the

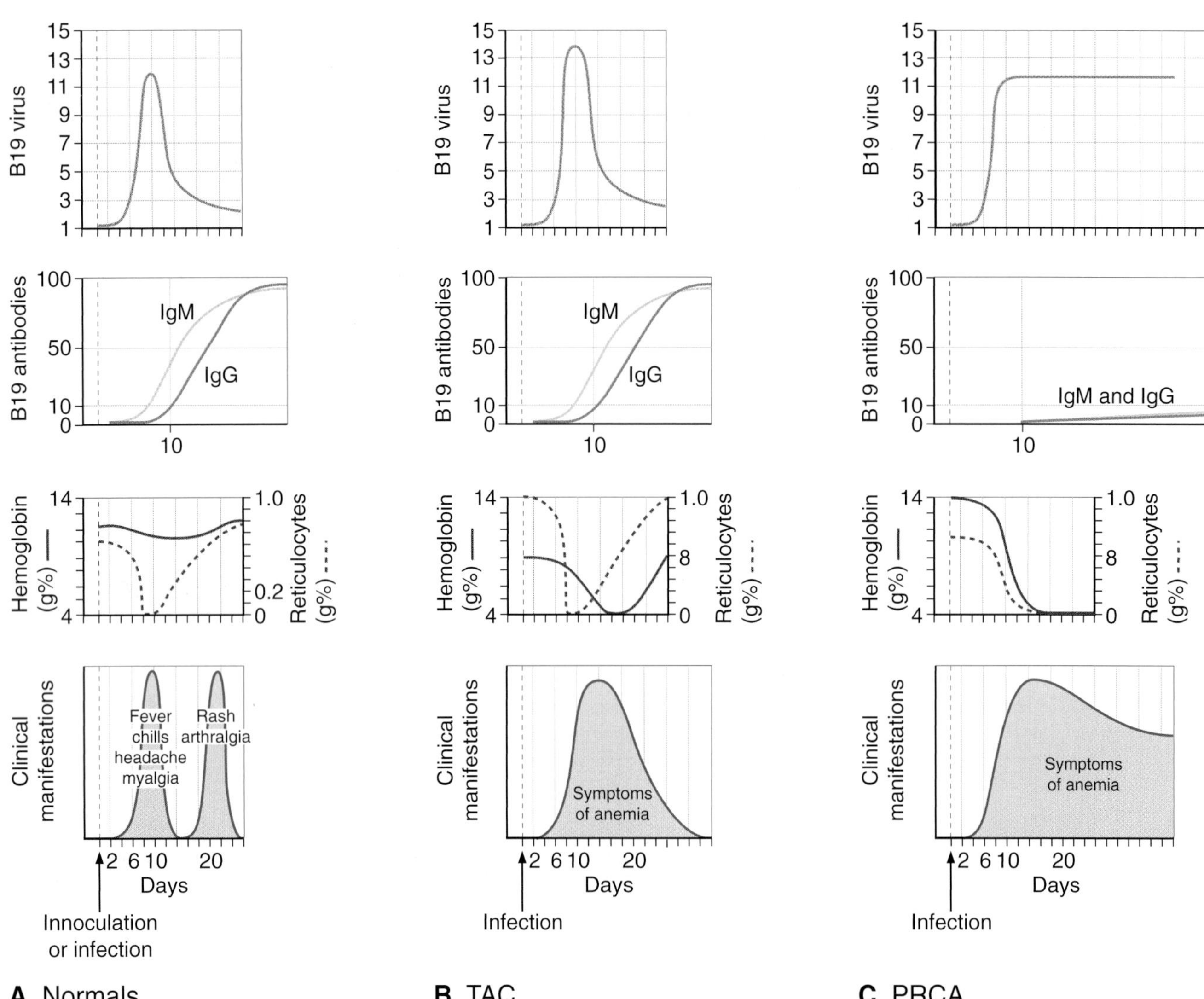

■ **Figure 76–6.** Schematic of the time course of B19 infection in fifth disease *(A)*, transient aplastic crisis *(B)*, and persistent anemia *(C)*. (From Young NS, Brown KE: Parvovirus B19. N Engl J Med 350:586–597, 2004, with permission.)

appearance of circulating specific antivirus antibody, and administration of commercial immunoglobulins can cure or ameliorate persistent parvovirus infection in immunodeficient patients (see later).

Pathogenesis

In normal volunteers, B19 infection was followed by an acute but self-limited (4–8 days) cessation of red cell production and a corresponding decline in hemoglobin levels (Figs. 76–6*A* and 76–7). When erythroid turnover is normal, this transient interruption of red cell production prior to the onset of the neutralizing antibody response does not lead to anemia. When the demand for erythrocytosis is high, most usually as a result of hemolysis, the erythroid progenitor compartment is large, leading to higher B19 viral titers; with a shortened red blood cell lifespan, even a brief interruption in red cell production can precipitate an aplastic crisis (Fig. 76–6*B*; see also Fig. 76–7). The crisis resolves with a disappearance of viremia on the development of a specific humoral immune response. In patients with immune compromise, the lack of a neutralizing antibody response results in prolonged viremia and chronic pure red cell aplasia (Fig. 76–6*C*; see also Fig. 76–7).

The infected fetus may suffer severe effects both because red blood cell turnover is high and because the immune response is deficient, especially during the second trimester. In infected fetuses, parvovirus particles can be detected by electron microscopy within the hematopoietic tissues of the liver and thymus. B19 DNA and capsid antigen have been observed in the myocardium,[46] and the fetus may develop myocarditis to compound the severe anemia and secondary cardiac failure (see Fig. 76–7). By the third trimester, a more effective immune response to the virus protects against fetal loss.

Although parvoviral DNA can be found in the skin and joints of affected patients, the pathogenesis of the rash in erythema infectiosum and of the polyarthropathy is immune complex-mediated. In inoculated volunteers,

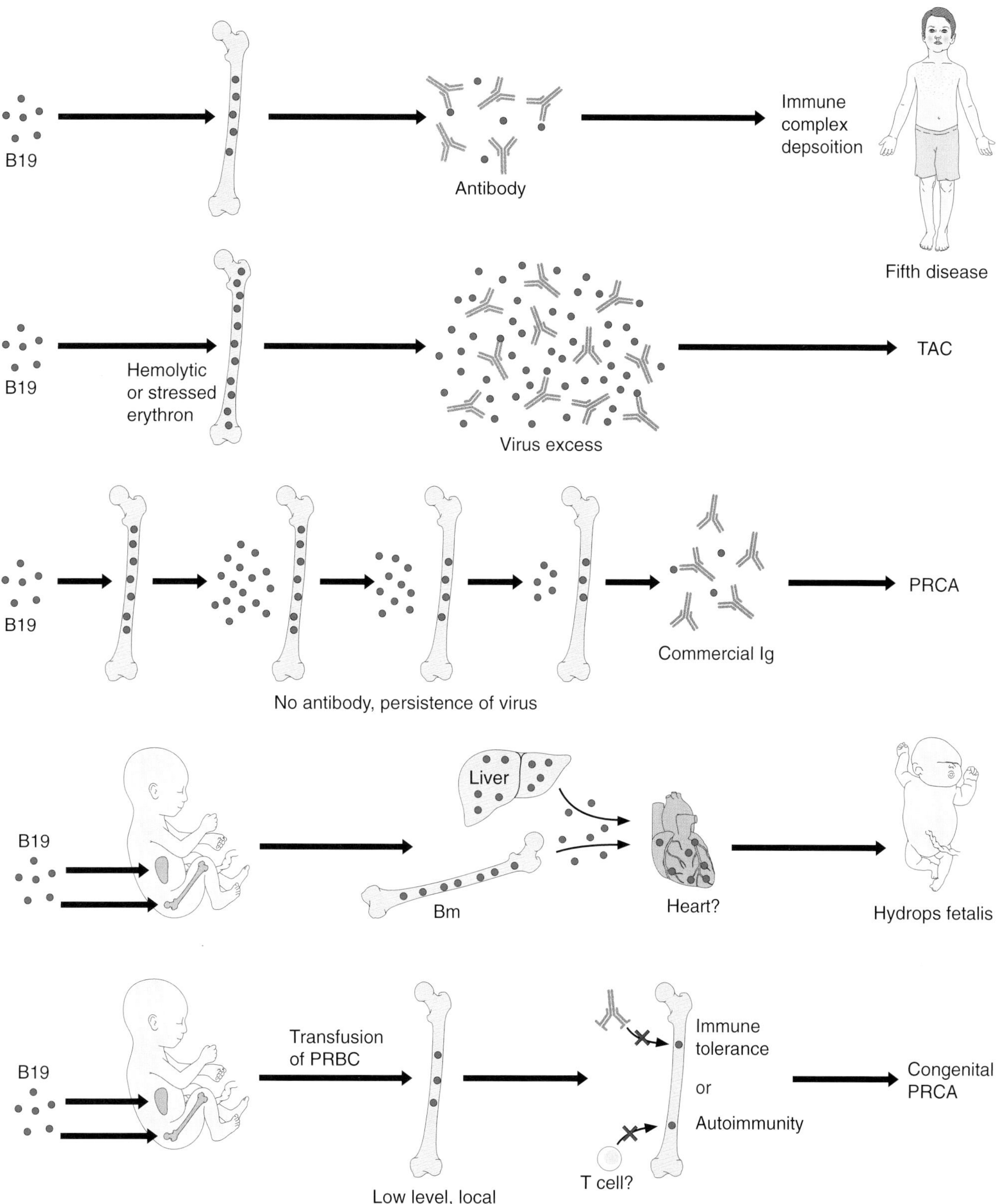

Figure 76–7. Pathogenesis of parvovirus B19 infection.

TABLE 76–2. Hematologic and Nonhematologic Diseases Caused by Parvovirus B19

Disease	Acute/Chronic	Host
Hematologic Diseases Caused By Parvovirus B19		
Transient aplastic crisis	Acute	Patients with increased erythropoiesis
Pure red cell aplasia	Chronic	Immunodeficient/immunocompromised patients
Hydrops fetalis/congenital anemia	Acute/chronic	Fetus (<20 wk)
Hemophagocytosis	Acute/chronic	?
Neutropenia/pancytopenia	Acute/chronic	?
Nonhematologic Diseases in Which Parvovirus B19 Is Etiologic or Suspected		
Fifth disease	Acute	Normal children
Polyarthropathy syndrome	Acute/chronic	Normal adults
Hepatitis	?	?
Myocarditis	?	?
Vasculitis/endothelial infection	?	?
Neurologic	?	?

rash and joint symptoms appeared when viremia was no longer present and at the time of development of a detectable immune response.[47] Fifth disease has been precipitated in chronically infected individuals by immunoglobulin therapy.[48]

As noted previously, B19 DNA can be also detected in other cell types, including endothelial cells, hepatocytes, and synovial tissue. It is unclear whether the virus actively replicates in these tissues, and whether the persistence of low levels of viral DNA in these tissues could be a target for a local inflammatory response.

CLINICAL DISEASE

Parvovirus B19 is the known or suspected cause of a number of hematologic and nonhematologic diseases (Table 76–2). These disorders occur in patients of all ages and may be acute or chronic.

Hematologic Manifestations

Transient Aplastic Crisis

The term *aplastic crisis* was coined by Owren[49] to describe the abrupt onset of severe anemia with absent reticulocytes in patients with hereditary spherocytosis, in contrast to hemolytic crises, in which bone marrow turnover is increased and elevated. TAC occurs as a single episode in the patient's life. In TAC cases, there often is a history of a preceding prodromal illness, and mini-epidemics in large kindreds of hereditary spherocytosis early suggested an infectious etiology.

TAC was the first clinical illness associated with B19 infection. When stored sera from over 800 children admitted to a London hospital were examined, 6 patients had evidence of recent infection with B19 (either antigenemia or seroconversion)—all were Jamaican immigrants with sickle cell disease presenting with TAC. Aplastic crisis was diagnosed by the combination of reduced hemoglobin, absent circulating reticulocytes, and erythroid hypoplasia in the bone marrow.[2] In a retrospective study of sera from sickle cell patients in Jamaica, 86% of TAC cases were associated with recent parvovirus infection.[50]

TAC has been described in a wide range of hemolytic disorders, including hereditary spherocytosis, thalassemia, red cell enzymopathies such as pyruvate kinase deficiency, and autoimmune hemolytic anemia.[51] TAC can also occur under conditions of erythroid "stress," such as with hemorrhage or iron deficiency anemia and following kidney or bone marrow transplantation. Aplastic crisis can be the first presentation of an underlying hemolytic disease (usually hereditary spherocytosis) in a hematologically well-compensated patient. Acute anemia has been described in hematologically normal persons, and a decrease in hemoglobin levels and reticulocytes was seen in healthy volunteers.[47] Although suffering from an ultimately self-limiting disease, patients with TAC can be severely ill.[52] Symptoms include dyspnea, lassitude, and confusion resulting from the worsening anemia; congestive heart failure and bone marrow necrosis may develop, and the TAC can be fatal.

Community-acquired aplastic crisis is almost always due to parvovirus B19, and parvovirus should be the presumptive diagnosis in a patient whose anemia worsens due to an abrupt cessation of erythropoiesis, as documented by reduced reticulocytes and the characteristic bone marrow morphology. In contrast to patients with erythema infectiosum, TAC patients are viremic at the time of presentation, with concentrations of virus as high as 10^{14} genome copies/mL. The diagnosis is readily made by detection of B19 DNA in the serum. As virus is cleared from the blood, B19-specific IgM becomes detectable. TAC is a unique event in the patient's life, and, following acute infection, immunity is lifelong.

Transient erythroblastopenia of childhood (TEC) (see Chapter 12), the temporary failure of red cell production in hematologically normal children, does not appear to be associated with parvovirus B19.[53] Sporadic cases of TEC with thrombocytopenia have been described with evidence of recent B19 infection, but classical TEC is associated with high platelet counts.

Neutropenia, Thrombocytopenia, Pancytopenia, and Hemophagocytosis

Both TAC and B19 infection in hematologically normal patients are often associated with changes in the other blood lineages, varying degrees of neutropenia, and thrombocytopenia,[54,55] and frank agranulocytosis.[56,57] Some cases of idiopathic thrombocytopenic purpura and Henoch-Schönlein purpura have been blamed on parvovirus B19[58–61]; in a recent study, 13% of patients (6 of 47) with idiopathic thrombocytopenia had evidence of recent B19 infection.[62] Pancytopenia is much less common.[63,64] Hemophagocytosis, which is a rare complication of many different viral infections, has been described in acute and persistent B19 infection, usually with a favorable outcome.[65–68]

Pure Red Cell Aplasia

Persistent B19 infection resulting in pure red cell aplasia can occur in a wide variety of immunosuppressed states: congenital immunodeficiency,[4] acquired immunodeficiency (human immunodeficiency virus infection or acquired immunodeficiency syndrome),[48] lymphoproliferative disorders,[5] and after organ transplantation. The degree of immunosuppression may be subtle, and pure red cell aplasia may be the presenting illness of patients with human immunodeficiency virus infection or with very limited immune dysfunction.[69] In all cases, the stereotypical presentation is persistent anemia associated with reticulocytopenia; other blood lineages may also be affected, and patients rarely may present with pancytopenia. Examination of the bone marrow usually reveals scattered giant pronormoblasts but no other erythroid precursors. B19-specific antibody is absent or low, but there is persistent or recurrent parvoviremia as detected by B19 DNA in the serum, with titers greater than 10^6 genome copies/mL. Administration of intravenous immunoglobulin can be ameliorative of the anemia and sometimes curative.[5] Temporary cessation of maintenance chemotherapy may also lead to resolution of anemia, because decreasing the level of iatrogenic immunosuppression allows the host to produce antibody and resolve the virus infection.

Fetal Infection

The fetus is at particular risk of persistent B19 infection, especially during the early middle trimester when the immune response has not matured and there is a rapid expansion of the erythroid compartment. B19 infection in pregnancy can lead to an adverse outcome, either miscarriage or hydrops fetalis (Fig. 76–8). In epidemiologic studies in the United Kingdom[70] and in the United States,[71] the risk of fetal parvovirus B19 infection was calculated at 30%, and the risk of fetal loss following confirmed B19 infection was 5–9%.

Parvovirus B19 probably causes 10–15% of all cases of nonimmune hydrops; approximately one third of the cases of B19-induced hydrops will resolve spontaneously.[72] Generally, if the fetus survives the hydrops, there are no long-term sequelae resulting from congenital B19 infection. However, rare cases of congenital red cell aplasia or dysplasia following in utero B19 infection have been reported[73–75]; all were treated with intravenous immunoglobulin, but in two of four survivors, anemia persisted even though B19 DNA could no longer be detected, suggesting that the anemia is not simply due to direct viral cytotoxicity.

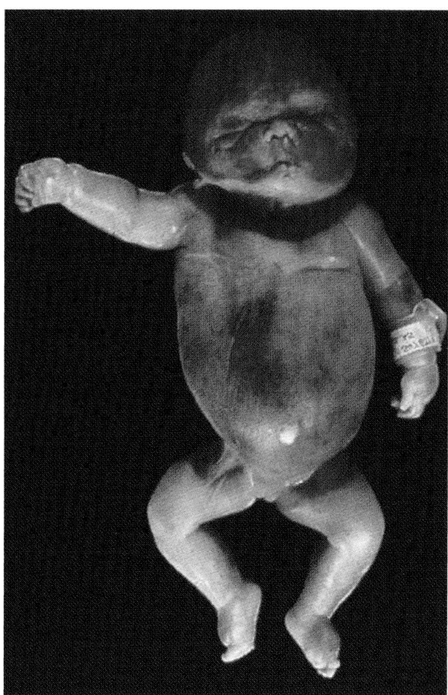

Figure 76–8. Hydrops fetalis in an infant infected with parvovirus B19 in utero.

Nonhematologic Disease

About 50% of B19 infections are asymptomatic or so minor as not to warrant medical attention. The most common clinical presentation of parvovirus infection is the rash illness called erythema infectiosum, fifth disease, or slapped cheek rash. Infection begins with a minor febrile illness about a week after exposure, with mild hematologic abnormalities during the second week and the classical facial cutaneous eruption at 17–18 days. The rash may spread to the extremities in a lacy reticular pattern and can be exacerbated by exercise, emotion, bathing, or sunlight. There may be great variation in the appearance of the skin findings, and especially in adults the characteristic slapped cheek may not be apparent.

Although in children B19 infection is usually mild and of short duration, in adults and especially in women there is arthropathy in approximately 50% of patients.[76] The joint distribution is often symmetrical, with arthralgia and even frank arthritis affecting the small joints of the hands and occasionally the ankles, knees, and wrists. Resolution usually occurs within a few weeks, but persistent or recurring symptoms can continue for years.[77] In the absence of a history of a rash, the symptoms may be mistaken for acute rheumatoid arthritis, especially because prolonged symptoms do not correlate with serologic studies, such as the duration of B19 IgM response, or persistent viremia. In addition, B19 infection can be associated with autoantibody production, including transient rheumatoid factor.[78] In one study of patients attending an "early synovitis" clinic in the United Kingdom, 12% had evidence of recent infection with B19,[77] with three patients fulfilling diagnostic criteria for definite rheumatoid arthritis.

The virus has been more tenuously linked to other symptoms (see Table 76–2).[79] That B19 DNA can be detected by polymerase chain reaction (PCR) for years in a variety of normal tissues, including bone marrow,[80] synovial tissue,[81] liver,[82] kidney,[83] and skin,[19,84] is of unknown clinical significance, but confounds many case reports claiming disease association.

DIAGNOSIS

Parvovirus B19 should be considered in the differential diagnosis of anemia with low or absent reticulocytes, especially in patients who are immunodeficient or immunosuppressed (see Chapter 12). Bone marrow should be examined if feasible. In B19 infection, there is a marked decrease or absence of erythroid precursors, with sparing of other bone marrow lineages. If seen, giant pronormoblasts are highly suggestive of B19 infection.

Parvovirus B19 can only be cultured with difficulty in the laboratory, in late erythroid progenitor cells and in some erythro-megakaryoblastoid cell lines—methods impractical for routine use. Detection of virus in tissues, cells, or serum for diagnostic purposes relies on DNA hybridization or PCR techniques. Most patients with symptomatic infection have greater than 10^6 B19 virions/mL of serum, detectable by simple DNA hybridization assays[85] (Table 76–3). In acute B19 infection, B19 DNA is only present at these levels for 2–4 days; B19 DNA at high titer in serial serum samples or more than 2 days after the onset of anemia implies chronic infection.

The sensitivity level of detection of B19 is greatly increased by the use of PCR but at the risk of possible contamination and false-positive results that confuse interpretation. Even in immunocompetent persons, B19 DNA may be detectable in serum by PCR for months following an acute infection,[85] and in most symptomatic chronic B19 infections PCR is unnecessary. However, a sensitive PCR assay may be required in patients who have been treated with immunoglobulin and for the diagnosis of congenital B19 infection.[73] Testing by quantitative PCR for B19 is now more widely available.[86] In addition to the value of these assays in screening blood and blood products, these methods allow quantitation of viremia, and help to determine if intervention is warranted and to follow the response to treatment. B19 DNA also can be detected in bone marrow by dot-blot hybridization, in situ hybridization, and in situ PCR, but, except for cases of suspected congenital infection, a bone marrow sample is not usually required to confirm the diagnosis.

TABLE 76–3. Diagnosis of Parvovirus B19

Disease	IgM	IgG	B19 DNA Direct Hybridization	B19 DNA PCR
Fifth disease	+++	++	+	+
Polyarthropathy syndrome	++	+	−	+
Transient aplastic crisis	+/−	+/−	++	++
Persistent anemia	+/−	+/−	++	++
Hydrops/congenital infection	+/−	+	+/−	++
Previous infection	−	++	−	+/−

The best test to detect recent infection with B19 remains the IgM capture assay.[87] In a radioimmunoassay or enzyme-linked immunosorbent assay, IgM can be detected in over 90% of cases by the third day of TAC (or at the time of rash in fifth disease). IgM remains detectable for 2–3 months following infection.

Parvovirus B19 IgG also can be detected in similar enzyme-linked immunosorbent assays, and an international standard (IU/mL) has been set by the World Health Organization Expert Committee on Biological Standardization for anti–parvovirus B19 testing and reporting.[88] IgG is detectable by the seventh day of illness, and then for life; titers greater than 5 IU/mL indicate previous infection. In persistent parvovirus infection, serologic studies for B19 antibodies are unhelpful, except that high titers of B19 IgG make a diagnosis of chronic B19 infection unlikely.

TREATMENT

Most parvovirus infections do not require specific treatment. TAC is self-limited and is readily treated by blood transfusion and supportive therapy. Administration of anti-inflammatory drugs usually is beneficial in B19 chronic arthropathy.

In patients with chronic anemia caused by persistent B19 infection, administration of immunoglobulin is indicated[5,48]; if renal failure is not present, IgG is infused at a dose of 0.4 gm/kg for 5 days. Patients should respond within 1–2 weeks with a marked reduction in the level of B19 viremia, reticulocytosis, and resolution of the anemia. Relapse can be monitored by observation of reticulocyte counts and assays for B19 DNA, but it is not unusual for low levels of virus to remain detectable by PCR following successful intravenous immunoglobulin treatment. If clinical relapse occurs less than 6 months after the initial treatment, especially in human immunodeficiency virus–positive patients, maintenance by a single-day infusion of 0.4 gm/kg IgG every 4 weeks may control the B19 viremia.[48]

PREVENTION

An effective vaccine against parvovirus B19 infection could prevent TAC of sickle cell disease and in other hemolytic disorders and prevent pure red cell aplasia in immunodeficient persons. Vaccination of women prior to pregnancy would avert hydrops fetalis. B19 capsid proteins, generated by VP2 and VP1 genes in expression systems, will self-assemble to form virus-like particles (lacking B19 DNA), and these empty particles can be used to generate immune responses, especially when engineered to overexpress the highly immunogenic VP1.[89] A single dose of 2.5 μg of virus-like particles elicited neutralizing antibody responses in

CURRENT CONTROVERSIES & FUTURE DIRECTIONS

Parvovirus B19

- The diagnosis of parvovirus infection can be confusing. IgG only indicates infection in the past; IgM is useful to document recent infection. Detection of DNA by hybridization methods is most reliable for parvovirus-induced hematologic diseases. Gene amplification may be too sensitive, because small amounts of virus can be detected in normal persons for months following infection.
- Many diseases have been associated with parvovirus by gene amplification studies alone. More data are necessary to establish the role of the virus in myocarditis, nephritis, and neurologic and rheumatic conditions.
- Nonproductive infection and destruction of target cells by parvoviruses is theoretically possible but difficult to establish as clinically important.
- The significance of molecular variants of B19 parvovirus is still unclear.
- A recombinant vaccine is effective in eliciting neutralizing antibodies, but its commercial viability and extent of application must be determined.

normal volunteers[90]; this recombinant vaccine is in development.

Suggested Readings*

Anderson LJ, Young NS (eds): Human Parvovirus B19. Basel: Karger, 1997.

Brown KE, Anderson SM, Young NS: Erythrocyte P antigen: cellular receptor for B19 parvovirus. Science 262:114–117, 1993.

Brown KE, Hibbs JR, Gallinella G, et al: Resistance to parvovirus B19 infection due to lack of virus receptor (erythrocyte P antigen). N Engl J Med 330:1192–1196, 1994.

Kurtzman G, Frickhofen N, Kimball J, et al: Pure red-cell aplasia of 10 years' duration due to persistent parvovirus B19 infection and its cure with immunoglobulin therapy. N Engl J Med 321:519–523, 1989.

Mortimer PP, Humphries RK, Moore JG, et al: A human parvovirus-like virus inhibits haematopoietic colony formation in vitro. Nature 302:426–429, 1983.

Full references for this chapter can be found on accompanying CD-ROM.

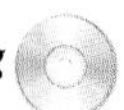

CHAPTER 77

Human Immunodeficiency Virus: Hematologic Complications

Elaine M. Sloand, MD

> **KEY POINTS**
>
> **Human Immunodeficiency Virus: Hematologic Complications**
>
> - Bone marrow failure associated with human immunodeficiency virus (HIV) infection is related to cytokine and immune dysregulation as well as to progenitor cell depletion. Bone marrow is not a significant reservoir for HIV-1.
> - In treating anemia, exclude drug toxicity and check erythropoietin levels—treat with erythropoietin if levels are low.
> - For immune thrombocytopenic purpura, adminster corticosteroids acutely and optimize antiviral therapy. For thrombotic thrombocytopenic purpura, treat with plasmapheresis, and consider vincristine if chronic.
> - The coagulopathy associated with HIV infection is generally not clinically significant. In case of thrombosis, free protein S levels should be measured, and anticoagulate as in uninfected patients.

INTRODUCTION

Since acquired immunodeficiency syndrome (AIDS) was first identified in the United States, a cumulative total of over 800,000 cases have been reported to the Centers for Disease Control and Prevention (CDC). The first test for human immunodeficiency virus (HIV) became available a year following the identification of the retrovirus in 1984. More than 40 million individuals are infected worldwide[1]; 95% of them are in developing countries.

The current CDC definition of AIDS includes HIV-infected adults and adolescents who have less than 200 $CD4^+$ T lymphocytes/μL or a $CD4^+$ T-lymphocyte count as a percentage of total lymphocytes of less than 14. The virus is transmitted sexually, parenterally, and vertically from an infected mother to her infant (Table 77–1). Without treatment, CD4 cells gradually decline, opportunistic infections develop, and there is an increased risk of HIV-related malignancies. Although highly active antiretroviral therapy (HAART) has led to vast improvements in prognosis and quality of life for infected persons in the United States and Europe, in Africa and much of Asia the disease remains untreated[2,3] and represents the leading cause of death.[4–6] In the early years after recognition of the syndrome and the etiologic agent, cytopenias and other hematologic abnormalities were common. These complications have greatly diminished with routine treatment of immunocompromised individuals with triple antiretroviral therapy, but anemia and non-Hodgkin's lymphomas in AIDS patients are still problems encountered by the consulting hematologist.

EPIDEMIOLOGY AND RISK FACTORS

The first American patient with AIDS was reported in 1981 but was retrospectively recognized to have been infected in the 1970s. Since the early 1990s, there has been a decline in the incidence of new AIDS cases related to public health measures, which have limited new infections as well as widespread use of HAART, which has slowed the progression of the disease and improved long-term survival.

Men who have sex with men constitute the greatest number of cases, although the incidence in this population, which peaked in the early 1980s (5–20 per 100 person-years), has since declined (2–4 per 100 person-years). Injection drug users constitute the next largest proportion of cases (<0.5 per 100 person-years).[7] Heterosexual transmission comprises the most cases worldwide but is less frequent in the United States, where minority women are overrepresented.

Genetic Factors

Chemokine receptor expression can influence viral infection and may be responsible for the susceptibility of hematopoietic cells of different lineages to HIV infection.

TABLE 77–1. Modes of Transmission of HIV-1

Sexual Intercourse—Anal and Vaginal
Contaminated needles
Injection drug use
Needle injuries
Injections
Mother to Child
In utero
Peripartum
Breast milk
Transfusion/Transplantation
Blood
Semen
Kidneys, bone marrow, corneas, heart valves

Inherited mutations in the gene coding for the CCR5 receptor confer relative resistance to infection and are present in long-term nonprogressing patients.[8–10]

PATHOPHYSIOLOGY

Similar to other retroviruses, the HIV-1 genome contains *gag, pol,* and *env* genes that encode, respectively, for viral core proteins, enzymes controlling replication (reverse transcriptase, integrase, and a viral protease), and envelope glycoproteins. Viral *rev* and *tat* genes encode proteins that regulate transcription and processing of viral messenger RNA. HIV-1 also contains a number of other genes (*nef, vif, vpr,* and *vpu*) that mediate interaction with the host cell and infectivity.

The virus gains entry into the cell when HIV glycoprotein (gp)120 binds to the cell membrane via the CD4 receptor and a second chemokine receptor (Fig. 77–1). Cells that express the CD4 receptor include T helper lymphocytes, macrophages, and dendritic cells, as well as CD34 cells.[11] Although several chemokine receptors can function as coreceptors for HIV cell entry, CCR5 and CXCR4 are the most relevant. Their cognate ligands are capable of inhibiting viral entry by these receptors and are secreted by monocytes and CD34 cells themselves.[9,12,13] Modulation of expression of the chemokine receptors is affected by cytokines. Binding of HIV gp120 to CD4 leads to a conformational change in the envelope that creates a high-affinity binding site for the chemokine receptor. After the interaction among gp120, CD4, and the chemokine receptor, structural changes occur in gp41 that allow it to anchor to and subsequently fuse with the host cell membrane.

Following entry into the cell, HIV is uncoated in the cytosol, viral RNA is transcribed into double-stranded DNA by reverse transcriptase, and the RNA is transported to the nucleus, where it circularizes and inserts randomly into host chromosomes. Expression of new virus involves transcription of the provirus into genomic RNA and then translation into viral proteins. Gag and Pol precursor proteins are cleaved and the virus assembles at the inner surface of the plasma membrane, ultimately budding from the cell to release an infectious particle (see Fig. 77–1).

The low numbers of both CD4 and CD8 cells in HIV infection result primarily from a combination of increased apoptosis and decreased lymphopoiesis.[14–16] The relative number of infected CD4 cells is small, but infection is not a prerequisite for CD4 cell apoptosis. Products of HIV infection (gp120, Fas-L, cytokines) and/or the immune dysregulation accompanying infection directly or indirectly result in CD4 and CD8 cell death.[14,15,17] Defects in CD8 cell function and impaired antigen presentation, as well as deficiencies in B-cell function and antibody generation, are also seen in HIV-infected persons.

HIV-1 INFECTION

Clinical Features

Initial infection is frequently associated with an illness that resembles acute aseptic viral meningitis, but more than 50% of individuals are asymptomatic. A cellular immune response to the virus follows rapidly, resulting in increased populations of cytotoxic T cells; a humoral response with appearance of immunoglobulin (Ig)M and then IgG follows within 4–12 weeks (Fig. 77–2). Despite a vigorous immune response that may result in clearing of the virus from the circulation, viral replication continues in the lymph nodes and spleen, and these sites act as a reservoir for infection even in the presence of apparently effective antiviral therapy.[18,19]

Cytopenia, bone marrow failure, thrombosis, immune and thrombotic thrombocytopenia, and malignancies are all increased in frequency in patients infected with HIV-1.[20–23] Historically, many of these complications were a reflection of drug toxicity,[24] but others were directly or indirectly due to viremia and its immunologic consequences.[25–27] At least in the industrialized world, significant advances made in development and institution of triple antiretroviral therapy have substantially modified all the clinical manifestations of HIV.

Diagnosis

Standard HIV testing historically has been based on detection of HIV-specific antibodies by an enzyme-linked immunosorbent assay (ELISA) with a confirmatory Western blot. A person is classified as HIV-1 seropositive when a blood sample is positive in two successive ELISAs and in one Western blot (or an equally sensitive and specific test); on immunoblot, two of the three bands of p24, gp41, and gp120/160 must be present (Fig. 77–3). Only a fraction of tests positive by ELISA are actually confirmed by immunoblot, although newer antibody assays are now very sensitive and specific.

Antibody pretransfusion testing may be negative early in infection; the donor is infectious and the humoral immune response is not yet evident. The time from infection to the first positive test for HIV is the "window period."[28] A small number of recipients have been infected following transfusion of blood that was negative for HIV-1 antibody. Although adequate for diagnosis, efforts to improve on serology for pretransfusion testing

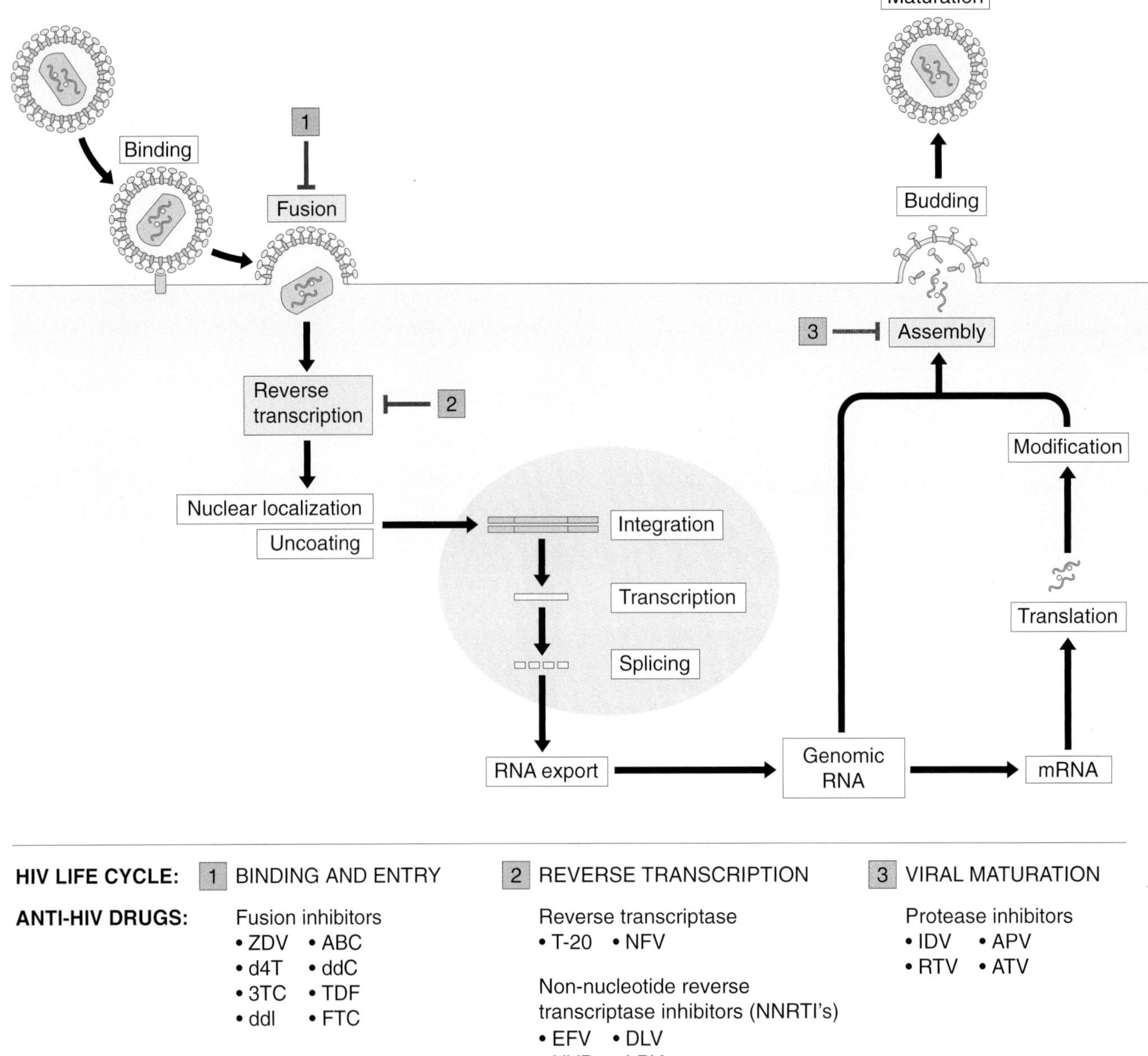

Figure 77–1. Life cycle of HIV-1 and sites of action of antiretroviral medications. New therapies include fusion inhibitors that compete with receptor binding of HIV-1.

have led to the development and implementation of the first antigen detection tests and subsequently nucleic acid–based testing.[29] These assays, which are not dependent on an antibody response, usually become positive at day 16 (viral antigen) and 11 (viral nucleotides) following infection, a significant improvement over the window period of 4–6 weeks for standard ELISA. The risks for all transfusion-transmitted infections have decreased dramatically as a result of extensive pretransfusion questioning and the introduction of these supplemental HIV tests. Using current antibody testing alone, the transfusion risk of HIV is under 1 per 1 million units transfused.[29] More recently, tests based on detection of HIV nucleic acids have been used to identify HIV in pools of blood samples; "NAT technology" can push these risks yet closer to zero.[30]

Treatment

In the absence of antiviral therapy, HIV infection progressively destroys CD4 lymphocytes with the consequence of severe immunodeficiency (see Fig. 77–1). CD4 cells die either as a result of apoptosis (programmed cell death) or direct cytolysis by the virus, although the latter appears to be an infrequent mechanism.[14,16] Apoptosis of CD4 cells may result from cytokine dysregulation, continued immune stimulation, or exposure to viral proteins.

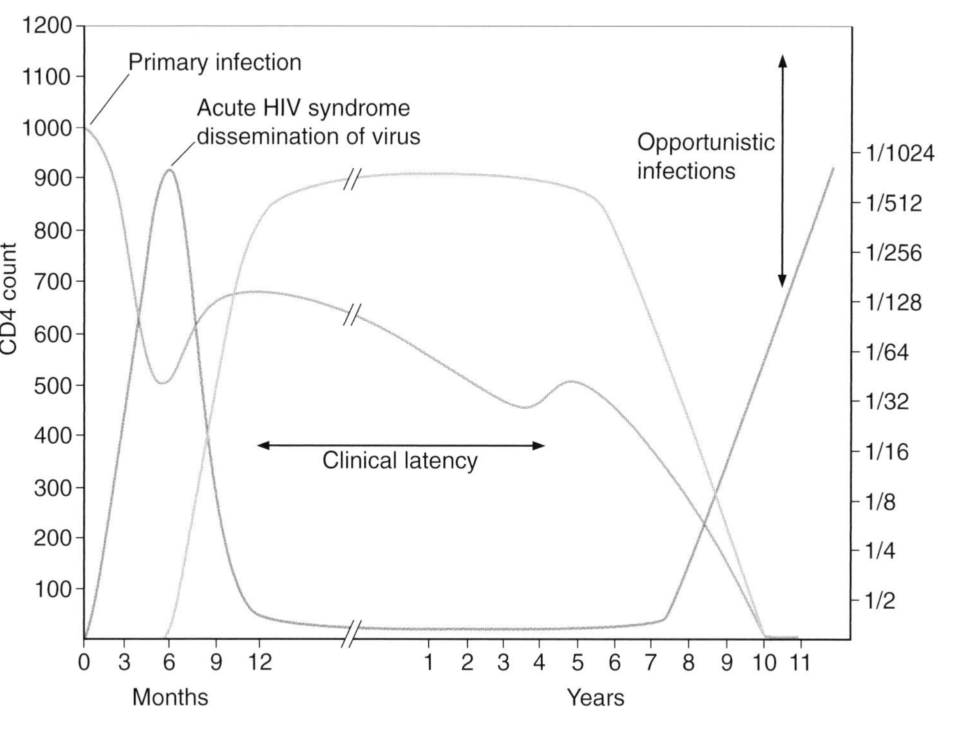

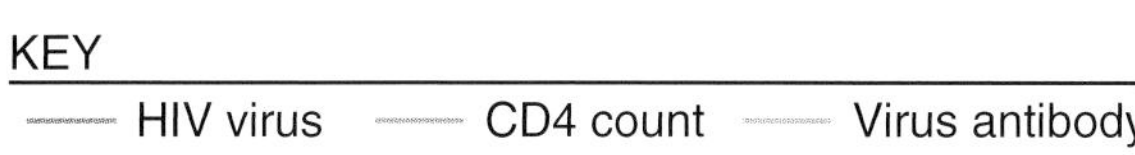

Figure 77–2. Immune response to HIV and relationship to clinical symptomatology and development of AIDS. After primary HIV infection, there is a period of viremia followed by development of IgM and then IgG antibody 4–7 weeks later. Development of antibody is accompanied by disappearance of the virus from the circulation. Eventually CD4 counts decrease, viral antibody titers decline, and viremia recurs.

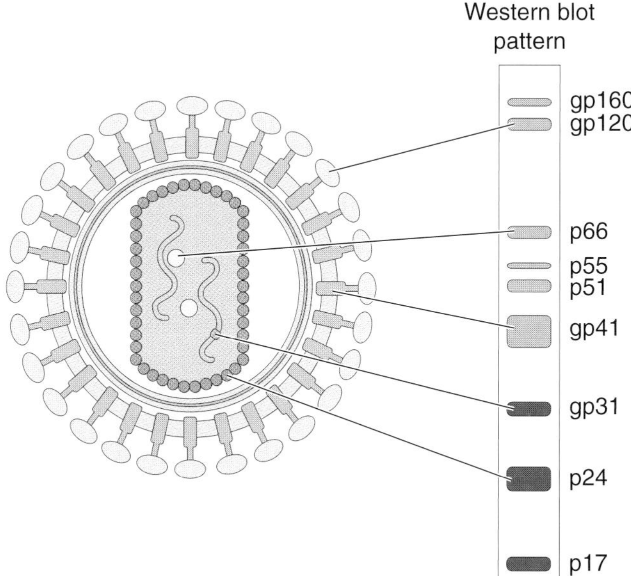

Figure 77–3. Schematic of Western blot to detect viral antibodies. Viral antigens are separated by electrophoresis into Gag (p17) or core proteins (p55, p24, and p17), envelop proteins (gp160, gp120, and gp41), and polymerase proteins (p66, p51, and p31). Reactivity of the test serum is measured.

In the HIV-infected individual, the half-life of peripheral blood T cells is markedly shortened, from approximately 82 to 23 days. Although increases in CD8 cells compensate, CD4 cell production is not increased and CD4 counts decline. Antiretroviral therapy increases production of CD4 cells without affecting their survival.

The life cycle of the virus and the sites targeted by antiretroviral therapy are depicted in Figure 77–1. Both the nucleoside reverse transcriptase inhibitors (including zidovudine, didanosine, zalcitabine, stavudine, and lamivudine) and the non-nucleoside reverse transcriptase inhibitors (nevirapine, delavirdine) block reverse transcription of the viral RNA genome into DNA (Table 77–2). The protease inhibitors suppress viral production by decreasing viral protease activity; enzyme inhibition leads to aborted viral formation, with defective particles lacking intact core protein being released instead of infectious virus. The development of resistance to any of the currently licensed non-nucleoside reverse transcriptase inhibitors invariably leads to cross-resistance to other drugs in that class. Non-nucleoside reverse transcriptase inhibitors with activity in the presence of such mutations are in development. A new class of drugs, fusion inhibitors, block union of the virus with the membrane, and one has been licensed.[31] Antivirals generally are given in combinations to avoid the emergence of resistance. HAART has resulted in a reduction of AIDS-defining illnesses in patients with advanced immunodeficiency and in death rates. During HAART the viral load should be repeatedly measured in order to assess the potency of the drug regimen. Variability in bioavailability and viral resistance make response rates different even in individ-

TABLE 77–2. Drugs Employed in the Treatment of HIV Infection

NRTIs	NNRTIs	PIs	Fusion Inhibitors
Zidovudine (ZDV)	Efavirenz (EFV)	Indinavir (IDV)	Enfuvirtide (T-20)
Stavudine (d4T)	Nevirapine (NVP)	Ritonavir (RTV)	
Lamivudine (3TC)	Delavirdine (DLV)	Nelfinavir (NFV)	
Didanosine (ddI)		Amprenavir (APV)	
Abacavir (ABC)		Lopinavir (LPV)	
Zalcitabine (ddC)		Atazanavir (ATV)	
Tenofovir (TDF)			
Entricitabine (FTC)			
Treatment usually consists of two NRTIs along with			
A single PI			
A PI enhanced with a low dose of a second PI, RTV			
An NNRTI			
One or two NRTIs			

Abbreviations: NNRTIs, non-nucleoside reverse transcriptase inhibitors; NRTIs, nucleoside reverse transcriptase inhibitors; PIs, protease inhibitors.

uals with similar degrees of immunosuppression. Viral load increasing over time signals the development of drug resistance and the need to alter drug combinations.

Viral load reduction begins rapidly with HAART, but T cells only gradually increase over months to years. These regenerated CD4 cells are generally of the memory type ($CD45RO^+$ or $CD34RA^+$), with naive T-cell numbers recovering very slowly. Naive cells bearing the T-cell receptor excision circle do eventually appear; thymic function improves in patient on HAART and is an important step in immune reconstitution.[32,33] Recovery of T-cell number and function following HAART initially correlates with improvement in viral load, but sustained improvements are seen even in the face of virus resistance and increases in viremia.[34] Protease inhibitors result in decreased apoptosis of CD4 cells,[35] a feature exhibited in cultures of drug-treated normal T cells as well; this characteristic of the protease inhibitors may account for stable CD4 counts despite high viral loads.

Even with optimal antiretroviral therapy, total eradication of infected CD4 cells is not possible and infected lymphocytes form sizable reservoirs in lymph nodes and spleen.[36,37] Alternative strategies attempt to gain access to these reservoirs. Short "drug holidays" are advocated by some for patients early in the course of their disease. Periods of viremia that follow drug discontinuation are associated with increased CD8 cytotoxic cell activity against HIV, but the benefits of this approach have not been validated and the theoretical advantage of structured treatment interruption must be weighed against the risk of developing resistance. CD8 cell dysfunction can partially be corrected in vitro after co-culture with interleukin-2, suggesting a role for impaired HIV-specific CD4 T helper function.[38] Interleukin-2 also partially blocks lymphocyte apoptosis.[37–40] These salutary properties led investigators to conduct clinical trials of interleukin-2 in HIV-infected patients[37,41,42]: administration of doses of 1–5 million U/m^2, two to three times weekly, resulted in modest but sustained increases in CD4 counts and improvement in natural killer cell activity in patients with CD4 counts greater than 400 cells/μL for 3–6 months. Higher doses might result in even greater increments in CD4 counts but are associated with more substantial toxicity.[43] Nevertheless, long-term interleukin-2 administration is still unable to eradicate HIV entirely.[37,44]

Opportunistic infections are the hallmark of the immunodeficiency associated with HIV infection. Prophylaxis has improved the morbidity and mortality associated with AIDS. The widespread use of HAART led to a decline in the incidence of and improved clinical outcomes of many opportunistic infections. Immune reconstitution might make prophylaxis against some opportunistic infections unnecessary; this question is addressed in ongoing clinical studies.

HEMATOLOGIC COMPLICATIONS AND THEIR TREATMENT

Anemia

Anemia is the most frequent cytopenia observed in HIV-1 infection (Fig. 77–4), often as a complication of antiviral drug therapy[24] (Table 77–3). Striking anemia with transfusion-dependence was common early in the epidemic, when high doses of zidovudine were in use, but severe depression of hemoglobin levels is now rare, except in patients with advanced disease.[45] Nucleoside analogues other than zidovudine do not cause anemia. Zidovudine is commonly associated with marrow toxicity, particularly with its long-term administration. Use of lower zidovudine doses in combination with other non-myelosuppressive antiviral drugs (such as the protease inhibitors or other nucleoside analogues) has reduced the frequency of anemia, although patients with advanced disease on doses of zidovudine of less than 500 mg/day still demonstrate significantly lower hemoglobin levels when compared to similarly immunosuppressed HIV-infected patients not taking the drug.[46] Although the mechanism responsible for zidovudine-associated anemia, inhibition of thymidine kinase and DNA chain termination, should theoretically also affect cells of other

TABLE 77–3. Hematologic Toxicities of Drugs Used to Treat HIV-1–Infected Patients

Medication	Type of Activity	Hematologic Toxicity
Zidovudine	Nucleoside analogue	Anemia (most common), neutropenia (dose dependent)
Stavudine	Nucleoside analogue	Anemia, neutropenia (dose dependent)
Ganciclovir	CMV infection	Anemia, neutropenia, thrombocytopenia
Valganciclovir	CMV infection	Anemia, neutropenia, thrombocytopenia
Primaquine	*Pneumocystis* pneumonia	Rare agranulocytosis, thrombocytopenia Methemoglobinemia, especially in G6PD deficiency
Pentamidine	*Pneumocystis* pneumonia	Infrequent anemia, thrombocytopenia, leukopenia
Sulfadiazine	Toxoplasmosis	Leukopenia (40%), thrombocytopenia (12%)
Clindamycin/ pyrimethamine	Toxoplasmosis	Anemia, leukopenia, thrombocytopenia in 34%
Amphotericin B	Antifungal	Anemia

Abbreviations: CMV, cytomegalovirus; G6PD, glucose-6-phosphate dehydrogenase.

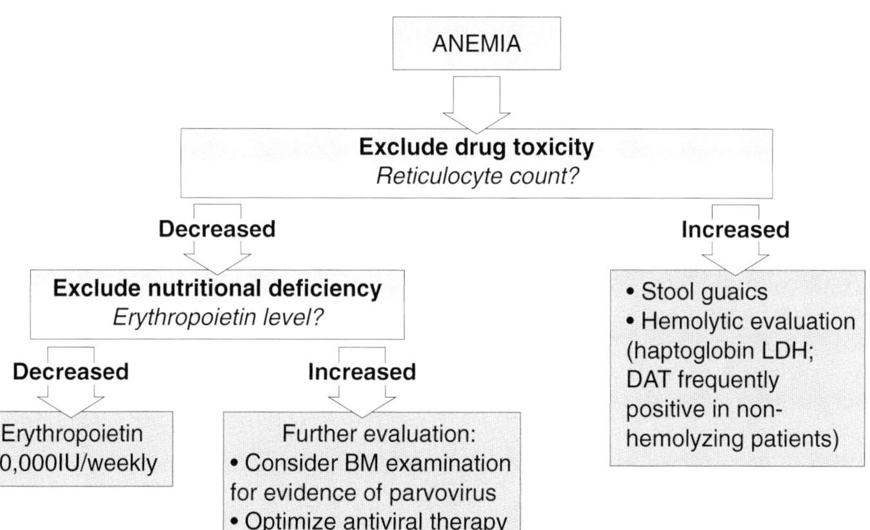

Figure 77–4. Algorithm for evaluation and treatment of anemia in HIV after exclusion of drugs. Abbreviations: BM, bone marrow; DAT, direct antiglobulin testing; LDH, lactate dehydrogenase.

lineages, neutropenia is less frequent and thrombocytopenia is very uncommon. The factors responsible for the preferential suppression of erythropoiesis by zidovudine are not known. Other nucleoside analogues such as didanosine, dideoxycytidine (zalcitabine), lamivudine, and stavudine do not have significant bone marrow toxicity. Protease inhibitors, such as indinavir, ritonavir, and nelfinavir, alone or in combination with zidovudine or other nucleoside analogues, have little or no effect on hematopoiesis.[47,48] In several large multicenter studies, persistent anemia was associated with shorter survival, independent of the degree of immunosuppression.[24,49]

Treatment

Treatable causes of anemia include nutritional/vitamin deficiency, gastrointestinal losses, parvovirus B19 infection[50,51] (discussed in Chapter 76), and inadequate erythropoietin production (Table 77–4). In HIV infection, erythropoietin levels are low in some patients, in part because tumor necrosis factor-α acts to blunt erythropoietin release in the response to anemia.[52] Patients with low erythropoietin levels respond better to its administration than do patients with normal or elevated levels of the hormone. In one meta-analysis, patients with erythropoietin levels below 500 IU/L demonstrated significant increases in hemoglobin levels, decreases in transfusion requirements, and improvement in quality of life with erythropoietin replacement, which was ineffective in patients with high erythropoietin levels.[53]

Some patients with HIV infection have severe anemia, requiring frequent transfusion. Clinical evidence suggests that transfusion may be associated with substantial morbidity in HIV-infected patients. In one study, transfused patients with advanced disease had an increased incidence of cytomegalovirus infection and death.[54] Laboratory data suggest that transfusion may cause viral activation: allogeneic lymphocytes present in transfused blood components stimulate viral production by HIV-infected lymphocytes in vitro.[55] When quantitative polymerase chain reaction was used to measure circulating HIV, viral load was found to be increased in HIV-infected

TABLE 77–4. Causes of Anemia in HIV-Infected Patients

Drugs (most common offenders)
- Zidovudine
- Trimethoprim-sulfamethoxazole
- Amphotericin B
- Ganciclovir
- Dapsone
- Delavirdine

Malnutrition
- Iron
- Folate
- Vitamin B_{12}

Infectious
- HIV
- Parvovirus B19
- *Mycobacterium avium* complex
- *Mycobacterium tuberculosis*
- *Histoplasma capsulatum*

Decreased erythropoietin production

Neoplasia
- Non-Hodgkin's lymphoma

Gastrointestinal blood loss

Hemolysis (rare despite positive direct antiglobulin test)

Cirrhosis (concurrent hepatitis B or C)

Hypersplenism

patients 5 days after transfusion.[56] There appeared to be no significant differences in viremia or infectious complications when leukocyte-depleted blood components were used, however.[57]

For parvovirus infection, commercial immune globulin infusion (400 mg/kg/day × 5–10 days) almost always results in marked improvement in hemoglobin levels and resolution of anemia.[51,58] HIV-infected patients often develop recurrent episodes of B19 infection and need repeated treatments with intravenous immunoglobulin.

Thrombocytopenia

Thrombocytopenia may be related either to decreased platelet survival or to compromised bone marrow function. Opportunistic infection, splenomegaly, fever, and autoimmune causes all can contribute to reduce the life expectancy of the platelet. Platelet-associated antibodies are not usually of value because the frequent detection of cell-associated antibody fails to correlate with platelet count in HIV-infected patients.[59] Thrombocytopenia in mildly immunosuppressed individuals is due to increased destruction of platelets, whereas decreased thrombopoiesis relating to disordered marrow function accounts for low platelet counts late in the course of the disease.[60,61]

Immune Thrombocytopenic Purpura

Once a common presenting symptom in the asymptomatic HIV-infected person, immune thrombocytopenic purpura (ITP) is now much less frequent in this population. HIV should still be sought in all adults with newly diagnosed ITP. Although the pathophysiology of ITP in HIV-infected patients is unclear, viremia decreases the platelet count. Treatment with antiretroviral drugs results in lowering of the viral load and improvement in platelet counts.[62–64] The exact role played by antibody is unclear. Platelet-specific antibodies are often present in HIV-1–infected hemophiliacs, a 7S platelet–reactive IgG has been quantitated in serum and inversely related to the platelet count.[65] In HIV-1–infected intravenous drug users presenting with ITP, immune complexes on the platelet surface were identified.[66] An antibody directed against HIV gp160/120 may cross-react with platelet GPIIb/IIIa, a mechanism of molecular mimicry.[67,68]

Treatment

Treatment of patients with HIV-related ITP is as for uninfected individuals (Fig. 77–5); HIV patients exhibit similar rates of responses to corticosteroids,[69] intravenous immunoglobulin,[70] and RH_0(D) immune globulin (WinRho).[71,72] The potent immunosuppressive effects of glucocorticoids have led to their short-term use as temporizing agents. Intravenous immunoglobulin is expensive, in short supply, requires intravenous administration, and improves the platelet count only for a few days. WinRho has advantages of cost and supply and can be self-administered subcutaneously; unfortunately, responses also are of relatively short duration. Vincristine can be effective but continued administration causes neuropathy in patients already at risk for this problem.[73] Institution of antiviral therapy in treatment-naive patients and optimization of antiviral therapy in others will increase platelet counts to safe levels in most.[74,75] For patients failing all other measures, splenectomy is safe and does not lead to reduction of CD4 counts or to progression of the disease, while producing good platelet increments.[76–78] Antiviral agents and corticosteroids generally do not have a large affect on platelet survival; better platelet counts result more from increased marrow production.[61,62,79]

Thrombotic Thrombocytopenic Purpura

Thrombotic thrombocytopenic purpura (TTP) occurs with increased frequency in HIV-infected patients. The clinical presentation is more subtle than with classic TTP and the response to therapy better.[80] With moderately decreased platelet counts and mild anemia, the diagnosis may only be suggested by the microangiopathic picture evident on blood smear,[81,82] red cell fragments and schistocytes. The etiology of TTP in AIDS is unknown. TTP in a cohort of patients undergoing experimental treatment for cytomegalovirus suggested that this herpesvirus might be involved,[81] perhaps by a mechanism of cytomegalovirus-mediated destruction of endothelial cells, decreased prostacyclin production, and release of prothrombotic high-molecular-weight von Willebrand factor multimers (see Chapter 75).[83–85] Endothelial cells from small but not large blood vessels undergo apoptosis when exposed to plasma from patients with TTP associated with HIV infection.[86] Antibodies directed to von Willebrand factor–cleaving pro-

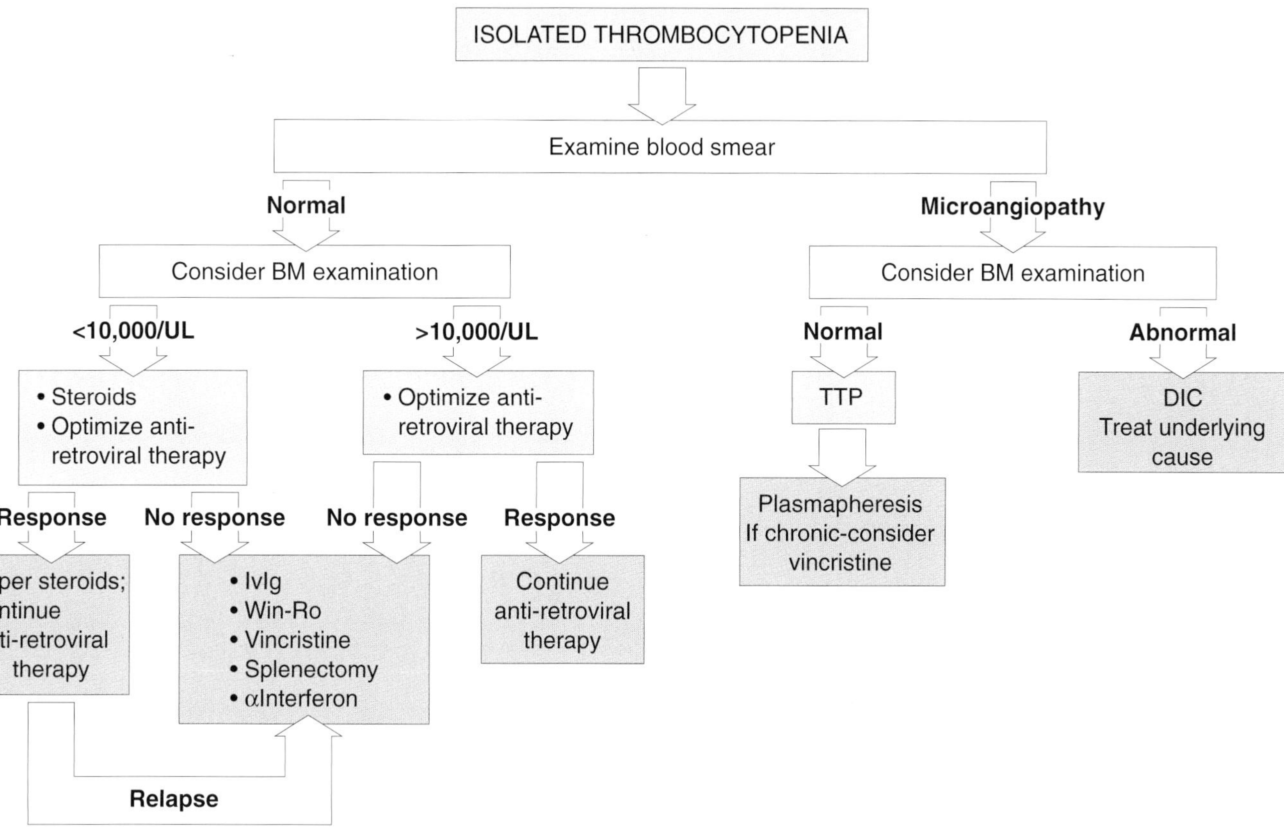

Figure 77–5. Algorithm for work-up and treatment of thrombocytopenia in HIV.

tease occur in HIV-infected patients with TTP as in TTP from other causes.[81,87]

Treatment

Therapy is similar to that of TTP unrelated to HIV.[88] Although well-controlled trials are lacking, plasmapheresis with plasma rather than albumin as replacement is generally regarded as the treatment of choice; plasma exchange designed to replace 35–40 mL/kg per exchange is recommended. The frequency of exchanges should be governed by the clinical course; lactate dehydrogenase values are useful to assess the hemolysis. Successes with aspirin, antiplatelet agents, and vincristine have been reported, usually as components of multiple treatments. Monthly vincristine injections may be performed for the rare patient with chronic TTP unwilling to undergo regular plasmapheresis.[89]

Neutropenia

Neutropenia in HIV infection results from shortened survival and diminished bone marrow production of neutrophils. Neutrophil-associated antibodies are frequent in all HIV-infected persons but their presence rarely correlates with the degree of neutropenia.[59] Early in the epidemic, granulocyte-macrophage and granulocyte colony-stimulating factors were shown to decrease the number of bacterial infections in HIV-infected patients with mild neutropenia (absolute neutrophil count < 1000), but no study ever showed that they improved patient survival. Better antiretroviral medications and antibiotics have greatly diminished infectious risk, and these cytokines[34] are now infrequently employed. However, AIDS patients are less tolerant of chemotherapy and myelosuppressive drugs in general and they often require dose adjustments for neutropenia. Because chemotherapy dose adjustments correlate with diminished responses and increased relapses, efforts are appropriately directed to decrease the depth of the nadir by administering hematopoietic growth factors (Table 77–5).

Treatment

Granulocyte-macrophage colony-stimulating factor can ameliorate the myelotoxicity of ganciclovir[91] therapy of cytomegalovirus, resulting in decreased therapy interruptions and prolonging time to progression of cytomegalovirus disease. In HIV-infected patients receiving chemotherapy, granulocyte colony-stimulating factor decreased the frequency of fever and neutropenia, and the need for dose reductions[92–94] (see Table 77–5).

Bone Marrow Failure

Bone marrow dysfunction in HIV is related to many factors, including cytokine and immune dysregulation as well as progenitor cell depletion. That progenitor cells might represent a significant reservoir for HIV was pos-

TABLE 77–5. Hematologic Growth Factors Used in Treatment of HIV-Associated Cytopenias

Drug	Dose	Therapeutic Effect	Adverse Effects
GM-CSF	0.25–8 μg/kg/day	Improvement of leukocyte count and function	Back pain, myalgia, chills, nausea, headache, fever, rash ? Increase HIV replication
G-CSF	150 μg/m²/day	Improvement of proliferation and differentiation of committed progenitor cells	Bone pain
Erythropoietin	40,000 IU weekly	Improvement in Hgb in patients with low erythropoietin levels	None
Stem cell factor	In vitro studies: 10 ng/mL	Improvement of white cell count when used with G-CSF	None
IL-3	0.5–5.0 μg/kg/day	Increase in erythropoiesis, ANC	Rash, fevers
Interferon-α	3 × 10⁶ units SC every other day	Variable response in prolonging platelet survival	Fever, myalgias, fatigue
IL-2	1.5 million U/m², 2–3 times weekly	Increase in lymphopoiesis and decreased lymphocyte apoptosis, increase in CD4 count	↑PTT, proteinuria, fever, rash Capillary leak

Abbreviations: ANC, absolute neutrophil count; G-CSF, granulocyte colony-stimulating factor; GM-CSF, granulocyte-macrophage colony-stimulating factor; Hgb, hemoglobin; IL, interleukin; PTT, prothrombin time; SC, subcutaneously.

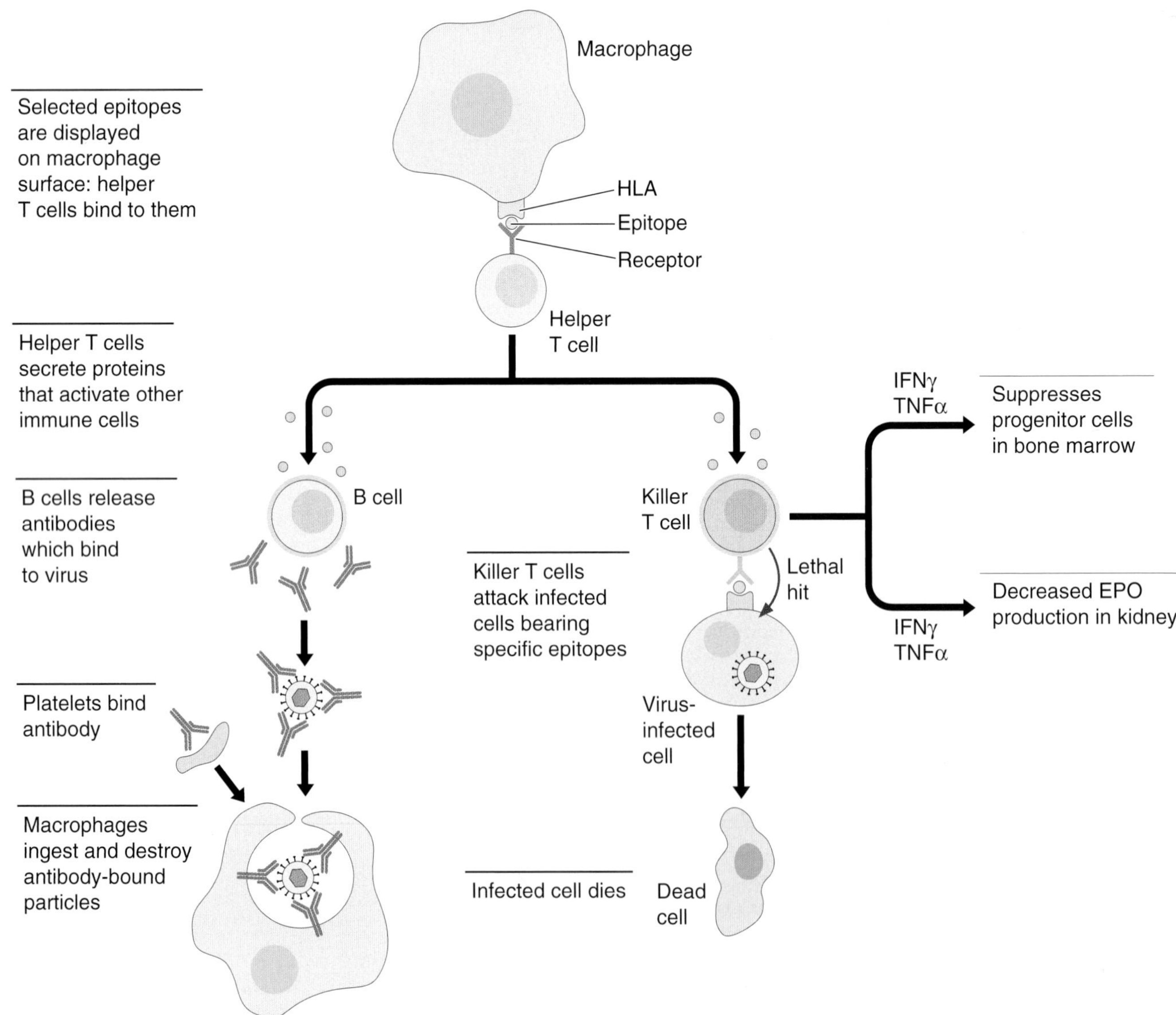

Figure 77–6. Mechanisms of cytopenias in HIV infection.

tulated early in the AIDS epidemic, but subsequent laboratory data showed these cells to be rarely infected.[94,95] CD34 cells are susceptible to infection in vitro when exposed to certain strains of HIV, but more primitive progenitor cells are resistant to infection.[96] In an extensive examination of HIV-infected patients, CD34 cells were tested by polymerase chain reaction, but infection could be demonstrated in only a small proportion of the sickest patients.[97] Similarly, stromal cells can be infected with HIV[98] but do not appear to harbor large amounts of virus in vivo.[99]

Assessments of the effects of HIV infection on progenitor cell function have yielded equivocal results.[100–105] Diminished colony formation by normal cells infected with HIV appears to be strain-specific.[104–106] Differences among laboratories may be related to techniques of assaying colony growth (total bone marrow vs. purified $CD34^+$ cells), culture conditions (use of specific cytokines or growth factors), and patient selection. Stromal cell function is decreased minimally after infection with HIV,[107,108] but when normal CD34 cells and stroma from HIV-infected patients are co-cultured, normal numbers of colonies result.[109] Cytokine release by infected lymphocytes likely leads to bone marrow compromise. Both tumor necrosis factor-α and interferon-γ induce Fas expression on the CD34 cell surface, apoptosis, and hematopoietic cell depletion.[110] Even when primitive progenitor cells were shown to be decreased in patients with HIV, the magnitude of the differences was smaller than in patients with other bone marrow failure states with comparable blood counts.[109] Inhibition of apoptosis resulted in enhanced colony formation by marrow cells from HIV-infected patients.[111] Protease inhibitors have a direct effect on apoptosis of hematopoietic progenitor cells, an effect also seen in colony culture of uninfected cells.[112]

The bone marrow findings in HIV are nonspecific; examination generally gives little diagnostic information except for the presence of opportunistic infection.[113–117] Foamy histiocytes and granulomas are typical of *Mycobacterium avium-intracellulare. Histoplasma, Cryptococcus,* and mycobacteria can be identified in granulomas, often without special stains,[118] but the diagnosis of these organisms ordinarily does not require bone marrow examination. Occasionally frankly dysmorphic cells mimic myelodysplasia.[117] A true myelodysplastic syndrome should be diagnosed by abnormal cytogenetics or repeated and consistently abnormal bone marrow morphology (Fig. 77–6).

Coagulation Abnormalities

The diverse coagulation abnormalities occurring in the setting of HIV infection do not substantially add to the risk of thrombosis, as compared to an equally ill group of patients who suffer inactivity after surgery, the presence of indwelling catheters, cancer, lymphedema, and hypoalbuminemia.[119] Antiphospholipid syndrome occurs[120,121]: in one study, antiphosphatidylcholine antibodies were present in 50% of HIV-1–infected patients and anticardiolipin autoantibodies in 64%.[121] With severe

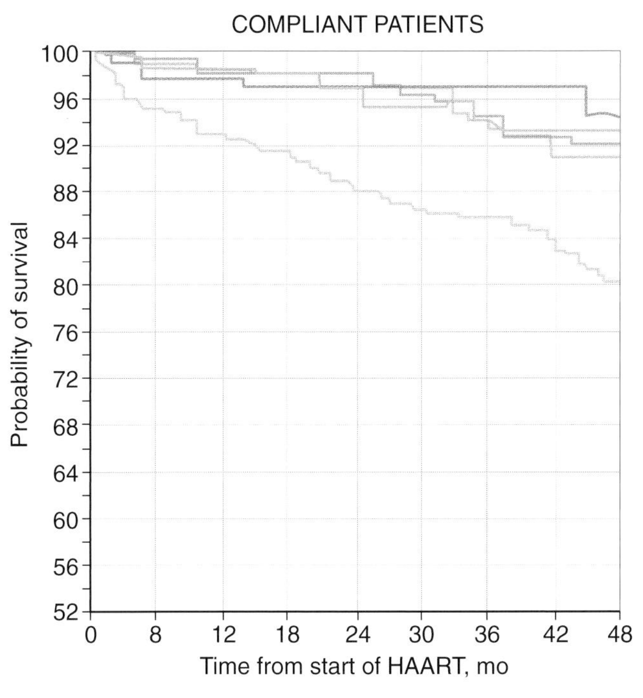

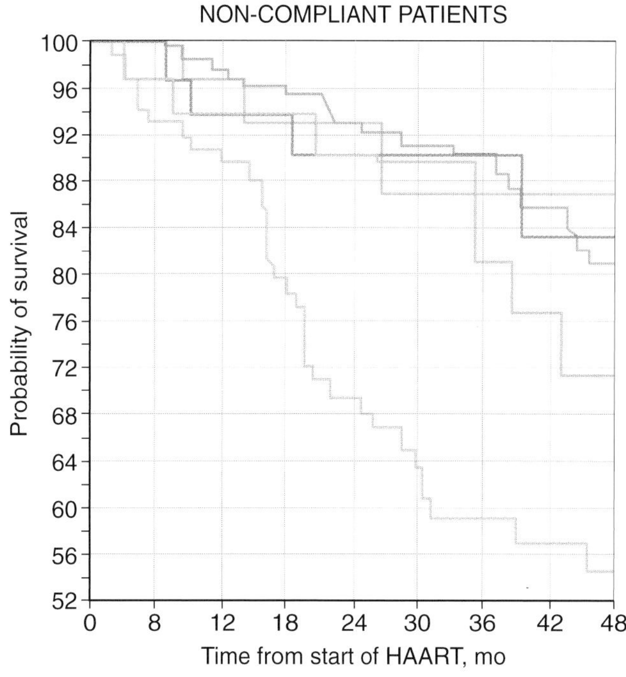

KEY

≤0.350 x 10^9 cells/L — 0.300–0.349 x 10^9 cells/L — 0.250–0.299 x 10^9 cells/L — 0.200–0.249 x 10^9 cells/L — <0.200 x 10^9 cells/L

Figure 77–7. Survival of patients who are compliant and noncompliant with a HAART regimen.

immunocompromise, antibody can disappear. However, unlike in patients without HIV infection, the presence of lupus anticoagulant is not associated with increased risk of thrombosis.[21,122]

Levels of functional protein S are decreased in some proportion of HIV-infected patients, with estimates varying from 27% to 73%, and as many as 12% of deficient patients develop thrombotic complications.[123,124] Increased levels of complement-binding protein 4, which binds protein S, may account for decreased functional protein S. There is statistical association of diminished protein S with thrombotic events in AIDS.[125,126] Decreases in heparin cofactor II have also been described,[127] but without correlation to a thrombotic tendency.

Treatment

No clear guidelines are available for treatment of coagulation abnormalities in HIV infection. Long-term anticoagulation of patients with protein S deficiency would seem prudent.

HIV-Related Malignancies

Hodgkin's lymphoma, non-Hodgkin's lymphoma, and Kaposi's sarcoma occur at increased frequency in patients with AIDS (see Chapter 44). The development of these malignancies is facilitated by immunosuppression, infection with human herpesvirus 8 and Epstein-Barr virus, and cytokine dysregulation. HAART has changed the epidemiology of these malignant lymphoproliferative syndromes, decreasing the incidence of many lymphomas and especially Kaposi's sarcoma. The presentation and treatment of these cancers are very different in the HIV-infected patient compared to other affected individuals. Effective chemotherapeutic regimens must be individualized, especially in consideration of potentially limited bone marrow reserve. A panoply of drug toxicities and interactions must be balanced. Despite dismal initial results, prognosis for the HIV cancer patient has improved in the last decade as a result of better antiretroviral therapy and chemotherapy regimens designed specifically for this population.

PROGNOSIS

HAART has greatly improved the prognosis of AIDS. Patients compliant with their antiviral regimen do not require opportunistic infection prophylaxis unless the CD4 count declines to 200 cells/μL (Fig. 77–7).

CURRENT CONTROVERSIES & FUTURE CONSIDERATIONS

Human Immunodeficiency Virus: Hematologic Complications

- What is the role of antiretroviral "drug holidays" and cytokine therapy in eliminating residual viral reservoirs?
- What is the utility of cellular and gene therapy in effecting immune reconstitution?

Suggested Readings*

Moroni M, Antinori S: HIV and direct damage of organs: disease spectrum before and during the highly active antiretroviral therapy era. AIDS 17(Suppl 1):S51–S64, 2003.

Scaradavou A: HIV-related thrombocytopenia. Blood Rev 16:73–76, 2002.

Volberding PA, Baker KR, Levine AM: Human immunodeficiency virus hematology. Hematology (Am Soc Hematol Educ Program) 294–313, 2003.

Volberding P: The impact of anemia on quality of life in human immunodeficiency virus-infected patients. J Infect Dis 185(Suppl 2):S110–S114, 2002.

Yeni PG, Hammer SM, Carpenter CC, et al: Antiretroviral treatment for adult HIV infection in 2002: updated recommendations of the International AIDS Society–USA Panel. JAMA 288:222–235, 2002.

Full references for this chapter can be found on accompanying CD-ROM.

CHAPTER 78

Hepatitis C Virus

Harvey J. Alter, MD, and Juan I. Esteban, MD

KEY POINTS

Hepatitis C Virus

- On average, hepatitis C virus (HCV) infects 1–2% of the world's population; in some endemic areas prevalence reaches 20%. By far the major route of transmission is percutaneous inoculation, particularly through intravenous drug abuse and blood transfusion. Many other shared needle/instrument exposures also exist, including folk medicine practices and mass immunizations. Sexual transmission is very inefficient, but on a global scale even a low rate of transmission may account for many cases.
- The hallmark of HCV infection is its ability to persist in 75–85% of infected individuals. Persistence is related to the virus' high mutation rate and its ability to exist as a swarm of distinct variants (quasispecies) that can readily escape host immune responses. Further, host immune responses may be specifically blunted by interactions with HCV-encoded proteins.
- Although persistent infection occurs in the majority of patients, spontaneous recovery is more common than previously estimated, occurring in 20–25% of infected adults and in up to 50% of infected children. Spontaneous recovery generally occurs within the first 6 months of infection. Infection that persists beyond 1 year does not resolve except through antiviral therapy.
- The key to spontaneous recovery is a vigorous cell-mediated immune response, particularly a strong T_H1 CD4 T helper cell response.
- Although HCV infection can evolve from mild hepatitis without fibrosis to severe chronic hepatitis leading to cirrhosis, this evolution is not inevitable; even in the absence of treatment, the incidence of cirrhosis is no more than 20–30%. Twenty or more years are required for cirrhosis to develop. Hepatocellular carcinoma (HCC) can also be a consequence of HCV infection and almost always evolves in the setting of preexisting cirrhosis. The onset of HCC is generally 30–60 years after first infection. In the absence of cirrhosis, hepatitis C is usually asymptomatic and without physical signs. A small proportion of patients have extrahepatic syndromes such as cryoglobulinemia that are due to immune complex formation.
- Optimal current therapy is a combination of pegylated interferon alfa plus ribavirin given for 6–12 months, depending on viral genotype. This combination results in sustained virologic response (SVR) in about 50% of HCV genotype 1 and 4 patients and 75% of genotype 2 and 3 patients. SVR, defined as the absence of viral RNA 6 months after cessation of therapy, appears equivalent to "cure." There is currently no HCV vaccine.

INTRODUCTION

In the early 1970s, prospective studies of transfusion-associated hepatitis showed that, even prior to hepatitis B donor screening, only 25% of transfusion-associated hepatitis as hepatitis B virus–related,[1] nor could hepatitis A virus be implicated.[2] Evaluation of transfusion-acquired non-A, non-B hepatitis (NANBH) cases over many years revealed that at least 50% became chronic, based on alanine aminotransferase (ALT) elevations; that some asymptomatic patients had advanced hepatic inflammatory disease; and that 20% of NANBH evolved into cirrhosis. Chimpanzee studies proved that NANBH was a blood-transmissible agent.[3] Attempts to develop an assay for this common blood-transmitted agent proved to be uncommonly difficult until 1989, when Houghton and associates at Chiron Corp.[4] applied the then relatively new science of molecular biology and blindly cloned the NANBH virus—hence discovering hepatitis C virus (HCV) without the virus being visualized, grown in culture, or detected immunologically. A single immunoreactive clone was identified among some 6 million tested; the expressed protein became the antigenic target of the first immunoassay to detect antibody to HCV. Repository samples showed that 90% of transfusion-associated NANBH cases[5] and 82% of community-acquired cases[6] were HCV-related. The anti-HCV antibody assay was mandated for blood screening in 1990, and this test has prevented over 1 million transfusion-associated hepatitis cases in the first decade of its use. Posttransfusion hepatitis C has been virtually eradicated, and the current estimated risk is 1 case for every 2 million transfused products.

STRUCTURAL BIOLOGY AND GENETIC VARIATION OF HCV

Viral Structure

HCV is a small virus, with an estimated diameter between 40 and 50 nm,[7,8] and a lipid-containing envelope.[9] HCV shares partial sequence homology, and a very similar genomic organization, with members of the family *Flaviviridae*,[10] which includes the human flaviviruses (dengue, West Nile, and yellow fever viruses) and the animal pestiviruses. HCV has been classified as a new genus, *Hepacivirus*, within the family *Flaviviridae*.

The HCV genome (Fig. 78–1) is a single-stranded, positive-sense RNA molecule of about 9500 kb containing a single open reading frame, encoding a large polyprotein of about 3000 amino acids that is cleaved into two envelope glycoproteins, E1 and E2; the core (C) protein, which along with genomic RNA forms the nucleocapsid[11,12]; and a series of nonstructural proteins designated NS2 to NS5. The specific hepatocyte receptor for HCV has not been identified, but the extensively glycosylated envelope proteins E1 and E2 are thought to be the site of viral attachment, resulting in cell entry by receptor-mediated endocytosis.[13–16] The E2 protein contains a hypervariable domain of 27 amino acids (HVR1)[17] which includes neutralizing antibody epitopes that are under strong immune selection. The nonstructural proteins NS2 to NS5 have multiple enzymatic functions, including proteinase, helicase, and RNA-dependent RNA polymerase, which are critical to viral assembly and function and may serve as new targets for antiviral therapy. NS5A has an "interferon sensitivity determining region," encoding a protein proposed to play a role in modulating response to both endogenous and therapeutic interferon-α.[18]

HCV Genotypes

Phylogenetic analysis has identified six major HCV genotypes (designated by Arabic numbers) and more than 50 subtypes (identified by lower case letters; genotypes 1a, 1b, 2a, 3a, etc.).[19,20] Genotypes, subtypes, and isolates can be distinguished by sequence divergences averaging 30%, 20%, and 10%, respectively. Genotypes 1, 2, and 3 show a broad geographic distribution, whereas others are mostly confined to specific geographic regions; in the United States, genotype 1a predominates. Despite differences in epidemiology, no correlates for pathogenicity have been clearly established between the distinct HCV

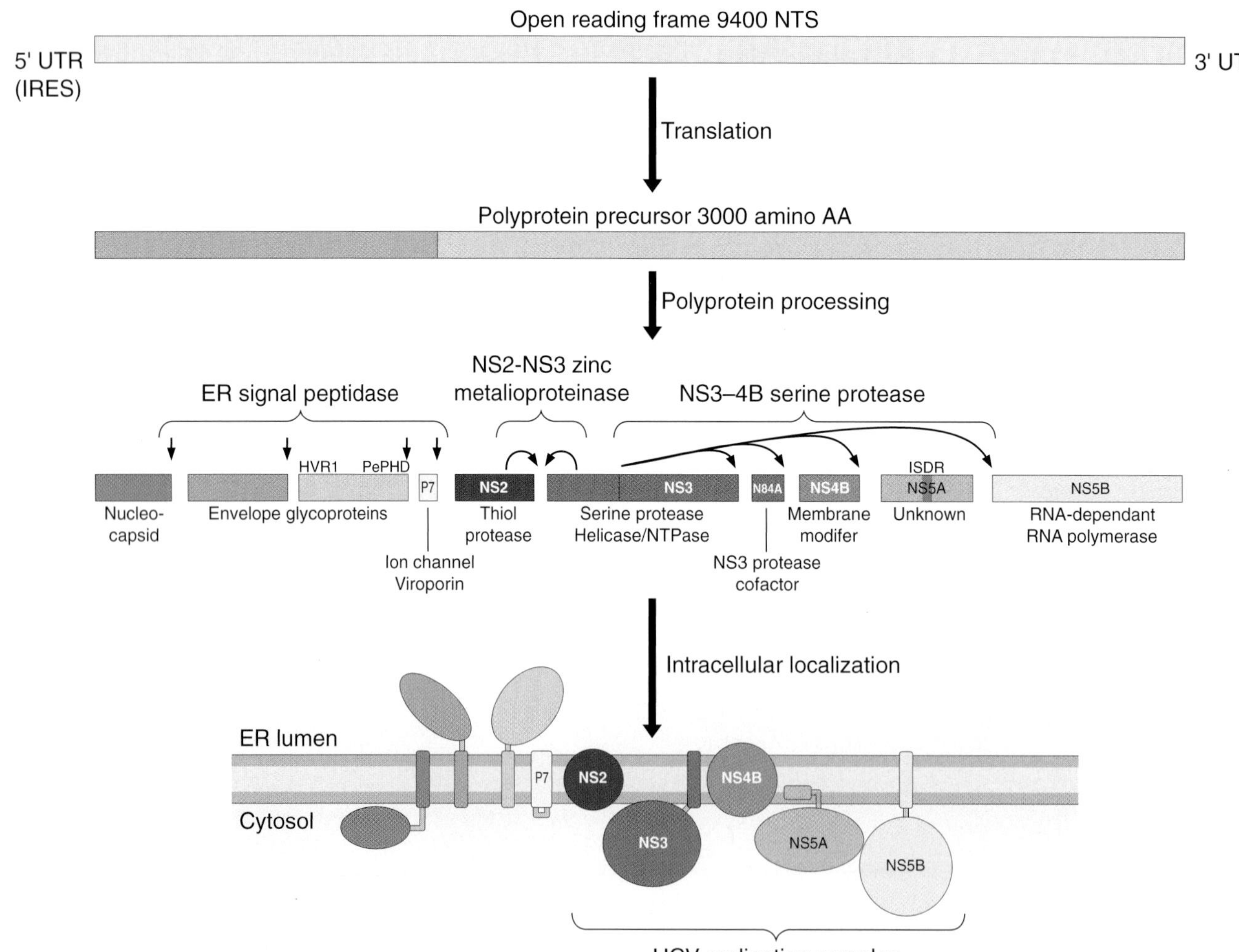

Figure 78–1. HCV genome and gene products. The HCV genome (~9500 kb) codes for a single polyprotein which is cleaved by the combined action of host and viral-encoded proteases into 10 different structural (envelope, core) and nonstructural proteins. The 5′ end of the HCV genome begins with a highly conserved region of 341 nucleotides (5′ untranslated region [UTR]) containing the internal ribosome entry site (IRES) that initiates translation of the polyprotein precursor and is the primary target for HCV polymerase chain reaction assays. Protease and helicase enzymes are potential targets for new antiviral therapies.

genotypes or subtypes. Most striking is the different sensitivity of genotypes to interferon alfa: patients infected with genotypes 2 or 3 have a significantly higher chance of clearing infection under treatment than those infected with genotypes 1 or 4.[21–26]

HCV Quasispecies

HCV, like most RNA viruses, circulates not as a homogeneous population of identical viral particles but as a complex mixture of related mutants, differing from each other by one or more nucleotides, a genomic distribution referred to as quasispecies.[26–30] Its existence as a mixed RNA virus population provides a significant adaptation advantage to the virus, allowing for the rapid selection of the mutant(s) best fit for a new environmental condition.[31] The complexity of the quasispecies plays an important role in the establishment of persistent infection[32] and in response to interferon[33–36]; in general, the more diverse and complex the quasispecies, the greater the likelihood of persistent infection and treatment failure. The mutation rate is unevenly distributed throughout the genome, with the 5′ untranslated region, core, and NS3 being most conserved and the hypervariable region of E2 (HVR1) being the most diverse.

EPIDEMIOLOGY

HCV infects 1–3% of the world's population, an estimated 200 million persons, and yet its modes of spread are relatively limited. HCV is principally transmitted by overt and covert parenteral routes, including blood transfusion and injection drug use, and, to a much lesser degree, from patient to health care worker through accidental needlestick. Prior to modern-day medical practices, infection also occurred through improperly sterilized medical and dental instruments, reused needles and common-use medicinal vials. In Egypt, where prevalence rates reach 20% in some areas, HCV infection has been traced to shared-needle treatments for schistosomiasis. Other incriminated practices have included tattooing, acupuncture, ear piercing, and possibly cocaine snorting.[37] In developed nations, most of these parenteral risks have been eliminated; the lingering risk is injection drug use, wherein rates of HCV transmission remain high and recurrent HCV infections in the same individual have been documented.[38] In developing nations, and particularly primitive populations, there are other sources of parenteral spread—scarification practices, ritual surgeries, and folk medicine practices,[39] which all utilize shared instruments.

Sexual transmission of HCV has been difficult to document but undoubtedly occurs. The strongest evidence comes from case-control studies, performed primarily in persons with acute, clinically apparent hepatitis C,[40] approximately 10% of whom have no risk factor except multiple sexual partners, sex with a prostitute, or a sexually transmitted disease within the 6 months preceding the onset of hepatitis. Sexual transmission is most likely to occur in the very early stages of HCV infection, when viral titers are at their highest and virus circulates unbound to antibody, or when partners engage in traumatic sex or sex during menstruation, when there is the potential for direct exchange of blood as well as sexual fluids. There is minimal evidence for sexual spread from persons who are chronically infected with HCV; long-term sexual partners of HCV-infected index cases are rarely anti-HCV antibody positive unless they also have an established parenteral risk factor.[37] Because data on sexual transmission are inconclusive, there is no public health guidance that specifically proscribes unprotected sex for HCV carriers. Rather, condoms or other barrier protection are recommended for all individuals who have multiple sexual partners, irrespective of HCV status. In monogamous couples in which one partner is unexpectedly found to be anti-HCV antibody positive, a rational policy is to test the other partner; if he or she is found to be anti-HCV antibody negative despite years of exposure, counseling can emphasize the low probability of sexual transmission and leave the decision for barrier protection to the affected couple. HCV is highly inefficient compared to most sexually transmitted viruses, but the sheer magnitude of the HCV-infected global population could result in a large number of sexually transmitted HCV infections, adding significantly to the disease burden.

Maternal-fetal transmission of HCV has been well documented, but the risk is much lower than for hepatitis B and estimated to be less than 5%; risk increases when the mother is newly infected near the time of delivery and when maternal viral titers are high in chronic carriers. As the risk of vertical transmission is low, in the absence of effective vaccines or hyperimmune HCV globulins, and because infants do well with neonatal HCV infection, there are no guidelines that recommend against pregnancy for HCV-infected woman and no specific obstetric practices are indicated. Because passively transferred maternal antibody can persist in the infant long after delivery, the best means to assess perinatal infection is to perform a qualitative test for HCV RNA 4 weeks post-partum; if HCV RNA is negative at 1 month postdelivery, it is unlikely to become positive subsequently. Anti-HCV can be validly measured in the infant at age 8–12 months.

IMMUNOPATHOGENESIS OF HCV INFECTION

Mechanisms of Persistence

HCV is not directly cytopathic, as evidenced by the lack of correlation between viral load and the extent of liver damage in both acute and chronic infection. Hepatocyte injury is predominantly immune mediated, but an insufficient immune response leads to persistent infection in 60–85% of exposed individuals. The immunopathogenesis of HCV infection is schematized in Figure 78–2. Following acute exposure, viral replication becomes detectable within the first 1–2 weeks, reaching peak levels (10^6–10^8 genomes/mL) in about 4 weeks.[41–47] Within days of exposure, HCV activates a set of innate immune responses that appear dependent on upregulation of interferon response genes, interferon-regulated transcriptional factors, and cytokine genes that activate resident macrophages (Kupffer cells) and natural killer cells. A cytotoxic CD8 T-cell response coincides with the

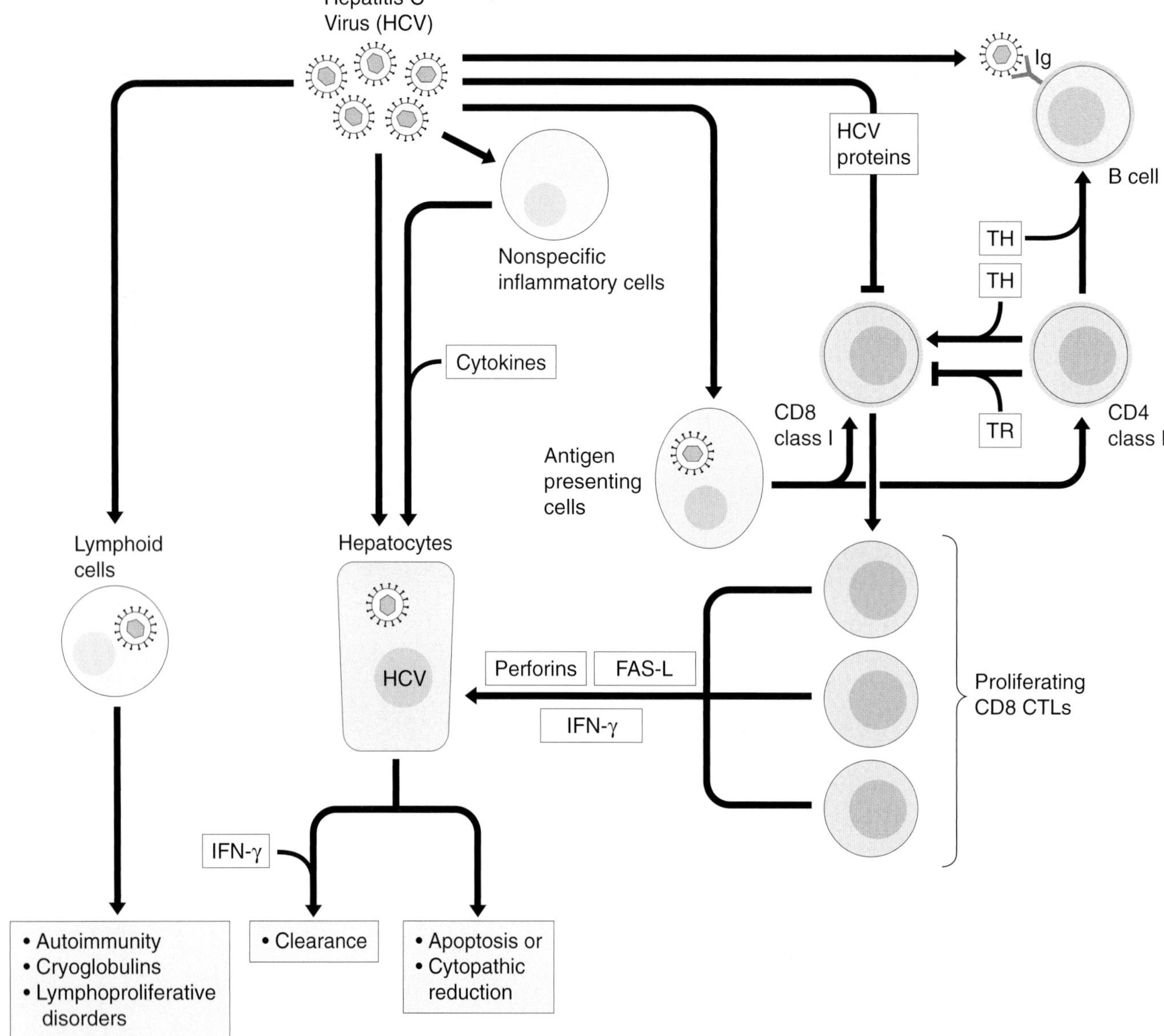

Figure 78–2. Immunopathogenesis of hepatitis C. This figure demonstrates the central role of major histocompatibility complex (MHC) class II–directed CD4 type 1 T helper (T_H1) cells that enhance the effector functions of MHC class I–directed CD8 cytotoxic T-lymphocyte (CTLs). Impaired T_H1 CD4 cell function characterizes persistent HCV infection. The death of liver cells occurs both by direct CTL killing and by apoptotic mechanisms. Generation of interferon-γ (IFN-γ) effects viral clearance even in the absence of liver cell death. Viral proteins can inhibit HCV-specific CTLs, as can T-regulatory cells (TR). Although abundant antibodies are produced, they do not seem to play an important role in either immunopathogenesis or viral clearance. HCV invasion of lymphoid cells can lead to autoimmunity, cryoglobulinemia, and, rarely, lymphoma.

TABLE 78–1. Interpretation of Serologic and Molecular Assays for HCV

Anti-HCV Antibody	RIBA	HCV RNA	Interpretation	Indicated Action
Positive	Negative	Not indicated	False + antibody	None
Positive	Indeterminate	Negative	False + antibody	None
Positive	Indeterminate	Positive	Active, probably early, HCV infection	Medical follow-up for acute or chronic hepatitis C; repeat assays in 2–4 wk
Positive	Positive	Negative	Recovered from prior HCV infection	Optional repeat HCV RNA to confirm interpretation; no further evaluation required
Positive	Positive	Positive	Active HCV infection	Medical evaluation for acute or chronic hepatitis C; consider liver biopsy and possible treatment pending clinical status

first biochemical evidence of hepatitis, about 7 weeks after exposure. These early cytotoxic T-lymphocyte effectors do not produce interferon-γ but are efficient at destroying infected hepatocytes. In some, but not all, patients, a multispecific CD4 type 1 T helper cell (T_H1) response subsequently appears and coincides with a sharp decrease in HCV RNA level, normalization of ALT, and a shift of the cytotoxic T-lymphocytes toward an interferon-γ–producing population that inhibits viral replication.[45,47] Sustained persistence of the T_H1 response leads to viral eradication, whereas its abrogation is followed by viral breakthrough and persistence.[42,48–50] Overall, viral persistence has been associated with impaired innate immunity,[50] dendritic cell dysfunction, diminished T_H1 CD4 activity,[49,52–54] dysfunctional cytotoxic CD8 cells,[54] increased complexity of the viral quasispecies, the presence of very-high-level viremia that overwhelms the immune response, the induction of suppressive T-regulatory cells,[55,56] and virus-specific stunting of the T-cell response.

Antibodies to a wide number of HCV antigens become detectable after the appearance of the cellular immune response and ALT elevation. There is some evidence for a protective role of HCV-specific antibodies from in vitro and chimpanzee inoculation studies,[57,58] but the virus can persist despite high levels of antibody to diverse antigens. Recently, HCV pseudoparticle assays[59] have identified neutralizing antibodies to E1 and E2 proteins in most chronically infected patients. However, these antibodies seem to be ineffective in viral clearance and are not present in spontaneously resolving acute infection. Durable, protective antibodies have not been identified in recovered patients. Thus, among individuals who resolve the infection, specific cellular immune responses are maintained indefinitely, while antibodies progressively decline and eventually may disappear decades after exposure.[60]

Despite the relative dysfunction of $CD8^+$ T cells in chronic HCV infection, the intrahepatic cytotoxic T-lymphocyte response is still sufficiently potent to recognize individually infected hepatocytes and to cause low-level persistent hepatic inflammation—the main factor in the induction of liver fibrosis and cirrhosis—through activation of hepatic stellate cells that generate myofibroblasts producing collagen and other extracellular matrix proteins.[61–63] In addition, liver damage occurs through generation of perforins and Fas ligand that induce apoptotic death, even of cells that do not contain virus.[64]

Molecular and Serologic Detection

The first commercial assay for HCV antibody detection became available in 1990. Presently, most blood banks screen with a third-generation enzyme immunoassay (EIA) that detects antibody to HCV core and three nonstructural proteins (NS-3, -4 and -5). The anti-HCV antibody assay has high sensitivity (99%) among chronic carriers, but its specificity varies with the population tested. In patients with known liver disease or in high-risk populations such as drug addicts, the specificity is high (98%), but in low-risk, asymptomatic populations such as blood donors, approximately 40% of repeat reactive EIAs prove to be false positives. The specificity of the anti-HCV assay is determined by a supplemental recombinant immunoblot assay (RIBA), in which four HCV proteins are embedded in a cellulose strip and overlaid with patient serum. Persons who are repeat EIA reactive and RIBA positive have true antibody to HCV, indicating current infection or prior exposure. Persons with EIA reactivity, but negative or indeterminate (one band) RIBA generally have not been exposed to HCV, with the exception of a small number who are tested relatively early in the evolution of their antibody response. Appropriate interpretations and indicated actions are summarized in Table 78–1. Increasingly, clinical decisions are based primarily on HCV RNA testing. In an individual who is both anti-HCV antibody and HCV RNA positive, the RIBA provides no additional useful information; in those who test HCV RNA negative, RIBA can distinguish between a false-positive assay and true antibody consequent to spontaneous recovery from prior HCV infection.

The HCV RNA assay is available in both qualitative and quantitative formats. Qualitative assays are performed by polymerase chain reaction (detection limit, 50–100 IU/mL) or transcription-mediated amplification (detection limit, 5–6 IU/m). Although analytic sensitivity of these assays varies, their clinical sensitivity is roughly equivalent. Quantitative assays are based on target amplification (polymerase chain reaction) or signal amplification (branched-chain DNA assay), in which the signal is enhanced by the use of multiple hybridization probes. Polymerase chain reaction–based assays are more sensitive, but the branched-chain DNA assay has a wider dynamic range. Because each quantitative assay expresses the result in different units (copies, molecular equivalents, genome equivalents), results are now expressed in international units (IU) based on comparisons with an international standard.

HCV genotyping requires HCV RNA amplification as a first step. The genotype of the amplified HCV RNA is determined using any of three methods: a reverse hybridization line probe assay, which probes for regions of the genome that are genotype-specific; direct sequencing; or restriction fragment length polymorphism assay. Determination of HCV genotype has prognostic implications for treatment response but does not predict the clinical course or outcome of untreated subjects (Fig. 78–3).

CLINICAL FEATURES OF HCV INFECTION

Hepatitis C is characterized by a mild and generally asymptomatic acute infection, an indolent chronic phase that may be asymptomatic and nonprogressive for many decades, and a devastating end stage of cirrhosis and liver failure. Attention has focused on the end-stage outcomes, but the reality is that only a minority of patients develop such severe liver disease and perhaps 70% either recover spontaneously early in their infection or remain clinically stable, especially in our age of effective treatments. In the absence of cirrhosis, hepatitis C is generally a benign and often unrecognized disorder. The three major outcomes of HCV infection and their relative frequency are depicted in Figure 78–4.

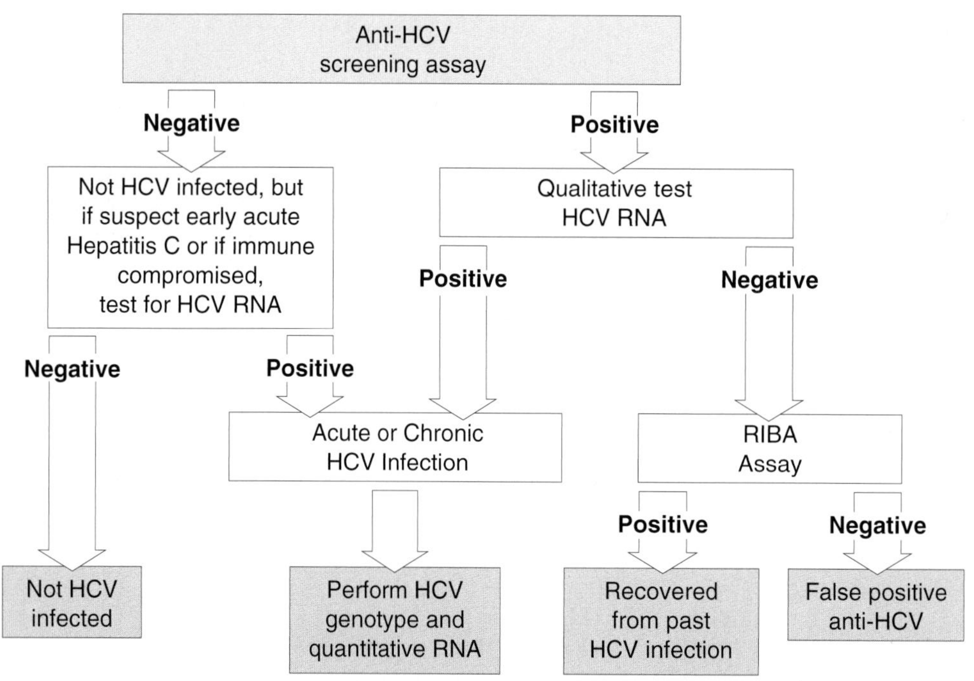

■ **Figure 78–3.** HCV testing algorithms.

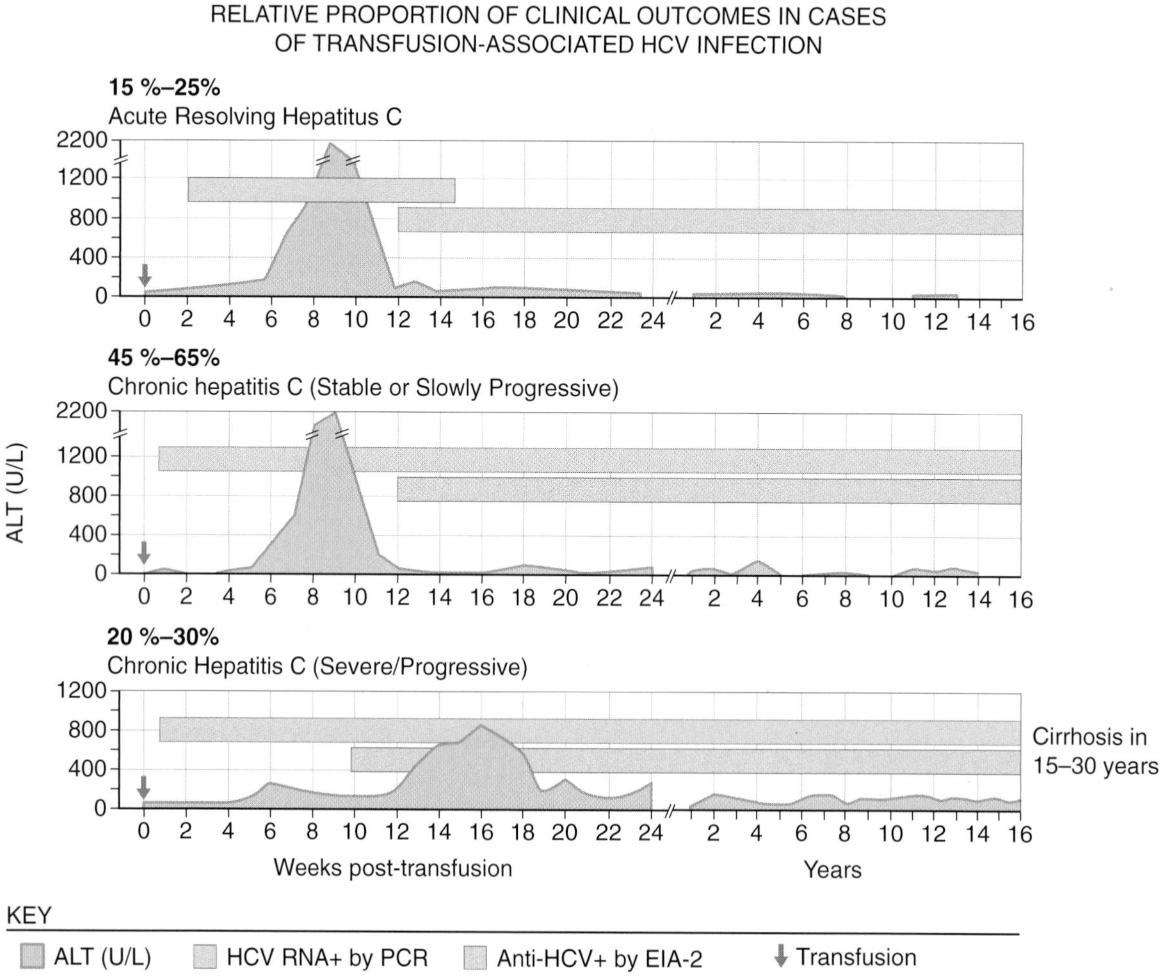

RELATIVE PROPORTION OF CLINICAL OUTCOMES IN CASES OF TRANSFUSION-ASSOCIATED HCV INFECTION

15 %–25%
Acute Resolving Hepatitus C

45 %–65%
Chronic hepatitis C (Stable or Slowly Progressive)

20 %–30%
Chronic Hepatitis C (Severe/Progressive)

Cirrhosis in 15–30 years

ALT (U/L)

Weeks post-transfusion

Years

KEY

ALT (U/L) HCV RNA+ by PCR Anti-HCV+ by EIA-2 Transfusion

■ **Figure 78–4.** Major patterns of HCV infection. Three general patterns occur after HCV exposure. All begin similarly with early detection of HCV RNA, followed by alanine aminotransferase (ALT) elevation and then the appearance of anti-HCV antibody. In 15–25% of patients, HCV RNA clears, ALT returns to normal, and anti-HCV antibody persists. The majority (45–65%) have persistent viremia, low-level ALT elevations, and either nonprogressive or very slowly progressive chronic hepatitis C. In 20–30%, the chronic hepatitis C will eventuate in cirrhosis in 20 or more years (more rapidly in the presence of human immunodeficiency virus or another immunodeficiency state or alcoholism).

Acute Hepatitis C

HCV accounts for only 15% of acute symptomatic hepatitis in the United States; this low proportion reflects clinical benignity rather than incidence. In acute HCV infection, ALT elevations generally begin 6–10 weeks after exposure and are usually modest (<10 times normal), but rare patients (<1%) develop fulminant hepatitis that may be fatal. When symptoms and signs occur during acute infection, they are indistinguishable from those resulting from hepatitis A or B: anorexia, nausea, vomiting, severe fatigue, hepatic tenderness, and jaundice in approximately 25% of cases. Historically, it was estimated that approximately 15% of persons spontaneously resolved acute HCV infection, but more recent studies indicate that spontaneous clearance may occur in 20–25% of infected adults[65,66] and in as many as 40–50% of infected children.[67] Some recovering subjects (7% in one prospective study)[65] lose not only HCV RNA but also anti-HCV antibodies; this absence of residual HCV markers leads to a further underestimate of HCV recovery rates. Spontaneous recovery generally occurs within the first 6 months and has not been observed once chronic infection is established.

Chronic Hepatitis C

The vast majority of HCV infections are first detected in persons with long-standing chronic infection. When patients with chronic hepatitis C are symptomatic, the most common symptom is fatigue, but at a level difficult to distinguish from that found in the general population and only occasionally debilitating. There are HCV-specific extrahepatic syndromes probably caused by immune complex formation: cryoglobulinemia, glomerulonephritis, nephrotic syndrome, and arthritis.[68] Very rarely, lymphoma may develop, presumably as a result of HCV replication within lymphocytes. Although porphyria cutanea tarda is rare in HCV infection, most cases are HCV-associated (see Chapter 54).[69] Physical signs in HCV infection relate to cirrhosis, at which point signs and symptoms are indistinguishable from cirrhosis due to any cause. The clinical relevance of chronic HCV infection stems from the magnitude of the infected global population, such that even a small proportion of serious sequelae of infections results in a massive disease burden.

There are no specific biochemical or histologic markers that can distinguish those patients who will develop cirrhosis from individuals with stable disease, but data from long-term prospective follow-up studies,[70] and from analysis of retrospective-prospective studies[65,71] that trace patients for as long as 50 years, suggest that no more than 20–30% of patients with chronic hepatitis C progress to cirrhosis and possible end-stage liver disease. Figure 78–5 depicts the likelihood of developing severe liver disease in a theoretical cohort of 100 immunocompetent, nonalcoholic adults prospectively followed from the onset of acute HCV infection. By projection based on spontaneous resolution, nonprogressive infections, and treatment responses, only 28% will have severe outcomes; the proportion of severe cases will further decrease as treatments improve. Indeed, using a similar algorithm, the risk of cirrhosis for genotype 2 and 3 patients is already reduced to 11% because 80% respond well to current therapies. Other groups of patients will not do as well because of comorbid conditions such as alcoholism or coexisting immunosuppression (see later).

Hepatocellular Carcinoma

HCV infection is now the first or second leading cause of hepatocellular carcinoma (HCC) in the world, its relative position depending on the geographic region and the competing incidence of hepatitis B virus–associated HCC. HCV is not directly oncogenic but rather exerts its effect through its causal role in the development of cirrhosis. Almost all viral-associated HCC evolves in the setting of cirrhosis and generally develops 30 or more years after the onset of infection and 10 or more years after the onset of cirrhosis. The risk of developing HCC in patients with cirrhosis is less than 1–3% per year.

The frequency of HCC in relation to age and the duration of infection is illustrated in comparisons of the occurrence rates in the United States and Japan. Although both countries have a comparable HCV prevalence, the frequency of HCC in Japan is six- to eightfold higher. As shown in Figure 78–6*A*, there is a cohort effect wherein a time-limited past exposure, with minimal new infections, continues to move the curve to the right as the infected population ages. The curves suggest that the primary exposure occurred 30 years earlier in Japan than in the United States, a hypothesis now confirmed by phylogenetic tree analysis.[72] The global incidence of HCC has increased in the past 2 decades (Fig. 78–6*B*), and the rates of HCC in the United States will increase considerably over the next 3 decades as the population ages.[73] Fortunately, the actual number of HCC cases will be less than predicted because improved antiviral treatments, given to an increasingly large segment of the HCV-infected population, will eradicate the infection in many individuals before they develop cirrhosis and the potential for HCC.

Cofactors That Influence the Outcome of HCV Infection

There are certain co-moribund conditions with which HCV disease progression is more rapid and serious outcomes are more frequent. A prime example is human immunodeficiency virus–HCV co-infection.[74] Indeed, as highly active antiretroviral therapy has dramatically reduced short-term mortality from acquired immunodeficiency syndrome, HCV has become the leading cause of death in cohorts in which both infections are common. More severe hepatitis C is also observed among patients with hereditary T-cell immune defects or acquired T-cell disorders other than acquired immunodeficiency syndrome. Further, immunosuppressed liver transplant recipients, all of whom become reinfected with HCV, may develop cirrhosis in only 5–10 years.[75] The common denominator of accelerated HCV disease is defective cell-mediated immunity. T-cell defects may also account for more severe disease in patients who are infected after age 60 compared to those infected early in life. Why immune deficiency should foster worsening

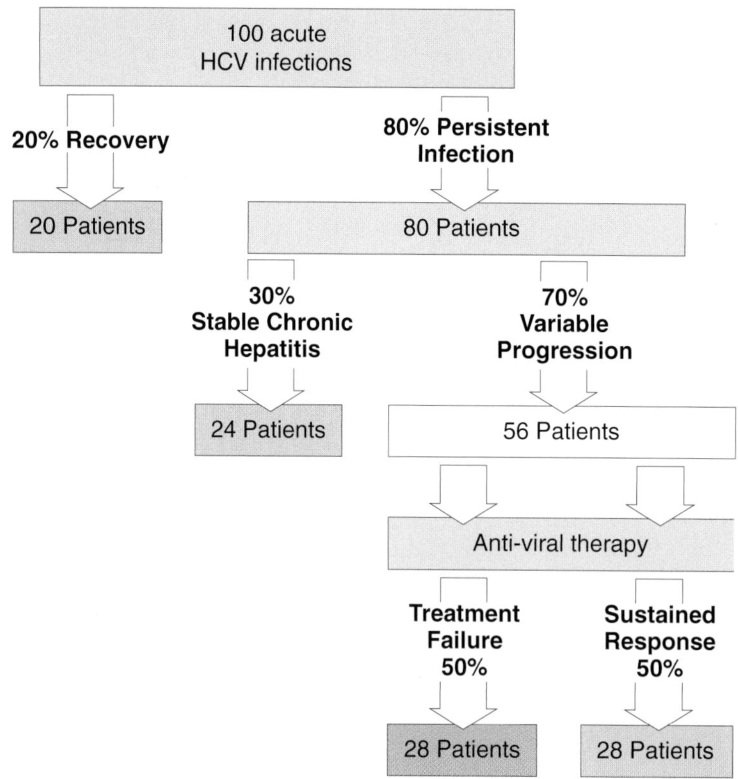

Figure 78–5. HCV outcomes in a theoretical cohort of 100 acute infections. Among 100 acutely infected individuals, approximately 20% will have spontaneous recovery during the first 6 months and 80% will become chronic HCV carriers. Of the 80 patients with chronic infection, 30% (24 patients) will have normal or low-level ALT elevations and mild, nonprogressive liver disease, whether or not they are treated. The outcome in the other 70% cannot be accurately predicted. Presently, most of these patients will be treated with therapies that provide a 50% sustained viral response that appears to be equivalent to a cure. Hence, of the residual 56 patients, 28 will be "cured" and 28 will be treatment failures. In composite, 72% will do well (20 with spontaneous recovery +24 with mild stable infection +28 treatment responders) and 28% will be at continued risk for developing cirrhosis.

disease is unclear because HCV-associated liver damage is thought to be immune mediated. Immune suppression may remove some protective response in preference to the T-cell cytotoxicity.

Excessive alcohol consumption greatly worsens the outcome of HCV infection: excess alcohol intake (>40 gm alcohol [4 drinks/day] in men and >20 gm alcohol/day in women) leads to more severe hepatitis C and a greater likelihood of developing cirrhosis.[76] The combined effects of alcohol and HCV are synergistic, and some studies[77] have shown a greater than hundredfold increased risk of cirrhosis in HCV-infected patients who abuse alcohol compared to those who are HCV-infected alone. HCV-infected patients should be advised to abstain from alcohol or to limit their intake to no more than one drink per day (10 gm alcohol).

TREATMENT OF HCV INFECTION

Because only a fraction of untreated patients develop cirrhosis, and current therapy is only effective in half the patients and is poorly tolerated, treatment decisions must be individualized based on disease severity, risk of side effects, and likelihood of response (Fig. 78–7*A*). The goal of treatment is a sustained virologic response (SVR), defined as undetectable serum HCV RNA at the end of treatment and 6 months thereafter. SVR leads to long-term improvement in quality of life[78] and liver histology,[79–81] and a reduced incidence of HCC.[82]

Pegylated Interferon-α Plus Ribavirin

SVR rates have increased considerably, first through the use of interferon alfa in combination with the nucleoside analogue ribavirin (Fig. 78–7*B*), and recently with the introduction of pegylated interferon alfa.[83,84] Pegylated interferon alfa has an extended serum half-life of several days and can be administered by subcutaneous injection once weekly. Figure 78–7*B* depicts composite responses according to genotype. In genotype 1 infections, the best SVR rate (44%) was achieved with the higher dose of ribavirin (1200 mg/day) and the longest treatment schedule (48 weeks).[85] In contrast, for genotypes 2 and 3, a 24-week regimen with 800 mg of ribavirin was as effective as other schedules, with response rates as high as 79%.[85]

Adverse Events

Side effects occur in over 75% of treated patients and can severely impact quality of life. Interferon alfa causes

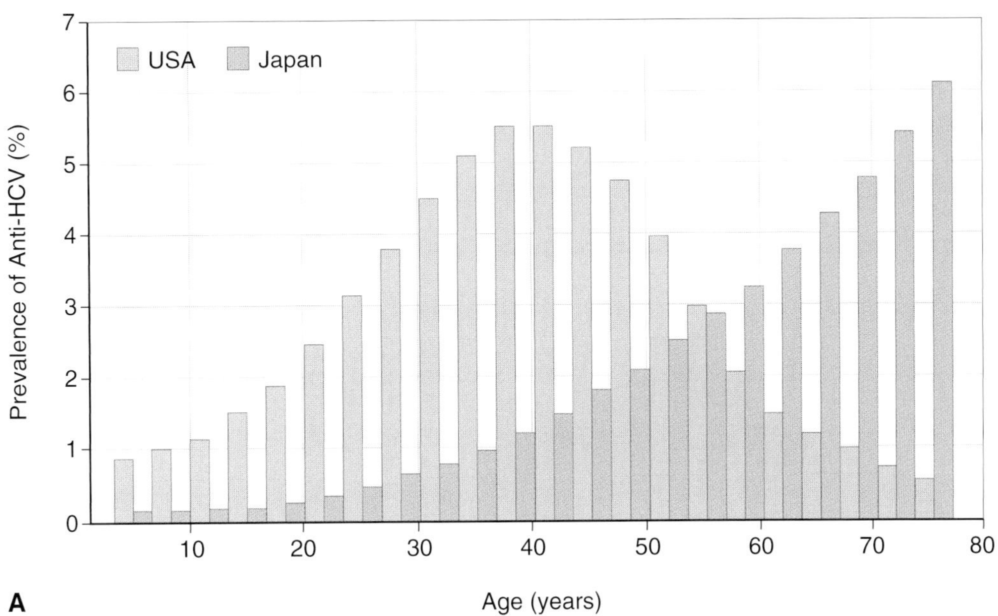

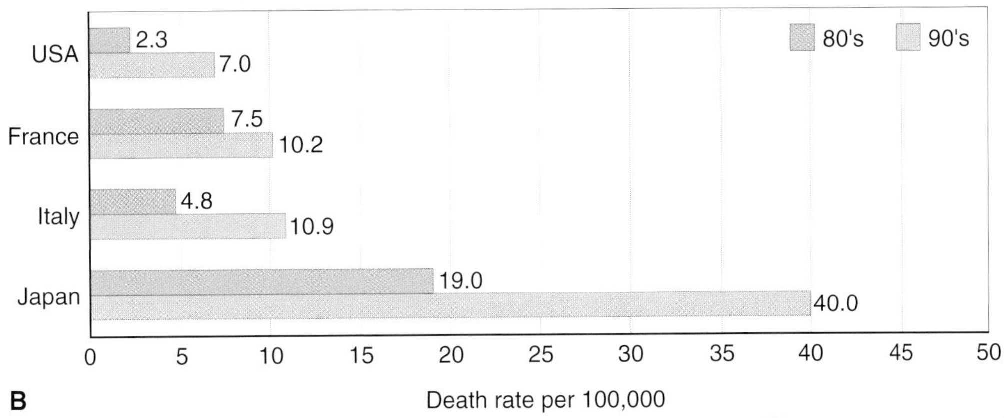

Figure 78–6. *A,* Age-adjusted prevalence of anti-HCV antibody in the United States and Japan. This pattern suggests a cohort effect wherein new infections are rare and the Japanese cohort was infected about 30 years earlier than the U.S. cohort. This correlates with the current higher incidence of hepatocellular carcinoma (HCC) in the Japanese population, which has been infected for a longer duration. The age-adjusted prevalence of anti-HCV antibody in Japan peaks in the population older than 70 years, whereas the frequency in those less than 20 is very low; in the United States, the peak prevalence is at age 40. (Modified from Yoshizawa H: Hepatocellular carcinoma associated with hepatitis C virus infection in Japan: projection to other countries in the foreseeable future. Oncology 62[Suppl 1]:8–17, 2002.) *B,* Increasing global incidence of HCC in the past two decades. (Modified from El-Serag HB, Mason AC: Rising incidence of hepatocellular carcinoma in the United States. N Engl J Med 340:745–750, 1999 and Higuchi M, Tanaka E, Kiyosawa K: Epidemiology and clinical aspects on hepatitis C. Jpn J Infect Dis 55:69–77, 2002.)

fatigue, muscle aches, headache, fever, weight loss, nausea, vomiting, insomnia, concentration and memory disturbances, irritability, depression, hair thinning, neutropenia, thrombocytopenia and hyper- or hypothyroidism. Side effects associated with ribavirin are hemolytic anemia, fatigue, itching, rash, sinusitis, nausea, and vomiting. Ribavirin is teratogenic, and strict contraception during treatment is mandatory. Adverse events are often managed with analgesics and antidepressants but sometimes require dose reduction or discontinuation.

Predictors of Response Before and During Treatment

Baseline variables associated with a higher likelihood of SVR include genotype 2 or 3, viral load less than 2 million copies/mL, young age (<40 years), low body weight (<75 kg), and absence of cirrhosis, but none of these factors is sufficiently reliable to anticipate response in the individual patient. The best predictor of SVR is the early virologic response during treatment. Early virologic response, defined as a 2-log or greater decline of HCV

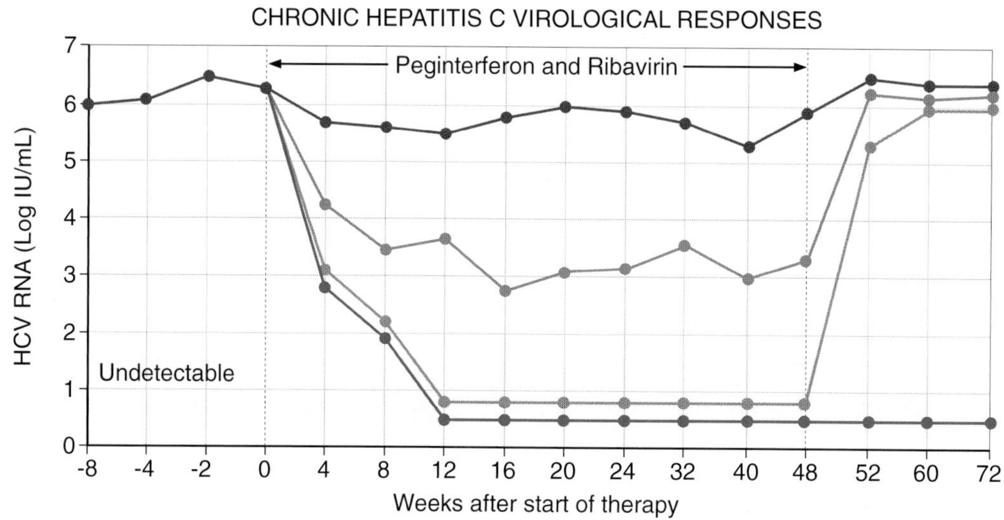

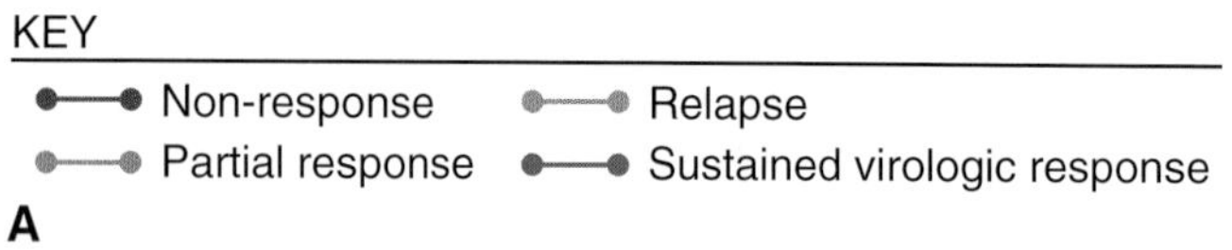

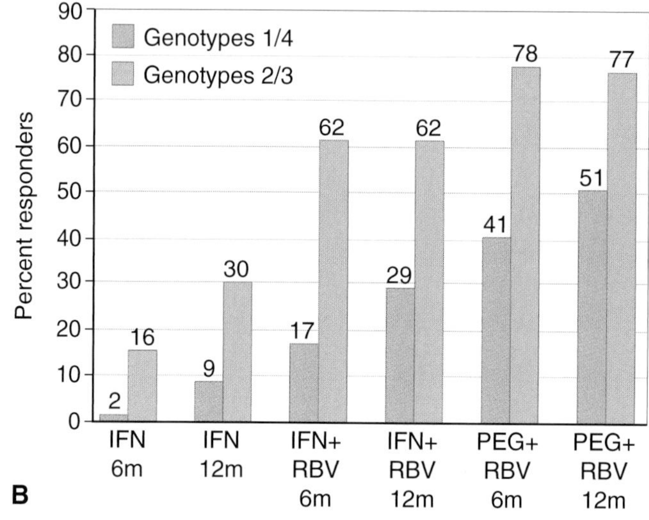

Figure 78–7. *A*, Patterns of HCV treatment response. There are four primary patterns of response to combination interferon-ribavirin therapy: (1) nonresponse; (2) partial response with a lowered viral load, but one that does not become undetectable (viral load returns to baseline during therapy [breakthrough] or just after cessation of therapy); (3) relapse: viral level becomes undetectable during therapy, but returns to baseline when treatment stops; and (4) sustained virologic response, in which viral level remains undetectable 6 months after cessation of treatment (probable "cure"). *B*, Viral response rates according to viral genotype and type and duration of therapy. The combination of pegylated interferon alfa plus ribavirin for 12 months in genotype 1 and 4 infections and 6 months in genotype 2 and 3 infections provides the best response rates.

RNA at 12 weeks, has a positive predictive value for SVR of 70%. Moreover, patients who fail to achieve such early virologic response have virtually no chance of SVR (negative predictive value 97–100%),[84,86] and in these nonresponders treatment can be discontinued after 3 months.

Selection of Patients for Treatment

HCV RNA–positive patients with elevated ALT and no major contraindication should be offered treatment. Treatment is optional for patients with persistently normal ALT, especially if liver biopsy confirms mild inflammation and no fibrosis. Patients with HCV genotypes 2 and 3 should be offered therapy irrespective of ALT level because treatment efficacy is so high. Current guidelines[87,88] for treatment and monitoring of adult patients with chronic hepatitis C are summarized in Figure 78–8. In patients with compensated cirrhosis, the interferon alfa–ribavirin combination is less well tolerated and efficacy is lower, with SVR rates less than 20%[89–91]; hepatic decompensation under therapy is a major concern.

Liver Transplantation

Orthotopic liver transplantation is the treatment of choice for end-stage HCV cirrhosis, which is the most common indication for such transplantation. Short-term prognosis after transplantation is relatively good, with 5-year survival rates of 65%.[92] HCV reinfection of the graft is inevitable, and progressive liver disease occurs in greater than 90% of patients, with cirrhosis developing in 10–30% at 5 years.[93–96]

Treatment of Acute Hepatitis C

Although HCV infection is infrequently detected during the acute stage, when detected, early treatment should be considered. Data from small and often uncontrolled studies of early treatment have shown SVR rates in response to interferon alfa of 30–100%,[98–101] but the optimal treatment strategy remains to be defined. Because spontaneous recovery is more common in patients who present with symptomatic acute hepatitis and spontaneous clearance usually occurs during the first 12 weeks,[101] patients with acute hepatitis C should be observed untreated for at least 3 months. Those who fail to resolve their infection should be treated with pegylated interferon alfa, with or without ribavirin, for at least 6 months.

PREVENTION

Intensive efforts to develop an HCV vaccine have been only partially successful. Classic vaccine approaches such as viral inactivation or attenuation cannot be applied because the virus does not grow in tissue culture. The largest vaccine effort has used the recombinant envelope proteins E1 and E2, with and without adjuvant and in various dosing schedules. Recombinant vaccines, although they induce antibody, have failed to produce a sterilizing, fully protective immune response in chimpanzees; they do appear to reduce the proportion of

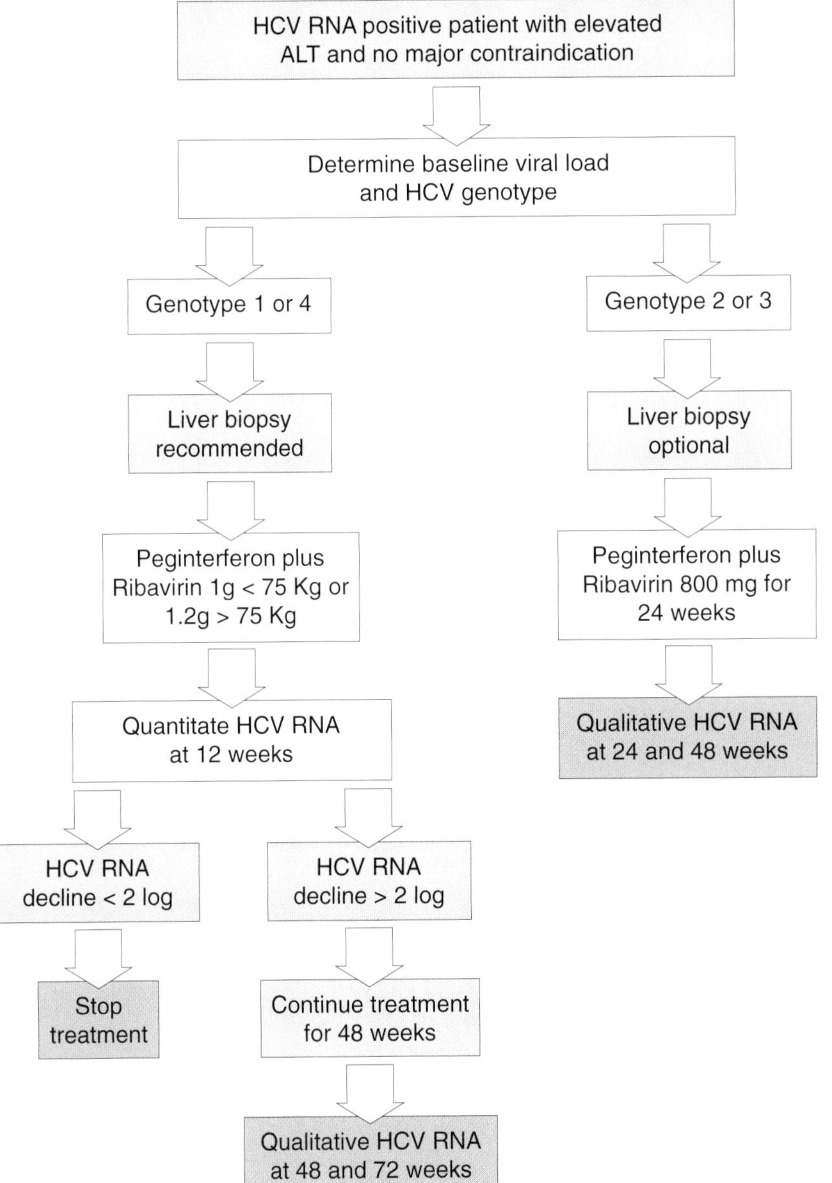

Figure 78–8. Algorithm for treating and monitoring HCV-infected patients according to viral genotype.

CURRENT CONTROVERSIES & FUTURE CONSIDERATIONS

Hepatitis C Virus

Epidemiology

- Despite its inefficient transmission by sexual routes, there is need to ascertain the extent to which sexual intercourse contributes to the global burden of HCV infection.
- Cocaine snorting with shared devices has been reported as a significant covert risk for HCV transmission. However, this transmission route has not been widely acknowledged nor experimentally proven. Given the frequency of this mode of drug abuse, this mechanism needs to be explored further.

Pathogenesis

- Is the impaired HCV-specific T-cell immune response seen in those with persistent infection the cause or the consequence of the persistent carrier state?
- What are the major pathways by which HCV subverts (tolerizes) the immune response, and are these amenable to therapeutic intervention?
- Are there host susceptibility genes that foster viral persistence?

Natural History

- Will the pace of fibrosis progression increase as persons with previously stable disease reach the 6th to 8th decades of life when their immune systems are progressively weakened? If such age dependent acceleration is shown, early treatment, even of milder cases, would be increasingly indicated.
- Are persons who spontaneously clear the virus or have a sustained treatment response truly cured or do they harbor small amounts of residual virus that could become clinically relevant under conditions of immunosuppression?

Treatment and Prophylaxis

- There is need for treatments that specifically target critical steps in the viral life cycle. In development are viral protease and helicase inhibitors. These will allow treatment cocktails with interferon and ribavirin that should considerably increase efficacy.
- Treatments that are not interferon-based since up to 50% of subjects are insensitive to or intolerant of interferon.
- Immune based therapies that enhance Th-1-biased T cell immunity are a novel approach.
- A neutralizing hepatitis C immune globulin, particularly for use in the transplant setting, should be developed.
- As for HIV, for HCV vaccine development the highly mutable nature of the virus and the absence of a strong neutralizing antibody response are major impediments. If developed, a vaccine's optimal use will be controversial because, in the developed world, hepatitis C currently does not pose a major infectious risk except for those who share needles. Needle exchange programs could be nearly as effective as vaccination.

Transplantation

- What are the mechanisms of accelerated post-transplant fibrosis progression in 30% of transplanted subjects? Is this related to transplant-associated immunosuppression? Immunosuppressive strategies that do not enhance viral replication are needed.
- How can the supply of organs be increased for the anticipated increase in HCV-related end-stage liver disease over the next two decades? Are there feasible alternatives to liver transplantation for end-stage liver disease?

experimentally infected animals that develop persistent infection. It is unknown whether these outcomes in the chimpanzee can be translated to humans. Vaccines that use a broader spectrum of structural and nonstructural HCV proteins, and DNA vaccines followed by an HCV protein boost, are in development.[102] Many other vaccine approaches are being considered, including a virus-like particle vaccine produced in baculovirus,[103] but all face the formidable challenge of an extremely mutable virus and highly diverse quasispecies. HCV is a virus that is well adapted to evade a vaccine-generated immune response. Nonetheless, there is hope that a vaccine will ultimately be effective because there is a mechanism for spontaneous viral clearance and because HCV does not integrate into the host genome. Even if a fully protective HCV vaccine cannot be achieved, a therapeutic vaccine would be a major adjunct to antiviral therapy by allowing a simultaneous assault on viral replication and a strong stimulus to adaptive immunity.

Suggested Readings*

Alter HJ, Holland PV, Purcell RH, et al: Posttransfusion hepatitis after exclusion of commercial and hepatitis-B antigen-positive donors. Ann Intern Med 77:691–699, 1972.

Alter HJ, Purcell RH, Shih JW, et al: Detection of antibody to hepatitis C virus in prospectively followed transfusion recipients with acute and chronic non-A, non-B hepatitis. N Engl J Med 321: 1494–1500, 1989.

Alter MJ, Margolis HS, Krawczynski K, et al: The natural history of community-acquired hepatitis C in the United States. The Sentinel Counties Chronic non-A, non-B Hepatitis Study Team. N Engl J Med 327:1899–1905, 1992.

Choo Q-L, Kuo G, Weiner AJ, et al: Isolation of cDNA clone derived from blood-borne non-A, non-B viral hepatitis genome. Science 244:359–362, 1989.

Gerlach JT, Diepolder HM, Zachoval R, et al: Acute hepatitis C: high rate of both spontaneous and treatment-induced viral clearance. Gastroenterology 125:80–88, 2003.

**Full references for this chapter can be found on accompanying CD-ROM.*

CHAPTER 79

Dengue and Hemorrhagic Fever Viruses

Timothy P. Endy, MD, MPH, Khin Saw Aye Myint, MD, and Siripen Kalayanarooj, MD

KEY POINTS

Dengue and Hemorrhagic Fever Viruses

Diagnosis

- Diagnosis of viral hemorrhagic fever requires a high clinical suspicion based on travel history, epidemiologic risk factors, and elimination of other potential viral, bacterial, and parasitic causes that may present similarly, such as measles, rickettsia, leptospirosis, and malaria.
- Fever is present with external manifestations of bleeding, including petechiae, ecchymoses, oozing at puncture site, gingival bleeding, epistaxis, and hemorrhagic conjunctivitis; and internal manifestations, such as melena, hematemesis, and severe vaginal bleeding.
- Hematologic abnormalities and multiorgan involvement are characteristic: thrombocytopenia, leukopenia, prolongation of prothrombin and partial thromboplastin times, hepatitis, renal failure, and encephalitis.
- Laboratory diagnosis is made by viral isolation, virus genome detection by polymerase chain reaction, or virus-specific antibody–based serologic assays, which are available only through specialized reference laboratories.

Treatment

- Treatment includes early recognition and supportive care with appropriate correction of volume, blood loss and electrolytes using normal saline, Ringer's lactate or equivalent, plasma or plasma expanders, platelets, and dialysis in the case of severe renal failure.
- The antiviral drug ribavirin or immune plasma may be useful in select viral infections.
- Specific viruses may be highly contagious, with nosocomial outbreaks common. Patients suspected as infected with these viruses should be placed in strict isolation in rooms with separate ventilation, chemical disinfection of body fluids, appropriate handling of patient specimens, and barrier protection of health care providers.

INTRODUCTION

Infections by a variety of pathogens can be complicated by fever, coagulopathy, and hemorrhage. Hemorrhagic fever, or more specifically viral hemorrhagic fever, has acquired a more specific meaning as an arthropod- or rodent-borne viral infection that results in hemorrhage and shock. The coagulopathy is manifested externally by hemorrhage into the skin as petechiae or ecchymoses, oozing at puncture sites, epistaxis, gingival bleeding, and hemorrhagic conjunctivitis; internally, hematemesis, melena, and severe vaginal bleeding can occur (Fig. 79–1). Cardiovascular collapse and shock syndrome result from blood loss or intravascular plasma leakage into the extravascular space.

This chapter emphasizes the exemplary viral hemorrhagic fever viruses, particularly dengue virus because of its current global epidemic and economic impact, and its most serious complications, dengue hemorrhagic fever (DHF) and dengue shock syndrome.

THE ORGANISMS

The viral hemorrhagic fever viruses are ribonucleic acid (RNA) viruses with differing vectors of transmission, epidemiology, pathogenesis, and case-fatality rates (Table 79–1). Hematologic and cardiovascular system manifestations vary, but the viruses share an ability to produce direct cellular activation, cell damage, and cell death, leading to derangements in the coagulation and complement pathways and plasma leakage.

The viral hemorrhagic fever viruses as RNA viruses lack a DNA polymerase–like editing activity and thus are highly susceptible to point mutations.[1] During replication, homologous and heterologous recombination, gene reassortments, and the formation of quasispecies can occur.[2] The high mutation and recombination rates, resultant competition among mutant genomes, and the natural selection of strains adapted to the host environment explain the great diversity seen among the RNA viruses.[3] An RNA genome that undergoes rapid evolution can become highly adaptable to its host and environment. An example of genetic reassortments producing

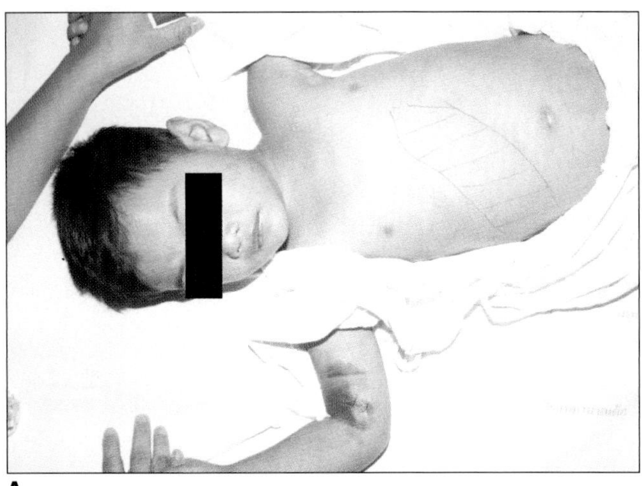

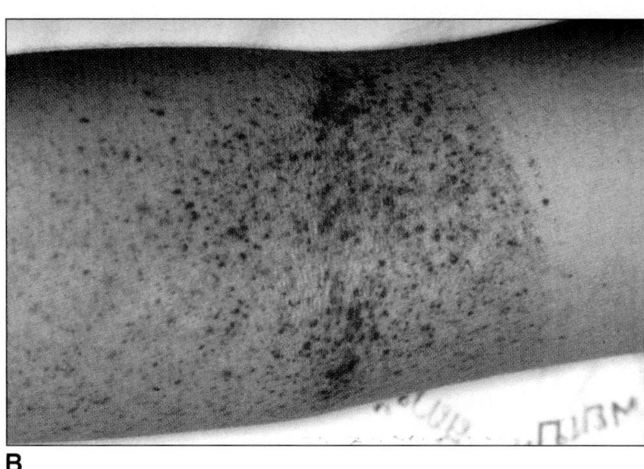

A

B

Figure 79–1. *A,* A 7-year-old Thai child with DHF, demonstrating an enlarged liver and ecchymosis of the right upper arm. *B,* Petechiae in a child with DHF following inflation of a sphygmomanometer cuff on the right upper extremity.

TABLE 79–1. Etiology, Transmission, Case-and Treatment of the Viral Hemorrhagic Fevers

Disease and Mode of Transmission	Virus		Case-Fatality Rate	Treatment
	Family	Genus		
Mosquito-Borne				
Dengue hemorrhagic fever	Flaviviridae	*Flavivirus*	1–50%	Supportive care
Rift Valley fever	Bunyaviridae	*Phlebovirus*	<1% (?)	Supportive care
Yellow fever	Flaviviridae	*Flavivirus*	15–80%	Supportive care
Chikungunya	Togaviridae	*Alphavirus*	<1% (?)	Supportive care
Tick-Borne				
Crimean-Congo hemorrhagic fever	Bunyaviridae	*Nairovirus*	30–50%	Ribavirin [141,142,146–148]
Kyasanur Forest disease	Flaviviridae	*Flavivirus*	5–10%	Supportive care
Omsk hemorrhagic fever	Flaviviridae	*Flavivirus*	0.4–2.5%	Supportive care
Rodent-Borne				
Junin hemorrhagic fever	Arenaviridae	*Arenavirus*	30%	Supportive care
Machupo hemorrhagic fever	Arenaviridae	*Arenavirus*	30%	Supportive care
Hemorrhagic fever with renal syndrome	Bunyaviridae	*Hantavirus*	10–15%	Ribavirin [141–143]
Lassa fever	Arenaviridae	*Arenavirus*	16.5%	Ribavirin [141,142,144,145,151]
Unknown				
Ebola hemorrhagic fever	Filoviridae	*Filovirus*	90%	Supportive care
Marburg hemorrhagic fever	Filoviridae	*Filovirus*	22–90%	Supportive care

Adapted from Viral haemorrhagic fevers: report of a WHO Expert Committee. World Health Organ Tech Rep Ser 721:5–126, 1985.

a pathogenic virus occurred during an outbreak of Rift Valley fever (RVF) in East Africa during 1997 and 1998[4]: in 14 patients with hemorrhagic fever, virus isolates were not RVF virus but a reassorted new bunyavirus subsequently named Garissa virus.

Three of the viruses discussed in this chapter are in the family *Bunyaviridae*: RVF virus (genus *Phlebovirus*), Crimean-Congo hemorrhagic fever (CCHF) virus (genus *Nairovirus*), and the viruses that cause hemorrhagic fever with renal syndrome (HFRS; genus *Hantavirus*). They share similar morphologic features, a spherical virion and a size between 80 to 120 nm.[5] The *Bunyaviridae* contain a lipid envelope with two or three glycoproteins that determine cell tropism and host pathogenicity and are sites for viral neutralization by antibody.[6–9] The genetic organization is a single negative strand of RNA organized into three segments named large (L), medium (M), and small (S) segments, which encode for the virus nucleocapsid, glycoproteins, and polymerase proteins, respectively.[10,11] Viral factors that are associated with human disease are illustrated by the CCHF virus M-segment–encoded polyprotein that contains a mucin-like domain and the presence of a furin cleavage site,[12] implicated in causing endothelial damage, cytotoxicity, and interferon antagonism.[13] The effect on host gene regulation of hantavirus illustrates viral regulation of host genes as a mechanism to produce severe disease. In general, pathogenic strains suppress early cellular interferon responses that instead are activated by nonpathogenic strains.[14]

Marburg and Ebola viruses of the family *Filoviridae* are unique among the hemorrhagic fever viruses in their morphology: long filamentous forms, 80 nm in diameter and a length of 790 nm for Marburg virus and 970 nm for Ebola virus.[15,16] A single strand of negative-sense RNA contains seven genes coding for the structural proteins, nucleoprotein (NP), VP30, VP35, and the polymerase (L) protein.[16] Membrane-associated proteins are the matrix protein (VP40), VP24, and the glycoprotein (GP). Genetic analysis of the L gene demonstrates homology with the paramyxoviruses suggests the *Paramyxoviridae* as a common ancestor for the filoviruses.[17] GP is the structural protein that makes up the virion surface spikes and mediates virus entry into susceptible cells.[18] The GP protein may be one of the major determinants of pathogenicity, inducing cytotoxicity of endothelial cells through its mucin domain.[13]

The dengue viruses consist of four serologically and genetically distinct viruses, DENV-1, DENV-2, DENV-3, and DENV-4.[19] Each can produce human infection and result in lifelong protective immunity to the infecting serotype—but not to the other dengue serotypes. Thus an individual can develop multiple infections from dengue virus. Dengue is typical of the genus *Flavivirus* in its spherical nucleocapsid outer structure, 30 nm in diameter, surrounded by a lipid bilayer.[20] At the virion core is a positive-sense single-stranded RNA consisting of a long open reading frame containing the coding regions for the structural proteins (C, prM, and E) and the nonstructural proteins (NS1, NS2A, NS2B, NS3, NS4A, NS4B, and NS5).[21] Virus tropism and early events are directed by the outer E glycoprotein utilizing a mammalian cellular receptor, a highly sulfated type of heparan sulfate[22,23]; in insect cells, the E protein uses a different non–heparan sulfate receptor.[24] The utilization of different cellular receptors for mammalian and insect cells is an example of the arboviruses' strategic adaptability. The E outer protein is the major site for viral neutralization by antibody.[25] For tick-borne encephalitis, eight distinct epitopes on the E glycoprotein differ in location, function, and serologic specificity, and there is a complex interaction among neutralizing antibody, heterologous non-neutralizing antibody, and enhancing antibody on the conformational structure of the E protein.[26] This interaction and resultant changes in conformational structure can result in a sixfold increase in antibody avidity; fusion is driven by conformational changes in the E protein.[26,27]

Dengue virus serotypes differ in their ability to produce large outbreaks of human disease and severe clinical disease.[28] As observed over decades in Thailand, DENV-3 was associated with large epidemics, all serotypes caused DHF, and DENV-4 was more likely to lead to secondary infections.[28] Genetic characterization of DENV-2 strains in Thailand revealed that many different variants circulated simultaneously as quasispecies.[29] Distinct genotypic groups correlated with dengue fever and DHF, implying both a common viral progenitor and that DHF-producing DENV-2 viruses segregate into only one genotypic group that has evolved independently in Southeast Asia.[29] Based on comparison of Southeast Asian genotypes of DENV-2 with non–DHF-producing American strains of DENV-2, unique genotype and nucleotide sequence in the E-NS1 region are associated with more severe dengue disease and DHF.[30,31]

EPIDEMIOLOGY AND RISK FACTORS

Considerable differences in mode of transmission, geographic distribution, and seasonality among the viral hemorrhagic fever viruses translate to diverse epidemiologic patterns and risk factors for infection[32] (Table 79–2). In general, the viruses can be classified as either arthropod-borne or rodent-borne, but for the filoviruses Ebola and Marburg, the mode of transmission is unknown. The vector can be urban mosquitoes, as for dengue virus, or both urban and sylvatic mosquitoes, as for yellow fever virus. Ticks can remain infected for years, infect their progeny transovarially, and maintain a continuous virus burden in the environment. Among the rodent-borne viruses, a small field mouse that can reside in a house will have different transmissibility as compared to the rodent in the field. For some of the viral hemorrhagic fever viruses, an intermediate vertebrate can serve as a reservoir in nature, resulting in viral amplification, as monkeys do for yellow fever and Kyasanur Forest disease, and sheep and cattle do for RVF. For dengue viruses, there is no reservoir except humans, with the transmission cycle entirely dependent on human-to-mosquito-to-human passage. The diversity in the vector, mode of transmission, and reservoir are reflected in the range of disease patterns in humans, which can be sporadic, endemic, or epidemic with an enzootic and/or epizootic transmission cycle. Human-to-human transmission can occur by direct contact, as for Crimean-Congo, Lassa, Marburg, and Ebola viruses, or only through arthropods, as for dengue and yellow fever viruses, or humans may be a dead-end host.

Specificity in the mode of transmission might imply a well-defined geographic distribution, but many of these viruses are considered emerging pathogens. Dengue fever has become a major pandemic in the last 40 years, extending from Southeast Asia to most of the tropical and subtropical regions of the world, because of the spread of its primary mosquito vector, *Aedes aegypti,* through commercial shipping and air transportation. CCHF may be increasing in the Middle East, and RVF has spread outside of sub-Saharan Africa into the Middle East.[33–35] Ebola virus produces large epidemics in equatorial Africa and is a major cause of death among gorillas in Gabon and Congo.[36]

RVF is an acute zoonotic disease that affects ruminant animals and humans. Human infections occur as an epizootic and transmission occurs primarily from infected mosquitoes (*Culex, Aedes,* and *Anopheles* species) and secondarily from the handling of infected animal carcasses.[37] RVF virus was originally isolated in 1930 in the Rift Valley of Kenya and has been responsible for many large outbreaks of animal and human disease in East

TABLE 79–2. Incidence, Geographic Distribution, Age, and Risk Factors of the Viral Hemorrhagic Fevers

Disease	Incidence	Geographic Distribution	Age	Risk Factors
Dengue hemorrhagic fever (DHF)	Globally, 50–100 million cases of infection, 500,000 cases of DHF. Seasonal incidence dependent on breeding of mosquito vector, *Aedes aegypti*. During severe outbreaks, incidence for total dengue infection as high as 12/1000, that for DHF 0.4/1000.	Tropical and subtropical regions of the world. Endemic in Southeast Asia, Southwest Asia, Central America and parts of South America.	Any age at risk for infection. Primarily a childhood disease in endemic countries.	Previous dengue virus infection. Host genetic factors: may be increased for HLA-B*51, HLA-A2, HLA class I alleles A*0203, A*0206, and A*0207; decreased for HLA-B44, B62, B76 and B77. Increased for females; decreased for blacks. Viral factors, decreased for American genotype of dengue-2. Behavior that increases chances of being bitten by daytime feeding vector, such as urban residence, lack of window screens, failure to use insect repellants.
Rift Valley fever	Sporadic seasonal outbreaks in domestic animals with human infections. In Egypt during 1977, 18,000 human cases and 598 deaths.	Africa, sub-Saharan Africa, Middle East.	All age groups.	Primarily a disease of domestic animals. Adults at greatest risk during epizootics: those working or living around domestic animals, from the bite of the mosquito or handling infected carcasses. Laboratory worker infection common. May be viral strains that produce more severe disease.
Yellow fever	Seasonal incidence. Annual number of cases in South America between 50 and 300, and approximately 4000 cases in Africa. Large outbreaks in Africa involving 100,000 cases and 30,000 deaths.	Tropical regions of Africa (between 15° N and 10° S) and South America in the Amazon region, Orinoco and Magdalena Valleys (10° N and 40° S), Bolivia, Brazil, Colombia, and Peru.	All age groups.	Sylvatic and urban cycle. During sylvatic cycle, agriculture and forest workers at greatest risk. Behavior that increases chances of being bitten by feeding mosquito vector, such as lack of window screens, failure to use insect repellants. May be cross-protection from previous flavivirus infections.
Chikungunya	Seasonal incidence with sporadic outbreaks.	Tropical Africa, Southeast Asia, Southwest Asia.	All ages. Primarily a pediatric disease in Thailand during the 1960s.	Sylvatic and urban cycle in Africa, primarily urban in Asia. During sylvatic cycle, agriculture and forest workers. Behavior that increases chances of being bitten by feeding mosquito vector, such as lack of window screens, failure to use insect repellants.
Crimean-Congo hemorrhagic fever	Seasonal incidence with sporadic outbreaks.	Asia, Middle East, Europe, Africa.	All ages. Adult workers in agriculture, with domestic animals at particular risk.	Behavior that increases chances of being bitten by feeding tick vector, such as failure to use insect repellants. Health care and laboratory workers at high risk from hospitalized patients.
Kyasanur Forest disease	Seasonal incidence with sporadic outbreaks.	Shimoga, North Kanara, South Kanara, and Chikamagaloor Districts Karnataka State, India.	Primarily adults.	Workers in and around the forest. Behavior that increases chances of being bitten by feeding tick vector and failure to use insect repellants. Laboratory workers at high risk.
Omsk hemorrhagic fever	Seasonal incidence with sporadic outbreaks.	Omsk, Novosibirsk, and Tyumen regions of western Siberia, Russia.	All ages.	Agricultural workers. Behavior that increases chances of being bitten by feeding tick vector, such as failure to use insect repellants, direct contact with infected muskrats.
Junin hemorrhagic fever	Annual occurrence of cases.	Buenos Aires, Santa Fé, Córdoba, and La Pampa Provinces, Argentina.	All ages susceptible, cases primarily in . male adults	Restricted to agricultural region where *Calomys* species of rodents live. Behavior that increases exposure to rodent excrement. Human-to-human transmission cases have occurred, and laboratory workers are at risk.
Machupo hemorrhagic fever	Sporadic cases.	Beni region of Bolivia.	All ages.	Same as for Junin hemorrhagic fever.
Hemorrhagic fever with renal syndrome	Several hundred cases per year to 42,000 cases in large outbreaks.	Disease in Asia, Scandinavia, Europe. Antibody prevalence in the Americas, Western Pacific, Africa, Eastern Mediterranean.	Adults.	Higher prevalence in males. Behavior that increases risk to exposure to rodent *Apodemus*, *Clethrionomys*, *Rattus* excreta. Farmers, soldiers, laboratory personnel, animal-room workers, and rodent breeders are at particular risk.
Lassa fever	Sporadic outbreaks.	West Africa.	All ages.	Persons living in rural or urban areas infested with the *Mastomys* species rat. Behavior that increases exposure to rat excreta. Health care and laboratory workers at high risk from hospitalized patients.
Ebola and Marburg hemorrhagic fevers	Sporadic outbreaks of hundreds of cases.	Equatorial Africa: Sudan, Zaire, Ivory Coast, Congo for Ebola; Uganda, Zimbabwe, Kenya for Marburg.	All ages.	Nonhuman primates may be source of some outbreaks from contact with carcasses. Person-to-person, nosocomial transmission have occurred, and laboratory workers are at risk.

Africa. Age-specific mortality for RVF is greatest for the elderly (57% in those ≥ 90 years, 22% in those ages 80–89 years, and 19% in those ages 70–79 years), with overall mortality of 14%.[34] Factors responsible for the spread of RVF include migration of infected livestock and mosquito vectors; global weather pattern changes, such as periods of heavy rainfall; and economic development resulting in environmental conditions favoring mosquito breeding, such as the building of dams and the associated flooding of plains.[38,39]

CCHF, first clinically described in 1944 in Western Crimea of the former Soviet Union, has a wide geographic range, producing human disease in Africa, Asia, the Middle East, and Europe.[40] Unlike RVF, CCHF is transmitted to humans by the bite of infected *Hyalomma* species ticks. Domestic animals serve in the transmission cycle as the viral-amplifying host or reservoir. Ticks maintain the virus in the environment, remain infected for long periods, and infect their progeny by transovarial transmission.[37,41,42] Risk for human infection involves behavior that increases potential exposure to bites from ticks, handling of infected carcasses, and nosocomial transmission.

HFRS was described the early 1900s in China, the former Soviet Union, Scandinavia, Eastern Europe, and Korea.[37,43] During the Korean War, over 3000 United Nations soldiers developed hemorrhagic disease with renal failure, shock, and death in 10–15% of cases.[37,43] The etiologic agent was isolated in 1967 from the rodent *Apodemus agrarius* and named Hantaan virus, after the Hantaan River. There are over 20 genotypes of the genus *Hantavirus*. The virus is maintained in the environment by specific rodent species[44]; human infection occurs by inhalation of infected rodent excreta. The genotype determines the severity of clinical disease.

Ebola and Marburg hemorrhagic fevers represent two dramatic agents because of their severe hemorrhagic disease and high mortality. Marburg hemorrhagic fever was first described and the virus isolated during an outbreak of hemorrhagic fever that occurred in Marburg and Frankfurt, Germany, and in Belgrade, Yugoslavia, from imported African green vervet monkeys.[45] Both types occur in central Africa, Ebola hemorrhagic fever the rain forests of central and western Africa and Marburg hemorrhagic fever in the drier areas of central and eastern Africa.[46] Marburg hemorrhagic fever has produced several outbreaks since its initial description in Zimbabwe, Kenya, and the Democratic Republic of the Congo. Ebola hemorrhagic fever and its serotypes have been responsible for numerous outbreaks of human disease in Côte d'Ivoire, Sudan, Uganda, Congo, and Gabon.[46] Risk factors for transmission were contact within the family or in the hospital with the patient's body fluids.[47] The natural reservoir and mode of transmission to humans for both Marburg and Ebola viruses are unknown.

Dengue virus infections have been recognized since the 1700s with major epidemics in Asia, North America, and Africa.[48–50] Dengue was responsible for large outbreaks of illness in Japanese and Allied soldiers in Southeast Asia during World War II, and the virus was isolated during the war in both Japan and the United States.[51–54] Philippine hemorrhagic fever and Thai hemorrhagic fever, described in the 1950s, were shown by viral isolation to be complications of dengue virus infection[55–58] and were renamed dengue hemorrhagic fever. Dengue virus infection and DHF have spread to become an endemic disease with periodic large outbreaks of disease throughout the tropical and subtropical regions of the world.[50,59–61] Dengue is the second most important tropical infectious disease globally, after malaria, with over half the world's population living in areas at risk for transmission[62]: annually there are 50–100 million cases of dengue infection, 500,000 cases of severe dengue disease (DHF), and 25,000 deaths.[62] The dengue viruses are transmitted by a mosquito vector, *A. aegypti*. Transmission is from infected mosquitoes to humans back to mosquitoes, with maintenance of the virus by overwintering in mosquitoes and transovarial transmission of the virus to the mosquito's progeny.[63,64] *Aedes aegypti* is an urban mosquito with preferential feeding on humans by the female, which requires a blood meal to lay eggs.[65] Breeding occurs in urban potable water containers, used vehicle and bicycle tires, empty bottles, and household planters. Dengue disease and transmission has been studied extensively in Thailand[66] (Fig. 79–2). Most adults in endemic regions are seropositive for dengue virus, reflecting the high burden of virus transmission in the population. Continuous transmission of dengue virus within a population is due to the different dengue serotypes that become predominant in any given year.[67,68] Because immunity is conferred from the infecting dengue serotype but does not protect against other serotypes, an individual may become infected from two or more dengue serotypes during a lifetime. There may be marked spatial and temporal clustering of virus transmission of each dengue serotype. The constant influx of virus-susceptible children, the spread of differing dengue serotypes, and intrinsic population dynamics provide an environment of continuous transmission without the development of herd immunity.[69]

PATHOPHYSIOLOGY

The hemorrhagic fever viruses produce bleeding manifestations either by direct effects on cellular function or by activation of host immune and inflammatory pathways. Dynamic interplay between viral and host factors results in a spectrum of disease severity from an asymptomatic to mild illness to its most severe manifestation, hemorrhagic disease.[70] Our knowledge of the host factors responsible for severe disease is limited because of the lack of appropriate animal models and prevalence of the disease in areas of the world where well-controlled human studies are difficult to perform. Common characteristics for the viral hemorrhagic fever viruses include an initial infection in dendritic or monocytes/macrophages followed by disseminated viremia. Viremia induces immune activation with derangement in the host response, either directly by the virus or indirectly by downregulation of cell-mediated T helper cell type 1 (T_H1) responses. There is activation of the complement pathway followed by endothelial damage directly by the

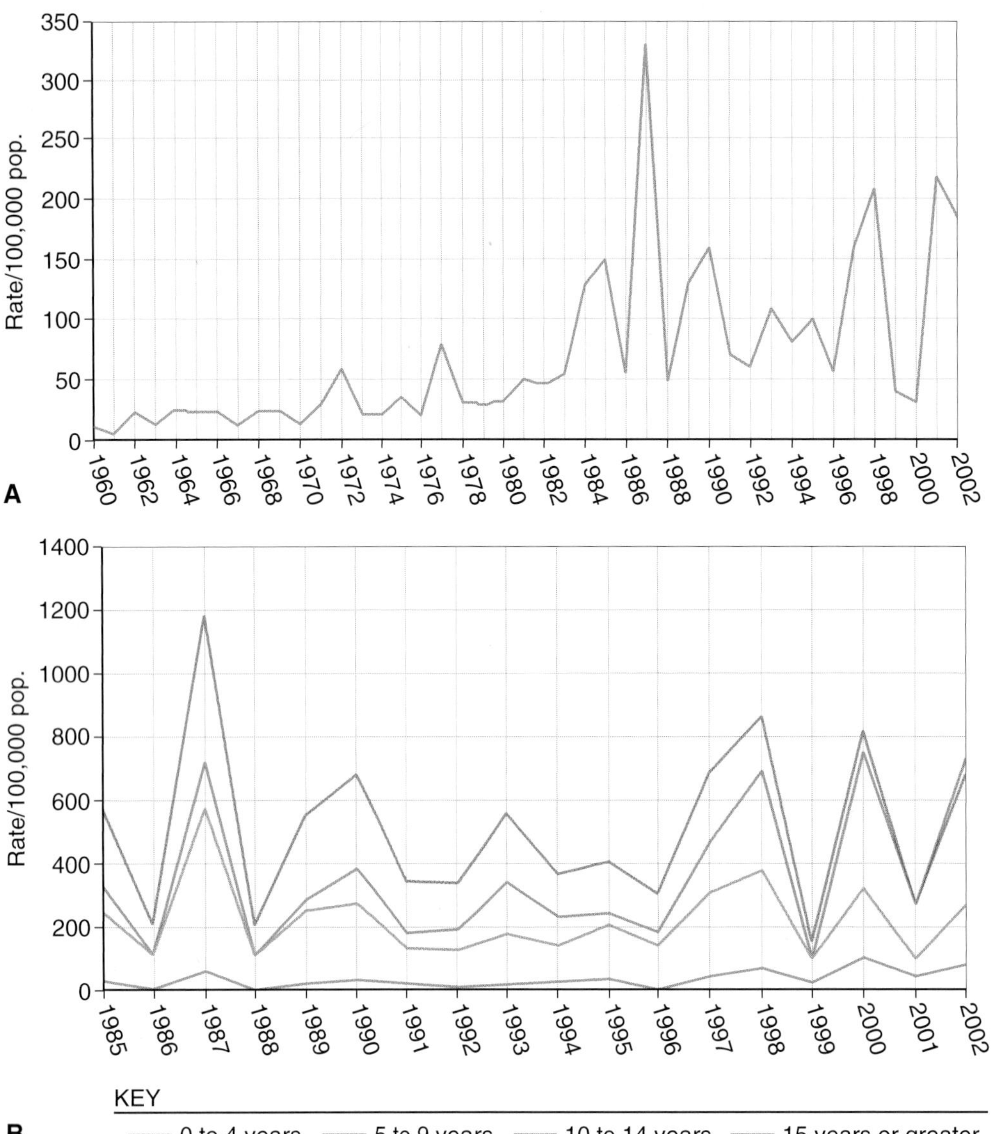

Figure 79–2. *A,* Thai Ministry of Health data displaying the annual incidence of DHF in Thailand from 1960 to 2002. DHF incidence grew from 10 per 100,000 population during 1960 to 24 per 100,000 by 1969. DHF incidence continued to increase with large outbreak years in 1984 and 1985, followed by the largest outbreak in Thailand during 1987, with an incidence of 330 per 100,000. Dengue disease and DHF are primarily childhood diseases in endemic regions, though all ages are at risk of dengue infection and severe dengue disease. ***B,*** Thai Ministry of Health data displaying the age-specific incidence of DHF in Thailand from 1985 to 2002 demonstrate that children ages 5–9 years are at greatest risk for DHF, followed by those in the 10- to 14-year age category.

virus or indirectly by the host immune response, leading to coagulopathy, plasma leakage, and shock or death.[71]

Acute infection with the hantaviruses is associated with activation of $CD8^+$cells and production of interferon-γ.[72,73] Inflammatory cytokines (tumor necrosis factor-α [TNF-α] as well as the T helper cell type 2–associated cytokines interleukin-6 and interleukin-10) are elevated during acute infection, correlating to increased levels of immunoglobulin (Ig)E.[74] Circulating immune complexes may be responsible for the renal dysfunction produced during HFRS.[75]

The immune response during acute symptomatic Ebola virus infection was studied during two large outbreaks in Gabon.[76] In patients who survived, there was an early and increased level of IgG antibody directed against the nucleoprotein and the 40-kDa viral protein of Ebola virus, followed by clearance of circulating viral antigen, activation of cytotoxic T cells, and upregulation of FasL, perforin, CD28, and interferon-γ messenger RNA in peripheral blood mononuclear cells (PBMCs). The immune response in fatal infection was characterized by an impaired humoral response, with lack of IgG antibody production and high levels of interferon-γ, intravascular apoptosis, and activation of monocytes/macrophages prior to death.[76,77] The presence of interleukin-1β and elevated concentrations of interleukin-6 was associated with nonfatal infection, and the presence of high levels of interleukin-10 and neopterin was indicative of fatal disease. The immune response during acute asymptomatic Ebola virus infection was studied in seven 7 close family contacts of symptomatic Ebola-infected patients: inflammatory cytokines peaked 7 days postexposure; there were high levels of interleukin-1β, TNF-α, interleukin-6, interleukin-1 receptor antagonist, and two soluble TNF receptors, and high plasma interleukin-10 and cortisol concentrations.[78,79] Expression of interferon-γ messenger RNA as well as the apoptosis markers Fas and FasL in PBMCs were increased. Cytotoxic T-cells were activated. Even during asymptomatic Ebola virus infection, the host produces a rapid inflammatory response without clinical symptoms and with upregulation of cytotoxic T cells to clear virus-infected cells.

In nonhuman primates infected with Ebola and Marburg virus, dendritic cells were early and sustained targets of infection, becoming functionally impaired and unable to produce cytokines or to become activated.[80,81] Coagulation abnormalities were associated with a rise in tissue factor and a subsequent decline in protein C.[82] Endothelial cells during acute infection demonstrated absence of a direct infection by Ebola virus, suggesting a host-mediated cellular injury.[82]

Severe Dengue Disease (DHF)

The pathogenesis of severe dengue disease differs from that of the other viral hemorrhagic fevers because the risk of DHF is greatest during the second dengue infection. Severe disease is a manifestation of enhancement by antibody from a previous dengue infection, high dengue viral load, and a robust immune response based on cross-reactive memory T cells.[83] The end result, however, is similar to that in other viral hemorrhagic fevers: derangements in the host response either directly by the virus or indirectly by downregulation of cell-mediated T_H1 responses, and activation of the complement pathway followed by coagulopathy, endothelial damage, plasma leakage, and intravascular volume depletion with shock and/or death. Priming of the host innate immune response after the first dengue infection triggers an immunologic cascade similar to that seen in other viral hemorrhagic fever viruses on first infection.

In the current model of the pathogenesis of severe dengue disease, the host response starts when an infected mosquito takes a blood meal and dengue is introduced into a human (Fig. 79–3).[84] Resident skin dendritic cells are highly permissive for dengue and are the initial targets of infection.[85,86] The dengue receptor is an ICAM-3–grabbing nonintegrin (DC-SIGN) molecule.[87,88] Infected dendritic cells undergo maturation and produce TNF-α and interferon-α, which induces activation in uninfected bystander dendritic cells.[89]

Antibody enhancement was first inferred epidemiologically, because DHF in children largely occurred with a secondary dengue virus infection.[90] In the "sequential infection" hypothesis, priming of the immune system occurs during a first dengue infection, leading to DHF on subsequent dengue infections.[91] In a series of elegant experiments using human monocytes and patient sera, antibody-dependent enhancement of dengue virus growth was found primarily in children with DHF, and this enhancing activity was a significant risk factor for severe illness.[92,93] Dengue viruses replicate in mononuclear phagocytic cells; subneutralizing concentrations of dengue antibody increase dengue virus infection in these cells through an Fc receptor, antibody-virus complex mechanism.[94] The result of antibody enhancement is a high dengue viral load with increased direct viral cellular damage and/or a greater activation of the host immune response. Peak dengue viral load correlates with both dengue disease severity and immune activation.[95] DHF was associated with higher mean plasma viremia levels as compared to those in children without DHF, and correlated to peak plasma interferon-γ levels, the severity of plasma leakage, and thrombocytopenia.[96] Early immune activation in acute dengue infection predicted the development of severe dengue illness.[97] Soluble TNF receptors were higher in children who developed DHF as compared to children with dengue fever and nondengue illness, and related to the degree of subsequent plasma leakage; other cytokines higher in DHF were soluble CD8, soluble interleukin-2 receptor, and interferon-γ.[97] The observation of a greater cytokine response associated with severe dengue disease has supported the hypothesis that excessive T-cell activation from preexisting dengue-specific memory T cells is a contributing cause of DHF.[98]

Primary dengue virus infections result in the production of both serotype-specific and serotype–cross-reactive CD4 and CD8 memory cytotoxic T lymphocytes. This important immunologic response by the host results in lifelong protective immunity to another infection from the same dengue serotype. In secondary dengue infection from another dengue serotype, there is activation of these preexisting cross-reactive CD4 and CD8 memory cytotoxic T lymphocytes, resulting in a rapid release of cytokines, generalized T-cell activation, and cytotoxic T lymphocyte–mediated lysis of dengue virus–infected monocytes.[98] Monocyte lysis releases chemokines that lead to endothelial damage, plasma leakage, and hemorrhage.[98] T-cell activation is an important determinant of DHF.[99] The role of preexisting memory T cells in the development of DHF in secondary dengue infections was explored in a prospective study of dengue disease in schoolchildren in Thailand. PBMCs were collected prior to asymptomatic, mild, or severe (DHF) dengue illness and stimulated with inactivated dengue antigens: cells that secreted interferon-γ and TNF-α in the presence of dengue antigen were found primarily in children who subsequently developed DHF.[68,100]

Apoptosis has been a consistent observation in human and animal studies of the viral hemorrhagic fever viruses and also observed in vitro and in animal models.[76,101,102] Sera from patients with DHF induced endothelial cell apoptosis by a caspase-dependent pathway.[103] Apoptosis has been demonstrated in children with DHF (Fig. 79–4).[104] The mean number of apoptotic cells per 10^5 cells was higher in children with more severe disease and peaked on the day of defervescence (Fig. 79–5). Programmed cell death, either induced by a direct viral effect or as part of the host immune response, may play a role in the pathophysiology of severe dengue disease.[104]

A marked coagulopathy and thrombocytopenia are cardinal hematologic features of DHF. Circulating immune complexes are present, the complement pathway is activated at the time of shock in DHF, and there are decreased serum levels of C3, C4, and C5 and increased C3a, correlating to disease severity.[105] Dengue antibody complexes on the surface of platelets from patients with DHF likely produce rapid clearance and destruction of platelets in the spleen.[106] The development of plasminogen cross-reactive antibodies in secondary dengue infections may be another explanation of the coagulopathy.[107]

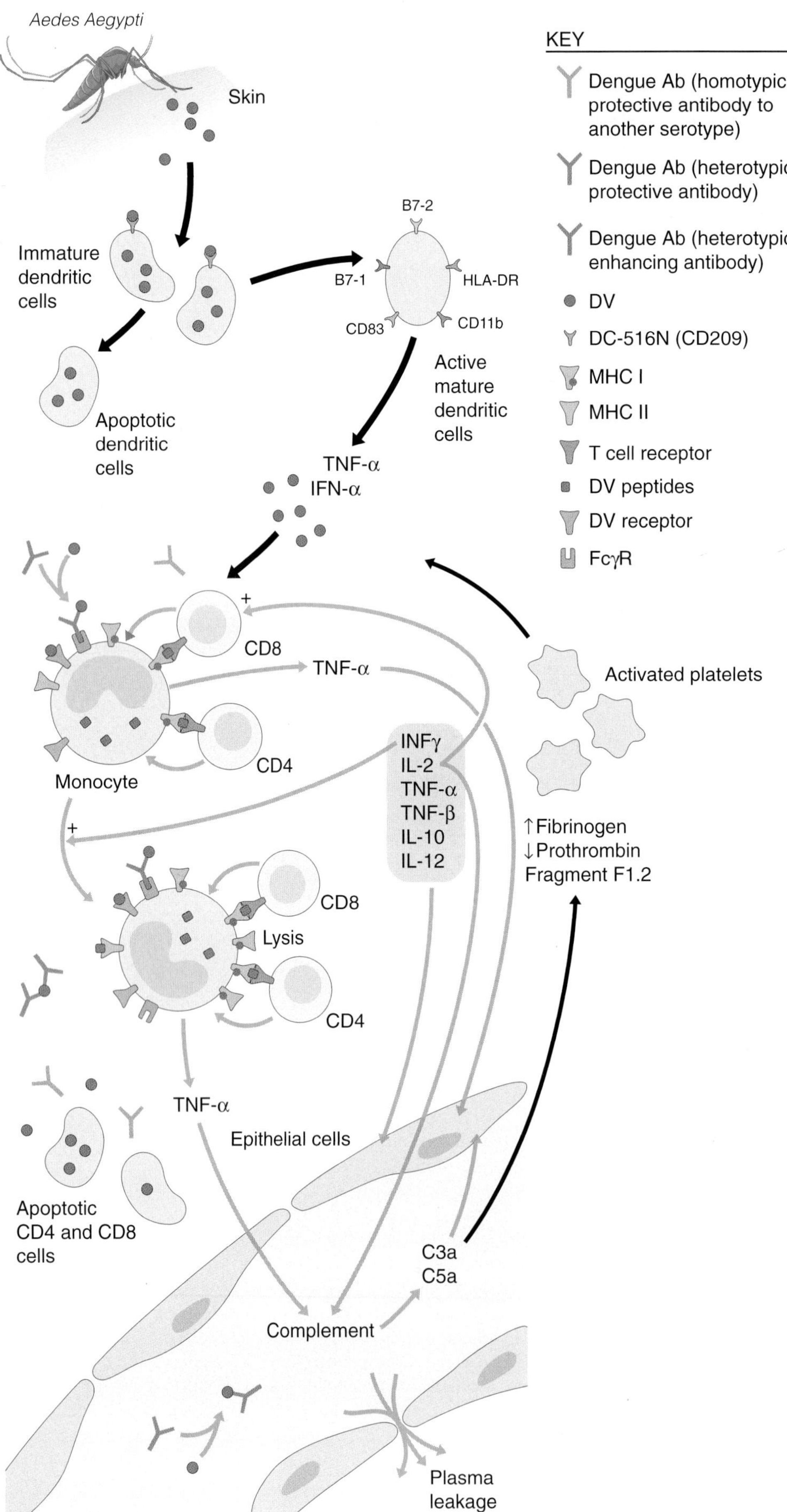

Figure 79–3. Model of the immunology and pathogenesis of severe dengue disease (DHF). (Adapted in part from Kurane I, Ennis FA: Immunopathogenesis of dengue virus infections. *In* Gubler DJ, Kuno G [eds]: Dengue and Dengue Hemorrhagic Fever: Its History and Resurgence as a Global Public Health Problem. New York: CAB International, 1997, p 273.)

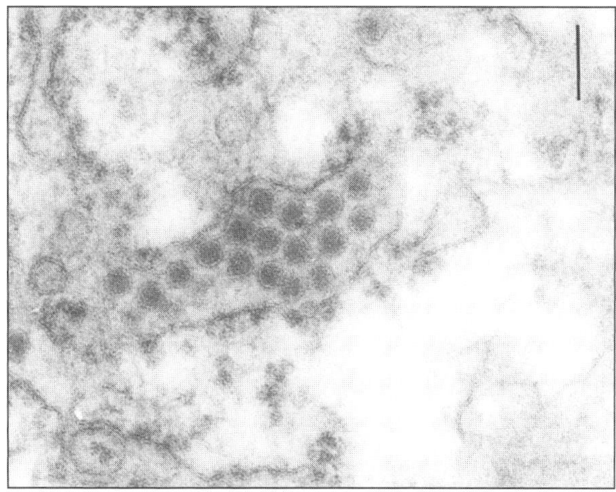

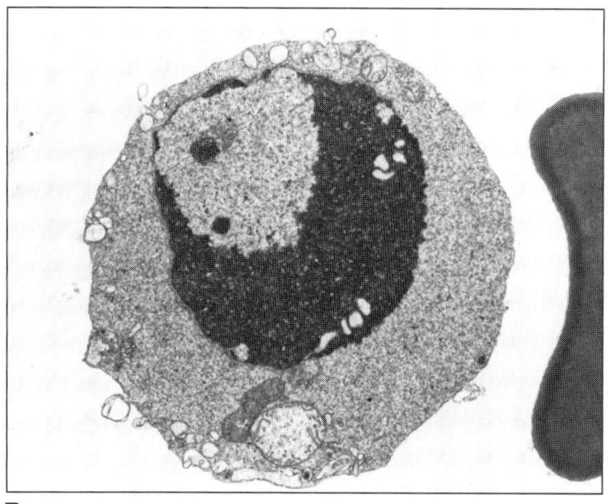

A B

Figure 79–4. *A,* Electron micrograph of dengue virus in cell culture (dengue virus–infected Vero cell). Numerous mature virions are seen in the dilated endoplasmic reticulum. (Bar = 100 nm.) ***B,*** Electron micrograph of apoptosis of circulating white blood cells in a dengue patient. Lymphocyte showing early apoptosis with peripheral margination of nuclear chromatin. (Magnification × 15,400.) (Photographs courtesy of Dr. Ludmila Asher, Division of Pathology, Walter Reed Army Institute of Research, Silver Spring, MD.)

Monocytes produce fibrinolytic and coagulation enzymes such as urokinase, plasminogen activator, plasminogen activator inhibitor, and a procoagulant activity that has been characterized as tissue factor.[108] Monocytes infected with dengue virus in vitro demonstrated a threefold increase in plasminogen activator inhibitor without an increase in urokinase, plasminogen activator, or procoagulant activity, and they may be responsible for the coagulopathy of DHF.[108] In children hospitalized with severe dengue disease in Thailand, activated partial thromboplastin time was consistently prolonged, fibrinogen levels were decreased, and levels of prothrombin fragment F1.2 were increased.[109] In Vietnamese children with DHF, there was moderate to severe depression of plasma fibrinogen, and low concentrations of the anticoagulant proteins C, S, and antithrombin III; levels of thrombomodulin, tissue factor, and plasminogen activator inhibitor type 1 were high.[110] These data indicate a consumptive coagulopathy; activation of the coagulation pathway may be the main culprit in the association of thrombocytopenia and hemorrhage with severe dengue illness.[109]

Genetic factors also may determine why certain patients develop DHF on their second dengue infection. In studies of Thai children with DHF, human lymphocyte antigen (HLA) A and B typing showed a positive association for DHF with HLA-A2 and a negative relationship for HLA-B13.[111] HLA class I alleles A*0203, A*0207, and A*02011 were more associated with dengue fever, whereas the A*0203, A*0206, and A*0207 alleles were associated with DHF.[112] In a case-control study of Thai patients with dengue, HLA class I associations were detected with secondary infections but not in patients with primary infections.[113] Less severe dengue illness was associated with HLA-A*0203, and HLA-A*0207 was associated with DHF patients. HLA-B44, B62, B76, and B77 appeared to be protective against developing clinical disease after secondary infection.

CLINICAL DISEASES AND HEMATOLOGIC MANIFESTATIONS

Initial Evaluation

The early clinical presentation of a viral hemorrhagic fever is protean and often indistinguishable from other viral or nonviral infectious causes of illness. The initial differential diagnosis is extensive and includes viruses, bacteria, fungi, protozoans, rickettsia, and spirochetes that can be complicated by a hemorrhagic state resulting in fever, coagulopathy, and hemorrhage. Infectious diseases, especially fulminant *Neisseria meningitidis, Rickettsia rickettsii* (Rocky Mountain spotted fever), *Rickettsia tsutsugamushi* (scrub typhus), and *Leptospirosis,* can be particularly difficult to distinguish clinically from the viral hemorrhagic fevers. In hospitalized children admitted with a diagnosis of DHF in northern Thailand, 7.5% were found to have leptospirosis[114] (a distinguishing characteristic of leptospirosis was the higher white blood cell and absolute neutrophil counts).

Fever is universal in viral hemorrhagic fever. A travel history, which includes an assessment of activities as a risk for exposure to rodents and insect vectors as well as pretravel vaccination and prophylactic medication, is crucial in the evaluation of a febrile patient. Understanding of the geographic distribution of the viral hemorrhagic fever viruses, mode of transmission, and seasonality guide the history and physical examination, later evaluations, and biocontainment. An estimate of the day of clinical illness is based on the date of exposure, a 5- to 10-day incubation period, and the first day of fever. Clinical manifestations and complications of infection begin to diverge after the febrile period, providing clues as to etiology and for clinical management. For DHF, the day of defervescence is the hallmark for the occurrence of plasma leakage and shock. Of the viral hemorrhagic fever viruses, four viruses—Crimean-Congo,

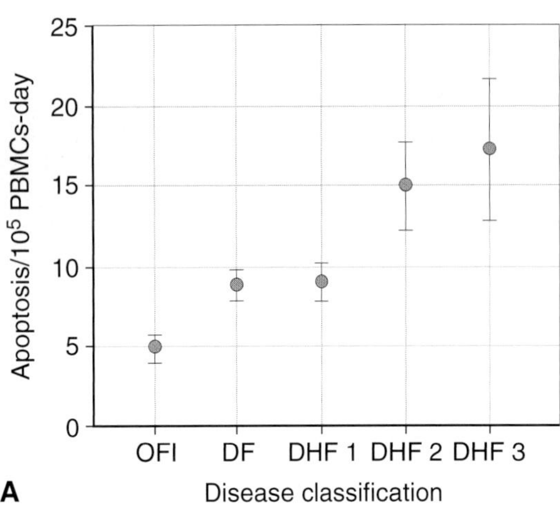

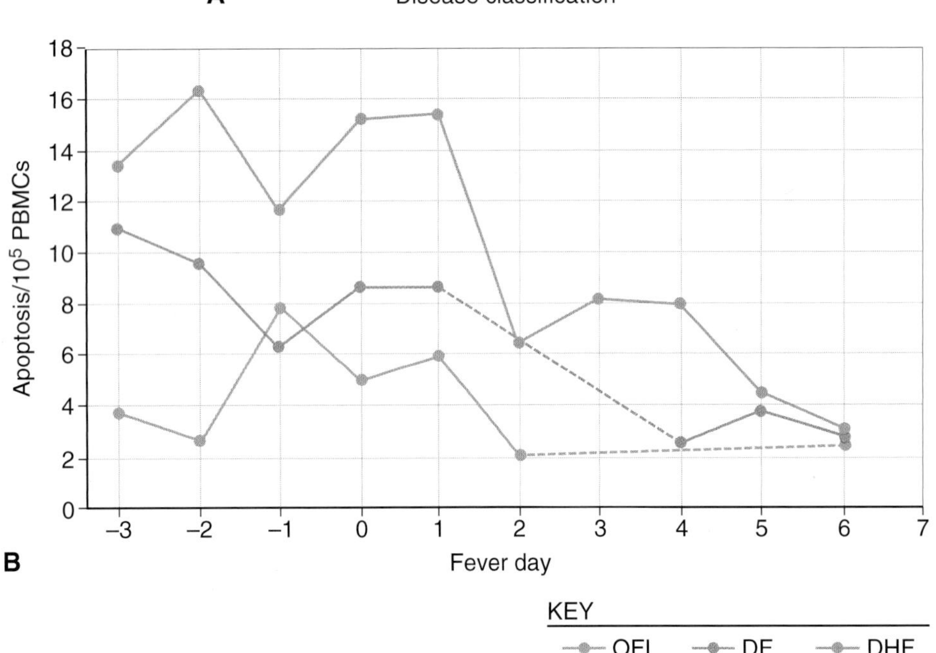

Figure 79–5. *A*, Apoptic cells correlated with increase dengue severity and peaked prior to defervesence in a prospective study of hospitalized children with DHF, *B*.

Lassa, Ebola, and Marburg—pose significant risk for direct transmission through contaminated blood or body fluids, fomites, and (less likely) aerosol transmission. Biocontainment precautions include a negative-pressure room, safety goggles, N-95 mask, and disposable gown, gloves, and shoe coverings. Great care must be taken in obtaining and transporting blood and body fluid samples, and testing of samples should be performed in a biocontainment laboratory.

Symptoms, Signs, and Clinical Course

Early symptoms and signs of the viral hemorrhagic fever viruses include high fever, headache, myalgia, arthralgia, anorexia, and varying degrees of nausea, vomiting, and diarrhea.

In a study of 124 patients, the major clinical characteristics for RVF included hepatocellular failure (75%), acute renal failure (41%), and hemorrhagic manifestations (19%).[35] Development of retinitis, unique to RVF, was seen in 16 patients, and 7 experienced meningoencephalitis as a late complication. A third of patients died. Hepatorenal failure, shock, and severe anemia were all factors associated with mortality.[35]

In CCHF, the time between the onset of fever and hemorrhagic manifestations can be brief[115]: progression from onset of fever, chills, headache, and muscle pains to severe hemorrhage can occur in 3 days, with death on the sixth day of illness.[115] Also associated with CCHF are vomiting, diarrhea, and throat pain.[116]

The initial presentation of HFRS can be abrupt onset of fever with severe headache, myalgia, and back and belly pain mimicking an acute abdomen. Following an initial febrile period, there is onset of hemorrhage, elevation of liver enzymes, and acute renal failure. In 24 children with HFRS in Korea, 38% were in the initial febrile phase and 56% were in the oliguric phase of renal failure on hospital admission.[117] All had fever and abdominal pain; headache and vomiting were the most common symptoms, and backache, hemorrhage in the conjunctiva of the eyes, and hypertension occurred in one-third. Unlike in the other viral hemorrhagic fever viruses, leukocytosis was common. Common causes of death were shock, respiratory failure, and pulmonary hemorrhage.[117] In a retrospective analysis of HFRS in 26 American soldiers, 2 had an initial presentation of severe shock and hemorrhage and the rapid onset of death,[118] 18 presented with acute renal failure, several developed acute pulmonary edema requiring hemodialysis, and retroperitoneal hemorrhage was a major complication, 6 patients had a febrile illness with normal renal function, thrombocytopenia, abnormal urinalysis, and transient elevation of liver enzymes.[118]

Marburg hemorrhagic fever presents with sudden onset of fever, headache, vomiting, and initially non-bloody diarrhea.[119,120] Patients may develop myalgia, conjunctivitis, lymphadenopathy, and a maculopapular rash by the seventh day of clinical illness, leading to desquamation. External and internal hemorrhage occurs between 6 and 12 days of illness, correlating with severe thrombocytopenia and coagulopathy. Laboratory abnormalities seen in acute Marburg virus infection include leukopenia, thrombocytopenia, and elevation of liver function tests[119]; amylase may be elevated as well as blood urea nitrogen, and there may be urinary proteinuria.

Ebola hemorrhagic fever is clinically indistinguishable from Marburg hemorrhagic fever in the initial phases of the acute illness. Common symptoms include fever, headache, myalgia, arthralgia, diarrhea, vomiting, and abdominal pain.[121] Severe asthenia is common and distinguishes Ebola from Marburg virus infection. Other features of acute Ebola infection include conjunctivitis, sore throat, rash, and late desquamation. Hemorrhagic manifestations were seen in less than 45% of the cases during the 1995 outbreak of Ebola hemorrhagic fever in the Democratic Republic of the Congo.[121] Poor prognostic signs on presentation were obtundation, anuria, shock, tachypnea, and absence of fever. Convalescent complications included arthralgia and eye disease with complaints of ocular pain, photophobia, hyperlacrimation, and loss of visual acuity, consistent with a uveitis.[122] Acute Ebola virus infection during pregnancy is associated with severe bleeding, spontaneous abortion, and an even higher case-fatality rate (96%, as compared to 77% in nonpregnant patients).[123]

Acute dengue virus infection can manifest in a spectrum ranging from asymptomatic to a subclinical mild febrile illness to a more severe nonhemorrhagic illness termed dengue fever and to DHF.[124] Depending on the population and serotype of the outbreak, the incidence of asymptomatic dengue infections ranges from 1.4% to 4.3% per year, or approximately one to two times the incidence of symptomatic dengue infection.[68] During the initial febrile illness, both dengue fever and DHF lead to fever, headache, myalgia, arthralgia, fatigue, and anorexia.[125] A "saddle-back" fever is typically present and heralds defervescence, the onset of rash, and recovery in dengue fever.[126] A nonproductive cough is frequent. Convalescence can be prolonged and associated with postinfection depression and lethargy.[125] The presenting symptoms of both dengue fever and DHF are similar to those of other viral hemorrhagic fevers, difficult to distinguish from each other and from other causes of febrile illnesses.[68] A tourniquet test (inflating a blood pressure cuff on the upper arm beginning between the diastolic and systolic pressures and lasting for 5 minutes) is often positive (more than 10 petechiae per 2.5 cm^2 below the blood pressure cuff). Its predictive value is a function of the incidence of dengue infection in the population at the time of evaluation; the tourniquet test is not useful in distinguishing between dengue fever and DHF but may differentiate dengue from other febrile illnesses.[127,128]

Laboratory Evaluation

Common laboratory findings during the initial phase of illnesses for both dengue fever and DHF include leukopenia, mild anemia, mild thrombocytopenia, and elevations in liver function tests.[128] The hematologic manifestations of acute dengue virus infection may be a direct viral effect on infected bone marrow and lymphocytes or an indirect effect of the acute-phase response and cytokine cascade. Dengue-infected B lymphocytes can be demonstrated during acute illness.[129] In 61 children with DHF, the absolute total lymphocyte counts and CD3, CD4, CD8 and HNK-1 cell counts were decreased during the febrile illness and reached their lowest values on the day of defervescence and during plasma leakage.[130] The total lymphocyte, B, and CD8 cell counts rapidly increased after shock, whereas CD3, CD4, and HNK-1 cell counts increased gradually, returning to normal during convalescence. Absolute lymphopenia on the day of shock was due to a relative decline in T cells (both CD4 and CD8 cells) and HNK-1 cells.[130]

Dengue virus infection may induce transient bone marrow suppression, in part accounting for the hematopoietic findings during clinical illness[131] (Fig. 79–6). In experiments using dengue virus infection of long-term marrow cultures as a model, early blast cells and hematopoietic elements were infected, killed, and eliminated by phagocytosis by specialized marrow macrophage dendritic cells; stromal cells rather than hematopoietic precursors were selectively infected and failed to functionally support hematopoiesis.[131]

Dengue Hemorrhagic Fever

DHF is the most severe form of acute dengue virus infection and differs from dengue fever because of plasma leakage and hemorrhage[132] (Fig. 79–7). The World Health Organization case definition of DHF requires the following: fever or a history of acute fever lasting from 2 to 7 days; hemorrhagic tendencies as manifested by a positive tourniquet test or petechiae, ecchymoses, purpura, or external bleeding or hematemesis or melena; thrombocytopenia (100,000 cells/μL or less); evidence of plasma leakage by a rise in the hematocrit of 20% or greater, or a decrease in the hematocrit following volume replacement equal to 20% or greater of baseline; or signs of plasma leakage as demonstrated by pleural effusion, ascites, or hypoproteinemia.[133] Children with DHF before the onset of plasma leakage are more likely to manifest

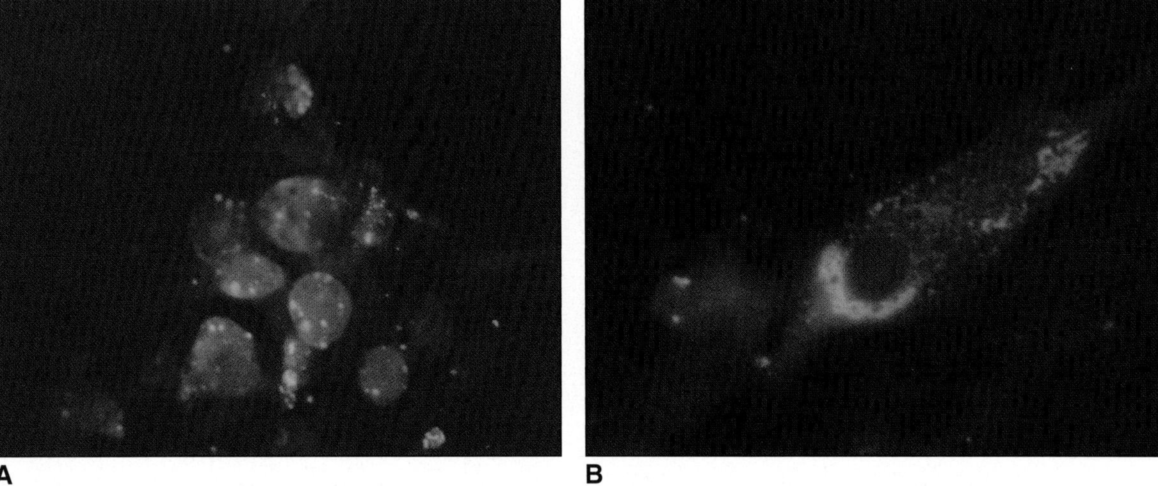

Figure 79–6. Virus infection of bone marrow *(A)* and stromal cells *(B)*, using dengue-2 virus and long-term human bone marrow cultures, and green fluorescent–tagged dengue antibody. (Photographs courtesy of Dr. Stephen Rothwell, Division of Medicine, Walter Reed Army Institute of Research, Silver Spring, MD.)

higher liver enzyme abnormalities and an elevated erythrocyte sedimentation rate than are children with dengue fever.[128,134] The acute febrile phase lasts between 2 and 7 days, with hemorrhagic manifestations limited to petechiae, hemorrhage, or easy bruising.[132,135] The liver may be enlarged but the spleen is normal, and generalized lymphadenopathy may be present.[136] Defervescence is the classic sign of impending plasma leakage, and the patient is frequently restless with cold extremities. Thrombocytopenia, coagulopathy, and hemorrhage occur during this time, and the onset of shock is acute. Plasma leakage manifests as a pleural effusion, ascites or swollen extremities, intravascular hemoconcentration, and an increase in the hematocrit. The World Health Organization criteria define DHF in increasing severity from grades I to IV, with grade I characterized by a fever with constitutional symptoms and the hemorrhagic manifestation a positive tourniquet test or easy bruising, and grade IV by profound shock with undetectable blood pressure or pulse.[133] Unusual manifestations of dengue virus infection can include severe hepatitis with jaundice, metabolic acidosis, and disseminated intravascular coagulation, producing a hepatic encephalopathy and a Reye-like syndrome.[137,138] Encephalitis and a neurologic disorder similar to poliovirus infection can also occur during acute dengue virus infection.[139]

TREATMENT

The treatment of the viral hemorrhagic fevers is largely supportive, using fluid and electrolyte replacement for volume depletion and shock, and blood component replacement with whole blood, packed red blood cells, platelets, plasma, plasma expanders, or albumin. The effects of supportive treatment on reducing the morbidity and mortality from these infections can be dramatic, and the high mortality observed in the viral hemorrhagic fevers may be largely due to the lack of such care in developing countries. For example, during the 1995 Ebola outbreak in Kikwit, Democratic Republic of the Congo, the use of blood transfusions in a subgroup of acute Ebola infections reduced mortality to 12.5%, as compared to 80% in those who did not receive blood transfusions.[140]

For three of the viral hemorrhagic fevers, CCHF, HFRS, and Lassa fever, the antiviral drug ribavirin may be effective in reducing mortality.[141] Ribavirin (1-β-D-ribofuranosyl-1,2,4-triazole; Virazole as the intravenous formulation, Rebetron as the oral formulation) is a nucleoside (guanosine) analogue that has activity against a range of RNA and DNA viruses.[142] The mechanism of action of ribavirin is alteration of the cellular nucleotide pools and induction of lethal mutagenesis of RNA virus genomes.[142] Information on the role of ribavirin therapy in reducing mortality is limited because of a lack of well-controlled clinical trials. The only double-blind, placebo-controlled study of intravenous ribavirin was conducted in 242 patients with HFRS in China[143]: mortality was reduced sevenfold in the ribavirin-treated patients and therapy resulted in a significant reduction in the risk for the oliguric renal phase and for developing hemorrhagic manifestations.[143] In nonhuman primates given a lethal dose of Lassa fever virus, the efficacy of ribavirin alone was 50%, and, when combined with Lassa virus immune nonhuman primate serum, the effectiveness was 100%.[144] In a clinical study of Lassa fever patients in Sierra Leone, mortality in patients given intravenous ribavirin within the first 6 days after onset of fever was 9% as compared to 47% in patients receiving therapy after 7 days or more of illness.[145] The use of ribavirin in CCHF has been limited, and its reported effectiveness is based largely on in vitro and limited clinical data.[146,147] In a large study of 139 treated patients, the efficacy of oral ribavirin was 70% in patients suspected of having CCHF and 89% in patients with confirmed CCHF.

Oral administration of ribavirin is a 30-mg/kg initial loading dose, followed by 15 mg/kg every 6 hours for 4

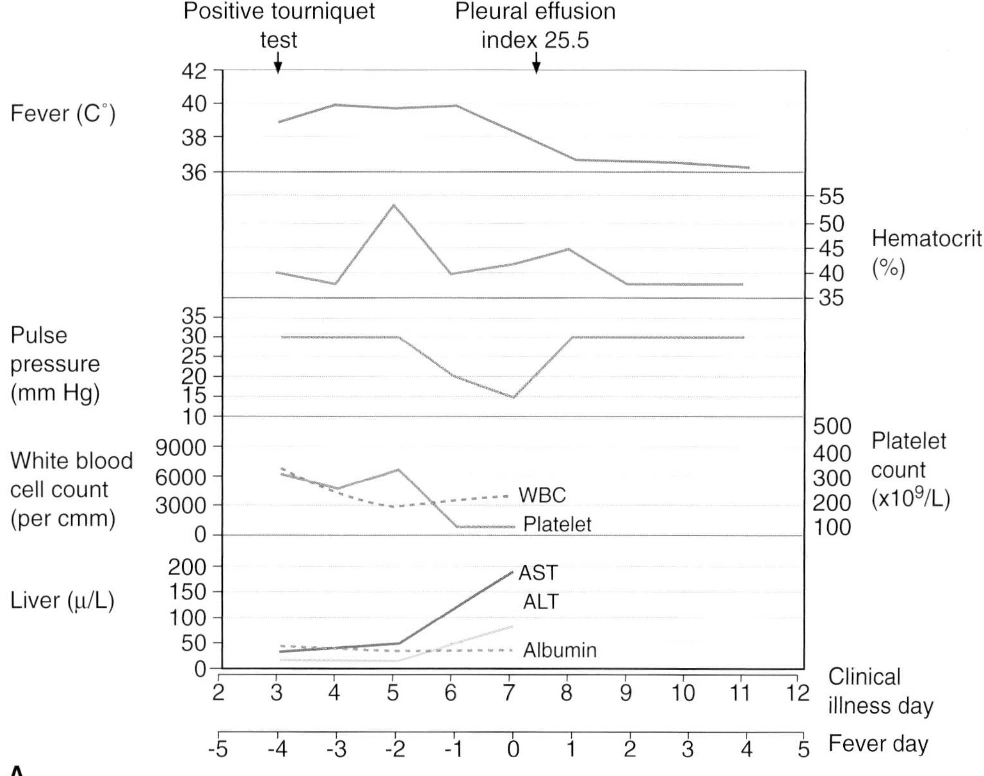

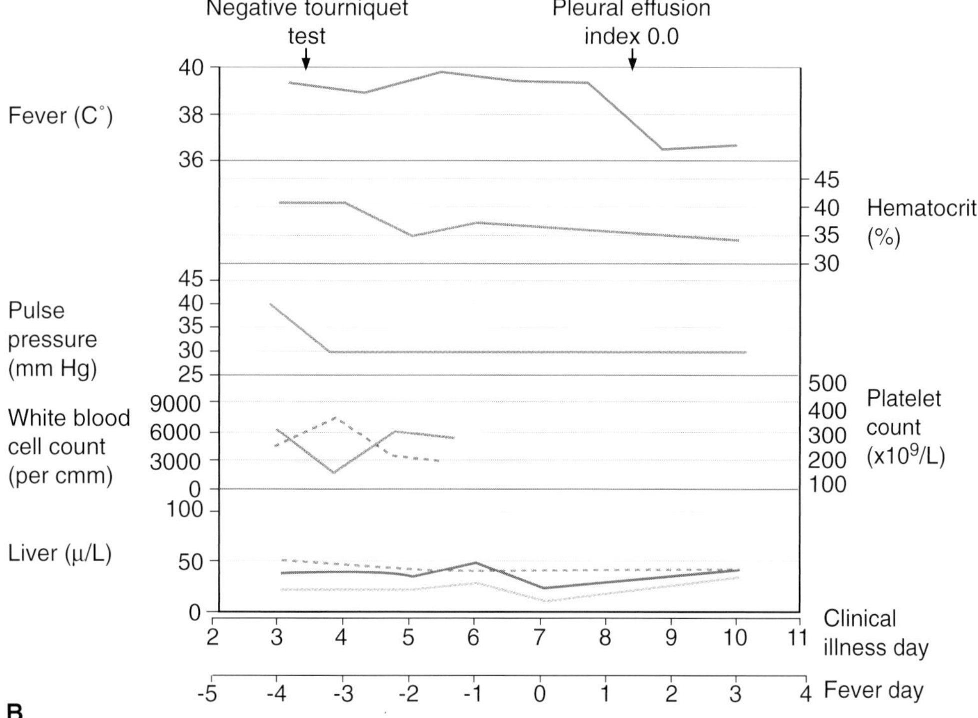

Figure 79–7. *A*, Clinical course of a child with secondary dengue virus infection and grade III DHF. *B*, Clinical course of a child with acute primary dengue fever without DHF.

days, then by 7.5 mg/kg every 8 hours for 6 days, for a total treatment duration of 10 days.[148] For intravenous ribavirin, the 7-day treatment course is a loading dose of 33 mg/kg (maximum dose of 2.64 g), followed by 16 mg/kg (maximum dose of 1.28 g) every 6 hours for the first 4 days, and 8 mg/kg (maximum dose of 0.64 g) every 8 hours for the subsequent 3 days.[143]

The management protocol for DHF stresses the effectiveness of early recognition and appropriate supportive care in significantly reducing mortality. During the 1960s, the case-fatality rate from DHF ranged from 3.5% in 1960 to 7.8% in 1963. The institution of an educational program for all Thai physicians in the recognition of DHF and the development of a treatment algorithm based on volume replacement during plasma leakage reduced the case-fatality rate of DHF to 0.2% in 2001 (Fig. 79–8). The initial phase of treatment of DHF, prior to the onset of plasma leakage, is to monitor for hemorrhage and shock and provide symptomatic care. Paracetamol can relieve high fevers, but salicylates or nonsteroidal anti-inflammatory drugs should be avoided because of their antiplatelet effects and the risk of Reye's syndrome. Early oral rehydration may decrease the risk for hospitalization.[149] Signs of shock should be sought, especially during the critical phase of defervescence. Daily serial hematocrit determination is an essential laboratory parameter because it is a direct indicator of plasma leakage and determines the amount of intravenous fluid

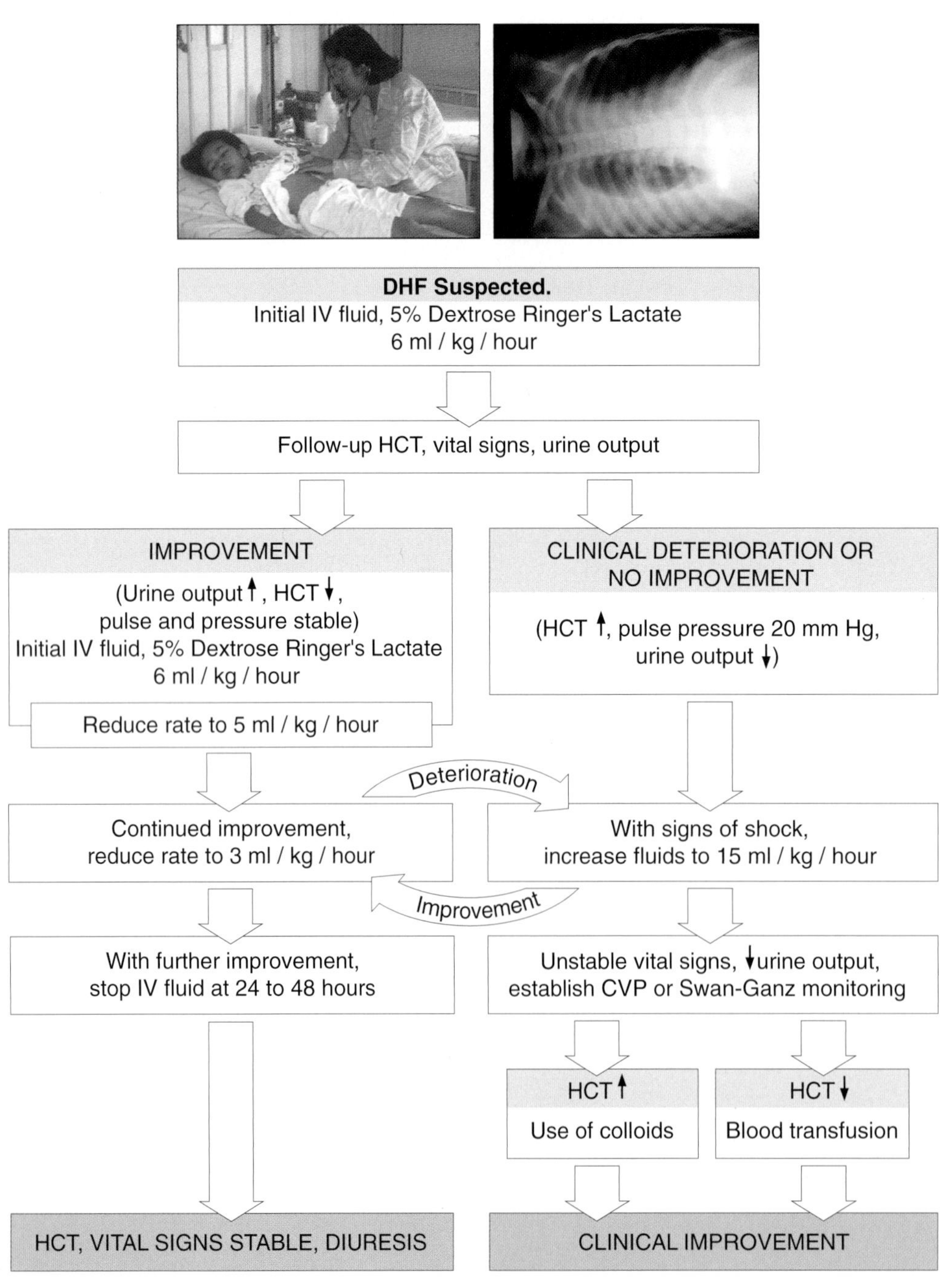

Figure 79–8. Treatment algorithm for dengue hemorrhagic fever. (Adapted from Nimmannitya S: Management of dengue and dengue haemorrhagic fever. *In* Thongcharoen P [ed]: Monograph on Dengue/Dengue Haemorrhagic Fever New Delhi: World Health Organization Regional Office for South-East Asia, 1993, p 55.)

replacement (see Fig. 79–8). Physiologic saline, Ringer's lactate, Ringer's acetate, glucose solution diluted in physiologic saline, plasma, or plasma expanders such as dextran or albumin may be used for rapid volume expansion. Whole-blood transfusion should be administered for a falling hematocrit and suspicion of internal hemorrhage. Colloids (dextran or the protein digest gelafundin) can restore the cardiac index and blood pressure and normalize hematocrit more rapidly than do crystalloids.[150]

CURRENT CONTROVERSIES & FUTURE CONSIDERATIONS

Dengue and Hemorrhagic Fever Viruses

- Though much is known about the pathophysiology of the viral hemorrhagic fevers, the exact mechanisms and dynamic interplay between viral and host-factors in inducing a hemorrhagic state are still unknown.
- Dengue hemorrhagic fever is unique amongst the viral hemorrhagic viruses as a hemorrhagic state largely influenced by pre-existing immunity to heterologous dengue virus serotypes which suggests an inducible condition that makes the host-immune system susceptible to hemorrhage upon a secondary infection. The factors associated with this predisposition towards hemorrhage are still unknown.
- Very few clinical trials have been performed to assess the effectiveness of therapies such as antivirals, plasma expanders, intravenous solutions and blood products on improving survivability from a viral hemorrhagic fever virus.
- New products are being evaluated that act to down-regulate the coagulation cascade as seen during viral hemorrhagic fever infection and has demonstrated promise in animal models. Potentially new interventions may be available to reduce mortality from these viruses.
- Several vaccines against the viral hemorrhagic fever viruses are in pre-clinical or human clinical vaccine trials, holding promise of a licensed vaccine that could be used to induce protective immunogenicity against these viruses.

PREVENTION

For viral hemorrhagic fevers that are transmitted to humans by insect vectors, the mainstay for prevention is in the use of personal protective measures against insect bites: insect repellants containing *N,N*-diethyl-*m*-toluamide (DEET) and permethrin-impregnated clothing are effective against mosquitoes and ticks. Bed netting is effective, but the vector for dengue and yellow fevers, *A. aegypti,* is a daytime-feeding mosquito. The use of window screens and the elimination of potential mosquito breeding sites around urban dwellings are important for controlling the transmission of dengue fever. Spraying indoors or drift sprays using malathion eliminate adult mosquitoes; larvicides kill mosquito larva in drinking water. Eradicating rodents in the household and avoiding them in the field are important preventive measures for the rodent-borne viral hemorrhagic fever viruses.

Vaccines can prevent viral infection; however, the only currently licensed vaccine against the viral hemorrhagic fever viruses is that against yellow fever virus. Vaccines against dengue, RVF, chikungunya, Junin, hantavirus, Ebola, and Marburg viruses are in development.

Suggested Readings*

Centers for Disease Control: Management of patients with suspected viral hemorrhagic fever. MMWR Morb Mortal Wkly Rep 7(S-3):1–16, 1988.

Gear JHS (ed): Handbook of Viral and Rickettsial Hemorrhagic Fevers. Boca Raton, FL: CRC Press, 1988.

Gubler DJ, Kuno G (eds): Dengue and Dengue Hemorrhagic Fever: Its History and Resurgence as a Global Public Health Problem. New York: CAB International, 1997.

Viral haemorrhagic fevers: report of a WHO Expert Committee. World Health Organ Tech Rep Ser 721:5–126, 1985.

World Health Organization: Dengue Haemorrhagic Fever: Diagnosis, Treatment, Prevention and Control (ed 2). Geneva: World Health Organization, 1997.

Full references for this chapter can be found on accompanying CD-ROM.

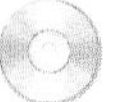

CHAPTER 80
MALARIA

James W. Kazura, MD

KEY POINTS

Malaria

Diagnosis

- Malaria should be suspected in an acute febrile illness accompanied by anemia and modest thrombocytopenia; other signs and symptoms include lethargy, neurologic dysfunction such as confusion and seizures, and splenomegaly.
- Nonimmune travelers to and infants and pregnant women living in malaria-endemic areas are most susceptible to severe malaria morbidity.
- A pertinent history that includes the place and times of travel to malaria-endemic areas and use of chemoprophylaxis is essential.
- Inspection of peripheral blood smears for the presence of intraerythrocytic malaria parasites is the standard for diagnosis. Repeated smears may be needed because of the cyclic nature of parasite growth and because *Plasmodium falciparum*–infected red blood cells may be sequestered in deep vascular beds.
- *Plasmodium falciparum* malaria in a nonimmune traveler should be considered a medical emergency because rapid progression to hyperparasitemia can cause profound anemia, coma, and death.

Treatment

- Antimalarial drugs recommended by the Centers for Disease Control and Prevention (currently either weekly mefloquine or daily atovaquone plus proguanil) are the mainstay of malaria prophylaxis in the nonimmune traveler.
- Routine intermittent antimalarial drugs are recommended to reduce morbidity in pregnant women and newborns living in malaria-endemic areas where transmission of the infection is stable and high.
- Treatment of acute severe anemia caused by malaria includes blood transfusion in combination with antimalarial drugs (quinine or quinidine in combination with tetracycline) that rapidly kill blood-stage parasites.

INTRODUCTION

Definition

Malaria is a paradigm of the role of infectious diseases in the natural selection of the human genome, particularly of genetic pathways involved in regulating the erythron. Inherited disorders of hemoglobin and red blood cell enzymes now recognized to protect against malaria have arisen in populations in which this infectious parasite has been a major cause of childhood death: hemoglobin S and C, α- and β-thalassemias, and glucose-6-phosphate dehydrogenase deficiency in sub-Saharan Africa and tropical regions of Asia and the Pacific (see Chapters 20, 21, and 23). Thought to be eradicable in the mid-20th century through vector control with insecticides and mass treatment with chloroquine, the impact of malaria on global health instead has increased for the past 50 years as a result of the emergence of drug-resistant parasites and biologic and political barriers to the use of DDT.[1] There are 300–500 million incident cases of malaria per year in the world, and about 1 million children per year currently die from malaria in sub-Saharan Africa alone.[2]

Parasite Biology

Plasmodium species are unicellular eukaryotic apicomplexan parasites that are phylogenetically related to other human pathogens such as *Leishmania* and *Toxoplasma*. The malaria life cycle involves obligatory development in both an invertebrate vector and a definitive vertebrate host. The four malaria species that infect humans—*Plasmodium falciparum, P. vivax, P. malariae,* and *P. ovale*—are transmitted by *Anopheles* species of mosquitoes. Each species has unique biologic features related to its ability to grow in red blood cells and hepatocytes (Table 80–1). Humans are infected when female mosquitoes inoculate haploid sporozoites into the bloodstream during blood feeding. These extracellular parasites have tropism for the liver and invade hepatocytes within 30 minutes of inoculation, where they undergo asexual reproduction (hepatic schizogony), such that a single sporozoite is progenitor to thousands of intracellular merozoites. After 1–2

TABLE 80–1. Biologic Features of Various *Plasmodium* Species That Infect Humans

	P. vivax	*P. falciparum*	*P. malariae*	*P. ovale*
Incubation period (days)	12–17	9–14	16–40	16–18
Merozoites per hepatic schizont	10,000	40,000	15,000	15,000
Duration of intraerythrocytic cycle (hr)	48	48	72	50
Average parasitemia (per μL blood)	20,000	20,000–100,000	6000	9000
Duration of untreated infection (yr)	1–3	<1	3–50	1–2
Latent liver stage	Yes	No	No	Yes

weeks (or longer in the case of some species), merozoites are released from the hepatocyte and parasitize erythrocytes. Through a complex process of adherence, then reorientation of the apical aspect of the merozoite toward the red blood cell surface, followed by progressive fusion of the parasite and erythrocyte membrane, the merozoite enters the erythrocyte and is contained within a newly formed space termed the *parasitophorous vacuole*. Digesting hemoglobin as its primary energy source, the parasite undergoes a 48- to 72-hour cycle of asexual reproduction (erythrocytic schizogony), progressing from an early ring stage to trophozoite and finally schizont. Each schizont contains 6–24 merozoites that are released when the red blood cell ruptures. This event is repeated multiple times and results in approximately 10-fold growth of the parasite biomass with each cycle of erythrocytic schizogony. A small number of young rings do not undergo asexual reproduction but differentiate into sexual forms termed *gametocytes*. Female and male gametocytes are ingested by the mosquito during blood feeding and mate to form diploid zygotes in the midgut of the insect. Through meiotic reduction division and differentiation in the hemolymph, the *Plasmodium* life cycle is continued when infectious sporozoites appear in the mosquito salivary gland.

Erythrocyte receptors and merozoite invasion ligands have been well characterized for *P. vivax*.[3,4] The Duffy blood group expressed on the surface of reticulocytes is required, and its ligand is the Duffy-binding protein (see Chapter 3). Evidence for the remarkable selective force of malaria on the human genome includes the single nucleotide polymorphism that silences expression of the Duffy blood group required by *P. vivax* for invasion of red blood cells. Nearly 100% of Bantus are homozygous for this mutation. In the case of *P. falciparum*, two or more alternative invasion pathways have evolved. These pathways involve several merozoite surface proteins with epidermal growth factor–like motifs similar to the *P. vivax* Duffy-binding ligand.[5] Polymorphisms of erythrocyte membrane glycoproteins and band 3 apparently have been selected by falciparum malaria, but the molecular mechanisms by which they afford protection against malaria are poorly understood.

EPIDEMIOLOGY AND RISK FACTORS

Plasmodium falciparum malaria is endemic in tropical and subtropical areas of Africa, Asia, the South Pacific, and Latin America. Vivax malaria is found widely in Latin America and Asia but only in focal regions of Africa because of the high frequency of Duffy blood group negativity. *Plasmodium malariae* and *P. ovale* exist in many areas of Africa and Asia but have much lower frequencies than do *P. falciparum* and *P. vivax*. Liver-stage *P. vivax* and *P. ovale* are capable of becoming dormant, and completion of hepatic schizogony may be delayed for months to years. *Plasmodium vivax* may thus be endemic in temperate areas where mosquito vectors temporarily disappear during periods of cold weather, as in Russia and Afghanistan. Both falciparum and vivax malaria were endemic in the United States until the early part of the 20th century; they disappeared because of changes in ecology related to urbanization and water management. Because mosquitoes hospitable to malaria still exist in the United States, transmission is theoretically possible: local mosquito vectors may take a blood meal from travelers who have acquired infection outside the United States. Indeed, transmission of *P. vivax* by this route has been described in the last decade.

Infants and children younger than 3–5 years of age experience most of the malaria infections in areas of sub-Saharan Africa and tropical Asia and the Pacific, where transmission of *P. falciparum* is stable year round or has predictable seasonal variation. Blood-stage infection rates of 80% and greater are typical. In addition to high infection rates, the youngest age groups also have the greatest burden of malaria-related illnesses (see later). With repeated exposure to malaria, immunity against blood-stage parasites and clinical or "antidisease" immunity eventually develop. Acquired immunity is manifested by less frequent and lower density blood-stage infection and reduced frequencies of uncomplicated and severe malaria morbidity. The temporal profile of acquired protection against uncomplicated and severe malaria differ, suggesting two distinct mechanisms.[6–8] Antiparasite and antidisease immunity persist into adulthood but wane if exposure to malaria ceases, as when residents temporarily migrate to nonendemic areas.

In contrast to adults and older children living in malaria-endemic regions, malaria infection represents a life-threatening illness in the nonimmune individual, such as travelers and military personnel from nonendemic areas who lack immunity. Chemoprophylaxis and other precautions to prevent infection are critical in these individuals. The risk of acquiring malaria according to area of travel is greatest for Papua New Guinea and the Solomon Islands, with progressively lower risks in West Africa, East Africa, India, and rural areas of Southeast Asia, East Asia, South America, and Central America.[9] In the United States, approximately 1500 malaria cases are reported to the Centers for Disease Control and Prevention every year: two thirds are American travelers, and the remainder are immigrants from malaria-endemic regions and military personnel. One hundred eighty-five malaria-related deaths were recorded in the United States between 1963 and 2001; 123 involved travelers.[10] Over 90% of the deaths were due to *P. falciparum*. Fatal outcomes of malaria infection were related to failure to undertake chemoprophylaxis, lack of adherence to the prescribed drug regimen, or delay in seeking medical attention.

Malaria may be acquired by transfusion of infected red blood cells. Routine screening of blood donors for malaria is not performed in the United States, and there are occasional cases of transfusion-related malaria.[11] The risk of malaria transmission can be minimized by following the recommendations of the Food and Drug Administration and American Association of Blood Banks related to deferral of blood donation: exclusion of travelers from malaria-endemic areas who are residents of nonmalarious areas for 1 year, if they have been free of malaria symptoms (irrespective of chemoprophylaxis), and exclusion of donation by immigrants or visitors from malaria-endemic areas or any individual who has had a diagnosis of malaria for 3 years.

Congenital malaria may develop in newborns if their mothers have blood-stage infection at the time of delivery.[12]

CLINICAL FEATURES AND HEMATOLOGIC MANIFESTATIONS

Uncomplicated Malaria

The clinical presentation depends on previous malaria exposure, the age of the patient, and the infecting malaria species. Uncomplicated malaria morbidity is most common. Fever, chills, and headache develop when rupture of the red blood cell releases merozoites at the completion of their intraerythrocytic development. "Malaria paroxysms" recur every 48 hours with *P. vivax* and *P. ovale* and every 72 hours with *P. malariae*. Fever occurs more irregularly with *P. falciparum* because lysis of red blood cells is not synchronized for this species despite the 48-hour period of intraerythrocytic development. In addition to the classical malaria paroxysm, nonspecific symptoms such as myalgia, diarrhea, and lethargy also may be present. Lassitude is particularly common in infants and children living in malaria-endemic areas.

Anemia and splenomegaly commonly develop, especially with *P. vivax* and *P. ovale* infection. Splenic rupture has been observed in *P. vivax* malaria. In contrast to *P. falciparum*, malaria symptoms caused by *P. vivax* and *P. ovale* may present years after exposure to infected mosquitoes, because these species have a dormant hepatic stage that may lead to late relapse. *Plasmodium malariae* infection is characterized by chronic low-level parasitemia and mild symptoms such as fatigue, weakness, and low grade fever. This species also can cause glomerulonephritis through immune complex formation.

Complicated or Severe Malaria

The greatest risk of severe illness and death occurs with *P. falciparum* infection, although morbidity and occasional deaths are caused by *P. vivax*. *Plasmodium falciparum* can reach an extraordinarily high biomass because red blood cells of any age may be infected by the parasite (*P. vivax* merozoites invade only mid- to late-stage reticulocytes). Unlike other malaria species, *P. falciparum*–infected red blood cells also adhere to endothelial cells and cause microvascular obstruction and tissue hypoxia. Cytoadherence and sequestration of infected red blood cells in deep vascular beds is the cause of the severe pathology in the brain, placenta, lung, and other organs in falciparum malaria.[13–15]

Travelers to and children and pregnant women resident in malaria-endemic regions are at greatest risk of severe malaria. The clinical presentations of severe malaria may include altered mental status, seizure, coma, severe anemia, respiratory distress, hypotension, and high fever, similar to that observed in bacterial sepsis.[16,17] Syndromes are categorized according to the major organ system involved:

- Cerebral malaria: The patient presents with generalized seizures and coma. The onset is usually rapid with few premonitory symptoms. Parasitemia may exceed 10,000 asexual *P. falciparum* per μL blood with more than 20% infected red blood cells. Cerebral malaria is likely due to sequestration of infected red blood cells in brain capillaries and deposition of hemozoin, a byproduct of hemoglobin digested by the parasite.
- Severe anemia: The patient presents with a marked drop in hemoglobin level, often to less than 5 gm/dL, and hyperparasitemia. The pathogenesis of severe malaria anemia is discussed later.
- Hypoglycemia and lactic acidosis
- Acute renal failure
- Pulmonary edema
- Diarrhea, particularly in infants and young children

Hematologic Manifestations

Erythrocytes

Mild Anemia

Infants and pregnant women commonly have mild anemia in areas where malaria transmission is stable and high, as in sub-Saharan Africa and Papua New Guinea. This chronic, nonacute anemia with hematocrit less than 25–30% has a complex etiology, with additional contributing factors of iron deficiency (often secondary to intestinal helminth infections such as hookworm or inadequate iron stores in postpubertal women), folic acid deficiency, micronutrient deficiency, and parvovirus B19 infection.[18–24] In infants living in a highly endemic area of Tanzania, 60% of mild anemia episodes were due to malaria and 30% were attributable to iron deficiency.[25] Population-based studies of childhood anemia and anemia in pregnancy have evaluated iron supplementation and intermittent presumptive treatment with antimalarial drugs: both interventions have benefit by decreasing the degree and frequency of anemia in infants and in pregnant women. There is controversy surrounding routine iron supplementation as a public health intervention, because some observations suggest that mild iron deficiency is associated with a decreased frequency of attacks of uncomplicated malaria.

The peripheral blood smear in mild anemia typically shows red blood cells that are normocytic and normochromic unless there is iron deficiency. Morphologic features of inherited red blood cell conditions common in African or Asian populations may be present, such as target cells with hemoglobin C and various thalassemias. Markers of iron status, such as soluble transferrin receptor and serum ferritin levels, should be interpreted cautiously because they may be affected by acute-phase responses to malaria and other infectious diseases that are common in these populations. Haptoglobin levels are frequently decreased secondary to the intravascular hemolysis that accompanies blood-stage parasitemia.

Mild anemia also occurs in incompletely immune populations in areas of Asia and Latin America where malaria transmission is less intense and seasonal. A prospective study of 4000 persons presenting with mild malaria in a rural area of Thailand showed that 18% had a hematocrit less than 30% and 1% required a blood transfusion.[26] Risk factors for anemia were age less than 5 years, palpable spleen or liver, recrudescent infections after antimalarial drug administration, and female sex. Pure *P. falciparum* infection, as opposed to mixed-species infection that included *P. vivax* and *P. falciparum*, was more likely to cause anemia. Anemia in this setting is largely related to resistance to antimalarial drugs.

Severe Anemia

Profound and potentially life-threatening anemia with hemoglobin levels less than 5–7 gm/dL may occur in the nonimmune traveler[27] and in infants in malaria-endemic areas.[28] A particularly serious compounding problem in sub-Saharan Africa and other areas of the world, with a high prevalence of human immunodeficiency virus infection, is the requirement for blood transfusion. Severe anemia is seen primarily with high-level *P. falciparum* infection (>20% of red blood cells infected, >10,000 parasites/μL blood). The precise prevalence of severe malaria anemia is not known but is markedly lower than the mild anemia described previously. Unlike in mild anemia, genetic susceptibility likely plays a major role in susceptibility to profound malaria anemia. Mouse malaria models have implicated various cytokine polymorphisms.[29–32] Case-control studies of human malaria have identified tumor necrosis factor-α, inducible nitric oxide synthase, and interleukin-10 promoter polymorphisms as risk factors.[33]

Severe anemia with falciparum malaria generally appears within 48 hours of presentation with a febrile illness. The hemoglobin and hematocrit often continue to decline during the initial 4–5 days of administration of antimalarial drugs. Hematologic values recover over the next 6–7 weeks.

Pathogenesis of Malaria Anemia

Destruction and decreased production of red blood cells both contribute to the anemia of malaria[28] (Fig. 80–1). Loss of red blood cells occurs through several mechanisms. Intravascular hemolysis that accompanies the cyclical pattern of intraerythrocytic growth of blood-stage parasites accounts for only a small proportion of total red blood cell loss, because the degree of anemia observed in the individual patient is disproportionate to the level of parasitemia. Phagocytosis of infected and uninfected cells contribute to erythrocyte loss. Malaria antigens transported to the infected red blood cell surface may lead to opsonization by circulating antimalaria antibodies and removal of erythrocytes by reticuloendothelial cells that express Fc receptors. Uninfected red blood cells may also develop abnormally rigid membranes in the malaria-infected patient and be similarly susceptible to elimination.[34,35] This pathophysiology may underlie the progressive decrease in red blood cells that occurs after drug-mediated clearance of malaria parasites. Finally, there may be increased pooling and removal of red blood cells (and other cellular elements of the blood) in malaria patients with splenomegaly and hypersplenism.

Underproduction of red blood cells is explained by inflammatory cytokines such as tumor necrosis factor-α which are frequently elevated and suppress erythropoiesis by inhibiting optimal bone marrow responses to erythropoietin or impairing the growth of early erythroid progenitors, burst- and colony-forming cells.[36] Erythropoietin levels have been inappropriately low for the degree of anemia in some studies but are elevated in others, a variability likely due to the heterogeneity of underlying factors that contribute to anemia in economically poor settings, such as iron, folic acid, and micronutrient deficiency. Bone marrow examination of a limited number of patients has shown modest dyserythropoiesis that is independent of folate deficiency.[37,38]

Platelets and Leukocytes

Mild thrombocytopenia, platelet counts of 90,000–140,000/μL, is common in both *P. falciparum* and *P. vivax* malaria. The platelet count may be a prognostic indicator of the severity of clinical malaria,[39] but thrombocytopenia rarely reaches a level that predisposes to bleeding. The pathogenesis of malaria-related thrombocytopenia is poorly understood but may be due to pooling of platelets in the spleen and a shortened platelet lifespan. Elevated leukocyte counts to greater than 10,000/μL are common in mild malaria and predict increased mortality in severe malaria anemia.[40]

Coagulation Factors

Antithrombin III, protein C, and protein S activities tend to be low in patients with severe malaria and increase with recovery. Bleeding with disseminated intravascular coagulation has occurred in nonimmune individuals with severe malaria, but bacterial infection is also often present.

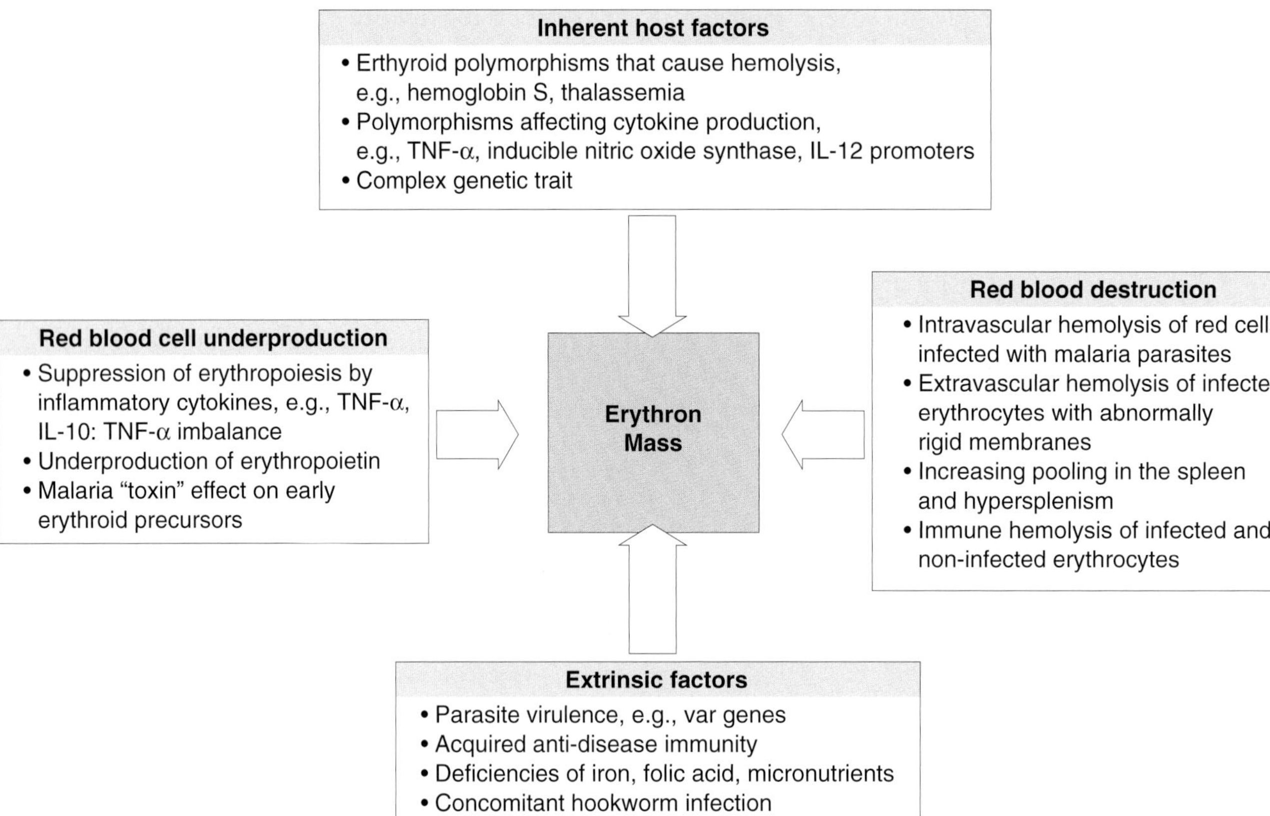

Figure 80–1. Pathogenesis of malaria-associated anemia.

DIAGNOSIS

Consideration of malaria in the differential diagnosis is critical in the traveler presenting with a febrile illness and anemia or other signs and symptoms of acute malaria. A thorough history, including dates and places of travel and the use of chemoprophylaxis, should be obtained. Because of the high frequency of drug-resistant *P. falciparum* in most areas of the world, malaria should not be excluded even in persons who have complied with the appropriate preventative recommendations.

Inspection of thin and thick blood smears for intraerythrocytic malaria parasites is the standard for parasitologic diagnosis. A positive blood smear in a resident of an endemic area should be considered in the context of age and clinical presentation, because older semi-immune children and adults may have asymptomatic blood-stage infection. A microscopist skilled in malaria diagnosis must inspect blood smears because artifacts and platelets are easily confused with malaria parasites. A blood smear showing typical asexual ring stages of *P. falciparum* is presented in Figure 80–2. Other tests aid in malaria diagnosis, including commercial kits that detect histidine-rich protein 2 or parasite lactate dehydrogenase in serum. These assays are highly sensitive in nonimmune individuals but of less value for residents of endemic areas who frequently have asymptomatic parasitemia.

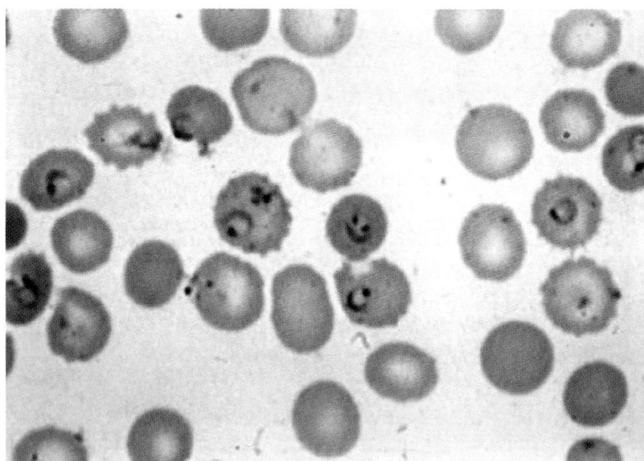

Figure 80–2. Peripheral blood smear of patient with *Plasmodium falciparum* infection. Multiple red blood cells contained ring-stage parasites. (Obtained from the World Health Organization website by permission.)

ACUTE AND CHRONIC MANAGEMENT

Prevention

Nonimmune individuals traveling to malaria-endemic regions should self-administer chemoprophylaxis and take measures to limit exposure to infected mosquitoes.

Diagnosis

- History of travel to endemic area
- Use of appropriate chemoprophylaxis?
- Acute drop in hemoglobin to <5–7 g/dL
- Blood smear to determine malaria species

P. falciparum

- Chroloquine resistant strains: quinine plus doxycyline, tetracycline, pyrimethamine/sulfadoxine, or clindamycin OR atovaquone/ proguanil
- Choloroquine sensitive strains: chloroquine

Transfusion?

- Evidence of appropriate erythropoietic response?
- Evaluate reticulocyte count over time
- Bone marrow exam to exclude other causes of anemia
- Follow hemolgobin/hematocrit, consider fluid volume shifts

P. vivax, P. malariae, P. ovale

- Chloroquine EXCEPT where *P. vivax* is chloroquine-resistant, then use quinidine plus doxcycline
- Primaquine to eliminate liver stage *P. vivax* and *P. ovale*

Evaluate progress of treatment

- Twice daily or more frequent smears to determine parasitemia and hematologic response
- Replace folic acid and iron stores as needed

Figure 80–3. Treatment algorithm for malaria-associated anemia.

Briefly, the current recommendation for Americans traveling to *P. falciparum*–endemic areas of the world exclusive of the Middle East are mefloquine weekly or the combination of atovaquone and proguanil daily. Updated information is available in the Traveler's Health section of the Centers for Disease Control and Prevention website (*http://www.cdc.gov*). For hematologists, it should be noted that primaquine, which is occasionally recommended for prophylaxis when mefloquine or atavaquone plus proguanil are not tolerated, may induce hemolysis in persons with glucose-6-phosphate dehydrogenase deficiency; screening for deficiency of this enzyme should be performed prior to use of primaquine. Prophylaxis for *P. vivax* infection is chloroquine, but chloroquine-resistant *P. vivax* exists in Papua New Guinea and parts of Asia. Despite intense efforts to develop vaccines against malaria, none currently exists.

Treatment

The primary treatment of severe anemia caused by *P. falciparum* infection is administration of antimalarial drugs such as quinine that rapidly eliminate blood-stage parasites (quinidine is used in the United States because parenteral quinine is not available) and blood transfusion (Fig. 80–3). The level of parasitemia and reticulocyte counts should be monitored closely to confirm appropriate hematologic responses. Folic acid stores depleted by increased erythropoiesis should be replaced. Treatment of anemia caused by *P. vivax* or another malaria species is less urgent and may include oral chloroquine, except when drug resistance is suspected based on travel history. Current recommendations for the use of various antimalarial drugs approved for use in the United States are posted on the website of the Centers for Disease Control and Prevention.

PROGNOSIS

Complete recovery from the hematologic complications of malaria is certain in patients administered appropriate antimalarial drugs and supportive care.

CURRENT CONTROVERSIES & FUTURE CONSIDERATIONS

Malaria

- What is the molecular pathogenesis of severe anemia caused by *Plasmodium falciparum* infection?
- What genetic polymorphisms confer susceptibility to severe malaria anemia?
- The role of iron supplementation in preventing and mitigating malaria-associated anemia during childhood must be determined.
- What is the impact of intermittent presumptive treatment with antimalarial drugs on malaria-related anemia in childhood and during pregnancy?

Suggested Readings*

Breman JG: The ears of the hippopotamus: manifestations, determinants, and estimates of the malaria burden. Am J Trop Med Hyg 64(1–2 Suppl):1–11, 2001.

Cowman AF, Crabb BS: The *Plasmodium falciparum* genome—a blueprint for erythrocyte invasion. Science 298:126–128, 2002.

Hill AV: The genomics and genetics of human infectious disease susceptibility. Annu Rev Genomics Hum Genet 2:373–400, 2001.

Menendez C, Fleming AF, Alonso PL: Malaria-related anaemia. Parasitol Today 16:469–476, 2000.

Miller LH, Baruch DI, Marsh K, Doumbo OK: The pathogenic basis of malaria. Nature 415:673–679, 2002.

Warrell DA: Pathophysiology of severe falciparum malaria in man. Parasitology 94(Suppl):S53–S76, 1987.

Full references for this chapter can be found on accompanying CD-ROM.

SECTION 3
HEMATOLOGIC PROBLEMS OF MEDICAL PRACTICE

CHAPTER 81
DIFFERENTIAL DIAGNOSIS OF ANEMIA

Geraldine P. Schechter, MD

KEY POINTS

Differential Diagnosis of Anemia

- The initial clues to the etiology of an anemia are most often provided by the laboratory evaluation.
- In patients with anemia without abnormal concentrations of white blood cells or platelets, the size of the red cells (the mean corpuscular volume [MCV]) is a powerful tool for focusing the laboratory evaluation.
- In patients with a low MCV, iron parameters (serum iron, total iron-binding capacity, and serum ferritin) and the red cell concentration will readily distinguish among iron deficiency anemia, thalassemia trait, anemia of chronic disease, and sideroblastic anemia.
- In patients with a high or normal MCV, the serum creatinine assesses adequacy of erythropoietin production, the serum cobalamin measures tissue vitamin B_{12} availability, and the reticulocyte concentration differentiates whether the anemia reflects a hypoproliferative or hyperproliferative marrow process. Iron parameters again are important to indicate anemia of chronic disease or early iron deficiency.
- Examination of red cell and white cell morphology offers important clues to the etiology of hemolytic anemias and may raise suspicion of a marrow replacement processes.
- Elevated reticulocytes or indirect bilirubin levels should always suggest hemolysis, but these parameters, along with other indirect measures of shortened red blood cell survival, may result from other processes.
- Hemolytic anemias are uncommon. The initial screens to elucidate the usual causes should include microscopic evaluation of red blood cells for shape abnormalities (spherocytes, schistocytes, bite cells, and sickle cells among others), the direct Coombs test for the presence of immunoglobulin and complement on the red cell membrane, and an assay for glucose-6-phosphate dehydrogenase.
- In patients with anemia in combination with an abnormal white blood cell or platelet count, the history and physical findings figure prominently, as does the morphology of the peripheral blood cells. A bone marrow aspirate and biopsy are frequently required to yield a diagnosis.

INTRODUCTION

The requirements for physiologic erythropoiesis include a normal erythroid progenitor cell and bone marrow microenvironment, adequately supplied with erythropoietin, iron, folate, cyanocobalamin, and thyroid and other hormones.[1] Failure, absence, or inadequacy of any of these factors will lead to anemia of varying severity. Defining the etiology of a patient's anemia must take into consideration epidemiologic factors as well as the patient's history and the physical examination, but laboratory evaluation is usually needed to arrive at a specific diagnosis. This chapter addresses these issues and promotes an efficient, cost-effective approach to the evaluation of anemia.

EPIDEMIOLOGY

There are generally accepted criteria for anemia in adolescent and adult males and females[2] (Table 81–1). Using these standards, data collected between 1988 and 1994 in the U.S. third National Health and Nutrition Examination Survey (NHANES III) showed that the prevalence of anemia in community-living individuals varied with gender and ethnicity, and after the fifth decade increased in both men and women. Over the age of 65, the prevalence of anemia reached 10.6%, with a striking level of 27.6% in African Americans.[3]

The most common cause of anemia in the world is iron deficiency (see Chapter 17). In chronically ill

TABLE 81–1. Criteria for a Diagnosis of Anemia in Adults

	Women	Men
Red blood cells ($\times 10^{12}$/L)	<4.0	<4.5
Hemoglobin (gm/dL)	<12	<14
Hematocrit (%)	<37	<40

patients, particularly in the hospital setting, the most frequent etiology is the so-called anemia of chronic disease or, more precisely described, erythroid hypoproliferation resulting from the effects of inflammatory cytokines and hepcidin on iron reutilization and erythropoietin responsiveness[4–7] (see Chapter 19). Renal insufficiency with subsequent inadequate erythropoietin production is often the explanation for anemia in patients with chronic illnesses. Anemias caused by hemolysis, megaloblastosis, bone marrow infiltration, and stem cell disorders are much rarer, although they present interesting challenges to the consulting hematologist. In NHANES III, fully one third of anemias in patients over the age of 65 were unexplained, even after serum values for iron, folate, and vitamin B_{12} and a history of chronic inflammation or renal insufficiency were assessed.[3]

DIAGNOSTIC CLUES

History and Physical Examination

A history of excessive bleeding, usually menorrhagia or bleeding of gastrointestinal origin, is an obvious clue to iron deficiency. Hematuria is an uncommon cause of anemia unless extremely heavy and prolonged over weeks to months, as may occur with hemoglobin SS or SC disease. Multiple pregnancies or frequent blood donations may lead to depletion of iron stores. A family history of anemia and jaundice suggests hemolysis, and a report of dark urine raises the possibility of red cell destruction that is intravascular. Chronic infections, serious acute infections, and connective tissue disorders are often accompanied by the anemia of inflammation. Symptoms of neuropathy or glossitis and a history of other evidence of excessive alcohol use point to megaloblastic anemia or cirrhosis. Weight loss and night sweats raise concerns of an occult malignancy, granulomatous disease, or human immunodeficiency virus infection.

Physical findings of importance in the diagnosis of anemia include fever, jaundice, glossitis, lymphadenopathy, hepatosplenomegaly, neuropathy, and evidence of inflammation, such as cutaneous ulcers or decubiti.

Laboratory Findings

Three simple laboratory tests organize the approach to the diagnosis of isolated anemia (anemia without leukocyte or platelet count abnormalities): (1) mean corpuscular volume (MCV), (2) reticulocyte percentage or concentration, and (3) examination of the peripheral blood smear. Even when abnormalities of the white blood cell count and differential and/or the platelet count are present, this testing triad remains a useful starting point.

With the hemoglobin and the red blood cell count, the MCV is a red cell parameter that is measured directly by electronic counters. The calculated mean corpuscular hemoglobin, which is derived from the measured hemoglobin and red cell count, correlates closely with the MCV and provides little additional information. The mean corpuscular hemoglobin concentration is calculated from the hemoglobin/hematocrit ratio and is primarily helpful in suggesting spherocytosis if elevated (see later). Another red blood cell parameter reported by electronic counters is the red blood cell distribution width (RDW). An elevated RDW reflects significant red cell size heterogeneity and should prompt microscopic examination of the peripheral blood smear, but the RDW otherwise has limited utility for diagnosing the causes of anemia. Typically, but not always, the RDW is elevated in nutritional anemias and normal in other types of anemia.

Structuring the approach to the diagnosis of anemia based on the initial assessment of the MCV leads to a classification of microcytic anemias (MCV < 80 fL), macrocytic anemias (MCV > 100 fL), and normocytic anemias (MCV 80–100 fL). More complex anemias with associated white blood cell or platelet abnormalities are discussed separately.

MICROCYTIC ANEMIAS

The most common causes of microcytic anemia include iron deficiency anemia and thalassemia trait (see Chapter 21). Typically in iron deficiency, the extent of the decrease in MCV correlates with the severity of the fall in red blood cell count and hemoglobin. In contrast, in α- or β-thalassemia trait, the hemoglobin and hematocrit levels may be close to normal despite a very low MCV, reflecting the high red cell count typical of this disorder[8] (Table 81–2). A syndrome that may mimic the low MCV/normal or almost normal hemoglobin pattern of thalassemia trait occurs in the polycythemia vera patient who has been made iron deficient by numerous phlebotomies but has persistent red cell proliferation. The anemia of chronic inflammation is microcytic in about 25% of cases, reflecting very low serum iron values that lead to impaired reutilization of iron. Sideroblastic anemia may also be microcytic, usually in the inherited form[9] but occasionally also in the acquired type (see Chapter 55). However, acquired sideroblastic anemias are usually macrocytic or normocytic because of the accompanying abnormal DNA synthesis. The most useful laboratory parameter to distinguish these four entities is the pattern of serum levels of iron, total iron-binding capacity (TIBC), and ferritin (Table 81–3). Figure 81–1 describes an algorithm for evaluating microcytic anemia based on these parameters. Figure 81–2 shows photomicrographs of peripheral blood smears from patients with microcytic anemias.

TABLE 81–2. Differentiating Thalassemia Trait from Other Microcytic Anemias

	MCV	Hemoglobin	Red Blood Cell Count	RDW
Thalassemia trait	Low	Normal/slightly low	Normal/high	Normal*
Iron deficiency anemia	Low	Low	Low	High
Anemia of chronic inflammation	Low	Low	Low	Normal*

*Occasionally high.

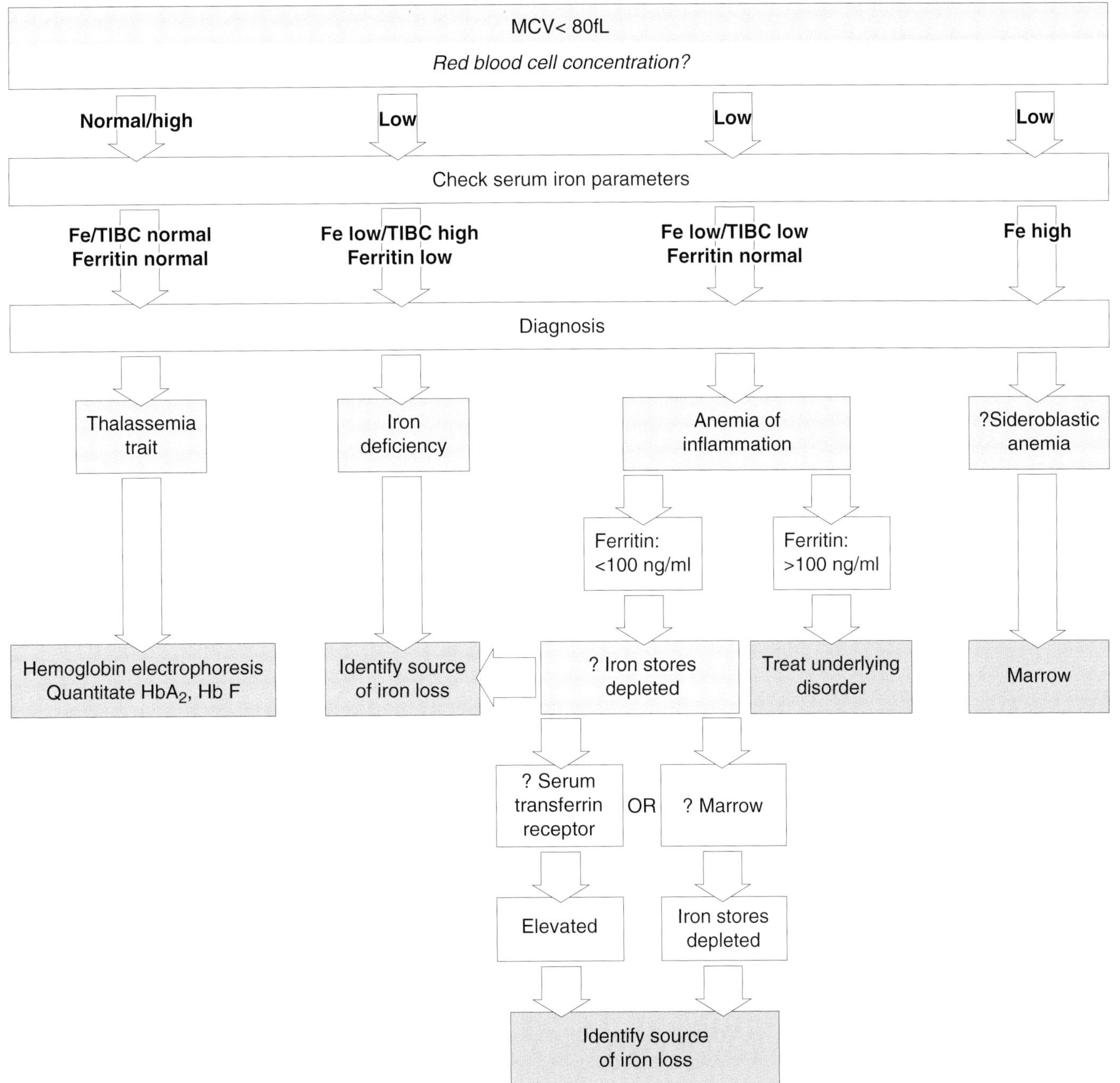

Figure 81–1. Algorithm for evaluation of microcytic anemia.

TABLE 81–3. Differentiating Microcytic Anemias (MCV < 80 fL) Using Iron Studies

Disorder	Serum Iron	Serum TIBC	Serum Ferritin
Iron deficiency anemia	Low (<45 μg/dL)	High (>300 μg/dL)	Low (<20 ng/mL)
Anemia of inflammation	Low (<45 μg/dL)	Low or normal (<250 μg/dL)	High (>100 ng/mL)
Anemia of inflammation + iron depletion	Low (<45 μg/dL)	Low or normal (<250 μg/dL)	Normal (<100 ng/mL)
Thalassemia trait	Normal	Normal	Normal
Sideroblastic anemia	High	Normal	Normal

Abbreviation: TIBC, total iron-binding capacity.

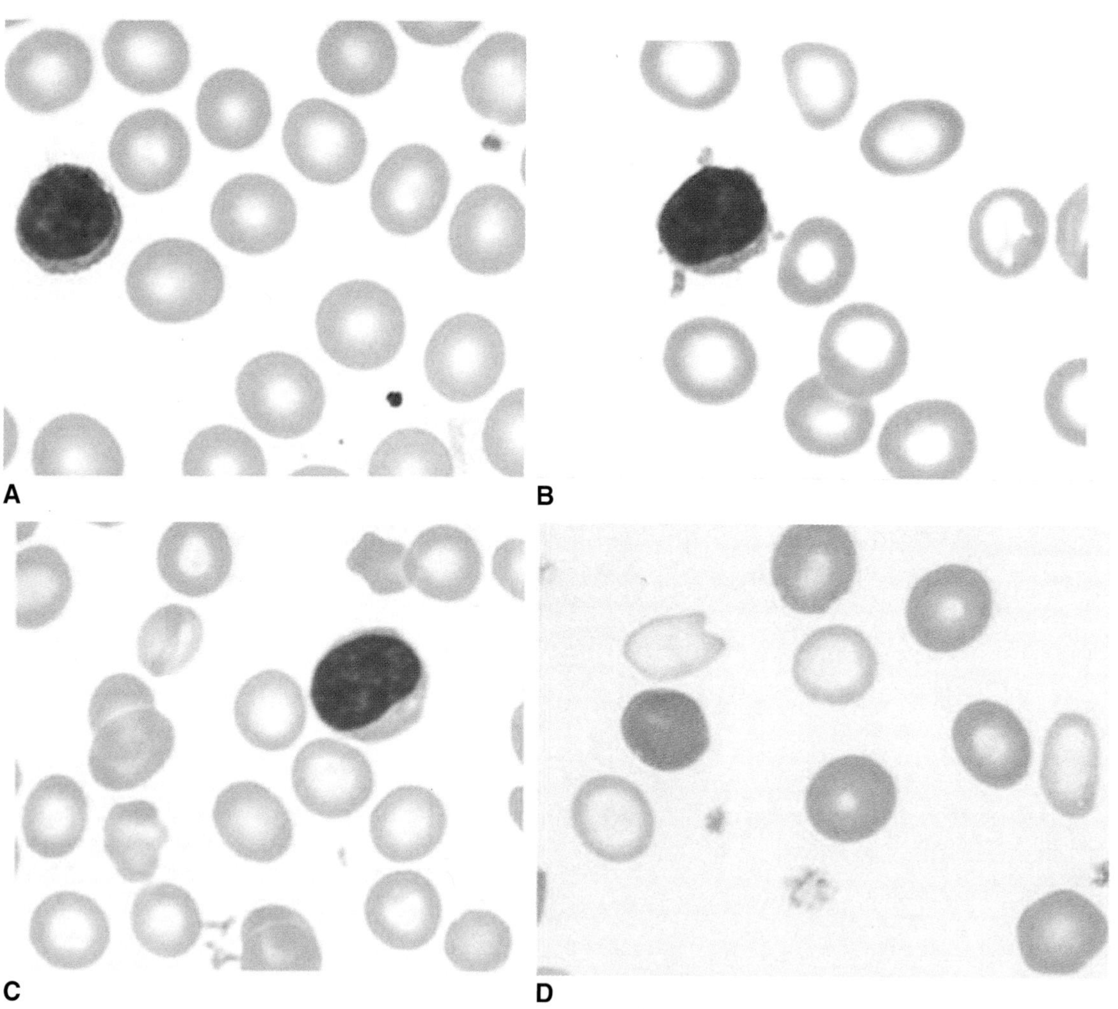

Figure 81–2. Peripheral blood smear photomicrographs (×1000) from patients with microcytic anemias. ***A,*** Normal red blood cells. ***B,*** Microcytosis and hypochromia (MCV 70 fL) caused by iron deficiency. ***C,*** Microcytosis and hypochromia resulting from β-thalassemia trait (MCV 67). ***D,*** Dimorphic red blood cells caused by sideroblastic anemia.

Iron Deficiency Anemia

The characteristic pattern of iron parameters in patients with iron deficiency anemia is low serum iron, high serum TIBC (>300 μg/dL), and low serum ferritin (<20 ng/mL). Once this pattern is identified, no further hematologic evaluation is necessary; required instead is to identify the source of iron loss—most commonly occult bleeding from gastrointestinal lesions or excessive vaginal bleeding, and more rarely malabsorption of iron or chronic hemoglobinuria from intravascular hemolysis. When the source of blood loss has been corrected, anemia should completely resolve with adequate oral iron replacement within a month. If anemia does not resolve, either the patient is not compliant, the prescribed form of iron is not absorbed well (frequently because of an enteric coating), bleeding is continuing, or the diagnosis is incorrect or complicated by additional factors.

Anemia of Chronic Inflammation

Patients with anemia of chronic inflammation may have levels of serum iron as low as those found in iron deficiency, but serum ferritin, an acute-phase reactant, will be high while TIBC levels are normal or low. When serum ferritin levels are below 100 ng/mL, iron depletion likely coexists[10] (see Table 81–3). Some investigators have reported that the serum level of a truncated form of the transferrin receptor can be utilized to confirm the presence of iron deficiency in such patients, without resorting to bone marrow aspiration to determine iron stores.[10–12] In patients with iron deficiency as well as those with an expanded erythroid mass resulting from hemolytic anemia, thalassemia, or megaloblastosis, the serum transferrin receptor level is higher than levels found in patients with anemia of chronic inflammation and adequate iron stores. Not infrequently, however, iron stain of the marrow in anemia of inflammation with elevated serum transferrin receptor levels will show macrophage iron stores to be present.[13] The elevated transferrin receptor level in these cases may indicate a "functional" iron deficiency, most likely related to their markedly low serum iron levels reflecting the increased level of hepcidin activity which reduces intestinal absorption of iron, and inhibits release of macrophage iron into the blood.

Microcytosis of Thalassemia Trait

Normal iron studies indicate that the microcytosis of thalassemia trait is not due to iron deficiency (Table 81–3). A number of mathematical formulas have been used to attempt to distinguish thalassemic from nonthalassemic microcytosis, but in general they do not offer any more information than does the MCV alone.[8] To define the type of thalassemia or a hemoglobinopathy associated with microcytosis (such as hemoglobin E), the required next steps are quantitation of the minor hemoglobins A_2 and fetal hemoglobin as well as hemoglobin electrophoresis. Elevated levels of A_2 and/or fetal hemoglobin will confirm β-thalassemia trait (Table 81–4). To define α-thalassemia trait requires molecular analysis, and such studies are generally not necessary for most clinical purposes. Hemoglobin electrophoresis is important to establish sickle β-thalassemia or heterozygous or homozygous hemoglobin E, all of which are associated with microcytosis.

Sideroblastic Anemias

Sideroblastic anemias are characterized by a persistently high serum iron and high iron saturation of the TIBC. Microcytic anemia associated with a high serum iron should prompt examination of the marrow to determine the presence of ringed sideroblasts, the morphologic hallmark of these heterogeneous disorders (see Chapter 55).

TABLE 81–4. Evaluating Microcytosis Consistent with Thalassemia Trait

	Hb A_2	Hb F	Hb Electrophoresis Patterns
β-Thalassemia	Increased	Normal or increased	AA or SA or CA or EA*
α-Thalassemia	Normal	Normal	AA or AS or AC or AE†

*In individuals heterozygous for hemoglobin (Hb) S or C or E and β-thalassemia, the percentage of Hb S, C, or E will be greater than that of Hb A.

†In individuals heterozygous for Hb S or C or E who also have α-thalassemia, the percentage of Hb A will be greater than that of Hb S or C or E and is usually higher than in the heterozygous individual without α-thalassemia.

MACROCYTIC ANEMIAS

Common causes of macrocytic anemias are listed in Table 81–5; abnormalities of DNA synthesis accounts for the macrocytosis noted in many. The MCV in nutritional megaloblastic anemias often exceeds 110 fL. Cobalamin or folic acid deficiency must be considered in the diagnosis when macrocytosis is reported (see Chapter 18), but they were present in less than 10% of hospitalized cases with an MCV greater than 100 fL in a large prospective study.[14] The most common cause of macrocytosis in these 300 hospitalized patients was medications that inhibit DNA synthesis, including cancer chemotherapy, antiretroviral agents, and anticonvulsants. (The macrocytosis induced by zidovudine and stavudine antiretroviral drugs is sufficiently frequent to be used to monitor compliance![15]) Alcoholism with or without liver disease was the second most frequent cause of macrocytosis. Macrocytosis is a well-recognized feature of the myelodysplastic syndromes; other marrow disorders, such as aplastic anemia, leukemia, myeloma, and carcinomatous involvement also may exhibit large red blood cells.[14] Reticulocytosis often elevates the MCV into the macrocytic range but rarely above 110 fL. Other less frequent causes include nonalcoholic liver disease, hypothyroidism, and rarely familial macrocytosis.[14] Spurious elevation of the MCV may occur as a result of clumping of red cells (as in cold agglutinin hemolytic anemias, or with rouleaux formation due to monoclonal gammopathies).

The useful initial screening tests for patients with macrocytosis, together with the history and physical examination, include a reticulocyte count, serum cobalamin level, and evaluation of thyroid function (Fig. 81–3; see also Table 81–5). Folic acid levels are not helpful because of the rapidity of onset of folic acid deficiency, particularly in the alcoholic, and the ease with which folate can be quickly replaced.[16] A review of the peripheral smear while awaiting the screening laboratory results can narrow possible diagnoses: polychromasia indicates reticulocytosis; hypersegmented neutrophils and macro-ovalocytes favor cobalamin or folic acid deficiency; and hyposegmented Pelger-Huët cells suggest myelodysplasia (Fig. 81–4). If the laboratory results are uninforma-

TABLE 81–5. Differentiating Macrocytic Anemias

	Characteristic Findings on Initial Screening Evaluation*
Nutritional megaloblastic anemias	
Cobalamin deficiency	Low serum cobalamin[‡]; hypersegmented neutrophils
	Increased serum methylmalonic acid and/or homocysteine[‡]
	Low red cell folate
	High serum iron that falls with specific therapy
	Intrinsic factor antibody is positive in <50% of pernicious anemia patients
Folic acid deficiency	Alcoholism, inadequate diet, or increased requirement (hemolysis, pregnancy)
	Hypersegmented neutrophils; increased serum homocysteine[‡]
	Low serum and red cell folate[†]
	Normal serum cobalamin and methylmalonic acid
	High serum iron that falls with specific treatment
Myelodysplastic syndromes	Abnormalities of white blood cells and platelets frequently present
	Hyposegmented neutrophils (Pelger-Huët cells) may be present
	Persistent high serum iron (sideroblastic anemia)
Other marrow disorders	Leukocyte and platelet count abnormalities
	"Leukoerythroblastic" blood smear: immature white blood cells, nucleated red blood cells
Drugs or substances	Alcohol, cancer chemotherapy, phenytoin, zidovudine, stavudine
Liver disease	Targeted red blood cells, abnormal liver function tests
	Low white blood cell and platelet counts frequently present
Hypothyroidism	High thyroid-stimulating hormone
"Spurious" macrocytosis	Reticulocytosis; cold agglutinins
	Rouleaux resulting from monoclonal gammopathy

*Reticulocyte count, serum cobalamin, thyroid function test, and peripheral blood smear.

[†]Serum and red cell folate studies are not recommended. If serum cobalamin is normal and folate deficiency is suspected, it is more cost-effective to treat with folic acid.

[‡]Tissue cobalamin levels are usually low when serum levels are less than 200 pg/mL, almost always low when levels are below 100 pg/mL, and rarely low when levels are 200–300 pg/mL. Elevated methylmalonic acid levels confirm tissue cobalamin deficiency (if renal function is normal). Both methylmalonic acid and homocysteine are elevated in renal insufficiency.

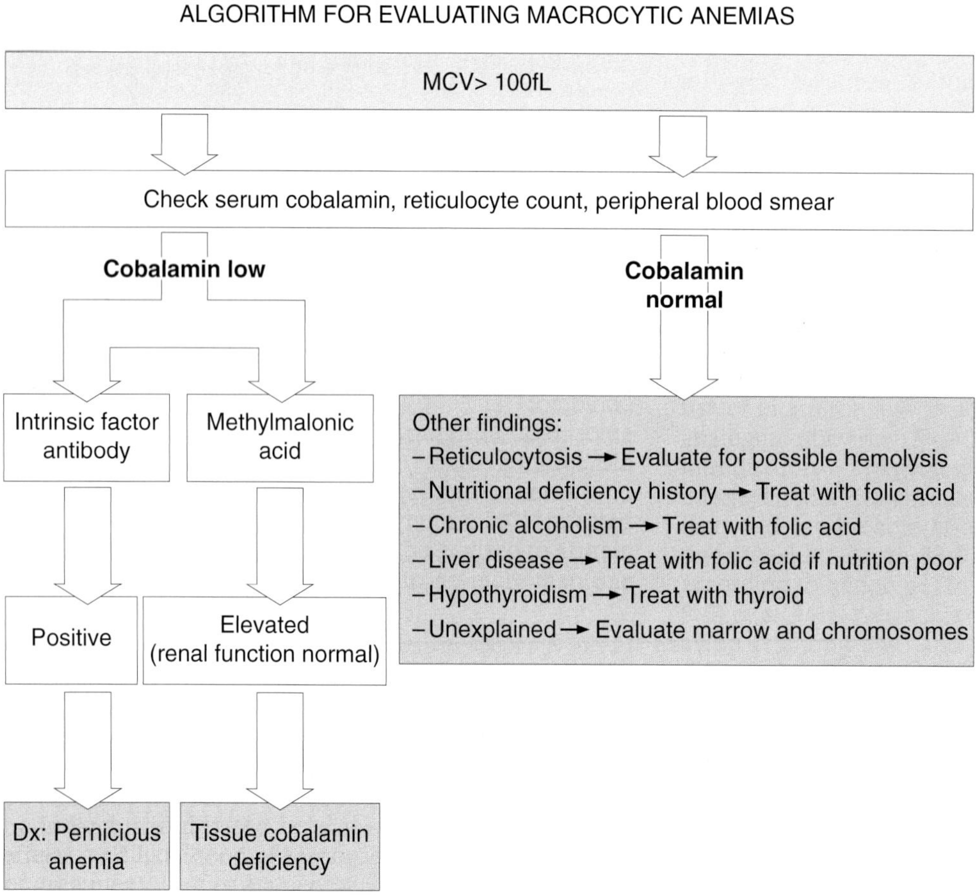

ALGORITHM FOR EVALUATING MACROCYTIC ANEMIAS

MCV> 100fL

Check serum cobalamin, reticulocyte count, peripheral blood smear

Cobalamin low

Intrinsic factor antibody → Positive → Dx: Pernicious anemia

Methylmalonic acid → Elevated (renal function normal) → Tissue cobalamin deficiency

Cobalamin normal

Other findings:
- Reticulocytosis → Evaluate for possible hemolysis
- Nutritional deficiency history → Treat with folic acid
- Chronic alcoholism → Treat with folic acid
- Liver disease → Treat with folic acid if nutrition poor
- Hypothyroidism → Treat with thyroid
- Unexplained → Evaluate marrow and chromosomes

Figure 81–3. Algorithm for evaluation of macrocytic anemia.

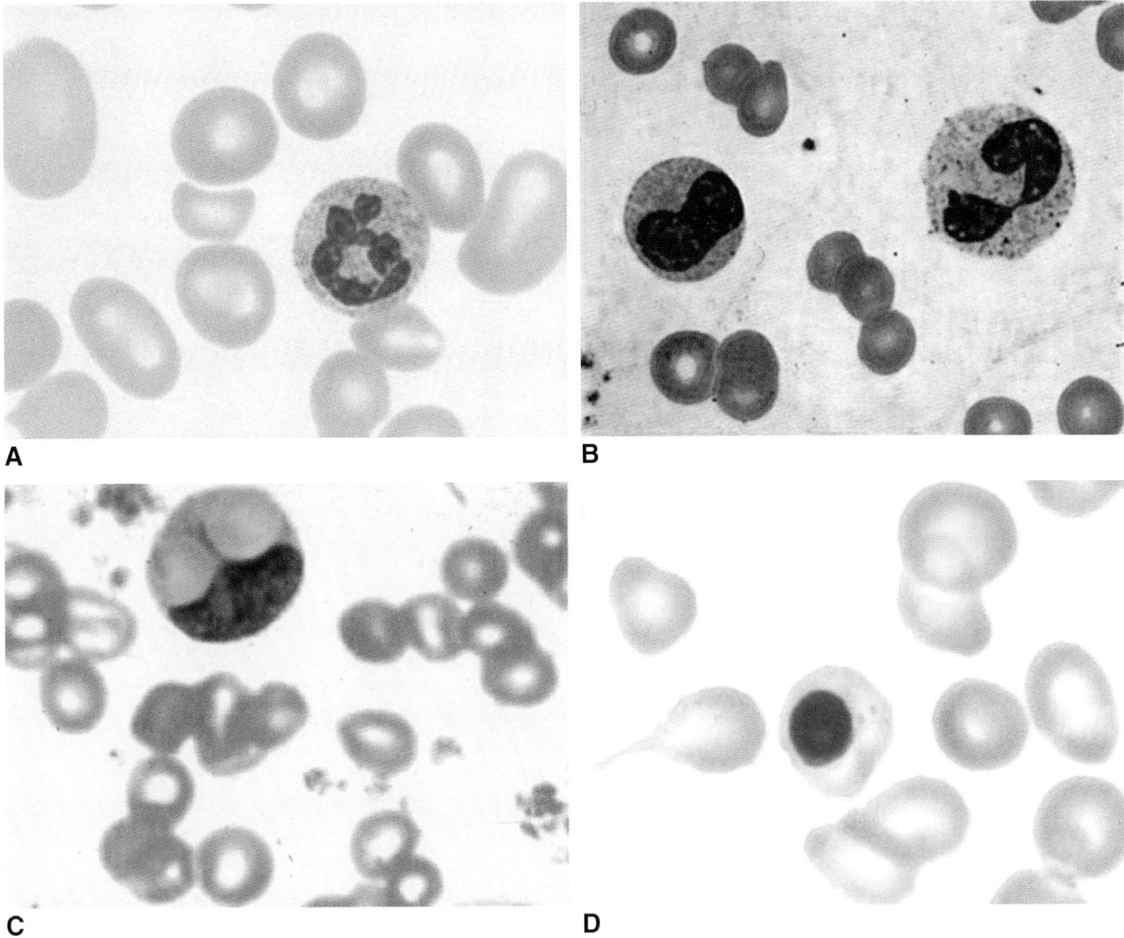

Figure 81–4. Peripheral blood smear photomicrographs (×1000) from patients with macrocytic anemia. *A,* Macrocytes and hypersegmentation resulting from nutritional megaloblastic anemia. *B,* Bilobed neutrophil (Pelger-Huët cell) and a metamyelocyte associated with myelodysplastic syndrome. *C,* Erythrophagocytosis and spurious macrocytosis caused by agglutinated red cells in a patient with *Mycoplasma*-associated cold agglutinin hemolytic anemia. *D,* Nucleated and teardrop red cells associated with myelofibrosis.

tive, a marrow aspirate and biopsy should be obtained, particularly in patients with symptomatic anemia or abnormalities also in white blood cell or platelet counts. Review of the marrow cellular morphology for evidence of abnormal maturation, dysplasia, or ringed sideroblasts, as well as cytogenetic evaluation, may resolve the etiology of macrocytic anemia. Less commonly, other marrow disorders such as aplastic anemia and leukemias may be discovered to be responsible for the macrocytosis.

Some clinicians include serum methylmalonic acid and homocysteine levels in the evaluation of macrocytosis[14]; when renal function is normal, elevation of both is specific for tissue cobalamin deficiency, and only homocysteine will be high in folic acid deficiency. Historically, a low serum cobalamin level led to a Schilling test to confirm malabsorption caused by pernicious anemia or ileal dysfunction or to uncover maldigestion. In the last condition, the patient can absorb crystalline cobalamin but not food cobalamin and thus can be treated with small oral doses of medicinal vitamin B_{12}. Unfortunately, the Schilling test is no longer readily available, and treatment for cobalamin deficiency now must assume the presence of malabsorption. Serum intrinsic factor antibody is specific for malabsorption caused by pernicious anemia, but the test has a low sensitivity.

NORMOCYTIC ANEMIAS

The three best initial screens for normocytic anemias are the reticulocyte number, serum creatinine as a surrogate for erythropoietin secretion, and microscopic examination of the peripheral blood smear. The reticulocyte response is useful in classifying anemias as hypo- or hyperproliferative (Table 81–6). Normal or low reticulocyte percentage or concentration indicates an inadequate marrow response to the anemia. The absolute reticulocyte concentration, now measured reliably with automated counters (normal range, 25,000–125,000/μL), is preferred because, unlike the reticulocyte percentage, this value will not be spuriously increased by a low red blood cell count.

TABLE 81–6. Differentiating Normocytic Anemias*

Low Reticulocyte Count (Hypoproliferative Anemias)	High Reticulocyte Count (Hyperproliferative Anemia)
Acute bleeding or hemolysis (at onset)	Response to recent acute bleeding or hemolysis
Anemia of chronic inflammation/disease	Chronic hemolytic anemia Response to specific therapy for a deficiency
Early iron deficiency anemia	Response to withdrawal of a marrow toxin
Erythropoietin deficiency (anemia of renal disease)	
Mixed nutritional anemias	
Anemia of liver disease[†]	
Anemia of hypothyroidism, hypoadrenalism	
Myelodysplastic syndromes[†]	
Red cell aplasia or aplastic anemia[†]	
Marrow replacement (myelophthisic) anemias[†,‡]	

*A screening evaluation should be performed, including reticulocyte count, peripheral blood smear, serum creatinine, iron studies, cobalamin, and thyroid function.
[†]Anemia frequently accompanied by abnormalities of white blood cells or platelets. These disorders may also be macrocytic.
[‡]Serum and urine protein electrophoresis may be considered part of the screening process in the older population.

Hypoproliferative Anemias

Common disorders associated with hypoproliferative anemias include chronic inflammation, early iron deficiency, erythropoietin deficiency resulting from renal insufficiency, liver disease, hypothyroidism, and marrow replacement disorders. Acute blood loss from either bleeding or hemolysis usually is not associated with a high reticulocyte count early, although polychromasia from reticulocytes ejected from the marrow by erythropoietic stress ("shift" reticulocytes) may be seen on the peripheral blood smear. A few days are required for the increased production of erythropoietin stimulated by tissue hypoxia to effect sufficient erythroid marrow proliferation and differentiation to produce an absolute reticulocytosis. The rise in reticulocytes becomes evident approximately 5 days after a bleeding episode and peaks at about 10 days. Mixed nutritional anemias, such as combined cobalamin and iron deficiencies, may also show a normal MCV, blurring the usefulness of the MCV classification of anemia, but an elevated RDW can suggest the heterogeneous size of the red cells (see Chapter 76). A very low reticulocyte count (<0.1%) suggests the uncommon entity of pure red cell aplasia (or aplastic anemia if the white blood cell and platelet counts also are low). Pure red cell aplasia may occur secondary to parvovirus B19 infection, or due to drug toxicity, or as a result of an autoimmune process.

The anemias resulting from marrow replacement by leukemias, lymphomas, myeloma, metastases from solid tumors, and clonal myeloid disorders such as myeloid metaplasia and myelofibrosis are collectively termed myelophthisic; these anemias are usually normocytic. Stem cell disorders such as myelodysplasia and acute leukemias that manifest erythropoietic failure often produce macrocytic red blood cells. In some circumstances, particularly myeloma and lymphomas and solid tumors such as renal carcinoma, inflammatory cytokines play a role in the pathophysiology of the anemia, and serum iron studies may suggest anemia of inflammation. The history and physical examination often implicates the etiology of anemia in these disorders. A history of breast or prostate cancer, the presence of unexplained splenomegaly, or a diagnosis of lymphoma strongly suggests marrow replacement with tumor and are indications to perform a bone marrow aspiration and biopsy. The peripheral blood smear can be very helpful in the recognition of these disorders. Immature myeloid cells or atypical lymphoid cells suggest clonal myeloid or lymphoid disorders. Nucleated red blood cells and immature myeloid cells, "leukoerythroblastic" peripheral blood findings, suggest a myelophthisic process caused by carcinomatous involvement or marrow fibrosis. Multiple myeloma frequently presents with anemia, with few clues in the physical examination or the peripheral blood smear; serum and urine protein electrophoresis may be a useful screen in the older individual with an unexplained normocytic anemia.

Not uncommonly, particularly in the elderly, the evaluation of a mild normocytic hypoproliferative anemia does not yield a satisfactory diagnosis even after multiple laboratory studies, including iron and cobalamin levels, renal and thyroid function tests, serum and urine protein electrophoresis, and review of the peripheral blood smear and even bone marrow evaluation. In older males, mild anemias may relate to low testosterone levels, but hemoglobin levels are often lower than expected for testosterone deficiency; a more likely explanation is mildly decreased renal function resulting from treatment of hypertension and diabetes with angiotensin-converting enzyme (ACE) inhibitors or angiotensin receptor blockade agents. Indeed, ACE inhibitors have been used to prevent high-altitude erythrocytosis and to treat erythrocytosis following renal transplant. The renin-angiotensin system may help to sustain erythropoietin secretion, and angiotensin II may be a directly acting growth factor for erythroid progenitor cells. ACE inhibitors and particularly ACE receptor blockade could account for the mild anemia often seen in patients treated with these agents.[17,18]

Hemolytic Anemias

Hemolytic anemias are usually normocytic, but the associated reticulocytosis may elevate the MCV into the macrocytic range, as noted earlier. The combination of an elevated reticulocyte count and an increased unconjugated bilirubin fraction immediately implicates a hemolytic process (Fig. 81–5). A very high serum lactate dehydrogenase may be due to an intravascular hemolytic process such as a microangiopathic hemolytic anemia or paroxysmal nocturnal hemoglobinuria, or, alternatively, may indicate a very severe extravascular hemolytic anemia. The serum haptoglobin, an acute-phase reactant,

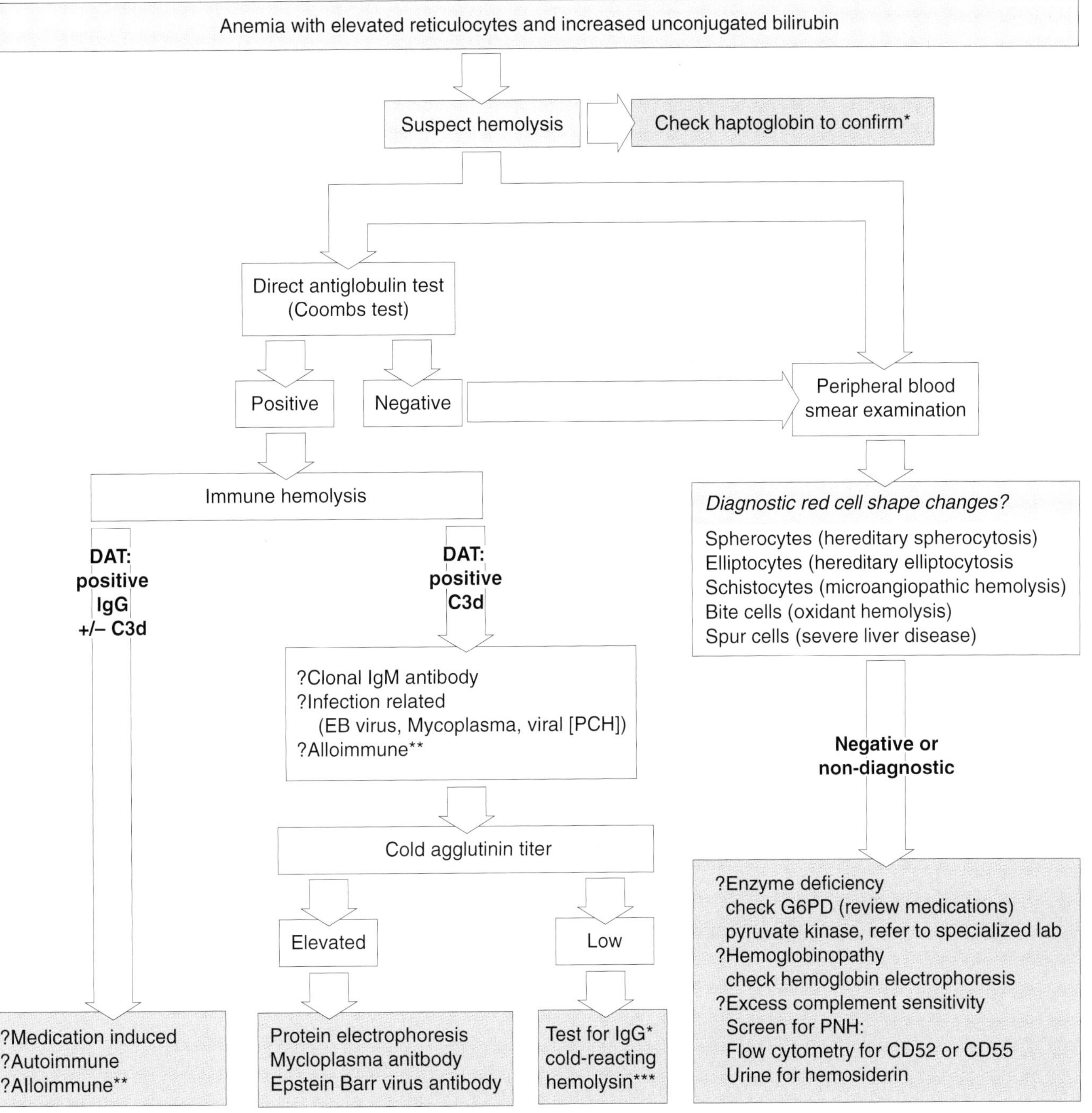

*Other parameters that may be useful: serum lactic dehydrogenase which is markedly increased in intravascular hemolysis and plasma hemoglobin which is elevated in severe hemolysis.
**Hemolytic transfusion reactions, mismatched red blood cell transplants
***Donath-Landsteiner test
PCH, paroxysmal cold hemoglobinuria; G6PD, glucose-6-phosphate dehydrogenase;
PNH, paroxysmal nocturnal hemoglobinuria; EB, Epstein-Barr; rbc, red blood cell
DAT, Direct antiglobulin test

Figure 81–5. Algorithm for the evaluation of hemolytic anemia.

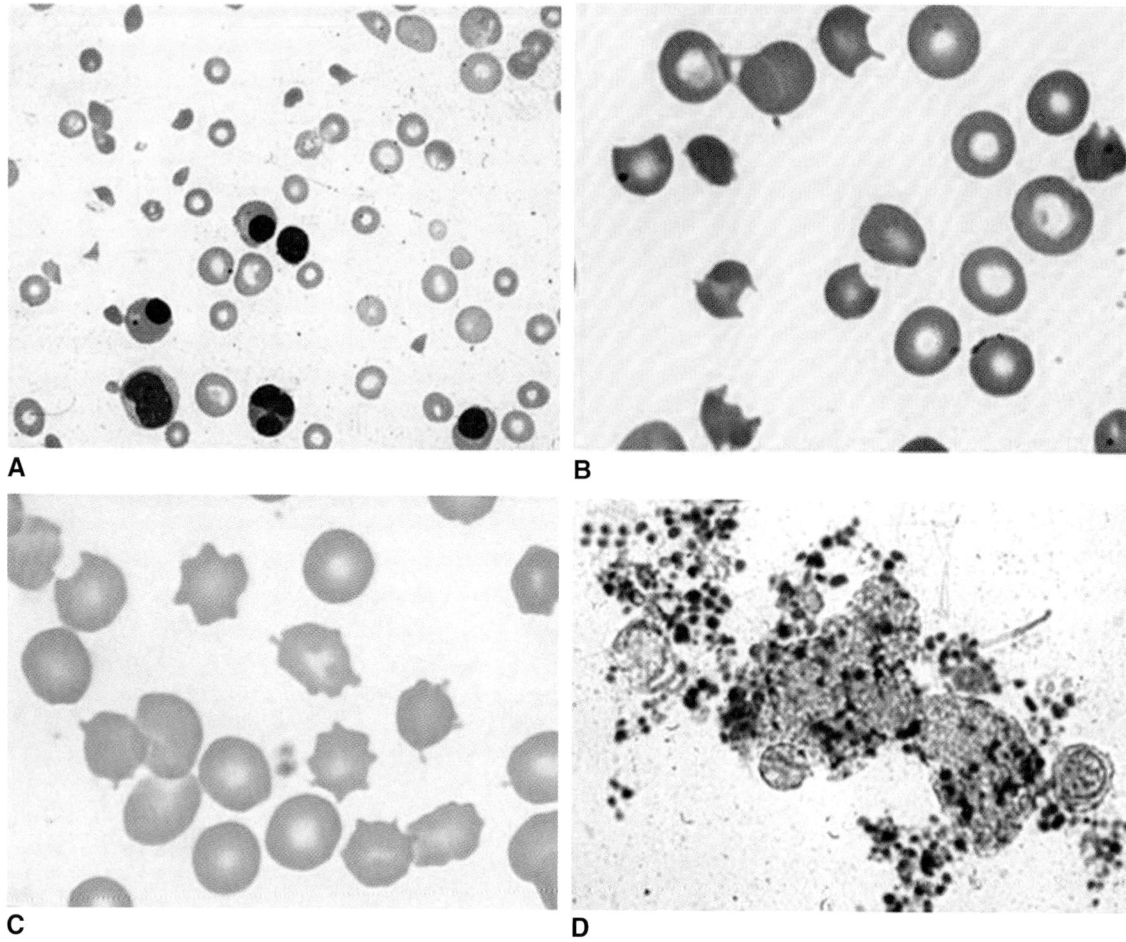

Figure 81–6. Photomicrographs from patients with acquired hemolytic anemias. ***A,*** Red cell fragmentation and nucleated red blood cells indicating microangiopathic hemolytic anemia caused by thrombotic thrombocytopenic purpura (×400). ***B,*** Bite cells caused by severe drug-induced oxidant hemolysis (×1000). ***C,*** Spur cells from a patient with advanced cirrhosis (×1000). ***D,*** Urinary hemosiderin stained with Prussian blue (×400) resulting from intravascular hemolysis in a patient with paroxysmal nocturnal hemoglobinuria.

TABLE 81–7. Recognizing Hemolytic Anemia

Laboratory Findings Consistent with Hemolysis	Alternative Explanations for the Findings
Reticulocytosis	Response to bleeding or exogenous erythropoietin Recovery after specific therapy of nutritional anemia or withdrawal of a marrow toxin
Elevated serum unconjugated bilirubin	Gilbert disease Internal bleeding (large hematoma) Megaloblastosis (ineffective erythropoiesis)
Low serum haptoglobin	Congenital low haptoglobin Severe liver disease Internal bleeding (large hematoma)
Elevated serum lactate dehydrogenase	Megaloblastic anemia Malignancy Tissue infarction
Red cell shape abnormalities: spherocytes, elliptocytes, sickled cells, fragmented cells, bite cells, spur cells	Elliptocytosis may not have a shortened survival Normal red cell shape does not rule out hemolysis (e.g., normal red cells in mild G6PD deficiency hemolysis, and paroxysmal nocturnal hemoglobinuria)
Nucleated red cells in peripheral blood	Marrow infiltration; severe hypoxia or acidosis
Positive direct antibody test (Coombs test)	Antibody on red cells may not necessarily initiate hemolysis Immunoglobulin on red cells may be adsorbed nonspecifically
Hemoglobinemia	In vitro hemolysis caused by phlebotomy technique or other mishap
Hemoglobinuria	Myoglobinuria
Hemosiderinuria	Hemosiderinosis or hemochromatosis

Abbreviation: G6PD, glucose-6-phosphate dehydrogenase.

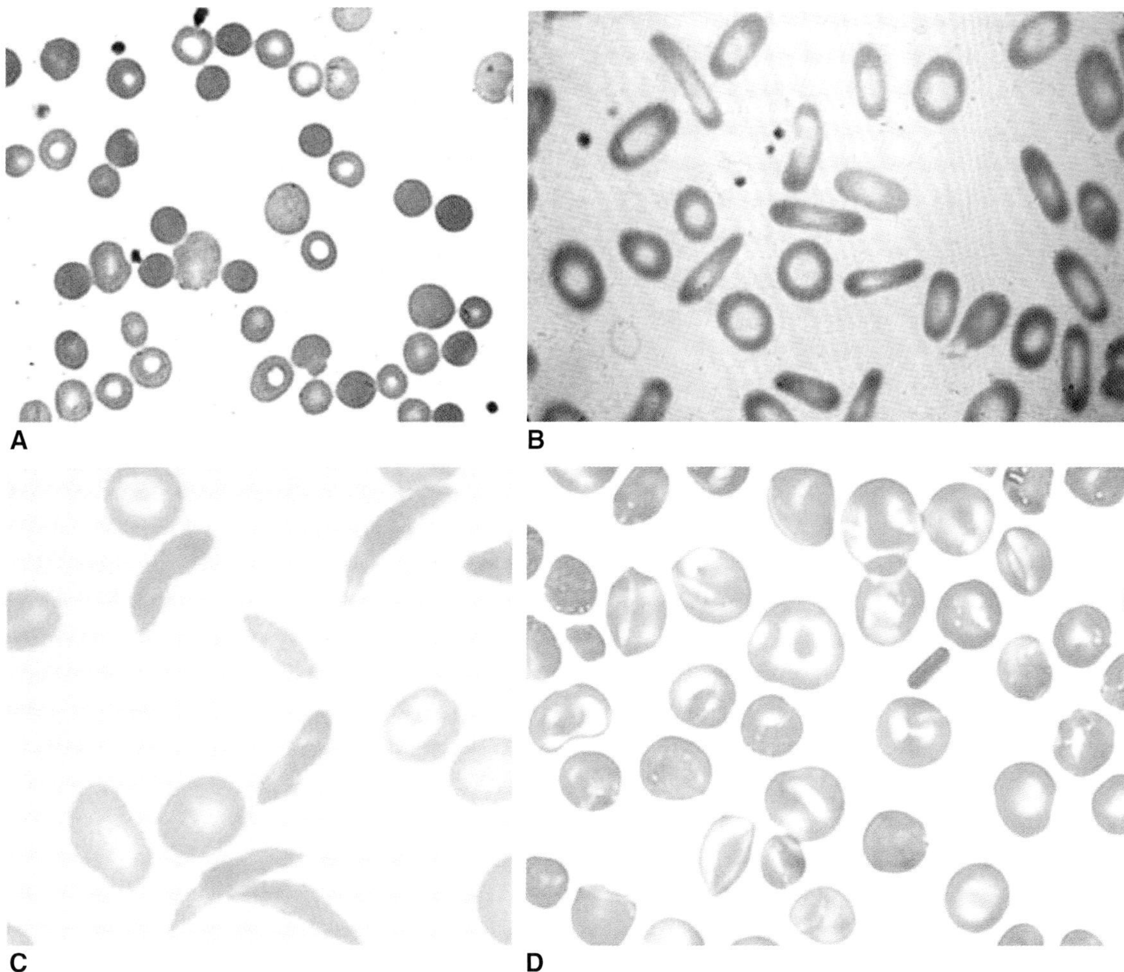

Figure 81–7. Photomicrographs from patients with hereditary hemolytic anemias. *A*, Spherocytes and reticulocytosis (×400) resulting from hereditary spherocytosis. Acquired autoimmune hemolytic anemia would show similar findings. *B*, Elliptocytes from a patient with hereditary elliptocytosis (×1000). *C*, Irreversibly sickled cells from a patient with sickle cell anemia (×1000). *D*, Target cells and a hemoglobin C crystal from a patient with hemoglobin C disease (×1000).

Current Controversies & Future Considerations

Differential Diagnosis of Anemia

- Will the transferrin receptor assay be a useful and cost-effective method to determine iron deficiency in the presence of the anemia of chronic disease?
- Will an assay for hepcidin improve the current assays to diagnose the anemia of inflammation/chronic disease?
- How should we change our approaches to older patients with unexplained anemia?
- Will a simple assay or procedure be developed that will confirm that an anemia is caused by drug-induced blockade of the renin-angiotensin system?
- Can an easily performed test be developed to detect a shortened red blood cell survival?
- Serum tests to evaluate nutritional megaloblastic anemias have essentially eliminated the need for bone marrow aspirations in these disorders. Does the future hold peripheral blood assays to evaluate other diseases, such as the myelodysplastic syndromes, that will obviate the need for invasive studies?

will almost always be low but may be normal in mild hemolysis in the setting of infection or inflammation. An elevated plasma hemoglobin indicates severe intravascular hemolysis, such as in acute transfusion reactions, and is not usually helpful in less severe forms. Hemosiderinuria is found in chronic intravascular hemolysis, as in red cell destruction caused by an abnormal heart valve (see Chapter 24), or in paroxysmal nocturnal hemoglobinuria (see Chapter 25). Sloughed renal tubular cells that have taken up hemoglobin filtered through glomeruli will form casts that stain for iron with Prussian blue (Fig. 81–6*D*). Frequently, confirmation of the presence of hemolysis comes from recognizing characteristic abnormal red cell shapes found in both acquired and hereditary disorders (Figs. 81–6 and 81–7).

Laboratory features of hemolysis may be present in other nonhematologic conditions (Table 81–7), especially if an abnormality occurs in isolation, rather than in combination with the other laboratory markers of erythrocyte destruction. For example, a reticulocytosis can occur a few days after discontinuing an alcoholic binge, as recovery from a marrow toxin (rather than hemolysis). Similarly, an isolated elevated unconjugated bilirubin fraction may be related to the inherited Gilbert syndrome or due to the resorption of blood from a large hematoma.

CONCLUSION

The evaluation of anemia using the classification described in this chapter can proceed in an orderly way and will often lead to the appropriate diagnosis and management without necessarily resorting to invasive studies.

Suggested Readings*

Andrews NC: Disorders of iron metabolism. N Engl J Med 341:1986–1995, 1999.

Beutler E, Hoffbrand AV, Cook JD: Iron deficiency and overload. Hematology (Am Soc Hematol Educ Program) 40–61, 2003.

Ganz T: Hepcidin, a key regulator of iron metabolism and mediator of anemia of inflammation. Blood 102:783–788, 2003.

Nemeth E, Rivera S, Gabayan V, et al: IL-6 mediates hypoferremia of inflammation by inducing the synthesis of the iron regulatory hormone hepcidin. J Clin Invest 113:1271–1278, 2004.

Savage DG, Ogundipe A, Allen RH, et al: Etiology and diagnostic evaluation of macrocytosis. Am J Med Sci 319:343–352, 2000.

Full references for this chapter can be found on accompanying CD-ROM.

CHAPTER 82
ERYTHROCYTOSIS

Jerry L. Spivak, MD

KEY POINTS

Erythrocytosis

- Red cell mass and plasma volume measurements are the only ways to identify absolute erythrocytosis and contracted plasma volume syndromes.
- An elevated serum erythropoietin level supports the diagnosis of secondary erythrocytosis.
- A normal serum erythropoietin level does not exclude polycythemia vera or inappropriate erythropoietin production as a cause of erythrocytosis.
- Phlebotomy is a safe, effective, and rapid method for reducing an elevated red cell mass in any condition causing erythrocytosis.
- Phlebotomy therapy is also effective in reversing plasma volume contraction syndromes not caused by fluid loss.

INTRODUCTION

Transport of oxygen from the lungs to other tissues is a major function of the blood, and an elegant but complex mechanism has evolved in higher organisms to ensure its success. Given the complexity of this mechanism, it is not surprising that it is vulnerable to suppression, leading to anemia and tissue hypoxia. At the same time, given the essential role of oxygen in body metabolism, it is also not surprising that physiologic restraints on this mechanism are few, leading frequently to situations in which erythropoietin is inappropriately produced and, not infrequently, harmful.

Mechanisms Controlling Erythropoiesis

Figure 82–1 illustrates the mechanisms involved in the control of red cell production. Normally, the red cell mass is maintained at a constant level that may vary between individuals of the same age and gender by more than 30%[1] and between genders by the same amount based on the hemoglobin or hematocrit. Erythropoiesis, the orderly continuous process by which primitive committed erythroid progenitor cells proliferate and differentiate into the mature circulating non-nucleated erythrocytes that transport oxygen from the lungs to the tissues and carbon dioxide in the opposite direction, is primarily regulated by the glycoprotein hormone erythropoietin. Erythropoietin is a 165–amino acid polypeptide that has an apparent molecular mass of 30,400, of which 40% consists of carbohydrate residues; the most abundant and important of these is sialic acid, which accounts for acidic pI of the protein.[2] The carbohydrates of erythropoietin are responsible for its solubility, stability, secretion, and protection from premature destruction in the liver; however, although necessary for physical survival of the protein, they are unnecessary for its biologic activity.[3]

In common with other members of the hematopoietic growth factor superfamily to which it belongs,[4] the tertiary structure of erythropoietin is a four-α-helix bundle with two disulfide bonds that are essential for biologic activity. Erythropoietin has two binding sites for its cognate receptor that differ in their affinity, and it is these sites, not the protein's tertiary structure, that dictate its receptor specificity.[5] Erythropoietin is a highly conserved protein from an evolutionary prospective and has no significant homology with any other protein except for the hematopoietic growth factor thrombopoietin, with which it shares 21% sequence identity.[6]

Erythropoietin interacts with its target cells by binding to the erythropoietin receptor, a type 1 transmembrane protein that is a member of the hematopoietic growth factor receptor superfamily.[7] These receptors share in common four positionally conserved cysteines and a WSXWS motif in their extracellular domain, a single transmembrane domain, and a lack of intrinsic tyrosine kinase activity in their cytoplasmic domain. Erythropoietin receptors exist as homodimers, the conformation of which is changed by coupling with erythropoietin.[8] This change in conformation is associated with autophosphorylation of the JAK2 tyrosine kinase that is responsible for intracellular signal transduction involving cell proliferation and survival through protein tyrosine phosphorylation.[9] Given the ubiquity of erythropoietin receptor expression, the relative importance of these two functions appears to be cell-context specific.

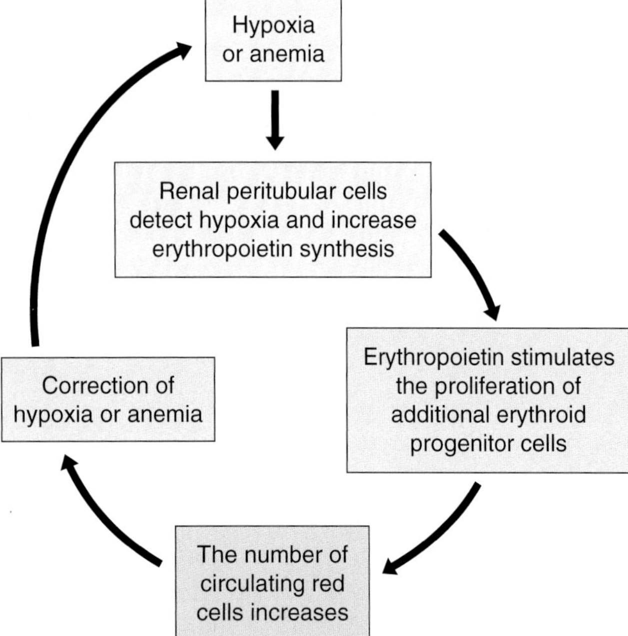

Figure 82–1. An elegant feedback mechanism exists for maintaining tissue oxygenation. Hypoxemia or anemia is detected by peritubular interstitial cells in the kidney, which begin making erythropoietin. The erythropoietin travels to the bone marrow, where it increases erythropoiesis, resulting in an increase in the number of circulating red cells transporting oxygen to the tissue.

With respect to erythropoiesis, erythropoietin acts at several differentiation stages and in different ways during red cell development. Hematopoiesis is normally a stochastic process but is subject to environmental modulation.[10] Thus, interleukin-3 is required for the production of the most primitive committed erythroid progenitor cells,[11] the burst-forming units–erythroid (BFU-E), so named because of the large and distinctive colonies they form when cultured in vitro. BFU-E are largely dormant and require erythropoietin to trigger them into cell cycle.[12] Because BFU-E express low numbers of erythropoietin receptors, a high concentration of erythropoietin is required to activate them.[13,14] BFU-E then give rise to erythroid progenitor cells designated colony-forming units–erythroid (CFU-E) on the basis of the small colonies they form when cultured in vitro. These erythroid progenitor cells lack self-renewal capacity and have limited proliferative capacity. CFU-E express high numbers of erythropoietin receptors and over 90% are in cell cycle. Thus, CFU-E are sensitive to lower concentrations of erythropoietin and require it not for DNA synthesis but to maintain their survival as they differentiate into proerythroblasts and mature red cells.[15] Erythropoietin is not required for hemoglobin synthesis in the CFU-E but only for cell viability, because erythroid progenitor cells overexpressing the antiapoptotic protein Bcl-x_L are capable of autonomous differentiation into mature, fully hemoglobinized, enucleate erythrocytes in the absence of erythropoietin.[16]

Regulation of Erythropoietin Production

Hypoxia is the only physiologic regulator of erythropoietin gene expression, and hypoxic signaling is mediated by a ubiquitous mechanism involving a heterodimeric transcription factor complex of basic helix-loop-helix proteins designated hypoxia-inducible factor-1 (HIF-1) types α and β.[17] The HIF-1α/β heterodimeric transcriptional complex interacts with a specific hypoxia response element in the erythropoietin gene to activate its transcription. HIF-1β is also a component of the aryl hydrocarbon receptor nuclear translator. Both HIF-1 proteins are constitutively expressed, but the intracellular concentration of HIF-1α is tightly controlled by the level of tissue oxygenation.[18] During normoxia, hydroxylation of two specific proline residues in HIF-1α by three prolyl hydroxylases occurs in an oxygen-, iron-, and 2-oxoglutarate–dependent fashion. This posttranslational modification, together with acetylation of lysine residue 532, permits binding of the von Hippel-Lindau protein (VHL) to HIF-1α, which targets the protein for ubiquitination and proteasomal degradation (Fig. 82–2). Oxygen-dependent hydroxylation of asparagine residue 803 in the HIF-1α transcriptional activation domain also blocks binding of other transcription cofactors involved in HIF-1α–mediated gene transcription.[19]

Normally, the half-life of HIF-1α is approximately 5 minutes. With hypoxia, intranuclear accumulation of HIF-1α occurs in less than 2 minutes,[20] indicating that the intracellular HIF-1α level is regulated by reducing its degradation rather than by increasing its synthesis. With increasing hypoxia, the HIF-1α protein level and DNA-binding activity increase exponentially, with the greatest increase occurring at the threshold of tissue hypoxia.[21]

In adults, under normal circumstances the bulk of erythropoietin is produced in the kidneys by circumscribed peritubular interstitial fibroblasts in the inner renal cortex and outer medulla.[22,23] With hypoxia, additional cells are recruited to produce the hormone. Changes in plasma erythropoietin reflect changes in its production. Erythropoietin is also produced constitutively in the liver in both hepatocytes and interstitial fibroblasts.[24] In contrast to the kidneys, intrahepatocyte erythropoietin production can be up- or downregulated by significant hypoxia. The contribution of other tissues to plasma erythropoietin is negligible.

The plasma half-life of erythropoietin is approximately 6 hours in humans,[25] which is much longer than for most hematopoietic growth factors and a direct reflection of the glycoprotein's function as a hormone. Erythropoietin is metabolized by erythroid progenitor cells,[26] which have the highest concentration of erythropoietin receptors, which are saturable.[27] Less than 10% of the hormone is excreted in the urine.[28]

Under normoxic conditions, the plasma erythropoietin level reflects the balance between erythropoietin production and catabolism and is normally constant in a given individual, though variable between individuals without respect to age or gender.[29] This individual variability, which is also seen with respect to the hemoglobin and hematocrit levels, results in a wide normal range for the plasma erythropoietin concentration, from 4 to

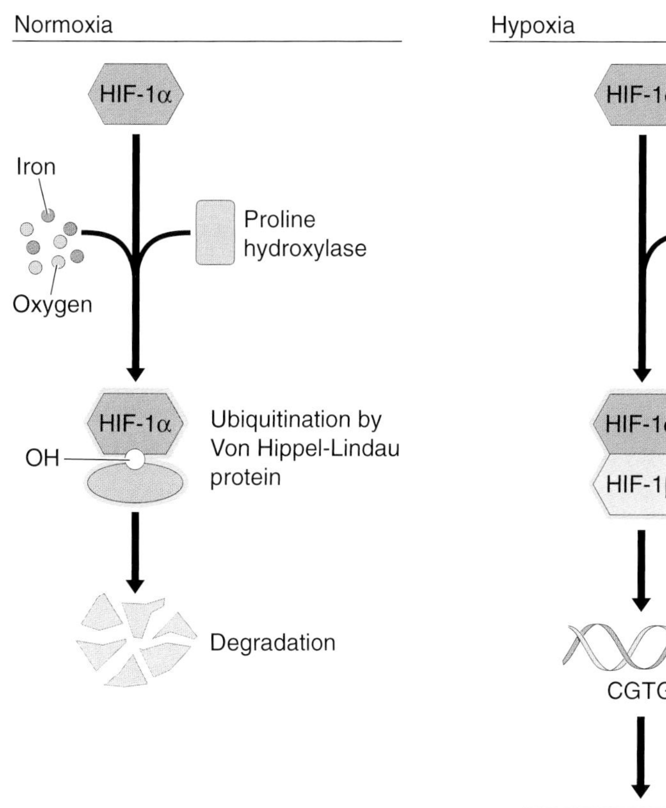

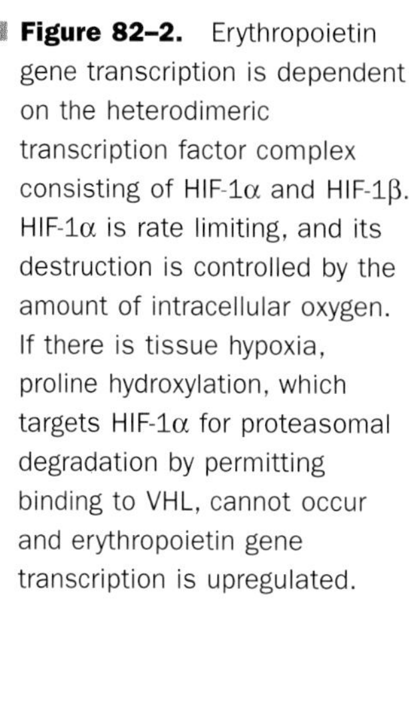

Figure 82–2. Erythropoietin gene transcription is dependent on the heterodimeric transcription factor complex consisting of HIF-1α and HIF-1β. HIF-1α is rate limiting, and its destruction is controlled by the amount of intracellular oxygen. If there is tissue hypoxia, proline hydroxylation, which targets HIF-1α for proteasomal degradation by permitting binding to VHL, cannot occur and erythropoietin gene transcription is upregulated.

26 mU/mL. Because tissue hypoxia is the physiologic regulator of erythropoietin production, it follows that there will be an inverse correlation between the hemoglobin or hematocrit level and the plasma erythropoietin level (Fig. 82–3).

Erythropoietin is a potent hormone, active at the picomolar level, and expansion of the erythroid progenitor cell pool by erythropoietin is exponential. Thus, erythropoietin production is tightly regulated. With tissue hypoxia, there is a rapid increase in erythropoietin production, exceeding catabolism, permitting its plasma level to rise sharply.[30] However, unless the hypoxic insult is severe, the plasma erythropoietin concentration levels off and gradually falls back into the normal range before the red cell mass increases.[31] The wide normal range of erythropoietin levels may obscure a slight increase from baseline.

The downregulation of erythropoietin production after hypoxia involves several mechanisms. Tissue hypoxia per se generates a number of compensatory changes, such as an increase in minute ventilation and heart rate, leading to an increase in arterial oxygen saturation (Sa_{O_2}), tissue perfusion, and tissue oxygen delivery. Hyperventilation also causes respiratory alkalosis, and the change in blood pH stimulates red cell synthesis of 2,3-bisphosphogylcerate (2,3-BPG), the concentration of which in red cells is stoichiometric with hemoglobin.[32] When 2,3-BPG binds to hemoglobin, it reduces hemoglobin oxygen

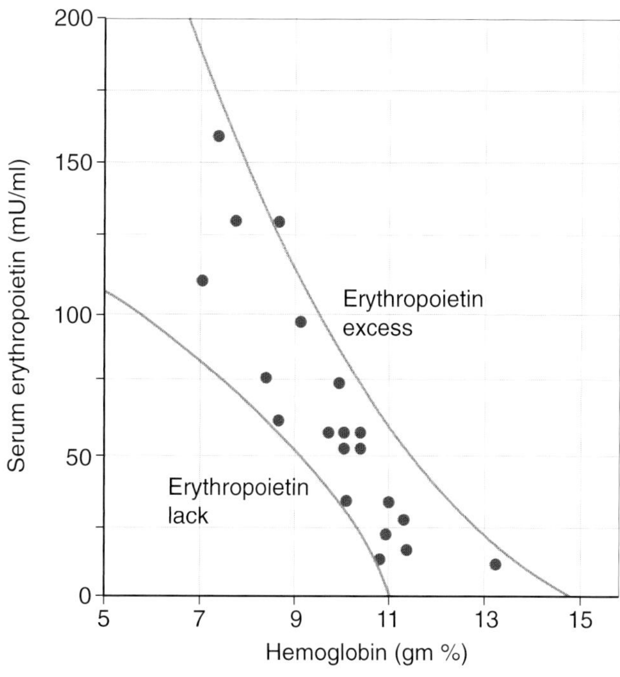

Figure 82–3. The inverse relationship between plasma erythropoietin and the hemoglobin level plotted arithmetically with 95% confidence limits. Erythropoietin levels outside the 95% confidence interval indicate inappropriate erythropoietin production.

affinity, offsetting the effect of the respiratory alkalosis to increase it and enhancing tissue oxygenation. In addition, even before there is an increase in the number of circulating red cells, there is an increase in erythropoietin catabolism associated with the expansion of the erythroid progenitor cell pool.[26] Furthermore, hyperventilation or high altitude is associated with fluid loss and plasma volume shrinkage.[33] The resulting increase in blood viscosity also serves, by a mechanism as yet undefined, to reduce erythropoietin production.[34] This effect is, of course, augmented by the subsequent increase in red cell mass. Indeed, in humans, only in chronic mountain sickness or in certain patients with large right-to-left cardiac shunts, where the existing cause for hypoxia is coupled with impaired ventilation, is there failure to downregulate erythropoietin production.

CLINICAL FEATURES AND DIAGNOSIS

Signs and Symptoms

The causes of erythrocytosis are outlined in Table 82–1. The symptoms and signs associated with erythrocytosis are due to the underlying disorder and red cell mass elevation. If the development of erythrocytosis is gradual, there may be no symptoms. The most common symptoms include headache, blurred vision, tinnitus, dizziness, scotomata, anorexia, vertigo, weakness and reduced mental activity. Cough or dyspnea point to a respiratory or cardiac cause for the erythrocytosis; insomnia, snoring, and daytime somnolence suggest sleep apnea. Paresthesias, extremity pain, epigastric distress or abdominal fullness, and aquagenic pruritus frequently accompany polycythemia vera.

Systemic hypertension, conjunctival and mucous membrane hyperemia, facial plethora, and palmar erythroid are due to the increased red cell mass. Cyanosis and clubbing indicate the presence of right-to-left shunting but do not define its location. Spider angiomata suggest that the erythrocytosis is due to the hepatopulmonary syndrome. Splenomegaly, in the absence of liver disease, suggests that the erythrocytosis is due to polycythemia vera. If the erythrocytosis is extreme, a cerebrovascular accident, myocardial infarction, or venous thromboembolism may be its presenting manifestation; intra-abdominal venous thrombosis is a presenting manifestation of polycythemia vera, particularly in women.

TABLE 82–1. Causes of Erythrocytosis

Relative Erythrocytosis

Hemoconcentration resulting from dehydration; diuretics; androgens, ethanol, or tobacco abuse

Absolute Erythrocytosis

Hypoxia

Carbon monoxide intoxication
High-oxygen-affinity hemoglobin
High altitude
Pulmonary disease
Right-to-left cardiac or vascular shunts
Sleep apnea syndrome
Hepatopulmonary syndrome

Renal Disease

Renal artery stenosis
Focal sclerosing or membranous glomerulonephritis
Renal cysts
Renal transplantation

Tumors

Hypernephroma
Hepatoma
Cerebellar hemangioblastoma
Adrenal tumors
Pheochromocytoma
Meningioma
Uterine myoma

Drugs

Androgens
Recombinant erythropoietins
SU5467

Familial (with Normal Hemoglobin Function)

Erythropoietin receptor mutations
VHL mutations
2,3-BPG mutation

Polycythemia Vera

Laboratory Findings

Measurement of the Red Cell Mass and Plasma Volume

A high hematocrit or hemoglobin level is usually the first abnormality to suggest the presence of erythrocytosis. However, unless the hematocrit is over 60% in a man (hemoglobin greater than 20 gm/dL) or over 50% in a woman (hemoglobin greater than 16 gm/dL), there is no assurance that the elevation of the hematocrit or hemoglobin is not due to simple plasma volume contraction.[35] Indeed, some of the same disorders that cause erythrocytosis are also responsible for plasma volume contraction syndromes (see Table 82–1). To assess acuity, prior blood counts are helpful. The only way to distinguish an absolute elevation of the red cell mass as the cause of a high hematocrit, as opposed to plasma volume contraction, is to measure both the red cell mass and the plasma volume directly.

The use of formulas to derive these values or extrapolation of the red cell mass from a plasma volume measurement are unacceptable surrogates[36] for the following reasons: the red cell mass and plasma volume vary independently and red cell distribution is not uniform in small vessels.[37] Therefore, the whole-body hematocrit derived from independent measurements of the red cell mass and plasma volume, divided by the peripheral venous hematocrit, equals 0.92 on average.[38] Additionally, the hematocrit in individual organs varies widely, for example, from 80% in the spleen to 40% in the liver.[39] The whole-body hematocrit/peripheral blood hematocrit ratio can be decreased with splenomegaly owing to the attendant increase in plasma volume or increased if the splenomegaly is due to pooling of red cells, as in polycythemia vera.[40] Examples of red cell mass and plasma volume measurements are provided in Table 82–2.

TABLE 82–2. Red Cell Mass (RCM) and Plasma Volume (PV) Measurements in the Evaluation of Suspected Erythrocytosis

	A: Androgen Therapy (S = 2.15), 52-yr-old Man (Hct = 56.0%)		B: Chronic Renal Disease (S = 1.99), 37-yr-old Woman (Hct = 47%)		C: Polycythemia Vera (S = 1.41), 55-yr-old Woman (Hct = 46.0%)	
	Expected*	Observed	Expected*	Observed	Expected*	Observed
RCM (mL)	2370	2661	1675	1976	1209	1640
PV (mL)	3393	1824	2776	2230	1967	2169
TBV (mL)	5763	4485	4451	4206	3176	3809

*The expected values were derived from the formulas in Pearson et al.[1] Patient A illustrates the profound plasma volume contraction and minimal erythrocytosis that can occur with androgen administration. Patient B illustrates the secondary erythrocytosis associated with renal cysts in a patient with end-stage renal disease with elevation of the red cell mass and contraction of the plasma volume. Patient C illustrates the plasma volume expansion occurring in polycythemia vera that masks the increase in the red cell mass.

Abbreviations: Hct, hematocrit; S, body surface area in m^2; TBV, total blood volume.

With respect to erythrocytosis, the ratio of plasma to red cells varies according to the cause of the erythrocytosis. With tissue hypoxia from any cause, as the red cell mass increases, the plasma volume shrinks. This phenomenon occurs in high-altitude erythrocytosis,[33] hypoxic erythrocytosis resulting from right-to-left cardiac or vascular shunts,[41] chronic carbon monoxide intoxication,[42] and impaired pulmonary gas exchange.[43] Iatrogenic causes include administration of recombinant erythropoietin,[44] androgenic steroids,[45] and blood transfusion.[46] Thus, as the red cell mass is increased, there is a tendency for plasma reduction.

In contrast, in polycythemia vera, in which erythropoiesis is autonomous, erythropoietin production is suppressed, and tissue oxygenation is satisfactory, as the red cell mass increases, the plasma volume either stays the same or increases. The net results are first, an expansion of the total blood volume with a reduction in peripheral vascular resistance, and second, because of the expanded plasma volume, masking of the actual extent of red cell mass expansion as measured by the hematocrit regardless of whether the spleen is enlarged.[47] Importantly, because the increase in red cell mass is insidious and plasma volume expansion keeps peripheral vascular resistance low, it is not until the vascular space is literally engorged that patients become symptomatic. At this juncture, however, they are also at great risk of thrombosis or hemorrhage. Indeed, a catastrophic presentation with hepatic vein thrombosis, particularly in women, is not infrequently the presenting manifestation of polycythemia vera. As a corollary, because plasma volume expansion can mask expansion of the red cell mass as measured by the hematocrit or hemoglobin level, and because erythrocytosis is the only feature that separates polycythemia vera from its companion myeloproliferative disorders, idiopathic myelofibrosis and essential thrombocytosis, direct measurement of the red cell mass and plasma volume is mandatory if polycythemia vera is a diagnostic possibility, as indicated in Figure 82–4.

Blood Gas Measurements

The Sao_2, if measured directly, is the most sensitive measure of tissue hypoxia because it directly correlates with the red cell mass, unlike the partial pressure of arterial oxygen (Pao_2).[43] This is because allosteric heme-heme interactions as a consequence of oxygen binding ensure that hemoglobin is fully saturated with oxygen over a wide Pao_2 range. Pao_2 correlates with the red cell mass only when it falls below 67 mm Hg.[43] An arterial oxygen saturation of greater than 92% excludes tissue hypoxia as a cause of erythrocytosis with two exceptions[48]: first, the Sao_2 will be normal with a high-oxygen-affinity hemoglobin, and second, if the Sao_2 is not measured but calculated from the Pao_2, hemoglobin oxygen desaturation resulting from chronic carbon monoxide intoxication will be missed. In this regard, it is important to remember that the timing of the Sao_2 measurement and corroborating carboxyhemoglobin measurements are important. In patients with sleep apnea or positional (supine) hypoxemia, arterial oxygen desaturation and tissue hypoxemia can be episodic yet still cause erythrocytosis.[49] The half-life of carboxyhemoglobin is 4–6 hours, and, if measurements for carboxyhemoglobin are remote from the cessation of exposure, both it and the Sao_2 will be normal. Thus, measurements of both must be performed under the appropriate conditions to obtain clinically valid results.

Measurement of Plasma Erythropoietin

As discussed earlier, the plasma erythropoietin level is a relatively insensitive measure of tissue hypoxia. As illustrated in Figure 82–5, many patients with hypoxic causes for erythrocytosis have a normal plasma erythropoietin level. Even in polycythemia vera, the plasma erythropoietin level can be normal as opposed to reduced. In this regard, like measurement of the Sao_2, measurement under the appropriate clinical circumstances may be necessary to document increased erythropoietin production.

Given the many causes for relative and absolute erythrocytosis (see Table 82–1), it is important that the diagnostic evaluation be methodical (see Fig. 82–4). Thus, in patients with a normal erythropoietin level without a family history of erythrocytosis who fail to meet the diagnostic criteria for polycythemia vera, a urinalysis, renal ultrasound, and abdominal computed tomography

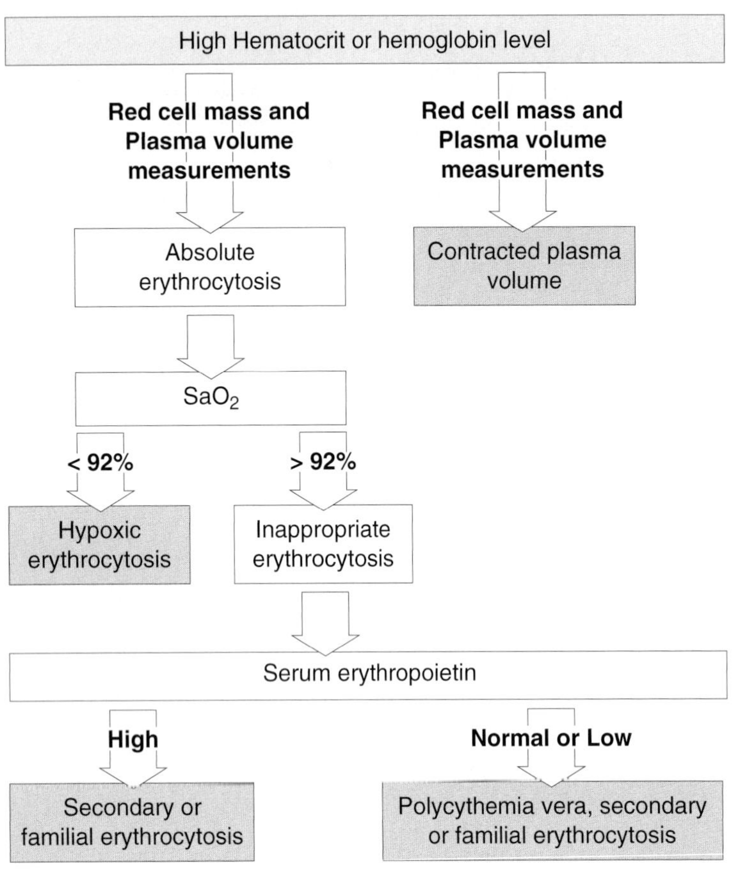

Figure 82–4. Diagnostic algorithm for erythrocytosis. Direct measurement of the red cell mass and plasma volume is the only accurate method for distinguishing absolute erythrocytosis from plasma volume contraction. The diagnostic process then proceeds serially to identify hypoxic and nonhypoxic causes for erythrocytosis with or without an elevation in serum erythropoietin.

will be necessary to exclude secondary causes for the erythrocytosis.

SPECIFIC CAUSES OF ERYTHROCYTOSIS

Tissue Hypoxia

Hypobaric Hypoxia

The erythrocytosis that develops with ascent to high altitude as a result of the attendant reduction in ambient oxygen tension is just one adaptive mechanism to enhance tissue oxygen delivery. Others include hyperventilation, increase in pulmonary diffusing capacity, a reduction in hemoglobin oxygen affinity, and an increase in circulating red cell number. An increase in pulmonary artery pressure that is associated with hypoxemia of any cause is also an adaptive response in humans.

Chronic mountain sickness, a disorder associated with right heart failure and thrombotic events, can be considered as a loss of the adaptive response to hypobaric hypoxia with excessive erythrocytosis, pulmonary hypertension, and a reduction in ventilatory drive. Cobalt toxicity may be responsible for chronic mountain sickness affecting Peruvian miners[50] by inhibiting the oxygen-dependent hydroxylation of HIF-1α, enhancing its accumulation, and promoting continuous erythropoietin gene transcription and uncontrolled red cell mass expansion.[51] Hyperuricemia, hypertension, and proteinuria are other consequences of the chronic hypoxia and erythrocytosis.[19]

Chronic Obstructive Lung Disease

Impaired ventilatory function resulting from anatomic pulmonary disease regardless of cause produces the same erythropoietic response seen when normal individuals are subjected to hypobaric hypoxia.[43] In patients with concomitant congestive heart failure or in whom there is plasma volume expansion, the true extent of the erythrocytosis may be masked and an increase in the plasma erythropoietin level may not be apparent because of downregulation by the expanded erythroid progenitor cell pool. The plasma volume expansion may reflect a reduction in renal blood flow and glomerular filtration rate, both of which can be restored by therapeutic phlebotomy.[52]

Sleep Apnea

Intermittent nocturnal hypoxemia, whether caused by mechanical airway obstruction or positional pulmonary hypoventilation, can stimulate sufficient erythropoietin production to cause erythrocytosis.[49] Systemic as well as pulmonary hypertension, biventricular cardiac hypertro-

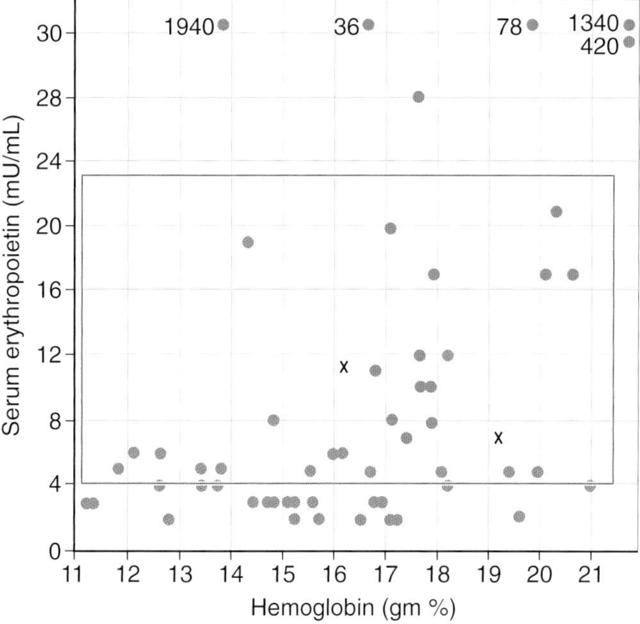

KEY

P Vera   2 erythrocytosis

Figure 82–5. Serum erythropoietin levels in patients with polycythemia vera (o), secondary erythrocytosis (◻), or spurious erythrocytosis (x). As indicated by the box, in each of these situations, the erythropoietin level can be normal.

phy, and plasma volume contraction are also features of severe sleep apnea, whose victims are not often aware of the cause of their malady.[53] Although hypogonadism is not uncommon in men with the sleep apnea syndrome, testosterone administration can also cause this syndrome.[54] Sleep apnea is more common in men, but women with polycystic ovary disease are particularly susceptible not only because of obesity but also because of increased testosterone production.[55] Testosterone may alter upper airway patency during sleep,[56] and ethanol may facilitate airway musculature hypotonia while depressing arousal mechanisms.[57] Daytime somnolence, decreased cognitive performance, and snoring are important clues to the presence of sleep apnea, which may be present without the characteristic physiognomy.

Chronic Carbon Monoxide Intoxication

Erythrocytosis resulting from carbon monoxide intoxication is most commonly a consequence of tobacco abuse[42] or inadvertent environmental exposure.[58] The affinity of carbon monoxide for hemoglobin is 200 times greater than that of oxygen as a consequence of its slower rate of dissociation from the protein. Carbon monoxide also shifts the hemoglobin-oxygen dissociation curve to the left, reducing the release of oxygen to the tissues. The increase in hemoglobin oxygen affinity caused by carbon monoxide binding is similar to that of high-oxygen-affinity hemoglobins. Carboxyhemoglobin also has a reduced affinity for 2,3-BPG, and, at high concentrations, carbon monoxide depresses red cell 2,3-BPG production. Finally, by an unknown mechanism, carbon monoxide intoxication causes a reduction in the plasma volume.[42] Spurious or stress erythrocytosis is actually a manifestation of tobacco-related chronic carbon monoxide intoxication.[59] Remember that the half-life of carboxyhemoglobin is 4–6 hours and, unless the carboxyhemoglobin measurements are made during or close to the time of exposure, the carboxyhemoglobin level will not be elevated.

Cyanotic Congenital Heart Disease

Anatomic shunting of blood from the right side of the heart to the left results in hypoxemia, cyanosis, and erythrocytosis with a diminished plasma volume.[41] In addition, there may be an associated coagulopathy with hypofibrinogenemia and thrombocytopenia.[60,61] The chronic hypoxemia also leads to impaired renal function, proteinuria, and hyperuricemia associated with a reduced glomerular filtration rate and renal plasma flow and an increased filtration fraction.[62,63] Similar abnormalities have been observed in patients with cor pulmonale[52] and high-altitude erythrocytosis,[19] and not surprisingly, they, as well as the coagulopathy associated with the erythrocytosis,[64] are reversible with correction of the hypoxemia or with phlebotomy.[63]

The Hepatopulmonary Syndrome

The hepatopulmonary syndrome is characterized by liver disease, intrapulmonic capillary dilation, hypoxemia ($Pao_2 < 70$ mm Hg), cyanosis, and clubbing.[65] In addition to the dilated pulmonary capillaries that prevent uniform hemoglobin oxygenation and also increase red cell transit time, further exacerbating the problem, intrapulmonary and pleural arteriovenous anastomoses and portopulmonary anastomoses have been documented,[66] especially at the lung bases, and may be exacerbated by pleural effusions or ascites. A challenge of 100% oxygen, contrast-enhanced echocardiogram (bubble study) and pulmonary angiography will define the severity and mechanisms for the hypoxemia.[65] Patients exhibit platypnea and orthodeoxia. Liver transplantation is the only effective remedy for the hepatopulmonary syndrome.[65]

High-Oxygen-Affinity Hemoglobins

Hemoglobin tetramers normally exist in equilibrium between two conformations, a "tense" or deoxygenated state and a "relaxed" or oxygenated state.[67] Amino acid substitutions that prevent the appropriate intramolecular heme-heme interactions necessary to maintain the stability of the deoxygenated or tense state will shift the equilibrium to the oxygenated or relaxed state. Most amino acid substitutions causing an increase in hemoglobin oxygen affinity occur in the $\alpha_1\beta_2$ interface, the carboxy-terminal end of the β chain, or the binding site for 2,3-BPG.[67] The amount of erythrocytosis depends on the extent of the increase in hemoglobin oxygen affinity caused by the amino acid substitution. (The hemoglobinopathies are discussed in Chapter 20.) The serum erythropoietin level can also be normal, because these patients compensate for increased hemoglobin oxygen affinity by increasing red cell mass.[68] The diagnosis of a high-oxygen-affinity hemoglobin, once the presence of an elevated red cell mass is established, requires the demonstration of a low hemoglobin P_{50} (the partial pressure of oxygen at which hemoglobin is half-saturated with oxygen).

Inappropriate Erythropoietin Production

Renal Disease

The kidneys are normally the major site of erythropoietin production in adults and, therefore, a potential site for inappropriate production of the hormone. Erythrocytosis in association with renal artery stenosis is uncommon because the degree of kidney hypoxia is usually not severe.[69] Similarly, renal cysts can be a site of unregulated erythropoietin production[70,71] and can cause erythrocytosis even in patients with end-stage renal disease, but there may only be amelioration of anemia rather than erythrocytosis. Focal sclerosing[72] or membranous[73] glomerulonephritis have been associated with erythrocytosis.

Posttransplantation Erythrocytosis

Postrenal transplantation erythrocytosis is defined as a persistent elevation in hematocrit of greater than 51% following renal transplantation. Its prevalence varies from 2% to 22% and it occurs 8–24 months after surgery. Erythrocytosis is persistent in 75% of cases.[74] There is a striking male predominance, suggesting that androgens are an important permissive factor. Smoking, hypertension, and diuretic use are predisposing factors. Patients with this complication have increased erythropoietin production from their native kidneys,[75] but increased bioavailable insulin-like growth factor-I (IGF-I)[76] and an altered renin-angiotensin axis may also be involved, because erythroid progenitor cells have receptors for angiotensin II.[77]

Tumor-Associated Erythrocytosis

Erythrocytosis as a paraneoplastic syndrome is a rare entity and, like posttransplantation erythrocytosis, is most often seen in men, presumably because of the erythropoiesis-enhancing effects of androgens. Although most erythropoietin-producing tumors have been malignant (see Table 82–1), benign tumors such as uterine myoma[78] and meningiomas[79] also have been implicated. Tumors of the kidneys and liver are most common. A common denominator may be a mutation in the tumor suppression gene *VHL*, which is responsible for targeting HIF-1α for proteasomal destruction (see Fig. 82–2). Patients with the von Hippel-Lindau syndrome, in which this gene is mutated, develop erythrocytosis in association with tumors of the cerebellum, liver, kidneys, and adrenal glands as well as pheochromocytomas.[80] These tumors produce erythropoietin,[81,82] although plasma erythropoietin may not be increased above the normal range (see Fig. 82–5). This may in part be due to feedback inhibition in the form of hormone catabolism to keep plasma erythropoietin within the normal range. As proof of principle, successful tumor removal will alleviate the erythrocytosis.

Familial Erythrocytosis

Familial erythrocytosis, also known as primary familial and congenital polycythemia, although leukocytes and platelets are not involved, is characterized by an elevated red cell mass with a normal or low plasma erythropoietin level and a normal hemoglobin P_{50}.[83] Many causes have been identified through molecular genetics, including those caused by high-oxygen-affinity hemoglobins or the von Hippel-Lindau syndrome. Indeed, the most common causes are mutations in the erythropoietin receptor that result in truncation of its carboxy-terminal domain[84] or *VHL* mutations (Chuvash polycythemia).[85,86]

Erythropoietin receptor mutations, usually with autosomal dominant inheritance, have been localized to the exon VIII portion of the cytoplasm domain. These mutations uniformly result in truncation of the tyrosine residue that serves as a binding site for the negative regulatory phosphatase SHP-1. Murine hematopoietic cells forced to express this mutant erythropoietin receptor are hyporesponsive to erythropoietin in serum-free medium[87] but are hypersensitive to IGF-I,[87] suggesting that erythrocytosis is due to IGF-I, and not directly to erythropoietin.

Currently, the most common cause of familial erythrocytosis appears to be an autosomal recessive disorder caused by mutations in the *VHL* gene.[85] First discovered as an endemic form of erythrocytosis in the Chuvash region of Russia, the syndrome has been widely identified elsewhere.[86] Among Chuvash natives with erythrocytosis, there was a mutation (Arg200Trp) on both *VHL* alleles, but in other populations different mutations have been observed. In addition to erythrocytosis, affected individuals have elevated plasma erythropoietin, varicose veins, vertebral hemangiomas, low blood pressure, and a hypercoagulable state.[88] Surprisingly, despite homozygosity for the defective *VHL* gene, the hemangioblastic cerebellar, renal, and adrenal tumors characteristic of the von Hippel-Lindau syndrome[80] have not been observed.

Drug-Induced Erythrocytosis

Alterations in the red cell mass can be induced pharmacologically either secondarily through changes in plasma volume or directly through enhancement of erythropoiesis. Diuretics should always be considered as a possible cause of apparent erythrocytosis resulting from plasma volume contraction in patients with renal impairment or after renal transplantation. Ethanol intoxication as a consequence of binge drinking has also been associated with severe plasma contraction caused by inhibition of antidiuretic hormone release, leading to hemoconcentration with hematocrits greater than 20 gm/dL and arterial or venous thrombosis.[89,90]

Less well recognized is the erythrocytosis associated with testosterone replacement therapy by any route and with anabolic steroid use to boost athletic performance.[91,92] Androgens not only increase the red cell mass, presumably through an erythropoietin-mediated mechanism, they also cause plasma volume contraction,[45] which only serves to magnify the increase in blood viscosity. Either effect can predominate, and thrombosis or sudden death can be the outcome. Testosterone therapy can, of course, precipitate sleep apnea, and other exposures such as diuretic therapy, tobacco use, or ethanol ingestion will also aggravate the situation.

The introduction of recombinant erythropoietin as a therapeutic agent was accompanied by its surreptitious use as an effective surrogate for blood doping in athletes. These athletes are at risk for sudden death because, like androgenic steroids, recombinant erythropoietin causes plasma volume contraction as it expands the red cell mass.[44] This is the antithesis of the physiologic response to high-level exercise conditioning, in which there is plasma volume expansion with little or no increase in the red cell mass.[93] To prevent erythropoietin abuse, effective techniques have been developed to detect recombinant erythropoietin in body fluids because of its unique signature on isoelectric focusing.[94]

Finally, an absolute erythrocytosis was an unexpected complication of the use of the vascular endothelial growth factor receptor antagonist SU5416.[95]

Polycythemia Vera

Polycythemia vera, discussed in detail in Chapter 36, is the only clonal or malignant cause of erythrocytosis. Although erythrocytosis is the only feature that separates polycythemia vera phenotypically from its companion myeloproliferative disorders, idiopathic myelofibrosis and essential thrombocytosis, it, like these disorders, involves a multipotent hematopoietic stem cell. Polycythemia vera, in contrast to all other forms of erythrocytosis, is usually associated with an increase in the plasma volume, which can be exacerbated by splenomegaly.[47] This leads to masking of the erythrocytosis when the hematocrit or hemoglobin is relied upon alone. A normal hemoglobin or hematocrit level in the presence of significant splenomegaly suggests that the red cell mass is actually increased. Similarly, microcytic erythrocytosis is also a clue to the presence of an absolute increase in red cell mass, although not absolutely diagnostic for polycythemia vera.[96] The important conclusion is that, because erythrocytosis is the only specific phenotypic feature of polycythemia vera, the diagnosis of this disorder requires a demonstration that there is an absolute increase in red cell mass established by direct measurement of the red cell mass and plasma volume by isotope dilution. A number of diagnostic tests have been proposed for polycythemia vera but none are specific (Table 82–3).

Newer surrogate epigenetic markers indicative of polycythemia vera include overexpression of granulocyte messenger RNA for PRV-1 (CD177),[97] impaired expression of the platelet thrombopoietin receptor Mpl[98] and the JAK2 V617F mutation; however, none are specific for polycythemia vera.[99]

TABLE 82–3. Diagnostic Issues in Polycythemia Vera

Serum erythropoietin	Not specific
Cytogenetics	Abnormal in less than 25% of patients at diagnosis
Clonal assays	Applicable only in informative women
Bone marrow aspiration and biopsy	Can be normal; not specific
Erythroid progenitor cell assays	Not widely available, not standardized, not specific
Computed tomography scanning for spleen size	Not standardized, not specific

MANAGEMENT

Therapeutic phlebotomy is a safe and immediately effective therapy that not only reduces the red cell mass but also quickly expands the plasma volume. Thus, with the exception of plasma volume contraction caused by excessive diuresis or impaired antidiuretic hormone production, phlebotomy is as appropriate when plasma volume contraction is the problem as when there is absolute erythrocytosis. The exception is erythrocytosis caused by a high-oxygen-affinity hemoglobin. In these instances, red cell mass reduction by phlebotomy would be inappropriate in the absence of symptoms or signs of hyperviscosity.

The use of therapeutic phlebotomy has also been a matter of debate in patients with primary familial or congenital erythrocytosis caused by erythropoietin receptor mutations. This debate has been fueled in part by the athletic prowess of the propositus in the first described kindred, who was an Olympic cross-country skiing champion.[100] However, thrombotic events have been observed in other kindreds with erythropoietin receptor mutations. Patients with so-called Chuvash polycythemia in whom *VHL* gene mutations permit unregulated survival of HIF-1α also have an increase in thrombotic events.[88] Any doubt that congenital erythrocytosis predisposes to adverse events should be dispelled by observations in transgenic mice forced to overexpress erythropoietin, in which heart failure, hypertension, hemorrhage resulting from impaired clot formation, and shortened survival were major features.[101,102]

Therapeutic phlebotomy has also been successfully employed in patients with chronic lung disease. Although it does not improve airway function, it does improve cerebral blood flow and cognition; it also reduces blood viscosity.[103] In patients with cyanotic congenital heart disease, because the risk of cerebrovascular thrombosis has been considered to be low,[104] and because this complication has been associated with microcytic erythrocytosis,[105] it has been argued that phlebotomy should only be employed to alleviate symptoms of hyperviscosity, such as headache, dizziness, confusion, tinnitus, scotomata, fatigue, and paresthesias.[104] This is, of course, a

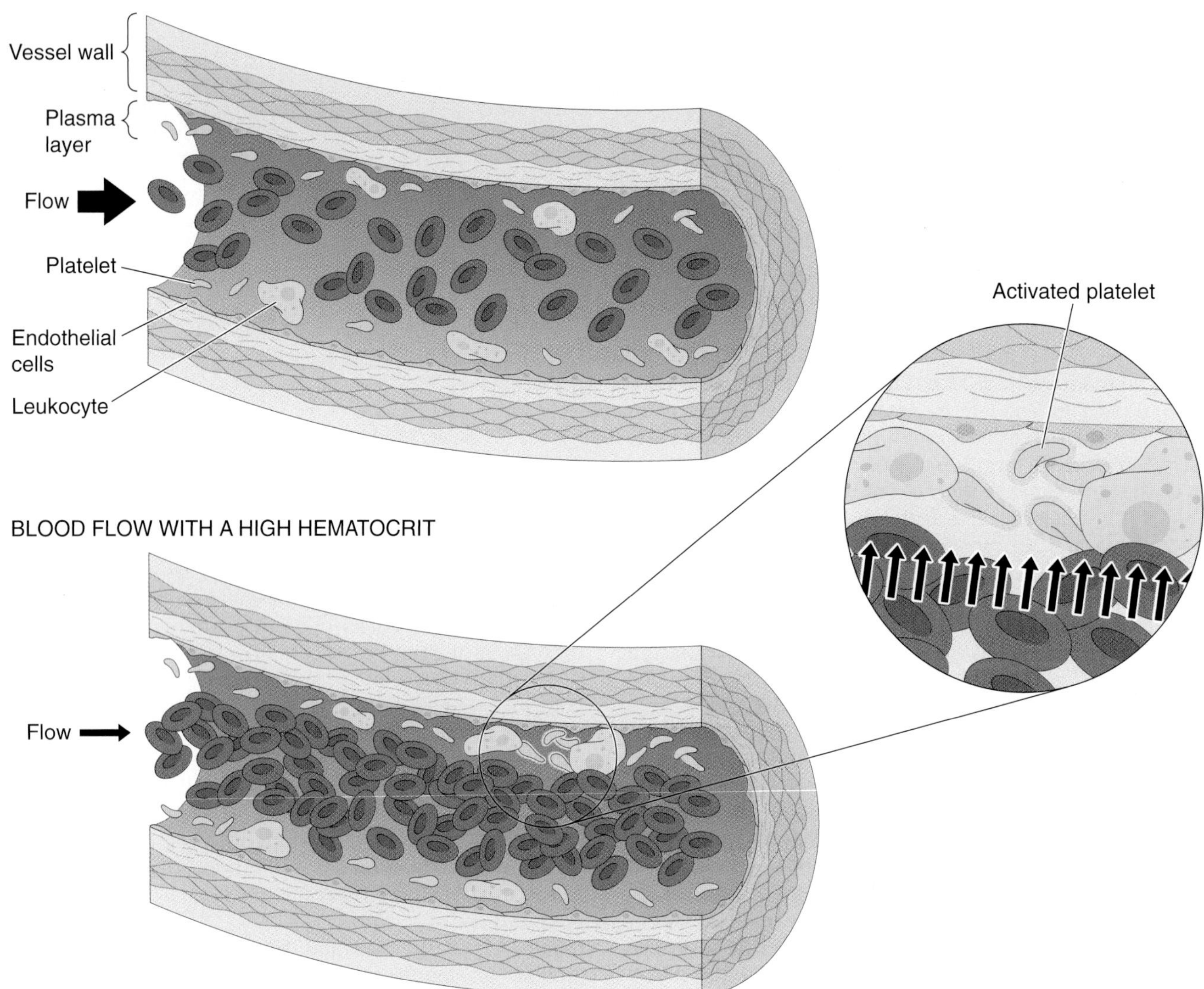

Figure 82–6. Effect of the red cell mass on intravascular cell-cell interactions. As the red cell mass expands, platelets, leukocytes, and endothelial cells are brought in to closer contact, enhancing the opportunity for interactions and thrombogenesis.

circular argument because, by alleviating hyperviscosity, thrombosis will be prevented and cardiac output and tissue perfusion will be improved.[106] What are also missing in this argument are the observations that, in addition to alleviating symptoms of hyperviscosity, phlebotomy improves hemostasis in a situation in which the risk of hemorrhage is increased, and, by reducing the red cell mass, may serve to limit infarct size if a thrombosis does occur.[107] Likewise, a reduction in red cells will reduce vessel wall–platelet interactions (Fig. 82–6) and platelet aggregation.[108] Phlebotomy also improves renal function in hypoxic patients with erythrocytosis. In cases of cyanotic congenital heart disease, phlebotomy may induce hypovolemia. For the erythrocytosis associated with chronic pulmonary disease, a hematocrit of no greater than 55% is a reasonable target, and in cyanotic congenital heart disease, a hematocrit of 65% is commonly used. In both, the response of the patient is the best criterion.

In polycythemia vera, where tissue hypoxia is not an issue and thrombosis or hemorrhage resulting from hyperviscosity are major and often life-threatening complications, phlebotomy is a cornerstone of therapy. Phlebotomy improves platelet function, reduces the risk of hemorrhage, and does not accelerate the disease.[109] Iron deficiency in an adult in the absence of anemia does not impair aerobic function.[110] Perhaps the reluctance to use phlebotomy therapy is a consequence of the Polycythemia Vera Study Group's major clinical trial in which an inappropriately high hematocrit value (50%) was selected as the target.[111] This target hematocrit was not only too high for women, it was also too high for most men. Because there is often plasma volume expansion, which masks the true hematocrit even in the absence of splenomegaly, the optimal hematocrit target is less than 42% in a woman or less than 45% in a man, which not only improves cerebral perfusion but reduces thrombotic events.[112]

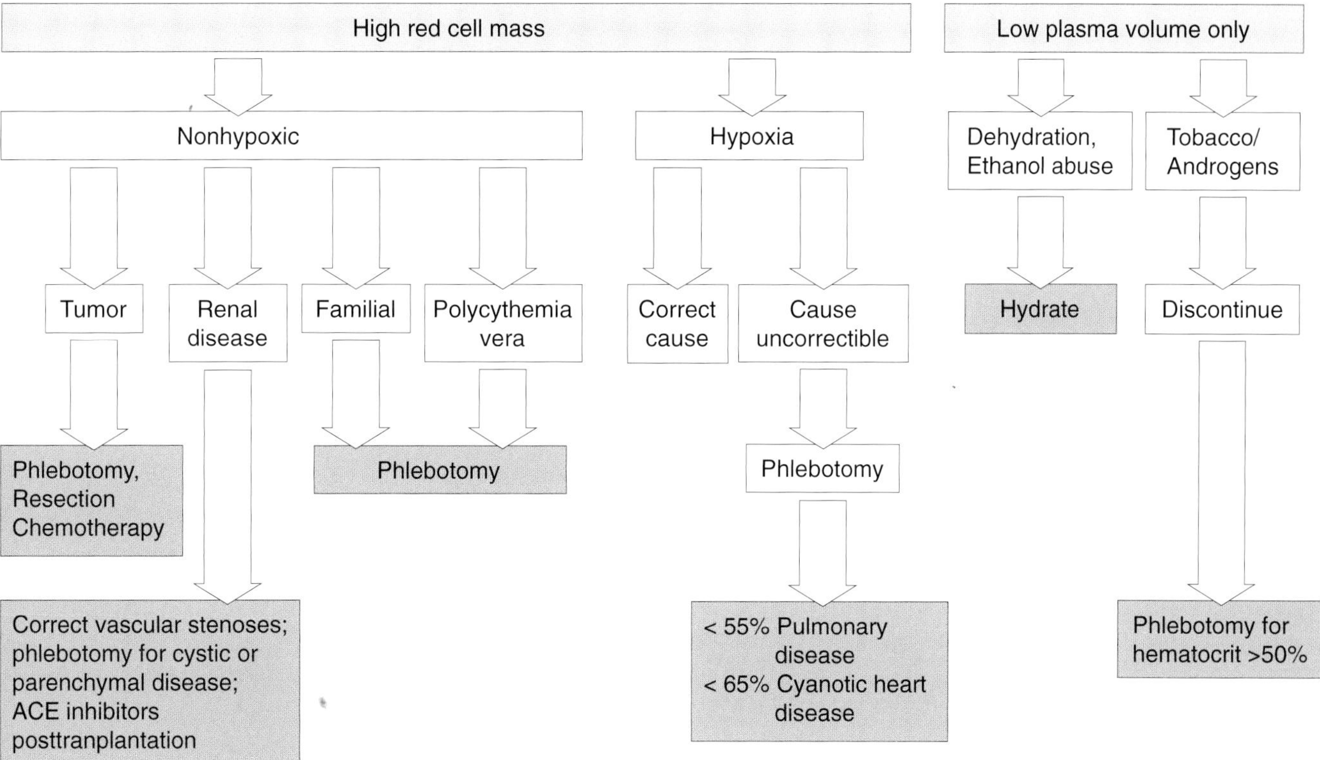

Figure 82–7. Management algorithm for erythrocytosis.

Once the red cell mass has been mechanically controlled by phlebotomy and the diagnostic evaluation has identified the etiology of the erythrocytosis, specific therapy can be instituted as outlined in the management algorithm in Figure 82–7.

Suggested Readings*

Eisensehr I, Noachtar S: Haematological aspects of obstructive sleep apnoea. Sleep Med Rev 5:207–221, 2001.

Gordeuk VR, Sergueeva AI, Miasnikova GY, et al: Congenital disorder of oxygen-sensing: association of the homozygous Chuvash polycythemia VHL mutation with thrombosis and vascular abnormalities but not tumors. Blood 103:3924–3932, 2004.

Lamy T, Devillers A, Bernard M, et al: Inapparent polycythemia vera: an unrecognized diagnosis. Am J Med 102:14–20, 1997.

Pearson TC, Guthrie DL, Simpson J, et al: Interpretation of measured red cell mass and plasma volume in adults. Expert Panel on Radionuclides of the International Council for Standardization in Haematology. Br J Haematol 89:748–756, 1995.

Pearson TC, Weatherly-Mein G: Vascular occlusive episodes and venous haematocrit in primary proliferative polycythaemia. Lancet 2:1219–1221, 1978.

Scott VL, Dodson SF, Kang Y: The hepatopulmonary syndrome. Surg Clin North Am 79:23–41, 1999.

Semenza GL: HIF-1: mediator of physiological and pathophysiological responses to hypoxia. J Appl Physiol 88:1474–1480, 2000.

Spivak JL: The clinical physiology of erythropoietin. Semin Hematol 30:2–11, 1993.

Spivak JL: Polycythemia vera: myths, mechanisms, and management. Blood 100:4272–4290, 2002.

Vlahakos DV, Marathias KP, Agroyannis B, Madias NE: Posttransplant erythrocytosis. Kidney Int 63:1187–1194, 2003.

Full references for this chapter can be found on accompanying CD-ROM.

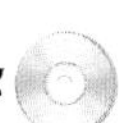

CHAPTER 83

Hematologic Abnormalities in Chronic Kidney Disease

Arrigo Schieppati, MD, Anna Falanga, MD, and Giuseppe Remuzzi, MD

KEY POINTS

Hematologic Abnormalities in Chronic Kidney Disease

- Anemia is a common feature of chronic kidney disease and is associated with cardiovascular morbidity and mortality.
- The cause of anemia of renal failure is mainly the erythropoietin deficiency, but a role is played by the uremic condition, the bleeding tendency of uremia, hemolysis, and iron and folic acid deficiency.
- The development of recombinant human erythropoietin has been one of the major breakthroughs in the cure of patients with renal failure, providing them with an effective means to correct anemia.
- Chronic kidney disease is associated with an increased susceptibility to infections, which can be in part attributed to a number of abnormal functions of leukocytes in uremia.
- Uremia is complicated by a bleeding tendency, which once was a major cause of morbidity and mortality.
- There are a number of treatments available that correct the bleeding tendency of uremia. They include improved dialysis schedules, correction of anemia, and administration of agents that improve platelet–vessel wall interaction.

INTRODUCTION

In his *Epistola Anatomico-medica XLI,* the Italian anatomist and pathologist Giambattista Morgagni (1682–1771) described a woman with severe bleeding (epistaxis and hematemesis) who had the odor of urine on her breath.[1] This is probably the first description of the association of uremia and bleeding tendency, one of several hematologic manifestations associated with renal diseases. Other abnormalities include reduced production of red blood cells, altered platelet function and coagulation abnormalities, and white blood cell dysfunction. This chapter reviews the pathogenesis, diagnosis, and treatment of the hematologic disorders associated with renal diseases.

EFFECTS OF CHRONIC KIDNEY DISEASE ON ERYTHROPOIESIS

Anemia is a common consequence of chronic kidney disease and develops well before the stage of uremia is reached.[2] The correction of anemia by recombinant human erythropoietin (rhEPO) has shown that erythropoietin deficiency is the primary underlying defect in anemia of chronic kidney disease.[3,4] Prior to the introduction of rhEPO, approximately a quarter of chronic uremic patients were blood transfusion dependent. It has now become apparent that many symptoms previously attributed to uremia are in fact due to anemia. The most common cause of death among dialysis patients is cardiovascular disease, and anemia significantly contributes to the development of heart failure in chronic uremia.[5–7]

There is a direct relationship between the severity of anemia and the degree of renal function impairment. Anemia is virtually a constant feature of acute or chronic kidney disease. As renal function progressively deteriorates, the hematocrit continues to decline and may reach concentrations as low as 15–20%. In a cohort study of 604 patients with renal disease of different severity, a significant direct correlation between predicted glomerular filtration rate and hematocrit was found, along with a significant inverse correlation between serum creatinine and hematocrit.[8] In this study, anemia was noted early in renal disease: 45% of patients with serum creatinine of 2 mg/dL or less had a hematocrit of less than 36%, and 8% had a hematocrit less than 30%.

The anemia associated with renal disease is normocytic and normochromic. Reticulocyte count is low for the degree of anemia, and the erythroid bone marrow appears hypoplastic, without interference with leukopoiesis or megakaryocytopoiesis.[9]

Pathophysiology of Anemia in Chronic Kidney Disease

The anemia of chronic kidney disease is a complex disorder determined by a variety of factors. The primary defect is decreased erythropoiesis, although a number of other factors may play contributory roles, such as hemolysis, which is frequently present, bleeding, and iron or folic acid deficiency (Fig. 83–1).

The Uremic Milieu

In the predialysis era, it was thought that uremic waste products could play a role in the pathogenesis of anemia,[10] but the persistence of anemia with the advent of dialysis suggested other causes. The importance of the uremic milieu in red blood cell survival is documented by the shortened half-life of red blood cells from normal subjects after transfusion into uremic patients.[11,12] Lipid peroxidation of the cell membrane also contributes to shortened red cell survival, through a mechanism of defective antioxidant activity.[13] The increased bleeding tendency of the uremic state, frequent blood samplings, occult blood loss, and blood loss during hemodialysis are additional factors contributing to the anemia in patients with chronic kidney disease.

The Role of Erythropoietin

The existence of a factor that stimulates erythropoiesis was first suspected by Carnot and Deflandre in 1906, when they demonstrated that an increase in red blood cell count could be induced by injecting serum from anemic rabbits into normal rabbits. They suggested that the serum contained a substance called "hémopoietine" capable of stimulating the bone marrow to produce red blood cells. In 1958, Gurney and coworkers reported that patients with renal disease and anemia lacked an erythropoietic stimulating factor in their plasma.[14] In 1977, Miyake and coworkers purified human erythropoietin,[15] and in 1986 Lai and colleagues[16] characterized its molecular structure. The current knowledge of the structure and function of erythropoietin is described in several reviews.[17,18]

Hypoxia causes the production of a protein named hypoxia-inducible factor-1.[19] This factor binds to an oxygen-sensitive enhancer located immediately downstream from the transcription stop site of the gene for erythropoietin (located on chromosome 7), and activates the transcription of the *EPO* gene. An in situ hybridization technique for *EPO* messenger RNA has shown that the site of production is in the interstitial cells of the renal cortex close to the base of the proximal tubule cells.[20] In vitro experiments suggest that the same cell sensible to hypoxia may produce erythropoietin. Oxygen deficiency may be sensed effectively in the renal cortex, and reduced capillary flow also might induce increased erythropoietin production (Fig. 83–2).

Several other factors, besides anemia and hypoxia, may play a role in either the production or the action of erythropoietin. Cobalt, androgens, and insulin-derived growth factor seem to work as agonists, and inflammatory cytokines as antagonists. The underlying kidney disease does not seem to influence erythropoietin production, with one notable exception. In autosomal dominant polycystic kidney disease, plasma erythropoietin levels are roughly twice as high as those seen in other renal diseases.[21] This is associated with a higher than average hemoglobin concentration and hematocrit.

Treatment of Anemia in Chronic Kidney Disease

Hematopoietic Growth Factors

Recombinant Human Erythropoietin

The cloning and expression of the human *EPO* gene was reported in 1985,[22] and in 1986 the first clinical experience with recombinant human erythropoietin in patients with chronic kidney disease and anemia was published.[23] rhEPO given by intravenous bolus to 10 patients

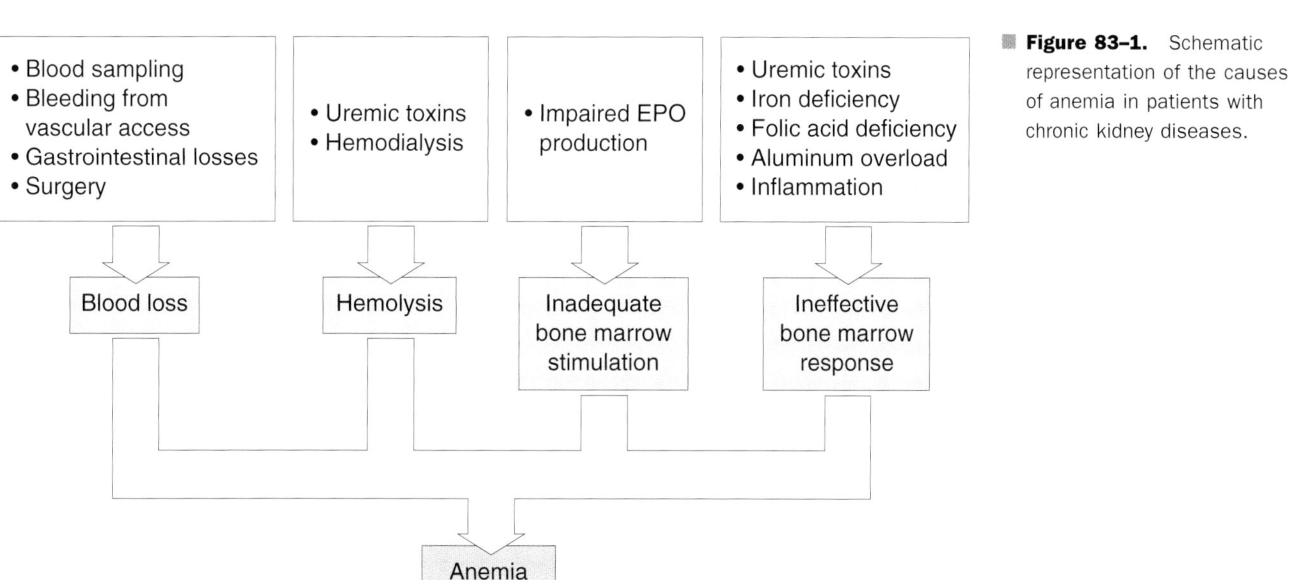

Figure 83–1. Schematic representation of the causes of anemia in patients with chronic kidney diseases.

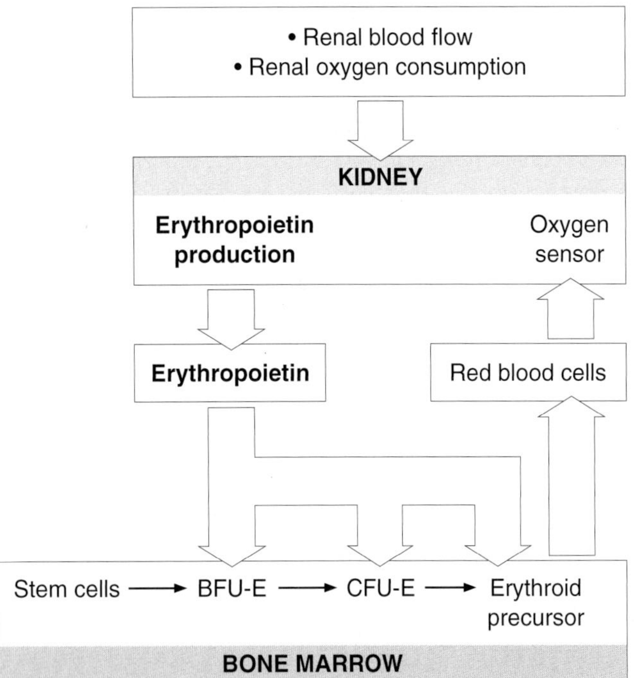

Figure 83–2. Feedback control of red cell production by erythropoietin. The surface of maturing progenitor cells in bone marrow contains erythropoietin receptors that first disappear at the early precursor-cell stage. The receptors close a feedback loop, between a renal oxygen sensor and bone marrow progenitor cells, that ensures that under normal conditions the rate of red cell production matches the need for oxygen-carrying red cells in the circulation. BFU-E, burst-forming units–erythroid; CFU-E, colony-forming units–erythroid. (Modified from Erslev AJ: Erythropoietin. N Engl J Med 324:1339–1344, 1991.)

three times per week raised the mean hemoglobin concentration from 6.1 to 10.3 gm/dL within 12 weeks. The efficacy results of combined Phase I and II clinical trials with rhEPO were reported in 1987[24] and demonstrated a dose-dependent response. The efficacy of rhEPO therapy was demonstrated also in uremic patients not yet on dialysis,[25–27] and in patients receiving continuous ambulatory peritoneal dialysis.[28] In 1989, the Food and Drug Administration (FDA) approved the human use of rhEPO. The drug became rapidly a mainstay of the management of patients on chronic dialysis.

rhEPO contains the identical 165–amino acid sequence of natural erythropoietin, but the glycosylated moiety is different. There are two forms of rhEPO: erythropoietin alpha and erythropoietin beta. The first one is produced by genomic DNA and the second one by complementary DNA; they differ from each other in the oligosaccharide component. Both forms of rhEPO are available for clinical use; they do not show any difference in pharmacokinetics and efficacy.[29] The half-life of rhEPO ranges from 4 to 13 hours after intravenous administration, and is greater than 24 hours when administered subcutaneously. With the subcutaneous route, levels peak at 8–12 hours and decline slowly thereafter; maximum levels with subcutaneous administration are only about 10% of those achieved after the same intravenous dose.

TABLE 83–1. Recommendations for Erythropoietin Administration

Hemodialysis	
Erythropoietin*	Subcutaneous route (preferred by most guidelines): 80–120 units/kg/wk, two or three doses per week Intravenous route (more comfortable for patients): 120–180 units/kg/wk, two or three doses per week
Darbepoetin	Subcutaneous or intravenous route: 0.45 µg/kg/wk once a week
Peritoneal Dialysis, Chronic Kidney Disease in Predialysis Phase	
Erythropoietin*	Subcutaneous route (preferred by most guidelines): 80–120 units/kg/wk, two or three doses per week
Darbepoetin	Subcutaneous or intravenous route: 0.45 µg/kg/wk once a week

*Note of caution: In many Europe countries, erythropoietin alpha is not licensed for subcutaneous administration because of the risk of pure red cell aplasia.

Both alpha and beta rhEPO preparations appear to be eliminated by primarily nonrenal routes.

Darbepoetin (Novel Erythropoiesis Stimulating Protein)

Darbepoetin alpha, also named novel erythropoiesis stimulating protein (NESP), is a molecule that stimulates erythropoiesis by the same mechanism as erythropoietin.[30] Darbepoetin contains 5 N-linked carbohydrate chains, two more than rhEPO, and has increased molecular weight and greater negative charge.[31] The first pharmacokinetic study of darbepoetin reported that the half-life after a single injection is approximately three times longer than that of rhEPO (25.3 vs. 8.5 hours) following intravenous administration.[32] For subcutaneous administration, the mean half-life of darbepoetin is 48.8 hours. Clinical studies in more than 1500 patients have concluded that darbepoetin is as effective and safe as rhEPO in the treatment of anemia of chronic kidney disease.[33]

Treatment with Recombinant Erythropoietin

The U.S. Renal Data System (USRDS) collects data on all patients on renal replacement therapy. It reported that, in 1991 (2 years after the FDA approval of rhEPO), more than 50% of patients on dialysis had a hemoglobin less than 10 gm/dL.[34] In 2001, this had fallen to less than 10% of dialysis patients. According to the USRDS, the mean hemoglobin level in the dialysis population is 11.7 gm/dL, and weekly rhEPO doses are 17,000 units. The response to erythropoietin is dose dependent, but varies among patients.[35] The response is dependent on the route of administration (intravenous vs. subcutaneous) and the frequency of administration (daily, twice weekly, three times weekly). Response should be expected within 3 months, although the dose of erythropoietin required to reach a target hematocrit may vary (Table 83–1).

The National Kidney Foundation Kidney Disease Outcomes Quality Initiative (K/DOQI) work group guidelines[36] recommend subcutaneous administration of rhEPO for the treatment of anemia in predialysis, peritoneal dialysis, and hemodialysis patients. The recommended subcutaneous dose for adult patients is 80–120 units/kg/wk (given in two to three doses). Several investigators, including the K/DOQI work group, suggest relying upon target hemoglobin (Hb), rather than hematocrit (Hct), values.[37] The currently recommended target hemoglobin concentration ranges between 10 and 12 gm/dL, with the K/DOQI work group recommending target values at the higher end of this range (11–12 gm/dL). The median intravenous maintenance dose necessary for maintaining target Hb/Hct at approximately 12 gm/dL and 36% is on average 75 units/kg three times per week, with a wide range (25–200 units/kg three times per week). In some studies, the subcutaneous administration of erythropoietin appeared more effective and less expensive than the intravenous one,[38,39] requiring on average a 32% smaller dose to achieve the same target.[40,41]

Subcutaneous administration of rhEPO is the preferred route of treatment also in patients on peritoneal dialysis. However, intraperitoneal administration may be considered in some of these patients in whom intravenous or subcutaneous administration cannot be performed.[42] To maintain adequate hemoglobin levels, intraperitoneal administration appears to require higher doses of erythropoietin than intravenous or subcutaneous dosing, and it is therefore not convenient.

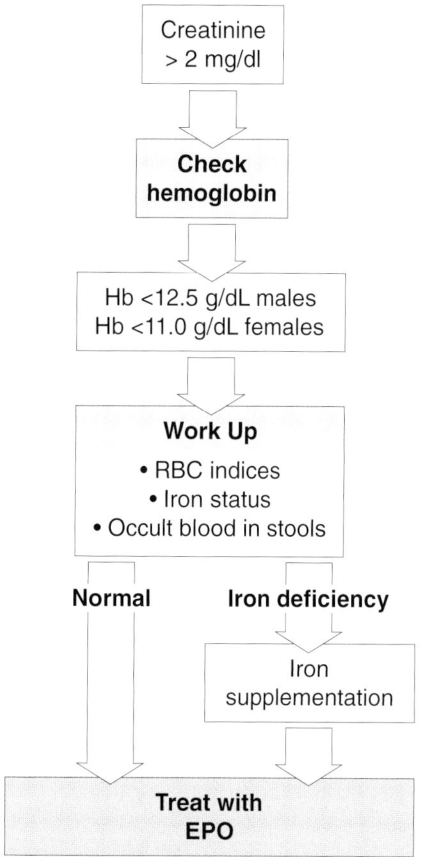

Figure 83–3. Simplified algorithm of anemia treatment in patients with chronic kidney diseases.

Treatment in Predialysis Phase

rhEPO is increasingly used to treat the anemia in patients with chronic renal disease before they reach end-stage renal failure (Fig. 83–3). Increased hemoglobin levels in such patients may provide several benefits, including the amelioration of anemia-induced symptoms, cardiovascular improvement, and decreased mortality.[43–47] The correction of anemia in the predialysis phase is not associated with significant changes in the rate of progression of renal disease, provided that blood pressure is maintained at the target levels.[48] There is some evidence that anemia correction may slow the rate of progression.[49]

The Role of Dialysis

There has long been the impression that removal of more small or mid-sized "toxic" molecules results in higher hemoglobin. However, the data are controversial. Analysis of a very large population of 2094 rhEPO-treated hemodialysis patients from the USRDS Dialysis Morbidity and Mortality Study (DMMS) showed that the effect of the delivered dose of dialysis on the response to rhEPO was evident only for those who were dialyzed with a synthetic dialyzer.[50] Apart from the specific effect of a better removal of uremic toxins, an adequate dialysis may ameliorate the anemia as a consequence of improvements in red cell survival, blood coagulation, nutritional status, and well-being.

Correction of Anemia in Transplanted Patients

After renal transplantation, anemia is rapidly corrected by the erythropoietin produced by the graft. Erythropoietin serum levels double within 7 days after transplantation and remain elevated until the anemia is corrected. In some recipients, iron deficiency secondary to increased iron utilization may occur,[51] but it spontaneously corrects.

Posttransplantation erythrocytosis defines a condition of increased hemoglobin (16–17 gm/dL) that develops in some transplant patients[52,53]—7.6% in a recent study.[52] It is due to increased erythropoietic activity independent of the erythropoietin plasma level. Erythroid burst-forming unit sensitivity in vitro to increasing erythropoietin concentrations can also be shown.[52] Angiotensin-converting enzyme inhibitors and losartan, an angiotensin II type 1 receptor antagonist, diminish posttransplantation erythrocytosis without altering erythropoietin plasma levels.[54]

Treatment with Darbepoetin

The recommended starting dose of darbepoetin in patients with chronic renal insufficiency or peritoneal dialysis is 0.45 μg/kg administered once weekly by subcutaneous injection.[55] The recommended starting dose for patients on hemodialysis is 0.45 μg/kg administered once weekly by either the intravenous or subcutaneous route.[55] Patients who are being treated with rhEPO may be switched to darbepoetin by determining the equivalent dose of darbepoetin on a simple dose conversion chart, based upon the results of clinical experience.[56] As a rule of thumb, the conversion rate from rhEPO to darbepoetin is 200 : 1, but the rate of conversion may be much different (e.g., 900 : 1).

Darbepoetin should be given once weekly to patients who previously received rhEPO two or three times weekly, and once every 2 weeks to patients who previously received rhEPO once weekly.[57] The same route of administration (intravenous or subcutaneous) may be maintained when switching patients from rhEPO to darbepoetin. The dose of darbepoetin should be adjusted to achieve and maintain a target hemoglobin level of 11–12 gm/dL. Doses should not be adjusted more than once per month because the achievement of a steady-state hemoglobin response to darbepoetin may require a period of 2–6 weeks. Maintenance doses may be as infrequent as once a month.[57,58]

Side Effects of Treatment

The incidence of some of the most frequently reported adverse events has been reported as follows: arterial hypertension (0.75 events per patient-year), clotted vascular access (0.25), and hyperkalemia (0.11). The relationship of rhEPO therapy to seizures is uncertain. The real incidence of these events is difficult to ascertain because seizures are not infrequent in the dialysis population. However, the rate of seizures during the first 90 days of rhEPO therapy appears to be higher than that during the subsequent 90 days.[59,60] Strict control of the rate of hemoglobin rise (no more than 1.5 gm/dL in a 4-week period) and close monitoring of the blood pressure appear warranted.

Clotting of Vascular Access

Clotting of the vascular access and the artificial kidney are frequently reported in rhEPO-treated patients.[61] In patients treated with either erythropoietin alpha or erythropoietin beta, increases in factor VIII, von Willebrand factor antigen, fibrinogen, and whole blood platelet aggregation have been observed. These effects favor a tendency to thrombosis. Increased anticoagulation with heparin may be required. Other thrombotic events of concern are cerebrovascular accidents and transient ischemic attacks, and myocardial infarction. A statistically certain relationship has not been established between the rate of rise in hemoglobin and the incidence of thrombotic events. Neither higher hemoglobin concentrations nor higher rhEPO doses adversely affect the survival of a prosthetic arteriovenous access graft.

Hyperkalemia

Hyperkalemia may be more frequent in patients on dialysis after the initiation of rhEPO therapy. Mechanisms of the increased tendency to hyperkalemia may be a less efficient dialysis (blood flow being equal, a higher hematocrit means less plasma available for correction) and lesser compliance with dietary prescriptions because patients on rhEPO experience improved well-being and quality of life, with enhanced appetite.

Hypertension

Hypertension is the most commonly reported side effect of rhEPO therapy in end-stage renal failure patients. In a review of 47 publications including 3428 patients, development or worsening of hypertension was found in 785 of them (23%) during rhEPO treatment.[62] Increased blood pressure levels have been reported more often during the first 90 days of therapy. The following risk factors for developing hypertension associated with rhEPO therapy have been identified: preexisting hypertension, rapid correction of anemia, and high doses of rhEPO. Intravenous administration of rhEPO is not considered a risk factor.

High blood pressure in rhEPO-treated patients can be effectively managed by reducing dry body weight, starting or increasing antihypertensive therapy, and reducing the dose of rhEPO. Regression of left ventricular hypertrophy and normalization of cardiac index and other hemodynamic and functional parameters are evident during treatment with rhEPO, and are maintained afterward, providing adequate control of blood pressure.[61] The beneficial effects of rhEPO therapy on the cardiovascular system outweigh the risk of increased blood pressure.

Pure Red Cell Aplasia

A most alarming side effect of rhEPO use is the development of antierythropoietin antibodies in association with severe transfusion-dependent anemia, caused by a pure red cell bone marrow aplasia.[63,64] Only three cases had been reported in the literature before the publication of the seminal work of Casadevall and colleagues in early 2002,[65] which described and characterized 13 patients with pure red cell aplasia who had developed antibodies able to block the formation of erythroid colonies by normal bone marrow cells. Anemia developed on average 10 months after therapy initiation, with a range of 1 to 92 months. To date, the total number of cases of rhEPO-induced pure red cell aplasia known from the literature is 250.[66] Only four cases of antibody-mediated pure red cell aplasia associated with darbepoetin have been reported despite its use in thousands of patients, some of whom have been treated for nearly 4 years with this agent. In these four patients, other forms of rhEPO were used prior to darbepoetin. No cases have been reported in patients treated only with darbepoetin.

When pure red cell aplasia is suspected, rhEPO administration should be immediately interrupted. It is also recommended to avoid switching patients to other forms of erythropoietin or to darbepoetin, because the antierythropoietin antibodies cross-react with all commercially available recombinant erythropoietic products.[67] Treatment with immunosuppressive therapy is associated with recovery from aplasia.[68]

TABLE 83–2. Causes of Inadequate Response* to Erythropoietin Therapy

Infection/inflammation
Chronic blood loss
Malnutrition, folate or vitamin B_{12} deficiency
Aluminum toxicity
Osteitis fibrosa
Malignancies
Hemolysis
Pure red blood cell aplasia

*Definition of inadequate response: failure to achieve target hemoglobin at a dose of 450 units/kg/wk IV, within 4–6 months, after iron supplementation.

Causes of Inadequate Response to Erythropoietin

Hyporesponsiveness to rhEPO has been defined as the failure to achieve target hemoglobin in the presence of adequate iron stores at a dose of 450 units/kg/wk intravenously within 4–6 months,[62] or the failure to maintain it subsequently at that dose.[69] Several conditions have been associated with inadequate response to rhEPO. Iron deficiency (both absolute and functional) is the most common cause and is discussed in detail.[70–75] Other factors are listed in Table 83–2.

Iron Deficiency

A suboptimal response to rhEPO most commonly results from failure of delivery of an adequate amount of iron to the erythron. Enhanced iron utilization resulting from rhEPO-induced red blood cell formation can quickly deplete iron stores previously reduced by poor iron absorption, occult gastrointestinal bleeding, or dialysis-related blood losses.[20] Treatment with rhEPO is, at this time, the most common cause of iron deficiency.

The most accurate assessment of the iron stores is by staining the bone marrow aspirate for iron with Perls Prussian blue stain.[73] In the absence of this reliable, but invasive, reference standard, the iron status is commonly assessed by serum iron concentration, serum ferritin, transferrin saturation, and red blood cell indices.[74] Serum iron concentration fluctuates during rhEPO administration, but the serum ferritin is a good indicator of iron stores; the transferrin saturation index appears to be even better (higher sensitivity and similar specificity).[75]

The failure to make enough iron available to meet the demands of enhanced erythropoiesis despite the presence of adequate iron stores, as reflected by the level of serum ferritin, has been defined as "functional iron deficiency" (in contrast to "absolute iron deficiency"). The red blood cells appear hypochromic (with a mean corpuscular hemoglobin concentration <28 gm/dL) when mobilization of iron from stores and its transport to the erythron become inadequate. A percentage of circulating hypochromic red blood cells greater than 10% (normal range: <2.5% of circulating red cells), in the presence of adequate iron stores and the absence of hemoglobinopathies or inflammatory diseases, should be diagnostic of functional iron deficiency.[76,77]

The primary goal is to ascertain whether an inadequate response to rhEPO is due to iron deficiency or another cause. By first replenishing and then maintaining iron stores, it is possible to achieve the target hematocrit with the lowest necessary dose of rhEPO. In the presence of adequate response to rhEPO, iron supplementation should be targeted at keeping the level of serum ferritin greater than 100 ng/mL, the transferrin saturation more than 20%, and hypochromic red cells less than 10% (Box 83–1).

The intravenous route is mandatory in the presence of absolute or functional iron deficiency; oral iron supplementation is often unsuccessful, because rapid replacement of the iron consumed is not well tolerated, and gastrointestinal absorption is diminished by the presence of phosphate binders or histamine H_2 receptor blockers. In the maintenance phase, oral iron alone can only rarely sustain the response to rhEPO, as has been suggested by the experience on a national scale in the United States when iron dextran was unavailable for an extended time. The intravenous administration of iron enhances the erythropoietic response despite apparently adequate iron stores.

The availability of new, well-tolerated, parenteral iron preparations—iron dextran, iron saccharate, and sodium ferric gluconate complex—is a factor promoting the use of the intravenous route in the maintenance phase of rhEPO therapy.[78] Supplementation of intravenous iron

Box 83–1. Recommendation for Iron Support

- Iron status should be checked and maintained at a transferrin saturation greater than 20% and serum ferritin greater than 100 ng/mL.
- Oral iron is the preferred supplementation route for predialysis patients, at a daily dose of at least 200 mg of elemental iron in two divided doses.
- Hemodialysis patients usually are not able to achieve adequate iron status with oral iron, and are given intravenous iron. A variety of schedules are used:
- 100 mg of iron gluconate or 125 mg of iron dextran for 8–10 dialysis sessions has been recommended by guidelines.
- When target iron levels are reached (transferrin saturation >20%, serum ferritin >100 ng/mL), 25–125 mg of iron is given once a week.
- A test dose of 25 mg of intravenous iron dextran or iron gluconate is recommended prior to initiating intravenous therapy.

on a regular basis at a dose of 25–125 of iron dextran or gluconate at the end of each hemodialysis session[79] seems to be superior to bolus therapy[80] in maintaining target hematocrit while requiring significantly less rhEPO.[80,81] Guidelines and treatment schedules for iron supplementation in predialysis, hemodialysis, and continuous ambulatory peritoneal dialysis patients have been published.[79,82]

Resistance to rhEPO sometimes occurs in iron overload (transferrin saturation >50%, and serum ferritin >500–1000 ng/mL), and ascorbate supplementation may prevent it.[83] Iron overload is treated by withholding iron, increasing rhEPO, and performing phlebotomy[62]; the administration of deferoxamine could improve hemosiderosis and maintain the response to rhEPO without iron administration.

Aluminum Overload

In hemodialysis patients, aluminum toxicity may cause microcytic anemia despite normal iron deposits.[84] Aluminum and iron utilize common pathways for intestinal absorption, transport in the plasma, and binding to transferrin; aluminum overload may interfere with iron utilization in the response to rhEPO.[85] The sources of the aluminum accumulation are primarily both gastrointestinal aluminum absorption from antacids used to bind dietary phosphorus and improperly processed water for dialysate. During the last decade, the water for dialysate has been properly processed, and aluminum salts have been widely replaced by calcium-containing phosphate binders, so at present lower serum aluminum levels are generally observed in the dialysis population.

Other Causes

Infectious and inflammatory chronic diseases, malignancies, and secondary hyperparathyroidism may also account for an inadequate response to erythropoietin. For more extensive discussions of these conditions, see Chapter 19 or the literature.[86]

The Effect of Correction of Anemia in Chronic Kidney Disease

Quality of Life

The correction of anemia with rhEPO has virtually eliminated the need for transfusion in most patients with anemia of chronic kidney disease. It has also improved the quality of life as measured by several different parameters. Exercise capacity and tolerance have been measurably increased,[87–89] and surveys of both objective and subjective quality-of-life indicators have shown significant improvement.[90–92]

Survival

The age-adjusted mortality rate for dialysis patients is 3.5 times that of the general population. The most common cause of death is cardiovascular disease. Anemia and hypertension are independent predictors of mortality; anemia is also independently predictive of heart failure. In a study on clinical and laboratory data of 21,899 hemodialysis patients collected in dialysis centers throughout the United States in 1993, hemoglobin concentrations (Hb/Hct = 10/30) less than or equal to 8 gm/dL were associated with a twofold increase in the odds of death when compared with concentrations of 10–11 gm/dL; no improvement in the odds of death was observed for hemoglobin concentrations higher than 11 gm/dL.[93] Conversely, in another study, the relative risk of death was significantly decreased with a hematocrit of 33–36%.[94] In a study of 3111 adult hemodialysis patients in 17 prospective clinical trials, a reduction in mortality risk (of about 20% after 1 year on rhEPO therapy), in comparison with 246 untreated patients, was observed, and in the long term the percentage of total mortality caused by cardiovascular disease was reduced as well.[95]

Target Hematocrit

Significant relief of symptoms, with a low risk of side effects, has been observed when the Hb/Hct in hemodialysis patients is between 9.5/29 and 11/33.[96] Additional improvements in the quality of life, cardiac function, physical work capacity, cognitive function, and sexual function have been reported at a hematocrit of 36–39%.[61] The benefits and risks of complete correction of anemia (hematocrit 38–42%) and the optimal target concentration have not yet been established. Clinicians are reluctant to totally correct anemia in end-stage renal disease because (1) the morbidity of anemia is not well appreciated, (2) there is a bias that moderate anemia is acceptable for dialysis patients, (3) the principles of rhEPO therapy are not followed, (4) there is an inordinate amount of concern about the side effects of therapy, and (5) the cost of the treatment is high.

EFFECTS OF CHRONIC KIDNEY DISEASE ON WHITE BLOOD CELLS

Chronic kidney disease is associated with an increased susceptibility to infections. Many studies have found that leukocyte chemotaxis is impaired in uremia.[97–102] Impairment of chemotactic function may be associated with a circulating inhibitor of chemotaxis,[99,102] a decreased intracellular cyclic GMP/cyclic AMP ratio,[103,104] or a plasma factor blocking granulocyte membrane receptors. Interestingly, the chemotactic activity of granulocytes is diminished further, rather than corrected, by hemodialysis.[105] Studies of granulocyte phagocytosis and respiratory burst in uremia are conflicting, with some demonstrating normal phagocytic and bactericidal activities in uremic granulocytes,[106] and others showing depressed phagocytic activity[107] and respiratory burst.[108]

Hemodialysis has a profound effect on granulocyte kinetics. During the first 2 hours of hemodialysis, all patients develop peripheral neutropenia mediated by complement activation on the dialysis membrane[109] and sequestration of granulocytes in the lung. In the hours following hemodialysis, the release of neutrophils from the bone marrow and sites of sequestration produces rebound neutrophilia.

Several laboratories have studied the effects of hemodialysis on white blood cell integrins, a family of transmembrane glycoproteins that interact with endothelial cell ligands as well as with complement components.[110–112] Mac-1, an integrin primarily expressed on granulocytes and macrophages, is a receptor for C3b1[112–114] and is involved in the adhesion of white cells to dialysis membranes.[115–118] During cuprophane hemodialysis, there is a rapid increase in the surface expression of Mac-1 associated with a consistent decrease in granulocyte counts.[119] By contrast, the use of hemophane or polysulfone membranes produces less Mac-1.[119] The finding that surface expression of Mac-1 remains elevated with cuprophane membranes, even when the granulocyte count normalizes, suggests that more than one molecule may be implicated in the mechanism of granulocytopenia during cellulose membrane dialysis. A new family of leukocyte adhesion molecules has been described, and the structure of one of them, LAM-1, has been elucidated.[120] LAM-1 is shed during leukocyte activation by chemotactic factors. LAM-1 shedding associated with decreased endothelial cell binding has also been exhibited by granulocytes harvested early during the first use of a cellulose dialysis membrane. This suggests that, during cellulose hemodialysis, complement activation upregulates Mac-1, producing cell adhesion and sequestration. This is followed by LAM-1 shedding. Possibly, the increased susceptibility to infection exhibited by hemodialysis patients is the consequence of "low" LAM-1 granulocytes and the loss of their capacity to transmigrate to sites of infection. This suggestion is concordant with the higher incidence of infection seen in patients receiving chronic cuprophane hemodialysis as compared to polysulfone hemodialysis.[121]

Monocytes are markedly activated by contact with dialysis membranes, as documented by transient increases in plasma levels of interleukin (IL)-1 and tumor necrosis factor (TNF)[122] during hemodialysis.[123–125] Thus, within 5 minutes of cuprophane hemodialysis, monocytes initiate transcription of IL-1 and TNF in large amounts.[126] In addition, macrophage colony-stimulating factor[127]—the growth factor for monocytes—accumulates in uremia and provides a further stimulus for the synthesis and secretion of IL-1 and TNF by monocytes. Candidate factors for monocyte activation during hemodialysis include complement activation and a component of the dialysis buffer, such as acetate, but also bacterial and endotoxin contaminations and the direct contact of monocytes with the dialysis membrane.

Because IL-1 and TNF upregulate cell metabolism in different systems and increase the expression of genes encoding for various biologically active proteins,[128] the functional consequences of monocyte activation during hemodialysis may be of some importance. The possibility that cytokines released by activated monocytes might augment susceptibility to infections, immune dysfunction, and atherosclerosis has been investigated.[129] It has been known for many years that uremic patients suffer from an acquired form of immunodeficiency characterized by abnormal T-cell proliferation in response to antigenic challenges. This defect could well be the consequence of monocyte dysfunction, because T-cell activation is monocyte dependent. The monocytes in uremic nonresponders to hepatitis B vaccination are unable to deliver to T lymphocytes the necessary signal required for triggering IL-2 synthesis. Consistently, exogenous IL-2 normalizes the proliferative response of uremic T lymphocytes. More recent studies[130,131] have shown that purified IL-1, the monocyte-derived signal for T-cell activation, is unable to normalize the T-cell proliferative response. However, exogenous IL-2 eliminates the defect.[124] This observation is consistent with other studies[131,132] that document reduced IL-2 production by uremic T cells.

Normal T-cell activation is followed by the release of a soluble form of IL-2 receptor (IL-2R) into the circulation.[133] Uremic serum markedly inhibits the release of IL-2R.[131] Further studies are needed to clarify the true clinical impact of reduced surface expression of IL-2R on the immunodeficiency of uremic patients.

EFFECTS OF CHRONIC KIDNEY DISEASE ON HEMOSTASIS

Bleeding in uremia was originally described by Morgagni[1] and beautifully described in a case report by Richard Bright.[134] Ecchymoses and epistaxis are the major bleeding manifestations seen today, with gastrointestinal bleeding, hemopericardium, or subdural hematoma occurring only occasionally.[135] However, the underlying bleeding diathesis remains. Uremic patients who undergo surgery or invasive procedures are always at risk for serious bleeding.

Causes of Uremic Bleeding

Over the past 20 years, research has partially clarified the nature of uremic bleeding. (Table 83–3). The pathogenesis is multifactorial, and the major defects involve platelet–vessel wall and platelet-platelet interactions. The skin bleeding time is the best predictor of clinical bleeding in uremia.[136–138] It depends on platelet number and function, vascular integrity, and the hematocrit and thus gives an excellent overall assessment of primary hemostasis. The platelet count in uremia is usually normal,[139,140] whereas platelet function is impaired. Dense granule content is decreased[141,142] and a storage pool defect with reduction in platelet ADP and serotonin is present. Decreased subnormal platelet ATP release in response to stimuli indicates a defect in granule secretion.[143] Calcium content is increased in uremic platelets,[144] which also mobilize calcium abnormally in response to stimulation.[145]

Several abnormalities of platelet-platelet interaction have also been reported in uremia. They include defective platelet aggregation in vitro in response to various stimuli[141,146–148] and defective platelet thromboxane A_2 production in response to endogenous and exogenous stimuli,[149,150] not correctable by thrombin.[144] In a subpopulation of uremic patients, irreversible platelet aggregation does not occur in response to platelet-activating factor.[151,152] This abnormality is independent of a plasma factor or factors but is probably due to the platelets'

TABLE 83–3. Causes of Uremic Bleeding

Platelet Abnormalities
Subnormal dense granule content
Reduction in intracellular ADP and serotonin
Impaired release of the platelet α-granule protein and β-thromboglobulin
Enhanced intracellular cyclic AMP
Abnormal mobilization of platelet Ca^{2+}
Abnormal platelet arachidonic acid metabolism
Abnormal ex vivo platelet aggregation in response to different stimuli
Defective cyclooxygenase activity
Abnormality of the activation-dependent binding activity of the glycoprotein IIb/IIIa complex
Uremic toxins, especially parathyroid hormone
Abnormal Platelet–Vessel Wall Interactions
Abnormal platelet adhesion
Increased formation of vascular prostaglandin I_2
Altered von Willebrand factor
Anemia
Altered blood rheology
Erythropoietin deficiency
Abnormal Production of Nitric Oxide
Drug Treatment
β-Lactam antibiotics
Third-generation cephalosporins
Nonsteroidal anti-inflammatory drugs

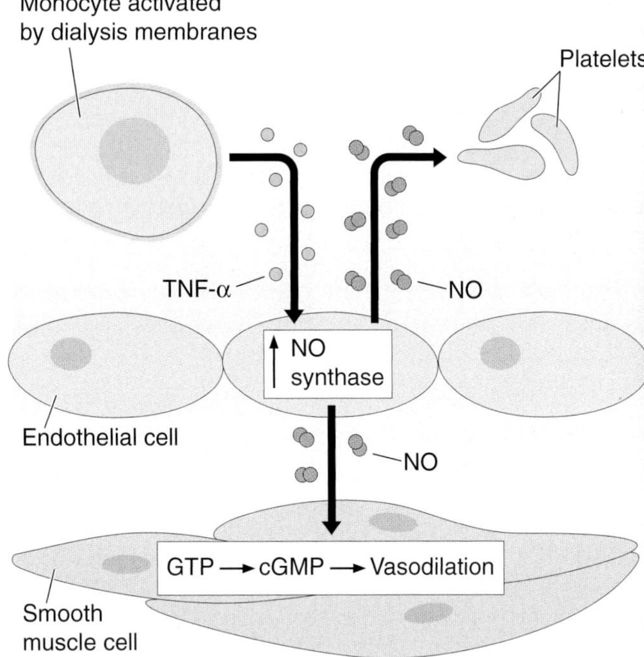

Figure 83–4. Nitric oxide (NO)–mediated disorders in uremia. The contact with dialysis membrane or acetate dialysis buffer activates circulating monocytes that release cytokines, such as tumor necrosis factor-α (TNF-α). TNF-α causes the transcription of inducible NO synthase messenger RNA in vascular endothelial cells that release a large amount of NO either in the circulation or within the vessel wall. NO enters target cells (platelets and smooth muscle cells), where it activates soluble guanylate cyclase, causing impairment of platelet function (hence the bleeding tendency) and relaxation of smooth muscle cells (hence vasodilation).

reduced capacity to form thromboxane A_2 in response to platelet-activating factor.

Experimental and clinical data suggested the possibility that the bleeding tendency in uremia is associated with excessive formation of nitric oxide (NO)[153] (Fig. 83–4). Prolongation of skin bleeding time was observed in healthy volunteers given NO by inhalation.[154] The possibility that high systemic NO may play a role in the abnormal primary hemostasis in uremia is supported by the observation that *N*-monomethyl-L-arginine, a competitive inhibitor of NO synthesis, normalized the prolonged bleeding time in uremic rats.[153] Experimental findings were confirmed by human studies; thus, patients with chronic kidney disease have a defective platelet aggregation associated with higher than normal platelet NO synthesis.[155] It has been suggested that substances accumulate in the plasma of uremic patients that are capable of upregulating vascular NO synthesis. The stimulatory activity was attributed to cytokines such as TNF-α and IL-1β, which are potent inducers of the inducible isoform of NO synthase and circulate in increased amounts in the plasma of patients with chronic kidney disease who either do not receive dialysis or are on maintenance hemodialysis.[155,156–159]

Two adhesive proteins, fibrinogen and von Willebrand factor (vWF), and two adhesion receptors, glycoprotein (GP) Ib and the GPIIb/IIIa complex, play a vital role in the formation of platelet thrombi at the sites of injury.[160] Binding of GPIb to vWF is normal in uremic patients,[161] as is the surface expression of the receptor.[162,163] In patients with chronic kidney disease, a decrease in the total content of platelet GPIb has been documented,[162,163] accompanied by an increase in soluble glycocalicin (a soluble proteolytic fragment of GPIb), probably as a result of proteolytic damage to membrane GPIb. The normal surface expression of this receptor and the total decrease in content account for a redistribution from the intraplatelet pool to the surface pool.[161,162] The activation-dependent receptor function of the GPIIb/IIIa complex is defective in uremia, as shown by decreased binding of both vWF and fibrinogen to stimulated platelets.[161] The number of GPIIb/IIIa receptors expressed on the platelet membrane is normal. Removal of substances present in uremic plasma markedly improved the GPIIb/IIIa defect. Thus, a reversible abnormality of the activation-dependent binding activity of GPIIb/IIIa, caused by a dialyzable toxic substance or substances[162,164] or by receptor occupancy by fibrinogen fragments present in uremic plasma,[165] is probably a major component of the altered platelet function in uremia. The impaired GPIIb/IIIa activation in uremia may explain aggregation defects as well as reduced VWF-dependent adhesion and thrombus formation.[166–168]

In an investigation of vWF and platelet adhesion with the use of blood from uremic patients with a bleeding tendency, evidence was found of both platelet and plasma abnormalities.[166] Quantitative and functional abnormalities of the vWF molecule, which promotes platelet adhesion and aggregation to subendothelial collagen,[169] have been reported, although the vWF multimer pattern is normal.[170] The observation that cryoprecipitate,[171] a plasma derivative rich in factor VIII and vWF, and desmopressin,[172] a synthetic derivative of antidiuretic hormone that releases autologous vWF from storage sites, significantly shorten the bleeding time of uremic patients suggests that a functional defect in the vWF-platelet interaction may indeed play a role in the abnormal hemostasis of these patients.

Platelet adhesion and aggregation in flowing systems[173,174] are markedly potentiated by red blood cells. Erythrocytes enhance platelet function by releasing ADP,[175] by inactivating prostaglandin I_2[176] and by increasing platelet–vessel wall contact by displacing platelets away from the axial flow and toward the vessel wall.[173] The independent role of anemia in the bleeding tendency of uremia has been extensively investigated. A significant negative correlation was found between bleeding time and packed cell volume in 52 patients on chronic hemodialysis.[177] The bleeding time was longer than 270 seconds in 90% of patients with packed cell volumes less than 30% but in only 45% of patients with packed cell volumes greater than 30%. Despite a shorter bleeding time, a significant negative correlation between hematocrit and bleeding time was still demonstrable in 15 nonuremic anemic patients. These results were subsequently confirmed by other studies[178,179] that found that anemia was the main determinant of the prolonged bleeding time in uremic patients. Uremic bleeding time has been shortened and symptomatic hemostatic improvement achieved by treatment with rhEPO.[180,181] In one randomized study,[182] the bleeding time became normal in all patients on erythropoietin as hematocrits increased to 27–32%. Thus, partial correction of anemia was sufficient to correct defective primary hemostasis in uremia.

Consequences of the Bleeding Tendency in Uremia

Gastrointestinal bleeding occurs with greater frequency and higher mortality in uremic patients than in the general population.[183,184] Upper gastrointestinal bleeding is the second leading cause of death in acute renal failure.[185] The most common causes of bleeding are peptic ulcers, hemorrhagic esophagitis, gastritis, duodenitis, and gastric telangiectasias.[186–188] Angiodysplasia with gastrointestinal bleeding has been observed in the stomach, duodenum, jejunum, and colon.[189,190] This abnormality, affecting the microcirculation of the gastrointestinal mucosa and submucosa, occurs most often in hemodialysis patients.[191]

Although now rare, hemorrhagic pericarditis with cardiac tamponade can occur in uremia.[192,193] Subdural hematoma has been reported to occur in 5–15% of hemodialysis patients.[194] Head trauma, hypertension, and systemic anticoagulation are risk factors.[194] Anticoagulation during dialysis may be a major risk factor in causing bleeding in patients with fibrinous pleuritis.[195,196] Spontaneous retroperitoneal bleeding is a rare complication in patients receiving chronic hemodialysis.[197,198] Trauma, anticoagulation, and the presence of polycystic kidneys are predisposing factors. Spontaneous subcapsular hematoma of the liver is a newly recognized complication in uremia.[199]

Intraocular hemorrhage can also occur in uremia, and spontaneous hyphema has been reported during dialysis.[200] There is no visual loss, and the hemorrhage generally resolves without any therapy. Intraocular bleeding with only temporary visual loss has also been reported in a large percentage of transplant and dialysis patients after cataract surgery. Another risk of bleeding in uremic patients is associated with aspirin given to prevent vascular access thrombosis[201] or platelet activation on dialyzer membranes.[202] The beneficial effect of aspirin on vascular access thrombosis can be achieved with a moderate dose (160 mg/day), which inhibits platelet thromboxane A_2 generation without affecting vascular prostaglandin I_2 formation.[201] However, even a moderate dose of aspirin prolongs the bleeding time,[203] and this fact may explain the frequency of gastrointestinal bleeding in uremic patients.[190,204] Thus, the use of aspirin in uremic patients treated with rhEPO to prevent the thrombotic complications associated with an increasing hematocrit is highly questionable.

Abnormalities of Coagulation and Fibrinolysis

Activated partial thromboplastin, prothrombin, and thrombin times are generally normal in uremia[205–213]; fibrinogen and factor VIII:C are usually increased. Changes in the major natural inhibitors of coagulation have been found. Conflicting results regarding antithrombin III levels have been reported; previous reports demonstrated increased levels of this natural anticoagulant,[203,214–216] but reduced levels have also been found in uremic patients.[217,218] This together with the observed decrease in protein C anticoagulant activity with normal protein C amidolytic activity and antigen[219,220] and decreased protein S,[221] may further contribute to the thrombotic tendency. Thrombin is continuously formed, as demonstrated by increased levels of thrombin–antithrombin III complex,[162,222–224] D-dimer,[218,222,223,225] and fibrinopeptide A.[222,223,226,227] These findings suggest that a hypercoagulable state exists in chronic uremia.

Contrasting results regarding the fibrinolytic system have been obtained. Previous reports described decreased fibrinolytic activity in uremia either absolutely[228–231] or relative to the extent of activation of coagulation,[216] and this has been used as an explanation for the thrombotic tendency. Studies found, instead, activation of fibrinolysis in uremia, with an increase of plasmin-antiplasmin complexes and fibrinogen and fibrin degradation products[232–235] as well as a decrease in the activity of plasminogen activator inhibitor in end-stage renal disease and after hemodialysis sessions.[236] These findings probably reflect a fibrinolytic response secondary to fibrin deposition, which may take place also if the overall fibrinolytic activity is depressed.

These abnormalities of coagulation or fibrinolysis partially corrected by dialysis[228,237] predispose the uremic patient to thrombosis, rather than bleeding.

Thrombotic Complications

Thrombosis of the arteriovenous shunt is a frequent occurrence in uremic patients undergoing hemodialysis. Plasma levels of lipoprotein(a), an independent risk factor for atherosclerotic cardiovascular disease, are markedly increased in chronic uremic patients either on hemodialysis[238,239] or continuous ambulatory peritoneal dialysis.[239] Because platelet aggregation plays a major role in thrombus formation, antiplatelet agents have been used, with encouraging results. Sulfinpyrazone, aspirin, and/or dipyridamole have proved useful in several studies.[240] Fibrinolytic agents, such as streptokinase[241,242] or urokinase,[243] have produced contrasting results. More studies are needed to determine the most effective treatment for this complication.

Therapeutic Strategies

Although some investigators have found that both hemodialysis and peritoneal dialysis partially improve the hemostatic abnormality of uremia, both forms of dialysis can potentially produce adverse effects on hemostasis. For all patients with hemorrhagic complications or undergoing major surgery, the adequacy of dialysis should be appropriately checked (Box 83–2).

Anemia can contribute to the prolongation of the bleeding time in uremia.[177–179] Thus, the correction of anemia with rhEPO may contribute significantly to the prevention and control of bleeding in uremic patients (Table 83–4).

Desmopressin (1-deamino-8-D-arginine vasopressin)—a synthetic derivative of antidiuretic hormone—induces the release of autologous vWF from storage sites.[244] In a randomized, double-blind, crossover trial, desmopressin given intravenously at a dose of 0.3 μg/kg body weight in 50 mL of physiologic saline over a period of 30 minutes temporarily corrected the prolonged bleeding time in patients with chronic kidney disease.[171] The shortening of bleeding time was significant 1 hour after the end of the infusion, and the effect lasted 6–8 hours. Desmopressin loses efficacy with repeated administration.[245]

Desmopressin also can be given by the intranasal route,[246] which is well tolerated and quite safe. At 10–20 times the intravenous dose (3 μg/kg), intranasal desmo-

Box 83–2. Guidelines for the Management of Hemorrhagic Complications of Uremia

- For all patients with hemorrhagic complications or undergoing major surgery, the adequacy of dialysis should be appropriately checked.
- It is also advisable to change the dialysis schedule for 1 or 2 months in patients who have experienced severe hemorrhages (such as major gastrointestinal bleeding, hemorrhagic pericarditis, or subdural hematomas) or who have undergone recent cardiovascular surgery so that heparin can be avoided.
- Acute bleeding episodes may be treated with desmopressin at a dose of 0.3 μg/kg, intravenously (added to 50 mL of saline over 30 minutes) or subcutaneously. Intranasal administration of this drug at a dose of 3 μg/kg is also effective and well tolerated.
- Because a favorable effect of cryoprecipitate on bleeding time has not been uniformly observed, we do not recommend its use.
- The effect of desmopressin lasts only a few hours, a major limitation to its use in treating severe hemorrhage. Desmopressin appears to lose efficacy when repeatedly administered.
- The ideal treatment of persistent chronic bleeding should have a long-lasting effect.
- Conjugated estrogen treatment given by intravenous infusion in a cumulative dose of 3 mg/kg as daily divided doses (i.e., 0.6 mg/kg for 5 consecutive days) is the most appropriate way to achieve long-lasting hemostatic competence.

TABLE 83–4. Therapeutic Options for Uremic Bleeding

Treatment	Indication	Dose	Start	Peak	End
Packed red blood cells transfusion	Prophylaxis of bleeding in patients with anemia	To correct hematocrit >30%			Related to red blood cell blood
rhEPO	Prophylaxis of bleeding in patients with anemia	80–120 units/kg/wk			
Desmopressin*	Acute bleeding	0.3 μg/kg intravenously 3.0 μg/kg intranasally	1 hr	2–4 hr	6–8 hr
Conjugated estrogens	Major surgery or long-lasting effect required	0.6 mg/kg/day intravenously for 5 consecutive days	6 hr	5–7 days	21 days

*Desmopressin effect is lost after repeated administrations.

pressin shortens the bleeding time and decreases clinical bleeding. Desmopressin has also been given subcutaneously,[247] with the dose the same as that used for intravenous administration. Peak responses are achieved after a 30- to 90-minute delay when the subcutaneous route is employed. Adverse effects include facial flushing, mild transient headache, nausea, abdominal cramps, and mild tachycardia. Protein C anticoagulant activity decreases after desmopressin infusion.[248,249] In one case report, an elderly uremic patient with atherosclerosis suffered a stroke immediately after desmopressin infusion.[250] Nonetheless, desmopressin is useful in the treatment of bleeding, and in the prevention of bleeding during surgery or invasive procedures.

Heparin

Heparin may also present a problem. "Regional" heparinization has been used to minimize the effects of systemic anticoagulation.[251–253] Heparin is given by constant infusion through the inlet line of the dialyzer. Simultaneously, protamine sulfate is infused into the outlet port before the blood returns to the patient. Even this schedule of heparin administration, however, may be associated with a high incidence of bleeding.[254] As an alternative, frequent injections of low-dose heparin can be given during dialysis to maintain a lower and more constant level.[255] Usually, 40–50 IU/kg of heparin is given at the beginning of hemodialysis, followed by 60% of the initial dose after 1 hour and 2 hours, and 30% of the initial dose after 3 hours. The activated partial thromboplastin time is measured hourly and should be maintained at 1.5–2 times the basal value.

Low-molecular-weight (LMW) heparin has been proposed as an alternative to unfractionated heparin in patients receiving chronic hemodialysis who are at high risk for bleeding.[256] LMW heparins have a mean molecular mass of 4000–5000 Da. Like unfractionated heparin, LMW heparins inactivate factor Xa, but they have a lesser effect on thrombin. As a result, LMW heparins do not prolong the activated partial thromboplastin time.[257–250] LMW heparins are at least as effective as unfractionated heparin for the treatment and prevention of venous thromboembolism. They are also equally effective for preventing thromboembolism prior to long-term anticoagulation after a mechanical heart valve replacement and for patients with a mechanical valve who have a contraindication to oral anticoagulation.[261,262] They have greater bioavailability when given by subcutaneous injection. The duration of the anticoagulant effect is greater because of reduced binding to macrophages and endothelial cells, permitting once- or twice-daily administration. The anticoagulant response (anti-Xa activity) to LMW heparin is highly correlated with body weight, permitting administration of a fixed dose.

LMW heparins are cleared by the kidney, and they are excreted unchanged in the urine. Therefore, clearance of these drugs is reduced in subjects with reduced creatinine clearance. The pharmacokinetics of the LMW heparin enoxaparin[263] was evaluated in 12 healthy volunteers and 36 patients with mild, moderate, or severe renal impairment. Enoxaparin was administered once daily by subcutaneous injection at a dose of 40 mg for 4 days, and venous blood samples were taken over a 5-day period to determine anti–factor Xa and anti–factor IIa activity and the activated partial thromboplastin time. The results for anti-Xa activity showed that the rate of absorption of enoxaparin was similar across the four groups of study participants. The elimination half-life increased with the degree of renal impairment, and this relationship was more evident after repeated dosing. Anti-Xa exposure was not significantly different between healthy volunteers and patients with mild or moderate renal impairment, but was significantly increased in patients with severe renal impairment (creatinine clearance <30 mL/min). The authors concluded that the clearance of enoxaparin is reduced in patients with severe renal impairment. Dose adjustment of enoxaparin may need to be recommended in these patients, but no recommendation can be made in patients with mild or moderate renal impairment.

A recent report described serious adverse incidents with the use of LMW heparins in patients with chronic renal disease.[264] A systematic analysis of case records at the Hope Hospital, Salford, UK, from July 2002 to March 2003 disclosed ten patients that experienced an adverse

Current Controversies & Future Considerations

Hematologic Abnormalities in Chronic Kidney Disease

- Although the current indications for erythropoietin treatment in end-stage renal disease patients are well established and agreed upon, the issue of the stage of renal dysfunction at which erythropoietin treatment should be started in order to prevent cardiovascular complications is still a matter of debate.
- The optimal iron supplementation therapy, in term of dose and iron formulation, is not yet established and requires further studies.
- In the future, development of new erythropoiesis-stimulating molecules will improve treatment of renal anemia.
- Correction of anemia in patients with end-stage renal disease by erythropoietin has significantly reduced the bleeding complications of uremia.
- Interest is now focused on the cardiovascular complications of uremia, and the role of thrombogenic factors is a matter of investigation.

incident on LMW heparin therapy. Five patients were on maintenance hemodialysis therapy, and one patient was on continuous ambulatory peritoneal dialysis therapy. Four patients had calculated creatinine clearances between 5 and 33 mL/min. The dose was 1 mg/kg twice daily in most cases. Patients experienced a variety of major bleeding events: retroperitoneal bleeding (one patient), spontaneous soft tissue bleeding (three patients), gastrointestinal bleeding (two patients), dialysis catheter and cannula site bleeding (two patients), hemorrhagic pericardial effusion (one patient), and intracranial bleeding (one patient). Three patients died despite aggressive resuscitation, including packed red blood cell infusions and protamine sulfate administration.

Prostaglandin I_2 showed some promise as an alternative.[265–266] Given in a continuous infusion during dialysis at a mean dose of 5 ng/kg/min, prostaglandin I_2 completely inhibited platelet aggregation without causing bleeding.[267] However, it was associated with headache, flushing, tachycardia, and chest and abdominal pain, which required careful monitoring and a physician's supervision.[267–269] Thus, the use of prostaglandin I_2 should be limited to patients at high risk for hemorrhage.

Peritoneal dialysis, when applicable, avoids the risk of bleeding associated with heparin or anticoagulants.

Suggested Readings*

Alexiewicz JM, Smogorzewski M, Fadda GZ, et al: Impaired phagocytosis in dialysis patients: studies on mechanisms. Am J Nephrol 11:102–111, 1991.

Farooq V, Hegarty J, Chandrasekar T, et al: Serious adverse incidents with the usage of low molecular weight heparins in patients with chronic kidney disease. Am J Kidney Dis 43:531–537, 2004.

Livio E, Benigni A, Remuzzi G: Coagulation abnormalities in uremia. Semin Nephrol 5:82–90, 1985.

Lohr YW, Schwab S: Minimizing hemorrhagic complications in dialysis patients. J Am Soc Nephrol 2:961–975, 1991.

Macdougall IC: An overview of the efficacy and safety of novel erythropoiesis stimulating protein (NESP). Nephrol Dial Transplant 16(Suppl 3):14–21, 2001.

Macdougall IC: Erythropoietin and renal failure. Curr Hematol Rep 2:459–464, 2003.

Moia M, Mannucci PM, Vizzotto L, et al: Improvement in the haemostatic defect of uraemia after treatment with recombinant human erythropoietin. Lancet 2:1227–1229, 1987.

NKF-DOQI: Clinical practice guidelines: treatment of anemia of chronic renal failure. Am J Kidney Dis 30(Suppl 3):S192–S237, 1997.

Pereira AA, Sarnak MJ: Anemia as a risk factor for cardiovascular disease. Kidney Int Suppl 87:S32–S39, 2003.

Full references for this chapter can be found on accompanying CD-ROM.

CHAPTER 84

Hematologic Abnormalities in Liver Disease

Franklin A. Bontempo, MD

> **KEY POINTS**
>
> **Hematologic Abnormalities in Liver Disease**
>
> - Severe liver disease can result in multiple morphologic abnormalities of red cells, including macrocytosis, stomatocytosis, target cells, acanthocytes, and schistocytes.
> - Anemia is common in patients with liver disease and is usually mild to moderate in severity. The etiology is multifactorial and can include hemodilution, iron deficiency, folic acid deficiency, hypersplenism, bone marrow suppression from alcohol, and anemia of chronic disease.
> - Pancytopenia can occur particularly in patients with severe liver disease.
> - Thrombocytopenia and reduced levels of clotting factors resulting from impaired liver synthetic function can contribute to clinically significant bleeding tendencies in patients with liver disease.

INTRODUCTION

The liver plays a central role in the maintenance of the blood vascular system, including the circulating red blood cells, white blood cells, and platelets, as well as the bone marrow, coagulation factors, and other plasma proteins. Alterations in liver function lead directly or indirectly to abnormalities in hematologic parameters that need to be recognized to make a diagnosis of liver disease or that need to be managed when liver disease is already known to be present. In addition, the close association of the liver with the spleen and lymphatic system causes further hematologic effects when the liver is abnormal. Because the liver serves many synthetic and metabolic functions, hematologic abnormalities may occur by a variety of mechanisms. Analysis of the hematologic abnormalities associated with liver disease is complicated by the fact that many of the causes of the liver disease may also be associated with hematologic abnormalities.

RED BLOOD CELL ABNORMALITIES

Red blood cells (RBCs) are commonly affected in a variety of ways as outlined in Table 84–1.

Morphologic Changes

Morphologic changes of RBCs are common in patients with liver disease and may occur by a variety of mechanisms. They deserve particular attention because they may offer important clues to the diagnosis of suspected or unsuspected liver disease (Fig. 84–1). Unfortunately, many of these morphologic abnormalities may also be seen in other disorders that may or may not be present in patients with liver disease and may need to be differentiated from the latter. As many as two thirds of patients with liver disease, with or without anemia, have macrocytic RBCs, particularly when the liver disease is associated with alcoholism. The etiology of the macrocytic cells may be unclear because of accompanying nutritional deficiencies but even in the absence of these, RBC size tends to be above average and above the normal range, approximately 100–110 fL.[1] Target cells, with their characteristic "bull's-eye" appearance, are common in liver disease and are due to an increased red cell surface area that results from an increase in the cholesterol/phospholipid ratio and the uptake of cholesterol by the red cell membrane, leading to a bell-shaped surface that appears as a central dense area on light microscopy. Despite this morphologic abnormality, target cells have a normal lifespan and may actually be protective against the effects of hemolysis. Stomatocytes also occur in liver disease and are characterized by the appearance of a mouthlike wide slit across the surface of the red cell.

Table 84–1. Changes in Red Blood Cells Caused by Liver Disease

Morphologic Abnormalities
Macrocytes
Target cells
Stomatocytes
Acanthocytes/spur cells
Schistocytes
Anemia
Dilutional
Blood loss
Nutritional
Iron
Folate
Vitamin B_{12}
Sideroblastic
Chronic disease
Hypersplenism
Hemolytic
Aplastic/bone marrow suppression
Reticulocytosis
Erythrocytosis

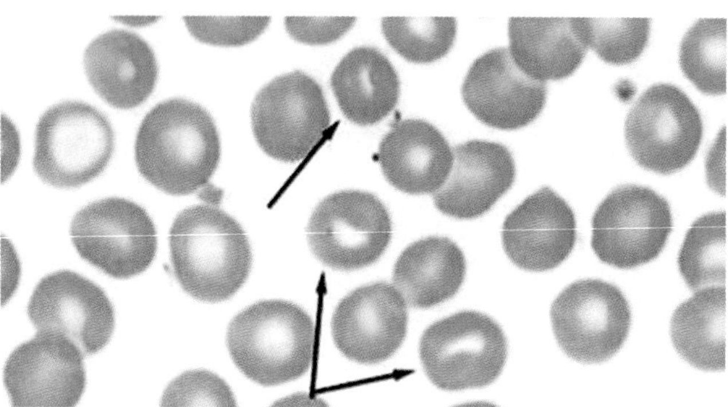

Figure 84–1. Stomatocytes in patient with liver disease.

What causes them is unknown, but they may be associated with abnormalities of membrane permeability. In patients with liver disorders, they are commonly, but not exclusively, associated with alcoholism. Acanthocytes, or spur cells, are RBCs with spiny projections of varying width and length that occur particularly in alcoholic liver disease and are usually associated with hemolysis and shortened RBC survival. They may also be seen in several other rare disorders, including abetalipoproteinemia, chorea-acanthocytosis syndrome, and McLeod syndrome which are not related to liver disease. Schistocytes may be seen in liver disease when disseminated intravascular coagulation is present as a result of the liver disease.

Anemia

Older estimates of the frequency of anemia in patients with liver disease are approximately 75%, but recent surveys are lacking. The severity of the anemia bears some relationship to the severity of the liver disease but also to the type and cause of liver disease as well as the presence of other anemia-causing conditions. The degree of anemia caused by liver disease itself is usually mild to moderate, with a fall in the hemoglobin to approximately 12 gm/dL and in the hematocrit to 36%. The anemia may be exaggerated by the effect of hemodilution resulting from an increased blood volume without substantial change in the red cell mass, likely due to renal sodium retention and subsequent retention of water. In addition, the metabolism of both iron and folic acid are altered in liver disease, and these changes may affect RBCs. Iron deficiency may occur as a result of blood loss from esophageal, gastric, or duodenal varices secondary to portal hypertension, but the usual indicators of iron deficiency anemia may be lacking.

Alternatively, in alcoholism, iron absorption may actually be elevated. This may be due to the iron content of the beverage, which may vary depending on how it is prepared, with beer and stout tending to have higher iron content than wine, or it may be due to the increased absorption of iron because of the alcohol itself. These effects may be further confounded by decreased iron intake in severe alcoholics whose dietary intake is poor. Further complicating the picture seen in liver disease is the elevation of the serum ferritin level, which may occur as a result of an acute-phase reaction or release from the diseased liver, which is the site of ferritin production. Even in chronic liver disease, iron stores may be mildly elevated unless hemorrhage is ongoing. As a result, liver disease may be associated with a tendency toward either iron deficiency or iron overload depending on multiple factors. An additional alteration of iron, particularly in alcoholic liver disease, is sideroblastic anemia, arising from impaired synthesis of heme (see Chapter 55). This leads to an anemia with a characteristic dual population of both macrocytic and normocytic RBCs, commonly referred to as a dimorphic erythron; this may occur in 25–30% of anemic alcoholic patients[2,3] and may also complicate the anemia of liver disease. A final alteration of iron metabolism that may occur in liver disease is the anemia of chronic disease, which may cause a normochromic, normocytic appearance on the peripheral smear with a normal or decreased total iron-binding capacity and increase in transferrin saturation depending on the stage of liver disease (see Chapter 19).

Folate is normally secreted by hepatocytes in bile and reabsorbed in the intestine, although this cycle can be interrupted in liver disease. In particular in patients with alcohol abuse, who frequently have concomitant poor oral folate intake, the enterohepatic circulation of folate may be disrupted because alcohol diminishes secretion of folate. This causes loss of folate into the serum, and antagonizes the effects of folate on erythropoiesis,[4] commonly leading to a macrocytic anemia that may be clinically significant and may occur rapidly. As a result, folate deficiency is the most likely cause of macrocytic anemia in patients with liver disease. Interruption of the enterohepatic cycle for vitamin B_{12} in liver disease may occur but is less dramatic and less likely to be clinically significant for a variety of reasons.

RBC survival is estimated to be moderately decreased in most patients with liver disease but is poorly understood. It may again be seen frequently in patients with alcoholic liver disease, but may also be due to hypersplenism in patients with portal hypertension and in those with hemolysis. The degree of anemia caused by hypersplenism is related to the size of the spleen, with a larger spleen causing increased pooling of RBCs as well as the shortened RBC survival that may result from removal of abnormal RBCs. Anemia caused by hypersplenism is modulated by the ability of the patient's bone marrow to compensate for the lowered hematocrit.

Hemolysis is common in patients with liver disease; in patients with alcoholic liver disease, it may occur intermittently with binge drinking. Zieve described a syndrome of hemolysis in alcoholic liver disease patients with cirrhosis, jaundice, and hypertriglyceridemia that bears his name, although the physiologic association between its components has remained uncertain.[5] Spur cell anemia, as mentioned previously, may frequently complicate liver disease and is associated with hemolysis and shortened RBC survival. It occasionally has responded to splenectomy. Of note, however, transfusion of RBCs from patients with liver disease and shortened RBC survival into normal recipients has been shown to result in improved RBC survival, suggesting in general the effects of the milieu on RBC survival rather than an intrinsic RBC defect.[6,7] Less common causes of hemolysis in liver disease patients include metabolic defects caused by significant hypophosphatemia[8] and copper-induced damage of RBCs in patients with Wilson's disease.[9] The latter has been successfully treated with plasmapheresis.[10]

A final cause of anemia in patients with liver disease is bone marrow suppression and aplastic anemia. Alcohol may have a direct marrow suppressive effect, but patients with liver disease caused by viral hepatitis, particularly hepatitis C, are reported to have an incidence of mild to severe aplastic anemia of 0.1–0.2%. The mechanism is unknown.[11]

Reticulocytosis

Reticulocytes may be increased to 8–10% in anemic patients with liver disease, particularly after withdrawal of an offending agent such as alcohol.[12–14] In one study of anemic patients with cirrhosis, the mean reticulocyte percentage was 2.8%.[1] The reticulocyte level in liver disease patients will depend on the relative effects of suppressed marrow function and the degree of anemia.

Erythrocytosis

Occasionally, patients with liver disease are found to have erythrocytosis associated with inappropriate production of erythropoietin. Of primary concern is the possibility that the cause is hepatocellular carcinoma, although rare patients with hepatitis alone[15] or arteriovenous shunts caused by cirrhosis with resulting hypoxia have also been found to have erythrocytosis.[16]

ABNORMALITIES OF PLATELETS

Both platelet number and function may be decreased in patients with liver disease, with the severity of the abnormalities depending on both the severity and type of liver disease.

Thrombocytopenia is one of the most common abnormalities in patients with liver disease. When patients with severe hepatocellular disease are considered, the incidence of thrombocytopenia ranges from at least 70% to 90% when defined as a platelet count of less than 150,000; whereas patients with biliary tract disorders such as primary biliary cirrhosis and sclerosing cholangitis have an incidence of thrombocytopenia of 38–63%. Patients with hepatocellular carcinoma usually have no thrombocytopenia unless there is underlying hepatocellular disease.[17] Shortened platelet survival, decreased platelet production, hypersplenism, splenic sequestration and disseminated intravascular coagulation (DIC) can all contribute to thrombocytopenia (Box 84–1). Normally, about one third of the platelets are sequestered in the spleen, but in patients with splenomegaly, this may increase to as high as 90%.[18] Shortened platelet survival may be exacerbated by hypersplenism causing the active removal of platelets, in contrast to pooling, wherein platelets may be recoverable and available for clotting. In addition, significant reductions in platelet survival with resulting thrombocytopenia may occur in patients with autoimmune liver disease, in which autoimmune destruction of platelets may be significant, as in antibody-positive autoimmune hepatitis, or in patients with autoimmune "overlap" syndromes, in which there is an autoimmune component to other diseases, such as primary biliary cirrhosis or sclerosing cholangitis. Although decreased production of thrombopoietin, which is made in the liver, has been postulated as a cause of reduced platelet production, evidence to support this contention is conflicting. DIC may also decrease platelet counts in liver disease due to consumption and is discussed below.

Definitive analysis of platelet function in patients with liver diseases is lacking, with some studies showing minimal platelet dysfunction even with severe liver disease and others showing mild dysfunction that is of questionable clinical significance. Especially in patients with alcoholic liver disease, there may be a prolongation of bleeding time out of proportion to the degree of

Box 84–1. Factors Contributing to Thrombocytopenia in Liver Disease

- Severity of liver disease
- Splenomegaly
- Bone marrow dysfunction/? depressed thrombopoietin
- Shortened platelet survival
- Disseminated intravascular coagulation (DIC)

thrombocytopenia. In most clinical situations, the bleeding time will begin to rise when the platelet count falls to approximately 50,000–75,000, but in patients with platelet dysfunction caused by liver disease, bleeding times may be long even without thrombocytopenia. In cirrhotics, prolonged bleeding times have been found to respond significantly to desmopressin (DDAVP),[19] suggesting an enhancement of platelet function with its use. The mechanisms responsible for the presumed abnormalities of platelet function remain unclear, and differentiating platelet defects caused specifically by liver disease from those caused by the underlying condition causing the liver disease, particularly alcohol, has been difficult. Closure times using whole blood aggregometers have replaced bleeding times in some centers, and these more automated tests of platelet function may also be abnormal in patients with liver disease.

WHITE BLOOD CELL ABNORMALITIES

White blood cells may be abnormal in number and function in patients with liver disease.[20] Neutropenia may occur as a result of the effects of a production defect mediated by alcohol, viral hepatitis, other infection, or an associated deficiency of folic acid or vitamin B_{12}. Commonly hypersplenism and/or splenic sequestration in patients with portal hypertension and cirrhosis may be an additional cause. In patients with acute alcoholism, even without the foregoing, neutropenia may be present and some studies have suggested a decrease in granulocyte marrow reserve and production.[20] In addition, studies have shown an increase in the risk of infection in alcoholics, particularly pneumococcal pneumonia, and neutrophil adherence, motility, and chemotaxis have been shown to be impaired in this patient population. However, the specific contribution of liver disease versus the effect of alcohol is unclear. Lymphopenia has been noted in most alcoholics with leukopenia,[21] and blastogenic transformation and dermal hypersensitivity have been found to be impaired in patients with alcohol abuse.[20]

BONE MARROW ABNORMALITIES

There may be morphologic and hematopoietic changes in the bone marrow in patients with liver disease in general, but the abnormalities are most striking in patients with alcoholic liver disease. The bone marrow may be suppressed by the effects of alcohol and infection as noted previously, leading to a hypoproliferative bone marrow aspirate and biopsy. Occasionally, in viral hepatitis the marrow may be aplastic, with all cell lines depressed. The bone marrow effects of alcoholic liver disease commonly include hypocellularity, macrocytic RBCs, and megaloblastic changes in RBC precursors even without folate deficiency probably as a direct result of alcoholism. In addition, there may also be ringed sideroblasts, an increased number of plasma cells, and vacuolization of RBC and myeloid precursors. Further evidence for bone marrow dysfunction in alcoholism is provided by abnormalities of in vitro colony formation.

COAGULATION ABNORMALITIES

The liver plays a major role in the maintenance of adequate hemostasis, and many coagulation changes occur in liver disease as outlined in Box 84–2. Most of the clotting factors are made in the hepatocyte (exceptions are von Willebrand factor, prostacyclin, tissue factor pathway inhibitor, tissue plasminogen activator, plasminogen activator inhibitor, thrombomodulin, and thrombin-activatable fibrinolysis inhibitor). Although factor VIII:C is probably made in the liver, as suggested by liver transplantation in patients with hemophilia A,[22] it may have a second production site in the hepatic endothelial cell. The classic coagulation cascade is shown in Figure 84-2, with the prothrombin time (PT) pathway beginning at factor VII and the activated partial thromboplastin time (aPTT) pathway beginning at factor XII. Factors II, V, VII, IX, X, XI, and XII are all made in the liver, are not acute-phase reactants, and are frequently depressed in patients with hepatic synthetic defects. Factors II, VII, IX, and X are also vitamin K dependent and may be depressed in vitamin K deficiency without liver disease. If no vitamin K deficiency is present, however, the factors tend to be reduced sequentially in the order of their half-lives from shortest to longest (VII, IX, X, and II).

Factors V and VII have the shortest half-lives (about 6–8 hours) and are frequently reduced in early liver disease, with consequent prolongations of the PT and aPTT. However, a lower level of factor V may be necessary to prolong the aPTT than the level of factor VII required to prolong the PT, causing the PT to be more often prolonged in early liver disease prior to any change in the aPTT. In severe liver disease, most of the clotting factors are depressed; depression of clotting factor levels sufficient to prolong the PT and aPTT is associated with an increased risk of bleeding at the time of surgery. Exceptions are factor VIII:C and fibrinogen (factor I), which are acute-phase reactants and tend to be signifi-

Box 84–2. Coagulation Abnormalities in Liver Disease

- Prolongation of the prothrombin time and activated partial thromboplastin time
- Decreased clotting factor levels
- Dysfibrinogenemia
- Prolongation of the thrombin and reptilase times
- Decreased levels of antithrombin III, protein C, protein S, and plasminogen
- Disseminated intravascular coagulation
- Fibrinolysis
- Low levels of factor XIII

cantly elevated in patients with many acute and chronic disorders, including liver diseases. Factor VIII:C levels were observed to be elevated in pre–liver transplant patients to a mean of 2.30 units/mL,[17] and fibrinogen tends to be relatively spared and remain in the lower limits of the normal range in all but the most severe cases of disorders of hepatocellular synthetic function or direct hepatotoxicity. In addition, liver diseases are associated with dysfunctional fibrinogen molecules as a result of abnormal quaternary structures of the fibrinogen molecules with increased sialic acid residues or fibrin molecules with abnormal polymerization, leading to an acquired dysfibrinogenemia that is unlikely to be associated with clinical bleeding. However, with either a dysfibrinogenemia or a depressed fibrinogen level, prolongation of the thrombin time and reptilase time may occur, because both of these clotting times depend primarily on the rate of conversion of fibrinogen to fibrin.

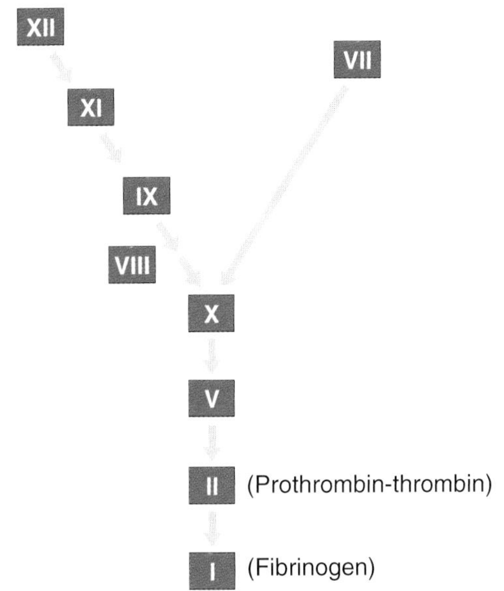

Figure 84–2. The basic clotting cascade.

Although bleeding is the usual consequence of the abnormalities of the clotting cascade seen in liver disease, other coagulation proteins that inhibit clotting, including antithrombin III, protein C, protein S, and plasminogen, may also be abnormal in patients with liver disease. The place of these proteins in the clotting cascade is shown in Figure 84–3. It should be recognized that deficiencies of these proteins rarely lead to clinical thrombosis in the setting of liver disease; rather, the clear clinical consequence of liver disease is bleeding, not thrombosis.

A further complication of liver disease may be the presence of disseminated intravascular coagulation (DIC) with its associated thrombocytopenia, consumptive coagulopathy, and formation of fibrin degradation products. Unfortunately, studies of liver disease have shown that fibrin degradation products are seen in 15–20% of patients with severe liver disease,[17] and the features of consumption are often virtually indistinguishable from the decreased synthesis of clotting factors and thrombocytopenia seen in hepatic disease. This makes the differentiation of DIC from the coagulopathy of liver disease one of the most difficult diagnoses in coagulation unless the clinical history and time course for the clotting parameters, particularly thrombocytopenia, are known. Often, the distinction can only be made after serial DIC clotting profiles are obtained. DIC may be more clearly seen and expected, however, in patients with ascites-induced LeVeen shunts, in whom the incidence of DIC may be as high as 90%[23] (Box 84–3).

Another disorder sometimes found in patients with liver disease, particularly during liver resection surgery or

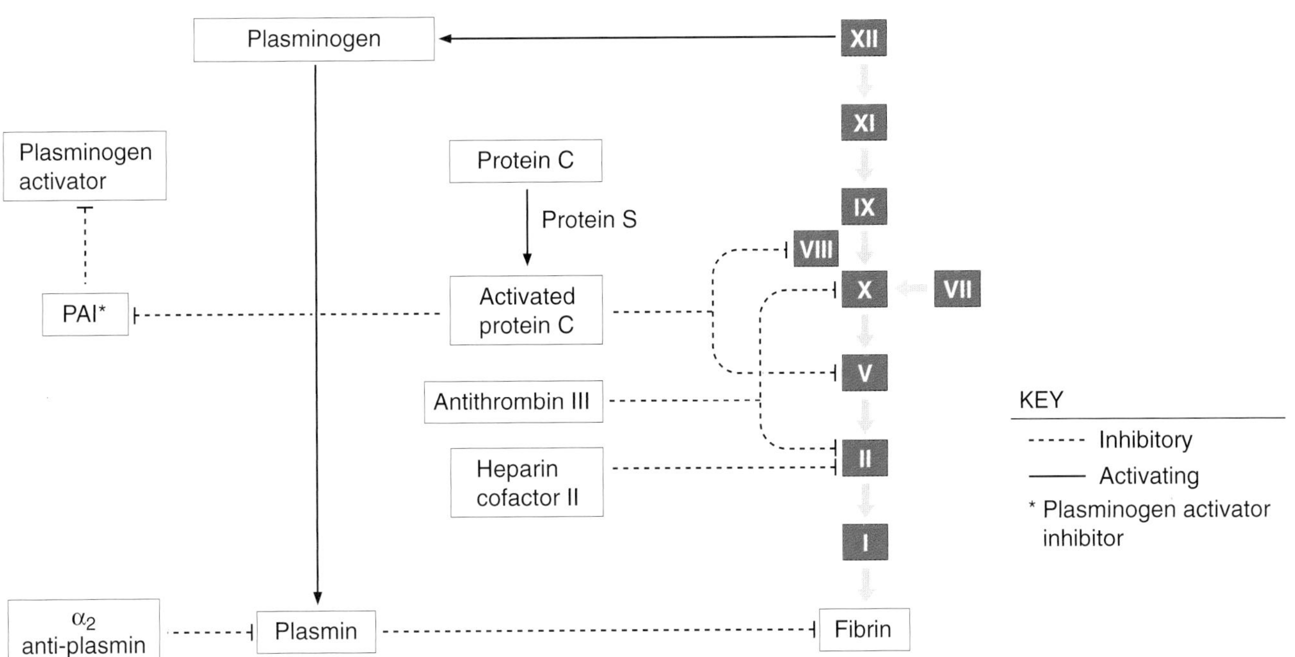

Figure 84–3. The coagulation and fibrinolytic pathways with inhibitors.

Box 84–3. Bleeding Symptoms and Signs in Liver Disease

- Hematemesis
- Melena
- Bright red rectal bleeding
- Easy bruising
- Oozing from venipuncture sites
- Prolonged PT and APTT
- Long bleeding time or closure time
- Thrombocytopenia

liver transplantation, is primary fibrinolysis. This may be due to release of plasminogen activators during surgery and excessive activation of plasminogen to plasmin and/or to decreased production of α_2-antiplasmin.[24,25] This disorder is also characterized by prolongation of clotting parameters and decreased levels of fibrinogen, as in DIC, but without thrombocytopenia, and may be treated with fibrinolytic inhibitors. Unfortunately, a secondary form of fibrinolysis may be found in 25-30% of patients with DIC, and care must be taken before treating with fibrinolytic inhibitors if DIC is present.

Fibrin clots are stabilized by factor XIII, which may also be depressed in patients with liver disease, but the reduced levels are not usually indicative of congenital factor XIII deficiency and are not usually clinically significant. They must, however, be regarded in context when liver disease is present.

The treatment of bleeding in patients with liver disease largely depends on identifying the severity of the coagulation dysfunction and replacing with plasma for depression of clotting factors, cryoprecipitate for low fibrinogen, platelets for thrombocytopenia, and platelets and/or DDAVP for platelet dysfunction (Box 84–4). In the rarer case of bleeding associated with fibrinolysis, ε-aminocaproic acid or tranexamic acid could be used.[26]

Box 84–4. Treatment Options in a Bleeding Patient with Liver Disease

- Fresh frozen plasma
- Platelets
- Cryoprecipitate
- Desmopressin (DDAVP)
- Antifibrinolytic agents

ABNORMALITIES OF OTHER PROTEINS

Other proteins of hematologic significance that may be abnormal in liver disease are haptoglobin and immunoglobulins. Haptoglobin is a molecule produced by the liver that acts as a scavenger for intravascular hemoglobin and decreases rapidly in the face of hemolysis, which makes it an excellent marker for the presence of the latter. Although studies yield conflicting evidence, the haptoglobin level may be elevated early in liver disease as an acute-phase reactant, but may subsequently fall as hepatocellular disease worsens, complicating its usefulness in detecting hemolysis.

Immunoglobulins are frequently measured on serum protein electrophoreses for a variety of reasons. Many patients with liver disease, particularly those with cirrhosis or autoimmune liver disease, have a polyclonal hypergammaglobulinemia often accompanied by a pattern of β-γ "bridging" on electrophoresis, which should not be confused with a monoclonal disorder.

Suggested Readings*

***Full references for this chapter can be found on accompanying CD-ROM.**

CHAPTER 85

Chronic Bruising and Bleeding Diathesis

Karen L. LoRusso, MD, and B. Gail Macik, MD

KEY POINTS

Chronic Bruising and Bleeding Diathesis

- Evaluation of a bleeding disorder requires a basic understanding of hemostatic processes.
- A description of bleeding events, personal and family history of bleeding, comorbidities, medications, and physical findings provide clues to diagnosis.
- Initial laboratory studies screen for evidence of malfunction of the major pathways of hemostasis: primary hemostasis, secondary hemostasis, and clot stability/fibrinolysis.
- The history, physical examination, and screening laboratory studies are used to establish an algorithmic approach to the chronic bruising/bleeding patient.
- Effective management is dependent on identifying and linking a defective hemostatic pathway to a specific bleeding disorder.

INTRODUCTION

Consultations for excessive bleeding are sought for many reasons, including a history of bleeding after surgery or trauma, a coagulation laboratory abnormality, or a personal or family history of bleeding or bruising. A bleeding diathesis is an inherent problem of blood coagulation, and such inborn states are rare in the population, but acquired defects of hemostasis are common. A hemostatic evaluation starts with a relevant history, physical examination, and initial screening laboratory tests to guide more specific laboratory studies. The goal of the evaluation is to identify the defective hemostatic component and to link the defect to specific symptoms and signs. This chapter discusses the components of a hemostatic evaluation and provides an algorithm for developing a differential diagnosis and management plan for a patient with a bleeding tendency.

OVERVIEW OF THE HEMOSTATIC SYSTEM

The first challenge is the localization of the bleeding problem to an individual component of the complex hemostatic pathway. Bleeding disorders may affect the structure and function of the vasculature, the number and function of platelets, the quantity and function of coagulation proteins, the stabilization of the clot, the process of fibrinolysis, or any combination of these individual components. To approach the problem in an organized manner, coagulation can be thought of in three stages: the initiation, propagation, and maintenance of a blood clot. Disorders of clot initiation and propagation are categorized into problems of primary and secondary hemostasis, respectively. Disorders of clot maintenance are divided into problems of stabilization resulting from improper processing and cross-linking of fibrin strands and problems of inappropriate fibrinolysis. A detailed overview of the hemostatic properties of blood vessels, platelets, and the enzymatic reactions and control mechanisms for clot formation and dissolution are beyond the scope of this chapter, but are covered more extensively in Chapters 7, 8, and 9. A simplified overview to assist in defining a bleeding disorder is presented here.

The steps of primary hemostasis include all the interactions of vascular elements, proteins, and platelets that are necessary for the formation of a platelet plug.[1–4] After injury, the vessel contracts to reduce blood flow and increase the interaction of platelets with the components of the vessel wall. Platelets adhere to the vascular defect, activate, and bind to each other to form the platelet plug. Platelet adhesion occurs when receptors on the platelet surface interact with components of the exposed matrix of the vessel wall. Proteins involved in the process of adhesion include von Willebrand factor (vWF), the platelet glycoprotein Ib-IX-V complex, the platelet glycoprotein Ia/IIa complex, other integrin proteins, and collagen. The process of platelet activation can occur through several mechanisms: the binding of matrix proteins, the binding of soluble signal compounds (e.g., ADP or epinephrine), and the binding of the surface proteins of other platelets.[3–5] Activated platelets produce through the intrinsic prostaglandin pathway a potent stimulant for platelet aggregation, thromboxane A_2. In addition, activation promotes release of platelet granules. The dense granules contain ADP, serotonin, and calcium that stimulate further activation. The α-granules contain fibrinogen, vWF, and thrombospondin that support aggregation and adhesion.[3–5] Primary hemostasis ends with the formation of the platelet plug and the transformation of the platelet surface into a phospholipid platform appropriate to support the enzymatic reactions of secondary hemostasis.

Secondary hemostasis encompasses all the reactions of the clotting cascade leading to the formation of fibrin clot.[1,6,7] Coagulation in vivo is initiated by trauma to the endothelium, prompting exposure of tissue factor to factor VII with the resultant complex activating factors X and IX. Activated factor X binds with its cofactor, factor V, and prothrombin (factor II) to create the prothrombinase complex that generates thrombin, the enzyme that cleaves fibrinogen to fibrin. Thrombin also amplifies the coagulation cascade by activating factor XI. In turn, factor XI creates more activated factor IX that, with its cofactor, factor VIII, generates even more activated factor X to continue the loop of thrombin generation. Adequate quantities of properly functioning clotting factor proteins are required for the series of reactions and amplifications to occur. Secondary hemostasis is completed with the production of fibrin strands.

Once secondary hemostasis has generated fibrin, the strands must be cross-linked to stabilize the clot and the clot must be retained long enough for vessel repair to occur. Thrombin activates factor XIII, and this enzyme covalently cross-links fibrin strands to form a stable clot. The cross-linked clot is relatively resistant to protease degradation except for the action of the designated fibrinolytic pathway. Tissue plasminogen activator (tPA) or urokinase converts plasminogen to plasmin, the primary fibrinolytic enzyme. Inhibitors of plasmin generation (plasminogen activator inhibitor-1 [PAI-1]) and plasmin function (α_2-plasmin inhibitor) control fibrinolytic activity and prevent too rapid clot lysis.[8] A stable fibrin clot is the end product of coagulation, but the timely dissolution of the clot is important for the maintenance of hemostasis.

EVALUATION OF CHRONIC BRUISING/BLEEDING–INITIAL APPROACH

A detailed history and physical examination reveal bleeding characteristics and suggest which of the hemostatic pathways may be defective. The signs and symptoms are categorized into disorders of primary hemostasis, secondary hemostasis, or clot stabilization and fibrinolysis. Screening laboratory assays confirm suspicions and direct advanced testing. The hemostasis consultant must combine elements of the history and physical findings and interpretations of specialized laboratory evaluations to diagnose the bleeding disorder and to construct a management plan. An algorithm outlining an overview of the approach is provided in Figure 85–1.

The Hemostatic History

A bleeding history starts with the characterization of bleeding episodes, looking for evidence of a disorder of primary hemostasis, secondary hemostasis, or clot maintenance (clot stability and fibrinolysis).[9–12] Specific questions about the amount, location, timing, and response to treatment help define the type and magnitude of the bleeding disorder. The hematologist must confirm a measurement of loss and not rely on subjective accounts.[13] A description of the type and location of the bleed can narrow the search for the dysfunctional hemostatic element. Bruises or mucosal bleeding suggest a disorder of primary hemostasis, whereas hemarthroses or large hematomas suggest a disorder of secondary hemostasis. Delayed or recurrent bleeding for days after an injury is more likely a defect of secondary hemostasis or clot maintenance. A spontaneous hemarthrosis without history of trauma suggests a severe clotting factor deficiency. Occasionally, response to a particular therapy may provide a clue to the bleeding disorder. For example, improvement after receiving desmopressin suggests von Willebrand disease (vWD), mild hemophilia A or possibly platelet dysfunction—conditions distinguishable by appropriate laboratory testing.

Inquiry about past hemostatic challenges provides additional, albeit occasionally conflicting, information about the possible bleeding disorder. Clues are uncovered to determine if the disorder is congenital or an acquired defect. A primary bleeding disorder may be distinguished from a systemic disorder presenting with bleeding or from a factitious syndrome. Did the patient bleed or not bleed in response to similar hemostatic challenges of the same magnitude? Contact sports, dental procedures, minor trauma, menses, and childbirth are common challenges.[14] If the response to similar hemostatic challenges changes over time, then an acquired bleeding disorder is suggested. A full hemostatic evaluation that reveals no abnormalities is suspicious for a primary systemic or organ defect or possibly Munchausen syndrome.

Concurrent medical problems, medications, aging, and social or lifestyle issues may contribute to a bleeding tendency or worsen a preexisting disorder.[1,5,15-17] Cirrhosis impacts all pathways of hemostasis. Poor liver function results in low coagulation factor levels. Portal hypertension contributes to splenomegaly with platelet sequestration. Both cirrhosis and uremia adversely effect platelet function.[15] Myeloproliferative diseases, plasma cell dyscrasias, or malignancies may produce paraproteins that interfere with fibrin polymerization and stabilization.[16,17] Hypersensitivity reactions or a paraneoplastic manifestation of an underlying malignancy can present with characteristic "palpable purpura" resulting from vasculitis. A list of prescribed and over-the-counter medications or supplements is essential. Nonprescription products that contain aspirin affect platelet function.[5]

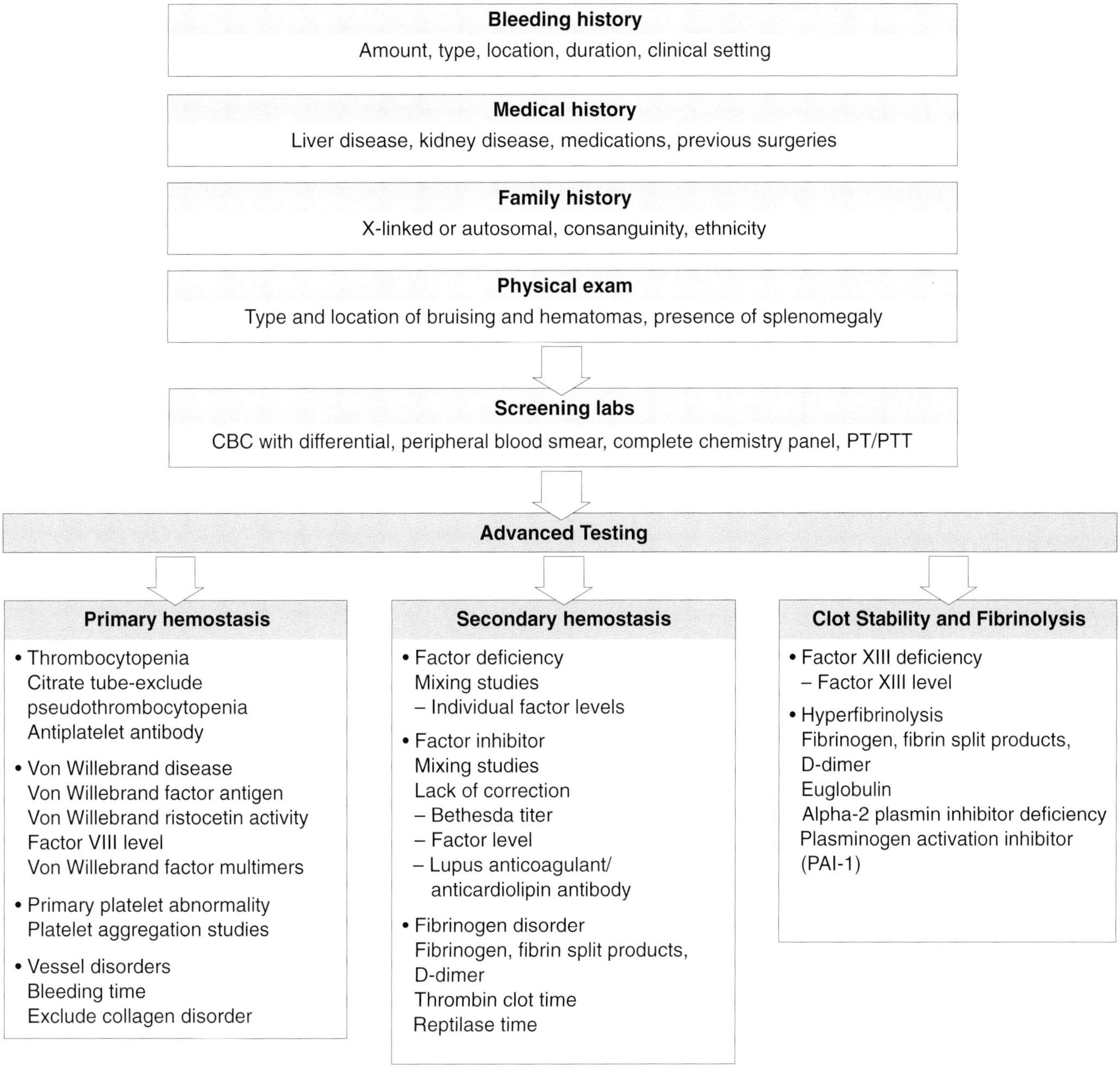

Bleeding history
Amount, type, location, duration, clinical setting

Medical history
Liver disease, kidney disease, medications, previous surgeries

Family history
X-linked or autosomal, consanguinity, ethnicity

Physical exam
Type and location of bruising and hematomas, presence of splenomegaly

↓

Screening labs
CBC with differential, peripheral blood smear, complete chemistry panel, PT/PTT

↓

Advanced Testing

Primary hemostasis

- Thrombocytopenia
  Citrate tube-exclude pseudothrombocytopenia
  Antiplatelet antibody
- Von Willebrand disease
  Von Willebrand factor antigen
  Von Willebrand ristocetin activity
  Factor VIII level
  Von Willebrand factor multimers
- Primary platelet abnormality
  Platelet aggregation studies
- Vessel disorders
  Bleeding time
  Exclude collagen disorder

Secondary hemostasis

- Factor deficiency
  Mixing studies
  – Individual factor levels
- Factor inhibitor
  Mixing studies
  Lack of correction
  – Bethesda titer
  – Factor level
  – Lupus anticoagulant/ anticardiolipin antibody
- Fibrinogen disorder
  Fibrinogen, fibrin split products, D-dimer
  Thrombin clot time
  Reptilase time

Clot Stability and Fibrinolysis

- Factor XIII deficiency
  – Factor XIII level
- Hyperfibrinolysis
  Fibrinogen, fibrin split products, D-dimer
  Euglobulin
  Alpha-2 plasmin inhibitor deficiency
  Plasminogen activation inhibitor (PAI-1)

Figure 85–1. Algorithm for evaluation of a bleeding diathesis.

Medications may damage the liver or kidney. Vessel fragility induced by long-term steroid therapy, sun damage to the skin (solar purpura), or normal age-related changes of the skin (senile purpura) manifests as increased bruising. An eating disorder may present as scurvy or vitamin K deficiency. Alcohol abuse contributes to bleeding by damage to organs and direct interference with platelet function. Domestic violence can present as chronic bruising. If bleeding is due to an underlying systemic, organ, or psychosocial disorder, one must treat the primary disorder.

A family history is vital for establishing an inherited bleeding disorder. At least two generations must be reviewed to determine ethnicity, inheritance patterns, and the presence of consanguinity.[18–20] An X-linked bleeding disorder occurring only in males of the family except for sons of affected individuals is a classic family history for hemophilia A or B. Hemophilia is found among all ethnicities, but some disorders are more common in a single subpopulation (e.g., factor XI deficiency in Ashkenazi Jewish families). A disorder that skips generations is likely autosomal recessive and less likely to be vWD, an autosomal dominant disorder. Lack of family history usually suggests an acquired disorder, but undetermined parentage or disorders such as hemophilia A that have a high spontaneous mutation rate may mislead the investigation. Box 85–1 reviews the essential components of a hemostatic history.

Box 85-1. Components of Hemostatic History

- Type, amount, location, and timing of bleeding episodes
- Response to other hemostatic challenges
- Response to treatment for previous bleeding episodes
- Current health history, especially liver or kidney problems
- Medications, both prescription drugs and over-the-counter supplements
- Bleeding tendencies in at least two generations of family members

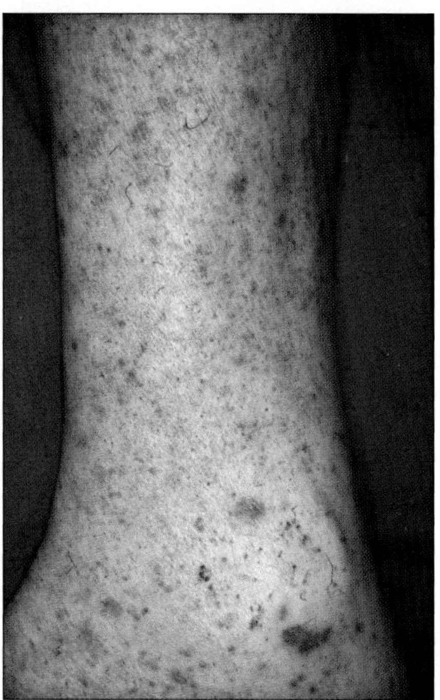

Figure 85–2. Lower extremity petechiae associated with thrombocytopenia.

Physical Examination Findings in a Bleeding Disorder

The physical examination provides clues to the type of bleeding disorder.[10–12] Bleeding into the skin or soft tissues is a common complaint. Accurate characterization of bleeding is necessary to decipher the particular disease process. *Purpura* is commonly used as a generic term for bruising, but precise definitions are associated with unique etiologies and characteristics. Petechiae are dermal lesions less than 2 mm in size, purpuras are lesions 2 mm to 1 cm, and ecchymoses are greater than 1 cm. These dermal lesions are often seen with platelet or primary hemostasis problems. Ecchymoses of differing ages or petechiae particularly of the palate or on the anterior tibial surface of the lower extremities suggest a platelet problem (Fig. 85–2). Lesions that may be confused with purpura or ecchymoses include hematoma (Fig. 85-3), a deep, soft tissue hemorrhage often seen in hemophilia A or B, and telangiectasia, dilated superficial capillaries that blanch. Mucosal telangiectasia and a history of epistaxis and gastrointestinal blood loss suggest hereditary hemorrhagic telangiectasia (Osler-Weber-Rendu disease) (Fig. 85-4). Hepatosplenomegaly, jaundice, lymphadenopathy, and joint deformity are other physical findings that suggest a possible etiology for a bruising/bleeding tendency. Body habitus, joint hyperextensibility, and changes in skin turgor suggest a connective tissue disorder such as Ehlers-Danlos syndrome, a disorder characterized by abnormal collagen that interferes with the blood vessel response to injury and may not support platelet adhesion or aggregation.

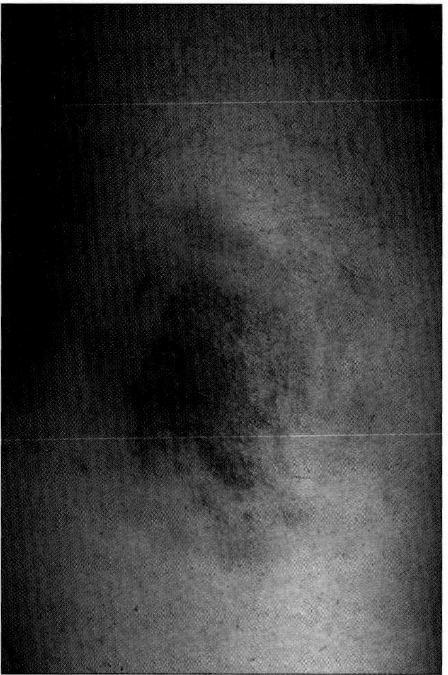

Figure 85–3. Deep hematoma associated with muscular bleed.

Screening Laboratory Tests for Evaluation of Bruising and Bleeding

All patients with bleeding and bruising tendencies require a complete blood count, including platelet count, peripheral blood smear, complete chemistry panel, prothrombin time (PT), and activated partial thromboplastin time (aPTT), to screen for abnormalities that may contribute to disruption of hemostasis.[9,21–23] The complete blood count measures the hemoglobin, hematocrit, and platelets to exclude myeloproliferative disorders or thrombocytopenia. The peripheral smear allows inspection of the leukocyte, erythrocyte, and the platelet morphologies. Chemistry panels provide information on related medical problems such as kidney or liver dysfunction. The PT and aPTT are clot-based assays that screen for quantitative or functional abnormalities of the coagulation factor proteins and fibrinogen. The PT reflects the activity of the extrinsic pathway, especially factor VII, and the common pathway (factors V, X, II, and fibrinogen). The aPTT reflects the activity of the factors in the intrinsic pathway (factors VIII, IX, XI, XII, prekallikrein, and high-molecular-weight kininogen) and the common pathway. Care should be taken when collecting the sample because heparin contamination and inappropriate sample handling may lead to false results. These initial laboratory studies plus the clinical suspicion gathered from the history and physical examination differentiate between disorders of primary hemostasis, secondary hemostasis, clot stability, and fibrinolysis, or suggest a possible combined disorder. Review of past laboratory studies, including old complete blood counts and coagulation studies, establishes the time of onset of the disorder.

DISORDERS ASSOCIATED WITH BRUISING/BLEEDING—DIFFERENTIAL DIAGNOSIS AND MANAGEMENT OVERVIEW

Disorders of Primary Hemostasis

Table 85–1 provides an overview of the major categories of hemostatic disorders. If the initial history, physical examination, and screening laboratory tests suggest a primary hemostatic disorder, the next step is to differentiate between vascular abnormalities, platelet abnormalities, and vWD, the most common inherited bleeding disorder.

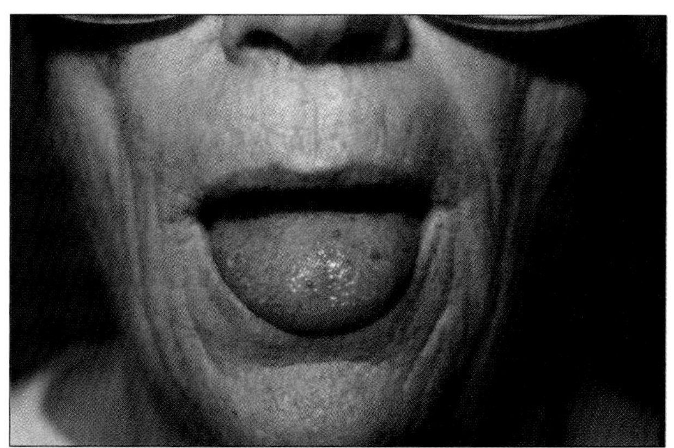

Figure 85–4. Oral telangiectasia associated with hereditary hemorrhagic telangiectasia (Osler-Weber-Rendu disease).

Hemorrhagic Vascular Disorders

Presenting features of vascular disorders mimic those of platelet disorders, with petechiae and ecchymoses. If platelet tests are normal, the vascular disorders are often diagnoses of exclusion without a confirming laboratory test available. Physical examination findings supporting the diagnosis of a vascular abnormality are the primary means of differentiating this class of disorders and may be diagnostic for the condition. Ehlers-Danlos syndromes have characteristic joint and skin findings.[24] Hereditary hemorrhagic telangiectasia (Osler-Weber-Rendu disease) presents with telangiectasias of the oral, nasal, and gastrointestinal tract that become more numerous with age.[25] Onset of the bleeding symptoms (lifelong vs. older age) distinguishes between the inherited and acquired disorders. A thickened tongue, "raccoon eyes," and monoclonal gammopathy suggest vascular infiltration with amyloid as a cause of bleeding. Palpable purpuras are most commonly seen with a concurrent vasculitis. Box 85–2 provides a list of inherited and acquired forms of vascular disorders to be considered when a patient pres-

Box 85–2. Vascular Disorders

Hereditary Disorders

- Ehlers-Danlos syndrome
- Osler-Weber-Rendu disease/hereditary hemorrhagic telangiectasia
- Marfan syndrome
- Pseudoxanthoma elasticum
- Amyloidosis

Acquired Disorders

- Scurvy
- Amyloidosis
- Cushing's syndrome
- Arteriovenous malformations

TABLE 85–1. Major Categories of Most Common Hemostatic Disorders

Pathway	Major Components	Salient Clinical Features	Classic Disorder
Primary hemostasis	Blood vessels Platelets von Willebrand factor	Oozing from mucosa Bruising/ecchymoses Petechiae Telangiectasia	Osler-Weber-Rendu disease Thrombocytopenia Dysfunctional platelets (aspirin/uremia/ congenital) von Willebrand disease
Secondary hemostasis	Clotting proteins—factors II–XIII Fibrinogen	Delayed hematomas	Hemophilia A and B Vitamin K deficiency Liver disease
Fibrinolysis	tPA α_2-Plasmin inhibitor PAI-1	Delayed bleeding Poor wound healing	Dysfibrinogenemia α_2-Plasmin inhibitor Liver disease

ents with a primary hemostatic bleeding defect but no evidence of platelet or vWF abnormalities.

Management of vascular bleeding disorders is uniformly difficult. Because the bleeding is linked to structure or function defects of the blood vessels themselves, no "replacement product" is available. To compound the problem, sutures may not hold in the defective tissue. Treatment options vary depending on the condition. Acquired disorders such as amyloidosis caused by multiple myeloma or vasculitic purpura benefit from treating the underlying disorder. An antifibrinolytic drug such as ε-aminocaproic acid slows the dissolution of clot and may aid in clot retention at a site of injury. Antifibrinolytic drugs are also used to promote thrombosis of telangiectasia and arteriovenous malformation with varying success.[26] Embolization of bleeding vessels with various substances can control a difficult bleeding site, but, in conditions such as hereditary hemorrhagic telangiectasia, new lesions will continue to form. Conjugated estrogens decrease bleeding from gastrointestinal arteriovenous malformation, but side effects preclude long-term treatment.[26] The best management for many of these disorders is to avoid unnecessary procedures.

Platelet Disorders

Platelet disorders disrupt the formation of a platelet plug, leading to poor initial localization of clot to the site of injury.[1,3,4] The hemostatic history includes bruising and bleeding that is evident as continued oozing from an injured or surgical site. Capillary bleeding is particularly evident and is manifest as bleeding from mucosal surfaces. Epistaxis, gum bleeding, and menorrhagia are common manifestations, and hematoma formation is rare except with severe injury. Box 85–3 displays six major subcategories of platelet disorders, including inherited and acquired thrombocytopenia, inherited and acquired platelet function defects, and inherited and acquired combined thrombocytopenia and platelet function disorders. Bleeding is typically more severe with functional defects of the platelet, either acquired or congenital.[1,3-5,19,20] Platelet counts as low as 10,000-30,000/μL

Box 85–3. Categories of Platelet Disorders

Thrombocytopenia–Quantitative Disorders

Inherited/Congenital

- Epstein's syndrome
- Fechtner syndrome
- Mediterranean macrothrombocytopenia
- Sebastian syndrome
- *AML1* gene mutation
- Arteriovenous malformation

Acquired

- Immune thrombocytopenic purpura
- Splenomegaly
- Medications
- Infection
- Human immunodeficiency virus infection
- Alcohol
- Posttransfusion purpura
- Myelodysplastic syndrome
- Myelofibrosis
- Aplastic anemia
- Bone marrow infiltration

Functional Defects–Qualitative Disorders

Inherited/Congenital

- Glanzmann's thrombasthenia
- δ- and/or α-Storage pool deficiencies
- Arachidonic acid metabolism dysfunctions
- Platelet-type von Willebrand disease

Acquired

- Medications
- Uremia
- Dysproteinemias
- Myelo- and lymphoproliferative disorders

Combined Quantitative & Qualitative Disorders

Inherited/Congenital

- May-Hegglin anomaly
- Bernard-Soulier syndrome
- Gray platelet syndrome

Acquired

- Immune thrombocytopenic purpura
- Cirrhosis

may be well tolerated, especially in immune thrombocytopenic purpura (ITP)[27,28] or congenital thrombocytopenic conditions,[29] as long as the platelets function normally and no additional defects of the hemostatic system are evident. Thrombocytopenia resulting from decreased production is either primary, resulting from bone marrow disorders, or secondary, resulting from marrow suppression by malignancy, infections, drugs, or nutritional deficiencies. Peripheral destruction or sequestering of platelets is common; etiologies include consumption caused by active bleeding, disseminated intravascular coagulation, thrombotic thrombocytopenic purpura/hemolytic-uremic syndrome, immune destruction (ITP), or sequestration from splenomegaly. A positive family history guides the differential diagnosis toward an inherited quantitative or combined quantitative and qualitative disorder.

Laboratory evaluation of platelet disorders utilizes routine tests and tests specific to platelet structure and function.[1,4,9,23] The platelet count is easily confirmed by an automated count, and review of the blood smear identifies cellular abnormalities. Enlarged platelets are found with Bernard-Soulier syndrome, a congenital quantitative and qualitative disorder (see Chapter 59), and in disorders associated with rapid platelet turnover, such as ITP. Bone marrow biopsy identifies primary production defects such as aplastic anemia, myelodysplasia, or infiltrative processes of the marrow. Antiplatelet antibody may identify immune mechanisms for platelet destruction, but specificity and sensitivity of the assays are poor.

Advanced testing for platelet disorders involves specialized platelet function studies. The oldest study is the bleeding time, a controlled 1-mm-deep incision of the skin monitored for the time the incision takes to stop bleeding. The test is controversial because of the wide normal range (2–10 minutes), the lack of correlation with bleeding at sites other than the skin, the technical difficulty associated with consistent performance of the test, and interference from medications, systemic disorders affecting the skin, and low hematocrit.[30,31] The bleeding time is particularly unsuitable in patients with skin damage (e.g., solar purpura, senile purpura) or edematous states because the local defect interferes with assessment of hemostatic potential. The bleeding time neither predicts nor excludes surgical bleeding; therefore, it is not indicated as a preoperative screening test. A bleeding time test performed by an experienced technologist on a patient who has normal skin and is on no medication (including caffeine) may be used as an initial screen for a primary hemostatic defect, but confirmatory studies of platelet function and vWF are required, thus questioning the usefulness of first performing this invasive study. The PFA-100 is an instrument that monitors platelet plug formation by blockage of flow through a small aperture in a membrane containing collagen/epinephrine or collagen/ADP. The instrument is rapidly replacing the bleeding time as an initial screen for primary hemostatic disorders because of its ease of use and lack of invasiveness. Studies suggest that it is superior to the bleeding time in vWD and at least as good for primary platelet disorders.[32] However, similar to the bleeding time, the instrument cannot predict or exclude bleeding and should not be used as a preoperative screening test or as a generalized determination of bleeding tendency.

Other instruments that monitor global function of the primary hemostatic system are increasingly available and growing in popularity, but these instruments are not yet fully tested or routinely available. Platelet aggregation studies are most useful for evaluating inherent platelet abnormalities. They are performed using either whole blood or platelet-rich plasma and utilize various activators of platelets, including ADP, collagen, epinephrine, ristocetin, and arachidonic acid to assess platelet response to stimulation. Accurate studies are technically difficult and can vary with age, gender, and ethnicity. Different functional disorders are manifest by failure to respond to one or more of the activators. If granules are not present or cannot be released, platelets will fail to react to collagen and have only partial response to epinephrine and ADP. Electron microscopy to identify platelet granules differentiates between storage pool disorders (lack of granules) and release defects. Currently, laboratory testing to adequately evaluate disorders of adhesion proteins or granule release defects is not available.

Identification of the specific platelet defect is important for effective management. Detailed therapy for various platelet disorders is addressed in separate chapters; however, common treatment modalities are reviewed here. When possible, non-blood products should be used to control bleeding or treat the underlying disorder. Antifibrinolytic agents such as ε-aminocaproic acid decrease bleeding caused by both quantitative and qualitative platelet disorders by slowing fibrinolysis.[26] Desmopressin decreases bleeding in some qualitative bleeding disorders, although the mechanism of action is unclear.[33,34] Steroids, immunoglobulin preparations, immune-modulating drugs, and chemotherapeutic agents are used to treat platelet disorders depending on the underlying etiology.[3,5,27,28] With the exception of heparin-induced thrombocytopenia and thrombotic thrombocytopenic purpura, platelet transfusion remains the mainstay of therapy for treatment of platelet disorders associated with active bleeding. Even in heparin-induced thrombocytopenia, thrombotic thrombocytopenic purpura, and ITP, which may be exacerbated by or unresponsive to transfusion, platelet therapy is indicated for severe, life-threatening hemorrhage. Platelet concentrates are the leading cause of transfusion reactions and, despite aggressive screening, transmission of infectious material remains a concern.[35] Allergic reactions and transfusion-related acute lung injury are rare but serious complications of platelet transfusion. Repeated platelet transfusions for patients with congenital qualitative platelet disorders or bone marrow production disorders lead to alloantibody production, decreasing the effectiveness of transfusions. For all platelet disorders, first-line therapy consists of hemostatic drugs or drugs that alter the underlying defect, with platelet transfusion reserved for severe bleeding or disorders without a non–blood product treatment option.

Von Willebrand Disease

vWD is the most common inherited bleeding disorder, affecting all races and both genders.[36] vWF tethers the platelet to the site of vessel injury by attaching to the platelet glycoprotein 1b-IX-V receptor and receptors in the matrix of the disturbed blood vessel wall. Factor VIII is unable to circulate unless bound to vWF; therefore, vWF contributes indirectly to formation of the fibrin clot by delivering one of the required cofactors of the coagulation cascade to the site of injury. Childhood epistaxis, easy bruising, heavy menses, and intermittent bleeding with surgical procedures are the hallmarks of vWD presentation.[36,37] Other than ecchymoses, there are no salient physical findings. vWD is an autosomal dominant disorder and should be evident in several family members and generations; however, with mild type 1 deficiencies, significant bleeding may never occur.[38]

Laboratory documentation of vWD consists of testing for the antigen level, activity level, and factor VIII activity to assess the ability of vWF to perform its carrier function.[36,39] Ristocetin cofactor activity is the most common activity test, but other activity assays, including collagen-binding studies, are available. The aPTT will be prolonged if factor VIII levels are low. Obtaining multimer analysis provides qualitative assessment of the protein and allows differentiation between two major subtypes, type 1 (normal protein but decreased levels), and type 2 (abnormal protein but low or normal levels). Provocative testing by desmopressin challenge may be necessary to determine if a normal-appearing protein functions appropriately—all dysfunctional proteins are considered type 2 disorders regardless of the multimeric evaluation. vWF is an "acute-phase reactant"; therefore, several sets of laboratory data may be needed to confirm a true nadir vWF level. Stress and estrogen contribute to elevated levels of vWF, but patients with type O blood have lower baseline levels that may be confused with mild vWD.

Management of vWD consists primarily of desmopressin and antifibrinolytic agents for type 1 patients or a vWF blood concentrate for patients not responsive to desmopressin.[1,26,33,36,40] Desmopressin is administered intravenously or by nasal spray. Two nasal sprays are available; vWD patients should use only a brand that delivers 150 μg per spray, not the more dilute spray developed to treat diabetes insipidus. If fluid intake is not restricted, monitoring of sodium levels after desmopressin administration is necessary to prevent dilutional hyponatremia. Cryoprecipitate is an excellent source of vWF if virally attenuated clotting factor concentrates such as Humate-P are not available. Estrogen elevates vWF levels and may decrease excessive menses or improve bruising. Chapter 64 contains a complete review of vWD.

Disorders of Secondary Hemostasis

Failure to create a strong fibrin clot results in continued bleeding and poor wound healing.[1,6] Fibrin is both a bandage and scaffolding to support infiltration of fibroblasts that begin the process of tissue repair. Decreased or dysfunctional clotting factor proteins impair secondary hemostasis. A single clotting protein may be decreased, or multiple clotting proteins may be defective. Factor VIII is unique in requiring a cofactor, vWF, to travel to the site of clot formation. A low factor VIII level may be due to lack or dysfunction of the carrier protein vWF, and not due to a defect in factor VIII production. Delayed bleeding, deep muscle hematomas, and hemarthroses are the cardinal features, but surgical bleeding and menses may be life-threatening. Bleeding is out of proportion to the inciting trauma or may even be spontaneous. Box 85–4 lists secondary hemostasis disorders according to inherited or acquired status.

The patient's history allows the clinician to distinguish between congenital and acquired disorders, and inheritance patterns narrow the differential diagnosis. Congenital factor VIII and IX deficiencies, the most common inherited defects, are sex-linked disorders, but most other inherited clotting factor deficiencies are autosomal recessive conditions.[18,41,42] Severe deficiencies of clotting factors are usually diagnosed in childhood. The diagnosis of mild factor deficiencies (5–40% of normal) can be delayed into adulthood if there has been no major challenge to hemostasis. Vitamin K deficiency and severe liver dysfunction are acquired disorders that decrease clotting factor levels and contribute to excessive bruising and bleeding.[1,15,43] Autoimmune acquired inhibitors to coagulation factors occur infrequently but can be associated with severe bleeding complications.[44,45] They are frequently idiopathic, but may be associated with pregnancy, surgery, malignancies (particularly myelo- or lymphoproliferative disorders), medications (antibiotics or valproic acid), or autoimmune disease states. Not all acquired deficiencies are due to synthetic defects or autoantibodies. For example, in amyloidosis, factor X deficiency results because factor X binds to amyloid, resulting in lower circulating levels.[46]

Box 85–4. Disorders of Secondary Hemostasis

Inherited/Congenital Disorders

- Hemophilia A (Factor VIII deficiency)
- Hemophilia B (Factor IX deficiency)
- Factor deficiencies II, V, VII, X, XI, XIII
- Inherited dysfibrinogenemia/afibrinogenemia/hypofibrinogenemia

Acquired Disorders

- Autoantibodies to clotting factors
- Vitamin K deficiency
- Liver disease
- Anticoagulant administration
- Factor X deficiency related to amyloid

Historical clues are joined by laboratory screens to create a pathway to specific secondary hemostasis defects or diagnoses. The hallmark laboratory finding in disorders of secondary hemostasis is a prolongation of the PT (extrinsic pathway) and/or the aPTT (intrinsic pathway).[1,9,21,22] An isolated PT prolongation is seen with factor VII deficiency. An isolated aPTT increase can be seen with factors VIII, IX, XI, XII, prekallikrein, and high-molecular-weight kininogen. If both the PT and aPTT are prolonged, then there are either multiple coagulation factor defects (e.g., vitamin K deficiency) or a defect in a single common pathway protein (factor V, X, II, or fibrinogen). Advanced testing for problems of secondary hemostasis includes mixing studies, specific clotting factor levels, thrombin clot time, reptilase time, and antibody titers if an inhibitor is present. Mixing studies combine one part patient plasma with one part normal plasma, with a PT and/or aPTT test performed on the mixture. Mixing studies that result in the complete and persistent correction of the PT/aPTT indicate a factor deficiency, and the next step is to perform appropriate factor level tests. Lack of correction indicates interference with clot formation because of a clotting factor antibody, paraprotein, lupus anticoagulant, or anticoagulant such as heparin or a thrombin inhibitor drug. History directs the appropriate next line of testing to find the inhibiting substance. A partial correction may indicate a combination of factor deficiency and weak inhibitor. Again, history and associated physical findings guide additional evaluation. If the aPTT prolongs with incubation, a time- and temperature-dependent factor inhibitor is present, most likely an inhibitor of factor VIII or V. If an antibody to a clotting factor is detected, a Bethesda titer helps to design appropriate therapy (see Chapter 63). The thrombin clot time and reptilase time assess fibrinogen function if a dysfibrinogenemia is suspected, but heparin may also prolong the thrombin clot time.

Once the clotting factor defect is identified, treatment can begin. In the majority of secondary hemostasis disorders, the cornerstone of treatment is replacement of the missing clotting factor.[1,18,47-49] Fresh frozen plasma contains all clotting factors but usually in concentrations too low to effectively replace any single factor fully. Factor concentrates made by purifying specific clotting factors from plasma or by recombinant technology are available for several but not all clotting proteins. Plasma-derived concentrates include factor VIII and IX products and prothrombin complex concentrates, which contain varying amounts of the vitamin K–dependent clotting factors (II, VII, IX, and X). Cryoprecipitate contains enriched amounts of vWF, factor VIII, factor XIII, and fibrinogen. Each unit of cryoprecipitate derived from a single unit of plasma contains 100–250 mg of fibrinogen and will increase the fibrinogen level by 5–7 mg/dL. Fresh frozen plasma is the only readily available product in the United States for replacement of factor XI and factor V. Recombinant clotting factors are available for factors VIII, IX, and VII. As a rule, recombinant or the most concentrated form of factor available should be used for treatment. Bypassing products, including an activated prothrombin complex concentrate such as FEIBA or recombinant activated factor VII, may control bleeding by compensating for lack of a specific clotting factor that is being neutralized by an inhibitor.[50,51]

In some cases, treatment with non-blood products is possible. Desmopressin releases vWF, which will result in modest increases of its passenger protein, factor VIII. Patients with mild hemophilia A and minor bleeding may respond to desmopressin therapy by doubling the baseline level of factor VIII. In addition, antifibrinolytic agents may promote better clot retention and decrease the requirement for specific clotting factor replacement. Finally, the best treatment of a factor deficiency may be treatment of the underlying disorder that caused the decrease in factor. Vitamin K replacement is easy to administer by oral (preferred) or intravenous routes and will result in correction of factor deficiencies within 24–48 hours in most patients. Immune-modulating products such as prednisone, chemotherapeutic agents, or intravenous gamma globulin may help decrease antibody production in patients with inhibitors to clotting factors.[52,53] These general guidelines for treatment of disorders of secondary hemostasis are addressed in greater detail in other chapters.

Disorders of Clot Stabilization and Fibrinolysis

A fibrin clot must remain in place long enough to allow repair of the vessel injury. Difficulties in the stabilization of the clot can arise from abnormalities of fibrin or lack of proper cross-linking of the fibrin strands by factor XIII.[54-57] Even a well-formed clot is subject to premature dissolution if regulation of fibrinolysis is impaired.[58-60] PAI-1 controls tPA activity and prevents overproduction of plasmin.[60] α_2-Plasmin inhibitor binds free plasmin and prevents excessive fibrin(ogen)olysis. Dysfibrinogenemia, factor XIII deficiency, and disorders of fibrinolysis are often not considered until after disorders of primary or secondary hemostasis have been excluded, primarily because these disorders are rare and have few defining historical or physical examination findings. Poor wound healing or excessive scar formation may be an indicator of factor XIII deficiency or excessive fibrinolysis that destroys the fibrin scaffolding before fibroblasts can complete repair of the wound. Acquired defects in clot maintenance occur with cirrhosis as a result of production of abnormal fibrinogen, decreased production of factor XIII and α_2-plasmin inhibitor, and failure to clear tPA. Medication-related hyperfibrinolysis is seen after administration of thrombolytic agents.

Laboratory evaluation begins with assessment of the PT, aPTT, fibrinogen level, and fibrin degradation products. With abnormalities of fibrinogen, the PT and aPTT are usually prolonged, although the fibrinogen level may be normal. Advanced testing to evaluate fibrinogen function includes the reptilase time and the thrombin clot time. These assays assess the ability to cleave fibrinogen into fibrin; prolongation indicates a structural defect in fibrinogen. If the defect prevents fibrin formation, then bleeding occurs. The PT and aPTT are normal in factor XIII deficiency, and determination of a factor XIII level should be considered in patients with delayed bleeding, poor wound healing, and a totally normal laboratory evaluation. The euglobulin clot lysis time is a global screen for disorders of fibrinolysis, with short times seen with defects of the fibrinolytic system. Direct assays for PAI-1, tPA, plasminogen, and α_2-plasmin inhibitor are available to identify the specific defect in the fibrinolytic system. Finally, D-dimer and fibrin (fibrinogen) degradation products indicate increased fibrin breakdown resulting from either increased clot production or excessive fibrinolysis. Because factor XIII is responsible for creating the cross-linked D-dimer, patients who lack factor XIII will have elevated degradation products without D-dimer present.

Disorders of clot stability are primarily treated by blood products that replace the abnormal component. Fibrinogen and factor XIII are contained in cryoprecipitate, and specific concentrates of these proteins are occasionally available. Plasma is the only source for α_2-plasmin inhibitor and plasminogen. Platelets contain large quantities of PAI-1 in the α-granules and may be helpful in increasing local concentrations of this inhibitor at the injury site. Non–blood product treatment consists of antifibrinolytic drugs such as ε-aminocaproic acid. These drugs slow the activation of plasminogen to plasmin and interfere with plasminogen binding to fibrin.

Bruising Without Identifiable Bleeding Disorder

The final and most perplexing patient to categorize is the patient for whom no bleeding disorder can be found. If all coagulation laboratory studies are normal or negative, then it is necessary to reassess for other causes of bleeding. The patient has either a primary blood vessel or skin defect, a systemic disorder affecting blood vessels, a platelet or clotting factor defect that cannot be identified by current methodology, or a factitious bleeding disorder. A thorough history and physical examination can identify risk factors or symptoms suggestive of the underlying disorder. Blue toes or fingers may be secondary to hemorrhage at sites of thrombotic emboli and not a bleeding disorder at all. Bleeding limited to a single organ system such as the skin or gastrointestinal tract is more likely a tissue defect. With time, sun exposure, aging, and steroid use may all lead to skin damage resulting in chronic bruising. Screening tests for vasculitis, cryoglobulinemias, plasma cell dyscrasias, liver disease, uremia, or lymphoproliferative disorders may identify the etiology of the systemic illness presenting as bruising. Factitious purpura as a manifestation of Munchausen syndrome is a diagnosis of exclusion that taxes the skill of the clinician to rule out a true physical disorder. The bleeding may be created by self-injury, ingestion of anticoagulant medications, or mimicking bleeding by swallowing, instilling, or letting of blood. There is no specific diagnostic test for the factitious disorder. A history that seems almost unbelievable or, conversely, "too good to be true" or a contradictory history, physical findings, or laboratory tests are clues to the disorder.

SUMMARY

Patients frequently present to the hematologist with a complaint of easy bruising or excessive bleeding with previous trauma or surgery. A detailed hemostasis history and pertinent physical examination together with screening laboratory tests start the process of identifying the bleeding diathesis or abnormality. A solid understanding of the hemostatic pathways, including primary hemostasis, secondary hemostasis, clot stabilization, and fibrinolysis, enables a systematic approach to identifying the underlying disorder and designing a reasonable management plan. Ultimately, not all chronic bruising or bleeding can be explained, but the guidelines in this chapter are designed to help initiate an appropriate hemostatic evaluation.

CURRENT CONTROVERSIES & FUTURE CONSIDERATIONS

Chronic Bruising and Bleeding Diathesis

- Not all patients who complain of bruising have an identifiable bleeding disorder as defined by current laboratory tests.
- The bleeding time is a poor diagnostic tool for assessment of primary hemostasis and should not be used for preoperative screening for bleeding risk.
- Global assessment of hemostatic potential of blood may prove more useful than individualized tests of the components of hemostasis.

Suggested Readings*

Acharya SS, Coughlin A, Dimichele DM, for the North American Rare Bleeding Disorder Study Group: Rare Bleeding Disorder Registry: deficiencies of factors II, V, VII, X, XIII, fibrinogen and dysfibrinogenemias. J Thromb Haemost 2:248–256, 2004.

Kitchens CS: Approach to the bleeding patient. Hematol Oncol Clin North Am 6:983–989, 1992.

Liu MC, Kessler CM: A systematic approach to the bleeding patient. *In* Kitchens CS, Alving BM, Kessler CM (eds): Consultative Hemostasis and Thrombosis. Philadelphia: WB Saunders, 2002, pp 27–39.

Sham RL: Evaluation of mild bleeding disorders and easy bruising. Blood Rev 8:98–104, 1994.

Triplett DA: Coagulation and bleeding disorders: review and update. Clin Chem 46:1260–1269, 2000.

Full references for this chapter can be found on accompanying CD-ROM.

CHAPTER 86

Venous and Arterial Thrombosis

Charles W. Francis, MD, and Karen L. Kaplan, MD, PhD

KEY POINTS

Venous and Arterial Thrombosis

- Venous thromboembolism is common, with an annual incidence of about 1 in 1000 that increases with age.
- The presentation of deep vein thrombosis and pulmonary embolism is nonspecific, and the diagnosis should be confirmed by laboratory and imaging tests.
- Prophylaxis is effective in preventing venous thromboembolism during high-risk periods, and selection requires appropriate risk stratification.
- Most patients with acute deep vein thrombosis or pulmonary embolism can be treated with 5 or more days of heparin or low-molecular-weight heparins followed by several months of an oral vitamin K antagonist, with INR monitoring and adjustment to 2–3.
- The optimal duration of therapy must be individualized based on clinical factors determining risk of recurrence and bleeding and also patient preferences.
- The pathogenesis of arterial thrombosis is complex and depends on progression of atherosclerosis, plaque instability and rupture, and embolization of plaque-associated thrombus.
- Approximately 20% of strokes are caused by cardiogenic emboli, and their occurrence can be significantly reduced by long-term oral anticoagulant therapy in patients with atrial fibrillation, severe left ventricular dysfunction, and valvular disease or prosthetic valves.
- Aspirin is highly effective in both primary and secondary prevention of myocardial infarction, treatment of acute myocardial infarction, and prevention of stroke.
- Clopidogrel is more effective than aspirin for the combined outcome of new myocardial infarction, new stroke, or vascular death, especially in patients with peripheral arterial disease.

VENOUS THROMBOEMBOLISM

Introduction

Because of their expertise in hemostasis, hematologists are frequently consulted for evaluation of possible hypercoagulability in patients presenting with venous thrombosis. Additionally, problems in diagnosis frequently arise because of the protean presenting symptoms and need for careful, objective diagnosis. Other issues include the choice of anticoagulants, the duration of treatment, and the very difficult problem of managing thrombosis in patients with active bleeding or at high risk for bleeding.

Epidemiology and Pathogenesis

Venous thromboembolic disease is a common medical problem with an annual incidence of approximately 1 in 1000.[1–3] Thrombosis most commonly affects leg veins, resulting in acute symptoms, and also causes structural damage that can result in chronic venous insufficiency in up to one third of patients associated with varying degrees of chronic leg swelling, pain, and ulceration.[4–6] Nearly all pulmonary emboli derive from deep leg vein thrombi and result in 50,000 to 100,000 deaths per year in the United States.[7–9]

The pathogenesis of thrombosis involves abnormalities in the blood, its flow, and the vessel wall, a combination termed *Virchow's triad* (Fig. 86–1). Venous stasis is a common contributor to thrombosis, as are intrinsic abnormalities in the hemostatic system that result in "hypercoagulability" (see Chapter 67). The normal endothelium is thromboresistant, but vessel wall disease contributes to thrombotic potential, particularly in atherosclerosis. Endothelial injury can also contribute to venous thrombosis following trauma or surgical injury.

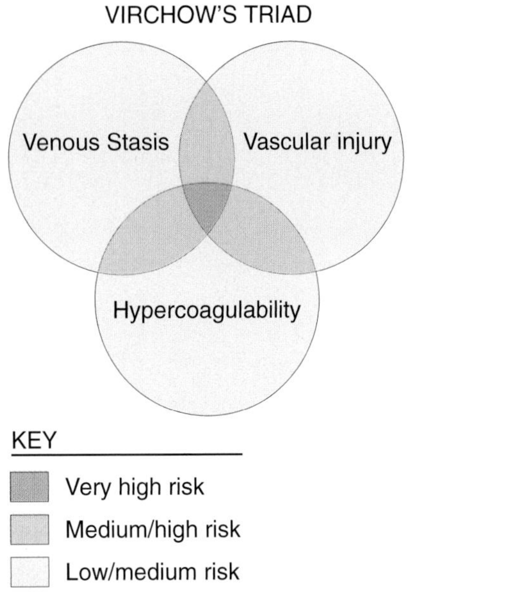

Figure 86–1. Virchow's triad. Venous stasis, vascular injury, and hypercoagulability all contribute to risk of venous thromboembolism.

Clinical Features and Diagnosis

Presentation

Venous thrombosis presents typically with leg pain and swelling, which may be quite variable in its severity and rate of progression. Frequently, patients notice tightness, aching, or pain in the calf with some degree of swelling that develops over 1 or several days. An acute onset may lead to an office or emergency room visit within the first day, but this may be delayed for several days when mild pain or swelling is gradually progressive. Symptoms may be limited to the calf, or the whole leg may be involved with swelling and tenderness. Symptoms are often attributed to muscle strain or excessive exercise. Physical findings include swelling, edema, localized tenderness, and dilated superficial collateral veins. Although the presentation may be very suggestive of deep vein thrombosis, other diagnoses should be considered, including cellulitis, hematoma, bruise, muscle strain, and ruptured Baker's cyst. Also, deep vein thrombosis must be distinguished from superficial vein thrombosis, which presents with a painful and tender area localized along the course of a superficial vein. If superficial thrombosis does not extend to deep veins, it is of less consequence and usually requires only symptomatic therapy. It is important to recognize that deep vein thrombosis can be entirely asymptomatic in nonambulatory or hospitalized patients. Diagnosis then requires a high degree of suspicion, and the only findings may be mild leg swelling and tenderness, or the initial presentation may be pulmonary embolism.

Diagnosis

Because of the important therapeutic implications, the diagnosis of deep vein thrombosis should always be objectively confirmed. Overall, only approximately 25% of patients in whom deep vein thrombosis is suspected will have the diagnosis confirmed. The diagnostic approach should begin with a careful clinical assessment to establish the likelihood of deep vein thrombosis, and this is followed by laboratory studies and imaging[10,11] (Fig. 86–2). Useful and verified systems for establishing pretest probability based on readily available clinical parameters have been published.[12–17] Ultrasound has become the preferred imaging test and is sensitive and specific in symptomatic patients with proximal thrombosis.[18–22] Several studies in recent years have demonstrated the diagnostic value of D-dimer measurement.[23–28] D-dimer is a fibrinolytic degradation product of cross-linked fibrin, and nearly all patients with deep vein thrombosis will have an elevated level. It is, however, not specific, and an elevated D-dimer is found in many other conditions. Therefore, a normal D-dimer is useful in excluding the diagnosis of deep vein thrombosis, particularly in patients with a low pretest probability. In patients with a moderate to high clinical suspicion of deep vein thrombosis, the pretest probability of deep vein thrombosis is sufficiently high that an imaging test should be the initial choice, and the noninvasive compression Doppler ultrasound is the first choice. A positive ultrasound establishes the diagnosis, but in patients with a negative ultrasound, a normal D-dimer provides confirmatory evidence to exclude the diagnosis. A positive D-dimer in this setting, however, leads to diagnostic uncertainty, which can be resolved with repeat ultrasound or venography. The incorporation of D-dimer testing into the diagnostic algorithm results in the need for fewer ultrasound examinations, because the diagnosis can be excluded in low-risk patients. Also, fewer moderate- to high-risk patients need repeat ultrasound or venography.

The diagnosis of pulmonary embolism is also difficult.[29,30] Presenting symptoms are nonspecific and typically include chest pain and dyspnea, leading to a differential diagnosis that includes muscle strain, myocardial ischemia, pneumonia, pleuritis, pericarditis, or esophagitis. Physical findings are also nonspecific and include tachypnea, tachycardia, localized crackles, and signs of right heart failure in severe cases. Electrocardiographic findings of right heart strain, hypoxia, chest radiographic findings typical of infarction or a major vessel cutoff, and echocardiographic features of right heart dilation and pulmonary hypertension can be useful. However, specific diagnostic testing is required (Fig. 86–3). As with diagnosis of deep vein thrombosis, establishment of the pretest probability is the initial step in planning diagnostic testing.[25,31–33] Because of its high sensitivity, measurement of D-dimer is useful,[24,25,34,35] and a normal value can exclude the diagnosis in patients with a low pretest probability. Imaging is required in patients with a moderate or high pretest probability, and either ventilation-perfusion lung scanning or spiral computed tomography (CT) scanning is appropriate.[29,36–39] There is more experience with the former, and a normal perfusion scan excludes the diagnosis of pulmonary embolism. A high-probability lung scan leads to treatment as does a CT showing filling defects in proximal vessels. If the results of imaging are low probability or negative, further

DIAGNOSTIC TESTING FOR DEEP VENOUS THROMBOSIS

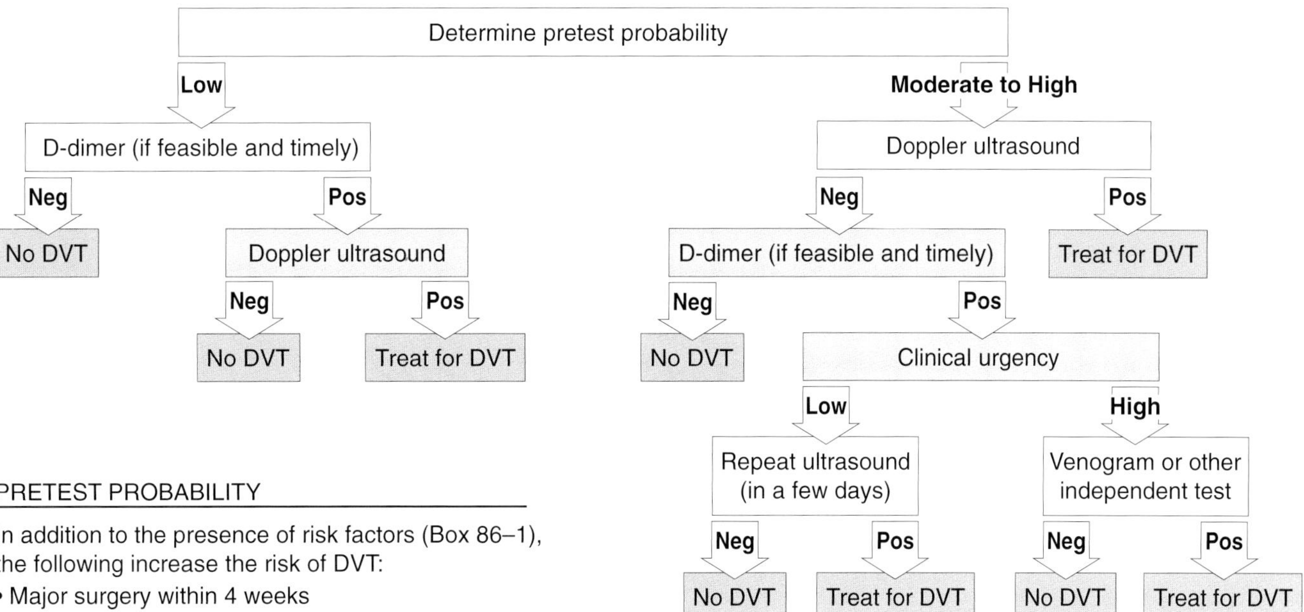

PRETEST PROBABILITY

In addition to the presence of risk factors (Box 86–1), the following increase the risk of DVT:

- Major surgery within 4 weeks
- Localized tenderness along the distribution of the deep venous system
- Entire leg swollen
- Calf swelling 3 cm more than asymptomatic side (measured 10 cm below tibial tuberosity)
- Pitting edema confined to the symptomatic leg
- Collateral superfical veins (nonvaricose)
- DVT more likely than alternative diagnoses

Figure 86–2. Strategy for diagnostic testing for deep vein thrombosis.

imaging tests can be avoided if a D-dimer measurement is normal. Unfortunately, the results of the ventilation-perfusion scan or spiral CT scan in many patients with a moderate or high pretest probability are indeterminate, and this requires further evaluation.[40–44] Because most pulmonary emboli result from deep vein thrombosis, a bilateral Doppler ultrasound may be positive, leading to therapy. Clinical suspicion is an important determinate of further diagnostic testing, and pulmonary angiography may be needed in patients with a high clinical suspicion.

Difficult problems arise in diagnosis of recurrent disease, because the findings must be interpreted in relation to both the initial event and also new findings. New leg symptoms may signal a recurrence, and this can be established by showing thrombus extension by ultrasound in comparison with the initial study. Typically, thrombi regress over weeks to months during treatment, but up to 50% remain abnormal at 1 year.[45,46] Obtaining a "baseline" repeat ultrasound after several months or at the end of therapy may provide a useful comparison when symptoms subsequently develop in the same area. Likewise, D-dimer levels return to baseline, and sustained or recurrent elevation can be a marker of recurrence.[47] Pulmonary vascular occlusions also resolve over several weeks, and recurrence can be established by identification of new areas of ventilation-perfusion mismatch on a ventilation-perfusion scan or by new intravascular occlusions on CT scans.

Chronic venous insufficiency presents with variable degrees of chronic leg swelling, skin thickening, aching, hyperpigmentation, and ulceration in the most severe form. This is more common after ileofemoral thrombosis and may develop within the first year, but more commonly is progressive over several years.[4,48] The fully developed syndrome is easily recognizable, but the differential diagnosis may include localized cellulitis and arterial insufficiency. The latter, however, is less commonly associated with edema and presents with pain on exercise or at rest in its severe form, with associated evidence of arterial obstruction.

Prophylaxis

Primary prophylaxis is used to prevent venous thromboembolism in patients at high risk. As with any preventive strategy, the adverse effects must be minimal because the majority of patients receiving prophylaxis would never develop disease, and the strategy is most effective when applied to patients at highest risk. Prophylaxis is recommended for short periods during which patients are at high risk, typically during hospitalizations or following surgical procedures. The rationale for prophylaxis derives from the high risk of venous thromboembolic disease and the serious consequences, including sudden death, which is a frequent presentation

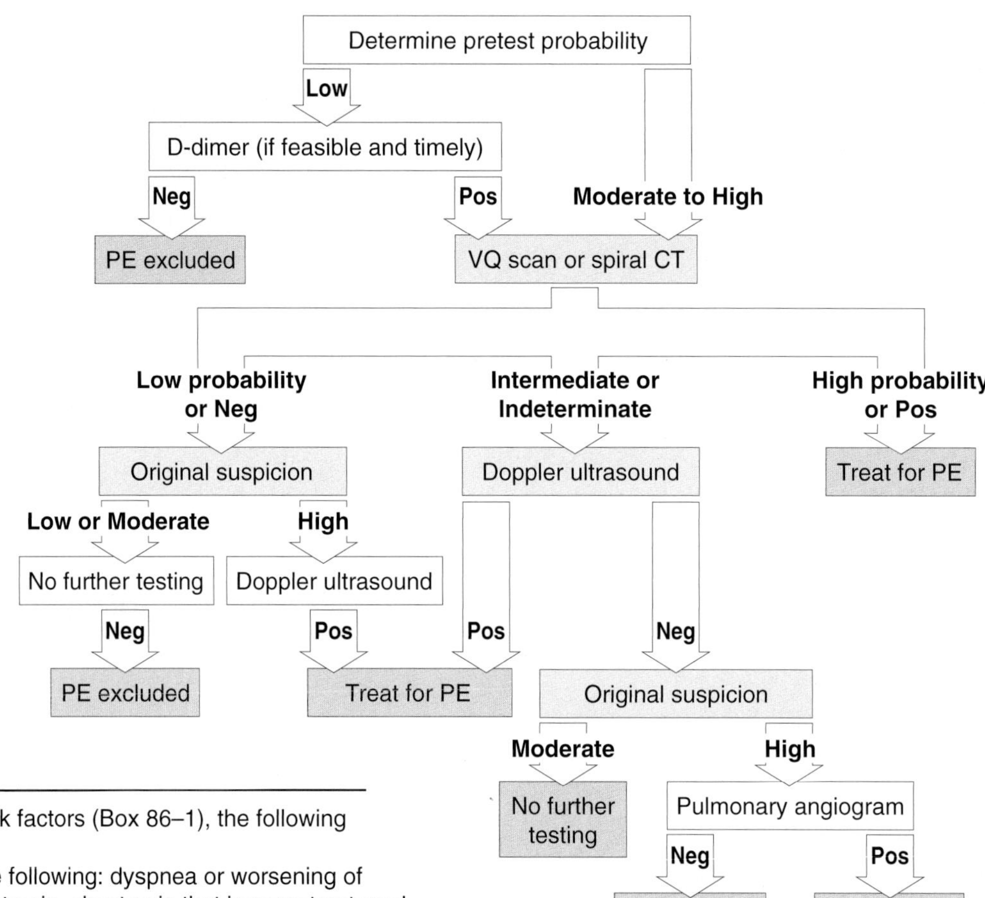

PRETEST PROBABILITY

In addition to the presence of risk factors (Box 86–1), the following increase the liklihood of PE:

- Respiratory: two or more of the following: dyspnea or worsening of chronic dyspnea, pleuritic chest pain, chest pain that is nonretrosternal and nonpleuritic, an arterial oxygen saturation less than 92% while breathing room air that corrects with oxygen supplementation less than 40%, hemoptysis, or pleural rub
- Heart rate > 90 bpm
- Leg symptoms
- Low grade fever
- Chest radiography compatible with PE
- Syncope
- Blood pressure < 90 mm Hg and heart rate > 100 bpm
- Ventilation or oxygen supplementation > 40%
- New onset right heart failure (elevated JVP and new S1, Q3 and T3 sounds or RBBB)

Figure 86–3. Strategy for diagnostic testing for pulmonary embolism.

of pulmonary embolism. In patients found at autopsy to have died primarily from pulmonary embolism, 75% succumbed within the first hour after developing symptoms,[49] too short a time for accurate diagnosis and effective therapy. Thus, the choice of appropriate prophylaxis can prevent morbidity and mortality from venous thromboembolic disease with a low frequency of serious complications.

The choice of prophylaxis depends on understanding the level of risk in an individual patient. A number of clinical factors contributing to elevated risk have been identified[50] (Box 86–1). The risk increases progressively with age, particularly over age 60. Surgery or trauma greatly increases risk, but this risk is temporary and decreases progressively over days to weeks. Other frequent major risk factors include prior venous thromboembolism, active malignancy, immobilization, and paralysis. Thrombophilic states are increasingly identified (see Chapter 67), and they contribute to varying levels of additional risk. Most patients who develop venous thromboembolic disease have multiple risk factors.[51] For example, an elderly patient having major surgery for colon cancer would be at very high risk.

For hospitalized patients, the choice of prophylaxis is based on the level of risk (Table 86–1). Among surgical patients, the level of risk is determined by the type of surgery and additional factors such as those listed in Box 86–1. Thus, patients having minor surgery and no risk factors are at low risk. Longer duration of surgery and the presence of additional risk factors move the patient into a higher risk category. For medical patients, the level of risk and choice of prophylaxis are dependent on the number of risk factors present. Age over 60 is a major risk factor, and most hospitalized patients will be in the high-risk category.

Suggested prophylactic methods are chosen to reduce risk with an acceptable frequency of side effects and cost.[52,53] The incidence of venous thromboembolic disease is less than 5% in patients at minimal risk, and simple measures of ambulation and leg exercises that carry no adverse effects are recommended (Table 86–2). The risk increases significantly in the moderate category, and the use of low-dose unfractionated heparin or low-molecular-weight heparin is recommended. A large number of clinical trials have documented the effectiveness of both strategies. Because of its short half-life, unfractionated heparin must be administered two or three times daily, and this reduces deep vein thrombosis and pulmonary embolism by approximately two thirds.[54] This benefit is associated with increased bleeding complications, mostly wound hematomas, in surgical patients. The longer half-life of low-molecular-weight heparins permits more convenient once-daily administration, and multiple studies and meta-analyses have shown this to be equivalent to unfractionated heparin for general surgery.[52,53,55]

TABLE 86–1. Levels of Risk for Venous Thromboembolism

	Risk		
	All VTED	**Proximal DVT**	**PE**
Minimal	2	0.5	0.2
Ambulatory patients			
Minor outpatient surgery			
Moderate	5–20	1–4	1–2
Minor surgery with risk factors			
Major surgery, <40 yr, no risk factors			
Medical inpatients, <40 yr, with single risk factor			
High	20–40	4–8	2–4
Major surgery, >40 yr			
Minor surgery, >60 yr, with additional risk factors			
Myocardial infarction			
Stroke with paralysis			
Highest	40–80	10–20	4–10
Knee or hip replacement			
Hip fracture			
Spinal cord injury			
Major trauma			

Abbreviations: DVT, deep vein thrombosis; PE, pulmonary embolism; VTED, venous thromboembolic disease.

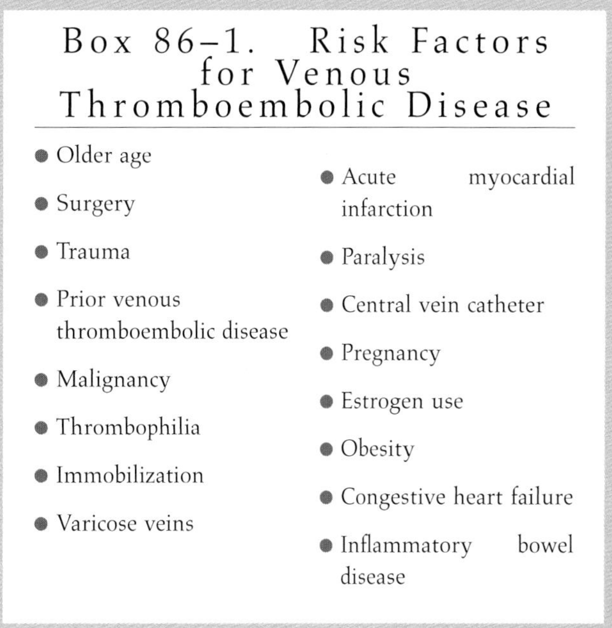

Box 86–1. Risk Factors for Venous Thromboembolic Disease

- Older age
- Surgery
- Trauma
- Prior venous thromboembolic disease
- Malignancy
- Thrombophilia
- Immobilization
- Varicose veins
- Acute myocardial infarction
- Paralysis
- Central vein catheter
- Pregnancy
- Estrogen use
- Obesity
- Congestive heart failure
- Inflammatory bowel disease

TABLE 86–2. Recommended Prophylaxis for Venous Thromboembolic Disease

Surgical Patients	**Risk Class and Prophylaxis**	**Medical Patients**
Minor surgery*; no risk factors	**Minimal** Ambulation, leg exercises	Fully ambulatory
Minor surgery with ≥1 risk factor Major surgery,* <40 yr, with no risk factors	**Moderate** LDUH q12h; LMWH†	Inpatient, ≥40 yr, with a single risk factor
Major surgery, ≥40 yr Minor surgery, ≥60 yr, with additional risk factors	**High** LDUH q8h; LMWH‡	Inpatient, ≥40 yr, with ≥1 risk factor Inpatient, ≥60 yr, with 1 or more additional risk factors
Total hip or knee replacement	LMWH,‖ warfarin,§ fondaparinux	

*Minor surgery: <45 minutes. Major surgery: ≥45 minutes.
†Dalteparin 2500 units, 1–2 hr preoperatively and once daily postoperatively; enoxaparin 20 mg, 1–2 hr preoperatively and once daily postoperatively; tinzaparin 3500 units, 1–2 hr preoperatively and once daily postoperatively.
‡Dalteparin 5000 units, 10–12 hr preoperatively and once daily postoperatively; enoxaparin 40 mg, 10–12 hr preoperatively and once daily postoperatively.
§Dosage. Adjusted to INR 2–3.
‖Dalteparin 5000 units, once daily; enoxaparin 30 mg, q12h; fondaparinux 2.5 mg, once daily.
Abbreviation: LDUH, low-dose unfractionated heparin.

Several specific patient groups are at a particularly high risk of venous thromboembolism, especially those undergoing major lower extremity orthopedic procedures. Prospective clinical trials have identified optimal prophylactic approaches that generally require a higher level of anticoagulation. In these high-risk patients, low-dose unfractionated heparin is not as effective as low-molecular-weight heparin.[55–61] Carefully controlled anticoagulation with warfarin to achieve the target International Normalized Ratio (INR) of between 2 and 3 in the immediate postoperative period is also effective.[52,53,62–66] Patients with spinal cord injury and those with multiple trauma are also in the highest risk category, and the use of low-molecular-weight heparins has been demonstrated to be highly effective in preventing venous thromboembolism.[67,68]

Venous stasis is an important contributor to risk, and mechanical measures to reduce stasis are also effective. Intermittent pneumatic devices rhythmically squeeze the legs, increase blood flow, and also stimulate fibrinolytic activity.[69–72] They are effective and particularly appropriate in patients at high risk of bleeding or if bleeding complications would be particularly serious, as in neurosurgery. Although pneumatic compression devices are effective, compliance is problematic because they are frequently removed for physical therapy, movement in and out of bed, or nursing care. Thus, they may not be operative much of the time and this diminishes effectiveness. A smaller number of studies have shown moderate effectiveness of graduated compression stockings, which are fitted to provide graded compression that is greatest at the ankle.[73]

The duration of prophylaxis and timing of initiation in surgical patients are matters of controversy and investigation. Most commonly, prophylaxis has been initiated 1–3 hours preoperatively because evidence indicates that the period during surgery is one of particularly high risk and that thrombi begin to form during the procedure. However, this practice results in peak levels of anticoagulant during the surgical procedure and may result in an increase in bleeding complications.[74,75] In Europe, prophylaxis is often initiated the evening before surgery, which results in a low but detectable level of anticoagulation during the procedure. In North America, it is common practice to initiate anticoagulation 12–24 hours after surgery, particularly with orthopedic surgery patients, and this has been demonstrated to be effective in prospective trials. Evidence indicates that better results, however, can be achieved by initiating prophylaxis closer to surgery, and some regimens begin 6–8 hours postoperatively.[75,76]

Opinion also differs regarding duration of prophylaxis in high-risk orthopedic patients. Initial guidelines were based on older studies that administered prophylaxis for 7–14 days, which corresponded to the period of hospitalization. This approach is commonly used, and prophylaxis is typically administered during hospitalization for surgery or acute illness. This practice is now being reconsidered as hospital stays have been progressively shortened. For example, patients undergoing hip or knee replacement are commonly hospitalized for approximately 4 days, a period too brief for adequate prophylaxis. Therefore, extending prophylaxis into the postdischarge period is necessary because a minimum duration of 7–14 days is needed. Several studies, however, have demonstrated that the risk of thrombosis extends even longer into the postoperative period.[77–81] Studies have clearly demonstrated that new deep vein thromboses develop following discharge, and up to 10% of patients may develop proximal deep vein thrombosis following discharge after hip replacement surgery if prophylaxis is not provided. Surgeons have raised questions regarding the clinical relevance of these findings because the rate of symptomatic venous thromboembolism is less than 4% at 3 months following 7–10 days of prophylaxis.[82–85] A meta-analysis, however, indicates that the rate of symptomatic postdischarge venous thromboembolism can be reduced with prophylaxis for up to 30 days,[86] and a large population-based study indicates that the risk extends up to 3 months.[87] Practice is evolving to extend the period of prophylaxis following high-risk surgery for up to 30 days postoperatively.[88,89] Comparable studies are not available in medical patients at high risk, but this information is critically needed.

Treatment

Patients presenting with symptoms of acute deep vein thrombosis or pulmonary embolism require immediate treatment to provide symptomatic relief, prevent disease extension or recurrence, and minimize structural damage to deep leg veins. Anticoagulant therapy is appropriate for most, but fibrinolytic therapy and surgical interventions are occasionally needed. Important initial considerations in planning therapy include the extent of cardiopulmonary compromise in patients with pulmonary embolism, the choice of inpatient versus outpatient therapy, and the ability to comply with acute and long-term treatment. Frequently, patients have coexisting medical illnesses that need to be considered in planning therapy. For example, pulmonary embolism may worsen preexisting congestive heart failure. Patients with active malignancy present difficult challenges because of the high risk of recurrence and impact of treatment-related thrombocytopenia and anorexia on warfarin management. Careful evaluation of bleeding risk is especially important because of the risks associated with either anticoagulant or fibrinolytic therapy.

Anticoagulation

Rapid anticoagulation with a short course of unfractionated or low-molecular-weight heparin followed by a longer period of oral anticoagulation with warfarin is the best treatment for most patients with deep vein thrombosis or pulmonary embolism[10] (Box 86–2; see also Chapter 88). Treatment should be initiated as soon as the diagnosis is established or prior to diagnostic testing in patients with a high clinical suspicion. Thrombus extension and recurrent embolization often occur during the period of initial presentation and can be minimized by administering full anticoagulant doses as rapidly as possible. Delay in therapy or subtherapeutic anticoagulation

Box 86–2. Anticoagulant Therapy for Venous Thromboembolic Disease

Initial Therapy

- LMWH subcutaneously once or twice daily:
- enoxaparin (Lovenox): 1 mg/kg q12h; or 1.5 mg/kg once daily
- dalteparin (Fragmin): 100 units/kg q12h; or 200 units/kg once daily
- tinzaparin (Innohep): 175 units/kg once daily

or

- Heparin 80 units/kg, and start an infusion of 18 units/kg/hr
- Check aPTT after 4–6 hr and adjust infusion to prolong the aPTT 1.5–2.5 times control

or

- fondaparinux once daily (5 mg <50 kg, 7.5 mg 50–100 kg, 10 mg >100 kg)

Maintenance Therapy

Oral Anticoagulation

- Give warfarin 5–10 mg during the first hospital day
- Check INR daily
- Adjust dose to prolong INR to 2–3 times control
- Discontinue LMWH or heparin after a minimum of 5 days when INR is therapeutic
- Continue warfarin with regular monitoring for desired period

LMWH

- Continue subcutaneous injections q12h or once daily as for initial therapy

Heparin

- Heparin subcutaneously q12h in a dose adjusted to prolong the midinterval aPTT to 1.5 times control

aPTT, activated partial thromboplastin time; INR, International Normalized Ratio; LMWH, low-molecular-weight heparin.

increases the risk of recurrence.[90,91] Appropriately managed anticoagulation therapy is highly effective, with symptomatic recurrence rates of 3–5%. In contrast, patients with pulmonary embolism not treated with anticoagulation have a high rate of recurrence and death.[95]

Either low-molecular-weight or unfractionated heparin can be used for initial treatment. For most patients, however, low-molecular-weight heparin is preferable because it has a longer half-life and better bioavailability, so that patients can be managed as outpatients with subcutaneous injections. Unfractionated and low-molecular-weight heparins have been compared in randomized controlled trials of patients with proximal deep vein thrombosis.[93–98] These trials[99,100] are discussed in Chapter 88 and indicate that low-molecular-weight heparin is at least as effective as unfractionated heparin and may be associated with slightly less bleeding. Outpatient management results in both cost savings and improved patient satisfaction.[93,94,101,102] The choice of outpatient therapy must be considered carefully, however, because venous thromboembolic disease is a serious and sometimes fatal disease unless managed appropriately. Inpatient treatment is a better choice for patients with severe symptoms, complex coexisting medical problems, and high risk of bleeding or with large pulmonary emboli. Outpatient therapy is appropriate for those who are stable with satisfactory understanding of the disease and therapy, and with adequate control of acute symptoms. There must be good medical follow-up and education provided for subcutaneous injections to be administered by the patient, family member, or visiting nurse.

Three low-molecular-weight heparins are available in the United States for treatment of venous thromboembolic disease. Twice-daily treatment may be better in more severely symptomatic patients with larger thrombus burden.[97,98,103–105] Warfarin should be started on the first day of treatment in a dose of between 5 and 10 mg, with lower doses appropriate for smaller individuals or those with poor nutrition. The INR should be checked daily in hospitalized patients or at least every other day in outpatients. Low-molecular-weight heparin can be stopped when the INR is over 2 on 2 consecutive days. This usually requires a 5- to 7-day course of treatment with low-molecular-weight heparin. Recent studies show that fondaparinux is also effective for initial treatment of deep vein thrombosis or pulmonary embolism.[105a,105b]

Treatment with continuous intravenous unfractionated heparin may be preferable for selected patients. These include patients who may need to undergo an invasive procedure requiring normal hemostasis. Because of its short half-life, the anticoagulant effect of unfractionated heparin is gone within several hours after stopping the infusion. In contrast, anticoagulant levels of low-molecular-weight heparin persist for more than 12 hours after administration. Also, unfractionated heparin may be preferable because of its short half-life in patients with a recent bleeding event or a high risk of bleeding. Additionally, the anticoagulant effects of unfractionated heparin can be completely reversed with protamine sulfate, whereas the effect on low-molecular-weight heparin is incomplete. Because treatment with intravenous unfractionated heparin gives more constant anticoagulant levels that can be monitored using the activated partial thromboplastin time (aPTT), many physicians prefer unfractionated heparin for patients with large pulmonary emboli.

Treatment with unfractionated heparin requires careful laboratory monitoring (see Box 86–2 and Chapter 88). The success of treatment depends on rapidly achieving a therapeutic aPTT, and recurrences are more frequent in patients with subtherapeutic values.[90,91] Heparin dosing nomograms have been developed that facilitate rapid achievement of therapeutic anticoagulant levels.[106,107] Because commercially available reagents and laboratory systems vary in sensitivity to heparin, optimal monitoring requires that laboratories standardize the therapeutic aPTT range for heparin to correspond with plasma heparin levels of 0.2–0.4 units/mL using protamine titration or to 0.3–0.7 units/mL using an anti–factor Xa assay.[53] Another consideration in heparin monitoring is the effect of the acute-phase response that elevates levels of heparin-binding proteins and factor VIII during acute illness. These changes can result in a decrease of aPTT during therapy and lead to a perception of "heparin resistance." Most patients with "subtherapeutic" aPTTs despite receiving over 1500 units/hr will have adequate plasma levels if measured directly by using an anti-Xa assay.[108] As with treatment using low-molecular-weight heparin, warfarin should be initiated on the first day, and the heparin infusion can be stopped when the INR is in the therapeutic range for 2 consecutive days. Platelet counts should be monitored in patients receiving heparin because of the serious consequences of heparin-induced thrombocytopenia (see Chapter 69).

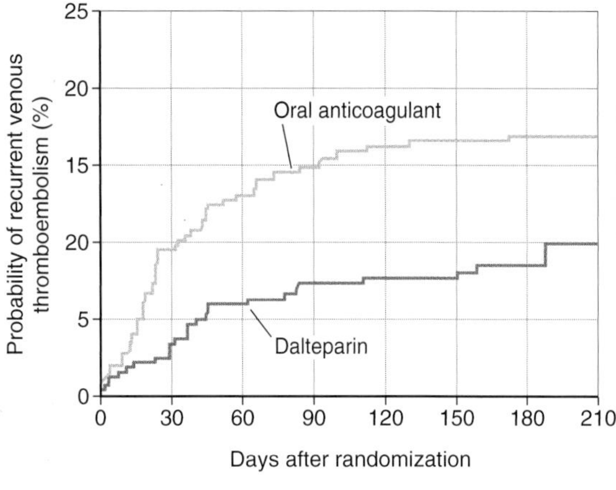

Number at risk							
Dalteparin	336	310	274	248	237	220	206
Oral anticoagulant	336	301	268	240	240	211	194

Figure 86–4. Kaplan-Meier estimates of the probability of symptomatic recurrence of venous thromboembolism among patients with cancer, according to whether they received secondary prophylaxis with dalteparin or oral anticoagulant therapy for acute venous thromboembolism. (From Lee AY, Levine MN, Baker RI, et al: Low-molecular-weight heparin versus a coumarin for the prevention of recurrent venous thromboembolism in patients with cancer. N Engl J Med 349:146–153, 2003, with permission.)

Duration of Anticoagulation

The risk of recurrence decreases with time after the initial presentation but persists for a prolonged period. Therefore, long-term anticoagulation is necessary. The vitamin K antagonist warfarin is the only currently available oral anticoagulant and is highly effective. Because of biologic variability in response and interactions with food and other medications,[109,110] monitoring of anticoagulant levels using the INR is required. Keeping the INR in the range of 2–3 minimizes the risk of recurrent thrombosis and bleeding complications, and this usually requires weekly or biweekly monitoring in stable patients.

Heparin or low-molecular-weight heparin can also be used satisfactorily for long-term treatment in patients who are intolerant of warfarin or pregnant patients in whom warfarin is contraindicated (see Chapter 88).[111–117] In some groups, long-term low-molecular-weight heparin may be more effective than warfarin. For example, patients with active malignancy are at high risk of recurrence and bleeding,[118] and warfarin therapy is difficult because of bleeding risk, multiple medications, and changes in diet and appetite. A recent clinical trial by Lee and colleagues demonstrated a significantly lower rate of recurrence with low-molecular-weight heparin than with warfarin[119] (Fig. 86–4).

The optimal duration of anticoagulation remains a topic of controversy and investigation and must be individualized for each patient. Critical considerations include the risk of recurrence, risk of bleeding complications, and issues of patient compliance and preference. Generally, the risk of recurrence is less in patients who develop deep vein thrombosis following surgery or in association with another transient risk factor, and risk is also less with calf vein thrombosis than proximal deep vein thrombosis. Several studies have specifically addressed the issue of duration of therapy with idiopathic or recurrent deep vein thrombosis in prospective trials.[120–126] Generally, recurrence rates are very low during warfarin therapy. The highest rates of recurrence are early in treatment or in the period immediately following discontinuation of anticoagulation. The risks of bleeding complications must also be considered, because the clinical consequences of a major bleeding episode are often greater than those of recurrent deep vein thrombosis. Rates of bleeding on long-term oral anticoagulation are generally between 2% and 3% per year, and they are strongly dependent on the adequacy of quality control and on patient-specific factors that influence bleeding.[7,127] Long-term rates of recurrence in patients with idiopathic deep vein thrombosis are high, reaching 15–20% at 2–4 years in patients after anticoagulation has stopped.[123–125,128] Idiopathic venous thromboembolic disease appears to be associated with an ongoing risk of recurrence. For example, Agnelli and associates[125] showed a rate of recurrence of approximately 5% per patient per year when therapy was discontinued either after 3 months or after an additional 9 months of therapy, suggesting that the recurrence rate after discontinuation of treatment was not reduced by a longer initial treatment period (Fig. 86–5).

Decisions regarding length of treatment should be individualized and based on the extent of thrombosis, coexistence of acquired or inherited risk factors, and

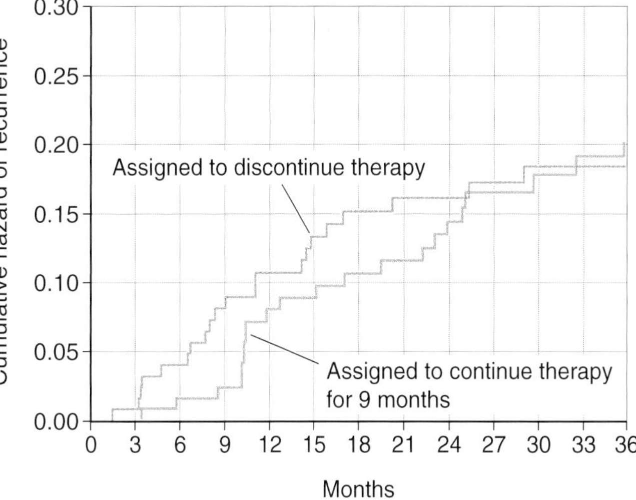

Figure 86–5. Cumulative hazard of recurrent venous thromboembolism in patients assigned to discontinue oral anticoagulant therapy and those assigned to continue oral anticoagulant therapy. (From Agnelli G, Prandoni P, Santamaria MG, et al: Three months versus one year of oral anticoagulant therapy for idiopathic deep venous thrombosis. Warfarin Optimal Duration Italian Trial Investigators. N Engl J Med 345:165–169, 2001, with permission.)

TABLE 86–3. Recommendations for Duration of Anticoagulation

Presentation	Modifying Factors	Duration
Calf DVT*	Following surgery or transient risk factor	6–12 wk
	Idiopathic	3–6 mo
Proximal DVT or PE	Following surgery or transient risk factor	3–6 mo
	Idiopathic	6–12 mo
	Recurrent disease or with major ongoing risk†	Indefinite

*Management without anticoagulation using serial ultrasound to monitor for proximal extension is also recommended.
†Example of major risks include active malignancy or congestive heart failure.
Abbreviations: DVT, deep vein thrombosis; PE, pulmonary embolism.

whether the event was provoked or idiopathic (Table 86–3). Patients with recurrent thrombosis or with significant ongoing risk factors such as malignancy need long-term anticoagulation. Inherited thrombophilia also influences the duration of therapy. The risk of recurrence is high with antithrombin deficiency or with lupus anticoagulant/antiphospholipid antibody and probably also with protein C or protein S deficiency. The presence of factor V Leiden or the prothrombin 20210 mutation is associated with less ongoing risk.[129–131]

Calf Vein Thrombosis

Approximately 10% of patients will present with deep vein thrombosis isolated to the calf veins only. If the thrombus remains confined to the calf, the likelihood of significant pulmonary embolism is low.[132] However, approximately 20% will extend into proximal veins with more serious implications.[133] Two approaches to management are appropriate. Patients can be monitored with repeated compression ultrasonography, and treatment withheld if there is no evidence of proximal extension. Only symptomatic management would be provided. Alternatively, if serial monitoring is unavailable or the patient is noncompliant, treatment is indicated. Anticoagulation may also be preferable in patients who are very symptomatic.

Recurrent Thrombosis

Diagnosis and management of recurrence after an initial episode of deep vein thrombosis can be difficult. Symptoms of pain and swelling associated with recurrence may be similar to those with postphlebitic syndrome. Also, the presence of residual thrombus may make interpretation of a repeat ultrasound difficult, and the compression ultrasound remains abnormal 12 months after an acute episode in nearly 50% of patients.[45,134] It is therefore helpful to obtain a baseline ultrasound during a stable interval after resolution of initial symptoms for comparison if recurrent symptoms develop. If recurrence develops after treatment is discontinued, the approach is similar to initial treatment. However, a longer duration of anticoagulation may be indicated, and an indefinite duration may be needed in patients with multiple recurrences. Patients who have documented recurrence while receiving adequate anticoagulant therapy present difficult challenges. Options include increasing the INR to a higher level, placement of an inferior vena cava filter, or changing anticoagulation from warfarin to chronic low-molecular-weight heparin.

Pregnancy

Pregnancy and parturition increase the risk of venous thromboembolism, and management of venous thromboembolism during pregnancy raises difficult problems with risks to the fetus as well as the mother from diagnostic tests and anticoagulant treatment.[135–137] Warfarin should be avoided during pregnancy because it crosses the placenta and can cause a distinctive embryopathy if administered in the first trimester.[138–140] If necessary, warfarin may be used during the second trimester when the risk is less, but use of heparin or low-molecular-weight heparins is preferable for women who need anticoagulation during pregnancy. Management of pregnant women needing anticoagulation because of a prosthetic heart valve is discussed in Chapter 88. Additionally, anticoagulant effects can cause fetal hemorrhage. Unlike warfarin, heparin and low-molecular-weight heparins do not cross the placenta or affect the fetus. The hemorrhagic risk in pregnant women seems to be similar to that in other patients,[141,142] although long-term administration is associated with osteoporosis.[143,144] This may be less with low-molecular-weight heparins. Heparin should be discontinued at the beginning of labor or 24 hours before elective delivery to avoid bleeding complications. It can be reinstituted 24–48 hours after delivery if adequate hemostasis has been achieved. Warfarin can be used after delivery and is safe in nursing mothers because it is not excreted in breast milk and results in no infant anticoagulation.[145–147]

Fibrinolytic Therapy

Anticoagulant therapy is very effective in preventing recurrence, but residual clot persists for long periods, and vein scarring with valve dysfunction is common. Fibrinolytic therapy can result in rapid clot dissolution and should be considered in selected patients (Box 86–3) who are markedly symptomatic with extensive ileofemoral thrombosis of acute onset and with low risk of bleeding complications. Both streptokinase and urokinase are approved for treatment of deep vein thrombosis, and they are often administered for 1–3 days. This acute treatment is then followed by heparin or low-molecular-weight heparin and warfarin.[148] The use of catheter-directed thrombolysis has become more popular and results in a high rate of venographic and clinical improvement,[149] although there are no direct randomized comparisons of catheter-directed and systemic fibrinolytic therapy. The strongest indication for fibrinolytic therapy for venous thromboembolic disease is in patients with large pulmonary emboli associated with hemodynamic compromise. It can result in rapid improvement and can be life-saving. Treatment can be administered with infusions of streptokinase or urokinase, and 100 mg of tissue plasminogen activator administered as a constant infusion over 2 hours is also effective.

Box 86–3. Selection of Individuals for Thrombolytic Therapy

Treat Those Most Likely to Respond and Benefit

- Deep vein thrombosis: large proximal thrombi with symptoms for less than 7 days
- Pulmonary embolism: massive or submassive embolism, especially with hemodynamic compromise

Select Individuals to Avoid Bleeding Complications

Major Contraindications

- Risk of intracranial bleeding: recent head trauma or central nervous system surgery, history of stroke or subarachnoid bleeding, intracranial metastatic disease
- Risk of major bleeding: active gastrointestinal or genitourinary bleeding, major surgery or trauma within 7 days

Relative Contraindications

- Remote history of gastrointestinal or genitourinary bleeding or of peptic ulcer or other lesion with potential for bleeding: recent minor surgery or trauma; severe, uncontrolled hypertension; coexisting hemostatic abnormalities

Surgical Approaches

Surgical approaches to preventing pulmonary embolism include ligation of veins proximal to a thrombus or placing a "filter" in the inferior vena cava. The latter approach is frequently used, and several devices can be placed in the inferior vena cava through a vascular catheter introduced into the jugular or femoral vein under local anesthesia and guided fluoroscopically to the appropriate position. The most frequently used devices are variants of the umbrella-shaped Greenfield filter, which consists of metal struts fixed to the vein wall by prongs. The filter traps embolizing clots centrally and maintains flow near the vein periphery. A high long-term patency rate can be achieved, and the most frequent complications are sequelae of venous stasis, which can occur in up to 40% of patients. A device that can be removed after brief placement has been introduced.

A recent randomized controlled trial investigated the efficacy and safety of vena cava filters in the prevention of pulmonary embolism.[150] The results showed that pulmonary emboli were less frequent in the initial 12 days in patients assigned to receive filters in addition to anticoagulants. Over 2 years, however, a greater proportion of patients with filters had recurrent deep vein thrombosis, although data were not provided on anticoagulation in those with late pulmonary embolism. Indications for placement of an inferior vena cava filter include patients with proximal deep vein thrombosis with absolute contraindications to anticoagulant therapy or who have recurrent venous thrombosis or pulmonary embolism despite optimal anticoagulation. Other relative indications include patients with venous thromboembolism and a high risk of bleeding, pulmonary embolism with hemodynamic instability, and pulmonary hypertension resulting from recurrent pulmonary embolism. The presence of the filter increases risk of recurrent deep vein thrombosis. Therefore, most patients will require continued anticoagulant therapy or resumption of therapy after the contraindication is resolved.

ARTERIAL THROMBOEMBOLISM

Pathogenesis

Arterial occlusive disease has three main causes: (1) atherosclerotic lesions that completely occlude a vessel; (2) atherosclerotic lesions with thrombi superimposed, usually on a ruptured plaque; and (3) embolism of a fibrin thrombus, platelet thrombus, or portion of atherosclerotic plaque.

Evidence suggests that atherosclerotic plaque forms when there is arterial endothelial injury. The normal arterial wall has an intimal layer composed of endothelium and subendothelium, with the internal elastic lamina

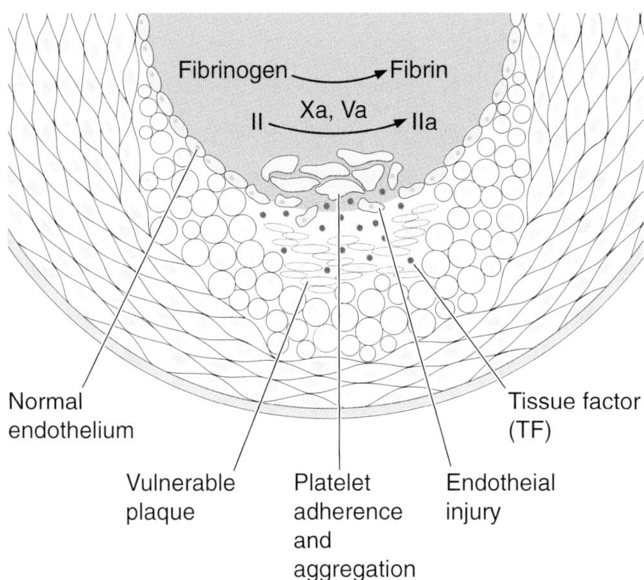

Figure 86–6. Injury to the vessel wall predisposes to development of atherosclerotic lesions. Initially, platelets adhere to a damaged endothelium and aggregate. Thrombin is formed locally, resulting in conversion of fibrinogen to fibrin, which stabilizes the thrombus adherent to the vessel wall.

immediately beneath the intima. The medial layer is located beneath the internal elastic lamina and is composed of smooth muscle cells, and the adventitia (connective tissue and fibroblasts) is beneath the media. The injury hypothesis for atherogenesis[151] suggests that, when the intima is disrupted and the endothelium is denuded, platelets adhere to the subendothelium, secrete their dense and α-granule contents (several of which have biologic activity relevant to plaque formation and progression), and form aggregates (Fig. 86–6). Fibrin then forms over and through the platelet plug, and this fibrin-platelet thrombus becomes incorporated into the arterial wall, covered by a fibrous cap. It is now thought that loss of endothelium is not necessary for formation of atherosclerotic plaque, which can result from endothelial dysfunction, with abnormal vasoregulation and local inflammation causing a pro-inflammatory, proliferative, and procoagulant milieu.[152–155] Dysfunctional endothelial cells express chemoattractant cytokines that stimulate the directed migration of monocytes[156,157] and T lymphocytes[158] into the vessel wall and other cytokines that lead to expression of scavenger receptors on monocyte-macrophages[154] and proliferation of macrophages in the developing plaque.[159] Thus, a thickened intima composed of smooth muscle cells, lipid-laden macrophages, and the fibrin and platelets develops beneath the fibrous cap. Components of the thrombus and modified lipoproteins[160] stimulate further inflammatory cytokine release, and platelet-derived growth factor and transforming growth factor-β released from activated platelets stimulate collagen synthesis and migration of smooth muscle cells into the neointima of the plaque.[159] When a break occurs in the fibrous cap as a result of thinning of the cap by the action of collagenases and matrix metalloproteinases,[161] tissue factor–rich macrophages and microparticles derived from apoptosis of macrophages[162] and subendothelial collagen are exposed to blood (see Fig. 86–6). Exposed tissue factor interacts with factors VII and X in plasma, leading to thrombin generation, more platelet activation, and new fibrin formation on the plaque surface.[163] Embolization of platelet or platelet-fibrin thrombi from the plaque surface can occur in either the early or later stages. The fibrin thrombus may completely occlude the vessel, leading to myocardial infarction or stroke. Thrombotic occlusion of very small arteries by platelet and/or fibrin thrombi is thought to be the mechanism of lacunar infarcts.[164]

When a platelet aggregate, platelet-fibrin thrombus, or piece of atherosclerotic plaque breaks off and enters the circulation, it may lodge anywhere in the arterial tree distal to its site of origin; Figure 86–7 shows potential sites of thrombus and paths of embolism. Carotid plaque or associated thrombi lodge in vessels in the brain. Emboli arising from atrial or ventricular thrombi in the setting of atrial fibrillation, following myocardial infarction, or with cardiomyopathy may go to the carotid circulation or peripherally. Atrial thrombi occur in the setting of atrial fibrillation, with ineffective contraction of the atria leading to stasis, an important feature of Virchow's triad (see Fig. 86–1). Ventricular thrombi occur primarily in aneurysms following myocardial infarction or with severe congestive heart failure. Thrombi also occur on diseased native or prosthetic valves, especially mechanical valves.

Risk Factors

Risk factors for arterial thromboembolism fall into two groups: those that increase the risk of development of atherosclerosis and those that increase the risk of thrombus formation on an atherosclerotic plaque. There are important interactions between the processes of atherosclerosis and arterial thrombosis, with thrombus formation contributing to plaque development through incorporation of thrombus into developing plaque and thrombosis occurring on disrupted plaques.[163] Box 86–4 lists both established and newer risk factors suggested to be important in atherosclerosis and arterial thrombosis.

Many recent studies have shown that the C-reactive protein, an acute-phase protein synthesized in the liver in response to interleukin-6,[165] both reflects existing atherosclerosis and also is active in the development of atherosclerotic lesions through induction of monocyte chemoattractant protein-1, intercellular adhesion molecule-1, vascular cell adhesion molecule-1, and E-selectin; mediation of macrophage uptake of low-density lipoprotein; and stimulation of monocyte production of tissue factor.[166] Elevated C-reactive protein levels are predictive of clinical events.[167]

Elevated fibrinogen has been recognized as a risk for myocardial infarction, based on several large epidemiologic studies.[168,169] Like C-reactive protein, fibrinogen is an acute-phase reactant, and its synthesis by hepatocytes can increase by about fourfold in response to inflammatory cytokines.[170] In addition to providing the bulk of the

Box 86–4. Risk Factors for Atherosclerosis/Atherosclerotic Vascular Disease

Conventional Risk Factors for Atherosclerosis

- Hyper/dyslipidemia
- Hypertension
- Diabetes
- Smoking
- Obesity

Novel Risk Factors for Atherosclerotic Vascular Disease

Inflammatory Markers

- C-reactive protein
- Interleukins
- Vascular and intercellular adhesion molecules
- Soluble CD40 ligand
- Leukocyte count

Hemostasis/Thrombosis Markers

- Fibrinogen
- von Willebrand factor
- Plasminogen activator inhibitor-1
- Tissue plasminogen activator
- Factors V, VII, and VIII
- D-dimer
- Fibrinopeptide A
- Prothrombin fragment 1+2

Platelet-Related Factors

- Platelet hyperactivity

Lipid-Related Factors

- Lipoprotein(a)
- Small, dense low-density lipoprotein
- Oxidized lipoproteins

Other Factors

- Homocysteine
- Insulin resistance
- Lipoprotein-associated phospholipase A_2
- Infectious agents (*Chlamydia pneumoniae, Helicobacter pylori*, herpes simplex, cytomegalovirus)
- Peroxisome proliferator-activated receptors

thrombus, fibrinogen is necessary for platelet aggregation in low-shear settings[171]; regulates cell adhesion, chemotaxis, and proliferation[172]; and is a determinant of blood viscosity. Fibrinogen and fibrin are found within atherosclerotic plaques,[173,174] and recently, elevated fibrinogen has been reported to be a risk factor for venous thrombosis.[175]

Homocystinemia occurs in certain inherited disorders of homocysteine metabolism,[176] in renal failure,[177] and in vitamin B_{12} and folate deficiencies.[178] In vitro studies in the 1970s demonstrated direct cytotoxicity for endothelial cells.[179] Recent reviews have discussed other mechanisms of homocysteine toxicity to the vessel wall.[180] Retrospective case-control studies and cross-sectional studies have supported an association between elevated plasma homocysteine and atherosclerosis, as have meta-analyses of prospective longitudinal studies.[181] Other data support an association between elevated homocysteine levels and venous thrombosis.[182] Plasma homocysteine levels can be lowered with B vitamins, especially folic acid.[178]

Lipoprotein(a) is an acute-phase reactant[183] whose apoprotein is a combination of apolipoprotein B and another polypeptide (apolipoprotein A) with high homology to plasminogen, although it lacks the site for activation to plasmin.[184] The size of apolipoprotein A varies among individuals because of a varying number of repeats of one of the kringle structures of the protein.[185] Lipoprotein(a) binds to several vessel wall cells and to subendothelial matrix.[186,187] Because of its structural homology to plasminogen, it binds to the plasminogen receptor on endothelial cells and thereby inhibits plasminogen activation to plasmin by tissue plasminogen activator or urokinase on the cell surface, thus inhibiting fibrinolysis.[188] There are reports that elevated levels of lipoprotein(a) are more detrimental in the presence of other risk factors such as diabetes and high levels of low-density lipoprotein,[189,190] fibrinogen,[191] or homocysteine.[192]

Infectious agents were first implicated in atherogenesis in 1911,[193] and there were reports of herpesvirus involvement in atherosclerosis in the 1970s.[194] More recently, attention has focused on infection with *Chlamydia pneumoniae* as a risk factor,[195] based on epidemiologic data.[196] *Chlamydia* may modulate effects of lipids and inflammation on monocytes and the vessel wall, leading to increased expression of inflammatory cytokines and adhesion molecules.[195]

Intriguing information suggests that the CD40-CD40 ligand interaction induces adhesion molecule expression on endothelial cells and macrophages.[197] CD40 ligation can also induce tissue factor expression in macrophages,[198] which may be important in thrombus formation. These interactions may be of particular importance in early atherosclerosis in patients with systemic lupus erythematosus because their cells express abnormally high levels of CD40 ligand.[199]

Management

Management of patients with arterial emboli or thrombosis with potential for embolization is with anticoagulation and/or antiplatelet therapy. Clearly, preventing development of atherosclerotic plaque is important in preventing arterial occlusion and embolization, but that discussion is beyond the scope of this chapter. Topics to be emphasized here include prevention of embolization from cardiac thrombi, particularly in the setting of atrial fibrillation, and use of antiplatelet agents to prevent arterial occlusion.

Prevention of Embolism in Patients with Cardiac Disease

Approximately 20% of ischemic strokes are due to cardiogenic emboli,[200] and systemic embolization is also a potential consequence of cardiac or valvular thrombi (see Fig. 86–7). Evidence for anticoagulation use is discussed in the following sections.

Atrial Fibrillation

Atrial fibrillation is a strong risk factor for stroke because of the high incidence of development of left atrial thrombus and cerebral embolization. Several studies examined prophylaxis against stroke in the setting of atrial fibrillation in patients with or without valve disease.

A meta-analysis of 16 randomized trials of oral anticoagulant or aspirin in nonvalvular atrial fibrillation compared adjusted-dose warfarin (INR 2–3) versus placebo, aspirin versus placebo, and warfarin versus aspirin.[199] Warfarin was significantly better than placebo in four of the six studies, with a 65% risk reduction in ischemic strokes overall. There was a small but nonsignificant increase in intracranial hemorrhage with warfarin, and a significant relative risk of 2.4 for extracranial hemorrhage (absolute risk of 0.3% per year). The combined analysis of the aspirin versus placebo trials also showed a significant 22% decrease in the incidence of stroke, but only one of the six trials was significant on its own. Bleeding was rare, without difference between aspirin and placebo, for either intra- or extracranial bleeding. Warfarin was compared with aspirin in 5 nonblinded, randomized trials. Warfarin reduced the overall relative risk for all stroke by 36% compared with aspirin, and reduced the relative risk of ischemic stroke by 46%. There was, however, an increase in the relative risk of intracranial hemorrhage on warfarin, particularly in the Stroke Prevention in Atrial Fibrillation (SPAF) II study.[201]

To guide therapy, a scoring system has been developed ($CHADS_2$) for the risk of stroke in patients with

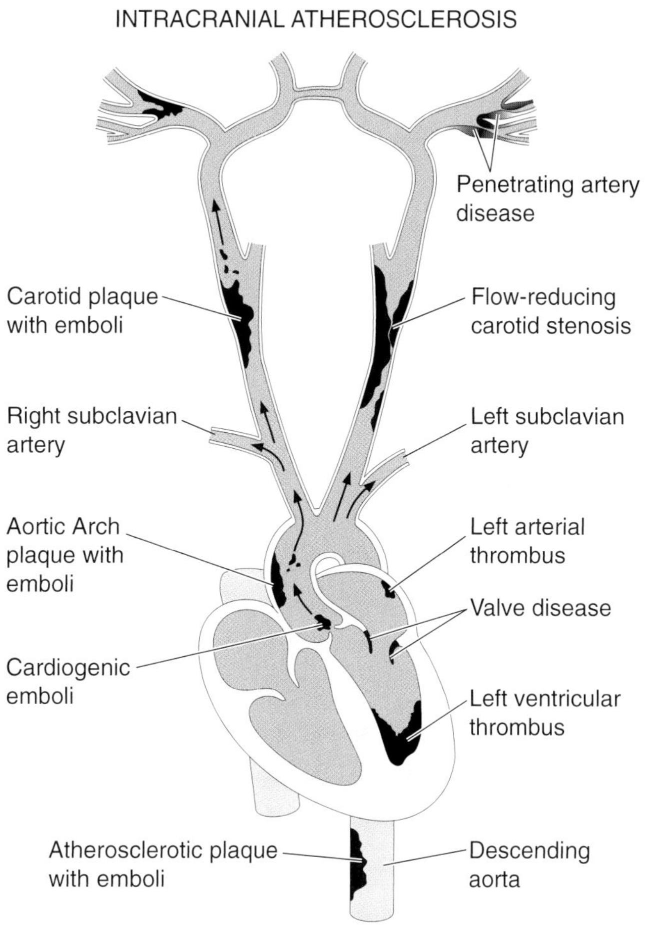

INTRACRANIAL ATHEROSCLEROSIS

■ **Figure 86–7.** Sites from which thromboemboli can originate and result in thromboembolic vascular occlusion are indicated.

atrial fibrillation.[202] One point each is assigned for recent congestive heart failure, hypertension, age 75 years or older, and diabetes mellitus. Two points are given for history of stroke or transient ischemic attack. Scores of 0–1 are considered low risk, 2–3 moderate risk, and 4, 5, or 6 high risk. Clinical guidelines for management of newly detected atrial fibrillation based on the score recommend rate control and chronic anticoagulation using adjusted-dose warfarin unless patients are in the low-risk category or have a contraindication to warfarin. An analysis of all the SPAF trials[203] and analyses of groups of over 13,000[204,205] and over 11,000[202] patients with nonvalvular atrial fibrillation have been published recently, with similar findings of reduction in stroke with warfarin at an INR of 2–3 as compared with placebo or aspirin. Thus, adjusted-dose warfarin (INR 2–3) should be given to patients with nonvalvular atrial fibrillation who are at a moderate to high risk of stroke and who do not have a contraindication to warfarin.

Left Ventricular Dysfunction

Patients with left ventricular dysfunction are at increased risk of stroke,[206] with several studies reporting that the risk increases as left ventricular function worsens.[207,208] The mechanism of stroke is thought to be embolism of left ventricular thrombus formed secondary to stasis or asynergy.[208,209] Patients with ejection fractions of less than 30% were reported to have a first stroke rate of 1.5% per year, with a cumulative rate of 8.1%.[207] Recurrent strokes occur at a higher rate, up to 45% over 5 years.[210] Stroke risk reduction with warfarin was reported to be 83% (95% confidence interval [CI], 71–91%).[207] Anticoagulation with warfarin to an INR of 2–3 has been recommended following myocardial infarction when the ejection fraction is 28% or less,[211] and it appears to be beneficial. Two large studies (WATCH and WARCEF) are underway to determine the efficacy of warfarin in other types of heart failure. Warfarin anticoagulation also decreases systemic embolism in heart failure.[212]

Valvular Disease

Patients with mitral valve disease may develop enlargement of the left atrium and are at risk for atrial thrombus formation and for atrial fibrillation. The American College of Chest Physicians (ACCP) recommendations for anticoagulation for native mitral and aortic valve disease are shown in Box 86–5.[213] Prosthetic valves in either the mitral or aortic position are at risk for developing thrombosis on the valve, with mechanical valves at higher risk than bioprosthetic valves. ACCP recommendations for prosthetic valves are shown in Box 86–6.[214] A meta-analysis of the risks and benefits of adding antiplatelet drugs to anticoagulation concluded that low-dose aspirin decreases the risk of thromboembolic events (odds ratio, 0.41; $P < .001$) or death (odds ratio, 0.49; $P < .001$) with a slight increase in the risk of major bleeding (odds ratio, 1.50; $P < .033$).[215]

Peripheral Arterial Occlusion

Systemic anticoagulation with heparin followed by warfarin is recommended in the ACCP guidelines for acute peripheral arterial insufficiency resulting from systemic embolization from cardiac sources or from in situ thrombosis on atherosclerotic plaque.[216] The duration was not specified, but if the source of emboli is still present or the underlying atherosclerotic disease is unchanged, long-term anticoagulation with warfarin is reasonable. Thrombolytic therapy should be considered if occlusion has been present for less than 14 days as long as the risk of bleeding is low.[216]

Antiplatelet Therapy to Prevent Arterial Occlusion

The first antiplatelet drug used in arterial disease was aspirin, which is still used widely for both primary and secondary prevention of myocardial infarction, treatment of acute myocardial infarction, and stroke prevention. Its antiplatelet action derives from its ability to inhibit cyclooxygenase,[217] the enzyme necessary to convert arachidonic acid into prostaglandins G_2 and H_2, from which thromboxane A_2 is generated. Other classes of antiplatelet drugs shown to be effective in arterial disease include phosphodiesterase inhibitors (e.g., dipyridamole), which lead to accumulation of cyclic AMP in platelets,[218] and the ADP receptor inhibitors, including ticlopidine and clopidogrel. ADP binding to its receptor

Box 86–5. ACCP Recommendations for Native Valve Disease[63]

Mitral Valve Disease Recommendations

Rheumatic Mitral Valve Disease

- Long-term warfarin with target INR of 2.5* if history of systemic embolism or of chronic or paroxysmal atrial fibrillation, or if left atrial diameter is greater than 5.5 cm
- Long-term warfarin with target INR of 3.0 if recurrent systemic embolism; may add aspirin (80–100 mg/day)
- Alternative strategies (aspirin, dipyridamole, clopidogrel) if unable to take warfarin

Mitral Valve Prolapse

- No anticoagulation if no history of systemic embolism, transient ischemic attacks (TIAs), or atrial fibrillation
- Aspirin at 160–325 mg/day if unexplained TIAs
- Long-term warfarin with target INR 2.5 in place of aspirin if documented systemic embolism, chronic or paroxysmal atrial fibrillation, or recurrent TIAs.

Mitral Annular Calcifications (MAC) and Nonrheumatic Mitral Regurgitation (MR)

- MAC with noncalcific systemic embolism: warfarin with target INR of 2.5
- MAC with atrial fibrillation: warfarin with target INR of 2.5
- MR with atrial fibrillation or history of systemic embolism: warfarin with target INR 2.5

Aortic Valve and Aortic Arch Disorders

- No warfarin for aortic valve disease without another indication for anticoagulation
- Warfarin for mobile aortic atheromas and aortic plaques greater than 4 mm by transesophageal echocardiography

Patent Foramen Ovale (PFO) and Atrial Septal Aneurysm

- Patients with unexplained systemic embolism or TIAs and demonstrable venous thrombosis or pulmonary embolism should be treated with warfarin unless venous interruption or PFO closure is done

*Target 2.5 with range 2.0–3.0.

Box 86–6. ACCP Recommendations for Mechanical and Bioprosthetic Heart Valves[64]

Mechanical

- All patients with mechanical prosthetic heart valves should receive warfarin.
- Unfractionated heparin or low-molecular-weight heparin should be used until the INR is therapeutic for at least 2 days. (*NOTE:* There is a recent black box warning, especially in pregnancy, against low-molecular-weight heparin.)

Target INRs

- 2.5 for St. Jude Medical bileaflet valve, Carbomedics bileaflet valve, or Medtronic-Hall tilting-disk mechanical valve in the aortic position, if left atrial size is normal and the patient is in sinus rhythm
- 3.0 for tilting-disk valves and bileaflet valves in the mitral position
- 3.0 for bileaflet mechanical aortic valves if atrial fibrillation
    - Alternative for tilting-disk and bileaflet valves is a target INR of 2.5 with addition of 80–100 mg aspirin daily
- 3.0 for patients with caged-ball or caged-disk valves, plus aspirin 80–100 mg/day
- In patients with mechanical valves and additional risk factors, recommend target INR of 3.0 plus aspirin 80–100 mg/day
- For patients with mechanical prosthetic valves who develop systemic embolism on warfarin, recommend target INR of 3.0 plus aspirin 80–100 mg/day

Bioprosthetic

- Mitral position: warfarin for 3 months with target INR 2.5 definitely; evidence less strong for aortic position but recommended there as well.
- Heparin may be used until INR is therapeutic for at least 2 days.
- Patients with a bioprosthetic valve and atrial fibrillation should receive long-term warfarin with target INR of 2.5.
- Patients with a bioprosthetic valve with left atrial thrombus seen at surgery should receive long-term warfarin with a target INR of 2.5. This is optional for a patient with a bioprosthetic valve and a permanent pacemaker.
- Patients with a bioprosthetic valve and a history of systemic embolism should receive warfarin with a target INR of 2.5.
- For patients with bioprosthetic valves in sinus rhythm, recommend long-term aspirin at 80 mg daily.

exposes the platelet fibrinogen receptor glycoprotein IIb/IIIa, needed for fibrinogen binding and platelet aggregation.[219] Other potent antiplatelet agents are the glycoprotein IIb/IIIa inhibitors, used in interventional cardiology procedures, but these drugs are not further discussed in this chapter.

The Antiplatelet Trialists Collaboration[220] reviewed 145 randomized trials of long-term antiplatelet therapy versus placebo and 29 randomized trials of aspirin versus other antiplatelet regimens. End points were vascular events (nonfatal myocardial infarction, nonfatal stroke) or vascular deaths. The trials reviewed included about 70,000 individuals with preexisting vascular disease (high risk) and about 30,000 subjects from the general population (low risk). Direct comparisons of different antiplatelet regimens involved about 10,000 high-risk patients. Aspirin (75–325 mg/day) showed a significant benefit over placebo ($P < .00001$) in reducing new events in 20,000 subjects with acute myocardial infarction, a history of stroke or transient ischemic attack, or a history of other vascular disease (unstable angina, angioplasty, atrial fibrillation, peripheral vascular disease, vascular surgery, or valvular disease). Significant reductions of about one third were reported in nonfatal myocardial infarction and nonfatal stroke, and of one sixth in vascular death. Similar reductions were seen for middle-aged and elderly subjects, in men and women, in the presence or absence of hypertension, and in diabetic and nondiabetic subjects. For the low-risk subjects, there was also a one-third reduction in nonfatal myocardial infarction ($P < .0005$). There was a nonsignificant increase in ischemic or unknown-etiology stroke in this group, and there was a significant increase in hemorrhagic stroke (0.37 vs. 0.27; $P < .05$). There was no effect on vascular death. The groups available for the comparisons of different antiplatelet regimens were much smaller. A comparison of low-dose (75–325 mg/day) to higher dose (500–1500 mg/day) aspirin did not show a significant difference, nor did comparisons of aspirin to aspirin plus dipyridamole, sulfinpyrazone, or ticlopidine. Data on antiplatelet therapy in high-risk patients were updated in 2002 and are shown in Figure 86–8.[221]

A second report from the Antiplatelet Trialists Collaboration[222] analyzed randomized trials of antiplatelet therapy for maintenance of arterial or vascular graft patency. There were 46 trials of antiplatelet therapy versus control (8000 patients) and 14 trials in which two antiplatelet regimens were compared (4000 patients).

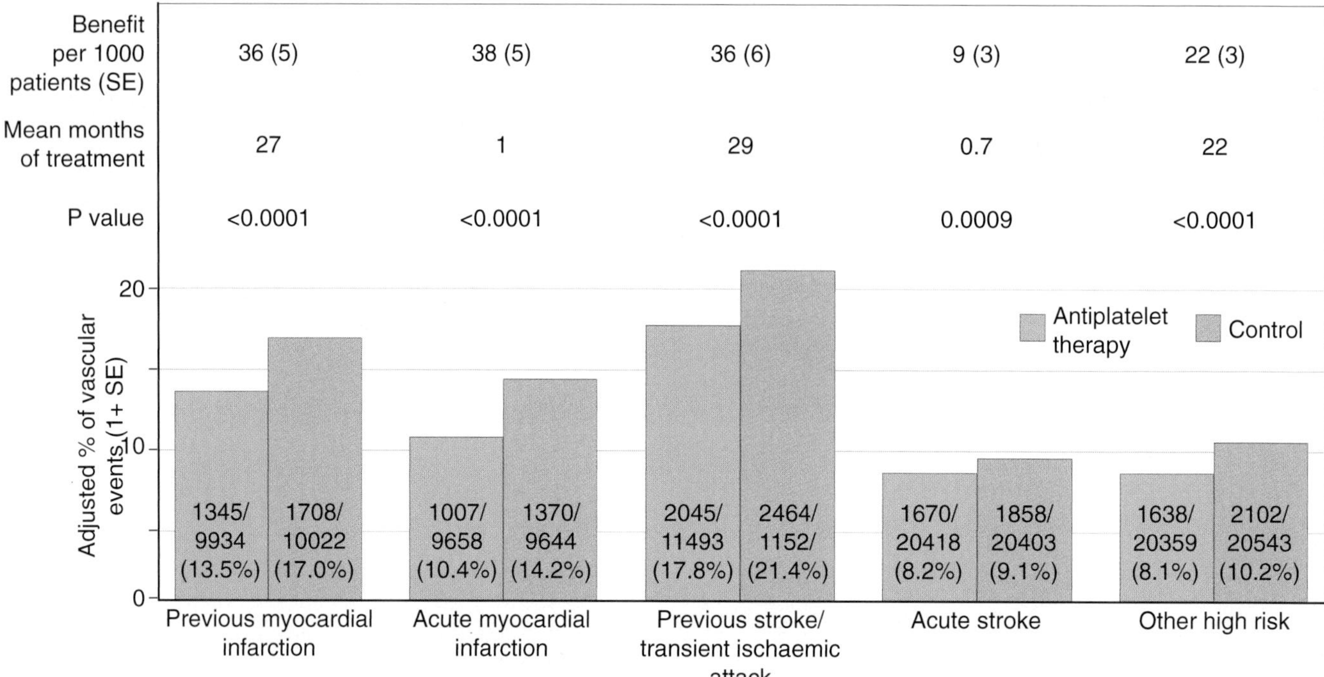

Figure 86–8. Absolute effects of antiplatelet therapy on vascular events (myocardial infarction, stroke, or vascular death) in five main high-risk categories. Adjusted control totals have been calculated after converting any unevenly randomized trial to even ones by counting control groups more than once. Abbreviation: SE, standard error. (Adapted from Collaborative overview of randomised trials of antiplatelet therapy—III: reduction in venous thrombosis and pulmonary embolism by antiplatelet prophylaxis among surgical and medical patients. Antiplatelet Trialists' Collaboration. BMJ 308:235–246, 1994, with permission.)

There was a highly significant decrease ($P < .00001$) in coronary artery graft occlusion with antiplatelet therapy versus control (4000 patients), in peripheral artery procedures or disease (3000 patients), and in hemodialysis patients with a shunt or fistula (400 patients). A smaller benefit was seen in patients after coronary angioplasty ($P < .01$; 800 patients). There was no clear evidence that one antiplatelet regimen was superior to any other. Overall, there was a slight increase of 1 fatal bleed per 1000 when antiplatelet therapy was started just before a procedure (95% CI, 0–3; not significant), and there was a significant excess of nonfatal major bleeds (2.2% vs. 0.9%).

Dipyridamole together with aspirin was reported to reduce the stroke rate by 37% in patients with previous stroke or transient ischemic attack compared to placebo, and by 18% or 16% compared to aspirin or dipyridamole alone, respectively, in the ESPS-2 study.[223] A recent review of 19,000 patients in randomized trials of dipyridamole for nonembolic arterial disease concluded that dipyridamole with or without aspirin was not better than other antiplatelet drugs (primarily aspirin) in preventing vascular death (relative risk 1.02; 95% CI, 0.90–1.17), although with aspirin it was better than other antiplatelet agents in preventing vascular events, largely because of the results of the ESPS-2 study.[224]

The Caprie study is the largest evaluating clopidogrel in arterial disease.[225] It was a randomized, blinded comparison of clopidogrel versus aspirin for atherosclerotic vascular disease, and it included patients with recent myocardial infarction, recent ischemic stroke, or symptomatic peripheral arterial disease, with approximately 6300 patients in each group. The primary outcome was the occurrence of ischemic stroke, myocardial infarction, or vascular death. After a mean follow-up of 1.91 years, there were 1960 first events, with an annual risk of 5.32% in the clopidogrel group and 5.83% in the aspirin group (relative risk reduction, 8.7%; $P = .043$). There were no major differences in bleeding or adverse events. Rash and diarrhea were slightly more frequent with clopidogrel, but upper gastrointestinal discomfort, gastrointestinal bleeding, intracranial hemorrhage, and neutropenia were all more frequent with aspirin. There were no significant differences in any of the secondary end points in the study (stroke, myocardial infarction, amputation, or death) individually. There was a significant benefit of clopidogrel in the patients who entered with peripheral arterial disease ($P = .0028$). A subsequent publication analyzed the effect of clopidogrel in preventing myocardial infarction in the Caprie trial.[226] New myocardial infarction developed in 5.04% of those treated with aspirin versus 4.2% of those treated with clopidogrel ($P = .008$).

A systematic review of antiplatelet therapy for the prevention of the combined end point of myocardial infarction, stroke, or vascular death in patients with peripheral vascular disease included patients from the Caprie study.[227] In patients with stable peripheral vascular disease, antiplatelet therapy was superior to control ($P = .02$) for the combined end point. Death from vascular or unknown causes was also significantly less with antiplatelet therapy. There was no significant benefit from antiplatelet treatment in patients undergoing lower limb bypass surgery or in those undergoing percutaneous balloon angioplasty. When aspirin was compared with other antiplatelet therapy (ticlopidine, clopidogrel, or dipyridamole plus aspirin), the second regimen was better than aspirin ($P = .003$). Most of the patients in the "other" antiplatelet group were from the Caprie study.[225]

ACCP recommendations for management of chronic peripheral arterial insufficiency[216] are to use aspirin, with or without dipyridamole, in patients with a history of intermittent claudication, although they state that clopidogrel may be superior to aspirin in reducing ischemic complications. Pentoxifylline is not recommended, but a trial of cilostazol may be indicated if there is disabling claudication.

Although this chapter has not focused on treatment of acute myocardial infarction, recent literature indicates that clopidogrel has beneficial effects in patients with non–ST segment elevation acute coronary syndromes.[228,229] Many patients with coronary artery disease undergo stenting currently, and glycoprotein IIb/IIIa inhibitors are used routinely during stenting.[230] Clopidogrel has been shown to prevent stent thrombosis if used for 30 days or more after stent placement.[231–234]

Summary

Two mechanisms of arterial thromboembolism have been discussed in this section: cardioembolism and arterial thrombosis. Cardioembolism is most effectively treated with warfarin, with the recommended target INR determined by the nature of the cardiac disease—atrial fibrillation, diseased native valves, prosthetic valves, or severe heart failure. Platelet inhibitors are generally used for arterial thrombosis. Aspirin has been shown to be clearly superior to placebo in preventing nonfatal myocardial infarction, nonfatal stroke, or vascular death in patients with underlying coronary, cerebrovascular, or peripheral arterial disease. One large study suggested that the combination of aspirin and dipyridamole was superior to aspirin alone, but other studies have not confirmed this. Most recently, clopidogrel has been shown to be superior to aspirin for prevention of nonfatal myocardial infarction, nonfatal stroke, or vascular death. In general practice, aspirin is still used initially in most situations, with substitution of clopidogrel if aspirin fails, although for stents, clopidogrel is preferred, at least for the initial post-stent period.

Current Controversies & Future Considerations

Venous and Arterial Thrombosis

- What is the optimal duration of antithrombotic prophylaxis during periods of high risk, such as following major or orthopedic surgery?
- What is the optimal duration of oral anticoagulant therapy following an episode of deep vein thrombosis or pulmonary embolism? Should this be modified by the presence of a hypercoagulable state, the rate of thrombus resolution, or persistent elevation of D-dimer?
- Does fibrinolytic therapy significantly improve outcomes in patients with pulmonary embolism and right heart strain or in patients with large proximal deep vein thrombosis?
- Which patients with transient ischemic attack or stroke should receive aspirin and which should receive clopidogrel?

Suggested Readings*

Agnelli G, Prandoni P, Santamaria MG, et al: Three months versus one year of oral anticoagulant therapy for idiopathic deep venous thrombosis. Warfarin Optimal Duration Italian Trial Investigators. N Engl J Med 345:165–169, 2001.

De Schryver EL, Algra A, van Gijn J: Cochrane Review: dipyridamole for preventing major vascular events in patients with vascular disease. Stroke 34:2072–2080, 2003.

Gould MK, Dembitzer AD, Doyle RL, et al: Low-molecular-weight heparins compared with unfractionated heparin for treatment of acute deep venous thrombosis. Ann Intern Med 130:500–509, 1999.

Hart RG, Halperin JL, Pearce LA, et al: Lessons from the Stroke Prevention in Atrial Fibrillation trials. Ann Intern Med 138:831–838, 2003.

Hirsh J, Lee AY: How we diagnose and treat deep vein thrombosis. Blood 99:3102–3110, 2002.

Lee AY, Levine MN, Baker RI, et al: Low-molecular-weight heparin versus a coumarin for the prevention of recurrent venous thromboembolism in patients with cancer. N Engl J Med 349:146–153, 2003.

Rosendaal FR: Venous thrombosis: a multicausal disease. Lancet 353:1167–1173, 1999.

Ross R: Atherosclerosis—an inflammatory disease. N Engl J Med 340:115–126, 1999.

**Full references for this chapter can be found on accompanying CD-ROM.*

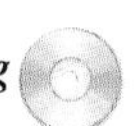

CHAPTER 87

Thrombotic Complications in Patients with Malignancy

Agnes Y. Y. Lee, MD, BSc, Catie E. Kobbervig, MD, and John A. Heit, MD

KEY POINTS

Thrombotic Complications in Patients with Malignancy

- Venous thromboembolism is a common complication in patients with cancer that increases the morbidity and mortality of these patients.
- Patients with malignant brain tumors and cancer of the ovary and pancreas have the highest risk of venous thromboembolism. The exact risk in an individual patient is likely dependent on the tumor type, stage of disease, and presence of extrinsic risk factors such as chemotherapy, hormonal therapy, and surgery.
- Routine screening for occult cancer in patients presenting with idiopathic venous thromboembolism has not been shown to improve cancer-related survival and is not warranted in the absence of clinical features and abnormal basic laboratory findings suggestive of underlying malignancy.
- Prophylaxis with anticoagulants is indicated in patients undergoing surgery for malignancy and those hospitalized for medical reasons, but routine prophylaxis in patients with an indwelling central venous catheter is not recommended.
- For treatment of venous thromboembolism, monotherapy with low-molecular-weight heparin is more efficacious than traditional therapy with heparin and vitamin K antagonists and has comparable safety with respect to bleeding.

INTRODUCTION

Although the association between malignant neoplasm and venous thromboembolism was first noted by Armand Trousseau some 140 years ago,[1] many issues regarding the epidemiology, pathophysiology, prevention, and management of venous thromboembolism among patients with malignancy remain unresolved. Recent recognition of the unique natural history of venous thromboembolism among cancer patients has stimulated many clinical trials addressing primary and secondary prevention of venous thromboembolism in cancer patients. Additional studies also have addressed the most appropriate investigation for occult cancer among patients presenting with idiopathic venous thromboembolism, the incidence and primary prevention of central venous catheter–associated venous thrombosis, and the effect of anticoagulation on cancer patient survival. In this chapter, we review the limited information regarding the epidemiology and pathophysiology of cancer-associated venous thromboembolism. In addition, we review selected data from clinical trials investigating prevention and management of cancer-associated venous thromboembolism.

Funded, in part, by grants from the U.S. Public Health Service, National Institutes of Health (HL66216 to J.A.H.). Dr. Lee is a recipient of a New Investigators Award from the Canadian Institutes of Health Research Rx & D Research Program.

EPIDEMIOLOGY

Risk of Venous Thromboembolism

Active malignancy is an independent risk factor for venous thromboembolism, with a four- to sixfold increased risk of deep vein thrombosis and pulmonary embolism (Table 87–1).[2–5] Consequently, venous thromboembolism is one of the most common complications seen in cancer patients.[6,7] Furthermore, active cancer accounts for almost 20% of all new venous thromboembolism events occurring in the community.[8]

Cancer is also an independent risk factor for death within 7 days after venous thromboembolism. The 1-week risk of death is increased 7- and 2.4-fold among female and male cancer patients not receiving chemotherapy, respectively, and 4- and 8.5-fold among female and male cancer patients receiving chemotherapy.[9] Moreover, cancer patients with venous thromboembolism have worse survival than cancer patients without venous thromboembolism (Fig. 87–1).[10,11]

TABLE 87–1. Independent Risk Factors for Deep Vein Thrombosis or Pulmonary Embolism

Baseline Characteristic	Odds Ratio	95% CI
Institutionalization with or without recent surgery		
No institutionalization or recent surgery	1.00	
Institutionalization without recent surgery	7.98	4.49–14.18
Institutionalization with recent surgery	21.72	9.44–49.93
Trauma	12.69	4.06–39.66
No malignancy	1.0	
Malignancy without chemotherapy	4.05	1.93–8.52
Malignancy with chemotherapy	6.53	2.11–20.23
Prior central venous catheter or transvenous pacemaker	5.55	1.57–19.58
Prior superficial vein thrombosis	4.32	1.76–10.61
Neurologic disease with extremity paresis	3.04	1.25–7.38
Serious liver disease	0.10	0.01–0.71

Abbreviation: CI, confidence interval.
Adapted from Heit JA, Silverstein MD, Mohr DN, et al: Risk factors for deep vein thrombosis and pulmonary embolism: a population-based case-control study. Arch Intern Med 160:809–815, 2000.

TABLE 87–2. Relative Risk of Venous Thromboembolism by Tumor Site Compared with Patients without Malignancy

Type of Cancer	Relative Risk (95% CI)
Head/neck	0.29 (0.20–0.40)
Bladder	0.42 (0.36–0.49)
Breast	0.44 (0.40–0.48)
Esophagus	0.76 (0.58–0.97)
Cervix	0.90 (0.68–1.18)
Liver	0.92 (.076–1.10)
Prostate	0.98 (0.93–1.04)
Patients without malignancy	1.0
Rectum	1.11 (1.00–1.22)
Lung	1.13 (1.07–1.19)
Colon	1.36 (1.29–1.44)
Renal	1.41 (1.25–1.59)
Stomach	1.49 (1.33–1.68)
Lymphoma	1.80 (1.65–1.96)
Pancreas	2.05 (1.87–2.40)
Ovary	2.16 (1.93–2.41)
Leukemia	2.18 (2.01–2.37)
Brain	2.37 (2.04–2.74)
Uterus	3.4 (2.97–3.87)

Abbreviation: CI, confidence interval.
Modified from Thodiyil PA, Kakkar AK: Variation in relative risk of venous thromboembolism in different cancers. Thromb Haemost 87:1076–1077, 2002.

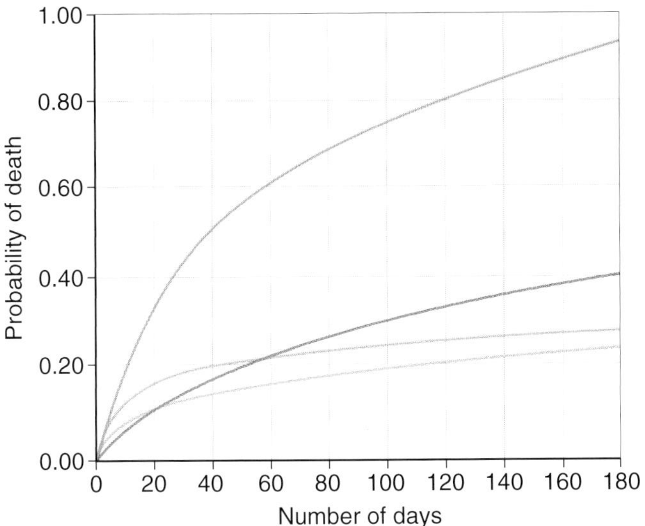

Figure 87–1. Probability of death according to hospital admission diagnosis. (From Levitan N, Dowlati A, Remick SC, et al: Rates of initial and recurrent thromboembolic disease among patients with malignancy versus those without malignancy: risk analysis using Medicare claims data. Medicine [Baltimore] 78:285–291, 1999, with permission.)

Compared to deep vein thrombosis alone, pulmonary embolism is an independent predictor for reduced survival for up to 3 months.[9] Thus, prevention of venous thromboembolism will improve cancer patient survival.

Unfortunately, there are few data that allow one to predict which cancer patient will develop venous thromboembolism. Although the risk of venous thromboembolism by tumor type remains uncertain, the risk appears to be higher for patients with malignant brain tumors and cancer of the ovary, pancreas, colon, stomach, lung, and kidney (Table 87–2).[10,12,13] Among patients with high-grade glioma, the presence of extremity paresis increases the risk of venous thromboembolism.[14] However, the risk by tumor histology, stage, and site of local invasion or metastases is still largely unknown.

Chemotherapy increases the risk for venous thromboembolism. Compared to those without cancer, patients receiving cytotoxic or immunosuppressive therapy have a 6.5-fold increased risk of venous thromboembolism.[2] Cancer patients receiving chemotherapy account for 13% of the overall burden of venous thromboembolism disease in the community.[8] Chemotherapy combined with the angiogenesis inhibitors has been shown to increase the risk of venous thromboembolism.[15–17]

Hormonal therapy also increases the risk of venous thromboembolism.[18–20] For example, the risk is increased two- to fivefold among women with breast cancer treated with tamoxifen.[19] The risk is further increased in post-menopausal women[21] and when tamoxifen is combined with chemotherapy.[19,22] Conversely, women with breast cancer treated with the aromatase inhibitor anastrozole have approximately half the risk of venous thromboembolism compared to tamoxifen.[23,24]

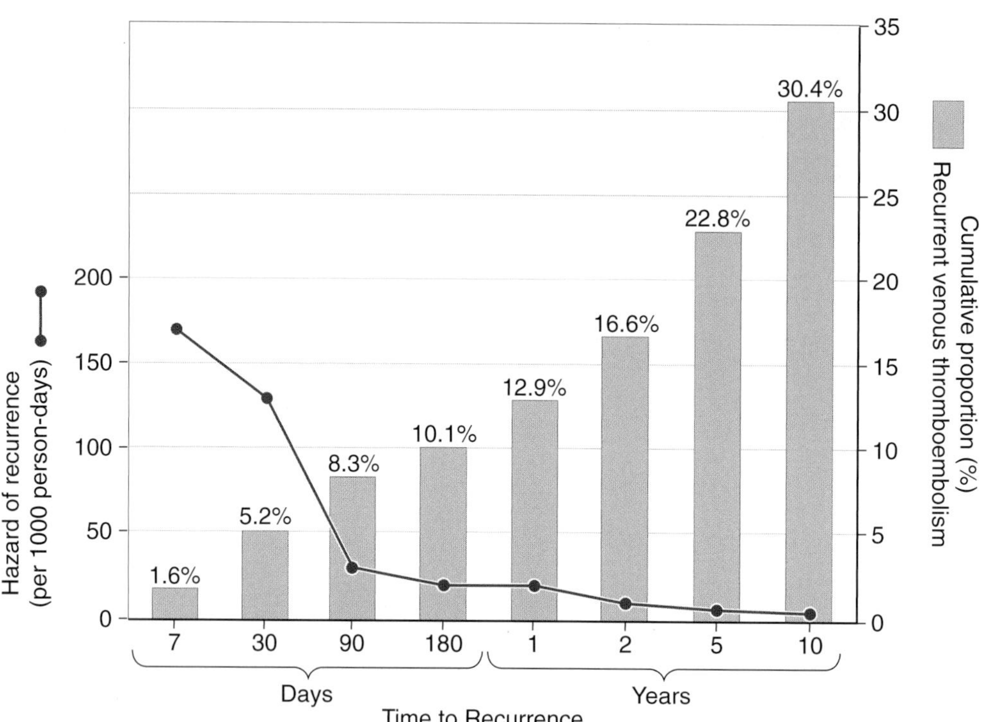

Figure 87–2. Cumulative incidence (%) and hazard (per 1000 person-days) of first venous thromboembolism recurrence.

A central venous catheter or transvenous pacemaker increases the risk of upper extremity deep vein thrombosis about sixfold (see Table 87–1).[2] Historical studies have reported incidences as high as 60%,[25] but contemporary studies have found a much lower risk of symptomatic catheter-related thrombosis of 3–4% (1.14 per 1000 catheter-days) without thromboprophylaxis.[26–28] This reduction in risk is likely due to improvement in catheter design, insertion techniques, and maintenance care, and to differences in study design.

Cancer patients undergoing surgical procedures have twice the risk of postoperative deep vein thrombosis and over three times the risk of fatal pulmonary embolism compared to noncancer patients, despite prophylaxis with anticoagulants.[29,30] The exact risk varies depending on the tumor type and extent of surgery.

The cumulative incidence and hazard of venous thromboembolism recurrence are shown in Figure 87–2.[31] Active malignant neoplasm is an independent predictor of venous thromboembolism recurrence.[10,31] Patients with malignancy have over a twofold increased risk of recurrence, and patients receiving concurrent chemotherapy have over a fourfold increased recurrence risk.[31]

Occult Malignancy

It has long been recognized that venous thromboembolism may be a sign of occult malignancy. In one study, the standardized incidence ratio (SIR, or observed-to-expected case ratio) of a cancer diagnosis within 1 year after the first episode of a venous thromboembolic event was 3.4, with subsequent rates for the following 5 years ranging from 1.3 to 2.2.[32] In a large population-based study, the SIR for the first year for all cancers was 4.4 and the risk remained elevated at 1.3 for more than 10 years.[33] Other studies have also demonstrated an increased risk of malignancy in association with venous thromboembolism, but the risk declines almost to baseline levels after 6 months to a year after the thromboembolic event (Table 87–3).[34–36]

TABLE 87–3. Standardized Incidence Ratios (SIR), or Observed-to-Expected Case Ratio, of Cancer Diagnosis within 6 Months or 1 Year of First Episode of a Venous Thromboembolic Event

Study	SIR (at 1 yr Unless Noted)	95% CI
Schulman and Lindmarker (2000)[32]	3.4	2.2–4.6
Baron et al. (1998)[33]	4.4	4.2–4.6
Sorenson et al. (1998)[36]	2.1 (DVT)	1.9–2.4
	2.3 (PE)	2.0–2.7
Nordstrom et al. (1994)[35]	5.27 (<6 mo)	4.10–6.74
	1.01 (≥6 mo)	0.81–1.26

Abbreviations: CI, confidence interval; DVT, deep vein thrombosis; PE, pulmonary embolism.

A subsequent cancer diagnosis is more likely in patients with idiopathic venous thromboembolism compared to those who develop a deep vein thrombosis or pulmonary embolism in association with a transient, reversible risk factor such as surgery, and in patients with recurrent venous thromboembolism.[33,36–39] Extensive cancer screening after an idiopathic or recurrent venous thromboembolic event is not warranted based on current data.[40–43] Studies have shown that comprehensive radiologic and laboratory testing at the time venous thromboembolism is diagnosed will increase the detection of occult malignancies, but screening does not improve cancer-related mortality outcomes. This is largely because effective treatment is not available for many malignancies associated with venous thromboembolism, such as pancreatic, stomach, and liver cancers.[44,45] Patients with idiopathic or recurrent venous thromboembolism should have a thorough history and physical examination as well as routine blood work, and a chest radiograph should be obtained in smokers. More extensive investigation is warranted only if initial findings suggest the presence of an underlying malignancy. This strategy has been shown to identify the majority of occult cancers that are present at the time of the thromboembolic event.[39,42,46,47]

PATHOPHYSIOLOGY

Active cancer is associated with a hypercoagulable state that involves the interaction of multiple complex mechanisms (Fig. 87–3).[48,49] Tumors can produce procoagulant molecules that can activate coagulation either directly or indirectly by initiating an inflammatory response, which in turn induces further release of procoagulants from tumor cells.[50] In addition, extrinsic factors, such as surgery and chemotherapy, can further enhance this hypercoagulable process through venous stasis, perturbation of coagulation proteases, or direct endothelial injury. Although laboratory evidence of coagulation activation is common in patients with cancer (Box 87–1), such changes have not been predictive of clinical disease.[51]

The two best characterized tumor procoagulants are tissue factor and cancer procoagulant.[49] Many different solid tumor cells, as well as leukemia blast cells, constitutively express tissue factor. Expression of tissue factor on tumor cells, tumor-associated macrophages, and endothelial cells is also upregulated in response to cytokines. In addition to its primary function in hemostasis, tissue factor also has a role in the cellular signaling that is involved with angiogenesis, tumor growth, and the metastatic potential of some cancers.[52–54] Evidence suggests that cancer procoagulant is a cysteine protease that directly activates factor X in the absence of activated factor VII, but the complementary DNA encoding this protein has not been isolated nor is the protein sequence known.[55] Recent evidence also suggests that cancer procoagulant can induce dose-dependent platelet activation by a mechanism that appears to be similar to that of thrombin. Cancer procoagulant is found exclusively on malignant cells and its expression in acute promyelocytic leukemia blasts parallels their degree of malignant transformation and response to all-*trans* retinoic acid.[56] Tumor cells also release inflammatory cytokines and

Box 87–1. Changes in Coagulation Laboratory Markers Associated with Malignancy

- Shortening or prolongation of prothrombin time or partial thromboplastin time
- Elevated levels of fibrinogen and activated coagulation factors
- Mild to moderate thrombocytosis
- Upregulated expression of platelet activation markers (e.g., platelet factor 4, CD62)
- Suppression of fibrinolytic activity (e.g., elevated levels of plasminogen activator inhibitor type 1)
- Elevated levels of prothrombin fragment 1 + 2 and thrombin-antithrombin complex

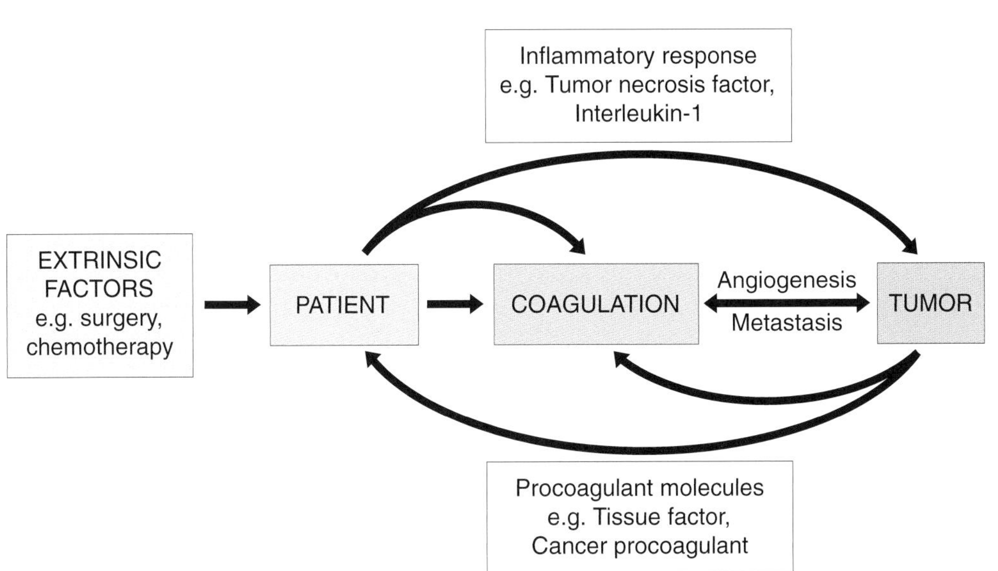

Figure 87–3. Activation of coagulation in patients with malignancy. (Modified from Lee AY: Cancer and thromboembolic disease: pathogenic mechanisms. Cancer Treat Rev 28:137–140, 2002.)

chemokines, such as tumor necrosis factor, interleukin-1, and vascular endothelial growth factor, that act on leukocytes and endothelial cells to further enhance the procoagulant activity.[49]

Besides tumor cell activity, an inflammatory response involving monocytes and other immune regulatory cells can further fuel the prothrombotic process.[57,58] Release of potent inflammatory mediators such as tumor necrosis factor and interleukin-1 can elicit downstream responses that can promote thrombin generation. However, as for coagulation markers, elevated levels of inflammatory markers have not correlated directly with the development of clinical thromboembolic disease.

DIAGNOSIS

Diagnosing venous thromboembolism in the presence of malignancy can be more challenging than in noncancer patients. Although the presence of a risk factor such as malignancy increases the pretest probability that a patient has venous thromboembolism,[59,60] the typical signs and symptoms of deep vein thrombosis and pulmonary embolism are nonspecific and are not uncommon in patients with cancer. Therefore, as it is in patients without cancer, objective testing is necessary to support or refute clinical suspicions for venous thromboembolism. To date, few studies have tested the accuracy and determined the predictive values of diagnostic investigations specifically in patients with cancer. Consequently, patients with or without cancer presenting with suspected venous thromboembolism are evaluated using similar algorithms (see Chapter 86, Figs. 86–2 and 86–3).

For suspected deep vein thrombosis, compression duplex ultrasound is the most appropriate initial screening test in most patients. In contrast, D-dimer testing has limited usefulness in patients with cancer because many of these patients test positive in the absence of thrombosis,[61–64] and one study has shown that the negative predictive value is too low to safely exclude deep vein thrombosis in this high-risk population.[62] Although other retrospective studies have suggested that D-dimer testing remains clinically useful in cancer patients,[63,64] prospective management studies are needed to support these findings. Contrast venography, the "gold standard" test, may be necessary to confirm the diagnosis in difficult cases. In patients with contraindications to traditional venography, magnetic resonance venography is an accurate though expensive alternative.[65]

For suspected pulmonary embolism, either helical (spiral) computed tomography, pulmonary angiography, or ventilation-perfusion lung scintigraphy should be the test of first choice. Spiral computed tomography is often preferred in patients with malignancy because of the potential for coexisting pulmonary or pleural lesions, which may make ventilation-perfusion scans difficult to interpret. In addition, spiral computed tomography may provide alternate diagnoses to explain clinical signs and symptoms in cancer patients. Pulmonary angiography remains the reference standard for the diagnosis of pulmonary embolism but is not readily available in many institutions.[65,66] Magnetic resonance angiography is a promising technique, particularly when gadolinium-enhanced imaging is used.[67]

PROPHYLAXIS OR PRIMARY PREVENTION

Venous thromboembolism is common in cancer patients and often more difficult to diagnose than in patients without cancer. In addition, the risks of complications from anticoagulant therapy for the treatment of venous thromboembolism are higher than in the general population. Therefore, it is essential that patients with known malignancies receive appropriate prophylaxis to decrease their risk of venous thromboembolism.

Medical Patients

Two studies have evaluated the role of thromboprophylaxis in cancer patients without another indication for prophylaxis. Levine and colleagues randomly assigned low-dose warfarin (International Normalized Ratio [INR] 1.3–1.9) or placebo to women with stage IV breast cancer who were receiving chemotherapy. Seven of 159 patients in the placebo group developed venous thrombosis versus 1 of 152 in the low-dose warfarin group.[68] This statistically significant difference was not associated with an increase in bleeding. The FAMOUS trial evaluated the efficacy of dalteparin in improving survival in patients with advanced solid malignancies and also followed patients for symptomatic venous thromboembolism.[69] A significant difference in the incidence of venous thromboembolic events between the groups was not observed, but the study was underpowered for this end point.

Although there is a lack of evidence to support routine prophylaxis in medical outpatients with cancer, it remains important to consider the overall risk of venous thromboembolism in individual patients. Thromboprophylaxis with either low-dose warfarin or low-molecular-weight heparin should be considered in cancer patients with multiple risk factors, such as a history of venous thromboembolism or prolonged immobilization, and in patients receiving combined chemotherapy and hormonal therapies or antiangiogenic agents.

Surgical Patients

Both low-dose unfractionated heparin and low-molecular-weight heparin are effective at reducing the risk of postoperative venous thromboembolism in cancer patients.[30] However, despite prophylaxis, cancer patients still have a significantly increased risk of venous thromboembolism compared to patients without malignancy.[29,30] Whether patients with cancer would benefit from higher intensity prophylaxis remains unclear.[70–72]

The use of thromboprophylaxis beyond hospitalization for surgery in patients with malignancy has been studied. Bergqvist and coworkers administered 1 week of low-molecular-weight heparin enoxaparin to cancer patients undergoing planned curative abdominal or pelvic surgery and then randomized them to receive either placebo or enoxaparin for 3 additional weeks. At 1 month, the rate of venographically detected deep vein thrombosis was 12% in the placebo group versus 4.8% in the enoxaparin group, and the difference in thrombotic risk persisted at 3 months.[73] The rates of bleeding and overall mortality were the same in both groups. However, extended thromboprophylaxis cannot be recommended routinely in patients undergoing cancer surgery prior to confirmatory results from other studies. Furthermore, it remains controversial whether venographically detected thrombosis is clinically relevant and serves as sufficient evidence to change clinical practice. Nonetheless, as in medical oncology patients, it is reasonable to consider extending prophylaxis in those patients who have additional risk factors for venous thromboembolism.

Patients with Catheters

Early studies indicated that the risk of thrombosis with long-term central venous catheters was as high as 14%, or 1 event per 1000 device days.[25,74] Consequently, prophylaxis with either low-dose warfarin or low-molecular-weight heparin was recommended based on two small, open-label, randomized trials that used venography to screen for catheter-related thrombosis.[75–77] However, recent studies suggest that the overall thrombotic risk is low and probably insufficient to warrant prophylaxis.[26–28] Moreover, pharmacologic prophylaxis has been shown to be relatively ineffective in reducing symptomatic events.[27,28,78] In a study of 425 cancer patients receiving chemotherapy through a central venous catheter who were randomized to low-molecular-weight heparin prophylaxis or placebo, the incidence of symptomatic catheter-related thrombosis was 3.7% and 3.4%, respectively.[28] In a similarly designed study, a difference in symptomatic events was not detected between patients randomized to warfarin 1 mg daily and those assigned to placebo.[27] In addition, the safety of warfarin has been questioned in patients receiving fluorouracil-based chemotherapy and warfarin at 1 mg daily. One third of the patients in this study had elevated INRs, and the bleeding risk was significant and correlated with high INR values.[79] Based on current data, neither warfarin 1 mg nor prophylactic doses of low-molecular-weight heparin can be recommended as prophylaxis for cancer patients with indwelling central venous catheters.[30]

TREATMENT OR SECONDARY PREVENTION

Initial Therapy

The standard regimen for the treatment of acute venous thromboembolism consists of initial therapy with unfractionated heparin or low-molecular-weight heparin followed by long-term therapy with a coumarin derivative for secondary prophylaxis. Studies have shown that low-molecular-weight heparins are at least as efficacious as unfractionated heparin and are likely to be associated with a lower risk of major bleeding.[80–86] Furthermore,

TABLE 87–4. The Efficacy of Low-Molecular-Weight Heparin (LMWH) and Unfractionated Heparin (UFH) for Initial Therapy of Venous Thromboembolic Event (VTE) in Patients With and Without Cancer

	3-Month Incidence of Recurrent VTE			
	No. Patients	**LMWH (%)**	**UFH (%)**	***P* Value**
Cancer	546	9.2	9.2	NS
No cancer	2275	4.0	4.2	NS

Combined results from four randomized trials[80–83] showing the 3-month rates of recurrent VTE separately for patients with and without cancer. NS, not significant.

low-molecular-weight heparins can be given in an outpatient setting without the need for laboratory monitoring and have a lower risk of heparin-induced thrombocytopenia.[87,88] In most developed countries, outpatient low-molecular-weight heparin has become the standard of care for the initial treatment of patients with deep vein thrombosis or hemodynamically stable pulmonary embolism, and it has been used successfully in selected cancer patients.[87–90]

Whether low-molecular-weight heparins and unfractionated heparin perform comparably in patients with cancer has not been formally investigated. Based on published data extracted from trials that reported on the outcomes of the subgroup of cancer patients, it appears that low-molecular-weight heparins and unfractionated heparin have similar efficacy in patients with and without cancer (Table 87–4). There have been no published data on the bleeding risk of therapeutic doses of low-molecular-weight heparin compared with unfractionated heparin in cancer patients.

For several low-molecular-weight heparins, both once-daily and twice-daily injections are available or approved for use, but there are few direct comparison data regarding the efficacy of once- versus twice-daily low-molecular-weight heparin among cancer patients. A subgroup analysis of cancer patients from a randomized trial comparing once- versus twice-daily low-molecular-weight heparin (enoxaparin) suggested that twice-daily administration was associated with a lower risk of recurrence compared with once-daily administration, but the difference was not statistically significant.[83] Given the hypercoagulable status of cancer patients, it is possible that twice-daily administration of low-molecular-weight heparin is required in order to provide a more steady state of anticoagulation, but this hypothesis has not been tested.

Long-Term Therapy

Coumarin derivatives are the mainstay of long-term anticoagulant treatment for preventing recurrent venous thromboembolism.[91] These vitamin K antagonists are started within the first 24 hours of diagnosis and are continued for a minimum of 3 months. Because of differences in the anticoagulant response between patients

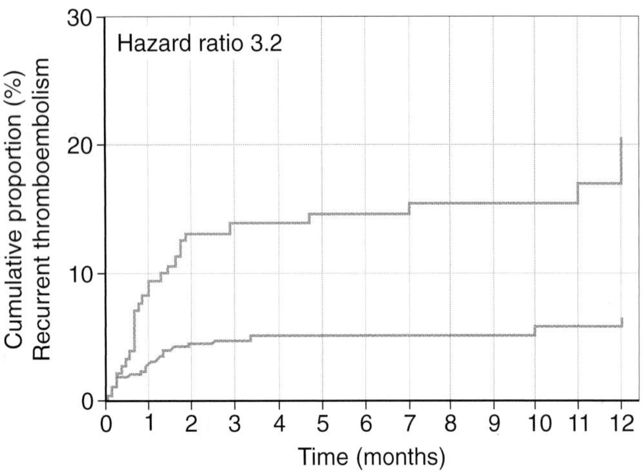

KEY

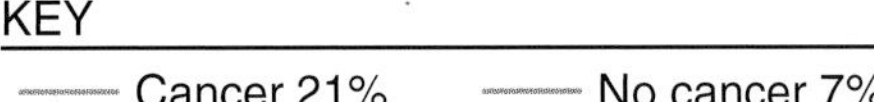

Figure 87–4. Cumulative incidence of recurrent thrombosis in patients with and without cancer while on oral anticoagulant therapy. (From Prandoni P, Lensing AW, Piccioli A, et al: Recurrent venous thromboembolism and bleeding complications during anticoagulant treatment in patients with cancer and venous thrombosis. Blood 100:3484–3488, 2002, with permission.)

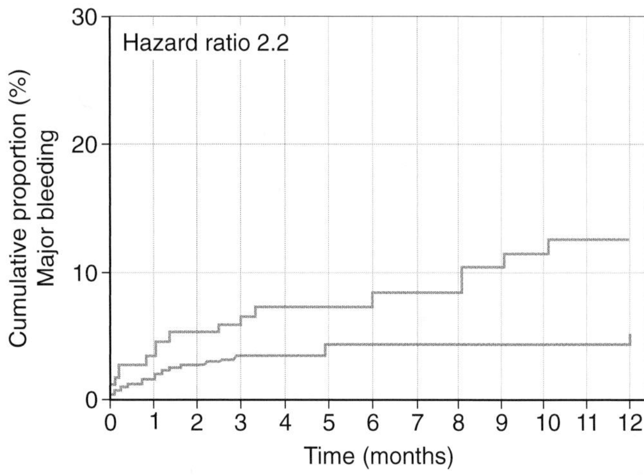

KEY

Cancer 12% No cancer 5%

Figure 87–5. Cumulative incidence of major bleeding in patients with and without cancer while on oral anticoagulant therapy. (From Prandoni P, Lensing AW, Piccioli A, et al: Recurrent venous thromboembolism and bleeding complications during anticoagulant treatment in patients with cancer and venous thrombosis. Blood 100:3484–3488, 2002, with permission.)

and within patients over time, dose adjustments are needed based on the INR. For the majority of patients with venous thromboembolism, the target therapeutic range is 2.0–3.0.[92] The anticoagulant response to vitamin K antagonists is affected by drug-drug interactions, changes in vitamin K status, liver dysfunction, gastrointestinal disturbances such as vomiting and diarrhea, and consumption of alcohol. Furthermore, because vitamin K antagonists have a delayed onset of action and prolonged clearance of the anticoagulant effect, it is difficult to manage in patients who require frequent interruption of their anticoagulant therapy. For cancer patients who require periodic invasive procedures or experience frequent episodes of chemotherapy-induced thrombocytopenia, treatment with warfarin is very problematic. Switching to or bridging with heparins may be indicated in these circumstances to provide more thorough and flexible coverage when invasive procedures are necessary.[93–95]

Recent studies have shown that cancer patients have a two- to threefold higher risk of recurrent venous thromboembolism compared with patients without cancer.[96,97] Although treatment failures may be related to subtherapeutic anticoagulation, recurrent venous thromboembolism also occurs commonly while the INR is maintained within the therapeutic range. The annual risk of recurrent venous thromboembolism in cancer patients treated with warfarin is approximately 25%,[96,97] with the highest incidence reported during the first month of treatment (Fig. 87–4). It also varies somewhat depending on the INR control. Based on results from two large randomized trials, the incidence of venous thromboembolism recurrence is 18.9 per 100 patient-years for INRs within the therapeutic range, but this increases to 54.0 per 100 patient-years for INRs below 2.0.[97] A higher level of INR (>3.0) did not appear to lower the risk of recurrent venous thromboembolism.

Cancer patients on oral anticoagulant therapy also have a high risk for major bleeding. In a large cohort study, the annual risk for major bleeding was 12.4%, compared with 4.9% in patients without cancer.[96] This study also showed that the risk continues to accumulate over time (Fig. 87–5). In contrast to the direct correlation between INR and recurrent venous thromboembolism, the incidence of major bleeding in patients with cancer appears to be independent of the intensity of anticoagulation as reflected by the INR.[97,98]

The efficacy and safety of long-term low-molecular-weight heparin have been evaluated in a number of small studies that included primarily patients without cancer.[99–106] Meta-analyses of these studies have not found a statistically significant difference in the incidence of recurrent venous thromboembolism between low-molecular-weight heparin and oral anticoagulant therapy,[107,108] but low-molecular-weight heparin was associated with a significant reduction in the risk of bleeding.[108]

To date, two published clinical trials have examined the use of long-term low-molecular-weight heparin as an alternative to warfarin therapy in cancer patients with acute venous thromboembolism.[109,110] The CANTHANOX trial compared 3 months of standard warfarin therapy with enoxaparin therapy at 1.5 mg/kg once daily in cancer patients with proximal deep vein thrombosis, pulmonary embolism, or both.[109] A total of 15 of 75 patients had recurrent venous thromboembolism or major bleeding in the warfarin group, compared with 7 of 71 patients assigned to enoxaparin. The difference was not statistically significant (P = .09). There was also no difference in mortality. Notably, six patients in the warfarin group died of bleeding. Based on these results, the investigators concluded that warfarin is associated with a high bleeding risk in cancer patients with venous thromboembolism and that prolonged treatment with low-molecular-weight heparin may be as effective as and safer than oral anticoagulant therapy.

The CLOT trial evaluated the use of long-term dalteparin in 676 cancer patients with proximal deep vein thrombosis, pulmonary embolism, or both.[110] Patients were randomized to usual treatment with dalteparin initially followed by oral anticoagulant therapy or dalteparin alone for 6 months. In the dalteparin group, patients received therapeutic doses at 200 units/kg once daily for the first month and then 75–80% of the full dose for the next 5 months. Over the 6-month treatment period, the cumulative risk of recurrent venous thromboembolism at 6 months was reduced from 17% in the oral anticoagulant group to 9% in the dalteparin group, resulting in a statistically significant risk reduction of 52% (P = .002). Accordingly, one episode of recurrent venous thromboembolism was prevented for every 13 patients treated with dalteparin. Overall, there were no differences in major or any bleeding between the groups; major bleeding was reported in 6% of patients in the dalteparin arm and 4% in the oral anticoagulant arm. By 6 months, 39% of the patients had died in each group; 90% of the deaths were due to progressive cancer. These figures are not surprising given that 67% of the patients had metastatic cancer at the time of study enrollment.

In summary, there is strong evidence that long-term low-molecular-weight heparin is efficacious and safe for preventing recurrent venous thromboembolism in cancer patients. Bleeding does not appear to be increased compared with warfarin therapy, but this remains a major concern in cancer patients receiving long-term anticoagulant therapy because of their comorbid conditions.

Recurrent Venous Thromboembolism

Few studies have addressed treatment of recurrent venous thromboembolism. Traditionally, insertion of an inferior vena caval filter has been recommended. However, a randomized trial in patients with proximal deep vein thrombosis has shown that filters reduce the short-term incidence of pulmonary embolism at the expense of a higher long-term risk of recurrent deep vein thrombosis and postphlebitic syndrome.[111] Low-molecular-weight heparin has been reported in a retrospective study to be effective and safe for treating patients who recur with venous thromboembolism while on warfarin therapy.[112] Although the available evidence is weak, it is reasonable to use low-molecular-weight heparin for recurrent venous thromboembolism and reserve the use of filters for patients who also have serious bleeding.

Duration of Therapy

The most appropriate duration of anticoagulant therapy has not been studied in cancer patients. It is generally recommended that anticoagulant treatment should be continued for as long as the cancer is "active" and while the patient is receiving antitumor therapy. For patients with metastases, "indefinite" therapy is the accepted approach. However, patients should be evaluated frequently to assess the risk-benefit ratio of ongoing anticoagulant therapy, taking into consideration the overall clinical status of the patient, including the quality of life and life expectancy.

Suggested Readings*

Baron JA, Gridley G, Weiderpass E, et al: Venous thromboembolism and cancer. Lancet 351:1077–1080, 1998.

Geerts WH, Pineo GF, Heit JA, et al: Prevention of venous thromboembolism: The Seventh ACCP Conference on Antithrombotic and Thrombolytic Therapy. Chest 126(Suppl 3):338S–400S, 2004.

Gomes MP, Deitcher SR: Diagnosis of venous thromboembolic disease in cancer patients. Oncology (Huntingt) 17:126–135, 139, 2003.

Heit JA, O'Fallon WM, Petterson TM, et al: Relative impact of risk factors for deep vein thrombosis and pulmonary embolism: a population-based study. Arch Intern Med 162:1245–1248, 2002.

Hutten BA, Prins MH, Gent M, et al: Incidence of recurrent thromboembolic and bleeding complications among patients with venous thromboembolism in relation to both malignancy and achieved International Normalized Ratio: a retrospective analysis. J Clin Oncol 18:3078–3083, 2000.

Lee AY, Levine MN: Venous thromboembolism and cancer: risks and outcomes. Circulation 107(Suppl I):I-17–I-21, 2003.

Lee AY, Levine MN, Baker RI, et al: Low-molecular-weight heparin versus a coumarin for the prevention of recurrent venous thromboembolism in patients with cancer. N Engl J Med 349:146–153, 2003.

Prandoni P, Lensing AW, Piccioli A, et al: Recurrent venous thromboembolism and bleeding complications during anticoagulant treatment in patients with cancer and venous thrombosis. Blood 100:3484–3488, 2002.

Sorensen HT, Mellemkjaer L, Olsen JH, Baron JA: Prognosis of cancers associated with venous thromboembolism. N Engl J Med 343:1846–1850, 2000.

Sorensen HT, Mellemkjaer L, Steffensen FH, et al: The risk of a diagnosis of cancer after primary deep venous thrombosis or pulmonary embolism. N Engl J Med 338:1169–1173, 1998.

Full references for this chapter can be found on accompanying CD-ROM.

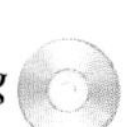

CHAPTER 88

Anticoagulant and Thrombolytic Therapy

Theodore E. Warkentin, MD, and Mark A. Crowther, MD, MSc, FRCPC

KEY POINTS

Anticoagulant and Thrombolytic Therapy

- Anticoagulants can be classified based on their mechanism(s) of action: (1) reduction of functional levels of the vitamin K–dependent coagulation factors (coumarins); (2) catalysis of antithrombin-mediated inhibition of several coagulation enzymes (heparins, danaparoid) or factor Xa alone (fondaparinux); (3) direct inhibition of a coagulation enzyme (direct thrombin inhibitors such as hirudin); or (4) direct proteolysis of coagulation factors (recombinant activated protein C).
- The "classic" anticoagulants, heparin and warfarin, have well-defined antidotes (protamine and vitamin K, respectively), whereas newer anticoagulants do not.
- Low-molecular-weight heparins and fondaparinux have minimal or no effect on routine coagulation assays; thus, the prothrombin time and activated partial thromboplastin time cannot rule out their presence even at therapeutic levels.
- Low-molecular-weight heparin has a lower risk of causing immune heparin-induced thrombocytopenia compared with unfractionated heparin, but low-molecular-weight heparin should not be used to treat heparin-induced thrombocytopenia caused by unfractionated heparin.
- Direct thrombin inhibitors differ in their elimination: hirudin derivatives (renal), bivalirudin (enzymic), argatroban (hepatobiliary), and melagatran (renal).
- Low initial doses of coumarin (e.g., first dose of warfarin, 5 mg or less) may reduce the risk of acute protein C depletion and associated microvascular thrombosis (coumarin necrosis).
- Management of severe bleeding during pharmacologic fibrinolysis includes (at least) stopping the fibrinolytic agent, giving antifibrinolytic therapy (ε-aminocaproic acid or tranexamic acid), and giving fibrinogen (e.g., cryoprecipitate).

INTRODUCTION

Anticoagulants inhibit coagulation by preventing generation of thrombin, or by inhibiting thrombin directly, or both. The ultimate effect is reduced fibrin (thrombus) formation.[1,2] Anticoagulants are widely used to treat and prevent thrombosis involving arteries, veins, intracardiac chambers, and prostheses, such as mechanical heart valves. Because these agents only prevent thrombus accretion, clinical resolution of thrombus occurs via endogenous proteolysis of fibrin (thrombolysis). This chapter also reviews pharmacologic thrombolysis.

The agents we discuss range from the "classic" drugs (heparin, warfarin) to those introduced more recently, such as the direct thrombin inhibitors (DTIs). Ironically, whereas the former have well-defined antidotes, the latter usually do not. Bleeding is the most common adverse event caused by anticoagulants, and is usually associated with high drug levels. When bleeding occurs despite anticoagulation within the target therapeutic range, factors such as recent surgery or occult gastrointestinal lesions may coexist.

Overview of Coagulation

Figure 88–1 presents a simplified scheme of the coagulation cascade.[2] Coagulation is most often triggered when tissue factor (TF), usually found in extravascular sites, binds to circulating factor VIIa following vessel injury. TF-VIIa complexes activate factor X, generating factor Xa, which together with a cofactor (factor Va) forms "prothrombinase" on the altered phospholipid surfaces of activated platelets. Factor Xa within prothrombinase generates the key procoagulant enzyme, thrombin (factor IIa), from prothrombin (factor II). Various positive feedback loops help to convert a small procoagulant stimulus into a "thrombin burst." For example, TF-VIIa

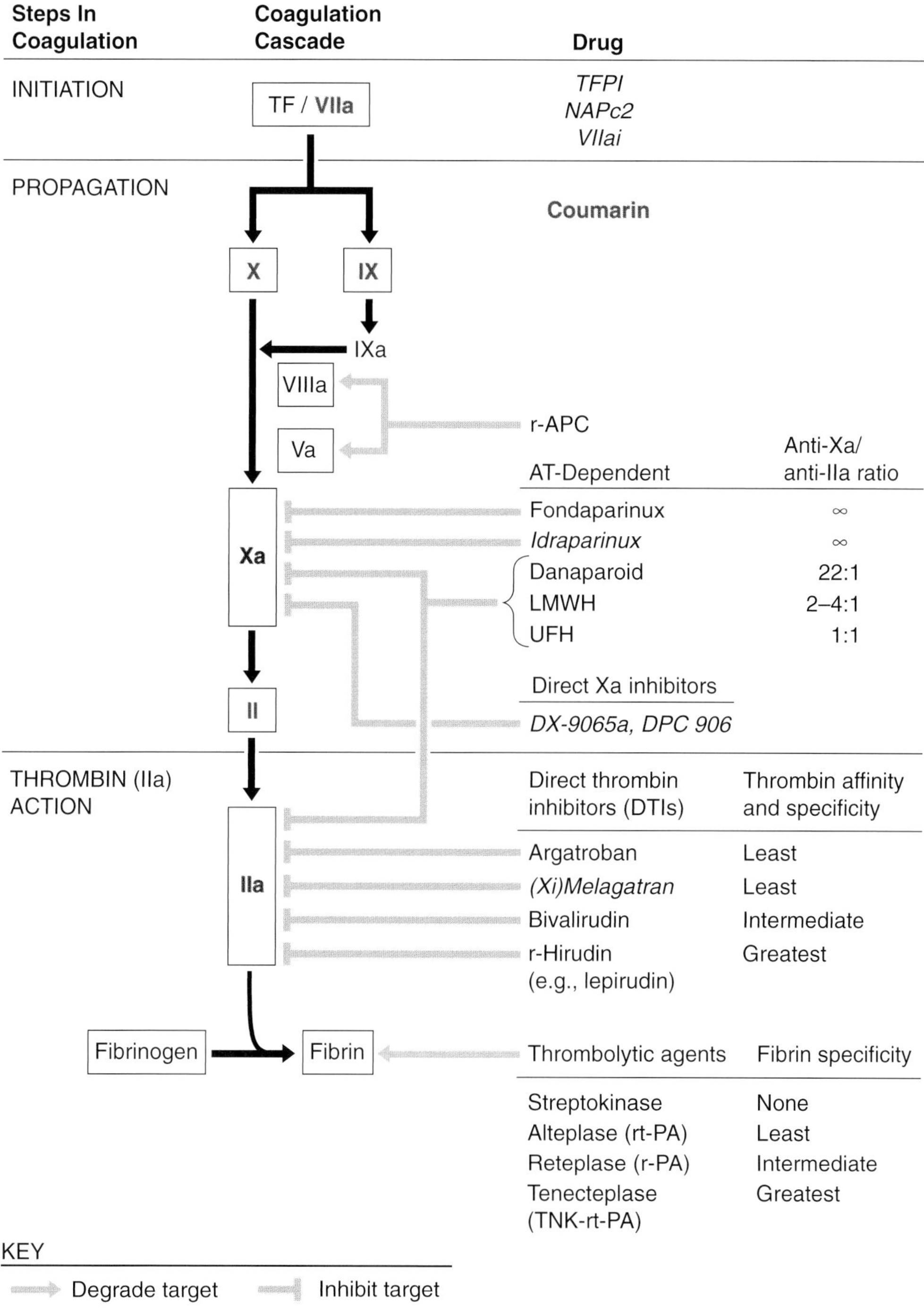

Figure 88–1. Effects of anticoagulants on the coagulation cascade. Coumarins (e.g., warfarin) alter the synthesis of four procoagulant zymogens, factors VIIa, X, IX, and II (prothrombin), shown in *red*. The other anticoagulants degrade *(blue arrow)* or inhibit *(tan blunted arrow)* various coagulation factors. Anticoagulants indicated using *italics* are not approved, except for *(Xi)Melagatran*, which has limited approval in Europe. Abbreviations: AT, antithrombin; DTIs, direct thrombin inhibitors; LMWH, low-molecular-weight heparin; NAPc2, nematode anticoagulant protein c2; rAPC, recombinant activated protein C; TF, tissue factor, TFPI, tissue factor pathway inhibitor; UFH, unfractionated heparin; VIIai, active site–blocked VIIa. (Modified from Hirsh J, Weitz JI: New antithrombotic agents. Lancet 353:1431–1436, 1999.)

complexes also activate factor IX to factor IXa, which acts with a cofactor (factor VIIIa) to form the "tenase" complex that activates factor X to Xa. Other thrombin-initiated positive feedback loops (not shown in Fig. 88–1) include activation of factors V to Va, VIII to VIIIa, and XI to XIa.

Coagulation is regulated by at least four inhibitory systems: (1) tissue factor pathway inhibitor (TFPI); (2) the protein C anticoagulant pathway; (3) antithrombin (formerly antithrombin III); and (4) heparin cofactor II (which plays a minor role). Protein Z, a vitamin K–dependent protein, acts as a cofactor for protein Z–dependent protease inhibitor to inhibit Xa, although its physiologic role is debated.[3]

Anticoagulants work in one of four ways, either by (1) reducing functional levels of the vitamin K–dependent coagulation factors (coumarins); (2) catalyzing antithrombin-mediated inhibition of coagulation enzymes, either several (heparins, danaparoid) or a specific coagulation factor (Xa inhibition by fondaparinux); (3) directly inhibiting a coagulation factor (e.g., inhibition of thrombin by hirudin, or inhibition of TF-VIIa by TFPI); or (4) direct proteolysis of coagulation factors (recombinant activated protein C [APC]).

INDIRECT THROMBIN AND FACTOR Xa INHIBITORS

This section discusses heparin, both unfractionated heparin and low-molecular-weight heparin; fondaparinux (and its derivative, idraparinux); and danaparoid. These are *indirect* inhibitors of coagulation factors, most importantly thrombin and/or factor Xa, because they require the cofactor *antithrombin* to exert their inhibitory effect.

Unfractionated Heparin and Low-Molecular-Weight Heparin

Unfractionated heparin was first approved in 1939 for the prevention and treatment of postoperative thrombosis and embolism[4]; multiple other indications followed (Box 88–1).[5] Open-heart surgery, usually performed using unfractionated heparin, began in 1953.[6] In 1993, the low-molecular-weight heparin enoxaparin was first approved in the United States for antithrombotic prophylaxis after hip replacement surgery.[7] Subsequently, enoxaparin has been approved for antithrombotic prophylaxis in several clinical settings (after knee replacement surgery, after general [abdominal] surgery, for unstable angina and non-q wave myocardial infarction [given together with aspirin], and in medical patients at risk for deep vein thrombosis and pulmonary embolism), as well as for treatment (together with warfarin) of acute deep vein thrombosis, with or without pulmonary embolism.[7]

Box 88–1. Approved Indications for Unfractionated Heparin in the United States

- Prophylaxis and treatment of deep vein thrombosis and its extension
- Prophylaxis and treatment of pulmonary embolism
- Prevention of postoperative deep vein thrombosis and pulmonary embolism in patients undergoing major abdominothoracic surgery who are at risk of developing thromboembolic disease (low-dose regimen)
- Treatment of atrial fibrillation with embolization
- Diagnosis and treatment of acute and chronic consumptive coagulopathies (disseminated intravascular coagulation)
- Prevention of clotting in arterial and cardiac surgery
- Prophylaxis and treatment of peripheral arterial embolism

From Physicians' Desk Reference: Antiplatelet & antithrombotic prescribing guide. Montvale, NJ: Thomson Medical Economics, 2003.

Pharmacology

Heparin is a highly sulfated glycosaminoglycan.[8] Usually obtained from pig intestinal mucosa, unfractionated heparin contains polymers varying from 3000 to 30,000 Da (mean, 15,000 Da; range, 9 to 90 monosaccharide units). Chemical or enzymatic depolymerization techniques can be used to make low-molecular-weight heparin preparations that vary from 2000 to 9000 Da (mean, 4500 Da; range, 6 to 27 monosaccharide units). All unfractionated or low-molecular-weight heparin molecules that retain significant anticoagulant activity contain a specific five-saccharide sequence ("antithrombin-binding pentasaccharide") present within up to one third of heparin chains, greatly increasing the efficiency with which antithrombin inactivates thrombin, factors Xa, IXa, and XIa, and the TF-VIIa complex.[9] Antithrombin is most efficient at inactivating thrombin and factor Xa, as shown by higher second-order rate constants (8900 and 2500 $mol^{-1}\ sec^{-1}$, compared with values ranging from 300 to 450 for VIIa-TF complex and factors IXa and XIa). Catalysis by unfractionated heparin increases antithrombin-mediated inhibition 1000-fold.

Besides containing the specific antithrombin-binding pentasaccharide sequence, heparin molecules must be at least 18 saccharide units long to bind to both antithrombin and thrombin; in contrast, antithrombin bound to any pentasaccharide-containing heparin—even with a chain length fewer than 18 saccharide units—will inhibit factor Xa (Fig. 88–2). Thus, whereas unfractionated heparin catalyzes inhibition of thrombin and factor Xa equally well, low-molecular-weight heparin preferentially inhibits factor Xa (usual anti-Xa/anti-IIa ratio, 2–4 : 1). Low-molecular-weight heparin preparations (e.g., ardeparin [Normiflo], dalteparin [Fragmin], enoxaparin [Lovenox], reviparin [Clivarin], tinzaparin [Innohep]) differ in both jurisdictional availability and composition. Table 88–1 lists the low-molecular-weight heparin preparations (enoxaparin, dalteparin, tinzaparin) in predominant use in the United States. Both unfractionated and low-molecular-weight heparin inhibit factors IXa and XIa, although with substantially less avidity than thrombin and/or factor Xa.

The biologic half-life of heparin when administered by intravenous bolus at a dose of 100 units/kg is about 1 hour; however, the half-life decreases in a nonlinear fashion at lower doses.[8] These complex pharmacokinetics result because heparin binds to and is cleared by endothelial cells and macrophages in a rapid, saturable fashion, whereas heparin in solution is cleared more slowly through the kidneys. Thus, molecules of larger size are cleared more rapidly than lower molecular-weight forms. Furthermore, heparin (especially unfractionated heparin) can bind to and be neutralized by proteins such as platelet factor 4, histidine-rich glycoprotein, fibronectin, and vitronectin. Increased levels of these inflammatory proteins cause heparin "resistance."[10,11] Because plasma levels of these heparin-binding proteins vary among patients, the anticoagulant response to unfractionated heparin is unpredictable, and careful laboratory monitoring is mandatory.

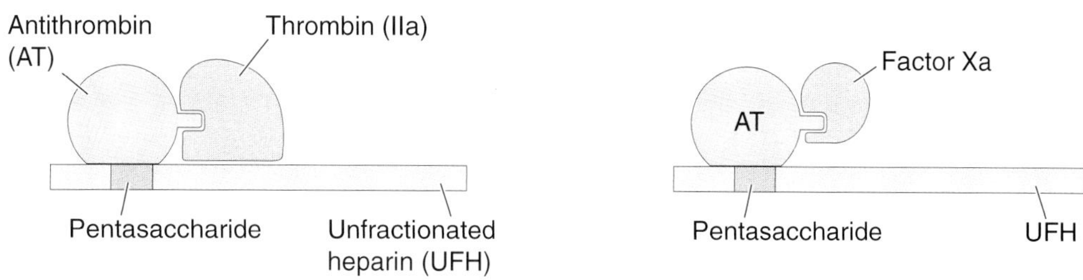

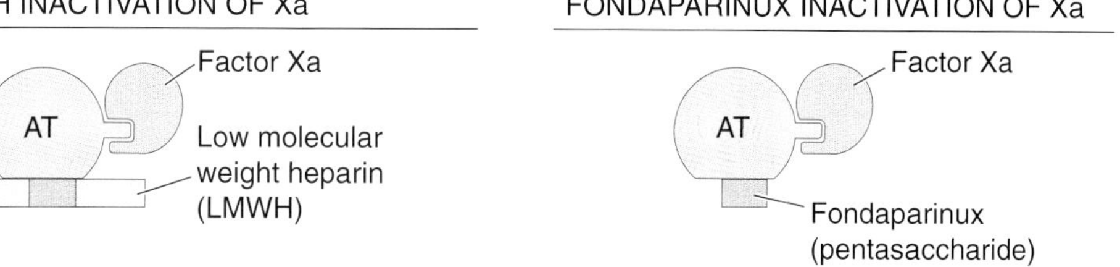

Figure 88–2. Relative effects of unfractionated heparin (UFH), low-molecular-weight heparin (LMWH), and fondaparinux on antithrombin (AT)-mediated inhibition of factor Xa (Xa) and thrombin (IIa). A five-saccharide region ("pentasaccharide") within UFH and LMWH is required for binding to AT (see also Fig. 88–3). Whereas UFH catalyzes inhibition of factor Xa and thrombin equally well, only LMWH chains 18 saccharide units or longer catalyze thrombin inhibition (not shown), and smaller LMWH chains (that contain the pentasaccharide sequence) or fondaparinux (pentasaccharide) catalyze inhibition of factor Xa alone.

TABLE 88–1. Low-Molecular-Weight Heparin Preparations Marketed in North America

Name	Mean Mol. Wt. (Da)	Degradation Method	Dosing for Approved Prophylactic Indications	Dosing for Approved Therapeutic Indications
Enoxaparin (Lovenox)	4500 (68% 2000–8000)	Benzoylation and alkaline β-elimination	30 mg SC bid (often, 40 mg od in Europe) *Abdominal surgery*: 40 mg SC od beginning 2 hours pre-surgery *Hip/knee replacement*: 30 mg SC q12h beginning 12–24 hr postsurgery (for hip surgery, 40 mg SC od beginning 12 ± 3 hours presurgery can also be considered) *Medical patients in acute illness*: 40 mg SC od	*ACS*: 1 mg/kg SC q12h (together with oral aspirin 100–325 mg od)* *DVT ± PE*: 1 mg/kg SC q12h (outpatient) or 1.5 mg/kg SC od given at the same time (outpatient or inpatient)
Dalteparin (Fragmin)	5000 (90% 2000–9000)	Nitrous acid	*Hip replacement*: 2500 IU 4–8 hours SC postsurgery, then 5000 IU SC od beginning the day after surgery[†] *Abdominal surgery*: 2500 IU SC od beginning 1–2 hours before surgery, and resuming the day after surgery[‡]	*ACS*: 120 IU/kg SC q12h (not more than 10,000 IU per dose) together with oral aspirin 75–165 mg od
Tinzaparin (Innohep)	5500–7500	Enzymatic (heparinase)	Not indicated in the United States; in Canada, generally given in a fixed dose (3500–4500 units SC od)	*DVT ± PE*: 175 IU/kg SC od (in- or outpatients)[§]

*To reduce risk of bleeding with vascular instrumentation, the vascular access sheath should remain in place for 6–8 hours following a dose of enoxaparin, and the next scheduled dose should be given no sooner than 6–8 hr after sheath removal.
[†]Other options are (1) to give 2500 IU SC beginning within 2 hours prior to surgery, followed by 2500 IU 4–8 hours postsurgery, then 5000 IU SC od beginning on the first postoperative day; or (2) to give 5000 IU SC beginning the evening before surgery, then 5000 IU 4–8 hours postsurgery, and then 5000 IU SC od beginning on the first postoperative day (allowing approximately 24 hours between doses).
[‡]Other options, particularly for patients at high risk (e.g., malignancy), are (1) 5000 IU SC beginning the evening before surgery, then 5000 IU SC od postoperatively; or (2) to give 2500 IU SC beginning 1–2 hours prior to surgery, followed by 2500 IU SC 12 hours later, and then 5000 IU SC od postoperatively.
[§]Package insert notes that safety and efficacy of treatment were determined in inpatients, but does not restrict setting within which therapy is delivered.
Abbreviations: ACS, acute coronary syndrome (defined here as unstable angina or non–Q wave myocardial infarction); bid, twice daily; DVT ± PE, deep vein thrombosis with or without pulmonary embolism; IU, international units (anti-Xa); od, once daily; SC, subcutaneously.

Low-molecular-weight heparin preparations overcome many of these pharmacokinetic limitations; their smaller size, and lesser charge, result in less nonspecific binding and endothelial/macrophage metabolism, and thus slower clearance (vis-à-vis unfractionated heparin) via the kidneys.[12] Because low-molecular-weight heparin preparations given by subcutaneous injection exhibit near-100% bioavailability, predictable drug levels, and an elimination half-life of about 3–6 hours, this permits once- or twice-daily injection without the need for anticoagulant monitoring in patients without renal dysfunction. Peak levels are reached about 4 hours postinjection.

Clinical Use

Unfractionated heparin or low-molecular-weight heparin is often given when rapid therapeutic-dose anticoagulation is needed, such as for venous thromboembolism (i.e., acute deep vein thrombosis and/or pulmonary embolism),[13] acute coronary syndrome (i.e., acute myocardial infarction or unstable angina),[14,15] percutaneous coronary intervention,[16] acute limb ischemia secondary to thromboembolism,[17] and cerebral venous sinus thrombosis.[18] Unfractionated heparin is also used for intraoperative anticoagulation during cardiac surgery (with or without cardiopulmonary bypass) and vascular surgery. Unfractionated heparin is commonly used to prevent thrombosis of other extracorporeal circuits, including during intermittent or continuous hemodialysis and during extracorporeal membrane oxygenation.

Treatment of deep vein thrombosis or pulmonary embolism consists of therapeutic-dose heparin, given as intravenous unfractionated heparin[19] or subcutaneous low-molecular-weight heparin,[20–22] with overlapping oral anticoagulation. Until the early 1990s, unfractionated heparin was usually given alone for 5 days, followed by at least 5 days of unfractionated heparin/coumarin overlap, then several months of coumarin alone.[23] Now, coumarin is routinely started within 24 hours of initiating unfractionated heparin or low-molecular-weight heparin.[13] Although unfractionated heparin was once the only initial therapy for acute venous thrombosis, the majority of patients in Canada (and many in the United States) are now treated with weight-adjusted outpatient low-molecular-weight heparin without laboratory monitoring.[24] The duration of warfarin typically ranges from as little as 6 to as long as 12 weeks (small calf-vein deep vein thrombosis in a patient with a reversible risk factor for deep vein thrombosis, such as plaster cast immobilization) to indefinite (recurrent deep vein thrombosis or deep vein thrombosis occurring in selected high-risk patients, e.g., those with metastatic cancer). Increasingly, treatment of deep vein thrombosis or pulmonary embolism employing low-molecular-weight heparin followed by oral anticoagulants occurs entirely in an outpatient setting,[25] with considerable cost savings.[26,27]

Prevention of venous thromboembolism (antithrombotic prophylaxis) is another common indication for unfractionated heparin and low-molecular-weight heparin, especially following surgery or immobilizing trauma,[28] or in patients with acute medical disorders,[28,29] such as acute stroke.[18] Extended-duration low-molecular-weight heparin can be appropriate after certain orthopedic procedures,[28,30–32] and for patients with cancer-associated hypercoagulability,[33] or to prevent or treat venous thromboembolism in certain high-risk pregnant patients.[34–36]

Many but not all of these indications were established through randomized clinical trials. For example, efficacy of the low-molecular-weight heparin dalteparin (120 IU/kg/12 hr subcutaneously plus aspirin) in acute coronary syndrome was established in a placebo-controlled randomized clinical trial in which the end point of death or myocardial infarction at 6 days was significantly reduced from 4.8% to 1.8%.[37] Two other studies[38,39] of therapeutic-dose enoxaparin found reduced rates of death, myocardial infarction, or recurrent angina compared with intravenous unfractionated heparin.[40] In contrast, the recommendation to treat acute limb ischemia secondary to acute thromboembolism is based on long-standing clinical practice, despite the absence of formal studies establishing an unequivocal benefit of anticoagulation.[17]

Dosing and Monitoring

Initial dosing of therapeutic-dose unfractionated heparin is weight based (80 units/kg bolus; initial infusion, 18 units/kg/hr).[8,41] Nomograms such as the one shown in Table 88–2[42] that utilize standardized dose adjustments to activated partial thromboplastin time (aPTT) values reduce the time required to attain therapeutic anticoagulation for venous thromboembolism,[43] acute coronary syndrome,[43–45] and stroke/transient ischemic attacks.[46] For antithrombotic prophylaxis, unfractionated heparin is usually given by subcutaneous injection as 5000 units two or three times daily, depending upon whether thrombotic risk is moderate or high.[28]

The *activated partial thromboplastin time* is usually used to monitor the anticoagulant effect of therapeutic-dose unfractionated heparin, with the target aPTT level corresponding to an anti-Xa level of 0.35–0.70 units/mL (i.e., a ratio of patient/control aPTT of 1.5–2.5 for many

TABLE 88–2. Weight-Based Nomogram for Therapeutic-Dose Unfractionated Heparin

aPTT*	Dose
Initial dose	80-unit/kg bolus, then infusion at 18 units/kg/hr
<35 s	80-unit/kg bolus, then increase infusion by 4 units/kg/hr
35–45 s	40-unit/kg bolus, then increase infusion by 2 units/kg/hr
46–70 s	No change
71–90 s	Decrease infusion by 2 units/kg/hr
>90 s	Hold infusion 1 hour; then decrease infusion by 3 units/kg/hr

*The aPTT values indicated need to be determined for each individual laboratory based upon anti-Xa levels.

Adapted from Hirsh J, Raschke R: Heparin and low-molecular-weight heparin. The Seventh ACCP Conference on Antithrombotic and Thrombolytic Therapy. Chest 126(Suppl):188S–203S, 2004.

aPTT reagents).[8] It is important for the laboratory to determine the aPTT therapeutic range appropriate for their coagulation instrument and thromboplastin reagent.[8] In some patients, high doses of unfractionated heparin (>40,000 units/24 hr) are required to attain the therapeutic range ("heparin resistance").[47] This is often related to acute inflammation or malignancy, with increased levels of unfractionated heparin–binding proteins (e.g., vitronectin, von Willebrand factor).[48,49] "Pseudo heparin resistance" describes patients receiving high doses of heparin who have therapeutic anti-Xa levels despite subtherapeutic aPTT levels. This can be caused by high factor VIII levels, which tend to decrease the aPTT.[47,50–52] Monitoring by anti-Xa levels may be appropriate in situations when aPTT monitoring is judged to be unreliable (e.g., baseline elevation of the patient's aPTT as a result of coagulopathy or "lupus anticoagulant"), or if heparin resistance occurs.[8]

Table 88–1 indicates dosing of low-molecular-weight heparin. Prolongation of the aPTT by low-molecular-weight heparins is not sufficiently predictable to permit monitoring by this assay. Using anti-Xa levels to monitor low-molecular-weight heparin may be needed in certain situations, such as renal failure or in the elderly (because low-molecular-weight heparin can accumulate),[53] or during pregnancy (because the volume of distribution of heparin can change during pregnancy).[54,55] Monitoring at 4 hours postinjection (when low-molecular-weight heparin levels peak) is recommended.[56] Platelet count monitoring during heparin therapy is discussed later.

Box 88–2. Protamine Dosing for Reversing Unfractionated Heparin

A patient with acute deep vein thrombosis and recent gastric bleeding received a 5000-unit intravenous (IV) bolus of unfractionated heparin (UFH) at 6 AM. The patient then received IV UFH by infusion at 1200 units/hr. At 9 AM the patient developed brisk gastrointestinal bleeding. What dose of protamine sulfate should be given?

Assume:

- Half-life of UFH is 60 min
- 1 mg of protamine neutralizes 100 units of heparin

At 9 AM:

Half-Lives (or hr) Since Administration	Approximate Residual Anticoagulant Effect
5000 (3)	625 units
1200 (2.5)	225 units
1200 (1.5)	450 units
1200 (0.5)	900 units
Total	2200 units

Estimated protamine dose = 22 mg

Note: Efficacy of neutralization should be assessed by an aPTT, with additional protamine delivered if the aPTT remains prolonged.

Adverse Effects and Antidote

Bleeding

Bleeding in patients who are therapeutically anticoagulated can be broadly divided into two types: *predictable* bleeding (e.g., in association with surgery,[23] trauma,[57] or menses), and *unpredictable* bleeding (e.g., gastrointestinal or intracerebral bleeding). Predictable bleeding is dose related, and in some situations is preventable, for example, by stopping intravenous unfractionated heparin 4 hours before elective surgery. Unpredictable bleeding is not necessarily dose related, and has a higher likelihood of adverse outcome, such as mortality or long-term morbidity in the case of intracerebral bleeding. Older age, renal failure, and concomitant thrombolytic therapy are other risk factors for heparin-associated bleeding.[58,59]

Major and minor bleeding includes events requiring medical intervention for assessment or treatment. Major bleeding includes bleeding that is fatal or requires hospitalization, occurs in a closed space (e.g., intracranial, retroperitoneal, intraocular), or results in transfusion of 2 or more units of blood. Other bleeding requiring medical intervention that fails to meet the criteria for major bleeding is considered minor. Overt bleeding that does not require intervention is called trivial bleeding, which despite its name can be troubling for the patient (e.g., recurrent epistaxis).

If unknown, the source of bleeding of sufficient intensity to warrant therapy should be investigated. All anticoagulants should be withheld, and red blood cells transfused as needed. In exceptional situations, pharmacologic adjuncts may be appropriate (e.g., tranexamic acid, desmopressin [DDAVP], intravenous conjugated estrogen). Transfusion of plasma or coagulation factor concentrates is not appropriate for bleeding caused only by heparin. Reversal of anticoagulation has been recently reviewed.[60]

Antidotes for unfractionated heparin and low-molecular-weight heparin are appropriate in certain cases of clinically important bleeding. Protamine sulfate (1 mg/100 units of circulating unfractionated heparin) will neutralize completely the anticoagulant effect of unfractionated heparin (Box 88–2). When administered to patients receiving low-molecular-weight heparin, protamine neutralizes only about half its anti-Xa effect.[61] Protamine (derived from fish) should be avoided in patients with serious fish allergy. Hypotension and bronchoconstriction are potential side effects associated with prior use of protamine insulin or history of serious fish allergies.[62] Risk of dose-related hypotensive reactions are minimized by giving protamine slowly (over 10–20 minutes).

Heparin-Induced Thrombocytopenia

Heparin-induced thrombocytopenia occurs in as many as 3–5% of postoperative patients (and a smaller proportion of patients in other situations) who receive unfractionated heparin for 1–2 weeks (see Chapter 69).[63–65] This hypercoagulability state is caused by immunoglobulin G antibodies that recognize platelet factor 4 (a platelet α-granule protein) when it is bound to heparin.[66–68] Despite a reduced platelet count, heparin-induced thrombocytopenia patients remain at high risk for thrombosis, even if heparin is stopped or replaced with low-molecular-weight heparin or warfarin.[69] To minimize these and other complications (e.g., warfarin-induced venous limb gangrene[70]), rapidly acting alternative anticoagulants that do not cross-react with the heparin-induced thrombocytopenia antibody (e.g., lepirudin, argatroban, or danaparoid [where available]) should be given, and coumarin delayed until substantial resolution of thrombocytopenia has occurred.[71] Heparin-induced thrombocytopenia should be suspected in any patient who develops thrombosis during (or soon after) heparin therapy, or who develops unexpected thrombocytopenia 5 or more days after starting heparin (or less than 1 day on restarting heparin, if heparin had been used within the past few weeks or months[72]). The frequency of platelet count monitoring for heparin-induced thrombocytopenia depends on the risk of this adverse drug reaction (Table 88–3).[71,73] Heparin-induced thrombocytopenia occurs less frequently with low-molecular-weight heparin than with unfractionated heparin.[63–65]

TABLE 88–3. Platelet Count Monitoring for Heparin-Induced Thrombocytopenia*

Type of Patient	Heparin, Dose	Intensity of Platelet Count Monitoring†
HIT "Common" (>1%)		
Surgical	UFH, prophylactic or therapeutic dose	At least every other day until day 14‡
Medical	UFH, therapeutic dose	At least every other day until day 14‡
HIT "Uncommon" ("Infrequent") (0.1–1%)		
Surgical	LMWH, prophylactic or therapeutic dose	Two or three times from days 4 to 14‡
Medical	UFH, prophylactic dose	Two or three times from days 4 to 14‡
HIT "Rare" (<0.1%)		
Medical	LMWH, prophylactic or therapeutic dose	Routine monitoring is not recommended, unless UFH was given before LMWH (then see HIT "uncommon")
Pregnancy	LMWH, prophylactic or therapeutic dose	Routine monitoring is not recommended, unless UFH was given before LMWH (then see HIT "uncommon")

*The table contents are a summary that reflects recent consensus conference recommendations.[71,73]

†Looking for greater than 50% platelet count fall from day 4 to day 14 of heparin treatment.

‡Platelet count monitoring can be discontinued before day 14 when heparin is stopped.

Abbreviations: HIT, heparin-induced thrombocytopenia; LMWH, low-molecular-weight heparin; UFH, unfractionated heparin.

Osteoporosis

Long-term unfractionated heparin treatment can cause osteoporosis, likely because heparin both decreases bone formation by osteoblasts and increases bone resorption by osteoclasts.[74] The risk of osteoporosis with long-term low-molecular-weight heparin therapy is unknown, but is likely to be lower than that found with long-term unfractionated heparin treatment.[75,76]

Fondaparinux and Idraparinux

Pharmacology

Fondaparinux (Arixtra; molecular weight 1728 Da) is a synthetic, homogeneous analogue of the antithrombin-binding pentasaccharide region of heparin.[77] It differs from heparins, which are obtained from animal sources, and are thereby heterogeneous and polydisperse. Given its small size, it catalyzes inhibition of free (soluble) factor Xa, but not thrombin (see Fig. 88–2). Fondaparinux appears also to inhibit activated factor IX.[78] Peak levels occur 2 hours following subcutaneous injection, and its terminal half-life ranges from 17 to 21 hours (healthy young and elderly volunteers, respectively).[79]

Idraparinux is a long-acting variant pentasaccharide under clinical development.[77,80] Administered once per week by subcutaneous injection, its half-life is 80 hours. Its prolonged half-life results from high binding affinity to antithrombin.

Clinical Use

Fondaparinux is approved for antithrombotic prophylaxis after hip and knee surgery, and for the treatment of deep vein thrombosis and pulmonary embolism. The dose for antithrombotic prophylaxis is 2.5 mg once per day by subcutaneous injection beginning 6 hours after surgery.[81–84] Reduced bleeding (with comparable efficacy) is seen if the drug is started 6–8 hours after surgery, rather than 4–6 hours after.[85] In a meta-analysis of four orthopedic surgery trials,[86] the common odds reduction of venous thromboembolism (compared with enoxaparin) was 55.2% (95% confidence interval, 45.8–63.1%; $P < .001$). Major bleeds occurred somewhat more often in the fondaparinux-treated patients, however (2.7% vs. 1.7%; $P = .008$).

Fondaparinux (7.5 mg subcutaneously once daily; 5.0 mg if patient weight is <50 kg and 10.0 mg if >100 kg) was compared with enoxaparin (1 mg/kg subcutaneously twice daily) in a randomized clinical trial of 2205 patients with deep vein thrombosis. Patients received the study drug for at least 5 days, stopping it when therapeutic levels of oral anticoagulation were achieved for 2 consecutive days. Recurrent thrombosis occurred in 43 (3.9%) and 45 (4.1%) patients assigned to fondaparinux and enoxaparin, respectively. Major bleeding occurred in 1.1% of patients receiving fondaparinux and 1.2% of patients receiving enoxaparin. Mortality rates were 3.8% and 3.0%, respectively.[87] In a study of patients with pulmonary embolism, fondaparinux was equivalent to enoxaparin.[88] These studies led (in May 2004) to the licensing of fondaparinux for the treatment of acute deep vein thrombosis and pulmonary embolism in the United States.

In addition to its use to treat and prevent venous thromboembolism, fondaparinux should be effective for the prevention and treatment of thrombosis in patients with immune heparin-induced thrombocytopenia. However, only anecdotal use is reported to date,[71,89] and dosing appropriate for heparin-induced thrombocytopenia is not established.

Dosing and Monitoring

Neither anticoagulant nor platelet count monitoring is recommended. Although platelet factor 4/heparin–reactive antibodies have been generated in patients receiving fondaparinux, the absence of reactivity of these antibodies against platelet factor 4/fondparinux suggests that risk of immune thrombocytopenia is negligible.[90] If required, fondaparinux can be monitored using a factor Xa inhibition assay, generated using known concentrations of fondaparinux, in a manner similar to that used for low-molecular-weight heparin.[91]

Adverse Effects and Antidote

Bleeding may occur in patients treated with either fondaparinux or idraparinux. Bleeding with the latter agent could be particularly problematic given its long half-life. No specific antidotes exist for either pentasaccharide, although a specific antidote for idraparinux is currently in development. Studies in normal volunteers receiving either fondaparinux[92] or idraparinux[93] suggest that recombinant factor VIIa improves hemostatic function, as measured by certain surrogate measures. Bleeding should be managed supportively and the source of bleeding identified and corrected, if possible.

Danaparoid

Pharmacology

Danaparoid (Orgaran; mean molecular weight, 6000 Da) is a mixture of nonheparin glycosaminoglycans derived from pig gut, namely heparan sulfate (84%), dermatan sulfate (12%), and chondroitin sulfate (4%). Its anti-Xa/anti-IIa ratio (22 : 1) is higher than seen with low-molecular-weight heparin (2–4 : 1).[94] The anti-IIa effect may be mediated in part by dermatan sulfate, which catalyzes thrombin inhibition by heparin cofactor II. Its bioavailability approaches 100% with subcutaneous injection, with plasma anti-Xa levels peaking 4–5 hours later. Its anti-Xa half-life is 25 hours, whereas the half-life of its anti-IIa activity is shorter (2–4 hr). Danaparoid undergoes partial renal elimination, and the dose should be reduced by about one third in patients with severe renal insufficiency.

Clinical Use

Danaparoid is effective for prevention of thrombosis following orthopedic surgery (approved indication). In a randomized clinical trial of hip fracture patients, danaparoid (750 units q12h subcutaneously) was associated with a lower frequency of deep vein thrombosis than warfarin (7% vs. 21%; $P < .001$).[95] Danaparoid also compared favorably against unfractionated heparin in clinical trials of deep vein thrombosis[96] and elective cancer surgery.[97]

The predominant use of danaparoid in jurisdictions where it remains available (Canada, European Union; it was withdrawn from the United States market in April 2002) is for treatment of heparin-induced thrombocytopenia. In a randomized, open-label trial versus dextran-70 for patients with heparin-induced thrombocytopenia, danaparoid was associated with significantly improved outcomes, particularly in the subgroup with severe thrombosis.[98] In vitro cross-reactivity for heparin-induced thrombocytopenia antibodies does not predict for adverse outcomes,[99] and testing for cross-reactivity is not recommended.

Dosing and Monitoring

For antithrombotic prophylaxis (e.g., after orthopedic surgery), danaparoid is usually given as 750 anti-Xa units either two or three times daily by subcutaneous injection. When given in therapeutic doses (e.g., when treating heparin-induced thrombocytopenia[100]), it is usually given by initial bolus (2250 units for an average-sized adult), followed by 400 units/hr for 4 hours, then 300 units/hr for 4 hours, and then 200 units/hr. Although anticoagulant monitoring (by anti-Xa units) is not usually required, it may be desirable in certain situations, such as life- or limb-threatening thrombotic problems associated with heparin-induced thrombocytopenia, renal insufficiency, or in very small or large patients.[94] Therapeutic doses of danaparoid can also be given by twice-daily subcutaneous injection; the usual dose is 2250 units twice daily, which resembles the dose (2000 units twice daily) shown to be more effective than intravenous unfractionated heparin in a study of non–heparin-induced thrombocytopenia patients with venous thromboembolism.[96] If required, danaparoid levels may be measured using an anti-Xa level employing a standard curve calibrated using known concentrations of danaparoid.

Adverse Effects

As with all anticoagulants, danaparoid causes bleeding. Bleeding may be exacerbated in patients with renal insufficiency, if danaparoid accumulates.

DIRECT THROMBIN INHIBITORS

DTIs are named for their ability to inhibit thrombin without the requirement for a cofactor (cf. *indirect* thrombin inhibition via antithrombin by heparin).[2,101] There are two major classes of DTIs (Fig. 88–3): (1) *bivalent* DTIs such as hirudin derivatives (lepirudin,

THROMBIN

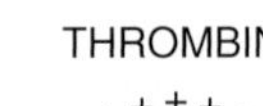

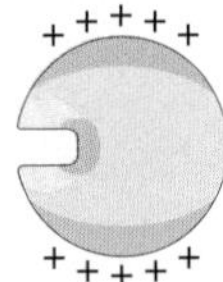

SOLUBLE THROMBIN

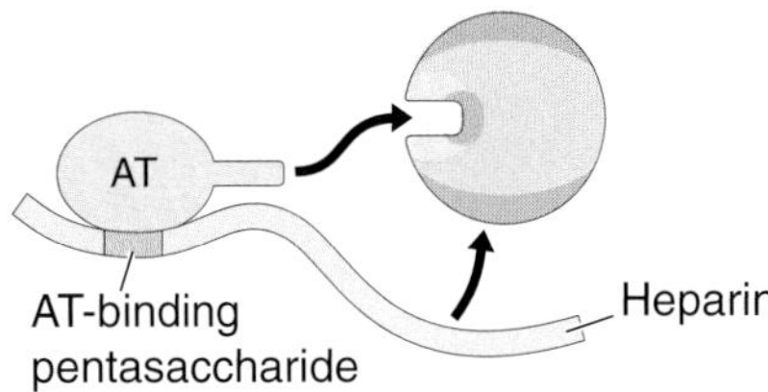

FIBRIN-BOUND THROMBIN

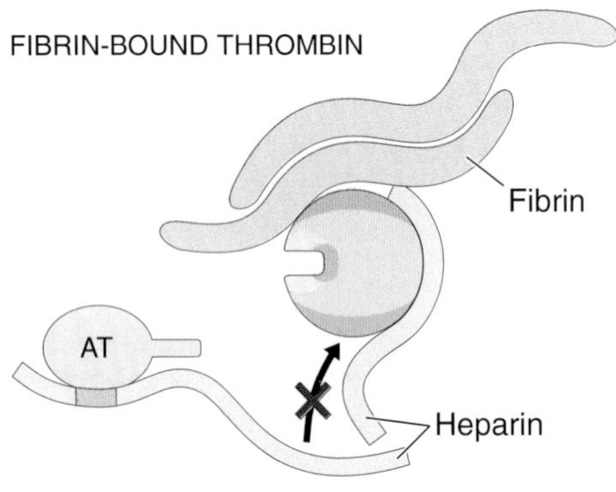

BIVALENT DTIs

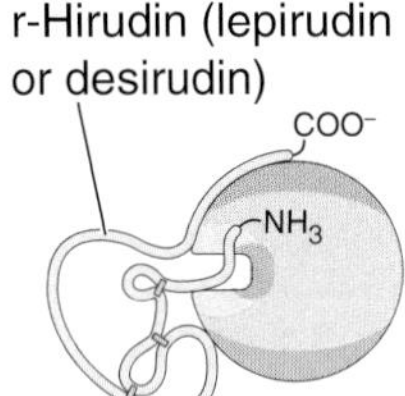

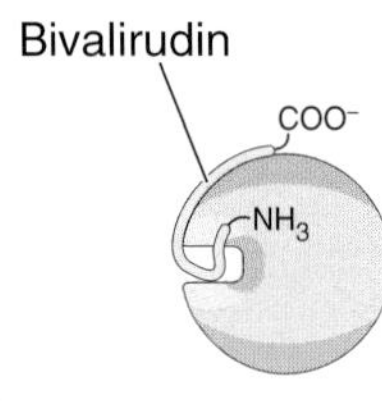

UNIVALENT DTIs

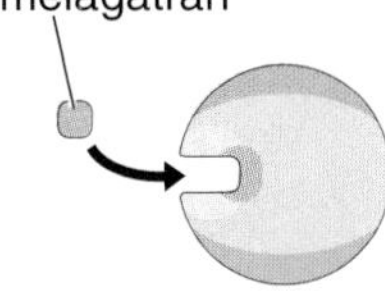

KEY

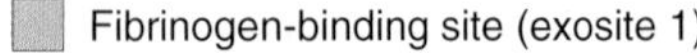

desirudin) and the hirudin analogue ("hirulog") bivalirudin, all of which are prepared by recombinant biotechnology; and (2) *univalent* small-molecule thrombin active site inhibitors (argatroban, ximelagatran).

Recombinant Hirudin

Pharmacology

Hirudin is a 65–amino acid polypeptide produced by the medicinal leech that binds noncovalently and with high affinity (K_i, ~10^{-14} M) to both the active site and exosite I (fibrinogen binding site) regions of thrombin, resulting in stable hirudin-thrombin complexes.[102] Hirudin inhibits both soluble and clot-bound thrombin. Lepirudin (Refludan; molecular weight 6980 Da) and desirudin (Revasc; molecular weight 6960 Da) are marketed hirudin derivatives.

Clinical Use

Lepirudin is approved for anticoagulation in patients with heparin-induced thrombocytopenia and associated thromboembolic complications. Historically, controlled studies[103–106] in patients with serologically confirmed heparin-induced thrombocytopenia suggest a relative risk reduction for new thrombosis of about 0.63–0.78.[71,107] Lepirudin is effective for preventing thrombosis in patients with "isolated heparin-induced thrombocytopenia" (an "off-label" use).[108] Desirudin, a variant hirudin, is available in Europe for antithrombotic prophylaxis after hip replacement surgery.[109] Although hirudins underwent clinical evaluation for treatment of acute coronary syndrome, limited therapeutic benefit and high bleeding rates, including some studies with excess intracerebral hemorrhage, resulted in failure to obtain approval, and routine use in this setting is not recommended.[14]

Dosing and Monitoring

The approved therapeutic-dose regimen for treatment of heparin-induced thrombocytopenia in a patient with normal renal function is an intravenous bolus of 0.4 mg/kg (maximum dose, 40 mg) over 15–20 seconds,

Figure 88–3. Comparison of the structure-function relationship of the DTIs with heparin. A schematic representation of thrombin shows its two positively charged exosites: fibrin(ogen)-binding exosite I and heparin-binding exosite II; also shown is the active (catalytic)–site cleft flanked by the apolar (noncharged) region. Heparin bridges binding of antithrombin (AT) to soluble thrombin and thereby catalyzes AT-mediated thrombin inactivation. In contrast, heparin binds simultaneously to fibrin and thrombin, making it difficult for AT-heparin to inactivate clot (fibrin)–bound thrombin. The four DTIs all inhibit thrombin directly, without requirement for a cofactor such as AT. Bivalent DTIs bind to two sites on thrombin, whereas univalent DTIs bind only to the active site cleft. Bivalirudin also is cleaved by thrombin at the Arg3-Pro4 peptide site, leading to reversibility of thrombin inhibition (not shown).

followed by an intravenous infusion of 0.15 mg/kg/hr (maximum initial dose, 15 mg/hr). However, some experts advise omitting the bolus (especially in the elderly) in the absence of life- or limb-threatening thrombosis.[110,111] Drastic dose reductions for renal insufficiency are required (see Table 69–3 in Chapter 69). Monitoring is usually by aPTT, with target aPTT usually 1.5–2.5 times the patient baseline or mean laboratory normal range. It has been suggested[102] that a standard curve (lepirudin-aPTT) be prepared using normal pooled plasma, because some aPTT reagents exhibit flattening of the lepirudin-aPTT relation at high therapeutic levels; if this is the case, the target aPTT of 1.5–2.0 times should be used, because the assay will not reliably distinguish overdosing at higher aPTT levels (see Chapter 69). The aPTT ratio should be determined at 4-hour intervals until steady state is achieved.[108]

TABLE 88–4. Pharmacologic Features of Bivalirudin

Feature of Bivalirudin	Comment
Short half-life (25–36 min)	Avoids need for initial IV bolus; rapid reversal upon stopping
Predominantly enzymic metabolism	Less risk of overdosing in renal failure than with lepirudin (only 20% of excretion is renal)
	Does not require dose adjustment with hepatic impairment (cf. argatroban)
Minimal prolongation of PT/INR	Simplifies transition to warfarin anticoagulation
Low immunogenicity	Low (?negligible) risk of anaphylaxis (cf. lepirudin)

Abbreviations: INR, International Normalized Ratio; IV, intravenous; PT, prothrombin time.

Adverse Effects

The major adverse effect is bleeding, which was severe in 15–20% of patients receiving lepirudin for heparin-induced thrombocytopenia.[102] Refludan is cleared renally, and accumulates in patients with renal insufficiency. Antihirudin antibodies develop often,[112,113] which on occasion alter pharmacokinetics (leading either to increased or, more often, decreased clearance). Anaphylaxis following bolus administration has been estimated to occur in 1 in 625 patients who has previously received lepirudin,[114] providing another reason to avoid bolus administration.[71]

Bivalirudin

Pharmacology

Bivalirudin (Angiomax; molecular weight 2180 Da) is a 20–amino acid oligopeptide consisting of the active site and exosite 1–binding regions of hirudin connected by a short tetraglycine spacer (K_i for thrombin, ~2 nM).[101,115] It is a "designer" molecule with favorable pharmacologic features (Table 88–4).

Clinical Use

Bivalirudin is approved for use as anticoagulant in patients with unstable angina undergoing angioplasty,[115] based upon comparative studies with unfractionated heparin.[116,117] It is under study for anticoagulation during cardiac surgery.[118,119] Early favorable off-label use for acute heparin-induced thrombocytopenia has also been reported.[120]

Dosing and Monitoring

The approved dose for percutaneous coronary intervention is a 1.0-mg/kg bolus followed by 2.5 mg/kg/hr for 4 hours.[116,117] More recent studies[121–124] evaluated a reduced bolus (0.75 mg/kg) with infusion (2.5 mg/kg/hr) for the duration of the angioplasty. No monitoring is routinely performed. In contrast, dosing for heparin-induced thrombocytopenia usually begins at about 0.15 mg/kg/hr by constant intravenous infusion (no initial bolus), and adjusting by aPTT (target 1.5–2.5 times baseline aPTT) (note: dosing efficacy and safety for heparin-induced thrombocytopenia is not established). Dosing for "off-pump" and "on-pump" cardiac surgery is discussed elsewhere.[115,118,119,124]

Adverse Effects

Bleeding is a potential complication, although this occurred less often with bivalirudin than in unfractionated heparin–treated patients in some of the percutaneous coronary intervention trials.[116,117,122] There was a trend to lower bleeding when used for off-pump cardiac surgery, compared with controls receiving heparin with protamine reversal.[119] Patients who have received lepirudin can have antihirudin antibodies that cross-react with bivalirudin,[125] but the clinical significance of this remains unclear.

Argatroban

Pharmacology

Argatroban (U.S. and Canadian trade name, Argatroban; non-U.S. trade name, Novastan; molecular weight 527 Da) is a small-molecule, nonpeptidic arginine derivative that binds reversibly to the active site pocket of thrombin (K_i for human thrombin, ~40 nM).[126,127] It inhibits both free (soluble) and clot-bound thrombin.[128] It is administered exclusively by the intravenous route. The drug is excreted by the hepatobiliary route and may be preferred over hirudin derivatives in patients with renal dysfunction.

Clinical Use

Argatroban is approved for use as an anticoagulant in patients with heparin-induced thrombocytopenia with or without thrombosis,[126] based upon improved outcomes in a composite end point (death, amputation, new throm-

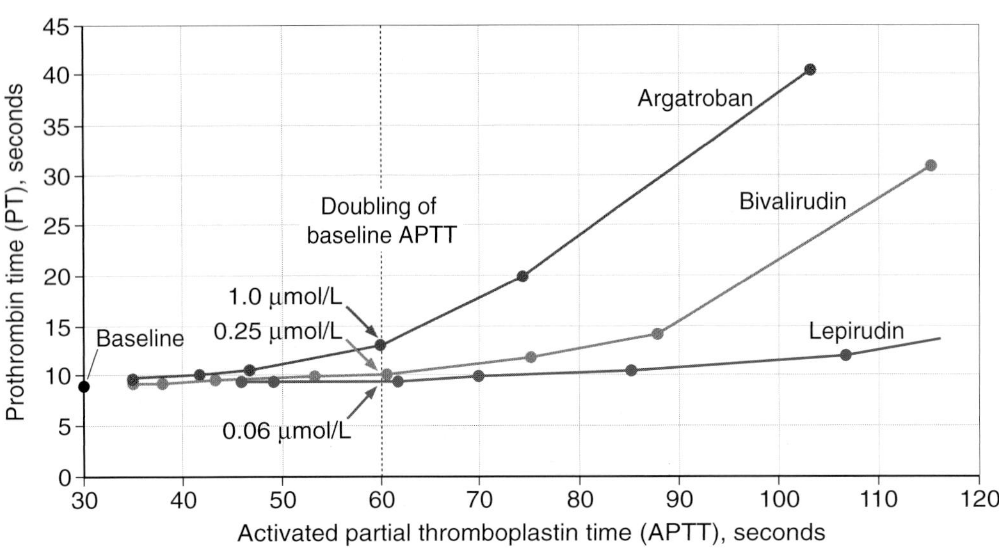

Figure 88–4. INR-aPTT relationship for three DTIs. The lower the affinity and specificity for thrombin (argatroban < bivalirudin < recombinant hirudin), the higher the drug concentration required to double the aPTT, and the greater the prolongation of the INR. (Modified from Warkentin TE: Bivalent direct thrombin inhibitors: hirudin and bivalirudin. Best Pract Res Clin Haematol 17:105–125, 2004.)

bosis) compared with historical controls.[129,130] Argatroban is also approved for percutaneous coronary intervention in heparin-induced thrombocytopenia patients.[126,131]

Dosing and Monitoring

Argatroban is usually administered as a constant intravenous infusion with a recommended initial dose of 2 μg/kg/min. Some physicians prefer to start with a lower dose (0.5–1 μg/kg/min), especially in intensive care unit settings, to reduce risk of over-anticoagulation. The drug is monitored using the aPTT (target, 1.5–3.0 times baseline), beginning 2 hours after starting the infusion; stable plasma levels are achieved 1–3 hours after the infusion is started. The drug should be avoided in patients with significant hepatic impairment, or its starting dose reduced to 0.5 μg/kg/min.

Adverse Effects

Bleeding is a potential complication. Argatroban also prolongs the prothrombin time and International Normalized Ratio (INR) more than does lepirudin and bivalirudin (Fig. 88–4),[101,132] perhaps because of the high molar concentrations of argatroban required for therapeutic effect (relative to the bivalent DTIs).[133] This can complicate overlapping warfarin anticoagulation, which is another reason to postpone initiation of warfarin in a patient receiving DTI therapy such as argatroban during treatment of acute heparin-induced thrombocytopenia (see Chapter 69).[134] Argatroban is not advised for use in cardiac surgery, because dosing and efficacy are not established.

Ximelagatran/Melagatran

Pharmacology

Ximelagatran (Exanta) is an orally available prodrug of melagatran, a 430-Da mimetic of fibrinopeptide A that blocks the active (catalytic) site of thrombin.[135,136] Melagatran is a rapid, competitive, selective, and reversible DTI (K_i = 2 nM); both free and clot-bound thrombin are inhibited. Ximelagatran is well absorbed in the small intestine (20% bioavailability), and following ingestion is biotransformed into melagatran. Blood levels of ximelagatran and melagatran peak within 30 and 120 minutes of ingestion, respectively. Melagatran has a half-life of 4–5 hours in patients, and thus is given twice daily by the subcutaneous route. Ximelagatran is also given twice daily by mouth.

At least 80% of melagatran is eliminated unchanged via the kidneys. The half-life of ximelagatran is prolonged in the elderly and in patients with renal dysfunction, and thus (xi)melagatran is contraindicated in patients with severe renal failure (creatinine clearance <30 mL/min).[137] Its pharmacokinetics and pharmacodynamics are not influenced by aspirin, and there is no interference with drugs that are metabolized by cytochrome P-450 isozymes (cf. warfarin).[138]

Clinical Use

Ximelagatran received limited approval in Europe for antithrombotic prophylaxis after orthopedic surgery; typically, perioperative subcutaneous melagatran is followed by oral ximelagtran.[139–141] In contrast, North American studies have studied only postoperative oral ximelagatran.[142–145] In these studies, (xi)melagatran proved as, or more, effective than the comparator anticoagulant regimen (low-molecular-weight heparin or warfarin). Other potential indications include long-term secondary prophylaxis of venous thromboembolism (THRIVE III trial),[146,147] atrial fibrillation (SPORTIF III trial),[148–151] and, possibly, treatment of acute deep vein thrombosis[152] and secondary prophylaxis after myocardial infarction.[153] However, (xi)melagatran failed to win U.S. Food and Drug Administration (FDA) approval for any of its sought indications (atrial fibrillation, long-term secondary prevention of deep vein thrombosis, and orthopedic prophylaxis) in 2004.

Dosing and Monitoring

In Europe, the approved dose for post–orthopedic surgery antithrombotic prophylaxis is melagatran 3 mg (started 4–8 hours after surgery) given twice daily by subcutaneous injection (usually for 1–2 days), followed by oral ximelagatran 24 mg twice daily. Optimal dosing in other clinical settings remains to be determined. No anticoagulant monitoring is required, because ximelagatran produces a predictable anticoagulant response. Although immunoassays can determine drug levels, these are unlikely to become routinely available. Ximelagatran prolongs the aPTT, INR, and thrombin times. However, these effects are assay reagent dependent, do not correlate well with blood levels, and have not been evaluated with respect to efficacy or safety.

Adverse Effects

Given the lack of antidote, the short half-life of ximelagatran is an advantage. Serious bleeding is managed symptomatically with red cell transfusions, as appropriate. Although not well studied, dialysis or hemoperfusion likely removes melagatran from the circulation. Activated coagulation factor complexes or recombinant factor VIIa reduces some of the anticoagulant activity of melagatran in animals and in human volunteers,[154] but evaluation of ximelagatran-induced bleeding has not been reported. About 15–20% of patients develop at least a doubling of liver enzymes (transaminases) that occurs about 2–6 months into treatment, with spontaneous recovery within 2–3 months with or without continuing the drug.[135,153] Occasionally, reversible jaundice occurs. Whether transaminitis is a "signal" for risk of potentially serious hepatotoxicity remains uncertain.

MISCELLANEOUS ANTICOAGULANTS

Recombinant Activated Protein C

Recombinant APC (drotrecogin alfa, activated; Xigris) degrades activated factor V (Va) and VIII, and can thus be classified as an "anticoagulant" (although it has not been evaluated for this purpose). Recombinant APC decreases mortality in adults with severe sepsis.[155] Fatal bleeding events during the 4-day infusion period occurred in 0.4% of patients enrolled in Phase 2 and 3 clinical trials.[156] Invasive procedures and severe thrombocytopenia were risk factors for bleeding. Recombinant APC variably prolongs the prothrombin time/INR and APTT.[157] Whether recombinant APC has clinically useful antithrombotic effects is unknown.

Experimental Anticoagulants

Inhibitors of Factor VIIa-TF Complex

Three inhibitors of factor VIIa-TF complex have undergone evaluation (see Fig. 88–1).[2] Recombinant TFPI (tifacogin) directly inhibits VIIa-TF complexes. However, unlike recombinant APC, recombinant TFPI did not reduce mortality (though it did increase bleeding) in a clinical trial of sepsis.[158] Recombinant nematode anticoagulant protein c2 (NAPc2) is a small protein derived from a hookworm that binds to a noncatalytic site on both factors X and Xa, thus inhibiting VIIa-TF; the half-life of NAPc2 is long (48 hours), resembling that of factor X. Recombinant NAPc2 was evaluated in a dose escalation study of patients undergoing elective total knee joint replacement.[159] Active site–blocked VIIa (factor VIIai) competes with factor VIIa for binding to tissue factor.[160] This anticoagulant is in early preclinical development.

Direct Factor Xa Inhibitors

Drugs with predominant direct factor Xa–inhibiting properties (e.g., DX-9065a, DPC 906) are undergoing clinical testing.[2] Unlike fondaparinux, these drugs also inhibit surface-bound factor Xa within prothrombinase. DPC 906 is an orally active agent.

VITAMIN K ANTAGONISTS

Coumarins

Pharmacology

Vitamin K antagonists are derived from coumarin.[161] Vitamin K is required for posttranslational modification of glutamate (Glu) residues in four procoagulant factors (factors II, VII, IX, and X). Addition of a carboxyl group (COO–) to each Glu residue (to form γ-carboxyglutamate, or Gla, residues) causes these vitamin K–dependent factors to become functional zymogens (proenzymes), because they now can bind to phospholipid surfaces. Protein C and protein S are vitamin K–dependent *anti*coagulant factors. Figure 88–5 shows that vitamin K antagonists interfere with vitamin K epoxide reductase[162]; resulting inability to regenerate reduced vitamin K (vitamin KH_2) leads to failure of posttranslational modification of Glu to Gla in the amino-terminal regions of the vitamin K–dependent coagulation factors.[163] Lack of Gla residues results in failure of calcium-dependent bridges between the protein and the phospholipid surface; this, in turn, results in an inability to form conformationally dependent coagulation factor complexes, thus preventing activation of coagulation.

Warfarin is the most widely used coumarin in the United States, Canada, and the United Kingdom, whereas phenprocoumon and acenocoumarol are also used in continental Europe. Warfarin is rapidly absorbed from the gastrointestinal tract (peak levels at 90 minutes postingestion),[164] has a long half-life (36–42 hours),[165] and circulates bound mostly to albumin. Warfarin is a racemic mixture of *S* and *R* isomers, with metabolism of the more potent *S* isomer influenced by common mutations in the cytochrome P-450 hepatic microsomal enzyme, 2C9. In comparison with the wild-type enzyme (CYP2C9*1), patients with *CYP2C9**2 and *CYP2CP**3 mutations (8–19% and 6–10% of whites, respectively[161]) require lower

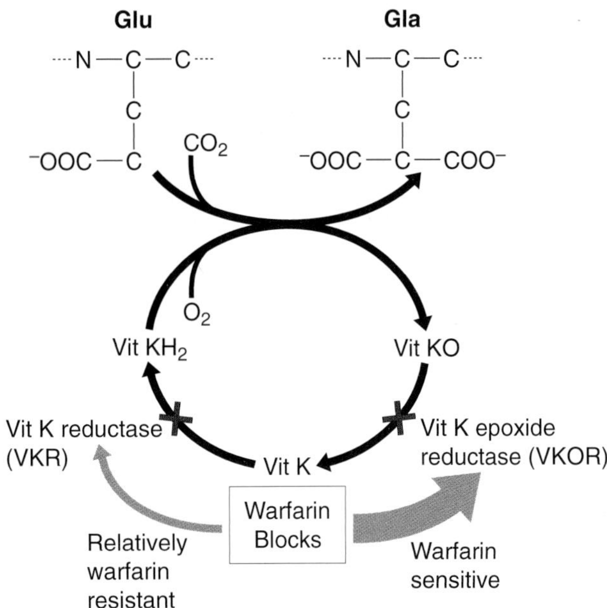

Figure 88–5. Coumarin (warfarin) and the vitamin K cycle. Giving vitamin K can regenerate vitamin KH_2 because vitamin K reductase is relatively resistant to the effect of coumarin. Abbreviations: Gla, γ-carboxyglutamate; Glu, glutamate. (Modified from Ansell J, Hirsh J, Poller L, et al: Management of the vitamin K antagonist. The Seventh ACCP Conference on Antithrombotic and Thrombolytic Therapy. Chest126[Suppl]:204S–233S, 2004.)

doses of warfarin and have a higher frequency of bleeding complications.[166,167] A rare mutation in the factor IX gene can cause marked warfarin sensitivity in affected males,[168] although, in the absence of warfarin, factor IX antigen and activity levels are normal.

Box 88–3 lists the putative half-lives of the vitamin K–dependent factors.[163] The antithrombotic effect of vitamin K antagonists depend mostly on achieving hypoprothrombinemia (reduced factor II levels).[169] Prothrombin's long half-life (60–72 hours) means that vitamin K antagonists cannot achieve therapeutic anticoagulation for *at least* 5 days following initiation. Thus, for patients with acute thrombosis, vitamin K antagonists are usually started only when the patient is therapeutically anticoagulated on unfractionated heparin or low-molecular-weight heparin (otherwise, there is considerable risk of progressive thrombosis[170]). This also explains why intermediate (6–10 mg) or large (>10 mg) warfarin loading doses are inappropriate, because they do not speed the achievement of "therapeutic hypoprothrombinemia" but do increase risk of excessively prolonged INR values and disproportionately reduced protein C levels (Fig. 88–6),[171] with at least theoretically increased risk of coumarin necrosis.[70,172,173]

Box 88–3. Putative Terminal Half-Lives of the Vitamin K–Dependent Procoagulant and Anticoagulant Factors

Procoagulant Factors (Half-Life)

- Factor II (prothrombin) (60 hr)
- Factor X (40 hr)
- Factor IX (24 hr)
- Factor VII (4–6 hr)

Anticoagulant Factors (Half-Life)

- Protein C (9 hr)
- Protein S (60 hr)

There are six vitamin K–dependent hemostatic factors, four with procoagulant activity and two with anticoagulant activity. (Protein Z, another vitamin K–dependent coagulation factor that inhibits factor Xa, is of unknown clinical importance.) Treatment with coumarin anticoagulants reduces functional levels of these factors. The paradoxic procoagulant effect of warfarin can be explained by the different half-lives[163] of these factors following onset of action of coumarin: the time to a therapeutically significant reduction of the major procoagulant factor, prothrombin (half-life, ~60 hr), is much longer than the time to a clinically important reduction in the major anticoagulant factor, protein C (half-life, ~9 hr). Thus, within the first several days of coumarin anticoagulation, and under certain clinical circumstances (see text), there can arise transient, but clinically important, procoagulant effects that can result in skin necrosis or other thrombotic complications.

Clinical Use

Coumarin is widely used for long-term primary and secondary prevention of thrombosis in diverse settings.[161,174] It is indicated for the prevention of stroke in patients with atrial fibrillation,[175] to prevent first or recurrent deep vein thrombosis or pulmonary embolism in certain high-risk patients (e.g., patients with congenital protein C deficiency or prior deep vein thrombosis[176,177]), to prevent prosthetic valve thrombosis,[178] or to prevent atherothrombosis in arteriopathic patients.[179,180]

Dosing and Monitoring

Warfarin was traditionally administered using large loading doses; doses as large as 1 mg/kg appear to produce "therapeutic" anticoagulation in as little as 24 hours. However, such large doses increase the risk of prohemorrhagic or prothrombotic adverse effects. Relatively high loading doses of 10 mg[161,181] to 15 mg[174] daily for the first 2 or 3 days of therapy are still used by some physicians, but we disagree with this practice. Besides increasing risk of early over-anticoagulation, large initial doses predispose certain at-risk patients to coumarin

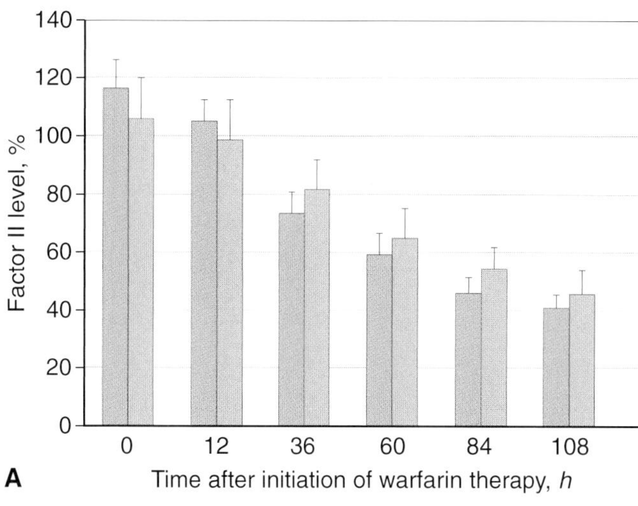

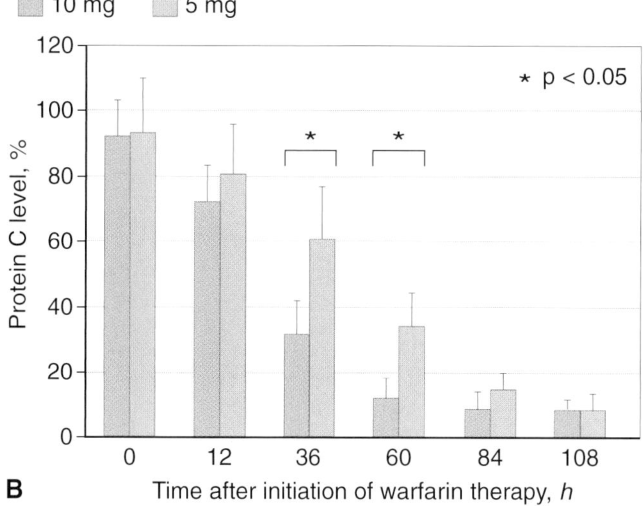

Figure 88–6. Effects of warfarin loading dose of 10 mg versus 5 mg. Although a higher loading dose of warfarin had no significant effect on prothrombin levels (*A*), significantly lower levels of protein C (*B*) and factor VII (not shown) were seen at 36 and 60 hours in patients who received 10 mg, with greater potential for elevated INR, bleeding (low factor VII) and/or hypercoagulability (low protein C). (From Harrison L, Johnston M, Massicotte MP, et al: Comparison of 5-mg and 10-mg loading doses in initiation of warfarin therapy. Ann Intern Med 126:133–136, 1997, with permission.)

necrosis related to rapid depletion of protein C natural anticoagulant. We recommend that patients be started on warfarin at the expected maintenance dose, which for most patients is 5 mg/day[172]; a 5-mg maximal initial dose is also recommended by the manufacturer of warfarin.[182] This strategy reduces the likelihood of excessive prolongation of the INR, thus reducing the need for very frequent INR determinations in the first week of therapy. Indeed, most patients started on a 5-mg dose of warfarin will only require INR determinations on day 4 or 5 and day 7.

TABLE 88–5. Conceptual Approach to Warfarin-Drug Interactions*

Mechanisms of Interaction Between Warfarin and Other Drugs	Selected Examples
Reduced Warfarin Effect (Lowers INR)	
Enhanced clearance of warfarin as a result of P-450 hepatic enzyme induction	Alcohol (chronic use), barbiturates, carbamazepine, rifampin
Reduced absorption of warfarin from the gastrointestinal tract	Cholestyramine
Enhanced Warfarin Effect (Raises INR)	
Reduced production of endogenous (gut bacteria) vitamin K	Antibiotics
Decreased clearance of warfarin by interfering with hepatic metabolism	Alcohol (acute use), amiodarone, erythromycin, fluconazole
Unknown mechanism	Sulfonamide antibiotics

*Many drugs have been described to interact with warfarin, most as small case series. Only selected examples are listed; interactions may vary between patients, and may be modified if patients are taking more than one drug that interacts with warfarin. Whenever a drug is started in a patient on warfarin therapy, the INR should be rechecked within a week.

Monitoring is performed using the prothrombin time, which is usually expressed as the INR. The INR was developed to standardize laboratory monitoring, because it was realized that systematic targeting of 1.5- to 2.0-fold above the baseline prothrombin time led to systematic over-anticoagulation of patients who were being monitored by insensitive thromboplastin reagents.[183] Calibration of the INR is ensured by comparing reagents with a standard thromboplastin maintained by the World Health Organization; the ratio of this standard to the test thromboplastin is known as the International Sensitivity Index.

Disadvantages of vitamin K antagonists include a narrow therapeutic index (with a risk of thrombosis if the INR falls below the therapeutic range, and bleeding if the INR is above the usual therapeutic range), as well as highly variable dose-response relationships mandating ongoing regular INR monitoring even after a stable dosing has been achieved. Maintenance doses vary widely among patients (from 3 to 150 mg/wk for warfarin), and are influenced by diet (variable vitamin K intake) and medication intake (Table 88–5).[161,184] Physicians should consider warfarin-drug interactions when drugs are added (or subtracted) from a patient's medication list; at this time increased frequency of INR monitoring is appropriate.

Adverse Effects

Warfarin has three principal side effects: bleeding, microvascular thrombosis (coumarin necrosis), and teratogenicity.

TABLE 88–6. Management of Elevated INR Values Secondary to Warfarin*

Situation	Recommended Management
Nonbleeding Patient with INR Above Therapeutic Range	
INR 4.5–6.0	Withhold warfarin and recheck INR in 24–48 hours; *or* withhold warfarin, administer 1 mg oral vitamin K, and recheck INR in 24–48 hours; *or* reduce warfarin dose and recheck INR in 24–48 hours.
INR 6.1–10.0	Withhold warfarin and recheck INR in 24 hours; *or* withhold warfarin, give 1 mg oral vitamin K, and recheck INR in 24 hours; *or* withhold warfarin, administer 1–2.5 mg of oral vitamin K, and consider using plasma or PCCs *only* in patients judged to be at high risk of hemorrhage, and recheck INR in 24 hours.
INR >10	Withhold warfarin, give 1–5 mg of oral vitamin K and recheck INR in 24 hours; *or* withhold warfarin, administer 0.5–1.0 mg of IV vitamin K, and recheck INR in 24 hours; *or* withhold warfarin, give 1–5 mg of oral vitamin K, consider using plasma or PCCs only in patients judged to be at high risk of hemorrhage, and recheck INR in 24 hours; *or* withhold warfarin, give 0.5–1 mg of IV vitamin K, consider plasma or PCCs only in patients judged to be at high risk of hemorrhage, and recheck INR in 24 hours.
Bleeding Patient or Urgent Surgery Required (with or without INR Above Therapeutic Range)	
INR at therapeutic or supratherapeutic level and urgent surgery required (within 24 hours)*	Hold warfarin; give vitamin K_1, 2–4 mg intravenously (for INR 5.0–9.0), with the expectation that a reduction of the INR will occur in 24 hours. If the INR is still high, administer an additional dose of vitamin K_1, 1–2 mg intravenously.
INR at therapeutic or supratherapeutic level and emergent surgery (within 1–2 hours) needed*	Hold warfarin; give vitamin K_1, 2–5 mg intravenously, and administer FFP, CSP, or PCC. Recheck INR after coagulation factor replacement.
Major but non–life-threatening bleeding with any increase in INR	Hold warfarin; consider giving plasma or PCCs; give intravenous vitamin K (1–10 mg, depending on the INR*); correct mechanical causes of bleeding; provide medical support, including red cell transfusions, as appropriate.
Life-threatening bleeding with any increase in INR	Hold warfarin; give PCCs or plasma; give intravenous vitamin K (5–10 mg, depending on the INR*); correct mechanical causes of bleeding; provide medical support, including red cell transfusions, as appropriate; consider recombinant factor VIIa if no adequate response is achieved.

*Generally, it takes 4 hours before vitamin K_1 begins to lower the INR; thus, if surgery is required very soon, plasma or PCCs should be given in addition to vitamin K_1.

Abbreviations: CSP, cryosupernatant plasma; FFP, fresh frozen plasma; IV, intravenous; PCC, prothrombin complex concentrates.

Adapted from Ginsberg JA, Crowther MA, White RH, Ortel TL: Anticoagulation therapy. Hematology (Am Soc Hematol Educ Program) 339–357, 2001.

The risk of major hemorrhage is about 2.5% per year, with about one in six such bleeds being fatal.[185] Bleeding has an element of predictability: for every 1.0 increase in INR above the usual therapeutic range, bleeding risk approximately doubles.[186,187] Bleeding that occurs after trauma or surgery also is considered to be *predictable*; the risk can be reduced by reversing vitamin K antagonist effect prior to elective surgery or at the time of emergency surgery. *Unpredictable* bleeding (most seriously intracerebral or gastrointestinal) often occurs with little or no warning. Endoscopy usually reveals an explanation for gastrointestinal bleeding in warfarin-anticoagulated patients.[188] Risk factors include older age, alcohol abuse, renal insufficiency, and prior history of gastrointestinal bleeding.[189,190] Prompt medical attention of a substantially increased INR is important, because early treatment may lessen bleeding severity (see later). Bleeding complications tend to be more common during the first days or weeks of therapy than later.

Table 88–6 lists principles for management of an elevated INR caused by coumarin.[60,191] When a patient presents with an unanticipated, excess anticoagulant effect, and has no clinical evidence of bleeding, he or she can be managed with simple warfarin withdrawal, with or without oral vitamin K. If the elevated INR is less than 4.5, warfarin can be withheld; if the INR is between 4.5 and 10.0, a single 1-mg oral vitamin K dose should be considered, because this will reduce the INR to the usual therapeutic range within 24 hours in most patients.[192,193] If the INR is more than 10.0, a single 2.5-mg oral vitamin K dose should be administered.[194] In all cases, the INR should be checked in 24–48 hours. The etiology of the prolonged INR should be determined. If the cause is temporary (e.g., course of antibiotics), warfarin can be reintroduced at a lower dose. If the explanation is ongoing (e.g., new ongoing medication), the dose of warfarin should be reduced with more frequent INR monitoring until stable dosing is achieved. Some patients have very difficult-to-control INR values (e.g., patients with hepatic metastases, chronic fungal infections requiring frequent courses of antifungal drugs, poor compliance). In such cases, necessity for anticoagulation should be reviewed, and other treatments with more favorable risk-benefit ratios should be considered (e.g., low-molecular-weight heparin or aspirin in suitable patients).

More urgent treatment is needed for actively bleeding patients, or those judged to be at high risk of bleeding, including admission for observation, identification, and (if possible) correction of the bleeding source. Vitamin K should be given as slow intravenous infusion in a dose of 2.5–5 mg; this will normalize the INR in many patients within 24 hours.[195,196] With serious bleeding, coagulation

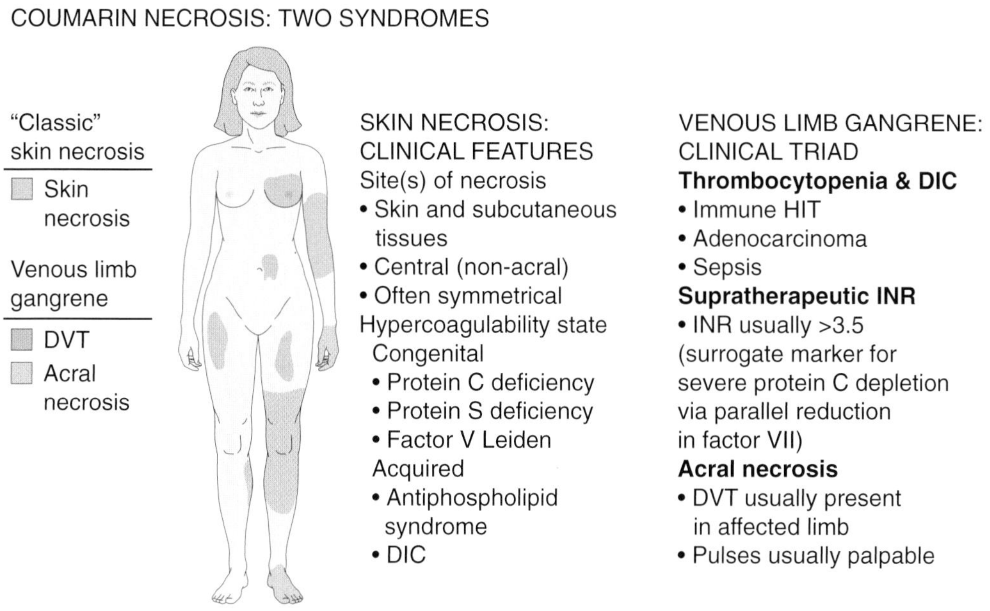

Figure 88–7. Coumarin necrosis: two syndromes.

factor replacement should be considered.[197] Fresh frozen plasma remains the "standard" treatment in North America, although it may be less effective for this indication than clotting factor concentrates (such as prothrombin complex concentrates), which contain high levels of the deficient factors.[197] Although formulas exist to predict the amount of fresh frozen plasma, in most cases, 2–4 units are given and the INR rechecked; if it remains prolonged, additional fresh frozen plasma is administered. Fresh frozen plasma can cause volume overload and (rarely) anaphylaxis (in some patients with congenital immunoglobulin A deficiency). Although recombinant factor VIIa has also been used in this situation,[198] it is very expensive and has not been evaluated in prospective studies.

Coumarin necrosis denotes one of two paradoxical prothrombotic complications of vitamin K antagonist therapy: coumarin-induced skin necrosis and venous limb gangrene (Fig. 88–7).[173,199] These are rare complications characterized by microvascular thrombosis that typically begin 2–6 days after commencing vitamin K antagonist therapy. Skin necrosis typically affects central tissue sites such as the breast, abdomen, buttocks, thigh, and calf, and predominantly involves skin and subdermal tissues. Congenital abnormalities of the protein C natural anticoagulant pathway are implicated in many patients. In contrast, venous limb gangrene affects acral (distal extremity) sites, and can cause extensive necrosis necessitating limb amputation.[70,134,200] Patients typically have a hypercoagulability syndrome associated with thrombocytopenia, such as heparin-induced thrombocytopenia or cancer-associated disseminated intravascular coagulopathy (or both[201]). Typically, the INR is prolonged, which represents a surrogate marker for severe depletion in protein C via concomitant reduction in factor VII.[200]

Coumarins are contraindicated during the first trimester of pregnancy.[36] This is because γ-carboxyglutamate (Gla)-containing proteins are found in bone, and pharmacologic vitamin K antagonism can cause embryopathy (chondrodysplasia punctata).[202] Warfarin use in pregnancy has also been associated with a poorly defined condition of neurologic injury. There is wide jurisdictional variation in the acceptability of warfarin use during the second and early third trimesters of pregnancy.

SPECIAL SITUATIONS

Pregnancy and Anticoagulation

Low-molecular-weight heparin is probably the best anticoagulant option during pregnancy: it has known advantages over coumarin (reduced teratogenicity) and unfractionated heparin (superior predictability; reduced osteoporosis). Ironically, because of paucity of prospective data in pregnant women with prosthetic heart valves, and because of anecdotal evidence of treatment failures in these patients, the manufacturer warns against use of low-molecular-weight heparin in these patients.[34] This warning does not represent a specific contraindication, however.[178] Warfarin is an important option during the second and early third trimester[55]; later during pregnancy, transition to low-molecular-weight heparin is often made to facilitate obstetric considerations. Thus, a typical treatment approach for a woman with a prosthetic valve contemplating pregnancy would be transition from coumarin to low-molecular-weight heparin for conception and the first trimester, transition to warfarin for the second and early third trimester, and later transition to low-molecular-weight heparin during the third trimester. Optimal peripartum management is controversial, but for patients on therapeutic-dose low-molecular-weight heparin, one of two strategies is likely optimal: either an elective induction at 37 weeks' gestation with the low-molecular-weight heparin having been held for fully 24 hours (and restarted immediately after delivery) or switching from low-molecular-weight heparin to unfractionated heparin administered in therapeutic doses, with aPTT and platelet count monitoring, beginning at 37 weeks. The unfractionated heparin is discontinued at the time of onset of labor.

Sometimes the hematologist is asked to contribute to the discussion about choice of prosthetic valve in a young woman who is planning future pregnancies. In this situation, either bioprosthetic or mechanical valves may be considered. Bioprosthetic valves will not require (in most cases) indefinite anticoagulation, but will require eventual replacement; mechanical valves necessitate long-term anticoagulation but will likely require infrequent replacement.

Neuraxial Anesthesia

The risk of permanent disability from spinal/epidural hematomas means that special precautions are required for use of neuraxial anesthesia in anticoagulated patients. In some centers, neuraxial anesthesia is used both for intraoperative anesthesia and postoperative pain control, especially in the elderly and those undergoing lower limb orthopedic surgery, that is, patients in whom low-molecular-weight heparin is appropriate. Beginning in the 1990s, there were reports of epidural hematomas in low-molecular-weight heparin–treated patients undergoing neuraxial anesthesia, resulting in the FDA advising strongly against their combined use. Many clinicians were troubled by this, because both neuraxial anesthesia (which improves postoperative pain control and mobility) and low-molecular-weight heparin (a highly effective anticoagulant for such patients) are beneficial. There is evidence[203] that the risk of epidural hemorrhage may be related to a residual anticoagulant effect persisting 12 hours (but not 20–24 hours) after the last dose. This unanticipated residual anticoagulant effect may have implications for the observation that epidural hematomas were observed in North America (where twice-daily dosing is routine) but were very rare in Europe (where once-daily dosing is routine). Thus, it seems appropriate to use once-daily low-molecular-weight heparin prophylaxis when neuraxial anesthesia is given, and to remove the catheter 20 hours after the preceding dose of low-molecular-weight heparin, and to resume the low-molecular-weight heparin 4 hours later. With this strategy, no cases of epidural hematoma have been reported. In general, the first dose of low-molecular-weight heparin should be delayed after insertion, manipulation, or removal of an epidural catheter; although no firm guidelines exist, the dose should be delayed for a minimum of 4, and preferably as long as 12, hours. If warfarin is planned for long-term postoperative prophylaxis, its initiation should be withheld until removal of the epidural catheter. These strategies have recently been endorsed by the American Academy of Regional Anesthesia.[204]

Catheter Flushing

Central venous catheters and other intravascular catheters are frequently "locked" with unfractionated heparin–containing solutions in an attempt to reduce thrombotic complications. However, there is no standardized dose, frequency, or concentration, and efficacy remains uncertain. Potential complications of heparin "locking" include heparin-induced thrombocytopenia initiation or potentiation, inadvertent heparin overdosing,[205] and infection resulting from frequent accessing of the central venous catheter.

Semipermanent central venous catheters are being used with increasing frequency for patients requiring frequent intravenous therapy (e.g., hemodialysis, antineoplastic chemotherapy, total parenteral nutrition, or extended antimicrobial therapy). Such catheters were reported to have a thrombotic failure rate approaching 10%, and early trials suggested that low-dose warfarin may prevent these complications.[206] However, subsequent large studies suggest that the thrombotic failure is less than 5% and that prophylactic anticoagulation does not appear to reduce this risk.[207–209]

THROMBOLYTIC THERAPY

Pharmacology

Table 88–7 lists four fibrinolytic (thrombolytic) agents licensed in the United States, including indications and doses: streptokinase, alteplase, reteplase, and tenecteplase.[210,211] Figure 88–8 illustrates their mechanism of action. None of the agents directly lyses fibrin, but rather they activate plasminogen to the fibrin-cleaving protease, plasmin. Streptokinase (a purified product of streptococcus) achieves this indirectly; when bound to plasminogen, the resulting "activator complex" converts other plasminogen molecules to plasmin. This reaction does not require fibrin, and thus streptokinase is not "fibrin-specific."

The other fibrinolytic agents listed (all produced by recombinant biotechnology) directly activate plasminogen to plasmin, thus mimicking the two physiologic activators of plasminogen, tissue plasminogen activator (tPA) and urokinase (see Fig. 88–8). Indeed, alteplase is identical to human wild-type tPA, whereas reteplase is a deletion mutation of tPA, and tenecteplase has glycosylation-altering amino acid substitutions that confer greater resistance to plasminogen activator inhibitor type 1 (PAI-1).[212] Their plasminogen-activating reactivities are enhanced in the presence of fibrin, leading to the following relative fibrin specificity: alteplase < reteplase < tenecteplase (see Fig. 88–1). Pharmacokinetic advantages of tenecteplase include its administration as a single, patient weight–adjusted bolus over 5 seconds (see Table 88–7).

Plasminogen activators are inhibited by PAIs, most importantly PAI-1. After administration of therapeutic-dose streptokinase, PAI-1 is rapidly depleted, resulting in a systemic "lytic state" due to the unregulated circulating plasmin. This predisposes to hemorrhage if circulating

TABLE 88–7. Thrombolytic Agents

Medication (Trade Name)	Indication	Treatment Regimen: [Bolus or Accelerated Infusion] and Subsequent Infusion
Streptokinase (Streptase)	AMI*	**[no bolus]** 1,500,000 IU over 60 minutes IV
	AMI*	*Intracoronary protocol* **[20,000 IU IC]** 2,000 IU/min over 60 minutes IC
	PE	**[250,000 IU over 30 minutes IV]** 100,000 IU/hr for 24 hours IV
	DVT	**[250,000 IU over 30 minutes IV]** 100,000 IU/hr over 72 hours IV
	ATE	**[250,000 IU over 30 minutes IV]** 100,000 IU/hr for 24–72 hours IV
	AV fistula occlusion	**[250,000 IU in 2 mL into *each* limb of the catheter]** dwell time, 2 hours
Alteplase, recombinant (Activase); rtPA	AMI*	**[15 mg IV]** >67 kg: 50 mg over 30 minutes IV, then 35 mg over 60 minutes IV; <67 kg: 0.75 mg/kg over 30 minutes IV, then 0.50 mg/kg over 30 minutes IV
	AMI*	**[6–10 mg IV]** 60 mg (less bolus) over 60 minutes IV, then 20 mg/h for 2 hours IV
	CVA†	**[10% of total dose over 1 minute IV]** 0.9 mg/kg (maximum dose 90 mg) less bolus over 1 hours IV
	Massive PE	**[no bolus]** 100 mg over 2 hours IV
Alteplase, recombinant (Cathflo Activase); rtPA	CVC occlusion	**[2 mg in 2 mL into CVC]** attempt to withdraw blood after 30 and 120 minutes
Reteplase (Retevase)	AMI*	**[10 units over 2 minutes IV at time 0 and 30 minutes]** no infusion
Tenecteplase (TNK-tPA)	AMI*	**[weight-adjusted bolus given IV over 5 seconds: <60 kg, 30 mg; 60–70 kg, 35 mg; 70–80 kg, 40 mg; 80–90 kg, 45 mg; >90 kg, 50 mg]** no infusion

[**Bold** text in brackets] indicates bolus (and/or accelerated infusion) dose.
*Initiation as soon as possible after onset of symptoms
†Within 3 hours of symptoms, and after excluding hemorrhagic CVA.
Abbreviations: AMI, acute myocardial infarction; ATE, arterial thromboembolism; AV, arteriovenous; CVA, (thrombotic) cerebrovascular accident; CVC, central venous catheter; DVT, deep vein thrombosis; IC, intracoronary; IU, international units; IV, intravenous; PE, pulmonary embolism.

plasmin degrades hemostatic "plugs." Fibrin-specific thrombolytics (which, by definition, bind to fibrin at sites of thrombosis) normally do not systematically deplete PAI-1; thus, they produce lesser degrees of such a lytic state. Nevertheless, these agents can produce bleeding complications, probably because they lead to lysis of fibrin at sites of physiologic hemostasis.

Thrombin normally binds to fibrin, an effect that helps to localize thrombin within a thrombus. However, this binding to fibrin, or to fibrin degradation products generated during pharmacologic fibrinolysis, protects thrombin from physiologic (or heparin-catalyzed) inhibition by antithrombin.[213] (This protection might explain why bivalirudin—which inactivates clot-bound thrombin—is more effective than unfractionated heparin in settings such as percutaneous coronary intervention.[214]) Despite evidence that heparin is relatively ineffective at neutralizing thrombin bound to fibrin(ogen), it is usually given to patients receiving fibrinolytics.[215]

Clinical Use

Accepted indications for one or more of the fibrinolytic agents include acute myocardial infarction, thrombotic stroke, deep vein thrombosis, massive pulmonary embolism,[216] arterial thromboembolism, and occlusions of central venous catheters and arteriovenous fistulas (see Table 88–7). Fibrinolytic agents are also used in clinical settings lacking formal approval, such as peripheral arterial occlusion and deep vein thrombosis.[212] Indeed, alteplase is the most widely used thrombolytic agent for peripheral arterial occlusion, even though streptokinase is approved for this indication. Clinical experience and prospective outcome data for many of these indications are limited. However, in highly selected patients, thrombolytic therapy can be limb salvaging (and surgery sparing).[217–219] Although rapid lysis of venous thrombi likely improves acute symptoms more rapidly than anticoagulation alone, whether thrombolysis reduces long-term complications, such as postphlebitic syndrome, is unknown. Given the lack of good-quality prospective data, the optimal doses, infusion strategies, and the need for supplemental device-based therapies cannot be determined (or recommended) at this time.

Dosing and Monitoring

Table 88–7 lists recommended dosing in various clinical situations.

Adverse Effects

Bleeding is the main complication of thrombolytic therapy. Intracranial hemorrhage occurs in 0.5–1.0% of patients. Risk factors include age over 75 years, female gender, and low body weight.[220] Despite expectations to the contrary, the fibrin-specific thrombolytic alteplase caused more intracranial bleeding than did streptokinase (although greater efficacy in restoring coronary flow gave a survival advantage to alteplase-treated patients).[221] Alteplase also was associated with greater (non-intracranial) bleeding than tenecteplase in one trial.[222]

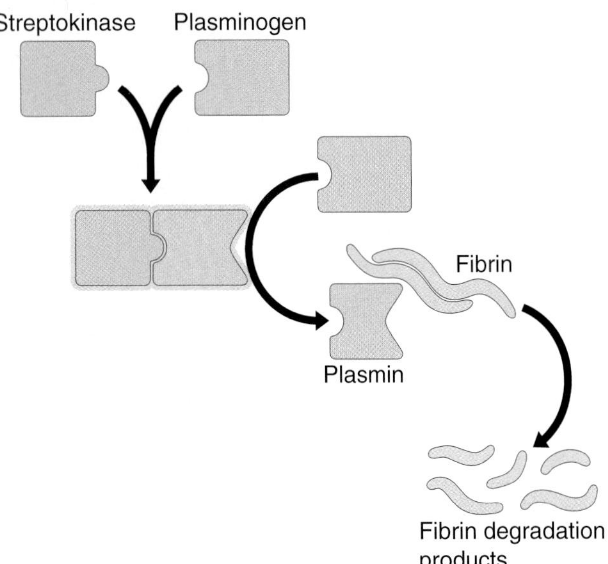

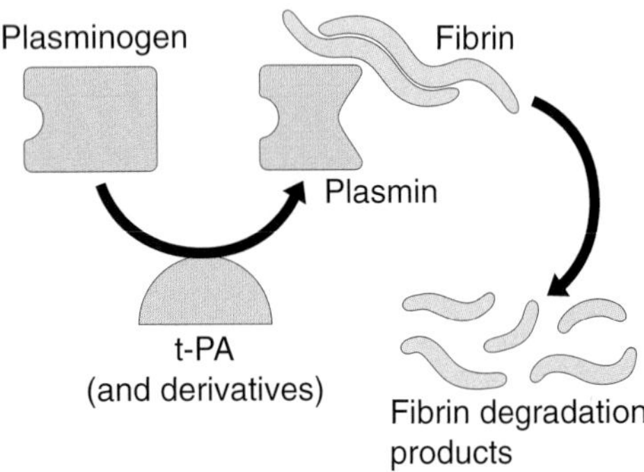

Figure 88–8. Mechanism of action of thrombolytic agents. t-PA (and derivatives) refers to alteplase, reteplase, and tenecteplase.

TABLE 88–8. Management of Serious Bleeding Secondary to Thrombolytic Therapy

Strongly Consider

1. STAT: Stop thrombolytic agent, heparin, and any other antithrombotic agent.
2. STAT: Draw blood for CBC, INR, aPTT, thrombin times, clottable fibrinogen.*
3. STAT: Give at least 10 units of cryoprecipitate.†
4. STAT: Give antifibrinolytic therapy, either ε-aminocaproic acid (Amicar), 0.1 gm/kg over 30 minutes by IV route, followed by infusion at 0.5–1 gm/hr until bleeding subsides; or tranexamic acid (Cyklokapron), 10 mg/kg IV every 6–8 hours until bleeding subsides.
5. STAT: Give protamine sulfate if patient received heparin bolus or IV infusion within past 4 hours.‡
6. Recheck blood work after giving above treatment.

Possibly Indicated

7. Consider red cell concentrates for anemia.§
8. Consider platelet transfusions,‖ especially if patient is thrombocytopenic, antiplatelet agents have been given, and bleed is life-threatening.
9. Consider FFP transfusions‖ (initial dose, 2 units), especially if INR is increased or bleed is life-threatening.

*In urgent situations, cryoprecipitate, an antifibrinolytic drug, and protamine sulfate should be given without waiting for laboratory results or radiologic imaging.

†Cryoprecipitate contains fibrinogen, factor VIII/von Willebrand factor, and factor XIII; 10 units of cryoprecipitate will raise the fibrinogen by 0.7 gm/L in the average-sized adult.

‡Give 1 mg protamine sulfate per 100 units heparin administered as a recent bolus. For a patient receiving a constant heparin infusion, give 1 mg of protamine sulfate for each 100 units given in the previous 4 hours; reduce protamine dose by 50% if heparin has been stopped for 30 minutes. Protamine should be infused slowly, without exceeding 50 mg in any 10-minute period.

§Primary hemostasis improves with higher hematocrit.

‖Platelets and FFP both contain factor V, which can be depleted by thrombolytic therapy.

Abbreviations: aPTT, activated partial thromboplastin time; CBC, complete blood count; FFP, fresh frozen plasma; INR, International Normalized Ratio; IV, intravenous.

Adapted from Sane[221] and Warkentin and Crowther.[60]

An important disadvantage of streptokinase is its immunogenicity: many patients have neutralizing anti-streptokinase antibodies either from previous bacterial infections or from previous treatment with streptokinase. As a result, streptokinase should always be administered as a bolus followed by an infusion; the bolus is designed to overcome the inhibitory antibodies. Allergic reactions (urticaria, fever, bronchospasm, anaphylaxis) are uncommon but important complications of streptokinase. The impact of neutralizing antibodies on the efficacy of streptokinase is controversial. However, reexposure within a short time of prior exposure is not recommended given the potential for reduced efficacy.

Table 88–8 lists an approach for managing serious hemorrhage caused by thrombolytic therapy.[60,223]

CURRENT CONTROVERSIES & FUTURE CONSIDERATIONS

Anticoagulant and Thrombolytic Therapy

- What are the optimal initial doses of warfarin and other coumarins?
- What is the target INR therapeutic range for selected populations (e.g., antiphospholipid syndrome)?
- Should routine anticoagulation be employed after cardiac surgery? If so, with which agent?
- Dosing and monitoring of DTIs must be optimized.

Suggested Readings*

Ansell J, Hirsh J, Poller L, et al: Management of the vitamin K antagonist. The Seventh ACCP Conference on Antithrombotic and Thrombolytic Therapy. Chest 126(Suppl):204S–233S, 2004.

Crowther MA, Julian J, McCarty D, et al: Treatment of warfarin-associated coagulopathy with oral vitamin K: a randomised controlled trial. Lancet 356:1551–1553, 2000.

GUSTO Investigators: An international randomized trial comparing four thrombolytic strategies for acute myocardial infarction. N Engl J Med 329:673–682, 1993

Harrison L, Johnston M, Massicotte MP, et al: Comparison of 5-mg and 10-mg loading doses in initiation of warfarin therapy. Ann Intern Med 126:133–136, 1997.

Hirsh J, Raschke R: Heparin and low-molecular-weight heparin. The Seventh ACCP Conference on Antithrombotic and Thrombolytic Therapy. Chest 126(Suppl):188S–203S, 2004.

Raschke RA, Reilly BM, Guidry JR, et al: The weight-based heparin dosing nomogram compared with a "standard care" nomogram: a randomized controlled trial. Ann Intern Med 119:874–881, 1993.

Warkentin TE, Crowther MA: Reversing anticoagulants both old and new. Can J Anesth 49(Suppl):S11–S25, 2002.

Warkentin TE, Elavathil LJ, Hayward CPM, et al: The pathogenesis of venous limb gangrene associated with heparin-induced thrombocytopenia. Ann Intern Med 127:804–812, 1997.

Wells PS, Holbrook AM, Crowther NR, Hirsh J: Interactions of warfarin with drugs and food. Ann Intern Med 121:676–683, 1994.

Full references for this chapter can be found on accompanying CD-ROM.

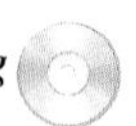

CHAPTER 89
DISSEMINATED INTRAVASCULAR COAGULATION

Cheng Hock Toh, MD, FRCP (London), FRCPath (UK)

KEY POINTS

Disseminated Intravascular Coagulation

- Disseminated intravascular coagulation (DIC) is caused by the enhanced and abnormally sustained generation of thrombin in vivo.
- DIC indicates the transition from localized, adaptive, and compensated coagulation processes into maladaptive responses.
- Identifying circulating biomarkers that propagate thrombin generation may indicate the timing of dissemination and be a tool for therapeutic targeting.
- DIC exemplifies multifaceted interactions between the inflammatory and coagulation pathways, involving the blood–endothelial vasculature interface.
- The pathologic and clinical manifestations of DIC are dependent upon the host/genetic responses to thrombin generation.

INTRODUCTION

Disseminated intravascular coagulation (DIC) represents a departure from the neat compartmentalization of the hemostatic response to local injury that has been crucial for human survival and its evolution.[1] Classically conceptualized by the triad involvement of coagulation factors, platelets, and the vessel wall, hemostatic plug formation is exquisitely controlled and continues as an adaptive response even as the injury increases in intensity. The "equal and opposite" host reaction to injury aims to maintain overall homeostatic re-equilibration, and this level of coagulation activation is typically not dysfunctional. However, this response may turn maladaptive depending on individual susceptibility thresholds to either the increasing intensity or nature of the insult. It is this dysfunctional form of systemic hemostatic activation, which can lead to hemodynamic and metabolic derangements, that is considered DIC. The emerging evidence points to a pathogenesis that is not just "coagulation gone haywire" but that fully involves all components of the classical triad of hemostasis. Events go beyond the fluid and blood–endothelial cell interface to involve critical subendothelial and constitutive neuronal processes.[2,3] The importance of this is borne out clinically, for DIC is well validated as an independent predictor of mortality.[4,5] Its presence doubles the risk of mortality in severe sepsis and trauma.[5,6] DIC therefore represents hemostatic dysfunction that has net liability to the host.

DEFINITION

DIC arises as a complication of a variety of clinical disorders and is characterized by the increasing loss of localization or compensated activation of coagulation. This continuum in clinicopathologic severity has definable phases that characterize patients at risk for increased mortality. The International Society on Thrombosis and Hemostasis (ISTH) Standardisation Sub-Committee has therefore proposed working definitions to facilitate earlier detection and treatment of DIC.[7] The new emphasis is on recognizing a nonovert stage of hemostatic dysfunction rather than an overt, frankly decompensated stage that is usually too late for therapeutic rescue.

PATHOPHYSIOLOGY

Several themes in DIC pathogenesis are important to consider in approaching the diagnosis, management, and relevant therapeutic strands. First is the central role played by thrombin generation in vivo.[8,9] Second, mechanisms that fuel and perpetuate thrombin generation are responsible for its dissemination. Third is the parallel and con-

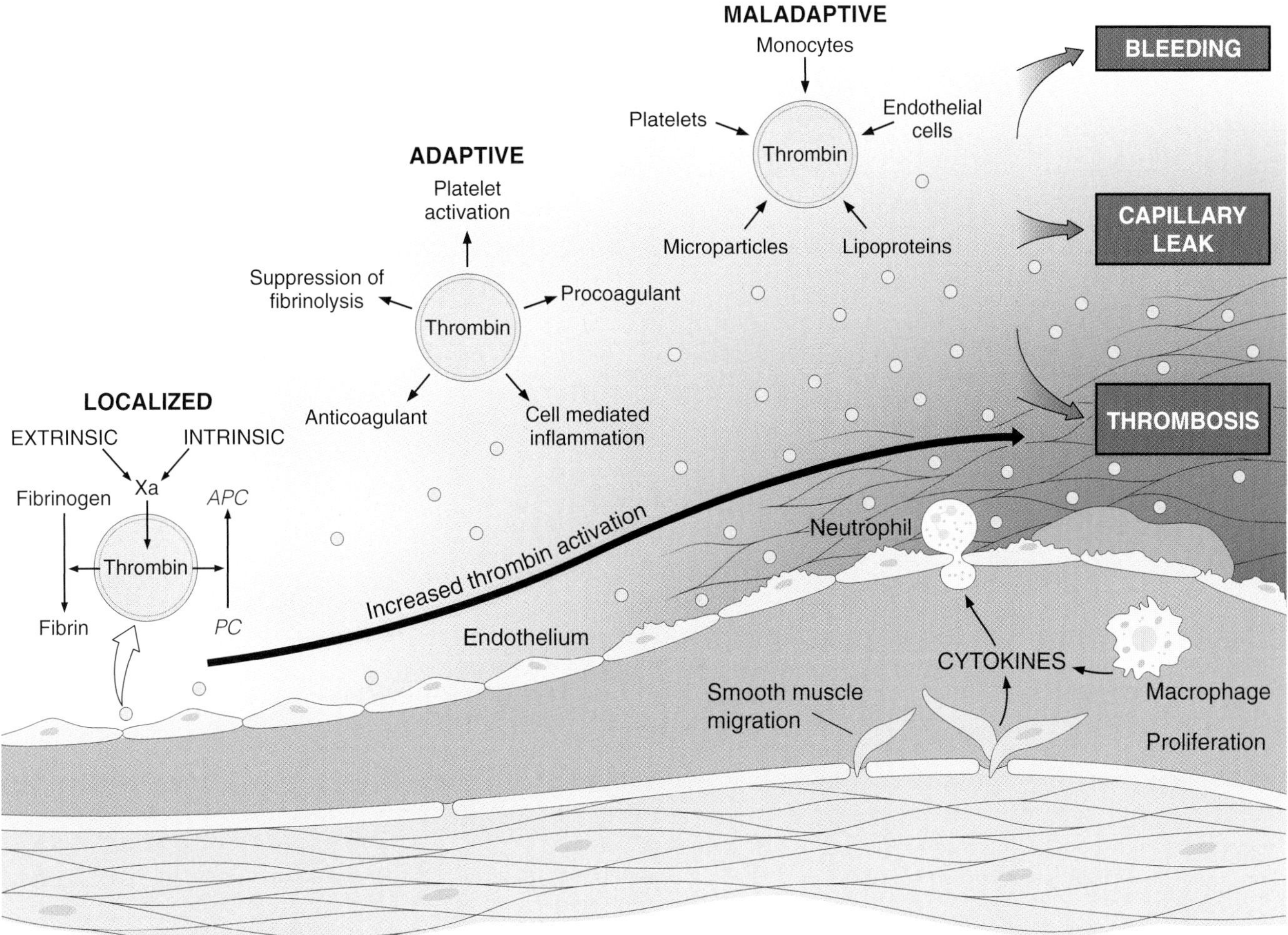

Figure 89–1. Thrombin generation in vivo: sequence from adaptive to the maladaptive events of DIC. Localized hemostatic activation leads to the homeostatic effects of thrombin in balancing the procoagulant conversion of fibrinogen to fibrin and in activating the protein C (PC) anticoagulant pathway to negatively feed back on further thrombin generation. In adaptation to a more generalized insult, thrombin's ubiquitous and often opposing actions continue to be overall protective to the host. The maladaptive phase, characterizing the onset of DIC, sees mechanisms that enhance and abnormally sustain thrombin generation. This is exemplified by the provision of increased negatively charged phospholipid surfaces in the circulation. The consequences for coagulation and inflammation, with direct involvement of white blood cells and cytokine release, play out on the endothelial vasculature. The clinicopathologic manifestations will depend on host/genetic responses in terms of predominant microvascular thrombosis, bleeding, capillary leak, or a spectrum of these.

comitant activation of the inflammatory cascade. Fourth is the importance of the endothelial microvasculature in this process. These themes are summarized in the Key Points and illustrated in Figure 89–1.

Thrombin Generation in Vivo

The process of generating thrombin in vivo is pivotal to hemostatic control, since it synchronizes and balances both pro- and anticoagulant forces as well as pro- and antifibrinolytic activities. Clot formation by way of the conversion of fibrinogen to fibrin is simultaneously controlled by thrombin activation of the protein C anticoagulant regulatory pathway (see Fig. 89–1).[10] This also serves a number of potential roles, including the walling off of pathogens, recruitment of cellular processes, and the activation of appropriate endothelial response signals.[11] Platelet activation, in addition to facilitating platelet aggregation, also leads to the release of chemokines and growth factors.[12] Although fibrinolysis can be directly promoted via thrombin-induced tissue plasminogen activator release from endothelial cells to generate plasmin, the process is held in check at the site of thrombin burst through the actions of thrombin-activatable fibrinolysis inhibitor in preventing binding of plasminogen to partially digested fibrin for its conversion to the fibrinolytic enzyme plasmin, and at a second level by plasminogen activator inhibitor-1 complexing to tissue plasminogen activator.[13,14]

This fine, exquisite homeostatic balance of controlled thrombin generation is lost in DIC. An appreciation of the many thrombin-mediated activities, which may either be cooperative or antagonistic to each other, is fundamental to understanding the different clinical manifestations and the management of this condition (Fig. 89–2).

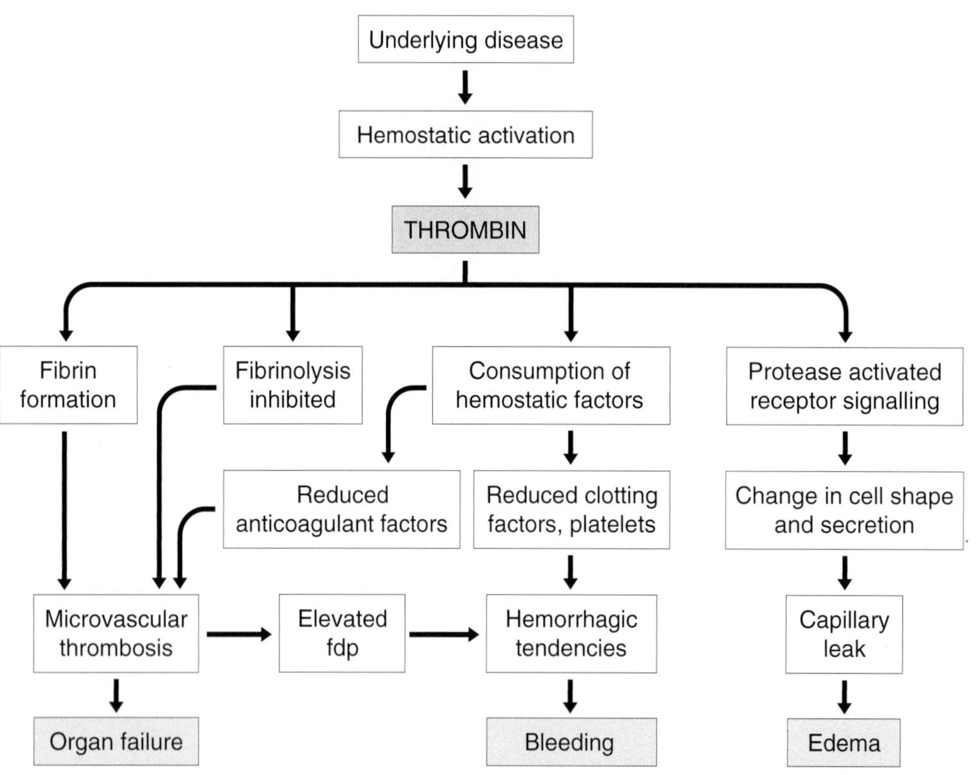

Figure 89–2. Mechanisms in DIC. Systemic activation of hemostatic processes leads to thrombin generation and its consequences, which include intravascular fibrin deposition, depletion of hemostatic factors, and protease-activated receptor-mediated cell signaling responses. As a result, there may be thrombosis of small vessels contributing to organ failure, severe bleeding, capillary leakage and edema. Abbreviation: fdp, fibrin degradation products.

Mechanisms Disseminating and Sustaining Thrombin Generation

Although tissue factor is an important initiator, it may not be as relevant in sustaining thrombin generation in DIC. Its exposure rapidly induces tissue factor pathway inhibitor expression, which increases with increasing DIC severity.[15] Secondary bursts of thrombin formation are provided by the intrinsic pathway of coagulation and this leads to depletion of the anticoagulant regulatory proteins: protein C, protein S, and antithrombin.[16] Apart from continuous consumption by ongoing protease-inhibitor complex formation, such as thrombin-antithrombin and activated protein C (APC)–protein C inhibitor interactions,[17] these can be further decreased by elastase degradation as well as by reduced synthesis through liver dysfunction.[18] In addition to an impaired anticoagulant system, increased exposure of negatively charged or anionic phospholipid surfaces further propagates coagulation kinetics.[19] In vitro, the availability of such surfaces accelerates the prothrombinase reaction dramatically by 250,000-fold.[20] In vivo, this relevance is demonstrated by the observation that factor Xa infusions alone are not thrombogenic unless co-infused with anionic phospholipid surfaces.[21] Such surfaces, mainly rich in phosphatidylserine, can arise from externalization of the inner cell membrane leaflet upon activation and apoptosis.[22] Cell damage also leads to microparticle release, which increases anionic phospholipid availability to sustain in vivo thrombin generation. These microparticles are less readily cleared by the reticuloendothelial system in comparison to the rapid phagocytotic removal of apoptotic cells.[23] Of relevance too is phospholipid surface provision by oxidized low-density lipoprotein and very-low-density lipoprotein, the latter of which can increase severalfold in severe sepsis to further enhance thrombin generation.[24] The very-low-density lipoprotein generated is relatively deficient in apolipoprotein E, which results in an increased circulating half-life because the clearance mechanism is largely apolipoprotein E dependent.[25,26] This procoagulant effect is compounded by the loss of circulating high-density lipoprotein with its natural anticoagulant-promoting properties.[27,28] Taken together, these mechanisms form a spatially and temporally expansive response that is the hallmark of DIC (Box 89–1).

Links Between Inflammation and Coagulation

Once activated, the inflammatory and coagulation pathways interact to amplify the response.[29] Whereas cytokines and pro-inflammatory mediators can induce coagulation, thrombin as well as factor Xa and probably tissue factor–factor VIIa complex can interact with protease-activated receptors on cell surfaces to promote further activation and additional inflammation.[30] Protease-activated receptor signaling upregulates adhesion molecules and triggers production of chemokines that activate neutrophils and monocytes, whose products can directly injure tissues.[31] Concomitant subendothelial perturbation further recruits macrophages to drive the inflammatory reaction.[32,33] When this process generalizes, it results in a dysregulated, undirected response that fuels the vicious cycle between inflammation and coagulation.

Endothelial Cell Activation and Dysfunction

The normal adaptive response of endothelial surfaces regulates coagulation and inflammation.[34] Natural anticoagulant mechanisms at the endothelial surface dampen this inflammatory-coagulant interface, and sensory neurons, when stimulated, can increase prostacyclin production from the endothelium to reduce injury.[3,29] Dysfunction and failure of this large, physiologic endothelial organ beyond its adaptive responses can lead to significant collateral damage and is indicated by the development of DIC. The degree of this relates to the triggering insult, and the dominance of thrombotic versus bleeding sequelae or capillary leakage depends on genetic and host-related factors (see Fig. 89–1).[35] Because of its higher endothelial cell surface–to–blood volume ratios, the microvasculature is particularly affected in DIC.[36]

Box 89–1. Mechanisms Sustaining Thrombin Generation

- Activation of intrinsic pathway of coagulation
- Reduction in endogenous anticoagulant activation:
    - reduction in circulating proteins C, S, and antithrombin
    - reduced endothelial protein C receptor and thrombomodulin expression
    - increased inhibition by serine protease inhibitors
- Increased availability of negatively charged phospholipid surfaces:
    - externalization of inner cellular membrane leaflet
    - cellular microparticle formation
    - circulating lipoproteins
    - reduced reticuloendothelial clearance
- Circulating tissue factor on monocytes and microparticles

PRESENTATION, CLINICAL FEATURES, AND DIAGNOSIS

Presentation

The perturbed hemostatic consequences of DIC can manifest clinically at any point in the spectrum from bleeding to thrombosis (see Fig. 89–2). Bleeding is the archetypal physical manifestation as a result of (1) reducing platelets, (2) reduced coagulation factors, and (3) inhibition of platelet function by fibrin(ogen) degradation products (FDPs), which are ineffectively cleared when the reticuloendothelial system is saturated.[37] However, the occurrence of organ failure is much more common. Microvascular thrombosis is potentiated by (1) increased fibrin formation, (2) inhibition of fibrinolysis, and (3) reduced anticoagulant factors (protein C, protein S, and antithrombin). Simultaneous bleeding and thrombotic signs would be a key feature, with purpura fulminans as an extremely gross manifestation involving both hemorrhagic skin necrosis and gangrene (Fig. 89–3). Typically, however, the features of DIC are not clinically overt because of predominant microcirculatory localization of the pathologic process. Autopsy findings have shown both diffuse bleeding at various sites, with hemorrhagic tissue necrosis, and thrombi, particularly in small blood vessels.[38] A point of emphasis is that the clinician must repeatedly assess for both physical and laboratory changes of organ failure as evidence of a rapidly evolving disturbance of hemostatic dysfunction.

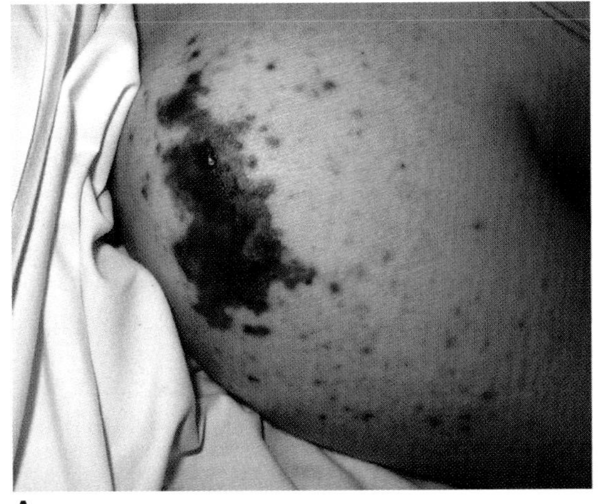
A

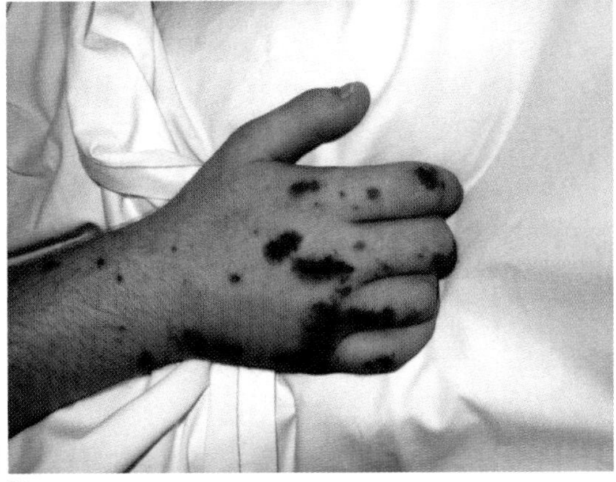
B

Figure 89–3. Purpura fulminans in a patient with DIC resulting from meningococcal septicemia in the shoulder *(A)* and hand *(B)*. (From Toh CH, Dennis M: Disseminated intravascular coagulation: old disease, new hope. BMJ 327:974, 2003. Copyright BMJ Publishing Group, used by permission.)

TABLE 89–1. Clinical Conditions Associated with DIC

Clinical Condition	Examples
Sepsis/severe infection	Potentially any microorganism, be it bacterial, viral, or protozoal
Trauma	Serious tissue injury Head injury Fat embolism
Organ destruction	Severe pancreatitis
Malignancy	Solid tumors Hematologic malignancies (e.g., acute promyelocytic leukemia)
Obstetric calamities	Placental abruption Amniotic fluid embolism
Vascular abnormalities	Giant hemangiomas (Kasabach-Merritt syndrome) Large vessel aneurysms (e.g., aortic)
Acute hepatic failure	Necrosis Fatty liver of pregnancy
Severe toxic or immunologic reactions	Snakebites Recreational drugs Severe transfusion reactions Transplant rejection

Clinical Features

As indicated previously, the triggering insult influences the nature of the hemostatic complication. As such, knowledge of the different disease associations with DIC is important. These are listed in Table 89–1, and the more frequently encountered ones are discussed here.

Severe infection and sepsis, irrespective of the underlying organism, is the most common cause of DIC. Both gram-negative and gram-positive bacteria are involved.[39,40] So are systemic fungal infections and viral disorders, including severe acute respiratory syndrome (SARS), influenza, and herpes.[41,42] Parasitic causes such as malaria are also highly relevant. The generalized inflammatory consequence is caused by the cytokine storm primarily from activated mononuclear cells, which drives the interconnection with coagulation processes. These can be directly provoked by specific cell membrane components or toxins secreted by the organism.[43,44]

This same inflammatory response also occurs in trauma, wherein the initiating trigger is severe endothelial damage.[6] Penetrating brain injury can introduce highly tissue factor–rich or thromboplastic tissue into the systemic circulation, with massive activation of intravascular coagulation.[45] About a third of patients who have sustained sufficient head trauma to lose consciousness develop DIC. Likewise, burns and pancreatitis cause similar consequences to this inflammation-coagulation cascade.[46,47]

Although malignancies can be complicated by DIC, such cases are usually far less overt with the exception of acute promyelocytic leukemia and disseminated prostatic carcinomas, in which disproportionate hyperfibrinolysis occurs.[48] The inflammatory involvement in the DIC of cancer is far less than that of the previously noted causes, and the etiology includes tissue factor expression by solid tumor cells and direct prothrombinase activation via mucin or possibly by a putative cysteine protease with factor X–activating properties.[49,50] Likewise, snake venoms can have specificity for different components of the coagulation cascade. *Echis carinatus* venom directly activates prothrombin to thrombin, and the venom of *Vipera russelli* (Russell viper) directly activates factor X.[51,52] The DIC that ensues following the bite of such snakes reflects these specific activities.

Among obstetric complications causing DIC, placental separation or abruptio placentae is the most common because of the release of thromboplastin-rich placental tissue.[53] Amniotic fluid embolism, which tends to occur in unusually vigorous deliveries in older multiparous women, causes DIC via direct prothrombinase activation.[54] Less overt DIC occurs in women with preeclampsia and can be a surrogate marker of progression of this obstetric pathology.

Although vascular disorders such as giant hemangiomas can show a laboratory picture indistinguishable from the DIC of sepsis or trauma, the distinction that they are somewhat different pathogenic entities is important. Local activation and consumption of coagulation processes leading to overflow into the systemic circulation is causative and the concomitant activation of inflammation is negligible.[55] This also relates to large aortic aneurysms.[56] However, when aneurysms rupture, a DIC akin to that of severe trauma typically ensues. Likewise, the coagulopathy of liver disease is also not maladaptive, with little inflammatory overlay.[57] The DIC-like picture exemplifies reduced synthesis of coagulation factors as well as consumption. Acute hepatic necrosis and fatty liver of pregnancy can, however, cause acute DIC.

Diagnosis

DIC should always be considered if there is a defect in hemostatic parameters (coagulation screen or platelet count) arising in any of the underlying diseases. Thrombocytopenia is the most common laboratory abnormality, followed by a prolonged prothrombin time. There should be clear consideration for the extent of coagulopathy versus microangiopathic red cell fragmentation in the differentiation of diagnoses (Fig. 89–4). Thrombotic thrombocytopenic purpura can be distinguished through its neurologic involvement, a relative excess of microangiopathy, and paucity in coagulation defects.[58] Likewise, hemolytic-uremic syndrome has end-organ predilection for the kidneys.[59] Of note, a laboratory profile indistinguishable from typical DIC can be seen during rapid volume replacement with colloids. This is due not only to plasma dilution but to direct colloid interference with fibrin polymerization to prolong clot times.[60] Because this is often the same patient group predisposed to DIC (i.e., with hypovolemic shock), care must be taken in interpretation of laboratory findings.

Laboratory diagnostic tests in DIC need to keep pace with the acute setting, and the parameters need to be simple, rapid, and robust in performance.[61] Blood smear changes (Box 89–2) revealing some degree of schisto-

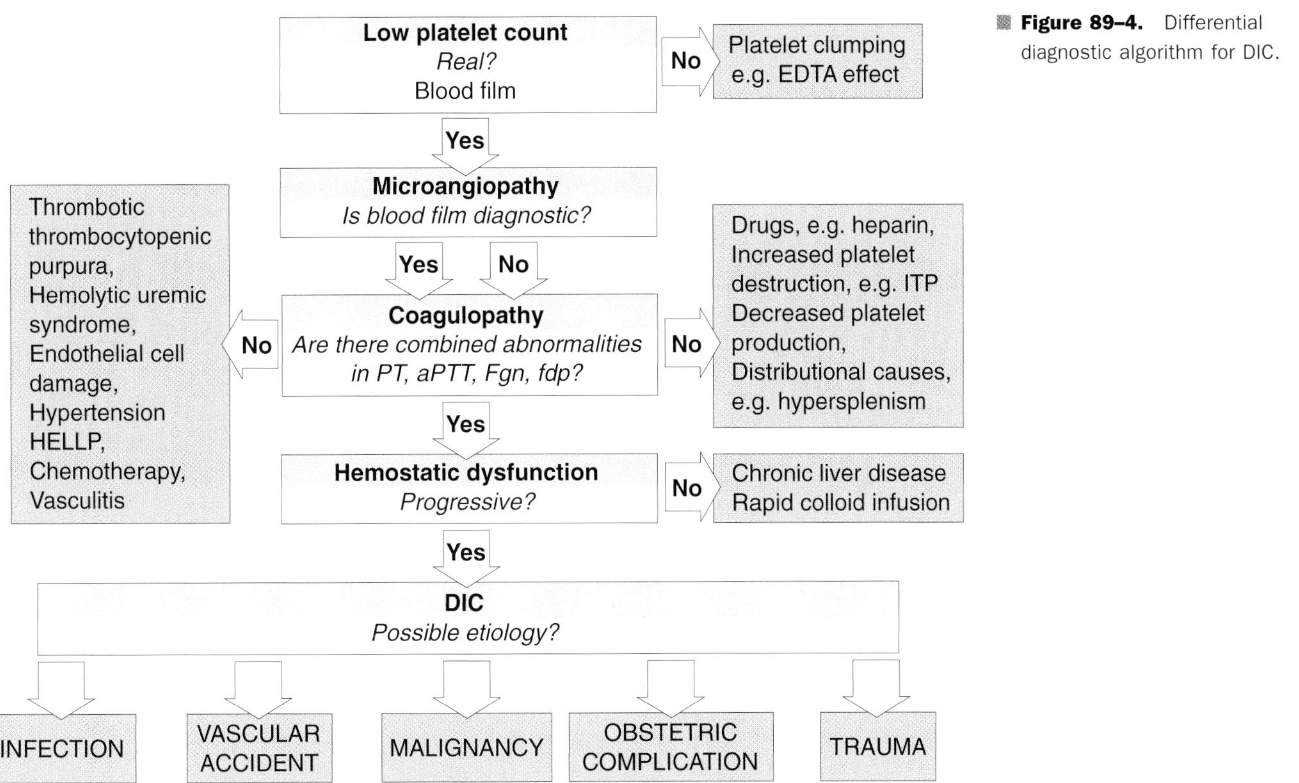

Figure 89–4. Differential diagnostic algorithm for DIC.

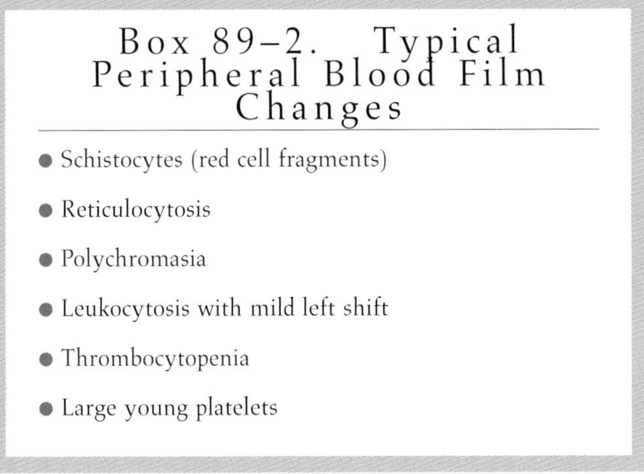

Box 89–2. Typical Peripheral Blood Film Changes

- Schistocytes (red cell fragments)
- Reticulocytosis
- Polychromasia
- Leukocytosis with mild left shift
- Thrombocytopenia
- Large young platelets

cytes in over half of cases (Fig. 89–5) are helpful but not specific. With regard to the global tests of coagulation, the characteristic findings are prolongation in clotting times [e.g., prothrombin time, activated partial thromboplastin time (aPTT)] reflecting depleted coagulation factors; low platelet counts; reduced fibrinogen levels representing conversion to fibrin or fibrinogenolysis; and elevated FDPs, including D-dimer. Whereas FDPs may be either fibrinogen or fibrin derived, D-dimer is formed as a result of plasmin degradation of cross-linked fibrin and is therefore more specific for fibrin degradation.[62]

None of these tests is sufficiently specific as a single determinant, and a diagnosis of DIC requires the scoring of these parameters within a diagnostic algorithm (Fig. 89–6).[7,63] However, changes in all parameters do not occur simultaneously, and results within the normal range do not exclude significant consumptive coagulopathy. The acute-phase response can shorten the activated partial thromboplastin time via elevations particularly in factors VIII, IX, and XI of the intrinsic pathway and in increasing fibrinogen levels.[64,65] As such, the ISTH guidance on identifying early, nonovert DIC scores not only for abnormal results but for abnormal trends in these results (Table 89–2).[66]

Although the recognition of the pivotal role played by sustained thrombin generation in vivo in DIC pathogenesis has led to the development of numerous assays centered around detection of its generation (e.g., prothrombin fragment 1 + 2, thrombin-antithrombin complexes), or its activation of the protein C pathway (e.g., APC–inhibitor complexes, such as APC–α_1-antitrypsin) and the consequences of its activity (e.g., fibrinopeptide A, soluble fibrin), a major drawback of most of these molecular markers of coagulation activation relates to their impracticality in the acute care setting.[17,67] Many are based on the enzyme-linked immunosorbent assay technology and require a level of stringency in either sample handling, processing, or testing that is beyond the scope of the routine diagnostic laboratory testing. Chromogenic-based assays measuring antithrombin and protein C can be more practical and useful. Depletion of these proteins has been related to outcome in sepsis.[68,69] However, their sensitivity for the early phase of DIC is unclear because DIC is usually already rampant when these levels are below 50% of normal.

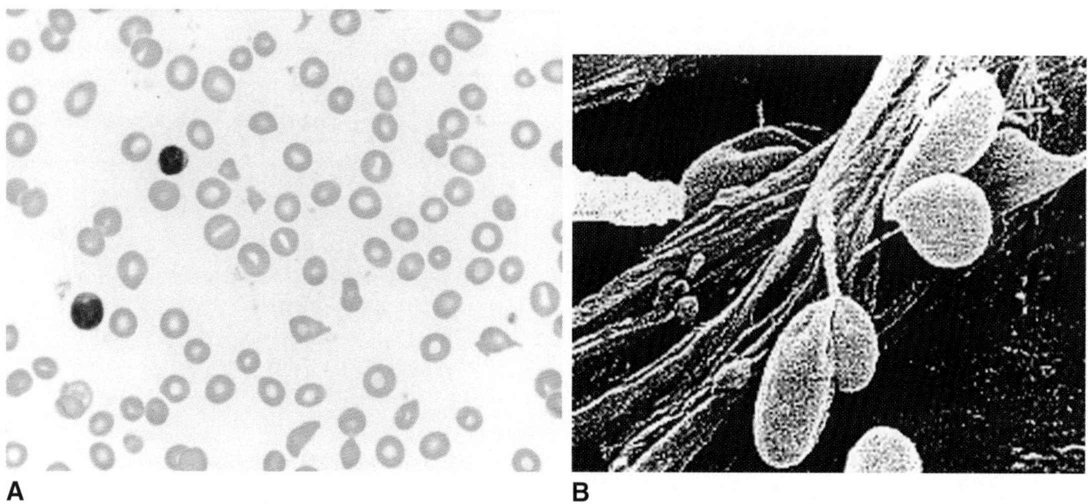

Figure 89–5. Red cell fragmentation in DIC. ***A,*** The peripheral blood film from a patient with DIC secondary to disseminated malignancy. ***B,*** The near-severing of red cells by fibrin strands. (From Bull BS, Kuhn IN: The production of schistocytes by fibrin strands [a scanning electron microscope study]. Blood 35:104, 1970. Copyright American Society of Hematology, used by permission.)

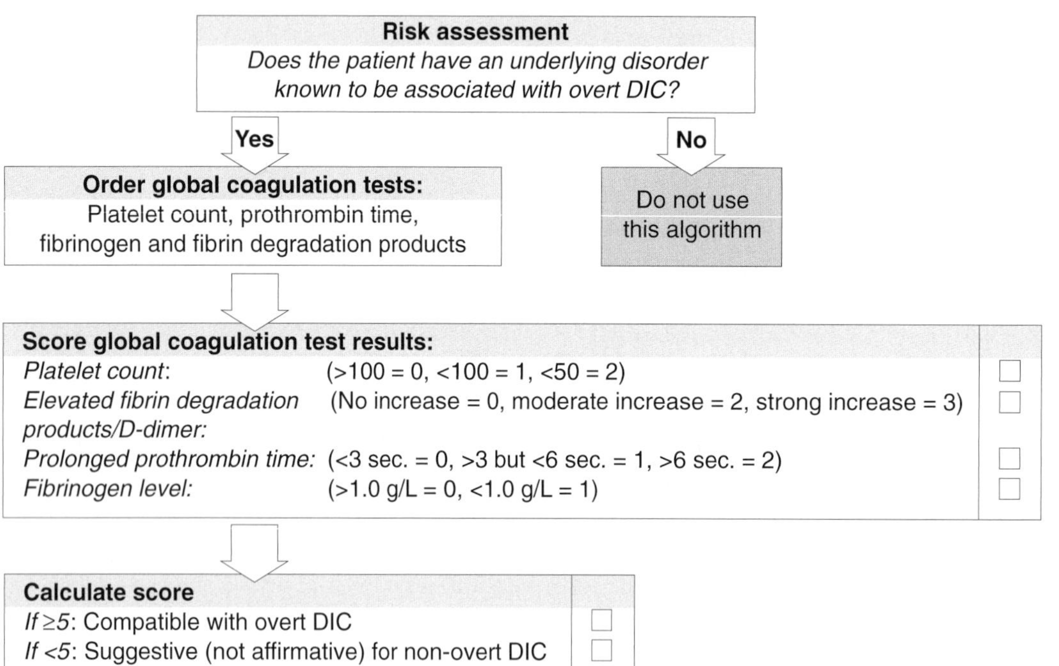

Figure 89–6. Laboratory testing and diagnosis of overt DIC.

A further note of concern centers on specificity issues, especially with regard to the standardization of assays between different manufacturers. The classic example is that of cross-reactivity between soluble fibrin and D-dimer assays.[70] Although it would theoretically be advantageous to identify the precursor of fibrin as an early marker of DIC, the present assays are not sufficiently specific or discriminatory.[71] The growing appreciation of the link between inflammation and coagulation has raised awareness of the need for more specific assays that can directly link these processes in vivo but that also fulfill practical simplicity, rapidity in performance, and robustness as evidence for identifying DIC (see Table 89–2).[24,72]

ACUTE MANAGEMENT VERSUS CHRONIC MANAGEMENT

Acute Management

The cornerstone of managing DIC is the treatment of the underlying disorder. In the acute setting, this tends to be fairly obvious, for example, in the context of the patient

TABLE 89–2. Phases and Laboratory Data of Coagulation Activation Leading to Disseminated Intravascular Coagulation

Clinical Findings	Laboratory Analysis	Laboratory Data
Compensated Hemostatic Activation		
No symptoms	No measurable consumption in global hemostatic tests Increased molecular markers of coagulation Mild changes in regulatory factors	PT, aPTT, Fgn, Plt: within normal limits SF, TAT, F_{1+2}: elevated PC, AT: slightly decreased
Nonovert DIC: Early Decompensation of Hemostatic System		
Mild bleeding Decreased organ function (e.g., kidneys, lungs, liver)	Continuous consumption in global hemostatic tests Increasing molecular markers of coagulation Reduced regulatory factors Increase in thrombin-enhancing biomarkers	PT: increasing prolongation Plt: falling aPTT, Fgn: often within normal limits SF, TAT, F_{1+2}: elevated PC, AT: decreased Microparticles, VLDL: increased
Overt DIC: Fully Decompensated Hemostatic Dysfunction		
Skin bleeding Multiorgan failure	Consumption of hemostasis components	PT, aPTT: greatly prolonged Plt: diminished Fgn: reduced, often still within normal limits SF, TAT, F_{1+2}: elevated PC, AT: markedly reduced

Abbreviations: aPTT, activated partial thromboplastin time; AT, antithrombin; F_{1+2}, prothrombin fragment 1 + 2; Fgn, fibrinogen; PC, protein C; Plt, platelets; PT, prothrombin time; SF, soluble fibrin; TAT, thrombin-antithrombin complex; VLDL, very-low-density lipoproteins.

with severe trauma. In the postoperative patient with overwhelming infection, prompt attention in instituting broad-spectrum antibiotics intravenously is requisite.[73] Shock should be vigorously treated to maintain the blood volume and correct vascular stasis, hypoxia, or acidosis. In obstetric situations, rapid complete evacuation of the uterus may be life-saving.[53] Plasma and platelet substitution therapy needs to be considered for those patients at risk of bleeding complications, although the efficacy of such treatment is not based on randomized controlled trials. Neither is there evidence that these might "add fuel to the fire."[42] As such, judicious use along the lines suggested in Figure 89–7 appears rational. In terms of snakebites, specification of their precise nature is of major relevance in the use of corresponding antivenoms.

Critically ill patients may develop a coagulopathy because of vitamin K deficiency, and 10 mg of vitamin K should be given before coagulopathy is attributed exclusively to DIC.[74] Likewise, patients with DIC can also become vitamin K depleted. Treatment with coagulation factor concentrates is not recommended because traces of activated coagulation factors could exacerbate the coagulation disorder.[75] Antifibrinolytic agents such as tranexamic acid are also not recommended generally. Because there can often be insufficient fibrinolysis, further inhibition would be inappropriate. A clear exception is in predominant hyperfibrinolysis, typified by the disproportionately low fibrinogen and very high FDPs resulting from indiscriminate fibrin(ogen)olysis. D-dimers are usually only modestly elevated as a result of a relative lack of formally cross-linked fibrin. Examples of this situation are acute promyelocytic leukemia and disseminated prostate cancer.[48,76] Fibrinogen replacement to maintain levels above 1.0 gm/L may be necessary, but laboratory interpretation must be tempered with the knowledge that clot-based methods for fibrinogen determinations can give artifactually lower results compared to immunologic methods because high FDP levels interfere with fibrin polymerization.

As to the use of aprotinin, which can broadly inhibit serine proteases including plasmin and elastase, this has had mixed results and has therefore not entered mainstream consideration.[77] A synthetic protease inhibitor with a similar activity spectrum called gabexate mesylate has also been used for treating DIC, but this has not yet undergone the rigors of a randomized controlled trial setting.[78]

Although it might seem reasonable to use heparin to inhibit excess thrombin generation, benefit on clinically important outcome measures in patients with DIC has never been demonstrated in controlled clinical trials.[79] As indicated before, a spectrum of hemostatic dysfunction is usually present even when not clinically obvious, and the patient could be further compromised toward bleeding through heparin treatment.[80]

The clinician should also be aware that eradication of the primary provocative stimulus might not be sufficient. This is mostly the case when there are systemic inflammatory responses; sepsis is the prime example when appropriate antibiotics fail to deliver clinical improvement.[73,81,82] The coagulopathy may not be florid in the fluid phase, but the extent of inflammatory-coagulation cycling can be ongoing at the endothelial and vascular level. It is at this juncture in the clinical course that modulatory therapy should be considered (see Fig. 89–7).[83] In the setting of severe sepsis, the strongest evidence is for the use of recombinant human APC by continuous infusion over 96 hours at 24 μg/kg/hr.[84] This regimen has been shown to significantly reduce the relative and absolute risk of mortality by 19.4% and 6.1%, respectively, in patients with sepsis. This APC effect is believed to be mediated through combined anticoagulant and anti-

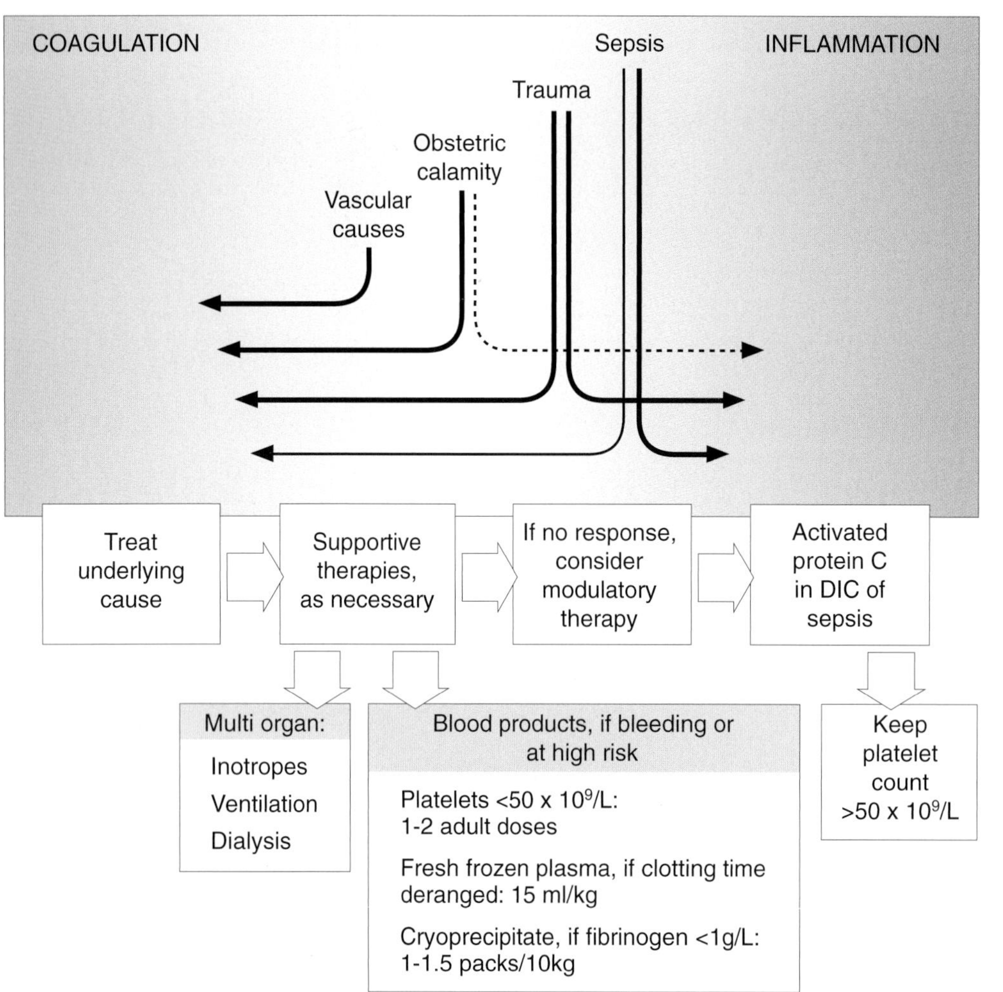

Figure 89–7. Management principles in DIC. The heterogeneity in clinical sequelae for the different causes of DIC reflects the extent of crossover between coagulation and inflammation processes. In the main, DIC arising from vascular and obstetric calamities has minimal inflammatory dysfunction, and these cases respond particularly well to treatment of the underlying cause, with use of supportive circulatory and blood product therapy as necessary. The DIC of trauma and sepsis involves far greater systemic inflammatory responses. These cases can resolve with treatment of the underlying cause, but, not uncommonly, this may be inadequate. Modulatory treatment with recombinant human activated protein C would be indicated in sepsis, and adequate circulating platelet numbers are required to prevent bleeding complications.

inflammatory properties. The latter are evident in attenuating the inflammatory response via modulation of nuclear factor-κB and direct antiapoptotic, cytoprotective effects.[85,86] In short, the mechanistic evidence suggests that the therapeutic efficacy of APC is as a counter to thrombin in re-equilibrating the pitfalls of excessive thrombin activity in vivo. In practical terms, care should be exercised when recombinant human APC is used in the presence of thrombocytopenia. Platelet transfusion is important when platelet counts are less that 50×10^9/L because of reports of intracranial bleeding.[87]

There is less evidence for the use of zymogen blood-derived protein C replacement therapy, and, because zymogen protein C has to bind to the endothelial protein C receptor for conversion to APC by the thrombin-thrombomodulin complex, the efficiency of this therapy would depend on adequate thrombomodulin and endothelial protein C receptor cell surface levels.[88] This may, however, be rather diminished in severe sepsis.[89]

Antithrombin has also been shown to have anti-inflammatory properties.[90] However, a large randomized controlled trial of high-dose antithrombin in sepsis failed to demonstrate a significant mortality reduction, although subgroup analysis suggests that this was primarily due to the adverse outcome of heparin co-infusion with antithrombin.[80] The use of tissue factor pathway inhibitor, another endogenous anticoagulant, has also not shown benefit.[91]

In all these decisions, close joint consultation with critical care specialists is essential. Timing of targeted modulatory treatment is at present difficult, but evidence of increasing thrombin generation via increasing abnormalities in the DIC score or detection of thrombin-enhancing biomarkers might be useful, although these approaches remain to be validated. Efforts to improve perfusion and strategies such as improved glucose control and low-dose steroid usage are part of current best practice, and nutritional aspects should also be considered, especially with regard to the information that specific lipids can augment thrombin generation.[92–94]

Chronic Management

In the event of an unexpected laboratory finding suggestive of DIC in an otherwise stable patient, a search for an underlying etiology is imperative. The process is usually not as disseminated as the coagulation results might suggest, for example, in asymptomatic aortic aneurysms. The relevance of recognizing this is that such patients can respond dramatically to surgical correction.[95] A further consideration is chronic liver disease. As already highlighted, liver-related coagulopathy is not DIC in the maladaptive context of hemostatic dysfunction.

A concern is always the possibility of an occult malignancy. Because of the increasing number of patients on warfarin for stroke prevention and the link between covert malignancy and venous thromboembolism, increased warfarin sensitivity should alert the clinician to order a full DIC screen.[96] Mucin-secreting adenocarcinomas are most commonly associated with chronic DIC and, although usually disseminated by this time, it is worthwhile recognizing that the pathology involves platelet-mucin–rich thrombi that respond therapeutically to heparin via preventing P-selectin interaction with its ligand on tumor products.[97]

PROGNOSIS

The comment that the letters "DIC" could stand for "Death Is Coming" is a reminder of the progress that remains to be made in understanding and managing this not uncommon condition.[98] There, are however, reasons for cautious optimism. First, the emerging efficacy of drugs that suppress both coagulation and inflammation is promising.[99] Second, the improved understanding of the complexities of DIC and the recognition that it is not solely about coagulation disturbances have been important insights, especially because clotting end points represent only 10% or less of thrombin's pleiotropic activity![100] Third, the laboratory diagnosis of DIC has improved in that it now allows identification of an earlier stage in the decompensating process through simple, rapid, and robust tools.[7,66] This will ensure better triaging of care, more appropriate timing of intervention, and rapid monitoring of response. It is therefore the author's expectation that a cohesive clinical strategy embracing diagnostic and therapeutic advances holds immediate promise for improving survival in DIC.

CURRENT CONTROVERSIES & FUTURE CONSIDERATIONS

Disseminated Intravascular Coagulation

- Will targeting the early maladaptive and nonovert phase of DIC provide the therapeutic window of opportunity for modulatory treatment in conditions such as severe sepsis and trauma?
- Can we develop a single, simple, rapid, and widely applicable diagnostic test to recognize this nonovert phase of DIC?
- Is the therapeutic benefit of APC due to greater anti-inflammatory than anticoagulant properties? If so, could tailored analogues of APC possessing greater anti-inflammatory properties be more efficacious?
- Can functional tests of thrombin's nonclotting activity be developed and applied to gain a better handle on its pathologic consequences?

Suggested Readings*

Aird WC: The role of the endothelium in severe sepsis and multiple organ dysfunction syndrome. Blood 101:3765–3777, 2003.

Coughlin SR: Thrombin signalling and protease activated receptors. Nature 407:258–264, 2000.

Esmon CT: New mechanisms for vascular control of inflammation mediated by natural anticoagulant proteins. J Exp Med 196:565–577, 2002.

Levi M, ten Cate H: Disseminated intravascular coagulation. N Engl J Med 586:586–592, 1999.

Taylor FB, Toh CH, Hoots WK, et al: Towards definition, clinical and laboratory criteria and a scoring system for disseminated intravascular coagulation. Thromb Haemost 86:1327–1330, 2001.

Full references for this chapter can be found on accompanying CD-ROM.

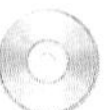

CHAPTER 90
CHEMOTHERAPY TOXICITIES AND COMPLICATIONS

Doru T. Alexandrescu, MD, Peter H. Wiernik, MD, and Janice P. Dutcher, MD

> **KEY POINTS**
>
> **Chemotherapy Toxicities and Complications**
>
> - The vast majority of chemotherapeutic agents also target various normal biologic processes. Actively dividing cells in the bone marrow, gastrointestinal tract, hair follicles, and gonads are most susceptible to growth inhibition, usually in a dose-dependent manner.
> - Substantial overlapping toxicity may result from combination regimens.
> - Bone marrow suppression and peripheral blood cytopenias are the most common and dose-limiting toxicities of the chemotherapy agents used in treatment of hematologic malignancies. Severe myelosuppression can occur in patients with decreased marrow reserve (e.g., old age, myelodysplasia, previous chemotherapy or radiotherapy).
> - A thorough evaluation of comorbid conditions is necessary in order to avoid additional toxicities with the use of chemotherapy (e.g., vinca alkaloid neurotoxicity in patients with diabetes or hereditary neurologic disease, use of anthracyclines or arsenic trioxide in patients with preexisting cardiac dysfunction, bleomycin in the presence of pulmonary disease or chest irradiation).
> - Better control of toxicities through use of growth factors, antiemetic agents, and antibiotics may allow for increased dose intensity of chemotherapeutic regimens.

INTRODUCTION

Whereas newer targeted therapeutics for hematologic malignancies have specific and often unintended side effects, most chemotherapy agents for hematologic malignancies broadly target biologic processes of normal cells, with systemic toxicities. With cytotoxic chemotherapeutic agents, actively proliferating cells in the bone marrow, gastrointestinal epithelium, hair follicles, and gonads are particularly susceptible to inhibition of growth, but idiosyncratic reactions can occur virtually in any organ system. This chapter reviews commonly encountered toxicities of chemotherapy, along with their treatment.

CUTANEOUS TOXICITY

Skin and mucosal membranes are particularly susceptible to the side effects of chemotherapy by virtue of their rapid rate of division. Common toxicities include alopecia, either of anagen (active mitotic growth phase) or telogen effluvium (dormancy phase) types, and stomatitis. Severe anagen alopecia usually occurs within 2 weeks of drug administration, and is commonly seen with anthracyclines, alkylating agents, and nitrosoureas; it is reversible after discontinuation of chemotherapy. Various patterns of pigmentation in the nails, skin, and mucous membranes are most commonly produced by anthracyclines and alkylating agents.[1] Characteristically, busulfan can induce a generalized cutaneous darkening, similar in aspect to Addison's disease ("busulfan tan"),[2] while bleomycin has been associated with flagellate hyperpigmentation,[3] and hydroxyurea has a predilection for pigmentation of traumatized zones. Nail involvement commonly manifests as pigmentation or Mees' lines after treatment with anthracyclines (Fig. 90–1*A*),[4] as transverse leukonychia after chemotherapy treatment for Hodgkin's disease,[5] or as its variant Beau's lines (onychomadesis) during treatment of lymphoma or Hodgkin's disease.[6,7] Moreover, a phenomenon of photo-onycholysis has been described after the use of 6-mercaptopurine.[8]

Photosensitivity reactions consist of painful erythema, pruritus, edema, and occasional desquamation and blistering, of a sunburn-like appearance, distributed in the sun-exposed areas. A particular photoreactivation phenomenon ("ultraviolet recall") is associated with methotrexate,[9] in which enhancement of a prior sunburn occurs 1–3 days after the ultraviolet light exposure, at a

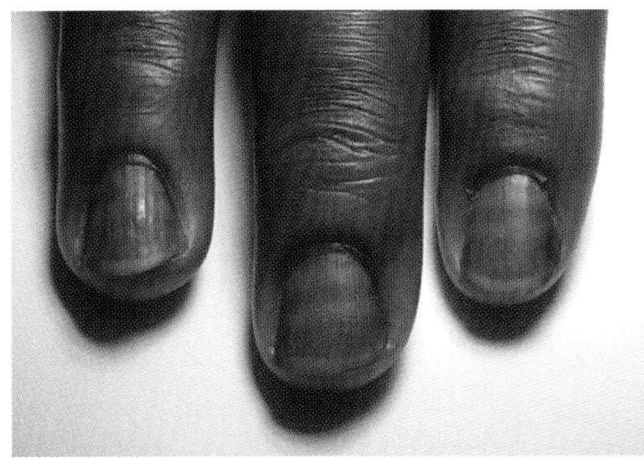

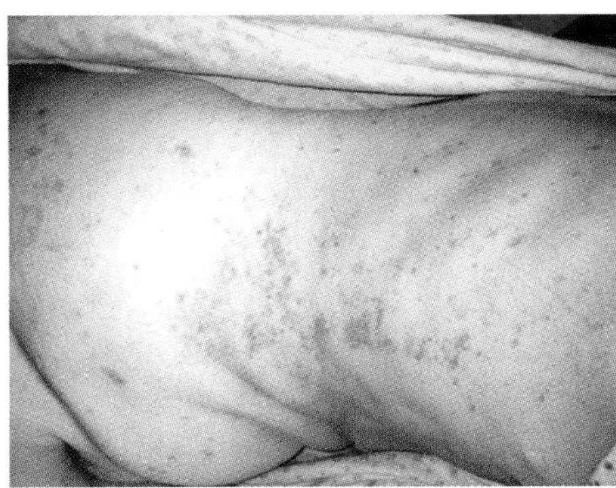

Figure 90–1. *A,* Nail changes after administration of cyclical doxorubicin/cyclophosphamide. *B,* Morbilliform rash after topotecan given for myelodysplasia.

TABLE 90–1. Chemotherapy Agents Producing Phototoxicity, Radiation Recall, and Radiation Enhancement

Agents Causing Phototoxicity	Agents Causing Radiation Enhancement	Agents Causing Radiation Recall
Dacarbazine	Bleomycin	Arsenic trioxide
Doxorubicin	Chlorambucil	Bleomycin
Hydroxyurea	Cyclophosphamide	CCNU
Methotrexate	Doxorubicin	Cyclophosphamide
Procarbazine	Etoposide	Cytarabine
Thioguanine	Hydroxyurea	Daunorubicin
Vinblastine	Interferon	Doxorubicin
	6-Mercaptopurine	Etoposide
	Methotrexate	Hydroxyurea
		Idarubicin
		Melphalan
		Methotrexate
		Vinblastine

time when the initial erythema starts to subside. Augmentation of radiation toxicity by concurrent or within 7 days administration of chemotherapy is commonly referred to as radiation enhancement, but a delayed effect of radiation recall, most commonly described with the use of anthracyclines,[10] manifests as an inflammatory dermatitis. Both can extend to unirradiated surrounding skin.[11] Photosensitivity also occurs after treatment with photodynamic agents, or psoralen plus ultraviolet A light (Table 90–1).

The hand-foot syndrome consists of involvement of palms and soles with edema and erythematous plaques associated with a burning sensation (acral erythema). Most cases occur in adults with lymphoma and acute myeloid leukemia (AML),[12–15] commonly associated with doxorubicin and high-dose cytarabine administration. Other less common toxicities occurring after the use of chemotherapy agents are listed in Table 90–2. Occasional reports describe the occurrence of telangiectasia with carmustine and hydroxyurea,[16] erythema nodosum with busulfan,[17] exfoliative dermatitis with methotrexate and busulfan/chlorambucil,[18] or furunculosis with methotrexate.[19] A particular acneiform rash is associated with gefitinib, a small molecule tyrosine kinase inhibitor; cetuximab, an endothelial growth factor antibody; and imatinib, a small molecule inhibitor of bcr/abl tyrosine kinase.

Extravasation occurs in up to 5% of chemotherapy infusions. Based on their local destructive potential, chemotherapeutic agents can be classified into irritants (e.g., producing pain, inflammation, or phlebitis) and vesicants (e.g., having the potential to induce more severe and permanent damage, such as necrosis). Lesions produced by vesicants can manifest immediately after the extravasation takes place, or be delayed for many days. With a significant amount of extravasation, a vesicant agent can produce ulceration, necrosis, and eschars.[20]

CUTANEOUS AND SYSTEMIC HYPERSENSITIVITY REACTIONS

Hypersensitivity or allergic reactions (HSRs), such as rash, urticaria, angioedema, or contact dermatitis, may occur with almost all the chemotherapy drugs, with the notable exception of nitrosoureas (Table 90–3). Such reactions are relatively commonly associated with the use of natural products and derivatives such as L-asparaginase and paclitaxel (Taxol), but may also be seen during administration of teniposide, etoposide, cisplatin, and procarbazine. Occasionally, alterations in hemodynamics and wheezing, dyspnea, or back pain can occur. Type I reactions are the most common, frequently occurring within 60 minutes of chemotherapy administration.[21] The incidence of HSRs is similar between the *Escherichia coli* and *Erwinia* types of L-asparaginase, with an estimated risk of 4–8% per individual dose, progressively increasing with the number of doses.[22,23] However, pegasparaginase is less immunogenic; the incidence of HSRs is 13%, but the reactions are less severe.[24,25] Although recommended by the manufacturer, administration of a test dose or skin testing has a poor positive and negative predictive value.[23,26] With repeated use of cytarabine, patients can develop an acute "flulike" syndrome characterized by fever, chills, arthralgias, myalgias, macular rash, conjunctivitis, and, uncommonly, hypotension, known as "cytarabine syndrome."[27] "Cytarabine lung" may also occur, with pulmonary infiltrates and an acute respiratory distress syndrome.

Infusion of monoclonal antibodies is even more frequently accompanied by HSRs, which usually present as mild, transient, nonallergic phenomena produced by

TABLE 90–2. Agents Producing Acral Erythema, Flushing, Inflammation of Keratosis, Neutrophilic Eccrine Hidradenitis, Eccrine Squamous Syringometaplasia, and Eruption of Lymphocyte Recovery

Agents Causing Acral Erythema	Agents Causing Flushing	Agents Causing Inflammation of Keratosis*	Agents Causing Neutrophilic Eccrine Hidradenitis†	Agents Causing Eccrine Squamous Syringometaplasia‡	Agents Causing Eruption of Lymphocyte Recovery§
Cisplatin	Asparaginase	Cisplatin	Bleomycin	BCNU	Cytarabine
Cyclophosphamide	BCNU	Cytarabine	CCNU	Busulfan	Daunorubicin
Cytarabine	Bleomycin	Dacarbazine	Chlorambucil	Cisplatin	Etoposide
Daunorubicin	Carboplatin	Doxorubicin	Cyclophosphamide	Cyclophosphamide	
Doxorubicin	Carmustine	Pentostatin	Cytarabine	Cytarabine	
Etoposide	Cisplatin	Vincristine	Doxorubicin	Doxorubicin	
Hydroxyurea	Cyclophosphamide		Mitoxantrone	Etoposide	
Idarubicin	Dacarbazine			Methotrexate	
Melphalan	Doxorubicin				
6-Mercaptopurine	Etoposide				
Methotrexate	Procarbazine				
Vincristine	Teniposide				

*Selective inflammation of actinic and seborrheic keratoses.
†Erythematous or violaceous macules, papules, nodules, plaques, or pustules on the trunk, limbs, neck, or head occurring 2 days to 2 weeks after chemotherapy.
‡Squamous metaplasia of the eccrine glands in the dermis, manifested by macules, papules, vesicles, or plaques occurring 2 days to 6 weeks after chemotherapy.
§Rash caused by lymphocyte recovery 1–3 weeks after chemotherapy suppression in patients with acute leukemia.

TABLE 90–3. Hypersensitivity Reactions

Type I			
Itching, urticaria, angioedema	L-Asparaginase Bleomycin Busulfan Carboplatin Chlorambucil Cisplatin Cyclophosphamide	Cytarabine Daunorubicin Doxorubicin Epirubicin Etoposide Filgrastim Mechlorethamine	Melphalan Methotrexate Mitoxantrone Procarbazine Sargramostim Teniposide Vincristine
Localized urticaria	Doxorubicin	Epirubicin	Idarubicin
Type II			
Hemolytic anemia	Carboplatin	Cisplatin Chlorambucil	Interferon alfa Teniposide
Type III			
Cutaneous vasculitis	Busulfan Cyclophosphamide Cytarabine	Hydroxyurea 6-Mercaptopurine	Methotrexate Mitoxantrone
Erythema multiforme	Busulfan Bleomycin Cisplatin Chlorambucil	Cyclophosphamide Etoposide Hydroxyurea Imatinib	Mechlorethamine Methotrexate Vinblastine
Pneumonitis	Methotrexate	Rituximab	
Type IV			
Allergic contact dermatitis	Cisplatin (T) Daunorubicin (T)	Doxorubicin (T)	Mechlorethamine (T)
Nonspecific			
Exanthematous drug rashes	Bleomycin Bortezomib Carboplatin Chlorambucil Cyclophosphamide Cytarabine Etoposide	Gefitinib Hydroxyurea Idarubicin Imatinib Methotrexate Mitoxantrone	Pentostatin Procarbazine Thalidomide 6-Thioguanine Thiotepa Vincristine
Toxic epidermal necrolysis	L-Asparaginase Bleomycin Chlorambucil	Cytarabine Doxorubicin Methotrexate	Procarbazine Thalidomide Rituximab
Infusion-related reactions	Alemtuzumab	Gemtuzumab	Rituximab

Abbreviation: T, topical.

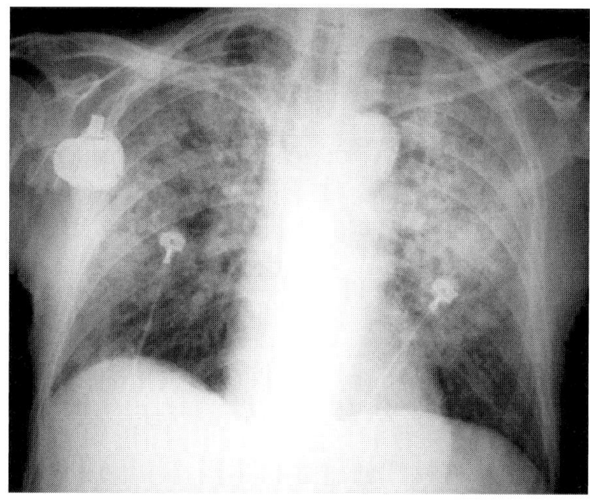

Figure 90–2. Hypersensitivity pneumonitis (HP) complicated by alveolar hemorrhage, after treatment with rituximab.

cytokine release as a result of antigen-antibody interaction on the surface of leukocytes. Murine antibodies, humanized murine antibodies, and human antibodies, including human intravenous immunoglobulin, all are associated with a variety of HSRs. Severe, life-threatening reactions can occur, including organ failure. In some instances, the intensity of the HSR is difficult to differentiate from manifestations of tumor lysis syndrome, and the two may overlap early during the first treatment doses, perhaps because of a high tumoral burden.[28] If the innate hypersensitivity axis is not suppressed with prednisone or dexamethasone and diphenhydramine (Benadryl), as is recommended, many patients treated with rituximab would experience an acute hypersensitivity reaction consisting of flulike symptoms (fever, chills, itching, urticaria, rash, nasal congestion) within the first 2 hours of the infusion, but shortness of breath, bronchospasm with wheezing, or hypotension can occasionally develop.[29] Rarely, lung interstitial disease (Fig. 90–2), sometimes progressing to adult respiratory distress syndrome[30] and cardiogenic shock, can occur.[31] Cutaneous hypersensitivity can occur in the form of Stevens-Johnson syndrome and toxic epidermal necrolysis,[32] and Schamberg's disease has also been described.[33] Similar acute flulike reactions develop in up to 90% of patients during infusion of alemtuzumab, despite premedication, but these HSRs diminish in intensity and often do not recur after the first 2 weeks of treatment.[34] Subcutaneous administration is associated with a decreased incidence and severity of events.[35] Fever and chills, which can be accompanied by signs of hemodynamic instability, occur commonly during or after the infusion of gemtuzumab[36,37]; however, severe anaphylaxis and cases of adult respiratory distress syndrome are rarely observed.

MYELOTOXICITY AND OTHER HEMATOLOGIC COMPLICATIONS

Bone marrow suppression and blood cytopenias represent the most common toxicity of the cytotoxic agents used to treat hematologic malignancies. The acute interaction between chemotherapy agents and hematopoietic cell lines commonly results in different degrees of suppression, generally more severe in patients with a preexisting decreased marrow reserve (old age, myelodysplasia, previous use of chemotherapy), and peripheral macrocytosis is very common with the antimetabolites, such as methotrexate, and with hydroxyurea.[38,39] The most frequent and dose-limiting form of myelotoxicity is granulocytopenia, followed by thrombocytopenia.[40,41] Agents associated with renal toxicity, such as cisplatin and carboplatin, reduce erythropoietic production, resulting in anemia.[42–45] Supportive treatment with blood product transfusions and use of growth factors, predominantly granulocyte colony-stimulating factor and erythropoietin, either first- or second-generation long-acting agents, are commonly used to treat chemotherapy-induced cytopenias. Following an episode of severe cytopenia, use of pharmacologic doses of hematopoietic growth factors is indicated, but treatment may also require chemotherapeutic drug dose delay or dose reduction. However, for curative-intent treatment, dose delivery should be preserved. The time interval between drug exposure and maximal myelosuppression varies with the class of agents. It is typically 6–12 days for anthracyclines and cyclophosphamide, but may be delayed to 3–5 weeks for temozolomide and nitrosoureas, such as carmustine (BCNU). For cell cycle–specific agents, such as methotrexate and cytarabine, the myelosuppression occurs earlier, usually within 3–5 days. Methotrexate myelotoxicity is largely prevented or reduced by leucovorin administration within 48 hours. However, modest benefit may also occur using amifostine after cyclophosphamide.[46,47]

Factor IX Specifics of Cytokine Use

Imatinib can also cause cytopenias by interfering with proliferative STAT (signal transducers and activators of transcription), Raf, and other cytokine receptor signaling. Although typically mild, dose-related pancytopenia can occur, especially in patients with marrow fibrosis. It can also occur early on in treatment of chronic myelogenous leukemia.

Secondary Myelodysplastic Syndrome and AML

Delayed development of myelodysplastic syndrome and AML[48–73] are the result of DNA-damaging chemotherapy. These secondary malignancies are discussed in detail in Chapter 29.

Thrombosis and Hemostasis Disorders

Mild coagulation abnormalities, consisting in deficiencies of factors IX and XI and a decrease in serum fibrinogen, are relatively frequently caused by treatment with L-asparaginase,[74,75] which less often causes bleeding. However, during L-asparaginase treatment, maintaining the fibrinogen level over 100 mg/dL with the use if human cryoprecipitate is recommended. A deficiency in antithrombin III caused by L-asparaginase has been related to the development of thrombosis.[76]

Although most commonly reported with the use of fludarabine for chronic lymphocytic leukemia (CLL),[77,78] immune-mediated hemolytic anemia and thrombocytopenia may occur and respond poorly to steroids. Hemolytic anemia can also occur with interferon preparations,[79] cisplatin,[80] 2-chlorodeoxyadenosine,[81] and monoclonal antibodies (rituximab).[82] Drug discontinuation will help resolve the active cell destruction, although antibodies to either red cells or platelets may circulate for a prolonged period, likely as a result of immune dysfunction.

Drug-Induced Immunosuppression

A particular concern is development of immunosuppression after both cytotoxic and targeted therapies. Although most of the chemotherapy agents that cause myelosuppression are associated with variable grades of immunosuppression, alkylating agents and antimetabolites have more pronounced effects. Fludarabine is associated with opportunistic fungal, viral, parasitic, and mycobacterial infections, as a result of myelosuppression and alterations in T-cell subsets. In a retrospective review of 402 patients, 49% developed infections, with *Pneumocystis jiroveci* (*carinii*) infection or listeriosis occurring in up to 7% of patients on fludarabine and prednisone. Cutaneous zoster developed in 26% of the patients with a CD4 count of less than 50/μL.[83] Similarly, treatment with bortezomib was followed by an 11% rate of development of herpes zoster.[84] Patients treated with these agents should receive antifungal and antimicrobial prophylaxis.

There is also a high degree of immunosuppression with the newer agents. Rituximab, an anti-CD20 antibody, induces a B-cell depletion in all patients that is sometimes profound. Courses of treatment are often associated with decreased serum immunoglobulins, sometimes to below the normal range. These processes should be periodically monitored given the variable patient response. Although the incidence of infections does not appear to be significantly increased, 31% of patients have been reported to have infections, of which 19% were bacterial, 10% viral, and 1% fungal, with only 2% serious events.[85] Such patients are also often given antifungal and antimicrobial prophylaxis. Unusual viral infections, such as progressive multifocal leukoencephalopathy and cytomegalovirus, have been reported in association with the use of rituximab in the peritransplant period.[86] Most importantly, reactivation of hepatitis B has been reported, and it is advisable to identify patients with prior hepatitis B infection and use prophylaxis in this cohort as well. Combining immunosuppressive agents can lead to more profound risk of infections, as evidenced by the documentation of a higher incidence of infections (44% vs. 29%) seen in patients with CLL treated with concurrent as opposed to sequential administration of fludarabine and rituximab.[87] Alemtuzumab is associated with infection in up to 45% of cases, and gemtuzumab produces lymphopenia and infection in up to 30%, including opportunistic infections, sepsis, pneumonia, and herpes simplex virus infection. Because of these risks, prophylaxis is recommended with antifungal, anti-*Pneumocystis*, and antiviral agents tailored to the patient and the treatment regimen.

CARDIOTOXICITY

Cardiac toxicity is most commonly a complication of anthracycline treatment and occasionally is seen with high doses of cyclophosphamide. An acute form of anthracycline toxicity consists of electrocardiographic changes, rhythm disturbances, and immediate ventricular dysfunction,[88] but is usually transitory, and therefore cardiac monitoring during infusion is only indicated for patients with symptoms or a history of cardiac disease. Rare cases of cardiac death have been reported and likely reflect a predisposition to DNA damage from a genetic polymorphism.[89] A cumulative dose-related cardiomyopathy occurs, and is commonly, but not always, irreversible (Fig. 90–3). Clinical heart failure occurs in 3%, 7%, and 18% of patients receiving doxorubicin at cumulative doses of 400, 550, and 700 mg/m^2, respectively,[90] but a higher incidence of up to 62% of subclinical heart disease has been detected using exercise stress radionuclide ventriculography.[91] Prior radiation increases the incidence and reduces the dose at which cardiotoxicity can be seen.[92] Mortality secondary to progressive heart failure can occur.[93,94] The overall incidence and severity is less with regimens utilizing prolonged continuous infusions of anthracyclines.[93] Although the co-administration of the antioxidant dexrazoxane is clearly associated with a decrease in cardiotoxicity in nonhematologic malignancies,[95,96] concerns were raised regarding interference with the efficacy of antineoplastic therapy.[97] Idarubicin was estimated to have a 0.53 relative cardiotoxicity comparative to rapid-infusion doxorubicin,[98] and a total cumulative dose of 150 mg/m^2 appeared to be safe in acute leukemia and myelodysplasia patients without previous use of anthracyclines.[99] Daunorubicin-related cardiotoxicity was estimated to be 0.75 on a dose-equivalent basis compared to doxorubicin, based on small numbers of patients.[98] Mitoxantrone appears to have a relative cardiotoxicity of 0.5 compared to rapid-infusion doxorubicin, equivalent with the 96-hour continuous infusion of doxorubicin.[100]

Acute cardiomyopathy can occur with high doses of cyclophosphamide. A severe hemorrhagic form[101] has been reported in patients receiving individual rather than cumulative doses of 5–6 gm/m^2, and can be fatal, whereas the milder forms undergo clinical progression infrequently.[102] Other agents are associated with other forms of cardiac toxicity. Prolongation of the Q-Tc interval and arrhythmias, including ventricular tachycardia, have been observed during treatment with arsenic trioxide.[103] Bortezomib bolus infusion results in mild to moderate hypotension in 12% of patients, but rare arrhythmic and ischemic episodes have been reported.[84] A reversible bradycardia has been reported with thalidomide, as have instances of complete heart block.[104] Development of myocardial ischemia is uncommon, and has occasionally been described in patients receiving cisplatin, bleomycin,

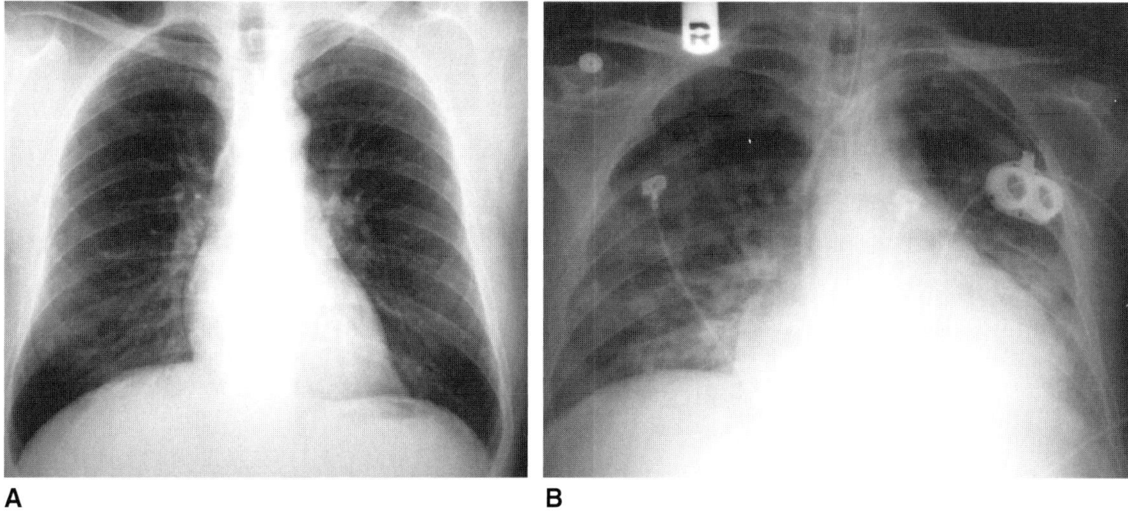

Figure 90–3. Cardiac silhouette *(A)* before treatment with anthracyclines, and *(B)* after treatment, corresponding to the development of intractable congestive heart failure.

cyclophosphamide, vinca alkaloids, and etoposide.[105–110] Acute myocardial infarction occurs most frequently in patients with preexisting coronary artery disease or coronary risk factors, but occasional coronary events were reported in patients with normal angiograms and no risk factors.[111] Prior mediastinal radiation appears to play an important role, particularly in patients with lymphoma.[112]

PULMONARY TOXICITY

Lung toxicity during and following chemotherapy has a complex etiology and clinical course. Some instances are due to direct cytotoxicity, others to oxygen-induced exacerbation of DNA damage, and others to immune responses, cytokine and chemokine recruitment of inflammatory cells, and synergistic toxicity following radiation. A syndrome of chronic pulmonary fibrosis is a final common pathway associated with lung injury. Bleomycin-induced pulmonary fibrosis occurs in up to 10% of patients,[113] and, although dose related, can occur at doses of only 100 mg/m^2.[114] Exposure to high concentrations of oxygen, age, radiation, and the use of growth factors may act synergistically in triggering bleomycin-associated lung injury. Symptoms of dry cough, exertional dyspnea, low-grade fever, and chest pain develop insidiously or acutely, with patchy pulmonary infiltrates that may be progressive and even lead to pulmonary failure.[113] Early use of steroids and avoidance of supplemental oxygen, if possible, can limit the degree of progression and, if the condition is recognized early, may lead to substantial improvement.

Other chemotherapeutic agents also cause acute and chronic pulmonary toxicity. With methotrexate, an acute pulmonary fibrosis resembling hypersensitivity pneumonitis occurs, predominantly involving the lung bases. Rash and eosinophilia are commonly present,[115] and the use of steroids appears to be beneficial. Acute pulmonary fibrosis also results from cyclophosphamide. With all-*trans* retinoic acid treatment of acute promyelocytic leukemia, pulmonary infiltrates can occur with fever, shortness of breath, and hypoxemia, either alone or as the presenting symptoms of retinoic acid syndrome.[116] Carmustine (BCNU) is associated with the occurrence of cumulative pulmonary inflammation followed by pulmonary fibrosis. After high-dose therapy administered prior to autologous stem cell transplantation for lymphoma, BCNU may result in development of late-onset fibrosis, especially in doses exceeding 475 mg/m^2.[117] Ground-glass infiltrates are predominantly present in the subpleural regions. Early prophylaxis with pulsed steroids can prevent the syndrome, and early treatment with steroids results in decreased morbidity and mortality.[118] The pulmonary fibrosis generated by busulfan is of late onset and appears to be independent of the dose administered. Other rare causes of chronic pulmonary fibrosis are ifosfamide,[119,120] fludarabine,[121] 6-mercaptopurine,[122] chlorambucil, and melphalan.[123]

Hypersensitivity pneumonitis occurs with a variety of chemotherapeutic agents and appears not to be dose related; it can occur either early or late during the course of treatment. It manifests as sudden-onset shortness of breath, cough, and fever and should be anticipated even after initial doses of treatment. On radiographs, mediastinal and hilar lymphadenopathy are common but ground-glass appearance can occur as well.[124] Most commonly, the drugs associated with idiosyncratic hypersensitivity pneumonitis are bleomycin, used for lymphomas; methotrexate maintenance treatment for leukemia[125]; and procarbazine, fludarabine, and rituximab, used for lymphomas and CLL (see Fig. 90–2).[33]

Other rare complications of chemotherapy include bronchiolitis obliterans with organizing pneumonia, which has been rarely recognized in relation with cytarabine treatment,[126] and formation of lung nodules, which can result sporadically from the use of bleomycin.[127] A vascular leak syndrome has been proposed as the etiology of noncardiogenic pulmonary edema produced by doxorubicin and, more commonly, by high-dose cytarabine in leukemia.[128]

GASTROINTESTINAL TOXICITY

Prior to the use of potent antiemetics, acute nausea and vomiting were commonly observed after administration of cisplatin, mechlorethamine, anthracyclines, and dacarbazine, often in a dose-dependent fashion. Other drugs induce variable degrees of nausea, including cyclophosphamide, 5-azacytadine, L-asparaginase, methotrexate, etoposide, bleomycin, and vincristine. The efficacy of antiemetic therapy in hematologic malignancies is summarized in Table 90–4.

Diarrhea is common after the use of methotrexate, cytarabine, and cisplatin.[141] The mainstay of treatment is the use of selective opiates (e.g., loperamide),[142] along with maintenance of bowel rest and adequate hydration; more refractory cases usually benefit from the use of octreotide, kaolin, or anticholinergics. Constipation, sometimes severe, often occurs as a noncumulative toxicity after vinca alkaloids, and is more severe after individual doses exceeding 2 mg.[143] Up to 60% of myeloma patients treated with thalidomide at maximum doses develop constipation, although administration of 200 mg/day produces it in one third of cases.[144] Instances of intestinal obstruction have been reported with the use of bortezomib[84] and imatinib.[145]

Mucositis is common after treatment with cytotoxic agents that are designed to ablate the marrow or cytoreduce lymphomas and leukemias and myeloma. Mucositis is very common in the settings of high-dose therapy for leukemia and preparative regimens for stem cell transplantation.[146] The drugs causing mucositis include methotrexate, cytarabine, doxorubicin, etoposide, mechlorethamine, cisplatin, carboplatin, melphalan, busulfan, thiotepa, and procarbazine. Maximal mucosal damage is usually seen 4–10 days after the agent is administrated, often during severe neutropenia and exacerbated by bacterial overgrowth.[147] A frequent complication of chemotherapy for acute leukemias, especially after high-dose cytarabine, is neutropenic enterocolitis; when it occurs in the terminal ileum, it is termed *typhlitis*. Clinical symptoms include fever, abdominal pain, and diarrhea. This condition can be associated with a 50–68% mortality rate.[148] Medical management consists of bowel rest and appropriate use of systemic antibiotics and antifungals. Early surgical management may be required in patients who do not respond quickly because of the potential for bowel perforation.[149]

Although uncommon, acute pancreatitis can occur with the use of L-asparaginase in the treatment of acute lymphocytic leukemia (ALL), or after high-dose cytarabine or steroids, or with 6-mercaptopurine, ifosfamide, or cisplatin. Conservative management consists of bowel rest, analgesics, and hydration. If pancreatitis is seen with L-asparaginase, it is standard to discontinue treatment.

TABLE 90–4. Efficacy of Antiemetic Drugs or Combinations in Treatment of Malignancy

Drug	Efficacy
Dexamethasone	48% PR with cisplatin administration[129]
HiD Metoclopramide	42% CR or near-CR of cisplatin-induced emesis[130]
	30% vs. 0% CR of emesis with low-dose vs. high-dose cisplatin administration[131]
	40% PR with cisplatin[129]
HiD Metoclopramide + dexamethasone	67% CR of cisplatin-induced emesis[132]
	25% CR over 5 days in NHL patients treated with CHOP[133]
Metoclopramide, dexamethasone + lorazepam or diphenhydramine	60% CR in cisplatin-induced emesis; 83% ≤ 2 emetic episodes[134]
Granisetron	70% CR of cisplatin-induced emesis P gi 27[135]
	89.5% CR of vomiting in patients with hematopoietic malignancies[135]
	66% CR × 24 hours for moderately emetogenic cyclophosphamide-based ALL therapy in children[136]
Granisetron + dexamethasone	75% CR of N/V over 5 days in NHL patients treated with CHOP[133]
Ondansetron	75% CR or near-CR of cisplatin-induced emesis[130]
	65% vs. 20% CR with low-dose vs. high-dose cisplatin[131]
	45.5% CR × 24 hours for moderately emetogenic cyclophosphamide-based ALL therapy in children[136]
	68.6% CR during moderately emetogenic chemotherapy[137]
Ondansetron + dexamethasone	91% CR of cisplatin-induced emesis
Ondansetron + methylprednisolone	46% CR of emesis × 3 days in treatment of hematologic malignancies and breast cancer[138]
Ondansetron + methylprednisolone + lorazepam	69% CR of emesis × 3 days in treatment of hematologic malignancies and breast cancer[138]
Palonosetron	81% CR during moderately emetogenic chemotherapy[137]
	40–50% complete control × 24 hours during highly emetogenic therapy[139]
Aprepitant	63–73% CR of emesis with highly emetogenic chemotherapy (review of 3 randomized studies)[140]

Abbreviations: ALL, acute lymphocytic leukemia; CHOP, cyclophosphamide, doxorubicin, vincristine, and prednisone; CR, complete response; HiD, high-dose; NHL, non-Hodgkin's lymphoma; N/V, nausea and vomiting; PR, partial response.

HEPATOTOXICITY

The majority of hepatotoxic reactions produced by chemotherapy agents are idiosyncratic drug sensitivities with evidence of acute toxic hepatitis. Dose-dependent hepatotoxicity also occurs, as does veno-occlusive disease of the liver.[150] A summary of the hepatotoxic effects of chemotherapy agents and combinations of drugs for hematologic malignancies is presented in Table 90–5. Because these agents may need to be given in the setting of liver disease, Table 90–6 summarizes the dose reductions commonly employed with the use of chemotherapy agents in the presence of liver dysfunction.

Significant hepatotoxicity results from the utilization of antimetabolites. In one study, high doses of methotrexate in the treatment of ALL were associated with a reversible elevation of hepatic transaminases in all

TABLE 90–5. Hepatic Toxicities* of Chemotherapy Agents

Transaminitis	Cholestasis	Fibrosis/Steatosis	Necrosis	VOD
Cyclophosphamide+	Chlorambucil+	Chlorambucil+	Busulfan+	BCNU+ (HiD)
Doxo/epirubicin+	Cytarabine+ (HiD)		Chlorambucil+	Busulfan+ (HiD)
Etoposide+ (HiD)	Doxo/epirubicin+	L-asparaginase+++	Cyclophosphamide+	Cyclophosphamide+ (HiD)
Hydroxyurea+	Etoposide+ (HiD)	Methotrexate+++	Etoposide+	Cytarabine+
Melphalan+ (HiD)	6-Mercaptopurine+ (HiD)		Methotrexate+	Dacarbazine+
6-Mercaptopurine+ (HiD)	Mitoxantrone+		Vincristine+ (with RT)	6-Mercaptopurine+
Mitoxantrone+	BCNU++ (HiD)			
Vincristine+	L-asparaginase++			
BCNU++ (HiD)				
L-asparaginase++				
Cytarabine+++ (HiD)				
Methotrexate+++ (HiD)				

*Likelihood of toxicity: +, low; ++, medium; +++, high.
Abbreviations: HiD, high-dose; RT, radiotherapy.

TABLE 90–6. Dose Reductions for Commonly Used Agents in Patients with Hepatic Dysfunction

Agent	Bilirubin 1.5–3 mg/dL AST 2–4× normal	Bilirubin 3.1–5 mg/dL AST >4× normal	Bilirubin >5 mg/dL
Cyclophosphamide	100%	75%	Hold
Daunorubicin	75%	50%	Hold
Doxorubicin	50%	25%	Hold
Epirubicin	50%	25%	Hold
Etoposide	50%	25% or Hold	Hold
Methotrexate	100%	75%	Hold
Vinca alkaloids	50%	25% or Hold	Hold

Dose reductions based on Shrier and colleagues,[151] Anderson and colleagues,[152] *Physicians' Desk Reference*,[153] Dobbs and colleagues,[154] and King and Perry.[155,156]

patients, exceeding 300 IU/L in 92% of cases.[157] Furthermore, maintenance therapy for acute leukemia with long-term use of oral methotrexate is associated with a high incidence of liver fibrosis and cirrhosis,[158] and sporadic cases of hepatocellular carcinoma have occurred in the setting of hepatic fibrosis after methotrexate treatment for ALL.[159]

Hepatic veno-occlusive disease is a known complication of autologous bone marrow transplantation, with a frequency of 10–15%. It consists of nonthrombotic obliteration of the small hepatic veins,[160] and manifests clinically by hepatomegaly, ascites, and abdominal pain. Although most cases are reversible with supportive care, the potential to progress toward fatal liver necrosis is present. Most cases appear to be drug induced, occurring in the setting of autologous bone marrow transplantation,[161,162] although acute graft-versus-host disease can produce an indistinguishable picture. Different combinations used for transplantation, especially those including high-dose cyclophosphamide[163] and busulfan,[164] but also conventional doses of 6-thioguanine,[165] cytarabine, or dacarbazine, have been implicated. Reports of hepatic veno-occlusive disease are increasing in frequency with the use of with gemtuzumab therapy for AML.[166]

NEUROTOXICITY

Peripheral neuropathy is commonly encountered with the use of systemic chemotherapy, because peripheral nerves lack the protective effect of the blood-brain barrier. Both motor and sensory fibers can be involved. Sensory neuropathy is the usual presenting complaint, with a "stocking-and-glove" distribution in the extremities associated with the sensation that the patient is feeling through a "wad of cotton." Progressive neuropathy is associated with pain, decreased sensation, and a burning dysesthesia.

Vincristine disrupts the microtubules and transport processes within axons, resulting in a dose-limiting sensory and motor neuropathy, which particularly affects the small sensory fibers. Most patients treated with vincristine experience neurotoxicity, but severe symptoms occur more commonly in older patients, those with prior radiation to an extremity, or use of growth factors.[167] Loss of deep tendon reflexes is a sign of cumulative toxicity. Transient cranial neuropathies can involve the oculomotor, optic, facial, or auditory nerves, and some patients experience jaw pain lasting for several days.[168] Symptoms of autonomic neuropathy are seen in up to half of patients treated with vincristine, especially colicky abdominal pain and/or constipation, but postural hypotension, bladder atonia, and impotence also can develop. A paralytic ileus can develop,[169] especially in children and the elderly.

The other vinca alkaloids, such as vinblastine and vindesine, have less neurotoxicity, often manifested by lower extremity muscle pain and jaw cramps.[170] A particular type of neurotoxicity is produced by cisplatin, secondary to accumulation in the dorsal root ganglions, and is dose related; peripheral nerve fibers are less affected.[171] As a result of principal involvement of large myelinated sensory fibers,[172] alterations in deep tendon reflexes and proprioceptive sensation dominate the clinical picture, with relative preservation of temperature

TABLE 90–7. Common Neurologic Complications of Commonly Used Chemotherapy Agents

Agent	Neuropathy	Myelopathy	Acute Encephalopathy	Chronic Encephalopathy	Aseptic Meningitis	Seizures	Cerebellar Syndrome
Asparaginase			+			+	
5-Azathioprine	+		+				
BCNU	+ (CN)		+	+		+	
Bortezomib	++	+				+	
Busulfan						+++ (HiD)	
Cisplatin	+++ (HiD), + (LD), + (CN)	+	+			+	
Cytarabine	+	+ (IT)	+ (HiD)		+ (IT)		++ (HiD)
Etoposide	+ (CN)		+			+	
Fludarabine	+		+	+ (HiD)			
Ifosfamide	+		+			+	
Interferon-α	+		+, ++ (IT)			+	
Mechlorethamine	+		+			+	
Methotrexate	+	+ (IT)	++ (HiD)	+	++ (IT)	+	
Procarbazine	+		+				+
Vinca alkaloids	+++, + (CN)		+ (IV), +++ (IT)			+	+

Abbreviations: CN, cranial neuropathy; HiD, high-dose; IT, intrathecal; IV, intravenous; LD, low-dose.

and pinprick sensation and motor strength. Autonomic neuropathy is uncommon,[168] and recovery of cisplatin-induced neuropathy is slow in the majority of patients. Insufficient data support the use of amifostine to prevent cisplatin neuropathy[173]; however, use of vitamin E in one study significantly reduced the neurotoxicity.[174] Ototoxicity is common with the use of cisplatin, is more severe in children, and manifests by tinnitus and a dose-dependent loss of hearing in the high frequencies in up to 20% of patients.

Neurotoxicity with other agents is also seen (Table 90–7). Cytarabine in high doses has rarely been associated with peripheral neuropathies similar to the Guillain-Barré syndrome, or cranial nerve dysfunction. A moderate peripheral neuropathy develops after high doses or prolonged administration of arsenic trioxide in up to 20% of patients.[175,176] Thalidomide causes an irreversible, predominantly sensory peripheral distal neuropathy, sometimes with a proprioceptive deficit, that appears dose related. It may be associated with lightheadedness and dysesthesias.[177] Bortezomib causes frequent sensory and occasionally motor neuropathy,[178] with up to 6% of patients discontinuing the medication because of neuropathy, although dose reduction often ameliorates the intensity of symptoms.[84] Central nervous system toxicity occurs with a number of agents. Long-term central nervous system toxicities have been observed mostly with high-dose therapy with agents that pass the blood-brain barrier and after intrathecal administration. Methotrexate in high systemic doses (more than 1 gm/m^2) may cause acute confusion, somnolence, and seizures that develop in the first 24 hours after administration.[168] A transient subacute strokelike picture with confusion and transient focal neurologic deficits has been described,[179] as has chronic leukoencephalopathy.[180] Intrathecal methotrexate can produce a myelopathy, but more commonly it results in the development of aseptic meningitis. Infrequent occurrences of sudden death, seizures, neurologic deficits, or acute encephalopathy have been reported often when both intrathecal and high-dose methotrexate are combined alone or in combination with brain irradiation. Treatment includes rapid cerebrospinal fluid drainage, ventriculolumbar perfusion, alkaline diuresis, and high-dose leucovorin rescue. Repeated high doses of parenteral cytarabine, exceeding 2–3 gm/m^2, as used in the treatment of AML, can cause acute cerebellar degeneration,[181] which is usually reversible but more likely in patients over the age of 50, or with liver and renal dysfunction.[182–184] Cisplatin is associated with development of Lhermitte's sign in up to 40% of patients, which usually resolves spontaneously within several months after discontinuing cisplatin, but a true myelopathy is extremely unusual.[168] A spontaneously resolving encephalopathy in up to 20% of patients occurs with the use of ifosfamide.[185] At high doses, BCNU may cause seizure and a subacute-onset encephalomyelopathy.[186] Thalidomide commonly produces somnolence in up to half of the patients taking it extensively, but tolerance usually develops after a couple of weeks.[177]

Less common neurotoxicity occurs with hydroxyurea, which at high doses can cause sedation, seizures, and confusion,[168] and with chlorambucil, which at high doses produces myoclonus with stiffness and encephalopathy.[187] Interferon alfa use has been associated with irritability, insomnia, somnolence, and confusion in up to 25% of patients and with severe depression during prolonged use. Intrathecal interferon can produce a transient acute reaction, with dizziness, vomiting, and headache, but occasionally a dose-dependent severe encephalopathy can develop.[188] Retinoic acid is an uncommon cause of pseudotumor cerebri,[189] especially in children.

OCULAR TOXICITY

Although the ocular side effects of chemotherapy are relatively rare, their evolution has the potential to lead to irreversible deficits. Perhaps most common is late-onset cataracts after steroid use. Cytarabine in high doses causes conjunctivitis, blurred vision, photophobia, and ocular pain, occurring several days after commencing the treatment.[190] Artificial tears and glucocorticoid eyedrops are effective in controlling this syndrome.[191] Furthermore, blepharoconjunctivitis can be caused by cyclophosphamide,[192] with blurring of vision manifested at doses of 750 mg/m^2.[193] Cataracts induced by busulfan occur probably as a direct effect on lens proliferating cells, at doses between 1 and 6 mg daily for several years.[194] Various degrees of retinopathy can be induced by nitrosoureas, from asymptomatic leaks of small retinal vessels to optical atrophy and progressive blindness,[195] and use of cyclosporine after bone marrow transplantation for ALL also can induce a retinopathy[196] and cortical blindness.[197] Optic neuroretinitis was reported in a myeloma patient treated with BCNU, procarbazine, and cyclophosphamide,[198] and progressive visual loss with nerve fiber-layer infarcts and intraretinal hemorrhages was noted following intravenous high-dose BCNU (800 mg/m^2), with autologous transplantation.[199] Ocular toxicities occur even more commonly with high-dose methotrexate therapy, consisting of blurring of vision, sensation of burning, and dryness.[200] Optic nerve atrophy occurred in patients with ALL who received methotrexate along with brain irradiation and intrathecal cytarabine.[201] Vinca alkaloids used in the treatment of leukemia commonly produce corneal hypoesthesia[202] and a reversible cranial neuritis,[203] and vincristine also produces optical neuropathy.[204]

RENAL TOXICITY

Acute renal failure usually occurs when cisplatin is used with inadequate hydration. A slower and delayed decrease in glomerular filtration can present with various degrees of renal dysfunction.[205] Dose-related hypomagnesemia resulting from a proximal tubule defect is common,[206] but hyponatremia and hypocalciuria can occasionally occur. Successful prophylaxis of cisplatin-induced nephropathy is accomplished by administering an appropriate level of hydration, usually 2.5–3 L of saline.[207] Late development of azotemia and proteinuria has been described in patients who received doses of at least 1 gm/m^2, with a considerable percentage of patients requiring hemodialysis.[208] High doses of methotrexate can produce acute nephrotoxicity by precipitating in the renal tubules, which is usually reversible in a couple of weeks.[209] Prevention of this condition can be accomplished by alkalinization of the urine, and methotrexate doses must be adjusted to the degree of preexisting renal insufficiency. Acute reversible hyponatremia occurs most frequently in patients receiving high-dose cyclophosphamide, apparently through an increased secretion of antidiuretic hormone.[210] The principal urologic complication of cyclophosphamide, however, is hemorrhagic cystitis. Treatment, as well as prevention, of cystitis involves frequent voiding, vigorous hydration, and bladder irrigation. Additional renal toxicity can result from the effects of ifosfamide on the proximal renal tubule, but cystitis can also develop. Mesna has been shown to reduce the incidence of hematuria with use of both drugs,[211,212] but appears to be ineffective against the tubular defect produced by ifosfamide.[213] Vincristine and cyclophosphamide can induce the syndrome of inappropriate secretion of antidiuretic hormone.[214] A proximal tubular defect can be produced by 5-azacytadine.[215] With interferon alfa, glomerular dysfunction can manifest as proteinuria and increase in serum creatinine, although interstitial toxicities can occur.[216] Dose adjustments for the degree of renal insufficiency are performed for several drugs.[217–220] No dose modifications are necessary for anthracyclines and mitoxantrone, vinca alkaloids, procarbazine, 6-mercaptopurine, and oral melphalan.

VASCULAR TOXICITY

Chemotherapy for lymphoma and myeloma is associated with a significant incidence of thrombotic and thromboembolic events (Table 90–8). Combinations of agents such as cyclophosphamide, doxorubicin, and etoposide, followed by cytarabine, bleomycin, vincristine, and methotrexate, can induce thrombosis,[221] with an incidence after treatment for Hodgkin's disease or non-Hodgkin's lymphoma of 6–13%[222,223]; the incidence with thalidomide may be 13–20% during treatment for myeloma. Treatment of lymphoma with combination chemotherapy may also result in thrombotic microangiopathy syndromes, occasionally after achievement of remission.[224,225] Thrombotic thrombocytopenic purpura and hemolytic-uremic syndrome have been reported after the use of cytarabine plus daunorubicin for AML,[226] after interferon alfa for chronic myelogenous leukemia,[227,228] and after high-dose therapy for transplantion.[229] A thrombotic thrombocytopenic purpura–like syndrome also is seen in patients receiving immunosuppressive agents such as cyclosporine and FK-506 after allogeneic transplantation.[229] Thrombotic microangiopathy has also been reported after bleomycin,[230] high-dose cisplatin,[231] or carboplatin[232] administration.

Pulmonary veno-occlusive disease is the result of a gradual obliteration of venules and veins in the lungs by collagenous or fibrinous tissue, with consequent development of pulmonary hypertension. IT has been reported with the use of etoposide, cyclophosphamide, and total-body irradiation for transplantation in hematologic malignancies,[233] with MOPP (mechlorethamine, vincristine, procarbazine, and prednisone) and COPP (cyclophosphamide, vincristine, procarbazine, and prednisone) for Hodgkin's disease,[234] and with bleomycin for lymphocytic lymphoma.[235]

GONADAL TOXICITY

In the testicle, germinal epithelium cells have a very high mitotic rate and thus are susceptible to the cytotoxicity of chemotherapy.[236–254] Therapy for hematologic malignancies has various effects on gonadal function, depending upon the age of the patient, cumulative dose, and individual agents employed. Although mechlorethamine is the most gonad-suppressive, other agents or combi-

TABLE 90–8. Vascular Complications of Chemotherapy Agents

Myocardial Ischemia & Infarction	Intravascular Thrombosis	Microangiopathic Hemolytic Anemia	Raynaud's Phenomenon	Pulmonary Veno-occlusive Disease	Hypertension	Hypotension	Vasculitis
Bleomycin	Bortezomib	Bleomycin	Bleomycin	BCNU	Bleomycin	BCNU	Ara-C
Bortezomib	Cyclophosphamide	Carboplatin	Cisplatin	Bleomycin	Cisplatin	Dacarbazine	Busulfan
Carboplatin	Doxorubicin	Cisplatin	Doxorubicin		Procarbazine	Etoposide	Hydroxyurea
Cisplatin	Methotrexate		Vincristine		Vinblastine	Teniposide	Methotrexate
Etoposide	Thalidomide		Vincristine			Vincristine	
Vinblastine	Vincristine					Thalidomide	
Vincristine							

nations of drugs are also variably gonadotoxic. In comparison with adults, prepubertal and pubertal males generally sustain less toxicity on the seminiferous tubules, and their endocrine function is only minimally altered. Adult males experience a marked impairment in spermatogenesis, more so with MOPP or MOPP-like regimens for Hodgkin's disease than with ABVD (doxorubicin, bleomycin, vinblastine, and dacarbazine).[251] Regimens omitting the procarbazine appear to be less toxic than COPP and MOPP[255] (see Chapter 40). More gonadal damage can be seen in non-Hodgkin's lymphoma patients, because the age at diagnosis is higher than that of their Hodgkin's disease counterparts. However, treatment of acute leukemias appears to result in less gonadotoxicity.[256] In females, follicular damaging effects are commonly encountered as a result of cyclophosphamide- or cytarabine-containing regimens[257,258]; however, the hormonal axis in prepubertal females appears relatively spared, with ALL survivors usually having a normal or accelerated puberty.[259] In mature women, amenorrhea can occur especially with alkylating agents. Mechlorethamine, cyclophosphamide,[260] and drug combinations used in treatment of Hodgkin's disease result in variable degrees of infertility and hormonal disturbances.[261–263]

Current Controversies & Future Considerations

Chemotherapy Toxicities and Complications

- Integration of new targeted therapies with standard agents is currently under investigation; unexpected and additive toxicities of these agents may occur.
- More careful studies of drug toxicities in specific ethnic groups and studies of drug-drug interactions are warranted.
- Long-term monitoring must be undertaken for the hematologic cancers with a substantial curability rate.

Suggested Readings*

De Vita VT Jr, Hellman S, Rosenberg SA (eds): Principles and Practice of Oncology (ed 5). Philadelphia: Lippincott, 1997.

Holland JF, Frei E, Kufe DW, et al (eds): Cancer Medicine (ed 6). Hamilton: BC Decker, 2003.

Perry MC (ed): The Chemotherapy Source Book (ed 3). Philadelphia: Lippincott Williams & Wilkins, 2001.

Rose BD (Editor-in-Chief): Up To Date Online 12.2, 2004. (Available at: *http://www.uptodate.com*)

Wiernik PH: Complications of treatment. *In* Wiernik PH, Steele GD, Phillips TL, et al (eds): Adult Leukemias. Hamilton: BC Decker, 2001, pp 263–274.

Full references for this chapter can be found on accompanying CD-ROM.

CHAPTER 91
Cytokine Therapy and Its Complications

Arnold Ganser, MD, and Michael Heuser, MD

KEY POINTS

Cytokine Therapy and Its Complications

- Recombinant human granulocyte colony-stimulating factor (rhG-CSF) or recombinant human granulocyte-macrophage colony-stimulating factor (rhGM-CSF) is recommended in chemotherapy-associated neutropenia as primary prophylaxis in patients at a high risk of febrile neutropenia (≥40%), in circumstances with an increased risk for adverse outcomes, and in patients age 65 or older with non-Hodgkin's lymphoma, small-cell lung cancer, or urothelial tumors.
- rhG-CSF or rhGM-CSF is recommended for mobilization of peripheral blood progenitor cells and for reconstitution after autologous or allogeneic peripheral blood progenitor cell or bone marrow transplantation.
- Recombinant human erythropoietin (rhEPO) is recommended in chemotherapy-associated anemia with hemoglobin of 10 gm/dL or less.
- Recombinant human interleukin-11 (rhIL-11) may be used to accelerate platelet reconstitution after intensive chemotherapy.
- Recombinant human keratinocyte growth factor (rhKGF) effectively alleviates symptoms of oral mucositis after myeloablative chemotherapy.

BIOLOGIC ACTIVITY OF HEMATOPOIETIC GROWTH FACTORS

All cells found in peripheral blood are derived from multipotent stem cells, which reside primarily in the bone marrow. The process leading to proliferation and differentiation of hematopoietic stem cells into progenitor cells and the cellular blood elements is tightly regulated by hematopoietic growth factors. Some factors, such as Steel factor and Flk-2, appear to have effects mainly on stem and progenitor cells, whereas more lineage-restricted factors such as erythropoietin and granulocyte colony-stimulating factor (G-CSF) predominantly affect progenitor and mature cells. The effects of hematopoietic growth factors are mediated through receptors of the hematopoietic growth factor superfamily,[1] and these are expressed on hematopoietic cells and leukemia cell lines, and some are also expressed on other tissues.[2–6] The effects of hematopoietic growth factors are negatively regulated by at least two different protein families, the Scr-homology 2–containing protein tyrosine phophatases[7,8] and the protein family of suppressors of cytokine signaling.[9–12]

Granulocyte-Colony Stimulating Factor

Endogenous G-CSF induces neutrophil maturation and may enhance neutrophil function.[13–15] G-CSF knockout mice are severely neutropenic, whereas effects on other lineages are minimal.[16] G-CSF is produced by monocytes, fibroblasts, and endothelial cells in response to inflammatory signals. Early clinical studies with recombinant human G-CSF (rhG-CSF) demonstrated a dose-dependent increase in circulating neutrophil counts over the dose range of 1–60 µg/kg/day.[17] Neutrophil counts increased between 1.8- and 12-fold, whereas eosinophils and basophils remained unchanged and monocytes increased only at the highest doses.[18] During rhG-CSF administration, a left shift is seen in white blood cell differentials that may include the appearance of promyelocytes and myeloblasts. If G-CSF is discontinued, peripheral neutrophil counts decrease by approximately 50% per day and return to baseline in 4–6 days in healthy subjects.[19] In the United States, two recombinant proteins are currently approved, filgrastim and pegfilgrastim. Filgrastim differs from endogenous G-CSF by the addition of an amino-terminal methionine and is not glycosylated.[20] The elimination half-life is approximately 3.5 hours after either intravenous or subcutaneous dosing. Pegfilgrastim is a pegylated form of filgrastim and thus has a longer half-life than filgrastim (15–80 hours in cancer patients). Outside of the United States, additional preparations of G-CSF are approved for clinical use: lenograstim, a glycosylated rhG-CSF, and nartograstim, an amino-terminal–mutated rhG-CSF.

Granulocyte-Macrophage Colony Stimulating Factor

Endogenous granulocyte-macrophage colony-stimulating factor (GM-CSF) enhances growth and differentiation in various cell lineages, including neutrophils, monocytes, eosinophils, dendritic cells, and, in cooperation with erythropoietin, erythrocytes. GM-CSF knockout mice do not develop defects in hematopoiesis but instead show a severe lung disorder similar to pulmonary alveolar proteinosis.[21] GM-CSF is induced by inflammatory stimuli and can be produced by T cells, macrophages, fibroblasts, and endothelial and epithelial cells.[22] Administration of recombinant human GM-CSF (rhGM-CSF) increases the number of neutrophils and eosinophils as well as macrophages and lymphocytes. In vitro, rhGM-CSF increased the chemotactic, antifungal, and antiparasitic activities of neutrophils and monocytes.[23] After 5 days of GM-CSF administration, granulocytes increased 3-fold in healthy volunteers compared to 7.2-fold after G-CSF administration.[24] Recently, various immunomodulatory effects of GM-CSF have been described[25] and are currently under investigation for a variety of clinical applications.[26,27] In the United States, sargramostim is the only rhGM-CSF approved for clinical use. It differs from the endogenous GM-CSF by one amino acid at position 23 and by O-glycosylation. The mean terminal half-life is approximately 2.7 hours if administered subcutaneously. Outside of the United States, molgramostim and regramostim are available, which are nonglycosylated and fully glycosylated, respectively.

Erythropoietin

Endogenous erythropoietin regulates red blood cell production and is produced primarily in the kidney. Erythropoietin knockout mice develop severe anemia,[28] as do humans deficient in erythropoietin as a result of chronic kidney disease. Normal serum erythropoietin levels range from approximately 4 to 30 units/L. Levels can rise 100- to 1000-fold with severe anemia. During the last decade, the role of erythropoietin in nonhematopoietic tissues became evident. The erythropoietin receptor is expressed in human endothelial cells,[29] and erythropoietin stimulates migration, proliferation, and differentiation of endothelial cells.[30] The erythropoietin receptor is also expressed in the central nervous system, where erythropoietin has trophic and cell-protective effects in injury states.[31,32] In 1989, the U.S. Food and Drug Administration (FDA) first approved the recombinant human form of erythropoietin, epoetin alfa (rhEPO), as a pharmaceutical for anemia of chronic renal failure. Epoetin alfa contains the identical amino acid sequence as endogenous human erythropoietin and has a half-life of approximately 3–10 hours in healthy individuals after intravenous administration. Recently, darbepoetin alfa has been approved as a pharmaceutical. It is a rhEPO modified by the addition of two N-glycosylation sites, thus giving it an approximately threefold longer half-life than epoetin alfa.[33] Outside the United States, epoetin beta is available, which differs from epoetin alfa only in terms of glycosylation and sialic acid content.[34] rhEPOs appear to be similarly effective as endogenous erythropoietin in stimulating the maturation of erythroid progenitors to mature erythrocytes.

Interleukin-11

Endogenous interleukin-11 exhibits a wide variety of biologic activities in hematopoietic, hepatic, adipose, neuronal, and osteoclast tissues and has been implicated as a multifunctional hematopoietic cytokine. In both normal and myelosuppressed mice, it significantly reduced the period of thrombocytopenia and increased the number of megakaryocyte, erythroid, and granulocyte progenitors in bone marrow, spleen, and platelets in peripheral blood.[35,36] However, disruption of interleukin-11 affects neither megakaryocyte development nor platelet production,[37,38] indicating a redundant role of growth factors in hematopoiesis. Oprelvekin is the only recombinant human interleukin-11 (rhIL-11) approved for clinical use and differs from the endogenous interleukin-11 by lack of the amino-terminal proline residue. This alteration has not resulted in measurable differences in bioactivity compared to endogenous interleukin-11. The mean terminal half-life is approximately 7 hours after subcutaneous administration.

Keratinocyte Growth Factor

A member of the family of fibroblast growth factors, initially known as fibroblast growth factor-7, keratinocyte growth factor has keratinocyte-stimulating activity and has been evaluated for alleviating chemotherapy-induced oral mucositis. Keratinocyte growth factor induces proliferation and differentiation in epithelial cells.[39] The keratinocyte growth factor receptor was found on various tissues, including tumor cells and tumor cell lines, but expression was limited to nonhematopoietic tissues.[40–42] Mice expressing a dominant-negative keratinocyte growth factor receptor developed epidermal atrophy and a delayed reepithelialization of wounds.[43] In mouse models of chemotherapy-induced gastrointestinal injury, recombinant human keratinocyte growth factor (rhKGF) improved survival and ameliorated weight loss in the treatment group.[44] In 2004, the first rhKGF—palifermin, which is a truncated version of endogenous keratinocyte growth factor—was approved for clinical use by the FDA.

CLINICAL USE OF RECOMBINANT HUMAN HEMATOPOIETIC GROWTH FACTORS

Recombinant Human G-CSF and GM-CSF

Neutropenia itself is not associated with symptoms and does not affect quality of life. However, it is a risk factor for infection typically associated with fever and accompanied by considerable morbidity and mortality. The risk of infection begins to increase as the absolute neutrophil count (ANC) declines below 1000/μL and is especially high if the ANC is below 100/μL. The duration of chemotherapy-associated neutropenia is another risk factor for infection, with an increased risk if neutropenia exceeds 10–14 days. In addition, neutropenia in cancer patients may delay timely delivery of chemotherapy and may thus compromise treatment outcome. Several options have been tried in cancer patients to prevent these adverse outcomes, including use of colony-stimulating factors, prophylactic antibiotic use, granulocyte transfusion, and dose reduction or delay of chemotherapy. To prove beneficial, the treatment must reduce the incidence of febrile neutropenia and its associated morbidity or mortality, allow timely application of the full chemotherapy dose, or reduce overall costs compared to conventional treatment. In the following sections, data on the use of colony-stimulating factors in comparison to other treatment modalities in neutropenic cancer patients, in acute leukemias and myelodysplastic syndrome, in hematopoietic stem cell transplantation, and in bone marrow failure syndromes are presented (see Table 91–2 later for summary).

Indications, Dosing and Adverse Events

FDA-approved indications for colony-stimulating factors and recommended doses are listed in Table 91–1. Nonlicensed uses of colony-stimulating factors include neutropenia in a variety of hematologic diseases and are discussed briefly. Colony-stimulating factors should not be used 24–48 hours before and must not be started until 24 hours after cytotoxic therapy in cancer patients. Treatment with filgrastim (rhG-CSF) or sargramostim (rhGM-CSF) in the chemotherapy setting is recommended by the manufacturer until the ANC has reached 10,000/μL following the neutrophil nadir. However, a shorter duration of administration that is sufficient to achieve clinically adequate neutrophil recovery is a reasonable alternative.[45] In patients receiving bone marrow transplantation, rhG-CSF is started 24 hours after and rhGM-CSF 2–4 hours after bone marrow infusion. However, based on available clinical data, starting colony-stimulating factors up to 5 days after peripheral blood progenitor cell reinfusion is reasonable.[45] In the transplantation setting, colony-stimulating factor dose should be adjusted to keep the ANC above 1000/μL. The longer acting rhG-CSF, pegfilgrastim, has been shown to be equally effective as filgrastim in a single dose per chemotherapy cycle by either weight-based dosing (100 μg/kg)[46] or a fixed dose.[47] It should not be administered between 14 days before and 24 hours after administration of cytotoxic chemotherapy. Concurrent use of colony-stimulating factors with cytotoxic chemotherapy may increase proliferation of myeloid cells and thus the sensitivity to cytotoxic chemotherapy. Clinical trials investigating concurrent use of colony-stimulating factors with cytotoxic chemotherapy have shown an increase of thrombocytopenia and neutropenia.[48–50] Therefore, the above-mentioned restrictions for the use of colony-stimulating factors before or during chemotherapy should be strictly followed outside of clinical trials.

Colony-stimulating factors are generally well tolerated. Twenty percent to 30% of patients experience bone or musculoskeletal pain, which is attributed to the rapid proliferation of myeloid cells in the bone marrow, and fever or skin rash may occur. Adverse events such as fatigue, diarrhea, injection site reactions, and edema were less frequently reported in patients treated with rhG-CSF compared to patients receiving rhGM-CSF.[51] Some patients treated with sargramostim reported dyspnea, likely resulting from transient accumulation of granulocytes in the pulmonary vasculature.[52] Some data suggest that molgramostim may have a more unfavorable adverse event profile than sargramostim.[53] Thus, in clinical practice G-CSF is mostly preferred to GM-CSF. However, well-controlled comparative trials evaluating relative colony-stimulating factor efficacy are not available and the strength of evidence to support the use of rhG-CSF or rhGM-CSF varies based on the specific indication for colony-stimulating factor administration.[45] Asymptomatic splenic enlargement has been frequently observed with long-term use of colony-stimulating factors,[54] and atraumatic splenic rupture has been very rarely reported.[55,56] Other rare adverse events of G-CSF use are Sweet's syndrome[57] and flare-up of rheumatoid arthritis in patients with Felty's syndrome.[58,59]

In patients with sickle cell disease, the use of rhG-CSF has been associated with sickle cell crisis.[60,61] After repeated administration of the rhGM-CSF produced in yeast, the development of non-neutralizing and neutralizing antibodies has been reported.[62,63] Patients with acquired aplastic anemia have an inherent risk to develop myelodysplastic syndrome or acute myeloid leukemia, and concern has been raised about a possible contributory role from long-term G-CSF therapy.[64–66] However, no evidence exists for other diseases that use of colony-stimulating factors increases the risk for cancer.

Chemotherapy-Associated Neutropenia in Cancer Patients

Different strategies in the use of colony-stimulating factors have been investigated to reduce the incidence of febrile neutropenia and its sequelae in cancer patients undergoing cytotoxic therapy. Colony-stimulating factors can be used as primary prophylaxis (i.e., directly after the first cycle of chemotherapy in treatment-naive patients and without any episode of febrile neutropenia); as secondary prophylaxis (i.e., directly after subsequent cycles following an episode of febrile neutropenia); or therapeutically (i.e., after the onset of febrile neutropenia to reduce its duration and improve the outcome of infection). The American Society of Clinical Oncology (ASCO) published guidelines for the use of colony-stimulating factors in cancer patients in 2000, which are discussed with more recent data in the following section (Table 91–2).

Primary prophylaxis of febrile neutropenia by use of colony-stimulating factors is not recommended for most patients treated with myelosuppressive chemotherapy.[45] Although colony-stimulating factors reduce the risk of febrile neutropenia and documented infections, no effect on mortality from infection, response rate to antibiotics, or overall survival could be demonstrated.[67–69] Because febrile neutropenia is associated with considerable health care costs, a reduction in the incidence of febrile neutropenia by use of colony-stimulating factors may be

TABLE 91–1. Licensed Indications and Recommended Dosage for Hematopoietic Growth Factors

Generic name (Brand Name)	Indication	Dosage
Erythropoietin		
Epoetin alfa (Epogen, Procrit)	Anemia related to	
	• Cancer in patients with chemotherapy for ≥2 mo (nonmyeloid malignancies)	• 150 units/kg tiw SC or 40,000 units qw SC
	• Surgery (elective, noncardiac, nonvascular) if hemoglobin >10 to ≤13 gm/dL	• 300 units/kg qd SC from 10 days before until 4 days after
	• Chronic renal failure	• 50–100 units/kg tiw IV or SC
	• Zidovudine-treated, HIV-infected patients	• 100 units/kg tiw IV or SC
Epoetin beta (Neorecormon)	Anemia related to	
	• Solid tumors in patients with platinum-based chemotherapy or MM, low-grade NHL, or CLL in patients with chemotherapy and low serum erythropoietin	• 450 units/kg qw in 3–7 doses
	• Surgery (autologous blood donation)	• Dosage determined individually
	• Chronic renal failure	• 20 units/kg tiw SC or 40 units/kg tiw IV
	• Prematurity in infants	• 250 units/kg tiw SC
Darbepoetin alfa (Aranesp)	Anemia related to	
	• Cancer in patients with chemotherapy for ≥2 mo (nonmyeloid malignancies)	• 2.25 μg/kg qw or q2w
	• Chronic renal failure	• 0.45 μg/kg qw IV or SC
Granulocyte Colony-Stimulating Factor		
Filgrastim (Neupogen)	• Cancer patients receiving myelosuppressive chemotherapy; patients with AML receiving induction or consolidation therapy	• 5 μg/kg qd SC or IV
	• Cancer patients receiving BMT	• 10 μg/kg qd IV over 4–24 hr or SC over 24 hr
	• Peripheral blood progenitor cell mobilization	• 10 μg/kg qd SC or 5 μg/kg bid SC
	• Congenital neutropenia	• 6 μg/kg bid SC
	• Idiopathic or cyclic neutropenia	• 5 μg/kg qd SC
Lenograstim (Granocyte)	• Cancer patients receiving myeloablative chemotherapy with stem cell rescue (nonmyeloid malignancies) or receiving myelosuppressive chemotherapy	• 5 μg/kg qd SC
	• Peripheral blood progenitor cell mobilization	• After chemotherapy: 5 μg/kg qd SC; without prior chemotherapy: 10 μg/kg qd SC
Pegfilgrastim (Neulasta)	• Cancer patients receiving myelosuppressive chemotherapy (nonmyeloid malignancies)	• 6 mg once per chemotherapy cycle SC
Granulocyte-Macrophage Colony-Stimulating Factor		
Sargramostim (Leukine)	• Older patients with AML receiving induction chemotherapy	• 250 μg/m^2 qd IV (on day 11)
	• Peripheral blood progenitor cell mobilization	• 250 μg/m^2 qd IV over 24 hr or SC
	• Patients with NHL, ALL, or Hodgkin's disease receiving autologous BMT, patients receiving BMT from HLA-matched related donors, or patients with BMT failure or engraftment delay	• 250 μg/m^2 qd over 2 hr
Molgramostim (Leucomax)	• Cancer patients receiving myelosuppressive chemotherapy	• 5–10 μg/kg qd SC
	• Patients receiving autologous or syngeneic BMT	• 10 μg/kg qd IV
Interleukin-11		
Oprelvekin (Neumega)	• Cancer patients receiving myelosuppressive chemotherapy (nonmyeloid malignancies)	• 50 μg/kg qd SC
Keratinocyte Growth Factor		
Palifermin (Kepivance)	• Patients with hematologic malignancies receiving myelotoxic therapy requiring hematopoietic stem cell support	• 60 μg/kg qd IV

Abbreviations: ALL, acute lymphoblastic leukemia; AML, acute myeloid leukemia; bid, twice daily; BMT, bone marrow transplantation; CLL, chronic lymphocytic leukemia; HIV, human immunodeficiency virus; HLA, human leucocyte antigen; IV, intravenously; MM, multiple myeloma; NHL, non-Hodgkin's lymphoma; qd, once daily; qw, once weekly; q2w, once every 2 weeks; SC, subcutaneously; tiw, three times weekly.

cost-effective. Early economic analyses found colony-stimulating factors to be cost-effective when the risk of febrile neutropenia with a particular regimen exceeded 40%.[70] The ASCO guidelines therefore recommend primary prophylactic use of colony-stimulating factors as a treatment option if the risk of febrile neutropenia equals or exceeds 40%.[45] However, recently it has been proposed that costs are neutral if the risk of febrile neutropenia is between 18% and 25%.[71,72] For reasons of cost-effectiveness and depending on local costs, colony-

TABLE 91–2. Recommendations for the Use of rhG-CSF and rhGM-CSF

Indication	Recommendation
Chemotherapy-associated neutropenia in solid tumors and lymphoma	
Primary prophylaxis	Not generally recommended* May be considered in special circumstances with increased risk for adverse outcomes* May be cost-effective depending on risk of febrile neutropenia (≥40%) and local costs* Recommended in patients age 65 or older with NHL, SCLC, or urothelial tumors
Secondary prophylaxis	Not generally recommended* May be considered in tumors in which a decrease in dose intensity would compromise long-term outcome (e.g., germ cell tumors)*
Treatment of febrile neutropenia	Not generally recommended* May be considered in patients with high risk for adverse outcomes or prolonged hospitalization as a result of febrile neutropenia*
Treatment of afebrile neutropenia	Not recommended*
Increase of dose intensity	Not recommended*
Increase of dose density	Effective in elderly patients with high-grade NHL and lymph node–positive breast cancer
Concomitant radiation therapy	Should be avoided*
Radiation therapy in solid tumors	May be considered if large fields are involved*
Chemotherapy-associated neutropenia in AML	Not recommended for postinduction therapy unless proven to be cost-effective* Recommended for postconsolidation therapy depending on dose intensity* Not recommended in refractory or relapsed AML* Not recommended concurrent with chemotherapy (priming) outside of clinical trials*
MDS	Not generally recommended in patients with MDS; no data exists for long-term use of CSFs* CSFs may be used in patients with severe neutropenia and recurrent infections* Combination of CSFs with erythropoietin should be limited to clinical trials
Chemotherapy-associated neutropenia in ALL	Recommended after the initial induction or first postremission course of chemotherapy to reduce the duration of neutropenia by approximately 1 wk* Concomitant use during induction chemotherapy should be limited to clinical trials However, in regimens containing topoisomerase II inhibitors and alkylating agents, an increased risk of therapy-related myeloid leukemias and MDS has been documented
Hematopoietic stem cell transplantation	Recommended for mobilization of autologous or allogeneic PBPCs* Recommended for hematopoietic reconstitution after autologous or allogeneic PBPC or bone marrow transplantation as well as for delayed or failed engraftment*
Bone marrow failure syndromes	Recommended for certain bone marrow failure syndromes when improvement of neutrophil count is appropriate

*According to the ASCO guidelines for the use of hematopoietic colony-stimulating factors (2000).
Abbreviations: ALL, acute lymphoblastic leukemia; AML, acute myeloid leukemia; CSFs, colony-stimulating factors; MDS, myelodysplastic syndrome; NHL, non-Hodgkin's lymphoma; PBPC, peripheral blood progenitor cell; SCLC, small-cell lung cancer.

stimulating factors may be used more often for primary prophylaxis in the future. In addition, primary prophylaxis of febrile neutropenia may be indicated in special circumstances with a high risk of febrile neutropenia, such as poor performance status, bone marrow compromise, or other comorbidity.[45] Patients age 65 years and older are at increased risk of febrile neutropenia and prolonged hospitalization.[73,74] A recent review by the European Organization for Research and Treatment of Cancer (EORTC) found evidence that prophylactic use of G-CSF reduced the incidence of febrile neutropenia and infections in elderly patients treated with myelotoxic chemotherapy for non-Hodgkin's lymphoma, small-cell lung cancer, or urothelial tumors and recommended primary prophylactic use of G-CSF in this patient population.[75] Secondary prophylaxis of febrile neutropenia is recommended only in patients in whom a treatment delay or dose reduction may compromise survival (e.g., those with germ cell tumors).[45]

Primary and secondary prophylaxis of (afebrile) neutropenia with colony-stimulating factors has been used to prevent dose reduction or dose delay in cancer patients. However, for most tumors, maintaining dose intensity has not resulted in improved disease-free or overall survival.[76,77] Thus, use of colony-stimulating factors is not recommended as primary or secondary prophylaxis to maintain dose intensity except for tumors in which a decrease in dose intensity would compromise long-term outcome (e.g., germ cell tumors).[45] Whereas dose-intense chemotherapy has not been shown to improve outcome in several malignancies,[78–81] some evidence exists with regard to dose-dense (every 2 weeks) chemotherapy. In older patients with aggressive non-Hodgkin's lymphoma, 14-day cycles of cyclophosphamide, doxorubicin, vincristine, and prednisone (CHOP) with colony-stimulating factors support improved event-free and overall survival compared to 21-day cycles of CHOP.[82] This benefit has not been seen in younger patients with aggressive non-Hodgkin's lymphoma.[83,84] In addition, dose-dense adjuvant chemotherapy in lymph node–positive breast cancer patients improved disease-free and overall survival compared to the usually used schedule (every 3 weeks).[85] Use of colony-stimulating factors to increase dose intensity is not recommended outside of clinical trials[45]; it may, however, be useful to allow dose-dense chemotherapy in special settings.

Therapeutic use of colony-stimulating factors has been investigated with regard to whether it reduces the mortality from febrile neutropenia. A meta-analysis of eight randomized trials found no benefit in mortality for patients treated with antibiotics and a colony-stimulating factor compared to patients treated with antibiotics alone.[86] As in primary prophylaxis, treatment of febrile neutropenia with a colony-stimulating factor may reduce the risk of prolonged hospitalization and its costs, but cost-effectiveness has not been proven yet. Certain patients with fever and neutropenia are at higher risk for infection-associated complications, and several risk factors have been described.[87,88] These include profound neutropenia (ANC < 100/μL), uncontrolled primary disease, pneumonia, hypotension, multiorgan dysfunction, and invasive fungal infection. The ASCO guideline states that colony-stimulating factor treatment may be considered in these patients, but the benefits have not been proven.[45] Treatment of afebrile neutropenia with a colony-stimulating factor is not supported by current data.[89] According to the ASCO guideline, colony-stimulating factors should be avoided in patients receiving concomitant chemotherapy and radiation therapy, particularly involving the mediastinum.[45] In patients receiving radiation therapy involving large fields, therapeutic use of colony-stimulating factors may be considered if prolonged delays secondary to neutropenia are expected.[45]

Neutropenia in Acute Myeloid Leukemia and Myelodysplastic Syndromes

Induction and consolidation treatment in acute myeloid leukemia is associated with a high incidence of febrile neutropenia. In myelodysplastic syndromes, the rate of infection is directly related to the degree of neutropenia, and infections are a major cause of morbidity and mortality. Colony-stimulating factors have therefore been evaluated for their efficacy in reducing infectious complications in induction and consolidation therapy of acute myeloid leukemia and in neutropenic myelodysplastic syndrome patients. However, concern has been raised that colony-stimulating factors may promote leukemia growth and the conversion from myelodysplastic syndrome to overt leukemia. Randomized trials of colony-stimulating factor administration after induction chemotherapy in acute myeloid leukemia all demonstrated a consistent reduction (by 2–6 days) in time to neutrophil recovery.[90–99] In most trials this was accompanied by a reduction in the duration of hospital stay and antibiotic usage. However, the majority of trials have not found an increased response rate or patient survival. It has been proposed that elderly acute myeloid leukemia patients (>55 years), who are at increased risk for serious complications from febrile neutropenia, may be better candidates for colony-stimulating factors.[100] Use of colony-stimulating factors in acute myeloid leukemia patients after consolidation treatment has markedly decreased the duration of neutropenia and the use of antibiotics compared to controls.[94,101] However, outcome parameters were not improved. Interestingly, no accelerated growth or increased drug resistance has been noted in any of these studies. In 2000, the ASCO recommended the use of colony-stimulating factors in acute myeloid leukemia for *postinduction* therapy only if it appears to be cost-effective.[45] This mainly depends on local treatment schedules and local costs. Colony-stimulating factor use in acute myeloid leukemia for *postconsolidation* therapy appeared to be cost-effective and thus was recommended by the ASCO in 2000[45] and by the Haemato-Oncology Task Force of the British Committee for Standards in Haematology in 2003.[102] Use of colony-stimulating factors in refractory or relapsed acute myeloid leukemia is not recommended.[45]

In vitro studies proposed that colony-stimulating factors may sensitize acute myeloid leukemia blasts to S-phase–specific agents such as cytarabine,[103,104] and several "priming" studies have investigated the effect of concurrent use of colony-stimulating factors with chemotherapy in acute myeloid leukemia. However, concern has been raised that stimulation and sensitization of normal hematopoietic progenitors may prolong the duration of neutropenia. Several trials failed to detect a difference for either remission rate or duration of neutropenia if colony-stimulating factors were used concurrent with induction chemotherapy.[93,95,96,98,105–109] However, a recently published randomized trial in adult patients (≤60 years) found a significantly increased event-free survival (P = .01) and overall survival at 4 years (45% compared to 35% without G-CSF priming; P = .02) in patients with standard-risk acute myeloid leukemia.[110] Priming of acute myeloid leukemia blasts with colony-stimulating factors still remains experimental and should be used under controlled conditions in clinical trials only.

In neutropenic myelodysplastic syndrome patients, colony-stimulating factors used alone were shown to increase the neutrophil count.[111–116] Later studies confirmed this finding in high-risk myelodysplastic syndrome patients treated with chemotherapy and rhG-CSF or no rhG-CSF.[117,118] These studies provided some evidence of an improved response rate with rhG-CSF compared to controls, but duration of response or survival was not influenced. No published data for the long-term and continuous use of colony-stimulating factors in myelodysplastic syndrome patients exist, although in an early report of a randomized trial comparing G-CSF with best supportive care, overall survival was shorter in the G-CSF group with refractory anemia and excess blasts.[119] However, the ASCO guideline recommends that *intermittent* administration of colony-stimulating factors may be considered in a subset of patients with severe neutropenia and recurrent infection.[45] Combination therapy with a colony-stimulating factor plus rhEPO has been proposed and showed neutrophil responses in up to 100% of patients.[120] Synergy of the combination therapy so far has been shown for the erythroid response,[121,122] but the benefit in terms of infection rate, survival, and cost-effectiveness remains to be determined. Combination therapy in myelodysplastic syndromes therefore should be limited to clinical trials.

Neutropenia in Acute Lymphoblastic Leukemia

Several randomized trials in children and adults with acute lymphoblastic leukemia showed that the administration of rhG-CSF during or after induction or post-remission chemotherapy can reduce the duration of neutropenia by up to 8 days.[123–129] Some studies found a decreased rate of infections, reduced usage of antibiotics, shortened hospitalization, or higher complete response rate in the rhG-CSF group. However, no difference was found with respect to disease-free or overall survival. Based on these results, in 2000, the ASCO guidelines recommended the administration of rhG-CSF begun after completion of the first few days of chemotherapy of the initial induction or first postremission course.[45] However, recently published data on 412 children with acute lymphoblastic leukemia reported a higher incidence of therapy-associated myeloid leukemia or myelodysplasia in children treated with rhG-CSF following remission induction therapy (median duration of use, 9 days) compared with those not receiving rhG-CSF (11% vs. 2.7%; $P = .019$).[130] The chemotherapy protocol contained topoisomerase II inhibitors and alkylators, which are known risk factors for the development of secondary myeloid leukemias. In the absence of outcome-related benefits, colony-stimulating factors should not be used with treatment protocols containing topoisomerase II inhibitors or alkylators in acute lymphoblastic leukemia. No recommendations can be given for the use of colony-stimulating factors in refractory or relapsed acute lymphoblastic leukemia.[45]

Use of Colony-Stimulating Factors in Hematopoietic Stem Cell Transplantation

Nonrandomized studies provided evidence that patients receiving colony-stimulating factor–mobilized autologous peripheral blood progenitor cells had more rapid neutrophil recovery with reduced red blood cell and platelet transfusion requirements and shorter hospital stay,[131–134] with similar results in randomized studies including allogeneic transplantation.[135–137] Moreover, in the allogeneic setting, peripheral blood progenitor cell donors spent fewer nights in the hospital and had fewer days with restricted activity compared with the marrow donors.[138] A randomized comparison of rhG-CSF and rhGM-CSF showed similar efficacy for cell yield but a shorter time to hematopoietic recovery with rhG-CSF compared to rhGM-CSF in one trial.[139,140] Thus, the ASCO guidelines recommended the use of colony-stimulating factors for mobilization of peripheral blood progenitor cells; recombinant human G-CSF should be used at higher doses (10 µg/kg once daily) and may be combined with rhGM-CSF or administered after cytotoxic agents.[45]

After transplantation of colony-stimulating factor–mobilized autologous or allogeneic peripheral blood progenitor cells in patients receiving myeloablative conditioning regimens, colony-stimulating factors accelerate hematopoietic reconstitution and may reduce the need for red blood cell and platelet transfusions and duration of hospitalization.[134,141,142] Similarly, the use of colony-stimulating factors after reinfusion of bone marrow cells accelerates hematopoietic reconstitution and reduces costs.[143,144] Delayed administration of colony-stimulating factor after reinfusion of peripheral blood progenitor cells or bone marrow cells (day +5 to +7) has been equally effective as early administration[145–147] and further reduces costs.[145] The ASCO guidelines recommend use of colony-stimulating factors for accelerated reconstitution after autologous or allogeneic peripheral blood progenitor cell or bone marrow transplantation as well as for delayed or failed engraftment.[45]

Neutropenia in Bone Marrow Failure Syndromes

In acquired aplastic anemia, neutrophil responses to rhG-CSF and rhGM-CSF with or without immunosuppressive therapy have been reported,[148,149] but overall response and survival were not changed by colony-stimulating factor treatment.[149] Concern exists that colony-stimulating factors promote the development of myelodysplastic syndrome and acute myeloid leukemia, but it has been shown that myelodysplastic syndrome and cytogenetic abnormalities occur with a similar incidence in patients with aplastic anemia treated with rhG-CSF as in those not treated with rhG-CSF.[150] Although colony-stimulating factors can prove clinically helpful during episodes of infection, their continuous use in aplastic anemia should be restricted to clinical trials.

In Fanconi's anemia, rhG-CSF can raise the neutrophil count but in general does not affect hemoglobin or platelets.[151] Evidence exists that colony-stimulating factors may promote the development of acute myeloid leukemia with monosomy 7[152] and therefore should be limited to clinical trials.

Severe chronic neutropenia refers to conditions associated with an average ANC less than 500/µL. It may occur in isolation, as in infantile agranulocytosis (Kostmann's syndrome) or cyclic, idiopathic, or autoimmune neutropenia, or in combination with other symptoms, as in Shwachman-Diamond syndrome, Chédiak-Higashi syndrome, or glycogen storage disease type 1b. Recurrent infections with considerable morbidity and mortality most likely occur in Kostmann's syndrome but may compromise patients with other forms of severe chronic neutropenia. In various forms of severe chronic neutropenia, rhG-CSF has become the primary therapeutic to treat neutropenia and prevent serious infectious complications. Clinical trials confirmed a remarkable increase in the neutrophil count in approximately 95% of patients and virtually abolished episodes of serious bacterial and fungal infection.[54,153–155] Although initial reports on GM-CSF were promising,[156] rhGM-CSF is considered to be less effective.[157] Often, rhG-CSF has to be administered chronically. Kostmann's syndrome and Shwachman-Diamond syndrome may progress to acute myeloid leukemia and myelodysplastic syndrome, and concern has been raised that this risk may be increased by administration of rhG-CSF. However, based on the data of the severe chronic neutropenia international registry, myelodysplastic syndrome or acute myeloid leukemia occurred without a predictable relationship to the duration or dose of rhG-CSF treatment, and no patients with cyclic or idiopathic neutropenia developed myelodysplastic syndrome or acute myeloid leukemia.[157] Thus, use of rhG-CSF in bone marrow failure syndromes has been recommended when improvement of neutrophil count is appropriate.[102]

Recombinant Human Erythropoietin

Anemia is a widespread and significant clinical problem accompanied by fatigue, dyspnea, tachycardia, and a reduced quality of life. Anemia can have a multitude of causes, including poor red cell production due to an impaired erythropoietic progenitor cell or deficiency in iron, vitamins, or erythropoietin; decreased red cell survival; blood loss; or hypersplenism. Alternatively, in patients with cancer or chronic disease, anemia can occur without any underlying known cause other than these diseases themselves and is termed *anemia of cancer* or *anemia of chronic disease.* Probable mechanisms for this type of anemia include impaired iron use, suppressed erythroid progenitor cell differentiation, insufficient erythropoietin production, and shortened red blood cell survival,[158] which may be mediated by inflammation-associated cytokines such as interleukin-6, interleukin-1, interferon, and tumor necrosis factor-α.[159] In patients with anemia of cancer, an impaired erythropoietin response with low endogenous erythropoietin levels has been reported.[160,161]

Diagnostic work-up in anemic patients aims at identifying correctable causes of anemia. If no specific treatment is available, transfusions or stimulants of erythropoiesis may be indicated. Transfusions, although necessary in acute situations, are a limited resource and carry the risk of transfusion-related reactions or infection. Therefore, a great array of indications have been investigated for rhEPO since its introduction into the clinic in 1989. Clinical trials are ongoing to identify more accurately the true benefits of these products. Primary outcome measures are improvement in hemoglobin concentration, reduction of transfusion requirements, and symptomatic improvement, including quality of life. Secondary outcome measures include disease-free and overall survival, especially in solid tumors. Cost-benefit calculations are increasingly performed to establish the role of rhEPO in the treatment of anemia. The following sections discuss data on the use of rhEPO in anemia of cancer patients with and without treatment; in bone marrow and peripheral blood progenitor cell transplantation; in myelodysplastic syndromes, idiopathic myelofibrosis, bone marrow failure syndromes, and some hemoglobinopathies; and in patients undergoing surgery (see Table 91–3 for summary).

TABLE 91–3. Recommendations for the Use of rhEPO, rhIL-11, and rhKGF

rhEPO	Recommended in patients with chemotherapy-associated anemia and hemoglobin ≤10 gm/dL (including multiple myeloma, NHL, or CLL if not responding to cytoreductive treatment).* Treatment of chemotherapy-associated anemia with hemoglobin >10 to <12 gm/dL should be based on clinical circumstances.* Hemoglobin level can be raised to and should be kept at 12 gm/dL.* Intravenous iron substitution may be beneficial.* Non–treatment-related anemia in cancer is only marginally affected by rhEPO. Not generally recommended in bone marrow transplantation. Some evidence supports the use of rhEPO in low-risk MDS with low levels of endogenous erythropoietin.* Epoetin beta may be used in anemic patients (hemoglobin 10–13 gm/dL) undergoing major surgery to increase the amount of preoperatively donated autologous blood.
rhIL-11	May be used in patients with intensive chemotherapy leading to low platelet counts.
rhKGF	Effective in patients with hematologic malignancies receiving myeloablative chemotherapy to alleviate symptoms of oral mucositis.

*According to the ASCO/ASH guidelines for the use of epoetin (2002).
Abbreviations: CLL, chronic lymphocytic leukemia; MDS, myelodysplastic syndrome; NHL, non-Hodgkin's lymphoma.

Indications, Dosing, and Adverse Events, Including Pure Red Cell Aplasia

FDA-approved indications for rhEPO and recommended doses are listed in Table 91–1. Off-label and investigational use includes treatment of anemia of a variety of hematologic diseases and is discussed briefly. In patients with cancer and concomitant chemotherapy evidence of clinical benefit for epoetin was largely obtained by weight-based dosing of epoetin three times weekly.[162] Recent evidence from a randomized, double-blind study supports application of 40,000 units of epoetin alfa once weekly,[163] which has been common use in clinical practice. In 2001, a longer acting derivative of epoetin alfa, darbepoetin alfa, was approved by the FDA. Darbepoetin alfa has a threefold longer terminal half-life than epoetin alfa. It may be administered weekly in patients having received epoetin alfa thrice weekly and has been used effectively with a single monthly dose in 30 of 36 patients with chronic renal failure.[164] However, preliminary data from a randomized, open-label study comparing epoetin alfa 40,000 units once weekly with darbepoetin alfa 200 μg once every 2 weeks in 305 cancer patients with chemotherapy-induced anemia (hemoglobin ≤11 gm/dL) showed that patients with epoetin alfa have a significantly greater hemoglobin response rate during the first 4 weeks of therapy compared to patients with darbepoetin alfa (P = .0078).[165] Further trials are evaluating the appropriate dosage and dosing interval of darbepoetin including use of higher doses in patients with myelodysplasia.[166,167]

For most indications, the recommended target hemoglobin is 12 gm/dL and the hematocrit should not exceed 36%. In general, rhEPO dose should be reduced by 25% when hemoglobin approaches 12 gm/dL or hemoglobin increases more than 1 gm/dL in any 2-week period. The dose may be increased if hemoglobin does not increase more than 1–2 gm/dL after 4–8 weeks of therapy. If response remains absent beyond 6–8 weeks after appropriate dose increase has been attempted, continuing epoetin treatment does not appear to be beneficial.[168]

rhEPO is generally well tolerated. Hypertension has been reported in 20–30% of patients with chronic renal failure.[169] In cancer patients treated with epoetin alfa, diarrhea and edema were significantly more frequent in the epoetin group than in the placebo group.[170] However, a recent meta-analysis for rhEPO in cancer patients has not found an increased risk of adverse events in the treatment group compared to placebo.[171] Use of rhEPO may increase the risk of thrombotic events and death in patients with cardiovascular comorbidity or if hemoglobin is raised above the target value of 12 gm/dL. A randomized, prospective trial of 1265 hemodialysis patients with clinically evident cardiac disease compared epoetin alfa treatment targeted to a maintenance hematocrit of either 42% ± 3% or 30% ± 3%. Increased mortality was observed in patients randomized to a target hematocrit of 42% compared to patients with target hematocrit of 30% (35% vs. 29% mortality). The incidences of nonfatal myocardial infarction (3.1% vs. 2.3%) and of all other thrombotic events (22% vs. 18%) were also higher in the group randomized to achieve a hematocrit of 42%.[172] In a randomized, placebo-controlled trial in 939 women with metastatic breast cancer and a target hemoglobin level of 12–14 gm/dL in the epoetin alfa group, the incidence of fatal thrombotic vascular events was higher in the group randomized to receive epoetin alfa as compared to placebo (1% vs. 0.2%), and the proportion of subjects surviving at 12 months after randomization was lower in the epoetin alfa group than in the placebo group (70% vs. 76%; P = .012 by log-rank test).[173]

Antibody-mediated pure red cell aplasia, a profound anemia characterized by the absence of reticulocytes and the virtual absence of erythroid precursors in the bone marrow, has been reported in a significant number of patients exposed to rhEPO.[174–176] Between 1998 and April 2004, 175 cases with documented epoetin-associated antibodies were reported for Eprex (epoetin alfa), 11 cases for Neorecormon (epoetin beta)—both manufactured and distributed outside the United States—and 5 cases for Epogen (epoetin alfa).[177] Nearly all patients had chronic renal failure, and nearly all had received epoetin administered by the subcutaneous route.[177] Several factors related to the production, handling, storage, and route of administration of epoetin may be responsible for the increased incidence of Eprex-associated pure red cell aplasia beginning in 1998. In that year, the stabilizing agent for Eprex was changed from human serum albumin to polysorbate 80 and glycine because of concern that human serum albumin could transmit a variant of Creutzfeldt-Jakob disease.[178] Although not specifically studied with epoetin, subcutaneous administration of other proteins has been associated with greater immunogenicity than with intravenous administration.[179] In cancer patients treated with epoetin, the absence of reports on pure red cell aplasia may be due to chemotherapy-associated immunosuppression.[177] By instituting a "best handling practice" and a change in labeling in which subcutaneous administration of Eprex is contraindicated in patients with chronic renal failure in most countries, the exposure-adjusted incidence of pure red cell aplasia caused by Eprex could be reduced by more than 80%.[177] No controlled data are available for the treatment of epoetin-associated pure red cell aplasia. In general, transfusions for symptomatic anemia and cessation of all erythropoietic stimulating agents is recommended[175]. Patients should not be switched to an alternative epoetin preparation, because antibodies cross-react with all commercially available rhEPO products.[180] A retrospective study evaluated the response to immunosuppressive treatment in 47 patients with chronic renal failure and epoetin-associated pure red cell aplasia.[181] Without immunosuppressive treatment, no spontaneous remissions were observed. Among 37 patients who received an immunosuppressive agent (e.g., steroids, cyclophosphamide, cyclosporin, or intravenous gamma globulin) or immunosuppression associated with renal transplantation, 29 recovered (78%). Response to treatment was mostly seen within 3 months, and remission was stable in all responders after cessation of immunosuppression.

Treatment-Associated Anemia in Cancer Patients

The incidence of anemia in patients with solid tumors varies greatly depending on tumor type and treatment, but for mild anemia often is above 50%.[182] Anemia invariably induces fatigue, which is a major determinant of quality of life. Anemia in cancer patients has been associated with poorer survival.[183] However, in most cancers it is not an independent prognostic factor but rather correlates with advanced tumor stages. Nevertheless, hypoxia may impair the efficacy of radiation therapy, thus compromising patient survival.[184] The use of rhEPO in anemic cancer patients is discussed in the following section.

The ASCO and the American Society of Hematology (ASH) collaborated to produce guidelines in 2002 for the appropriate use of rhEPO in cancer patients with chemotherapy-associated anemia.[168] Based on evidence from well-controlled trials of patients with a baseline hemoglobin concentration of ≤10 gm/dL or less, epoetin therapy significantly increased hemoglobin compared with placebo, with an absolute difference in change of mean hemoglobin ranging between 1.6 and 3.1 gm/dL. Data are inconclusive for patients with baseline hemoglobin of more than 10 gm/dL. A meta-analysis of all randomized studies published between 1985 and 1998 found that epoetin therapy reduced the relative odds of receiving red blood cell transfusions by an average of 62% (odds ratio 0.38; 95% confidence interval, 0.28–0.51).[185] The absolute risk reduction corresponded to a number-needed-to-treat of 4.4 or, based on higher quality studies, 5.2 (95% confidence interval, 3.8–8.4). This meta-analysis did not stratify for baseline hemoglobin. However, in a recent Phase III randomized trial of weekly epoetin alfa, in patients with mild anemia (≥9 gm/dL), the incidence of transfusion was reduced from 29% in the placebo group to 19% in the epoetin alfa group.[163] The ASCO/ASH guideline provides no clear evidence as to whether epoetin therapy translates into clinically meaningful symptomatic improvement. However, a recent review identified 41 studies addressing quality-of-life improvement in epoetin therapy. Thirty-six studies, including 11 well-controlled trials, reported statistically significant improvements in quality of life.[186] One meta-analysis found a significant effect of epoetin on quality of life only in patients with baseline hemoglobin of 10 gm/dL or less.[185] Four studies did not observe a significant difference in quality of life between epoetin-treated patients and controls.[186] Taken together, the effect of rhEPO on quality of life appears to be positive. ASCO/ASH guidelines recommend epoetin as a treatment option in cancer patients with chemotherapy-associated anemia if the hemoglobin has declined to 10 gm/dL or less.[168] For anemic patients with declining hemoglobin levels that are still in the range of greater than 10 but less than 12 gm/dL, the decision to use epoetin should be based on clinical circumstances such as advanced age or comorbid conditions.[168]

These recommendations apply as well for patients with multiple myeloma, non-Hodgkin's lymphoma, and chronic lymphocytic leukemia experiencing chemotherapy-associated anemia if cytoreductive treatment has failed to induce a hemoglobin response.[168,187,188] Patients with myeloid malignancies have typically been excluded from epoetin trials because of concerns regarding growth-promoting effects of rhEPO, and therefore no data are available to give recommendations for rhEPO use.[168] At present, evidence is insufficient to give recommendations for cancer patients with radiotherapy-associated anemia.[186]

Similar efficacy of the longer acting darbepoetin alfa compared to epoetin has now been reported.[189,190] At present, it is typically administered once every 2 or 3 weeks, but the true benefits in convenience compared to epoetins have to be determined in further studies.

It is recommended to monitor iron, total iron-binding capacity, transferrin saturation, or ferritin levels and to institute iron repletion when indicated in patients treated with rhEPO.[168] Recent evidence from a prospective, open-label, randomized trial demonstrated a higher percentage of patients with hematopoietic response if iron was administered intravenously compared to no and oral iron supplementation (68% vs. 25% and 36%, respectively; $P < .01$).[191] However, in anemic cancer patients, guidelines for optimal timing and periodicity of monitoring and the optimal dosing regimen for iron repletion are not available.[168]

A considerable number of patients will not respond to rhEPO therapy. To separate responders from nonresponders, predictors of response have been evaluated. Serum erythropoietin levels less than 100 units/L, an increase in hemoglobin of 0.5 gm/dL or more after 4 weeks of treatment, serum ferritin levels less than 400 ng/mL at 4 weeks, and others have been proposed as predictive factors for response to epoetin alfa.[163,192,193]

Anemia in Cancer Patients Not Associated with Treatment

Epoetin use in "anemia of cancer" has been studied in several trials.[194–197] Although studies consistently found an increase in hemoglobin, results are inconclusive with respect to reduction of the need for red blood cell transfusions and quality-of-life improvement. The ASCO/ASH guideline does not provide firm recommendations for the use of rhEPO in cancer patients with anemia not associated with treatment. However, for anemic patients with multiple myeloma, non-Hodgkin's lymphoma, and chronic lymphocytic leukemia not receiving chemotherapy, limited data are available for the use of epoetin,[198,199] and it is recommended to initiate chemotherapy and/or corticosteroids and await the hematologic outcome achieved solely by tumor reduction before considering epoetin.[168]

Anemia Caused by Bone Marrow or Hematopoietic Progenitor Cell Transplantation

Three randomized, controlled trials investigated the effect of rhEPO in patients receiving an autologous transplant. The need for red blood cell transfusions could not be reduced by administration of rhEPO,[200,201] and thus it cannot be recommended in this setting. However, autologous transplantation was performed safely in patients denying allogeneic blood transfusions for religious reasons with posttransplant support of rhEPO, G-CSF, intravenous iron, and ε-aminocaproic acid.[202]

In allogeneic transplantation, conflicting data exist with respect to improved hemoglobin concentration and reduced transfusion requirements.[186] In a randomized, placebo-controlled trial, the median time to transfusion independence was reduced from 27 to 19 days, but transfusion requirements were similar for the rhEPO and the placebo groups.[200] Another randomized, placebo-controlled study found an increase in hemoglobin in the epoetin group compared to the placebo group, but transfusion requirements were not different between the groups.[203] Recent guidelines from the EORTC do not recommend the general use of rhEPO in allogeneic transplantation.[186]

Anemia in Myelodysplastic Syndromes

A double-blind, placebo-controlled trial investigating the effect of epoetin (150 units/kg once daily) in patients with myelodysplastic syndrome found that significantly more patients who were treated with epoetin achieved a hematologic response compared with placebo controls (37% vs. 11%; $P = .007$).[204] Interestingly, in a subgroup analysis, this difference remained significant only in patients with refractory anemia. Unfortunately, transfusion requirements and quality-of-life improvements were not reported. Another study found a delayed response to rhEPO in myelodysplastic syndrome. At 26 weeks, response rates for patients with refractory anemia, refractory anemia with ringed sideroblasts, and refractory anemia with excess blasts type I and type II were 48%, 58%, 34%, and 13%, respectively.[205] Moreover, a hemoglobin response was reported in 101 of 428 patients with myelodysplastic syndrome (24%) treated with rhEPO.[206] Baseline serum erythropoietin levels below 100 mU/L[207] or below 150 mU/L[205] were predictive for response. Thus, the ASCO/ASH guideline proposed the use of epoetin in patients with refractory anemia and a low level of endogenous erythropoietin.[168] Combination therapy with epoetin (150–300 units/kg once daily) and G-CSF (1 μg/kg once daily) showed clinically meaningful responses in myelodysplastic syndrome patients (increased hemoglobin level and reduced transfusion requirements) in 36–48% of patients.[120–122,208,209] Responses generally occurred within 6–8 weeks and may have persisted for several months. However, a recent trial including 50 low-grade anemic myelodysplastic syndrome patients found no difference in quality of life but significantly higher costs in patients treated with rhEPO and rhG-CSF compared to patients with best supportive care.[209] A hemoglobin response was only seen in 4 of 45 patients, if epoetin was combined with GM-CSF.[210]

Anemia in Idiopathic Myelofibrosis

rhEPO has been investigated in anemia of idiopathic myelofibrosis. Except for one study,[211] rhEPO was unable to reduce transfusion requirements in idiopathic myelofibrosis.[212–214] rhEPO may be added to a combination of androgen preparation and corticosteroid in anemic patients with myelofibrosis, although at a low level of evidence that this may be effective.[215]

Anemia in Bone Marrow Failure Syndromes

Diamond-Blackfan anemia is a congenital form of pure red cell aplasia in which the erythroid precursors are reduced or absent. Data indicate that the erythroid stem/progenitor cells are partly or completely refractory to erythropoietin,[216] and consistently with this finding no hematologic response has been observed in patients treated with high doses of rhEPO.[217] However, other hematopoietic growth factors such as interleukin-3 may be effective.[218] In Fanconi's anemia, rhEPO failed to induce a hematologic response.[219]

In acquired aplastic anemia, the addition of high doses of rhEPO (400 units/kg once daily) to G-CSF has led to an improved erythroid response (>1 gm/dL or >50% decrease in red blood cell transfusion requirements) compared to lower doses or control (36.8% vs. 14.6% and 12.9%, respectively) in a randomized, controlled study with 131 patients.[150] Responses were seen in patients with nonsevere aplastic anemia and therefore might be due to stimulation of residual normal erythropoiesis. Similar effects were reported in a smaller study.[220] Recently, a retrospective analysis of six patients diagnosed with paroxysmal nocturnal hemoglobinuria and treated with rhEPO reported one patient who became transfusion independent and another with a mean rise in hemoglobin of 1.5 gm/dL.[221] Further studies are needed to confirm the use of rhEPO in aplastic anemia and paroxysmal nocturnal hemoglobinuria.

Anemia in Sickle Cell Disease and β-Thalassemia

In sickle cell disease, rhEPO has been investigated as an alternative to hydroxyurea for induction of hemoglobin F production. When used in combination with hydroxyurea, rhEPO produced an increase in the number of reticulocytes containing hemoglobin F compared to hydroxyurea alone from 64% to 78%.[222] Other studies showed conflicting results.[223–225] Thus, further studies are needed to clarify the role of rhEPO in sickle cell disease. Individual hematologic responses to rhEPO were also reported in β-thalassemia patients.[226–228]

Anemia in Patients Undergoing Surgery

Outside the United States, epoetin beta has been approved to increase the amount of donated autologous blood at the time of an elective surgery. Eligible patients should have hemoglobin levels of 10–13 gm/dL, no iron deficiency, and a need for transfusion during surgery of 4 or 5 units of red blood cells for women or men, respectively. In a randomized, placebo-controlled trial, 71% of patients treated with epoetin beta were able to donate six times or more compared to 32% of the placebo patients. The period of anemia after blood donation was shortened.[229] These benefits have to be weighed against an increased risk of thromboembolic events.

In the United States, epoetin alfa has been approved in a subpopulation of patients undergoing elective, noncardiac and nonvascular surgery to reduce the need for allogeneic blood transfusions. In anemic patients (hemoglobin >10 to <13 gm/dL), the proportion of perioperatively transfused patients was significantly reduced from 13 of 29 (45%) in the placebo group to 5 of 31 (16%) in the epoetin alfa group.[230] Importantly, patients were expected to require 2 or more units of blood and were not able or willing to participate in an autologous blood donation program. All patients received oral iron and coagulation prophylaxis. In patients undergoing coronary artery bypass graft surgery, the risk of death from thrombotic/vascular events was increased in the epoetin alfa group compared to the placebo-treated group.[231]

Controversies and Future Directions of rhEPO Use

Concern has been raised that rhEPO treatment may promote tumor growth because erythropoietin receptors are found on many tumor cell lines. Conversely, it has been postulated that rhEPO may sensitize tumors to radio- and/or chemotherapy and thus may be used for better tumor control.[232,233] A recent review has found no consistent evidence from multiple, well-controlled studies that treatment with rhEPO improves survival.[186] Another recent meta-analysis from the Cochrane Database of Systematic Reviews found inconclusive evidence as to whether rhEPO improves tumor response (fixed effect: relative risk 1.36; 95% confidence interval, 1.07–1.72;

seven trials, n = 1150; random effects: relative risk 1.21; 95% confidence interval, 0.92–1.59).[171] However, concern with respect to the safety of rhEPO arose from two studies with increased mortality in the rhEPO groups compared to controls.[173,234] A randomized, double-blind, placebo-controlled trial in patients with metastatic breast cancer receiving chemotherapy was terminated early due to a statistically significant difference in 12-month survival in favor of the placebo group (70% in the epoetin group vs. 76% placebo controls; P = .0117).[173] This was mainly due to an increase of disease progression in the epoetin group compared to the placebo group (6% vs. 3%) and an increase in the incidence of thrombotic and vascular events in the epoetin group (1% vs. 0.2%). In a second trial, patients with head and neck cancer and mild anemia were randomized to receive epoetin beta or placebo before and during radiation therapy. Patients randomized to epoetin had a higher risk of locoregional tumor progression (relative risk 1.69; 95% confidence interval, 1.16–2.47; P = .007) and poorer survival (relative risk 1.39; 95% confidence interval, 1.05–1.84; P = .02).[234] Both trials have been widely discussed and criticized[235] for a high target hemoglobin in the epoetin group, a high percentage of protocol violators, and imbalances in baseline characteristics between treatment and control groups. In 2004, the FDA held a public hearing of which full details are available online (*http://www.fda.gov/ohrms/dockets/ac/04/briefing/4037b 2.htm*). The FDA did not place any restrictions on the use of rhEPOs but agreed that more studies are required to answer the questions of whether rhEPOs affect tumor progression or survival in cancer patients.

Several important questions related to the optimal use of rhEPO remain to be answered in the future. In addition to safety and efficacy in cancer patients, the efficacy in myelodysplasia and other benign hematologic diseases has to be addressed. Similarly, the use of iron supplementation in the cancer setting has to be investigated. Economic evaluations of rhEPO consistently report that this treatment is not cost-effective in cancer patients[236] and in patients with myelodysplastic syndrome.[209] Therefore, predictors of epoetin response have to be investigated to identify in advance patients who will benefit from treatment with rhEPO.

Recombinant Human Interleukin-11

Thrombocytopenia is a common adverse event in a wide variety of chemotherapy protocols, bringing thrombopenic patients at risk of fatal hemorrhage. In 2001, the ASCO published guidelines on the use of platelet transfusions. The authors recommended a platelet threshold of 10 × 10^9/L for prophylactic platelet transfusions for most cancer patients receiving chemotherapy and a threshold of 20 × 10^9/L if comorbid conditions are present, such as high fever or signs of hemorrhage.[237] The prophylactic use of stimulants of megakaryopoiesis and platelet production has the potential to avoid transmission of infectious agents through allogeneic platelet transfusions and to reduce costs. To this end oprelvekin, a rhIL-11, has been approved by the FDA for cancer patients with nonmyeloid malignancies receiving myelosuppressive chemotherapy (see Table 91–1 for indications and dosage and Table 91–3 for summary). Common adverse events include fluid retention that can result in peripheral edema, dyspnea on exertion, capillary leak syndrome, atrial arrhythmias, papilledema, and dilutional anemia. In addition, allergic reactions including anaphylaxis have been reported.

Two randomized placebo-controlled trials have shown efficacy of oprelvekin for reducing platelet transfusion requirements in patients receiving intensive chemotherapy. Primary prophylactic use of rhIL-11 was investigated in patients with advanced breast cancer receiving intensive chemotherapy and G-CSF support. In the rhIL-11 group, 27 of 40 patients (68%) did not require transfusions compared with 15 of 37 patients (41%) in the placebo group (P = .04).[238] Use of rhIL-11 for secondary prophylaxis of thrombocytopenia has been investigated in patients with various solid tumors who had recovered from an episode of severe chemotherapy-induced thrombocytopenia (platelet count ≤20 × 10^9/L). Of 27 patients in the treatment group, 8 (30%) did not require transfusions compared with 1 of 27 patients (4%) in the placebo group (P < .05).[239] The median number of platelet transfusions in the treatment and control groups was 1 and 3, respectively (P = .06), whereas the mean number did not differ between groups. Whereas ecchymosis occurred in 21% of rhIL-11-treated patients compared to 37% of placebo patients, no other differences among the groups in the incidence or severity of bleeding events were evident. It should be mentioned that the studies were performed at a time when the recommended threshold for platelet transfusions was 20 × 10^9/L or less. A recent economic analysis found that rhIL-11 treatment is not cost-effective compared to platelet transfusions in patients receiving myelosuppressive chemotherapy.[240] Thus further trials are needed that define the true benefits of rhIL-11 in the era of an even more restricted use of platelet transfusions.

In autologous transplantation with peripheral blood progenitor cells in patients with breast cancer, the platelet transfusion requirement was not reduced with oprelvekin compared to placebo.[241]

In patients with myelodysplastic syndrome, aplastic anemia, or graft failure, oprelvekin was evaluated at a low dose of 10 μg/kg. Six of 16 patients (38%), including five patients with myelodysplastic syndrome and one with aplastic anemia, showed a platelet response with a median increase in peak platelet counts of 95 × 10^9/L above baseline.[242] These results await confirmation in a larger patient cohort. An investigation of rhIL-11 in patients with refractory idiopathic thrombocytopenic purpura was terminated early because of a decrease in hemoglobin levels, lack of platelet response, and toxic side effects.[243]

Recently, rhIL-11 has been investigated for its effects on the mucosal barrier. In patients with hematologic malignant disease undergoing chemotherapy, oprelvekin was shown to reduce the frequency and load of bacteremia.[244] Further trials will investigate if this is associated with a decreased rate of infectious complications.

Recombinant Human Keratinocyte Growth Factor

Myeloablative chemotherapy with stem cell support is associated with a high rate of severe mucositis. In these cases, high doses of analgesics and total parenteral nutrition are needed, and the risk of infectious complications is increased by compromise of the mucosal barrier. To circumvent these sequelae, a rhKGF, palifermin, has been investigated in the setting of myeloablative chemotherapy (see Table 91–1 for indications and dosage and Table 91–3 for summary). Palifermin is administered intravenously for 3 days before and for 3 days after myelotoxic therapy beginning shortly after stem cell reinfusion. A Phase I study showed good tolerability of palifermin.[245] The most common side effects of palifermin are skin rash; unusual sensations in the mouth, such as tingling; and increases in amylase and lipase, although these enzymes may be salivary in origin. No data on the long-term use of rhKGF exist. Thus the role of rhKGF in promoting epithelial tumor growth has not been established and palifermin has not been approved for nonhematologic malignancies. In a recent trial, palifermin was used in 212 patients with lymphoma, myeloma, or leukemia undergoing autologous peripheral blood progenitor cell transplantation with intensive conditioning radio/chemotherapy to investigate its effect on oral mucositis. In this randomized, placebo-controlled, double-blind study, the incidence of grade 3 or 4 oral mucositis was reduced from 98% in the placebo group to 63% in the treatment group ($P < .001$). Moreover, the median duration of oral mucositis in patients with grade 3 or 4 mucositis was reduced from 9 days in the placebo group to 6 days in the treatment group ($P < .001$). The use of opioid analgesics and the incidence of use of total parenteral nutrition were significantly lower in the rhKGF group compared to placebo. Interestingly, palifermin recipients had a lower incidence of febrile neutropenia than did placebo recipients (75% vs. 92%; $P < .001$). In an exploratory analysis, a trend toward a lower incidence of blood-borne infections in the palifermin group than in the placebo group was seen (15% vs. 25%).[246] Based on these data, it is expected that the use of palifermin will be rapidly adopted by clinicians; however, to establish the long-term safety, close monitoring of patients will be required.

CYTOKINES IN DEVELOPMENT

Several hematopoietic growth factors are under investigation for clinical purposes but have not been approved yet. Thrombopoietin, the c-Mpl ligand, is the primary physiologic regulator of megakaryocyte and platelet development. Two recombinant forms of thrombopoietin have been evaluated for clinical use. Recombinant human thrombopoietin is a glycosylated, full-length thrombopoietin that leads to an increase in platelet count by day 5 after a single dose.[247] It has been effective in nonmyeloablative chemotherapy settings, whereas no beneficial effect was seen in stem cell transplantation or leukemia chemotherapy.[248] A nonglycosylated, pegylated, and truncated form of thrombopoietin, megakaryocyte growth and development factor (PEG-MGDF), has been shown to induce antibody formation cross-reacting with the endogenous thrombopoietin, and subsequent thrombocytopenia.[249] In addition, PEG-MGDF was unable to improve platelet recovery after myelosuppressive chemotherapy in acute myeloid leukemia,[250,251] and further development has been terminated. Currently, the role of thrombopoietin in various diseases with non–chemotherapy-induced thrombocytopenia is investigated.[248]

Interleukin-3, also called multicolony-stimulating factor, promotes the survival, proliferation, and development of multipotential hematopoietic progenitor cells.[252] In spite of promising initial results,[253,254] in larger clinical trials the degree of hematopoietic stimulation has been disappointing.[255–257] However, combination of interleukin-3 with GM-CSF resulted in increased mobilization of progenitor cells compared to interleukin-3 alone.[258] The combination of interleukin-3 with other cytokines is currently being investigated by use of chimeric proteins. Leridistim (myelopoietin) is an interleukin-3/G-CSF dual receptor agonist increasing both neutrophil and platelet counts. In a Phase III trial of patients with breast cancer receiving chemotherapy, however, Leridistim has been clearly inferior to G-CSF alone.[259] In addition, promegapoietin has been developed as an interleukin-3/thrombopoietin dual receptor agonist that has stimulatory effects on both neutrophil and platelet counts in nonhuman primates.[260]

FMS-like tyrosine kinase 3 (FLT-3) ligand has little direct effect on progenitor cell proliferation but synergizes with other cytokines to enhance proliferation.[261,262] FLT-3 ligand induces mobilization of hematopoietic progenitor cells when administered in mice and demonstrated synergy when used in combination with G-CSF or GM-CSF.[263] Thus progenipoietin-1 has been developed as a FLT-3/G-CSF dual receptor agonist.[264] Recently FLT-3 ligand has been shown to increase numbers of monocytes and dendritic cells in patients with peritoneal carcinomatosis or mesotheliomas.[265] A potential stimulatory effect of FLT-3 ligand on immune function needs further study.

Recombinant human stem cell factor (rhSCF, ancestim) has been used in combination with G-CSF to mobilize progenitor cells to the peripheral blood.[266,267] Interestingly, in patients who have failed a prior mobilization with G-CSF, the administration of rhSCF led to successful progenitor harvests in approximately half of the patients,[268] although accompanied by a high rate of adverse events. In Australia, ancestim has been approved for mobilization of peripheral blood progenitor cells in combination with filgrastim. In summary, recent development of hematopoietic growth factors aims at targeting early or multiple hematopoietic progenitors to induce multilineage responses.

CONCLUSION

Cytokines constitute a special weapon in a hematologist's armament of drugs because they are "constructive" agents, in contrast to the vast majority of "destructive"

CURRENT CONTROVERSIES & FUTURE CONSIDERATIONS

Cytokine Therapy and Its Complications

- There is still a need to have better predictive parameters for the selection of patients who might benefit from the use of hematopoietic growth factors. This is especially important for anemic patients who are candidates for treatment with erythropoietin.[269]
- The potential stimulation of tumor cell growth by erythropoietin—albeit it seems to be a rare event—requires additional data collection and analysis.[269]
- The possible induction of a higher rate of graft-versus-host disease by the administration of G-CSF after allogeneic stem cell transplantation has not yet been completely resolved.[270,271]
- The use of G-CSF or GM-CSF as a priming agent in the treatment of acute myeloid leukemia remains controversial and might very much depend on the way it is combined with chemotherapy.[272]
- A clinically effective thrombopoietic agent is needed. Probably a stimulation of accelerated platelet recovery will not be achieved by using a single agent but requires the combination of at least two early and late acting factors.[273]
- Advances in our understanding of cell signalling should permit to develop orally applied cytokine mimetics for every clinically useful cytokine, thus replacing the parenteral administration.[274,275]

cytotoxic drugs in hematology or oncology practice. Colony-stimulating factors are an integral part of hematopoietic stem cell transplantation and reduce the incidence of febrile neutropenia. Other cytokines are able to reduce the use of red blood cell and platelet transfusions, and to alleviate symptoms from mucositis. However, these beneficial effects are accompanied by high expenses. Cytokine development mirrors the great advances that have been achieved in our understanding of the regulatory mechanisms in hematopoiesis. As this understanding grows, new drugs and new applications will emerge.

Suggested Readings*

Bokemeyer C, Aapro MS, Courdi A, et al: EORTC guidelines for the use of erythropoietic proteins in anaemic patients with cancer. Eur J Cancer 40:2201–2216, 2004.

Ozer H, Armitage JO, Bennett CL, et al: 2000 update of recommendations for the use of hematopoietic colony-stimulating factors: evidence-based, clinical practice guidelines. American Society of Clinical Oncology Growth Factors Expert Panel. J Clin Oncol 18:3558–3585, 2000.

Pagliuca A, Carrington PA, Pettengell R, et al: Guidelines on the use of colony-stimulating factors in haematological malignancies. Br J Haematol 123:22–33, 2003.

Repetto L, Biganzoli L, Koehne CH, et al: EORTC Cancer in the Elderly Task Force guidelines for the use of colony-stimulating factors in elderly patients with cancer. Eur J Cancer 39:2264–2272, 2003.

Rizzo JD, Lichtin AE, Woolf SH, et al: Use of epoetin in patients with cancer: evidence-based clinical practice guidelines of the American Society of Clinical Oncology and the American Society of Hematology. J Clin Oncol 20:4083–4107, 2002.

Full references for this chapter can be found on accompanying CD-ROM.

SECTION 4
HEMATOLOGIC COMPLICATIONS IN SURGERY

CHAPTER 92
EVALUATION OF THE ACUTELY BLEEDING PATIENT

Herbert H. Watzke, MD

KEY POINTS

Evaluation of the Acutely Bleeding Patient

- Medical history, physical examination, and targeted laboratory investigations are the key elements in the evaluation of an acutely bleeding patient.
- A conclusive but negative history of bleeding during surgery has a high negative predictive value for an inherited coagulation defect.
- Persistent bleeding even after reoperation points toward a systemic hemorrhagic disease.
- Many commonly used medications (heparins, platelet-inhibitory drugs, antibiotics) may cause bleeding perioperatively but are not readily detected by routine coagulation screening.
- Measures to counteract bleeding (protamine in the case of heparin overdosage, massive transfusions) may cause bleeding.
- Spontaneous bleeding from the gastrointestinal tract is almost always caused by an anatomic lesion.
- Spontaneous bleeding in soft tissues or organs is usually accompanied by severely altered, diagnostic laboratory tests.

INTRODUCTION

Evaluation of an acutely bleeding patient is a complex process that has several unique features. First, it is usually carried out under considerable constraints of time because immediate measures to stop bleeding are expected from this evaluation in order to prevent severe damage to the patient or even to preserve life. Second, it usually takes place in the setting of acute bleeding occurring as an unexpected complication of surgery, and therefore is of utmost medical and legal importance. Finally, it involves evaluation of blood coagulation, a multivariant system with numerous, largely interdependent and interacting variables that frequently obscure identification of the major cause of bleeding.

Surgery is still the ultimate test of the hemostatic system. Accordingly, underlying defects of hemostasis frequently may remain asymptomatic and unrecognized and yet will bleed excessively during surgery. Nevertheless, the vast majority of intraoperative and early postoperative bleeding is caused by technical problems of surgery, such as inefficient or undone ligatures or cauterizations.[1] It is therefore important to constantly include the surgeon in the work-up of such bleeding. The readiness to reoperate on a patient for acute postoperative bleeding is inversely correlated with the suspicion of an underlying defect. The strength of this suspicion and the subsequent readiness of the surgeon to reoperate may vary over time depending on the results of the ongoing evaluation by the hematologist.

Evaluation of an acutely bleeding patient is best carried out using a systematic approach. This includes a detailed history, a thorough physical examination, and a targeted laboratory investigation. Although these activities can be easily carried out step by step in a chronically bleeding patient, it can be difficult to use this stepwise approach in an acutely bleeding surgical patient who requires an acute medical intervention: a reliable history is occasionally not obtainable, a meaningful physical examination can be hampered by bandages or casts, and technically complex coagulation tests are frequently necessary but often not acutely available. It is important in this situation that at least sufficient material for coagulation testing (citrated plasma, EDTA plasma) is obtained before any nonspecific therapy to improve coagulation, such as platelets, prothrombin complex concentrates, DDAVP, or factor VIIa, is initiated.

This chapter focuses on evaluation of acutely bleeding patients with a view to establishing a diagnosis. For details of treatment, the reader is referred to the relevant chapters.

TABLE 92–1. Functional Half-Life, Time of First Administration Postoperatively, Prophylactic Doses, and Laboratory Tests for Antithrombotics Used to Prevent Venous Thromboembolism in Surgery

	Functional Half-Time	Time of Administration after Surgery	Prophylactic Dose/Day	Laboratory Tests
Unfractionated heparin (SC)	2 hr	10–12 hr	3 × 5000 IU	Anti-Xa
Low-molecular-weight heparin (SC)	4 hr	10–12 hr	1 × 2000–5000 IU	Anti-Xa
Coumarin (oral)	Days	1st postoperative day		INR
Fondaparinux (SC)	15 hr	6 hr	1 × 2.5 mg	Anti-Xa
Melagatran (SC)	3 hr	Beginning of surgery	1 × 2 mg	Not available
Ximelagatran (oral)	3 hr	12 hr	1 × 24 mg	Not available

Abbreviations: Anti-Xa, anti–factor Xa antibody; INR, International Normalized Ratio; SC, subcutaneous.

HISTORY OF AN ACUTELY BLEEDING PATIENT

The history of an acutely bleeding surgical patient includes the follow key elements:

- History of antithrombotic or platelet-inhibitory medication
- Underlying medical problems
- Timing of bleeding during the acute event
- List of measures to treat bleeding during the acute event
- History of bleeding before the acute event

History of Antithrombotic or Platelet-Inhibitory Medication

Antithrombotic agents and platelet aggregation inhibitors are widely used medications that can cause severe acute bleeding during and after surgery. The history of an acutely bleeding patient must therefore include questions regarding these substances.

Antithrombotics

Medical prophylaxis of postoperative venous thromboembolism is required in the majority of patients undergoing major surgery. It is carried out using several different agents such as unfractionated heparins, low-molecular-weight heparins, heparinoids, vitamin K antagonists, selective thrombin inhibitors, and factor Xa inhibitors.[2] These substances are given in close proximity to surgery based on the concept that blood clots develop during the actual process of surgery itself and can be best inhibited by an early onset of prophylactic measures or even by a preoperative initiation of prophylaxis. These substances effectively reduce postoperative thromboembolism but increase bleeding at the same time. The bleeding tendency is usually moderate and clinically not apparent. However, if timing or dosing is incorrect, severe clinically overt bleeding can occur[3] (Table 92–1). The actual timing of antithrombotic prophylaxis can usually be retrieved from the patient's chart and the personal history. The correct dosing can be checked by a simple laboratory test in only a minority of instances (i.e., using the prothrombin time for a vitamin K antagonist). The dose intensity of the widely used unfractionated heparins and low-molecular-weight heparins is more difficult to assess[4] and has a major drawback: the half-life of these substances is so short (see Table 92–1) that their anticoagulant activity may be below the detection limit shortly after an overdose has caused bleeding. Only if the half-life of low-molecular-weight heparin is prolonged, such as in patients with renal failure, will accumulation lead to long-lasting altered tests for anticoagulant activity.

Antiplatelet Agents

Platelet aggregation inhibitors such as acetylsalicylate, clopidogrel, ticlopidine, dipyridamole, glycoprotein IIb/IIIa inhibitors, and the so-called nonsteroidal anti-inflammatory drugs are widely prescribed for a broad spectrum of indications and are compounds of many over-the-counter drugs, in particular analgesics. They cause a mild bleeding diathesis that rarely leads to spontaneous bleeding, is usually not apparent even in the majority of surgical interventions, but can cause severe bleeding in special situations such as open cardiac surgery, neurosurgery, prostatic surgery, and ophthalmologic surgery. Although the patient's list of medications will clearly indicate drugs with platelet-inhibitory activity, it is more difficult and sometimes impossible to get precise information on over-the-counter drugs in an acutely bleeding patient, because patients do not always remember the kind of medication, and rarely remember the exact time of last intake, which can be important because the functional half-life of most of these substances is several days.

Several antibiotics cause bleeding by decreasing the synthesis of vitamin K–dependent clotting factors. These include cephalosporins, trimethoprim/sulfamethoxazole, and levofloxacin.[5] Other substances such as penicillins, sulfonamides, and tricyclic antidepressants have been reported to cause bleeding through development of factor VIII antibodies.[6] Various "alternative medications" such as large quantities of garlic, vitamin E, vitamin C,

TABLE 92–2. Acquired Causes of Bleeding

Diagnosis	Clinical Manifestation	Confirmation
Thrombocytopenia	Petechial bleeding	Platelet count <20,000/μL
Platelet inhibitors	None	Long template bleeding time, long capillary closure time
Heparin administration	Soft tissue hemorrhage	Anti-Xa (units/mL); long aPTT
Liver failure	Soft tissue hemorrhage	Long PT; low factors II, V, VII, IX, X
Coumarin intake	Soft tissue hemorrhage Hematuria	Drug history; PT; low factors II, VII, IX, X
Acquired hemophilia	Soft tissue hemorrhage	Long aPTT, low factor VIII
Acquired vWD	Mucosal bleeding	Analysis of vWF multimers; myeloma, lymphoma, MGUS
Inhibitors against factor V and/or factor II	Soft tissue hemorrhage	Low levels of factor V and/or factor II, history of "fibrin glue"
Uremia	None	Long template bleeding time, long capillary closure time
DIC	Soft tissue hemorrhage	Long aPTT, long PT, high D-dimer, low platelets, low fibrinogen
Amyloidosis	Soft tissue hemorrhage Skin bleeding	Low factor X, prolonged PT
Dysproteinemia	Soft tissue hemorrhage	Long PT, low platelets

Abbreviations: Anti-Xa, anti–factor Xa antibody; aPTT, activated partial thromboplastin time; DIC, disseminated intravascular coagulation; MGUS, monoclonal gammopathy of uncertain significance; PT, prothrombin time; vWD, von Willebrand disease; vWF, von Willebrand factor.

and ginger have been associated with increased risk for bleeding.[7]

Underlying Medical Problems

A broad variety of acute or chronic medical conditions are associated with increased bleeding as a result of acquired defects of blood coagulation (Table 92–2). Some of them affect only one specific structure, such as the factor X molecule, which is specifically absorbed by amyloid fibrils in amyloidosis, or the factor VIII molecule when it is blocked by a specific antibody. Other medical conditions may affect more than one component of blood coagulation, as is the case in severe liver disease. Deficiency in coagulation factors may arise from impaired protein synthesis by the liver and/or low-grade disseminated intravascular coagulation caused by impaired clearance of activated coagulation factors and/or decreased synthesis of α_2-antiplasmin.[8] In addition, thrombocytopenia is frequently observed in chronic liver disease and is caused by enhanced sequestration of platelets in the enlarged spleen.[9] Other medical conditions associated with increased bleeding are uremia, acute promyelocytic leukemia, systemic lupus erythematosus, and dysproteinemias.

Timing of Bleeding During the Acute Event

Timing of the hemorrhagic complication can give important information on the nature of a possible underlying coagulation disorder (Box 92–1). Intraoperative oozing at the surgical site is often due to defects in primary hemostasis, caused by impaired formation of the primary platelet-rich clot as a result of abnormalities in platelet count or platelet function. It is characterized by the development of multiple submucous or subepithelial flat hematomas after minimal mechanical trauma (such as suction devices) and by constant oozing from usually "dry" operative sites.

Box 92–1. Onset and Underlying Causes of Perioperative Hemorrhage

Intraoperative Onset of Hemorrhage

- Thrombocytopenia
- Intake of platelet inhibitors
- Heparin overdosage

Immediately Postoperative Onset of Hemorrhage

- Structural or technical defects
- Mild but multiple acquired coagulation factor defects

Delayed Postoperative Onset of Hemorrhage

- Severe hereditary coagulation factor deficiencies
- Multiorgan failure
- Disseminated intravascular coagulation
- Nonsteroidal anti-inflammatory drug administration

Delayed postoperative bleeding is characteristic of inherited deficiencies of coagulation factors, multiorgan failure, disseminated intravascular coagulation, intake of nonsteroidal anti-inflammatory drugs, or connective tissue disorders. Formation of the primary platelet-rich clot is not affected by these defects. Thus, blood initially clots normally. However, subsequent stabilization of the primary clot is impaired and delayed bleeding will occur.

Deficiencies in factor XIII or fibrinogen or collagen may also be associated with defects in wound healing.

List of Measures to Treat Bleeding During the Acute Event

An important feature of the consultative process in an acutely bleeding patient is to get a clear picture of all measures that have already been taken to stabilize the patient and/or stop bleeding. These include specific measures such as targeted replacement of blood products (red blood cells, platelets, and coagulation factors), infusion of antidotes such as protamine or vitamin K, and more nonspecific measures such as infusion of DDAVP, activated clotting factor concentrates, or recombinant factor VIIa.

Massive transfusion is an imprecise term that implies that most of the patient's blood volume has been replaced with transfused blood within minutes or hours. Coagulation abnormalities occur in 30% of such patients and typically will become apparent after anatomic bleeding sites are controlled. The majority of the bleeding abnormalities are caused by the fact that stored blood does not contain functional platelets, which results in platelet deficiency in the recipient of large transfusion volumes. Transfusion of 20 units will lower the platelet count to approximately 100,000/μL.[10] Deficiencies in factor VIII and factor V have been reported following massive transfusions.[11] However, their decrease in activity does not correlate with the number of units transfused and is usually not sufficient to indicate replacement. Prolongation of the prothrombin time and the partial thromboplastin time has been reported in massive transfusions in association with cardiovascular shock and disseminated intravascular coagulation.

Protamine is commonly used to neutralize the effect of heparin, particularly in the setting of hemodialysis or cardiopulmonary bypass. One milligram of protamine sulfate will neutralize 80–100 USP units of heparin. Bleeding following therapy with protamine can have two causes. First, a rebound of heparin can occur because protamine sulfate is cleared from the blood more rapidly than heparin. Second, excessive amounts of protamine sulfate can induce thrombocytopenia and interfere with fibrin formation.[12]

Nonspecific measures such as therapy with factor VIIa or DDAVP may mask a severe bleeding tendency that becomes clinically apparent when their effect ceases as a result of a short half-life (as with factor VIIa) or exhaustion of the therapeutic effect of the substance used (as with DDAVP).

History of Bleeding Before the Acute Event

A conclusive but negative history of bleeding has an extremely high negative predictive value for the presence of an inherited defect in hemostasis.[13] It is even superior to laboratory screening tests in preoperative prediction of surgical bleeding. Its value in the exclusion of an inherited defect in acutely bleeding patients has not been formally proven but seems likely to be similar. Several authors have proposed comprehensive questionnaires in order to simplify and standardize the evaluation of patients with regard to bleeding disorders.[14] The questions usually are binary and make little use of quantitative evaluations. They focus on signs and symptoms of bleeding following surgery and/or trauma and on spontaneous bleeding. The following key questions are common elements in such standardized evaluations.

Bleeding Complication Following a Surgical Procedure?

This is probably the single most important question when taking a history for bleeding. If conclusive and positive, it is a strong indicator for an inherited hemostatic defect. However, it is obviously of no value in patients without a previous surgical intervention and thus frequently inconclusive in children and young adults. Furthermore, its value in the exclusion of an underlying genetic abnormality of coagulation is largely dependent on the kind of surgery performed in the past. There are interventions such as cardiothoracic surgery or prostate surgery that have a high risk of bleeding even in patients with a normal hemostatic system and therefore are generally not good indicators for a defect in hemostasis. Other major operations, such as renal transplantations, have been performed without bleeding complications in fully anticoagulated patients, indicating little dependence on normal hemostasis during this procedure. However, severe genetic defects of coagulation may very well manifest themselves during such procedures. Excessive bleeding following circumcision, extraction of wisdom teeth, or tonsillectomy is generally a good indicator for a severe hemostatic defect, particularly because these procedures are usually performed early in life and their prevalence is high.

Estimation of the blood loss is important to discriminate between "normal" and excessive surgical bleeding. Excessive bleeding should be suspected when significantly more blood transfusions are required than expected, when reoperation does not control bleeding, or when a prolonged hospital stay is required.

Spontaneous Bleeding?

Spontaneous bleeding by definition is bleeding that occurs without any identifiable trauma. It can manifest throughout the body. If it occurs in the mucosa (epistaxis, menorrhagia, melena) and skin (petechiae), it is usually associated with moderate to severe thrombocytopenia, qualitative platelet disorders, or severe von Willebrand disease. Easy bruising in the skin of the abdomen and thighs, as is frequently observed in obese premenopausal women, is typically not associated with a generally increased bleeding tendency or with abnormalities in coagulation. Spontaneous hemarthroses, bleeding into muscles, or soft tissue hematomas are characteristic for severe deficiencies of coagulation factors, particularly factor VIII and factor IX. Spontaneous bleedings from surfaces inside the body, such as macrohematuria, hematochezia, hemoptysis, hematemesis, and melena, can be associated with severe hemostatic defects but are more frequently caused by preexistent anatomic lesions.

Prolonged Bleeding or Exaggerated Bruising After Minor Trauma?

Prolongation and particularly reoccurrence of bleeding after minor trauma such as razor cuts or paper cuts that requires exertion of pressure for prolonged periods may indicate an underlying hemostatic defect. Similarly, bleeding complications requiring medical help during the loss of deciduous teeth may also be indicative of an impaired hemostatic system.

Persistent Menorrhagia Without Uterine Abnormalities?

Menstrual histories can occasionally be very helpful when a genetic hemostatic disorder is suspected in an acutely bleeding patient, particularly if menorrhagia is associated with persistent microcytic anemia despite regular iron supplementation and/or the use of oral contraceptives, if hysterectomy or other surgical interventions had been performed to treat menorrhagia, or if otherwise unexplained anemia is present. However, *menorrhagia* simply denotes increased menstruation and is an imprecise term with regard to the actual blood loss. Therefore, various bleeding scales have been developed in an attempt to better quantify menstrual blood loss.[15] They monitor the duration of maximal blood loss (normally 3 days or less), the duration of menstruation (normally 7 days or less), and the number of tampons or pads used during menstruation.

Family History of Bleeding?

Congenital bleeding disorders are relatively rare compared with acquired bleeding disorders. Their pattern of inheritance is either autosomal recessive (deficiencies in factors II, V, VII, XI, X, and XII; platelet defects such as Bernard-Soulier syndrome or Glanzmann's thrombasthenia), autosomal dominant (von Willebrand disease), or X-chromosomal recessive (hemophilia A, hemophilia B, Wiskott-Aldrich syndrome). Autosomal recessive disorders are characterized by mild deficiencies in heterozygous persons, most of them being asymptomatic. Autosomal dominant disorders affect half of the family members, usually in each generation. Their clinical picture is more variable compared with the recessive disorders as a result of variable penetrance and expressivity of the latter defects. Although a family history may be of great value in the diagnosis of a hemostatic defect, one has to bear in mind that a negative history does not exclude a genetic defect: patients may not be able to obtain relevant information on family members, the family history might be negative when the defect is mild, or the mutation may have occurred de novo in a parental germ cell.

PHYSICAL EXAMINATION

A thorough physical examination in an acutely bleeding patient is absolutely required. It not only can give an idea of the amount of internal blood loss but, more importantly, can help to discriminate between surgical and nonsurgical causes of bleeding (Box 92–2). Such evidence includes petechiae, ecchymoses, telangiectasia, hemarthroses, or hematomas.

Petechiae are small, circular (no more than 2 mm in diameter), painless, nonitching, red dots that are located in the dermis and—in contrast to hyperemic allergic lesions—do not disappear with application of local pressure. They represent minimal, probably capillary skin bleeds. Their color is bright red and subsequently changes to dark red over time. Petechiae are in close proximity to each other but are not confluent. Their distribution throughout the body is typical: they are found in the skin of the lower extremities, particularly the calves and feet in ambulatory patients. They also may occur on the forearm following the use of a sphygmomanometer or on the back in bedridden patients. Petechiae are pathognomonic for severe thrombocytopenia (usually <20,000/μL) but may occur at platelet counts as high as 50,000/μL when platelet inhibitors are taken. Petechiae usually disappear within 1–2 weeks after resolution of the initial thrombocytopenia. Mucosal bleeding in the oral cavity ("wet purpura") is occasionally associated with petechiae and is a sign of very severe thrombocytopenia (<10,000/μL). These lesions are larger, are usually not circular, and predominantly are located in the buccal mucosa, probably as a result of increased mechanical stress in this area.

Ecchymoses are flat, cutaneous lesions that are considerably larger (up to several centimeters) and usually not circular. They can occur spontaneously in females in relation to menses (purpura simplex), are typically located in the skin of the abdomen and thighs, and are not associated with a systemic bleeding tendency. Ecchymoses on the extensor surfaces of the upper extremities with a reddish purple color typically occur in elderly people (senile purpura) and are presumably caused by decreased elasticity of blood vessels and subcutaneous fat with age. Ecchymoses in psychogenic purpura (factitious purpura) have a bizarre pattern, repeatedly occur in areas accessible to the patient, and may persist for months with a denial of repeated trauma. Splinter hemorrhages are small (1- to 2-mm) longitudinal bleeds underneath the nails of fingers and toes and are fre-

Box 92–2. Clinical Features of Perioperative Hemorrhage

Defect of Hemostasis Likely

- Intraoperative onset of unusual bleeding
- Multiple bleeding sites aside from area of surgery
  - Vascular access sites
  - Mucosal membranes
  - Skin
  - Soft tissues
  - Hematuria
  - Melena
- Delayed hemorrhage

Surgical Problem Likely

- Isolated bleeding from the surgical site
- Early and sudden onset of massive bleeding
- Pulsatile, bright red bleeding from surgical site

quently associated with small, circular hemorrhagic lesions similar to petechiae on the fingertips. They are caused by cardiac, mostly valvular, microemboli in patients with endocarditis. Large and often confluent ecchymoses with bleeding manifestations in the subcutaneous tissues are frequently observed during severe impairment of blood coagulation together with low platelet counts, as seen in disseminated intravascular coagulation. These lesions are located on the back and the gluteal region, areas that are mechanically altered in bedridden patients.

Bleeding into joints and/or soft tissues is a hallmark of the hemophilias. Interestingly, hemarthrosis is not a feature of a bleeding diathesis caused by acquired inhibitors of factor VIII. Cerebral bleeds and bleeding in the mucosa and lamina propria of the colon are typical of overdosing of coumarins. Retroperitoneal bleeds are also occasionally observed during intensive heparin therapy.

Telangiectasias are blanching lesions that predominantly are located in the face, under the tongue, and in the oral and nasal mucosa, the lips, and the chest wall. They can occur in association with underlying systemic disease, such as Osler-Weber-Rendu syndrome (mucosal and visceral telangiectasia) or the CREST syndrome (*c*alcinosis, *R*aynaud's phenomenon, *e*sophageal disease, *s*clerodactyly, and *t*elangiectasia), or simply can be associated with normal aging, pregnancy, or the use of oral contraceptives or estrogen replacement therapy. Telangiectasias of spider-like appearance (spider nevi) predominantly located on the chest are typically associated with liver disease.

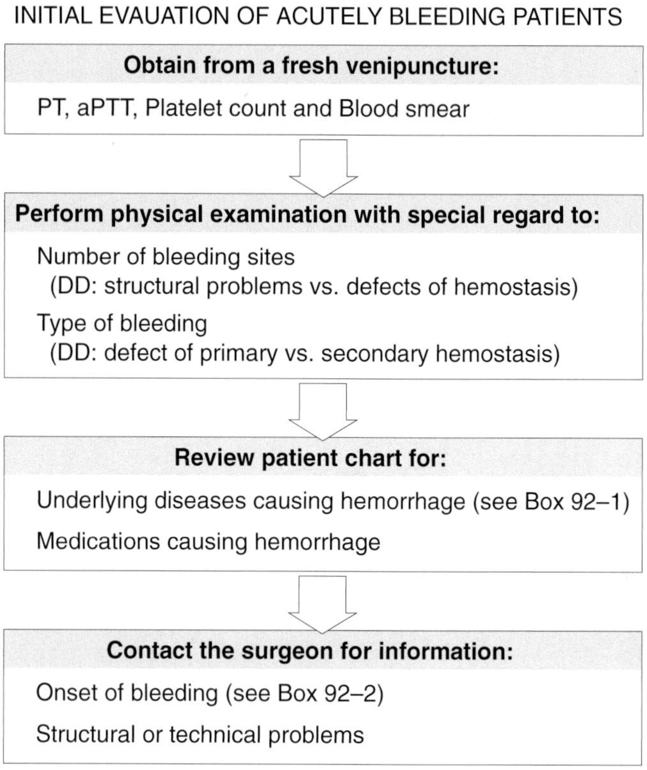

INITIAL EVAUATION OF ACUTELY BLEEDING PATIENTS

Obtain from a fresh venipuncture:

PT, aPTT, Platelet count and Blood smear

↓

Perform physical examination with special regard to:

Number of bleeding sites
(DD: structural problems vs. defects of hemostasis)

Type of bleeding
(DD: defect of primary vs. secondary hemostasis)

↓

Review patient chart for:

Underlying diseases causing hemorrhage (see Box 92–1)

Medications causing hemorrhage

↓

Contact the surgeon for information:

Onset of bleeding (see Box 92–2)

Structural or technical problems

Figure 92–1. Initial evaluation of acutely bleeding patients.

LABORATORY INVESTIGATION

Laboratory investigation is the final and decisive step in the evaluation of an acutely bleeding patient. It will finally allow the identification of a hemorrhagic diathesis and will guide the treatment. The algorithm of laboratory investigation is largely dependent on the results of the patient history and clinical examination, which may give clues to the reason for bleeding. Basic screening tests, which are readily available or can even be performed as bedside tests, can be used to distinguish between defects in primary hemostasis (caused by thrombocytopenia) or secondary hemostasis (caused by a deficiency in coagulation factors). More sophisticated tests will be necessary to differentiate among the various disorders in each of the two main categories of defects.

Blood should be drawn from a fresh peripheral venipuncture as early as possible in the process of evaluation. Blood samples drawn from vascular devices are totally unsuitable because they will frequently yield false abnormal results due to contamination with anticoagulants or plasma, or dilution of the patient's blood by saline or other fluids. The results obtained from a blood sample that are used to guide further measures in an acutely bleeding patient must be free of suspicion of any preanalytical error (Fig. 92–1).

Basic Laboratory Tests

Platelet Count

Thrombocytopenia can be expected when a bleeding tendency is already evident during surgery, when bleeding is manifest immediately after surgery, when frequent spontaneous mucosal bleedings have occurred, or when typical petechiae are present. Thrombocytopenia, defined as a platelet count less than 150,000/μL, can easily be detected on an automated blood cell count. Pseudothrombocytopenia should be suspected whenever moderate to severe thrombocytopenia is present without any corresponding clinical manifestation such as petechiae or mucosal bleeding. It is caused by in vitro aggregation of platelets in the presence of EDTA, which is routinely added to blood collection tubes to prevent coagulation of blood. The mean platelet volume is increased because smaller platelet clumps are automatically counted as single platelets with increased size. A blood smear showing platelet aggregates will increase the suspicion of pseudothrombocytopenia. The (pseudo) thrombocytopenia disappears when platelets are collected in citrate.

Direct observation of platelet morphology on the blood smear can be helpful to differentiate among the various congenital causes of thrombocytopenia such as α-granule deficiency, May-Hegglin anomaly, or Wiskott-Aldrich syndrome (Fig. 92–2).

WORKUP OF AN ACUTELY BLEEDING PATIENT WITH CLINICAL SUSPICION OF A DEFECT IN PRIMARY HEMOSTASIS

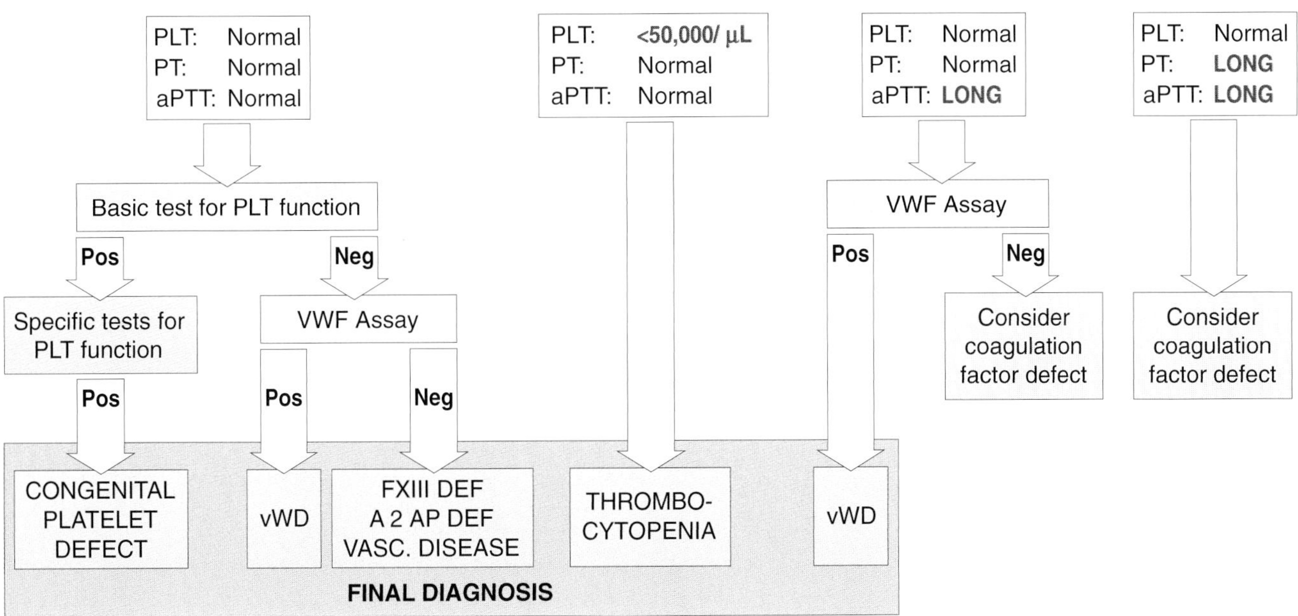

Figure 92–2. Defects in primary hemostasis.

Prothrombin Time

The prothrombin time is the oldest basic test of blood coagulation. It is now available in numerous variations. It is basically performed by the addition of a commercial source of tissue factor and calcium to the patient's plasma, which has been anticoagulated by the addition of citrate. The time until formation of a fibrin clot is a global measure for activities of coagulation factors involved in the tissue factor–dependent pathway and the common pathway of blood coagulation (i.e., factors II, VII, V, X, and fibrinogen). Reduction of coagulant activity by more than 40% in a single factor is necessary to affect the prothrombin time. Less reduction is necessary to prolong the prothrombin time in the case of multiple factor deficiencies. Spontaneous bleeding and exaggerated surgical bleeding will occur only if the prothrombin time is severely prolonged.

Box 92–3. Causes of Bleeding Despite Normal Prothrombin Time and Activated Partial Thromboplastin Time

- Mild hemophilia A or B
- Mild von Willebrand disease
- Thrombocytopenia
- Acquired or inherited platelet abnormalities
- α_2-Antiplasmin deficiency
- Factor XIII deficiency
- Paraproteinemia
- Vascular abnormalities

Activated Partial Thromboplastin Time

The activated partial thromboplastin time globally reflects activities of coagulation factors in the intrinsic pathway (factors VIII, IX, XI, and XII, prekallikrein, and high-molecular-weight kininogen) and the common pathway (factors II, V, X, and fibrinogen) of blood coagulation. It is carried out by the addition of phospholipids, a surface activating agent (such as kaolin), and calcium to citrate-anticoagulated plasma. The time until formation of a fibrin clot is a global measure for activities of coagulation factors involved in the two pathways. The association of bleeding with a prolongation of the activated partial thromboplastin time is dependent on the degree of deficiency and the specific deficient factor. Deficiencies in factor XII, prekallikrein, and high-molecular-weight kininogen have no association with increased bleeding despite the fact that they lead to an extreme prolongation of the activated partial thromboplastin time. Deficiencies in factors IX and VIII of no more than 30% may only slightly prolong the activated partial thromboplastin time (or result in a normal value), but may very well cause severe hemorrhagic complications during surgery or trauma (Box 92–3). Deficiency of factor XI will prolong the activated partial thromboplastin time but is very variable with regard to its association with increased perioperative bleeding. Prolongation also can be caused not only by deficiencies of coagulation factors but also by other conditions, such as the antiphospholipid antibody syndrome (which is a thrombophilic condition and not associated with increased bleeding); elevated levels of split products from fibrinogen or fibrin; antibodies against factors VIII, IX, and V; or anticoagulants such as heparin.

Misunderstanding of some of the basics of heparin monitoring can lead to acute bleeding episodes. The intensity of therapy with the so-called unfractionated heparins is monitored using the activated partial thromboplastin time. It is commonly recommended to increase the dose of unfractionated heparins until a prolongation of 1.5–2.5 times the "control" value is reached. However, there are many limitations regarding the reliability of an activated partial thromboplastin time in the therapeutic range (i.e., 1.5- to 2.5-fold prolongation of the control value). The therapeutic range of unfractionated heparins was established in clinical studies of patients with thromboembolism that related the clinical outcome (prevention of thromboembolic events vs. induction of bleeding events) to plasma heparin concentration: unfractionated heparin levels of 0.2–0.4IU/mL by the protamine titration method and anti–factor Xa levels of 0.3–0.6IU/mL by the use of amidolytic assays were used to delineate the therapeutic range. Therefore, each laboratory must adjust its activated partial thromboplastin time to yield a prolongation of 1.5–2.5 with the above-mentioned heparin concentrations.

Confusion in clinical practice also arises from definition of the control value. By standard definition, the control value is the mean of the laboratory range of the activated partial thromboplastin time, and not the patient's activated partial thromboplastin time, before starting heparin. This control value is useless in patients with a prolongation of the activated partial thromboplastin time before starting heparins, particularly in patients with the lupus anticoagulant. The correct dose of unfractionated heparin must be established using heparin assays in these patients.

A further practical limitation of the reliability of the activated partial thromboplastin time is in the situation of so-called heparin resistance, a state in which extremely high doses of heparins are necessary to adequately prolong the activated partial thromboplastin time. This may be due to high levels of heparin-binding proteins such as platelet factor 4 or elevated levels of factor VIII, an acute-phase reactant that shortens the activated partial thromboplastin time but does not reduce the anticoagulant activity of heparin. Increasing the dose of heparin in the latter case may cause bleeding while the activated partial thromboplastin time is in the normal range.

Finally, low-molecular-weight heparins lead to a prolongation of the activated partial thromboplastin time only when excessively overdosed, and then are associated with a severe bleeding diathesis (Fig. 92–3).

Specialized Laboratory Tests

Platelet Function

The template bleeding time is an in vivo test and is a measure of primary hemostasis, which depends upon platelet number and function and upon normal function of the microvasculature. It is helpful to globally detect deficiencies in the number and/or function of platelets, and is helpful in the diagnosis of von Willebrand disease in patients with a history of easy bruising. However, it does not reliably predict/exclude surgical bleeding when performed preoperatively.[16]

The capillary closure time is an automated in vitro test that estimates the aggregability of platelets upon activation with various agonists such as ADP or epinephrine. It is useful as a global screening test when abnormalities in platelet function are suspected. It is of limited value in the prediction of surgical bleeding.[17]

Platelet aggregation studies are necessary to define the exact nature of a platelet defect in patients with a history suggesting a platelet disorder and/or abnormal screening test results such as template bleeding time or capillary closure time. They are time-consuming laboratory tests and thus usually not available in time in the situation of an acutely bleeding patient.

Coagulation Factors

Abnormalities of the prothrombin time or activated partial thromboplastin time require further work-up. Mixing studies of patient plasma and normal plasma (1:1) are performed initially. Correction of the abnormal test in the mixing study is indicative of a coagulation factor deficiency, because it is sufficient to raise all factor levels in the mix to approximately 40% in order to obtain normal clotting times. Failure to temporarily or permanently correct prolongation of the prothrombin time or activated partial thromboplastin time is consistent with the presence of inhibitors to specific coagulation proteins or a lupus anticoagulant. The further work-up is dependent on the results of the mixing test and may include analysis of the activity of coagulation factors reflected by the prolonged tests or further work-up of possible inhibitors.

Thrombin Time

Prolongation of activated partial thromboplastin time together with prothrombin time without any evidence of a deficiency in coagulation factors and in the absence of an inhibitor strongly suggests the presence of a quantitative or qualitative fibrinogen disorder. The thrombin time monitors the conversion of fibrinogen to fibrin. It will be prolonged when fibrinogen levels are reduced to less than 100mg/dL, when dysfibrinogenemia and/or elevated levels of fibrinogen-fibrin degradation products are present, and in the case of an acquired antibody against thrombin. In addition, heparin will also prolong the thrombin time.

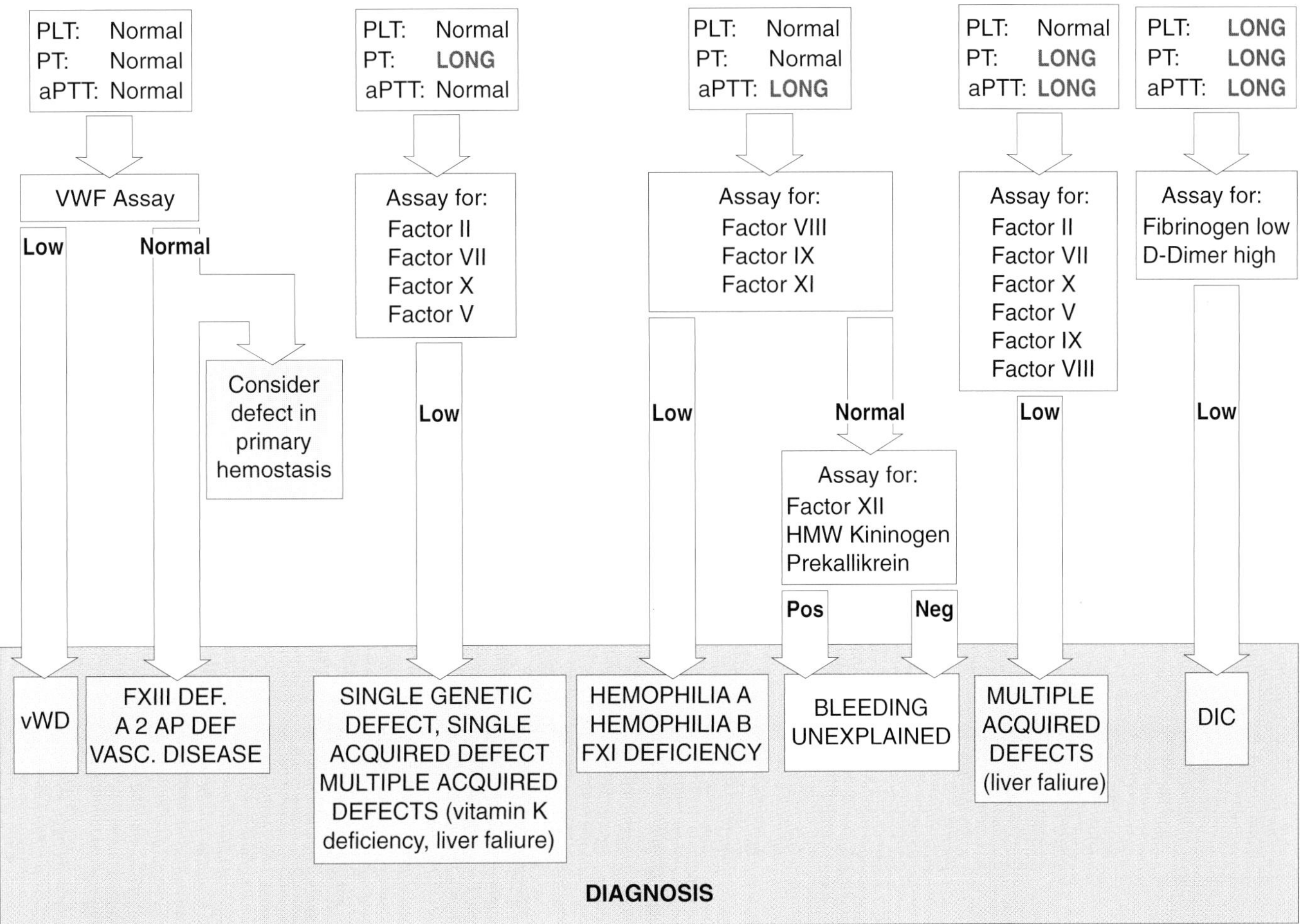

Figure 92–3. Defects in coagulation.

Reptilase Time

The reptilase time measures the conversion of fibrinogen into fibrin after the addition of a fibrinogen-converting venom. It is prolonged when fibrinogen is low and/or fibrinogen-fibrin degradation products are present. In contrast to the thrombin time, it is not prolonged in the presence of heparin. Thus it is used to distinguish between the effects of heparin and fibrinogen-fibrin degradation products in a heparinized patient with prolonged thrombin time and with suspected or proven elevation of fibrinogen-fibrin degradation products, a situation frequently encountered in patients with disseminated intravascular coagulation.

Heparin Assay

Assays detecting the presence of low-molecular-weight heparin should be performed whenever otherwise unexplained exaggerated bleeding occurs after surgery in the presence of normal prothrombin and activated partial thromboplastin times. Accumulation of low-molecular-weight heparin in patients with renal failure or high doses of low-molecular-weight heparin given by mistake will lead to a significant bleeding diathesis that is undetectable by screening tests. Concentration of low-molecular-weight heparin should be less than 0.1 anti–factor Xa units/mL when determined 4 hours after the last subcutaneous dose to prevent postoperative bleeding.

Fibrinogen-Fibrin Degradation Products and D-Dimer

Fibrinogen-fibrin degradation products and D-dimer are generated during fibrinogen conversion and cross-linking of fibrin. They are helpful in establishing the diagnosis of disseminated intravascular coagulation when elevated.

Suggested Readings*

Bowie EJW, Owen CA Jr: The significance of abnormal preoperative hemostatic tests. Prog Hemost Thromb 5:179–209, 1980.

Burk CD, Muller L, Handler SD: Preoperative history and coagulation screening in children undergoing tonsillectomy. Pediatrics 89:691–695, 1992.

Coller B, Schneiderman PI: Clinical evaluation of hemorrhagic disorders: bleeding history and differential diagnosis of purpura. *In* Hoffmann R, Benz EJ, Shattil SJ, et al (eds): Hematology: Basic

Principles and Practice (ed 2). New York: Churchill Livingstone, 1995, pp 1252–1266.

Levine MN, Hirsh J, Kelton JG: Hemorrhagic complications of antithrombotic therapy. *In* Colman RW, Hirsh J, Marder VJ, Salzman EW (eds): Hemostasis and Thrombosis—Basic Principles and Clinical Practice. Philadelphia: Lippincott, 2000, pp 873–882.

Liu MC, Kesser CM: A systematic approach to the bleeding patient. *In* Kitchens CS, Alving BM, Kessler CM (eds): Consultative Hemostasis and Thrombosis. Philadelphia: Saunders, 2002, pp 27–38.

Ratnoff OD: Why do people bleed? *In* Wintrobe MM (ed): Blood, Pure and Eloquent. New York: McGraw-Hill, 1980, pp 600–657.

Full references for this chapter can be found on accompanying CD-ROM.

CHAPTER 93

Surgery in Specific Hematologic Conditions

Richard B. Hostetter, MD, Peter Mattei, MD, and Douglas J. Schwartzentruber, MD

KEY POINTS

Surgery in Specific Hematologic Conditions

- The surgical oncologist often plays a key role in diagnosis of hematologic malignancies by obtaining tissue for diagnosis. He or she must understand the type and amount of tissue needed, and how it must be collected (i.e., in saline, in formalin, or cryopreserved).
- A first consideration is whether the tissue for biopsy is palpable by physical examination or if image-guided techniques are needed.
- The differential diagnosis of abdominal pain in the cancer patient is extensive, and is influenced by concomitant factors such as the use of narcotics, use of antitumor drugs with gastrointestinal side effects, immobilization, dehydration, and electrolyte imbalances. Symptoms of diffuse peritonitis may not be manifest in patients receiving chemotherapy or steroids.
- Lymphoma accounts for almost 50% of malignant causes of intestinal perforation.
- Splenectomy is carried out for relief of symptoms of splenomegaly, for correction of cytopenias, to establish a diagnosis or stage of disease, or to alter the course of disease. The general consensus is in favor of laparoscopic versus open procedures, particularly for smaller spleens.
- Sickle cell patients who undergo surgery are at risk for vaso-occlusive disease in the perioperative period. The risk is increased for patients who are older, are pregnant, have a recent increase in the activity of their disease, or have chronic organ dysfunction as a result of the cumulative effects of multiple acute vaso-occlusive crises.
- Sickle cell patients undergoing surgery should be screened for risk factors, which should be minimized, and should undergo the least invasive surgical approach. Consideration should be given to transfusion therapy to raise the hemoglobin to 10 gm/dL preoperatively.
- Hemophilia patients can undergo surgery safely following replacement of clotting factor to appropriate levels. For major procedures, patients should be replaced to 100% perioperatively, 40–50% in the first 3–5 days postoperatively, and greater than 30% for up to 2 weeks after surgery.

INTRODUCTION

The specialties of surgery and hematology are interdependent in many aspects of the care of patients with hematologic diseases. Good communication between the medical and surgical care providers is essential to function as a unified team and provide optimal integrated care to the patient with hematologic disease. The team approach provides continuity of care such that the patient's diagnosis, treatment, and symptom management are carried out in a timely and cost-effective way. In the first part of this chapter we discuss the various approaches for the diagnosis of hematologic malignancies. We discuss the surgical aspects of tissue procurement and the surgical complications and implications of hematologic malignancy. In the second part, we discuss surgical considerations in sickle cell disease, hemophilia, and von Willebrand disease. This is by no means an exhaustive review of the role of surgery in the care of hematologic and oncologic patients, but rather is an attempt to give a clear, compelling argument for the necessity of multimodality treatment that crosses all aspects of the care of these patients.

SURGICAL CONSIDERATIONS IN HEMATOLOGIC MALIGNANCY

The role of a surgical oncologist in hematologic diseases is a critical one. Surgeons who have a special interest, special training, and demonstrated expertise in oncology will greatly enhance the diagnosis, staging, therapeutic intervention, and palliation of the cancer patient. The establishment of an effective multimodality, multidisciplinary care team ensures that clinical issues will be handled in an efficient, cost-effective, and patient-friendly manner. Of utmost importance is the need for continued multidisciplinary communication as the patient progresses through treatment.

Frequently the surgical oncologist is consulted for assistance in obtaining tissue for diagnosis, or in gaining venous access for infusion of chemotherapy. Aside from diagnostic procedures, surgical intervention in hematologic malignancies is rarely curative and frequently is performed for palliative reasons. The ability to provide significant and long-term improvement in a patient's symptoms while minimizing his or her hospital stay and postoperative risk is critical in balancing the role of the surgical oncologist and the hematologist.

Probably the most notable indications for palliative surgery include relieving emergent spinal cord compression, control of significant hemorrhage, treatment of bowel obstruction, or repairing a bowel perforation, all of which may be secondary to malignancy or the result of therapy. The unique knowledge of the surgical oncologist and awareness of the underlying malignancy will greatly improve the surgeon's ability to make appropriate decisions and interventions. Equally important is the timing of surgical intervention, which must be carefully considered in the setting of neutropenia or recent chemotherapy.

Performing a Biopsy for Diagnosis

The first role that a surgical oncologist frequently plays in assisting the medical oncologist and hematologist is in establishing a patient's diagnosis. It is important for a surgeon to understand that some conditions require multiple diagnostic steps in order to obtain the correct diagnosis and stage of disease. Certain diagnoses require additional amounts of tissue for additional studies such as flow cytometry, as well as for cryopreservation for future studies and/or research studies; diagnosis may also require assessment of multiple sites to rule out the possibility of heterogeneous diseases or multiple cell types present within one disease state. The ease with which this tissue is obtained might impact treatment and/or subsequent patient quality of life. There are times as well when the diagnostic intervention will be coordinated with the simultaneous placement of a port or central venous access catheter, or with bone marrow aspiration/biopsy.

As the surgical oncologist obtains tissue for diagnosis, it is imperative that he or she understand the type and amount of tissue needed, and how the tissue needs to be collected, whether fresh in saline solution, cryopreserved, or placed in formalin solution. Communication between the pathologist, hematologist, and surgeon is essential in planning and obtaining tissue for the diagnosis. The surgical oncologist should review the radiologic imaging and positron emission tomography scan (if available) to verify that the planned tissue biopsy will provide the greatest degree of information with the least amount of morbidity to the patient. The amount and location of tissue needed for diagnosis will determine which approach can be used, ranging from the very simple diagnosis made by fine-needle aspiration in the clinic to the more aggressive and invasive procedure performed in the operating room (Fig. 93–1). The simple drainage of a suspicious fluid accumulation might be diagnostic as well as provide information about the stage of a malignancy and possibly relieve symptoms. The goal in all biopsies is to facilitate a rapid diagnosis in the least morbid way so patients may begin therapy. Percutaneous fine-needle aspiration and core biopsy of gastrointestinal and splenic lesions are effective and safe despite the general concern for complications.[1–4] With modern advances in minimally invasive approaches, the surgical oncologist is capable of obtaining a greater volume of

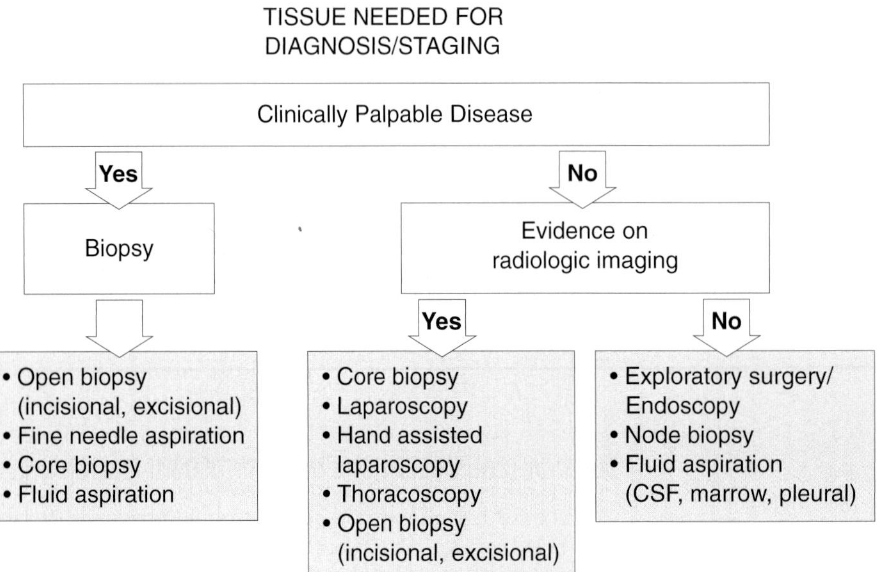

Figure 93–1. Approach to biopsy for diagnosis. Abbreviation: CSF, cerebral spinal fluid.

tissue with a lesser degree of invasiveness, morbidity, and cost as well as shorter hospital stay. Laparoscopy is effective in the diagnosis and staging of lymphoproliferative diseases.[5,6] Special circumstances that highlight the utility of laparoscopy are biopsy of focal intra-abdominal lesions when percutaneous biopsy fails, primary diagnosis and staging of abdominal adenopathy in the absence of peripheral adenopathy, or when splenectomy is required.[5]

In summary, when contemplating a biopsy, the first consideration is whether the tissue to biopsy is palpable by physical examination or image-guided techniques are needed (see Fig. 93–1). The second consideration is what information is needed from the biopsy, and whether it can be obtained by cytology with fine-needle aspiration or requires histology (core biopsy, surgical incision or excision). The third consideration is the volume of tissue required, recognizing that additional tissue may be needed for special studies and research purposes. Last, yet very important, is the concern of selecting a method that is safe for the patient, provides the most information for staging, and will not delay institution of cancer therapy.

Obtaining Venous Access

The surgeon plays a critical role in obtaining long-term venous access for systemic therapy as well as blood sampling for measurement of various parameters. There are many types of venous access devices.[7,8] Communication with the hematologist/oncologist about the various needs and length of need will allow for the most appropriate choice. Ensuring that a surgical oncologist is well experienced with multiple types of lines and devices, management of complications, and the ongoing care of such a device will greatly improve a patient's quality of life during treatment of cancer. All of these devices should be very familiar to the nursing staff, the emergency room staff, and hospital staff so as to allow optimal care, leading to preservation and function of these devices in a safe, cost-effective means.

The use of port devices is a frequent choice for many patients. Many of the newer devices allow flushing at longer intervals when not in use, and can be flushed with saline. Selecting a device that can be flushed with saline and does not require heparin is particularly advantageous in patients with thrombocytopenia. Furthermore, saline-flushed lines can be used to draw blood for measurement of coagulation parameters without the concern for artifactual results that can occur in heparin-flushed lines.

Evaluating Abdominal Pain

Gastrointestinal symptoms of nausea, emesis, diarrhea, constipation, and abdominal pain are frequently experienced by patients receiving therapy for hematologic/oncologic problems. Abdominal pain is one of the most common reasons for a surgical consultation and is an important indicator of acute abdominal disease in the immune-compromised patient.[9] Steroids may blunt the symptoms and delay the diagnosis of an acute abdominal process. Pain is the most consistent symptom in patients who experience bowel perforation while receiving steroids.[10]

The differential diagnosis of abdominal pain in cancer patients is quite extensive. Constipation is a frequent cause of generalized abdominal pain. Vincristine is one of the drugs most frequently associated with paralytic ileus, which may occur in up to one half of patients receiving this vinca alkaloid.[11–13] Patients may experience intense colicky abdominal pain, constipation, and abdominal distention within several days of receiving vincristine. Intervention is generally conservative, but the patient may require nasogastric tube decompression. Constipation may also be the result of the use of narcotics, immobilization, dehydration, and electrolyte imbalances. When treating constipation, all of these factors need to be addressed. Ideally, constipation should be prevented by the prudent use of narcotics; maintaining adequate hydration, including roughage in the diet; and consistent use of bulk-forming agents and stool softeners. Maintaining normal bowel habits is also important in preventing hemorrhoid and anorectal complications.

Pain in the right upper quadrant is not always gallbladder disease, and other causes must be considered, such as diffuse hepatic infiltration by tumor, or veno-occlusive disease. Veno-occlusive disease occurs in 4–22% of patients following intensive chemotherapy and bone marrow transplantation.[14–16] Clinical manifestations include severe right upper quadrant pain (mimicking cholecystitis), hepatomegaly, ascites, jaundice, and in some cases encephalopathy. Veno-occlusive disease usually occurs within 3 weeks of marrow infusion and when patients are severely leukopenic and thrombocytopenic.[17] The diagnosis is usually made clinically after ruling out other entities such as cholecystitis, pancreatitis, and ulcer disease. Treatment is supportive.

Left upper quadrant pain or tenderness may be a manifestation of splenomegaly in patients with lymphoma. Exacerbation of pain and referral of pain to the left shoulder may be indicative of a splenic infarct. Isolated abdominal wall tenderness may be caused by a rectus sheath hematoma occurring in patients with thrombocytopenia or those receiving anticoagulants. Another cause of focal abdominal wall pain that mimics an acute abdomen is herpes zoster prior to the appearance of skin lesions.

Bulky retroperitoneal adenopathy or bleeding may cause abdominal pain. Tumor invasion of the pancreas may occasionally lead to pancreatitis. Drugs that can result in pancreatitis include L-asparaginase, 6-mercaptopurine, and corticosteroids.[18–21] Pancreatitis after high-dose cyclophosphamide has been attributed to tumor lysis in patients with lymphoma.[22]

Genitourinary causes of abdominal pain include ureteral obstruction from cancer, scarring, stones (from postchemotherapy hyperuricemia), cystitis, and/or pyelonephritis. In women, gynecologic causes of abdominal pain include tubo-ovarian pelvic abscess, ectopic pregnancy, and hemorrhage from ovarian cysts.[23]

Diagnosing and Treating Gastrointestinal Lymphoma

Patients with gastrointestinal lymphoma are frequently diagnosed by the surgeon who is operating emergently for bowel obstruction, bleeding, or perforation. In this circumstance, resection of the tumor and diseased bowel is generally performed. However, the resection should not be extensive if it will result in a short gut syndrome. If the diagnosis of gastrointestinal lymphoma is made preoperatively, the decision to treat the patient initially with surgery or with systemic therapy is controversial and needs to be carefully addressed in a multidisciplinary setting. This topic is addressed later.

Surgical Intervention

Obstruction

Obstruction is a frequent reason for emergency abdominal surgery in patients with lymphoma. Primary small bowel lymphoma should be suspected in patients with abdominal pain, weight loss, and occult gastrointestinal bleeding[24] (Fig. 93–2). As many as 6% of patients with gastrointestinal lymphoma present with obstruction, either complete or, more commonly, partial.[25] The surgical management of malignant small bowel obstruction is resection with primary anastomosis, or bypass if resection is not warranted or possible. Though lymphoma can occur in the large bowel, it very rarely is a cause of complete obstruction.[26]

Perforation

Lymphoma is one of the malignant causes of intestinal perforation, accounting for almost one half of all tumor perforations.[27–29] Primary gastrointestinal lymphoma is rare, comprising only 2% of non-Hodgkin's lymphomas in one series of 4234 patients.[30] It is reported that less than 20% (generally less than 10%) of patients with primary gastrointestinal lymphoma (of the stomach, small bowel, or colon) develop perforation on presentation or during chemotherapy.[11,25,30–34] Perforation of tumors involving the stomach and colon are less frequent than tumors involving the small bowel.[32,34] Perforation appears to be less frequent in patients with leukemia than in patients with lymphoma.[27,28,35–37]

Gastrointestinal perforation generally manifests symptoms of diffuse peritonitis: intense constant abdominal pain, guarding, abdominal distention, fever, hemodynamic instability (requiring fluid resuscitation), and leukocytosis. It is important to keep in mind, however, that patients receiving chemotherapy or steroids may not be able to manifest the typical clinical findings associated with perforation. In a series of 79 patients receiving steroids, symptoms of perforation were blunted, resulting in significant delays in diagnosis.[10] Abdominal pain was the most consistent finding and it occurred in all but one of these patients. Free intra-abdominal air was visualized radiographically in about half of these patients, consistent with other series.[38,39] When free intraperitoneal air is present, urgent abdominal exploration is generally required. However, 14% of patients with free intraperitoneal air do not have an obvious perforated abdominal viscus and may not require surgery.[39]

The surgical treatment of intestinal perforation in cancer patients should be the simplest, life-saving procedure that controls sepsis, establishes gastrointestinal continuity, and allows for prompt therapy of the underlying malignancy. In some circumstances, curative surgical therapy may be indicated. In precarious clinical situations, simple closure of a perforated lymphoma has been performed successfully, though this is not generally advocated.[40] Small bowel perforations are best managed by resection and primary anastomosis, reserving exteriorized stomas for cases of severe peritonitis.[41] Large bowel perforations with peritoneal contamination are generally managed by resection, colostomy, and Hartman procedures or mucous fistula.

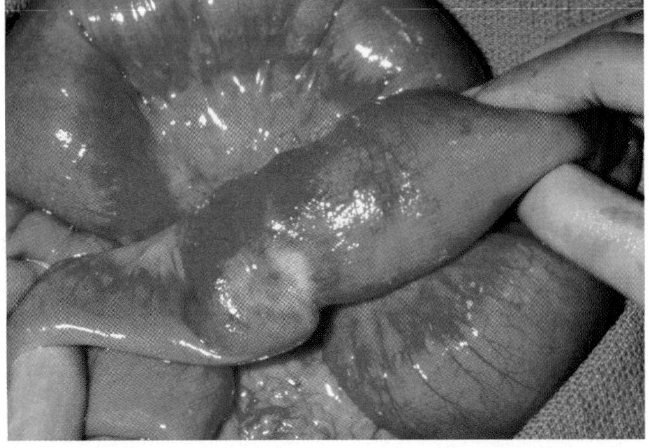

A

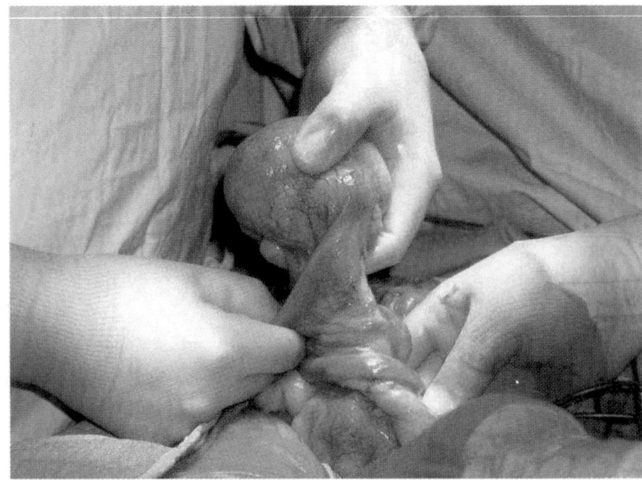

B

Figure 93–2. *A,* Small bowel primary lymphoma, diagnosed at laparotomy for bowel obstruction. Bowel proximal to obstruction is dilated, whereas distal bowel is decompressed. Treatment was surgical resection and primary anastomosis. *B,* Small bowel primary lymphoma, diagnosed at laparotomy for symptoms of bowel obstruction. Treatment was resection of segment of bowel with tumor and primary anastomosis.

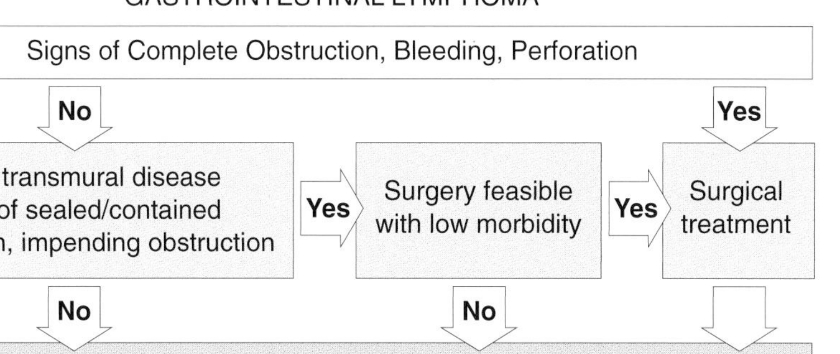

Figure 93–3. Algorithm for management of gastrointestinal lymphoma.

Bleeding

Up to 20% of patients with primary gastrointestinal lymphoma may present with bleeding or develop bleeding during chemotherapy.[31–33,42,43] In one surgical study of gastrointestinal lymphoma, bleeding was the presenting symptom in 39% of small bowel and 21% of gastric lymphomas.[25] Bleeding is generally more frequent in gastric than in intestinal lesions.[32,43] When emergent surgery is performed for bleeding, the goal is to resect the bleeding lesion and perform a primary anastomosis if possible. Gastric surgical devascularization has been successful in treating bleeding after chemotherapy.[42,44] An infrequent source of intra-abdominal hemorrhage in patients with hematologic malignancies is spontaneous splenic rupture.[45] The treatment for this condition is urgent laparotomy and splenectomy.

Surgery Versus Chemotherapy as Initial Therapy

Patients with bleeding, perforation, obstruction, or infection/phlegmon require surgery first to address the urgent surgical condition. The controversy arises in patients with uncomplicated gastrointestinal involvement with lymphoma. Whether to surgically treat or start treatment with chemotherapy is frequently a dilemma that requires multidisciplinary decision making.[34,46] In the subset of patients with low-grade mucosa-associated lymphoid tissue lymphoma of the stomach and concomitant *Helicobacter pylori* infection, eradication of the infection may be sufficient to eradicate the tumor.[46] The ability to correctly diagnose lesions with endoscopy or percutaneous needle biopsy has made more patients eligible for systemic therapy first. The major concern of using chemotherapy first is spontaneous perforation[25,47,48] or bleeding[42] following a response to therapy. This finding, however, is infrequent. In general, the trend in practice and in the literature for patients with gastric lymphoma is to favor the systemic or nonoperative approach if there are no urgent indications for surgery.[34,42,47,49–52] This approach may also be followed in patients with intestinal lymphoma if the lesion can be identified and biopsied preoperatively. However, because many of the patients with intestinal lymphoma present with symptoms that prompt surgical treatment, the diagnosis is usually made at the time of surgical treatment, which generally requires resection of the tumor. Hence, many patients with intestinal lymphoma are managed surgically first. An algorithm for the management of patients with gastrointestinal lymphoma is summarized in Figure 93–3.

Other Conditions Requiring Surgery

Neutropenic Colitis

Neutropenic colitis is an inflammatory abdominal process characteristically occurring in patients with hematologic malignancies (principally leukemia) receiving chemotherapy. The true incidence of this disease entity is unknown because of the many similar clinical syndromes and lack of pathologic confirmation, but it is generally reported in 3–11% of patients with leukemia[37,53,54]; the incidence has been reported to be as high as 32%.[55] The clinical syndrome is characterized by abdominal distention, pain (often localized to the right lower quadrant), watery diarrhea (sometimes bloody), and fever in the setting of neutropenia and thrombocytopenia.[56,57] It most commonly develops 7–10 days after treatment and during profound neutropenia. The pathogenesis of this process is not clear but involves loss of the bowel mucosal barrier and subsequent infection. It generally localizes in the terminal ileum and right colon.[56,57] When confined to the cecum, it is termed *typhlitis*.[53,58] The diagnosis of enterocolitis is made clinically, and the differential diagnosis includes pseudomembranous colitis, appendicitis, and diverticulitis.[57,59,60] Differentiating appendicitis from enterocolitis may be very difficult preoperatively. Both entities may have similar clinical findings and a similar frequency in leukemic children with right lower quadrant pain.[61,62]

Management of neutropenic colitis is usually nonoperative and consists of bowel rest, decompression, hydration, nutritional support, broad-spectrum antibiotics, and correction of coagulopathy and neutropenia[54–57,59,60] (Fig. 93–4). Patients who have evidence of free intraperitoneal perforation, peritonitis, uncontrollable bleeding despite correction of coagulopathy, increasing fluid or vasopressor requirements, or failure to improve after 2–3 days of medical management should undergo surgery. The preferred surgical treatment is right hemicolectomy and ileostomy.

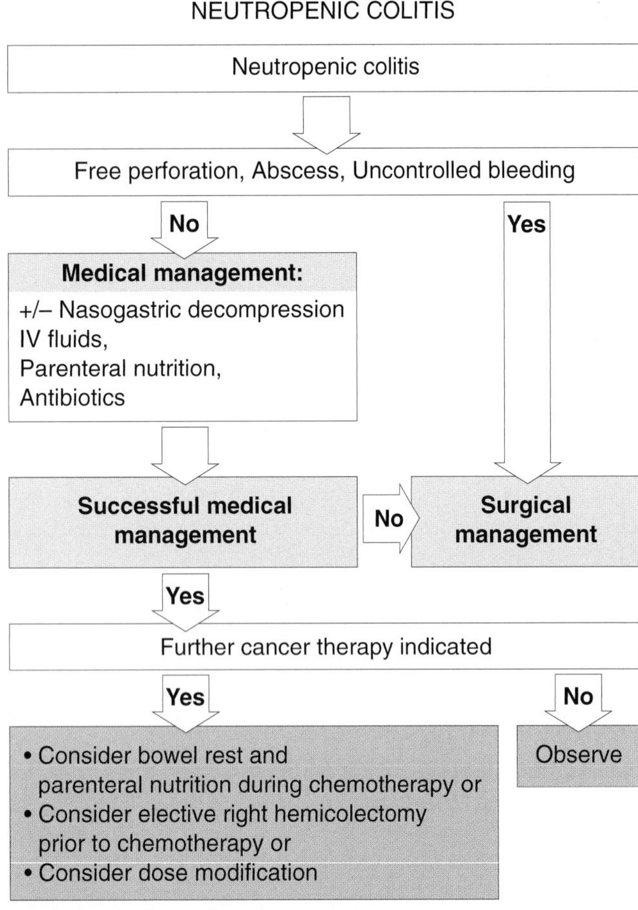

Figure 93–4. Management of neutropenic colitis. Abbreviation: IV, intravenous.

Patients who have been successfully managed without surgery may be at increased risk of recurrence during subsequent chemotherapy. One author has recommended that subsequent chemotherapy should be given in the settings of bowel rest and total parenteral nutrition.[59] Another has advocated performing an elective right hemicolectomy.[63]

Indications for Splenectomy

Splenectomy has been advocated for the relief of symptoms of splenomegaly, for correction of cytopenias, to establish a diagnosis or stage of disease, and occasionally to alter the disease course. A splenectomy may also be performed in selected individuals at risk of life-threatening bleeding from splenic rupture following accidental trauma. It is important to remember that the spleen is a critical lymphoid organ and therefore a splenectomy should not be attempted until it has been ruled out as a principal lymphopoietic site. Adequate preparation of the patient includes preoperative vaccination and correction of abnormal bleeding parameters.

Whether the surgical approach is laparoscopic, hand-assisted, or open laparotomy is best determined on an individual basis. Though no randomized trials of open versus laparoscopic splenectomy have been performed, the general consensus is in favor of the laparoscopic approach, particularly for smaller spleens. Laparoscopic splenectomy has been safely performed in multiple benign and malignant hematologic conditions, such as idiopathic thrombocytopenic purpura, thrombotic thrombocytopenic purpura, hemolytic anemia, splenomegaly, hereditary spherocytosis, sickle cell disease, myelofibrosis, non-Hodgkin's and Hodgkin's lymphoma, chronic lymphocytic leukemia, hairy cell leukemia, and lymphoproliferative and myeloproliferative disorders.[64–67] Though there is debate in the literature about the role of laparoscopic splenectomy in large spleens (variably defined as >500–2000 gm), many experienced centers advocate the laparoscopic approach.[65,68–73] There is general agreement that patients with larger spleens have greater operative times, larger blood loss, longer hospital stays, and greater morbidity. The technique of hand-assisted laparoscopic splenectomy may be necessary or beneficial in larger spleens.[66,72–74]

Often debated is the need for and safety of cholecystectomy for gallstones during splenectomy for hematologic disease. Both procedures may be performed safely during the same surgery in children with sickle cell disease.[75]

Gallbladder Disease

Gallstones that are asymptomatic generally do not require surgical treatment, regardless of the phase of cancer therapy. However, a careful history should be obtained, and patients with symptoms attributable to gallstones should undergo elective cholecystectomy. The best timing of this intervention is prior to initiating chemotherapy, emphasizing the need for a carefully focused history pertinent to the biliary system.

If biliary symptoms develop in the midst of cancer therapy, it is preferable to delay intervention until resolution of neutropenia, as long as the patient improves with conservative management. An interval cholecystectomy should then be performed prior to initiating the next cycle of chemotherapy.

Acalculous cholecystitis in critically ill patients can be quite challenging to diagnose and treat. If a HIDA (hepatoiminodiacetic acid) scan with morphine stimulation does not enable visualization of the gallbladder, cholecystectomy or cholecystostomy may be necessary. The temporary drainage with a cholecystostomy may be lifesaving and a bridge to eventual cholecystectomy after systemic recovery from the effects or complications of chemotherapy.

Soft Tissue Infection

Perianal conditions occurring in patients receiving chemotherapy include cellulitis, abscess, ulcers, fissures, and thrombosed/bleeding hemorrhoids.[11] Diarrhea and constipation contribute to these abnormalities and should be treated aggressively. Perianal infections requiring surgical intervention have been reported in 1–8% of patients with leukemia.[37,76,77]

Preexisting anorectal conditions should be carefully evaluated before chemotherapy and treated if necessary.

Digital rectal examinations, instrumentation, and enemas should be avoided during neutropenic periods. When symptoms develop during chemotherapy, a careful perianal inspection and gentle external palpation should be performed. Fissures or thrombosed hemorrhoids may be evident on examination and rarely if ever require surgical intervention acutely unless complicated by uncontrolled hemorrhage. Perirectal infection in febrile and neutropenic patients manifests with intense pain, swelling, and induration. If no abscess is evident on external palpation, medical therapy is initiated. Recommended therapy includes broad-spectrum antibiotics, warm compresses, Sitz baths, topical and/or systemic analgesics, and stool softeners or antidiarrheal agents as appropriate. If the initial examination is suspicious for an abscess or the patient fails to improve after 24–48 hours of conservative therapy, a pelvic computed tomography scan is helpful to rule out a perianal abscess or inflammatory process that requires surgical drainage. In rare circumstances, proximal fecal diversion may be needed for severe local infection and failure to heal.[37,77,78] Radiation therapy to treat perianal complications is not recommended.[11,79]

Necrotizing soft tissue infections in cancer patients are rare. Gangrenous cellulitis of the extremity, clostridial myonecrosis, and Fournier's gangrene of the scrotum and perineum have been described in case reports of patients with hematologic malignancies.[80–82] These entities present initially with subtle pain, swelling, and fever but then rapidly progress to fulminant tissue necrosis. Early recognition, aggressive surgical débridement, and broad-spectrum antibiotics (including anaerobic coverage) are necessary to reduce the high mortality of these infections.

SURGICAL CONSIDERATIONS IN BENIGN HEMATOLOGIC CONDITIONS

Sickle Cell Disease

Patients who are homozygous for sickle cell (SS disease) or doubly heterozygous for sickle cell and either hemoglobin C (SC disease) or β-thalassemia (Sβ disease) have severe alterations in erythrocyte function that result in increased red blood cell rigidity and adherence and the tendency for the defective hemoglobin to polymerize, causing the cells to elongate into a "sickle" shape.[83] Sickle-shaped red blood cells cannot pass through capillaries normally, resulting in vaso-occlusion and hemolysis. The result of this process is a vaso-occlusive *crisis*, which is extremely painful and can cause tissue ischemia and organ dysfunction.

Patients may require an operation either for complications of sickle cell disease, such as gallstones, or for an unrelated indication, such as appendicitis. Regardless of the indication for a given operation, patients with sickle cell disease are at increased risk of postoperative complications, principally related to sickle crises. Acute chest syndrome is a particularly serious form of vaso-occlusive crisis that affects the lung and can cause severe and potentially life-threatening respiratory decompensation.[84]

Perioperative Management

The factors that cause red blood cells to sickle in experimental models include hypoxia, acidosis, hypothermia, and dehydration. This has resulted in the widespread conventional teaching that correcting these precipitating factors is therapeutic for sickle cell patients who are in the midst of a crisis and, by further extrapolation, that avoiding these conditions will minimize the risk of developing a crisis in the perioperative period. Nevertheless, although they remain useful guidelines for all patients who undergo an operation, there is no conclusive evidence that supplemental oxygen, alkalosis, hydration, or maintenance of normothermia can prevent a sickle crisis from occurring in any given patient.[85]

Although all patients with sickle cell disease are at some risk for complications, several factors have been identified in large retrospective studies that correlate with increased risk.[85,86] These are summarized in Table 93–1. Age is a risk factor in that older patients tend to have more complications. The incidence of complications is also increased with certain surgical procedures. Low-risk procedures include tonsillectomy/adenoidectomy, myringotomy tube placement, and hip replacement. Intermediate risk is associated with nonobstetric intra-abdominal procedures and thoracic surgery, and high-risk procedures include cesarian section and dilation and curettage. Minimally invasive surgery has several advantages that make it the preferred approach in most patients, but it might not result in fewer serious vaso-occlusive complications in patients with sickle cell disease.[87–89] Pregnancy increases the risk of postoperative complications regardless of the procedure being performed. The presence of organ dysfunction secondary to chronic sickle cell disease–related tissue injury also increases the risk of complications and the mortality of a surgical procedure. Patients being prepared for surgery should be screened especially for evidence of chronic lung disease, renal insufficiency, and neurologic deficits, all of which can result from repeated ischemic insults to

TABLE 93–1. Risk Factors for Complications in Patients with Sickle Cell Disease

Risk Factor	Characteristics
Age	Increased risk in older patients
Type of procedure	Low risk: tonsillectomy, myringotomy, hip replacement Intermediate risk: nonobstetric abdominal surgery High risk: cesarean section, dilation and curettage
Chronic organ dysfunction	Chronic lung disease, renal insufficiency, and neurologic deficits are especially worrisome
Acute increase in disease severity	Recent complications and hospitalizations
Acute infection	Increased risk
Pregnancy	Increased risk

the end organs involved. It is characteristic of patients with sickle cell disease to have episodic periods during which the disease is quite active, with many painful crises and frequent hospitalizations, separated by periods of relative quiescence of the disease. Patients with a recent history of increased disease severity are also at higher risk of postoperative complications. This is sometimes attributable to factors that are correctable, such as a recent drop in the hematocrit or an acute infection, but is most often inexplicable.

These known risk factors form the basis for the preoperative screening that is recommended for all but very minor operations in patients with sickle cell disease.[86,90] This should include a detailed history and physical examination, with special attention paid to signs and symptoms of increased recent disease activity and chronic organ dysfunction. Laboratory data should include at minimum a complete blood count, serum chemistry panel with blood urea nitrogen and creatinine measurements, and, if a history of liver dysfunction or gallstones is suspected, a liver function panel. A sample should also be sent for blood type and crossmatch. Urinalysis should be performed, looking for evidence of renal injury such as hematuria and proteinuria, and evidence of urinary tract infection. Oxygen saturation should be measured by pulse oximetry to rule out hypoxia, and a chest radiograph should be obtained to rule out evidence of chronic lung disease or acute pulmonary infiltrates. In addition, sexually active females should have a qualitative urine or serum human chorionic gonadotropin determination.

The risk of serious postoperative complications related to sickle crises and acute chest syndrome is known to correlate with the percentage of sickle hemoglobin. In the past, standard preoperative preparation included exchange transfusion or transfusions with packed red blood cells to decrease the level of hemoglobin S to less than 30%. More recent studies have shown that patients treated with a more conservative approach, including transfusion to a hemoglobin level of 10 gm/dL, have a similar incidence of sickle cell disease–related complications and have fewer complications related to transfusion.[91,92]

Intraoperative management of the patient with sickle cell disease is generally no different from that of any patient under general anesthesia. Again, careful attention should be paid to the standard parameters that guide all operations but that may be more important in patients with sickle cell disease—hydration status, temperature regulation, end-organ perfusion, and tissue oxygenation—all of which help to avoid local tissue acidosis and sickling of red blood cells. Significant blood loss should be replaced with packed red blood cell transfusions to maintain a hemoglobin of 10 gm/dL or higher. Patients with a history of frequent painful crises may have a relative tolerance of opioids and certain anesthetics because of frequent exposure to narcotic analgesics.

Patients with sickle cell disease need to be monitored carefully for postoperative complications that would ordinarily be considered minor. Atelectasis and hypoxia should be avoided whenever possible, and should be treated aggressively with respiratory therapy and supplemental oxygen when they do occur. The real significance of these signs, however, is that they may be an indication of an impending episode of acute chest syndrome. This potentially deadly process is usually marked by chest pain, tachypnea, and pulmonary infiltrates. Treatment is supportive and may require intensive respiratory measures and exchange transfusion. Other sickle cell disease–related complications include painful crises and stroke. Patients with sickle cell disease are also at increased risk of severe sepsis in the postoperative period.

Operative Procedures

Patients with sickle cell disease require surgery for many of the same indications as the rest of the population, but are more likely to require certain operations. These include cholecystectomy, splenectomy, diagnostic laparotomy/appendectomy, and hip replacement.

Patients with sickle cell disease are at high risk for the development of pigmented gallstones, presumably because of increased red blood cell lysis and turnover. The gallstones are generally asymptomatic and are frequently identified in patients who present with abdominal pain. It can sometimes be very difficult to distinguish a hepatic sickle crisis from biliary colic or acute cholecystitis. In general, serum activities of lactate dehydrogenase and aspartate aminotransferase are elevated during a hepatic crisis, whereas they typically remain normal with acute gallbladder disease.[93] There is also typically an abrupt drop in hemoglobin in patients with crisis. Nuclear medicine biliary scans can sometimes help to identify the patient with acute cholecystitis or impacted gallstone. Nevertheless, it can be very difficult to distinguish the two disorders. Patients with asymptomatic gallstones should probably undergo cholecystectomy on an elective basis to avoid the potential need for an emergent operation, though the risks of anesthesia and surgery for any given patient should be weighed carefully.

The cholecystectomy procedure itself is usually fairly straightforward. The operation is generally best done laparoscopically, which has been shown to be safe for patients with sickle cell disease.[94] Patients are usually prepared preoperatively with transfusion, if necessary, to a hemoglobin of 10 gm/dL or greater. Prophylactic intravenous antibiotics are recommended. In patients with jaundice or clinical suspicion of cholangitis or pancreatitis, cholangiography may be indicated to rule out common bile duct stones. This can be done by endoscopic retrograde choledochopancreatography or intraoperatively. Patients generally tolerate the operation quite well, but typically have a longer average hospital length of stay because of concern about potential complications and pain control issues.

In some children with sickle cell disease, acute splenic sequestration crises are a source of severe and sometimes recurrent abdominal pain, often associated with severe hemolysis requiring transfusion. Splenectomy is indicated for patients with frequent painful splenic crises or hypersplenism. With proper preoperative preparation, often including transfusion of platelets, the conduct of the operation is usually straightforward. Splenectomy should be performed laparoscopically whenever possible, to avoid the postoperative complications inherent with a large flank incision. In patients with splenic crises and gallstones who are otherwise healthy, both laparoscopic cholecystectomy and laparoscopic splenectomy may be performed during the same general anesthesia with minimal increase in risk. In fact, patients with a history of abdominal crises should probably undergo simultaneous prophylactic appendectomy as well, although this is more controversial. Diagnostic laparoscopy alone, usually combined with empirical appendectomy, may be indicated in patients with sickle cell disease and severe abdominal pain to help resolve an acute diagnostic dilemma or, in the patient with frequent episodes of abdominal pain, to avoid diagnostic uncertainty in the future by removing the appendix.

Adults with sickle cell disease are at increased risk of osteonecrosis of the hip.[95] This painful and potentially debilitating disorder is a frequent indication for prosthetic hip replacement. Large retrospective studies have suggested that hip replacement is relatively safe in patients with sickle cell disease, with a life-threatening complication such as acute chest syndrome occurring in fewer than 5%.[85]

In summary, all patients with sickle cell disease are at risk for vaso-occlusive disease in the perioperative period. The risk is increased for patients who are older, are pregnant, have a recent increase in the activity of their disease, have chronic organ dysfunction as a result of the cumulative effects of multiple acute vaso-occlusive crises, and/or have current acute infection. Factors that may precipitate a vaso-occlusive crisis include dehydration, hypothermia, acidosis, and hypoxia, though there is no evidence that avoiding these factors in the clinical setting will prevent its occurrence. Patients with sickle cell disease may require surgery because of a complication of their disease, such as cholecystectomy, splenectomy, diagnostic laparoscopy, or hip replacement. Guidelines for sickle cell patients who require surgery include screening for risk factors and minimizing their impact with specific therapy, using a minimally invasive surgical approach whenever feasible, and transfusion with packed red blood cells to maintain a hemoglobin level of 10 gm/dL or greater. With meticulous attention to current guidelines for transfusion therapy and risk factor management, the majority of sickle cell patients can safely undergo elective surgical procedures, although the risk for a serious complication is never zero.

Hemophilia

Factor VIII deficiency (hemophilia A) is the most common inherited coagulation factor deficiency. It is an X-linked recessive disorder that affects approximately 1 in 10,000 males in the United States. The severity of the disease is dependent on an individual's factor VIII level. Those with greater than 30% of the normal level of factor VIII have essentially normal hemostasis and a normal activated partial thromboplastin time; levels below 2% lead to spontaneous bleeding into joints and soft tissues. Patients with factor VIII levels between 5% and 30% rarely develop spontaneous hemorrhage but usually have a significantly prolonged partial thromboplastin time and are at risk for significant bleeding during surgery and after major injury. Patients with levels between 2% and 5% exhibit an intermediate syndrome with less frequent spontaneous bleeding episodes.

Patients with hemophilia are at risk of bleeding not only during an operation, but for several weeks after the operation as well. Replacement therapy with human recombinant factor VIII has largely replaced the use of blood-derived products such as plasma, cryoprecipitate, and factor VIII concentrate used in the past. There is some debate as to how much factor VIII is necessary for surgical prophylaxis, with most printed guidelines erring on the side of caution.[96,97] For elective major surgery, the recommendations are to achieve a factor VIII level that is near 100% of normal during the procedure, between 40% and 50% of normal for the first 3–5 days, and greater than 30% of normal for 2 weeks after the operation.[98]

The half-life of circulating factor VIII is approximately 12–16 hours, but may be considerably shorter in children.[99] Dosing is usually by intermittent bolus infusion given every 6–8 hours, although some have suggested that continuous infusion may provide more reliable factor VIII levels with less expense.[100] It is necessary to monitor factor VIII levels carefully throughout the treatment period. A commonly used formula for determining the appropriate dose for intermittent bolus dosing is

Body weight (kg) × (0.5 IU/kg) × Desired percent increase of factor VIII level = No. IU of factor VIII required

The second most common inherited coagulation factor deficiency is factor IX deficiency. Hemophilia B is clinically indistinguishable from hemophilia A and is also transmitted as an X-linked recessive trait. It is approximately one quarter as common as hemophilia A. The goal of prophylaxis for elective surgery is a factor IX level of at least 50% of normal during surgery and at least 30% of normal for 7–10 days after surgery. The half-life of factor IX is between 18 and 30 hours. Dosing is based on the following formula:

Body weight (kg) × (1 IU/kg) × Desired percent increase of factor IX level = No. IU of factor IX required

Factor IX is given every 12–24 hours, and levels are monitored frequently during the course of treatment.

All patients with hemophilia should be screened for the presence of serum inhibitors of the factor in question before an elective operative procedure. The issue of serum inhibitor activity eventually affects approximately 15% of patients with hemophilia A and up to 5% of patients with hemophilia B who have the severe form of the disease.[101] Patients who have inhibitors sometimes respond to immune tolerance protocols. Recombinant factor VIIa has been used with some success in these patients, as well.[101]

In summary, patients with hemophilia require factor replacement therapy before, during, and after surgery. For major surgery, the goal is to achieve factor levels of

100% of normal during the operation, and between 30% and 50% of normal for 1–2 weeks after surgery. Patients should be evaluated for the possibility of coagulation factor inhibitors, the presence of which poses a significant challenge for proper replacement therapy in a small but significant percentage of affected patients.

von Willebrand Disease

Von Willebrand disease (see Chapter 64) is the most common inherited disorder of hemostasis, affecting approximately 1% of the general population.[83] Most affected patients have a mild form of the disease, and the severe form is quite rare. Several types have been described, most of which are inherited as an autosomal dominant trait. The disorder is caused by a qualitative or quantitative defect in von Willebrand factor (vWF), which mediates platelet aggregation and adhesion. It also serves as a plasma carrier protein for coagulation factor VIII. The diagnosis is suspected on the basis of a personal or family history of bleeding and a prolonged bleeding time and/or partial thromboplastin time. The diagnosis is confirmed by measuring levels of vWF activity (ristocetin cofactor), vWF antigen, and factor VIII. Further classification is by vWF multimer analysis.

Patients with von Willebrand disease can safely undergo elective surgery, with the aggressiveness of prophylactic therapy varying with the severity of the disease and the magnitude of the surgical procedure.[97,102] Patients with mild disease undergoing minor operations need no specific therapy. Desmopressin acetate (DDAVP) improves hemostasis in some forms of von Willebrand disease by inducing the release of factor VIII from hepatic stores and vWF from endothelial cells. It is useful in most patients with the most common subtypes of the disease (types I and 2A) but not effective in patients with type 3 and contraindicated in patients with type 2B disease. Maximum effect is within 1 hour and lasts for approximately 6 hours. The typical dose is 0.3–0.4 μg/kg intravenously over 20 minutes; an intranasal spray is also available. In patients for whom DDAVP is not useful, a vWF-containing plasma-derived concentrate is used. Cryoprecipitate is no longer recommended because of the risk of virus transmission.

CURRENT CONTROVERSIES & FUTURE CONSIDERATIONS

Surgery in Specific Hematologic Conditions

- Surgery vs. chemotherapy as initial therapy for gastrointestinal lymphoma.
- Optimal preoperative hemoglobin for patients with sickle cell anemia.
- Utility of routine coagulation studies in children being prepared for surgery versus selective screening on the basis of detailed history and physical examination.
- Level of factor replacement necessary in the perioperative period in patients with hemophilia.
- Safer and more effective laparoscopic techniques allow for greater complexity of surgery to be done with minimal morbidity.
- Gene therapy for sickle cell anemia and inherited coagulation disorders.
- Development of a safe and reliable blood substitute for patients who require transfusion.
- Prenatal genetic testing and counseling for inherited hemoglobinopathies and coagulation disorders.

Suggested Readings*

Crump M, Gospodarowicz M, Shepherd FA: Lymphoma of the gastrointestinal tract. Semin Oncol 26:324–337, 1999.

Koch P, del Valle F, Berdel WE, et al: Primary gastrointestinal non-Hodgkin's lymphoma: II. Combined surgical and conservative or conservative management only in localized gastric lymphoma—results of the prospective German Multicenter Study GIT NHL 01/92. J Clin Oncol 19:3874–3883, 2001.

Rosen M, Brody F, Walsh RM, et al: Outcome of laparoscopic splenectomy based on hematologic indication. Surg Endosc 16:272–279, 2002.

Williams N, Scott AD: Neutropenic colitis: a continuing surgical challenge. Br J Surg 84:1200–1205, 1997.

Full references for this chapter can be found on accompanying CD-ROM.

PART IV

Tools for the Hematologist

CHAPTER 94
ALLOGENEIC BONE MARROW TRANSPLANTATION

John Barrett, MD, FRCP, FRCPath

KEY POINTS

Allogeneic Bone Marrow Transplantation

- Allogeneic bone marrow transplantation involves transfer of stem cells and lymphocytes from bone marrow, peripheral blood, or umbilical cord blood.
- Bone marrow transplantation is used to treat a wide spectrum of hematologic malignancies and nonmalignant hematologic disorders as well as rare inborn errors of metabolism and storage diseases. Treatment of solid tumors by allografting is investigational.
- Progress in understanding allograft immunology and stem cell biology and the introduction of new antimicrobial and immunosuppressive agents over the last 30 years has resulted in continuing improvement in transplant outcome.
- Best results are obtained in younger patients with less advanced primary disease receiving transplants from well-matched family donors.
- Major limitations are availability of suitably matched donors, complications of graft-versus-host disease, slow recovery of immune function, and recurrence of advanced malignant diseases after transplant.

INTRODUCTION

Marrow transplantation has its origins in the discovery that mice could be protected from radiation-induced marrow aplasia by transfer of hematopoietic cells. In the mid-1950s, clinical investigators first used autologous marrow cell infusions to restore hematopoiesis in patients with malignant diseases given myelosuppressive treatments for their malignancy.[1] Successful allogeneic bone marrow transplantation began following the development of tissue typing in the 1960s. The first successful human lymphocyte antigen (HLA)–identical sibling transplants, in children with immune deficiency diseases, were reported by clinical investigators in the United States and Holland in 1968.[2–4] Reports of successful transplants for leukemia and aplastic anemia from HLA-identical siblings quickly followed.[5,6] By 1980, bone marrow transplantation had progressed from an experimental salvage treatment to an elective treatment of high-risk leukemias, and a spectrum of otherwise fatal malignant and nonmalignant disorders.[7–10] The International Bone Marrow Transplant Registry (IBMTR), formed in Milwaukee in 1972 by Mortimer Bortin, became an important resource for the collection of data on transplants and outcomes worldwide. The publications from this organization have done much to define risks and benefits and to refine outcome prediction for transplants for specific diseases and for transplant approaches. In the last 2 decades, the development of unrelated donor panels made it possible to perform increasing numbers of unrelated donor transplants.[11] Over the last few decades, disease- and transplant-specific outcomes have become well defined and survival following transplant improved, with the introduction of better antibiotics, new antivirals and antifungals, and new immunosuppressive agents (cyclosporine, monoclonal antibodies) to prevent graft-versus-host disease The 1990s saw the introduction of cord blood transplantation[12] and peripheral blood stem cell (PBSC) transplantation,[13] and the gradual decline in the use of bone marrow as a stem cell source. Conceptual and technical advances led to the use of stem cell transplants to cure malignant diseases (including solid tumors) by an allogeneic graft-versus-malignancy effect.[14–16] It is estimated that over 10,000 allogeneic stem cell transplantations are performed annually in over 800 specialty centers worldwide (Fig. 94–1).

ELEMENTS OF CLINICAL ALLOGENEIC STEM CELL TRANSPLANTATION

HLA Typing

HLA typing involves molecular or serologic typing of blood leukocytes to determine the major histocompatibility loci of the major histocompatibility (MHC) gene complex on chromosome 6. In HLA-identical siblings,

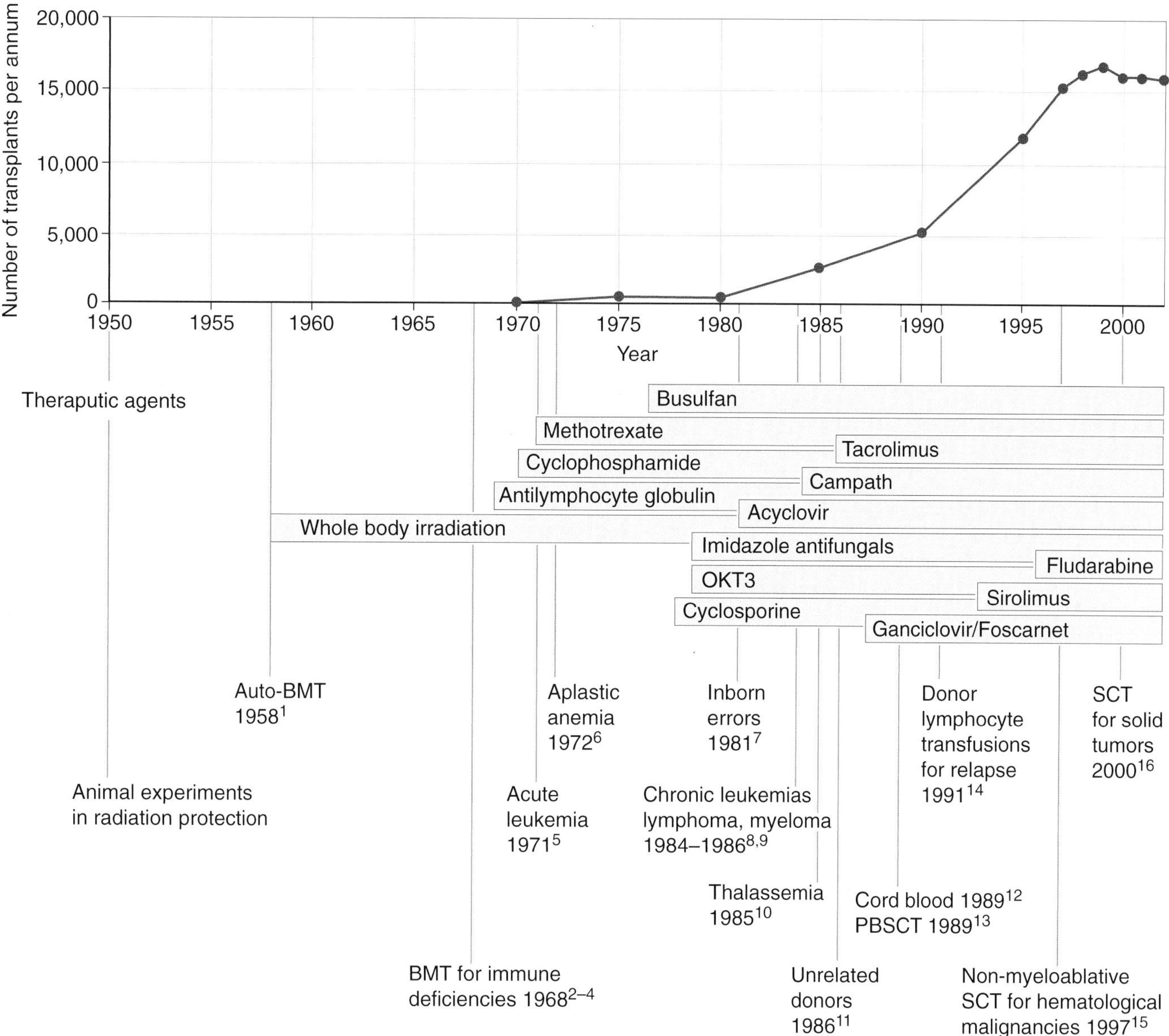

Figure 94–1. Milestones in the development of blood and marrow stem cell transplantation and introduction of important therapeutic agents, 1950–2000.

identity at the three major loci, HLA-A, -B, and -DR, is sufficient to determine HLA compatibility between donor and recipient, because the MHC complex is passed from parent to child in a single haplotype and only rarely (<2% of cases) do crossovers occur, creating mismatches usually at the A locus. Further typing for HLA-C, -DQ, and -DP is also performed on unrelated donors, because the MHC locus within a population undergoes multiple recombinations, and HLA-A, -B, and -DR identity is no guarantee that other minor loci are also matched.[17]

Finding Donors

Because the best transplant outcome occurs with the closest matched donor, the aim of the donor search is to find a donor who is fully HLA-A, -B, and -DR identical, preferably from the family, by HLA-typing the patient, siblings, and parents. There is a 25% chance that any sibling will be a complete, six-locus match with the recipient, and occasionally, through shared family alleles, parents may be compatible with their children. In the absence of an HLA-identical sibling donor, the choice rests between an unrelated HLA-identical donor, a mismatched (haplotype-identical) family donor, or a cord blood transplant. The National Bone Marrow Donor Panel (NMDP) has typed around 5 million potential bone marrow or peripheral blood stem cell donors and connects internationally with another 5 million potential donors who can be contacted for detailed compatibility testing. It is estimated that fully HLA-A, -B, and -DR matched unrelated donors are available for about 25% of the patient population seeking an unrelated donor. In the remaining 50% of patients, the choice falls between a partially matched unrelated or family donor or a cord blood transplant. The process of accessing the NMDP and making donor stem cells available to the transplant center takes approximately 6 weeks. In some situations, this time lag may rule out the possibility of an unrelated marrow donor and favor a cord blood or family donor transplant. In the United States, HLA-A, -B, and -DR typed cord blood for transplantation is available cryopreserved at the New York Blood Center, the National Marrow Donor Panel, and numerous smaller facilities. For patients weighing over 35 kg, adult donors are preferable to cord blood because the latter contains too few stem cells for rapid engraftment. After the best donor has been identified, the final decision to transplant, and which stem cell source to use, depends upon an informed comparison of predicted survival and quality of life for the patient with or without the proposed transplant (Fig. 94–2).

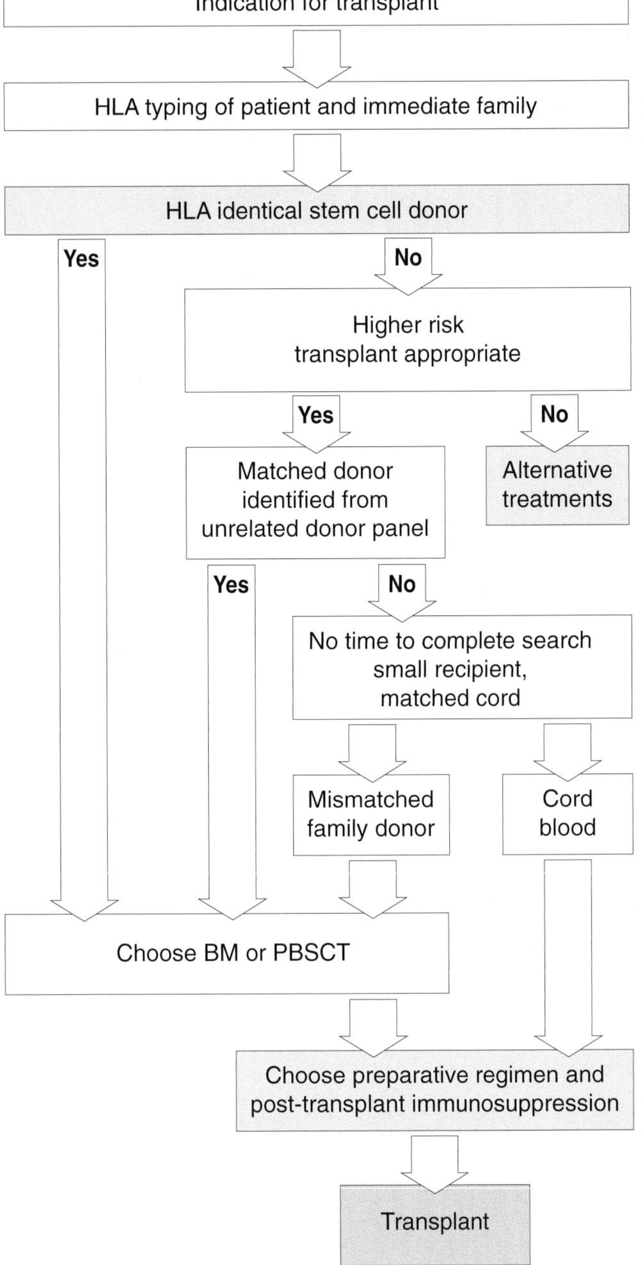

Figure 94–2. Decision tree for donor selection and allogeneic stem cell transplantation.

Sources and Preparation of Stem Cells for Transplant

The CD34 marker defines a population of stem cells that contains the self-renewing hematopoietic progenitors required for long-term (lifelong) maintenance of hematopoiesis. Bone marrow, peripheral blood, and umbilical cord blood are the tissue sources of the $CD34^+$ stem cell routinely used for transplantation. Stem cells can also be obtained from fetal liver tissue, and this source has in the past been used for correction of immune deficiencies in infants. The characteristics of bone marrow, peripheral blood stem cell, and cord blood transplants are compared in Figure 94–3.[18]

Bone Marrow

Stem cells are collected for transplant by multiple (several hundred) needle aspirations from the posterior and anterior iliac crests and sternum of an anesthetized donor. The samples are aspirated directly into heparin to prevent coagulation and pooled in a collection bag. A 1- to 2-hour procedure provides about 1 L of bone marrow, which is filtered to remove bony spicules and aggregates before use. In addition to $CD34^+$ cells, bone marrow transplants contain the entire repertoire of maturing and mature hematopoietic cells, stromal cells, and lymphocytes derived from circulating blood.

Peripheral Blood

The frequency of circulating stem cells is normally too low to collect a sufficient amount for transplant purposes. However, large numbers of stem cells can be mobilized from the marrow into the blood by administration of granulocyte colony-stimulating factor. Stem cell donors receive six daily subcutaneous injections of granulocyte colony-stimulating factor. Circulating stem cells are then collected during a 1- to 2-hour apheresis procedure. PBSC transplants also contain large numbers of lymphocytes and monocytes.

Umbilical Cord Blood

Cord blood is rich in CD34 cells and is being increasingly used as a transplant source.[19] However, the relatively small total number of stem cells available in a 200-mL cord blood transplant unit has in the past restricted its use to recipients weighing less than 35 kg. The numerical disadvantage in CD34 cells is offset by a greater self-renewing capacity of a population of immature, highly proliferative cord blood stem cells. T cells are largely naive (antigen inexperienced) and natural killer (NK) cells are also immature.[18] Recent data has shown the potential use of cord blood in adults, with similar outcomes to those observed with mismatched unrelated donors. Furthermore, using reduced intensity conditioning, results may improve further.[19a]

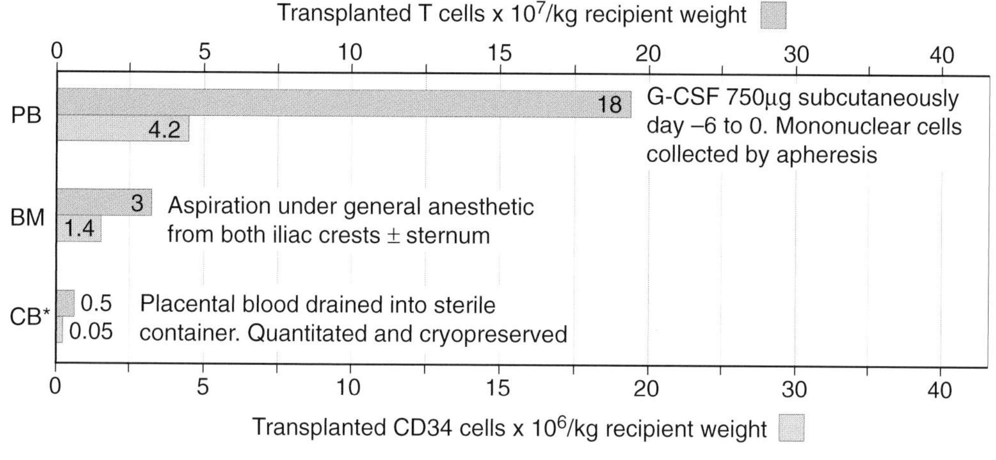

Figure 94–3. Characteristics of transplants derived from marrow, peripheral blood and umbilical cord blood showing relative amounts of stem cells and lymphocytes available to the recipient. (Cell doses in cord blood transplants are adjusted for a recipient of 25 kg body weight.)

Cell Processing and Transplantation

Manipulations of stem cells prior to transplant include simple maneuvers (volume reduction, filtration to remove bone spicules and particles from bone marrow harvests, red cell removal to prevent transfusion reactions, addition of 10% dimethylsulfoxide for cryopreservation in liquid nitrogen), and complicated techniques to select CD34 cells and deplete lymphocytes with antibody-coated magnetic beads. Cells for transplant are given intravenously, usually through a central line, either as fresh preparations (less than 24 hours elapsed from collection to transfusion) or as cryopreserved, thawed products. The precautions used with any blood product administration are also applied during stem cell transfusions. Contaminating dimethyl sulfoxide can be safely transfused but can cause flushing and headache. The problem can be avoided by restricting the volume of transplanted cells to less than 100 mL. ABO incompatibility is not a barrier to stem cell transplantation provided mismatched donor red cells are removed to prevent their destruction by recipient antibodies.[20]

Conditioning Regimens

The aim of the conditioning regimen is to immunosuppress the recipient sufficiently to prevent rejection of the transplant, to make space in the marrow for healthy donor stem cells, and to cytoreduce malignant cells in patients transplanted for leukemias and malignant disorders. Conditioning regimens, therefore, vary with the underlying disease to be treated and with the degree of immunosuppression required to achieve engraftment.[21]

Immunosuppressive conditioning is required to establish engraftment in all recipients, except infants with severe combined immune deficiency receiving an HLA-identical sibling transplant. Recipients of a transplant from an identical twin donor do not require immunosuppression to achieve engraftment, but recipients with aplastic anemia or malignant disease receive conditioning as treatment of the underlying condition. The most commonly used immunosuppressive agents are cyclophosphamide in doses up to 200 mg/kg, fludarabine in doses around 125 mg/m^2, antilymphocyte globulin, and anti-CD52 (alemtuzumab).

Myelosuppression is used to "make space" for engrafting donor stem cells in transplants for nonmalignant disorders. Busulfan has been widely used to achieve marrow ablation in a range of disorders, including the thalassemias and metabolic diseases.

Treatment to control malignant disease involves standard- to high-dose chemotherapy and may include whole-body radiation. Many regimens are disease specific, but typical generally applicable preparative regimens include total-body irradiation to a total of 12–15 Gy given in twice-daily fractions over 4–5 days or busulfan up to 12 mg/kg intravenously over 2–4 days in association with an immunosuppressive agent (cyclophosphamide or fludarabine). It is important to note that, although cyclophosphamide is an alkylating agent, it is not myeloablative even in high doses because it spares nondividing stem cells.

Reduced-intensity conditioning regimens are increasingly used in older or debilitated patients.[22] These regimens use highly immunosuppressive but nonmyeloablative combinations of chemotherapy, radiation, and antibodies, designed to achieve engraftment while minimizing regimen-related toxicity and preserving the immune-mediated graft-versus-malignancy effect of the transplant. Typical regimens employ fludarabine with or without cyclophosphamide as immunosuppression, with or without addition of reduced doses of alkylating agents or radiation to add antileukemic potential. Common regimens and their applications in allogeneic stem cell transplantation are shown in Figure 94–4.[23–33]

Preventing Graft-Versus-Host Disease

To prevent graft-versus-host disease, either transplants must be almost completely depleted of functioning T

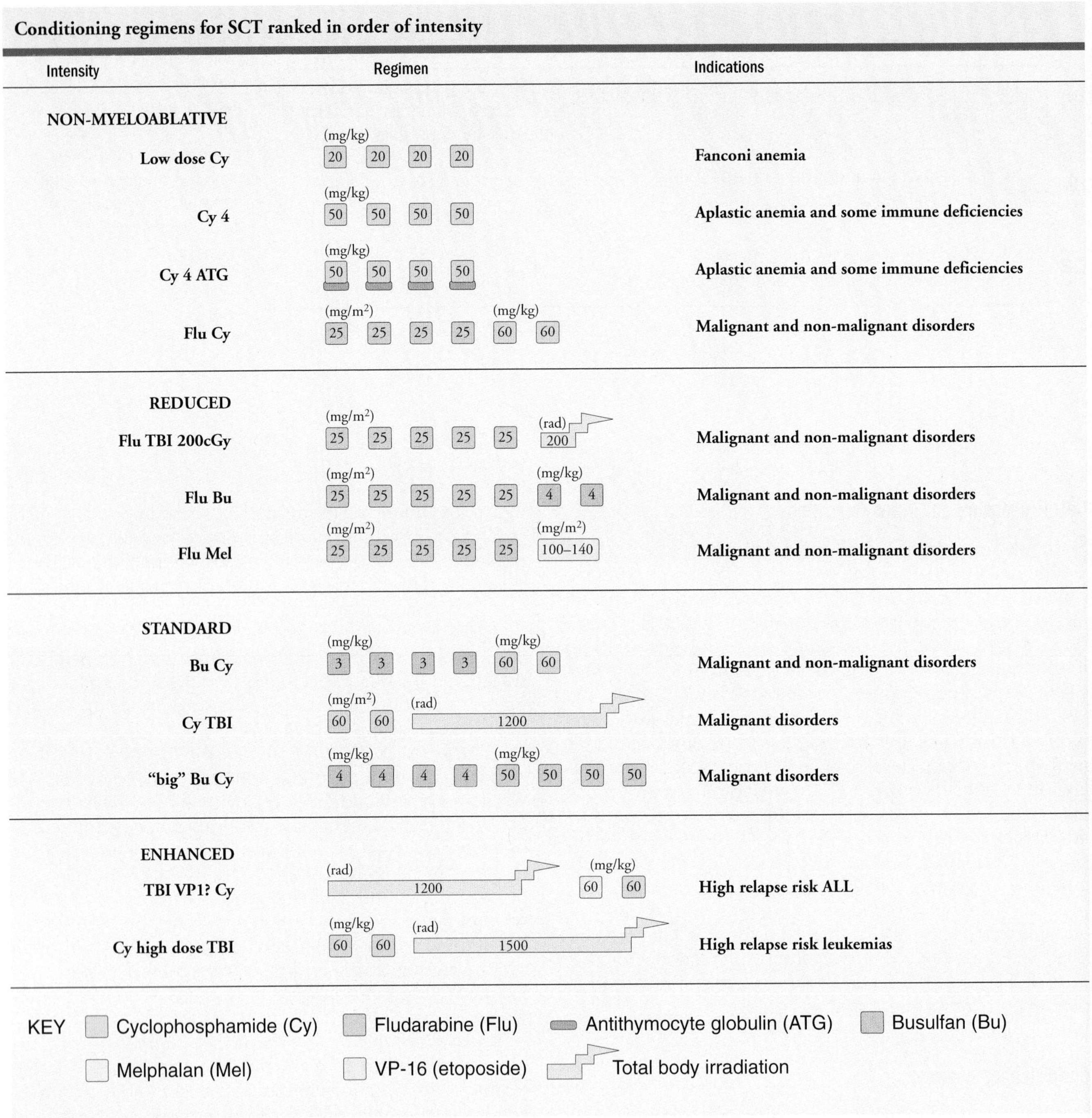

Conditioning regimens for SCT ranked in order of intensity

Intensity	Regimen	Indications
NON-MYELOABLATIVE		
Low dose Cy	(mg/kg) 20 20 20 20	Fanconi anemia
Cy 4	(mg/kg) 50 50 50 50	Aplastic anemia and some immune deficiencies
Cy 4 ATG	(mg/kg) 50 50 50 50	Aplastic anemia and some immune deficiencies
Flu Cy	(mg/m²) 25 25 25 25 (mg/kg) 60 60	Malignant and non-malignant disorders
REDUCED		
Flu TBI 200cGy	(mg/m²) 25 25 25 25 25 (rad) 200	Malignant and non-malignant disorders
Flu Bu	(mg/m²) 25 25 25 25 25 (mg/kg) 4 4	Malignant and non-malignant disorders
Flu Mel	(mg/m²) 25 25 25 25 25 (mg/m²) 100–140	Malignant and non-malignant disorders
STANDARD		
Bu Cy	(mg/kg) 3 3 3 3 (mg/kg) 60 60	Malignant and non-malignant disorders
Cy TBI	(mg/m²) 60 60 (rad) 1200	Malignant disorders
"big" Bu Cy	(mg/kg) 4 4 4 4 (mg/kg) 50 50 50 50	Malignant disorders
ENHANCED		
TBI VP1? Cy	(rad) 1200 (mg/kg) 60 60	High relapse risk ALL
Cy high dose TBI	(mg/kg) 60 60 (rad) 1500	High relapse risk leukemias

KEY Cyclophosphamide (Cy) Fludarabine (Flu) Antithymocyte globulin (ATG) Busulfan (Bu) Melphalan (Mel) VP-16 (etoposide) Total body irradiation

Figure 94–4. Conditioning regimens for stem cell transplantation ranked in order of intensity. **Key: cyclophosphamide (Cy); fludarabine (Flu); antithymocyte globulin (ATG); total-body irradiation; busulfan (Bu); melphalan (Mel); VP-16 (etoposide). Relative doses of agents are indicated by size of the corresponding symbol.**

lymphocytes, or steps must be taken to suppress the alloreaction posttransplant. After non–T-cell–depleted, HLA-identical, sibling transplants, a combination of immediate posttransplant methotrexate and long-term cyclosporine or tacrolimus is the standard approach.[34] Combinations of T-cell depletion with posttransplant immunosuppression are required for mismatched transplants.

HEMATOLOGIC AND IMMUNOLOGIC OUTCOMES POSTTRANSPLANTATION

Engraftment

Once established, the transplant is capable of maintaining hematopoiesis and immunity lifelong. The pattern and degree of engraftment can vary and are determined by the ability of the conditioning regimen to suppress recipient resistance to engraftment, the donor-recipient match, the T-cell content of the transplant, and the posttransplant immunosuppression. Donor and recipient cells can be separately identified by differences in DNA fingerprinting (using mini-satellite probes) or in appropriate cases by fluorescent in situ hybridization analysis for sex chromosomes. By coupling such techniques with lineage-specific chimerism determination, a complete picture of immune and myeloid engraftment can be created. Studies find that T-cell and myeloid cell engraftment occur independently. However, it is the degree to which donor T cells engraft that determines the durability and completeness of the graft.[21] With adequate immunosuppressive conditioning, donor T lymphocytes rapidly dominate the peripheral lymphocyte compartment, and subsequently eliminate residual host immune cells and hematopoietic cells (including B cells) by a powerful "graft-versus-marrow" effect. The graft-versus-marrow effect is best seen after reduced-intensity ("nonmyeloablative") transplants in which the marrow recovery is initially of recipient origin, switching to donor about 3 months later. In T-cell–depleted transplants, or with less effective immunosuppression in the conditioning regimen, the recovery of donor T cells is slower and mixed chimeric states can persist, sometimes indefinitely.[35] Falling donor T-cell chimerism is an indication of impending graft rejection and requires intervention—donor lymphocyte transfusion and maintenance of posttransplant immunosuppression.[25,36] The kinetics of hematologic and immune recovery are illustrated in Figure 94–5.

Hematopoietic Recovery

After an uncomplicated stem cell transplantation, the appearance of monocytes in the blood heralds recovery of the blood count, which occurs around the 10th to 14th posttransplant day. Neutrophil recovery usually precedes that of platelets and reticulocytes, but dependence on red cell and platelet transfusion is normally lost within 3 weeks. Hematopoietic recovery is slower in the presence of splenomegaly, marrow fibrosis, and circulating antibodies to blood cells. Some recipients of ABO-incompatible stem cells continue to destroy regenerating donor red cells for months after transplant and remain red cell transfusion dependent until residual recipient antibody production dwindles.[37] Potentially more serious

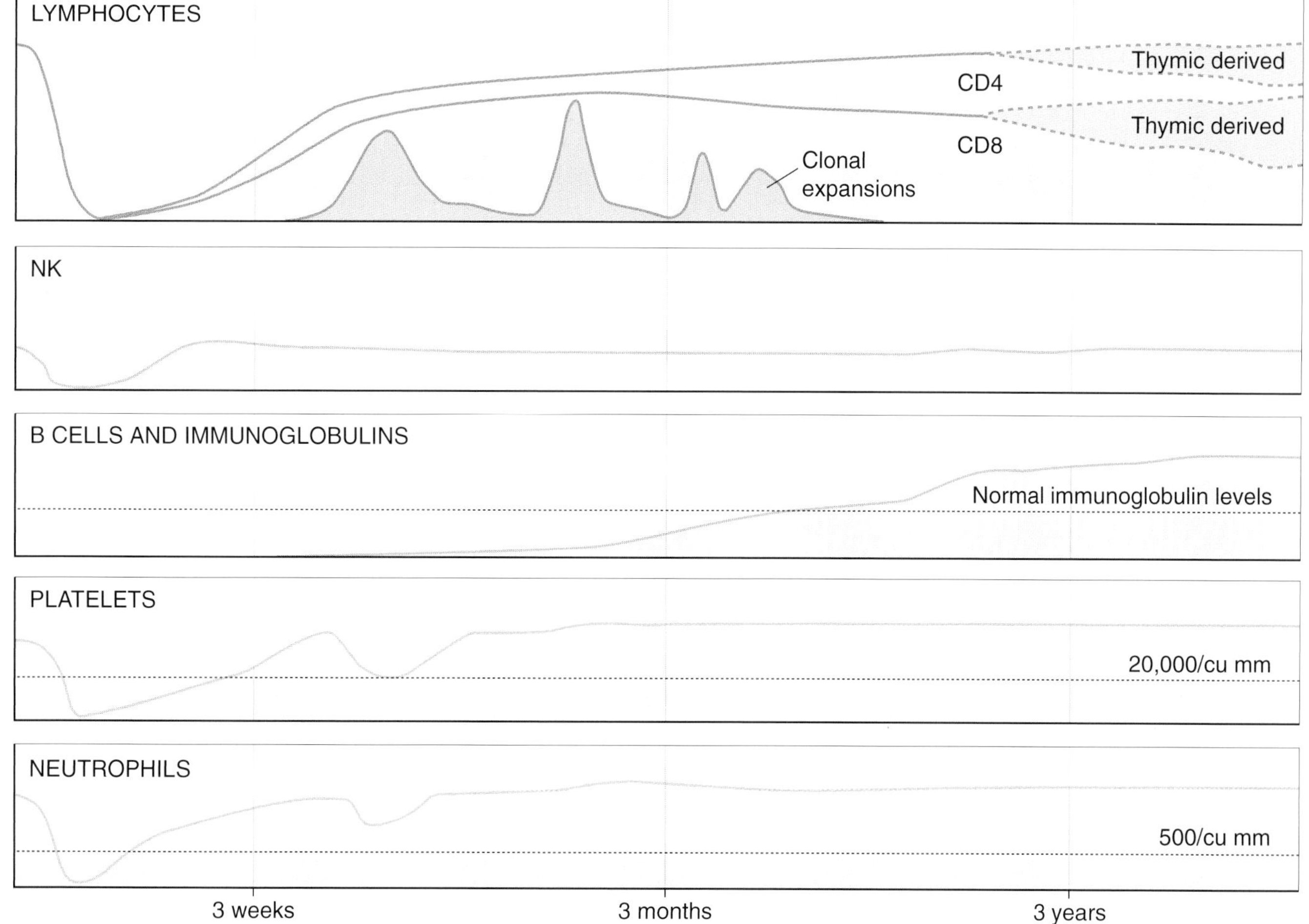

Figure 94–5. Kinetics of hematologic and immune recovery after stem cell transplantation. Figure shows expansion of individual lymphocyte subsets, immunoglobulins, platelets, and neutrophils posttransplant relative to lower limits of normal ranges.

is a minor ABO blood group mismatch (e.g., donor group O, recipient group A). Rarely, such minor mismatches induce rapid and life-threatening hemolysis of recipient red cells within 2 weeks of the transplant. The problem (caused by the activation of donor B-cells producing anti-A and -B) occurs particularly in PBSC trans-plant recipients not receiving methotrexate for graft-versus-host disease prophylaxis.[38] Despite the establishment of ultimately complete and stable hematopoiesis, it is not uncommon for patients to develop reversible cytopenias during the first few months after transplant, as a result of a myelosuppressive effect from ganciclovir used to treat cytomegalovirus reactivation, and in association with graft-versus-host disease.

Immune Reconstitution

The profound lymphopenia that follows the conditioning regimen is a powerful stimulus for expansion of incoming donor lymphocytes, through a poorly understood homeostatic mechanism. Circulating lymphocyte numbers can normalize within 3 months, but lymphocyte counts are extremely variable after stem cell transplantation. NK cells recover to normal or increased numbers within the first few weeks. Whereas $CD8^+$ recovery is prompt, $CD4^+$ T cells remain below 200/mm^3 for months. Thus, although cell counts may be normal, functional tests of immunity remain abnormal for months, even in uncomplicated transplants.[39] Donor B-cell recovery and antibody production is particularly slow to recover, and levels of immunoglobulins, especially immunoglobulin A, can remain low for years after transplantation.[40] Stem cell source affects the quality of immune recovery, with PBSC transplants having a more rapid and complete immune recovery than bone marrow transplants.[41]

T-Lymphocyte Abnormalities

Early posttransplant, the T-cell repertoire is irregular because of clonal expansions of T cells responding to recipient and viral antigenic stimuli. This initial T-cell expansion is dominated by the donor's post-thymic antigen-experienced memory and effector lymphocytes, which cause graft-versus-host disease but also provide graft-versus-leukemia responses and antiviral immunity. Much later, around a year or more posttransplant, new, thymus-derived T cells begin to populate the peripheral T-cell compartment with naive T cells, normalizing the balance of T-cell subsets.[42]

NK Cell Abnormalities

Early recovering NK cells show functional immaturity, with incompletely developed killer immunoglobulin–like receptor inhibitory molecules and a greater propensity for cytotoxicity.[43]

Factors Influencing Immune Recovery

Many factors, such as immunosuppression and graft-versus-host disease, influence the pace and completeness of immune recovery, but recipient age is the most important factor[44] (Table 94–1). Transplants performed in recipients with a functioning thymus (typically below the age of 20 years) normalize lymphocyte subsets and function more rapidly, and eventually reconstitute a tolerized T-cell repertoire of donor prethymic cells maturing through the recipient thymus. Older recipients show incomplete and delayed acquisition of thymic-derived lymphocytes.[42]

TABLE 94–1. Factors Affecting Immune Recovery after Transplant

Factor	Effect
Immunosuppression to prevent or treat GVHD	Impairment of GVL and antiviral responses
GVHD	Immunodeficiency, thymic damage delays tolerance
Recipient age	Younger age favors full and rapid thymic recovery
T-lymphocyte dose	High doses increase T-cell repertoire diversity
Profound host immunoablation	Favors donor T-cell clonal expansion
Growth factors IL-2, IL-12, IL-7	Favor T-cell expansion and thymic recovery
Lymphoid chimerism	Mixed chimerism reduces GVL response and GVHD
HLA mismatching	NK cell alloreactivity favors GVL response without GVHD
Cytokine gene polymorphisms	Affect GVHD, GVL response, immune reconstitution

Abbreviations: GVHD, graft-versus-host disease; GVL, graft-versus-leukemia; IL, interleukin; NK, natural killer.

Mechanisms of Cure of Nonmalignant Disorders

A transplant of healthy donor stem cells can be used not only to correct the bone marrow stem cell failure of severe aplastic anemia, but also to replace defective hematopoietic lineages (e.g., erythropoiesis in sickle cell disease). The transplantation of pluripotent lymphohematopoietic progenitors also provides the cells necessary to correct congenital and acquired immune deficiencies. Reconstituted immunity is derived both from post-thymic T cells given with the transplant, and from lymphocytes generated by donor-derived CD34 cells, maturing in the thymus and B-cell developmental areas to generate a new adaptive immune system. The replacement of the recipient lymphohematopoietic system with that of a healthy donor also provides a means of correcting genetic errors of metabolism caused by defective enzymes (storage diseases, mucopolysaccharidoses, etc.). Correction relies upon the penetration of non-hematopoietic tissue by enzyme-competent donor–derived macrophages, dendritic cells. and glial cells,[45] which deliver enzyme to affected cells by diffusion and pinocytosis or by direct cell-cell exchange.[46] The spectrum of disorders correctable by stem cell transplantation is wide. Figure 94–6 shows correctable genetic disorders according to their cell of origin and their relationship to

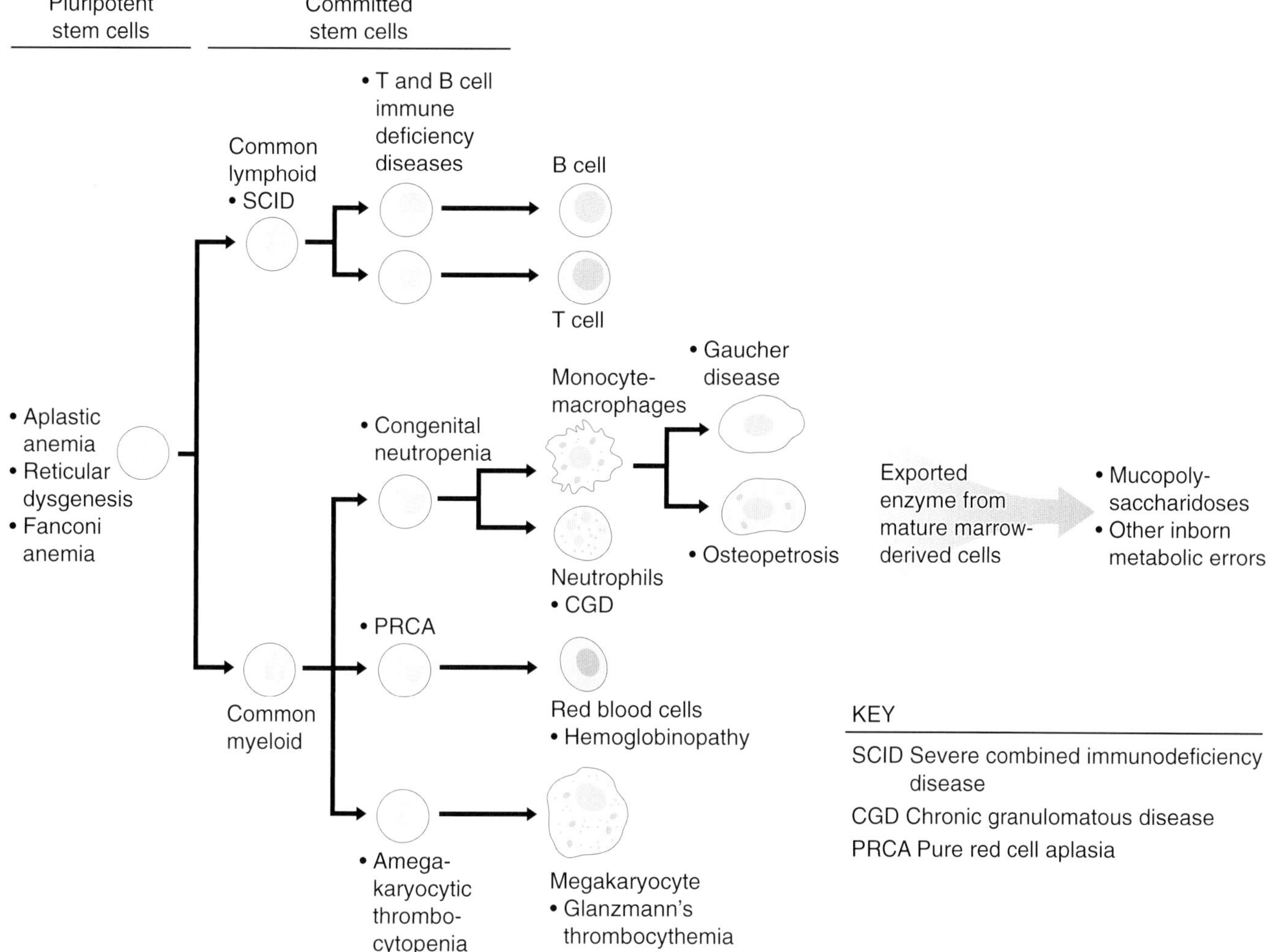

Figure 94–6. Correction of genetic disorders by replacement with hematopoietic stem cells and their progeny. Abbreviations: CGD, chronic granulomatous disease; SCID, severe combined immunodeficiency disease.

the transplanted stem cell. It has recently been found that bone marrow contains rare populations of primitive multipotent stem cells capable of giving rise not only to hematopoietic cells but also fibroblasts, neural, muscle, and endothelial cells, cartilage, and bone progenitors.[47] Although these findings have enormous implications for the future use of adult stem cells to repair or replace nonhematopoietic tissues, multiple studies after conventional allogeneic stem cell transplantation have not identified significant numbers, if any, of nonhematopoietic tissue cells of donor origin.[48]

Mechanism of Cure of Malignant Disorders

Two mechanisms are involved in the cure of malignant disease by stem cell transplantation. The first is the conditioning regimen, which confers a powerful antitumor effect from myeloablative doses of chemotherapy or radiotherapy. The second is the graft-versus-leukemia (or graft-versus-tumor) effect exerted by transplanted donor T cells and NK cells against malignant tissue.[49]

Cellular Basis of Graft-Versus-Leukemia Effect

T lymphocytes recognize antigens presented by HLA molecules on malignant cells. They destroy tumor cells by direct cytotoxicity, inducing death by lysis through the perforin-granzyme pathway and by apoptosis through activation of Fas on the cell surface.[50] Graft-versus-leukemia effects from NK cells have only been detected in HLA class I mismatched transplants from haploidentical family donors or unrelated donors. NK cells use the perforin-granzyme pathway to kill their targets, but are only activated when inhibitory signals from self-MHC class I molecules on the target are missing or overcome by powerful activating signals through their NKG2D receptor.[51] Cytokines may modulate graft-versus-leukemia reactivity, and genetic variability in the pattern of cytokine production is believed to underlie individual differences in the quality of the graft-versus-leukemia response. Detection of favorable or unfavorable cytokine gene polymorphisms may in future be important for individualizing transplant conditions to optimize the graft-versus-leukemia response[52] (Fig. 94–7*A*).

Clinical Manifestation of Graft-Versus-Leukemia Effect

The graft-versus-leukemia effect can occur within months after transplant. T-cell–mediated graft-versus-leukemia response has mainly been studied in patients in whom residual leukemia can be followed with molecular markers, such as BCR/ABL expression in chronic myelogenous leukemia. The lymphocyte response to chronic myelogenous leukemia seen after donor lymphocyte infusion to treat posttransplant relapse is similar to that seen during a viral infection: brief but massive expansion (up to 10% of circulating T cells) of single clones of $CD8^+$ effector T cells, specific for chronic myelogenous leukemia antigens, is followed by prompt disappearance of the BCR/ABL marker.[53] The graft-versus-leukemia effect requires donor immune competence—it often accompanies graft-versus-host disease,[54] it correlates with the ability to handle cytomegalovirus reactivation,[55] and it requires full donor lymphocyte engraftment.[25] Immunosuppression with steroids or cyclosporine negatively affects graft-versus-leukemia responses and there are many documented cases of patients whose residual disease increases during immunosuppressive treatment and diminishes when immunosuppression is withdrawn[56,57] (Fig. 94–7*B*). Once established, graft-versus-leukemia effects are probably sustained lifelong. Cure of leukemia by stem cell transplantation may, therefore, represent an ongoing equilibrium between a competent immune system suppressing an undetectably small but persisting leukemic clone.

COMPLICATIONS OF BONE MARROW TRANSPLANTATION

Complications after stem cell transplantation follow a predictable pattern (Fig. 94–8). The first 100 days mark the period of greatest risk after transplant, and consequently 100-day mortality is widely used as a benchmark for comparing transplant outcome; thereafter, the transplant-related mortality risk diminishes progressively (Fig. 94–9). In the first few weeks after transplant, the clinical picture is dominated by infectious complications from neutropenia, the immediate effects of the conditioning regimen, and complications related to engraftment—graft-versus-host disease, graft rejection, or complete graft failure. Complications after day 100 include the development of chronic graft-versus-host disease, and continuing problems with infections, including those induced by high-dose steroids and other immunosuppressive therapy. Late effects, occurring years after transplant, are the consequence of the preparative regimen or chronic graft-versus-host disease. Leukemia recurrence can occur at any time, but the risk diminishes with time.

Graft Rejection and Failure

Early graft rejection should be assumed in a patient who fails to show hematopoietic recovery by day 21 posttransplant. Graft rejection is usually asymptomatic, but may be accompanied by fever and minimal splenomegaly. In engrafted patients who later reject, the blood counts fall precipitously in a few days, sometimes in association with a brief lymphocytosis (of recipient origin). Diagnosis of graft failure is established by finding a low or falling blood count with an aplastic marrow, and chimerism analysis demonstrating loss of donor-derived myeloid and lymphoid cells. Rejection can sometimes be suppressed by increasing immunosuppression if initiated before the onset of complete graft failure. However, complete marrow aplasia is usually only correctable with a second stem cell transplantation. High-dose methylprednisolone, prolonged treatment with OKT3, and stem cell transplantation can salvage some patients, but unless a nonmyeloablative transplant has been performed, there is a high mortality from persisting failure to engraft.[58]

Acute Graft-Versus-Host Disease

Acute graft-versus-host disease can occur as early as 10 days after the transplant (see Chapter 97 for a detailed account of pathophysiology and clinical features). The disease is manifest by rash, diarrhea, and liver function abnormalities. The expression of acute graft-versus-host disease varies widely; some patient have no evidence or a minimal and localized skin rash, and others develop life-threatening damage to the endothelium of the gastrointestinal tract, or hepatic failure from intrahepatic biliary obstruction.[59] Acute graft-versus-host disease and its treatment is associated with immune dysfunction, and is often accompanied by cytomegalovirus reactivation.

Chronic Graft-Versus-Host Disease

Chronic graft-versus-host disease can present in the third month posttransplant with dryness and lichenoid changes of the skin and buccal mucosa, conjunctival irritation and dryness, and a mixed hepatitic-obstructive pattern of liver enzymes (see Chapter 97). Chronic graft-versus-host disease can progress to severe scleroderma with loss of hair, poor nail growth, marked fasciitis with muscle trapping, chronic liver damage, profound immune deficiency with recurrent infections, bronchiolitis obliterans, and rarely nephrotic syndrome. Most chronic graft-versus-host disease evolves on a background of the acute form, but about 40% of cases occur de novo. Patients with diffuse erythroderma from acute graft-versus-host disease have a higher risk of progressing to a debilitating exfoliative dermatitic form of chronic graft-versus-host disease.[60]

Infections

Viral Infections

Infection or reactivation of viruses is especially dangerous in the first 3–6 months posttransplant.

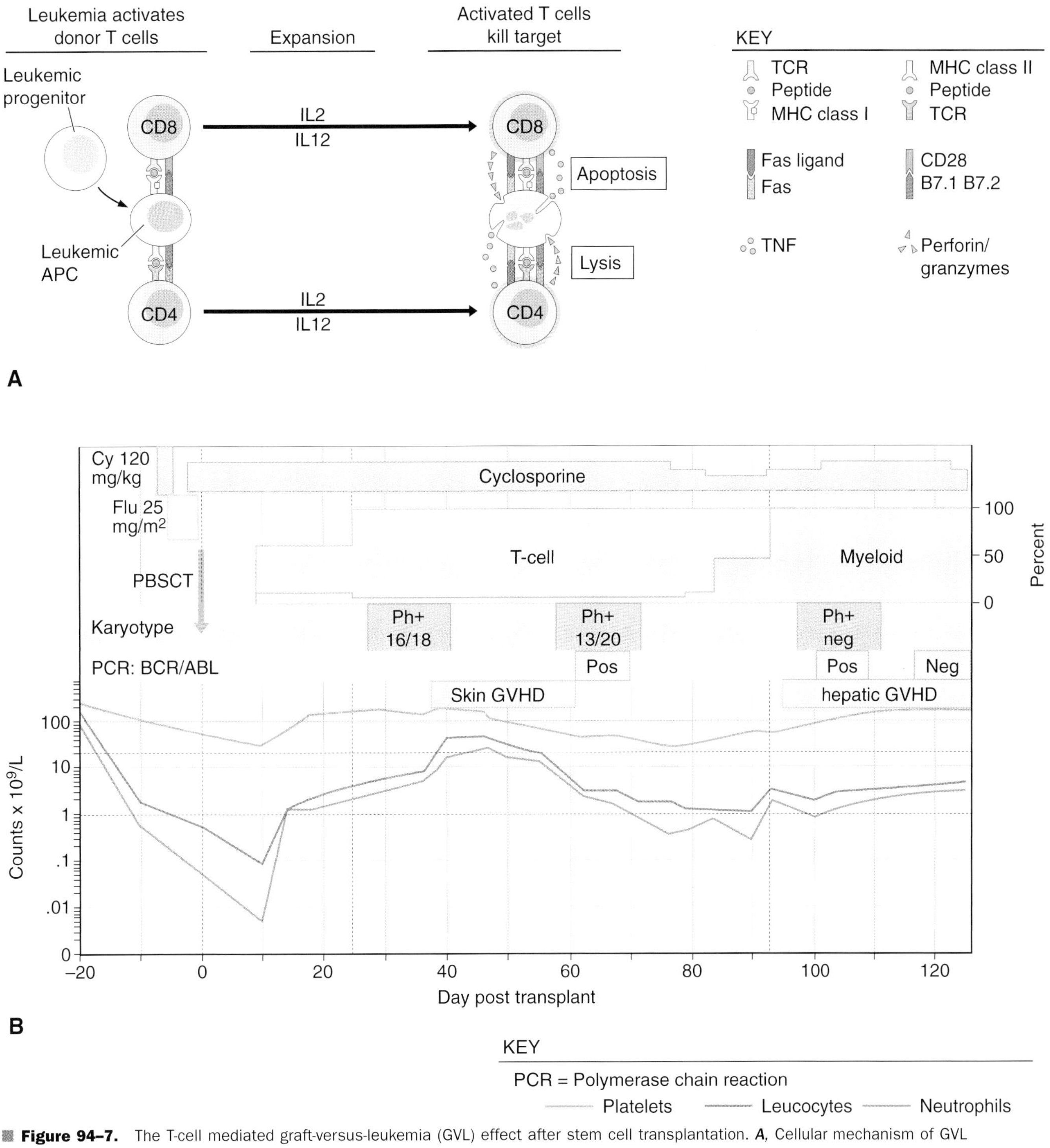

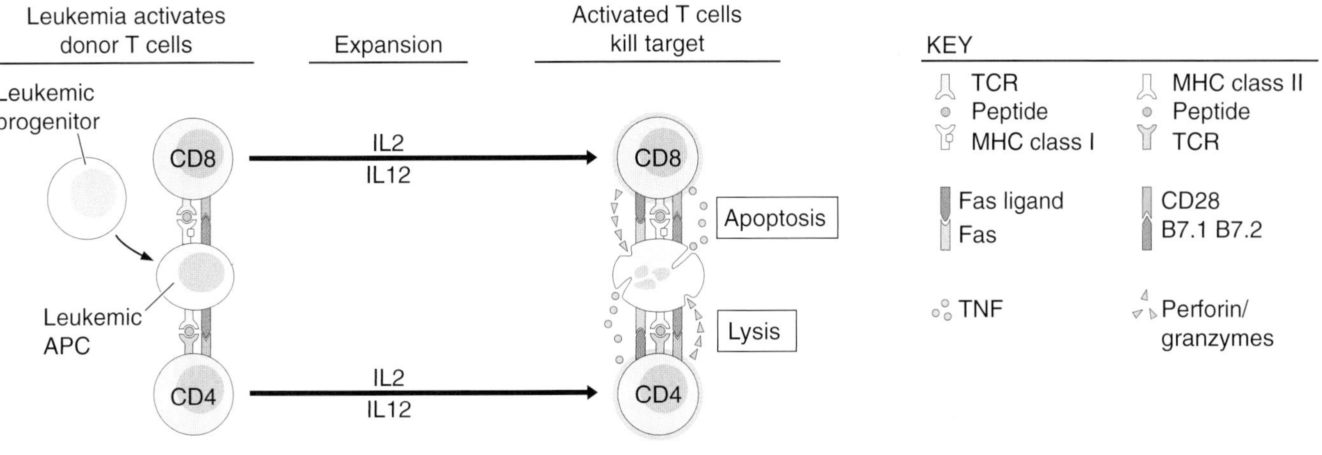

Figure 94–7. The T-cell mediated graft-versus-leukemia (GVL) effect after stem cell transplantation. ***A,*** Cellular mechanism of GVL response showing key molecules involved in allogeneic T-cell activation, expansion, and effector function against the leukemic target. Abbreviations: DC, dendritic cell; IL, interleukin; TNF, tumor necrosis factor, +, stimulatory effect; –, inhibitory effect; ***B,*** GVL effect from engrafting lymphocytes in a patient with chronic myelogenous leukemia. The patient, in chronic phase, received an HLA-identical stem cell transplant following a nonmyeloablative regimen, which allowed engraftment but did not prevent recovery of the leukemia following a chemotherapy-induced cytopenia. The later full engraftment of donor T cells resulted in the full eradication of the leukemia and a molecular cure. The figure shows changes in platelet and leukocyte counts, slow but complete engraftment of donor T cells and myeloid cells, and conversion of bone marrow from 100% Philadelphia chromosome positive to molecular cure (polymerase chain reaction for BCR/ABL was negative on day 120 posttransplant).

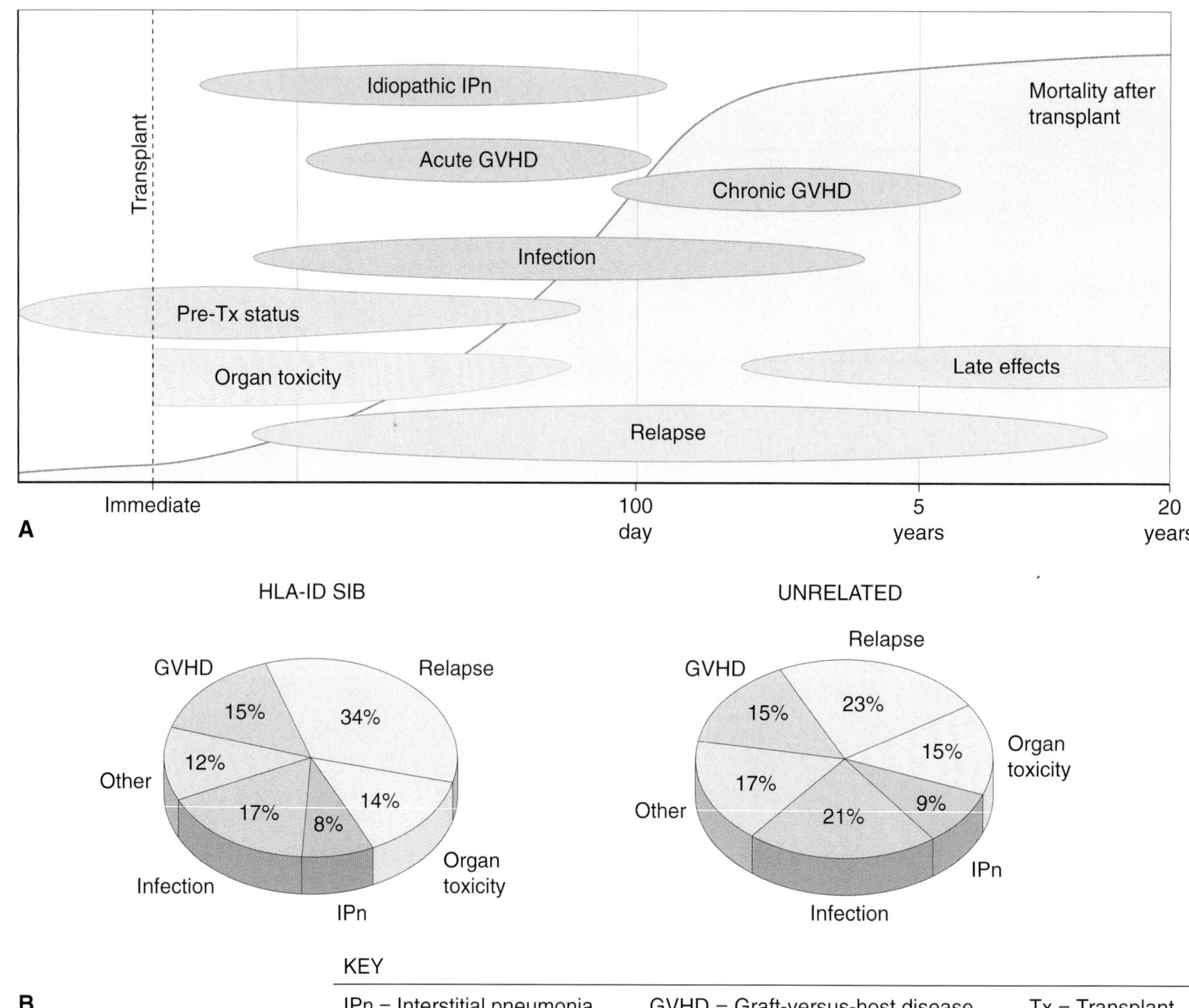

Figure 94–8. *A*, Time scale of complications following stem cell transplantation illustrating the timing of adverse events. *B*, Mortality. Pie diagrams break down the causes of treatment failure for HLA-identical sibling and unrelated donor transplants.

Cytomegalovirus reactivation carries a high risk of fatal interstitial pneumonia if untreated. Cytomegalovirus and herpes simplex virus reactivation are best treated by preemptive antiviral prophylaxis and early treatment of viral antigenemia in the case of cytomegalovirus.[61,62] Potentially lethal complications in the early months posttransplant occur from respiratory syncytial virus and human herpesvirus 6 pneumonia, adenoviral hepatitis, gastroenteritis and hemorrhagic cystitis, and BK viral hemorrhagic cystitis. Varicella-zoster reactivation in the form of zoster typically occurs beyond 6 months from transplant.[63] Epstein-Barr virus reactivation causes a rapidly proliferating B-cell lymphoma, usually in mismatched T-cell–depleted transplants, which requires prompt treatment with the anti-CD20 monoclonal rituximab or infusion of Epstein-Barr virus–specific T cells from the donor.[64]

Bacterial, Fungal, and Protozoal Infections

Predisposition to bacterial infection after stem cell transplantation is multifactorial. Early posttransplant infections resulting from neutropenia and infected intravenous lines predominate.[65] Later, prolonged use of steroids predisposes mainly to fungal infection.[66] Delayed recovery of immunoglobulins, especially in association with chronic graft-versus-host disease, renders patients at long-term risk from pneumococcal and *Haemophilus* pneumonia and sepsis.[67] Pulmonary infection from *Pneumocystis jiroveci* (*carinii*) is a potentially fatal complication of stem cell transplantation. Fortunately, prophylaxis with weekly trimethoprim-sulfonamide or monthly inhalation of pentamidine has all but eradicated this complication.[67] Toxoplasmosis is also rarely encountered as a consequence of this prophylactic regimen.[68]

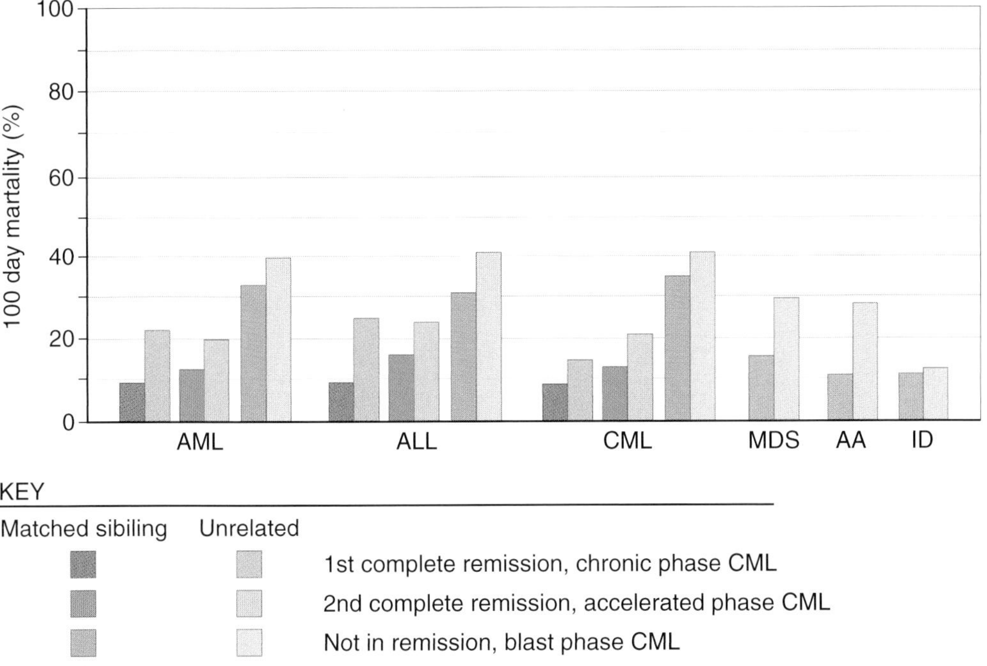

Figure 94–9. Risk of transplant-related mortality (TRM) according to disease status and transplant matching, showing higher TRM in malignant versus nonmalignant diseases, unrelated versus related donor transplants, and advanced versus early elective transplantation. (Data from the IBMTR.[87])

Delayed Effects from the Preparative Regimen

Intensive chemotherapy and radiation have a number of delayed consequences. Radiation therapy in particular predisposes to cataracts, gonadal failure, thyroid failure, and second malignancies.[69,70]

Disease Recurrence

Although transplant survival has continued to improve, recurrence of the malignant disease for which the transplant was performed stands out as the single biggest cause of treatment failure. The most predictive factor for disease relapse is the status of the malignancy prior to transplant. Regardless of the specific disease, transplants performed electively, early in the course of the disease when it is still susceptible to chemotherapy, have the greatest likelihood of success (e.g., acute leukemia in remission, chronic myelogenous leukemia in chronic phase, and myelodysplastic syndrome without excess of blasts). Such transplants have a low rate of disease recurrence and of transplant-related mortality. At the other extreme, patients treated late in the course of disease, with malignancy refractory to treatment, have a high rate of disease recurrence and a high transplant-related mortality (see Fig. 94–9, and see disease-specific outcomes for details). Relapse can be treated immunologically with donor lymphocytes, preceded if necessary by therapy to reduce tumor bulk, or more aggressively with high-dose conditioning and a second transplant, taking advantage of a different donor if available, and minimizing graft-versus-host disease prophylaxis in order to maximize graft-versus-leukemia effects.[71,72] Apart from spectacular success in obtaining sustained molecular remissions from donor lymphocyte infusion in chronic myelogenous leukemia, the results of donor lymphocyte infusion have been otherwise disappointing, with sustained remissions occurring only in a minority of acute myeloid leukemia and fewer acute lymphoblastic leukemia transplant recipients.[73] Second transplants sometimes have prolonged disease-free survival but with a high risk of transplant-related mortality and disease recurrence. Favorable factors for survival after second transplants are a long interval between transplant and relapse, development of chronic graft-versus-host disease, and leukemia type; chronic myelogenous leukemia patients have the best outcome.[74,75]

Factors Determining Transplant Outcome

Transplant outcome is determined by inherent characteristics of the disease, the patient, and the donor, and specific treatment choices of the transplanter (Table 94–2). Although stem cell transplantation is performed with many variations in diverse centers worldwide, the outcomes for particular patient, disease, and transplant types are remarkably similar. A study showed that unfavorable center effects were only identifiable in units performing less than 20 allografts per annum.[80] Thus the predominating factors determining success or failure of the transplant are intrinsic to the patient's age and performance and disease status.

Monitoring and Prevention of Posttransplant Complications

The principle of good posttransplant management is to anticipate and prevent complications that could prove fatal. Figure 94–10 illustrates standard regimens for prophylaxis of graft-versus-host disease and bacterial, fungal,

TABLE 94–2. Factors Affecting Transplant Outcome

Factor		Impact			
Favorable	**Unfavorable**	**TRM**	**GVHD**	**Relapse**	**Reference**
Patient and donor variables					
HLA = sib D	unrelated D	+	+		
Identical twin D	HLA = sib D	+	+		
Patient age >60 yr	>60 yr	+	+		76
Karnofsky score >90	<90	+			
Non-malignant disease	malignant disease	+			
Early disease status	advanced disease	+		+	
Elective transplant	salvage transplant	+		+	
KIR mismatched	KIR matched		+	+	51
CMV serology $D^+/R^{+/-}$	D^-, R^+	+			77
Transplant variables					
CD34 dose 3–6 × 10^6/kg	$<3 \times 10^6$/kg	+		+	
PBSCT	BMT	+		+	18
Unmanipulated SCT	T cell depletion		+	+	78
Regimen intensity high	low			+	28
Immunosuppression low	high			+	79

Abbreviations: CMV, cytomegalovirus; D, donor; GVHD, graft-versus-host disease; HLA = sib, HLA-identical sibling; KIR, killer immunoglobulin–like; PBSCT, peripheral blood stem cell transplant; R, recipient; SCT, stem cell transplant; TRM, transplant-related mortality.

and viral infection and for treatment of graft-versus-host disease. A typical follow-up schedule includes the monitoring of disease recurrence, chronic graft-versus-host disease, endocrine function, growth and development in children, and psychosocial adaptation.

OUTCOME OF STEM CELL TRANSPLANTATION IN SPECIFIC DISEASE STATES

Nonmalignant Disorders

The majority of patients transplanted for nonmalignant disorders are infants and children. Because they have a greater chance than adults of surviving stem cell transplantation, it has been possible to safely extend transplants to infants and children with mismatched donors. Results of transplants for nonmalignant disorders are also generally superior to those for malignant disease, because it has proved much easier to eliminate nonmalignant conditions than malignant diseases with stem cell transplantation. In general, transplant outcomes are better for inherited disorders if the transplant is performed early, before irreversible tissue damage occurs. The decisions to transplant in nonmalignant disorders rests upon balancing possible outcomes of stem cell transplantation with nontransplant treatments. Outcomes can be predicted from standard risk factors described earlier. Examples of nontransplant alternatives include immunosuppression for severe aplastic anemia, lifelong transfusion for thalassemia, and enzyme therapy for some inborn errors of metabolism. The nonmalignant disease categories that are transplanted are listed in Box 94–1.

Outcomes for transplants in more common immune deficiency diseases are listed in Table 94–3. Of note is the very favorable outcome for severe combined immune deficiency, exceeding 90% disease-free survival overall. Transplants for bone marrow failure states are summarized in Table 94–4 and Figure 94–11. Younger age and acquired aplastic anemia are favorable factors. Transplants for hemoglobinopathies are summarized in Table 94–5 and illustrated in Figure 94–11. Allogeneic stem cell transplantation for thalassemia has dramatically changed the outlook for individuals fortunate enough to have an HLA-identical sibling donor. Although very favorable survival with disease correction can be achieved in young individuals, the decision to transplant patients with sickle cell anemia is complicated because of the difficulty of identifying precisely which individuals are at high risk of mortality from sickle cell complications.

Hematologic Malignancies

For malignant diseases, successful outcome of stem cell transplantation (disease-free survival) is the resultant of transplant-related mortality and probability of disease relapse or progression (see Fig. 94–9). The patient's disease characteristics tend to influence both curability and transplant-related mortality, such that patients transplanted electively when the malignancy is in remission, well controlled, or not advanced have both lower transplant-related mortality and lower relapse rates than those transplanted when the disease has progressed or is more aggressive. Conversely, the intensity of the transplant approach tends to affect relapse and transplant-related mortality in opposite ways such that attempts to improve the curability of the transplant negatively impact on survival and attempts to reduce transplant-related mortality increase disease relapse. In high-risk advanced malignancy, different transplant approaches that may increase

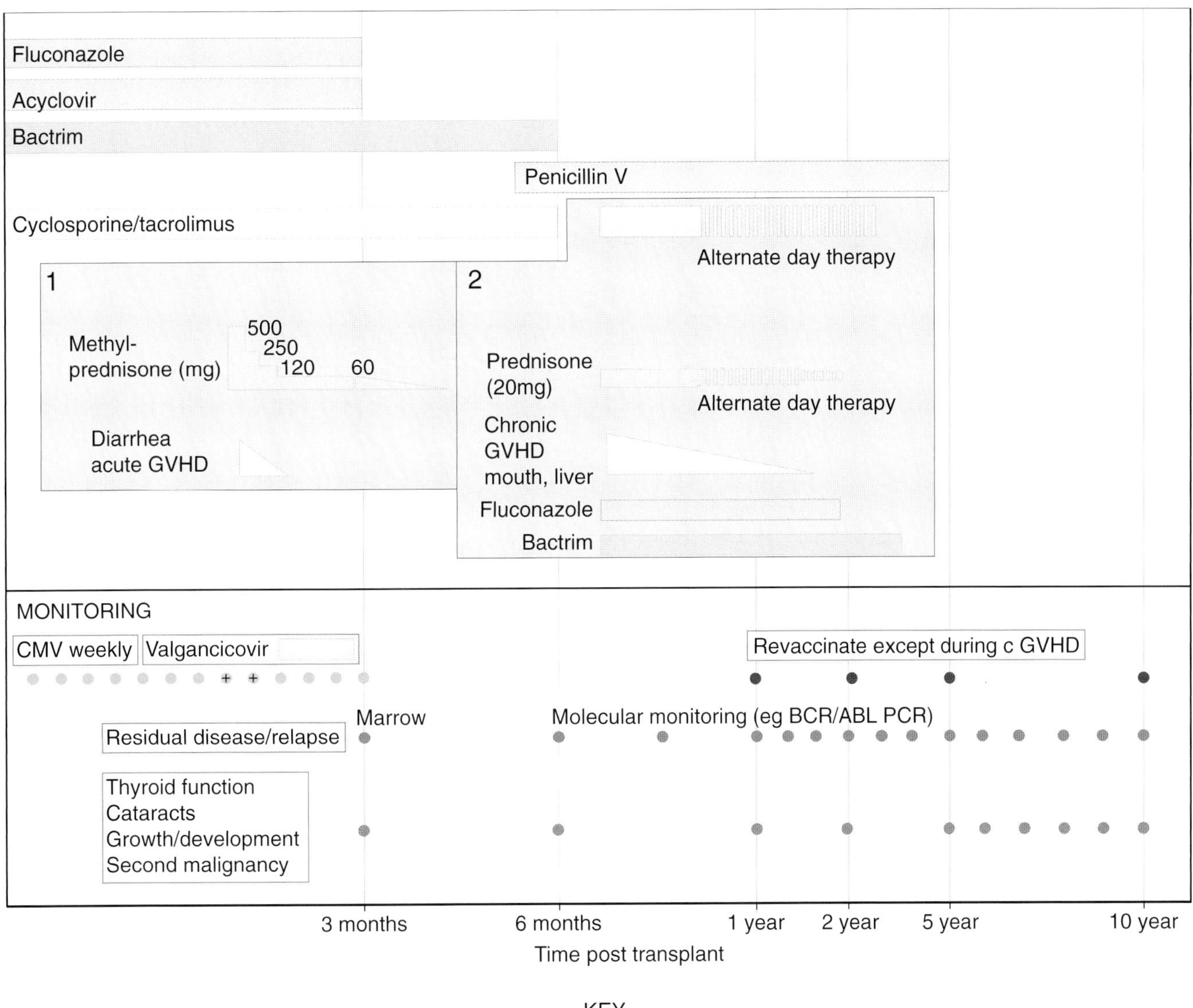

Figure 94–10. A typical posttransplant monitoring schedule showing prophylaxis of infection and graft-versus-host disease (GVHD), and regular monitoring for relapse and delayed organ damage. *Inset 1,* Decrescendo methylprednisolone treatment schedule for acute GVHD. *Inset 2,* Typical alternate-day treatment schedule with cyclosporine and low-dose prednisolone, and accompanying infection prophylaxis.

TABLE 94–3. Bone Marrow Transplantation for Common Immune Deficiencies

Disease	Donor	*n*	% Survival	Reference	Comments
SCID	HLA = sib	21	96 at 5 yr	82	Only one patient died. All others corrected.
	Unrelated	89	75 at 5 yr	83	Series includes 12 related donors.
					PEG-ADA for patients with SCID-ADA is an alternative.
WAS	HLA = sib	55	87	84	Survivors had complete disease correction. Unfavorable outcome for older recipients.
	Other related	48	85		
	Unrel. recip. <5 yr	52	50		
	Unrel. recip. >5 yr	15	25		
CGD	HLA = sib	10	70	36	SCT only indicated in patients not responding to standard antibacterial prophylaxis.
CN	HLA = sib	8	100	85	Treatment with G-CSF usually effective.

Abbreviations: CGD, chronic granulomatous disease; CN, congenital neutropenia; G-CSF, granulocyte colony-stimulating factor; HLA = sib, HLA-identical sibling; PEG-ADA, pegylated adenosine deaminase; SCID, severe combined immune deficiency; SCID-ADA, SCID with adenosine deaminase deficiency; SCT, stem cell transplant; WAS, Wiskott-Aldrich syndrome.

Box 94–1. Diseases Treated by Stem Cell Transplantation (SCT)

Corrected by SCT

Immune Deficiencies [36,81–85]

- Severe combined immune deficiency disease (SCID), SCID with adenosine deaminase deficiency, Wiskott-Aldrich syndrome, lymphocyte function-associated antigen-1 deficiency, reticular dysgenesis, other rare T-cell disorders
- Chronic granulomatous disease, congenital neutropenia, Chédiak-Higashi syndrome, other rare granulocyte disorders
- Chronic Epstein-Barr virus infection

Bone Marrow Disorders [86–91]

- Aplastic anemia
- Fanconi's aplastic anemia
- Dyskeratosis congenita
- Schwachman-Diamond syndrome
- Histiocytoses
- Osteopetrosis

Red Cell Disorders [92–97]

- Thalassemia syndromes
- Sickle cell anemia
- Diamond-Blackfan syndrome
- Pure red cell aplasia
- Paroxysmal nocturnal hemoglobinuria
- Dyserythropoietic anemias
- Sideroblastic anemia
- Severe inherited and acquired hemolytic anemias
- Congenital erythropoietic porphyria

Platelet Disorders

- Glanzmann's thrombasthenia
- Congenital amegakaryocytic thrombocytopenia

Metabolic Disorders [98–100]

- Mucopolysaccharidoses: type 1 (Hurler), type V (Maroteaux-Lamy)
- GM_1 gangliosidosis, metachromatic leukodystrophy
- Cerebrosidosis types 1, 2, and 3 (Gaucher)

Not Corrected by SCT [101]

Variable or No Significant Benefit—Not Standard Indications for SCT

- Mucopolysaccharidosis type II (Hunter syndrome), type III (San Filippo disease), type IV (Morquio disease)
- Osteogenesis imperfecta

No Benefit

- Hypoxanthine-guanine phosphoribosyltransferase deficiency (Lesch-Nyhan syndrome)
- Type IIA glycogen storage disease (Pompe's disease)
- Niemann-Pick disease
- Infantile globoid cell leukodystrophy (Krabbe's disease)

TABLE 94–4. Recent Results of Bone Marrow Transplantation for Marrow Failure States

Disease, Donor Type	n	% Survival	Reference	Comments
Severe aplastic anemia				
HLA = sib				
1–20 yr	844	76 ± 4	87	IBMTR data (diverse regimens, multiple centers)
20–40 yr	845	67 ± 3		
1–50 yr	1699	75	86	EBMT multicenter study (diverse regimens)
2–59 yr	94	88	88	Four centers, all received Cy ATG.
Unrelated donor				
≤20 yr	358	53 ± 6	87	IBMTR data (diverse regimens, multiple centers)
>20 yr	114	32 ± 10		
Identical twin	34	91	86	
Fanconi aplasia				
HLA = sib	151	66	89	IBMTR multicenter analysis (mainly low dose Cy regimen)
Other donor	48	29	89	

Abbreviations: ATG, antithymocyte globulin; Cy, cyclophosphamide; HLA = sib, HLA-identical sibling.

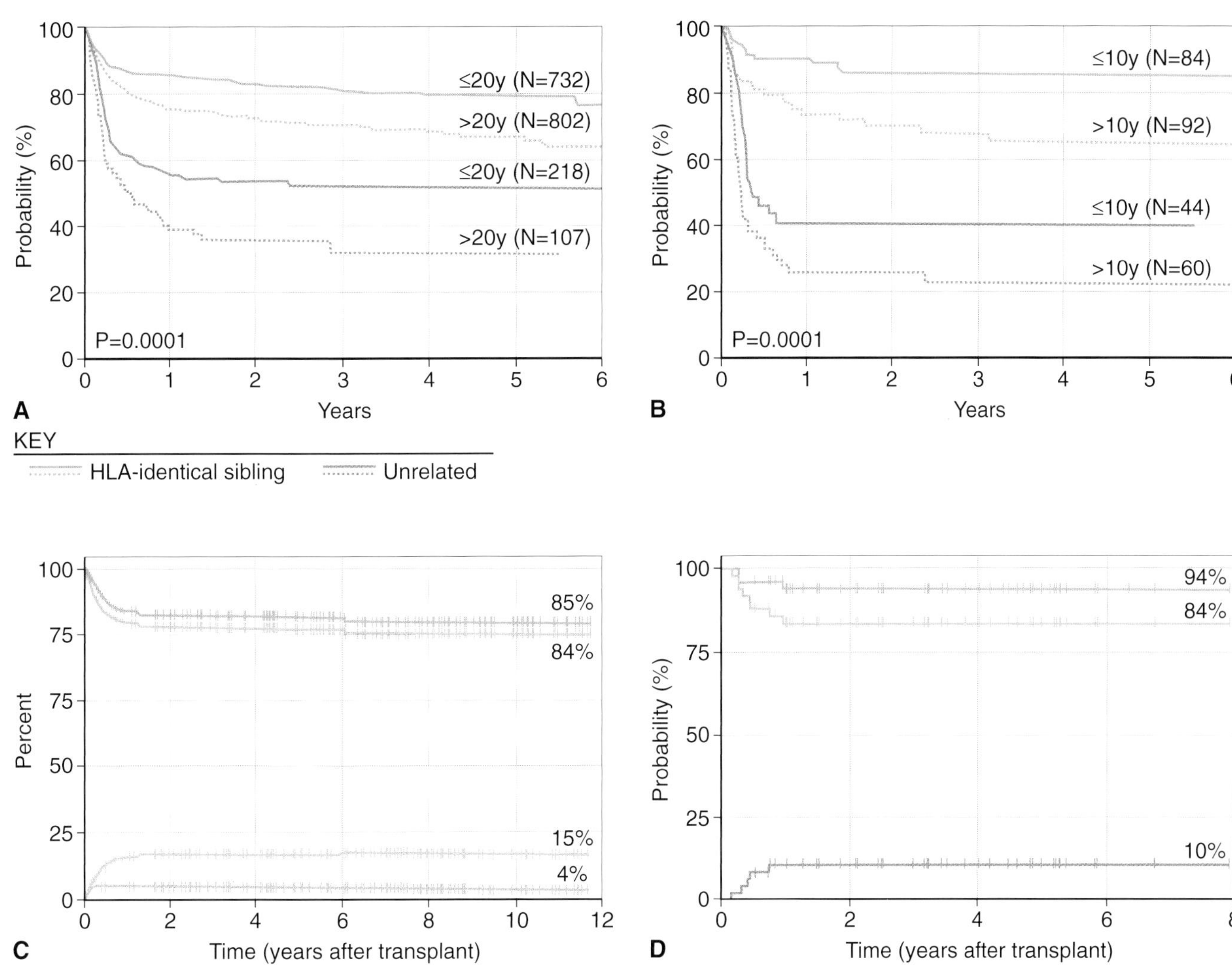

Figure 94–11. Outcomes after stem cell transplantation (SCT) for nonmalignant marrow disorders. *A,* SCT for severe aplastic anemia, showing impact of donor status and age on transplant survival. (Data from the IBMTR.[87]) *B,* Allogeneic SCT for Fanconi's aplastic anemia showing impact of patient age and donor type on survival. (Data from the IBMTR.[87]) *C,* Thalassemia-free survival following allogeneic SCT from an HLA-identical sibling (good risk, younger patients). (Data from Giardini and Lucarelli.[92]) *D,* Sickle cell anemia survival following allogeneic SCT from an HLA-identical sibling. (Data from a multicenter study.[96])

TABLE 94–5. Recent Results of HLA-Identical Sibling Bone Marrow Transplantation for Hemoglobinopathies

Disease, Donor Type	*n*	% DFS	Reference	Comments
Thalassemia, <17 yr				
Class I (no risk factors)	124	91	92	Thalassemia-free survival, Bu/Cy conditioning
Class II (1–2 risk factors)	297	84		Risk based on hepatomegaly, degree of liver damage on biopsy, chelation efficiency
Thalassemia, >17 yr				
Mainly Class III (high risk)	109	62	93	High mortality for older individuals
Thalassemia, 9 centers	21–102	76–91	94	Worldwide experience (Italy, USA, UK, Iran, India, Singapore, Hong Kong)
Sickle cell anemia (SCA), >95% HLA = sib				
Group 1 elective	14	93	95	Single center Belgian experience
Group 2 SCA morbidity	36	88		
Median age 9.4 yr (mixed group 1&2)	50	84	96	Multicenter USA experience

Abbreviations: Bu/Cy, busulfan and cyclosporine; DFS, disease-free survival; HLA = sib, HLA-identical sibling.

TABLE 94–6. Recent Results of Large Analyses of Stem Cell Transplantation for Myeloid Malignancies

	HLA = sib		URD			
	n	% DFS	*n*	% DFS	Reference	Comments
AML Myeloablative Transplants						
CR1 all	3419	62 ± 2	–	–	104	Multicenter
children	388	66 ± 3	334	43 ± 8		
adults	2306	58 ± 1	109	47 ± 6		
all ages	3193	61 ± 1	586	41 ± 2	87	3yr DFS, IBMTR
CR2 all ages	659	45 ± 5	735	42 ± 2	87	3yr DFS, IBMTR
>CR2 all ages	717	23 ± 4	–	–		
primary induction failure	88	15–21	–	–	105,106	Related + unrelated SCT
AML Reduced Intensity Transplants						
<5% blasts at transplant		49	–	–		
5–20% blasts at transplant	113	24	–	–	107	Related + unrelated SCT
>20% blasts at transplant		14	–	–		
MIDS						
<20yr, RA RARS	48	77	49	45	87	3yr DFS, IBMTR
more advanced	88	60	110	46		
≥20yr, RARS	254	50	92	37		
more advanced	648	40	257	33		
Median age 38yr						
IPPS low		60	–	–		Related + unrelated SCT, single center 5yr DFS
Intermediate-1	251	36	–	–	109	
Intermediate-2		28	–	–		
Median age 59yr						
RA		59 ± 8	–	–		Mainly HLA identical sibs single center 3 yr DFS
RAEB	50	46 ± 16	–	–	110	
RAEB-t/AML/CMML		33 ± 28	–	–		
Median age 2yr, CMML	43	32	–	–	111	Infants (14 unrel.) multicenter, 5yr DFS
CML Myeloablative Transplants						
CP ≤1yr	2876	69 ± 2	613	54 ± 4	87	3yr DFS IBMTR
CP >1yr	1391	57 ± 3	936	46 ± 3		
CP < 1 <30yr		68		61		
30–40yr	450	67	2464	57	114	NMDP
>40yr		57		46		
AP		50	–	–	87	3yr DFS IBMTR
BC		20	–	–		
CML Reduced Intensity Transplants						
All stages (84 in CP)	153	60–83%	–	–	115	7 centers in USA, Italy, UK, Hungary, Israel

Abbreviations: AML, acute myeloid leukemia; AP, accelerated phase; BC, blast crisis; CMML, chronic myelomonocytic leukemia; CP, chronic phase; CR, complete remission; DFS, disease-free survival; HLA = sib, HLA-identical sibling; IPSS, International Prognostic Staging System; RA, refractory anemia; RAEB, refractory anemia with excess blasts; RAEB-t, refractory anemia with excess blasts in transition; RARS, refractory anemia with ringed sideroblasts; SCT, stem cell transplant; URD, unrelated donor.

or reduce transplant-related mortality have relatively little impact on outcome, which is largely determined by treatment failure from disease recurrence. In general, the allograft typically offers a distinctly better opportunity for cure of disease, compared with either chemotherapy or autologous stem cell transplantation.[102] However, the associated higher transplant-related mortality of a curative transplant necessarily restricts the allograft to situations in which the transplant offers a higher disease-free survival than competing strategies. Appropriate transplant selection requires reliable data on disease-free survival for a particular donor-recipient match and transplant approach, which must be compared with contemporaneous outcomes using the best nontransplant treatment.

Numerous retrospective, and some prospective, analyses compare outcome for allogeneic stem cell transplantation with that for autotransplants, or chemotherapy. Because both stem cell transplantation and alternative treatments are constantly improving, the indications for stem cell transplantation require constant revision.[103] An example of a changing indication is illustrated by the impact of imatinib mesylate on the treatment of chronic myelogenous leukemia. The success of this new treatment has been so great that few patients with chronic myelogenous leukemia receive stem cell transplantation as primary elective treatment.[114] Conversely, the improved results for treating older patients with lower intensity conditioning regimens have increased the indication for

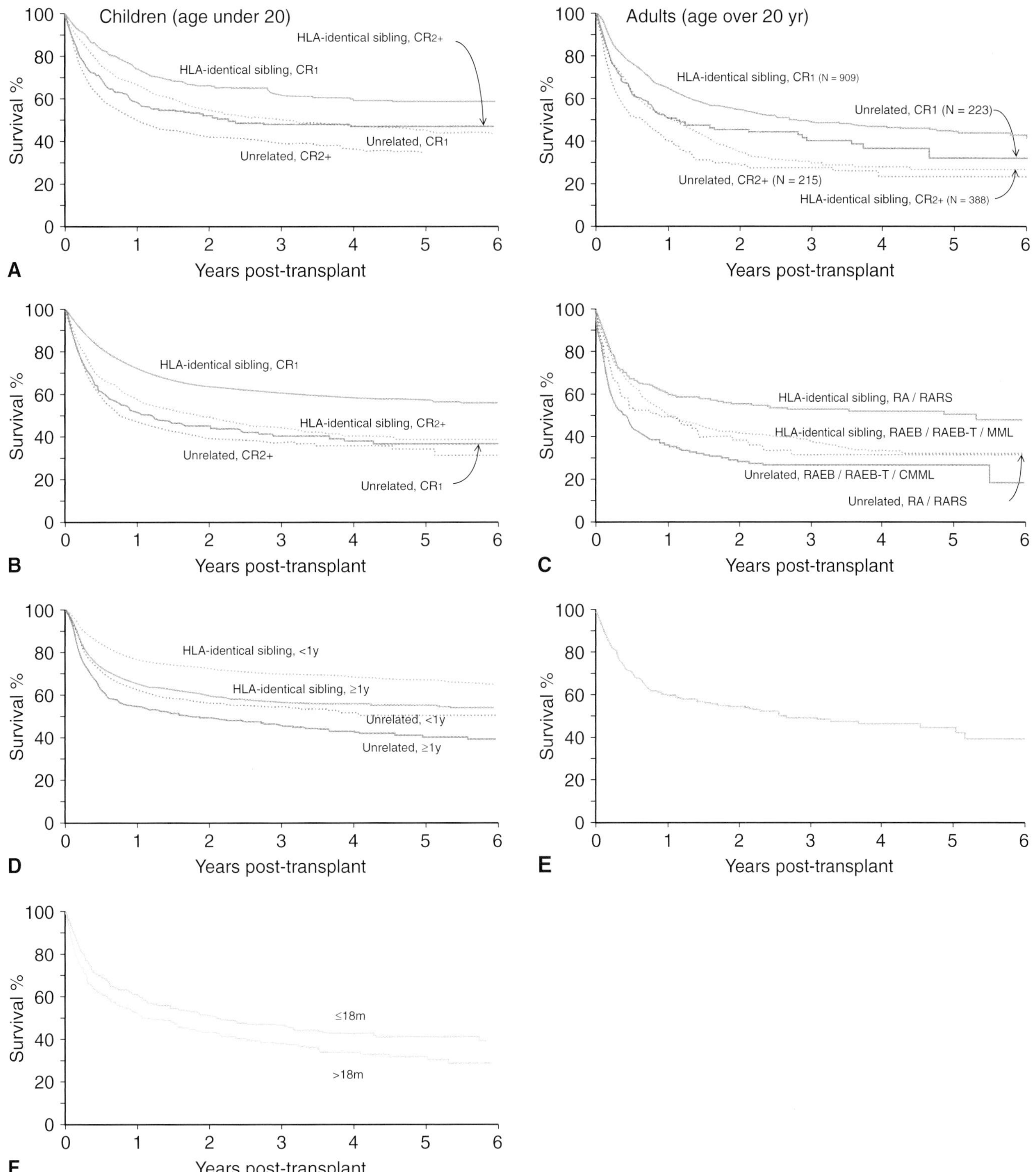

Figure 94–12. Outcomes after stem cell transplantation (SCT) for hematological malignancies. ***A,*** Survival according to disease status for children and adults with acute lymphoblastic leukemia. ***B,*** Survival according to disease status and donor type for patients with acute myeloblastic leukemia. (Data from the IBMTR.[87]) ***C,*** Survival following allogeneic SCT for adults with myelodysplastic syndrome showing impact of disease status on survival. (Data from the IBMTR.[87]) ***D,*** Survival following allogeneic SCT for chronic myelogenous leukemia showing impact of transplant timing and donor type on outcome. ***E,*** Survival after allogeneic SCT for chronic lymphocytic leukemia. ***F,*** Survival following allogeneic SCT for multiple myeloma showing superior survival for patients transplanted within 18 months of diagnosis. (Data from the IBMTR.[87])

TABLE 94–7. Stem Cell Transplantation for Acute Lymphoblastic Leukemia

	HLA = sib		URD			
	n	**DFS**	**n**	**DFS**	**Reference**	**Comments**
Childhood ALL (<20 yr, mostly under 15 yr)						
CR1	30	58.5	–	–	116	
	76	45	–	–	117	
	561	61 ± 4	280	50 ± 3	87	IBMTR
CR2: all	962	47 ± 6	805	39 ± 4	87	IBMTR
all	38	62	–	–	118	Single center
CR1 <18 mo	91	29 ± 5	–	–	119	Retrospective comparison BMT vs chemotherapy
CR1 18–36 mo	88	41 ± 6	–	–		
CR1 >36 mo	76	53 ± 7	–	–		
Adult ALL (>20 yr)						
CR1	909	48 ± 4	223	40 ± 8	87	IBMTR > 20 yr
	43	68	77	26	120	3 yr DFS
CR2	388	30 ± 5	215	28 ± 7	87	IBMTR > 20 yr

Abbreviations: BMT, bone marrow transplant; CR, complete remission; DFS, disease-free survival; URD, unrelated donor.

TABLE 94–8. Stem Cell Transplantation for Other Lymphoid Malignancies (Mainly HLA Identical Siblings)

Disease		n	% DFS	Reference	Comments
CLL		54	47	121	Median age 41 yr
		316	47 ± 7	87	3 yr DFS, IBMTR
MM	Stage I		50	122	3 yr DFS, EBMT
	Stage II–III		30		
NHL	Low (median 38 yr)	113	49	87	3 yr DFS, IBMTR
	Intermediate (median 39 yr)	225	29		
	High (median 26 yr)	205	38		
	Reduced intensity				EBMT
		188	46	123	48% had received a prior autologous SCT
		113	40–84	124,125	Indolent and aggressive lymphomas
HD	Advanced refractory disease	100	15	126	IBMTR, 65% relapse

Abbreviations: CLL, chronic lymphocytic leukemia; DFS, disease-free survival; HD, Hodgkin's disease; MM, multiple myeloma; NHL, non-Hodgkin's lymphoma.

transplantation in selected patients with chronic lymphocytic leukemia and myelodysplastic syndrome, in whom other treatments offer little or no chance of survival and cure.[108,115] Recent results for stem cell transplantation in myeloid and lymphoid malignancies are summarized in Tables 94–6, 94–7, and 94–8 and illustrated in Figure 94–12.

Bone Marrow Transplantation for Solid Tumors

Despite continuing advances in the treatment of nonhematologic malignant diseases, most patients with metastatic cancer have a very poor prognosis. Disappointingly, the opportunity to dose-intensify anticancer treatment using autologous stem cell rescue has not produced much benefit. The realization that leukemia could be controlled by graft-versus-leukemia effects raised the possibility that other cancers might also be susceptible to an analogous graft-versus-tumor effect. The development of immunosuppressive nonmyeloablative conditioning regimens opened the door to experimental studies exploring the potential of the allograft to confer a graft-versus-tumor effect.[127] The largest experience has been with stem cell transplantation to treat metastatic renal cell cancer and metastatic melanoma. These diseases are notable for spontaneous regressions and response to interleukin-2 treatment—features suggestive of immune-mediated disease regulation. It is now clear that modest but well-defined graft-versus-tumor effects can be seen in renal cell (Fig. 94–13), breast, ovarian, and prostate

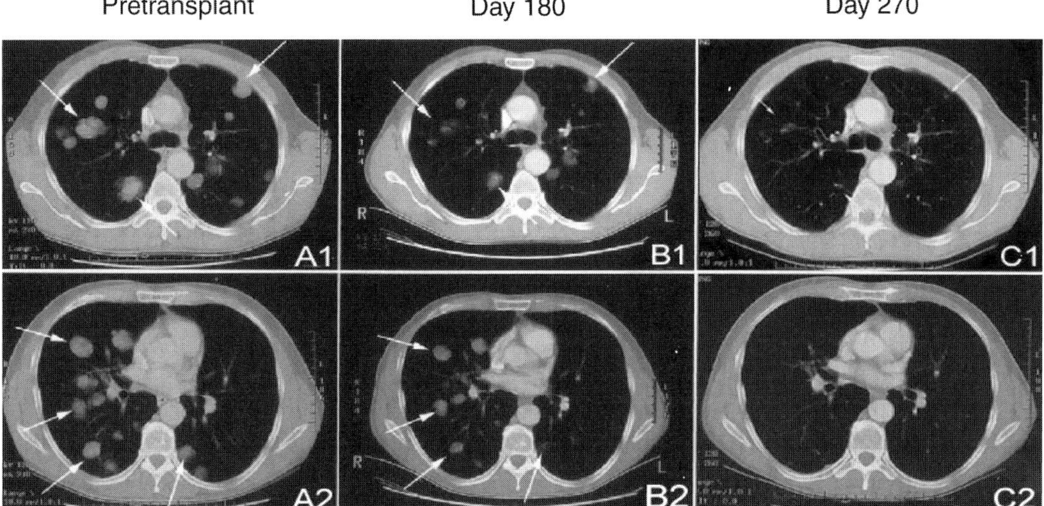

Figure 94–13. Graft-versus-tumor effect: Complete remission of pulmonary metastases 280 days following a nonmyeloablative stem cell transplant for metastatic renal cell carcinoma. (From Childs RW, Barrett J: Nonmyeloablative allogeneic immunotherapy for solid tumors. Annu Rev Med 55:459–475, 2004, with permission.)

TABLE 94–9. Stem Cell Transplantation for Metastatic Tumors

Disease	n	GVT Effect	Reference
Renal cell carcinoma	>60	10% CR, 40% PR	16,128
	10	3 PR	131
Breast cancer	1	1 PR	132
	14	5 PR	133
Ovarian carcinoma	5	1 CR, 2 PR	134
Colon	6	1 PR	133
Melanoma	25	1 PR	135

Abbreviations: CR, complete remission; GVT, graft-versus-tumor; PR, partial remission.

Current Controversies & Future Considerations

Allogeneic Bone Marrow Transplantation

- Several issues regarding transplantation must be resolved:
- Choice of stem cell source: peripheral blood versus bone marrow
- Choice of donor for patients with no available HLA-identical family member: mismatched or unrelated donor
- Conditioning regimen selection: low versus higher intensity
- Best approach to graft-versus-host disease prevention: immunosuppressive agents versus T-cell depletion
- Indications for transplant require constant revision to take into account improved outcomes for transplant or improved alternative treatments.

cancer but not in melanoma.[16,128–135] Notably, complete and durable disease regressions occur in about 10% of patients with metastatic renal cell carcinoma.[16] Table 94–9 lists reported studies using allogeneic stem cell transplantation in various metastatic malignancies. Currently there are insufficient data to determine precise indications for allogeneic stem cell transplantation in these disorders.

Suggested Readings*

Donors and Histocompatibility Testing

Bosse R, Kulmburg P, von Kalle C, et al: Production of stem-cell transplants according to good manufacturing practice. Ann Hematol 79:469–476, 2000.

Gluckman E, Rocha V, Chevret S: Results of unrelated umbilical cord blood hematopoietic stem cell transplantation. Rev Clin Exp Hematol 5:87–99, 2001.

Schmitz N, Barrett J: Optimizing engraftment—source and dose of stem cells. Semin Hematol 39:3–14, 2002.

Schreuder GM, Oudshoorn M, Claas FHJ: Histocompatibility typing procedures for stem cell transplantation. *In* Atkins, K, Champlin R, Ritz J, et al (eds): Clinical Bone Marrow and Blood Stem Cell Transplantation (ed 3). Cambridge: Cambridge University Press, 2004, pp 101–112.

Conditioning Regimens

Barrett AJ: Conditioning regimens for allogeneic stem cell transplants. Curr Opin Hematol 7:339–342, 2000.

Storb RF, Champlin R, Riddell SR, et al: Non-myeloablative transplants for malignant disease. Hematology (Am Soc Hematol Educ Program) 375–391, 2001.

Immune Reconstitution and Graft-Versus-Leukemia Effects

Barrett AJ: Basis of the alloresponse. Cytotherapy 4:419–422, 2002.

Kolb HJ, Schmid C, Barrett AJ, Schendel DJ: Graft-versus-leukemia reactions in allogeneic chimeras. Blood 103:767–776, 2004.

Mackall CL, Gress RE: Pathways of T-cell regeneration in mice and humans: implications for bone marrow transplantation and immunotherapy. Immunol Rev 157:61–72, 1997.

Storek J, Ferrara S, Ku N, et al: B cell reconstitution after human bone marrow transplantation: recapitulation of ontogeny? Bone Marrow Transplant 12:387–398, 1993.

Posttransplant Infections

Blijlevens NM, Donnelly JP, de Pauw BE: Empirical therapy of febrile neutropenic patients with mucositis: challenge of risk-based therapy. Clin Microbiol Infect 7(Suppl 4):47–52, 65, 2001.

Ljungman P: Immune reconstitution and viral infections after stem cell transplantation. Bone Marrow Transplant 21(Suppl 2):S72–S74, 1998.

Momin F, Chandrasekar PH: Antimicrobial prophylaxis in bone marrow transplantation. Ann Intern Med 123:205–215, 1995.

Wagner HJ, Rooney CM, Heslop HE: Diagnosis and treatment of post-transplantation lymphoproliferative disease after hematopoietic stem cell transplantation. Biol Blood Marrow Transplant 8:1–8, 2002.

Wingard JR: Fungal infections after bone marrow transplant. Biol Blood Marrow Transplant 5:55–68, 1999.

Transplants for Nonmalignant Diseases

Fischer A, Haddad E, Jabado N, et al: Stem cell transplantation for immunodeficiency. Springer Semin Immunopathol 19:479–492, 1998.

Giardini C, Lucarelli G: Bone marrow transplantation for beta-thalassemia. Hematol Oncol Clin North Am 13:1059–1064, 1999.

Gluckman E: Bone marrow transplantation in children with hereditary disorders. Curr Opin Pediatr 8:42–44, 1996.

Horowitz MM: Current status of allogeneic bone marrow transplantation in acquired aplastic anemia. Semin Hematol 37:30–42, 2000.

Shah A, Kapoor N, Crooks G, et al: Allogeneic hematopoietic stem cell transplantation for metabolic disease. *In* Atkinson K, Champlin R, Ritz J, et al (eds): Clinical Bone Marrow and Blood Stem Cell Transplantation (ed 3). Cambridge: Cambridge University Press, 2004, pp 963–973.

Walters MC, Storb R, Patience M, et al: Impact of bone marrow transplantation for symptomatic sickle cell disease: an interim report. Multicenter investigation of bone marrow transplantation for sickle cell disease. Blood 95:1918–1924, 2000.

Transplants for Malignant Diseases

Bacigalupo A, Galbusera V, Frassoni F: Allogeneic hematopoietic stem cell transplantation for acute myelogenous leukemia. *In* Atkinson K, Champlin R, Ritz J, et al (eds): Clinical Bone Marrow and Blood Stem Cell Transplantation (ed 3). Cambridge: Cambridge University Press, 2004, pp 783–798.

Barrett AJ, Horowitz MM, Pollock BH, et al: Bone marrow transplants from HLA-identical siblings as compared with chemotherapy for children with acute lymphoblastic leukemia in a second remission. N Engl J Med 331:1253–1258, 1994.

Barrett J: Allogeneic stem cell transplantation for chronic myeloid leukemia. Semin Hematol 40:59–71, 2003.

Bellucci R, Ritz J: Allogeneic stem cell transplantation for multiple myeloma. Rev Clin Exp Hematol 6:205–224, 2002.

Champlin R, van Besien K, Giralt S, Khouri I: Allogeneic hematopoietic transplantation for chronic lymphocytic leukemia and lymphoma: potential for nonablative preparative regimens. Curr Oncol Rep 2:182–191, 2000.

Childs RW, Barrett J: Nonmyeloablative allogeneic immunotherapy for solid tumors. Annu Rev Med 55:459–475, 2004.

Gajewski JL, Phillips GL, Sobocinski KA, et al: Bone marrow transplants from HLA-identical siblings in advanced Hodgkin's disease. Clin Oncol 14:572–578, 1996.

Gokbuget N, Hoelzer D: Recent approaches in acute lymphoblastic leukemia in adults. Rev Clin Exp Hematol 6:114–141, 2002.

Grimwade D, Walker H, Oliver F, et al: The importance of diagnostic cytogenetics on outcome in AML: analysis of 1,612 patients entered into the MRC AML 10 trial. The Medical Research Council Adult and Children's Leukaemia Working Parties. Blood 92:2322–2333, 1998.

Michallet M, Archimbaud E, Bandini G, et al: HLA-identical sibling bone marrow transplantation in younger patients with chronic lymphocytic leukemia. European Group for Blood and Marrow Transplantation and the International Bone Marrow Transplant Registry. Ann Intern Med 124:311–315, 1996.

Toze CL, Barnett MJ: Allogeneic haemopoietic stem cell transplantation for non-Hodgkin's lymphoma. Best Pract Res Clin Haematol 15:481–504, 2002.

Wayne AS, Barrett AJ: Allogeneic hematopoietic stem cell transplantation for myeloproliferative disorders and myelodysplastic syndromes. Hematol Oncol Clin North Am 17:1243–1260, 2003.

Wheeler KA, Richards SM, Bailey CC, et al: Bone marrow transplantation versus chemotherapy in the treatment of very high-risk childhood acute lymphoblastic leukemia in first remission: results from Medical Research Council UKALL X and XI. Blood 96:2412–2418, 2000.

Full references for this chapter can be found on accompanying CD-ROM.

CHAPTER 95

Autologous Transplantation of Hematopoietic Stem Cells

Edward A. Stadtmauer, MD

> **KEY POINTS**
>
> **Autologous Transplantation of Hematopoietic Stem Cells**
>
> - Autologous hematopoietic stem cell transplantation is based on the dose-response relationship of many chemotherapy agents and radiation: the greater the dose, the greater the response. Infusion of autologous stem cells allows for substantial dose escalation of these agents.
> - Successful autologous stem cell transplantation requires (1) proper patient selection; (2) adequate stem cell harvest, processing, and storage; (3) appropriate high-dose therapy; (4) intravenous stem cell reinfusion; and (5) supportive care and follow-up.
> - Autologous stem cell transplantation improves survival for selected groups of patients with multiple myeloma, non-Hodgkin's and Hodgkin's lymphoma, germ cell cancer, and acute myeloid leukemia.

INTRODUCTION

Use of autologous (self) hematopoietic stem cells as a source of cells to reconstitute the marrow after high-dose therapy now exceeds that of allogeneic sources. The goal of the allogeneic transplantation is eradication of disease by replacement of the bone marrow and hematopoietic tissue with healthy donor cells while also initiating a graft-versus-tumor reaction. Autologous transplantation, in contrast, is based on the dose-response relationship of many chemotherapies and radiation: the higher the dose, the greater the response. Bone marrow suppression becomes the dose-limiting toxicity when doses of most antineoplastic agents are increased. Infusion of autologous hematopoietic stem cells and the use of myeloid growth factors allows for substantial chemotherapy dose escalation as well as the potential for multiple cycles of high-dose therapy. Approximately 20,000 hematopoietic stem cell transplants were conducted in North America in the year 2002.[1] The most common indications for autologous stem cell transplantation are multiple myeloma, non-Hodgkin's and Hodgkin's lymphoma, and acute myeloid leukemia, whereas transplantation for breast cancer, previously a common indication, is infrequently performed today (Fig. 95–1). The successful autologous stem cell transplantation consists of a number of steps, including (1) proper patient selection; (2) stem cell harvest, processing, and storage: (3) high-dose antineoplastic chemotherapy with or without radiation therapy; (4) stem cell reinfusion; and (5) supportive care and follow-up posttransplant (Fig. 95–2).

PATIENT SELECTION

Indications for Autologous Stem Cell Transplantation

The indications for autologous stem cell transplantation, listed in Box 95–1, are prioritized by the degree of evidence for clinical benefit:

- Level 1: evidence from at least one well-designed comparative trial
- Level 2: consistent evidence from multiple nonrandomized clinical trials (standard of care)
- Level 3: promising evidence from multiple noncomparative trials
- Level 4: evidence from case reports and small series
- Level 5: numerous trials show little or no evidence for clinical benefit

Level 1 indications include multiple myeloma, intermediate-grade non-Hodgkin's lymphoma, and Hodgkin's disease. Level 2 indications include germ cell cancer, acute myeloid leukemia, low-grade lymphoma, and neuroblastoma. Level 3 indications are acute lymphoid leukemia, high-grade lymphoma, mantle cell lymphoma, ovarian cancer, and autoimmune disease. Level 4 indications are chronic myeloid and lymphoid leukemia, primitive neuroectodermal tumors, Ewing's sarcoma, desmoplastic round cell tumor of the peri-

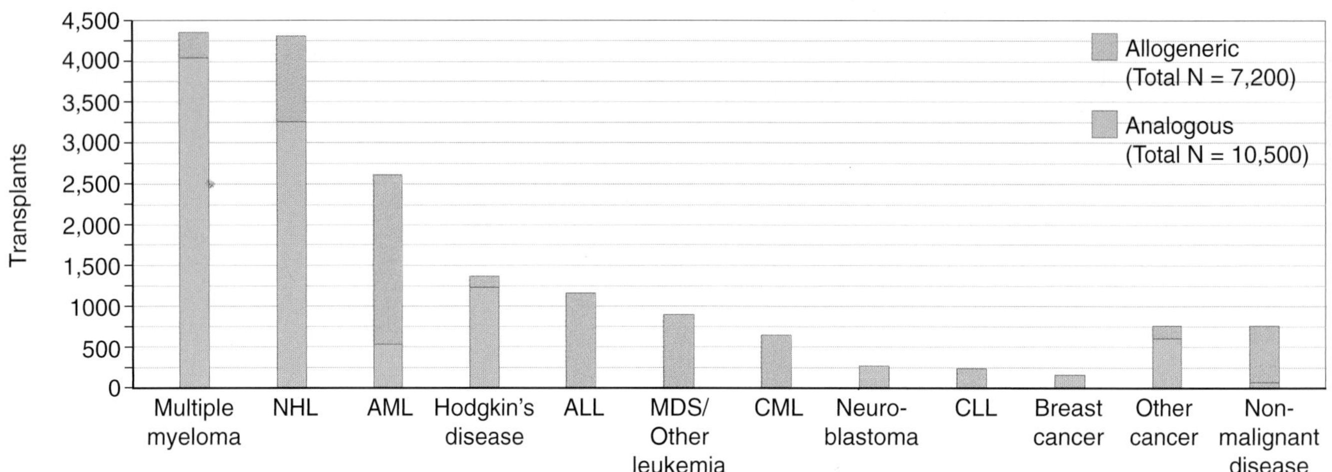

Figure 95–1. The International Bone Marrow Transplant/Autologous Bone Marrow Transplant Registry receives information from over 450 bone marrow transplant centers throughout the world. In 2002, approximately 18,000 hematopoietic stem cell transplantations were reported to the registry. Over 9000 of the 10,500 autologous stem cell transplantations were for multiple myeloma, non-Hodgkin's lymphoma, and Hodgkin's lymphoma. Solid tumors, the most common indications in the 1990s, are now treated only in selected circumstances.

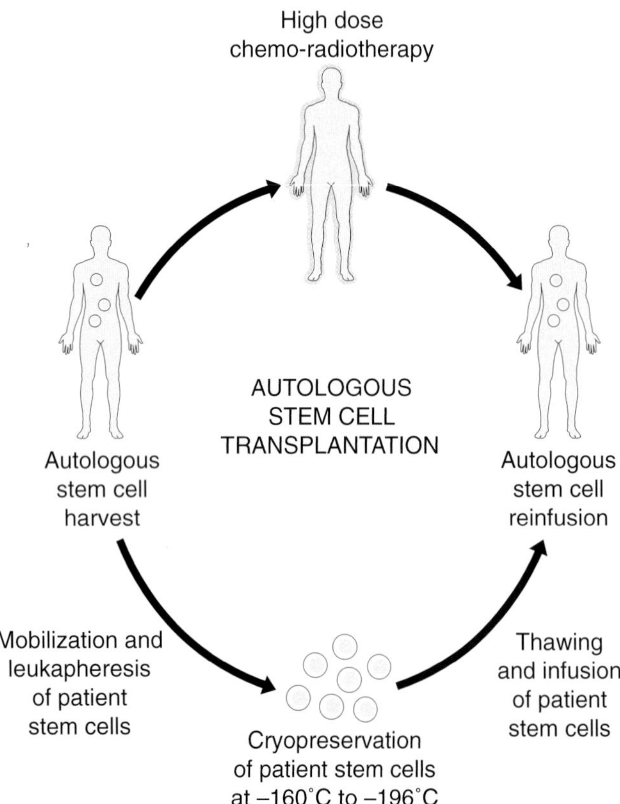

Figure 95–2. The autologous hematopoietic stem cell transplantation process requires completion of a number of steps: *(1)* proper patient selection, *(2)* mobilization and collection of hematopoietic stem cells from bone marrow or blood, *(3)* cryopreservation and storage of the stem cell product in liquid nitrogen freezers, *(4)* high-dose chemoradiotherapy, *(5)* thawing and infusion of the stem cell product into the patient, *(6)* supportive care during the period of pancytopenia, and *(7)* long-term follow-up.

toneum, and small-cell lung cancer. Finally, Level 5 data exist to suggest against autologous stem cell transplantation for glioma and both high-risk and metastatic breast cancer.

Patient Evaluation Prior to Transplantation

Radiation and chemotherapy, when given in the high doses allowed by hematopoietic stem cell infusion, are associated with significant extramedullary toxicity. Patients undergo a pretransplant evaluation to assess cardiac, renal, hepatic, and pulmonary function. A poor performance status, defined by Karnofsky and colleagues[2] as less than 70% or by the Eastern Cooperative Oncology Group as a score of less than 2 (unable to live at home and care for most personal needs), is the best general predictor of poor outcome following autologous stem cell transplantation.[3] Disease status at time of transplantation is also an obvious predictor of outcome, with those in remission faring better in almost all cases than those with progression or less than complete response.

Comorbid conditions and organ dysfunction are considered prior to selection for autologous stem cell transplantation (see Chapter 96). Most patients evaluated for transplantation have had prior anthracycline drug exposure. Examples include CHOP and ABVD for Hodgkin's and non-Hodgkin's lymphoma, VAD or DVD for myeloma, and idarubicin, mitoxantrone, or daunorubicin for acute leukemia. Fortunately, high doses of anthracycline are rarely used as a component of the autologous stem cell transplantation regimen, and life-threatening cardiomyopathy is rare after transplantation.[4] High-dose cyclophosphamide as part of the preparative regimen results in the highest reported likelihood of posttransplant cardiomyopathy, which is usually mild when

Box 95–1. Evidence-Based Indications for Autologous Stem Cell Transplantation

Level 1: At Least One Comparative Clinical Trial Shows Survival Benefit

- Multiple myeloma
- Intermediate-grade non-Hodgkin's lymphoma (NHL)
- Hodgkin's disease

Level 2: Multiple Noncomparative Trials Consistently Show Survival Benefit (standard of care)

- Germ cell cancer
- Neuroblastoma
- Acute myeloid leukemia
- Amyloidosis
- Low-grade NHL

Level 3: Multiple Noncomparative Trials Show Promise for Survival Benefit

- Acute lymphocytic leukemia
- High-grade NHL
- Mantle cell lymphoma
- Ovarian cancer

Level 4: Small Series and Case Reports Suggest Possible Survival Benefit

- Primitive neuroectodermal tumors
- Autoimmune disease
- Chronic myeloid leukemia
- Chronic lymphoid leukemia
- Small-cell lung cancer

Level 5: Numerous Series Show No Clear Survival Benefit

- Breast cancer
- Glioma

Box 95–2. Patient Selection Criteria for Autologous Bone Marrow Transplantation

- Adequate performance status: Karnofsky > 60, ECOG < 3
- Appropriate disease and disease status
- Left ventricular ejection fraction: > 40%
- Pulmonary function tests (FVC, FEV, DL_{CO}): > 50%
- Creatinine, creatinine clearance: < 2.0 mg/dL, > 50 mL/min
- Bilirubin, ALT, AST: <3 times upper limit of normal
- Adequate home caregiver support
- Lack of active infection
- Adequate understanding and psychological stability

Abbreviations: ALT, alanine aminotransferase; AST, aspartate aminotransferase; DL_{CO}, diffusion capacity; ECOG, Eastern Cooperative Oncology Group; FEV, forced expiratory volume; FVC, forced vital capacity.

recorded, although it may primarily reflect cardiac damage from the original anthracycline exposure rather than new damage from the high-dose regimen.[5] In light of this, a pretransplant left ventricular ejection fraction greater than 45% is usually advised.[6]

Pulmonary function tests, including diffusion capacity, forced expiratory volume, and forced vital capacity, are frequently conducted prior to autologous stem cell transplantation. The preparative regimen frequently contains pulmonary toxins (e.g., carmustine [BCNU], busulfan, and total-body irradiation), and interstitial pneumonitis and pulmonary fibrosis are infrequent but can lead to significant morbidity and death after autologous bone marrow transplantation. Patients with pulmonary function test results less than 50% of predicted require thoughtful decision making prior to transplantation.[7]

Both hepatic and renal dysfunction predict for inferior outcome of transplantation as a result of further organ toxicity. In addition, many agents used in the preparative regimen and supportive care require metabolism and clearance by liver and kidneys. Thus, aspartate aminotransferase, alanine aminotransferase, bilirubin, or creatinine levels two to three times above normal usually preclude transplantation.[8]

Other considerations in the selection of patients include nutritional status, age, prior infections, and psychosocial status (Box 95–2). A normal albumin predicts adequate nutritional reserve, although patients with cachexia or morbid obesity fare worse than more nutritionally average patients.[9] Recent evidence indicates that standard criteria for patient selection identify older patients in the 65- to 80-year age group who tolerate autologous stem cell transplantation without increased morbidity,[10–12] especially for diseases such as lymphoma and myeloma. Although most prospective candidates have had prior periods of prolonged neutropenia, active bacterial, viral, and fungal infections should be treated prior to consideration of autologous stem cell transplantation. For these patients, excessive use of corticosteroids, particularly as part of antinausea prophylaxis, should be avoided. Substance abuse can worsen outcome with autologous bone marrow transplantation.[13] For this reason, strategies to manage drug, nicotine, and alcohol dependence during the transplantation period will substantially improve patient outcomes.

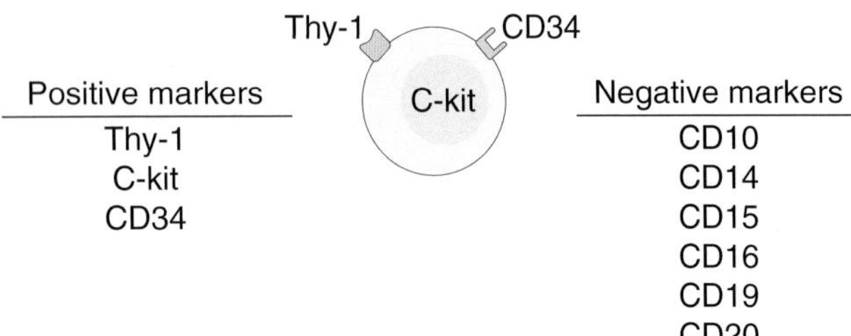

Figure 95–3. The hematopoietic stem cell phenotype: Thy-1$^+$, absence of lineage markers (lin$^-$), CD34$^+$ with expression of *c-kit*. Cells of this phenotype have properties of self-renewal and the ability to restore full hematopoiesis in mice and humans.

HEMATOPOIETIC STEM CELL COLLECTION, PROCESSING, STORAGE, AND INFUSION

Identification of the Hematopoietic Stem Cell

The bone marrow contains hematopoietic cells at all levels of differentiation that are derived from a small pool of pluripotent precursor cells or hematopoietic stem cells capable of self-renewal and differentiation. These cells have been isolated and characterized in mice and humans and have been shown to have the following properties: Thy-1$^+$, lineage markers negative (Lin$^-$; e.g., CD10, CD14, CD15, CD16, CD19, and CD20 negative), and CD34$^+$ with expression of *c-kit*.[14–17] Hematopoietic stem cells with CD34$^+$Thy-1$^+$Lin$^-$ phenotype have been shown to self-renew and restore full hematopoiesis[18] (Fig. 95–3).

Bone Marrow Collection

Collection and storage of adequate numbers of hematopoietic stem cells are necessary prior to proceeding with high-dose therapy and stem cell infusion. Hematopoietic stem cell transplantation differs from transplantation of solid organs in that donors do not suffer a permanent organ loss, because removed hematopoietic stem cells are replaced within a short period of time.

The original method for acquiring hematopoietic stem cells and more differentiated precursors is bone marrow harvest. The patient is brought to the operating room and placed in the prone position and general or regional anesthesia is induced. The patient then undergoes numerous bilateral posterior iliac crest percutaneous bone marrow aspirations, removing 5–10 mL of marrow per aspiration. Approximately 1–2 L of bone marrow containing 1–2 × 10^8 mononuclear cells/kg body weight (approximately 2 × 10^6 CD34$^+$ cells/kg body weight) is collected. The procedure takes between 1 and 2 hours, and patients can be discharged that evening or the next day. Transfusion is common during or soon after the procedure for autologous donation, because these patients frequently start with borderline hemoglobin.

Blood Stem Cell Collection

It has been known for decades that pluripotent hematopoietic stem cells circulated in the blood, and since the 1980s these "peripheral blood stem cells" have been demonstrated to reliably and completely reestablish hematopoiesis when infused after marrow ablative therapy.[19,20] Peripheral blood stem cells are collected using a continuous-flow cell separation device, rarely via bilateral antecubital veins and more commonly via tunneled or temporary double- or triple-lumen central venous apheresis catheters. The blood is withdrawn in the apheresis device at a rate of 30–70 mL/min and the continuous-flow centrifuge is set to separate a fraction composed predominately of mononuclear cells from other blood elements. This fraction contains the hematopoietic stem cells and is retained, while the remainder is reinfused into the patient via the return lumen.

A usual collection processes 10–15 L of whole blood over 2–4 hours, and each apheresis procedure is assayed for CD34$^+$ cell content. The CD34$^+$ cell/kg collection goal depends on the number of transplants planned and the intensity of the preparative regimen, but generally the target is 4–6 × 10^6 CD34$^+$ cells/kg body weight. Values below 2 × 10^6 CD34$^+$ cells/kg result in delayed engraftment of both platelets and granulocytes. For the majority of patients this goal is accomplished by 2–3 aphereses, but may require as few as 1 or as many as 10 collections depending on the underlying disease, the prior treatment, and the collection goal. Currently, the vast majority of patients undergoing stem cell harvest prior to autologous transplantation undergo peripheral blood stem cell rather than bone marrow harvest, with bone marrow harvest reserved for those who are poor blood collectors.

Blood Stem Cell Mobilization

Current Understanding

Hematopoietic stem cells originate in the bone marrow and under physiologic conditions circulate at low levels in the blood. Recruitment of larger numbers of stem cells into the blood, or "mobilization," allows for efficient collection of adequate numbers for transplantation. Mobilization appears to mimic physiologic release of stem cells and progenitors from the bone marrow as would occur in response to injury and inflammation. The bone marrow microenvironment (Fig. 95–4) consists of hematopoietic cells at all levels of differentiation surrounded by stromal cells, including mesenchymal progenitors, osteoclasts, endothelial cells, macrophages, fibroblasts, and adipocytes, as well as the extracellular matrix composed of collagen, glycoproteins, and glycosaminoglycans that they produce. These cells communicate via specific cell surface receptors and cytokines and chemokines. In particular, adhesion molecules such as integrins and very-late antigens (VLA-4 and -5) maintain hematopoietic progenitor cells in the bone marrow.[21] VLA-4, for instance, binds to vascular cell adhesion molecule-1 (VCAM-1) on stromal cells.[22] Anti–VLA-4 has been shown to prevent binding of surface

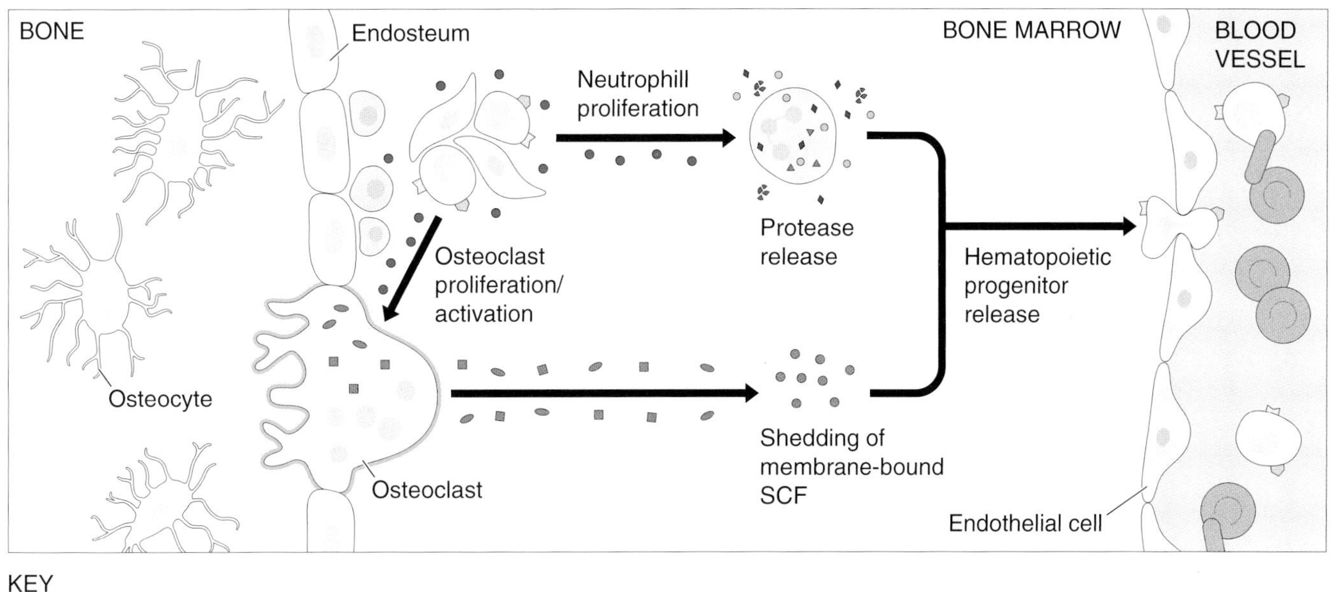

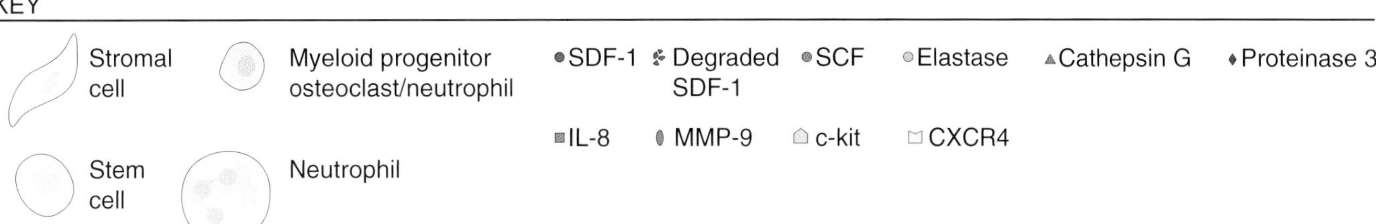

Figure 95–4. A model for hematopoietic stem cell mobilization. Chemotherapeutic agents such as cyclophosphamide and the cytokine G-CSF induce increased SDF-1 levels in the bone marrow. G-CSF and SDF-1 trigger neutrophil proliferation and release of proteases such as elastase, cathepsin G, and proteinase 3. Also, SDF-1 stimulates proliferation and activation of osteoclasts and release of the mobilizing chemokines interleukin-8 and matrix metalloproteinase-9. This activity leads to degradation of stem cell adhesion, including shedding of membrane-bound stem cell factor and CXCR4 inactivation. These events are central to the release of hematopoietic progenitors for bone marrow into the blood. (From Cottler-Fox MH, Lapidot T, Petit I, et al: Stem cell mobilization. Hematology [Am Soc Hematol Educ Program] 419–437, 2003, with permission.)

adhesion molecules to VCAM-1, inducing rapid mobilization of stem cells into the blood.[23] The circulating mobilized CD34$^+$ cells differ from the bone marrow CD34$^+$ cells by lower levels of VLA-4 and *c-kit* expression.

Cytokines are secreted cellular proteins. Granulocyte colony-stimulating factor (G-CSF) is the most potent single agent for hematopoietic stem cell mobilization, and the mechanisms for this action are only now becoming apparent.[24] Stem cell factor in the steady state is membrane bound and not active. Shedding and release of stem cell factor results in stem cell proliferation.[23] Chemokines, a second class of mobilizing agents, are classified based on the position and spacing of the first two conserved cysteine (C) residues. Stromal-derived factor-1 (SDF-1) is a C-X-C (CXC) chemokine. SDF-1 binds CXC chemokine receptor 4 (CXCR4), which is found on CD34$^+$ cells.[25,26] Osteoclasts appear to be the source of a number of chemokines and proteolytic enzymes as part of the mobilization process. SDF-1 induces osteoclasts to secrete another CXC chemokine, interleukin-8, as well as matrix metalloproteinase-9.[27] These chemokines and other osteoclast- and neutrophil-derived proteolytic enzymes such as elastase, proteinase 3, and cathepsin G lead to degradation of the extracellular matrix, adhesion molecules, and cytokines and facilitate the egress of stem cells from bone marrow into the blood.[28] Alkylating agents and other DNA-damaging chemotherapy with inflammatory cytokines such as G-CSF first induce myelosuppression, which itself induces stem cell proliferation that is significantly augmented by administration of G-CSF.[28] Cyclophosphamide and G-CSF, for example, induce increased SDF-1, interleukin-8, and other factors to trigger neutrophils and osteoclasts to proliferate and release proteases and matrix metalloproteinase-9. This disrupts and degrades the usual bone marrow stem cell adhesion and retention mechanisms (VLA-1 binding to VCAM-1 and SDF-1 binding to CXCR4) and permits release of stem cells from the bone marrow microenvironment. This process appears to result primarily from the degradation of the chemokine (VLA-1 and SDF-1) rather than the receptor. Additionally, matrix metalloproteinase-9 mediates the shedding of membrane-bound stem cell factor, which, together with proteinase 3, induces stem cell proliferation.

Clinical Mobilization Techniques

Current stem cell mobilization regimens include single- or multiple-agent cytokines as well as the combination of single- or multiple-agent chemotherapies with cytokines. The choice depends on various factors, including disease status, timing, and target number of cells, with the goal to minimize the number of pheresis procedures and minimize toxicity, while maximizing the likelihood of achieving the desired target cell dose. The optimal goal of 4–6 × 10^6 CD34$^+$ cells/kg per transplant can reduce the likelihood of a subset of patients with prolonged neutrophil and platelet recovery.[29–31] A strong predictor of the ability to collect sufficient CD34 cells on a particular day after mobilization treatment is the circulating CD34 count. A value of 10 predicts a good mobilization.[32,33]

G-CSF at 10–20 µg/kg/day by subcutaneous injection has become the standard mobilization regimen. G-CSF mobilizes more CD34$^+$ stem cells with less toxicity than granulocyte-macrophage colony-stimulating factor (GM-CSF). A dose response to G-CSF has been seen, with higher doses resulting in increased peripheral CD34$^+$ cells[34] and twice-daily doses more effective than daily dosing.[35] Bone pain is the most frequent toxicity; gastrointestinal toxicities (nausea, diarrhea, vomiting) and constitutional symptoms (fevers, chills, night sweats) are less common and usually of low severity. Bone pain usually responds to acetaminophen or ibuprofen. Prophylactic use of these agents prior to G-CSF dose can ameliorate symptoms. When G-CSF 10 µg/kg/day is used, cell yield is optimized when pheresis is begun on day 5 within 3–7 hours after G-CSF administration. The pegylated form of G-CSF, pegfilgrastim, has not yet been shown to be an adequate single agent for stem cell collection. Combinations of cytokines, including G-CSF with GM-CSF, stem cell factor, erythropoietin, interleukin-3, and interleukin-2, have been used to enhance stem cell mobilization.[36] Although some trials have shown marginal increases in cell yields, the increased expense and toxicity have not warranted routine use when compared to G-CSF alone. In particular, the stem cell factor and G-CSF combination has led to increased cell yield, but allergic reactions and the need for close observation during administration limit the use of this combination.[37,38]

A new factor, AMD3100, is a reversible inhibitor of the binding of SDF-1 to the CXCR4 receptor allowing release of stem cells from the microenvironment. This more targeted approach to stem cell mobilization has been shown to mobilize stem cells in humans when used alone or in combination with G-CSF, and clinical trials are ongoing.[39]

The majority of patients in preparation for autologous stem cell transplantation have active disease requiring active antineoplastic therapy. The combination of chemotherapy and cytokine-induced mobilization affords both increased CD34$^+$ cell yield versus G-CSF alone and continued disease-specific chemotherapy to maintain remission or response. The most commonly used regimens include cyclophosphamide in doses of 2–7 gm/m^2 in combination with G-CSF or GM-CSF.[40,41] This has been used most often with the most common current indication for stem cell transplantation, multiple myeloma. The addition of etoposide or taxanes can improve cell yield and has been active for solid tumor patients.[42,43] In patients with Hodgkin's and non-Hodgkin's lymphoma, regimens containing ifosfamide, carboplatin, etoposide, cis-platinum, cytosine arabinoside, and corticosteroids (ICE or ESAP) with G-CSF have been successful mobilization regimens while continuing disease cytoreduction.[44–46] High-dose cytarabine with G-CSF can also be used prior to collection for acute leukemia. In choosing a mobilization regimen, stem cell toxins such as melphalan, carmustine, radiation, and nitrogen mustard should be avoided.

Tumor Contamination of Stem Cell Collections

Tumor cells have been detected in the stem cell products from patients with multiple myeloma, lymphoma, leukemia, breast cancer, neuroblastoma, and small-cell lung cancer. Whether and to what degree infusion of contaminated stem cells into patients after high-dose therapy alters outcome after autologous stem cell infusion remains to be determined. A number of approaches toward stem cell purging of tumor contamination have been pursued. These are listed in Box 95–3. All can be very effective at removal of occult or overt neoplastic cells, but no approach has been shown in randomized prospective trials to improve survival. The most informative clinical trials of three common purging approaches follow.

One approach has been the use of anti-CD34 monoclonal antibodies to positively select and enrich for hematopoietic stem cells while substantially depleting non-CD34$^+$ cells, including contaminating tumor cells. A prospective randomized trial in 190 patients with multiple myeloma using purged versus unpurged autologous blood stem cells has been performed using CD34$^+$ selection.[63,64] After CD34 selection, plasma cell contamination was reduced by a median of 3.1 logs, with 54% of CD34-selected products without detectable tumor. The unselected products contained a median of 2 million plasma cells that were infused. Nevertheless, after 5 years of follow-up, no difference in disease-free or overall survival was detected. No difference in hematopoietic engraftment, infection, or immune reconstitution was observed, though the purging procedure added cost. CD133, a newly identified stem cell antigen, may provide an alternative to CD34.[69]

A second approach is immunologic purging.[70] In a study of 114 patients with B-cell non-Hodgkin's lymphoma and Bcl-2 overexpression, bone marrow stem cell collections underwent three cycles of ex vivo immunologic purging using a cocktail of three anti–B-cell monoclonal antibodies (anti-CD10, anti-CD20, and B5) that induced complement-mediated B-cell lysis. Polymerase chain reaction amplification of the t(14;18) detected no residual lymphoma cells in the infused stem cell product in 50% of the patients. The incidence of relapse was significantly lower and long-term survival longer compared to that in patients with residual lymphoma cells detected.

Third, 4-hydroperoxycyclophosphamide (4-HC) has been used to kill tumor cells with relative sparing of hematopoietic stem cells. Stem cells contain high levels of aldehyde dehydrogenase, which inactivates the active metabolites of 4-HC. A number of promising clinical trials

Box 95–3. Methods for Purging Tumor Cells from Stem Cell Products in Vitro Successfully Utilized in Clinical Trials

Pharmacologic Purging

- Exposure of bone marrow to active chemotherapeutic agents (cyclophosphamide analogues)
  - 4-hydroperoxycylophosphamide
    - AML[47,48]
    - NHL[49]
  - Mafosphamide
    - AML[50]

Immunologic Purging

- Complement-mediated lysis
  - AML[51,52]
  - NHL[53–55]
- Immunomagnetic bead depletion
  - Neuroblastoma[56]
  - ALL[57]
  - NHL[58]
- Immunotoxins
  - Ricin[59,60]

CD34 Cell Selection

- Autoimmune disease[61,62]
- Multiple myeloma[63–65]
- Breast cancer[66,67]
- Neuroblastoma[68]

Molecular Inhibition of Gene Expression

- c-*myb* antisense[72]

Abbreviations: ALL, acute lymphocytic leukemia; AML, acute myeloid leukemia; NHL, non-Hodgkin's lymphoma.

have been conducted using 4-HC–purged bone marrow for the treatment of acute myeloid leukemia. Although no randomized trial of purged versus unpurged autologous transplantation has been carried out, a registry analysis of 294 patients with acute myeloid leukemia undergoing autologous stem cell transplantation with either 4-HC–purged or unpurged bone marrow, all transplanted within 6 months of first or second remission, was conducted.[71] Patients receiving 4-HC–treated bone marrow had longer time to recovery, though transplant-related mortality was similar in the two groups. Multivariate analysis demonstrated improved leukemia-free survival for the 4-HC–purged group. This benefit has not been sufficient when compared to delayed engraftment and the results of alternate treatment methods to recommend pharmacologic purging as a routine approach.

Stem Cell Processing, Storage, and Reinfusion

Cryopreserved hematopoietic stem cells may be stored for many years prior to their use. Room-temperature or refrigerated storage can be used for products to be used within hours to a few days, but a progressive loss of viable stem cells occurs during nonfrozen storage. Cryopreservation of cells in liquid nitrogen results in much less progressive loss of stem cells over months or years if proper storage conditions are maintained. Cryopreservation allows for multiple-day transplantation preparative regimens, planned courses of tandem or multiple transplantations, and elective storage of cells for patients to undergo successful transplantation procedures years after harvest.

Cells can be damaged during cryopreservation as a result of ice crystal formation during cooling.[73] At rapid rates of cooling, intracellular ice crystals form and result in mechanical disruption of the cell membrane and cell death. At slower rates of cooling, ice crystals of free water form in the extracellular space, resulting in increased concentration of extracellular solutes, such as sodium, that do not pass freely across the cell membrane. The increased extracellular osmolality leads to dehydration injury of cells and cell death.[74] To decrease cell damage, stem cell labs now use a slow rate of cooling in controlled-rate freezers, and cryoprotectants. Cryoprotectants prevent dehydration injury by moderating the increased concentration of non–cell membrane–penetrating extracellular solutes during ice formation and by decreasing the amount of free water absorbed by the ice crystals.[75] Dimethylsulfoxide is a hygroscopic polar cryoprotectant that rapidly and freely diffuses through the cell membrane and is nontoxic to the cells at freezing temperatures.[76] A 10% dimethylsulfoxide solution contributes about 10 times the molality of sodium chloride. The addition of dimethylsulfoxide thereby markedly reduces the osmotic gradient across the cell membrane during freezing by reducing the relative contribution of the nonpenetrating solutes such as sodium. Most laboratories store hematopoietic stem cells in the liquid phase of liquid nitrogen (below −120° C), though particularly for patients who will undergo transplantation within a short period of time, storage at −80° C is safe and easy.

Dimethylsulfoxide may be directly toxic to hematopoietic stem cells at physiologic temperatures. Also, if warming is slow during the thawing process, intracellular ice recrystallization can occur. At the time of stem cell reinfusion, the frozen bags of cells are thawed in 37° C water baths just before infusion to reduce potential stem cell damage. The cells from each bag are drawn up into syringes and infused over a few minutes intravenously, usually via unfiltered central venous catheters. The majority of recipients experience some mild, infusion-related morbidity, though serious toxicities are rare. Dimethylsulfoxide-lysed blood cells, contaminants from purging procedures or reagents, and cold temperature are responsible for these (Box 95–4). Patients should be closely monitored during the procedure and kept well hydrated with adequate blood counts. Patients are frequently pretreated with antihistamine, antiemetic,

Box 95–4. Common Toxicities Associated with Hematopoietic Stem Cell Infusion

- Anaphylactic/allergic reaction
- Histamine release
  - Hypotension
  - Skin flushing
  - Dyspnea
  - Abdominal cramps
  - Nausea
  - Diarrhea
- Cardiovascular effects
  - Hypertension
  - Bradycardia
  - Heart block
- Headache
- Hemoglobinuria

antipyretic, and antianxiolytic agents prior to infusion. The increasing use of blood pheresis products has decreased the likelihood of red blood cell contamination in the infused product, making alkalinization and mannitol diuresis to decrease renal toxicity less necessary. Dimethylsulfoxide has a serum half-life of 20 hours. A small proportion of dimethylsulfoxide is reduced to dimethylsufide, which is volatile and is released through the lungs for up to 48 hours after administration, accounting for a common "creamed corn" or garlic-like odor after stem cell infusion.[77]

High-Dose Regimens

In the context of allogeneic stem cell transplantation, the high-dose regimen is truly preparative; that is, it prepares the patient for the donor stem cell infusion. Regimens such as total-body irradiation and cyclophosphamide or busulfan and cyclophosphamide were designed as profoundly immunosuppressive and marrow destructive, enabling donor cells to engraft. In autologous stem cell transplantation, the high-dose regimen is the therapy, and the stem cell transplant is supportive care during the myelosuppression. Whereas a limited number of preparative regimens are needed for allogeneic transplantation, numerous high-dose regimens have been designed for autologous transplantation, each specifically chosen to destroy maximally the particular disease being targeted. The diseases treated with autologous stem cell transplantation tend to be resistant to conventional doses and regimens of radiation and chemotherapy. Dose escalation, particularly of alkylating agents and radiation, can overcome this resistance. Agents chosen for high-dose regimens are those that can be substantially dose-escalated before nonhematologic toxicities occur, resulting in maximally tolerated doses. The likelihood of drug

TABLE 95–1. Agents Used in High-Dose Therapy Regimens with Dose-Limiting Toxicity

Agent	Dose-Limiting Toxicity
Total-body irradiation	Mucositis, hepatitis, pneumonitis
Busulfan	Mucositis, hepatitis, pneumonitis
Carmustine (BCNU)	Pneumonitis, hepatitis
Melphalan	Mucositis
Thiotepa	Encephalopathy, mucositis
Cyclophosphamide	Myocarditis
Ifosfamide	Cystitis, encephalopathy
Etoposide	Mucositis
Carboplatin	Neuropathy, hepatitis, renal failure

resistance to any given single agent mandates the use of multiple drugs with or without radiation in each high-dose regimen. When combining multiple agents, the guiding principle is to combine agents with different dose-limiting toxicities (Table 95–1).

Table 95–2 shows various regimens that have been commonly used for autologous transplantation. These agents are usually given in an inpatient unit. Patients can be treated in regular single rooms but can be sent home after stem cell infusion with either close home care nursing service support or frequent return to the outpatient clinic, where physical and laboratory assessment, transfusions, and infusions can be conducted. Patients are usually administered prophylactic antibacterial, antifungal, and antiviral antibiotics and myeloid growth factors (G-CSF, GM-CSF) in an attempt to reduce duration of neutropenia and incidence of infections. In addition, a number of potential organ toxicities can occur during transplantation and these are listed in Table 95–1. These and the tremendous advances in the supportive care of patients undergoing autologous stem cell transplantation are discussed in further detail in Chapter 96. Currently, autologous stem cell transplantation has become a common procedure with acceptable and manageable toxicity and low expectation for transplant-related mortality (<5%).

CLINICAL APPLICATION OF AUTOLOGOUS STEM CELL TRANSPLANTATION

Plasma Cell Disorders

Multiple myeloma has become the most common indication for autologous stem cell transplantation despite the fact that little evidence exists that the patients so treated are cured. The rationale includes a dose-response relationship between melphalan and radiation in myeloma disease response, the relative low toxicity of melphalan other than severe marrow suppression, and improvements in supportive care for older patients. These factors have overcome concerns about the contamination of stem cell products with malignant plasma cells, and frequent organ dysfunction in this patient population. Early studies in patients with advanced disease, however, clearly demonstrated high response rates with 20–50%

TABLE 95–2. Representative High-Dose Regimens

Agent	TBI/CY (NHL)	Mel/TBI (MM)	Bu/CY (AML)	Cb/VP-16 (Germ Cell)	TBI/VP-16 (MM)/ Mel (ALL)	BCV (NHL, HD)	BEAM (NHL)	CTCb (Solid)
Cyclophosphamide (C; CY)	120 mg/kg		120–200 mg/kg			6000		6000
Melphalan (M; Mel)		100–140				100–200		140
Etoposide (E; V; VP-16)				1200	60 mg/kg	1200–2400	400–800	
Carmustine (B)						300–600	300–600	
Busulfan (Bu)			16 mg/kg (PO) 14 mg/kg (IV)					
Thiotepa (T)								500
Carboplatin (Cb)				1200				800
Fractionated total-body irradiation (fTBI)	1200 cGy	800–1200 cGy			1200–1320 cGy			

All doses are mg/m^2 unless otherwise indicated.
Abbreviations: ALL, acute lymphocytic leukemia; AML, acute myeloid leukemia; HD, Hodgkin's disease; IV, intravenous; MM, multiple myeloma; NHL, non-Hodgkin's lymphoma; PO, oral.

achieving virtual complete remission with less than 5% treatment-related mortality. This led to the use of high-dose therapy and stem cell transplantation earlier in the course of myeloma therapy. The seminal observation published in 1996 from the InterGroupe Francophone du Myelome (IFM) in France evaluated 200 previously untreated patients under 65 years who were randomly assigned to either 1 year of conventional-dose chemotherapy or 4–6 months of the same therapy followed by high-dose therapy with melphalan 140 mg/m^2 and TBI 800 cGy and unpurged bone marrow infusion, both followed by interferon alfa maintenance therapy.[77] The autologous bone marrow transplantation arm was superior in inducing complete remission (22% of the transplantation patients versus 5% of the chemotherapy patients). At 5-year and 7-year follow-up, both event-free and overall survival were superior for the autologous bone marrow transplantation arm, and mortality rates were similar in both groups. These results have recently been confirmed in another prospective randomized clinical trial, and in three nonrandomized comparative trials (Table 95–3, Fig. 95–5).

TABLE 95–3. Conventional Therapy (CT) versus High-Dose Chemotherapy (HDC) for Myeloma*

Author	*N*	CT	HDC	*P* Value
Historical				
Barlogie [78]	246	48	62+	.01
Lenhoff [79]	548	44	NR	.001
Palumbo [80]	144	48	56+	<.01
Randomized				
French IFM [77]	200	44	57	.03
MRC VII [81]	401	42	54	.04

*Summary of comparative trials (median survival in months).

The optimal timing of transplantation is under active investigation. One published study randomly assigned patients to early autologous bone marrow transplantation after three to four cycles of conventional-dose therapy or to late autologous bone marrow transplantation after disease progression after a median of eight cycles of conventional-dose therapy.[82] Early transplantation significantly improved event-free survival, but did not impact overall survival with a median follow-up of 6 years. Other studies reported only in abstract form corroborate this result.[83,84] An Autologous Bone Marrow Transplant Registry (ABMTR) analysis from over 4000 patients registered in North America suggests transplantation within 18 months of diagnosis leads to superior survival versus later transplantation.[85] Thus, current data favor early transplantation.

Because many patients relapse after autologous bone marrow transplantation for myeloma, double or tandem transplantations have been evaluated. The IFM assigned 399 patients with untreated myeloma who were under 60 years to receive three or four courses of conventional therapy and randomly assigned single or double transplantation.[86] Patients in the single-transplantation group received a high-dose regimen of melphalan 140 mg/m^2 and TBI 800 cGy. Those in the double-transplantation group underwent the first transplantation after receiving melphalan 140 mg/m^2 and received melphalan 140 mg/m^2 and TBI 800 cGy prior to the second transplantation. After a median follow-up of 6 years, response rates in the two groups were not significantly different, but probabilities of event-free survival and overall survival were doubled with tandem transplantation. These benefits were not evident in interim analyses conducted with less than 5 years' follow-up however, suggesting the need for long-term follow-up to assess overall benefit[87] (Fig. 95–6).

Other attempts to improve outcome for patients with myeloma after autologous bone marrow transplantation have been explored, but none has yet improved outcome. Thus, removing plasma cells or selecting CD34 cells has not improved survival. Posttransplant maintenance therapies, including interferon alfa, thalidomide, corticosteroids, and chemotherapy, have been utilized with variable evidence for improvement in progression-free survival but not overall survival. Combinations of

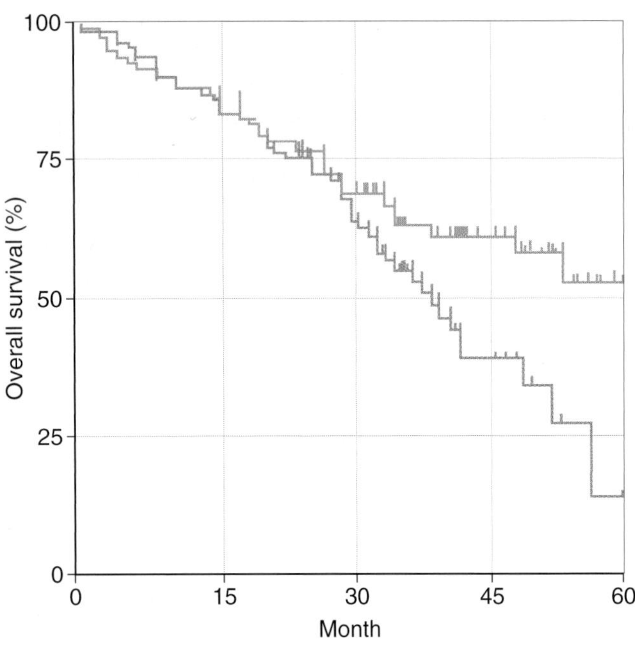

KEY

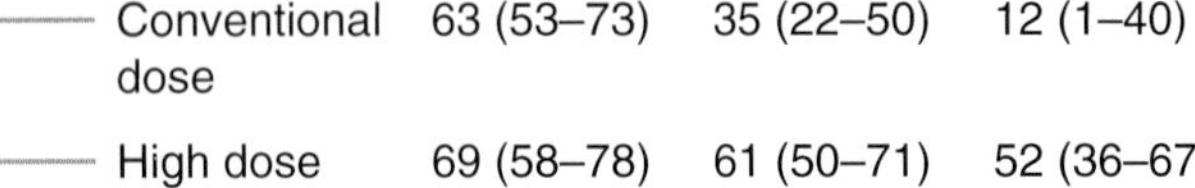

Conventional dose	63 (53–73)	35 (22–50)	12 (1–40)
High dose	69 (58–78)	61 (50–71)	52 (36–67)

■ **Figure 95–5.** IFM90 compared conventional dose therapy for myeloma for 12 months to 4–6 months of the same therapy followed by an autologous bone marrow transplantation (ABMT). Currently, with 7 years' median follow-up, event-free (EFS) and overall survival (OS) were significantly improved for ABMT: 7-year EFS 16% versus 8%, median EFS 28 months versus 18 months (P = .01); 7-year OS 43% versus 25%, median OS 57 months versus 44 months (P = .03).

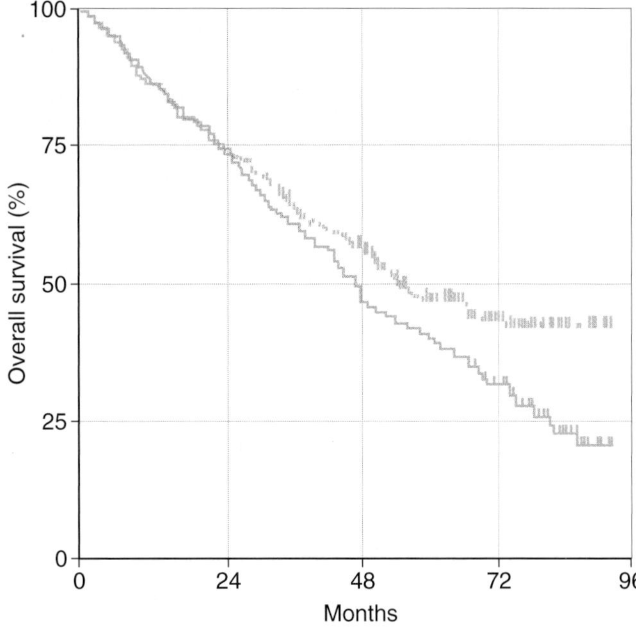

KEY

Probability of Overall survival (95% CI)

Single-transplant group	50 (43–57)	31 (24–38)	20 (13–29)
Double-transplant group	57 (49–64)	42 (35–50)	42 (34–49)

■ **Figure 95–6.** The probabilities of overall survival are shown with their 95 percent confidence intervals (CIs) below for three time points. Tick marks indicate patients at risk.

autologous stem cell transplantation followed by non-myeloablative allogeneic stem cell transplantation are promising and the subject of a national clinical trial (see Chapter 94). In conclusion, the favorable results of autologous stem cell transplantation for myeloma in patients under 65 years has led to the routine incorporation of this modality into the initial treatment plan.

Lymphoma

Diffuse large B-cell lymphoma enters complete remission readily, and the majority of patients are cured with conventional-dose chemotherapy combined most recently with rituximab. However, relapsed or primary refractory disease has a low progression-free survival with conventional-dose salvage chemotherapy therapy. Salvage chemotherapy followed by high-dose therapy and autologous stem cell transplantation was first applied to this disease setting in the late 1970s, and by the 1980s it was clear that 35–40% of these patients were long-term survivors with low mortality. A prospective, randomized clinical trial reported in 1995 by the PARMA Group was the first comparative trial in any disease demonstrating the efficacy of autologous stem cell transplantation.[88] Patients were all treated with DHAP salvage chemotherapy (cisplatin, cytarabine, and dexamethasone). A total of 215 patients were enrolled and 109 (58%) responded. This group was then randomized to either a further cycle of DHAP or high-dose BEAC chemotherapy (carmustine, etoposide, cytarabine, and cyclophosphamide) with autologous bone marrow transplantation. At 5 years, the event-free survival was 46% in the transplant group and 12% in the chemotherapy group (P = .001). The overall survival at 5 years was 53% and 32%, respectively (P = .038). Currently, relapsed responding intermediate-grade non-Hodgkin's lymphoma is the second most common indication for autologous stem cell transplantation.

The use of high-dose therapy and autologous stem cell transplantation as part of initial therapy for high-risk intermediate-grade lymphoma is much more controversial. In the Groupe d'Étude des Lymphomes de Adulte (GELA) trial, 916 patients with responding intermediate- or high-grade lymphoma with at least one unfavorable prognostic factor were randomized to cycles of conventional-dose chemotherapy or high-dose CBV (cyclophosphamide, carmustine, and etoposide) with autologous bone marrow transplantation.[89] At 5 years, event-free and overall survivals were no different. Another GELA study randomized patients with high International Prognostic Index scores to cycles of conventional-dose chemotherapy or three dose-intensive cycles of chemotherapy followed by BEAM and autologous stem cell transplantation. The study was closed prematurely after 270 patients were enrolled because of inferior results in the transplant arm. Most recently, the GOELAMS group (Groupe Ouest-Est des Leucemies et des Autres Maladies du Sang) reported the results of a prospective randomized trial of CHOP versus CHOP followed by BEAM and autologous stem cell transplantation for patients with untreated intermediate-grade lymphoma who had low-, low intermediate–, or high intermediate–risk International Prognostic Index scores.[90] With a median follow-up of 4 years, 5-year event-free survival favored the transplant group (55% vs. 37%, P = .037), whereas overall survival was not different (71% vs. 56%, P = .076). The lack of overall survival advantage was attributed to successful salvage in the CHOP group with autologous stem cell transplantation. Also, recent data suggest that the addition of rituximab improves the long-term survival with CHOP beyond that seen in these trials. The current results of comparative trials, therefore, are insufficient to recommend incorporation of high-dose therapy and stem cell transplantation into the initial therapy of intermediate-grade lymphoma.

Follicular lymphoma has been the subject of numerous Phase II trials of autologous bone marrow transplantation consolidation of responding relapsed disease or first remission.[91–97] As noted earlier, this disease has been the subject of clinical trials of stem cell purging. With median follow-up of 4–5 years, survival ranges from 60% to 90%. However, the long natural history of follicular lymphoma and the lack of comparison trials to conventional-dose therapies make it difficult to determine the true benefit of the procedure.

The short survival and lack of effective salvage therapies for mantle cell lymphoma have fostered the investigation of autologous bone marrow transplantation in that disease. Limited data are available. Initial results suggest that survival may be improved in a manner similar to myeloma, but a continuous pattern of relapse makes cure elusive.

High-grade lymphoma (lymphoblastic and Burkitt's) has benefited from more intensive but nonmyeloablative chemotherapy regimens. The incremental benefit of a single course of high-dose therapy and autologous stem cell transplantation remains to be demonstrated. Certainly, autologous stem cell transplantation has not been able to salvage relapsed high-grade lymphoma, and these patients are best considered for investigational or allogeneic transplant treatment approaches.

High-dose therapy followed by autologous stem cell transplantation has been widely used for patients with recurrent and responding Hodgkin's disease. Approximately 30–50% of these patients can be salvaged using chemotherapy-based regimens such as BCV or BEAM. Two randomized trials have now been reported comparing conventional-dose salvage chemotherapy to autologous stem cell transplantation for relapsed and refractory Hodgkin's disease. The British National Lymphoma Investigation (BNLI) randomized 40 patients with relapsed or refractory Hodgkin's disease to receive cycles of conventional-dose carmustine, etoposide, cytarabine, and melphalan (mini-BEAM) or high-dose BEAM with autologous stem cell transplantation.[98] Three-year event-free survival was improved in the autologous stem cell transplantation arm (53% vs. 10%; P = .025) but overall survival was similar. Similar results were seen with a larger trial from the German Hodgkin's Lymphoma Study Group (GHSG).[99] Both studies were closed early because of poor accrual. In the absence of more robust comparative data, autologous stem cell transplantation remains the best available therapy for relapsed or primary refractory Hodgkin's disease, but further data need to be accumulated.

Leukemia

Autologous stem cell transplantation has found a role in the treatment of acute myeloid leukemia since the 1970s. Numerous Phase II trials have shown leukemia-free survival 20–30% for patients transplanted in second or subsequent complete remission and 35–70% for patients transplanted in first complete remission. Interpretation of these results is hindered by inconsistent high-dose regimens, purging techniques, and uncertain prognostic characteristics of the study populations. Throughout the 1990s, three comparative trials of autologous transplantation versus allogenic transplantation or conventional-dose chemotherapy consolidation were conducted. Results are summarized in Table 95–4. Though relapse was decreased in the autologous transplant arms when compared to conventional-dose chemotherapy, overall survival was not improved. Additionally, up to 50% of patients never received the assigned autologous transplant. Finally, the studies were of insufficient size to analyze by cytogenetic risk group. Likewise, when autologous bone marrow transplantation was compared to allogeneic transplantation, disease-free survival was

TABLE 95–4. Conventional Therapy versus High-Dose Therapy and Autologous Stem Cell Transplantation for Acute Myeloid Leukemia in First Complete Remission

Author	Treatment	DFS	OS	Relapse
Zittoun [100]	Allo-BMT	55%	59%	24%
	ABMT	48%	56%	41%
	Chemotherapy	30%	46%	57%
		P = .05	P = .43	
Harousseau [101]	Allo-BMT	45%		38%
	ABMT	47%		44%
	Chemotherapy	53%		43%
		P = NS		P = NS
Cassileth [102]	Allo-BMT	42%	46%	29%
	ABMT	37%	47%	48%
	Chemotherapy	35%	54%	61%
		P = .70		P = .10

Abbreviations: ABMT, autologous bone marrow transplantation; BMT, bone marrow transplantation; DFS, disease-free survival; NS, not significant; OS, overall survival.

TABLE 95–5. Prospective Randomized Trials of High-Dose Chemotherapy in Metastatic Breast Cancer

		Assignment		EFS (%)		OS (%)		
Trial	**Randomized**	**ABMT**	**Control**	**ABMT**	**Control**	**ABMT**	**Control**	***P* Value**
Philadelphia [103,104]	199	110	89	4	4	15	14	NS
Pegase 3 [105]	180	89	91	19	46	30	38	NS
Pegase 4 [106]	61	32	29	49*	21*	55*	28*	.06
Canada [107]	224	112	112	9	9	30	18.5	NS

*At 3 years.
Abbreviations: ABMT, autologous bone marrow transplantation; EFS, event-free survival; NS, not significant; OS, overall survival.

TABLE 95–6. Published Randomized Trials of High-Dose Chemotherapy in High-Risk Primary Breast Cancer

		Assignment		EFS (%)		OS (%)		
Trial	**Randomized**	**ABMT**	**Control**	**ABMT**	**Control**	**ABMT**	**Control**	***P* Value**
Netherlands [108]	885	442	443	59	65	70	72	.38
CALGB [109]	783			68	64	79	79	NS
Anglo-Celtic [110]	605	307	298	57	54	62	64	.38
ECOG [111]	540	270	270	48	46	58	61	.45
Scandinavian [112]	525	274	251	72	63	83	77	.12

Abbreviations: ABMT, autologous bone marrow transplantation; EFS, event-free survival; NS, not significant; OS, overall survival.

improved for allogeneic transplantation, but treatment-related mortality precluded overall survival advantage. General practice standards based on these results include consideration of allogeneic donor transplantation for young patients with human lymphocyte antigen–matched donors. Otherwise, autologous stem cell transplantation in first remission is suggested. In some instances, a stem cell harvest can be stored with transplantation in subsequent remission.

The data to support autologous transplantation in other forms of leukemia, including acute lymphocytic leukemia, chronic myelogenous leukemia, chronic lymphocytic leukemia, and myelodysplastic syndrome, are much more limited. Patients with these diseases who enter complete morphologic and cytogenetic remission and are older or do not have histocompatible donors should be considered for clinical trials.

Solid Tumors

Throughout the 1990s, breast cancer was the most common indication for hematopoietic stem cell transplantation. This was based on numerous Phase II trials reporting high response rates in metastatic breast cancer and disease-free survival at 2 years in 20–30% of patients. Patients with high-risk primary breast cancer had autologous stem cell transplantation incorporated into the initial therapy of mastectomy, adjuvant chemotherapy, radiation, and hormonal therapy, with 60–70% progression-free survival at 5 years. Ultimately, no randomized prospective trial showed a long-term survival benefit in any setting of breast cancer when compared to conventional-dose therapy (Tables 95–5 and 95–6). Progression-free survival was minimally improved in a number of trials, generally in younger patients with hormone receptor–positive and otherwise better prognostic disease, but this result has not translated into sufficient benefit to warrant the increased cost and toxicity of autologous stem cell transplantation.

No randomized comparative trial of high-dose therapy versus conventional-dose therapy has been successfully completed in ovarian cancer. Several comparisons of results with conventional-dose therapy to results in the ABMTR transplant database have been made. In the largest analysis, 422 patients with high-risk ovarian cancer underwent autologous stem cell transplantation.[113] Patients in second complete remission or partial remission with platinum-sensitive disease had 2-year survival of 45%, whereas those with nonresponsive disease had 2-year survival of 19%. In light of the lack of prospective randomized trials, these data are sufficient to consider high-dose therapy and autologous stem cell transplantation for selected patients with resistant or relapsed disease now in remission after salvage therapy.

Germ cell cancers in men and women are uncommon and fortunately very curable with conventional-dose therapy. Despite this, 20–30% of patients with advanced disease will progress and approximately half of these will fail conventional-dose salvage chemotherapy. Numerous Phase II trials have now shown that 15–20% of these patients can achieve long-term relapse-free survival after one to three courses of high-dose chemotherapy (usually carboplatin and etoposide based) with autologous stem cell rescue.[114–117] The use of autologous stem cell transplantation as part of the initial therapy for high-risk patients has now been compared to conventional-dose chemotherapy in a completed prospective randomized trial that has yet to be reported. Autologous stem cell transplantation has also been used for rare tumors such as neuroblastoma, primitive neuroectodermal tumors, Ewing's sarcoma, and desmoplastic small-cell tumor of the retroperitoneum with promising results.

Autoimmune Disease

Autoimmune diseases such as multiple sclerosis, scleroderma, rheumatoid arthritis, systemic lupus erythematosus, and refractory autoimmune cytopenia all benefit from immunosuppression or immune modulation in their treatment. A subset of these patients are resistant to conventional-dose therapy and experience substantial morbidity and mortality. A number of cases have been reported of patients undergoing autologous stem cell transplantation for malignant disease in which a coincidental autoimmune disease improved. High-dose regimens of cyclophosphamide with or without other immunosuppressive agents such as antithymocyte globulin, radiation, or busulfan and with or without stem cell lymphocyte depletion have been used. Small series have shown low treatment-related mortality, and some long-term progression-free survivors.[118,119] A number of National Institutes of Health–sponsored randomized trials comparing high-dose therapy to conventional-dose therapy are underway.

CONCLUSIONS

High-dose therapy with autologous hematopoietic stem cell transplantation has lived up to its promise as an effective therapy for a number of poor-prognosis malignancies. Autologous stem cell transplantation is now a standard consideration as part of the early therapy for all patients under age 70 years with multiple myeloma, and is part of the standard of care for patients with relapsed Hodgkin's and non-Hodgkin's lymphoma, acute myeloid leukemia, and relapsed and refractory germ cell cancer. The active investigation of the role of this treatment modality in other hematologic malignancies, solid tumors, and autoimmune diseases and the continued enhancement of stem cell collection and processing techniques hold promise for further advances in the future.

CURRENT CONTROVERSIES & FUTURE CONSIDERATIONS

Autologous Transplantation of Hematopoietic Stem Cells

- Find the optimal methods for stem cell harvesting incorporating newer targeted agents.
- Define the role of autologous stem cell transplantation in such diseases as low-grade lymphoma, ovarian cancer, and autoimmune disease.
- Clarify the role of autologous stem cell transplantation for acute myeloid leukemia and acute and chronic lymphoid leukemia with respect to allogeneic transplantation and other treatment modalities.
- Evaluate and optimize new stem cell mobilization strategies.

Suggested Readings*

Attal M, Harousseau JL, Stoppa AM, et al: Autologous bone marrow transplantation versus conventional chemotherapy in multiple myeloma: a prospective, randomized trial. N Engl J Med 335: 91–97, 1996.

Freedman AS, Neuberg D, Mauch P, et al: Long-term follow-up of autologous bone marrow transplantation in patients with relapsed follicular lymphoma. Blood 94:3325–3333, 1999.

Philip T, Guglielmi C, Hagenbeek A, et al: Autologous bone marrow transplantation as compared with salvage chemotherapy in relapses of chemotherapy-sensitive non-Hodgkin's lymphoma. N Engl J Med 333:1540–1545, 1995.

Rowley S: Cryopreservation of hematopoietic cells. *In* Blume K, Forman SJ, Appelbaum FR (eds): Thomas' Hematopoietic Cell Transplantation (ed 3). Boston: Blackwell, 2004, pp 599–612.

Stadtmauer EA, O'Neill A, Goldstein LJ, et al: Conventional-dose chemotherapy compared with high-dose chemotherapy plus autologous hematopoietic stem-cell transplantation for metastatic breast cancer. N Engl J Med 342:1069–1076, 2000

Zittoun RA, Mandelli F, Willemze R, et al: Autologous and allogeneic bone marrow transplantation compared with intensive chemotherapy in acute myelogenous leukemia. N Engl J Med 332:271–323, 1995.

Full references for this chapter can be found on accompanying CD-ROM.

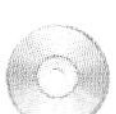

CHAPTER 96

Supportive Care for the Hematopoietic Stem Cell Transplant Patient

Hillard M. Lazarus, MD, FACP

> **KEY POINTS**
>
> **Supportive Care for the Hematopoietic Stem Cell Transplant Patient**
>
> - Patient selection
> - Visceral organ dysfunction
> - Transfusion support
> - Diagnosis and treatment of cytomegalovirus infections
> - ABO incompatible transplants
> - Mucositis prevention and treatment
> - Graft failure and rejection
> - Donor lymphocyte infusion
> - Late complications
> - Anti-infective vaccinations

INTRODUCTION

Hematopoietic stem cell transplantation has evolved into one of the most effective therapeutic modalities for the treatment of malignant, immunologic, and genetic disorders.[1–6] In the decades since clinical hematopoietic stem cell transplantation procedures were performed initially, overall and disease-free survival rates have dramatically improved as a result of a greater understanding of histocompatibility in humans, advances in platelet transfusion support, improved antibiotics, more effective anticancer drugs, the development and implementation of recombinant hematopoietic growth factors, and use of alternative sources of hematopoietic stem cells.[7] It is estimated that more than 25,000 people now have survived 5 or more years after a hematopoietic stem cell transplantation, a stark contrast to one of the first reports in which none of the first 200 transplant recipients had survived.[8] The use of this modality, however, requires extremely sophisticated supportive care in order to achieve a successful outcome, the topic of this review.

PATIENT ELIGIBILITY AND SELECTION

Hematopoietic stem cell transplantation clearly is associated with potential cardiac, pulmonary, hepatic, and renal toxicities. Although there is concern about performing stem cell transplantation in patients with clinical evidence of visceral organ dysfunction, data are limited for excluding relatively asymptomatic patients on the basis of noninvasive testing (Table 96–1). Several studies have shown that pretransplant cardiac testing using techniques such as multiple gated acquisition scans, echocardiograms, and exercise tolerance testing did not predict adverse transplantation outcome.[9–17] In one large, single-institution study, there was no difference in early treatment-related mortality and 5-year overall survival when comparing patients with a left ventricular ejection fraction less than 50% as assessed by echocardiography ($N = 20$) versus those whose left ventricular ejection fraction was greater than 50% ($N = 288$).[9] However, the combination of prior exposure to anthracyclines (cumulative doses $\geq 300\,mg/m^2$) with decreased left ventricular ejection fraction may be associated with the development of clinical congestive heart failure after transplantation.[10] Resting and exercise-induced ejection fraction may be predictive in younger patients.[11]

In contrast, asymptomatic decrements in pulmonary function testing (forced expiratory volume in 1 minute and diffusion capacity) appear to correlate with adverse transplantation outcome.[12–14] Goldberg and coworkers[12] reported that a reduced forced expiratory volume in 1 minute is associated with a higher 100-day posttransplant treatment-related mortality and may predict an increase

TABLE 96–1. Pretransplant Evaluation Assessment

Issue	Comments
Transplant risk discussion	Need for discussion of immediate, early, and late complications
Disease assessment	Physical examination, radiologic tests appropriate for tumor, marrow and blood biopsy, cytogenetics, flow cytometry
Red blood cell ABO/Rh & HLA typing*	Consideration for allogeneic transplantation and facilitate platelet transfusions in highly alloimmunized thrombocytopenic patients
Viral serology studies	HIV, hepatitis B & C, CMV, HSV, VZV, EBV
Quality of life/activities of daily living	Performance status, pretransplantation interview(s)
Dental	Panorex, cleaning, extractions (if indicated)
Cardiac	MUGA scan or echocardiogram for left ventricular ejection fraction
Pulmonary	DL_{CO}, FEV_1, arterial blood gas determination
Renal	Urinalysis, creatinine clearance
Hepatic	Transaminases, total/direct bilirubin
Psychologic	Psychology evaluation & consultation
Special	Pharmacokinetic determinations of busulfan and other appropriate agents

*Patient and prospective donor.

Abbreviations: CMV, cytomegalovirus; DL_{CO}, diffusion capacity; EBV, Epstein-Barr virus; FEV_1, forced expiratory volume in 1 minute; HIV, human immunodeficiency virus; HLA, human lymphocyte antigen; HSV, herpes simplex virus; MUGA, multiple gated acquisition; VZV, varicella-zoster virus.

Box 96–1. Central Venous Catheters: Properties and Complications

- Type: single, multilumen, apheresis, hemodialysis, infusional
- Names: Hickman, Quinton, Bard, Vygon, Secalon, Groshong, Raaf, Davol, Vas-Cath, Pellethane, Arrow-Howes, Mahurkar, Quinton-Raaf PermCath, Broviac, Leonard, Bard-Hickman
- Uses: apheresis, chemotherapy administration, infusion, transfusion, blood drawing
- Duration in situ: long and short term (e.g., 1–1715 days)
- Complications as reported in 19 separate series:
  - Local or tunnel infections: 1–25%
  - Bacteremia: 0–31%
  - Thrombosis rates: 2–74%
  - Overall dysfunction: 7–58%
  - Other complications: migration, extremity pain and swelling, bleeding, emboli, leakage, fracture

Data from Lazarus HM, Trehan S, Miller R, et al: Multi-purpose Silastic dual-lumen central venous catheters for both collection and transplantation of hematopoietic progenitor cells. Bone Marrow Transplant 25:779–785, 2000.

in cytomegalovirus interstitial lung disease. However, defining the lower limit of pulmonary function needed to survive stem cell transplantation has not been addressed. Likewise, renal insufficiency is a relative contraindication, but many patients will tolerate preparative regimens and high-dose therapy.[15,16] Conversely, patients who have visceral organ injury such as hepatic dysfunction may be at increased risk for hepatic veno-occlusive disease, and the risks versus benefits of transplantation must be weighed on an individual patient basis.[17]

SPECIAL CONSIDERATIONS

Pharmacokinetics and Drug Dosing

High-dose therapy may be affected by interpatient variability in pharmacokinetics.[18,19] Oral administration of drugs may be suboptimal because food or other medications may interfere with the intestinal microenvironment and alter absorption; in addition, ingestion of pills may be difficult if the patient is nauseated or has difficulty swallowing.[20] Large deviation from normal body weight also challenges dosing strategies based on actual or ideal weight.[21,22]

One agent commonly used in transplantation, busulfan, until recently was available only in oral form. Bioavailability for this drug has been noted to vary sixfold in children and twofold in adults.[23] High blood concentrations are associated with hepatic veno-occlusive disease, and suboptimal concentrations are associated with increases in relapse and graft rejection.[24] One approach has been to administer a very small "test" dose and modify therapy based on pharmacologic results.[25,26] Parenteral busulfan preparations have overcome this issue and may reduce the incidence of hepatic veno-occlusive disease.[24] Similar data are being generated for individual dose adjustment for cyclophosphamide.[27]

Central Venous and Pheresis Catheters

A successful transplant depends heavily on the use of a long-term, Silastic, multilumen, small-bore, flexible catheter for chemotherapy administration, infusion of hematopoietic cells, and supportive care management, including frequent blood sampling and intravenous administration of antibiotics, analgesics, antiemetics, blood components, and parenteral nutrition (Box 96–1). In autologous transplant recipients, a hybrid catheter that embodies the properties of a pheresis catheter and long-term supportive care catheter often is used.[28–30] Catheters generally are inserted in the upper, anterior chest, although femoral catheters tunneled along the abdominal wall can be used in those patients with large chest tumors or vascular abnormalities that preclude insertion in the chest.[31] The placement of central venous catheters can be accomplished even in thrombocytopenic pa-

TABLE 96–2. Recommended Approaches for Administering Serotonin Antagonists* for Prevention of Chemotherapy-Induced Nausea and Vomiting

Antiemetic Prophylaxis Agents	Route of Administration	Potentially Severe Emetogenic Agent† Exposure	Potentially Intermediate Emetogenic Agent Exposure
Dolasetron‡	Oral	100 mg	100 mg
Dolasetron‡	IV bolus	100 mg	100 mg
Granisetron	Oral	1–2 mg	1 mg
Granisetron	IV bolus	1–2 mg	1 mg
Ondansetron	Oral	12–16 mg ODT	8 mg ODT
Ondansetron	IV bolus	12–16 mg	8 mg
Palonosetron	Oral preparation NOT AVAILABLE	–	–
Palonosetron	IV bolus	0.25 mg	

*In combination with dexamethasone 16 mg IV or oral.
†For a given dose range, select the lower dose first and escalate as necessary.
‡Requires metabolic activation for efficacy, hence administer 30–60 minutes before chemotherapy.
Abbreviations: IV, intravenous; ODT, oral disintegrating tablet.

tients after platelet transfusion therapy. Despite use of sophisticated insertion techniques, however, massive hematomas, pneumothoraces, hemothoraces, and other surgical problems are not uncommon. Complications associated with routine use of central venous catheters during the transplantation and posttransplantation periods include local pain, extremity swelling, migration, leakage, bleeding at the exit site, emboli, local and disseminated infection, occlusion, and thrombosis. Catheters may remain in situ for many months or longer after transplantation, but often are removed for problems such as infection such as bacteremia or fungemia. In one recent study of these catheters, the in situ duration was a median of 63 days (range, 7–190 days), the local/tunnel infection rate was 2%, and bacteremia rate was 15%; 9% of patients experienced catheter-related thrombosis, and in 29% of patients catheter dysfunction was reported at some time.[28] Blood cultures obtained simultaneously from a catheter and a peripheral vein helped discriminate whether the bacteremia was catheter related; when cultures from the catheter turned positive at least 120 minutes sooner than cultures from a peripheral vein ("differential time to positivity"), the odds that the bacteremia was catheter related increased substantially.[32]

Nausea and Vomiting

Nausea and vomiting are the most common acute adverse events arising from high-dose chemotherapy and radiation therapy used in the stem cell transplant setting.[33] The use of 5-hydroxytryptamine (serotonin) receptor blockers revolutionized the treatment of chemotherapy-associated nausea.[34] A serotonin blocker in combination with dexamethasone now is the most frequently prescribed prophylaxis for emesis associated with high-dose cytotoxic therapy.[35–41] The American Society of Clinical Oncology recommends more intensive use of antiemetics in transplant patients because the high-dose chemotherapy regimen is more highly emetogenic, frequently total-body irradiation is a component of the

TABLE 96–3. Approaches for "Breakthrough" Emesis

Antiemetic Agent	Route	Dose	Frequency
Metoclopramide	IV	2 mg/kg	Every 2 hr
Metoclopramide	IV/PO	*10 mg	Four times a day
Haloperidol	IV	1–2 mg	Every 4 hr
Marinol	Oral	2.5–7.5 mg	Every 4–6 hr
Lorazepam	IV	1–2 mg	Every 4–6 hr

*Low dose improves gastroparesis.
Abbreviations: IV, intravenous; PO, oral.

therapy, the cytotoxic treatments are given for a number of consecutive days, and most transplant patients are not chemotherapy naive.[42] Table 96–2 lists recommended approaches for the use of a serotonin antagonist in combination with dexamethasone for the prevention of chemotherapy; the approach for "breakthrough" emesis is shown in Table 96–3.

Hepatic Veno-occlusive Disease

Hepatic injury in the course of a stem cell transplant may affect nearly half of recipients as a result of infection, high-dose chemoradiotherapy, malignancy, antibiotics, parenteral alimentation, immunosuppressive agents, graft-versus-host disease (GVHD), and hepatic veno-occlusive disease. The latter syndrome, a result of chemotherapy-induced liver injury, often is fatal and is characterized by jaundice, fluid retention, and painful hepatomegaly; it may occur commonly in patients who undergo a myeloablative preparative regimen and stem cell transplantation. The onset of hepatic veno-occlusive disease is usually within the first 2 weeks after initiating the preparative regimen, although "late-onset hepatic veno-occlusive disease" has been described.[43–45] The progressive concentric occlusion of lumina of small intrahepatic veins and necrosis of hepatocytes in the centrilobular area of injury lead to portal hypertension, ascites, and hepatic failure. Whenever possible, the diagnosis of hepatic veno-occlusive disease should be verified histologically, because many patients who have a "veno-occlusive disease–like syndrome" may have other entities.[46] A variety of factors are associated with the development of hepatic veno-occlusive disease. These may include a history of previous hepatocellular disease, busulfan-containing preparative regimens, advanced patient age, presence of GVHD, type of GVHD prophylaxis, fungal infection within 1 week of initiating the preparative regimen, and poor performance status at the start of transplantation.[43,45,47] Various agents have been given as prophylaxis against hepatic veno-occlusive disease, including intravenous and subcutaneous heparin, oral ursodiol, *N*-acetylcysteine, and glutamine, but the results of such interventions have been mixed. In these reports, the patient populations studied often were small and not at high risk for veno-occlusive disease; although the incidence of hepatic veno-occlusive disease may have been reduced in some studies compared to placebo or historical controls, severity and mortality did not differ between groups.[48–54]

Several antithrombotic agents, including tissue plasminogen activator (TPA), antithrombin III, and defibrotide, a single-stranded polydeoxyribonucleotide that possesses anti-ischemic, antithrombotic and thrombolytic activity, have been administered as therapy for established or suspected hepatic veno-occlusive disease.[55–58] Unlike the other agents, defibrotide does not appear to cause significant anticoagulant effects and may function by repairing endothelial damage. Richardson and coworkers treated 75 severe hepatic veno-occlusive disease patients, most of who also had ascites and evidence of multisystem organ failure.[58] A 35% complete response rate without significant toxicity was attained in 67 patients who received four or more days of therapy.

Neutropenic Fever

Neutropenic fever, a common complication of cancer therapy, is a medical emergency. Although hematopoietic stem cell transplant patients are at considerable risk for this toxicity, in part as a result of the intensity of the preparative regimen, a detailed discussion is beyond the scope of this chapter; the reader is referred to several up-to-date reviews.[59–63] Many patients undergoing transplantation are receiving antiviral agent prophylaxis and sometimes antibacterial agent prophylaxis at the start of transplantation, although use of the latter has been associated with the emergence of resistant organisms such as vancomycin-resistant *Enterococcus*.[64] When a neutropenic patient develops fever, a prompt evaluation must be undertaken that includes a chest radiograph and cultures of blood, urine, and other body fluids (as appropriate). Broad-spectrum antibacterial agent therapy must be initiated quickly, with the choice of agents designed to reflect the type of infecting organisms and their microbiologic sensitivities that predominate at each center. The initial antibacterial agent therapy is expanded accordingly for positive culture results. For example, intravenous vancomycin is added to the regimen as coverage for a bacteremia caused by gram-positive cocci. About 15% of patients who become afebrile may develop a second or subsequent infection, and such patients continue to require close scrutiny. Although many patients will become afebrile within 72–96 hours of initiating antibacterials, neutropenic fever may persist and various antifungal therapies are added in empirical fashion because occult infection rates are quite high.[65,66] Newer treatment strategies are being developed to address the use of preemptive antifungal therapy and include the use of techniques such as the blood galactomannan assay.[67,68]

TRANSFUSION SUPPORT FOR THE TRANSPLANT PATIENT

General Blood Banking Considerations

Most hematopoietic stem cell transplant patients develop some degree of anemia and thrombocytopenia requiring transfusion. All blood component transfusions must be irradiated routinely (1200–3000 cGy) to prevent inadvertent lymphoid engraftment and proliferation leading to transfusion-associated GVHD; this preparation usually must continue until full immunologic reconstitution returns at 6–9 months after transplantation. Further, transfusions from blood relatives must be avoided for all potential allogeneic transplant candidates, and most centers utilize a formal protocol to prevent such occurrences.

Red blood cell transfusions should be considered if the hemoglobin is less than 8 gm/dL or the hematocrit less than 25%, or if the patient has clinical symptoms of severe fatigue, headache, tachycardia, cardiac ischemia, or hypotension. The cause of anemia in the course of an allogeneic or autologous stem cell transplantation is multifactorial, but may reflect a relative endogenous erythropoietic deficiency.[69] Recombinant human erythropoietin treatment has been used successfully to correct anemia in stem cell transplant recipients; the effect is more pronounced in the allograft compared to the autograft patient,[69,70] but erythropoietin is not effective until there is evidence of hematopoietic recovery.

Spontaneous bleeding is greatest at platelet counts of 20,000/μL or less.[71] Several investigators have advocated lower threshold levels for prophylactic transfusion in view of heighten concerns about transfusion costs and risks of infection and alloimmunization.[72–77] At least three prospective, randomized studies demonstrated that a prophylactic platelet transfusion "trigger" of 10,000/μL was as effective as the previous 20,000/μL threshold based on hemorrhagic morbidity and mortality. Conversely, the optimal quantity of platelets to be given per transfusion remains a controversial subject. Two studies compared isolated transfusion of different doses of platelets to be given to the same thrombocytopenic patient and demonstrated that "higher dose" platelet transfusions resulted in greater transfusion increments and longer intervals between transfusion than predicted.[78–80] In another study comparing "low-dose" versus "high-dose" platelet transfusions, fewer transfusion events were observed in the former situation, supporting the concept that reducing the number of platelets transfused rather than the number of transfusion events might be most cost-effective.[81,82] Platelets, however, express thrombopoietin receptors, and use of frequent low-dose platelet transfusions may substantially decrease thrombopoietin blood concentration. This effect might actually increase platelet transfusion use because less thrombopoietin would be available to stimulate return of marrow megakaryocyte production. This issue is the subject of a recently activated study undertaken by the newly formed Transfusion Medicine/Hemostasis Clinical Trials Network.

Red blood cell and platelet transfusion requirements in patients given nonmyeloablative peripheral blood stem cell transplants from human lymphocyte antigen–matched siblings are reduced compared to myeloablative allografts.[83] One center retrospectively compared 40 hematologic malignancy patients ages 21–67 years given 200 cGy with/without fludarabine conditioning and nonmyeloablative allografts with 67 concurrent patients ages 23–66 years given myeloablative peripheral blood stem cell transplants. Sixty-three percent of reduced-conditioning recipients required red blood cell transfusions (median 2 units; range, 0–50 units) compared to 96% of the myeloablative regimen transplants (median 6 units; range, 0–34 units) (P = .0001). Similarly, only 23% of those patients given nonmyeloablative transplants required platelet transfusions compared with 100% among the myeloablative allograft recipients (median 24 units; range, 4–358 units) (P < .0001).

Granulocyte Transfusions

Neutropenic patients who develop infection continue to experience significant morbidity and mortality despite use of effective antimicrobial agents. Granulocyte transfusions have been used for prevention and treatment of this problem, but efficacy has been hampered by lack of suitable related donors, a relatively small quantity of granulocytes that can be obtained from normal donors, the short "shelf life" of the granulocyte product, and the potential complications of this therapy, including alloimmunization, pulmonary injury, and transmission of infectious disease.[84,85] Recently, granulocyte colony-stimulating factor (G-CSF) given to normal subjects has been shown to dramatically increase the number of circulating granulocytes and can increase collection yields 2- to 10-fold compared to previous techniques. Further, G-CSF-stimulated neutrophils survive in vivo much longer after transfusion than unmobilized cells.[86–88] The addition of G-CSF to orally administered dexamethasone substantially increased the numbers of granulocytes collected to approximately 8×10^{10}.[89–93] Recipients of granulocyte transfusions obtained in this fashion routinely achieve blood neutrophil counts in excess of 1500/μL; transfusion reaction events such as hypoxemia and fever are uncommon. Infused cells can be demonstrated to appear in sites of infection, and invasive bacterial infection and candidemia have resolved.[94,95] One group recently demonstrated successful prophylaxis in a small series of hematopoietic stem cell transplant recipients at high risk for reactivation fungal infection.[96]

Granulocyte transfusions from unrelated donors appear as efficacious as those obtained from related donors, and without appearance of antineutrophil antibodies,[94,95,97] but the procurement time is significantly shorter, potentially resulting in improved patient outcome.[98] The Transfusion Medicine/Hemostasis Clinical Trial Network soon will begin a prospective, multi-institutional trial to assess survival and antimicrobial response using granulocyte transfusions in neutropenic, hematopoietic stem cell transplant patients who have documented invasive bacterial and fungal infection.

Cytomegalovirus Infection and Disease

Cytomegalovirus is a leading cause of infectious morbidity and mortality in the allogeneic setting but is significantly less common in autografts, except in recipients of $CD34^+$-enriched autografts. These autografts are designed to eliminate tumor yet also result in low autologous T-cell graft content.[99] Both multiple myeloma and lymphoma patients who are cytomegalovirus seropositive appear to be at increased risk for cytomegalovirus reactivation during autotransplantation.[100]

Cytomegalovirus disease is defined as symptomatic infection (seroconversion or isolation of virus and clinical signs/symptoms) or a positive culture from a deep tissue or histologic evidence of viral infection.[101] Interstitial pneumonitis is the most severe form of infection (50% mortality rate), most often resulting from reactivation infection. The incidence of primary cytomegalovirus infection in cytomegalovirus-seronegative patients has been reduced markedly by exclusive use of cytomegalovirus-seronegative blood products (and leukocyte filtering of blood products to remove cytomegalovirus-infected white blood cells) in cytomegalovirus-seronegative patients. Antiviral agents and intravenous immunoglobulin prophylaxis can prevent reactivation cytomegalovirus disease in seropositive patients but can suppress marrow function. Practitioners often chose to monitor patients using sensitive, sophisticated assays such as blood polymerase chain reaction testing and begin therapy as soon as infection is documented (i.e., preemptive therapy).[101–103]

Intravenous Immunoglobulin

Randomized trials have failed to demonstrate a reduction in bacterial infection and GVHD associated with the use of intravenous immunoglobulin.[102] Intravenous immunoglobulin may be useful as a component of preemptive therapy and treatment of cytomegalovirus disease, but not prevention of reactivation of cytomegalovirus infection. Extended intravenous immunoglobulin therapy during GVHD prevention beyond 3 months after transplantation may impair recovery of humoral immunity, and its role in prophylaxis and therapy of GVHD has not been clearly defined.[92] The benefits of intravenous immunoglobulin therapy must be weighed against the marked increase in severe thrombotic events associated with its use.[104,105]

ABO-Incompatible Transplants

Red blood cell antigens are not expressed on hematopoietic stem cells; as a result, allogeneic transplants can be performed successfully across either major or minor ABO-incompatible barriers between donor and recipient without an increase in GVHD or graft rejection. Other red blood cell antigens may lead to immediate or delayed hemolytic transfusion reactions.[106,107]

Major ABO incompatibility between donor and recipient can lead to a clinically significant risk of hemolysis. Blood stem cell transplant grafts collected by apheresis are associated with a lower risk of hemolysis compared to a marrow graft because of a lower red cell burden. This risk is reduced by removal of red cells from the graft using any of a variety of techniques. Occasionally, it is necessary to deplete recipient isoagglutinin titers by large-volume plasma exchange.[108–110] Rarely, host isoagglutinins may persist for years because of the presence of mature recipient B lymphocytes or plasma cells that survived the preparative regimen, necessitating continuing red blood cell transfusions until complete resolution.

If there is a minor ABO incompatibility in the transplant, plasma contained in the donor graft is removed to prior to infusion to prevent hemolysis. These patients may experience delayed but life-threatening hemolysis mediated by viable donor lymphocytes in the stem cell graft.[111] These cells may transiently produce isoagglutinins to result in potentially life-threatening hemolysis of recipient red blood cells 7–14 days after transplantation, sometimes requiring hemodialysis.[111,112] This situation is more likely to occur in red blood cell group A recipients given group O donor grafts, although hemolysis may occur after transfusion of group O red blood cells used in transfusion support, possibly through passive absorption of group A or B antigens from donor plasma onto the red blood cell membrane.[111] Minor ABO-incompatible hemolysis is less likely with posttransplantation immunosuppression when agents such as methotrexate or mycophenolate mofetil are used. Thus, most reported cases involve patients treated with cyclosporine alone without either methotrexate, prednisone, or antithymocyte globulin. Blood stem cell recipients are at greater risk of this complication than marrow recipients because of the greater number of lymphocytes in the graft.[113–115]

Transfusion-Related Issues in Stem Cell Transplantation

Even though use of blood products during transplantation has declined, blood component transfusions remain an important aspect of supportive care for the patient undergoing transplantation despite complications such as hemolytic, febrile, and allergic reactions, transfusion-related acute lung injury, and alloimmunization that account for clinically significant morbidity and mortality after transplantation.[116] Although the risks of transmission of viral illnesses, including human immunodeficiency virus, hepatitis B virus, and non-A, non-B hepatitis virus, have decreased dramatically,[117] other transfusion-related infections, including cytomegalovirus, parvovirus, and human T-lymphotrophic virus types 1 and 2, remain concerns. In addition, even more rare transmissible illnesses such as agents associated with the spongiform encephalopathies and parasitic infections have been associated with acute and chronic complications.[118] Bacterial contamination of red blood cells and platelets, although rare, can account for significant transfusion-related morbidity and potential mortality.[119] It remains unclear whether the risk of transfusion-related infections is reduced by using in-line and other types of leukofilters.[120]

In the autologous setting, dimethylsulfoxide used for the cryopreservation of stem cells has been associated with a variety of clinically significant toxicities, including nausea, fever, cardiopulmonary complications, hypertension, and, rarely, anaphylaxis; these toxicities appear to be related to the amount of dimethylsulfoxide present in the graft.[121,122] Patients must be monitored closely for changes in vital signs and urine output, and some centers routinely employ electrocardiographic monitoring. Premedications often are given, including corticosteroids, antiemetics, diuretics, and other supportive medications, to decrease the risk of complications during stem cell infusion.

MUCOSITIS DURING TRANSPLANTATION

Oral mucositis is a frequent and significant debilitating and painful complication in patients undergoing stem cell transplantation. It occurs as a consequence of epithelial injury from cytotoxic drugs, radiation therapy, and preexisting infection.[123–127] Extensive evaluation and treatment of the patient's oral cavity by a dental specialist before transplantation is essential before initiating the preparative regimen; optimal management is outlined in Table 96–4.[127–131] A randomized Phase II study using amifostine 740 mg/m^2 prior to stem cell collection (after receiving DHAP salvage chemotherapy) noted a higher stem cell count during collection, and others link amifostine use to a lower rate of mucositis.[133–135] Recombinant human keratinocyte growth factor is a heparin-binding member of the fibroblast growth factor family and represents a promising approach for the effective management of acute radiation reactions in oral, gastrointestinal, and cutaneous epithelia after radiation exposure.[136] In a Phase II, double-blind, placebo-controlled prophylaxis study conducted in the autologous transplant setting, keratinocyte growth factor reduced the duration of severe oral mucositis and improved quality of life.[137] Further, in a preclinical animal model, keratinocyte growth factor-1 reduced epithelial damage, severity of GVHD, and pulmonary injury after allogeneic transplantation.[138–140] The glucagon-like peptides, including ALX-0600 (NPS Pharmaceuticals, Parsippany, NJ), which stimulate the growth and repair of the

TABLE 96–4. Mucositis Prevention

Maneuver/Agent	Comment
Dental evaluation/ cleaning	Prophylactic antibiotics may be necessary, as well as dental extractions
Ice chips	Hold in mouth for 15 min before, during, & after chemotherapy; effective only for short half-life chemotherapy (i.e., melphalan)
Interleukin-11	Animal model supports GI tract protection
Glutamine	Animal model supports GI tract protection
Anticholinergics	Decreased salivation may reduce drug oral concentrations
Amifostine	Given 24 hr and immediately before therapy; bolus infusion to avoid hypotension
Chlorhexidine	Prevents oropharyngeal bacterial infections
KGF-1	Investigational agent
Antiviral agents	Prophylaxis may decrease HSV-I or -II infections
Glucagon-like peptides	Reduce cytotoxic injury to intestines in preclinical animal models; await clinical trial use

Abbreviations: GI, gastrointestinal; HSV, herpes simplex virus; KGF, keratinocyte growth factor.

intestine, are attractive targets for reducing the injury associated with cytotoxic agent exposure.[141,142]

GRAFT FAILURE AND REJECTION

Engraftment failure after a myeloablative hematopoietic stem cell transplantation is a life-threatening situation occurring at an overall frequency of less than 5%.[143] Primary reasons for graft failure are outlined in Box 96–2. In the autologous stem cell setting, data suggest a dose-response relationship between number of $CD34^+$ cells infused and engraftment kinetics, especially for platelet recovery.[144] Minimum levels of 2.0–2.5 × 10^6 $CD34^+$ cells/kg patient weight are needed, and optimal levels are greater than 5.0 × 10^6 $CD34^+$ cells/kg.[145,146]

Graft dysfunction is much more likely with use of blood and marrow grafts obtained from haploidentical related donors, matched unrelated donors, and umbilical cord blood; after T-cell–depleted marrow transplants; or with reduced-intensity preparative regimens.[147–156] Other factors may also contribute to graft failure. Abnormal marrow environment, splenomegaly, inadequate GVHD prophylaxis, and occurrence of cytomegalovirus, human herpesvirus 6 and 8, and parvovirus infections have been implicated in causing graft failure.[157–159]

Management of graft failure includes withdrawal of potentially marrow-suppressive agents such as antibiotics, administration of recombinant hematopoietic growth factors, infusions of additional hematopoietic stem cells (if available), and, in the case of a failed allograft, the decision to perform a second transplantation.[143] Guardiola and associates[160] reviewed 82 leukemia and aplastic anemia patients who underwent second allografts for graft failure or rejection. Most patients were given second conditioning regimens and the initial (same) regimen usually was used a second time. Overall survival at 3 years was 30%, but 100-day treatment-related mortality was 53%.

Box 96–2. Issues To Be Addressed Regarding Engraftment Failure

- Adequacy of initial stem cell dose: number $CD34^+$ cells/kg recipient weight infused, loss of cells during collection or processing, or inadequate cell collections
- Hindrance to engraftment: splenomegaly (sequestration) or marrow fibrosis or malignancy
- Previous exposure of recipient to donor antigens or cells (i.e., immediate family member transfusion), or heavy exposure of patient to blood transfusions previously (i.e., aplastic anemia)
- Intensive ex vivo graft manipulation (T-cell depletion)
- Human lymphocyte antigen or ABO disparity between host and recipient
- Use of reduced-intensity conditioning regimen
- Development of infection such as cytomegalovirus, human herpesvirus 6 and 8, parvovirus
- Adequacy of graft-versus-host disease prophylaxis regimen
- Primary engraftment failure versus secondary failure (i.e., loss after initial engraftment)
- Demonstration of residual host immunity directed against donor cells mediated via natural killer or cytotoxic T lymphocytes
- If and when should a different donor be used?
- Should additional cytotoxic or immunosuppressive therapy be given before a second graft infusion?
- Should the cellular rescue product constitute a donor lymphocyte infusion, stem cell infusion, or both?

DONOR LYMPHOCYTE INFUSIONS: ADOPTIVE IMMUNOTHERAPY

Adoptive immunotherapy with effector T cells, either in bulk or selected for specific antitumor activity, can overcome regulatory mechanisms that prevent in vivo generation of specific antitumor effectors. A variety of studies have explored the infusion of donor T cells, also known as donor lymphocyte infusion, into an allograft recipient who has a functioning donor graft (Box 96–3). In general, such cells are collected from the same allograft donor (either in steady state or after cytokine stimulation) using standard apheresis techniques. Donor lymphocyte infusion appears to be most effective as a therapeutic intervention when administered to a host who has minimal residual disease (i.e., molecular relapse) and a more indolent malignancy (e.g., chronic myelogenous leukemia [CML] in chronic phase or indolent non-Hodgkin's lymphoma). Most centers administer donor

Box 96–3. Donor Lymphocyte Infusion

Efficacy

- Significant activity in chronic myelogenous leukemia, multiple myeloma, indolent non-Hodgkin's lymphoma
- Significant activity in cytomegalovirus, Epstein-Barr virus
- Modest activity in acute leukemia, aggressive lymphoma

Toxicity

- Graft-versus-host disease
- Marrow suppression

Unanswered Questions

- Collection in steady state or after cytokine exposure/mobilization
- Optimal cytotoxic agent type, dose, interval before donor lymphocyte infusion

Future Strategies

- Cellular engineering (e.g., photoinactivation, suicide gene insertion, ex vivo expansion)

lymphocyte infusion after cytotoxic therapy in those subjects who have a larger tumor burden (clinical relapse) or biologically more aggressive disease (CML in accelerated phase or blast crises). Donor lymphocyte infusion after matched sibling stem cell transplantation may be complicated by GVHD, marrow aplasia, and failure to eradicate the malignant disorder.

Responses, however, are largely disease specific. Collins and associates[161] reported a survey of 140 North American patients given donor lymphocyte infusion for a variety of diseases. Complete responses were observed in 60% of CML patients; the most durable and highest response rates were in patients in chronic-phase relapse (75.7%) rather than accelerated-phase (33.3%) or blast-phase (16.7%) relapse. However, donor lymphocyte infusion was less efficacious in acute myeloid leukemia and acute lymphocytic leukemia (15.4% and 18.2% response rate, respectively). Complete remissions also were observed in multiple myeloma and myelodysplasia patients. Donor lymphocyte infusion infusions were associated with acute and chronic GVHD in about 60% of patients and pancytopenia in nearly 20%.

CML and multiple myeloma have the best antitumor responses after infusion of sibling matched donor lymphocyte infusion.[162,163] More recently, donor lymphocyte infusions have been demonstrated to have efficacy as therapy for patients with indolent non-Hodgkin's lymphoma and myelodysplastic syndrome experiencing relapses after nonmyeloablative allografts.[164,165] Other groups have reported that, despite potential logistic problems, donor lymphocyte infusion can be useful to prevent or treat relapsed disease in the matched unrelated donor setting.[166] One group recently reported molecular remission in CML patients who underwent autograft followed by adoptive transfer of costimulated autologous T cells.[167]

Other groups have utilized T-cell therapy to treat infections such as cytomegalovirus, Epstein-Barr virus, and human herpesvirus 6,[168–171] including the use of genetically modified T cells. T-cell proliferation is not required, at least in a mouse model, raising the possibility of preventing GVHD by treatment with ultraviolet light in vitro.[172] Finally, pretreatment of donor cells with a patient-specific myeloma idiotype protein in multiple myeloma patients receiving reduced-conditioning allografts was effective in a preliminary study.[173] Additional studies are likely to improve the prospects of effector immune cell therapy alone and in addition to allogeneic cells.[174]

LATE COMPLICATIONS AFTER TRANSPLANT

Complications occurring many months to years after transplant are caused by the preparative regimen, late infection, chronic GVHD, recurrence of malignancy, and secondary malignancy (Table 96–5). Common complications from the preparative regimen, from infections, and from GVHD and its prevention and treatment include pulmonary fibrosis and bronchiolitis obliterans, chronic hepatitis and iron overload, endocrine dysfunction such as hypothyroidism, hypogonadism and growth retardation in children, cataracts, avascular necrosis of joints, late-onset leukoencephalopathy, and cognitive function impairment.[175] More recently, increased use of monoclonal antibodies such as rituximab may impair B-cell reconstitution for many months, and an associated late-onset neutropenia may develop. Patients may develop a potentially fatal infection about 3–4 months after transplantation, at a time when the patient often has been returned to the care of the local oncologist.[176,177]

Quality of Life

Numerous studies document the late impact of transplantation on normal activity, including employment, relationships with others, and sexuality.[178–186] Patients report altered body image, sexual difficulties, fatigue, lack of physical strength, inability to work at their chosen employment, and financial problems. Because many of these issues may antedate the transplantation, recognizing them early will benefit the patient later on. A reduced quality of life more often persists in older patients, those with less formal education, subjects with a more advanced disease state at transplantation, and those in whom there is evidence of active chronic GVHD and chronic visceral organ dysfunction. Autologous transplant recipients tend to report an improved quality of life versus subjects who underwent an allogeneic procedure.

TABLE 96–5. Surveillance for Late Effects of Hematopoietic Transplantation

Organ	Complication	Treatment	Monitoring Tests	Comments
Heart	Atherosclerotic cardiovascular disease	Standard	Routine screening; stress testing	
	Congestive heart failure	Standard	Physical examination	
Lung	Bronchiolitis obliterans	Immunosuppressants	Physical examination; pulmonary function tests	Rapid diagnosis and treatment essential
	Pulmonary fibrosis	Corticosteroids	Pulmonary function tests	Restrictive; onset at 3–6 mo; recovery or stabilization often by 2 yr
	Bronchitis; bronchiectasis	Prophylactic antibiotics; treatment of acute exacerbations	Physical examination	Obliterative bronchiolitis is best characterized; occurs in 2–14% of allografts, 50% mortality
Liver	Chronic hepatitis	Antiviral therapy; avoid excess alcohol	Liver function tests	Prevalence of hepatitis B infection: 2.0–3.1% Prevalence of hepatitis C infection: 6.0–7.4%
	Iron overload	Phlebotomy; deferoxamine	Ferritin	Affects up to 88% of long-term survivors; assess all survivors (even if asymptomatic) using serum ferritin, or ratio serum transferrin receptor to serum ferritin
Kidney	Renal insufficiency	Avoid nephrotoxins	Renal function tests	7–15% develop subclinical hypothyroidism; overt hypothyroidism, onset median 50 mo, in about 15% of patients after fractionated TBI (lesser after non-TBI regimens)
Endocrine	Hypothyroidism; autoimmune thyroiditis (rare)	Thyroid hormone replacement	Thyroid-stimulating hormone and thyroid function tests	
	Hypogonadism	Hormone replacement	Physical examination and blood sex hormone concentration	
Skin	Damage/skin cancer	Moisturizers; sunscreens; avoid direct sunlight	Physical examination	
Eyes	Cataracts; sicca syndrome	Extraction; lubricants; immunosuppressants	Yearly eye examination	Risk factors: higher TBI dose, age >23 yr, allograft, corticosteroid use
	Microvascular retinopathy, disc edema, hemorrhage, infectious retinitis			Fungal infections, onset about 4 mo; nonfungal infections later
Mouth	Increased caries; impaired development (child); gingival disease; sicca syndrome	Oral moisturizing agents; immunosuppressants, oral fluoride rinse; dental care	Dental examination	Prevention with twice-daily tooth brushing, fluoride application, antiseptic mouthwashes, frequent dental examinations
Bone	Avascular necrosis	Surgical intervention and pain control		Prevalence 4–10%; onset 18 mo (range, 4–132 mo), hip most common joint
	Low bone density, osteopenia, osteoporosis	Calcium; exercise; bisphosphonates	Bone density measurements	Nearly 50% low bone density, one third osteopenia, 10% osteoporosis at 12–18 mo posttransplant; cumulative dose/no. days glucocorticoid therapy and cyclosporine, tacrolimus therapy associated with loss of bone mineral density
Reproductive system	Infertility; gonadal failure		Blood sex hormone and gonadotropin concentration; fertility work-up, including sperm count	TBI conditioning usually causes gonadal failure; recovery only 10–14% in women (pregnancy <3%) and <20% in men; higher recovery rates in transplants for nonmalignant conditions
Quality of life	Fatigue; sleeping disorder	Symptomatic therapy	Psychology follow-up	Prevalence up to 65%; risk factors include older age, advanced disease at transplantation, lower level of education, development of chronic GVHD
	Sexual dysfunction	Andrology and gynecology consultations	Psychology follow-up	Prevalence 25%; women may have higher rates than men
General	Secondary cancer	Oncologist evaluation	Pelvic examination; PAP smear; breast examination; mammogram; colon cancer screening; prostate-specific antigen	

Abbreviations: GVHD, graft-versus-host disease; PAP, Papanicolaou; TBI, total-body irradiation.

Patients who survive beyond 5 years, particularly those who are disease free, generally perform at a level at least equal to age-matched comparison groups. These individuals, however, still may experience difficulties in areas pertaining to close relationships, sexual functioning, and fear of recurrence. Controlled studies using instruments sensitive to quality of life are being developed to determine whether interventions aimed to enhance positive outcomes of traumatic experiences such as transplantation will lead to meaningful improvements for the individual patient.

Secondary Malignancies

Secondary malignancy is among the most serious of late effect in hematopoietic stem cell transplant recipients. Acute myeloid leukemia and myelodysplastic syndromes are most common and have the shortest latency.[187–191] The risk of solid tumors also continues to increase and can become significant 5–10 years after transplantation,[192,193] and both are difficult to treat.[194] Risk factors for developing a second cancer include alkylating agent exposure, radiotherapy during the preparative regimen, acute GVHD (grade II–IV), use of antithymocyte globulin in the posttransplant setting, and chronic GVHD.[187,194] The use of etoposide in autologous transplant patients at doses greater than $2 gm/m^2$ has shown a variably slightly increased (up to 3% at 5 year) cumulative incidence of acute myeloid leukemia and myelodysplastic syndrome.[191,195]

Epithelial and cutaneous solid tumors arise at a rate four- to eightfold higher than in the general population.[193,196,197] Curtis and coworkers[197] studied over 19,000 allogeneic transplant recipients between 1964 and 1992 at 235 centers and reported an eightfold increase in solid tumors among subjects who survived 10 or more years after transplantation (cumulative incidence rate, 2.2% at 10 years and 6.7% at 15 years). The most commonly observed cancers were malignant melanoma and cancers of the liver, central nervous system, thyroid, bone, connective tissue, and buccal cavity; the latter tumors were strongly linked to male gender and patients with chronic GVHD. The risk was higher for younger recipients who were given higher doses of total-body irradiation.

Posttransplantation lymphoproliferative disorders are of particular concern and arise early in the posttransplant setting, usually peaking at 1–5 months, followed by a sharp decline after the first year.[198] These disorders appear to be related to the immunosuppression used in the prophylaxis and treatment of GVHD, or T-cell depletion of the graft, and do not appear to be a result of the preparative regimen. Many reflect Epstein-Barr virus reactivation, and evidence of the Epstein-Barr virus genome is often present in the lymphoma cells.

All patients undergoing hematopoietic stem cell transplantation should be informed of the potential risk of developing a second cancer and should be monitored on a continuous basis. The trend toward an increased risk over time after transplantation and the greater risk among younger patients indicate the need for lifelong surveillance.

POSTTRANSPLANTATION VACCINATION

Hematopoietic stem cell transplant recipients frequently experience many years of immune dysfunction associated with an increased risk for bacterial, fungal, and viral infections.[199–201] Clearly, neutropenia remains a significant risk for infection. One recent single-center, prospective 54-month trial in 351 autograft and allograft recipients showed that 234 nosocomial infections occurred in 169 recipients; 71.5% of these infections occurred while the patients were neutropenic.[202] Natural killer cells are the first to reconstitute (within 1 month) and achieve near-normal blood concentrations and function by 3 months after transplantation, because these cells do not require a functional thymus.[203] Although $CD3^+$ cell numbers recover soon after transplantation, patients remain immunosuppressed as a result of prolonged inversion of the CD4/CD8 ratio (relative absence of $CD4^+$ helper cells and the increased presence of $CD8^+$ suppressor cells). Cellular dysfunction can be demonstrated for 6–12 months after transplantation using in vitro assays and the demonstration of anergy to recall antigens.[203–206] Further, in allograft recipients, donor lymphoid cells cannot be reeducated in the absence of a functional thymus, and patients continue to receive immunosuppressive agents as prophylaxis for GVHD. In the autograft setting and in allograft recipients in whom GVHD does not occur, mature blood B-cell populations expressing CD19 and CD20 return to normal levels 3–6 months after transplant. Overall, immune reconstitution appears to occur more rapidly in autograft and allograft recipients receiving blood stem cell grafts compared to marrow grafts.[207–210]

Infections caused by encapsulated bacterial organisms such as *Streptococcus pneumoniae* and *Haemophilus influenzae* type B may pose a significant hazard in the late posttransplantation period, and response to anti-infective vaccines may be suboptimal.[211–214] Further, European and U.S. surveys indicate considerable variability in the practice guidelines with respect to vaccination after transplantation, because few large multicenter trials have been conducted[215,216] (Box 96–4). Effective vaccination is most difficult in hematopoietic stem cell transplant recipients given the limited capacity of a regenerating immune system, often still under immunosuppression (in the case of an allograft). Further, use of the more potent live, attenuated viral vaccines compared to inactivated or killed vaccines is contraindicated because of the risk of disseminated infection.[214] Finally, polysaccharide-based vaccines such as pneumococcal vaccine frequently fail to elicit a sufficient response. In contrast, the protein-conjugated vaccines, such as anti–*Haemophilus influenzae* type b, frequently confer protection.[217–219] A number of strategies are being developed to improve anti-infective vaccination and reduce late infectious.[220] Current recommendations and timing for vaccination in the posttransplant setting have been published.[221]

Box 96–4. Issues Relating to Anti-infective Vaccines

- Few published multicenter trials
- Potentially compromised host response
- Continued immunosuppression and need to avoid live vaccines (with exceptions; see below)
- Anti-infective vaccinations usually initiated at 1 year after transplantation, to include:
  - Pneumococcal vaccine
  - *Haemophilus influenzae* type b vaccine
  - Recombinant hepatitis B vaccine
  - Killed, enhanced, inactivated poliovirus vaccine
  - Diphtheria/tetanus toxoid
- Use live, attenuated mumps/measles/rubella at 2 years when patient is withdrawn from immunosuppressive therapy and has no evidence of active graft-versus-host disease
- Yearly influenza A vaccination
- Assess response to anti-infective vaccines using blood antibody studies
- Consider protein conjugated vaccines (i.e., protein conjugated pneumococcal vaccine) in poor responders
- Investigational approaches include immune enhancers (i.e., granulocyte-macrophage colony-stimulating factor) in poor responders

SUMMARY

Both autologous and allogeneic hematopoietic stem cell transplantations have resulted in an increasing number of patients who are cured of their underlying disease, and are surviving greater than 5 years after transplantation. Late complications can occur in many organ systems, including the heart, lungs, liver, kidney, endocrine glands, eyes, skin, and oral cavity. Secondary cancers, reactivation or recurring infections, and psychiatric problems can also occur. Most of the late effects are related to chronic GVHD and immunosuppression or the late effects of high-dose chemotherapy, radiation therapy, and corticosteroids.

Current Controversies & Future Considerations

Supportive Care for the Hematopoietic Stem Cell Transplant Patient

- Mucositis prevention
- Enhancement of antifungal prophylaxis and treatment
- New antiviral diagnostic testing and therapy
- Enhancement of anti-infective vaccines
- Reducing second malignancies

Suggested Readings*

Dykewicz CA; Centers for Disease Control and Prevention (U.S.); Infectious Diseases Society of America; American Society of Blood and Marrow Transplantation: Summary of the guidelines for preventing opportunistic infections among hematopoietic stem cell transplant recipients. Clin Infect Dis 33:139–144, 2001.

Lazarus HM, Creger RJ: Special care of blood and marrow stem cell transplant patients. *In* Wiernik P, Dutcher J, Goldman J, Kyle R (eds): Neoplastic Diseases of the Blood. Cambridge, UK: Cambridge University Press, 2003, pp 1096–1122.

Sepkowitz KA: Antibiotic prophylaxis in patients receiving hematopoietic stem cell transplant. Bone Marrow Transplant 2002; 29: 367–371.

Socie G, Salooja N, Cohen A, et al, for the Late Effects Working Party of the European Study Group for Blood and Marrow Transplantation: Nonmalignant late effects after allogeneic stem cell transplantation. Blood 101:3373–3385, 2003.

Spielberger R, Stiff P, Bensinger W, et al: Palifermin for oral mucositis after intensive therapy for hematologic cancers. N Engl J Med 351:2590–2598, 2004.

Full references for this chapter can be found on accompanying CD-ROM.

CHAPTER 97

Graft-Versus-Host Disease

James L. M. Ferrara, MD, Gregory Yanik, MD, and Riccardo Valdez, MD

KEY POINTS

Graft-Versus-Host Disease

Acute Graft-Versus-Host Disease

- Principal risk factors: donor-recipient histocompatibility differences, number of T cells, increased age (donor or recipient), intensity of conditioning
- Prevention: calcineurin inhibitor ± methotrexate/steroids, reduced-intensity conditioning
- Three principal targets: skin, liver, gastrointestinal tract; lungs are also a target (idiopathic pneumonia syndrome)
- Scoring: overall severity grades I–IV; severity correlates with mortality
- Pathology: epithelial apoptosis, variable lymphocytic infiltrate
- Pathophysiology: three-step process
- Primary therapy: high-dose steroids

Chronic Graft-Versus-Host Disease

- Principal risk factors: donor-recipient histocompatibility differences, increased age (donor or recipient), peripheral blood stem cell source
- Scoring: limited (skin only) or extensive
- Principal targets: skin, eyes, mucosal surfaces, lungs, liver, gastrointestinal tract, bone marrow, immune system
- Pathophysiology: poorly understood
- Primary therapy: calcineurin inhibitor + steroid

ACUTE GRAFT-VERSUS-HOST DISEASE

Classification

Graft-versus-host disease is the major cause of morbidity and mortality following allogeneic hematopoietic stem cell transplantation. Graft-versus-host disease has traditionally been classified by the time of its clinical manifestations. Acute graft-versus-host disease occurs within the first 100 days after hematopoietic stem cell transplantation, whereas chronic graft-versus-host disease occurs after day 100. This simple classification is increasingly unsatisfactory, particularly as reduced-intensity conditioning regimens gain wider acceptance. The clinical manifestations of acute graft-versus-host disease after such conditioning often occur much later, blurring the sharp day 100 demarcation between the acute and chronic forms. Nevertheless, extensive clinical data have been codified according to this classification and it will be used throughout this chapter.

Pathophysiology

The pathophysiology of acute graft-versus-host disease after hematopoietic stem cell transplantation can be considered as a three-step process wherein the innate and adaptive immune systems interact (Fig. 97–1). The three steps are (1) tissue damage to the recipient by the radiation/chemotherapy pretransplantation conditioning regimen, (2) donor T-cell activation and clonal expansion, and (3) cellular and inflammatory factors. In step 1, the conditioning regimen (irradiation and/or chemotherapy) leads to damage and activation of host antigen-presenting cells by inflammatory cytokines. In step 2, host antigen-presenting cells present alloantigen to the resting T cells and activate them. Donor T-cell activation is characterized by cellular proliferation and the secretion of cytokines, including interleukin-2 and interferon-γ. In step 3, mononuclear phagocytes and neutrophils cause inflammation and are triggered by mediators such as lipopolysaccharide that leak through the intestinal mucosa damaged during step 1. The inflammation recruits effector cells into target organs, amplifying local tissue injury with further secretion of inflammatory

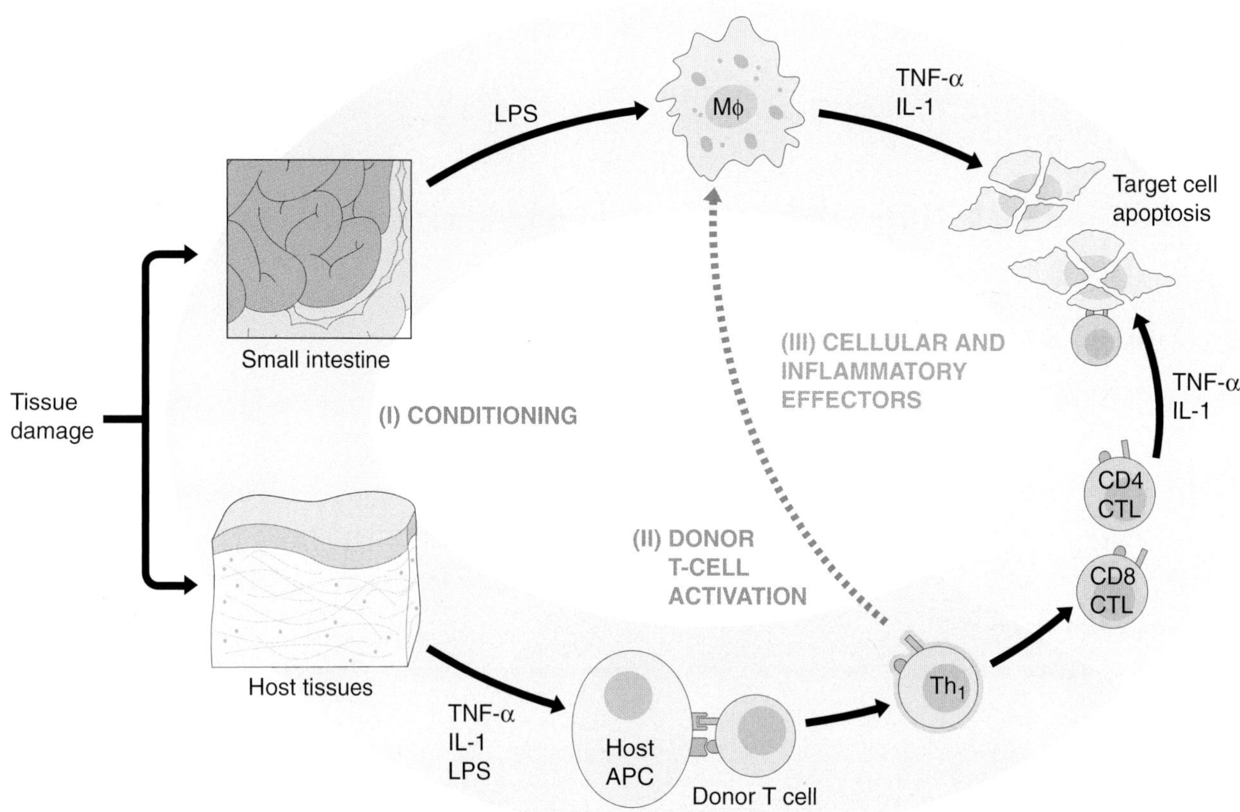

Figure 97–1. The pathophysiology of acute graft-versus-host disease can be summarized in a three-step process. In step 1, the conditioning regimen (irradiation, chemotherapy, or both) leads to the damage and activation of host tissues, especially the intestinal mucosa. This allows the translocation of lipopolysaccharide from the intestinal lumen to the circulation, stimulating the secretion of the inflammatory cytokines TNF-α and interleukin-1 from host tissues, particularly macrophages. These cytokines increase the expression of major histocompatibility complex antigens and adhesion molecules on host tissues, enhancing the recognition of major and minor histocompatibility antigens by mature donor T cells. Donor T-cell activation in step 2 is characterized by the predominance of T_H1 cells and the secretion interferon-γ, which activates mononuclear phagocytes. In step 3, effector functions of activated mononuclear phagocytes are triggered by the secondary signal provided by lipopolysaccharide and other stimulatory molecules that leak through the intestinal mucosa damaged during steps 1 and 2. Activated macrophages, along with cytotoxic T lymphocytes, secrete inflammatory cytokines that cause target cell apoptosis. $CD8^+$ cytotoxic T lymphocytes also lyse target cells directly. Damage to the gastrointestinal tract in this step, principally by inflammatory cytokines, amplifies lipopolysaccharide release and leads to the "cytokine storm" characteristic of severe acute graft-versus-host disease. This damage results in the amplification of local tissue injury, and it further promotes an inflammatory response.

cytokines in a response that, together with cytotoxic T lymphocytes, leads to target tissue destruction.[1,2]

Step 1: Effects of Hematopoietic Stem Cell Transplantation Conditioning

The first step of acute graft-versus-host disease starts before donor cells are infused. Prior to hematopoietic stem cell transplantation, a patient's tissues have been damaged by a number of factors, including the underlying disease and its treatment, infection, and transplantation conditioning. High-intensity chemoradiotherapy, characteristic of many hematopoietic stem cell transplantation conditioning regimens, activates host antigen-presenting cells that are critical to the stimulation of donor T cells infused in the stem cell inoculum. Total-body irradiation is particularly important in this process because it activates host tissues to secrete inflammatory cytokines, such as tumor necrosis factor-α (TNF-α) and interleukin-1, and it induces endothelial apoptosis that leads to epithelial cell damage in the gastrointestinal tract.[3,4] This damage to the gastrointestinal tract amplifies graft-versus-host disease by allowing the translocation of microbial products such as lipopolysaccharide into the systemic circulation. This scenario helps to explain the increased risk of graft-versus-host disease associated with intensive conditioning regimens.[5–7]

Step 2: Donor T-Cell Activation and Cytokine Secretion

Murine studies have demonstrated that host antigen-presenting cells alone are both necessary and sufficient to stimulate donor T cells to proliferate as early as day 3 after hematopoietic stem cell transplantation, preceding the engraftment of donor stem cells.[8–10] Inflammatory cytokines and microbial products such as lipopolysaccharide may all be considered "danger signals"[11] that help to activate T cells and may make the difference between an immune response and tolerance.[12] When T cells are exposed to antigens in the presence of adjuvant such as lipopolysaccharide, their migration and survival are dramatically enhanced in vivo.[13] The effect of advanced age in enhancing allostimulatory activity of host antigen-presenting cells may also help explain the increased incidence of acute graft-versus-host disease in older recipients.[14] The elimination of host antigen-presenting cells by activated natural killer (NK) cells can prevent graft-versus-host disease in experimental models.[15] This suppressive effect of NK cells on graft-versus-host disease has been confirmed in humans: human leukocyte antigen (HLA) class I differences driving donor NK-mediated alloreactions in the graft-versus-host direction, mediate potent graft-versus-leukemia effects, and produce higher engraftment rates without causing severe, acute graft-versus-host disease.[15,16]

Cytokines secreted by activated T cells are generally classified as T_H1 (secreting interleukin-2 and interferon-α) or T_H2 (secreting interleukin-4, -5, -10, and -13).[17] Dendritic cells can help modulate the function of T cells, which, in turn, have multiple effects, including (1) amplification of cytokine secretion, (2) lysis of target cells by Fas/Fas ligand (FasL) interactions, (3) activation of macrophages, (4) activation of endothelium to induce macrophage binding and extravasation, and (5) recruitment of macrophages by secreting monocyte chemoattractant protein-1 (MCP-1).[13,15,18,19]

Monoclonal antibodies against interleukin-2 or its receptor can prevent graft-versus-host disease when administered shortly after the infusion of T cells,[20–22] but this strategy was only moderately successful in reducing established graft-versus-host disease.[23,24] Cyclosporine and FK506 dramatically reduce interleukin-2 production and effectively prevent graft-versus-host disease. Interleukin-15 is another critical cytokine in initiating allogeneic T-cell division in vivo,[25] and elevated serum levels of interleukin-15 are associated with acute graft-versus-host disease in humans.[26] Interferon-α increases the expression of numerous molecules involved in graft-versus-host disease, including adhesion molecules, chemokines, major histocompatibility complex antigens and Fas, resulting in enhanced antigen presentation and the recruitment of effector cells into target organs.[27–29] Interferon-α also alters target cells in the gastrointestinal tract and skin so that they are more vulnerable to damage during graft-versus-host disease; the administration of anti–interferon-α monoclonal antibodies prevents gastrointestinal graft-versus-host disease,[30] and high levels of both interferon-α and TNF-α correlate with the most intense cellular damage in skin.[31] Interferon-α mediates the immunosuppression associated with graft-versus-host disease that was seen in several experimental hematopoietic stem cell transplantation systems, in part by the induction of nitric oxide,[32–37] and primes macrophages to produce pro-inflammatory cytokines and nitric oxide in response to lipopolysaccharide.[38,39] Paradoxically, at early time points after hematopoietic stem cell transplantation, interferon-α can reduce graft-versus-host disease by enhancing Fas-mediated apoptosis of activated donor T cells.[8,9,40]

Subpopulations of regulatory donor T cells can prevent graft-versus-host disease. Repeated in vitro stimulation of donor $CD4^+$ T cells with alloantigens results in the emergence of a population of regulatory T-cell clones (Treg cells) that secretes high amounts of interleukin-10 and transforming growth factor-β (TGF-β).[41] The immunosuppressive properties of these cytokines are explained by their ability to inhibit antigen-presenting cell function and to suppress proliferation of responding T cells directly.[42–44] Natural suppressor cells and $NK1.1^+$ T cells can also prevent graft-versus-host disease in experimental models.[45–47]

Step 3: Cellular and Inflammatory Effectors

The pathophysiology of acute graft-versus-host disease culminates in the generation of multiple cytotoxic effectors of target tissue injury, including several inflammatory cytokines, specific antihost cytotoxic T lymphocytes, NK cells, and nitric oxide. Significant experimental and clinical data suggest that soluble inflammatory mediators act in conjunction with direct cell-mediated cytolysis by cytotoxic T lymphocyte and NK cells to cause the full spectrum of deleterious effects seen during acute graft-versus-host disease. As such, the effector phase of graft-versus-host disease involves aspects of both the innate and adaptive immune response and the synergistic interactions of components generated during step 1 and step 2.

The Fas/FasL and the perforin/granzyme (or granule exocytosis) pathways are the principal effector mechanisms used by cytotoxic T lymphocytes and NK cells to lyse their target cells.[48,49] Perforin is stored together with granzymes and other proteins in cytotoxic granules of cytotoxic T lymphocytes and NK cells; perforin inserts itself into the target cell membrane, forming "perforin pores" that allow granzymes to enter the cell and induce apoptosis through various downstream effector pathways.[50] FasL binds Fas, which results in the formation of the death-inducing signaling complex and the subsequent activation of caspases.[51] A number of T-cell surface proteins also possess the capability to trimerize tumor necrosis factor receptor–like death receptors that also induce apoptosis in their targets.[52–54] $CD4^+$ cytotoxic T lymphocytes preferentially use the Fas/FasL pathway during acute graft-versus-host disease, whereas $CD8^+$ cytotoxic T lymphocytes primarily use the perforin/granzyme pathway, consistent with other conditions involving cell-mediated cytolysis. FasL-defective donor T cells cause markedly reduced experimental graft-versus-host disease in liver, skin, and lymphoid tissue. The Fas/FasL pathway is particularly important in hepatic graft-versus-host disease, consistent with the marked sensitivity of hepatocytes to Fas-mediated cytotoxicity in models of murine hepatitis.[55]

In the effector phase of acute graft-versus-host disease, inflammatory cytokines synergize with cytotoxic T lymphocytes, resulting in the amplification of local tissue injury and the development of target organ dysfunction in the transplant recipient. A central role for inflammatory cytokines in acute graft-versus-host disease was confirmed by a recent murine study using bone marrow chimeras in which target organ injury was induced, even in the absence of epithelial alloantigens, and mortality and target organ injury was prevented by the neutralization of TNF-α and interleukin-1.[2] TNF-α plays a central role in intestinal graft-versus-host disease in murine and human studies.[42,56,57] Two recent studies demonstrated that neutralization of TNF-α alone or in combination with interleukin-1 resulted in a significant reduction of graft-versus-host disease.[2,43] Although neutralization of interleukin-1 with an interleukin-1 receptor antagonist was able to prevent graft-versus-host disease in mice, its use in a randomized clinical trial in humans was not.[44,54]

Macrophages secrete cytokines after ligation of Toll-like receptors by lipopolysaccharide and other microbial products that have leaked though a damaged intestinal mucosa. Because the gastrointestinal tract is known to be particularly sensitive to the injurious effects of cytokines,[56,58] damage to the gastrointestinal tract incurred during the effector phase can lead to a positive feedback loop wherein increased translocation of lipopolysaccharide results in further cytokine production and progressive intestinal injury. Thus, the gastrointestinal tract may be critical to propagating the "cytokine storm" characteristic of acute graft-versus-host disease.[59] Elevated serum levels of lipopolysaccharide have been shown to correlate directly with the degree of intestinal histopathology occurring after allogeneic hematopoietic stem cell transplantation,[58,60,61] and gram-negative gut decontamination during hematopoietic stem cell transplantation has been shown to reduce graft-versus-host disease.[62–65]

Lipopolysaccharide can stimulate inflammatory chemokines that are expressed in inflamed tissues and are specialized to recruit effector cells, such as T cells, neutrophils, and monocytes.[66] Chemokine receptors are differentially expressed on activated T cells that can rapidly switch chemokine receptor expression to acquire new migratory capacity.[13,67] $CCR5^{+}CD8^{+}$ T cells migrate into the liver, lung, and spleen during graft-versus-host disease,[68,69] and levels of several chemokines are elevated in graft-versus-host disease–associated lung injury.[70] The expression of chemokines and their receptors may help to explain the unusual cluster of target organs (skin, gut, and liver).

Clinical Manifestations

Historically, there are three primary target organs of acute graft-versus-host disease: the skin, the gastrointestinal tract, and the liver. Many authorities now believe that the lung is also a target organ, with disease manifesting itself as idiopathic pneumonia syndrome. Acute graft-versus-host disease affects each of these target organs in close temporal proximity. The most common, and often the earliest, clinical sign is a maculopapular skin rash (Fig. 97–2). The rash is often pruritic and can first appear on the upper back, nape of the neck, or torso. It may spread confluently over the entire epidermis, involving the palms and soles in particular. In some cases, the skin may degenerate.

Histologic changes of the skin (Fig. 97–3) involve primarily the epidermis; lymphocytic infiltration of the dermis is often not prominent. Dyskeratotic cells in the epidermis are a characteristic finding, sometimes observed adjacent to lymphocytes in a process called "satellite cell necrosis" (see Fig. 97–3*C*). Complete separation of the epidermis and dermis can be seen in the most severe form.

The gastrointestinal tract is also commonly involved during acute graft-versus-host disease, and may be extremely difficult to treat. The primary manifestation is diarrhea, which is secretory in nature and often exceeds several liters per day. Abdominal cramping frequently accompanies diarrhea. Histologically, apoptotic cells often cluster near the base of the crypts. Discontinuous involvement of the epithelium is the rule, with some areas of completely denuded mucosa that may be adjacent to normal epithelium. Endoscopies or colonoscopies are often performed to sample tissues for diagnosis.

The primary manifestation of graft-versus-host disease in the liver is cholestasis, with predominantly increased conjugated bilirubin. Hepatic enzymes, particularly alkaline phosphatase, may also be elevated, but their involvement is quite variable and they are not included in the standard grading systems. Histologic confirmation of hepatic graft-versus-host disease by biopsy is often not possible, because of thrombocytopenia. Many other complications of hematopoietic stem cell transplantation may elevate serum bilirubin, particularly veno-occlusive disease; thus, hepatic graft-versus-host disease tends to be overdiagnosed. Histologic evidence includes lymphocytic infiltration of the portal triads and bile duct atypia, generation, and dropout.

The overall grade of acute graft-versus-host disease is assigned on a scale of I to IV based on the highest stage in each of these three target organs (Fig. 97–4). Small modifications were made in 1995 to produce consensus criteria. These systemic criteria do not include pulmonary manifestations. The predominance of experimental and clinical evidence favors the inclusion of the lung as a target organ of acute graft-versus-host disease. The primary objection has been the lack of epithelial apoptosis on biopsy. The unique epithelial histology of the lung, which lacks the stratified layers of the skin or the intestine, may help explain this difference. Idiopathic pneumonia syndrome, defined as acute lung injury of noninfectious origin after hematopoietic stem cell transplantation, is currently considered a separate category. Idiopathic pneumonia syndrome occurs in 5–15% of patients, is frequently fatal, and currently has no clear grading system (Fig. 97–5). Histologic findings include perivascular and periluminal infiltrates, as well as alveolar inflammation.

Risk Factors and Prevention

Graft-versus-host disease can thus be considered an exaggerated and dysregulated response of a normal immune system (that of the donor) to tissue damage that

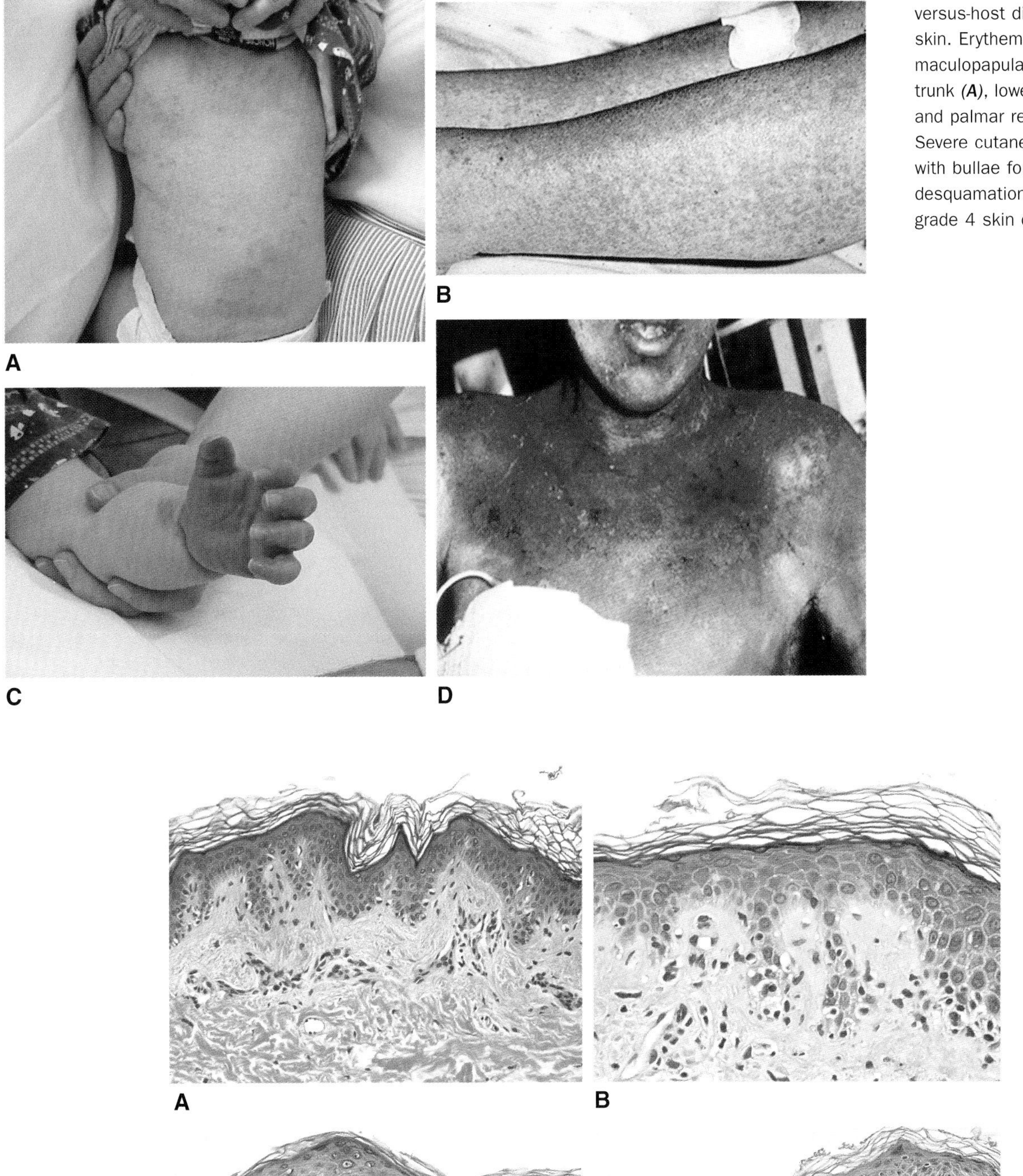

Figure 97–2. Acute graft-versus-host disease of the skin. Erythematous maculopapular rash on the trunk *(**A**)*, lower extremity *(**B**)*, and palmar region *(**C**)*. ***D,*** Severe cutaneous involvement with bullae formation and skin desquamation, as seen with grade 4 skin disease.

Figure 97–3. *A,* Histopathology of normal skin. ***B,*** Histopathology of skin in grade 1 acute graft-versus-host disease. Interface/basal vacuolar change with sparse perivascular lymphocytic infiltrate and exocytosis of inflammatory cells into the dermis. ***C,*** Histopathology of skin in grade 2 acute graft-versus-host disease. Interface vacuolar change, lymphocytic infiltrate, and dyskeratotic cells in the epidermis. Damaged epithelial cells occasionally are surrounded by two or more lymphocytes in a process known as "satellite cell necrosis" *(inset)*. ***D,*** Histopathology of skin in grades 3 and 4 acute graft-versus-host disease. Fusion of the basal vacuoles results in the formation of clefts and microvesicles, characteristic of grade 3 lesions *(inset)*. Subsequent separation of the epidermis from the dermis is seen in grade 4 disease.

ACUTE GVHD STAGING

Stage	Skin[1]	Hepatic[2]	Gastro-intestinal[3]
Stage 1	Maculo-papular rash <25% BSA	Bilirubin 2–3 mg/dl	Diarrhea 500–1,000 ml/day
Stage 2	Maculo-papular rash <25–50% BSA	Bilirubin 3–6 mg/dl	Diarrhea 1,000–1,500 ml/day
Stage 3	Diffuse erythema >50% BSA	Bilirubin 6–15 mg/dl	Diarrhea >1,500 ml/day
Stage 4	Bullae or desquamation	Bilirubin >15 mg/dl	Severe abdominal pain, +/– ileus, or hematochezia

A

Glucksberg et al, Transplantation 18:295–304, 1974

CONSENSUS GRADING CRITERIA: ACUTE GVHD

Grade	Stage
Grade I	Stage 1–2 rash and no liver or gut involvement
Grade II	Stage 3 rash, or stage 1 liver involvement, or stage 1 GI
Grade III	Stage 0–3 skin, with stage 2–3 liver, or stage 2–4 GI
Grade IV	Stage 4 skin, or stage 4 liver involvement

KEY:

BSA = Body surface area

1 For skin staging: Rule of "9's" used

2 For hepatic staging: Bilirubin measurements based upon serum total bilirubin

3 For GI staging: use 3 day averages for stool output. Upper GI involvement present if nausea/vomiting + abdominal endoscopic biopsy present

B

Figure 97–4. Clinical staging and grading of acute graft-versus-host disease. *A,* Modified Glucksberg criteria for staging of individual target organs (skin, liver, gastrointestinal tract) affected by acute graft-versus-host disease. *B,* Consensus criteria for overall grading of acute graft-versus-host disease.

IDIOPATHIC PNEUMONIA SYNDROME (IPS)
Non-infectious, diffuse lung injury following BMT

- Diagnosis criteria:
  a. Diffuse bilateral lung injury on chest radiograph
  b. Clinical signs and symptoms of pneumonia
  c. Abnormal respiratory function (oxygen support)
- Onset: <100 days post transplant
- Histology: Interstitial pneumonitis
- Therapy: Supportive care, +/– corticosteroids
- Clinical trials: Anti-TNF agents, CVVH
- Response rates: Historically poor. Mortality 50–80%

KEY:

TNF = Tumor necrosis factor
CVVH = Continuous veno-venous hemofiltration

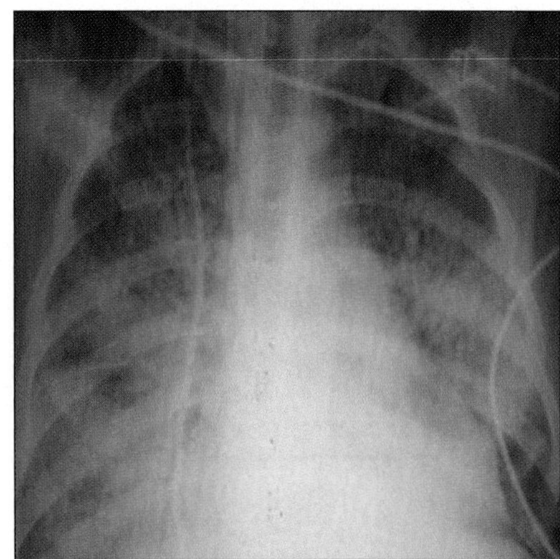

Chest radiograph, IPS

Figure 97–5. Idiopathic pneumonia syndrome: diagnostic criteria, clinical features, and chest radiograph exhibiting diffuse interstitial involvement.

is intrinsic to transplantation. The donor's immune system reacts as if there is a massive and uncontrolled infection, and its efforts to deal with this injury result in the clinical manifestations of graft-versus-host disease. It is quite possible that the tissue injury intrinsic to the administration of high-dose chemoradiotherapy initiates the breakdown of mucosal barriers, allowing endotoxin into the tissues. Toll-like receptors on dendritic cells bind to endotoxin and activate signal transduction pathways that lead to dendritic cell maturation and induce inflammation.[71] The upregulation of costimulatory molecules, major histocompatibility complex molecules, adhesion molecules, cytokines, chemokines, prostanoids, and other inflammatory mediators primes and triggers attack on target tissues, fueling the fire. Thus, it is likely that the danger hypothesis[11] contributes to the "cytokine storm," making graft-versus-host disease a disorder of dysregulated innate and adaptive immune responses. Risk factors for acute graft-versus-host disease can be considered according to the three-step model, as can the prophylactic strategies designed to reduce its morbidity.

Reduced-Intensity Conditioning Regimens

One common thread among target organs is their exposure to the environment. Skin and gut have very obvious barrier functions and a well-developed reticuloendothelial system. Similarly, the liver is the first line of defense downstream of the gut. The lung's less intense exposure to organisms, particularly gram-negative rods, reduces the frequency of its involvement. All these organs are subject to injury from conditioning and breaches of a protective barrier that allows organisms or endotoxin into the circulation. The three-step model predicts that less intense conditioning regimens will be associated with less severe graft-versus-host disease, and that including increased total-body irradiation dose in the conditioning regimen causes worse graft-versus-host disease. Similarly, advanced disease status usually receives additional or more intensive preparative therapy and, thus, indirectly causes more severe graft-versus-host disease. Available data also suggest that the severity of graft-versus-host disease after reduced-intensity regimens is less than that seen after conventional-dose conditioning despite the fact that these patients are at risk for a much more severe form of graft-versus-host disease.[72–75] Increased recipient age is also a risk factor for acute graft-versus-host disease, and this increased risk is due, at least in part, to enhanced activation of host antigen-presenting cells as a function of age.[14]

Modulation of Donor T Cells

Histocompatibility differences between donor and recipient are major determinants of donor T-cell activation and, thus, increased HLA disparity is one of the most important risk factors for acute graft-versus-host disease. Female donors, particularly those with multiple pregnancies, cause greater graft-versus-host disease in male recipients because proteins encoded on the Y chromosome can serve as minor histocompatibility antigens in male recipients.

The number of T cells in the donor marrow is directly associated with the severity of acute graft-versus-host disease, and T-cell depletion is one of the most effective forms of prophylaxis; a T-cell dose of 10^5/kg or less was associated with complete control of graft-versus-host disease if an HLA-identical sibling served as the donor.[76] The combination of very high stem cell numbers and CD3 T-cell numbers less than 3×10^4/kg allowed haploidentical transplantation without graft-versus-host disease.[77] Unfortunately, the nonspecific removal or clearance of T cells results in increased fatal opportunistic infections, resulting in equivalent overall survival.[78–80]

The first generally prescribed preventive regimen was the administration of intermittent low-dose methotrexate immediately after bone marrow transplantation, when T cells will have started to divide after exposure to allogeneic antigens.[44] The introduction of cyclosporine in the late 1970s was a significant advance in graft-versus-host disease prevention. As a single agent, cyclosporine is about as effective as methotrexate alone; however, in combination with methotrexate, cyclosporine significantly reduces graft-versus-host disease and improves survival.[81,82] Inability to deliver optimal doses of cyclosporine and methotrexate because of organ toxicity is also a risk factor for mucosal graft-versus-host disease. More recently, a similar agent, tacrolimus, has shown similar control. Both drugs inhibit T-lymphocyte activation by binding to immunophilins; cyclosporine binds cyclophilin and tacrolimus binds FKBP-12. The net result is the inhibition of T-lymphocyte activation (reviewed by Vander Woude and Bierer[83]). Subsequent comparisons of tacrolimus versus cyclosporine in combination with methotrexate showed no advantage for either combination.[84,85] The addition of prednisone to the conventional two-drug regimen also did not improve protection against graft-versus-host disease.[86]

More recently, mycophenolate mofetil, an inhibitor of the de novo pathway of guanosine nucleotide synthesis, has been studied. Because T lymphocytes are dependent on de novo synthesis of purines, mycophenolate mofetil inhibits proliferative responses of T cells to both mitogenic and allogeneic stimulation. Myeloid and mucosal cells can utilize salvage pathways, so the drug is less toxic to mucosa and myeloid recovery. Mycophenolate mofetil does not inhibit the activation of T cells as such, but blocks the coupling of activation to DNA synthesis and proliferation.[87] Recent limited trials of the combination of mycophenolate mofetil with cyclosporine or tacrolimus are promising.[75,88–90] The most common approaches to chemical control of donor T cells as prophylaxis for graft-versus-host disease are schematized in Figure 97–6.

Blockade of Inflammatory Stimuli and Effectors

Elimination of intestinal colonization with bacteria reduces graft-versus-host disease by minimizing the triggering signal for monocytes and macrophages, as well as minimizing the actuation of antigen-presenting cells. The first indication that elimination of exposure to microor-

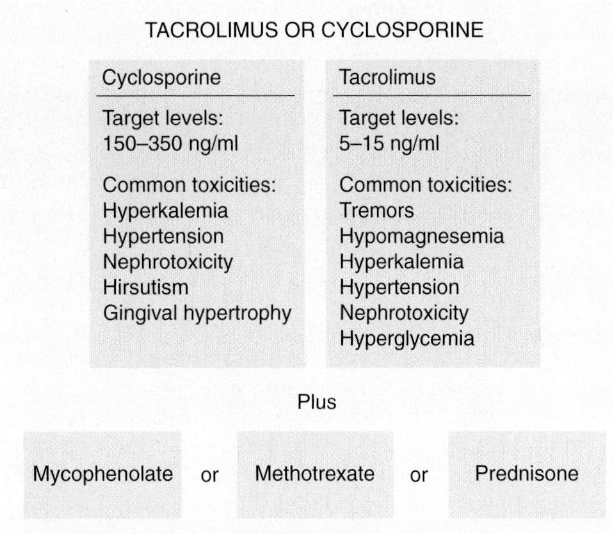

Figure 97–6. Common methods of prophylaxis for acute graft-versus-host disease include either tacrolimus or cyclosporine combined with one of the following: methotrexate, or mycophenolate, or prednisone. Common toxicities associated with tacrolimus and cyclosporine are included.

ganisms could prevent graft-versus-host disease was in germ-free experiments in mice, wherein graft-versus-host disease was not observed until the mice were colonized with gram-negative organisms.[91] In a later study, gut decontamination and use of a laminar airflow environment was associated with less graft-versus-host disease and better survival in patients with severe aplastic anemia.[62]

As alluded to earlier, an important role for TNF-α in clinical acute graft-versus-host disease was suggested by studies demonstrating elevated levels of TNF-α in the serum of patients with acute disease and other endothelial complications, such as veno-occlusive disease.[92–94] Recently, therapy of graft-versus-host disease with humanized anti–TNF-α (infliximab)[95,96] or a dimeric tumor necrosis factor receptor fusion protein (etanercept) has shown some promise.[97] More studies are required to understand the pharmacokinetics and proper use of these agents after allogeneic transplantation, because tumor necrosis factor inhibition may increase the risk of opportunistic infections.

Two Phase I/II trials showed promising data that specific inhibition of interleukin-1, with either the soluble interleukin-1 receptor or interleukin-1 receptor antagonist, could result in remissions in 50–60% of patients with steroid-resistant graft-versus-host disease.[98,99] However, a randomized trial of the addition of interleukin-1 receptor antagonist or placebo to cyclosporine and methotrexate did not show any protective effect of the drug, despite attaining very high plasma levels.[44] Interleukin-11 was able to protect the gastrointestinal tract in animal models and prevent graft-versus-host disease,[100,101] but it did not prevent clinical disease.[102] Thus, not all preclinical data successfully translate to new therapies.

Primary Therapy

High-dose corticosteroids are the backbone of primary therapy for significant (grade II–IV) acute graft-versus-host disease. Calcineurin inhibitor (cyclosporine or tacrolimus) levels should be optimized, prior to the initiation of steroid therapy. A wide variety of corticosteroid doses and schedules have been utilized, with the majority of patients receiving at least 2 mg/kg/day of prednisone equivalent. Systemic corticosteroid therapy has generally been reserved for patients with Glucksberg grade II (or higher) acute graft-versus-host disease.[103–105] Recent trials comparing 2 mg/kg to 10 mg/kg/day of corticosteroids have not shown a survival advantage with higher dosing.[104] Complete response rates of 25–35% have been reported using corticosteroids as front-line therapy.[106,107] Extended taper schedules of several months do not appear to provide a long-term survival advantage. Topical therapy, without the use of systemic corticosteroids, is often employed in the treatment of grade I graft-versus-host disease that is limited to the skin.

Salvage Therapy

Patients with progressive graft-versus-host disease and those who remain steroid dependent (i.e., their disease flares during their steroid taper) require additional therapy. A number of agents have been utilized in this scenario, including (1) immunosuppressants with broad anti–T-cell specificity (mycophenolate, rapamycin, antithymocyte globulin); (2) blockade of inflammatory cytokines (TNF-α antagonists, interleukin-1 receptor antagonist); and (3) agents targeting T-cell activation molecules (anti-CD25 antibodies, interleukin-2 antagonists).

Substitution of one calcineurin inhibitor for another, such as tacrolimus for cyclosporine, is occasionally successful in patients with unresponsive disease or with toxic side effects.[108] The development of tacrolimus-related neurotoxicity or nephrotoxicity is a common reason for switching to cyclosporine. Horse or rabbit antithymocyte globulin has been widely used as a second-line agent, with response rates of 30–70%.[109–112] However, infectious complications of antithymocyte globulin are common, and long-term survival rates remain poor. OKT3, a broad anti-CD3 monoclonal antibody, has some efficacy but is associated with frequent infectious complications.[113]

Drugs that target activation molecules are generally more specific and cause fewer side effects than agents with broad anti–T-cell activity. Agents such as daclizumab, etanercept, and infliximab are currently being studied for their role in this clinical setting. Daclizumab, a humanized anti-CD25 monoclonal antibody, has shown promise in recent trials. High response rates (50–70%) and long-term survival of 30–50% has been reported.[114,115] A trial of recombinant interleukin-1 receptor antagonist resulted in rapid responses in patients with cutaneous or gastrointestinal graft-versus-host disease, but without long-term survival benefits.[99] Infliximab, a murine-human chimeric IgG1κ monoclonal antibody, binds tightly to both the soluble and transmembrane forms of TNF-α.[116] As a result, TNF-α cannot bind to its cellular receptor, thereby inhibiting an important inflammatory effector pathway of acute graft-versus-host disease. Recent clinical trials using this agent have been promising, especially in the setting of gastrointestinal graft-versus-host disease.[95,117] Etanercept, a soluble tumor necrosis factor receptor antagonist, has likewise shown promise in preclinical and clinical trials, with responses noted in patients with acute graft-versus-host disease and/or idiopathic pneumonia syndrome posttransplantation.[43,97,118–120]

Impact on Survival and Quality of Life

Despite the use of broad immunosuppressive agents and target-specific therapy, the prognosis for patients with severe (grade III/IV) acute graft-versus-host disease remains poor. Limited progress has been made in the treatment of steroid-refractory graft-versus-host disease. Only 10% of patients who develop grade IV graft-versus-host disease will survive longer than 1 year, and acute disease often progresses to become extensive chronic graft-versus-host disease, which has significant effects on quality of life (see later). The identification of high-risk patients based upon cytokine genotype polymorphisms, the development of novel preemptive strategies, and newer therapies targeting not just T cells but other effector cells, including endothelial cells and donor-derived macrophages, are active areas of investigation.

CHRONIC GRAFT-VERSUS-HOST DISEASE

Classification

Chronic graft-versus-host disease is a leading cause of morbidity and mortality in long-term survivors of allogeneic hematopoietic stem cell transplantation.[121] It is traditionally defined to occur at least 100 days following an allogeneic transplantation, but the temporal definition is increasingly unsatisfactory, especially in the context of the low-intensity regimens that are now being widely used. Many symptoms of acute graft-versus-host disease are recognized to appear later than 100 days after hematopoietic stem cell transplantation, or following donor lymphocyte infusion. Approximately 40% of patients who survive more than 100 days following receipt of an HLA-identical sibling transplant, and over 50% of patients surviving receipt of an alternative donor transplant, will develop clinically significant chronic graft-versus-host disease.[122,123] The clinical course is variable, ranging from limited cutaneous involvement to protracted, multiorgan dysfunction and a significant impairment in quality of life.

The histologic findings and clinical features characteristic of chronic graft-versus-host disease may develop as early as 50 days posttransplantation, and those of acute graft-versus-host disease may begin following day 100. The classification schema presented here incorporates a number of additional factors: (1) the extent of organ involvement, (2) the presence or absence of prior acute graft-versus-host disease, and (3) the number of high-risk features (Fig. 97–7). In the majority of cases, chronic graft-versus-host disease develops as a progression or consequence of prior acute graft-versus-host disease. In approximately 20% of cases, however, chronic graft-versus-host disease may develop de novo, without prior acute disease.[123] De novo chronic graft-versus-host disease typically carries a more favorable prognosis than other forms.

The Seattle staging system of "limited versus extensive" chronic graft-versus-host disease is the most widely used[124] (Box 97–1). In this classification, limited chronic graft-versus-host disease is defined as localized skin involvement with or without concurrent hepatic dysfunction. Extensive chronic graft-versus-host disease is defined as either generalized skin involvement or limited

CHRONIC GVHD
Classification Schema

A BY PRIOR HISTORY
- De novo chronic GVHD
- Prior acute GVHD

B BY ORGAN CRITERIA

Limited:
- Limited skin +/– hepatic

Extensive:
- Generalized skin, or
- Limited skin, plus
  - Ocular, or
  - Oral, or
  - GI, or
  - Hepatic (+ biopsy)

C BY PROGNOSTIC RISK FACTORS

High risk:
- >50% skin involvement
- Progressive acute GVHD
- Platelet count <100 X 10^9/L

Low risk:
- <50% skin involvement
- No prior acute GVHD
- Platelet count >100 X 10^9/L

Figure 97–7. Classification schema for chronic graft-versus-host disease, based upon *(A)* prior history of timing of onset, *(B)* by the extent of organ involvement, or *(C)* the number of prognostic risk factors present.

TABLE 97–1. Diagnostic Evaluation for Chronic Graft-Versus-Host Disease

Organ System	Clinical Examination Findings & Symptoms	Diagnostic Testing
Cutaneous	Dyspigmentation, scleroderma, morphea, alopecia, onychodystrophy, lichen planus	Skin biopsy—punch
Hepatic	Jaundice, rare hepatomegaly	ALT, bilirubin
Hematologic	Immune-mediated thrombocytopenia	Complete blood counts
	Immune-mediated hemolytic anemia	Coombs testing
Gastrointestinal	Diarrhea, anorexia, weight loss	Endoscopy, colonoscopy
	Odynophagia, dysphagia, abdominal pain	Calorie counts
Immunodeficiency	CMV disease, varicella reactivation, fungal disease, oral thrush, sinusitis, streptococcal pneumonia	Serologic testing
Musculoskeletal	Scleroderma, fasciitis, myositis	Range-of-motion tests
	Weakness, cramps, joint contractures	CPK, muscle biopsy
Performance status	Disability, depression, anxiety	Karnofsky status, "quality of life" assessment
Pulmonary	Dyspnea on exertion, hypoxemia, fatigue, cough, wheezing	Pulmonary function tests, high-resolution chest CT, bronchoalveolar lavage
Ocular	Ocular "sicca," keratoconjunctivitis, cataracts (steroid related), photophobia	Schirmer test, slit-lamp examination
Oral	Lichenoid changes, xerostomia	Lip biopsy
Vaginal	Vaginal dryness, vaginal strictures	Gynecologic examination

Abbreviations: ALT, alanine aminotransferase; CMV, cytomegalovirus; CPK, creatine phosphokinase; CT, computed tomography.

Box 97–1. Classification of Chronic Graft-Versus-Host Disease by Organ Criteria

Limited Chronic Graft-Versus-Host Disease

- Localized skin involvement, *and/or*
- Hepatic dysfunction resulting from chronic graft-versus-host disease

Extensive Chronic Graft-Versus-Host Disease

- Generalized skin involvement, *or*
- Localized skin involvement and/or hepatic dysfunction, *PLUS*
  - Histology with chronic aggressive hepatitis, bridging necrosis, or cirrhosis, *or*
  - Ocular involvement (by Schirmer testing), *or*
  - Involvement of minor salivary glands or oral mucosa on labial biopsy, *or*
  - Involvement of any other target organ

skin disease in addition to involvement of other organs, including eyes, oral cavity, lungs, and liver. Unfortunately, the application of these criteria is inconsistent, reflecting the difficulties in using nonquantitative end points.

The diagnosis of chronic graft-versus-host disease requires the presence of at least one manifestation of the disorder. Biopsies or other diagnostic tests (i.e., pulmonary function testing, Schirmer testing) should be performed, if possible, in order to rule out alternative (especially infectious) etiologies (Table 97–1). The clinical manifestations of chronic graft-versus-host disease often parallel those seen in autoimmune conditions, and include keratoconjunctivitis and xerophthalmia (ocular sicca), xerostomia, lichen planus, scleroderma, fasciitis, morphea, serositis, esophageal strictures, obstructive hepatic disease, and obstructive lung disease (bronchiolitis obliterans). The skin and oral mucosa are the most common sites of involvement, often involved in 50–75% of cases.[123,125,126] Gastrointestinal/esophageal disease and bronchiolitis obliterans have been reported in approximately 10–20% of cases.[123,125,126]

Recently, grading criteria for chronic graft-versus-host disease based upon survival parameters have been proposed.[123,127–129] Factors reported in association with poor survival include thrombocytopenia (<100 × 10^9/L), extensive skin involvement (>50% body surface area), impaired performance status (Karnofsky score), gastrointestinal involvement, and a progressive onset from acute graft-versus-host disease.[123,127–129] Incomplete or partial response to therapy has also been associated with poor survival, with patients surviving less than 6 months post-transplantation.[127] The Hopkins group has recently proposed stratifying patients by the number of risk factors, with the presence of one or more being associated with increasing non–relapse-related mortality.[129]

Pathophysiology

Whereas our understanding of the pathophysiology, prevention, and treatment of acute graft-versus-host disease has grown significantly in recent years, similar gains have not been made in chronic graft-versus-host disease. Mechanistic pathways have yet to be clearly identified, in part because animal models have been significantly less informative. Experimental chronic graft-versus-host disease exhibits features similar to autoimmune conditions, with a predominant lymphocyte shift from a T_H1 toward a T_H2 phenotype.[130] T cells from animals with

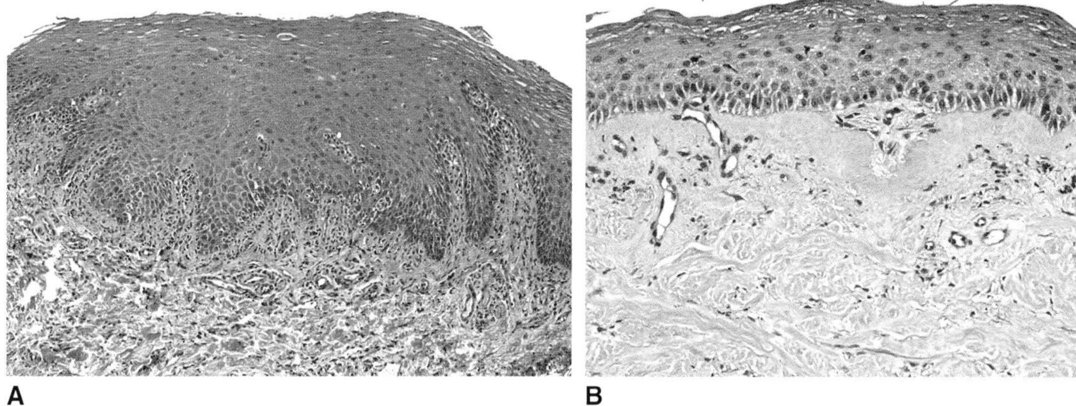

Figure 97–8. *A,* Histopathology of skin in early chronic-phase graft-versus-host disease. Lichenoid lesions display acanthosis, satellite cell necrosis, basal cell degeneration, and a lymphocytic infiltrate that is mainly below the epidermis. Lesions may closely resemble lichen planus or show features similar to those seen in acute graft-versus-host disease. ***B,*** Histopathology of skin in late chronic-phase graft-versus-host disease. Sclerodermoid pattern with epidermal atrophy, thick and hyalinized collagen bundles in the dermis with extension into subcutis, and resultant atrophy of adnexal structures.

chronic graft-versus-host disease produce unusual patterns of cytokines, such as interleukin-4 or interferon-γ (in the absence of interleukin-2,) and can stimulate collagen production by fibroblasts. Interestingly, eosinophilia is often present as an early manifestation of chronic graft-versus-host disease, further supporting the notion that cells with a T_H2 cytokine profile are important mediators of this problem.[131] Donor $CD4^+$ T-cell activation in the absence of $CD8^+$ T-cell activation can result in impaired elimination of autoreactive B cells, and humoral autoimmunity.[132] Anti-CD20 monoclonal antibody (rituximab) has recently been used clinically to treat severe autoimmune disorders,[133] and recently chronic graft-versus-host disease.[134] Autoimmune phenomena may be explained by the massive apoptosis of T cells early in acute graft-versus-host disease, the disposal of which overwhelms the macrophage/dendritic cell system, resulting in inappropriate presentation of autoantigens.[135] The autoreactive immune cells of chronic graft-versus-host disease are associated with a damaged thymus, which may be injured by acute graft-versus-host disease, by the conditioning regimen, or by age-related involution and atrophy. Thus, the normal ability of the thymus to delete autoreactive T cells and to induce tolerance may contribute to chronic graft-versus-host disease, although such a relationship has not been demonstrated clinically.

Clinical Manifestations

Skin

Cutaneous chronic graft-versus-host disease presents as either a lichenoid eruption, sclerodermatous involvement (Fig. 97–8), or a combination of both. Lichenoid changes are common early in the course of chronic graft-versus-host disease, and are best characterized as patchy, erythematous rashes resembling lichen planus (Fig. 97–9).

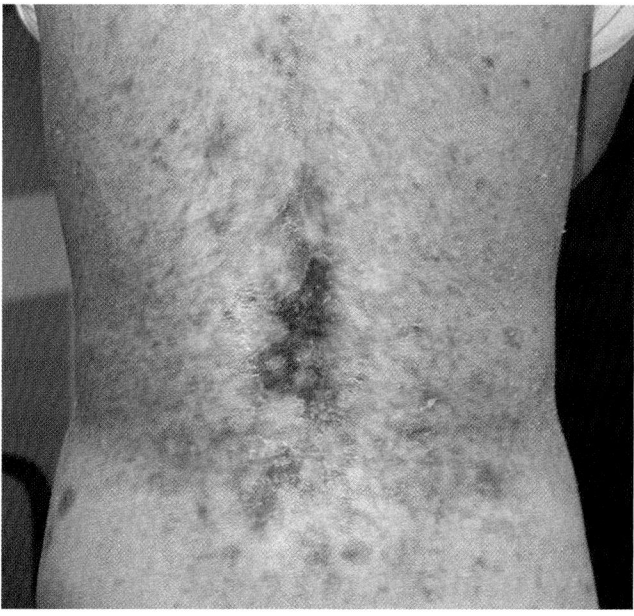

Figure 97–9. Extensive lichen planus with ulcerations on the posterior truncal surface.

Lichenoid changes are often noted in the facial region (periorbital), palms/soles, and genitourinary region (vaginal or glans penis). Sclerodermatous changes typically develop later, and may resemble those seen in systemic sclerosis. Thickened skin with marked dyspigmentation, especially in pressure areas such as the bra or belt line, is commonly noted. Areas of both hypopigmentation (morphea) and hyperpigmentation are described, often in close association with each other (Fig. 97–10). Sclerotic changes may affect other epithelial structures, including hair growth, nail beds, and sweat glands. Periungual erythema with cracking and linear ridges over the nail surface is common (Fig. 97–11).

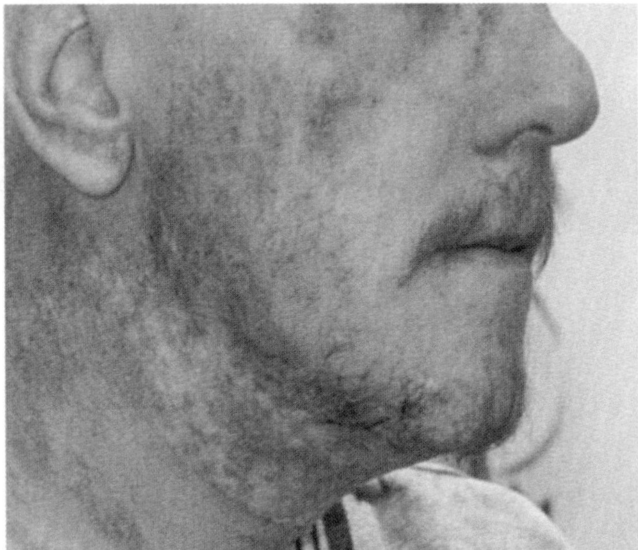

■ **Figure 97–10.** Dyspigmentary changes associated with chronic graft-versus-host disease. Patches of hypopigmentation (morphea) and hyperpigmentation are noted in the mandibular region, in close association with each other.

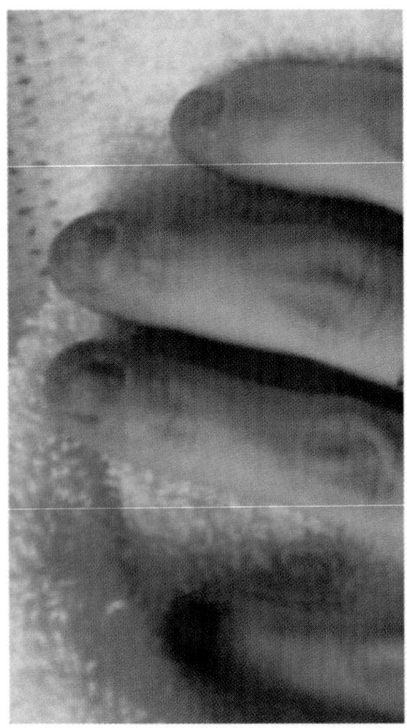

■ **Figure 97–11.** Periungual erythema and dyskeratotic nail changes.

Fasciitis, leading to a "cobblestone appearance of the skin," may develop as a result of subcutaneous tissue inflammation and subsequent fibrotic changes within the subcutaneous tissue.

Oral Cavity

Oral graft-versus-host disease may range from mild buccal erythema to significant leukoplakia, lichen planus, xerostomia, and perioral restriction. Xerostomia occurs as a consequence of salivary gland dysfunction. Histologically, lymphocytic changes in labial salivary glands may lead to inflammation, and eventual xerostomia. Such xerostomia may persist for months or years, even when other sites of chronic graft-versus-host disease are quiescent. The loss of salivary gland function greatly increases the risk of dental caries. Nystatin, with its high glucose content, may also increase this risk, and should be avoided in such patients. Oral salivary preparations, oral corticosteroid rinses, and even pilocarpine have been utilized for xerostomia with various amounts of success.[136–141] Secondary viral infections, such as herpes simplex, are common, and should be suspected in individuals with significant oral mucositis developing after primary engraftment. Antibiotic prophylaxis should be considered in all patients with chronic graft-versus-host disease who are undertaking dental procedures, even if a central line is no longer present.

Eyes

Ocular chronic graft-versus-host disease presents with signs of keratoconjunctivitis (ocular sicca). Signs and symptoms include corneal dryness, photophobia, and pain as a result of progressive lacrimal gland dysfunction. Ocular involvement in chronic graft-versus-host disease is quite common and may occur in over 50% of patients. The keratopathy must be recognized early in order to prevent corneal abrasions and scarring. A Schirmer tests for ocular dryness should be performed routinely in all patients with chronic graft-versus-host disease. Patients should be treated with protective eyewear, ocular lubricants, and ophthalmic ointments at night. As lacrimal gland dysfunction progresses, punctual occlusion/plugs may prevent corneal dryness. Moisturizing contact lens or moisture chamber eyeglasses have been developed and may provide symptomatic relief.[142]

Lungs

Obstructive lung disease is a well-recognized posttransplantation complication, occurring in up to 25% of allogeneic transplant recipients.[143–146] Patients typically present 3–12 months posttransplantation with cough, wheezing, or dyspnea on exertion as the predominant presenting features. Recurrent bronchitis and sinusitis are common complications. Frequent infections and colonization with fungal or *Pseudomonas* species are seen as a result of poor mechanical clearance in patients with compromised immunologic function.

Obstructive lung disease is identified on pulmonary function testing (spirometry) by a forced expiratory volume or forced expiratory volume/forced vital capacity less than 80% of predicted, together with a 10% decline from baseline. These changes reflect enhanced airflow resistance upon expiration, and correlate with narrowing or destruction of smaller airways and terminal bronchioles. Bronchiolitis obliterans remains the most common histopathology associated with obstructive lung disease (Fig. 97–12*A*). The clinical course of this syndrome is variable, ranging from a gradual decline in function over several years to a rapid pulmonary deterioration

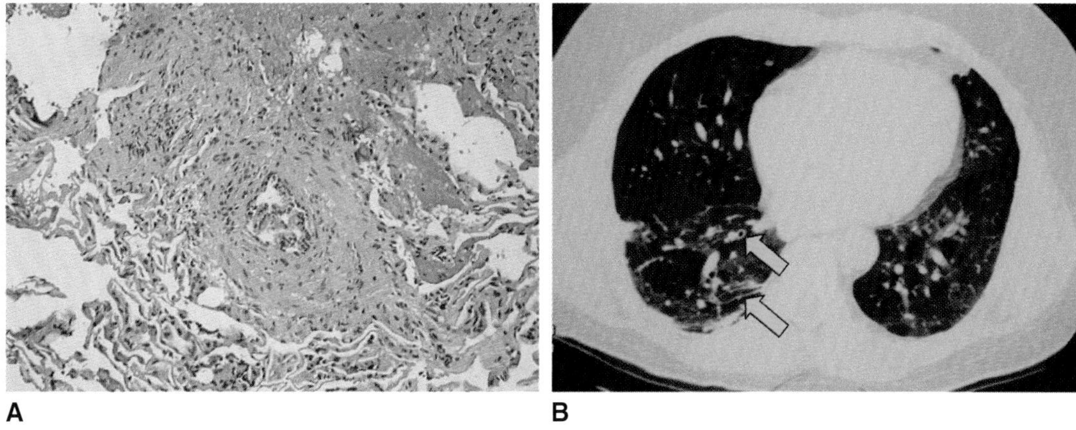

Figure 97–12. *A,* Histopathology (transbronchial biopsy) of the cicatricial form of obstructive lung disease (bronchiolitis obliterans), characterized by concentric, periluminal fibrous bands, with complete obliteration of small airways (100×). *B,* High-resolution computed tomography scan of patient with bronchiolitis obliterans syndrome. Note bronchiectasis *(arrows)*, air space disease, and peripheral centrilobular nodules.

over a few months. Responses to immunosuppressive therapy have been limited, usually resulting in preservation of existing lung function.[147,148] Historically, the mortality of patients with bronchiolitis obliterans syndrome is high.[147] In severe cases, lung allografts have been successfully performed.

Plain films of the chest in patients with bronchiolitis obliterans syndrome are often unremarkable, with hyperinflation on end-expiratory films as the primary radiographic feature. High-resolution computed tomography is required to optimally define the severity of disease (Fig. 97–12*B*). Common computed tomography findings include (1) bronchiectasis, (2) air trapping, (3) the presence of centrilobular nodules, and (4) ground-glass opacifications. Bronchiectasis and air trapping are characteristic of small airway disease, whereas centrilobular nodules represent peribronchiolar inflammation or fibrosis pathologically.

The pathophysiology of bronchiolitis obliterans syndrome has yet to be clearly defined (Fig. 97–13). The development of obstructive lung disease and bronchiolitis obliterans syndrome is characterized by bronchiolar leukocyte recruitment leading to fibrinous obliteration of the airway.[144,149–151] The mechanism of injury likely involves small airway epithelial injury followed by an ongoing inflammatory response. The severity of the injury parallels the duration of this inflammatory response. Compared to healthy transplant recipients, bronchoalveolar lavage fluid from patients with bronchiolitis obliterans syndrome reveals elevations in interleukin-1 receptor antagonist, interleukin-8, TGF-β, and MCP-1, all of which have been implicated in other fibroproliferative processes.[152–155]

Bone Marrow

The hematologic findings of chronic graft-versus-host disease include thrombocytopenia, hemolytic anemias, and neutropenias.[156,157] The hematologic abnormalities may be a consequence of immune-mediated stromal injury or peripheral destruction. As earlier described, the presence of thrombocytopenia ($<100 \times 10^9$/L) has been associated with a poor long-term outcome.[129] Coombs-positive hemolytic anemias are not uncommon, with variable response to corticosteroids or anti-CD20 antibody therapy.[158]

Liver

Hepatic manifestations of chronic graft-versus-host disease may include cholestatic jaundice, with increased serum conjugated bilirubin levels. In other cases, an acute hepatitis with elevations in serum transaminases is observed.[159] Ursodiol prophylaxis has been used in an attempt to minimize posttransplantation hepatic cholestasis. Hepatic biopsies often reveal biliary ductal damage or bridging necrosis,[126,160] and are often required to differentiate the hepatic findings of chronic graft-versus-host disease from infectious or noninfectious etiologies, including iron overload and drug effects.

Gastrointestinal Tract

Distinguishing the manifestations of acute versus chronic graft-versus-host disease in the gastrointestinal tract can sometimes be quite problematic. Gastrointestinal involvement developing in acute graft-versus-host disease, including diarrhea and abdominal discomfort, may persist past day 100. Gastric dysmotility and malabsorption may result from either form, though more commonly they are associated with acute graft-versus-host disease. Esophageal involvement (dysphagia and odynophagia) may be reflected by a number of pathologic findings, including esophagitis, ulcerations, esophageal webs, and/or stricture formation. Anorexia is also a common finding associated with chronic graft-versus-host disease, often pronounced in patients undergoing a prolonged corticosteroid taper during their course of therapy.

Immune System

Infectious complications that develop because of the prolonged immune dysfunction of chronic graft-versus-host

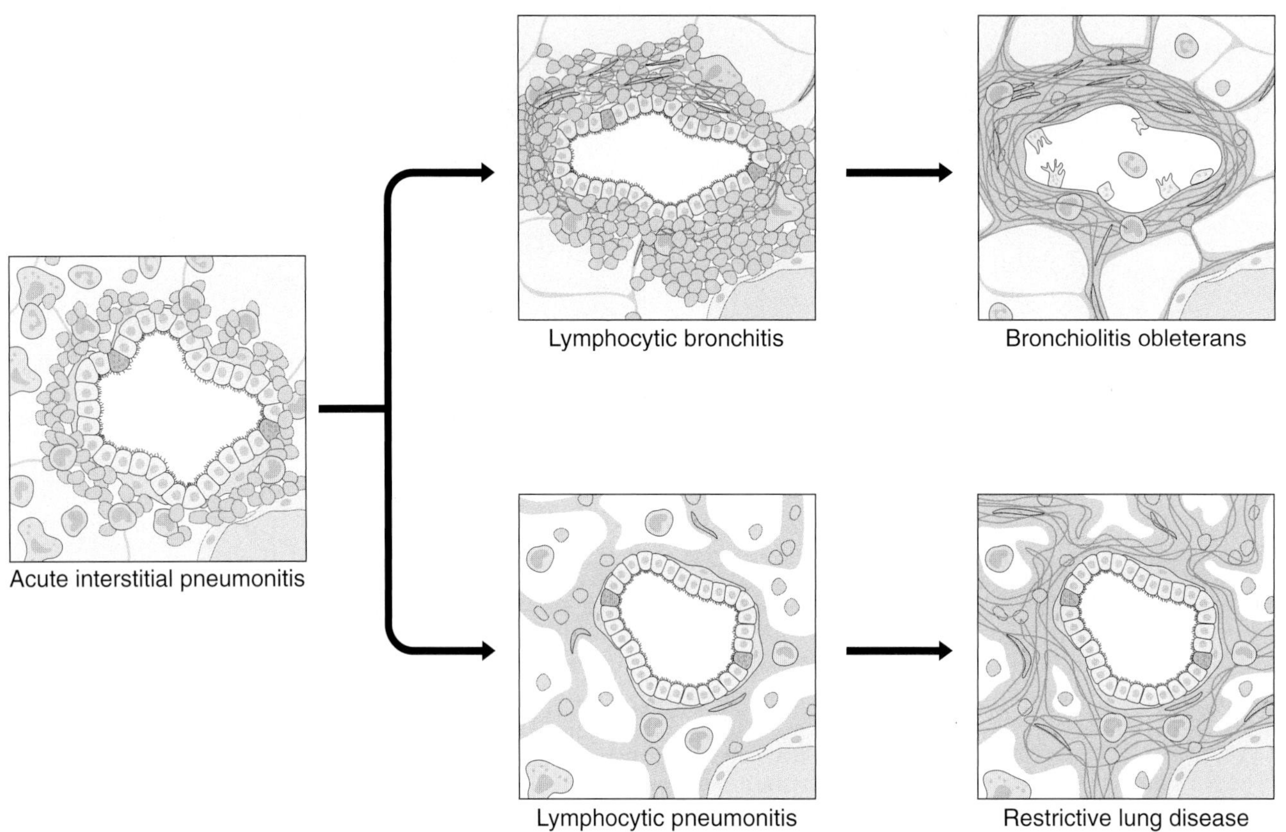

Figure 97–13. The development of chronic lung injury, both restrictive and obstructive lung disease, may be viewed from a triphasic model. ***A,*** The first phase of disease, occurring early after allogeneic transplantation, is characterized by an acute interstitial pneumonitis with peribronchial inflammation, initiated by the production of pro-inflammatory cytokines. ***B*** and ***C,*** In the second stage, a chronic lymphocytic bronchitis/pneumonitis develops as a consequence of this persistent pro-inflammatory milieu. During this phase, alterations in the normal reparative capacity of the lung occur, thereby promoting the transition from acute to chronic lung injury. This transition is accompanied by a change in the character of the interstitial infiltrate to one that is predominantly lymphocytic in nature, along with a shift to a profibrotic environment. ***D,*** When inflammation of the airway epithelium predominates, an obstructive lung disease develops. ***E,*** When epithelial cells in the alveolar septa are the principal targets of injury, interstitial thickening, septal fibrosis, and loss of alveolar architecture occur, leading to the development of a restrictive lung process.

disease are a source of significant morbidity and mortality.[161–167] These infections include cytomegalovirus, varicella reactivation, bacteria (especially in the sinopulmonary tract), invasive fungi, and atypical mycobacteria. *Pneumocystis jiroveci* (*carinii*) also occurs, and prophylaxis is required and should be administered while patients remain on immunosuppressive therapy. Functional asplenia leads to an increased risk of encapsulated bacterial infections, including *Streptococcus pneumoniae* and invasive *Haemophilus influenzae* type B. Antipneumococcal prophylaxis therefore should be strongly considered in all patients receiving prolonged immunosuppressive therapy, and is mandatory if circulating Howell-Jolly bodies are noted on peripheral blood smear. A combination of impaired epithelial integrity (cutaneous/gastrointestinal), abnormal pulmonary clearance mechanisms, diminished T- and B-cell numbers and function, and immunosuppressive therapy increases the risk of opportunistic infections in patients with chronic graft-versus-host disease.[163–165]

Other Organs

Anasarca, peripheral edema, pleural effusions, joint effusions, and pericardial effusions have all been associated with extensive chronic graft-versus-host disease. The pathophysiology behind these processes is unclear. Pericardial and pleural effusions may be associated with local complications, necessitating drainage procedures. Peripheral neuropathies, myositis, and myasthenia gravis are well-recognized neuromuscular complications.[168–170] It may be difficult to differentiate the neuromuscular effects of chronic graft-versus-host disease from effects of medications such as corticosteroids, tacrolimus, or cyclosporine. Vaginal involvement with lichenoid vulvar changes, vaginal dryness, and often vaginal strictures may

TABLE 97–2. Risk Factors Associated with the Development of Chronic Graft-Versus-Host Disease

Generally Accepted Factors	Factors under Consideration
Alternative donor sources	Increased CD34 cell count in graft
Use of peripheral stem cells	Lower incidence with cord blood
Increased patient age	Increasing donor age
Presence of acute graft-versus-host disease	Busulfan in conditioning regimen
Use of T-cell–depleted grafts	Female donor to male recipient
Donor lymphocyte infusions	

TABLE 97–3. Cumulative Incidence of Chronic Graft-Versus-Host Disease (GVHD) in Recipients of Peripheral Blood or Bone Marrow, Related-Donor Transplants

			Chronic GVHD	
Author	Randomized	No. Patients	Allogeneic PSC	Bone Marrow
Blaise (2001)	Yes	111	54%	30%
Bensinger (2001)	Yes	172	46%	35%
Schmitz (2002)	Yes	350	67%	54%
Couban (2002)	Yes	228	40%	30%
Flowers (2002)	Yes	126	63%	52%
Anderson (2003)	No	194	37%	28%
Total		986	55% ± 7	42% ± 7

*P value < .0001.
Abbreviation: PSC, peripheral stem cells.

develop. Topical corticosteroids or surgical dilation can produce symptomatic relief. Endocrine dysfunction, including hypothyroidism, irregular menses, and growth delays, has been reported. In particular, children may develop significant morbidity related to prolonged corticosteroid use, with growth arrest/short stature, delayed secondary sexual characteristics, and avascular necrosis.[171]

Risk Factors and Prevention

A number of factors have been identified that are associated with the development of chronic graft-versus-host disease (Table 97–2). HLA disparity, the presence of prior acute graft-versus-host disease, older patient age, the use of alternative donors (mismatched or unrelated), the use of peripheral stem cells as the donor source, the administration of donor lymphocyte infusions posttransplantation, and the use of non–T-cell–depleted grafts have all been identified by one or more groups.[125,126,172,173] In particular, the use of peripheral stem cells has been associated with chronic graft-versus-host disease rates in excess of 50% among recipients of HLA-matched sibling transplants.[174–180] Data combined from 16 studies noted a relative risk of extensive chronic graft-versus-host disease of 1.66 (95% confidence interval, 1.35–2.05; $P < .001$) for peripheral stem cell grafts compared to bone marrow grafts.[181] Higher CD34 cell counts in peripheral stem cell grafts (<8.0 × 10^6 CD34 cells/kg) have been reported in association with increased extensive chronic graft-versus-host disease rates.[182] Of note, CD34 counts did not correlate with CD3 counts in this report. Overall, chronic graft-versus-host disease rates in recipients of peripheral stem cells appear to be approximately 15% higher than observed among bone marrow recipients (Table 97–3).

The impact of the conditioning regimen upon the incidence of chronic graft-versus-host disease remains controversial. A meta-analysis of five prospective, randomized trials that compared busulfan-based regimens to total-body irradiation–based regimens found no significant differences in chronic graft-versus-host disease rates.[183] In contrast, Ringden and associates noted an increased risk of chronic graft-versus-host disease (59% vs. 47%) and obstructive bronchiolitis (26% vs. 5%) in recipients of a busulfan-based regimen.[184] The issue remains somewhat controversial, because other trials have failed to show similar differences in chronic graft-versus-host disease rates.[185]

Factors that do not appear to impact chronic graft-versus-host disease rates include the use of tacrolimus versus cyclosporine prophylaxis,[85] the deletion of the day 11 methotrexate dose,[186,187] or the use of non-busulfan conditioning regimens.

In contrast to advances in the management of acute graft-versus-host disease, advances in chronic graft-versus-host disease therapy have been slow. Strategies to reduce the severity of acute graft-versus-host disease, the primary risk factor for the development of the chronic form, have not always led to decreased rates of chronic graft-versus-host disease. T-cell depletion reduces the risk of chronic graft-versus-host disease by approximately 50%, though increases in overall survival have not been noted.[188] Cord blood transplantation has been associated with less acute and chronic graft-versus-host disease.[189,190] By contrast, preemptive therapy, based upon early screening tests (day 100 skin and lip biopsies) for chronic graft-versus-host disease, has not led to improvements in response.[191]

Primary Therapy

Historically, cyclosporine (or tacrolimus) plus prednisone have been the primary therapy for extensive chronic graft-versus-host disease. Alternating-day azathioprine and prednisone was superior to prednisone alone (5-year survival rates 50% vs. 26%).[192] However, a randomized trial comparing cyclosporine plus prednisone to prednisone alone as front-line therapy for chronic graft-versus-host disease did not show an improvement in response, survival, need for salvage therapy, or relapse rate. Though treatment with the two-drug regimen reduced the incidence of steroid-related complications, it did not reduce transplant-related mortality. In fact, survival without recurrent malignancy was lower in the two-drug arm.[193] Two large randomized trials of front-line therapy for chronic graft-versus-host disease are currently in progress, one using cyclosporine and prednisone with or without hydroxychloroquine, and a second with mycophenolate mofetil (or placebo) in combination with a calcineurin inhibitor and prednisone.

Salvage Therapy

Patients whose chronic graft-versus-host disease inadequately responds to corticosteroid-based therapy should be considered for salvage using any number of available regimens. Trials using thalidomide,[194] mycophenolate mofetil,[195] pentostatin,[196] hydroxychloroquine,[197] etrinate,[198] rituximab,[158] clofazimine,[199] etanercept,[97] and extracorporeal photopheresis[200] have all been published, with response rates ranging from 25% to 50%. Many of these trials contained 50 or fewer patients, thus necessitating the need for larger, multicenter trials. Localized therapies, such as topical tacrolimus (0.1% ointment) for oral lichen planus chronic graft-versus-host disease, have likewise shown promise in single-center reports.[201,201]

In recent years, extracorporeal photopheresis has become an increasingly powerful tool for the treatment of steroid-refractory chronic graft-versus-host disease, with response rates approximating 50% reported in several trials.[200,203,204] Responses are most often observed with cutaneous graft-versus-host disease, and are infrequent for patients with bronchiolitis obliterans.[200,205] The frequency and duration of extracorporeal photopheresis therapy for individual patients vary between centers, with a minimum of 4–6 months used in most trials.[200,203–205] Infectious complications, primarily catheter-related events, have been noted. The mechanism of action of extracorporeal photopheresis remains poorly understood. In one report, CD4/CD8 ratios normalized following extracorporeal photopheresis therapy, lymphocytes shifted to a predominantly T_H2 phenotype, and $CD56^+$ NK cells increased in numbers.[102] However, similar changes in lymphocyte function and CD4/CD8 ratios have not been confirmed by others.[200,205]

Supportive Care Measures

Infection remains the leading cause of death in patients with chronic graft-versus-host disease. Permanent functional asplenia occurs with extensive chronic graft-versus-host disease, and lifelong prophylaxis for encapsulated organisms (*S. pneumoniae*, *H. influenzae* type b) should be administered. Prophylaxis for *P. jiroveci* is required for 3–6 months after discontinuation of immunosuppressive therapy. Appropriate cytomegalovirus prophylaxis should be given to all patients with chronic graft-versus-host disease. Prophylactic acyclovir should be administered for the prevention of varicella-zoster reactivation for a minimum of 1 year posttransplantation, or longer if the patient is still on immunosuppressive therapy. Patients on topical steroids for oral graft-versus-host disease should receive anti-candidal coverage with nystatin swishes or clotrimazole troches. Intravenous immunoglobulin should be administered to patients with subtherapeutic immunoglobulin G levels (<400 mg/dL). After the first year posttransplantation, vaccinations should be given per guidelines from the Centers for Disease Control and Prevention, regardless of immunosuppressive therapy.[206]

Hepatic dysfunction has decreased with the addition of ursodeoxycholic acid.[171] Estrogen replacement therapy, calcium supplementation, and the use of osteoclast inhibitors should be considered for individuals at high risk for osteopenia and bone fractures, especially those receiving chronic corticosteroid therapy. The development of avascular necrosis, a common complication of young adults/teenagers on chronic corticosteroid therapy, remains problematic. Permanent joint dysfunction, with subsequent need for joint replacement when older, is often required. Ocular sicca symptoms have responded to retinoid therapy and pilocarpine.[207,208] Punctual plugs, ocular lubricants, and moisture chamber contact lenses have been used with varying success.

Impact on Survival and Quality of Life

Chronic graft-versus-host disease is the leading cause of non–relapse-related mortality in patients surviving greater than 1 year after allogeneic bone marrow transplantation. Such mortality is increased among older patients, those with HLA mismatching, older donors, and those with thrombocytopenia.[209] Whereas chronic graft-versus-host disease that progresses from the acute form clearly impacts long-term survival, de novo chronic graft-versus-host disease has much less impact.[210] Increasing severity of chronic graft-versus-host disease is associated with higher non–relapse-related mortality.[121] Infectious complications and progressive organ failure are the two principal causes of death from chronic graft-versus-host disease. Infections by invasive fungi, cytomegalovirus, *Pseudomonas* species, *S. pneumoniae*, and vancomycin-resistant *Enterococcus* are common in patients with chronic graft-versus-host disease, and each is associated with significant mortality.

Freedom from relapse is generally greater in patients with chronic graft-versus-host disease than in those without it (Fig. 97–14). However, very severe, extensive chronic graft-versus-host disease does not further reduce relapse rates in these patients.[123,211–213] Chronic graft-versus-host disease in patients with nonmalignant diseases adversely affects survival.[122,214]

With increased numbers of long-term survivors of allogeneic BMT, studies focusing on quality-of-life issues have gained importance. Functional, physical, and psychosocial impairments have been well described.[123,185,215–218] Functional impairments, including joint contractures and avascular necrosis, visual impairments from steroid-induced cataracts, esophageal dysmotility, sclerodermatous changes, and ocular and oral sicca symptoms all greatly impact quality of life. Growth impairment, ovarian or gonadal dysfunction, chronic fatigue, anorexia/weight loss, and alopecia are common. Psychosocial issues, such as loss of employment, poor school performance, and depressive disorders, are likewise common. Increased pain, immobility, and impaired activities of daily living have been reported in recipients of peripheral blood stem cells compared to marrow.[219] This dysfunction was primarily attributable to the higher

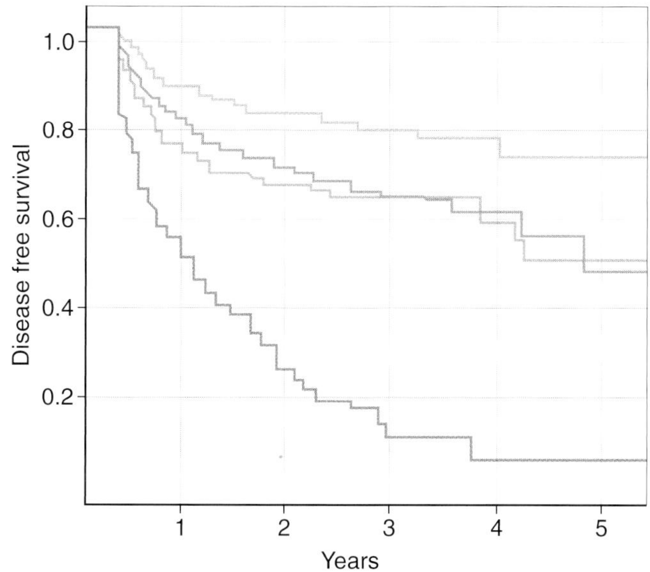

Figure 97–14. Association of severity of chronic graft-versus-host disease with disease-free survival in patients with low, intermediate, and high risk, or no chronic graft-versus-host disease. (From Lee SJ, Klein JP, Barrett AJ, et al: Severity of chronic graft-versus-host disease: association with treatment-related mortality and relapse. Blood 100:406–414, 2002, with permission.)

rate of chronic graft-versus-host disease in stem cell recipients.

In summary, although significant progress has been made in the treatment of both acute and chronic graft-versus-host disease, much work remains to be done. Better understanding of the pathogenesis of these complex disorders should lead to trials of new cellular and molecular therapies with potential for improved long-term outcome.

Current Controversies & Future Considerations

Graft-Versus-Host Disease

- Nature of graft-versus-host disease after low-intensity conditioning
- Cytokine modulation of acute graft-versus-host disease
- Extracorporeal photopheresis for treatment and/or prophylaxis
- Double cord blood units as alternative donor source

Suggested Readings*

Chao NJ, Holler E, Deeg HJ: Prophylaxis and treatment of acute graft-vs.-host disease. *In* Ferrara JLM, Cooke KR, Deeg HJ (eds): Graft-vs.-Host Disease (ed 3). New York: Marcel Dekker, 2005, pp 459–479.

Ferrara JLM, Antin JH: The pathophysiology of graft-vs.-host disease. *In* Blume KG, Forman SJ, Appelbaum FR (eds): Thomas' Hematopoietic Cell Transplantation (ed 3). Oxford: Blackwell Publishing Ltd, 2004, pp 353–368.

Mineishi S, Schuening FG: Graft-versus-host disease in mini-transplant. Leuk Lymphoma 45:1969–1980, 2004.

Petersdorf EF, Sasazuki T: Advances in tissue typing and their potential impact on GVHD incidence and severity. *In* Ferrara JLM, Cooke KR, Deeg HJ (eds): Graft-vs.-Host Disease (ed 3). New York: Marcel Dekker, 2005, pp 401–426.

Sullivan KM: Graft-vs.-host disease. *In* Blume KG, Forman SJ, Appelbaum FR (eds): Thomas' Hematopoietic Cell Transplantation (ed 3). Oxford: Blackwell Publishing Ltd, 2004, pp 635–664.

Full references for this chapter can be found on accompanying CD-ROM. 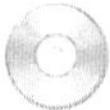

CHAPTER 98

Practice of Blood Component Transfusion

Firoozeh Alvandi, MD, and Harvey G. Klein, MD

KEY POINTS

Practice of Blood Component Transfusion

General Concepts

- Informed consent should be obtained and documented in the patient's medical record indicating that the patient has voluntarily accepted or refused transfusion after having been advised of the benefits and risks of as well as potential alternatives to transfusion.
- Red blood cells, whole blood, and plasma should be ABO compatible.
- Blood components should be infused through standard infusion filters (170–260 μ) to remove clots.
- Blood components should be administered slowly and under close patient observation for the first 15 minutes of transfusion.
- Cellular blood components must never be infused with hypertonic or hypotonic solutions or solutions containing glucose or calcium.
- To avoid hemolysis, only approved infusion pumps should be used when strict control of infusion rate is required.
- Uncertified blood warming methods should never be used lest thermal hemolysis occur.
- Medications should not be administered in the same line as or mixed with blood components because these may result in hemolysis or agglutination or confound transfusion reactions.
- Transfusion should not exceed 4 hours because risk of bacterial contamination increases with increasing time at room temperature.
- If transfusion of a unit of blood is anticipated to take longer than 4 hours, the transfusion service can divide the unit into smaller aliquots.
- Leukoreduction filters must never be used for granulocytes.
- Leukoreduction does *not* prevent transfusion-associated graft-versus-host disease. *Only irradiated blood components are indicated for use for the prevention of transfusion-associated graft-versus-host disease.*
- Gamma irradiation does *not* substitute for leukoreduction for preventing febrile reactions or alloimmunization, and does *not* reduce the risk of pathogen transmission by blood.

Compatibility Testing and Release of Blood Components for Transfusion

- Red blood cells, whole blood, and plasma should be ABO compatible.
- Patient blood specimens should be submitted well in advance of elective procedures for a "type and screen," which will identify most compatibility difficulties, particularly for alloimmunized patients.
- For patients who have been transfused or pregnant within 30 days prior to the date of blood product transfusion, type and screen must be performed on a sample that has been drawn within 3 days of the scheduled transfusion in order to detect newly formed antibodies.
- Fully tested red cells require 45–60 minutes to prepare; cryopreserved red blood cells and fresh frozen plasma may take even longer.
- Group-specific red cells (group A for group A patient, etc.) and an "abbreviated crossmatch" can be prepared in 15 minutes.
- After transfusion of one or more blood volumes (massive transfusion), an abbreviated red blood cell crossmatch can be performed to provide red blood cells more rapidly.
- In an emergency, group O red blood cells may be released uncrossmatched—with the consent of the requesting physician—although testing will be completed following release.
- In emergency situations, group O, Rh-negative or Rh-positive blood (depending on age and gender of patient), or ABO/Rh-specific blood is an effective and relatively safe way to shorten the time required to obtain urgently needed blood.

Management of Immune-Mediated Platelet Refractoriness

- When a 1-hour post–platelet transfusion corrected count increment (CCI) is less than 5000 after each of two platelet transfusions, ABO compatible fresh (less than 72 hours in storage) platelets should be used for two subsequent transfusions.

- If the CCI does not exceed 5000, human leukocyte antigen (HLA) antibody screening to detect alloantibodies or commercial platelet compatibility tests should be performed.
- If HLA antibodies are detected, HLA-compatible platelets should be tried.
- When alloantibodies with broad specificity are found (for HLA A and B loci), platelets from HLA-matched donors are indicated.
- Crossmatched compatible platelets may be beneficial when HLA antibody status of the recipient cannot be determined, HLA-matched platelets cannot be obtained, or the patient is refractory to HLA-matched platelets (up to 40–50% of cases).
- Administration of corticosteroids, washed platelets, or intravenous immunoglobulin has not proved useful in the management of refractoriness.

INTRODUCTION

The introduction of the closed-system plastic bag and use of simple centrifugation has made component therapy the standard of care for blood transfusion support. With the availability of components, the need for transfusion is based on the evaluation of laboratory findings in the context of a patient's clinical status and physiologic needs. Reliance solely on a "transfusion trigger" (i.e., a specific hemoglobin level, platelet count, or prothrombin time at which transfusion takes place irrespective of the patient's physiologic requirements) substitutes an algorithmic approach to management for good medical judgment. The transfusion of blood components based on absolute values may expose patients to additional potential complications of transfusion (infectious, cardiopulmonary, hemostatic, immunologic) without additional benefit. As with any medical treatment, blood transfusion requires informed consent.[1] For a discussion of complications of transfusion, the reader is referred to Chapter 99.

According to the latest survey, almost 29 million blood components are transfused annually in the United States. More than half of the components are red blood cells, with some 14 million units transfused to 4.9 million patients. About 12 million platelet units are transfused, approximately 70% of which are prepared by plateletpheresis. The remainder is pooled individual platelet units derived from whole blood. Some 2.5 million units of plasma are transfused and the balance is composed of cryoprecipitate and granulocytes.[2]

BLOOD COMPONENT PREPARATION AND COMPATIBILITY

Blood Component Preparation

Blood is collected into an interconnected series of sterile, disposable plastic bags containing anticoagulant, preservative, and additives to optimize viability during storage. Blood components are routinely separated from whole blood by centrifugation (Fig. 98–1).

Increasingly blood components are prepared by apheresis, a process by which selected components or substances in blood are removed from the circulation and the remainder of the blood is returned to the individual. Apheresis is used for routine blood component collection (red cells, platelets, plasma, stem cells) and therapeutic removal of undesirable components and substances from circulation, achieved through automated machines. This is discussed further in the section on apheresis (see Fig. 98–7 later).

Blood Component Storage and Modification

The development of citrate anticoagulant (1914) and preservatives (1916) led to the establishment of blood depots during World War I where blood could be stored for several days following collection. Depending on the additives used and storage conditions, whole blood and red blood cell concentrates may be stored refrigerated at 1°–6°C for up to 42 days. Platelets are currently stored at room temperature for no more than 5 days, and fresh frozen plasma and cryoprecipitate may be stored frozen for as long as 1 year. Granulocytes, the most labile component, may be stored for no more than 24 hours after collection. These varying shelf lives account for occasional difficulties with component availability and inventory management.

Blood components are often modified for special purposes, and such modifications may result in changes in composition and storage characteristics of the products. Some of the commonly used procedures include leukocyte reduction to limit the contaminant white blood cells that may cause alloimmunization, transmission of cell-associated viruses, and febrile reactions; gamma irradiation to inactivate lymphocytes to prevent transfusion-associated graft-versus-host disease; washing to remove antibodies, cytokines, and other plasma proteins responsible for allergic reactions; and cryopreservation for long-term storage of rare blood. Any modification or manipulation that violates the integrity of the closed container of a blood component (such as washing, pooling, and some methods used for deglycerolization or thawing) presents a risk of bacterial contamination and shortens the component expiration date. Once the closed seal is broken, refrigerated storage is limited to 24 hours and storage at room temperature (e.g., for pooled platelets) may be as short as 4 hours (Table 98–1).

Blood Compatibility

The scientific basis for compatible transfusions was the identification of ABO blood groups in the early 1900s by

TABLE 98–1. Indications for Additional Modifications of Cellular Blood Components

Leukoreduction	Irradiation (Red Blood Cells, Platelets, Granulocytes)	Washing (Plasma Removal)	Volume Reduction	Freezing-Deglycerolization (Red Blood Cells)
Description				
Filtration of component after collection, at bedside, or removal of WBC during automated collection for a 3- to 4-log reduction (99.9%) of WBC; final WBC content ≤5 × 10^6	Gamma irradiation (cesium or cobalt) of component with 2500 cGy (centigrays) to inactivate viable lymphocytes within the component	Component washed with sterile normal saline to remove >98% of plasma proteins, electrolytes, and antibodies; WBC content 5 × 10^8	Removal of plasma from cellular components (mainly platelets; RBC concentrates contain very little plasma)	Addition of glycerol and freezing generally within 6 days of collection depending on the additive solution used at the time of collection and glycerolization-freezing method used
Purpose				
Reduction of febrile nonhemolytic transfusion reactions (FNHTR) Reduction of CMV transmission (CMV-safe) Reduction of HLA alloimmunization	Prevention of transfusion-associated graft-versus-host disease	Prevention of allergic reactions Decrease in risk of hyperkalemia	Reduction of circulatory overload Removal of antibodies	Long-term storage of autologous or allogeneic rare blood phenotypes
Indications				
Patients who have experienced an episode of FNHTR Alternative to CMV-seronegative components (from donor tested negative for CMV): • Neonates • Transplant patients	Recipients of allogeneic hematopoietic or solid organ transplants Recipients of transfusion from blood relatives Patients on immunosuppressive regimens Patients with congenital immunodeficiencies and certain malignancies Premature infants (especially those undergoing extracorporeal membrane oxygenation)	Patients who experience recurrent severe allergic reactions (not responsive to premedication with antihistamines) IgA-deficient patients when IgA-deficient component is not available Recipients at risk from hyperkalemia: • Newborns • Intrauterine transfusions May be effective when ABO-identical blood is not available for patients with paroxysmal nocturnal hemoglobinuria (PNH)	Patients with expanded plasma volume: • Normovolemic chronic anemia • Thalassemia major • Sickle cell disease • Congestive heart failure Pediatric, elderly, and other patients susceptible to volume overload	Patients with rare blood phenotypes or multiple alloantibodies
Comments				
Equivalent to CMV seronegative components *Not effective and not indicated for prevention of transfusion-associated graft-versus-host disease* *Filtration results in a 10–15% loss of the cellular component*	*Not* indicated for prevention of FNHTR and unnecessary for aplastic anemia patients (despite ATG therapy) or HIV patients in the absence of other indications for irradiation (see above) RBC shelf life is decreased to 28 days (if greater than the original expiration date) but platelet or granulocyte shelf life is not affected	Washing results in a 15–20% loss of red cells or platelets *Not* equivalent to "leukoreduced" Red blood cells must be used within 24 hr and platelets must be used within 4 hr of washing (because of opening of the closed system)	*Not* equivalent to washing for prevention of allergic reactions Results in a 4-hr post–volume-reduction expiration time because of the decreased plasma/volume needed for optimal platelet metabolism	May *not* be feasible for red blood cells with certain abnormalities (such as Hgb S, hereditary spherocytosis, PNH) *Not* equivalent to "leukoreduced" *(may remove >95% of WBC)* Depending on the method of glycerolization-freezing used (open or closed system), the post-deglycerolization shelf life may be 24 hr or 2 week (respectively)

Abbreviations: ATG, antithymocyte globulin; CMV, cytomegalovirus; Hgb, hemoglobin; HIV, human immunodeficiency virus; HLA, human leukocyte antigen; IgA, immunoglobulin A; RBC, red blood cells; WBC, white blood cells.

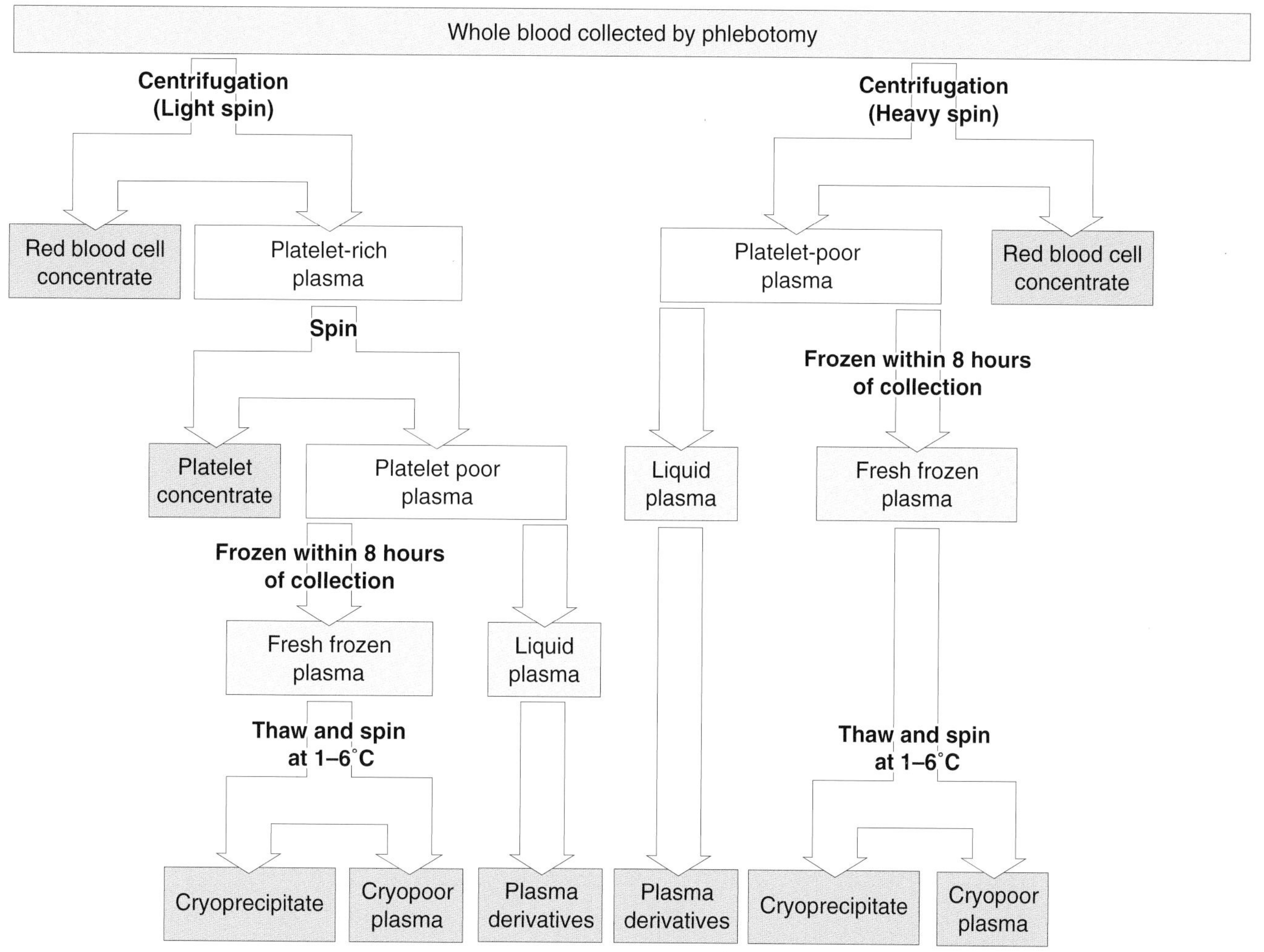

Figure 98–1. Component preparation by centrifugation (light or heavy spin). Red blood cell concentrate, platelet concentrate, cryoprecipitate, and cryo-poor plasma are final products; fresh frozen plasma can be used as a final product or further processed to obtain cryoprecipitate and cryo-poor plasma. Cryo-poor plasma has little fibrinogen, factor VIII, factor XIII, and von Willebrand factor and may be used as the replacement fluid of choice for the treatment of thrombotic thrombocytopenic purpura that is refractory to plasma exchange with fresh frozen plasma. Liquid plasma can be used as a final product or further processed to make plasma derivatives. Liquid plasma has reduced factor V and factor VIII (labile factor) activity.

Karl Landsteiner.[3] Further characterization of red cell antigens, discovery of numerous additional blood group systems, compatibility testing, analysis of transfusion reactions, and a basic understanding of hemolytic disease of the newborn and autoimmune hemolysis were made possible by the discovery of the direct antiglobulin (Coombs) test in 1945.[4,5]

Antiglobulin Test

The antiglobulin or Coombs test provides a method by which alloantibodies may be detected and compatible blood units identified. When a clinically important alloantibody is present in a recipient's serum, *antigen-negative* blood must be selected. If the alloantibody is against a very high-frequency antigen (present in greater than 90% of individuals) or when multiple alloantibodies are present, procurement of compatible blood may be difficult or impossible. In some cases, the presence of red cell autoantibodies makes all units (including those of the patient) appear incompatible and masks the presence of alloantibodies.

The antiglobulin test makes use of antibodies to human globulins to detect the presence of antibody (or complement) on the red blood cell surface, or the presence of antibody in a patient's serum. The *direct antiglobulin test*, or the direct Coombs test, detects antibody or complement that is coating red blood cells and may be positive in hemolytic transfusion reactions (for which it is the single most important assay), hemolytic disease of the newborn, autoimmune hemolytic anemia (including hemolysis associated with medications), extrinsically administered immune globulins (passively acquired), and post-marrow or organ transplantation settings (donor's lymphocytes producing antibody to red cells of the recipient). False-positive results may occur

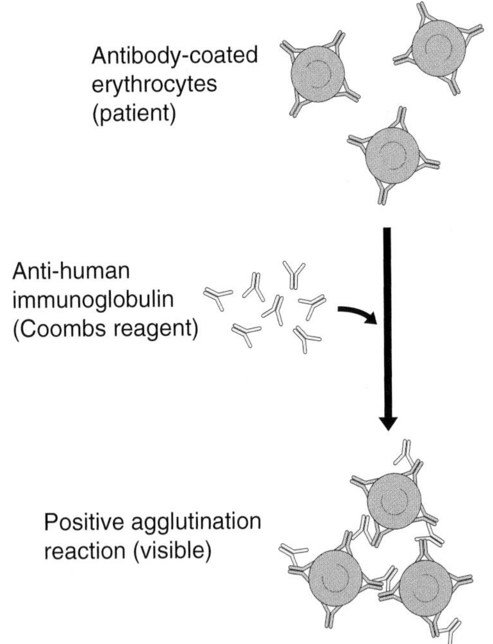

■ **Figure 98–2.** Positive direct Coombs test (direct antiglobulin test). Anti–human immunoglobulin (reagent) is added to the patient's red blood cells, which have been coated with antibody (in vivo). The reagent anti–human immunoglobulin attaches to the antibodies coating the patient's red blood cells, causing visible agglutination.

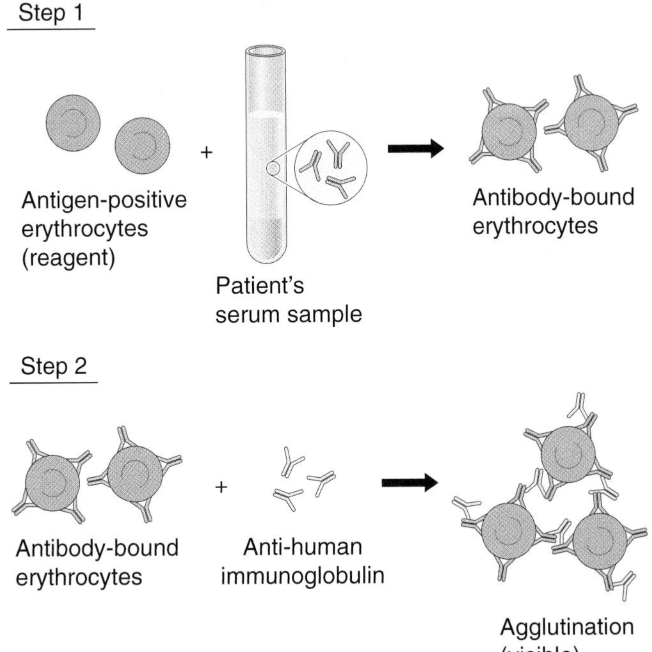

■ **Figure 98–3.** Positive indirect Coombs test (indirect antiglobulin test). In step one, reagent red blood cells coated with antigen are added to the patient's serum, which contains antibody. In the presence of antigen-antibody specificity, the antibody from the patient's serum coats the reagent red blood cells (in vitro); this does not result in visible agglutination. In step two, reagent anti–human immunoglobulin is added to the antibody-bound reagent red blood cells. The reagent anti–human immunoglobulin attaches to the antibodies that are coating the reagent red blood cells, causing visible agglutination.

with hypergammaglobulinemia when rouleaux formation may be mistaken for agglutination (Fig. 98–2).

The *indirect antiglobulin test*, or indirect Coombs test, is the method used in the antibody screen portion of a "type and screen" and in the serologic crossmatch (patient serum and donor "reagent" red cells), and detects antibody present in the serum, but not bound to the red blood cells (Fig. 98–3). When the indirect antiglobulin test is positive, antibody specificity must be identified and the corresponding antigen always avoided in transfusions. A negative antibody screen (indirect antiglobulin test) does not necessarily indicate absence of alloantibodies because the titer of antibody may be below the level of detection or the antibody might be directed against a low-incidence antigen (present in less than 10% of individuals) not present on reagent testing cells, yet present on some patient cells. A negative indirect antiglobulin test does not guarantee that blood is compatible, nor does a weak test indicate that hemolysis is likely to be mild. Although a positive indirect antiglobulin test does not indicate that the alloantibody will have clinical importance, it demands further investigation (Table 98–2).

The best known and clinically most important blood groups include ABO, Rh, Kell, Kidd, and Duffy. Naturally occurring antibodies such as anti-A and/or anti-B are present in the absence of prior sensitizing stimulus. Development of most other alloantibodies requires prior sensitization. In general, blood components that contain more than 2 mL of red blood cells must be compatible with the patient's plasma. Particular attention is paid to Rh type because less than 1 mL of red blood cells, a volume found in most platelet concentrates, is sufficient to sensitize an Rh-negative patient.[6,7]

Plasma-containing components, including platelet preparations, should be ABO compatible with the patient's red blood cells when possible lest passive antibodies in the plasma hemolyze the recipient red cells (Table 98–3).

COMPONENT DESCRIPTION AND INDICATIONS FOR TRANSFUSION

Whole Blood

Most of the whole blood collected is separated into components. Whole blood is rarely available and infrequently used. A unit of whole blood typically has a volume of 450–500 mL and a hematocrit of 35–45%. Table 98–4 presents suggested administration guidelines.

TABLE 98–2. Direct Antiglobulin Test (DAT) and Indirect Antiglobulin Test (IAT)

Direct Antiglobulin Test	Indirect Antiglobulin Test
Direct antiglobulin test detects antibody or complement that is *coating* red blood cells *Positive in: • Hemolytic transfusion reaction • Hemolytic disease of the newborn • Autoimmune hemolytic anemia • Passively acquired (immune globulins) • Associated with drugs (extensive list of medications, including penicillins, cephalosporins, quinidine, methyldopa) • Post-marrow or organ transplant (donor antibodies against recipient red cells) A positive DAT does not necessarily indicate in vivo hemolysis or shortened survival of red blood cells False positives may result from conditions resulting in rouleaux formation	*Indirect antiglobulin test* detects antibody present in the *serum*, not bound to the red blood cells *Positive in: • Presence of immunoglobulin G or M antibodies in serum, such as antibodies in recipient serum against donor cells in a crossmatch • May be detected in sera from previously transfused patients or previously pregnant women • Autoimmune hemolytic anemia • Associated with drugs that cause autoantibody formation or immune complex formation A positive IAT may not be clinically significant A negative IAT does not guarantee blood compatibility

*In autoimmune hemolytic anemias, the antibody may be present in the serum and on the red blood cells of the patient and therefore both DAT and IAT may be positive.

TABLE 98–3. Compatibility of Recipient Blood with Donor Blood Components

Patient ABO Group	Whole Blood	Red Blood Cells	Platelets	Plasma	Cryoprecipitate
O	O	O	Any (O preferred)	O, A, B, AB	N/A
A	A	A or O	Any (A preferred)	A or AB	N/A
B	B	B or O	Any (B preferred)	B or AB	N/A
AB	AB	AB, A, B, or O (in order of preference)	Any (AB preferred)	AB, A, or B	N/A

Modified from Brecher ME (ed): Technical Manual (ed 14). Bethesda, MD: AABB Press, 2003, pp 454, 467.

- *Indications:* acute hypovolemia with red cell loss, massive transfusion, and exchange transfusion
- *Nonindications:* chronic anemia (where blood volume is often increased)

Whole blood is not a source of functional platelets or granulocytes, which deteriorate in less than 24 hours at refrigerator temperatures and should not be administered for nutritional purposes.

Red Blood Cells

Red blood cells ("packed" red cells) are separated from whole blood by centrifugation. A unit of red blood cells has a volume of approximately 250–350 mL and contains 200 mL of red blood cells plus anticoagulant at a hematocrit of 60% (with additive solution) to 80% (without additive solution).

- *Indications:* Treatment of symptomatic anemia

In general, clinicians transfuse if the hemoglobin falls below 6 gm/dL and rarely consider transfusion when it exceeds 10 gm/dL. The interval between these values is the area of controversy. Practice guidelines support a hemoglobin level of less than 7 gm/dL as generally acceptable for the initiation of red blood cell transfusion in symptomatic patients.[8–10]

- *Nonindications:* Volume expansion or nutritional purposes

Red blood cell transfusion is rarely indicated in otherwise treatable anemias, including anemias associated with vitamin B_{12}, iron, or folate deficiency; if symptoms are severe, these patients may benefit from a single-unit transfusion.

In general, 1 unit of packed red blood cells will increase the hemoglobin by 1 gm/dL in an average-size adult. In the average pediatric patient, transfusion of 8–10 mL/kg of red blood cells is expected to increase hemoglobin by 3 gm/dL. Hemoglobin determination is frequently used to determine the "transfusion trigger." However, the decision to transfuse should be based on a careful assessment of a patient's clinical symptoms, coexisting or underlying medical conditions, and the cause of the anemia. The single adequately powered prospective study (intensive care unit patients)[11] and

TABLE 98–4. Suggested Blood Component Administration Guidelines

	Whole Blood*	Packed RBC	Granulocytes	Platelets	Plasma
Adults					
First 15 min	2 mL/min	2 mL/min	2 mL/min	2–5 mL/min	2–5 mL/min
Subsequently	100–230 mL/hr	100–230 mL/hr	75–100 mL/hr	200–300 mL/hr	200–300 mL/hr
Children					
First 5 min	N/A	N/A	N/A	5% of total volume† ordered for transfusion	5% of total volume† ordered for transfusion
First 15 min	5% of total volume† ordered for transfusion	5% of total volume† ordered for transfusion	5% of total volume ordered for transfusion	N/A	N/A
Subsequently	Variable (as tolerated)	2–5 mL/kg/hr	Over 2–3 hr (for a 200-mL product)	As tolerated	1–2 mL/min

*Generally unavailable and rarely used.
†Volume ordered for pediatric transfusion should be based on the child's weight (10–15 mL/kg); excludes granulocyte transfusion.
Abbreviations: N/A, not applicable; RBC, red blood cells.
Modified from Blood Product Administration Procedure Manual, Nursing and Patient Care Services, Clinical Center, October 2004 revision. Bethesda, MD: National Institutes of Health, 2004.

numerous observational studies indicated that patients with cardiovascular disease are particularly sensitive to anemia and fare better at a higher level.[8,12,13]

Effectiveness of therapy with red blood cells should be assessed with a posttransfusion complete blood count to help guide subsequent transfusion therapy.

Platelets

Platelets that are separated from whole blood shortly after collection are referred to as "whole blood–derived platelets," "random-donor platelets," or "platelet concentrates" and contain less than 70 mL of plasma. Platelets collected by apheresis are "single-donor platelets" or "apheresis platelets." One bag of platelets collected by apheresis contains a total volume of greater than 100 mL (up to 500 mL) of plasma. A therapeutic dose of platelets for an average adult is 1 unit of platelets (5.5×10^{10} platelets) per 10 kg body weight. Each unit is expected to increase the platelet count in an average-sized adult by approximately 5000/μL. Each apheresis (single-donor) platelet product is expected to contain approximately 3×10^{11} platelets, which is roughly equivalent to 4–6 units of random donor platelets. Table 98–4 presents suggested administration guidelines.

- *Indications:* Bleeding associated with thrombocytopenia, rapid fall in platelet counts, qualitative platelet defects, or as prophylaxis for major bleeding in severely thrombocytopenic patients.

Indications for use are the same for both preparations, except for immunized refractory patients who may require single-donor human leukocyte antigen (HLA)–matched and compatible platelets. Single-donor platelets offer the additional advantage of decreased donor exposure and a lower risk of bacterial sepsis.[14]

- *Nonindications:* Bleeding unassociated with thrombocytopenia (except for the unusual patient with a clinically significant platelet function defect), other defects in hemostasis (such as factor deficiencies), or platelet dysfunction caused by many common medications (aspirin, penicillins, nonsteroidal anti-inflammatory drugs)

Platelet transfusion is usually contraindicated in thrombotic thrombocytopenic purpura (TTP) because most of these patients suffer from thrombosis rather than hemorrhage, and platelet transfusion may place them at increased risk of thrombosis.[15–18] Patients with TTP who develop life-threatening hemorrhage may benefit from a cautious trial of platelets.

The threshold for prophylactic platelet transfusion varies based on the patient's underlying condition and likelihood of hemorrhage.[8,19] A threshold of 10,000/μL is effective in preventing morbidity and mortality from bleeding in stable oncology patients undergoing chemotherapy.[19–23] A platelet count greater than 50,000/μL is desirable prior to invasive procedures and in the immediate postprocedure period[19,24–26]; procedures such as intramuscular injection, intravenous catheter insertion, skin biopsy, and marrow aspirate and biopsy are routinely accomplished at platelet counts lower than 50,000/μL. The location of a procedure (internal jugular vein) and concurrent hemostatic defects may modify this decision.[19,27] Platelet counts closer to 100,000/μL, may be prudent for patients at high risk of intracranial hemorrhage, such as those with cerebral leukostasis, or for those undergoing neurosurgical or ocular procedures.[28] Stable chronically thrombocytopenic patients (such as those with aplastic anemia or myelodysplasia) may tolerate platelet counts as low as 5000/μL in the absence of complicating factors such as fever, infection, and additional defects in hemostasis.[29] More aggressive support is indicated for patients who are unstable—those who are febrile, infected, or receiving multiple medications, especially if the platelet counts are falling[19] (Table 98–5).

Platelet transfusions should be monitored by a posttransfusion platelet count (1–24 hours) to assess response and guide subsequent transfusion therapy. A corrected count increment (CCI) may be used to determine the increase in platelet count in an individual after platelet transfusion[30] (Box 98–1). Some suggest that a more effective, scientific approach than CCI or expected posttransfusion increment provides a more accurate assessment of response to platelet transfusion[31]; however, this level of precision is rarely necessary. An absolute posttransfusion increment of 10,000/μL or greater (2000 per unit of random-donor platelets) in an average-sized adult corresponds to a CCI of 5000.

Platelet Refractoriness

Patients who respond poorly to repeated platelet infusions are considered "refractory." Posttransfusion platelet counts (1 hour and 24 hour) are critical in the management of refractory patients. Failure to achieve a CCI of 5000 or greater is cause to suspect platelet refractoriness. Refractoriness may be immune or non-immune mediated. *Non–immune-mediated* causes of platelet refractoriness include fever, infection, splenomegaly, disseminated intravascular coagulation, massive bleeding, and medications that enhance platelet destruction. Platelets and granulocytes also have antigens to which an antigen-negative individual may become alloimmunized.[32–35] *Immune-mediated* causes of platelet refractoriness include repeated transfusions, especially with non–leukocyte-reduced platelets, and multiparity (alloimmunization to HLA and human platelet antigens).[36] In practice, the distinction between immune- and non–immune-mediated platelet refractoriness is less clear.[19,36–39]

TABLE 98–5. Guidelines for Platelet Transfusion per National Institutes of Health Practice

Patient Population	Threshold
Stable aplastic anemia patient	<5000/μL or bleeding
General oncology patient	<10,000/μL
Stable non-oncology patient	<10,000/μL
Post–hematopoietic stem cell transplant	<10,000/μL
Aplastic anemia patient receiving ATG	<20,000/μL
Patients undergoing invasive procedures	<50,000/μL
Neurosurgery patients	<100,000/L

Abbreviation: ATG, antithymocyte globulin.

Granulocytes

Granulocytes are collected by apheresis for specific patients, from donors who are mobilized prior to collection with corticosteroids and/or cytokines (granulocyte colony-stimulating factor) in order to enhance collection[40,41] (Fig. 98–4). Granulocytes have a volume of 250 mL and contain plasma, approximately 30 mL red blood cells, and variable amounts of mononuclear leukocytes and platelets and can be stored up to 24 hours postcollection.[42] Granulocyte concentrates should be ABO, Rh, and red blood cell crossmatch compatible, and a minimal therapeutic dose should contain greater than 1×10^{10} granulocytes.[43] Table 98–4 presents suggested administration guidelines.

- *Indications:* Neutropenia in patients with expected marrow recovery who have an absolute neutrophil count of less than 0.5×10^9/L, and documented infection not responding to appropriate antibiotic treatment for 24–48 hours, or defective granulocyte function despite normal counts (e.g., chronic granulomatous disease)

Once initiated, in the absence of development of contraindication to ongoing granulocyte transfusions (such as severe reactions stemming from alloimmunization), therapy should continue until recovery of marrow function (absolute neutrophil count), resolution of infection, or progression of infection despite administration of adequate doses of granulocytes.[43,44]

- *Nonindications:* Absence of above-mentioned criteria

Granulocyte transfusion is generally contraindicated in patients with prior severe pulmonary reactions to HLA or human neutrophil antigen (HNA) or alloimmunization (serologic HLA or HNA incompatibility).

Pulmonary toxicity may be exacerbated when granulocytes and amphotericin B are administered in close temporal proximity. Administration of amphotericin B

Box 98–1. Calculation of Corrected Count Increment (CCI)

$$\text{CCI} = \frac{(\text{Posttransfusion platelet count} - \text{pretransfusion platelet count}) \times \text{body surface area}}{\text{Number of platelets transfused}}$$

- Posttransfusion platelet count is best obtained 15 minutes to 1 hour posttransfusion.
- Body surface area = the square root of [(height in cm × weight in kg)/3600].
- The number of platelets transfused is expressed as multiples of 1×10^{11}.

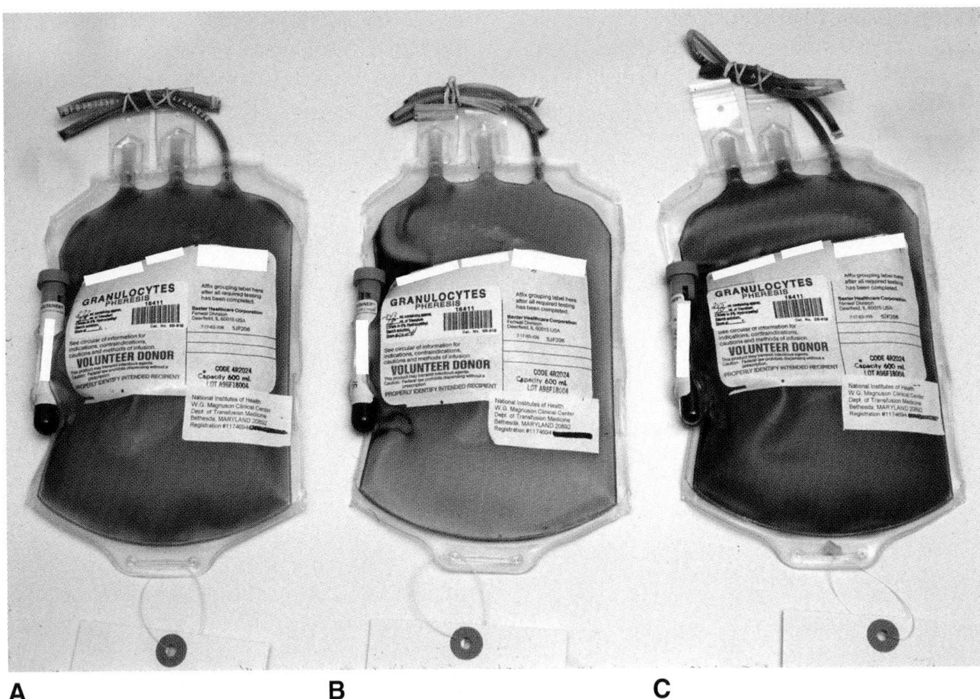

Figure 98–4. Granulocyte concentrates prepared using three different donor preparative regimens: *(A)* granulocyte colony-stimulating factor (G-CSF) alone; *(B)* G-CSF plus dexamethasone; and *(C)* dexamethasone alone. G-CSF 5 μg/kg was given at 16–24 hours and dexamethasone 8 mg orally was given 12 hours prior to collection. Components were left undisturbed on a countertop at room temperature for 4 hours. The starch effect allowed the red cells to sediment rapidly, resulting in a sharply demarcated, easily visible buffy coat layer in the bags containing larger amounts of white cells. Granulocyte content in components prepared using G-CSF and dexamethasone stimulation *(B)* were three- to fourfold higher than in the other two components. (Courtesy of Susan F. Leitman, MD, Chief, Blood Services Section, Department of Transfusion Medicine, Clinical Center, National Institutes of Health.)

and granulocytes should be separated temporally as much as possible[45] (i.e., one administered in the morning, the other in the evening, or, as per National Institutes of Health practice, at least 4 hours apart).

Granulocyte concentrates may contain large doses of leukocyte-associated pathogens such as cytomegalovirus. This is of particular concern to immunosuppressed individuals such as stem cell transplant recipients, solid organ transplant recipients, neonates undergoing extracorporeal membrane oxygenation, and low-birth-weight and premature infants.

Response to Granulocyte Therapy

Although granulocyte transfusions decrease the length of bacterial infection, proof that granulocyte transfusions decrease mortality in any situation has been elusive.[44] Higher granulocyte doses, however, have been correlated with more favorable outcomes in reviews of various studies.[44,46,47] Granulocyte transfusion therapy should be evaluated after an initial course of at least 4 days of therapy.[48]

A 1- to 6-hour posttransfusion complete blood count with differential for determination of absolute neutrophil count to help assess efficacy of granulocyte transfusions should accompany each granulocyte transfusion. The posttransfusion increment in absolute neutrophil count varies based on the granulocyte content of the transfused unit. To detect increments in peripheral blood, a dose three to four times above the minimal therapeutic dose may be needed. Because granulocytes traffic to the lungs before equilibrating in peripheral blood,[49–51] a posttransfusion increment several hours after transfusion may be higher than a 1-hour posttransfusion absolute neutrophil count. If the patient's absolute neutrophil count fails to reach expected levels or if a reaction occurs, an investigation, including an HLA antibody screen and tests for antibodies to HNA, is indicated. Because it may not be possible to obtain HLA- or HNA-compatible granulocytes to support a complete course of granulocyte therapy for patients with specific HLA or HNA alloantibodies, alloimmunization to HLA or HNA antibodies generally precludes subsequent granulocyte transfusions, as further therapy with (non–HLA- or non–HNA-matched) granulocytes may not be effective and may cause severe pulmonary reactions.[34] However, use of HLA- or HNA-compatible granulocytes does not guarantee effectiveness and does not necessarily prevent additional adverse reactions.[43,52] Intravenous administration of meperidine (Demerol) 25–50 mg may abort the severe rigors that occasionally complicate granulocyte infusions.[43]

Fresh Frozen Plasma

Plasma separated from whole blood or collected by apheresis and frozen within 8 hours is labeled fresh frozen plasma. Fresh frozen plasma contains most plasma proteins at the time of thaw at about the same concentration as at the time of collection. A unit of fresh frozen plasma collected from whole blood contains approximately 200 mL of plasma (mixed with anticoagulant). Fresh frozen plasma prepared by apheresis contains approximately 400–600 mL of plasma (mixed with anticoagulant). By convention, 1 mL of fresh frozen plasma is expected to provide 1 unit of activity of all factors (except labile factors V and VIII). In practice, individual units may vary in content. If multiple factors are consumed, plasma factor levels of above 30% can be achieved with a fresh frozen plasma dose of 10–15 mL/kg (equivalent to approximately 4–6 units of fresh frozen plasma).[8] Table 98–4 presents suggested administration guidelines.

- *Indications:* Correction of multiple clotting factor deficiencies in patients who are bleeding or scheduled for an invasive procedure; replacement of factors consumed in disseminated intravascular coagulation, coagulation factor deficiencies caused by liver disease, and coagulation factors diluted by replacement fluids during massive transfusion; as replacement fluid in the treatment of TTP (plasma exchange); rapid reversal of warfarin (Coumadin) effect; and replacement of congenital factor deficiencies when the specific factor concentrate is not available (i.e., replacement of factors II, V, X, XI)[53]

Specific concentrated or recombinant factor preparations are preferable to fresh frozen plasma because these products have been treated to reduce the risk of viral transmission and are labeled for potency. An International Normalized Ratio greater than 1.6 or an activated partial thromboplastin time 1.5 times the upper range of normal (factor level activity less than 30%) is a guide to consider treatment.[8,53,54]

- *Nonindications:* Volume expansion and protein replacement in nutritional deficiencies
  Crystalloids and colloids (synthetic volume expanders) can be used for that purpose without exposing the recipient to infectious disease risks and immune-mediated effects such as transfusion-related acute lung injury.

Cryoprecipitate

Cryoprecipitate ("cryo") is the cold-insoluble portion of plasma containing high-molecular-weight glycoproteins. Ordinarily stored frozen, cryoprecipitate can be kept at room temperature for up to 6 hours; upon pooling, it must be transfused within 4 hours. Compatibility testing is unnecessary. A unit of cryoprecipitate usually contains less than 15 mL of plasma and is expected to contain greater than 80 IU (international units) of factor VIII (antihemophilic factor), greater than 150 mg of fibrinogen, and about 30% of the factor XIII of the original plasma. Cryoprecipitate also contains von Willebrand complex activity. One unit of cryoprecipitate can increase fibrinogen in an average adult by 5–10 mg/dL. A therapeutic dose for an adult is 80–150 mL of cryoprecipitate (8–10 units pooled).[53] Table 98–4 presents suggested administration guidelines.

- *Indications:* Treatment of fibrinogen deficiency, dysfibrinogenemia, factor XIII deficiency, disseminated intravascular coagulation, and urgent treatment of hemophilia A and von Willebrand disease in the absence of factor VIII concentrate or recombinant factor VIII

Cryoprecipitate has also been used to correct the platelet defect of uremic bleeding, although with variable success.[55]

The dosage of cryoprecipitate needed depends on the underlying deficiency and on the plasma volume of the patient. The number of bags of cryoprecipitate needed to replace fibrinogen can be calculated as follows:

$$\frac{(\text{Desired} - \text{initial fibrinogen level [mg/dL]}) \times \text{patient's plasma volume [dL]}}{250 \text{ mg (fibrinogen per cryo bag)}}$$

The plasma volume for an average adult = (1 − [Hct%/100]) × patient weight (kg) × 70 mL/kg.

For infants and children under 40 kg, the plasma volume = ([1 − hematocrit%]/100) × patient weight in kg × 80–85 mL/kg.

- *Nonindications:* Absence of specific hemostatic abnormality for which it is indicated (as noted previously) or for which specific factor concentrates (factor VIII) or recombinant factor preparations are available

HEMATOPOIETIC PROGENITOR CELLS

Hematopoietic progenitor cells and umbilical cord blood are commonly collected and stored by blood banks. *Progenitor or "stem" cells* that were originally derived from bone marrow harvests are now more often collected from the peripheral blood (referred to as peripheral blood stem cells [PBSCs]) via apheresis for reconstitution of hematopoiesis and immune function in patients with a variety of malignancies and immune disorders. The number of circulating progenitor cells is increased by mobilizing the donor with hematopoietic growth factors, most often granulocyte colony-stimulating factor, or, in the case of autologous transplants, a combination of chemotherapy and growth factors (Fig. 98–5). The degree of mobilization, and the probability of a successful collection, is best predicted by measuring circulating cells that express the membrane glycoprotein CD34, a marker for committed PBSCs. Where this assay is not available in real time, total white blood cell and mononuclear cell counts have been used.[56–58]

Standard collections of allogeneic PBSCs involve 3–4 hours per apheresis procedure, during which about 10 L of blood are processed. Two to four collections are usual; however, large-volume procedures in which 25–30 L are processed are being used increasingly to allow complete collections with a single procedure. Although PBSC collections are generally well tolerated, side effects associ-

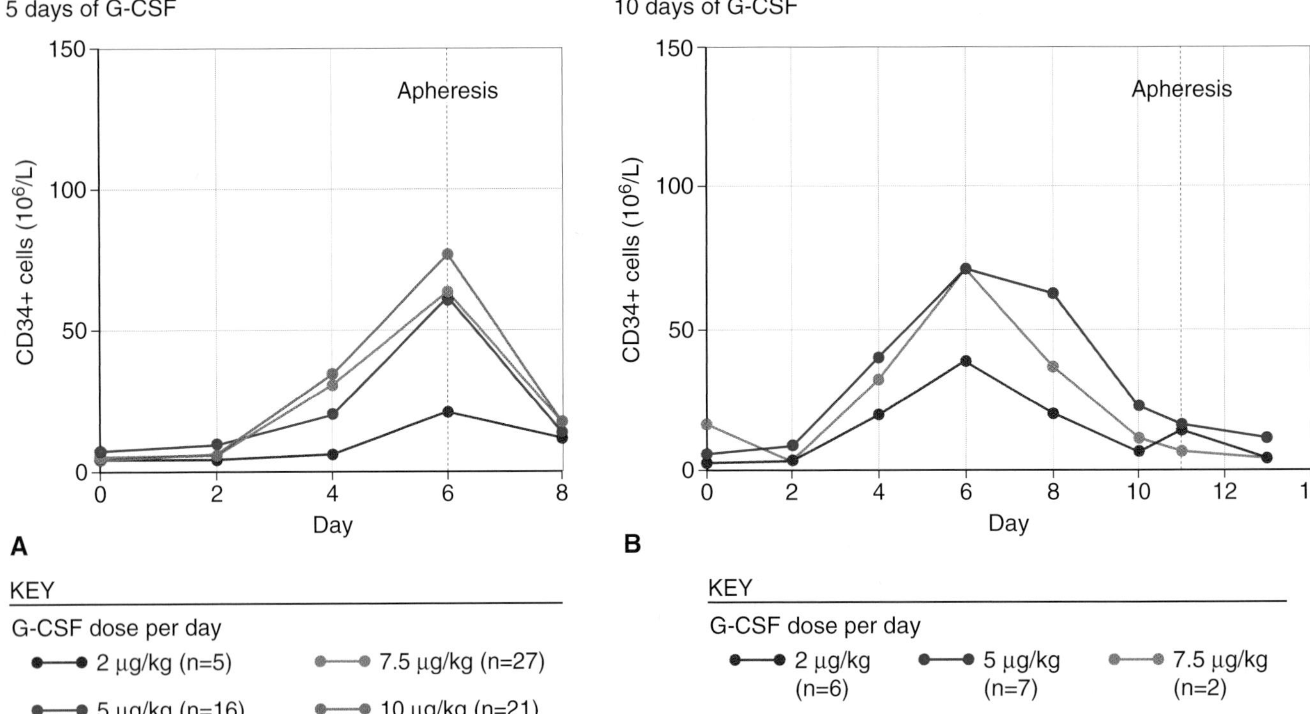

Figure 98–5. Number of CD34[+] cells mobilized as a function of dose of daily granulocyte colony-stimulating factor administered for *(A)* 5 days and *(B)* 10 days; CD34 counts were obtained every other day and on the day of apheresis. (Modified from Stroncek DF, Clay ME, Petzoldt ML, et al: Treatment of normal individuals with granulocyte-colony-stimulating factor: donor experiences and the effects on peripheral blood CD34+ cell counts and on the collection of peripheral blood stem cells. Transfusion 36:601–610, 1996.)

ated with the several-day administration of growth factor are common. Bone pain, headache, fatigue, insomnia, and gastrointestinal disturbances occur, usually respond to administration of acetaminophen or nonsteroidal anti-inflammatory drugs, and vanish once growth factor injections cease.[59] With longer collections, symptomatic hypocalcemia becomes a problem and calcium chloride infusion is advisable.[60] Vascular complications and citrate toxicity are not unlike those experienced in other long apheresis procedures (see later). With cell mobilization, splenomegaly occurs in most donors[61] and splenic rupture has been reported.[62] PBSC donors should be advised to refrain from contact sports for a few weeks after the last mobilization.

PBSC grafts are infused as fresh collections or stored frozen with the cryoprotectant dimethylsulfoxide in liquid nitrogen. Thawed cells infused with dimethylsulfoxide may cause nausea, vomiting, fever, dyspnea, and anaphylaxis. Reactions are dose dependent and may be lessened by prophylactic administration of antihistamines.[63]

PBSCs carry the same risks as other blood components, including risks of transfusion-transmitted infectious agents, and are tested in the same manner as other blood components. However, given their highly specialized use and their life-saving potential, exceptions are made to donor selection criteria normally used for allogeneic blood collections with concurrence of the treating physician and the recipient.

Adequate cell dose for engraftment depends on whether the procedure is an autograft, a related allograft, or an unrelated transplant. Cell dose, cell source, and patient characteristics are all important variables.[64] A minimum CD34[+] cell dose of 5×10^6 cells/kg recipient weight is targeted[65] for unrelated PBSC transplants, although a minimum dose of $2–4 \times 10^6$ CD 34[+] cells/kg recipient weight ($2–4 \times 10^8$ nucleated cells/kg recipient) is ordinarily infused by clinicians and may be sufficient.[66] Lower doses may be adequate in related donor settings; however, engraftment of both leukocytes and platelets correlate with CD34 cell content.[67–71]

Umbilical cord blood is obtained from the placenta during the third stage of delivery or postdelivery with the consent of the mother, and is stored frozen in liquid nitrogen. The component volume is usually 50–100 mL and may be further reduced by processing to remove nucleated red cells and plasma. The HLA type is determined and used as a search criterion for cord blood. The estimated likelihood of using cord blood stored for a family member (related bank) is approximately 1 in 10,000 to 1 in 200,000. There is a longer engraftment period associated with use of cord blood progenitor cells, although the risk of graft-versus-host disease is reduced.[72–75] The small volumes and yields of CD34-positive progenitor cells currently make cord blood most suitable for children and smaller adults.[76–78] Units from more than one cord have been infused into larger recipients with apparent success.[79]

PBSCs stored in liquid nitrogen likely remain stable for many years; however, the maximum safe storage period has not been determined.

INCOMPATIBILITY IN TRANSPLANT SETTINGS

ABO Incompatibility

Transplantation of hematopoietic progenitor cells relies on compatibility at the major histocompatibility locus, so that selection of the recipient-donor pair is determined by HLA similarity at the expense of ABO compatibility. Because HLA and ABO genes are inherited independently, some (10–30%) of these transplants will be ABO incompatible. Although ABO incompatibility does not appear to impact graft failure, mismatches can cause immediate hemolysis, delayed red blood cell engraftment, or delayed hemolysis based on the nature of ABO incompatibility between the recipient and donor.[80–82]

Minor Incompatibility

Minor incompatibility exists when the *donor's serum* contains antibodies against red blood cell antigens of the recipient (e.g., recipient group A, B, or AB and donor group O). Prior to infusion of the hematopoietic progenitor cells, plasma containing anti-A and anti-B can be removed to prevent immediate postinfusion hemolysis of the recipient's red blood cells.[83] Ten percent to 15% of minor ABO-incompatible transplant recipients may experience abrupt onset of hemolysis 7–10 days posttransplant when immune-competent B lymphocytes in the graft mount a response against the recipient red blood cell antigens. Patients must be monitored carefully and transfused aggressively at the first sign of hemolysis.[81] Hemolysis may be severe or even fatal unless recognized promptly.

Major Incompatibility

In major incompatibility, the *recipient's serum* contains antibodies against the red blood cell antigens of the donor (e.g., recipient group O and donor group A, B, or AB; recipient group A or B and donor group AB). Hemolysis of red blood cells in the hematopoietic progenitor cells upon infusion may occur if the graft is not processed to remove red blood cells prior to infusion. After transplantation, the recipient may produce antibodies against donor red cell antigens for months, especially with the use of nonmyeloablative regimens. Red blood cell engraftment and erythropoiesis may be delayed, resulting in red cell aplasia.[84]

Minor and major (bidirectional) incompatibility between the donor and recipient occurs when each has antibodies against the ABO blood group antigens of the other (e.g., the recipient's blood group is A and that of the donor is B or vice versa) (Fig. 98–6).

All transfusions must be irradiated to prevent transfusion-associated graft-versus-host disease. Table 98–6 reviews appropriate transfusion management during phases of transplantation.

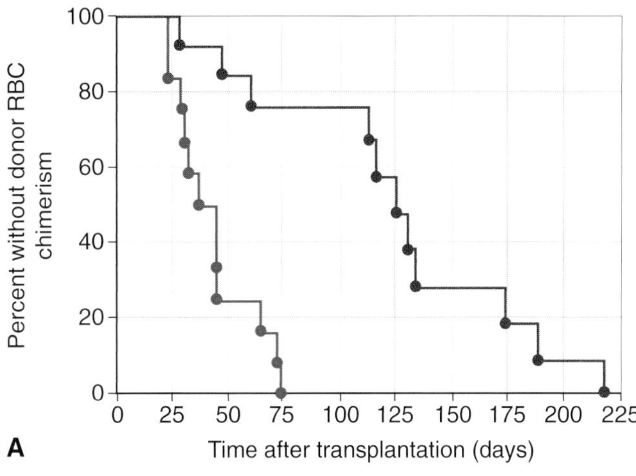

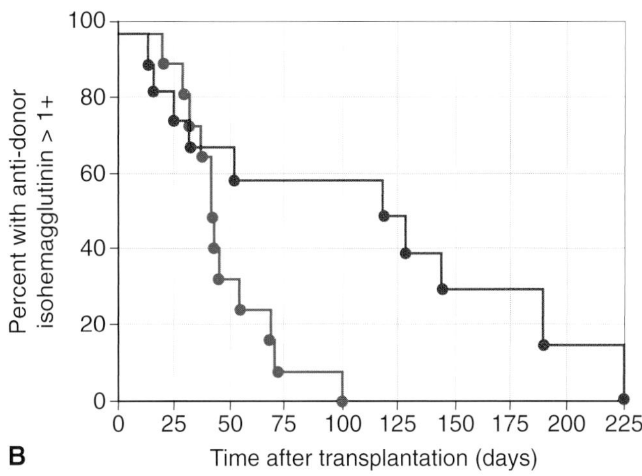

Figure 98–6. Onset of donor red blood cell chimerism and decline in anti–donor isohemagglutinin levels after reduced-intensity nonmyeloablative stem cell transplant (NST) compared with myeloablative stem cell transplant (SCT). ABO-incompatible NST resulted in delayed decline in anti–donor isohemagglutinins and delayed onset of donor chimerism compared with myeloablative SCT. ***A,*** Percentage of patients with no detectable donor red blood cell chimerism. ***B,*** Percentage of patients with persistent host anti–donor isohemagglutinins as a function of days posttransplantation. (Modified from Bolan CD, Leitman SF, Griffith LM, et al: Delayed donor red cell chimerism and pure red cell aplasia following major ABO-incompatible nonmyeloablative hematopoietic stem cell transplantation. Blood 98:1687–1694, 2001.)

Rh Incompatibility

Rh incompatibility occurs in 10–15% of hematopoietic progenitor cell transplantations. Transfusion practice is analogous to that of major and minor ABO incompatibility,[85] although the consequences are less severe. With myeloablative conditioning, anti-D formation in Rh-negative recipients of Rh-positive hematopoietic stem cells usually does not occur. Anti-D is more likely to develop from immune-competent lymphocytes of Rh-negative donor hematopoietic stem cells transplanted to Rh-positive recipients undergoing myeloablative conditioning.[86] Similar findings in Rh-incompatible hematopoietic stem cell transplant recipients undergoing nonmyeloablative

TABLE 98–6. Transfusion in Minor and Major ABO-Incompatible Transplants

		Phase I*	Phase II†			Phase III‡
Recipient	**Donor**	**All Components**	**RBC**	**Platelets**	**FFP**	**All Components**
Minor Mismatch						
A	O	Recipient group	O	A; *AB; B; O*	A; *AB*	Donor group
B	O	Recipient group	O	B; *AB; A; O*	B; *AB*	Donor group
AB	O	Recipient group	O	AB; *A; B; O*	AB	Donor group
AB	A	Recipient group	A	AB; *A; B; O*	AB	Donor group
AB	B	Recipient group	B	AB; *B; A; O*	AB	Donor group
Major Mismatch						
O	A	Recipient group	O	A; *AB; B; O*	A; *AB*	Donor group
O	B	Recipient group	O	B; *AB; A; O*	B; *AB*	Donor group
O	AB	Recipient group	O	AB; *A; B; O*	AB	Donor group
A	AB	Recipient group	A	AB; *A; B; O*	AB	Donor group
B	AB	Recipient group	B	AB; *B; A; O*	AB	Donor group
Minor and Major and Mismatch						
A	B	Recipient group	O	AB; *A; B; O*	AB	Donor group
B	A	Recipient group	O	AB; *B; A; O*	AB	Donor group

*Phase I: From time patient is prepared for hematopoietic progenitor cell transplant.
†Phase II: From initiation of myeloablative therapy from the time direct antiglobulin test is negative and isohemagglutinins against donor are no longer detectable (for RBC) or when recipient erythrocytes are no longer detectable (for FFP).
‡Phase III: After the forward and reverse types of the patient are consistent with donor ABO group.
Italicized blood groups indicate next best choice in order of preference.
Abbreviations: FFP, fresh frozen plasma; RBC, red blood cells.
Modified from Brecher ME (ed): Technical Manual (ed 14). Bethesda, MD: AABB Press, 2003, p 556; and from Friedberg RC: Transfusion therapy in hematopoietic stem cell transplantation. *In* Mintz PD (ed): Transfusion Therapy Clinical Principles and Practice. Bethesda, MD: AABB Press, 1999.

conditioning and immunosuppression with fludarabine and/or Campath 1H have been reported.[87]

Red blood cells may be removed from the donor hematopoietic progenitor cells to decrease risk of alloimmunization (similar to ABO major incompatibility) for Rh-negative recipients of Rh-positive hematopoietic progenitor cells. Rh-positive recipients of hematopoietic progenitor cells from Rh-negative donors previously alloimmunized to the Rh antigen should be monitored for signs of delayed hemolysis (as in minor incompatibility). In either situation, Rh-negative blood components are the first choice for transfusion.

Administration of Rh Immune Globulin with Rh-Incompatible Blood Components

Rh immune globulin is a plasma derivative that is obtained by fractionation of pooled plasma from hyperimmunized donors and treated to reduce the risk of virus transmission. It is available in intramuscular and intravenous forms and is indicated for prevention of alloimmunization of Rh-negative recipients exposed to Rh-positive red blood cells through transfusion or pregnancy. Use of Rh immune globulin has resulted in a greater than 90% decrease in the incidence of alloimmunization to the Rh antigen in pregnant Rh-negative females with Rh-positive fetuses and thus similarly reduced Rh antibody–mediated hemolytic disease of the newborn[88] (Table 98–7). The remaining cases result primarily from inadequate administration or failure to administer Rh immune globulin. The need for the use of Rh immune globulin in postmenopausal females and in males depends mostly on the magnitude of exposure, the possibility the individual may require transfusion in the future, and the likelihood that the individual will form antibody (anti-D).[92,97] Studies indicate that debilitated and immunocompromised individuals are less likely to form anti-D.[98–100]

For large exposures requiring many doses of Rh immune globulin, treatment may not be feasible, especially if the patient is unlikely to become pregnant, to form antibody (leukemia, solid tumors) or to be retransfused.[92] Rh immune globulin is not indicated for use in Rh-positive individuals, Rh-negative individuals who have developed anti-D from prior exposure, pregnancy in Rh-negative female with a known Rh-negative fetus or newborn, or Rh-negative patients with immune thrombocytopenic purpura.

MASSIVE TRANSFUSION

Massive transfusion is the transfusion of blood components over a 24-hour period in amounts that equal or exceed the total blood volume of the patient. Initially, adequate intravascular blood volume and blood pressure may be maintained with colloids (albumin, plasma protein fraction) or crystalloids (lactated Ringer's solution

TABLE 98–7. Rh Immune Globulin (RhIg)

Indications	Dosage
• Prevention of development of anti-D and subsequent hemolytic disease of the newborn in pregnant Rh-negative women with an Rh-positive fetus • Exposure of Rh negative individuals to Rh-positive red blood cells *Based on likelihood of alloimmunization, magnitude of transfusion, and likelihood of need for subsequent transfusion* IM RhIg: used in Rh-negative subjects after exposure to small-volume of Rh-positive red blood cells IV RhIg: used for large-volume exposures *>90% success in preventing Rh alloimmunization in pregnancy*[88,89] *Failure is usually the result of missed or insufficient injection (failure to follow recommendations or failure to detect event that may have led to alloimmunization), or large spontaneous fetomaternal hemorrhages not adequately covered by the residual amount of standard anti-D in the absence of additional RhIg administration*[89–91] *If RhIg has not been given within 72 hours of a sensitizing event, it should still be administered as soon as the need is recognized for up to 28 days*[92] *The mechanism of action is unknown.* • Treatment of ITP in Rh-positive patients only (IV RhIg)[93–96]	Full dose contains 300 μg anti-D to cover an exposure of 15 mL of Rh-positive RBC • Pregnant or postpartum women—within 72 hr of delivery[88,92,97] • After amniocentesis and chorionic villus sampling performed at gestational age >34 wk • Minidose contains 50 μg anti-D to cover an exposure of 2.5 mL of Rh-positive RBC • Fetus delivered or aborted up to 12 wk of gestation[90,97] • After amniocentesis and chorionic villus sampling at less than 34 wk of gestation In cases of erroneous transfusions, RhIg dose should be calculated based on the RBC volume transfused. *Half-life of RhIg is 21 days. Additional RhIg should be administered when there is expected ongoing risk of fetomaternal hemorrhage or additional transfusion of products containing Rh-positive red blood cells 21 days or more after the last dose of RhIg is given*[90,92,97]

Abbreviations: IM, intramuscular; ITP, immune thrombocytopenic purpura; IV, intravenous; RBC, red blood cells.

or normal saline). Generally a platelet count of greater than 50,000/μL, or 80,000–100,000/μL for neurologic surgery, ophthalmologic surgery, or cardiopulmonary bypass, a prothrombin time or partial thromboplastin time of less than 1.5 times the normal range, and a fibrinogen concentration of greater than 80–100 mg/dL are considered adequate for maintenance of hemostasis.[8] Transfusion of packed red blood cells may become necessary after a loss of more than 30% of the blood volume, depending on the rate of blood loss, tissue perfusion, and oxygenation status of the patient.[101] Usually massive transfusion, even in trauma settings, requires only replacement of platelets.[54] Combinations of low values seen during massive transfusion may require replacement therapy.[8,101,102]

Massive transfusion can be associated with a variety of adverse sequelae, including dilution of hematostatic constituents,[54,103] disseminated intravascular coagulation,[54] hypothermia, acidosis, hypocalcemia (secondary to citrate accumulation that may occur when large volumes of blood are administered at rapid rates, such as more than 100mL/min, especially in the presence of liver and renal dysfunction[104,105]), hyperkalemia (associated in part with accumulation of potassium in stored blood, hypothermia, and metabolic acidosis, especially in newborns and patients with renal disease), hypokalemia (possibly resulting from metabolic alkalosis, edema, increased diuresis, and β-adrenergic stimulation),[111] and other biochemical disturbances[104,105] (also see Chapter 99).

Disseminated intravascular coagulation probably complicates massive transfusion less often than suspected, and is associated with shock, independent of blood loss or transfusion. Transfusion management of disseminated intravascular coagulation is supportive while the underlying cause is being addressed. Treatment includes administration of cryoprecipitate when fibrinogen levels are below 80 mg/dL. Other components such as platelets may be necessary, especially if bleeding is severe.[54]

Whenever possible, dilution and/or consumption of hemostatic constituents of blood, such as platelets, coagulation factors, and fibrinogen, and electrolyte levels should be determined frequently and evaluated in the context of the patient's clinical status. Transfusion of blood components based on fixed ratios or algorithms should be avoided, and prophylactic platelet administration is usually not justified.[106]

ALTERNATIVES TO ALLOGENEIC BLOOD TRANSFUSION

Alternatives to the use of blood component therapy are available and may be particularly useful for bleeding patients who refuse allogeneic blood transfusions, such as Jehovah's Witnesses, or bleeding patients unresponsive to appropriate transfusion therapy. Patients with religious concerns about blood transfusion must be informed and allowed to make an informed decision regarding acceptance of any human-derived contents in any products that may be administered.[1,107]

Examples of alternatives to allogeneic blood transfusion are listed in Table 98–8. A discussion of pharmacologic hemostatic agents such as vitamin K, protamine sulfate, conjugated estrogens, 1-deamino-8-D-arginine vasopressin (DDAVP), recombinant factor VIIa, ε-aminocaproic acid, and tranexamic acid, which may be useful in some settings as alternatives or adjuncts to

TABLE 98–8. Alternatives to Allogeneic Blood Transfusion

Preoperative	Intraoperative	Postoperative
Autologous Blood Collection The donor's hemoglobin should meet or exceed 11 gm/dL. The donor must be at no increased risk of bacterial infection. Donations can take place up to every 5 days with the last collection no later than 72 hr prior to the procedure. Autologous blood is subject to the same shelf-life limitations as allogeneic blood components. *The unit may be frozen until the time it will be used.* Transfusion-transmitted disease (e.g., viral), red cell alloimmunization, and some transfusion reactions are prevented. *Risk of bacterial contamination and of clerical error leading to transfusion of ABO incompatible units is not decreased significantly.*[108] **Erythropoietin Therapy** To improve hematocrit prior to elective surgery **Correction of Nutritional Anemias** Iron, vitamin B_{12}, folate, etc. therapy prior to elective surgery	**Blood Salvaged from a Sterile Surgical Field** Blood is salvaged by devices that collect, centrifuge, wash, and concentrate the red blood cells. Blood collected in this manner may be stored at room temperature for 4 hr from the end of the collection and at 1°–6°C for up to 24 hr if refrigeration began within 4 hr from initiation of collection.[109] *Use of intraoperative blood recovery in oncologic procedures is controversial.* *Gross contamination of the surgical field with malignant cells constitutes a relative contraindication to the use of this technique.* **Acute Normovolemic Hemodilution (ANVH)** In cases in which intraoperative transfusion is likely, ANVH may be considered if the patient has a preoperative hemoglobin level of ≥12 gm/dL, is not infected or bacteremic, and does not have clinically significant cardiovascular, pulmonary, renal, or liver disease. Whole blood is collected from the patient during surgery, prior to anticipated significant blood loss, and the volume replaced with crystalloid (3 mL crystalloid for 1 mL whole blood withdrawn) or colloid (1 mL colloid for 1 mL whole blood withdrawn). Blood collected in this manner may be kept at room temperature for up to 8 hr or stored at 1°–6°C for up to 24 hr from the time of collection (if refrigeration started within 8 hr of collection)[109] and reinfused (usually in the operating room) after cessation of major blood loss or sooner if indicated.[110]	**Blood Recovered from Drainage** This procedure has been used primarily with cardiac and orthopedic surgery.[108] Blood recovered in this manner is generally dilute (hematocrit of approximately 20%) and may be partially hemolyzed. Transfusion with blood recovered in this manner should start within 6 hr of initiation of collection.[109]

component transfusion,[111] is beyond the scope of this chapter.

APHERESIS

Overview

Apheresis is the process by which selected components or substances in blood are removed from the circulation and the remainder of the blood is returned to the individual (Fig. 98–7). Apheresis is used for routine blood component (red cell, platelet, plasma, stem cell) collection and therapeutic removal of undesirable components and substances from circulation, achieved through automated machines. The kinetics of most intravascular substances indicate that exchange of one to one and one-half plasma volumes results in the highest efficiency removal, with progressively decreased efficiency with each additional consecutive exchange (Fig. 98–8). The volume of blood processed in order to attain the desired apheresis effect (for therapeutic component collection) depends on the nature of the substance of interest, including its intravascular distribution and its concentration in the particular patient. The patient's total blood volume determines the safe extracorporeal blood volume (which should not exceed 15% of blood volume). Small patients may require that the instrument be primed with blood. Table 98–9 lists the types of apheresis procedures and indications for treatment of hematologic disorders.

Apheresis procedures are generally safe, especially for normal component donors.[112] Complications are mainly related to vascular access (central venous catheters), hemodynamic changes (especially for patients with cardiovascular disease), anticoagulant toxicity, and a variable loss of blood components. Risks associated with apheresis are usually related to a patient's underlying disease.[113,114] More than 50 deaths (a rate of approximately 3 in 10,000) have been reported, although mostly in the setting of preexisting cardiopulmonary disease.[114,115]

A plasma exchange may result in a 30% or more decrease in platelet counts,[116] and platelet transfusion may be required for patients with low platelet counts and hemostatic problems. Hematocrit may decrease by 5–20%. Generally, cellular blood component counts return to normal after a few days and proteins and electrolytes reequilibrate within hours, although fibrinogen may remain below baseline levels after 72 hours.[117,118] Hypotension may occur as a result of both volume shifts and potentiation of bradykinin activity (as a result of enhancement of activation and accumulation of kinins in patients receiving angiotensin-converting enzyme inhibitors) or blood contact with filters and plastic separation pathways. Thus it is important to withhold angiotensin-converting enzyme inhibitors from patients for at least 24 hours prior to a therapeutic apheresis pro-

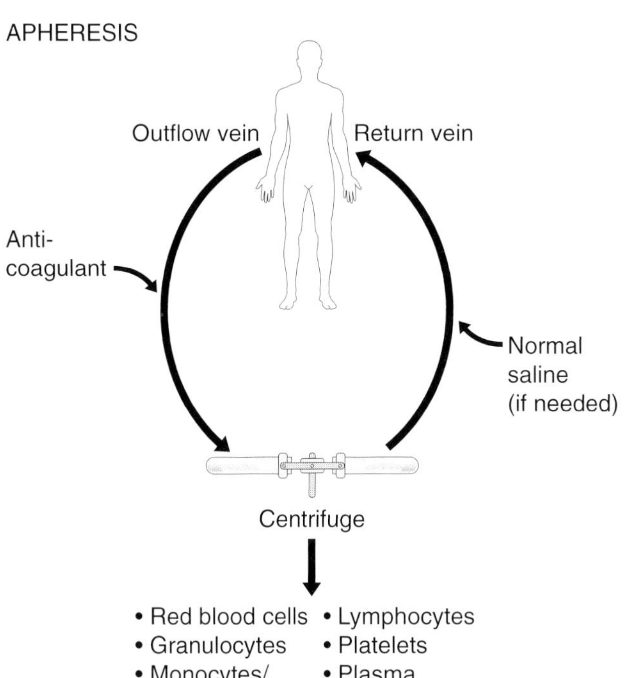

Figure 98–7. Centrifugal separation of blood components during apheresis.

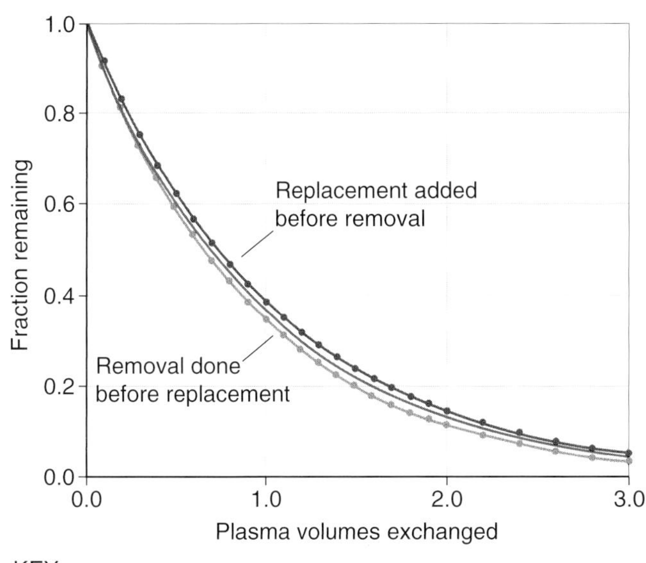

Figure 98–8. Percent remaining intravascular substance after processing from a multiple-lumen or dual-venipuncture (continuous) apheresis and after batch processing from a single-line venipuncture (discontinuous) apheresis with replacement fluid added before or after removal of intravascular substance. (Modified from Chopek M, McCollough J: Protein and biochemical changes during plasma exchange. *In* Berkman EM, Umlas J [eds]: Therapeutic Hemapheresis. Washington, DC: AABB Press, 1980, pp 13–52.)

cedure, especially when accompanied with albumin or plasma protein fraction replacement, which contains bradykinin and prekallikrein activator.[119–123]

Certain medications, especially those bound to plasma proteins (e.g., phenytoin [Dilantin]) or those with a long plasma half-life, may be decreased by plasma exchange procedures,[124] and the levels of these medications should be adjusted accordingly or they should be administered after the procedure when possible. Citrate is infused to prevent coagulation of blood in the extracorporeal circuit and may result in "citrate toxicity": binding of calcium and decreased levels of ionized calcium.[124,125] Symptoms of citrate toxicity include mild perioral tingling and discomfort, chest tightness, and tetany in severe cases. If these symptoms do not subside with adjustment of citrate and whole blood flow rates, administration of oral calcium (as chewable tablets) or intravenous calcium chloride (for large-volume apheresis procedures) helps prevent hypocalcemia and the accompanying syndromes.[60,126,127]

Therapeutic Apheresis Indications in Hematologic Disorders

Thrombocytapheresis

Thrombocytapheresis is a first-line therapy for thrombocytosis (platelet counts greater than 500,000/μL) in symptomatic patients with myeloproliferative disorders in which the platelets are qualitatively abnormal as well as increased in number (hemorrhage or thrombosis) such as seen in essential thrombocytosis, polycythemia rubra vera, chronic myelogenous leukemia, and myelofibrosis.[128–131] Prophylactic thrombocytapheresis in asymptomatic patients with thrombocytosis is generally not indicated, and hemorrhage and thrombosis do not nec-

TABLE 98–9. Recommendation for Therapeutic Apheresis in Hematologic Disorders

Category I—Accepted as Standard First-Line or Primary Therapy
ABO-mismatched marrow transplant (red cell removal from marrow)
Cutaneous T-cell lymphoma (photopheresis)
Erythrocytosis or polycythemia vera (phlebotomy)
Leukocytosis/thrombocytosis (cytapheresis)
Posttransfusion purpura (plasma exchange)
Sickle cell disease (red blood cell exchange)
Thrombotic thrombocytopenic purpura (plasma exchange)
Category II—Generally Accepted as Adjunctive or Supportive Therapy
ABO-mismatched marrow transplant (plasma exchange in recipient)
Erythrocytosis or polycythemia vera (erythrocytapheresis)
Coagulation factor inhibitors (plasma exchange)
Cryoglobulinemia (plasma exchange)
Cryoglobulinemia with polyneuropathy (plasma exchange)
Hyperviscosity (plasma exchange)
Idiopathic (autoimmune) thrombocytopenic purpura (immunoadsorption)
Myeloma, paraproteins, or hyperviscosity (plasma exchange)
Myeloma or acute renal failure (plasma exchange)
Polyneuropathy with IgM, with or without Waldenström's macroglobulinemia (plasma exchange)
Category III—No Clear Indication Based on Conflicting or Insufficient Evidence of Efficacy or Favorable Risk-to-Benefit Ratio; Sometimes Used as a Last Resort
Aplastic anemia or pure red cell aplasia (plasma exchange)
Autoimmune hemolytic anemia (plasma exchange)
Cutaneous T-cell lymphoma (leukapheresis)
Hemolytic disease of the newborn (plasma exchange)
Hemolytic-uremic syndrome (plasma exchange)
Platelet alloimmunization and refractoriness (plasma exchange or immunoadsorption)
Malaria or babesiosis (red blood cell exchange)
Multiple myeloma with polyneuropathy (plasma exchange)

Modified from Smith JW, Weinstein R, Hillyer KL, for the AABB Hemapheresis Committee: Therapeutic apheresis: a summary of current indication categories endorsed by the AABB and the American Society for Apheresis. Transfusion 43:820, 2003.

essarily correlate with the extent of thrombocytosis.[132,133] Cytapheresis is acutely beneficial (each procedure will lower the count 30–50%).[134,135] Patients should begin cytoreductive chemotherapy simultaneously, because plateletpheresis is not an effective long-term measure.[136]

Leukocytapheresis (Leukapheresis)

Leukocytapheresis is a first-line therapy for malignant leukocytosis, or "hyperleukocytosis" (immature white blood cell counts of greater than 100,000/μL or rapidly rising blast cells at counts less than 100,000/μL) in symptomatic patients with leukemias that may result in leukostasis in the central nervous system, kidneys, and lungs. The syndrome occurs mainly with acute nonlymphocytic leukemias. Leukocytapheresis has also been used in the treatment of leukostasis associated with acute lymphoblastic/lymphocytic leukemias,[137–139] acute myelocytic leukemia,[140] chronic lymphocytic leukemias,[141] and chronic myelomonocytic leukemias.[142] The size and physical characteristics of the cells, as well as the absolute count, may help predict those patients who will suffer from this syndrome and those that might benefit from acute leukapheresis. The "leukocrit" can be a helpful measurement.[143] Leukapheresis does not modify the course of the underlying disease.[140,144,145]

Leukocytapheresis may prove useful in the short-term control of chronic myelogenous leukemia and myeloproliferative disorders in early pregnancy when chemotherapy is not feasible.[146,147] Changes in mentation, dizziness, blurred vision, hypoxia, or respiratory symptoms constitute a medical emergency and an indication for immediate treatment. Therapeutic leukapheresis can reduce the leukocyte count by 30–50% in a matter of hours and symptoms may abate promptly.[143,148] If the white cell count is significantly higher than 100,000/μL, then a 50% reduction may not be sufficient and the patient may continue to be symptomatic. In this case additional leukocytapheresis procedures may be necessary. Reduction of the white cell count may permit cytoreductive chemotherapy to be given with less concern about the fever, increased uric acid, renal failure, and electrolyte imbalances common to the acute cytolysis syndrome. Chemotherapy with hydroxyurea or a similar agent should be initiated concurrently because repeated leukocytapheresis may not control hyperleukocytosis and does not reduce mortality.[140,145]

Erythrocytapheresis/Red Cell Exchange

Erythrocytapheresis is used to reduce red cell mass acutely in the treatment of symptomatic excessive polycythemia (visual disturbances, confusion, lethargy, hemorrhage, threatened stroke, thrombosis of abdominal vasculature). Saline or colloid volume replacement is administered to maintain isovolemia.[124,149,150]

Red cell exchange, the removal of abnormal red cells and replacement with stored red blood cells, is used acutely in the treatment of complications of sickle cell disease, including acute chest syndrome, stroke, retinal infarction, priapism, and hepatic crisis, or as protracted or chronic treatment for the prevention of recurrent complications such as stroke, severe painful crises, and reduction of iron overload associated with transfusion[151–154] (also see Chapter 99 for a discussion of iron overload). The goal is to achieve a hemoglobin A level of greater than 50%.[152,155] Exchange transfusion can effect levels of hemoglobin A difficult to achieve with simple transfusion and may benefit patients in the third trimester for preeclampsia, sepsis, and preoperative management.[124,151] Transfusion and exchange have been used to treat sickle complications during pregnancy; however, routine use is unnecessary.[156]

Red cell exchange may be used in conjunction with antiparasitic treatment in malaria to decrease circulating parasite load in symptomatic patients (cerebral malaria, severe anemia, pulmonary edema, renal failure, disseminated intravascular coagulation, shock, acidosis, malaria hemoglobinemia) when it exceeds 5% (especially in nonimmune individuals), with the goal to decrease parasitemia to less than 5%.[157–160]

TABLE 98–10. Category I and II Recommendations for Therapeutic Plasma Exchange in Various Disorders

Category I	Category II
Acute inflammatory demyelinating polyradiculoneuropathy	ABO-mismatched marrow transplant* (recipient)
Antiglomerular basement membrane antibody disease	Acute central nervous system inflammatory demyelinating disease
Chronic inflammatory demyelinating polyradiculoneuropathy	Coagulation factor inhibitors
Demyelinating polyneuropathy with immunoglobulin (Ig)G and IgA	Cryoglobulinemia
Familial hypercholesterolemia (selective adsorption)	Cryoglobulinemia with polyneuropathy
Myasthenia gravis	Familial hypercholesterolemia
Posttransfusion purpura	Hyperviscosity
Phytanic acid storage disease	Idiopathic (autoimmune) thrombocytopenic purpura
Thrombotic thrombocytopenic purpura	Lambert-Eaton myasthenia syndrome
	Myeloma, paraproteins, or hyperviscosity
	Myeloma or acute renal failure
	Pediatric autoimmune neuropsychiatric disorders (PANDAS)
	Polyneuropathy with IgM (with or without Waldenström's macroglobulinemia)
	Rapidly progressive glomerulonephritis
	Rheumatoid arthritis (lymphoplasmapheresis)
	Sydenham's chorea

*Removal of red blood cells from the marrow is the preferred method.

Modified from Smith JW, Weinstein R, Hillyer KL, for the AABB Hemapheresis Committee: Therapeutic apheresis: a summary of current indication categories endorsed by the AABB and the American Society for Apheresis. Transfusion 43:820, 2003.

Therapeutic Plasma Exchange/Plasmapheresis

Therapeutic plasma exchange is used as a first-line emergency treatment of thrombotic microangiopathies (as a first-line therapy in TTP and as a last resort in hemolytic-uremic syndrome) and of hyperviscosity syndrome complicating the paraproteinemias of multiple myeloma, Waldenström's macroglobulinemia, and cryoglobulinemia.[161,162] Therapeutic plasma exchange may be used to lower coagulation factor (VIII, IX) inhibitor levels in patients with uncontrollable bleeding or undergoing invasive procedures[161,163] and as a last-resort treatment in immune (autoimmune) thrombocytopenic purpura in adults refractory to steroids and high-dose intravenous immunoglobulin.[164,165] TTP- and hemolytic-uremic syndrome–like presentations associated with administration of immunosuppressive agents (e.g., vinca alkaloids, mitomycin, bleomycin, BL22, cisplatin, tacrolimus, and cyclosporin A) do not respond well to therapeutic plasma exchange.[166,167]

The effectiveness of therapeutic plasma exchange in TTP seems to depend upon the removal of ultra-large von Willebrand factor multimers and reduction of the immunoglobulin G antibodies against von Willebrand factor–cleaving protease (ADAMS13).[168–171] In therapeutic plasma exchange for TTP, plasma is administered to maintain isovolemia, remove autoantibody to, and supply additional ADAMTS13. Colloids or saline can be used for this purpose for conditions other than TTP. Plasma depleted of the ultra-large von Willebrand factor multimers (cryoprecipitate-reduced plasma) may be beneficial for patients refractory to therapeutic plasma exchange with fresh frozen plasma as replacement fluid,[172,173] although this remains controversial.[174] Therapeutic plasmapheresis used in combination with steroids and immunosuppressive therapy may result in fewer relapses and decreased need for splenectomy.[175]

Therapeutic plasma exchange is often performed daily, then tapered until platelet counts stabilize at greater than 100,000/μL for 2 consecutive days. Response to therapy can be monitored by clinical assessment and laboratory measurements (platelet count, lactate dehydrogenase, extent of schistocytosis).[176] Tapering of treatment to prevent relapse is controversial. A multicenter survey found no difference in relapse rate between patients undergoing tapering of therapeutic plasma exchange and those whose therapeutic plasma exchange was terminated without a tapering (to every other day prior to termination).[177]

Hyperviscosity responds to even small volume exchanges, although procedures will need to be repeated until the paraprotein can be controlled with chemotherapy[162] (Table 98–10).

EXCHANGE TRANSFUSION FOR THE TREATMENT OF HEMOLYTIC DISEASE OF THE NEWBORN

Hemolytic disease of the newborn refers to the destruction of fetal red blood cells by maternal immunoglobulin G antibodies that cross the placenta and react with a paternally derived antigen present on the fetal red blood cells. Hemolytic disease of the newborn has been traditionally associated with Rh antibodies (anti-Rh_0D), although other antibodies including anti-A, anti-B, and anti-Kell have been implicated and may cause significant hemolytic disease of the newborn. Mild cases present with asymptomatic laboratory findings of a positive direct antiglobulin test and mild bilirubinemia. Severe cases may result in intrauterine death (hydrops fetalis, erythroblastosis fetalis) or high risk of kernicterus as a result of high concentrations of unconjugated bilirubin.

The first line of therapy in severe cases is intrauterine red blood cell transfusion using compatible (with the mother's antibody), irradiated, cytomegalovirus-negative, sickle-negative red blood cells suspended in 5% albumin or fresh frozen plasma. With enhanced prevention of Rh alloimmunization and Rh hemolytic disease of the newborn, most cases currently requiring exchange transfusion are a result of ABO hemolytic disease of the newborn.[178] Exchange transfusion may be considered in patients refractory to other therapies. Simultaneous removal of excess bilirubin, antibody, and red cells coated with antibody, and the administration of albumin to which excess bilirubin can bind, preventing kernicterus,[178–180] can be achieved through exchange transfusion. Usually a two-blood-volume exchange removes about 25% of the excess bilirubin and 70% of the red blood cells coated with antibody. Additional exchange transfusions may be necessary if bilirubin continues to rise.[179,180]

Exchange transfusion may result in a rapid rise of antibody to levels higher than prior to the exchange (as a result of plasma replacement without replacement of globulins) as evidenced by studies in autoimmune disorders treated with exchange transfusion.[181,182]

Suggested Readings*

American College of Obstetrics and Gynecology: ACOG Practice Bulletin: Prevention of Rh D Alloimmunization, Number 4, May 1999 (replaces Educational Bulletin Number 147, October 1990). Clinical management guidelines for obstetrician-gynecologists. Int J Gynecol Obstet 66:63–70, 1999.

CURRENT CONTROVERSIES & FUTURE CONSIDERATIONS

- Whole blood is seldom available for allogeneic use. ABO identical whole blood may be beneficial in settings of massive transfusions in patients who require concomitant oxygen-carrying capacity and volume expansion; it also contains stable coagulation factors. Should it be more readily available for use in the massive transfusion setting?
- Red cells age during storage. The standard for acceptable red cells is in vivo survival of 75% of radiolabelled cells at 24 hours. Are fresh(er) red cells better for transfusion?
- While platelets do not have Rh antigens, a unit of platelets contains small amounts of red blood cells that may result in alloimmunization of Rh-negative recipients. Should Rh-negative patients, particularly immunocompetent females of childbearing potential, routinely receive Rh-negative platelets? Should RhIg be routinely administered with every Rh-positive platelet transfusion to an Rh-negative patient?
- ABO compatible platelets may still contain antibodies that cause hemolysis. Should all platelet transfusions be ABO identical?
- Leukoreduction of cellular blood components decreases alloimmunization; it is associated with a 10% loss of platelets and increased cost. Likewise, ultraviolet B (UV B) irradiation has been effective in decreasing the incidence of alloimmunization; however UV B is not currently licensed for use in the United States. Would it be safe and cost effective to use UV B as a means of leukoreduction?
- Alloimmunization and transmission of cell-associated viruses can be reduced by universal leukoreduction of blood components. Transfusion-associated graft-versus-host disease can be prevented by gamma irradiation of blood components. Should all blood components be leukoreduced and gamma irradiated?
- Plasma transfusions containing HLA alloantibodies have been implicated as one cause of transfusion-related acute lung injury (TRALI). Plasma from multiparous women frequently contain such alloantibodies. Should all plasma be screened for HLA antibodies, or should fresh frozen plasma be prepared from male donors only?
- Granulocyte therapy is indicated for neutropenic patients (neutrophil count $<0.5 \times 10^9$/L) with active bacterial infection who do not respond to 48 hours of appropriate antimicrobial therapy and in whom marrow recovery is likely. Patients with granulocyte dysfunction may also benefit from granulocyte therapy. Granulocyte therapy decreases the length of bacterial infection, but does it decrease mortality? Should it be used prophylactically?
- Red cell substitutes are intended to deliver oxygen without need for compatibility testing and exposure of the recipient to infectious and immune risks associated with transfusion. These may have a role in trauma and resuscitation when there may be no access to compatible blood immediately, may serve as an adjunct to autologous hemodilution during surgery, or in the management of cancer-related vascular occlusive syndromes. However adverse side effects and short half-life of the various red cell substitutes in circulation limit their use. None are licensed for routine use. Various preparations are under investigation to minimize side effects and maximize oxygen carrying capacity and persistence in circulation.
- Pathogen inactivation techniques have been used successfully in nearly eliminating transmission of pathogens in plasma-derived protein fractions. These techniques have not been equally successful when applied to cellular blood components and have side effects that preclude their use currently. Various techniques of cellular pathogen inactivation are under investigation to balance effectiveness with decreased side effects.

McLeod BC, et al (eds): Apheresis Principles and Practice (ed 2). Bethesda, MD: AABB Press, 2003.

Practice guidelines for blood component therapy: Report by American Society of Anesthesiologists Task Force on Blood Component Therapy. Anesthesiology 84:732–747, 1996.

Roseff SD (ed): Pediatric Transfusion: A Physician's Handbook. Bethesda, MD: AABB Press, 2003.

Schiffer CA, Anderson KC, Bennett CL: Platelet transfusion for patients with cancer: clinical practice guidelines of the American Society of Oncology. J Clin Oncol 19:1519–1538, 2001.

Smith JW, Weinstein R, Hillyer KL: Therapeutic apheresis: a summary of current indication categories endorsed by the AABB and the American Society for Apheresis. Transfusion 43:820, 2003.

Snyder EL, Haley NR (eds): Hematopoietic Progenitor Cells: A Primer for Medical Professionals. Bethesda, MD: AABB Press, 2000.

Starr D: Blood—An Epic History of Medicine and Commerce. New York: Perennial Press, 2002.

Triulzi DJ (ed): Blood Transfusion Therapy: A Physician's Handbook (ed 7). Bethesda, MD: AABB Press, 2002.

Full references for this chapter can be found on accompanying CD-ROM.

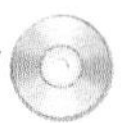

CHAPTER 99

Complications of Transfusion: Transfusion Reactions and Transfusion-Transmitted Diseases

Lynne Uhl, MD, and Margot S. Kruskall, MD

KEY POINTS

Complications of Transfusion: Transfusion Reactions and Transfusion-Transmitted Diseases

- Blood transfusions are associated with measurable but largely manageable complications and risks.
- Immune-mediated hemolysis is the most frequently reported transfusion-associated fatality; the majority of cases are due to ABO-related clerical errors.
- Febrile nonhemolytic transfusion reactions are largely due to recipient antibodies directed against donor leukocytes in the blood component. The incidence of these reactions has been substantially reduced by the use of leukoreduced blood.
- Any unexpected sign or symptom in association with a blood transfusion should be considered as a possible reaction. Unusual complications such as transfusion-associated acute lung injury, posttransfusion purpura, and transfusion-associated graft-versus-host disease should be kept in mind.
- Risks of transfusion-transmitted viral diseases have fallen dramatically in the last two decades with the implementation of improved donor history screening and new tests for the presence of implicated organisms in donor blood.
- Bacterial contamination of platelets has surfaced as an important risk, related to the room-temperature storage of this component prior to transfusion. A high fever and hypotension in a transfusion recipient should raise immediate suspicion.
- Parasitic infections transmitted through blood are uncommon, but of growing importance in an increasingly mobile blood donor population.

INTRODUCTION

A blood transfusion is a potentially treacherous undertaking, involving the infusion of living allogeneic cells collected in an imperfectly sterilized environment, immersed in a chemical storage medium, surrounded by leachable plastic, and run through a synthetic filter. In actual practice, the risks are of a low and largely manageable magnitude (Fig. 99–1), provided that appropriate practices and precautions are employed.[1] This chapter reviews the risks of transfusion—transfusion reactions and transmitted diseases—and strategies for circumventing them.

TRANSFUSION REACTIONS

Immune-Mediated Transfusion Reactions

Immune-Mediated Hemolysis

Any transfusion that results in the shortened survival of red cells can be considered a hemolytic transfusion reaction. Reactions caused by antibody-mediated destruction are discussed here; nonimmune causes of red cell destruction are discussed later in this chapter.

Frequency

Deaths from hemolytic transfusion reactions are the most frequent transfusion-associated fatalities reported to the Food and Drug Administration (FDA); the majority are due to ABO antibodies and occur at a rate between 1 in 300,000 and 1 in 700,000 transfusions.[2,3] Clerical, rather than technical, errors—mislabeling of the crossmatch specimen, or infusion of the unit to an unintended recipient—cause nearly all of these deaths.

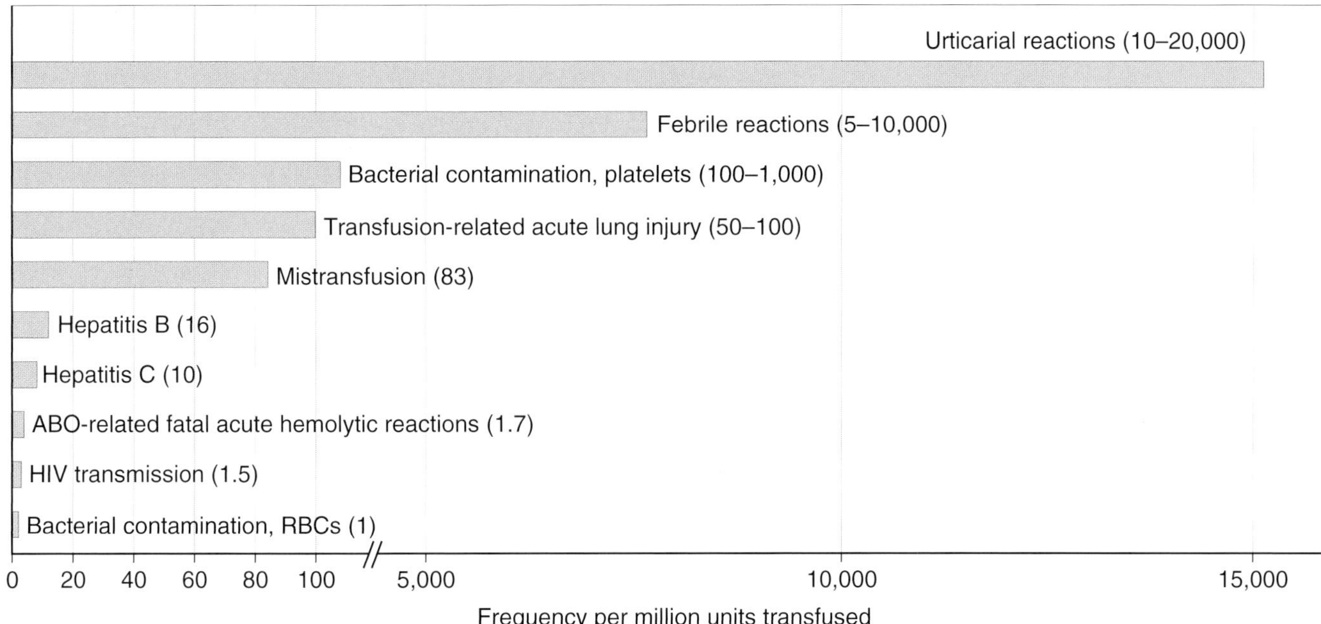

Figure 99–1. The risks of various complications of transfusion, expressed as frequency per million units transfused. (Redrawn from AuBuchon JP, Kruskall MS: Transfusion safety: realigning efforts with risks. Transfusion 37:1211–1216, 1997.)

Pathophysiology

A hemolytic transfusion reaction usually occurs within minutes to hours of a transfusion of allogeneic red cells, in a patient who has formed clinically significant (i.e., hemolytic) antibodies to the donor's (foreign) antigen(s). Some antibodies are present even in the absence of previous blood exposure—notably anti-A and anti-B in the ABH blood group system. Such antibodies are directed at carbohydrate epitopes, and develop in the first year after birth in response to exposure to similar epitopes in the environment, such as are present on bacteria, viruses, and plants. Historically, these antibodies have been called "naturally occurring,"[4] are present in high-titer mixtures of immunoglobulin (Ig)M and IgG classes, and fix complement. As a result, the hemolysis is brisk, and often intravascular (Fig. 99–2).

Alternatively, hemolysis can be caused by antibodies formed following exposure to red cells: through transfusion, from the fetal-to-maternal hemorrhage that occurs during pregnancy and parturition, or less frequently, through other unusual sources of exposure such as shared intravenous needles. The development of red blood cell alloantibodies is a fairly common event, occurring in as many as 30% of patients following transfusion; the frequency of alloimmunization may be even higher in patients with underlying autoimmune disorders, but lower in individuals who are immunosuppressed, and extremely rare in neonates.[5–7] The antigens that stimulate antibody formation are typically glycoproteins, the antibodies produced are usually IgG, and complement fixation is less impressive. Red cell destruction is typically extravascular, and the sequelae less extreme, although striking hemolysis may occur (see Fig. 99–2). These antibodies are detected through compatibility testing, and in particular the antibody screen (an assay that detects red cell alloantibodies in plasma); thus transfusion of antigen-incompatible blood, and acute hemolysis, can nearly always be avoided. However, "delayed hemolysis," involving leisurely red cell destruction over the first 2 weeks following the transfusion, is a more common complication (Fig. 99–3).[8] This distinct picture results from the tendency of red cell alloantibodies to diminish in titer over time, often becoming undetectable. In this setting, reexposure to a foreign antigen in an ostensibly compatible transfusion leads to an anamnestic antibody response. Newly formed antibody is deposited on the transfused red blood cells gradually, in keeping with the rate of antibody production. In more than 80% cases, the timing and amount of antibody produced are so modest that clinically detectably shortened red cell survival cannot be documented.[9] Common red cell antigen targets for hemolysis are listed in Table 99–1; note that not all antibodies are clinically significant (hemolytic).[10]

In contrast to donor red cell antigens, passively acquired alloantibodies rarely cause problems, because blood banks screen and eliminate alloimmunized donors. However, passively transfused ABO antibodies can occasionally cause hemolytic mischief, typically when a group O apheresis platelet product with a high-titer anti-A is transfused into a group A recipient.[11,12]

Clinical Features

Fever, probably related to activation of a network of cytokines (interleukin-1, -6, and -8; tumor necrosis factor-α),[13] and pain at the intravenous site, resulting from vein inflammation from the complement byproducts c3a and c5a, are often the earliest signs of trouble. Less predictable events include flushing, nausea, and cardiovascular symptoms, such as chest pain, hypotension,

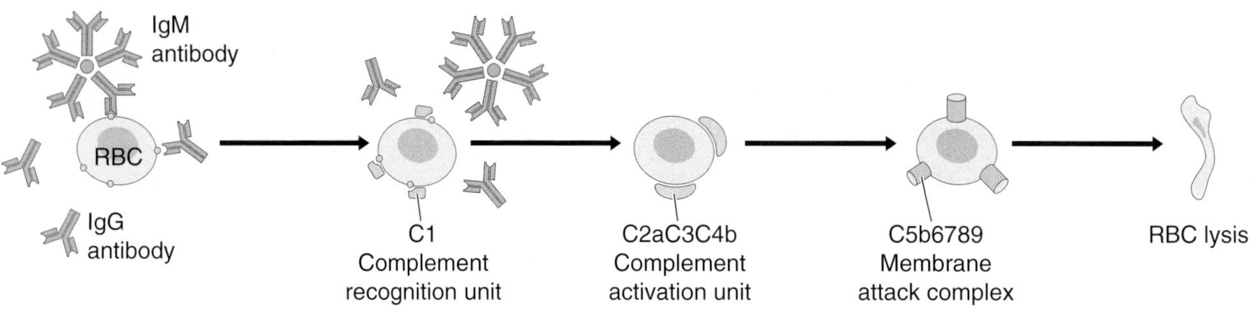

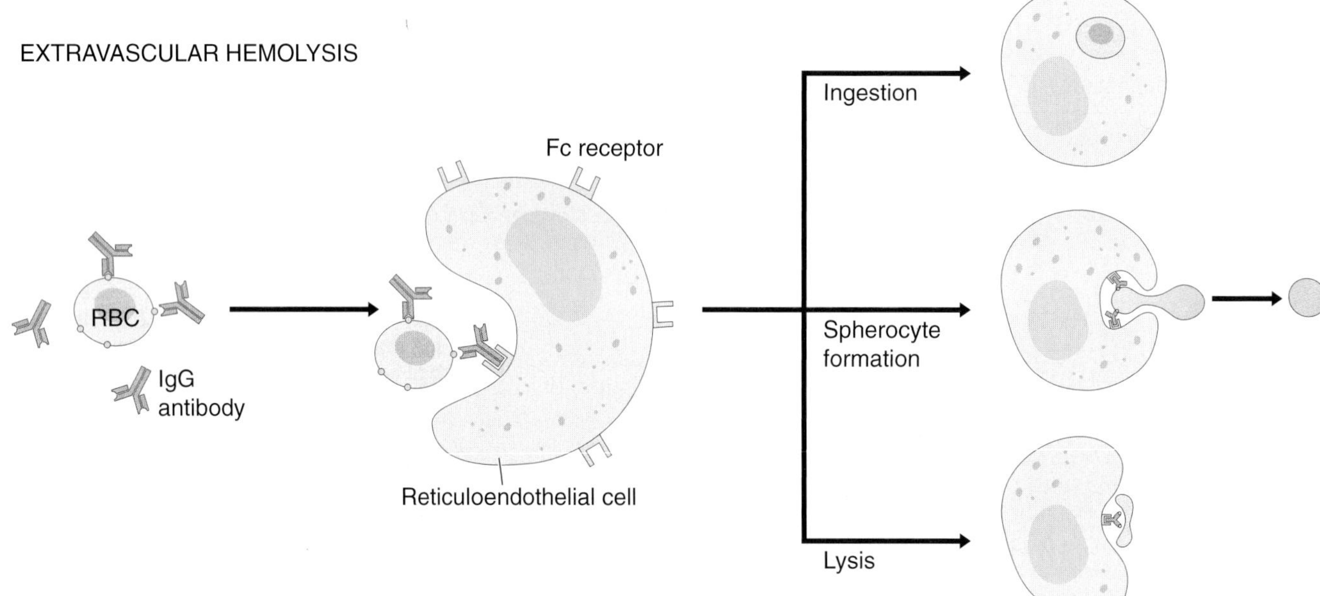

Figure 99–2. Mechanisms of immune-mediated hemolysis following transfusion.

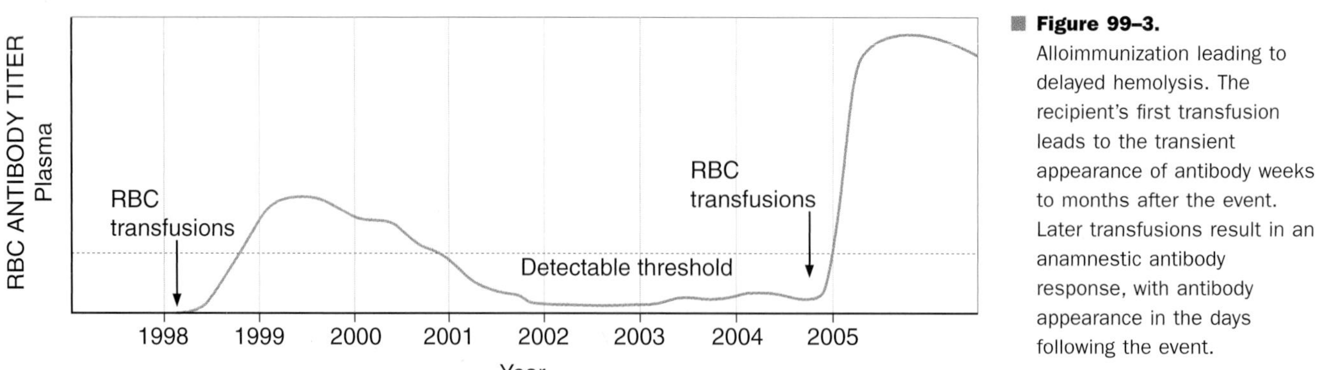

Figure 99–3. Alloimmunization leading to delayed hemolysis. The recipient's first transfusion leads to the transient appearance of antibody weeks to months after the event. Later transfusions result in an anamnestic antibody response, with antibody appearance in the days following the event.

dyspnea, and a sense of impending doom. Costovertebral tenderness may occur as a result of acute tubular necrosis induced by the combined effects of antigen-antibody complexes and complement.[14] Concomitant kidney swelling causes symptoms because the organ's covering (Glisson's capsule) is innervated. Disseminated intravascular coagulation is noted in some cases, and may be one of the only signs of a hemolytic reaction in the anesthetized patient, manifested by excessive bleeding during the surgical procedure. In the patient with sickle cell anemia, a hemolytic transfusion reaction may also induce a pain crisis and life-threatening anemia, the latter a combination of donor red cell destruction, recipient reticulocytopenia, and possibly recipient bystander red

TABLE 99–1. Clinical Significance of Antibodies to Blood Group Antigens

Blood Group System	ISBT Number	Major Antigens	Hemolytic Transfusion Reactions
ABO	001	A, B, AB, O	Severe, sometimes fatal
MNS	002	M, N	None
		S, U	Severe
		s	Rare
P	003	P_1	Rare
Rhesus (Rh)	004	D, C, C^w, E, c, e	Severe
Lutheran (Lu)	005	Lu^a	None
		Lu^b	Mild
Kell	006	K, k, Kp^b, Js^a, Js^b	Severe
		Kp^a	Mild
Lewis	007	Le^a	Rare
		Le^b	None
Duffy	008	Fy^a, Fy^b	Severe
Kidd	009	Jk^a, Jk^b	Severe
Diego	010	Di^a, Di^b, Wr^a	Severe
Cartwright (Yt)	011	Yt^a	Rare
		Yt^b	None
Xg	012	Xg^a	None
Chido/Rogers	017	Ch, Rg	None

Adapted from Reid ME, Øyen R, Marsh WL: Summary of the clinical significance of blood group alloantibodies. Semin Hematol 37:197–216, 2000.

cell destruction.[15] Autoantibody formation may develop in association with, or in the weeks following, a transfusion; this is usually manifested as a positive direct antiglobulin test, although in rare cases frank autoimmune hemolysis can result.[16,17]

Laboratory Diagnosis

The hallmark laboratory finding of immune-mediated hemolysis is the positive direct antiglobulin test (also known, more informally and less informatively, as the "direct Coombs test"). A posttransfusion sample of the recipient's red cells is mixed with rabbit antihuman globulin, containing activity against human IgG and complement components (at least C3d). If the transfused cells have been sensitized by a recipient antibody, and IgG and/or complement is present on the red cell surface, the rabbit antiserum will cross-link the substances on neighboring red cells, resulting in visual agglutination of the transfused cell population. Other supportive tests include rises in the levels of lactate dehydrogenase and indirect bilirubin, and in severe cases, the presence of hemoglobin and breakdown products such as methemoglobin in the plasma, the disappearance of haptoglobin, and the appearance in the urine of hemosiderin. Other causes of hemolysis should also be considered and ruled out (Table 99–2).

Treatment

Because acute hemolytic transfusion reactions are rare, and no good animal model exists, treatment strategies are empirical and symptom based. Stopping the transfusion as soon as possible is important, because the risk of mortality is correlated with the volume of blood infused. The unit of blood, and blood-filled tubing, should be disconnected, leaving the intravenous catheter for venous access. A serious risk from immune hemolysis is renal failure. Treatment of hypotension with crystalloids is important to maintain renal function, and intravenous furosemide (20–80 mg) to maintain renal flow has also been advocated.[14] Dopamine in low doses ("renal-dose" dopamine, 1–3 μg/kg/min) promotes renal vasodilation and increases urine output; however, its role in ameliorating the risk of anuric renal failure is controversial.[18,19] Alkalinization of the urine with intravenous sodium bicarbonate (to a urine pH of >6.5) makes hemoglobin more soluble, and may prevent tubular obstruction by hemoglobin casts. Hyperkalemia may result from massive release of intracellular red cell stores, and potassium levels should be monitored closely, especially in the setting of renal impairment, wherein dialysis may be required to control the level. Although disseminated intravascular coagulation may occur, heparin treatment is rarely necessary. In the absence of complications within the first 24 hours, long-term sequelae are unlikely. Delayed hemolytic reactions are nearly always mild or asymptomatic, and treatment is not usually needed.

Prevention

Compatibility testing—ABO and Rh typing of the donor and recipient, antibody screening and identification, and in complex situations a crossmatch of the donor's red cells against recipient plasma—is the mainstay against immune hemolysis. Because most acute immune hemolysis is due to clerical errors, improved methods are needed for outwitting human nature through the prevention of mislabeled samples used for the crossmatch, and better explicit identification of the patient for whom a unit of blood is intended.[20–22] Although delayed hemol-

TABLE 99–2. Other Clinical Pictures That Can Be Confused with a Hemolytic Transfusion Reaction

		Examples Caused by Factors in:	
Sign/Symptom	**Other Explanations**	**Donor Unit**	**Recipient**
Hemolysis	Thermal injury to red cells	Overheating, freezing	
	Osmotic injury to red cells	Admixture of blood with hypotonic solutions or drugs; transfusion of inadequately deglycerolized red cells	Infusion of hypotonic solutions; water irrigation of bladder
	Mechanical injury to red cells	Infusion through a small-bore needle or with excess pressure	Microangiopathy (DIC, TTP, HUS); extracorporeal circulation
	Infections	Infected blood unit	Malaria, *Clostridium welchii*
	Congenital and acquired hemolytic anemias	G6PD deficiency	G6PD deficiency; sickle cell anemia; autoimmune hemolytic anemia; drug-induced hemolysis
Hyperbilirubinemia	Nonimmune red cell lysis	Transfusion of lysed or aged red cells	Resorption of large hematoma
Fever	Other immune and nonimmune etiologies	Transfusion of infected blood	Febrile nonhemolytic transfusion reaction; fever caused by other underlying condition
Hypotension or shock	Other immune and nonimmune etiologies	Infusion of infected blood product; infusion of blood product with high levels of vasoactive mediators	IgA deficiency

Abbreviations: DIC, disseminated intravascular coagulation; G6PD, glucose-6-phosphate dehydrogenase; HUS, hemolytic-uremic syndrome; IgA, immunoglobulin A; TTP, thrombotic thrombocytopenic purpura.

Adapted from Beauregard P, Blajchman MA: Hemolytic and pseudo-hemolytic transfusion reactions: an overview of the hemolytic transfusion reactions and the clinical conditions that mimic them. Transfus Med Rev 8:184–199, 1994.

ysis is largely unavoidable, a patient's antibody history should always be used in choosing red cells, even if the antibody screen has become negative.

White Cell-Associated Transfusion Reactions (Febrile Nonhemolytic Transfusion Reactions)

These reactions typically involve a rise in temperature of 1°C or more (≥2°F), or chills, or both in a patient during or in the hours following a transfusion.

Frequency

Although febrile reactions are not usually serious, and long-term complications do not occur, they are common in leukocyte-containing blood products (approximately 1% of red cell transfusions and up to 30% of platelet transfusions).

Pathophysiology

Most febrile reactions occur with transfusion of cellular components, especially red cells and platelets, and are related to the presence in the component of leukocytes, or leukocyte-associated cytokines such as interleukin-1β, interleukin-6, and tumor necrosis factor-α released from the white cell during storage. Of historical importance, the discovery, in the 1960s, of leukocyte antibodies in patients experiencing febrile reactions to red cells led to the recognition of the human leukocyte antigen (HLA) system.[23] Febrile reactions to red cell components usually involve recipient antibodies directed against donor white cell antigens, most commonly HLA specific. This reaction is more common in female recipients, because of the frequent occurrence of immunization to paternal HLA antigens during pregnancy.[24] Reactions to platelet components are further aggravated by the accumulation in the plasma of cytokines and other bioreactive substances during the component's room-temperature storage.[25–27]

Clinical Features

Chills, and in severe cases rigors, associated with a rise in temperature, usually begin a half an hour or more after the onset of the transfusion. The delay in symptoms may be due to the buoyant density of white cells, which move to the top of the blood bag, and are therefore infused later in the transfusion. In a platelet donor, chills and rigors predominate, and fever is less common.[28]

Laboratory Diagnosis

As for any reaction to a transfusion, the blood should be discontinued immediately, and clinical and laboratory investigations initiated to rule out hemolysis or sepsis, two other important etiologies for posttransfusion fever.

Treatment

Fever can be treated with an antipyretic, customarily acetaminophen 325–650 mg. Chills and rigors associated with platelet transfusions respond promptly to intravenous meperidine (50 mg), which reduces shivering, although a second dose may need to be given after 2 hours.[29]

Prevention

Although a largely benign reaction, fever and chills are hallmark signs of two other transfusion complications, acute immune hemolysis and bacterial contamination, and curtailing these white cell–related reactions is desirable. Although studies are limited, the use of acetaminophen or diphenhydramine as "premedication" to prevent these reactions has not been shown to be efficacious.[30] Filtration of blood components to reduce the number of residual white blood cells to below 5×10^6 cells (leukoreduction) can eliminate more than three quarters of febrile reactions. Leukoreduction is most effective when the white cell reduction step takes place right after collection from the donor, before storage, because cytokine accumulation is prevented.[31–34] The nature of the residual cases of fever and chills in leukoreduced products remains uncertain.[34]

Allergic Reactions

Frequency

These common reactions occur in as many as 3% of recipients of plasma-containing components.[31] Rare, severe reactions resembling anaphylactic shock (interchangeably called "anaphylactoid" shock) occur in between 1 in 20,000 and 1 in 47,000 transfusions.[35]

Pathophysiology

In many cases, the allergic reaction is triggered by a donor allergen (e.g., penicillin or haptoglobin) or an alloantigen (e.g., albumin or IgA) interacting with a recipient's mast cell–bound IgE antibodies.[36] Far less commonly, donor antibodies cause the problem in a recipient containing the respective antigen.[37] The interaction between immunogen and antibody results in antibody cross-linking and mast cell activation, and then release of a variety of mediators that contribute to the symptom complex, including histamine, leukotrienes, and platelet-activating factor.

Clinical Features

Allergic reactions usually begin within the first 45 minutes of administration of a plasma product. Over 90% involve a dermatologic manifestation, usually urticaria, and may be limited to one or a handful of pruritic wheals on the skin. Other manifestations such as maculopapular rash, pruritus, and periorbital edema occur as well.[38] Less frequent scenarios involve erythema, bronchospasm, angioedema, and systemic symptoms such as dyspnea, abdominal cramping, hypotension, tachycardia, and even cardiac and respiratory arrest.[39,40] Fatalities can occur, but are fortunately rare (<1 per year).[2]

Laboratory Diagnosis

Except for detection of antibodies to IgA (see later), no specific laboratory tests are useful in this situation.

Treatment

Treatment of a mild dermatologic reaction includes slowing or stopping the transfusion, and administering an antihistamine such as diphenhydramine, 25–50 mg orally or intravenously. Because urticaria is rare in the setting of acute hemolysis or other life-threatening transfusion complications, this is the only situation in which continuing the transfusion while investigating the symptom is acceptable.

For more serious anaphylactic reactions, the transfusion should be discontinued, and the patient treated as for any allergic reaction. IgA deficiency in a recipient with anti-IgA is a specific case in point. Approximately 1 person in 700 lacks IgA antibodies; a very small proportion of these individuals have made antibodies to IgA, usually in response to a previous exposure to blood.[35] Even very small amounts of transfused plasma containing IgA can result in facial flushing, wheezing, dyspnea, and cyanosis; chest or abdominal pain; and sometimes profound hypotension. This life-threatening reaction must be treated immediately, by stopping the blood transfusion and administering epinephrine (0.3 mL of a 1 : 1000 dilution subcutaneously, or, if shock has already occurred, intravenous epinephrine in a 1 : 10,000 dilution).[39] Laboratory evaluation, including demonstration of IgA deficiency and class-specific anti-IgA, is helpful in defining the nature of the anaphylaxis, but only in retrospect.

Prevention

In patients with recurrent dermatologic reactions, antihistamines are sometimes useful when given prophylactically just prior to the transfusion. An alternative strategy, when cellular components are used, is to wash the plasma out of the component.

In the IgA-deficient individual with anti-IgA who has had an allergic reaction, future transfusions must be administered with care. Red cells can be rendered free of plasma using automated cell-washing technology. Plasma can also be removed from platelets; here the use of citrate-buffered saline as a wash solution, and relatively fresh (<48 hour old) components may be necessary for thorough removal of IgA.[41] Alternatively, IgA-deficient donors can be recruited; this is especially valuable for fresh frozen plasma.

Transfusion-Related Acute Lung Injury

Rapid development of shortness of breath during a blood transfusion should prompt consideration of this immune-orchestrated assault on the lungs.

Frequency

The incidence of transfusion-related acute lung injury, once considered rare, is actually on the order of 1 : 1000 to 1 : 5000 transfusions, and is now one of the three most commonly reported reasons to the FDA for death following a transfusion.[42] Mortality may be as high as 20%. The syndrome is frequently underdiagnosed; in one study of a fatal case of transfusion-related acute lung injury involving a frequent blood donor, 15 additional reactions in 36 other recipients of this donor's blood were identified in retrospect, the majority of which had not been reported to the transfusion service.[43]

Pathophysiology

The syndrome is associated, in the majority (70%) of cases, with antibodies to leukocytes in a donor's plasma. Using agglutination techniques, these antibodies can be shown to be directed against HLA class I or II epitopes,

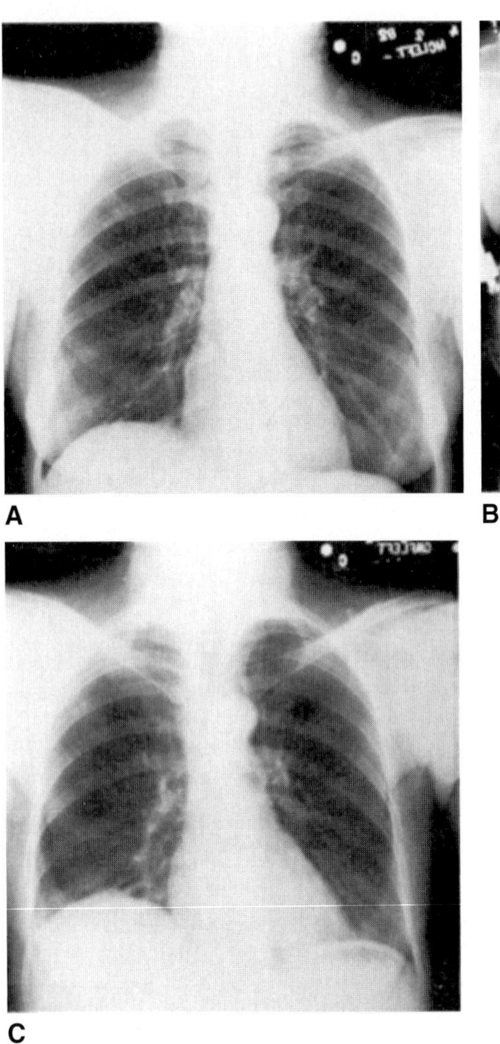

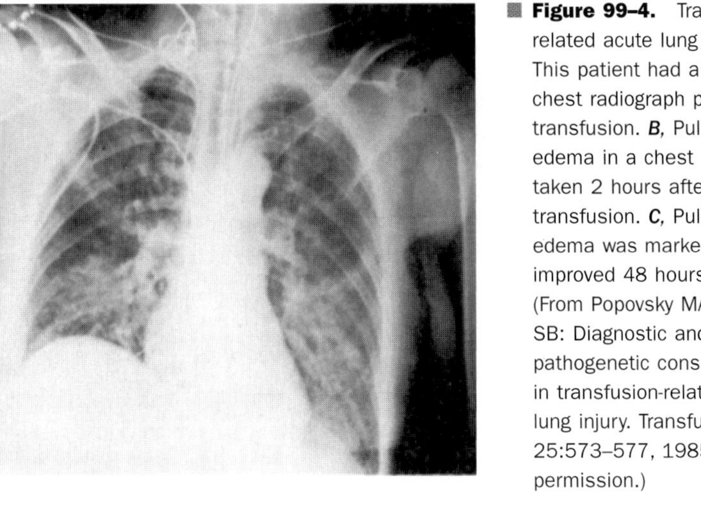

A B C

Figure 99–4. Transfusion-related acute lung injury. *A,* This patient had a normal chest radiograph prior to transfusion. *B,* Pulmonary edema in a chest radiograph taken 2 hours after a transfusion. *C,* Pulmonary edema was markedly improved 48 hours later. (From Popovsky MA, Moore SB: Diagnostic and pathogenetic considerations in transfusion-related acute lung injury. Transfusion 25:573–577, 1985, with permission.)

or other epitopes on granulocytes or monocytes.[44] Less commonly (5–20% of cases), the implicated antibody is present in the recipient,[44,45] and in the remainder of reports, no antibody can be identified in either donor or recipient. Additional antibodies may be detected with tests of improved sensitivity, such as flow cytometry.[46] Creative research may be necessary; a case of transfusion-related acute lung injury was proven in a lung transplant recipient, involving only the transplanted lung, following a transfusion of blood containing an HLA antibody directed against the lung donor's class I antigen.[47] Additional factors may be necessary for the reaction to occur. A "two-event" model proposes an underlying physiologic injury or stress resulting in pulmonary sequestration of polymorphonuclear leukocytes; subsequently, the infusion of biologically active lipids and/or cytokines in a transfused plasma-containing blood component prime the sequestered white cells, resulting in endothelial cell injury and a capillary leak syndrome.[48]

Clinical Features

The clinical problems begin within 6 hours after the initiation of a transfusion, with respiratory symptoms ranging from dyspnea and hypoxia to frank respiratory failure. Fever, chills, hypotension (often refractory to intravenous fluids) and tachycardia may also develop.[43] The chest radiograph reveals diffuse pulmonary infiltrates consistent with pulmonary edema; however, in contrast to heart failure, the central venous pressure is low because the etiology of the edema is increased vascular permeability rather than high filling pressures[45] (Fig. 99–4). At autopsy, aggregates of neutrophils are found adherent to vascular endothelium. Fresh frozen plasma is the most common product implicated in these reactions, although all plasma-containing components have been reported, including even intravenous immunoglobulin.[49] Neutrophil-rich products may also rarely initiate the syndrome, as was recently described in an allogeneic bone marrow transplant recipient.[50]

Laboratory Diagnosis

The diagnosis can be supported in retrospect by the identification of HLA or granulocyte-specific antibodies in either the implicated donor or the recipient, and, if found, evidence of the target antigen (antigen typing or cross-matching) in the corresponding recipient or donor, but such findings are not necessary for the diagnosis to be made on clinical grounds.

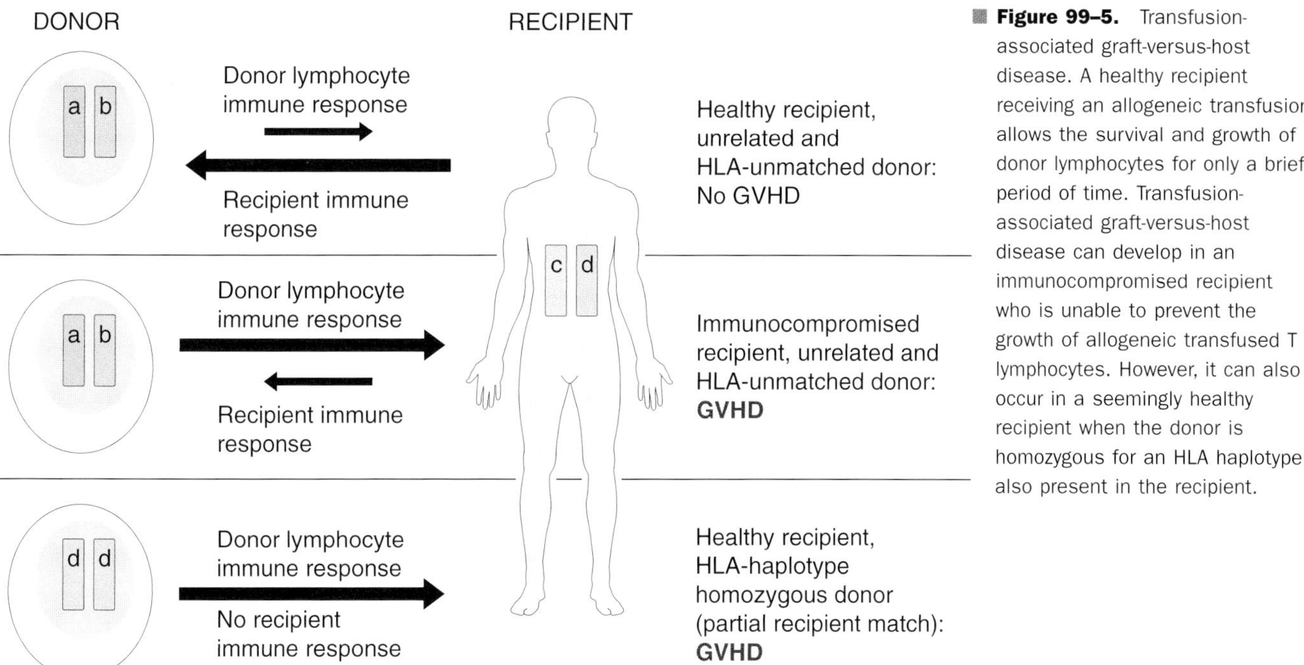

Figure 99–5. Transfusion-associated graft-versus-host disease. A healthy recipient receiving an allogeneic transfusion allows the survival and growth of donor lymphocytes for only a brief period of time. Transfusion-associated graft-versus-host disease can develop in an immunocompromised recipient who is unable to prevent the growth of allogeneic transfused T lymphocytes. However, it can also occur in a seemingly healthy recipient when the donor is homozygous for an HLA haplotype also present in the recipient.

Treatment

Treatment is largely supportive, and includes discontinuing the blood component, and providing hemodynamic and respiratory support as needed, which in many patients includes the need for mechanical ventilation. The vast majority of patients will have recovered within 4 days.

Prevention

Steps to help the individual recipient are of no help, because the problem usually lies with an immunized donor. Attention has recently focused on multiparous female donors, because in those women with three or more births, the likelihood of developing HLA antibodies may exceed 25%.[51,52] In a suggestive recent study, transfusion of plasma from such donors, versus plasma from subjects without a history of pregnancy, was associated with poorer pulmonary function in recipients.[53] A variety of donor deferral strategies have been proposed along these lines, including the deferral of multiparous or HLA-alloimmunized women.[54] Taking a more extreme stand, at the end of 2003, the United Kingdom stopped the distribution for transfusion of plasma donated by women.

Posttransfusion Purpura

A rare but profound and life-threatening thrombocytopenia may develop within days of a transfusion of a cellular blood component. For a complete discussion, the reader is referred to Chapter 60.

Transfusion-Associated Graft-Versus-Host Disease

This rare, but nearly always fatal, complication of blood transfusion occurs when viable donor lymphocytes in a transfused cellular blood component proliferate in the recipient.

Frequency

Although now rare, this picture was until recently bafflingly frequent, as in Japan, where the incidence of transfusion-associated graft-versus-host disease in the 1980s was as high as 1 in 685 otherwise healthy patients undergoing cardiac surgery.

Pathophysiology

The attacking lymphocytes are an oligoclonal expansion of cytotoxic T cells, whose targets include foreign HLA antigens. Critical features that determine whether transfusion-associated graft-versus-host disease will occur include the number, and viability, of transfused lymphocytes; the immune status of the recipient; and the extent of HLA antigen sharing between donor and recipient (Fig. 99–5). In immunologically healthy blood recipients, transfused lymphocytes survive and may even replicate, but usually for only a few days.[55,56] However, in immunocompromised patients, resistance to allogeneic cell growth is impaired (Table 99–3). Such situations include congenital immune disorders, including severe combined immunodeficiency; fetuses and small newborns; some malignancies, including Hodgkin's disease and some solid tumors; bone marrow transplant recipients; and others who have undergone immunomodulatory therapy. Drugs such as fludarabine (Fludara)[57] and cladribine (Leustatin)[58] create marked lymphopenia and immunosuppression, and even in the nonmalignant setting can render a patient susceptible to fatal transfusion-associated graft-versus-host disease.[59] For as yet unclear reasons, human immunodeficiency virus (HIV) infection in a recipient does not predispose to transfusion-associated graft-versus-host disease.[60] Transfusion-associated graft-

TABLE 99–3. Patients/Conditions at Risk of Developing Transfusion-Associated Graft-Versus-Host Disease

Disorder/Condition	Examples/Comments
Congenital immune disorders	For example, severe combined immunodeficiency
The fetus and newborn	Intrauterine transfusions, transfusions to premature and small infants
Malignancies	Transfusions to patients with Hodgkin's lymphomas, non-Hodgkin's lymphomas, other hematologic cancers, some solid tumors
Bone marrow transplant recipients	
Immunosuppressant drugs	Transfusions to patients taking fludarabine, cladribine
Partially HLA-matched transfusions	Transfusion from haplotype-homozygous donor into recipient with the same haplotype (especially likely in blood from relatives, or in a homogeneous population)

versus-host disease has also occurred in seemingly immunocompetent individuals who received blood from donors who were highly HLA matched, and often related by blood. Such HLA matching frequently involves a donor homozygous for an HLA genotype common to the population (such as A1, B8, or DR3 in northwestern Europe, and A26, B38, or DR2 in Japan), and a recipient heterozygous for the same genotype.[61–64]

Clinical Features

The clinical picture begins 3–30 days following the transfusion of a white cell—containing blood product—whole blood, red cells, platelets, granulocytes, and rarely even liquid (but not frozen) plasma. Initial symptoms include fever and a skin rash, which begins as a maculopapular exanthem and progresses to a diffuse desquamating erythroderma. Gastrointestinal symptoms, including watery or even bloody diarrhea, with anorexia, nausea, and vomiting, and liver function abnormalities, including elevated transaminases and hyperbilirubinemia, ensue.[65] Because the marauding donor cells also attack the recipient's bone marrow, profound aplastic anemia develops and regularly leads to death, in the weeks after onset of symptoms, as a result of hemorrhage or infection. By comparison, graft-versus-host disease associated with bone marrow transplantation does not lead to aplasia, because here the marrow cells are also of donor origin.

Laboratory Diagnosis

The diagnosis can be suspected on clinical grounds, but is often missed because the picture may be difficult to distinguish from that of a severe drug eruption or viral exanthem. Skin, liver, or bone marrow biopsies may be helpful, especially when evidence of cell death (epidermal basal cell vacuolization, degeneration of bile ducts, or bone marrow aplasia) is coupled with a mononuclear infiltrate.[66] Testing to prove the existence of two cell populations usually requires time-intensive molecular approaches, such as comparison of the HLA typing of the recipient's peripheral blood, now populated by donor lymphocytes, versus another tissue such as hair, reflective of the recipient's genes.[67]

Treatment

Many attempts at treatment have been reported, including antithymocyte globulin, T-cell—specific monoclonal antibodies, steroids, cyclophosphamide, cyclosporine, and most recently serine protease inhibitors such as nafamostat mesylate. However, although useful in the graft-versus-host disease that occurs after bone marrow transplantation, these maneuvers are only rarely successful in transfusion-associated graft-versus-host disease.[68,69]

Prevention

The syndrome can be prevented with the use of gamma irradiation of any cellular transfusion component. A dose of 2500 cGy completely inhibits T-cell proliferation, with minimal effects on platelets, granulocytes, and red cells. Red cell irradiation does cause a chronic leak of potassium and hemoglobin, with a cumulative increase in their concentrations in the component supernatant. In light of this membrane injury, the American Association of Blood Banks recommends that red cells not be stored for longer than 28 days following irradiation,[70] and, to prevent hyperkalemia in a small recipient, irradiation should be performed just prior to use for in utero, neonatal, and pediatric transfusions. Note that transfusion-associated graft-versus-host disease has been reported following leukocyte-depleted (nonirradiated) components; leukocyte depletion techniques do not guarantee sufficient cell reduction to prevent the syndrome, and should not be used in lieu of irradiation.[67,71] Irradiation has proven extremely effective. More than 95% of blood products in Japan are irradiated prior to transfusion, and no cases of transfusion-associated graft-versus-host disease were found in 2000 and 2001.[66] As more potent therapeutics are developed that can modify the immune system, the need to recognize the risk of transfusion-associated graft-versus-host disease becomes more important, and some authors in other parts of the world have called for universal, rather than patient-specific, irradiation of cellular blood components to prevent future cases.[72]

Transfusion-Related Immune Modulation

Blood transfusions can cause not only alloimmunization, but also immunosuppression. In the mid-1960s, an animal model of kidney transplantation documented improved organ survival in recipient animals given blood from their respective kidney donors.[73] This same effect was subsequently demonstrated in human kidney transplants,[74] and although partially eclipsed by improved immunosuppressant agents such as cyclosporine, continues to be noted.[75,76] Other beneficial examples of immunomodulation include a reduction in fetal loss in habitual aborters following donor-specific transfusions from marital partners,[77] and a reduced rate of recurrence in Crohn's disease following perioperative transfusions.[78,79]

More ominously, a role for transfusion in the spread of cancer or infection may also exist. The role of donor leukocytes in this form of immunosuppression, and the value of their depletion in circumventing this, have been shown in animal models. Allogeneic blood transfusions in a mouse tumor model, for example, enhance both growth of the primary tumor and the formation of metastatic nodules,[80] and leukodepletion of the blood product prior to transfusion abrogates the tumor-enhancing effect.[81] Similarly, in animal models of infection, allogeneic transfusions increase mortality.[82–84]

Neither the pathophysiology of transfusion-induced immunomodulation, nor, in humans, a causal relationship between transfusion and cancer recurrence or postoperative infection has been established. An array of randomized controlled trials have yielded contradictory results not resolved by careful meta-analyses.[85] Possible explanations for this include patient selection biases, observational biases, and other confounding variables. In addition, the adverse effect of transfusion-related immune modulation may be small in comparison to other factors that alter risk for infection or tumor recurrence.[85] Thus, a role for leukoreduction to address this complication has not been proven.

Nonimmune Transfusion Complications

Circulatory Overload

Frequency

Congestive heart failure is rare in an otherwise healthy patient receiving transfusions, even in the setting of massive blood loss. In some investigators' reports, however, as many as 1 in 100 transfusions recipients develops volume overload; such individuals are usually older, and already in positive fluid balance for other reasons, such that even a modest increment with a transfusion of 1 or 2 units is the final straw.[86]

Pathophysiology

Blood transfusions may compromise the cardiac status of patients with underlying cardiac disease, or those who, with high cardiac output resulting from anemia, are already struggling with elevated central venous pressures.[87] A tightrope must be walked, because increasing anemia has, in some studies, been associated with increased mortality in these patients.[88]

Clinical Features

Transfusions can cause classical congestive heart failure, including dyspnea, orthopnea, cyanosis, jugular venous distention, tachycardia, hypertension, and peripheral edema.

Laboratory Diagnosis

Radiographic evidence of congestive heart failure is typical. Respiratory distress also occurs with transfusion-related acute lung injury, but a distinguishing feature is the central venous pressure, which is elevated in congestive heart failure and normal or low in transfusion-related acute lung injury.

Treatment

Treatment of transfusion-associated congestive heart failure is similar to that for heart failure of other etiologies, and includes oxygen and diuretics; in extreme circumstances, phlebotomy may be necessary.

Prevention

A more modest transfusion rate and prophylactic administration of diuretics may be helpful with subsequent transfusions. Note that the diuretic, or any drug, should be administered orally or by peripheral vein, but never added directly to the blood bag, because medications may cause hemolysis or clotting.

Hypothermia and Electrolyte Abnormalities

Hypothermia, a core body temperature below 35°C,[89] is a complication of massive transfusion that can occur when large volumes of recently refrigerated blood are transfused rapidly to a patient, typically in the emergency room or operating room. Hypothermia can result in serious complications for the recipient, including metabolic derangements, abnormal hemostasis, and ventricular arrhythmias.[90–93] This complication can be circumvented with the use of in-line blood-warming devices designed for controlled heating to temperatures less than 42°C (a level of heat that does not cause heat injury to red blood cells).[94]

In liver transplantation during the anhepatic phase, massive transfusion can lead to *hypocalcemia,* because the citrate anticoagulant present in blood products, especially plasma, binds calcium. Citrate is metabolized in large part, and rapidly, by the liver and kidneys.[95] When this metabolic pathway is overwhelmed, citrate levels rise and hypocalcemia results, with neurologic and neuromuscular symptoms (paresthesias, cramps, and seizures) as well as cardiorespiratory complications, including prolongation of the Q-T interval, cardiac arrhythmias, and respiratory arrest.[96] Hypocalcemia is very rare in other clinical scenarios, although it can be precipitated by transfusion in patients who are already hypocalcemic for other reasons.[97] Treatment involves the infusion of supplemental calcium; this must be given judiciously so as to avoid overcompensation and hypercalcemia.[95]

Infusions of large volumes of citrate do not cause acidosis (and therefore, the routine administration of bicarbonate is an unnecessary urban myth), but rather *metabolic alkalosis,* because the metabolism of citrate results in accumulation of bicarbonate. Treatment of the acid-base disturbance is not usually required.

Extracellular potassium concentrations rise in stored red cell components as a result of disruption of the sodium-potassium pump mechanism. However, the extracellular content of potassium usually does not exceed 7 mEq/unit; as a result *hyperkalemia,* although reported in pediatric massive transfusion recipients[98] (especially with irradiated blood[99]) and in adults with end-stage kidney disease,[100] is uncommon.[101]

Iron Overload

Each unit of red blood cells contains 200–250 mg of iron. Much of this iron is stored in reticuloendothelial cells and, when these are saturated, in other less accommodating tissues, including the liver, the pancreas and other endocrine organs, and the heart. Signs and symptoms of hemochromatosis may begin with iron accumulations of 400 mg/kg body weight, or 100–150 units of red cells; levels in excess of 1000 mg/kg body weight may be lethal.[102] Chelation treatment using subcutaneous or intravenous desferrioxamine can reverse tissue damage, and even prevent it when started early in a patient with predictable needs for long-term transfusions (e.g., sickle cell anemia and thalassemia). An adjunctive, but cumbersome, strategy is the transfusion of a red cell product enriched with less-mature cells ("neocytes"). Because these cells have a longer posttransfusion survival in the recipient, the interval between transfusions can be increased, and the overall transfusion requirement and iron load reduced.[103]

Plasticizer Toxicity

The main component of a blood bag is polyvinyl chloride, a rigid plastic made more malleable by the addition of chemical plasticizers such as di-2-(ethylhexyl)pthalate (DEHP). DEHP leaches out of the bag during red cell storage, and is thus transfused. DEHP, and its metabolite MEHP, accumulate in fat, and have been implicated in organ damage, including to the liver and heart, and in carcinogenesis in animal models.[104] Paradoxically, however, these plasticizers also are incorporated into the red cell membrane, and improve transfused red cell survival.[105] A movement to replace DEHP with other, less leachable, plasticizers such as butyryl tri-*n*-hexyl citrate (BTHC) is underway.[106–108]

Hypotensive Reactions

Hypotension as a complication of blood transfusion is an uncommon observation. In many cases the use of angiotensin-converting enzyme inhibitor drugs to treat hypertension is involved. Angiotensin-converting enzyme breaks down bradykinin, a peptide with vasodilatory activity; angiotensin-converting enzyme inhibitor drugs impair bradykinin metabolism. Adverse events with these drugs have been reported following platelet and plasma transfusions using bedside leukodepletion filters,[109] probably because the patient's endogenous kallikrein-kinin cascade is activated through contact with the filter's synthetic, frequently negatively charged, surface, and bradykinin is produced. Because bradykinin breakdown is impaired in patients taking angiotensin-converting enzyme inhibitors, severe hypotension can result. Additional symptoms may include flushing, nausea, abdominal pain, respiratory distress, and loss of consciousness.[110] These reactions have not been reported in prestorage leukodepleted products, probably because the bradykinin generated during filtration is broken down during storage.[111] Fortunately, the reactions occur quickly following the start of the transfusion, usually within 1 hour, and abate just as quickly when the transfusion is stopped.[112]

TABLE 99–4. Required Viral Screening Tests for Whole Blood and Plateletpheresis Donors and Residual Risk for Transfusion-Transmitted Disease

Disease	Blood Donor Screening Test	Risk of Transfusion-Transmitted Disease*
HIV	Anti–HIV-1/2 P24 antigen NAT	1:1,8000,000
HBV	HBsAg; anti-HBcAg	1:220,000
HCV	Anti-HCV; NAT	1:1,600,000
HTLV-1/2	Anti–HTLV-1/2	1:64,000
WNV	NAT	1:10,000

*Risk per unit transfused.
Abbreviations: anti-HBcAg, antibodies to hepatitis B core antigen; HBsAg, hepatitis B surface antigen; HBV, hepatitis B virus; HCV, hepatitis C virus; HIV, human immunodeficiency virus; HTLV, human T-lymphotrophic virus; NAT, nucleic acid testing; WNV, West Nile virus.
Adapted from Busch MP, Kleinman SH, Nemo GJ: Current and emerging infectious disease risks of blood transfusions. JAMA 289:959–962, 2003.

TRANSFUSION-TRANSMITTED VIRAL DISEASES

The commonly recognized viruses transmitted by transfusion include HIV, hepatitis B and C viruses, human T-lymphotrophic virus types 1 and 2, and West Nile virus. Disease transmission occurs largely from collections from infected but asymptomatic donors. Fortunately, the risk for transmission of these viruses has dramatically fallen over the last 20 years, in large part as a result of improved donor screening assays, including the introduction of nucleic acid testing (Fig. 99–6 and Table 99–4).[113–115]

Introduction of new and improved technologies for blood component preparation has further reduced the risk for disease transmission. Examples include universal leukoreduction, which reduces the burden of cytomegalovirus and potentially other leukotropic viruses,[116] chemical viral inactivation (e.g., solvent-detergent treatment), and nanofiltration.[117] The introduction of solvent-detergent treatment of pooled plasma has virtually eliminated the risk of clotting factors transmitting HIV and hepatitis.[118]

HIV infection is discussed here as an important example of transfusion-transmitted viral disease, and West Nile virus as the newest viral challenge in transfusion practice; the reader is referred to Tables 99–4 and 99–5 and other chapters in this text that review hepatitis C, cytomegalovirus, Epstein-Barr virus, and the human herpesviruses (see Chapters 74, 75, and 78).

Human Immunodeficiency Virus

HIV, a lentivirus (among the most complex groups of retroviruses), was identified as the causative agent of

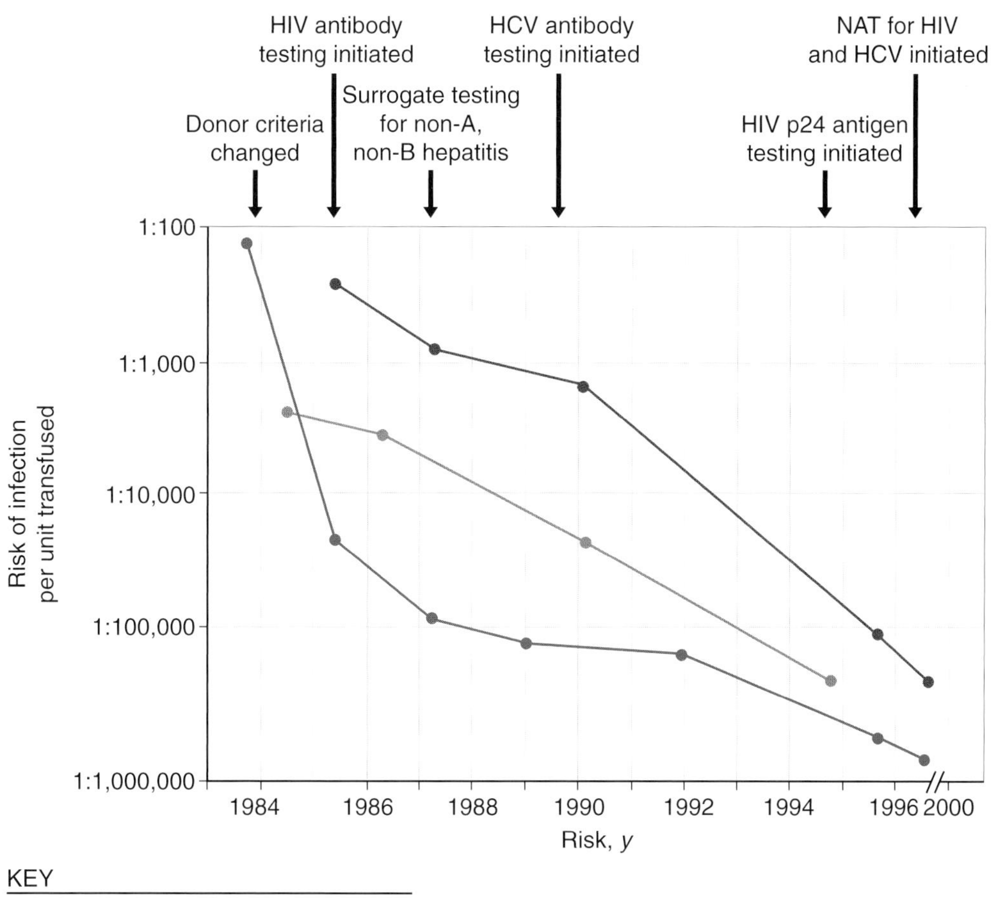

Figure 99–6. The changing risk for transfusion-associated viral infections—HIV, hepatitis B (HBV), and hepatitis C (HCV)—in the United States. The risk for transfusion-transmitted viral infections has dramatically declined over the last 2 decades, attributable to (1) changes in donor exclusion criteria and (2) introduction of new infectious disease screening tests. (Redrawn from Uhl L: Infectious risks of blood transfusion. Curr Hematol Rep 1:157, 2002; data from AuBuchon and colleagues[114] and Uhl.[113])

TABLE 99–5. Other Viruses with Known or Theoretical Risks of Transmission through Transfusion

Agent	Transfusion-Transmitted Disease: Y/N	Risk Factor for Clinically Significant Disease	Blood Component	Clinical Manifestation	Management/Risk Reduction Related to Blood Components
CMV	Y	Immunocompromised patient and premature babies	Red cells, platelets, granulocytes, hematopoietic stem cells	Posttransfusion hepatitis, retinitis, pneumonitis, colitis, bone marrow suppression	CMV-seronegative blood products; leukoreduced blood products
EBV	Y	Immunocompromised patient	Red cells, platelets, granulocytes, hematopoietic stem cells	Posttransfusion hepatitis, lymphoproliferative disorders	Leukoreduced blood products
Parvovirus B19	Y	Immunocompromised patient; hematologic disorders (e.g., sickle cell disease)	Clotting factors	Erythroid aplasia	IVIG; donor screening being considered
HHV-8	No known cases reported	Immunocompromised patient	None reported	Kaposi's sarcoma, cavity-based lymphomas	Not applicable

Abbreviations: CMV, cytomegalovirus; EBV, Epstein-Barr virus; HHV, human herpesvirus; IVIG, intravenous immunoglobulin.

acquired immunodeficiency syndrome in 1983. This virus preferentially infects CD4-positive T lymphocytes in lymph nodes and other lymphoid tissue. Clinical manifestations of acute HIV infection at the time of seroconversion are nonspecific and include fever, lymphadenopathy, sore throat, headache, myalgias, arthralgias, and nausea/vomiting.[119] A transfusion recipient may thus be unaware of the infection for many months unless incidentally tested or notified by a blood collection facility.

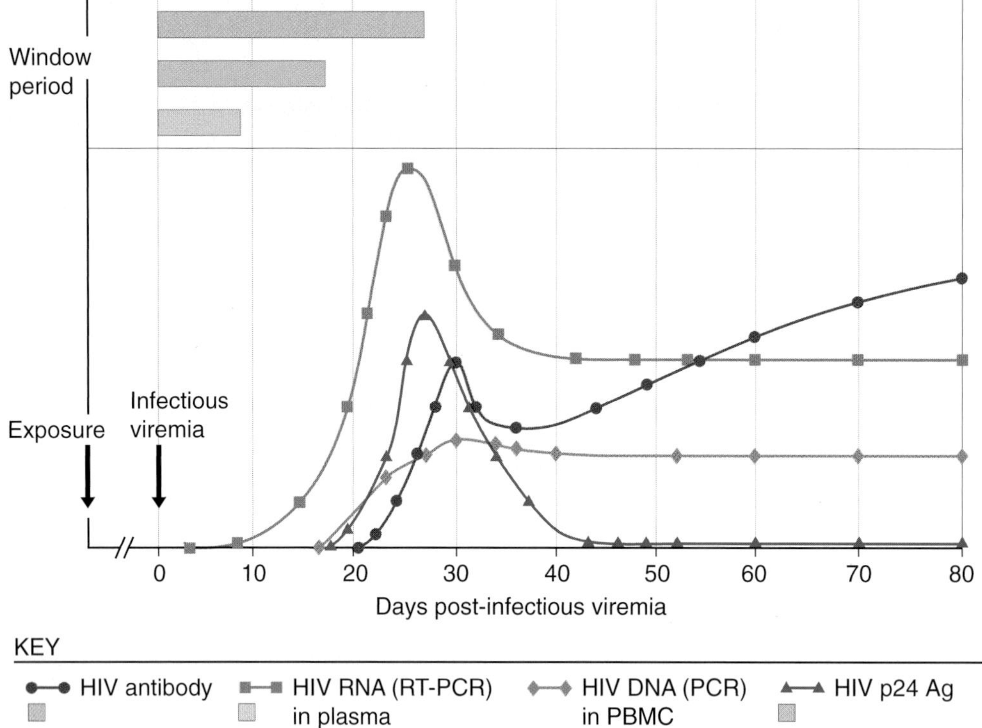

Figure 99–7. Primary HIV infection: time sequence of plasma viremia and immune response. Following exposure, local viral replication in regional lymphoid tissue takes place (over 7 days to 6 months). Subsequently, infectious viremia develops (day 0). The graph depicts the time course for the earliest detection of specific viral markers using plasma or whole blood assays. The interval between onset of viremia and earliest detection of a viral marker defines the "window" period, a measurement that has significant implications for blood safety because identification of an infectious donor can be missed during this interval. With HIV-antibody screening alone, the window period is approximately 3 weeks. The introduction of p24 antigen testing reduced this period to 15 days, and nucleic acid testing (e.g., HIV RNA testing) to 10 days. (Redrawn from Busch MP, Satten GA: Time course of viremia and antibody seroconversion following human immunodeficiency virus exposure. Am J Med 102:123, 1997.)

The recognition that this virus is transmitted by blood and blood derivatives has been the biggest driving force for changes in donor evaluation in the history of transfusion medicine.[120] Understanding the epidemiology as well as the biologic factors of the infection has led to improved strategies for eliminating the risk of introduction of an infected unit into the donor pool. These include donor exclusion based on risk of exposure to infection (beginning in 1983), testing for antibody to the virus (1985), and direct testing for circulating virus using protein and, later, nucleic acid detection assays (1995). The combined use of these strategies has resulted in a remarkable reduction in the risk of transfusion-transmitted HIV from an estimated 1 in 100 units transfused at the height of the problem to 1 in 1,800,000 units today.[115] Possible explanations for the rare but residual risk of transfusion-transmitted infections include[121]:

1. Collection of a unit during the "window period" of infection—the interval after HIV infection during which the donor is infectious, but the infection is not detectable by current assays[122] (Fig. 99–7).
2. Infection with variant strains of HIV not detectable by current assays. Current assays are capable of detecting antibodies directed against the main groups of the HIV-1 family; however, the assays are less robust in detection of antibodies directed against, for example, HIV-1 group O. To compensate for this, individuals born in Africa (where HIV-1 group O is endemic) or with a history of transfusion or sexual contact while traveling in Africa are deferred from blood donation in the United States.
3. Technical error. Analytical error is a concern for any assay. Survey data from the Centers for Disease Control and Prevention and the National Institutes of Health–sponsored Retrovirus Epidemiology Donor Study suggest that 0.5–2 HIV-seropositive donors/year might be missed as a result of technical errors, although most should be picked up by nucleic acid detection.

West Nile Virus

This mosquito-borne flavivirus, with a primary avian host, was first isolated from the blood of a Ugandan woman in 1937.[123] The virus appeared in the United States in 1999, and by 2002, reports of documented transfusion-transmitted West Nile virus had been published.[124]

The majority of infections in humans are subclinical. Manifestations in a minority of patients include fever, headache, anorexia, and myalgias. Central nervous system complications, usually meningoencephalitis, occur in approximately 1 in 150 infected individuals. Cases of acute flaccid paralysis have also been reported, some of which were initially confused with Guillain-Barré syndrome. However, West Nile virus acute flaccid paralysis is typically associated with elevated cerebrospinal fluid protein and cellular content, whereas albuminocytologic dissociation is characteristic of acute Guillain-Barré syndrome.[123]

During the peak summer season in areas with the highest incidence of West Nile virus infection, the risk of potentially infectious units is between 10 and 15 per 10,000 units. The prompt recognition of high incidence of the virus, and the morbidity and mortality of transfusion-associated infection, have resulted in a remarkably rapid development—within 4 years of first recognition of the illness in the United States—of detection assays for the purpose of blood donor screening, including an RNA detection assay introduced in July 2003.[125]

TRANSFUSION AND BACTERIAL CONTAMINATION

Bacterial contamination of donated blood is a recognized risk of transfusion, but until recently was considered a rare and unavoidable problem of far less urgency than viral transmission. However, with the accumulation of impressive improvements in screening of donor blood for viral diseases, and an increasing focus on risk reduction of transfusions, bacterial contamination has taken center stage. Particularly notable is that the relative risk of transfusion of a bacterially contaminated blood product (most commonly platelets) may be up to 250 times the combined risk for transfusion-associated HIV-1, hepatitis B and C viruses, and human T-lymphotrophic virus types 1 and 2.[126]

The patient experiencing a septic transfusion reaction may present with chills/rigors and fever (typically, ≥2°C rise over the pretransfusion temperature). In severe cases, hypotension and disseminated intravascular coagulation develop.[127] Because many of the patients receiving transfusion (e.g., patients on chemotherapy who, as a result, are neutropenic and thrombocytopenic) are at risk for infection secondary to underlying disease, such reactions may not be readily recognized as a complication of transfusion, but, rather, ascribed to the underlying medical condition. Bacteria may be introduced into a blood component at any of a number of points, including contamination of the blood bag during its manufacture,[128] collection of blood from an asymptomatic bacteremic donor,[129,130] inadequate sterilization of the donor venipuncture site,[131] or inoculation during component processing. Approaches to curtail these risks include new donor exclusion criteria and development of technologies for bacterial detection and elimination.[132–134]

Bacteria in Red Blood Cells

Bacterial contamination of red cells is rare, in large part because refrigerated storage conditions are not conducive to bacterial growth. Most reported cases involve psychrophilic (cold-loving) organisms such as *Yersinia enterocolitica, Serratia marcescens,* and *Pseudomonas aeruginosa*[135] (Fig. 99–8). Based on fatality data reported to the FDA, the estimated risk of death following transfusion of a bacterially contaminated red cell or whole blood product is 10 per million components transfused.[136] However, a recent report from New Zealand described a much higher incidence of transfusion-associated *Y. enterocolitica* infection (1:65,000) and fatality rate (1:104,000 red cell units transfused).[137] Regional variations may be involved, although realistic concerns have been raised about underrecognition and underreporting of this complication.[138]

Bacteria in Platelets

Transfusion-associated sepsis occurs more frequently following platelet transfusion than red cell transfusion and is related to the required storage environment. Unlike red cells, which are refrigerated at 0°–10°C, the optimal storage temperature for platelets (22°C) is also ideal for a variety of bacteria. The organisms most commonly identified in contaminated platelet products are skin commensals (e.g. *Staphylococcus epidermidis, Staphylococcus aureus,* and *Streptococcus* species), which are thought to contaminate the product at the time of collection as a result of incomplete disinfection of the phlebotomy site or through introduction of a skin core during the venipuncture procedure.[131] In rare instances, bacterial contamination may be the result of occult bacteremia in the donor.[129]

Data derived from prospective surveillance studies show that the prevalence of bacterial contamination in whole blood–derived platelets (also known as random-donor platelets) is 34 per 100,000 units manufactured, and in apheresis platelets, 51 per 100,000 units manufactured.[139] The incidence of severe cases of transfusion-associated bacterial sepsis has not been established, largely because of the difficulties in diagnosis as described earlier. However, it has been estimated to occur in approximately one sixth of transfused contaminated platelet products.[136] Thus, given that approximately 4–6 million platelet products are transfused annually in the United States, the expected incidence for clinically significant (and, potentially, fatal) transfusion-associated sepsis is 300–1000 cases.[126]

Strategies to Reduce Risk of Transfusion-Related Sepsis

Careful assessment of the donor's health and fastidious arm sterilization are critical but not sufficient to prevent bacterial contamination of a collected product. A new thrust is the detection of bacteria in the product itself, with a focus on platelets; however, this has so far proved to be a challenging goal. In most instances the bacterial inoculum introduced at the time of collection is below

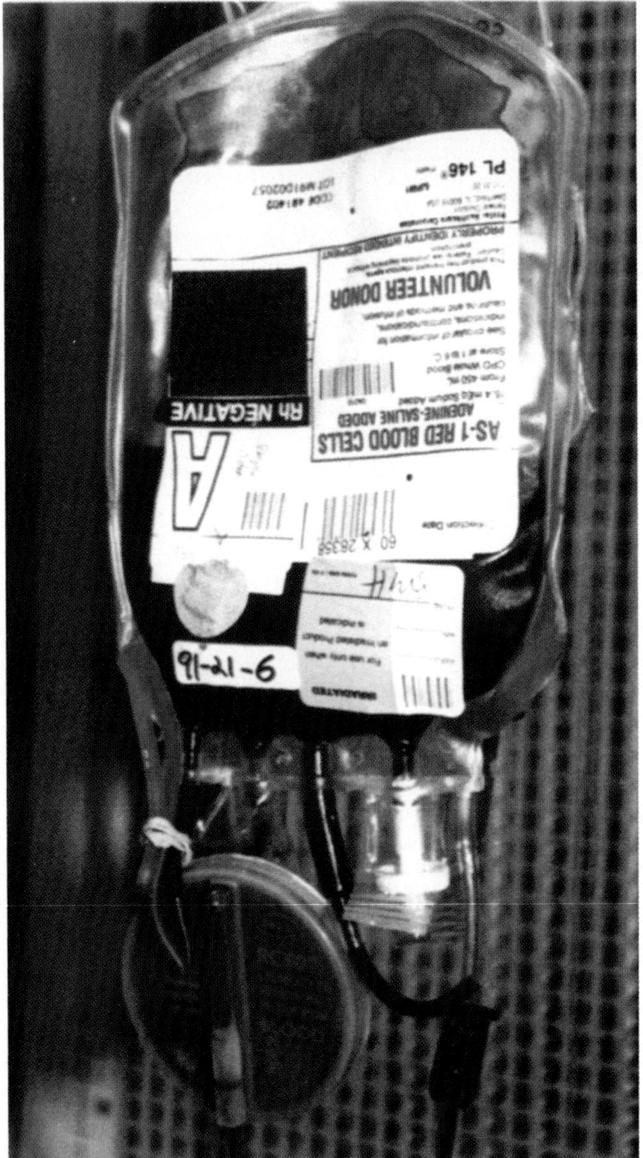

Figure 99–8. Bacterially contaminated red blood cell component. The unit is darker in color than the blood component segments. A gram-negative rod was cultured from the red cell component; the associated segments were culture negative. (From Kim DM, Brecher ME, Bland LA, et al: Visual identification of bacterially contaminated red cells. Transfusion 32:221–225, 1992.)

the recognition threshold of today's bacterial detection systems (but perhaps also below the dose that causes human illness). During room-temperature storage, however, the organisms can multiply to levels that may be clinically significant for at-risk patients.[133,140] Several bacterial detection strategies have been designed to identify contaminated platelet components after storage but before release for transfusion. These include, in increasing order of sensitivity, evaluation of altered biochemical (e.g., change in pH) or physical (e.g., disappearance of normal platelet swirling) properties[141]; screening for bacteria by Gram stain or fluorescent microscopy using acridine orange[142]; detection of bacteria through use of RNA probes or multiplex polymerase chain reaction testing[132]; and use of automated culture detection systems.[143] Logically, sensitivity of detection is higher the longer the storage period; thus, for maximum sensitivity, the ideal test would be employable just prior to release of the product for transfusion, with a rapid turnaround time. Such testing could potentially also extend the storage time for platelets, which was reduced from 7 days to 5 by the FDA specifically out of concern about bacterial overgrowth.[143]

TRANSFUSION-TRANSMITTED PARASITIC INFECTION

Transfusion-transmitted parasitic infections are well documented in regions of the world endemic for the organisms, and are a growing problem in our mobile global community[144] (Fig. 99–9). They occur as a result of collection of blood from asymptomatic donors who, in most instances, are unaware of their parasitemia. Medical history screening questions are only partially effective, and new diagnostic testing and inactivation strategies are under study.[118,144–146]

Malaria

Although rare in temperate zones, malaria is widespread globally, affecting an estimated 300–500 million individuals.[118] The disease is caused by infection with one of four *Plasmodium* species: *P. falciparum, P. vivax, P. ovale,* and *P. malaria;* infections with *P. falciparum* and *P. vivax* constitute the majority. The parasite is introduced into its host through the bite of the female *Anopheles* mosquito and subsequently travels to the liver, where the immature sporozoites invade hepatocytes. Here the organisms divide and mature into schizonts, each of which contains many thousand merozoites. Eventually, the tissue schizonts rupture, releasing the merozoites into the circulation, where they invade red cells. The clinical manifestations of the disease are associated with the erythrocytic stage of the life cycle and are the result of altered red cell metabolism and membrane integrity, leading to red cell hemolysis. Lysis of the red cells induces the release of a host of pro-inflammatory cytokines that contribute to the fever, anemia, and thrombocytopenia seen in infected individuals.[147]

Transfusion-transmitted malaria is rare in the United States, with an estimated rate of 1 case per 4 million transfusions.[148] Currently, potential donors who have traveled to a malaria-risk area are deferred from donation for 1 year, and for 3 years if they have lived or emigrated from an endemic area.[149,150] No blood-based screening test exists. Epidemiologic studies suggest that current donor screening policies, particularly those related to travel history, provide a fairly sound barrier against introduction of potentially infected blood components into the blood supply.[148] However, these data may be challenged in the future given the recent reports of seven cases of locally acquired malaria in the state of Florida.[151,152]

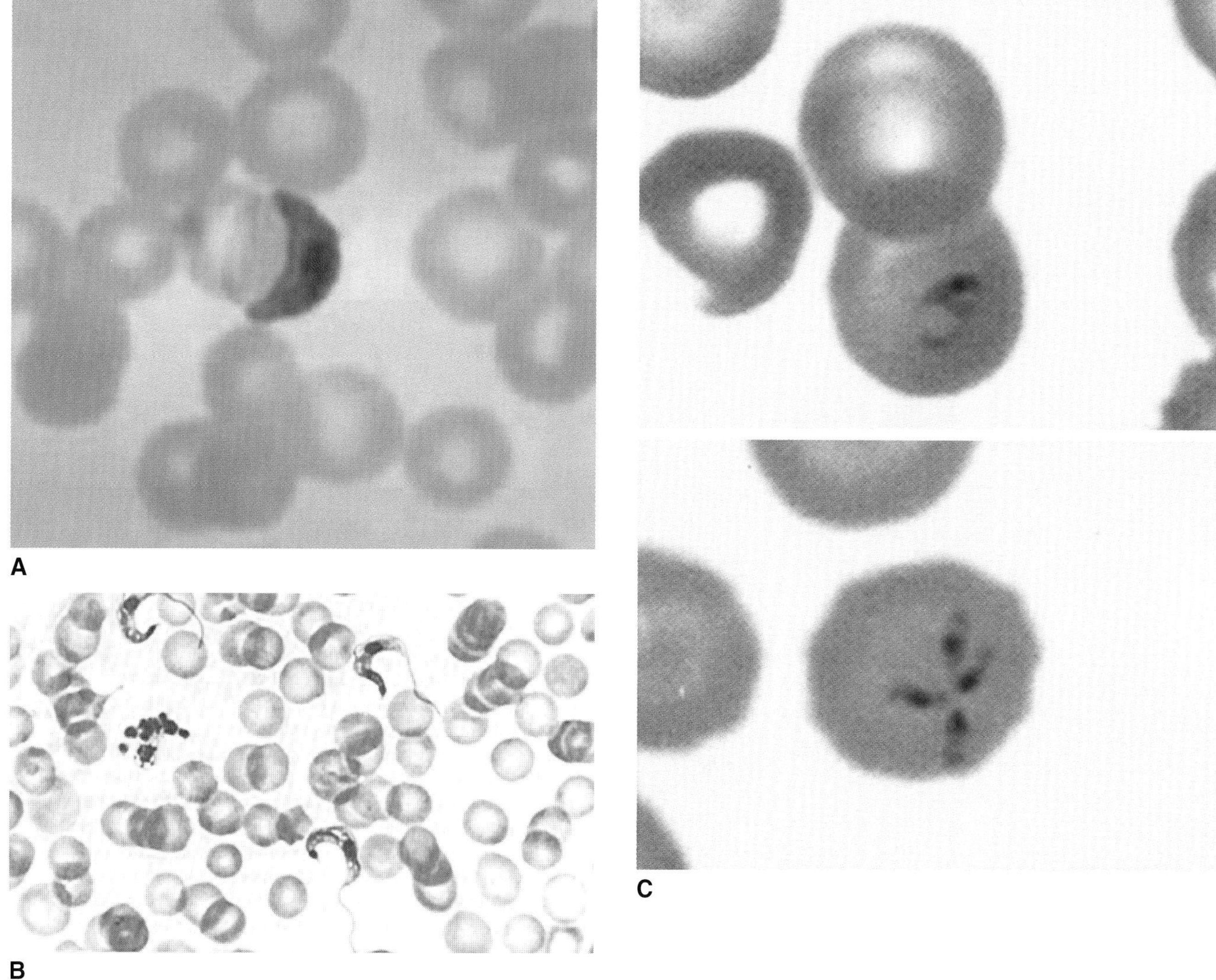

Figure 99–9. Transfusion-transmitted parasitic infections. *A,* Peripheral blood smear from a patient infected with *Plasmodium falciparum*. *B,* Peripheral blood smear with *Trypanosoma cruzi* trypomastigotes. *C,* Peripheral blood smear with the intraerythrocytic merozoites of *Babesia microti.* (*C* from Herwaldt BL, Neitzel DF, Gorlin JB, et al: Transmission of *Babesia microti* in Minnesota through four blood donations from the same donor over a six-month period. Transfusion 42:1154–1158, 2002, with permission.)

Chagas' Disease

Also known as American trypanosomiasis, Chagas' disease is endemic in Latin America and is the result of accidental infection of humans by the protozoan parasite, *Trypanosoma cruzi.*[146,153] The predominant mode of infection is through self-inoculation via introduction of parasite-laden feces into the bite of the reduviid bug, the primary vector for this organism. Vertical transmission from mother to fetus and infection through blood transfusion also occurs.[146] In the acute phase of the disease, the organisms multiply and invade muscle tissue, including cardiac and esophageal muscle. Fever, malaise, lymphadenopathy, and hepatosplenomegaly frequently develop. Resolution occurs within 4–6 weeks and is followed by a chronic phase of infection that may remain clinically silent for up to 30 years.[146] The development of cardiac, esophageal, and colonic abnormalities, including arrhythmias, cardiomyopathy, altered gastrocolonic motility, and megacolon, marks termination of the latent phase. Pathologic analysis suggests that these functional abnormalities are the result of inflammatory responses evoked by parasitic invasion.

Because this disease has a relatively protracted quiescent phase, during which hematogenous parasitism occurs, the risk for obtaining blood from an infected, otherwise asymptomatic donor exists. There have been six reported cases of transfusion-transmitted *T. cruzi* in the United States and Canada within the last 10 years, all in immunocompromised recipients.[153–157] More recently, analysis of blood donors in the Los Angeles and Miami areas established seropositive rates of 1 in 7500 and 1 in 9000 blood donors, respectively.[158] However, look-back analysis of recipients of seropositive blood components showed no evidence of seroconversion. This raises the question of whether there are important cofactors, such as coincident immunosuppressive therapy, which make certain blood recipients susceptible to infection.[157]

Despite the apparent low risk for transfusion-transmitted *T. cruzi,* many within the transfusion community are concerned that the frequency may be underestimated because of the mild acute symptoms and protracted interval until manifestations of chronic disease appear. At this time, there are no approved laboratory tests to screen blood donors for the presence of Chagas' disease. However, a new enzyme-linked immunosorbent assay for antibodies against a recombinant polyvalent *T. cruzi* antigen (TcF) is undergoing evaluation.[159]

Babesiosis

The parasite *Babesia microti* is transmitted to humans by the deer tick *Ixodes dammini.* Following introduction into the systemic circulation at the time of the tick's "blood meal," the parasite invades red cells. During this intraerythrocytic phase, rapid production of intraerythrocytic trophozoites and merozoites occurs, with eventual cell lysis and subsequent infection of additional erythrocytes.[160] Most cases of babesiosis are diagnosed by the clinical history of tick bite and identification of the intracellular parasites on peripheral blood smear.

Although the majority of individuals infected with babesia experience no clinical symptoms, infection has been associated with life-threatening hemolysis and death. Those at risk for severe disease include splenectomized patients, the elderly, and the immunocompromised.

Babesia is second only to malaria in frequency as a cause of transfusion-transmitted parasitic infection.[161] The annual incidence in the United States is probably less than 1 per million donated units of blood. However, the risk may be higher in areas endemic for the organism (specifically the Northeast).[162] At this time, there are no effective methods for donor testing; a modest step has been taken by avoiding blood collection in endemic areas during the summer months when humans are at highest risk for tick bites.[144]

Creutzfeldt-Jakob Disease

The transmissible spongiform encephalopathies are a group of fatal neurodegenerative disorders afflicting both animals and humans in which the putative etiologic agent, a protease-resistant prion protein (PrP), accumulates in nervous tissue.[163] In humans, the resulting clinical syndrome, sporadic Creutzfeldt-Jakob disease, is characterized clinically by progressive dementia, ataxia, and myoclonus, and eventual mutism and death. The estimated annual incidence of sporadic Creutzfeldt-Jakob disease is 1 per million population and the mode of acquisition is undefined.[163] Inherited cases (secondary to coding mutations in the prion protein gene [*PRNP*]) and iatrogenic cases (resulting from exposure to contaminated tissue via dura transplant or growth hormone injections) were thought to make up the balance of affected individuals.[163,164] More recently, however, a new form of transmissible spongiform encephalopathy has been described, so-called variant Creutzfeldt-Jakob disease. It differs from the sporadic form in that patients are younger, have more prominent psychiatric symptoms, and demonstrate an electroencephalographic pattern that is not typical of sporadic Creutzfeldt-Jakob disease.[165,166] Furthermore, unlike sporadic Creutzfeldt-Jakob disease, it has been suggested that variant Creutzfeldt-Jakob disease is causally linked to the consumption of foodstuffs contaminated with neural tissue derived from cattle afflicted with bovine spongiform encephalopathy.[163] Murine animal models support the proposal that the prion agents of bovine spongiform encephalopathy and variant Creutzfeldt-Jakob disease are of the same strain; transgenic and wild-type mice inoculated with isolates obtained from cattle or humans with the clinical diagnosis of variant Creutzfeldt-Jakob disease demonstrated similar incubation times for disease manifestation, similar clinical features, and a biochemical profile of the prion protein (PrP^{SC}).[167,168] To date, more than 125 individuals from the United Kingdom and 5 patients from France have been diagnosed with variant Creutzfeldt-Jakob disease. No case of variant Creutzfeldt-Jakob disease has been identified in the United States.[169]

Infectivity of Blood and Risk Reduction Strategies

Epidemiologic and surveillance studies of affected and control populations show no evidence for transfusion-associated sporadic Creutzfeldt-Jakob disease.[170] Additionally, the infectious agent has never been isolated from the blood of animals with naturally occurring transmissible spongiform encephalopathy infections. Recently, however, Llewelyn and colleagues reported on a patient who died of variant Creutzfeldt-Jakob disease subsequent to a blood transfusion donated by an individual who later developed the disease.[171]

Experimental models of transmissible spongiform encephalopathy demonstrate that blood and its components are infectious during both the incubation and clinical phases of disease.[170] Furthermore, experiments in which blood was spiked with the infective agent reveal that the prion particles partition preferentially into the buffy coat fraction of whole blood; low to no infectivity was noted in plasma and red cell components, respectively.[170] These observations as well as the recognition that patients diagnosed with variant Creutzfeldt-Jakob disease have PrP in their lymphoreticular tissue (a tissue that is intimately associated with circulating blood) have prompted several changes within the blood banking community in an effort to minimize the possible risk of variant Creutzfeldt-Jakob disease transmission through blood transfusion.[164,166] Such measures include leukoreduction of both cellular and noncellular blood products as well as nanofiltration of fractionated plasma derivatives, the goal being to reduce the load of the potentially infectious agent.[172] Based on the epidemiologic characteristics of variant Creutzfeldt-Jakob disease, additional measures have included new donor exclusion criteria such as indefinite deferral of individuals who have spent 3 or more months, cumulatively, in the United

Kingdom from 1980 through 1996, indefinite deferral of donors who have spent 5 or more years, cumulatively, in France since 1980; recipients of blood transfusion or blood components while in the United Kingdom between 1980 and the present; and donors who have injected bovine insulin since 1980, unless it is confirmed that the product was not manufactured from U.K. cattle.[166] Development of a screening assay for prions has been hampered by the level of sensitivity required for a robust screening assay.[170]

CONCLUSION

Blood and blood component transfusion can be a lifesaving intervention when used in the appropriate setting. However, as with all medical therapeutics, there are associated risks for morbidity and mortality. The risks of many complications and transfusion-transmitted diseases have been greatly reduced, but the task is not complete: unsolved immunologic issues, limits of detection of known infectious agents, new emerging infections, and human foibles remain challenges to a zero-risk blood supply.

Suggested Readings*

Busch MP, Satten G: Time course of viremia and antibody seroconversion following human immunodeficiency virus exposure. Am J Med 102:117–124, 1997.

Heddle NM, Klama L, Singer R, et al: The role of the plasma from platelet concentrates in transfusion reactions. N Engl J Med 331:625–628, 1994.

Petz LD, Garratty G: Hemolytic transfusion reactions. *In* Petz LD, Garratty G (eds): Immune Hemolytic Anemias. Philadelphia: Churchill Livingstone, 2004, pp 541–572.

Sampathkumar P: West Nile virus: Epidemiology, clinical presentation, diagnosis, and prevention. Mayo Clinic Proc 78:1137–1144, 2003.

Sazama K: Reports of 355 transfusion-associated deaths: 1976 through 1985. Transfusion 30:583–590, 1990.

Full references for this chapter can be found on accompanying CD-ROM.

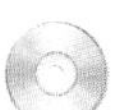

CHAPTER 100

BLOOD AND BONE MARROW MORPHOLOGY

John K. Choi, MD, PhD, and Jay L. Hess, MD, PhD

KEY POINTS

Peripheral Blood Smear

- The peripheral blood smear is easily made and results are quickly available, permitting rapid generation of a differential diagnosis.
- Blood smear findings are seldom pathognomonic but must be combined with laboratory data and clinical features.
- Most acute and chronic leukemias, some lymphomas, and rare specific infections are first diagnosed in the peripheral blood.
- Cytochemical stains, flow cytometric immunophenotyping, and often cytogenetics may be performed on peripheral blood.

Bone Marrow Aspirate Smear

- Advantages of the bone marrow aspirate smear include ability to enumerate specific hematopoietic cell types and identification of subtle cytologic abnormalities.
- Aspiration cannot be performed in many diseases with increased fibrosis, typically myelofibrosis and also metastatic tumors, and some infectious diseases.
- Most leukemias are best evaluated on the aspirate smear. Occasion nonhematopoietic tumor cells may be present in the smear but not in the biopsy.
- Cytochemical stains, flow cytometric immunophenotyping, and cytogenetic analysis are best evaluated from the marrow aspirate. Immunoperoxidase staining also can be performed.

Bone Marrow Biopsy

- The marrow biopsy allows examination of an inaspirable marrow, better quantification of marrow cellularity, evaluation of marrow architecture, and identification of focal lesions.
- Differentiation of specific cell types such as blasts, promyelocytes, and myelocytes is more difficult in biopsy specimens compared to aspirate smears. Iron is often lost during biopsy processing.
- Focal lesions such as lymphoma, metastatic tumors, and granulomas are best evaluated on the biopsy.
- Many special stains are available for the identification of specific tumors and microorganisms.
- Touch preparations of core biopsies are helpful for cytologic evaluation if an aspirate is not obtainable. In addition, cells from core samples may be dissociated for immunophenotyping and cytogenetic studies.

Optimal Evaluation

- Ideal evaluation includes examination of the blood smear, the marrow aspirate smear, and the biopsy.
- Proper evaluation of both blood and bone marrow specimens involves a systematic qualitative and quantitative evaluation of each lineage, correlation with clinical data and laboratory findings, and selection of appropriate ancillary studies to generate a clinically useful interpretation.

INTRODUCTION

Specimen Preparation and Processing

Morphologic examination of the peripheral blood smear, bone marrow aspirate, and bone marrow biopsy is a cost-effective and valuable tool for the diagnosis and evaluation of blood disorders.[1,2] Proper interpretation of the blood smear requires correlation with enumeration of red blood cells, white blood cells, and platelets, performed manually or now more routinely using automated electronic machines. The bone marrow aspirate allows optimal cytologic examination of cells and provides material for cytogenetic analysis and immunophenotyping by flow cytometry. The trephine biopsy is useful for accurate estimate of overall cellularity and to assess the architecture of the marrow. Examination of the biopsy is of crucial importance when the marrow cannot be aspirated.

Automated machines provide blood counts and the leukocyte differential by measuring and combining size, electromagnetic properties, light scattering, and the chemical reactivity of blood cells.[3-7] Electronic evaluation is much more rapid (15–45 minutes) than is manual counting and more precise, because thousands of cells are assessed compared to the 100–200 cells usually examined by eye. Some problems with automated leukocyte differential counting include insufficient cell numbers, abnormal cells that need visual confirmation or assessment, and, in rare cases, misclassification of blasts as normal cells. Unlike blood, there is no electronic replacement for microscopic examination of bone marrow aspirate and biopsy, and therefore knowledge of blood and bone marrow morphology and of the special techniques available for detailed study is a necessity for the hematologist.

The peripheral blood smear is made by pushing or pulling a drop of blood along the surface of a glass slide with a spreader in order to produce a thin smear, which is air-dried and stained with the dyes eosin and methylene blue (Wright) with or without Giemsa (Giemsa Wright). The bone marrow aspirate and biopsy are usually obtained from adjacent sites from the iliac crest. One or 2 mL of marrow are typically collected into EDTA-anticoagulated tubes ("purple tops") and the spicules are spread on glass slides. The bone marrow aspirate is dried in air and then stained. The bone marrow biopsy is fixed in formalin or B5-formalin for a minimum of 2 hours, decalcified using either acid or EDTA, and then processed overnight by automated machines. In the event of a "dry tap"—an inability to collect marrow by aspiration—it is advisable to perform touch preparations by lightly touching the bone marrow core a few times against several glass slides. Another 2–4 hours are needed to manually embed the processed bone marrow biopsy in paraffin, cut sections onto glass slides, and stain the slides. The stained slides are microscopically examined by pathologists or, in some hospitals, by hematologists.

Even in large institutions that manually examine over 100,000 peripheral blood smears per year, the vast majority are completed within 2–4 hours.[8,9] Urgent samples can be prepared and examined within an hour. The bone marrow aspirate is usually available within the same time frame. Processing of the bone marrow biopsy requires a minimum of 16 hours.

Landmarks for Bone Marrow Examination Procedure

The posterior iliac crest is the most common and preferred site for bone marrow examination. Biopsy and aspiration performed at this site have only rare complications (<1%), even in pancytopenic patients, usually hemorrhage or local infection (Fig. 100–1). The exact order of the biopsy and aspirate procedures usually does not affect the qualities of the specimens, provided that different entry sites or needle angle directions are used (more difficult to accomplish in small children) and artifacts are often visible in the second sample, usually replacement of marrow elements with peripheral blood.

In current practice the sternum is rarely chosen to obtain an aspirate (and never biopsied). The bone and the marrow cavity are easily accessed; the risk is a catastrophic complication due to the sternum's proximity to the great vessels and the chest cavity. The procedure should be avoided in young children and uncooperative subjects, and if the physical landmarks or sternum itself is distorted, as for example from a prior surgery, or osteopenic.

The anatomic landmarks must be correctly located and the procedure should be cautiously executed. If only a small area of the sternal periosteum is anesthetized, a complaint of sharp pain can be a signal of mislocation. The needle is directed at a 90° angle to the surface of the chest, then carefully and slowly advanced the few millimeters from the surface of the bone into the marrow space, avoiding excessive forcefulness. The needle can be grasped in the operator's dominant hand and, if the guard is removed, guided between the fingers of the opposite hand, with frequent assessment of position relative to the intercostal spaces and depth below the skin, to prevent slippage. In contrast to the iliac crest, a perceptible "give" in pressure signals entry into the cavity, and gentle aspiration—usually the most painful part of the procedure—yields marrow cells.

Basics of Using a Microscope

A high-quality clinical microscope is a delicate instrument. Depending on the configuration, its cost is comparable to an expensive automobile ($25K to $100K). Like a car, a microscope should be serviced regularly by a knowledgeable technician and "driven" responsibly. Unfortunately, many inexperienced drivers are on the road and doing much damage. Two basic recommendations will help to prevent mishaps:

1. Properly illuminate the specimen to produce an image that is uniformly bright without glare or refractions. A method of optimal illumination was first described in 1893 by August Kohler and is still used today. Kohler illumination consists of proper focusing (1) of the light source (the bulb filament) and (2) of the light onto the specimen slide. The first is best left to a technician; the second should be performed routinely by the microscopist (Fig. 100–2). A good virtual tutorial is presented at *http://www.microscopyu.com/tutorials/java/kohler/* (also see *http://www.olympumicro.com/primer/index.html*).
2. Use care when working with oil, which can permanently damage microscope objectives. Minimal amounts of oil (usually one drop) should be place on the slide and used with only oil immersion objectives. These objectives are labeled with "oil" and are typically 50× and 100×, with some 63×. Almost all 40× objectives are air dried and are easily damaged by inexperienced operators. Excess oil and oil spills should be cleaned or reported because early intervention prevents permanent damage.

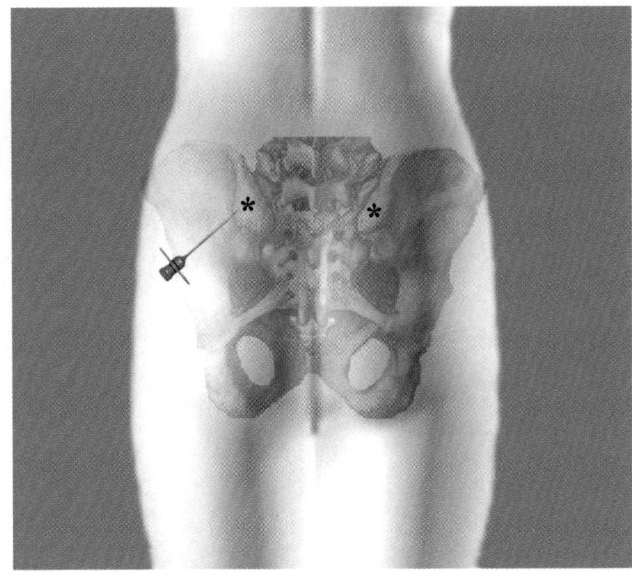

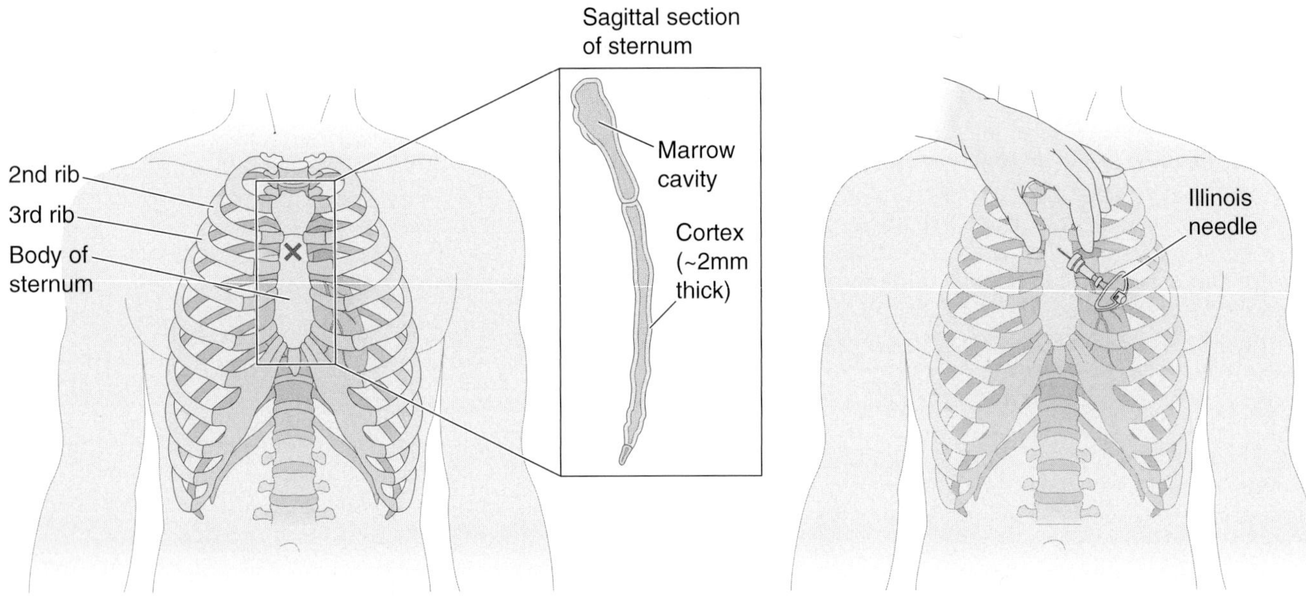

Figure 100–1. A, Aspiration and biopsy at the posterior iliac crest. Most packaged kits provide an antiseptic solution and a xylocaine anesthetic. The Jamshidi needle is placed at the posterior superior iliac spine (*), an easily palpated bony prominence 1–5 cm lateral to the spine and 0–2 m above the top of the buttock. The angle of the needle should be perpendicular to the bone surface and directed downwards or outwards, in the direction of the ipsilateral anterior superior iliac spine; a common problem is to "shave" the cortex, uncomfortable for the patient and resulting in an inadequate specimen to the pathologist. The 1 cm core specimen and aspirations are usually obtained from separate sites at slightly different angles of entry. B, Sternal aspiration. Preferred is the small area from the manubrium to the first sternal segment where the bone is thickest (red X); lower portions of the sternum are avoided because the depth of bone narrows and may be replaced by cartilage in younger individuals, and the proximity to the right ventricle which lies immediately beneath. The midline is located by identifying the sternal notch, and the aspiration site is chosen above the level where the second rib intersects the sternum. The safety of the procedure requires that these anatomic landmarks be correctly located. After infiltrating skin and periosteum with local anesthesia, the Illinois needle is positioned just off the midline (to avoid the occasional anatomical variant of a midline septum). If only a small area of the sternal periosteum is anesthetized, a complaint of sharp pain can be a signal of mislocation. The needle is directed at a 90° angle to the surface of the chest, then carefully and slowly advanced the few millimeters from the surface of the bone into the marrow space, avoiding excessive forcefulness. The Illinois needle is provided with a guard to prevent deep penetration, but can also be employed with the guard removed. The needle can be grasped in the operator's dominant hand and guided between the fingers of the opposite hand, with frequent assessment of position relative to the intercostal spaces, to prevent slippage. In contrast to the iliac crest, a perceptible "give" in pressure signals entry into the cavity, and gentle aspiration—usually the most painful part of the procedure—yields marrow cells. Rotation of the needle can sometimes improve the yield if no cells are immediately aspirated.

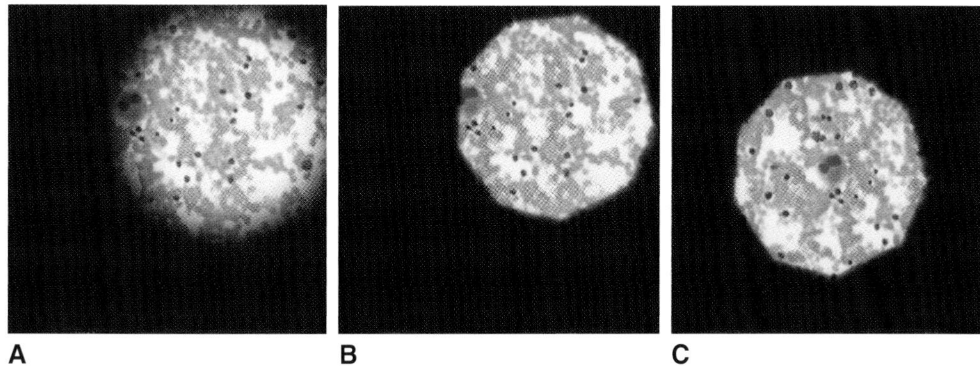

Figure 100–2. Steps during Kohler illumination for optimizing specimen image:

1. View and focus the specimen using the 10× objective.
2. Decrease the diaphragm opening size until the edges can be seen *(A)*.
3. Focus the edges by adjusting the condenser vertically *(B)*.
4. Center the diaphragm opening by adjusting the condenser laterally *(C)*.
5. Open the diaphragm to light the whole field.

Morphology of Normal Cells in Smears

Usually only fully differentiated blood cells are present on the peripheral blood smear. Immature cells are observed in certain physiologic states, as in neonates and during pregnancy, and in disease, such as infections and leukemia. Recognition of all cells at different stages of maturation, in addition to frankly abnormal cells, is required to properly evaluate both the peripheral blood smear and bone marrow aspirate. A constellation of characteristics permits classification of a cell to its lineage and differentiation stage. Some features can be altered or even absent in some diseases, such as myelodysplastic syndrome, complicating the classification of stage; sometimes, even the lineage is uncertain and a cell is classified by best fit, or the most number of correct features. Occasional cells defy precise classification—so-called "skipocytes."

Important morphologic features include the (1) pattern of chromatin condensation, (2) shape of the nucleus, (3) type of cytoplasmic granules, (4) size and shape of the cytoplasm, and (5) size and number of nucleoli. In general, as cells mature, the chromatin becomes more condensed and appears darker with Wright stain. Nuclei become irregular in shape with maturation of granulocytes, monocytes, and megakaryocytes. Maturing myeloid cells accumulate primary (red or azurophilic) granules, followed by secondary granules, and then lose their primary granules. All maturing cells have increasing amounts of cytoplasm relative to the nucleus, expressed as the nucleus/cytoplasm ratio; the terms *scant*, *moderate*, or *abundant* cytoplasm are defined as cytoplasm that is less than, equal to, or greater than the area of the nucleus, respectively. Nucleoli appear as negative-staining, round areas and are seen most prominently in myeloblasts; smaller nucleoli are present in activated mature lymphocytes and macrophages, but nucleoli are quite inconspicuous in lymphoblasts and mature myeloid cells.

Erythrocytes

Erythrocytes without nuclei are the most prevalent cell type in the peripheral blood, typically 400–1000 times the number of white blood cells. Nucleated red blood cells are rare in normal peripheral blood but are second in frequency only to granulocytes in the marrow. Nucleated red blood cells undergo orderly differentiation from pronormoblasts (or rubriblasts; 14–19 μm), to basophilic normoblasts (prorubricytes; 12–17 μm), to polychromatic normoblasts (rubricytes; 12–15 μm), and finally to orthochromatic normoblasts (metarubricytes) (Fig. 100–3*A*). Maturation is characterized by increasing round chromatin condensation to a pyknotic nucleus and accumulation of hemoglobin that converts the cytoplasm from a deep blue color to a mixture of blue and red (polychromasia) to red.

Granulocytes

Granulocytes include neutrophils, eosinophils, and basophils. Except in neonates, neutrophils are the most prevalent nucleated cells in normal peripheral blood and marrow. The stages of differentiation from most immature to most mature are myeloblasts (12–20 μm), promyelocytes (15–25 μm), myelocytes (10–20 μm), metamyelocytes (10–12 μm), bands (10–16 μm), and segmented neutrophils (10–16 μm). Maturation is characterized by increasing round chromatin condensation, nuclear lobulation, acquisition of primary granules followed by secondary granules, increasing cytoplasm, and loss of nucleoli (Fig. 100–3*B*).

Eosinophils and Basophils

Eosinophils and basophils also undergo a similar orderly differentiation. The major distinction among the granulocytes is the characteristic secondary granule: very fine red-brown for neutrophils, large orange for eosinophils, and large black for basophils. Eosinophil myelocytes can have occasional large basophilic granules and resemble the atypical eosinophils seen in acute myeloid leukemia (AML) of the French-American-British (FAB) class AML-M4eo. Mature eosinophils have bilobed nuclei and only large orange granules. Basophils lose variable amounts of granules during the staining process and thus may have only a few granules for purposes of identification. Eosinophils and basophils can be staged like neutrophils but usually are reported without subclassification (Fig. 100–3*C*).

Lymphocytes

Lymphocytes, the second most common nucleated cell type in normal peripheral blood and third in the marrow, undergo orderly morphologic maturation from lymphoblasts (10–20 µm) to immature lymphocytes (9–18 µm) to mature lymphocytes (8–10 µm) (Fig. 100–3*D*). Maturation is characterized by increasing round chromatin condensation and decreasing size. Normal lymphoblasts and immature lymphocytes are usually seen only in the pediatric population; these early B cells are

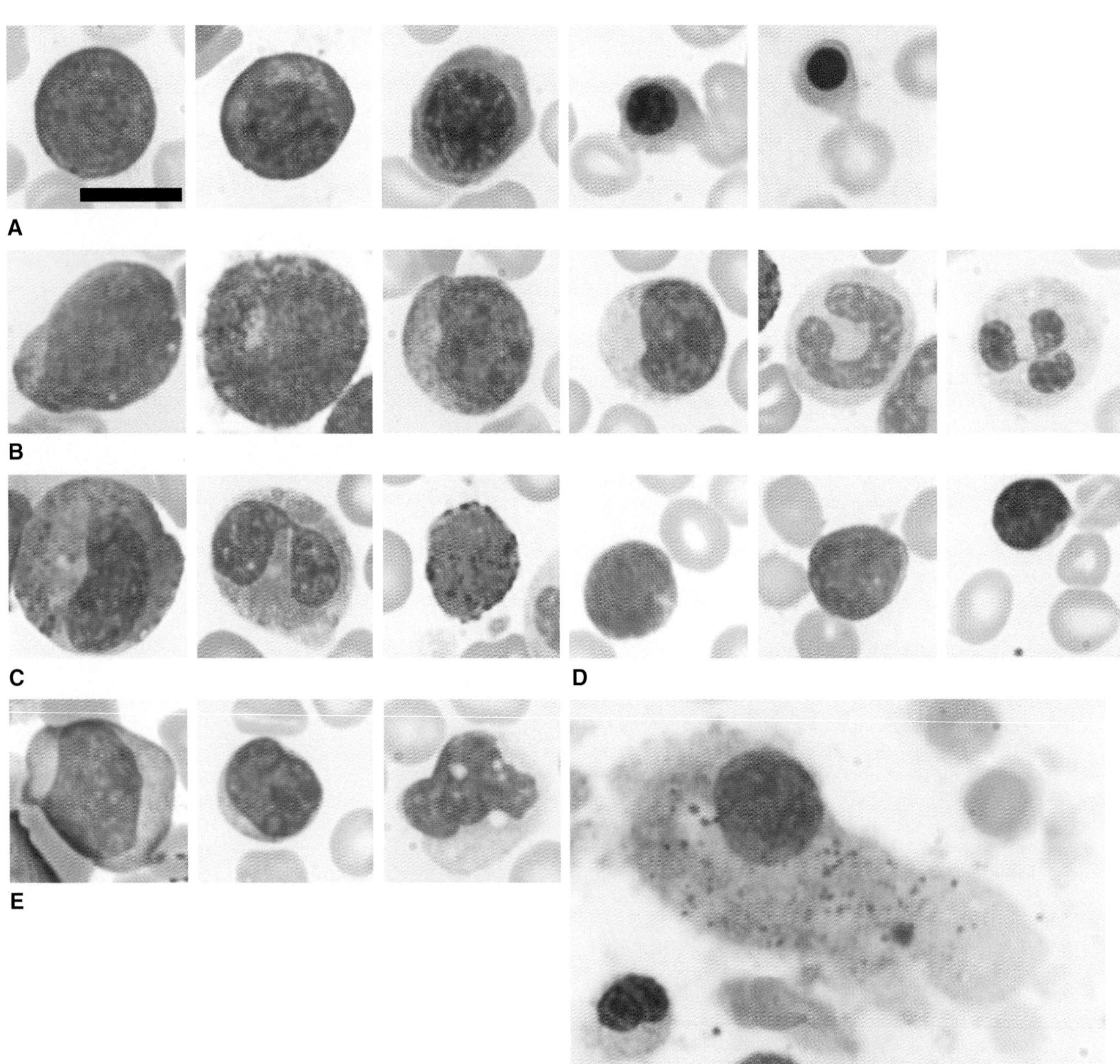

Figure 100–3. Morphology of normal blood cells. (Black bar = 10 µM.) ***A,*** Pronormoblast, basophilic normoblast, early polychromatic normoblast, late polychromatic normoblast, and orthochromatic normoblast in aspirate smears (×1000). ***B,*** Myeloblast, promyelocyte, myelocyte, metamyelocyte, band, and segmented neutrophil in aspirate smears (×1000). ***C,*** Immature eosinophil, eosinophil, and basophil (×1000). ***D,*** Lymphoblast, immature lymphocyte, and lymphocyte (×1000). ***E,*** Monoblast, immature monocyte, monocyte, and macrophage (×1000).

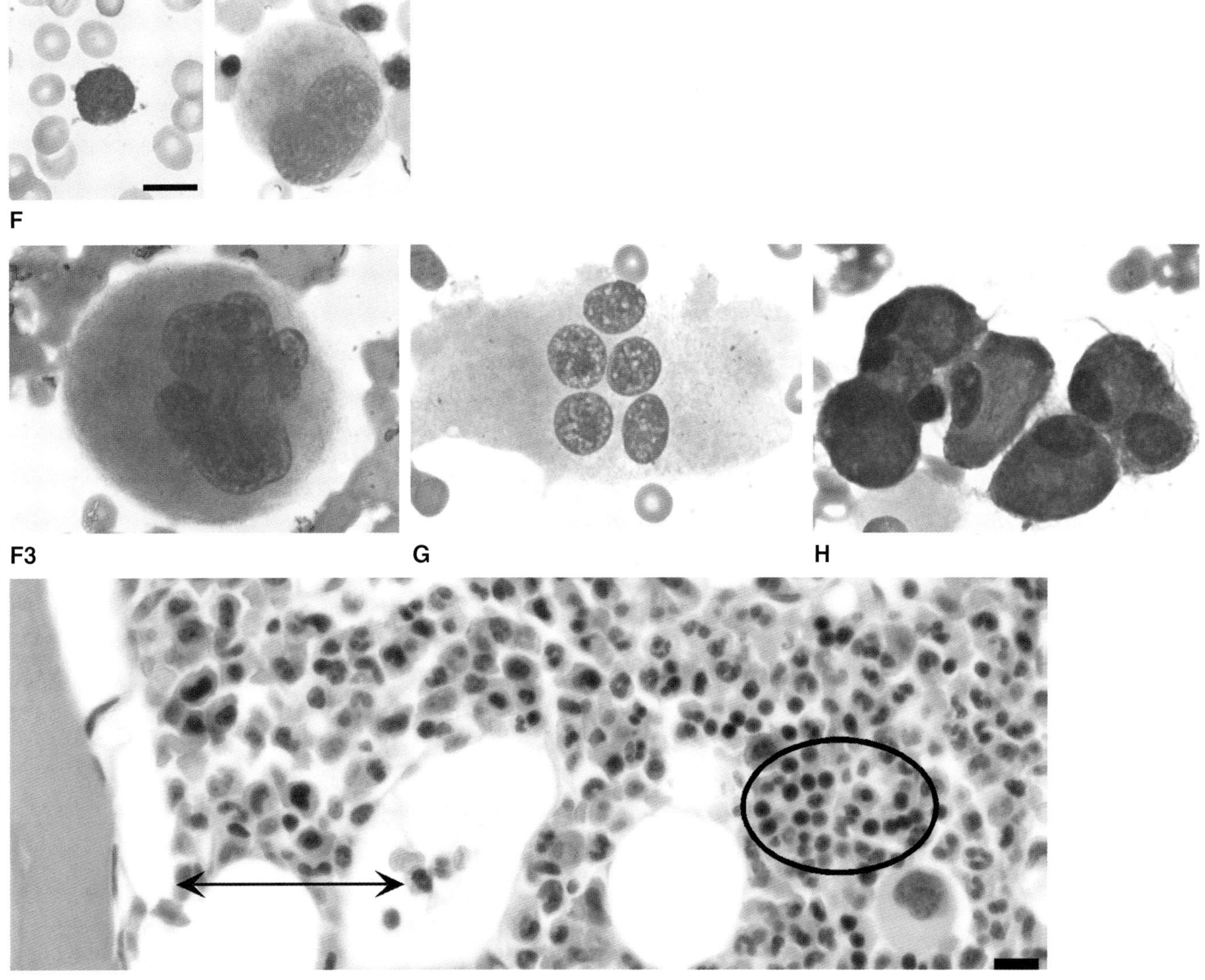

■ **Figure 100–3, cont'd** *F,* Megakaryoblast, early megakaryocyte, and megakaryocytes in aspirate smears (×500). *F3,* Mature megakaryocyte (×500). *G,* Osteoclast (×500). *H,* Osteoblast (×500). *I,* Bone marrow biopsy (×400). Leftmost = bone trabecula; ↔, paratrabecular space with immature myeloid cells; ○, circled erythron (a megakaryocyte is below the circle).

collectively called hematogones. Plasma cells are B cells differentiated to produce immunoglobulin; plasma cells are rare in the circulation but are present in variable numbers in the marrow. Mature lymphocytes, mostly T cells, are the predominant lymphocytic cell type in the peripheral blood and in adult marrow. Their nuclei are round but can be irregular and even cleaved in neonates and infants. As many as 10% of normal peripheral lymphocytes are large granular lymphocytes of natural killer or cytotoxic T-cell lineage; they are typically reported as lymphoid variants (see Fig. 100–8*B* later).

Monocytes

Monocytes are the third most common nucleated cell type in the peripheral blood but are rare (<1%) in the bone marrow. Monocytes mature from monoblasts (12–20 μm) to promonocytes or immature monocytes (12–20 μm) to monocytes (12–20 μm). Maturation is characterized by linear chromatin condensation, nuclear folding, increasing cytoplasm, and cytoplasmic vacuolization (Fig. 100–3*E*). After migration into tissue, monocytes undergo further changes to become macrophages/ histiocytes with even lower nucleus/ cytoplasm ratios. The designations "histiocyte" and "macrophage" are often used interchangeably, except in certain specific morphologic variants; tingible body macrophages, multinucleated giant cell histiocytes, epithelioid histiocytes, histiocytes of granulomas, and histiocytes of hemophagocytosis are examples.

Megakaryocytes

Megakaryocytes are mostly restricted to the bone marrow, but rare naked megakaryocytic nuclei occasionally can be identified in the peripheral blood. Megakaryocytes are the largest normal hematopoietic cells of the marrow, with a wide range in size (35–160 μm); they are best evaluated in a biopsy but are present in the aspirate, often embedded in bone marrow fragments or "spicules." Maturation is characterized by increasing cytoplasm and multilobation of the nuclei (Fig. 100–3*F*).

Miscellaneous Cells

Rare, miscellaneous cells are present in the normal bone marrow but do not circulate; they are important to recognize because they can mimic other hematopoietic cells. Osteoclasts (Fig. 100–3*G*) are confused with megakaryocytes because of their similar size and cytoplasmic granules. Osteoclasts are multinucleated, but their round to oval nuclei are similar in size and not connected. Osteoblasts (Fig. 100–3*H*) can be confused with plasma cells because of their similar size, eccentric nuclei, and basophilic cytoplasm. They differ in that the osteoblasts have fine chromatin, polygonal cytoplasm and eccentric nuclei that partially protrude from the cytoplasm. Also, osteoblasts lack a perinuclear halo. Occasionally, a cluster of osteoblasts in a bone marrow aspirate can mimic metastatic tumor. Mast cells (20–30 μm) have numerous basophilic granules that obscure their nuclei; they resemble basophils but their finer granules resist degranulation during staining.

Morphology of Normal Cells in Marrow Biopsies

Erythroid Cells

In core biopsies of normal marrow, erythroid elements cluster in cohesive units called erythrons. Early proerythroblasts are large and tend to have very round nuclei and linear or comma-shaped nucleoli. Late normoblasts are recognizable by their pale, evenly spaced cytoplasm and jet-black, perfectly round nuclei (see Fig. 100–3*A*). Several abnormalities of erythroid cells may be detected on core biopsies. Disorganized and scattered erythroid elements with loss of erythrons may be seen in myelodysplasia. Nuclei may show nuclear blebs, a key finding in myelodysplasia but also sometimes seen in liver disease, severe infections, and arsenic poisoning.[10,11] Giant proerythroblasts with violaceous inclusions are typical of parvovirus B19 infections. Erythroblasts that are difficult to recognize on dysplastic core biopsies can be identified with immunoperoxidase stains for hemoglobin A or glycophorin A.

Myeloid Cells

Normally, the most immature myeloid cells are aligned along the bone trabeculae. Myeloblasts in normal marrow are infrequent (typically only about 1%). In biopsies, myeloblasts are recognized by their scant to moderate eosinophilic cytoplasm and vesicular nuclei with prominent, eosinophilic nucleoli. In contrast to erythroblasts, nucleoli in myeloblasts tend to be eosinophilic, not basophilic, and round, not comma-shaped. As progenitors mature, they move from the trabeculae to the center of the intertrabecular space.[12] In normal marrow, neutrophils are the most abundant cell type (see Fig. 100–3*B*). Eosinophils are easily identified but comprise only 1–2% of normal cells. Basophils are not easily visualized on tissue sections because their granules dissolve during processing. One common abnormality is a left shift in myeloid maturation, manifested by a relatively reduced number of neutrophils and an increase in early forms. Myeloblasts are best quantitated in aspirate smears, but in biopsies particular attention should be paid to myeloblasts in clusters, as seen in myelodysplasia and leukemia. Hemopoietic growth factor (granulocyte and granulocyte-macrophage colony-stimulating factor) administration can increase the myeloid/erythroid (M:E) ratio and relative numbers of early myeloid elements, usually associated with more immature and maturing myeloid cells adjacent to bone trabeculae. Abnormal localization of immature progenitors, or immature myeloid cells located away from marrow trabeculae, is a finding that is most commonly associated with myelodysplasia.[13] Staining for chloracetate esterase helps to identify myeloid elements in difficult cases, but the stain is inhibited by mercury-based fixatives as well as acid decalcification. Immunoperoxidase stains useful for identifying myeloid cells include those for myeloperoxidase, CD15, and CD43. Monoblasts are usually negative for myeloperoxidase but are positive for lysozyme and KP-1 (CD68) (Table 100–1).

Megakaryocytes

In normal marrow sections cut at 3 μM, three to five megakaryocytes are present per high-power (40×) field; normal megakaryocytes have three to five nuclear lobes that are connected by a thin thread of chromatin (see Fig. 100–3*F*) (osteoclasts have separate nuclei with distinct nucleoli). Emperipolesis is a normal finding in which other hematopoietic elements (often neutrophils) are found coursing their way through the megakaryocyte cytoplasm. A single occasional megakaryocyte with unilobated nuclei is not abnormal, but significant numbers of megakaryocytes with hypolobated nuclei are suggestive of myelodysplasia, particularly the 5q− syndrome. Megakaryocytes usually are not proximate; clusters of megakaryocytes may be seen in myeloproliferative and myelodysplastic disorders, and also following thrombopoietin administration and after cancer chemotherapy.[14] Megakaryocytes (and other hematopoietic elements) localized in dilated bone marrow sinusoids are highly suggestive of idiopathic myelofibrosis. Frequent small megakaryocytes also are common in both myeloproliferative and myelodysplastic disorders. Increased numbers of exceptionally large megakaryocytes are typical of essential thrombocytosis. Mature megakaryocytes are periodic acid–Schiff (PAS) positive and stain for CD42b, CD61, and von Willebrand factor on immunoperoxidase assays.

CYTOCHEMICAL STAINS

Specific chemical reactions to cellular molecules can be applied to peripheral blood and bone marrow aspirate

TABLE 100–1. Immunoperoxidase Stains Useful in the Evaluation of Hematopoietic and Nonhematopoietic Tumors

A: Hematopoietic Tumors

	B-Cell Lymphoma	Hodgkin Lymphoma (Classical)	T-Cell Lymphoma	Pre-B-Cell Lymphoma/ Pre-B-ALL	T-Lymphoblastic Lymphoma/ T-ALL	AML M0-M5	AML M6	AML M7	Myeloma
LCA*	+	– (RS)	+	+	+	+/–	+/–	+/–	–
CD20	+	+/– (RS)	–	–	–	–	–	–	+/–
CD79a	+	+/– (RS)	–	+	–	–	–	–	+
CD3	–	– (RS)	+	–	+	–	–	–	–
UCHL1	–	– (RS)	+	–	+/–	+/–	+/–	–	–
TdT	–	–	–	+	+	–	–	–	–
Hgb	–	–	–	–	–	–	+	–	–
Gly A	–	–	–	–	–	–	+	–	–
κ/λ	–	–	–	–	–	–	–	–	+
CD138	–	–	–	–	–	–	–	–	+
CD15	–	+ (RS)	–	–	–	+/–	–	–	–
CD30	–	+ (RS)	–	–	–	–	–	–	–
CD34	–	–	–	+/–	+/–	+[†]	+	+/–	–
Lys	–	–	–	–	–	+/–[‡]	–	–	–
MPO	–	–	–	–	–	+[§]	+/–	+/–	–
KP-1	–	–	–	–	–	+[‡]	–	–	–
vWF	–	–	–	–	–	–	–	+/–	–
CD61	–	–	–	–	–	–	–	+/–	–

B: Nonhematopoietic Tumors

	Carcinoma	Melanoma	Neuroblastoma	Ewing's Sarcoma	Osteosarcoma	Rhabdomyosarcoma	Seminoma
LCA*	–	–	–	–	–	–	–
LMW, keratin							
AE1	+	–	–	+/–	–	–	–
HMW, keratin							
AE3/Cam5.2	+	–	–	–	–	–	–
S100	–	+	–	–	+/–	–	–
HMB45	–	+	–	–	–	–	–
MART	–	+	–	–	–	–	–
CD99 (MIC2)	–	–	–	+	–	+/–	–
NSE	–[‖]	–	+	+/–	–	–	–
Synaptophysin	–[‖]	–	+	–	–	–	–
Desmin	–	–	–	–	+/–	+	–
Myoglobin	–	–	–	–	–	+	–
PLAP	–	–	–	–	–	–	+

*Leukocyte common antigen (LCA) is very helpful in the preliminary assessment of whether of hematopoietic origin but combinations of markers are required for definitive classification.

[†]CD34 is usually negative in acute promyelocytic leukemia and acute monocytic leukemia.

[‡]Lysozyme and KP-1 are usually positive in monocytic and myelocytic leukemias and acute monocytic leukemia.

[§]MPO is frequently negative in monocytic leukemias.

[‖]Carcinomas with neuroendocrine differentiation often express these antigens.

Abbreviations: Gly A, glycophorin A; Hgb, hemoglobin; HMW, high molecular weight; κ/λ, immunoglobulin κ and λ light chains (used to assess clonality of cytoplasmic immunoglobulin); LMW, low molecular weight; Lys, lysozyme; MPO, myeloperoxidase; NSE, nonspecific esterase; PLAP, placental alkaline phosphatase; Pre-B, precursor B; RS, Reed-Sternberg cells; TdT, terminal deoxynucleotidyl transferase; vWF, von Willebrand factor.

smears. Cytochemistry employs supravital stains, iron stain, Sudan black B, myeloperoxidase, nonspecific esterase, periodic acid–Schiff reaction, and terminal deoxynucleotide transferase (TdT). Supravital and iron stains are routinely used to identify reticulocytes and sideroblasts. Less commonly used stains include tartrate-resistant acid phosphatase for hairy cell leukemia and leukocyte alkaline phosphatase (LAP) for chronic myelogenous leukemia, both now largely replaced by more specific and sensitive tests (flow cytometry for hairy cell leukemia and cytogenetics and molecular studies for chronic myelogenous leukemia) (see Chapters 31 and 35).

Sudan black B, myeloperoxidase, nonspecific esterase, PAS, and TdT are used to determine the lineage of leukemias (Table 100–2, Fig. 100–4) and to subclassify acute myeloid leukemia. These stains, in combination with morphology, defined the original FAB criteria to subclassify acute myeloid leukemia.[15,16] TdT detection by immunofluorescence has been replaced by flow cytometric analysis of bone marrow aspirate or immunohistochemistry of bone marrow biopsy using anti-TdT antibodies.[17] With the incorporation of flow cytometric immunophenotyping, the FAB classification added AML-M7 and M0 in 1985 and 1991.[18,19] The World Health Orga-

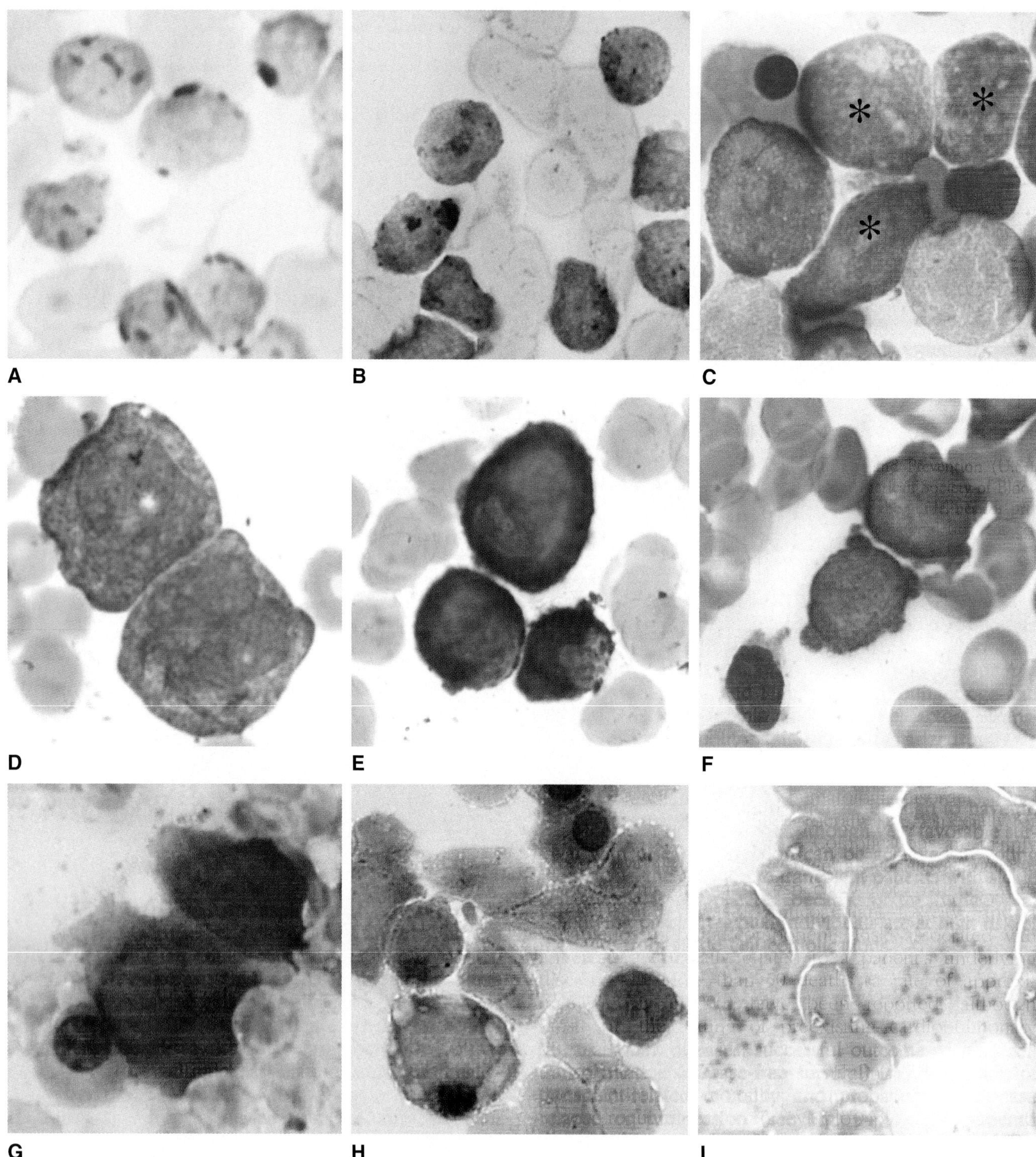

■ **Figure 100–4.** Cytochemistry of blasts. ***A,*** Coarse PAS positivity in precursor B-cell acute lymphoblastic leukemia. ***B,*** Focal Sudan black B positivity in myeloblasts. ***C,*** Focal myeloperoxidase positivity in myeloblasts (*); note the strong positivity in the maturing myeloid cells. ***D–F,*** Wright-stained blasts of acute promyelocytic leukemia, with Auer rods ***(D)*** with strong positivity for Sudan black B ***(E)*** and myeloperoxidase ***(F)***. ***G,*** Diffuse nonspecific esterase positivity in monoblasts. ***H,*** Focal nonspecific esterase positivity in erythroblast. ***I,*** Multipunctate α-naphthyl acetate esterase positivity in megakaryoblasts.

TABLE 100–2. Cytochemical Staining Pattern in Blasts of Various Leukemias

	Pre-B-ALL*	Burkitt	Pre-T-ALL	Myeloid	APML	Monocyte	Erythroid	Megakaryocyte
SBB	–	–	–	+	++	–/+	–	–
MPO	–	–	–	+	++	–	–	–
CAE	–	–	–	+/–	++	–	–	–
NSE	–	–	focal +	–	–/+	++	focal +/–	–
ANA	–	–	focal +	–	–	diffuse + (S)	focal +/–	punctate + (PR)
PAS	coarse +	–	–	fine +	fine +	fine/coarse +	coarse +	coarse +
APhos	NF	NF	focal +	NF	NF	NF	focal +	NF
TdT	+	–	+	–	–	–	–	–

*Rare pre-B-ALL can be SBB- and NSE-positive hematopoietic tumors.
Abbreviations: ANA, α-naphthyl acetate esterase; APhos, acid phosphatase; CAE, chloroacetate esterase; MPO, myeloperoxidase; NF, nonfocal; NSE, nonspecific esterase; PAS, periodic acid–Schiff reagent; (PR), partially resistant to fluoride; Pre-B, precursor B; Pre-T, precursor T; (S), sensitive to fluoride; SBB, Sudan black B; TdT, terminal deoxynucleotidyl transferase.

nization classification[20] has significantly changed the FAB system and incorporated clinical, cytogenetic, and molecular findings. Nevertheless, cytochemistry for acute leukemias remains useful because it can be performed on touch imprints of bone marrow biopsies in inaspirable cases and may help identify acute leukemias that lack immunophenotypical markers.

Very strongly Sudan black B– and myeloperoxidase-staining cells often represent normal myeloid precursor cells. Myeloblasts usually show minimal focal staining of mononuclear cells with scant cytoplasm (see Fig. 100–4*B* and *C*), with the important exception of the strong, intense staining seen in acute promyelocytic leukemia (see Fig. 100–4*E* and *F*).

Supravital Stains

Supravital stains, brilliant cresyl blue or new methylene blue, identify reticulocytes; the stains precipitate the ribosomes present in young red blood cells still producing hemoglobin. Reticulocytes correlate with polychromatic red blood cells but also with some orthochromatic red blood cells, which retain fewer ribosomes.[21,22] These stains can also highlight Pappenheimer bodies (iron-containing inclusions), Heinz bodies (denatured hemoglobin), and Howell-Jolly bodies (DNA). Reticulocytes can also be counted by machine using dyes that fluoresce when bound to RNA or by supravital stains that scatter or absorb light. Automated examination of larger numbers of red blood cells allows greater precision in the reticulocyte count[23,24] but requires a greater volume of blood compared to the single drop sufficient for manual determination.

Iron

Iron is commonly detected using Perls Prussian blue, in which ferric ions react with ferrocyanide in acid solution to form an insoluble precipitate, ferric ferrocyanide. Iron from hemoglobin destruction is stored in macrophages as hemosiderin, ferric hydroxide polymers, or ferritin. Acid treatment for decalcification of bone marrow biopsies solubilizes metal ions and can produce an artifactual lack of iron. Iron is better evaluated in aspirate smears or un-decalcified clot sections. Low to absent staining is commonly seen in normal young children less than 5 years of age,[25] in menstruating or pregnant women,[26,27] and in patients with polycythemia vera.[28] Sideroblasts are erythrocytes that contain stainable iron; they are increased during high iron turnover as in chronic hemolytic anemia,[29] thalassemia,[30] megaloblastic anemia,[31] congenital dyserythropoietic anemia,[32] and hemochromatosis. Sideroblasts also can be seen in lead poisoning, in alcoholism,[33] with drugs such as chloramphenicol, in myelodysplastic syndrome,[34] and in congenital sideroblastic anemia (see Chapter 55). Sideroblasts with abundant iron encircling the nucleus are termed *ringed sideroblasts* and are useful in the subclassification of myelodysplastic syndrome. Iron is occasionally seen in plasma cells,[35,36] particularly in alcoholism.[33]

Sudan Black B

Sudan black B is a lipophilic dye relatively specific for granulocytes; it stains both primary and secondary granules in neutrophils, eosinophils, and basophils. The method is very sensitive: normal and neoplastic myeloblasts without morphologic evidence of granules stain positive. Monocytes are negative or have weak scant positivity, whereas normal lymphocytes and erythroid and megakaryocytic cells are negative. Strongly staining lymphoblasts suggest a biphenotypic leukemia; other features of myeloid differentiation of these cells can be detected. Neoplastic lymphoblasts are negative, and the rare positive cases express no other myeloid differentiation markers.[37,38] Oil red O is less frequently employed lipophilic dye that can aid in the diagnosis of Burkitt's lymphoma[39]; oil red O staining is also positive in precursor B lymphoblasts, which are usually also PAS positive.[40]

Myeloperoxidase

Myeloperoxidase is a specific peroxidase found in granulocytes and promonocytes and localized to the endoplasmic reticulum, Golgi apparatus, and cytoplasmic granules. In general, the reactivity of myeloperoxidase is similar to that of Sudan black B, but the myeloperoxidase functional assay is less sensitive and more specific, because reactivity is seen only in the granulocytic lineage. Myeloperoxidase is often decreased to absent in the mature granulocytes of acute myeloid leukemia, chronic myelogenous leukemia, and myelodysplastic syndrome. The MPO protein can also be detected by antibodies but moderate positivity is detected in monocytes and in some precursor B-cell acute lymphoblastic leukemia,[41] suggesting that flow cytometry may be less specific (or more sensitive) than is cytochemistry.

Platelet Peroxidase

Platelet peroxidase is localized to the endoplasmic reticulum and nuclear membranes but not seen in the Golgi apparatus or cytoplasm. Platelet peroxidase is present in megakaryocytes but not in granulocytes and monocytes. The enzyme is detected using the substrates 3,3′-diaminobenzidine or 4-chloro-naphthol, leading to insoluble colored precipitates followed by electron microscopy for precise intracellular localization. Platelet peroxidase is a sensitive marker of normal and neoplastic megakaryoblasts, and very early megakaryoblasts have platelet peroxidase activity prior to expression of surface glycoproteins (CD41, CD42a, CD61) as detected by flow cytometry.[42] However, very early erythroblasts, macrophages, and hairy cell leukemia may also register positive in this assay.[43]

Nonspecific Esterase

Nonspecific esterase is a class of enzymes that includes carboxyl esterases, aryl esterases, and acetyl esterases that hydrolyze nitrogen-free alcohols and organic acids. Nonspecific esterase hydrolyzes naphthyl ester–based substrates, leading to an insoluble colored precipitate. Three main substrates are used to detect monocytic differentiation. Naphthol AS acetate is hydrolyzed in most cells but very strongly in monocytes; fluoride inhibits the activity in monocytes but not in lymphoblasts, myeloblasts, and promyelocytes.[44] α-Naphthyl acetate and α-naphthyl butyrate can be employed under conditions that lead to strong diffuse cytoplasmic staining of monocytes and single focal staining in T lymphocytes, resulting in a cytochemical assay that is more sensitive for determining monoblastic differentiation than is flow cytometry. Normoblasts can also contain nonspecific esterase in vitamin B_{12} deficiency, folate deficiency, myelodysplastic syndrome, and erythroleukemia. Granulocytic precursors of myelodysplastic syndrome and acute promyelocytic leukemia also may be positive in this test. Under different conditions, the α-naphthyl acetate substrate can produce staining of normal and neoplastic megakaryocytes in a characteristic multipunctate pattern that is partially inhibited by fluoride, a pattern useful in the diagnosis of AML-M7.[45] Naphthol AS-D chloroacetate substrate can be used to detect chloroacetate esterase, which is present in all neutrophilic granulocytes at the promyelocyte or later stages of differentiation. All other hematopoietic cells are negative, including myeloblasts, eosinophils, and basophils.

Periodic Acid–Schiff

PAS identifies 1,2-glycol groupings and their derivatives, present in most carbohydrates but not in lipids, nucleic acids, or proteins. PAS normally stains granulocytic and monocytic cells as well as megakaryocytes in a fine granular pattern.

Most precursor B-cell acute lymphoblastic leukemias have variable coarse and inclusion-like blocks of PAS-positive granules. A similar pattern can be seen in leukemic erythroblasts and in metastatic nonhematopoietic malignancies such as rhabdomyosarcoma, Ewing's sarcoma, and neuroblastoma. Normoblasts normally do not stain but may be positive in myelodysplasia, acute myeloid leukemia, iron deficiency,[46] hemolytic anemia, thalassemia,[47,48] and megaloblastic anemia.[46]

Acid and Alkaline Phosphatases

Acid phosphatase is relatively nonspecific enzymatic activity present in all hematopoietic cells. At low pH, the phosphatase incubated with an α-naphthyl phosphate substrate produces an insoluble colored precipitate. Acid phosphatase activity is weak in lymphocytes, strong in granulocytes, stronger in eosinophils, monocytes, and platelets, and strongest in histiocytes, plasma cells, megakaryocytes, mast cells, and osteoclasts. Intracellular localization of activity has been useful in the diagnosis of T-cell lymphoma/leukemia, because a single focal perinuclear pattern is seen with normal and neoplastic T cells, including T lymphoblasts.[49,50] Erythroblasts but not other blasts share this staining pattern. Strong acid phosphatase activity that is resistant to inhibition by tartrate is seen in most but not all hairy cell leukemia cases,[51] and the test can be positive in other B- and T-cell hematopoietic malignancies.[52] Most of these stains have been replaced by flow cytometric immunophenotyping.

Alkaline phosphatase activity historically was important for the diagnosis of chronic myelogenous leukemia, before techniques were developed to detect the *BCR/ABL* translocation. Unlike normal reactive neutrophils in a leukemoid reaction, the neutrophils of chronic myelogenous leukemia have low to absent levels of LAP. Eosinophils, basophils, myeloid progenitors, lymphocytes, monocytes, normoblasts, and megakaryocytes are negative. Faint staining can be seen in some platelets and rare lymphocytes. In abnormal hematopoiesis, LAP activity can be increased in myeloblasts of chronic myelogenous leukemia in blast crisis, acute myeloid leukemia of monocytic lineage, and occasional chronic lymphocytic leukemia cases. LAP scores are calculated from a 100-neutrophil cell count, assigning a staining intensity of 0 to 4 with lymphocytes as 0 and the strongest staining neutrophil in the positive control as 4. The 100 intensities are summed to calculate the LAP score, which is highly laboratory- and observer-dependent. Despite its

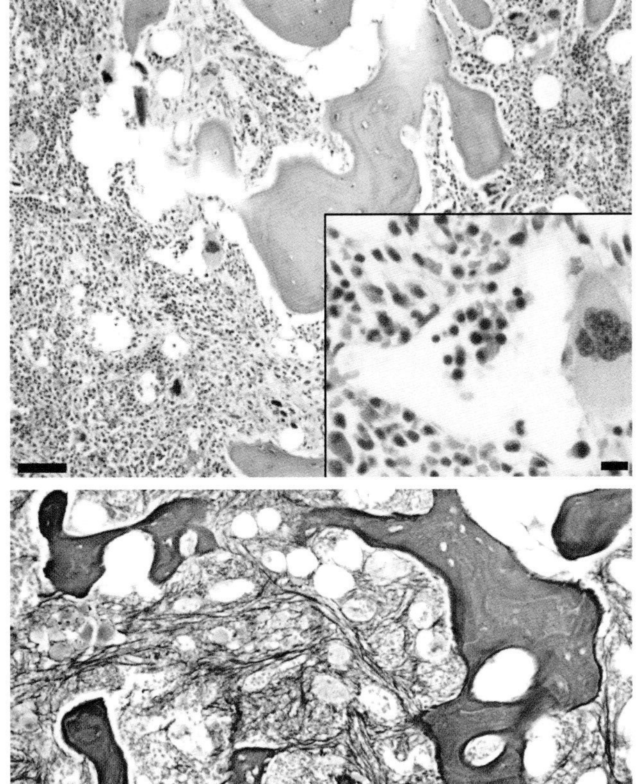

Figure 100–5. Reticulin stain in chronic idiopathic myelofibrosis. The hematoxylin and eosin–stained section (*top*; ×100, black bar = 100μM) shows hypercellularity and osteosclerosis. *Inset* shows a dilated bone marrow sinusoid containing maturing erythroid cells and a megakaryocyte (*right*; ×400, black bar = 10μM). The reticulin stain shows marked reticulin fibrosis (*bottom*; × 100, black bar = 10μM).

subjectivity, normal values between institutions are similar. A low LAP score is not specific for chronic myelogenous leukemia and can be seen in chronic myelomonocytic leukemia and juvenile myelomonocytic leukemia, while atypical chronic myelogenous leukemia can show normal to increased levels. LAP scores are normal or elevated in many other diseases, such as polycythemia vera, chronic idiopathic myelofibrosis, and Down's syndrome.

Reticulin

The reticulin stain on biopsy sections highlights newly formed collagen before it becomes highly cross-linked; normally, only a delicate collection of fibrils is present around blood vessels. The amount of reticulin is graded as normal or mildly, moderately, or markedly increased, or on a 1 to 4 scale. Increased reticulin is observed with elevated numbers of megakaryocytes and in a variety of myeloproliferative disorders (Fig. 100–5). Reticulin fibrosis is also common in lymphomas (particularly follicular lymphomas and Hodgkin's lymphoma) and metastatic carcinoma.

Immunohistochemistry

A multitude of antibodies now make it possible to detect a wide range of antigens in paraffin sections (see Table 100–1); many of the markers can be adapted for use on aspirate smears or cytologic fluids. Most commonly, the primary antibody is detected with a peroxidase-conjugated secondary antibody and diaminobenzidine, resulting in a brown insoluble reaction product. Not all epitopes are preserved after formalin fixation, and flow cytometry of fresh tissue is more sensitive for detection of antigens and for the determination of immunoglobulin light chain clonality of lymphocytes.

PERIPHERAL BLOOD SMEAR EVALUATION

The patient's identification should be confirmed. At low power (10×), initial scan of the slide locates a region near the feathered edge for morphologic examination; under higher magnification (50× or 100×) the ideal region should contain red blood cells that are proximate but not touching. Lateral edges of the smear should be avoided because they can have falsely elevated numbers of immature myeloid cells.

Rough quantification of cells can be performed on the smear, but more accurate manual counts of white blood cells and red blood cells require a hemocytometer. With a normal hematocrit, the red blood cells occupy approximately 50% of the surface area of the smear. In contrast, severe anemia produces a larger empty surface area and polycythemia produces overlapping red blood cells throughout the smear. White blood cell counts are estimated by determining the number of myeloid cells, including degenerating nuclei, viewed using a 50× oil lens; multiple fields are counted and the counts averaged. Each white blood cell in a field is equivalent to 3000–4000/μL. Platelet counts are similarly estimated using a 100× oil lens; each platelet in a field is equivalent to a concentration of 10,000–15,000/μL. Aggregates of platelets or white blood cells suggest the possibility of incorrect automated results and should initiate repeat manual counts or further automated counts using heparinized instead of EDTA-anticoagulated blood.

Qualitative Abnormalities

Qualitative abnormalities of red blood cells (Fig. 100–6, Table 100–3)[6,53–55] include variation in size (anisocytosis), small red blood cells (microcytes) and large red blood cells (macrocytes); shape (poikilocytosis), especially the presence of teardrop cells (dacryocytes), target cells (leptocytes), sickle cells, spherocytes, schistocytes, acanthocytes, and echinocytes; hemoglobinization, including decreased hemoglobin concentration (hypochromia); polychromasia (young reticulocytes resulting from increased RNA); and cell inclusions, such as nuclear fragments (Howell-Jolly bodies), ribosomal RNA aggregates (basophilic stippling), abnormal iron accumulation (Pappenheimer bodies), and microorganisms such as malaria.

Myeloid cells (Fig. 100–7, Table 100–4) can show abnormal differentiation, such as a left shift in neutrophil

TABLE 100–3. Partial List of Abnormal Red Blood Cell Morphologies and Their Associated Disorders

	Spherocyte	Target Cell	Acanthocyte	Echinocyte	Dacryocyte	Schistocyte	Macro-ovalocyte	Elliptocyte	Hypochromasia	Polychromasia	Basophilic Stippling	Pappenheimer Body
Microcytic Anemia												
Thalassemia	+	++	+	+	+	+		+	+	+	+	+
Sideroblastic anemia (subset)	+	+	+			+			++		+	+
Iron deficiency	+	+		+	+	+		+	++			
Lead poisoning									+		++	+
Pyropoikilocytosis	+		+	+	+	++		+		+		
Normocytic Anemia												
Sickle cell disease	+	++								++	+	+
Autoimmune hemolytic anemia	++		+	+	+	+				++		+
Microangiopathic hemolytic anemia	+		+	+		++				+		
Hereditary spherocytosis	++									++		
Marrow fibrosis/infiltration	+			+	++	+		+			+	
Pyruvate kinase deficiency			+	+				+		+	+	
Macrocytic Anemia												
Megaloblastic anemia	+			+	+	+	++	+			+	+
Myelodysplastic syndrome			+				++					
Liver disease	+	++	++	+								
Unrelated to Anemia												
Healthy neonates	+	+	+			+				+		+
Hyposplenism/splenectomy	+	+	+			+				+		+
Transfusion	+			+								
Storage artifact				+								

Data from Bain,[6] O'Connor,[53] Smith,[54] and Bessis.[55]

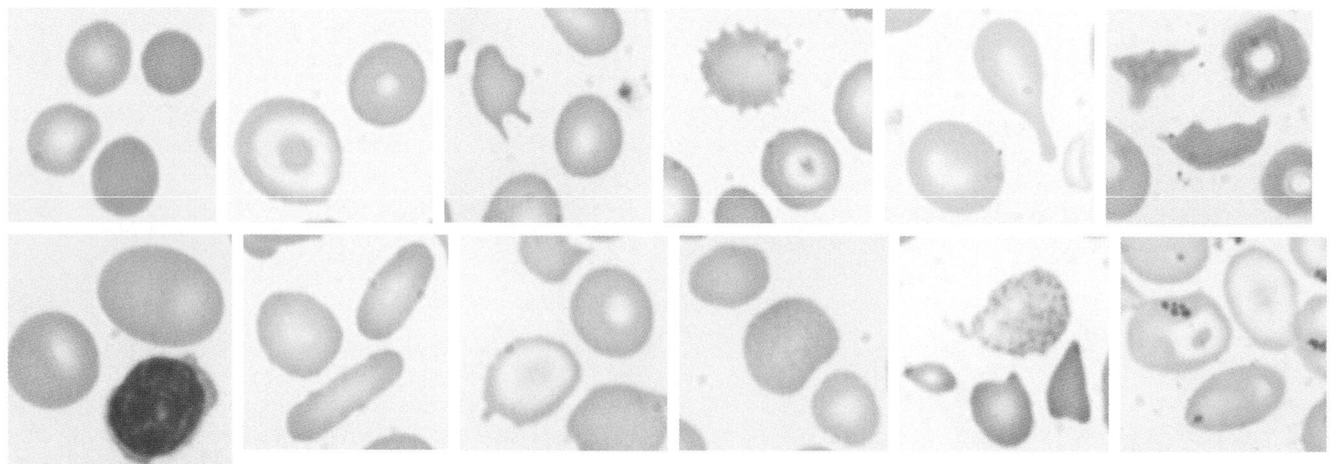

■ **Figure 100–6.** Abnormal morphology of red blood cells. *Top row, left to right:* spherocyte, leptocyte, acanthocyte, echinocyte, dacryocyte, and schistocyte. Note that the schistocyte pattern shows red blood cells with refractile rings indicative of water artifact. *Bottom row, left to right:* macro-ovalocyte, elliptocyte, hypochromasia, polychromasia, basophilic stippling, and Pappenheimer bodies.

maturation or "arrest" at the blast stage as in acute leukemia; nuclear segmentation, such as hypersegmented, hyposegmented, or ringed neutrophils; granulation, such as Auer rods, Chédiak-Higashi granules, toxic granulation, hypogranulation, and uneven cytoplasmic distribution of granules; and cytoplasmic inclusions, such as vacuoles, Döhle bodies, and microorganisms (bacteria, yeast, or aggregates of viral particles).

Qualitative abnormalities of lymphoid cells (Fig. 100–8) can affect maturation, including plasmacytoid

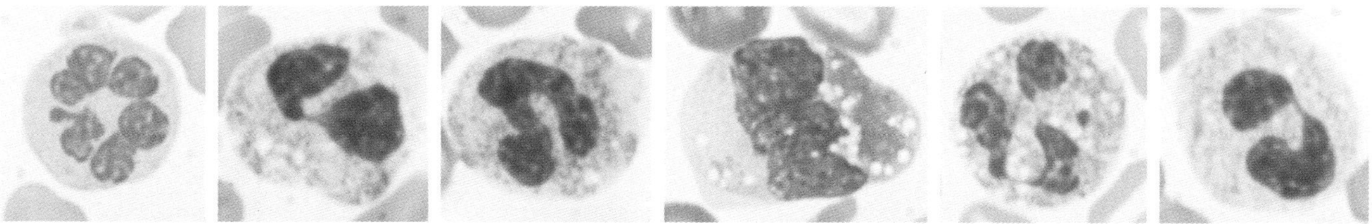

Figure 100–7. Abnormal morphology of granulocytes. *Left to right:* hypersegmented, hyposegmented, hypergranular, hypogranular, vacuoles, and Döhle bodies.

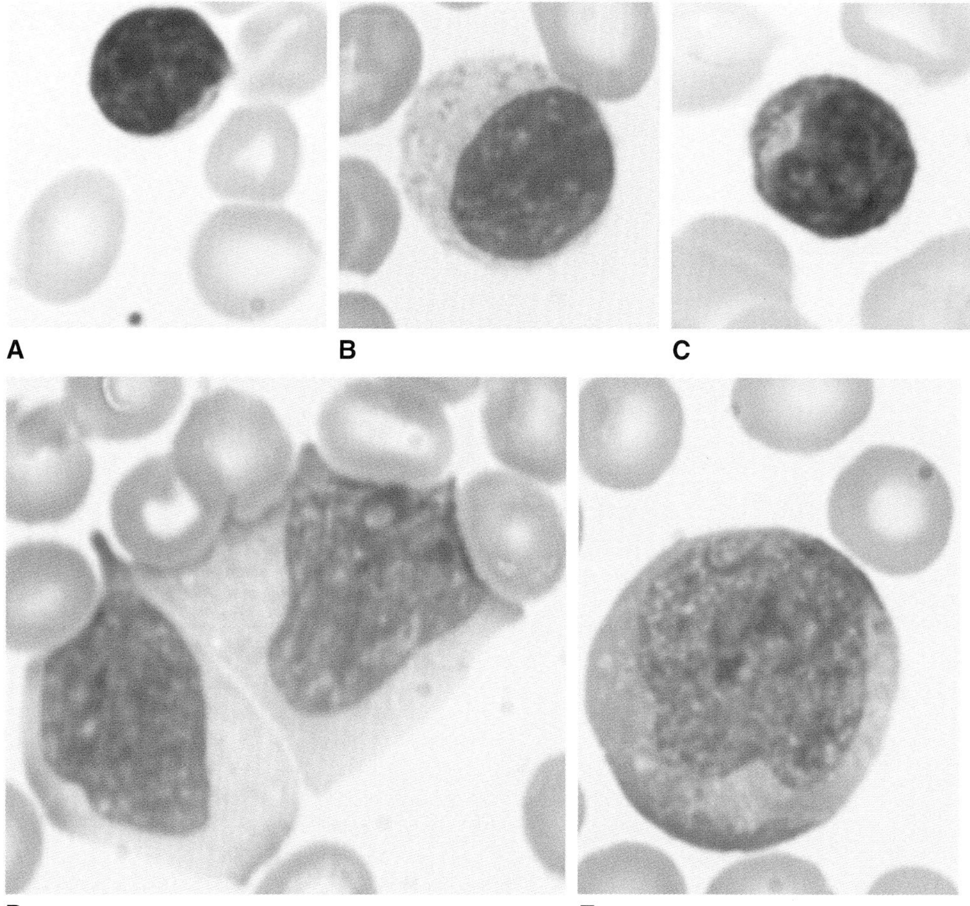

Figure 100–8. Lymphoid variants/atypical lymphocytes. ***A,*** Normal lymphocyte. ***B,*** Large granular lymphocytes are cytotoxic T or natural killer (NK) cells that are normally present in the peripheral blood smear and increased in number with viral infections. ***C,*** Plasmacytoid lymphocytes are typically B cells with some but not all of the features of plasma cell. The depicted cell has the basophilic cytoplasm, eccentric nuclei, and perinuclear hof but lacks the abundant cytoplasm and peripheral nuclear chromatin condensation ("clockwork face" nuclei) of a plasma cell. ***D,*** Atypical lymphocytes (Downey type II) are activated cytotoxic T or NK cells and are characterized by wedge-shaped nuclei, round and linear chromatin condensation, and abundant gray to light blue cytoplasm that wraps around surrounding red blood cells. They can have small granules and vacuoles. ***E,*** Immunoblasts (Downey type III) can be either activated B or T cells and are characterized by large round to irregular nuclei, some round chromatin condensations, multiple nucleoli, basophilic cytoplasm, and a perinuclear halo.

activation, atypical large granular lymphocytes, or an immunoblastic stage of differentiation, or arrest at the blast stage, as in acute leukemia; nuclear morphology, such as a wedge or cleaved shape; or cytoplasmic inclusions, including granules or vacuoles.

Qualitative abnormalities of platelets (Table 100–5) are usually detected by functional or flow cytometric assays but may occasionally manifest as abnormalities in size or granulation. Gray platelet syndrome can be associated with gray granulocytes.[56]

TABLE 100–4. Abnormal Neutrophil Morphologies and Their Associated Disorders

	Left Shift in Maturation	Isolated Blasts	Hypersegmented	Hyposegmented	Hypergranular	Hypogranular	Vacuoles	Döhle Bodies
Infection/inflammation	+				+		+	+
Pregnancy	+				+			+
G-CSF	+				+		+	+
Megaloblastic anemia			+		+		+	
Alder-Reilly anomaly					+		+/−	
May-Hegglin anomaly							+	+
Pelger-Huët anomaly				+				
MDS		+	+	+		+	+	
CML	+		+					
AML		+						

Abbreviations: AML, acute myeloid leukemia; CML, chronic myelogenous leukemia; G-CSF, granulocyte colony-stimulating factor; MDS, myelodysplastic syndrome.

TABLE 100–5. Some Abnormal Platelet Morphologies and Their Associated Disorders

Abnormal Morphology	Associated Disorders
Giant platelets	Increased platelet destruction (ITP, TTP, DIC) Hyposplenism Myelodysplastic/myeloproliferative disorder/ acute myeloid leukemia May-Hegglin anomaly (Fechtner syndrome, Sebastian syndrome) Bernard-Soulier syndrome Marfan syndrome
Small platelets	Wiskott-Aldrich syndrome
Agranular platelets	Gray platelet syndrome Cardiopulmonary bypass Hairy cell leukemia Myelodysplastic/myeloproliferative syndrome

Abbreviations: DIC, disseminated intravascular coagulation; ITP, immune thrombocytopenic purpura; TTP, thrombotic thrombocytopenic purpura.

Artifacts

Artifacts may confuse the interpretation of the peripheral blood smear. Degenerating nuclear debris, termed "smudge" cells, represents abnormally fragile leukocytes that circulate intact in the peripheral blood; they are associated with chronic lymphocytic leukemia. Artifacts also can be introduced in the collection and transport of the blood sample. With selective binding of methylene blue to heparin-coated cells, the Wright-stained smear will be a uniform blue color without eosin contrast, resulting in unclassifiable mononuclear blue cells (segmented neutrophils can still be recognized). With EDTA, prolonged storage of a blood sample can lead to echinocytes, apoptosis of neutrophils, nuclear lobulation of lymphocytes, and cytoplasmic vacuoles in leukocytes. As a result, lymphocytes can be mistaken for lymphoma cells, vacuoles for signs of sepsis, and apoptotic neutrophils as nucleated red blood cells. Transport at elevated temperatures can cause abnormal red blood cell fragmentation that is morphologically indistinguishable from pyropoikilocytosis.

Occasionally a blood smear shows a refractile ring encircling the central pallor of a red blood cell, which represents either incomplete drying of the smear before staining or water contamination of the methanol used during staining. An old Wright solution can precipitate on a smear, producing numerous small blue-black particles that can be mistaken for platelets or bacteria. True bacterial and fungal organisms are uniform in size and shape, but artifactual organisms can appear as a result of contamination of the staining solution; the septic patient's smear should show organisms within neutrophils or monocytes, toxic granulation, Döhle bodies, vacuoles, and apoptosis of neutrophils.[57,58]

Infectious Organisms

Infectious organisms can circulate in the blood; identification of organisms within cells is the strongest evidence of true sepsis rather than artifact secondary to contamination. The most commonly occurring organism on the blood smear is malaria; more rarely, bacteria and fungi can be seen (Fig. 100–9). Bacteria are characterized by the uniform size and shape of the organisms, which stain purple to black in color and appear singly or in small aggregates. Many bacterial strains have been reported on the peripheral smear, including *Bacteroides*,[59] *Borrelia*,[60] *Clostridium*,[61] *Corynebacterium*,[61] *Ehrlichia*,[62] *Klebsiella*,[63] *Legionella*,[64] *Neisseria*,[65] *Pseudomonas*,[66] *Streptococcus*, and *Yersinia*.[67] *Mycobacteria* appear as negative-staining rods in macrophages in the peripheral

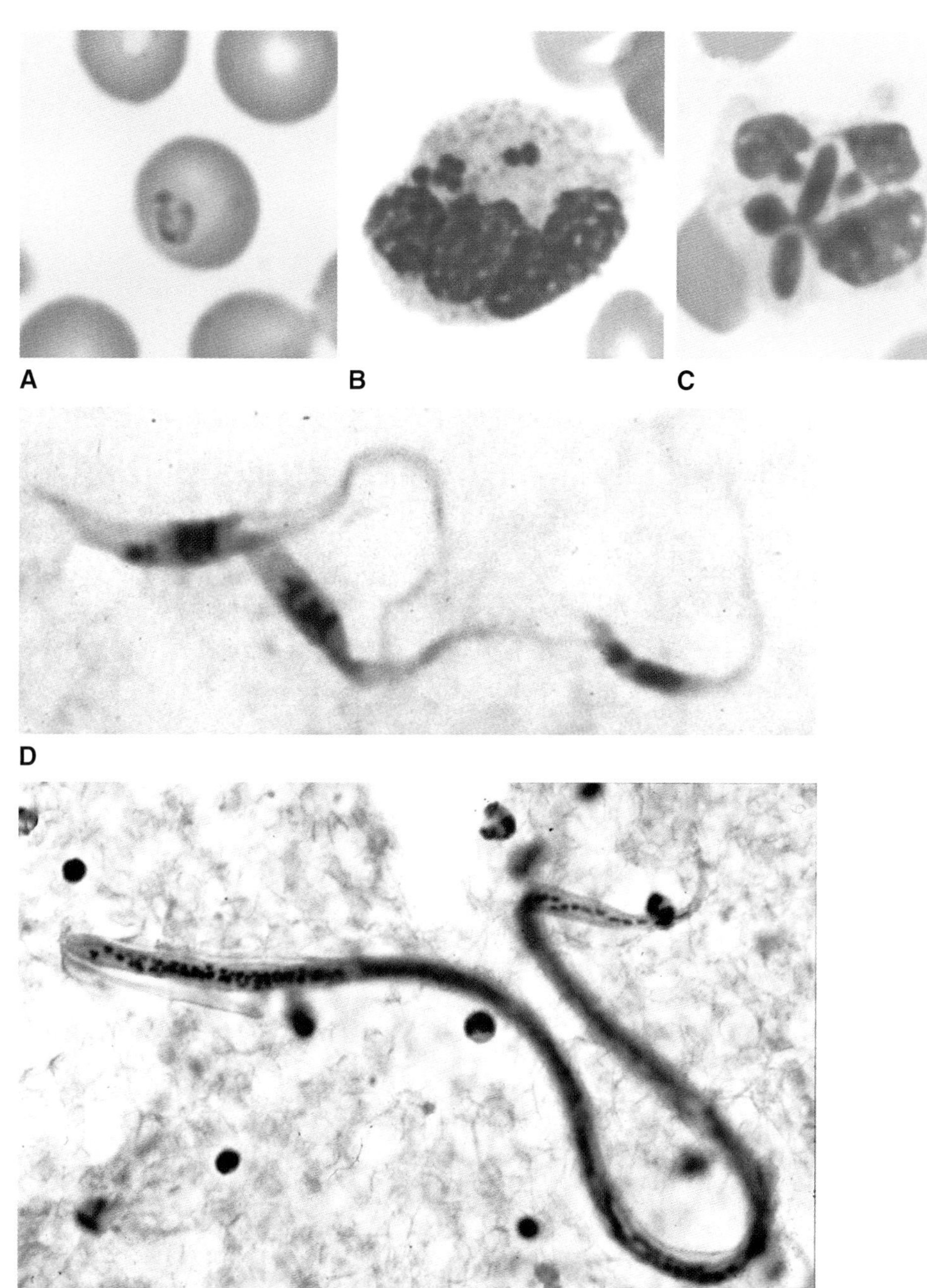

Figure 100–9. Infectious organisms in peripheral blood smears. ***A,*** *Plasmodium falciparum*. ***B,*** *Streptococcus mitis*. ***C,*** *Candida albicans*. ***D,*** *Trypanosoma cruzi* in thick film preparation. ***E,*** *Wuchereria bancrofti* in thick film preparation. (***A–D,*** ×1000; ***E,*** ×100.) (Courtesy of Ms. Marybeth Helfrich, Children's Hospital of Philadelphia, Pennsylvania *[**B**]*, Dr. Dennis Cornfield, Lehigh Valley Hospital *[**C**]*, and Dr. Karin L. McGowan, Children's Hospital of Philadelphia *[**D, E**]*).

blood but more often on bone marrow aspirate smears.[68] Fungi detected include *Candida*,[69,70] *Cryptococcus*,[71,72] *Histoplasma*,[73] and *Penicillium*.[74,75] Parasites include *Plasmodium*, *Babesia*,[76] *Leishmania*,[77,78] *Trypanosoma*,[79] and assorted filarias.[80] Of these, only *Babesia* is endogenous to Western countries, but all can be seen in patients with exposure from international travel.

Cancer Cells

Cells of many cancers circulate in the peripheral blood but usually at so low a concentration that sensitive detection or purification methods are required for their identification.[81–84] Circulating neuroblastoma,[82,85,86] rhabdomyosarcoma,[82,87] melanoma,[88] and carcinoma[89,90] cells can mimic circulating blasts. After blasts of acute leukemias, the mature appearing lymphocytes of B and T lymphoma are the most frequent circulating cancer cells; cells from all lymphomas, including multiple myeloma, have been reported in the peripheral blood.[91] Circulating lymphoma cells have morphology similar to that in the lymphomatous node; for example, follicular lymphomas tend to be irregular to cleaved,[92,93] but normal lymphocytes in neonates and infants can mimic this appearance. Mantle cell lymphoma cells are round to irregular, and in some cases have blastic morphology that can be confused as acute leukemia.[94,95] Large-cell lymphoma and anaplastic large-cell lymphoma produce large atypical cells.[96–98] The Sézary cells of mycosis fungoides are large lymphocytes with hyperchromatic, convoluted nuclei.[99] Burkitt's and lymphoblastic lymphoma cells can circulate and are indistinguishable from their leukemic counterparts; a leukemic classification is assigned when greater than 25% of the marrow is involved by the tumor.

BONE MARROW BIOPSY AND ASPIRATE EVALUATION

Examination of the Bone Marrow Aspirate

Aspirate smears are first examined at low power, noting the presence or absence of spicules and the cellularity of the spicules. After ensuring that no sheets of blasts, lymphoid aggregates, or other abnormalities are present, thin areas adjacent to spicules are selected for examination under high magnification with an oil immersion lens. An estimate is made of the M:E ratio, and the maturation and number of erythroid and myeloid cells and megakaryocytes are assessed. Other cell types are noted and a differential cell count is performed, usually of 200 cells. The aspirate smear also is evaluated for the presence of stainable iron, including careful examination under oil for ringed sideroblasts.

Examination of the Clot Section

The approach to the clot section is similar to that of the core (see later). Generally the findings are similar to those in the core, so that its description can be brief, except when the clot section has more evaluable marrow.

Examination of the Bone Marrow Biopsy

The core should first be examined at low power (4×) to assess cellularity and its overall architecture. Typically the M:E ratio and organization of other hematopoietic elements can be assessed at 20×, with examination of cytologic features at 40× where needed. Five to six intertrabecular spaces (at least 1 cm and preferably 2 cm or more of core) or more are ideally obtained and scanned[100]; a statement on the adequacy of the sample should be made. Larger biopsies and/or bilateral biopsies are particularly important for cancer or lymphoma staging where involvement may be local.[101,102]

Cellularity

Cellularity is expressed as a percentage of total intratrabecular space, typically in increments of 5%. The first 2 mm of subcortical marrow are often hypocellular and not representative. Normal cellularity varies with age from 80% at birth, with a roughly 10% decrease each subsequent decade,[103] but the normal cellularity at 5–18 years of age is 60% ± 20%.[104] Marrows are judged as normocellular, mildly hypo- or hypercellular, moderately hypo- or hypercellular, and markedly hypo- or hypercellular. Marrows may be hypocellular without other pathologic findings. Alternatively, the interstitial areas in hypocellular marrows sometimes contain proteinaceous material that constitutes serous atrophy; common causes include malnutrition, human immunodeficiency virus infection, and chemotherapy or radiation effect.

M:E Ratio

The M:E ratio is age dependent, ranging from 4–5:1 at birth to 1–2:1 during infancy and then rising again so that adolescents and adults typically show ratios of 2–3:1. Large deviations may be seen. Myeloproliferative disorders, particularly chronic myelogenous leukemia and some leukemoid reactions, are accompanied by M:E ratios greater than 10:1. Hemolytic anemias, megaloblastic anemias, and some myelodysplastic disorders may show dramatically reversed M:E ratios.

Erythroid, Myeloid, and Megakaryocytic Maturation

The quality and quantity of each lineage is assessed. The degree of differentiation and dysplasia, if present, are noted.

Other Cell Types and Abnormalities

Lymphoid Aggregates or Infiltrates

The number of lymphocytes in bone marrow varies greatly with age, ranging from about 80% in the first few months of life to 50% at 18 months and then decreasing to about 10–20% in children and adults.[105] Lymphocytes are usually scattered rather than clustered. Lymphoid aggregates should be described by their location, cytology, and percentage of marrow involvement. Reactive lymphoid aggregates are common in adults after age 50; they tend to be small and non-paratrabecular and composed of small T lymphocytes with round nuclei.[106] Similar aggregates may occur in chronic lymphocytic leukemia and other lymphoproliferative disorders. Immunophenotyping can be helpful to evaluate aggregates in suspicious cases. Reactive lymphoid aggregates composed of a mixture of T and B lymphocytes with germinal centers are uncommon but often accompany autoimmune diseases such as rheumatoid arthritis. Paratrabecular lymphoid aggregates are more frequently the result of lymphomatous involvement. Most common is a follicular lymphoma aggregate composed of small to intermediate-sized lymphocytes with irregular to cleaved nuclei. Bone marrow involvement may be discordant, because the cytology of the cells differs from extramedullary sites; for a mixed or large-cell follicular lymphoma, the bone marrow may primarily be involved by small cleaved cells.[107–109] Hairy cell leukemia shows a diffuse interstitial pattern, rather than lymphoid aggregates, with mononuclear cells with pale cytoplasm imparting a "fried egg" appearance. Immunoperoxidase stains for B-cell markers (especially DBA.44) are helpful in confirming the diagnosis in subtle cases.[110]

Involvement of bone marrow by classical Hodgkin's lymphoma may be difficult to distinguish morphologically from some large-cell non-Hodgkin's lymphomas, particularly T-cell–rich B-cell lymphoma.[111] Both processes typically fill the intertrabecular space in a patchy pattern, with a heterogeneous infiltrate of small lymphocytes, plasma cells, histiocytes, eosinophils, and variable numbers of cytologically atypical cells with very prominent nucleoli; usually there is marked fibrosis. Immunohistochemical staining is helpful: Reed-Sternberg cells and mononuclear variants are characteristically CD15- and CD30-positive and negative for leukocyte common antigen; they usually lack other B- and T-cell markers except for the occasional cell staining for CD20. In contrast, the malignant cells in T-cell–rich B-cell lymphoma are usually leukocyte common antigen- and CD20-positive and CD15- and CD30-negative.

Plasma Cells

Plasma cells do not deserve comment unless they are increased. The number of plasma cells rises with age, from less than 1% in children to 1–2% in adults.[112] Plasma cells may be much elevated in autoimmune conditions such as rheumatoid arthritis and secondary to infections, including human immunodeficiency virus. Clonality of plasma cells is readily assessed by immunoperoxidase staining for intracellular κ and λ light chains and can be further defined by staining for immunoglobulin heavy chains.

Granulomas

Granulomas are observed in about 10% of bone marrow biopsies. Most common are lipogranulomas, recognizable as clusters of histiocytes with small lipid vacuoles, often with associated small lymphocytes, and of no clinical significance. Epithelioid granulomas are less frequent (Fig. 100–10) and have many possible etiologies. They should be evaluated with special stains for acid-fast bacteria and fungi (Gomori silver stain) to exclude infectious causes. Granulomas, often with Langerhans giant cells, are seen in about a third of cases of miliary *Mycobacterium tuberculosis*.[113] Because acid-fast organisms are rare in these granulomas, a diligent high-power survey of the entire core is required. Granulomas in *Mycobacterium avium-intracellulare* infections most commonly occur in human immunodeficiency virus–infected patients; the granulomas are diffuse and ill defined but contain very numerous acid-fast, PAS-positive organisms.[114] "Donut-shaped" granulomas are characteristic of Q fever.[115,116] Some fungal organisms seen in bone marrow of immunosuppressed patients include *Histoplasmosis capsulatum*, which usually is associated with diffuse lymphohistiocytic aggregates; the budding yeast are small (2–5 µM), round, Gomori silver stain–, and PAS-positive forms that show unequal budding.[117] *Cryptococcus neoformans* is a 5- to 10-µM round organism with a clear halo and narrow-based, unequal budding, within histiocytes that are often diffusely scattered; *Cryptococcus* is PAS-positive and Gomori silver-positive and characteristically has a capsule that stains pink on mucicarmine stains and blue on Alcian blue stain. Protozoal causes of granulomas include *Leishmania donovani* and *Toxoplasma gondii*[118]; immunoperoxidase stains can identify the *T. gondii* trophozoites. Small granulomas may also be seen incidentally in infectious mononucleosis, which is usually diagnosed on clinical and serologic grounds; immunoperoxidase stains for Epstein-Barr virus latent membrane protein and in situ hybridization for Epstein-Barr early region protein-1 are available to confirm the viral origin of the granulomas.

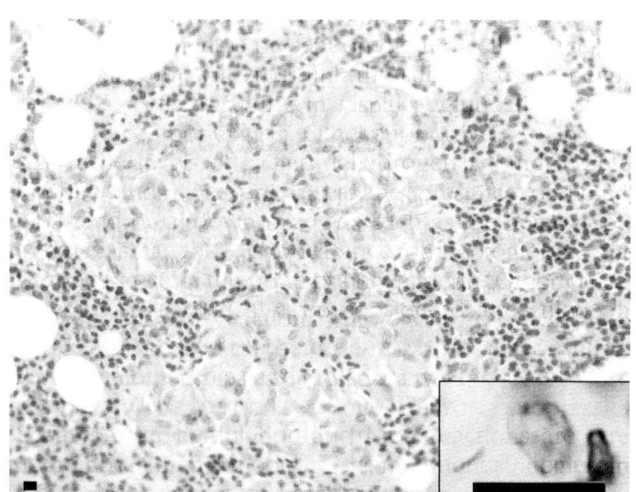

Figure 100–10. Epithelioid granuloma in bone marrow clot section (×100). Lower right *insert* shows acid-fast mycobacterium at ×1000 magnification. (Black bar = 10 µm.)

Among noninfectious etiologies, granulomas occur with both non-Hodgkin's and Hodgkin's lymphomas. In Hodgkin's lymphoma, lymphomatous involvement is usually accompanied by considerable fibrosis, and the mononuclear cells that are diagnostic for bone marrow involvement must be sought with diligence. Paraneoplastic granulomas in bone marrow may be associated with both lymphomas and other malignancies without actual involvement by tumor.[119,120]

The bone marrow contains well-formed epithelioid granulomas in about 50% of all cases of sarcoidosis.[113] Characteristically these granulomas are "naked" and lack both the necrosis and surrounding lymphocytes more common in infectious granulomas. Poorly formed lymphohistiocytic aggregates, often in association with eosinophils, may be seen in drug reactions. However, in a significant number of cases, the etiology of the granulomas is never established.

Storage Histiocytes

Storage histiocytes have a variety of appearances and many etiologies. The most common inherited disorder showing storage histiocytes is Gaucher's disease: deficiency of glucocerebrosidase leads to the accumulation of glucocerebroside in macrophages, imparting a linear striated pattern resembling crumpled tissue paper. Gaucher cells stain positively in PAS, nonspecific esterase, and Sudan black B tests, and are weakly positive for iron.[121] Pseudo-Gaucher cells are also filled with glucocerebroside but occur in a variety of disorders, including chronic myelogenous leukemia, thalassemia, congenital dyserythropoietic anemia, and, rarely, myelodysplastic syndrome. Gaucher and pseudo-Gaucher cells

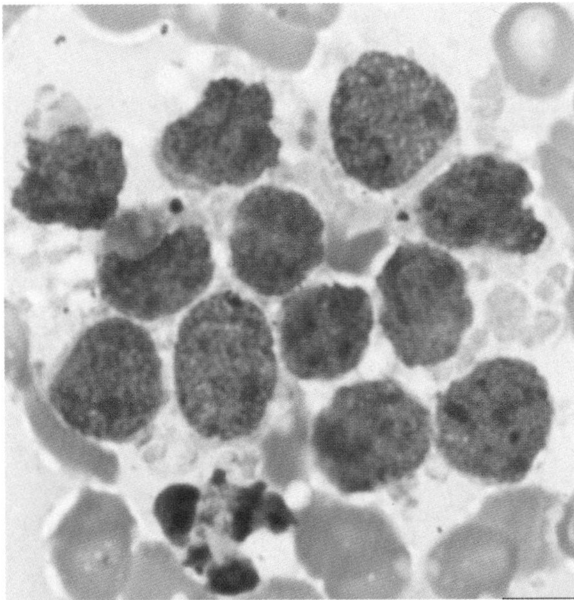

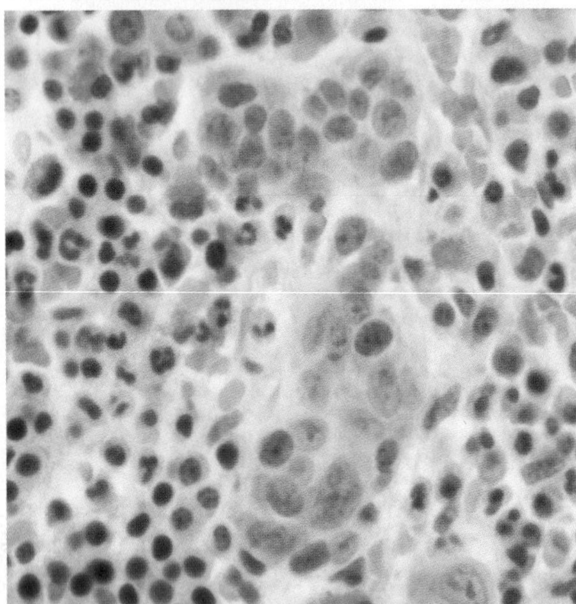

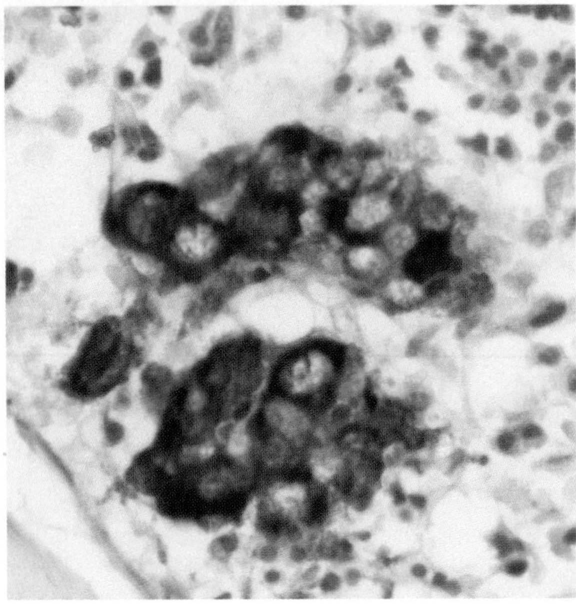

are distinguished by measuring glucocerebrosidase levels in peripheral blood leukocytes. Niemann-Pick disease types A and B (sphingomyelinase deficiency) or types C and D (mutations in *NPC1* leading to defects in cholesterol esterification) show frequent macrophages with microvesicular lipid droplets.[122] Other storage disorders, including Tangier disease, Batten's disease, and Fabry's disease, show collections of storage macrophages in bone marrow. Lipid-laden macrophages also arise from nonstorage causes, such as hypercholesterolemia and traumatic fat necrosis.[123]

Mast Cells

Mast cells in tissue sections often have a plump fusiform or spindled morphology. In systemic mastocytosis, increased numbers of mast cells are paratrabecular in location and seen in association with lymphocytes, eosinophils, and reticulin fibrosis.[124,125] The small purplish granules so characteristic of mast cells on marrow aspirate smears are often difficult to appreciate on biopsies. Mast cells are readily stained by toluidine blue and can be definitively identified by immunoperoxidase stains for tryptase.[125]

Tumor Cells

Bone marrow is host to a variety of metastatic nonhematopoietic tumors. In children, neuroblastoma, Ewing's sarcoma, rhabdomyosarcoma, and other primitive neuroectodermal tumors commonly spread to bone. In adults, the most frequent cancers invading the marrow are prostate, breast, and lung. The bone marrow examination is critical because tumor cells often elicit a desmoplastic reaction, making aspiration impossible. Fibrosis of the bone marrow is extremely common, especially with the carcinomas, and often is patchy, filling one intertrabecular space while sparing another. Tumor cells may be rare, so the finding of fibrosis should prompt an assiduous search for them. Extensive osteoclastic activity is frequently provoked by tumor invasion and there may be osteoblastic activity as well, particularly with prostate cancer. Small-cell carcinoma may mimic acute leukemia (Fig. 100–11). Immunoperoxidase studies are very helpful in the evaluation of metastatic tumors (see Table 100–1). Specific identification of metastatic tumors is often not possible nor necessarily of clinical utility, but estrogen and progesterone receptor status may be helpful for prognosis and therapeutic decisions in breast cancer.

Figure 100–11. *Top,* Bone marrow aspirate showing involvement by small-cell carcinoma closely resembling acute lymphoblastic leukemia (×100). The tumor cells are slightly cohesive, an important clue to the nonhematopoietic origin of the tumor. *Middle,* Metastatic carcinoid tumor. The tumor cells form cohesive nests associated with a desmoplastic (fibrotic) reaction (×40). *Bottom,* A chromogranin immunoperoxidase stain shows that the tumor cells stain strongly (brown reaction product) and therefore are of neuroendocrine origin (×40).

Eosinophilic Inclusions

Eosinophilic inclusions in proerythroblasts are characteristic of parvovirus B19 infection. Eosinophilic intranuclear inclusions, usually in endothelial cells, also are seen in cytomegalovirus infection, which sometimes results in marked bone marrow hypocellularity. Immunoperoxidase stains are available for cytomegalovirus and common herpes simplex viruses 1 and 2.

Deposits and Debris

Amyloid deposits may be seen in multiple myeloma, lymphoplasmacytic lymphoma, or even in a morphologically otherwise unremarkable marrow. Amyloid appears as acellular eosinophilic deposits that are PAS-positive, localized both interstitially and in the walls of blood vessels. Amyloid is definitively stained with Congo red, which appears dark pink on light microscopy and birefringent in polarized light. A variety of other metabolic disorders may result in crystalline deposits, including cystinosis and oxalosis.[126,127] Eosinophilic necrotic debris, particularly in an apparently hypercellular marrow, often represents necrotic tumor. Although a specific diagnosis may not be possible, immunoperoxidase stains for keratin, B-cell, and T-cell markers also may bind to necrotic tissue, providing a clue to the underlying pathology.

Assessment of Bone

The superficial few millimeters of the bone marrow biopsy are composed of dense cancellous bone, and the remainder of trabecular bone. The bone trabeculae should be examined for osteoclastic and osteoblastic activity. The cement lines in bone normally have a lamellar pattern well seen on reticulin staining. A jigsaw or mosaic pattern with extensive remodeling and giant osteoclasts is highly suggestive of Paget's disease. Primary disorders of bone generally require correlation with radiographic findings. Thin bone trabeculae are common in osteoporosis, renal failure, and multiple myeloma. Less commonly, the trabeculae are thickened, a process terms osteosclerosis, as seen in osteopetrosis, some metastatic carcinomas, myeloma, and chronic idiopathic myelofibrosis.

Suggested Readings*

Bain BJ: Blood Cells: A Practical Guide (ed 2). London: Blackwell Science, 1995.

Bain BJ, Clark DM, Lampert IA, Wilkens BS: Bone Marrow Pathology (ed 3). London: Blackwell Science, 2001.

Foucar K: Bone Marrow Pathology (ed 2). Chicago: ASCP Press, 2001.

Hayhoe FGJ, Flemans RJ: Color Atlas of Hematological Cytology (ed 3). St. Louis: Mosby, 1992.

Jaffe ES, Harris NL, Stein H, Vardiman JW (eds): WHO Classification of Tumours: Pathology and Genetics of Tumours of Haematopoietic and Lymphoid Tissues. Lyon: IARC Press, 2001.

Full references for this chapter can be found on accompanying CD-ROM.

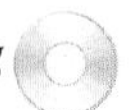

CHAPTER 101

Flow Cytometry

João B. Oliveira, MD, Maryalice Stetler-Stevenson, MD, PhD, Margaret Brown, BS, ASCP, and Thomas A. Fleisher, MD

KEY POINTS

Flow Cytometry

- Flow cytometry has become an integral part of the laboratory assessment of many hematologic disorders.
- The technology provides a powerful tool to assess a host of cell surface and intracellular characteristics.

Flow Cytometry Parameters

- Nonfluorescent signals
  - Forward scatter: correlates with cell size
  - Side scatter: correlates with cell granularity
- Fluorescent signals
  - Light emitted from a fluorochrome passing through the excitation beam
  - Typically based on binding of fluorochrome-conjugated monoclonal antibody

Data Presentation

- Reflects light intensity versus cell frequency
- The histogram yields a single parameter (color) versus cell frequency
- Dot or contour plot yields two parameters (colors) versus cell frequency

Gating

- Method to focus study on a cell population or subpopulation
- Achieved with nonfluorescent parameters (three-part differential) and/or specific reagents

Immunophenotyping

- Identifies cell subsets, establishes lineage, stage differentiation, assess activation, and determines clonality.
- Lymphocyte results should be checked to confirm that T cells + B cells + NK cells = 100%.

This work was supported by the Intramural Research program of the NIH.

INTRODUCTION

Flow cytometry is an important analytical tool in the evaluation of hematopoietic cells. The clinical use of this technology has been expanded, in part due to the large number of monoclonal antibody reagents developed over the past two decades. These reagents serve as biomarkers that identify different cell types and often are linked to functional characteristics. The development of monoclonal reagents has been paralleled by improvements in fluorochrome chemistry, which has made "multicolor" analysis by bench-top clinical cytometers feasible. The combination of an array of reagents and the simplified operation of modern flow cytometry has facilitated this approach for the evaluation of peripheral blood and bone marrow. As a result, flow cytometric studies have extended our understanding of normal hematopoietic cell development, differentiation, activation, and apoptosis. They have also provided important information in hematologic malignancies, insight into reconstitution following stem cell transplantation, and of the specific cell defects associated with immune deficiencies and the defining characteristic features of a number of hematologic disorders.

The basic elements of a flow cytometer are shown in Figure 101–1. As illustrated, the excitation source consists of one or more focused monochromatic light beams generated by one or more lasers. The collection side of the optical bench includes filters and dichroic mirrors set in prescribed locations to capture specific wavelengths. These "tuned" light signals are directed to photodetectors (photodiodes and photomultiplier tubes) that quantify the light output at the specific wavelengths defined by the filters or dichroic mirrors.[1,2]

The key to consistent and reproducible data is that each cell intersects the excitation beam in the same location. Hydrodynamic focusing accomplishes this process by injecting the cell suspension into a flowing stream of sheath fluid, generating a single-file stream of cells within the sheath fluid stream.[1,2] The cells flow in a very constant location, and thus each cell consistently intersects the excitation beam. Upon encountering the excitation beam, all cells generate nonfluorescent, light scatter signals that are collected in the plane of (forward light scatter) and at a right angle to (side scatter) the excita-

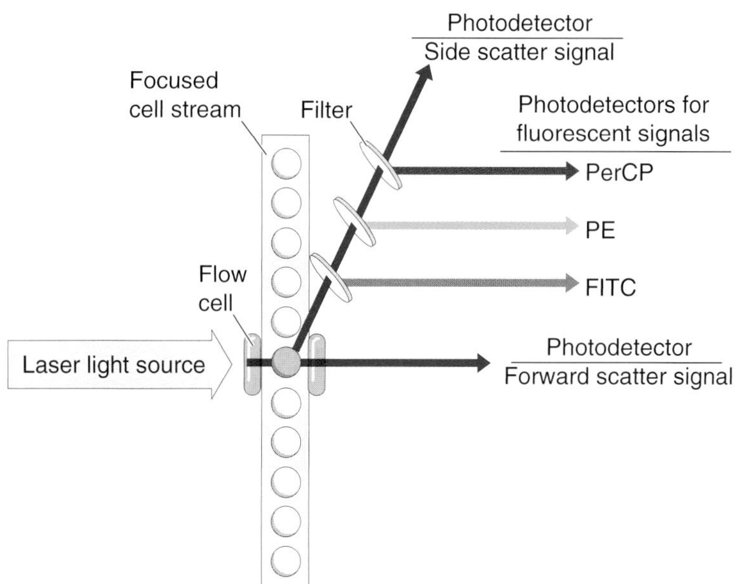

Figure 101–1. Schematic view of a flow cytometer, demonstrating the intersection of the focused cell flow by the laser beam with generation of scattered (forward and side [right angle]) and emitted (fluorescence) light. The various light signals are directed to the appropriate photodetectors (photodiodes and photomultiplier tubes) using filters (and dichroic mirrors) to "tune" the wavelength, and these optical signals are converted into electronic signals and directed to a computer for data analysis.

tion beam. The former is an index of cell size/refractile index and the latter an index of cellular regularity/granularity. The combination of these two nonfluorescent signals yields a three-part leukocyte differential (Fig. 101–2) and also discriminates among leukocytes, red blood cells, and platelets.[3] Evaluating unique cell characteristics depends on fluorescent signals that are generated by the binding of specific monoclonal antibody reagents directly conjugated with a fluorochrome. Alternatively, the primary reagent may be unconjugated and detected using an indirect method that employs a secondary fluorochrome-conjugated detection antibody. Fluorochromes are compounds that absorb light (energy) of a defined wavelength and emit light of longer wavelength (lower energy). A host of different fluorochromes are used in clinical flow cytometry, including fluorescein isothiocyanate, phycoerythrin, peridinin chlorophyll protein, and allophycocyanin (Table 101–1). More recently, combinations of two linked fluorochromes have been designed to transfer the emitted light (energy) from the first fluorochrome to excite the second fluorochrome (see Table 101–1). The availability of multiple fluorochromes that absorb light of the same wavelength but emit light at different wavelengths allows multiple reagents to be combined in a multicolor study. A second light source is present in most clinical instruments, further extending the range of multicolor protocols. Cell populations can be divided into multiple subpopulations (five different conjugated reagents in one tube generate up to 2^5 or 32 different cell subpopulations). The disadvantage of expanded numbers of subpopulations identified in one tube relates to data management and interpretation. In addition, color compensation can be very complex.

Flow cytometry first moved from a research tool to a clinically useful method when applied as a supplement to the morphologic classification of leukemias and lymphomas.[4–7] The human immunodeficiency virus (HIV) pandemic introduced the need for an absolute CD4 T-cell count as a prognosticator in acquired immunodeficiency syndrome.[8] More recently, flow cytometry has proven to be an important tool in quantifying and characterizing hematopoietic stem cells, defining immune deficiencies, characterizing certain red blood cell–related disorders, evaluating platelets, and assessing the cell cycle and apoptosis.[9–15] Flow cytometry also can evaluate the inside of the cell as well as evaluate proteins on the cell surface. Fixation and permeabilization are required to permit intracellular entry of reagents. The presence of specific proteins within the cell can be used to assess their functional characteristics.[16–19]

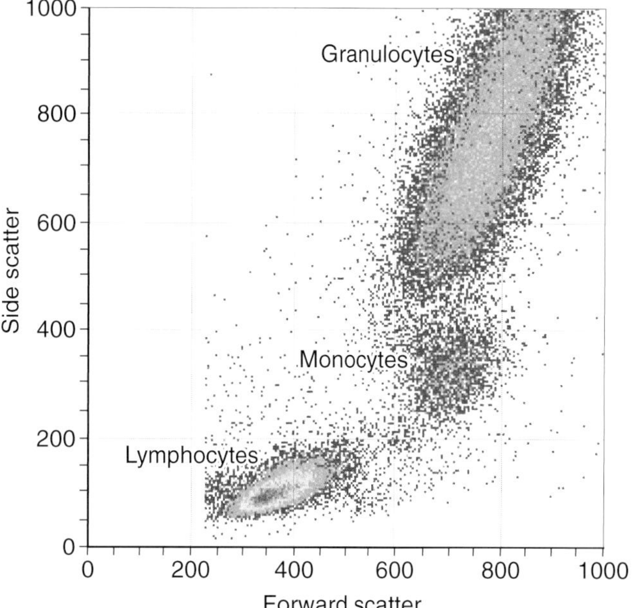

Figure 101–2. Dot plot of forward scatter (*x* axis) versus side scatter (*y* axis) on lysed whole blood sample demonstrating a three-part leukocyte differential.

TABLE 101–1. Fluorochromes Commonly Used in Clinical Flow Cytometry

Fluorochrome	Excitation (nm)	Flow Cytometer	Emission (nm)
Fluorescein isothiocyanate (FITC)	490	488	525
Phycoerythrin (PE)*	480/565	488	578
Peridinin chlorophyll protein (PerCP)	488	488	677
Allophycocyanin (APC)	650	633	660
CY5	649	633	674
PE-CY5*	480/565	488	674
PE-CY7*	480/565	488	784
PE-Texas Red*	480/565	488	620

*Dual (tandem) fluorochrome–first of pair excites the second fluorochrome.

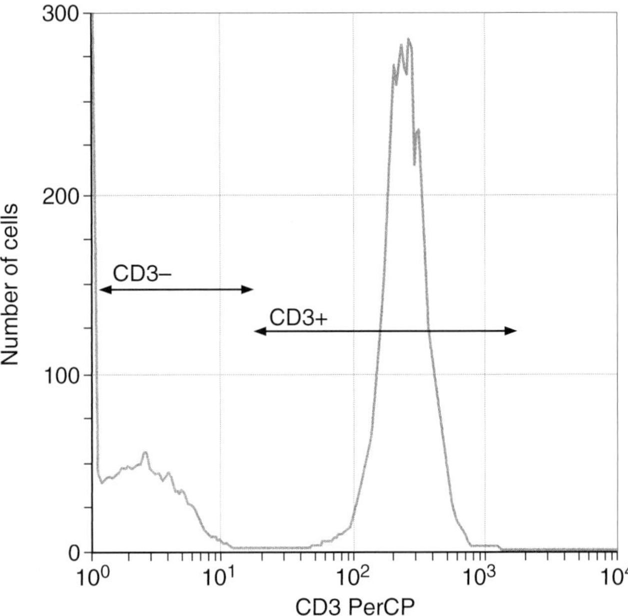

Figure 101–3. Single-parameter histogram, a distribution plot of CD3 expression by lymphocytes based on fluorescence intensity (*x* axis) versus number of events/cells (*y* axis).

DATA COLLECTION, PRESENTATION, AND INTERPRETATION

Clinical flow cytometers typically generate data in graphic form based on cell frequency versus one or more measurements of light intensity (signal strength). The relationship can be plotted as a single-parameter histogram (Fig. 101–3) that presents the quantitative distribution of cells (*y* axis) versus signal strength of a single parameter (*x* axis; e.g., side scatter, forward scatter, fluorochrome fluorescence). Alternatively, the signal intensity of two parameters can be plotted versus cell frequency using dot (Fig. 101–4*A*), density (Fig. 101–4*B*), or contour (Fig. 101–4*C*) plots. These two-parameter displays include the third dimension of cell frequency, and thus evaluation of more than two parameters requires sequential graphic representation to demonstrate all subpopulations in a data set. Clinical evaluation requires collection of 10,000–20,000 events (cells) in order to yield meaningful data for standard cell populations and subpopulations. However, in rare-event evaluations, such as peripheral hematopoietic $CD34^+$ stem cell enumeration or minimal residual disease detection, larger total numbers of cells must be collected; often 100,000 or more cells are required to generate a statistically reliable measurement.[10]

The distinction between positive and negative for a given parameter is not always easily determined. Typically, the signal from cells that have been incubated with an irrelevant fluorochrome-conjugated antibody (control stained cells) or background autofluorescence signals from unstained cells (control unstained cells) can be considered background; a marker (cursor) set to include 98–99% of all cells being evaluated, serving as the starting point for negative-positive discrimination (Fig. 101–5). However, there are circumstances when this approach may require modification or alternative interpretation, as when evaluating the expression of markers that do not result in baseline separation between negative and positive cells. These issues require an experienced operator and laboratory to ensure that the data reported are valid.

Ultimately, the results generated reflect the quality of the reagents, cell preparation, instrument settings, and approach to data evaluation used in the study. That data can always be produced does not ensure their validity. As with any clinical laboratory test, optimal instrument performance requires rigorous quality control and complete records. The preparation of cells and the reagents must be monitored and are best assessed using a control sample whenever possible. In the clinical laboratory setting, compliance with the Clinical Laboratory Improvement Amendment of 1988 is mandated and requires regular participation in proficiency surveys.

The most common approach used by clinical laboratories involves whole blood analysis, which enables evaluation of any major blood cell type. Cell discrimination is most easily determined based on forward and side light scatter, parameters that define platelets (smallest blood cell), erythrocytes, and leukocytes (three distinct patterns of scattered light with lymphocytes overlapping significantly with erythrocytes). Owing to the frequency difference between erythrocytes and leukocytes, there is no real concern of lymphocyte contamination when evaluating red blood cells (10,000 erythrocytes would include <20 leukocytes under normal circumstances). However, the reverse is not true because the presence of significant numbers of erythrocytes makes evaluation of lymphocytes virtually impossible owing to their overlapping scatter properties. Consequently, the study of leukocytes in a whole blood sample (or bone marrow) usually requires a lysis step to eliminate erythrocytes; some more automated approaches to CD4 quantitation and basic immunophenotyping utilize a no-lyse method based on CD45 staining plus light scatter characteristics. Evaluation of a lysed whole blood sample yields a three-part differential with normal lymphocytes the smallest (forward angle scatter) and most regular/agranular (side scatter)

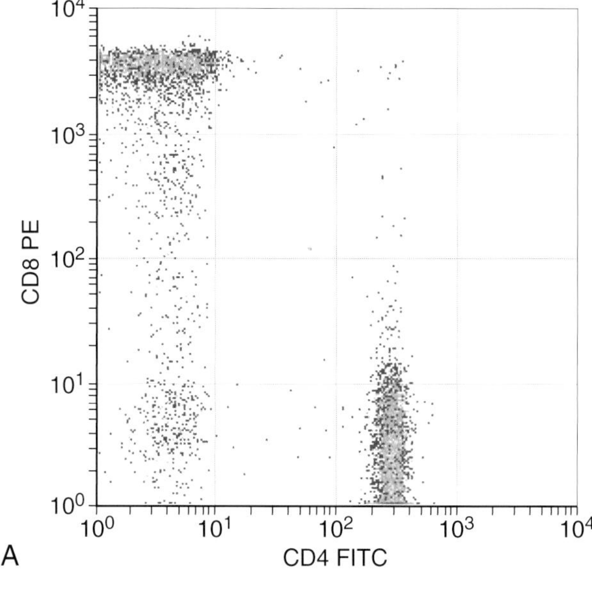

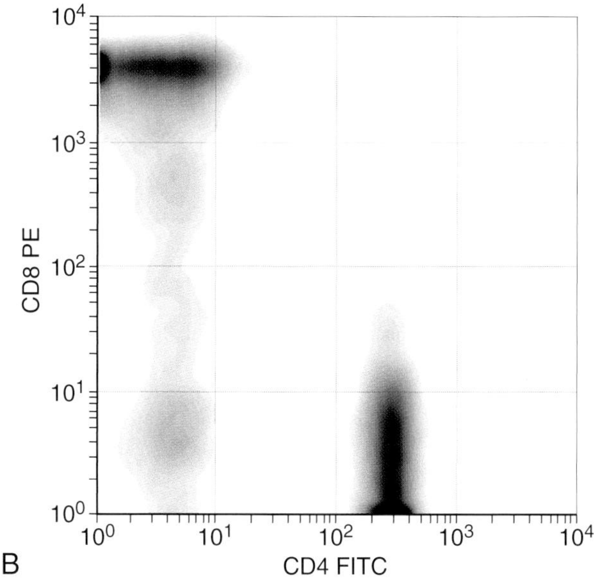

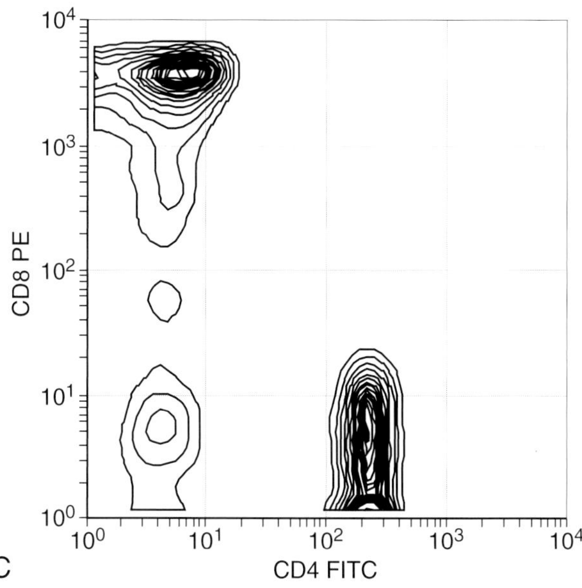

cells, while granulocytes are slightly larger but also show substantial granularity, and monocytes fall between these two cell types (see Fig. 101–2). The two less prevalent granulocyte populations are found within the three scatter areas: eosinophils within the granulocyte population while basophils overlap with lymphocytes. Hematopoietic stem cells are typically found in the "lymphocyte" part of the scatter plot. All of these relationships are derived from normal blood cells, but in hematopoietic malignancy the tumor cells may not follow normal cell characteristics.[5–7,20] Standard practice in most clinical laboratories is to confirm the accuracy of the three-part differential using the pan-leukocyte monoclonal antibody CD45,[3,21] a reagent that stains lymphoid cells more brightly than myeloid or monocytic cells. Used in combination with the myelomonocytic specific antibody CD14, this method provides an excellent check of cell gating[3,21] (Fig. 101–6), although in malignant conditions the level of CD45 expression can vary significantly.[5–7] Under certain circumstances, it may be necessary to include CD45 in each tube to assure consistent evaluation of cells.[21]

Gating focuses a flow cytometry study to a specific cell type. Usually nonfluorescent parameters, forward and side scatter, are used to define the gate. As previously noted, these parameters separate the three major blood cell types and also generate a three-part leukocyte differential in red cell–lysed blood samples. Most clinical studies of lymphocytes, monocytes, eosinophils, platelets, erythrocytes, and hematopoietic stem cells use this method. There is no single guideline for the evaluation of all data. When a monoclonal reagent exclusively identifies one cell population, data interpretation is unambiguous, as is the case for the pan–T-cell marker CD3 shown in Figure 101–3. In this example, the evaluation is confined to lymphocytes based on forward and side scatter, and two distinct populations can be identified, the CD3-positive T cells and the CD3-negative lymphocytes that include B and NK cells. In other situations, biologic variability in the level and/or range of cell surface protein expression affect the interpretation of data. Examples of this are shown in Figures 101–7 and 101–8, where in both examples there are at least three cell populations: cells negative for the antibody, cells showing intermediate fluorescence, and cells that are strongly positive. In Figure 101–7, the intermediate-staining cells are predominantly NK cells that express a lower level of CD8 expression while the bright-staining cells are primarily T cells. In Figure 101–8*A*, the intermediate-staining cells are monocytes and the bright-staining cells are $CD4^+$ T cells, with the former being present only in very small numbers if proper gating techniques are used that exclude the majority of monocytes (Fig. 101–8*B*).

Figure 101–4. *A*, Dot plot of two-color (CD4 and CD8) staining evaluating lymphocytes. The number of dots reflects the frequency of events. ***B***, Density plot using the same parameters. The color intensity reflects the frequency of events. ***C***, Contour plot using the same parameters, in which each contour line represents approximately 5% of the events.

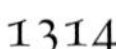

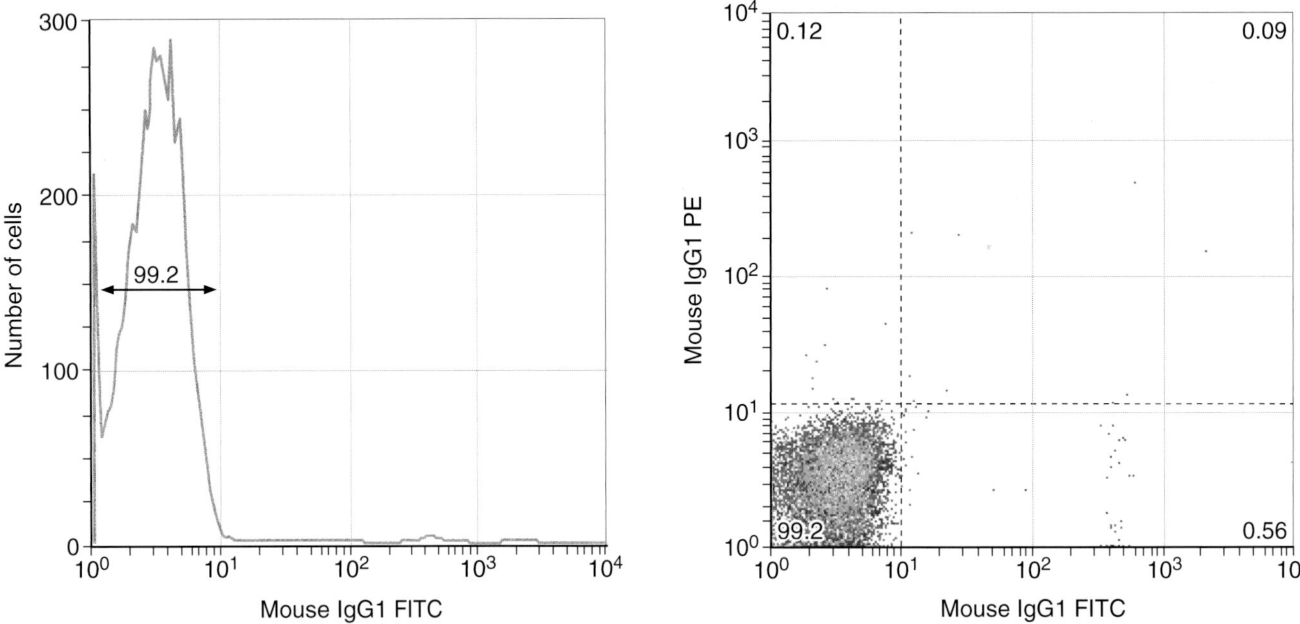

Figure 101–5. Strategy to establish a negative parameter in a flow cytometry study using control cells stained with an irrelevant conjugated monoclonal antibody. *Left,* Histogram with the cursor set to include 99% of the cell population as unstained. *Right,* Dot plot in which over 99% of the cells are set in the left lower quadrant, which is considered negative for both fluorochromes.

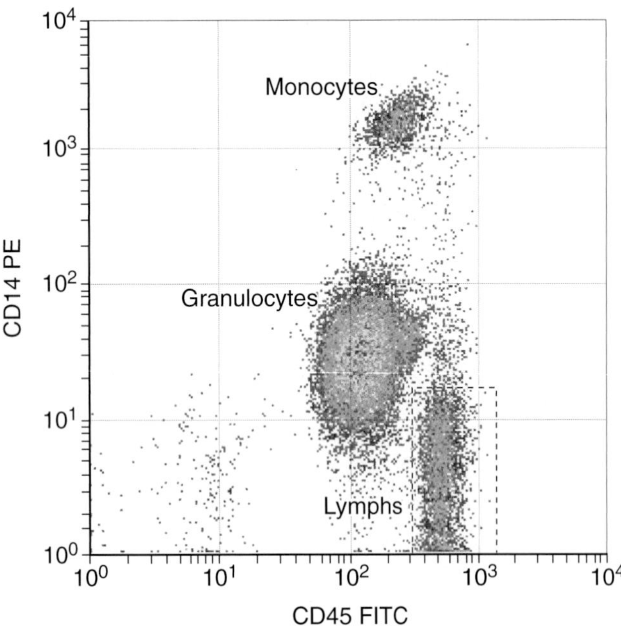

Figure 101–6. Dot plot demonstrating the use of the "gating" monoclonal reagents CD14 and CD45 to confirm the three-part differential.

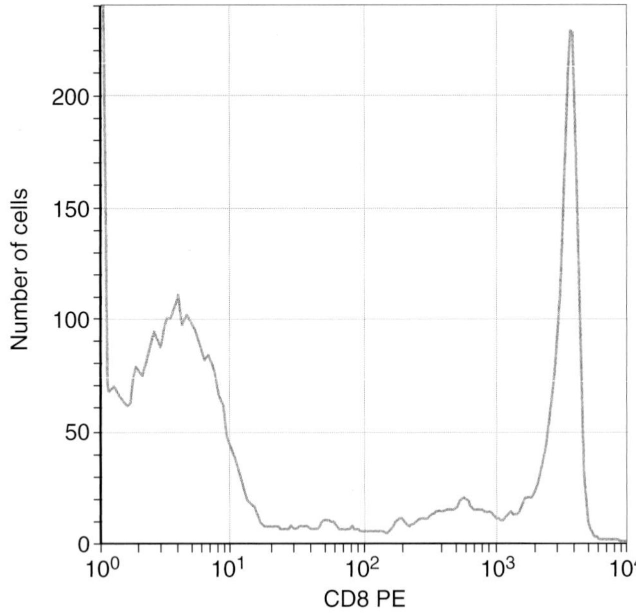

Figure 101–7. CD8 histogram evaluating gated lymphocytes.

The finding of low-density CD4 expression on monocytes helps explain the capacity of HIV to gain entry into this cell type.

A large number of monoclonal antibodies distinguish cells of a specific lineage (Table 101–2). These reagents are assigned a CD (cluster of differentiation) number after consensus is reached regarding the specificity of the antibody by international workshops. Monoclonal antibody binding can be used to identify cells based on either specific or differential binding. For example, cells of the erythroid lineage show exclusive expression of glycophorin. Within the granulocyte population, neutrophils and eosinophils are discriminated based on expression of the

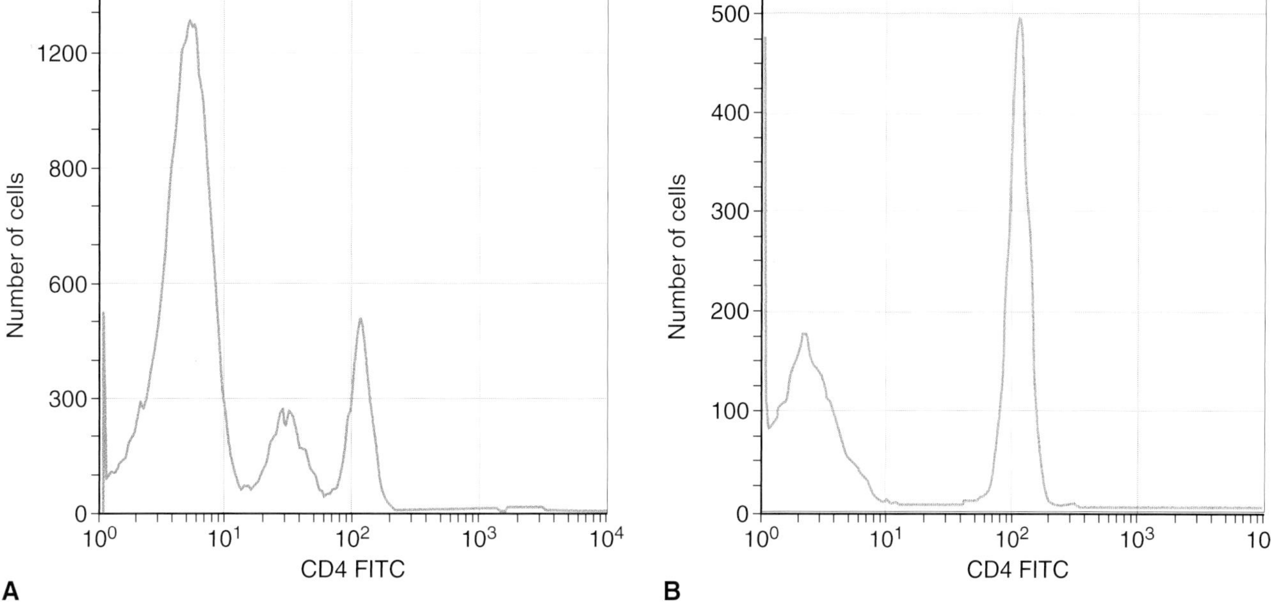

Figure 101–8. *A*, CD4 histogram evaluating mononuclear cells (lymphocytes and monocytes). ***B***, CD4 histogram evaluating only lymphocytes.

complement receptor CD16.[22] Lineage-specific antibodies can distinguish populations and subpopulations of lymphocytes as well as stages in specific cell differentiation. Hematopoietic stem cells can be identified by the expression of the cell surface protein CD34, and further subdivided by additional markers that are acquired sequentially during stem cell differentiation.[10] Results from flow cytometry have facilitated evaluation of the stem cell compartment in peripheral blood, cord blood, and bone marrow.

Many of the monoclonal antibodies used to evaluate hematopoietic elements identify antigens not exclusively expressed on one specific cell type. Understanding these expression patterns is the basis for effective data interpretation. Often combining antibodies can clarify the relative expression of a specific surface protein on different cell types. The expression of many surface proteins changes during the life cycle of a cell. For example, some proteins are expressed preferentially early and/or late during cell development and differentiation. Others may only be expressed following cell activation or with the acquisition of a particular functional state. When the expression of a specific protein changes depending on cell conditions, a range of expression from negative to clearly positive is expected, as shown in Figure 101–9 for the α chain of the interleukin-2 receptor (CD25) on T cells. Varied molecular species (isoforms) of a protein may be expressed under different conditions based on alternative RNA splicing, which can result in a mixture ranging from cells that express one or the other isoform to cells that express both while in the process of undergoing isoform switch (Fig. 101–10). Such biologic variability requires reporting results with an interpretation more sophisticated than simple negative versus positive. A surface protein also may be expressed at a low level on an entire cell population (Fig. 101–11). Our laboratory commonly notes the geometric mean channel (GMC) fluorescence of the unstained and stained cells and then reports the increased fluorescence over control cells (based on the quotient of the GMC of stained cells divided by the GMC of unstained cells). For many markers used in evaluating malignant cells, the expression level may be strikingly heterogeneous.

Flow cytometry has recently emerged as a powerful tool to study intracellular characteristics,[16–19] and intracellular flow cytometry can be used to assess the functional properties of cells. Intracellular flow cytometry is a real-time method, and intracellular staining can be linked to cell surface staining, thereby providing cell subset discrimination while assessing specific cellular properties.

FLOW CYTOMETRY IN HEMATOLOGY

Characterization of lymphocytes by flow cytometry (immunophenotyping) in nonmalignant states is one of the most common applications of this technology in the clinical laboratory.[11] As previously noted, flow cytometry is a critical tool in monitoring disease progression and therapy in HIV infection.[8] In addition, distinctive lymphocyte findings characterize most primary immune deficiency disorders. Specific lymphocyte populations and subpopulations also are investigated in disorders characterized by inflammation, with attention to expression of activation markers. The reconstitution of the immune system can be monitored by flow cytometry following intensive chemotherapy and after stem cell transplantation,[9] in immunotherapy and vaccine therapy in experimental protocols for malignancies. Functional testing of intracellular cytokines following cell activation by either nonspecific or antigen-specific stimulation has found

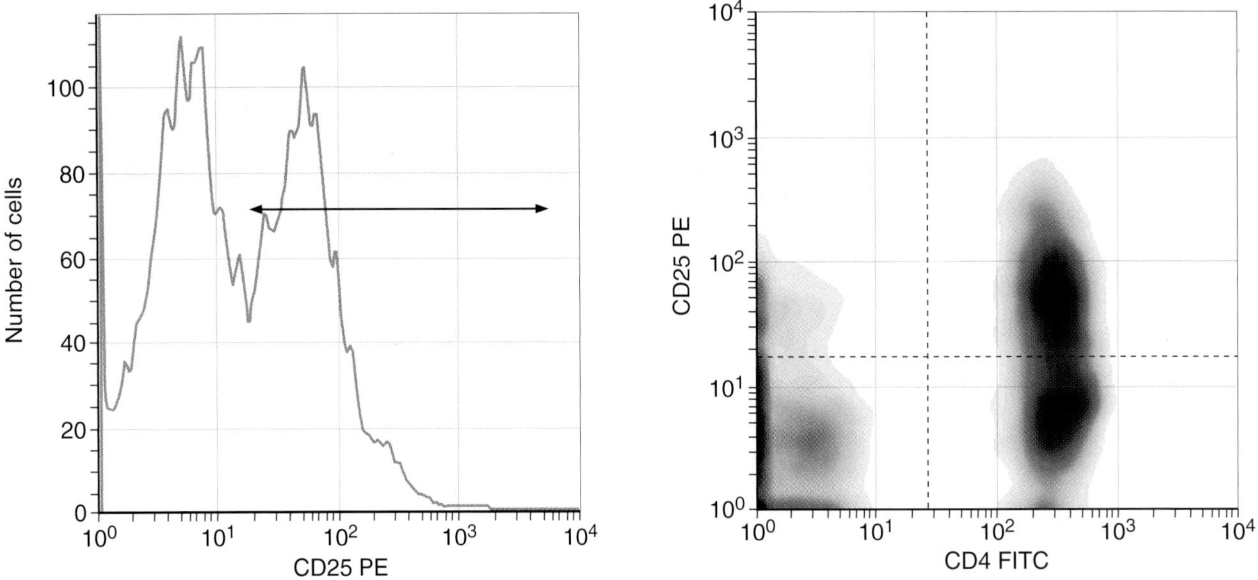

■ **Figure 101–9.** *Left,* Single-parameter histogram of CD25 expression on lymphocytes. *Right,* Density "two-color" plot of CD25 (*y* axis) and CD3 (*x* axis) expression.

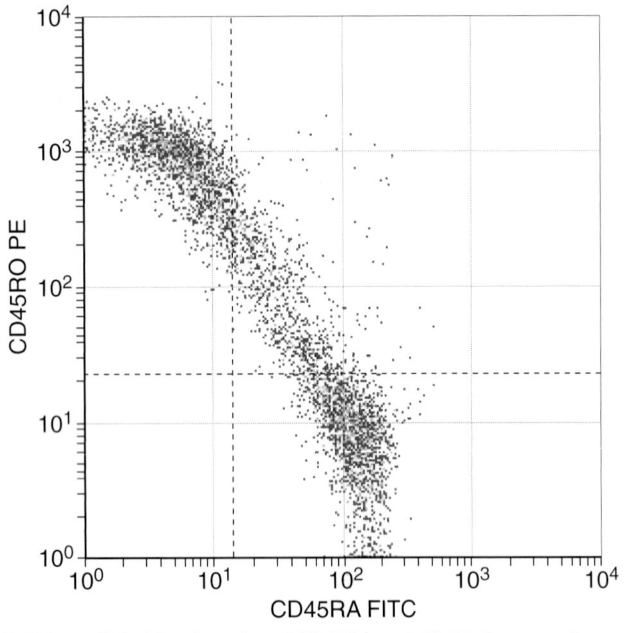

■ **Figure 101–10.** Dot plot of CD45RA and CD45RO expression on $CD4^+$ T cells.

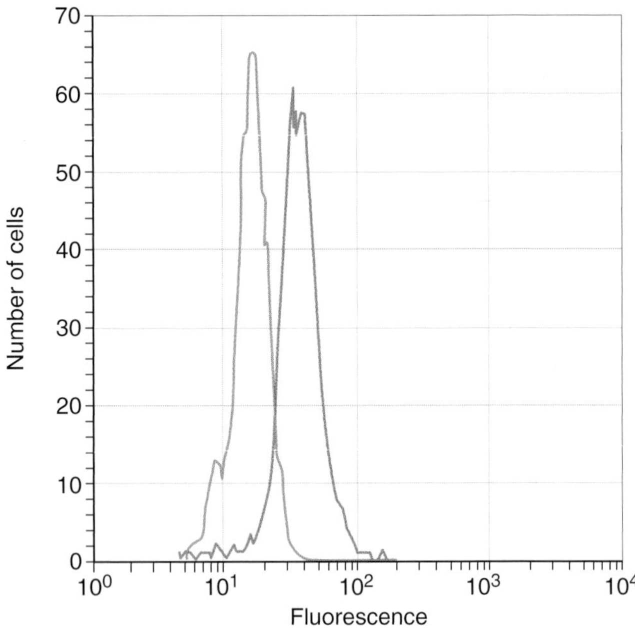

■ **Figure 101–11.** Overlapping negative control and positive histograms.

TABLE 101–2. Leukocyte Antigens Commonly Used in Clinical Flow Cytometry Based on CD (Cluster of Differentiation) Designation

CD Designation	Antigens
CD1a	Cortical thymocytes, dendritic cells, Langerhans cells
CD2	T cells, thymocytes, NK-cell subset
CD3	T cells, thymocytes
CD4	T-cell subset, thymocyte subset, monocytes/macrophages
CD5	T cells, B-cell subset
CD7	Thymocytes, T cells, NK cells, early myeloid cells
CD8	T-cell subset, thymocyte subset, NK-cell subset
CD9	Eosinophils, basophils, platelets, pre-B cells, activated T cells
CD10	Early B cells, neutrophils, bone marrow stromal cells
CD11b	Monocytes, granulocytes, NK cells
CD11c	Myeloid cells, monocytes
CD13	Myelomonocytic cells
CD14	Monocytes, myelomonocytic cells
CD15	Granulocytes, monocytes, endothelial cells
CD16	NK cells, granulocytes, macrophages
CD19	B cells (from pre-B-cell stage)
CD20	B cells
CD21	Mature B cells, follicular dendritic cells
CD22	Mature B cells
CD23	Activated B cells
CD25	Activated T cells, activated B cells
CD33	Myeloid cells, myeloid progenitor cells, monocytes
CD34	Hematopoietic precursor cells, capillary endothelium
CD36	Platelets, monocytes/macrophages
CD41	Megakaryocytes, platelets
CD42b	Megakaryocytes, platelets
CD45	Leukocytes
CD45RA	T-cell (naive) subsets, B cells, monocytes
CD45RO	T-cell (memory) subsets, B-cell subsets, monocytes/macrophages
CD55	Hematopoietic cells, some nonhematopoietic cells
CD56	NK cells, NK/T cells
CD57	NK cells, T-cell subsets, B cells, monocytes
CD59	Hematopoietic cells, nonhematopoietic cells
CD61	Platelets, megakaryocytes, macrophages
CD79a	B cells
CD103	Intestinal epithelial lymphocytes
CD117	Myeloid blast cells, mast cells
Glycophorin	Erythrocytes, erythrocyte precursors

Abbreviations: NK, natural killer; pre-B, precursor B.

application in atopic and autoimmune disease[18,19] (Fig. 101–12). Methods to evaluate lymphocyte activity and proliferation have evolved based on measurement of activation markers and changes in DNA content.[15,16,23] More recent approaches accurately quantitate antigen-specific T cells based on antigenic peptide–major histocompatibility complex multimers.[24]

Assessment of leukocytes other than lymphocytes is now performed in the clinical laboratory. Evaluation of monocytes by flow cytometry now has greater clinical significance with the definition of immune deficiencies associated with defective monocyte surface receptor expression, such as interferon (IFN)-γ receptor deficiency (Fig. 101–13*A*). Functional assessment of an intracellular signaling pathway of the IFN-γ receptor involves stimulation of monocytes with IFN-γ and intracellular staining with antibodies to detect the phosphorylated form of STAT-1[17] (Fig. 101–13*B* and *C*). Kits dependent on protein phosphorylation using similar methods are now commercially available.

Granulocytes can be evaluated for the expression of critical adhesion molecules and functionally for the capacity to generate reactive oxygen species.[16,25] Assessment of the oxidative burst in granulocytes is a diagnostic screening test for chronic granulomatous disease and provides information about the underlying genetic defect (Fig. 101–14), but its availability is restricted to specialized laboratories. Granulocyte-specific autoantibodies can be detected by flow cytometry. Flow cytometric methods can consistently identify and characterize eosinophils[22] and basophils have been studied for intracellular cytokine production in atopic disease.[18]

Hematopoietic stem cell enumeration and isolation are dependent on flow cytometry. The use of CD34 as a marker is central, and specific methods are recommended to quantitate CD34$^+$ hematopoietic stem cells.[9,10] Additional markers have been studied to identify the pluripotent stem cell. Stem cells are purified from either bone marrow or peripheral blood utilizing CD34 selection methods, followed by flow cytometry to assess the effectiveness of the separation.

The evaluation of erythrocytes by flow cytometry has been applied to a number of disorders, including the assessment of autoantibody in hemolytic anemia and the detection of fetal hemoglobin–containing red cells (F cells) in fetomaternal hemorrhage and sickle cell anemia.[12] Flow cytometry allows accurate detection of fetal red blood cells based on staining with antibodies directed to hemoglobin (Hb) F, i antigen, and D antigen; this approach is essential for the management of patients with fetomaternal hemorrhage because the classical Kleihauer-Betke test for the detection of F-cells lacks sensitivity and demonstrates poor reproducibility.[12] In sickle cell anemia and thalassemia, increased levels of Hb F are associated with better outcome, and Hb F levels may be used to monitor response to therapy (Fig. 101–15*A*). F-cell analysis is useful in the measurement of F reticulocytes; the youngest circulating reticulocytes. This population can be recognized by double staining with a nucleic acid dye, such as thiazole orange, and antibody to Hb F (Fig. 101–15*B*). Quantitation of F-cells correlates with the rate of red blood cell production in anemia.[12] Precise blood type phenotyping after multiple transfusions can be practically accomplished by flow cytometry, when standard methods such as rosetting or agglutination give mixed, imprecise results.

The detection of glycosylphosphatidylinositol (GPI)-anchored proteins, such as CD55 and CD59, on erythrocytes and leukocytes by flow cytometry is now the method of choice to diagnose paroxysmal nocturnal hemoglobinuria (see Chapter 25). Diagnosis by flow cytometry has a high degree of sensitivity, allowing detection of as few as 0.1% abnormal cells, facilitating classification of paroxysmal nocturnal hemoglobinuria

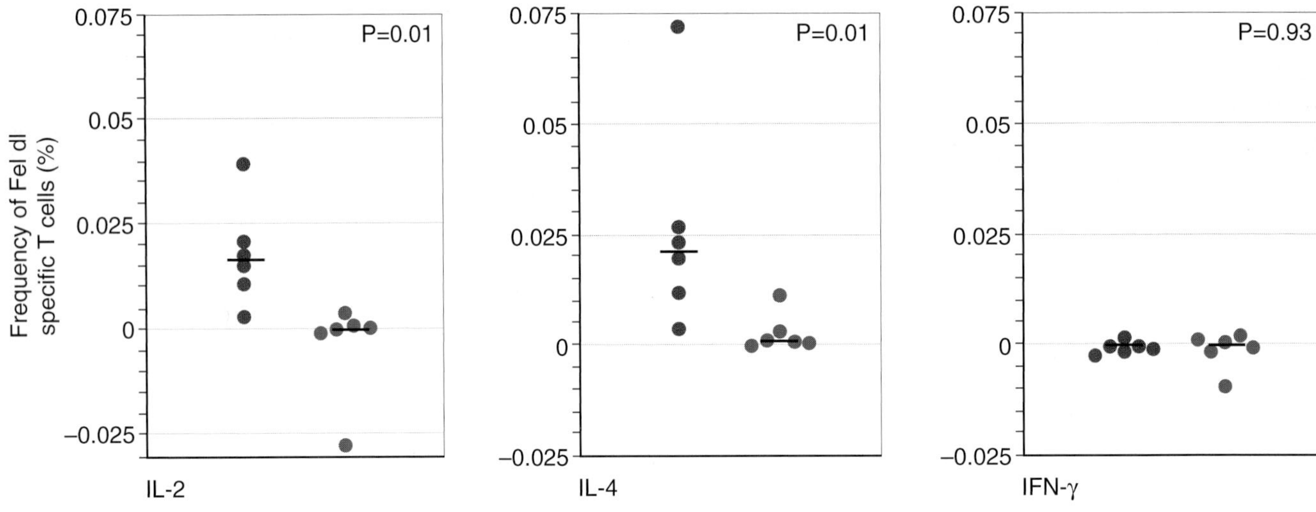

Figure 101–12. Frequency of intracellular cytokine (interleukin [IL]-2, IL-4, IFN-γ)–expressing CD4 T cells following in vitro exposure to Fel d1 in a group of cat allergic (AA) and nonatopic (NA) subjects. Results demonstrate that the cat-allergic subjects' CD4 T cells produce IL-2 and IL-4 but not IFN-γ following allergen exposure, whereas the controls do not respond. (Courtesy of Calman Prussin, MD, Laboratory of Allergic Diseases, National Institute of Allergy and Infectious Diseases, National Institutes of Health.)

cells into type I (normal GPI–anchored protein expression), type II (reduced expression), or type III (absent expression).

Flow cytometric evaluation of platelets potentially offers a major advantage by allowing study of whole blood, eliminating the need for cell isolation and thus minimizing cell manipulation.[13,14] Detection of reticulated platelets, assessment for states of platelet activation and aggregation, and detection of platelet-associated immunoglobulin can be accomplished by cytometric methods. Using specific monoclonal antibodies, platelets can be counted without losing accuracy in the very low range.[26] The technique is simple, involving staining of whole blood and determining the number of platelets and red blood cells in the sample. The ratio of platelets to blood cells, when linked to the red blood count obtained by standard methods, is used to calculate platelet number.[14] Multicenter studies sponsored by the International Society for Laboratory Hematology demonstrated that this method is precise and reliable.[24] Reticulated platelets are identified by increased RNA content (stained by nucleic acid dyes such as thiazole orange). The measurement of reticulated platelets is a sensitive and specific method to distinguish between destructive thrombocytopenia (caused by hypersplenism or autoimmune thrombocytopenia, as examples) and bone marrow failure.[13] The combination of reticulated platelet number with flow detection of platelet-associated immunoglobulin helps in the evaluation of immune thrombocytopenia, although the latter method alone has low specificity.[13] Platelet immunophenotyping can support the diagnosis of rare genetic disorders associated with abnormal expression of surface receptors, such as Bernard-Soulier syndrome and Glanzmann's thrombasthenia.[13,27]

Box 101–1. Clinical Applications of Flow Cytometry

- Immunophenotype lymphocytes
- Characterize hematopoietic malignancies
- Quantitate hematopoietic stem cells
- Study other hematopoietic cells (monocytes, eosinophils, neutrophils, red cells, platelets)
- Assess in vitro lymphocyte activation and/or proliferation
- Evaluate mitogen/antigen-induced intracellular cytokine production
- Detect antigen-specific lymphocytes

FLOW CYTOMETRY IN HEMATOLOGIC MALIGNANCIES

Flow cytometric immunophenotyping is vital in the diagnostic evaluation of hematolymphoid neoplasms[7,28,29] (Box 101–1). Diagnosis of a B-cell neoplasm requires the identification of a neoplastic B-cell population and then subclassification into an appropriate diagnostic category. Markers of chronic B-cell leukemia or lymphoma include light chain restriction, absence of normal antigens, and the detection of antigens not normally present on mature B cells. A B-cell population with restricted light chain expression is, with rare exceptions, a B-cell neoplasm. The expression of a single immunoglobulin light chain by a B-cell population results in a unimodal pattern of

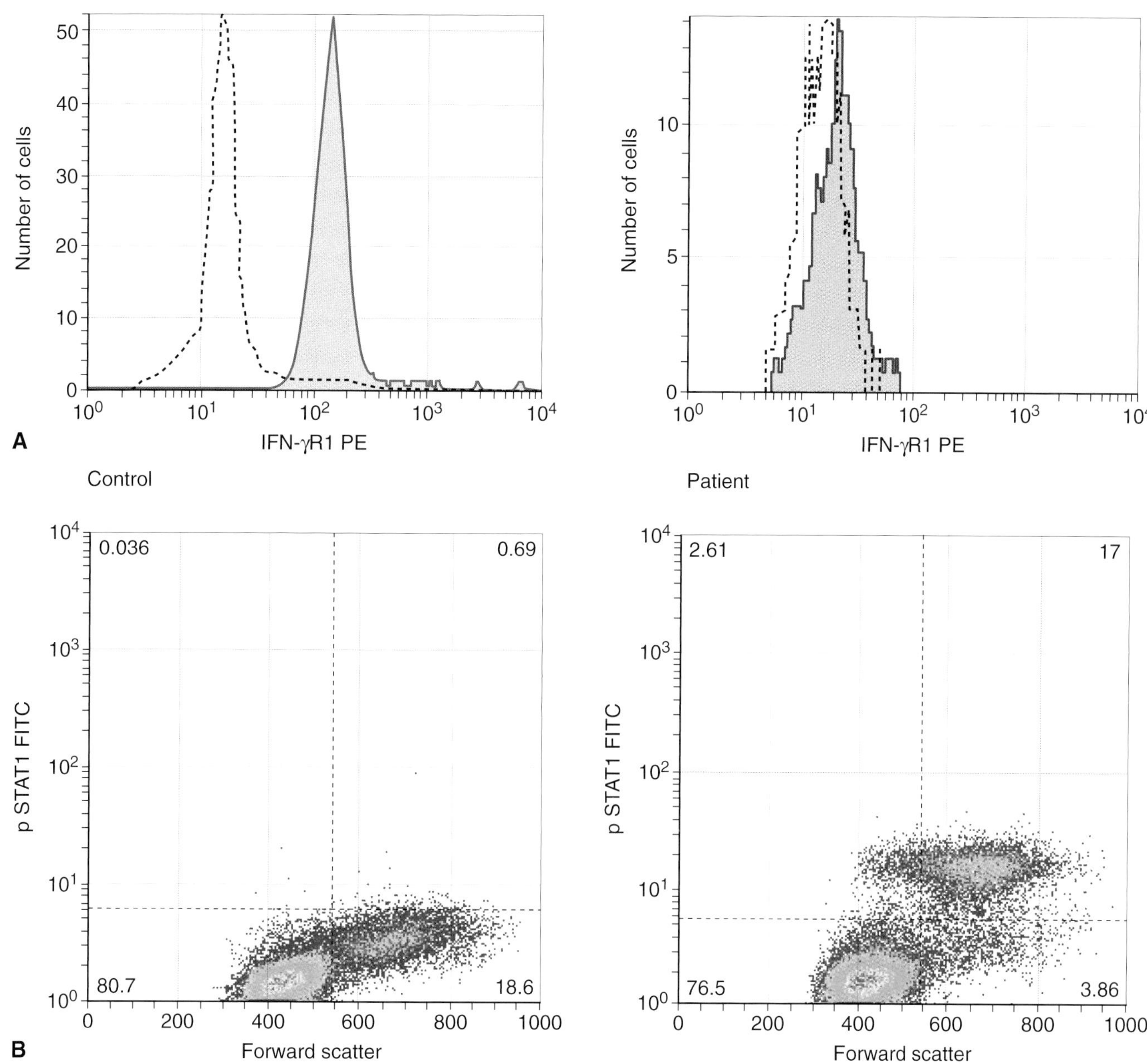

Figure 101–13. *A,* Assessment of the expression of the IFN-γ receptor α chain on monocytes from a control subject and a patient with recurrent *Mycobacterium avium* complex infection. *B,* Intracellular expression of phosphorylated STAT-1 (pSTAT1) before *(panel A)* and after *(panel B)* incubation of monocytes with IFN-γ.

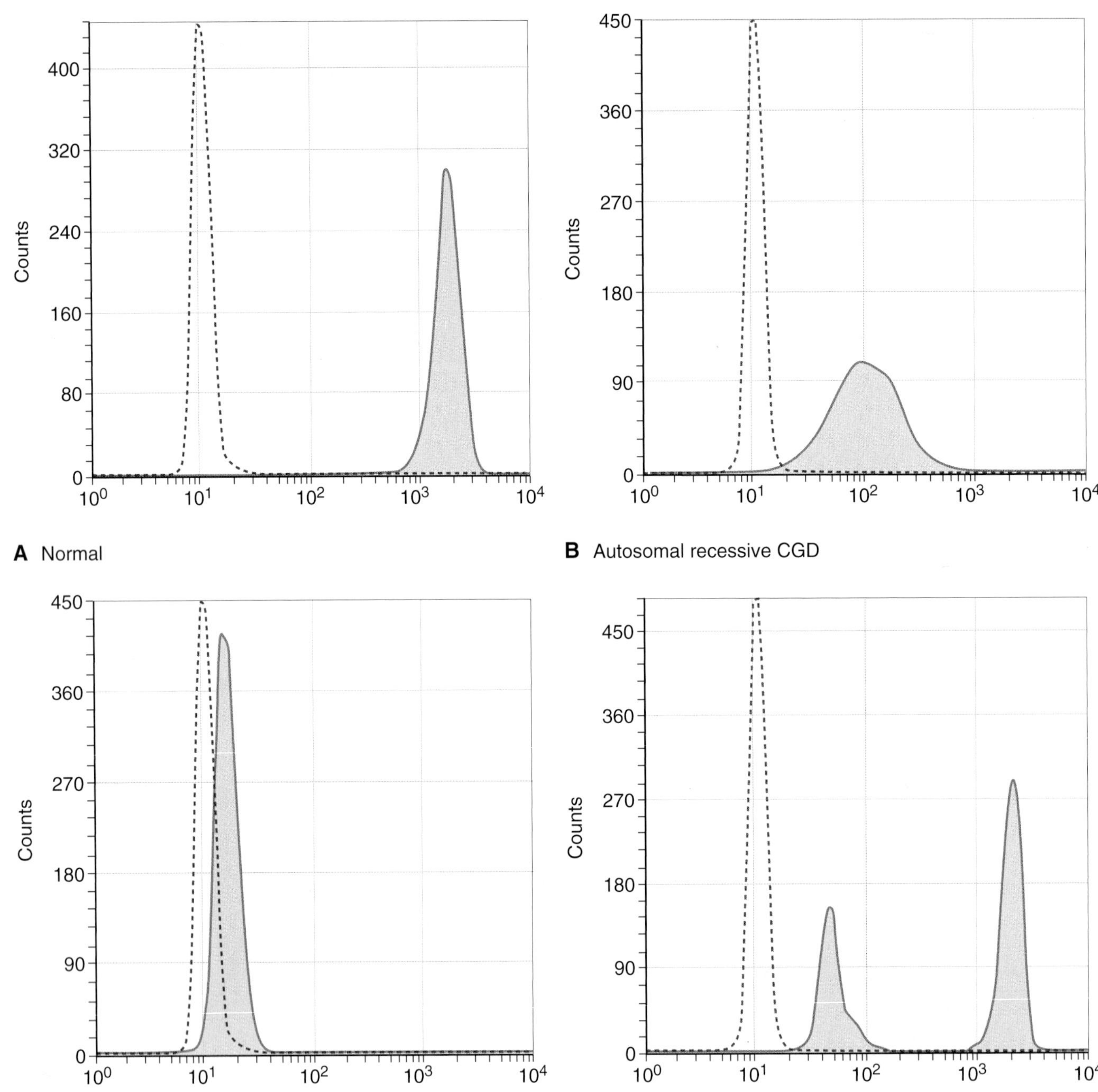

■ **Figure 101–14.** Histograms depicting typical patterns of oxidative burst following PMA stimulation in a normal donor ***(A)***, in a patient with autosomal recessive chronic granulomatous disease (CGD) ***(B)***, in a patient with X-linked CGD ***(C)***, and in an asymptomatic female carrier ***(D)***. *Dotted lines* represent unstimulated control cells. X axis plots fluorescent intensity. Solid histogram represents PMA stimulated cells.

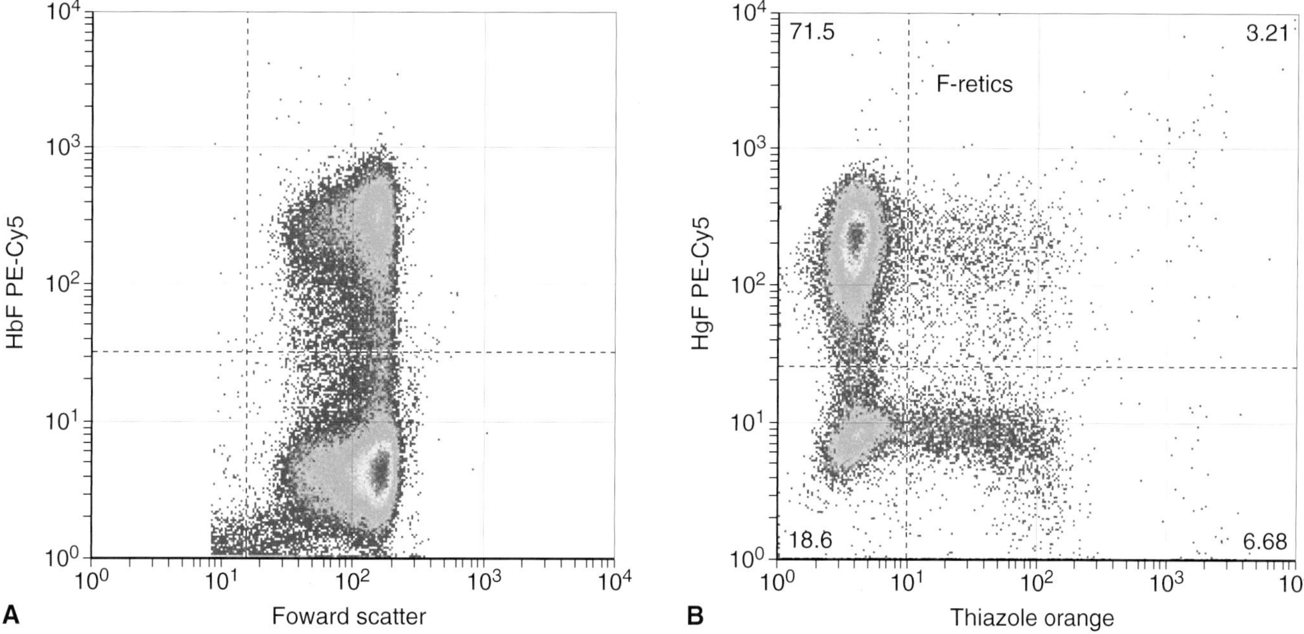

Figure 101–15. (*A*) Hemoglobin F–containing red blood cells and (*B*) F reticulocytes in a patient with sickle cell anemia under treatment. (Courtesy of Jennifer Studdard, Clinical Center, National Institutes of Health.)

staining, wherein one light chain reagent (anti-κ or anti-λ) is positive and the other is negative in all of the malignant cells (Fig. 101–16*A*). In normal or benign lymph node tissue, virtually every B cell expresses κ or λ; lack of expression of either of these in mature B cells also indicates the presence of a malignant B-cell population[7,28] (Fig. 101–16*B*). In samples containing monoclonal B cells admixed with polyclonal B cells, the simultaneous analysis of size and markers that are differentially expressed among benign and malignant elements facilitates the identification of lymphoma cells, allowing minimal residual disease detection.[7,28,30] For example, the CD11c$^+$ B cells in the peripheral blood specimen of a patient with hairy cell leukemia may be monoclonal, while the CD11c$^-$ B cells are polyclonal; simple examination of numbers of cells staining with λ and μ would not be useful in this case. Delineating an abnormal pattern of expression of antigens of malignant B cells also allows subclassification into discrete diagnostic categories: CD5 and CD23 in chronic lymphocytic leukemia and mantle cell lymphoma, CD10 in follicular lymphoma and Burkitt's lymphoma, and CD11c as well as CD103 in hairy cell leukemia are examples.[7,28]

Flow cytometric indicators of T-cell neoplasia include subset restriction, absence of normally expressed antigens, the presence of abnormal antigens, and abnormal levels of T-cell antigen expression.[7,28,29,31,32] In normal reactive lymphoid populations, there is a mixture of CD4- and CD8-positive cells. T-cell leukemias and lymphomas, however, are restricted in CD4 or CD8 expression (the majority are CD4$^+$CD8$^-$, although CD4$^-$CD8$^+$, CD4$^-$CD8$^-$, and CD4$^+$CD8$^+$ types can also be observed), analogous to light chain restriction in B-cell neoplasms (Fig. 101–17). Because 75% of mature T-cell neoplasms fail to express at least one T-cell antigen (Fig. 101–18), analysis for absence of a T-cell antigen is more useful than is subset restriction analysis: CD7 is most frequently absent, followed by loss of CD2, CD5, and CD3.[7,26] In evaluating T-cell antigen expression, the small percentage of peripheral blood CD3$^+$ T cells are CD7$^-$ and a subset of normal γ/δ T cells that do not express CD5 must be considered. Detection of abnormal or inappropriate antigen expression is useful in the diagnosis of T-cell malignancy, and neoplastic T cells may be visualized as a homogeneous population with an abnormal level of antigen expression. For example, CD3 may be expressed at a higher or lower level than normal as measured by staining with anti-CD3 antibody[32,33] (see Fig. 101–17).

Immunophenotypic markers of lineage and stages of differentiation allow precise classification of an acute leukemic process.[6] Because acute leukemias can have a heterogeneous pattern of antigen expression, tumor cells must be differentiated from normal populations in order to accurately define the immunophenotype. From the CD45 expression versus side scatter (SSC) pattern for bone marrow elements, cells can be segregated into distinct populations, including lymphocytes, monocytes, granulocytes, nucleated red cells, and blasts (see Fig. 101–18*A*). Thus these two parameters can be used to define a blast gate (characterized by low SSC and dim CD45) that contains few mature normal cells.[5,34]

Flow cytometry is essential for determination of lineage in acute lymphoblastic leukemia. Acute lymphoblastic leukemia cells typically occupy the blast gate on CD45 versus SSC plots (see Fig. 101–18*B*), although in select cases CD45 expression may be dimmer or brighter than normal. Acute lymphoblastic leukemia blasts have an immature T- or B-cell immunophenotype and may express terminal deoxynucleotidyl transferase (TdT) and CD34. However, classification of acute

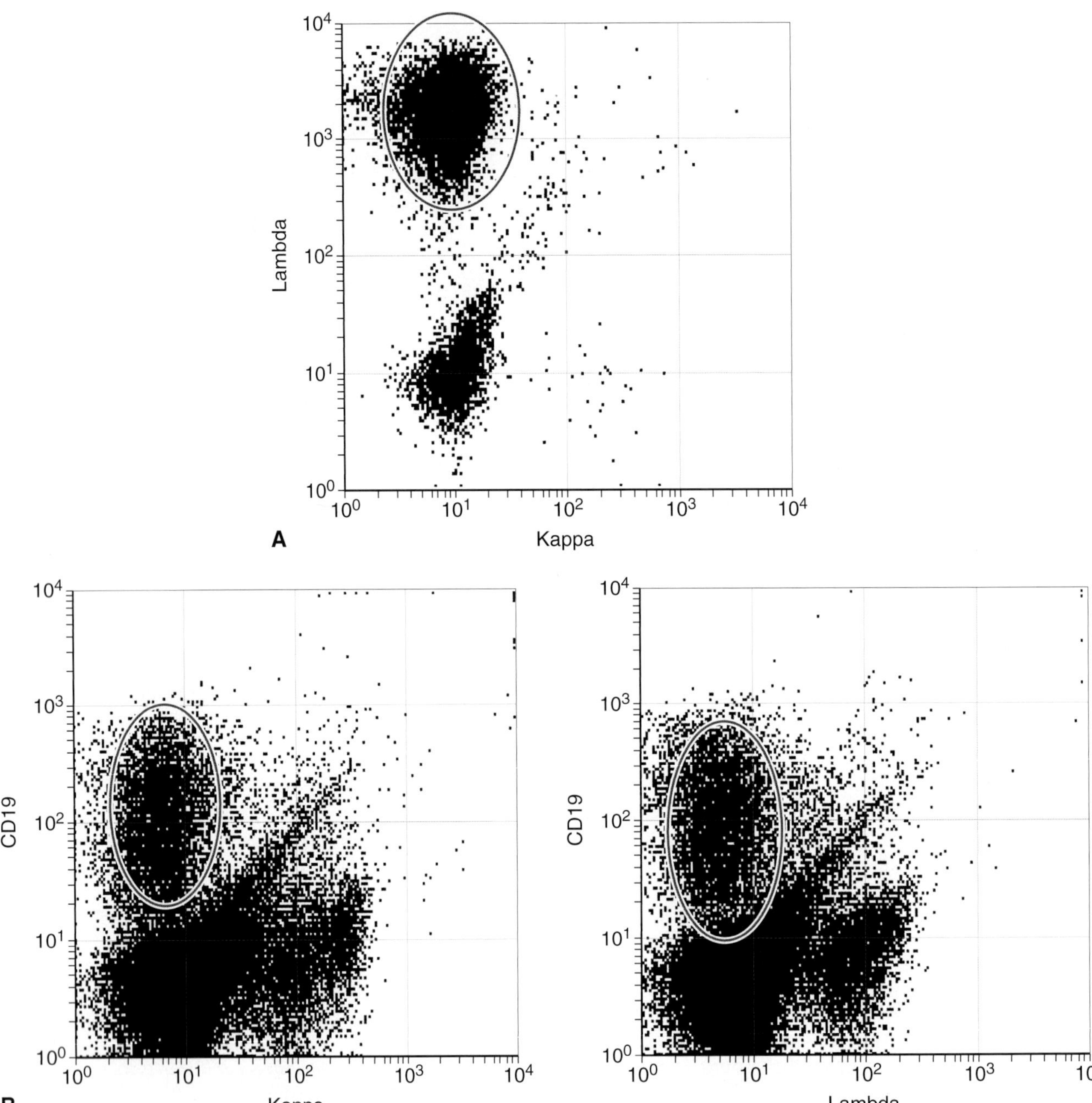

Figure 101–16. *A,* Monoclonal light chain population in a B-cell neoplasm. The oval contains the λ-positive, κ-negative monoclonal B cells. *B,* Surface light chain–negative B-cell lymphoma, all of the B cells are κ and λ negative (in *ovals*).

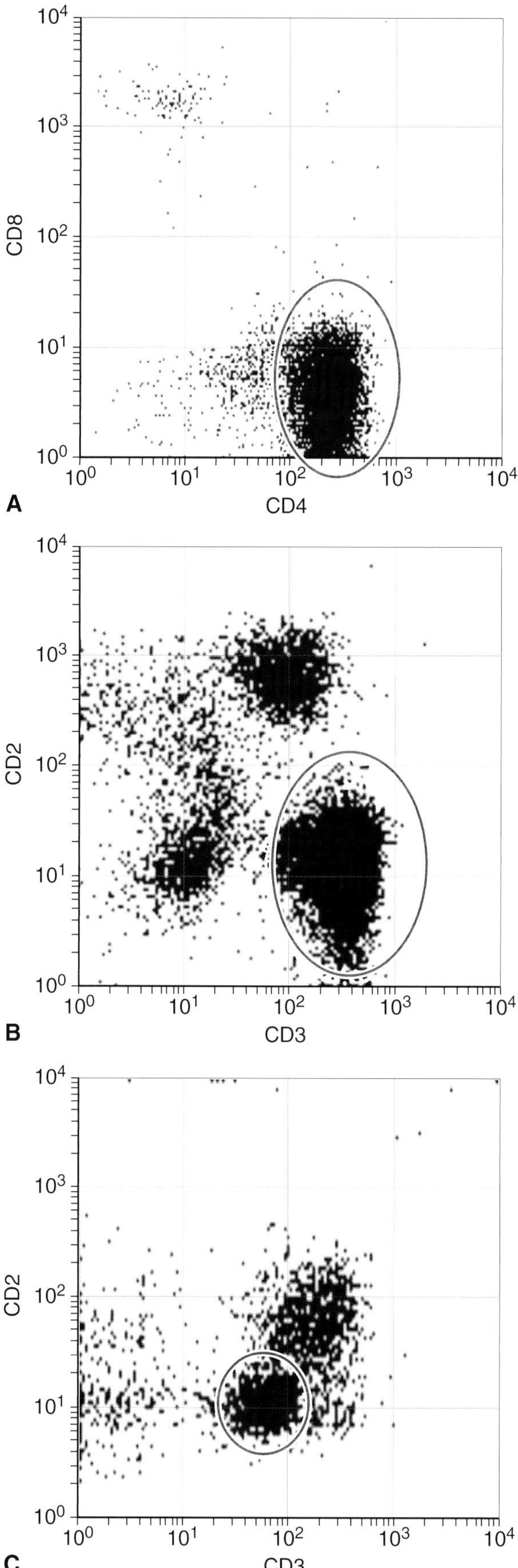

leukemia is based upon a complete panel of T, B, and myeloid antibodies because expression of myeloid antigens is common in acute lymphoblastic leukemia. B-precursor acute lymphoblastic leukemia typically expresses CD19, CD10, CD34, HLA-DR, and TdT and is usually positive for CD22 and CD24 (see Fig. 101–18*C* and *D*). The blasts in T-lineage acute lymphoblastic leukemia often overlap with the brighter CD45 mature lymphocyte and monocyte gates. The most specific marker for T-cell lineage in acute lymphoblastic leukemia is intracytoplasmic staining for CD3, as surface CD3 is usually negative. CD7 is the most sensitive marker for T-lineage acute lymphoblastic leukemia but is less specific because it is frequently expressed by myeloid leukemias. CD2, CD1a, CD5, TdT, and CD34 are also observed in T-lineage acute lymphoblastic leukemia. CD4 and CD8 are typically double positive or double negative.

Flow cytometry is useful in identifying granulocytic, monocytic, erythroid, and megakaryocytic differentiation in acute myeloid leukemia. Both the pattern of antigen expression and the location of the blasts on a CD45 versus SSC data plot help in subclassification. Blasts in acute myeloid leukemia have an immature phenotype and may express CD13, CD33, CD117, and myeloperoxidase. CD34 and HLA-DR may be positive but are not lineage-specific. In addition, blasts may express the lymphoid antigens TdT, CD56, or CD7. In acute myeloid leukemia with monocytic differentiation, the blasts can overlap with normal monocytes on the CD45 versus SSC data plot and express monocytic antigens, such as CD14 and CD36. Erythroid differentiation can be determined by bright expression of CD71 and glycophorin, and megakaryocytic differentiation is characterized by bright CD61 and CD41 expression.

CURRENT CONTROVERSIES & FUTURE CONSIDERATIONS

Flow Cytometry

- The increasing range of reagents and expanded understanding of cell biology should mean that flow cytometry will play an even larger role in the laboratory assessment of blood cells.
- In the future, far more extensive approaches to cell characterization will be based on extensive "polychromatic" approaches that currently have been extended to 17-color studies. Whether the power of this type of flow cytometry will have a practical place in the clinic must be demonstrated.[35]

Figure 101–17. Flow cytometric analysis of T-cell neoplasms. ***A,*** Malignant T cells are $CD4^+$ and $CD8^-$ (in *oval*). ***B,*** Malignant T cells (in *oval*) expressing CD3 but negative for CD2. ***C,*** Malignant T cells (in *oval*) expressing abnormally dim CD3 and negative for CD2.

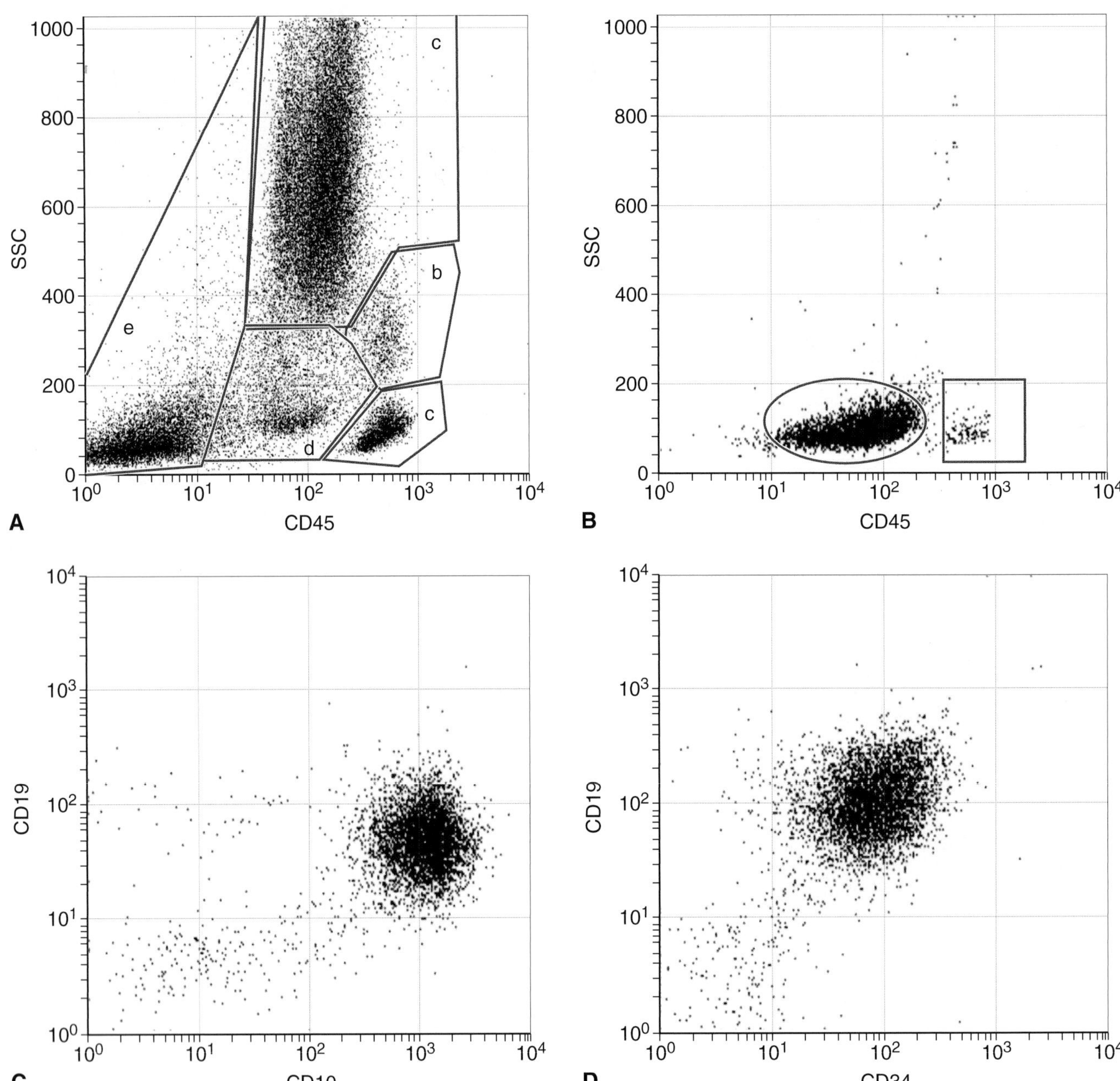

■ **Figure 101–18.** *A,* Staining pattern of CD45 versus side scatter for normal bone marrow: *a,* mature granulocytes; *b,* mature monocytes; *c,* mature lymphocytes; *d,* blasts; *e,* nucleated red cell precursors. ***B,*** Staining pattern of CD45 versus side scatter for acute lymphoblastic leukemia (ALL). *Box,* mature lymphocytes; *oval,* lymphoblasts. ***C,*** $CD10^+$ and $CD19^+$ ALL cells. ***D,*** $CD34^+$ and $CD19^+$ ALL cells.

Suggested Readings*

Basic Concepts of Flow Cytometry

Givan AL: Flow Cytometry: First Principles (ed 2). New York: Wiley-Liss, 2001.

Clinical Applications of Flow Cytometry

Ault KA: The clinical utility of flow cytometry in the study of platelets. Semin Hematol 38:160–169, 2001.

Bleesing JJ, Fleisher TA: Immunophenotyping. Semin Hematol 38:100–110, 2001.

Bleesing JJH, Fleisher TA: Cell function-based flow cytometry. Semin Hematol 38:169–178, 2001.

Gratama JW, Sutherland DR, Keeney M: Flow cytometric enumeration and immunophenotyping of hematopoietic stem and progenitor cells. Semin Hematol 38:139–147, 2001.

Stetler-Stevenson M, Braylan R: Flow cytometric analysis of lymphomas and lymphoproliferative disorders. Semin Hematol 38:111–123, 2001.

Weir EG, Borowitz MJ: Flow cytometry in the diagnosis of acute leukemia. Semin Hematol 38:124–138, 2001.

Future Directions in Flow Cytometry

Perfetto SP, Chattopadhyay PK, Roederer M: Seventeen-colour flow cytometry, unraveling the immune system. Nat Rev Immunol 4:648–665, 2004.

CHAPTER 102

Human Leukocyte Antigen and Transplantation

Effie W. Petersdorf, MD

KEY POINTS

Human Leukocyte Antigen and Transplantation

Facts

- With HLA-matched unrelated donors, graft rejection, graft-versus-host disease, and mortality are increased compared to HLA-matched sibling transplants.

Hypotheses

- HLA loci other than HLA-A, -B, and -DR are important determinants of transplant outcome.
- HLA-"matched" patients and donors are mismatched for alleles detectable by high-resolution DNA methods.
- Genes other than *HLA* are important to transplant outcome.

Data

- High-resolution HLA typing methods can identify allele differences between patients and donors who are serologically identical.
- HLA class I and class II alleles are functional; donor mismatching for alleles is associated with increased graft rejection, graft-versus-host disease, and mortality.
- The total number of HLA mismatches is a determinant of post-transplant complications; as the number of HLA mismatches increases, the risk of complications increases.
- Key epitopes or residues of the HLA molecule that are involved in peptide binding or contact with the T-cell receptor may define tolerability of a mismatch.
- Nongenetic factors, including stage of disease at the time of transplantation, can influence the tolerability of HLA mismatching.

INTRODUCTION

The major histocompatibility complex is the most comprehensively studied multi-megabase region of the human genome. Elucidation of the structure and function of the major histocompatibility complex has been motivated by its biomedical importance in transplantation, autoimmunity, and infectious diseases. More than 224 genes are now identified within the 3,673,800 bases of the major histocompatibility complex,[1] an estimated 40% of which are involved in immune function. The classical transplantation genes, human leukocyte antigen (*HLA*)-*A*, *-B*, *-C*, *-DR*, *-DQ*, and *-DP*, share structural properties and encode polypeptides that are critical in controlling T-cell recognition and determining histocompatibility in transplantation.[2,3] The class I region encodes nonclassical *HLA* genes capable of antigen presentation[4] and class I–related *MIC* genes that participate in stress and serve as ligands for NKG2D.[5] The class II region contains at least seven genes whose functions include loading and assembly of class II gene products (*DM*), peptide editing (*DN/DO*), transport of cytosolic proteins for presentation by class I (*TAP* in association with calnexin, calreticulin, tapasin, and Erp57 protein), and proteasome degradation genes (*LMP*).[6–15] The class III region encodes genes involved in inflammation and has direct significance in transplantation.[16,17] The clustering of genes that share similar function within the major histocompatibility complex is striking and likely represents developmental reduplication.[18–20]

Investigators today are equipped with an array of DNA-based methods that provide a high level of discrimination of *HLA* genes. The ability to detect single nucleotide differences between two unique HLA alleles has propelled the field of histocompatibility to a new level of clinical testing in support of allogeneic transplantation. The goal of histocompatibility testing and matching for donor selection is to reduce the risk of post-transplant complications resulting from HLA incompatibility. This entails not only the identification of matched donors, but also an understanding of tolerable mismatches. In this chapter, state-of-the-art molecular typing

TABLE 102–1. HLA Class I Antigens and Alleles*

HLA-A		HLA-B		HLA-C			
Antigen	**Allele**	**Antigen**	**Allele**	**Antigen**	**Allele**	**Antigen**	**Allele**
A1	A*0101-10	B7	B*0702; 0704-38	B52(5)	B*5201-05	Cw1	Cw*0102-10
A2	A*0201-68	B703	B*0703	B53	B*5301-09	Cw2	Cw*0202-09
A3	A*0301-14	B8	B*0801-21	B54(22)	B*5401-02	Cw10(w3)	Cw*0302; 0304
A23(9)[†]	A*2301-12	B13	B*1301-13	B55(22)	B*5501-16	Cw9(w3)	Cw*0303
A24(9)	A*2402-42	B14	B*1401-06	B56(22)	B*5601-12	Cw3	Cw*0305-16
A9	A*2410	B15	B*1501-83	B57(17)	B*5701-09	Cw4	Cw*0401-15
A25(10)	A*2501; 03-04	B18	B*1801-19	B58(17)	B*5801-06	Cw5	Cw*0501-09
A26(10)	A*2601-20	B27	B*2701-07; 2709-25	B59	B*5901	Cw6	Cw*0602-11
A10	A*2502	B2708	B*2708	B67	B*6701-02	Cw7	Cw*0701-26
A11	A*1101-17	B35	B*3501-49	B73	B*7301	Cw8	Cw*0801-12
A29(19)	A*2901-11	B37	B*3701-05	B78	B*7801-05	–[‡]	Cw*1202-12
A30(19)	A*3001-12	B38(16)	B*3801-09	B81	B*8101-02	–	Cw*1402-05
A31(19)	A*3101-09	B39(16)	B*3901-28	–[‡]	B*8201-02	–	Cw*1502-12
A32(19)	A*3201-08	B40	B*4001-48	–	B*8301	–	Cw*1601-02; 1604
A33(19)	A*3301-07	B41	B*4101-06			–	Cw*1701-03
A34(10)	A*3401-05	B42	B*4201-05			–	Cw*1801-02
A36	A*3601-04	B44(12)	B*4402-39			–	
A43	A*4301	B45(12)	B*4501-06				
A66(10)	A*6601-04	B46	B*4601-02				
A68(28)	A*6801-02; 6804-11; 6813-25	B47	B*4701-04				
A69(28)	A*6901	B48	B*4801-08				
A28	A*6803; 12	B49(21)	B*4901-03				
A74(19)	A*7401-10	B50(21)	B*5001-02; 5004				
A80	A*8001	B51(5)	B*5101-34				

*Allele names updated as of July 2004. Allele designations can be found at *http://www.ebi.ac/uk/imgt/hla.*
[†]Antigens listed in parentheses are public specificities.
[‡]Defined by DNA typing methods; no corresponding antigen is defined by sera or cellular typing.

methods are described, and the immunogenetic variables that affect outcome after unrelated donor hematopoietic stem cell transplantation are reviewed.

THE MAJOR HISTOCOMPATIBILITY COMPLEX

Class I Genes: HLA-A, HLA-B, and HLA-C

Classical class I genes (*HLA-A, -B,* and *-C*) show sequence and structural homology with one another. The role of class I molecules in antigen presentation helps to explain the extensive polymorphism. As of January 2004, over 309 HLA-A, 563 HLA-B, and 167 HLA-C alleles have been defined in racially and ethnically diverse human populations[21] (*http://www.ebi.ac.uk/imgt/hla*). In addition to *HLA-A, -B,* and *-C,* three nonclassical class I genes, *HLA-E, -F,* and *-G,* have been defined.[22–24] These genes encode cell surface molecules that have different patterns of expression. HLA-F and HLA-G molecules are found on the placental trophoblast, whereas HLA-E molecules are ubiquitously expressed. The function of HLA-E, -F, and -G molecules is not fully known, but they in part serve as ligands for natural killer (NK) cell receptors and thus may regulate NK function.[25,26]

HLA-A, -B and *-C* genes are each composed of eight exons. Exon 1 is a leader sequence; exons 2, 3, and 4 encode the α1, α2, and α3 domains of the class I molecule, respectively; exon 5 encodes the transmembrane portion of the molecule; and exons 6, 7, and 8 encode the cytoplasmic tail. The majority of DNA-based methods target polymorphisms encoded in exons 2 and 3 of HLA-A, -B, and -C alleles. Nucleotide substitutions within exons 2 and 3 are concentrated in discrete hypervariable regions, impacting binding of peptide fragments for presentation to the T-cell receptor.[4] These polymorphic sites also determine the allospecificity of the molecule and form the basis for the classification as HLA alloantigens (Table 102–1).

Class II Genes: HLA-DR, HLA-DQ, and HLA-DP

The class II region of the major histocompatibility complex encodes the three classical loci, HLA-DR, HLA-DQ, and HLA-DP. These loci encode nine distinct genes: *DRA, DRB1, DRB3, DRB4, DRB5, DQA, DQB, DPA,* and *DPB*. Like the class I genes, class II genes are highly polymorphic, with more than 317 DRB1, 39 DQB1, and 107 DPB1 alleles currently known[21] (Table 102–2).

Each class II molecule consists of a single α chain (encoded by *DRA, DQA,* or *DPA*) that is noncovalently bound to a polymorphic β chain.[2] The β chains of HLA-DR, -DQ and -DP antigens are encoded by exon 2 of the *DRB1, DQB1,* and *DPB1* genes, respectively. The polymorphic second exon defines the specificity of the class II antigen. Within DRB, DRB1 is distinct but DRB3, DRB4, and DRB5 are inherited as a genetic unit, or *haplotype*. For example, the DR1 haplotype is encoded by two functional genes: a polymorphic *DRB1* gene and a nonpolymorphic *DRA* gene. In contrast, the DR3 haplotype

TABLE 102–2. HLA Class II Antigens and Alleles*

Antigen	Allele	Antigen	Allele	Antigen	Allele
DR1	DRB1*0101-11	DQ5(1)	DQB1*0501-04	DPw1	DPB1*0101
DR15(2)[†]	DRB1*1501-14	DQ6(1)	DQB1*0601-21	DPw2	DPB1*0201-02
DR16(2)	DRB1*1601-08	DQ2	DQB1*0201-03	DPw3	DPB1*0301
DR17(3)	DRB1*0301; 0304-05	DQ7(3)	DQB1*0301;0304	DPw4	DPB1*0401-02
DR18(3)	DRB1*0302-03	DQ8(3)	DQB1*0302;0305; 0310-13	DPw5	DPB1*0501
DR3	DRB1*0306-26	DQ9(3)	DQB1*0303	DPw6	DPB1*0601
DR4	DRB1*0401-50	DQ3	DQB1*0306-09	–[‡]	DPB1*0801-9901[§]
DR11(5)	DRB1*1101-49	DQ4	DQB1*0401-02		
DR12(5)	DRB1*1201-09				
DR13(6)	DRB1*1301-63				
DR14(6)	DRB1*1401-48				
DR7	DRB1*0701-08				
DR8	DRB1*0801-28				
DR9	DRB1*0901-03				
DR10	DRB1*1001				

*Alleles of B1 genes only (alleles of A1 genes not shown). Allele names updated as of July 2004. Allele designations can be found at *http://www.ebi.ac/uk/imgt/hla*.
[†]Antigens listed in parentheses are broadly defined public specificities subsequently split into two or more subtypic antigens.
[‡]Defined by DNA typing methods; no antigen has been defined by sera or cellular typing.
[§]Additional DPB1 alleles have been defined (DPB1*0801-9901) for which no corresponding antigens have been defined.

is encoded by three genes: a polymorphic *DRB1* gene, a nonpolymorphic *DRA* gene, and a polymorphic *DRB3* gene. Polymorphism within the class II region can result from *trans* pairing of a polymorphic DQ α chain encoded by one parental chromosome with a polymorphic DQ β chain encoded by the other parental chromosome.

HLA Nomenclature: Phenotype and Genotype; Antigens and Alleles; Vector of Incompatibility

HLA gene products have traditionally been characterized and classified by their reaction with anti-HLA antibodies, and are hence referred to as *antigens*. For a given locus, the antigens encoded by each of the two *HLA* genes are codominantly expressed. Heterozygous individuals will possess two different antigens at that locus, the combination of which is termed the *phenotype*. Because of the broadly reactive nature of anti-HLA antibodies, the same serologically defined antigen may be encoded by two or more unique sequences or *alleles*. The naming of HLA alleles and antigens is updated monthly by the World Health Organization Nomenclature Committee for Factors of the HLA System[21] (*http://www.ebi.ac.uk/imgt/hla*). Early nomenclature used the serologic phenotype to designate the antigen. With the elucidation of HLA polymorphism at the sequence level, both phenotype and genotype information is incorporated into the name of a given determinant. Using HLA-A2 as an example, the allele HLA-A*0201 encodes a molecule recognized serologically as A2. *HLA-A* defines the genetic locus and the *asterisk* separates the locus name from the allele name. The digits *02* indicate the broadly defined serologic specificity (A2), and the digits *01* identify the unique allele sequence that encodes the alloantigen.

HLA alleles encoded on a single chromosome 6 are termed a *haplotype*. The combination of two parental haplotypes inherited by an individual comprises that individual's HLA *genotype*. HLA haplotypes are determined by typing as many members of a family as are available in order to establish the gametic assignment.[27] In the absence of family study, haplotype frequencies can be estimated.[28,29] Through the efforts of the MHC Haplotype Consortium, eight common human haplotypes are being sequenced.[30] The most well-known and studied haplotype, HLA-A1, -B8, -DR3, demonstrates conservation of HLA and non-HLA markers in the class I, class III, and class II regions. The effect of the A1, B8, DR3 haplotype on both humoral and cellular immunity has been demonstrated (reviewed by Price and colleagues[31]). The A1, B8, DR3 haplotype is best studied as a disease susceptibility determinant for type 1 diabetes, pemphigus vulgaris, myasthenia gravis, systemic lupus erythematosus, scleroderma, celiac disease, and human immunodeficiency virus progression.[31] More generally, HLA alleles and haplotypes are known to influence responsiveness to vaccines,[32–34] and are informative for analysis of anthropologic and evolutionary studies,[35,36] as well as in forensic medicine.[37]

Major histocompatibility complex haplotypes display a high degree of nonrandom association of alleles at two or more HLA loci. This phenomenon is known as *linkage disequilibrium* and represents an evolutionary advantage to maintain alleles together, possibly to confer survival advantage to the organism.[38] Linkage disequilibrium of HLA class I and II alleles has profound implications in the search for suitably matched unrelated donors for hematopoietic stem cell transplantation. For the purposes of finding a donor, strong linkage disequilibrium between two or more HLA loci (e.g., HLA-A1, -B8, -DR3 in Caucasian Americans) can be of major benefit to a patient, because matching for two of the loci (e.g., A1, B8) will very often determine matching for the third (e.g., DR3). Patients possessing HLA haplotypes with less strongly

TABLE 102–3. Vector of HLA Incompatibility

		Examples	
Vector*	Definition	Recipient	Donor
HVG	Presence of donor alleles or antigens not present in the recipient	A*0201,6802†	A*0201,6801†
		A*0201,0201‡	A*0201,6801‡
GVH	Presence of recipient alleles or antigens not present in the donor	A*0201,6802†	A*0201,6801†
		A*0201,6802‡	A*0201,0201‡

*HVG, host-versus-graft; GVH, graft-versus-host.
†These combinations contain bidirectional (both HVG and GVHD) mismatch vectors.
‡Unidirectional mismatches.

linked alleles will have more difficulty finding donors. In the field of transplantation, haplotype frequencies have been used to estimate the probability of identifying suitable donors[39,40] and to determine the ideal size of unrelated donor registries.[41–45]

Assessing the HLA matching between the recipient and the prospective donor is termed the *vector of incompatibility* and accurately predicts posttransplant complications of graft failure and acute graft-versus-host disease in related haploidentical transplants.[46] The vector (also known as the direction of the mismatch) describes both host-versus-graft and graft-versus-host alloreactivity. The presence of donor antigens or alleles not shared by the recipient determines host-versus-graft allorecognition and visa versa. Mismatching between a donor and recipient can be described as *bidirectional* if both host-versus-graft and graft-versus-host vectors are present at a given HLA locus. *Unidirectional* mismatching occurs if one but not the other vector is present. Unidirectional mismatching in the graft-versus-host vector occurs when the donor is homozygous and the recipient is heterozygous and shares one allele or antigen with the donor (e.g., patient A*0201, *0205 vs. donor A*0201, *0201). Unidirectional mismatching in the host-versus-graft vector occurs when the patient is homozygous and the donor is heterozygous and shares one allele with the patient (e.g., patient A*0201, *0201 vs. donor A*0201, *0205) (Table 102–3).

HLA TYPING METHODS

Serology

Serologic testing is based on the complement-dependent microcytotoxicity assay using panels of alloantisera.[47] Serologic reagents can discriminate epitopes shared by more than one distinct antigen (*public specificities*) and epitopes unique to a single antigen (*private specificities*, or *splits* of the public antigen). The public specificity A19, for example, is shared by several distinct antigens: A29, A30, A31, A32, A33, and A74 (see Table 102–1). Clusters of serologically cross-reactive HLA-A and -B antigens can be broadly classified as belonging to *cross-reactive epitope groups* (CREGs). Antigens within a CREG are presumed to share one or more public epitopes in addition to their individual and unique private epitope(s). When a donor and recipient differ by their serologically defined antigens, these mismatches may be defined as *minor* CREGs if the antigens share serologic cross-reactive epitopes. Examples of CREG mismatches include HLA-A2 and -A28, and HLA-B60 and -B61. An equivalent nomenclature is not yet available for HLA-C.[48] A *major* HLA antigen mismatch occurs when the antigens do not show serologic cross-reactivity. Examples of major mismatches are HLA-A1 and -A2, and HLA-B8 and -B44. The classification of public and private antigens into CREGs constitutes a basis for donor-recipient matching in hematopoietic stem cell transplantation. New software tools have integrated phenotype with genotype to aid in permissible HLA mismatch searches.[49] To bridge the transition in nomenclature from serologic to DNA-based typing methods, "serologically equivalent" designations have been defined.[48]

Cellular Typing

Historical methods for assessing compatibility between two individuals include the mixed lymphocyte culture, a test that primarily measures proliferation of $CD4^+$ T cells responding to class II antigens.[50,51] Cells that proliferate in a mixed lymphocyte culture reaction belong to the helper T lymphocyte subset. The strength of the proliferation measured in a mixed lymphocyte culture test correlates roughly with the degree of class II region incompatibility.[52] Alloimmune responses to class I antigens occur among $CD8^+$ cytotoxic T lymphocytes and can be measured in bulk culture using the cell-mediated lympholysis assay. This assay is a two-step procedure beginning with an activation phase in which responder cells are cultured with irradiated stimulator cells. After incubation for 6–10 days, the responder cells are tested against chromium-labeled target cells.[51] Cytotoxicity is measured by chromium release and used to assess the degree of functional class I disparity between two individuals.

DNA-Based Techniques

Most DNA HLA typing methods use polymerase chain reaction amplification of *HLA* genes from genomic DNA followed by hybridization to known oligonucleotide probes or sequencing. The latter is more accurate, but polymerase chain reaction probe hybridization is commonly used to infer the HLA allele. Probe hybridization may discriminate alleles at a level equivalent to serologically defined epitopes (e.g., HLA-A2), or *low-resolution* discrimination. DNA typing methods that identify polymorphisms short of the full nucleotide sequence are termed *intermediate resolution*. For example, a probe-based method that employs a wider array of probes might identify the presence of either the HLA-A*0201 *or* the HLA-A*0209 allele ("HLA-A*0201/09"), but is unable to discriminate one allele from the other. Typing methods that discriminate the complete nucleotide sequence of a unique HLA allele (e.g., HLA-A*0201) are termed *high* *resolution.* High-resolution typing results may be achieved by sequencing an *HLA* gene or by the use of comprehensive panels of oligonucleotide probes that describe all known polymorphic positions.

DNA Amplification Strategies for HLA Typing

Locus-specific, group-specific, or allele-specific amplification of *HLA* genes is used based on the needed level of antigen or allele information. *Locus-specific* primers amplify all alleles encoded at a given locus, including those of a heterozygous sample. In an HLA-A1,2–positive sample, both the A1 and the A2 alleles are coamplified. *Group-specific* primers amplify a group of alleles that share a common polymorphism. For example, a primer specific for the HLA-A2 group of alleles will only amplify the HLA-A2 allele in a heterozygous HLA-A1,2-positive sample). *Allele-specific* primers amplify a single allele by taking advantage of a unique polymorphism. For example, in an HLA-A2 homozygous sample that is heterozygous for two different HLA-A2 alleles (e.g., HLA-A*0201, 0205), the HLA-A*0205 allele can be amplified and analyzed independently of the HLA-A*0201 allele. A stepwise process is used to first identify the loci in both alleles, graduating to group-specific or allele-specific amplification to isolate one of the two alleles for further characterization as required to match donor and recipient; this process can provide the user with flexibility in the appropriate level of resolution required for clinical testing.

Sequence-Specific Primers

The sequence-specific primer method employs a panel of amplification primers whose sequence is complementary to known polymorphisms encoded by an HLA locus or group of alleles.[53–58] Following PCR amplification, the products are electrophoresed on a gel (Fig. 102–1). The HLA type is assigned by the composite pattern of positive and negative polymerase chain reactions. The sequence-specific primer method provides cost-effective, rapid determination at low resolution. With the use of expanded primer panels, this approach can also achieve high-resolution typing.

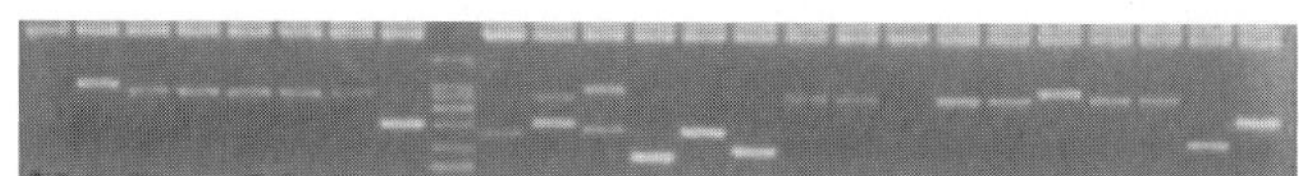

Figure 102–1. Sequence-specific primer methods were used to amplify exon 2 of HLA-DPB1. The primer sets included control primers and DNA ladders to allow identification of the size of the amplified HLA-DPB1 fragments. Positive and negative amplification of the appropriate-sized fragments are shown in this figure; the allele assignments can be interpreted with the aid of software programs.

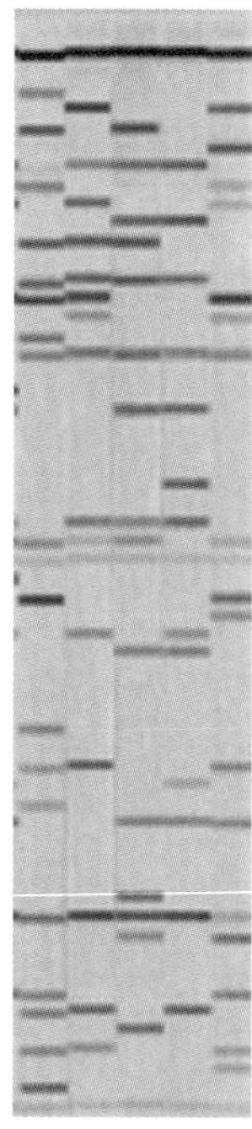

Figure 102–2. Line strip. This figure displays a reverse probe format of sequence-specific oligonucleotide probe hybridization using the Dynal RELI system. In brief, biotinylated locus-specific primers amplify HLA-B exons 2 and 3. Amplified samples are allowed to hybridize to a nylon membrane that is imprinted with probes specific for nucleotide substitutions in exons 2 and 3.

Oligonucleotide Probe Hybridization Methods

Both low- and high-resolution typing of HLA alleles can be achieved using sequence-specific oligonucleotide primer hybridization methods[59–69] using biotinylated primers. The amplified biotinylated amplicon products are incubated with membrane strips imprinted with sets of probes specific for each HLA locus and washed so that only matching sequences remain. These are identified using streptavidin. Positive and negative probe reactions are analyzed for the HLA type (Fig. 102–2). Because only known polymorphic sites in an *HLA* gene are probed, no information is obtained for other regions of the gene.

Sequencing

Automated sequencing has emerged as a powerful approach to typing *HLA* genes because it provides the highest resolution typing of HLA alleles and is definitive for verifying novel alleles.[70–74] HLA alleles can be sequenced from cloned templates (complementary DNA) or directly from polymerase chain reaction–amplified genomic DNA and analyzed on an automated sequencer (Fig. 102–3). Assignment of the HLA allele(s) is based on alignment to consensus sequences.

Oligonucleotide Arrays

Oligonucleotide array technology combines standard nucleic acid hybridization approaches with high-density DNA array technology. Oligonucleotide array technology is particularly well suited for the detection of complex polymorphisms in heterozygous individuals,[75] because multiple regions of polymorphisms in many *HLA* genes can be simultaneously assessed. Oligonucleotide probes can be designed to all known substitutions, or to all four

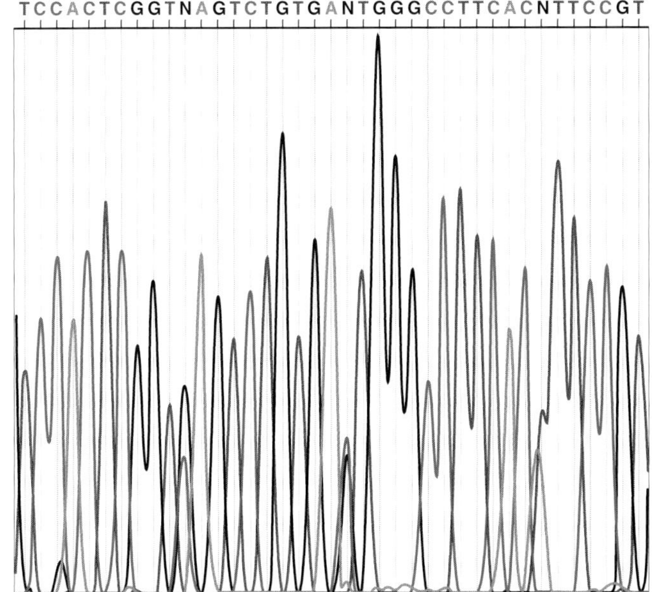

■ **Figure 102–3.** Sequence-based typing. This HLA-A*0201,0301 direct automated sequencing trace depicts polymorphic positions ("N") of exon 2 when both alleles are coamplified (methods described by Petersdorf and associates [91]).

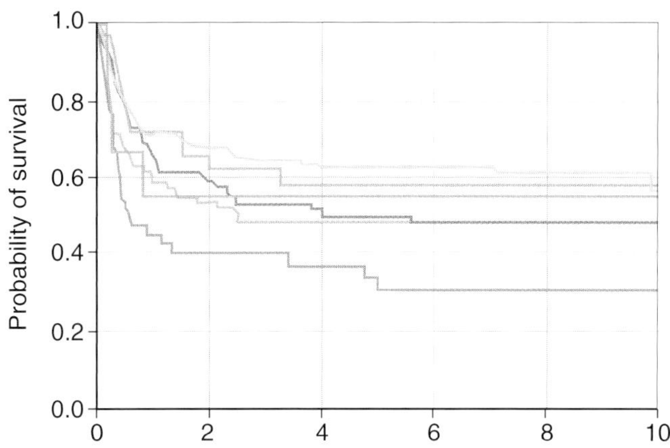

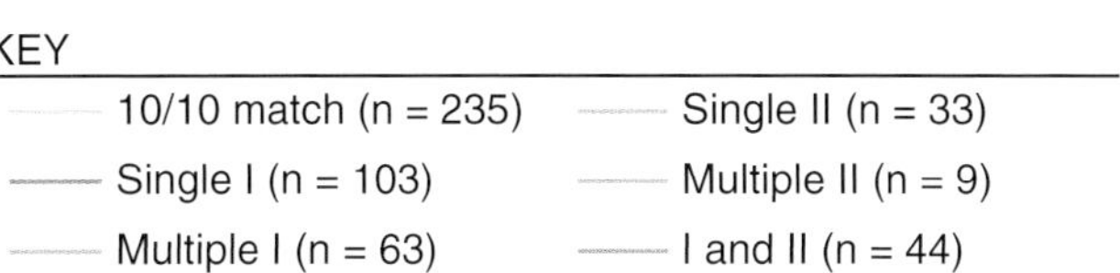

■ **Figure 102–4.** Kaplan-Meier survival curve for patients undergoing unrelated donor hematopoietic cell transplantation for the treatment of chronic myeloid leukemia (E. Petersdorf, unpublished data). HLA-A, -B, -C, -DRB1, and -DQB1 were retrospectively typed using high-resolution DNA methods. Six groups are displayed: 5-locus, 10-allele matches; one HLA-A, -B, or -C allele mismatch; two or more HLA-A, -B, or -C mismatches in any combination; one HLA-DRB1 or -DQB1 mismatch; two or more -DRB1 and -DQB1 mismatches in any combination; combinations of two or more HLA-A, -B, -C, -DRB1, and -DQB1 mismatches.

potential nucleotides, and thereby enable detection of new sequence polymorphisms. Redundancy of probe sequences allows combinations of alleles to be distinguished in heterozygous individuals.

HLA TYPING IN SUPPORT OF UNRELATED HEMATOPOIETIC STEM CELL TRANSPLANTATION: DONOR MATCHING IN THE DNA ERA

Comprehensive and precise donor HLA matching is a key factor in the overall safety of unrelated donor hematopoietic stem cell transplantation as a cure for hematologic disorders, despite improvements in transplantation preparative regimens, immunosuppressive regimens, and supportive care.[76–83] Improvements in polymerase chain reaction–based typing technology have resulted in improved resolution for a greater number of *HLA* genes,[84–86] have equipped investigators with powerful tools for identifying the functional importance of HLA diversity[87–110] (Fig. 102–4), and have improved outcomes. Although the importance of complete and precise donor HLA matching cannot be overstated, demands of a 5-locus, 10-allele–matched donor are unrealistic for many patients for two major reasons: (1) there may be a lack of HLA-matched donors (because the patient's genotype has less common alleles or alleles not found in strong linkage disequilibrium), and (2) the patient's disease status may not afford the time for a lengthy search. In both of these clinical situations, understanding the limits of HLA mismatching is of paramount importance. As more information becomes available on tolerable mismatches, relaxation of HLA donor selection criteria may be possible so that suitable donors are available for all patients in need of a transplant.

From the published literature, five major concepts of unrelated donor HLA matching have emerged from retrospective analysis of transplant populations worldwide: (1) class I and class II allodeterminants both confer biologically important effects after transplantation; (2) alleles defined by high-resolution HLA typing methods are functionally relevant; (3) the total number of HLA mismatches is a determinant of posttransplant outcome; (4) residues of the class I and II molecule that are involved in peptide binding or T-cell receptor contact may define permissibility of a mismatch; and (5) the tolerability of an HLA mismatch may be influenced by non-HLA factors, including stage of the disease at the time of transplantation.

HLA Class I and II: Classical Transplantation Genes

Class I HLA-A, -C and -B and class II HLA-DR alleles predict engraftment outcome.[79,88,92,99,105,107,111] In one of the first descriptions of graft failure in class I mismatched unrelated transplantation, cytotoxic T lymphocyte clones capable of recognizing a mismatch between HLA-B*4402 and HLA-B*4403 were uncovered.[111] HLA-C mismatching was identified as a risk factor for graft failure in chronic myeloid leukemia unrelated donor hematopoietic stem cell transplantation,[99] and subsequently shown to be related to the total number of class I mismatches as well as whether the mismatch involved an HLA-C antigen or HLA-C allele.[107]

Early studies uncovered class II allele mismatching as an important risk factor for acute graft-versus-host disease.[87,89,94,96,97,101,106] HLA class I allele differences may also evoke donor antihost responses that may correlate with the development of acute graft-versus-host disease. Donor-derived cytotoxic T lymphocytes have been shown to recognize a disparity in the recipient HLA-B allele.[112] With the availability of allele typing for HLA-A, -B and -C, recent studies have demonstrated the importance of class I disparity in graft-versus-host disease risk.[92,103,108] The Japan Marrow Donor Program (JMDP) published the first large study describing the effect of class I alleles on graft-versus-host disease risk.[92] HLA-A and HLA-C allele disparities were each independent risk factors for severe acute graft-versus-host disease; interestingly, no contribution from class II was found. In a recent update of the JMDP experience, HLA-A, -C, -B, and -DRB1 were each found to be independent risk factors for grades III–IV acute graft-versus-host disease.[108] In a new analysis by the National Marrow Donor Program, adverse effects of HLA-A, -B, -C, and -DRB1 mismatching on graft-versus-host disease and survival were observed.[103] Class I mismatches had deleterious effects similar to DRB1 mismatches with respect to risk of grades III–IV acute graft-versus-host disease and mortality.

HLA-DP remains an enigma. Its role as a classical transplantation alloantigen has been shown in some studies,[100,104,106] but not in others.[103,108] Retrospective examination of HLA-DP has required very large numbers of donor-recipient pairs because more than 80% of HLA-A, -B, -DRB1, and -DQB1–matched unrelated donor pairs are mismatched for HLA-DP. Analysis of HLA-DPB1 indicates increased risks associated with two-DPB1 allele mismatching compared to one-DPB1 mismatching in HLA-A, -B, -C, -DRB1, and -DQB1–matched pairs,[100,104,106] particularly in the polymorphic DPB1 exon 2. A recent analysis employed donor alloreactive T-cell clones to identify permissive and nonpermissive HLA-DP epitopes.[113] The authors retrospectively evaluated 118 transplant patients who were categorized according to their DPB1 alleles in this fashion, and demonstrated that nonpermissive HLA-DPB1 mismatches were associated with increased risks of acute graft-versus-host disease and transplant-related mortality. Taken together, if HLA-DPB1 typing and matching is attempted, the clinical challenge is the relative lack of HLA-DPB1–identical donors despite comprehensive matching for other class I and II genes. When the search process identifies several potential HLA-A, -C, -B, -DR, and -DQ–matched donors, and when the patient's clinical course affords sufficient time to evaluate donor compatibility, then prospective evaluation of potential donors for HLA-DP may be considered.

Allele and Antigen Effects: Alleles Confer Clinical Significance

The location and the number of amino acid residues mismatched in class I molecules encoded by HLA alleles has been shown to define risk of graft failure specifically in regions involved in either peptide binding or T-cell receptor contact.[107] Among donor-recipient pairs mismatched for a single allele, graft failure occurred in 1 of 2 homozygous recipients and in none of 47 heterozygous recipients ($P = .04$). Among pairs mismatched for a single antigen, graft failure occurred in 4 of 5 homozygous recipients and in 7 of 51 heterozygous recipients ($P = .004$). These data suggest that multiple mismatches for residues that affect peptide binding and T-cell receptor contact might have been instrumental in evoking T-cell responses that led to graft failure in these patients.

In a large retrospective study of 1874 pairs typed for HLA-A, -B, -C, -DRB1, -DQB1, and -DPB1 alleles, adverse effects on transplant outcome were measured for HLA-A, -B, -C, and -DRB1.[103] A worse outcome was observed among antigen-mismatched pairs than among antigen-matched but allele-mismatched pairs. However, when allele mismatches at HLA-A, -B, -C, and -DRB1 were considered together, the risks of acute graft-versus-host disease and mortality were each increased.

In a second retrospective analysis, risks associated with allele versus antigen mismatches were determined.[109] Using matched low-risk patients (chronic myeloid leukemia transplanted in chronic phase within 2 years of diagnosis) as the reference group, the hazard of mortality was statistically significantly increased among patients with a single allele mismatch or a single antigen mismatch compared to patients with matches. This suggests that allele and antigen mismatches have similar effects on mortality.

Relationship of the Number of HLA Mismatches to Risk of Graft Failure and Graft-Versus-Host Disease

The risks of graft failure, graft-versus-host disease, and mortality increase in parallel with the number of HLA disparities. The JMDP examined the impact of allele disparity on engraftment in 1298 patients.[108] The overall incidence of graft failure increased with increasing numbers of mismatched HLA loci (1.7% failure in matched transplants; 4.8%, 4.1%, and 4.8% in HLA-A/B, HLA-C, and HLA-DR/DQ single-locus incompatible transplants, respectively; 10.4%, 8.9%, and 6% in HLA-A/B plus -C, HLA-A/B plus -DR/DQ, and HLA-C plus -DR/DQ two-locus incompatible transplants, respectively; and 10.6% in three-locus incompatible transplants). In a study by the Seattle program, the dose effect of allele mismatches was evaluated in 300 patients who underwent unrelated donor hematopoietic stem cell transplantation for the treatment of chronic myeloid leukemia.[91] A single allele mismatch at HLA-A or -B or -C did not increase the risk of graft failure compared to matched recipients (2%); however, multiple HLA-A, -B, and/or -C allele mismatches were associated with a 29% incidence of graft failure.

Graft-versus-host disease and mortality increase with increasing numbers of class I and II mismatches between the donor and recipient.[91,92,103,106,108,110] This effect is observed not only with two or more class I mismatches among class II–matched transplants, but also among class I–matched transplants mismatched for two or more class

II alleles, and transplants mismatched for combinations of two or more class I plus class II alleles. Class I disparities are a risk factor for graft-versus-host disease; HLA-C disparity in the presence of mismatching at any other HLA locus (class I and/or class II) is associated with significantly increased incidence of grades II–IV graft-versus-host disease compared to matched, HLA-A/B mismatched, HLA-C mismatched, or HLA-DR/DQ mismatches.[108,109]

Permissive and Nonpermissive Mismatches

With the availability of complete sequence information on donor and recipient pairs, it is now feasible to link mismatching at specific nucleotide positions, and the putative amino acid residues or epitopes of the molecule, to define clinically relevant epitopes and thereby establish "safe" or permissible combinations of mismatches.[102,107,113] For instance, substitutions at residue 116 a site participating in peptide binding (residue P9 of the peptide) have been found to be associated with a significantly increased risk of graft-versus-host disease and transplant-related mortality.[102] Ongoing research is defining epitopes of the HLA-DP molecule important to clinical outcome,[113] provides an alternative approach, and may relieve the need to match the entire exon 2 of DPB1.

Non-HLA Variables of Clinical Importance

The relationship between HLA mismatching, disease stage, and outcome after unrelated hematopoietic stem cell transplantation has been evaluated recently by the Seattle program in order to define the limits of HLA mismatching.[109] Among 948 patients who received a T-cell–replete unrelated donor transplant after myeloablative conditioning and the combination of cyclosporine/methotrexate as postgrafting immunosuppression, a single allele or antigen mismatch was found to confer a significantly increased risk of mortality for low-risk patients (chronic myeloid leukemia in chronic phase transplanted within 2 years of diagnosis). This effect was not present in higher risk patients. These results demonstrate that, when a fully matched donor is not available, higher risk patients may benefit from earlier transplantation from a mismatched donor and avoid the risk of disease progression during a prolonged search for a fully matched donor. As more information on the importance of non-HLA factors in shaping the permissibility of HLA mismatching becomes available, future patients should benefit from a tailored approach to their transplant, which would include not only the match of the potential donor, but also the timing of the transplant and the specific transplant regimens used for conditioning and immunosuppression.

ROLE OF MINOR HLA ANTIGENS AND KIRS

This chapter has focused on the classical class I and II *HLA* genes and their central role in the immune response in the transplant model. The study of the major histocompatibility complex in host-versus-graft and graft-versus-host allorecognition in transplantation would not be complete without consideration of *minor histocompatibility antigens* and the *killer cell immunoglobulin-like receptors* (KIRs). Although it is beyond the scope of this chapter to provide an in-depth review of these disciplines, an overview of current topics is presented below and a bibliography is included in the Suggested Reading list.

Minor Histocompatibility Antigens

Minor histocompatibility antigens are encoded by genes outside the major histocompatibility complex and are endogenous polymorphic peptides that are recognized by T cells in a major histocompatibility complex–restricted manner. In HLA-matched sibling transplantation, there is no major HLA disparity in the recipient. However, graft-versus-host disease can develop as a result of donor T-cell recognition of different recipient-derived peptides that are bound to the HLA molecules of recipient antigen-presenting cells. Although the genes that encode minor histocompatibility antigens are much less polymorphic than the classical *HLA* genes, the total number of minor histocompatibility antigen–encoding loci is predicted to be large.[114]

Several minor histocompatibility antigens have been identified.[115–124] One such antigen, termed HA-1, has been investigated in HLA-identical sibling transplants and shown to correlate with risk of acute graft-versus-host disease in some patient populations[116] but not others.[125] The CD31 platelet–endothelial cell adhesion molecule was found to be associated with an increased risk of graft-versus-host disease among patients receiving hematopoietic stem cell transplantation from HLA-identical sibling donors in some series[126,127] but not in others.[128] The clinical applications of minor histocompatibility antigens include leveraging donor antihost recognition as a means to induce graft-versus-leukemia alloreactivity.[129–133] At this time, prospective typing and matching of potential unrelated donors for minor histocompatibility antigens might be advantageous for transplant outcome; however, it has practical limitations and may reduce the number of available donors for many patients.[134]

Killer Cell Immunoglobulin-like Receptors

The killer cell immunoglobulin-like receptors (KIRs) have recently been elucidated.[135] KIRs are a family of inhibitory and activating receptors expressed on most NK cells and subpopulations of T cells. KIR genes are encoded on human chromosome 19 and thus segregate independently of the *HLA* genes on chromosome 6. KIR haplotypes and genotypes can differ in their gene content, in the number of activating and inhibitory receptors, and in the allelic polymorphism in ethnically and racially diverse populations.[136–141]

Inhibitory KIR receptors interact with class I molecules; the critical points of interaction are the amino acid residues at positions 77 and 80 of HLA-C, and the Bw4 epitope of HLA-B molecules. Because *KIR* genes and *HLA* genes segregate independently, matched unrelated donor-recipient pairs are predicted to be KIR mismatched. Studies in related and unrelated transplants have demonstrated that lack of expression of the correct inhibitory HLA class I ligands by the recipient can trigger donor NK cell alloreactivity and thereby lead to killing of recipient cells, including leukemic cells. If donor NK cells can destroy patient antigen-presenting cells, the target of graft-versus-host disease is removed. Likewise, if donor NK cells can destroy residual patient tumor cells, then this should lead to reduced posttransplant relapse. Based on the patient's HLA-C genotype at residues 77 and 80 and presence of Bw4, it is feasible to predict the pattern of donor KIR recognition and therefore theoretically possible to determine whether potential unrelated donors are KIR matched (undesirable because the donor NK cells are not activated) or KIR mismatched (desirable because donor NK cells kill patient's malignant cells).

In a study of patients who underwent T-cell–depleted haploidentical mismatched transplantation for high-risk acute myeloid leukemia or acute lymphoblastic leukemia, acute myeloid leukemia patients transplanted from KIR-mismatched donors had significantly improved 5-year survival compared to patients who received KIR-matched transplants.[142] KIR mismatching was associated with no graft failure, no acute graft-versus-host disease, and a 0% five-year probability of relapse, whereas KIR matching was an independent risk factor for poor transplant outcome. Patients carrying the diagnosis of acute lymphoblastic leukemia were not protected against relapse with the use of KIR-mismatched donors. The patients in this study received T-cell–depleted grafts, a high CD34-positive cell dose, and no postgrafting immunosuppression, a regimen that promotes rapid NK recovery. Donor-recipient KIR genotype differences have been correlated with increased risk of acute graft-versus-host disease after related or unrelated hematopoietic stem cell transplantation.[143] In HLA-matched sibling transplantation, patients homozygous for the HLA-C group 2 epitope had lower survival compared to patients who were homozygous for the HLA-C group 1 epitope, particularly when the donor had the *KIR2DS2* activating gene.[144]

However, in other studies of T-cell–replete transplants receiving postgrafting immunosuppression, no protective effects of KIR ligand mismatching were found.[109,145] As a larger, ethnically diverse transplant experience with T-cell–replete and T-cell–depleted allogeneic transplantation becomes available, it is anticipated that the clinical effects of the HLA-KIR axis to lower posttransplant relapse and graft-versus-host disease will become evident.

CONCLUSIONS

The safety and efficacy of unrelated hematopoietic stem cell transplantation are optimal when the recipient and donor are HLA matched, and when the patient's disease is under control at the time of transplantation. Because most patients do not have HLA-matched donors, and many patients have high-risk disease, more information on the tolerability of HLA mismatching is needed in order for all patients to benefit from unrelated hematopoietic stem cell transplantation. Permissible mismatches include HLA molecules that mediate host-versus-graft and graft-versus-host allorecognition by T cells, and class I molecules that serve as ligands for NK-mediated recognition of host tumor and antigen-presenting cells. Future applications of minor histocompatibility antigens include induction of graft-versus-leukemia alloreactivity to lower posttransplant relapse.

CURRENT CONTROVERSIES & FUTURE CONSIDERATIONS

Human Leukocyte Antigen and Transplantation

- Despite matching for HLA-A, -B, -C, -DRB1, and -DQB1, patients experience higher risk of graft-versus-host disease after unrelated donor transplantation compared to HLA-matched sibling transplantation. What is the role for minor histocompatibility antigens? Are there other genes that play a role in graft-versus-host disease?
- Donor disparity for HLA-DPB1 may increase post-transplant complications. Are there approaches to matching for this locus that would increase the pool of available donors without increasing the search time?
- The tolerability of HLA mismatching may be influenced by nongenetic factors, including the stage of disease at the time the transplant is performed. For high-risk patients, how can the donor search process be optimized to increase their chances of a successful transplant?
- Are there approaches to identify tolerable mismatches based on location of the mismatched residue in the HLA molecule? Based on the amino acid substitution?
- What is the impact of HLA mismatches with different conditioning and immunosuppressive regimens? Are the HLA effects that have been observed in patients undergoing myeloablative conditioning the same for patients conditioned with nonmyeloablative regimens? Are the HLA effects the same for T-cell–replete and T-cell–deleted grafts?
- What is the role of the NK-KIR gene family in host-versus-graft and graft-versus-host recognition?
- What is the role of minor histocompatibility antigens in inducing graft-versus-leukemia effects to lower posttransplant relapse?

Suggested Readings*

Beatty PG, Boucher KM, Mori M, Milford EL: Probability of finding HLA-mismatched related or unrelated marrow or cord blood donors. Hum Immunol 61:834–840, 2000.

Bleakley M, Riddell SR: Molecules and mechanisms of the graft-versus-leukemia effect. Nature Rev Cancer 4:371–380, 2004.

Flomenberg N, Baxter-Lowe LA, Confer D, et al: Impact of HLA class I and class II high resolution matching on outcomes of unrelated donor bone marrow transplantation: HLA-C mismatching is associated with a strong adverse effect on transplant outcome. Blood 104:1923–1930, 2004.

Lanier LL: Natural killer cell receptor signaling. Curr Opin Immunol 15:308–314, 2003.

Parham P, Adams EH, Arnett KL: The origins of HLA-A, B, C polymorphism. Immunol Rev 143:141–180, 1995.

Full references for this chapter can be found on accompanying CD-ROM.

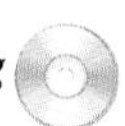

CHAPTER 103

Cytogenetics/Fluorescent In Situ Hybridization

Katrin M. Carlson, PhD, and Michelle M. Le Beau, PhD

KEY POINTS

Cytogenetics/Fluorescent In Situ Hybridization

- Recurring numerical and structural chromosomal abnormalities are associated with distinct subtypes of leukemias, which have unique morphologic, immunophenotypical, and clinical features, such as response to therapy.
- Cytogenetic and genetic abnormalities are better predictors of clinical behavior and outcome than is morphology alone; the World Health Organization has incorporated cytogenetic data into a new classification schema for acute myeloid leukemia.
- Cytogenetic analysis should be requested for any patient with a suspected or confirmed hematologic malignant disease. Cytogenetic results can aid in the diagnosis and subclassification of the disease and in the selection of the appropriate therapy. In addition, chromosomal abnormalities serve as a biologic marker to monitor response to therapy or to detect residual disease.
- Fluorescent in situ hybridization (FISH) provides increased sensitivity over cytogenetic analysis, because chromosomal abnormalities can be detected in samples that appear to be normal by conventional cytogenetic analysis.
- In chronic lymphocytic leukemia and multiple myeloma, FISH should be performed in conjunction with cytogenetic analysis in all cases.
- In other diseases, FISH is most powerful when the analysis is targeted toward abnormalities that are associated with a particular disease or are known to occur in a particular patient's tumor. Cytogenetic analysis should be performed at the time of diagnosis to identify the chromosomal abnormalities in an individual patient's malignant cells. FISH may be useful in detecting minimal residual disease or early relapse and to assess the efficacy of therapeutic regimens.

INTRODUCTION

Although chromosomes were first visualized through the microscope over 100 years ago, technical limitations prohibited the accurate determination of the chromosome number for many years. In 1923, Painter reported that the chromosome number in humans was 48, and this remained the paradigm for over 30 years. It was not until Tjio and Levan combined the use of colchicine to arrest cells in mitosis (1937) and hypotonic treatment to increase cell volume (1952) that the human chromosome number was established unequivocally to be 46.[1] In 1959, the first chromosome abnormality in a human disease was described in patients with Down syndrome and, shortly thereafter, in 1960, Nowell and Hungerford described an unusually small G-group chromosome (the Philadelphia [Ph] chromosome) in cells from patients with chronic myelogenous leukemia.[2] Prior to 1971, chromosomes were visualized by solid staining, which did not allow for the definitive identification of each individual chromosome. Rather, the chromosomes were organized into seven groups, A through G. A revolutionary advancement in the field of cytogenetic analysis was the introduction by Caspersson and colleagues of a staining method that resulted in a unique pattern of horizontal bands along the length of each chromosome.[3] Using this new banding method, Rowley reported in 1973 that the Philadelphia chromosome was the product of a reciprocal translocation between chromosome 9 and chromosome 22.[4] The identification of this chromosome abnormality led to the search for similar abnormalities in other types of hematologic malignant diseases. Other specific abnormalities soon were found to be associated with certain types of leukemia and lymphoma, and cytogenetic analysis of human tumors became one of the most rapidly progressing and exciting areas of the laboratory sciences and of cancer research.

In hematologic malignant diseases, specific numerical and structural chromosomal abnormalities are associated with distinct subtypes of leukemia or lymphoma that have unique morphologic, immunophenotypic, and clinical

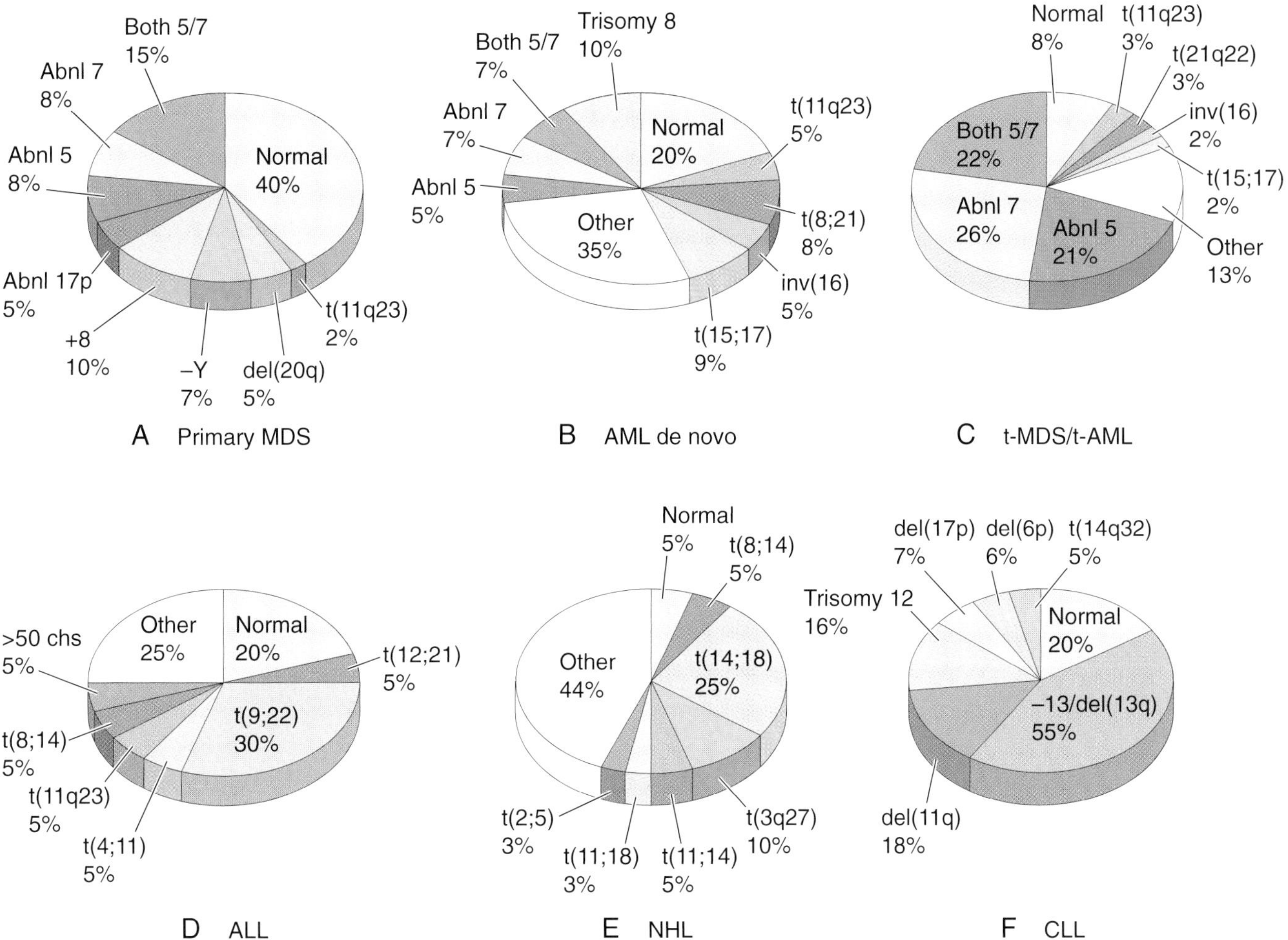

Figure 103–1. Frequency of recurring abnormalities in hematologic malignant diseases. *A*, Primary myelodysplastic syndromes. *B*, Acute myeloid leukemia de novo. *C*, Therapy-related myelodysplastic syndrome/acute myeloid leukemia. *D*, Acute lymphoblastic leukemia. *E*, Non-Hodgkin's lymphoma. *F*, Chronic lymphocytic leukemia.

features, such as response to therapy (Fig. 103–1). The recurring chromosomal abnormalities result in altered function of cellular oncogenes or tumor suppressor genes; thus, chromosomal abnormalities represent one class of genetic change involved in the pathogenesis and progression of human tumors. In the most recent classification system of tumors of hematopoietic and lymphoid tissues, the World Health Organization (WHO) has recognized that cytogenetic abnormalities are often better predictors of clinical behavior and outcome than is morphology alone and, therefore, have incorporated genetic data into the classification scheme.[5] The new classification of acute myeloid leukemia includes acute myeloid leukemia with t(8;21), inv(16) or t(16;16), t(15;17), and 11q23 abnormalities, and clearly illustrates the major role of cytogenetic analysis in the diagnosis and subclassification of a hematologic neoplasm, in the selection of the appropriate therapy, and in monitoring the effects of therapy. Here we review cytogenetic methods, such as banding, fluorescent in situ hybridization (FISH), and spectral karyotyping (SKY) analysis, and outline how these techniques can be applied to the diagnosis and treatment of neoplastic disease.

CONVENTIONAL CYTOGENETIC ANALYSIS

Specimen Collection

Detailed methods for the cytogenetic analysis of hematologic malignant diseases have been described.[6] Cytogenetic studies are performed on spontaneously dividing cells that are typically cultured for short periods (24–72 hours). The dividing cells are collected by arresting them in metaphase using a spindle fiber inhibitor, usually colcemid. A hypotonic solution is added to increase cell volume, which aids in chromosome spreading, and the cells are preserved using a methanol–acetic acid fixative. The cell suspension is applied to microscope slides, which ruptures the cell membrane and spreads the chromosomes, followed by histologic staining (Fig. 103–2). Conventional cytogenetic studies can be performed on almost any tissue containing actively dividing cells. Bone marrow is chosen for cytogenetic studies of both chronic and acute leukemias, but peripheral blood, pleural fluid, or effusions also serve if dividing leukemia cells are present. Lymph node or tumor mass biopsies are pre-

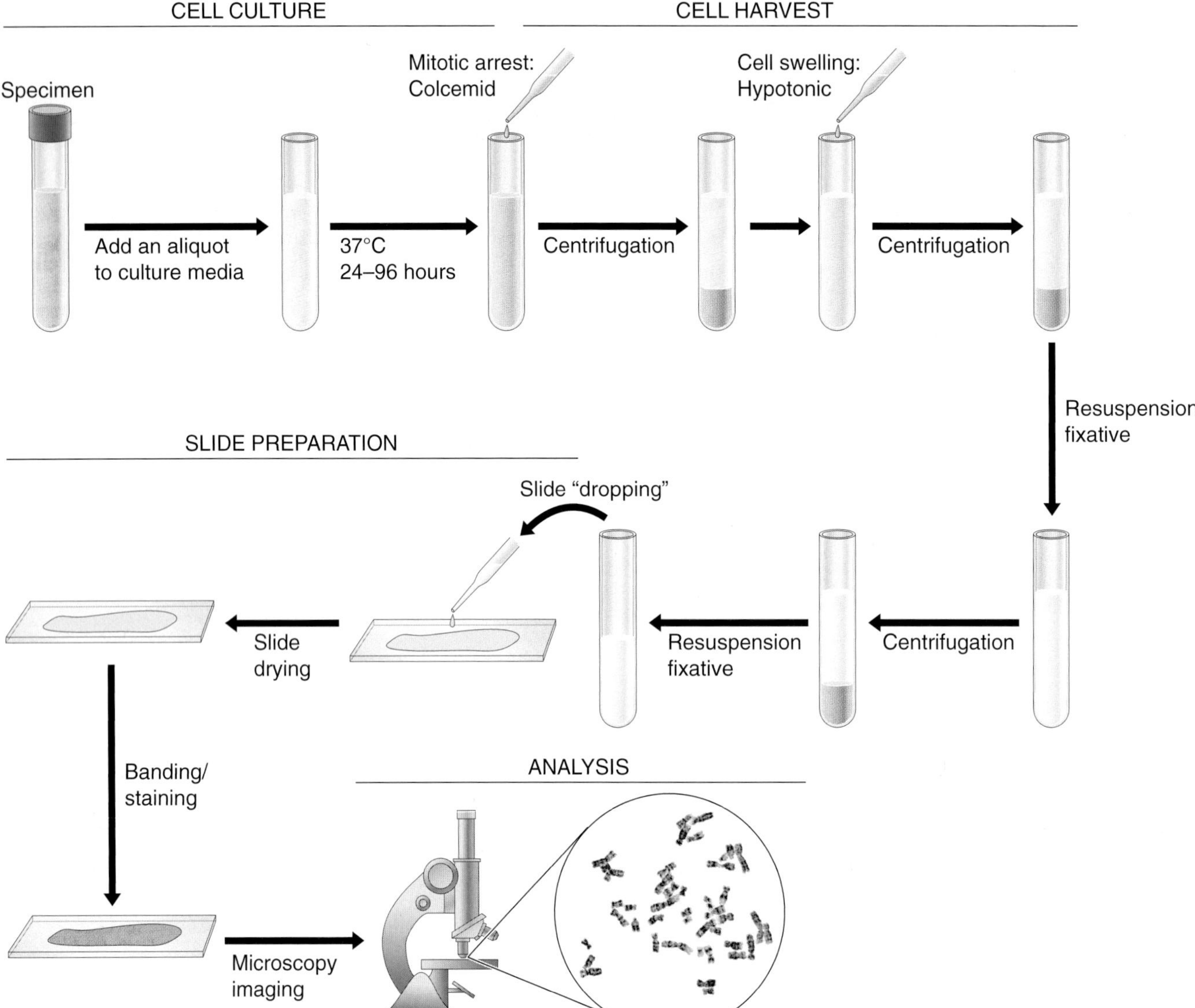

Figure 103–2. Schematic diagram outlining the steps involved in cytogenetic analysis. ***Cell Culture:*** An aliquot of the specimen is added to culture medium containing serum and antibiotics. Culturing methods vary, but typically involve 24- to 96-hour incubations at 37°C in a 5% CO_2/95% air atmosphere. ***Harvest:*** The harvest procedure is a multistep process that begins by arresting the cells in metaphase using a spindle fiber inhibitor such as colcemid. Cell cycle arrest is followed by exposure to a hypotonic solution, which increases cell volume, allowing the chromosomes to disperse within the cytoplasmic membrane. Fixative (3:1 methanol/acetic acid) is then added, which removes water from the cells, extract lipids and proteins from cell membranes and cytoplasm, and enhances the morphology of the chromosomes. ***Slide Preparation:*** Slides are prepared by placing a drop of fixative containing the cells in suspension on a microscope slide. As the fixative dries, the surface tension flattens the cells and the chromosomes spread out. When the cytoplasmic membrane breaks, chromosomes may spread too far and result in a hypodiploid metaphase spread. Random loss of chromosomes as a result of the technical aspects of slide preparation is commonly observed, and should be interpreted appropriately. Once the metaphase cells have dried, the chromosomes are stained so that they can be viewed with a brightfield microscope. A number of banding methods are available; the most commonly used is an enzymatic treatment with trypsin followed by staining with Giemsa, resulting in the "G" banding pattern. ***Analysis:*** Analysis typically involves the evaluation of 20 metaphase chromosome spreads using brightfield microscopy and digital imaging.

ferred for lymphoma studies. The analysis of bone marrow samples from patients with lymphoma is not optimal, even when marrow involvement has been confirmed by morphologic analysis, because dividing lymphoma cells are usually not identified. Tissue should be collected in cell culture media with heparin to prevent clotting and with antibiotics to avoid bacterial contamination, and transported to the laboratory immediately. EDTA and sodium citrate affect cell viability and should not be used for the collection of cells intended to undergo mitosis (Box 103–1).

Box 103–1. Specimen Collection Guidelines

- Tissues processed for hematologic malignancies: 1–5 mL of bone marrow aspirate, 0.5–2.0 cm of bone core biopsy, 10–15 mL of peripheral blood, approximately 0.5–1 cm^3 of lymph node biopsy. Ascites fluid, pleural fluid, and other fluids can also be used. The volume required will depend on the cellularity.
- Collect the specimen using sterile techniques in a syringe coated with preservative-free sodium heparin.*
- Rotate the syringe if a previous aspirate was obtained before aspirating a second sample for cytogenetic analysis.
- Transfer the specimen to a sterile 15-mL conical centrifuge tube containing 5 mL culture medium (RPMI 1640, 100 units sodium heparin, 100 units/mL penicillin, 100 μg/mL streptomycin). If culture medium is not available, substitute with sterile saline. For tissue specimens, substitute with sterile saline.
- Transport the specimen to the cytogenetics laboratory as quickly as possible.†

*The use of preservative-free heparin is essential, because preservatives in heparin suppress cell growth. The use of Vacutainer tubes should be avoided because the heparin contains preservatives.
†To avoid loss of cell viability, it is critical that the specimen be transported at room temperature to the cytogenetics laboratory without delay. Overnight shipment of specimens frequently results in loss of cell viability, and most laboratories experience a high proportion (25–50%) of inadequate analyses using such specimens. Specimens from lymphoid malignancies are particularly susceptible to loss of viability during shipping.

Banding and Nomenclature

The first chromosomal banding technique (Q-banding) was described in 1970, allowing investigators to distinguish each human chromosome and to identify rearranged chromosomes.[3] Different methods are available for chromosome staining. The most widely used involves Giemsa stain and produces the "G" banding pattern or G bands. A band is defined as a part of a chromosome that is distinguishable from its adjacent segments by appearing darker or lighter with one or more banding techniques. Once banded, chromosomes are identified by three major features: chromosome length, centromere position, and banding pattern. The written description of the chromosomal complement of a cell is termed the *karyotype*. The International System of Human Cytogenetic Nomenclature (ISCN 1995), developed from several international conferences, allows results to be expressed consistently.[7] In this system, abnormalities are described with abbreviated terms for the rearrangement, followed by a numerical description of the chromosome(s), chromosome arm(s), and bands involved (Fig. 103–3). A glossary of the most commonly used terms to describe chromosomal abnormalities is given in Box 103–2.

Reporting and Interpretation of Results of Cytogenetic Analysis

A typical cytogenetic study includes the complete analysis of at least 20 banded metaphase cells. A full examination may not always be possible, depending on the cellularity, mitotic index, and quality of the specimen. An analysis of less than 20 cells is still informative if a clonal abnormality is detected. Cytogenetic evaluation should include the analysis of cells from more than one preparation, preferably two short-term cultures (for 24 and 48 hours). Direct preparations, in which metaphase cells are prepared without prior culturing in vitro, are less suitable. Genetic mutations accumulate during the progression of a normal cell to a malignant state. Therefore, multiple, related subpopulations of cells derived from a single progenitor may be present in any one specimen. A chromosomal abnormality is considered clonal if a structural abnormality or gain of a chromosome is identified in two or more cells. Chromosome loss can occur as a technical artifact during metaphase cell preparation; a loss of a chromosome is clonal when it occurs in three or more cells. The number of cells observed in each clone is listed after the clone description in brackets: [*n*]. The simplest clone is termed the *stemline*. The stemline is listed first, and related clones are listed in order of increasing complexity. To describe subclones, the term *idem* followed by any additional changes as compared to the stemline can be used; "idem" always refers to the abnormalities described in the stemline clone. This type of karyotypic progression is referred to as clonal evolution.

Applications of Conventional Cytogenetic Analysis

Cytogenetic analysis should be requested for any patient with a suspected or confirmed hematologic malignant disease for several reasons. First, because recurring chromosomal abnormalities are correlated with distinct subtypes of leukemia or lymphoma, cytogenetic results aid in diagnosis. Second, cytogenetic abnormalities also represent independent predictors of response to therapy and outcome. Third, any abnormality noted at the time of diagnosis can be used as a biologic marker to monitor the response to therapy or to detect residual disease in later specimens, and the absence of a biologic marker can be interpreted to represent a cytogenetic remission. Likewise, if the abnormal chromosome(s) is detected in a follow-up specimen, it is indicative of residual disease, relapse, or, in the case of karyotypic evolution, disease progression. Finally, in some cases, cytogenetic results can be used to select risk-adapted therapies that target the abnormal protein resulting from the cytogenetic rearrangement: all-trans retinoic acid for acute promyelocytic leukemia, and imatinib for chronic myeloid leukemia are examples.

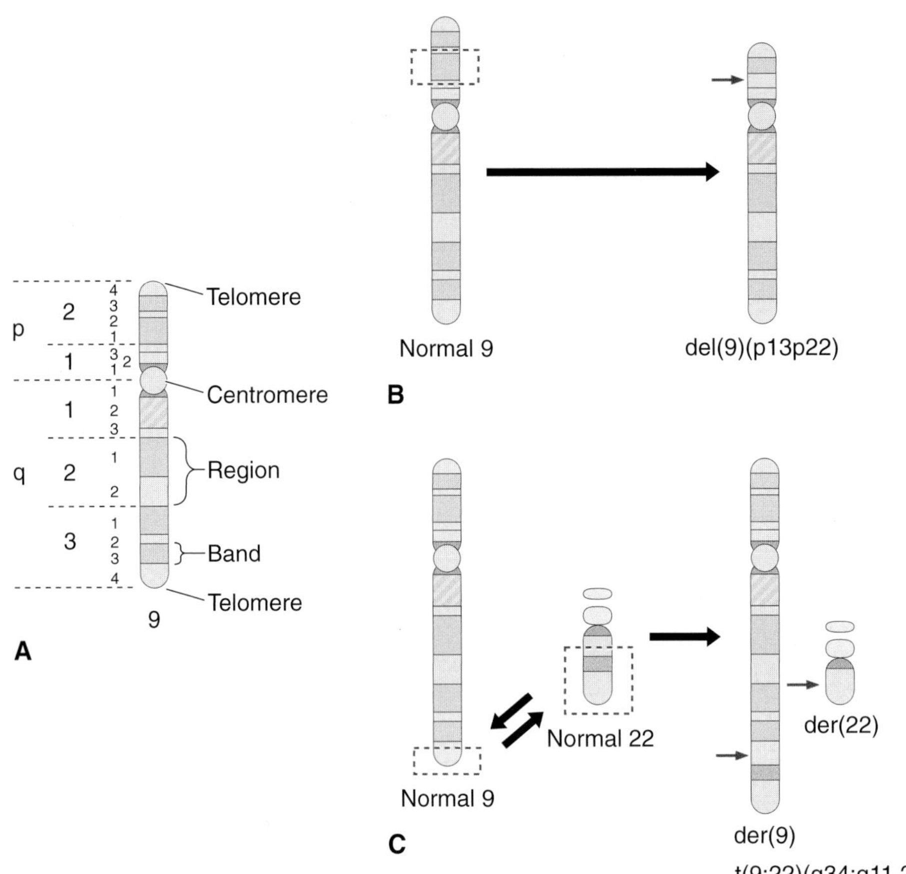

Figure 103–3. Schematic diagram illustrating a normal chromosome, and two recurring chromosomal abnormalities observed in human leukemias. ***A,*** Diagram of the banding pattern of a normal chromosome 9. Using the International System for Human Cytogenetic Nomenclature (ISCN 1995), each chromosome, chromosome arm, and band is uniquely identified with a detailed lettering and numbering system, resulting in a universal nomenclature system for describing chromosomal abnormalities.[7] The autosomes are numbered 1 to 22, with chromosome 1 being the largest and chromosome 22 the smallest; the sex chromosomes are designated as the X and Y chromosomes. Relative to the location of the centromere, the shorter portion of the chromosome is termed the *petite arm* or "p-arm" and the longer portion the "q-arm." By convention, chromosomes are oriented with the "p-arm" up and the "q-arm" down. Each chromosome arm is divided into regions that are bordered by prominent features, such as the centromere, telomere, or a distinct chromosome band. Regions are numbered in ascending order, with region 1 being closest to the centromere. Within each region, each band and subband is numbered sequentially; numbers increase as the distance from the centromere increases. The convention for designating a chromosome location identifies the involved chromosome, followed by the chromosome arm, region, band, and subband (if applicable). For example, the breakpoint of the t(9;22) in chronic myeloid leukemia is designated as 9q34 (chromosome 9, q arm, region 3, band 4). ***B,*** Diagram of the mechanism of an interstitial deletion of the short arm of chromosome 9, a common abnormality in acute lymphoblastic leukemia. Chromosome breaks occur in 9p13 and 9p22, and the intervening chromosomal segment is lost [del(9)(p13p22)]. ***C,*** Diagram of the mechanism of the reciprocal t(9;22)(q34;q11.2) in chronic myeloid leukemia. Breaks occur in bands q34 and q11.2 of chromosomes 9 and 22, respectively, followed by a reciprocal exchange of chromosomal material. This rearrangement results in the translocation of the *ABL* oncogene, normally located at 9q34, adjacent to the *BCR* gene on chromosome 22, giving rise to the fusion *BCR/ABL* gene, whose protein product plays a role in the transformation of hematopoietic cells.

FLUORESCENT IN SITU HYBRIDIZATION

Background and Theory

FISH is based on the same principle as Southern blot analysis, the ability of single-stranded DNA to anneal to complementary DNA. In the case of FISH, the target is the nuclear DNA of interphase cells, or the DNA of metaphase chromosomes affixed to microscope slides (Fig. 103–4). The test probe is labeled through incorporation of a fluorescently tagged reporter nucleotide. The test probe anneals to its complementary sequences on fixed metaphase chromosomes or interphase nuclei and is visualized by fluorescence microscopy as a brilliantly colored signal at the hybridization site. FISH can be performed using standard cytogenetic cell preparations, bone marrow or peripheral blood smears, or fixed and sectioned tissue.

FISH Probes

A variety of probes are used to detect chromosomal abnormalities by FISH (Table 103–1). In general, these

Box 103–2. Glossary of Cytogenetic Terminology

Aneuploidy—An abnormal chromosome number resulting from either gain or loss of chromosomes.

Banded chromosomes—Chromosomes with alternating dark and light segments caused by special stains or pretreatment of metaphase cells with enzymes before staining. Each chromosome pair has a unique pattern of bands.

Breakpoint—A specific site on a chromosome containing a DNA break that is involved in a structural rearrangement, such as a translocation or deletion.

Centromere—The constriction along the length of the chromosome that is the site of the spindle fiber attachment. The position of the centromere determines whether chromosomes are *metacentric* (X-shaped, e.g., chromosomes 1–3, 6–12, X, 16, 19, 20) or *acrocentric* (inverted V-shaped, e.g., chromosomes 13–15, 21, 22, Y). During mitosis, the two exact copies of the DNA in each chromosome are separated by shortening of the spindle fibers attached to opposite sides of the dividing cell.

Clone—In the cytogenetic sense, this is defined as two cells with the same additional or structurally rearranged chromosome or three cells with loss of the same chromosome.

Deletion—A segment of a chromosome is missing as the result of two breaks and loss of the intervening piece (interstitial deletion). Molecular studies of many recurring chromosomal deletions have shown that, in each case, the deletions were interstitial, rather than terminal (single break with loss of the terminal segment).

Diploid—Normal chromosome number and composition of chromosomes.

Haploid—Only one half the normal complement (i.e., 23 chromosomes).

Hyperdiploid—Additional chromosomes; therefore, the modal number is 47 or greater.

Hypodiploid—Loss of chromosomes with a modal number of 45 or less.

Inversion—Two breaks occur in the same chromosome with rotation of the intervening segment. If both breaks were on the same side of the centromere, it is called a *paracentric inversion*. If they were on opposite sides, it is called a *pericentric inversion*.

Isochromosome—A chromosome that consists of identical copies of one chromosome arm with loss of the other arm. Thus, an isochromosome for the long arm of chromosome 17 [i(17)(q10)] contains two copies of the long arm (separated by the centromere) with loss of the short arm.

Karyotype—Arrangement of chromosomes from a particular cell according to an internationally established system such that the largest chromosomes are first and the smallest ones are last. A normal female karyotype is described as 46,XX and a normal male karyotype is 46,XY. An *idiogram* is an idealized representation (diagram) of the chromosomes.

Pseudodiploid—A diploid number of chromosomes accompanied by structural chromosomal abnormalities.

Recurring Abnormality—A numerical or structural abnormality noted in multiple patients who have a similar neoplasm. Such abnormalities are characteristic or diagnostic of distinct subtypes of leukemia and lymphoma that have unique morphologic and/or immunophenotypic features. Recurring abnormalities represent genetic mutations that are involved in the pathogenesis of the corresponding diseases; many recurring abnormalities have prognostic significance.

Translocation—A break in at least two chromosomes with exchange of material. In a reciprocal translocation, there is no obvious loss of chromosomal material. Translocations are indicated by t; the chromosomes involved are noted in the first set of brackets and the breakpoints in the second set of brackets. The Ph translocation is t(9;22)(q34;q11.2).

Nomenclature Symbols

p—short arm

q—long arm

+—If before the chromosome, indicates a gain of a whole chromosome (e.g., +8).

−—If before the chromosome, indicates a loss of a whole chromosome (e.g., −7), and if after the chromosome, indicates loss of part of the chromosome (e.g., 5q−, loss of part of the long arm of chromosome 5).

?—Indicates uncertainty about the identity of the chromosome or band listed just after the ? symbol.

t—translocation

del—deletion

inv—inversion

i—isochromosome

mar—marker chromosome

r—ring chromosome

Modified from Rowley JD: Chromosome abnormalities in human cancer. *In* De Vita VT, Hellman S, Rosenberg S (eds): Practice and Principles of Oncology (ed 3). Philadelphia: JB Lippincott, 1991.

TABLE 103–1. FISH Probes to Detect Recurring Chromosomal Abnormalities

Disease[*]	Abnormality	Probe	Format[†]	Vendor[‡]
AML-M2	t(8;21)	*RUNX1/ETO*	Two-color dual fusion	Vysis
AML-M4Eo	inv(16)/t(16;16)	*CBFB*	Two-color break-apart	Vysis, Ventana
AML-M3	t(15;17)	*PML/RARA*	Two-color dual fusion	Vysis, Ventana
AML	t(11q23)	*MLL*	Two-color break-apart	Vysis
			Single color	Ventana
AML/MDS	−5/del(5q)	*EGR1/D5S23/D5S72*	Two-color deletion	Vysis
		CSF1R/D5S23/D5S72	Two-color deletion	Vysis
	−7/del(7q)	*D7S522/CEP7*	Two-color deletion	Vysis
		D7S486/CEP7	Two-color deletion	Vysis
	del(20q)	*D20S108*	Single color	Vysis
	+8	*CEP8*	Single color	Vysis; Cytocell, Ltd
CML	t(9;22)	*BCR/ABL*	Two-color single fusion	Vysis
		BCR/ABL ES	Two-color extra signal	Vysis
		BCR/ABL	Two-color dual fusion	Vysis
		MBCR/ABL	Two-color single fusion	Ventana
		BCR/ABL	Two-color dual fusion	Ventana
	+8	*CEP8*	Single color	Vysis; Cytocell, Ltd
	i(17q)	*HER2/CEP17*	Two color (17q/centromere)	Vysis, Ventana
ALL	t(12;21)	*TEL/AML1*	Two-color extra signal	Vysis
	t(11q23)	*MLL*	Two-color break-apart	Vysis
	t(8;14)	*IGH/MYC/CEP8*	Tricolor dual fusion	Vysis
	t(9;22)	*BCR/ABL* ES	Two-color extra signal	Vysis
		BCR/ABL	Two-color single fusion	Vysis
		BCR/ABL	Two-color dual fusion	Vysis
		MBCR/ABL	Two-color single fusion	Ventana
		mBCR/ABL	Two-color single fusion	Ventana
	del(9p)/t(9p)	*CDKN2A*(p16)/*CEP9*	Dual color	Vysis
CLL, myeloma	+12	*CEP12*	Single color	Vysis
	del(13q)	*D13S319*/13q34	Two color	Vysis
		RB1/13q34	Two color	Vysis
	del(11q)	*ATM*	Single color	Vysis
	−17/del(17p)	*TP53*	Single color	Vysis
	t(14q32)	*IGH*	Two-color break-apart	Vysis
Myeloma	t(4;14)	*IGH*/FGFR3	Two-color dual fusion	Vysis
	t(14;16)	IGH/*MAF*	Two-color dual fusion	Vysis
	Hyperdiploid	*D5S23/D5S721/CEP9/CEP15*	Three color	Vysis
NHL	t(11;18)	*BIRC3/MALT1*	Two-color dual fusion	Vysis
	t(14;18)	*IGH/BCL2*	Two-color dual fusion	Vysis
	t(8;14)	*IGH/MYC*	Two-color dual fusion	Vysis
	t(14q32)	*MYC*	Two-color break-apart	Vysis
		IGH	Two-color break-apart	Vysis
ALCL	t(2;5)	*ALK*	Two-color break-apart	Vysis
MCL, myeloma	t(11;14)	*CCND1/IGH*	Two-color dual fusion	Vysis
Miscellaneous				
Bone marrow transplants		*CEPX/CEPY*	Single color or two color	Vysis
Subtelomeric–each chromosomal arm			Single color	Vysis
			Two-color	Cytocell, Ltd

[*]ALCL, anaplastic large cell lymphoma; ALL, acute lymphoblastic leukemia; AML, acute myeloid leukemia; CLL, chronic lymphocytic leukemia; CML, chronic myeloid leukemia; MCL, mantle cell lymphoma; MDS, myelodysplastic syndrome; NHL, non-Hodgkin's lymphoma.

[†]In two-color break-apart probes, DNA sequences from the 5′ and 3′ regions of a single gene are labeled and detected with red and green fluorochromes. In the germline configuration, a yellow fusion signal is observed, whereas individual red and green signals are observed when the sequences are separated as a result of a translocation.

With two-color fusion probes, DNA sequences flanking the breakpoints of the involved genes are brought together to form either one (single-fusion probes) or two (dual-fusion probes) yellow fusion signal(s).

With the two-color, extra-signal probes, DNA sequences flanking the breakpoint on the partner chromosomes are brought together to form a fusion yellow signal; however, part of the DNA sequences recognized by one of the probes may remain at the original site, giving rise to an extra signal in a single color.

[‡]Vysis, Inc., Downers Grove, IL (*http://www.vysis.com*); Ventana Medical Systems, Tucson, AZ (*http://www.ventanamed.com*); Cytocell, Banbury, England (*http://www.cytocell.co.uk*).

FISH METHODS

PROBE LABELING

Probe DNA + Label → Probe

DENATURATION

DNA template Probe

HYBRIDIZATION

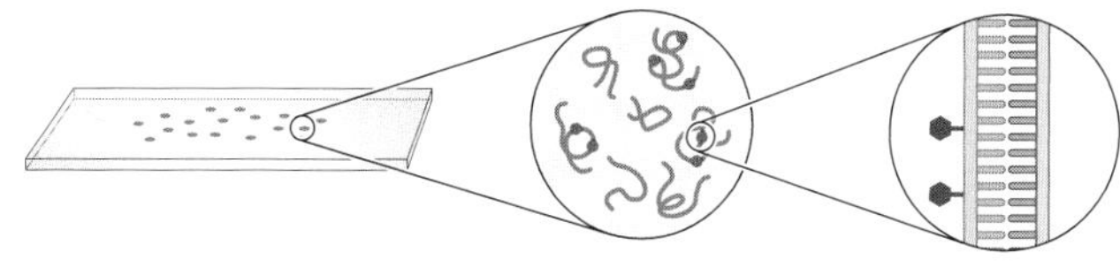

INTERPRETATION

Disomy Trisomy

Figure 103–4. Schematic diagram illustrating FISH (fluorescent in situ hybridization). A test probe is directly labeled through incorporation of fluorescently tagged nucleotides. To allow hybridization of complementary sequences, both the labeled test probe and the cellular DNA are denatured by heating in a formamide solution to form single-stranded DNA. The hybridization solution containing the denatured, labeled test probe is applied to the microscope slide, covered with a coverslip, and sealed. The hybridization proceeds for 4–24 hours at 37°–40°C. Subsequently, the coverslip is removed and the unbound probe is removed through multiple washes in a sodium chloride/sodium citrate solution. Analysis is performed using fluorescence microscopy.

probes can be divided into three groups: (1) probes that identify a specific chromosome structure, (2) probes that hybridize to multiple chromosomal sequences, and (3) probes that hybridize to unique DNA sequences.[8]

Centromere Probes

Examples of probes that hybridize to a specific chromosome structure include α- and β-satellite probes. These probes represent tandemly repeated DNA sequences that flank the centromeres of human chromosomes. In most instances, these sequences are distinct, such that an α-satellite probe derived from one chromosome will hybridize to that chromosome only. At present, specific probes are available for chromosomes 1–4, 6–12, 15–18, and 20, as well as the X and Y chromosomes. Hybridization of chromosome-specific repetitive sequence probes is particularly suitable for the detection of monosomy, trisomy, and other aneuploidies in both leukemia and solid tumors (Fig. 103–5*E*).[9–11]

Chromosome Painting Probes

Chromosome painting probes utilize cloned DNA libraries derived from whole, flow-sorted human chromosomes.[12,13] After hybridization and detection, the result is the fluorescent staining or "painting" of an entire chromosome. Chromosome-specific painting probes are available for each of the human chromosomes. They are particularly useful in characterizing marker chromosomes (a rearranged chromosome of unknown origin), or additional material of unknown origin translocated to other chromosomes.

Locus-Specific Probes

Probes that hybridize to unique DNA sequences are usually genomic clones, which vary in size depending on the nature of the cloning vector. Probes in this group are particularly useful for detecting structural rearrangements. Using multicolor FISH, recurring translocations can be identified in interphase or metaphase cells by using genomic probes that are derived from the breakpoints.[14,15] For example, a locus-specific probe for the *BCR* gene at 22q11.2 detected with a green fluorochrome, and a locus-specific probe for the *ABL* gene at 9q34 detected with a red fluorochrome, will appear as a bright yellow spot (the combination of green and red fluorochromes) in leukemia cells containing the *BCR/ABL* fusion gene resulting from the t(9;22)(q34;q11.2) (Fig. 103–5*A* and *B*). The same strategy currently serves to detect the *PML/RARA* product of t(15;17) and *TEL/AML1* (*ETV6/RUNX1*) fusion gene produced by the t(12;21) translocation (see Table 103–1).

FISH Strategies

Dual-Color/Single-Fusion Probes

Different strategies have been developed for the detection of recurring translocations in interphase cells, each with variable sensitivity. The selection of a particular probe configuration depends on the application. In the initial method, a *single fusion signal* is detected by the hybridization of dual-color locus-specific probes to their target sequences at the junction of the translocation breakpoints. In the example of t(9;22), the directly labeled probe contains the 5′ portion of the *BCR* gene at 22q11.2 (Spectrum Green), and the 3′ portion of the *ABL* gene (Spectrum Orange) at 9q34 (LSI bcr/abl dual-color probe; Vysis, Inc., Downers Grove, IL). In cells with t(9;22), one green and one red signal are observed on the normal homologues, and a yellow fusion signal is seen on the Ph chromosome [der(22)t(9;22)] as a result of the translocation of the *ABL* sequences to chromosome 22. Probes of this type have a relatively high number of false-positive fusion signals (1.5–5.6%), because of the close proximity and random juxtaposition of target chromosomes in interphase nuclei. The sensitivity of single-fusion FISH probes is 5–10% (mean number of fusion signals in normal samples plus 2 standard deviations), thus limiting their utility for the detection of minimal residual disease.[8,16] Recent efforts have resulted in the generation of other probe strategies that have increased sensitivity, such as the dual-color/dual-fusion probes (described later).

Dual-Color/Extra-Signal Probe

The next generation of FISH probes are termed *extra-signal probes* (Vysis, Inc). Similar to single-fusion probes, extra-signal probes use DNA sequences flanking the breakpoints on the chromosomes to form a fusion yellow signal. However, in the example of the t(9;22), one of

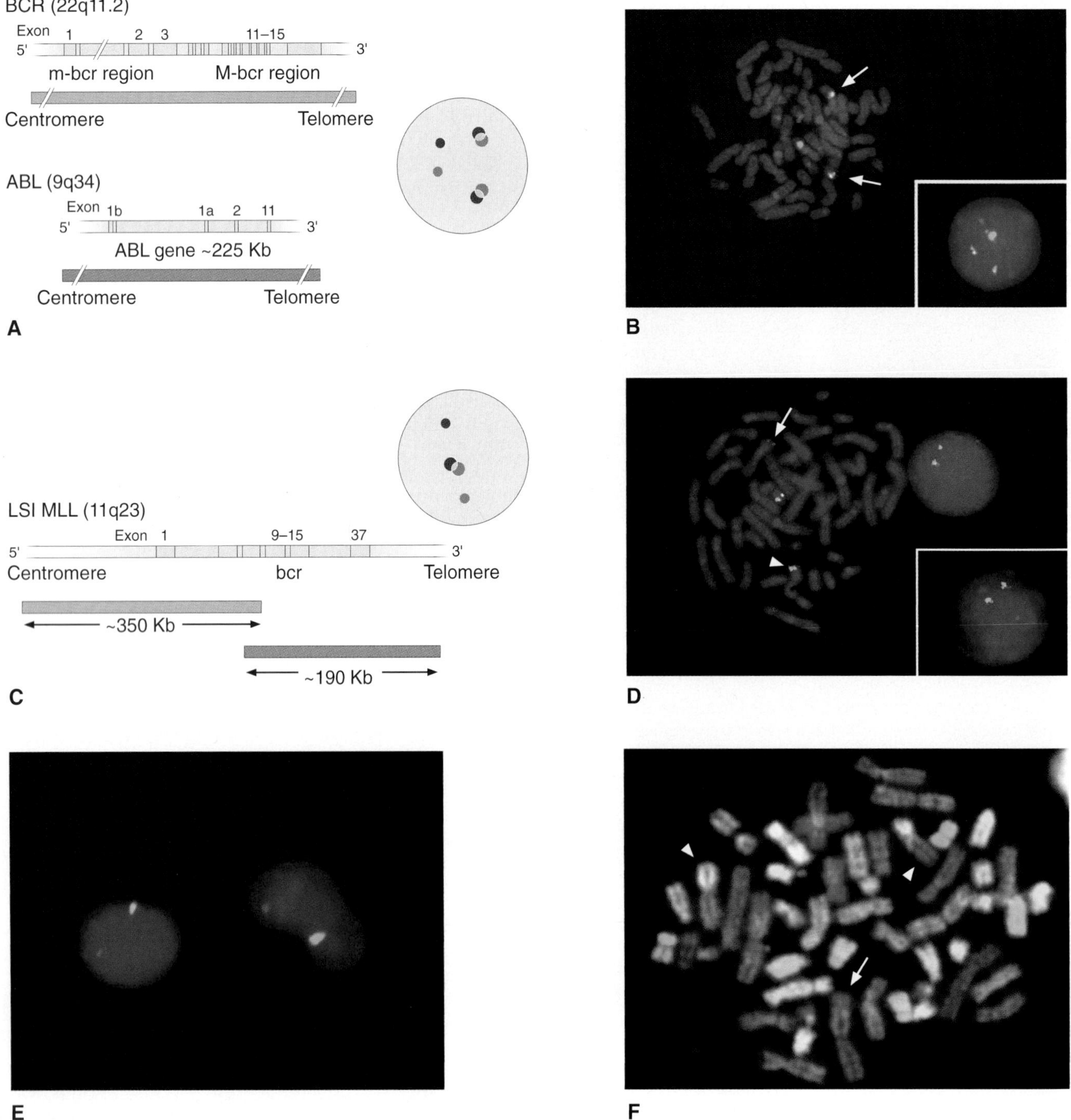

the probes (*ABL*) has been modified to include a larger segment of DNA, so that when the translocation occurs, a portion of the DNA sequences recognized by the *ABL* probe remain at the original site, giving rise to an extra signal in a single color (red). False-positive signals can be distinguished from genuine fusion signals resulting from the t(9;22) by the absence of this extra red signal for the 5′ *ABL* sequences. These probes improve sensitivity, and they can detect Ph-positive cells in less than 1% of nuclei in a sample.[17] However, that 5′ *ABL* sequences, and therefore the "extra signal," are deleted in approximately 15% of patients as a result of complex submicroscopic deletions occurring in conjunction with the translocation.[18] For this group of patients, the extra-signal probe has the same sensitivity as the original single-fusion probe (5–10%).

Dual-Color/Dual-Fusion Probe

A third type of probe for detecting translocations is a *dual-fusion signal BCR/ABL* probe (Vysis, Inc). In the example of the t(9;22), both probes have been modified to include larger regions so that cells with the t(9;22) have one red and one green signal observed on the normal homologues, and yellow fusion signals observed on both the der(22) and der(9) homologues (see Fig. 103–5*A* and *B*). This type of probe has a substantially lower rate of false-positive cells, and the threshold value for a positive result is approximately 1%.[19] In a recent study, quantitative analysis of 6000 nuclei could detect minimal residual disease with a sensitivity of approximately 0.2%.[19]

Dual-Color Break-Apart Probe

A fourth type of probe is referred to as a *two-color break-apart probe*. Two-color break-apart probes are designed such that DNA sequences from the 5′ and 3′ regions of a single gene are differentially labeled and detected with red and green fluorochromes. In the germline configuration, a yellow fusion signal is observed, whereas separate red and green signals are seen when the sequences are separated as a result of a translocation (Fig. 103–5*C* and *D*). Knowledge of the partner gene is not necessary and, therefore, the method is most useful for loci that are translocated to multiple sites, such as *MLL* and *IGH*. The sensitivity of this type of probe is exceedingly high (cutoff value of ~1.7%), with very high specificity.

Reporting and Interpretation of FISH Results

When interpreting FISH results, the probe strategy provides a general indication of the sensitivity of the specific test. The specific laboratory reference range for the probe in use should be provided. The Laboratory Practice Committee of the American College of Medical Genetics has established the "Standards and Guidelines for Clinical Genetics Laboratories" (2nd ed, 1999) (available through *www.faseb.org/genetics/acmg*). The guidelines for clinical FISH analysis establish procedures for probe validation, assay validation, and assay analytical sensitivity. Each laboratory must have its own normal and abnormal reference ranges; without this information, it is not possible to interpret FISH results accurately. FISH nomenclature, much like chromosome banding nomenclature, is outlined in the ISCN (1995).[7] However, because of the relative novelty of the FISH technique, the nomenclature system is still in the development stages and not yet widely applied.

Applications of FISH

The applications of FISH in cancer diagnosis are summarized in Table 103–2, and have been described in depth in several recent reviews.[8,20–22] In many cases, FISH

Figure 103–5. Fluorescent in situ hybridization (FISH) and spectral karyotyping (SKY) analysis of hematologic malignant diseases. Panels ***B, D,*** and ***E*** illustrate images of metaphase and interphase cells following FISH; the cells are counterstained with 4,6-diamidino-2-phenylindole-dihydrochloride (DAPI). ***A,*** Schematic diagram of the *BCR* and *ABL* loci, location of the *BCR* and *ABL* dual-fusion probe (Vysis, Inc.), and configuration of signals in interphase cells. ***B,*** Hybridization of the *BCR/ABL* dual-fusion probe to metaphase and interphase cells with the t(9;22). In cells with the t(9;22), only one green and one red signal is observed on the normal 9 and 22 homologues, and two yellow fusion signals *(arrows)* are observed on the der(9) and the der(22) (Ph) chromosomes as a result of the juxtaposition of the *ABL* and *BCR* sequences. ***C,*** Schematic diagram of the *MLL* gene, location of the *MLL* break-apart probe (Vysis, Inc.), and configuration of signals in interphase cells. ***D,*** Hybridization of the *MLL* break-apart probe to metaphase and interphase cells with a t(11q23). In cells with an *MLL* translocation, a yellow fusion signal is observed for the germline configuration on the normal chromosome 11 homologue, a green signal is observed on the der(11) chromosome *(arrowhead)*, and a red signal is observed on the partner chromosome *(arrow)*. ***E,*** Hybridization of directly labeled centromere-specific probes for the X (CEPX™ Spectrum Orange; Vysis, Inc.) and Y (CEPX™ Spectrum Green; Vysis Inc.) chromosomes to interphase cells from a marrow aspirate of a female patient with acute myeloid leukemia who received a marrow transplant from a male donor. Centromere-specific probes hybridize to the repetitive DNA sequences that are present at the centromeres of human chromosomes. ***F,*** SKY analysis of a metaphase cell from an M7 acute myeloid leukemia. Twenty-four differentially labeled probes representing each human chromosome are co-hybridized, and imaging analysis software assigns a unique color to each. A complex karyotype was identified by conventional cytogenetic analysis, including a derivative chromosome 1 with additional material of unknown origin on 1p, a deletion of 8p, a derivative chromosome 11 resulting from an unbalanced translocation involving 1 and 11, and a derivative chromosome 12, consisting of 11q and 12q. The results of SKY confirmed the identity of the rearranged chromosome 12 *(arrowhead)*, but also clarified the other abnormalities. The additional material on 1p was derived from chromosome 8 (*long arrow*, blue signal), and the der(11) actually consisted of material from chromosomes 1, 11, and 12 (*short arrow:* 11p, white signal; chromosome 12, brown signal; 1p, blue-pink signal).

analysis provides increased sensitivity, in that cytogenetic abnormalities have been detected in samples that appeared to be normal by morphologic and conventional cytogenetics. FISH is most powerful when targeted toward abnormalities associated with a particular disease, or known to occur in a particular patient's tumor. For example, cytogenetic analysis is often performed at the time of diagnosis to identify the chromosomal abnormalities in an individual patient's malignant cells; thereafter, FISH can be used to detect residual disease or early relapse and to assess the efficacy of therapeutic regimens.

SPECTRAL KARYOTYPING/M-FISH

Background and Theory

The latest achievement in cytogenetic analysis is the complete, simultaneous color karyotyping of all of the human chromosomes, termed *spectral karyotyping* (SKY) or *multiplex-FISH* (M-FISH). SKY is based upon the technique of combinatorial or ratio-labeling,[23,24] in which a probe is labeled with more than one reporter molecule in varying ratios and detected with more than one fluorochrome, allowing for an increase in the detectable targets beyond the number of available fluorochromes. Useful combinations of N fluorochromes is equal to $2^N - 1$; thus, increasing the number of fluorochromes to four allows for the detection of 15 different target sequences, increasing to five fluorochromes allows for 31 combinations, and so on. The two techniques of combinatorial multicolor karyotyping, SKY and M-FISH, differ by the method of image acquisition and by the analysis algorithms used to make the correct chromosome designation based on the emitted spectra. With both methods, the end result is an impressive color display (Fig. 103–5*F*). Although relatively new, spectral karyotyping has already impacted on the cytogenetic analysis of neoplastic diseases: it is often possible to completely characterize marker chromosomes (rearranged chromosomes of unknown origin) and complex karyotypes in tumors with a single hybridization.

Applications of SKY/M-FISH

SKY offers advantages over standard G-band analysis (see Table 103–2). For example, SKY can detect many subtle translocations, such as cryptic translocations involving telomeric material, which can be visualized as obvious color exchanges; telomeric rearrangements have been neglected in neoplastic diseases.[25] A second obstacle facing cancer cytogeneticists has been the characterization of homogeneously staining regions (hsrs) and double minute chromosomes (dmins), the cytogenetic manifestations of oncogene amplification. SKY allows for the identification of the chromosome of origin of these small pieces of genetic material, based simply on color, and provides a starting point from which the amplified gene can be identified. Discovery of new oncogenes using this method would improve our understanding of neoplastic disease and provide important diagnostic and prognostic correlations, as has been the case for *NMYC* in childhood neuroblastoma.[26]

Since its introduction, SKY, used predominantly as a research tool, has been applied to the analysis of over 400 primary hematologic malignancies.[27] In almost all

TABLE 103–2. Applications and Limitations of Cytogenetic, Fluorescent In Situ Hybridization (FISH), and Spectral Karyotyping (SKY) Analysis

	Cytogenetic Analysis	FISH Analysis	SKY Analysis
Specimens*	BM, PB, LN, Mass	BM, PB, LN, Mass	BM, PB, LN, Mass
Sensitivity	1:20–1:100	1:20–1:1000	1:20–1:100
Rapid technique	No	Yes	No
Labor intensive	Yes	No	Yes
Detects numerical abnormalities	Yes	Yes	Yes
Detects structural abnormalities	Yes	Yes	Yes
Monitor therapeutic response, minimal residual disease	Yes	Yes	No
Cells required:			
Metaphase	Yes	Yes	Yes
Interphase	No	Yes	No
Terminally differentiated (nondividing)	No	Yes	No
Detects all abnormalities with a single test	Yes	No	Yes†
Identification of:			
Multiple clones/evolution	Yes	No	No‡
Marker (rearranged) chromosomes	No	Yes	Yes
Cryptic rearrangements	No	Yes	No
Gene amplification	No	Yes	Yes
Lineage of neoplastic cells	No	Yes	No
Automated systems available	Yes (Interactive)	Yes	Yes (Interactive)
Cost	High	Low	High§

*BM, bone marrow aspirate or biopsy; LN, lymph node; PB, peripheral blood.
†Does not detect some structural rearrangements (e.g., small cryptic translocations, paracentric inversions, small deletions, and small duplications). In addition, SKY does not provide information on breakpoints or involved chromosomal segments, unless used in conjunction with a banding method (e.g., DAPI staining).
‡Because of the labor-intensive nature of SKY, analysis of more than 10 cells per case becomes prohibitive, limiting the ability to define multiple clones.
§Requires a dedicated SKY imaging and analysis system ($80,000).

cases, the karyotype derived from G-banding was refined to more accurately describe chromosomal abnormalities; in some instances, SKY resulted in the identification of new, previously undetected abnormalities. SKY should result in the recognition of new recurring abnormalities in diseases that have already been well characterized, such as leukemias and lymphomas, as well as in tumors that have been less amenable to conventional cytogenetic studies.

Advantages and Limitations of Cytogenetic, FISH, and SKY Analyses

The advantages and limitations of cytogenetic, FISH, and SKY analysis are described and contrasted in Table 103–2. Perhaps the most critical parameters are the sensitivity and specificity of each method, and the speed with which each can be accomplished. Cytogenetic and SKY analysis have a relatively low sensitivity (1:20 to 1:100 cells) as compared to FISH (1:20 to 1:1000). Moreover, both cytogenetic analysis and SKY require highly skilled personnel, and they are labor intensive; results are not available for 1–3 weeks in all but exceptional cases. In contrast, material for FISH can be processed in 4–24 hours, and analysis of 1000–2000 cells can be accomplished in 15–45 minutes. FISH is such a rapid technique that cytogenetic patterns of tumor cells can be obtained in a time frame sufficient for chromosome data to be considered in treatment decisions. All three methods can be used to detect both numerical and structural chromosomal abnormalities. Cytogenetic and SKY analyses require dividing cells from which metaphase chromosomes can be examined, whereas FISH may be applied to both metaphase cells and interphase cells, allowing for the accurate and informative analysis of specimens for which no metaphase spreads were isolated.

The specificity of cytogenetic analysis is very high, and conventional testing can detect the presence of virtually all chromosomal abnormalities with a single study. In contrast, the major limitation of FISH is that the detection of abnormalities is restricted to those loci tested, and to those probes that are currently available (see Table 103–1). With the exception of several probes marketed by Vysis, Inc. (Abbott Laboratories), most of the commercially available FISH probes have not yet received U.S. Food and Drug Administration approval for diagnostic use. This limitation compels laboratories to continue to use both cytogenetic analysis and FISH methods to analyze the same clinical sample, rather than FISH alone. Other constraints to FISH are technical. First, the technique is highly sensitive for the detection of trisomy, but less sensitive in detecting chromosome loss.[10] The false-monosomy rate (presence of only one signal in a diploid cell) can vary from 3% to 9% of all nucleated cells in preparations from bone marrow or peripheral blood; therefore, the application of FISH to detect monosomy in a small percentage of the cell population, as in minimal residual disease, is limited. Second, processing of bone marrow and peripheral blood cells is relatively simple; the preparation of other tissues, such as paraffin-embedded tissues or frozen sections from lymph node biopsies, is much more difficult. Artifacts created by crushing and sectioning of tissue and incomplete penetration of the probe into the cell nucleus may produce misleading results. In these tissues, the percentage of cells showing false monosomy may be very high (>50%).

SKY is limited because each individual chromosome is painted along its length uniformly, preventing discrimination of one subregion or band of the chromosome from another. Rearrangements that do not alter the appearance of the chromosome, such as paracentric inversions and microdeletions, will not be detected. Moreover, the specific breakpoints of any rearrangement cannot be determined without the aid of another method, such as traditional banding. Likewise, although the chromosomal origins of double minute chromosomes and homogeneously staining regions are easily discernible by SKY, the origin of the amplified material cannot be determined without a second in situ hybridization method, such as reverse painting or comparative genomic hybridization. Maximal precision is obtained by combining SKY with conventional analysis of banded metaphase cells, or the hybridization of specific single-copy probes (see Table 103–1).

RECURRING ABNORMALITIES

Chronic Myeloid Leukemia

The first consistent chromosome abnormality in any malignant disease, the Ph chromosome, was identified in chronic myeloid leukemia (see Chapter 31). The t(9;22)(q34;q11.2) arises in a pluripotent stem cell that gives rise to both lymphoid and myeloid lineage cells. The standard t(9;22) is identified in about 92% of chronic myeloid leukemia patients, whereas 6–8% have variant translocations that involve a third chromosome in addition to numbers 9 and 22. The t(9;22) and resultant *BCR/ABL* fusion classically define chronic myeloid leukemia.[28] A minority of patients have a rearrangement involving *ABL* and *BCR* that is detectable only at the molecular level (<1% of cases).[28,29] The BCR/ABL fusion protein is located on the cytoplasmic surface of the cell membrane and acquires a novel function in transmitting growth-regulatory signals to the nucleus via the RAS/MAPK, PI3K/AKT, and JAK/STAT signal transduction pathways. The tyrosine kinase activity of the BCR/ABL fusion protein can be specifically inhibited by imatinib mesylate (Gleevec/STI571).[30] Imatinib has shown remarkable activity in all phases of chronic myeloid leukemia and is the preferred therapy for most patients with newly diagnosed disease.[31,32] Patients on treatment with imatinib may acquire chromosomal abnormalities in Ph negative cells that herald disease progression or that may be of unclear clinical significance. In a recent series, 15% of patients who had achieved a complete cytogenetic response to imatinib showed clonal karyotypic abnormalities, most commonly +8, −7, or del(20q), and some had clinical features of a myelodysplastic syndrome.[33]

As they enter the more aggressive stages of accelerated and blast phase disease, most chronic myeloid leukemia patients (80%) show karyotypic evolution with the appearance of new chromosomal abnormalities in very distinct patterns in addition to the Ph chromosome.[29] A change in karyotype is a grave prognostic sign.[29] A gain of chromosomes 8, 19, or a second Ph (by gain of the first), or an i(17q) frequently occur in combination to produce modal chromosome numbers of 47–50.

Primary Myelodysplastic Syndromes

The myelodysplastic syndromes are a heterogeneous group of diseases (see Chapter 15). Clonal chromosome abnormalities can be detected in marrow cells of 40–100% of patients with primary myelodysplastic syndrome at diagnosis (in 25% of patients with refractory anemia; in 10% with refractory anemia with ringed sideroblasts; in 50% with refractory cytopenias with multilineage dysplasia; in 50–70% with refractory anemia with excess blasts types 1 and 2; and in 100% with myelodysplastic syndrome with isolated del(5q).[34,35] The common chromosome changes, +8, −5/del(5q), −7/del(7q), and del(20q), are similar to those seen in acute myeloid leukemia de novo (see Fig. 103–1*A* and *B*). Myelodysplastic syndrome with isolated del(5q) occurs in a subset of older patients with refractory anemia, frequently women, who have low myeloblast counts and normal or elevated platelet counts.[36] The interstitial deletion of 5q is typically the sole abnormality; deletions vary in size but are similar to those noted in acute myeloid leukemia. However, the relatively benign course of the 5q− syndrome can extend over several years.[36] Cytogenetic abnormalities in myelodysplastic syndrome are predictive of survival and progression to acute myeloid leukemia.[35] Patients with a "good outcome" have normal karyotypes, −Y alone, del(5q) alone, or del(20q) alone; those with an "intermediate outcome" have other abnormalities, and those with a "poor outcome" have complex karyotypes (≥3 abnormalities, typically with abnormalities of chromosome 5 and/or 7) or chromosome 7 abnormalities.[35]

Acute Myeloid Leukemia De Novo

Clonal chromosomal abnormalities are detected in 80–90% of patients with acute myeloid leukemia (see Fig. 103–1*B*) (see Chapter 28). The most frequent abnormalities are +8 and −7, seen in most subtypes of acute myeloid leukemia.[37,38] A new classification system established by the WHO uses cytogenetic abnormalities as one of the main criteria for disease classification.[5]

The t(8;21)(q22;q22) is observed in 5–10% of all acute myeloid leukemia cases with an abnormal karyotype and in 15% of M2 patients.[39] Acute myeloid leukemia with t(8;21) has a favorable prognosis in adults (overall 5-year survival of 70%), whereas the outcome in children is poor.[40] Molecularly, the t(8;21) involves the *RUNX1/AML1* gene on chromosome 21, which encodes a transcription factor, also known as core-binding factor, which is essential for hematopoiesis.[39,41,42] Transformation by the AML1/ETO fusion protein probably results from transcriptional repression of normal *AML1* target genes through aberrant recruitment of nuclear transcriptional corepressor complexes.

Inv(16)(pl3.1q22) or t(16;16)(pl3.1;q22) is observed in acute myelomonocytic leukemia with abnormal eosinophils (M4Eo), including large and irregular basophilic granules, and which show positive reactions with periodic acid–Schiff and chloroacetate esterase (5% of acute myeloid leukemia and 25% of acute myelomonocytic leukemia patients).[37,40,43] These patients have a good response to intensive chemotherapy, with a complete remission rate of approximately 90% and an overall 5-year survival of 60%.[40] The breakpoint at 16q22 occurs within the *CBFB* gene, which encodes one subunit of the RUNX1/CBFB transcription factor. Thus, like t(8;21), inv(16) disrupts the RUNX1/AML1 pathway regulating hematopoiesis.[39]

The t(15;17)(q22;q11.2-12) is highly specific for acute promyelocytic leukemia and has not been found in any other disease.[44] Rare variant translocations (<2% of cases) include the t(11;17)(q23;q11.2-12) and t(5;17)(q34;q11.2-12). Establishing the diagnosis of acute promyelocytic leukemia with the typical t(15;17) is important, because this disease is sensitive to therapy with all-*trans* retinoic acid. The t(15;17) results in a fusion retinoic acid receptor-α protein (PML/RARA). The oncogenic potential of the acute promyelocytic leukemia fusion protein results from the aberrant repression of RAR-α–mediated gene transcription through histone deacetylase–dependent chromatin remodeling.[45,46]

Recurring translocations involving 11q23 occur in approximately 35% of acute myelomonocytic and acute monoblastic leukemia patients.[37,47,48] There are at least 47 different recurring rearrangements that involve 11q23, and thus, along with 14q32, 11q23 is one of the bands most frequently involved in rearrangements in human tumor cells.[37,48] The breakpoints in the translocation partners include 1p32, 4q21, and 19p13.3 in acute lymphoblastic leukemia and 1q21, 2q21, 6q27, 9p22, 10p11.2, 17q25, 19p13.3, and 19p13.1 in acute myeloid leukemia. Translocations involving 11q23 have a very unusual age distribution, comprising about three quarters of the chromosome abnormalities in leukemia cells of children under 1 year of age.[48] With the exception of the t(9;11), which may have an intermediate outcome, translocations of 11q23 are associated with a poor prognosis.[40] Translocations of 11q23 involve *MLL,* which encodes a histone methyltransferase that assembles in protein complexes that regulate gene transcription by chromatin remodeling.[47]

Acute Myeloid Leukemia and Myelodysplastic Syndrome Associated with Prior Cytotoxic Treatment

Therapy-related myelodysplastic syndrome or acute myeloid leukemia is a late complication of cytotoxic therapy used in the treatment of both malignant and nonmalignant diseases[49] (see Chapter 29). Following alkylating agents, the characteristic recurring chromosomal abnormalities are loss of part or all of chromosomes 5 and/or 7 (−5/del(5q) or −7/del(7q); see Fig. 103–1*C*).[50,51] In our experience, 92% of therapy-related myelodysplastic syndrome/acute myeloid leukemia patients had an abnormal karyotype, and 70% had an abnormality of chromosomes 5 and/or 7[51] (confirmed in other series).[52] In contrast, only about 16% of patients with acute myeloid leukemia de novo have a similar abnormality of chromosomes 5 or 7, or both.[37,43]

A second subtype of therapy-related acute myeloid leukemia is distinctly different from the more common leukemia that follows alkylating agents or irradiation. In therapy-related acute myeloid leukemia following drugs that inhibit topoisomerase II, such as etoposide, teniposide, and doxorubicin,[49–51] there is a shorter latency period (1–2 years); presentation with overt leukemia, often with monocytic features, without a preceding myelodysplastic phase; and a more favorable response to intensive induction therapy. Balanced translocations involving the *MLL* gene at 11q23 or the *RUNX1/AML1* gene at 21q22 are common in this subgroup.[49]

Acute Lymphoblastic Leukemia

Acute lymphoblastic leukemia is the most frequent leukemia in children (see Chapter 32). The most useful prognostic indicators are karyotype (including ploidy), age, white blood cell count, sex, and response to initial therapy.[37,53] In both childhood and adult acute lymphoblastic leukemia, the identification of prognostic subgroups based on recurring cytogenetic abnormalities and molecular markers has resulted in the application of risk-adapted therapies (see Fig. 103–1*D*).[37,53]

The incidence of the t(9;22) in acute lymphoblastic leukemia is 30% in adults (and may approach 50% in adults over 60 years of age) and 5% in children. Thus, the Ph chromosome is the most frequent rearrangement in adult acute lymphoblastic leukemia. About 70% of the patients show additional abnormalities, much more commonly than in chronic myeloid leukemia: +der(22)t(9;22), +21, abnormalities of 9p, +8, −7, and +X occur in descending order of frequency. Monosomy 7 is associated with a poorer outcome.[54] A chromosomally normal cell line is frequently present in the marrow of Ph$^+$ acute lymphoblastic leukemia patients (70%) but is rare in untreated chronic myeloid leukemia. The disease in both adults and children is characterized by an early precursor-B-cell phenotype, elevated white blood cell counts, a high percentage of circulating blasts, and a poor prognosis. As in chronic myeloid leukemia, the t(9;22) in acute lymphoblastic leukemia results in a *BCR/ABL* fusion gene. However, in over half of the patients, the break in *BCR* is more proximal, resulting in a smaller fusion protein with greater tyrosine kinase activity (BCR/ABL^{p190}).

Translocations involving the *MLL* gene at 11q23 occur in 5% of acute lymphoblastic leukemia patients.[37,55] Of these, the most common is the t(4;11)(q21;q23). The t(11;19)(q23;p13.3) is second in frequency; however, this rearrangement is not limited to acute lymphoblastic leukemia in that approximately 50% of these cases have acute myeloid leukemia, usually monoblastic. Translocations involving 11q23 are found in infant acute lymphoblastic leukemia (60–80%). Patients with the t(4;11) have a pro-B-cell phenotype (CD10$^-$CD19$^+$), with coexpression of monocytic (CD15$^+$) or, less commonly, T-cell markers. Clinically, they have aggressive features with hyperleukocytosis, extramedullary disease, and a poor response to conventional chemotherapy.[55] Rearrangements affecting *MLL* represent a major class of mutations in acute leukemia and identify patients with a poor outcome.

The t(12;21)(p12;q22) has been identified in a high proportion (~25%) of childhood precursor-B-cell leukemia.[56] The translocation is not easily detected by cytogenetic analysis because of the similarity in size and banding pattern of 12p and 21q; the rearrangement can be reliably identified using reverse transcriptase–polymerase chain reaction or FISH analysis. The t(12;21) defines a distinct subgroup of patients characterized by an age between 1 and 10 years, B-lineage immunophenotype (CD10$^+$CD19$^+$HLA-DR$^+$), and a favorable outcome. The t(12;21) is not seen in T-cell acute lymphoblastic leukemia and is uncommon in adults (~4% of acute lymphoblastic leukemia cases). In a recent series, patients with the t(12;21) had a 5-year event-free survival of 91%, as compared to 65% for patients without this rearrangement; however, t(12;21) may be associated with late disease recurrences.[38] The translocation results in a fusion protein containing the amino-terminus of ETV-6/TEL, a transcriptional repressor of the ETS family, and most of the RUNX1/AML1 transcription factor.[38]

The leukemia cells of some patients with acute lymphoblastic leukemia are characterized by a gain of many chromosomes. Two distinct subgroups are recognized: a group with 1–4 extra chromosomes (47–50), and the more common group with more than 50 chromosomes. Chromosome numbers usually range from 51 to 60, and a few patients may have up to 65 chromosomes. Hyperdiploidy (>50 chromosomes) is common in children (~30%) but rare in adults (<5%). Certain additional chromosomes are common (the X chromosome and chromosomes 4, 6, 10, 14, 17, 18, and 21); chromosome 21 is gained most frequently (100% of cases). Patients who have hyperdiploidy with greater than 50 chromosomes have all of the previously recognized clinical factors that indicate a good prognosis, including age between 1 and 9 years, low white blood cell count, and favorable immunophenotype (early pre-B or pre-B cell).[57] The favorable prognosis associated with high hyperdiploidy has been associated with gains of chromosomes 4, 10, 6, and 17, but a gain of chromosome 5 and i(17q) are associated with a poor outcome.[57]

Non-Hodgkin's Lymphoma

Cytogenetic analyses of non-Hodgkin's lymphoma have been reported in a number of large series (see Fig. 103–1*E*)[58,59]: more than 90% of cases are characterized by clonal chromosomal abnormalities and, more importantly, many of the recurring abnormalities correlate with histology and immunophenotype (see Chapter 43). For example, the t(14;18) is observed in a high proportion of follicular small cleaved cell lymphomas (70–90%), most patients with a t(3;22)(q27;q11.2) or t(3;14)(q27;q32) have diffuse large B-cell lymphomas, and patients with a t(8;14)(q24.1;q32) have either small noncleaved cell or diffuse large B-cell lymphomas. Another example, the t(11;14) (q13;q32), is observed in virtually all mantle cell lymphomas.[60] Band 14q32, the location of *IGH,* is frequently involved in translocations in B-cell neoplasms (~70%). In contrast, a large proportion of T-cell neoplasms are characterized by rearrangements that involve 14q11.2, 7q34, or 7p14, the locations of the T-cell receptor genes.

Chronic Lymphocytic Leukemia

Chromosomal abnormalities associated with chronic lymphocytic leukemia recently have been delineated by FISH (see Fig. 103–1*F*)[61] (see Chapter 34). When conventional cytogenetic techniques are used, only 50% of chronic lymphocytic leukemia patients have detectable abnormalities; most common is trisomy 12 (20–60%), followed by structural abnormalities of 13q and 14q.[62] With FISH, chromosomal alterations can be detected in more than 80% of patients.[62] The most frequent chromosomal changes are deletion of 13q (55%); deletion of 11q, the location of the *ATM* gene (18%); trisomy of 12q (16%); deletion of 17p, the location of the *TP53* gene (7%); and deletion of 6q (6%).[62] Mortality correlates with cytogenetic subtype, with a shorter median survival observed for 17p (32 months) or 11q (79 months) deletions than with no detectable abnormality (111 months), trisomy of 12q (114 months), or −13/del(13q) (133 months).[62] FISH probes capable of detecting the deletions of 11q, 13q, and 17p, trisomy 12, and *IGH* translocations are commercially available and should facilitate risk-adapted treatment strategies.

Multiple Myeloma

As in chronic lymphocytic leukemia, the application of molecular cytogenetic tools such as FISH has led to the discovery of numerous chromosomal abnormalities in multiple myeloma, in its precursor, monoclonal gammopathy of undetermined significance, and in plasma cell leukemia[63,64] (see Chapter 47). Monoclonal gammopathy of undetermined significance is characterized by chromosomal aneuploidy, *IGH* translocations (45%), and deletions of 13q (15–50%). Loss of chromosome 13 or a del(13q) are the most frequent chromosomal losses in multiple myeloma (40–50%) and confer a poor prognosis.[64] *IGH* translocations deregulate the expression of oncogenes located near the translocation breakpoints; they are detectable by interphase FISH analysis in 50% of patients with monoclonal gammopathy of undetermined significance, 60–75% of patients with multiple myeloma, and more than 80% of patients with plasma cell leukemia.[64] The t(11;14)(q13;q32), found in 15% of cases, results in cyclin D1 overexpression and deregulated expression of the *MYEOV* (myeloma overexpressed) gene. The t(4;14)(p16;q32), which is present in about 15% of patients, deregulates the expression of the fibroblast growth factor receptor-3 gene *(FGFR3)* on the der(14) chromosome and *MMSET* on the der(4) chromosome. The t(4;14) is associated with a poor clinical outcome, whereas the t(11;14) confers a favorable prognosis. Translocations involving unknown partners confer an intermediate prognosis.

T-Cell Acute Lymphoblastic Leukemia

Precursor-T-cell neoplasms have a distinct pattern of recurring karyotypic abnormalities[37] (see Chapter 32). Rearrangements involving 14q11.2 and two regions of chromosome 7 (7q34 and 7p14) are particularly common in T-cell malignancies: the t(11;14) (p13;q11.2) (~3%;

CURRENT CONTROVERSIES & FUTURE CONSIDERATIONS

Cytogenetic Analysis/Fluorescent In Situ Hybridization

- What is the significance of the clonal abnormalities arising in cells without the t(9;22) in chronic myeloid leukemia patients treated with imatinib?
- Should cytogenetic analysis be performed on all patients with acute leukemia at diagnosis, followed by FISH without accompanying cytogenetic studies for those cases with a clonal abnormality for which FISH probes are available? Does the detection of multiple abnormalities within an abnormal clone, the presence of multiple clones, and clonal evolution provided by cytogenetic analysis (but not by FISH) provide additional information of clinical value?
- Should FISH be performed on all specimens from patients with chronic lymphocytic leukemia, myeloma, or monoclonal gammopathy of undetermined significance, without accompanying cytogenetic analysis?
- How should cytogenetic analysis be integrated with emerging technologies that are likely to play a major role in the future diagnosis and management of hematologic disorders, including quantitative reverse transcriptase–polymerase chain reaction, microarray-based gene expression profiling, and proteomic analysis?
- Will the development of risk-adapted, targeted therapies alter the role of cytogenetic analysis in the management of patients with hematological malignant diseases?

RBTN2 gene), t(10;11)(q24;q11.2) (~3%; *HOX11* gene), and t(7;9)(q34;q34) (~2%; *NOTCH1* gene). Patients with T-cell acute lymphoblastic leukemia are most often young males with a mediastinal tumor mass, high white blood cell count, and leukemia cells in the cerebrospinal fluid. These same clinical characteristics are associated with lymphoblastic lymphoma, another T-cell malignancy.

Suggested Readings*

Biogen: Atlas of Genetics and Cytogenetics in Oncology and Haematology. Available at: *http://www.infobiogen.fr/services/chromcancer*

Heim S, Mitelman F: Cancer Cytogenetics (ed 2). New York: Wiley-Liss, 1995.

Jaffe ES, Harris NL, Stein H, Vardiman JW (eds): The World Health Organization Classification of Tumours: Pathology and Genetics of Tumours of Haematopoietic and Lymphoid Tissues. Lyon: IARC Press, 2001.

Le Beau MM, Larson RA: Cytogenetics and Neoplasia. *In* Hoffman R, Benz EJ, Shattil SJ, et al (eds): Hematology: Basic Principles and Practices (ed 3). New York: Churchill-Livingstone, 2000, pp 848–870.

Mitelman F (ed): ISCN (1995): An International System for Human Cytogenetic Nomenclature. Basel: Karger, 1995.

Full references for this chapter can be found on accompanying CD-ROM.

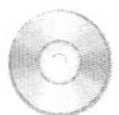

CHAPTER 104

Gene Expression Methods

Sandeep S. Dave, MD, MS, and Louis M. Staudt, MD, PhD

KEY POINTS

Gene Expression Methods

- Every somatic cell in the body contains the same complement of genomic DNA, but only a fraction of the roughly 30,000 genes encoded in the genome are expressed as messenger RNA (mRNA) in any given cell. The gene expression profile of a cell determines its lineage, structure, and function.
- DNA microarray technology can simultaneously measure the mRNA expression of thousands of genes in a biopsy sample, providing a molecular profile of the tumor.
- Gene expression can be used to distinguish tumors that belong to different diagnostic categories. In addition, gene expression profiling has revealed that some current diagnostic categories are composed of multiple molecularly and clinically distinct diseases.
- In many cancers, the gene expression profile of the diagnostic biopsy sample can be used to predict length of survival and the response to treatment.
- The large amount of data generated by DNA microarray analysis poses significant analytical challenges. A variety of pattern recognition algorithms and statistical methods can be used to derive biologically and clinically significant insights from these data sets.
- "Unsupervised" methods of analysis are used to uncover patterns in gene expression data. "Supervised" methods of analysis are used to identify genes whose expression patterns are associated with external data such as length of survival or response to therapy.
- A "gene expression signature" is a set of genes whose expression reflects a particular biologic characteristic of a cell, such as lineage and stage of differentiation, proliferation rate, and activity of particular intracellular signaling pathways. Gene expression signatures can be used to extract biologic insights from gene expression profiling data.
- DNA microarrays show great promise as a tool to provide reproducible molecular diagnoses and prognoses to patients with hematologic malignancies.

INTRODUCTION

The sequencing of the human genome has created opportunities for a comprehensive characterization of the molecular mechanisms underlying pathogenesis and outcome in hematologic disease. Techniques are evolving rapidly to study oncogenic changes that occur at each level of the genome in hematologic malignancies. Gene expression profiling using microarrays has emerged as a widely applied genomics technique for the study of cancer. Only a fraction of the genes encoded in the genome are transcribed into messenger RNA (mRNA). The transcribed (expressed) fraction of genes depends upon the lineage of the cell and its stage of differentiation, the activity of intracellular regulatory pathways and the influence of extracellular stimuli. The expressed genes can also influence whether a cell is normal or malignant. Microarrays provide a powerful method of measuring, in parallel, the expression of thousands of genes that together constitute a tissue or tumor's gene expression profile.

MICROARRAY METHODOLOGY

Microarray Platforms

Although there are many methods of constructing microarrays, two formats have been mainly employed: spotted DNA and oligonucleotide microarrays.

Spotted DNA microarrays are constructed by using a robotic arm to place DNA fragments representing thousands of genes at a predetermined position on a glass slide.[1] To measure gene expression, mRNA is extracted from the cells of interest (such as a tumor biopsy), reverse-transcribed into complementary DNA (cDNA), and fluorescently labeled with a "red" dye (Cy5). Similarly, mRNA from a reference sample (typically prepared from related cell lines or normal tissues) is reverse-transcribed to cDNA and fluorescently labeled with a "green" dye (Cy3). The fluorescently labeled cDNAs from the two sources are then combined and placed on the surface of the DNA microarray. During the incubation, each cDNA molecule hybridizes to the microarray element corresponding to its gene of origin. The extent of hybridization (binding) of the fluorescent cDNA (red vs. green) to each microarray feature is quantified using a scanning fluorescence microscope. Thus, a single experiment can simultaneously provide information on the relative expression levels of the thousands of genes represented on the microarray (Fig. 104–1*A*).

The oligonucleotide microarray is sold commercially by Affymetrix as Genechip.[2] The technology used to create oligonucleotide microarrays is analogous to the manufacture of semiconductor chips. The DNA sequence corresponding to expressed regions of each gene is divided into 25-nucleotide-long oligonucleotide segments. These oligonucleotides are synthesized in situ at defined positions on a quartz substrate by a modification of the photolithography process used in the computer industry. To measure gene expression, mRNA is extracted from the cells of interest and reverse-transcribed into cDNA; cDNA is then transcribed to RNA using biotin-labeled ribonucleotides. The biotin-labeled RNA is fragmented, allowing it to hybridize efficiently with the 25-nucleotide oligonucleotides on the surface of the microarray. The hybridized array is then washed and stained with streptavidin-phycoerythrin and incubated with biotinylated anti-streptavidin antibody. A laser scanner is used to measure the fluorescence associated with each microarray element and the information is integrated by a computer to generate a signal for each gene represented on the microarray (Fig. 104–1*B*).

The two microarray platforms differ in the method by which they measure gene expression, but data generated using either platform lead to similar conclusions.[3–5]

Data Analysis

Analyzing the thousands of data points generated by each microarray experiment can be daunting and presents significant challenges for interpretation. Therefore, a variety of approaches have been developed to analyze microarray data,[6] broadly classified as either "unsupervised" or "supervised" analyses.[7,8]

In an unsupervised analysis, pattern recognition algorithms are used to identify underlying structure in the gene expression data sets; the most commonly used algorithm is hierarchical clustering.[7] Hierarchical clustering can be used to group genes together that are coordinately expressed across samples (Fig. 104–2*A*), or to group samples such as tumor biopsies based on the similarity in their expression of a set of genes. Hierarchical clustering can also be used to define gene expression signatures.

Gene expression signatures are sets of coordinately expressed genes that reflect a biologic characteristic of a sample, such as its lineage, stage of differentiation, or activity of an intracellular signaling pathway.[9] The relative expression of gene expression signatures in a tumor sample can provide important insights into its cellular composition and biologic processes. Applied to hematologic malignancies, biologic features of tumors can be correlated with differences in clinical outcome[10–14] (Fig. 104–2*B*).

Supervised analyses of gene expression data employ statistical methods to relate gene expression data to pathologic and/or clinical data; statistics can distinguish diagnostic groups based on gene expression (also known as "class prediction"). Supervised methods have also been used to create gene expression–based prognostic models (also known as "outcome prediction").[15] Examples of such supervised analyses applied to the prediction of prognosis in diffuse large B-cell lymphoma and follicular lymphoma, as well as in the application to molecular diagnosis, are detailed later.

Validation of Microarray Data

Supervised analysis of microarray data requires validation. When comparing expression data across tens of thousands of genes represented on a microarray, a large number of genes can differ in expression between samples purely by chance[16–18]—the "multiple comparisons problem." For this reason, statistical techniques of cross-validation must be applied to supervised analyses in order to ensure that the findings are reproducible in an independent set of data.

Two methods of cross-validation are commonly employed: the training set–test set method and leave-out-one cross-validation.[19,20] In the training set–test set method, the samples are divided into independent training and test sets. All aspects of supervised analyses and model development are then performed using only data from the training set. The optimal model developed on the training set is then tested on the test set in order to verify the reproducibility of the model (Fig. 104–3*A*). Leave-out-one cross-validation entails removing samples of a known type from the data set one at a time, and then determining whether the model can predict the category of the missing sample (Fig. 104–3*B*). The training set–test set methods of validation can be applied to class prediction as well as outcome prediction; leave-out-one cross-validation is generally applied only to class prediction.

MOLECULAR MECHANISMS OF PATHOGENESIS IN HEMATOLOGIC MALIGNANCIES

Diffuse Large B-Cell Lymphoma

Diffuse large B-cell lymphoma is the most common form of non-Hodgkin's lymphoma, accounting for nearly a third of the cases (see Chapter 39). Although the disease is responsive to chemotherapy, only about 40% of patients are cured of lymphoma. This observation raised the probability that this single diagnostic category might be composed of multiple molecularly distinct diseases that are indistinguishable morphologically but respond differently to treatment.

Gene expression profiling was used to explore whether the diagnosis of diffuse large B-cell lymphoma encompasses more than one molecular disease.[21] Lymph-node biopsy specimens from patients with diffuse large B-cell lymphoma were profiled for gene expression

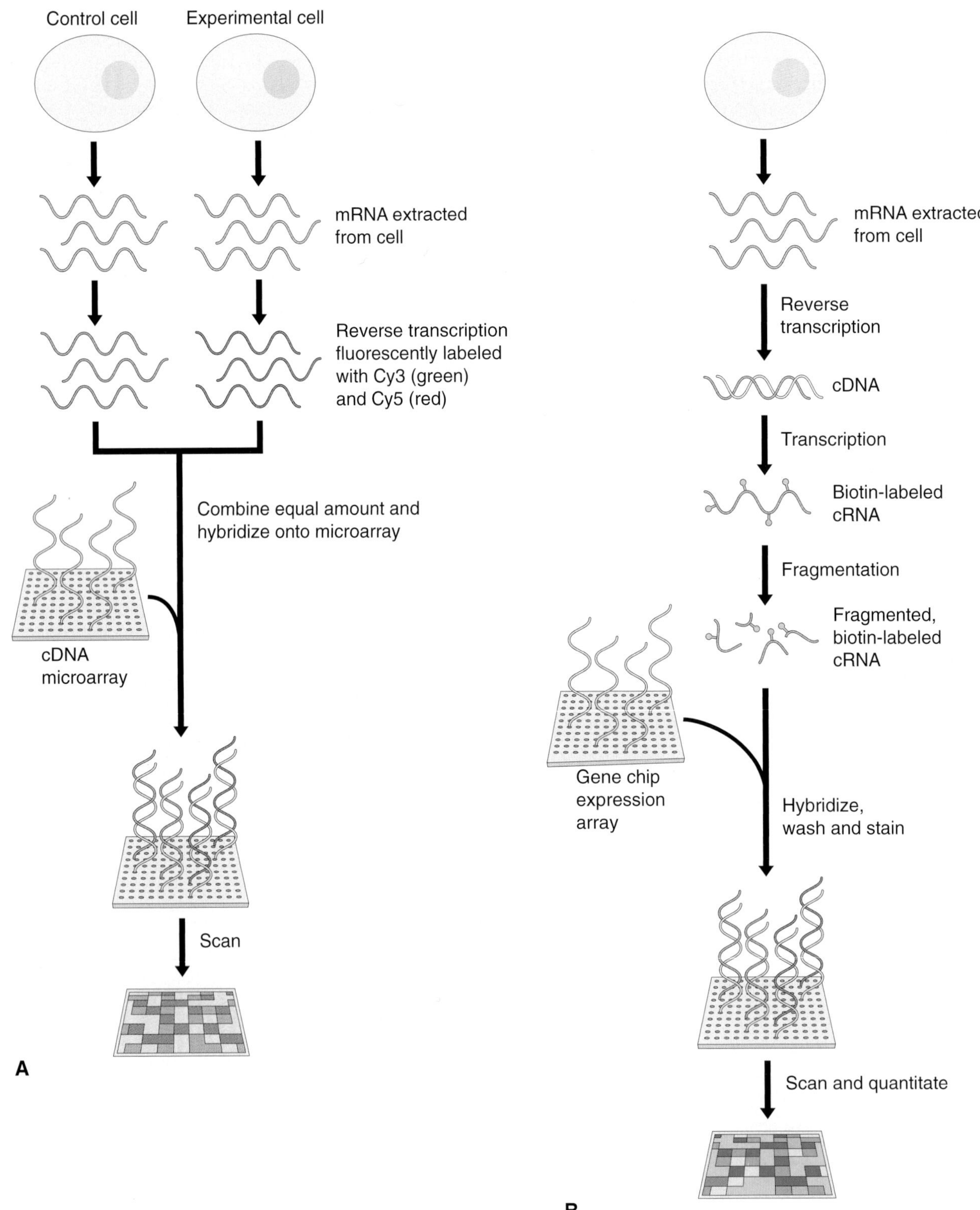

Figure 104–1. Two formats to measure gene expression by microarray. **A**, cDNA microarrays. ***B***, Oligonucleotide microarrays. (Courtesy of Jiang Long and Bioteach, University of British Columbia, Vancouver, Canada.)

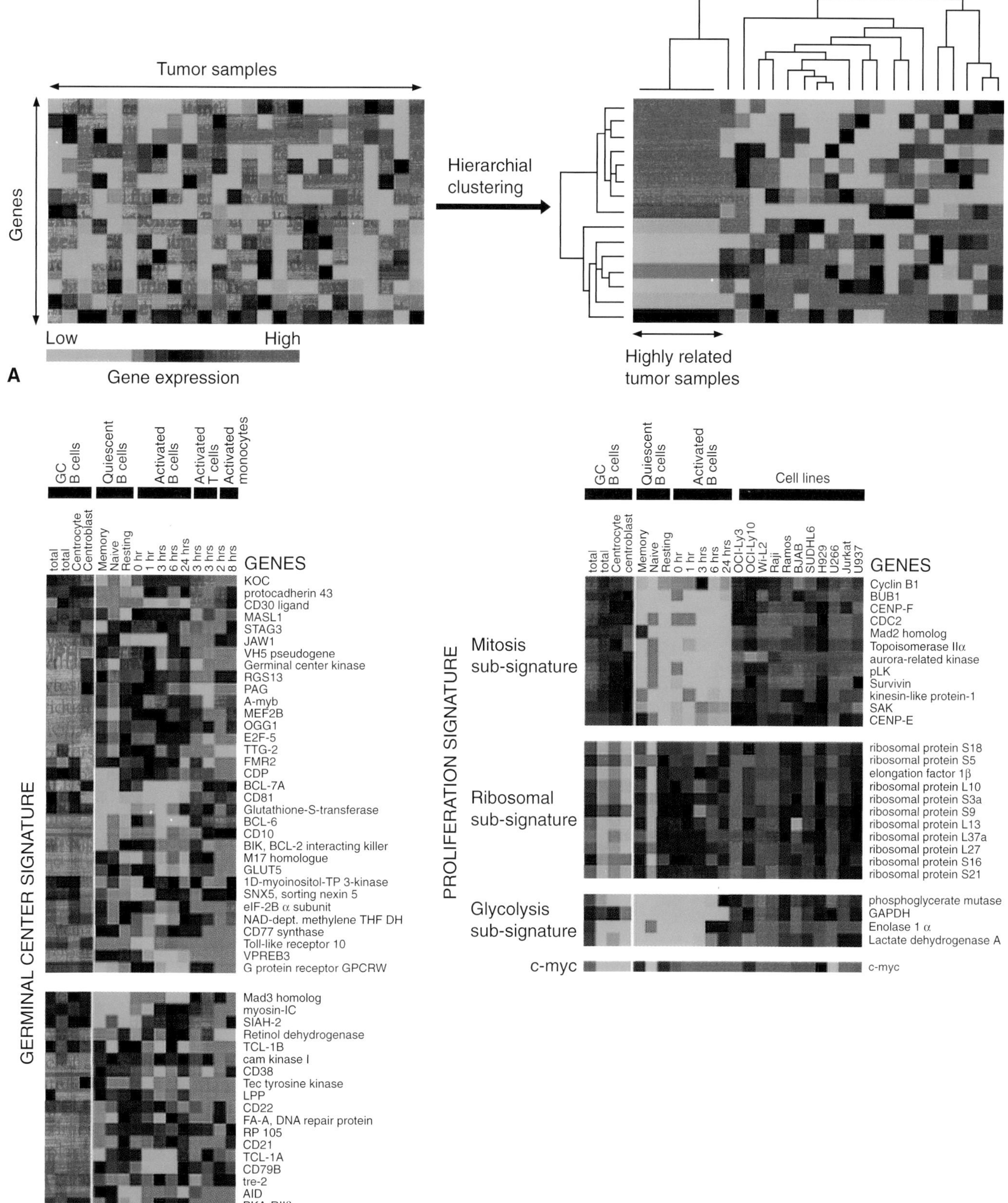

Figure 104–2. Analysis of gene expression data. ***A,*** Hierarchical clustering to group tumor samples. The dendrograms in the *right* figure show the degree of relatedness of adjoining genes and tumor samples. The length of the branch is inversely proportional to the correlation of the sample or gene; short branches are associated with highly correlated genes. ***B,*** Two gene expression signatures that are commonly encountered in B-cell lymphomas. Overexpression of the germinal center signature is characteristic of B cells of germinal center origin, including centrocytes and centroblasts as well as malignant cells derived from germinal center B cells. The proliferation signature consists of several components that can be differentially expressed in different cell populations.

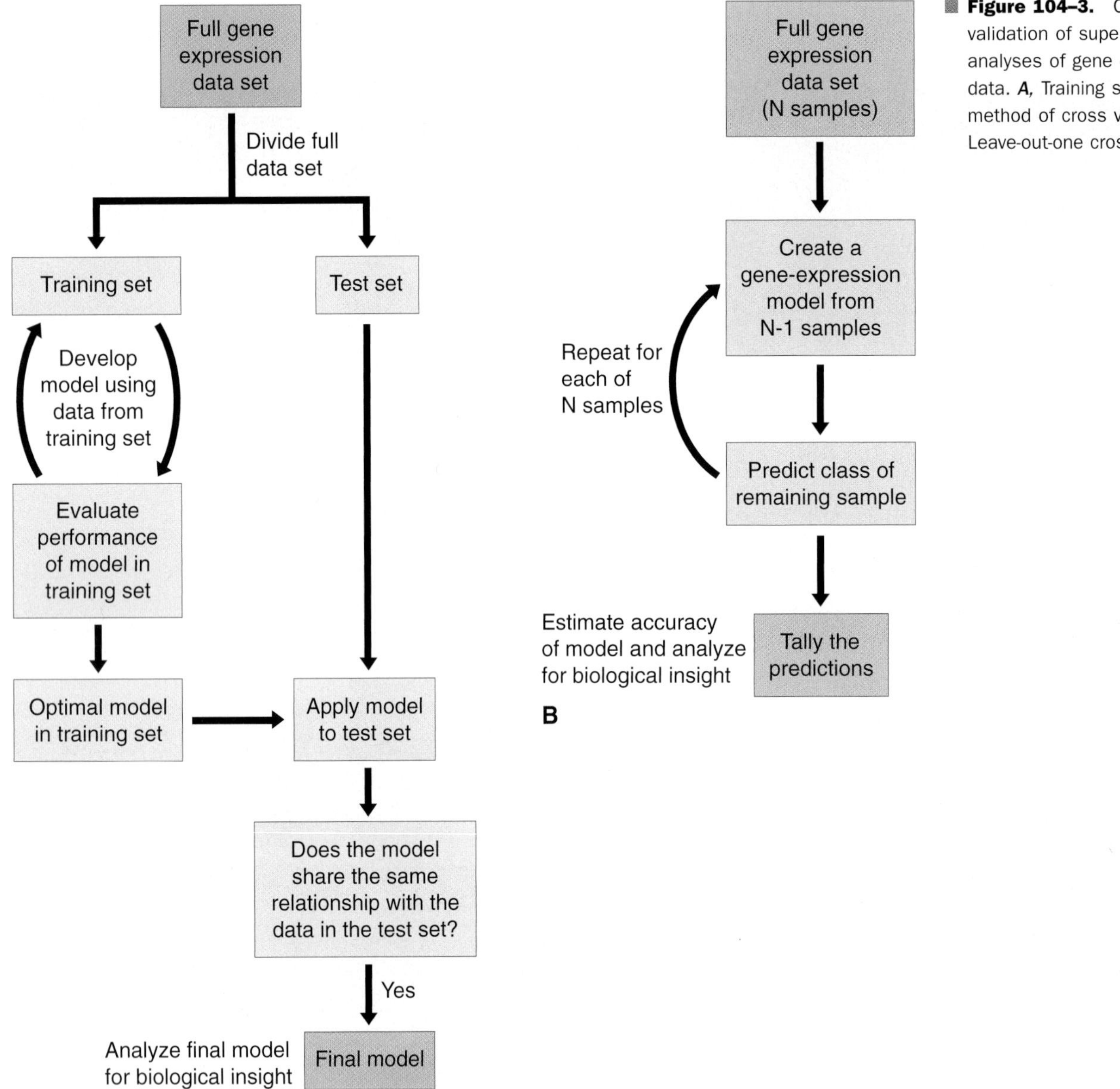

Figure 104–3. Cross-validation of supervised analyses of gene expression data. ***A,*** Training set–test set method of cross validation. ***B,*** Leave-out-one cross-validation.

using "Lymphochip" DNA microarrays, a type of spotted DNA microarray constructed from genes that are known to be expressed by lymphoid cells and neoplasms.[22] Among diffuse large B-cell lymphomas, the germinal center B-cell signature was found to vary significantly.[21] This signature characterizes normal B cells that are responding to stimulation with a foreign antigen in the germinal centers of secondary lymphoid organs (Fig. 104–2*B*). Using unsupervised methods, two major molecular subgroups of diffuse large B-cell lymphoma were identified (Fig. 104–4*A*). The germinal center B cell–like (GCB) subgroup expressed genes in the germinal center B-cell signature highly, but the activated B cell–like (ABC) group did not. Instead, ABC diffuse large B-cell lymphomas expressed genes that are induced by mitogenic stimulation of peripheral blood B cells. A classifier was constructed to distinguish the ABC and GCB subgroups of diffuse large B-cell lymphoma using Bayesian statistics[3]; a small proportion that do not express genes characteristic of either group were "unclassified." The subgroups defined using the gene expression signature were clinically distinct, showing strikingly different survival rates following treatment with anthracycline-containing regimens. Patients with the GCB form of diffuse large B-cell lymphoma have a significantly higher 5-year survival rate (60%) than do patients with the ABC form (31%). The classifier was used to identify the GCB and ABC subgroups within an independent set of diffuse large B-cell lymphoma tumors that had been profiled using Affymetrix microarrays[23]; again, these subgroups had distinct survival rates (see Fig. 104–4*B*). The prognostic distinction based on gene expression was statistically independent of the International Prognostic Index (derived from the patient's age, stage, performance status, number of extranodal sites, and serum lactate dehydrogenase concentration), a well-established

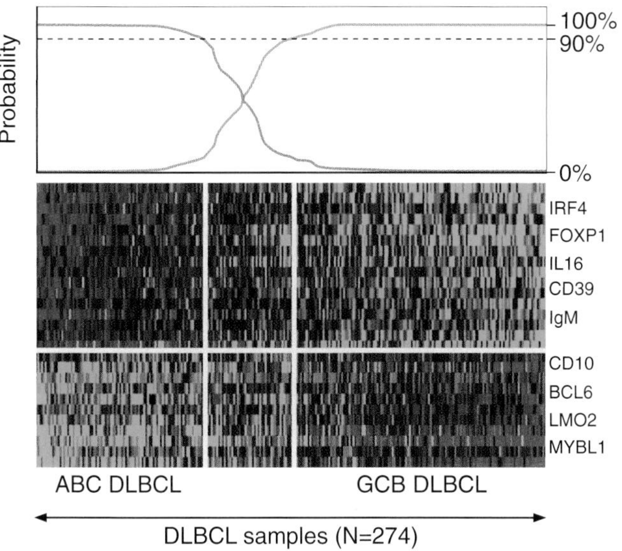

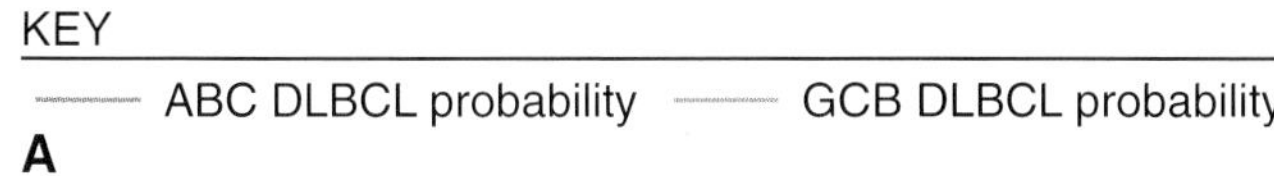

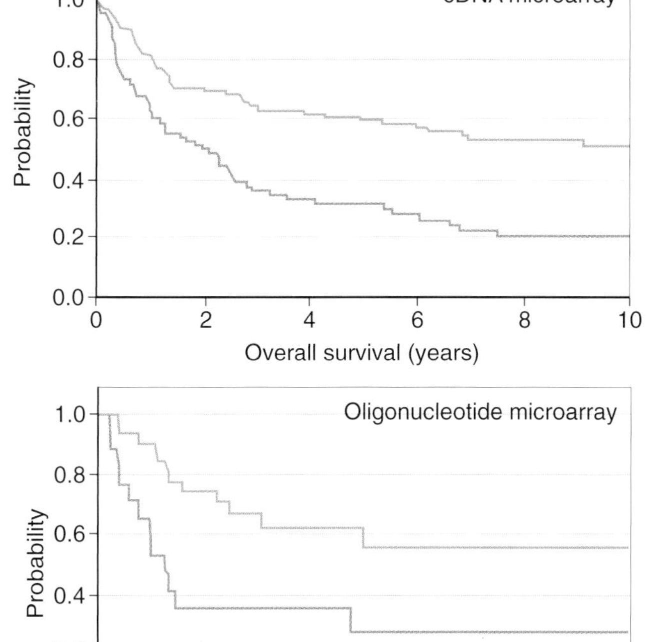

predictor of outcome in diffuse large B-cell lymphoma.[24]

A study of recurrent chromosome abnormalities further supported the existence of these distinct molecular subgroups of diffuse large B-cell lymphoma. The t(14;18) translocation involving the *BCL2* gene and amplification of the c-*rel* locus on chromosome 2p were found to be recurrent oncogenic events in the GCB subgroup tumors but were never observed in the ABC subgroup tumors.[25,26] Constitutive activation of the nuclear factor-κB signaling pathway was a feature of the ABC but not of the GCB subgroup.[27] Interruption of the nuclear factor-κB pathway in ABC diffuse large B-cell lymphoma cell lines causes apoptosis, suggesting that this pathway is a potential therapeutic target.

Follicular Lymphoma

Follicular lymphoma is the second most common form of non-Hodgkin's lymphoma, accounting for nearly a quarter of all cases.[28] The disease is generally indolent, with a median survival of nearly a decade, but the course is highly variable. Some patients can have slow progression or even spontaneous remission, whereas others experience rapid progression or transformation to an aggressive lymphoma and early death from the disease.[29,30] A variety of treatments have been employed, including different chemotherapy regimens, high-dose chemotherapy with autologous stem cell rescue, allogeneic stem cell transplantation, and newer agents such as rituximab and idiotype vaccines. Most therapies result in significant regression of the tumor in the majority of patients, but relapse is usual. No treatment has been convincingly shown to improve overall survival, and there is no agreement regarding in the best initial approach to the disease.[31]

Follicular lymphoma usually arises as a result of the t(14;18) translocation that leads to constitutive expression of BCL-2, a protein that blocks apoptosis. The malignant cells then subsequently acquire additional genomic mutations, which lead to disease progression and/or transformation to aggressive lymphoma, resulting in early death.[32]

To explore the molecular mechanisms that affect the length of survival in follicular lymphoma, gene expression profiling was performed on biopsy samples from 191 untreated patients with newly diagnosed follicular lymphoma (Fig. 104–5*A*). To create a gene expression–based model of survival in follicular lymphoma, a method of supervised analysis and cross-validation called "survival signature analysis" (Fig. 104–5*B*) was devised.

Figure 104–4. Diffuse large B-cell lymphoma comprises more than one molecular subgroup. ***A,*** Development of a Bayesian predictor to distinguish the activated B-cell and germinal center B-cell subgroups, with a small number of unclassified samples. ***B,*** Distinct survival differences between the molecular subgroups of diffuse large B-cell lymphoma. The survival differences are demonstrable, regardless of the microarray used to measure gene expression.

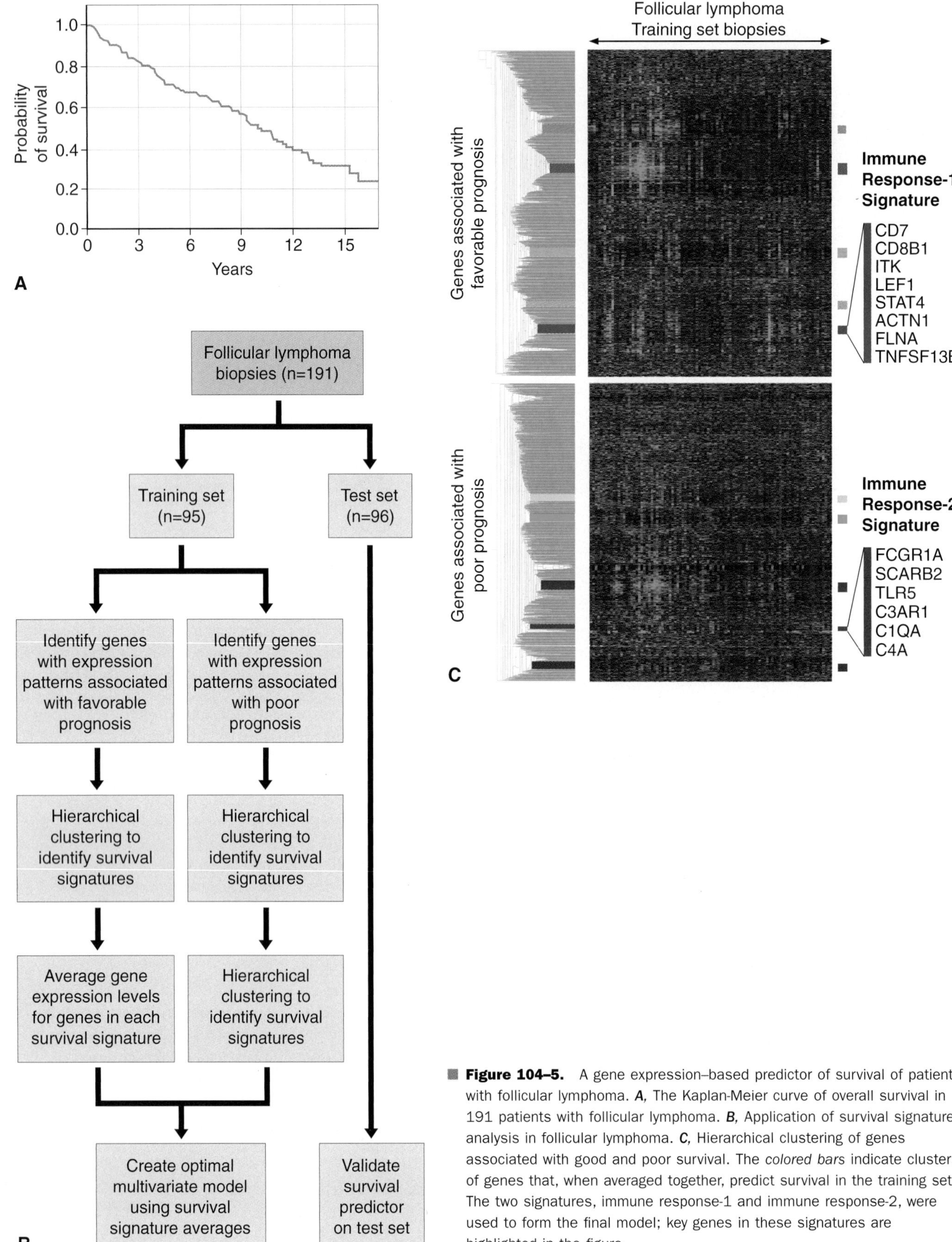

Figure 104–5. A gene expression–based predictor of survival of patients with follicular lymphoma. ***A,*** The Kaplan-Meier curve of overall survival in 191 patients with follicular lymphoma. ***B,*** Application of survival signature analysis in follicular lymphoma. ***C,*** Hierarchical clustering of genes associated with good and poor survival. The *colored bars* indicate clusters of genes that, when averaged together, predict survival in the training set. The two signatures, immune response-1 and immune response-2, were used to form the final model; key genes in these signatures are highlighted in the figure.

Survival signature analysis begins with the division of the samples into equal training and test sets; model development proceeds only with data from the training set. The Cox proportional hazards model is used to identify genes from the training set biopsy samples that are associated with survival. Hierarchical clustering is applied separately to the genes associated with good and bad prognoses, aiming to identify survival-associated gene expression signatures. The expression levels of genes in each signature are then averaged to create a single "survival signature average." These survival signature averages are used in multivariate models of survival using the training set cases, and the optimal model is then applied to the test set to determine its reproducibility. In follicular lymphoma, 10 survival-associated gene expression signatures were identified, 5 from the genes associated with good prognosis and 5 from those associated with poor prognosis (Fig. 104–5*C*).

The predictive power of the model was illustrated by dividing the patients in the test set into four equal quartiles based on their survival predictor scores. These quartile groups had strikingly disparate median survival rates of 3.9 years, 10.8 years, 11.1 years, and 13.6 years (Fig. 104–6). Consistent with previous studies in follicular lymphoma, the components of the International Prognostic Index as well as the presence of B symptoms (fevers, night sweats, and/or weight loss) predicted survival of patients in the study. However, gene expression–could independently predict survival when combined in a multivariate model with the International Prognostic Index or any single clinical variable ($P < .001$). The gene expression–based model was not a surrogate for any clinical variables but rather identified distinct biologic attributes of the tumors that are associated with survival.

Tumor biopsies typically include both malignant and nonmalignant cells. To directly identify which cells expressed the survival-associated gene expression signatures in follicular lymphoma, the malignant $CD19^+$ cells were separated from the nonmalignant $CD19^-$ cells by flow sorting and each subpopulation was profiled for gene expression (Fig. 104–7). These gene expression studies revealed the origin of the immune response-1 and immune response-2 signatures from the nonmalignant immune cells within the biopsy samples.[33]

That molecular features of nonmalignant cells can influence survival in follicular lymphoma implies an important interplay between the host immune system and the malignant cells in the disease. These features are present at diagnosis, suggesting that the stochastic acquisition of oncogenic abnormalities is not a primary determinant of overall survival in follicular lymphoma. Clinically, the survival predictor could be used to identify a quartile of patients with an extremely indolent form of this disease, in which the median survival is more than 13 years following diagnosis. In the absence of a reliably curative treatment, this is a group of patients for whom observation may be most appropriate and for whom the survival predictor would provide valuable prognostic information. The least favorable quartile had a median survival of only 3.9 years, and these patients should be considered for newer treatments in clinical trials.

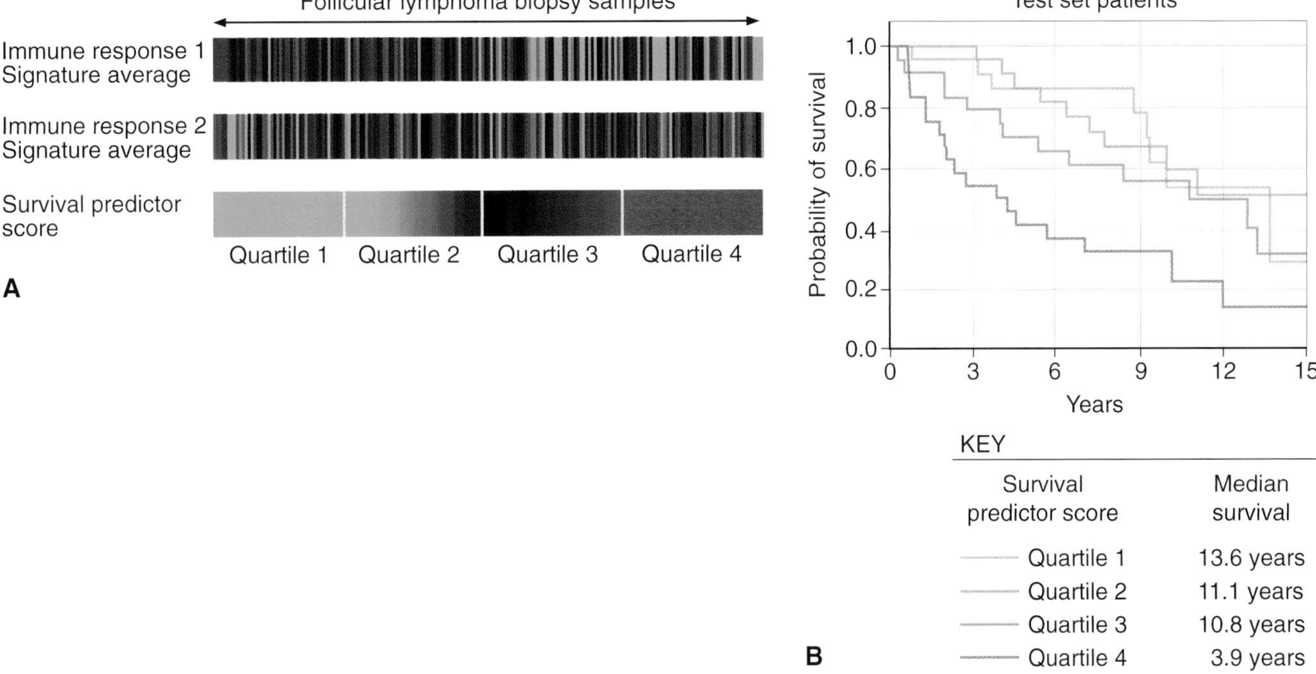

Figure 104–6. Gene expression signatures and survival in follicular lymphoma. *A,* Association of the survival predictor score generated by the gene expression model for each patient with the survival-associated immune response signatures. *B,* Kaplan-Meier curve of overall survival of patients in the test set for each quartile of the survival predictor score.

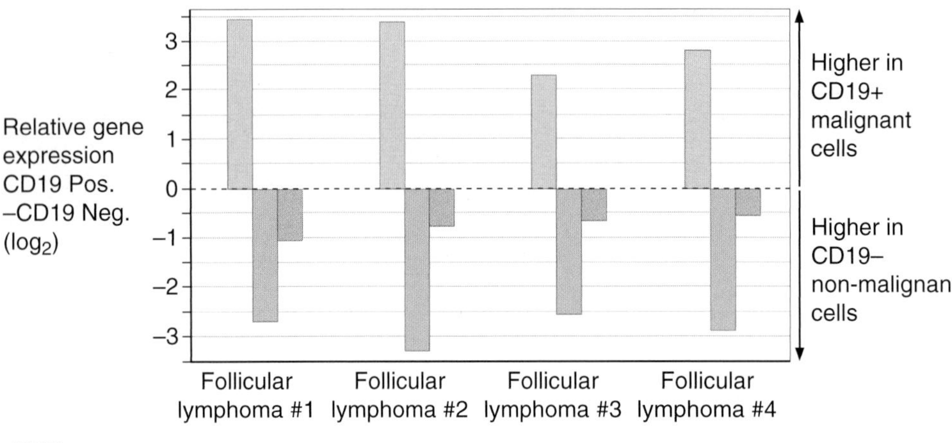

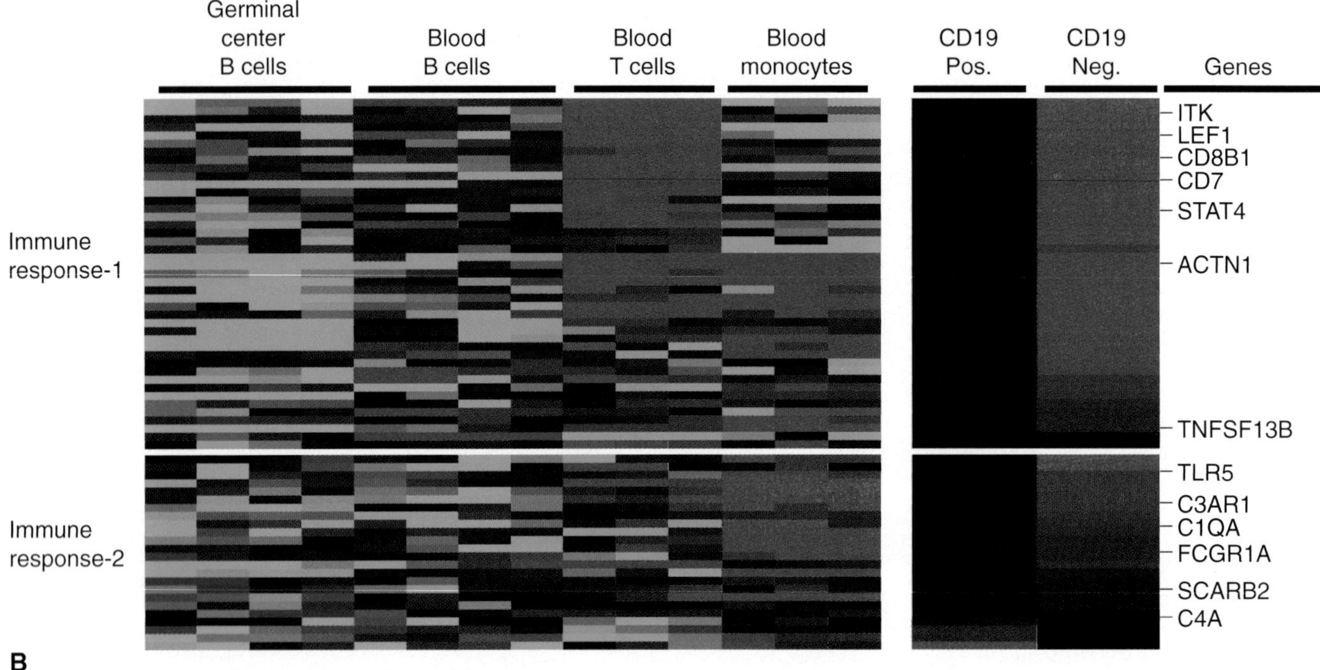

Figure 104–7. The survival signatures in follicular lymphoma are derived from nonmalignant cells. *A*, Distribution of gene expression signatures in the malignant and nonmalignant cells. *B*, Expression of the survival signatures in purified populations of normal germinal center or peripheral blood B cells, T cells, and monocytes.

Other Hematologic Malignancies

Ease in obtaining malignant cells and their ready purification from normal cells by flow cytometric methods facilitated the analysis of leukemias and lymphomas by microarrays. Gene expression has been used to uncover important molecular pathways, to make fine discriminations within accepted diagnostic categories, and to provide practical information regarding survival outcomes, susceptibility to relapse, and likelihood of therapy-related toxicity (Table 104–1).

One of the earliest applications of microarrays was in the distinction of acute myelogenous leukemia from acute lymphoblastic leukemia. In a seminal study, Golub and colleagues[8] demonstrated that over 1000 of nearly 7000 genes, measured using an oligonucleotide microarray, were differentially expressed in the two entities; a weighted predictor of 50 of these genes accurately assigned the correct diagnosis in an independent set of patients. This early analysis was an important proof of the concept that gene expression using microarrays could make diagnostic distinctions and provide insights into the

TABLE 104–1. Gene Expression Analysis Studies of Leukemias and Lymphomas

Disease Entity	Selected Studies
Myelodysplastic Syndrome/Leukemia	
Myelodysplastic syndrome	Chen G, et al: Blood 104:4210–4218, 2004 [48]
Chronic myelogenous leukemia	McLean LA, et al: Clin Cancer Res 10(1 Pt 1):155–165, 2004 [49]
Acute myelogenous leukemia	Bullinger L, et al: N Engl J Med 350:1605–1616, 2004 [4]
	Valk PJM, et al: N Engl J Med 350:1617–1628, 2004 [5]
Chronic lymphocytic leukemia	Wiestner A, et al: Blood 101:4944–4951, 2003 [50]
Acute lymphoblastic leukemia	Holleman A, et al: N Engl J Med 351:533–542, 2004 [51]
	Ross ME, et al: Blood 102:2951–2959, 2003 [39]
T-cell leukemia	Ferrando AA, et al: Cancer Cell 1:75–87, 2002 [52]
Non-Hodgkin's Lymphoma	
Diffuse large B-cell lymphoma	Rosenwald A, et al: N Engl J Med 346:1937–1947, 2002 [25]
Follicular lymphoma	Dave SS, et al: N Engl J Med 351:2159-2169, 2004 [33]
Mantle cell lymphoma	Rosenwald A, et al: Cancer Cell 2:185–197, 2003 [53]
Primary mediastinal B-cell lymphoma	Rosenwald A, et al: J Exp Med 198:851–862, 2003 [54]
	Savage KJ, et al: Blood 102:3871–3879, 2003 [55]
Multiple myeloma	Davies FE, et al: Blood 102:4504–4511, 2003 [56]
	Zhan F, et al: Blood 101:1128–1140, 2003 [57]

underlying biology. Further investigations of patients who had translocation of the mixed lineage leukemia (*MLL*) gene showed overexpression of the *FLT3* gene.[34] FMS-like tyrosine kinase-3 (FLT-3) is a tyrosine kinase receptor, and aberrations of the gene are leukemogenic.[35,36] *FLT3* mutations in patients with acute myelogenous leukemia have suggested its role in the pathophysiology of the disease. Pharmacologic inhibition of FLT-3 using a small-molecule inhibitor (PKC412) was found to be effective in a mouse xenograft model.[37] Thus gene expression profiling served as a starting point in the delineation of a pathway with a therapeutic goal.

In pediatric acute lymphoblastic leukemia, the six known clinical groups, largely defined by their characteristic cytogenetics (T-cell derived, E2A/PBX-1, Philadelphia chromosome positive, TEL/AML-1, MLL rearranged, and hyperdiploid), could be discerned by gene expression using both cDNA and oligonucleotide microarrays with an accuracy of greater than 95%.[38,39] Similarly, in pediatric acute myelogenous leukemia, genes were identified for each of the major prognostic subtypes, including t(15;17) (*PML/RARA*), t(8;21) (*AML1/ETO*), inv(16) (*CBFB/MYH11*), *MLL*-chimeric fusion genes, and cases classified as M7 in the French-American-British classification.[40] A predictor developed using these genes was over 90% accurate in classifying the leukemia types. The predictor developed using the pediatric samples was also highly accurate in discriminating the major cytogenetic subgroups in adult patients.

Although chromosome examination represents the current standard method in leukemia, assessment of cytogenetics is technically difficult and laborious, the sample size is often small, and reproducibility may be inconsistent. Automated microarrays potentially would provide a more reliable and rapid, as well as less expensive, means of discerning molecular abnormalities that guide diagnostic and therapeutic decisions.

GENE EXPRESSION AND MOLECULAR DIAGNOSIS

Conventional pathologic diagnosis involves the integration of diagnostic information from several sources: tissue morphology, expression of selected protein markers, and cytogenetic aberrations. The process can be subjective, time intensive, and expensive. Non-Hodgkin's lymphoma is a particularly challenging area in conventional pathologic diagnosis. Clinical management differs significantly for the various types of non-Hodgkin's lymphoma, and distinguishing them can be difficult using existing methods. Furthermore, as discussed earlier, certain non-Hodgkin's lymphoma categories include molecular subgroups that differ substantially in gene expression, response to therapy, and overall survival. Present diagnostic categories of cancer can be distinguished using gene expression.[8,39,41–43] In addition, information from DNA microarrays is well correlated with results from other methods such as flow cytometry, and immunohistochemistry.[44,45] By providing a complete molecular profile of a tumor, DNA microarrays potentially can replace a number of tests that are currently performed to obtain a diagnosis. The results obtained using microarrays are quantitative and highly reproducible and thus have the potential to provide an objective, molecular diagnosis of cancer.[46]

As a first step toward the clinical use of microarrays, a custom oligonucleotide microarray named LymphDx was designed for molecular diagnosis and outcome prediction in non-Hodgkin's lymphoma. Biopsy specimens were obtained from over 500 patients with a variety of lymphomas and lymphoproliferative conditions. Genome-wide gene expression profiles of the specimens were obtained using Affymetrix U133 microarrays. The genes most differentially expressed among non-Hodgkin's lymphoma types were the starting point for the LymphDx microarray. In addition, genes used in outcome predictors for diffuse large B-cell lymphoma, follicular lymphoma, and mantle cell lymphoma were included, and genes were added from the genomes of the Epstein-Barr and human herpesvirus 8 viruses, which are known to be important in the pathogenesis of several types of non-Hodgkin's lymphoma. Roughly 2500 genes are represented as oligonucleotide features on the LymphDx microarray.

Many different methods have been formulated using gene expression to distinguish cancer subgroups.[8,19,42,47] The LymphDx microarray has been employed to profile gene expression in 434 biopsy samples from a variety of malignant and benign lymphoproliferative disorders (Fig.

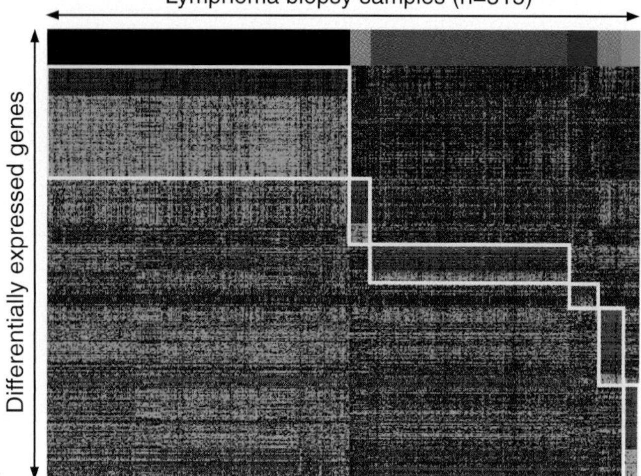

Figure 104–8. Using gene expression to distinguish non-Hodgkin's lymphoma subtypes.

104–8). Thus the LymphDx microarray offers a single diagnostic platform that can provide a comprehensive molecular diagnosis of a tumor as well as prognostic information for the major forms of non-Hodgkin's lymphoma. By replacing the large number of current diagnostic assays, it may become a cost-effective clinical tool.

POTENTIAL SHORTCOMINGS OF MICROARRAYS

DNA microarrays cannot be used as the sole source of diagnostic information, because biopsy samples with inadequate representation of malignant cells will not yield a reliable gene expression profile. Therefore, the sample should be examined by a pathologist before gene expression profiling. Current DNA microarray technology requires frozen tissue, which poses a significant limitation because specimens are generally preserved in formalin; a major change in the processing of biopsy samples will be required before the use of microarrays can become standard. These problems could be overcome by the widespread adoption of centralized tissue banking and specialized centers that perform microarray analysis for diagnosis.

CURRENT CONTROVERSIES & FUTURE CONSIDERATIONS

Gene Expression Methods

- Given the novelty of the technology, almost all microarray data are retrospective. Prospective validation of microarray-derived clinical data remains to be undertaken.
- Will frozen tissue capabilities become available more widely? Will specialized centers emerge for tissue banking and microarray processing?
- Other technologies are maturing that measure other molecular features of tumors, such as protein expression and chromosomal aberrations. How will these technologies be integrated with gene expression profiling?

Suggested Readings*

Alizadeh AA, Eisen MB, Davis RE, et al: Distinct types of diffuse large B-cell lymphoma identified by gene expression profiling. Nature 403:503–511, 2000.

Dave SS, Wright G, Tan B, et al: Prediction of survival in follicular lymphoma based on molecular features of tumor-infiltrating immune cells. N Engl J Med 351:2159–2169, 2004.

Golub TR, Slonim KD, Tamayo P, et al: Molecular classification of cancer: class discovery and class prediction by gene expression monitoring. Science 286:531–537, 1999.

Ransohoff DF: Rules of evidence for cancer molecular-marker discovery and validation. Nat Rev Cancer 4:309–314, 2004.

Staudt LM: Molecular diagnosis of the hematologic cancers. N Engl J Med 348:1777–1785, 2003.

Full references for this chapter can be found on accompanying CD-ROM.

CHAPTER 105

Coagulation Testing

Margaret E. Rick, MD

KEY POINTS

Coagulation Testing

Coagulation Studies

- Screening coagulation assays
- Monitoring of oral anticoagulation with International Normalized Ratio
- Monitoring heparin with activated partial thromboplastin time
- Lupus anticoagulant testing
- Specific coagulation factor assays and inhibitors
- Von Willebrand factor assays
- Assays in bleeding patients who have normal screening tests

Assays for Disseminated Intravascular Coagulation and Fibrinolysis

- Euglobulin clot lysis
- Fibrinogen/fibrin degradation products and D-dimer
- Tissue plasminogen activator, plasminogen activator inhibitor-1, plasminogen

Assays of Platelet Quantity and Function

- Quantitation of platelets
- Platelet aggregation
- Platelet function analyzers
- Bleeding time
- Assays for heparin-induced thrombocytopenia
- Assays for thrombotic thrombocytopenic purpura
- Assays for antibodies to platelets

Evaluation of Thrombophilia

- Inhibitor proteins: protein C, protein S, antithrombin
- Inherited defects in coagulation factors: factor V Leiden, prothrombin gene mutation 20210, high levels of circulating coagulation factors
- Lupus anticoagulants and thrombosis
- Factors contributing to arterial thrombosis

INTRODUCTION

Laboratory testing is essential for the diagnosis of hemostatic and thrombotic diseases. The clinical presentation of a number of these diseases is identical, and they can be identified only by specific tests that differentiate them from one another. This chapter addresses the tests that are useful in patients with bleeding disorders first and then addresses the diagnostic assays for diseases that result in thrombophilic states.

We have learned a good deal about the physiology of the hemostatic system in the past 2 decades. Our ability to test for aberrations in this system has also improved, but we still depend on a number of laboratory assays that have been available for many years because they are relatively inexpensive and have a fast turnaround time, the latter being a property that is particularly important when evaluating a patient with acute life-threatening bleeding. Automated instruments have been developed for assessing samples for coagulation and thrombophilic defects and for screening platelet function more rapidly and simply than was possible with previous tools.

SCREENING COAGULATION ASSAYS

A simplified coagulation cascade and its relation to the screening coagulation tests are shown in Figure 105–1. The circulating coagulation factors are zymogens and cofactors that are activated by proteolytic cleavage, usually at the membrane of cells that provide a phos-

Dr. Rick wrote this chapter in her private capacity and no official endorsement or support by the National Institutes of Health is intended or should be inferred.

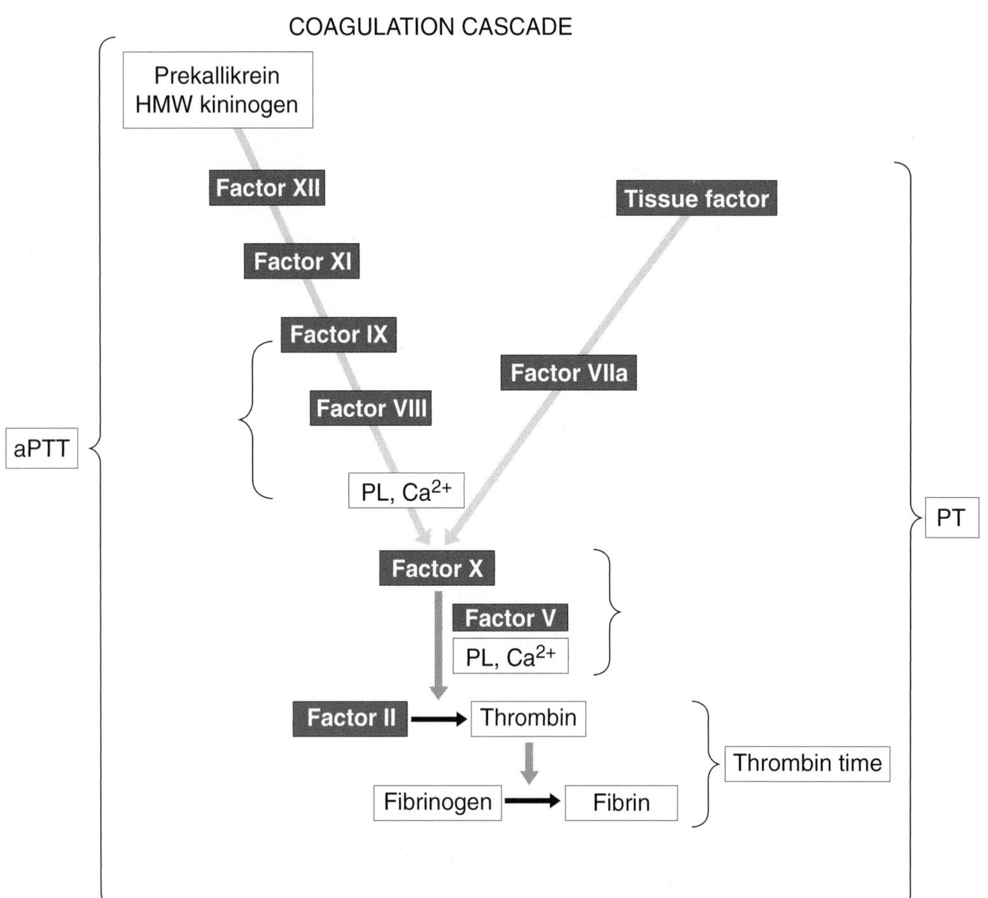

Figure 105–1. Simplified coagulation cascade indicating the intrinsic pathway measured by the activated partial thromboplastin time (aPTT), the extrinsic pathway measured by the prothrombin time (PT), and the conversion of fibrinogen to fibrin, which is measured by the thrombin time. Other proteins—prekallikrein and high-molecular-weight (HMW) kininogen—participate in the contact activation phase but are not considered to be coagulation factors. Abbreviations: Ca^{2+}, calcium ions; PL, phospholipid.

TABLE 105–1. Screening Coagulation Assays

Assay	Pathway Measured	Factors Measured
Prothrombin time	Extrinsic and final common pathway	Tissue factor, factors VII, II, V, X, fibrinogen
Activated partial thromboplastin time	Intrinsic and final common pathway	Factors VIII, IX, XI, XII, II, V, X, fibrinogen
Thrombin time	Fibrinogen conversion to fibrin (final step in common pathway)	Fibrinogen and potential inhibitors of thrombin
Fibrinogen (functional)	Fibrinogen conversion to fibrin (final step in common pathway)	Concentration and ability to form fibrin clot

pholipid surface for the reactions. Activation of the cascade begins with cellular injury, exposing tissue factor and initiating the "extrinsic pathway." There are a number of interactions between the intrinsic and extrinsic coagulation systems that are not shown in this figure for simplicity.

For all coagulation assays, the clinician should check the normal reference range of the laboratory used by the hospital. It should be noted that coagulation samples that are sent to an outside laboratory may encounter conditions (temperature, storage) that affect the results. If in doubt about a clinical result, it is best to repeat the assay.

Coagulation screening tests are often done before invasive procedures (most commonly, the prothrombin time and activated partial thromboplastin time [aPTT]), and these tests are also used in the initial evaluation of the bleeding patient (Table 105–1). For the screening assays, as well as for most other functional coagulation assays, the sample is anticoagulated by collecting blood into one-tenth volume of sodium citrate, which chelates the calcium that is necessary in several of the coagulation reactions. Calcium chloride is added back to the plasma during the assay. The assays measure different pathways and have differing sensitivities to coagulation factor deficiencies: in general, the aPTT will become abnormal when one of the factors in the pathway is less than 40–50%, and the prothrombin time will become abnormal when one of the factors is less than 20–25%. When one of the screening tests is abnormal, a mixing study is performed to help in the further testing of the sample.

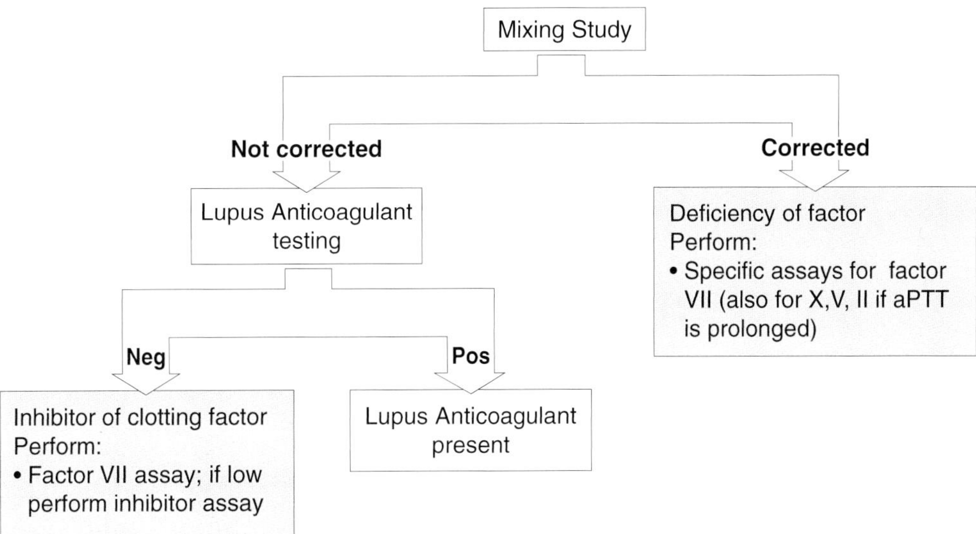

Figure 105–2. Algorithm for evaluation of an isolated prolonged prothrombin time (PT). Liver disease and vitamin K deficiency are the most common causes of a prolonged PT. Lupus anticoagulants (LACs) may prolong the PT by 1–2 seconds, but a greater prolongation should be investigated with a specific assay for prothrombin. Dysfibrinogenemia occasionally causes a prolongation of the PT without a prolongation of the aPTT. (Redrawn from Noel P, Rick ME: Laboratory Testing. *In* Williams ME, Kahn MJ [eds]: ASH-SAP American Society of Hematology Self-Assessment Program [ed 2]. Boston: Blackwell Publishing, 2005.)

Mixing Studies

Mixing studies are performed as an initial step when a screening study is abnormal in order to help determine whether the patient has a deficiency (the normal plasma will "correct" the abnormal clotting test when a factor deficiency is present), or the patient has an inhibitor to a factor (usually the abnormal assay remains in the abnormal range, though in practice low-titer inhibitors may "correct" in a 1:1 mixing study). The test is carried out by mixing the patient sample with pooled normal plasma (1:1) and then repeating the test within 5 minutes of mixing the plasmas. In a mixing study for a prolonged aPTT, the mixture of patient and normal sample is also held at 37°C for 1–2 hours, and the aPTT is repeated a second time in order to detect a potential slow-acting inhibitor to factor VIII.

Prothrombin Time

The prothrombin time, which measures the extrinsic pathway, is performed by adding tissue factor to citrated plasma, recalcifying, and measuring the time to clot formation. Automated instruments commonly depend on end points measured by a change in optical density or on a mechanical change as the clot forms. Commercial sources of tissue factor include both tissue extracts and recombinant molecules.

Causes for a prolonged prothrombin time include the following (Fig. 105–2):

- Vitamin K deficiency or oral anticoagulant therapy with a coumarin
- Liver disease with decreased synthesis of factor VII
- Anticoagulation with lepirudin or argatroban
- Early disseminated intravascular coagulation
- Inherited deficiency or inhibitor of factor VII (rare)
- Dysfibrinogenemia (rare)

Monitoring Oral Anticoagulant Therapy (Coumarins) with the Prothrombin Time—the INR

A calculated value that is derived from the prothrombin time, the International Normalized Ratio (INR), is used to determine dosing of coumarin therapy. It is useful in making comparisons in different laboratories and when reagent lots are changed within a laboratory. The INR is the ratio of the patient's prothrombin time to the normal mean prothrombin time for the laboratory that incorporates a value for the particular tissue thromboplastin being used in the laboratory. It is essentially a ratio of the prothrombin times (PTs) performed as though the laboratory's thromboplastin was the international reference preparation of thromboplastin. Each commercial preparation of thromboplastin is assigned an International Sensitivity Index (ISI) score by its manufacturer, and the INR includes it in the calculation:

$$\mathrm{INR} = \left(\frac{\text{PT of patient}}{\text{Mean normal PT of lab}}\right)^{\mathrm{ISI}}$$

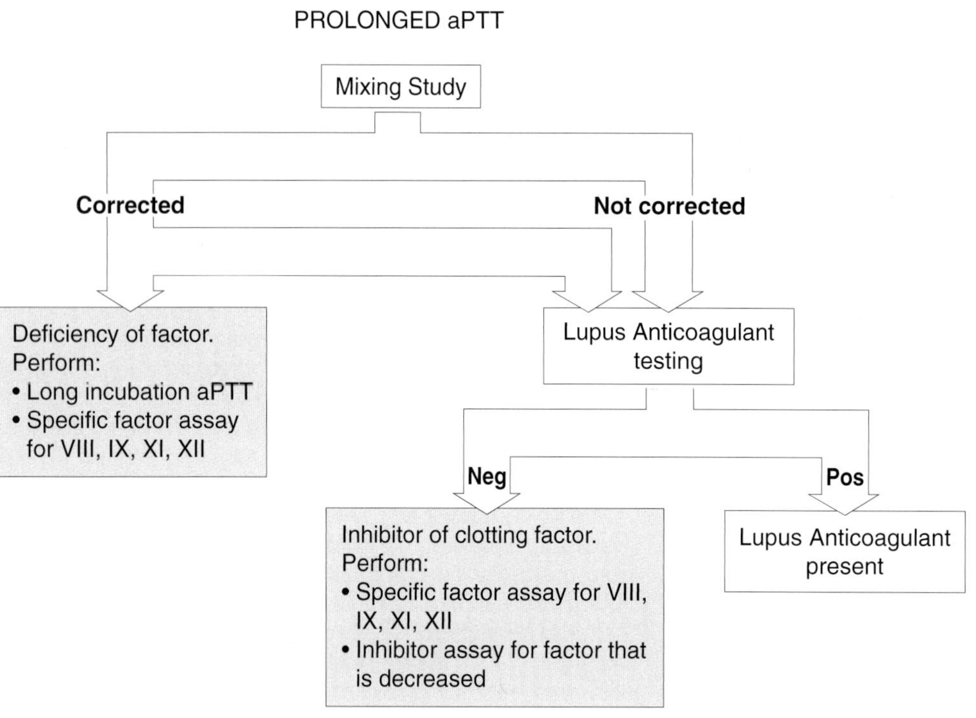

Figure 105–3. Algorithm for evaluation of an isolated prolonged activated partial thromboplastin time (aPTT). Because a minority of plasmas with lupus anticoagulants (LACs) show correction in the 1:1 mixing study, many laboratories perform a LAC assay before or concomitantly with the factor assays. (Redrawn from Noel P, Rick ME: Laboratory Testing. *In* Williams ME, Kahn MJ [eds]: ASH-SAP American Society of Hematology Self-Assessment Program [ed 2]. Boston: Blackwell Publishing, 2005.)

The INR values are meant to be used for a patient who has been stabilized on an established dose of coumadin and should *not* be used to assess other diseases such as hepatic failure. The INR is not standardized for levels of factors that are not affected by vitamin K antagonists, such as factor V and fibrinogen.

Activated Partial Thromboplastin Time

The aPTT measures the intrinsic pathway and is performed using citrated plasma. Both phospholipids and a "surface" such as kaolin on which to bind and activate factor XII are added, and the plasma is recalcified; the time to clot formation is the end point. The test is performed by instruments that measure the end point by methods described previously for the prothrombin time.

Causes for a prolonged aPTT include the following (Figs. 105–3 and 105–4):

- Lupus anticoagulants
- Inherited or acquired deficiencies of factor VIII, IX, XI, or XII
- Inherited or acquired von Willebrand disease
- Inhibitors to any of the factors listed above
- Heparin contamination of sample (especially if drawn from an indwelling catheter)
- Anticoagulation with lepirudin or argatroban
- Deficiency of prekallikrein or high-molecular-weight kininogen (rare, see Long-Incubation aPTT below)

Unfractionated heparin is monitored using the aPTT. The target is a prolongation of 1.5–2.5 times the mean normal aPTT for the laboratory. One may also assess the heparin concentration using an anti–factor Xa assay (heparin range approximately 0.3–0.7 units/mL). *Low-molecular-weight* heparin does not usually require monitoring unless renal function is abnormal; one may use an anti-Xa assay with a standard curve specific for low-molecular-weight heparin (low-molecular-weight heparin range approximately 0.5–1.2 IU/mL for a sample drawn 4–6 hr after subcutaneous injection of low-molecular-weight heparin).

Long-Incubation aPTT

A long-incubation aPTT is performed to assess whether a deficiency is present that interferes with the contact activation of factor XII. A prekallikrein deficiency will prolong the aPTT assay because there is a positive feedback loop between the activation of factor XII and the conversion of prekallikrein to kallikrein. If prekallikrein is deficient, the aPTT will be prolonged. This test is performed like the aPTT except that the initial incubation/activation stage is prolonged from 3–4 minutes to 10 minutes before recalcifying and measuring the time to clot formation. If the aPTT is corrected to the normal range by the longer incubation time, a presumptive diagnosis of prekallikrein deficiency can be made. Prekallikrein deficiency does not cause bleeding, and finding a shortening to normal of the aPTT with prolonged incubation may obviate further work-up in a patient with a negative bleeding history and a prolonged aPTT.

Thrombin Time

The thrombin time is performed by adding exogenous purified human or bovine thrombin to plasma and measuring the time to clot formation. Causes for a prolonged thrombin time include the following (Fig. 105–5):

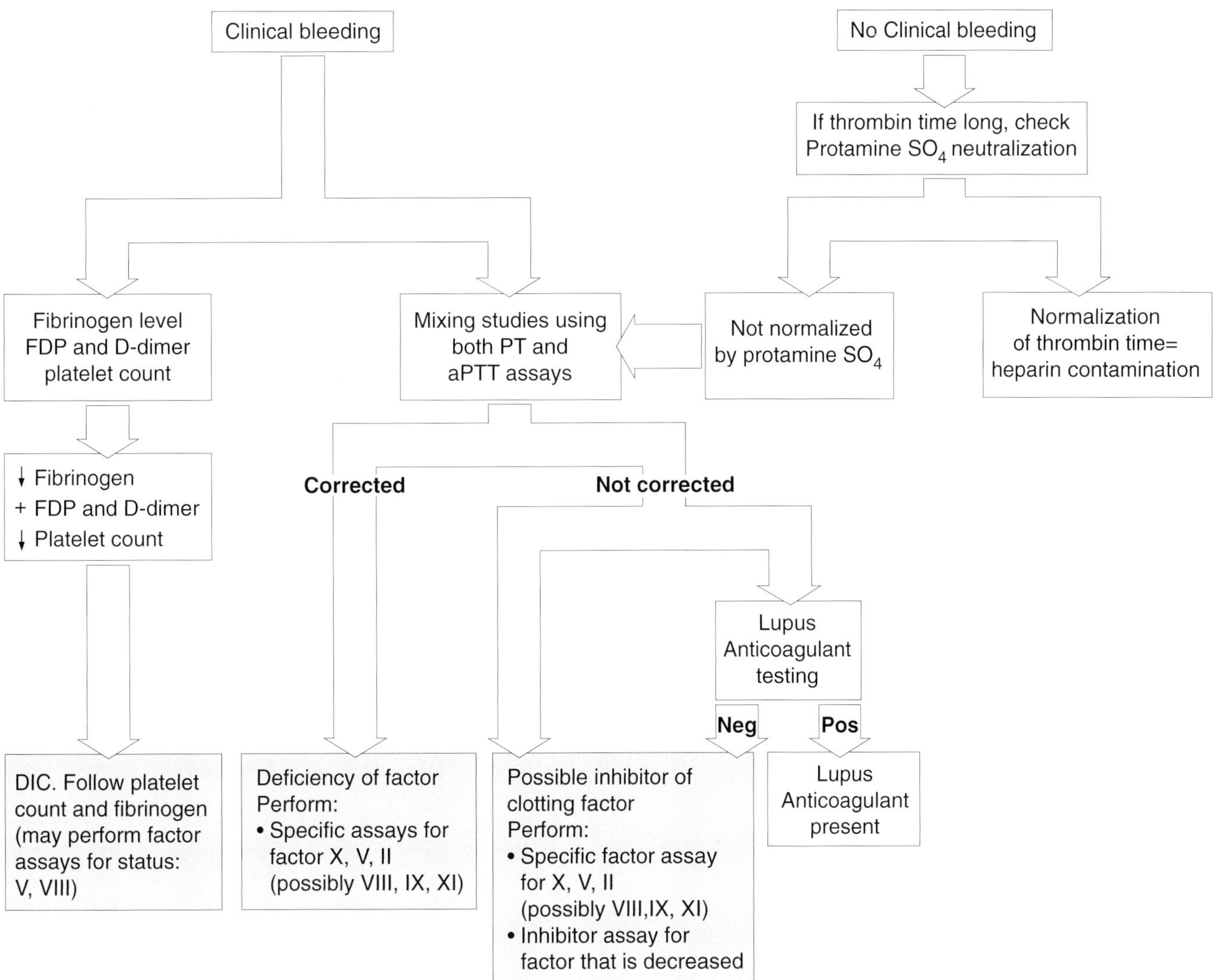

Figure 105–4. Algorithm for evaluation of a prolonged prothrombin time (PT) and aPTT. This algorithm considers unified causes for prolonged PT and aPTT, and a patient may have two different diseases that account for the prolongation of each respective test (e.g., liver disease [PT] and a lupus anticoagulant [aPTT]), or the patient may have thrombocytopenia causing the bleeding and a lupus anticoagulant causing an incidental prolonged aPTT. (Redrawn from Noel P, Rick ME: Laboratory Testing. *In* Williams ME, Kahn MJ [eds]: ASH-SAP American Society of Hematology Self-Assessment Program [ed 2]. Boston: Blackwell Publishing, 2005.)

- Low concentration of fibrinogen (less than 50–70 mg/dL)
- Dysfibrinogenemia
- Anticoagulation with heparin or other antithrombin agent (lepirudin, argatroban)
- Antibody to thrombin (rare)
- Fibrinogen/fibrin degradation products at high concentrations

Heparin can be neutralized by adding protamine sulfate (or heparinase) to the plasma, and the thrombin time will normalize. Another reagent, reptilase, can also convert fibrinogen to fibrin, and it is not inhibited by heparin. If both the thrombin time and reptilase time are prolonged, it may indicate that the patient has a dysfibrinogenemia, and further testing can be carried out to confirm this diagnosis (see later) (see Fig. 105–5).

Fibrinogen Assays

Functional concentrations of fibrinogen are assayed using very high concentrations of thrombin, so the concentration of functional fibrinogen is the limiting element. In this assay, the time to clot formation is dependent on the functional fibrinogen concentration. Causes for an abnormally low functional fibrinogen assay include the following:

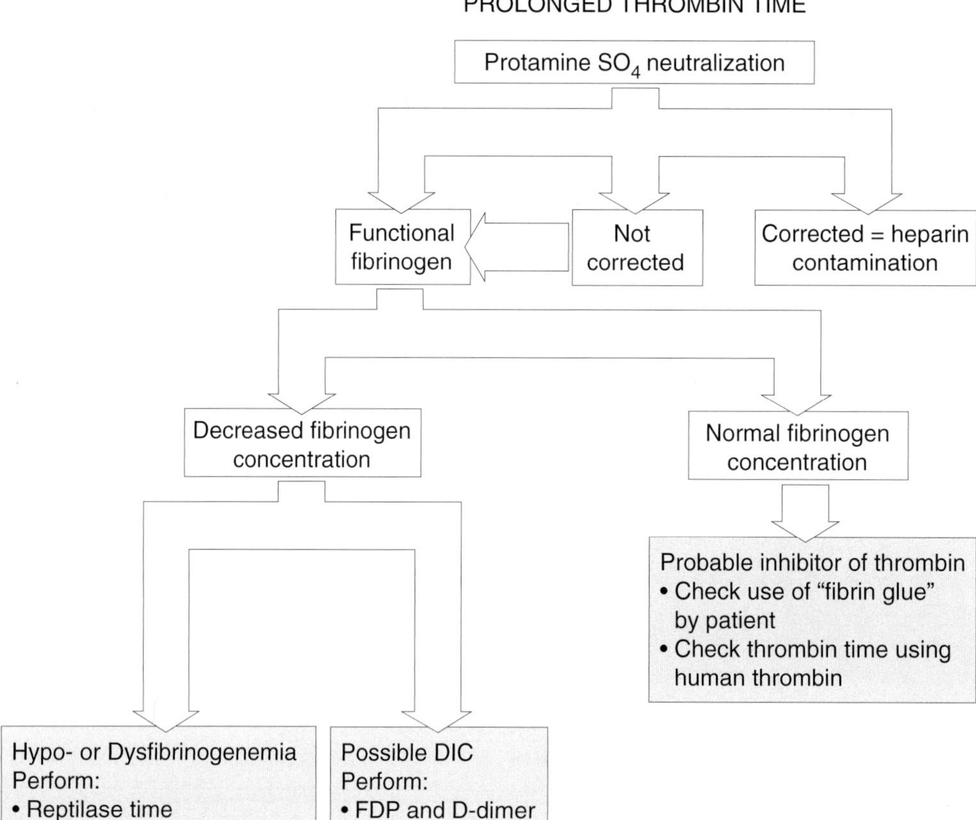

Figure 105–5. Algorithm for evaluation of a prolonged thrombin time. Most abnormal thrombin times in hospitalized patients are due to heparin contamination of a sample drawn from an indwelling line.

- Low concentration of fibrinogen (less than 50–70 mg/dL)
- Dysfibrinogenemia

Immunologic concentrations of fibrinogen are assessed using an antibody to fibrinogen in techniques such as immunodiffusion. In normal individuals, the immunologic fibrinogen concentration is approximately 25–30% higher than the functional fibrinogen. If there is a greater discrepancy between the two assays (more than ~30–35% higher immunologic than functional fibrinogen), a presumptive diagnosis of a dysfibrinogenemia can be made. Further testing requires specialized assays, such as fibrin monomer polymerization studies and protein or gene sequencing.

Antiphospholipid Antibody Testing

Lupus anticoagulants are antibodies that bind to phospholipid-protein complexes and inhibit phospholipid-dependent steps in the coagulation cascade. They are one class of antiphospholipid antibody. The aPTT is usually prolonged by lupus anticoagulants in the screening assays, and most often the 1:1 mixing study using the aPTT does not correct to the normal range in these patients; low-titer lupus anticoagulants, however, may correct in mixing studies. The prothrombin time may also be prolonged 1–2 seconds in patients with lupus anticoagulants. If the prothrombin time is more prolonged, a factor II level (prothrombin) should be measured, because 5–10% of patients with lupus anticoagulants also have (additional) antibodies to factor II. The specific tests for lupus anticoagulants are based on assays that include the phospholipid-dependent steps in either the intrinsic pathway, the extrinsic pathway, or the final common pathway of coagulation. These tests are all two-step procedures in which excess phospholipid is added in the second step (often called the platelet or phospholipid neutralization step) to bind the lupus anticoagulant and still leave sufficient phospholipid for the coagulation reactions. The clotting time of the second step is compared to the clotting time in the first step. If a lupus anticoagulant is present, there will be significant shortening of the clotting time in the second step. Representative lupus anticoagulant assays for each of these pathways include:

- Staclot—aPTT pathway
- Dilute thromboplastin inhibition time—prothrombin time pathway

- Dilute Russell's viper venom time—final common pathway

If a deficiency of a clotting factor is present or if the patient is on coumadin, normal plasma is first added to the patient's plasma to correct the deficiency (1:1 mix), and then both steps of the assay are performed. If an inhibitor to a specific clotting factor, rather than a lupus anticoagulant, is present, the clotting time in step 2 will not shorten significantly. It is important that the patient's plasma sample be processed to remove any phospholipid (platelet or platelet membrane) fragments in the plasma before testing and before freezing by filtering the plasma or by a "hard spin"; otherwise, these fragments can bind the lupus anticoagulant and result in a false-negative test.

Lupus anticoagulants are a diverse group of antibodies, and one assay may not detect a patient's lupus anticoagulant. It has been shown that testing for lupus anticoagulants with one assay picks up approximately 75% of cases, while performing two different assays increases the ability to detect a lupus anticoagulant to over 90%.

A second class of antiphospholipid antibody that does not interfere with the coagulation cascade is directed to a different phospholipid-protein complex and is called *anticardiolipin antibody*. Although different protein components can be complexed with phospholipid as the antigen in this test, the most commonly identified protein component is β_2 glycoprotein I. The assay is done in an enzyme-linked immunosorbent assay (ELISA) format, and the wells are coated with phospholipid that complexes with serum β_2 glycoprotein I. Patient serum is added, and any antibody that is bound from the patient's serum is measured after washing the plate by using an antibody to either immunoglobulin G, M, or A. Immunoglobulin G anticardiolipin antibody is most common, immunoglobulin M is less common, and immunoglobulin A anticardiolipin is very uncommon. The immunoglobulin G anticardiolipin antibody appears to be most frequently associated with clinical problems.

The significance of a positive lupus anticoagulant test is greater if the test remains positive for at least 6 weeks. To diagnose the antiphospholipid syndrome (a thrombotic syndrome; see later), one must have (1) a history of a clinical thrombotic event or multiple pregnancy losses plus (2) a persistent lupus anticoagulant or anticardiolipin antibody (elevated to greater than 3 standard deviations) that remains positive for at least 6 weeks.

COAGULATION FACTOR ASSAYS

Most functional assays for specific coagulation factors are based on a clot end point using a modification of the prothrombin time or aPTT. A factor-deficient substrate is used that provides all the factors except for the one being measured, which is to be supplied by the patient's plasma. If the patient's plasma supplies the factor that is missing from the deficient substrate plasma, the clotting time will be shortened into the range comparable to normal plasma. A standard curve is prepared using dilutions of normal plasma, and the concentration of the factor in the patient's plasma is quantitated by relating the patient clotting time to the clotting times of the normal plasma curve. Most normal reference ranges are approximately 50–150%; however, these ranges do not reflect the levels necessary for hemostasis because coagulation factors circulate in excess. Chromogenic assays, which are based on the ability of a factor to cleave a small chromogenic substrate specific for that factor, are commercially available for factor VIII and factor X. They are more expensive and less widely used for quantitation of specific factors.

Tests for inhibitors of specific factors are based on the same assays used to measure their concentrations (see earlier). These assays evaluate the ability of the patient's plasma to inhibit the factor present in normal plasma and thus prolong the expected clotting time. They use a 1:1 (vol:vol) mixture of patient and normal plasma and are quantitated by testing several dilutions of the patient's plasma mixed with undiluted normal plasma, searching for the dilution that inhibits approximately 50% of the factor in normal plasma. The titer (in Bethesda units) is reported as the reciprocal of the dilution that inhibits 50% of the factor present in normal plasma. Assays for factor VIII inhibitors must include an incubation at 37°C for 2 hours to ensure that a "slow-reacting" inhibitor is not missed; other factors can be tested after an incubation of the mixture of approximately 5 minutes.

Von Willebrand Factor Assays

Von Willebrand factor is a large glycoprotein that functions as a bridging molecule between platelets and vascular subendothelium and binds and protects factor VIII in the circulation. It circulates as a series of multimers formed from a dimer by disulfide linkages.

The diagnosis of von Willebrand disease can be difficult because of the wide normal range of von Willebrand factor levels, the variation in levels as a response to acute and chronic stress or illness and physiologic conditions such as pregnancy, the recognized lower level of von Willebrand factor in individuals with blood type O (25% lower than other ABO blood types), and the lack of correlation of von Willebrand factor levels with bleeding. At the present time, the hematology community is becoming somewhat more conservative in its willingness to make a diagnosis of von Willebrand disease in patients with borderline values unless there are definite clinical symptoms and/or a positive family history of the disease. A number of assays are used to measure the various functions of von Willebrand factor (Table 105–2).

The concentration of von Willebrand factor (*von Willebrand factor antigen*) in plasma is measured by specific antibodies in an ELISA format. Functional assays for von Willebrand factor are based on its ability to bind to platelet or subendothelial substrates and on its ability to bind and protect factor VIII in plasma. Platelet binding is measured in the *ristocetin cofactor* assay, which measures the binding of plasma von Willebrand factor to its platelet receptor by measuring the aggregation that follows by aggregometry or by a visual end point. Antibody-based assays that detect the von Willebrand factor

TABLE 105–2. Von Willebrand Factor (VWF) Assays

VWF Function	Assay	Property of VWF	Value of Assay
VWF concentration	VWF antigen	Concentration (determined by specific antibody to VWF; ELISA format)	Initial diagnostic screening
VWF platelet or matrix-related activities	Ristocetin cofactor	Ability to bind to platelet receptor, GPIb, at ~1.2 mg/mL ristocetin	Initial diagnostic screening
	Collagen binding	Ability to bind to collagen (ELISA format)	Initial or later diagnostic test
Factor VIII binding	Factor VIII activity	Functional clotting activity assay	Initial diagnostic screening
	Binding assay for factor VIII	Direct measurement of ability of patient VWF to bind normal factor VIII	Analysis of subtype of VWD (2N)
Ristocetin-induced platelet aggregation	RIPA	Ability to bind to platelet receptor, GPIb, at 1.2 and <0.6 mg/mL ristocetin	Analysis of subtype of VWD (2B)
VWF multimer study	Agarose gel electrophoresis	Multimer size distribution	Analysis of subtype of VWD (2A and 2B)

Abbreviations: ELISA, enzyme-linked immunosorbent assay; GPIb, glycoprotein Ib; RIPA, ristocetin-induced platelet aggregation; VWD, von Willebrand disease.

TABLE 105–3. Von Willebrand Disease (VWD) Classification

VWD Type	Ristocetin Cofactor	VWF Antigen	Factor VIII Activity	RIPA	VWF Multimers
Type 1	↓	↓	↓/Normal	↓/Normal	Normal
Type 2					
2A	↓/↓↓	↓/Normal	↓/Normal	↓	↓ HMW/IMW
2B	↓/↓↓	↓/Normal	↓/Normal	↑	↓ HMW/Normal
2M	↓	↓/Normal	↓/Normal	↓	Normal
2N	Normal	Normal	↓	Normal	Normal
Type 3	↓↓↓	↓↓↓	↓↓	↓↓↓	None detected

Abbreviations: HMW, high molecular weight; IMW, intermediate molecular weight; RIPA, ristocetin-induced platelet aggregation; VWF, von Willebrand factor.

binding site domain for the platelet receptor are also available, but they do not display the functional aggregation end point. The *collagen-binding* function of von Willebrand factor is assessed by exposure of plasma von Willebrand factor to collagen-coated wells; the bound factor is measured using a specific antibody in an ELISA format. *Factor VIII activity* levels reflect the binding ability of von Willebrand factor for factor VIII; factor VIII activity is decreased when there is a moderate or severe decrease in von Willebrand factor or when there is a qualitative defect in its binding site for factor VIII. The qualitative defect in binding can be measured in a specific *factor VIII binding assay* that uses the patient's von Willebrand factor to capture normal purified factor VIII. *Ristocetin-induced platelet aggregation* assesses whether the patient's von Willebrand factor might have a qualitative "gain of function" abnormality and bind more readily to the platelet receptor glycoprotein Ib; the assay uses several concentrations of ristocetin that are added to the patient's platelet-rich plasma, including a low concentration (<0.6 mg/mL) that does not cause aggregation in normal plasma. The test has an aggregation end point (all or none). If the patient's platelet-rich plasma aggregates at the low concentrations of ristocetin, this indicates a qualitative abnormality in von Willebrand factor (or, very rarely, in the patient's platelet receptor for von Willebrand factor, which is a platelet disease called platelet-type von Willebrand disease). *Von Willebrand factor multimers* are visualized after electrophoresis in low-concentration agarose gels (~1%); the von Willebrand factor bands are visualized after Western blotting using immunofluorescence developing techniques. The absence of large multimers is characteristic of two of the qualitative subtypes of von Willebrand disease (type 2A and 2B) (Table 105–3, Box 105–1).

Assays for Patients Who Have Bleeding, but Normal Coagulation and Platelet Tests

Factor XIII deficiency is very rare, and it is not detected in the screening coagulation tests. Both screening assays (testing for dissolution of clot in monochloroacetic acid or in urea) and specific assays are available for factor XIII. A deficiency of an inhibitor of fibrinolysis, *α_2-antiplasmin,* can lead to bleeding, often with invasive procedures. A specific factor assay is available for α_2-antiplasmin and has been automated. A third, rare, cause of bleeding in a patient with normal screening tests is a *deficiency of plasminogen activator inhibitor-1;* both activity and antigen assays are available to measure this protein.

Abnormalities that cause bleeding in patients with normal screening tests:

Box 105–1. Von Willebrand Disease Classification

- Type 1: Quantitative defect
- Type 2: Qualitative defects
  - 2A: Decreased function as a result of ↓ high-molecular-weight multimers (proteolysis or decreased multimerization)
  - 2B: Gain of function; ↑ binding of von Willebrand factor to platelet glycoprotein Ib, with removal of von Willebrand factor as a result of binding, platelet aggregate formation, and clearance (patient may be thrombocytopenic)
  - 2M: Defect in binding to platelets resulting from abnormality in the von Willebrand factor domain that binds platelet glycoprotein Ib
  - 2N: Decreased binding to factor VIII with rapid clearance of VIII
- Type 3: Severe quantitative defect (homozygous/doubly heterozygous)

- Factor XIII deficiency
- α_2-Antiplasmin deficiency
- PAI-1 deficiency

ASSAYS FOR DISSEMINATED INTRAVASCULAR COAGULATION AND FIBRINOLYSIS

We lack sensitive screening assays for the fibrinolytic system. *Euglobulin clot lysis time* measures the ability of a fraction of the patient's serum to lyse an endogenous clot formed from a plasma fraction that is depleted of the normal inhibitors of the fibrinolytic system. Normal euglobulin clot lysis times are greater than 2 hours. *Fibrinogen/fibrin degradation products* measure for the presence of products of fibrinogen and/or fibrin that result from cleavage by plasmin. *D-dimer tests* are specific for plasmin cleavage products from fibrin (not fibrinogen) and imply that fibrin has been formed and that secondary fibrinolysis, rather than primary fibrinolysis, is occurring (as seen in disseminated intravascular coagulation).

Fibrinogen/fibrin degradation products and D-dimer tests can be carried out quickly using semiquantitative latex bead assays; these tests are usually performed for evaluation of possible disseminated intravascular coagulation. False positives may be present in patients with rheumatoid factors. Recent or active bleeding will cause elevated levels of both assays, and renal failure will elevate the fibrinogen/fibrin degradation products. Results must be interpreted within the clinical situation. Levels of factor V and factor VIII are decreased in advanced disseminated intravascular coagulation, and these tests may be ordered for further confirmation.

Box 105–2. Assays of Fibrinolytic System Activity and Proteins

- Euglobulin clot lysis time—screening assay for fibrinolytic activity
- Fibrinogen/fibrin degradation products and D-dimer assays—cleavage products of fibrinogen and/or fibrin
- α_2-Antiplasmin—protease that inhibits circulating plasmin
- Tissue plasminogen activator (activity and antigen)—protein that activates plasminogen
- Plasminogen activator inhibitor-1 (activity and antigen)—protein that inhibits tissue plasminogen activator
- Plasmin activity—activity of enzyme that cleaves fibrinogen and other coagulation factors

ELISA methods for measuring D-dimer are utilized for more quantitative assays. The latter test has been used to "rule out" the presence of thromboembolic disease (when the test is negative).

α_2-Antiplasmin is an important inhibitor of circulating plasmin, and a decrease in its activity is associated with bleeding from unchecked fibrinolysis. Other assays that are available include assays for specific proteins in the fibrinolytic pathway, *tissue plasminogen activator, plasminogen activator inhibitor-1,* and *plasminogen,* by both functional and antigen assays (Box 105–2).

ASSAYS OF PLATELET QUANTITY AND FUNCTION

Quantitation of Platelets

Platelet counts are usually measured in automated cell counters by methods that use electrical impedance or light scatter. They are very sensitive methods and generally have good linearity even at the 5000–10,000/μL range. It is also important to examine the peripheral smear from the patient to ensure that platelet clumps, which may not be measured as platelets in the instrument because of their larger size, are not falsely lowering the count. EDTA-induced platelet clumps may be avoided by drawing the blood into citrate or heparin. Direct fingerstick smears may also be helpful in estimating the platelet count in these patients.

Platelet Aggregation

Platelet aggregometry evaluates the ability of platelets (in either whole blood or platelet-rich plasma) to respond to several known platelet agonists with the formation of aggregates. The agonist initially causes platelets to undergo a shape change and internal signaling with "activation" accompanied by aggregation; this is followed by a release of dense granule contents, some of which are agonists for aggregation, and a second wave ensues. The agonists used are classified as "weak" (epinephrine and ADP) and strong (collagen and thrombin). Arachidonic acid is also a stronger agonist that bypasses the need for platelet membrane receptors. Using platelet-rich plasma, one can see the primary wave (formation of platelet aggregates) caused by the agonist that is added to the platelet-rich plasma (with the exception of collagen, which does not cause aggregation directly), followed by a second wave that occurs because of the release of dense granule contents. In the platelet-rich plasma system, the end point is based on the increase in light transmittance that occurs when platelet aggregates are formed and fall by gravity from the light path because of their large size. The platelet release reaction may also be monitored in the platelet-rich plasma system using a lumi-aggregometer, which detects the released granule ATP by a fluorescent indicator pair such as luciferin-luciferase. These assays aid in the diagnosis of qualitative granule and release defects. In the whole blood system, the end point is a change in conductance when aggregates are formed. Platelet aggregation testing is time consuming and requires special instruments and a knowledgeable technologist as well as a fresh blood sample from the patient. It is also quite sensitive and requires careful interpretation.

Platelet Function Analyzers

Several instruments have been developed in the last decade that allow automated testing of platelet function by simpler and less time-consuming methods. Although these instruments generally are not as sensitive or specific as platelet aggregation, the tests can be completed rapidly and are simple to perform. As an example, one of the analyzers (the platelet function analyzer-100™, or PFA-100), works by aspirating a fresh citrated whole blood sample through an aspiration tube to a membrane with an aperture in it. Either epinephrine plus collagen or ADP plus collagen is added to the sample, and the platelets respond by adhering and aggregating at the membrane surface, ultimately forming a plug that occludes the aperture in the membrane and decreases the pressure in the aspiration line. The end point is the time to the decrease in the pressure as a result of the occluded aperture. This methodology will detect abnormalities associated with intrinsic platelet defects and the effects of nonsteroidal anti-inflammatory drugs and other platelet inhibitors if the abnormality is severe enough; it will also detect the platelet "defects" of von Willebrand disease.

Bleeding Time

The bleeding time depends on platelet numbers, platelet function, vascular integrity, hemoglobin concentration, and to some extent coagulation factors. It is a difficult test to standardize and does not predict bleeding during surgical procedures. The test is performed in the forearm by making a small incision of standard length and depth while maintaining a standard venous pressure in the arm (a blood pressure cuff is inflated to and kept at 40 mm Hg). Handheld templates or spring-loaded commercial devices are used to make the standard incision. A clean filter paper is brought to the edge of the wound every 30 seconds to carefully blot the blood without disturbing the forming clot, and the length of time until bleeding stops is noted. The normal range is generally 2–9.5 minutes, though some normal subjects who have been studied extensively for bleeding disorders have recorded bleeding times as long as 11.5 minutes. Currently the main use of the bleeding time is for the diagnosis of von Willebrand disease and intrinsic platelet defects. Platelet function analyzers are being used in some centers in place of the bleeding time to assess platelet function.

Assays for Heparin-Induced Thrombocytopenia

Most assays for heparin-induced thrombocytopenia assess whether an *antibody to a heparin–platelet factor 4 complex* is present in the patient's plasma (ELISA format). This test is very sensitive, and it is positive in some patients who do not have the clinical syndrome of heparin-induced thrombocytopenia; the results must be interpreted within the context of the clinical situation. The "gold standard" laboratory procedure for assessing whether a patient has heparin-induced thrombocytopenia is the *serotonin release assay*. It is performed with a low (therapeutic) and a high concentration of heparin, and it is less likely to report false positives. This test requires the use of radioactivity and is not widely available. Another similar functional test is available that measures the release of ATP at high and low concentrations of heparin; it does not require the use of radioactivity, but requires a lumi-aggregometer.

Assays for Thrombotic Thrombocytopenic Purpura

Antibodies that inhibit the activity of the von Willebrand factor cleaving protease (ADAMTS13) are responsible for a large number of "spontaneous" acquired cases of thrombotic thrombocytopenic purpura, and mutations in the protease account for the rare congenital recurrent familial syndromes. The activity of ADAMTS13 can be measured by assays that test for a decrease in the high-molecular-weight multimers of von Willebrand factor after exposure to conditions that allow the protease to cleave von Willebrand factor. Detection of a decrease in high-molecular-weight multimers can be performed by a number of methods: direct visualization of the plasma von Willebrand factor multimers in gel electrophoresis, ristocetin cofactor assay, and collagen binding assay. A different method assesses the increased products of von Willebrand factor proteolysis by polyacrylamide gel electrophoresis and densitometry, and an ELISA test measures the increase in the products using specific monoclonal antibodies. Most of these assays can also detect an inhibitor to ADAMTS13 with the use of 1:1 mixing studies with normal plasma. Detecting an inhibitor to

ADAMTS13 activity is more definitive for the diagnosis of spontaneous acquired thrombotic thrombocytopenic purpura than is measuring a low level of protease activity in the plasma, which occurs in a number of inflammatory states and in renal and hepatic failure.

Assays for Antibodies to Platelets

Antibodies to platelet membrane glycoproteins play a pathogenic role in the development of thrombocytopenia in immune thrombocytopenic purpura. They are difficult to measure, but can be detected in approximately 50–70% of immune thrombocytopenic purpura patients by specific assays for antibodies directed to platelet glycoproteins Ib or IIb/IIIa. The most reliable of these tests uses a format called monoclonal antibody immobilization of platelet antigen; the test requires sufficient platelets with bound antibody from the patients, and often the platelet numbers are limited in this setting. The antibody quantitation does not always correlate well with the changing clinical status in some patients with immune thrombocytopenic purpura.

EVALUATION OF THROMBOPHILIA

The hemostatic system has a number of naturally occurring inhibitor proteins that prevent the formation and extension of thrombi; these include protein C, protein S, and antithrombin, which are described in more detail in Chapter 67. Inherited or acquired deficiencies of these factors can lead to life-threatening thrombosis. In contrast to the screening studies of coagulation that are often performed before invasive procedures, the tests for the inhibitor proteins are usually assessed after a thrombosis occurs. Because they can be consumed during the thrombotic process, and some can also be lowered by anticoagulant therapy, the timing of testing for the activity of these inhibitors is important. Most often, it is recommended that assays for these proteins be performed well after the acute thrombotic event and several weeks after the completion of anticoagulant therapy. This is not true for the abnormalities that are measured by DNA-based testing; these studies can be done at any time.

In most cases, deficiencies of the inhibitor proteins have been shown to lead to venous thrombotic disease and not to arterial thrombosis. This is true for protein C, protein S, and antithrombin. Lupus anticoagulants, which are an acquired abnormality, are an exception because they are associated with both venous and arterial thrombosis. Although lupus anticoagulants prolong coagulation tests in vitro, they lead to thrombosis in vivo (by mechanisms discussed later).

Inhibitor Proteins of Hemostasis

Protein C

Protein C is a vitamin K–dependent protein that acts by cleaving factor V and factor VIII, inactivating them and limiting ongoing fibrin formation. Both functional (detection of fibrin clot formation) and antigen assays are available for the protein. In type 1 protein C deficiency, both activity and antigen are decreased; in type 2, more antigen than activity is present, indicating a qualitative defect in the molecule. Protein C activity should not be measured in patients who are taking coumadin because the factor is dependent on vitamin K for its synthesis and will be decreased.

Protein S

Protein S is a vitamin K–dependent cofactor that enhances the activity of protein C. Approximately 60% of protein S circulates in an inactive form that is bound to a complement-binding protein, C4b-binding protein. Functional and immunologic assays are available for the protein, and one needs to know whether the assay being used measures the total or free (active) fraction of protein S. As with protein C, there are both quantitative (type 1) and qualitative (type 2) abnormalities of protein S. The level of protein S will also be decreased in patients who are taking coumadin.

Antithrombin

Antithrombin is an important inhibitor of the activated forms of several coagulation factors. Therapeutic heparin and the heparan sulfates that are structural parts of cell membranes bind to antithrombin, enhancing its activity and making it a much more rapid-acting inhibitor. Both activity and antigenic assays are available for antithrombin, and both quantitative and qualitative defects are described.

Inherited Defects in Coagulation Factors Predisposing to Thrombosis

Inherited mutations present in some coagulation factors and high levels of some coagulation factors render them prothrombotic.

Factor V Leiden

Factor V Leiden is an inherited abnormality occurring in a cleavage site of factor V (R506Q) that prevents normal proteolysis of factor V by activated protein C. When this mutation is present, fibrin is formed to a greater extent than normal. Approximately 5% of the white population in the Western world is heterozygous for this mutation, and it confers a relatively low risk for thrombotic disease compared to the abnormalities in the inhibitors discussed previously. DNA-based techniques are used to identify the mutation. A functional test that is not specific for factor V Leiden, but identifies most carriers of the gene, is called the *activated protein C resistance assay*. It is a clotting assay based on either the aPTT or a factor V assay that compares the clotting time of a baseline test with the clotting time of the test done after activated protein C is added to the plasma. In normal individuals, the time to clot formation is prolonged with the added protein C, whereas in carriers of factor V Leiden (and other unidentified defects), the clotting time is much less prolonged. Some patients with a lupus anticoagulant will have a positive activated protein C resistance assay, and other unknown defects may also cause an abnormal assay.

Prothrombin Gene Mutation 20210

A mutation in the 3′ end of the prothrombin gene promotes synthesis of prothrombin and leads to high levels of the factor in the circulation. This predisposes to venous thrombosis. The mutation is identified using DNA-based techniques.

Other Circulating Factors Predisposing to Thrombosis

Unusually high levels of some clotting proteins, including factors VIII, IX, XI, and fibrinogen, are associated with venous thrombosis. Mutations of fibrinogen that result in fibrin clots that are resistant to plasmin, and mutations of plasminogen that inhibit normal activation to plasmin, can lead to thrombosis. High levels of homocysteine and of lipoprotein(a) have also been associated with venous thrombosis. In some cases, high homocysteine levels may be due to a heat-labile variant of methylenetetrahydrofolate reductase, and treatment with folic acid may lower the plasma homocysteine to normal levels.

Elevated Homocysteine Levels

Increased circulating homocysteine levels are associated with both venous and arterial thrombosis. They are measured by chemical methods such as high-performance liquid chromatography in the clinical laboratory. Generally a fasting level of greater than 13–15 μmol/L is considered a risk factor, though it appears that there is an increasing risk of thrombotic disease as the level of homocysteine progressively increases. Elevations are considered moderate between 15 and 30, intermediate between 30 and 100, and severe above 100 μmol/L. When fasting levels are normal, an oral methionine challenge can be administered, but this test has not been shown to have prognostic value for arterial thrombotic disease. Several different enzyme defects can lead to elevated homocysteine levels, including a heat-labile methylenetetrahydrofolate reductase enzyme and cystathionine β-synthase deficiency. The former can often be treated simply with folate supplementation.

Lupus Anticoagulants and Thrombosis

Although lupus anticoagulants prolong clotting times in vitro, they are associated with both arterial and venous thrombosis in vivo. A number of mechanisms leading to thrombosis have been proposed, including inhibition of the activation of protein C, activation of platelets, interference with the protective "anticoagulant" coating of annexin V at cell surfaces, and damage to endothelial cell surfaces. Assays for lupus anticoagulants are discussed earlier in the chapter.

Factors Contributing to Arterial Thrombosis

Arterial thrombosis is caused by a more complex array of both environmental and genetic factors than is venous thrombotic disease. High levels of fibrinogen or homocysteine, on a congenital basis, have been associated with arterial thrombosis, and the acquired antibodies associated with lupus anticoagulants and heparin-induced thrombocytopenia also predispose to arterial thrombosis. Polymorphisms and mutations in genes encoding coagulation factors and platelet proteins and the enzymes related to nitric oxide have also been identified as possible contributors to arterial thrombosis, but their contribution remains uncertain.

Suggested Readings

Ansell J, Hirsh J, Dalen J, et al: Managing oral anticoagulant therapy. Chest 119(1 Suppl):22S–38S, 2001.

Giles A, Verbruggen B, Rivard G, et al: A detailed comparison of the performance of the standard versus the Nijmegen modification of the Bethesda assay in detecting factor VIII:C inhibitors in the haemophilia A population of Canada. Thromb Haemost 79:872–876, 1998.

Laffan M, Brown SA, Collins PW, et al: The diagnosis of von Willebrand disease: A guideline from the UK Haemophilia Centre Doctors' Organization. Haemophilia 10:199–217, 2004.

Posan E, McBane RD, Grill DE, et al: Comparison of PFA-100 testing and bleeding time for detecting platelet hypofunction and von Willebrand disease in clinical practice. Thromb Haemost 90:483–490, 2003.

Seligsohn U, Lubetsky A: Genetic susceptibility to venous thrombosis. N Engl J Med 344:1222–1231, 2001.

Triplett DA: Lupus anticoagulants: diagnosis and management. Curr Hematol Rep 2:271–272, 2003.

INDEX

Note: Page numbers followed by the letter b refer to boxed material. Page numbers followed by the letter f refer to figures; those followed by the letter t refer to tables.

B

C

E

I

J

K

L

M

O

P

Q

R

S

T

U

V

W

X

Y

Z